U0268730

第 11 版

斯莱森杰 - 福特伦
Sleisenger and Fordtran's

胃肠病学和肝病学
Gastrointestinal and Liver Disease

病理生理学、诊断、治疗和管理
Pathophysiology | Diagnosis | Management

上 卷

主编

MARK FELDMAN, MD
Chairman of Internal Medicine
Texas Health Presbyterian Hospital Dallas
Clinical Professor of Internal Medicine
University of Texas Southwestern Medical School
Dallas, Texas

LAWRENCE S. FRIEDMAN, MD
Professor of Medicine
Harvard Medical School
Professor of Medicine
Tufts University School of Medicine
Boston, Massachusetts
The Anton R. Fried, MD, Chair
Department of Medicine
Newton-Wellesley Hospital
Newton, Massachusetts
Assistant Chief of Medicine
Massachusetts General Hospital
Boston, Massachusetts

LAWRENCE J. BRANDT, MD
Professor of Medicine and Surgery
Albert Einstein College of Medicine
Emeritus Chief
Division of Gastroenterology
Montefiore Medical Center
Bronx, New York

副主编

RAYMOND T. CHUNG, MD
Director of Hepatology, Vice Chief, Gastroenterology
Division of Gastroenterology
Massachusetts General Hospital and Harvard Medical School
Associate Member, Broad Institute
Boston, Massachusetts

DAVID T. RUBIN, MD
Joseph B. Kirsner Professor of Medicine
Chief, Section of Gastroenterology, Hepatology, and Nutrition
Department of Medicine
University of Chicago
Chicago, Illinois

C. MEL WILCOX, MD, MSPH
Division of Gastroenterology and Hepatology
University of Alabama at Birmingham
Birmingham, Alabama

人民卫生出版社

·北 京·

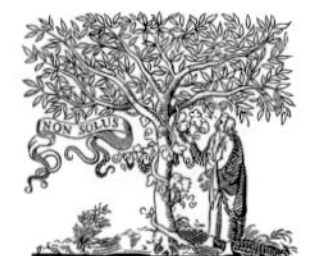

ELSEVIER
Elsevier (Singapore) Pte Ltd.
3 Killiney Road
#08-01Winsland House I
Singapore 239519
Tel: (65) 6349-0200
Fax: (65) 6733-1817

Sleisenger and Fordtran's Gastrointestinal and Liver Disease: Pathophysiology/Diagnosis/Management, 11/E

ISBN: 978-0-323-60962-3

This translation of Sleisenger and Fordtran's Gastrointestinal and Liver Disease: Pathophysiology/Diagnosis/Management, 11/E by Mark Feldman, Lawrence S. Friedman and Lawrence J. Brandt was undertaken by People's Medical Publishing House and is published by arrangement with Elsevier (Singapore) Pte Ltd.

Sleisenger and Fordtran's Gastrointestinal and Liver Disease: Pathophysiology/Diagnosis/Management, 11/E by Mark Feldman, Lawrence S. Friedman and Lawrence J. Brandt 由人民卫生出版社进行翻译,并根据人民卫生出版社与爱思唯尔(新加坡)私人有限公司的协议约定出版。

斯莱森杰-福特伦胃肠病学和肝病学:病理生理学、诊断、治疗和管理(第 11 版/上卷)(袁农、孙明瑜、李鹏、闫秀娥、鲁晓岚、王立主译)
ISBN: 978-7-117-35188-1

第 11 版

斯莱森杰 - 福特伦
Sleisenger and Fordtran's

胃肠病学和肝病学
Gastrointestinal and Liver Disease

病理生理学、诊断、治疗和管理
Pathophysiology | Diagnosis | Management

上 卷

主 编 Mark Feldman Lawrence S. Friedman Lawrence J. Brandt

副主编 Raymond T. Chung David T. Rubin C. Mel Wilcox

主 审 张澍田 季 光 贾继东 黄永辉

主 译 袁 农 孙明瑜 李 鹏 闫秀娥 鲁晓岚 王 立

人民卫生出版社

·北 京·

图书在版编目（CIP）数据

斯莱森杰-福特伦胃肠病学和肝病学：病理生理学、诊断、治疗和管理. 上卷/（美）马克·费尔德曼（Mark Feldman），（美）劳伦斯·S. 弗里德曼（Lawrence S. Friedman），（美）劳伦斯·J. 布兰特（Lawrence J. Brandt）主编；袁农等主译. —北京：人民卫生出版社，2023. 12

ISBN 978-7-117-35188-1

Ⅰ. ①斯… Ⅱ. ①马…②劳…③劳…④袁… Ⅲ. ①胃肠病学②肝疾病-诊疗 Ⅳ. ①R57

中国国家版本馆 CIP 数据核字(2023)第 194462 号

图字：01-2021-1476 号

斯莱森杰-福特伦
胃肠病学和肝病学：病理生理学、诊断、治疗和管理
Silaisenjie-Futelun
Weichangbingxue he Ganbingxue：Bingli
Shenglixue、Zhenduan、Zhiliao he Guanli
（上卷）

主　　译：袁　农　孙明瑜　李　鹏
　　　　　闫秀娥　鲁晓岚　王　立
出版发行：人民卫生出版社（中继线 010-59780011）
地　　址：北京市朝阳区潘家园南里 19 号
邮　　编：100021
E - mail：pmph @ pmph. com
购书热线：010-59787592　010-59787584　010-65264830
印　　刷：人卫印务（北京）有限公司
经　　销：新华书店
开　　本：889×1194　1/16　　印张：68. 5
字　　数：2907 千字
版　　次：2023 年 12 月第 1 版
印　　次：2023 年 12 月第 1 次印刷
标准书号：ISBN 978-7-117-35188-1
定　　价：780. 00 元
打击盗版举报电话：010-59787491　E-mail：WQ @ pmph. com
质量问题联系电话：010-59787234　E-mail：zhiliang @ pmph. com
数字融合服务电话：4001118166　E-mail：zengzhi @ pmph. com

主 编

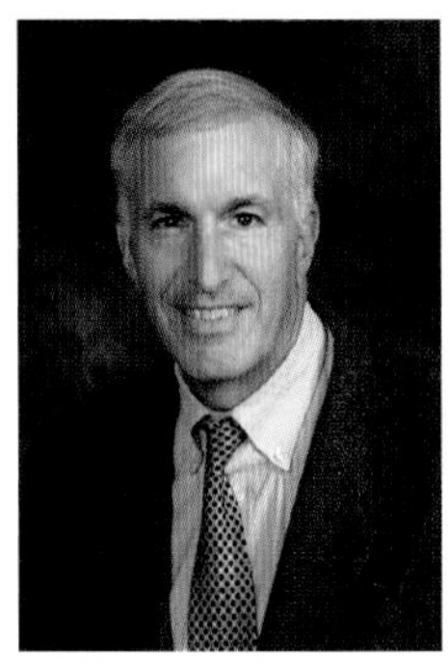

Mark Feldman, MD

第5~11版

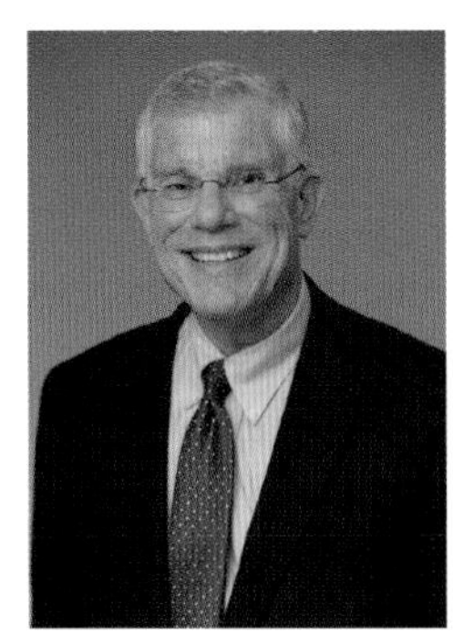

Lawrence S. Friedman, MD

第7~11版

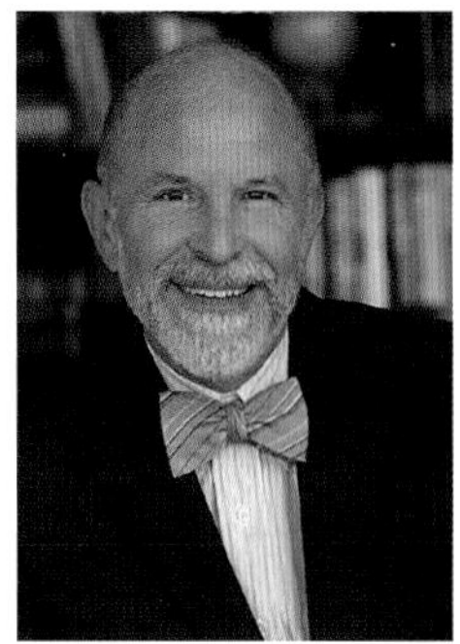

Lawrence J. Brandt, MD

第8~11版

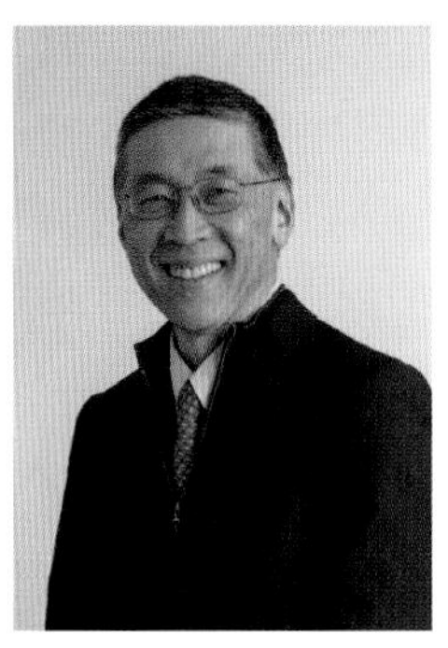

Raymond T. Chung, MD

第11版

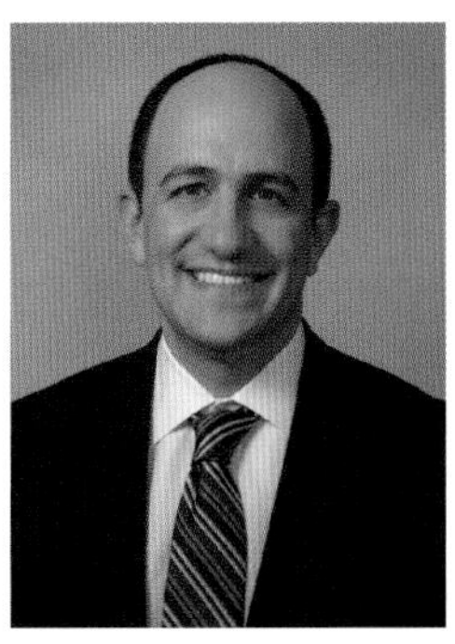

David T. Rubin, MD

第11版

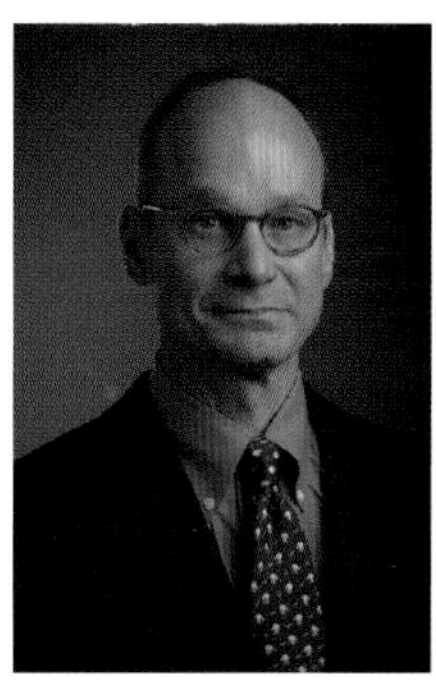

C. Mel Wilcox, MD

第11版

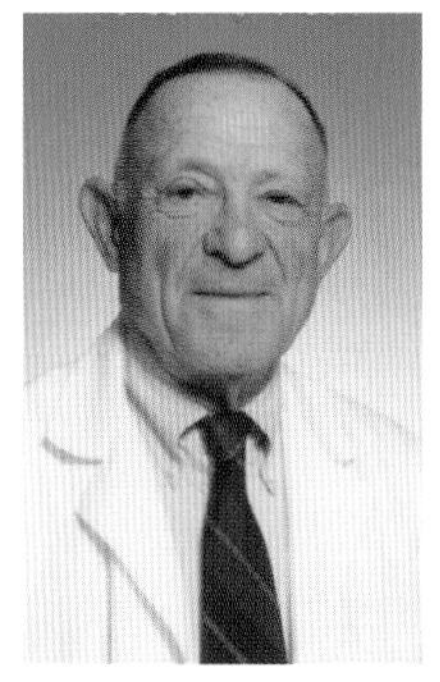

Marvin H. Sleisenger, MD

第1~7版

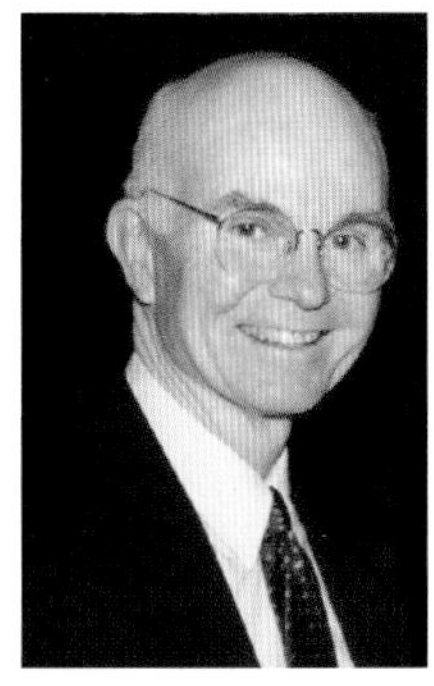

John S. Fordtran, MD

第1~5版

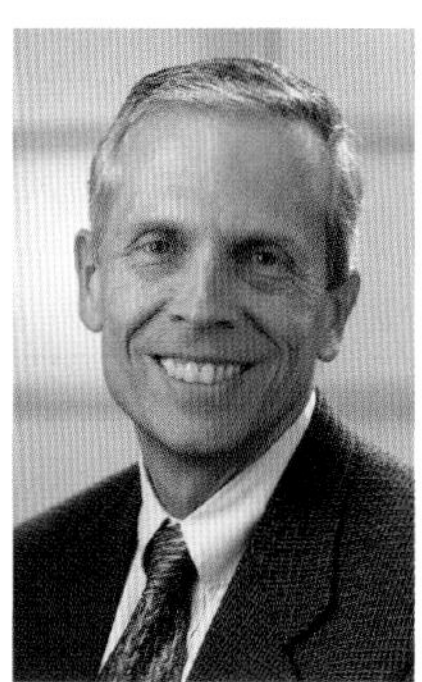

Bruce F. Scharschmidt, MD

第5和6版

主审和主译

主　审

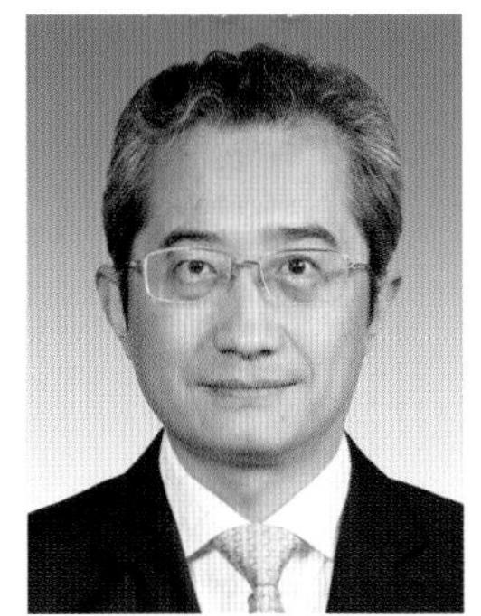
张澍田

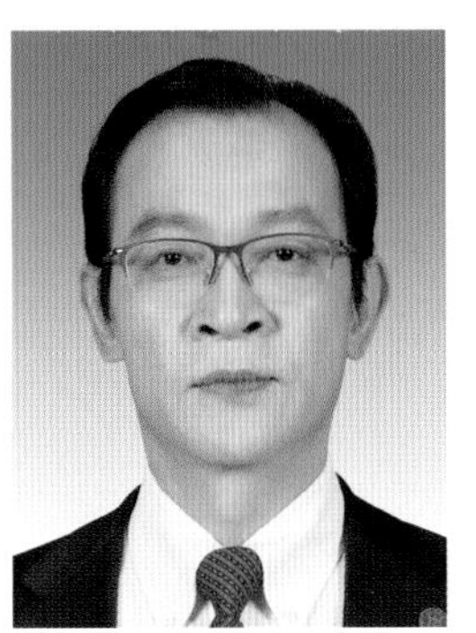
季　光

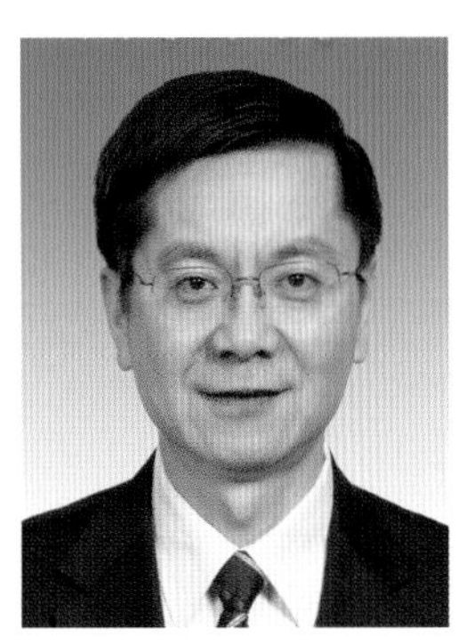
贾继东

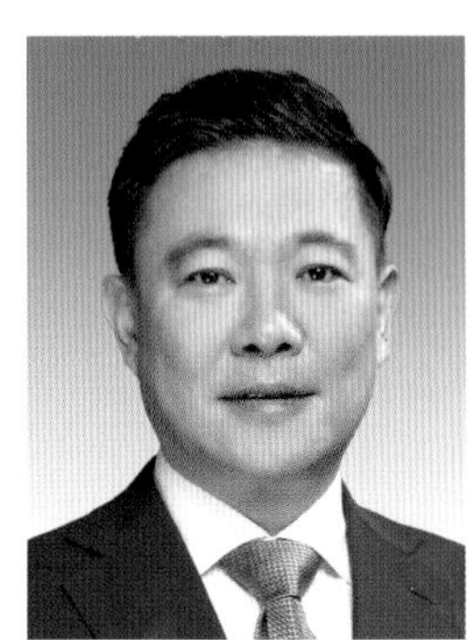
黄永辉

主　译

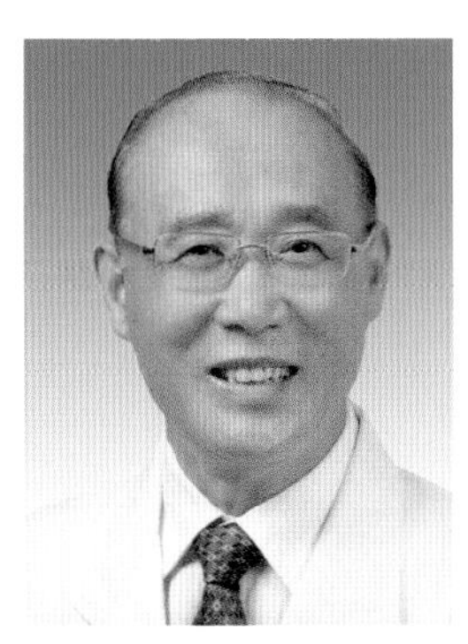
袁　农

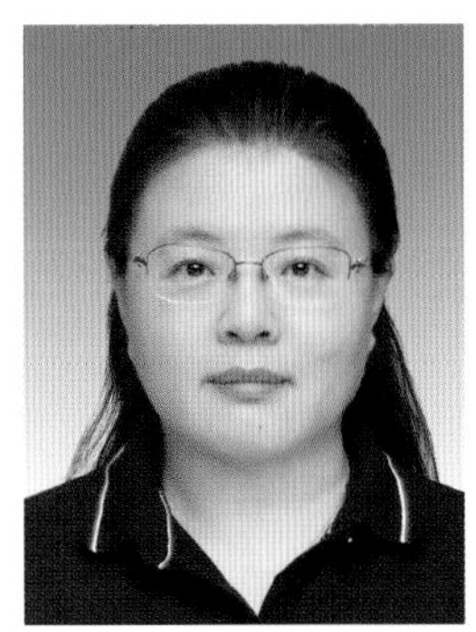
孙明瑜

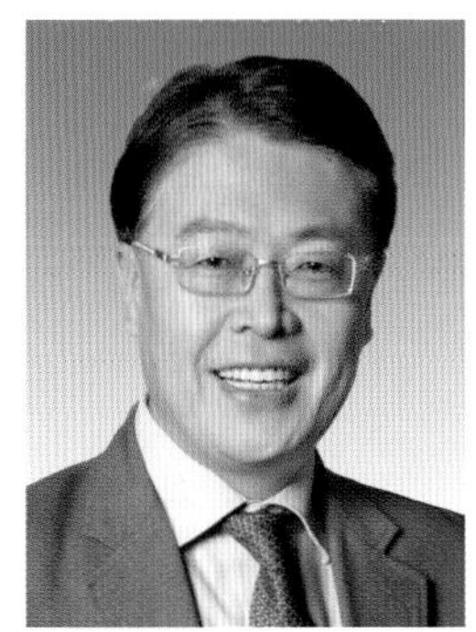
李　鹏

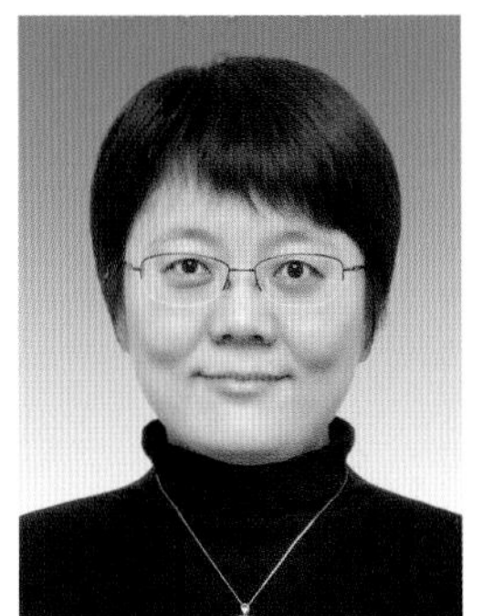
闫秀娥

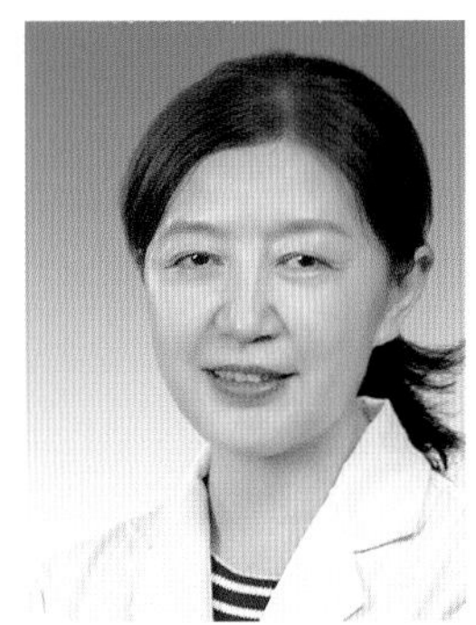
鲁晓岚

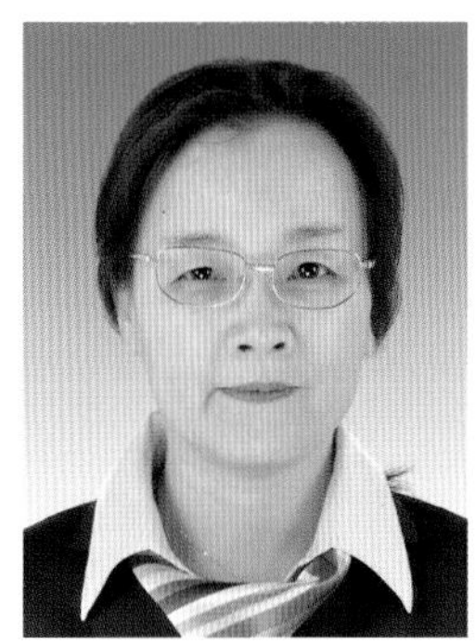
王　立

译者名单

主　审　张澍田　首都医科大学附属北京友谊医院
季　光　上海中医药大学
贾继东　首都医科大学附属北京友谊医院
黄永辉　北京大学第三医院

主　译　袁　农　孙明瑜　李　鹏　闫秀娥　鲁晓岚　王　立

译　者（以姓氏笔画排列为序）

王　立	重庆医科大学附属第一医院	消化科	主任医师
王　萍	陕西省人民医院	消化科	主任医师
王迎春	北京大学第三医院	消化科	副主任医师
王欣欣	首都医科大学附属北京佑安医院	病理科	主任医师、副教授
王俊雄	首都医科大学附属北京友谊医院	消化分中心	副主任医师
叶　蔚	浙江中医药大学附属杭州市中医院	脾胃病科	主任医师、教授
刘　军	陕西省人民医院	儿科	主任医师
刘　晖	首都医科大学附属北京佑安医院	病理科	主任医师
刘文正	北京大学第三医院	消化科	主治医师
闫秀娥	北京大学第三医院	消化科	主任医师、副教授
汤善宏	中国人民解放军西部战区总医院	消化科	副主任医师、副教授
祁兴顺	中国人民解放军北部战区总医院	消化科	副主任医师
孙明瑜	上海中医药大学附属曙光医院	肝病研究所	主任医师、教授
李　鹏	首都医科大学附属北京友谊医院	消化分中心	主任医师、教授
张　烁	浙江中医药大学附属第二医院	消化科	主任医师、教授
张　莉	西安交通大学第二附属医院	消化科	副主任医师、讲师
陈立刚	厦门大学附属中山医院	消化科	主任医师、副教授
郑　炜	北京大学第三医院	消化科	主治医师
胡伟玲	浙江大学医学院附属邵逸夫医院	消化科	主任医师
施海韵	首都医科大学附属北京友谊医院	消化分中心	副主任医师
袁　农	上海中医药大学附属曙光医院	肝病研究所	主任医师、教授
郭晓燕	西安交通大学第二附属医院	消化科	主任医师、教授
郭雪艳	陕西省人民医院	消化科	副主任医师
韩跃华	浙江大学医学院第二附属医院	消化科	主任医师
程　芮	首都医科大学附属北京友谊医院	消化分中心	副主任医师
程　妍	西安交通大学第二附属医院	消化科	副主任医师、副教授
鲁晓岚	上海复旦大学附属浦东医院	消化科	主任医师、教授
曾翔俊	首都医科大学	病理生理教研室	教授
谢　咚	上海中医药大学附属曙光医院	肝病研究所	博士后

学术秘书　程　芮　谢　咚

编者名单

Nezam H. Afdhal, MD, DSc
Senior Physician in Hepatology
Department of Gastroenterology
Beth Israel Deaconess Medical Center
Boston, Massachusetts, United States

Rakesh Aggarwal, MD, DM
Director
Jawaharlal Institute of Postgraduate Medical Education and Research
Puducherry, India

Taymeyah Al-Toubah, MPH
Gastroenterology and Oncology
H. Lee Moffitt Cancer Center
Tampa, Florida, United States

Jaime Almandoz, MD
Assistant Professor
Department of Internal Medicine, Division of Endocrinology
University of Texas Southwestern
Dallas, Texas, United States

Ashwin N. Ananthakrishnan, MD, MPH
Associate Professor of Medicine
Harvard Medical School
Division of Gastroenterology
Massachusetts General Hospital
Boston, Massachusetts, United States

Karin L. Andersson, MD, MPH
Assistant Professor of Medicine
Harvard Medical School
Hepatologist
Division of Gastroenterology
Massachusetts General Hospital
Boston, Massachusetts, United States

Farshid Araghizadeh, MD, MBA
Colon and Rectal Surgeon
Texas Digestive Disease Consultants (TDDC) and The GI Alliance (TGIA)
Dallas–Fort Worth, Texas, United States

Louis J. Aronne, MD
Sanford I. Weill Professor of Metabolic Research
Department of Medicine
Weill Cornell Medicine
New York, New York, United States

Fernando Azpiroz, MD, PhD
Chief
Department of Gastroenterology
University Hospital Vall d'Hebron
Professor of Medicine
Universitat Autònoma de Barcelona
Barcelona, Spain

Bruce R. Bacon, MD
Professor of Internal Medicine
Division of Gastroenterology and Hepatology
Saint Louis University School of Medicine
St. Louis, Missouri, United States

William F. Balistreri, MD
Director, Pediatric Liver Care Center
Gastroenterology, Hepatology, and Nutrition
Cincinnati Children's Hospital Medical Center
Cincinnati, Ohio, United States

Todd H. Baron, MD
Professor of Medicine
Division of Gastroenterology and Hepatology
University of North Carolina
Chapel Hill, North Carolina, United States

Bradley A. Barth, MD, MPH
Professor
Department of Pediatrics
University of Texas Southwestern
Dallas, Texas, United States

Lee M. Bass, MD
Associate Professor of Pediatrics
Gastroenterology, Hepatology, and Nutrition
Ann and Robert H. Lurie Children's Hospital of Chicago
Northwestern University Feinberg School of Medicine
Chicago, Illinois, United States

Alex S. Befeler, MD
Professor of Internal Medicine
Medical Director of Liver Transplantation
Department of Internal Medicine
Saint Louis University
St. Louis, Missouri, United States

Mark Benson, MD
Associate Professor of Medicine
Section of Gastroenterology and Hepatology
University of Wisconsin School of Medicine and Public Health
Madison, Wisconsin, United States

William Bernal, MD
Professor
Liver Intensive Therapy Unit
King's College Hospital
London, United Kingdom

Adil E. Bharucha, MBBS, MD
Professor of Medicine
Division of Gastroenterology and Hepatology
Mayo Clinic
Rochester, Minnesota, United States

Taft P. Bhuket, MD
Associate Clinical Professor of Medicine
Division of Gastroenterology
University of California, San Francisco
San Francisco, California
Chief of Gastroenterology and Hepatology
Director of Endoscopy
Alameda Health System
Oakland, California, United States

Yangzom D. Bhutia, DVM, PhD
Assistant Professor
Cell Biology and Biochemistry
Texas Tech University Health Sciences Center
Lubbock, Texas, United States

J. Andrew Bird, MD
Associate Professor
Pediatrics, Division of Allergy and Immunology
University of Texas Southwestern Medical Center
Director
Food Allergy Center
Children's Medical Center
Dallas, Texas, United States

Boris Blechacz, MD, PhD
Clinical Associate Professor of Internal Medicine
Gastroenterology and Hepatology
Palmetto Health—University of South Carolina
Columbia, South Carolina, United States

Diego V. Bohórquez, PhD
Assistant Professor
Departments of Medicine and Neurobiology
Duke University Medical Center
Durham, North Carolina, United States

Jan Bornschein, MD
Translational Gastroenterology Unit
John Radcliffe Hospital
Oxford University Hospitals
Oxford, United Kingdom

Christopher L. Bowlus, MD
Professor and Chief
Division of Gastroenterology and Hepatology
University of California Davis
Sacramento, California, United States

Lawrence J. Brandt, MD
Professor of Medicine and Surgery
Albert Einstein College of Medicine
Emeritus Chief
Division of Gastroenterology
Montefiore Medical Center
Bronx, New York, United States

Robert Scott Bresalier, MD
Professor of Medicine
Lydia and Birdie J Resoft Distinguished Professor in GI Oncology
Gastroenterology, Hepatology, and Nutrition
The University of Texas MD Anderson Cancer Center
Houston, Texas, United States

Simon J.H. Brookes, PhD
Professor
Human Physiology
College of Medicine, Flinders University
Adelaide, South Australia, Australia

Alan L. Buchman, MD, MSPH
Professor of Clinical Surgery
University of Illinois at Chicago
Medical Director
Intestinal Rehabilitation and Transplant Center
Chicago, Illinois, United States

Ezra Burstein, MD, PhD
Professor
Departments of Internal Medicine and Molecular Biology
UT Southwestern Medical Center
Dallas, Texas, United States

Andres F. Carrion, MD
Assistant Professor of Clinical Medicine
Program Director, Transplant Hepatology Fellowship
Division of Gastroenterology and Hepatology
University of Miami
Miami, Florida, United States

Scott Celinski, MD
Surgical Oncologist
Department of Surgery
Baylor University Medical Center
Dallas, Texas, United States

Francis K.L. Chan, MBChB(Hons), MD, DSc
Professor of Medicine
Department of Medicine and Therapeutics
Chinese University of Hong Kong
Hong Kong, China

Eugene B. Chang, MD
Martin Boyer Professor
Department of Medicine
University of Chicago
Chicago, Illinois, United States

Joseph G. Cheatham, MD
Associate Professor of Medicine
Department of Medicine
Uniformed Services University
Bethesda, Maryland
Program Director
Gastroenterology Fellowship
Naval Medical Center San Diego
San Diego, California, United States

Shivakumar Chitturi, MD
Associate Professor
Australian National University
Senior Staff Hepatologist
The Canberra Hospital
Australian Capital Territory, Australia

Daniel C. Chung, MD
Associate Professor of Medicine
Harvard Medical School
Division of Gastroenterology
Massachusetts General Hospital
Medical Co-Director
Center for Cancer Risk Analysis
Massachusetts General Hospital Cancer Center
Boston, Massachusetts, United States

Raymond T. Chung, MD
Director of Hepatology, Vice Chief, Gastroenterology
Division of Gastroenterology
Massachusetts General Hospital and Harvard Medical School
Associate Member, Broad Institute
Boston, Massachusetts, United States

Marcello Costa, MD
Matthew Flinders Distinguished Professor and Professor of Neurophysiology
Physiology
Flinders University
Adelaide, South Australia, Australia

Thomas G. Cotter, MD
Gastroenterology Fellow
Section of Gastroenterology, Hepatology, and Nutrition
University of Chicago Medicine
Chicago, Illinois, United States

Albert J. Czaja, MD
Professor Emeritus of Medicine
Gastroenterology and Hepatology
Mayo Clinic College of Medicine and Science
Rochester, Minnesota, United States

Brian G. Czito, MD
Professor
Radiation Oncology
Duke University Medical Center
Durham, North Carolina, United States

Paul A. Dawson, PhD
Professor
Pediatrics— Gastroenterology, Hepatology, and Nutrition
Emory University
Atlanta, Georgia, United States

Gregory de Prisco, MD
Diagnostic Radiologist
Department of Radiology
Baylor University Medical Center
Director of Medical Education
American Radiology Associates
Dallas, Texas, United States

Jill K. Deutsch, MD
Clinical Fellow
Department of Internal Medicine
Section of Digestive Diseases
Yale New Haven Hospital—Yale University School of Medicine
New Haven, Connecticut, United States

Kenneth R. DeVault, MD
Professor of Medicine
Mayo Clinic College of Medicine
Jacksonville, Florida, United States

Adrian M. Di Bisceglie, MD
Professor of Internal Medicine
Department of Internal Medicine
Saint Louis University
St. Louis, Missouri, United States

John K. DiBaise, MD
Professor of Medicine
Division of Gastroenterology and Hepatology
Mayo Clinic
Scottsdale, Arizona, United States

Philip G. Dinning, PhD
Flinders Medical Centre
Human Physiology
Flinders University
Adelaide, South Australia, Australia

J. Marcus Downs, MD
Program Director
Colon and Rectal Surgery
Texas Health Resources
Clinical Professor of Surgery
Colon and Rectal Surgery
University of Texas Southwestern Medical School
Dallas, Texas, United States

Douglas A. Drossman, MD
Professor Emeritus of Medicine and Psychiatry
Division of Digestive Disease and Nutrition
University of North Carolina
President
Center for Education and Practice of Biopsychosocial Care
Chapel Hill, North Carolina
President
Drossman Gastroenterology PLLC
Durham, North Carolina, United States

Kerry B. Dunbar, MD, PhD
Section Chief, VA Gastroenterology Section
Department of Medicine–Gastroenterology and Hepatology
VA North Texas Healthcare System–Dallas VA Medical Center
Associate Professor of Medicine
Department of Medicine–Division of Gastroenterology and Hepatology
University of Texas Southwestern Medical School
Dallas, Texas, United States

John E. Eaton, MD
Assistant Professor of Medicine
Department of Internal Medicine
Division of Gastroenterology and Hepatology
Mayo Clinic
Rochester, Minnesota, United States

Steven A. Edmundowicz, MD
Professor of Medicine
Interim Director, Division of Gastroenterology and Hepatology
University of Colorado Anschutz Medical Campus
Aurora, Colorado, United States

David E. Elliott, MD, PhD
University of Iowa Carver College of Medicine
Department of Internal Medicine
Division of Gastroenterology and Hepatology
Iowa City VAHCS
Department of Internal Medicine
Veterans Administration Health Care System
Iowa City, Iowa, United States

B. Joseph Elmunzer, MD, MSc
Peter B. Cotton Professor of Medicine and Endoscopic Innovation
Division of Gastroenterology and Hepatology
Medical University of South Carolina, Charleston
Charleston, South Carolina, United States

Charles O. Elson, MD
Professor of Medicine and Microbiology
Basil I. Hirschowitz Chair in Gastroenterology
University of Alabama at Birmingham
Birmingham, Alabama, United States

Grace H. Elta, MD
Professor Emeritus
Formerly the H. Marvin Pollard Collegiate Professor
Division of Gastroenterology
University of Michigan
Ann Arbor, Michigan, United States

Michael B. Fallon, MD
Professor of Medicine
Gastroenterology, Hepatology, and Nutrition
University of Arizona
Chair
Department of Internal Medicine
University of Arizona—Phoenix
Phoenix, Arizona, United States

Geoffrey C. Farrell, MD
Professor, Hepatic Medicine
Australian National University
Senior Staff Hepatologist
The Canberra Hospital
Australian Capital Territory, Australia

Jordan J. Feld, MD, MPH
Associate Professor of Medicine
University of Toronto
Research Director
Toronto Centre for Liver Disease
Senior Scientist
Sandra Rotman Centre for Global Health
Toronto General Hospital
Toronto, Ontario, Canada

Mark Feldman, MD
Chairman of Internal Medicine
Texas Health Presbyterian Hospital Dallas
Clinical Professor of Internal Medicine
University of Texas Southwestern Medical School
Dallas, Texas, United States

Nielsen Q. Fernandez-Becker, MD
Clinical Associate Professor of Medicine
Division of Gastroenterology and Hepatology
Stanford University
Redwood City, California, United States

Paul Feuerstadt, MD
Attending Physician
Gastroenterology
Gastroenterology Center of Connecticut
Hamden, Connecticut
Assistant Clinical Professor of Medicine
Gastroenterology
Yale University School of Medicine
New Haven, Connecticut, United States

Peter Fickert, Prof
Division of Gastroenterology and Hepatology
Medical University of Graz
Graz, Austria

Robert E. Fleming, MD
Professor of Pediatrics
Saint Louis University School of Medicine
St. Louis, Missouri, United States

Alexander C. Ford, MBChB, MD
Professor of Gastroenterology and Honorary Consultant Gastroenterologist
Leeds Institute of Medical Research
St. James's University of Leeds
Leeds Gastroenterology Institute
Leeds Teaching Hospitals Trust
Leeds, West Yorkshire, United Kingdom

John S. Fordtran, MD
Internal Medicine, Division of Gastroenterology
Baylor University Medical Center
Dallas, Texas, United States

Chris E. Forsmark, MD
Professor and Chief
Division of Gastroenterology, Hepatology, and Nutrition
University of Florida
Gainesville, Florida, United States

Lawrence S. Friedman, MD
Professor of Medicine
Harvard Medical School
Professor of Medicine
Tufts University School of Medicine
Boston, Massachusetts
The Anton R. Fried, MD, Chair
Department of Medicine
Newton-Wellesley Hospital
Newton, Massachusetts
Assistant Chief of Medicine
Massachusetts General Hospital
Boston, Massachusetts, United States

Scott Fung, MD
Associate Professor
Department of Medicine
University of Toronto
Staff Hepatologist
University Health Network
Toronto General Hospital
Toronto, Ontario, Canada

Vadivel Ganapathy, PhD
Professor
Cell Biology and Biochemistry
Texas Tech University Health Sciences Center
Lubbock, Texas, United States

John J. Garber, MD
Instructor in Medicine
Harvard Medical School
Assistant in Medicine
Division of Gastroenterology
Massachusetts General Hospital
Boston, Massachusetts, United States

Praveen Ramakrishnan Geethakumari, MD, MS
Assistant Professor
Division of Medical Oncology
Department of Internal Medicine
University of Texas Southwestern Medical Center
Dallas, Texas, United States

Marc G. Ghany, MD, MHSc
Liver Diseases Branch
National Institute of Diabetes and Digestive and Kidney Diseases
National Institutes of Health
Bethesda, Maryland, United States

Pere Ginès, MD, PhD
Chairman
Liver Unit
Hospital Clinic Barcelona
Full Professor of Medicine
University of Barcelona
Principal Investigator
Institut d'Investigacions Biomediques August Pi i Sunyer (IDIBAPS)
Barcelona, Spain

Robert E. Glasgow, MD
Professor and Vice Chairman
Surgery
University of Utah
Salt Lake City, Utah, United States

Gregory J. Gores, MD
Executive Dean for Research, Professor of Medicine
Division of Gastroenterology and Hepatology
Mayo Clinic
Rochester, Minnesota, United States

Peter H.R. Green, MD
Phyllis and Ivan Seidenberg Professor of Medicine
Columbia University Medical Center
New York, New York, United States

David A. Greenwald, MD
Director of Clinical Gastroenterology and Endoscopy
Division of Gastroenterology
Mount Sinai Hospital
New York, New York, United States

C. Prakash Gyawali, MD, MRCP
Professor of Medicine
Division of Gastroenterology
Department of Medicine
Washington University in St. Louis
St. Louis, Missouri, United States

Hazem Hammad, MD
Assistant Professor of Medicine
Division of Gastroenterology and Hepatology
University of Colorado Anschutz Medical Campus
Aurora, Colorado, United States

Heinz F. Hammer, MD
Associate Professor of Medicine
Department of Internal Medicine
Medical University
Graz, Austria

Stephen A. Harrison, MD
Visiting Professor of Hepatology
Radcliffe Department of Medicine
University of Oxford
Oxford, United Kingdom

David J. Hass, MD
Associate Clinical Professor of Medicine
Division of Digestive Diseases
Yale University School of Medicine
New Haven, Connecticut, United States

David M. Hockenbery, MD
Member
Clinical Research
Fred Hutchinson Cancer Research Center
Professor of Medicine
Division of Gastroenterology
University of Washington
Seattle, Washington, United States

Christoph Högenauer, MD
Associate Professor of Medicine
Department of Internal Medicine
Medical University of Graz
Graz, Austria

Jacinta A. Holmes, MBBS, PhD
Division of Gastroenterology
Massachusetts General Hospital
Boston, Massachusetts, United States
Gastroenterology
St. Vincent's Hospital
University of Melbourne
Fitzroy, Victoria, Australia

Colin W. Howden, MD
Hyman Professor of Medicine
Division of Gastroenterology
University of Tennessee Health Science Center
Memphis, Tennessee, United States

Patrick A. Hughes, PhD
Centre for Nutrition and Gastrointestinal Diseases
Adelaide Medical School
University of Adelaide
South Australian Health and Medical Research Institute
Nutrition and Metabolism
Adelaide, South Australia, Australia

Sohail Z. Husain, MD
Professor of Pediatrics
Division of Gastroenterology, Hepatology, and Nutrition
Stanford University School of Medicine
Stanford, California, United States

Christopher D. Huston, MD
Professor
Medicine, Microbiology, and Molecular Genetics
University of Vermont College of Medicine
Attending Physician
Medicine and Infectious Diseases
Fletcher Allen Health Care
Burlington, Vermont, United States

M. Nedim Ince, MD
University of Iowa Carver College of Medicine
Iowa City, Iowa, United States
Department of Internal Medicine
Division of Gastroenterology and Hepatology
Iowa City VAHCS
Department of Internal Medicine
Veterans Administration Health Care System
Iowa City, Iowa, United States

Rachel B. Issaka, MD, MAS
Assistant Member
Clinical Research and Public Health Science Divisions
Fred Hutchinson Cancer Research Center
Assistant Professor
Department of Medicine, Division of Gastroenterology
University of Washington
Seattle, Washington, United States

Johanna C. Iturrino, MD
Assistant Professor of Medicine
Harvard Medical School
Beth Israel Deaconess Medical Center
Boston, Massachusetts, United States

Theodore W. James, MD
Fellow
Division of Gastroenterology
University of North Carolina
Chapel Hill, North Carolina, United States

Harry L.A. Janssen, MD, PhD
Professor of Medicine
Gastroenterology and Hepatology
University of Toronto
Toronto, Ontario, Canada

Dennis M. Jensen, MD
Professor of Medicine
Professor of Medicine–Gastrointestinal
David Geffen School of Medicine at UCLA
Staff Physician
Medicine-Gastrointestinal
VA Greater Los Angeles Healthcare System
Key Investigator
Director, Human Studies Core and Gastrointestinal Hemostasis Research Unit
CURE Digestive Diseases Research Center
Los Angeles, California, United States

Pamela J. Jensen, MD
Department of Pathology
Texas Health Presbyterian Hospital Dallas
Dallas, Texas, United States

D. Rohan Jeyarajah, MD
Chair of Surgery
Assistant Chair of Clinical Sciences
Head of Surgery
TCU and UNTHSC School of Medicine
Fort Worth, Texas
Director, Gastrointestinal Services
Methodist Richardson Medical Center
Director, HPB/UGI Fellowship
Associate Program Director, General Surgery Residency Program
Methodist Richardson Medical Center
Richardson, Texas, United States

Peter J. Kahrilas, MD
Gilbert H. Marquardt Professor of Medicine
Feinberg School of Medicine
Northwestern University
Gastroenterology and Hepatology
Northwestern Medicine
Chicago, Illinois, United States

Vishal Kaila, BS, MD
Resident
Internal Medicine
Texas Health Presbyterian
Dallas, Texas, United States

Patrick S. Kamath, MD
Professor of Medicine
Division of Gastroenterology and Hepatology
Consultant
Gastroenterology and Hepatology
Mayo Clinic College of Medicine and Science
Rochester, Minnesota, United States

Gilaad G. Kaplan, MD, MPH
Professor of Medicine
University of Calgary
Calgary, Alberta, Canada

Purna Kashyap, MBBS
Associate Professor of Medicine
Physiology and Biomedical Engineering
Mayo Clinic
Rochester, Minnesota, United States

Jennifer Katz, MD
Assistant Professor of Medicine
Division of Gastroenterology
Montefiore Medical Center
Bronx, New York, United States

David A. Katzka, MD
Professor of and Consultant in Medicine
Gastroenterology
Mayo Clinic
Rochester, Minnesota, United States

Debra K. Katzman, MD, FRCPC
Professor of Pediatrics
Department of Pediatrics
The Hospital for Sick Children and University of Toronto
Toronto, Ontario, Canada

Jonathan D. Kaunitz, MD
Professor of Medicine and Surgery
UCLA School of Medicine
Attending Gastroenterologist
West Los Angeles Veterans Affairs Medical Center
Los Angeles, California, United States

Laurie Keefer, PhD
Professor
Medicine and Psychiatry
Icahn School of Medicine at Mount Sinai
New York, New York, United States

Ciarán P. Kelly, MD
Professor of Medicine
Gastroenterology
Harvard Medical School
Fellowship Program Director
Gastroenterology
Beth Israel Deaconess Medical Center
Boston, Massachusetts, United States

Sahil Khanna, MBBS, MS
Associate Professor of Medicine
Gastroenterology and Hepatology
Mayo Clinic
Rochester, Minnesota, United States

Arthur Y. Kim, MD
Associate Professor of Medicine
Harvard Medical School
Division of Infectious Diseases
Massachusetts General Hospital
Boston, Massachusetts, United States

Kenneth L. Koch, MD
Professor of Medicine
Department of Medicine
Section on Gastroenterology and Hepatology
Wake Forest University School of Medicine
Winston-Salem, North Carolina, United States

Benjamin Kulow, MD
Colon and Rectal Surgeon
Saint Luke's Health System
Kansas City, Missouri, United States

Rekha B. Kumar, MD, MS
Assistant Professor of Medicine
Endocrinology, Diabetes, and Metabolism
Weill Cornell Medical College
Attending Physician
Endocrinology, Diabetes, and Metabolism
New York Presbyterian Hospital
New York, New York, United States

Vidhya Kunnathur, MD
Assistant Professor
Division of Digestive Diseases
University of Cincinnati
Cincinnati, Ohio, United States

Joann Kwah, MD
Assistant Professor of Medicine
Albert Einstein College of Medicine
Gastroenterology
Montefiore Medical Center
Bronx, New York, United States

Brian E. Lacy, MD, PhD
Senior Associate Consultant
Division of Gastroenterology
Mayo Clinic
Jacksonville, Florida, United States

Anne M. Larson, MD
Professor of Medicine
Division of Gastroenterology/Hepatology
University of Washington
Seattle, Washington, United States

James Y.W. Lau, MD
Professor of Surgery
Department of Surgery
The Chinese University of Hong Kong
Director
Endoscopy Centre
Prince of Wales Hospital
Hong Kong, China

Ryan Law, DO
Assistant Professor
Division of Gastroenterology
University of Michigan
Ann Arbor, Michigan, United States

Benjamin Lebwohl, MD, MS
Assistant Professor of Medicine and Epidemiology
Columbia University Medical Center
New York, New York, United States

Anthony J. Lembo, MD
Professor of Medicine
Department of Medicine
Beth Israel Deaconess Medical Center
Boston, Massachusetts, United States

Cynthia Levy, MD
Professor of Medicine
Division of Hepatology
University of Miami
Miami, Florida, United States

Blair Lewis, MD
Medical Director
Carnegie Hill Endoscopy
Clinical Professor of Medicine
Mount Sinai Medical Center
New York, New York, United States

James H. Lewis, MD
Professor of Medicine
Director of Hepatology
Division of Gastroenterology
Georgetown University Medical Center
Washington, DC, United States

Rodger A. Liddle, MD
Professor of Medicine
Department of Medicine
Duke University Medical Center
Durham, North Carolina, United States

Steven D. Lidofsky, MD, PhD
Professor of Medicine
University of Vermont
Director of Hepatology
University of Vermont Medical Center
Burlington, Vermont, United States

Keith D. Lindor, MD
Senior Advisor and Professor
Office of the University Provost
Arizona State University Medicine
Gastroenterology and Hepatology
Mayo Clinic Hospital
Phoenix, Arizona, United States

Mark E. Lowe, MD, PhD
Harvey R. Colton Professor of Pediatric Science and Vice Chair
Department of Pediatrics
Washington University School of Medicine
St. Louis, Missouri, United States

Cara L. Mack, MD
Professor of Pediatrics
University of Colorado School of Medicine
Children's Hospital Colorado
Aurora, Colorado, United States

Ryan D. Madanick, MD
Assistant Professor of Medicine
Division of Gastroenterology and Hepatology
University of North Carolina School of Medicine
Chapel Hill, North Carolina, United States

Willis C. Maddrey, MD
Special Assistant to the President
Professor of Internal Medicine
Arnold N. and Carol S. Ablon Professorship in Biomedical Science
Adelyn and Edmund M. Hoffman Distinguished Chair in Medical Science
University of Texas Southwestern Medical Center
Dallas, Texas, United States

Matthias Maiwald, MD, PhD
Senior Consultant in Microbiology
Department of Pathology and Laboratory Medicine
KK Women's and Children's Hospital, Singapore
Adjunct Associate Professor
Department of Microbiology and Immunology
Yong Loo Lin School of Medicine
National University of Singapore
Adjunct Associate Professor
Duke-NUS Graduate Medical School
Singapore, Singapore

Lawrence A. Mark, MD, PhD
Associate Professor of Clinical Dermatology
Department of Dermatology
Indiana University School of Medicine
Indianapolis, Indiana, United States

Paul Martin, MD, FRCP, FRCPI
Chief, Division of Gastroenterology and Hepatology
University of Miami
Miami, Florida, United States

Ricard Masia, MD, PhD
Associate Director, Translational Pathology
Surface Oncology
Cambridge, Massachusetts, United States

Joel B. Mason, MD
Professor of Medicine and Nutrition
Divisions of Gastroenterology and Clinical Nutrition
Tufts University
Director
Vitamins and Carcinogenesis Laboratory
USDA Human Nutrition Research Center at Tufts University
Boston, Massachusetts, United States

Jeffrey B. Matthews, MD
Dallas B. Phemister Professor and Chairman
Department of Surgery
The University of Chicago Medicine
Chicago, Illinois, United States

Craig J. McClain, MD
Professor of Medicine and Pharmacology and Toxicology
Vice President for Health Affairs and Research
University of Louisville
Director
Gastroenterology
Robley Rex VA Medical Center
Louisville, Kentucky, United States

Stephen A. McClave, MD
Professor and Director of Clinical Nutrition
Department of Medicine
University of Louisville School of Medicine
Louisville, Kentucky, United States

Shilpa Mehra, MD
Assistant Professor of Medicine
Department of Medicine
Division of Gastroenterology
Albert Einstein College of Medicine
Bronx, New York, United States

Megha S. Mehta, MD
Assistant Professor of Pediatrics
University of Texas Southwestern Medical Center
Dallas, Texas, United States

Shivang S. Mehta, MD
Pediatric Gastroenterology Fellow
Department of Pediatric Gastroenterology
University of Texas Southwestern Medical Center
Dallas, Texas, United States

Joanna M.P. Melia, MD
Assistant Professor of Medicine
Johns Hopkins University School of Medicine
Baltimore, Maryland, United States

Frederick H. Millham, MD, MBA
Chair, Surgery
South Shore Hospital
Weymouth, Massachusetts
Associate Professor of Surgery (Part Time)
Harvard Medical School
Boston, Massachusetts, United States

Ginat W. Mirowski, DMD, MD
Adjunct Clinical Professor
Department of Oral Pathology, Medicine, and Radiology
Indiana University School of Dentistry
Professor of Clinical Dermatology (Clinical Track)
Department of Dermatology
Indiana University School of Medicine
Indianapolis, Indiana, United States

Joseph Misdraji, MD
Associate Professor of Pathology
Harvard Medical School
Associate Pathologist
Massachusetts General Hospital
Boston, Massachusetts, United States

Daniel S. Mishkin, MD, CM
Chief of Gastroenterology
Atrius Health
Boston, Massachusetts, United States

Bijal Modi, MD
Department of Internal Medicine
Division of Hematology and Oncology
Texas Health Presbyterian Hospital Dallas
Dallas, Texas, United States

John Magaña Morton, MD, MPH, MHA
Vice Chair for Quality
Department of Surgery
Chief
Bariatric and Minimally Invasive Surgery
Yale School of Medicine
Department of Surgery
New Haven, Connecticut, United States

William Conan Mustain, MD
Assistant Professor of Surgery
Division of Colon and Rectal Surgery
University of Arkansas for Medical Sciences
Little Rock, Arkansas, United States

Filipe Gaio Nery, MD
Physician
Departamento de Anestesiologia, Cuidados Intensivos e Emergência
Centro Hospitalar do Porto–Hospital Santo António, Porto
Researcher, EPIUnit
Instituto de Saúde Pública, Universidade do Porto, Porto
Researcher, Ciências Médicas
Instituto de Ciências Biomédicas de Abel Salazar
Porto, Portugal

Siew C. Ng, MBBS (Lond), PhD (Lond)
Professor of Medicine
Department of Medicine and Therapeutics
State Key Laboratory of Digestive Disease
LKS Institute of Health Science
The Chinese University of Hong Kong
Hong Kong, China

Mark L. Norris, BSc (Hon), MD
Associate Professor of Pediatrics
Pediatrics
Children's Hospital of Eastern Ontario
University of Ottawa
Ottawa, Ontario, Canada

John O'Grady, MD, FRCPI
Professor
Institute of Liver Studies
King's College Hospital
London, United Kingdom

Manisha Palta, MD
Associate Professor
Radiation Oncology
Duke University
Durham, North Carolina, United States

Stephen J. Pandol, MD
Professor
Medicine
Cedars-Sinai Medical Center
Los Angeles, California, United States

John E. Pandolfino, MD, MSCI
Hans Popper Professor of Medicine
Feinberg School of Medicine
Northwestern University
Division Chief
Gastroenterology and Hepatology
Northwestern Medicine
Chicago, Illinois, United States

Darrell S. Pardi, MD, MS
Vice Chair
Division of Gastroenterology and Hepatology
Associate Dean
Mayo School of Graduate Medical Education
Mayo Clinic
Rochester, Minnesota, United States

Michelle Pearlman, MD
Professor of Medicine
Department of Internal Medicine, Division of Digestive and Liver Diseases
University of Texas Southwestern
Dallas, Texas, United States

Vyjeyanthi S. Periyakoil, MD
Director, Palliative Care Education and Training
Department of Medicine
Stanford University School of Medicine
Stanford, California, United States

Patrick R. Pfau, MD
Professor, Chief of Clinical Gastroenterology
Section of Gastroenterology and Hepatology
University of Wisconsin School of Medicine and Public Health
Madison, Wisconsin, United States

Angela K. Pham, MD
Clinical Assistant Professor
Gastroenterology, Hepatology, and Nutrition
University of Florida
Gainesville, Florida, United States

Kimberly L. Pham, MD
St. George's University Grenada
West Indies, Grenada

Daniel S. Pratt, MD
Clinical Director, Liver Transplantation
Division of Gastroenterology
Massachusetts General Hospital
Assistant Professor of Medicine
Harvard Medical School
Boston, Massachusetts, United States

David O. Prichard, MB, BCh, PhD
Gastroenterologist
Gastroenterology and Hepatology
Mayo Clinic
Rochester, Minnesota

Michael Quante, PD, Dr
Technische Universität München
II Medizinische Klinik
Klinikum rechts der Isar
München, Germany

Eamonn M.M. Quigley, MD
Professor of Medicine and Chief, Gastroenterology and Hepatology
David M. and Lynda K. Underwood Center for Digestive Disorders
Houston Methodist Hospital
Weill Cornell Medical College
Houston, Texas, United States

Balakrishnan S. Ramakrishna, MBBS, MD, DM, PhD
Head
Institute of Gastroenterology
SRM Institutes for Medical Science
Chennai, Tamil Nadu, India

Mrinalini C. Rao, PhD
Professor
Department of Physiology and Biophysics
University of Illinois at Chicago
Chicago, Illinois, United States

Satish S.C. Rao, MD, PhD
Professor of Medicine
Harold J. Harrison, MD, Distinguished University Chair in Gastroenterology
Medicine-Gastroenterology/Hepatology
Augusta University
Augusta, Georgia, United States

Christopher K. Rayner, MBBS, PhD
Professor
Adelaide Medical School
University of Adelaide
Consultant Gastroenterologist
Department of Gastroenterology and Hepatology
Royal Adelaide Hospital
Adelaide, South Australia, Australia

Ahsan Raza, MD
General and Colorectal Surgery
Rapides Surgical Specialists
Alexandria, Louisiana, United States

Miguel D. Regueiro, MD
Chair and Professor of Medicine
Department of Gastroenterology and Hepatology
Cleveland Clinic, Digestive Disease and Surgery Institute
Cleveland, Ohio, United States

John F. Reinus, MD
Professor of Medicine
Department of Medicine
Albert Einstein College of Medicine
Medical Director of Liver Transplantation
Montefiore-Einstein Center for Transplantation
Montefiore Medical Center
Bronx, New York, United States

David A. Relman, MD
Thomas C. and Joan M. Merigan Professor
Departments of Medicine and Microbiology and Immunology
Stanford University
Stanford, California
Chief of Infectious Diseases
Veterans Affairs Palo Alto Health Care System
Palo Alto, California, United States

Arvind Rengarajan, MD
Barnes-Jewish Hospital
Department of Internal Medicine
Washington University in St. Louis
St. Louis, Missouri, United States

Joel E. Richter, MD
Professor and Director
Division of Digestive Diseases and Nutrition
University of South Florida
Director
Joy McCann Culverhouse Center for Swallowing Disorders
University of South Florida
Tampa, Florida, United States

Sumera H. Rizvi, MD
Assistant Professor of Medicine
Division of Gastroenterology and Hepatology
Mayo Clinic
Rochester, Minnesota, United States

Syed Mujtaba Rizvi, MD
Assistant Professor
Division of Medical Oncology
Department of Internal Medicine
UT Southwestern Medical Center
Dallas, Texas, United States

Eve A. Roberts, MD, PhD
Adjunct Professor
Pediatrics, Medicine, and Pharmacology and Toxicology
University of Toronto
Adjunct Scientist
Genetics and Genome Biology Program
Hospital for Sick Children Research Institute
Associate
Division of Gastroenterology, Hepatology, and Nutrition
The Hospital for Sick Children
Toronto, Ontario, Canada
Associate Fellow
History of Science and Technology Program
University of King's College
Halifax, Nova Scotia, Canada

Martin D. Rosenthal, MD
Assistant Professor
Surgery
University of Florida
Gainesville, Florida, United States

Marc E. Rothenberg, MD, PhD
Professor of Pediatrics
Cincinnati Children's Hospital Medical Center
Cincinnati, Ohio, United States

Jayanta Roy-Chowdhury, MBBS
Professor
Departments of Medicine and Genetics
Director, Genetic Engineering and Gene Therapy Core Facility
Albert Einstein College of Medicine
New York, New York, United States

Namita Roy-Chowdhury, PhD
Professor
Departments of Medicine and Genetics
Albert Einstein College of Medicine
New York, New York, United States

David T. Rubin, MD
Joseph B. Kirsner Professor of Medicine
Chief, Section of Gastroenterology, Hepatology, and Nutrition
Department of Medicine
University of Chicago
Chicago, Illinois, United States

Jayashree Sarathy, PhD
Associate Professor
Department of Biological Sciences
Program Director of Master of Science in Integrative Physiology
Benedictine University
Lisle, Illinois
Visiting Research Professor
Department of Physiology and Biophysics
University of Illinois at Chicago
Chicago, Illinois, United States

George S. Sarosi Jr., MD
Robert H. Hux MD Professor and Vice Chairman for Education
Department of Surgery
University of Florida College of Medicine
Staff Surgeon
Surgical Service
NF/SG VAMC
Gainesville, Florida, United States

Thomas J. Savides, MD
Professor of Clinical Medicine
Division of Gastroenterology
University of California San Diego
La Jolla, California, United States

Lawrence R. Schiller, MD
Attending Physician
Gastroenterology Division
Baylor University Medical Center
Dallas, Texas, United States

Mitchell L. Schubert, MD
Professor of Medicine and Physiology
Virginia Commonwealth University Health System
Chief, Division of Gastroenterology, Hepatology, and Nutrition
McGuire Veterans Affairs Medical Center
Richmond, Virginia, United States

Cynthia L. Sears, MD
Professor of Medicine and Oncology
Johns Hopkins University School of Medicine
Baltimore, Maryland, United States

Joseph H. Sellin, MD
Professor Emeritus
Division of Gastroenterology
Baylor College of Medicine
Chief of Gastroenterology
Ben Taub General Hospital
Houston, Texas, United States

M. Gaith Semrin, MD, MBBS
Associate Professor
Pediatric Gastroenterology and Nutrition
UT Southwestern Medical Center
Children Medical Center Dallas
Dallas, Texas, United States

Vijay H. Shah, MD
Professor
Medicine, Physiology, and Cancer Cell Biology
Chair
Division of Gastroenterology and Hepatology
Associate Chair of Research Medicine
Mayo Clinic College of Medicine and Science
Rochester, Minnesota, United States

G. Thomas Shires, MD
John P. Thompson Chair
Surgical Services
Texas Health Presbyterian Hospital Dallas
Dallas, Texas, United States

Maria H. Sjogren, MD, MPH
Senior Hepatologist
Department of Medicine
Walter Reed National Medical Center
Bethesda, Maryland, United States

Phillip D. Smith, MD
Professor of Medicine and Microbiology
University of Alabama at Birmingham
Birmingham, Alabama, United States

Elsa Solà, MD, PhD
Liver Unit
Hospital Clinic
Associate Professor
University of Barcelona
Researcher
Institut d'Investigacions Biomediques August Pi i Sunyer (IDIBAPS)
Barcelona, Spain

Rhonda F. Souza, MD
Co-Director, Center for Esophageal Diseases
Department of Medicine
Baylor University Medical Center
Co-Director, Center for Esophageal Research
Baylor Scott and White Research Institute
Dallas, Texas, United States

Cedric W. Spak, MD, MPH
Clinical Assistant Professor
Infectious Diseases
Baylor University Medical Center
Staff Physician
Infectious Diseases
Texas Centers for Infectious Disease Associates
Dallas, Texas, United States

Stuart Jon Spechler, MD
Chief, Division of Gastroenterology
Co-Director, Center for Esophageal Research
Department of Medicine
Baylor University Medical Center at Dallas
Co-Director, Center for Esophageal Research
Baylor Scott and White Research Institute
Dallas, Texas, United States

James E. Squires, MD, MS
Assistant Professor
Department of Pediatrics
UPMC Children's Hospital of Pittsburgh
Pittsburgh, Pennsylvania, United States

Neil H. Stollman, MD
Associate Clinical Professor
Department of Medicine, Division of Gastroenterology
University of California San Francisco
San Francisco, California
Chief
Division of Gastroenterology
Alta Bates Summit Medical Center
Oakland, California, United States

Sarah E. Streett, MD
Clinical Associate Professor
Director IBD Education
Division of Gastroenterology and Hepatology
Stanford University
Redwood City, California, United States

Jonathan R. Strosberg, MD
Associate Professor
Gastrointestinal Oncology
Moffitt Cancer Center
Tampa, Florida, United States

Frederick J. Suchy, MD
Children's Hospital Colorado
Professor of Pediatrics and Associate Dean for Child Health Research
Pediatrics
University of Colorado School of Medicine
Aurora, Colorado, United States

Aravind Sugumar, MD
Instructor
Gastroenterology and Hepatology
Cleveland Clinic Foundation
Cleveland, Ohio, United States

Shelby Sullivan, MD
Associate Professor of Medicine
Director, Gastroenterology Metabolic and Bariatric Program
Division of Gastroenterology and Hepatology
University of Colorado Anschutz Medical Campus
Aurora, Colorado, United States

Gyongyi Szabo, MD, PhD
Mitchell T. Rabkin, MD Chair
Chief Academic Officer
Beth Israel Deaconess Medical Center and Beth Israel Lahey Health
Faculty Dean for Academic Affairs
Harvard Medical School
Boston, Massachusetts, United States

Jan Tack, MD, PhD
Head, Division of Gastroenterology and Hepatology
Leuven University Hospitals
Professor of Medicine
Translational Research Center for Gastrointestinal Disorders (TARGID)
Department of Clinical and Experimental Medicine
University of Leuven
Leuven, Belgium

Nicholas J. Talley, MD, PhD
Distinguished Laureate Professor
Faculty of Health and Medicine
University of Newcastle, Australia
Newcastle, New South Wales, Australia

Jarred P. Tanksley, MD, PhD
Resident
Radiation Oncology
Duke University
Durham, North Carolina, United States

Narci C. Teoh, MD
Professor of Medicine
Australian National University
Senior Staff Hepatologist
The Canberra Hospital
Australian Capital Territory, Australia

Dawn M. Torres, MD
Program Director GI Fellowship
Department of Medicine
Walter Reed National Military Medical Center
Associate Professor of Medicine
Department of Medicine
Uniformed Services University of the Health Sciences
Bethesda, Maryland, United States

Kiran Turaga, MD, MPH
Associate Professor
Department of Surgery
The University of Chicago
Chicago, Illinois, United States

Richard H. Turnage, MD
Executive Associate Dean for Clinical Affairs
Professor of Surgery
University of Arkansas for Medical Sciences Medical Center
University of Arkansas for Medical Sciences
Little Rock, Arkansas, United States

Michael F. Vaezi, MD, PhD, MS
Professor of Medicine and Otolaryngology
Division of Gastroenterology and Hepatology
Vanderbilt University
Director
Center for Swallowing and Esophageal Disorders
Vanderbilt University Medical Center
Director
Clinical Research
Vanderbilt University Medical Center
Nashville, Tennessee, United States

Dominique Charles Valla, MD
Professor of Hepatology
Liver Unit
Hôpital Beaujon, APHP, Clichy-la-Garenne
France
CRI, UMR1149
Inserm and Université de Paris
Paris, France

John J. Vargo II, MD, MPH
Associate Professor of Medicine
Gastroenterology and Hepatology
Cleveland Clinic
Cleveland, Ohio, United States

Santhi Swaroop Vege, MD
Professor of Medicine and Director Pancreas Group
Gastroenterology and Hepatology
Mayo Clinic
Rochester, Minnesota, United States

Axel von Herbay, MD
Professor of Pathology
Faculty of Medicine
University of Heidelberg
Heidelberg Hans Pathologie
Hamburg, Germany

Margaret von Mehren, MD
Professor
Department of Hematology/Oncology
Fox Chase Cancer Center
Philadelphia, Pennsylvania, United States

David Q.-H. Wang, MD, PhD
Professor of Medicine
Departments of Medicine and Genetics
Director, Molecular Biology and Next Generation Technology Core
Marion Bessin Liver Research Center
Albert Einstein College of Medicine
Bronx, New York, United States

Sachin Wani, MD
Associate Professor of Medicine
Division of Gastroenterology and Hepatology
University of Colorado Anschutz Medical Campus
Aurora, Colorado, United States

Frederick Weber, MD
Clinical Professor
Division of Gastroenterology and Hepatology
University of Alabama Birmingham
Birmingham, Alabama, United States

Barry K. Wershil, MD
Professor
Pediatrics
Northwestern University Feinberg School of Medicine
Chief, Division of Gastroenterology, Hepatology, and Nutrition
Pediatrics
Ann & Robert H. Lurie Children's Hospital of Chicago
Chicago, Illinois, United States

David C. Whitcomb, MD, PhD
Professor
Medicine, Cell Biology and Molecular Physiology, and Human Genetics
University of Pittsburgh and UPMC
Pittsburgh, Pennsylvania, United States

C. Mel Wilcox, MD, MSPH
Division of Gastroenterology and Hepatology
University of Alabama at Birmingham
Birmingham, Alabama, United States

Christopher G. Willett, MD
Professor and Chairman
Radiation Oncology
Duke University
Durham, North Carolina, United States

Joseph C. Yarze, MD
Assistant Professor of Medicine
Harvard Medical School
Associate Physician
Division of Gastroenterology
Massachusetts General Hospital
Boston, Massachusetts, United States

Anahit A. Zeynalyan, MD
Resident
Internal Medicine
Baylor University Medical Center
Dallas, Texas, United States

中文版序言（一）

《斯莱森杰-福特伦胃肠病学和肝病学：病理生理学、诊断、治疗和管理》（第 11 版）是最权威的消化领域专著之一，涵盖胃肠病学、肝病学相关病理生理学、诊断、治疗、管理等综合内容，提供了消化领域在临床及基础方面全面、前沿的理论知识，是全球消化医生手中宝贵的经典教科书。

本书分为上、下两卷，首先从胃肠道生理、营养、症状体征、多器官消化系统疾病等角度进行了知识点总结，其次，通过解剖部位划分，细致地将每一个消化脏器相关疾病逐一概述，包含定义、流行病学、病理机制、临床表现、诊断与鉴别诊断、诊断路径、相关并发症、治疗、随访、患者教育等，在上一版教材内容基础上，全面更新相关知识点，书中插图典型、精美、引用最新研究进展，在启发读者进行基本知识回顾同时，进行拓展阅读，鼓励深入阅读，巩固和提高消化医生临床诊治、综合分析、掌握先进技术的能力，是消化医生手中最有力的工具书之一。

本书将消化系统疾病细致分类，对于消化专业年轻医生是一本真正可以全面、系统化的获得前沿知识的经典专著，引用了较多基础研究、临床实例，启发读者进行思考，鼓励阅读更多更新的研究进展和规范的诊疗措施，旨在提高在年轻医师成长过程中能够发现问题、分析问题、解决问题的能力，内容实用性很强，同时，书中附有大量真实的、彩色的、典型的临床病例图片，可以加深读者对疾病的理解和认识，特别是对各方面知识进行总结、归纳，绘制流程图、三线表、要点框，有助于对知识点的整体掌握、记忆。

本书翻译审校人员包括国内消化领域学科学术带头人、知名专家、中青年骨干，编译过程中，多次进行修改、审核、校稿，最终在专家、教授的群策群力下，在繁忙的临床工作之余，高效、高质量、高要求地完成了所有工作，付出了巨大努力。最后，衷心希望大家通过本书的学习，能有所收获，并提出宝贵的意见和建议。

张澍田　教授

首都医科大学附属北京友谊医院院长

国家消化系统疾病临床医学研究中心主任

中华医学会常务理事

中国医师协会常务理事

中国医师协会消化医师分会会长

2023 年 7 月

中文版序言（二）

《斯莱森杰-福特伦胃肠病学和肝病学：病理生理学、诊断、治疗和管理》（第11版）是一本涉及消化系统包括胃、肠、肝、胆和胰等的病理学、生理学、诊断学和疾病管理学的权威著作。十几代数百名世界著名消化病学专家对本书进行了更新迭代和补充，才铸就了这本全面、权威和实用的专著。

现今是一个期刊数量呈指数级爆炸增长的时代，对于临床医师和科研人员来说，这无疑令人感到兴奋。但是，也正因如此，时间的限制和信息的冗杂，全面地评估和吸收第一手信息可能变得愈加困难，获得一个更可靠的、更全面的、更新的综合类书籍和指南变得尤为重要。

本人对推荐这部新书感到非常兴奋和荣幸。这本世界巨著，是一本专门针对医学专业人士撰写的消化疾病学参考书籍，旨在提供关于消化疾病的发生发展、病理生理、诊断和治疗等方面的深入信息。本书力求系统、全面地介绍消化疾病学领域的知识，既有理论的深度，又有实践的指导，以帮助医学专业人士更好地了解和应对消化疾病。

本书共分为上、下两卷，每个部分涵盖了不同的主题，并按照逻辑顺序展开。上卷介绍胃食管胰胆病学，下卷包括肝脏和肠道病学，不但介绍了各系统的生理病理学，同时详细梳理了常见食管、胰、胆、肝脏、肠道相关疾病的病因发病机制，包括遗传因素、环境因素、生活方式等方面的影响，以帮助读者全面了解疾病的全过程。以大篇幅叙述了相关的临床表现、诊断和分型方法，包括症状、体征、实验室检查、影像学和病理学等方面，以帮助读者准确诊断和分类患者的疾病；同时深入介绍疾病经典和新的治疗方法，包括药物治疗、手术治疗和综合治疗等，帮助医生更好地制订治疗计划。另外，也涉及了相应的预防和管理策略，包括生活方式干预、饮食调节和心理支持等方面，以帮助患者减轻症状、预防复发和提高生活质量。

本书的特点之一是非常注重实用性。每个章节都配有丰富的临床案例和实用技巧，帮助读者更好地理解和应用所学知识。

本书也非常注重前沿性，介绍了新的研究成果和治疗方法，包括基因治疗、免疫治疗等前沿技术。此外，本书还介绍了各种新型诊断工具和治疗设备，包括内镜、影像导航系统等先进设备。

尤其是这本书还采用了大量精美、生动的插图和图表。这些插图不仅展示了疾病的发展过程和相关机制，还通过详细的示意图和病例分析帮助读者更直观地理解病情。同时，注重对重要概念的强调和讲解，使得读者能够轻松理解并且快速掌握重点知识。

此外，本书还配备大量的参考文献，方便读者深入学习和研究。这些参考文献的来源广泛，包括了研究论文、临床指南及专业学术期刊，为读者提供了更新、更深入的领域知识。

总之，本书是一部不可多得的肝胆肠胃疾病领域的权威著作。它不仅具有高度概括性、专业性、引导性和前瞻性，还具有一定的科普性和实用性，是极为宝贵的工具书。

我衷心地感谢整个翻译团队的辛勤努力和杰出贡献。该团队是由30多位全国知名医学院校的高年资医师和研究人员组成，他们的专业知识和丰富经验使得这部中译版巨著得以成功问世，并成为国内消化医学界的一件可赞誉的盛事。

无论您是临床医生，还是科研人员，我相信本书将是您不可或缺的学习和工作得力助手和良师，愿您能借助这部权威著作，进一步认识和探索消化和肝病领域的前沿知识，为我们共同的事业做出更大的贡献。

希望本书能够广泛传播，造福更多的读者和患者！

季　光
消化内科学教授
上海中医药大学校长
2023年7月

中文版序言（三）

久负盛名的第 11 版 *Sleisenger and Fordtran's Gastrointestinal and Liver Disease：Pathophysiology/Diagnosis/Management* 于 2021 年由 Elsevier 出版社出版了。这部首版于 1973 年的消化病学名著的第一个特点是系统、全面，不仅包括了常见消化系统症状的诊断思路、检查方法和治疗手段及所有空腔和实质性器官的疾病，还包括了其他系统疾病及社会心理因素对消化系统的影响。第二个特点是注重对消化疾病相关基础知识的总结，对每个疾病的病因、发病机制及病理生理进行了深入浅出的描述。第三个特点是主编、副主编及 230 多位作者多是该疾病领域里的顶级专家。以本人较熟悉的肝脏疾病部分为例，负责编写乙型肝炎的专家为 Harry L. A. Janssen 教授，负责编写自身免疫性肝炎的专家为 Albert J. Czaja 教授，负责编写原发性胆汁性胆管炎的专家为 Keith D. Lindor 教授，负责编写血色病的专家为 Bruce R. Bacon 教授，负责腹水及其并发症部分的是 Pere Ginès 教授，负责编写急性肝衰竭的专家为 John O'Grady 教授。这些长期致力于相应疾病临床和科研工作的权威学者的亲自参编，保障了本书的学术水准和权威性。

在信息技术高度发达的今天，专业知识的获取也更加便捷。各种网络资源及移动终端的普及更使得各种专业信息唾手可得。这些信息获取方式的优势是能够超越时空的限制而对临床工作供即时帮助，但其局限性也不言而喻，其最主要的缺点是知识碎片化，而且文献质量良莠不齐。因此，对于年轻临床医生，特别是住院医生和专业学位研究生而言，必须认真研读一本临床专业经典名著，才能真正系统了解和掌握本专业的知识体系，包括本学科的基本范畴（学科内涵和外延）、疾病的基本概念、临床基本特征及基本诊疗原则等。

为便于更多的中国医生阅读这部消化病学名著，人民卫生出版社邀请上海中医药大学附属曙光医院袁农教授等消化界知名专家担任主译（6 位）和主审（4 位），并组织来自国内 7 家知名高等医学院校附属医院的 23 位中青年医生（其中 21 位副高级职称以上）将本书全文翻译成中文。学术著作的翻译历来是一项极为艰辛的智力活动，需要广博的专业知识，熟练的英文阅读能力，流畅的中文表达能力，而且还需要付出宝贵的时间、精力和耐心。作为本译著的主审之一，本人感谢全体译校者及编辑所付出的心血和汗水！

本书译稿经过多次审校及编辑加工，以尽量准确表达原文的真实内容。因翻译、审校本书的工作量巨大（上、下两卷共 132 章），不当甚至谬误之处在所难免，更难真正达到"信、达、雅"的最高翻译境界。在此，我们恳请广大读者不吝指教，对于阅读中发现的问题提出意见和建议，以便我们在重印或再版时尽量改进和提高。

贾继东　教授
首都医科大学附属北京友谊医院肝病中心
中华医学会肝病学分会前主任委员（2006—2012 年）
亚太地区肝病学会前主席（2009—2010 年）
国际肝病学会前主席（2013—2016 年）
2023 年 7 月

中文版序言（四）

我非常有幸能与张澍田教授、袁农教授等共同翻译《斯莱森杰-福特伦胃肠病学和肝病学：病理生理学、诊断、治疗和管理》这部消化系统经典名著。此书作为消化系统的旷世著作，其在消化界的地位和影响可与《史记》对中国文学史的影响相媲美。《史记》素有“史文学，双合璧，树正史，把典立”的文学特征，被赞誉为“史家之绝唱”。而本书则具有“全覆盖，样俱全，析秋毫，寻微幽”的撰写特点，堪称另一种“无韵之离骚”。但由于各种原因，目前这部消化巨著并未有中文版上市，也使国内很多医务人员不能尽享其魅力，不能不说是一种遗憾。幸好在袁农教授的大力倡导和精心组织下，着手翻译此书最新版，承蒙抬爱，我惶恐接下此翻译和审核任务。希望通过翻译团队的共同努力，为广大读者传递最准确的原著内容，并希望能在巩固基础、拓宽视野、提出创新等方面发挥其作用。

首先，本书具有“全覆盖”的特点，以脏器为横轴，不同疾病种类为纵轴，涵盖了几乎所有涉及消化脏器的疾病种类，勾画了一幅全面的消化系统疾病网格图。其次，本书具有“样俱全”的特点，体现在不仅仅包含了常见病，也详尽描述了很多少见病的发病机制，临床表现，诊断和治疗进展等，同时也全面描述了解剖、组织胚胎等基础知识，为读者能够正确理解疾病奠定基础。再次，本书具有“析秋毫”的特点，本书各个章节的撰写非常详细，对于疾病的“细枝末节”可以说做到了细致入微，可以帮助读者结合临床实践，理解临床少见表现。最后，本书具有“寻微幽”的特点，不仅仅是已达成共识的基本内容，本书还提供了很多疾病机制和疾病治疗方面的进展性内容，尤其是近年来靶向治疗和消化内镜等方面的飞速发展，为消化系统疾病的诊断和治疗打开了另一扇窗户，而本书也涉猎了很多此方面的内容。

一本好书如同一架梯子，可以引导我们登上知识的殿堂，衷心希望此中文版能让每一位读者获益，提高自身的专业技术水平，在消化系统疾病的探索中走得更高，更远！

黄永辉　教授

北京大学第三医院北方院区执行院长

中华医学会消化内镜分会常务委员

北京医学会消化内镜分会副主任委员

2023 年 7 月

中文版前言

早在 1994—1996 年，我在美国加州大学旧金山分校(University of California，San Francisco，UCSF)附属 Moffit-Long 医院做访问学者。当时 Marvin H. Sleisenger 教授任 UCSF 另一所附属医院——退伍军人事务医学中心(Veterans Affairs Medical Center)消化中心主任，那时我与他相识。当时 UCSF 附属 3 个医院的消化科医生、研究生及进修医生，每周三上午在 Moffit-Long 附属医院的 HSW300 进行消化疾病专题研讨会(Medical Grand Round)。Sleisenger 教授几乎逢会必到，并在会上积极讨论发言。在讨论会上能经常聆听到他精辟的讲解和分析，当时给我留下了深刻的印象，对他非常敬佩。那时阅读到他与美国达拉斯西南医学中心消化科教授 John S. Fordtran 联合主编的 *Gastrointestinal Disease* 一书，受益匪浅。我学习期满后回国，在重庆医科大学附属第一医院消化科工作期间，一次偶然的机会，在医院临街的医学书店翻阅到了 Sleisenger 和 Fordtran 主编的由国内出版的英文影印版 *Gastrointestinal and Liver Disease*：*Pathophysiology/Diagnosis/Management* 一书，这是该书第 6 版，是在原胃肠病学基础上增加了肝脏病学后的首版。我购买了一套(上、下卷)，此后对历次修订版本也不断参阅学习，对自己从事消化专业临床与教学工作帮助很大。

该书是一部消化病学世界级水平的经典权威著作，是美国及世界许多国家医学院校选读的消化病学教科书和参考书，特别是研究型医生更新知识、开拓思维、找准科研创新的切入点与突破口的参考著作。该书首版于 1973 年，由 Marvin H. Sleisenger 教授和 John S. Fordtran 教授领衔、联合全球消化病专家编著而成。该书出版发行之后，引起全世界消化专业同仁的广泛好评和赞誉，被公认是当代最具影响的消化病学经典著作。此后，该书每 4~5 年修订再版一次，至 2021 年已出版第 11 版。

该书第 11 版的学术价值和实用性概括为以下几点：

1. 全书共 132 章，是一部巨著，分上、下两卷。上卷共 70 章，从第 1 章至第 42 章讲述了消化病生物学、营养及消化各器官病变的症状体征等专题(相当于总论部分)。从第 43 章至第 70 章讲述了食管、胃、胆、胰疾病。下卷共 62 章，从第 71 章至第 132 章讲述了肝脏及大、小肠疾病。本书每章内容均密切联系基础理论和前沿知识，并突出论述了病理生理学。通过阐述各种疾病的发病机制，揭示疾病发生、发展和转归的规律，为消化疾病的诊断、治疗、预防提供了理论依据。

2. 全书 132 章，由来自北美、欧洲、澳大利亚及亚洲 230 多位著名消化病学专家编写而成。可以说每一章节都是各位专家长期从事临床、科研及教学工作的经验总结，有些还是专家长期从事的研究课题，是一生心血的积累！因作者来自世界各地，所以其理论与经验更具有国际性。

3. 本书不仅全面论述了消化系统的基础理论，包括胃肠生物学、分子生物学、免疫学、遗传基因学的前沿知识，而且对消化器官的解剖学、组织学、胚胎学及病理学均有详细的论述，并系统介绍了消化系统各种疾病的诊断、治疗、护理及预防。书中内容还涉及消化外科、小儿消化疾病，甚至涉及与消化系统疾病有关的口腔、皮肤、神经内分泌及传统医学等学科的疾病。

4. 书中讲述的消化系统疾病的流行病学、诊断、治疗药物和技能，均采用了随机对照试验、系统评价、meta 分析等循证医学的方法进行评估。重视收集和分析原创性研究资料，明确哪些问题已基本解决，哪些问题尚未阐明，对指导临床研究选择最佳课题具有较好的参考价值。

5. 该书各章在文字论述的同时，均有精美的图表，共计 1 100 多幅。这些图表形象地解读了文章中论述的重点内容，为读者理解内容要点起到“看图识文”的效果。

将这部第 11 版原著翻译为中文在国内首次出版，无疑有助于国内消化专业内、外科医师及研究人员学习专业理论、更新学科知识、提高技术水平，同时也为学习消化专业的研究生、医学生们提供了一部经典的教科书和参考书，对推动国内胃肠病学和肝脏病学的临床、教学、科研的发展有所裨益。为此，我们与人民卫生出版社讨论协商同意后，组建了由北京、上海、西安、杭州、重庆等高等医学院校附属医院的 33 位消化专家组成的翻译团队，经过两年多的认真翻译、反复审校，现将上卷 70 章先期出版，下卷 62 章随后出版。在此，我对各位译、校、审专家表示衷心的感谢！

常言道“翻译”是遗憾之作，达到“信、达、雅”并非易事。有时我们翻译时，对原著中的不少英文词句审之又审、慎之又慎，但最终仍不如意。其原因可能与译者的专业知识、实践经验、医学英语水平和中文程度存在差别有关。因此译书中难免有不足之处，甚至错误。在此，恳请各位读者特别是国内消化界同仁指正！

袁　农

本书主译(执行)

西安交通大学第三附属医院原主任医师、教授

重庆医科大学附属第一医院原主任医师、教授

上海中医药大学附属曙光医院主任医师、教授

2023 年 7 月

原著序言

试图为第 11 版 *Sleisenger and Fordtral's Gastrointestinal and Liver Disease: Pathophysiology/Diagnosis/Management* 一书撰写序言。这本教科书几十年来一直致力于为读者做好应对胃肠道和肝脏病患者提出挑战的准备。编著此书是一项艰巨的任务，但也是一种极大的乐趣。仅仅完成第 11 版教科书本身就是一个了不起的成就。一代又一代的胃肠病学家和肝病学家，一直依靠本书为读者提供了全面、最新、可靠的信息。

第 11 版是在以前版本基础上进行了扩充，本书既往的版本一直被是相关领域的重要参考书。在过去的半个世纪里，本书也是该领域图书馆的重要藏书。自出版以来，这本经典教科书一直在呈现各专业领域的学术进展。如今，我们这些对胃肠病学和肝脏病学感兴趣的人，有越来越多的方式获得激励、了解、教育和更新。举办讲座、与同事交流以及参加当地、地区和全国性的学术会议都有其作用。我们都要向广大的患者学习。在现有期刊数量显著增加的时代，对医学期刊中相关文章的阅读变得越来越困难。在当今时间有限的情况下，执业临床医生将比以往任何时候都更觉得这本教科书可靠、信息丰富和实用。在这两卷书中，概述了现在已知的情况，以及未来可能带来的情况。为了实现这些目标，作者需要具备技能、知识、实践经验和教学的综合能力。总的来说，这些努力成功地在我们感兴趣的领域提供了准确和全面的最新信息，有助于我们对过去和现在进行反思，并勾划出有待解决的问题。

我们有幸生活在胃肠病学和肝脏病学日新月异的时代。多份期刊上发表的大量新观点令人振奋，且往往势不可挡。我们每个人都必须评估和吸收新的信息，同时应努力将新的进展融入我们的实践中。要跟上时代保持领先并实现我们的目标，需要付出相当大的努力和奉献。有一个可靠和可信赖的指南来更新和激励我们是一种宽慰。

本书为我们提供了一个关于既定知识的坚实、权威的平台，并确定了在哪些方面正在取得进展，使我们在可预见的未来能够更好地武装起来。我们都需要了解新观察结果可能的有效性和有用性。至关重要的是，我们必须认识到导致我们得出结论的数据的确定程度。已经(也将有)明确的改变游戏规则的进展，还有许多看似不错的想法和方法结果却被回避了。新的概念必须被认识、反复检查、处理，然后融入我们的思维中，从而影响我们的行动。

本书涵盖主题的广度和深度令人印象深刻。我有幸为 2010 年出版的第 9 版撰写了序言。当比较从那时到现在知识的拓展时，人们可以理解我们所拥有的成就，以及我们希望(和期望)在未来实现的目标。

本书提供了一个有用且可信的指南，可供读者随时查阅。如果将过去版本中的章节与现在的章节进行比较，可以进一步验证我们的专业正在取得进展，其未来令人鼓舞。第 11 版的 3 位资深主编和 3 位副主编是最重要的权威专家，他们在确定感兴趣的主题和说服这些领域的专家分享知识方面的能力得到了广泛认可。撰写一篇关于自己所从事专业领域的最新评论可能是一项艰巨的任务，不仅需要知识，而且需要勇气。主编们肯定成功了。精心挑选各个章节的作者，使他们都能就需要强调什么内容提出自己的观点，阐述我们所知道的和我们需要知道的内容，以诊断和有效治疗特定的疾病，并就如何管理患者提供建议和指导，同时将新的观察结果融入实践中。

关于肝脏部分，目前对导致肝炎的病毒和药物诱导的肝脏疾病的了解，以及对肝脏中过多脂肪累积在慢性肝病病因中的许多后果的关注，令人惊叹。这些成果已被记录在案，在不久的将来有机会(和希望)获得更有效的治疗药物。就在这个版本出版之前，我们对几种类型的病毒性肝炎进行了有效、可普遍应用的治疗，我们所希望的大部分已经实现。现在很可能会发现有利于影响广泛脂肪性肝损伤的治疗方法，包括它们与心血管疾病的关系。广泛使用先进的内镜检查改变了许多胃肠道、胆管和胰腺疾病的评估和治疗方法。此外，就在几年前，谁能预见到生物疗法和微创手术的进步，将如何重新引导我们对一系列疾病的治疗，或肠道微生物菌群在许多疾病的发病机制中有多么重要。一旦我们了解了如何有利地改变肠道微生物菌群，就有望取得重大的进展。

下一步是什么？基因组编辑和对肠道微生物菌群的认识，目前还处于起步阶段，在未来的几年里，它们将受到广泛的关注。随着时间的推移，人类基因组工程和肠道微生物菌群的研究会越来越精确，需要不断进行深思熟虑的监督，以确保我们做我们应该做的事情，而不仅仅是我们能做的事情。在本版本中，对我们专业的许多方面都有未来的蓝图和预测。重要的是要摒弃那些没有被证明是有效的旧观念，同时要不断地重新审视我们认为自己所掌握的东西的基础，并适当地改变我们所做的事情。

当我们看到医学上已经(和正在)发生的事情，以及这些进展在胃肠病学和肝脏病学中的影响时，我们都感到惊讶。当然，最好的前景还没有到来，我们都希望用现在所掌握和应用的知识与技能，激励我们创造一个更美好的未来。

Willis C. Maddrey, MD
Dallas, Texas

原著前言

1971 年夏天，美国旧金山的 Marvin H. Sleisenger 博士和达拉斯的 John S. Fordtran 博士开始了一项新的计划：为胃肠病学家规划、编写和出版一本新的教科书——*Gastrointestinal Disease: Pathophysiology/Diagnosis/Management*。该书因包含了对所讨论疾病的病理生理学的最新论述而受到广泛赞誉，这在医学教科书中是第一次。自该书问世以来，后续版本每 4~5 年出版一次，我们很高兴这本受人尊崇的第 11 版教科书延续了创始主编们设定的传统和标准。可以肯定的是，自第 1 版出版以来已经进行了无数次的改进，例如增加了关于肝脏疾病的章节，在网络上和手持设备上提供了每月更新以引起人们关注版本之间发生的重要新进展，纳入了新的诊断和治疗流程的视频，以及来自世界各地作者的参与，使本书具有真正的国际风范。

2017 年夏天，现任主编与出版商会面协商，详细审阅了该书的第 10 版。最重要的是，由 3 名资深主编组成的核心小组邀请了 3 名副主编（Raymond T. Chung 博士、David T. Rubin 博士和 C. Mel Wilcox 博士）加入他们的行列，以促进对各章节的批判性审查，帮助选择最专业的作者，并提供内容更丰富的专业知识。每位副主编都与一位资深主编密切合作。我们希望这是一部易于阅读、精心编写、高度准确和全面的对胃肠道和肝脏疾病研究现状进行综述的著作。本书的目标读者主要是胃肠病学和肝脏病学家以及胃肠病学学员。我们希望这本书也能对普通内科医生、其他专业医生和各级学生都有所帮助。

回顾 50 年来，由于严格的基础科学和临床研究，我们在该领域取得的进展确实非常显著，而且未来将有更大的发展前景。第 11 版讨论的特色进展包括：改善慢性乙型和丙型肝炎的诊断和治疗；幽门螺杆菌感染的诊断和治疗进展及其对预防和治疗消化性溃疡病和胃肿瘤的益处；通过筛查和监测改进结、直肠癌的预防工作；Barrett 食管的识别和治疗以及食管腺癌预防的新方法；扩大使用生物制剂和新型小分子治疗和预防炎症性肠病复发；认识到越来越多的免疫和自身免疫性疾病不仅影响胃和肝胆系统，而且还影响胰腺和肠道；提高了对胃肠道出血患者进行风险分层和治疗的能力；以及肝脏、胰腺和小肠移植的持续进展。我们在对肠道微生物菌群的了解方面取得了显著进展，肠道微生物菌群正成为各种领域关注的焦点，如肠易激综合征、炎症性肠病、肥胖、肝性脑病和其他疾病，包括非胃肠道疾病。我们特别高兴的是，通过重新组织和更新病理生理学、临床表现和管理的讨论，完全重新设计了炎症性肠病章节，所有这些都在迅速发展。

不幸的是，这本教科书的最初联合创始主编 Marvin H. Sleisenger 博士于 2017 年 10 月 19 日逝世，享年 93 岁。我们非常怀念 Marvin！我们相信第 11 版的出版会得到他的认可和赞扬！

Mark Feldman，MD

Lawrence S. Friedman，MD

Lawrence J. Brandt，MD

原著致谢

第 11 版 *Sleisenger and Fordtral's Gastrointestinal and Liver Disease：Pathophysiology/Diagnosis/Management* 的主编和副主编们非常感谢来自北美、欧洲、亚洲和澳大利亚的 230 多位作者，他们为全书贡献了自己的知识、专业技能和智慧。我们也十分感谢爱思唯尔有才华的工作人员，他们帮助这本书获得了新的生命，特别是 Nancy Duffy、Dolores Meloni 和 Deidre Simpson。Cindy Thom 负责监督这本书的制作。特别感谢我们的助理——Sherie Strang、Alison Sholock、Amy Nash 和 Amy Majkowski，他们为我们提供了出色的秘书支持。还要感谢得克萨斯大学西南分校的 Willis C. Maddrey 博士的精彩序言，这是他第二次被邀请为本书做序。深情地缅怀 Marvin H. Sleisenger 博士，他在共同主编本书第 11 版的过程中不幸与世长辞。对 John S. Fordtran 博士持续不断的研究和贡献表示敬意。还非常感谢我们的爱人——Barbara Feldman、Mary Jo Cappuccilli、Lois Brandt、Kim Wilcox、Diane Abraczinskas 和 Rebecca Rubin 的爱和支持。最后，要感谢本书的读者，感谢他们对这本教科书的信心和信任。

我们将第 11 版献给你们，我们的读者，因为在我们编写、编辑和制作这本教科书的过程中，始终是以你们为中心。希望我们的书能满足你们的教育需要。

缩略词表

AASLD	American Association for the Study of Liver Diseases	美国肝病研究学会
ACG	America College of Gastroenterology	美国胃肠病学会
ACTH	Corticotropin	促肾上腺皮质激素
AE	Angioectasia	血管扩张
AFP	Alpha fetoprotein	α-胎甲蛋白
AGA	American Gastroenterological Association	美国胃肠病学会
AIDS	Acquired immunodeficiency syndrome	获得性免疫缺陷综合征
ALF	Acute liver failure	急性肝衰竭
ALT	Alanine aminotransferase	丙氨酸转氨酶
AMA	Antimitochondrial antibodies	抗线粒体抗体
ANA	Antinuclear antibodies	抗核抗体
ANCA	Antineutrophil cytoplasmic antibodies	抗中性粒细胞胞浆抗体
APACHE	Acute physiology and chronic health examination	急性生理学和慢性健康检查
APC	Argon plasma coagulation	氩离子血浆凝固
ASGE	American society for Gastrointestinal Endoscopy	美国胃肠内镜学会
AST	Aspartate aminotransferase	天门冬氨酸转氨酶
ATP	Adenosine triphosphate	三磷酸腺苷
BICAP	Bipolar electrocoagulation	双极电凝
BMI	Body mass index	体重指数
BRBPR	Bright red blood per rectum	经直肠鲜红血
CBC	Complete blood count	全血细胞计数
CCK	Cholecystokinin	胆囊收缩素
CEA	Carcinoembryonic antigen	癌胚抗原
CDI	*Clostridioides difficile* infection	梭状芽孢杆菌感染
CF	Cystic fibrosis	囊性纤维化
CFTR	Cystic fibrosis transmembrane conductance regulator	囊性纤维化跨膜转导调节因子
CMV	Cytomegalovirus	巨细胞病毒
CNS	Central nervous system	中枢神经系统
CO_2	Carbon dioxide	二氧化碳
COX	Cyclooxygenase	环氧合酶
CT	Computed tomography	计算机断层扫描
CTA	Computed tomography angiography	计算机断层血管造影
DAA	Direct-acting antiviral agent	直接作用抗病毒制剂
DIC	Disseminated intravascular coagulation	弥散性血管内凝血
DILI	Drug-induced liver injury	药物诱导的肝损伤
DNA	Deoxyribonucleic acid	脱氧核糖核酸
DU	Duodenal ulcer	十二指肠溃疡
DVT	Deep vein thrombosis	深静脉血栓形成
EBV	Epstein-Barr virus	EB 病毒
EGD	Esophagogastroduodenoscopy	食管胃十二指肠内镜
EGF	Epidermal growth factor	表皮生长因子
EMG	Electromyography	肌电图
ERCP	Endoscopic retrograde cholangiopancreatography	内镜逆行胰胆管造影

ESR	Erythrocyte sedimentation rate	红细胞沉降率
EUS	Endoscopic ultrasonography	超声内镜检查
FDA	U. S. Food and Drug Administration	美国食品药品管理局
FNA	Fine-needle aspiration	细针穿刺
GAVE	Gastric antral vascular ectasia	胃窦血管扩张
GERD	Gastroesophageal reflux disease	胃食管反流病
GGTP	Gamma glutamyl transpeptidase	γ-谷氨酸转肽酶
GI	Gastrointestina	胃肠道
GIST	GI stromal tumor	胃肠道基质瘤
GU	Gastric ulcer	胃溃疡
H & E	Hematoxylin and eosin	苏木精-伊红染色(HE 染色)
H2RA	Histamine-2 receptor antagonist	组胺-2 受体拮抗剂
HAV	Hepatitis A virus	甲型肝炎病毒
HBV	Hepatitis B virus	乙型肝炎病毒
HCC	Hepatocellular carcinoma	肝细胞癌
HCG	Human chorionic gonadotropin	人绒毛膜促性腺激素
HCV	Hepatitis C virus	丙型肝炎病毒
HDL	High-density lipoprotein	高密度脂蛋白
HDV	Hepatitis D virus	丁型肝炎病毒
HELLP	Hemolysis, elevated liver enzymes, low platelets	溶血、肝酶升高、血小板减少
HEV	Hepatitis E virus	戊型肝炎病毒
Hgb	Hemoglobin	血红蛋白
HHT	Hereditary hemorrhagic telangiectasia	遗传性出血性毛细血管扩张症
HIV	Human immunodeficiency virus	人免疫缺陷病毒
HLA	Human leukocyte antigen	人白细胞抗原
HPV	Human papillomavirus	人乳头状瘤病毒
HSV	Herpes simplex virus	单纯疱疹病毒
HP	Helicobacter pylori	幽门螺杆菌
IBD	Inflammatory bowel disease	炎症性肠病
IBS	Irritable bowel syndrome	肠易激综合征
ICU	Intensive care unit	重症监护室
IMA	Inferior mesenteric artery	肠系膜下动脉
IMT	Intestinal microbiota transplantation	肠道微生物群移植
INR	International normalized ratio	国际标准化比值
IV	Intravenous	静脉注射
IVIG	Intravenous immunoglobulin	静脉注射免疫球蛋白
LDH	Lactate dehydrogenase	乳酸脱氢酶
LDL	Low-density lipoprotein	低密度脂蛋白
LGI	Lower gastrointestinal	下胃肠道
LGIB	Lower gastrointestinal bleed	下胃肠道出血
LLQ	Left lower quadrant	左下象限
LT	Liver transplantation	肝移植
LUQ	Left upper quadrant	左上象限
MELD	Model for end-stage liver disease	终末期肝病模型
MEN	Multiple endocrine neoplasia	多发性内分泌瘤
MHC	Major histocompatibility complex	主要组织相容性复合物
MRA	Magnetic resonance angiography	磁共振血管造影
MRCP	Magnetic resonance cholangiopancreatography	磁共振胰胆管造影
MRI	Magnetic resonance imaging	磁共振成像
NAFLD	Nonalcoholic fatty liver disease	非酒精脂肪性肝病
NASH	Nonalcoholic steatohepatitis	非酒精脂肪性肝炎

NG	Nasogastric	鼻胃管
NPO	Nil per os(nothing by mouth)	禁食
NSAID	Nonsteroidal	非甾体抗炎药
O_2	Oxygen	氧
PBC	Primary biliary cholangitis	原发性胆汁性胆管炎
PCR	Polymerase chain reaction	聚合酶链反应
PET	Positron emission tomography	正电子发射断层摄影
PPI	Proton pump inhibitor	质子泵抑制剂
PSC	Primary sclerosing cholangitis	原发性硬化性胆管炎
PSE	Portosystemic encephalopathy	门体脑病
PUD	Peptic ulcer disease	消化性溃疡病
RA	Rheumatoid arthritis	类风湿性关节炎
RLQ	Right lower quadrant	右下象限
RNA	Ribonucleic acid	核糖核酸
RUQ	Right upper quadrant	右上象限
SBO	Small bowel obstruction	小肠梗阻
SBP	Spontaneous bacterial peritonitis	原发性细菌性腹膜炎
SIBO	Small intestinal bacterial overgrowth	小肠细菌过度生长
SOD	Sphincter of Oddi dysfunction	奥迪括约肌功能障碍
TB	Tuberculosis	结核
TG	Triglyceride(s)	甘油三酯
TIPS	Transjugular intraheptic portosystemic shunt	经颈静脉肝内门体分流术
TNF	Tumor necrosis factor	肿瘤坏死因子
TNM	Tumor node metastasis	肿瘤转移结节
TPN	Total parenteral nutrition	全肠外营养
UC	Ulcerative colitis	溃疡性结肠炎
UDCA	Ursodeoxycholic acid	熊去氧胆酸
UGI	Upper gastrointestinal	上胃肠道
UGIB	Upper gastrointestinal bleed	上胃肠道出血
UGIS	Upper gastrointestinal series	上胃肠道系列检查
UNOS	United Network for Organ Sharing	器官共享联合网
US	Ultrasonography	超声检查
USA	United States of America	美利坚合众国
VLDL	Very-low-density lipoprotein	极低密度脂蛋白
WBC	White blood cell	白细胞
WHO	World Health Organization	世界卫生组织
ZES	Zollinger-Ellison syndrome	佐林格-埃利森综合征

目　录

上　卷

第一部分　胃肠道生物学 …… 1

第 1 章　细胞生长与肿瘤 …… 1
第 2 章　黏膜免疫与炎症 …… 13
第 3 章　肠道微生物群 …… 24
第 4 章　胃肠道感觉转导 …… 33

第二部分　胃肠道营养 …… 51

第 5 章　营养原则和胃肠病患者的营养评估 …… 51
第 6 章　营养管理 …… 72
第 7 章　肥胖 …… 88
第 8 章　肥胖的外科和内镜治疗 …… 96
第 9 章　喂养和进食障碍 …… 112
第 10 章　食物过敏 …… 127

第三部分　症状、体征和生物心理社会学问题 …… 139

第 11 章　急性腹痛 …… 139
第 12 章　慢性腹痛 …… 152
第 13 章　食管疾病症状 …… 161
第 14 章　消化不良 …… 169
第 15 章　恶心和呕吐 …… 182
第 16 章　腹泻 …… 194
第 17 章　肠道气体 …… 213
第 18 章　大便失禁 …… 221
第 19 章　便秘 …… 238
第 20 章　胃肠道出血 …… 262
第 21 章　黄疸 …… 296
第 22 章　胃肠病学的生物心理社会问题 …… 306
第 23 章　人为胃肠疾病 …… 321

第四部分　多器官相关问题 …… 331

第 24 章　口腔疾病及胃肠道和肝脏疾病的口腔表现 …… 331
第 25 章　胃肠道和肝脏疾病的皮肤表现 …… 340
第 26 章　咽、食管、胃和小肠憩室 …… 352
第 27 章　腹部疝和胃扭转 …… 360
第 28 章　胃肠道异物、胃石和腐蚀物摄入 …… 377
第 29 章　腹腔内脓肿和胃肠道瘘 …… 389
第 30 章　胃肠道嗜酸性粒细胞性疾病 …… 401
第 31 章　蛋白丢失性胃肠病 …… 411
第 32 章　胃肠道淋巴瘤 …… 418
第 33 章　胃肠道间质瘤 …… 433
第 34 章　神经内分泌肿瘤 …… 446
第 35 章　人类免疫缺陷病毒感染的胃肠道后果 …… 472
第 36 章　实体器官和造血细胞移植的胃肠道和肝脏并发症 …… 483
第 37 章　系统性疾病的胃肠道和肝脏表现 …… 503
第 38 章　胃肠道血管病变 …… 531
第 39 章　外科腹膜炎及其他腹膜、肠系膜、网膜和横膈膜疾病 …… 549
第 40 章　妊娠期患者的胃肠道和肝脏疾病 …… 561
第 41 章　放疗的急性和慢性胃肠道副作用 …… 574
第 42 章　胃肠内镜检查的准备及并发症 …… 586

第五部分　食管 …… 595

第 43 章　食管解剖学、组织学、胚胎学和发育异常 …… 595
第 44 章　食管神经肌肉功能及动力障碍疾病 …… 606
第 45 章　药物、创伤和感染引起的食管疾病 …… 627
第 46 章　胃食管反流病 …… 635
第 47 章　Barrett 食管 …… 655
第 48 章　食管肿瘤 …… 663

第六部分　胃和十二指肠 …… 683

第 49 章　胃和十二指肠解剖学、组织学及发育异常 …… 683
第 50 章　胃神经肌肉功能与神经肌肉病变 …… 696
第 51 章　胃分泌 …… 723
第 52 章　胃炎和胃部疾病 …… 739
第 53 章　消化性溃疡疾病 …… 762
第 54 章　胃腺癌和其他胃肿瘤 …… 776

第七部分 胰腺……795
第 55 章 胰腺解剖学、组织学、胚胎学和发育异常…795
第 56 章 胰腺分泌……805
第 57 章 胰腺遗传性疾病和小儿胰腺疾病……813
第 58 章 急性胰腺炎……842
第 59 章 慢性胰腺炎……864
第 60 章 胰腺癌、囊性胰腺肿瘤和其他非内分泌胰腺肿瘤……890
第 61 章 胰腺疾病的内镜治疗……906

第八部分 胆道……913
第 62 章 胆道解剖学、组织学、胚胎学、发育异常和小儿疾病……913
第 63 章 胆道运动功能和功能障碍……932
第 64 章 胆汁分泌和肠肝循环……937
第 65 章 胆囊结石疾病……950
第 66 章 胆结石疾病的治疗……978
第 67 章 非结石性胆源性疼痛、急性非结石性胆囊炎、胆固醇贮积病、腺肌瘤病和胆囊息肉……993
第 68 章 原发性和继发性硬化性胆管炎……1004
第 69 章 胆管、胆囊和壶腹部肿瘤……1021
第 70 章 胆道疾病的内镜和放射治疗……1036

索引……1050

第一部分　胃肠道生物学

第 1 章　细胞生长与肿瘤

Ezra Burstein 著

章节目录

一、正常组织的稳态机制 …… 1
（一）细胞增殖 …… 1
（二）凋亡 …… 3
（三）衰老 …… 3
（四）调节细胞生长的信号通路 …… 4
二、肠道肿瘤的发生 …… 5
（一）多步骤形成 …… 5
（二）克隆扩增 …… 6
（三）癌干细胞 …… 6
（四）上皮-间充质转化 …… 6
三、肿瘤相关基因 …… 6
（一）癌基因 …… 6
（二）致癌生长因子和生长因子受体 …… 6
（三）核原癌基因 …… 7
（四）肿瘤抑制基因 …… 7
（五）DNA 修复基因 …… 9
（六）非编码 RNA …… 9
（七）致癌信号通路 …… 9
四、肿瘤微环境 …… 9
五、肿瘤代谢 …… 10
（一）炎症和癌症 …… 10
（二）微生物群 …… 10
六、肿瘤转移的生物学特征 …… 10
血管和淋巴管新生 …… 10
七、环境影响 …… 10
（一）化学致癌 …… 10
（二）饮食因素 …… 11
八、分子医学：胃肠肿瘤学当前和未来的研究方法 …… 11
（一）二代测序 …… 11
（二）分子诊断 …… 11

正常的细胞增殖和分化对包括消化道在内的所有器官的组织稳态至关重要。肿瘤形成过程涉及这些机制的基本破坏，从而导致癌症发展和转移，并额外获得癌的其他标志物。作为一个群体，胃肠道恶性肿瘤是癌症相关死亡的主要原因。因此，了解肿瘤形成的基础生物学至关重要。本章对正常细胞生长的机制以及促进恶性转化的基本细胞和分子改变进行了综述。本章中讨论的基本概念将为后面章节中特定胃肠肿瘤的讨论提供了一个框架。

一、正常组织的稳态机制

（一）细胞增殖

组织稳态的维持是通过细胞增殖和分化的精确平衡来维持的。作为正常组织功能的一部分或在组织修复过程中，细胞增殖和分化为替代濒死细胞提供了新的细胞成分。在基本水平上，当细胞增殖逃避了维持衰老和程序性细胞死亡平衡的稳态机制时，肿瘤就会发生。细胞增殖发生在细胞分裂的过程中，这一过程是通过一系列有序的步骤发生的，被称为细胞周期（图 1.1）。在细胞准备分裂时，有一段生物合成活跃期称为 G_1 期，通常与细胞大小的增加有关。这个阶段之后是基因组的精确复制，称为 S 期。之后是被称为 G_2 期的中间间隙期，最后是有丝分裂发生在 M 期。

继续进行 DNA 复制发生在 G_1/S 检验点或限制（R）点。细胞在到达 R 点之前，可能会退出这种活跃增殖的周期，进入被称为 G_0 的静止期。细胞随后可以从 G_0 状态重新进入细胞周期（见图 1.1）。G_2 期和 M 期之间的边界存在另一个检查点。G_2/M 检查点确保有丝分裂在基因组复制后修复任何受损 DNA 之前不会进行。在癌症中经常观察到这些检查点的功能受损。

细胞周期进程的调节，主要由一组被称为细胞周期蛋白和细胞周期蛋白依赖性激酶（cyclin-dependent kinase，CDK）实现的。这些蛋白在细胞周期的特定部分表达，参与调节 G_1/S 和 G_2/M 检查点。在 G_1 期，细胞周期蛋白 D 和 E 最活跃[1]。在成纤维细胞中细胞周期蛋白 D1 的过度表达导致细胞更快地进入 S 期，并且与其在癌症中的作用一致，细胞周期蛋白 D1 在许多胃肠道和非胃肠道恶性肿瘤中频繁过表达[2]。在 S 期，细胞周期蛋白 A 主要表达，G_2 期，细胞周期蛋白 B 是主要调节因子（见图 1.1）。

每个细胞周期蛋白与 CDK 形成复合物，并以细胞周期依赖的方式作为 CDK 活性的催化剂发挥作用（见图 1.1）。细胞周期蛋白-CDK 复合物通过关键靶蛋白的磷酸化来调节细胞周期进程。例如，细胞周期蛋白 D1 依赖的从 G_1 期到 S 期

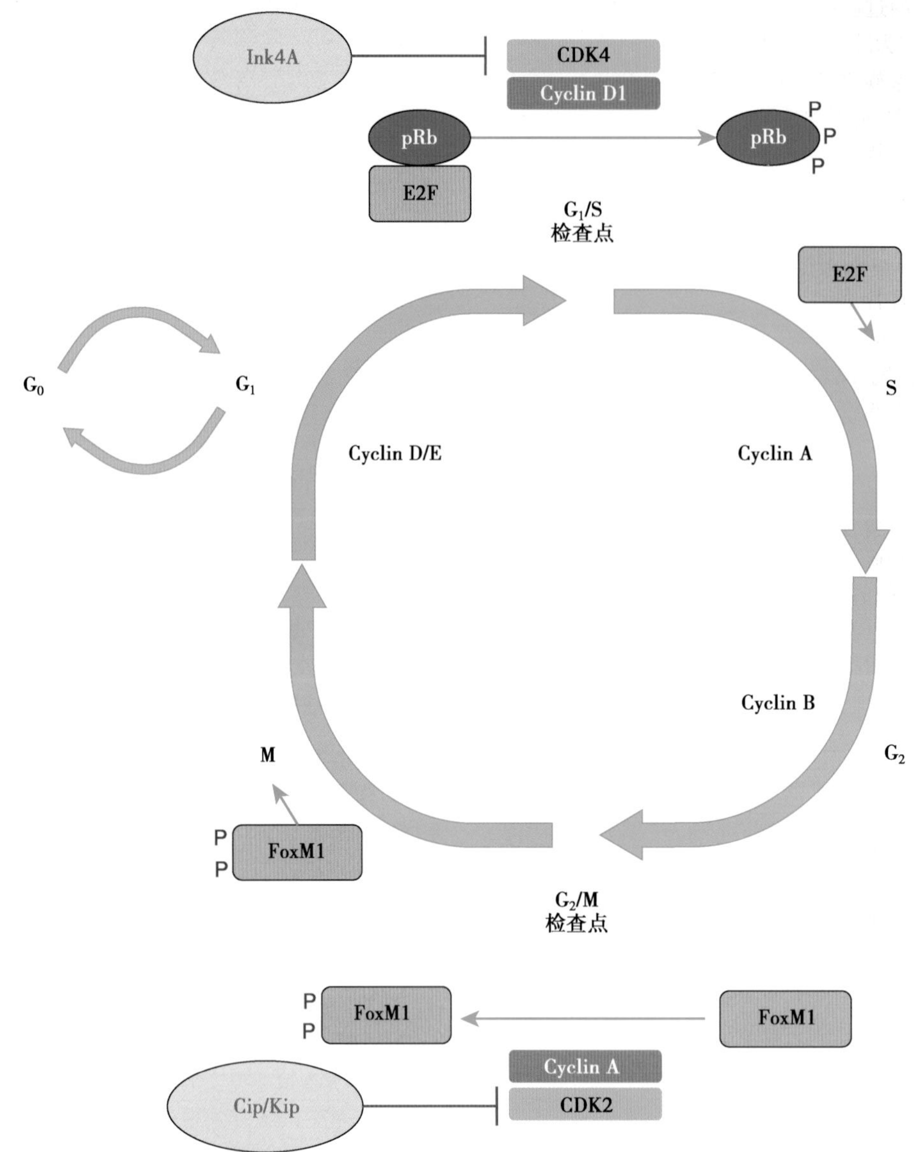

图 1.1 细胞周期蛋白(cycs)、细胞周期蛋白依赖性激酶(cdk)和 cdk 抑制剂对细胞周期的调节。在正常细胞周期中,DNA 合成(染色体中 DNA 复制)发生在 S 期,而有丝分裂(细胞核首先分裂形成一对新的细胞核,随后实际细胞分裂形成一对子细胞)发生在 M 期。S 期和 M 期由两个间隙期分隔;有丝分裂后和 DNA 合成前的 G_1 期,以及 S 期后的 G_2 期。在这些间隙期,细胞合成蛋白质和代谢物,增加其质量,并为 S 期和 M 期做准备。细胞周期进程主要通过细胞周期蛋白和 CDK 的协调活动在 G_2/M 和 G_1/S 两个检查点进行调节,反过来 CDK 抑制剂(Ink4 和 Cip/Kip 家族)又对其进行负调节。Ink4A,Ink4A 抑制剂;CDK4,细胞周期蛋白依赖激酶 4;Cyclin D1,细胞周期蛋白 D1;pRb,成视网膜母细胞瘤蛋白;E2F,细胞周期相关转录因子 E2F;Cyclin A,细胞周期蛋白 A;Cyclin B,细胞周期蛋白 B;Cyclin D/E,细胞周期蛋白 D/E;FoxM1,细胞周期相关转录因子 FoxM1;CDK2,细胞周期蛋白依赖激酶 2;Cip/Kip,细胞周期蛋白依赖激酶抑制因子;S,DNA 合成期;G_2,DNA 合成后期;M,有丝分裂期;G_0,静止期(细胞停止分裂);G_1,DNA 合成前期(细胞周期第一阶段)

的进展是肿瘤抑制蛋白 pRb(视网膜母细胞瘤基因的产物)以及 Rb 家族成员 p130 和 p107 的细胞周期蛋白 D1/CDK4 磷酸化的结果[3],这些蛋白隔离 E2F 转录因子,促进 S 期所需因子的表达,并被 CDK4 磷酸化导致其功能受到抑制。因此,Rb 表达的缺失也会导致更快速的进展到 S 期,这是在许多肿瘤中观察到的另一种基因病变。在 G_2/M 转换中也发现了一个类似的通路,其中细胞周期蛋白 A/CDK2 介导另一个转录调节因子 FoxM1 的激活,该转录调节因子是参与有丝分裂的因子表达所必需的[4]。

细胞周期也受多种 CDK 抑制剂的调节,这些抑制剂被归类为不同的类别,并有多个名称[5]。CDK4 和 CDK6 受到 Ink4 抑制剂家族成员的抑制,这些抑制剂被称为 p16INK4a(*Cdkn2a* 基因编码)、p15INK4b(*Cdkn2b* 基因编码)、p18INK4c(*Cdkn2c* 基因编码)及 p19INK4d(*Cdkn2d* 基因编码)[6]。因此,这些因素也影响了细胞周期蛋白 D1/CDK4 对 pRb 的调节,以及随后的 E2F 的激活及进入 S 期。p16INK4A 在癌症中的缺失导致 CDK4 的过度激活，并且在胃肠道癌症中经常失活，这一发现与其作为肿瘤抑制基因的功能相一致[7,8]。CDK 抑制剂的 Cip/Kip 家族成员被称为 p21Cip1（*Cdkn1a* 基因编码）、p27Kip1（*Cdkn1b* 基因编码）和 p57Kip2（*Cdkn1c* 基因编码），它们更混杂，干扰多个细胞周期蛋白/CDK 复合物，包括 CDK2。

（二）凋亡

凋亡是一种程序性细胞死亡的形式，由被称为半胱天冬酶（caspases）的特定蛋白酶进行基因编程和执行[9]。与其他蛋白酶（如凝血酶系统）级联反应相似，半胱天冬酶在无活性的前体形式裂解后获得活性，通常是由于另一种半胱天冬酶的作用或无活性半胱天冬酶的局灶性积累。细胞凋亡是对抗细胞增殖的重要机制，因此，逃避正常的凋亡机制在肿瘤发生中起着关键作用。形态学上，细胞凋亡的特征包括染色质致密化、细胞质浓缩、核碎裂和质膜的明显改变，导致紧密化的凋亡小体最终被吞噬和消除。

细胞凋亡可能由内部或外部刺激而触发。内部刺激可能包括营养缺乏、缺氧、DNA 损伤或其他应激源，包括特定毒素、化学信号和病原体。细胞凋亡通常发生在正常发育过程中，以促进组织模式形成。同样，包括组织炎症在内的许多应激情况，都会触发细胞凋亡。细胞凋亡也可由肿瘤坏死因子受体超家族的特异性细胞表面受体刺激发生，这些细胞表面受体包括被称为死亡受体的肿瘤坏死因子 R1 和 Fas（图 1.2）。

在细胞内水平上，所有形式的细胞凋亡的最后一个常见的事件是所谓的执行者半胱天冬酶（半胱天冬酶-3 和半胱天冬酶-7）的激活，它们介导了大量下游靶标的剪切，最终促发细胞死亡。促凋亡信号经常汇集在线粒体水平，在那里它们破坏线粒体膜的稳定性并破坏有氧呼吸所需的电梯度（见图 1.2）。除了导致细胞能量学的效应外，这一过程还导致一些存在于线粒体膜间隙中的蛋白质释放到细胞溶胶中，包括细胞色素 c（呼吸链的一个组成部分）。在胞质溶胶中，细胞色素 c 帮助组装一种被称为凋亡小体的多蛋白复合体，它含有 Apaf1，有利于激活半胱天冬酶 9，后者可直接激活半胱天冬酶-3 和半胱天冬酶-7。另一方面，死亡受体通过受体启动的细胞内信号事件激活执行者半胱天冬酶，最终导致半胱天冬酶 8 的上游激活。

导致凋亡小体形成的线粒体膜通透性增加是由 Bcl-2 家族蛋白控制的。一方面，Bax 和 Bak 帮助线粒体膜形成孔隙，而另一方面 Bcl-2、Bcl-xL 和 Mcl-1 则抑制孔隙的形成。Bcl-2 家族中促凋亡和抗凋亡成员之间的化学计量比可以决定细胞存活和细胞死亡之间的平衡[10]。在癌症中，促凋亡和抗凋亡因子间（包括 Bcl-2 家族成员）平衡的改变是常见的事件。

（三）衰老

衰老是细胞永久性丧失分裂能力的过程。衰老可能发生在对癌基因激活或 DNA 损伤诱导的应激或固定数量的细胞分裂（复制性衰老）之后。衰老不仅与退出细胞周期有关，还与包括多种促炎症因子的分泌表型相关。作为一种生理事件，衰老限制了失调或过度增殖。然而，当失调时，衰老也会导致干细胞的衰老和耗竭[11]。在癌变过程中，衰老经常被绕过或缺失。

复制性衰老是触发端粒的缩短，端粒是染色体末端保护基因组完整性的重复序列。端粒随着每次细胞的分裂而缩短，当它们达到极短的长度时，就会启动 DNA 损伤信号和细胞衰老。当原代细胞经历重复轮次的复制，最终获得关键的短端粒时，这种现象在体培养可以常规看到[12]。为了防止持续复制触发的衰老，癌细胞会激活端粒酶，在染色体末端增加额外的端粒[13]。

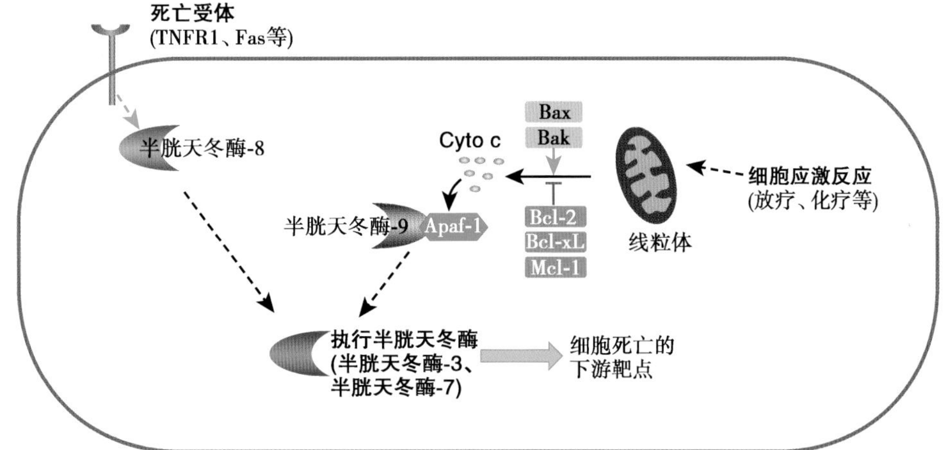

图 1.2　细胞凋亡（程序性细胞死亡）平衡细胞增殖以调节整体组织生长。促凋亡分子和抗凋亡分子的复杂相互作用，导致介导细胞死亡的半胱天冬酶下游激活。其中一些信号是通过细胞应激启动的，细胞应激可使线粒体膜不稳定，一些信号是通过死亡受体启动的，包括 TNFR1 和 Fas。线粒体途径受促凋亡（Bax，Bak）和抗凋亡（Bcl-2，Bcl-xL）分子之间的相互作用调节。在线粒体通透性化后，细胞色素 c 释放促进凋亡小体复合物（APAF1、半胱天冬酶-9 和细胞色素 c）的形成。半胱天冬酶-8（死亡受体下游）或半胱天冬酶-9（凋亡小体形成的结果）的激活，导致执行者半胱天冬酶（半胱天冬酶-3 和半胱天冬酶-7）的激活，后者靶向负责细胞死亡的下游靶点。TNFR1，肿瘤坏死因子受体 1；Fas，一种表达于细胞表面的受体（与相应配体结合能启动死亡信号转导）；Apaf-1，凋亡酶激活因子；Cyto c，细胞色素 c；Bax，促凋亡 Bax 分子；Bak，促凋亡 Bak 分子；Bcl-2，抗凋亡 Bcl-2 分子；Bcl-xL，抗凋亡 Bcl-xL 分子；Mcl-1，抗凋亡 Mcl-1 分子

(四) 调节细胞生长的信号通路

细胞增殖是通过细胞从 G_0 期停滞过渡到活跃的细胞周期来实现的(见图 1.1)。尽管细胞周期的增殖受上述机制的调控,但整体增殖也受到外部刺激的调节。与细胞膜表面特异性跨膜受体结合的生长因子尤为重要。通过跨膜细胞表面受体,细胞外基质和细胞间黏附分子(即整合素、钙黏蛋白、选择素、蛋白聚糖)发挥作用也会对细胞增殖产生显著影响。细胞-基质或细胞-细胞相互作用的改变在促成恶性细胞的侵袭表型中尤为重要。

与配体结合后,这些跨膜受体蛋白的细胞质尾部激活细胞内信号级联反应,改变基因转录和蛋白表达。根据这些受体启动的细胞内信号级联反应的性质,它们可分为三大类:①酪氨酸激酶;②丝氨酸和苏氨酸激酶;③G 蛋白偶联受体(G protein-coupled receptor,GPCR)。

许多肽生长因子的受体在其胞内尾部含有酪氨酸激酶活性。与配体结合后,激发酪氨酸激酶活性,导致细胞内靶蛋白中酪氨酸残基磷酸化。大多数受体还通过自身磷酸化受体酪氨酸残基来放大信号,在某些情况下,这也会导致自身活性的减弱,从而影响分子内反馈调节机制。许多肽生长因子受体,包括表皮生长因子及其相关生长因子受体,均属于这一类受体。

细胞表面的其他受体具有直接作用于丝氨酸或苏氨酸残基而非酪氨酸的激酶活性。这些受体还可使细胞内多种细胞蛋白磷酸化,导致生物反应的级联反应。包括酪氨酸激酶受体在内的许多生长因子受体上存在多个丝氨酸和苏氨酸磷酸化位点,这表明存在于单个细胞上的各种受体之间存在显著的相互作用[14]。转化生长因子(TGF-α)受体复合物是含丝氨酸-苏氨酸激酶的跨膜受体的一个重要例子。

许多受体是所谓的 7-膜受体家族的成员。这些受体与鸟嘌呤核苷酸结合蛋白(也称为 G 蛋白)偶联,因此,这些受体被称为 G 蛋白偶联受体。G 蛋白的构象变化依赖于磷酸鸟苷的存在[15]。G 蛋白的激活可触发多种细胞内信号,包括刺激磷酸酯酶 C 和通过膜磷脂水解生成磷酸肌醇(最重要的是 1,4,5-三磷酸肌醇)和甘油二酯,也可以调节第二信使环磷酸腺苷和单磷酸鸟苷[16]。以生长抑素受体为代表的 G 蛋白偶联受体普遍存在于胃肠道内。

生长因子和细胞因子与细胞表面受体的结合通常会引起影响生长的各种细胞功能的改变。这些功能包括离子转运、营养摄取和蛋白质合成。然而,配体-受体的相互作用最终必须改变一种或多种影响细胞增殖的稳态机制。

Wnt 通路是信号通路的一个重要例子,其通过调节多种稳态机制来调控肠上皮细胞的增殖(图 1.3)。Wnt 信号在多

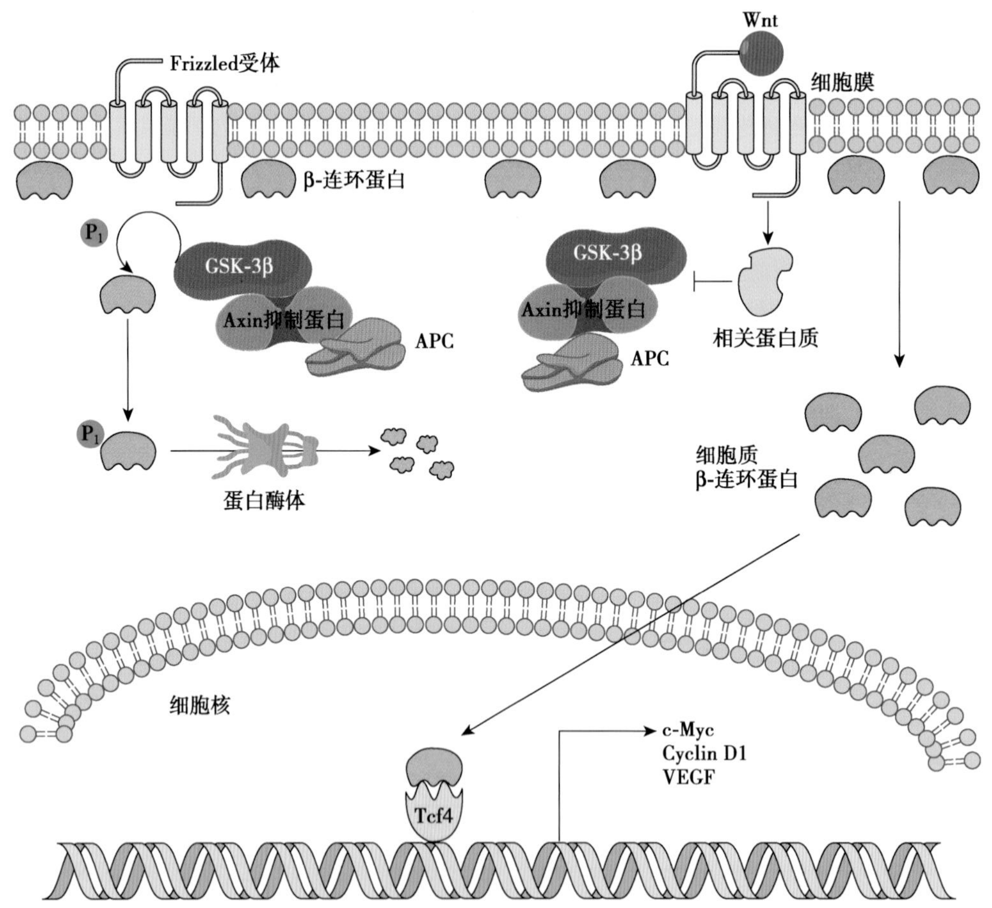

图 1.3　Wnt 信号通路是肠上皮细胞增殖和肿瘤发生的重要调节因子。在缺少 Wnt 信号(左上)的情况下,胞质 β-连环蛋白受到破坏复合体的调节,该复合体由 APC、Axin 和糖原合成酶激酶-3β(GSK-3β)组成。破坏复合体磷酸化 α-连环蛋白,并通过泛素-蛋白酶体途径靶向降解。在 Wnt 信号活跃的情况下(右上),α-连环蛋白降解被阻止,蛋白被稳定,导致过量的细胞质 α-连环蛋白转移到细胞核。核 α-连环蛋白与转录因子 4(Tcf-4)相互作用调节多种关键靶基因的表达。APC,腺瘤性结肠息肉病;Cyclin D1,细胞周期蛋白 D1;P,磷酸基团;VEGF,血管内皮生长因子

物种进化过程中被保守留下来，其作用通常是调节干细胞微环境中的增殖，对维持胃肠道上皮稳态至关重要。从信号角度来看，其作用在很大程度上依赖于 α-连环蛋白在细胞核内的积累，它与转录因子 Tcf-4 结合激活一组靶基因[17]。在正常细胞中，α-连环蛋白在很大程度上与细胞黏附连接相关，该蛋白的胞质池通过磷酸化和泛素化途径迅速降解。这是由所谓的破坏复合体介导的，其中包括肿瘤抑制因子 APC。当分泌的 Wnt 配体与 Frizzled 家族的细胞表面受体结合时，α-连环蛋白的组成性降解被抑制，从而导致该因子在核内聚积，随后促进细胞增殖基因的转录激活。小鼠 Wnt 信号的抑制可通过 Tcf-4 的缺失或 Wnt 抑制剂 Dickkopf-1 的过表达来实现，从而导致肠上皮细胞急剧的低增殖[18,19]。Wnt 信号在隐窝底部最活跃，随着分化的发生，组织内环境稳态由生长抑制信号维持，生长抑制信号可对抗增殖信号并促进其分化，包括 TGF-α 家族的成员，如 BMP-4[20]。该家族的特定成员具有独特的组织稳态的功能，包括促进间充质细胞的分化和纤维化表型、诱导特定的 T 细胞亚型和多种其他活性。从广义上讲，TGF-α 家族成员的作用是通过 Smad 蛋白家族在细胞内介导的，Smad 蛋白家族是在配体-受体结合后被激活的转录因子[21]。TGF-α 可诱导细胞周期抑制剂 p15INK4B 和 p21CIP1/WAF1 的转录，是一种强效的生长抑制因子，介导细胞周期阻滞在 G_1 期。此外，它还增强了 p27KIP1 对细胞周期蛋白 E/CDK2 复合物的抑制活性[22]。

二、肠道肿瘤的发生

（一）多步骤形成

正常肠上皮向肿瘤的转化需要多个连续的基因改变。结肠肿瘤形成过程中发生的累积变化最直接地说明了肿瘤发生的多步骤性质（见第 127 章）。从正常上皮到腺瘤性息肉再到恶性肿瘤的进展与基因改变的积累是相平行的，基因改变使控制增殖和组织稳态的关键途径发生了改变。对结肠癌分子发病机制的研究已成为阐明其他胃肠道癌（包括胃癌和胰腺癌）基因改变的范例。

几乎所有胃肠道癌症都存在基因组不稳定性。这种基因方面不稳定的环境促进了胃肠道癌症多步骤改变积累的特征。基因组的不稳定性可能是由多种机制引起的，包括基因组 DNA 序列的变化或通过核苷酸的修饰改变其功能，这一过程称为表观遗传变化。在结肠癌中，目前有 3 种公认的促进癌变的遗传/表观遗传不稳定类型（图 1.4），它们被称为染色体不稳定型、微卫星不稳定型（microsatellite instability，MSI）和 CpG 岛甲基化表型（CpG island methylator phenotype，CIMP）[23,24]。染色体不稳定性是指染色体结构的改变，导致染色体大片段缺失、重复和易位，从而导致非整倍体状态。相反，微卫星不稳定性是指重复 DNA 序列片段（指微卫星 DNA）的频繁改变，通常在染色体水平上是二倍体或近二倍体（见下文 DNA 修复的讨论）。CpG 岛甲基化表型是指表观遗

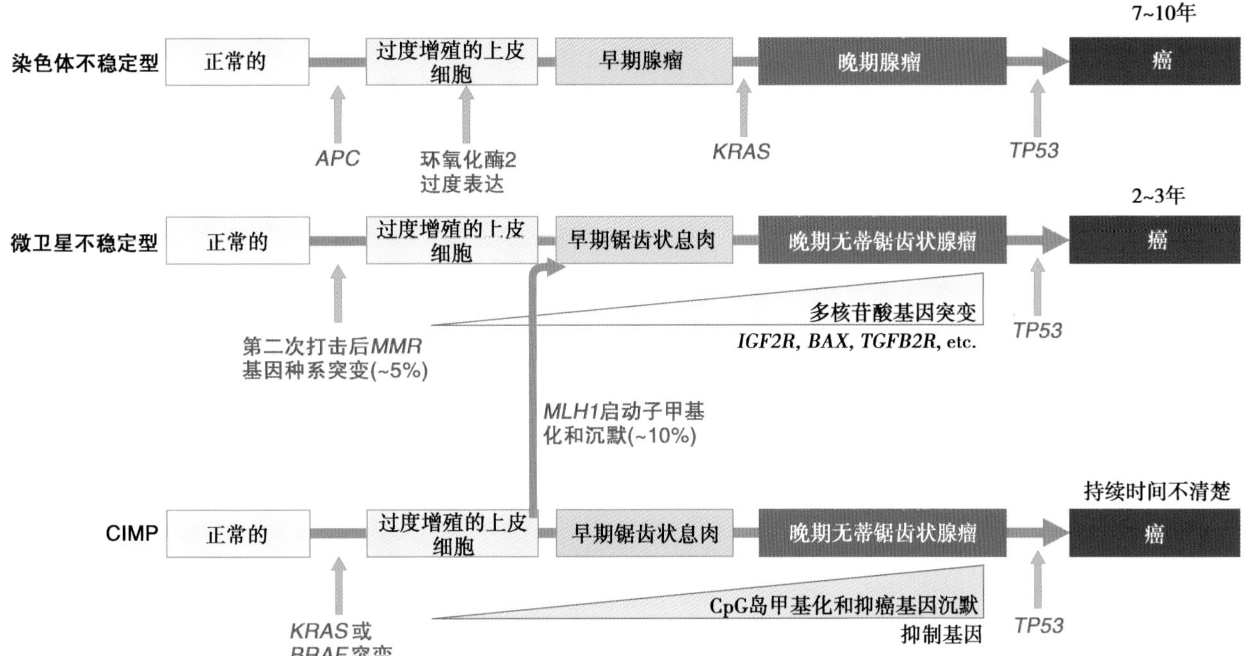

图 1.4　基于潜在遗传不稳定性的结直肠癌多步骤形成模型。如左图所示，有 3 条主要通路：染色体不稳定型（上通路）、微卫星不稳定型（中通路）和 CpG 岛甲基化或 CIMP（下通路）。从正常结肠上皮进展为癌与获得几种遗传和表观遗传学改变有关。在染色体不稳定型途径中（顶部途径），这些改变包括腺瘤性结肠息肉（*APC*）的早期丢失，随后通过点突变激活致癌基因（如 *KRAS*），并通过点突变或缺失灭活肿瘤抑制基因（如 *APC*、*TP53*）。根据息肉大小的分析，突变总数的增加可能与早期良性腺瘤进展为癌症有关。在微卫星不稳定型中（中间通路），DNA 错配修复（*MMR*）基因的突变产生突变表型，其中突变累积在特定靶基因的（见 DNA 错配修复章节）。肿瘤通过该途径比通过染色体不稳定型途径发展得更快（2~3 年 vs 7~10 年）。*MMR* 基因的种系突变占所有结直肠肿瘤的 5%。在 CIMP 通路中（下通路），起始事件被假定为 *BRAF* 或 *KRAS* 激活突变，以某种方式触发广泛的 CpG 岛甲基化，特别是基因启动子，导致基因沉默。其中潜在的基因靶标是 MMR 通路的组成部分 *MLH1*，当 *MLH1* 作为 CIMP 通路的一部分沉默时，肿瘤沿着与微卫星不稳定型癌症（MSI-H）相似的分子进化。散在性 *MLH1* 甲基化和沉默占散在性结直肠癌的近 10%。另外，发生于 CIMP 通路的锯齿状腺瘤可以经历类似于染色体不稳定型的途径成为微卫星稳定的肿瘤

传修饰的积累,即鸟嘌呤残基在所谓的 CpG 岛上的甲基化,即基因启动子位点富含胞苷和鸟嘌呤的区域。这种修饰对基因转录具有强效作用,可导致基因沉默。其他形式的表观遗传学变化涉及组蛋白的化学修饰,这些组蛋白是核小体组装所必需的,控制染色质致密化和 DNA 进入。尽管组蛋白本身的突变在癌症中是罕见,但修饰组蛋白的酶的突变正在成为一组重要的肿瘤相关突变。值得注意的是,这些途径的参与并不是相互排斥的。

（二）克隆扩增

克隆扩增对于肿瘤的发展至关重要[25]获得可能为细胞提供生长或存活优势的突变后,这些突变细胞会进行克隆扩增。随着该群体的生长,特别是随着遗传/表现遗传不稳定性的获得,当该群体内的细胞维持另一种基因改变,使其生长特性进一步增强时,即发生第二轮克隆扩增。这种迭代的选择过程,随着基因改变的不断积累,导致恶性肿瘤发生。由于克隆扩增过程的性质,一旦发生明显的恶性肿瘤,通常在同一肿瘤中存在多个克隆,各种癌细胞中存在不同类别的突变,被称为肿瘤异质性,这一持续的过程可能赋予某些细胞选择的优势[26]。肿瘤转移可能是由于肿瘤细胞亚群的进化所促进的,这些肿瘤细胞亚群具有穿过循环系统的能力,并能在新环境中兴旺生长。

（三）癌干细胞

识别肿瘤异质性形成了癌症干细胞(cancer stem cell, CSC)的假说,其断言存在一个具有干细胞样特性的肿瘤细胞亚群。癌症干细胞被认为是发生克隆扩增的肿瘤起始细胞。此外,设想彻底根除这些细胞是肿瘤治疗的一个关键目标,根除失败可能导致疾病复发。在癌症干细胞的假设中有两个模型[27]:第一个是分层模型,癌症干细胞作为肿瘤中所有细胞的祖细胞,而其他细胞的长期生殖潜能有限。该模型的基本依据是:在异种移植实验中发现,只有具有特异性表面标记的细胞才能重新填充肿瘤。在胃肠道中,对假定的癌症干细胞的分析证明了,其与正常肠道干细胞共享的转录程序和标志物,如 Lgr5 和 EphB2,它们可鉴定和纯化结肠癌干细胞[28]。第二个随机模型,假设每个癌细胞都具有成为癌症干细胞的相同潜能,但是,这种认为是随机基于排除外部环境线索外的内部因素。

（四）上皮-间充质转化

已经注意到,在上皮来源的肿瘤中,一些细胞获得间充质细胞的特征。在正常胚胎形成过程中也会发生类似的过程,此时极化的上皮细胞不再识别相邻上皮细胞或其基底膜施加的边界,而是采用迁移间充质细胞的特征。这种现象被称为上皮-间充质转化(epithelial-mesenchymal transition, EMT),赋予细胞穿过通常作为上皮细胞边界的组织平面的能力,如基底膜、致密胶原蛋白、糖蛋白和蛋白聚糖基质。肿瘤细胞通过基底膜的移行可能涉及关键蛋白水解活性的产生。另外,肿瘤细胞可能产生能够激活细胞外基质中存在的酶原因子。例如,肿瘤可能产生尿激酶,其本身是一种蛋白酶或纤溶酶原激活剂。在获得进入间充质间隙后,肿瘤细胞可进入淋巴管和血管进行转移。

除了这些特征,人们已经认识到发生上皮-间充质转化不仅可获得侵袭性特征,还可获得癌症干细胞样特征[29]。

上皮-间充质转化的一个关键特征是,丢失了保持正常上皮细胞-细胞相互作用的黏附连接性。这种现象的相关性是黏附连接的关键分子成分 E-钙黏蛋白(E-cadherin)的表达缺失[30]。E-钙黏蛋白的突变在许多胃肠道癌中很常见,特别是胃癌,其中 E-钙黏蛋白的种系突变也与遗传性弥漫性胃癌相关。

三、肿瘤相关基因

在肿瘤形成过程中,发生改变的基因属于两个不同的组别:①癌基因,它主动赋予细胞促生长的特性;②肿瘤抑制基因,其产物通常抑制肿瘤生长或增殖。肿瘤抑制基因中的一个重要类别包括 DNA 修复基因,它可防止新突变的积累。癌基因的激活或肿瘤抑制基因的失活有助于肿瘤恶性转化。尽管这些基因中大多数编码蛋白质,但许多具有致癌和肿瘤抑制功能的促癌基因并不编码蛋白质,而是编码调节基因组功能的 RNA,即所谓的非编码 RNA。

（一）癌基因

根据《癌症体细胞突变目录》(Catalog of Somatic Mutations in Cancer, COSMIC)[31],有强有力的证据表明,有近 80 个致癌基因参与癌症。编码正常细胞蛋白的基因,其功能可能促进肿瘤形成过程(如抗凋亡功能、刺激细胞增殖等),当其以不适当的高水平表达时,可能作为癌基因发挥作用。这种现象的典型机制是基因扩增,当肿瘤获得多个正常基因拷贝时,会产生剂量效应,从而导致基因表达增加。

在其他情况下,各种突变可能导致正常基因不适当的活化,从而导致促癌活动。点突变或融合蛋白中产生的大基因重排,是导致癌基因激活的突变示例。例如,编码含酪氨酸激酶的生长因子受体的几个基因突变,导致酪氨酸激酶活性不受调节而成为致癌基因,不再依赖于适当配体[如表皮生长因子(epidermal growth factor, EGF)]的存在。由于其促肿瘤活性,这些突变倾向于在特定的癌症类别中复发。将来源于正常细胞基因的癌基因命名为原癌基因。这些基因大多广泛表达于多种不同类型的肿瘤细胞中。

最后,癌基因的另一个来源是病毒编码的蛋白,可能影响细胞生长或存活[32]。这些因素虽然进化为有利于病毒循环,但在某些情况下可能也有利于肿瘤的发生,这就是特定病毒与癌症风险增加相关的原因。此外,以逆转录病毒为例,病毒基因组能够将自身插入宿主的基因组中,会导致插入位点附近基因表达的破坏,有时可能具有致癌活性。

癌基因编码的蛋白可能影响癌症的任何标志,如刺激生长因子途径、促进肿瘤侵袭、防止细胞死亡或具有其他促肿瘤作用。关于促进生长因子通路方面,癌基因可能编码:①生长因子或其受体;②受体自身下游的细胞内信号转导分子,包括在细胞核水平上介导生长因子作用的转录因子。

（二）致癌生长因子和生长因子受体

多种生长因子表达增强的转化作用已在体外和体内得到

证实。一些由癌基因编码的生长因子相关蛋白目前已被公认,包括编码血小板源性生长因子 α 链的 Wnt 和 Sis 蛋白家族。癌细胞可能参与自分泌信号以促进其生长,或诱发邻近基质高分泌这类生长刺激因子。更常见的是,多种受体表达上调或失调导致的构成作用。其中包括 EGF 受体家族(ERBB 1~4)的受体酪氨酸激酶,在多种胃肠道肿瘤中表达上调。

信号转导相关癌基因

有效地将配体-受体结合转化为细胞内信号的中间步骤对于介导细胞的功能反应是至关重要的。编码参与信号转导的关键蛋白的基因突变也可导致细胞转化(图 1.5)。在这方面,最大的癌基因编码具有蛋白激酶活性的蛋白质。这个大的癌基因组的许多成员在胃肠道肿瘤中表达,其中包括与质膜内表面相关的 Src 非受体酪氨酸激酶。

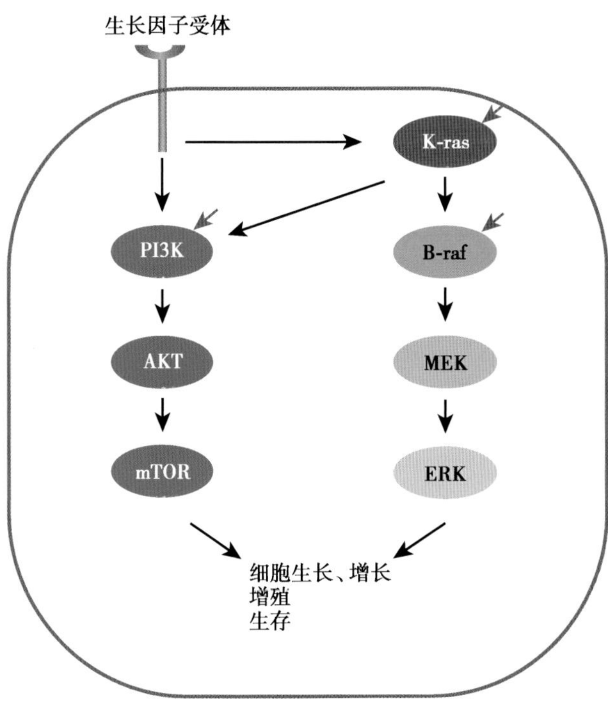

图 1.5 *K-ras* 起主要作用的生长因子受体下游的信号转导。癌基因 *K-ras* 可激活多种信号通路。结直肠癌中经常发生突变的分子,用红色箭头标出,包括 K-ras(40%)、B-raf(10%)和 PI3K(15%)。AKT,v-AKT 癌基因的细胞同源物;ERK,细胞外信号调节激酶;MEK,MAPK/ERK 激酶;mTOR,哺乳动物西罗莫司靶蛋白;PI3K,磷酸肌醇-3 激酶

G 蛋白通过三磷酸鸟苷(GTP)与二磷酸鸟苷(GDP)的交换来调节 GPCR 大家族的信号转导。在这方面,编码 G 蛋白相关蛋白家族的 *ras* 基因家族是胃肠道癌症中最常检测到的致癌基因之一。*ras* 家族包含 3 个基因:*H-ras*、*K-ras* 和 *N-ras*。这些因子对于转导来自各种生长受体信号级联和点突变的信号至关重要,点突变导致关键热点位置的氨基酸替换被激活,从而将正常基因转化为致癌基因。

迄今为止,几乎所有胃肠道恶性肿瘤中的 *ras* 突变都发生在 *K-ras* 致癌基因中。突变频率最高的是胰腺外分泌肿瘤(>90%)[33]。通过点突变激活的 *ras* 基因已在大约 50% 的结肠癌和锯齿状肿瘤的一个子集被确定(见图 1.4)[34]。

大多数 *ras* 基因致癌突变引起的生化改变,通过降低三磷酸鸟苷酶活性或使无活性的二磷酸鸟苷结合形式不稳定,使其维持在有活性的三磷酸鸟苷结合状态。然而,仍有一些 *ras* 基因突变体保留了显著的三磷酸鸟苷酶活性,因此,可能涉及将 *ras* 转变为转化蛋白的其他机制[35]。

Ras 激活的一个功能性结果是,关键下游丝氨酸/苏氨酸激酶的磷酸化和活化。Ras 的另一个重要靶点是 B-raf。在没有可识别的 *K-ras* 突变的结肠癌中,20% 具有活化的 *B-raf* 突变[36]。这与癌基因通路可通过特定通路的任何一个连续组分改变而被激活的概念相符(见图 1.5)。

(三) 核原癌基因

许多细胞致癌基因编码定位于细胞核的蛋白质。从本质上讲,这些核癌基因产物是信号转导途径的最终介质,也受细胞质和质膜结合的癌蛋白的影响,因为它们作为转录因子,调节某些基因的表达,从而促进细胞增殖和抑制正常分化。

Myc 家族阐明了核癌基因的作用。c-Myc 蛋白产物参与关键的细胞功能,如增殖、分化、凋亡、转化和关键基因的转录激活[37]。通常,c-Myc 在许多胃肠道癌中过度表达或扩增。研究发现 c-Myc 是结直肠癌中 α-连环蛋白/TCF-4 复合物的转录靶点(见图 1.3),这可以解释 c-Myc 在这种类型癌症中的过度表达[38]。

(四) 肿瘤抑制基因

肿瘤抑制基因的突变与所有胃肠道癌症相关,其中许多肿瘤抑制基因及其产物已被鉴定和描述,(见表 1.1)。与癌基因特有的功能性获得性突变不同,肿瘤抑制基因的突变是功能丧失性突变,因此是双等位基因。

表 1.1 与遗传性胃肠道癌综合征疾病相关基因的突变

疾病	突变基因
家族性腺瘤性息肉病(FAP),衰减型家族性腺瘤性息肉病(AFAP),Gardner 综合征	*APC*
遗传性非息肉病性结直肠癌(HNPCC)(林奇综合征)	*MLH1*,*MSH2*,*PMS2*,*MSH6*,*EP-CAM*(通过中断相邻的 *MSH2* 基因)
MUTYH-相关性息肉病(MAP)	*MUTYH*
黑斑息肉综合征(Peutz-Jeghers 综合征)	*STK11*
Cowden 病	*PTEN*
幼年型息肉病	*SMAD4*,*BMPR1A*
遗传性弥漫性胃癌	*CDH1*
遗传性胰腺癌	*ATM*, *BRCA1*, *BRCA2*, *PALB2*, *PALLD*, *CDKN2A*, *PRSS1*, *SPINK1*,*PRSS2*,*CTRC*,*CFTR*
多发性内分泌肿瘤 1 型(MEN1)	*Menin*

APC,结肠腺瘤样息肉病;MEN1,多发性内分泌肿瘤 1 型;MUTYH,mutY 同源物。

肿瘤抑制基因存在的最初识别来源于对易患癌症家族的遗传分析。在胃肠道中,遗传性肠癌、胃癌和胰腺癌综合征的论述最多,并在本文外其他章节进行讨论(见第 54 章、第 60 章和第 127 章)。在这些综合征中,在没有其他易感环境因素的情况下,特定肿瘤的患病风险显著增加。肿瘤的发生通常比一般人群年龄更小,靶组织内可发生多种原发性肿瘤。

从遗传学角度来看,癌症遗传综合征通常具有孟德尔遗传的常染色体显性遗传模式。基于对遗传性视网膜母细胞瘤的研究,Knudson 提出了"二次打击"假说[39],该假说解释了散发性和家族性癌症之间的关系。散发性肿瘤是由肿瘤抑制基因体细胞双等位基因失活突变引起的,而家族性癌症综合征中的肿瘤,是受累家族成员中所有细胞中存在的肿瘤抑制基因的单等位基因突变遗传加速导致的。当这种种系突变被抑癌基因剩余正常等位基因的体细胞突变所降低时,就会引起肿瘤克隆的发展,最终形成肿瘤(图 1.6)。由于种系突变,肿瘤抑制基因完全失活的可能性大大降低,因为只需要一次额外的打击,从而导致发病年龄较小,并有可能这些综合征伴随肿瘤的多样性。

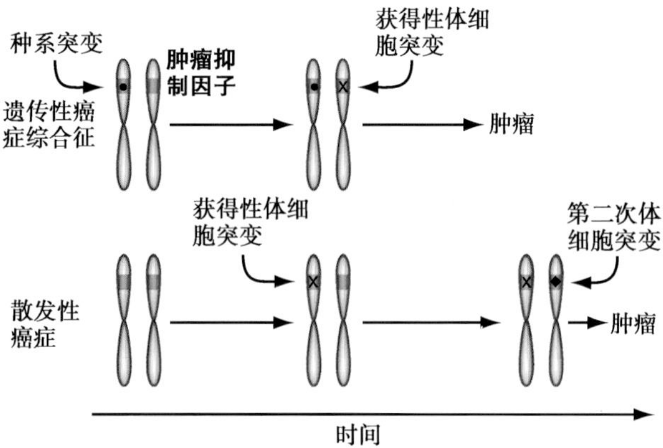

图 1.6 Knudson 二次打击假设。在遗传性癌症综合征中,由于种系突变,一条染色体具有无活性的肿瘤抑制基因(*TSG*)位点。剩余配对染色体上的对应 TSG 位点随后被体细胞突变灭活,导致肿瘤形成。相反,在散发性癌症中,*TGS* 的两个等位基因位点需要通过两次独立的体细胞突变而失活,这一事件不太可能发生在单个细胞内

尽管,这种二次打击模型已被普遍观察到,但也有例外。当只有一个等位基因发生突变时,一些肿瘤抑制因子可能具有增加癌症风险的功能。而且,一些癌症遗传综合征表现出体细胞隐性遗传方式,因为只有当存在双等位基因失活突变时,才会发生遗传风险。肿瘤抑制基因的另一个重要特征是,它们在每种组织类型中的功能并不完全相同。因此,特定肿瘤抑制基因的失活仅在某些组织中具有致瘤性。例如,肿瘤抑制基因 *RB1* 和 *VHL* 分别在视网膜母细胞瘤和肾细胞癌中起着重要作用,但在胃肠道恶性肿瘤中很少发生突变。在胃肠道恶性肿瘤的发病机制中起着关键作用的肿瘤抑制基因,*APC*、*TP53* 和 *SMAD4* 将在后面描述。此外,我们将讨论 DNA 修复途径,当其丢失时,可引起肿瘤形成,因此也作为肿瘤抑制因子发挥作用。

1. 结肠腺瘤性息肉病基因

遗传连锁分析显示,家族性腺瘤性息肉病(familial adenomatous polyposis,FAP)和 Gardner 综合征家族受累成员中,5q21 上的标志因子与息肉发生密切相关[40]。进一步的工作鉴定出了导致 FAP 发病的 *APC* 基因[41-43]。在第 126 章详细讨论了 APC 引起腺瘤性息肉综合征的全部疾病谱。在大多数散发性结肠息肉和癌症中也发现了 *APC* 体细胞突变[44,45]。*APC* 突变被鉴定出是最早腺瘤发生的特征,表明从正常上皮细胞到结肠癌的多步骤进展中 *APC* 起着"守门人"的关键作用(见图 1.4)。

APC 基因由 15 个外显子组成,预测编码的蛋白质含有 2 843 个氨基酸,分子量约 310KDa。大多数种系和体细胞 *APC* 基因突变导致终止密码子提前,从而使 APC 蛋白产物被截断并丧失功能。如前所述,*APC* 是 Wnt 信号通路的负调节因子,它的失活可导致类似 Wnt 组成性激活的状态。在细胞内表现为 α-连环蛋白的稳定,它介导 Wnt 激活的转录效应和随后的致癌表型(见图 1.3)。有趣的是,实现这一信号转导结果的另一个机制是 α-连环蛋白本身的突变,使该蛋白不受 *APC* 降解的影响。

2. *TP53*

TP53 是人类癌症中最常见的突变基因[46],在所有胃肠道的癌症中,发现 *TP53* 点突变频率都很高[47]。事实上,*TP53* 点突变已在多达 50% ~ 70% 的散发性结肠癌中被确定(见图 1.4)。有趣的是,这些突变在致癌过程中出现得相对较晚,因为该基因仅在一小部分结肠腺瘤中发生突变[48]。

以 53kDa 大小的基因产物而命名,p53 是一种在细胞周期调控和细胞凋亡中起关键作用的核磷酸化蛋白[47]。在细胞核中,p53 作为一种转录因子发挥作用,可由细胞应激条件诱导,如电离辐射、生长因子撤除或细胞毒治疗。p53 的诱导使细胞阻滞在 G_1 期,以利于 DNA 修复、衰老或触发细胞凋亡。这些反应部分由其转录靶标介导,如细胞周期的 p21CIP1/WAF1 抑制因子或促凋亡基因 *PUMA*[49]。有趣的是,*TP53* 突变通常作为包含一个等位基因的基因组缺失的组合发生的,以及第二个等位基因中针对蛋白质内特定热点的错义突变。最近研究的证据表明,基因组缺失不仅通过去除 *TP53* 发挥作用,而且通过丢失具有肿瘤抑制活性的相邻基因发挥作用[50]。此外,第二类突变,特定的错义突变可能通过获得致肿瘤活性功能发挥作用[51]。除了散发性癌症中的 *TP53* 点突变外,在 Li-Fraumeni 综合征中还观察到种系 *TP53* 突变,Li-Fraumeni 综合征是一种常染色体显性遗传性家族性疾病,受累者可能患乳腺癌、软组织肉瘤、骨肉瘤、白血病、脑肿瘤、结肠癌和肾上腺皮质癌[52]。

3. *SMAD4*

SMAD4 是位于染色体 18q 上的肿瘤抑制基因,在大多数胰腺癌和结肠癌的一个亚群中缺失或突变。Smad4 是该基因编码的蛋白,是 TGF-α 超家族因子的必需细胞内介质。Smad4 作为转录因子发挥作用,是 Smad4 蛋白家族其他成员的专性伴侣[53]。突变体 Smad4 缺乏这些特性和其他作用,导致 TGF-α 抑制增殖的功能丧失。*SMAD4* 的种系突变可引起幼年型息肉病综合征(见第 126 章)。

（五）DNA 修复基因

DNA 复制本身和各种类型的 DNA 损伤剂会将错误引入基因组。这些错误包括正常 DNA 复制过程中核苷酸的自发错配、核苷酸的氧化损伤和完全的双链断裂。因此，已经进化出多种细胞机制来防止或纠正 DNA 错误。复制过程中产生的一类错误可能发生在 DNA 的重复单核苷酸或二核苷酸延伸中，即所谓的微卫星区域[54]。这些重复区域容易出现 DNA 错配，如果不解决，可能导致短插入或缺失。用于纠正这些错误的细胞机制称为错配修复系统。酶结合错配的 DNA，用错配的核苷酸切断 DNA 链，解开 DNA 片段，用正确的核苷酸填补缺口，最后重新连接封闭剩余的缺口。DNA 错配修复基因家族包括两个基本的分子组分：由 MSH2 和 MSH6 组成的错配识别复合体；由 MLH1 和 PMS2 组成的诱导剪切复合体。这些基因中的任何一个突变都会导致错配修复缺陷，当其作为种系突变而遗传时，会引起 Lynch 综合征，也称为遗传性非息肉病性结直肠癌[55,56]。错配修复因子的完全缺失会导致非常高的 DNA 突变率，而错配修复缺失的肿瘤积累了大量的肿瘤体细胞突变，通常超过 2 000 个体细胞突变，导致大量肿瘤特异性新抗原[57]。受影响的细胞称为复制错误阳性细胞，与复制错误阴性表型相反[58,59]。由于微卫星 DNA 序列受到这类遗传不稳定性的影响，与非肿瘤组织相比，肿瘤细胞在这些 DNA 片段延伸中表现出插入或缺失，这种现象被称为微卫星不稳定性。从机制上讲，DNA 修复缺失并不会直接导致癌症，而是创造了一种环境，允许在含有重复 DNA 序列的多种基因中突变积累，如 TGF-α Ⅱ 型受体、IGF Ⅱ 型受体、BAX 和 E2F-4 等。

错配修复基因的缺失是肿瘤内突变累积的重要机制（见图 1.4）。虽然，5% 的结肠癌是由于 Lyach 综合征（遗传性非息肉病性结直肠癌）所致，即错配修复系统中的种系突变，但有两倍的肿瘤（10%）表现出相似的分子特征，而任何错配修复基因均无种系突变。这些肿瘤通常是由该系统中的体细胞功能丧失驱动的，最常见的是由于该基因启动子区被称为 DNA 甲基化的表观遗传变化，导致 *MLH1* 基因表达沉默。*MLH1* 启动子超甲基化最常见于组织学上表现为锯齿状腺瘤且也携带 *B-Raf* 突变的病变（见图 1.4）。最后，人们已经认识到，另一种可导致高突变负荷状态的机制是，复制型 DNA 聚合酶 Pol-ε 或 Ⅱολ-δ 通过多种错义突变失去核酸外切酶校对活性[60]。

另一个参与癌症发生的重要 DNA 修复途径是由 *MUTYH* 基因介导的。*MUTYH* 基因编码一种 DNA 糖基化酶，参与氧化鸟嘌呤核苷酸（如 8-氧鸟嘌呤残基）的修复，可能与腺嘌呤不适当地配对，如果未校正，最终导致体细胞 G∶C→T∶A 突变。*MUTYH* 的双等位基因突变导致类似 FAP 的腺瘤性息肉病综合征，只是其遗传方式为常染色体隐性遗传（见第 126 章）[61,62]。有趣的是，*APC* 基因的 G∶C→T∶A 突变几乎普遍存在于种系 *MUTYH* 突变患者的息肉中，这表明 MUTYH 和 FAP 综合征在息肉分子发病机制上有重要的相似性。

（六）非编码 RNA

人类基因组包含多种基因，其产物为不编码蛋白质的 RNA。这些 RNA 的产物被称为非编码 RNA，由一大类能介导多种效应具有广泛活性的 RNA 分子组成。非编码 RNA 的类别正在迅速扩大，包括所谓的微小 RNA（micro-RNA）和长非编码 RNA，它们在癌症中经常失调。微小 RNA 通过 RNA 降解或翻译抑制在其他 RNA 转录沉默中发挥关键作用，通常一次调节几十个靶 RNA。它们的生物起源涉及常规的基因转录，随后通过多种核酸酶切割事件处理产生的 RNA，最终通过蛋白核糖核酸内切酶产生小干扰 RNA（siRNA）。这些 siRNA 与互补的 mRNA 序列结合，这种结合决定了 RNA 靶标的特异性。长非编码 RNA 可能具有多种功能，如基因沉默、剪接和端粒延伸。

（七）致癌信号通路

单个致癌基因或肿瘤抑制基因不一定直接诱导细胞转化，但作为已讨论的更大致癌信号通路的组分，通常彼此协同发挥作用。一些与胃肠道肿瘤发生特别相关的通路包括 Wnt 和 Ras 信号通路。这些信号通路是调节正常组织稳态的通路，但当信号以异常或扩增的方式转导时就会致癌。Wnt 信号的主要特征如图 1.3 所示。α-连环蛋白从内质膜转移到细胞质。在那里，它与 APC 蛋白 Axin 和糖原合成酶激酶-3α 形成大分子复合物。糖原合成酶激酶-3α 使 α-连环蛋白磷酸化触发其降解。在 Wnt 信号活跃的情况下，α-连环蛋白被稳定并进入细胞核，在那里它与转录因子 Tcf-4 相互作用上调许多关键靶基因，包括 c-Myc、细胞周期蛋白 D1 和血管内皮生长因子（vascular endothelial growth factor，VEGF）。如前所述，Wnt 信号通路对调节正常肠上皮的增殖至关重要，而 Wnt 信号通路失调几乎是所有结直肠癌的普遍特征。后者可由 APC、Axin 或 α-连环蛋白基因突变引起，但最常见的仍是肿瘤抑制基因 APC 的改变。其中一个组分的改变就足以激活整个通路。因此，有必要在其发挥功能的整体信号通路背景下，考虑个体基因改变。

由于信号通路通常不是线性的，因此会出现额外的复杂性水平。信号通路之间经常存在重叠，通路之间的区别可能是任意的。例如，*K-ras* 癌基因的突变导致多种不同信号通路的激活，包括 Raf/ERK/MAPK、PI3K/Akt 和核因子-κB，所有这些通路均在肿瘤发生中起重要作用（图 1.5）。这些效应通路之间的串扰可进一步调节细胞反应。例如，作为 PI3K 靶点的 Akt 可以磷酸化 Raf，从而通过 MAPK 通路调节信号[63]。最后，这些信号转导通路中的每一条都调节与肿瘤发生相关的多个生物学过程[64]，包括细胞周期过程、细胞凋亡、衰老、血管生成和侵袭。

在胃肠道肿瘤发生中起特别重要作用的另一条途径是环氧合酶-2（COX-2）通路。COX-2 酶是炎症和肿瘤诱导前列腺素合成的关键调节因子。虽然有关 *COX-2* 突变的阐述尚少，但 COX-2 在结直肠腺瘤和癌症中的过度表达与肿瘤进展和血管生成有关（见图 1.4），主要通过诱导前列腺素 E_2 合成。发现使用多种药物（阿司匹林、非甾体抗炎药或 COX-2 选择性抑制剂如塞来昔布等），抑制 COX-2 与结直肠腺瘤和癌症的风险降低有关[65]。

四、肿瘤微环境

癌症最终是一个复杂的组织，不仅由包含许多基因病变的肿瘤细胞组成，如前所述，而且由许多赋予肿瘤所有特性的细胞成分组成。事实上，非肿瘤细胞对肿瘤行为和演变的影响越来越被人们所认识。对肿瘤行为有公认影响的细胞成分包括：间充质细胞、脉管系统、募集到肿瘤中的各种免疫细胞（尤其是在肠道肿瘤中），以及对肿瘤微环境有显著影响的肿瘤相关微生物群。此外，这些要素的协同作用形成了代谢环境，如肿瘤的氧气和营养供应，这对原发部位肿瘤的演变及其向远处转移的潜力起着重要作用。

五、肿瘤代谢

肿瘤细胞表现出异常的代谢特征，以促进其生长和合成代谢的需要。1924 年诺贝尔奖得主德国科学家 Otto Heinrich Warburg 的观察发现，肿瘤细胞表现出需氧糖酵解的显著增加和线粒体呼吸的减弱。这种被称为 Warburg 效应的代谢状态已得到验证，是大多数恶性肿瘤代谢的标志性特征[66]。越来越清楚的是，表征癌症形成的基因病变的整体是伴随细胞转化发生的细胞代谢改变的原因。许多与胃肠道癌症有关的基因（*p53*、*K-Ras*、*PI3K*、*mTOR*、*HIF*、*Myc*）实际上可以调节细胞代谢途径。此外，代谢调节因子（如琥珀酸脱氢酶亚基）内的种系突变不是经典的致癌基因或肿瘤抑制基因，与肿瘤发生的高风险相关（嗜铬细胞瘤和副神经节瘤）[67,68]。在癌细胞中糖酵解增加的选择优势可能包括对缺氧环境的耐受性更强，以及将代谢副产物（如乳酸）分流到其他生物合成途径。这些改变的代谢途径有希望成为治疗的新靶点。

（一）炎症和癌症

免疫细胞募集到肿瘤微环境中会导致多种效应。一方面肿瘤免疫监视是公认的，免疫抑制状态增加了癌症发生的风险。另一方面，许多造血来源的细胞成分可以促进原发性肿瘤生长，阻止有效的免疫监视，或促进肿瘤细胞获得有利于转移的特征。具有未成熟特征的髓系细胞，即所谓的髓源性抑制细胞，就是这种现象的一个重要例子[69]。

此外，许多慢性炎症会增加癌症的部位特异性风险；例如溃疡性结肠炎（见第 115 章）、慢性胃炎（见第 52 章）、慢性胰腺炎（见第 59 章）、Barret 食管（见第 47 章）和慢性病毒性肝炎（见第 79 和 80 章）。炎症对肿瘤形成的影响是多方面的和复杂的。炎症细胞产生的细胞因子可导致转录因子（如核因子-κB 和 STAT3）[70,71]介导的肿瘤细胞中抗凋亡和促增殖信号的激活。免疫细胞也可能促进血管的重塑并促进血管生成（稍后讨论），炎症也可能通过细胞因子刺激产生活性氧诱导 DNA 损伤。

（二）微生物群

人体拥有超过 100 万亿的微生物，这些微生物的最大浓度存在于胃肠道中。这些微生物与宿主之间的相互作用是一个备受关注的领域，特别是对广泛的自身免疫、代谢和肿瘤疾病[72]。有意思的是，结肠肿瘤与特定的细菌亚群相关，肿瘤相关的微生物物种群具有诱导特定动物模型中发生结肠肿瘤[73]。具核梭形杆菌是一种通常存在于口腔内的生物体，就是这种行为的一个例子，因为发现它与结肠肿瘤相关，当将具核梭形杆菌引入到由种系 APC 突变驱动的结肠癌模型中时，可以驱动结肠肿瘤的发生[74]。

六、肿瘤转移的生物学特征

肿瘤远处转移的建立需要多个过程，其中许多过程涉及肿瘤细胞和正常宿主细胞之间相互作用的改变。要转移，一个细胞或一组细胞必须脱离原发肿瘤，获得淋巴或血管间隙的通路，在远处黏附于内皮表面，穿透血管壁侵入第二组织部位，最后增殖为第二肿瘤病灶。血管生成是原发肿瘤增殖和肿瘤转移的必要条件。肿瘤细胞也必须克服宿主免疫细胞的杀伤。因此，很少有循环肿瘤细胞（<0.01%）成功地启动转移灶。有人提出了转移的“适者生存”观点，其中选择性竞争有利于原发部位细胞亚群的转移[75]。有利于这一观点的是，原发部位和转移到远处部位肿瘤的突变状态往往截然不同，这表明只有特定的肿瘤细胞克隆才能获得转移的能力。

血管和淋巴管新生

血管生成对于维持原发性肿瘤的持续生长至关重要。如果随着原发肿瘤的扩大，而新生血管不发育，那么距现有血管最远的肿瘤细胞就不能获得足够的营养和氧气，就会发生中心性坏死。因此，新生血管的形成是促进肿瘤转移播散的重要的因素[76]。研究发现，恶性肿瘤细胞和基质细胞产生的许多蛋白生长因子是血管生成的强效刺激物，包括 VEGF-A、碱性成纤维细胞生长因子和 TGF-α。VEGF-A 可能是包括结直肠癌在内的大多数肿瘤类型中表达上调的最关键因素。与胃肠道癌变密切相关的多种遗传途径参与调节 VEGF-A 的表达，包括 Wnt 和突变型 ras[77]。

血管生成发生在一系列有序的事件中。刺激载瘤血管中的内皮细胞，降解内皮基底膜，迁移到血管周围基质中，启动毛细血管芽，血管芽胚发育成管状结构，进而发育成毛细血管网。模拟血管生成早期事件的体外模型表明，这一过程涉及蛋白酶和蛋白酶抑制剂之间的平衡，其方式与肿瘤侵袭过程相似。事实上，肿瘤侵袭和血管生成之间的功能相似之处在于它们对细胞运动、基底膜蛋白水解和细胞生长的相互需求方面是显而易见的。

除血管生成外，淋巴管生成在肿瘤转移过程中也起着重要作用。对肿瘤淋巴管生成的分子基础已获得了一些重要线索。VEGF-C 或 VEGF-D 与淋巴管内皮细胞上的 VEGF 受体-3 结合，刺激新淋巴管的形成[78]，这导致肿瘤团块内出现新的淋巴通道，从而促进肿瘤细胞向局部淋巴结的播散[79]。

七、环境影响

从根本上讲，癌症是一种遗传性疾病，基因突变是导致肿瘤形成的因素或机制的共同特征。另外，环境因素在肿瘤的发生中也起着重要作用，因为它们影响潜在基因病变的进展。

（一）化学致癌

许多具有致癌潜力的化合物通常需要宿主酶的代谢修饰，这一过程称为代谢激活。最初的化合物，即前致癌物，通过宿主酶转化为亲电衍生物，然后对 DNA 进行化学修饰。突变是由于碱基对扭曲导致 DNA 复制过程中发生的错配所致。影响任何化学致癌物效力的因素包括前致癌物的激活与致癌物失活或降解之间的平衡[80]。致癌物失活通常是通过在肝脏中发生的偶联反应实现的。

这些原理通过实验性结肠癌得以证实：给啮齿动物喂食苏铁素（cycasin）后可导致结肠癌发生，苏铁素是苏铁属植物坚果中的一种糖基化合物。苏铁素的葡萄糖残基在大鼠肝脏中被 α-葡萄糖苷酶裂解形成甲基偶氮氧基甲醇，随后在肝脏和结肠中被酶降解产生甲基重氮，甲基重氮是一种致癌物质。这些相同的代谢物是通过化合物二甲基肼的转氨酶修饰形成的，并导致大鼠发生结肠癌。

在人类中，经常吸烟与多种胃肠道癌（包括胰腺癌和结肠癌）的患病风险密切相关。在长期主动吸烟者中，患胰腺癌的风险会增加两倍。在烟草中已发现包括砷、苯和环氧乙烷在内的多种致癌物质。但与胰腺癌或结肠癌的发生密切关联的化学物质尚未确定。

（二）饮食因素

化学诱变在胃肠道和相关器官内癌症的发展中可能尤其重要。胃肠道中大多数原发性癌发生于黏膜，而此黏膜表面暴露于具有潜在致癌物或前致癌物的膳食成分的复杂混合物中。1995 年的研究已经直接证明了饮食因素在人体中作为诱变剂的致癌作用。例如，食物被真菌代谢产物黄曲霉毒素污染的频率与世界各地区肝细胞癌的发病率相平行[81]。研究还表明，黄曲霉毒素可引起肝细胞癌中 *TP53* 基因突变，这为基因与环境之间提供了令人信服的联系[81]。

许多食物中存在的硝酸盐似乎是额外的膳食成分，可能在胃肠道中作为前致癌物存在。饮食来源的硝酸盐可在低胃酸的胃中，通过细菌作用转化为亚硝酸盐，随后转化为具有致突变的亚硝胺[82]。这些事件可能是记录在案的高硝酸盐食物的摄入量与不同人群中胃癌发病率之间相关性的基础。

其他饮食因素也可能参与调节饮食中前致癌物的生物效力。膳食脂肪的相对和绝对含量的变化可能导致结肠微生物群组成及其代谢特征的改变，从而调节将膳食成分转化为潜在致突变化合物的酶的生成。膳食纤维含量的变化可改变肠内容物在肠道中的传递时间，从而改变黏膜暴露于潜在诱变剂的持续时间。胆盐含量可能是调节前致癌物生物学效应的另一个管腔因素，非结合型胆汁酸盐可通过损伤肠黏膜和加快肠上皮增生促进癌变。

这些机制可以解释某些人群中，不同膳食成分的摄入与结直肠癌发病率之间的相关性（见第 127 章）。高纤维摄入量可致快速结肠通过，显示结直肠癌的发病率低于低纤维摄入量和延迟通过的人群。调查发现，食用西方饮食的日本移民，在美国结直肠癌的发病率远高于食用传统日本饮食的本土人群[83]。

八、分子医学：胃肠肿瘤学当前和未来的研究方法

（一）二代测序

DNA 测序依赖于聚合酶介导的链合成，以及通过各种理化方法检测在化学反应的连续步骤中掺入的核苷酸。同时监测数十亿个反应的能力，即所谓的大规模平行测序，以及将短序列读取通过计算组装成连续长序列读取的能力，彻底改变了测序技术。这些新的方法，通常被称为二代测序（next generation sequencing，NGS），正在逐步应用到癌症患者的临床医疗的多个环节中[84]。首先，种系 DNA 的测序越来越多地用于确定患者是否可能患有癌症遗传综合征。其次，这些技术还可应用于确定肿瘤的突变前景，以指导治疗决策。

DNA 测序的范围可能涉及整个基因组。无需任何步骤的富集或选择，即可使用来自特定来源的 DNA 进行全基因组测序，另一种方法是对样本进行初步富集，富集过程可利用杂交方法和引物库从样本中提取感兴趣的区域，其目的是降低样本的复杂性并增加测序反应过程中可能的读取次数。随着可获得的读取次数的增加，即所谓的读取深度，测序的准确性提高，成本也降低了。最常见的富集方法是关注基因组中已知隐藏基因的区域，统称为外显子组，它相当于整个基因组的 1% 左右。对于某些应用，来自整个外显子组的基因子集可能是唯一富集测序的基因亚群，这是基于 NGS 的诊断检测的基础，重点是与癌症相关的基因面板。因为 NGS 涉及短读段，通过计算组装成预测的长读段，这项技术对影响一个等位基因的基因倒位、大片段插入或一般拷贝数变异不敏感。

癌症与肿瘤基因组学

随着遗传信息从测序分析中获得，了解观察到的基因变化的潜在影响成为一项重要挑战。单核苷酸变异是指与参考序列相比，遗传密码的单个碱基对发生的变化。无义突变是指引入提前终止密码子。剪接受体或供体位点的单核苷酸变异，可能导致外显子序列丢失或内含子序列的错误表达。这些类型的变化相对容易解释和裁定，错义突变是指导致密码子编码的氨基酸发生变化。考虑到人群中存在的正常遗传变异，因此了解这些变化是否缺失是相当困难的。当这类变异的影响尚不清楚时，这些被称为“意义不明的变异”。目前外显子组测序的主要局限性包括意义不明的变异、检测拷贝数变异和大范围序列重排以及外显子组捕获策略无法检测到的内含子或启动子突变的可能性。

（二）分子诊断

基因检测是识别癌症高危家庭和评估家庭成员中个体癌症风险的有力工具。如今，评估大多数与家族性癌症综合征相关基因的测序面板已经上市。基因检测的应用必须考虑检测的灵敏度和特异性，以及患者信息的保密性和对医疗保险的潜在影响问题。由于这检测依赖于靶标富集，因此了解其潜在局限性非常重要。基于这些原因，遗传咨询也成为基因检测过程中必不可少的组成部分。

除了基因种系检测外，肿瘤分子表型分析对于指导治疗决策也是很重要的。为了检测错配修复缺陷引起的肿瘤，可以对存档的结肠肿瘤样本进行肿瘤 MSI 检测[85]。此外，错配修复所需的 4 种蛋白（MLH1、PMS2、MSH2、MSH6）的免疫组化染色缺失可能提供相似的信息。研究表明，结肠肿瘤的 MSI 状态可预测对基于 5-氟尿嘧啶的化疗反应[86,87]。

最近研究表明，错配修复缺陷肿瘤由于其体细胞突变和肿瘤新抗原的高负荷，对免疫检查点抑制治疗具有良好的

反应[88]。

随着我们对胃肠道癌分子机制理解的深入,靶向特定信号通路疗法很可能也会随之增加。靶向 EGF 受体并阻断 EGF 受体信号通路的抗体,已被证明对结直肠癌的治疗是有益的。然而,它们的益处仅在缺乏 *K-ras* 激活突变的癌症中显示。因此,结直肠癌中 *K-ras* 突变的检测,现在是此类靶向治疗前的一个标准流程。此外,目前 *c-KIT* 癌基因的小分子酪氨酸激酶抑制剂目前已成为胃肠道间质瘤的常规治疗方法(见第 33 章)[89]。分子生物学技术也可能在疾病分期中发挥作用。例如,在发现癌转移之前,捕获少量的循环肿瘤细胞可能会使预后和治疗获益[90]。最后,随着更多遗传标志物的检测成为可能,这些方法将成为癌症术后复发监测的另一个重要的手段。

(郭雪艳 袁农 译,曾翔俊 校)

参考文献

第 2 章 黏膜免疫与炎症

Charles O. Elson, Phillip D. Smith 著

章节目录

一、黏膜表面免疫球蛋白 …… 14
二、黏膜免疫细胞生理学 …… 15
三、黏膜免疫系统的功能解剖学 …… 15
（一）派尔斑（派尔集合淋巴结）和 M 细胞 …… 15
（二）肠上皮细胞 …… 16
（三）模式识别受体对病原体相关分子模式的识别系统 …… 18
四、肠道抗原递呈 …… 18
五、肠道免疫系统内的效应区室 …… 18
（一）上皮内淋巴细胞 …… 19
（二）固有层淋巴细胞和单核细胞 …… 19
（三）T 细胞分化 …… 19
（四）固有淋巴样细胞 …… 20
（五）树突状细胞 …… 20
（六）巨噬细胞 …… 20
（七）口服耐受性 …… 21
（八）趋化因子在体内稳态和炎症中的作用 …… 22

黏膜免疫是指发生在黏膜部位的免疫反应。对黏膜免疫系统的需求与相对全身免疫系统的需求截然不同。在黏膜部位，“外部世界”通常通过单层上皮与内部世界分开。黏膜免疫系统存在于许多部位，包括肠道、呼吸道（尤其是上呼吸道）、泌尿生殖道、乳腺、眼睛和耳朵。这些位点中的每一个都会遇到一系列不同的环境刺激，并进化出自己特有的一组细胞群。尽管如此，这些不同的隔室可以相互作用并共享一些细胞群，形成一个共同的黏膜免疫系统。本章重点介绍肠黏膜免疫系统[1]。

肠黏膜形成黏膜免疫系统最大的隔室，在几个方面具有独特性[2]。不同于其他黏膜部位，肠道中有数十亿至万亿的微生物，主要是细菌。这些微生物及其产物，连同摄入的食物，形成了一种庞大的抗原负荷，机体必须耐受这种负荷以维持黏膜内稳定。这种不寻常的环境和与之相关的需求形成了一种独特的免疫系统，它由诱导淋巴滤泡组成，命名为肠道相关淋巴组织（gut-associated lymphoid tissue，GALT）和分布在上皮中的效应细胞［上皮内淋巴细胞（intra-epithelial lymphocyte，IEL）］和固有层（lamina propria，LP）中作为单核细胞。总的来说，这些细胞构成了免疫系统中数量最多的细胞。

黏膜免疫细胞的具体特征和特殊性反映了细胞发挥功能的独特环境。为了维持肠黏膜内的黏膜稳态，免疫系统中最重要的任务之一是将潜在的有害抗原（如致病细菌和毒素）与可能有益于身体的产品，（如来自食物或共生细菌的分子）区分开来。为了实现体内稳态，黏膜独特的细胞类型、免疫球蛋白（Igs）和分泌介质以协调的方式发挥作用。与全身免疫系统相反，其重点是在遇到外来抗原后数秒钟内迅速发挥作用，黏膜免疫系统准备做出反应，但主要是耐受性的[3,4]，排斥有害抗原，允许有益/无害的抗原持续存在，而不引起过敏反应或炎症等有害的免疫反应。

数十亿活化浆细胞、记忆 T 细胞、记忆 B 细胞、巨噬细胞和树突状细胞存在于 LP 中，但不存在明显的活动性炎症。这种现象被称为控制性或生理性炎症（图 2.1）。重要的是，免疫细胞进入 LP 和细胞活化是抗原驱动的。因此，无菌小鼠的 LP 中几乎没有免疫细胞，但在肠道共生菌正常定植后的数小时至数天内，细胞发生大量内流和活化[5-7]。类似的过程开始于人类新生儿，其肠道在出生时定植，开始启动黏膜免疫系统的发育，刺激先天性和适应性系统免疫。微生物群在婴儿期扩大和变化，导致数以万亿计的肠道细菌与每个胃肠道器官的宿主细胞产生交集，对肠道血管、神经和免疫系统产生深远的影响。人类与其共生的肠道微生物群共同进化，并发展出多种反应机制，包括肠道上皮细胞和先天性、适应性和调节性免疫成分[8]。

肠道微生物群的异常组成与多种代谢和免疫性疾病有关，包括炎症性肠病（inflammatory bowel disease，IBD）。许多（如果不是大多数）赋予 IBD 易感性的基因变异与参与调节宿主-微生物群相互作用的每个组分的细胞和功能有关[9]。肠道微生物群本身是下一章的主题。尽管肠道菌群的抗原驱动持续存在，但肠道淋巴细胞效应细胞未能发育成侵袭性炎症细胞。细菌或其产物在这种持续的暂停激活状态中发挥作用[10]。有助于控制肠黏膜炎症。

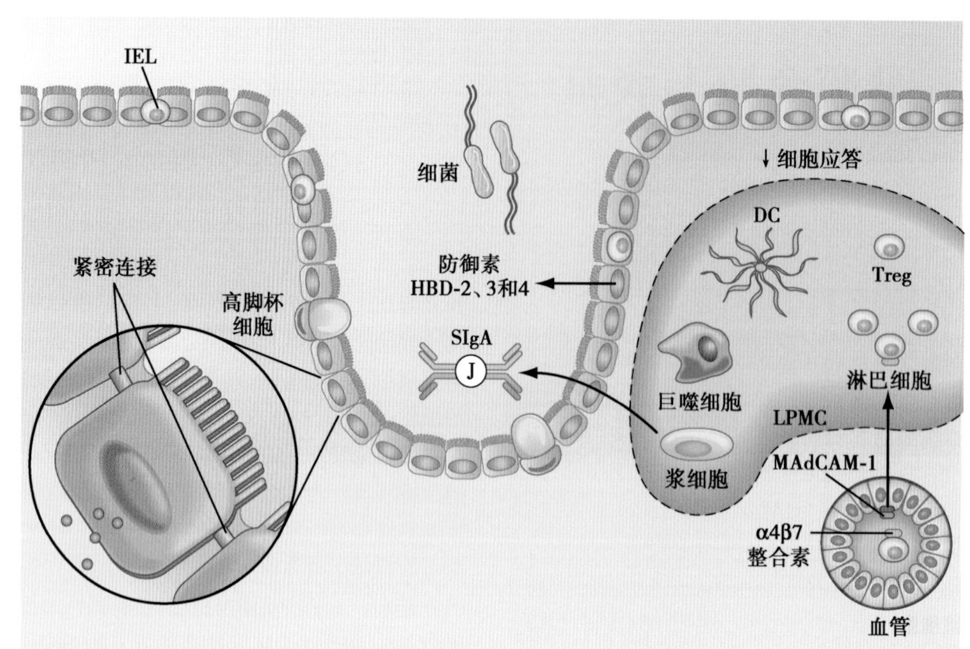

图 2.1　抑制黏膜免疫反应的机制。肠道使用许多不同的机制抑制黏膜免疫反应。肠道内抗原的主要来源是共生菌群，但先天性和适应性免疫反应都控制局部反应。杯状细胞分泌的黏蛋白和上皮细胞之间的紧密连接等物理屏障可防止腔内菌群的侵袭（圆形插图）。如防御素 HBD-2、3 和 4 被认为可维持隐窝的无菌性，而由局部浆细胞产生的分泌性免疫球蛋白 A 可以防止肠腔细菌的附着和侵袭，从而降低抗原负荷。即使在抗原激发下，由于模式识别受体（如 Toll 样受体）的表达减少和淋巴细胞通过其抗原受体被激活的能力降低，肠道淋巴细胞、巨噬细胞和树突状细胞也被编程为无反应。整合素 α4β7 可引导循环淋巴细胞从血管（如高内皮小静脉）流出，它还可以识别地址素 MAdCAM-1。DC，树突细胞；HBD 人 β 防御素；IEL，上皮内淋巴细胞；LPMC，固有层单核细胞；MAdCAM，黏膜地址素细胞黏附分子；SIgA，分泌型免疫球蛋白 A，一种具有连接 J 链的二聚体；Treg，调节性 T 细胞（以前称为抑制性 T 细胞）

一、黏膜表面免疫球蛋白

免疫球蛋白 A，一种免疫调节抗体。分泌型 IgA（secretory IgA，SIgA）是黏膜免疫反应的标志（图 2.2）。IgG 是全身免疫系统中最丰富的同种型抗体，但 IgA 是黏膜分泌物中含量最丰富的抗体[3,11,12]。考虑到人类每天产生的 IgA⁺浆细胞的数量和分泌的 3~5g IgA，IgA 应是人体内最丰富的抗体。

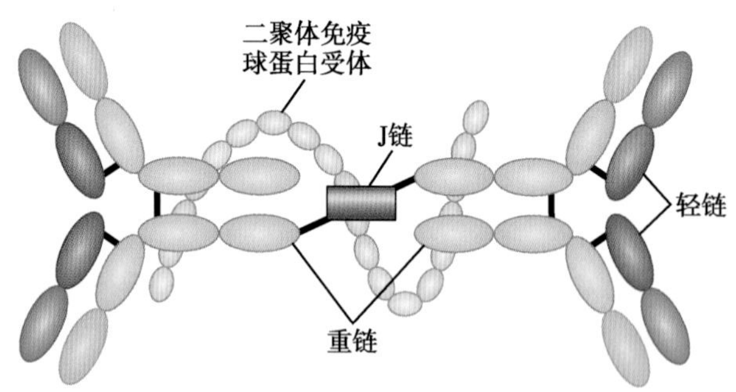

图 2.2　分泌型免疫球蛋白（Ig）A 复合物。两个 IgA 分子通过 J 链连接，并通过聚合 Ig 受体（pIgR）稳定，形成二聚体分泌型 IgA

SIgA 是 LP 中浆细胞产生的 IgA 的二聚体形式，通过特殊途径经肠腔上皮转运到肠腔（图 2.3）。两个 IgA 分子（同源二聚体）通过 J 链（由浆细胞产生）结合在一起。随后，同源二聚体与一种高度特化的糖蛋白结合，即聚合免疫球蛋白受体（polymeric Ig receptor，pIgR），以前称为分泌成分，是一种由上皮细胞产生的 55kD 糖蛋白[11]。pIgR 在肠上皮细胞的基底外侧膜上表达[13]。并且仅与二聚体 IgA 或 IgM 结合（也与 J 链聚合形成多聚体）。SIgA 一旦与肠上皮细胞上的 pIgR 结合，就会在囊泡内主动转运至肠上皮细胞的顶膜。囊泡与顶膜融合，pIgR/IgA 复合物释放到肠腔内。在肠腔内 pIgR 用于保护 SIgA 二聚体不被腔内蛋白酶和胃酸降解[13]。

SIgA 与黏液结合，增强其结合和捕获微生物产物的能力[14]。除了其独特的形式外，SIgA 还具有抗炎的性质，这一点也不寻常。它不与经典的补体成分结合，而是与肠腔内细菌抗原结合，阻止其被上皮细胞摄取，促进其凝集和随后的清除[12,15-18]。这一过程称为“免疫排斥”（immune exclusion），包括由于与分泌抗体的特异性相互作用而导致的抗原凝集、包埋和清除[14]，而不是上皮产生的非特异性排除机制（如黏液的产生、蛋白水解消化、防御素分泌）。SIgA 还可通过更直接的机制对某些病原体产生特异性保护性免疫，如抑制细菌毒力[19]，以及非抗原特异性结合游离或结合 pIgR 上的细菌聚糖残基或 SIgA 复合物。派尔集合淋巴结中的 M 细胞[20,21]（稍后讨论）选择性地结合 SIgA 和 SIgA 免疫复合物[22,23]，通过 M 细胞摄取抗原 IgA 复合物是抑制局部炎症反应的潜在机制[24]。

IgM 是另一种能够结合 pIgR 的抗体。与 IgA 一样，IgM 利用浆细胞产生的 J 链形成多聚体，（IgM 是一种五聚体）。pIgR 与聚合过程中形成抗体的 Fc 部分结合。IgM 结合 pIgR

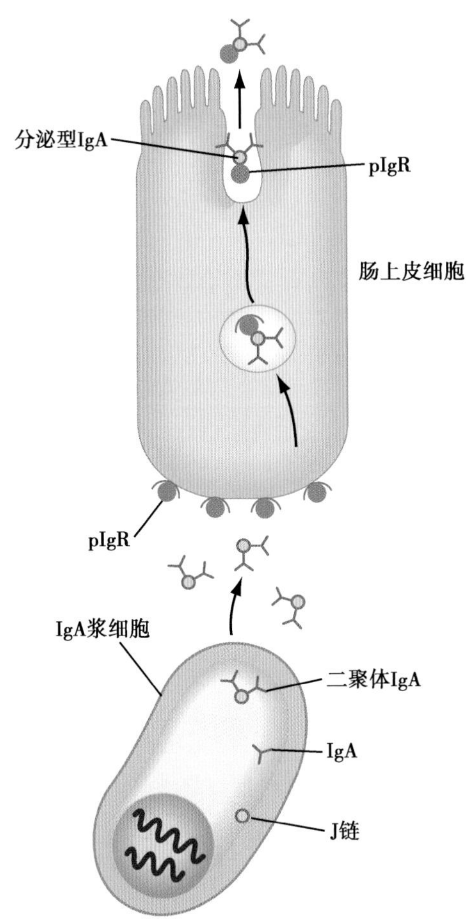

图 2.3　二聚体免疫球蛋白 A(IgA)的组装和分泌。IgA 浆细胞(下图)产生的 IgA 和 J 链二聚化形成聚合 IgA,其与肠上皮细胞(上图)产生的膜结合聚合 Ig 受体共价结合。该复合物内化,转运至上皮细胞顶端表面,并分泌至管腔中。pIgR,聚合免疫球蛋白受体

的能力在 IgA 缺乏的患者中可能很重要,分泌型 IgM 可弥补管腔内 IgA 的缺失。

SIgA 是黏膜产生的主要抗体同种型,但黏膜中也存在 IgG[25,26]。由肠上皮细胞表达的新生儿 Fc 受体(neonatal Fc receptor,FcRN)可作为 IgG 的双向转运蛋白[27,28],IgG 的转运体在控制某些新生儿感染和 IgG 代谢中很重要。在 IBD 患者中,检测到 LP 和腔内 IgG 显著增加[29]。

IgE 的产生可能在肠道对蠕虫的反应和食物过敏中起重要作用(见第 10 章)。据报道,CD23(低亲和力 IgE Fc 受体)由肠上皮细胞表达,一个动物模型表明,它可能促进抗原摄取,并导致食物过敏中的肥大细胞脱颗粒。在这种情况下,IgE 转胞吞作用和肥大细胞脱颗粒可能与进入腔内的液体和电解质流失有关,这一事件与肺部和肠道的过敏反应密切相关[30,31]。

二、黏膜免疫细胞生理学

将肠腔与固有层(LP)分开的细胞、结构和介质与不断变化的肠腔环境相互作用,起到物理屏障的作用。肠道屏障不仅每天发生变化,而且随着时间的推移不断变化。许多屏障机制在出生时尚未完全发育成熟,动物研究的证据表明,新生儿肠道抗原转运明显高于成年人。

由杯状细胞产生的黏液层包被排列在肠道内表面,它是由与 O-连接寡糖高度糖基化的糖蛋白(黏蛋白)和与蛋白质骨架连接的 N-聚糖链混合物组成[32],在人类基因组中已经鉴定出至少 21 种不同的黏蛋白基因,这些基因分别编码分泌型和膜结合型黏蛋白,每种黏蛋白都由不同的碳水化合物和氨基酸组成[33,34]。结肠内主要的黏蛋白是 MUC1、MUC2、MUC3A、MUC3B、MUC4、MUC13 和 MUC17。MUC2 是一种分泌型黏蛋白,作为肠黏液的主要成分,而其他黏蛋白是膜结合黏蛋白。膜结合黏蛋白参与细胞信号转导、黏附、生长和免疫调节等过程。黏液通过多种机制保护肠上皮,包括黏液的黏性及其与糖蛋白受体的竞争性结合,以减少微生物向肠黏膜的渗透[35]。结肠中有两个黏液层,一层松散的外层含细菌,一层致密的内层无细菌[36]。黏液流可使肠腔内容物离开上皮细胞。此外,肠道感染和炎症与黏液屏障的破坏和功能障碍有关,这可能伴随着宿主对微生物群的先天性和适应性免疫反应的改变[37]。

在黏液层下面,上皮作为物理屏障,通常阻止抗原通过上皮细胞(跨细胞途径)和细胞间隙(细胞旁途径),后者由紧密连接(TJ)复合体(如封闭带)和连接下间隙调节[38]。紧密连接在阻止大分子跨上皮细胞扩散方面具有更大的作用,因为这些连接排除了管腔中存在的几乎所有分子[39]。紧密连接形成的屏障是一种动态结构,可能被各种细胞因子和生长因子修饰。细胞因子 IFN-γ、TNF-α、IL-1β、IL-4、IL-6 和 IL-13 可增加肠道紧密连接的通透性,而 IL-10、IL-17 和 TGF-β 可降低肠道紧密连接的通透性[40],可能具有限制肠道炎症的特征,如同 IBD 炎症一样[41]。

三、黏膜免疫系统的功能解剖学

黏膜免疫系统的几个关键特征有助于维持体内平衡和清除病原体。黏膜免疫系统由诱导区室和效应区室两部分组成。派尔集合淋巴结和其他淋巴滤泡构成诱导区室,称为肠道相关淋巴组织(GALT)。上皮内淋巴细胞和固有层淋巴细胞是先天的和经历抗原刺激的记忆细胞,构成效应室。上皮、上皮下区域、LP、派尔集合淋巴结和肠系膜淋巴结(mesenteric lymph node,MLN)中的细胞群和免疫应答可能存在显著差异。位于这些区室中的细胞不仅在位置上存在差异,而且在表型和功能上也有所不同。

(一) 派尔斑(派尔集合淋巴结)和 M 细胞

滤泡相关上皮(follicle-associated epithelium,FAE)是一种特殊的上皮细胞,覆盖在派尔集合淋巴结和孤立的淋巴滤泡上。FAE 中的 M(微折叠)细胞与邻近的吸收上皮相反,微绒毛很少,黏蛋白覆盖层有限,细胞质细长,形成一个包围上皮下淋巴细胞、巨噬细胞、T 细胞、B 细胞和树突状细胞的囊袋(图 2.4)。M 细胞的吞噬作用和转胞吞作用具有高度特异性,能够从肠腔内摄取大颗粒抗原,并将其完整地转运至上皮下空间[42-45]。这些细胞溶酶体的含量很少,因此很少或根本没有对抗原进行加工[46]。M 细胞的顶端表面表达几种独特

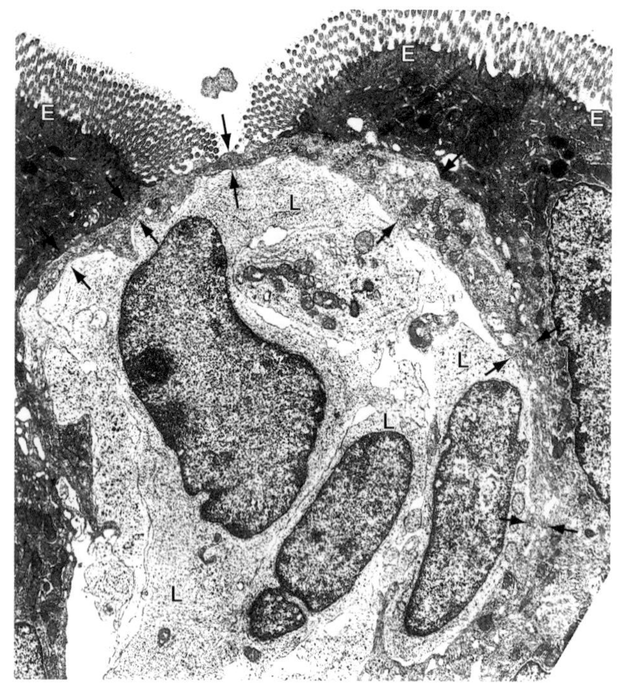

图 2.4　M 细胞。派尔集合淋巴结上皮非柱状区域的透射电子显微图显示了微折叠细胞（M）以及相关的微绒毛覆盖的肠上皮细胞和至少 3 个淋巴细胞（L）的横截面图。请注意 M 细胞减少的细胞质（箭头之间），它桥接微绒毛覆盖的上皮细胞之间的表面，与微绒毛形成紧密连接，并在淋巴细胞和肠腔之间形成屏障（×9 600）。B，B 细胞；E，肠上皮细胞。（From Owen RL，Jones AL. Epithelial cell specialization within human Peyer's patches：an ultrastructural study of intestinal lymphoid follicles. Gastroenterology 1974；66：189-203.）

的凝集素样分子，有助于促进与特定病原体的结合，如与脊髓灰质炎病毒的结合[47]。与 M 细胞结合并转运至底层派尔集合淋巴结的抗原，通常会引起阳性（SIgA）反应。因此，M 细胞似乎在黏膜免疫的初始阳性方面至关重要[48,49]。然而，某些病原体或其毒素可能利用 M 细胞并使用 M 细胞的转胞吞作用穿透肠黏膜。

M 细胞是派尔集合淋巴结和淋巴滤泡的导管。穿过 M 细胞进入上皮下囊袋的抗原，被巨噬细胞和树突状细胞摄取并携带到派尔集合淋巴结中。一旦抗原进入派尔集合淋巴结，分泌 TGF-β 的 T 细胞就会促进 B 细胞向同型 IgA 转换。M 细胞分化的诱导依赖于上皮细胞和派尔集合淋巴结淋巴细胞之间的直接接触[45,50]，至少部分通过 NOTCH 受体和配体的表达介导[51]。在缺乏派尔集合淋巴结 B 细胞的情况下，不存在 M 细胞，因为在缺乏派尔集合淋巴结的 B 细胞缺陷的动物中，尚未鉴定出 M 细胞。典型的派尔集合淋巴结具有 T 细胞依赖区和 B 细胞依赖/生发中心，但只有输出淋巴管。

在派尔集合淋巴结活化后，诱导淋巴细胞表达特异性整合素（α4β7），为内皮配体 MadCAM-1 的黏膜部位提供归巢信号[52,53]。淋巴细胞离开派尔集合淋巴结，流向 MLN，然后进入胸导管，再进入主要的肠淋巴引流系统，最后排入循环系统中（图 2.5）。在那里，黏膜活化的细胞及其黏膜“地址素”进入血液循环中，并在不同部位黏膜的高内皮小静脉中排出[54]。携带 α4β7 分子的细胞从 LP 中排出，并在 LP 中进行终末分化。趋化因子及其受体（稍后讨论）和黏附分子及其配体有助于引导这种运输模式。

（二）肠上皮细胞

肠上皮是由单层柱状上皮细胞组成。这些肠上皮细胞（ntestinal epithelial cell，IEC）来源于隐窝基部的干细胞区，从干细胞区向绒毛迁移，分化为吸收上皮细胞或分泌细胞，包括杯状细胞、肠内分泌细胞、帕内特细胞和簇状细胞[45]。除了作为物理屏障的功能外，IEC 还有助于肠道黏膜的固有免疫和适应性免疫，并在维持肠道稳态中发挥关键作用[45]。

吸收性上皮细胞通过紧密连接维持物理屏障，紧密连接由紧密连接蛋白、带状闭塞物、其他闭塞物和连接黏附分子组成。紧密连接密封上皮细胞之间的空隙，动态调节溶质运输。一些树突状细胞可以表达紧密连接蛋白，可以在上皮细胞之间延伸突起，以采集腔内的抗原样本[55]。如图 2.6 所示，IEC 与免疫细胞进行传递，特别是肠上皮淋巴细胞，并产生各种趋

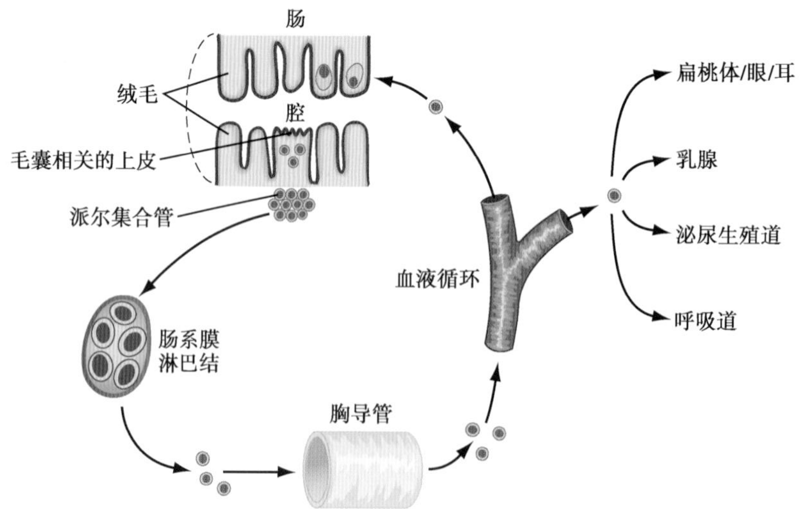

图 2.5　黏膜淋巴细胞迁移。抗原刺激后，T 和 B 淋巴细胞从肠道（派尔集合淋巴结）迁移到引流肠系膜淋巴结，在那里它们进一步分化，然后经胸导管到达体循环。然后，携带适当黏膜地址素的细胞选择性地回到构成共同黏膜相关淋巴组织（包括肠免疫系统）的黏膜表面

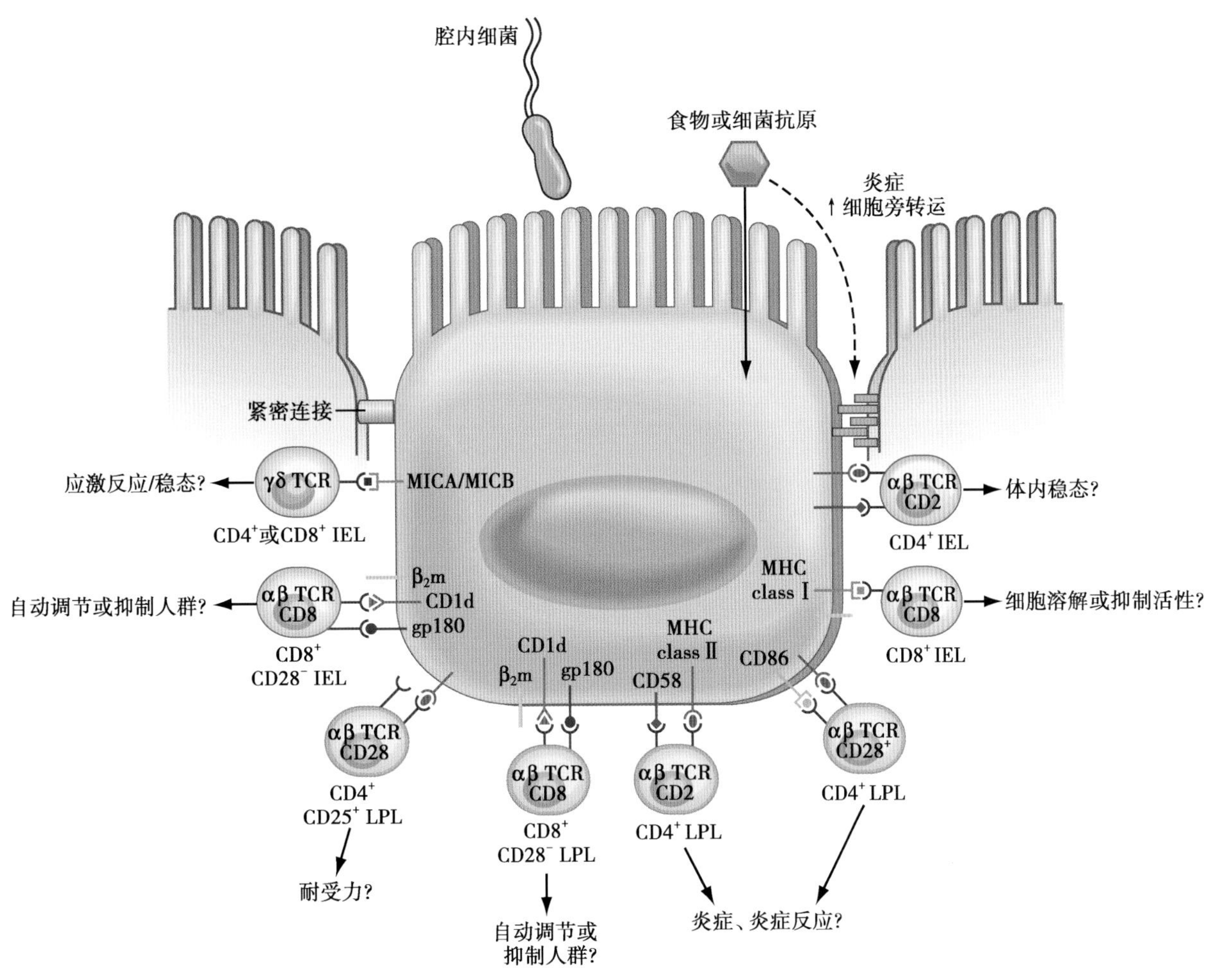

图 2.6　正常肠上皮细胞（IEC）。IEC 显示经典的 MHC 分子（Ⅰ类和Ⅱ类），有可能将传统抗原递呈给局部 T 细胞群及广泛排列的非经典Ⅰ类分子（例如 CD1d、MICA/MICB 和 β_2m（如图所示）和 MR-1、ULBP 和 HLA-E）。也有可能将非常规抗原递呈给独特的 T 细胞群。除此之外，其他活化途径似乎在肠道中显现功能（例如，通过 CD58-CD2 相互作用活化），经典的共刺激分子在 IEC 上不表达，但 CD86 可能在 UC 患者中被诱导。B7 家族的其他成员也有表达，如 PO-L1（CD274）和 ICOS-L（CD275），可能在局部 T 细胞活化中起作用。β_2 微球蛋白（β_2m）与 MHC Ⅰ类、CD1d、HLA-E、HLA-G 和 FcRn 相关。β_2m，β_2 微球蛋白；gp180，膜糖蛋白 180（CD8 配体）；IEL，上皮内淋巴细胞；LPL，固有层淋巴细胞；MHC，主要组织相容性复合体；MICA/MICB，MHC Ⅰ类相关链 A 和 B；TCR，T 细胞受体

化因子，调节细胞转运到黏膜，如同以下讨论。

1. 帕内特细胞

帕内特细胞（Paneth cell）是一种来源于上皮干细胞的分泌细胞群，位于小肠的隐窝底部[45]。由于大的嗜酸性颗粒占据其大部分细胞质，这些细胞在染色后很容易被识别出来（见第 98 章）。这些颗粒含有高浓度的抗菌肽，包括 α-防御素、溶菌酶、c 型凝集素和磷脂酶-A2。它们将这些抗菌肽分泌到隐窝的管腔中，从而保持隐窝相对无菌。防御素在各种细菌配体（包括内毒素）的刺激下释放，内毒素通过 Toll 样受体（Toll-like receptor，TLR）和核寡聚化结构域 2（nuclear oligomerization domain，NOD2）诱导帕内特细胞。帕内特细胞与干细胞共定位在隐窝底部，除提供抗菌肽外，还可提供维持干细胞功能的重要因素。帕内特细胞的发育受 WNT 通路中的转录因子和 NOD 信号级联反应中的转录因子的调控（如转录因子 MATH-1）。转录抑制因子 GFI-1 通过抑制促肠内分泌细胞转录因子神经元素-3（NEUROG3）在帕内特细胞发育中起重要作用。帕内特细胞和防御素 5 和 6 数量的减少与回肠克罗恩病有关。由于帕内特细胞具有高度分泌性，各种分子的合成较强。因此，帕内特细胞依赖于未折叠的蛋白质反应来维持细胞内稳态。干扰小鼠的未折叠蛋白质反应会导致回肠炎[56,57]。

2. 杯状细胞

杯状细胞（goblet cells）是一种分泌型上皮细胞，在黏蛋白和其他分子的产生中具有特异性。肠道中存在两种类型的黏蛋白层。一种是未附着或疏松层，这是小肠的特征。在远端结肠中存在第二种黏液层，也称附着层，细菌无法穿透。除了其物理特性外，黏蛋白还与抗菌肽相互作用以维持抗菌肽靠近上皮的高浓度。有多种细胞因子增加 Muc-2 的表达，包括 IL-1β、IL-4、IL-6、IL-13 和 TNF-α。几种金属蛋白酶，包括 ADAM-10 和 ADAM-17 及 meprin23，参与黏蛋白释放到肠腔中。杯状细胞还选择性地产生三叶因子-3（trefoil factor-3，TFF-3），它可影响黏液的黏稠度，在损伤后的上皮修复中起重要作用。TFF-3 缺乏的小鼠由于不能愈合病变，因而对右旋糖酐硫酸钠（dextran sulfate sodium，DSS）结肠炎高度敏感。固有免疫细胞也与杯状细胞相互作用，通过刺激肠细胞分化为杯状细胞来增加其数量。2 型先天性淋巴组织细胞（type 2 innate lymphoid cell，ILC2）衍生的 IL-13 和 ILC3 衍生的 IL-22

与杯状细胞增生和黏蛋白生成增加有关。

杯状细胞也可以通过杯状相关抗原通道(goblet-associated antigen passage,GAP)传输抗原穿过上皮层。已证明可溶性抗原和细菌能穿过杯状细胞,并呈递给底层的 $CD103^+$ $CX3CR1^-$ 耐受树突状细胞。随后 $CD103^+$ 树突状细胞迁移至肠系膜淋巴结,诱导抗原特异性 T 调节(T regulatory,Treg)细胞。因此,GAP 似乎有助于维持肠道内环境的稳态[58]。

3. 簇状细胞

簇状细胞(tuft cells)是一种上皮细胞,在正常肠道中不常见,但在寄生虫感染过程中数量增加。簇状细胞可通过独特的形态(以从顶膜突出的一丛微绒毛为特征)和一种独持的表型(以 ATOH1 和 Neurog 3 表达为特征)进行鉴定。簇状细胞表达与味觉受体相关的基因(见第 4 章),能够通过这些化学传感器辨别肠腔中的蠕虫。簇状细胞促发细胞因子 IL-25,可激活 ILC2 产生 IL-13,进而刺激黏蛋白产生,有助于清除寄生虫。ILC2 产生 IL-13 通过增加簇状细胞的数量提供正反馈回路[59,60]。

(三)模式识别受体对病原体相关分子模式的识别系统

全身免疫系统中的经典抗原呈递细胞(antigen-presenting cell,APC),具有识别细菌和病毒上高度保守的病原体相关分子模式(pathogen-associated molecular pattern,PAMP)的固有能力。PAMP 受体在 APC 表面(如 TLR)和细胞内[如核寡聚结构域(nuclear oligomerization domain,NOD)受体]均有表达。尽管 IEC 暴露于大量的管腔细菌中,但它们仍具有识别这些细菌一些成分的能力。在正常情况下 IEC 促炎反应下调。例如,由于缺乏细菌脂多糖(lipopolysaccharide,LPS)受体 TLR4,IEC 对细菌脂多糖无反应。然而,其他模式识别受体的表达得以维持,包括识别细菌鞭毛蛋白的 TLR5 的表达[61]。TLR5 在基底外侧表达,定位于识别已侵入上皮层的沙门氏菌属等生物[62]。在 TLR5 入侵和参与后,诱导肠上皮分泌大量的细胞因子和趋化因子,将炎性细胞吸引到局部环境中,以控制感染的扩散。

细胞内的 NOD1 和 NOD2 已被证明有助于肠道炎症。大约 25% 的克罗恩病患者存在 *NOD2/CARD15* 基因突变,从而干扰了其对细菌刺激产生适当的免疫应答的能力(见第 115 章)[63-68]。除此之外,在正常 IEC 弱表达的 TLR 在 IBD 患者 IEC 上表达水平较高[69]。在 IEC 上表达不同的 TLR,以及它们在肠道炎症和体内稳态中对先天和适应性 T 细胞和 B 细胞应答的作用,已在几种小鼠模型中得到证实[70,71]。

相反,一些细菌诱导 IEC 产生抗炎细胞因子(如 IL-10),和增加过氧化物酶体增殖物激活受体-γ(PPAR-γ)的表达[72,73]。此外,其他细菌产品(如来自噬菌体的调理素)有助于促进屏障和 IEC 分化[74]。

四、肠道抗原递呈

对抗原蛋白的有效免疫应答需要 T 淋巴细胞的帮助。这反过来取决于 APC 呈递的抗原,APC 将抗原的一小片段内化、消化与表面主要组织相容性复合体(major histocompatibility comple,MHC)异源二聚体偶联,最终与 $CD4^+$ T 细胞受体(MHC Ⅱ类)或 $CD8^+$ T 细胞受体(MHC Ⅰ类)相互作用。肠黏膜中的多个细胞可作为 APC,包括树突状细胞、巨噬细胞和 B 细胞。这些细胞将抗原递呈给 CD4 T 细胞的能力取决于其表面 MHC Ⅱ类的表达。在人类和啮齿类动物中,MHC Ⅱ类分子也存在于正常小肠上皮和较小范围的结肠细胞上。在体外研究表明,从大鼠和人小肠中分离出的肠细胞可以将抗原递呈给先前准备好的 T 细胞[75,76],这提示肠道 IEC 可能将肽递呈给位于上皮下方的 T 细胞的可能性。因此,IEC 能够在适当的背景下将抗原加工和递呈至 LP 内的细胞。有趣的是,LP 中存在双向淋巴细胞-上皮细胞串扰,LP 淋巴细胞(LP lymphocyte,LPL)通过 Notch-1 信号和诱导 IEC 分化、极化和屏障功能诱导促进黏膜屏障功能[77]。重要的是,在 IBD 中已报告 IEC 可增加 MHC Ⅱ类分子的表达[78,79],这可能增加 IEC 激活淋巴细胞的潜力[80,81]。

有趣的是,用于治疗 IBD 的药物(如 5-氨基水杨酸制剂)可能会降低 IEC MHC Ⅱ类分子的表达[82]。在正常受试者和 IBD 患者除表达 MHC Ⅱ类分子外,还表达 T 细胞活化所需的多种共刺激分子(见图 2.6)。这些分子包括细胞间黏附分子(intercellular adhesion molecule,ICAM)-1,它们可与 T 细胞上的白细胞功能相关抗原(leukocyte function associated antigen,LFA)-1 以及 ICOS 配体和 PD-L1 结合。CD86(B7-2),与 CD28 和 CTLA-4[83]结合,在溃疡性结肠炎 IEC 中表达。有趣的是,IEC 对这些共刺激分子的独特表达可能参与了黏膜反应的不同调节。小肠 IEC 不表达 CD80(B7-1)[84],因此 IEC 激活幼稚 T 细胞是不可能的,有助于 T 细胞反应的下调。然而,肠道炎症过程中表达的增加可能有助于增强 T 细胞刺激[85]。

MHC Ⅰ类和非经典Ⅰ类分子也由 IEC 表达。因此,IEC 将抗原呈递给某些 T 细胞群是可能的,这已被多个研究组报道[86-88]。具体而言,在人类 IEC 上表达的 CD1d 能够将抗原(与 CEACAM5 形成复合物)递呈至 $CD8^+$ T 细胞[89-91]。CD1d 限制性自然杀伤 T 细胞(natural killer T,NKT),具有固有性和适应性淋巴细胞特征的效应记忆细胞,是免疫反应最早的应答者之一,影响 NK 细胞、T 细胞和 B 细胞等其他免疫细胞谱系的活化。NKT 细胞参与感染性、恶性和免疫介导性疾病的免疫应答[92]。IEC 还表达其他非经典Ⅰ类分子。MICA 是一种应激诱导的 MHC 相关分子,在正常 IEC 上表达,并被 $CD8^+$ T 细胞、T 细胞和 NK 细胞上的 NKG2D 激活受体识别,其作用可能具有特别重要的意义,因为克罗恩病患者肠黏膜中具有 Th1 细胞因子谱的 $CD4^+NKG2D^+$ T 细胞数量增加[93]。

在人类中,IEC 特异性激活 $CD8^+$ 调节性 T 细胞,后者参与局部耐受和与 $CD8^+$IEC 的相互作用。IEC 在黏膜免疫调节中的作用在 IBD 组织研究中得到了最好的证实。来自 IBD 患者的 IEC 与来自正常受试者的 IEC 相反,在体外可刺激 $CD4^+$ T 细胞,而不是调节性 $CD8^+$ 细胞[80,81,94]。此外,口服抗原不会导致 IBD 患者耐受,但会引起主动免疫[95]。

五、肠道免疫系统内的效应区室

两种淋巴细胞群,即上皮内淋巴细胞和固有层淋巴细胞,存在于肠黏膜中。这两种不同细胞群的区室化与它们对不同微环境线索的反应能力相关。

（一）上皮内淋巴细胞

上皮内淋巴细胞（intra-epithelial lymphocyte，IEL）是肠道免疫系统的主要分支之一，可平衡保护性免疫和维持上皮屏障完整性。在小肠中，98% 以上的 IEL 是 T 细胞，且多为 $CD8^+$[96-98]，包括 $CD8^+$ αT 细胞，以及 $CD4^+CD8^+$ 双阳性和 $CD4^-CD8^-$ 双阴性细胞。与全身免疫系统中 $CD8^+$ T 细胞表达的 αβTCR 相比，更多的这些细胞也表达 γδT 细胞受体（TCR）[99]。大约有一半小鼠小肠 IEC 表达 γδ T 细胞受体[100]，而小鼠和人类大肠主要含有与全身免疫系统相似的 $αβCD4^+$ 或 $αβCD8^+$ T 细胞。

根据它们的表型，将 IEL 分为两个亚组：诱导 IEL（iIEL），包括常规 MHC Ⅰ类和Ⅱ类在胸腺中选择的 TCRαβT 细胞；天然 IEL，包括 $TCRαβCD8^+αα$、TCRγδ 双阳性和 TCRγδ 双阴性细胞。这两个亚群都具有细胞溶解性，通过颗粒酶或 Fas 的结合而被杀死，并分泌 Th1 细胞因子。然而，iIEL 可以转移对多种病原微生物的保护，而天然 IEL 不能转移这种免疫保护，不具有免疫记忆。这种差异可能是由于非经典 MHC 分子在原位通过 IEC 自然激活 IEL，而不是由专业 APC 上多态 MHC 表达的分子激活 iIEL[100]。两个 IEL 亚群均表达存在于自然杀伤细胞（NK）上的分子。IEL 表达多种活化标志物，为 $CD45RO^+$（记忆细胞）。IEL 也表达整合素，整合素是由 TGF-β 和 E-钙黏蛋白在 IEL 上诱导的[102]。分离的 IEC 很难通过其 TCR 激活，即使在强烈刺激下也几乎不增殖[98]，并且可能通过交替途径（例如，通过 CD2）激活。

iIEL 分泌一系列不同于外周血对应分泌的细胞因子[98,103-105]。IEL 产生的广谱细胞因子，包括 IFN-γ、TNF-α、IL-2、IL-4、IL-6、IL-10、TGF-β、角质细胞生长因子（KGF）和 IL-17 等，对肠道屏障功能和局部免疫应答具有重要影响[106]。

在功能上，IEL 可能杀死由于感染、转化或其他细胞侵袭而处于应激状态的上皮细胞[100]。另外，尽管 IEL 在管腔抗原识别中的实际功能的证据很少，但仍然被认为可以抑制局部免疫细胞。IEL 不会进出上皮，相反，当上皮细胞从隐窝移动到绒毛表面时，上皮细胞在 IEL 上移动。因此，IEL 很可能充当上皮完整的哨兵。

（二）固有层淋巴细胞和单核细胞

LP 是肠黏膜中的主要效应位点，含有丰富的抗原记忆 T 细胞。固有层淋巴细胞（lamina propria lymphoid cell，LPL）比其外周成分更容易发生凋亡，这是一种限制活化淋巴细胞炎症作用的潜在调节机制。在克罗恩病等炎症性肠病中，LPL 具有抵抗细胞凋亡的能力。

很明显，与全身免疫系统相比，黏膜 LP 在一组独特的规则下运行，反映在其功能解剖（无组织的结构）及其反应和调节中。高度特化的细胞介导了这些效应，有些仅在 LP 中检测到。

固有层单核细胞（lamina propria mononuclear cell，LPMC）是一组异质性细胞[107]（见图 2.1）。一种常见的细胞类型是 IgA^+ 浆细胞，但除巨噬细胞和树突状细胞外，50% 以上的 LPMC 是 T 细胞和 B 细胞（共同构成 LPL 群）。与 IEL 相反，LPL 表达黏膜地址素，但与 IEL 相似，LPL 表达活化的记忆表型，并且不会因 TCR 的参与而增殖。LPL 活化的替代途径主要是通过 CD2 和 CD28[103,108]。

在健康黏膜中，LPMC 通过 TCR 对抗原刺激的反应能力下调，如果不适当地活化，则发生凋亡的趋势增加，抑制对正常肠腔内容物的反应。细胞凋亡增加的机制可能与死亡受体 Fas 及其配体参与活化的 LPL，以及细胞内抗凋亡和促凋亡因子 Bcl2 和 Bax 之间的不平衡有关。在克罗恩病中已经报告了这种促凋亡平衡的缺陷[109,110]。

总之，上述机制有助于控制/生理性炎症，其特征为健康肠黏膜。当调节机制被破坏时，就会发生不受控制的炎症，如同 IBD 患者的黏膜一样。

（三）T 细胞分化

肠道相关淋巴组织（GALT）（见图 2.5），B 和 T 淋巴细胞与通过覆盖滤泡相关上皮（FAE）中的 M 细胞采样的抗原相互作用。T 淋巴细胞从幼稚 Th0 细胞到不同 Th 亚群的活化和成熟受到微环境（尤其是微生物群）和对病原体反应的强烈影响。病毒感染诱导 CD4 Th1 细胞，而寄生虫定植诱导 $CD4^+$ Th2 亚群。$CD4^+$ Th17 效应细胞对细胞外细菌和真菌产生反应。微生物群影响了黏膜 T 细胞的反应。例如，在小鼠中，被称为分段丝状细菌（关节假丝酵母）的共生菌选择性地诱导 $CD4^+$Th17 细胞[8]。

树突状细胞、GALT 内的专职 APC 及其分泌的介质使 T 淋巴细胞向几种效应细胞之一倾斜。当树突状细胞分泌 IL-12/p35-40 异源二聚体时[111]，产生分泌 IL-2、IFN-γ 和 TNF-α 的 Th1 细胞，并诱导转录因子 STAT-4（信号转导因子和转录因子激活剂 4）的活化和磷酸化。STAT-4 反过来诱导 IFN-γ 的表达和产生。IFN-γ 诱导 STAT-1 活化，进而诱导 T 细胞表达的 T 盒（T-bet）活化，T-bet 是诱导 Th1 细胞因子和 IL-12 受体 β2 生成的主要转录因子，同时抑制 Th2 细胞因子的生成。因此形成了促进 Th1 和抑制 Th2 应答的周期循环。T-bet 的激活可能是 TH1 介导的黏膜疾病的一个重要步骤，如一些克罗恩病患者中观察到的黏膜疾病。另一个重要的促 Th1 细胞因子是 IL-18。IL-18 通过增强 AP-1（c-fos/c-jun）依赖的 IL-12Rβ2 链表达，介导其对 T 细胞的作用，使 IFN-γ 启动子反式激活和核因子 κB（NF-kB）的激活[111]。

相反，当树突状细胞或其他黏膜细胞分泌 IL-4 时，Th2 细胞因子（IL-4、IL-5、IL-6、IL-9、IL-10、IL-13）通过激活 STAT-6 然后激活主转录因子 GATA-3 而产生。GATA-3 能够促进多种 Th2 细胞因子的表达，包括 IL-4、IL-5 和 IL-13。除了 IL-4 外，IL-13 还以 IL-4 非依赖性的方式在 Th2 发育和 IgE 合成中发挥重要作用。这些细胞因子似乎促进了食物过敏的发生（见第 10 章）。IL-5 诱导表达表面 IgA 的 B 细胞分化为产生 IgA 的浆细胞。IL-6 引起 IgA 分泌明显增加，对 IgM 或 IgG 合成影响不大。

第三个重要的 LP CD4 亚群是 Th17 细胞。Th1 极化细胞 IL-12 由 p40 和 p35 亚单位组成，与 Th17 极化细胞因子 IL-23 相似，后者由 p40 和独特的 p19 亚单位组成。以前归因于 IL-12 驱动的 Th1 途径的某些炎症活动，实际上可能是 IL-23 驱动的 Th17 通道的可能性得到了研究的支持，研究显示，当 IL-12 被抑制时，肠道炎症仍然可能存在，抑制 IL-23 而不是 IL-12 可改善炎症[112-116]。在克罗恩病中，IL-12 和 IL-23 的表达增加，而且在克罗恩病患者的临床研究中，抑制 IL-12 和 IL-23 的共同 p40 亚单位是有益的[117,118]。Th17 细胞表达维甲酸相关孤儿受体-γt（RORγt），这是这些细胞的主要转录因子。除 RORγt 外，人类 Th17 细胞还表达 IL-23R、CCR6 和 CD161，而缺乏 Th1 细胞特有的趋化因子受体 CXCR3[119-122]。Th17 细胞分泌的主要效应细胞因子是 IL-17A、IL-17F、IL-21、IL-22、IL-26、TNF-α 和趋化因子 CCL20。人类 Th17 细胞在 IL-1β、IL-6、IL-21、IL-23 和 TGF-β 的影响下分化[121]。在人类中，并非所有 Th17 细胞都产生 IL-22，并且已鉴定出产生 IL-22 但不产生 IL-17 的 CD4 辅助性 T 细胞的 Th22 亚群[122]。IL-17 促进中性粒细胞的募集和活化，而 IL-22 通过上皮增生和增加黏液分泌促进黏膜愈合[123]。

调节性 T 细胞（regulatory T cell，Treg）在肠道中大量存在，与 CD4 效应细胞相似，也由亚群组成，亚群沿肠道长度分布不均匀，反映了不同的微环境[124]。主要的 Treg 亚群表达转录因子 Foxp3。Foxp3$^+$调节性 T 细胞在胸腺（t-Treg）生成，也被称为“天然 Treg”。Foxp3$^+$调节性 T 细胞也由初始 CD4 T 细胞在外周组织生成，被称为“外周 Treg”（peripheral Treg，pTreg）或诱导 Treg。pTreg 的一个亚群存在于人和小鼠的结肠黏膜中，表达 Th17 细胞典型的转录因子 RORγt[125]。有趣的是，Foxp3$^+$ RORγt$^+$ Treg 细胞在哺乳期小鼠中被微生物诱导，该微生物群通过杯状相关通道被摄取[58]。Foxp3-T 调节 1 细胞（T regulatory 1 cell，Tr1）也以高丰度存在于肠黏膜中，并选择性产生大量 IL-10。Foxp3$^+$ Treg 仅产生 TGF-β 或 TGF-β 加 IL-10 作为其抑制性效应细胞因子。

某些微生物群或它们的产物可在小鼠中诱导不同类型的 Treg。例如，脆弱拟杆菌的多糖 A 成分可选择性地诱导 Foxp3$^+$IL-10$^+$CD4T 细胞[126,127]。相关微生物群梭状芽孢杆菌已被证明在小鼠结肠黏膜中诱导 Foxp3$^+$ Treg[128]，这种效应至少部分是由于这些器官在发酵过程中产生的短链脂肪酸（short-chain fatty acid，SCFA；乙酸盐、丙酸盐、丁酸盐）所致。SCFA 在小鼠的先天和适应性免疫细胞上有基因组编码的受体，它们倾向于抑制免疫反应[129]。人类具有相同的 SCFA 受体，很可能有相似的 Treg 应答[129-131]。SCFA 如丁酸盐等是肠细胞的主要营养物质，而不是葡萄糖。因此，在 IBD 中发现的产生 SCFA 的细菌耗竭可能对上皮和 Treg 功能产生多种有害影响。在小鼠中，Treg 的效应细胞因子，如 TGF-β 和 IL-10 的缺乏会导致结肠炎。IL-10 和/或其受体的缺乏，通过人类的失活突变，导致早期 IBD[132]。因此，Treg 及其效应细胞因子对于通过潜在控制致病性的先天和适应性反应来维持肠道内稳态至关重要。

LP 中 T 细胞谱系的生物学是复杂的，部分与这些细胞群的可塑性有关。在特定的情况下，Th17 细胞可能成为 Th1 细胞。而且，最近在人类中发现了表达 Th17 细胞因子并在体外具有强效抑制活动的调节性 Foxp3$^+$细胞[125]。这些发现表明，所有已知的 T 细胞亚群在体内都存在一定程度的可塑性，反映在它们根据微环境产生特定细胞因子的能力上。Th17 细胞在肠黏膜中发挥稳态作用[133]，这可能归因于活动性克罗恩病中抗 IL-17A 单克隆抗体治疗失败[134,135]。解决 LP 环境的复杂性及其介质和效应器，包括微生物群，将可能有助于更好地设计治疗策略来改变肠道炎症。

（四）固有淋巴样细胞

最近发现的固有淋巴样细胞（innate lymphoid cell，ILC）产生辅助性 T 细胞（T helper，Th）相关的细胞因子，但不表达与其他免疫细胞谱系相关的 T 细胞受体或细胞表面标志物。因此，ILC 是谱系标记阴性的，其免疫应答无抗原特异性。ILC 是固有性免疫的效应器和组织建模的调节因子。ILC 有几个亚群，均具有不同的细胞因子表达模式，类似于辅助性 T 细胞亚群 Th1、Th2 和 Th17[136]。

第一组 ILC 包括 ILC1 细胞和 NK 细胞。ILC1 细胞表达转录因子 T-bet，并通过产生 IFN-γ 对 IL-12 作出反应。它们与 NK 细胞不同之处在于它们不表达 NK 细胞标志物 CD16 和 CD94，缺乏穿孔素和颗粒酶 B。ILC1 细胞在克罗恩病患者发炎的肠道中增多，表明 ILC1 细胞在肠道炎症发病机制中起作用。

第二组 ILC 包括 ILC2 细胞，也称为天然辅助细胞、核细胞和先天性辅助细胞 2。它们的转录因子是维甲酸受体相关孤儿受体-α（related orphan receptor-α，RORα）和 GATA3，它们在驱虫反应和过敏性肺部炎症中起关键作用。

第三组 ILC 包括 ILC3 和淋巴组织诱导剂（lymphoid tissue inducer，LTi）细胞。该组的一些细胞表达 NK 细胞活化受体 NKp46，该受体依赖于转录因子 RORγt，缺乏细胞毒性效应性穿孔素和颗粒酶。第三组 ILC 表达 IL-22，而不表达 IFN-γ 或 TNF。ILC3 的一个子集表达 MHC Ⅱ类分子，并用于调节适应性 CD4$^+$ T 细胞对微生物群抗原的反应[137]。ILC 对黏膜稳态和肠道炎症的作用是一个需要深入研究的课题。

（五）树突状细胞

树突状细胞（dendritic cell，DC）在肠黏膜的耐受和免疫中起着核心作用。DC 在淋巴组织内不断迁移，并呈现很可能来自濒死的凋亡细胞的自身抗原以及非自身抗原，以维持自身耐受[138]。在小鼠远端小肠的 LP 中，DC 表达趋化因子受体 CX3CR1 并形成跨上皮树突，允许直接采样管腔内的抗原[139]。表达 CCL25（CCR9 和 CCR10 的配体）的 IEC 可将 DC 吸引到小肠黏膜，而 CCL28（CCR3 和 CCR10 的配体）可将 DC 吸引到结肠黏膜[140-142]。

树突状细胞处理内化抗原的速度比巨噬细胞慢[80,143]，可能有助于局部耐受[81,144]。树突状细胞诱导的耐受性与下列因素有关：①抗原呈递给 T 细胞时的成熟程度有关（未成熟树突状细胞激活调节性 T 细胞）；②共刺激分子 CD80 和 CD86 的下调；③产生抑制性细胞因子 IL-10、TGF-β 和 IFN-α；④与共刺激分子 CD200 相互作用[145,146]。小鼠 CD103$^+$树突状细胞能够执行抗原处理的所有阶段，包括细菌抗原的摄取、运输和呈递[147]。在小鼠 LP 中，CD103$^+$树突状细胞与 CX3CR1$^+$巨噬细胞具有相同的免疫监测负荷（共同承担免疫监视的责任），这些亚群的功能受损可能有助于 IBD 的发展[148]。

（六）巨噬细胞

固有层（LP）巨噬细胞是固有免疫系统的一部分，协调对微生物及其产物的初始应答。在所有身体组织中，巨噬细胞在胃肠黏膜中数量最多，位居于 LP 中的数量最高。在这个关键位置，巨噬细胞的功能有：①防范病原体和破坏上皮的有毒物质；②有助于耐受共生细菌和食物抗原；③通过清除凋亡和死亡细胞维持组织稳态。肠道巨噬细胞通过强大的吞噬作用和杀菌能力介导这些固有功能。

固有细胞对微生物的反应在几分钟内启动，并指向 PAMP，即存在于微生物上的保守碳水化合物、脂质和核酸分子。巨噬细胞通过预先确定的模式识别受体（pattern recognition receptor，PRR）识别 PAMP，PRR 包括典型的种系编码的跨膜 TLR 和胞质感受器，包括核苷酸结合寡聚化结构域（nucleotide-binding oligomerization domain，NOD）样受体。PRR 的预定性质促进了对微生物抗原的快速固有反应，但限制了巨噬细胞能反应的配体的多样性。

婴儿期后，肠道巨噬细胞来源于循环中的促炎性单核细胞并由其补充，后者募集到 LP。然而，在肠道 LP 中，巨噬细胞表现出独特的固有受体表型，尽管存在强效的吞噬和杀菌活性，但其促炎症能力非常有限，称为炎症无能。3 个重要特征导致炎症无能。首先，健康黏膜中的肠巨噬细胞不表达 LPS（CD14）、IgA（CD89）、IgG（CD16，32 和 64）、CR3（CD11b/CD18）、CR4（CD11c/CD18）、IL-2（CD25）和 IL-3（CD123）的生长因子受体、整合素白细胞功能相关抗原-1（LFA-1）（CD11a）和 TREM-1。肠巨噬细胞也表达很低水平的趋化因子受体 CCR5 和 CXCR4，这是 R5 和 X4 HIV-1 的共受体。这些受体表达受到抑制的机制尚不清楚，但由于肠道巨噬细胞来源的单核细胞表达这些受体，局部因素可能是通过诱导表观遗传调控导致这种独特的表型，因为新招募的单核细胞驻留在固有层。尽管如此，肠巨噬细胞表达一些受体，这些受体参与识别潜在的有害微生物并与之相互作用，特别是 TLR1 和 TLR3-9，以及 TGF-β R Ⅰ 和 R Ⅱ，它们介导 Smad 信号的募集和激活。肠道巨噬细胞独特的受体表型具有深远的功能意义。例如，CD14 的缺失与肠道巨噬细胞不能识别 LPS 是一致的，这一特征非常适合位于富含免疫刺激 LPS 的微环境中的巨噬细胞。

肠道巨噬细胞炎症无能特征的第二个机制是 NF-κB 信号失调。LP 基质细胞因子，特别是 TGF-β，强效下调单核细胞 TRIF、MyD88 和 TRAF6 蛋白，导致新招募到固有层的单核细胞不能磷酸化 NF-κB p65。肠道巨噬细胞还表达细胞因子信号转导抑制因子（suppressor of cytokine signaling，SOCS1）mRNA 水平的增加，后者促进 MAL（MyD88 接头样蛋白）的降解，以及抑制其 TRIF 信号转导的不育犰狳基序包含蛋白（sterile Armadillo motif-containing protein，SARM）水平增加。MyD88 是 NF-κB 活化通路中除 TLR3 外所有的 TLR 的关键元件，TRIF 介导 TLR3 诱导的 RANTES 和 IFN-γ 产生，以及 TLR4 介导的 MyD88 非依赖性信号。此外，肠道巨噬细胞不能通过丝裂原活化蛋白激酶（mitogen-activated protein kinase，MAPK）通路激活 NF-κB，涉及磷酸化（p）p38、p-ERK 或 p-JNK，依赖于 TRAF6 通路。这些失调导致肠道巨噬细胞明显不能激活 NF-κB，从而释放 NF-κB 通路依赖性促炎细胞因子。

炎症无能的第三个机制成分是活跃的 TGF-β 信号。肠巨噬细胞 TGF-β R Ⅰ 和 R Ⅱ 被局部基质 TGF-β 激活，诱导 Smad 信号级联反应。Smad4 是级联反应的关键组分，与磷酸化异二聚体 Smad2/3 复合物结合，然后转位到细胞核中，启动 IκBα 的基因转录，其将 NF-κB 隔离在细胞质中。与血液单核细胞相反，肠道巨噬细胞不表达通路抑制分子 Smad7，引起 IκBα 组成型表达和 NF-κB 信号转导的阻断，从而抑制 NF-κB 介导的反应。

总之，这些主要由基质 TGF-β 诱导的重叠机制，在人类固有肠道巨噬细胞中引起严重的炎症无能。最近的研究还表明，刺激暴露的肠道巨噬细胞不会极化为经典的和交替激活的（M1 和 M2）巨噬细胞，这些巨噬细胞是小鼠组织巨噬细胞的特征。在感染或上皮破坏的情况下，免疫刺激微生物和微生物产物被肠巨噬细胞迅速吞噬，提供强有力的但非炎症的宿主防御。同样，肠巨噬细胞以非炎症方式清除凋亡细胞和碎片。因此，肠巨噬细胞在促进健康人肠黏膜无或几乎无炎症中起基础作用。

（七）口服耐受性

高度调节的黏膜免疫系统的表现之一是口服耐受[149,150]。口服耐受是对口服抗原的特异性无应答[150]。这也发生在其他黏膜表面，称为黏膜耐受。

免疫系统可调节对通过口服途径大量引入的抗原的反应，特别是能够避免完全消化的抗原。值得注意的是，高达 2% 的膳食蛋白质全部完整地进入肠道脉管系统。对这些抗原无应答状态是通过口服耐受所实现的。人类的肠黏膜免疫系统具有区分有害和无害抗原，甚至有益抗原，并对每种类型抗原产生不同免疫应答的能力，并已在动物模型中进行了广泛的研究[95,151,152]。口服耐受/黏膜耐受的破坏，可能导致食物过敏、腹腔疾病（乳糜泻）和 IBDs，并与系统性免疫介导疾病有关。

口服耐受食物抗原和黏膜耐受微生物群之间的一个重要区别是，前者减弱肠道和系统性免疫应答，而后者仅减弱黏膜免疫应答[150]。影响口服耐受的因素包括宿主的年龄、遗传因素、抗原的性质以及耐受原的形式和剂量。对口服耐受性的解释部分与消化本身有关，在消化过程中，大分子被降解，从而使潜在的免疫原性物质变成无免疫原性或耐受性物质。

新生儿很难实现口服耐受，这可能与新生儿肠道屏障相对通透，以及黏膜免疫系统不成熟有关。在 3 月龄内，可诱导口服耐受，以往对食物抗原的许多抗体反应受到抑制。新生儿有限的饮食可进一步保护婴儿对食物抗原产生强烈的免疫反应。有趣的是，肠道微生物群已被证明会影响口服耐受的发展。妊娠期和婴儿早期持续暴露于微生物分子如 LPS 与儿童特应性反应和哮喘发病率较低相关[153,154]。微生物群对口服耐受的影响可能是通过调节细胞因子反应介导的[155]、对肠屏障功能和恢复紧密连接的积极作用[156]、通过下调 TLR 表达抑制肠道炎症和分泌可能抑制单核细胞产生炎性细胞因子的代谢物生成。

抗原的性质和形式也会影响耐受性的诱导。与碳水化合物和脂质相比，蛋白质抗原的耐受性最强[156]。关于抗原的形式，以可溶性形式的卵清蛋白（ovalbumin，OVA）具有相当高的耐受性，而聚集的 OVA 诱导耐受性的能力明显降低。抗原采样部位也可能影响耐受性，因为通过肠外途径暴露抗原（预先致敏）可降低黏膜耐受性的发展。

认为给予抗原的剂量对产生口服耐受形式也至关重要。在小鼠模型中,高剂量的抗原与T细胞的克隆缺失或无能有关。在这种情况下,将T细胞从耐受动物转移至不耐受动物不会导致耐受转移。另一方面,已发现低剂量抗原可激活调节性/抑制性T细胞[157-159],但抗原剂量对口服耐受的影响仍有待确定。CD4和CD8谱系的Treg细胞均具有口服耐受的作用。$CD4^+$ Treg细胞似乎在派尔集合淋巴结中被激活并分泌TGF-β,TGF-β是T细胞和B细胞反应的强效抑制因子,同时通过诱导B细胞从IgM到IgA的基因切换来促进IgA的产生[160,161]。低剂量抗原给药引起的Treg细胞产生TGF-β和IL-10,有助于解释被称为旁观者抑制的口服耐受的相关现象。口服耐受具有抗原特异性,但效应臂无抗原特异性。当不相关(旁观者)的抗原与耐受抗原系统联合给予时,也会抑制T细胞和B细胞对不相关抗原的应答(因此是旁观者抑制),因为分泌的TGF-β和IL-10可抑制对联合给予抗原的应答。仅产生IL-10(一种强效免疫抑制细胞因子)的Treg1细胞也可能参与旁观者抑制和口服耐受[162-164]。在小鼠中,$CD4^+$ Treg细胞活性的缺失导致IBD,而其扩增可改善鼠结肠炎[165-167]。在IBD患者中,Treg细胞的数量通常大于对照组,并提示有外周-肠道转移[168-170]。这些细胞不能预防IBD是否是由于内在缺陷或微环境效应仍在研究中[171]。

抗原特异性$CD8^+$ T细胞可能在口服耐受性[172,173]以及黏膜免疫应答调节中发挥作用。具体来说,通过正常IEC体外激活人$CD8^+$外周血T细胞,导致具有调节活性的$CD8^+$ $CD28^-$ T细胞扩增[174]。此外,在IBD病患者的LP中,此类细胞的数量显著减少,支持这些上皮诱导的T调节细胞在控制肠道炎症中的作用[175]。

最后,口服耐受性也可能受到作为抗原呈递细胞的细胞作用以及抗原摄取位点的影响。在小鼠中,口服给予的Ⅲ型呼肠孤病毒,被表达Ⅲ型呼肠孤病毒特异性受体的M细胞摄取(见图2.2)[11]。从而诱导了活跃的IgA反应。相反,呼肠孤病毒I感染IEC并可诱导耐受性。因此,特异性抗原是否通过M细胞或IEC进入黏膜,可能决定产生的免疫应答类型(IgA vs耐受性)。有趣的是,脊髓灰质病毒疫苗是为数不多的对人类有效的口服疫苗之一,可与M细胞结合,这可能解释了其刺激肠道产生主动免疫的能力[176]。

(八)趋化因子在体内稳态和炎症中的作用

肠道相关淋巴组织(GALT)中IEC可分泌许多趋化因子,这证明上皮细胞参与调节肠道免疫应答。在分泌的趋化因子中,IEC产生的趋化因子具有吸引炎性细胞,如淋巴细胞、巨噬细胞和树突状细胞的能力,从而有助于正常的黏膜稳态(表2.1)。在感染和炎症过程中,其中大多数趋化因子的产生会增加。

表2.1　趋化因子及其受体、产生趋化因子的细胞和靶细胞

趋化因子	受体	产生趋化因子的细胞	靶细胞	参考文献
CCL5(RANTES)		IEC Mϕ	T细胞 嗜酸粒细胞 白细胞	177
CXCL9(MIG)	CXCR3	结肠IEC 内皮细胞 淋巴细胞	Th1CXCR3$^+$ NK DC	183,184
CXCL10(IP10)	CXCR3	结肠IEC 内皮细胞 淋巴细胞	Th1XCXR3$^+$	183,184
CXCL11(ITAC)	CXCR3	结肠IEC 内皮细胞 淋巴细胞	Th1XCXR3$^+$	183,184
CCL25(TECK)	CCR9	IEC	$CD8^+$E7	188-191
CX3CL1(Fractalkine)	CX3CR1	IEC	CD8>CD4单核细胞 NK细胞	192-194,200
CCL28(MEC)	CCR3 CCR10	结肠IEC	CD4Tm嗜酸性细胞	200
CCL22(MDC)	CCR4	结肠IEC	CD4Th1	195
CCL20(MIP3α)	CCR6	IEC	DC、CD4Tm	196-199
CXCL12	CXCR4 CXCR7	IEC	CD4Th1CD45RO$^+$ 浆细胞	201-205
CXCL8(IL-8)	CXCR1>CXCR2	IEC Mϕ 嗜中性粒细胞	嗜中性粒细胞	206

DC,树突状细胞;IEC,肠上皮细胞;Mϕ,巨噬细胞;NK,自然杀伤细胞。

趋化因子 CCL5[活化调节,正常 T 细胞表达和分泌(regulated on activation,normal T cell expressed and secreted,RANTES)]主要由巨噬细胞分泌,但也可由人类 IEC 产生[177]。RANTES 可能在固有和适应性黏膜免疫中发挥作用[178],并在溃疡性结肠炎患者黏膜中证实 RANTES 表达增加[179-182]。CXC 趋化因子,包括干扰素-γ(MIG,CXCL9)诱导的单核因子、似乎促进 Th1 反应的趋化因子 IFN-γ 诱导蛋白 10(IP-10,CXCL10),以及 IFN-γ 诱导的 T 细胞 α-趋化因子(ITAC,CXCL11)由淋巴细胞、内皮细胞和人结肠 IEC 组成性表达[183,184]。IFN-γ 刺激后,其表达和极化的基底外侧分泌增加。CXC 趋化因子吸引高表达水平 CXCR3 的 Th1 细胞[185],有助于 NK T 细胞趋化和增加细胞溶解反应[186],并激活树突状细胞亚群[187]。

与炎症相关的 CXCR3 受体相反,组织特异性趋化因子受体 CCR9 在小肠 IEL 和 LPL 上呈组成性表达[188-190]。其配体趋化因子胸腺表达的趋化因子(TECK,CCL25)在空肠和回肠上皮中存在差异表达,据报告,从隐窝到绒毛的表达水平逐渐降低[191]。研究显示,在克罗恩病患者发炎的小肠中,IEC 表达的 CCL25 增加,外周血淋巴细胞的 CCR9 表达也增加,而 LPL 的表达减少[189]。

神经趋化因子[Fractalkine(CX3CL1)]是 IEC 表达的一种独特趋化因子,具有结合趋化因子和黏附分子的特性。CX3CL1 吸引表达特异性受体 CX3CR1NK 的细胞,包括 NK 细胞、单核细胞、$CD8^+$ T 淋巴细胞和较小范围的 $CD4^+$ T 淋巴细胞[192]。其在克罗恩病中的表达增加,尤其是在 IEC 的基底外侧[193,194]。

巨噬细胞源性趋化因子(MDC,CCL22)由结肠 IEC 组成性表达和分泌,吸引产生 $CCR4^+$ Th2 细胞因子的淋巴细胞。已有报告,结肠 IEC 细胞系在受刺激后可由极化的基底外侧分泌 MDC/CCL22[195]。对优先分泌抗炎细胞因子的淋巴细胞的特异性募集,支持肠上皮在调节正常黏膜稳态中的重要作用,并增加了越来越多的证据表明,这些细胞具有调节黏膜免疫应答的能力。

趋化因子巨噬细胞炎性蛋白-3α(MIP3,CCL20)的独特之处在于,能够特异性吸引未成熟树突状细胞以及记忆 $CD4^+$ T 淋巴细胞[196-198]。CCL20 也由人小肠 ECs(主要在滤泡相关上皮)和结肠 IEC 表达和产生,可能是淋巴细胞黏附于 α4β7 配体 MAdCAM-1[196] MIP3α 的介质,在 IBD 患者的结肠 IEC 中表达和分泌增加[199]。黏膜记忆 T 细胞,以及 IEC,表达 MIP3α 的同源受体 CCR6。

黏膜防御,包括微生物群本身,提供对肠道病原体的防卫。微生物群与食物和水中的临时细菌和病原体竞争,并阻止其在肠道内定殖。一些肠道病原体诱发宿主炎症,进而杀死肠道中的厌氧菌,从而为耐氧菌病原体打开了一个生态位。某些细菌是病原体,因为它们已经进化出破坏黏膜屏障的机制。在健康黏膜中,固有巨噬细胞以非炎性的方式强效地吞噬和杀死这些微生物,但在疾病条件下,导致炎症无能的机制被破坏,使巨噬细胞保留其单核祖细胞的促炎特征。然而,一旦 IEC 受到侵袭,就会产生大量的趋化因子如 IL-8,这些趋化因子会将血液中的中性粒细胞和单核细胞吸引到感染部位的肠道中。这些吞噬细胞是炎性的,可产生更多的趋化因子和其他细胞因子,并迅速获得临界质量杀死入侵的细菌,从而消除感染。

(胡伟玲 袁农 译,曾翔俊 校)

参考文献

第 3 章　肠道微生物群

Eugene B. Chang，Purna Kashyap 著

章节目录

一、人类肠道微生物群的特征 ………………………… 24
（一）肠道微生物群的空间变异 ………………… 24
（二）肠道微生物群的时间变化和恢复力 ……… 27
二、影响肠道微生物群变异性和恢复力的因素 ……… 27
（一）年龄 ……………………………………… 27
（二）性别 ……………………………………… 27
（三）遗传 ……………………………………… 27
（四）地理与饮食 ……………………………… 27
（五）运动 ……………………………………… 28
（六）药物 ……………………………………… 28
（七）其他生活方式因素 ……………………… 28
（八）微生物-微生物信号 ……………………… 28
三、宿主-肠道微生物群相互作用对宿主生理功能的影响 ……………………………………… 29
（一）肠道微生物群与免疫系统的相互作用 …… 29
（二）肠道微生物群与胃肠道的相互作用 ……… 29
（三）微生物群-肠-脑轴 ……………………… 29
四、肠道微生物群在人类疾病中的作用 ……………… 29
代谢功能 ……………………………………… 29
五、炎性疾病 ……………………………………… 30
（一）炎症性肠病 ……………………………… 30
（二）乳糜泻（Celiac 病） …………………… 30
六、癌症 …………………………………………… 31
结直肠癌 ……………………………………… 31
七、功能性胃肠疾病 ……………………………… 31
八、肠道微生物群在药物反应调节中的作用 ………… 31
九、肠道微生物群的治疗调节 ……………………… 31
十、肠道微生物群的非细菌成员 …………………… 32
十一、未来发展方向 ……………………………… 32

一、人类肠道微生物群的特征

肠道微生物群是一个多样化的生态系统，包括微生物（细菌、古细菌、真菌和病毒，包括噬菌体）、微生物基因组（即基因）和周围的环境条件。特定生态位中单独的微生物群被称为微生物种群（框 3.1），通常与微生物组（包括微生物的基因组）的概念互换使用。每一种群都有助于肠道生态系统的稳定，并驱动与宿主产生特定的相互作用。尽管我们主要关注的是细菌，但我们在理解这些成分中的每一种的作用方面都取得了进展。随着新一代测序和先进的实验工具的出现，我们在微生物群特征及其对宿主影响的能力方面，取得了长足的进步（框 3.2）。肠道微生物群的组成在个体之间差异显著，因此就特定微生物成员方面而言，很难鉴定出一种通用的“健康”肠道微生物群并不奇怪。这种差异主要反映在 4 个优势门类相对丰度的差异：拟杆菌门、厚壁菌门、变形菌门和放线杆菌门[4,5]。与组成相比，微生物功能特性的一个子集似乎在个体间是保守的，包括中心代谢途径和营养代谢，例如碳水化合物和蛋白质。然而，微生物功能仍存在显著的个体间差异，如药物代谢、致病岛和营养转运蛋白。塑造肠道微生物群的因素有几个（图 3.1），但没有一个关键因素。饮食似乎具有最突的影响，但肠道微生物群的成员和功能是由不同因素之间复杂的相互作用导致的。

（一）肠道微生物群的空间变异

微生物群的组成沿胃肠道变化，从口腔到肛门沿纵轴和径向轴有所不同[6]。有几个因素决定了细菌在肠道不同生态位中的定位，包括氧化还原电位、化学和营养梯度、宿主免疫活性和黏液层（图 3.2）[7]。结肠中的细菌密度最高，这可能是由于营养利用率增加且转运较慢所致（见图 3.1）。相比之下，小肠部位恶劣的化学环境和相对快速的转运速度，导致微

框 3.1　描述微生物群内单个生物之间及微生物群与宿主之间关系的术语表

外来生物：在非原产地发现的微生物。

本土生物：现生存于其原来生长地的微生物。

共栖：严格地说，术语共栖（源自 cum mensa，“共享一张桌子”）描述了两种微生物之间的关系，其一种微生物获益，另一种不受影响。在大多数情况下，共栖一词用于描述定植在特定生态位且不造成危害的原位微生物，但可能包括对彼此或宿主有益的微生物。

微生物群：微生物及微生物基因组（即基因）和周围环境条件[181]。

微生物种群：在特定生态位的微生物群（细菌、古生菌、低等和高等真核生物、病毒）[180]。

致病共生菌：通常指一种潜在的生物病原体，在微生物群受到干扰等特定的情况下具有致病性。例如艰难梭菌，它可以存在于健康人的肠道，但通常会在抗生素治疗后发生问题。

病原体：任何病理（致病）的有机体。

制药生物：提取自人类微生物群，经证实具备生物学效应的生物实体，包括活的或死的微生物、细胞壁成分、纯化的蛋白质或脂质、个别代谢物（如神经递质）或活性酶。

益生元：一种不易消化的化合物，通过其在肠道内的微生物代谢，发挥调节微生物群落的功能，从而对宿主产生有益的生理作用[182]。

共生体：任何参与共生（互利）关系的有机体。

合生元：一种不易消化的化合物，包含益生元和益生菌，并结合适当的营养素，以刺激合生元中的特定有益微生物。

框 3.2　评估微生物群组成和微生物功能的技术

微生物群组成

1. 微生物培养

对微生物群组成的研究早期在技术上受到基于培养技术的限制，即需要依赖于不同条件下的专用培养基来识别特定的微生物。这限制了我们的识别能力，使我们仅能鉴定一小部分已确定培养条件的微生物，这些微生物占肠道微生物菌群的 5%~15%[183,184]。因此，由于无法培养出常驻细菌，多样性有限的细菌常被认为是无菌的。如今，由于基于非培养依赖性序列的认证技术，人体内几乎所有的部位均被描述为具有特征性的常驻微生物[185-187]。基于测序的数据也提高了我们培养以前被认为无法培养的细菌的能力。我们现在能够利用各种培养条件，培养出相当大比例的个体粪便微生物群[188,189]，这使得我们能够利用无菌小鼠等模型，确定微生物组成变化的相关性以及单个或群体细菌对宿主表型的相互作用和影响。

2. 显微镜检查

早期研究方法包括肠道组织的扫描和透射电子显微镜检查，根据单个细菌的形态学和高分辨率图像提供多样性估计，但不能进行细菌鉴定[190,191]。如革兰氏等普通染色提供了形态学以外的分辨率，但还不足以进行鉴定。荧光显微镜提供了通过荧光原位杂交技术对特定微生物 16S rRNA 细菌的鉴定[192]。测序数据可用性的增加，开发出更精准的荧光原位杂交探针，具有不需要培养的优点。固定方法与保存黏液兼容，同时可使用多个探针可检测样品中的多种细菌[193,194]。此外，显微镜是确定肠道内微生物的生物地理学及黏膜表面细菌与宿主的相互作用的主要工具。荧光成像与计算工具的进步，显著提高了我们在体内和体外可视化微生物的能力。传统的荧光探针需要氧气限制其在体内的应用，但采用"点击"化学新工具，用非氧荧光标记细菌，进行体内跟踪[195]。

3. 第二代测序

早期培养独立成分分析工具是采用变性梯度凝胶电泳分离大小不同的条带，其中 7 个代表不同的分类群。在第二代测序技术（如 Illumina、454、Ion Torrent、SOLiD 等）中，基于标记（16S rRNA）和团体内所有基因的鸟枪法测序已取代变性梯度凝胶电泳，特别是考虑到测序成本的下降。基于标记的方法利用了在所有微生物中发现的编码 16S rRNA 亚基的基因中 DNA 序列的保守性，插入的可变区通过聚合酶链反应靶向扩增，可以同时识别样本中的不同分类群。然而，考虑到扩增子的长度较小，基于标记的测序在识别种属水平以外分类群的能力上受到限制。第三代测序技术，如单分子实时测序技术（single-molecule real-time）已经出现，考虑到其产生 10 千碱基的读长的潜力（来自单个 DNA 片段的连续序列），这将可能取代目前的方法[183]。

微生物功能

组成数据洞察宿主-微生物间相互作用的能力有限。因此，重要的是详细说明存在哪些微生物来确定其作用、功能和其代谢产物对肠道微生物群落和宿主的影响。尽管人类种群的组成存在异质性，考虑到核心微生物功能似乎是保守的，这一点尤其重要。

1. 宏基因组学

宏基因组学通常被称为全基因组测序或鸟枪法测序，宏基因组学能使微生物群落中的所有基因表现出来，并提供了群落的广泛功能的潜力，但无法在给定的一组条件下提供特定的功能。

2. 转录组学

转录组学方法如 RNAseq（即转录组测序技术）提供了给定条件下微生物群落基因表达谱的快照。该数据可用于进一步推断使用分析工具，如 HUMAnN2 的代谢途径的差异表达[196]。

3. 蛋白质组学与代谢组学

蛋白质组学可提供微生物群落蛋白质的全面表征，而代谢组学提供了微生物群落小分子及其代谢产物的全面表征。这两种方法都可以描述复杂群落的整体代谢状态，这是由于不同群落或同一群在不同条件下的基因表达差异所致。对于蛋白质组学，可以使用液相色谱法（liquid chromatography，LC）直接基于疏水性、电荷、或两者直接分离蛋白质，也可在色谱分离之前通过蛋白酶（如胰蛋白酶）消化为肽，然后通过质谱法（mass spectrometry，MS）对亲本肽进行分离，并通过串联质谱法（MS-MS）获得片段化信息。目前最大的挑战是下游的生物信息学处理，因为需要根据宏基因组信息构建预测蛋白质数据库，以将获得的肽序列信息分配给蛋白质。此外，由于小分子的巨大多样性，以及性质和浓度的差异，需要使用多种方法来涵盖大量的代谢产物，这些方法包括使用 LC、气相色谱法、高压液相色谱法、超高压液相色谱法、耦联质谱法分析和质子磁共振光谱学（proton nuclear magnetic resonance spectroscopy，^{1}H-NMR）等来分离生物群落相关的大量代谢物[197]。代谢组学检测以靶向或非靶向的方式进行，并使用统计学方法进行下游处理以识别特征。仍然存在的挑战是准确识别 MS 光谱中的代谢物，尽管 HMDB、METLIN 和 ChemSpider 等多个光谱数据库已取得了重大进展，所有这些数据库都在不断更新，但准确鉴定 MS 光谱中的代谢物仍是目前存在的挑战之一。

4. 微生物的体外和体内模型

类器官

类器官源于组织干细胞或多能干细胞，可在培养基中维持，在培养基中它们保持其极性并再现细胞的组成和结构，因此，代表研究特定疾病背景下宿主-微生物相互作用的理想体外模型系统。研究宿主-微生物动力学的方法包括共培养；将类器官来源的单层组织细胞暴露于微生物/微生物制品中，以及显微注射。这些方法对于研究腔内相互作用及模拟厌氧微生物建模尤为相关[198]。

无菌小鼠

尽管人类是研究微生物的理想生物系统，但仍需要动物模型来帮助解构宿主-微生物组间复杂的相互作用，并阐明其相互作用的潜在机制。传统的小鼠模型提供了概念性知识，但它们的可转移性和研究定植状态的能力有限。采用无菌和悉生生物（以前为无菌小鼠，但现已被确定的相关微生物群所定植）动物模型允许对单个微生物以及来自小鼠或其他物种（人类；人源化小鼠）的复杂群落进行建模，以研究微生物-微生物之间以及微生物-宿主之间的相互作用。微生物群落转移后重述疾病状态的表型特征，有助于鉴定微生物驱动的表型。它们也是在受控环境中研究宿主、环境和饮食因素对微生物组影响的理想选择。在可转移性方面，人源化小鼠忠实地再现了人类微生物群落的结构和功能[199]，代表了一种可转移的临床前模型。

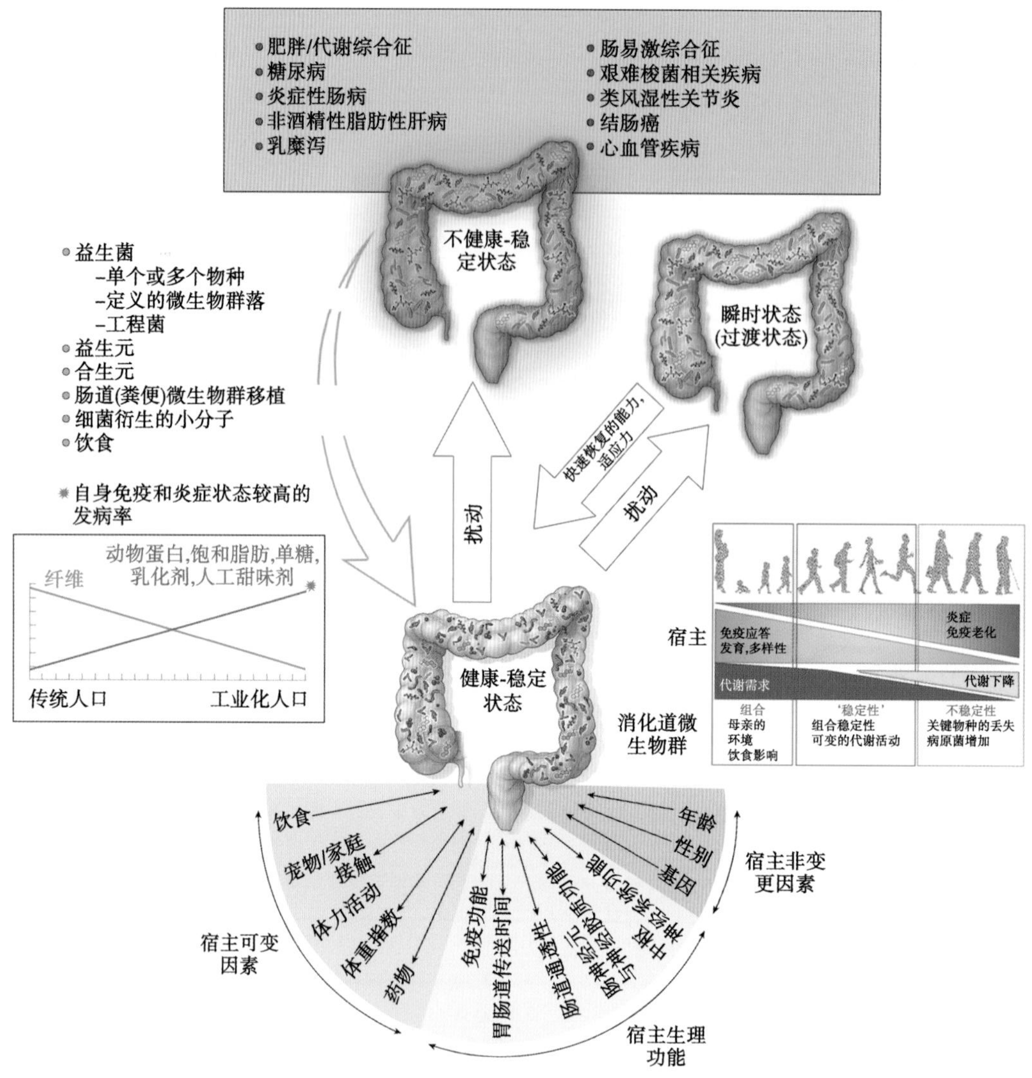

图 3.1　肠道微生物群的特征。该图概述了影响肠道微生物群的可改变和不可改变的宿主因素、肠道微生物群与宿主生理之间的相互作用、微生物群的恢复力以及微生物群有害转变的后果和控制微生物群的潜在机制

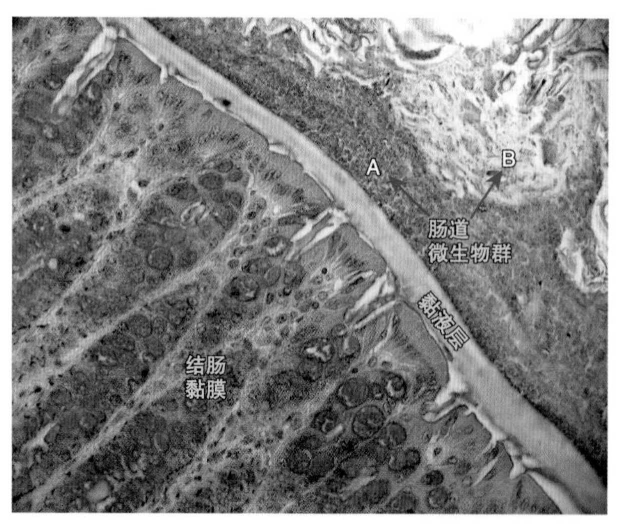

图 3.2　显微照片(20×)显示 C57BL/6J 小鼠近端结肠标本中分布在黏膜上的细菌。组织被固定在能保留黏液的卡诺固定液中(60% 乙醇,30% 氯仿,10% 冰醋酸),并用显示黏液的阿尔新蓝染色,突出黏液。结肠黏液正上方的一层是与黏膜相关的微生物群——一个相对稳定的群落,可能形成生物膜基质,即使在结肠灌洗后也能保持群落稳定性。微生物群有微弱的分层,表明该群落的组织不是随机的。黏膜相关微生物区上方的过渡区是肠道微生物和食物颗粒的混合物。(图片由以色列 Lev Lichtenstein 博士提供)

生物群的丰度和多样性降低。此外,结肠和小肠表面上皮与细菌的接触方式不同。结肠黏液层有两层:内层完全没有细菌,而较疏松的外层由细菌填充[8]。相反,小肠只有一层不完整的黏液层,其内的抗微生物因子(如 REGIIIγ)在将微生物与上皮分离出来方面似乎比黏液更重要[9,10]。氧气从黏膜到管腔内的径向梯度,导致了黏膜相关微生物和管腔内相关微生物在成员分类、遗传学和功能上的差异[11]。黏膜中的变形菌门和放线菌门中耐氧生物的比例增加,突出了氧有效性的影响。此外,主要使用氨基酸的细菌群与黏液层有关[12],黏液层是驱动肠道营养差异的来源。

肠道微生物群特征的研究大多数采用粪便样本,将粪便微生物作为结肠中存在的微生物的替代物。尽管这种方法较为简易,但被更广泛的科学界所接受,但其仅从微生物方面洞察宿主-微生物的相互作用。尚需要一种更有区域针对性的抽样方法,来了解微生物在调节宿主代谢、消化和吸收、局部免疫系统,以及引起或促成炎症性肠病、肠易激综合征、食物过敏、乳糜泻和结肠癌等疾病方面的作用[11]。

(二) 肠道微生物群的时间变化和恢复力

健康稳定状态的特征是由生命早期的组成和功能变化发展而来的多样化的肠道菌群。然而,由于存在显著的人际差异,以至于很难给出“健康”状态的确切定义。也许这一定义的最佳近似值是肠道菌群通过向宿主提供必要的关键功能来促进健康[13]。基于宏基因组测序结果,将肠道健康菌群分为 3 组(拟杆菌、普雷沃特菌或瘤胃球菌),但当扩展到更大的“健康”人群时,基于健康群落分为 3 组的宏基因组测序的肠型概念并不成立,很明显,人际变异性的范围是稳定构型的连续谱[13]。随着时间的推移,肠道微生物生态系统大体是稳定的,即肠道菌群从个体纵向获得的样本中的组成比从不同个体获得的样本中的组成更相似。因此,尽管个体微生物的相对丰度可以发生改变,但整体群落功能和成员群落仍保持完整。同样,一个能导致慢性病或健康状况不佳的“不利”的微生物群落也可以是稳定的。恢复力是微生物群落状态的一个关键特性,它被定义为微生物群落在转变为不同的稳态之前能够承受的压力或扰动量(见图 3.1)。高度的恢复力是维持健康状态的理想选择,但不是在不健康的情况下。微生物之间的竞争以及进一步维持单个微生物水平的正反馈和负反馈有助于稳定性[13]。某些扰动,如短疗程的抗生素,可会导致微生物群落结构的短暂破坏(见图 3.1),通常会恢复到原来的状态[14]。持续的扰动,如长期的饮食改变/抗生素给药(见图 3.1),或在脆弱阶段(如幼儿期或围生期)的持续扰动[15,16],可导致微生物群落无序组装,并转变为抵抗变化的促疾病状态。

二、影响肠道微生物群变异性和恢复力的因素

(一) 年龄

肠道微生物组成的最显著和最有影响的变化发生在生命的最初几年。尽管有一些证据表明微生物是在子宫内获得的,但大多数微生物的获得始于婴儿出生时,那时婴儿的肠道中植入了来自母亲阴道的微生物[17]。相反,剖宫产婴儿的肠道被定植了其母亲皮肤的细菌[17]。喂养方式也与微生物群组成的差异有关,与母乳喂养婴儿相比,配方奶喂养导致双歧杆菌数量降低[18]。婴儿继续从环境和母亲身体的不同部位获得微生物,有趣的是,从母亲身体上获得的微生物更适合婴儿肠道,存活时间更持久[19]。

肠道微生物群的早期发育对于培育黏膜免疫[20,21]和全身免疫反应至关重要[22-24]。在免疫系统成熟阶段,即在婴儿期使用抗生素,干扰宿主-微生物的相互作用,与晚年患哮喘、1 型糖尿病和肥胖等疾病的风险较高有关[17]。

肠道微生物群的组成和功能在一生中都在不断变化。到 3 岁时,个体的微生物群已与成年人基本相似[25,26],尽管青春期前肠道微生物群充实了支持发育的维生素合成等功能[27]。一般而言,微生物成员和功能多样性随年龄的增长而增加[4]。而生活在长期护理设施中的老年人,往往携带与社区居民不同且多样性较低的肠道微生物群[28]。

(二) 性别

女性微生物群的多样性和功能丰富程度高于男性[4],而拟杆菌和普雷沃特菌的丰度降低[29]。尽管这些差异的意义尚不清楚,但动物研究提供了一些线索。共生菌的定植可预防易患 1 型糖尿病的雄性而非雌性小鼠发生糖尿病[30,31]。这种保护作用依赖于雄激素受体的活性,可通过将肠道微生物从成年雄性移植到未成熟的雌性小鼠,即可将该保护作用转移到雌性小鼠身上。这说明了肠道微生物群中性别依赖性差异的一个潜在影响,其中的差异可影响自身免疫的激素依赖性调节。

(三) 遗传

单卵双胞胎的肠道微生物群组成比双卵双胞胎的更为相似,这表明宿主基因在选择肠道某些微生物分类群中的作用[32]。其中一些关联已经被揭示,如 FUT2 多态性、免疫相关的基因变异[33]以及改变胆汁酸水平的基因[34]。尽管并非所有分类群都受到宿主遗传的影响,而遗传度似乎是驱动大约 10% 微生物分类群的一个因素[34]。事实上,拟杆菌门类中的成员似乎更易受到环境因素的影响。有趣的是,克里斯滕森菌科家族(*Christensenellaceae*)中的一个高度可遗传的分类群,与其他可遗传的分类群共同出现,在瘦的个体中富有,与消瘦相关,这表明某些宿主性状的遗传力可能是关键细菌代际转移的结果[34]。

(四) 地理与饮食

肠道微生物群组成随地理位置的不同而具有显著差异,这体现了文化、饮食和环境因素对肠道微生物群的综合影响。例如,生活在美国和欧洲的个体的微生物群组成与生活在非西方、非城市环境中的个体的微生物群组成不同——并且多样性较低,如马拉维农村、坦桑尼亚、布基纳法索或亚马逊[26,35-37]。特别是非城市环境中的居民普雷沃特菌属的比例更大,拟杆菌的比例更低[38]。与西方饮食文化相关的肠道微生物群表达了更多的能够降解氨基酸和单糖的酶,这些酶反

映了西方饮食中的高蛋白和简单碳水化合物的特点，而与传统饮食文化相关的肠道微生物群表达了更多的能够降解淀粉的酶，因为这些饮食包括高淀粉主食，如玉米和木薯[26]。饮食在形成相同人群中肠道微生物群组成和功能方面起着重要作用[39]，这可能在一定程度上导致地理差异，而对不同地理区域之间的差异，还应考虑其他因素的作用。美国纯素食者和其他农业文化个体的肠道菌群存在明显差异，这表明除了饮食之外，很可能还存在影响微生物群组成和功能的地理特异性因素[40]。

饮食的影响不仅局限于微生物群组成，因为即使在没有组成成分变化的情况下，也可以观察到功能差异的存在[40]，这强调了在评价饮食影响时，多组学分析评估微生物群组成和功能的重要性。部分肠道微生物群是由长期饮食习惯形成的，但短期的饮食习惯变化也会引起肠道微生物群的快速但可逆的变化[41]。这可能有助于解释在与肠道微生物群改变相关的胃肠道疾病中观察到的症状间歇性恶化。在膳食成分中，可供微生物利用的纤维中的碳水化合物（microbiota-accessible carbohydrate，MAC）是肠道微生物营养物质的关键来源之一。在发酵的 MAC 中，微生物代谢产生的短链脂肪酸（short-chain fatty acid，SCFA），SCFA 有助于减轻炎症，可作为上皮细胞的能量来源，并改善胃肠道转运功能[42]。西方饮食中 MAC 含量较低，与发生炎症和代谢相关疾病的风险有关[42]。低 MAC 饮食的长期影响很难在人类中进行评估，因为其需要对多代基因验证进行研究。在小鼠模型中的实验表明，低 MAC 饮食诱导的肠道菌群的有害变化在高 MAC 饮食的早期大部分是可逆的[43]，尽管在多代动物中给小鼠喂食低 MAC 饮食会导致微生物多样性的进行性丧失，微生物分类群的消失是饮食不能挽救的，需要移植缺失的细菌[43]。低膳食纤维导致肠道微生物对宿主上皮和黏液的依赖性增加，导致上皮屏障破坏和炎症易感性增加。在高蛋白饮食中也观察到类似的效应，其导致微生物密度增加以及微生物群引起结肠炎的可能性增加[44]。除膳食中的大量营养素外，乳化剂等添加剂和人工甜味剂等替代品，也会对肠道微生物群产生有害影响，有增加代谢和炎症性疾病的倾向[45]。

膳食成分作为微生物代谢途径的底物，因此可影响特定微生物代谢产物的生成，从而影响宿主生理。例如与炎症有关的色氨酸衍生物吲哚乙酸和吲哚丙酸；来自膳食碳水化合物的短链脂肪酸，可以影响肠道 5-羟色胺能途径，从而改变胃肠道运动；以及膳食脂肪相关的游离脂肪酸和脂多糖，它们与肠道神经退行性病变、胃肠道动力改变和导致肥胖的全身效应有关。除了直接转化饮食成分外，细菌尿素酶还可以将宿主来源的尿素转化为氨，导致肝脏疾病患者发生高氨血症相关脑病[46]，还可引起与克罗恩病相关的微生物群组成的改变[47]。

（五）运动

迄今为止，关于运动对人体肠道微生物群的直接影响的研究很少，因为很难将运动的影响从饮食影响中隔离开来。例如，研究发现与体型、年龄和性别相匹配的非运动员对照组相比，运动员的肠道微生物群更为多样化，炎症标志物水平更低[48]。然而，与对照组相比，运动员的饮食含有更多的蛋白质、水果和蔬菜，这使结果的解释变得复杂。在动物模型中可分析运动的影响，发现与运动相关的肠道微生物群组成的变化，可以降低对炎症的易感性[49]和体重增加[50]。与运动相关的肠道微生物群变化的幅度可能是类似的，但在组成上与饮食变化不同[51]；这就提出了一种可能性，即尽管运动通常用于对抗肥胖，但它不可能减轻进食西方高脂肪饮食带来的所有不良影响。

（六）药物

抗生素可显著降低微生物多样性[52]，并且在生命早期似乎通过干扰肠道微生物群的成熟产生更深远的影响，甚至发现生命早期阶段使用亚治疗水平的抗生素可增加生命后期肥胖的发生[53]。同样，在猪模型中，早期抗生素应用改变了肠道微生物群，改变了葡萄糖调节，最终导致 SCFA 信号和胰腺发育的持久变化[54]。接受过多疗程抗生素治疗的幼儿肠道微生物群组成的多样性低于未接受治疗的儿童[55]，早期抗生素使用与微生物群的成熟延迟、菌群组成和功能的持久改变有关[56]。此外，围生期使用抗生素可导致肠道微生物群的持续变化，并增加后代对炎症的易感性[15,16]，这些观察结果也支持早期使用抗生素与克罗恩病风险增加的相关性[57]。

多种其他类型的药物，包括质子泵抑制剂（proton-pump inhibitor，PPI）、泻药、二甲双胍、他汀类药物、激素、苯二氮䓬类药物、抗抑郁药、非甾体抗炎药和抗组胺药等，都与肠道微生物群组成的变化有关[4,58,59]。常用于治疗 2 型糖尿病和非酒精性脂肪性肝病的二甲双胍与肠道微生物群的显著变化有关，这些变化部分是二甲双胍相关的葡萄糖代谢改善的原因[60]。质子泵抑制剂是世界上使用最广泛的 10 种药物之一[61]，与细菌丰度水平降低、口腔微生物丰度增加以及肠道中存在的潜在病原体相关[61]。

（七）其他生活方式因素

吸烟、饮酒等习惯以及心理应激[62]都与肠道微生物群的变化有关，尽管现在得出这些变化会导致应激或酒精有害作用的结论还为时过早。吸烟对微生物群多样性的不利影响，可以从戒烟后观察到的多样性增加中直接推断出来[4,63]。家庭接触者也会对微生物群组成产生影响。同一个家庭中的成员可共享皮肤微生物菌群，有趣的是，家庭宠物显著增加了家庭接触者之间的皮肤微生物群的共享[64]。

重要的是要认识到，上述任何一个单独的因素都不是孤立存在的。事实上，微生物结构上的选择压力可能是由于它们中许多因素之间的相互关系驱动的，在具有不同遗传背景或 *FUT2* 基因发生单一突变的小鼠中，进行的两项研究证实了这一点，其中通过饮食克服了对肠道微生物群的遗传影响[33,65]。

（八）微生物-微生物信号

有几种机制可以决定微生物的自我选择，并使用群体感应分子，如自动诱导剂（高丝氨酸内酯）、细菌素和孢子形成刺激因子，促进群落动态变化和稳定性[66,67]。这些群体感应分子，尤其是细菌素，可以为防止感染提供保护[68-70]。

三、宿主-肠道微生物群相互作用对宿主生理功能的影响

人类与其肠道微生物之间的相互作用是双向的：肠道微生物群与免疫系统、胃肠道甚至神经系统之间都会发生相互信号传递。因此，仅从因果关系方面考虑是不明智的，因为与疾病状态相关的肠道微生物群的变化可能会进一步使疾病状态持续存在。目前微生物介质影响宿主生理的机制是一个活跃的研究领域。肠道微生物群对色氨酸代谢产生的几种生物活性分子，如吲哚乙酸和吲哚丙酸，可作为芳基碳氢化合物受体（aryl hydrocarbon receptor，AhR）和色胺的配体（色胺是5-羟色胺受体4的配体）。已发现微生物群衍生的AhR配体无论是在外周还是在中枢神经系统均对炎症有保护作用，这表明它们在炎症性肠病、多发性硬化症和神经精神疾病中的作用[71]。肠道微生物还产生与人类N-酰基酰胺类似的N-酰基酰胺，后者与G蛋白偶联受体（G protein-coupled receptor，GPCR）相互作用以调节胃肠道生理功能[72]。与人类N-酰基酰胺相互作用的GPCR与糖尿病、肥胖、癌症和炎症性肠病等疾病有关。目前尚不清楚这类分子模式是否常见，但该领域正在迅速发展。在这里，我们简要地论述了已知的肠道微生物群和宿主各个区室之间存在的双向相互作用。

（一）肠道微生物群与免疫系统的相互作用

肠道微生物群决定了免疫系统的成熟，而反过来免疫系统又可以调节微生物群的组成及其促炎症的潜能。上皮细胞和树突状细胞是与肠道微生物群接触的第一道防线。宿主细胞利用模式识别受体，如Toll样受体（Toll-like receptor，TLR）、NOD样受体和C型凝集素，识别两种共生微生物和病原体表面的微生物相关分子模式。肠道微生物通过免疫耐受在肠道中生存。例如，脆弱拟杆菌产生“共生因子”（多糖A），通过TLR直接在调节性T细胞上发出信号，以促进特定生态位的黏膜免疫耐受[73]。微生物还产生大量的其他免疫调节分子，包括作用于TLR9受体的CpG（胞嘧啶磷酸二酯酶鸟嘌呤）DNA；作用于特定的传感器（P2X和P2Y）促进肠Th17细胞生成ATP[74,75]；以及作用于GPCR下调炎症反应的SCFA[76]。

反过来宿主免疫系统有助于控制和塑造肠道微生物群的组成。上皮细胞产生抗菌蛋白，如α-防御素，限制细菌与上皮细胞之间的接触[10]。宿主-微生物信号转导的紊乱与微生物群中一些组分的异常扩增有关，可能对炎症反应和疾病风险产生不利影响[77]。信号系统不同程度的缺陷，包括参与先天性免疫的特异性TLR和转录因子，可导致“大肠菌源性”微生物群的出现[78,79]。上皮细胞通过动员NLRP6（含6个吡喃结构域的NOD样受体家族）炎症小体和最终释放IL-18的分子级联反应，IL-18模拟γ-干扰素和杀菌免疫反应，对病原体侵袭作出反应[80,81]。

（二）肠道微生物群与胃肠道的相互作用

胃肠道促进营养物质消化和吸收的关键功能包括胃肠动力、分泌和感觉。胃肠道传输时间在全世界人群之间存在差异[82]。然而，传输时间的变化可能与不同的疾病状态有关，包括感染、炎症性疾病和功能性疾病，如肠易激综合征（IBS）伴有便秘或腹泻[83]。胃肠道传输是肠道微生物群和胃肠道之间双向相互作用的一个示例。将来自健康人的复杂粪便微生物群落移植到无菌（germ-free，GF）小鼠体内，可刺激神经递质5-羟色胺的产生，显著缩短胃肠道传输时间，这表明肠道微生物在调节胃肠道传输中的作用。或者在人源化小鼠（人类细菌定植的ex-GF小鼠）中使用聚乙二醇或洛哌丁胺等药物，增加或减少胃肠道传输时间可显著改变肠道微生物群落[83]，以及类似的肠道微生物群组成和功能的改变，这些在腹泻和便秘患者中已有报道[84,85]。影响胃肠道传输时间的一些微生物介质示例包括：可影响肠神经元存活的脂多糖和刺激肠道合成5-羟色胺的SCFA，而反过来SCFA在胃肠道动力、分泌和感觉方面发挥重要作用并不奇怪[86]。对胃肠道传输的影响强度在很大程度上取决于喂食人源化小鼠的饲料[83]，因为饲料会影响下游介质，如SCFA。除传输外，肠道微生物群还可影响胃肠道感觉，表现为将肠微生物群从IBS患者转移到GF大鼠后，GF大鼠内脏可发生超敏反应得到证实。除了在生命早期破坏肠道微生物群外[87]，还论述了内脏超敏与大肠埃希菌扩增之间也存在相关性。肠道微生物群在维持肠上皮屏障以及液体和电解质转运方面起着重要作用。肠道微生物群的特定成员可改变上皮内紧密连接蛋白的表达，像丁酸盐等这样的微生物代谢产物在维持上皮屏障方面起着重要作用。胆汁酸的微生物解离和代谢可改变胆汁酸池，如鹅去氧胆酸和脱氧胆酸，其在结肠中起着促分泌素作用。

（三）微生物群-肠-脑轴

肠道微生物的影响远远超出了胃肠道。信息可以以“自上而下”的方式传播，因为我们的经验——通过大脑过滤——有助于塑造我们的肠道微生物群。例如，将小鼠暴露在各种形式的压力下会改变其微生物群的组成[88,89]。相反，肠道微生物群也可以通过多种途径以“自下而上”的方式影响神经系统。首先，它们可以改变肠道神经系统的功能[90]，而肠道神经系统又通过迷走神经与中枢神经系统相连，肠道微生物群通过激活迷走神经通路激活大脑的应激回路[89]。其次，微生物的代谢产物可以损害中枢神经系统中不受血脑屏障保护的区域，如下丘脑-垂体-肾上腺轴[91]。动物模型表明，某些肠道微生物可以在生命早期帮助编程下丘脑-垂体-肾上腺轴，从而影响整个生命过程中的应激反应[89]。最后，微生物群衍生的小分子如SCFA可以通过血脑屏障扩散[91]。

肠道微生物群对神经系统的发育有影响，影响从血脑屏障形成到髓鞘形成再到神经发生的一切[92]。研究表明肠道微生物群会影响小鼠的行为[92,93]。这些发现激发了人们对肠道微生物群与人类心理健康之间关系的兴趣，包括与自闭症谱系障碍、焦虑症、抑郁症、疼痛敏感性、学习和记忆的联系[93,94]。

四、肠道微生物群在人类疾病中的作用

代谢功能

1. 肥胖（见第7章）

大量证据表明肠道微生物群与肥胖之间存在联系。有大量的观测数据显示，肥胖患者的微生物群组成在多个分类水

平上发生了变化,肠道微生物多样性降低。支持微生物群与肥胖之间联系的实验数据包括:GF 小鼠缺乏饮食诱导的肥胖,和 GF 小鼠与来自肥胖人类双胞胎的肠道微生物群定植相比来自瘦双胞胎的定植有更大的体重增加[95]。已提出支持肠道微生物群在肥胖症和糖尿病中作用的几种假定机制:例如通过微生物糖苷水解酶增加能量的获取、通过活化蛋白激酶减少介导的肌肉脂肪酸氧化减少、肝脏脂肪生成增加、饱食感激素改变,并诱导慢性低度炎症。小肠微生物群在脂质消化和吸收中起着重要作用,并可能导致肥胖[96]。生物过程中的昼夜波动(昼夜节律)是生物代谢过程中的关键调节因子,与肠道微生物群呈现双向沟通作用。肠道微生物群表现出组成和功能(如,丁酸盐的生成)的昼夜波动,并向分子时钟发出信号,导致基因表达的变化,这种变化可在肝脏和大脑等远处器官中见到。反过来,昼夜节律又可以改变肠道微生物群组成。生物钟对饮食的变化作出反应,很可能是饮食诱导肥胖中微生物群相关效应的重要介质[97-100]。

2. 2 型糖尿病

与肥胖相似,有观察性和实验数据支持肠道微生物群在 2 型糖尿病中的作用。在一项初步人体研究中,来自瘦供体的肠道微生物群移植(粪菌移植)[IMT(FMT)]改善了肥胖受体的胰岛素敏感性、增加了微生物多样性和丁酸盐产生菌的数量[101,102]。肠道微生物群也是血糖对不同膳食营养素反应的重要决定因素[103],这进一步支持其作为 2 型糖尿病的决定因素和治疗靶点的作用。

3. 心血管疾病

除了对肥胖和代谢综合征的影响外,膳食成分的微生物代谢也会影响心血管疾病。肠道微生物群的不同成员(氢化厌氧球菌、天冬酰胺梭菌、哈氏梭菌、产孢梭菌、大肠埃希菌、彭氏变形杆菌、雷氏普罗维登斯菌和迟缓爱德华菌)将胆碱、磷脂酰胆碱和左旋肉碱(在红肉中发现的)等代谢底物转化为三甲胺(TMA),随后通过宿主黄素单加氧酶 3(FMO3)转化为三甲胺氧化物(TMAO),被发现是小鼠动脉粥样硬化斑块形成的主要驱动因素[104]。发现血浆中左旋肉碱水平与同时增高的 TMAO 水平可预测人类受试者心血管疾病增加的风险[104],验证了动物模型的结果[105]。小分子 3,3-二甲基-1-丁醇通过抑制广泛的 TMA 裂解酶(包括来源于人粪便的裂解酶)可转化为 TMA 的多种底物,降低 TMAO 水平,可预防易感小鼠中胆碱饮食诱导的动脉粥样硬化[106]。这为通过操纵宿主-微生物共代谢来治疗微生物群相关疾病提供了一个重要的范例。

4. 非酒精性脂肪性肝病(见第 87 章)

非酒精性脂肪性肝病(NAFLD)是肝脏脂肪代谢综合征的一种表现,与其他代谢紊乱疾病相似,与微生物群组成和代谢功能的变化相关。动物研究表明,NAFLD 可通过操纵肠道微生物群来诱导[107]。尽管 NAFLD 肝功能异常的具体机制仍不清楚,但除了上述肥胖和 2 型糖尿病的作用外,还提出了脂多糖和肠道细菌产生乙醇的作用。

五、炎性疾病

(一) 炎症性肠病(见第 115 和第 116 章)

肠道微生物群在炎症性肠病(IBD)中的作用已被广泛研究。遗传学研究将 IBD 与作为细菌感受器的基因中的宿主多态性联系起来,如核苷酸结合寡聚化结构域所含蛋白 2(domaincontaining protein 2,NOD2)和 TLR4[53],提示肠道微生物群的病因学作用。抗生素治疗后 IBD 患者亚群的改善进一步支持了这种关系[108]。易感 GF 动物无炎症表明,肠道微生物群是 IBD 发病机制的重要组成部分。鉴于 IBD 是一种多因素疾病,并已知如遗传、早期生活暴露和饮食等多种因素也会影响肠道微生物群的组成,因此,IBD 患者肠道微生物群的变化具有显著的异质性,这是可以预期的。α 多样性的减少被认为是 IBD 患者一致的趋势,但在 IBD 患者中也描述了肠杆菌科细菌(包括大肠埃希菌和梭杆菌)丰度的相对增加。黏膜相关微生物群的特征一直是个重要的研究方向,它被认为在病原体产生中起更重要的作用。在 IBD[110] 中黏膜相关细菌丰度更高[109],黏膜相关细菌可能随着疾病严重程度的变化和时间的推移而变化[111]。对新诊断的克罗恩病初治儿童的回肠和直肠活检显示,肠杆菌科、巴斯德菌科、韦荣球菌科和梭杆菌科的相对丰度增加,拟杆菌科和梭状芽孢杆菌科相对丰度降低[112]。总之,这些发现支持黏膜相关微生物群在 IBD 中的潜在作用,但很难确定其因果关系。最近的一项 meta 分析发现,肠道微生物群组成发生的非特异性变化与多种疾病有关,因此很难单独归因于微生物群组成[113]。

动物研究为肠道微生物群在 IBD 中作用的潜在机制提供了证据。抗菌防御基因缺陷的小鼠容易自发或对肠道损伤作出反应而发生微生态失调和结肠炎,强有力地支持了宿主-微生物相互作用在 IBD 中的重要性[110]。虽然将 IBD 患者的肠道微生物群移植到 GF 小鼠体内不会引起自发性结肠炎,但它确实增加了化学诱导或遗传易感小鼠对结肠炎的易感性[110]。高蛋白质膳食引起的肠道微生物密度增加会加重结肠炎,而高纤维膳食则会增加肠内微生物的多样性,改善肠道屏障功能,缓解了结肠炎[44]。

(二) 乳糜泻(Celiac 病)(见第 107 章)

乳糜泻是一种免疫介导的疾病,由遗传易感性个体中的麸质(含谷蛋白)触发的[114]。根据观察到的肠道微生物群组成和功能变化,人们越来越关注肠道微生物群及其在乳糜泻中的潜在作用。与 IBD 相似,研究之间存在显著的异质性。尽管在最近使用二代测序检测的研究中,微生物 α 多样性的显著降低和变形菌门的扩增似乎是最为一致的[115]。生命早期的暴露可能有一定作用,因为与无此遗传倾向的婴儿相比,有乳糜泻遗传倾向的婴儿厚壁菌门的丰度更高,拟杆菌目内缺乏细菌。还观察到微生物群的异常成熟:与无易感性的婴儿不同,即使在 2 岁时,微生物群特征仍然与成人不同。遗传易感婴儿暴露于麸质后,早期发生自身免疫性乳糜泻的频率高于麸质暴露延迟至 12 月龄时的频率,这表明不成熟的微生物群可能进一步加速免疫过程[116]。在人体研究中很难确定因果关系,但与共生肠道微生物群定植的相同小鼠相比,在遗传上易患乳糜泻的 GF 小鼠,要经历更严重的麸质诱导的乳糜泻病理变化,表明健康的微生物群可能具有保护作用[114]。另外,当暴露于胶质蛋白时,定植乳糜泻患者肠道细菌的 GF 大鼠表现出肠道通透性降低,这是乳糜泻的标志,表明不健康的微生物群在乳糜泻发病机制中的致病作用[117]。然而,肠道微生物群在乳糜泻中作用的潜在机制仍在研究中。

六、癌症

结直肠癌(见第127章)

肠道微生物群可能直接(通过产生致癌分子)或间接(通过创造促炎症微环境)触发致癌[118]。支持这一假设的小鼠研究表明,无论是在GF状态下还是使用抗生素,消耗微生物群都会降低发生结直肠癌的发病风险[119]。已发现结直肠癌患者个体的肿瘤组织中含有核梭杆菌[119],有趣的是,在转移灶中也发现了核梭杆菌以及其他相关的结直肠癌微生物群。发现使用窄谱抗生素消除核梭杆菌,可以减少结直肠癌异种移植物小鼠的癌细胞增殖和肿瘤生长[120]。最近发现,在肠道中形成生物膜的两种微生物,即产肠毒素的脆弱拟杆菌和产生大肠埃希菌机动蛋白的结肠埃希菌菌株之间的合作,可触发导致结直肠癌的DNA损伤。在一项已发表研究的meta分析中,确定了幽门螺杆菌感染与结直肠癌之间的相关性,尽管结肠癌的发病率并不能反映胃癌的发病率,但这表明了这种相关性的其他机制或复杂的相互作用[121]。解没食子酸链球菌(原名牛链球菌)菌血症也与结直肠癌相关,但目前尚不清楚它是结直肠癌的结果还是驱动因素[121]。

七、功能性胃肠疾病(见第122章)

肠道细菌在功能性胃肠疾病(如IBS)中的作用,是基于微生物群的组成变化及其在调节宿主生理学(包括胃肠道转运、上皮屏障功能、肠道分泌、内脏感觉和肠-脑轴调节)中的作用提出的。虽然没有统一的"IBS-微生物群"模式,但在不同分类水平上似乎存在微生物多样性的降低和改变[122,122a]。已证实几种微生物代谢物如SCFA、硫化氢、甲烷、色胺和胆汁酸对宿主生理学的影响[122]。微生物群靶向治疗已广泛应用于功能性胃肠疾病。现有数据表明,益生菌的应用可使腹胀和胃肠胀气症状有所改善[123],但不支持任何特定益生菌、益生元或合生元的治疗作用(见第130章)。IMT(FMT)也被用于治疗腹泻型IBS患者,但治疗效果存在差异[122b]。与治疗其他疾病一样,在确定IMT(FMT)对IBS的治疗作用(如果有的话)之前,还需要进行更严格的试验。

八、肠道微生物群在药物反应调节中的作用

肠道微生物群是观察到的药物治疗反应和不良事件个体间差异的重要因素。肠道微生物群编码基因不仅增强宿主的代谢能力[124],而且在包括药物在内的肠腔化合物的生物转化中发挥作用[125]。微生物群的可塑性使其成为一个更相关的因素,因为与基因相比,微生物群是可以改变的。微生物群已被确定为在药物反应、介导药物作用和某些药物代谢方面发挥作用,从而影响药物疗效和不良反应[126]。尽管已经确定了几种这样的相互作用,但有些是在动物模型中阐述的,因此还需要在人体中进行证实,并在不同队列中进行验证。次级胆汁酸和粪甾醇是微生物代谢的产物,可能预测他汀类药物的反应[127];某些拟杆菌属于免疫治疗癌症使用的CTLA-4抗体的成功相关[128];给予双歧杆菌可能会增强程序性细胞死亡蛋白1配体1(PD-L1)的反应——用于治疗黑色素瘤的抗体[129]。肠道微生物群也可能对二甲双胍抗糖尿病起一定作用[130]。迟缓爱格特菌携带强心苷还原酶(cgr)操纵子,可灭活地高辛,具有狭窄的治疗窗[131]。肠道微生物群也可以解释对复方镇痛剂对乙酰氨基酚反应的个体间差异[132],因为某些细菌(如梭状芽孢杆菌)产生的对甲酚,可与作为磺基转移酶家族1A成员1(SULT1A1,一种人类肝酶)底物的对乙酰氨基酚竞争[132],并导致N-乙酰-p-苯醌亚胺蓄积,进而导致肝毒性。用于治疗结肠癌和胰腺癌的化疗药物伊立替康(CPT-11)在肝脏中失活,但无活性的代谢产物可被细菌β-葡萄糖醛酸酶转化为活性药物,进而导致腹泻,这种明显的副作用可能迫使一些患者停药[133]。靶向抑制这类细菌酶可显著提高对化疗方案的依从性,而不影响疗效。这些例子只是冰山一角,鉴于肠道微生物群巨大的代谢潜力[134],它可能在大多数治疗药物的生物转化和反应中起到十分重要的作用。

九、肠道微生物群的治疗调节

肠道微生物群是一个重要的研究领域,因为它代表了疾病病理生理学和药物反应中的一个可变因素。目前有几种方法用于调节微生物群(见图3.1),范围从IMT中的生态系统方法、单独使用选定的细菌菌株或与益生菌联合使用、通过益生元刺激特定的细菌群落功能及与合生元和饮食一样的联合方法。IMT在艰难梭菌感染(*Clostridioides difffcile* infection,CDI)的处理中具有最显著的作用,CDI目前是美国医疗保健中最常见的感染[135,136]。有几种机制与IMT在CDI中的有效性相关,包括次级胆汁酸生成增加;微生物多样性的恢复和开放营养生态位的填充;以及随着丁酸盐生成增加,微生物群落结构的变化。总体而言,复发性CDI中IMT的缓解率范围为80%~95%[137],在一项meta分析(观察性研究)中,一级治愈率为91.2%,总复发率为5.5%[138]。针对万古霉素耐药肠球菌(VRE)定植患者中进行的初步研究表明,IMT可能有利于VRE的净化[139,140]。目前正在研究粪便替代品,并可能在不久的将来取代IMT。使用IMT的类似方法也正在多种慢性疾病中进行测试,从胃肠道疾病(如IBD、IBS)到代谢性疾病(如肥胖症、2型糖尿病)。骨髓移植后自体IMT的早期数据显示,似乎有希望在移植后减少腹泻疾病,一些研究也显示了移植物抗宿主病中同种异体IMT的益处[141]。

改善生态系统方法的另一种选择是单一细菌或细菌组合,如益生菌,以改善疾病状态。尽管有趋势支持某些益生菌菌株或制剂可使腹泻状态、坏死性小肠结肠炎、IBD、IBS患者从中获益[142,143],但益生菌的临床研究仍存在较大缺陷,难以得出临床有用的信息(见第130章)。微生物联合体治疗方法似乎更有前景,研究表明,确定含有梭状芽孢杆菌簇ⅩⅣa菌种,Blautia产品和博尔特梭状芽孢杆菌(*Clostridium bolteae*)的共生细菌联合体,可以恢复机体对VRE的定植抗性[144];梭状芽孢杆菌目中的共生细菌联合体,可赋予单核细胞增强李斯特菌耐药性[145];而含有梭状芽孢杆菌的共生细菌联合体,可

恢复对艰难梭菌的定植耐药性[146]。鉴定特定的微生物介质和提高对肠道细菌作用机制的理解，将有助于开发下一代更有针对性的益生菌，包括基因工程共生菌/益生菌生物，以提供疫苗或治疗的分子[147,148]。益生元最初是用于增强某些有益细菌的，如乳酸杆菌和双歧杆菌，然而，这种方法从此逐渐进化为关注微生物群落的整体功能及其对宿主功能的影响，因此，这组不再局限于特定的低聚糖，而是包括一系列广泛的膳食成分。合生元是指益生元与益生菌的结合，理论上应该放大益生菌的益处，这实际上已经在婴儿预防败血症的大型研究中看到[149]。微生物群靶向疗法的安全性记录良好[150,151]，然而，这些数据缺乏与药物安全性监测相关的严谨性[152]。肠道微生物群也是一类相对较新的治疗药物的丰富来源，通常被称为药物生物学，其中包括胞外多糖衣[153,154]和某些双歧杆菌的菌毛[155]；抗细菌分子，被称为抑菌素；抗菌噬菌体；甚至细菌DNA，均被证明具有抗炎活性[69,156-160]。

十、肠道微生物群的非细菌成员

目前认为被称为真菌群落的真菌集合代表了肠道微生物群落的一个次要组分部分，但鉴于缺乏完整注释的基因组数据库，例如可用于细菌的数据库，这可能是被低估的结果[161]。利用标记基因18S及其内转录间隔区的测序估计真菌群落的多样性，与细菌的多样性相似[162]。真菌普遍存在，念珠菌是最普遍的真菌属，约有160种[163,164]，其中白色念珠菌、热带念珠菌、光滑念珠菌和近平滑念珠菌在人类中占主导地位[161]。真菌生物体受环境[165]和饮食的影响。念珠菌的存在与免疫缺陷状态和高碳水化合物的饮食有关，但与高氨基酸、蛋白质和脂肪酸的动物源性饮食无关[166]。使用抗生素后真菌的过度生长证明了细菌和真菌之间的竞争关系[165,167]。真菌过度生长的生物学效应仍在研究中，但真菌生物群与胃肠道内（如IBD）和胃肠道外（如过敏性气道反应）的免疫应答有关。先天性免疫系统的某些成分，如TLR 2和4、dectin-1（一种C型凝集素受体）、CD5、CD36和SCARF1（清道夫受体家族成员），以及补体系统的成分可被真菌糖蛋白细胞壁成分、β-葡聚糖、几丁质和甘露聚糖激活，通过白细胞介素-17（IL-17）、IL-22和NF-κB等分子产生免疫信号转导[161]。针对真菌细胞壁表位的抗酿酒酵母抗体（anti-*Saccharomyces cerevisiae* antibody，ASCA）与白色念珠菌具有显著交叉反应性，被认为是克罗恩病的生物标志物[168-171]。ASCA也可能是预测发生克罗恩病的早期免疫标志物（见第115章）[171]。

病毒体代表了最多样化的生物系统之一，主要由噬菌体组成，噬菌体是感染细菌细胞的病毒，真核细胞病毒只占病毒体的一小部分。噬菌体具有毒力（裂解）循环和温和（溶原性）循环。在溶原性阶段，它们可以将其遗传物质整合到细菌基因组中或作为染色体外质粒存在，这一机制是细菌间抗生素耐药性或毒力因子转移的基础。噬菌体的数量超过细菌，可以塑造肠道细菌群落的组成[172]。与细菌相似，病毒体在个体间存在差异，但在个体内相对稳定，对饮食变化有反应[39,173,174]。噬菌体可通过刺激巨噬细胞产生白细胞介素-1b（IL-1b）和肿瘤坏死因子-α[175]，刺激干扰素产生[176]，并增强DNA疫苗的效力，直接影响免疫系统[177]。噬菌体在黏附胃肠黏液和提供一种非宿主来源的先天性免疫中也发挥了作用。结果发现，噬菌体衣壳蛋白与黏液黏蛋白结合[178]导致噬菌体在黏液中富集，这可能为细菌感染黏膜表面提供了防御。噬菌体对细菌的作用可以在治疗上加以利用，特别是随着多重耐药菌的增加，噬菌体可能代表一种新的重要的治疗模式。

真核生物病毒也可以影响免疫系统，如诺如病毒，已被证明可以塑造小鼠的黏膜免疫。共生菌群可以在决定病毒感染的结果中发挥重要作用。与细菌脂多糖结合的小鼠乳腺肿瘤病毒与微生物群相互作用，诱导免疫逃逸途径，触发TLR4，诱导IL-10的产生[179]。反过来病毒可以通过影响微生物群的其他成员来影响宿主，但尚需做大量的工作来鉴定这样的跨界相互作用，包括更好的注释病毒DNA序列数据库和深入分析病毒特征的技术。

十一、未来发展方向

随着我们扩大对微生物群途径以及由此产生的微生物代谢产物，与宿主生理学机制相互作用的理解进一步加深，我们将能够使用综合系统生物学方法开发更精确的干预措施，该方法可能是针对微生物群的个体专门制作的。有必要更好地了解微生物群的组装以及围生期和生命早期暴露的潜在有害影响，因为它们可能会对微生物群和人们的健康产生持久的影响。此外，我们刚刚开始认识到除细菌以外的微生物（如真菌、噬菌体、寄生虫）的重要作用以及微生物和宿主之间的信号传递，这将证明对微生物群的有效操纵至关重要。除了微生物群的研究前景之外，我们在样本的收集、测序和分析方面还面临着异质性形式的重大挑战，干预措施中使用的菌种和菌株的差异、依赖于特定微生物与疾病状态的关联，以及在临床研究和药物试验中，对微生物群作为一个重要的生物学变量缺乏更深入的认识。

（徐琳　袁农 译，曾翔俊 校）

参考文献

第 4 章　胃肠道感觉转导

Diego V. Bohorquez，Rodger A. Liddle 著

章节目录

一、激素和神经递质 …… 33
（一）激素和神经递质的定义 …… 33
（二）递质释放模式 …… 34
二、胃肠腔内的转导信号 …… 36
（一）通过细胞表面受体识别信号 …… 36
（二）G 蛋白偶联受体 …… 37
（三）酶偶联受体 …… 37
（四）离子通道偶联受体 …… 37
三、营养化学感应 …… 38
（一）脂质 …… 38
（二）蛋白质和氨基酸 …… 38
（三）味觉 …… 38
（四）感知微生物群 …… 38
（五）刺激递质释放的其他因素 …… 39
四、传递介质 …… 39
（一）肠神经肽 …… 40
（二）胃泌素 …… 40
（三）胆囊收缩素 …… 40
（四）胰泌素 …… 40
（五）血管活性肠肽 …… 41
（六）胰高血糖素 …… 41
（七）葡萄糖依赖性促胰岛素多肽 …… 42
（八）胰多肽家族 …… 42
（九）P 物质和速激肽 …… 42
（十）生长抑素 …… 42
（十一）胃动素 …… 43
（十二）瘦素 …… 43
（十三）生长激素释放肽 …… 43
五、神经递质 …… 43
（一）乙酰胆碱 …… 43
（二）儿茶酚胺 …… 44
（三）多巴胺 …… 44
（四）血清素(5-羟色胺) …… 44
（五）组胺 …… 45
（六）一氧化氮 …… 45
六、大麻素和其他化学递质 …… 46
（一）大麻素 …… 46
（二）腺苷 …… 46
（三）细胞因子 …… 46
七、激素和神经递质的重要性 …… 46
（一）胃肠道生长和异常生长 …… 46
（二）生长因子受体 …… 46
（三）表皮生长因子 …… 47
（四）转化生长因子-α …… 47
（五）转化生长因子-β …… 47
（六）胰岛素样生长因子 …… 47
（七）成纤维细胞生长因子和血小板衍生生长因子 …… 47
（八）三叶因子 …… 47
八、糖尿病与胃肠道 …… 47
九、食欲的胃肠调节 …… 48

胃肠道依赖于激素和神经递质将腔内产生的信号与全身稳态结合起来。例如，大脑中人的饱腹感在很大程度上是由肠道中存在的食物引起的。这一过程始于摄入营养物质刺激肠上皮中的感觉细胞，通过释放特定的化学信使调节食物的摄入。胃肠激素和神经递质与消化过程的各个方面都密切相关，包括营养物质的摄入和吸收。因此，这些递质对生命至关重要并不奇怪[1,2]。在本章中，将通过以下几个方面来分析调节性递质在胃肠功能中的关键作用：这些递质由感觉上皮细胞合成和分泌；食物或其他胃肠道因素如何触发其释放；最具代表性的成员；以及它们在疾病背景下的重要性。

一、激素和神经递质

胃肠道上皮的感觉细胞、肠内分泌细胞以及肠道神经系统的神经元是化学信使的主要产生者[34]，这些化学信使以激素或神经递质的形式释放。肠内分泌细胞以单细胞的形式存在于肠黏膜中，分散在众多的肠细胞——肠道的吸收细胞中。大多数肠内分泌细胞的顶端表面开口于肠腔，在肠腔内暴露于食物和其他内容物中。受到刺激后，肠内分泌细胞从其基底外侧表面释放激素，进入细胞旁间隙，并被摄取到血液中。与肠内分泌细胞不同，在黏膜上皮下方发现肠神经元，虽然绒毛和隐窝具有丰富的神经支配，但肠神经元并不被认为是直接暴露于肠道中的食物中。

与内分泌细胞集中在单个器官中的其他内分泌器官不同，胃肠道散在的分泌激素细胞的功能受到质疑，因此区分激素和神经元的作用变得十分重要。

（一）激素和神经递质的定义

定义激素和神经递质的标准，是确定候选递质是真正的激素还是神经递质。第一个被发现的激素是胰泌素，实验证

明,将这种肠提取物注射入血液后可以刺激胰腺分泌[3]。从那时起,建立了以下标准来证明一种物质可作为激素发挥作用。第一,对一个器官的刺激必须通过血液发挥作用引起远处反应。第二,反应必须独立于神经刺激。第三,在没有分泌器官的情况下不应发生反应。第四,将纯量的候选激素应用在靶组织上,反应应该是可重复的。已有 30 多种胃肠激素符合这些标准,它们的奇特性将在本章的"递质"章节中讨论。

证明化学物质是神经递质是一个更具有挑战性的事件,但同意使用以下标准定义神经递质。第一,候选分子必须存在于突触前神经元内。第二,递质必须在突触前去极化的反应中释放。第三,特定的候选受体必须存在于突触后细胞上。

通常认为激素只存在于内分泌系统和神经系统的神经递质中。然而,这些概念是在没有任何技术可视化单个细胞与其周围环境沟通信息时提出的。如今,越来越清楚的是,认识到这两个系统之间有着紧密的协同关系。事实上,一些细胞同时发挥内分泌和神经作用。比如,外周感觉细胞,如舌的味觉细胞和鼻的孤立性化学感受嗅觉细胞被称为副神经元,可以向血液中释放激素,并在突触连接处释放神经递质[4]。越来越多的证据表明,肠内分泌细胞具有相似的双重功能[5,6]。这些观察结果还扩展了内分泌系统和神经系统之间的联系。

此外,一个递质可同时作为激素或神经递质,这取决于它所在的位置。例如,摄入食物后,胆囊收缩素(cholecystokinin,CCK)通常从肠内分泌细胞释放到血液中,起到激素的作用。然而,CCK 在胃肠道和大脑神经中也大量存在,其在突触末端释放,起到神经递质的作用。这种递质的保守性,允许相同的信使在不同的位置具有不同的生理作用,并通过递质递送到其靶组织的方式使其成为可能。

(二) 递质释放模式

肠内分泌递质可以通过以下方式释放到其靶点上:内分泌、旁分泌、自分泌或通过突触神经传递(图 4.1)。

(1) 内分泌:当递质被分泌到血液中时,就会发生这种类型的传递。最常见的内分泌递质是多肽、脂类和单胺类,统称为激素。在胃肠道中,最主要的激素类型是肽形式(例如肽 YY、胃泌素、促胰液素)。激素在远隔部位与靶细胞表面的特异性受体结合,调节代谢过程[7]。

(2) 旁分泌:与通过血液到达远处靶点的内分泌机制相反,胃肠道的信号转导细胞也可以产生作用于邻近细胞的递质。这一过程被称为旁分泌信号,是产生生长抑素的肠内分泌细胞的典型特征[8]。旁分泌递质在局部分泌,不能弥散很远,它们与附近细胞上的受体结合发挥其生物学作用。一旦释放,递质就会迅速被靶细胞摄取,被胞外酶分解代谢,或与细胞外基质黏附,从而限制了递质在远处发挥作用的能力。由于旁分泌信号作用于局部,其起效一般较快,可突然终止。相比之下,内分泌信号转导需要更长的时间,且信号转导的终止需要清除循环中的激素。旁分泌递质可以是多肽(如生长抑素)或单胺(如组胺)。

(3) 自分泌:一些细胞拥有自身信使的细胞表面受体。这样,当一个信使被释放后,它可以作用于同一个分泌细胞,这种传递方式被称为自分泌,已被证实有几种生长因子。自分泌信号与某些癌症的生长有关,包括结直肠癌(见第 1 章)[9]。

(4) 神经传递:胃肠道信号转导的第四种形式是神经传递。这种形式的信号主要存在于肠神经系统。它是一个复杂的神经细胞网络,必须有效地交流来调节众多的胃肠道功能(图 4.2)。当胃肠道神经元被激活时,神经递质形式的信号在被称为突触的神经-神经连接处释放。这种结构帮助神经

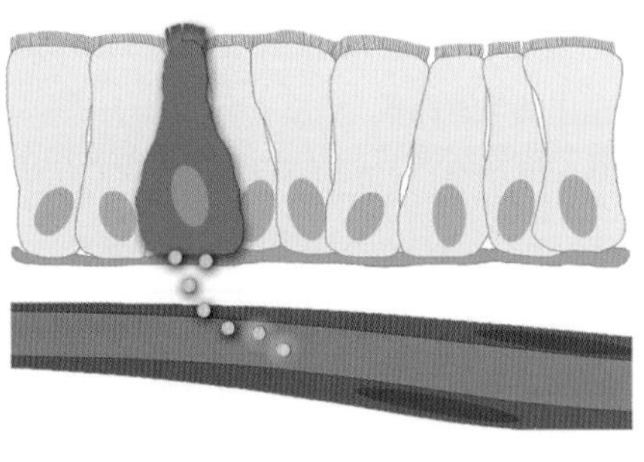

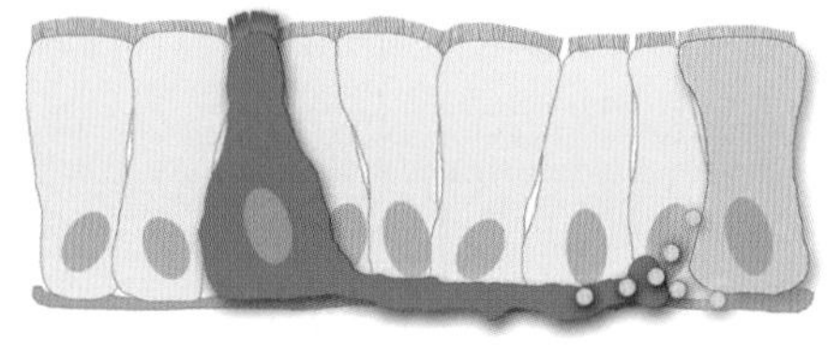

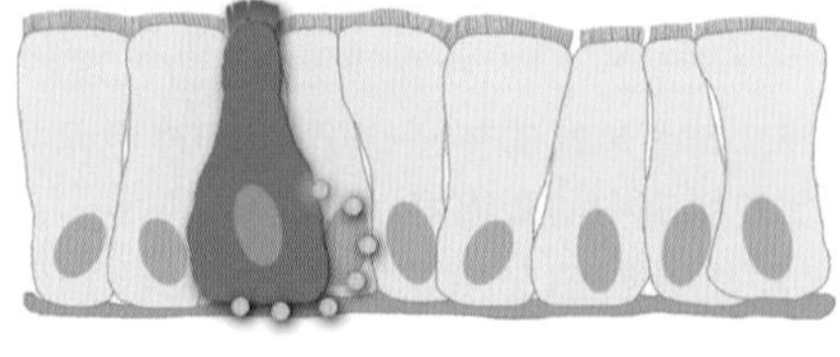

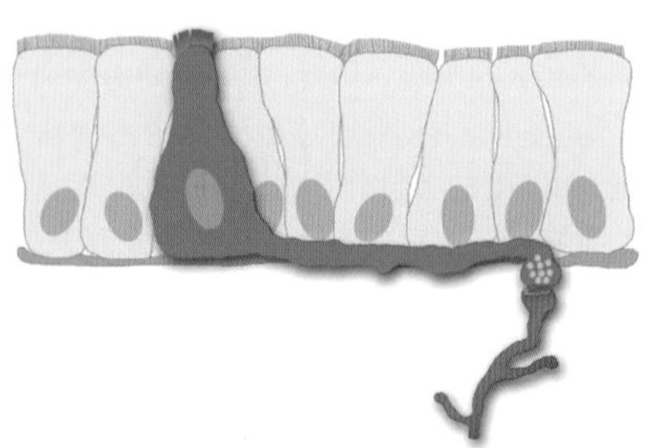

图 4.1　递质释放模式。化学感受细胞和神经元可通过血液内分泌;细胞旁间隙局部旁分泌;自分泌作用于同一释放细胞或经突触神经传递等途径分泌递质

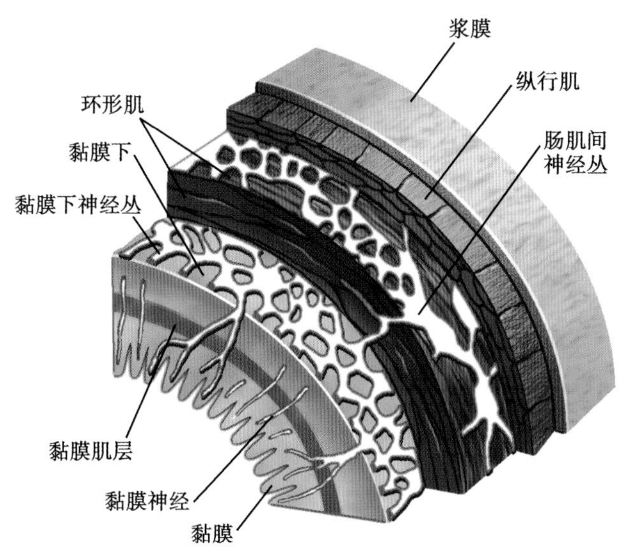

图 4.2 肠神经系统的组织。肠神经系统由两大神经丛组成，一个为黏膜下神经丛，另一个位于环形和纵向平滑肌层之间。这些神经元接受并协调胃肠道和中枢神经系统的神经传递

元在靶细胞的特定位置递送神经递质，并影响其他神经元、肌肉细胞、上皮细胞和分泌细胞以及胃肠道其他特殊细胞（如肠神经胶质细胞）的功能。神经递质对消化过程至关重要，包括肠道运动和分泌的协调。尽管胃肠道可以分泌多种神经递质，但最常见的是血管活性肠肽等多肽，或小分子物质，如乙酰胆碱和去甲肾上腺素。其他分子，如一氧化氮（nitric oxide，NO），可以简单地弥散到突触间隙对突触后细胞产生作用。有些神经实际上也会直接向血液中释放多肽和神经递质。这一过程被称为神经内分泌信号转导，可能用于根据释放的递质引起全身效应。

胃肠道的主要激素和神经递质列于框 4.1。它们的作用依赖于靶组织上的特异性受体。例如，神经递质作用的特异性取决于神经与靶细胞突触的精确位置。调节其合成、分解代谢或分泌可调节释放细胞内的递质浓度。一旦分泌，递质的浓度可以通过分解代谢迅速调节，或者再将神经递质摄取到分泌神经元中。许多肽类递质的半衰期非常短，一般在 2~5 分钟的范围内，这便于快速启动和终止信号转导。

框 4.1 胃肠道激素和递质

主要作为激素功能的肽
胃泌素
葡萄糖依赖性促胰岛素肽（GIP）
胰高血糖素和相关基因产物（GLP-1，GLP-2，肠高血糖素，胃泌酸调节素）
胰岛素
胃动素
胰多肽
酪酪肽（PYY）
分泌素（胰泌素）

可作为激素、神经肽或旁分泌因子
胆囊收缩素（CCK）
促肾上腺皮质激素的释放因子（CRF）
内皮素
神经降压素
生长抑素

主要作为神经肽的肽类
降钙素基因相关肽（CGRP）
强啡肽和相关基因产物
脑啡肽和相关基因产物
甘丙肽
胃泌素释放肽（GRP）
神经调节肽 U
神经肽 Y
组氨酸异亮氨酸肽（PHI）或组氨酸甲硫氨酸肽（PHM）
垂体腺苷酸环化酶激活肽（PACAP）
P 物质和其他速激肽（神经激肽 A，神经激肽 B）
促甲状腺激素释放激素（TRH）
血管活性肠肽（VIP）

作为生长因子的肽
表皮生长因子
成纤维细胞生长因子
胰岛素样因子
神经生长因子
血小板衍生生长因子
转化生长因子-β
血管内皮生长因子

作为炎症介质的肽类
干扰素
白细胞介素
淋巴因子
单核细胞因子
肿瘤坏死因子-α

作用于神经元的肽类
胆囊收缩素
胃泌素
胃动素

肠道内产生的非肽类递质
乙酰胆碱
三磷酸腺苷（ATP）
多巴胺
γ-氨基丁酸（GABA）
组胺
5-羟色胺（血清素）
一氧化氮
去甲肾上腺素
前列腺素和其他二十烷酸

新发现的激素或神经肽
胰淀素
生长素
鸟苷素和尿鸟苷素
瘦素

二、胃肠腔内的转导信号

营养传递过程涉及细胞表面受体激活,触发递质的释放。然后,递质进入血液或激活感觉传入神经。尽管释放递质的细胞,即肠内分泌细胞,被认为通过旁分泌或内分泌信号间接与神经相互作用,但一种新的概念正在出现,即肠内分泌细胞和神经实际上通过突触连接进行交流的[5,6]。随着转基因技术和先进的光学工具的使用,肠内分泌细胞在神经元中观察到几个解剖学特征,包括树突样棘、轴突样突起。这些轴突样胞质突起长度,从隐窝到绒毛、从小肠近端到远端长短不一(图4.3)。此外,肠道内分泌细胞具有突触的分子成分、基因和蛋白质,并通过突触样连接与感觉神经元相连(图4.4)。这些联系可能在胃肠功能生物学中有广泛的应用,包括从营养物质和胃肠微生物群传递感觉信号。参与信号从肠腔向身体其余部分转导的一些关键成分介绍如下。

(一)通过细胞表面受体识别信号

胃肠道上皮细胞使用膜结合受体识别管腔内的分子。当受体被激活时,受体将信号从细胞外传到细胞质中。虽然这个过程相当复杂,但有一些关键的检查点可以调节信号级联反应。其中一些检查点发生在受体激活、脱敏、内化和/或再致敏的瞬间。由于其调节潜力,它们是治疗干预的有吸引力的靶点。

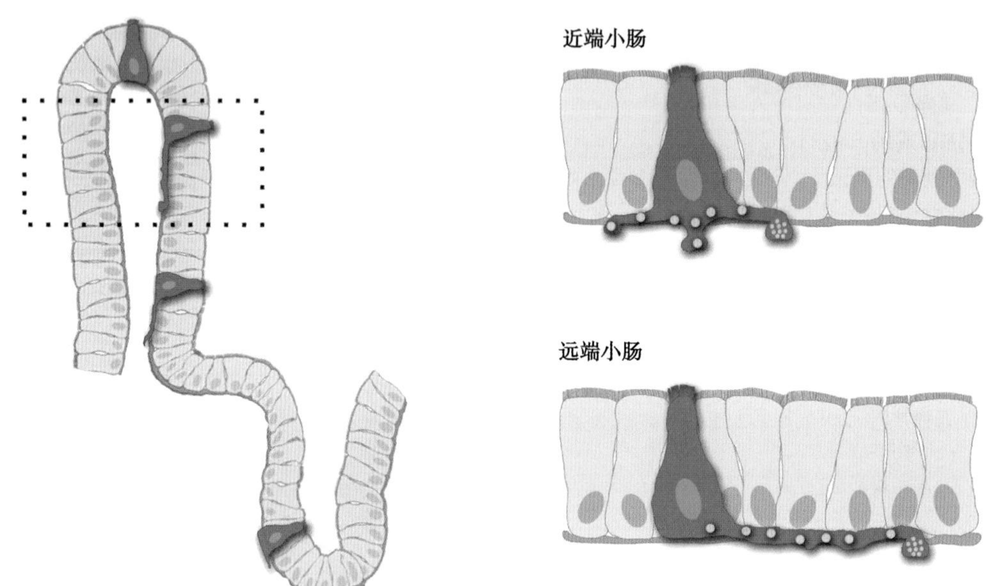

图4.3　肠内分泌细胞轴突样突起。肠内分泌细胞有类似神经元轴突的细胞质延伸。其中一些作为旁分泌调节器,如同生长抑素分泌细胞中的旁分泌调节器;然而,在其他细胞中,这些轴突样基底突用于连接支配肠道的神经元

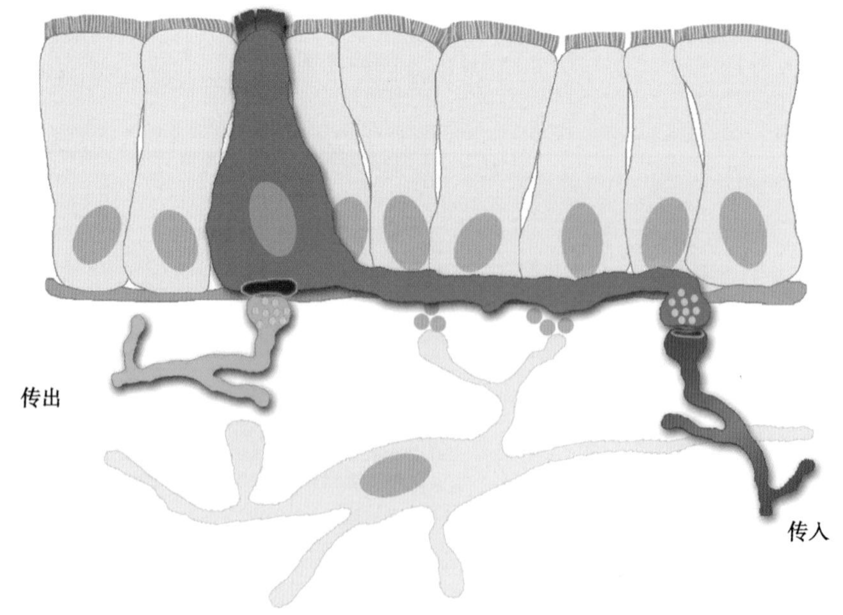

图4.4　肠内分泌细胞为副神经元。肠内分泌细胞与传入和传出神经元连接,显现能够发送和接收神经元信号

受体根据其结构和信号机制分为主要家族。细胞表面受体的主要家族包括:G 蛋白偶联受体、酶偶联受体和离子通道。以下是每个受体家族的一些主要方面。

(二) G 蛋白偶联受体

G 蛋白偶联受体(G protein-coupled receptor,GPCR)的典型特征是其 7 个跨膜结构域。它们是最常见的蛋白质受体家族,具有广泛的生理作用,从感知视网膜中的光产生视觉,到感知胃肠道中的营养物质来调节食物摄入。当受到特定配体的刺激时,GPCR 发生构象变化,导致其与 G 蛋白相结合,因此得名。这些 G 蛋白与细胞膜的细胞内表面结合[10,11],由 3 个不同的亚基(α、β 和 γ)组成。是 Gα 亚基赋予 G 蛋白的名称(表 4.1)。例如,刺激效应器(如腺苷酸环化酶)的 G 蛋白被归类为 Gs(用于刺激),而抑制效应器的 G 蛋白被称为 Gi(用于抑制)[12-14]。当 G 蛋白作用于效应器时,会导致细胞内第二信使(如 C-AMP 或钙)浓度快速升高,随后第二信使改变一种或多种蛋白激酶的活性,以催化现有蛋白的磷酸化,并最终改变其生理活性。

表 4.1 G 蛋白 α 亚基的分类及其信号通路

分类	信号
Gαs	腺苷酸环化酶、钙通道
Gαi 和 Gαo	腺苷酸环化酶、环单磷酸鸟苷、磷酸二酯酶,c-Src,STAT 3
Gαq	磷脂酶 C-β
Gα12 和 Gα13	钠-氢交换

一般而言,GCPR 信号机制涉及以下事件。当配体或第一信使与受体结合时,受体改变其构象并与 G 蛋白复合物结合。在静息状态下,G 蛋白复合物不与受体相互作用。然而,一旦结合,Gα 亚基中发生分子替代——二磷酸鸟苷(GDP)被三磷酸鸟苷(GTP)取代。这种替代引起 Gα 亚基的激活。然后激活的 Gα 亚基与 β 和 γ 亚基分离,并在膜中横向移动以激活效应器。通过不同的 Gα 亚基工作,效应器的活性可上调或下调。当与效应器相互作用完成时,与 Gα 亚基结合的 GTP 被水解回 GDP 并与 Gα 分离。通过这种方式 Gα 移回到原位与其他两个亚基重新结合。然后效应器诱导细胞内第二信使浓度增加。两个最常见的第二信使是环磷酸腺苷和钙。涉及每个第二信使的机制简要概述如下。

(1) 通过环磷酸腺苷(cyclic adenosine monophosphate,cAMP)信号转导。第二信使是 β 肾上腺素能受体的经典下游效应因子,β 肾上腺素能受体是 GPCR 家族,其特征已被很好地描述。这些受体与 Gαs 偶联并激活腺苷酸环化酶,该酶催化 ATP 转化为 cAMP。然后,高浓度的 cAMP 改变蛋白激酶 A(PKA)的活性,最终调节参与重要生理功能的限速酶。例如,糖原磷酸化酶的调节增加了糖原向葡萄糖-1 磷酸盐的转化,导致血糖水平的升高。

(2) 通过钙(Ca^{2+})信号转导。与 Gαq 亚基相关的 GPCR 使用 Ca^{2+} 作为第二信使。细胞内 Ca^{2+} 浓度的增加可由电压门控 Ca^{2+} 通道、配体门控 Ca^{2+} 通道的激活或由膜磷脂激活引起胞质 Ca^{2+} 的释放所致。后者是由与 Gαq 相关的 GPCR 激活触发的。当激活时,Gαq 沿细胞膜移动以激活磷脂酶 Cβ。然后,磷脂酶 Cβ 将膜磷脂磷脂酰肌醇二磷酸裂解为甘油二酯和 1,4,5-三磷酸肌醇(IP3),生成两个潜在的信号分子。在 Ca^{2+} 存在的情况下,二酰基甘氨酸可激活蛋白激酶 C。此外,来自内部储存的 Ca^{2+} 水平升高,也可激活 Ca^{2+}-钙调素激酶。通过这种方式,两种不同的激酶被激活:通过增加胞质 Ca^{2+} 的钙调蛋白激酶和通过甘油二酯和 Ca^{2+} 作用的蛋白激酶 C。然后,这些激酶催化细胞内靶蛋白的磷酸化。受体激活后,IP3 从质膜进入细胞质中,与位于内质网和线粒体上的 IP3 受体结合。IP3 受体结合引起细胞内细胞器释放 Ca^{2+},进一步增加细胞质 Ca^{2+} 浓度。最终细胞质 Ca^{2+} 浓度通过主动转运出细胞或再摄取进入细胞内 Ca^{2+} 储备,Ca^{2+} 细胞质浓度恢复正常。

如果细胞受到过度刺激,会发生一个适应过程,以防止细胞过度反应。信号衰减通过配体诱导的受体脱敏或受体内化来实现。通过磷酸化方式使受体脱敏。磷酸化还可以进一步标记受体进行内化,内化是通过激活特定的受体激酶和募集抑制蛋白样分子完成的,使受体与 G 蛋白解偶联[15]。解偶联和随后的受体内化结束信号传递,最终恢复细胞反应性。

(三) 酶偶联受体

酶偶联受体中最具代表性的是酪氨酸激酶受体家族。这些受体主要是生长因子的靶点,如表皮生长因子。这些受体的独特之处在于它们既是受体又是酪氨酸激酶。当被激活时,受体催化磷酸盐从 ATP 转移到靶蛋白。酶偶联受体由 3 个结构域组成:即配体结合细胞外结构域、跨膜结构域和胞质结构域。胞质结构域包含蛋白酪氨酸激酶区域和激动剂激活受体磷酸化的底物区域。通过这种方式,可以发生来自其他激酶的磷酸化或自身磷酸化来调节酪氨酸激酶受体的活性[16]。一般情况下,受体酪氨酸激酶以单体形式存在于细胞膜中。然而,随着配体结合,这些受体发生二聚化、自身磷酸化,并启动其他细胞内信号转导通路,最终调节生理功能[17]。在第一章中已经讨论了受体酪氨酸激酶与细胞生长和肿瘤形成的关系[18]。

还有几种其他类型的酶偶联受体,包括受体鸟苷酸环化酶、非受体酪氨酸激酶、受体酪氨酸磷酸酶和受体丝氨酸/苏氨酸激酶。尽管这些受体通过不同的酶发挥作用,但信号转导原理仍与酪氨酸激酶受体相似。

(四) 离子通道偶联受体

离子通道偶联受体参与细胞间的快速信号传递。这类受体在电脉冲驱动信号的组织中很重要,如神经细胞和肌肉。例如,在神经细胞中,离子通道对相对数量较少的神经递质作出反应而开放或关闭,并允许特定离子流过质膜。流动动力学取决于细胞内外的浓度。这种离子流调节靶细胞的兴奋性,最终触发神经传递、肌肉收缩、电解质和液体分泌或激素释放等过程。

这类受体的一个例子是瞬时受体电位阳离子通道 M5,或称之为 TRPM5。该离子通道受体被细胞内 Ca^{2+} 浓度升高激活,是味觉信号苦味、甜味和鲜味转导的关键成分[19]。此外,最近的研究表明,它可介导肠内分泌细胞释放阿片类物质和激素(如 CCK)[20]。因此,离子通道偶联受体可能是调节胃肠道上皮感觉细胞功能的有吸引力的靶点。

三、营养化学感应

(一) 脂质

肠腔内的脂类是饱腹感的强效诱导剂和全身代谢的调节剂。虽然其机制尚不完全清楚,但最近研究已证明,细胞表面受体可识别特定的脂质,从而激活几种激素的释放,包括 CCK、YY 肽和胰高血糖素样肽-1。

脂质可以是甘油三酯形式或不同链长的游离脂肪酸形式。不同的受体识别不同的脂质。例如,Gq 偶联的 GPCR40(即 FFAR1)和 GPCR120 对中链和长链脂肪酸发生反应;而 Gαi 偶联的 GPCR41(即 FFAR3)和 GPCR43(即 FFAR2)与 2~5 个碳的短链脂肪酸结合[21]。一些 GPCR 可能对肠腔中的脂质产生反应。其他非 GPC Rs 也参与脂质感应,如含免疫球蛋白样结构域的受体(ILDR)。ILDR 在 CCK 细胞中表达,并被脂肪酸和脂蛋白的组合激活,这表明必须吸收脂肪酸以刺激 CCK 分泌。尽管大多数营养受体的具体位置尚未确定,但可能是至少一些脂质需要在激活激素释放之前被消化吸收。这一假说得到了研究的支持,在研究中向肠道内注入脂质,只有在形成乳糜微粒(由吸收的脂质形成的脂蛋白颗粒)的情况下,才会触发激素分泌[22]。

一些脂质产生的感觉信号似乎是通过迷走神经的传入纤维传递的。例如,将脂质注入十二指肠可增加棕色脂肪温度,如果将脂质与丁卡因(一种用于阻断迷走神经传入激活的强效局部麻醉剂)一起输注,该作用则会消失[23]。通过传入神经或血流传递的信号,最终诱导体内稳态变化(例如饱腹感、体温、胃肠动力),对胃肠腔中营养物质的存在作出反应。

(二) 蛋白质和氨基酸

蛋白质可能是胃肠道激素分泌的强效刺激物。大多数蛋白质只有在被消化为蛋白胨和氨基酸时才会刺激激素分泌。最近发现肠内分泌细胞表达几类介导激素分泌的氨基酸受体。例如,钙感知受体(calcium sensing receptor,CaSR),最初被认为具有检测和对细胞外 Ca^{2+} 的反应,以及调节肾脏和甲状旁腺中的钙稳态[24],还可识别 L-氨基酸以及二肽、三肽[25]。CaSR 在调节 L-氨基酸刺激的胃泌素和胃酸分泌中的作用已被确立[26,27]。芳香族氨基酸苯丙氨酸和色氨酸是刺激 CaSR 的最有效的氨基酸。也是刺激 CCK 分泌最有效的氨基酸。在 CCK 细胞中 CaSR 的发现及其与分泌的联系,支持其作为胃肠道营养传感器的生理重要性。除 CCK 外,CaSR 还介导葡萄糖依赖性促胰岛素肽(glucose-dependent insulinotropic peptide,GIP)、胰高血糖素样肽-1(glucagon-like peptide 1,GLP-1)和酪酪肽(peptide tyrosine tyrosine,PYY)的分泌[28-30]。

另一个与 CaSR 密切相关的氨基酸感应受体是 G 蛋白偶联受体 GPRC6A。GPRC6A 对碱性氨基酸有反应,并在远端小肠的味觉细胞和肠内分泌细胞中表达,从而介导 GLP-1 的分泌[31]。GPRC6A 的基因缺失可导致饮食诱导的肥胖,这意味着该受体对代谢调节很重要[32]。最后,味觉受体 T1R1/T1R3 也可识别酸性氨基酸,似乎并不局限于舌的味觉细胞,而是分布在全身的化学感受细胞中。总之,CaSR、GPFC6A 和 T1R1/T1R3 共同对所有 20 种 L-氨基酸均有反应,代表了感知氨基酸营养刺激的综合机制。

部分消化蛋白形成的蛋白胨也能刺激激素的分泌。G 蛋白偶联受体 GPR93 不仅是溶血磷脂酸受体,而且还能被蛋白胨激活[33]。GPR93 在肠细胞和肠内分泌细胞中表达,其活化与 CCK 分泌偶联[34]。因此,GPR93 可能是蛋白胨在餐后刺激 CCK 释放的机制。

一些完整的蛋白通过一类内源性管腔活性激素释放因子间接刺激激素分泌,包括管腔胆囊收缩素释放因子[35]和苯甲二氮䓬结合抑制剂[36]。最有效的蛋白是那些竞争胰蛋白酶结合的蛋白,从而使内源性释放因子逃避肠腔内的蛋白水解和消化。

(三) 味觉

对各种食物中的味觉感知,对于调节欣快、满足感、食物摄入和其他主要的代谢功能是非常重要的。胃肠道通过专门的化学感受细胞表达的特定受体检测化学物质和毒素。这些细胞在舌中最具特征性,它们集中在味蕾中。味觉感受细胞可以检测产生 5 种不同味道的化学物质:甜、咸、酸、苦和鲜味—酱油的香味。虽然这是一个活跃的研究领域,但只有对甜味、苦味和鲜味的感知机制有很好的了解。这 3 种味道是由两个 GPCR 家族的激活介导的:味觉-1 受体(taste-1 receptor,T1R)和味觉-2 受体(taste-2 receptor,T2R)。在人类中,有 30 种 T2R 蛋白和 3 种 T1R 蛋白,分别命名为 T1R1、T1R2 和 T1R3[37-39]。

甜味和鲜味被 T1R 识别。在舌中 T1R1 和 T1R2 在不同的味觉感知细胞中表达,但始终与 T1R3 一起表达。通过这种方式,受体形成异原二聚体,允许在 T1R2+T1R3 的情况下检测甜味配体,在 T1R1+T1R3 的情况下检测鲜味[40],T1R 也在肠内分泌细胞中表达[41]。葡萄糖与肠内分泌细胞中的 T1R2+T1R3 受体的结合导致肠促胰岛素激素的分泌,如 GLP-1。GLP-1 最终调节多种功能,包括胰岛素分泌、营养吸收和肠道运动[42]。因此,肠道表达的味觉信号系统,已成为开发治疗与饮食相关疾病(如 2 型糖尿病)的活跃研究领域[43]。

苦味感知通过直接味觉厌恶、诱导咽部呕吐反射和恶心,作为防止摄入有毒物质的一种警告信号。存在于舌及肠道中的大量 T2R 可识别苦味化合物,如植物中的有毒生物碱[44]。人们认为,绕过舌中 T2R 的苦味化合物可被肠道中的 T2R 识别,作为诱导呕吐等保护性反应的备用机制[45]。T2R 及其相关的 Gα-胃蛋白的激活导致细胞质内 Ca^{2+} 迅速增加,从而刺激细胞膜去极化和激素释放。在肠道中,苦味化学物质可刺激肠内分泌细胞释放 CCK,使胃排空减慢、食欲下降,从而有降低毒素吸收的可能性[42,45,46]。

(四) 感知微生物群

肠内分泌细胞有一个典型的小而狭窄的开口通向管腔表面。尽管长期以来人们一直认为营养素刺激其顶端部位的肠内分泌细胞,但有一些报道认为,吸收而非肠腔营养素刺激肠道激素释放[22]。因此,开放到肠腔的肠内分泌细胞的顶端部分可能有助于感知细菌输入。支持这种假说的证据来自于一些细菌 Toll 样受体(如 TLR4、5 和 9)仅在肠内分泌细胞中专一表达[47]。当细菌配体(如 LPS 或鞭毛蛋白)刺激这些特异性 TLR 时,肠内分泌细胞会分泌 CCK 和几种趋化因子。值得注意的是,细胞因子和防御素仅在肠内分泌细胞系中(如 STC-1)分泌,只对细菌配体而不是脂肪酸的反应。此外,沉默 TLR 信号的中心介质 MyD88,可减少细菌配体而不是脂肪酸刺激的 CCK 分泌[48]。这一证据表明,肠内分泌细胞中可能存在两种不同的感知途径:一种是细菌,另一种是营养素。

长期以来,人们一直认为肠内分泌细胞上的化学感受受体位于顶端表面,顶端表面对肠腔开放。然而,这一点尚未得到证实,最近的证据表明,当暴露在基底侧表面时,一些营养素会刺激肠内分泌细胞。因为肠道微生物群驻留在胃肠道的管腔中,所以 Toll 样受体很可能位于微绒毛上。未来,阐明肠内分泌细胞上受体的位置可能有助于设计靶向特定受体的药物,调节参与食欲调节和胰岛素分泌的激素的分泌。

(五) 刺激递质释放的其他因素

有证据表明,胃肠激素可以被存在于肠腔中的某些非营养因子释放(图 4.5)。CCK 是第一个被发现可由腔内释放因子调节的激素[49,50]。从肠道冲洗液中纯化出[49,50]管腔 CCK 释放因子,当注入动物管腔时显示可刺激 CCK 释放。引起 CCK 释放的其他管腔内因素是地西泮结合抑制剂和胰腺监测肽[51,52]。有人提出,促胰液释放因子以酸敏感的方式调节胰泌素的分泌[53]。胰腺分泌性胰蛋白酶抑制剂,也称为监测肽,是由胰腺腺泡细胞产生的内源性胰蛋白酶抑制剂[54]。当分泌到十二指肠时,监测肽直接刺激 I 细胞分泌 CCK。这些蛋白直接作用于肠内分泌细胞,最有可能是通过细胞表面受体。这些释放因子的存在突出了肠腔内还存在未被充分认识的生物活性分子。

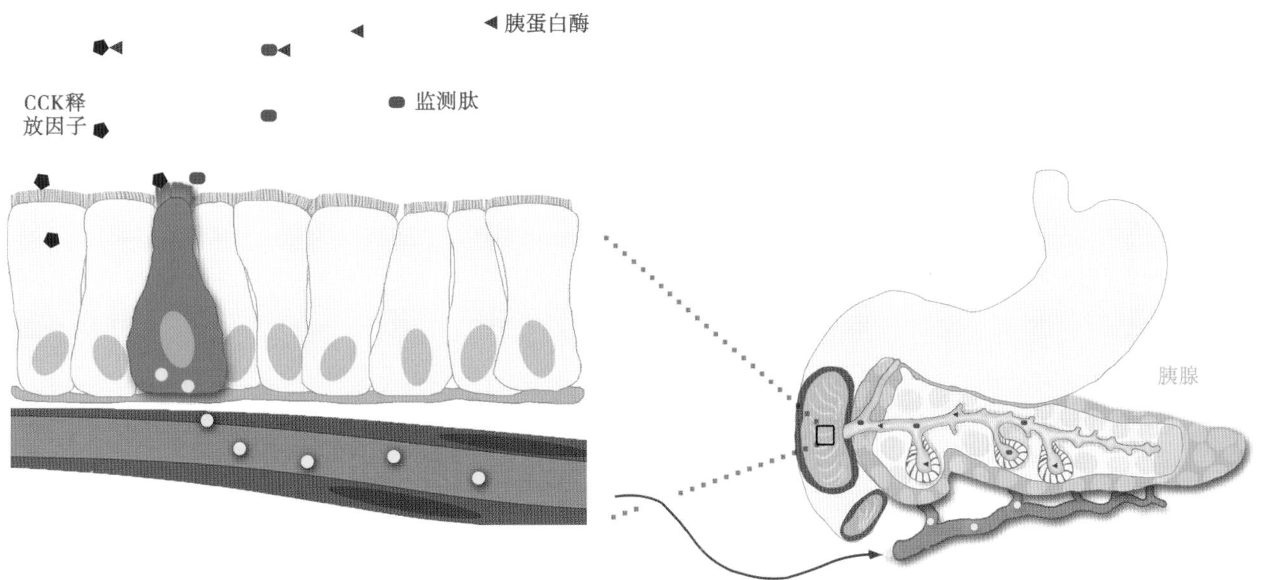

图 4.5　肠腔内释放因子对胆囊收缩素(CCK)分泌的调节。肠上皮细胞分泌因子,因其能够刺激肠内分泌细胞释放 CCK,而被称为 CCK 释放因子(绿色)。CCK 被释放到血液中,刺激胰腺分泌监测肽和胰蛋白酶。监测肽进一步刺激 CCK 的释放,构成前馈机制。反过来,肠道中的胰蛋白酶消化食物,抑制监测肽和 CCK 释放因子的作用。因此,胰蛋白酶作为反馈调节剂发挥作用

四、传递介质

刺激递质释放的相同因子通过特定的基因调控元件同时调节特定递质基因的表达。肠道激素基因的表达通常与肽的产生有关,并根据生物体的生理需要进行调节。例如,一旦引起生物反应,信号可能随后被发回内分泌细胞“关闭”激素分泌。这种负反馈机制是许多生理系统所共有的,避免了激素的过量产生与分泌。

所有的胃肠肽均通过 DNA 转录合成信使 RNA,信使 RNA 随后被翻译成前体蛋白,也称为前激素原。新翻译的蛋白含有一个信号序列,该信号序列指向内质网,为结构修饰准备肽前体[55]。这些前体被转运到高尔基体,在将肽包装成分泌颗粒之前,进一步的结构修饰就会发生。分泌颗粒可靶向立即释放或储存在靠近准备释放的质膜处。虽然许多激素是由单个基因产生的,但在组织和血液中可以有多种分子形式。不同的分子形式是源于翻译前或翻译后加工的差异所致。一种常见的翻译前加工机制是 mRNA 的选择性剪接,它来自同一基因产生独特的肽。

翻译后修饰可通过前体分子的裂解发生,其中信号肽的酶裂解产生激素原。导致成熟胃肠肽的其他翻译后特征包括:肽裂解为较小形式(如生长抑素)、羧基端酰胺化(如胃泌素)和酪氨酸残基硫酸化(如 CCK)。这些加工步骤对激素的生物活性至关重要。例如,硫酸化 CCK 的效力是未硫酸化形式的 100 倍。胃肠胰激素的大量生化学复杂性在分泌这些肽的不同组织中十分明显。由于胃肠肽由内分泌及神经组织分泌,因此所涉及的不同组织常常决定了肽生成的加工步骤。许多激素基因能够制造选择性剪接的 mRNA 或经历不同翻译后加工的蛋白质,最终产生不同大小的激素。这些修饰对于受体结合、信号转导和随后的细胞反应都非常重要[56]。以下我们概述胃肠道递质的主要特征,包括神经肽、神经递质和

其他递质。

（一）肠神经肽

以前认为单个肠内分泌细胞(enteroendocrine cell, EEC)只产生一种激素。然而，通过纯化 EECs 的转录组学分析，现在已知 EEC 产生多种类型的肽类激素和神经递质[57-59]。因此，根据产生的激素对 EEC 进行分类并不像用传统的单字母命名那样简单。很明显，刺激单个 EEC 可引起多个递质的释放，从而发挥多种生理反应。我们将肠道主要递质的主要生物学作用总结如下。

（二）胃泌素

如第 51 章详细讨论的，胃泌素(gastrin)是刺激胃酸分泌的主要激素。随后发现胃泌素可能有促进胃黏膜生长和一些胃癌生长的作用[60]。人胃泌素是位于 17 号染色体上的单个基因的产物。这种活性激素是由一种称为前胃泌素原的前体肽产生的。人前胃泌素原含有 101 种氨基酸，但通过连续酶裂解加工成两种主要形式的胃泌素：G34 和 G17 以及一些小分子形式。所有胃泌素的共同特征是酰胺化四肽(Try-Met-Asp-Phe-NH2)羧基端，具有完整的生物活性。一种称为甘氨酸延伸胃泌素的非酰胺化胃泌素形式由结肠黏膜产生。已在动物模型中证明，甘氨酸延伸的胃泌素可刺激正常结肠黏膜增殖，并促进结直肠癌的发展。目前尚不清楚这种形式局部产生的胃泌素是否有助于人类结肠癌发生，并且甘氨酸延伸胃泌素的受体尚未确定[61]。

大多数胃泌素是在胃窦内分泌细胞中产生的[62]。在胃肠道其他区域产生的胃泌素量要少得多，包括近端胃、十二指肠、空肠、回肠、结肠和胰腺。另外还在胃肠道外发现了胃泌素，包括脑、肾上腺、呼吸道和生殖器官，但其在这些部位的生物学作用尚不清楚。

胃泌素和 CCK 的受体是相关的，构成所谓的胃泌素-CCK 受体家族。分别从胰腺和脑中克隆出 CCK-1 和 CCK-2(以前称为 CCK-A 和-B)受体互补 DNA，之后认识到 CCK-2 受体与胃的胃泌素受体完全相同[63]。

人 CCK-1 受体存在于胆囊中，而在大多数种属中存在于胰腺中。CCK-1 受体对 CCK 的亲和力比对胃泌素的亲和力高 1 000 倍。CCK-1 和 CCK-2 胃泌素受体具有大于 50% 的序列同源性，对各种受体拮抗剂和胃泌素的反应不同。

进食后，胃泌素从特殊的内分泌细胞(G 细胞)释放到血液循环中。刺激胃泌素释放的膳食特定成分包括蛋白质、肽类和氨基酸。胃泌素释放受胃 pH 的极大影响。空腹和胃酸增加可抑制胃泌素释放，而高胃 pH 是其分泌的强烈刺激物。

高胃泌素血症发生在与产酸减少相关的病理状态下，如萎缩性胃炎。在长期服用抑酸药物(如组胺受体拮抗剂和质子泵抑制剂)的患者中，血清胃泌素水平也会升高。在这种情况下，高胃泌素血症是由碱性 pH 环境刺激胃泌素产生引起的。高胃泌素血症的另一个重要但不太常见的原因是产生胃泌素的肿瘤，也称为 Zollinger-Ellison 综合征(见第 34 章)。

（三）胆囊收缩素

胆囊收缩素(CCK)是一种肽类递质，主要由近端小肠的肠内分泌细胞产生，并在进食后分泌到血液中。循环中的 CCK 与胆囊、胰腺、胃平滑肌和周围神经上的特异性 CCK-1 受体结合，以刺激胆囊收缩和胰腺分泌，调节胃排空和肠道运动，并诱导饱腹感[64]。这些作用有助于协调膳食营养素的摄入、消化和吸收。摄入的脂肪和蛋白质是刺激 CCK 释放的主要食物成分。

CCK 最初被鉴定为一个由 33 个氨基酸组成的多肽。然而，自从 CCK 被发现以来，已经从血液、肠道和脑中分离出大小不同形式的 CCK。所有形式的 CCK 都是由单个基因通过前激素原的翻译后加工产生的。从 CCK-58 到 CCK-8 大小不同形式的 CCK 具有相似的生物活性[65]。

CCK 是胆囊收缩的主要激素调节因子。它还在调节膳食刺激引起的胰腺分泌中起重要作用(见第 56 章)。在许多物种中，后一种效应直接通过胰腺腺泡细胞上的受体介导，但在人类中，胰腺 CCK-1 受体的丰度较低，CCK 似乎通过存在 CCK-1 受体的肠胰腺神经元间接刺激胰腺分泌。在一些物种中，CCK 对胰腺具有营养作用，尽管其在人类胰腺肿瘤中的潜在作用是推测性的。CCK 也能延迟对胃的排空[66]，这一作用可能对协调食物从胃输送到肠道很重要。CCK 被认为是调节饱腹感和摄食量的主要介质，当食物在胃或肠道时，这种效应尤其明显。CCK 通过与胃窦和泌酸黏膜中生长抑素(D)细胞上的 CCK-1 受体结合抑制胃酸分泌。生长抑素在局部可抑制邻近 G 细胞释放胃泌素，并直接抑制壁细胞分泌胃酸[67]。

临床上 CCK 已经与胰泌素一起用于刺激胰腺分泌，进行胰腺功能的检测。还可通过放射成像或同位素成像来评估胆囊的收缩能力。目前，尚未发现已知的 CCK 过量引起的疾病。据报道，在肠黏膜表面积减少的乳糜泻患者和神经性贪食症患者中 CCK 水平降低[68,69]。在一些慢性胰腺炎患者中，有 CCK 水平升高的报道(见第 59 章)，推测可能是由于胰酶分泌减少和 CCK 释放负反馈调节中断所致[70]。

（四）胰泌素

胰泌素(secretin)是第一个发现的胃肠激素，是观察到将肠提取物经静脉注射到狗的体内，引起胰腺分泌时发现的[71]。胰泌素在十二指肠中通过酸刺激释放，其刺激胰液和碳酸氢盐的分泌，导致肠道内酸性食糜中和(见第 56 章)。胰泌素还可抑制胃酸分泌(见第 51 章)和肠动力。

人胰泌素是一种由 27 个氨基酸组成的肽类，与许多其他胃肠肽相似，在羧基端被酰胺化。它是结构相关胃肠激素的胰泌素-胰高血糖素-血管活性肠肽家族的创始成员。胰泌素在小肠的肠内分泌细胞中含量最多，但几乎在所有的 EECs 中均有表达[72]。

胰泌素受体是 G 蛋白偶联受体(GPCR)大家族的一个成员，它在结构上与胰高血糖素、降钙素、甲状旁腺激素、垂体腺苷酸环化酶激活肽(pituitary adenylate cyclase-activating peptide, PACAP)和血管活性肠肽的受体相似。

胰泌素的主要生理作用之一是刺激胰液和碳酸氢盐分泌(见第 56 章)。胰腺碳酸氢盐在到达十二指肠后，可中和胃酸并升高十二指肠 pH，从而“关闭”胰泌素的释放(负反馈)。有人认为，酸刺激胰泌素释放受内源性肠胰泌素释放因子的调节[73]。这种肽刺激胰泌素的释放，直到胰蛋白酶的流动足以降解释放因子并终止胰泌素的释放。

虽然促胰泌素的主要作用是刺激胰液和碳酸氢盐分泌，但它是一种肠抑胃泌素（enterogastrone），当胃肠道腔中存在脂肪时释放，并抑制胃酸分泌。在生理浓度下，胰泌素抑制胃泌素释放、胃酸分泌和胃动力[74]。临床常用胰泌素试验来诊断胃泌素肿瘤[75]（第 34 章）。

（五）血管活性肠肽

血管活性肠肽（Vasoactive Intestinal Polypeptide，VIP）是一种在肠道生理学中具有广泛意义的神经调节剂。VIP 是一种强效血管扩张剂，可增加胃肠道血流量，引起平滑肌舒张和上皮细胞分泌[76,77]。作为一种化学信使，VIP 从神经末梢释放，并局部作用于携带 VIP 受体的细胞。VIP 属于胃肠肽家族，包括结构相关的胰泌素和胰高血糖素。VIP 受体是一种 G 蛋白偶联受体，可刺激细胞内 cAMP 的生长。

与其他胃肠肽一样，VIP 作为前体分子合成，是裂解为 28 种氨基酸的活性肽。VIP 主要在外周肠神经系统和中枢神经系统的神经元中表达，并与其他肽一起释放，主要包括肽组氨酸异亮氨酸（peptide histidine isoleucine，PHI）和/或肽组氨酸蛋氨酸（peptide histidine methionine，PHM）（见框 4.1）[78]。

VIP 是整个中枢和外周神经系统的重要神经递质[79]。由于其广泛分布，VIP 对许多器官系统都有影响，最值得注意的是，在胃肠道中，VIP 可刺激肠上皮和胆管细胞分泌液体和电解质[80,81]。

VIP 与 NO 一起，是肠道非肾上腺素能、非胆碱能神经传递的主要成分[82]。胃肠道平滑肌表现的基础张力或持续动力，是由平滑肌膜电位节律性去极化引起的。VIP 作为这种节律活动的抑制性递质，引起膜超极化和随后的胃肠道平滑肌舒张。因此，VIP 是胃肠道括约肌的重要神经调节剂，包括食管下括约肌和 Oddi 括约肌。在某些病理状态下，如贲门失弛缓症和先天性巨结肠，VIP 神经支配的缺乏被认为分别在食管松弛缺陷和肠动力障碍中起主要作用[83,84]。

与肠黏膜内衬的胃肠内分泌细胞不同，VIP 由神经元产生和释放，血清中大多数可测量的 VIP 可能来源于神经元。正常情况下，血清 VIP 水平较低，进餐无明显变化。然而，在胰性霍乱中（又称为 Vemer-Morrison 综合征，表现为水样腹泻、低钾血症和胃酸缺乏）[85]，VIP 水平可极高[80]。分泌 VIP 的肿瘤通常会引起大量腹泻[86]（见第 34 章）。

（六）胰高血糖素

胰高血糖素（glucagon）是由胰腺 α 细胞以及回肠和结肠的肠内分泌细胞合成并释放的。胰高血糖素是一种由 29 个氨基酸组成的肽类，其通过糖原异生、糖原分解和脂解调节葡萄糖稳态，并与胰岛素反向调节。胰高血糖素基因不仅编码前胰高血糖素源，还编码胰高血糖素样肽（GLP）。这种前体肽由信号肽、胰高血糖素相关多肽、胰高血糖素以及 GLP-1 和 GLP-2 组成。组织特异性肽加工通过激素原转化酶发生，在胰腺中产生胰高血糖素，在肠道中产生 GLP-1 和 GLP-2（图 4.6）[87,88]。

胰高血糖素和 GLP-1 调节葡萄糖稳态[89]。在进餐后，胰腺内分泌细胞释放胰高血糖素，并与骨骼肌和肝脏上的 G 蛋白偶联受体结合，发挥其血糖调节作用。GLP-1 刺激胰岛素分泌，并增强葡萄糖对胰腺 β 细胞的胰岛素释放作用（见后文的“肠-胰岛轴”）。GLP-1 类似物已被开发用于治疗 2 型糖

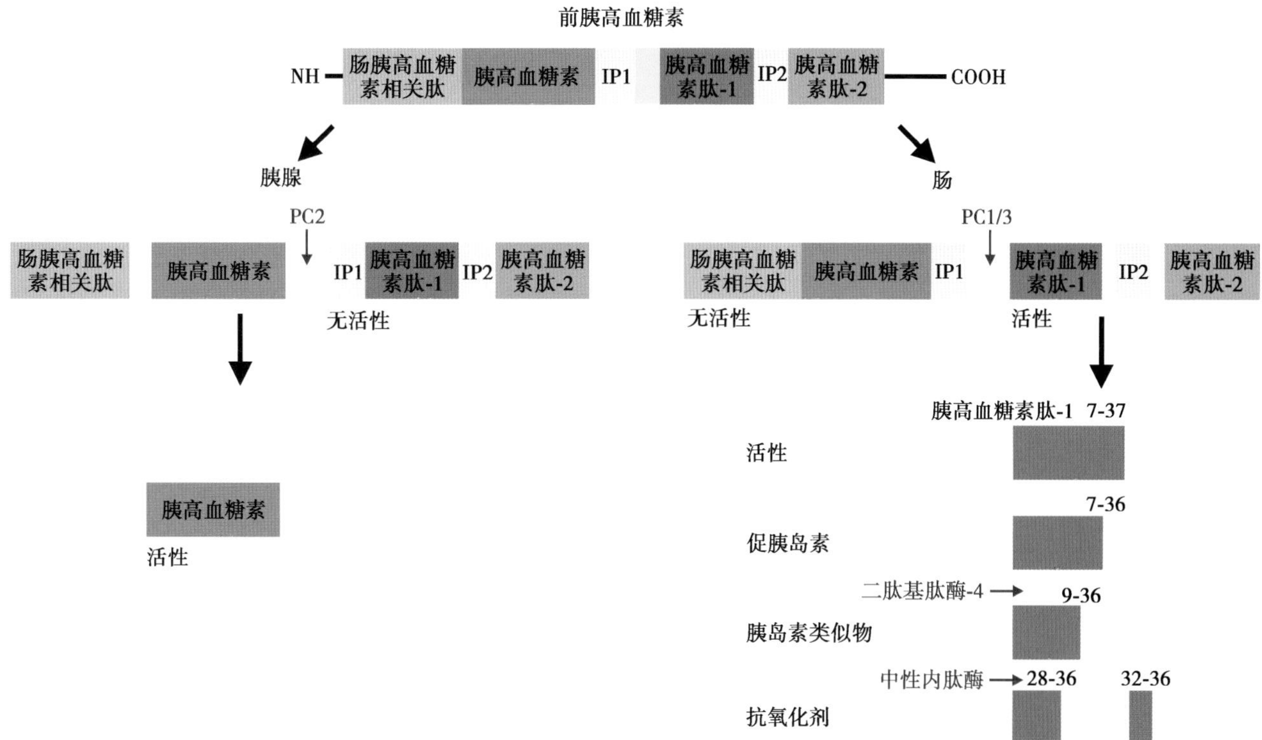

图 4.6　胰高血糖素的翻译后加工。胰高血糖素基因被转录并翻译成一种前体肽——前胰高血糖素原。前胰高血糖素原进行酶裂解（黄框），裂解的产物类型取决于酶的类型。例如，胰腺中表达的 PC2 可将前胰高血糖素原裂解为活性胰高血糖素；而在肠道中表达的 PC1/3 将胰高血糖素原裂解成不同的肽片段，产生胰高血糖素样肽-1（GLP-1）和胰高血糖素样肽-2（GLP-2）。在肠道中，GLP-1 被进一步加工成具有不同生物活性功能的小片段。参与这一过程的酶有二肽基肽酶-4（DPP4）和中性内肽酶（NEP）

尿病。一种长效人类 GLP-1 类似物可改善 β 细胞功能,并可降低 2 型糖尿病患者的体重[90,91]。GLP-2 是一种肠道生长因子,可增加绒毛高度、刺激肠隐窝增殖、并阻止肠细胞凋亡的。基于这些作用,GLP-2 激动剂用于治疗短肠综合征。

(七) 葡萄糖依赖性促胰岛素多肽

葡萄糖依赖性促胰岛素多肽(GIP)因其具有抑制胃酸分泌的能力(肠抑胃素效应)而被发现,最初被称为胃抑多肽。随后发现,对胃酸分泌的影响仅发生在高于生理范围的极高浓度时。然而,GIP 对胰岛素释放具有强效作用(如 GLP-1),可增强葡萄糖刺激的胰岛素分泌[92]。基于这一作用,GIP 被重新定义为葡萄糖依赖性促胰岛素多肽。

GIP 是由小肠黏膜细胞产生的 42 种氨基酸组成的肽,在摄入葡萄糖或脂肪后,GIP 被释放到血液中。在血糖水平升高的情况下,GIP 与其胰腺 β 细胞上的受体结合,激活腺苷酸环化酶和其他增加细胞内钙浓度的途径,导致胰岛素分泌。然而,重要的是,GIP 只有在高血糖时才会对胰岛素分泌产生影响,在血糖正常的条件下,不会刺激胰岛素释放。

GIP 受体也在脂肪细胞上表达,通过脂肪细胞 GIP 增加甘油三酯的储存,这可能有助于脂肪积累。基于 GIP 的促胰岛素特性,再加上其对脂肪细胞的作用,有人提出 GIP 可能在肥胖和发生与 2 型糖尿病相关的胰岛素抵抗中发挥作用[93]。与这一提议相一致的是,实验发现缺乏 GIP 受体的小鼠在接受高脂饮食时体重不会增加[94]。但能否使用 GIP 拮抗剂治疗肥胖尚待观察。在极少数的情况下,GIP 受体可能在肾上腺皮质异常表达,导致食物依赖性库欣综合征[95,96]。

(八) 胰多肽家族

胰多肽(pancreatic polypeptide,PP)最初是在胰岛素制备过程中分离得到的,是 PP 家族的创始成员[97]。PP 肽家族包括神经肽 Y(NPY)和酪酪肽(PYY),它们是由于存在 C 末端酪氨酸酰胺而被发现的[98,99]。PP 由特殊的胰腺内分泌细胞(PP 细胞)储存和分泌[100],NPY 是在中枢和外周神经系统中发现的主要神经递质[101]。PYY 已定位于整个胃肠道的肠内分泌细胞,但在回肠和结肠中的浓度最高,它在合成 GLP 的相同细胞中产生[102]。

PP-PYY-NPY 肽类家族作为内分泌、旁分泌和神经内分泌递质发挥作用,调节因与五种受体亚型之一结合而产生的许多作用[103]。PP 抑制胰腺外分泌、胆囊收缩和肠蠕动[104]。PYY 可抑制迷走神经刺激的胃酸分泌及其他运动和分泌功能[105]。缺乏正常产生的 36 个氨基酸肽的前两种氨基酸的 PYY 的缩写形式,PYY3-36 已被证明在给人类服用时可以减少摄食量,这表明肠释放的肽可能在调节进餐量方面发挥作用[106]。许多 PYY 细胞具有沿相邻肠细胞基底表面运行的神经肽,这些肠细胞具有 Y1 和 Y2 两种 PYY 受体亚型,局部释放的 PYY 很可能具有结肠抗分泌作用[107]。NPY 是中枢神经系统中含量最丰富的肽之一,与 PYY3-36 相比,NPY 是一种强效的食物摄入刺激物[108]。在外周,NPY 影响血管和胃肠道平滑的肌功能[109]。

(九) P 物质和速激肽

P 物质属于速激肽家族的多肽,其中包括神经激肽 A 和神经激肽 B。速激肽遍布于外周和中枢神经系统,是神经病理性炎症的重要介质[110]。速激肽作为一个类群,由产生前速激肽原 A 和前速激肽原 B 的两个基因编码,两者共有的是一个保守性很好的 C 末端五肽。转录和翻译加工产生 P 物质、神经激肽 A 和/或神经激肽 B,它们在很大程度上是通过选择性剪接进行调节的。这些肽主要作为神经肽发挥作用。P 物质是初级感觉传入神经元的神经递质,与脊髓 I 层的特定受体结合[111]。该肽家族的三种受体已被确定——NK-1、NK-2 和 NK-3[112]。P 物质是 NK-1 受体的主要配体,神经激肽 A 是 NK-2 受体的主要配体,神经激肽 B 是 NK-3 受体的主要配体。然而,所有这些肽都可以通过与所有 3 种受体亚型结合并发出信号。

P 物质被认为是神经源性炎症的主要介质。在肠道中,艰难梭菌引起的实验性结肠炎是由毒素诱导的 P 物质释放和随后的 NK-1 受体的活化所致[113]。这些炎症后遗症可被 P 物质受体拮抗剂阻断。P 物质受体在溃疡性结肠炎和克罗恩病患者的肠道中含量更为丰富[114]。

(十) 生长抑素

生长抑素(somatostatin)是一种由 14 个氨基酸组成的环肽,最初被确定为生长激素分泌的抑制剂。自发现以来,几乎在身体的每个器官和整个胃肠道中都发现了它。在消化道中,生长抑素可由胃和肠黏膜中的 D 细胞和胰腺的胰岛 D 细胞以及肠神经元产生[115]。生长抑素具有许多药理学作用,大多具有抑制性作用。

在胃中,生长抑素在调节胃酸分泌中起着重要作用[116]。在胃窦中,D 细胞向管腔内开放,直接暴露于酸中。胃内 pH 的降低会刺激 D 细胞分泌生长抑素,抑制胃泌素的释放(见第 51 章)。胃泌素分泌减少降低了对产酸的刺激,胃内容物的 pH 升高。因此,胃酸对胃泌素释放的一些抑制作用(见前文的"胃泌素")是由生长抑素介导的。

生长抑素的释放也受机械刺激、膳食成分(包括蛋白质、脂肪和葡萄糖)以及其他激素和神经递质的影响[117]。毒蕈碱样刺激似乎是生长抑素分泌最重要的神经刺激。

已发现至少有 5 种生长抑素受体可解释不同的药理学特性[118]。例如,受体亚型 2 和 3 与抑制性 G 蛋白偶联,但受体亚型 1 不与之偶联。此外,只有生长抑素受体亚型 3 可抑制腺苷酸环化酶。生长抑素的抑制作用是通过降低 cAMP 减少、抑制 Ca^{2+} 通道、或 K^+ 通道开放介导的。

在消化道中,生长抑素具有广泛的抑制作用。除了对胃酸的作用外,生长抑素还可以减少胃蛋白酶原的分泌。生长抑素能显著地抑制胰酶、胰液和碳酸氢盐分泌,减少胆汁流量[119]。生长抑素对肠道动力的影响在很大程度上是抑制性的,但它可能通过对胃动素的作用刺激移行性复合运动,生长抑素还可减少肠道对营养物质和液体的转运,减少内脏血流量,并对组织生长和增殖有抑制作用[120,121]。

由于生长抑素具有多种生理作用,因此具有一些临床重要的药理学用途。许多内分泌细胞拥有生长抑素受体,对抑制性调节敏感。因此,生长抑素和最近开发的生长抑素类似物,用于治疗内分泌肿瘤产生的激素过量的疾病,如肢端肥大症、类癌和胰岛细胞瘤(包括胃泌素瘤)[122]。生长抑素还能降低内脏血流量和门静脉压,因此生长抑素类似物被用于治疗食管静脉曲张出血(见第 92 章)[123]。利用其对分泌的抑制作用,通过使用生长抑素类似物治疗某些类型的腹泻和减少胰瘘的液体排出量。许多内分泌肿瘤表达丰富的生长抑素受体,这使应用放射性标记的生长抑素类似物,如奥曲肽,定位全身的小肿瘤成为可能。

(十一) 胃动素

胃动素(motilin)是一种由十二指肠上皮内分泌细胞产生的一种含有 22 个氨基酸的肽类[124]。胃动素不是通过食物刺激释放的,而是以周期性和反复的模式分泌到血液中,在禁食状态下与移行性复合运动同步。血液胃动素水平的升高,可调节由胃窦十二指肠区域开始并向远端肠道进展的Ⅲ期收缩。

胃动素与食管、胃以及小肠和大肠平滑肌细胞上的特定受体结合,通过这些受体发挥推进作用[125]。胃动素受体激动剂,如红霉素,对胃肠道动力有明显影响,偶尔会产生痉挛腹痛和腹泻等不良副作用[126]。然而,胃动素激动剂可能有助于治疗胃和肠动力障碍,目前正在研究用于治疗便秘型肠易激综合征[127]。

(十二) 瘦素

瘦素(leptin)是一种由 167 个氨基酸组成的蛋白,主要由脂肪细胞分泌。血中瘦素水平反映了全身的脂肪储备[128]。其主要作用似乎是减少食物摄入量。瘦素是信号分子细胞因子家族的一员。瘦素受体的 5 种不同形式已被报道[129]。一种短形式的瘦素受体似乎通过血脑屏障将瘦素从血液中转运进入下丘脑。一种长型的瘦素受体位于下丘脑核区,瘦素与瘦素受体结合并激活 Janus 激酶信号转导和翻译系统(JAK STAT)[130]。少量瘦素由胃的主细胞和胎盘产生,存在于母乳中。

外周给予瘦素可以减少食物摄入量。然而,随着动物变得肥胖,这种效应就会降低。有趣的是,当将瘦素注射到中枢神经系统时,肥胖动物对瘦素的反应正常,食物摄入量减少,推测肥胖中的瘦素"抵抗",发生在转运瘦素通过血脑屏障的瘦素受体水平[131]。瘦素通过降低 NPY(一种强效的食物摄入刺激物)和增加 α-促黑色素细胞刺激素(α-MSH,一种食物摄入抑制剂),在大脑内发生减少食物摄入的能力。在外周,瘦素通过与 CCK 的协同作用减少进餐量[133]。在缺少瘦素受体的肥胖小鼠中,瘦素加 CCK 减少进餐量的协同效应消失,但可以通过脑中瘦素受体的基因重建得到恢复[134]。在瘦素受体缺陷甚至瘦素抵抗引起的罕见人类肥胖病例中,人们可能会预期瘦素-CCK 协同效应对餐量上的损失。

随着肥胖的发展,瘦素的血液水平增加,瘦素似乎反映了总脂肪含量[135]。在细胞水平上,大脂肪细胞比小脂肪细胞产生更多的瘦素。由于其对摄食量的影响,人们最初认为外源性瘦素可用于治疗肥胖。然而,在临床试验中,仅证实了外源性瘦素对体重减轻的效果非常有限。据报道,瘦素缺乏是少数家族中肥胖的一个原因,但这种情况极为罕见[136,137]。瘦素受体突变被认为是导致家族中肥胖的另一个原因[138]。

(十三) 生长激素释放肽

生长激素释放肽(ghrelin)是由胃产生的一种由 28 个氨基酸组成的肽,是生长激素促分泌素受体的天然配体[139]。当中枢或外周给药时,生长激素释放肽刺激生长激素的分泌,增加食物摄食量,导致体重增加[140,141]。循环中的生长激素释放肽水平,在禁食期间或与能量负平衡相关的条件下增加,如饥饿或厌食会增加。相反,在进食后和肥胖患者中生长激素释放肽水平较低。生长激素释放肽似乎在摄食和能量平衡的神经激素调节中起着核心作用。

胃底是生长激素释放肽最丰富的来源,在肠道、胰腺、垂体、肾脏和胎盘中也有少量的生长激素释放肽。生长激素释放肽是由独特的内分泌细胞产生的,该细胞被称为 P/D1 细胞[142,143],其分为开放和闭合两种类型。开放型暴露于胃腔,与胃内容物接触,而闭合型位于胃固有层的毛细血管网附近[144]。这两种细胞类型都会分泌激素进入血液。基于其结构,生长激素释放肽是胃动素家族多肽的一员,和胃动素一样,生长激素释放肽刺激胃收缩、增强胃排空。

观察发现,循环中的生长激素释放肽水平在餐前急剧升高,餐后突然下降,这表明它是开始进餐的信号。食物对血浆生长激素释放肽水平的影响可通过摄入葡萄糖重现,似乎与膳食对胃膨胀的物理影响无关。在正能量平衡状态下(如肥胖),循环中的生长激素释放肽水平较低,并与体重指数呈负相关[145,146]。相反,生长激素释放肽水平在禁食、恶病质和厌食症患者中较高。重要的是,体重减轻增加了循环中的生长激素释放肽水平[147]。

胃释放的生长激素释放肽作用于迷走神经发挥其对摄食的作用。然而,当它被递送到中枢神经系统时仍具有很强的活性,在中枢神经系统生长激素释放肽激活下丘脑弓状核内的 NPY 和豚鼠相关的蛋白产生神经元,这些神经元参与摄食的调节[141,148]。

胃旁路术患者并未表现出正常个体餐前血浆生长激素释放肽的升高[149]。这种生长激素释放肽释放的缺乏可能是胃旁路手术诱导体重减轻的整体有效性的机制之一。

Prader-Willi 综合征是一种先天性肥胖综合征,其特征为严重的食欲亢进、生长激素缺乏和性腺功能减退。尽管肥胖通常与较低的生长激素释放肽水平相关,但普瑞德-威利综合征患者的循环生长激素释放肽水平较高,餐后不会下降[150,151]。该综合征的生长激素释放肽水平与接受输注外源性生长激素释放肽个体,在刺激食欲和增加摄食量上相似,这表明生长激素释放肽分泌异常可能是普瑞德-威利综合征食欲亢进的原因[152]。

五、神经递质

在整个胃肠道的神经传递中,仅描述了有限数量的递质。尽管它们的分布广泛,但由于其局部释放和再摄取或失活的特性,使它们只能在精确部位产生特定的和有时间限制的作用。

(一) 乙酰胆碱

乙酰胆碱(acetylcholine)在胆碱能神经元中合成,是胃肠运动和胰腺分泌的主要调节因子。乙酰胆碱储存在神经末梢,通过神经去极化释放。释放的乙酰胆碱与突触后毒蕈碱和/或烟碱受体结合。烟碱型乙酰胆碱受体属于配体门控离子通道家族,是由 α、β、γ、δ 和 ε 亚基组成的同源五聚体或异源五聚体[153]。α 亚基被认为是乙酰胆碱受体结合后突触后膜去极化的介质。毒蕈碱受体属于七次跨膜螺旋 GPCR 家族。已知有 5 种毒蕈碱胆碱能受体(M1 至 M5)。毒蕈碱受体可根据受体信号转导进一步分类,M1、M3、和 M5 刺激腺苷酸环化酶,M2 和 M4 抑制腺苷酸环化酶。乙酰胆碱被乙酰胆碱酯酶降解,其降解产物可通过神经末梢上的高亲和力转运蛋白再循环。

(二) 儿茶酚胺

肠神经系统的主要儿茶酚胺(catecholamines)类神经递质包括去甲肾上腺素和多巴胺。去甲肾上腺素由酪氨酸合成,由支配肠神经节和血管的节后交感神经末梢释放。酪氨酸通过酪氨酸羟化酶转化为多巴。多巴最初通过多巴脱羧酶转化为多巴胺,并包装成分泌颗粒。去甲肾上腺素由多巴胺通过分泌颗粒中的多巴胺*β*-羟化酶的作用形成。在适当的刺激后,神经末梢释放含有去甲肾上腺素的分泌颗粒,并与肾上腺素能受体结合。

肾上腺素受体是 G 蛋白偶联的受体,有 7 个典型的跨膜结构域,分为 α 和 β 两种基本类型。α-肾上腺素受体进一步分为 α1A、α1B、α2A、α2B、α2C 和 α2D。同样 β 受体包括 β1、β2 和 β3。已知肾上腺素能受体通过各种 G 蛋白发出信号,从而导致腺苷酸环化酶和其他效应系统受到刺激或抑制。细胞内单胺氧化酶或胺转运蛋白的快速再摄取可终止去甲肾上腺素信号转导。肾上腺素能受体刺激的作用可调节平滑肌收缩、肠血流量和胃肠道分泌。

(三) 多巴胺

多巴胺(dopamine)是胃肠道分泌、吸收和运动的重要介质,是中枢和外周神经系统的主要儿茶酚胺神经递质。在中枢神经系统中,多巴胺调节食物摄入、情绪和内分泌反应,并在外周控制激素分泌、血管张力和胃肠运动。胃肠道多巴胺的特征因几个原因一直具有挑战性。首先,多巴胺对胃肠动力能产生抑制性或兴奋性的影响[154]。一般而言,由突触前受体介导的兴奋性反应的激动剂浓度,低于由突触后受体介导的抑制作用。其次,在似乎具有种属特异性的位置鉴定多巴胺受体,阻碍了多巴胺受体的定位[155]。第三,多巴胺在胃肠道运动中的研究,通常使用该激动剂的药理学用量。因此,多巴胺在高剂量下激活肾上腺素能受体的能力混淆了对结果的解释。

通常认为,多巴胺通过 1 型和 2 型两种不同的受体亚型发挥作用。目前,分子克隆已经证实了 5 种多巴胺受体亚型,每种亚型都具有独特的分子结构和基因位点[155]。多巴胺受体是完整的膜 GPCR,当暴露于激动剂和拮抗剂时,每种受体亚型都具有特定的药理学特征。多巴胺从神经末梢释放后,通过一种特定的多巴胺转运蛋白从突触间隙中清除。

(四) 血清素(5-羟色胺)

长期以来已知血清素(即 5-羟色胺)在胃肠道神经传递中发挥作用[156]。胃肠道含有 95% 以上的全身 5-羟色胺,5-羟色胺在上皮分泌、肠动力、恶心和呕吐等各种生理过程中都很重要[157]。5-羟色胺由必需氨基酸色氨酸合成,在神经末梢转化为其活性形式。分泌的 5-羟色胺通过 5-羟色胺特异性转运蛋白再摄取在突触间隙中失活。大多数血浆 5-羟色胺来源于肠道,存在于黏膜肠嗜铬细胞和肠神经系统中。5-羟色胺通过与特定受体结合来介导其作用。在肠神经元、肠嗜铬细胞和胃肠平滑肌上发现了 7 种不同的 5-羟色胺受体亚型(5-HT1 至 5-HT7)。

5-羟色胺的作用是复杂的(图 4.7)[158]。可通过刺激胆

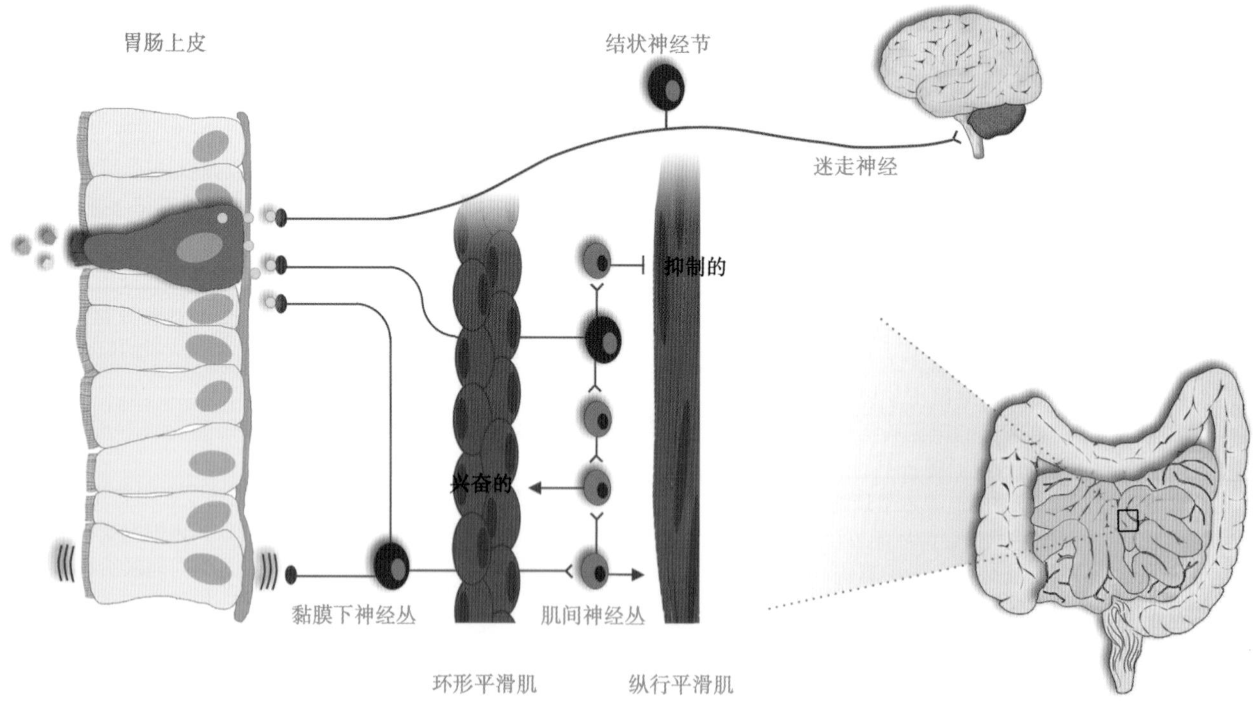

图 4.7　肠神经系统中的 5-羟色胺(血清素)。体内约 90% 的 5-羟色胺是由肠上皮的嗜铬细胞(绿色)产生。与肠内分泌细胞一样,肠嗜铬细胞是一种感觉细胞,对胃肠腔内容物作出反应,能释放血清素,也称为 5-羟色胺(5-HT)。释放的 5-HT 刺激迷走神经的传入纤维,将感觉信号传递入脑。这些迷走神经神经元的胞体聚集在结状神经节中。此外,5-HT 还可刺激黏膜下神经丛和肌间神经丛神经元的神经纤维。在这些神经丛整合的信息最终调节环形平滑肌和/或纵向平滑肌的兴奋或抑制。这两层平滑肌的同步收缩,最终搅动和推动食糜(部分消化的食物)

碱能神经使平滑肌收缩或通过刺激抑制性含 NO 的神经元使平滑肌舒张[157]。黏膜细胞释放的 5-羟色胺刺激感觉神经元,启动蠕动反射和分泌(通过 5-HT4 受体),并通过激活 5-HT3 受体调节感觉。肌间神经丛含有 5-羟色胺能的中间神经元,能投射到肠壁外的黏膜下神经丛和神经节。由 5-羟色胺激活的外源性神经元参与肠道感觉,可能引起腹痛、恶心和肠易激综合征相关的症状。5-羟色胺激活的固有神经元是正常胃肠功能蠕动和分泌反射的主要成分。5-羟色胺也可以激活迷走神经传入通路,在中枢神经系统中调节食欲、情绪和性功能。由于这些不同的作用,通常用于治疗抑郁和焦虑的选择性 5-羟色胺再摄取抑制剂,与安慰剂治疗相比具有显著的胃肠道副作用并不奇怪。

5-羟色胺及其受体与胃肠动力障碍性疾病的发病机制有关[159]。特异性 5-羟色胺受体亚型导致了选择性激动剂和拮抗剂的开发,用于治疗肠易激综合征和慢性便秘与腹泻。例如,5-HT3 受体拮抗剂可减少肠道分泌,用于治疗腹泻型肠易激综合征。5-HT4 受体激动剂可引起促动力作用,用于治疗便秘型肠易激综合征和其他动力障碍[160,161]。

5-羟色胺也可通过 5-羟色胺 N-乙酰转移酶促转化为褪黑素[162]。除松果体外,胃肠道是人体褪黑素的主要来源。美洛托宁(melatonin,即褪黑素)在肠嗜铬细胞中产生,进食后释放到血液中。已知褪黑素对胃肠道有许多作用,包括减少胃酸和胃蛋白酶的分泌、诱导平滑肌松弛以及通过抗氧化作用预防上皮损伤[163]。有人提出,餐后释放的褪黑素可有助于餐后嗜睡[164]。

(五) 组胺

在胃肠道中,最广为人知的是组胺(histamine)在调节胃酸分泌(见第 51 章)和肠动力方面的核心作用。组胺由胃和肠的嗜铬样细胞以及肠神经产生。组胺由 L-组氨酸经组氨酸脱羧酶合成,并激活 3 种 GPCR 亚型。H1 受体存在于平滑肌和血管内皮细胞上,与磷酸脂肪酶 C 活化有关。因此,H1 受体介导了组胺诱导的许多过敏反应。胃壁细胞、平滑肌和心脏肌细胞上存在 H2 受体。H2 受体结合刺激 Gs(刺激腺苷酸环化酶的 G 蛋白)并激活腺苷酸环化酶。H3 受体存在于中枢神经系统和胃肠道肠嗜铬细胞中。这些受体通过 Gi(抑制性 G 蛋白)发出信号并抑制腺苷酸环化酶[165]。组胺还可以与 N-甲基-D-天冬氨酸(N-methyl-D-aspartate,NMDA)受体相互作用,并独立于 3 种已知的组胺受体亚型,增强 NMDA 神经元的活性。与其他神经递质不同,没有已知的转运蛋白能终止组胺的作用。然而,组胺在组胺 N-甲基转移酶的作用下代谢为替甲基组胺,然后在单胺氧化酶 B 和乙醛脱氢酶的作用下降解为替甲基咪唑乙酸。

(六) 一氧化氮

一氧化氮(nitric oxide,NO)是 L-精氨酸通过一氧化氮合酶(nitric oxide synthase,NOS)产生的一种独特的化学信使[166]。目前已知 3 种类型的 NOS。Ⅰ型和Ⅲ型又分别称为内皮型 NOS 和神经元型 NOS,并具有结构性活性。NOS 活性的微小变化可通过细胞内钙的升高而发生。只有当细胞被特异性炎性细胞因子激活时,NOS(Ⅱ型)的诱导形式才明显。这种形式的 NOS 能够产生大量的 NO,并且不依赖于钙。NOS 经常与肠神经系统神经元中的 VIP 和 PACAP 共定位[167]。

NO 作为一种不稳定的气体,半衰期相对较短。与大多数神经递质和激素不同,NO 不通过膜结合受体发挥作用。相反,NO 容易扩散到邻近细胞中直接激活鸟苷酸环化酶(图 4.8),NO 活性因其氧化为硝酸盐和亚硝酸盐而终止。许多肠神经利用 NO 向邻近细胞发出信号,诱导上皮细胞分泌、血管舒张或肌肉松弛。NO 也由巨噬细胞和中性粒细胞产生,帮助杀死入侵的生物体[168]。

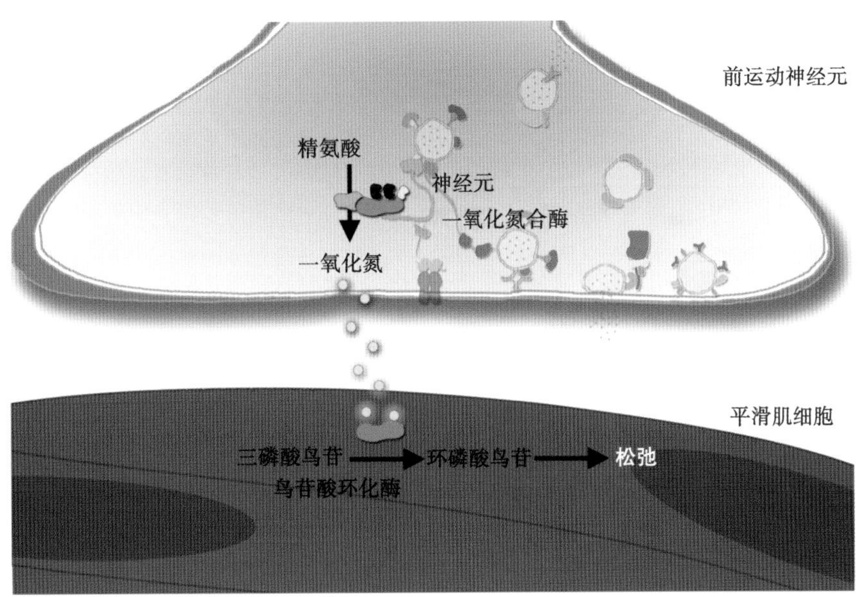

图 4.8　通过一氧化氮(NO)松弛平滑肌张力。NO 由精氨酸经一氧化氮合酶合成,穿过质膜弥散进入平滑肌细胞。NO 结合并激活鸟苷环化酶,将鸟苷三磷酸转化为 cGMP。cGMP 可引起平滑肌松弛。(Modified from Alberts B,Bray D,Lewis J,et al,eds. Molecular Biology of the Cell. 4nt ed. New York:Garland Science;2002,P. 831.)

六、大麻素和其他化学递质

（一）大麻素

大麻素（cannabinoids）有3类：人工合成的大麻素、植物中发现的大麻素和内源性大麻素。特别是内源性大麻素，其具有与神经递质相似的功能，因为它们参与突触传递[169]。然而，与典型的神经递质相比，内源性大麻素信号的流动是逆行到传统的神经递质[170]。由于其亲脂性，内源性大麻素是一种膜结合分子，被认为富集在突触后神经元。因此，当释放时，内源性大麻素从突触后移动，作用于突触前大麻素受体，抑制突触前功能[171]。通过这种方式，内源性大麻素信号有助于突触后神经元调节感觉细胞递质的分泌。

有几种类型的内源性大麻素配体，包括花生四烯酸乙醇胺（anandamide）、2-花生四烯酸酰基（2-AG）、2-花生四烯酸甘油醚（Noladin ether）、N-花生四烯醇基多巴胺（NADA）、维罗汉明（virodhamine，OAE）和溶血磷脂酰肌醇。内源性大麻素以及其他大麻素通过作用于GPCR大麻素受体CB1和CB2来调节代谢和行为。这两种受体均分布于全身，但CB1主要存在于神经元和上皮化学感受细胞中，CB2主要存在于免疫系统的细胞中。

在胃肠道中，CB1受体也参与对抗促炎反应和预防结肠炎的发生[172]。内源性大麻素除了激活经典的大麻素受体外，还可以刺激GPR119等GPCR。重要的是，GPR119是在小肠内分泌细胞中发现的一种受体，其被内源性大麻素激活后触发像CCK和PYY这样的饱腹感诱导激素的释放[172]。这些发现使胃肠道内源性大麻素研究领域成为开发治疗方法的活跃领域。

（二）腺苷

腺苷（adenosine）是一种内源性核苷，通过4种GPCR亚型中的任何一种发挥作用[173]。腺苷可引起肠道平滑肌松弛，并刺激肠道分泌。腺苷还可引起外周血管舒张和参与神经疼痛通路的伤害感受器激活。

（三）细胞因子

细胞因子（cytokines）是由各种免疫调节细胞产生的一组多肽，参与细胞增殖、免疫和炎症反应。细胞因子是由特定刺激诱导的（如病原体产生的毒素），通常引起涉及其他细胞介质的复合反应，以清除异物。细胞因子可分为白细胞介素（interleukin，IL）、肿瘤坏死因子（tumor necrosis factor，TNF）、淋巴毒素、干扰素、集落刺激因子（colony-stimulating factor，CSF）和其他[174]。白介素亚型可进一步分为至少35种单独的物质，从IL-1到IL-35。肿瘤坏死因子有TNF-α和TNF-β两种，又称为淋巴毒素-α。干扰素是在病毒或细菌感染时产生的，有干扰素-α（又称白细胞源性干扰素或干扰素-β）和干扰素-γ两个品种。干扰素-α由T淋巴细胞产生，临床上用于治疗病毒性肝炎（见第79章和第80章）。主要的CSF是粒细胞单核吞噬细胞CSF、单核吞噬细胞CSF和粒细胞CSF。这些制剂被用于化疗诱导的中性粒细胞减少症和骨髓移植后的骨髓支持。趋化因子可诱导和传播炎症，分为CXC（α趋化因子）和CC（β趋化因子）两组。其他细胞因子，如转化生长因子-β（transforming growth factor，TGF-β）和血小板衍生生长因子（platelet-derived growth factor，PDGF），具有增殖作用。

七、激素和神经递质的重要性

（一）胃肠道生长和异常生长

胃肠道组织的生长是细胞增殖和衰老之间的平衡。许多因素参与了胃肠黏膜的维护。营养素和其他肠腔内因素刺激肠黏膜的生长，是维持正常消化和吸收功能所必需的。激素和递质作为第二信使，通常在食物摄入后分泌，并介导对胃肠道的许多营养作用。它们在细胞增殖中起着关键作用。肠增生的改变主要表现为萎缩、增生、异型增生或恶性肿瘤（见第1章）。除了前面提到的GLP-2外，还有几种对胃肠道具有重要促生长作用的生长因子，包括表皮生长因子（epidermal growth factor，EGF）、TGF-β、胰岛素样生长因子（insulin-like growth factor，IGF）、FGF、PDGF家族的肽、肝细胞生长因子、三叶因子和许多细胞因子（包括IL）[175]。以下列出了其中一些受体的重要特性。

（二）生长因子受体

生长因子通过与特定的细胞表面受体相互作用来调节细胞增殖。这些受体是膜蛋白，具有生长因子配体的特异性结合位点。当配体与其受体在同一细胞内相互作用时，就会出现一种不寻常的信号形式。例如，存在于成纤维细胞系细胞内表面的PDGF受体被细胞内配体激活。这一过程被称为胞内分泌信号转导。然而，大多数肽生长因子与不同细胞上的受体相互作用以调节增殖。

生长因子受体可以是含有一个跨膜区域的单个多肽链，如EGF的受体，也可以由两个亚基异二聚体组成，其中一个亚基含有跨膜结构域，另一个亚基位于细胞内，但与跨膜亚基共价结合。异二聚体也可以二聚化形成由4个亚基组成的受体（如IGF受体）。配体与其受体的结合通常引起两个或多个受体的聚集并激活内在酪氨酸激酶的活性。生长因子受体与配体结合时也具有自身磷酸化的能力。此外，受体酪氨酸激酶活性可能使信号转导中重要的其他细胞内蛋白磷酸化。自身磷酸化减弱了受体的激酶活性，通常导致受体下调和内化。受体自身磷酸化位点的突变可能导致构成型受体活性和细胞转化。生长因子受体可能与各种细胞内信号通路偶联，包括腺苷酸环化酶、磷脂酶C、钙-钙调素蛋白激酶、MAP激酶和核转录因子。因此，生长因子在胃肠道的大多数细胞中发挥着重要和不同的作用。因此，生长因子受体或下游信号蛋白的突变，会导致细胞生长不受调节和肿瘤形成并不奇怪（见第1章）。

生长因子的一个重要作用是调节转录因子表达的能力，转录因子可以调节许多其他基因的表达[176]。早期反应基因如jun和fos在配体结合后被迅速激活，并控制许多其他参与细胞增殖的基因的表达。其他重要的转录因子包括c-myc和核因子κB（NF-κB）。后者以无活性形式存在于细胞质中，与配体结合后转移至细胞核，在那里激活其他转录因子。NF-κB 是调控细胞增殖和炎症的关键靶点。最初在视网膜母细胞瘤中发现的磷酸化形式的 Rb-1，是一种与转录因子 p53 复合的细胞增殖抑制剂。Rb-1 的去磷酸化释放 P53，从而激活导致细胞增殖的其他基因。

几乎胃肠道的所有生长因子都具有旁分泌作用。然而，许多生长因子也具有自分泌甚至内分泌作用。很明显，分泌到肠腔中的生长因子和其他信号分子可具有重要的局部生物学作用。在循环中发现的生长因子的远距离效应可能对某些类型癌的生长非常重要，特别是肺癌和结肠癌。

（三）表皮生长因子

表皮生长因子（EGF）是第一个被发现的生长因子。它是一个结构相关且具有类似相关受体的生长因子家族的原型。该家族的其他成员包括 TGF-α、双调蛋白和肝素结合 EGF。EGF 与尿抑胃素（urogastrone，最初从尿液中分离出来）结构相同，尿抑胃素可抑制胃酸分泌并促进胃溃疡愈合。EGF 由颌下腺和十二指肠的 Brunner 腺分泌。EGF 可能与胃肠道管腔细胞相互作用以调节增殖。EGF 对胃黏膜具有重要的营养作用，EGF 受体的广泛分布表明，EGF 对整个肠道的各种细胞具有促有丝分裂的作用。据报道，EGF 受体与梅特里埃病患者（Minitrier 病、巨大肥厚性胃炎）的胃黏膜增生相关[177]。而且，两名患者进行了阻断配体与 EGF 受体结合的单克隆抗体的有效治疗[178]。

基于 EGF 受体在某些肿瘤的生长和存活中起着关键作用的证据，EGF 受体被认为是人类癌症实验性治疗的重要靶点。已对单克隆抗体以及小分子酪氨酸激酶抑制剂治疗人类肿瘤进行了临床评估[179]。

（四）转化生长因子-α

转化生长因子-α（TGF-α）由胃肠道的大多数上皮细胞产生，并通过 EGF 受体发挥作用。因此，它与 EGF 具有相同的营养特性。认为其在黏膜损伤后胃重建中起着关键作用。此外，它似乎在肠道肿瘤中很重要，因为大多数胃癌和结肠癌均产生 TGF-α（见第 54 章及第 127 章）。

（五）转化生长因子-β

转化生长因子-β（TGF-β）肽家族具有多种生物学作用，包括刺激增殖、分化、胚胎发育和细胞外基质的形成[180]。与 TGF-α 受体相比，有三种不同的 TGF-β 受体[181]。TGF-β 在几乎所有的细胞类型中调节细胞生长和增殖，并能增强自身从细胞中产生。TGF-β 很可能在炎症和组织修复中起着关键性作用。TGF-β 通过其化学诱导特性募集成纤维细胞增加胶原生成。这种作用可能产生有益或有害的影响，这取决于其沉积部位和产生的丰度。例如，TGF-β 可能在手术后粘连的发生中起关键作用[182]。

（六）胰岛素样生长因子

胰岛素基因的选择性剪接产生两种结构相关的肽，IGF Ⅰ和 IGF Ⅱ[183]。IGF 至少通过 3 种不同的 IGF 受体发出信号。IGF Ⅰ受体是一种酪氨酸激酶，IGF Ⅱ受体与甘露糖 6-磷酸受体相同。虽然 IGF 在胃肠道中的确切功能尚不清楚，但它们在肠上皮中具有强效的促有丝分裂活性。IGF Ⅱ似乎对胚胎发育至关重要。

（七）成纤维细胞生长因子和血小板衍生生长因子

至少已确定有 7 种相关的 FGF[184]。这些肽类对包括间充质细胞在内的各种细胞类型具有促有丝分裂作用，并可能在器官形成和新生血管形成中发挥重要作用[185]。尽管 PDGF 并非胃肠道所特有的，但它是研究最透彻的生长因子之一。它对成纤维细胞的生长十分重要，其受体在肝脏和整个胃肠道中表达，似乎能促进伤口愈合。

（八）三叶因子

三叶因子（trefoil factor）（pS2、解痉素和肠三叶因子，也分别称为 TTF1、2 和 3）是在整个胃肠道中表达的蛋白质家族[186]。它们具有共同的结构，具有 6 个半胱氨酸残基和 3 个二硫键，形成了三叶草外观，稳定了肠腔内的肽。pS2 肽在胃黏膜中产生，解痉素在胃窦和胰腺中发现，肠三叶因子在整个小肠和大肠中产生。这些肽由胃中的黏液颈细胞或肠道中的杯状细胞产生，并分泌到肠道的黏膜表面。三叶因子很可能作用于上皮细胞的顶端表面，在那里它们对胃肠黏膜具有促生长的特性。

其他多肽信号也可能通过 GPCR（C 蛋白偶联受体）具有促生长作用。3 个重要的例子包括胃泌素、CCK 和胃泌素释放肽（GRP）。胃泌素刺激胃的肠嗜铬样细胞生长，并诱导含有壁细胞的泌酸黏膜增殖[187]。胃泌素与胃的 CCK-2 受体结合，激活磷酸脂肪酶 C 和 Ras 通路，最终分别导致蛋白激酶 C 和 MAP 激酶的激活。MAP 激酶也可被生长因子典型的酪氨酸激酶受体激活，引起参与细胞增殖的转录因子磷酸化。在一些细胞中，cAMP 和 PKA 通过激活核转录因子，如 cAMP 反应元件结合（蛋白、CREB）对细胞生长发挥协同效应。然而，在其他细胞中，cAMP 拮抗增殖。因此，根据细胞类型，刺激 cAMP 产生的激素可能会增强 EGF、IGF 和 PDGF 等生长因子的作用。某些结肠癌细胞拥有 CCK-2 受体，并对胃泌素的增殖效应作出反应。而且，胃泌素可能由一些结肠癌产生，使其能够发挥自分泌作用促进癌的生长[188]。但循环胃泌素是否会引起结肠癌的发生尚不清楚。

八、糖尿病与胃肠道

胃肠激素在胰岛素分泌和葡萄糖稳态调节中发挥着重要作用。这些激素控制着促进营养物质消化和吸收的过程，以及对进入血液的营养物质的处置。特别是，肠肽通过 3 种不同的机制控制餐后血糖水平：①刺激胰腺 β 细胞分泌胰岛素；②通过抑制胰高血糖素分泌抑制肝糖原异生；③通过抑制胃排空延迟碳水化合物向小肠的输送[189]。这些作用中的每一个都能减少正常情况下进食后发生的血糖波动。

餐后释放的胰岛素中约 50% 是胃肠激素促进胰岛素分泌的结果[190]。这种相互作用被称为肠-胰岛轴，刺激胰岛素释放的肠肽被称为肠促胰岛素。主要的肠促胰岛素为 GLP-1 和 GIP。GLP-1 不仅刺激胰岛素分泌，还可增加 β 细胞数量，抑制胰高血糖素分泌,延缓胃排空。当葡萄糖水平升高时,GIP刺激胰岛素分泌,并减少胰高血糖素刺激的肝糖原生成[191]。因此,当摄入膳食时,葡萄糖被吸收,刺激GLP-1和GIP分泌。然后血液循环中的葡萄糖刺激β细胞产生胰岛素,肠促胰岛素与葡萄糖共同作用增加胰岛素水平,从而显著增强了这种作用。

餐后高血糖也可以通过延迟食物从胃到小肠的输送来控制,使胰岛素的升高与葡萄糖的吸收速度同步。一些延迟胃排空的肠道激素已被证明可以降低餐后血糖水平(框4.2)[189]。胰淀素(胰岛淀粉样多肽)是一种由37个氨基酸组成的肽,主要与胰岛素一起在胰岛的β细胞中合成。尽管最初人们认识到它能够形成与β细胞丢失相关的淀粉样沉积物,但最近发现它能抑制胰高血糖素分泌、延缓胃排空和诱导饱腹感[192]。肥胖患者的胰岛素抵抗与胰岛素和胰淀素水平均升高有关。

框4.2 调节餐后血糖水平的胃肠肽

刺激胰岛素释放
胰高血糖素样肽-1
葡萄糖依赖性促胰岛素肽
胃泌素释放肽
胆囊收缩素(增强氨基酸刺激的胰岛素释放)
胃泌素(存在氨基酸时)
血管活性肠肽(增强葡萄糖刺激的胰岛素释放)
垂体腺苷酸环化酶激活肽(增强葡萄糖刺激的胰岛素释放)
胃动素
延缓胃排空
胆囊收缩素
胰淀素
胰泌素
抑制胰高血糖素释放
胰淀素

2型糖尿病的特征是高循环胰岛素水平和胰岛素抵抗。此外,餐后胰岛素水平未适当升高,发生显著的高血糖,这与肠促胰岛素效应受损一致。在2型糖尿病中,保留了GIP的分泌,然而,GIP的促胰岛素分泌作用降低[193]。尽管确切的原因尚不清楚,但GIP刺激的胰岛素释放缺陷在胰岛素分泌的晚期最为明显。与GIP相反,胰岛素抵抗2型糖尿病患者的GLP-1分泌减少。较低的GLP-1水平是由分泌受损而不是激素降解增加引起的[194]。与GIP不同,胰岛素对GLP-1输注的反应得以保留,表明β细胞可以对这种肠促胰岛素激素作出正常反应。这些观察结果表明,应用GLP-1给药可能是治疗与糖尿病相关高血糖症的可行方法[195]。越来越多的证据表明,在2型糖尿病中可能发生β细胞衰竭,支持使用肠促胰岛素激素,如GLP-1,或通过二肽基肽酶-4(DPP-4)延缓GLP-1降解的药物来增强β细胞功能[196,197]。目前临床上已有几种肠促胰岛素类似物用于糖尿病的治疗[198]。

九、食欲的胃肠调节

进餐期间,摄入的营养物质与口腔和胃肠道细胞相互作用。胃和小肠的内分泌细胞具有与胃肠激素分泌相关的受体。然后胃肠肽(见第7章和第9章)被释放到周围空间,在那里它们发挥旁分泌作用或被摄取到血液循环中,作为激素发挥其功能[199]。这些递质中的每一种都有利于生物体所必需的营养物质的摄入、消化、吸收或分布。一些胃肠激素控制摄入食物量的大小,被称为饱腹感信号。饱腹感激素具有几个特性[200]。第一,它们减少进餐量。第二,阻断其内源性活性导致进餐量增加。第三,食物摄入量的减少并不是厌恶食物的结果。第四,激素的分泌是由摄入通常会导致停止进食的食物引起的(表4.2)。大多数饱腹感信号与从胃肠道到后脑的神经上的特异性受体相互作用。肠内分泌细胞与神经突触的发现提出了一种可能性,即饱腹信号最初受到神经传递信号的调节,随后受到激素信号的加强[57,201]。其他感觉系统,如味觉,整合了两种机制来完成短期和长期的感觉信号。

表4.2 调节饱腹感和摄食量的胃肠肽类

减少摄食量	增加摄食量
胆囊收缩素(CCK)	生长激素释放肽
胰高血糖素样肽-1	
肽酪氨酸-酪氨酸(PYY3-36)	
胃泌素释放肽	
胰淀素	
载脂蛋白(A-IV)	
生长抑素	

CCK是研究最广泛的饱腹感激素之一。CCK以时间和剂量依赖性的方式减少动物和人类的摄食量[202],这种效应是由位于迷走神经末梢的CCK-1受体介导的[203]。CCK对摄食量的影响是一种已证实的生理作用,因为给予CCK受体拮抗剂可诱导饥饿并导致进餐量增加。CCK还能延迟食物从胃中排空的速度,这可以解释为什么当胃膨胀时,CCK的饱腹感作用最明显。总之,这些发现表明CCK为终止进餐提供了信号。

GLP-1由回肠和结肠中的肠内分泌细胞产生,随着对肠道中的食物发生反应而释放。尽管GLP-1的主要作用是刺激胰岛素分泌,但它也会延迟胃排空。而且,输注GLP-1会增加饱腹感,产生饱腹感,从而减少食物摄入,而不会引起厌恶感[204]。GLP-1受体存在于脑室周围核、下丘脑背内侧核和下丘脑弓状核中,这些核是调节饥饿的重要区域。与CCK一样,GLP-1的中枢给药可抑制食物摄入。

PYY也由回肠和结肠的肠内分泌细胞产生。两种形式的PYY被释放到循环中,PYY1-36和PYY3-36。PYY1-36与神经肽Y受体家族的所有亚型结合,而PYY3-36对Y2受体具有很强的亲和力。当给予动物时,PYY3-36会导致摄食量减少,缺乏Y2受体的小鼠对PYY3-36的厌食作用具有抵抗力,表明PYY3-36通过该受体传递饱腹感信号[205]。PYY3-36在人体中被证明可降低饥饿评分和热量摄取量[206]。有趣的是,大多数参与饱腹感的胃肠肽受体也在脑中发现,它们在脑中介导相似的饱腹感效应。这可能代表了用于类似目的的肽信号的保守性。

瘦素被称为肥胖信号,因为它释放到血液中的量与体脂的量成比例，被认为是能量平衡的长期调节因子。与 CCK 一起，瘦素能减少摄食量，比单独使用任何一种药物都能更大程度地降低体重[133]。因此，能量平衡的长期调节因子似乎可以通过减少进餐量影响短期调节因子，从而促进体重减轻。

饥饿与开始进餐是密切相关的。生长激素释放肽是唯一已知的具有促食欲作用的循环胃肠激素[149]。胃饥饿素由胃产生，其水平在开始进餐前突然升高，进食后迅速降低，表明它是开始进餐的信号。与此作用相一致的是，研究证明给予抗饥饿素抗体或饥饿素受体拮抗剂可抑制摄食[207]。目前尚不清楚胃饥饿素是否对饥饿者发生的饥饿痛和可闻及的肠鸣音有反应。

减肥手术，尤其是 Roux-en-Y 胃旁路手术，是病态肥胖长期减肥最有效的手术。尽管认定与该方法伴随的体重减轻是胃容量减少和热量吸收不良的结果，但最近的证据表明，餐后胃饥饿素释放减少和 PYY 释放过多，可能是由激素因素导致的热量摄入减少。

（张莉　袁农 译，曾翔俊 校）

参考文献

第二部分　胃肠道营养

第 5 章　营养原则和胃肠病患者的营养评估

Joel B. Mason 著

章节目录

一、基本营养概念 …… 51
（一）能量存储 …… 51
（二）能量代谢 …… 52
（三）蛋白质类 …… 54
（四）碳水化合物 …… 55
（五）脂类 …… 55
（六）主要矿物质 …… 56
二、微量营养素 …… 56
（一）维生素 …… 60
（二）微量元素 …… 60
（三）影响微量营养素需求量的生理学和病理生理学因素 …… 61
三、饥饿 …… 62
四、营养不良 …… 63
（一）蛋白质能量营养不良 …… 63
（二）蛋白质能量营养不良引起的生理损害 …… 65
五、营养评估技术 …… 66
（一）病史 …… 66
（二）体格检查 …… 66
（三）人体测量学 …… 67
（四）蛋白质热量状态的功能测量 …… 68
（五）蛋白质热量状态的生物化学检测 …… 68
（六）评估目标人群的快速筛查工具 …… 69
六、住院患者积极的营养支持 …… 70
（一）接受大手术的营养不良患者 …… 70
（二）与酒精相关的失代偿肝病住院患者 …… 71
（三）放射治疗患者 …… 71

关注患者的营养需求会对医疗结局产生重要的积极影响，这在胃肠道疾病和肝脏疾病的治疗中尤其重要。因为这些疾病不仅会改变机体营养物质的代谢和需求，而且还会干扰营养物质的摄入和吸收。患者的营养管理仍是一个在临床治疗中尚未得到充分重视和有效解决的问题。

对营养问题的关注不足或错误理解，其部分原因是没有区分出从营养治疗中获益的患者和对营养治疗无反应的患者，这也是很多临床试验未能证明营养支持对住院患者有益的原因所在。本章的主要目的是提供必要的科学性原则和实用性工具，从而识别出能够受益于营养管理的患者并为其制定恰当的营养计划提供必要的指导。营养摄入过量或不足都可能影响临床结局，因此，明确患者需要的热量和蛋白质是制定最适宜营养计划的前提。

一、基本营养概念

（一）能量存储

机体内储存的能量会持续氧化提供能量，储存在脂肪组织中的甘油三酯（triglyceride，TG）是人体主要的能量储备，其在禁食状态下对生存至关重要（表 5.1）。TG 的高能量密度和疏水特性使其每单位质量释放的能量是糖原的 5 倍。TG 以油脂的形式紧密地储存在脂肪细胞中，每克 TG 氧化后释放的热量为 9.3kcal/g。糖原以胶体的形式储存在细胞内，每克糖原约含 2g 水，氧化时产生的热量仅为 4.1kcal/g。但是脂肪组织不能为骨髓、红细胞、白细胞、肾髓质、眼部组织和周围神经等组织提供能量，因为这些组织不能氧化脂质，因此它们需要葡萄糖提供能量。在耐力运动中，肌肉组织中的糖原和甘油三酯为运动中的肌肉提供了重要的能量来源。

表 5.1　体重 70kg 男子的内源性能量储存

组织	能量底物	质量	
		g	kcal
脂肪贮存组织	TG	13 000	121 000
肝脏	蛋白质	300	1 200
	糖原	100	400
	TG	50	450
肌肉	蛋白质	6 000	24 000
	糖原	400	1 600
	TG	250	2 250
血液	葡萄糖	3	12
	TG	4	37
	游离 FA	0.5	5

FA，脂肪酸；TG，甘油三酯。

（二）能量代谢

机体各器官功能的正常运行、代谢的平衡维持、热量的产生和机械运动的进行都需要持续的能量供给。机体每日总能量消耗（total energy expenditure，TEE）由 3 部分组成：静息能量消耗（resting energy expenditure，REE）（约占 TEE 的 70%）、体力活动能量消耗（约占 TEE 的 20%）以及食物热效应（约占 TEE 的 10%）。在计算门诊患者的能量需求时，应该将 TEE 的后两个组成部分考虑在内。但是对于住院的重症患者而言，体力活动所消耗的能量通常可以忽略，进食热效应所消耗的能量可以通过下文的预测方程进行计算。

1. 静息能量消耗

REE 表示一个人在两餐之间、非饮食状态下、安静清醒时的能量消耗。在这种情况下，健康成年人每小时消耗的热量约为 1kcal/kg 体重。机体不同组织的能量需求差异显著（表 5.2）比如肝脏、肠道、大脑、肾脏和心脏的质量约占机体总体重的 10%，而它们的能量消耗却占了 REE 的 75%。相比之下，静息状态下骨骼肌的能量消耗约占 REE 的 20%，其质量却占了体重的 40%。脂肪组织消耗的 REE 不到 5%，质量却占了体重的 20% 以上。

表 5.2 70kg 体重男性各组织的静息能量需求

组织	组织质量		消耗能力		
	g	%体重	kcal/d	kcal/（g 组织·d）	%REE
肝脏	1 550	2.2	445	0.28	19
胃肠道	2 000	3.0	300	0.15	13
大脑	1 400	2.0	420	0.30	18
肾脏	300	0.4	360	1.27	15
心脏	300	0.4	235	0.80	10
骨骼肌	28 000	40.0	400	0.014	18
脂肪贮存组织	15 000	21.0	80	0.005	4

REE，静息能量消耗。

通过间接测热法可以对 REE 进行准确的评估，具体方法是测量受试者休息时二氧化碳的产生量和氧气的消耗量，从而估计体内的能量消耗情况。虽然间接热量测定是计算 REE 的金标准，但是这种方法的实用性和必要性尚有待商榷。此外，可以使用一些经验方程式来估算静息能量需求（表 5.3）[1-4]。其中 Harris-Benedict 和 Mifflin 方程主要是针对成人设计的，而世界卫生组织（WHO）公布的计算公式则适用于儿童和成人，这些方程适用于健康受试者。对于身体成分异常的超重人群可采用间接测热法[5]。

表 5.3 静息能量消耗的常用计算公式

Harris-Benedict 方程式		
男性	66+（13.7×W）+（5×H）-（6.8×A）	
女性	665+（9.6×W）+（1.8×H）-（4.7×A）	
Mifflin 方程式		
男性	（10×W）+（6.25×H）-（5×A）+5	
女性	（10×W）+（6.25×H）-（5×A）-161	
WHO 公式		
年龄/岁	**男性**	**女性**
0~3	（60.9×W）-54	（60.1×W）-51
3~10	（22.7×W）-495	（22.5×W）+499
10~18	（17.5×W）+651	（12.2×W）+746
18~30	（15.3×W）+679	（14.7×W）+996
30~60	（11.2×W）+879	（8.7×W）+829
>60	（13.5×W）+987	（10.5×W）+596

注：按 kcal/d 计算。A，年龄（岁）；H，身高（cm）；W，体重（kg）。

对于急性病患者而言，大部分情况下可以使用预测方程进行计算，但是由于炎症反应和代谢应激对能量消耗具有显著影响，因此有必要在计算公式中加入相应的校正因子。蛋白质能量营养不良（PEM）和无叠加疾病的低热量饮食均能使 REE 比实际体型的预期值降低 10%~15%，而急性病或创伤则导致机体的能量消耗显著增加（见下文）。

2. 体力活动的能量消耗

体力活动对能量消耗的影响取决于日常活动的强度和持续时间。专业运动员在比赛中能够将 TEE 增加 10~20 倍。表 5.4 所示的活动系数均以 REE 的倍数表示，可用于估算患者活动时的 TEE。某一特定体力活动所消耗的能量等于（每小时 REE）×（活动系数）×（活动持续时间，以小时为单位）。TEE 表示所有日常活动（包括休息期间）所消耗能量的总和。

表 5.4 不同水平体力活动的相对热效应

活动水平	示例	活动因子
静息		1.0
非常轻	站立、驾驶、打字	1.1~2.0
轻度	步行 3.3~4.8km/h，购物，轻松的家务活动	2.1~4.0
中度	步行 4.8~6.4km/h，骑自行车，园艺、擦洗地板	4.1~6.0
重度	跑步，游泳，攀登，打篮球	6.1~10.0

Adapted from Alpers DA，Stenson WF，Bier DM. Manual of nutritional therapeutics. Boston：Little，Brown；1995.

3. 食物的热效应

进食或摄入营养物质会增加机体的新陈代谢。日常饮食中蛋白质对代谢率的影响最大,其次是碳水化合物,然后是脂肪。一餐包含所有这些营养物质的膳食通常会使机体的代谢率增加 5%~10%。

4. 住院患者推荐的能量摄入

为住院患者制定营养计划时,通常不需要使用床边间接热量测定仪来获得能量消耗的实际值。我们可以用一些简单的计算公式来解决其实用价值和准确性不足的问题,兹举例说明如下。

(1) 结合代谢应激因素的方法

代谢应激(即任何引起一定程度全身炎症的损伤或疾病)将通过多种机制增加代谢率(见后文)。能量消耗的增加与应激的大小大致成正比[6]。因此,可通过将预测的 REE(由 Harris-Benedict 或 WHO 方程确定)乘以应激因子来估计急性病患者的每日总能量需求:

$$TEE = REE \times 应激因子$$

表 5.5 描述了住院患者中伴随一些常见疾病和临床情况的代谢应激因素。由于 Mifflin 方程并非设计用于估计 TEE 与应激因子,因此在本文中不建议使用。在急性病住院患者中,通常无须纳入活性因子。

成人住院患者的另一种简单的替代公式是(虽然准确性有一些降低):

- 无应激或轻度应激患者实际体重(actualbody weight, ABW):20~25kcal/(kg·d)
- 中度应激患者:25~30kcal/(ABW·d)
- 严重应激患者:30~35kcal/(ABW·d)

表 5.5　估计住院患者总能量消耗的代谢应激因素

损伤或疾病	相对应激因子*
二度或三度烧伤,>40% BSA	1.6~2.0
多发性创伤	1.5~1.7
二度或三度烧伤,20%~40% BSA	1.4~1.5
严重感染	1.3~1.4
急性胰腺炎	1.1~1.2
二度或三度烧伤,10%~20% BSA	1.2~1.4
长骨骨折	1.2
腹膜炎	1.2
单纯性术后状态	1.1

*假设健康对照组的应激因子为 1.0。

BSA,体表面积。

From Psota T, Chen KY. Measuring energy expenditure in clinical populations:rewards and challenges. Eur J Clin Nutr 2013;67:436-42.

需要注意的是,当 ABW 不能正确反映去脂体重时,需要对上述公式进行调整。对于超出理想体重(ideal body weight, IBW)30%以上的肥胖者,需要使用校正后的 IBW 代替 ABW(理想体重见表 5.6)。因为使用校正后的 IBW 有助于避免高估患者的能量需求,具体的计算公式为:校正后的 IBW = IBW +0.5(ABW-IBW)[6]。对于因细胞外液体潴留(如腹水)而导致体重明显增加的患者,需要使用 IBW 计算患者的能量需求。

表 5.6　25 岁男性和女性的理想体重与身高的关系

男性,中等身材			女性,中等身材		
身高/(ft/inch)	体重/lb		身高/(ft/inch)	体重/lb	
	范围	中位数		范围	中位数
5′1″	113~124	118.5	4′8″	93~104	98.5
5′2″	116~128	122	4′9″	95~107	101
5′3″	119~131	125	4′10″	98~110	104
5′4″	122~134	128	4′11″	101~113	107
5′5″	125~138	131.5	5′0″	104~116	110
5′6″	129~142	135.5	5′1″	107~119	113
5′7″	133~147	140	5′2″	110~123	116.5
5′8″	137~151	144	5′3″	113~127	120
5′9″	141~155	148	5′4″	117~132	124.5
5′10″	145~160	153	5′5″	121~136	128.5
5′11″	149~165	157	5′6″	125~140	132.5
6′0″	153~170	161.5	5′7″	129~144	136.5
6′1″	157~175	166	5′8″	133~148	140.5
6′2″	162~180	171	5′9″	137~152	144.5
6′3″	167~185	176	5′10″	141~156	148.5

注:通过假设男性 1inch 鞋跟、女性 2inc 鞋跟以及男性和女性室内服装重量分别为 5lb 和 3lb,校正裸体体重和身高。

1ft≈0.3m;1inch≈2.54cm;1lb≈0.45kg。

Data from Metropolitan Life Insurance Company. New height standards for men and women. Statistical Bulletin 1959;40:1-4.

(2) **无应激因素的计算方法**

预测患者每日能量消耗的最准确和广泛验证的公式是不包含应激因素的计算公式。然而,这个公式需要患者的每分钟通气量,因此仅限于使用机械通气的患者[4],这个公式是:TEE=(用 Mifflin 方程计算出的 REE 值×0.96)+(T_{max}×167)+(V_e×31)-6 212,其中 T_{max} 表示过去 24 小时内的最高体温(以摄氏度为单位),V_e 是以升为单位的每分钟呼气量。

表 5.7 是基于 BMI 估算住院患者每日总能量需求的简化替代方法[7],虽然该方法的可靠性和准确性有所不足,但是其不需要计算每分钟通气量,因此更简单更实用。当使用这种不精确的方法来估算住院患者的能量消耗时,需要结合临床经验,因为疾病会影响计算结果(如腹水、全身性水肿等)。

表 5.7　基于体重指数(BMI)估计的住院患者的能量需求

BMI/(kg/m²)	能量需求量*/[(kcal/(kg·d)]
<15	35~40
15~19	30~35
20~29	20~25
≥30	15~20

注:在计算胰岛素抵抗或重症患者的能量需求时,应考虑每个 BMI 类别内的较低范围,以降低与过度喂养相关的高血糖和感染风险。*建议将这些值用于重症患者和所有肥胖患者,在估计非重症患者的能量需求时,需要增加总热量的 20%。

(3) **热量补充与避免高血糖症**

在过去的 20 年里,急性病患者的热量补充趋向于使用更保守的计算方法,其原因之一是急性病及其治疗方案往往会加重原有的糖尿病或产生新的葡萄糖耐量异常。高血糖是肠内营养和肠外营养的常见不良后果,尤其是肠外营养。这个问题对于重症监护室(ICU)患者更为重要,因为即使是轻微的高血糖也会导致严重的临床结局。在外科 ICU(SICU)[8]和内科 ICU(surgical ICU,MICU)[9]患者的高质量临床试验发现,与血糖值维持在 215mg/dL 以下的患者相比,随机接受强化胰岛素治疗且血糖水平维持在 111mg/dL 以下的患者的发病率显著降低。随机接受严格血糖调控的 SICU 患者的死亡率也显著降低。尽管在 MICU 研究中,严格血糖控制导致的死亡率降低仅在入住 MICU 超过 3 天的患者中实现。同样,在儿科 ICU(pediatrics,surgical ICU,PICU)患者的临床试验中,通过强化年龄特异性血糖控制,继发性感染、PICU 住院时间和死亡率均降低[10]。这些观察结果几乎可以肯定是急性高血糖在先天免疫系统中产生的众多机制损害的临床表现[11]。然而,在 ICU 严格控制血糖的临床获益并不一定总能产生[12],而是以更频繁的低血糖发作为代价的[8-10,12]。因此如何严格控制血糖的问题仍然存在争议。

一项 ICU 患者的大型多中心试验中,极度严格控制(目标血糖范围为 81~108mg/dL)产生的低血糖风险增高 13 倍,死亡率也显著增加[13]。因此,这是过度的血糖控制。一个专家小组最近建议制定相应的临床方案,使 ICU 患者的血糖水平保持在 150mg/dL 或者更低,最好是通过连续输注胰岛素,每 1~2 小时监测一次,以便进行适当的调整,并避免血糖值低于 70mg/dL[14]。在重症患者中进行的 29 项试验的荟萃分析结果概括了之前观察到的 SICU 和 MICU 患者之间的差异[15]。总体而言,在随机接受严格血糖控制的患者中,败血症的相对风险降低了约 25%,尽管这种获益主要归因于 SICU 患者,在 SICU 患者中,其败血症的减少几乎近 50%,在 MICU 患者中未观察到获益,在任何类别的重症患者中也未观察到总死亡率的明显差异。

超重和肥胖患者在 ICU 患者中所占的比例越来越高,如何给这些患者补充适当的能量尚有争议。目前主流的策略是低热量进食,即每天供给估算能量需求的 60%~70%(或 11~14kcal/kg ABW),同时每天摄入蛋白质 2~2.5g/kg IBW,后者能够降低净蛋白分解代谢和去脂体重损失风险。临床实践发现,"低热量进食"策略能够有效控制血糖、预防代谢并发症的发生(如高碳酸血症、高甘油三酯血症)。有文献对 ICU 中肥胖患者的低热量进食和一些重要的临床终点指标(包括死亡率、住院时间、机械通气持续时间和感染性并发症)进行系统的回顾性研究发现,与正常热量营养支持相比,尚未就支持低热量营养支持的净效益或风险达成一致的共识[16]。因此,这个问题仍然悬而未决。

(三) 蛋白质类

在人类蛋白质中常见 20 种不同的氨基酸(amino acid,AA)。一些氨基酸的碳骨架不能由机体合成(包括组氨酸、异亮氨酸、亮氨酸、赖氨酸、蛋氨酸、苯丙氨酸、苏氨酸、色氨酸、缬氨酸和精氨酸)因此被称为必需氨基酸。其他氨基酸(包括甘氨酸、丙氨酸、丝氨酸、半胱氨酸、酪氨酸、谷氨酰胺、谷氨酸、天冬酰胺和天冬氨酸)在大多数情况下是非必需的,因为它们可以由内源性前体或必需氨基酸制成。在疾病状态和早产儿中,某些非必需氨基酸的细胞内和(或)血浆浓度通常非常低,被认为是条件必需氨基酸。长期以来,在全胃肠外营养中加入超元素谷氨酰胺,以补充危重疾病期间该 AA 的细胞内耗竭。然而,严格进行的临床试验显示,静脉补充谷氨酰胺无相关获益[17-19]。在一项多器官衰竭重症成人的随机安慰剂对照多中心、多国试验中,补充谷氨酰胺与死亡率增加相关[18]。显然,在急性疾病期间补充条件必需的 AA 不一定意味着获益[20]。然而,人们仍然对确定危重疾病(如早产儿)的临床情况感兴趣,其中补充条件必需的氨基酸可能改善临床结局[20]。精氨酸、半胱氨酸、甘氨酸、谷氨酰胺、脯氨酸和酪氨酸是属于这一类氨基酸。

平均体重为 75kg 的人体内大约含有 12kg 蛋白质。与脂肪和碳水化合物相比,人体中没有蛋白质储存库,过量的蛋白质摄入会被分解代谢,之后以氮的形式排出体外。蛋白质摄入不足会导致氮含量出现净损失。在美国,蛋白质的每日推荐摄入量为 0.8g/(kg·d),这是根据平均需求量[0.6g/(kg·d)]加上在健康人群中观察到的生物学差异性需求之后得出的结果。在维持机体氮平衡方面,静脉注射 AA 与口服相同 AA 成分的蛋白质一样有效。

个体蛋白质的需求量主要受到以下几个因素的影响,如非蛋白质热量、总能量需求、蛋白质质量和患者的营养状况(表 5.8)。当机体的能量摄入不能满足能量需求时,蛋白质的需求随之增加。这种能量需求增加的幅度与能量供应不足的程度成正比。因此,氮平衡同时反映了蛋白质摄入量和能量平衡。如果总热量不足,有时仅通过补充热量就可以纠正负氮平衡。

表 5.8　推荐的每日蛋白质摄入量

临床状况	每日蛋白质需求量/(g/kg IBW)
正常	0.80
代谢应激	1.0~1.6
血液透析	1.2~1.4
腹膜透析	1.3~1.5

注:需要额外的蛋白质需求来补偿特定患者人群(例如烧伤、开放性伤口、蛋白丢失性肠病或肾病患者)中过量的蛋白质损失。对于未接受透析治疗的肾功能不全患者以及某些肝病和肝性脑病患者,可能需要降低蛋白质的摄入量。

IBW,理想体重。

随着机体代谢应激和代谢率的增加,氮排泄量相应的成比例增加,两者的定量关系为"2mg(N)/kcal REE"。某种程度上,氮排泄量的增加是机体代谢应激消耗更多蛋白质的结果,这对于管理患者的营养需求有两个重要的启示:一是疾病通过提高分解代谢和新陈代谢率,增加了对蛋白质的绝对需求量(表 5.8),即需求量与应激程度成正比;二是由于急性病患者中有更多的能量底物来自蛋白质,因此如果总热量中有更大比例的热量来自蛋白质,那么就能更容易地实现氮平衡。在健康成年人中,大约 10% 的总热量来自蛋白质;而在患者中,如果有 15%~25% 的总热量来自蛋白质,那么氮平衡就更容易实现。此外,蛋白质的需求量也取决于蛋白质来源中必需 AA 是否充足。必需 AA 的不足会降低机体对营养的摄取效率,进而导致机体的蛋白质需求量增加。在正常成年人中,蛋白质总需求量中大约 15%~20% 应为必需 AA。

特殊的患者(如烧伤、开放性伤口、蛋白质丢失性肠病或肾病患者)需要补充额外的蛋白质以补充蛋白质的流失。对于没有进行充分透析的急性肾功能衰竭患者,则需要减少蛋白质的摄入量。因为在这种情况下,氮质血症的增加与蛋白质供给之间存在正相关关系。急性肾功能衰竭患者在进行充分的透析后,可根据实际的需求量增加蛋白质摄入量,包括摄入额外的蛋白质以补充透析造成的蛋白质损失(见表 5.8)。对于肝性脑病患者而言,基础的药物治疗就可以实现氮平衡,因此不需要限制蛋白质摄入量;对药物干预没有应答的患者可从适度的蛋白质限制中获益[0.6g/(kg·d)]。

氮平衡

氮平衡通常作为蛋白质平衡的替代指标(即摄入的蛋白质或氨基酸是否足以补充蛋白质的净损失)。氮平衡可以通过计算氮摄入量与氮损失量(尿液、粪便、皮肤和体液中)之间的差值进行评估。临床上,成年人可用以下公式进行计算:氮平衡=(营养物质中氮含量(g))-(尿素氮(g)+4)。每 6.25g 蛋白质(或 AA)中含有大约 1g 氮。尿素氮占尿氮总量的大约 80%,该公式中额外增加的 4g 氮是为了补充其他途径的氮损失。氮平衡可以替代蛋白质平衡,因为无论机体健康与否,人体中约 98% 的氮都存在于蛋白质中。

正氮平衡(即摄入量>消耗量)代表蛋白质合成代谢和净增加,而负氮平衡代表蛋白因分解代谢发生了净损失。例如,每天 1g 的负氮平衡表示每天 6.25g 蛋白质损失,这相当于每天 30g 的含水肌肉组织损失。临床上,由于饮食中的氮摄入量被高估,而不完整的尿液收集等造成的氮损失量被低估,因此氮平衡在大多数情况下表现为正平衡。此外,由于机体中存在一个不稳定的"氮池",这往往会抑制和延缓因蛋白质摄入量改变而观察到的相应变化,因此最好在蛋白质供应发生实质性变化的 4 天之后再进行氮平衡评估。

(四) 碳水化合物

日常膳食中主要的可消化碳水化合物(包括淀粉、蔗糖和乳糖)需要经过完全消化后才能产生单糖(葡萄糖、果糖和半乳糖)。此外,机体每天还需要摄入 5g~20g 不可消化的碳水化合物(包括可溶性纤维和不可溶性纤维)。通过糖酵解过程,细胞可以将葡萄糖代谢为三碳化合物,或者通过糖酵解和三羧酸循环(tricarboxylic acid,TCA)将葡萄糖代谢为水和二氧化碳并产生三磷酸腺苷(adenosine triphosphate,ATP)。

在碳水化合物的摄入方面,人们无须选择特定的饮食模式,这是因为葡萄糖可以由 AA 或甘油内源性合成。由于碳水化合物和蛋白质代谢之间的相互作用,碳水化合物也是一种重要的能量来源。碳水化合物的摄入能够刺激胰岛素分泌、抑制肌肉蛋白分解、刺激肌肉蛋白合成以及减少氨基酸产生的内源性葡萄糖。此外,葡萄糖也是红细胞、白细胞、肾髓质、眼组织、周围神经和大脑所必需的能量物质。当这些组织的葡萄糖需求得到满足时(大约为 150g/d),碳水化合物和脂肪对于节省蛋白质的效果是相似的[21]。

(五) 脂类

脂类主要由 TG、甾醇类和磷脂类组成,这些化合物不仅是机体重要的能量来源,而且是合成类固醇激素、前列腺素、血栓素和白三烯的前体物质,还是细胞膜的结构成分和必需营养物质的载体。膳食脂质主要由 TG 组成,TG 含有 16~18 个碳的饱和与不饱和长链脂肪酸(fatty acid,FA)。使用脂肪作为"燃料"时,需要水解内源性或外源性 TG 和细胞摄取释放的 FA(见第 102 章)。长链 FA 通过肉碱依赖性转运系统,通过线粒体外膜和内膜递送。一旦进入线粒体后,FA 通过 β-氧化降解为乙酰辅酶 A(coenzyme A,CoA),然后进入 TAC 循环。因此,利用脂肪作为燃料的能力取决于功能正常的线粒体。与机体衰老或失调相关的线粒体丰度或功能的降低有利于使用碳水化合物作为"燃料"[22,23]。

必需脂肪酸

人类缺乏产生 n-3 型(碳 3 和碳 4 之间的双键)和 n-6 型(碳 6 和碳 7 之间的双键)FA 系列所需的去饱和酶。亚油酸(C18:2、n-6)和亚麻酸(C18:3、n-3)均是必需脂肪酸,为防止这两类 FA 缺乏,其摄入量应分别占每日热量总摄入量的 2% 和 0.5%。在胃肠外营养出现之前,仅在婴儿中发现必需脂肪酸缺乏症(essential fatty acid deffciency,EFAD),表现为伴有血浆 FA 特征特异性变化的鳞屑性皮疹(见后文)。由于脂肪组织中的必需 FA 储备充足,所以成人很少出现 EFAD。然而,目前已知在接受长期全胃肠外营养(TPN)且缺乏肠外脂质的重度短肠综合征成人中,异常 FA 特征结合 EFAD 的临床综合征有时会发生[24]。患有其他原因引起的中度至重度脂肪吸收不良(脂肪排泄分数>20%)且不依赖TPN的成人也经常表现出EFAD的生化特征[25]。但这种生化状态是否会带来不良的临床后果尚不清楚。此外,如果没有外源性必需氨基酸(EFA)来源,缺乏任何脂肪来源的TPN可能导致成人EFAD。EFAD的血浆模式-2最早可在开始基于葡萄糖的TPN后10天和任何临床特征开始之前观察到。在这种情况下,EFAD可能是由于TPN引起的血浆胰岛素浓度升高所致,因为胰岛素抑制脂肪分解,从而抑制内源性必需脂肪酸的释放。EFAD的生化诊断标准为血浆脂肪酸谱中2种必需脂肪酸的绝对和相对缺乏,完整的临床EFAD综合征包括脱发、鳞屑性皮炎、毛细血管脆性增加、伤口愈合不良、感染易感性增加、脂肪肝和婴儿和儿童生长迟缓。

(六) 主要矿物质

主要矿物质是指机体大量需要的无机营养物质(>100mg/d),这些无机营养物质对维持机体的电解质平衡、体液平衡和正常细胞功能具有重要作用。营养不良和营养充足均会对主要矿物质平衡产生巨大影响。健康成年人的大量矿物质缺乏和矿物质推荐每日膳食供给量(recommended daily dietary allowance,RDA)的评估见表5.9。

表5.9 主要矿物质需求和缺乏评估

矿物质	肠溶性	肠胃外	缺乏的症状或体征	实验室评估	
				检测	备注
钙	1 000~1 200mg	5~15mmol	代谢性骨病、手足抽搐、心律失常	24小时尿钙双能X线吸收测量法	反映最近摄入量反映骨钙含量
镁	300~400mg	5~15mmol	虚弱,抽搐,心律失常、低钙血症	血清镁、尿镁	可能不会反映人体贮存
磷	800~1 200mg	20~60mmol	虚弱、疲劳、白细胞和血小板功能障碍、溶血性贫血、心力衰竭、氧合功能降低	血浆磷	可能不会反映人体贮存
钾	2~5g	60~100mmol	虚弱、感觉异常、心律失常	血清钾	可能不会反映人体贮存
钠	0.5~5g	60~150mmol	血容量减少,虚弱	尿氮	可能不会反映人体贮存 临床评估最佳

二、微量营养素

微量营养素(包括维生素和微量元素)是维持机体健康所必需的多种饮食成分。微量营养素的生理作用因其成分而异,一些微量营养素在生物酶中可作为辅酶或假体基团,另一些微量营养素则可作为生化底物或激素。而在某些情况下,微量营养素的功能无法进行准确定义。一般而言,维持机体生理功能所需微量营养素的平均每日膳食摄入量以毫克或更小的计量单位来衡量。通过这种方法,我们可以将微量营养素与常量营养素(如碳水化合物、脂肪、蛋白质)和常量矿物质(如钙、镁、磷)进行区分。

人体对饮食中微量营养素的需求由许多因素决定,如生物利用度、维持正常生理功能所需量、性别和年龄、影响营养物质代谢的疾病或药物以及某些生活习惯(如吸烟、饮酒)。美国国家科学院食品和营养委员会定期更新的饮食指南中推荐了每一种微量营养素的需求量,以满足所有健康人群的营养需求。1998年至2001年期间,该委员会对每种微量营养素的RDA进行了修订,成人微量营养素的需求量详见表5.10和表5.11。考虑到人群的个体差异,RDA的设定比平均需求量高出2个标准差,如此才能满足97%人口的需求量。因此,摄入略低于RDA的微量营养素就能够满足特定个体的健康需求。该指南还为大多数微量营养素划定了"可耐受上限(tolerable upper limit,TUL)",TUL指无不良健康风险的每日最大口服摄入量(见表5.10和表5.11)。对于进行TPN的个体而言,有关微量营养素推荐摄入量的相关数据远远少于RDA。因此,制定相关的指南非常必要,表5.12中提供了此类建议。

表5.10 维生素的显著特征

维生素种类	缺乏(RDA)	毒性(TUL)†	状态评估
维生素A	毛囊角化过度和夜盲为早期症状。结膜干燥症、角膜变性(角膜软化)和快速增殖的上皮去分化是后期缺乏指征。点滴状(Bitot)斑点(结膜或角膜局灶区域出现泡沫状外观焦)是干燥症的指征。角膜破坏和视网膜功能障碍引起的失明可能接踵而至。感染易感性增加也是一个结果(1μg视黄醇相当于3.33IU维生素A;女性,700μg;男性,900μg)	在成人中,>150 000μg可能引起急性毒性:致命性颅内高压、皮肤剥脱和肝细胞损伤。习惯性每日摄入量>10 000μg可发生慢性毒性:常见脱发、共济失调、骨骼和肌肉疼痛、皮炎、唇炎、结膜炎、假性脑瘤、肝纤维化、高脂血症和骨质增生较。单次大剂量维生素A(30 000μg)或妊娠早期习惯性摄入>4 500μg/d可致畸。类胡萝卜摄入过多引起以皮肤变黄为特征的良性病症(3 000μg)	血浆中的视黄醇浓度,以及乳汁和泪液中的维生素A浓度是合理准确的状态指标。毒性最好通过血浆中视黄醇酯水平升高来评估。夜视暗适应的定量测量和视网膜电图是有用的功能测试

表 5.10　维生素的显著特征(续)

维生素种类	缺乏(RDA)	毒性(TUL)†	状态评估
维生素 D	缺乏会导致新形成的骨矿化减少,这种情况在儿童期称为佝偻病,在成年人称为软骨病。缺乏也会导致晚年骨质疏松症,常见于胃旁路手术后。骨骺生长板的扩张和用未矿化的骨基质替代正常骨是佝偻病的主要特征,后者的特征也是骨软化症的特征。导致骨骼畸形和病理性骨折。可发生血清钙和磷酸盐浓度降低(1μg 相当于 40IU;15μg,年龄 19~70 岁;20μg,年龄>70 岁)	过量可导致血清中钙和磷酸盐浓度异常升高;可能发生转移性钙化、肾损伤和精神改变(年龄>9 岁为 100μg)	主要循环代谢物 25-羟基维生素 D 的血清浓度是全身状态的极好指标,但晚期肾病(4~5 期)除外,其肾 1-羟基化受损可导致单羟基和双羟基维生素 D 浓度解离,因此测量血清 1,25-二羟基维生素 D 是必需的
维生素 E	由饮食不足引起的缺乏在发达国家很少见。通常见于早产儿、脂肪吸收不良者和无 β 脂蛋白血症者。发生红细胞脆性,可产生溶血性贫血。神经元变性可产生周围神经病变、眼肌麻痹和脊髓后柱破坏。如果缺乏症不能及早纠正,神经系统疾病往往是不可逆的。可能导致早产儿发生溶血性贫血和晶状体后纤维增生。据报道可抑制细胞介导的免疫(15mg)	据报告,维生素 K 依赖性促凝血剂水平降低,口服抗凝剂增强和白细胞功能受损。据报告,每天 800mg 的剂量可略微增加出血性脑卒中的发生率(1 000mg)	α-生育酚的血浆或血清浓度最常用。通过将该值表示为每毫克总血浆脂质可获得额外的准确度。红细胞过氧化物溶血试验并不完全具有特异性,但可用于测量细胞膜对氧化的敏感性
维生素 K	除母乳喂养的新生儿(可能引起新生儿出血性疾病)、脂肪吸收不良或正在服用干扰维生素 K 代谢的药物(如华法林、苯妥英、广谱抗生素)的成年人以及服用大量维生素 E 和抗凝药物的个体外。缺乏综合征并不常见。通常表现为过度出血(女性 90μg,男性 120μg)	快速静脉输注维生素 K_1 与呼吸困难、潮红和心血管性虚脱相关;这可能与溶解溶剂中的分散剂有关。补充可能干扰基于华法林的抗凝治疗。服用大量维生素原甲萘醌的孕妇可能分娩时发生溶血性贫血、高胆红素血症和核黄疸(TUL 未确定)的婴儿	凝血酶原时间通常用作功能性维生素 K 状态的指标;其对维生素 K 缺乏既不敏感也无特异性。测定空腹血浆维生素 K 是一个准确的指标。羧基化不足的血浆凝血酶原也是一种准确的指标,但仅用于检测缺乏状态,应用不太广泛
维生素 B_1	经典缺乏症(脚气病)在食用精米饮食的亚洲人群中仍然流行。在全球范围内,酗酒、慢性肾透析和减肥手术后持续恶心和呕吐是常见的促发因素。高碳水化合物摄入量增加了人体对维生素 B_1 的需求。轻度缺乏通常会产生烦躁、疲劳和头痛。较明显的缺乏可产生周围神经病变、心血管和脑功能障碍。心血管受累(湿性脚气病)包括心力衰竭和外周血管阻力降低。脑部疾病包括眼球震颤、眼肌麻痹和共济失调(Wernicke 脑病),以及幻觉、短期记忆受损和虚构(Korsakoff 精神病)。缺损综合征在 24 小时内对肠外硫胺素有反应,但在某一阶段后部分或完全不可逆(女性为 1.1mg;男性为 1.2mg)	过量摄入主要经尿液排泄,尽管据报告每天>400mg/d 的肠外剂量可引起嗜睡、共济失调和胃肠道张力降低(TUL 未确定)	维生素 B_1 状态的最有效的测量指标是 RBC 转酮醇酶活性系数,其测量加入外源性 TPP 前后的酶活性;来自缺乏个体的红细胞在加入 TPP 后酶活性显著增加。也可对血液或尿液中的硫胺素浓度进行测量
维生素 B_2	缺乏通常与其他 B 族维生素缺乏同时存在。单独缺乏核黄素可引起鼻咽黏膜充血和水肿、唇炎、口角炎、舌炎、脂溢性皮炎和正色素性、正细胞性贫血(女性为 1.1mg;男性为 1.3mg)	目前尚无关于人体毒性的报道(TUL 尚未确定)	尚未在人体中报告毒性(未确定 TUL)最常见的评估方法是测定红细胞中谷胱甘肽还原酶的活性系数(该测试对葡萄糖-6-磷酸脱氢酶缺乏的个体无效)。测量血液和尿液浓度是不太理想的方法

表 5.10 维生素的显著特征(续)

维生素种类	缺乏(RDA)	毒性(TUL)[†]	状态评估
维生素 B_3	糙皮病是典型的维生素缺乏症,常见于以玉米为主要能量来源的人群。在中国、非洲和印度部分地区仍有流行。腹泻、痴呆(或伴有焦虑或失眠的症状)和在阳光暴露区域发生的色素性皮炎是典型的特征。舌炎、口腔炎、阴道炎、眩晕和烧灼样感觉迟钝是早期体征。偶尔发生于类癌综合征,因为色氨酸被转移到其他合成途径(女性,14mg;男性,16mg)	人体毒性主要是通过检查降血脂作用的研究而得知,包括潮红、高血糖、肝细胞损伤和高尿酸血症(35mg)	状态评估存在问题;维生素的血液水平不可靠。烟酸代谢物 N-甲基烟酰胺和 2-吡啶酮的尿排泄测量被认为是最有效的评估手段
维生素 B_5	缺乏症是罕见的;仅由于其喂食半合成饮食或食用已用于治疗阿尔茨海默病的拮抗剂(如高泛酸钙)而报道。人类实验性孤立性缺乏可产生疲劳、腹痛和呕吐、失眠和四肢感觉异常(5mg)	据报告,当剂量超过 10g/d(未确定TUL)时,会发生腹泻	泛酸的全血和尿液浓度是该状态的指标;血清水平被认为不准确
维生素 B_6	缺乏通常与其他水溶性维生素缺乏同时出现。中度至重度耗竭时出现口腔炎、口角炎、舌炎、易激怒、抑郁和意识模糊;也有 EEG 异常和婴儿惊厥的报道。异烟肼、环丝氨酸、青霉胺、乙醇和茶碱都是可抑制 B_6 代谢的药物(年龄 19~50 岁,1.3mg;>50 岁,女性 1.5mg,男性 1.7mg)	长期使用剂量超过 200mg/d(成人)可能引起周围神经病变和光敏反应(100mg)	有许多有用的实验室评估方法。血浆或红细胞 PLP 水平最常见。口服色氨酸负荷后黄嘌呤酸的尿排泄或红细胞转氨酶(ALT、AST)的活性指数均为维生素 B_6 依赖性酶活性的功能指标
维生素 B_7	孤立性缺乏罕见。通过饮食不足、长期给予缺乏维生素的 TPN 和摄入大量含有亲和素的生蛋清(亲和素是一种以高亲和力结合生物素的蛋白质,使其生物素不可用)。发生精神状态改变、肌痛、感觉过敏和厌食。以后出现,脂溢性皮炎和脱发。生物素缺乏通常伴有乳酸酸中毒和有机酸尿(30μg)	尚未报告人体毒性,儿童剂量高达 60mg/d(TUL 未确定)	在缺乏状态下,生物素的血浆和尿液浓度降低。在缺乏患者中也观察到柠檬酸甲酯、3-甲基巴豆酰甘氨酸和 3-羟基异戊酸的尿液浓度升高
维生素 B_9	育龄妇女最易发生缺乏。典型的维生素缺乏是巨幼细胞性贫血。骨髓中造血细胞增大,细胞核不成熟,反映 DNA 合成无效。外周血涂片显示大卵圆形细胞和多形核白细胞,平均超过 3.5 个核小叶。其他快速增殖的上皮(如口腔黏膜、胃肠道)的巨幼细胞变化分别产生舌炎和腹泻。柳氮磺胺吡啶和苯妥英钠抑制吸收,易致缺乏。习惯性低摄入量可能会增加患结直肠癌的风险[400μg 膳食叶酸当量(DFE);1μg 叶酸=1μg DFE;1μg 食物叶酸=0.6μg DFE]。	每日剂量>1 000μg 可部分纠正维生素 B_{12} 缺乏的贫血,因此掩盖(可能加重)相关的神经病变。据报告,大剂量可降低易发生癫痫发作个体的癫痫发作阈值。很少报告胃肠外给药可引起分散剂(1 000μg)的过敏现象	血清叶酸水平反映短期叶酸平衡,而红细胞叶酸更好地反映组织状态。血清同型半胱氨酸水平在缺乏早期升高,但无特异性,因为维生素 B_{12} 或 B_6 缺乏、肾功能不全和年龄较大也可能引起升高
维生素 B_{12}	除了严格的素食者外,饮食不足是一种罕见的缺乏导致原因。绝大多数缺乏病例来自肠道吸收丧失——恶性贫血、胰腺功能不全、萎缩性胃炎、SIBO 或回肠疾病的结果。巨幼细胞性贫血和其他上皮细胞的巨幼细胞变化(见叶酸)是持续耗竭的结果。可能发生周围神经、脊髓后柱和外侧柱以及脑内神经脱髓鞘。发生精神改变、抑郁和精神病。血液学和神经系统并发症可能独立发生。叶酸补充剂剂量超过 1 000μg/d 可部分纠正贫血,从而掩盖(或可能加重)神经病变并发症(2.4μg)	晶态 B_{12} 制剂很少报告过敏反应,可能是由于杂质,而不是维生素(TUL 未确定)	血清或血浆浓度通常是准确的。伴有神经系统并发症的轻微缺陷在≥60 岁的人群中越来越被认识,最好通过同时测量血浆维生素 B_{12} 和①血清甲基丙二酸(MMA)或②人全反钴胺素-Ⅱ(全 TC-Ⅱ)的浓度来确定,因为后者是细胞缺陷的敏感指标。正常低血浆维生素 B_{12} 浓度在 200~350pg/ml(=148~258pmol/L)伴 MMA 升高或全 TC-Ⅱ 降低,应视为缺乏状态

表 5.10　维生素的显著特征(续)

维生素种类	缺乏(RDA)	毒性(TUL)[†]	状态评估
维生素 C	显性缺乏症在发达国家并不常见。典型的维生素缺乏是坏血病,以疲劳、抑郁和结缔组织广泛异常为特征(如牙龈发炎、瘀点、毛囊周围出血、伤口愈合障碍、卷发、角化过度和体腔出血)。在婴儿中,可能发生骨化和骨生长缺陷。吸烟可降低血浆和白细胞维生素 C 水平(女性为 75mg;男性为 90mg;对吸烟者的需要量增加 35mg/d)	用量超过 500mg/d(成人)有时会引起恶心和腹泻。补充维生素 C 使尿液酸化,以及草酸盐合成增强的可能性,引起了人们对肾结石的关注,但这尚未得到证实。补充维生素 C 可能会干扰基于氧化还原电位的实验室检查(如粪便潜血试验、血清胆固醇、血清葡萄糖)。长期服用高剂量维生素 C 补充剂的戒断应在 1 个月内逐步进行,因为似乎确实发生了调节,引起了对反弹性坏血病的关注(2 000mg)	血浆抗坏血酸浓度反映了最近的饮食摄入量,而白细胞水平更密切地反映了组织储备。在任何给定的条件下,女性的血浆水平比男性高约 20%

RDA,推荐每日膳食供给量;由美国食品和营养委员会为女性(F)和男性(M)成人制定,1999—2001 年(2010 年更新维生素 D 和钙)。在某些情况下,数据不足以确定 RDA,在这种情况下,列出了委员会确定的适当摄入量(AI)。

[†]TUL,可耐受上限;由美国食品和营养委员会为成年人制定,1999—2001 年。

EEG,脑电图;PLP,5-磷酸吡哆醛;RBC,红细胞;TPP,焦磷酸硫胺素。

Adapted from Goldman L, Ausiello D, Arend W, et al, editors. Cecil textbook of medicine. 23rd ed. Philadelphia: WB Saunders; 2014.

表 5.11　微量矿物质特征

矿物质种类	缺乏(RDA)	毒性(TUL)[†]	状态评估
铬	人类缺乏仅在长期接受铬含量不足的 TPN 患者的人体中。统一观察高血糖或糖耐量受损。还报告了血浆游离脂肪酸浓度升高、神经病变、脑病和氮代谢异常。也有报道。改善在轻度葡萄糖不耐受但其他方面健康的个体中,补充铬是否可改善的葡萄糖耐量仍然存在争议(女性为 25μg;男性为 35μg)	经口摄入后的毒性并不常见,似乎仅限于对胃的刺激。在空气中暴露可引起接触性皮炎、湿疹、皮肤溃疡和支气管肺癌(未建立 TUL)	血浆或血清铬浓度是铬状态的粗略指标;当数值显著高于或低于正常范围时,似乎具有意义
铜	膳食缺乏罕见;在仅用牛奶喂养的早产儿和低出生体重儿以及接受不含铜的长期 TPN 的个体中观察到。临床表现包括皮肤和毛发脱色、神经功能障碍、白细胞减少和低色素性、小细胞性贫血、骨骼异常和伤口愈合不良。贫血由铁吸收障碍引起,因此是缺铁性贫血的一种继发性形式。除贫血和白细胞减少外,在 Menkes 病中也观察到铜缺乏的表现,这是一种与铜摄取受损(900μg)相关的罕见遗传性疾病	急性铜中毒在过量经口摄入和烧伤皮肤吸收铜盐后有报道。较轻的表现包括恶心、呕吐、上腹痛和腹泻;严重时可随之发生昏迷和肝细胞损伤。在低至 70μg/(kg·d)的剂量下可观察到毒性。还描述了慢性毒性。肝豆状核变性是一种罕见的遗传性疾病,与铜蓝蛋白水平异常降低和铜蓄积有关,特别是在肝脏和大脑中的积聚。最终导致这两个器官的损害(10mg)	目前还没有实用的检测边缘缺陷的方法。通过血清铜和铜蓝蛋白浓度降低,以及红细胞超氧化物歧化酶活性降低,可以可靠地检测到显著的缺乏
氟	婴儿摄入<0.1mg/d 和儿童摄入 0.5mg/d 与龋齿发生率增加有关。成年人的最佳摄入量为 1.5~4.0mg/d(女性为 3mg,男性为 4.0mg)	急性摄入>30mg/kg 体重的氟化物很可能引起死亡。长期过量摄入[0.1mg/(kg·d)]会导致牙齿斑驳(氟斑牙)、肌腱和韧带钙化以及外生骨疣,并可能增加骨骼的脆性[10mg/(kg·d)]	因为不存在可靠的实验室检查,因此使用摄入量或临床评估的估计值
碘	在缺乏补充的情况下,主要依赖低碘土壤食物的人群有地方性碘缺乏。母体碘缺乏会导致胎儿碘缺乏,从而产生自然流产、死胎、甲状腺功能减退、克汀病和侏儒症。大脑快速发育持续到第二年,在此期间,碘缺乏可能诱发永久性认知缺陷。在成人中,甲状腺发生代偿性肥大(甲状腺肿),同时并伴有不同程度的甲状腺功能减退(150μg)	大剂量(成人>2mg/d)可能通过阻断甲状腺激素合成而诱发甲状腺功能减退。对既往缺乏的个体补充>100μg/d 偶尔会诱导甲状腺功能亢进(1.1mg)	尿碘排泄是一种有效的实验室评估手段。血液中促甲状腺激素(TSH)水平是一种间接的、不完全特异性的评估手段。人群的碘营养状况可以通过甲状腺肿的患病率来评估

表 5.11 微量矿物质特征(续)

矿物质种类	缺乏(RDA)	毒性(TUL)[†]	状态评估
铁	世界上最常见的微量营养素缺乏。育龄妇女因为月经失血、妊娠、哺乳而构成高危险人群。钩虫感染是全球最常见的病因。典型的缺乏是低色素性小细胞性贫血。还观察到舌炎和凹甲[匙状指(趾)甲]。易疲劳常是贫血出现前的早期症状。在儿童中,严重程度不足以引起贫血的轻度缺乏与行为障碍和学习成绩差有关(绝经后女性 8mg;男性为 8mg;绝经前女性为 18mg)。	当习惯性饮食摄入量极高、肠道吸收过多、重复肠外给予铁或这些因素联合存在时,通常会发生铁超负荷。过多的铁储备通常在网状内皮组织中蓄积,几乎不会造成损伤(含铁血黄素沉着)。如果超负荷继续下去,铁最终将开始在肝实质、胰腺、心脏和滑膜等组织中蓄积,损伤这些组织(血色病)。遗传性血色病是一种常见隐性性状纯合性的结果。在纯合子中观察到肠道对铁的过度吸收(45mg)	负铁平衡最初导致骨髓中储存铁耗竭;骨髓活检和血清铁蛋白浓度是这种耗竭的准确和早期指标。随着缺铁乏变得更加严重,血清铁(SI)降低,总铁结合力(TIBC)增加;铁饱和度(=SI/TIBC)<16% 提示铁缺乏。在缺乏状态的后期会出现小红细胞症、低色素性和贫血。血清铁蛋白水平升高或铁饱和度>60% 可怀疑铁超负荷,尽管无论铁状态如何,全身性炎症均可升高血清铁蛋白水平
锰	锰缺乏尚未在人类中得到最终证实。据说可引起低胆固醇血症、体重减轻、毛发和指(趾)甲改变、皮炎和维生素 K 依赖性蛋白合成受损(女性,1.8mg;男性,2.3mg)	尚不清楚人类经口服摄入的毒性。中毒性吸入可引起幻觉、精神的其他改变和锥体外系运动障碍(11mg)	在锰缺乏得到更好的定义之前,适当的状态测量标准很难制定
钼	人类缺乏钼极为罕见;主要由缺乏该元素的 TPN 或亚硫酸盐胃肠外给药引起。报告导致高氧嘌呤血症、低尿酸血症、低尿硫酸盐排泄和中枢神经系统紊乱(45μg)	钼具有低毒性;在流行病学研究中,职业暴露和高饮食摄入与高尿酸血症和痛风相关(2mg)	不存在有效的临床可用评估方法。罕见的缺乏病例与低尿酸血症、高蛋氨酸血症和低水平的尿硫酸盐伴亚硫酸盐、黄嘌呤和次黄嘌呤排泄升高有关
硒	硒缺乏在北美罕见,但在长期接受缺乏硒的 TPN 的个体中观察到。这类患者有肌痛和(或)心肌病。世界上一些地区的人口,特别是中国的一些地区,硒的摄入量很少。正是在中国的这些地区,克山病呈地方性流行,这是一种以心肌病为特征的疾病。其可通过补硒(55μg)预防,但不治疗克山病	毒性与恶心、腹泻、精神状态改变、周围神经病变以及毛发和指甲脱落相关;在意外摄入 27~2 400mg(400μg)剂量的成人中观察到此类症状	红细胞谷胱甘肽过氧化物酶活性和血浆或全血硒浓度是最常用的评估方法。它们是相当准确的状态指标
锌	锌的缺乏对快速增殖的组织有其最深远的影响。轻度缺乏引起儿童生长发育迟缓。更严重的缺乏与生长停滞、致畸性、性腺功能减退和不育、味觉障碍、伤口愈合不良、腹泻、四肢和孔口周围皮炎、舌炎、脱发、角膜混浊、暗适应丧失和行为改变有关。还观察到细胞免疫功能受损。胃肠道分泌物的过度丢失(例如,通过慢性腹泻或瘘管)可能促发缺乏。肠病性肢端皮炎是一种罕见的隐性遗传性疾病,其肠道对锌的吸收受损(女性,8mg;男性,11mg)	急性锌中毒通常是由于在一天内摄入>200mg 的锌诱导(成人)。表现为上腹疼痛、恶心、呕吐和腹泻。吸入锌烟雾后可出现呼吸过度、出汗和虚弱。铜和锌竞争肠道吸收:长期摄入>25mg/d 锌可能导致铜缺乏。据报告,长期摄入>150mg/d 可引起胃糜烂、高密度脂蛋白胆固醇水平降低和细胞免疫功能受损(40mg)	常规临床使用中没有锌状态的准确指标。血浆、红细胞和毛发锌浓度经常会产生误导。尤其是已知急性疾病可降低血浆锌水平,部分是通过导致锌从血浆转移至肝脏。确定暗适应、味觉敏锐度和伤口愈合率的功能试验缺乏特异性

注:1999—2001 年美国食品和营养委员会为女性和男性成人制定的推荐每日膳食供给量(RDA)(2010 年更新了维生素 D 和钙)。在某些情况下,数据不足以确定 RDA,在这种情况下,列出了委员会发布的适当摄入量(AI)。

[†]1999—2001 年美国食品和营养委员会为成人确定的可耐受上限(TUL)。

Adapted from Goldman L, Ausiello D, Arend W, et al, editors. Cecil textbook of medicine. 22nd ed. Philadelphia: WB Saunders; 2004. With permission.

(一) 维生素

维生素分为脂溶性维生素(A、D、E、K)和水溶性维生素(详见表 5.10)两大类。脂溶性维生素不能作为辅酶,而几乎所有的水溶性维生素都能起到辅酶的作用。另外,脂溶性维生素主要通过微泡途径吸收,而水溶性维生素在肠道中的亲脂节段不会被吸收(详见第 103 章)。

(二) 微量元素

铁、锌、铜、铬、硒、碘、氟、锰、钼以及钴是人体必需的 10 种微量元素(见表 5.11)。与维生素不同,微量元素的生化功能目前尚无准确定义,但其主要的生理功能可能是作为辅基的组成部分或酶的辅助因子。

除缺铁之外,缺锌在临床中常见。胃肠道是锌排泄的主要部位,锌的缺乏对胃肠病学家来说是一个特别重要的问题。胃肠道分泌物的长期大量丢失(如炎症性肠病相关的慢性腹泻)是缺锌的常见病因之一。在这种情况下,机体对锌的需求量会成倍增加[26]。然而,缺锌的生化诊断存在不少困难(许多其他必需的微量元素也是如此)。因为人体的体液和组织中的锌浓度很低,对锌含量进行准确评估具有一定的难度。

此外,由于血清和红细胞中的锌含量与靶组织中的锌含量缺乏相关性,因此目前尚未设计出合理的检测方案。研究证实,在急性病患者中,锌从血清转移到肝脏,这又进一步弱化了测定血清中锌元素含量的价值[27]。碱性磷酸酶是一种锌元素依赖性蛋白,其在血清中的活性可以作为评估锌元素的一种功能性检测手段,但是它的临床实用价值很低。目前,对于锌缺乏的高风险患者,最好的干预措施是进行经验性补锌。需要注意的是,在TPN治疗方案中,锰元素的补充量比表5.12中的推荐量高出好几倍,这可能导致矿物质在基底神经节沉积,导致患者出现锥体外系反应和/或癫痫发作[28]。由于配置TPN使用的不同微量元素混合物中锰的含量差异很大,因此在制定相关的诊疗共识时需要特别注意。

表5.12 成人和儿童肠外微量营养素每日给药指南

微量营养素	成人	儿童
脂溶性维生素		
A	1 000μg(=3 300IU)	700μg
D	5μg(=200IU)	10μg
E	10mg(=10IU)	7mg
K	1mg	200μg
水溶性维生素		
C	100mg	80mg
B_6	4mg	1mg
B_{12}	5μg	1μg
生物素	60μg	20μg
叶酸	400μg	140μg
烟酸	40mg	17mg
泛酸	15mg	5mg
核黄素	3.6mg	1.4mg
硫胺素	3mg	1.2mg
微量元素		
铬	10~15μg	0.2μg/(kg·d)
铜	0.5~1.5mg	20μg/(kg·d)
碘*	—	—
铁	1~2mg	1mg/d
锰	0.1mg	1μg/(kg·d)
钼	15μg	0.25μg/(kg·d)
硒	100μg	2μg/(kg·d)
锌	2.5~4.0mg	50μg/(kg·d)

注:*肠外营养制剂的天然污染似乎可提供足量的碘。

成人维生素给药指南改编自 American Society of Parenteral and Enteral Nutrition (ASPEN). Board of Directors and the Clinical Guidelines Task Force. Guidelines for the use of parenteral and enteral nutrition in adult and pediatric patients. J Parenter Enteral Nutr 2002;26:144. Children's values adapted from Greene HL, Hambidge KM, Schanler R, Tsang RC. Guidelines for the use of vitamins, trace elements, calcium, magnesium, and phosphorus in infants and children receiving total parenteral nutrition: report of the Subcommittee on Pediatric Parenteral Nutrient Requirements from the Committee on Clinical Practice Issues of the American Society for Clinical Nutrition. Am J Clin Nutr 1988;48:1324; Am J Clin Nutr 1989;49:1332; and Am J Clin Nutr 1989;50:560.

(三)影响微量营养素需求量的生理学和病理生理学因素

1. 年龄

机体生理的进化贯穿着整个生命周期。随着年龄的不断增长,机体对某些微量营养素的需求也会发生相应的变化。目前已经研发出了针对老年人群的RDA。大多数人群的平均维生素 B_{12} 水平随着年龄增长而显著下降,主要是由于年龄相关性萎缩性胃炎的患病率逐渐升高以及由此导致的蛋白质结合维生素 B_{12} 吸收障碍所致[29]。大约10%至15%的老年流动人口存在维生素 B_{12} 缺乏,并且血浆中维生素 B_{12} 的水平低于正常范围(150pg/ml~300pg/ml)的老年人可能会发生神经变性。因此,建议使用细胞消耗维生素 B_{12} 的敏感检测指标(如血清甲基丙二酸、血清维生素 B_{12})进行诊断[30]。专家建议,老年人应该摄入晶体形式的维生素 B_{12} 作为补充剂,而不能仅仅依赖于食物中天然存在的蛋白质结合形式的维生素 B_{12}。从新修订的RDA中可以看出,与年轻人相比,老年人需要大量的维生素 B_6、维生素D和钙来维持健康(见表5.10和表5.11)。

2. 吸收不良和消化不良

维生素 B_{12} 主要在回肠中吸收,而其他的脂溶性和水溶性微量营养素则主要在小肠近端吸收。因此,胃肠道近端发生的弥漫性黏膜性病变可能导致多种微量营养素缺乏。然而,即使在没有近端小肠疾病的情况下,胆道疾病、小肠细菌过度繁殖和慢性胆汁淤积也可能影响胆汁酸浓度,从而影响脂溶性维生素的吸收。脂肪吸收不良通常与脂溶性维生素的选择性缺乏有关。很多维生素缺乏相关疾病的临床表现并不明显导致确诊困难,这对于维生素E缺乏导致的脊髓小脑退化具有灾难性、不可逆的影响[31]。此外,脂溶性维生素缺乏是囊性纤维化和先天性胆道闭锁症的常见并发症,这类患者通常存在着明显的脂肪吸收不良,但是也有一些例外情况(慢性胆汁淤积性肝病患者在晚期阶段出现不明显的脂肪吸收不良症状),这意味着对其进行监测十分必要[31]。当机体出现严重的脂肪吸收不良时,可能需要通过静脉输注维生素进行纠正。当出现严重的脂肪吸收不良时,口服使用经过化学修饰的维生素D和维生素E可以有效预防肠道对其进行破坏。聚乙二醇琥珀酸形式的维生素E(Nutr-E-Sol)对无法吸收常规α-生育酚的严重脂肪吸收不良患者非常有效[32]。同样,羟基化修饰的维生素D[1-羟基维生素D(Hectorol)和1,25-二羟基维生素D(Rocaltrol)]可用于对传统维生素D产生抗药性的患者。为预防和减少维生素D中毒的风险,在使用羟基化修饰的维生素D进行治疗的最初几周内,需要密切监测患者的血清钙水平,这是因为羟基化修饰的维生素D的临床疗效明显优于维生素 D_2 或维生素 D_3。相比之下,另外一种可用的脂溶性维生素水溶性制剂(将一种传统形式的维生素A或维生素E溶解在聚酯盐80(如Aquasol-E, Aquasol-A)之中,在改善机体吸收能力方面的功能尚不明确。

消化不良通常是由慢性胰腺功能障碍引起的,治疗不及时会导致脂肪吸收不良和脂溶性维生素缺乏。临床上,除了导致脂肪吸收减少的情况(如萎缩性胃炎或长期服用质子泵抑制药物),其他维生素 B_{12} 的缺乏罕见[33]。对于长期使用质子泵抑制剂(proton pump inhibitor,PPI)的患者是否需要检测维生素 B_{12} 水平,目前尚有争议[34]。萎缩性胃炎或 PPI 引起的维生素 B_{12} 吸收不良可通过补充少量的结晶型维生素 B_{12} 进行治疗。组胺-2 受体拮抗剂也能抑制蛋白质结合的维生素 B_{12} 吸收,但是其抑制作用比 PPI 要弱[35]。研究表明,许多药物可能对机体微量营养素的吸收产生不利影响,这是因为药物和微量营养素之间存在着复杂的相互作用,表 5.13 中论述了一些常见的作用机制。有关药物与微量营养素之间相互作用的内容请参考相关文献[36]。

表 5.13 药物对微量营养素状态的影响

药物	营养素	机制
氯乙胺嘧啶	维生素 D、叶酸	吸收养分,减少吸收
右旋安非他明,芬氟拉明,芬氟拉明,左旋多巴	潜在的所有微量营养素	导致厌食症
异烟肼	维生素 B_6	损害维生素 B_6 的摄取
NSAID	铁	消化道出血
青霉胺	锌	增加肾脏排泄量
PPI	维生素 B_{12}	中度促进细菌过度生长,减少胃酸/胃蛋白酶,损害吸收
柳氮磺胺吡啶	叶酸	损害吸收并抑制叶酸依赖酶

From Goldman L, Ausiello D, Arend W, et al, editors. Cecil textbook of medicine. 22nd ed. Philadelphia: WB Saunders; 2004.

三、饥饿

当出现能量缺乏和(或)蛋白质缺乏时,机体会启动一系列的代偿性机制从而减少能量缺乏造成的病理生理影响,这些代偿性机制包括了降低代谢率、维持葡萄糖稳态、保存体内氮、增加脂肪组织对 TG 摄取,从而满足机体的能量需求。

如果要了解急性病是如何破坏上述代偿性机制的,则需要了解机体在没有基础疾病的情况下是如何适应禁食的。禁食 24 小时内最容易获得的能量物质(包括循环葡萄糖、脂肪酸、甘油三酯、肝糖原和肌糖原)被用作能量来源。这些"能源商店"提供的能量总和大约为 5 000kJ(1 200kcal),对于一个体质量为 70kg 的个体而言,尚不能满足机体一天的能量需求。肝糖原的生成和氧化代谢减少,全身脂肪分解增加,进而提供额外的脂肪酸和酮体[37]。脂肪组织中 TG 氧化释放的脂肪酸约占禁食前 24 小时能量消耗的 65%。在禁食的最初几天里,大脑和血细胞等组织需要的葡萄糖(约占总能量消耗的 20%)只能通过糖酵解途径获得。由于脂肪酸不能被糖酵解转化为碳水化合物,因此它们必须使用葡萄糖或可以转化成葡萄糖的底物,来自骨骼肌的糖原载脂蛋白(主要是丙氨酸和谷氨酰胺)是其底物的主要来源,大约 15% 的 REE 是由蛋白质氧化提供的[38]。糖异生对肝糖原产量的贡献随着肝糖原分解速率的降低而增加。禁食 24 小时后,机体肝糖原的储备水平下降到正常水平的 15%。

在经历短期禁食状态(第 1~14 天)时,机体会产生多种减少瘦质量损失的适应性反应。首先是血浆中的胰岛素水平下降,肾上腺素水平增加,以及对儿茶酚胺敏感性的增加刺激脂肪组织分解[39,40]。此外,机体还会增加脂肪酸向肝脏转运的能力,血浆胰高血糖素与胰岛素浓度的比值也会增大,这些反应能够有效增加肝脏产生酮体的能力。当机体禁食第 3 天时,酮体生成率达到最高水平;在第 7 天时,血液中的酮体浓度增加了 75 倍。与脂肪酸不同,酮体能够通过血脑屏障,从而在禁食的 7 天中提供大脑所需的大部分能量[41]。酮体的供给明显降低了大脑对葡萄糖的需求,避免了降解肌蛋白来提供葡萄糖前体。

如果早期出现的蛋白质分解没有得到抑制,随着禁食状态的持续,在不到 3 周的时间内可能出现危及生命的情况。随着禁食状态的持续,心脏、肾脏和骨骼肌将其主要燃料底物变为脂肪酸和酮体。其他组织如骨髓、肾髓质和周围神经,则从葡萄糖的完全氧化转变为厌氧糖酵解,丙酮酸和乳酸生成增加,而后两种化合物可以在肝脏中通过 Cori 循环利用来自脂肪氧化的能量转化为葡萄糖,由此产生的葡萄糖可用于全身的能量消耗,这也使得以脂肪形式储存的能量能够用于葡萄糖合成。

在禁食的前几天,随着肝糖原显著减少,全身血糖产量下降幅度超过 50%。随着禁食的继续,肾脏中的谷氨酰胺转化为葡萄糖的比例占总葡萄糖产量的 50%。机体能量不足带来的疲劳感导致机体的活动量减少,而且随着激活状态的甲状腺激素越来越多地转化为不活跃的形式以及交感神经系统受到抑制等因素,REE 降低了大约 10%,从而保存了部分能量。在经历长期禁食时(第 14~60 天),机体表现出最大程度的适应性改变。此时体内的脂肪、碳水化合物和蛋白质代谢会经历一个平台期[42]。在此期间,机体的能量大部分来源于脂肪组织,脂肪组织为人体提供 90% 以上的能量供给。

随着禁食状态的持续,机体每天对肌肉蛋白的分解量会减少到 30g 以下,从而导致尿素氮的生成和排泄显著减少。渗透压负荷的减小使得尿液量减少到 200ml/d,从而减少了机体对液体的需求量。机体的总葡萄糖产量减少至大约 75g/d,为糖酵解组织(40g/d)和大脑(35g/d)提供了能量底物,同时维持了血糖浓度的相对稳定。当禁食 30 天时,机体的能量消耗减少 20%~25%。随着禁食状态的持续,机体的能量消耗仍然会维持在一个相对稳定的水平。需要注意的是,消瘦者和肥胖者对短期禁食和长期禁食的代谢反应有所不同。与消瘦者相比,肥胖者的脂肪分解过程受到抑制且与葡萄糖产量减低之间存在密切相关[43,44]。此外,肥胖者的蛋白质分解和氮损失减少有助于保存肌蛋白[45]。

目前,对禁食终末期事件的研究以动物实验为主。研究发现,禁食终末期动物的脂肪质量和肌肉蛋白含量减少,大多数器官的体积都会缩小。而大脑的重量和蛋白质含量仍然保持相对稳定。在禁食的终末期阶段,脂肪储存量达到临界水平,体脂产生的能量减少,肌肉蛋白分解代谢加速。当骨骼肌蛋白丢失达到 30%~50% 时会发生死亡事件[46]。对于人类而言,机体的能量供给低于某些阈值会导致死亡事件的发生,比如全身蛋白消耗量达到 30%~50%、脂肪消耗量达到 70%~95% 或男性 BMI 降低至 $13kg/m^2$ 以下、女性 BMI 降低至 $11kg/m^2$ 以下[47,48]。

四、营养不良

广义上讲,营养不良指的是营养供应和营养需求之间的持续不平衡,这种不平衡会导致代谢、器官功能和身体成分发生不同程度的病理生理改变。长期性是营养不良的主要特征,这是因为短期的营养失衡可通过机体的动态平衡机制和营养储备得到迅速纠正。一般而言,"营养不良"这个词主要用来描述蛋白质、卡路里或两者都不足的状态,更准确地称为蛋白质能量营养不良或蛋白质热量营养不良。在特定情况下,营养不良也被用于描述营养过度供应的状态,如持续向机体供给过量的热量导致的肥胖或维生素摄入过量产生中毒。

(一) 蛋白质能量营养不良

蛋白质能量营养不良(proteinenergy malnutrition,PEM)的演变过程存在差异,原发性 PEM 是由于蛋白质摄入不足、热量摄入不足或者两者同时摄入不足引起的。在某些情况下,摄入蛋白质的质量太差以至于机体无法获得特定的必需 AA 而发生 PEM。继发性 PEM 主要由疾病或损伤引起。急性病和损伤不仅导致机体对蛋白质和能量的需求增加,而且以各种方式损害了机体对营养物质的消化、吸收,例如广泛的回肠疾病或回肠切除直接导致脂肪吸收不良和热量缺乏。此外,急性病和损伤引起的厌食症也会引起 PEM(相关机制见后文)。

全身性炎症反应引起的蛋白质分解代谢和能量消耗显著增加是导致继发性 PEM 的常见病因。REE 与炎症反应的严重程度和急性程度呈显著正相关。与基线水平相比,炎症状态下机体的 REE 可能会增加 80%,而且炎症反应的程度与疾病的严重程度也呈显著正相关。对于广泛的二、三度烧伤患者而言,其 REE 水平可能是基线水平的 2 倍;败血症患者的 REE 水平约为基线水平的 1.5 倍;局部感染或长骨骨折患者的 REE 水平比基线水平高出 25%[6]。利用上述这些应激因子构建了一个计算患者热量需求的计算公式(见表 5.5)。当机体发生疾病或受伤时,蛋白质分解代谢显著增加,并且这种增加幅度与损伤的严重程度以及急性程度之间呈显著正相关。需要指出的是,蛋白质分解代谢的增幅明显大于能量消耗的增幅,因此,反映急性病蛋白质分解代谢程度的尿素氮损失大约是最大应激时水平的 2.5 倍[6]。分解代谢的增加会导致蛋白质出现净损失,因为蛋白质的合成速率通常不会随着分解代谢速率的增加而增加[49]。

人体内不存在已知的蛋白质储存形式,因此蛋白质的任何净损失都代表着功能活性组织的损失。一个健康成年人每天从尿液中排出的氮含量大约为 12g。在危重疾病情况下,每天从尿液中排出的氮含量增加到 30g。由于 1g 尿氮对应 30g 瘦体质量,因此在危重疾病情况下,机体每天会分解大量蛋白质,从而导致瘦体质量每天下降 500g,这些蛋白质损耗的大部分来自骨骼肌,其中 AA 的损耗在危重病患者中增加了 2~6 倍[50]。从骨骼肌动员 AA 是机体应对应激反应时的一种适应性表现,一旦被释放,这些 AA 就会部分脱氨基并用于糖异生,它们也能被肝脏和其他内脏器官吸收。因此,在应激情况下,肌肉的蛋白水解使机体能够将 AA 从骨骼肌转移到内脏器官,这对于生命的维持具有重要作用。然而,如果应激状态持续存在,这种适应性反应的局限性就会显而易见,甚至内脏器官的体积也会明显缩小[42]。

1. 原发性与继发性蛋白质-能量营养不良:从机体分区的角度看

随着营养不良的持续进展,组织损失的类型对于确定体重下降的病理结果至关重要。由于 95% 的能量消耗均发生在瘦体质量之中,因此瘦体质量对于维持能量的动态平衡和机体的健康具有重要作用。瘦体质量可细分为体细胞和内脏蛋白质、血液和骨细胞以及小叶外的瘦体质量,如血浆和骨基质(图 5.1)。当一个健康人处于完全禁食或半禁食状态时,脂肪组织是其主要的能量来源。因此,脂肪质量的减少与瘦体质量之间呈正相关[42]。需要注意的是,对于患者而言,由于机体新陈代谢的变化导致肌肉发生更大程度的消耗[51]。瘦体质量的损耗首先发生在骨骼肌,随着禁食状态的持续,内脏器官的体积也会因为蛋白质的损耗而缩小(如表 5.14 所示)。对于急性病和损伤导致的代谢增加而言,除非潜在的炎症反应得到及时纠正,否则仅仅通过营养支持很难恢复肌肉质量。外源性合成代谢药物与营养结合使用来减弱或逆转净分解代谢的方法得到越来越多的关注。目前,β-羟甲基丁酸、生长激素、氧甲氢龙、普萘洛尔等药物能否改善临床结果以及这些药物的治疗作用是否大于其潜在的副作用,目前尚不清楚[52]。此外,对于急性疾病患者而言,如果仅仅提供营养支持,那么由此增加的大部分体重都来源于脂肪和体液的增加。因此,如果炎症病灶不能消除,瘦体质量就不会明显增加[53]。

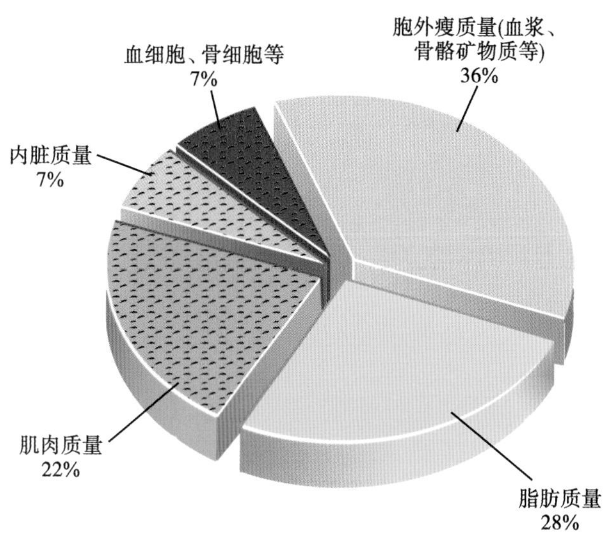

图 5.1　健康成人按体重进行的身体成分分析。斑点段和灰色段共同代表瘦体重,斑点段单独代表体细胞量。(Adapted from Mason JB. Gastrointestinal cancer: nutritional support. In: Kelsen D, Daly J, Kern S, et al., editors. Principles and practice of gastrointestinal oncology. Philadelphia: Lippincott Williams & Wilkins; 2002.)

表 5.14　单纯饥饿与代谢应激下的身体分区损耗

参数	骨骼肌消耗	内脏蛋白消耗	脂肪损失
禁食	+	+/-*	+++
代谢应激	+++	++/-*	+++

注:* 在这一过程的早期相对幸免,可能随着长期饥饿或代谢应激而变得明显。

细胞因子是伴随疾病和损伤的能量和蛋白质代谢改变最重要的介质。在患有全身性疾病的个体中，白细胞介素（IL）-1β、肿瘤坏死因子-α、IL-6 和干扰素-γ 水平的增加与能量消耗和蛋白质分解代谢增加以及 AA 进入内脏器官相关[54-56]，相关的细胞实验和动物模型也证实了这一观点（表 5.15）。在肿瘤相关的消耗综合征中发现，蛋白水解诱导因子和锌-α-2 糖蛋白是肿瘤恶病质特有的体液介质，这两种介质分别导致了蛋白质的分解代谢和脂肪组织的丢失[57]。肿瘤恶病质动物模型研究表明，如果能够设计出一种靶向肿瘤介导蛋白分解代谢的特异性抑制剂，这将会显著降低肿瘤恶病质相关的发病率和死亡率[58]。

2. 儿童蛋白质-能量营养不良

与成人营养不良不同的是，儿童营养不良会影响其生长和发育。放眼全球，儿童营养不良多见于发展中国家，主要原因有贫穷、食物供应不足和食物不洁。根据 Waterlow 营养不良分类表（如表 5.16 所示），儿童蛋白质能量营养不良会导致儿童消瘦和发育迟缓[59]。表 5.17 中概述了 3 种儿童蛋白质能量营养不良的常见综合征，包括了夸希奥科病、营养性消瘦症和营养性侏儒症[60]。虽然这三种综合征是单独分类的，但实际上它们的临床表现经常有重叠。

表 5.15 介导与代谢应激相关的高分解代谢和高代谢的主要细胞因子

细胞因子	细胞来源	代谢效应
IFN-γ	淋巴细胞、肺巨噬细胞	单核细胞增多呼吸爆发
IL-1β	单核/巨噬细胞、中性粒细胞、淋巴细胞、角质形成细胞、库普弗细胞	ACTH 和皮质醇水平升高急性期蛋白质合成增加肌肉中的 AA 释放胰岛素分泌减少高热
IL-6	单核/巨噬细胞，角质形成细胞，内皮细胞，成纤维细胞，T 细胞，上皮细胞	急性期蛋白质合成增加高热，食欲下降
TNF-α	单核/巨噬细胞、淋巴细胞、库普弗细胞、胶质细胞、内皮细胞、自然杀伤细胞、肥大细胞	游离脂肪酸合成减少脂解增加肌肉中释放的 AA 增加肝脏 AA 摄取增加高热

注：AA，氨基酸；ACTH，促肾上腺皮质激素。
Adapted from Smith M，Lowry S. The hypercatabolic state. In：Shils M，Olson J，Shike M，Ross AC，editors. Modern nutrition in health and disease. Baltimore：Williams & Wilkins；1999. p 1555.

表 5.16 儿童蛋白质-能量营养不良的 Waterlow 分类

参数	正常	轻微	中度	严重
身高标准体重（消瘦）				
NCHS 标准中位数百分比/%	90～100	80～89	70～79	<70
与 NCHS 中位数的标准差	+Z～-Z	-1.1Z～-2Z	-2.1Z～-3Z	<-3Z
年龄标准身高（发育迟缓）				
NCHS 标准中位数百分比/%	95～105	90～94	85～89	<85
与 NCHS 中位数的标准差	+Z～-Z	-1.1Z～-2Z	-2.1Z～-3Z	<-3Z

注：NCHS，国家卫生统计中心；Z，标准分数。

表 5.17 儿童蛋白质-能量营养不良综合征的特征

参数	综合征		
	夸希奥科病	营养性消瘦症	营养性侏儒症
食欲	差	好	好
水肿	存在	不存在	不存在
情绪	抱起时易怒，独处时冷漠	警觉	警觉
年龄对应的体重（%正常体重）	60～80	<60	<60
身高对应的体重	正常或降低	显著降低	正常

（1）恶性营养不良症（夸希奥科病）

夸希奥科病（kwahhiorkor）一词来自西非语，原意是“流离失所儿童所患的疾病”，多发于婴幼儿断奶后。外周水肿是鉴别恶性营养不良症与营养消瘦症、营养性侏儒症的要点所在。恶性营养不良症患儿表现出典型的皮肤和头发病理变化（详见下文）。由于腹部肌肉无力、肠胀气和肝大，患儿的腹部膨出，但腹水很少见。如果出现腹水，可能是并发症引起的（如肝病或腹膜炎）。恶性营养不良症患儿常常表现为嗜睡和淡漠，当患儿被抱起时又会出现烦躁不安的表现。恶性营养不良症多继发于营养不良儿童遭遇生理应激（如感染）。

与单纯消瘦症不同，恶性营养不良症患者多见白蛋白减少，其临床病理特点是细胞膜渗漏，细胞膜渗漏导致钾和其他细胞内离子渗透到细胞外导致水肿的发生。

（2） 营养性消瘦症

消瘦症患儿的临床表现主要有皮下脂肪几乎消失、肌肉明显萎缩、外观明显消瘦，肋骨、关节和面骨突出，皮肤浅薄松弛呈褶皱状。但是，内脏器官的蛋白质质量相对完好，患儿的血清白蛋白含量正常，从而维持着正常的血管渗透压，最大限度地减少水肿的发生，这也是消瘦症与恶性营养不良症的鉴别要点。

（3） 营养性侏儒症

营养性侏儒症患儿体形匀称，但身材矮小，性发育迟缓。通过使用适当的营养策略有助于刺激患儿成长和性成熟。成人 PEM 的诊断与儿童 PEM 的诊断有所不同，一是成人的身高一般不会增加，二是成人的 PEM 会导致消瘦而不是发育迟缓。成年人也会发生恶性营养不良症和消瘦症，但是在高收入社会中，对成人 PEM 的相关研究主要集中在继发性 PEM 住院患者、并发症以及恶性营养不良症和营养性消瘦症共有的临床表现方面。

（二） 蛋白质能量营养不良引起的生理损害

综上所述，除了大脑，几乎所有的器官和系统都可能受到 PEM 的不良影响。但是，通过及时合理的营养干预，大部分不良反应都能够逆转。下面，我们将重点围绕 PEM 相关的疾病及其危害性进行论述。

1. 系统性影响

（1） 胃肠道系统

PEM 不仅会对胃肠道的结构和功能产生不良影响，而且因为营养物质的摄入不足导致胃肠道受到的刺激减少。因此，如果仅仅依靠肠外营养支持，小肠黏膜会逐渐出现功能性萎缩，这种退变以刷状缘酶系的丧失和上皮屏障的完整性降低为主要的病理特征。此外，肠道缺乏营养物质的刺激也会导致肠绒毛萎缩。在肠道缺乏刺激的情况下也可以观察到绒毛萎缩，但在没有 PEM 的情况下，其结构萎缩的程度很小[61]。PEM 患儿的肠道、胰腺和肝脏的结构和功能也会发生病变，主要表现为肠绒毛明显萎缩，肠刷状缘水解酶部分或完全消失；胃液和胰液分泌量减少，胃液和消化酶浓度均会降低；胆汁分泌量和胆汁中的结合胆汁酸浓度降低。小肠上段的兼性厌氧菌数量增加，这些肠道菌群数量的增加可能是肠腔内游离胆汁酸比例增加的原因所在。患儿还会出现因碳水化合物、脂肪和水溶性维生素吸收不良导致的腹泻，腹泻的严重程度取决于 PEM 的程度，腹泻又加剧了营养不良的程度。此外，由于肠动力不足和肠胀气，晚期营养不良患者有时会出现腹部隆起。

（2） 心血管系统

中重度 PEM 会导致心肌质量下降。受损的心肌组织中可见肌原纤维萎缩、水肿、斑片状坏死以及慢性炎症细胞浸润（较少见），心功能减弱（如每搏输出量、心输出量和心脏做功量），而且常常伴随心动过缓、低血压等临床表现。

（3） 免疫系统

免疫系统最容易受到 PEM 的影响，因此临床上将多种免疫功能（如淋巴细胞总数、迟发性皮肤超敏反应）作为衡量机体营养不良的重要指标。有研究表明，PEM 患者的 T 淋巴细胞、多形核白细胞及其补体功能的完整性均受到不良影响，而且 B 淋巴细胞产生抗体的功能也受到不同程度的影响。由此可见，PEM 导致患者的免疫功能低下，感染风险增加，感染引起的炎症反应又会加剧 PEM，从而形成恶性循环。

（4） 呼吸系统

营养不良会导致患者的横膈肌和其他呼吸肌发生结构性和功能性萎缩，进而导致吸气量、呼气量和肺活量下降，加之肺通气动力不足导致患者的呼吸功能恶化。在行气管切开手术的患者中，PEM 与气管上皮定植的细菌之间存在着显著的相关性，细菌感染会进一步加剧 PEM 对免疫系统的损伤。

（5） 内分泌系统

适应性的激素水平变化在 PEM 患者中很常见。食物摄入不足导致循环葡萄糖和 AA 的可用性降低，循环胰岛素水平下降，生长激素水平升高。这些激素水平的变化常常伴随着 PEM 中生长激素水平的降低和皮质醇水平的升高，后两者共同促进了骨骼肌的分解代谢，从而释放更多的 AA 并转移至内脏器官。在严重营养不良的情况下，机体的尿素合成受到抑制，氮损失减少而氨基酸的再利用增加，促进了 AA 再利用。此外，脂肪分解和糖异生增强也为机体提供了必要的能量供给。血清三碘甲状腺原氨酸（T_3）和甲状腺素（T_4）水平通常随着反向 T_3 浓度的增加而降低，类似于在甲状腺功能正常疾病综合征中观察到的模式。T_3 浓度的降低可能在初级 PEM 中观察到的 REE 和蛋白质分解代谢率降低中起作用。

原发性性功能障碍常见于中重度的 PEM 成年患者并影响其生殖功能。男性睾酮和女性雌激素的循环水平明显下降，女性患者会出现闭经。当瘦体重下降到临界阈值以下时，会导致青春期延迟或月经量减少。需要指出的是，上述 PEM 相关的性功能障碍可能是机体为维持生命而进行的适应性改变，因为确保存活比儿童性成熟或成人生殖的需要更重要。

2. 其他影响

（1） 对伤口愈合的影响

对于营养状况良好的患者而言，其手术切口部位的胶原蛋白比营养不良的患者更充足。因此，对于营养不良的手术患者而言，术前进行营养支持比术后营养支持能够更快地促进伤口愈合。

（2） 对皮肤的影响

营养不良会导致皮肤干燥、变薄和起皱、表皮基底层萎缩和过度角化。严重的营养不良会导致皮肤蛋白和胶原蛋白大量消耗。恶性营养不良患者身体的不同部位会持续发生皮肤变化，首先是色素过度沉着，然后是表皮层开裂和剥离，变薄和萎缩的表皮会变得非常脆弱而且易于浸渍。

（3） 对毛发的影响

营养不良患者的头发会变得稀疏而且容易脱发，然而睫毛却变得长而繁茂，儿童可能会出现过多的胎毛。恶性营养不良症患儿的头发会出现色素减退，头发颜色呈红褐色、灰色或金色。成年患者会出现腋毛和阴毛脱落现象。

（4） 对肾脏的影响

营养不良一般不会影响肾脏的结构和功能。然而，当机体出现严重的营养不良时，患者的肾脏重量减轻，肾小球滤过率、肾脏排泄酸和钠的能力以及浓缩尿液的功能都会减弱，也可能出现轻度蛋白尿。

(5) 对骨髓的影响

严重的营养不良会抑制骨髓产生红细胞和白细胞的能力，从而导致贫血、白细胞减少和淋巴细胞减少。

五、营养评估技术

营养学评估旨在识别机体是否存在 PEM 以及其他类型的营养缺陷。PEM 的临床表现往往不明显，大多数 PEM 都是在进行系统的营养评估时发现的。例如，通过对 Child-Turcotte-Pugh（CTP）分级为 A 级的酒精性肝硬化患者进行营养学评估后发现，这些患者虽然没有 PEM 的典型临床表现，但是他们可能客观存在着轻微的 PEM 问题。CTP 分级为 A 级的患者血清白蛋白含量处于正常范围，但是通过体内中子活化分析方法对全身的氮含量进行研究后发现，超过 50% 的 CTP 分级为 A 级的患者的预期总蛋白低于 80%[62]，低于这一阈值的患者出现营养不良问题的概率会显著增加[63]。

对于其他健康人和慢性病患者而言，一般通过比较个体的实际测量数据（例如身高、体重）和已建立的标准数据（如表 5.6 所示）对其营养状况进行评估。目前尚缺乏对急性病患者 PEM 进行评估的金标准，这是因为大多数用于评估健康人 PEM 状况的参数都会随着疾病的不同而有所改变，例如体重和血清蛋白浓度。尽管评估急性病患者的 PEM 状况存在着上述的不确定性，但是营养评估的有效性已经得到证明。如果没有得到充分而有效的营养支持，急性病患者很容易出现营养不良的相关问题。因此，PEM 具有良好的预测价值。更重要的是，识别出营养不良患者并进行适当的营养干预能够有效改善患者的临床结局[64-68]。相关的荟萃分析结果表明，客观的营养学评估对于住院患者具有重要意义，营养学评估能够排除对强化营养支持无法获益的患者[69-71]。

全面的营养学评估需要结合病史、体格检查、人体测量学数据或营养状况的功能测量以及血液学检测。临床常用的营养评估工具包括体重、身高和其他人体测量学数据（如皮褶厚度和中臂测量）、功能测量（如握力或皮肤无反应性测试）、血清蛋白浓度（如白蛋白或前白蛋白）、全血细胞计数（包括绝对淋巴细胞计数）以及 24 小时尿肌酐和尿素氮水平。在特定的条件下，一些不容易获取的机体成分测量数据（如生物电阻抗和体内总钾量）对于营养学评估也具有重要的作用。

虽然一些营养学评估指标的特异性不高，但由于其对疾病预后的指导意义，因此在临床护理中仍然有用。目前尚缺乏一个具有高度特异性和敏感性的参数对 PEM 进行评估，综合运用上述营养学评估参数才是最佳选择。需要指出的是，如果临床医生进行营养学评估的目的仅仅是为了确定患者是否处于中、重度 PEM 进而采取强化营养支持措施，那么则不必要进行全面的营养学评估，因为通过简单的分类方法即可实现这一目标。

（一）病史

1. 体重减轻

体重在多长时间内减轻了多少？与疾病相关的无意识体重减轻是 PEM 临床显著程度的唯一实用预测指标。通过确定患者在过去 6 个月内是否持续存在着轻度（<5%）、中度（5%～10%）或重度（>10%）的体重变化情况可以对体重减轻进行有效的量化。

急性病会导致瘦体重大幅度减少，无意识的体重下降超过体重的 10% 与全身蛋白质减少 15%～20% 之间存在密切相关性[63]。这种程度的体重减轻不仅是衡量生理功能受损、临床预后不佳和住院时间延长的重要阈值[72-74]，而且还能够识别出可从强化营养支持治疗中获益的患者。然而，临床医生需要注意的是，根据患者的病史评估体重减轻程度的准确性有限。有研究发现，三分之一体重减轻的患者未能通过病史检查发现，四分之一体重正常的患者又被错误地归类为体重减轻[75]。此外，体重变化的营养学意义受到机体水合状态和细胞外液体潴留的影响。更重要的是，体重减轻并不是评估 PEM 的精确指标。因此，获取有助于准确识别患者 PEM 的其他病史资料很有必要（详见下文）。

2. 食物摄入

饮食习惯（如膳食的数量、分量和内容）是否发生了变化？食物摄入量发生改变的原因是什么（例如食欲、精神状态或情绪变化、准备食物的能力、咀嚼或吞咽能力以及胃肠道症状）？

3. 营养吸收不良的证据

是否有营养吸收不良的症状和（或）体征？或者症状、体征两者都与吸收不良的临床表现相一致？

(1) 特定营养素缺乏的证据

是否存在特定营养素（包括大量矿物质、微量营养素和水）缺乏的症状和（或）体征？（参见表 5.9～表 5.11）

(2) 疾病对营养需求的影响

潜在疾病是否增加了机体的营养需求或导致了营养损失？

(3) 功能状态

患者进行日常活动的能力是否影响了膳食的摄入量？患者能否购物和做饭？经济状况是否影响了患者购买食物的能力？

（二）体格检查

1. 水合状态

评估患者是否存在脱水的体征（如低血压、心动过速、血压和脉搏的体位性变化、黏膜干燥、腋汗减少、皮肤干燥）和体液过剩（如水肿或腹水）。

2. 组织耗竭

如果骨骼、肌肉和静脉轮廓清晰而皮肤皱褶松弛，则表明脂肪组织普遍缺失。示指和拇指之间的皮肤皱褶可以反映皮下脂肪的充足性。脸颊、臀部和肛周出现凹陷则表明身体的脂肪减少。通过检查颞肌、骨间肌和股四头肌，可以判断肌肉的损耗情况。

3. 肌肉功能

对单个肌群进行肌力测试，以确定是否存在全身或局部的肌无力。对心肌功能进行评估，使用肺活量测定法对患者的呼吸肌功能进行评估。

4. 特定的营养素缺乏

与增殖速度较慢的组织（如心脏、骨骼肌、大脑）相比较，增殖快速的组织（如口腔黏膜、头发、皮肤、胃肠道上皮、骨髓）对营养素的缺乏更加敏感（见表 5.9~表 5.11）。

（三）人体测量学

人体测量技术是通过对身体各部位的大小、重量或体积进行测量，以评估机体蛋白质和热量状况的一种技术。身高和体重是最常用的人体测量参数。当患者及其家属都不能提供可靠的病史信息时，身高和体重是很有用的测量参数，但它们的可靠程度不及无意识的体重减轻。因为身高和体重需要大样本的数据确定一定的生理区间值，而个体差异则会影响其准确性。

表 5.6 中列出了 Metropolitan Life Insurance 公司运用前瞻性死亡率数据建立的“理想体重”。需要指出的是，与 1983 年发布的“理想体重”数据相比较，1959 年发布的“理想体重”数据更具有指导意义，这是因为 1983 年发布的数据没有进行充分抽样导致数据存在偏倚。

一般而言，体重低于标准体重 85% 的个体存在着明显的 PEM。体重指数（BMI）（如表 5.18 所示）的计算公式为：体重（以“kg”为单位）除以身高（以“m”为单位）的平方。目前，BMI 已经取代了“身高-体重”这一指标。当 BMI 超出标准范围（18.5~24.9kg/m^2）时，患者出现不良临床结局的可能性更大。在许多外科疾病和酒精性肝病的治疗方面[76-78]，高于标准范围的 BMI 能够预测不良的临床结局[79]。在外科和内科患者群体中，BMI 偏低是一个独立危险因素[80]。BMI 偏低成年患者（BMI<14kg/m^2）的死亡风险很高，因此这类患者需要入院接受强化营养支持治疗。BMI 低于 18.5kg/m^2 表示 PEM，BMI 高于 24.9kg/m^2 则表示体内脂肪过多（超重或肥胖）。需要指出的是，尽管 BMI 指数适用于绝大多数的成年人，但它也可能与其他依赖于体重而不直接评估身体成分的测量方法一样具有误导性[81]。对于存在水肿的个体（实际脂肪和体细胞质量低于测得的 BMI 值）和肌肉发达的运动员（BMI 高通常表示瘦体重大）而言，BMI 有一定程度的误导性。此外，性别、种族也是混杂因素，但对临床治疗效果的影响不大。更重要的是，发育会导致身体成分发生显著变化。因此，需要通过多方面对儿童和青春期个体的营养状况进行评估[82]。

表 5.18　基于 BMI 列出的成年人营养状况分类

BMI/（kg/m^2）	营养状况
<16.0	严重营养不良
16.0~16.9	中度严重不良
17.0~18.4	轻度营养不良
18.5~24.9	正常
25.0~29.9	超重
30.0~34.9	肥胖（Ⅰ）
35.0~39.9	肥胖（Ⅱ）
≥40	肥胖（Ⅲ）

综上所述，对身体部位的测量能够提供一些有关营养状况的重要信息，而这些重要的信息可能是测量体重所无法获得的。目前，静水称重法、双能 X 射线吸收测量法、空气阻抗体积描记、全身钾和同位素标记水稀释法、体内中子活化分析法、计算机断层扫描以及磁共振成像技术均可通过非侵入性或微创方式对身体成分进行精准测定[82-89]。然而，这些检测技术存在着检测成本高、可及性和适用性低等局限性，因此，目前这些检测技术主要运用于临床研究领域。对上述检测技术的详细论述不属于本章范围，我们仅在表 5.19 中概述了每种测量工具的主要用途。

表 5.19　用于测量人体成分的先进技术

技术	主要用于身体成分分析
空气置换体积描记法[91]	身体中 FM 的比例，身体中 LM 的比例
CT[90]	局部 FM/LM
双能 X 线吸收法[92]	绝对 FM 和 LM；骨密度
体内中子活化分析[95]	总蛋白质，绝对 FM，绝对 LM
同位素标记水和 NaBr 稀释[94]	TBW，ICW，ECW
MRI[96]	局部 FM/LM
全身钾含量[93]	体细胞质量
水下称重法[89]	身体中 FM 比例，身体中 LM 比例

注：ECW，细胞外液；FM，脂肪量；ICW，细胞内液；LM，瘦体重；NaBr，溴化钠；TBW，总体重。

临床上，通常使用简单可操作但准确性不高的测量技术对身体成分进行评估。比如，通过评估皮下脂肪的厚度可以得出全身脂肪质量的近似值。在正常成年人中，皮下脂肪质量占了全身脂肪储备的大约 50%。人们也会通过肱三头肌和肩胛下皱褶对个体的营养情况进行评估。随着全身脂肪的变化，机体各个部位的皮下脂肪也会以不同的形式发生变化。中臂肌围（mid-arm muscle circumference，MAMC）也是一个评估机体骨骼肌质量的常用指标。表 5.20 中包含了前两次国家健康和营养调查（National Health and Nutrition Examination Surveys，NHANES Ⅰ和Ⅱ）获得的皮褶和手臂中部肌肉面积数据的解释性指南[90]。临床实践中，与“身高-体重”相类似，皮肤皱襞和附肢肌肉测量数据也存在着明显的个体差异。因此，这些测量数据在人群研究中的价值高于在个体研究中的价值[91]，但是这些数据的可重复性较差。尽管当前的数据库中不存在种族、年龄方面的偏倚，但仍缺乏机体水合作用和体力活动相关的校正数据。

临床上，可以在一段时间内对皮褶和肌肉面积两个指标进行连续测量从而增加其临床适用性，也可以对患者的恢复情况或临床干预的效果进行评估。这种策略的优势是对患者的相关临床指标进行前后比较，而不是与某个标准值进行比较。此外，上述两种指标在肝硬化患者的病情评估和管理方面具有重要价值，因为肝硬化会导致其他常见的营养状况评估标准失效。肱三头肌皮褶和中臂肌围的异常低值是肝硬化患者高死亡率的独立预测因子，将它们纳入 Cox 回归模型可提高 Child-Turcotte 评分的预后价值[92]。在重度酒精性肝炎患者接受合成类固醇治疗时，中臂肌围和瘦体重等指标的改善与治疗的积极反应性相关[93]。

表 5.20　上臂肌肉面积以及三头肌和肩胛下皮褶总和的标准

参数	年龄	百分比		
		5th	50th	85th
上臂肌肉面积*/cm^2				
男性	25~29	38	53	65
	45~49	37	55	66
	65~69	33	48	63
女性	25~29	20	30	38
	45~49	21	32	45
	65~69	22	35	46
三头肌和肩胛下皮褶总和/mm				
男性	25~29	12	24	41
	45~49	13	29	43
	65~69	12	27	42
女性	25~29	18	37	58
	45~49	21	46	68
	65~69	22	45	65

*上臂中部肌肉面积(cm^2)计算公式如下：

对于男性：面积=[臂围-(π×三头肌皮褶)]^2/4π-10

对于女性：面积=[臂围-(π×三头肌皮褶)]^2/4π-6.5

Adapted with permissio from Frisancho AR. Anthropometric standards for the assessment of growth and nutritional status. Ann Arbor, Mich：University of Michigan Press；1990.

生物电阻抗分析法作为一种廉价、方便、无创、安全的分析方法，在评估机体的瘦体重、体细胞质量和体内总水分方面具有明显优势，其中体细胞质量比瘦体重更有意义，因为它不包括非活体瘦体重［如血浆和骨骼矿物质(如图 5.1 所示)］。测量发现，身体的电流阻力与脂肪和骨骼中矿物质的含量成正比，因为这些身体成分的导电性较差。机体的其他部位富含导电性能良好的电解质，如果假设机体每个部位的含水量相同，我们就可以计算出身体中的总含水量、瘦体重和体细胞质量。对于接受肾脏透析的患者和 HIV 感染的患者而言，监测瘦体重具有更高的实用价值[94,95]。但是，急性病会导致体内水分总量及其分布发生显著变化，因此使用生物电阻抗分析方法并不能获得有价值的信息[96]。此外，用于计算身体成分的公式中包含着关于身体水分的假设，而这些假设会随着年龄、肥胖和疾病的变化而发生变化。因此，生物阻抗分析在使用之前必须经过特定验证。

(四) 蛋白质热量状态的功能测量

尽管目前已经开发出了几种针对 PEM 患者骨骼肌功能受损情况进行评估的技术，但只有握拳测力法(fist-grip dynamometry，FGD)得到广泛应用。FGD 使用握力计来测定最大握力。在拟行胃肠道手术的患者中，FGD 与通过体内中子活化分析和 MAMC 分析得到的全身蛋白结果之间存在很强的相关性[97]。FGD 在检测肝硬化患者的体内细胞量(body cell mass，BCM)耗竭方面也具有非常好的效用[98]。如前所述，评估中、重度 PEM 的有效指标是预测急性病患者临床结局的重要因素，而 FGD 也可以在其中发挥重要作用。研究发现，与握力正常的患者相比，术前握力低于标准值(经过年龄和性别校正)85%的患者，其发生围手术期并发症的风险会增加两倍[99]。在接受胃肠道肿瘤手术的患者中，FGD 在预测患者围手术期的发病率和死亡率方面具有更高的敏感性和特异性[100]。尽管 FGD 在快速、简便地评估住院患者和门诊患者的 PEM 方面具有很大的潜力，但是由于患者对该技术缺乏信任，因此其使用范围依然有限。呼吸肌肌力测定(通过床边肺活量计测量得到的最大持续吸气量和(或)最大持续呼气量进行衡量)也是测量蛋白质-卡路里状态的常用指标，但是由于受到多种因素的影响，其可靠性并不高。

综上所述，PEM 对机体的各个系统都有不良影响，其中免疫系统对 PEM 的影响最为敏感。迟发型皮肤超敏试验是评估细胞免疫功能完整性的常用方法。在危重病患者中，迟发型皮肤超敏试验在预测疾病的发病率和死亡率方面具有一定的价值，但其结果受到诸多因素的影响(如年龄、全身感染和大手术)。此外，皮肤的反应性会随着机体营养状态的恢复得到改善，因此，它对监测患者的疾病进展意义不大[101]。由此可见，最佳的选择是将迟发型皮肤超敏试验方法纳入一系列评估方法中，从而完成对机体营养状况的综合评估(详见下文“蛋白质-卡路里状态的鉴别分析”部分)。

(五) 蛋白质热量状态的生物化学检测

1. 血清蛋白

肝脏合成型蛋白质(如白蛋白、前白蛋白、转铁蛋白和视黄醇结合蛋白)的血清水平可以作为衡量蛋白质热量状态的生化指标(表 5.21)。在患者不存在并发症或其他损伤的情况下，上述任何一种蛋白质含量的降低都说明患者很可能存在 PEM。此外，由于前白蛋白、转铁蛋白和视黄醇结合蛋白的半衰期明显短于白蛋白的半衰期，因此它们比白蛋白可以更快地反映机体营养状态的变化。需要注意的是，导致血清蛋白质浓度发生变化的原因很多，例如慢性肾脏疾病或使用糖皮质激素(或口服避孕药)都可能导致前白蛋白水平异常升高。肝硬化患者中上述蛋白质血清水平的降幅与 Child 分级之间均存在着正相关。与健康人相比，Child 分级为 A 级患者的血清白蛋白水平也会有所下降[102]。当所有这些蛋白均表现为一种“消极”的急性时相反应物时，意味着这些蛋白质的血清浓度随着全身炎症反应程度呈现下降趋势，并且其下降幅度与炎症反应程度呈正相关。这种影响导致其可靠性下降，但是它们的作用却不可忽视。例如，对于住院患者而言，前白蛋白检测是一种快速有效的筛查 PEM 的方法[103]。

2. 肌酐-身高指数

临床实践表明，对身高进行校正后的 24 小时尿肌酐排泄量是一种评估总骨骼肌质量的有效方法。人体每天都会将恒定比例(大约为 2%)的肌肉肌酸转化为肌酐，所以身高与肌酐两者之间密切相关。对性别和身高进行调整后，如果肌肉肌酸转化为肌酐值低于正常值的 20% 以上，则表明存在着中、重度 PEM(如表 5.22 所示)。当前最新版的肌酐-身高指数(creatinine-height index，CHI)主要适用于 3 至 18 岁的儿童和青少年[104]。在对患者的营养状况进行评估时，可以将该方法与其他操作简便的方法联合使用(双能 X 线吸收

表 5.21 在肝脏中合成并用于评估营养状况的蛋白质

血清蛋白	正常值 均数±SD(范围)*	半衰期/d	功能	备注†
白蛋白	4.5(3.5~5.0)	14~20	维持血浆有效渗透压;小分子载体	多种非营养因素引起的血清水平变化
转铁蛋白	2.3(2.0~3.2)	8~9	结合血浆中的 Fe^{2+} 并将其输送到骨髓	铁营养影响血浆水平;在妊娠、雌激素治疗和急性肝炎期间升高;在蛋白缺失性肠病和肾病、慢性感染、尿毒症和急性分解代谢状态中降低;通常间接测量总铁结合能力
转甲状腺素蛋白(前白蛋白)	0.30(0.2~0.5)	2~3	结合 T_3,在较小程度上结合 T_4;是 RBP 的载体	慢性肾病透析患者服用皮质类固醇、糖皮质激素或口服避孕药后升高;甲状腺功能亢进症患者术后急性分解代谢降低;血清水平由总体能量和氮平衡决定
RBP	0.037 2±0.007 3‡	0.5	在血浆中转运维生素 A;与前白蛋白非共价结合	在肾近端小管细胞中分解代谢;随着肾脏疾病,RBP 增加,其半衰期延长;维生素 A 缺乏、急性分解代谢状态、手术后和甲状腺功能亢进症患者的血浆低水平

注:* 单位为 g/L。正常范围因中心而异;检查局部值。
†所有列出的蛋白质均受到水合作用和肝细胞功能障碍的影响。
‡正常值取决于年龄和性别。表中数值适用于集合受试者。
RBP,视黄醇结合蛋白;SD,标准差;T_3,三碘甲状腺原氨酸;T_4,甲状腺素。
Adapted from Heymsfield S, Tighe A, Wang Z-M. Nutritional assessment by anthropometric and biochemical means. In: Shils M, Olson J, Shike M, editors. Modern nutrition in health and disease. 8th ed. Philadelphia: Lea & Febiger; 1994. p 812.

表 5.22 基于身高计算的每日肌酐排泄量标准值

男性*		女性†	
身高/cm	理想肌酐/cm	身高/cm	理想肌酐/cm
157.5	1 288	147.3	830
160.0	1 325	149.9	851
162.6	1 359	152.4	875
165.1	1 386	154.9	900
167.6	1 426	157.5	925
170.2	1 467	160.0	949
172.7	1 513	162.6	977
175.3	1 555	165.1	1 006
177.8	1 596	167.6	1 044
180.3	1 642	170.2	1 076
182.9	1 691	172.7	1 109
185.4	1 739	175.3	1 141
188.0	1 785	177.8	1 174
190.5	1 831	180.3	1 206
193.0	1 891	182.9	1 240

*肌酐系数(男性)= 23mg/kg 的理想体重。
†肌酐系数(女性)= 18mg/kg 的理想体重。From Blackburn GL, Bistrian BR, Maini BS, et al. Nutritional and metabolic assessment of the hospitalized patient. J Parenter Enteral Nutr 1977;1:11-22.

法)[105]。对于接受长时间机械辅助通气的患者而言,CHI 是一个影响成功脱机率和存活率的独立预测因素[106]。为避免产生误导性结果,临床医生需要综合考虑诸多干扰因素,比如尿液采集不完整、肾功能异常、尿液采集前或采集过程中摄入过多的肉类或牛奶、使用糖皮质激素等,上述每一种因素都会直接影响肌酐的排泄量。

3. 蛋白质热量状态的判别分析

如上所述,用于评估 PEM 的各项参数都有其优势和不足。通过判别分析方法,已经开发出了包含这些不同参数以及不同参数组合的多因素指标体系。充分利用其优势,可以更准确地评估患者是否存在 PEM 并筛选出因 PEM 而产生不良临床结局的患者。在过去的几十年里,为了更好地评估急性住院患者的营养状态,人们已经开发出了多种评估指标,例如预后营养指数(包含血清白蛋白、转铁蛋白、迟发性皮肤超敏反应和三头肌皮褶厚度)用于预测接受胃肠道手术的患者术后发生并发症的可能性以及相关死亡率[107];老年营养风险指数(包括血清白蛋白、% IBW)用于预测老年住院患者发生感染并发症和死亡的可能性[108]。在紧急情况下,一些可以直接使用的 PEM 评估指标会受到疾病严重程度的显著影响,从而影响对营养不良程度的精确评估。多因素指标体系是衡量 PEM 并发症和致命性事件的最佳预测因子。最近,在急性护理环境指数列表中新增了两个指标,分别是营养风险评分-2002 年(Nutrition Risk Score-2002, NRS-2002)以及 NUTRIC 评分[109],需要明确的是,新增的这两个指标仅适用于 ICU 患者。引入 NRS-2002 和 NUTRIC 最重要的意义是研究这些评价指标能否区分出真正受益于强化营养支持的患者[110-112]。

(六) 评估目标人群的快速筛查工具

低成本、高效便捷而且准确性高的评估方法对于 PEM 患者的营养状况评估至关重要,在面对大量人群的营养状况评估时尤为明显。为此,人们已经开发出了主观总体评估法(subjective global assessment, SGA)和微型营养评定法(mini-nutritional assessment, MNA),并且对它们的性能进行了广泛的验证。

1. 主观总体评估

作为一种评估患者营养状况和预测术后感染的手段，SGA最初主要应用于外科住院患者（详见框5.1）。在预测术后感染方面，SGA优于血清白蛋白浓度、迟发性皮肤过敏、MAMC、CHI以及预后营养指数等指标[113]。根据病史和体格检查结果，可将患者分为三类：营养良好（A类）、轻度或中度营养不良（B类）及重度营养不良（C类）。尽管它的一些组成部分是主观的，但独立观察者之间有着良好的一致性[114]。临床实践表明，SGA的可靠性主要体现在其不依赖于住院医生的临床经验[115]，而且SGA可作为预测长期住院的老年患者以及其他疾病临床结局的一个重要指标[116-118]。

框5.1 营养状况的主观总体评估（SGA）

病史

体重变化：

过去6个月的体重减轻量：总量=________kg；

%损失=________

过去2周内的变化：________增加________无变化

________降低

膳食摄入量变化：

无变化________变化________

持续时间：________周

饮食状况：

________次优固体饮食

________低热量流体

________禁食

胃肠道症状（持续2周以上）：

________无________恶心________呕吐

________腹泻________厌食

功能容量：

________无功能障碍

________存在功能障碍

持续时间=________周

类型：

________以次优方式工作

________可移动但不能工作

________卧床不起

疾病对营养需求的影响：

主要诊断：________

代谢需求：________低应激________中应激

________高应激

体检（正常、中度或重度）

________皮下脂肪丢失（三头肌、胸部）

________肌肉萎缩（股四头肌、三角肌）

________踝关节或骶骨水肿

________腹水

SGA评级*

A=营养良好

B=轻度或中度营养不良

C=严重营养不良

*根据主观加权分配SGA中的A、B和C等级。目前进食良好且体重增加的体重减轻和肌肉萎缩的患者归类为营养良好。将中度体重减轻（5%～10%）、摄食量持续下降、体重持续减轻、进行性功能障碍和疾病引起的中度应激的患者归类为中度营养不良。体重严重减轻（>10%）、营养摄入不足、进行性功能损害和肌肉萎缩的患者归类为严重营养不良。

2. 微型营养评定

作为一种能够快速实施的筛查方法，MNA适用于评估老年人群的PEM。这种方法能够在几分钟内获得相关的病史、简单的体格检查以及人体测量（BMI、臂围、小腿围）数据。根据数据评分结果，将患者分类为营养状况良好、营养不良或存在营养不良风险。MNA是一种评估老年人PEM的有效方法，包括身体健康、活动自如的老年人、身体虚弱的老年人以及住院的老年患者[119,120]。此外，MNA在预测长期住院的老年患者的发病率方面也具有重要的价值[121]。需要指出的是，MNA不适用于超重或肥胖个体。尽管目前还有一些其他的营养状况筛选工具（比如用于筛查营养不足和营养过剩的营养筛查倡议），但是其应用价值和性能尚未得到广泛验证[122]。

六、住院患者积极的营养支持

在以下的章节中，我们将详细讨论在特定的胃肠道疾病和肝脏疾病中常用的营养管理方法。需要注意的是，在使用之前，我们首先要考虑这些方法能否给危重病患者带来实质性的益处。临床上，任何中、重度营养不良且不能在48h内满足自身营养需求的急性病患者，都是积极营养支持的适用对象。此外，积极营养支持的另一个常见适应证是营养良好或轻度营养不良的住院患者不能在未来10天内达到至少80%的热量和蛋白质需求。但是，截至目前，后一种适应证能否让患者获益尚缺乏足够的循证医学证据支持。伴随急性疾病而来的分解代谢使得机体的营养不足难以纠正，对于那些存在着严重持续代谢应激的患者，营养支持一般不会增加机体的蛋白质成分和体重。当体重增加时，主要是因为水分增加和脂肪团膨胀所致[123]。即使在体重没有增加或血清蛋白含量没有增加的情况下，为患者提供一个疗程的营养支持也能够改善其生理功能和临床结果[124]。在下面的内容中，我们列举了一些与胃肠病学相关的临床方案。与这些临床方案相关的临床研究表明，营养支持对住院患者能够产生积极的作用。

（一）接受大手术的营养不良患者

营养支持能够让计划进行大手术的中、重度营养不良患者获益，术前7天或更长时间的积极营养支持可减少围手术期的并发症，降低营养不良患者的死亡率[64-71,125-127]。一项退伍军人事务部TPN的合作研究对500名即将接受腹部或胸部大手术的受试者进行分层分析[64]，结果显示，严重营养不良的患者通过接受术前TPN可以将围手术期非感染性并发症的发生率减少近90%。但是，这种营养支持策略并不会对轻度营养不良或营养状况良好的个体产生任何益处。一项纳入90名胃癌或结直肠癌手术患者的临床试验表明，对于中、重度营养不良患者而言，术前营养支持不仅能够将并发症降低35%，而且能够显著降低死亡率[127]。需要说明的是，术前营养支持的益处仅限于严重营养不良的患者，这一结果与荟萃分析得出的结论相同[69,70]。术后营养支持并不能减少围手术期并发症的发生[128]。另有研究发现，肠内营养也能让这类患者获益。与术前TPN相比，术前进行肠内营养的临床实践较少，但是这两者所得出的结果具有良好的一致性[129,130]，即术前肠内营养和术前 TPN 都能让患者获益[131]。

（二）与酒精相关的失代偿肝病住院患者

在急性酒精性肝炎和其他形式的酒精性肝硬化失代偿期的住院患者中[62]，中、重度 PEM 的患病率非常高。对于急性酒精性肝炎患者而言，自主进食远远不能满足机体的营养需求。临床研究发现，及时实施肠内或肠外营养均可有效降低这类患者的发病率和死亡率并加速其身体康复[65-67,132]。

（三）放射治疗患者

目前，在接受放射治疗的头颈部肿瘤和食管恶性肿瘤的患者中，营养支持策略的有效性得到了广泛的研究。例如，在放射治疗过程中和放射治疗之后置入 PEG 管和鼻饲管能够有效抑制患者的营养状况进一步恶化[133,134]。头颈部肿瘤患者补充 PEG 能够明显改善其生活质量。目前，虽然尚无证据证实营养支持是否能够改善接受放射治疗患者的生存率并降低发病率，但是在改善患者的生活质量方面，营养支持策略值得推荐。

（张兆洲　译，孙明瑜　校）

参考文献

第 6 章 营养管理

Angela K. Pham, Stephen A. McClave 著

章节目录

一、特定疾病的营养 …… 72
(一) 肠衰竭 …… 72
(二) 胰腺炎 …… 73
(三) 克罗恩病 …… 73
(四) 肝病 …… 74
(五) 憩室病 …… 75
(六) 倾倒综合征 …… 75
(七) 癌症 …… 75
(八) 肥胖 …… 75
(九) 危重症 …… 76
二、营养治疗 …… 77
(一) 肠内营养 …… 77
(二) 肠外营养 …… 85
三、特殊饮食 …… 87

一、特定疾病的营养

营养评估和有指导的营养治疗在胃肠道疾病的治疗中非常重要。熟悉适当的营养干预措施在临床上取得良好疗效至关重要。上一章我们回顾了营养评估，本章将概述常见胃肠道疾病的营养问题以及经肠外营养（parenteral nutrition, PN）和肠内营养（enteral nutrition, EN）对营养缺乏的治疗。

（一）肠衰竭

肠衰竭（intestinal failure, IF）是指肠功能下降，不能满足机体营养需求的状态，导致依赖于肠外营养的使用[1]。肠衰竭的定义已被多次修订。欧洲临床营养与代谢学会（European Society for Clinical Nutrition and Metabolism, ESPEN）首次发表了关于肠衰竭的正式定义。在 ESPEN 的定义中，肠衰竭必须满足两个标准："①肠道功能下降不能满足大量营养素和（或）水和电解质吸收的最低需要量"和"②需肠外营养支持以维持健康和（或）生长"[2]。肠衰竭可分为Ⅰ型、Ⅱ型和Ⅲ型。Ⅰ型：急性、短期、自限性症状（如腹部手术后肠梗阻），可能需要短暂的营养支持[3]。Ⅱ型：长期急性状态的结果，常见于代谢不稳定的患者，需要数周或数月的静脉营养支持，可能是可逆或不可逆的[3]。Ⅱ型患者可能完全康复或进展为Ⅲ型肠衰竭。Ⅲ型是一种慢性状态，需要长期营养支持，通常需要家庭肠外营养支持[4]，病因包括克罗恩病（见第 115 章）、放射性肠炎（见第 41 章）、肠梗阻（见第 123 章）、动力障碍（见第 99、100 和 124 章）、肠外伤、先天性疾病（见第 98 章）、肠瘘（见第 29 和 115 章）和血管并发症（见第 118 章）。

短肠综合征（short bowel syndrome, SBS）是由于功能性小肠长度小于 200cm 导致肠道吸收不良引起的综合征，是肠衰竭的常见原因之一（见第 106 章）。广泛的小肠切除术后有 3 个临床阶段。第一阶段发生在切除术后的最初几周，特点是液体和电解质丢失紊乱，需要大量的静脉输液防止脱水。在第二阶段，可能持续两年，出现结构性代偿（细胞异常增生以增加细胞体积和吸收面积）和功能性代偿（减缓肠道传输以增加吸收时间）。第三阶段是稳定期，在此期间残留的肠管已最大限度地代偿，趋于稳定[5]。SBS 的营养管理取决于小肠切除的长度和部位，因为小肠具有代偿性地适应和增加吸收功能的能力。最初，质子泵抑制剂用于减少胃酸分泌，抗胆碱能药物和阿片类药物用于减缓肠道运动。SBS 患者口服药物的吸收功能受限，因此可能需要多于通常推荐剂量的抗胆碱药。在第一阶段就需要肠外营养以满足营养需求。

在第二阶段，逐渐开始口服饮食。随着口服饮食的耐受性越来越好，PN 的用量可以逐渐减少。患者应少食多餐，避免摄入单糖、膳食纤维和低营养的食物，液体和固体食物分开摄入。一般乳糖的耐受性良好，除非切除了近端空肠。多数病情稳定的成人 SBS 患者吸收的热量只有正常人的一半到三分之二，因此饮食摄入量应至少增加 50%。最能耐受的方案是暴饮暴食即每日进食 5~6 餐[6]。当经口饮食引起腹泻时，就不能完全脱离肠外营养。虽然经皮内镜下胃造口术（percutaneous endoscopic gastrostomy, PEG）在 SBS 治疗中的作用存在争议，但是连续 12~24 小时的管饲营养耐受性通常优于间断的推注式进食，其营养吸收更好和渗透性腹泻更少。EN 时通常进展缓慢，而 PN 时根据症状、食物和液体摄入量、大便和尿量的排出量、体重、机体对水的需要和微量营养素水平监测患者对营养的耐受性可在几个月内呈等热量减少[7]。

小肠广泛切除后，临床上将 SBS 分为 3 种类型。Ⅰ型：患者只剩下空肠，末端空肠造口术，没有结肠。这些患者会有大量的体液流失，不能代偿性适应，更有可能长期依赖 PN。Ⅱ型：患者的空肠长度不一，与部分结肠串联。临床上，Ⅱ型患者表现出更好的代偿性适应，但是如果没有长期的肠外营养支持，营养状况也会逐渐恶化。Ⅲ型：因为保留了完整的结肠和回盲瓣，并与小肠相连，所以残留小肠的代偿性适应可维持正常的肠道功能（意味着患者可以恢复饮食营养）[8]。回肠末端残端产生的胰高血糖素样肽（glucagon-like peptide, GLP）-1 具有营养效应，能促进短肠代偿性适应，因此这些患者很少需要肠内营养或肠外营养。临床上，有助于预测肠道康复成功与否的因素包括残余肠道中是否存在残余病变、肠道长度、代偿性适应的程度以及 PN 的持续时间。肠道自主性是指 SBS 患者在没有肠外营养的情况下生存的能力。如果患者有 70~90cm 的小肠和完整的结肠，或者在没有结肠的情

况下有130~150cm的小肠,则可以预期肠道能有自主性。在适应期内,摄入热量比摄入液体和电解质更容易实现肠道自主。瓜氨酸是一种由肠黏膜产生的非蛋白氨基酸,是永久性还是暂时性肠衰竭的预测因子[6]。一项研究显示,血浆瓜氨酸水平低于20μmol/L,提示永久性肠衰竭,阳性和阴性预测值分别为95%和86%[9]。

重度SBS患者(小肠剩余<200cm)通常需要葡萄糖电解质口服补液(oral rehydration solution,ORS)。摄入钠浓度至少为90mmol/L的含有葡萄糖的口服补液有助于利用空肠的钠-葡萄糖共转运蛋白吸收水分(见第101章)。一天内应口服2~3L口服补液盐,避免使用低渗透性液体,因其吸收主要依赖于被动扩散。SBS患者也应避免高渗液体,因为会导致液体转移进入肠腔,加重腹泻[6]。如果患者进行了保留结肠的回肠部分切除术(切除<100cm),可以使用胆汁酸结合树脂考来烯胺来减少胆盐引起的腹泻。然而,对于回肠残端有限(回肠切除>100cm)而结肠完整的患者,考来烯胺可通过消耗胆盐池而增加腹泻。一般来说,对于没有结肠的Ⅰ型SBS患者可以不限制脂肪摄入。但对于仍保留一定长度结肠的Ⅱ型和Ⅲ型SBS患者,脂肪限制可能有助于缓解腹泻[10],不过也可能不会改变腹泻量;如果不摄入高热量的高脂食物,多食也变得更困难。如果回肠末端切除超过50~60cm,应每月注射维生素B_{12}。生长抑素类似物奥曲肽可延缓肠内容物通过时间并抑制消化液分泌,但是它的使用仍然存在争议,因为它也与胆结石的形成和内脏蛋白质合成减少有关,并且还没有证明它可以替代PN的使用[11-14]。

使用生长激素和谷氨酰胺促进小肠黏膜增生和促进吸收是有争议的。一项单中心随机对照试验显示采用这种方法减少了肠外营养用量、热量和输注次数,尽管效果是短暂的,并且在停止治疗后测量参数恢复到基线水平[15,16]。有研究证实GLP-2类似物是小肠黏膜的营养刺激物,可改善肠道营养吸收。另一项随机对照试验显示Teduglutide(一种GLP-2类似物)可显著减少肠功能衰竭患者的PN的用量和天数,并使一小部分患者摆脱对PN的依赖(见第106章)[17]。

(二) 胰腺炎

营养治疗在急性胰腺炎(acute pancreatitis,AP)的治疗中经历过重大的模式转变。历史上,急性胰腺炎患者通过禁食以避免进一步刺激胰腺外分泌和炎症恶化的潜在风险。在过去的20年中,急性胰腺炎患者,包括所有重症患者都提倡早期使用EN。数据表明,与标准治疗(无EN/PN)或延迟EN相比,AP患者早期喂养(入院后24~36小时内开始)可以降低多器官衰竭(multiorgan failure,MOF)、手术干预、全身感染、脓毒症甚至死亡率。PYTHON[Pancreatitis, Very Early Compared with Selective Delayed Start of Enteral Feeding(胰腺炎,极早期与选择性延迟开始肠内营养相比)]研究是一项关于胰腺炎早期与选择性延迟肠内营养相关的研究,结果截然相反。该研究是一项随机对照试验,随机将患者分为两组,试验组在24小时内通过鼻空肠(nasojejunal,NJ)管接受EN,对照组在前4天内按需经口饮食(然后仅在经口饮食不耐受的情况下才开始EN),结果显示两组在严重感染率和死亡率上没有差异[19]。在这项研究中只有20%的患者收住ICU,并且不到8%的患者是重症急性胰腺炎(定义按照持续MOF>48小时)。营养治疗的关键是全身炎症反应综合征(systemic inflammatory response syndrome,SIRS)的严重程度。如果SIRS反应严重到需要入住ICU(特别是如果患者需要机械通气),应在入院后24~36小时内留置NG/NJ管并开始EN。如果SIRS不严重,患者可以在普通病房进行治疗,那么应该接受经口饮食,只有在4天后仍未改善饮食的情况下才考虑EN。在充分复苏之前,早期启动和推进EN应谨慎;因为需要肌力支持的血流动力学不稳定的患者,可能增加非闭塞性肠系膜缺血的风险(见第118章)[20]。

两项meta分析比较了EN和PN对于重症AP的影响,结果显示在接受EN治疗的患者中,总并发症和胰腺感染并发症的风险显著降低2倍,死亡风险降低2.5倍[21,22]。美国胃肠病协会(AGA)对12项随机对照试验技术审查发现,相对于PN,EN降低了感染性胰周坏死(OR 0.28,95% CI 0.15~0.51)、单器官衰竭(OR 0.25,95% CI 0.10~0.62)和多器官衰竭(OR 0.41,95% CI 0.27~0.63)的风险[23]。将重症AP患者与轻-中度患者进行分级管理有助于识别出那些需要入住ICU、大量补液、器官衰竭早期治疗和早期启动EN的患者[24]。此外有3项RCT研究比较了重症AP患者经胃营养和经空肠营养的影响,结果显示两组在耐受性和临床预后上没有显著差异[25,26]。

慢性胰腺炎(chronic pancreatitis,CP)患者常伴有与高代谢相关的体重下降,而腹痛、吸收不良和糖尿病进一步使患者的营养摄入减少[27,28]。空肠营养在此类患者中已被用于改善体重,减轻腹痛和胃肠道不良反应及减少镇痛药使用[29]。氧化应激参与了CP的病理生理过程,补充硒、维生素C、β-胡萝卜素、α-维生素E、蛋氨酸等抗氧化剂能缓解CP患者的疼痛[30]。

一项随机、安慰剂对照试验显示,用抗氧化剂治疗CP疼痛,虽然显著提高了血液中抗氧化剂的水平,但是对92名受试者的疼痛或生活质量没有任何改善[31]。这些发现反驳了另一项随机对照试验,127名CP患者进行抗氧化剂治疗,试验组有32%的患者疼痛缓解,而安慰剂组有13%的患者疼痛缓解;患者每月疼痛天数以及每月需要的镇痛药片数量也有所减少[30]。值得注意的是,在这项研究中患者的平均年龄为30岁,只有略多于四分之一的CP其病因是酒精。总体来说,相比于年轻的非酒精性CP患者,老年的酒精性CP患者受益于抗氧化治疗的可能性相对更小。CP患者应少食多餐,避免难以消化的食物(如豆类),不再推荐限制脂肪。对于体重减轻的患者,中链甘油三酯(medium-chain triglyceride,MCT)可能有助于提供额外的热量而不会引起脂肪泻。然而MCT的耐受性可能很差,因为味道难闻,可引起痉挛、恶心和腹泻[27,32]。脂溶性维生素、维生素B_{12}和钙的补充应该根据临床需要进行调整。

(三) 克罗恩病

克罗恩病(Crohn's disease,CD)(见第115章)相关的营养不良可能继发于厌食、吸收不良、肠道丢失增加和全身炎症的分解代谢效应[33]。镁、硒、钾、锌、铁和维生素B_{12}的缺乏很常见[34]。约50%的CD患者有维生素D缺乏。除骨质疏松症之外，维生素 D 也在 CD 的发病机制中起到了一定作用，因为它可能会下调 TNF-α 相关基因的表达[35-38]。虽然 IBD 的饮食疗法（如结肠炎五步疗法、Atkins 疗法、South Beach 疗法，特定的碳水化合物疗法、消除疗法或 Maker 疗法等商品化膳食）已被证实有助于减轻症状，但是缺少相关的安慰剂对照研究。然而，对于不能进食的患者，EN 是 IBD 治疗中非常重要的部分。来自亚洲的一项随机对照试验，比较了全天或半天口服肠内营养配方与即食饮食的作用，结果显示 EN 能明显改善 IBD 的症状[39]。糖皮质激素在诱导成人 CD 临床缓解方面比 EN 更有效，但是对于儿童 CD 患者 EN 与糖皮质激素一样有效能缓解临床症状[40]。一种专门针对 IBD 患者的含有转化生长因子-β 的肠内营养配方制剂已经上市销售，但是还没有有力证据支持使用[41]。

在活动性 CD 住院患者中，随机接受 EN 或 PN 治疗，在改善症状方面没有显著差异[42,43]，然而使用 PN 达到缓解的患者，一旦停止 PN 并恢复经口饮食，症状总会复发。应用 PN 仅限于对药物治疗无效或不能 EN 的 IBD 患者。肠道休息不是 CD 缓解的必要条件。营养不良是 CD 术后并发症的独立危险因素。ESPEN 2017 指南建议需要紧急手术的 CD 患者应接受 EN 或 PN 补充额外营养以改善术后预后。有关营养支持治疗来预防 CD 患者术后并发症相关的高质量研究还很少。一项 meta 分析显示，与术前不接受 EN 或 PN 的患者相比，术前接受 EN 或 PN 的 CD 患者术后并发症的发生率降低了 74%（分别为 20.0% 和 61.3%）[44]。另一项 meta 分析也显示了术前 PN 能改善营养状况，减少术后并发症和降低疾病严重程度[45]。

（四）肝病

营养不良在晚期肝病患者中很常见，依据不同的营养评估方法，在肝硬化患者中营养不良的患病率为 50%～90%[46]。营养不良会导致腹水、肝肾综合征等并发症，是生存率的独立预测因子。在伴有营养不良的肝硬化和门静脉高压患者中，粗略估计院内死亡率为 14.1%，而不伴有营养不良的患者为 7.5%[47,48]。肝病患者的营养缺乏是多种因素共同作用的结果，包括吸收不良、代谢改变、营养储存减少、营养需求增加以及因厌食、口味改变和饮食限制导致的饮食摄入减少。厌食症的病因是多因素的，包括腹水对胃的机械压迫以及调节炎症和食欲因子的改变（如 TNF-α 和瘦素的增加）[46]。镁缺乏会导致肝硬化患者出现味觉障碍[49]。因腹水和肝性脑病分别限制了饮食中的钠和蛋白质，会进一步限制食物的种类和量。此外，酒精性肝硬化患者常以酒精代替营养丰富的食物。胆汁盐生成减少会导致对高脂食物的不耐受和脂溶性维生素的吸收不良，尤其是在胆汁淤积性肝病患者中。低白蛋白血症进一步影响营养吸收，还会导致小肠水肿。酒精性肝硬化患者伴有慢性胰腺炎的，同时会导致蛋白质和脂肪的消化不良。

门体分流可导致营养物质绕过肝脏，阻止其代谢。糖异生和蛋白质分解代谢上调，糖原分解下调，胰岛素抵抗发生，导致作为能量来源的肌肉和脂肪被消耗。肝硬化患者需要更多的蛋白质，为了预防肝性脑病而限制蛋白质摄入，只会加重蛋白质-能量营养不良[46]。研究表明正常量的蛋白质摄入是合理的，不会加重肝性脑病（见第 94 章）[50]。患者应根据其蛋白质需求进行喂养，如果发生门脉高压性脑病，应使用药物进行治疗。虽然肝硬化患者中胰岛素抵抗很常见，但是不建议通过限制碳水化合物来预防与糖原合成和肝脏储备受损相关的低血糖。支链氨基酸（branchedchain amino acid，BCAA）缬氨酸、亮氨酸和异亮氨酸应优先作为肝衰竭患者的蛋白质来源，因其通过肌肉、肾脏、脂肪和脑组织代谢。与之相反，芳香族氨基酸（aromatic amino acid，AAA）酪氨酸、苯丙氨酸和蛋氨酸仅在肝脏代谢和脱氨。肝硬化时 AA 的血清浓度发生改变，AAA 升高，BCAA 降低。目前还不确定在肝硬化患者中 AA 浓度变化是否与门静脉高压相关。有假说认为 AAA 浓度的升高会导致肝性脑病，因为 AAA 是假神经递质。过去，补充 BCAA 可以降低高氨血症，因为 BCAA 通过骨骼肌的代谢提供合成 α-酮戊二酸的碳骨架，α-酮戊二酸与 2 个氨分子结合形成谷氨酰胺[46,51]。根据最新指南推荐，与标准的全蛋白配方相比，使用富含 BCAA 的配方没有改善危重症肝病患者的预后。一项针对门诊患者的随机对照试验表明，口服 BCAA 颗粒的长期营养补充方案可能有助于延缓肝病进展，延长无病生存率[52-54]。已接受抗生素和乳果糖治疗的肝性脑病患者，增加 BCAA 的治疗不会进一步改善其精神状态或昏迷等级[52-54]。

肝硬化患者会有微量营养素缺乏。酒精性和非酒精性肝病都可以出现复合维生素 B 和维生素 C 等水溶性维生素缺乏。维生素 B_1 缺乏会导致韦尼克（Wernicke）脑病和科萨科夫（Korsakoff）痴呆，这种情况不仅见于酗酒者而且也见于丙型肝炎相关的肝硬化患者。因此，建议所有的肝硬化患者补充维生素 B_1。丙型肝炎病毒感染时叶酸和维生素 B_6 水平下降，需要关注的是，在聚乙二醇干扰素和利巴韦林治疗丙肝时可进一步降低维生素 B_1、维生素 B_2 和维生素 B_6 水平[46]。与实质性肝病相比，脂溶性维生素缺乏更易发生在胆汁淤积性肝病中。在肝硬化患者中维生素 A 缺乏是癌症的一个危险因素（包括肝癌）[55]。肝病患者的维生素 D 水平较低，随着肝病的进展会进一步下降[56-58]。因此在胆汁淤积性和非胆汁淤积性肝病中，骨质疏松症的患病率都很高。对自身免疫性肝炎和肝移植患者使用的免疫抑制剂（包括糖皮质激素）会增加代谢性骨病的风险。慢性肝病患者发生骨质疏松症的其他危险因素包括高龄、低体重指数、性腺功能减退、雌激素缺乏、钙摄入量低、过度饮酒、吸烟和缺乏运动[59]。据报道，胆汁淤积性肝病和酒精性肝病中都存在维生素 E 缺乏，低水平的维生素 E 可能促进脂肪肝发展为脂肪性肝炎。缺锌也与肝病有关（尤其是酒精性肝病），可能会导致厌食、味觉和嗅觉改变、免疫功能障碍、蛋白质代谢改变、肝性脑病和糖耐量异常。补充锌可改善葡萄糖代谢，但有数据显示不能改善肝性脑病[55]。由于铜和锰排泄入胆汁，肝硬化或胆汁淤积性肝病患者的 PN 配方中，应减少或不加这些微量元素[60]。

随着肝功能恶化，腹水患者可能无法耐受因 PN 带来的大量液体，所以对于需要营养支持的肝硬化患者而言，EN 优于 PN[55]。过量的右旋糖和葡萄糖会导致脂肪变性，接受长期 PN 治疗的患者会发展成肝脏胆汁淤积、肝纤维化，甚至肝硬化[60]。继发于免疫功能紊乱和肠道通透性增加的导管相关脓毒症的风险也增加[61,62]。与肝硬化患者相比，那些热量摄入多的慢性肝病患者预后相对较好。肝糖原储存不足和糖异生能力降低可导致在延长禁食期间发生低血糖和瘦体重减少。因此,肝硬化患者禁食时间不应超过 3 小时,而且睡前需少量进食。合并严重营养不良的肝病患者在肝移植后易感染、ICU 住院时间延长和总住院时间延长,但目前没有 RCT 研究证明术前营养支持能改善肝移植术后的预后[63,64]。有研究显示早期的术后 EN 可以减少脓毒症的发生率,术后 PN 可以减少 ICU 住院时间[65,66]。两项随机对照研究表明肝移植术后给予肠道菌群共生治疗(益生菌和益生元)可减少细菌感染[67,68]。

(五) 憩室病

憩室病患者(见第 121 章)经常获得错误的营养信息。患者经常被告知避免食用坚果或含种子的食物,因为担心这些坚硬的小颗粒可能会滞留在憩室中并导致憩室炎,尽管已有证据显示这些食物没有伤害[69,70]。既往的回顾性研究和流行病学研究表明,膳食纤维有助于预防症状性憩室病,但没有相关的 RCT 研究[71]。纤维摄入量至少为 25g/d,以不溶性纤维为主,如麦麸、麸皮松饼和纤维谷物。益生菌也可以治疗和预防憩室炎[72]。迄今为止,研究最多的益生菌是各种乳酸杆菌菌株。一项纳入了 11 项益生菌治疗憩室病研究的 meta 分析,在 764 例接受评估的患者中,大多数患者的症状有所缓解或减轻[73]。然而,关于预防并发症和复发相关的高质量研究很少;目前 AGA 指南不推荐单纯性憩室炎患者使用益生菌[74]。肥胖和缺乏体育锻炼会增加症状性憩室病的风险,不管是男性还是女性[75-77]。

(六) 倾倒综合征

倾倒综合征,发生于胃切除术、迷走神经切断术或食管手术后,使食物快速进入小肠;随着减肥手术的日益普及,倾倒综合征越来越多(见第 8 章)。倾倒综合征有两种类型。早期倾倒综合征发生在饭后 30 分钟内,表现为腹痛、腹泻、肠鸣音异常、腹胀、恶心和血管舒缩性症状,包括潮红、出汗、心动过速、低血压和晕厥。这些表现是由于液体从血管内转移到十二指肠腔的高渗环境中,以及由于进入小肠的高碳水化合物负荷导致胃肠激素释放增加所致。肠胰高血糖素、胰多肽、YY 肽、血管活性肠多肽和神经降压素等激素引起全身和内脏血管舒张而出现相关的症状[78,79]。迟发性倾倒综合征发生在饭后 1~3 小时,其特征是低血糖、出汗,饥饿、疲劳和晕厥,这些症状可能是因为空肠中过量碳水化合物负荷引起 GLP-1 介导的胰岛素快速(较早)释放而出现的低血糖症状。倾倒综合征一般通过临床评估和改良的口服葡萄糖耐量试验诊断[78]。本章后面介绍倾倒综合征的营养治疗。

(七) 癌症

蛋白质-能量营养不良是癌症患者的常见问题。体重下降的发生率与肿瘤类型相关,肉瘤、乳腺癌和血液系统肿瘤患者发生率为 31% ~ 40%,结肠癌、前列腺癌和肺癌患者为 54% ~64%,而胰腺癌和胃癌患为 80%[80]。营养不良的发生不仅与癌症类型相关,还与特定的抗肿瘤治疗和患者的一般情况(年龄、性别和合并糖尿病、胃肠道疾病等)相关[81]。营养不良会降低抗癌治疗效果,导致治疗时间和住院时间延长、费用增加、发病率和死亡率增加。癌症患者营养不良的病因是多方面的,包括由肿瘤诱导的代谢异常引起的癌性恶病质、热量摄入不足、消化不良、吸收不良和癌症治疗本身引起的胃肠道毒性。癌性恶病质的重要介质被认为包括由肿瘤产生的蛋白水解诱导因子、脂质动员因子以及像神经肽 Y(食欲刺激)和阿黑皮素原(厌食刺激)这样的平衡神经激素的因子。蛋白水解诱导因子诱导蛋白质合成减少、蛋白质降解增加和促炎症细胞因子(IL-6 和 IL-8)增加。脂质动员因子可促进脂肪分解,导致体内脂肪减少和体重下降,而这与热量摄入无关[82]。

多数专家开始为癌症患者制定饮食方案,调整进食量和进食模式(即少食多餐)、添加辅食或补充剂,或改变食物配方(流质、泥状食物等)。采用糖皮质激素和醋酸甲地孕酮刺激食欲的方法,已经被成功用于轻度营养不良的癌症患者[83]。尽管这两种药物都能改善食欲和增加体重,但是醋酸甲地孕酮会增加深静脉血栓形成的风险[84,85]。对于不伴有营养不良的癌症患者,在接受化疗、放疗或手术治疗时不推荐常规的营养支持治疗,除非他们长时间不能摄取或吸收到足够的营养物质;已有研究表明常规营养支持治疗能改善这些患者的体重和氮平衡,但不能提高生存率[86]。虽然依赖于 PEG 喂养可能会延迟吞咽功能的恢复和经口进食,但在头颈部癌症患者中,EN 有效防止体重减轻、减少住院次数以及化疗和放疗的中断。化疗期间常规使用 PN 不能降低毒性、改善肿瘤反应或降低死亡率[86]。骨髓或造血干细胞移植后发生严重胃肠道黏膜炎症的患者会受益于 PN[87]。与 PN 相比,EN 与造血干细胞移植患者的发病率、腹泻、高血糖的增加和移植时间延迟相关,但与体重和体脂减少不相关[86]。癌症患者 PN 的使用应仅限于预期寿命合适且生活质量足够(Karnofsky 评分>50)的患者,因为这些患者不会长时间被动维持他们的营养需求(见第 132 章)。

(八) 肥胖

肥胖是"可预防性死亡"的第二大原因,它与 2 型糖尿病、高血压、冠状动脉疾病、脑血管疾病、阻塞性睡眠呼吸暂停、癌症、骨关节炎和抑郁症有关[88]。尽管严重肥胖的患者有丰富的脂肪组织,但是应尽早、及时接受营养治疗。对于严重肥胖患者的营养评估可能很困难。现行的估算能量消耗的公式在该人群中是无效的,间接测热法仍然是金标准(见第 5 章)。对于伴有糖耐量异常或糖尿病的肥胖患者,PN 中的浓缩葡萄糖溶液可导致高血糖,这会增加院内感染风险,抑制免疫反应,延迟伤口愈合及增加总体死亡率。在代谢应激期间,蛋白质分解导致糖异生。一些研究表明富含蛋白质的低热量喂养(即 2g 蛋白质/kg 理想体重/d 和 65% ~70% 的热量需求),也称为允许性低摄入,优于标准的营养方案,原因在于体内储备的脂质氧化可以提供能量来源,而补充的蛋白质则用于促进蛋白质合成代谢。然而这种方法仍有争议。在允许性低摄入的情况下很少发生高血糖,维持瘦体重会导致总体重下降[88]。对于严重肥胖患者,美国肠外和肠内营养学会推荐:BMI 在 30~50 之间时,每天推荐摄入热量为 11 ~ 14kcal/kg×实际体重;BMI>50,每天推荐摄入热量为 22 ~ 25kcal/kg×理想体重;BMI 在 30~40 之间时,推荐的蛋白质摄入量为 2g/kg×理想体重;BMI ≥40,推荐的蛋白质摄入量为 2. 5g/kg×理想体重。

美国预防服务特别工作组建议所有成年人都要进行肥胖筛查,BMI 在 30kg/m^2 或以上的人应该接受强化的多样性行为干预,对于 BMI 大于 40kg/m^2 或者 BMI 大于 35kg/m^2 且伴有肥胖相关并发症的个体,建议接受减肥手术(见第 8 章)。肥胖患者普遍存在微量营养素缺乏(尤其是铁和维生素 D),术前应予以纠正。减肥手术后患者从清淡的流质饮食逐渐过渡到固体饮食,同时特别鼓励由专门的减肥营养师进行营养指导。行 Roux-en-Y 胃分流术的患者,因为胃容量的缩小,需要限制经口进食。Roux-en-Y 胃分流术后共同通道的长度越短,出现微量营养素和常量营养素缺乏的可能性就越大[89]。腹腔镜可调节胃束带置入术是引起营养问题可能性最小的一种方法,但是并发症发生率高,超过 40% 的患者需要移除束带,这种方法逐渐被淘汰。垂直袖状胃切除术对胃肠道生理的破坏性较小,能有效减轻体重和降低糖尿病风险,因此得到越来越多的应用。了解患者的术后解剖结构和各种营养物质的吸收部位对于预防和诊断营养缺乏非常重要(表 6.1)。减肥术后营养缺乏分为 3 种类型:蛋白质-能量营养不良、维生素和矿物质缺乏和脱水。出院后不久就应开始终生补充维生素以防止出现营养不良。因为营养缺乏是一个渐进性过程,可能需要数年才会出现症状[88]。

表 6.1　胃和小肠的营养吸收部位

部位	营养物质
胃	水、乙醇、铜、碘化物、氟化物和钼
十二指肠	钙、铁、磷、镁、铜、硒、硫胺素、核黄素、烟酸、生物素、叶酸;维生素 A、维生素 D、维生素 E、维生素 K
空肠	二肽、三肽、氨基酸、钙、磷、镁、铁、锌、铬、锰、钼、硫胺素、核黄素、烟酸、泛酸、生物素、叶酸;维生素 B_6、维生素 C、维生素 A、D、维生素 E、维生素 K
回肠	叶酸、镁;维生素 B_{12}、维生素 C、维生素 D

Data from Kaafarani HM, Shikora SA. Nutritional support of the obese and critically ill obese patient. Surg Clin North Am 2011;91:837-55, viii-ix, Ret with permission。

减肥术后营养状况恶化的原因多种多样,包括胃空肠吻合口狭窄和胆胰侧旁路过长。微量营养素缺乏可导致贫血(铁、铜、锌、叶酸、维生素 B_{12}、维生素 A、维生素 E)、代谢性骨病(钙、维生素 D)、脑病(维生素 B_1)、多发性神经病变和肌病(维生素 B_1、铜、维生素 B_{12} 和维生素 E)、视觉障碍(维生素 B_1、维生素 A 和维生素 E)和皮疹(锌、必需脂肪酸、维生素 A)(见第 103 章)[89]。Roux-en-Y 胃旁路术后会出现铁、叶酸、钙和维生素 B_{12} 缺乏。胆胰分流后会出现锌、钠、氯化物、镁和脂溶性维生素缺乏。减肥手术后会经常出现脱水现象,尤其是在温暖的天气和剧烈运动之后。因为胃的容积缩小,患者大量饮水的能力受到限制,建议每天摄入约 2L 液体,饮水量因人而异及其日常活动量不同而有所不同[88]。

对于那些没有手术指征的肥胖患者,也可以采用药物疗法。根据 2013 年美国心脏病学会、美国心脏协会、成人超重和肥胖管理的肥胖协会的联合指南和肥胖药物治疗内分泌协会的临床实践指南推荐,如果患者的 BMI≥30kg/m^2 或 BMI≥27kg/m^2 且伴有高血压、血脂异常、2 型糖尿病或阻塞性睡眠呼吸暂停等肥胖相关并发症的[90,91],建议进行药物治疗。主要有 6 种减肥药物:芬特明、芬特明/托吡酯、奥利司他、氯卡色林、安非他酮/纳曲酮和利拉鲁肽(见第 7 章)。

芬特明在美国是治疗肥胖最常用的处方药。它是一种归类为肾上腺素能激动剂的Ⅳ级管控药品,具有增加静息能量消耗和抑制食欲的作用。因为没有长期安全性试验,作为单药治疗时建议短期使用(3 个月)。当与托吡酯缓释剂联合使用时,芬特明可长期使用。奥利司他通过抑制胰腺和胃脂肪酶的分泌来阻止脂肪的吸收,从而起到减肥作用。奥利司他还具有降低血糖和改善胰岛素敏感性的作用[92]。氯卡色林是一种选择性羟色胺-2C 受体激动剂,用于肥胖症的长期治疗。5-羟色胺 2C 受体在多巴胺系统的调节中发挥作用,被认为会影响饮食相关的行为。另外两种药品—安非他酮(一种多巴胺和去甲肾上腺素再摄取抑制剂)和纳曲酮(一种阿片类拮抗剂)分别被 FDA 批准用于治疗阿片类药物依赖和酗酒。纳曲酮/安非他酮作用于下丘脑弓状核和中脑边缘多巴胺系统"奖赏通路",调节食欲和对食物的渴望。利拉鲁肽获 FDA 批准用于慢性体重控制和 2 型糖尿病的治疗,它是 GLP-1 类似物,GLP-1 随着食物摄入而释放,起到减少饥饿感,减少食物摄入和延迟胃排空的作用[93]。

(九)危重症

评估危重患者的营养风险尤其重要,因为从营养角度来看,风险是双重的,营养状况恶化和疾病严重程度会共同导致病情加重。虽然营养风险较高的患者往往因存在胃肠道不耐受而难以完成规定的 EN 方案,但与营养风险较低的患者相比,他们更有可能从营养干预中获益。关于危重症患者营养治疗,美国肠外和肠内营养学会的指南建议所有入住 ICU 的患者均进行初步的营养风险筛查。虽然营养风险的概念非常重要,但是如何使用工具来确定此类风险(2002 年营养风险筛查或 NRS-2002 危重症患者营养风险评分或 NUTRIC 评分)还是存在困难。高营养风险患者(NRS-2002>5 或 NUTRIC 评分≥5)在入住 ICU 之后的 24~36 小时内应尽早开始 EN。需要在 3~4 天的时间达到目标剂量,尽量减少过度喂养的机会,因为外源性营养物质会增加肝脏的内源性糖异生作用。需要监测胃肠道的耐受情况,监测电解质以及时发现低磷血症。低血压患者可使用血管加压药物保持病情稳定。快速使蛋白质达标[2.0g/(kg·d)]比热量达标[20~25kcal/(kg·d)]更重要。为实现 EN 的临床获益,同时避免过度进食,需要尽力在住院的第一周内提供约 80% 的目标能量需求。对于低、中危的患者,营养性进食还获得了非营养性的获益如防止胃肠道黏膜萎缩和维持胃肠道完整性,但是这些不足以达到高危患者 EN 治疗的常用的治疗终点。为预防烧伤和骨髓移植患者肠道通透性增加和全身感染[95],促进颅脑损伤患者更快恢复认知功能[96]和降低高危患者的住院死亡率[97],需要增加 50%~60% 的目标能量。同样,一项对高危手术患者(NRS-2002≥5)的前瞻性研究表明,与接受不充分营养治疗的患者相比,术前接受充分营养治疗[10kcal/(kg·d),持续 7 天]在院内感染和总体并发症方面均有显著降低[98]。

一旦开始 EN,应该每天监测患者的耐受性。避免不适当的中断 EN,尽量减少禁食时间以避免肠梗阻和预防营养供应不足。胃残余容积(gastric residual volume,GRV)不应作为评价 ICU 患者是否进行 EN 的指标,GRV 与肺炎、反流或误吸的发生率不相关,也不能很好地反映胃排空情况。EN 方案的设计和实施要以尽可能提供更多的能量为目标,同时考虑基于容积的喂养方案,明确规定每天输注的目标容量。在血流动力学不稳定的情况下,需要适当调整治疗方案。如果正在升压治疗,应该减少 EN。在患者完全苏醒且病情稳定 24 至 36 小时后,可以谨慎开始或重启 EN,同时停用升压治疗。虽然危重症患者发生亚临床肠道缺血/再灌注损伤的风险增加,但是有研究显示肠道缺血是 EN 罕见的并发症。与不使用 EN 相比,对于应用稳定低剂量血管升压药物甚至多种血管升压药物的患者,使用 EN 降低 ICU 死亡率和住院死亡率[99]。

低营养风险的患者,如果不能保持自主进食且早期不适宜 EN 的,那么应在入住 ICU 的 7 天之内进行 PN[61]。高营养风险的患者,如果不适宜 EN,则应在入院后尽快启动 PN[61,100]。对于危重症患者,无论风险如何,对于已经在进行管内喂养但未达到目标方案的 60% 的,补充 PN 的添加应维持到入院后 7~10 天。随着对 EN 耐受性的提高,应该减少 PN。当患者可以从 EN 获得超过 60% 目标能量需求时,应该停止 PN。

对于需要 PN 的 ICU 患者,第一周需要高蛋白低热量 PN,提供的能量应为需求能量的 80%[20kcal/(kg·d)×实际体重]。与标准肠外营养相比,允许性低摄入可降低高血糖、感染、减少 ICU 和住院时间以及机械通气时间[61,101,102]。

所有接受营养支持的重症患者均需要通过肠内或肠外途径补充抗氧化维生素(包括维生素 E 和维生素 C)和微量元素(包括硒、锌和铜),这样能降低烧伤患者、创伤患者和需要机械通气的危重症患者的死亡率[61,100]。

二、营养治疗

(一)肠内营养

肠内营养(EN)能够维持胃肠道结构和功能的完整性。通过保持黏膜量和绒毛高度,刺激上皮细胞增殖,促进刷状缘酶的产生,保持能够分泌免疫球蛋白(Ig)A 的免疫细胞的数量(组成肠道相关淋巴组织)来维持结构完整性。通过维持上皮内细胞之间的紧密连接、维持黏液层的厚度、刺激血液流动以及诱导胃泌素、胆囊收缩素、铃蟾素和胆盐等各种内源性营养物质的产生和释放来维持功能完整性。供给的 EN 有助于危重症患者共生微生物群,防止出现致病的有害菌群[103]。

对于那些由于胃肠道功能障碍而不愿或不能进食的患者,需要通过一个喂养管提供食物。放射科医生、消化科医生或外科医生根据具体设备和专业知识可以在床边、X 线透视辅助下、内镜辅助下或手术室放置这些肠内营养管[104]。

1. 鼻肠管通路

使用经小肠喂养以预防误吸是一个复杂和争议的问题。对于误吸高风险或经胃喂养不耐受的危重患者,建议经小肠喂养[61,105]。床边鼻肠管(nasoenteric tube,NET)置入术(图 6.1)是医院和长期护理中最常用的肠内通道技术。应用带有 GPS 成像系统的导管有利于鼻肠管顺利通过幽门。另外内镜下经导丝 NET(endoscopic over-the-guidewire NET,ENET)置入术能实现直视下放置(图 6.2)。置入 ENET 后需要牵引绳固定(图 6.3)。

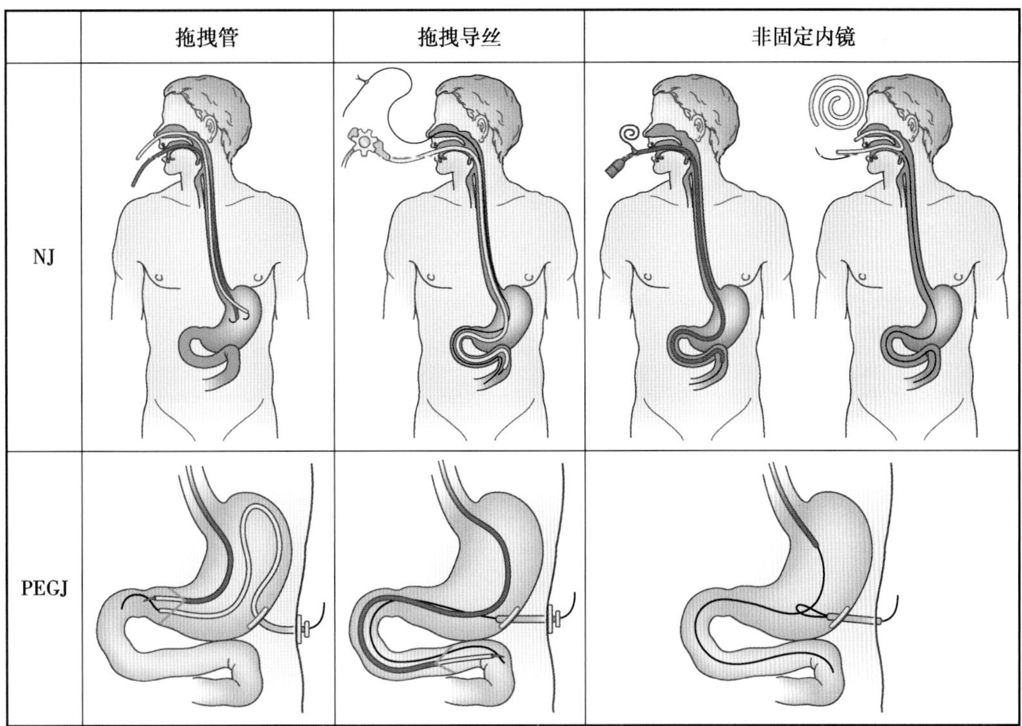

图 6.1　肠内通路的优先技术。将拖拽管拖动到位,会增加内镜撤回时发生近端位移的可能性。使用拖拽导丝更好,但导丝扭转仍会阻碍内镜检查。使用非固定内镜技术放置金属导丝,然后沿金属导丝将插管送至小肠,而无须使用内镜将其拖拽到位。NJ,鼻腔肠;PEGJ,经皮内镜下胃空肠造口术。(Reprinted with permission from Chandrasekhara V,Kochman M. Techniques in Gastrointestinal Endoscopy,Elsevier.)

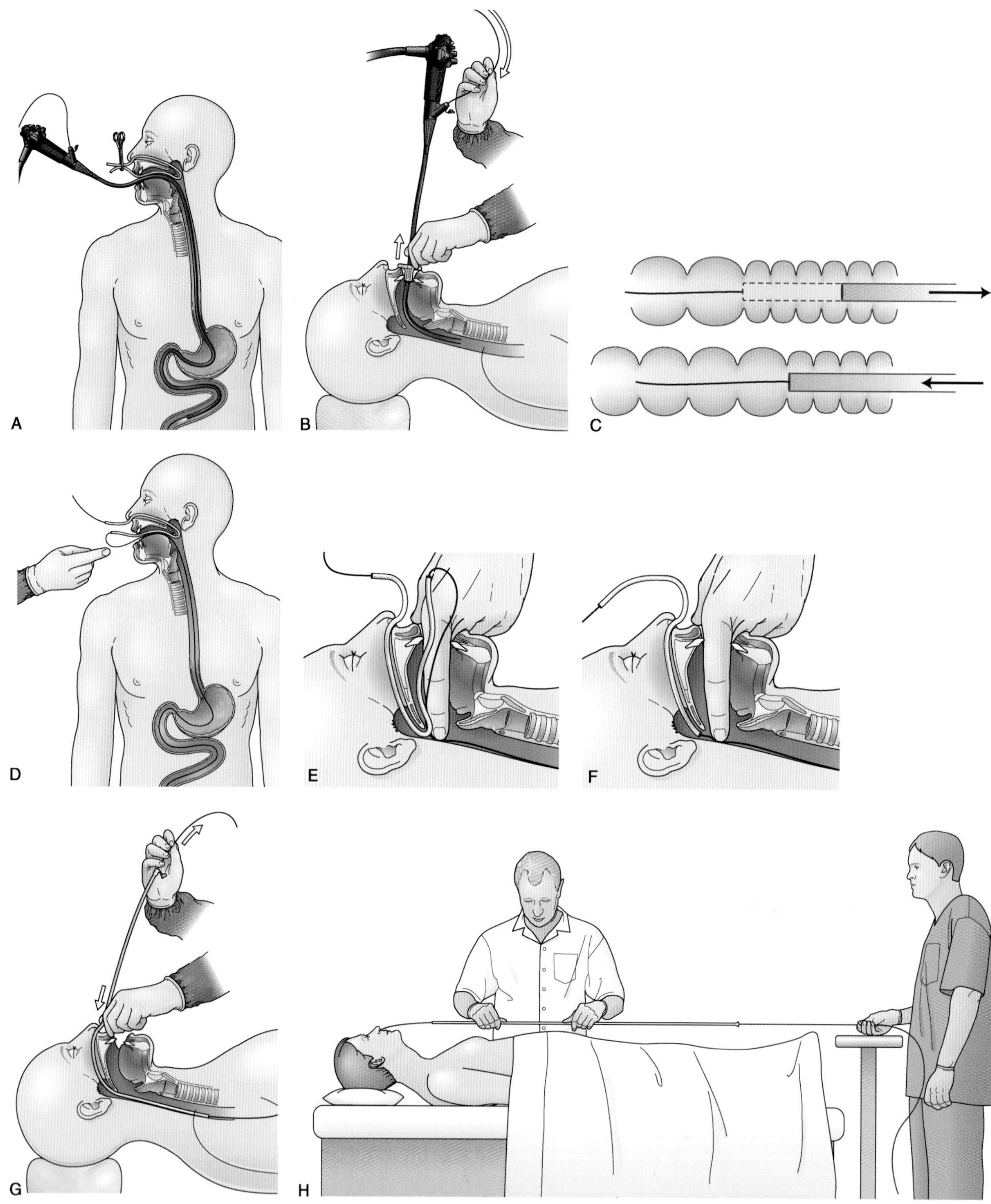

图 6.2　内镜下经导丝鼻肠管插入技术。A,将儿科结肠镜穿过 Treitz 韧带下方,导丝伸出内镜末端。B,在最初的导丝插入中,以导丝通过操作通道的相同速度将内镜从口腔中退出,以防止导丝尖端从其在小肠中的位置移位。C,使用锁孔技术将内镜从导丝上拔出。在内镜末端打褶的肠管,将内镜抽出 5~6cm。通过快速将内镜推回 2~3cm,肠管从内镜上脱落,1~2 次打折。D,导丝伸出口腔后,导丝尖端然后通过口鼻转移管。E 和 F,然后用示指将导丝固定在咽后壁上,同时对经鼻伸出的导丝施加牵引力,牵拉导丝至导丝伸直,在咽后壁手指感觉到抗力。G,在最终导丝转移的一项技术中,将饲养管沿导丝向下穿过鼻孔,速度与导丝从饲养管远端撤出完全相同,以避免导丝顶端移位。H,在最终导丝转移的替代技术中,助手将导丝固定在"空间点"(使用床旁工作台),然后将管子沿固定导丝滑入到最终位置。(Reprinted with permission from Chandrasekhara V, Kochman M. Techniques in Gastrointestinal Endoscopy, Elsevier.)

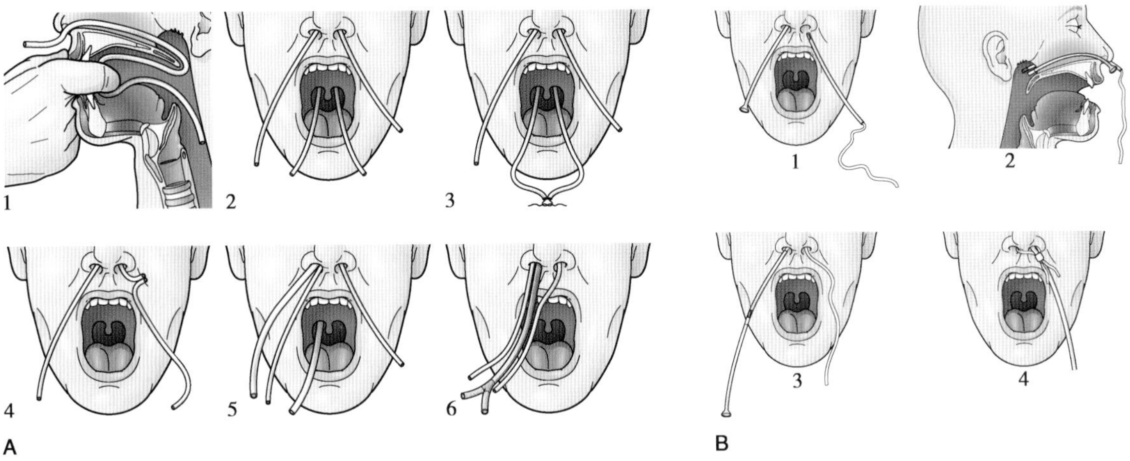

1 2 3 1 2
4 5 6 3 4
A B

图 6.3 内镜下鼻肠管固定的 Bridle 技术。A,使用两个 5Fr 新生儿饲养管。B,使用 2 个带有磁性末端的可屈式导管。(Reprinted with permission from Chandrasekhara V,Kochman M. Techniques in Gastrointestinal Endoscopy,Elsevier.)

一般选取 8~12Fr 的鼻胃管经润滑后在患者头部屈曲时进入胃部,可以嘱患者喝几口水帮助管子通过[106]。床边听诊确定鼻胃管的合适位置有一定困难。除那些能使用电磁 GPS 成像系统获得位置的导管之外,其他患者术后进行鼻饲前需要拍一张腹部平片以确认鼻胃管或鼻肠管的正确位置。令人意外的是,床边放置普通鼻肠管的成功率高于带磁重力珠的营养管(92% vs 56%),原因可能是营养管末端的重力珠实际上阻碍了管路自行通过幽门[107]。

我们也可以在床边,给患者适当的镇静剂,通过内镜下直视放置 NJ 营养管。用拖拉的方法将缝线连接到 NJ 管的末端,并用异物钳将其拖入小肠中。通常很难从异物钳上松开缝合线,而且很难在不移除相邻 NJ 管的情况下移除内镜,所以可以使用止血钳来拖拽该管,然后将其夹在小肠上。第二种常见技术就是"导线上方"技术,该技术需要使用能穿过鼻孔的 5mm 超细胃镜将导丝放入小肠中,退镜后导线留在原处,导丝引导下将鼻饲管放置小肠,成功率为 90%~100%[108-110]。该技术还可使用儿科结肠镜通过口腔向下进入小肠。一根导丝穿过肠腔,将内镜收回,导丝通过鼻子移出,最后将导管放置在导丝上[111,112]。

鼻肠管应用于那些需要经 NG 或 NJ 通路 EN,且需要 1 个月内的营养支持的患者。早期多次未能保持鼻胃管放置的患者或预计需要 1 个月以上喂养时间的患者应接受更持久的肠内通路,如 PEG、直接经皮内镜下空肠造口术(direct percutaneous endoscopic jejunostomy,DPEJ)、联合经皮内镜下胃空肠造口术(percutaneous endoscopic gastrojejunostomy,PEGJ)、外科胃造口术或手术空肠造口术。

2. 经皮内镜下肠内通路

经皮内镜下肠内营养管置入术通常需要在内镜室、手术室或床边进行,并中度或深度镇静。与鼻肠管通路相比,经皮肠内通路更为可靠,因为肠内通路较少出现导管功能障碍而使患者每天摄入更多的热量[113]。

(1) 经皮穿刺造口

经皮穿刺造口,如 PEG,适用于那些无法维持足够营养摄入超过 1 个月的患者,尽管其胃肠道功能正常。某些特定患者,如卒中患者在恢复吞咽功能和经口摄入营养前,PEG 是非常有用的。但在某些特定患者,如晚期痴呆患者、晚期恶性肿瘤患者,PEG 的作用是有限的[114-119]。对于高危患者,PEG 治疗后的高死亡率通常不是因为 PEG 的问题,而是与患者原发病和衰竭状态有关。PEG 除了能提供营养通道外,PEG 管还可用于补液、给药及胃减压。下面介绍一些常见的放置 PEG 的适应证。

癌症

头颈部癌症(head and neck cancer,HNC)患者由于肿瘤本身或抗肿瘤治疗引起吞咽困难,导致营养不良的风险很高。大约 50% 的 HNC 患者需要多种方式进行营养支持[120]。有研究显示可通过 PEG 的 EN 支持来减少 HNC 患者因脱水和营养不良导致的住院次数,防止体重减轻,避免治疗中断[121]。因 PEG 管导致肿瘤在造口部位种植转移是很罕见的。在一项回顾性研究中,304 例接受 PEG 管治疗的 HNC 患者,只有 2 例发生了吻合口转移(0.92%)[122]。但是,在 HNC 中放置 PEG 仍存在争议,因为依赖 PEG 喂养可能延迟吞咽功能的恢复和经口饮食的恢复。在肠梗阻的肠癌患者中,PEG 管还可以安全有效地用于肠减压。这种"通气性"经皮内镜下造口术,无须使用鼻胃管,不会产生恶心和呕吐,并可让那些临终患者出院,在一定程度上经口摄入部分软食[123]。

在晚期不能手术的癌症患者中应用 EN 或 PN 是有争议的。我们用远期生活质量评估(Karnofsky Performance Scale Index)来评估患者的生活质量(见第 132 章)。在晚期不能手术的恶性肿瘤患者中,使用 EN 或 PN 可提供更好的能量和心理安慰,如果患者的远期生活质量评估>50,或者营养支持可帮助患者完成放化疗方案,则应考虑使用 EN 或 PN[124]。最终,治疗策略应取决于患者的喜好和价值观,因为患者的自主性至关重要。PEG 放置的最终决定不仅根据科学事实,可能还需要基于患者的文化、个人、家庭、精神和宗教信仰等。

卒中

目前研究显示,对于卒中导致的吞咽困难,PEG 可作为患者在恢复吞咽功能和经口饮食前的营养支持"桥梁"。与 NG 饲喂相比,发现早期 PEG 可减轻呼吸机相关性肺炎的发生[125]。Cochrane meta 分析表明,与 NG 饲喂相比,PEG 饲喂可降低治疗失败率,并且能提高喂养的总体达标率。

痴呆

尽管,PEG 在痴呆患者中已得到了广泛的应用,但其获益的机制仍然不清楚。在一项前瞻性队列研究中,将 36 000 多名居住养老院且近期刚发生吞咽困难的痴呆患者随机分组,不管是否留置了 PEG 管还是留置的时间都不影响生存率[126]。痴呆症患者放置 PEG 最常见原因包括避免误吸、预防压疮、改善生活质量和延长生存期。痴呆患者放置 PEG 的获益也是有限的。当痴呆症患者由工作人员或家属手动喂养改为 PEG 管喂养时,他们会失去味觉、触觉、养育和社交互动[127]。超过 70% 痴呆症的患者需要管饲喂养[116]。由于活动能力下降和需要限制活动,PEG 管放置的养老院患者出现压疮的风险实际上可能会增加[119]。在另一项前瞻性研究中,对 150 名 PEG 管放置的患者进行随访发现,有 70% 的痴呆患者功能状态或总体主观健康状况没有得到改善[128]。虽然,这些患者的生活质量和健康状况可能无法直接改善,但他/她的护理变得更加易于管理。放置 PEG 后,家属和护理人员通常会减少挫败感和增加成就感[128]。放置 PEG 管对降低吸入性肺炎发生率的作用很小,因为患者仍然能够吸入口咽分泌物[129]。多个专业医疗机构,包括急性期后和长期护理学会、美国临终关怀与姑息医学会、美国老年医学会,均建议不采用经皮置管,支持首选经口辅助喂养方法。

(2) 经皮内镜下胃造口术

在 20 世纪 80 年代初期,Ponsky 和 Gauderer 发明了 PEG[130]。该手术包括在内镜检查胃壁后选择合适的胃造口位置后放置 PEG 管(图 6.4)。如果没有看到内镜透射光或手指按压点,则不应继续操作。有研究表明,术前预防性静滴抗生素对于预防术后造口感染非常重要[131,132]。术前 30 分钟应预防性静滴皮肤覆盖率高的抗生素,例如头孢唑林(1g)。

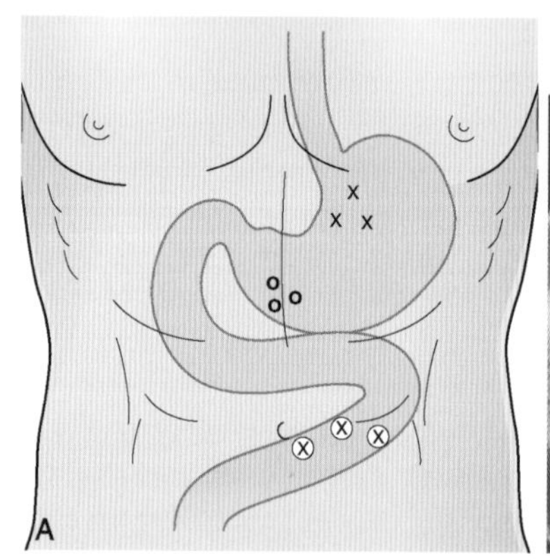

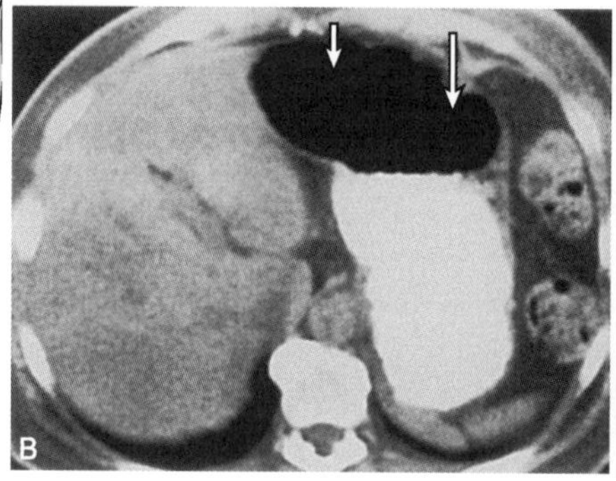

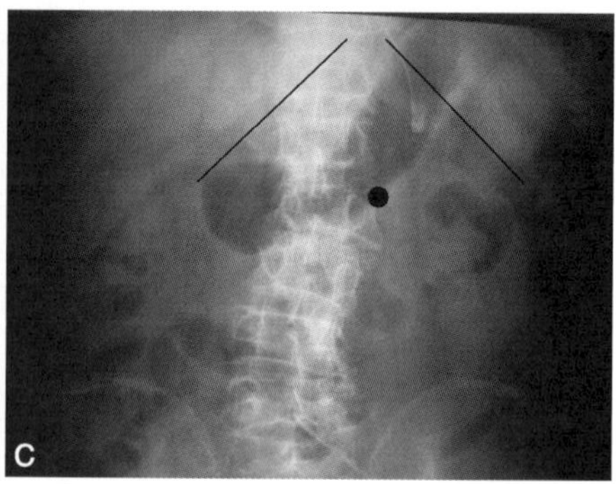

图 6.4 经皮内镜下胃造口术(PEG)、经皮内镜下胃空肠造口术(PEGJ)和直接经皮内镜下空肠造口术(DPEJ)部位定位的手术步骤。A,传统的 PEG 部位在左上腹用 x 标记。最佳的定位是在脐部上方,靠近中线或稍微靠近患者中线位置的右侧(圆圈)。PEG 在胃窦,如以后需要转换为 PEGJ 则是理想的。带圆圈的 x 显示了 DPEJ 置入部位的较大变化,这种变化可以选择在从左肋缘到左髂嵴的任何部位。B,CT 扫描显示,PEG 部位略高于或靠近患者脐部右侧与胃窦部最直接、垂直、最短的通道区相重合。而左上腹的传统部位有一个更长、更切线位的通道进入中体甚至更低的位置。C,在脐部放置硬币(黑圈),在放置 PEG 之前经鼻胃管注入 500mL 空气,有助于识别胃窦,方便选择 PEG 部位。(Reprinted with permission from Chandrasekhara V, Kochman M. Techniques in Gastrointestinal Endoscopy, Elsevier.)

PEG 管的放置可通过以下两种方式完成:Ponsky(拉)或 Sachs Vine(推)技术,取决于医生的偏好,因为两者同样有效[133]。第三种方式 Russell(插入)技术可能适用于外生性口咽癌、食管癌,因为近期头颈外科手术引起的口咽切口或食管狭窄阻碍内镜或 PEG 管的通过[134]。在 Russell 技术中,通过经皮放置 T 型固定件使胃壁紧贴腹壁;在腹壁做一切口,然后在胃内形成瘘管并逐层扩张;最后,将带有气球垫(在设计上类似气球替换管)的 PEG 管插入穿刺点[135]。PEG 放置的相对禁忌证为:胃底静脉曲张,胃大部切除,腹水和凝血障碍。成年患者最常用的 PEG 管为硅树脂管,尺寸为 16~20Fr[136]。不建议采用直径太大的 PEG 管,因为气孔道直径增大容易出现侧弯。

胃造口部位应用温和的肥皂水清洗,而不要用过氧化氢清洗,因为过氧化氢会刺激皮肤并导致造口渗漏。为了吸收水分并避免过度张紧,应在胃造口管外固定钮下面放一层纱布,而且不能用封闭性敷料,否则有出现造口周围皮肤浸软和溃疡的风险。

PEG 管装置大致分为两类,球囊型胃造口装置和低矮式球囊型胃造口装置。球囊型胃造口装置通常带有一个球囊做内部支撑(图 6.5)。球囊管可以通过胃造口术部位盲插入胃腔,球囊膨胀后用作内部支撑。因为球囊容易破裂,通常需要在 3~6 个月内更换。这种装置还带弹性的内部保险杠,由导丝引导,盲推导管进入胃造口部位,然后移除导丝,球囊扩张

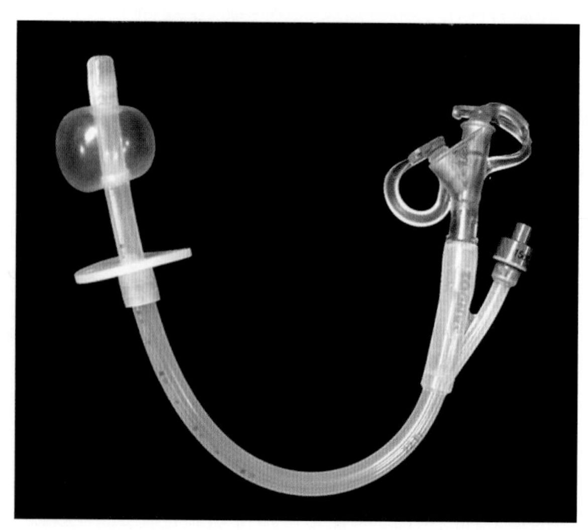

图 6.5 更换胃造口管

起到内部支撑作用。低矮式球囊型胃造口装置(图6.6)可直接经腹壁皮肤置入胃腔内,尤其适用于那些可能习惯性地拉扯床上用品并拔出自己管子接头的精神恍惚的患者。这个装置有一个内部支撑座是一种可充气的球囊或是一种有弹性的内部支撑座,需要导丝引导置入。这种低矮式的装置其管长有限,必须根据测量胃造口瘘管长度选择。通过低矮式球囊型胃造口装置喂养或胃肠减压时,必须使用单独的接入管将阀门连接在装置顶部。

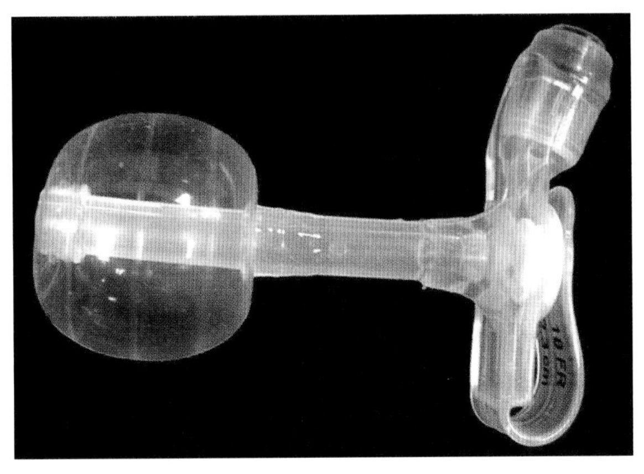

图6.6 小型经皮内镜下胃造口器械

(3) 经皮内镜下胃空肠造口术

对于需要肠内管饲的患者,可以通过2种方法建立内镜下经皮肠道通路。第一种方法为经皮内镜下空肠造口术(PEGJ),即首先以标准方式进行经皮内镜下胃造口术,然后可采用各种方法使空肠饲管穿过胃造口道进入小肠[108,137,138]。第二种方法是直接PEG(DPEJ),使用改进的Ponsky牵引技术,将小直径胃造瘘管直接置入近端空肠。

PEGJ置管有3种常用的技术。如图6.7的柯比技术是指内镜下,用一只长320cm活检钳抓住PEG末端丝线,并向下拖入近端空肠,随后将内镜撤回到PEG部位上方的近端胃部,然后用夹子将导丝固定在适当的位置。再将9~12Fr J管穿过导丝上PEG,一同送入小肠(图6.8和图6.9)。这种装置的管路平均使用寿命约为120天[137]。如图6.10显示的Johlin技术,从造口插入一根切除息肉常用的圈套管到胃内,将带有导丝的内镜插入圈套内,然后内镜通过开口并尽可能向下推进至空肠近端。0.035英寸标准的但有尖端的弹性导丝通过内镜通道进入小肠,然后将内镜缓缓地退回至胃的近端,导丝通过胃造口管抽出并形成一个钢丝环。拉动内镜中的导丝有助于判定钢丝环的近端,然后通过PEG取出。将J形管穿过导丝,直到其近端固定在胃造口管中,然后取下导丝。对于成熟的胃肠造口瘘管,也可使用一体式PEGJ系统替换。内镜检查时,还可以使用一种改进的Kirby技术,使该管通过导丝。该系统的内部支撑是一个球囊。

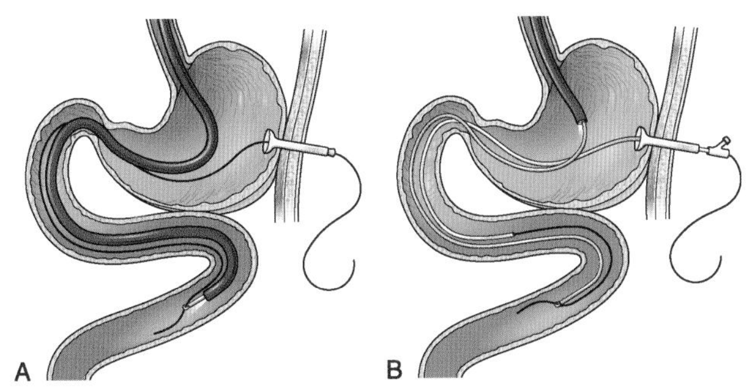

图6.7 沿导丝经皮内镜下胃空肠造口技术,又称Kirby技术。A,通过穿过固定在PEG内的瓣膜的单股导丝,再通过穿过儿科内镜的活检钳抓取。将活检钳推出内镜末端,将金属导丝固定在Treitz韧带下方。B,然后将内镜撤回到胃中,同时将活检钳推出内镜末端,将导丝固定在Treitz韧带下方。一旦内镜撤回到近端胃内,沿导丝穿过空肠延长管,直至远端接触导丝末端的活检钳。(Reprinted with permission from Chandrasekhara V, Kochman M. Techniques in Gastrointestinal Endoscopy, Elsevier.)

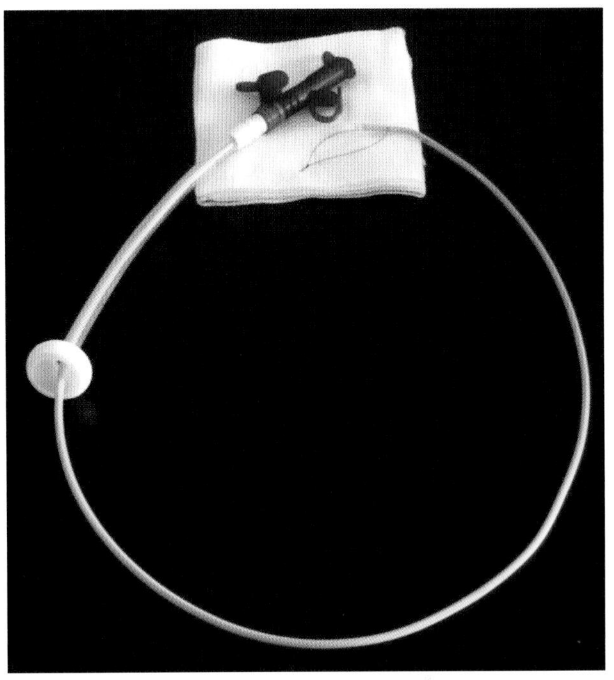

图6.8 胃空肠造口术(或经皮内镜下胃空肠造口术)喂养管。空肠喂养管末端的缝线有助于其放置,并且可以使用止血夹固定在空肠壁上

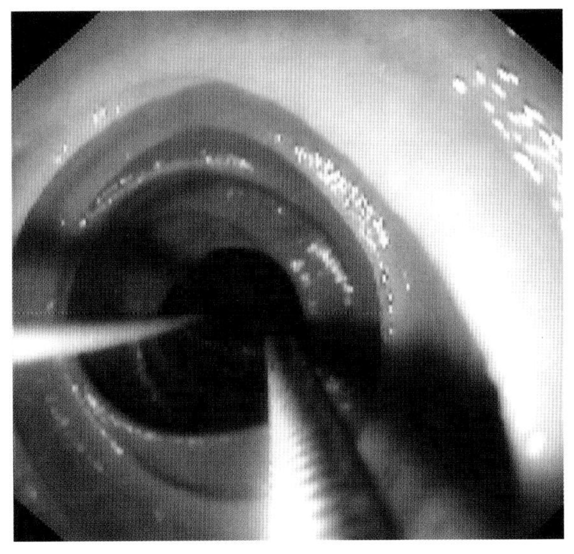

图6.9 显示经皮内镜下胃空肠造口术的导丝置入技术

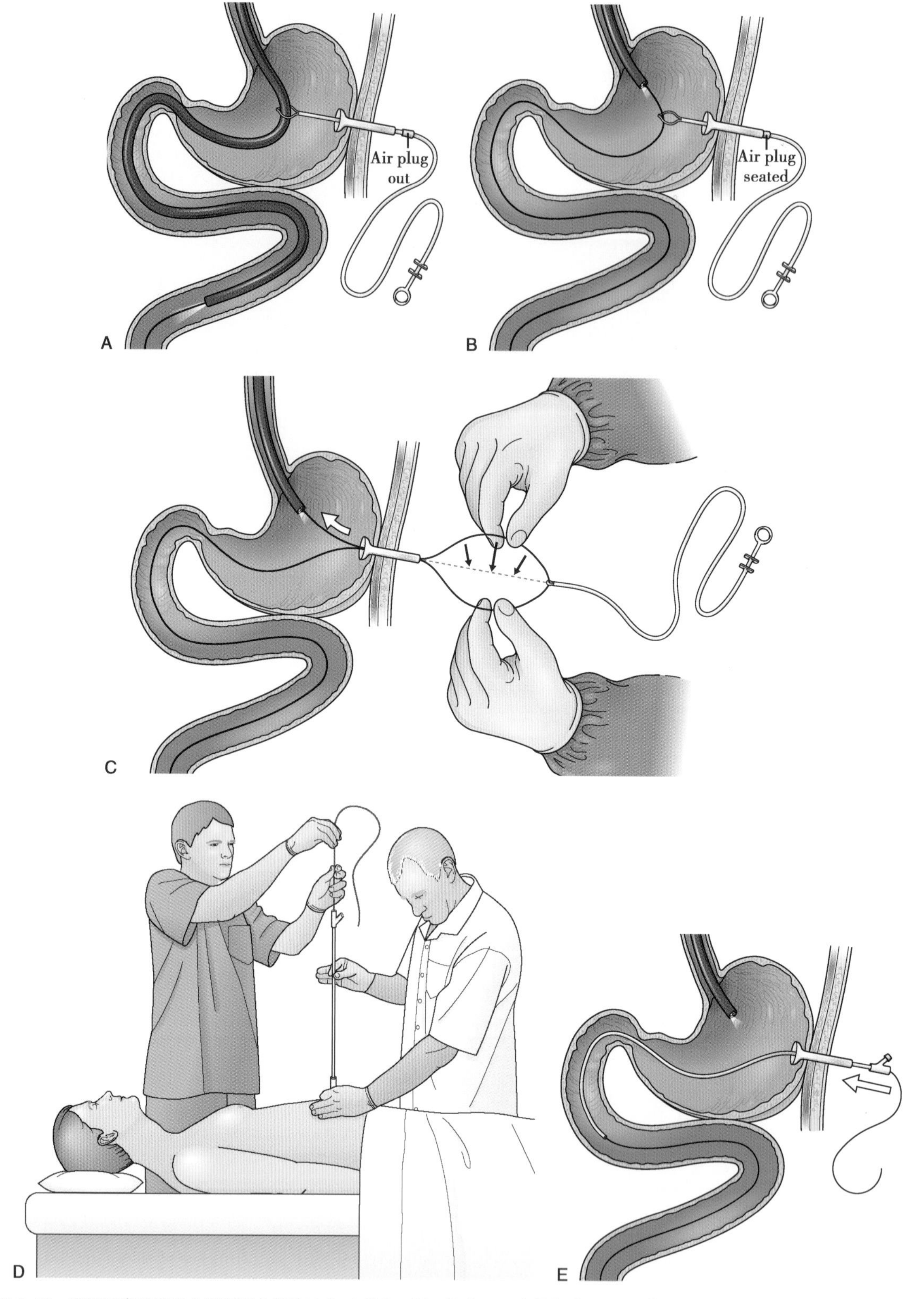

图 6.10　通过圈套器经皮内镜下胃空肠造口术，也称为 Johlin 技术。A，在最初放置 PEG 管之后，将 PEG 管切短至约 10cm，然后用自制或市售空气阀（图 6.11）放置圈套管进入胃内。小儿结肠镜通过圈套器进入胃内，然后向下进入 Treitz 韧带下方的小肠，然后再将金属导丝延伸到内镜末端之外。B，使用仔细的导丝转移技术，将内镜撤回到近端胃，保持导线尖端位于 Treitz 韧带下方。可将空气阀固定，以便观察胃内的圈套器。C，然后在导线上闭合圈套器，通过 PEG 拉出。当助手握住导丝圈从 PEG 中伸出时，术者牵拉从内镜操作通道中挤出的金属导丝，箭头指的哪一侧代表金属导丝的近端，然后通过 PEG 拉出导丝环。D，当术者将空肠管向下穿过 PEG 时，助手提供一个“空间点”来固定导丝。E，将空肠延长管向下进入最终位置，尖端位于 Treitz 韧带下方。（Reprinted with permission from Chandrasekhara V，Kochman M. Techniques in Gastrointestinal Endoscopy，Elsevier.）

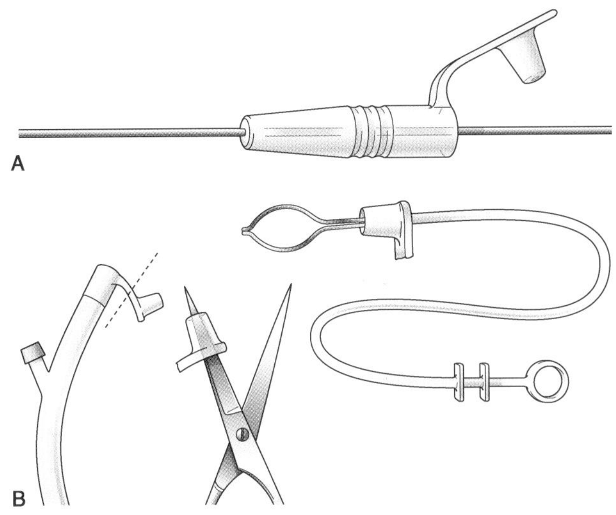

图6.11 市售和自制空气阀。A,上图显示了穿过导丝的市售空气阀,PEGJ转换过程中最常用。B,自制空气阀,可以切断喂养管上的阀塞,用剪刀取出阀芯,然后将圈套器或金属导丝穿过阀。(Reprinted with permission from Chandrasekhara V, Kochman M. Techniques in Gastrointestinal Endoscopy, Elsevier.)

(4) 直接经皮空肠造口术

直接经皮空肠造口术需要使用改良的Ponsky拖拉技术和儿科结肠镜将直径约14~16Fr PEG管直接放入小肠,达到Treitz韧带远端的穿刺部位(图6.12)。这种手术在技术上的成功率为68%~98%,在低体重指数或术后解剖结构改变(如将十二指肠和近端空肠带出腹腔的Billroth Ⅰ和Ⅱ手术)的患者中的成功率更高[139-142]。要保证DPEJ手术成功,就需要一支经验丰富的双人团队(1名"scope person",1名"skin person"),scope person避免胃腔过度膨胀,在内镜到达Treitz韧带下方后,skin person立即通过皮肤找内镜透光点并垂直指压定位并使用22G脊柱穿刺针刺破小肠,当套管针可以以相同的角度和位置通过时,套入22G探针并将其固定到小肠。

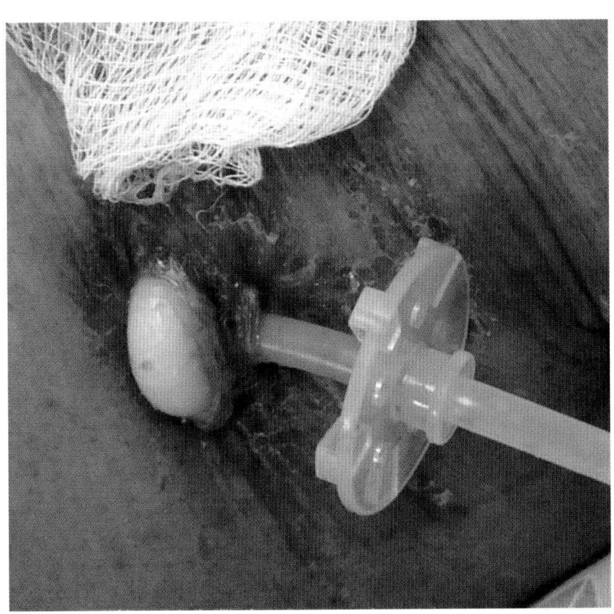

图6.12 直接经皮内镜下空肠造口术。双针穿刺技术中的探针插入和圈套器固定

一旦圈套住穿刺管,剩下的步骤实际上与Ponsky拖拉技术相同。DPEJ术不建议用Sachs-Vine推入技术和Russel穿刺技术。术后DPEJ管的护理类似于PEG管。

(5) 并发症

大多数PEG术后并发症来自患者的合并症,如伤口愈合不良、误吸或凝血障碍等。为了降低误吸风险,护理人员应在喂食期间和喂食后1小时将患者床头抬高30°~45°[105]。PEG的一种常见并发症是造口周围伤口感染[143]。造口周围感染的风险因素包括糖尿病、肥胖、营养不良、长期使用糖皮质激素、PEG插入部位切口小、缺乏抗生素预防性治疗以及PEG部位外部缓冲器压力过大[144]。PEG管外枕垫对腹壁过度收紧可引起埋藏缓冲器综合征(buried bumper syndrome, BBS)(图6.13),进而可导致黏膜溃疡、出血、造口漏、造口周围感染,甚至坏死性筋膜炎[145]。为了尽量减少BBS的机会,PEG管的外部枕垫应在放置后保持在皮肤上(无压痕)4天,之后应小心地将其从前腹壁后移1cm[145]。若出现造口周围伤口感染,通常使用口服抗生素(如头孢氨苄)治疗7天,以覆盖皮肤相关微生物。感染部位还应每日使用温和的肥皂和清水局部清洁。

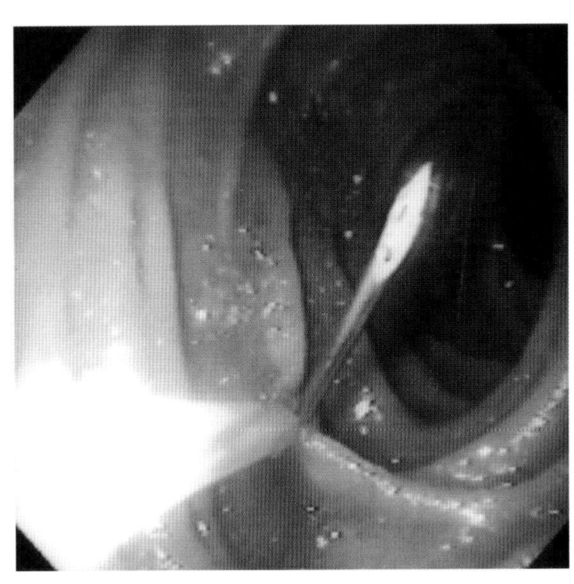

图6.13 埋藏缓冲器综合征

若真菌在聚硅氧烷PEG管定植,就会导致管子降解和损坏,需要及时更换[146]。若PEG管堵塞,可用温水、软饮料或在碳酸氢盐溶液中混合胰酶冲洗[147]。若冲洗不能解除堵塞,可能需要使用金属丝、标本刷、内镜清洁刷或市售的螺旋式清洁设备除垢。若PEG造口周围肉芽组织过度增生,提示造口管损伤过度反应,可在造口周围涂抹硝酸银软膏或烧灼和去除多余的肉芽组织[148]。

PEG术后其他常见的并发症还包括造口渗漏、发热、肠梗阻、皮肤溃疡、造口管移位[149-151]。胃造口周围渗漏是一个常见但又常被忽视的问题。导致造口渗漏的危险因素包括使用糖皮质激素、化疗、使用双氧水或碘过度清洗、饲管张力过度和侧扭及未使用外固定钮。PEG管周围渗漏的胃酸或胆汁可引起红斑和皮损,常被误认为是感染,其治疗方法有:保持局部干燥、频繁更换敷料、局部使用氧化锌、外固定钮与皮肤的距离保持 1cm,保持造口管固定同时防止过度牵拉,和质子泵抑制剂的使用[62,144]。放置 PEG 后气腹是常见的并发症,如果没有腹膜刺激征就不需处理。一旦有腹膜刺激征,应立即通过 PEG 管进行对比观察,以确定是否存在渗漏。一旦确认有渗漏,应进行手术探查[152]。

PEG 术后还有一些少见并发症,腹腔内出血或血肿形成、腹膜炎、坏死性筋膜炎、胃或结肠穿孔、肝胃瘘、胃结肠瘘、结肠皮肤瘘形成。结肠皮肤瘘是由于造口管在进入胃部之前不小心穿过结肠而产生的。尽管有时是急性的,但通常表现为慢性,如果在 PEG 管周围发现粪便或患者在通过 PEG 管进食后立即出现"腹泻",则要怀疑是否出现结肠皮肤瘘。

如果 PEG 管在放置后 7 天内脱落,应通过内镜在前腹壁的同一部位重新放置一个新的 PEG。没有必要通过同一胃壁穿刺点,因为靠近原来的胃穿刺点,新内固定钮的收紧和胃壁肌肉层的交叉可能有助于密封原来的入口道。这种情况时,建议患者短期服用广谱抗生素。如果 PEG 管在放置 4 周后移位,因为造口管已形成,这时不需要透视或内镜,可在床旁盲插更换 PEG 管。但建议在使用 PEG 管喂养前,拍片或透视以确认 PEG 管已放置在适当位置。

使用 PEGJ 管时,空肠管可能会向后方移动或扭结而致不能起作用。超过 50% 的 PEGJ 管需要在 6 个月内进行再更换[153]。PEG 管移位最常见于患者持续呕吐或 J 管放置不当时[137,154]。如果未能将 PEG 管切割至足够短的长度(<10cm),空肠管的长度缩短,PEG 管在胃底的位置过高,导致空肠管在胃内缠绕等情况,可能也会引起 PEG 管移位。将 PEG 管放置在胃窦内,可以避免空肠管在胃内缠绕,并用止血夹固定空肠管远端,可防止近端移位[144]。

3. 肠内喂养

患者可以通过弹丸式、间歇式或连续式接受管饲喂养。弹丸式喂养需要相对大容量(200~400mL)的喂养管,由注射器在短时间内注入。间歇式喂养是指在几个小时通过泵或使用床边营养液的重力滴注完营养液。连续喂食是指由机械泵在 12~24 小时内输送持续泵入营养液。临床上,接受小肠喂养的患者几乎都是给予连续式喂养,而不是快速弹丸式喂养,原因是避免管饲误吸。

我们通过评估患者是否有腹痛或腹胀、恶心和呕吐、排气排便等症状和腹部影像学上是否有肠袢扩张或空气/液体水平等,来监测肠内喂养的耐受性。胃残余容积(gastric residual volume,GRV)是衡量胃排空的一个很差的指标,与患者是否发生反流、误吸或肺炎不相关。目前已不推荐常规监测 GRV。目前,临床上减少误吸风险的措施包括:在插管的 ICU 患者中,喂养前后将床头抬高 30°~45°,从团注式改为连续式输注,使用促胃肠动力药(如甲氧氯普胺或红霉素)或麻醉性拮抗剂(纳洛酮或艾维莫潘)及将胃内输注改为幽门后输注。

(1) 肠内营养制剂

临床上,为成人住院患者长期使用 EN 而设计的基本喂养配方是不含乳糖和麸质的标准的多聚体膳。该膳食之所以被称为多聚体,是因为大量营养成分是完整的且未加工的。标准膳食中 15%~20% 的热量来自蛋白质,45%~60% 的热量来自碳水化合物,30%~40% 的热量来自脂肪。一般来说,这些配方提供 1kcal/ml,不过可以浓缩到 1.5~2.0kcal/ml。随着每毫升管饲量的能量含量增加,配方的含水量减少,渗透压增加。大多数肠内配方含有接近 80% 的游离水。而高氮配方是指蛋白质含量较高的配方。

要素膳内含有游离氨基酸形式的蛋白质,这种蛋白质几乎不含脂肪,即脂肪含量不到热量的 2%~3%。半要素膳内含有短肽蛋白质,主要由 3~5 个氨基酸长度的蛋白质组成。蛋白质的吸收率更高,因为短肽可以通过单个活性转运体完整地跨肠壁运输,而不像每个氨基酸都需要一个单独的转运体(见第 102 章)。脂肪以 MCT 的形式存在,可以直接吸收到门静脉,而不需要脂酶、辅脂肪酶或胆盐转运(见第 102 章)。半要素短肽/MCT 脂膳在很大程度上取代了原来的要素膳,并专为消化能力有限的患者设计。虽然从生理学角度的研究证明在肠功能受损的情况下,半要素膳比多聚体膳吸收得更多,但临床随机对照试验显示两者吸收率相当。

临床上,针对糖尿病、肾衰竭、肝衰竭、肺病、严重压力或创伤等某些特殊疾病的特殊患者设计了特殊配方。但是,很少或者没有数据表明,与标准多聚体膳相比,给这些特殊疾病患者特定的膳食能提高生存率,亦没有改善临床预后。有时使用这些特殊配方,主要是因为患者有低钾和低磷(肾病配方)或低钠(肝病配方)等电解质问题。但是,无论是肝功能衰竭还是肾功能衰竭的患者,都不应限制蛋白质的摄入。

免疫性组件配方是指在配方中添加精氨酸、谷氨酰胺、ω-3 脂肪酸、抗氧化剂和核苷酸,因为这些物质在免疫调节中起重要作用。精氨酸是细胞生长和增殖、伤口愈合、一氧化氮生成和淋巴细胞分化所必需的。重症患者对精氨酸的需求增加,所以补充精氨酸可能有助于伤口愈合[155]。鱼油可能有助于减少全身炎症反应。正在接受择期胃肠道手术的和术后在外科 ICU 中需要 EN 的患者,最有可能从精氨酸鱼油等免疫调节配方中获益。研究显示,在这些患者中使用免疫调节配方可减少感染、抗生素使用、机械通气持续时间、多器官功能障碍和住院时间[156]。虽然,在内科 ICU 患者中使用此类配方是安全的,但目前的数据显示并不能改变患者预后。同样,由于缺乏安全性和疗效等原因不建议对急性肺损伤或急性呼吸窘迫综合征患者使用含鱼油、抗氧化剂、抗炎配方。

(2) 肠内喂养的并发症

据报道,15%~30% 的患者出现管饲相关的胃肠道副作用,其中包括恶心、呕吐、腹胀、腹部痉挛和腹泻。腹泻最常见的原因是药物引起的,较少见的是艰难梭菌性小肠结肠炎(见第 112 章)。药物可以通过在山梨醇碱(一种已知的泻药)中溶解,由片剂变成液体,以便通过喂食管滴注。含镁药物、高渗药物和促胃肠动力药也可能促进腹泻。即使渗透压高达 600~700mOsm/L 的高渗 EN 膳食也很少引起腹泻。对于曾经对肠营养液耐受的新发腹泻患者,在改变其营养配方前,应对患者进行药物诱导和感染病原学评估。数据显示,不能通过稀释肠营养液浓度来改善患者胃肠道耐受性。对于肠功能受损的患者,使用半要素膳可能会改善吸收,减少腹泻。补充可溶性纤维或使用商品化的混合性可溶性/不溶性纤维膳食也可改善腹泻症状[157,158]。

比起 PN 喂养,EN 的代谢并发症少。高浓度配方可能会发生脱水和液体转移的情况,尤其是在脱水情况下。在糖耐量异常的患者中,高血糖可能与高碳水化合物的高输送率有关。同时管饲可能也影响药物的输送。苯妥英钠就受管饲的影响，因为苯妥英钠与肠内制剂可结合并形成黏附在饲管壁上的苯妥英钠喂养复合物[159]。环丙沙星也被证明与管饲结合，减少其吸收。许多肠营养配方中含有维生素 K，可使患者对华法林抵抗力增加。

（二）肠外营养

对于胃肠道功能异常的患者，营养素可通过肠外营养（PN）静脉输注。PN 提供的溶液包含大量营养素（碳水化合物、蛋白质、脂质等）、微量营养素（维生素、矿物质、微量元素等）、水电解质和药物。碳水化合物以葡萄糖的形式传递，蛋白质以氨基酸的形式传递，脂质以静脉脂肪乳剂（IV fat emulsions，IVFE）传递。当所有 3 种大量营养素合并为一种溶液时，称为总营养素混合物或 3 合 1 溶液。当单独给 IVFE 时，PN 公式称为 2 合 1 溶液。营养素输送可以通过中央静脉或周围静脉（PPN）。在大多数医院，PPN 的使用受到限制或禁止使用，因为 PPN 的适应证可能被滥用或导致静脉硬化，即使将营养液渗透压保持在 800~900mOsm/L 以下（这反过来导致通常需要 12~36 小时的短期治疗）。而中心静脉营养液可在 12~24 小时以上。PN 溶液的浓度是血液（1 800~2 400mOsm/L）的 6 倍，通常由大约 30~50g/L 的蛋白质和 1 000~1 200kcal/L 的蛋白质组成。

1. 胃肠外营养制剂

要配制 PN 制剂，首先必须根据先前的营养评估确定患者所需的热量和蛋白质（见第 5 章）[160]。除了危重症患者，蛋白质和热量需求随着患者代谢情况而调整。PN 的每种成分都有一定的热量，例如蛋白质 = 4kcal/g，碳水化合物（葡萄糖）= 3.4kcal/g，IVFE = 10kcal/g（脂肪 9kcal/g，乳化剂 1kcal/g）。根据患者不同代谢情况，蛋白质需要量通常在 1.2~2.0g/（kg · d）之间。即使患有严重肝性脑病或肾功能衰竭伴氮质血症需要立即透析的患者，蛋白质也不应受到限制。一般情况下，PN 制剂中脂肪含量通常为 1g/（kg · d），但对于甘油三酯血 > 400mg/dL 的高脂血症患者可能需要减少或限制脂肪摄入。尽管，这些患者需要限制脂肪摄入，但仍给予少量脂肪，通常给予 10% 预估的脂肪热量或每周 20% 的脂肪乳 500ml，以防止必需脂肪酸的缺乏。患者每日所需能量的其余部分以葡萄糖的形式给予。为防止高血糖和再喂养综合征（见下文代谢并发症），葡萄糖的量最初不应超过 200g。葡萄糖应在几天内滴定至目标值。补液量需根据患者的需求增加，而对于心肺衰竭的患者，其补液量应该受限。总需水量估计为 25~35ml/（kg · d）。

当 PN 配方中大量营养素组成确定后，就可以添加电解质、微量元素、多种维生素和胰岛素、肝素、质子泵抑制剂或 H2 受体拮抗剂等药物。可以根据患者的实验室检查结果和并发症情况来增加或减少任何肠外营养的成分。对于未进行监测的非 ICU 患者，PN 配方中的钾不应超过 10mmol/h。由于存在磷酸钙晶体沉淀的风险，还必须监测 PN 溶液中的钙和磷含量。一般来说，钙磷总和［（1/2mmol 钙 + mmol 磷）/L］应小于 45，以防形成晶体沉积。一般根据预设治疗方案添加维生素和微量元素，但也可根据实际需求额外补充。由于铜和锰经胆汁排出，因此在胆汁淤积患者中不得添加。肾功能不全患者应减少硒摄入量，而腹泻、高流量瘘或严重创伤患者应增加锌摄入量[161]。建议适度控制血糖，我们可通过胰岛素笔注射胰岛素或在液体中添加胰岛素，使血糖水平保持在 110~150mg/dL 之间[61]。框 6.1 列出了制订经中心静脉肠外营养处方的步骤及方法。

框 6.1　为 70kg 男性实施肠外营养医嘱的步骤方法

营养物质的热量含量

蛋白质：4kcal/g

脂肪：10kcal/g

碳水化合物：3.4kcal/g

该患者的估计每日需求

热量：25kcal/kg = 1 750kcal

蛋白质：1.2g/kg = 84g

液体量：30ml/kg = 2 100ml

制订步骤

1. 向 PN 混合液中加入蛋白质［1.2g/（kg · d）］
   需要 84g 蛋白质
   1g 蛋白质提供 = 4kcal，84g 提供总热量为 326kcal
   1 750kcal - 326kcal = 1 424kcal（仍需要）
2. 添加脂质［1~1.5g/（kg · d）］
   70g 脂肪 = 700kcal
   剩余 1 424kcal - 700kcal = 724kcal（仍需要）
3. 需添加碳水化合物［3~5g/（kg · d）］
   724kcal/3.4kcal/g 碳水化合物 = 212.9g
4. 总液体量
   30ml/kg = 2 100ml

其他添加剂

电解质、矿物质、维生素

药物添加剂：H_2 受体拮抗剂、胰岛素、肝素

2. 肠外营养的管理

开始时，肠外营养配方需要输注超过 24 小时。对于糖耐量异常的患者或具有再喂养综合征风险的患者（参见下文并发症部分），在最初 24 小时的肠外营养输注应仅提供每日热量需求的 25%。接下来的 48~72 小时内，逐渐增加至满足全热量需求，同时应监测患者血糖、镁、钾、磷和水容量[162]。肠外营养一般通过大中心静脉输注。任何一种情况下，用于输注 PN 的导管端口或管腔必须仅用于 PN 输注。使用 PN 端口或管腔来抽血或输注其他溶液，会增加导管感染的风险。

3. 实验室检测

开始肠外营养输注后，必须监测一些血清生化指标。肠外营养输注开始的最初几天，应密切监测血清中的电解质、镁、磷、钙、钾和血尿素氮水平。当这些指标达标后，可每周进行监测。对于长期家庭肠外营养输注的患者，进行这些常规血清生化指标的频率可降低到每月一次。每月还应检测全血细胞计数。在其他临床相关病例中，可能还需要监测血清锌、硒、铜、铬、维生素 B_{12} 和维生素 B_6 水平。因为，铁不是 PN 溶液的常规添加剂，PN 依赖患者需要监测是否出现缺铁性贫血。

4. 代谢并发症

由于肠外营养溶液中含有葡萄糖、氨基酸、脂质、维生素、电解质或矿物质，患者可能会出现代谢并发症[163]。高血糖

是最常见的代谢并发症，与PN葡萄糖含量、患者胰岛素敏感性和PN输注频率直接相关。危重病患者和糖耐量异常的患者，尤其需要密切监测血糖。出现高血糖的患者，首先应给予维持常规剂量的胰岛素对抗。在24小时所需的胰岛素总量中，2/3胰岛素应添加到第二天的PN配方中。可能需要每天对胰岛素剂量进行调整，ICU的患者可能需要单独滴注胰岛素。血糖水平失控会导致导管败血症等感染相关并发症。在住院患者中，即使静滴胰岛素也很难控制血糖，可以限制营养液摄入控制血糖。在这些患者中，高血糖及其导致的后果所带来的风险大于患者暂时营养不足所带来的风险。

再喂养综合征是指之前营养不良的患者突然大量提供葡萄糖热量，随着营养液摄入，这些患者的代谢异常导致一系列症状。大量葡萄糖摄入后刺激体内胰岛素分泌增加，会将钾、磷、镁和维生素 B_1 转移至细胞内，导致低钾血症、低磷血症和低镁血症[164]。除了神经系统后遗症外，还可能发生水钠潴留，引发心力衰竭[165]。血电解质的突然变化可能诱发心律失常。为防止再喂养综合征发生，应限制初始热量，然后在3~4天内从25%~80%到逐步增加大量营养素的摄入（尤其是葡萄糖）至100%目标能量，同时应仔细监测并维持电解质平衡。虽然PN或EN均有可能诱发再喂养综合征，但EN的风险更大。

在开始给予PN后出现肝功异常是很常见的，典型表现为血清转氨酶水平升高至正常值的两倍。转氨酶水平升高和相关的高胆红素血症值得研究。PN可导致3种PN相关的肝病：即脂肪变性、胆汁淤积和胆泥/胆结石，诊断前必须排除其他潜在的肝病。上腹部超声检查有助于排除胆管扩张、肝占位、胆石症或胆泥。因为PN喂养缺乏肠内刺激，因此可导致胆囊收缩素释放减少、胆汁流量减少和胆囊收缩力减弱。胆囊淤积可导致胆结石或胆泥形成，引起结石性和非结石性胆囊炎。与PN相关的脂肪变性表现为肝内脂肪浸润，尤其是门静脉区脂肪浸润更明显。在PN相关性脂肪变性患者中，血清转氨酶中度升高，通常发生于PN开始后2周内，并可能随时间的推移恢复正常；这些患者一般没有临床症状。PN相关脂肪变性常继发于喂养过度，若减少患者每日总输注热量，PN相关脂肪变性会逐渐减轻[166]。PN相关胆汁淤积是一种因胆汁分泌及排泄障碍引起的疾病，主要发生于儿童，表现为碱性磷酸酶、GGTP和胆红素升高。一小部分接受HPN治疗的患者中，长期PN相关胆汁淤积可能发展为肝硬化和肝衰竭。研究还显示，反复发作的导管相关脓毒血症可能加速PN诱导肝损伤加重。细菌和真菌感染与胆汁淤积症有关。小肠细菌过度生长是肝病发生的另一个危险因素，最有可能由发酵产生酒精或厌氧菌产生肝毒素引起[62]。

胆碱缺乏可能在长期PN相关的肝病发生有关[167]，其中脂质的来源是导致这种并发症的原因。在美国，PN溶液中的脂质成分以大豆为主，主要由亚油酸（一种ω-6脂肪酸）等长链甘油三酯组成，具有促炎症作用。这种脂质来源中的植物甾醇和甾烷醇可能对某些患者有肝毒性。与来源于大豆的长链甘油三酯不同，中链甘油三酯和橄榄油基本无促炎作用。鱼油含有丰富的ω-3脂肪酸，具有抗炎作用。在一些国家，可用含有中链甘油三酯、橄榄油和鱼油的IVFE静滴。对儿童进行的前瞻性和回顾性研究证明鱼油能有效逆转PN诱导的肝病[168]。在接受PN的成人患者中，肝脏生化指标的升高可通过适当的方式进行治疗，调整每天12~18小时内的循环PN方案，用间接热量测定以确认能量需求并调整以避免过量喂养，以及将基于大豆脂的IVFE转换为脂类混合物（含SMOF的大豆、MCT、橄榄油和鱼油）。

使用PN出现严重并发症的患者可能需要小肠移植（见第106章）。这些严重并发症包括进行性肝衰竭，反复发生的导管相关性败血症，主要静脉系统形成血栓影响了PN所需的中心静脉。目前，接受小肠移植的患者的5年生存率接近50%[169]，但仍低于接受家庭肠外营养治疗的患者的5年生存率。生活质量在家庭肠外营养和小肠移植患者中的差异有待进一步研究。

5. 血管通路装置

在解剖学上，通过锁骨下静脉和颈内静脉是最容易而且也是最安全的中心静脉通路。与其他中心静脉通路建立部位相比，锁骨下静脉常被选为长期中心静脉通路，因为这样可减少导管相关并发症。多腔导管允许同时输注多种液体和药物，但随着管腔数量的增加，感染风险随之增加。除非患者需要多个管路端口，否则首选单腔导管[170,171]。如果使用多腔导管，应指定1腔仅用于输注PN[172]。

有3种类型的中心静脉导管（central venous catheter，CVC）可用于肠外营养输注：经外周静脉穿刺的中心静脉导管（peripherally inserted central catheter，PICC）、隧道式留置CVC（Hickman、Broviac或Groshong导管）和植入式血管通路装置或"端口"。PICC已用于医院和家庭PN输注。PICC一般位于上肢，导管尖端位于上腔静脉和右心房交界处的中心静脉。与以前标准的中心插入导管相比，PICC导管可减少由插入导致并发症（如气胸）。而PICC只能用于预期短期需要PN的患者，而不适合长期PN患者，因为它们最多只能使用1~2月，更长时间使用可能会引起静脉硬化。

当导管需要使用时间超过1~3个月时，通常使用隧道式CVC。隧道式CVC是在皮下形成隧道留置导管，制造出一个物理屏障可预防细菌感染。他们有一个涤纶袖套，以诱导组织生长和局部纤维化，起到固定导管的作用，这样可以防止导管意外移位及细菌沿导管扩散[173]。这种导管的尖端应位于锁骨下静脉的远端1/3处，而可植入式静脉输液港的导管端口被放置在皮下，通常在胸壁上，无外部导管部分，因此无须每天进行肝素冲洗。植入式静脉输液港的端口需要一个专门的接入针，以便抽血或输液，而且留置寿命有限，床旁移除过程也比皮下隧穿导管更复杂。与隧道式（0.64/1 000导管日）和非隧道式（0.87/1 000导管日）导管相比，单腔PICC导管和可植入导管的导管相关血流感染（catheter related blood stream infection，CRBSI）发生率较低（0/1 000和0.19/1 000导管日）。与非隧道导管（17.8%）相比，单腔PICC导管和植入式导管也被证明具有更长的无故障持续时间，机械并发症更少（分别为13.9%和9.7%）[174]。

中心静脉导管并发症

中心静脉导管并发症的发生率为1%~20%[175]。锁骨下静脉导管置入的并发症包括血胸、气胸、臂丛神经损伤、血肿和皮下气肿。常见的长期导管并发症包括败血症、血栓形成和导管堵塞。还可能发生导管破裂、移位和空气栓塞。导管感染通常发生于接触性污染，分离出的主要病原微生物为凝固酶阴性葡萄球菌；其他病原微生物包括革兰氏阳性球菌的耐药菌株（例如，金黄色葡萄球菌、肠球菌属、链球菌属等）、革兰氏阴性杆菌（如肺炎克雷伯菌、大肠杆菌、阴沟肠杆菌等）和真菌（例如近平滑念珠菌、白色念珠菌、平滑念珠菌等）[176,177]。导管污染的主要原因为微生物从皮肤表面进入皮下组织，并到达导管尖端。花越多时间教居家使用中心静脉导管的患者进行中心静脉通路装置的护理和操作，患者发生感染性并发症的可能性就越小[178]。

导管感染很难诊断，如果患者免疫功能低下，感染时白细胞计数可能不会升高，并且外周血培养可能为阴性。导管尖端培养敏感性更高，可用于确诊导管感染。通常导管的细菌感染不用拔除导管。如果发生导管真菌感染和隧道感染，则需拔除导管才能有效治愈。一旦怀疑导管感染，就需要开始进行广谱抗生素或抗真菌治疗，并在确定病原微生物后进行针对性治疗。在每袋肠外营养液中加入肝素（1 000U/L）可防止细菌或真菌形成的亚临床血栓，从而降低导管相关败血症的风险。不建议常规使用抗凝治疗来降低导管相关感染的风险[179]。治疗中心静脉导管感染时，应注意导管中的细菌或真菌与抗生素或抗真菌剂的实际接触时间。有人认为，将抗生素封管在受感染的管路中（每次输液结束时）可能有助于减少中心管路的感染[180]。还有些人主张每天用 50%～70% 的乙醇冲洗导管，以消毒导管并减少感染事件[181]。已有研究提示，封管可降低 CRBSI 的风险，例如抗生素封管可以降低复发性 CRBSI 的发生率。乙醇具有杀细菌和杀真菌的特性，并且引起抗微生物耐药性的风险很低。一项随机对照试验将 38 名新开始 HPN 的患者分为两组，一组接受乙醇封管，另一组接受肝素封管的标准治疗，发现乙醇封管组有 4 名患者、对照组有 1 名患者出现 CRBSI[182]。对于有多次 CRBSI 病史的患者，建议使用预防性抗生素封管或乙醇封管，但是对于所有首次使用 HPN 的患者没有益处。值得注意的是，乙醇封管只能用于 Hickman 导管，不能用于聚氨酯导管。

导管刺激血管壁可诱发血栓形成。血栓通常由纤维蛋白组成。导管中药物沉积不太常见。中心静脉血栓形成可出现颈部疼痛、颈部肿胀、前胸壁静脉扩张症和导管功能障碍。事实证明，用生理盐水冲洗 CVC 与用肝素冲洗 CVC 一样有利于防止血栓阻塞导管[183]。静推或静滴链激酶等溶栓剂治疗纤维蛋白性血栓[184]。根据所用药物为酸性还是碱性，可输注少量氢氧化钠或盐酸治疗药物或沉积物导致的堵塞[185]。

三、特殊饮食

清流质饮食以产生最少量残渣的形式提供液体和能量，旨在避免胃肠道内产生高渗透压，避免因为高渗透压导致体液转移和相关的恶心和腹泻。清流质饮食通常含有丰富的碳水化合物，但蛋白质或脂肪含量很少，因此在营养上不足以满足基本的代谢需求。几乎没有证据表明，对于术后恢复患者而言，清流质饮食的耐受性优于任何其他饮食。在可能的情况下，不应开具清流质饮食的处方，因为使用清流质饮食没有生理学方面的依据，清流质饮食的钠含量往往很高，除了满足患者的个人愿望之外，没有证据显示提供清流质饮食是合理的。相反，腹部或胸部术后患者若早期给予肠内营养，可减少术后并发症、住院时间和死亡率（虽然可能会增加呕吐）[186,187]。

全流质饮食适用于不能咀嚼、吞咽或消化固体的患者。这种饮食以牛奶为主，不得用于乳糖不耐症患者。这种饮食中含有大量的单体碳水化合物，糖尿病患者应慎用。

胃肠道狭窄患者和胃轻瘫患者可用低纤维和少渣饮食，这样可以延长输注时间的同时减少梗阻的风险。减少碳水化合物的摄入量，改用煮熟的蔬菜、精制谷物和面包。对于胃轻瘫患者，也建议低脂肪摄入。

高纤维饮食包括可溶性和不溶性纤维，具有广泛的代谢和生理作用。这类饮食不但可用于降低憩室病患者的结肠腔内压力，还可能延缓糖尿病患者葡萄糖吸收，通过降低血清胆固醇和血清甘油三酯水平有益于心血管疾病。终身高纤维饮食可能有助于预防结肠癌。高纤维饮食主要包括蔬菜、水果、豆类、全麦面包和谷类等食品。

胃切除术后或防止倾倒综合征的饮食建议少食多餐、摄入高蛋白和高脂饮食，使小肠保持低渗透压；还应避免使用单糖，以防止快速吸收[188]。应限制液体摄入，且液体与固体食物应分开摄入，以避免胃快速排空。这类饮食还应包括香蕉和橙子等富含果胶的食物，以延缓胃排空。

低脂饮食用于减少与脂肪吸收不良相关的腹泻和脂肪泻，尤其是胰腺或胆囊功能障碍的患者。对于将长期摄入低脂饮食的患者，必须补充脂溶性维生素（A、D、E 和 K）。中链甘油三酯（MCT）可替代长链甘油三酯。MCT 具有 6～12 碳的脂肪酸链，水溶性高，并且无需胆汁盐就可在小肠吸收[189]。MCT 也不用形成乳糜微粒可直接被门静脉系统吸收。然而，大多数基于 MCT 的产品都不是很好吃。许多以 MCT 为基础的产品，例如含有 MCT 和短肽的半元素配方都具有药味。香草口味的产品能增加患者的口感。

消化科医师需要接受像临床营养师那样的技能培训，具备营养知识并能在临床应用到大多数胃肠道疾病患者的治疗中。消化科医师应该具备肠道营养通路的操作技能、评估肠内喂养患者消化道耐受性的能力和对疾病或损伤引起的代谢变化的评估能力，这样才能更好治疗患者。

（郭雪艳　黄燕萍 译，孙明瑜 校）

参考文献

第 7 章　肥胖

Rekha B. Kumar, Louis J. Aronne 著

章节目录

一、定义和流行病学 …… 88
二、病因 …… 88
（一）饮食 …… 88
（二）体力活动 …… 89
（三）宫内和母体因素 …… 89
（四）药物引起的体重增加 …… 89
（五）吸烟 …… 89
（六）微生物群 …… 89
（七）遗传 …… 90
三、预后 …… 90
四、病理生理学 …… 90
五、临床特点及诊断 …… 91
病史及体格检查 …… 91
六、并发症 …… 91
（一）糖尿病 …… 91
（二）血脂紊乱 …… 91
（三）心血管疾病 …… 91
（四）高血压 …… 91
（五）肾脏疾病 …… 91
（六）胆囊疾病 …… 92
（七）肝脏疾病 …… 92
（八）胃食管反流病 …… 92
（九）癌症 …… 92
（十）阻塞性睡眠呼吸暂停 …… 92
（十一）骨骼、关节、肌肉、结缔组织和皮肤疾病 …… 92
（十二）心理社会功能障碍 …… 93
七、医学治疗 …… 93
（一）饮食方法 …… 93
（二）药物治疗 …… 93

一、定义和流行病学

肥胖是一种慢性疾病，定义为导致疾病的体脂或脂肪组织过多。脂肪本身难以方便地测量，因此普遍采用体重指数(body mass index，BMI)作为肥胖的标志。BMI 的计算为所测量的体重[以千克(kg)为单位]除以身高[以米(m)为单位]的平方。正常的 BMI 为 18.5~24.9kg/m^2，超重为 25~29.9kg/m^2。BMI 为 30~34.9kg/m^2 属于Ⅰ度肥胖。BMI 为 35~39.9kg/m^2 属于Ⅱ度肥胖，BMI 超过 40kg/m^2 属于Ⅲ度肥胖[1]。然而使用 BMI 作为肥胖的衡量标准有其局限性，并且要特别考虑肌肉块较多，具有较高 BMI 值但可能在新陈代谢方面健康的个体。也要考虑到相反的情况，即部分具有低 BMI 值的人可能有代谢疾病，如来自亚洲和南亚地区的患者[2]。肥胖患病率迅速上升以及其对经济日益增长的影响使人们更加认识到治疗肥胖的重要性。美国肥胖医学委员会(American Board of Obesity Medicine)成立于 2011 年，是为医生获得肥胖医学认证的授权机构。肥胖医学是发展最快的亚专业之一，截至 2017 年，已有 1 500 多名医生获得认证。美国医疗保险和医疗补助中心(Centers for Medicare and Medicaid)从 2012 年开始覆盖了医生对肥胖的治疗[3,4]，并且美国医学会(American Medical Association)在 2013 年将肥胖列为一种疾病状态[5]。

肥胖在全球范围内的流行率正在上升。世界卫生组织(World Health Organization)和美国国立卫生研究院国家心肺血液研究所(the National Heart，Lung，and Blood Institute of the U. S. National Institutes of Health)都将肥胖列为流行病[6,7]。在美国超过 1/3(36.5%)的成年人是肥胖的[8]，如果肥胖趋势持续下去，到 2045 年，全世界将有 22% 的人超重或肥胖[9]。肥胖的并发症包括 2 型糖尿病、卒中、心脏病、非酒精性脂肪性肝病和某些癌症，这些都被认为是全球可预防的与肥胖相关的死因。2008 年，美国肥胖患者的年医疗费用估计为 1 470 亿美元，肥胖者的年医疗费用比正常体重者高 1 429 美元[10]。每年用于治疗与肥胖相关疾病的费用超过 1.4 万亿美元，包括医疗费用以及肥胖对工作效率和缺勤率影响相关费用。这些费用是美国国防开支花费的两倍以上[11]。

二、病因

肥胖很大程度上是由于能量的摄入和消耗不平衡引起的。这种不平衡可能由多种因素引起，包括饮食、体力活动、宫内影响、药物作用以及包括肠道微生物影响在内的遗传和环境因素之间共同作用的影响。遗传因素在肥胖的发展过程中扮演着重要的角色，并且已经发现一些基因与影响体重相关，但是肥胖流行的上升速度超出了遗传所能解释的。(见下文)。

(一) 饮食

在过去的几十年间，全球的饮食供应发生了显著的变化。除了份量的增加，精制碳水化合物、饱和脂肪和盐的消耗量也在增加。现在全世界包括新兴市场国家都可以方便地获得含糖饮料和快餐服务，超重和肥胖相关的并发症正在增加[12]。在年轻人冠状动脉风险发展研究中的报告表明，那些具有更

高的快餐摄入量的研究受试者,比那些摄入较少快餐的受试者平均重 6kg[13]。非传染性疾病联盟(Noncommunicable Disease Alliance)评估,水果和蔬菜的低摄入量会导致大约 19% 的胃肠道癌症,31% 的冠心病和 11% 的卒中[14]。目前有两种互相矛盾的观点,一个是来自不同大量营养素种类的所有热量是否对肥胖的增加相同,另一个是某些饮食模式和食物中大量营养素成分是否比其他的模式和成分对肥胖的增加更大。"卡路里是一种卡路里"的概念得到热力学定律和许多对照实验室研究的支持,在这些研究中,改变饮食中脂肪、蛋白质和碳水化合物的卡路里百分比不会影响减肥或增重[15]。大量营养素很重要的相互矛盾的论点得到了允许人们自由选择食物的研究支持。这些研究支持高蛋白、低碳水化合物的饮食可以避免体重过多增加。高蛋白食物有利的原因可能是增加饱腹感,增加了食物的热效应,并改善身体组成成分[16,17]。由于美国人减少了饮食中脂肪的摄入,增加了高糖碳水化合物(快速消化的碳水化合物,如白薯、含糖饮料、加工过的谷类食品)的摄入量,肥胖的流行变得更为严重[18]。以全谷物形式存在的碳水化合物,尤其是加工较少、消化较慢的谷物,可能会阻止体重增加。这些不太精细的碳水化合物,比如大麦和糙米,比那些可以被快速吸收的水果中的碳水化合物更有助于控制体重[19,20]。

(二) 体力活动

家里和工作场所的体力活动逐渐减少,能量消耗也相应地减少。在过去的 50 年中,工作场所和家中使用了越来越多的省力的设备,相应减少了体力消耗,并导致体重的增加。成人和儿童中,工作时体力消耗的减少,开车的增加,步行减少或骑自行车上学,都与肥胖率的上升有关[21,22]。在护士健康研究中,校正年龄、吸烟、运动水平和饮食因素后发现,每增加 2 小时看电视时间,肥胖率增加 23%(95% CI 为 17%~30%),糖尿病风险增加 14%(95% CI 为 5%~23%)[23]。看电视对体重增加的影响很可能是因为人们看电视时热量摄入增加,而不仅仅是单纯的久坐不动。

(三) 宫内和母体因素

宫内环境和妊娠期间发生的事件会影响产后体重、身体组成成分和患肥胖症的可能性。这些因素包括孕前母亲肥胖、母亲吸烟和妊娠糖尿病,这些都会增加个体日后体重增加和糖尿病的风险[24]。受孕期间吸烟的母亲的后代在出生后的前几十年中体重增加的风险增加,患糖尿病母亲生出的婴儿和小于胎龄的婴儿也是如此[25,26]。

(四) 药物引起的体重增加

几种常用的处方药会导致体重异常增加或干扰患者的减肥能力(表 7.1)。这些药物包括抗精神病药(如奥氮平、氯氮平)、抗抑郁药(如选择性 5-羟色胺再摄取抑制剂、帕罗西汀)、抗癫痫药(如丙戊酸钠、加巴喷丁)、胰岛素和胰岛素促泌剂(如噻唑烷二酮类)、糖皮质激素、孕激素和埋植剂、口服避孕药、β 受体阻滞剂等[27]。如果可能的话,这些药物应该被其他对体重有中性影响的药物或者可以同时治疗潜在疾病并导致体重下降的药物替代。应评估非处方药和补充剂的使用情况。有些药物如感冒药中的伪麻黄碱等能与抗肥胖药物治疗产生相互作用,如果使用兴奋剂减肥,则应该停止使用这类感冒药。

表 7.1 促进体重增加的药物

药品类别	与体重增加有关	与体重增加较少、体重不变或导致体重减轻有关的替代品
抗抑郁药	甲替林,阿米替林,帕罗西汀,西酞普兰,米氮平、氟西汀(>1 年)、舍曲林(>1 年)	氟西汀(<1 年) 舍曲林(<1 年) 安非他酮(可导致体重减轻)
抗精神病药	氯氮平,奥氮平,利培酮,喹硫平,锂	齐拉西酮,阿立哌唑
抗癫痫药	加巴喷丁,普瑞巴林,丙戊酸钠,卡马西平	托吡酯,唑尼沙胺,拉莫三嗪,左乙拉西坦,苯妥英
抗糖尿病的药物	胰岛素,磺脲类,噻唑烷二酮类	二甲双胍,胰高血糖素样肽-1(GLP-1)受体激动剂,DPP-4 抑制剂,SGLT-2 抑制剂,普兰林肽
抗高血压药	哌唑嗪,多沙唑嗪,特拉唑嗪,酒石酸美托洛尔,普萘洛尔	卡维地洛,奈比洛尔
避孕药具	复方醋酸甲羟孕酮 口服避孕药(上一代产品)	戴铜宫内节育器,低剂量口服避孕药
非处方感冒药	苯海拉明	根据需要短时间使用
类固醇	糖皮质激素,孕激素	使用最低剂量的糖皮质激素来控制潜在的疾病

(五) 吸烟

吸烟者的体重比不吸烟者低,戒烟通常与体重增加相关[28]。吸烟对体重的影响,有两种解释:第一,吸烟是产热的,也就是说,吸烟时的代谢率高于不吸烟时的代谢率;第二,吸烟减少饥饿感,改变味觉,因此吸烟者往往吃得更少[29]。

(六) 微生物群

肠道微生物群由数以万亿的微生物组成,这些微生物可能通过细菌代谢摄入的营养物质;或通过如短链脂肪酸等细菌代谢产物;或通过对细菌结构成分的免疫应答影响肥胖(见第 3 章)[30]。无菌非肥胖小鼠吞食了先天性肥胖小鼠的粪质后出现了体重增加的研究结果表明了微生物组在肥胖中的重要性[31]。将人类粪便转移到老鼠的类似研究已经进行。在一项研究中[32]，将4对不同肥胖程度双胞胎中的每个成员的粪便微生物菌群或来自瘦弱或肥胖的同卵双胞胎的保存菌群分别在不同组的无菌小鼠中进行定植。将肥胖双胞胎的粪便移植后，其体重和肥胖程度明显高于瘦双胞胎。身体组成的差异与短链脂肪酸发酵的差异（在瘦双胞胎中增加）和支链氨基酸代谢的差异（在肥胖双胞胎中增加）等相关。共同饲养瘦小鼠和肥胖小鼠，从而实现肠道微生物群的共享，防止肥胖和体重继续增加。肠道菌群和小鼠表型依赖于饮食，表明饮食和菌群之间的可传播和可改变的相互作用能影响宿主生物过程。

肥胖个体粪便微生物组中厚壁菌门的数量增加，而瘦弱个体中粪便中拟杆菌门和阿克曼菌的数量增加[33]。这些微生物在粪便中的比例受到遗传（见下文）和饮食的影响：拟杆菌门的含量在高碳水化合物饮食中比低脂饮食（low-fat diet，LFD）中增加的程度更大[34]。未来需要对人体微生物组进行研究，以了解医学干预如何影响体重、胰岛素抵抗和肥胖风险因素。

（七）遗传

有肥胖家族史会大大增加一个人患肥胖症的可能性。儿童肥胖的最大危险因素是父母或一级亲属有肥胖史。有患2型糖尿病的一级或二级亲属也是胰岛素抵抗的独立危险因素。尽管发展成肥胖的风险有很强的遗传成分，但只有不到2%的病例是由单基因缺陷导致的肥胖表型[35]。黑素皮素-4受体（*MC4R*）基因、瘦素基因、阿黑皮素原（*POMC*）基因、刺鼠基因对体脂和脂肪储存均有显著影响。MC4R基因异常可能占儿童早发性严重肥胖病例的6%[36]。瘦素缺乏或瘦素受体不足与啮齿动物和人类的严重肥胖有关[37]。瘦素具有减少食物摄入和增加能量消耗的双重作用，两者都有利于身体脂肪的丢失。用瘦素治疗瘦素缺乏的儿童可以降低他们的体重和饥饿感，这表明瘦素在正常群体中的重要性[38]。瘦素缺乏的杂合子在血清中可检测到较低水平的瘦素，并能增加肥胖症，这表明瘦素水平低与饥饿和体脂增加有关[39,40]。虽然遗传约占肠道微生物分类群的10%，但克里斯腾斯内尔科（*Christensenellaceae*）是一个高度可遗传的与消瘦相关的类群；遗传型肥胖相关的类群是一个需要进一步研究的领域。当发现早发性肥胖或肥胖综合征时，应考虑在儿童人群中对肥胖的单基因原因进行检测。表7.2显示了可能将肥胖作为其临床表现组成部分的其他遗传综合征[41]。

表7.2 肥胖遗传综合征

综合征名称	临床表现	基因突变/遗传
Albright遗传性骨营养不良/Ⅰa型假性甲状旁腺功能减退	肥胖，智力低下，短臂畸形，身材矮小	*GNAS1/GNAS*的错义、移码、无义、剪接位点、缺失、插入突变。常染色体显性
Alström综合征	儿童肥胖，胰岛素抵抗和2型糖尿病，失明，听力障碍	*ALMS1*移码、无义、错义突变。常染色体隐性遗传
Bardet-Biedl综合征/Laurence-Moon-Bardet-Biedl综合征	肥胖，视网膜色素变性，肾畸形，多指畸形，智力低下，性腺功能减退	*BBS1*、*BBS2*的错义、无义、剪接位点和移码突变。常染色体隐性遗传
Carpenter综合征/Ⅱ型尖头多趾并趾畸形	肥胖，脐疝，软组织并指，先天性心脏病，智力缺陷，性欲减退	*RAB23*的截短、错义、无义突变。常染色体隐性遗传
Prader-Willi综合征/Prader-Labhart-Willi综合征	肥胖症和贪食症，发育不良，肌张力减退，生殖器发育不全，智力低下，小手小脚	父系等位基因*KRN3/ZNF127/MAGEL2*删除、突变、缺失。常染色体显性遗传，X染色体连锁

From Kaur Y, de Souza RJ, Gibson WT, Meyre D: A systematic review of genetic syndromes with obesity. Obes Rev 2017; 18(6): 603-34.

三、预后

肥胖对患有这种疾病的儿童和成人的身体、精神和社会心理方面产生了巨大的影响。在对97篇关于BMI分类相关的全因死亡率风险比的文章进行meta分析后发现，与正常体重个体相比，所有类别肥胖的人有更高的全因死亡率[42]。在一项研究中，重度肥胖患者（BMI在40至50之间）的预期寿命减少了约10年，这与终生吸烟的影响相似[43]。一项使用国家健康和营养检测调查数据的研究发现，与正常体重的成年人相比，Ⅱ级和Ⅲ级肥胖的成年人提前3.7年死亡（全因死亡率），Ⅲ级肥胖的成年人提前5年死于心血管疾病[44]。

肥胖的一级和二级预防都可以改善预期寿命和合并症。适度的体重减轻5%~10%与心血管疾病危险因素如高血压、高脂血症和血糖控制的显著改善相关。在一项观察性研究中，观察"糖尿病健康行动"的参与者，体重减轻5%~10%的受试者实现了糖化血红蛋白降低0.5%，舒张压降低5mmHg，收缩压降低5mmHg，高密度脂蛋白（high density lipoprotein，HDL）胆固醇升高5mg/dL，甘油三酯降低40mg/dL[45]。

四、病理生理学

体重和脂肪量受到体内平衡的控制。在肥胖症中，由于神经激素信号传导受损，这种体内平衡受到破坏。下丘脑弓状核内有2个神经元体，它们整合来自脂肪细胞、肠和胰腺的外周信号，通过产热调节食欲和能量消耗。其中一个神经元体表达促食欲肽神经肽Y和刺鼠相关肽，每种都具有增加食物摄取和减少能量消耗的功能。另一神经元体表达POMC，以及可卡因和苯丙胺调节的转录本，这些是食欲减退的多肽通过激活下游通路，如激活下丘脑室旁核的MC4R，导致食欲减少和能量消耗的增加[46]。POMC神经元的损伤和伴随的炎症与饮食诱导的肥胖和对瘦素和胰岛素等体重调节激素的抵抗有关[47]。这种生理紊乱只是在肥胖疾病中调节体重的途径如何受到影响的一个例子。

包括胰高血糖素样肽(glucagon-like peptide,GLP)、缩胆囊肽、胰多肽、酪酪肽等肠肽,可以减少食物摄取量,而胃饥饿素是胃内产生的一种小肽,可以刺激食物摄取[48]。脑内脂肪酸代谢可能是另一个重要控制点。脂肪酸的氧化调节 5'-腺苷单磷酸激酶的活性,这种酶的激活或抑制取决于单磷酸腺苷和三磷酸腺苷的比值,被认为是食物摄入控制系统的潜在中心点[49]。

五、临床特点及诊断

病史及体格检查

肥胖患者的病史采集十分复杂,因为这是一种多因素的疾病,从子宫内因素到与工作相关压力源,这些因素可能跨越整个一生,并且随生命进程而发生的激素变化。诱发史应包括肥胖发病年龄、维持 1 年的最低成人体重、与体重增加相关的显著事件(如戒烟、受孕、围绝经期、药物使用等)。有厌食症、暴食症或暴饮暴食障碍等精神疾病史或饮食失调史,除了肥胖医学专家治疗外,通常还需要精神健康医生进行密切跟踪治疗。对严重酗酒和滥用药物的治疗应优先于肥胖治疗。应该包括吸烟和戒烟的详细病史,因为戒烟可能导致体重增加或减肥动力受挫。在开始锻炼计划之前,应详细记录患者目前的体育活动水平,包括生活方式和有组织的锻炼。最后,应该对睡眠障碍进行评估,包括打鼾、睡眠呼吸暂停、日间疲劳或晨起头痛。

应进行全面的体检,以评估肥胖的原因及其并发症。应测量身高和体重,并计算 BMI,以便对肥胖的类别和严重程度进行分类。应采用合适的方法在髂嵴正上方测量腰围,特别是对于 BMI 大于 25~35kg/m^2 的患者,且需要进一步进行风险分层[50]。测量血压时应使用尺寸合适的血压袖带,以避免袖带太紧或太松造成测量错误。其他需要注意的发现包括黑棘皮病和皮赘表明存在胰岛素抵抗;紫纹和颈背脂肪垫,提示高皮质醇症;甲状腺肿大和反射迟钝是甲状腺功能减退的症状。肥胖可能是其他内分泌疾病临床表现的一部分,如多囊卵巢综合征、库欣综合征、甲状腺功能减退、肢端肥大症。在发展为显性 2 型糖尿病之前的数月或数年内出现胰岛素抵抗和高胰岛素血症可导致显著的结果。长期肥胖患者可出现皮肤真菌感染、下肢水肿和足部畸形等症状。

某些肥胖并发症可能仅在实验室和调查检测中体现。应考虑使用糖化血红蛋白、空腹血糖或 75g 口服糖耐量试验来筛查 2 型糖尿病[51]。为了评估家族性高胆固醇血症等脂质代谢遗传性疾病,需要一个包括分级脂蛋白水平在内的完整血脂组合来评估。高尿酸血症、肝脂肪变性和胆汁淤积通常只有在实验室进一步检查后才被发现。因此,一个完整的实验室评估应包括血糖、尿酸、BUN、肌酐、ALT、AST、总胆红素和直接胆红素、碱性磷酸酶、总胆固醇、高密度脂蛋白胆固醇和低密度脂蛋白胆固醇、甘油三酯(TG)、全血细胞计数、促甲状腺激素检测、尿液分析。空腹血清胰岛素和葡萄糖测试值可用于计算胰岛素抵抗的稳态模型评估水平,方法是使用基于经过充分验证的方程式的在线计算器来测量胰岛素抵抗[52]。使用快速、廉价的方法(如生物电阻抗法或双能 X 射线吸收法)测量身体成分,可以提供更多有关体脂百分比、肌肉减少性肥胖和瘦体质的信息,并可在患者的治疗过程中进行纵向跟踪[53]。

六、并发症

当肥胖的明显并发症如高血压、2 型糖尿病、高脂血症或冠心病被诊断出来时,这些疾病应与医学监督下的减肥同时治疗。某些情况,如骨关节炎等情况,除非严重到需要关节置换,通常会随着患者体重减轻而改善。

(一) 糖尿病

与 2 型糖尿病患者有一级或二级亲属关系是胰岛素抵抗的一个独立危险因素(见上文),但糖尿病的风险也会随着 BMI 的增加而增加,当 BMI 大于 30kg/m^2 时,糖尿病的风险尤其大。中年时体重上升增加糖耐量受损和心脏病的风险,且与达到的总体重无关[54]。血压与体重指数呈线性相关,初次评估时,大约有一半的过度肥胖的人存在高血压[55]。

(二) 血脂紊乱

以低 HDL 胆固醇和高 TG 水平为特征的血脂异常,与非肥胖人相比,肥胖人群中更常见,特别是在有中心性肥胖的人群中[56]。当伴有高血压和高血糖时,这些紊乱符合国家胆固醇教育计划中代谢综合征的标准[57]。一项对 21 项队列研究的 meta 分析表明,肥胖对血压和血脂水平的不良影响(AEs)约占肥胖个体患冠心病额外风险的一半[58]。

(三) 心血管疾病

由于冠心病占我们社会死亡人数的近一半,它与肥胖的关系尤为重要。一项研究表明,BMI 增加 1.1kg/m^2 会使患主要心血管疾病的风险增加 6%[59]。肥胖还会增加心力衰竭和心房颤动的风险[60,61]。心脏病风险的增加很大程度上与中枢性肥胖有关。2004 年对来自 52 个国家的 29 000 多名患者进行的 INTERHEART 病例对照研究发现,腹部肥胖占人群首次心肌梗死的归因风险的 20%[62]。

(四) 高血压

超重或肥胖患者的血压通常升高。肥胖和高血压与心脏功能相互作用。超重和高血压的结合会导致心室壁增厚和心脏体积增大,从而导致心脏衰竭的可能性更大[63]。在瑞典肥胖受试者研究中,44% 到 51% 的受试者在基线时存在高血压[64]。舒张压每下降 1mmHg,心肌梗死的风险就降低 2% 至 3%。

(五) 肾脏疾病

肥胖可能会从几个方面影响肾脏。肥胖相关肾小球疾病的定义是 BMI≥30kg/m^2,肾脏活检显示肾小球肿大伴有或不伴有局灶节段性肾小球硬化。肥胖相关肾小球疾病的发病率显著上升，从 1986 年至 1990 年的 0.2% 上升到 2001 年至 2015 年的 2.7%[65]。由于酸碱代谢改变，超重患者患尿酸和草酸钙肾结石的风险也会增加[66]，BMI 增加与终末期肾病的风险有关。在一项来自北加州凯撒永久集团（Kaiser Permanente Group of Northern California）的研究中，Hsu 和他的同事发现，BMI 越高则越是终末期肾病的危险因素，这种情况即使在纠正了包括基线血压或糖尿病在内的多种潜在混杂因素后仍然存在[67]。

（六）胆囊疾病

胆石症是与超重有关的原发性肝胆疾病。肥胖患者体内增加的总胆固醇水平是通过胆汁排出的，胆汁中高胆固醇浓度（相对于胆汁酸和磷脂）可能增加胆固醇结石在胆囊中沉淀的可能性。在减肥期间，由于从脂肪中调动的胆固醇通过胆道系统的排出增加，胆结石形成的可能性会反常地增加[68]。含有中等水平脂肪的饮食会促使胆囊收缩，从而排空胆固醇含量，并可能降低与减肥相关的结石形成风险。同样，如果认为胆石形成的风险会增加，则使用胆汁酸治疗（如 UDCA）可能是明智的选择[69]。

（七）肝脏疾病

NAFLD 是用来描述与超重和肥胖相关的一系列肝脏异常的术语。这包括肝大，肝脏生化检测结果升高，肝脏组织学异常，其中包括脂肪变性、脂肪性肝炎、纤维化和肝硬化（见第 87 章）。

（八）胃食管反流病

超重和肥胖是导致胃食管反流病的因素，2014 年对 9 项研究的 meta 分析表明，胃食管反流病与 BMI 之间存在显著的统计相关性[70]。另一项 meta 分析表明，与正常体重组相比，超重组（BMI 25~29.9kg/m^2）胃食管反流病的优势比为 1.43，当 BMI 高于 30kg/m^2 时，胃食管反流病的优势比上升至 1.94。糜烂性食管炎和食管腺癌在肥胖人群中也更为常见，BMI 小于 25kg/m^2 的糜烂性食管炎的患病率为 12.5%，而 BMI 大于 30kg/m^2 的糜烂性食管炎的患病率为 26.9%，在食管癌病例对照和队列研究中的相对风险比为 2.27~11.3[71]。

（九）癌症

肥胖患者患某些类型的癌症明显增加。肥胖的男性患结肠癌、直肠癌和前列腺癌的风险增加，而肥胖的女性比正常体重的女性患生殖系统和胆囊癌的风险更大[72,73]。超重妇女患子宫内膜癌风险更高的一个解释是脂肪组织中芳构化反应产生的雌激素增多与身体脂肪过多的程度有关，而这是绝经后女性雌激素产生的主要来源[74]。乳腺癌不仅与全身脂肪有关，而且可能与中心体脂有更重要的关系，这可能有助于解释为什么 BMI 最高四分位数的女性在 75 岁时患乳腺癌的风险会增加。CT 测量的内脏脂肪增加表明与乳腺癌的风险有重要关系[75]。在护士健康研究中，18 岁后体重增加≥25kg 的女性患乳腺癌的风险增加（相对风险为 1.45；$P<0.001$）。与体重保持稳定的女性相比，绝经后体重增加≥10kg 的妇女患乳腺癌的风险也增加[76]。

（十）阻塞性睡眠呼吸暂停

颈围增加（男性≥43.2cm，女性≥40.6cm）、悬雍垂松软和扁桃体肥大是阻塞性睡眠呼吸暂停（obstructive sleep apnea，OSA）的预测因素[77]。相关的发现可能包括打鼾、睡眠紊乱、易怒和性欲下降。实验室检查可显示红细胞增多症。有白天疲劳、嗜睡和/或晨起头痛的患者应该接受阻塞性睡眠呼吸暂停综合征诊断性睡眠研究的筛查。阻塞性睡眠呼吸暂停综合征可能与体重进一步增加有关，而治疗睡眠呼吸暂停综合征可以促进体重减轻，但数据不太一致[78]。有证据表明，治疗阻塞性睡眠呼吸暂停综合征并不能促进体重减轻，因为一旦治疗阻塞性睡眠呼吸暂停综合征，夜间能量消耗减少[79]。随机对照试验证实阻塞性睡眠呼吸暂停综合征的治疗有助于体重减轻[80]。研究认为，阻塞性睡眠呼吸暂停综合征治疗改善体重调节的机制之一是通过改善皮质醇的调节[81]。

（十一）骨骼、关节、肌肉、结缔组织和皮肤疾病

骨关节炎在肥胖个体中显著增加。在膝关节和踝关节中的骨性关节炎可能与超重程度相关的创伤直接相关，但其他非负重关节的骨性关节炎的增加表明超重和肥胖的某些病症，如肌内脂肪浸润和全身炎症，可改变软骨和骨代谢，与负重无关[82]。骨关节炎在超重的健康成本中占有重要的一部分。体重增加也会造成关节疾病而导致残疾。

一些皮肤变化与超重有关。妊娠纹是很常见的，反映了小叶脂肪沉积扩张对皮肤的压力。黑棘皮病是指在许多超重个体的颈部、腋下、指关节和伸肌表面的皱襞中出现的加深的色素沉着（图 7.1）。黑棘皮病的发病机制被认为是由于高水平的循环胰岛素激活了胰岛素样生长因子 1 受体导致的[83]。

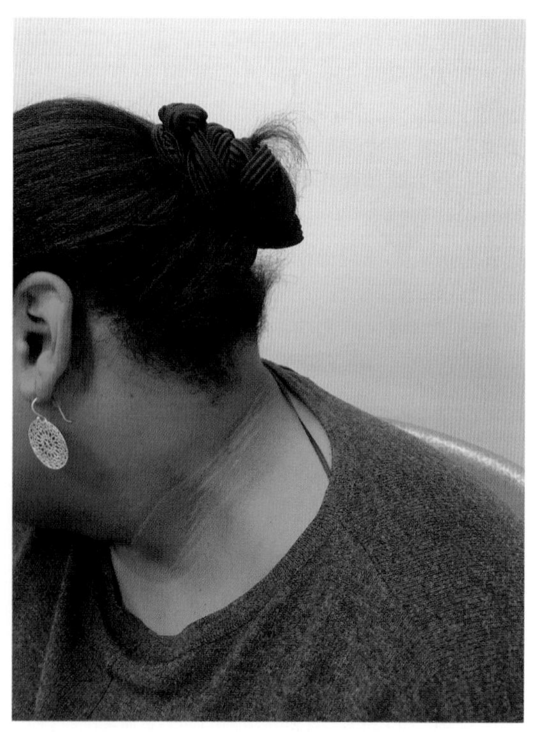

图 7.1　累及肥胖女性颈部的黑棘皮病

（十二）心理社会功能障碍

肥胖在儿童和成人中均被污名化，导致在社会交往过程中存在心理上的困扰[84]。与正常体重的儿童相比，超重儿童具有负面的自我形象消极，身体和社会功能也显著下降。与超重男性相比，超重女性出现心理障碍的风险更大，这可能是由于社会增加女性变瘦的压力所致[85]。肥胖合并抑郁症的患病率很高[86]。

七、医学治疗

（一）饮食方法

一般来说，没有一种饮食模式在临床试验中被证明是优越的。试验表明，任何一个特定的患者喜欢且最容易遵守的饮食，都会对该患者产生最大的减肥效果。

1. 低脂饮食

低脂饮食是帮助患者减肥的常用策略，大多数饮食指南建议将每天摄入的脂肪减少到能量摄入的30%或更少。在一项比较低脂饮食组（通常<25%来自脂肪的总热量）和一个常规饮食的对照组（占总热量的30%到40%）试验的meta分析中，与适当摄入脂肪组相比，低脂饮食组的体重减轻更大（差异3kg）[87]。

2. 低碳水化合物饮食

低碳水化合物饮食（low-carbohydrate diet，LCD）和极低的碳水化合物饮食在短期减肥方面比低脂饮食更有效，但对长期减肥却没有效果。5项试验的meta分析结果显示，在12个月的时间以内，低碳水化合物饮食的减肥效果优于低脂饮食[88]。低碳水化合物饮食可能还有减少2型糖尿病的发生等其他好处。原始人饮食（paleo diet）是低碳水化合物饮食的一种变体，因为它除了从饮食中除去乳制品之外，还去除了谷物。原始人饮食在这里没有进一步讨论，因为它被认为是一种“时尚”饮食，类似于阿特金斯饮食（Atkins diet）。

3. 膳食替代饮食

膳食替代饮食是一种导致热量不足的结构化方法。通过液体替代，一些患者可采用代餐来进一步减肥。这种方法可以在短期内使用，也可以在长期内作为部分流质饮食，如用低热量液体（蛋白奶昔）代替1~2餐，其余膳食作为能量平衡餐[89]。低热量液体的一个常见用途是在减肥手术前后的围手术期使用，但如果患者能够坚持下去，它可以持续更长时间[90]。减重的一个简单方法可以是用控制热量的单独包装食品进行膳食替代计划。每包含400kcal以下的冷冻低热量食品是一种方便且营养丰富的控制热量的方式。

4. 地中海饮食

对于首要问题是关注心血管健康的患者，可建议采用地中海饮食。地中海饮食（mediterranean diet，MD）没有单独的定义，但这些饮食富含水果、蔬菜、全谷类、豆类、坚果和种子，并将橄榄油作为单不饱和脂肪的重要来源。地中海饮食允许适度饮葡萄酒。有低到中等量的鱼、家禽和奶制品，很少有红肉。地中海饮食与总死亡率、心血管死亡率和癌症发病率的降低相关。

地中海饮食可以减少心血管疾病的发生。在一项对7 447名心血管疾病高风险成年人的随机试验中，与对照组（建议食用低脂饮食）相比，两组被分配到地中海饮食的组（补充特级初榨橄榄油或混合坚果）的总心血管事件（卒中、心肌梗死、心血管死亡）发生率较低；4.8年后，危险比为0.7（95% CI 0.5~0.9）。风险的绝对值降低约为每1 000人每年发生3次心血管事件[91]。

5. 间歇性禁食

长期的能量限制会导致代谢变化，从而使持续减肥变得困难[92]。长期减肥期间计划好的负能量平衡期似乎是代谢对减肥适应的关键。该理论支持间歇性能量限制（intermittent energy restriction，IER）作为一种刺激减肥或保持体重下降状态的方法。有几种IER模型已经被证明对长期的体重控制和长期的非平衡饮食一样有效。IER包括在规定的时间内限制热量摄入，在非能量限制期内随意进食（即饱腹感）。IER最常见的形式是“间歇性禁食”，即在短时间内（通常每周2~4天）严格限制热量摄入。能量平衡期（即1周的剩余时间）可能有限制，也可能没有限制。对IER的meta分析得出结论，尽管有些患者可能表现出更大的依从性，但这是一种替代方法，而不是优于慢性能量限制造成的体重下降。关于IER是否能减少饮食诱导的体重减轻后的体重增加的负向调节机制，数据是模棱两可的[93]。

（二）药物治疗

美国国立卫生研究院的国家心脏、肺和血液研究所建议，对于生活方式干预措施治疗6个月后无反应、BMI大于30kg/m^{2}或大于27kg/m^{2}并伴有体重诱发的合并症的患者，可以在治疗计划中加用减肥药物[94]。内分泌学会制定了第一个肥胖药物治疗指南，包括对药物引起的体重增加的管理[95]。这些指南回顾了美国食品药品管理局（FDA）批准的和超说明书的体重管理药物的现有证据。

在减肥治疗过程中（见第8章），一旦患者达到体重稳定期，需要额外减重以改善与体重相关的合并症，或者如果患者出现体重恢复，可以考虑进行减肥药物治疗。此外，它也可以作为快速减肥后（如胃内球囊）的一种维持策略[96]。

药物治疗的目标不仅是减轻体重，更重要的是改善如高血糖、高血脂和动脉粥样硬化性心脏病等与肥胖相关的合并症。患者和医生应该认识到肥胖是一种需要长期治疗的慢性病。患者应进一步了解，在大多数成功患者中，当前药物选择的疗效仅限于5%至10%的体重减轻，但同时使用几种方法可以实现更多的体重减轻。医生应该知道，所有的减肥药物都被列为妊娠X类，而不应该在妊娠期使用，且应当告知患者。

1. 芬特明/托吡酯

2012年，FDA批准了低剂量、控释型的芬特明/托吡酯作为一种长期治疗肥胖症的药物。芬特明是一种肾上腺素能激动剂，通过激活交感神经系统促进体重减轻，随后减少食物摄入和增加静息能量消耗。这种组合方式已被证明具有相加的减肥疗效[97]。芬特明/托吡酯有4种剂量：3.75/23mg（起始剂量）、7.5/46mg（最低治疗剂量）、11.25/69mg或15/92mg。大多数患者开始服用3.75/23mg，过渡到7.5/46mg，如果药物耐受性良好且需要最大疗效，则使用更高剂量，最高剂量为15/92mg。

FDA 要求制订风险评估和缓解策略，告知处方医生和育龄女性在妊娠早期有生殖能力的女性关于女性在受孕前 3 个月接触芬特明/托吡酯会导致婴儿发生先天性畸形，特别是口面部裂的风险增加[98]。芬特明/托吡酯缓释片最常见的不良事件包括：感觉异常、头晕、味觉障碍、失眠、便秘和口干。药物相互作用包括合用 MAO 抑制剂增加恶性高血压的风险，如果与其他类似交感神经胺类药物联合使用，心率和血压升高的概率增加。

这项为期 52 周的控释、芬特明/托吡酯联合用药对超重和肥胖成人体重及相关合并症的影响（CONQUER）试验，将 2 487 名体重指数平均为 36.6kg/m^2 的肥胖患者以及高血压、血脂异常、糖尿病或糖尿病前期、腹部肥胖等合并症患者随机分为安慰剂组、中剂量组（7.5/46mg），或最大治疗剂量（15/92mg）；结果显示，在低剂量组和最大剂量组中去除安慰剂后的体重减轻率分别为 6.6% 和 8.6%[99]。在重度肥胖成人中控释芬特明/托吡酯的随机对照试验和 CONQUER 试验两个 3 期临床试验中，与安慰剂相比，芬特明联合托吡酯治疗的肥胖和超重受试者可观察到收缩压、舒张压和 TG 的改善以及高密度脂蛋白的增加。在 CONQUER 试验延续 52 周的 SEQUEL 研究中，可见空腹血糖和胰岛素水平的改善，并且在基线时没有糖尿病的受试者中，两组治疗组进展为 2 型糖尿病分别降低了 54% 和 76%[100,101]。

2. 氯卡色林

氯卡色林是一种选择性 5-羟色胺 2C 受体激动剂，于 2012 年被 FDA 批准作为肥胖的长期治疗药物。氯卡色林通过 2A 和 2B 受体选择性激活中枢 5-羟色胺 2C 受体，并通过与下丘脑厌食性 POMC 神经元上的 5HT-2C 受体结合来降低食欲。由于氯卡色林对 5-羟色胺 2C 受体有选择性的兴奋作用，因此它能降低食欲，并被设计用于避免心脏瓣膜效应，例如先前报道的芬氟拉明通过 5HT-2B 受体介导二尖瓣或主动脉瓣关闭不全。到目前为止，该开发项目已经排除了两年内这种可能性，并在一项为期 5 年的心血管结局研究中收集了长期数据[102]。氯卡色林的推荐剂量为 10mg，每日两次，与食物同服或不同服。还有一种新的 20mg 缓释片，每天服用一次。如果 12 周后体重减少未达到≥5%，应停止用药。氯卡色林被列入《管制物质法》附表四（译者注：即定义为低滥用潜力和低依赖风险的药物）。临床实践中最常见的不良事件包括头痛、头晕、疲劳、恶心、口干和便秘。虽然在 3 期行为矫正和氯卡色林用于超重和肥胖管理（Behavioral Modiffcation and Lorcaserin for Overweight and Obesity Management，BLOOM）研究以及行为矫正和氯卡色林用于肥胖管理的第二项研究中没有报道，理论上，氯卡色林与其他 5-羟色胺药物存在相互作用（联合用药可能导致潜在的危及生命的 5-羟色胺综合征或神经阻滞剂恶性综合征样反应）。

BLOOM 试验包括了 3 182 名超重或肥胖的成年人，他们每天服用两次 10mg 氯卡色林或安慰剂治疗 52 周，并结合饮食和运动。在第 52 周，所有受试者被重新随机分为安慰剂组或氯卡色林组，为期 1 年。1 年时，除去安慰剂的平均减重率为 3.6%，服用氯卡色林的受试者中有 47% 减重率大于 5%，而对照组为 20.5%。第一年体重下降超过 5%，第二年继续使用氯卡色林治疗的受试者比那些改用安慰剂的受试者更能维持他们的体重下降[103]。在患有 2 型糖尿病的肥胖受试者中进行了 BLOOM-DM 研究。该试验结果表明，在 52 周时，每天服用 10mg 氯卡色林的患者中有 37.5% 体重下降超过 5%，是安慰剂组的两倍以上。氯卡色林组糖化血红蛋白降低 0.9%，安慰剂组降低 0.4%[104]。

3. 安非他酮/纳曲酮

在 2014 年 9 月，安非他酮/纳曲酮被 FDA 批准用于减肥。安非他酮的主要作用机制是作为多巴胺和去甲肾上腺素的再摄取抑制剂。抑制多巴胺和/或去甲肾上腺素的再摄取能够调节这条被各种食物所刺激的“奖赏路径”。纳曲酮是一种纯阿片类拮抗剂，阻断可能减缓体重减轻的阿片类途径。纳曲酮缓释片/安非他酮缓释片最常见的不良反应是恶心/呕吐、便秘、头痛、头晕、失眠、口干和癫痫发作风险增加。

与安非他酮/纳曲酮产生相互作用的药物包括 MAO 抑制剂（在给药期间或 14 天内使用）、阿片类药物、阿片类激动剂和阿片类局部激素。突然停止长期使用的酒精、苯二氮䓬类、巴比妥类或抗癫痫药物可能进一步增加癫痫发作的风险。有不受控制的高血压、癫痫史或近期有贪食或神经性厌食症的患者应避免使用安非他酮/纳曲酮。最近有过多呕吐的贪食症病史可能导致电解质异常，使人容易癫痫发作，如果服用安非他酮，会进一步增加癫痫发作的风险。对于近期有厌食性进食障碍病史的患者，不应给予减肥药，除非能与患者的精神科医生密切配合并监测复发情况。

进行了 4 项为期 56 周的多中心、双盲、安慰剂对照试验［CONTRAVE 肥胖研究，或 COR-Ⅰ[105]、COR-Ⅱ[106]、COR-BMOD（行为改变）[107] 和 COR-糖尿病[108]］，在 4 536 名患者的安慰剂对照队列中评估安非他酮/纳曲酮结合生活方式改变的效果。COR-Ⅰ、COR-Ⅱ和 COR-BMOD 试验纳入了 BMI≥30kg/m^2 或超重（BMI≥27kg/m^2）且至少有 1 种合并症的患者。糖尿病研究纳入了 BMI 大于 27kg/m^2、伴有或不伴有高血压和/或血脂异常的 2 型糖尿病患者。最终判定是相对于基线体重的百分比变化和体重至少减少 5% 的患者比例。在 56 周的 COR-Ⅰ试验中，服用安非他酮/纳曲酮 360/32mg 的患者体重平均变化为-5.4%，而安慰剂组为-1.3%。在 COR-Ⅰ试验中，42% 的治疗组患者体重从基线水平降低 5%，而安慰剂组患者为 17%；在 COR-Ⅱ试验中，50.5% 的治疗组患者体重从基线水平降低了 5%，而安慰剂组患者为 17.1%；在 COR-BMOD 试验中，66.4% 的治疗组患者体重从基线水平降低了 5%，而安慰剂组患者为 42.5%，以上数据均具有临床意义。

在 COR 糖尿病试验中，接受安非他酮/纳曲酮治疗的患者中，有 44.5% 的患者在 56 周后体重减轻≥5%，而安慰剂组为 18.9%（$P<0.001$）。使用安非他酮/纳曲酮的患者的糖化血红蛋白较基线水平降低了 0.6%，而安慰剂组降低了 0.1%。在所有的 COR 试验中，都达到了次要心血管终点，包括腰围、内脏脂肪、高密度脂蛋白胆固醇和甘油三酯等。

4. 利拉鲁肽

利拉鲁肽 3.0mg 于 2014 年 12 月获得美国 FDA 批准。利拉鲁肽是一种 GLP-1 受体激动剂，最多使用 1.8mg 剂量，已用于治疗 2 型糖尿病。在动物研究中，利拉鲁肽的外周给药会导致调节食欲的摄取。一项针对无糖尿病的肥胖个体的研究表明，利拉鲁肽 3.0mg/d 可以抑制急性食物摄入，减少主观饥饿感，延缓胃排空。相反，即使纠正了体重减轻，应用利拉鲁肽 3.0mg/d 的受试者的能量消耗也减少，这可能反映了代谢对体重减轻的适应[109]。

SCALE 肥胖和糖尿病前期研究以及 SCALE 糖尿病研究分别评估了利拉鲁肽 3.0mg 对超重和肥胖合并糖尿病前期以及糖尿病患者产生的效果。在 56 周、随机、安慰剂对照、双盲临床试验中，利拉鲁肽的平均减重显著高于安慰剂（8% vs 2.6%，SCALE 肥胖和糖尿病前期研究 5.9% vs 2%，SCALE 糖尿病研究，P<0.000 1）。在 SCALE 维持研究中检验了利拉鲁肽在维持体重方面的疗效。422 名体重减轻≥5% 的超重和肥胖受试者被随机分为每日 3.0mg 利拉鲁肽组或安慰剂组，为期 56 周。初始饮食的平均体重减轻为 6.0%。在研究结束时，利拉鲁肽组的受试者额外减少了 6.2%，而安慰剂组的受试者为 0.2%（P<0.000 1）[110,111]。

胃肠道症状，如恶心、呕吐和腹痛，是受试者退出试验的最常见原因。SCALE 肥胖和糖尿病前期研究的 11 名受试者发生了胰腺炎［利拉鲁肽组 2 841 人中有 10 人（0.4%），安慰剂组 1 242 人中有 1 人（<0.1%）］；在 SCALE 糖尿病研究或 SCALE 维持研究中患者均未发生胰腺炎。在所有的 SCALE Ⅲ期研究中也观察到胆囊炎和胆石症发生率的增加，但不清楚这些病例是否与药物治疗或体重减轻有关。虽然利拉鲁肽与血压和血脂的改善有关，但研究发现，在重度糖尿病患者中，利拉鲁肽可使心率增加 2.0/min。利拉鲁肽在啮齿类动物中与甲状腺髓样癌的相关性上带有黑框警告，但它与人类的相关性尚未确定。因此，利拉鲁肽禁忌用于有甲状腺髓样癌或有 MEN2 家族史的患者[112]。

5. 奥利司他

在 2012 年之前，唯一长期使用的减肥药是奥利司他，于 1999 年获 FDA 批准。奥利司他通过抑制胃肠道脂肪酶来促进减肥，从而减少胃肠道对脂肪的吸收。奥利司他不常用于肥胖治疗，因为有令人不快的大便紧迫感、油性便和大便失禁等不良反应，但对于服用其他抗肥胖药物治疗的便秘患者，奥利司他可以作为一种附加药物。每天 3 次，平均服用 120mg 奥利司他，会减少 30% 的脂肪吸收。奥利司他组 4 年后的平均体重减轻量（5.8kg）显著大于安慰剂组（3.0kg；P<0.001）[113]。

6. 研究方向

除了 5 种 FDA 批准的减肥药物和越来越多的治疗肥胖的内镜手术（即内镜下袖状胃成形术和胃内球囊）外，还有一些新的药物化合物正在临床试验中。临床试验中中枢作用靶点的一个例子是黑素肽，它是一种正在被评估是否可用于罕见遗传性肥胖综合征的 MC4R 激动剂[114]。其他试验性治疗的例子包括称为胃泌酸调节素的 GLP-1/胰高血糖素受体激动剂。研究表明，这种结合物有厌食效应。此外，正在研究的一种装置为 Gelesis 水凝胶胶囊，它在胃中膨胀，增加饱腹感，并可能改善血糖控制[115]。

肥胖症已成为一种全球流行病，是患糖尿病、心血管疾病和癌症等其他非传染性疾病的主要原因。其原因可以归因于遗传、表观遗传、环境和生活方式等现象的组合。目前的治疗包括饮食和行为干预，对更严重的病例，还包括药物和手术治疗。有几种具有不同作用机制的新药物疗法和一些新装置正在临床试验中。肥胖症的治疗手段正在发展，肥胖症现在被视为一种多因素的慢性疾病，需要联合使用药物治疗并且在适当情况下还需要行介入治疗。肥胖的外科手术和内镜治疗在第 8 章中讨论。

（王子元　孙明瑜 译，李鹏　袁农 校）

参考文献

第 8 章　肥胖的外科和内镜治疗

Shelby Sullivan, Steven A. Edmundowicz, John Magañ Morton 著

章节目录

一、肥胖病外科手术候选人的评估和选择 …… 96
二、肥胖的外科治疗 …… 97
（一）胃旁路术 …… 97
（二）袖状胃切除术 …… 97
（三）其他手术 …… 98
（四）手术并发症 …… 98
（五）营养缺乏 …… 100
（六）结果 …… 100
三、肥胖病手术并发症的内镜处理 …… 101
（一）溃疡病 …… 101
（二）手术后胃肠道出血 …… 101
（三）狭窄 …… 102
（四）异物并发症 …… 102
（五）渗漏和瘘管 …… 102
（六）胰胆管疾病 …… 103
（七）体重反弹及胃空肠吻合口扩张 …… 104
四、肥胖的内镜治疗 …… 104
（一）肥胖病内镜治疗候选人的评估和选择 …… 105
（二）美国目前内镜治疗肥胖病的实施 …… 105

重度肥胖是工业化国家首要的公众健康威胁（见第 7 章）。美国的肥胖患病率以惊人的速度持续上升，目前有三分之二的成年人体重超标，其中一半为肥胖患者[1,2]。肥胖的病因很复杂，且只有部分明确。遗传、环境和心理因素都有不同程度的参与，实际上，肥胖症是脂肪储存增加导致能量失衡紊乱，从而损害患者的器官功能和整体健康。已经证明肥胖患者易患多种疾病，包括心血管疾病、糖尿病、睡眠呼吸暂停和骨关节炎（见第 7 章）。

超重的诊断标准为体重指数（body mass index，BMI）>25kg/m^2；Ⅰ度肥胖，30～34.9kg/m^2；Ⅱ度肥胖，35～39.9kg/m^2；Ⅲ度肥胖，≥40kg/m^2；超病态肥胖，>50kg/m^2。在美国，无论性别、种族、民族和社会经济群体，肥胖症发生率均呈现上升趋势[3,4]。重度肥胖会使人的预期寿命减少 5～20 年，据预测，当代人的预期寿命可能有史以来第一次比上一代人短[5]。

神经和体液机制精细地调节能量摄入和消耗。能量调节的关键激素包括胰岛素、瘦素、胃促生长素和酪酪肽等。胰岛素是一种强效的合成激素，具有多种合成和促生长作用。脂肪细胞分泌的瘦素，可减少食物摄入并且增加能量消耗。由胃底细胞分泌的胃促生长素（瘦素的拮抗激素），促进合成代谢并诱发饥饿。回肠和结肠的内分泌细胞在进食后分泌的酪酪肽被认为是饱腹的信号。

肥胖是一种复杂的疾病，每个患者的根本病因各不相同。可以通过运动、药物和外科方法减重。然而，结合仔细的筛选评估和咨询，减重手术对于合适的患者人群是最有效的治疗选择[6]。减重手术自从 20 世纪 50 年代开展以来，一直在持续改进。当今，随着美国外科医师学会、美国代谢及减重手术学会新的代谢和减重手术认证和质量改进计划（Metabolic and Bariatric Surgery Accreditation and Quality Improvement Program，MBSAQIP）的不断努力、建立循证医学推荐，减重手术死亡率与常规外科手术（如腹腔镜胆囊切除术或胃底折叠术）相当[7,8]。

外科医生和医院的经验可以减少与减重手术相关的风险。在美国，MBSAQIP 及其要求认证的主要保险公司已经认可了容量结局效应[9,10]。有许多获得减重手术认证资格的标准，但目前的主要标准是一位外科医生完成手术数量超过 25 例，一家医院的每年完成患者数超过 50 例。获得认证资格的、有经验的外科医生和医院是最有效预防并发症证明[9,11-14]。

Roux-en-Y 胃旁路（roux-en-Y gastric bypass，RYGB）手术通过对食欲、能量调节、饱腹感等基础改变来调控代谢过程，从而诱导持续减重。长期随访研究表明，RYGB 通过逆转病态肥胖患者的一些代谢结果对患者的整体健康产生积极影响。RYGB 能够在术后 12 年甚至更久的时间里，通过改善血脂水平、糖尿病、高血压、阻塞性睡眠呼吸暂停和心血管事件（如心肌梗死）来降低死亡率[15]。

已证实减重手术无论在减重效果、生存率和治疗伴随疾病方面均优于药物治疗[16]。目前每年进行的减重手术数目超过 220 000 例，其中最常见的是腹腔镜袖状胃切除术[17]。下面将讨论手术适应证、术前评估、外科技术、结局、围手术期及术后并发症。

一、肥胖病外科手术候选人的评估和选择

减重手术的患者必须符合 1991 年美国国立卫生研究院（NIH）的统一标准，包括 BMI≥40kg/m^2，或 BMI≥35kg/m^2 伴有肥胖相关的合并症以及至少 6 个月在医学监督下尝试减重的档案记录[18]。最近的数据尝试扩展适应证至 BMI 为 30～35kg/m^2 的糖尿病患者[19]。肥胖相关的合并症包括高血压、糖尿病、高脂血症、胃食管反流病（GERD）、关节炎、肠易激综合征（IBS）、阻塞性睡眠呼吸暂停和非酒精性脂肪性肝炎（NASH）。术前的大量评估应尝试发现潜在的隐性合并症，如冠状动脉性疾病、睡眠呼吸暂停和肥胖低通气综合征（Pickwickian 综合征）。由于术前评估的复杂性，应该通过包括营养学家、心理学家、麻醉医生、减重外科医生和其他

可以解决任何胃肠道、心血管、肺脏或内分泌相关问题的亚学科专家在内的团队进行多学科综合评估。在该团队中,家庭和社会支持是必需的组成部分且不应被低估[20]。此外,向患者进行宣传教育对减重手术后的疗效至关重要。营养师、专科护士和减重外科医生需参与到健康宣教中,详细介绍术前和术后饮食及生活方式的改变并为患者做好术后准备。

一些减重外科医生要求患者在首次进行减重手术前,通过控制饮食和锻炼来减掉额外的体重,尤其是有体重反弹风险的患者[21]。术前减重是一种"降阶梯处理"的方法,类似于癌症的术前放化疗。这种额外的术前减重与合并症的缓解或并发症发生率无关[21,22]。然而,这与缩短手术时间、减小肝脏体积、术后 1 年减重效果更显著有关。因此,在平衡患者对医疗的可及性并不会延误治疗的情况下,应当鼓励所有患者术前减重[21]。

减重手术的适应人群受益于术前营养评估和咨询。患者在术后应根据指导循序渐进地从全流食开始,到半流食、糊状软食,最后添加常规质地的饮食。同样应当提醒患者减重手术是一种限制性的术式,所以更适合少食多餐[23]。

减重手术的禁忌证包括精神疾病,如精神分裂症、严重的双相情感障碍、精神活性物质滥用、近期因重度抑郁住院或存在自杀倾向以及发育迟缓。其他的禁忌证包括无法安全有效麻醉的严重心脏疾病,严重的凝血功能障碍,或不能遵守终身补充维生素等严格的术后营养要求。对伴有严重合并症的患者,年龄不是绝对禁忌证,且可以对 65 岁以上或 18 岁以下的患者行减重手术[24]。

术前患者必须进行筛查评估,包括外科医生会诊、心理评估、营养咨询、胸部 X 线片、心电图和上消化道内镜(EGD)检查。

欧洲内镜手术协会推荐术前 EGD 检查,以发现和治疗可能引起术后并发症或影响减重手术类型的上消化道病变[25]。一项纳入 272 例 RYGB 术前行 EGD 检查的研究中,12% 的患者的术前发现有临床意义,包括糜烂性食管炎(3.7%)、Barrett 食管(3.7%)、胃溃疡(2.9%)、糜烂性胃炎(1.8%)、十二指肠溃疡(0.7%)、胃类癌(0.3%);1.1% 的患者有 1 种以上的病变。

然而,在这些患者中有 2/3 会出现上消化道症状,而 RYGB 术后切除的远端胃无法被轻易评估,因此术前 EGD 检查非常重要[26]。此外,腹腔镜袖状胃切除术前筛查 GERD 非常关键,因为术前伴有 GERD 的患者术后出现 GERD 的风险最大。严重反流的发现可以引导外科医生和患者选择一致的手术流程[27]。

术前应完善心血管疾病、呼吸系统疾病和糖尿病的医学评估。心血管评估应包括近期胸痛史和运动耐受性评估。存在多个危险因素的患者,例如有深静脉血栓形成(deep vein thrombosis,DVT)或静脉淤滞性疾病史,术前可能需要临时放置下腔静脉滤器以预防静脉血栓栓塞[28]。识别隐匿性阻塞性睡眠呼吸暂停综合征也很重要,这样麻醉医生可以预测可能由麻醉性止痛药和术后体液转移加重的术后早期阶段出现的缺氧[29]。此外,术前必须控制好糖尿病,以降低围手术期的发病率(如伤口感染)[29]。

二、肥胖的外科治疗

(一) 胃旁路术

胃旁路术后,限制性结构和激素机制都可以限制食物摄入和营养吸收。1966 年 Mason 和 Iton 首次提出胃旁路手术,此后经过两次改进:一次是在 1966 年联合了 Roux-en-Y 吻合,而不是环式胃空肠吻合术;另一次是在 1994 年首次采用腹腔镜手术[30]。

腹腔镜方法优于开腹方案,且并发症的发生率明显降低。腹腔镜下 RYGB 手术可降低死亡率,降低伤口感染、肺部和血栓栓塞并发症、切口疝的发生率,且平均减少约 2 天的住院时间[31]。腹腔镜下 RYGB 手术有许多改进方式;最基本的组成部分包括构建胃囊、将胃囊与空肠相连以及改变消化酶的路线使其在到达空肠-空肠吻合口之前不与食物接触(图 8.1A)[8]。

术中应注意使患者处于适当的体位,以便于插管、防止神经压迫和皮肤破损。可以采取静脉水化,小剂量糖皮质激素和昂丹司琼等措施预防术后恶心呕吐。放置胃管防止胃胀和误吸。切开前应予预防性肝素(5 000U)皮下注射、持续压迫装置和给予头孢西丁(2g 静脉给药)。手术室中应当具备用以评估胃及深部肠道的内镜。

手术开始时,气腹针建立气腹后,将索引套管针置于剑突下方 18cm 的中线处。留置套管,腹腔镜下探查腹腔。抬起大网膜,找到 Treitz 韧带。将 Treitz 韧带远端 20cm 处空肠分为胆胰支和空肠支(Roux 袢)。下一步,在 Roux 袢远端 75~150cm 处行空肠-空肠吻合,可穿过横结肠系膜(结肠后位)或结肠(结肠前位)与近端胃囊相连,并且结肠后位手术可采取胃后或胃前路径。肠袢之间的任何肠系膜缺损都是疝气的易发部位,因此应当行永久连续性缝合。胃囊大小应在 15~30mL 之间,并根据胃小弯的大小构建。最后,胃空肠吻合口可采用环形缝合器、线形缝合器或手工缝合,也可放置手术引流管。

该手术的潜在不良事件包括出血,Roux 袢无法在无张力的情况下与胃囊连接,以及不可预料的解剖因素如肠管旋转不良、肝脏肿大、巨大网膜或腹壁过厚。尽管少见,但腹腔镜胃旁路手术中的意外发现可能会影响手术进程。这些发现可能包括既往手术遗留的需要松解的顽固性粘连,需要镜中像方法进行操作的 Treitz 韧带旋转不良,需要改变入路位置的疝;若肝脏有肝硬化表现则需要取活检,甚至发现腹腔静脉曲张或腹水则需要放弃手术。术前评估未发现的胃肠道间质瘤(GIST)需要完全切除,然后按原计划完成手术。

(二) 袖状胃切除术

袖状胃切除术(sleeve gastrectomy,SG,见图 8.1B)涉及切除 80% 的胃体组织,沿着胃小弯构建一个直径在 28~32Fr 的袖状胃。据推测,袖状胃越紧,越容易出现胃漏,胃漏是 SG 术后最常见的严重并发症;其他潜在的不良事件可能包括出血或狭窄。减少胃大弯的血供时需要小心。采用先进的双极切割设备或超声刀来闭合血管。在胃的近端,胃短血管可能靠近脾脏,外科医生必须避免对该区域过度牵拉,从

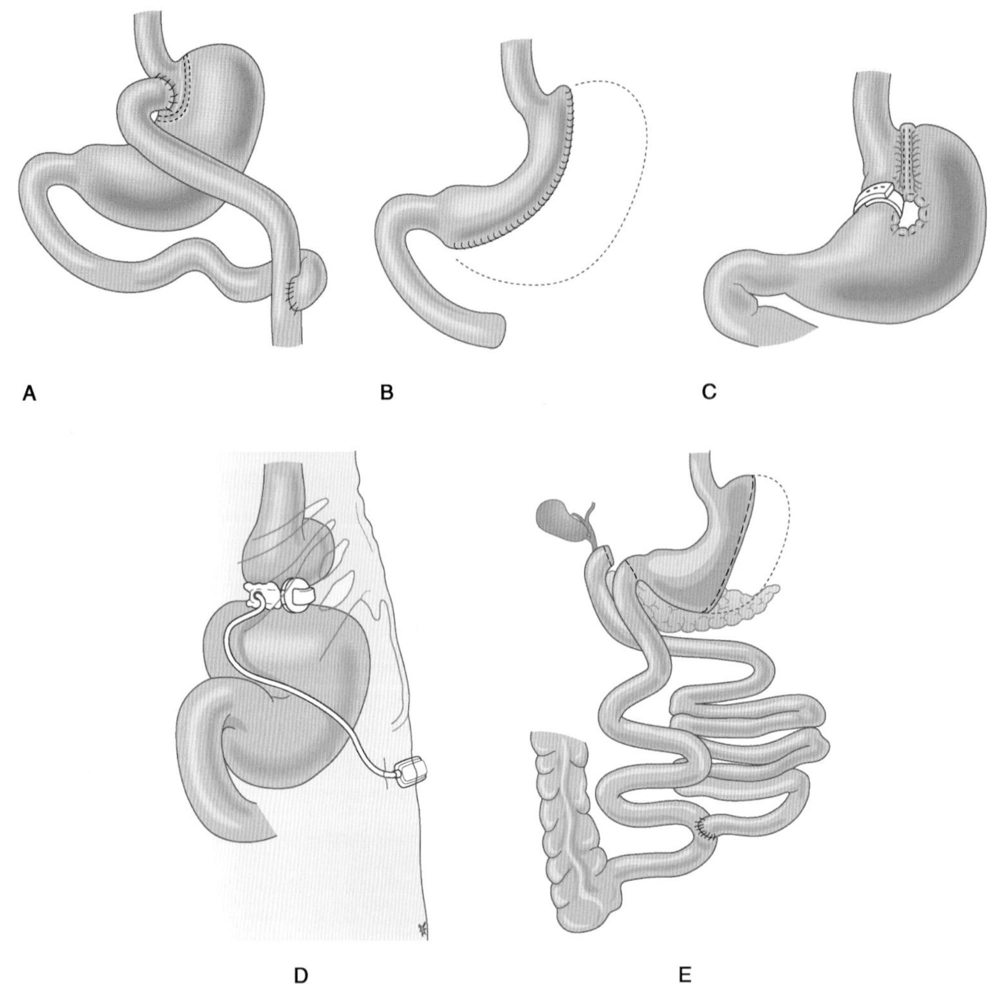

图 8.1　减重手术的类型。A，Roux-en-Y 胃旁路术。B，袖状胃切除术。C，垂直捆扎胃成形术。D，腹腔镜下可调节胃束带术。E，胆胰分流与十二指肠转位术。（A～C，from the American Society for Bariatric Surgery. The story of surgery for obesity，2005. Available at https://asmbs. Org.）

而避免剪切伤。可沿着袖状胃放置一个胃校正管（32～40Fr）来引导缝合。若袖状胃过于紧绷，尤其在胃角切迹处，可以导致流出道梗阻，并且使胃近端更易发生漏。许多外科医生使用空气或亚甲蓝进行术中密封性试验评估缝合效果。如果密封性试验结果为阳性，则在相应部位加固缝合线或重新缝合。

患者取仰卧位或分腿位。并根据外科医生的个人偏好放置五个套管针。然后，将肝脏牵开以暴露包括胃食管连接处在内的胃部。分离胃-结肠韧带，然后使用先进的双极切割设备或超声刀切割胃网膜弓的血管。沿胃大弯游离至近幽门 3～7cm 处，上至 His 角。然后胃体组织与其后小网膜囊内的附着物分离。在游离过程中应注意避免损伤脾静脉和脾动脉。通过胃校正管（32～40Fr）或内镜引导缝合。袖状胃通过从幽门近端到 His 角的多个钉仓构建。不宜离角切迹太近分隔胃体，以免造成此部位的狭窄。此外，外科医生在缝合时应确保前后边缘与胃小弯的距离相同，这样袖状胃才不会打弯或扭曲。一些外科医生可能会在缝合处使用支撑材料，施展各不相同的技术。外科医生也可能会在缝合线处连续缝合或使用间断缝合来使大网膜靠近新构建的胃大弯。手术过程中是否放置引流管取决于外科医生的习惯。术后患者住院 1 到 2 天，给予流食。

一些机构在术后第 1 天进行上消化道造影检查，明确造影剂可以自由通过袖状胃，没有造影剂外渗。患者在术后接受 6 个月的质子泵抑制剂（proton pump inhibitor，PPI）治疗，并终生服用复合维生素。

门诊患者饮食在 8 周内逐步进阶，从流食到糊状食物、软食，最终过渡到常规饮食。

（三）其他手术

其他常见的手术方式包括胃束带术（gastric banding，GB）（见图 8.1C 和 D）。由于减重效果不明显，且需要二次手术，因此 GB 手术量急剧下降[32]。GB 技术涉及“松弛部”或肝胃韧带技术，在此技术中，通过食管脂肪垫为分界，将柔软的可充气的硅胶胃带立即置于食管下括约肌下方。

十二指肠转位（duodenal switch，DS）的胆胰分流术（biliopancreatic diversion，BPD）现在占减重手术的 1% 以下（见图 8.1E）。

（四）手术并发症

RYGB 平均 30 天死亡率为 0.2%，垂直袖状胃切除术

(vertical SG,VSG)为 0.14%,GB 为 0.02%[33]。并发症分为 3 类:术中、术后早期(术后 30 天内)、术后晚期(>术后 30 天)。在监测结局和制定确保操作安全的标准和基准的循证医学指南方面取得了重大进展。如前所述,并发症的发生率与外科医生和医院的经验直接相关。

减重手术的并发症包括吻合口漏或狭窄、肺栓塞(pulmonary embolus,PE)和 DVT、胃肠道出血、营养缺乏、伤口并发症、肠梗阻、溃疡、疝以及呼吸系统和心血管并发症。在不同的外科手术中,并发症的发生率与每次手术产生的体重减轻量成正比。1 年时严重不良事件的概率为:SG,比值比(OR)= 3.22,95% 置信区间(CI)2.64~3.92;RYGB,OR = 4.92,95% CI 4.38~5.54;BPD+DS,OR = 17.47,95% CI 14.19~21.52[34]。

肠缺血可能是由于 Roux 肠袢扭转或肠系膜分离期间发生的肠疝所致[35]。肠缺血的症状是严重腹痛、便血和急腹症。

术后早期并发症为吻合口漏、肺和心血管并发症(包括 DVT、PE)以及死亡率。吻合口、胃袋漏或十二指肠瘘的发生率分别为 RYGB 2.2%、垂直捆扎胃成形术(vertical banded gastroplasty,VBG)1.0% 和 BPD 1.8%[33]。吻合口漏,最常发生于胃空肠吻合口或 SG 吻合钉线,通常位于裂孔附近,是死亡的独立风险因素[36]。已经证明,外科医生的经验对渗漏发生率有显著影响,经验丰富的医生的渗漏率为 1%~2%,职业生涯早期的外科医生的渗漏率高达 5%[37]。SG 渗漏很少发生,但治疗可能相对棘手。渗漏引流和静脉抗生素治疗是一线治疗。其他考虑因素包括支架置入和肠内营养。对于复杂的慢性渗漏,针对性治疗可能需要再次手术,将 SG 转化为 Roux-en-Y 食管空肠吻合术[38]。

PE 可占围手术期死亡的 50%[31]。目前,主要采用抗凝剂和序贯加压装置的组合用于 PE 预防。对于 DVT 或 PE 风险最高的患者,包括既往有静脉血栓形成事件、静脉淤滞、行动不便、肺动脉高压、严重睡眠呼吸暂停病史或 BMI 大于 60kg/m^2 的患者,可在术前临时置入下腔静脉滤过器,已在 330 例具有此类高风险因素的患者系列中证实,可将 PE 风险从 2.94% 降至 0.63%[31]。心肌梗死等心血管并发症也是术后早期死亡的重要原因。因此,对高危患者进行仔细的术前心脏评估并请心脏病专家会诊是非常重要的。男性患者、年龄大于 50 岁、医疗保险患者或慢性肺部疾病患者更容易出现肺部并发症[13]。造口狭窄导致持续呕吐增加吸入性肺炎或硫胺素缺乏的风险。腹腔镜减重手术后,肺不张发生率为 8.4%,因此患者术后宜早期活动[35]。

术后晚期并发症包括吻合口狭窄、胆结石形成、营养缺乏、肠梗阻、肠套叠、边缘溃疡、或残胃和十二指肠溃疡、瘘管、倾倒综合征和低血糖。在 2%~14% 的患者中报告了有胃空肠吻合口狭窄。狭窄通常在术后 4~6 周表现为呕吐和进行性食物不耐受。首先是固态食物,随后是液态食物[39]。当病态肥胖的患者经历手术诱导的体重快速减轻时,由于输送到胆囊的胆固醇增加,导致胆囊结石形成的发生率很高[40]。RYGB 术后高达 38% 的患者出现胆石症。如果患者术前患有胆结石,外科医生可以选择同时进行胆囊切除术,这在腹腔镜方法中不太常见,因为通过开放技术比腹腔镜更容易完成[41]。胆结石的形成继发于迷走神经损害、肠神经刺激改变、胆囊排空减少以及钙浓度和胆盐/胆固醇比值的变化[35]。在一项双盲随机安慰剂对照试验中显示,术后前 6 个月每日服用 600mg 熊去氧胆酸可使胆结石的发生率降至 2%[42]。为降低胆结石的发生率,对胆囊未预防性切除的患者,建议口服 6 个月疗程的熊去氧胆酸[42]。营养缺乏很常见,与术后解剖结构的改变和术后后遗症(如持续性呕吐)均有关。RYGB 患者中肠梗阻的发生率为 0.2%~7%,范围因手术技术而异。例如,如果 Roux 支以结肠后方式通过,则有 3 个潜在疝好发部位:结肠系膜、空肠-空肠以及结肠和 Roux 支之间[20]。大多数肠梗阻发生在术后 6~24 个月,但由于技术原因导致的肠系膜缺损,可能会发生得更早。早期发生的肠梗阻通常需肠切除,以避免胆胰支和远端胃逆行性膨胀,这可能导致远端胃缝钉线破裂和继发性腹膜炎[20]。在晚期肠梗阻中,仅在鼻胃管减压、静脉液体复苏和持续禁食状态失败后才需要手术干预。肠套叠常发生于术后数年。患肠套叠风险最高的患者是那些多余体重减少>90% 的人[35]。

靠近吻合口部位的空肠溃疡为吻合口溃疡。据估计,1%~16% 的 RYGB 患者会发生吻合口溃疡[43,44]。1% 的 RYGB 患者发生吻合口溃疡穿孔。溃疡穿孔与吸烟和使用非甾体抗炎药或糖皮质激素有关[45]。与可吸收缝线相反,胃空肠吻合口(gastrojejunal anastomosis,GJA)内层使用不可吸收缝线与溃疡发生率增加有关[46]。Hp 的存在也增加了吻合口溃疡的风险[47]。减重手术外科医生在术后 6 个月使用 PPI 治疗是一种常见的做法。如果吻合口溃疡药物治疗无效,就必须考虑胃-胃瘘管的可能性,并需要手术矫正。残余胃体的 pH 维持在 2~3,仍对迷走神经和激素刺激有反应;因此,残余胃体和十二指肠在术后数年仍可能发生溃疡,并且与 Hp 感染状态无关。对术后胃囊进行内镜评估具有挑战性;因此,不稳定的患者可能需要手术探查[35]。瘘管很少发生,常与吻合口溃疡伴随存在[35]。它们最常形成于胃囊和残胃之间,是由于胃囊到残余胃体的消化道瘘侵蚀所致[48]。大的未确诊的胃-胃瘘管可能导致体重反弹[20]。导致体重反弹的瘘管需选择内镜或外科手术修复。

多达 20% 的 RYGB 患者可能会发生倾倒综合征[49],依据餐后发生的时间早晚分为早期和晚期倾倒综合征。早期倾倒综合征会在进食后 15~30 分钟发生,常被认为是由于高渗透性食物快速进入空肠所致。这是由于进食时液体迅速进入肠腔,引起副交感神经反应,导致全身血管阻力减少,这种效应被称为“内脏血液池”[49]。症状包括腹部绞痛、大量腹泻、腹胀、头晕、恶心、面部潮红和心动过速;引起这些症状的原因是低血容量和随后的交感神经反应[35]。倾倒综合征是由摄入单糖、酸性食物和佳得乐等营养丰富的饮料引起的[49]。进食高蛋白质和高纤维食物避免这种不舒服的症状;其他可以改变的习惯包括少食、多餐、饭后躺下、避免过热和过冷食物[20],以减少与全身血管阻力降低有关的症状。早期倾倒常是自限性的,在术后 7~12 周左右可缓解。晚倾倒综合征发生在餐后 2~3 小时,继发于葡萄糖快速吸收,血糖升高,刺激胰高血糖素样肽-1 和肠抑胃肽释放。继而发生相对过度的胰岛素反应,导致低血糖和低钾血症。病人表现为出汗、虚弱、疲劳和头晕[49]。针对早期倾倒综合征提出的习惯改变同样可改善晚期倾倒综合征的症状[35]。治疗包括控制血糖水平的饮食和药物干预[35]。

2.0%的RYGB、0.7%的VBG、0.3%的腹腔镜可调节性胃束带术(laparoscopic adjustable gastric banding,LAGB)和0.2%的BPD术后可发生消化道出血。RYGB患者术后吞咽困难症状较术前相比并没有明显加重,可发展为食物不耐受、狭窄或其他梗阻[50]。

除手术类型外,明确的减重手术后并发症的危险因素包括老年、男性、BMI较高、合并症、医疗保险状况[51-53]。医疗保险状况带来的风险要高于年龄,因为没资格获得医疗保险可能会影响结局。虽然风险因素最多的患者手术风险最高,但考虑到他们所承受的疾病负担,他们也可能从减重手术中获得最大的好处[14]。值得注意的是,并发症可能不会影响减重手术长期效果,而减重手术长期效果是最能预测长期死亡风险的结果[21]。

(五) 营养缺乏

16.9%的RYGB患者存在营养和维生素缺乏以及电解质紊乱[33]。术后不能每日坚持口服维生素或频繁呕吐的患者发生营养缺乏的风险增加,最常见的营养缺乏是蛋白质、铁、维生素B_{12}、叶酸、钙和脂溶性维生素A、D、E、K缺乏[54]。

持续性呕吐可能导致硫胺素(维生素B_1)缺乏,进而可能导致韦尼克脑病,一种意识混乱、共济失调、眼肌麻痹和短期记忆受损综合征(见第103章)。可以通过适当服用硫胺素来预防这种神经功能缺陷。如怀疑硫胺素缺乏,应立即给予静脉注射或肌内注射硫胺素,以增加症状缓解的机会[55]。早期进行治疗很必要,因为即使延长给药时间,持续的严重症状可能也无法逆转。

胃壁细胞产生的内因子(intrinsic factor,IF)是回肠末端吸收维生素B_{12}所必需的(见第103章)。接受RYGB治疗的患者可能会出现维生素B_{12}缺乏,因为RYGB手术会将胃底的壁细胞与小胃囊分隔开。因此,摄入的食物和IF在空肠与Roux袢的交汇之前都没有接触[56,57]。此外,可能是因为胃底不再与食物接触,RYGB手术之后的胃壁细胞常常停止分泌IF[58]。研究表明,限制性减重手术不会导致维生素B_{12}缺乏,因为胃底的胃壁细胞仍与营养液保持接触[59]。

可能发生钙、铁和叶酸缺乏,因为它们大部分在十二指肠和空肠近端被吸收。在胃旁路手术后,食物常绕过消化道的这些部分。此外,钙的吸收需要脂溶性维生素D,而维生素D的缺乏会进一步加剧钙的缺乏[54]。

(六) 结果

减重手术的使用率之所以大幅上升,是因为它对病态肥胖的治疗效果得到了证实。两项meta分析有力地证明了减重手术可以成功地减少体重和降低死亡率[33]。Buchwald的meta分析纳入了22 094名患者,发现所有患者多余体重减少百分比的均值为61.2%[6]。BPD合并DS手术的体重减少指数最高(70.1%),其次是VBG(68.2%)、RYGB(61.6%),LAGB最低(47.5%)。Maggard的meta分析发现,术后3年或3年以上患者有相似的体重减少趋势,其中吸收不良型手术,BPD(53kg)和RYGB(42kg)术后患者的体重减少幅度最大;而限制型手术,LAGB(35kg)和胃成形术(32kg)术后患者的体重减少幅度较小[6,33]。

体重大幅度减少与长期死亡率明显降低有关。一项对9 949名RYGB患者和9 628名严重肥胖患者的回顾性队列对照研究发现,进行RYGB手术可使校正后的全因死亡率降低40%[60]。RYGB患者中,冠状动脉疾病相关死亡率降低了56%,糖尿病相关降低了92%,癌症相关降低了60%。另一项研究中,接受RYGB手术的患者癌症发病率降低了14%。在与肥胖相关的癌症类型中,癌症发病率下降幅度最大的是食管腺癌(减少2%)、结肠直肠癌(减少30%)、绝经后乳腺癌(4%)、子宫体癌(78%)、非霍奇金淋巴瘤(27%)和多发性骨髓瘤(54%)[61]。RYGB术后患者癌症风险较低可能是由于体重减少所致,许多研究表明体重减少可以降低癌症的发病率。此外,一旦肥胖患者减轻了体重,他们可能更容易获得所需的健康监测,如宫颈涂片检查和结肠镜检查。最后,考虑到BMI增加会导致外科肿瘤结局更差,可以推测随着体重的减少,手术结局可能会更好。

总的来说,减重手术极大地提高了生存率,降低了所有与疾病相关的死亡率。只有由非疾病引起的死亡率(例如,意外和自杀导致的死亡)在减重手术后增加,RYGB患者中增加了58%[60]。酗酒可能是为什么在外科手术组中意外和自杀发生率更高的一种原因。一项研究表明,胃旁路手术后酒精代谢发生改变可能是导致酗酒倾向的原因之一[62]。最近一项分析表明RYGB手术后酒精吸收速度增加,因此血液酒精浓度升高得更快、更早。这种高酒精浓度足以被定义为狂饮,这是导致酗酒的一个危险因素[63]。一项针对减重手术适应人群的研究发现,9%的人有自杀企图,19%的人术前酗酒。有人担心,这种脆弱的患者群体在减重的心理调整方面有额外的困难,这进一步支持了术前和术后进行心理咨询的必要性[64,65]。

减重手术除了降低患者死亡率外,还降低了发病率。相比正常体重患者,病态肥胖患者更容易出现胃肠道症状,如腹痛、胃灼热和睡眠障碍除了显著改善心脏危险因素外,减肥手术也为肥胖引起的许多医疗问题提供了巨大的益处。GERD症状的减轻可以明显减少术后使用PPI(9%~44%)和H_2受体拮抗剂(10%~60%)。事实上,GERD在RYGB后缓解效果极好,以至于RYGB被推荐用于治疗病态肥胖患者的顽固性GERD[50]。

近年来,许多临床试验表明,减重手术对2型糖尿病患者的血糖控制有显著的效果,以至于可以少用或不用药物治疗。此外,在瑞典一项前瞻性非随机病例对照试验中,与对照组相比较,接受减重手术的肥胖患者的2型糖尿病进展可能性显著降低[66]。尽管在肥胖症患者中,用减重手术防止2型糖尿病进展不是一项手术指征或药物治疗的替代方案,但这确实表明减重手术阻止糖代谢异常发展为糖尿病的机制是一个有待进一步探索的领域[66]。

肥胖的影响不仅仅是生理上的。SF36(健康状况调查简表)调查的管理显示RYGB手术后生活质量得到很大提高。术前,病态肥胖患者在一般健康状况、精力、生理功能、躯体疼痛、情感职能和社会功能等方面的得分明显低于美国健康人群标准。患者于RYG手术后最早3个月在这些方面中的得分与美国人群标准没有区别[67]。

随着减重手术的持续发展，人们逐渐意识到肥胖是一种慢性和复杂性疾病。因此，目前的治疗方法可能会有些变化，胃分流术是外科医生一致认同的[68]。基于这些变化就有对既往的减重手术进行改良的潜在可能。事实上，改良手术现在占所有减重手术的 15%。目前对改良减重手术的结局评估表明其发病率低，且具有足够的减重效果；然而，与首次减重手术相比，修复性减重手术发病率更高、体重减轻更少[69]。

三、肥胖病手术并发症的内镜处理

减重手术是治疗肥胖及其代谢合并症的一种有效手段，但这些手术会导致严重的并发症，胃肠病学专家必须能够识别和处理这些并发症。内镜在此类并发症的诊断和治疗中发挥着关键作用。

（一）溃疡病

胃空肠吻合口溃疡是 RYGB 手术的一种常见的晚期并发症。文献报道的发病率差异很大，但最近的一项系统回顾和管理数据库研究报道发病率为 4.6% ~6.28%（图 8.2）[70,71]。胃空肠吻合口溃疡在任何阶段都可以发生，但常发生在术后的前 3 个月。来自管理数据库的数据显示，对边缘溃疡的手术干预率随着时间的推移从 1 年的 6% 增加到 8 年的 17%，这表明多年后边缘溃疡的发病率更高[70]。患者常表现为上腹部疼痛、恶心、呕吐、食物不耐受及显性或隐匿性的出血；然而，高达 61% 的患者无症状[43]。此外，溃疡可发生在 RYGB 手术过程中形成的任一吻合口部位。

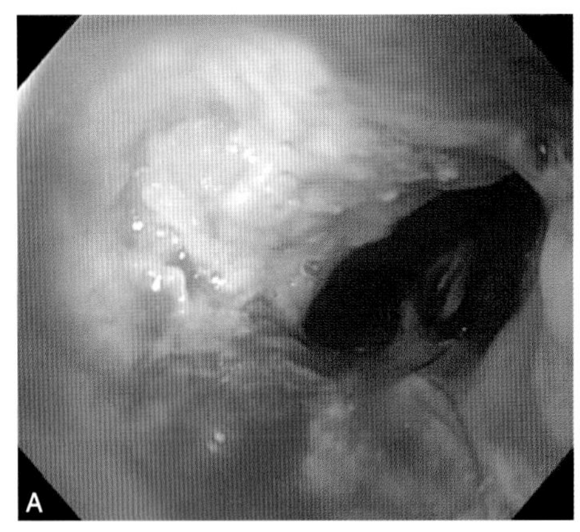

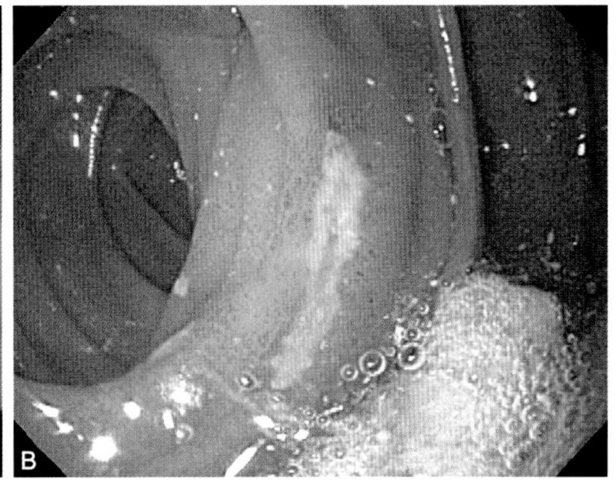

图 8.2　A，吻合口溃疡。B，空肠溃疡。（Images courtesy Christopher C. Thompson，MD.）

吻合口溃疡可能是由胃囊产生的少量胃酸、缺血、胆汁酸回流、Hp 感染、非甾体抗炎药（NSAID）、吸烟、酒精、异物（如不可吸收缝线或缝合钉）或 Roux 袢高张力等原因所致[46,72-76]。也可能由于胃-胃瘘管和缝合线中断，从而暴露于酸性环境中而导致溃疡。

术后任何时间段都可以采用水溶性造影剂（如泛影葡胺）或仔细的内镜检查评估吻合口溃疡。内镜评估应包括胃囊、GJA 和近端 Roux 袢。可以使用儿童结肠镜来完成。然而常需要加长内镜系统来对十二指肠和残余胃体进行观察。应该记录每个溃疡的大小、深度和潜在病因。Hp 粪便抗原检测可能是确认是否存在 Hp 的最简单和最准确的方法[77]。

溃疡的治疗可以是多方面的。对于 RYGB 患者，吻合口溃疡应采用可溶性质子泵抑制剂（PPI）或将肠溶胶囊打开后口服治疗，每日两次，逐渐减量直至超过 6 个月[78]。必要时可联合应用硫酸铝混悬液，一次 1g，每日 4 次；PPI 片剂效果似乎不显著。胆汁酸结合剂，如考来烯胺或考来替泊，可治疗胆汁反流。戒烟至关重要。需优化糖尿病的控制。如可能，应停用 NSAID；如需长期治疗，NSAID 应与 PPI 或前列腺素 E_1（PGE1）联合应用。如存在活动性 Hp 感染，应予以治疗。应清除溃疡内可见的缝合线或缝合钉。建议开始药物治疗 2~3 个月后复查上消化道内镜检查，以明确溃疡是否愈合。如果最大剂量的药物治疗无法使溃疡愈合，下一步的常规治疗应该是手术修复[70,79]。在有限的病例系列中，报道了使用内镜下缝合系统进行连续缝合并覆盖溃疡的治疗方法[80]。

（二）手术后胃肠道出血

减重手术后胃肠道出血的发病率和类型通常与手术方式密切相关。相比较 LAGB、SG、VBG 手术，减重术后上胃肠道出血更多见于 RYGB（一些病例报道 1.5% ~3.5%[81-83]）手术。多个部位可发生出血，包括胃囊、吻合口、缝合线、近邻的小肠、残余胃体或旁路小肠。此外，由于解剖结构的改变，患者在减重手术后可能会发生食管炎而继发出血。术后 24 小时内的早期出血常发生在的 GJA、残余胃体或空肠-空肠吻合口的缝合线处[82,84]。相当大一部分早期出血可能是胃肠道外出血，因此如果呕血和黑便症状不明显，应考虑胃肠道外出血；这些患者可能进展为血流动力学不稳定、少尿和腹胀，而没有明显的消化道失血体征。晚期出血常继发于吻合口溃疡出血；然而也应该考虑到残余胃体等其余部位的消化道失血[85]。

常规胃镜容易到达食管、胃囊和胃空肠吻合口。而残余胃体出血或空肠-空肠吻合口处出血是一个很大的挑战。这些情况则需要器械辅助式小肠镜进行检查。在早期出血的情况下，由于吻合口和缝合线尚未成熟，内镜检查的穿孔风险更大。若早期进行内镜检查，应尽量减少空气注入或采用 CO_2 注入。内镜治疗出血的效果显著。可以联合使用内镜下夹闭与注射肾上腺素来替代热效应治疗，以减少出血部位的组织损伤(图 8.3)[86-88]。新鲜的缝合线应避免电凝止血。可以选择使用止血粉,然而,减重手术后使用止血粉的数据仍有限。可以考虑血管造影介入治疗,但应当注意由此导致的患者新鲜吻合口缺血的情况。

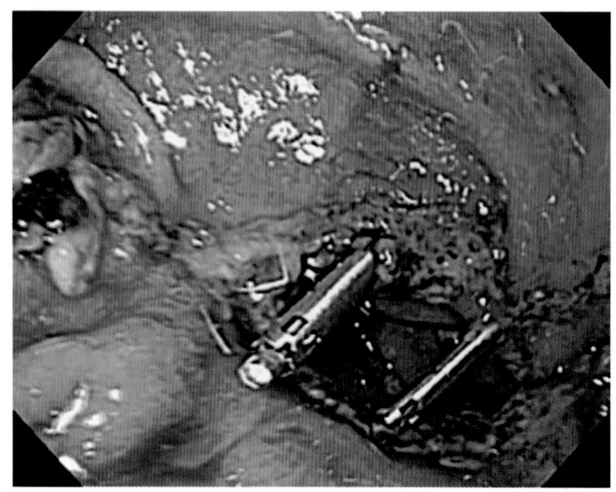

图 8.3　内镜下止血夹治疗术后出血。(Images courtesy Christopher C. Thompson, MD.)

(三) 狭窄

狭窄是减重手术后常见的并发症。患者表现为早饱、恶心、呕吐和吞咽困难,也可表现为餐后胸骨后或腹部疼痛。在既往存在 RYGB 手术史的患者中,狭窄常发生在 GJA 处,报道的 RYGB 术后发病率为 1.5% ~ 7.3%[89,92]。大多数 GJA 狭窄发生在术后 4 ~ 10 周。如果因溃疡或异物引起的狭窄,狭窄表现可延迟数月或数年。RYGB 术后狭窄较少见的部位包括空肠-空肠吻合处、肠粘连部位、穿过肠系膜所在的部位。

内镜检查是一种很好的诊断工具,因为通常可以识别病因(如异物),且可同时用于治疗。根据定义,如果标准 9.5mm 内镜无法通过吻合口,则存在造口狭窄。造口狭窄的治疗可以使用经内镜下(through-the-scope, TTS)球囊、Savary 扩张器或电外科切口进行。球囊扩张是最常用的技术,成功率超过 90%[91,92]。一些患者需从术后有症状开始即进行 2 ~ 3 次球囊扩张术,每 2 ~ 3 周重复一次。球囊导管应超出 GJA 推进,小心避免进入盲肢,当观察到导管推进为亚光学或遇到阻力时,则可使用导丝和/或 X 线透视成像。一旦球囊完全超出内镜,可开始充盈球囊,使其中点向狭窄部位施加径向压力至少 60 秒,或直至球囊"腰部"在 X 线透视下消失。尽管据报告直径 20mm 是成功的扩张,但首选最小有效扩张直径(2 ~ 12mm)。在几个疗程中逐渐扩张的方法可降低穿孔风险(据报告为 2.1% ~ 5%[91,92]),并降低因过度扩张而导致体重反弹的可能性。为了成功扩张可能必须取出 GJA 处的缝合材料[77]。

其他类型的减重手术也可能出现狭窄并发症。有 LAGB 手术史的患者可能由于束带部位水肿或组织增生而出现阻塞。可能对胃束带产生纤维反应;在这些患者中,如果完全松弛束带后狭窄仍然存在,可尝试内镜下扩张。若保守治疗不成功,也可考虑取出束带、更换束带或转换为 RYGB 手术。有 SG 手术史的患者可能在胃-食管连接处或胃角切迹处出现狭窄。可以尝试使用水压 TTS 球囊扩张进行连续的内镜下球囊扩张治疗,也有在狭窄部位进行气囊扩张的报道[77,93]。另一种治疗狭窄的方法是置入临时覆膜金属支架 8 周以上。最终,可能需要转换为 RYGB 手术[93]。

(四) 异物并发症

减重手术过程中常有异物(如缝合线、缝合钉、束带等)置入体内。异物及其继发的炎症反应,可导致疼痛、溃疡和梗阻。置入的异物(如胃束带、圈套等)也可被腐蚀或移位(图 8.4)。

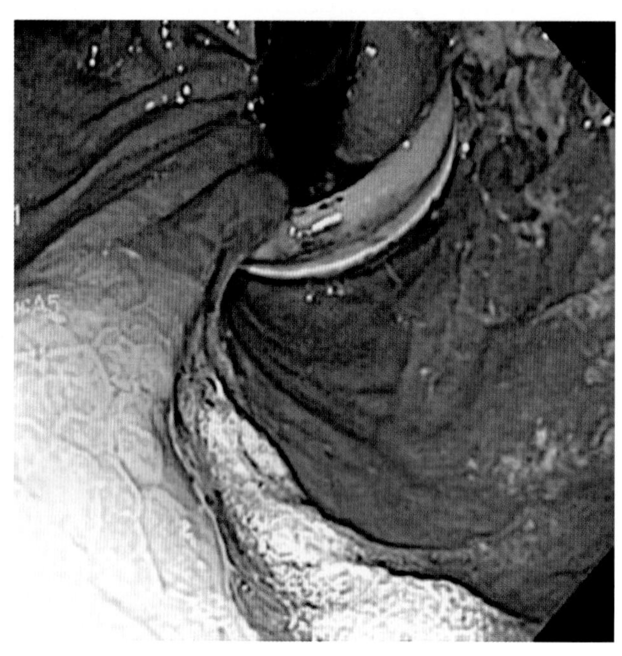

图 8.4　胃束带腐蚀。(From El-Hayek K, Timratana P, Brethauer SA, Chand B. Complete endoscopic/transgastric retrieval of eroded gastric band: description of a novel technique and review of the literature. Surg Endosc 2013; 27: 2974-9.)

减重手术后慢性疼痛患者应行内镜检查,清除可见残留异物。即使异物周围组织没有明显炎症,也可能与疼痛有关。缝线或缝合钉对周围组织的牵拉经常引起疼痛。Ryou 和同事发现 71% 的患者在异物取出后疼痛症状立即改善[94]。

(五) 渗漏和瘘管

渗漏是由于术后即刻组织对合不连续引起的。减重手术后渗漏的发生率在开放性 RYGB 后为 1.7% ~ 2.6%,在腹腔镜 RYGB 后为 0.3% ~ 4.2%,在 SG 后为 0.7% ~ 5.1%[94-99]。最近一项对 MBSAQUIP 数据库的回顾显示,36.4 万例减重手术的渗漏发生率为 0.3%[95]。RYGB 后渗漏可发生在以下几个部位:胃袋、GJA、空肠残端、空肠-空肠吻合、残余胃体、十二指肠残端(切除旁路中)和盲空肠支。当怀疑渗漏时,应考虑所有因素。最常见的部位是胃-空肠(68%)吻合或空肠-空肠(5%)吻合或胃袋缝钉线处(10%),剩下的 14% 涉及多个部位。一些部位的渗漏可能对定位极具挑战性,例如来自残余胃的渗漏,因为常规内镜检查和上消化道系列可能是正常的。

RYGB 分离患者的渗漏发生率最高。当胃袋与残余胃连续时，慢性胃-胃瘘的风险最高，与开放手术入路一样（图 8.5）。在 SG 患者中，大多数渗漏发生在胃-食管交界处附近的胃近端 1/3 处（85.7%），而其余渗漏发生在远端 1/3 处。

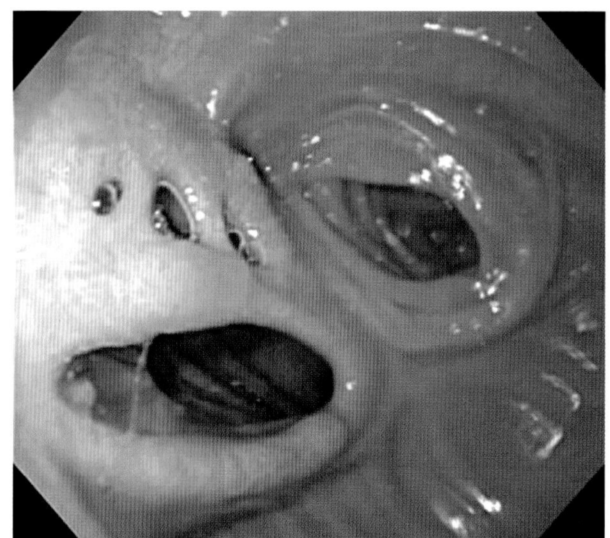

图 8.5　胃-胃瘘。（Images courtesy Christopher C. Thompson, MD.）

渗漏的死亡率为 3.3%～14%[96]。除 PE 外，它们是减重手术中危及生命的最严重并发症。除死亡风险加倍外，渗漏还导致住院时间增加了 6 倍。发生胃漏的患者发生伤口感染、败血症、呼吸衰竭、肾衰竭、血栓栓塞、内疝和小肠梗阻的风险将会增加。

渗漏常不伴发热、白细胞增高或疼痛。最常报告渗漏体征是心动过速[97]，存在于 72%～92% 的渗漏患者中。其他症状和结果包括恶心呕吐（81%）、发热（62%）、白细胞增多（48%），其中任何一种都需要高度怀疑减重手术后患者发生渗漏。客观结果包括引流量增加，以及术后两天 C 反应蛋白升高超过 22.9mg/dL（敏感性 1.00）。这与慢性胃-胃瘘不同，后者的病程更缓慢，通常表现为多食伴反酸、腹部不适和体重增加。由于胃酸可通过胃-胃瘘流入胃袋，因此当 RYGB 患者伴有胃灼热、酸反流或吻合口溃疡的时，应考虑瘘的形成[98]。

随着减重手术患者的内镜处理技术获得认可，它们得以在术后早期使用。应对远端狭窄进行扩张。支架置入等排除技术可闭塞或旁路渗漏。渗漏和瘘管也可以使用夹子、缝合器械或密封剂闭合。

支架置入以排除胃肠道渗漏是最确凿性证据支持内镜技术（图 8.6）。支架放置可在恢复肠内营养的同时愈合泄漏，且可能使胃漏的愈合速度增快且避免了肠外营养的需求。腹腔污染减少，腹痛可随之得到改善。采用前视内镜和 X 线透视引导，自膨式金属支架已成功使用。Pauli 及其同事对治疗减重手术后急性泄漏的支架植入进行了 meta 分析，发现渗漏成功闭合（定义为支架取出后泄漏闭合的放射学证据）的合并比例为 87.8%（95% CI 79.4～94.2）[99]。大多数泄漏经过 1 次治疗后可闭合，然而纳入的 7 项研究中 4 项报告了重新置入支架，9% 的患者无应答，需要翻修手术。在大多数研究中，支架是在 4～8 周之间取出的。16.9%（95% CI 9.3～26.3）的病例报告了支架移位。

内镜夹也被用于闭合瘘和渗漏。夹子用于对合缺损周围的组织以达到闭合效果，因此，最好垂直于缺损长轴释放。在夹子释放前对缺损边缘周围组织进行热消融或机械刮擦可获得更具弹性的封闭。Over-the-Scope 夹子，Padlock（US Endoscopy）或 OTSC（Ovesco Endoscopy AG, Tubingen, Germany），是一种镍钛合金夹，放置在内镜头端的帽上。可用组织锚和双夹钳器械，有助于放置夹子。与通过内镜插入的夹子对合黏膜不同，OTSC 可进行全层对合。胃肠道瘘闭合的病例系列显示成功率为 72%～91%[98,100-103]。其他小系列也显示纤维蛋白胶和各种瘘塞也有效[104]。

（六）胰胆管疾病

对于解剖结构改变的患者来说，使用超声内镜（EUS）和经内镜逆行胰胆管造影（ERCP）对胰腺和胆道疾病进行内镜下治疗十分具有挑战。LAGB、SG 和 VGB 术后的患者与正常解剖结构的患者一样，通常可以借助侧视内镜成功进行 EUS 或 ERCP。不幸的是体重减少过快可能容易形成结石：近 50% 的患者在 RYGB 术后会发生胆囊结石或泥沙样结石，其中超 25% 的患者可能需进行胆囊切除手术。有 RYGB 和 BPD+DS 手术史的患者通常需要特殊的工具和流程来完成

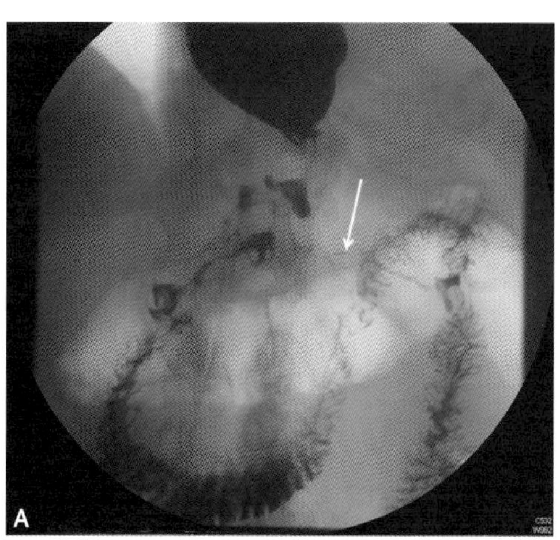

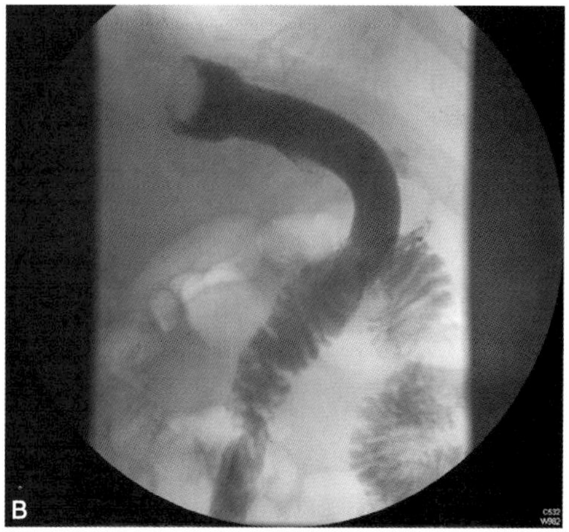

图 8.6　A，胃-皮肤渗漏（箭头）。B，支架置入治疗渗漏。（Images courtesy Christopher C. Thompson, MD.）

ERCP。虽然在大多数 RYGB 患者中球囊辅助小肠镜可以到达十二指肠乳头，但并不是每次都能调整到插管的最佳位置以及能够在必要时放置保护性胰腺支架。这就导致了各种进入分流的胃和使用十二指肠侧视镜完成 ERCP 的方法[105,106]。实施 ERCP 前，准备工作应包括明确是否需要 ERCP，以及通过断层成像了解解剖和病理特征。有些患者的解剖结构不适合单纯的内镜检查，甚至于通过装置辅助的小肠镜检查也同样不适用。通常情况下，如果计划手术，ERCP 可以在腹腔镜辅助下同时进行并到达胃部。如果没有手术计划，那么进行 ERCP 到达十二指肠大乳头的选择包括腹腔镜辅助 ERCP、肠镜辅助 ERCP、EUS 下直接胆道介入、使用 EUS 和双蘑菇头全覆膜金属支架在胃囊和旁路胃之间创建一个瘘管。EUS 引导下经胃 ERCP 是一种经腔内入路到达旁路胃的方式，可以使用双蘑菇头全覆膜金属支架一次性完成[107,108]。

（七）体重反弹及胃空肠吻合口扩张

减重手术可提供持久的减重效果，但是术后体重反弹是一个潜在的问题；体重反弹可再次出现肥胖相关的疾病风险，而且对生活质量产生重大的影响。尽管最开始术后体重减少是非常显著的，但 1～2 年内体重多会达到一个平台期。最近，美国退伍军人医疗保健系统的一项研究分析了 1 787 名减重手术后的患者，10 年随访率为 81.9%，发现 RYGB 术后 10 年，28.2% 的患者总体重减少百分比（%TBWL）小于 20%，3.4% 患者在基线体重的 5% 以内[109]。考虑到大量患者接受了减重手术，所以解决体重反弹疗法的需求将会持续增加。

减重手术后体重反弹可能是多因素导致的。在一项系统回顾中，这些因素包括不合规营养摄入和放牧式饮食模式、神经内分泌代谢调节、精神健康问题（暴食和药物滥用）、缺乏身体锻炼和解剖问题[110]。RYGB 术后出现体重反弹，可能伴有胃-胃瘘管，有研究表明胃囊尺寸过大和 GJA 直径与术后体重反弹有关[111,112]。同样地，SG 术后也可发生体重反弹，在有些患者中与袖状胃直径有关[113]。因为外科修复并发症的发生率高于首次减重手术，解决这些问题比较困难[114,115]。药物也可用于治疗体重反弹，然而，在一项回顾性分析中，只有一种超药品说明书使用的药物（托吡酯）显示体重下降显著，并且整个队列只有 56% 患者减重不足或体重反弹超过术后总减少体重的 5% 及以上[116]。然而，RYGB 术后腔内治疗已经显示出有效解决体重反弹和低发病率的前景。

已经在多平台上研究了经口出口缩窄术（transoral outlet reduction，TORe）（图 8.7）。一项随机双盲实验在 77 名胃空肠吻合口直径>20mm 的患者中比较了通过 Bard EndoCinch 进行 TORe 和假手术[117]。在 89.6% 的患者中，胃空肠吻合口直径缩小至<10mm，未发生穿孔及不良事件，这与假手术对照组的发生率相似；96% 的修复手术患者在术后随访 6 个月时体重减少或维持稳定。在意向性治疗分析结果中，与假手术对照组体重减少 0.2% 相比，进行修复手术的患者体重平均减少 3.9%（$P=0.014$）。Apollo OverStitch 装置也被证实在胃-空肠吻合口处采用全层缝合进行 TORe 是有效的[118]。最近一项纳入 3 项研究的针对 RYGB 术后体重反弹患者的 meta 分析发现，77%～100% 的患者停止体重反弹，12 个月体重下降了 5.83±11kg 到 10.5±12.5kg[119]。

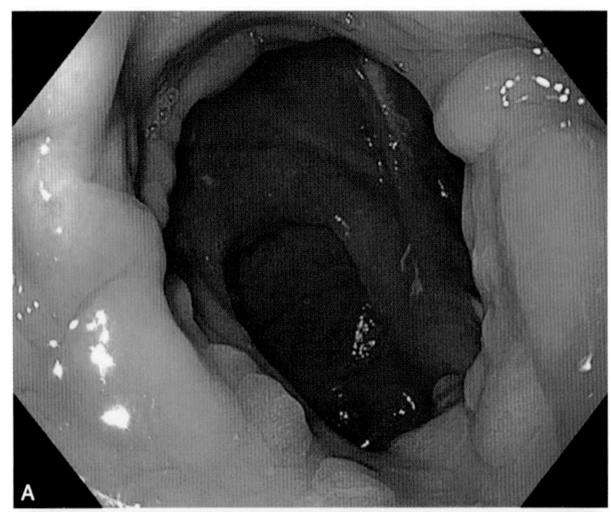

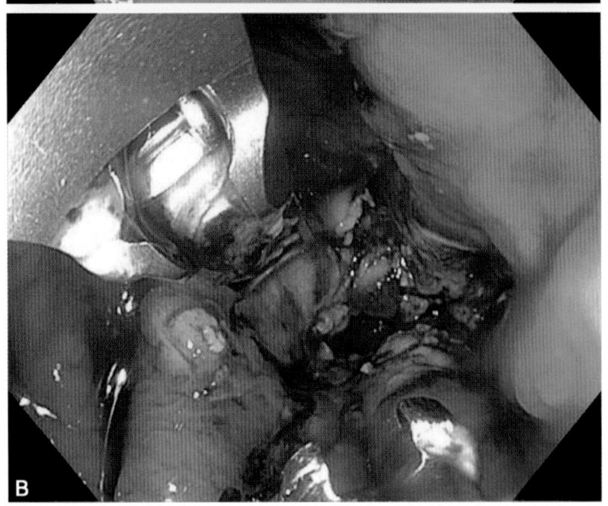

图 8.7　内镜下缝合扩张胃-空肠吻合。A，为缝合前。B，氩等离子凝固术和荷包缝合后。（Images courtesy Shelby Sullivan，MD.）

四、肥胖的内镜治疗

内镜减重治疗（endoscopic bariatric therapy，EBT）作为肥胖症首次治疗手段，在近几年进展迅速，多种设备已经被美国食品药品管理局（FDA）批准并且正在研究更多的疗法。虽然手术是有效的，但只有Ⅲ度肥胖（BMI 为 40kg/m^2）或有明显合并症的Ⅱ度肥胖（BMI 为 35～39.9kg/m^2）患者才符合手术条件。不仅许多患者不符合这一标准，而且每年符合这一标准的人群中接受减重手术的不到 2%[120]。手术率低是多种原因导致的，但要强调需要有更多的治疗选择。生活方式治疗应该作为其他任何肥胖治疗计划的基础，但其本身的有效性和持久性有限。近几年治疗肥胖的药物也有进展，并且有随机对照试验表明较之于单纯的生活方式治疗，药物治疗能适当改善减重效果[121]。然而，实际的临床结局可能不会像随机对照试验中观察到的体重减少或服药依从性相似[122,123]。

多中心随机对照试验已经表明，与仅接受生活方式治疗方法相比，迄今为止被批准的 EBT 具有显著的减重效果，这将在本节进行回顾。虽然 EBT 比减重手术少，但发生严重不良事件的风险也比减重手术少。此外，许多设备已被批准用于 BMI 在 30~40kg/m^2 之间的患者，增加了不符合减重手术患者的治疗选择。

EBT 可以分为胃部疗法和小肠疗法。胃部疗法是在胃部放置设备或进行操作。小肠疗法是在小肠放置设备或进行操作。胃和小肠的内镜减重治疗的两个显著特点是操作或放置设备的位置不同，以及不依赖于体重减少的影响 。虽然小肠疗法还没有被 FDA 批准，但是对于代谢结局，依赖或不依赖体重减少的影响均有数据支持。目前有数据支持体重降低对代谢结局的依赖影响，但没有数据表明胃部疗法对代谢结局有不依赖于体重减少的影响。在本章撰写之时，只有获得 FDA 批准或目前在美国实施的胃部 EBT，将是本节其余部分的重点。

（一）肥胖病内镜治疗候选人的评估和选择

美国消化内镜协会（ASGE）在 2015 年发表了一份关于 EBT 在临床实践中的立场声明[124]。ASGE 立场声明认可接受减重手术的肥胖患者的围手术期营养、代谢和非手术支持治疗的临床实践指南（2013 年由美国临床内分泌学家协会、肥胖协会和美国代谢与减重手术外科学会更新[125]），但也承认这些指南可能并不适用于所有 EBT。与减重手术相比，EBT 是微创手术，对于解剖结构的改变可能是短期的、可逆的，或长期变化最小。

可逆性、安全性和麻醉风险降低使得设备置入的术前评估标准降低。ASGE 立场声明建议至少进行病史、体格检查、肥胖相关疾病筛查，承诺改变生活方式，进行营养史和常规实验室检查。

基于 FDA 批准的设备和研究人群，EBT 的适应证各不相同。在一些案例中，有数据显示对于 FDA 标示适应证以外人群的安全性和有效性[126,127]，但任何 FDA 适应证以外的用途都被认为是超适应证使用。

（二）美国目前内镜治疗肥胖病的实施

FDA 已经批准了 4 种有减重适应证的胃部 EBT，包括 3 种胃内球囊（intragastric balloon，IGB）和 1 种用于抽吸疗法的设备。IGB 是一种通过注入生理盐水或混合氮气，从而占据胃内空间的设备，并且 6 个月后用内镜取出。这些设备通过占用胃内空间减重，并且液体水球还可以通过减缓胃排空来促进减重[128]。其他机制也可能增强饱腹感，但这一领域仍需进一步研究。表 8.1 包括所有目前 FDA 批准的 IGB 及其适应证。

抽吸治疗是用专门的内镜下经皮胃造口管进行的，带有可连接的组件，便于餐后抽吸部分胃内容物（图 8.8）。患者不仅可以吸出部分进食摄入的能量，而且该设备还可以促进饮食习惯的改变，从而减少进餐时的食物摄入量[129]。

目前美国正在实施的另一种治疗方法是内镜下袖状胃成形术，在内镜下对胃体进行一系列缝合将胃的形状改变成管状。尽管仅在 4 例患者中进行了研究，这种治疗可以减少胃容量，增加饱腹感，也可能延迟胃排空[130]。需要注意的是，FDA 尚未批准该操作，而是使用了一种获得 FDA 510（k）许可的设备，用于胃肠道组织对合。

1. 胃内球囊

目前 FDA 批准的两种注入生理盐水的 IGB，需在直视下置入内镜。单个液体充盈球囊（Orbera 胃球囊，Apollo Endosurgery，Austin，TX）通过导管输送，在不使用导丝的情况下置入，类似于口胃管。球囊进入胃后，在直视下用生理盐水充盈球囊，直至达到 400~700mL。充盈完成后，将导管拉到胃食管交界处以分离球囊，然后通过患者口腔取出。6 个月后，进行重复内镜检查，期间使用带有斜面针头的导管穿刺球囊，然后取出针头，将导管推进球囊，吸出液体。一旦球囊放气，使用双脚抓钳固定球囊，并通过患者口腔拉出球囊。

胃内双盐水填充球囊（ReShape 胃球囊，Apollo Endosurgery，Austin，TX）最近由与单液体填充球囊相同的制造商购买，但以后将不再制造。在内镜检查的初始阶段，通过放置的导丝将其输送到胃体。就位后取出导丝，用 375 或 450mL 与亚甲蓝混合的生理盐水填充近端球囊。球囊充盈完成后，用 6mL 矿物油密封球囊。对远端球囊重复该操作过程。操作完成后，将导管拉到胃食管交界处，使球囊与输送导管分离，然后通过口腔拉出。6 个月后，进行重复内镜检查，期间使用带有非斜面针头的导管在球囊上钻孔。然后缩回针头，将导管推进球囊吸出液体。对第二个球囊重复该过程。一旦两个球囊都放气了，使用 15mm 的鼠齿形鳄鱼钳在每个球囊上撕开一个孔，使用六角形圈套器固定器械的近端头端。然后通过患者口腔拔出器械。

可吞咽的充气 IGB（Obalon 球囊系统，Obalon Therapeutics，Carlsbad，CA）被吞咽在用亲水涂层拴在导管上的胶囊中。通过荧光透视或数字 X 线成像验证胶囊通过胃，患者口外连接到导管的气体分配器压力传感器上的压力下降表明此时气囊在胃的不受限制空间内展开。然后打开从气罐到球囊的流量调节阀，使气体流入球囊，球囊内最终压力为 9~13kPa，容积为 250mL。然后在注入导管的 1.5mL 水的压力下将球囊从导管中排出。在首次球囊给药后 2 周和 8 周重复该过程，使得 3 个球囊全部被置入胃内。在首次给予球囊 6 个月后，进行内镜手术取出气囊。用连接抽吸装置的注射器针头回缩每个球囊，然后使用 15mm 大鼠齿鳄鱼钳抓取，从口腔中取出，对剩余的两个球囊重复该过程。

（1）抽吸治疗设备

抽吸治疗设备（AspireAssist，Aspire Bariatrics，King of Prussia，PA）的植入式组件，是一种由医用级硅胶制成的气体造口管，采用标准牵拉 PEG 管置入技术置入[131]。放置时，同时放置外泵，1~2 周后患者返回，将胃造口管的外露部分转为皮肤造口，用于抽吸。与传统 PEG 管置入一样，患者应在术前 30 分钟静脉注射抗生素，还应该额外口服 24 小时预防性抗生素。

（2）内镜下袖状胃成形术

内镜下袖状胃成形术通过固定于内镜末端的缝合设备进行；目前唯一的商用缝合设备是 Overstitch（Apollo Endosurgery，Austin，TX）。首先使用标准的上消化道内镜评估胃，然后标记胃的前壁和后壁需缝合处。附有缝合装置的内镜可以带或不带外套管插入胃内。从靠近角切际的远端胃体前壁开始缝合，用螺旋装置抓取组织，向内镜方向牵拉，使针驱动器能将针穿过组织。以 U 形或 Z 形模式重复这个操作 5~8

表 8.1 美国食品药品管理局(FDA)批准的胃内球囊

设备	设备影像	FDA 批准状况
Reshape 双球囊系统 (ReShape Medical, San Celemente, CA)	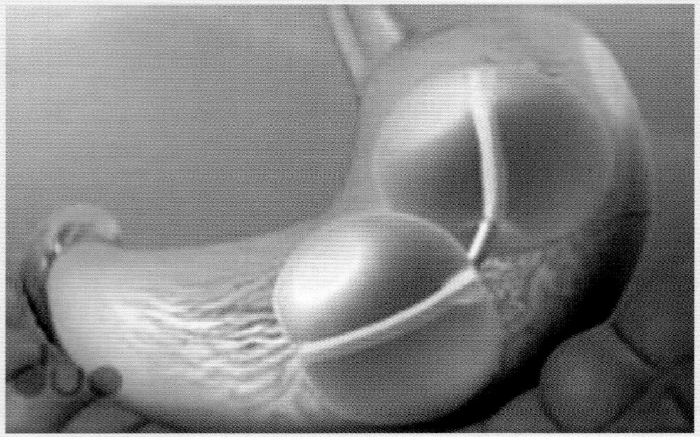	批准用于 BMI 30~40kg/m^2、肥胖伴 1 种相关共存病
Orbera 胃内球囊 (Apollo Endosurgery, Austin, TX)	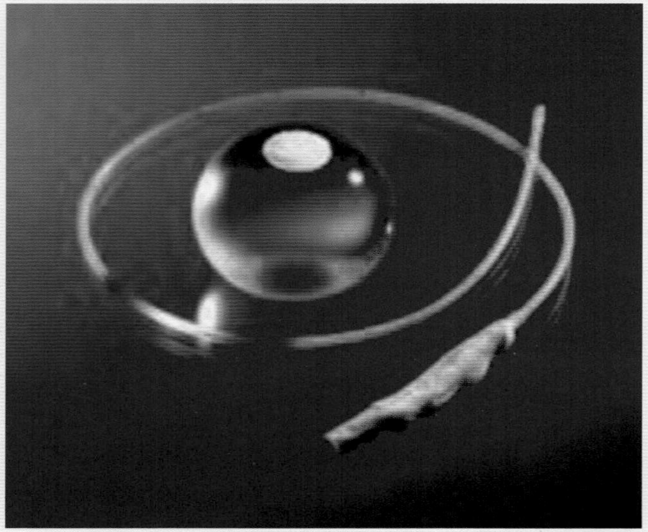	批准用于 BMI 30~40kg/m^2

表 8.1　美国食品药品管理局(FDA)批准的胃内球囊(续)

设备	设备影像	FDA 批准状况
Obalon 球囊系统 (Obalon Therapeutics, Carlsbad, CA)	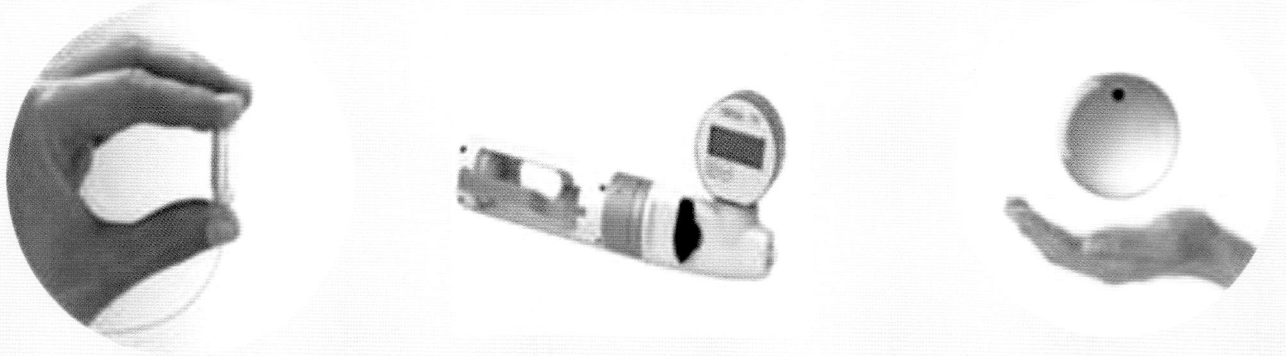	批准用于 BMI 30~40kg/m^2

Images from Abu Dayyeh BK, Edmundowicz SA, Jonnalagadda S, et al. Endoscopic bariatric therapies. Gastrointest Endosc. 2015;81(5):1073-86, with permission; and Sullivan S, Swain J, Woodman et al. Randomized sham-controlled trial of the 6-months swallowable gas-filled intragastric balloon system for weight loss. Surg Obes Relat Dis 2018;14(12):1876-89, with permission.

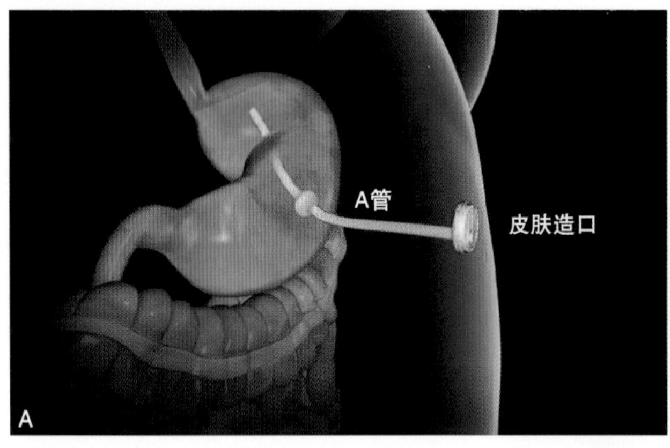

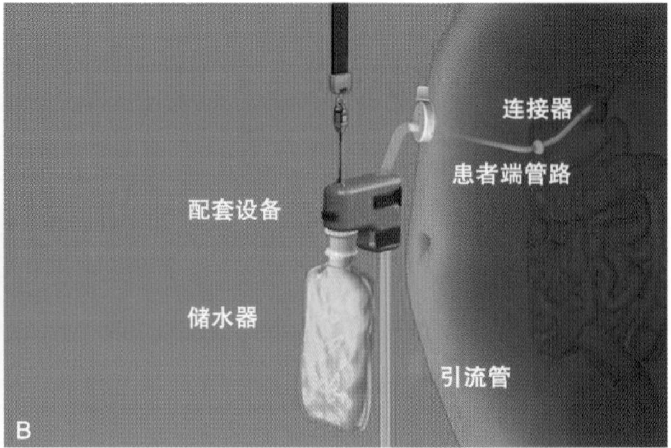

图 8.8　AspireAssist 系统的组件：A，固定组件；B，抽吸过程中使用的组件。（From Sullivan S. Aspiration therapy for obesity. Gastrointestinal Endoscopy Clinics of North America. 2017;27(2):277-88, with permission.）

次"咬合"，将针从换针导管中释放出来，并在缝线的另一端放置一个束带，使组织聚拢在针和束带中间。达到预期的松紧效果后切断缝线。向胃近端移动重复此操作，直至到达近端胃体（图 8.9）。有些医生会在第一层缝合线的基础上加固放置第二层缝合线，但这是可变的。通常手术时给予静脉注射抗生素。

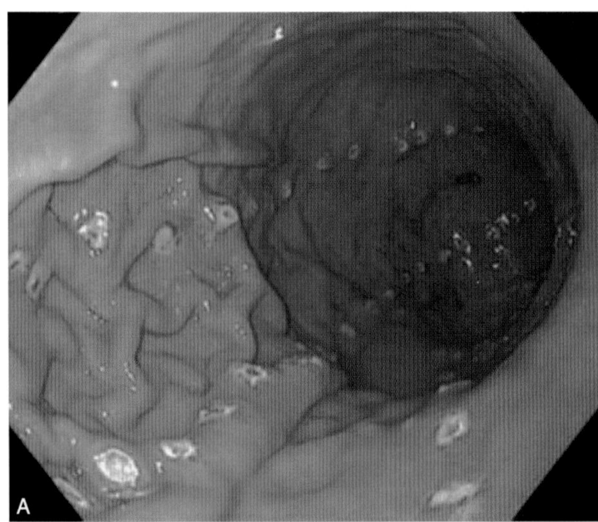

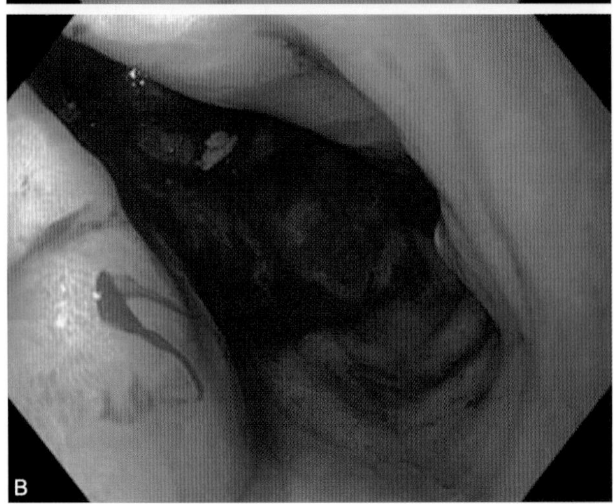

图 8.9　内镜下袖状胃成形术。A，术前胃体；B，术后胃体。（Images courtesy of Shelby Sullivan, MD.）

2. 内镜减重治疗并发症

（1）胃内球囊（IGB）

IGB 的不良事件很常见，但大多数非严重性不良事件的程度为轻到中度。表 8.2 展示了用于申请 FDA 批准的美国多中心关键性临床试验中报道的非严重性不良事件[132-135]。胃内注水球囊最常见的不良事件是恶心和呕吐，呕吐在吞入式胃内气囊系统中明显减少。这些症状与胃对 IGB 的适应性有关，通常在治疗后头几天至几周内缓解。胃内双注水球囊的关键性临床试验报道的胃溃疡发生率为 35%，明显高于 FDA 批准的其他 IGB，胃内单注水球囊与吞入式胃内气囊系统报道的发生率分别为 0% 与 0.9%；然而，这一结局差异主要是由于远尖端设计造成的，在试验中进行改进后可以使得溃疡

表 8.2　美国胃内球囊多中心试验中的非严重不良事件

不良事件	ReShape/%	Orbera/%	Obalon/%
呕吐	86.7	86.8	17.3
恶心	61.0	75.6	56.0
腹痛	54.5	57.5	72.6
胃溃疡	35.2*	0	0.9
消化不良	17.8	21.3	16.9†
嗳气	16.7	24.4	9.2
腹部不适	13.3	6.3	0
腹胀	11.0	17.5	14.6
糜烂性胃炎	9.1	0.6	7.1‡
GERD	6.8	30.0	见消化不良
糜烂性食管炎	0.4	0.6	1.8
便秘	5.3	0	2.7
腹泻	3.0	13.1	8.3

*在对 ReShape 球囊的远端头端进行设计改进后，溃疡发生率降低至 10%。

†消化不良和 GERD 的复合。

‡红斑、糜烂、炎症或息肉的复合。

From: Sullivan S, Edmundowicz SA, Thompson CC. Endoscopic bariatric and metabolic therapies: new and emerging technologies. Gastro 2017;152:1791-801, with permission.

范围变小,发生率降至 10%[136]。一篇随后发表的回顾性研究,分析了在美国 7 个不同中心接受临床治疗的 202 例患者数据,发现在 6 个月取出球囊时,溃疡发生率为 0.9%,糜烂发生率为 13.8%。胃内单注水球囊关键性临床试验的 GERD 发生率为 30%,显著高于其他两种 IGB[132],胃内双注水球囊的 GERD 发生率为 6.8%,吞入式胃内气囊系统 GERD 和消化不良的复合发生率为 16.9%。目前还没有使用吞入式胃内气囊系统进行临床治疗的回顾性分析发表。在美国关键实验和临床病例系列中,IGB 的早期取出率(症状相关和非症状相关)在胃内双注水球囊中为 15%[136] 和 6.4%[137],在胃内单注水球囊中为 18.8%[138] 和 16.6%[139]。尚未公布吞入式胃内气囊系统的早期取出率。

在美国关键性临床试验中,胃内双注水球囊的严重不良事件发生率(随机对照与交叉队列合并)为 10.6%[133,136],胃内单注水球囊为 10%[132,138],吞入式胃内气囊系统(随机对照与交叉队列合并)为 0.3%[134],因而 FDA 批准了这些设备(见表 8.2)。胃内双注水球囊和胃内单注水球囊最常见的严重不良事件是由适应性症状(恶心、呕吐和腹痛)导致的,伴或不伴脱水(胃内双注水和单注水球囊分别为 75% 和 71%)。胃内双注水球囊的其他严重不良事件包括:食管穿孔、食管撕裂、上消化道出血、胃溃疡、肺炎和肌痛。胃内单注水球囊的其他严重不良事件包括:胃出口梗阻、胃穿孔合并败血症、吸入性肺炎和 IGB 中污染液体引起腹部绞痛。在吞入式胃内气囊系统的关键性临床试验中,只有一项严重不良事件发生,即一例服用大剂量 NSAID 的患者发生出血性溃疡。

在随后的美国使用胃内单注水球囊治疗的回顾性分析中,没有系统地记录非严重不良事件。然而,7% 的患者在球囊取出后发现食管炎(基线为 3%),0.5% 有溃疡,0.5% 有食管撕裂。放置 IGB 后,8% 的患者脱水需门诊静脉输液,4% 的患者需住院治疗,1% 的患者在球囊取出后需住院治疗[139]。16.6% 的患者因恶心($n=11$)、呕吐($n=19$)、腹痛($n=4$)、反流($n=4$)、综合症状($n=2$)和患者要求($n=13$)而早期取出 IGB。此外,在一个关于胃内单注水球囊的临床病例系列中,发生 1 例吸入性事件和 1 例 IGB 放气,尽管最终该球囊顺利通过胃肠道自然排出。胃内双注水球囊报道的最常见的非严重不良事件是在球囊放置(8.4%)和取出($n=5$)时食管或胃黏膜撕裂(8.4%)、恶心(73.8%)、呕吐(49%)和术后疼痛(25.2%)。6.4% 的患者因症状($n=10$)早期取出 IGB;4 例患者胃内球囊自发性破裂,其中 2 例患者由于球囊迁移至小肠需手术取出。另外一例球囊放气患者,球囊取出前 1 周有机动车辆事故造成腹部钝性损伤病史[137]。已发表一项前瞻性收集数据的临床登记试验,该研究纳入 1 343 例接受吞入式胃内气囊系统治疗患者的安全性分析。14.22% 的患者发生非严重不良事件,最常见的是腹痛(5.29%)、恶心(4.69%)和呕吐(2.31%)。发生了 2 例严重的不良事件,包括 1 例患者脱水需静脉输液(0.07%),1 例胃穿孔接受球囊取出和穿孔修补术治疗(0.07%)[140]。

尽管在任何关键性临床试验或临床注册试验中未见死亡,但 FDA 于 2018 年 6 月 4 日更新发布了一篇致医疗保健提供者的信函,其中描述了胃内注水球囊在美国获批后发生的 12 例死亡,其中 7 例发生在美国。截至撰写本章节时,仍无法明确这些患者根本致死原因的数据。其他既往试验没有报道,但已确定与胃内注水球囊相关的事件包括过度填充液体和胰腺炎。制造商报告的胃内双注水球囊和胃内单注水球囊在美国的死亡率分别为 0.06%[141] 和 0.036%[142],这些不良事件的发生率仍然很低。截至撰写本章节时,在美国没有报道与吞入式胃内气囊系统相关的死亡报告。

(2) 抽吸疗法

在美国进行了两项比较抽吸疗法和生活方式治疗的随机对照试验,但只包括一项小型单中心初步研究和一项大型多中心试验。在初步研究中使用的先前旧的胃造口管设备与目前的胃造口管有很大区别,这与该研究中所有患者(治疗组 $n=10$)相比,胃造口管置入超过 4 周后腹部不适更多有关,促使了胃造口管设计的改进[129]。在美国多中心试验中(治疗组 $n=111$),最常见的不良事件是造瘘口边缘肉芽组织增生(40.5%)。5% 以上的患者发生的其他非严重不良事件包括:37.8% 胃造口管置入 4 周内有腹痛;17.1% 恶心/呕吐;17.1% 造口边缘刺激;16.2% 间断腹部不适;13.5% 潜在或明确的造口边缘细菌感染;8.1% 胃造口管置入 4 周后腹痛加剧;6.3% 消化不良;5.4% 造口边缘炎症。4 例患者(3.6%)报告了 5 例严重不良事件,包括严重腹痛(同一患者两次入院)、腹膜炎、幽门前溃疡和因功能障碍而更换胃造口管[143]。

(3) 内镜下袖状胃成形术

目前没有关于内镜下袖状胃成形术的随机对照试验。首次人体试验的 3 个研究阶段,包括第二阶段纳入 22 例患者(美国和多米尼加共和国)和第三阶段纳入 77 例患者(美国、多米尼加共和国和西班牙)。不良反应包括术后第一周出现频繁恶心、呕吐和突发的上腹痛,但在这些队列中均未报道严重不良反应[144]。包括美国和美国以外的地区并报告了不良事件的两项大型回顾性研究($n=248$ 和 $n=112$)已经发表[145,146]。两项研究都没有系统记录非严重不良事件,但在其中 1 项研究中,大量患者中描述了恶心、呕吐和腹痛症状[146]。在其中较大的回顾性分析中发生了 5 例严重不良事件(2%),包括 2 例需经皮引流和抗生素治疗的胃周炎性积液、脾挫裂伤导致的胃外出血、肺栓塞和气腹/气胸;该手稿未报道因适应性症状相关的住院[145]。在第二个回顾性系列中共发生 3 起需住院治疗的严重不良事件,包括 2 例出血患者(1 例患者术后第 1 天开始使用低分子量肝素和华法林),其中 1 例出血患者需内镜治疗。1 例患者发生胃周积液,采取了门诊口服抗生素治疗[146]。

3. 营养缺乏

目前还没有 IGB 或内镜下袖状胃成形术导致营养缺乏的报道。一项有关抽吸疗法影响对铁、维生素 D 和维生素 B_{12} 的初步研究,在纳入的 10 例患者中,需要补充铁、维生素 D(由于基线时维生素 D 低水平)和维生素 B_{12} 的患者分别是 4 例、3 例和 1 例,从而维持血液中这些微量元素的正常浓度。作为方案的一部分,所有受试者都接受了补钾和 PPI 治疗[129];而这治疗在美国多中心随机对照试验中并没有继续给予,111 例抽吸疗法组患者中,只有 4 例患者需要在试验的前 52 周补充治疗[143]。

4. 结局

(1) 胃内球囊

FDA 批准的 3 种 IGB 均进行了多中心随机对照试验。所有的研究都在前 6 个月采用了中等强度的生活方式干预治疗(6~13 个疗程);然而,只有胃内双注水球囊和吞入式胃内气囊系统有假对照组[134,136]。在一项减重设备研究中,已经证明事先了解小组分配可以使减重手术效果增加约 40%[147]。这与随机分组假对照试验设计的 IGB 试验组中所发现的体重减少差异相一致:在胃内单注水球囊的开放标签随机对照试验中,显示出了 35%~40%及以上的体重减轻(表 8.3)。此外,与关键性试验相比,来自胃内双注水球囊、胃内单注水球囊以及吞入式胃内气囊系统注册试验的临床疗效数据显示更多的减重手术效果。在胃内双注水球囊注册试验中,202 例患者(年龄 47.8±10.8 岁,女性 83.2%,BMI 36.7±6.6kg/m^2)放置球囊。6 个月时%TBWL(总体重减少)为 11.4±6.7%,但只获得 101 例患者随访数据[137]。在胃内单注水球囊注册试验中,321 例患者(年龄 48.1±11.9 岁,女性 80%,BMI 37.6±6.9kg/m^2)放置球囊。6 个月时%TBWL 为 11.8±7.5%,但只获得 199 例患者随访数据[139]。在吞入式胃内气囊注册试验中,1 387 例患者接受治疗,最终分析时 3.2%的患者被排除(36 例患者缺少最终体重,8 例患者基线 BMI<25kg/m^2)。1 343 名患者纳入意向治疗分析(45.7±10.8 岁,女性 78.6%,BMI 35.4±5.4kg/m^2),意向治疗分析的定义为至少放置 1 个球囊 1 天以上;82.1%的患者(n=1 103)被纳入完整分析,完整分析定义为正好放置 3 个球囊 20 周以上。完整分析的患者 6 个月时%TBWL 为 9.9%±6.2%,意向治疗分析的患者%TBWL 为 9.2%±6.3%。一项分析仅纳入按标签使用人群(BMI 30~40kg/m^2,放置 3 个球囊 20 周以上,n=787),结果显示%TBWL 为 10.0%±6.1%[140]。

表 8.3　美国多中心试验中调整意向治疗随机队列(前 6 个月)的受试者数量、体重指数、体重减轻百分比和应答率

设备	受试者数量		体重指数/(kg/m^2)		总体重减少百分比		试验组应答率*
	对照组	试验组	对照组	试验组	对照组	试验组	
Orbera	130	125	35.4±2.7	35.2±3.2	3.3%±5.0%	10.2%±6.6%	79.2%
Reshape	139	187	35.4±2.6	35.3±2.8	3.3%	6.8%	48.8%
Obalon	189	198	35.4±2.7	35.1±2.7	3.4%±5.0%	6.6%±5.1%	62.1%

*Orbera 和 Obalon 研究的应答率定义为:总体体重减轻≥5%,ReShape 研究的过度体重减轻≥25%。

From Sullivan S, Edmundowicz SA, Thompson CC. Endoscopic bariatric and metabolic therapies: new and emerging technologies. Gastro. 2017;152:1791-801, with permission.

(2) 抽吸疗法

美国的两项随机对照试验表明,抽吸疗法联合生活方式治疗的减重手术效果优于仅接受生活方式治疗。一项初步研究中,4 例患者仅接受 1 年的生活方式治疗[年龄 45.3±2.8 岁均数标准误(standard error of the mean,SEM),女性 100%,BMI 39.3kg/m^2±1.1SEM],10 例患者接受 1 年的抽吸疗法联合生活方式治疗(年龄 38.7±2.3SEM,女性 100%,BMI 42.0kg/m^2±1.4SEM)。仅接受生活方式治疗组 1 年的%TBWL 为 5.9%±5.0%,而抽吸疗法联合生活方式治疗组为 18.6%±2.3%(P=0.021)。抽吸疗法联合生活方式治疗组的 7 例受试者额外接受了 1 年治疗,在第 2 年结束时%TBWL 为 20.1%±3.5%[132]。

在 PATHWAY 研究中,优化后的意向治疗分析纳入了 60 例仅接受生活方式治疗的患者(46.8±11.6 岁,女性 88.3%,BMI 40.9±3.9kg/m^2)和 111 例抽吸疗法联合生活方式治疗的患者(42.4±10.0 岁,女性 86.5%,BMI 42.0±5.1kg/m^2)。在意向治疗分析中,仅接受生活方式治疗组和抽吸疗法联合生活方式治疗组的% TBWL 分别为 3.5%±6.0% 和 12.1%±9.6%,P<0.001;相比较之下,仅接受生活方式治疗组(n=31)和抽吸疗法联合生活方式治疗组(n=82)患者在完成 1 年治疗后结果分别为 4.9%±7.0% 和 14.2%±9.8%,P<0.001[143]。抽吸疗法联合生活方式治疗组中 55 例患者持续治疗超过 1 年,42 例患者、22 例患者和 15 例患者分别完成 2 年、3 和 4 年治疗,TBWL 分别为 15.3%±8.8%、16.6%±10.5%和 18.7±11.7%[148]。

(3) 内镜下袖状胃成形术

在一项纳入 248 例(年龄 44.5±10 岁,女性 73%,BMI 37.8±5.6kg/m^2)患者的多中心病例系列研究中减重数据首次被报道。87%患者术后 6 个月进行了随访,TBWL 为 15.2%(95% CI 14.2~16.3);62%的患者术后 24 个月进行了随访,TBWL 为 18.6%(95% CI 15.7~21.5)[145]。Sartoretto 等的病例系列研究共纳入 112 例患者(年龄 45.1±11.7 岁,女性 69%,BMI 37.9±6.7kg/m^2)。有 61.6%的患者在 6 个月时报告体重减轻 TBWL 为 14.9%±6.1%[146]。在美国患者中进行的多期首次人体试验,包括 2 期试验(n=22,年龄 39.2±1.2 岁,女性 91%,BMI 34.3±1.0kg/m^2)和 3 期试验(n=77,年龄 41.3±1.1 岁,女性 77%,BMI 36.1±0.6kg/m^2)[144]。2 期试验中,91%的患者 12 个月时报道的 TBWL 为 17.3%±2.6%;3 期试验中,57%的患者 12 个月时报告的 TBWL 为 17.4%±1.2%。目前为止,尚未有关内镜下袖状胃成形术的随机对照试验报道。

在美国,肥胖经常受到不公正的污名化,并被归咎于不良的饮食习惯或缺乏锻炼。实际上,肥胖的原因是多方面的,这些问题包括遗传、生理、社会经济地位、教育水平、健康食品的获取以及对食品如何直接影响健康的认知。肥胖的迅速增长问题必须通过一些方式解决从而取得更直接的效果。外科治疗病态肥胖比以往任何时候都安全有效。减重外科手术已成为普外科培训的常规组成部分,目前是该领域发展最快的一部分。内镜减重治疗是一种安全有效的新疗法。尽管这些操作比减重手术减少的平均体重要少,但风险也更低,并且为肥胖患者提供了重要的治疗选择。此外,内镜治疗减重手术并发症

不断进步，使得更多并发症在不需要额外手术即可得到治疗。无论是患者独自减重、正在考虑内镜或手术减重手术、还是已经接受了内镜或手术减重手术，医疗保健服务提供者必须共同努力，为这一人群提供最佳的支持和护理。最有效的内镜减重治疗或减重手术是选择合适的患者和经过专业培训的手术团队。虽然存在一定的风险，但减重外科手术和内镜肥胖治疗在合适的患者和合适的术者手上有可能是挽救生命的干预措施。

（祁兴顺 译，李鹏　袁农 校）

参考文献

第 9 章　喂养和进食障碍

Debra K. Katzman, Mark L. Norris 著

章节目录

一、流行病学 …… 112
二、致病因素 …… 113
（一）饱腹感 …… 113
（二）食欲 …… 113
（三）能量储存 …… 113
三、发病及病程 …… 114
四、评估 …… 114
五、特殊疾病的诊断 …… 114
（一）神经性厌食症 …… 114
（二）神经性贪食症 …… 115
（三）暴食症 …… 115
六、其他特殊性和非特殊性喂养或进食障碍 …… 115
（一）回避性/限制性摄食障碍 …… 116
（二）异食癖 …… 116
（三）反刍疾病 …… 116
（四）鉴别诊断 …… 116
（五）营养、医学和实验室评估 …… 117
七、胃肠道异常相关的进食障碍 …… 120
（一）功能性胃肠道疾病 …… 121
（二）食管症状 …… 121
（三）肝脏异常 …… 121
（四）胰腺并发症 …… 121
（五）肠系膜上动脉综合征 …… 121
（六）胃动力 …… 121
（七）便秘 …… 121
（八）药物和膳食补充剂 …… 121
（九）其他危及生命的胃肠道并发症 …… 122
（十）其他喂养和进食障碍中的胃肠道并发症 …… 122
八、成人进食障碍的管理 …… 122
（一）心理治疗 …… 122
（二）营养康复 …… 124
（三）胃肠道症状的医药管理 …… 125
九、进食障碍与肠道微生物群 …… 126

进食障碍（eating disorder，ED）是一种以体态、体重控制和/或饮食模式不同为特征的精神障碍。在《精神疾病诊断与统计手册（第 5 版）》（DSM-5）[1] 中，更新和扩展的章节总结了进食和进食障碍，包括：①神经性厌食症（anorexia nervosa，AN）；②神经性贪食症（bulimia nervosa，BN）；③暴食症（binge-eating disorder，BED）；⑤回避性/限制性食物摄入障碍（avoidant/restrictive food intake disorder，ARFID）；⑤异食癖（pica）；⑥反刍疾病；⑦其他特殊性喂养或进食障碍（other specified feeding or eating disorder，OSFED）；⑧非特殊性喂养或进食障碍（unspecified feeding or eating disorder，USFED）。本章的重点是成人 ED——AN、BN 和 BED；其他 ED 包括异食癖、反刍疾病和 ARFID，仅作简要讨论。虽然 ED 归类为精神疾病，但是相关行为通常会导致临床后遗症发生，大多与胃肠道相关。由于慢性营养不良、超重、催吐或排泄行为往往会导致严重、慢性和危及生命的并发症产生，所以 ED 患者可以从多学科治疗团队的持续护理中受益。事实上，AN 和 BN 是死亡率最高的精神疾病[2]。文献表明胃肠道并发症是 ED 患者最常见的并发症。

一、流行病学

虽然北美和欧洲人群的流行病学数据最为完善，但是全球不同地区都对 ED 进行了研究。大多数已发表的关于喂养和 ED 的流行病学数据早于 DSM-5 公布的修订诊断标准。早期研究表明 AN、BN 和 BED 的患病率和发生率更高，而剩余其他类别（既往 ED 未另行说明[NOS]，现为 OSFED 和 USFED）中的比例有所下降[3]，如预期一样，DSM-5 的变化旨在减少剩余其他类别患者的比例。值得注意的是，迄今为止很少有研究使用 DSM-5 调查 ARFID、异食癖或反刍疾病的发生率和患病率。

最近一项利用 DSM-5 研究 ED 人群的系统回顾表明，AN 的患病率范围为 1.7%～3.6%，点患病率为 0.67%～1.2%[4]。虽然 BN 传统上比 AN 更常见，但利用 DSM-5 群体研究还未能证实这一点。点患病率经常用于评估 BN。两项独立的研究报告表明，女童和妇女中 BN 的患病率几乎相同，约为 0.6%[4]。最近一项面访调查研究显示，BN 的终生患病率高于 AN（2.6% vs 0.8%）[5]，BED 患病率为 0.62%～3.6%（仅女性受试者或男性女性受试者混合）。据报道[4,6,7]，OSFED 终生患病率男性受试者为 0.3%，女性受试者为 0.6%[4,8]，在男性受试者中的点患病率为 0%，在男性和女性受试者样本中的点患病率为 2.4%[4,8]，在男性和女性受试者中，USFED 的终生患病率在 0.2% 到 0.9% 之间[8,9]。

与饮食失调相关的特定症状发生率也较高。2017 年，美国 6% 在校女青少年报告出现呕吐或使用泻药；5.9% 的人群在没有医生建议的情况下服用减肥药、粉剂或液体来减肥或防止体重增加；17.4% 的人群报告在前一个月内进行禁食减肥[10]。ED 发生在不同种族和社会经济的人群中，但每种人群均显示女性发病比男性更常见。过去，男性在 AN 患者中所占比例不足 10%，BN 患者中占 10%，在 BED 患者中占比

不到40%[11,12]。

研究表明[13,14]，约有14%的儿童和青少年接受了青少年ED住院治疗项目，而在儿科ED日间治疗项目中，多达22.5%的患者符合DSM-5对ARFID的诊断标准；与AN或BN相比，这些患者更年轻，病程更长，男性占比更多，并且通常合并精神症状和/或其他临床症状[13,14]。目前还没有异食癖在一般人群中的流行数据，在不同特定人群中可能存在很大差异。最近对符合DSM-5诊断标准的ED患病率的系统回顾未能确定任何包括异食癖或ARFID的研究[4]。在美国，异食癖似乎在健康儿童中罕见，相对普遍见于治疗镰状细胞病的儿童、缺铁的成人、习惯化的特殊个体、非洲的部分学龄儿童和孕妇（如非洲）[15]。反刍疾病的患病率尚不清楚，但在儿童和成人中都可能发生[15]。

二、致病因素

ED病因虽尚不完全清楚，但可以确定是多因素的结果，如心理变化[16]、社会文化[17]、基因[18]都与风险相关。如童年时期受到对自身体重及体型的负面评价会增加BED的患病风险一样[20]，作为风险因素，节食可能会增加AN和BN的风险[18,19]。在重视身体纤瘦[21,22]、自我效能和控制的社会背景下，开始节食以至随之而来的饮食态度和行为紊乱可能是解决对身体不满的重要手段。饮食限制可能会导致饥饿、暴食和排便三者的恶性循环[23]。一项回顾性研究发现，在众多风险因素中，儿童胃肠道疾病与较早的发病年龄和较严重的BN有一定关系[24]，而挑食和消化问题与青少年的AN有关[16]。

已有研究表明，生理易感性可能会增加ED的风险。神经生物学靶点可能在AN、BN和BED的发病机制中发挥作用。几十年来，研究人员致力于对ED的心理生物学，以及能量摄入、饥饿和饱腹感的神经生理学相关因素和决定因素的研究，研究结果强调了饮食行为的多因素和表型多样性的重要性。例如，能量摄入受到来自外周系统（如胃肠肽、迷走神经刺激）的信号分子与中枢神经肽和神经胺之间复杂相互作用的影响。如对肥胖症治疗的研究一样，单一机制不太可能成为ED治疗干预的基础。对摄食行为生理学的了解越多，就越有可能在未来建立综合治疗模式。有大量的文献讨论这方面的问题，下面对常见的研究机制进行简要概述。

（一）饱腹感

血清素长期以来一直是关注的焦点，可能在饱腹感紊乱中发挥作用。大量证据表明5-羟色胺功能的改变会导致ED患者食欲、情绪和冲动控制失调，这种改变在AN和BN患者恢复后仍会存在，也可能反映发病前的易感性[25,26]。也有证据表明ED人群中胆囊收缩素（CCK）水平会发生变化，但AN的结果不一致。虽然有证据表明年轻AN女性患者在餐前和餐后的CCK水平较高，可能会导致餐后恶心呕吐从而阻碍治疗进展[27,28]，但是其他报告显示与对照组相比，AN患者的CCK水平下降[29]。在BN患者中，有一致的证据表明饱腹反应受损，其特征是餐后CCK反应减弱和胃排空延迟[30-32]。相比之下，肥胖伴BED患者的餐后CCK反应与肥胖未患BED的人群没有差异[33]。CCK、暴食和体重指数（BMI）之间的关系需要进一步研究说明。

酪酪肽（peptide tyrosine-tyrosine，PYY）是一种引起饱腹感的肠道来源的食欲减退剂，在AN和BN患者中失调，但BED患者中没有。与对照组相比，AN年轻女性患者的PYY水平更高，这可能导致食物摄入量减少的原因[34,35]。在BN患者中，餐后PYY预期升高幅度减弱[36,37]，可能在饱腹感受损中起作用。最近研究发现BED患者组和非BED患者组的空腹PYY水平和餐后变化没有差异[38]。BN女性患者分泌的胃肠道饱腹多肽——胰高血糖素样肽1和胰多肽——呈异常低水平，研究认为这是以扩大胃容量和减少胃壁张力的形式以适应暴饮暴食的结果。这些饱腹多肽的分泌减弱，可能在维持暴食行为中发挥作用[39]。

（二）食欲

胃饥饿素是唯一已知的能刺激食欲和促进食物摄入的胃肠道激素，与ED有密切关系[40]。胃饥饿素会影响生长激素的分泌，诱导肥胖，并参与能量稳态的下丘脑核信号通路。胃饥饿素的分泌受神经（迷走神经）、机械（膨胀）、化学（渗透压；膳食中的热量和常量营养素）和激素（胰岛素）联合调节，但其优先次序未知[41]。研究关于AN患者中胃饥饿素的文献一致说明：①循环基础胃饥饿素的水平升高，这可能是长期饥饿的结果[40,42,43]；②生长激素和食欲对胃饥饿素的反应迟钝，表明胃饥饿素抗性或胃饥饿素敏感性的变化[41,44,45]；③部分体重恢复后胃饥饿素水平恢复正常，提示生理效应可以弥补营养摄入不足和能量储存的不足[40,46]。最近，一项随机、双盲、安慰剂对照试验在22名门诊AN患者中使用胃饥饿素激动剂，治疗后患者胃排空时间显著缩短，4周后体重增加趋势更明显[47]。

BN患者血浆胃饥饿素水平正常或升高，表明异常进食行为（包括暴饮暴食和排便）可能影响胃饥饿素分泌[36,37]。这些患者有餐后延迟反应（即胃饥饿素抑制降低）[48]，BN患者胃饥饿素的升高和暴饮暴食之间的关系需要进一步探索[46]。对BED患者胃饥饿素的功能进行研究的文献表明餐前和餐后胃饥饿素的循环水平较低，可以反映了慢性暴饮暴食导致的胃饥饿素下调和餐后胃饥饿素下降幅度较小[38]。

（三）能量储存

瘦素和脂联素是与身体脂肪储存的长期调节相关的激素信号。瘦素还通过与下丘脑腹侧内侧核的结合直接影响饱腹感，该区域称为饱腹感中心。瘦素和脂联素在ED患者中均有改变。许多研究发现，在体重减轻的AN患者群体中出现高血脂和低瘦素血症，体重恢复后出现逆转[49,50]，在食物不足的状态下，脂联素水平的升高可以起到保护性支持能量稳态的作用。BN患者血浆中瘦素水平降低和脂联素水平升高，与疾病持续时间延长和症状严重程度增加呈负相关[51,52]。BN患者中瘦素功能变化的机制尚不清楚，在BED患者中未观察到餐后瘦素水平降低[33]。

还有其他的机制，包括神经肽Y、胰高血糖素样肽-2、食欲素A和B、内源性大麻素、抵抗素（脂肪组织的特异性分泌因子）和脑源性神经营养因子等，需要更多的研究阐明在ED病理生理学中的作用。研究的首要任务是确认观察到的心理生物学异常是饮食失调行为的前因还是后果,这些信息将会阐明病因和可能的治疗靶点。患者经常报告进食后出现强烈的不适是他们持续限制食物的摄入的重要原因。在没有任何医学证据支持症状的情况下,不适感可能作为感性或心理的症状被忽略,但也可能是由于中枢神经系统或周围神经信号干扰而导致这一系列的症状。

三、发病及病程

AN 和 BN 最常见于青春期[53],BED 常见于二十多岁[54],ED 在任何年龄阶段均可发生,在中年和老年女性发病率增加[55,56]。ED 从一个类别到另一个类别的诊断改变是很常见的[57]。ARFID 通常在儿童期发病,可以持续到成年[1]。儿童和成人都有异食癖的报道,但对异食癖和反刍综合征的病程知之甚少[15]。

AN、BN 和 BED 与其他精神疾病的终生共病率分别高达 56.2%、94.5% 和 63.6%[58]。与 AN 和 BN 相关的死亡率比预期高 5 倍,是精神障碍疾病中死亡率最高的疾病之一[2]。一些数据支持 AN 为慢性病程,有报告称近一半的 AN 患者完全康复,60% 体重恢复正常,47% 饮食行为恢复正常,34% 病情实现部分恢复,21% 的患者则是长期慢性病程[59]。其他数据表明 AN 的治愈率可能比以前认为的更乐观[58],一项大型双队列研究报告的五年临床治愈率为 66.8%[60]。相反,在对 216 名 BN 和 EDNOS 患者进行 5 年随访中,74% 和 78% 的患者仍处于恢复状态[61]。在一项对 BED 患者的 6 年纵向研究中,43% 的患者仍有症状[62]。最近发表的一项针对 AN 和 BN 患者的 22 年纵向研究表明,暴饮暴食和清除行为的存在和持续性是治疗的不良预后指标,在初始评估时合并抑郁症提示 AN 会持续存在[63]。总之,虽然数十年的研究探讨了 ED 所有潜在的治疗方式,但是高达 50% 接受治疗的患者在随访中仍然会出现症状[64]。

四、评估

在美国,许多 ED 患者没有得到针对的特殊治疗[58]。虽然 ED 有明确的诊断标准,但是临床检测往往存在问题,多达 50% 的病例在临床环境中可能无法被识别。此外,ED 患者往往不愿透露自己的症状[65]。虽然根据定义,AN 患者体重不足,但在临床中很容易被忽略。即使在评估中注意到,体重过轻的临床严重性也常常得不到重视[66]。当怀疑或确诊 ED 时,患者可能拒绝或逃避临床或心理治疗,否认症状的严重性。因此,当患者无法或不愿透露自己的体型、体重、肥胖和体重增加或减少等问题时,确认这些问题尤其具有挑战性[67]。鉴于许多 ED 患者最初出现在初级保健或医疗亚专科机构,对不同卫生保健机构中患者临床体征和症状的识别将有助于适当的转诊,使诊断评估和治疗计划更加有效。一项研究报道 BN 患者在寻求 ED 治疗之前更有可能先寻求对胃肠道症状的治疗[68]。熟悉进食障碍的诊断和胃肠道并发症将帮助临床医生确定最适当的干预措施,包括可用于综合治疗计划的全部治疗资源。

当怀疑 ED 时,直接对限制性饮食或暴饮暴食或不适当的控制体重方式(框 9.1)进行临床调查,对于判断胃肠道症状的范围和严重程度和构成的医疗风险至关重要。准确及时地诊断 ED 是一个挑战。首先,患者主诉的病史可能是不可靠的,BN 和 BED 可能没有任何异常的阳性体征,异食癖和反刍综合征可能也没有。此外,一些饮食调整和运动行为当然是适当的,而识别与具有临床意义的 ED 相一致的病理性行为可能存在困难。ED 患者的症状有相当多的重叠,诊断的特异性是有效治疗的关键。

框 9.1 用于补偿过量食物摄入或预防体重增加的行为
清除行为
利尿剂滥用
泻药和/或灌肠滥用
自我诱导的呕吐(包括滥用吐根糖浆)
非清除行为
过度体力活动
禁食,限制饮食
不恰当的胰岛素暂停或剂量不足(在糖尿病患者中)
兴奋剂滥用(如咖啡因、麻黄、哌甲酯、可卡因)

考虑到患者经常不愿意承认或吐露 ED 的症状,有针对性地记录病史可能是作出及时诊断的关键。在某些情况下,出现阳性体征提示清除行为、体重出现变化,以及/或进行适当的营养治疗并排除其他潜在的体重降低原因后,仍难以增加体重时,才可能怀疑或确诊 ED。

五、特殊疾病的诊断

(一) 神经性厌食症

神经性厌食症(AN)的特征是体重显著降低(低于最小的正常值),担心体重增加(尽管体瘦),对体型或体重认知困扰(否认体重过轻或尽管消瘦但感觉肥胖的医学严重性)[1]。AN 患者在最初的评估中会经常否认或最小化对体重增加的恐惧(有时这种恐惧的明显消失会持续)[69]。即使患者不承认或不表现出对体重增加的强烈恐惧,也可以利用持续使用限制体重增加的行为证据(例如限制性进食、清除行为或过度运动)以用于诊断。AN 患者通常限制自己的食物选择和热量摄入,但是约一半 AN 患者也经常暴饮暴食和/或进行不适当的清除行为如催吐或使用泻药来防止体重增加(见框 9.1)。AN 进一步分为 2 种亚型:限制型(主要通过节食、禁食或运动控制体重的人)和暴食/清除型(经常清除热量以控制体重和/或经常暴饮暴食的人)[1]。在中老年妇女中,新发 AN 可能伴随着生活变迁的困难和对衰老的恐惧[56]。当患者在消化专科就诊中没有透露与体重有关的行为和担忧时,AN 的诊断可能会延迟。即使是真正的 ED 相关的症状或疾病,胃肠道不适的主诉有时会转移医生的注意力,从而延迟 ED 的诊断。一项对 20 名曾在消化科就诊并最终诊断为 ED 患者的研究发现,ED 的诊断平均延迟了 13 个月。值得注意的是,所有患者都表示有增重的愿望,并否认曾试图通过运动、清除行为或饮食限制来减肥[70]。AN 患者常不能或不愿将其维持健康体重的困难定义为故意的,所以诊断可能起初不准确和延迟。

（二）神经性贪食症

神经性贪食症（BN）的临床特征是反复暴饮暴食伴随着不恰当的补偿行为来控制体重或清除暴食期间的热量（见框 9.1）。平均而言，这些行为必须每周发生一次，持续至少 3 个月，以满足诊断标准[1]。体重和/或体型对自身形象的过度影响是诊断 BN 的内在因素。BN 患者心中的自我形象较差，这往往与他们的体重密切相关。AN 或 BN 患者经常每天称体重，甚至每天数次，自尊和情绪根据结果而波动。

根据定义，暴食是指在“不连续的一段时间内”（不是一整天都在过量饮食或素食）摄入异常大量的食物，同时伴有进食无法控制的感觉。许多患者在进食期间情绪麻木[1]。对一些人来说，这种状态似乎会刺激暴饮暴食。多数医生都熟悉自我催吐是主要清除行为，但是 BN 患者经常使用替代或其他手段防止体重增加，包括滥用泻药或灌肠剂、利尿剂、兴奋剂（如哌甲酯、可卡因、非处方“天然”补充剂和咖啡因），胰岛素剂量不足（糖尿病患者），禁食或限制性饮食，过度运动（见框 9.1）。在合并乳糜泻的青少年中，也有患者会有意识地摄入谷蛋白来促进减肥[71]。虽然大多数 BN 患者有清除行为，但那些仅使用过度运动或禁食的患者更难以识别。与暴饮暴食和节食一样，很难确定合理运动与病态过度运动行为之间的界限。一般来说，当一个人在受伤或生病的情况下仍继续锻炼，或日常锻炼超过了教练对团队的建议时，临床上应该引起怀疑。

如果怀疑 ED 时，建议临床医生询问其清除行为。虽然不能确定患者是否会坦率地回答，但是当被问及症状时，患者最终很可能会透露有关症状的信息[65]。一些患者表示，当临床医生提出这样的问题时，如果他们之前未能讨论自己的症状，他们会感到宽慰。然而，有时患者也会从临床医生的问题中学习技巧，因此建议临床医生提供有心理教育背景的问题（例如传达与行为相关的严重身体后果）并避免介绍有关危险行为的信息（如胰岛素剂量不足），根据临床情况酌情处理。患者可以从了解治疗可行性和有效性，以及感受到临床医生对自己的理解中受益。

所有这些旨在平衡热量摄入和控制体重的清除行为和其他行为在长期会造成医疗风险，其中一些行为甚至会造成更直接和潜在的致命后果。应告知患者这些危及生命的风险，并采取措施立即防止这种行为。例如，反复摄入吐根糖浆有严重的神经毒性、心脏毒性和死亡风险[72]，持续使用是一种临床急诊情况，需要立即住院治疗。许多患者没有意识到使用吐根糖浆的严重风险。同样，现在美国禁用的麻黄在年轻人中也会出现卒中或心脏不良事件的风险[73]。一些无麻黄的减肥药也可能导致心律失常[74]。虽然对患者来说难以戒除清除行为，但是在治疗开始时，他们可能愿意替代危害较小的行为。

（三）暴食症

暴食症（BED）的特点是反复和持续的暴饮暴食。暴食发作应该至少每周发生一次，平均持续 3 个月以上，才达到诊断标准。与 BN 不同的是，BED 症状与防止体重增加的经常性不适当补救行为无关。BED 与非病理性暴饮暴食的区别在于以下几种可能的相关症状，包括快速进食、不顾饥饿或饱腹而进食、因羞愧而独自进食以及暴饮暴食后的负面情绪[1]。除了常见的超重或肥胖，BED 患者常没有任何具体的阳性体征。在某些情况下，与 BED 相关的暴饮暴食可能导致或延续体重增加，但许多 BED 患者只有在超重后才会出现症状。BED 患者常常对自己的症状感到非常痛苦而寻求医疗帮助，但他们可能想解决的问题是如何解决体重增加而不是暴食症。寻求减肥治疗的患者中有相当一部分会有 BED，因此，专科医生很可能遇到这些尚未确诊为 BED 的患者。

六、其他特殊性和非特殊性喂养或进食障碍

其他特殊性喂养或进食障碍（OSFED）和非特殊性喂养或进食障碍（USFED）的表现不符合主要 ED 的标准，但由于患者出现痛苦或损伤（包括严重的医疗后果），仍然具有重要的临床意义。当不完全符合特定综合征诊断标准时（包括 DSM-5 中的 4 种情况），诊断为 OSFED，原因不明时诊断为 USFED。除了具有临床意义但未达到诊断标准的症状外，还有几种具有临时描述性质的命名性症状，包括非典型 AN、亚 BN、亚 BED，夜间进食综合征（night-eating syndrome，NES）和清除紊乱（purging disorder，PD）。

3 种变异型 OSFED 的特征是在存在其他标准的情况下，不能满足 AN、BN 或 BED 的所有临床综合征诊断标准，但是临床上出现显著的痛苦或损伤。非典型性 AN 是亚 AN 的一种形式，特征是在体重没有减轻情况下害怕肥胖和身体形象障碍。例如一些肥胖病史的人减重后（如胃旁路手术后）体重仍在正常范围内，但表现出对体重增加和身体形象困扰的极度恐惧。亚 BN 和亚 BED 也是变异型 OSFED。除频度和持续时间外，它们分别满足 BN 或 BED 的所有标准。复发性暴食症状的患者每月而不是每周发生，同时满足 BN 或 BED 的其他所有诊断标准的患者符合 OSFED 的诊断。

另外两个值得注意的变异型 OSFED 是 NES 和 PD。NES 首次描述于 1955 年[75]，特征是反复发作的傍晚或夜间暴饮暴食（不必需），以及没有相关不适当的补偿行为防止体重增加。尽管研究人员已经提出晨起厌食症、夜食癖（例如晚上或晚饭后摄入过多热量），以及睡眠障碍（各种方式包括入睡困难或维持睡眠困难），有研究人员提出了与睡眠障碍有关的额外进食标准，例如在夜间醒来时进食[76]，由于缺乏关于操作标准、患病率、病程、与其他 ED 的区别等方面的研究资料，NES 仍然缺乏一个正式的定义[77]。在 DSM-5 中 NES 定义是排除医学、药理学或社会背景的原因，一个人常在傍晚或夜间进食。与其他变异型 OSFED 一样，NES 必须要有临床相关的明显的损伤或痛苦，且不能用另外的 ED（如 BED 或 BN）更好地解释[1]。有研究表明与对照组平均每晚觉醒 0.3 次比较，肥胖的 NES 平均每晚 3.6 次觉醒。现有数据显示，NES 在夜间进食时摄入的热量，与因 BN 或 BED 而暴饮暴食的人相比要少得多[78]。NES 也可能发生在非肥胖者中[79]，但在肥胖者中更为常见，可能是减肥治疗方案效果不佳的原因[78,80]。

PD 是另一种变异型 OSFED，特征是在没有明显暴饮暴

食的情况下反复出现排泄症状。与其他 ED 一样,PD 在女性中更为常见,但发病高峰(20 岁)似乎比 BN 晚[81]。据估计,年轻成年女性一生中 PD 的患病率为 1.1%~5.3%。PD 的病程、预后及治疗方案有待进一步研究[82]。

(一) 回避性/限制性摄食障碍

在 DSM-4 中包含了“婴儿期或幼儿期喂养障碍”[11],在 DSM-5 中引入“回避性/限制性摄食障碍(ARFID)”,调整了先前的标准以包含更广泛的表述[83]。ARFID 在任何年龄均可发生。ARFID 的标志性特征是进食或喂养过程紊乱,导致严重的营养或社会心理问题,和/或需要特殊喂养措施(例如,通过膳食补充剂纠正营养缺乏或肠内营养补充热量)。进食障碍的原因通常是感觉缺失、对糟糕进食经历的恐惧或对进食缺乏兴趣。除非营养缺乏比预期的更为严重,并且需要额外的临床干预措施,否则不能将这种障碍称为 AN 或归因于某种疾病。ARFID 可与神经发育障碍(如智力障碍和自闭症谱系障碍)并存。与 AN 或 BN 患者相比,ARFID 和神经发育障碍疾病的并发在男性中更常见。与 ARFID 相关的营养缺陷可能对生长、发育和学习产生不利影响[1,84]。值得注意的是 ARFID 的诊断包含了一系列不同的临床表现。要诊断 ARFID,临床医生必须综合病史,以确定食物摄入量的范围和数量,同时确定营养缺乏是否与体重减轻、体重未能如预期增加或生长迟缓有关,是否与临床或实验室异常、对营养补充剂或管饲营养的依赖或个人社交和情感功能的障碍有关[84]。

(二) 异食癖

异食癖是一种周期性持续摄入非食物物质(如粉笔、纸张、油漆屑或洗衣粉)的进食障碍性疾病。虽然有些异食癖可能需要临床干预,但是发育正常的异食癖饮食(如婴儿吃土)不一定能确诊为异食癖。当异食癖被社会规范或文化认可时,就不符合异食癖的诊断标准。异食癖是唯一可以与其他 ED 同时发生的疾病,其他类型 ED 的诊断都相互排斥。

(三) 反刍疾病

反刍疾病的特征是不单纯由于身体状况出现的反复和持续的(至少超过 1 个月)不费力自发反刍。胃内容物有时会吐出来,也有可能被反复咀嚼和/或吞咽。有时反刍用于自我安慰或自我刺激。反刍疾病的患病率尚不清楚,但可以发生在儿童和成人[15]。反刍疾病的诊断可以被 AN 或 BN 所取代,这种行为可能与其他症状相叠加。

(四) 鉴别诊断

ED 的鉴别诊断包括评估和排除导致体重减轻、体重增加、厌食症、贪食、呕吐和其他相关症状的医学原因。在非典型表现或早发或晚发 ED 的情况下,这些考虑尤其重要[56]。ED 偶尔与其他疾病的诊断相混淆。然而,患有与体重减轻或食欲减退相关医学疾病的个体往往会表达对其体重减轻和体重、体形和大小变化的担忧,而 AN 个体则不然。ARFID 患者可能会对其食欲或营养差表示担忧或痛苦。食欲和/或体重减轻的医学原因包括甲状腺功能亢进症、Addison 病、糖尿病、恶性肿瘤、炎症性肠病、吸收不良、免疫缺陷、感染性疾病(如结核病、艾滋病)、胶原血管疾病、药物滥用、情绪和焦虑症、痴呆、谵妄和精神病(见第 35 和 37 章)。在表现与 ARFID 一致的患者中,应排除食物过敏或不耐受,以及可引起进食不适的其他胃肠道疾病[1]。与体重增加相关的疾病包括甲状腺功能减退症、库欣病和脑器质性疾病。

食欲亢进的鉴别诊断范围很广泛,包括 Prader-Willi 综合征(隐睾-侏儒-肥胖-低智能综合征)、痴呆(包括阿尔茨海默病)和颅内病变。食欲亢进也与某些药物的使用有关,尤其是许多精神类药物(如锂盐、丙戊酸钠、三环抗抑郁药、米氮平、传统和非典型抗精神病药物)、妊娠[85]和饥饿后再喂养[86]。与 BN、反刍疾病和 PD(有时是 AN)相关的反胃是意志性的(自我控制的),与胃食管反流病(GERD)或恶心伴呕吐不同[15]。

与食欲不振和体重减轻相关的精神疾病包括重度抑郁症、焦虑和物质使用障碍。此外,共病精神疾病在 ED 患者中很常见[58],且经常使诊断和治疗变得复杂化。因此,识别对体重和食物摄入的过度关注、不切实际或不适当的体重目标、或抵抗试图恢复正常的体重和/或限制过度运动,可以有助于区分 AN 与另一种精神疾病或揭示是否存在潜在的共病 ED。由于 BN、BED、OSFED 和 USFED 患者在就诊时的体格检查可能并不显著,因此在患者披露其症状或临床医生根据病史或病程的其他因素(如体重波动、月经不调)怀疑 ED 之前,诊断可能仍不明确。

虽然有一种针对 ED 之间共同维持机制的“跨诊断”ED 治疗方法[87],但是有证据表明不同 ED 的治疗反应存在差异,因此需要建立明确的诊断以优化治疗效果。尽管 ED 的许多表现重叠,患者在不同的诊断类别之间有交叉(表 9.1)[57],但是根据 DSM-5 诊断标准[1]是可以明确诊断的。异食癖是例外,可以与另一种 ED 同时发生。一般情况下,AN 的诊断优先于其他 ED,BN 可以取代除 AN 之外的所有其他诊断。在某些情况下低体重可将 AN 与 BN 区分开来。即使存在暴饮暴食、清除行为或两者兼有,那些体重严重不足并且符合其他 AN 标准的患者应该归类为 AN。AN 和 ARFID 都存在营养缺陷,在 ARFID 患者中可能表现为体重较轻、达不到体重预期、生长缓慢或营养缺乏,但是并没有身体形象障碍和对肥胖的恐惧。BED 或 BN 患者也可能有症状重叠。BN 的特点是反复的清除行为和其他行为以中和过多的热量摄入防止体重增加以及对体重的过度关注。与反刍综合征相关的呕吐很难与 BN 相关的清除行为区分开来。虽然所谓的反刍综合征相关的呕吐是有意识性的,但与典型 BN 的清除行为相比,这种呕吐毫不费力,所以从定义上来说不能称其为“呕吐”。患者和偶尔有医务人员常把两者弄错。与 AN 和 BN 不同的是,反刍综合征与身体形象障碍或过度体重或体型担忧无关。

OSFED 和 USFED 诊断只适用于不符合主要 ED 的完整的诊断标准,但仍具有相关临床显著损伤或痛苦的患者。例如,对体重增加和对自身形象问题有强烈恐惧的正常或超重个体不符合 AN 的标准,属于“非典型厌食症”。正常体重且反复清除行为但没有暴饮暴食的患者归类为 PD。正常体重或超重但经常夜间过量进食,既没有暴饮暴食也没有清除行为可能会诊断为 NES。

表 9.1 喂养和进食障碍特征的鉴别

进食障碍	诊断标准中的阳性体征	限制饮食	暴饮暴食	为控制体重或中和热量摄入的清除行为或其他行为	对体型和体重的过分关注
AN	明显体重不足	典型	可能出现	一半以上患者可能发生清除行为	是
ARFID	明显体重不足或其他营养缺乏	典型包括饮食不足,由于感官特征而避免吃某些种类的食物,由于创伤性进食经历(例如,呕吐、窒息)而害怕食物,或者对食物漠不关心	无	无	无
BED	无(多超重或肥胖)	无	必须平均每周发生一次,至少 3 个月	无	是
BN	无(多体重正常或超重)	可能有控制体重的行为	必须平均每周发生一次,至少 3 个月	必须平均每周发生一次才能符合诊断标准	是
反刍疾病	无	无	无	不以清除热量为目的的自发性反刍	无
异食癖	无	无	无	无	无

AN,神经性厌食症;ARFID,回避性/限制性摄食障碍;BED,暴食症;BN,神经性贪食症。

Data from American Psychiatric Association. Diagnostic and statistical manual of mental disorders. 5th ed. Arlington, VA: American Psychiatric Association 2013.

(五) 营养、医学和实验室评估

除了排除引起体重和食欲改变的器质性和精神性病因以外,对确诊或疑似 ED 的临床评估还包括获取患者饮食行为和症状的完整病史,关注每天摄取的热量,清除行为[如呕吐、泻药、利尿剂、减肥药、吐根糖浆、补充和替代药物(见第 131 章)]和运动模式。临床评估以营养状况评估为指导,包括确定体重与身高、年龄和性别是否相称。

1. 营养评估

一份包括个人 24 小时饮食回忆在内的详细的饮食史可以提供对热量摄入和营养质量的详细信息。临床医生还应该研究患者对饮食、食物、体重和健康的信念、态度和行为。评估为减少饥饿感而摄入的食物和饮料种类(含咖啡因的咖啡、茶、无糖苏打水)、分量、所使用的减肥产品、热量和脂肪摄入量、所摄入的低脂或无脂食物以及个人认为禁止(或有害)和安全(或有益)的食物。一些人报告未确诊的食物过敏,麸质敏感或乳糖不耐受,这些问题也在调查范围内。临床医生应该询问关于素食主义的问题以及患者成为素食者的原因。

ED 患者可能会经常称体重,有时一天几次。AN 患者会穿宽松的衣服以向别人隐藏体重下降。暴食症患者摄入大量食物。有清除行为的人会经常上厕所,尤其是饭后。

ED 患者能会表现出许多行为和进食习惯,包括将食物切成小块并在盘子周围移动,咀嚼食物并吐出,小口吃饭,每天吃同样的食物,并花很长时间吃饭。ED 患者为他人做饭而不吃任何准备好的食物并不少见。

摄入非食物物质的病史对于异食癖的评估是必要条件,通常还需要父母或看护者的附加病史。ARFID 患者避免进食可能与进食后出现不良后果的历史或恐惧有关(如呕吐史或"创伤性"胃肠道疾病或其他疾病)[1]。

2. 确定体重和体重状态时的特殊考虑

有几种公认的评估 ED 患者营养状况的方法,主要是测量体重、身高和计算体重指数(见第 5 章)。评估与身高相适应的体重是决定临床治疗和精神专科治疗紧迫性的关键因素。对于 AN 患者,重要的是不依赖自我报告的体重,因为报告很有可能不准确。AN 患者通常会竭尽全力隐瞒体重过轻,例如就诊之前增加"水负荷"、在身上增加或隐藏重物、穿着宽松的衣服产生体重正常的假象。因此,在评估体重时要考虑患者希望隐藏体重过轻或体重减轻的可能性。临床医生要在私人区域(不在走廊中)放置体重计,为 AN 患者制定清晰一致的称重方案。这包括要求患者在称重之前脱去衣服换成病号服,摘下沉重的首饰。当患者在就诊之前有饮水增加体重的历史时,检查尿比重和电解质可能会有所帮助;饮水过多或水负荷过重会出现低钠血症[88-90]。

评估成人体重与身高适宜性的标准方法之一是 BMI,计算公式如下:

$$\text{BMI}=\text{体重(kg)}/\text{身高(m)}^2$$

虽然 BMI 不适用于确定所有人的体重状况(例如有相对较高肌肉质量的人群和某些种族)[91],但是 BMI 是大多数 18 岁或以上的男性和女性的首要评估指标。男性和女性的正常 BMI 为 18.5~24.9kg/m^2;BMI 等于或小于 7.5kg/m^2 符合 ICD-10(国际疾病分类第 10 版)[11,92]中 AN 的体重过轻标准;BMI 在 25~29.9kg/m^2 之间为超重;BMI 超过 30kg/m^2 为肥胖[93]。

评估成人低体重的严重程度需要结合 BMI 的绝对值(例如 DSM-5 中 BMI<15kg/m^2 是极端严重程度)[1]和临床情况(包括体重史和临床并发症)。许多方法用于计算成人的预期体重百分比。较为广泛使用的公式之一是:

$$\text{预期体重(\%)}=(\text{患者实际体重}/\text{身高和性别的预期体重})\times 100\%$$

虽然这个线性方程(与 BMI 的二次方程相比)在极端身高下作用有限,但计算起来很简单。此外在概念上更容易让患者和家属理解，特别是在设定体重目标或限制时。体重在预期体重的 90%～110% 范围内是正常的，适合设为 AN 患者设置体重增加目标的良好开端。在此范围内，根据临床病史（包括患者的基线体重，最小体重和最大体重），是否及何时恢复月经，以及骨质流失逆转等医学参数以细化目标。对于超重或肥胖的患者（分别为>110% 或>120% 预期体重），将目标设定在 BMI 的正常范围可能不现实或不可取。

严重营养不良的患者需要住院治疗，以保证体重管理的有效性和安全性。对于体重过轻未达到这种程度的患者，营养管理的主要目标是增加体重恢复所需的热量，确保常量和微量营养素的充足摄入和平衡，并重新建立每日 3 餐和 1～3 份辅食的饮食模式。在这种情况下，应积极咨询经验丰富的 ED 专科医生，了解最佳的再喂养和治疗支持策略。患者还可以补充钙（如果饮食摄入不足）、维生素 D 和/或多种维生素。许多患者不仅限制热量，而且还限制特定食物或食物组，因此需要额外的饮食指导、调整和补充。对于 BN、BED 和 OSFED 所涵盖的亚 BN 和亚 BED，饮食干预包括控制过多的热量摄入，建立一种不易受情绪暗示和过度饥饿影响的饮食模式。许多 ED 患者对营养知识相当了解，通常希望避免与营养师见面，但是营养评估的信息对治疗团队来说是无价的。即使是见多识广的患者也可能从更健康的食物选择，膳食模式和适当的摄入中受益。

3. 医学评估

临床评估的目标是获取信息，有助于明确诊断，评估 ED 的急性和长期的临床情况和精神疾病情况，并确定综合全面的治疗计划。胰腺评估包括临床病史，要特别关注体重减轻，体重波动以及任何影响或旨在控制体重的暴饮暴食、清除行为或其他不当行为（见框 9.1）。应评估营养不良、营养过剩、清除行为和过度运动的临床并发症相关症状，明确完整的月经史。

体格检查包括对过低、过量或不正常饮食摄入的潜在并发症的全面评估，以及营养不良、体重不足、超重、过度运动和清除行为。如果怀疑 ED，体格检查可能会发现营养不良的迹象（如心动过缓、低血压、体温过低、毛发细幼、乳房组织萎缩、肌肉萎缩、周围神经病变）或慢性清除症状［如 Russell 征（长期刮擦中切牙引起自发呕吐导致的手背刮伤）］，肠鸣音减弱或活跃，呕吐反应减弱[94]，牙釉质腐蚀（牙冠硬组织破坏）[95]，或腮腺肥大[96]。

与进食障碍相关的并发症可能很严重，而且数目众多，无法在此详细回顾，主要的并发症列于表 9.2 中。应在体格检查和实验室检查中积极寻求常见或严重的并发症，以便采取适当的干预措施。重要和常见的发现包括异常生命体征（如低血压、血压和/或心率的直立性变化、心动过缓、体温过低）、低体重或超重、牙科病理学变化（如牙冠硬组织破坏、龋齿或两者兼有）[96-98]、骨质减少或骨质疏松症[99]。心脏并发症可能是致命的，包括 QT 间期延长，QT 分离，室性心律失常和心源性晕厥[100,101]。AN 的神经系统表现包括皮质萎缩和脑室增大[102]。内分泌异常包括月经紊乱、血清雌二醇水平降低、血清睾酮水平降低、皮质醇增多症和正常甲状腺功能亢进综合征，伴有低血压和寒冷不耐受[103]。重金属毒性是异食癖的潜在严重并发症[5,104]。

表 9.2　进食障碍患者行为的部分临床特征及并发症*

受影响系统	临床特征或并发症	
	AN、OSFED/USFED 患者中与减肥、饮食限制或暴饮暴食相关	AN、BN 或者 OSFED/USFED 患者与清除行为或再进食行为相关
心血管系统	心律失常 心动过缓 胸痛 心脏体积缩小 运动能力下降 呼吸困难 水肿 心脏衰竭 低血压 二尖瓣脱垂 直立性低血压 心悸 QT 间期延长 QT 离散度增加 晕厥	心肌病（使用吐根） 胸痛 水肿 直立性低血压 心悸 QT 间期延长 晕厥 室性心律失常
皮肤表现	手足发绀 头发和指甲变脆 皮肤干燥 脱发 高胡萝卜素血症 毛发细幼	Russell 标志（反复刮擦门牙造成的指关节病变）

表 9.2　进食障碍患者行为的部分临床特征及并发症*（续）

受影响系统	临床特征或并发症	
	AN、OSFED/USFED 患者中与减肥、饮食限制或暴饮暴食相关	AN、BN 或者 OSFED/USFED 患者与清除行为或再进食行为相关
内分泌与代谢	闭经和月经量过少 甲状腺功能亢进症 高胆固醇血症 低钙血症 低血糖 低镁血症 低钠血症 低磷血症 低温 血清雌二醇，血清睾酮水平低 骨质减少，骨质疏松症 青春期延迟，成长受限	闭经和月经量过少 高胆固醇血症 高磷血症 低氯血症 低血糖 低钾血症 低镁血症 低钠血症 低磷血症 代谢性酸中毒 代谢性碱中毒 继发性醛固酮增多症
胃肠道+	急性胃扩张、坏死和穿孔 肛门直肠功能障碍 便秘 胃排空延迟 早饱 肝脏酶学升高 血清淀粉酶升高 胃食管反流 肝损伤 肝大 胰腺炎 肠道传输时间延长 直肠脱垂 结肠传输减慢 肠系膜上动脉综合征	腹痛 急性胃扩张 Barrett 食管 腹胀 便秘 胃排空延迟 腹泻 吞咽困难 肝脏酶学升高 血清淀粉酶升高 食管出血 食管溃疡、糜烂、狭窄 食管黏膜撕裂 胃坏死和穿孔 胃食管反流 呕血 胰腺炎 肠道传输时间延长 直肠出血 直肠脱垂
一般情况	应激/情绪改变	应激/情绪改变 体重波动
泌尿生殖系统	急性肾损伤 闭经 萎缩性阴道炎 乳房萎缩 不孕不育 妊娠并发症（包括低出生体重儿、早产和围生期死亡）、母亲肾结石	月经异常 氮质血症 妊娠并发症（包括低出生体重儿）
血液系统	贫血 白细胞减少 中性粒细胞减少 血小板减少	

表 9.2 进食障碍患者行为的部分临床特征及并发症*(续)

受影响系统	临床特征或并发症	
	AN、OSFED/USFED 患者中与减肥、饮食限制或暴饮暴食相关	AN、BN 或者 OSFED/USFED 患者与清除行为或再进食行为相关
神经系统	认知变化 皮质萎缩 谵妄(再喂养综合征) 周围神经病变 脑室扩大	卒中(使用麻黄) 神经病变(使用吐根) 呕吐反射减弱或消失
口腔、咽喉	唇干裂 口臭	角膜炎 牙釉质侵蚀和龋齿 腮腺肿胀 牙冠硬组织破坏 咽和软腭损伤 唾液腺肥大 声带病理学改变

*不包括异食癖、反刍疾病和 ARFID(回避性/限制性摄食障碍)的特定并发症。
+在任何进食障碍中与暴食相关的胃肠道并发症均未列出,包括体重增加、急性胃扩张、胃破裂、胃食管反流、胃容量增加和排便量增加。
OSFED,其他特殊性喂养或进食障碍;USFED,非特殊性喂养或进食障碍。

1 型糖尿病患者为减轻体重而故意不使用胰岛素也可能造成相当大的风险。同样,一些 2 型糖尿病患者故意漏服降糖药,导致血糖控制不良和体重减轻。应引起怀疑的临床迹象包括血糖控制不佳,糖尿病酮症酸中毒反复发作,错过临床预约,自尊心差和饮食控制[105]。ED 和糖尿病的诊断,加上故意不用胰岛素,会造成糖化血红蛋白水平升高,低血糖发作增加,导致糖尿病酮症酸中毒住院,青春期发育迟缓和生长延迟以及微血管并发症增加[106,107]。

妊娠期 ED 并发症包括流产、母亲体重增加不足、胎儿宫内生长受限、早产、婴儿低出生体重和低 Apgar 评分,以及围生期死亡[108-111]。

4. 实验室评估

在初步评估时应进行实验室评估,以排除其他疾病和急性代谢紊乱。虽然有暴饮暴食和清除行为的人可能会表现出一些代谢异常,但是营养不良的 AN 患者有正常的实验室结果并不罕见[107]。在营养康复期间也应进行实验室检查以监测再次进食可能导致的各种严重和危及生命的代谢、心血管和神经系统异常(见第 5 和 6 章)[112]。

评估 ED 并发症的实验室检查项目取决于患者的病史、临床表现和营养不良的程度。AN 患者建议在初始评估时进行全血细胞计数以评估贫血、中性粒细胞减少症、白细胞减少症和血小板减少症。一项对 67 名 AN 患者的回顾性研究发现 27% 患者贫血,17% 存在中性粒细胞减少症,36% 存在白细胞减少症,10% 存在血小板减少症[113]。

对于怀疑或确诊 AN 或 BN 的患者,血清电解质水平检测很有用。在一项大规模 ED 研究中发现,有 4.6% 出现低钾血症[114],而另一项中等规模队列研究中,BN 患者低钾血症发生率为 6.8%[115];在后一项研究中,低钾血症在 BN 患者中明显更常见。虽然对低钾血症的评估可能无法识别出 BN 的隐匿性病例,但是有助于识别和监测继发于 ED 的心律失常风险。ED 患者也会出现低氯血症、低镁血症、低钠血症,高钠血症和低磷血症[106,107,115-117]。建议 AN 患者进行血糖测定以确定是否有低血糖发生,低血糖在这类人群中可能很严重[118]。虽然 25%~60% 的 BN 患者出现高淀粉酶血症,但是血清淀粉酶不能用于检测 BN 或评估暴饮暴食和清除行为的严重程度[119]。AN 或 BN 患者血清淀粉酶水平升高经常反映唾液淀粉酶活性增加[119,120],考虑到该患者人群中也会发生胰腺炎,临床上需要鉴别胰腺炎。还应进行肾脏和肝脏的生化检测和尿液分析。如果怀疑异食癖,应该检测血清是否存在重金属(如铅、汞、铜、锌)中毒的证据。

对于闭经的女性建议评估原因,有些会与体重减轻继发促性腺激素释放激素的波动性降低有关[103]。ED 的女性患者经常出现月经不调,但是有症状的 ED 患者可能会在就诊时处于月经期[121],AN 的女性患者可能受孕[122],因此建议检测定量 β-人绒毛膜促性腺激素和血清催乳素水平。在某些临床情况中,也会需要进行其他检测如评价卵巢功能的促卵泡激素或排除垂体病变的神经影像学检查。使用双能 X 线吸收扫描仪对髋关节和脊柱进行骨密度检测有助于识别骨量丢失,如果病情持续,可以在 1 年后再次进行复查评估进一步的骨量丢失情况。AN 女性患者的骨量减少和骨质疏松症分别高达 90% 和 40%,并且与骨折和脊柱后凸的风险相关[99,123]。

基线心电图可以识别 QTc 间期延长(AN 和无低钾血症的 BN 和 EDNOS)[124][125]。一些抗精神病药物和三环抗抑郁药可导致 QTc 间期延长,从而导致尖端扭转型室速和猝死。因此应该仔细选择精神类药物,并确定和监测患者的 QTc 间期。清除行为导致的低钾血症也有诱发心律失常的风险。吐根滥用可能导致致命的心脏毒性、心肌病和心律失常[126]。

七、胃肠道异常相关的进食障碍

胃肠道症状和体征在 ED 患者中很常见(框 9.2;见表 9.2)。受 AN 影响最明显器官是胃肠道[127]。在诊断或者寻求 ED 治疗之前，许多患者都会接受胃肠道疾病的治疗[128]。对 ED 住院患者的横断面研究表明，78% 至 98% 的患者同时有胃肠道症状[129-133]。此外，研究表明与 ED 相关的胃肠道异常可能与 ED 症状的活跃程度和持续时间有关[134,135]。与 ED 相关的胃肠道症状见表 9.2。

框 9.2 进食障碍患者常见的胃肠道症状
腹痛
嗳气
腹胀
肠鸣
食欲改变
便秘
腹泻
排便困难
胀气
恶心呕吐

（一）功能性胃肠道疾病

与正常对照组相比，胃肠道症状在节食者（尤其是腹痛、腹胀和腹泻）[136]和暴饮暴食者（恶心、呕吐和腹胀）中更为常见[137]。一项针对有胃肠道症状的肥胖患者的大规模研究发现，在调整 BMI 后，BED 与腹痛和腹胀之间有密切的相关性[138]。一项对 101 名的 ED 女性住院患者的研究发现，98% 的女性有功能性胃肠道疾病（functional gastrointestinal disorder，FGID），包括 IBS（52%）、功能性胃灼热（51%）、腹胀（31%）、便秘（24%）、功能性吞咽困难（23%）和肛门直肠疼痛（22%），52% 的女性符合 3 个及以上 FGID 的诊断标准[133]。另一项研究发现，在 ED 患者中，肠易激综合征（IBS）与饮食失调和心理感受密切相关[139]。Janssen 的研究组[140]认为一旦 ED 患者出现 FGID，心理和生理因素会相互加强，使得 FGID 和 FGID 相关症状可以独立于 ED 而持续存在。

（二）食管症状

食管症状在 ED 患者中常见。食管功能障碍可被贪食症状所掩盖[94,141]，并可被误诊为 AN[142]。在 23 例患者（11 例限制型和 12 例暴食/清除型）的病例对照研究中，15 例患者主诉反流（6 例限制型，9 例清除型），14 例主诉胃灼热（6 例限制型，8 例清除型），4 例主诉吞咽困难（3 例限制型，1 例清除型）[143]。AN 和 BN 患者也可见食管运动异常[144,145]。慢性 BN 患者常有轻度食管炎（例如在 37 例患者中占 22%），更严重的食管疾病罕见[146,147]。Barrett 食管、贲门黏膜撕裂（Mallory-Weiss tears）和 GERD 已被报道与 BN 慢性呕吐相关[148]。食管破裂有威胁生命的风险，可能使慢性呕吐复杂化[149]。食管自发性穿孔通常是由用力或呕吐引起的腹内压突然升高合并胸膜腔内压相对负压所致（Boerhaave 综合征）。

（三）肝脏异常

血清转氨酶水平升高、低血糖和凝血功能受损（在没有其他肝脏疾病的情况下）已在多项 AN 患者的研究中得到证实[150]。在一项研究中，879 名 ED 患者中有 4.1% 的肝脏生化检查结果升高[151]。在这些肝脏酶学异常的患者中，47% 找到了 ED 以外的病因，剩余 53% 没有发现除 ED 之外的其他原因。在体重不足和体重正常的研究参与者均有肝功异常的报道。研究结果表明肝脏生化检查异常不是 ED 的特异性指标，也不是常见指标；在归因于 ED 之前，应排除其他可能的原因[151]。AN 患者重新进食时也可观察到肝脏生化检查结果升高和肝脏肿大[149,151]。如果营养不良患者的间接胆红素水平升高，也应考虑其他诊断（如 Gilbert 综合征）。有一些病例报告称 AN 由于营养不良和相关的低灌注出现严重肝功能障碍或损伤[152-154]，也有报道称有重症 AN 患者因严重脂肪变性导致了致命的肝衰竭[155]。

（四）胰腺并发症

AN 患者、BN 患者[156-158]和 AN 患者再进食[159]均可能会出现急性胰腺炎。

（五）肠系膜上动脉综合征

肠系膜上动脉（superior mesenteric artery，SMA）综合征是一种罕见的疾病，可使 AN 复杂化。由于体重严重减轻导致主动脉和十二指肠的角度塌陷，导致 SMA 压迫十二指肠的水平部（见第 38 章）[160]。肠系膜上动脉综合征会有呕吐的症状，如果将呕吐单纯归因于 ED，可能会漏诊[161]。

（六）胃动力

近期一项系统综述表明 AN 患者有更明显的胃动力减弱、胃排空延迟和肠道传输延迟[150]。BN 患者肠道运输延迟和胃排空延迟也有报道[30,119,127,162,163]。

许多研究发现 ED 患者的胃功能异常，不仅包括前述的胃排空延迟[30,127,162-164]，而且还有胃舒张功能减弱（BN）[165]、胃动过缓（AN 和 BN）[134]和胃容量增加（BN）[135]的生理后遗症。进食障碍的生理后遗症，如胃容量收缩或扩大、胃动力改变、肠道传输延迟（通过反射途径）[166]和餐后 CCK 释放延迟，可能使症状长期存在，加剧患者对身体形象的过度关注，导致饮食模式异常。有证据表明 ED 患者的主观胃肠症状与客观生理数据没有很好的相关性[167]。

（七）便秘

便秘是 AN 和 BN 患者最突出的胃肠道症状。在一项对 28 名 ED 住院患者的研究中，100% 的 AN 患者和 67% 的 BN 患者有便秘[132]。AN 和 BN 的便秘与营养不良、肠道蠕动能力下降、脱水、因呕吐或滥用泻药等清除行为引起的低钾血症有关。AN 患者常出现恶心、呕吐、腹胀、腹泻、食欲下降和早饱，BN 患者常出现腹胀、食欲减退、腹痛、腹胀和恶心。在一项对 43 名严重 BN 住院患者的研究中，74% 有腹胀，63% 有便秘，47% 有恶心，肠鸣和腹痛的发生率也高于健康对照组[130]。AN 和 BN 患者也可能出现直肠出血和直肠脱垂的症状[168,169]。

（八）药物和膳食补充剂

临床医生应该意识到，ED 患者可以轻易获得许多产品，这些产品经常被作为控制或减轻体重的手段，这可能直接或间接导致严重的胃肠道症状和相关的毒性。泻药滥用在 ED 患者中仍然很常见,尤其是 BN 患者中。Neims 等人发现 BN 患者使用泻药的终生发生率为 14.94%[170]。其他研究表明 BN 患者滥用泻药的发生率在 10% 到 60% 之间。泻药并不是一种有效的减肥策略,因为在小肠中不起作用,而小肠是吸收营养最多的地方。即使用泻药,热量吸收也只减少 12% 左右。最常滥用的类型是刺激性泻药,副作用和毒性包括便秘、泻药性结肠炎、胃肠道出血、直肠脱垂、脱水和电解质异常。除此之外,患者还滥用容积型泻药、表面活性剂、高渗泻药和盐类泻药。

吐根是一种用于诱发呕吐的催吐剂。在一个郊区的 ED 专科诊所中,Greenfeld 等[171]发现 7.6% 的患者有使用吐根的经历,4.7% 有过短期的尝试,3.1% 的人长期使用,1.1% 定期规律使用。Steffen 等[172]报道在因暴食症状接受治疗的门诊患者中有 18% 会在某个阶段使用吐根。即使吐根很少使用,也可能会产生致命的后果,包括心肌病。

还有许多补充药、替代药及膳食补充剂,因潜在的通便和减肥功效而上市销售(见 131 章)。ED 患者需要接受减肥药,泻药,利尿剂,吐根和其他药物的筛查,了解滥用这些物质的不良后果。

(九) 其他危及生命的胃肠道并发症

在极少数病例中,ED 患者出现严重的并发症,包括急性胃扩张、胃肿胀、胃坏死、胃破裂、十二指肠梗阻、坏死性结肠炎和穿孔;隐匿性胃肠道出血(短暂肠道缺血)也有报道。在这种情况下,患者未告知或未确诊的 ED 会延迟或复杂化这些并发症的发现和诊断[156,173,183]。

(十) 其他喂养和进食障碍中的胃肠道并发症

与异食癖相关的胃肠道并发症包括胃石、胰腺炎、粪性结肠穿孔和便秘[184,185],食管穿孔可见于反刍综合征[186]。

八、成人进食障碍的管理

所有 ED 治疗的主要目标是达到饮食态度和行为的正常化、症状消失以及体重恢复(和调节)。积极的体重康复是 AN 治疗基石,体重增加对于减少或逆转严重营养不良的临床和认知并发症至关重要,但是对于成功治疗限制性 ED 也是巨大挑战之一。

ED 患者的最佳治疗方案需要整合心理治疗、营养治疗和初级临床治疗(图 9.1)。有时,根据 ED 症状的严重程度和营养不良的程度,临床专科的治疗和护理是有帮助的。出于多种原因,多学科治疗团队的模式也有用。首先,患者面对的是疾病的医学、心理和营养并发症的风险。其次,患者通常选择性逃避最终康复至关重要的护理。例如患者希望不被发现受伤以便可以继续参加运动;可能难以接受必要的心理治疗解决疾病原因;或可能希望逃过积极的体重管理。相反的是,患者可能试图寻求特定并发症的缓解,而排除适当的心理或营养治疗。

建立治疗协议对开始接受 ED 治疗的患者是有帮助的。虽然不是必需的,但是这对于病情严重可能会影响身体和心

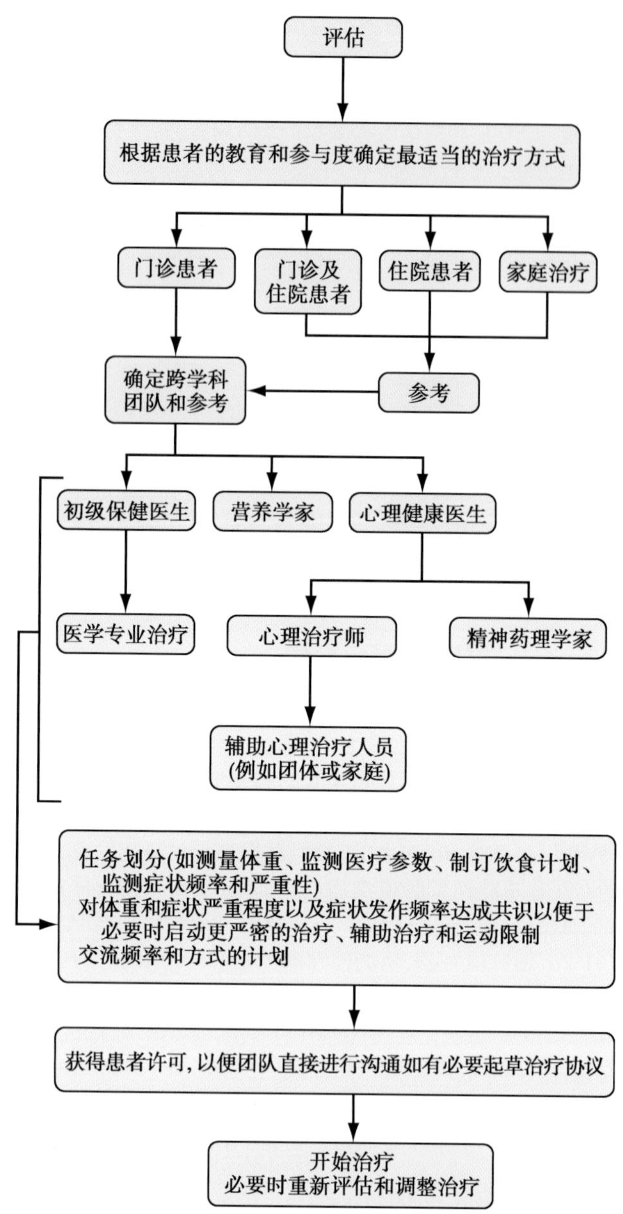

图 9.1　进食障碍成人患者的团队管理流程

理健康的患者尤为重要,因为他们需要住院治疗和护理。治疗协议允许医护人员建立初始治疗目标和标准,以调整治疗和护理的强度水平。这会将治疗预期透明化,对新出现的危机可以作出快速对应,并有助于避免在治疗过程中团队之间的意见分歧。治疗协议还为患者阐明了不坚持治疗或健康状况不佳的持续原因。作为治疗开始的一部分,应该要求患者同意临床团队成员之间的公开交流。如果患者不能同意这一点,则意味着在提供协调治疗方面存在潜在的困难,建议尽量得到患者的认同。根据患者的年龄和情况,还应制定计划明确与父母分享信息的内容和方式。

(一) 心理治疗

临床医生评估 ED 治疗的临床试验数据时,需要知道诊断标准最近已经经过修订,对于 BN 和 BED 现在包括了低于以往的临床试验的行为症状发生率和持续时间的疾病。其他

诊断的临床试验数据很少。事实上，对于多数曾经诊断为 EDNOS(现在是 OSFED 和 USFED)的 ED 患者来说，指导治疗决策的数据十分有限。然而，初步数据表明 CBT-E(强化认知行为疗法)对于有不同进食障碍症状的正常体重和超重成年人(包括以前属于 EDNOS 类别的患者)是有效的[187]。

在成人患者中，AN、BN、BED 和 OSFED 的心理治疗通常从心理治疗开始。在许多情况下，药物疗法可用作 BN 和 BED 的辅助治疗。主动体重管理可用于 AN。心理治疗可以用于支持患者达到体重管理的目标，最佳方案应该与团队中的营养师和初级保健临床医生努力相协调。无论选择何种心理治疗方式，针对建立正常饮食模式和引导患者注意异常模式的触发因素为目标的特定行为策略都可以增强治疗效果。

其中，鼓励患者识别并避免由情绪、日程和食物触发的暴饮暴食事件，计划 3 顿正餐和 2 顿餐间辅食以防止过度饥饿。一份在治疗期间可以回顾的饮食日志可以帮助患者更好识别心理压力、饥饿和症状之间的关系，并提供一个具体的框架，将症状与其他心理问题联系起来。缺乏具体经验性数据来指导治疗成人异食癖，反刍综合征或 ARFID 的。评估异食癖营养干预的两项随机对照试验不支持前述方法，没有关于反刍综合征治疗的随机对照试验[15]。加强对家庭环境的监督或调整对于防止异食癖幼儿或智力残疾人摄入有毒物质非常重要[15]，解决与 ARFID 相关回避性行为的行为性治疗可能会对患者有所帮助[188]。

1. 心理治疗的选择

各种心理治疗已确定对 ED 的疗效。最近的指南和综述总结了实证研究的结果，并强调缺乏治疗 AN、OSFED 和 USFED 的建议[189-193]。认知行为治疗(CBT)和人际关系治疗(IPT)对 ED 的治疗受到了很大的研究关注。CBT 是一种结构化的、基于手工的方法，可以处理思想，情感和行为之间的关系。IPT 是另一项短期治疗，主要关注当前的人际事件以及人际关系中的角色。心理治疗方式的选择依赖于诊断、临床和精神合并症、针对 ED 症状的治疗目标和延伸治疗目标、治疗史、患者体力和偏好以及护理级别。初步的治疗选择应尽可能以证据为基础，但是如果面临多种方案可供选择，医生基于临床的判断对于确定个体化治疗非常重要[190]。在实践中，许多 AN 或 OSFED 患者可以从灵活的治疗方法中受益，即选择适合于特定治疗环境的多种不同治疗方式，因为实证数据的缺乏来支持以证据为基础的循证医学治疗可能对于部分患者没有效果[194]。

现有证据表明，以家庭为基础的治疗(FBT)对青少年是有效的[195,196]。FBT 将父母定位为治疗团队的关键成员，帮助青少年从 ED 诊断中解脱出来，促进青少年的正常成长和发展。现在被认为是青少年的一线门诊治疗，尤其是那些年龄较小且病程较短的青少年[197]。FBT 可考虑用于与家人一起生活的年轻人，以及患者及其家人准备参与该治疗的年轻人[198,199]。

虽然现有的循证医学建议有限，但指南确实建议考虑 AN 患者的心理治疗：认知分析治疗(CAT)、CBT、IPT、焦点心理动力学治疗和明确关注 ED 的家庭干预[190]。一项比较 CBT、IPT 和非特异性支持性临床管理治疗体重过轻的 AN 门诊患者的研究发现，支持性治疗的总体效果优于 IPT，且在 20 周内对总体功能的影响也优于 CBT[200]，CBT 对低体重个体的疗效仍然不清楚，但作为 AN 的住院后治疗似乎是有用的，有助于改善成人体重恢复后的结局和预防复发[201]。能够持续预测治疗效果的因素尚未确定[191]。此外一些证据初步证明 CBT-E 可能对 AN 有效[202]。许多治疗 BN 的方法都有充分的证据支持。CBT 和 IPT 均有效，CBT 在减轻行为症状方面更胜一筹[192]，CBT 能更快地改善症状，治疗结束时效果更好，不过在随访评估中 CBT 与 IPT 无差异[203]。所有指南建议 CBT(16~20 个疗程持续 4~5 个月)作为 BN 的一线治疗[189,190,192]，但并非对所有患者都有效，IPT 可以作为替代疗法。CBT 和 IPT 两种疗法可以组合使用，也可以单独应用[204,205]。其他具有初步证据支持的其他的治疗方案包括辩证行为疗法(DBT，一种开发用于边缘型人格障碍的方法，重点是帮助患者发展调节情感的技能[206])和基于手册的引导式自我改变方法[207]。对于一部分患者来说，如果得不到其他治疗[209]，使用循证医学的 CBT 指南[208]进行自助或引导自助是阶梯式护理方法治疗的适当起点[190]。多种因素已被证明与 BN 的治疗结局相关，但有 2 种因素一致出现：严重程度(暴饮暴食频率较高)和疾病持续时间与预后较差相关[192]。

与 BN 一样，一些 BED 患者将从循证自助项目中获益，作为治疗的第一步或如果无法获得其他治疗[189,190,209]。研究发现，与对照组相比，以多种方式提供的自助干预(具有不同水平的专业或同伴支持)会产生更好的治疗结果，暴饮暴食的天数和与 BED 相关的心理问题减少[193]。在考虑自助后，美国精神病学协会(American Psychiatric association)[189]和国家临床疗效研究所(National Institute for Clinical excellence)[190]指南建议将适应 BED 的 CBT 作为初始治疗选择。团体 CBT 已被发现可有效治疗超重个体的暴饮暴食[210,211]。基于个体的 CBT 有一些支持，尽管方法学的局限性妨碍了明确的结论。如果 CBT 疗法与个体不匹配或不可用，则考虑联合 IPT 疗法和改良的 DBT 疗法。在一项研究中，发现 IPT 在 1 年随访时的禁欲率与 CBT 相似[211]，DBT 疗法显示了良好的结果，在一项随机对照试验中治疗后 6 个月时的恢复率为 56%[212]。值得注意的是，BED 的治疗通常不会导致体重减轻，但其益处可能在于防止体重进一步增加[193]。

最近对第三代疗法(主要的概念为针对认知和情绪的功能或意识)的系统回顾和 meta 分析纳入了 13 个随机对照试验，其中大多数集中在 BED[213]。虽然所有纳入的治疗方法(DBT、模式疗法、基于正念干预和以同情为中心的疗法)对于症状都有较大改善，但是没有一种疗法优于 CBT[214]。因此，研究认为在获得进一步证据之前，CBT 应继续作为 BN 和 BED 的首选疗法[214]。减重是 BED 合并肥胖的首要或次要治疗目标。暴饮暴食的模型提示饮食限制是暴食症的先决条件，因此关于同时解决暴饮暴食和肥胖的最佳方法和顺序一直存在争议。然而多数的数据表明，各种减肥方法不会加剧暴饮暴食，而且可能有助于减轻症状。一项前瞻性研究发现，没有证据表明低热量饮食会导致肥胖妇女暴饮暴食[215]。也有证据证明行为减肥疗法(BWLT)[216]和极低热量饮食[217,218]对减轻 BED 症状有效。在 2 年的随访中，IPT 和 CBT 指导下的自助疗法比 BWLT 更能有效地缓解 BED 暴饮暴食的症状[219]。不过在另一项研究报告中 BWLT 和 CBT 治疗 BED 肥胖患者的长期(6 年)疗效相当[220]。在 BED 的治疗中,增加锻炼会控制暴饮暴食与降低 BMI[221]。虽然许多研究认为治疗暴饮暴食并不意味着体重减轻,但是减少暴饮暴食有助于 BED 患者适度减肥,尤其在达到完全缓解的情况下[222]。

在所有诊断和治疗中,很少有人关注社会经济因素造成的不同结果。未来的研究应该探讨治疗效果是否因性别、年龄、种族,民族、社会经济地位或文化群体而有所不同[191,192]。鉴于与 ED 相关高发的精神病合并症以及社会心理学风险,一些 ED 患者将受益于从心理动力学疗法和灵活折中的治疗方法。这取决于患者的能力、治疗目标、治疗史和其他社会心理学因素。

2. 药物治疗

药物在治疗 BN 和 BED 方面有辅助作用。在研究的众多药剂中,只有氟西汀和利地塞米芬,获得美国 FDA 批准,分别用于 BN 和 BED。没有足够的证据支持治疗任何一种药物治疗 AN 主要症状的疗效。同样,没有临床试验数据支持异食癖、反刍综合征、ARFID、OSFED 或 USFED 的药物治疗,也没有足够的临床试验数据支持儿童和青少年 ED 的药物治疗[223]。

在评价治疗 AN 主要症状的药物中,有几种药物已在研究中。其中,没有任何证据能够为临床常规应用提供建议。一些数据表明奥氮平可能有助于 AN 的临床改善,但最近的一项 meta 分析未能证明非典型抗精神病药物在增加 BMI 或降低病理性饮食方面的优势[224]。

由于缺乏数据支持药物对于 AN 患者疗效和安全性,目前尚无推荐任何药物促进该类患者体重增加。对于其他适应证,应谨慎使用与体重增加相关的药物,并与患者坦诚讨论食欲和体重变化的预期风险和益处。如果选择这样的药物,应密切监测症状,以寻找暴饮暴食或清除行为的发作、复发或增加的证据。

氟西汀不能有效治疗体重不足 AN 患者的主要症状[225],对恢复期体重稳定的 AN 患者也没有明确益处[226,227],这些患者伴发精神类疾病很常见,可以通过药物治疗得到改善,但严重体重不足患者的抑郁症状对抗抑郁药物的反应可能不如正常体重患者。

精神类药物在 AN 治疗中的作用非常有限,但如果饮食来源不足,患者可能需要先优化钙和维生素 D 的补充[103]。虽然口服避孕药可能会减轻与 AN 的部分低雌激素血症的症状,但是不能防止该类患者的骨质流失[228,229],原因是胰岛素样生长因子(IGF-1)会抑制口服雌激素的作用。最近一项研究表明,对于年龄较大的女孩(骨龄≥15 岁)以 17β-雌二醇透皮贴剂的形式给药或者对于年龄较小的女孩(骨龄<15 岁,还未完全生长)起始口服小剂量乙炔雌二醇之后不断增加剂量,补充雌激素会增加脊柱和髋关节骨密度(Bone mineral density,BMD)。然而即使采取这些措施,骨密度也没有完全恢复[230]。临床医生必须牢记,为了医疗安全,也为了提高后续康复所需的心理认知,恢复体重是治疗低体重 AN 患者的重要且必需的选择。对于低 BMD 高风险的青少年患者可以考虑保守使用药物治疗[230]。

与 AN 药物治疗的局限性相反,许多治疗 BN 的药物已经明确了短期疗效,但是缓解率仍然较低[231,232]。CBT 在减轻 BN 相关症状方面比药物治疗更有效,但也有一些研究支持使用药物用于加强心理治疗。使用药物作为心理治疗的辅助手段(而非替代)是合适的,但可能不会对所有患者都有益处。一些证据支持在初级医疗机构中单独使用氟西汀(60mg/d)进行治疗[233],在对 CBT 或 IPT 没有充分反应的患者中,氟西汀对暴食症状的疗效优于安慰剂[234]。

地昔帕明和丙咪嗪(均为常规抗抑郁药的耐受剂量)对减轻 BN 患者的症状有效,而耐受性不佳[235]。关于 BN 患者的两项短期随机对照试验显示托吡酯对于减轻暴食和消除症状有效[236-238]。具有一定疗效(但数据较少)的其他药物包括曲唑酮[239]、昂丹司琼(严重 BN 患者)[240]和其他选择性 5-羟色胺再摄取抑制剂包括舍曲林、氟伏沙明和西酞普兰[232]。一些关于纳曲酮治疗暴食症状的研究显示[235],在减轻以前对其他药物没有反应的患者的症状方面,只有高剂量纳曲酮优于安慰剂[241]。使用该药物时,监测肝脏生化结果至关重要。考虑到潜在的不良反应,其他有效的药物对于 BN 患者来说都是相对禁忌。在一项临床试验中安非他酮与癫痫发作风险增加相关[242]。有病例报道称 BN 患者服用单胺氧化酶抑制剂存在诱发自发性高血压危象的风险[243]。虽然氟伏沙明在一项随机对照试验中显示出预防 BN 复发的疗效[244],但是另一项研究中,氟伏沙明联合分级心理治疗的随机对照试验没有显示该药物的疗效,反而报告一些服用活性药物的受试者出现了严重癫痫发作[245]。

与 BN 类似,抗抑郁药能减少 BED 患者的暴饮暴食并且耐受性良好。多种选择性 5-羟色胺再摄取抑制剂(如氟西汀、西酞普兰、舍曲林、氟伏沙明)以及 5-羟色胺-去甲肾上腺素再摄取抑制剂(如度洛西汀治疗合并抑郁症患者)显示出一定的疗效[232]。迄今为止,减肥药物对于 BED 患者的疗效也都是好坏参半。奥利司他(一种脂肪酶抑制剂)在 24 周的随机对照试验中显示能够降低 BED 患者体重,但与安慰剂相比,暴食发作频率没有变化[246]。最近一项针对 BED 患者的研究也未能证明能减少暴食发作[247]。托吡酯在减少 BED 患者的暴食症状和体重方面有一定的疗效,但副作用和高损失率限制了该研究结果在这类人群中的推广应用[232]。

2015 年初,右旋安非他明的前体药物利地塞米芬得到批准用于治疗成人中重度 BED。研究发现该药物有效且副作用很小[248]。然而,最近的一项长期研究(52 周)表明 84.5% 的入组患者出现轻度至中度不良反应,9% 的患者停药[249]。使用神经刺激性药物治疗 BED 的医生应密切监测患者的心率、血压和总体心血管健康状况。

(二) 营养康复

严重营养不良的成人患者,尤其是小于 70%～75% 预期体重的患者,需要住院治疗才能重新进食。AN 患者发生再喂养综合征的风险特别高。任何再进食的方式都可能发生这种情况,包括口服、肠内和肠外途径(见第 6 章)[250,251]。再喂养综合征的典型表现为低磷血症[也称为再喂养低磷血症(refeeding hypophosphatemia,RH)],在再喂养后的最初几周内出现耗竭和细胞转移,可导致多种医学并发症,包括谵妄、心力衰竭和死亡[112,252]。有证据表明 RH 的程度与入院时营养不良的程度(预期体重百分比或 BMI 中位数百分比)相关,而不是与低或高热量营养摄入有关[250,251,253]。最近的一项系统性回顾发现,对于轻度或中度营养不良的患者,采用高热量方法(>1 400~2 000cal/d)进行再喂养,无论是通过膳食还是联合鼻胃管喂养,都是有效和安全的[251]。一项研究发现 RH 也与入院前的体重减轻率相关,但与规定的热量摄入量无关[254]。这项研究表明,在促进 RH 发展的风险方面,营养不良的程度可能比能量摄入量更重要。因此,医生在对严重营养不良的患者(<70% 的 BMI 中值)重新摄食时应谨慎。然而,在严重营养不良的住院患者中,没有足够的证据来改变目前的医疗标准。有必要进一步研究以确定最佳的营养干预措施,可以使住院和非住院患者的安全增加体重。

目前,建议至少在再喂养的第一周内密切监测血清电解质,包括磷和镁的水平(开始喂养后 6~8 小时)[255]。每天评估心率、呼吸频率、下肢水肿和心力衰竭的迹象,至少持续一周,随着病情稳定,间隔更长时间进行间断评估。可以使用心脏遥测技术监测心律以便在出现 RH 或其他再喂养综合征时采取补充和其他适当措施。谵妄可能发生在再喂养的第二周或之后,可能持续数周[256-259]。

健康的节食干预可能有助于减少暴饮暴食[260],但是 BN 患者不鼓励进行减肥治疗,因为节食会刺激暴食和清除行为。在接受肥胖手术的患者中,BED 很常见,这些患者有部分但不是全部的临床综合征表现。

(三) 胃肠道症状的医药管理

ED 患者就诊时可能同时有胃肠道症状。在某些情况下,与 ED 相关的行为会导致严重的胃肠道并发症。在其他情况下,胃肠道症状可能是轻微的,与潜在的疾病无关,但也可能会影响营养康复的进程。鉴于限制饮食,暴饮暴食和清除行为可能导致或加剧某些胃肠道症状,同步治疗 ED 对于预防胃肠道表现的恶化是不可或缺的。细致的鉴别诊断也是必要的,能避免将有些症状归因为 ED,同时发现潜在的原发性胃肠道疾病。

依靠胃肠道症状的主诉无法准确地表明背后的病理性问题[146,261],因为可能受到情感[123]或身体形象困扰的影响[114]。当患者抱怨腹胀和便秘时,需要确定这些症状在多大程度上源于对体重增加的恐惧或是反映胃肠动力减弱。

许多研究评估了营养康复后胃肠道功能的改善情况。然而这些研究结果各异,结论受到小样本量和非随机设计的限制。在一项研究中,限制型 AN 患者的胃排空有所改善[146],但在饮食摄入量增加和 CBT 的 22 周治疗期后,暴食/清除型 AN 型患者的胃排空并未改善。同一研究中治疗后胃肠道症状自主评分有所改善,但仍然存在异常,与超声检查评估的胃排空无关[146]。对青少年和成人 AN 的另一项混合研究显示,体重增加后,尽管心率和血压均正常,但胃排空没有显著改善(N=6)[262]。其他研究表明营养康复会改善 AN 住院患者的胃排空,尚不清楚这种改善是否与再进食本身或体重增加有关[263]。便秘是 AN 和 BN 患者的常见症状,可能有多种原因。在有便秘的 AN 患者中,结肠转运延迟,但在住院 AN 患者中,再进食后 3~4 周内恢复正常[127,264]。然而在另一项研究中,严重便秘 AN 患者的肛门直肠功能障碍并未显著改善。AN 患者的异常感觉阈值和排便动力学改变可能是持续便秘的原因[264]。10% ~ 60% 的 AN[265] 和 BN[266] 患者滥用泻药,最常见的刺激性泻药[267]。部分患者使用泻药作为主要排便方法,可能逐渐将每日剂量增加至极量。虽然泻药滥用与结肠功能障碍的关系仍然存在争议(见第 128 章)[268-270],但是慢性泻药滥用患者在减少泻药用量的同时会出现便秘。直肠脱垂在 AN 和 BN 患者中常见,与便秘、泻药、过度运动和自我诱导的呕吐引起的腹内压增加有关[138,162]。与滥用泻药有关的其他医疗问题包括电解质和酸/碱变化,可能涉及肾脏和心血管系统并且危及生命。肾素-醛固酮系统在体液丢失时激活,停用泻药后,会导致水肿和急性体重增加。当患者感到臃肿或体重增加时又会进一步加剧泻药滥用[267]。

肠道转运延迟及其相关的临床症状对于 AN 和 BN 患者的治疗是一个特别有趣的临床挑战。现有数据表明,恢复正常饮食或体重增加将改善胃排空和结肠传输延迟,但是可能不足以恢复正常的胃肠功能。虽然有严重的 ED 和相关的胃肠道并发症,患者仍可能拒绝积极的体重管理或停止紊乱的饮食模式。这种抵抗可能因早期饱腹感、腹痛、腹胀或便秘而加剧,所有这些因素都可能强化对体重的过度担心或必须加强对饮食进一步限制。与病理不一致的主观症状进一步使治疗复杂化,部分主诉可能是由精神症状或疾病引起的,包括抑郁、焦虑或扭曲的身体形象。

重新进食和建立正常且健康的饮食模式既是治疗目标,又可以改善症状。对于胃排空延迟和结肠运输缓慢的 AN 或 BN 患者,精心的营养康复是合理保守规的治疗第一步。当饮食和体重恢复正常,许多与 ED 相关的胃肠道症状(如腹胀、便秘、恶心、呕吐、腹泻)会得到改善,这会使患者受益。其他治疗策略包括改变饮食以减少腹胀,如提倡少食多餐、鼓励在进餐早期饮用液体、最初以液体形式提供一定比例的热量(不超过 25% ~50%)[72,116]。

虽然现有数据不支持,但是各种促动力药物已经用于治疗 AN 患者的胃排空延迟[271]。

一些临床医生对于使用处方性泻药治疗便秘持保留意见。虽然在这种情况下,使用泻药治疗便秘是无效的,但是一些患者会受益于细致的肠道微生态恢复,以减少腹部不适和腹胀。增加液体摄入量、膳食纤维和添加大便软化剂和膨松剂是合理和保守的一线治疗方法。在某些情况下,渗透性泻药是缓解症状所必需的[272]。由于肛门直肠功能障碍引起的便秘需要进行肛门直肠功能再训练(见第 19、128 和 129 章)[264]。

一些患者可能受益于抗酸剂或 H_2 受体拮抗而缓解 GERD 和食管炎的症状,可能需要质子泵抑制剂缓解更严重的症状[72],虽然这种治疗在临床上是适当的,但应该向患者明确告知胃肠道疾病的根本原因和恶化程度,当与 ED 相关时,应积极进行心理治疗。

AN 患者因营养不良而继发的血清转氨酶轻度升高可能会随着体重恢复而正常。重症患者血清中肝脏酶学升高可能是再喂养综合征的征兆或反映 AN 相关的低灌注,需要进行紧急评估和干预[72,175]。

虽然许多与限制性饮食、暴饮暴食或清除行为有关的胃肠道症状可以保守治疗,但是部分胃肠道并发症需要进一步的诊断评估。有关ED灾难性胃肠道并发症报道，以及与ED同时发生或类似ED的原发性胃肠道疾病，应根据具体的临床背景评估患者主诉。

如果将呕吐仅归因于ED，则可能会漏诊SMA。ED相关的胃气肿由于胃肌肉萎缩、胃食管交界处“闭塞”和胃排空延迟[273]。急性胃扩张是AN暴食/清除亚型的罕见并发症，可由胃动力减弱和胃排空延迟引起[178]，但如果没有暴饮暴食的临床病史，则不需要怀疑[169]。如果在再喂养或有ED暴食史的情况下诊断为急性胃扩张时，需要紧急鼻胃管减压和液体复苏，因为如果治疗延迟会发生胃坏死、穿孔、休克和死亡[178]。在某些情况下，可能需要进行剖腹手术[133,136,169]。

需要更多的临床试验数据阐明进食障碍相关的胃肠道症状的治疗策略。然而，ED患者的胃肠道症状治疗可以依赖几个关键因素进行指导。首先应排除原发性胃肠道疾病，在适当情况下还要考虑ED会掩盖或模拟原发的胃肠道疾病。如果胃肠道的功能性症状与ED相关，那么第一步就是需要将营养康复与心理治疗相结合。AN患者的营养康复通常需要住院治疗，同时监测严重的潜在并发症(如再喂养综合征和急性胃扩张)。在ED治疗期间，患者对体重增加、正常进食以及停止暴饮暴食和清除行为的抵抗是常见的，因此在治疗计划中应考虑身体形象或情绪症状导致胃肠道症状的可能性。

九、进食障碍与肠道微生物群

最近的研究表明，肠道微生物群可能在ED的病因、进展和治疗中发挥重要作用。肠道微生物群是正常生理所必需的，这一点在代谢性疾病中的作用得到了强调。肠道微生物群可以被概念化为一个微生物群落，包括人类胃肠道内的细菌、古生菌、真菌、寄生虫和病毒(见第3章)[274]。个体肠道微生物群的组成是独一无二的，微生物群与人类健康和疾病的关系受到许多宿主因素的影响，包括但不限于遗传、营养、健康和营养状况、年龄、性别、地理位置和暴露情况[275]。涉及微生物群和ED的研究有限，不过最新的研究表明ED患者肠道微生物群发生了改变(失调)[275]。研究认为这种失调会改变肠-脑轴，对食欲控制和大脑功能产生影响，这可能导致ED的发展。异常进食行为和心理压力会反馈到肠道生态系统，再影响生理、认知和社会功能。这一相对较新的研究领域需要进一步探索以帮助了解肠道微生物如何影响人类宿主的ED病因以及肠道微生物群在疾病过程中如何变化。了解肠道生态系统在ED中的作用有助于研发新型的针对微生物组的靶向治疗药物，这些治疗可能会促进体重增加，改善再喂养期间的胃肠道耐受性，并通过脑-肠-微生物群轴改善精神健康问题[275]，最终改善ED的预后。

(谢咚 译，孙明瑜 校)

参考文献

第 10 章　食物过敏

J. Andrew Bird 著

章节目录

一、定义 …… 127
二、流行病学 …… 127
三、发病机制 …… 127
四、临床特征 …… 130
（一）免疫球蛋白 E 介导的疾病 …… 131
（二）免疫球蛋白 E 和非免疫球蛋白 E 共同介导的疾病 …… 131
（三）非免疫球蛋白 E 介导的疾病 …… 132
五、诊断 …… 134
六、预防 …… 136
七、治疗和自然史 …… 136

希波克拉底（Hippocrates）首次记载了食物过敏的现象，但直到 1921 年，Prausnitz 的经典实验才开始了对食物过敏的科学研究，并建立了过敏反应的免疫学基础[1]。在他的实验中，Prausnitz 将鱼过敏患者（Küstner）的血清注射到自己的皮下，第二天，他将鱼的提取液注射到相同的区域和对照部位。血清注射点的阳性局部反应（Prausnitz-Küstner 试验），证明敏感性可通过血清中的一种因子[如免疫球蛋白（immunoglobulin，Ig）E 抗体]从过敏个体转移到非过敏个体。1950 年 Loveless 首次对牛奶过敏患者进行的盲法安慰剂对照食物试验中证明，患者的病史和食物特异性 IgE 抗体的存在往往不足以诊断食物过敏[2]。在随后的 30 年中，制订了标准化方案来评估食物过敏，即双盲安慰剂对照口服食物试验[3]。

一、定义

有关食物过敏的定义，世界各地研究人员所使用的术语略有不同。以下是美国目前使用的术语[4]。食物不良反应是一个通用术语，表示摄入食物或食品添加剂后发生的任何不良反应的总称，可能是毒性或非中毒性反应的结果。任何暴露个体在摄入足够剂量后均会发生毒性反应。非毒性反应取决于个体敏感性，可能是免疫介导（食物过敏或食物超敏反应）或非免疫介导（食物不耐受）。食物不耐受包括大多数食物不良反应，可分为酶相关、药物性或特发性的。继发性乳糖酶缺乏是一种酶不耐受的成年人（见第 104 章），而大多数其他酶缺乏是罕见的先天性代谢缺陷，因此主要影响婴儿和儿童。药物性食物不耐受存在于对血管活性胺等物质有异常反应的个体中，血管活性胺通常存在于一些食物中（如过期奶酪中的酪胺）。生理机制尚不清楚的已证实食物不良反应通常归类为特发性不耐受。食物过敏通常表现为 IgE 介导的（立即反应），或非 IgE 介导（延迟反应）反应，后者被认为是细胞介导的。

二、流行病学

患病率约 8% 的儿童和 2% ~ 10% 的美国总人群有食物过敏[4,5]。食物过敏发的患病率在出生后的前几年最高，在前十年患病率下降。在幼儿中最常见的食物过敏原包括花生（2.2%）、牛奶（1.9%）、贝类（1.3%）、坚果（1.2%）、鸡蛋（0.9%）、鳍鱼（0.6%）、小麦（0.5%）、大豆（0.5%）和芝麻（0.2%）（参考 Gupta et al. PMID 30455345）。除花生和坚果外，大多数儿童食物过敏在前 10 年结束时都会消失。儿童在出生后 2 年或 3 年内易发生牛奶、鸡蛋和/或花生过敏[6]。花生、坚果、芝麻、鳍鱼和贝类过敏往往是终身的，但约 20% 的花生过敏幼儿可产生临床耐受性[4]。食物过敏可能在童年期后持续至成年期或在成年期发生。成人中最常见的食物过敏包括有贝类（2%）、花生（0.6%）、坚果（0.4%）和鳍鱼（0.4%）[7]。约 5% 的美国人群对生水果和蔬菜出现有限的口咽症状（如唇、舌、上颚和咽喉有瘙痒和/或刺痛感）。这些反应大多发生在患有季节性过敏性鼻炎的青少年或成人中，是由于花粉中的同源蛋白（如桦树或豚草花粉）与某些水果和蔬菜（如生苹果、李子、樱桃、猕猴桃、榛子、甜瓜、香蕉）之间的交叉反应所致，分别为花粉-食物过敏综合征或口腔过敏综合征[8,9]。食物过敏的患病率似乎在增加[10]。来自美国和英国的研究显示，在过去的 10 年里，花生过敏在幼儿中的患病率增加了 1 倍多[11,12]。此外，特应性疾病儿童的食物过敏患病率更高，例如 35% ~ 40% 的中度至重度特应性皮炎儿童有 IgE 介导的食物过敏[13]。

三、发病机制

与全身系统免疫能识别相对少量的抗原，并迅速通过炎症反应来中和潜在的病原体不同，黏膜免疫系统经常会遇到大量的抗原，一般会抑制对外来无害抗原（如食物蛋白、共生微生物）的免疫反应，只有在必要时才会对危险病原体产生快速保护性反应（见第 2 章）。胃肠道是人体最大的免疫细胞库，而胃肠道相关淋巴组织（gut-associated lymphoid tissue，GALT）是黏膜免疫系统的组成部分，它与外部环境密切接触，其作用是将潜在有害生物、外来蛋白质和无害的区分开，同时保持机体与微生物的隔离共生状态[14]。单层柱状上皮细胞将黏膜免疫系统与肠腔分离，可分泌许多有助于屏障功能的因子，包括黏蛋白、抗菌肽和三叶肽。上皮细胞还可以将抗体，特别是 IgA 抗体，转运到肠腔内，通过阻止对抗原或微生物的摄取，发挥其屏障功能。单层柱状上皮细胞层的下方是黏膜固有层，常驻有密集分布的各种免疫细胞，包括 $CD4^+$ 和 $CD8^+$ 效应 T 细胞、调节性 T 细胞(regulatory T cell,Treg)、分泌抗体的 B 细胞和单核吞噬细胞(巨噬细胞和树突状细胞)。这些散在于黏膜固有层的免疫细胞，组成了黏膜免疫系统的效应位点，发挥识别和清除来自环境致病原攻击的功能。位于肠黏膜内的集合淋巴结(Peyer 斑)、孤立淋巴滤泡，与附近的肠系膜淋巴结(mesenteric lymph node,MLN)组成感应位点，在此首次产生抗原特异性细胞和体液免疫反应。特异性上皮细胞(M 细胞)覆盖在集合淋巴结上，有助于选择性地摄入特定抗原进入此部位。相反，可溶性抗原主要经绒毛上皮细胞吸收，并被带入 MLN。缺乏对共生菌群的免疫反应，部分是因特定免疫调节环境实现的，这种环境也可影响对来自饮食中抗原的免疫反应。肠道黏膜的抗原呈递细胞和巨噬细胞对许多微生物配体反应低下[15]，并分泌高水平的免疫调节细胞因子，如白细胞介素(interleukin,IL)-10[16]。无论是先天的(自然杀伤细胞、多形核白细胞、巨噬细胞、上皮细胞和 toll 样受体)，还是获得性免疫反应[上皮内和固有层淋巴细胞、集合淋巴结、分泌型 IgA(secretory IgA,sIgA)和细胞因子]都为外来抗原提供了有效屏障。婴幼儿由于肠道屏障和免疫系统各组分的发育不成熟，其黏膜屏障功能差；新生儿各种酶活性不佳；sIgA 直到 4 岁才完全成熟。婴幼儿期这种不成熟的黏膜屏障，是胃肠道感染和食物过敏患病率高的原因之一。研究还表明，生理屏障功能的改变(如胃酸过多)可导致儿童和成人 IgE 敏感性增加[17]。

已发育成高效胃肠道黏膜屏障后，可以为处理和吸收摄入的食物以及排泄废物提供巨大的内表面积[18]。该屏障利用生理和免疫屏障来阻止外源性抗原的入侵(框 10.1)。生理屏障是由连接紧密的上皮细胞组成，并覆盖着一层厚厚的黏液，用来捕捉颗粒、细菌和病毒；三叶肽[trefoil factor,TFF；胃(TFF1 和 TFF2)和肠道(TFF3)黏液分泌细胞分泌的抗蛋白酶蛋白]有助于加强和促进屏障受损后的恢复；管腔和刷状缘的酶，胆盐和极低的 pH，这些都可以消灭病原体，使抗原失去免疫原性。尽管这种复杂的黏膜屏障在成人已发育成熟，但仍有大约 2% 摄入的食物抗原可以通过正常成熟的胃肠道黏膜屏障，被吸收和转运，以免疫完整性抗原形式播散全身[14]。75 年前 Walzer 和他的同事们进行了一系列严谨实验，用食物过敏患者的血清被动地使志愿者致敏，证明了免疫完整性抗原能穿过黏膜屏障并迅速播散至全身[19,20]。增加胃酸和肠道内食物的存在会降低抗原吸收，而胃酸降低(如 H_2 受体拮抗剂，或质子泵抑制剂所致)或摄入酒精会增加抗原吸收[21]。由于大多数人已经产生了耐受性，这些免疫完整的致敏蛋白质通常不会引起不良反应，但致敏个体则会发生过敏反应。虽然儿童 GALT 发育不成熟更易过敏，但显然由细胞和 IgE 介导的食物过敏反应可以发生在任何年龄阶段。

如前所述，GALT 主要产生抑制或耐受。正如 Osborne 和 Wells[22] 在 1911 年描述的那样，经口摄入的抗原会诱发一种全身性无免疫反应性，这种现象称为口服耐受。在动物实验中，先口服摄入后再注射抗原，并不能引起免疫反应。人类口服后再注射肿瘤抗原(血蓝蛋白)时，也表现出了类似的结果[23]。口服耐受被证明是一种主动调节反应，这种无反应状态可以通过 T 细胞迁移在幼鼠中成功诱导。MLN 对于口服耐受的产生至关重要，外科手术切除或免疫消融 MLN 后，口服耐受不能产生[24,25]。血液中的免疫细胞到肠道，和从肠道到 MLN 的转运受趋化细胞因子与其受体表达的调控。能从肠道摄取抗原的树突状细胞表达趋化因子受体 CCR7，这个受体的表达是树突状细胞从固有层迁移到 MLN 的关键要素，也是口服耐受性形成的必备条件[25]。肠道黏膜固有层树突状细胞的迁移可诱导幼稚动物产生免疫耐受性(图 10.1)[26]。

框 10.1　胃肠道的生理及免疫屏障
生理屏障
阻止摄入抗原的渗透
上皮细胞——单层柱状上皮细胞
糖萼——覆盖于捕获颗粒的复合糖蛋白和黏蛋白
肠微绒毛膜结构——阻止渗透
相邻肠细胞的紧密连接——即使是小肽也能阻止渗透
肠蠕动——将捕获的颗粒从粪便冲出
分解摄入的抗原
唾液淀粉酶和咀嚼
胃酸和胃蛋白酶
胰酶
肠酶
肠上皮细胞溶菌酶活性
免疫屏障
阻止摄入抗原的渗透
肠腔内特异性抗原 sIgA
清除跨越胃肠屏障的抗原
血清特异性抗原 IgA 和 IgG
网状内皮系统
IgG，免疫球蛋白 G；sIgA，分泌型免疫球蛋白 A。

从小鼠和人类 MLN 中分离到的 $CD103^+$ 树突状细胞，首先诱导初始 T 细胞分化为肠道归巢的 $CD4^+$ $Foxp3^+$ 调节性 T 细胞。这些 $CD103^+$ 树突状细胞可表达高水平的视黄醛脱氢酶 2(RALDH2)，该酶可以将视黄醛转化为维甲酸。效应 T 细胞的肠道归巢细胞活性和调节活性，都依赖于来自 $CD103^+$ 树突状细胞所产生的维甲酸。维甲酸前体的一个重要来源是含有维生素 A 的食物[27]。除了树突状细胞向初始 T 细胞传递信号外，MLN 的基质细胞也表达高水平的维甲酸生成酶，这都对因子印记效应如肠道归巢潜能具有很重要的意义[28]。

目前已明确肠道共生菌群(微生态)对黏膜免疫反应塑建起着主要作用。现在已经证明，人体中细菌数量与体细胞数量大致相同[29]。一个体重为 70kg 成年人，其体内细菌数量估计大约有 3.8×10^{13}。结肠中细菌的浓度约为 10^{11}/mL，四舍五入数量级达 10^{14}[29]。机体肠道微生态是在出生后 24 小时内就建立起来了，取决于母亲的菌群、遗传学和当地环境，包括剖宫产或阴道分娩(见第 3 章)。肠道微生态在 1 岁后达到成人模式，此后肠道微生态在一生中相对稳定[30]。在最近的一项研究中发现，食物过敏小鼠具有能转移疾病易感性的肠道微生物群，提示疾病相关微生物群可能参与了食

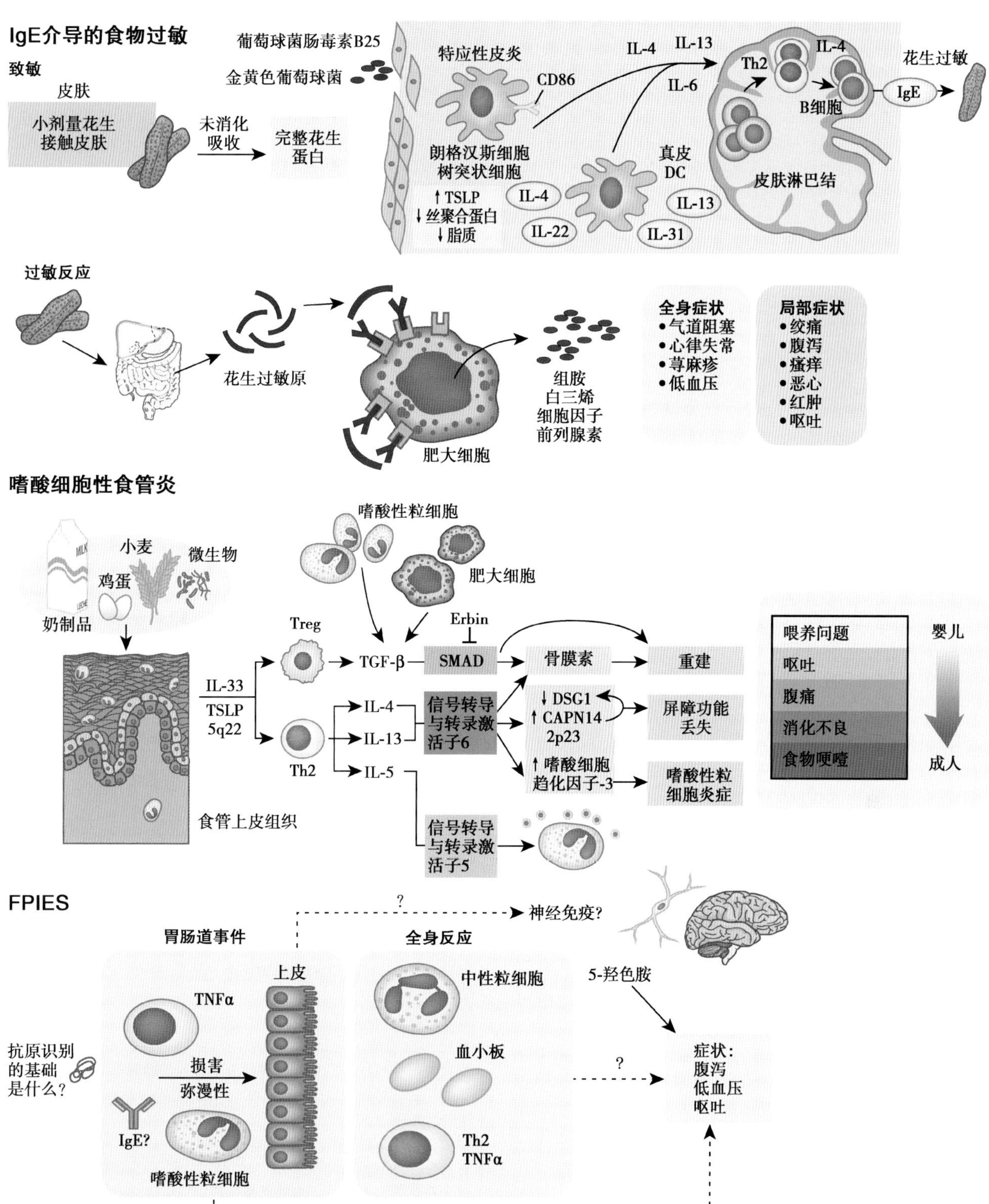

图 10.1 食物过敏的病理生理学。对食物的免疫反应性可能通过免疫球蛋白(Ig)E、非 IgE 和混合机制发生。在 IgE 介导的疾病中,食物过敏原的致敏作用主要是通过暴露于发炎的皮肤发生。一旦再次暴露于变应原后,可能会立即发生 IgE 介导的反应,导致过敏反应。已证实嗜酸性粒细胞性食管炎是由促特应性细胞因子(如 IL-33,TSLP)生成所致,这些细胞因子可激活 T 调节和 2 型辅助性 T 细胞(Th2),从而促进细胞因子分泌,导致食管屏障破坏、组织重塑和嗜酸性粒细胞炎症。人们对 FPIES 发生的潜在机制知之甚少。该图描述了 FPIES 患者中报告的各种相关结果,尽管缺乏对该病发病机制的统一认识。嗜酸性粒细胞、浆细胞和 $CD4^+$ T 细胞已被证实,但其在疾病发病机制中的相关性尚未确定。5-羟色胺与 FPIES 的触发症状有关,尽管尚不清楚它是反应的外周触发因素还是仅限于呕吐反射的中枢控制。FPIES,食物蛋白诱导的小肠结肠炎综合征;IL,白细胞介素;TGF-β,转化生长因子-β;TNF-α,肿瘤坏死因子-α;Treg,调节性 T 细胞;TSLP,胸腺基质淋巴细胞生成素

物过敏的病理发展过程[31]。给予哺乳期母亲及其后代食用乳酸杆菌的研究表明，益生菌在预防一些特定疾病如湿疹可能是有益的[32]，但其他学者的研究结果不支持这一结论。

肠上皮细胞(intestinal epithelial cell，IEC)也可能在决定摄取抗原的速度和方式上起着关键调节作用。对致敏大鼠的研究表明，肠道抗原转运分为两个阶段[33]。第一阶段，跨上皮转运是通过内含体实现的，具有抗原特异性，不依赖肥大细胞。致敏大鼠的转运速度比未致敏对照组快10倍。抗原特异性IgE抗体通过FcεRII结合到IEC)的黏膜面，加速过敏原进入体内。在第二阶段，细胞间转运占主导地位。肥大细胞在第一阶段被激活后，可以释放多种因子，导致细胞之间的紧密连接变松散。这种机制的第一阶段抗原特异性途径涉及抗体，第二阶段非特异性途径主要涉及细胞因子。与此概念一致的是，已发现肠上皮细胞表达多种细胞因子(如IL-1、IL-2、IL-6、IL-10、IL-12、IL-15、粒细胞-单核细胞集落刺激因子和干扰素-γ)受体，暴露于这些细胞因子之后，其功能会发生改变。

已经证明啮齿动物和人类均有体液和细胞免疫的口服耐受性。志愿者口服钥孔戚血蓝蛋白后，出现T细胞耐受，但启动了黏膜及全身B细胞免疫活性[34,35]。无法形成口服耐受性的婴儿，或口服耐受性破坏的老年人，都可能会出现食物过敏。婴儿更容易发生食物过敏反应，因为他们的免疫系统和胃肠道都没有成熟(见框10.1)。纯母乳喂养可促进口服耐受性的出现，并可预防某些食物过敏和特应性皮炎[36]。母乳的保护作用是由于其外源蛋白含量低，含有sIgA(被动防御外源蛋白质和病原体)和可溶性因子(如催乳素)，这些促进肠道黏膜屏障的早熟和婴儿免疫功能的建立。母乳的抗菌活性已被证实，但母乳中的sIgA阻止食物抗原渗透的程度尚不清楚。正常人血清中普遍存在低浓度的食物特异性IgG、IgM和IgA抗体。食物蛋白特异性IgG抗体往往在食用某种食物后的最初几个月上升。但随着时间的推移，即使这种食物蛋白质继续被摄入，其血中的IgG通常都会下降[37]。患有各种炎症相关肠病(如乳糜泻，食物过敏)的人往往有高水平的食物特异性IgG和IgM抗体，尽管没有证据表明这些抗体可致病。单纯体外抗原特异性T细胞增殖并不代表具有免疫致病性，而仅仅提示对抗原暴露有反应。

在具有遗传易感性的个体中，抗原呈递导致过度Th2反应(即分泌IL-4、IL-5、IL-10和IL-13的淋巴细胞)，使各种细胞产生过量的IgE，伴FcεⅠ受体过表达[38]。这些IgE抗体既可以结合肥大细胞、嗜碱性粒细胞和树突状细胞上高亲和力的FcεⅠ受体，又可以结合巨噬细胞、单核细胞、淋巴细胞、嗜酸性粒细胞和血小板上的低亲和力FcεⅡ(CD23)受体。当食物过敏原穿过黏膜屏障，触碰到与肥大细胞或嗜碱性粒细胞相结合的IgE抗体时，这些细胞就被激活并释放介质(如组胺、前列腺素、白细胞三烯)引起血管舒张，平滑肌收缩和黏液分泌，引发速发型超敏反应症状。这些被激活的肥大细胞还可以释放其他多种细胞因子(如IL-4、IL-5、IL-6、TNF-α、血小板激活因子)，诱导IgE介导的迟发炎症反应。由IgE介导的过敏反应症状有：全身症状(休克)；皮肤(荨麻疹，血管性水肿，瘙痒性麻疹样皮疹)；口腔(唇、舌及腭部瘙痒和水肿)；消化道(呕吐、腹泻)；以及上下呼吸道(鼻腔充血阻塞、喉头水肿和伴有眼部瘙痒及流泪的喘鸣)。盲食挑战试验显示，血浆组胺水平升高与进食后这些症状的出现有关[39]。IgE介导的胃肠道反应，内镜下可见局部黏膜血管扩张、水肿、黏液分泌和点状出血[40]。嗜酸性食管炎和嗜酸性胃肠炎是由细胞介导的超敏反应所致(见第30章)。活化T细胞分泌IL-5和其他细胞因子，引起嗜酸性粒细胞聚集，并诱导炎症反应，致使症状延迟出现[41]。从牛奶诱导嗜酸性食管炎患者的活检标本中扩增T细胞的研究显示，其组织内有大量的$CD4^+$ Th2细胞[42]。

总之，胃肠道将摄取的食物加工成一种可以被吸收的形式，并用于能量供给和细胞生长。在这一过程中，非免疫及免疫机制共同破坏或阻止外来抗原(如细菌、病毒、寄生虫、食物蛋白)进入人体内。尽管有这种优秀的屏障，完整性食物抗原蛋白仍能进入血液循环，但大部分不能被正常宿主免疫系统识别，免疫系统对这些非致病性物质处于一种“耐受”状态。

四、临床特征

许多胃肠道食物超敏反应已列入框10.2中。临床上这些疾病通常分为两大类：IgE介导型和非IgE(细胞)介导型超敏反应。许多其他疾病可能会出现类似于食物过敏反应的症状，这些在评估时必须排除(框10.3)。

早在IgE抗体被发现之前，对食物过敏症的研究集中在速发型超敏反应相关的放射影像学的变化上。在最早的一项研究中，进食小麦过敏的病人，横结肠和盆腔的结肠呈高张性改变，而盲肠和升结肠呈低张性改变[43]。在随后的一篇文章中，用X线钡餐透视检查，对12名食物过敏的儿童，进行了有食物过敏原和没有食物过敏原的对比研究[44]；发现有食物过敏原组胃张力下降、胃潴留、持续幽门痉挛、肠道蠕动增快或减慢。

框10.2 胃肠道食物超敏反应
免疫球蛋白E-介导的食物超敏反应
胃肠道过敏
婴儿肠绞痛(少见症)
花粉-食物过敏(口腔过敏综合征)
混合免疫球蛋白E和非免疫球蛋白E介导的超敏反应
嗜酸性粒细胞性食管炎
嗜酸性粒细胞性胃炎
嗜酸性粒细胞性胃肠炎
过敏性嗜酸细胞性结直肠炎
非免疫球蛋白E介导的食物超敏反应
膳食蛋白诱发的肠病
乳糜泻
疱疹样皮炎
食物蛋白诱导的小肠结肠炎综合征
机制不明
牛奶引起的婴儿隐匿性胃肠道出血和缺铁性贫血
胃食管反流病
婴儿肠绞痛(亚型)
炎症性肠病

框 10.3　必须与食物超敏反应相鉴别的疾病

可引起食物不良反应的细菌感染和疾病
产肠毒素细菌
　霍乱弧菌、产毒素大肠杆菌、艰难梭状芽孢杆菌
代谢紊乱
　肠病性肢端皮炎
　低 β 脂蛋白血症或无 β 脂蛋白血症
　原发性碳水化合物吸收不良：乳糖酶缺乏、蔗糖酶缺乏
　一过性果糖和/或山梨醇吸收不良
感染后吸收不良（继发性双糖酶缺乏、绒毛萎缩、胆盐解离）
　细菌：志贺氏菌、艰难梭菌
　寄生虫：贾第鞭毛虫、隐孢子虫
　病毒：轮状病毒
解剖异常
先天性巨结肠（尤其是伴有小肠结肠炎）
回肠狭窄
肠道淋巴管扩张
短肠综合征
其他疾病
婴儿期慢性非特异性腹泻
囊性纤维化
炎症性肠病
肿瘤
　神经母细胞瘤
　胃泌素瘤

20 世纪 30 年代末，应用硬式胃镜观察了过敏患者胃黏膜的改变。一项研究评估了因食物摄入而胃肠道过敏或哮喘加重的患者和对照受试者[45]。食物过敏原存在于胃黏膜上 30 分钟后，胃肠道食物过敏患者可观察到接触部位明显充血，斑块状水肿伴厚厚的灰色黏液和散在的瘀点，类似于 Walzer 之前报道过的被动致敏小肠黏膜的表现[21]。因摄入食物诱发哮喘的患者，还观察到胃黏膜轻微充血。随后的研究证实了这些早期的观察结果，并确定其为 IgE 介导的反应[40]。与正常对照相比，食物过敏患者在食物激发前表现出食物特异性 IgE 抗体和肠肥大细胞数量明显增加，而在食物激发阳性后，可染色肥大细胞和组织胺含量显著减少。

（一）免疫球蛋白 E 介导的疾病

由食物引起的 IgE 介导的胃肠道过敏反应包括两组主要综合征：花粉-食物过敏（口腔过敏）综合征和胃肠道过敏。这些疾病的特点是发作迅速，通常在摄入致病食物后数分钟至 1 小时内发生。检测食物特异性 IgE 抗体的简单实验室检查，例如皮肤点刺试验和血清食物特异性 IgE 抗体的体外检测[如 ImmunoCAP（ThermoFisher scientific，Waltham，MA）]通常有助于确定哪些食物引起患者的症状[4]。

1. 花粉-食物过敏综合征

花粉-食物过敏综合征（口腔过敏综合征）是一种直接接触性超敏反应，主要局限于口咽部，很少累及其他靶器官[28]。症状最常与摄入各种新鲜（未煮熟的）水果和蔬菜有关，包括唇、舌、上颚和咽喉的瘙痒迅速发作，伴或不伴血管性水肿，通常症状会迅速缓解。症状是由局部 IgE 介导的对保守的同源蛋白（结构相似的氨基酸序列，在进化过程中保持不变）的反应引起的，这些蛋白不耐热（即容易被烹饪破坏），并由某些水果、蔬菜和某些植物共有[46]。因对豚草或桦树花粉过敏所致的季节性过敏性鼻炎（花粉热）患者常受此综合征的困扰。在高达 50% 的豚草引起的过敏性鼻炎患者中，摄入甜瓜类（如西瓜、哈密瓜、蜜露）和香蕉会引起口腔症状[4]，而在桦树花粉过敏的患者中，摄入生马铃薯、胡萝卜、芹菜、苹果、榛子和猕猴桃之后出现症状。诊断是基于典型病史和阳性点刺皮肤试验（即"点刺和再点刺"：用针头点刺疑似的新鲜水果或蔬菜，然后再点刺患者的皮肤）即可确诊。

2. 胃肠道过敏

胃肠道过敏是由 IgE 介导的相对常见的超敏反应，通常伴随其他靶器官（如皮肤、气道）的过敏表现，并出现各种症状[4]。典型的症状是在进食后数分钟至两小时内出现，包括恶心、腹痛、腹部痉挛性绞痛、呕吐和/或腹泻。临床病史、食物特异性 IgE 抗体的证据（皮肤点刺试验阳性或血清食物特异性 IgE 抗体阳性），以及彻底清除疑似食物后，症状很快得以缓解，如果再次进食同样食物，症状再次出现就可以确定诊断。在 IgE 介导食物过敏中胃肠道过敏很常见，超过 50% 的儿童在双盲安慰剂对照进食诱发实验中，出现腹部症状[47]。

（二）免疫球蛋白 E 和非免疫球蛋白 E 共同介导的疾病

嗜酸细胞性食管炎、嗜酸细胞性胃肠炎及过敏性嗜酸粒细胞性结直肠炎可能是由 IgE 和/或非 IgE 介导的食物过敏反应，其特征是食管、胃和/或结直肠壁上有嗜酸性粒细胞浸润，多达 50% 患者伴随有外周血嗜酸性粒细胞增多（参见第 30 章）[4,13]。食管黏膜上可见基底细胞增生和固有层乳头状结构延长。这些嗜酸性粒细胞浸润可累及胃或小肠的黏膜层、肌层和/或浆膜层。嗜酸性粒细胞浸润肌层导致其增厚和僵硬，从而出现梗阻；而浆膜浸润通常表现为嗜酸粒细胞性腹水。在大多数患有嗜酸细胞性食管炎、嗜酸细胞性胃肠炎的儿童中，其发病机制与食物引起 IgE 和非 IgE 介导免疫反应有关[48,49]。具有 IgE 介导食物诱发症状的患者，通常有特应性疾病（特应性皮炎、特应性鼻炎，和/或哮喘）、血清 IgE 浓度升高、对多种食物和吸入物的皮肤点刺试验阳性、外周血嗜酸性粒细胞增多、缺铁性贫血和低白蛋白血症。

1. 嗜酸性粒细胞性食管炎

嗜酸细胞性食管炎（eosinophilic esophagitis，EoE）主要发生在儿童，尤其是男孩，表现为反流，呕吐、易怒、拒绝进食、早饱和发育停滞；这有别于成人反流、上腹痛或胸痛、吞咽困难和进食后哽噎感的症状[4,50]。食物诱发的 EoE 首次提出见于一组对 10 名儿童的研究中，这些儿童患有餐后腹痛、早饱或拒食、呕吐或干呕、发育停滞和对常规药物治疗无效（10 名儿童中有 4 名接受了尼森胃底折叠术）[51]。对这些儿童用以氨基酸为基础的配方奶（Neocate）加上玉米和苹果治疗 6~8 周后，8 例症状完全消失，另 2 例明显改善。食管黏膜活检显示嗜酸性粒细胞浸润明显减少或完全消失，基底细胞增生和固有层乳头结构延长明显改善。如果再次吃某种食物后，这些症状会重现。某些儿童的肺部和食管炎相关，有些为季节性食管炎症状[50]。在过去十年中，EoE 的患病率有所增加，一些作者认为，这可能与有反流症状的婴幼儿，过早使用抗酸剂

和促动力药物的比例增多有关。因为用抗酸剂可建立食物过敏反应的小鼠模型[52]，且抗反流药物可能会进一步损害婴儿的肠道屏障功能。在一组152名成年人使用H_2受体拮抗剂或质子泵抑制剂的队列研究中，发现用这些药物治疗3个月后，10%的患者出现食物特异性IgE升高，15%出现新的针对特定食物的IgE[53]。

EoE的诊断是基于有典型病史，食管黏膜嗜酸性粒细胞浸润(>15嗜酸性粒细胞/高倍视野[×40])，除外胃食管反流病(食管远端pH正常，或大剂量质子泵抑制剂治疗无效)[4,50]。由于病变呈斑块状分布，需要食管多块活检。单块食管活检的敏感性仅为55%，而5块活检的敏感性为100%。食管镜检查可见黏膜环(气管化，猫食管样)、纵行沟槽样改变、溃疡、白色丘疹(提示嗜酸细胞性脓肿)或狭窄，但至少有三分之一的EoE患者，内镜检查结果正常。有一些证据提示，特应性斑贴试验有助于鉴定引起过敏的食物，但需要进一步的研究来证实[4]。去除可疑食物3~6周后临床症状就会显著改善，而食管组织的病变要在6~10周后才有所改善，或恢复正常[54,55]。再次进食疑似食物过敏原后，症状复发和/或活检中有嗜酸性细胞浸润。当不能确定食物过敏的致敏原时，可口服糖皮质激素来缓解症状。糖皮质激素治疗通常有效，但停药后易复发[56]。局部糖皮质激素治疗包括吞咽氟替卡松喷雾剂或布地奈德，可使50%~80%患者的症状得到缓解，但使用这种方式治疗后，食管念珠菌病的发生可高达20%[4,57]。如果病情复发加重，每天服用低剂量的泼尼松或泼尼松龙，或隔天服用一次泼尼松可有效控制症状[50]。

2. 嗜酸性粒细胞性胃肠炎

嗜酸性粒细胞性胃肠炎(eosinophilic gastroenteriti，EG)表现为腹痛、恶心、呕吐、腹泻和体重减轻[58]。有蛋白质丢失肠病的婴幼儿可继发低白蛋白血症，导致全身性水肿，而通常其胃肠道症状很轻微[59]。少数EG婴儿也可表现为幽门狭窄、出口梗阻伴餐后喷射性呕吐[60]。

EG的免疫发病机制尚不清楚，但主要涉及细胞介导的机制。部分患者在摄入含有特异性IgE抗体的食物后出现症状加重，但大多数反应似乎与这一机制无关。体外试验显示，与正常对照相比，所有EG患者的外周血T细胞都过度分泌Th2细胞因子IL-4和IL-5，且EG患者十二指肠活检中扩增的T细胞在抗原刺激后可表达Th2细胞因子[42]。

EG的诊断依赖于典型病史，胃肠道黏膜活检显示明显的嗜酸性粒细胞浸润，外周血嗜酸性粒细胞增多(仅见于50%的患者)[58]。由于病变分布不均匀，需要多点活检。在某些情况下，皮肤过敏试验可能有助于识别致病食物，但通常需要进行为期6~10周的要素饮食治疗试验，以明确是否是食物诱发的这些疾病。在对儿童EG和蛋白丢失性肠病的研究中，发现采用以氨基酸为基础的配方治疗，可以改善症状和恢复肠道组织学改变[59]。与EoE一样，如果未发现明确的致敏原，建议给予糖皮质激素治疗，尽管停止使用糖皮质激素后，症状往往会出现复发。这种疾病的长期预后尚不明确。在一系列患有EG和蛋白质丢失性肠病的儿童中，随访2.5~5.5年，发现食物反应性疾病持续存在。

3. 过敏性嗜酸粒细胞性直肠结肠炎

过敏性嗜酸粒细胞性直肠结肠炎(allergic eosinophilic proctocolitis，AEP)通常发生在婴儿出生后几个月之内，最常见的原因是对牛奶或大豆蛋白过敏。目前报告的AEP患儿中半数以上为母乳喂养的婴儿，因为食物抗原可以通过母乳传递给婴儿[4,61]。受累及的婴儿常无临床表现，粪便往往成形，临床上出现便血或大便潜血阳性才被发现。失血通常是轻微的，但偶尔也会引起贫血。婴儿期的AEP已被确定为4岁后发生功能性胃肠病的潜在危险因素[62]。病变通常局限于远端结肠，表现为黏膜水肿，上皮层和固有层嗜酸性粒细胞浸润。严重的病例可出现隐窝破坏，中性粒细胞浸润为主。这种疾病的免疫发病机制尚不清楚，但可能与细胞介导的免疫反应有关。由于没有证据表明这种疾病与IgE抗体有关，皮肤点刺试验或血清食物特异性IgE抗体的测定对诊断没有帮助。去除致敏原后便血消失，就可诊断此病。停止进食可疑致敏食物72小时内，症状就会出现明显的改善，但症状完全消失、黏膜病变完全缓解可能需要一个月。如果再次接触同样的过敏原，会导致症状在数小时到几天内复发。乙状结肠镜的检查结果多种多样，从黏膜散在充血到黏膜脆性明显增加，并伴有小阿弗他样溃疡和出血。结肠黏膜活检显示隐窝上皮和固有层有明显的嗜酸性粒细胞浸润。牛奶和大豆蛋白诱导的儿童结肠直肠炎通常随着年龄增长逐渐免疫耐受(即在避免接触过敏原6个月到2年后，出现临床耐受)，但偶尔也会出现难治性病例[61]。

4. 婴儿肠绞痛

婴儿肠绞痛是一种定义不明的发作性哭闹综合征，其特征是难以安慰的极其痛苦的哭泣，抬起双腿，腹胀和产气过多。通常发生在婴儿出生后2~4周内，并持续到出生后3~4个月。多种社会心理和饮食因素都可能是婴儿肠绞痛的原因，但比较牛奶喂养和母乳喂养婴儿的研究显示，有10%~15%婴儿肠绞痛的病因是IgE介导的食物超敏反应。最近，对肠绞痛患儿与对照组患儿的粪便菌群进行了比较，结果表明，只有对照组的肠道微生物群多样性在出生后逐渐增加，第1周肠绞痛组的微生物群多样性显著低于对照组。在1~2周龄也是差异最显著的时候，肠绞痛婴儿变形菌门含量显著增加，而双歧杆菌和乳酸菌含量显著减少。此外，肠绞痛的表型还与变形菌门的特定菌属阳性有关，包括埃希氏菌属、克雷伯氏菌属、沙雷氏菌属、弧菌、耶尔森氏菌属和假单胞菌属。通过实施几次低过敏原性配方的简短试验，就可以诊断食物诱发的肠绞痛。食物过敏原引起的婴儿肠绞痛，通常是短暂的，因此没有必要长期限制饮食。应每3或4个月进行一次食物激发试验，以确定何时可以恢复婴儿正常饮食。

(三) 非免疫球蛋白E介导的疾病

一些胃肠道食物过敏性疾病显然不是IgE介导的，而是不同的异常抗原呈递，或与细胞介导的机制有关。在这些疾病中，检测食物特异性IgE抗体来寻找食物过敏原是没有意义的。非IgE诱导的超敏反应可分为2种综合征：食物蛋白诱导的小肠结肠炎和膳食蛋白诱导的肠病[4]。

1. 食物蛋白诱导的小肠结肠炎综合征

食物蛋白诱导的小肠结肠炎综合征(food protein-induced enterocolitis syndrome，FPIES)是一种紊乱性疾病，可能表现为慢性或急性症状。慢性 FPIES 是一种仅在接受牛奶或大豆婴儿配方奶粉喂养的 4 个月以下小婴儿中报告的疾病，表现为持续呕吐和腹泻，通常会导致脱水[4,65]。约三分之一的严重腹泻婴儿会发生酸中毒和一过性高铁血红蛋白血症。通过去除致病食物后数天内症状消退而确诊此病。再次进食后会发生急性 FPIES 反应（见下文），症状包括摄入后 1~4 小时内出现呕吐，伴或不伴 24 小时内出现腹泻（通常为 5~10 小时）[66]。如果在没有确定性挑战的情况下，慢性 FPIES 的诊断仍然是推定的。

急性 FPIES 通常在出生后第 1 年出现反复、迁延性呕吐，在进食后约 1~4 小时开始。呕吐伴有嗜睡和苍白，在进食后 24 小时内出现腹泻[66]。牛奶和大豆是最常见的诱因，但大米、燕麦、鸡蛋、小麦、花生、坚果、鸡肉、火鸡、和鱼等固体也有引发急性 FPIES 的报道[66,64]。母乳喂养的婴儿在哺乳时几乎从不出现症状，但他们可能会通过母乳中传递的食物蛋白而致敏，并在最初几次喂食全食物时出现反应[63]。很少报告成人 FPIES，常见的致敏食物是鳕鱼、贝类（如虾、蟹、龙虾）和鸡蛋[2]。

急性发作后获得的粪便通常含有隐血、黏液、白细胞和增加的碳水化合物量[66]。慢性 FPIES 婴儿的粪可能显示隐血、中性粒细胞、嗜酸性粒细胞、夏科-雷登晶体和/或还原性物质[66]。空肠活检发现绒毛变平，水肿，上皮内淋巴细胞、嗜酸性粒细胞及产生 IgM 和 IgA 的浆细胞数量增加，完整的肥大细胞数量减少，提示脱颗粒[67]。

该综合征的免疫发病机制仍不清楚。一些研究认为，食物抗原诱导的局部单核细胞（如巨噬细胞、树突状细胞）分泌 TNF-α 可能解释了该反应的原因[65]。其他研究表明，该疾病可能是由于 1 型转化生长因子-β（TGF-β）受体的表达低于 2 型受体引起的，表明每种受体对肠上皮中转化生长因子-β 的不同生物学活性的贡献不同。食物回避建议通常是基于共同反应性食物的经验（例如，如果对大米有反应，避免食用燕麦；如果对牛奶有反应，避免食用豆浆（表 10.1）。为了来扩大饮食，并确认耐受性是否已发展到之前确定的触发因素，通常需要进行口服食物激发试验。

表 10.1　食物蛋白诱导的小肠结肠炎综合征儿童的常见食物共过敏[66]

诱发 FPIES* 的食物	临床交叉反应/共同过敏原	观察到的发生率
牛奶	大豆	<30% ~40%
	任何固体食物	<16%
谷物：大米、燕麦等	其他谷物（包括大米）	大约 50%
豆科植物	大豆	<80%
家禽	其他家禽	<40%
	牛奶	<30% ~40%
任何固体食物	另一种固体食物	<44%
	牛奶或大豆	<25%
大豆	任何固体食物	<16%

*FPIES，食物蛋白诱导的小肠结肠炎综合征。

经口进食激发试验包括给予 0.3~0.6g/kg 体重，但整体不超过 3g 疑似蛋白变应原，同时监测外周血白细胞计数。结合阳性食物激发，出现症状后 4~6 小时内，外周血中的中性粒细胞绝对计数将至少增加 3500/mm^3，且粪便中可能发现中性粒细胞和嗜酸性粒细胞。约 15% 的食物抗原激发试验导致大量呕吐、脱水和低血压，因此必须在医疗监督下进行。

2. 食物蛋白诱导的肠病

食物蛋白诱导的肠病（不包括乳糜泻）通常发生在新生儿出生后的最初几个月，表现为腹泻（大约 80% 为轻至中度脂肪泻）和体重增加缓慢[61,68]。症状有迁延性腹泻、呕吐（可达 2/3）、生长迟滞、吸收不良（粪便有未消化食物、脂肪）和 D-木糖吸收异常。牛奶过敏是该综合征最常见的原因，不过它也与大豆、鸡蛋、小麦、大米、鸡肉和鱼类有交叉过敏性。在食物中找到过敏原，并停止进食可疑食物后，症状在几天到几周内很快缓解即可诊断。内镜下可见明显的斑片状绒毛萎缩，活检显示明显的圆形单核细胞浸润及少量嗜酸性粒细胞，类似于乳糜泻的病理改变，但范围一般没有乳糜泻广泛。直肠黏液、肉眼或显微镜下可见的便血等结肠炎表现不常见，但大约有 40% 的患儿存在贫血，多数有蛋白质丢失。停止接触过敏原约 6~18 个月后，肠道病变才有可能完全改善。不同于乳糜泻，该病多数临床治疗有效，可失去对蛋白的敏感性，但其自然病程尚有待研究。

3. 乳糜泻

乳糜泻（coeliac disease，CD）是一种病变广泛、可导致吸收不良肠病（见第 107 章）。表现为全部肠绒毛萎缩和广泛细胞浸润，主要是对麦胶蛋白（小麦、黑麦和大麦中麸质的醇溶性部分）过敏。CD 与人白细胞抗原 DQ2（α1*0501，β1*0201）密切相关，90% 以上表达阳性[69]。据报道，美国的乳糜泻发病率为 1/141[70]，而且在过去 10 年中呈上升趋势[71]。与基因相似的丹麦人相比，瑞典人乳糜泻发病率显著增高[72]，其流行病学的差异与瑞典不同的麸质喂养方式有关，为环境因素（如喂养习惯）也是导致这种疾病的原因提供了有力证据[73]。进食麦胶蛋白后，CD 患者肠道黏膜出现炎症，这些炎症与黏膜内组织型转谷氨酰胺转氨酶（tissue transglutaminase，TTG）活性增加有关。TTG 以一种有序和特定的方式脱酰胺麦胶蛋白，暴露能有效结合 DQ2 的抗原位点，并被 T 细胞识别[74]。

CD 的早期症状有腹泻或脂肪泻，腹胀和胃肠胀气，体重减轻，偶有恶心和呕吐。吸收不良导致的口腔溃疡和其他肠外症状不常见。因进食麸质所致乳糜泻的一个特征是小肠绒毛萎缩。未接受过治疗的乳糜泻病人，80% 以上成人和儿童体内存在针对麸质的 IgA 抗体[75]。此外，患者体内针对各种食物的 IgG 抗体含量常常增加，可能为食物抗原吸收增加所致。肠黏膜活检显示绒毛萎缩和炎性细胞浸润，停食麸质食物后 6~12 周病理组织学改善，再次食用麸质，肠黏膜组织再次出现之前的病理改变即可确诊。修订的诊断标准更多地依赖于血清学检查。IgA TTG 抗体定量测定可用于 2 岁以上儿童 CD 筛查。如果可疑 IgA 缺乏，就应测总 IgA，或者与 IgA 和 IgG 相关检测，如 IgG 脱氨基麦胶蛋白肽和 IgG TTG[76]。然而，乳糜泻的诊断，仍然必须有组织病理学证据，证明在进食麸质饮食期间，出现绒毛萎缩。停食麸质后症状缓解，血清学随访显示抗体消失以进一步确诊[77]。一旦确诊乳糜泻，就必须终生禁食含麸质食物以控制症状，及降低可能的胃肠道恶性肿瘤风险[77]。

4. 疱疹样皮炎

疱疹样皮炎是一种与麸质过敏性肠病相关的慢性疱疹性皮肤病。其特征是一种慢性、瘙痒严重、对称性分布于四肢外侧表面和臀部的丘疹、疱疹[78,79]。肠道黏膜组织学改变与CD基本相同，但该病的肠绒毛萎缩和炎性细胞浸润通常较轻，且其肠黏膜活检标本分离的T细胞株所产生的IL-4量，显著多于从CD分离出来T细胞株量[80]。虽然许多患者很少或没有胃肠道表现，但小肠活检通常提示肠道黏膜受损。除麸质饮食可以缓解皮肤症状，几个月后肠道功能也恢复正常。治疗以砜类药物为主，可迅速改善皮肤症状，但对肠道病变无效。

5. 其他胃肠道疾病

其他一些胃肠道疾病也被认为是由食物蛋白质超敏反应引起的。6个月以下的婴儿喂养巴氏杀菌的全脂牛奶可能会导致胃肠道隐匿性失血，偶尔甚至缺铁性贫血[81]。替换为热处理过的婴儿配方奶粉（包括牛奶衍生配方），通常症状在3天内就缓解。婴幼儿GERD可能是源于食物诱发的EoE。一项针对204例1岁以内GERD（24小时食管pH监测和食管活检确诊）婴儿的研究发现[82]，42%是由牛奶诱发的反流症状，一旦停止食用牛奶后，这些婴儿的反流症状缓解，pH恢复正常。据报道，牛奶过敏也可以引起便秘[84]，尽管其根本机制尚不清楚。循证医学证据表明，食物过敏参与IBD（克罗恩病和溃疡性结肠炎）发病，但确切的免疫病理学证据尚有待进一步研究。

五、诊断

食物过敏的诊断是临床诊断，包括详细病史、体格检查和有针对性实验室检查[4]。在某些情况下，病史就可诊断食物过敏（如单独进食花生后的急性过敏反应）。然而，在报道的食物过敏反应中，只有不到50%可以通过双盲安慰剂对照食物诱发试验来验证。明确为食物过敏反应和构建合适的口服食物诱发试验，需要收集的信息包括：①推测引发过敏反应的食物；②食用可疑食物的数量；③从摄入食物到出现症状的间隔时间；④引起症状的类型；⑤再次进食该食物时，是否再次出现类似症状。虽然任何食物都可引起过敏反应，但绝大多数过敏反应只由几种食物引起（框10.4）。

框10.4　大多数免疫球蛋白E介导的儿童食物超敏反应疾病的食物*

花生
牛奶
贝类
坚果
鸡蛋
鱼
小麦
大豆
芝麻

*按总体患病率顺序列出。

Adapted from Gupta RS, Warren CM, Smith BM, et al. The public health impact of parent-reported childhood food allergies in the United States. Pediatrics 2018;142(6):Epub 2018 Nov 19.

图10.2描述了评估和管理食物不良反应的标准方法。如果怀疑IgE介导的疾病，选择皮肤点刺试验或测定食物特异性IgE抗体（如ImmunoCAP法），然后，可采用适当的排除饮食法和单盲食物诱发试验。这些方法应仅限于可能引发过敏反应的疑似食物，因为，临床上常会出现无意义的结果，这样可能会导致过度限制饮食[85]。如果怀疑非IgE介导的胃肠道过敏反应性疾病，则需要实验室和内镜检查（±口服食物激发试验）才能得出明确的诊断（如前所述）。表10.2比较了4种非IgE介导食物过敏性疾病的主要特征。对于疑似IgE介导性疾病、食物诱导的小肠结肠炎和良性嗜酸性直肠结肠炎，需去除所有病史中可疑和/或皮肤试验（针对IgE介

表10.2　非IgE介导的胃肠道食物超敏反应的特征

流行病学特征	EoE和EG	食物蛋白引起的肠病	食物蛋白引起的小肠结肠炎	食物蛋白诱导的直肠结肠炎
发病年龄	1个月及以上	1~18个月	2周~9个月	1周~3个月
持续时间	≥1年	18~36个月	9~36个月	6~18个月
涉及的食物蛋白	牛奶，鸡蛋，大豆，小麦，大麦	牛奶，鸡蛋，大豆，小麦，大麦	牛奶，大豆，大米和燕麦	牛奶，大豆，母乳*
临床特征				
腹泻	轻度	中度	重度	罕见
生长停滞或体重减轻	中重度	中度	中度	无
便血	轻-中度	中度	中度	中-重度
呕吐/反流	显著†	不定	显著	无

*母乳中的食物蛋白质（通常为牛奶或鸡蛋蛋白）。
†干呕或胃食管反流。
EG，嗜酸性粒细胞性胃肠炎；EoE，嗜酸性粒细胞性食管炎。

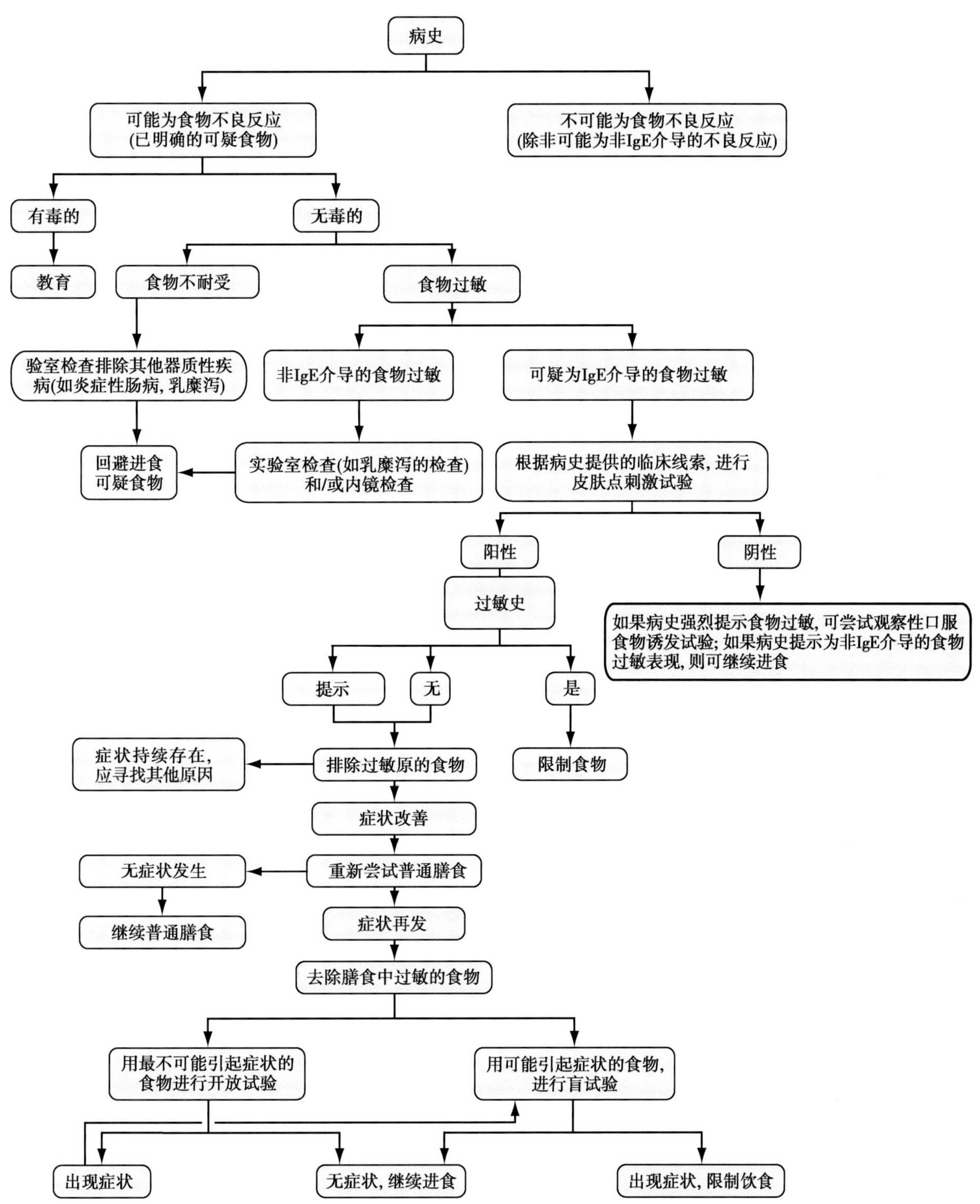

图 10.2　食物过敏的诊断及处理流程图。IgE，免疫球蛋白 IgE

导性疾病)阳性的食物 1~2 周。对于其他疑似胃肠道过敏的疾病(如食物蛋白诱导的肠病、EoE 或 EG),可能需要长达 12 周的筛选饮食,或接受要素饮食(如 Vivonex、Neocate 或 EleCare)以去除所有抗原。如果控制饮食后症状没有改善,并且确定进食依从性好,可除外食物过敏。对非 IgE 介导的食物过敏患者进行单盲或双盲食物诱发试验之前,须停止进食可疑食物 7~14 天或以上(后遗症时间超过 14 天时)。如同开药物处方一样,开筛选性饮食处方可能会有副作用(如营养不良或饮食失调),在没有证据表明它们可能有益的情况下不应这么做。

六、预防

在过去几十年中,有关如何预防 IgE 介导食物过敏的理论在不断改变。在 20 世纪 70 年代,普遍认为过早地将谷物引入婴儿的饮食中,可明显增加 CD 的发病率。而在 20 世纪 80—90 年代,专家一致认为延迟引入固体的致敏食物可能会减少 IgE 介导食物过敏的发病率;然而,在遵循这一建议后,IgE 介导食物过敏的发病率却进一步上升。这可能是由于还有许多其他未知因素参与食物过敏反应造成的。一个前瞻、随机对照研究和几项观察性研究得出了类似的结果,在易患过敏性疾病婴儿的饮食中尽早引入过敏原,可促进产生免疫耐受,而不是食物过敏[86]。

双重过敏原暴露假说是易患过敏性疾病婴儿食物过敏发病机制的主要理论依据[87]。在小鼠模型中,将过敏原先接触发炎皮肤,然后再经口喂服过敏原,可以使 Th2 细胞改变和致敏。而在小鼠的婴幼期,先口服过敏原,使胃肠道黏膜受首先接触过敏原,则会促进免疫耐受现象的发生。对人类的观察性研究也支持了这些小鼠实验的结果,并促成了一项随机对照试验即 LEAP 试验,早期识别花生过敏实验)的施行。

在 LEAP 试验中,将 4~11 个月龄没有发生花生过敏但具有过敏高危因素(即严重的湿疹和/或鸡蛋过敏)的婴儿分为两组,一组是有明确的花生过敏的证据,另一组是无花生过敏的证据[86]。然后将他们随机分配到不吃花生组,或摄入至少 6 克花生蛋白/周(至少分为 3 次)的小组,持续 60 个月,第 60 个月时,所有儿童进食花生。研究人员发现,每周摄入 6g 花生蛋白组的所有儿童,发生花生过敏的风险降低了 81%,即使停止食用花生,这种保护性反应也能维持 12 个月[88]。这些惊人的数据促使美国国家过敏和传染病研究所对指南进行了修改[89],建议如下:

(1) 患有严重湿疹和/或鸡蛋过敏的婴儿应在可进食花生产品的合适年龄(最早 4~6 个月),开始每周摄入 6g 花生蛋白,至少分 3 次。建议在摄入花生之前,应检测血清花生特异性 IgE 抗体或皮肤针刺试验,来评估 4~6 个月婴儿对花生的敏感性。

(2) 患有轻度到中度湿疹的婴儿应 6 个月左右,开始在饮食中加入适量的花生成分。在摄入之前需在卫生健康机构进行敏感性测试。

(3) 所有其他婴儿可以根据其家庭的喜好摄入固体过敏原包括花生,且在摄入前无须行敏感性测试。没有证据表明延迟引入致敏固体物质会对预防食物过敏反应有益。

最近的一项关于摄入其他固体致敏食物的荟萃分析发现(中度可信),4~6 个月婴儿摄入鸡蛋可以降低鸡蛋过敏的风险[90]。但对鱼和早期引入牛奶或水解配方奶所致免疫耐受的发现分别是“不确定”和“没有证据”[89,91,92]。鉴于此,过敏性固体食物可在 1 岁内与其他辅食一起食用,因为证据显示口服固体过敏原可促进免疫耐受的产生。

七、治疗和自然史

一旦确定食物过敏的诊断,严格消除致病变应原是唯一被证实有效的治疗方法。必须教会患者仔细检查食品标签,以便检测隐藏食物过敏原的潜在来源的[4]。H_1 和 H_2 抗组胺药和糖皮质激素等药物可以改变食物过敏原的症状,但疗效可能极小或副作用不可接受。必须常备肾上腺素,并用于治疗过敏反应。目前正在研究各种免疫治疗方法,以治疗 IgE 介导的食物过敏[如口服免疫治疗[oral immunotherapy,OIT)、表皮免疫治疗(epicutaneous immunotherapy,EPIT)][93]。

OIT 涉及将致敏食物混合到溶剂中,并摄入逐渐增加的剂量以提高反应性阈值。对于大多数能够遵守给药方案的患者,可实现脱敏。花生、牛奶和鸡蛋一直是研究最密切的用于 OIT 的食物。大多数方案从初始递增日开始,从极低的剂量开始,并以加倍剂量增加至食物蛋白的最大累积剂量 10~25mg[94]。在治疗日之后,通常每天在家中给药一次,每两周增加一次剂量。维持剂量为 300~4000mg 食物蛋白不等。

目前尚不清楚理想的治疗持续时间,大多数过敏个体可能需要无限期地继续接受治疗,以维持对意外摄入的保护。在长期避免过敏原后保持无反应性的能力称为持续无反应(sustained unresponsiveness,SU)。尚未在足够的人群规模中对 SU 进行深入研究,以便为大多数接受 OIT 的受试者提供准确的评估。现有数据表明 13%~50% 的受试者可以达到 SU[94];然而,由于存在有脱敏时间、脱敏前的治疗时间和食物过敏原不同,不同研究异质性明显,所以这些数据意义非常有限。

治疗的不良反应常见,通常为轻度。在本出版物出版时,尚无美国食品药品监督管理局批准的上市的疗法。一项二期临床试验已经完成,通过意向治疗分析显示,经过 20~34 周脱敏治疗后,大约有 79% 的花生过敏受试者能够安全摄入 443mg 或更多的花生蛋白,而安慰剂组受试者只有 19%[95]。3 期临床试验已经完成,尽管在本出版物发表时尚未对结果进行同行评审。

舌下免疫治疗(Sublingual immunotherapy,SLIT)是将溶解在液体培养基中的少量变应原置于舌下,通常保持 2 分钟,然后吞咽。使用 SLIT 研究的脱敏方法使用与 OIT 相似的构建方案,即每日含服一次,每 1~2 周逐渐加大剂量一次。SLIT 的起始剂量通常以微克为单位,维持剂量通常比 OIT 达到的维持剂量低 100 倍,变应原蛋白的最大剂量为 1~10mg。尽管 SLIT 的疗效研究不如 OIT 密切,但现有数据表明,高达 70% 的受试者可实现脱敏;然而,触发反应的阈剂量变化不如 OIT 测量的稳健[94]。治疗通常耐受性良好,报告的全身不良反应很少。

EPIT 通过将一种新型的含过敏原贴片贴在完整的皮肤

上，诱发皮肤免疫反应。局部皮肤的水分释放贴片上的过敏原，被朗格汉斯细胞摄入，随后下调效应细胞的反应[94]。一项针对花生过敏患者的 2b 期临床试验显示，EPIT 对 6~11 岁儿童的治疗效果显著[96]；3 期试验已经完成，但结果尚未公布。EPIT 的治疗效果不如 OIT 那样明显，诱发过敏反应的剂量阈值变化不大，类似于 SLIT。与 OIT 相比，EPIT 更容易出现免疫耐受。2 期临床试验中，最常见的不良事件是局部皮肤反应，只有一例受试者发生与治疗可能相关但并不严重的中度过敏[96]。165 名接受花生贴片治疗的受试者中，只有 3 人因为不良反应而退出了试验[96]。

食物过敏常发生于婴儿出生后的最初几年内，多数儿童随着年龄增长，10 岁以内食物过敏即消失，除了 IgE 介导的花生、坚果、鱼和贝类过敏[4]。虽然年纪小的幼儿更容易随年龄增长逐渐脱敏，但如果能找到致敏食物，并从饮食中去除一段时间，随着时间的推移，年龄较大的儿童和成年人也可能会脱敏（即临床耐受，摄入既往过敏食物也不会出现症状）[13]。

目前有关这一领域的研究为这些疾病的发病机制提供了新的信息，将会带来新的诊断和治疗方法。在此期间，必须仔细寻找特异性食物过敏原，指导患者避免摄入这些能引起症状的食物过敏原。

（王立　王俊雄 译，李鹏 校）

参考文献

第三部分　症状、体征和生物心理社会学问题

第 11 章　急性腹痛

Frederick H. Millham 著

章节目录

一、解剖及生理学 ······ 139
（一）内脏性疼痛 ······ 139
（二）躯体-腔壁性疼痛 ······ 142
（三）牵涉性疼痛 ······ 142
二、评估 ······ 142
（一）急诊处理方法 ······ 142
（二）病史 ······ 143
（三）体格检查 ······ 144
（四）实验室检查 ······ 145
（五）影像学检查 ······ 145
（六）其他诊断检查 ······ 145
三、病因 ······ 145
（一）急性阑尾炎 ······ 146
（二）急性胆源性疾病 ······ 147
（三）小肠梗阻 ······ 147
（四）急性憩室炎 ······ 148
（五）急性胰腺炎 ······ 148
（六）消化性溃疡穿孔 ······ 148
（七）急性肠系膜缺血 ······ 149
（八）腹主动脉瘤 ······ 149
（九）腹腔间隔室综合征 ······ 149
（十）腹腔内其他原因 ······ 150
（十一）腹腔外疾病和全身性疾病原因 ······ 150
（十二）特殊情况 ······ 151
四、药物治疗 ······ 151

急性腹痛是患者急诊就诊的常见主诉。2014 年美国 1 110 万急诊患者因腹痛就诊，占当年急诊患者总数的 8%[1]。大约有 40% 的患者不能立即找到腹痛的原因[2,3]，其余能找到急性腹痛病因的大多是外科疾病，需要进一步检查和外科干预[3]。少数病例存在有危及生命的病理改变。因此，有效快速且又准确地诊断急性腹痛的病因非常重要。以便对病情严重的患者能及时救治，同时不会对自限性疾病进行盲目的治疗。

一、解剖及生理学

许多生理因素决定了腹痛的感知。包括刺激物的性质，所涉及的神经感受器的类型，损伤部位到中枢神经系统的神经传导通路的解剖结构，以及对疼痛信号传递、解释和反应之间的相互影响及相互作用[4]。腹部病理状态引起的腹痛常由不同的感觉传入纤维以不同的方式传导，这些感觉传入纤维包括有自主神经和躯体神经[5,6]。这两种神经纤维以不同的方式传导信号，就出现不同的疼痛感觉。神经传导过程之间的相互影响会导致对腹痛感知的多样性[6]。这种特有的神经解剖学导致了三种不同类型的疼痛：内脏性疼痛、躯体-腔壁性疼痛和牵涉痛。内脏性疼痛通常起病缓慢和定位不准确，往往表现的是一种钝痛。躯体-腔壁性疼痛表现更剧烈、更尖锐、定位准确。牵涉性疼痛是一种感到远离病变刺激部位的体表痛。

腹部器官的感觉神经感受器位于空腔脏器的黏膜和肌层，浆膜结构表面（如脏腹膜）和肠系膜内（图 11.1）[6]。除了（对有害刺激的感知）痛觉外，感觉神经感受器还通过局部和中枢神经反射弧参与调节消化道的分泌、蠕动和血液流动的功能[7]。虽然不能感知这种方式传达的感觉信号，但这些胃肠道功能（分泌、运动、血液流动）的失调可引起疼痛。例如，肠易激综合征患者的腹痛，可能就是由于肠道传入神经元对正常内源性刺激物的敏感性过强，从而导致肠道运动和分泌功能异常，最终感受到腹痛[8]（见第 122 章）。

（一）内脏性疼痛

腹腔内脏由两个神经系统支配：迷走神经传入神经和脊髓内脏感觉神经[6]。脊髓内脏传入神经又称为内脏神经，包含有交感及副交感神经传出通路一起运行的盆腔内脏传入神经（图 11.2）[6]。内脏神经支配肠壁的所有层，包括绒毛膜和肠系膜。这些神经主要由无髓鞘 C 纤维组成，虽然可见很少量有髓鞘的 A-δ 纤维[9]。内脏疼痛在其源头由裸露的神经末梢传导，这些神经末梢缺乏躯体神经末梢的特殊结构，如包膜等。神经生理学研究已经确定了四种不同类型的内脏感觉神经：黏膜中的化学感受器、低阈值机械感受器、高阈值机械感受器和所谓的“沉默的”痛觉感受器[6,9]。黏膜化学感受器对腔内有害物敏感。低阈值机械感受器，也被称为“宽范围”感受器，具有相对高静息状态，可随管壁张力的增高而作出反应。高阈值机械感受器，也被称为“时相”感受器，其静息活性较低，仅对过度的机械扩张有反应。沉默的痛觉感受器只有在炎性介质存在时才会被激活[9]。

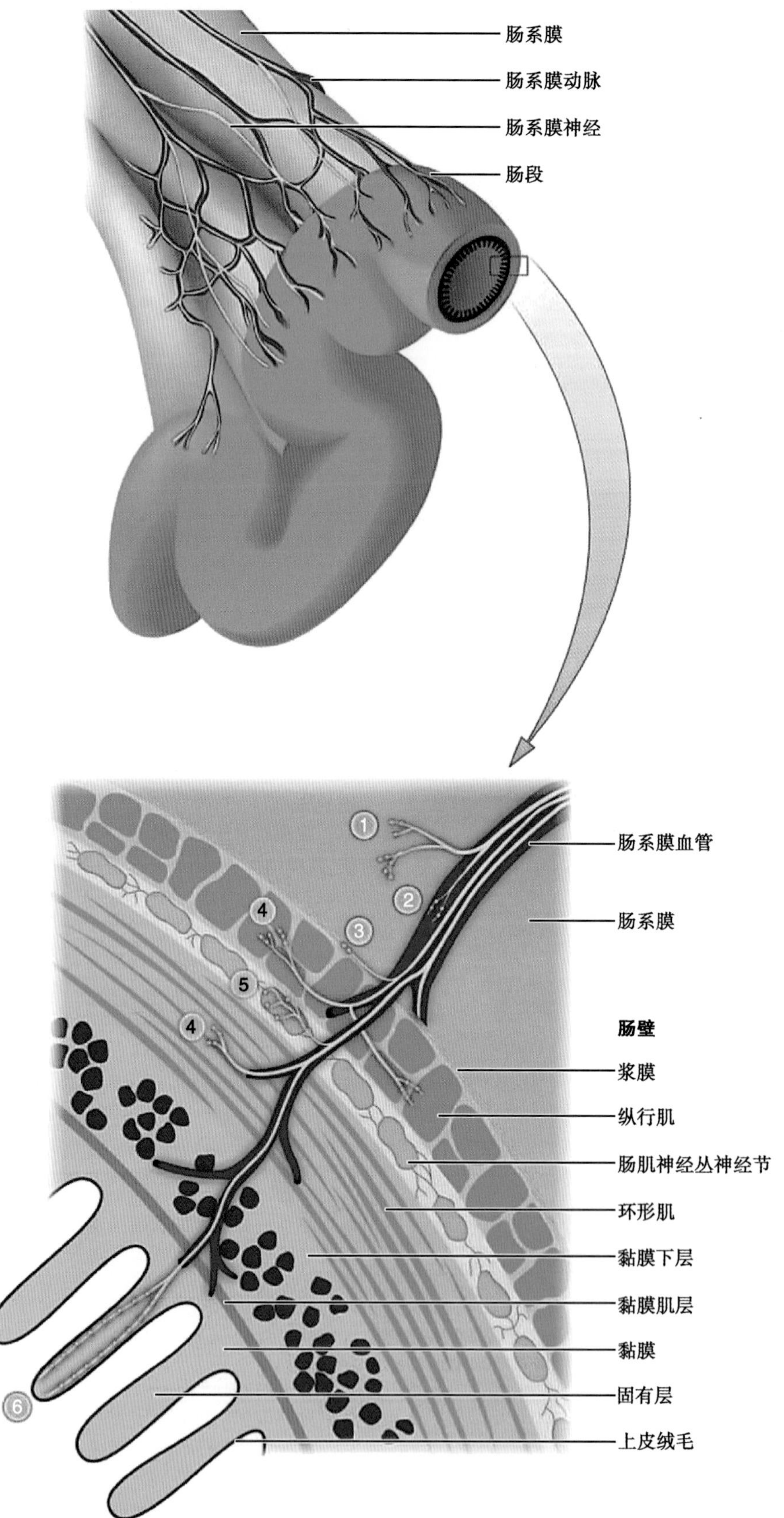

图 11.1 胃肠道的感觉神经支配。显示了传入感觉神经末梢在肠壁的分布,如下:1,肠系膜;2,肠系膜血管;3,浆膜;4,肌内排列(仅迷走神经);5,神经节内板层末梢(仅迷走神经和盆腔神经);6,黏膜。主要造成痛觉的是 1、2、3 和 6。(Modified from Knowles CH, Aziz Q. Basic and clinical aspects of gastrointestinal pain. Pain 2009;141:191-209.)。

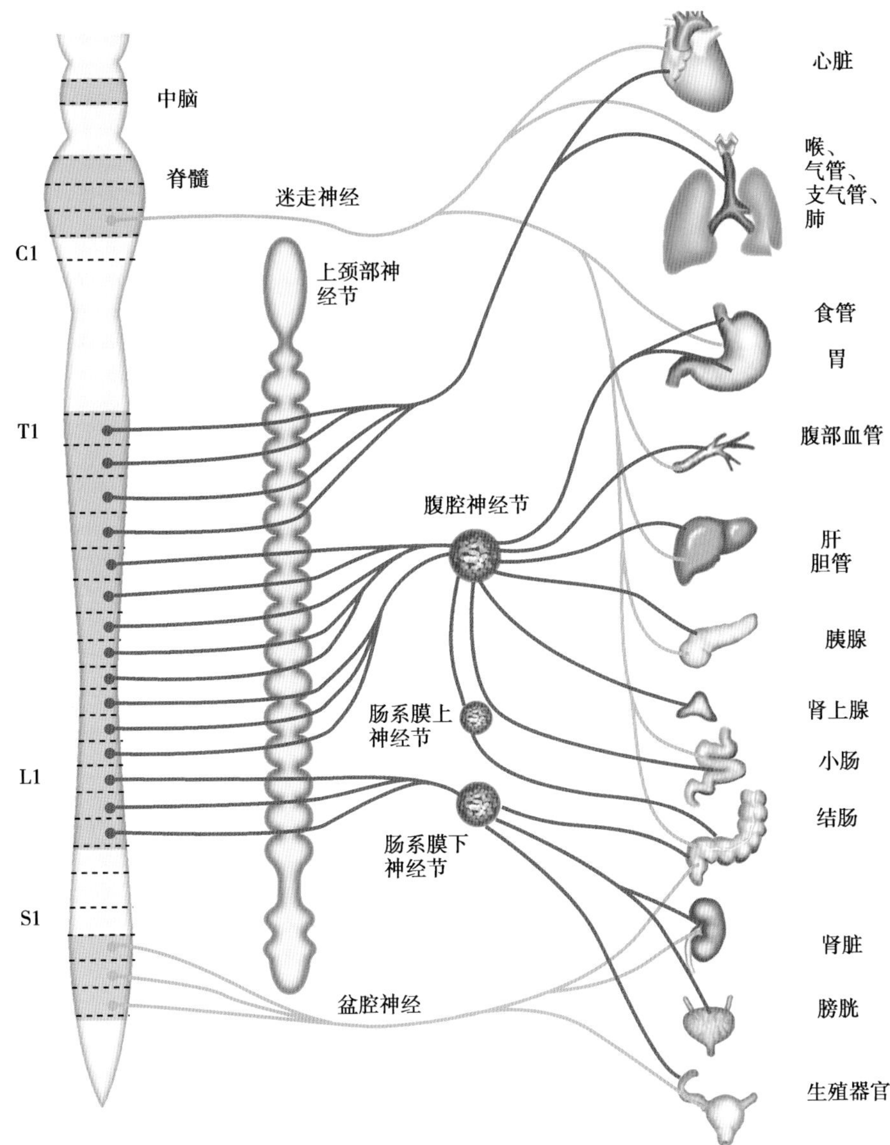

图11.2 内脏感觉神经支配通路。传导疼痛的内脏传入神经伴随有自主神经，将疼痛信号传入中枢神经系统。在腹部，这些神经纤维包括迷走神经、盆腔副交感神经以及胸腰交感神经。交感神经纤维（红线）；副交感神经（蓝线）。脊髓：C，颈椎；L，腰椎；S，骶骨；T，胸椎

高阈值感受器是转导输尿管和肾脏等器官的痛觉，因为这种疼痛是唯一能有意识感知的，而像膀胱和胃这样的器官，对于无害的刺激是没有痛觉的，对于有害的刺激可有意识地感知到，这些感觉是由低阈值和高阈值的感受器感知的[10]。脊髓内脏神经通过椎板Ⅰ、Ⅱ、Ⅴ和Ⅹ在脊髓中呈广泛传入分布[6]。下面4个解剖结构因素导致内脏性疼痛的定位不准确和牵涉性疼痛部位远离其起病源。第一，脊柱内脏传入神经分布于广泛的脊髓背根神经节，疼痛信号输入在脊髓水平呈弥散状态，导致解剖分辨能力差。第二，脊髓传入神经的内脏分布较为广泛和重叠，是双侧进入脊髓的。这种缺乏单侧特异性传入神经，导致内脏性疼痛定位在中线（图11.3）。第三，脊髓背根神经节的传入神经纤维与神经细胞体的比例较低；第四，脊髓背角的内脏传入神经元与躯体疼痛神经元之间存在相当大的汇聚或串扰。因此，内脏性疼痛常被模糊地划分为一个广泛的局部解剖区域。脊髓内的内脏传入神经纤维和腹壁上躯体神经纤维之间的相互干扰，可以产生远离病原部位体表处疼痛的感觉，或指牵涉性疼痛（见后文）。与脊髓内脏传入神经感觉系统不同，迷走传入神经主要传递无害性刺激，如饱足感[6]。

内脏性疼痛主要是由机械性感受器传导的脏器牵拉和扩张的结果，在严重的情况下，沉默的痛觉感受器神经末梢可检测到炎症介质导致疼痛加重。腹部脏器的切割和烧灼不会被认为是有害的。这些特性解释了为什么结肠镜检查时充气过多常常出现疼痛，而息肉切除术却没有疼痛。一旦疼痛信号经内脏痛觉神经元传入中枢神经系统，它们不仅将痛觉投射到作为同侧部分躯体神经感觉的大脑皮质（给信号指定位置和强度），而且还会投射到作为传导疼痛的一部分脑回内，引起不愉快的情绪行为（见第12章）[6]。

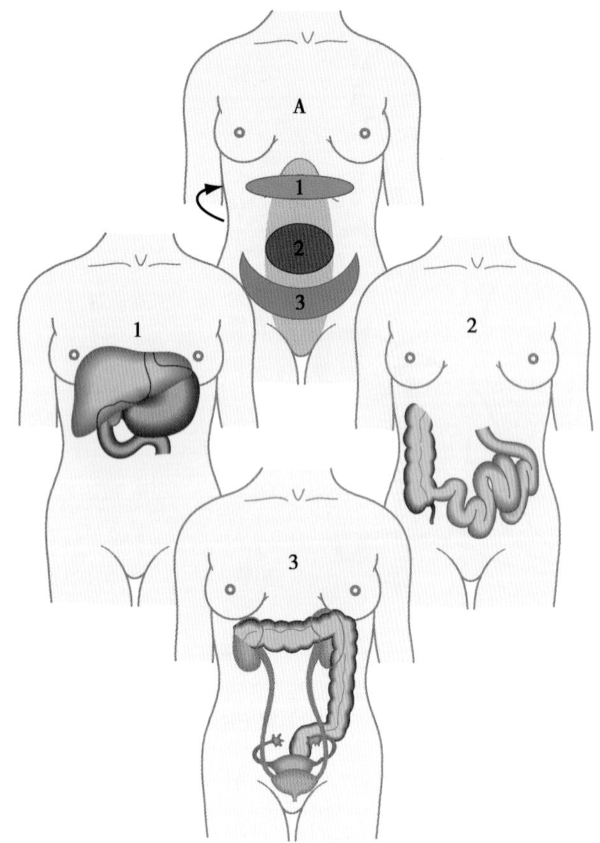

图 11.3 内脏疼痛的定位。分别在上腹部、中腹部和下腹部感觉到 1、2 和 3 中所示的器官区域引起的疼痛，如 A 所示。A 中的箭表示右肩胛区的胆道疼痛

（二）躯体-腔壁性疼痛

躯体-腔壁性疼痛由 A-δ 纤维传导，主要分布于皮肤和肌肉。这种神经通路感知的是尖锐、突发及定位明确的疼痛，例如急性损伤后的疼痛。传递这种痛觉至脊髓的神经就是躯体神经。刺激这些神经纤维可激活由肠神经系统诱导的局部调节反射，及由自主神经系统诱导的脊髓柱反射；除此之外还可以将这种疼痛感觉传递至中枢神经系统[11]。

由腹膜壁层的有害刺激引起的躯体-腔壁性疼痛比内脏性疼痛更强烈，定位更精确。急性阑尾炎就是一个例子，阑尾炎早期引起脐周定位不准确的内脏性疼痛，随后阑尾炎症波及邻近腹膜壁层，就出现定位准确的麦氏点躯体-腔壁性疼痛。躯体神经感知的腹痛通常因运动或振动而加重。传递这种疼痛的神经冲动是躯体感觉脊神经，这些神经是从第六胸（T6）到第一腰椎（L1）椎间发出来，同时支配相应节段的皮肤。因为这些神经纤维不穿过脊髓的中线，所以同侧腹壁疼痛的定位比内脏性疼痛精确得多。腹壁反射（例如，无自主保护，腹肌紧张）就是由躯体神经疼痛通路的脊柱反射弧所致的。脊髓水平段的抑制机制可调节疼痛传入神经冲动。传递皮肤触摸、振动和本体感觉的躯体 A-δ 神经纤维所在的脊髓节段，与受损脏器的内脏传入神经及脊髓胶质抑制性神经元的突触是在同一个脊髓节段内。此外，起源于中脑、脑室旁灰质和尾状核的抑制性神经元下降到脊髓内，调节传入疼痛通路（见第 12 章）[12]。

（三）牵涉性疼痛

当来自不同解剖区域的内脏传入神经元和躯体传入神经元，汇聚到脊髓同一节段的二级神经元时，在远离病变器官区域可感受到牵涉性疼痛。这种汇集可能是由于在胚胎发育早期，相邻结构的神经支配在同一部位，随后因发育改变，导致彼此迁移分开而引起的。因此，牵涉性疼痛可以被理解为是一种早期发育状态（例如，横膈膜的中心腱开始在颈部发育的，随着颅尾的移动，其神经分布及膈神经也随之变动）。图 11.4 显示膈下血肿或脾破裂，刺激膈肌后出现肩部疼痛（Kehr 征）[13]。

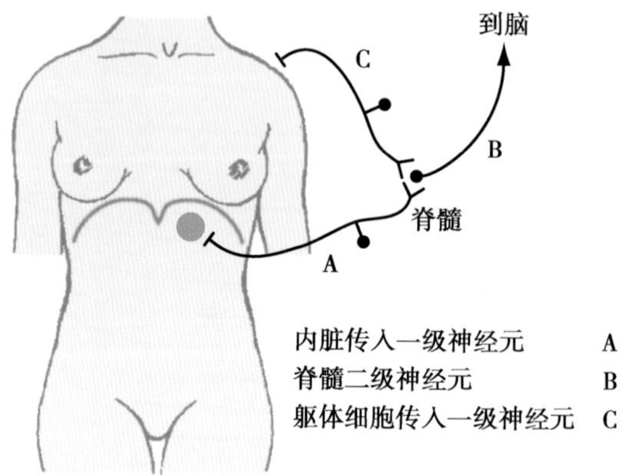

图 11.4 牵涉痛的神经解剖学基础。局部刺激可刺激支配膈肌的内脏传入纤维［如膈下脓肿（圆圈）］。这些内脏传入纤维（A）与脊髓中的二级神经元（B）以及起源于左肩区（颈根 3 至 5）的躯体传入纤维（C）形成突触。大脑将疼痛解释为躯体起源，并将其定位在肩部

二、评估

对急性腹痛患者的有效评估需要仔细而迅速的病史采集和体格检查（经常是连续反复多次检查），在许多情况，还需要选择性地做影像学检查。仔细询问病史和体格检查，配合适当及时的影像学检查，通常可以相对较快地作出准确的诊断。临床评估不充分或影像学方法选择不当，可能会出现不必要的病情延误，往往导致不良结果的发生。具有相似临床表现的疾病，如阑尾炎、胆囊炎和憩室炎，可以通过病史、体格检查及必要的影像学检查，几乎可以获得完全准确的诊断；其他疾病的患者也可以通过有序有效的评估和正确的选择影像学检查，获得初步诊断。

（一）急诊处理方法

腹痛有可能是危及生命的腹部疾患（“急腹症”）的表现。因此，当处理急性腹痛患者时。医生应首先快速评估患者的整体生理状态，寻找患者休克或血流动力学不稳定的原因。才能迅速治疗，从而获得满意的治疗效果。休克可表现为脸色苍白、发绀、花斑样改变、虚脱、低血压、心动过速或其他低灌注症状，如心动过速、呼吸急促和代谢性酸中毒。急性腹痛患者的评估除应包括心动过速、低血压等生命体征改变外，还应包括器官灌注评估，特别是血清乳酸、血小板计数、血清胆红素、格拉斯哥（Glasgow）昏迷评分、血清肌酐等。序贯器官

衰竭评估（Sequential Organ Failure Assessment，SOFA）（表 11.1）是评估败血症早期出现全身炎症反应的有用工具[14]。在急性腹痛的情况下，SOFA 评分大于或等于 2，血清乳酸水平大于 2，或需要升压药物支持的患者定义为感染性休克。如果有明显不稳定血流动力学表现，包括有休克的临床证据，应立即寻求外科会诊，气管插管和积极进行血流动力学复苏。急诊护理外科的格言是"死亡从放射学开始"，这提醒我们在影像诊断之前就应进行血流动力学复苏。

表 11.1　序贯器官衰竭评估（SOFA）

分数		1	2	3	4
器官系统	单位				
呼吸系统					
PaO_2/FiO_2	mmHg	<400	<300	<200*	<100*
凝血功能					
血小板	$000/mm^3$	<150	<100	<50	<20
肝脏					
胆红素	mg/dL	1.2~1.9	2.0~5.9	6.0~11.9	≥12
	μmol/L	20~32	33~101	102~204	>204
中枢神经系统					
Glasgow 昏迷评分		13~14	10~12	6~9	<6
肾脏					
肌酐	mg/dL	1.2~1.9	2.0~3.4	3.5~4.9	>5g
	μmol/L	110~170	171~299	300~440	>440
尿量	mL/d	—	—	<500	<200

*或需要呼吸支持。
SOFA 评分=个体器官系统评分之和。
如果在急性腹痛的情况下，SOFA 评分大于 2，则应怀疑败血症。
感染性休克定义为：SOFA 评分大于 2 且血清乳酸盐水平大于 2mmol/L 或在感染情况下需要使用血管升压药物。
Adapted from Singer M, Deutschman CS, Seymour CW, et al. The Third International Consensus Defnitions for Sepsis and Septic Shock (Sep-sis-3). JAMA 2016;315:801-10.

（二）病史

在 1921 年，Zachary Cope 爵士在他首次发表的关于腹痛论文中告诉我们，"可以自信地断言，即使不是绝大多数，也有大量的急性腹部疾病可以通过仔细询问病史，就可以对急性腹痛的病因作出诊断。"[15] 尽管，从那时起 1 个世纪以来，在临床影像学上取得了很大的进步，病史的询问或采集仍然是急性腹痛患者，最初评估最重要的组成部分。各种常见原因的急性腹痛相关疼痛的特征见表 11.2。关注这些疼痛特征可以帮助我们尽快作出临床诊断，或在鉴别诊断中排除重要疾病，从而可提高后续诊断性检查的可靠性和有效性。例如，当临床上高度怀疑有肠梗阻症状时，腹部平片对诊断就最有效[16]。

表 11.2　急性腹痛常见原因的比较

病因	起病	疼痛部位	特征	疼痛性质	放射痛	疼痛的强烈程度
急性阑尾炎	逐渐起病	早期在肚脐周围，后期在右下腹	早期范围弥散，后期定位准确	疼痛	无	++
胆囊炎	急性起病	上腹部中部，右上腹，右肩胛骨	定位明确	压痛	肩胛骨	++
胰腺炎	急性起病	上腹部，背部胸椎 10 至腰椎 2 区域	定位明确	钻顶样痛	中背部	++到+++
憩室炎	逐渐起病	左下腹部	定位明确	疼痛	无	++到+++
消化性溃疡穿孔	突发起病	上腹部	早期定位明确，后期范围弥散	烧灼痛	无	+++
小肠梗阻	逐渐起病	肚脐周围	范围弥散	痉挛性痛	无	++
肠系膜缺血、梗死	突发起病	肚脐周围	范围弥散	痛苦难忍	无	+++
腹主动脉瘤破裂	突发起病	腹部、背部、两侧腹	范围弥散	撕裂样痛	无	+++
胃肠炎	逐渐起病	肚脐周围	范围弥散	间歇性隐痛	无	+到++
盆腔感染性疾病	逐渐起病	下腹或盆腔	定位明确	疼痛	大腿	++
异位妊娠破裂	突发起病	下腹或盆腔	定位明确	尖锐性刺痛	无	++

+，轻度；++，中度；+++，重度。

1. 疼痛发展过程

几种常见急性腹痛病程如图 11.5 所示。起病的急缓往往可以帮助判断疾病的严重程度。疼痛出现突然，且为全腹剧烈疼痛，可能是腹内脏器出现了严重的病变，如空腔脏器穿孔、肠系膜血管梗死或动脉瘤破裂。这种患者通常能准确地回忆起疼痛发作准确时刻；腹痛的进展对判断疾病的病因也是一个重要的因素。某些疾病（如肠胃炎）所致腹痛有自限性，而在另一些疾病（如阑尾炎）的腹痛是进行性加重的。如果腹痛呈阵发性尤其伴随有恶心及呕吐，可诊断为空腔脏器梗阻；腹痛持续时间对疾病严重程度的判断也很重要。长期腹痛（例如，几周）往往在短期内不会危及生命，而那些数小时或数天内出现腹痛的患者更可能是有危及生命的急性疾病。

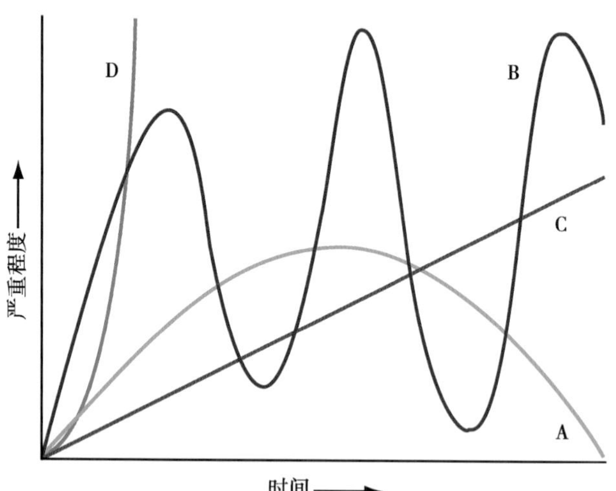

图 11.5　急性腹痛的类型。A，许多引起腹痛的病因，随时间的推移而自行消退（如肠胃炎）。B，有些疼痛是绞痛（即疼痛呈加剧，缓解交替出现），如肠、肾和胆道疼痛（绞痛）。时间过程可能差异很大，从肠道和肾脏疼痛的数分钟到胆道疼痛的数天、数周甚至数月。C，通常急性腹痛是进行性的，如急性阑尾炎或憩室炎。D，某些情况是灾难性发作，（呈突发、急剧严重过程），如腹主动脉瘤破裂

2. 疼痛部位

腹痛的部位可为解释病因提供线索。如前所述，一个伤害性刺激可能会导致内脏性、躯体-腔壁性和牵涉性疼痛的组合，因此，会出现疼痛部位不明确或多部位的疼痛感知，除非考虑神经解剖途径，否则会造成解释上的混淆。例如，左侧膈下脓肿引起的膈肌刺激疼痛，可牵涉到同侧肩部，并易被误解为缺血性心脏病引起的疼痛（见图 11.4）。胰腺或胆道疾病引起的背部放射性疼痛，可能与肌肉骨骼的病变相混淆，从而延误治疗。疼痛部位的变化，可代表从内脏刺激进展为局部壁腹膜刺激（如阑尾炎），或代表发生弥漫性腹膜刺激（如溃疡穿孔）。

3. 腹痛强度及特征

急性腹痛通常有 3 种形式出现。第一种是无法忍受剧烈疼痛，通常是由严重而又危及生命的疾病所导致的，如内脏穿孔、动脉瘤破裂或重症胰腺炎。第二种是空腔脏器梗阻的患者，如肠梗阻、肾绞痛或胆道疼痛，开始以逐渐加重痉挛性疼痛，随后出现阵发性剧烈疼痛，可以有缓解和加剧交替出现。往往伴随有恶心呕吐是这类疾病的典型症状。恶心或呕吐不一定是肠道梗阻，可以有其他脏器梗阻也会出现如肾结石。第三种方式是逐渐加重的不适感，通常开始时疼痛模糊不清，且疼痛部位不明确，但随着疼痛加剧，其疼痛部位逐渐明确。由炎症引起的急性阑尾炎或憩室炎，通常其疼痛特征就是这样的。而另一些疾病，如急性胆囊炎，开始时可能是因梗阻引起腹绞痛，随着病情的演变出现胆囊炎后，疼痛就变成持续性。临床医生应该谨慎，不要过分重视患者对疼痛的描述；异常是常见的，一个对疼痛准确的描述需要涉及诸多因素。而老年人即使可能存在有危及生命的病理因素，其症状可能很轻微，或不典型，所以对这群人疼痛的诊断具有一定难度。

4. 腹痛加重或缓解因素

疼痛与体位变化、饮食、排便和压力的关系，可为诊断提供重要线索。腹膜炎的患者躺着不动，而肾绞痛的患者可能会辗转不安，试图找到一个舒服的姿势。有时，某些食物会加剧疼痛，典型的例子就是，胆道疾病所致疼痛往往与摄入高脂肪食物有关。十二指肠溃疡所致疼痛常以进餐后可缓解；相反，胃溃疡或慢性肠系膜缺血性疾病往往出现进食时疼痛加剧。还可以根据患者常自行用药来缓解症状的线索来帮助其诊断。例如，慢性抗酸药或非甾体抗炎药使用史可能提示消化性溃疡的存在。随着患者和医生越来越多地依赖非甾体抗炎药来替代阿片类药物治疗慢性疼痛，这一问题得到越来越多的关注。

5. 相关症状

应了解患者有无全身症状（如发热、寒战、盗汗、体重减轻、肌痛、关节痛）、消化功能障碍（如厌食、恶心、呕吐、胀气、腹泻、便秘）、黄疸、排尿困难、月经周期的变化和是否受孕等方面的情况。仔细检查了解这些临床表现对诊断有重要价值。呕吐物为进食后的胃内容物，提示胃的出口梗阻；而含有粪质的呕吐物提示远端小肠或结肠梗阻。一系列发现的现象可帮助找到疾病的原因。

6. 既往病史

仔细询问患者的其他医疗问题往往能帮助诊断急性腹痛的原因。以前有过类似症状提示是一种复发性疾病。有部分小肠梗阻、肾结石或盆腔炎症可呈复发性。对于表现为肠梗阻且无手术史的患者，应给予特别关注，因为有可能是需要外科手术治疗的疾病，如疝气或肿瘤。全身性疾病的患者，如硬皮病、系统性红斑狼疮、肾病综合征、卟啉症或镰状细胞病，通常以腹痛表现来就诊。另外，在治疗某种疾病时，其所使用的药物副作用也可能引起腹痛。

（三）体格检查

如前所述，对急性腹痛患者的体格检查首先要评估患者的外貌，以及尽早了解有无脓毒症或休克的体征。应注意患者的对答能力、呼吸方式、床上的体位、有无强迫姿势、不适程度和面部是否有痛苦表情。如果患者以卷曲姿势一动不动地躺在床上，不愿移动或不想说话，面部表情痛苦，很可能患有急性腹膜炎。如果患者痉挛式疼痛并不断改变体位，仅仅是内脏性疼痛，很可能是肠梗阻或胃肠炎。有呼吸急促的表现，可能是休克引起的代谢性酸中毒的迹象。如果体格检查或心

电图发现有心房颤动，提示有肠系膜动脉血栓形成。无论病史提示何种诊断，所有患者都应进行详细的全身系统检查。

1. 腹部检查

评估急性腹痛的腹部检查至关重要，应将两乳头的连线到两大腿都应完全暴露，进行整个腹部的认真而仔细的检查。肥胖患者应询问腹壁突出程度是否大于既往正常状态。虚弱的患者可能会感到腹胀，但腹部突出相对不明显。在进行任何会干扰性腹部内容物的操作之前，应先了解肠鸣音是否存在及其活跃程度。如果无肠鸣音，检查者至少要在腹部的一个部位听 2 分钟，并在多个部位反复听诊。有经验的医师可以从中毒性巨结肠的空洞声里分辨出机械小肠梗阻（small intestine obstruction，SBO）的高音搅动声。然而，一些研究人员对 SBO 和其他疾病所致肠鸣音差异评估的可靠性提出了质疑[17]，临床医生在做出诊断时不应太过于依赖于肠鸣音的评估。然而，听诊可能是评估压痛的一种好方法，用听诊器听诊时，聪明的临床医生一边用听诊器头触诊腹部，一边同时仔细观察患者的面部表情。如果发现有压痛，接下来应进行反跳痛评估，以寻找腹膜炎的证据。震动患者的床或担架，或叩诊可能会引发反跳痛。接下来进行触诊时，应先检查远离疾病脏器周围，最后触诊疾病脏器投影的体表部位，以避免腹肌出现不自觉保护而致腹肌收缩张力增高，腹部张力增加后，体格检查时很难有其他的发现（如肿块）。由于这些患者通常有外科急诊，故麻醉开腹手术前，应彻底检查腹部。

2. 生殖器、直肠和盆腔检查

每个急性腹痛患者都应检查盆腔脏器和外生殖器。直肠指检和阴道检查可以帮助了解盆腔脏器是否有病变。所有急性腹痛的妇女都应排除妇科疾病。

（四）实验室检查

对于急性腹痛患者，仅有病史和体格检查通常不足以得到一个明确的诊断。所有急性腹痛患者，都应该做全血细胞及分类计数和尿检。测定血清电解质、血尿素氮、肌酐和葡萄糖水平对评估患者的血容量和酸碱状态、肾功能和代谢状态是有用的。所以对于每一位到急诊科就诊的急性腹痛患者都应做这些检查。育龄期妇女出现腹痛都必须进行尿或血清妊娠检查；对于有上腹痛或黄疸的患者，应进行肝功能、血清淀粉酶及脂肪酶检查。

白细胞总数增多，特别又有中性粒细胞分类增高，这些均是一个重要的发现。代谢性酸中毒、血清乳酸水平升高或碳酸氢盐水平降低与组织灌注不足和休克相关。出现这些现象的患者可能需要紧急手术干预，或进入重症室进行密切监护。

（五）影像学检查

1. 计算机断层扫描

高速螺旋计算机断层扫描（CT）的发展彻底改变了急性腹痛的评估。在许多情况下，如阑尾炎，CT 几乎可以消除诊断的不确定性。在无 CT 时代，仅病史和体格检查的特异性约为 80%；而 CT 对急性阑尾炎的敏感性和特异性分别是 94% 和 95%。急性腹痛的 CT 检查阴性，对于排除常见疾病具有相当大的价值。

有关能否将 CT 作为所有急性腹痛患者评估的标准检查法，人们提出了几个质疑[18]。第一，CT 有很多种检查方法，在特定临床环境下如何能选择最有效的方法。例如，怀疑有肾绞痛的患者，做平扫就可以诊断肾结石，在这种情况下，如果做增强 CT 就可能看不到结石而误诊。另外，怀疑为动脉闭塞性疾病的患者应使用造影剂进行 CT 动脉造影。对于就诊患者，选择最合适的 CT 检查应咨询放射科医生。第二，一些疾病，如急性胆囊炎和胆管炎，CT 并不是最佳的检查法。当出现右上腹疼痛的患者如果怀疑有这两种诊断中的任何一种时，上腹部超声检查才是主要诊断手段。第三，如前所述，当患者病情不稳定或有休克迹象时，应由外科医生进行评估，然后再考虑任何影像学检查。在怀疑有外伤或腹腔积血的患者中，腹部创伤超声重点评估是一个更好的检查方法，这可以在急诊科的床边完成。伴有休克或腹腔积液是剖腹探查手术的指征，而进一步的诊断手段，包括 CT 检查，或对患者的护理几乎没有价值。

另外，用 CT 评估急性腹痛，还应考虑 CT 是一种有放射辐射暴露检查。特别是 35 岁以下的患者和需要多次检查的患者，腹部 CT 可能会增加患癌症可能的风险[18]。此外，最好避免对孕妇进行 CT 检查，除非怀疑有危及生命的情况发生，这时的磁共振成像（MRI）是一个不错的选择[19]。

2. 超声

腹部创伤超声重点评估（focused abdominal sonogram for trauma，FAST）是一种快速、可靠、可床旁检测腹腔内积液的方法。虽然其主要用途是对外伤患者的评估，这种检查也有助于发现任何原因引起的腹腔内游离液体；可以增加主动脉成像，从而对主动脉瘤进行快速评估。对急性腹痛的评估，及时的腹部超声检查已经成为一个常规而又高度可信的检查手段[20]。

（六）其他诊断检查

其他诊断成像方式，如 MRI 和放射性核素扫描［如^{99m}Tc 标记的羟基亚氨基二乙酸（hydroxyl iminodiacetic acid，HIDA）］和内镜检查通常在急性腹痛患者的评估中起次要作用。这些测试的使用通常以 CT 或超声的结果为指导。血管造影可能不仅对内脏缺血的诊断有用，而且对改善或重建血液流动的治疗可提供有用的信息。诊断性腹腔灌洗，虽然现在很少使用，但在患者有心肺功能不太稳定，而又需要做影像学检查，这种方法还是有用的。在某些严重情况下，从病情不稳定的灌洗液中发现了白细胞，可能是剖腹探查手术的指征。对于病情不稳定、病情又恶化的急腹症患者，如果影像学检查有风险，应考虑剖腹探查手术。急性腹痛的整体处理方法如图 11.6 所示。

三、病因

急性腹痛通常定义为持续时间小于 1 周的疼痛。患者通常在最初的 24~48 小时内就医，尽管有些患者可能会忍受更长时间的腹部不适。患者寻求急诊评估腹痛最常见的原因是所谓的非特异性腹痛，在所有因腹痛到急诊科就诊的患者中，25%~50% 急诊腹痛的患者没有明确的特定疾病。急诊患者腹痛原因的构成比见表 11.3。

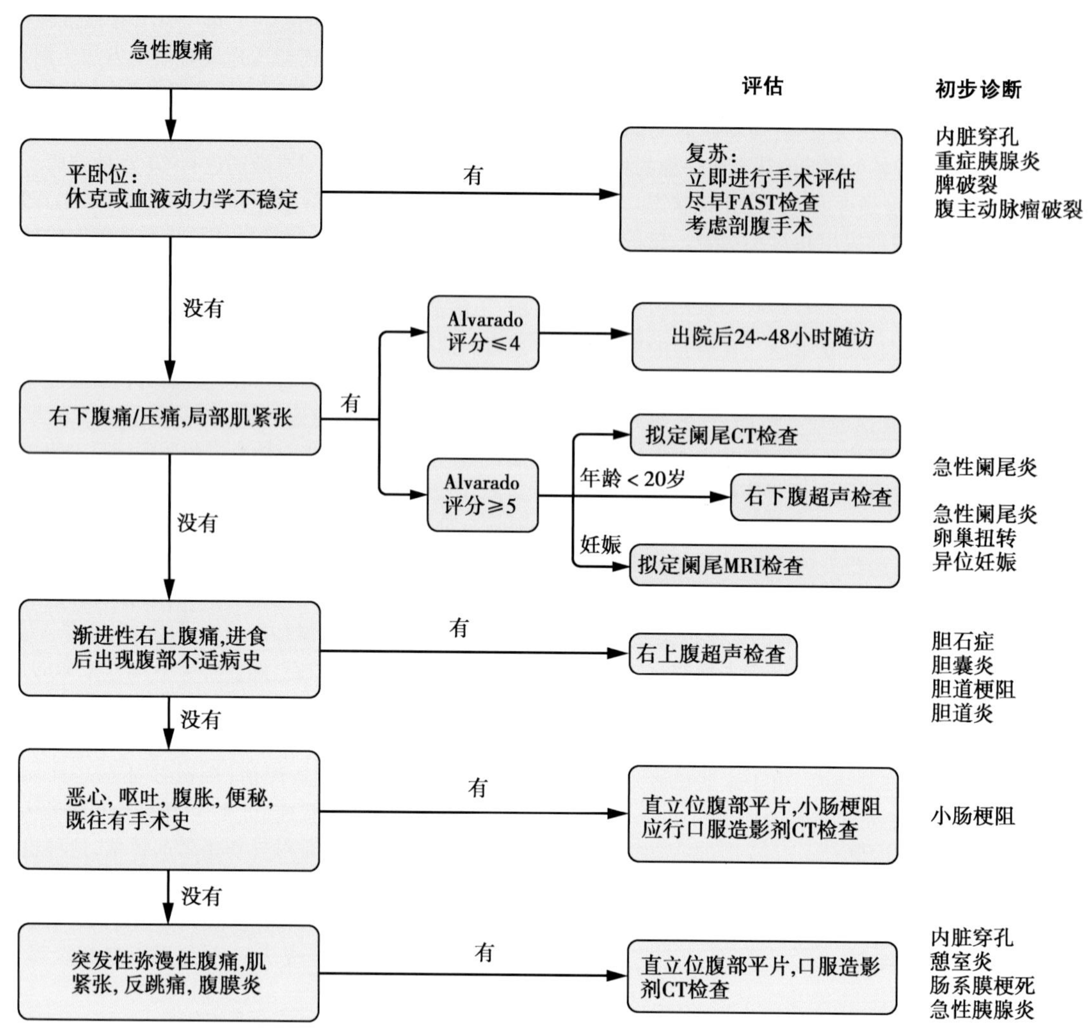

图 11.6　腹痛紧急评估方法。具体主诉和体格检查结果与适当的成像检查相结合。对于左下腹痛，最有可能的诊断是憩室炎。FAST，腹部创伤超声重点评估

表 11.3　急诊科就诊患者急性腹痛的原因构成比

病因	占比/%
非特异性腹痛	35
阑尾炎	17
小肠梗阻	15
泌尿系统疾病	6
胆道系统疾病	5
憩室疾病	4
胰腺炎	2
内科疾病	1
其他	15

From Irvin TT. Causes of abdominal pain in 1190 patients admitted to a British surgical service. Br J Surg 1989;76:1121-5.

（一）急性阑尾炎

急性阑尾炎是一种常见病，约占所有急诊 65 岁以下患者的 5%[21]，30% 的外科急症患者是在 50 岁以下[22]。2006 年美国因阑尾炎住院的患者有 318 000 人[23]，在北美的总发病率约为 82/10 万~110/10 万[24]。在西方国家[25]，男性一生中患阑尾炎的风险为 8.6%，女性为 6.7%，而在亚洲，这一风险可能是其两倍[26]。

急性阑尾炎的前驱症状常为厌食、恶心和脐周疼痛。6~8 小时内，疼痛转移至右下腹，腹膜体征出现。在无并发症的阑尾炎患者往往以低热至中度发热为主，通常为 38℃左右，轻度白细胞增多。较高的体温和白细胞计数明显增高，与穿孔和脓肿的形成有关。阑尾炎患者的病史、体格检查和白细胞计数的等特征，已纳入 Alvarado 评分法作为预测工具（表 11.4）[27]。对于男性来说，得分为 4 分或更低就可以排除阑尾炎，这个分数对妇女和儿童就没有那么有用了[28]。然而，急性阑尾炎的临床症状常常可表现为不典型，不能仅仅根据患者的病史和体格检查就否定急性阑尾炎的诊断，故有人提出了阑尾炎炎症反应的评分[29]。在儿童，肠系膜淋巴结炎（或淋巴结炎）经常被误诊为急性阑尾炎，但这种疾病通常有咽痛，并有自限性。肠系膜淋巴结炎也可能由耶尔森菌（*Yersinia enterocolitica*）引起的小肠结肠炎所致（见第 110 章）。

表 11.4　预测急性阑尾炎的 Alvarado 评分法

表现	分值
疼痛迁移	1
食欲不振	1
恶心	1
右下腹肌张力	2
反跳痛	1
发热	1
白细胞增多	2
白细胞核左移	1
总分	10

5~6 分提示阑尾炎；7~8 分阑尾炎的可能性比较大；9~10 分临床上可诊断阑尾炎。评分大于或等于 5 的患者应由外科医生进行评估或接受影像学检查以明确阑尾炎的诊断。

From Alvarado A. A practical score for the early diagnosis of acute appendicitis. Ann Emerg Med 1986；15：557-64.

CT 对急性阑尾炎有诊断价值，但腹部平片对急性阑尾炎的诊断没有意义。CT 上阑尾直径大于 10mm 通常就可以诊断为阑尾炎，尽管阑尾直径的正常范围可达 13mm[30]。急性阑尾炎的其他 CT 征象包括阑尾周围脂肪炎症，右下腹积液，以及增强扫描阑尾不显影[31]。CT 检查使阴性阑尾炎被切除率降低到 5% 左右[32]。因为 CT 有放射线辐射[18]，一些权威人士提倡避免对儿童和青少年进行 CT 检查[33]，在这些患者中，如果疑诊阑尾炎，需要检查建议用低放射性辐射的检查方法（见 120 章），如阑尾超声检查，其敏感性为 0.86，特异性为 0.81[34]。对于孕妇来说，也应避免放射线辐射暴露，MRI 已经成为孕妇首选的影像检查方法，其灵敏度和特异性接近 CT[35]。

（二）急性胆源性疾病

胆道疾病约占急诊科因腹痛而就诊的 7%，占 65 岁以上患者入院的 14%~121%[21,22]。受影响的患者通常在胆道疼痛（“胆绞痛”）和急性胆囊炎之间的疾病谱的某个点出现。胆道疼痛是一种右上腹（RUQ）或上腹疼痛综合征（通常在餐后），由胆结石引起的胆囊管一过性梗阻引起，具有自限性，一般持续不超过 6 小时。在大多数情况下，急性胆囊炎是由胆结石持续阻塞胆囊管引起的。急性胆囊炎的疼痛除了持续性外，几乎与胆源性疼痛没有区别，疼痛通常是局限于 RUQ 或上腹部的钝痛，可放射至背部及右肩胛骨，常伴有恶心、呕吐和低热等症状，检查时，可发现 RUQ 压痛、肌紧张和墨菲征（Murphy 征、RUQ 触诊时吸气骤停）是典型的。白细胞计数通常轻度升高，但也可能正常。血清总胆红素和碱性磷酸酶水平轻度升高很常见。

胆结石在胆道疼痛和急性胆囊炎病因学中的作用，使 RUQ 的超声检查成为关键的诊断手段。超声胆结石的显示可能提示胆道疼痛，而发现结石伴胆囊壁增厚、胆囊周围积液和超声探头压迫胆囊时出现的疼痛（超声墨菲征阳性），基本上可诊断急性胆囊炎，已取代肝胆闪烁显影（如 HIDA 扫描）在急性胆囊炎诊断中的应用[36]。虽然超声对结石的检测很敏感，但发现检测急性胆囊炎的灵敏度（73.4%）和特异度（85.5%）较差[37]。体格检查和实验室检查，再结合影像学检查对急性胆囊炎的准确诊断至关重要。急性胆囊炎东京共识诊断标准见表 11.5。急性胆囊炎患者最好在 48 小时内行胆囊切除术[38,39]。年龄较大、心动过速、超声表现有胆囊壁增厚的患者，特别是白细胞计数大于 13 000/mm^3 的患者，发生坏疽性胆囊炎的风险较高，通常需要紧急开腹胆囊切除术[40,41]。

表 11.5　急性胆囊炎东京诊断标准

A. 炎症的局部表现
墨菲征炎性
右上腹疼痛、包块、压痛
B. 全身感染表现
发热
C 反应蛋白升高
白细胞计数升高
C. 胆囊炎的影像学表现
明确诊断
临床上有 A 项，或有 B、C 中之一项，怀疑为急性胆囊炎时

Adapted from. Hirota J, Takada T, Kawarada Y, et al. Diagnostic criteria and severity assessment of acute cholecystitis; Tokyo Guidelines. Hepatobiliary Pancreat Surg 2007；14：78-82.

临床表现为 RUQ 疼痛、黄疸和败血症体征的患者，应怀疑胆结石阻塞胆管。RUQ 疼痛、发热、寒战以及黄疸（Charcot 三联征）提示上行性胆管炎[42]。这些患者需要静脉输液、抗生素和胆管引流，通常需要急诊内镜检查（见第 65、66、67 和 70 章）。

（三）小肠梗阻

无论在发达国家还是发展中国家[22]，肠梗阻都是引起腹痛的常见原因，各个年龄段的患者都可发生肠梗阻。在儿童以肠套叠、先天性畸形如旋转不良、梅克尔（Meckel）憩室为最常见原因[43]。成人约 70% 的病例是由术后粘连引起，还有很大一部分是因嵌顿疝，炎症性肠病和恶性肿瘤所致腹痛[44,45]。SBO 的特征是突然的，痉挛性脐周疼痛。伴有随后出现的恶心和呕吐，可以短暂缓解，而以反复发作为特点。体格检查显示病情急而严重、焦躁不安，常有发热、心动过速和血容积减少的迹象，包括直立性低血压。腹胀也很常见，但在肥胖的情况下可能很难辨别。尽管 SBO 患者的听诊常有肠鸣音亢进和气过水声，但这些体征并不能作为诊断的唯一条件[17]，需结合腹部叩诊和触诊。当腹部呈弥散性内脏疼痛时，体格检查往往没有一个定位明确的压痛点，这时应高度怀疑有肠缺血或穿孔。白细胞增多和乳酸酸中毒提示肠缺血或梗死。

腹部平片发现有扩张的小肠环、液气平及远端低张力的小肠和结肠，就可以诊断肠梗阻[46]。对于近端空肠梗阻的患者，腹部平片容易被误诊，因为有时候没有扩张的肠袢和“液气平”。CT 对肠梗阻的诊断和定位具有优势，低强化的肠壁是出现肠绞窄的征象,而无腹腔游离液体又明显降低了肠绞窄的可能性[47]。而其他征象如疼痛点移位,并不一定是缺血的可信征象。必要时可以进行干预检查[47]。

在有可靠的体检和实验室结果的 SBO 患者中,最初的治疗是让肠管休息,静脉输液,鼻胃肠减压术和密切观察[48,49]。对于入院接受非手术治疗的 SBO 患者,一个重要的检查手段就是经口或鼻胃管给 120ml 稀释造影剂,如果 12 小时在内盲肠出现造影剂,预示着梗阻已解除[50]。如果经保守治疗失败或有完全梗阻的证据,尤其怀疑肠缺血时需要急诊手术,而粘连性 SBO 需手术的比例不到 20%(见第 123 章)[48,50]。

(四) 急性憩室炎

急性憩室炎是一种常见病,大约 80% 的患者年龄大于 50 岁[51]。该疾病的总发病率增加了 50%,年轻人增加幅度更大[52,53]。憩室炎患者通常表现为左下腹(LLQ)持续性钝性疼痛和发热,可有排便困难或顽固性便秘,通常发现白细胞增多。体格检查显示 LLQ 压痛,部分病例有 LLQ 肿块。常在局部有腹膜刺激征。在严重情况下可出现全腹膜炎的表现,难以与其他原因所致空腔脏器穿孔鉴别,CT 可以帮助诊断,其灵敏度为 97%[54],对憩室炎患者的急诊评估,可常规进行 CT 检查。

急性憩室炎临床表现多样性,可有轻度腹部不适,也可出现粪源性腹膜炎的征象,这是外科急症。通过 CT 检查,可以确定憩室炎的严重程度,最好使用 Hinchey 分级系统来描述(见第 121 章表 121.2)。CT 无穿孔表现,且病情轻无并发症的患者,一般可门诊治疗。Hinchey Ⅰ型(局限性腹壁脓肿或炎症)患者常需要住院治疗,静脉注射抗生素。Hinchey Ⅱ型(盆腔、腹腔内或腹膜后脓肿)患者应该在 CT 引导下穿刺引流脓肿并接受一个疗程的广谱抗生素治疗。Hinchey Ⅲ型(化脓性全腹膜炎)和Ⅳ型(粪性全腹膜炎)患者常需急诊手术(见第 121 章)。尽管憩室炎分级具有诊断意义,但几乎没有证据支持其在选择手术或药物治疗之间有预测价值[55]。出现明显腹痛或压痛的患者可从早期的外科会诊中获益。

(五) 急性胰腺炎

在美国住院患者急性胰腺炎似乎正在增加[56]。急性胰腺炎典型症状是急性上腹疼痛,疼痛呈持续、剧烈,常放射至背部或左肩胛区域,可伴随有发热、厌食、恶心和呕吐,坐直位或身体稍前倾时通常腹痛略缓解。体格检查可有急性痛苦面容,常有心动过速和呼吸急促,上腹部叩诊和触诊有明显叩痛或压痛,肠鸣音减少,以及腹部肌张力增高。个别患者在两侧腹及脐周可出现瘀斑(分别为 Grey-Turner 或 Cullen 征),这说明胰腺大量坏死伴有出血;或四肢常冰冷和发绀,提示血液灌注不足。白细胞计数常常增高,可大至 12 000~20 000/mm^3。血清和尿淀粉酶水平升高通常出现在疼痛最初几小时内;血清脂肪酶也升高。根据胰腺炎的病因和严重程度,可出现血清电解质、钙、血糖水平、肝脏生化检查和动脉血气结果异常。超声有助于判断胰腺炎的病因是否由胆结石所致。CT 只适用于重症或胰腺炎并发症的诊断[57]。

虽然大多数急性胰腺炎病例是自限性的,但多达 20% 患者病情严重,并伴有局部或全身并发症,包括低血容量和休克、肾功能衰竭、肝功能衰竭和低钙血症。许多生理预后学量化表(如 SOFA 和 APACHE Ⅱ评分)已被作为衡量急性胰腺炎严重程度的指标[58]。Ranson 评分首次发表于 1974 年,至今仍是早期评估急性胰腺炎患者的有用且广泛采纳的检查表[59]。Ranson 评分包括 5 个早期因素和 6 个晚期因素,可提示有重症胰腺炎的倾向(见表 58.2)。急性胰腺炎严重程度(bedside index of the severity of acute pancreatitis,BISAP)的一个更简单的床边指标,包括血尿素氮大于 25mg/dL,男性,全身炎症反应综合征,年龄大于 60 岁,胸腔积液,这些指标也被证明是有用的[60]。急性胰腺炎亚特兰大分级系统在临床诊断中具有重要的应用价值[61],无器官衰竭或没有局部或全身并发症的患者分类为轻度,内科治疗效果好;器官衰竭持续时间少于 48 小时为中重度急性胰腺炎;当器官衰竭持续时间超过 48 小时,或影响多个系统时,考虑重症急性胰腺炎,通常需要重症监护室的多学科治疗。少数重症急性胰腺炎患者可出现严重的腹腔内脏器病变,通常是胰头附近的中结肠动脉或右结肠动脉血栓形成引起结肠梗死,病程早期这一过程 CT 可能看不清楚,临床上如果出现急速血流动力学不稳定为特征的病例,都应怀疑此症,这类患者需要立即开腹手术(见第 58 章)。

(六) 消化性溃疡穿孔

全世界有多达 400 万人受到消化性溃疡(peptic ulcer disease,PUD)的影响。其中有 5% 的患者出现穿孔[62]。PUD 的流行病学正在发生变化(见第 53 章)。自 20 世纪 90 年代末以来,*Hp* 感染的发生率显著下降[63]。PUD 的总发病率下降了一半之多,严重和复杂的 PUD,需要住院治疗的患者人数也减少了[22]。其发病率下降的原因可能与以下因素有关:质子泵抑制剂的发现及应用,Hp 的根除(见第 52 章),内镜下止血方法的增多(见第 20 章),明显减少了 PUD 手术治疗的病例数量[64],虽然老年人中复杂疾病的发生率增加,但与手术有关的发病率和死亡率也增加[65]。据作者经验发现,从用阿片类药物止痛转向滥用非甾体抗炎药物的流行,使得年轻患者中 PUD 穿孔的发生率越来越高。

消化性溃疡穿孔患者,通常会突然出现严重的弥漫性腹痛,这些患者能明确指出症状出现的确切时间,往往无征兆出现剧烈腹痛。腹部检查可发现全腹膜炎,伴有反跳痛、肌卫和腹肌强直。在这种情况下,可能无法将溃疡穿孔与其他脏器病变穿孔(如结肠憩室穿孔、阑尾炎穿孔)区别开来。年长或虚弱的患者可能临床症状不那么明显,通过腹部直立的平片或 CT 检查可见腹腔内有游离气体来诊断。

突然出现剧烈腹痛并伴有腹壁僵硬和腹腔内游离气的患者,应怀疑是消化性溃疡穿孔。75% 的患者在腹部平片上可检测到气腹(图 11.7)。可疑病例的腹部 CT 通常显示胃窦和十二指肠水肿,并有管腔外气体。当 CT 不能明确诊断时,患者又有弥漫性腹膜炎或血液灌注明显不足时应该立即手术探查。对于此类患者,剖腹手术是诊断的主要手段。当怀疑是消化性溃疡穿孔时,不建议使用内镜检查,因做胃镜时需充气,充气可以将已关闭的穿孔再次冲开。令人惊讶的是因

PUD 并发症而接受急诊手术的患者存活率低。在丹麦，按照脓毒症生存指南来临床操作，发现可以将消化性溃疡穿孔 30 天的患者，死亡率从 30% 降低到 25%[66]。这些患者的 2 年死亡率超过 40%（另见第 53 章）。

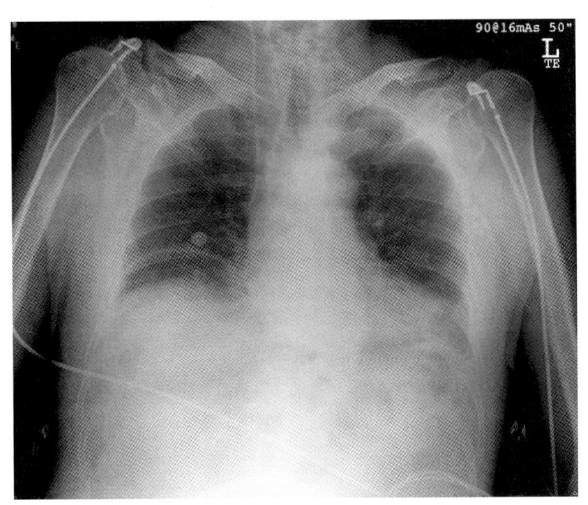

图 11.7 1 例 80 岁男性患者的直立位胸片，急性发作严重上腹痛，显示右侧横膈下腹腔内游离气体。患者因内脏穿孔出现了气腹。手术时发现十二指肠前壁溃疡穿孔

（七）急性肠系膜缺血

急性肠系膜缺血可由主动脉粥样硬化或心脏附壁血栓栓子脱落引起肠系膜血管阻塞，或肠系膜血管原发性血栓形成，通常发生在动脉粥样硬化性狭窄部位。栓子阻塞占了最大的比例，20 世纪 80 年代，肠系膜缺血的发生率为 50%，由于栓塞危险因素的处理取得了明显进展，到 2010 年，这一发生率不超过三分之一。其最常累及的是肠系膜上动脉，可能是因为肠系膜上动脉起始部位与腹主动脉的夹角较小[67]。肠系膜动脉粥样硬化性狭窄可导致原发性动脉血栓形成。患者通常有动脉粥样硬化病史，特别是有冠状动脉或脑血管上有粥样斑块史。原发性肠系膜血栓形成占肠系膜缺血病例的 68%[67]。非闭塞性肠系膜缺血是由于内脏灌注不足，可导致肠缺血和梗死，这种情况常发生在严重疾病如心源性休克或感染性休克。非闭塞性肠系膜缺血，又称“低流量”肠系膜缺血，大约有 10% 的病例。其余 10% 的肠系膜缺血是由静脉血栓形成引起的，常与有血栓形成倾向的疾病和小肠局灶性节段性缺血有关（第 118 章）。因为大多数肠系膜缺血性病例发生在有明显心血管疾病的患者，结局较差。围手术期死亡率从 50% 到近 100% 不等[67,68]。

急性肠系膜缺血临床特征，是突然出现的上腹部和脐周剧烈疼痛，但腹部体征轻微，疼痛程度与腹部查体完全不符，其他症状可以有腹泻、呕吐、腹胀和黑便。在体格检查中，大多数患者有急性痛苦面容，但腹部体征却不明显。休克大约占病例的 25%。

CT 血管造影是对疑似急性肠系膜缺血最好的初步诊断方法。肠系膜血管造影可能有助于确定肠缺血的原因和血管疾病的范围；然而，在这些病例中，CT 已经在很大程度上取代了正规的血管造影。急性栓塞性或血栓性肠缺血患者应立即进行血管重建术和肠切除术[69]。非闭塞性肠系膜缺血患者最好的治疗方法是抗休克。对于症状持续不减的患者，有必要剖腹切除梗死肠管。经介入导管扩张性治疗可能有助于内脏动脉造影发现血管痉挛的患者（见第 118 章）。

（八）腹主动脉瘤

腹主动脉瘤（abdominal aortic aneurysm，AAA）破裂的先兆是突然发作的急性、严重的腹痛，疼痛部位位于中腹部、脊柱旁或两侧腹。疼痛性质是撕裂性的，伴随有虚脱、头晕和多汗。如果患者在送往医院的过程中幸存下来，休克是最常见的表现。90% 患者在体格检查可以扪及一搏动微弱的包块，75% 的病例具有典型的临床表现，即：低血压、腹部搏动性肿块和腹痛三联征，需要立即手术治疗[69]。当病史中高度怀疑此病，临床上又有休克表现，急诊超声检查是诊断 AAA 的可靠方法，并可提供急诊干预的充分证据。尽管短期死亡率为 40%，但血管内修复腹主动脉夹层瘤的方法可以改善病情[70]，所有当怀疑 AAA 破裂的患者，需要紧急的血管外科会诊，以最大限度地提高生存率。

（九）腹腔间隔室综合征

虽然腹腔间隔室综合征（abdominal compartment syndrome，ACS）通常不表现为急性腹痛，但可以出现于任何急腹症。最初报道 ACS 发生在有严重腹腔内脏创伤后，出现病理性腹内压力升高。目前认为 ACS 是许多严重疾病过程中的常见并发症[71]。腹腔正常压力为 5～7mmHg，肥胖者可能更高[72]。在大容量复苏后幸存者，可能会出现内脏水肿而导致腹腔压力增高，或重症胰腺炎会引起内脏或腹膜后水肿，也可能会出现腹内压升高。腹内压力大于或等于 12mmHg 就为腹腔内高压（intra-abdominal hypertension，IAH）[71]。因腹内压升高影响了内脏器官灌注就定义为 ACS。在这种情况下，肾脏特别容易出现灌注不足，肾衰竭可能是 ACS 的首要表现[73]。

原发性 ACS 的定义是由腹腔内脏器官病理状况引起，如胃膨胀或急性胰腺炎引起的水肿[71]。更常见的是第二种 ACS，休克后出现肠壁广泛水肿导致 IAH 的发生。第三种形式，即在处理原发性或继发性 ACS 后，过度尝试闭合腹部伤口，可导致更糟糕的或反复出现的 ACS[72]。ACS 的危险因素列于框 11.1。

在仰卧位患者中，只需将传感器与导尿管连接，以腋中线为零参考点，即可测量腹内压。一次国际共识会议根据测量的膀胱压力建立了 ACS 分级方案，如表 11.6 所示[74]。膀胱压力的正常值小于 7mmHg。Ⅰ级 ACS 压力定义为 12～15mmHg，Ⅱ级 ACS 为 16～120mmHg，Ⅲ级为 21～125mmHg，Ⅳ等级大于 25mmHg。低级别 ACS 非手术治疗包括胃减压、镇静、神经肌肉阻滞剂、将患者置于头低脚高位，同时让髋部保持中立位置，以及应用利尿剂。对于严重 ACS 患者，尤其肾功能或呼吸功能开始受损时，开腹手术是最有效的治疗手段[75]。开腹手术的处理需要专科外科医师，通常需要转诊至医疗中心。值得庆幸的是，随着人们对 ACS 认识的不断提高和复苏技术的进步，ACS 发生率在 20 世纪初大幅下降[72,76]。

框 11.1 腹内高压和腹腔间隔综合征的风险因素

腹部手术,特别是有紧密筋膜闭合的
酸中毒(pH<7.2)
急性胰腺炎
菌血症
凝血病[血小板<55 000/mm³,或激活部分凝血酶时间为正常或更高的两倍,或凝血酶原时间<50%(INR>1.5)]
"控制损伤性"剖腹手术
腹部膨胀
胃轻瘫、胃胀或肠梗阻
腹腔积血/气腹
高体重指数(BMI>30kg/m²)
低体温(核心温度<33℃)
腹腔感染和脓肿
腹腔内或腹膜后肿瘤
腹腔镜过度充气致压力增加
肝功能障碍/肝硬化伴腹水
严重烧伤
严重创伤
大量液体复苏(>5L 胶体或晶体液/24h)
巨大切口疝修补术
机械通气
多次输血(>10U 红细胞/24h)
腹膜透析
腹膜炎
肺炎
俯卧位通气
脓毒血症
使用呼气末正压(PEEP)或"自主-呼气末正压"
肠扭转

Adapted from Malbrain MNG, Cheatham M, Kirkpatrick A, et al. Results from the International Conference of Experts on Intra-abdominal Hypertension and Abdominal Compartment Syndrome. I. Defnitions. Intensive Care Med 2006;32:1722-32.

表 11.6 腹腔内高压的分级体系*

分级	膀胱压力/mmHg
正常	<12
1	12~15
2	16~20
3	21~25
4	>25

*如果腹内高压并伴有器官功能障碍,则存在腹腔间隔综合征。

Adapted from Carr JA. Abdominal compartment syndrome: a decade of progress. J Am Coll Surg 2013;216:135-46.

(十) 腹腔内其他原因

引起急性腹痛的其他腹腔内原因包括:妇科疾病(如子宫内膜炎、伴或不伴输卵管-卵巢脓肿的急性输卵管炎、卵巢囊肿或扭转、异位妊娠);自发性腹膜炎(第 93 章);功能性消化不良(第 14 章);传染性肠胃炎(第 110~112 章);病毒性肝炎和其他肝脏感染(第 78 至 84 章);肾盂肾炎;膀胱炎;肠系膜淋巴结炎;炎症性肠病(第 115 和 116 章);以及其他肠道疾病,如肠易激综合征(第 122 章)和肠道假性梗阻(第 124 章)。由于胚胎发育时轴向扭转引起的网膜侧支血管变异可导致网膜阑尾炎综合征[77,78],该综合征临床表现类似于阑尾炎、憩室炎或其他病理情况,但有自限性自然史,通常只需要用非甾体抗炎药对症治疗[78],CT 上显示一个卵圆形炎性脂肪团位于非炎性结肠部分附近,就能证实此诊断[79]。

(十一) 腹腔外疾病和全身性疾病原因

急性腹痛可由腹外器官及全身性疾病引起。示例见框 11.2。除气胸、脓胸和食管穿孔外,很少需要对腹腔外或全身

框 11.2 急性腹痛的腹腔外及全身疾病原因

心脏病变
心内膜炎
心脏衰竭
心肌缺血和梗死
心肌炎
胸部病变
积脓症
食管破裂(Boerhaave 综合征)
食管痉挛
食管炎
胸膜痛(Bornholm 病)
肺炎
气胸
肺栓塞和梗死
血液系统疾病
急性白血病
溶血性贫血
过敏性发癜
镰状细胞病
代谢障碍
急性肾上腺功能不全(Addison 病)
糖尿病(尤其是酮症酸中毒)
高脂血症
甲状旁腺功能亢进
过敏反应(如昆虫叮咬、爬行动物毒液)
铅中毒
卟啉症
中毒
尿毒症
感染
带状疱疹
骨髓炎
梅毒
伤寒
神经系统病变
腹部癫痫
神经根病,脊髓或周围神经肿瘤,脊柱退行性关节炎,椎间盘突出
脊髓痨
其他杂症
血管性水肿
家族性地中海热
中暑
肌肉挫伤,血肿,肿瘤
戒毒
精神疾病

性疾病引起的急性腹痛患者进行手术干预。食管穿孔可能是医源性的，由钝性或穿透性创伤引起，也可以是自发性的（Boerhaave 综合征；见第 45 章）。

血管神经性水肿的特征是真皮、皮下组织、黏膜和黏膜下层的急性自限性水肿。水肿可影响面部皮肤，通常发生在口、舌、喉、四肢和生殖器周围。累及胃肠道可引起急性腹痛发作，有时还伴有恶心、呕吐和腹泻。肥大细胞介导的血管性水肿，常由食物、药物过敏或昆虫叮咬引起，其特征为荨麻疹、潮红、瘙痒、喉咙发紧、支气管痉挛和低血压。虽然血管紧张素转换酶抑制剂可引起这些症状，但缓激肽诱导的血管性水肿，病程较长，疾病的启动机制并不太清楚，与这些症状无关。在使用血管紧张素转换酶抑制剂的患者、先天遗传或后天缺乏 C1 酯酶抑制剂或功能障碍者中，可见肠壁血管性水肿，并可在腹部超声或 CT 检查中看到。发作的治疗取决于急性和严重程度，可能包括气道的建立和血流动力学支持，停用潜在诱因，抗组胺药和糖皮质激素的使用。对遗传性血管神经性水肿的患者，可使用纯化的 C1 酯酶抑制剂浓缩物、激肽抑制剂和缓激肽 B2 受体拮抗剂。

（十二）特殊情况

1. 极端年龄

评价极端年龄患者急性腹痛是一个挑战。有时候既往信息和体格检查结果通常很难得出或不可靠的腹痛原因。同样，在面对严重的腹腔内脏器疾病时，实验室数据有可能显示为正常。由于这些原因，极端年龄的患者往往在病程晚期才被诊断，从而导致发病率增加。例如，一般人群阑尾炎的穿孔率平均为 10%，但在婴儿中超过 50%。在这些人群中，急腹症的前兆具有高度变异性，需要高度怀疑指数。仔细询问病史、全面体格检查和高怀疑指数是最有用的诊断辅助手段。

在儿童中，急性腹痛的原因随年龄而变化。在婴儿期，肠套叠、肾盂肾炎、胃食管反流、梅克尔憩室炎以及细菌性或病毒性肠炎是急性腹痛的常见病因。儿童期急性腹痛常见于梅克尔憩室炎、膀胱炎、肺炎、肠炎、肠系膜淋巴结炎和炎症性肠病。在青少年中，以盆腔炎、炎症性肠病和成人常见的急性腹痛原因为主。在所有年龄的儿童中，最常见的两种疼痛原因是急性阑尾炎和继发于受虐待儿童的腹部创伤。

在老年人群中，胆道疾病几乎占急性腹痛病例的 25%，其次为非特异性腹痛、恶性肿瘤、肠梗阻、复杂性 PUD 和嵌顿疝。阑尾炎虽然在老年患者中罕见，但通常表现在病程晚期，与高发病率死亡率相关。

2. 妊娠

妊娠妇女急性腹痛的病因诊断比较困难。急性阑尾炎和胆囊炎的发生率在孕妇及非妊娠妇女是相同的。一些产科的疾病如胎盘早剥和阔韧带张力增加所引起的疼痛，应该加以鉴别。在计划进行影像学检查时，必须考虑放射性辐射对胎儿发育的危害。

妊娠期手术并不少见；大约每 500 名孕妇中就有 1 人需要进行非产科的普通外科手术[80]。手术之前首先应考虑的是母亲的安全问题。其次受孕期间的紧急外科干预，有胎儿丢失的风险，这与胎龄和手术干预方式有关。妊娠中期 3 个月以腹部手术治疗可能比较合适，这段时间致畸和自发早产的风险都最低。

阑尾炎的发生率在孕妇大约 1/2 000，并平均分布在妊娠早、中及晚期内。在妊娠后期，阑尾可能头侧移位，从而使腹膜刺激的征象远离麦氏点附近。在高度怀疑此病时，可选用超声或 MRI 可能对诊断有帮助。胆道疾病在受孕期间也很常见。开腹或腹腔镜治疗这些疾病是安全的，但约有 5% 的病例可出现不良结局[81]。

3. 免疫功能低下

除了一般人群中发生的阑尾炎和胆囊炎等疾病外，许多免疫功能低下宿主特有的疾病可能表现为急性腹部疼痛、中性粒细胞减少性小肠结肠炎、药物性胰腺炎、移植物抗宿主病、肠积气及巨细胞病毒和真菌感染（见第 36 章）。感染 HIV 的患者可能面临特殊挑战（见第 35 章）。当艾滋病晚期时，HIV 感染与其他一些疾病有关，可能表现为急性腹痛。在发展中国家，免疫缺陷患者最常见的腹部疾病之一是原发性腹膜炎（见第 39 章）。受累患者出现化脓性腹膜炎，但往往无明确的感染来源。自发性肠穿孔通常继发于巨细胞病毒感染，在晚期 HIV 感染者中也很常见。结核性腹膜炎是结核病常见地区患者的一个考虑因素[82]。免疫功能低下的患者，可能缺乏通常见于免疫功能正常者的急腹症危象的明确体征，在这些病例中，可能不存在体温升高、腹膜刺激征和白细胞增多。

四、药物治疗

急性腹痛患者治疗中的一个不适当做法是，在等待外科手术评估之前，延迟镇痛剂给药。Zachary Cope 爵士认为："吗啡对阻止严重的腹内疾病几乎没有作用，但它能有效地掩盖疾病的症状。"[83] 然而，延迟患者痛苦的做法似乎使其难以承受仔细的临床检查。在急性腹痛患者中比较早期给予镇痛药与给予安慰剂的 6 项研究表明，接受镇痛药的患者更舒服，不会出现诊断延迟[84,85]。

急腹症患者经常需要抗生素治疗急性腹膜炎。在适当的情况下，一旦获得初步诊断，应尽快给予针对可能致病病原体的抗生素治疗，但在确定可能的病原体之前，使用广谱抗生素治疗免疫功能正常的患者几乎没有益处。然而，对于免疫功能低下或中性粒细胞减少的患者，应在急性腹痛治疗早期接受广谱抗生素治疗。

（王立 译，李鹏　袁农 校）

参考文献

第 12 章　慢性腹痛

Joseph C. Yarze,Lawrence S. Friedman 著

章节目录

一、定义和临床方法 …… 153
二、腹壁疼痛 …… 153
　（一）前皮神经卡压和肌筋膜疼痛综合征 …… 153
　（二）滑脱肋骨综合征 …… 154
　（三）胸神经根病 …… 154
三、中枢介导的腹痛综合征 …… 154
　（一）流行病学 …… 154
　（二）病理生理学 …… 154
　（三）临床特点 …… 156
　（四）诊断和鉴别诊断 …… 157
　（五）治疗 …… 157
四、麻醉性肠综合征/阿片类药物诱导的胃肠道痛觉敏感 …… 159

评估任何主诉腹痛的患者都具有挑战性。腹痛可以是良性和自限性的，也可能是严重危及生命疾病的预兆（见第 11 章）。慢性腹痛是一个特别具有挑战性的临床问题。不仅是因为慢性腹痛的治疗是一项经常令人望而生畏的任务，临床医生还必须保持警惕，以避免忽视其他可治疗的结构性（“器质性”）疾病。本章和本教科书其他部分讨论的许多疾病都可引起慢性或复发性腹痛（框 12.1）。除了适当的诊断检测外，其中许多诊断都需要仔细考虑和临床询问，以判断疾病是否确实是患者疼痛的原因。一旦明确排除器质性慢性腹痛的潜在原因，通常会考虑功能性胃肠道疾病（functional gastrointestinal tract disorder，FGID）的诊断。尽管慢性腹痛的病因多种多样，但产生慢性疼痛的病理生理途径在许多人中是常见的。本章重点介绍慢性腹痛的神经肌肉原因、中枢介导性腹痛综合征（centrally mediated abdominal pain syndrome，CAPS）和麻醉性肠综合征（narcotic bowel syndrome，NBS）的神经肌肉性病因。CAPS 作为一种典型的疾病，说明了诊治慢性腹痛患者所涉及的许多复杂而相互关联的问题。

框 12.1　慢性或复发性腹痛的鉴别诊断

结构性（或器质性）疾病

炎症

阑尾炎（第 120 章）
乳糜泻和麸质敏感症（第 107 章）
大肠憩室症（第 121 章）
嗜酸性胃肠炎（第 30 章）
肠脂垂炎
炎症性肠病（第 115 和 116 章）
盆腔炎性疾病
原发性硬化性胆管炎（第 68 章）
硬化性肠系膜炎（第 39 章）

血管性

腹腔动脉综合征（第 38 章）
肠系膜缺血（第 118 章）
肠系膜上动脉综合征（第 15 章）

代谢性

糖尿病神经病变
铅中毒
卟啉症（第 77 章）

神经肌肉性

前皮神经卡压综合征
肌筋膜疼痛综合征
滑脱性肋骨综合征
胸神经根病

其他

腹部粘连（第 123 章）
腹部偏头痛（第 15 章）
腹部肿瘤（第 32~34、48、54、60、69、96 和 125~127 章）
速发型过敏反应（第 10 章）
血管性水肿（第 11 章）
大麻素呕吐综合征（第 15 章）
慢性胰腺炎（第 59 章）
周期性呕吐综合征（第 15 章）
Ehlers-Danlos 综合征
子宫内膜异位症（第 128 章）
家族性地中海热（37 章）
胆结石（第 65 章）
疝（第 27 章）
肠旋转不良（第 98 章）
肠梗阻（第 123 章）
乳糖不耐受（第 104 章）
神经源性腹痛（腹型偏头痛，腹型癫痫）（第 15 和 37 章）
消化性溃疡病（第 53 章）
小肠和骨盆腔脂肪增多症（第 39 章）

功能性胃肠病

胆囊疼痛（胆囊或括约肌功能障碍）（第 63 章）
中枢介导的腹痛综合征
功能性（非溃疡性）消化不良（第 14 章）
胃轻瘫（第 50 章）
肠易激综合征（第 122 章）
肛提肌综合征（第 129 章）
麻醉剂肠道综合征/阿片类药物诱导的胃肠道痛觉过敏

一、定义和临床方法

当腹痛持续或间断发生至少 6 个月时，被认为是慢性腹痛；当腹痛持续或间断发生不超过数日时，被认为是急性腹痛；当腹痛持续或间断发生超过数日但少于 6 个月时，被认为是亚急性腹痛。上述定义在制订诊断考虑列表时通常是有帮助的。临床医生最初必须采用广泛的方法，随后随着评价的进行，该方法也变得更加有针对性。重要的是，虽然典型的症状有助于记忆，但是一些患者，特别是免疫抑制和老年人，可能会表现出非典型特征。

与急性腹痛一样（见第 11 章），评估慢性腹痛患者的最初步骤是获取详细的病史。应确定疼痛的时间顺序，包括发作的突然程度和持续时间、疼痛的部位和可能的辐射区域。考虑到器官的双侧神经支配相对对称，在中线部位可感觉到消化道发出的内脏疼痛，但呈弥漫性，定位不佳[1]。牵涉痛通常位于与受累内脏传入相同的脊髓水平的皮肤皮区[2]。还应该询问患者疼痛的强度和性质，了解这些参数都是主观的。当考虑诊断可能性时，患者对诱发、加重或缓解因素的感知可能是有用的。

当最初试图确定患者的疼痛是器质性或功能性过程时，临床医生应在病史和体格检查中寻找支持或排除某些进行性、慢性基础疾病诊断的线索。病史中提示器质性病变过程的特征包括发热、盗汗、食欲改变、体重减轻和夜间觉醒。

全面的体格检查适用于寻找全身性疾病的证据。腹部检查应结合视诊、听诊、叩诊和触诊。在慢性腹痛急性加重的患者中，最关键的步骤是确定是否存在强制立即手术干预的过程（见第 11 章）。虽然慢性腹痛的大多数原因不需要立即手术治疗，但通常与慢性腹痛相关疾病过程中的相关并发症可能会急性出现（如炎症性肠病患者的肠穿孔）。此外，发生慢性腹痛的患者可能表现为与另一种疾病过程相关的急性疼痛（如基础肠易激综合征患者急性肠系膜缺血）。应听诊腹部以发现腹部杂音，这可能提示慢性肠系膜缺血。腹部触诊对是否存在脏器肿大、肿块、腹水以及疝的检查尤其相关。提示潜在器质性疾病的其他体格检查结果包括营养不良体征（如肌肉减少症、水肿）、维生素缺乏或肠外病变（如关节病、皮肤改变）。虽然不完全具体，但"闭眼征"常见于 CAPS 患者（见后文）。同样，卡奈特征（Carnett 征）和悬停征（hover sign）（后文描述）可见于腹壁疼痛的患者。

实验室检查可能是有帮助的，但临床医生必须首先提取病史和体格检查的相关方面，然后再聚焦实验室检查手段。不明智地使用实验室检测成本很高，会混淆临床表现，甚至可能导致并发症。值得强调的是，实验室检查结果异常并不一定证明与患者疼痛综合征相关的因果关系。临床医生在选择和解释实验室检查结果时必须十分谨慎。

内镜和影像学检查在诊断和排除慢性腹痛的许多病因方面具有重要作用。上消化道内镜检查、结肠镜检查、胶囊内镜检查和超声内镜检查可能适用于选定的病例。影像学检查包括钡剂和放射性核素研究、超声、CT、MRI、PET 和血管造影（CT、MR 和传统）。这些放射学检查的适应证不同，阐明个体临床情况的潜力也不同。特定疾病的内镜和放射学检查在本教科书的其他部分进行了详细讨论。

二、腹壁疼痛

（一）前皮神经卡压和肌筋膜疼痛综合征

据估计，10%～30% 以慢性腹痛为主诉就诊于胃肠病学医师的患者，其症状原因为慢性腹壁疼痛（chronic abdominal wall pain，CAWP）。前皮神经卡压综合征（anterior cutaneous nerve entrapment syndrome，ACNES）和肌筋膜疼痛综合征（myofascial pain syndrome，MFPS）是引起慢性腹壁疼痛的常见原因。这些综合征具有临床、诊断和治疗特征，识别他们的重要性在于为患者提供准确的诊断和有效的治疗，以及避免进一步昂贵的检查和不必要的手术干预。当主诉与进食或肠道功能无关但与运动明显相关的慢性和持续腹痛时，应怀疑腹壁是引起症状的原因。

CAWP 患者通常超重，且女性比男性更易罹患该病。尽管 ACNES 最初在 20 世纪 70 年代就被提出，但它仍然是慢性腹痛一个经常被漏诊、忽视和误诊的原因[3-5]。在 ACNES 中，当感觉神经的皮支被卡压时，疼痛就会发生，该感觉神经的皮支来源于脊柱 T7 至 T12 节段发出的神经血管束。神经卡压可能与腹内、腹外病变的压力或其他局部病变（如肥胖、纤维化或水肿）有关。腹壁发出的疼痛是离散的和局限性的，与起源于腹内来源的疼痛相反，其是弥漫性的、且局限性差。解剖学说明和神经卡压机制已在其他地方有详细介绍[6,7]。患者通常用一根手指指向其疼痛的位置，检查者常可将最大压痛区域定位在直径小于 2cm 的区域。体格检查时，患者通常将患处保护在不受检查者触及的部位（悬停征）[8]。患者常注意到与腹部肌肉系统收缩有关的活动会导致疼痛加重，在体格检查时，临床医生会注意到当患者绷紧腹部肌肉时，触诊的局部压痛增加（Carnett 征）[9]。

在 MFPS 中，疼痛来自骨骼肌的肌筋膜触发点。致病因素包括肌肉骨骼创伤、脊柱疾病、椎间盘疾病、骨性关节炎、过度使用、心理压力和相对不动等。MFPS 疼痛的确切病理生理学仍不清楚。MFPS 患者可能会发生 CAWP。疼痛可以从另一个部位转移来，确定疼痛触发点是一个有用的物理发现。当试图确定触发点时，检查者用单指触诊压痛区域。压痛点最常位于肌腹的中央部分，可感到僵硬或绷紧，并会引起跳跃征[10]。这一发现是指患者在检查到肌筋膜触发点时，通过眨眼、抽动或哭闹作出反应。触发点可能位于剑突、肋骨软骨连接处、或韧带和肌腱止点等一些少见的部位。

ACNES 和 MFPS 的成功治疗不仅能改善症状，而且可明确诊断[11,12]。治疗策略取决于症状的严重程度。对因某些反复运动引起的轻度和间歇性的症状，给予简单的安慰和避免这些运动的建议就足够了。急性加重期间可使用非麻醉性镇痛药、非甾体抗炎药（NSAID）和热敷。物理治疗也可能是有益的，尽管没有随机研究支持这种方法。对于重度和持续性症状，建议使用局部麻醉剂注射治疗，不论是否使用糖皮质激素[11-13]。已经介绍了各种注射技术[6]。一项随访 6～12 个月的回顾性调查研究显示，超声引导下触发点注射麻醉剂加糖皮质激素治疗，使超过 1/3 的患者症状显著改善[14]。不出所料，躯体化与治疗成功呈负相关。在一项纳入 136 例患者的研究中，病史和体格检查提示腹壁疼痛，接受注射治疗后获益，平均随访4年后，97%的病例诊断保持不变[15]。在仔细选择的注射治疗无效的症状患者中，一项前瞻性非随机研究表明，诊断性腹腔镜检查联合腹部触发点开放探查可能是有益的[16]。在本研究中，在松解靠近触发点的腹腔内粘连后，进行皮下神经切除术。在37个月的中位术后随访后，24例患者中有23例(96%)认为这种方法有利于治疗他们以前的难治性疼痛。来自同一研究者的一项回顾性观察性研究[17]和一项双盲、随机、对照试验[18]也显示，在对保守治疗无效的症状患者中，前神经切除术可长期获益。

（二）滑脱肋骨综合征

滑脱肋骨综合征（slipping rib syndrome，SRS）最初于20世纪初被提出[19,20]，是慢性下胸痛和上腹痛的一种不常见的公认原因。SRS通常会引起单侧肋下区剧烈的刺痛。急性剧痛后可有较持久的酸痛感。该综合征与第8、9或10肋骨前端肋软骨过度活动有关，在腹部肌肉收缩时，受累肋骨在邻近上肋骨后方滑脱。这种滑脱通过各种潜在机制引起疼痛，包括肋神经撞击和局部组织炎症。诊断的关键是对该综合征的临床认知，结合勾形手法的运用：临床医生用检查手指勾在患者最低肋骨下方，随着肋骨向前移动，疼痛重现，经常听到爆裂声或咔哒声[21]。保守治疗措施往往就足够了，但偶尔需要肋软骨神经阻滞（支持诊断的反应），甚至肋骨或肋软骨切除[22,23]。

在胸椎过度后凸和脊柱后侧凸的患者中，“肋骨尖综合征”（肋髂撞击）可能以类似SRS的方式引起疼痛。这种情况通常使用加权后凸矫形器（一种特殊重量的背部支撑装置，将身体中心置于腿上）和背部加固处理成功治愈[24]。

（三）胸神经根病

与胸神经根T7至T12相关的疾病可能是引起腹痛的原因。可引起该问题的疾病过程包括与背部和脊柱疾病相关的神经病变、糖尿病和带状疱疹感染[25,26]。获取患者完整的病史并进行仔细的体格检查，注意全身性疾病以及异常神经系统和皮肤病学结果的可能性，应得出正确的诊断。治疗取决于具体的基础疾病过程。

三、中枢介导的腹痛综合征

中枢介导的腹痛综合征（CAPS）以前被称为功能性腹痛综合征（functional abdominal pain syndrome，FAPS），是一种独特的疾病。将该综合征由FAPS更名为CAPS，以更准确地反映其病理生理。这种疾病也称为慢性特发性腹痛或慢性功能性疼痛，与腹型偏头痛[疼痛呈周期性（见第15章）]、慢性盆腔痛、恶病质或假装疼痛（见第23章）、肠易激综合征（irritable bowel syndrome，IBS）（见第122章）和功能性消化不良（functional dyspepsia，FD；见第14章）不同。有证据表明，该综合征与中枢神经系统扩增正常调节内脏信号有关，而与胃肠道的功能（即运动）异常无关[27]。该疾病的特征是连续的、几乎持续的或至少经常复发的腹痛，与排便习惯和进食的关系不大。CAPS的正确理解是正常（调节性）肠道功能的异常感知，而不是运动障碍。该综合征似乎与内源性疼痛调节系统的改变密切相关，包括下行和皮质疼痛调节回路的功能障碍。CAPS的罗马Ⅳ共识委员会诊断标准见框12.2[28]。纳入符合CAPS诊断标准的患者的研究表明，在长期随访中发现的慢性腹痛的器质性原因很少[29,30]。

框12.2　中枢介导的腹痛综合征† 罗马Ⅳ诊断标准*

必须符合以下所有条件：
1. 持续或几乎持续的腹痛。
2. 疼痛与生理事件（如进食、排便、月经）没有或仅有偶发的关系‡。
3. 疼痛限制了某些方面的日常功能§。
4. 疼痛不是假装的（如不是装病）。
5. 疼痛不能用其他结构性或功能性胃肠道疾病或其他医学状况来解释。

*过去3个月符合上述标准，诊断前症状发作至少6个月。

†中枢介导性腹痛综合征通常与心理社会共病相关，但没有可用于诊断的特定特征。

‡可能存在一定程度的胃肠功能紊乱。

§日常功能可能包括工作、亲密关系、社交/休闲、家庭生活、自我或他人照顾方面的障碍。

From Whorwell PJ，Keefer L，Drossman DA，et al. Centrally mediated disorders of gastrointestinal pain. In：Drossman DA，Chang L，Chey WD，Kellow J，Tack J，Whitehead WE，editors. Rome Ⅳ：functional gastrointestinal disorders：disorders of gut-brain interaction. I. Raleigh，NC：The Rome Foundation；2016. pp 1059-1116.

CAPS通常与其他不适的躯体症状有关，当CAPS持续存在或主导患者的生活时，通常与慢性疼痛行为和共病的心理障碍有关[31]。CAPS患者通常将其疾病定义为医学疾病，与IBS患者相比，其症状往往更严重，且与更大的功能障碍相关。如果存在心理障碍，则必须将其视为CAPS的共病特征，而不是原发精神疾患的一部分[32]。与慢性背痛的患者相比，慢性腹痛患者的身体功能显著更好，但对其健康的整体感知显著更差[33]。

（一）流行病学

虽然CAPS的流行病学尚不完全清楚，但认为该疾病比其他的功能性胃肠道疾病（FGID）更少见，估计患病率为2%[34]。以女性为主（女性：男性=1.5：1）。与无腹部症状的患者相比，CAPS患者因疾病而缺勤的天数更多，就诊次数也更多。相当大比例的患者被转诊到胃肠病学诊所和医疗中心，他们的医疗保健就诊次数不成比例，通常接受了大量的诊断程序和治疗。

（二）病理生理学

慢性疼痛是一种多维度（感觉、情绪、认知）体验。可解释为传入神经、脊髓和脑水平的神经生理功能异常。与外周或内脏损伤或疾病引起的急性疼痛不同，慢性功能性疼痛与结构异常和组织损伤引起的传入内脏刺激增加无关。CAPS被认为是一种与脑-肠轴功能障碍相关的生物心理社会疾病，伴有调节和动机性疼痛维度的改变（中枢敏化与疼痛信号的去抑制）[28,32]（见第22章）。如图12.1所示，CAPS的临床表达来源于心理和肠道生理的输入，通过中枢神经系统-肠神经轴以动态方式相互作用。该模型将CAPS的临床、生理和心

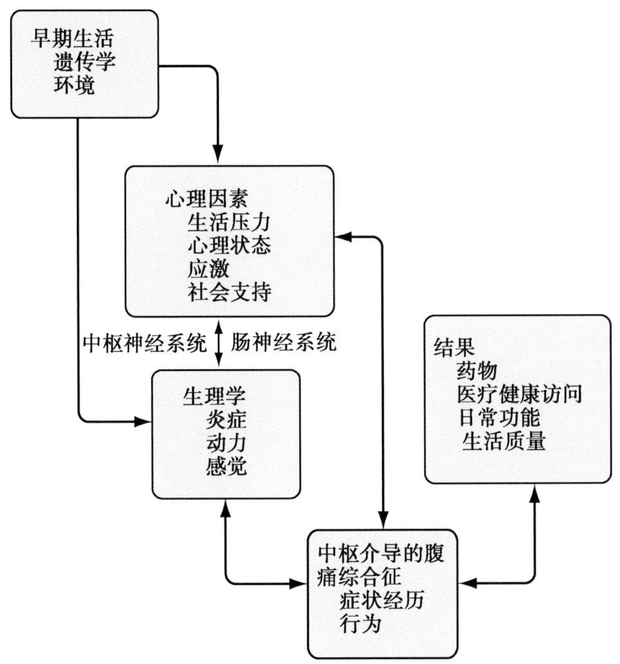

图 12.1　中枢介导的腹痛综合征(CAPS)的生物-心理-社会模型。与疾病的生物-心理-社会模型一致,由于生命早期的因素(如遗传、环境),一个人可能易感 CAPS。心理社会因素(如生活压力、社会支持)和胃肠道生理学(即炎症、运动和感觉)之间的相互作用导致症状和行为反应。CAPS 与脑肠神经轴的功能障碍相关,肠道传入信号的异常调节影响出现的症状,并导致医疗资源的使用增加和生活质量的降低

理社会特征整合为一种可理解的形式,为理解心理影响和应用精神药理学治疗提供了基础。

与疼痛性 FGID 病理生理学相关的研究集中于内脏超敏反应和脑-肠相互作用改变的概念。在 CAPS 中,脑-肠轴功能失调表现为传入内脏信号的中枢增强(与内脏高敏感性相反)[28,35]。CAPS 中的脑肠失调可由多种事件启动或改变,包括认知和情绪输入。对因非疼痛适应证接受妇科手术的女性发生慢性腹痛的前瞻性对照研究显示,手术组发生疼痛的频率显著更高[36]。仅通过心理社会变量预测术后慢性腹痛的发展,这意味着疼痛的发展与中枢配准和传入信号的放大密切相关。该研究强有力地支持了生物-心理-社会模式以及术后 CAPS 发生过程中认知和情绪输入的重要性。

1. 上行性内脏疼痛传递

内脏腹痛的传入涉及支配内脏的一级神经元,它将信号传递至胸腰交感神经系统,随后在脊髓背角形成突触。二级神经元通过脊髓丘脑和脊髓网状束从背角交叉上行。这些二级神经元在丘脑与三级神经元形成突触,三级神经元与躯体感觉皮层(感觉-辨别成分)和边缘系统(动机-情感激成分)形成突触;躯体感觉皮层与躯体特定区或点的精准定位以及传入信号的强度有关,边缘系统则包含前扣带回皮质[anterior cingulate cortex,ACC(图 12.2),也见于第 22 章]。岛叶皮质接收来自丘脑感觉区及孤束核的信号传入,并且将内脏感觉和情感信号整合[37]。根据个体的情绪状态,早期经历和对信号的认知解释,边缘系统可以调节疼痛感觉。这种中枢神经系统中疼痛感受信号的多成分整合解释了疼痛感觉和报道的差异性[38]。中枢神经系统中的情感产生区域通过

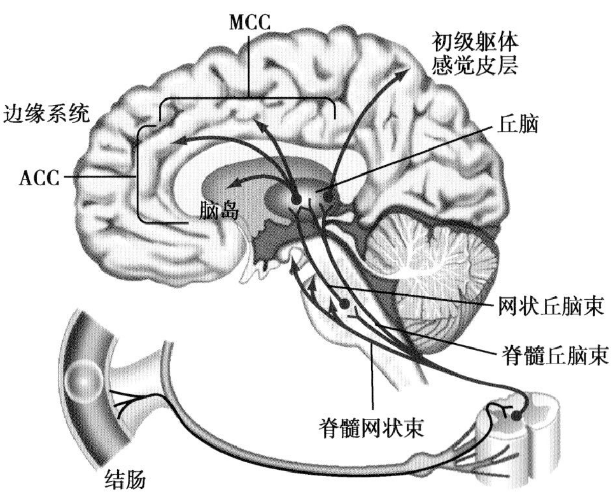

图 12.2　介导内脏痛觉的神经解剖学通路。内脏腹痛的传入涉及支配内脏的一级神经元,随后在脊髓背角形成突触。二级神经元从脊髓背角经脊髓丘脑束、脊髓网状束和网状丘脑束上行,在丘脑与三级神经元连接,然后在边缘系统[包含岛叶和前扣带回皮质(ACC)]和初级躯体感觉皮质形成突触。MCC,中扣带回皮质

调节来自肠道的传入感觉信号,对慢性疼痛感觉有着重要作用。

这种疼痛调控的概念构架已通过 PET 成像得到证实[39]。一群健康受试者将双手浸泡在热水中,一半人被催眠体验热水浸泡的痛苦,而另一半并未觉得疼痛甚至感到愉悦。两组受试者躯体感觉皮层的活动无明显差异;然而,那些经历过疼痛的受试者,大脑边缘系统前扣带回皮质(与疼痛经历的情感部分有关)的活化显著增强。脑功能成像研究比较了功能性胃肠病患者和正常对照组患者,发现异常的大脑活动主要集中在情感激发疼痛区域,包括前额叶皮质,前扣带回皮质,杏仁核和脑岛[40]。慢性疼痛患者的这些区域活化增加,提示异常的传入信号和中枢调节,某种程度上它们可由对内脏刺激关注的增加,异常的认知,传入信号的情感处理或共患精神疾病引起。

2. 疼痛的下行调节

根据"闸门控制学说"(门控理论),内脏疼痛的传入传递可通过从皮质向下至内脏神经的下行冲动调节[38]。在该模型中,门控系统的中央下行调控主要通过下行抑制系统进行[41]。该系统是一个以内啡肽或脑啡肽为基础的神经网络,它起源于大脑皮质和边缘系统,向下延伸至脊髓,主要与中脑(导水管周围灰质)和延髓[中缝尾核(图 12.3)]相联系。该系统可直接抑制二级神经元上的伤害性投射或通过脊髓中的抑制性中间神经元间接抑制伤害性投射(疼痛性投射)。然后脊髓背角作为闸门调节(即增加或减少),调控从外周疼痛位点传导至中枢神经系统的传入冲动传输。实际上,这种下行疼痛调节系统决定了从胃肠道上传至大脑的外周传入输入量。下行抑制系统可以扩散,并且当其被激活时,可以抑制全身的疼痛敏感性,这就是所谓的弥散性伤害抑制控制作用。慢性腹痛综合征患者,包括 CAPS,似乎存在激活弥散性伤害抑制控制作用的功能受损[42,43]。

3. 内脏敏感

反复的外周刺激上调传入信号或抑制下行疼痛调控机

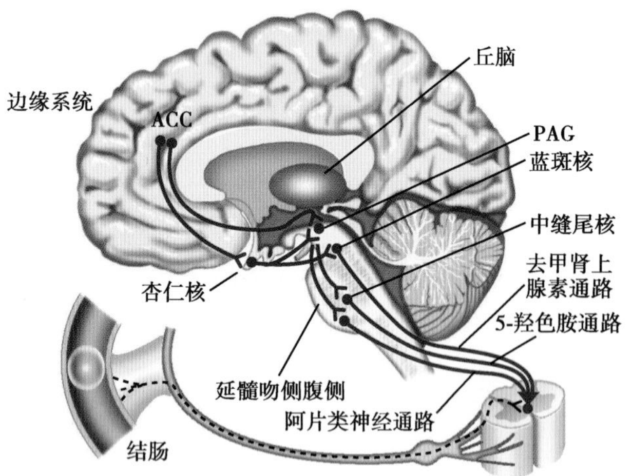

图 12.3　内啡肽或脑啡肽介导的下行抑制系统。该网络系统包含来自感觉皮层和边缘系统的连接（通过杏仁核和丘脑），主要与中脑导水管周围灰质（PAG）、蓝斑和延髓中缝尾核有主要联系。然后连接投射到脊髓背角的神经元上。当被激活时，该系统可抑制其从外周伤害性部位（疼痛部位）（如结肠）到大脑的传入冲动。通过释放 5-羟色胺（5-羟色胺能途径）和可能的去甲肾上腺素（去甲肾上腺素能途径）促进具有阿片类能特性的内啡肽活性。ACC，前扣带回皮质

制，从而使肠道致敏并且产生内脏痛觉过敏（对有害信号的疼痛反应增强）和慢性疼痛状态。临床研究支持这一观点，与健康受试者相比，功能性胃肠病患者似乎更容易出现痛觉增强[44]。术前使用局麻或 NSAID 治疗可减轻术后疼痛[45]，表明中枢神经系统对外周损伤的反应可通过预先减少传入中枢神经系统的输入量来调节。相反，复发性外周损伤（如重复腹部手术）可能使肠内受体敏感，从而使其甚至对基线传入活动的感觉也更疼痛（异常性疼痛）。内脏敏感可能通过神经轴的一个或多个水平层面的不同机制产生。反复疼痛性直肠扩张引起的直肠超敏反应见于肠易激综合征患者，而非 CAPS 患者[46]。这一观察结果支持了以下论点：肠易激综合征和 CAPS 是两种不同的疾病，其中肠易激综合征是一种传入刺激增强的疾病，而 CAPS 是一种以下行性疼痛调节改变为特征的疾病，具有明显的中枢性抑制。

4. 5-HT 的生物化作用

血清素[5-羟色胺（5-HT）]的生化作用受到公认的关注，因为胃肠道是其体内的主要来源[47]。5-HT 主要存在于黏膜肠嗜铬细胞中，是肠神经系统的一种神经递质，同时也是一种旁分泌分子，能发出其他（如迷走神经）神经活动的信号。5-HT 介导多种胃肠道功能，各种受体亚型（如 5-HT_1、5-HT_3、5-HT_4）的调节作用和 5-HT 再摄取影响胃肠道感觉运动功能。因此，5-HT 是脑-肠神经轴的重要调节器，其功能失调在中枢疼痛的增强中起着重要作用[48]。5-HT 系统的药理调控是一个引起关注的治疗靶点。

5. 中枢神经系统的作用

尽管外致敏可能会影响疼痛的发作，但由于中枢去抑制，中枢神经系统参与了慢性疼痛的易感性和持续性。在 CAPS 中，中枢神经系统的突出作用表现为缺乏外周运动或感觉异常，与心理社会障碍密切相关。此外，共病精神病诊断、主要生活应激源、性或身体虐待史、社会支持匮乏和不适应的应对策略都与较严重的慢性腹痛和较差的健康结局相关[49,50]。在 CAPS 患者和其他功能性胃肠道疼痛疾病患者中，这些因素可能损害或减少作用于背角神经元的下行抑制性疼痛通路，或可能放大内脏传入信号[32,42,51]。在 31 名健康志愿者中的研究使用功能性脑 MRI 显示，较高的神经质评分与预期疼痛期间负责情绪和认知评估的脑区参与相关[52]。这一发现支持了过度觉醒的不适应机制与对疼痛的预期，以及随后在神经质评分较高的人的疼痛体验中缺乏应对能力。感染后 IBS 患者（见第 122 章）和术后 CAPS 的前瞻性研究也支持大脑在胃肠道疼痛体验中的重要性[36,53]。粪便微生物群与脑-肠神经轴和 CAPS 的关系正在研究中[54]。

脑功能成像有助于阐明脑-肠相互作用，并已证实认知和情绪机制与慢性疼痛体验之间的联系可能通过损害边缘系统适当调节内脏体征的能力来介导。中枢神经系统的动机-情感成分，特别是 ACC（见图 12.2 和图 12.3），在 FGID（如 IBS）和其他慢性疼痛性疾病患者中功能失调[55-57]。一项对 IBS 和有虐待史患者的研究使用功能性脑 MRI 显示，在厌恶性内脏刺激（直肠球囊扩张）期间，ACC 区域发生了不同的激活[58]。这项研究证实了内脏疼痛报告和参与疼痛体验情感和动机方面的预定脑区的脑激活之间的密切相关性。抑郁症患者 ACC 活性恢复到基线水平与临床改善相关[59]，并可预测抗抑郁治疗的反应[60]。随着 IBS 患者的疼痛和情绪障碍的改善，ACC 内的活动也发生了相应的变化[59]。

其他研究表明，在功能性消化不良中，在 FD 患者中，即使在静息状态下，中枢神经系统区域的脑葡萄糖代谢也会增加，认为其对功能性肠道疾病很重要[61]。观察到的 IBS 和虐待史对不同 ACC 激活的协同作用，提示了有一种机制可解释中枢神经系统传入过程如何与该患者人群中更严重的疼痛和更差结局的报告相关。此研究和其他研究[62-66]表明，中枢疼痛调节失调至关重要，可能发生在各种医疗和心理状况下。一项研究使用功能性 MRI 显示，与正常对照组和缓解期 UC 患者相比，IBS 患者在安慰剂镇痛给药期间，未能有效参与直肠扩张诱导的疼痛的神经下调[67]。还探索了内源性大麻素系统在脑-肠神经轴中的作用和潜在的治疗意义[68]。通过多方面的方法逆转功能性脑成像研究的结果，同时改善患者的预后，仍然是一个挑战。CAPS 和其他功能性疼痛疾病中存在的脑结构变化仍未得到证实，但是如果存在这种变化，神经可塑性的潜力提高了可逆性的可能性[28]。

6. 临床意义

CAPS 作为各级脑-肠神经轴功能失调的概念具有重要的临床意义。通过将心理社会因素与慢性疼痛病理生理学相联系，这一概念方案将治疗方法从单纯的精神治疗方法转变为包括更广泛潜在治疗的范例。早期的药物和心理治疗最终可能被证明可以逆转与慢性疼痛相关的感觉输入和大脑结构变化的失调调节[69]，从而预防随后的慢性疼痛综合征的发生[70,71]。

（三）临床特点

1. 病史

通常 CAPS 患者为中年女性。慢性腹痛为病史之一，常超过 10 年，初次就诊时患者常处于痛苦中。疼痛通常被描述

为是重度、持续性和弥漫性的。疼痛往往是患者生活中的一个焦点，可以用情感或怪异的术语来描述，不受进食、排便或月经的影响。腹痛可能是几种疼痛症状之一，也许是连续疼痛经历的一部分，通常开始于儿童期，并随时间反复[29]。CPAS 有时与其他疾病共存，临床医生必须确定其中一种其他疾病对 CAPS 诊断的贡献程度。CAPS 通常会在患有一种定义明确的胃肠道疾病但接受过一次或多次手术，并在这些手术后发生慢性腹痛的患者中演变。此类患者经常因肠粘连引起的肠梗阻而重复进行手术。

CAPS 患者经常有焦虑、抑郁、躯体障碍和创伤后紧张症等精神疾病的诊断。可能有外伤史，包括军事创伤。性和身体虐待史很常见，预示着健康状况不佳、医疗不应、大量的诊断和治疗程序以及医疗保健就诊[50]。可能在孩童时期了解到，当被诊断为躯体疾病而不是精神疾病时，更可能受到关注，患者可能将心理因素的作用降至最低。有未解决的伤害史是一个共同的特征[72]。由于患者通常不愿承认虐待史，医生应就此进行询问[73]。

最后，CAPS 患者可能有较差的社交网络，并表现出无效的应对策略。他们感觉无法减轻症状，可能无法识别和表达情绪（述情障碍），并可能“灾难性”（即，以悲观和病态的方式看待自己的病情，对后果没有任何控制感）。慢性腹痛可能是自杀意念的独立危险因素[28]。这些认知与更高的疼痛评分相关，会导致一系列其他疾病的发生，更严重的心理痛苦和更差的临床结局的循环[74]。对许多人来说，这种疾病需要通过朋友、家人以及卫生保健提供者的关注来提供社会支持。

2. 患者行为方式

CAPS 患者常见某些行为特征。这些患者往往要求医生及时诊断出问题，并迅速缓解其慢性症状。他们同样否认他们的问题与心理上令人不安的问题之间的关系，并经常将抑郁归因于疼痛，而不认为抑郁是一个促成因素。通常陪同的配偶或父母负责汇报患者的病史，这一观察结果暗示了家庭功能障碍的可能性。致幻毒品使用史也并不少见（见下文），初次就诊时患者要求使用此类药物也是如此。这种类型的行为反映了患者将其情况视为需要立即缓解症状的急性疾病，而不认为是需要制订针对性强化和适应性治疗的慢性症状。

3. 体格检查

某些体格检查有助于支持 CAPS 的诊断。腹部触诊应该从远离症状最明显的部位开始。在腹部触诊时应注意患者的行为动作，重点是关注在触诊部位转移时患者行为动作是否有变化。CAPS 患者通常缺乏自主觉醒的体征。无明确适应证的多处腹部手术瘢痕的存在可能提示导致不必要手术的慢性疼痛行为。可以注意到闭眼征[75]，当腹部触诊时，CAPS 患者可能会畏缩，闭上眼睛，而那些由于器质性病变引起的急性疼痛的患者，往往会因害怕检查而睁大眼睛。通常，听诊器征（在腹部疼痛部位用听诊器的隔膜温和、分散注意力的按压）会引起 CAPS 患者的行为反应减弱，从而对疼痛强度进行更准确的评估。进行全面的体格检查可确保不会忽视其他诊断（如腹壁疼痛），并将患者的疼痛视为一种医学的状况。

（四）诊断和鉴别诊断

在获得完整的病史、进行全面的体格检查和适当关注患者生活中的心理社会因素后，医生会作出 CAPS 的诊断。未提示腹腔内器质性病变证据的体格检查，以及常规实验室检查的正常结果，支持患者的疼痛不是由可识别的结构性疾病所致的论点。认识到 CAPS 的诊断标准（见框 12.2），未能发现其他原因引起的慢性腹痛的证据（见框 12.1），医生应诊断为 CAPS。如果 CAPS 的特征不存在或不典型，或者如果在体格检查（如腹部肿块、肝脏肿大）或实验室筛查检查（如贫血、低蛋白血症）中发现相关异常，应考虑其他诊断并进行相应的检查。非特异性异常并不少见（如肝囊肿），需要确定其与患者症状的相关性。有一种诊断 CAPS 的临床方法已被提出（图 12.4）[27]。

（五）治疗

1. 建立成功的医患关系

一旦排除了其他的诊断，CAPS 患者与医生（或其他医疗

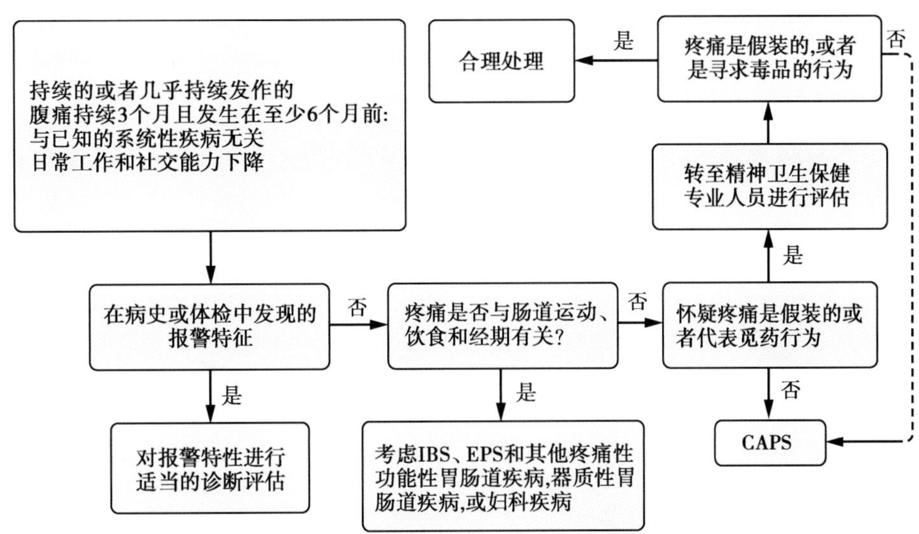

图 12.4　中枢介导的腹痛综合征（CAPS）的诊断算法。EPS，上腹痛综合征；IBS，肠易激综合征。（Adapted from Keefer L, Drossman DA, Guthrie E, et al. Centrally mediated disorders of gastrointestinal pain. Gastroenterology 2016;150:1408-19, with permission.）

保健提供者）之间建立成功的医患关系对于有效管至关重要。建立这种关系并走向成功的治疗需考虑几个因素（见第22章）。了解患者的心理社会背景是有益的，因为详细了解患者生活的这一方面有利于选择最有用的治疗方案。了解患者对疾病的理解程度非常重要，尤其是对于提高治疗计划的成功率。

在医患关系发展的早期，确定是否存在异常的疾病行为和相关的精神病诊断是很重要的，这些行为和诊断在高达60%的CAPS患者中存在[28]。同时还应了解家庭在患者疾病中的作用。正常情况下，家庭对疾病的经历会带来情感上的支持和关注其康复。在家庭互动功能失调的情况下，所有的压力都没有得到最佳的管理，将注意力转移到疾病上有助于减少家庭痛苦[76]。当家庭成员纵容患者时，对患者的管理承担不应有的责任，或成为患者的代言人时，就会出现功能障碍。如果观察到这样的家庭功能障碍，咨询可以帮助家庭制订更有用的应对策略。

还必须了解患者的文化信仰，因为患者可能不依从与其文化价值观不一致的治疗。重要的是要了解患者的心理社会资源（即社交网络资源），这可能有助于缓解压力的不利影响，并改善预后。

医生必须客观地承认疾病及其对患者生活的影响，向患者传达对疾病的确认。这一步骤对于确保患者理解医生认为CAPS是一种医学疾病非常重要。移情是首要的；它承认与患者疼痛相关的现实和痛苦，并可以提高对治疗计划的依从性、患者满意度和临床结局[77]。然而，这并不等同于对患者快速诊断和过度用药或进行不必要的诊断研究的愿望的过度反应。通过引导患者了解该综合征、解决任何问题、解释症状的性质，并确保理解所有已讨论过的问题来提供教育。需要重申的是，CAPS是一种医学疾病，通过改变疼痛控制中枢调节的药物或心理治疗可以减轻症状，这对患者来说是有帮助的。应提供保证，因为患者可能害怕严重疾病。评估完成后，医生应以清晰、客观和不带偏见的态度对患者关注的问题作出回应。然后，患者和医生必须协商治疗方案。这种方法使患者能够对治疗计划作出贡献并承担一定责任。在患者既往经验、利益和理解的背景下，医生应该提供选择而不是指令。当患者确信治疗计划将对其有益并且理解其基本原理时，更有可能依从治疗计划。最后，医生必须对花费的时间和精力以及对治疗的现实期望设定合理的限制。成功的关键是在设定适当界限的同时保持信任关系。

2. 制订治疗计划

一旦诊断出CAPS，主要的焦点应从测试和评估转移到开发有效的多方面的治疗计划，包括正在进行的患者访视以及药物和行为治疗。在认识通常需要组合和增强策略的情况下，临床情况必然会决定采用特定方法（图12.5）[27]。让患者了解治疗的目的是减轻症状并促进对这种慢性疾病的适应，而不是达到治愈是至关重要的。患者应通过识别疼痛发作的相关情况，包括情绪和认知反应，从而增加其对自身疾病的责任感。这种方法有助于患者深入了解病情加重的因素，并可反映出患者的应对方式。这些信息有助于确定行为治疗的策略。一般来说，除仔细选择的患者外，在无肠梗阻证据的CAPS患者中，不建议进行腹腔镜检查和粘连松解术[77a]。

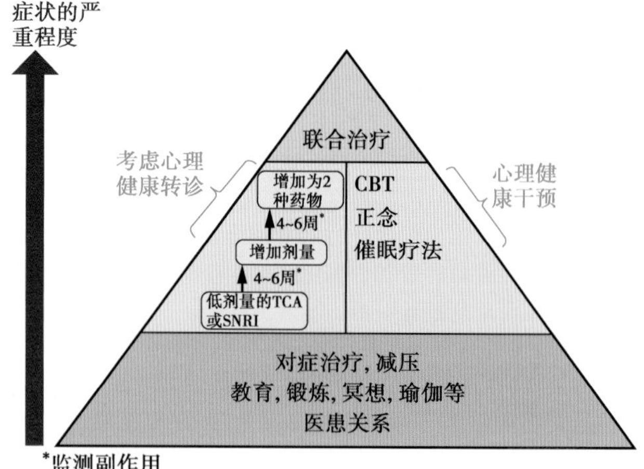

图12.5　基于症状严重程度的中枢介导的腹痛综合征管理概述。治疗的基础是建立牢固的医患关系和制订治疗计划，包括药理学和行为学方法，从针对特定症状的药物治疗和生活方式改变（如减压、运动）和教育开始。对于慢性疼痛，开始可使用低剂量三环类抗抑郁药（TCA）或5-羟色胺和去甲肾上腺素再摄取抑制剂（SNRI）。可以通过添加第二种药进行强化治疗（见正文）。可考虑进行心理健康干预，如认知行为疗法（CBT）或催眠疗法，以帮助管理疼痛和并减少由症状引起的心理压力。在重度病例中，药物和心理健康干预联合治疗是适当的。（Adapted from Keefer L，Drossman DA，Guthrie E，et al. Centrally mediated disorders of gastrointestinal pain. Gastroenterology 2016；150：1408-19，with permission.）

3. 药物治疗

目前缺乏前瞻性随机对照试验的证据支持CAPS的药物治疗。在功能性胃肠道疾病领域，特别是CAPS的药物开发一直很缓慢，部分原因是实验测试的经验过程必然发生在基于症状的综合征中[78]。此外，与其他功能性胃肠道疾病相比（如IBS、FD），CAPS不太常见。药理学脑成像方法有望成加速药物发现和后续开发的载体[79]。

尽管存在这些局限性，一些特定的药物已经被用于治疗CAPS（见下文）[79a]。可以预测的是，根据疾病的病理生理学（即，与脑-肠神经轴失调相关的生物心理社会疾病）、外周作用镇痛药（如对乙酰氨基酚、阿司匹林、其他非甾体抗炎药）对CAPS患者几乎没有益处。不应使用麻醉药和苯二氮䓬类药物治疗CAPS，因为这两种药物可能分别会增加疼痛敏感性和降低疼痛阈值，还必须牢记这些类型药物的药物依赖性的普遍性。处方此类药物有助于制订更复杂的治疗策略，而不仅仅是提供药物，并可能适得其反导致麻醉剂诱导的内脏疼痛强度增强，从而导致麻醉剂肠道综合征（见下文）[80]。

与治疗其他慢性疼痛疾病一样，三环类抗抑郁药物（tricyclic antidepressant，TCA）可能有助于CAPS[81-83]。这些药物通过抑制5-HT和去甲肾上腺素再摄取发挥作用，它们的获益来源于其能直接改善疼痛和（当以较高剂量使用时）治疗相关抑郁症的能力[84]。当目标是治疗疼痛时，TCA的给药剂量可低于治疗重度抑郁症的剂量（如地昔帕明，睡前25~100毫克/日）以尽量减少副作用。然而，治疗过程中剂量可能需要增加，特别是患者有精神疾病合并症时。在CAPS中使用选择性5-羟色胺再摄取抑制剂（selective serotonin reuptake inhibitor，SSRI，如西酞普兰）的证据较少，因为其缺乏去甲肾上腺素转运蛋白抑制会削弱其中枢镇痛作用的能力[85,86]。然而，当焦虑相关症状占主导地位时，可使用 SSRI[84,87]。5-羟色胺和去甲肾上腺素再摄取抑制剂(serotonin and norepinephrine reuptake inhibitor, SNRI)(如杜洛西汀、文拉法辛、米那普仑)对 CAPS 有益[78,84,88,89]。这类药物治疗便秘的作用低于 TCA，但中枢镇痛作用强于 SSRI。与 TCA 一样，SNRI 可同时用于治疗疼痛和抑郁[78,90]。当 TCA 或 SNRI 的临床反应欠佳时，可联合使用非典型(第二代)抗精神病药物(如喹硫平、阿立哌唑)、其他抗抑郁药或抗焦虑药(如米氮平、丁螺环酮)和 δ(delta)配体药物(如普瑞巴林、加巴喷丁)与其他药物(即所谓的强化治疗)[78,84,91]。药物强化治疗的获益来自于靶向不同脑区或受体的两种药物(每种药物通常以较低剂量给药)的使用，以达到最佳临床反应[91]。鉴于可能发生严重和复杂的不良事件，使用两种中枢神经调节剂的强化治疗，应由具有此类治疗的专业知识和经验的医生或多学科医生开具处方[27]。

对 IBS 的 TCA、SSRI 和 SNRI 和认知行为治疗(见下文)进行的系统综述和 meta 分析表明，所有这些治疗均有效(需要治疗的次数=4)[92]。已有文献综述了与使用中枢神经调节剂相关的潜在不良事件和停药注意事项。使用这些物的预防措施[84]。为了提高使用中枢神经调节剂的依从性，医师应解释这些药物是作为中枢镇痛药发挥作用，而不是简单地用于治疗精神疾病。

花时间向患者解释这些药物诱导大脑中神经递质的变化，从而改变疼痛感觉，并且剂量通常低于(在 TCA 治疗的情况下)用于治疗精神疾病的剂量，通常是有帮助的。需要强调的是，虽然药物临床获益可能滞后数周，但副作用会在治疗过程的早期出现。特别是使用三环类抗抑郁药后，大多数副作用在几天后减轻，可通过暂时降低药物剂量来减少。尽管如此，患者经常报告不良反应并提前停用新处方的药物，即使药物引起的症状通常在治疗前存在[93]。研究与个体对疾病的易感性和随后的药物反应相关的基因表达变异性(即药物基因组学)，有望成为优化一般慢性疼痛综合征和 FGID 管理的工具[94-96]。

4. 心理健康转诊和心理治疗

尽管上文已经介绍了使用两种药物的强化疗法，但另一种强化疗法是药物和心理治疗的联合治疗(见图 12.5)。后者在理论上很有吸引力，因为心理治疗作用于更高的皮层区域，而抗抑郁药物作用于皮层下区域[27,97]。患者可能不愿意去看精神卫生保健科医生，因为他们缺乏对转诊益处的了解，对被认为有精神问题而感到耻辱，或者将转诊视为医生的拒绝。心理干预最好是作为一种工具，与就医同时进行，可以帮助管理疼痛和减少症状引起的心理痛苦。

精神卫生保健提供者可以推荐任何一种用于疼痛管理的重度心理治疗[98,99]。这些心理治疗受益于促进高级脑功能的增强(如对既往创伤认知的适应和应对决策的改善)。认知行为治疗(cognitive behavioral treatment, CBT)识别适应不良的想法、观念和行为，结合心理教育和技能培训(如放松技巧)适用于 CAPS 的治疗[82]。证明 CBT 治疗有效的证据主要来自对 IBS 患者的研究[92,100,101]。来自功能性脑成像的证据表明，在慢性疼痛中，这种心理干预减少了直肠刺激所导致的中枢情绪区域(如杏仁核、ACC、额叶皮质)的激活[102]。CBT 已被证明对 CAPS 儿童的治疗特别有帮助，在一项研究中，父母参与治疗模式也产生了益处[103,104]。正念减压包括有意识地关注一个人的瞬间体验[105]。尽管这种疗法在 CAPS 中没有专门研究，但这种与冥想相关的心理逻辑结构显示出希望，并已被证明对 IBS 和其他慢性疼痛综合征患者有效[106]。催眠疗法的重点是松弛肠道，已在 IBS 患者中进行了主要研究，并发现对该疾病有益[107,108]。一项在儿童中进行的随机对照试验纳入了 31 例 CAPS 患者，得出的结论是，催眠治疗在一年时减轻疼痛方面优于标准药物治疗[109]。一项随访研究表明，平均持续 4.8 年后，催眠治疗仍明显优于传统药物治疗，表明肠道导向催眠治疗的有益作用是持久的[110]。一般情况下，诸如对治疗的信心和积极的认知等因素，大大有助于 CAPS 患者对各种治疗方式(药理学、CBT 和教育方法)的满意度[111]。

四、麻醉性肠综合征/阿片类药物诱导的胃肠道痛觉敏感

麻醉剂给药通常会引起胃肠动力障碍，继而引起便秘、肠梗阻和胃排空延迟，这种临床情况被称为阿片类肠道疾病或麻醉性肠道疾病。较少见的是麻醉性肠综合征(NBS)或阿片类药物引起的胃肠道痛觉过敏，这是一种独特的疾病，临床特征是与连续或递增剂量的麻醉剂相关的腹痛反常增加(框 12.3)[80,112]。NBS 是一种病理性疼痛亢进疾病，与阿片类药物对肠道分泌和运动的影响无关。NBS 越来越被认识，至少部分是由于宽松的处方麻醉药品治疗非恶性疾病变[113,114]。在一个普通慢性疼痛诊所中 NBS 的发生频率估计为 6%，在一项大型流行病学研究中的患病率估计为 4%[115,116]。一个大型病例系列表明，NBS 通常见于受过良好教育的年轻至中年女性，这些女性可能患有各种功能性或结构性胃肠道疾病[113]。该综合征也可见于术后患者。相关症状可能包括恶心、呕吐、胃灼热、便秘和腹泻。相关诊断可能包括胃轻瘫和肠假性梗阻。与 CAPS 一样，患者往往伴有焦虑或抑郁，频繁就医，导致相关医疗费用较高。正如预期的那样，这些患者通常残疾，有觅药行为，并认为自己一般健康状况非常差。

框 12.3　罗马Ⅳ麻醉性肠综合征/阿片类药物诱导的胃肠痛觉过敏诊断标准

必须包括以下所有内容：

1. 接受急性高剂量或慢性麻醉剂治疗的慢性或频繁复发的腹痛*。
2. 疼痛的性质和强度不能用当前或既往的胃肠道诊断来解释†。
3. 存在以下两种或以上情况：
   a. 继续或递增剂量的麻醉剂给药后疼痛加重或未完全消退。
   b. 当麻醉剂量减少时疼痛明显恶化，重新开始使用麻醉剂后疼痛改善("飙升和崩溃")。
   c. 发生频率、持续时间和疼痛发作强度。

*疼痛必须在大多数日期发生。

†患者可能有结构诊断(如炎症性肠病、慢性胰腺炎)，但疾病过程的特征或活动不足以解释疼痛。

From Whorwell PJ, Keefer L, Drossman DA, et al. Centrally mediated disorders of gastrointestinal pain. In: Drossman DA, Chang L, Chey WD, Kellow J, Tack J, Whitehead WE, editors. Rome Ⅳ: functional gastrointestinal disorders: disorders of gut-brain interaction. I. Raleigh, NC: The Rome Foundation; 2016. pp 1059-1116.

已描述 NBS 发生的各种假定机制[117]。提出的机制包括：阿片类药物诱导的神经胶质细胞（小胶质细胞和星形胶质细胞）激活[118]，通过 G-偶联的兴奋性阿片受体增强背角的疼痛信号[119]，通过激活髓质下行通路促进疼痛[120]，通过脊髓 N-甲基-D 天冬氨酸受体激活的疼痛易化途径[121]，以及中枢疼痛处理的异常（如在 CAPS 中）。

治疗这些患者对医生来说是一个挑战，需要牢固的医患关系和阿片类药物解毒。在 39 例特征明确的 NBS 患者的病例系列中[97]，90% 的患者成功完成了阿片类药物解毒项目，并与腹痛统计学显著减少 35% 相关[122]。对于戒毒后 3 个月仍停用麻醉药的患者，其腹痛评分比治疗前评分低 75%。不幸的是，到 3 个月时，近一半的患者已恢复使用麻醉剂。尽管疼痛得到缓解，但复发率如此之高的原因仍不清楚，但可能部分与医疗管理和处方实践通常几乎没有变化有关[123]。

（张烁 译，闫秀娥　刘军 校）

参考文献

第 13 章 食管疾病症状

Kenneth R. Devault 著

章节目录

一、吞咽困难 …… 161
（一）病理生理学 …… 161
（二）鉴别诊断及治疗方法 …… 162
二、吞咽痛 …… 164
三、癔球症 …… 164
（一）病理生理学 …… 164
（二）诊断及治疗方法 …… 165
四、呃逆 …… 165
五、食管源性胸痛 …… 165
（一）病理生理学 …… 165
（二）诊断及治疗方法 …… 166
六、胃灼热与反流 …… 166
（一）病理生理学 …… 167
（二）诊断及治疗方法 …… 167
七、胃食管反流病的食管外症状 …… 167

影响食管的常见症状包括吞咽困难、吞咽痛、癔球症、呃逆、胸痛、胃灼热、反流，以及一些由于胃食管反流引起的食管外症状。详细的病史采集可以辨别许多上述症状，再通过选择性检查和（或）试验性治疗亦可进一步辨别。吞咽困难可以表现在近端或远端，可能是单纯对固体或液体的吞咽困难，也可能两者皆有。吞咽困难患者应行钡餐造影、食管测压和胃镜检查。吞咽痛通常提示黏膜疾病，在大多数情况下应进行内镜检查。对癔球症和呃逆的评估通常不会出现明确的疾病，因此治疗具有挑战性。胸痛可能起源于食管，抑制胃酸治疗通常有效。如果没有反流，胸痛的评估和治疗就变得具有挑战性。胃食管反流病（gastroesophageal reflux disease，GERD）可能引起的典型症状（胃灼热和反流）和食管外症状，抑制胃酸试验性治疗有效，有助于诊断。动态 pH 测定是确定这些患者是否有反流的最佳方法。许多这些食管症状也可能发生在没有客观病理证据的患者身上，然后按照功能性疾病处理。

与食管有关的症状在普通内科和胃肠病专科实践中都是最常见的。例如，吞咽困难随着年龄的增长而变得更加常见，65 岁以上人群中有 15% 的人有吞咽困难[1]。胃灼热、反流以及其他 GERD 的症状也很常见。一项对明尼苏达州奥姆斯特德县健康受试者的调查发现，20% 的人，不论性别或年龄，至少每周有一次胃灼热[2]。轻微的 GERD 症状很少提示存在严重的潜在疾病，但必须予以关注，尤其是如果这些症状持续多年。频繁或持续的吞咽困难或吞咽疼痛提示存在食管问题需要检查和治疗。其他可能起源于食管但不具有特异性的症状包括癔球症、胸痛、嗳气、呃逆、反刍和食管外不适，如气喘、咳嗽、咽喉痛和声音嘶哑。评估食管症状的一个主要困难是，食管损伤的程度通常与患者或医生对症状严重程度的认知不相关[3]。在老年患者中，情况更特殊，尽管症状的总体严重程度下降，但胃食管反流导致食管黏膜损伤的严重程度却是增加的[4]。

一、吞咽困难

吞咽困难（dysphagia）一词来源于希腊语 dys（困难、障碍）和 phagia（吃），指的是食物在从口到胃的运输过程中受阻的感觉。大多数患者抱怨食物粘住、挂住或停在食管中，或者他们觉得食物“就是不能正常下咽”。他们偶尔会抱怨吞咽过程中有疼痛感。如果被问到：“你吞咽有困难吗？”一些食管下段吞咽困难的患者会说“不”，因为他们可能认为吞咽只是食物从口中转移到食管的过程。食管扩张的患者，尤其是由于贲门失弛缓症，可能会错误地将吞咽困难理解为反流甚至呕吐。吞咽困难通常表现为口咽或食管的某种类型的功能障碍，如有相关的精神疾病可以放大这种症状。

（一）病理生理学

吞咽困难是由于将食物从口腔运送到胃所需肌肉的力量或协调性出现问题，或者是口腔和胃部之间某个固定的梗阻造成的。偶尔有患者可能同时具有这两个病因。口咽吞咽机制和随后食管体部的初级和次级蠕动收缩，通常在 10 秒钟内将固体和液体团块从口腔输送到胃。如果这些有序的收缩不能形成或顺序进行，累积的食物团块会扩张食管腔，引起与吞咽困难有关的不适症状。对于一些患者，尤其是老年人，吞咽困难是初级或次级收缩振幅过低的结果，不足以清除食管内容物。高分辨率测压法已经确定了不同长度的蠕动减弱或缺失区域（蠕动间隙），这些或许可以解释一些常规测压结果正常的患者出现吞咽困难[5]。其他患者有原发性或继发性动力障碍，严重扰乱食管体部的有序收缩。因为这些运动异常可能不会出现在每一次吞咽中，吞咽困难症状可能时强时弱（仍见第 43 章）。

尽管有足够的蠕动收缩，食管机械性狭窄仍可能会中断食物团块的有序通过。症状随食管梗阻程度、相关食管炎及进食食物种类而有所不同。正常的食管在食物团块到达之前就会扩张。食管扩张不良（如由嗜酸性食管炎或放射性食管炎所致）的患者即使胃镜和消化道造影未见食管狭窄（见下文）[6]，也可能会出现吞咽困难。微小的阻塞性病变仅在进食大量未仔细咀嚼的食物团如肉类和干面包时才引起吞咽困难，而食管腔完全阻塞性病变进食固体和液体均有症状。

GERD可引起食管狭窄从而导致吞咽困难,但一些无明显食管狭窄的GERD患者也可出现明显吞咽困难症状,有些患者甚至可能没有食管炎[7]。即使食管中的团块已清除,食管感觉异常亦可导致吞咽困难的感觉。一些健康志愿者的远端食管被球囊状扩张以及被其他内容物刺激扩张时,也能体验到吞咽困难的感觉,因此内脏感觉异常可以解释那些病因不明的吞咽困难[8]。这一机制也适用于一些精神症状频发的痉挛性运动障碍患者,他们的吞咽困难症状被放大[9]。

(二) 鉴别诊断及治疗方法

当面对一个抱怨吞咽困难的患者时,医务工作者应该系统地处理这个问题。大多数患者可将这一症状定位在食管的上、下段,但偶尔有食管远端吞咽困难的患者,其症状仅出现在胸骨上切迹或更高位置。吞咽困难可以分为口咽和食管吞咽困难,当然两类患者会有重叠。首先应确定患者是仅在吞咽固体食物方面有困难,还是吞咽固体、液体都有困难。

1. 口咽吞咽困难

由于这一病变过程影响口腔、下咽和食管上段,患者往往不能下咽,并且必须反复尝试吞咽。患者通常以进食时咳嗽或窒息为主诉。无法将食物团块成功地从下咽区域经食管上括约肌(upper esophageal sphincter, UES)送入食管体内的表现,称为口咽或传输性吞咽困难。患者意识到团块没有离开口咽部,并将症状部位具体定位于颈段食管区域。在吞咽后立即发生或1秒内发生的吞咽困难提示口咽异常。有时,液体食物可能进入气管或鼻腔而不是食管。一些患者反复食物团块嵌塞,需要手动取出。病情严重的患者甚至因不能吞咽唾液而流口水。在这种情况下,家庭急救通常采用海姆利克氏操作法,但除非阻塞物位于气道内,否则这种方法是不合适的。患者家属需要被教育和告知,只要患者能说话,气道就是通畅的,强迫食管近端团块上移,反而可能导致而不是防止误吸。发音异常,如构音障碍或鼻音,也可能与口咽吞咽困难有关。系统性神经和神经肌肉疾病,如帕金森病、肌萎缩侧索硬化症和多发性肌炎可以吞咽困难为主要症状,甚至偶尔为唯一症状。口腔疾病也应考虑;牙齿不好或假牙不合适可能会影响咀嚼,导致患者去尝试吞咽过大或未充分咀嚼的食物团块。由于药物、辐射或原发性唾液功能障碍引起的唾液分泌减少,都有可能导致食物团块吞咽困难。

反复发作的肺部感染提示食物溢出进入气管(误吸),可能由于喉部保护不足。声音嘶哑可能是由喉返神经功能障碍或内在肌肉疾病引起的,这两种疾病都会导致声带的无效运动。软腭或咽部收缩肌无力可引起构音障碍、鼻音和咽鼻反流。Zenker憩室患者可出现吞咽时伴有咯咯声。不明原因的体重减轻可能是吞咽困难的唯一线索;患者因为吞咽困难而拒绝进食。口咽部吞咽困难的潜在原因见框13.1。

在获得详尽的病史后,应首先在吞咽治疗师(改良钡餐)的帮助下进行仔细的消化道造影(下咽部)检查。如果液体钡剂结果是正常的,尝试给予患者固体食物团块重复检查,以诱发患者吞咽困难症状,从而有助于病变定位。如果口咽部分检查正常,应检查食管的其余部分。经改良钡餐检查通常能发现问题并指导初步治疗。

框13.1 口咽吞咽困难的原因

神经肌肉原因*

肌萎缩侧索硬化(Lou Gehrig症)
中枢神经系统肿瘤(良性的或恶性的)
特发性UES功能障碍
UES或咽部测压异常†
多发性硬化
肌营养不良
重症肌无力
帕金森病
多发性肌炎或皮肌炎
产后综合征
脑卒中
甲状腺功能障碍

器质性原因

癌症
咽部或颈部感染
骨刺和其他脊柱疾病
手术或放射性治疗后
近端食管蹼
甲状腺肿大
Zenker憩室

*任何影响横纹肌或其神经支配的疾病均可能导致吞咽困难。
†尽管其与吞咽困难的真实关系尚不明确,但常常发现测压异常(UES压力过高或过低,协调异常,UES松弛不完全)
UES,食管上括约肌。

2. 食管吞咽困难

大多数食管吞咽困难患者的症状集中在胸骨下部,有时也可在上腹部。少数患者尽管食物团块停在下段食管,也出现胸骨上切迹或更高位置的症状。食管吞咽困难通常可以通过重复吞咽、抬举手臂过头顶、向后甩肩膀以及Valsalva动作来缓解。食管蠕动障碍或机械性梗阻性病变可导致食管吞咽困难。为明确食管吞咽困难症状的病因,以下3个问题的答案至关重要:

(1) 什么类型的食物或液体会引起症状?

(2) 吞咽困难是间歇性的还是进行性的?

(3) 患者有胃灼热的症状吗?

在这些答案的基础上,以器质(机械性)或神经肌肉(动力性)缺陷加以区分食管吞咽困难(框13.2),并推测其可能的具体原因(图13.1)。

固体和液体均吞咽困难的患者更可能是出现了食管动力障碍,而不是机械性梗阻。贲门失弛缓症是典型的食管动力障碍,除了吞咽困难外,许多贲门失弛缓症患者会出现未消化食物的轻微反流,尤其是在晚上,以及体重减轻。相比之下,像远端食管痉挛这样的痉挛性运动障碍患者,主要表现为胸痛和对液体冷热的过度敏感。硬皮病(系统性硬化)累及食管患者通常有Raynaud现象以及可能有胃灼热和反流。在这些患者中,轻微的吞咽困难可能是由于动力障碍或食管炎症,但严重的吞咽困难多提示存在消化性狭窄或恶性肿瘤(少见)(见第37、44、46章和48章)。

框 13.2　食管吞咽困难的常见原因

神经肌肉(动力性)疾病

原发性

贲门失弛缓症

食管远端痉挛

高收缩(jackhammer)食管

食管下括约肌高压

胡桃夹(高压)食管

其他动力异常*

继发性

南美锥虫病(Chagas 病)

反流相关动力障碍

硬皮病和其他风湿性自身免疫病

器质(机械性)性疾病

食管腔内

癌症和良性肿瘤

憩室病

嗜酸性食管炎

食管环和食管蹼(除 Schatzki 环外)

异物

下食管环(Schatzki 环)

药物所致狭窄

消化性狭窄

食管腔外

纵隔肿物

脊柱骨刺

血管压迫

*蠕动异常包括无蠕动和弱蠕动,以及高压性蠕动(胡桃夹食管)。

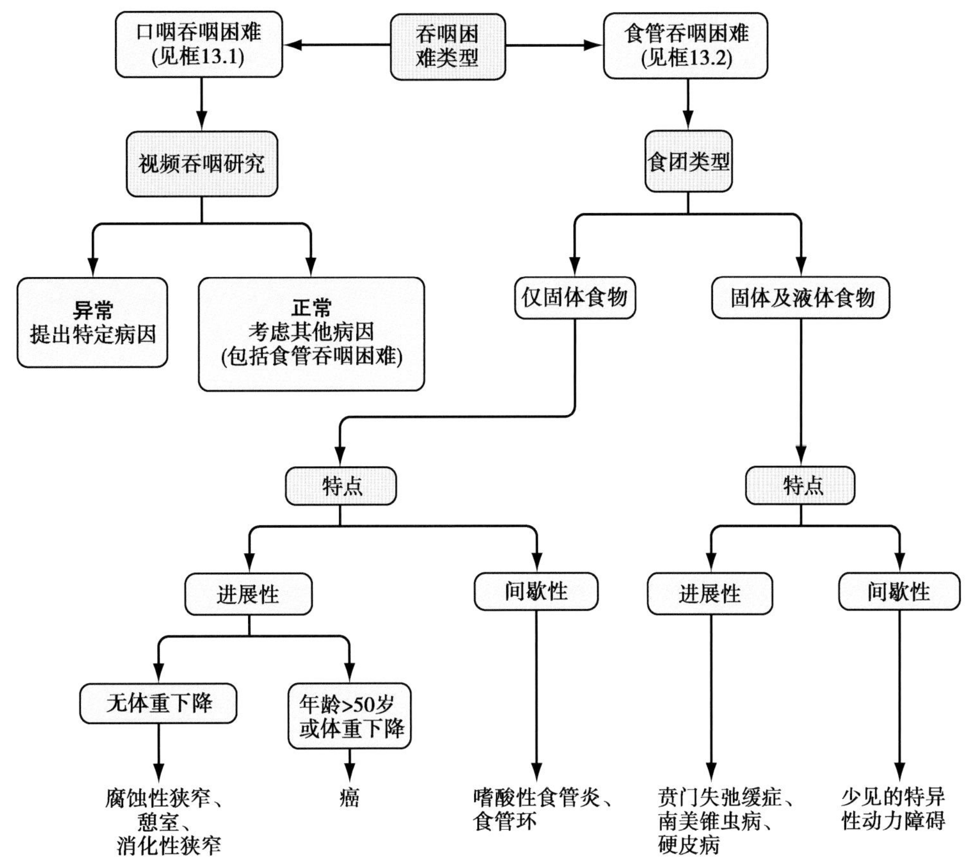

图 13.1　吞咽困难患者的诊断流程。关于每种类型吞咽困难诊断及治疗方法的详细信息,请参阅正文和框。少见的特异性动力障碍疾病包括胡桃夹食管、远端食管痉挛和其他无效食管动力障碍。(Modified from Castell DO, Donner MW. Evaluation of dysphagia: a careful history is crucial. Dysphagia 1987;2:65-71.)

对于仅在吞咽固体食物后才出现吞咽困难,而吞咽液体食物时没有症状的患者,应怀疑为机械性梗阻。当管腔内梗阻严重时,也会出现固体和液体同时吞咽困难。如果发生食物嵌塞,患者必须经常通过反胃来缓解。当患者在团块嵌塞后继续饮入液体,大部分液体可能会反流。在询问有液体反流的患者时,最重要的是将真正的液体吞咽困难患者(口服液体后即出现)与只有在进食过固体团块(可能阻塞)后才出现液体吞咽困难的患者区分开。在吞咽困难发作时,唾液分泌过多是很常见的,会造成更多的液体回流。

不伴有体重减轻的发作性和间歇性吞咽困难是食管蹼或

远端食管环(Schatzki 环)的特征性表现[10]。第一次发作通常发生在快速进食的时候,且常于饮酒后。患者感觉食物团块黏附在食管下部,通过喝大量的液体可以使食物下咽。多数患者在梗阻缓解后,可以继续顺利进食而无不适。最初一次距下次发作间期一般为数周或数月,但随后可能会频繁发生(详见第 43 章)。日常发生的吞咽困难一般不考虑由下食管环引起。

如果固体食物吞咽困难进展明显,需鉴别消化性食管狭窄和癌症。有些 GERD 患者可发展为良性食管狭窄(见第 46 章),这些患者大多有长期的胃灼热病史。良性病灶的患者很少出现体重减轻,因为这些患者食欲很好,并且会将他们的饮食结构转化为高热量软食和流质食物来维持体重。癌症患者与消化性狭窄患者在许多方面存在差异。癌症患者年龄更大,吞咽困难进展迅速,有或没有胃灼热的病史,或曾经出现过胃灼热症状但不是现在。大多数癌症患者都有纳差和体重减轻(见第 48 章)。真正的吞咽困难可能出现在药源性、腐蚀性或病毒性食管炎患者中,但这些急性食管损伤患者的主诉通常是吞咽疼痛(见第 45 章)。

当患者出现食物团梗阻伴吞咽困难时,需要鉴别嗜酸性食管炎(见第 30 章)[11]。嗜酸性食管炎最初在年轻成年男性中被描述,但是随后的一系列研究发现这种疾病在两性和所有年龄组中都存在[12]。

外科手术相关吞咽困难包括胃底折叠术后或其他食管胃交界处的手术,减肥手术后也可能出现吞咽困难(见第 8 章)。这种吞咽困难可能是由于机械性梗阻引起,但也有术后动力障碍的报道,可呈与贲门失弛缓症一致的测压表现[13]。

在获得患者重点的症状病史后,通常首先完成包含固体团块激发试验在内的消化道造影。另外,许多专家提倡内镜检查作为第一选择,特别是对于间歇性固体食物吞咽困难(提示下段食管环)或者有明显反流症状的患者。初始检查的选择应该基于当地的技术条件和首诊医生的偏好。如果消化道造影显示有梗阻性病变,通常会做内镜检查以确认和活检。内镜检查时也可以进行食管狭窄、环和肿瘤的扩张。这种经验性扩张常用于病史提示阻塞性吞咽困难且内镜检查结果正常的患者[14],但其安全性和有效性一直受到质疑[15]。如果消化道造影是正常的,可以做食管测压寻找食管运动障碍的原因。一些有反流和吞咽困难症状的患者,消化道造影、内镜检查结果正常,或两者均正常的情况下,可以对其进行诊断性抑酸治疗。

二、吞咽痛

和吞咽困难一样、吞咽痛是食管受累的特征性症状。吞咽痛的性质从吞咽时胸骨后隐痛到可放射至背部的刺痛(严重时患者无法进食甚至不能吞咽唾液)均可出现。吞咽痛通常反映食管黏膜炎症,在极少数情况下涉及肌层。引起吞咽痛的最常见病因包括食入腐蚀性物质、药物性食管炎、放射性食管炎和感染性食管炎[念珠菌、疱疹病毒、巨细胞病毒(框 13.3)](见第 41 和 45 章)。在这些疾病中,吞咽困难也可能存在,但疼痛是主要主诉。GERD 患者的很少出现吞咽痛,一旦出现通常存在严重食管溃疡。在少数案例中,非阻塞性食管癌可伴有吞咽痛的症状。由于许多引起吞咽痛的疾病都有相关的症状和体征,仔细研究病史通常可以帮助诊断。例如,一个青少年服用四环素治疗痤疮,在治疗过程中出现了吞咽痛,那么药物性吞咽困难是最有可能的;免疫功能受损的患者出现吞咽痛很可能是感染所致(见第 35、36 和 45 章);而 GERD 患者出现吞咽痛最可能是因为严重的消化性食管炎。食管胃十二指肠镜检查以观察食管黏膜并且活检是明确大多数吞咽痛患者诊断所必需的。

框 13.3 吞咽痛的原因
食入腐蚀性物质
酸
碱
药物性损伤
阿伦膦酸盐和其他双膦酸盐
阿司匹林和其他非甾体抗炎药
依美溴铵
铁制剂
氯化钾(特别是缓释型)
奎尼丁
四环素及其衍生物
齐多夫定
感染性食管炎
病毒
巨细胞病毒
埃博拉病毒
艾滋病毒
疱疹病毒
细菌
分枝杆菌(结核分枝杆菌或鸟分枝杆菌复合物)
真菌
白念珠菌
组织胞浆菌病
原虫
隐孢子虫病
肺孢子菌
严重反流性食管炎
食管癌

三、癔球症

癔球症是指喉间有异物或紧缩的感觉,与吞咽无关。高达 46% 的普通人群曾经历过至少一次癔球症[16]。这种感觉可以被描述为一种异物、紧缩、哽噎或窒息感,就好像东西卡在喉咙里。癔球症常发生在两餐之间,吞咽固体或大量液体食物可暂时缓解。频繁的干性吞咽和情绪压力会加重这种症状。癔球症可能发生在创伤事件后,比如吞下粗糙的团块(鱼骨),或者心理创伤性的内镜插管,即使没有严重的黏膜损伤仍可以出现上述症状[17]。有吞咽困难或吞咽疼痛症状时不能诊断为癔球症。

(一) 病理生理学

癔球症患者的生理和心理异常的检测一直是不一致和有

争议的。尽管经常有人提出，但压力测定异常的食管上括约肌功能障碍，食管上括约肌对食管扩张、酸化或精神压力高反应性，都不能证实是引起癔球症的直接原因[18]。此外，食管扩张可引起食管上括约肌压力不升高的癔球症，精神压力可引起正常受试者（无癔球症）、癔球症患者食管上括约肌压力升高。据报道，高达 90% 的癔球症患者有胃灼热症状[19]，但通过食管 pH 监测发现的食管炎或胃食管反流却不足 25%（见下文）。食管球囊扩张时，与对照组相比，癔球症患者在球囊体积较小的情况下即可诱发症状；这一发现表明，某些癔球症患者对食管牵张的感受性增强。

心理因素可能在癔球症的发生中起重要作用。最常见的相关精神疾病包括焦虑、惊恐障碍、抑郁、疑病症、躯体化障碍和内向[20]。实际上，癔球症是躯体化障碍患者第四常见的症状（见第 23 章）[21]。生物因素、疑病人格特征和窒息后学得的恐惧综合作用为症状的错误判读提供了一个框架，并加剧了癔球症或患者的焦虑症状[22]。

（二）诊断及治疗方法

癔球症患者首先需排除更危险的潜在疾病，然后提供对症治疗。鼻内镜、消化道造影检查可排除咽部病变[23]。癔球症患者经常在喉部出现红斑等变化，可能与喉咽反流相关。大多数反流专家认为这些改变是非特异性的，不能诊断为病理性反流[24]。如果患者有胃灼热，先进行抑酸治疗，但即使没有胃灼热，反流也可能是引起癔球症的原因。质子泵抑制剂（proton pump inhibitor，PPI）试验（通常餐前服用，每日两次）对一些患者具有诊断和治疗作用。动态反流监测可显示胃酸或非胃酸反流（见第 46 章）[25]。另外，如果患者有明显的焦虑，并且已经尝试抑酸治疗无效，应该考虑进行心理问题相关治疗。

四、呃逆

呃逆，又称打嗝，是由膈肌收缩和声门闭合共同引起的。因此，它不是经典的食管症状，但是基层医疗单位和胃肠道疾病专科中常见的主诉症状。大多数呃逆的病例都是特发性的，但与影响中枢神经系统，胸部或腹部的许多病症如创伤、肿物、感染、尿毒症等有关。与尿毒症相关的呃逆极难控制，胃肠道原因包括胃食管反流病、贲门失弛缓症、胃病和消化性溃疡。呃逆通常在饱餐后，由于大部分病例具有自限性，通常不需要干预。对慢性或疑难病例还需要包括能排除食管，胸部或全身性疾病的特定检查。胃食管反流病可引起呃逆，因此对某些患者进行试验性抑酸治疗是合理的[26]。许多药物可不同程度抑制呃逆：氯丙嗪、硝苯地平、氟哌啶醇、苯妥英钠、甲氧氯普胺、巴氯芬和加巴喷丁[27]。在难治性病例中也尝试了包括针灸在内的其他方式[28]。曾有膈神经消融和刺激治疗的报道，但只有在尝试多种低侵入性的治疗手段后仍无法控制，而生活质量严重受影响的顽固性病例中才使用[29]。

五、食管源性胸痛

对患者和初诊医生而言，食管源性胸痛与心绞痛很难区分。在解剖学位置上，食管与心脏相邻并由共同的神经支配。事实上，一旦排除了心脏疾病，食管疾病是胸痛最常见的病因。在美国，每年大约 100 万患者因考虑心源性胸痛行心脏冠状动脉造影检查，近 40% 患者的冠状动脉正常，其中大部分均是由食管疾病引起的[30,31]。

食管源性胸痛通常描述为挤压性或烧灼样胸骨后疼痛，可放射至背部、颈部、下颌或手臂。虽然并不总是与吞咽有关，但吞咽冷或热的液体可诱发疼痛。有些患者睡梦中会痛醒，情绪紧张还会加剧症状。疼痛的持续时间从几分钟到几小时不等，也可间歇性发作，持续数天。疼痛剧烈时患者可出现脸色苍白、大汗，但一般可自行或服用抑酸剂缓解，偶尔特别严重时则需要镇静剂或硝酸甘油来缓解。严格的问卷调查显示，大多数食管源性胸痛患者同时有其他食管症状，但在约 10% 的病例中胸痛是唯一的食管相关主诉[32]。

临床病史并不足以使医生确切地区分胸痛是心源性还是食管源性的。事实上，运动可以引起胃食管反流[33]呈现与心绞痛相似的劳累性胸痛，平板试验期间亦可诱发症状。提示食管源性胸痛的特征包括持续数小时的疼痛，胸骨后痛但不横向放射，影响睡眠或与进餐有关，且制酸剂可缓解症状。同时伴随其他食管症状有助于诊断，然而，多达 50% 的心源性胸痛的患者也存在一种或多种食管疾病症状[34]。此外，舌下含服硝基甘油可减轻疼痛已被证实对冠状动脉起源性疼痛不具特异性[35]。随着人们年龄的增长，心脏和食管疾病的发病率也随之增加，这两个问题可能不仅共存还相互作用产生胸痛。肌肉骨骼疼痛也可引起胸痛，因此检查应包括仔细的胸部触诊。

（一）病理生理学

引起食管源性胸痛的具体机制尚未明确，通常归因于化学感受器（通过酸、胃蛋白酶或胆汁）或机械感受器（通过扩张或痉挛）的刺激，也可能涉及温度感受器（受寒冷刺激）。胃食管反流主要通过酸敏感的食管化学感受器引起胸痛。酸引起的胃动力障碍也可能是食管性疼痛的原因。早期研究表明，向胃食管反流患者的食管灌注酸性物质会增加食管收缩的幅度和持续时间，诱发同步和自主收缩，同时伴有疼痛的发生[36]。自发性酸反流期间可观察到远端食管痉挛。但在随后使用现代设备进行的研究中，人们很少发现这种动力性变化[37]。此外，使用 24 小时动态食管 pH 和动力监测的研究结果显示，食管动力异常和胸痛之间的联系并不常见，并且自发性酸诱导型胸痛与食管动力异常也基本没有关联[38,39]。

与正常人相比，疑似食管源性胸痛的患者，高振幅食管收缩增加，同时同步收缩频率略有增加[40]。此外，食管腔内超声已经能够识别部分胸痛患者的纵行平滑肌的异常持续收缩[41]，但这种收缩引起疼痛的机制尚不清楚。一种可能的解释是，动力改变使食管壁张力升高，抑制食管血流量，形成肌局部缺血（即肌缺血）期，故而产生疼痛。Mac Kenzie 及其同事发现，与同龄对照组相比，有症状的食管动力障碍患者在将冷水注入食管后，食管复温率降低[42]。因为雷诺现象患者冷水灌注后复温率与血流量直接相关，故作者推测食管缺血是复温率降低的原因。然而在研究过程中，有症状的食管动力障碍患者均未出现胸痛。此外，食管具有广泛的动脉和静脉供血，这使得即使是极度异常的食管收缩也不太可能影响血流。食管源性胸痛与异常食管收缩之间的关系是复杂的，当确定收缩异常时，这些患者中的大多数是无症状的。而且食管收缩幅度的减少并不能预测胸痛的缓解[43]。与胸痛相关的动力改变可能是慢性疼痛综合征的表现，而不是疼痛的直接原因。事实上，在正常人和胃食管反流患者中，实验诱导加压可以产生测压变化并降低食管对球囊或酸刺激的耐受性[44]。

食管源性胸痛的其他潜在原因包括温度感受器被激发和管腔扩张。摄入热或寒冷的液体可导致严重的胸痛。这种关联以前被认为与食管痉挛有关，但随后的研究表明，寒冷诱发的疼痛使食管蠕动停止和扩张，而不是痉挛[45]。该观察结果表明，食管源性胸痛的原因可能是急性扩张激活牵张感受器所致。食管扩张和疼痛可见于急性食物嵌塞、饮用碳酸饮料（部分患者）和呃逆反射功能障碍者[46]。与无症状人群相比，相对低体积的食管球囊扩张即可诱发易感人群的食管源性胸痛[47]。因此，痛觉改变可能导致患者对疼痛刺激的反应不同。恐慌症是胸痛患者普遍被忽视的伴随症状[48]，应该在采集病史时特别询问。研究结果显示，抗焦虑药和抗抑郁药可以提高疼痛阈值，并能改善情绪状态，这可以解释为什么这些药物可以在没有压力变化的情况下改善食管源性胸痛[49,50]。

（二）诊断及治疗方法

多年来，治疗食管源性胸痛的处理方案不断发展[51]。在明确食管为胸痛病因前，必须通过运动压力测试，非侵入性心脏成像和冠状动脉造影等方法排除心源性病因。

冠脉结构正常但灌注血流量不足（微血管心绞痛）已被认为是一些患者胸痛的原因[52]。有报道显示改善微血管心绞痛的药物对食管也有作用，故难以根据治疗试验诊断微血管心绞痛；然而，大多数微血管性心绞痛患者的预后良好[53]。

目前公认对食管源性胸痛认识的重大进展为：胸痛与胃食管反流病存在关联。在排除了心脏病因的患者中，高达50%动态 pH 测试可检测到病理性酸反流或酸反流与胸痛相关[54]。这些患者试验性使用质子泵抑制剂治疗可以有效改善症状[55]。当患者同时存在反流症状时，胸痛和胃食管反流病之间的关联很容易识别，但在没有典型的反流症状的情况下就不那么明显。与动态食管内 pH 监测相比，每天两次口服 PPI 共 10~14 天的试验性抑酸治疗对食管源性胸痛的诊断具有很好的敏感性和特异性[56]。2013 年一项随机安慰剂对照试验的结果，支持基层医疗单位在排除心脏疾病的前提下，对有胸痛症状的患者进行 PPI 试验性治疗[57]。即使同时存在动力障碍，抑酸治疗也可缓解胸痛[58]。如果患者试验性抑酸治疗失败，则可尝试丙米嗪或曲唑酮等可提高疼痛阈值的药物[59]。

一些权威人士建议在此时使用静态食管测压以排除动力障碍，并用动态 pH 监测来排除 PPI 试验性抑酸治疗无效的胃食管反流。胸痛患者很少会有特定的动力障碍，如贲门失弛缓症或食管远端痉挛，更多的情况下是非特异性压力异常，很难解释单个患者的症状。胃食管反流监测无管无线系统的出现使得监测期更长、更舒适，这也增加了观察到疼痛和酸性事件之间相关性的可能性[60]。如果动态 pH 监测提示胃食管反流，则需要继续进行抑酸治疗。如果测压中发现痉挛性或高收缩性动力障碍，可尝试硝酸盐或钙通道阻滞剂降低食管压力，尽管一些胸痛和动力障碍患者对降低内脏敏感性的药物反应更好。以食管痉挛和胸痛为主的Ⅲ型贲门失弛缓症患者应避免手术（肌切开术）（见第 44 章）。

六、胃灼热与反流

胃灼热是西方人最常见的胃肠道主诉之一[2]。事实上，这个症状的普遍存在以至于很多人认为它是正常的而没向他们的医生告知相关症状。他们用非处方抗酸药来缓解症状，此类药物每年 10 亿美元的销售额中大部分都是用于控制胃灼热。尽管胃灼热的发病率很高，但经常被误解。它有许多同义词，包括消化不良、酸反流、胃酸过多和剧烈打嗝。如果患者没有主动提出胃灼热，医生应该仔细倾听患者描述的症状。一项来自欧洲的研究表明，使用“从胃或下胸部向颈部上升的燃烧感”的文字-图表描述可以增强识别患者胃食管反流的能力[61]。灼烧感通常从低处开始，沿胸骨后区域向上蔓延至颈部，偶尔向背部放射，很少会累及手臂。由胃酸反流引起的胃灼热可以通过服用抗酸剂、小苏打或牛奶得到暂时缓解。有趣的是，食管损伤的严重程度（食管炎或 Barrett 食管）与胃灼热的程度无关［例如，严重胃灼热患者在内镜检查时食管可能正常，严重食管炎或 Barrett 食管患者可能仅有轻微或甚至没有症状（见第 46 章和第 47 章）］[62]。

胃灼热通常发生在进食后 1 小时内，特别是在一天中最丰盛的一餐后。糖、巧克力、洋葱、消胀药和高脂肪食物可能会降低食管下括约肌压力，从而加重胃灼热。其他与胃灼热相关的食物由于其酸性或高渗透压而刺激炎性的食管黏膜，如柑橘类产品、番茄类食物、辛辣食物[63]。饮料包括柑橘汁、软饮料、咖啡和酒精，也可能引起胃灼热。酒精与胃灼热之间的关系复杂。研究表明，大多数与酒精有关的胃灼热与对酸敏感性增加有关，其原因是酒精破坏食管上皮细胞之间紧密连接，从而使正常量的胃酸深入黏膜并产生症状[64]。许多患者在晚餐或进食零食后不久就进入睡眠状态会加剧胃灼热，而有些患者则为右侧卧位时，胃灼热症状更加明显[65]。体重增加往往会导致胃食管反流病新症状的出现，并加重已有的 GERD 症状[66]。

弯腰、用力排便、抬举重物、静力训练等增加腹压的活动可加重胃灼热症状。对胃食管反流病患者来说，跑步也可能加重胃灼热，骑自行车可能是更好的运动方式[33]。由于尼古丁和吸入空气会降低食管下括约肌压力，因此吸烟会加剧反流症状[67]。情绪（如焦虑、恐惧、担忧）可能通过降低内脏敏感度阈值而不是增加胃食管酸反流量来加剧胃灼热[68]。某些药物可通过降低食管下括约肌压力和蠕动收缩（如氨茶碱、钙通道阻滞剂）或刺激炎性的食管（例如阿司匹林、其他非甾体抗炎药、双膦酸盐）来引发或加重胃灼热症状。

胃灼热可伴有口腔感觉到有苦味酸性物质或者咸性液体。反流可表现为苦味酸性液体回流到口腔，优势胃内食物、胃酸或胆汁很轻易反流。反流在夜间或患者弯腰时容易发作。无恶心、干呕、腹部收缩用力等表现的话，提示反流而不是呕吐（见第 15 章）。“吐清水”是一种不常见的但经常被误解的症状，它是用来形容口腔内突然充满清澈微咸的液体。这种液体不是反流物，而是唾液腺的分泌物，是食管远端迷走神经保护性反射引起的[69]。贲门失弛缓症患者可能有反流和类似吐清水的症状，而被误诊为胃食管反流病。

反流必须与反刍综合征区分开（见第 15 章）。反刍是依据罗马Ⅳ诊断标准的临床诊断。患者必须为持续或反复地将新近摄入食物反流至口腔内（之前没有干呕），之后再咀嚼并咽下。支持标准包括无恶心，回流物质变酸性时此过程停止，且反刍回流的是可识别且味道也不错的内容物[70]。在临床怀疑时，反刍实际上是一种排除诊断。有报道称，在长时间测压过程中经常会出现一种相当特殊的模式，但同时有反刍症状的发作才有意义[71]。贪食症患者有时也会出现反流，可能被误诊为胃食管反流病（见第 9 章）。反刍综合征和贪食症亦可引起食管炎，动态 pH 监测呈阳性或两者兼有，从而使临床鉴别更具挑战性。

夜间反流症状具有特别重要的意义。在对反流症状发作频繁的患者进行的一项调查中，74% 的患者有夜间发作[72]。这些夜间反流与仅有白天反流症状相比，在很大程度上影响睡眠和生活质量。夜间反流时间较长的患者发生严重的反流性食管炎和 Barrett 食管等 GERD 并发症风险也更高（见第 46 和 47 章）。

（一）病理生理学

胃灼热的发病机制目前知之甚少。虽然胃酸的反流最常与胃灼热相关，食管球囊扩张[73]、胆汁盐的反流[74]和酸诱导的动力紊乱也可引起相同的症状。疼痛的机制可能与黏膜化学感受器的刺激有关，最佳证据是食管对灌注进入食管黏膜内酸的敏感性以及 pH 监测显示的酸反流。这些化学感受器的位置未知。一种理论是食管经过反复酸暴露而变得敏感，导致在反复暴露于酸后即使较小的再次暴露也能产生症状。据报道，这种超敏状态可通过抑酸治疗控制[75]。

然而，酸反流的发散发作与症状之间的相关性很差。例如，餐后胃食管反流在健康人群中很常见，但症状并不常见。内镜表现为食管炎的患者的食管内 pH 监测通常表现出过度的胃酸反流，但这些反流发作中不到 20% 伴有症状[76]。此外，三分之一患有 Barrett 食管（最高级 GERD）的患者对酸不敏感[77]。食管酸敏感性随年龄的增长而下降，这一发现可以解释为什么老年 GERD 患者即使黏膜损伤相当严重，但表现出来的症状很轻微[78]。因此，症状的出现除了与暴露在酸性环境中相关，黏膜损伤和炎症也可能是促成因素，但大多数有症状患者的食管在内镜检查中看起来是正常的。其他可能影响胃灼热发生的因素包括酸清除机制、唾液碳酸氢盐浓度、酸反流量（通过反流发作的持续时间和近端范围来衡量）、胃灼热发生频率以及胃蛋白酶与酸的相互作用（见第 46 章）。超过 24 小时的酸反流监测研究证实，食管酸暴露的日变化相当大[79,80]。

如上所述，胃灼热强烈提示胃食管酸反流，但消化性溃疡、胃排空延迟，甚至胆囊疾病都会产生类似于酸反流的症状（见第 50、53 和 65 章）。反流不像胃灼热那样对酸反流更有特异性，且反流的鉴别诊断应该包括食管梗阻（例如食管环、食管狭窄、贲门失弛缓症）或胃疾病（例如胃轻瘫、胃出口梗阻）。罗马Ⅳ指南中提出，胃灼热也可以是一种功能性症状[81]。功能性胃灼热是指在没有胃食管反流病、黏膜组织病理学异常、动力性疾病或结构异常情况下的胸骨后烧灼不适或疼痛，且这种不适感或疼痛难以通过抑制胃酸分泌治愈。反流超敏是指有食管症状（胃灼热或胸痛）但在内镜检查中没有反流的证据（如食管炎），或在反流监测中酸负荷异常但出现生理性反流症状。

（二）诊断及治疗方法

对胃灼热和反流患者的诊疗方案在第 46 章已展开了广泛的讨论。简而言之，已发表的一系列指南支持首先试验性抑酸治疗的诊断和治疗策略，通常采用 PPI[82]。该方案有很好的成本效益，但敏感性和特异性不佳[83]。如果在试验治疗后症状的原因仍然不确定，那动态食管 pH 监测是确定有无病理性食管酸暴露的最佳方法。食管内镜检查仅在出现提示并发症的症状（例如吞咽困难、体重减轻、出血迹象）时使用，但症状对食管损伤的预测价值本身就是让人持怀疑态度的。虽然存在争议，但大多数指南建议慢性反流症状患者行内镜检查以筛查 Barrett 食管[84]；白人男性、老年人和肥胖患者的风险更高[85,62]。最新的 2012 年指南仍对 Barrett 食管筛查的效用提出质疑，尤其是女性[87]。

七、胃食管反流病的食管外症状

胃食管反流病的食管外症状列于框 13.4。虽然这些症状可能是由食管动力障碍引起的，但它们最常与胃食管反流病有关。在具有食管外症状的患者中，典型的胃灼热和反流症状程度通常很轻或不存在（见第 46 章）。

框 13.4　胃食管反流病的食管外表现
哮喘
慢性咳嗽
过多的黏液或痰
癔球症（食管神经官能症）
声音嘶哑
喉炎
肺纤维化
咽喉酸痛

胃食管反流可引起慢性咳嗽和其他食管外症状，这是由于胃内容物的反复微量误吸或迷走神经反射引起的，许多患者两者同时存在[88]。虽然支气管扩张剂会降低食管下括约肌压力，但大多数哮喘患者无论是否使用支气管扩张剂治疗的情况下都会出现胃食管反流。在动物实验研究中，在气管或声带中滴注少量酸[89]，可导致气道阻力显著变化，以及声带溃疡。误吸在成人中很难直接观察到，主要取决于痰中检测到含有脂肪组织的巨噬细胞[90]、置于胃中的示踪剂过夜后可在肺中探测到[91]、肺分泌物中胃蛋白酶水平增加[92]以及 24 小时双探针 pH 监测记录到的食管或喉咽酸反流[93]。来自动物和人类研究的数据表明，神经反射是这些症状的另一种病理生理基础。食管远端的酸灌注会增加所有受试者的气

道阻力，但变化最显著的还是同时患有哮喘和胃灼热的患者[94]。

通过长时间的食管内 pH 监测，确定了 35%～80% 的成人哮喘患者存在胃食管的异常酸反流[95]。提示反流性哮喘的症状包括：成年喘息发作但无过敏或哮喘病史，夜间咳嗽或喘息，饭后、运动或仰卧位时哮喘加重，支气管扩张剂加重或糖皮质激素依赖性的哮喘。在反流患者中，夜间咳嗽和胃灼热，反复肺炎，原因不明的发热和相关的食管动力障碍强烈提示存在误吸。肺移植后的安静误吸被认为是移植肺功能下降甚至出现排斥反应的重要原因[96]。除了反流，严重的食管动力障碍也可能发生在晚期肺部疾病患者中，包括那些肺移植术后恢复期的患者[97]。

与胃食管反流相关的耳鼻喉症状包括鼻涕倒流、声音改变、声音嘶哑、喉咙痛、持续性咳嗽、耳痛、口臭、牙酸蚀症和唾液分泌过多。许多胃食管反流病患者仅有头、颈部症状。对声带的检查可能有助于评估有疑似酸反流相关食管外症状的患者。一些患者出现声带和杓状软骨的红肿、充血和水肿。继发于胃食管反流病的声带溃疡、肉芽肿甚至喉癌的严重病例亦有报道。然而，喉部检查正常与出现酸反流相关的食管外症状之间并不矛盾，上述喉部症状也不是胃食管反流病发病的特异性体征。

疑似 GERD 食管外症状患者可以通过动态食管内 pH 监测，或试验性治疗来确诊并治疗（图 13.2）。这两种方法都是合理的，但许多专家首选每天服用两次 PPI 进行抑酸治疗[98]。PPI 试验性抑酸治疗无效的患者，应进行动态 pH 监测，但是进行该项检查时应该继续抑酸治疗还是中断抑酸治疗还不明确（见第 46 章）。具有食管外症状而 pH 监测提示正常酸暴露时，如何解释尤其具有挑战性。许多研究显示，当患者记录咳嗽时，反流事件与咳嗽之间的相关性较差，但当使用声学咳嗽监测（一种尚未批准的实验技术）来量化并计算咳嗽发作时间时，相关性更好[99]。

胃食管反流与食管外症状，特别是与喉部症状之间的关联有些争议。在一项研究中，对喉镜检查结果疑似胃食管反流的患者进行了下咽部和近端及远端食管的 pH 监测[100]，仅有 15% 的下咽探针、9% 的近端食管探针和 29% 的远端食管探针发现异常结果，表明大多数（70%）有症状和喉部反流征象的患者没有可检测到的异常酸暴露。该初步研究之后，对同一批患者进行了艾司奥美拉唑（40mg，每日两次）安慰剂随机对照试验，艾司奥美拉唑治疗组有效率为 42%，安慰剂治疗组有效率为 46%[101]。哮喘患者 PPI 治疗的随机对照试验结果与之相似[102]。尽管数据相互矛盾，但对疑似食管外 GERD 的患者进行 PPI 试验性治疗是合理的，但要想到有失败的可能性。

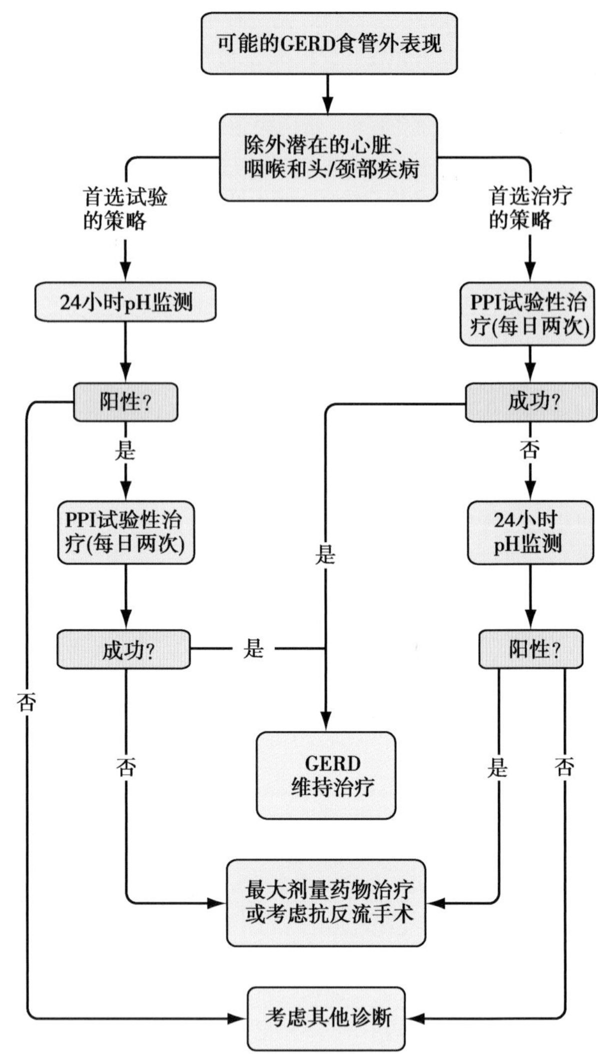

图 13.2　GERD 食管外表现患者治疗方法的流程图，包括非心源性胸痛。根据所评估的症状，排除基础疾病的方法各不相同（参见正文）。在早餐前和晚餐前给予质子泵抑制剂（PPI）。试验的持续时间取决于症状。例如，10～14 天的试验可能足以治疗非心源性胸痛，而慢性咳嗽可能需要 3 个月的试验周期

（叶蔚　闫秀娥 译，鲁晓岚　王立 校）

参考文献

第 14 章　消化不良

Jan Tack 著

章节目录

一、定义 …… 169
二、器质性原因 …… 170
（一）食物或药物不耐受 …… 170
（二）消化性溃疡 …… 170
（三）胃食管反流病 …… 170
（四）胃和食管癌 …… 170
（五）胆道和胰腺疾病 …… 170
（六）其他胃肠道疾病或系统性疾病 …… 170
三、功能性消化不良 …… 171
（一）复杂性消化不良 …… 171
（二）流行病学 …… 173
（三）病理生理学 …… 173
（四）致病因素 …… 174
四、初诊消化不良的处理方法 …… 175
（一）病史和体格检查 …… 175
（二）实验室检查 …… 175
（三）初始的管理策略 …… 175
（四）附加检查 …… 177
五、功能性消化不良的治疗 …… 177
（一）一般措施 …… 177
（二）药物治疗 …… 177
（三）心理干预 …… 180
六、建议 …… 180

一、定义

消化不良（dyspepsia）这个词来源于希腊语“δυς-”（dys-）和“πέψη”（pepse），字面意思是“难以消化”。在现代医学术语中，消化不良是指位于上腹部一组不同综合征。在文献中，消化不良广义上被定义为以上腹部为中心的疼痛或不适[1,2]，可包括各种症状，如上腹痛、餐后饱胀、早饱、厌食、嗳气、恶心呕吐、上腹胀气，甚至胃灼热和反流等。消化不良患者通常会同时存在上述几种症状[3]。

根据罗马共识委员会提出的最具影响力的分级，一些关于消化不良和功能性消化不良的共识定义已被提出。随着时间的推移，消化不良的定义变得越来越严格，越来越多集中于来源于胃十二指肠，而不是食管的症状[4,5]。

早期的定义认为消化不良包括所有上腹部和胸骨后感觉——实际上，上述症状都被认为与近端消化道有关[6]。罗马Ⅰ和Ⅱ共识委员会都将消化不良定义为以上腹部为中心的疼痛或不适[2,7]。其中不适包括餐后饱胀、上腹胀气、早饱、上腹灼热感、嗳气、恶心和呕吐。胃灼热可能是综合征的一部分，但罗马Ⅱ共识委员会定义当以胃灼热为主要症状时，患者应该被认为是胃食管反流病（gastroesophageal reflux disease，GERD），而不是消化不良。

罗马Ⅲ共识委员会将消化不良定义为起源于胃十二指肠的症状，并限定了其主要范围，这被罗马Ⅳ共识委员会所认同[4,6]。目前，尽管其他症状与消化不良可以共存，但仅有 4 种典型症状（餐后饱胀、早饱、上腹痛、上腹灼热感）被认为是起源于胃十二指肠的特定症状。

在消化不良的患者中，额外的临床检查可能会确定引起症状的潜在器质性疾病。在这些患者中，主要是器质性原因引起的消化不良症状（框 14.1）[8-12]，然而在大多数消化不良患者中，通过常规临床评估（包括上消化道内镜检查）并没有发现器质性异常，这些患者则被认为是功能性消化不良。术语“未检查的消化不良”指的是尚未进行诊断性检查，以及尚未确定解释消化不良症状的特定诊断的患者。

框 14.1　消化不良的器质性病因
消化道管腔病
慢性胃扭转
慢性胃或肠（肠系膜）缺血
食物不耐受
胃感染（巨细胞病毒、真菌、结核病、梅毒）
胃或食管肿瘤
胃食管反流
胃轻瘫（糖尿病，迷走神经切断术后，硬皮病，慢性假性肠梗阻，病毒性疾病后、特发性）
肠易激综合征
浸润性胃部疾病［巨大肥厚性胃炎（Menetrier 病），克罗恩病，嗜酸性胃肠炎，结节病，淀粉样变性］
寄生虫（蓝氏贾第鞭毛虫，粪类圆线虫）
消化性溃疡
药物
阿卡波糖
阿司匹林、其他非甾体抗炎药（包括 COX-2 选择性药物）
秋水仙碱
洋地黄制剂
雌激素
乙醇
糖皮质激素
铁剂、氯化钾
左旋多巴
麻醉剂
烟酸、吉非贝齐
硝酸盐类
奥利司他
奎尼丁

框 14.1 消化不良的器质性病因(续)
西地那非
茶碱
胰胆疾病
胆道疼痛:胆石症,胆总管结石,Oddi 括约肌功能障碍
慢性胰腺炎
胰腺肿瘤
系统性疾病
肾上腺皮质功能不全
糖尿病
心力衰竭
甲状旁腺功能亢进
腹腔内恶性肿瘤
心肌缺血
妊娠
肾功能不全
甲状腺疾病

二、器质性原因

引起消化不良最常见的器质性病因是消化性溃疡和胃食管反流病。上消化道恶性肿瘤和乳糜泻较少见,但在临床上是消化不良重要的器质性原因[8-11](见框 14-1)。有消化不良症状时通过内镜检查可以排除糜烂性食管炎、巴雷特食管、消化性溃疡、胃或十二指肠感染以及胃癌或食管癌。

系统研究表明,西方社会 20%~25% 消化不良患者有糜烂性食管炎,20% 据估计有内镜检查阴性的胃食管反流病;10% 有消化性溃疡;2% 有巴雷特食管;1% 或更少的患者有恶性肿瘤[9,12]。内镜或组织病理上微小改变的疾病,如十二指肠炎或胃炎,与有无消化不良症状无关。

(一) 食物或药物不耐受

与人们普遍认为的相反,摄入特定的食物(如香料、咖啡、酒精)或过量食物,从未被证实是引起消化不良的病因[13,14]。虽然摄入食物往往会加重消化不良症状,但这种影响可能与对食物的感觉运动反应有关,而不是对特定食物的不耐受或过敏。然而在健康人和功能性消化不良的患者中,辣椒素的骤然摄入均会诱发消化不良,其中后者的症状更为严重[15]。

消化不良是许多药物的常见副作用,包括铁剂、抗生素、麻醉剂、洋地黄、雌激素和口服避孕药、茶碱和左旋多巴。药物可能通过直接损伤胃黏膜、改变胃肠道感觉运动功能、激发胃食管反流或其他特异性机制引起消化不良症状。非甾体抗炎药因其可能在胃肠道中诱发溃疡而受到广泛关注。长期服用阿司匹林和其他非甾体抗炎药可能导致多达 20% 的患者出现消化不良,但消化不良的发生率与溃疡形成无明显相关性。在对照试验中,接受非甾体抗炎药治疗的患者中消化不良的发生率为 4%~8%,与安慰剂相比,优势比在 1.1~3.1 之间。这种效应的大小取决于非甾体抗炎药的剂量和类型[16]。与非甾体抗炎药相比,使用选择性 COX-2 抑制剂的患者较少出现消化不良症状和消化性溃疡(见第 117 章)[17]。

(二) 消化性溃疡

消化性溃疡是消化不良的明确病因,也是重要因素,但消化不良患者中消化性溃疡发生率仅有 5%~10%[8,9,12]。随着年龄增长,非甾体抗炎药使用和 Hp 感染是消化性溃疡的主要危险因素(见第 53 章)。

(三) 胃食管反流病

糜烂性食管炎是胃食管反流病的诊断标志,但大多数因胃内容物反流到食管而出现临床症状的患者,内镜下没有食管糜烂或非糜烂性的胃食管反流。大约 20% 的消化不良患者存在糜烂性食管炎,同样比例的患者可能是非糜烂性胃食管反流[8,9,12,18]。经验性抑酸治疗可降低消化不良患者出现糜烂性食管炎(见第 46 章)。

(四) 胃和食管癌

消化不良患者中患胃或食管恶性肿瘤风险估计低于 1%[11,12]。Hp 感染、胃恶性肿瘤家族史、胃手术史或来自胃癌流行区的移民患者罹患胃癌风险增加。男性、吸烟、酗酒以及长期存在胃灼热史的患者罹患食管癌的风险增加(见第 48 和 54 章)。

(五) 胆道和胰腺疾病

尽管成人消化不良和胆结石的患病率都很高,但流行病学研究证实,胆石症与消化不良无关。因此,消化不良的患者不应该常规检查胆石症,且因胆石症行胆囊切除术后也不一定有消化不良的临床表现。胆道疼痛的临床表现很容易与消化不良鉴别(见第 65 章)。

胰腺疾病虽不如胆石症普遍,但急慢性胰腺炎或胰腺癌的症状最初可能被误诊为消化不良。胰腺疾病通常有比较剧烈的疼痛,以及伴随厌食、体重迅速减轻或黄疸等症状(见第 58~60 章)。

(六) 其他胃肠道疾病或系统性疾病

几种胃肠道疾病可能引起类似消化不良的症状:①传染性疾病(如肠兰伯贾第虫、粪类圆线虫、结核病、真菌、梅毒);②炎症(乳糜泻、克罗恩病、结节病、淋巴细胞性胃炎、嗜酸性粒细胞性胃肠炎);③浸润性疾病(淋巴瘤、淀粉样变性、巨大肥厚性胃炎(Menetrier 病)。上述大多数可通过上消化道内镜检查和黏膜活检来识别。有复发性胃扭转和慢性肠系膜或胃缺血的人可能出现消化不良症状(见第 27、30~32、37、107、113、115 和 118 章)。以以前的定义标准来看,与胃轻瘫相关的症状(特发性、药源性或代谢性、全身或神经系统疾病)与消化不良相似,但特发性胃轻瘫与功能性消化不良伴胃排空延迟之间的区别仍是个持续讨论的问题(见后文和第 50 章)[18]。罗马Ⅲ和Ⅳ共识委员会认为恶心和呕吐是胃轻瘫的主要症状,并认为这不是消化不良的症状,因此可基于症状区分消化不良和胃轻瘫[3,5,18]。消化不良也可能是急性心肌缺血、妊娠、急慢性肾功能衰竭、甲状腺功能障碍、肾上腺功能不全或甲状旁腺功能亢进的临床表现或伴随症状。

三、功能性消化不良

根据罗马Ⅲ共识标准,功能性消化不良(functional dyspepsia,FD)定义为:在无器质性、全身性或代谢性疾病可以解释的情况下出现的早饱、餐后饱胀、上腹痛、上腹灼热感(框14.2)[5]。

框 14.2 功能性消化不良、餐后不适综合征和上腹部疼痛综合征的罗马Ⅳ标准

功能性消化不良[†]的诊断标准[*]	1. 包括以下一项或多项: 令人烦恼的餐后饱胀感 令人烦恼的早饱 令人烦恼的上腹疼痛 令人烦恼的上腹灼热感 和 2. 无可解释症状的器质性疾病(包括上消化道内镜检查)的证据
餐后不适综合征(PDS)的诊断标准[*]	必须包括以下一项或两项,每周至少 3 天: 1. 令人烦恼的餐后饱胀感(即,严重到足以影响日常活动) 2. 令人烦恼的早饱(即,严重到足以妨碍吃完常规餐量的膳食) 3. 常规检查中(包括上消化道内镜检查)无可能解释症状的器质性、系统性或代谢性疾病的证据 支持性标准 1. 也可出现餐后上腹疼痛或灼热,上腹部胀满,嗳气过度和恶心 2. 呕吐需要考虑另一种疾病 3. 胃灼热不是消化不良的症状,但通常可能与餐后不适综合征同时存在 4. 通过排便或排气缓解的症状通常不应被视为消化不良综合征的一部分 5. 其他个别消化症状或综合征(如胃食管反流病或肠易激综合征)可能与餐后不适综合征共存
上腹部疼痛综合征(EPS)的诊断标准[*]	必须包括以下一项或两项症状,每周至少 1 天: 1. 令人烦恼的上腹疼痛(即严重到足以影响日常活动) 2. 令人烦恼的上腹部烧灼感(即严重到足以影响日常活动) 无可能解释常规检查(包括上消化道内镜检查)症状的器质性、系统性或代谢性疾病的证据 支持标准 1. 疼痛可因进餐引起,也可因进餐缓解,也可在空腹时发生 2. 也可出现餐后上腹部胀满、嗳气,恶心 3. 持续呕吐可能提示另一种疾病 4. 胃灼热不是消化不良的症状,但常与上腹部疼痛综合征同时存在 5. 疼痛不符合胆道疼痛的标准 6. 通过排便或排气缓解的症状通常不应被视为消化不良综合征的一部分 7. 其他消化症状(如胃食管反流病、肠易激综合征)可与上腹部疼痛综合征并存

[*]在诊断前至少 6 个月症状发作的前 3 个月满足标准。
[†]必须符合餐后窘迫综合征和/或上腹部疼痛综合征的标准。

(一) 复杂性消化不良

1. 模式和异质性

复杂的消化不良综合征比罗马Ⅳ诊断标准定义的 4 种主要症状更广泛,它包括多种症状,如上腹痛、早饱、饱胀、上腹灼热感、上腹胀、嗳气、食欲不振、恶心和呕吐。功能性消化不良通常是慢性的,即使是症状高度明显时期,其症状多是间歇性的[1,8,19]。在临床就诊的功能性消化不良的患者中,最常见的症状是餐后饱胀和腹胀,其次是上腹痛、早饱、恶心和嗳气[3,20-23]。然而,如图 14.1 所述,功能性消化不良患者的临床症状存在较大的异质性。在一般人群中,最常见的消化不良症状是餐后饱胀、早饱、上腹痛和恶心[24-26]。

体重减轻传统上被认为是一种"报警"症状,预示着潜在严重的器质性疾病。然而,对临床就诊的功能性消化不良患者的研究,也显示出频发的不明原因体重减轻[20,21],在澳大利亚和欧洲的人群研究表明,未经检查的消化不良与不明原因的体重减轻之间存在联系[25,26]。

2. 亚组

消化不良综合征的异质性被广泛接受。普通人群和临床就诊的功能性消化不良患者,所进行的因素分析并未表明功能性消化不良是同种(即单一的)病症[25-27]。这些研究证实了复杂消化不良综合征的异质性,但没有提供具有临床意义的症状分类方法。

目前临床上已进行了若干尝试来鉴别具有临床意义的少数人群消化不良,以试图简化并指导治疗复杂的消化不良综合征异质性。罗马Ⅱ共识委员会以疼痛或不适作为主要症状提出了分类方法[2]。虽然该分类方法与是否存在 Hp 感染、胃排空延迟、对抑酸治疗反应均有相关性[28,29],但难以区分不适和疼痛、缺乏广泛接受的"主要"定义、少数症状之间重叠的不确定性、缺乏公认的病理生理机制的联系以及短期无稳定性主要症状,使该分类方法并未接受[4,30-33]。

罗马Ⅲ共识委员会提出了不同的分类方法(图 14.2)。对临床观察到的功能性消化不良患者和普通人群未经检查的消化不良患者的研究表明:40%~75% 的消化不良患者在进

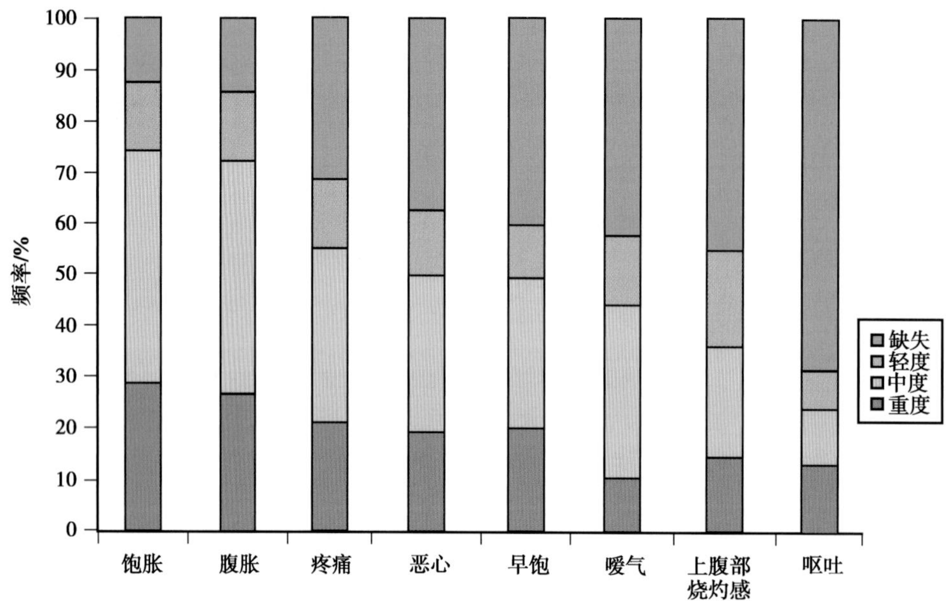

图 14.1　在三级转诊中心就诊的 674 例功能性消化不良患者的症状频率（患者百分比）及其严重程度评级。（Unpublished，University of Gasthuisberg，Leuven，Belgium.）

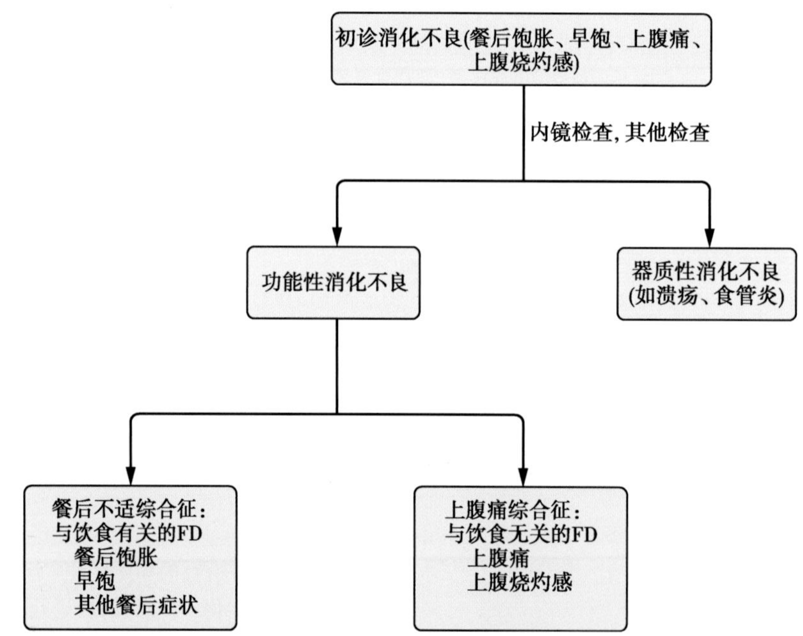

图 14.2　初诊消化不良、功能性消化不良（FD）和功能性消化不良亚型（根据罗马Ⅳ标准）分类的示意图

食后症状加重[26,34,35]。假设与饮食有关或无关的症状之间的区别，可能与病理生理和临床表现有联系，罗马Ⅲ共识委员会提出功能性消化不良可以作为一个概括性术语，分为餐后不适综合征（postprandial distress syndrome，PDS）——与饮食有关的消化不良症状，以餐后饱胀和早饱为特征；及上腹痛综合征（epigastric pain syndrome，EPS）——与饮食无关的消化不良症状，以上腹疼痛和上腹灼热感为特征[4]。在以人群为基础的研究中，基于罗马Ⅲ共识将功能性消化不良分为 EPS 和 PDS 的分类方法表现出了两者的具体情况，它们之间几乎没有重叠[36-38]。相比之下，研究表明在因功能性消化不良而向胃肠病学家咨询的患者中，罗马Ⅲ共识定义的 PDS 和 EPS 中有很大的重叠[1,39,40]。罗马Ⅳ共识委员会为了达到减少重叠的目的，将所有餐后发生的症状视为 PDS 的一部分[5]。因此，具有早饱或餐后饱胀感的患者出现餐后疼痛时，仍被归类为 PDS（见图 14.2）。流行病学研究和对患者队列的研究表明，PDS 是占主导的亚组，基于罗马Ⅳ共识的分类方法使其与 EPS 的重叠部分很小[5,41,42]。

3. 胃灼热与肠易激综合征重叠

消化不良和胃食管反流病之间的重叠问题一直是一个具有挑战性的问题。虽然早期研究者考虑到了一些类似于反流症状的消化不良患者[6]，但罗马委员会并不认为胃灼热主要来源于胃十二指肠，并将其排除在消化不良的定义之外[2,4,5,7]。在一般人群和功能性消化不良患者中，胃灼热与消化不良同时存在[18,26,29,43]，许多混杂因素阻碍了区分胃食管反流病和消化不良，例如许多胃食管反流病[18,26,44]患者中存在消化不良型症状以及患者和医生难以识别胃灼热[18,45,46]。

罗马Ⅱ共识委员会指出，以典型胃灼热为主要症状的患者几乎都有胃食管反流病，应与消化不良区分开来[2]。尽管这种鉴别方法有效[32,47,48]，罗马Ⅲ共识委员会提议需鉴别频繁胃灼热的患者，并通过文字-图片问卷来鉴别那些可以被识别出对抑酸治疗有效，及病理性食管酸暴露的功能性消化不良患者[47,48]。罗马Ⅲ和罗马Ⅳ共识意见指出胃灼热并不是胃十二指肠症状，尽管它通常与功能性消化不良症状有关，且其存在并不能排除功能性消化不良的诊断[4,5]。类似地，功能性消化不良与肠易激综合征[49]的频繁同时发生，在罗马Ⅲ和罗马Ⅳ共识指南中得到明确认可，但这并不排除功能性消化不良的诊断[4,5]。

（二）流行病学

消化不良症状在普通人群中很常见，发生率在 10%～45%之间[8,26,34,36-38,50-52]。女性略高于男性，年龄的影响在各研究中则各有不同。流行病学研究的结果受到消化不良定义标准的强烈影响，一些研究包括典型胃食管反流症状的患者，一些则未考虑许多胃食管反流患者中存在着消化不良症状。当排除胃灼热症状时，普通人群中未检查的消化不良的发生率在 5%～15%之间[26,34,36-38,50-52]。长期随访研究表明半数以上患者的症状可得到改善或缓解[19,53]。据估计，每年消化不良的发病率在 1%～6%之间[19]。

消化不良对生活质量的影响显著，尤其是功能性消化不良[50]。尽管大多数患者尚未寻求医疗救治，但其中多数人最终仍会寻求治疗，这会消耗大量费用[19,26,54-57]。影响就医的因素包括症状严重程度、对潜在严重疾病的恐惧、心理困扰以及缺乏足够的社会心理支持[56,57]。

（三）病理生理学

功能性消化不良的一些病理生理学机制是：胃排空延迟、胃对食物调节功能障碍、内脏高敏感性、轻度黏膜炎症、十二指肠对脂类或酸的敏感性改变、肠道动力异常和中枢神经系统功能障碍[3,8]。功能性消化不良异质性似乎可以通过上述一种或多种因素的影响来证实。关于功能性消化不良病理生理机制的研究早于罗马Ⅳ准则和分类，因此大多数研究是基于罗马Ⅰ和Ⅱ共识来定义消化不良的。

1. 胃排空延迟

一些研究调查了胃排空及其与功能性消化不良类型和严重程度的关系。胃排空延迟的发生率在 20%～50%之间（表 14.1）[3,8]。在一项涉及 868 名消化不良患者和 397 名对照患者的 17 项研究的 meta 分析中，近 40%的功能性消化不良患者存在对固体物质明显的胃排空延迟[58]。然而，其中大多数研究是以小样本进行调查的。在最大量的研究中，约 30%的 FD 患者胃排空延迟[3,23,59-61]。在一项大型研究中，使用呼吸试验测量罗马Ⅲ定义的亚组的胃排空，延迟排空仅占 23%，与 PDS 没有显著关联[61]。大多数研究未能在胃排空延迟和症状类型之间找到令人信服的关系。来自欧洲的 3 项大规模单中心研究显示，对固体物质产生胃排空延迟的患者更容易出现餐后饱胀、恶心和呕吐[23,59-61]，但另外两项来自美国的大型多中心研究并未发现，或仅发现微弱的关联[62,63]。胃排空延迟是否引起消化不良症状，或仅仅是偶然现象，仍然存在争议。

表 14.1 功能性消化不良患者研究中胃排空延迟的频率

研究者/年度	病例数	频率/%
Asano 2017	94	11
Jian 1989	28	59
Klauser 1993	69	35
Maes 1997	344	30
Perri 1998	304	33
Sarnelli 2003	392	23
Scott 1993	75	28
Stanghellini 1996	343	34
Talley 1989	32	30
Talley 1989	32	30
Talley 2001	551	24
Talley 2006	864	34
Vanheel 2017	560	23
Waldron 1991	50	42
Wegener 1989	43	30

2. 胃对进食的调节功能受损

胃近端和远端的运动功能差异显著。胃远端通过研磨和过筛内容物来调节固体的胃排空，直到颗粒小到可以通过幽门，胃近端主要在进食期间和之后储存食物。胃对饮食的调节是由于胃近端的迷走神经反射松弛，使胃可以在不增加胃内压力的情况下保持大内容量[64]。使用胃内测压法的研究表明进食与胃内压力下降有关，随后在持续性摄入营养物质的同时逐渐恢复压力，增加饮食引起的饱腹感[65]。

使用胃恒压计、闪烁成像术、超声、单光子发射计算机断层扫描（single photon emission CT，SPECT）或无创替代标志物（饱饮实验）的研究都表明大约 40%的功能性消化不良患者有胃调节功能障碍（表 14.2）[3,20,22,61,64]。一项关于罗马Ⅲ定义的 FD 亚型患者胃恒压调节研究发现，37%的患者胃容纳受损，但与 PDS 无明显联系。在进食过程中和进食后，胃近端的调节功能不足可能伴有胃内压升高和胃壁机械感受器的激活，从而诱发症状。虽然许多研究发现调节功能障碍与早饱和体重减轻之间存在联系，但也有研究尚未找到这种关联[3,20,22,61,64]。调节功能障碍引起消化不良症状的机制尚不清楚。在胃近端尚未适当放松的情况下进食，可能伴有胃近端的张力敏感机械感受器的激活。另一方面，胃近端的调节功能不足可迫使食物进入胃远端，从而引起胃窦扩张时张力敏感的机械感受器的激活[64]。

表 14.2 功能性消化不良患者与健康人相比出现调节功能受损的证据

研究者/年度	病例数	技术	与健康人群的差异
Asano 2017	94	闪烁成像术	15%调节受损
Boeckxstaens 2001	44	胃恒压器	无差异
Bredenoord 2003	151	SPECT 成像	43%调节受损
Caldarella 2003	30	胃恒压器	一组调节受损
Castillo 2004	35	SPECT 成像	无差异
Coffin 1994	10	胃恒压器	一组调节受损
Gilja 1996	20	超声	一组调节受损
Kim 2001	33	SPECT 成像	一组调节受损，41%异常
Piessevaux 2004	40	闪烁成像术	整体无差异；远端再分配高达 50%
Salet 1998	12	胃恒压器	一组调节受损
Tack 1998	40	胃恒压器	一组调节受损，40%异常
Thumshirn 1999	17	胃恒压器	70%调节受损
Troncon 1994	11	闪烁成像术	一组胃内分布改变
Vanheel 2017	560	恒压器	37%调节受损

SPECT，单光子发射计算机断层扫描。

3. 胃扩张的超敏反应

内脏高敏感性定义为对内脏刺激的感知异常增强，被认为是功能性胃肠道疾病的主要病理生理机制之一（见 22 章）[65]。多项研究已经确定，作为一个群体，功能性消化不良患者对等压胃膨胀高度敏感[3,21,61]。在罗马Ⅲ定义的 FD 亚组患者中进行的一项研究发现 37%的患者存在超敏反应，但与任何亚型均无优先相关性[60]。虽然内脏高敏感性产生的水平尚不清楚，但有证据表明张力敏感性机械感受器的参与以及内脏传入神经或中枢神经水平的改变与 FD 有关[66-69]。

4. 低度十二指肠黏膜炎症

十二指肠的低度黏膜炎症，由于十二指肠黏膜肥大细胞和嗜酸性粒细胞计数增加而引起的症状，已在功能性消化不良的患者中确定为一组[70-72]。对功能性消化不良引起免疫功能障碍的研究，最初是由感染后功能性消化不良的观察引起的[73]，而现在很明显的是，在功能性消化不良患者的很大一部分患者中，嗜酸性粒细胞和肥大细胞数量的增加是存在的，这些发现与早期饱腹感的症状具有明显相关性[70]。十二指肠的炎性细胞浸润（嗜酸性粒细胞和肥大细胞）与黏膜对黏液通透性增加和紧密连接蛋白表达有关，并与黏膜下神经丛神经元的活性和完整性受损有关[71,72]。轻度十二指肠炎症与胃感觉运动的变化在多大程度上相关，与前面描述的胃感觉运动功能的变化有关，或与之后讨论的对十二指肠肠腔内容物的敏感性增加有关，仍有待评估。

5. 十二指肠对脂质或酸的敏感性改变

在健康人和功能性消化不良患者中，十二指肠灌注营养脂质（非葡萄糖），并通过脂质消化和释放胆囊收缩素的机制增强胃胀感[74-76]。十二指肠输注胃酸后功能性消化不良患者会出现恶心，而健康受试者不会出现，这提示 FD 的十二指肠黏膜对酸反应具有高敏感性[77]。利用限制性 pH 电极对十二指肠进行 pH 监测，结果显示，与对照组相比，功能性消化不良患者的餐后十二指肠酸暴露增加，这种差异被认为与十二指肠酸清除能力的受损相关[78]。在以上观察的基础上，认为十二指肠对脂质或酸的敏感性增加可促进功能性消化不良患者产生相关症状，但对该领域内容仍需进一步深入研究。

6. 其他机制

一项关于功能性消化不良患者的研究报道，胃快速排空的高发生率与餐后症状相关[79]，而其他研究未能支持这一发现[23,35,61]。在功能性消化不良患者中发现位相性胃底收缩可引起胃壁张力短暂增加[67]。一项研究报道了部分功能性消化不良患者出现餐后胃近端阶段性收缩抑制缺乏[80]。多达三分之二的功能性消化不良患者发现胃肌电活动控制异常（经皮肤胃电图测量）[81,82]。消化不良症状类型与胃电图检查结果之间并未发现关联。研究报道了功能性消化不良患者存在小肠运动改变，最常见的是爆发性或团簇性运动过强，十二指肠逆行收缩比例增加（见第 99 章），但未发现与症状有明显关联[83]。

（四）致病因素

功能性消化不良患者的病因尚未确定，已被证实有遗传易感性，感染因素和心理因素。而潜在的致病因素与假定的病理生理机制之间的关系尚未得到深入研究。

1. 遗传易感性

遗传倾向人群研究表明遗传因素导致功能性消化不良。与配偶相比，患者的一级亲属发病率更高[84]。G 蛋白 β 多肽 3（*GNB3*）基因与患功能性消化不良的风险相关[85]；但在世界各地的不同研究中，该基因的特异性以及与消化不良患者之间的联系各不相同[86]。这就需要更多和更大规模的循证研究。

2. 感染

（1）Hp 感染

根据所研究的区域和人群的不同，功能性消化不良患者感染 Hp 的比例不同[3,8]。尽管 Hp 与一些器质性消化不良有关，但部分有限的证据证明 Hp 和功能性消化不良之间存在因果关系[87]。没有发现在 Hp 阳性和阴性受试者之间存在有消化不良症状类型或推定的病理生理机制的差异[3,8,88]。支持 Hp 在功能性消化不良发病机制中有作用的最佳证据是，根除 Hp 治疗后，功能性消化不良症状得到改善[87,89]。这些观察结果，导致了东京共识的建立，该共识将 Hp 相关性消化不良定义为，有 Hp 感染且内镜检查无其他疾病，根除 Hp 治疗后症状得到持续控制的消化不良[90]。这类人群在世界范围内有多少患病率以及其长期预后均需进一步的研究。

（2）感染后功能性消化不良

根据一个三级转诊中心的大型回顾性研究，首次提出感染后功能性消化不良是功能性消化不良的一种临床现象[22]。与未明确病因的功能性消化不良的患者相比，病史提示感染后功能性消化不良的患者更可能出现早饱、体重减轻、恶心、呕吐的症状，同时因为其胃氮能神经元的功能障碍而导致胃近端调节功能障碍的发生率亦显著增加[22]。在感染后功能性消化不良患者中，Hp 感染率并未增加，表明 Hp 不是致病的感染因子。功能性消化不良患者会有更显著的十二指肠黏膜炎症[73]。在一项前瞻性队列研究中，急性沙门菌胃肠炎 1 年后功能性消化不良的发病率较未感染受试者增加了 5 倍[91]。但仍需要进一步的研究来确定潜在的病理生理学和危险因素以评估其长期预后。

3. 心理社会因素

文献综述揭示了心理社会因素与功能性消化不良之间有明确关联[3,8,92]。功能性消化不良患者最常见的精神症状是焦虑、抑郁或躯体型障碍，以及近期或远期的身体或性虐待史。长期以来，心理困扰一直是功能性肠病，包括功能性消化不良（见第 22 章）患者寻求健康保健行为的公认特征。研究证实了一般人群中的消化不良症状与躯体化、焦虑和紧张的生活事件等心理社会因素之间的联系；这种联系反对单纯寻求医疗保健[27,36,92,93]。在临床上功能性消化不良患者的症状严重程度与心理社会因素（尤其是抑郁、虐待史和躯体化）的关系比与胃感觉运动功能异常的关系更为密切[94]。

尽管这些观察结果显示不同心理社会变量与功能性消化不良症状的存在和严重程度之间有着密切的联系，但并未确定心理社会因素和功能性消化不良是有共同易感性的单独表现，心理社会因素在消化不良的病理生理学中是否有因果作用也不明确。纵向研究支持这种普遍倾向的观点，是基于人群的研究中，在情绪障碍的发展前后，功能性消化不良都有被报道过，两者都会增加彼此的发病风险[95,96]。

社会心理并发症的存在也与功能性消化不良患者的症状严重程度有关，这些关联可能与内脏高敏感度有关[27,97]。然而，健康志愿者的急性焦虑与内脏高过敏的增加无关，但与胃顺应性的降低及膳食诱导调节明显受抑有关[98]。在功能性消化不良患者中，部分高敏感患者（不包含全部患者）的焦虑和胃敏感性之间存在联系[97]。遭受虐待的病史与功能性消化不良患者的内脏高敏有关[99]。

四、初诊消化不良的处理方法

考虑到消化不良的高患病率和大量因临床症状明显而就诊的患者，对这些患者的初始管理目标是为了确定哪些患者可以进行经验性治疗，哪些患者需要额外检查的诊断评估。

（一）病史和体格检查

临床医生应该对所有消化不良患者进行完整的临床病史采集和体格检查，同时应评估症状的性质、频率和持续时间。临床症状与膳食之间的关系以及特定饮食因素可能产生的影响均应在评估内容中。症状的发作可以呈现似急性胃肠炎也可以表现相对平稳。和失血、吞咽困难和贫血等其他报警症状一样，如果存在体重减轻，应该排除其他器质性疾病。根据罗马Ⅲ共识的分类，区分 EPS（上腹痛综合征）与 PDS（餐后不适综合征）症状亚群可能影响治疗的选择（见下文）[5]。对于长期存在症状的患者，医生此时必须了解求医的诉求，以便能够解决患者的恐惧和担忧。对全身性疾病（如糖尿病、心脏病、甲状腺疾病）症状或体征的进一步评估，以及患者的家族病史和个人病史，将提示患者是否有罹患可能表现为消化不良的特定器质性疾病的风险。体格检查发现腹部肿块、器官肿大、腹水或粪便隐血阳性均值得进一步的评估。

临床医生应该特别注意引起胃灼热症状的既往史，并通过图文问卷帮助患者确定典型的症状模式[45]。局限于上腹部的烧灼痛是消化不良的主要症状，但如表现为向胸骨后放射，则不认为是胃灼热。出现频繁、典型的反流症状应暂时诊断为 GERD 并进行初步治疗，而不是消化不良（见第 46 章）。GERD 与消化不良同时存在很常见（见前），如果对 GRED 恰当治疗后患者的症状没有改善，则应考虑消化不良。另外还应评估是否存在肠易激综合征，如果症状随着排便运动改善或与粪便频率一致，可推定诊断为肠易激综合征。一份包含胃灼热症状的图文结构化问卷可以帮助识别与恶心、胃食管反流和肠易激综合征不同的症状特征[100]。

一般要审核处方药和非处方药，尽量避免长期使用会引起消化不良的药物（尤其是非甾体抗炎药）。尽管许多指南建议，凡需非甾体抗炎药治疗的患者，应首先进行内镜评估以排除消化性溃疡，但对于不能停止使用非甾体抗炎药的患者，可以考虑进行质子泵抑制剂（proton pump inhibitor，PPI）试验。

（二）实验室检查

常规实验室检验的成本效益，特别是对于年轻无并发症的消化不良患者现尚未确定。然而，大多数临床医生会考虑对 45～55 岁的患者进行常规检查（全血计数、血清电解质、血钙、肝脏生化检查和甲状腺功能）。在特殊病例中，可以考虑选用其他检查项目，如血清淀粉酶水平，乳糜泻抗体，粪便检测虫卵和寄生虫，或贾第鞭毛虫抗原以及妊娠试验[3,5,8,11]

（三）初始的管理策略

在大多数情况下，患者的病史和体格检查可以将消化不良的症状与食管、胰腺或胆道疾病的症状区分开来，但初级保健医师和胃肠病学专家都应该知道，患者的病史和身体检查结果，甚至出现的报警症状，在区分功能性和器质性消化不良的方面是不可靠的[5,8,9,11,100-102]。因此，大多数指南和建议，提倡当引起消化不良的危险因素（例如，使用非甾体抗炎药，年龄在 45～55 岁，有报警症状）出现时应进行早期内镜检查[103-105]。对于大多数无器质性消化不良危险因素的患者来说，如何进行最佳管理仍然存在争议；目前专家已经提出了几种方法。可用的选择包括：①早期诊断性内镜检查，然后进行针对性药物治疗；②非侵入性 Hp 检测，根据结果进行治疗（“Hp 检测和治疗”策略）；③经验性抗胃酸分泌药物治疗。在后两种策略中，治疗无效或治疗后出现复发症状的患者可以进一步进行内镜检查。在理论上，可以首选使用促动力药物，但通常不推荐使用，因为尚缺乏广泛可用的具有既定疗效的促动力药物[104]。

1. 及时内镜检查和指导治疗

诊断性上消化道内镜检查可直接检测消化不良的器质性病因，如消化性溃疡、糜烂性食管炎或恶性肿瘤。在开始任何治疗之前，内镜检查仍然被认为是诊断上消化道疾病的金标准[106]。这个过程对患者和医生都有一定的安慰作用[107-109]。胃黏膜活检有助于 Hp 感染的诊断，如果结果为阳性，应进行根除治疗。通过患者症状发现早期胃癌是很少见的，但这种说法的证据也不充分[110-112]。内镜检查既昂贵又是侵入性，并且可能对治疗没有太大的影响。发现消化性溃疡或糜烂性食管炎的患者，应进行抗胃酸分泌药物治疗。内镜检查结果阴性的患者可能被诊断为功能性消化不良或非糜烂性食管炎，两者均可采用经验性抗胃酸分泌药物疗法。尽管如此，仍有人认为最初的经验性抗胃酸分泌药物治疗会延迟进行内镜检查，因为停止经验性治疗后，功能性消化不良和 GERD 患者都可能复发，这时患者应进行内镜检查。

一系列的随机对照试验将及时内镜检查和非侵入性的经验性治疗策略进行了对比。一项基于 5 项试验的 meta 分析将最初的内镜检查与“Hp 检测和治疗”策略进行比较，得出结论：早期内镜检查可能略降低消化不良症状复发的风险，但这种获益并不具有成本效益（表 14.3）[113]。大多数相关研究发现，及时内镜检查相关的直接和间接成本均高于经验疗法，而且不能被减少药物使用或随后就医次数抵消这些成本[104-116]。因此，对于所有无并发症的消化不良患者，现有数据不支持早期内镜检查作为一种初始治疗策略。

表 14.3 关于未经调查的消化不良患者初始管理策略的两项 meta 分析

研究者/年度	相对危险度(95% CI)
即时内镜检查与经验性抑酸治疗	
Bytzer 1994	0.99(0.61～1.63)
Delaney 2001	0.93(0.78～1.10)
Duggan 1999	0.86(0.63～1.18)
Lewin 1999	0.75(0.54～1.05)
平均	**0.89(0.77～1.02)**
HP 检测和治疗策略与内镜	
Arents 2003	1.05(0.90～1.21)
Duggan 1999	1.38(1.03～1.84)
Heany 1999	0.82(0.60～1.11)
Lassen 2001	0.84(0.59～1.19)
McColl 2002	0.78(0.51～1.19)
平均	**0.98(0.81～1.18)**

两项分析均未显示策略之间存在差异。CI，置信区间。

然而，大多数相关的临床实践指南提倡对年龄超过一定界限（通常在 45～55 岁）的患者进行早期内镜检查，以发现可治愈的上消化道恶性肿瘤[103-105]。其理由是绝大多数胃恶性肿瘤发生在 45 岁以上的患者中，并且 45 岁以上合并消化不良的患者，其癌症检出率也在上升[110-112]。大多数新诊断的胃癌患者在诊断时已经无法治愈，然而许多患者出现过提示应立即进行内镜检查的报警症状[112]。对于年龄在 45 岁以下有胃癌家族史的患者、从胃癌高发国家移民的患者、或有部分胃切除术的患者，也建议早期内镜检查。

2. Hp 感染的检测和治疗

Hp 与大多数消化性溃疡有关，是胃癌最重要的危险因素（见第 52～54 章）[117]。由于 Hp 与消化性溃疡相关，一些共识小组和指南提倡对无并发症的消化不良年轻患者（<45 至 60 岁）进行 Hp 检测[5,8,103-105]。检测结果为阳性的患者应接受根除治疗（PPI 和 2 种抗生素，如阿莫西林和克拉霉素，这取决于各人的耐药性，服用 14 天），而检测结果为阴性的患者应接受经验治疗，通常使用 PPI 治疗。对于一部分感染了 Hp 的功能性消化不良患者，这种“Hp 检测和治疗”策略的好处是可以治愈 PUD，或预防消化性溃疡和缓解症状（比安慰剂组高约 7%）[89,90,104,113,114,118]。根除 Hp 可以消除慢性胃炎，理论上可能有助于降低 Hp 相关胃癌的风险[119]。

另一方面，在西方国家，未行检查的消化不良患者的 Hp 感染率正在急剧下降，30 岁以下人群的感染率特别低（10%～30%）。广泛使用抗生素的缺点是会引起耐药性并偶尔引起药物过敏。长期以来，根除 Hp 是否会导致或使 GERD 加重一直存在争论[120]，但 2013 年一项针对 Hp 阳性 GERD 患者的随机对照根除试验未能证明根治治疗使 GERD 加重[121]。此外，非侵入性检测的准确性取决于人群中 Hp 的患病率以及检测的敏感性和特异性。Hp 的血清学检测是最便宜也是最不准确的。如果群体中 Hp 的患病率低于 60%，则优先选择 Hp 粪便抗原检测和尿素呼气试验检测；其更高的准确性减少了对非 Hp 感染患者的不恰当治疗（见第 52 章）[122]。

随机安慰剂对照试验表明，在初级治疗过程中采用“检测和治疗”方法后，消化不良症状仅略有减轻[123-125]。一项 meta 分析将“Hp 检测和治疗”策略和经验抗胃酸分泌药物治疗进行研究比较，发现两种方法在缓解症状或费用上几乎没有区别[126]。虽然早期的 Hp 高患病率假设模型提示“Hp 检测-治疗”策略有很大的益处[127-129]，但经济模型表明，与经验性抗胃酸分泌药物治疗相比，“Hp 检测和治疗”策略可能具有同等或更低的成本效益[130,131]。在 Hp 感染率高的地区，“Hp 检测和治疗”策略很可能对尚未调查研究的消化不良是有益的。

3. 经验性抗分泌药物治疗

初步经验性抗胃酸分泌药物治疗被广泛应用于未检查的消化不良患者的初步治疗中[132,133]。这种方法很有吸引力，因为这种治疗可以缓解大多数潜在的 GERD 或 PUD 患者的症状，并可能对多达三分之一的功能性消化不良患者有益。与 H_2RA（H_2 受体拮抗剂）相比，PPI 更能缓解症状，通常在治疗 2 周内起效[103-105]。经验性 PPI 治疗的缺点是停药后症状很快复发，并且可能出现反弹性胃酸分泌过多[134]，因此很多患者需要长期的 PPI 治疗。正如前面提到的，一项 Meta 分析将功能性消化不良患者分别应用“Hp 检测和治疗”策略和经验性抗胃酸分泌药物治疗进行分析研究比较，发现两种方法在症状解决有效率或费用上几乎没有区别[126]；然而，经济分析表明，经验性抗胃酸分泌药物治疗可能具有同等或更高的成本效益[130,131]。

4. 建议

初始治疗无并发症消化不良的最佳成本效益方法仍不清楚。临床决策应该考虑到每个患者的具体情况并权衡几个风险-收益因素。对于没有出现报警症状的消化不良年轻患者（年龄<50 岁至 60 岁），不建议早期内镜检查，因为检出阳性率低且不一定能带来更优的结果。但如果患者有癌症家族史，或者从胃癌或食管癌高发区移民，从担心潜在疾病角度考

虑,可以行早期内镜检查。在 Hp 感染高发人群(>20%)中,“Hp 检测和治疗”策略仍然很受欢迎,因为这种情况下 PUD 可以被治愈。Hp 检测方法有尿素呼吸试验或粪便抗原检测。Hp 阳性患者应接受 Hp 根除治疗(见第 52 章)。对于 Hp 阴性的患者,PPI 可以使用 1~2 个月。在 Hp 患病率较低的人群中,可以首选经验性抗胃酸分泌药物治疗(PPI 1~2 个月)。初步治疗无效的患者,以及那些在停止抗胃酸分泌药物治疗后症状复发的患者,仍应该接受内镜检查,尽管收益并不高。

对于年龄在 50 岁至 60 岁以上且没有报警症状的患者,大多数指南建议进行早期诊断性内镜检查,尽管这在发现早期恶性肿瘤方面的益处尚未得到证实。在这些病例中,内镜检查及 Hp 检测结果将会决定治疗方案的选择,但大多数患者很可能接受的是 PPI 治疗。

(四) 附加检查

对于初步治疗后进展性或难治性症状未缓解的患者,可进行其他检查。对于有顽固性症状的患者来说,尤其是伴有体重减轻的患者,检查乳糜泻和贾第鞭毛虫感染是有用的。对于有严重疼痛或体重减轻的患者,可以进行腹部超声或 CT 以排除胰胆管疾病和筛查腹腔动脉狭窄。

对于有严重的餐后饱胀感,尤其是难治性恶心和呕吐的患者,可以考虑使用显像法或呼气测试来进行胃排空试验。当发现胃排空严重延迟时,可以用小肠 X 光检查来排除机械性肠梗阻的可能。在难治性间歇性上腹部疼痛或灼烧的情况下,具有阻抗监测的食管 pH 检查有助于诊断非典型临床症状、经验性抗胃酸分泌药物治疗无效的 GERD。对于长期症状未缓解的患者,建议进行心理或精神方面的评估。胃电图、胃压力的检测或简单营养激发试验已用于病理生理学的研究,但目前并没有用于临床诊断或管理消化不良患者。

五、功能性消化不良的治疗

(一) 一般措施

在功能性消化不良患者中,医生的安慰和宣教是最重要的。尽管内镜检查结果正常,但仍应给予患者自信和一个积极的诊断。在肠易激综合征患者中,已经有证据显示积极的医患互动可以减少求医行为,这种方法可能也适用于功能性消化不良患者[135]。

生活方式和饮食干预适用于功能性消化不良患者,但饮食干预的影响尚未得到系统研究[14]。建议患者少食多餐似乎是合理的。由于十二指肠中存在脂质会增加胃敏感度,因此建议避免食用脂肪含量高的食物[75,76]。同样地,医生不建议食用含有辣椒素和其他刺激性辛辣食物[15]。在某些情况下[136],咖啡可能会加重症状,如果有影响,也应该避免饮用。戒烟和戒酒被认为有助于缓解症状,但这种观点还没有令人信服的证据[127]。尽管还没有确切的证据,但通常建议避免服用阿司匹林和其他非甾体抗炎药[8,16]。如果患者同时存在有明显的焦虑或抑郁状态,应选择适当的治疗方案。

(二) 药物治疗

并不是所有的患者都需要考虑药物治疗。药物治疗功能性消化不良的疗效是有限的。

1. 抑酸药物

对于 GERD 患者,抗胃酸分泌药物治疗往往具有治疗和诊断双重价值。基于对功能性消化不良患者治疗结果的 meta 分析中,抗酸药、硫糖铝和米索前列醇的疗效尚未得到证实[137]。一项 meta 分析汇总了 12 项随机安慰剂对照试验数据,报告评估了 H_2RAs 对功能性消化不良患者的疗效,结果提示 H_2RA 比安慰剂疗效显著,相对风险降低了 23%,其中对照组 7 例[137],这样看来,H_2RA 似乎对于治疗功能性消化不良是有效的,但是其中试验对象可能纳入了很多 GERD 患者,被误认为是功能性消化不良,因此显得治疗效果显著。

一项基于 15 例用 PPI 治疗功能性消化不良的安慰剂对照随机试验的 meta 分析也证实了这类药物效果优于安慰剂(10 例对照试验见表 14.4)[104,138]。相对风险降低(13%),这个数值低于 H2RA,但这可能反映了更严格的准入标准和更好地排除了 GERD 患者。标准剂量与低剂量 PPI 之间疗效无统计学差异,双剂量 PPI 治疗并不优于单剂量 PPI。患者的 Hp 状态不影响 PPI 的疗效。在以前的罗马分类中,对功能性消化不良的分组显示,反流症状重叠组中 PPI 治疗最有效;上腹痛组疗效较差,可能与上腹痛综合征相对应;消化动力障碍组的抗胃酸治疗与对照组无统计学差异,这组与餐后不适综合征对应[138]。根据罗马Ⅳ分类分组的 FD 患者 PPI 治疗缺乏前瞻性研究。

2. 根除 Hp 感染

一项 meta 分析报道,在随访的 12 个月里,与安慰剂相比,根治 Hp 感染治疗消化不良的发生率降低了 9%,需要治疗的次数为 12.5(见表 14.5)[104]。反对根除 Hp 的原因是应答者数量较少以及明显的症状缓解延迟出现。然而,少部分消化不良患者的症状在根除 Hp 后可以得到持续缓解[139]。根据全球会议“京都共识”的报告[90],这些病例被称为“HP 相关性消化不良”。其他支持使用根除疗法的理由是有根除 Hp 可以保护胃黏膜、预防治疗胃癌并且治疗时间短、费用相对较低。

3. 促胃动力剂

促胃动力制剂是一类通过不同类型受体对胃动力产生激动作用的异质性化合物。目前有关促动力药物在治疗功能性消化不良方面的疗效一直存在争议[104,137,140-142]。一项 meta 分析表明,在 FD 患者中,使用促动剂治疗优于安慰剂,需要治疗的次数为 7,但这种效应在很大程度上是由西沙必利驱动的,而去除西沙必利治疗,其治疗所需的次数增加到 12(见表 14.6)[142]。甲氧氯普胺和多哌立酮是多巴胺受体激动剂,对上消化道运动有刺激作用。与甲氧氯普胺可能会引起严重的神经系统不良反应不同,多哌立酮不穿过血脑屏障,但在心电图上与 QT 间期延长有关,并可能诱发心律失常,但缺乏多潘立酮对 FD 的安慰剂对照研究[104,142]。西沙必利通过 5-羟色胺 4($5\text{-}HT_4$)受体激动作用来促进肌间神经丛中的乙酰胆碱释放,并且促进胃排空。然而,这些药物的临床试验质量很差,人们担心这些公开发表的数据存在偏差,出于安全考虑,西沙比利已从美国市场撤出[141,142]。其他有疗效证据的药物还有替加色罗和阿考替胺(见下文)[142-144]。替加色罗的作用仅比安慰剂强一些,由于人们担心潜在的心血管风险,目前这种药在大多数国家被禁用[145]。

表 14.4　质子泵抑制剂治疗功能性消化不良患者的随机对照试验的meta分析

研究者/年份	质子泵抑制剂		安慰剂		风险比
	事件	总体	事件	总体	相对危险度(95% CI)
Blum 2000	272	395	170	203	0.82 [0.75, 0.90]
Bolling-Sternevald 2002	71	100	80	97	0.86 [0.74, 1.01]
Farup 1999	6	14	8	10	0.54 [0.27, 1.06]
Fletcher 2011	45	70	33	35	0.68 [0.56, 0.83]
Gerson 2005	16	21	9	19	1.61 [0.95, 2.74]
Hengels 1998	50	131	77	138	0.68 [0.53, 0.89]
Iwakiri 2013	194	253	71	85	0.92 [0.82, 1.03]
Peura 2004	474	613	271	308	0.88 [0.83, 0.93]
Suzuki 2013 (ELF)	16	23	28	30	0.75 [0.56, 0.99]
Talley 1998 (BOND)	242	423	162	219	0.77 [0.69, 0.87]
Talley 1998 (OPERA)	277	403	141	203	0.99 [0.88, 1.11]
Talley 2007	653	853	84	111	1.01 [0.90, 1.13]
Van Rensburg 2008	93	207	116	212	0.82 [0.68, 1.00]
Van Zanten 2006	84	109	100	115	0.89 [0.78, 1.00]
Wong 2002	231	301	107	152	1.09 [0.97, 1.23]
总体	—	3 916	—	1 937	0.87[0.82, 0.94]
总体事件	2 724	—	1 457	—	

事件表示有症状改善的患者的数量。总体表示接受治疗的患者总数。
CI, 置信区间
From Moayyedi PM, Lacy BE, Andrews CN, et al. ACG and CAG clinical guideline: management of dyspepsia. Am J Gastroenterol 2017;112:988-1013.

表 14.5　根除Hp治疗功能性消化不良随机对照试验的meta分析

研究者/年份	治疗组		对照组		风险比
	事件	总体	事件	总体	相对危险度(95% CI)
Ang 2006	49	71	45	59	0.90 [0.73, 1.12]
Blum (OCAY) 1998	119	164	130	164	0.92 [0.81, 1.03]
Froehlich 2001	31	74	34	70	0.86 [0.60, 1.24]
Gilbert 2004	13	34	8	16	0.76 [0.40, 1.46]
Gonzalez Carro 2004	22	47	31	46	0.69 [0.48, 1.00]
Gwee 2009	31	41	38	41	0.82 [0.67, 0.99]
HSU 2001	34	81	36	80	0.93 [0.66, 1.33]
Koelz 2003	67	89	73	92	0.95 [0.81, 1.11]
Koskenpato 2001	61	77	63	74	0.93 [0.80, 1.08]
Lan 2011	86	98	94	97	0.91 [0.83, 0.98]
Matfertheiner 2003	338	534	177	266	0.95 [0.85, 1.06]
Martinek 2005	5	20	12	20	0.42 [0.18, 0.96]
Mazzoleni 2006	39	46	40	43	0.91 [0.79, 1.06]
Mazzoleni 2011	166	201	175	203	0.96 [0.88, 1.04]
McColl 1998	121	154	143	154	0.85 [0.77, 0.93]
Mlwa 2000	33	48	28	37	0.91 [0.70, 1.18]
Ruiz 2005	46	79	64	79	0.72 [0.58, 0.89]
Sodhi 2013	164	259	188	260	0.88 [0.78, 0.99]
Talley (ORCHID) 1999	101	133	111	142	0.97 [0.85, 1.11]
Talley (USA) 1999	122	150	120	143	0.97 [0.87, 1.08]
van Zanten 2003	45	75	55	82	0.89 [0.70, 1.14]
Varannes 2001	74	129	86	124	0.83 [0.68, 1.00]
总体	—	2 604	—	2 292	0.91[0.88, 0.94]
总体事件	1 767	—	1 751	—	

事件表示有症状改善的患者的数量。总体表示接受治疗的患者总数。
From Moayyedi PM, Lacy BE, Andrews CN, et al. ACG and CAG clinical guideline: management of dyspepsia. Am J Gastroenterol 2017;112:988-1013.
CI, 置信区间

表 14.6　功能性消化不良患者选择的促动力药物的随机对照试验的meta分析

研究者/年份	促胃动力药		安慰剂		风险比	相对危险度
	事件	总计	事件	总计	相对危险度(95%CI)	95%CI
西沙比利 vs 安慰剂						
AJ-Quorain 1995	22	48	47	50	0.49 [0.36, 0.67]	
Champion 1997	43	83	26	40	0.80 [0.59, 1.08]	
De Groot 1997	26	61	35	60	0.73 [0.51, 1.05]	
De Nutte 1989	6	17	11	15	0.48 [0.24, 0.98]	
Francois 1987	8	17	14	17	0.57 [0.33, 0.99]	
Hanson 1998	101	109	99	110	1.03 [0.95, 1.12]	
Holtmann 2002	51	59	52	61	1.01 [0.88, 1.17]	
Kellow 1995	26	30	25	31	1.07 [0.86, 1.34]	
Rosch 1987	27	57	45	57	0.60 [0.44, 0.81]	
Teixeira 2000	9	22	11	16	0.60 [0.33, 1.09]	
Wang 1995	137	414	145	169	0.39 [0.33, 0.45]	
Yeoh 1997	46	52	47	52	0.98 [0.86, 1.12]	
小计	—	969	—	678	0.71 [0.54, 0.93]	
总体事件	502	—	557	—		
阿考替胺 vs 安慰剂						
Kusunoki 2012	15	21	18	21	0.83 [0.60, 1.15]	
Matsueda 2010-1	187	216	94	107	0.99 [0.90, 1.08]	
Matsueda 2010-2	290	346	99	116	0.98 [0.90, 1.07]	
Matsuoda 2012	383	452	405	445	0.93 [0.89, 0.98]	
Tack 2011	87	193	53	96	0.82 [0.64, 1.04]	
Talley 2008	195	312	71	104	0.92 [0.78, 1.07]	
小计	1 540	—	889	—	0.94 [0.91, 0.98]	
总体事件	1 157	—	740	—		
伊托必利 vs 安慰剂						
Holtmann 2006	175	406	86	142	0.71 [0.59, 0.84]	
Ma 2012	53	119	79	120	0.68 [0.53, 0.86]	
Shen 2014	14	40	22	40	0.64 [0.38, 1.06]	
Talley 2008-1	124	264	226	260	0.54 [0.47, 0.62]	
Talley 2008-2	288	315	309	830	0.98 [0.93, 1.02]	
Wong 2014	3	16	4	14	0.66 [0.18, 2.44]	
小计	1 160	—	906	—	0.70 [0.47, 1.03]	
总体事件	656	—	726	—		
替加色罗(6mg, 每日2次) vs 安慰剂						
Vakil 2008-1	423	685	452	675	0.92 [0.85, 1.00]	
Vakil 2008-2	356	652	420	655	0.85 [0.78, 0.93]	
小计	1 337	—	1 330	—	0.89 [0.82, 0.96]	
总体事件	779	—	872	—		
莫沙必利 vs 安慰剂						
Hallerback 2002	171	425	57	141	1.00 [0.79, 1.25]	
Lin 2009	21	30	26	30	0.81 [0.61, 1.06]	
小计	455	—	171	—	0.91 [0.73, 1.13]	
总体事件	192	—	83	—		
雅培-229 vs 安慰剂						
Talley 2000	253	488	47	121	1.33 [1.05, 1.70]	
小计	488	—	121	—	1.33 [1.05, 1.70]	
总体事件	253	—	47	—		
总计	—	5 949	—	4 095	0.81 [0.74, 0.89]	
总体事件	3 539	—	3 025	—		

0.2　0.5　1　2　5

偏向促胃动力药　偏向安慰剂

事件表示有症状改善的患者的数量。总计表示接收治疗的患者总数。

CI, 置信区间。

From Moayyedi PM, Lacy BE, Andrews CN, et al. ACG and CAG clinical guideline: management of dyspepsia. Am J Gastroenterol 2017;112:988-1013.

遗憾的是，对其他促动力药物的研究，通常不能为缓解功能性消化不良症状提供令人信服的证据[146]。基于系统性分析，促动力药物的疗效并不是由它们对胃排空的刺激作用产生的，而是由对调节功能和内脏超敏反应的影响而产生的[141,146]。虽然一些促动剂会损害胃的调节功能，增加胃的敏感性，但另一些促动剂也可能会增强胃的调节功能（见下文）[141]。

4. 增强胃调节作用的药物

胃调节功能受损是 FD 最常见的运动异常。在一项研究该病发病机制中，发现用抗焦虑 5-HT_{1A} 激动剂丁螺环酮，可改善早期饱腹感，并能调节胃的协调功能，却不影响焦虑状态。说明这类药物对改善症状是有益[147]。在另一项 5-HT_{1A} 激动剂（坦多螺酮）为期 4 周的多中心研究也显示，药物也可减轻上腹部疼痛和不适，而与焦虑和抑郁临床表现无关[148]。一类药物阿考替胺既是一种突触前毒蕈碱自受体抑制剂，也是一种胆碱酯酶抑制剂，可促进胃排空和调节[149]。在日本进行的一项为期 4 周的第 3 期研究表明，阿考替胺对 PDS 患者早饱、餐后饱腹感和上腹部胀满不适均有良好的疗效[144]。该药物耐受性良好，这一发现在欧洲的同一年开放性研究中得到了证实[150]。阿考替胺只在日本和印度有售。

5. 作用于中枢的神经调节剂

精神类药物如抗抑郁药、抗焦虑药和抗精神病药通常用于常规初始治疗疗效不佳的功能性胃肠道疾病。

使用这类药物的基本原理是其可能改变大脑中的疼痛处理途径，基于这一概念，这类药物被称为中枢神经调节剂（见第 12 和 22 章）[151]。一项 meta 分析证实，中枢神经调节剂可能对治疗 FD 有效，但有说服力的证据仅限于用非典型抗精神病药和三环类抗抑郁药治疗 FD，其他药物试验的临床研究在规模和数量上都不足以说服其有效性[151,152]。

在一项多中心试验中，FD 患者随机接受安慰剂、阿米替林或西酞普兰治疗 8 周，只有阿米替林导致症状改善，但仅限于以上腹部疼痛为特征的亚组（类 EPS 亚组）[153]。抗抑郁药治疗没有显著改变胃排空率或营养物体积耐受性，但通过单光子发射计算机断层成像评估，阿米替林增加了胃调节功能（见上文）[154]。阿米替林和西酞普兰治疗无法显著改善焦虑、抑郁或躯体化评分，但阿米替林能改善睡眠深度[155]。

一项关于选择性 5-羟色胺-去甲肾上腺素再摄取抑制剂文拉法辛（venlafaxine）的大型对照试验未能显示其对功能性消化不良患者有益，且患者耐受性较差[156]。米氮平是一种对多种神经递质受体具有活性的抗抑郁药，对 FD 和主要以体重减轻为症状的非抑郁和非焦虑患者有效。除了增加体重外，米氮平还改善了整体症状、早期饱胀恶心和营养耐受性。

6. 其他药物治疗

通过对 4 项 meta 分析的总结发现，铋盐似乎是有效的，但该分析的统计意义处于临界范围[137]。1 例对照试验显示西甲硅油优于安慰剂[158]。薄荷油对 FD 的治疗效果也得到了评价。在对照试验中，薄荷和香菜油胶囊在缓解 EPS 和 PDS 症状方面均优于安慰剂，且患者具有良好的耐受性[159]。其作用机制仍有待确定，但以往的机制研究表明，薄荷油可使近端胃松弛[160]。在一项来自香港的研究中，利福昔明，每天服用 3 次，每次 400mg，持续 2 周，患者对该药的耐受性很好，在缓解嗳气和餐后饱胀感方面优于安慰剂[161]。这一结论得到确认之前，不可吸收的抗生素可以推荐用于治疗 FD。

各种研究报告表明，使用混合草药制剂、日本汉方药、中草药或朝鲜蓟叶提取物可改善症状[162-167]。数据表明，其中一些制剂是有效的，但这种改进的机制有待确定。一项研究报道，在功能性消化不良患者中，长期食用红辣椒比服用安慰剂更能缓解消化不良的症状[168]。含有益生菌的产品在自我管理或处方治疗肠道症状上已被大众接受，但对于包括 PDS 在内的上腹部症状的研究较少。有限的数据支持其潜在的疗效，但需要更多的研究加以证明[169,170]。

（三）心理干预

虽然功能性消化不良患者社会心理并发症发病率较高，但社会心理因素在症状产生中的作用尚不清楚。由于这些心理社会共患病的产生，心理干预措施如团体支持与放松训练、认知疗法、心理疗法和催眠疗法已被用于治疗功能性消化不良的患者。对功能性消化不良心理干预临床试验的系统评价发现，目前已发表的试验均提出持续超过 1 年的心理干预是有益的，但所有的研究都受到统计分析不充分的限制[171]。因此作者由此得出结论来证实心理干预在功能性消化不良中疗效是不具说服力的。

六、建议

对于有轻度或间歇性症状的功能性消化不良患者，安慰、宣教和一些饮食改变可能就足够了。对于症状更严重的患者或进行安慰和生活方式改变效果不明显的患者来说，可考虑药物治疗。建议进行检测 Hp 感染，如果检测结果为阳性，则可进行 Hp 根除。症状的改善不太可能立即观察到，其潜在的益处常在长时间的随访中观察到（图 14.3）。初始药物治疗可以选用 PPI 或促动力药物。根据症状类型选择可能有助于确定最合适的初始治疗，如果疗效不佳，建议换用不同类别的药物。

所有并发胃灼热和 EPS 的患者均应进行 2~4 周（优选）的 PPI 治疗。在症状缓解的情况下，应中断治疗，对症状反复发作的患者进行间歇性或长期的 PPI（或 H_2RA）治疗。对于 PDS 患者，可以考虑使用改善胃肠道动力的药物（如阿考替胺）。由于存在严重不良事件的风险，不应使用甲氧氯普胺和西沙必利，同时临床医生应知道多哌立酮与 QT 延长有关。虽然从理论上讲，PPI 和促动力药物联合使用可能有更好的疗效，但更建议单药治疗。

对于那些经过初始治疗后上腹痛综合征的症状仍未改善的患者，即使没有明显的焦虑或抑郁，也可以考虑使用低剂量的三环抗抑郁药物；对于患有严重焦虑或抑郁的住院患者，可以考虑增加剂量。应该避免使用 5-羟色胺-去甲肾上腺素再摄取抑制剂；在 PDS 症状令人烦恼的患者中，5-HT_{1A} 激动剂可用于治疗难治性早期饱足感；对于症状持续的患者，可以测量其胃排空时间；在胃排空时间严重延迟的情况下，可以认为患者患有特发性胃轻瘫，可以考虑使用强效促动力药物，如红霉素或普鲁卡洛必利（见第 50 章）；在对照试验中，对于难治性患者，也可以使用西甲硅油、薄荷油，或有明显疗效的中草

未作调查研究的消化不良
经验性治疗：
“测试和治疗”
质子泵抑制剂
考虑加促胃动力药物
无效果
内镜检查
70%
30%
功能性消化不良
器质性消化不良
消化性溃疡
食管炎
乳糜泻
贾第鞭毛虫病
胰腺炎
胆道疾病
其他
餐后不适综合征
上腹疼痛综合征
如果Hp阳性且未进行治疗
则需进行根除性治疗
促胃动力药物
(可加质子泵抑制剂)
质子泵抑制剂治疗
(考虑加一种促胃动力药物)
通常可用阿考替胺*
早饱感则用5-HT受体部分激动剂
体重减轻则用来氮平
阿米替林及其他
三环类抗抑郁药
难治愈
难治愈
胃排空测定
正常
催眠疗法和/或
心理疗法、营养支持
延时的
当作胃轻瘫治疗

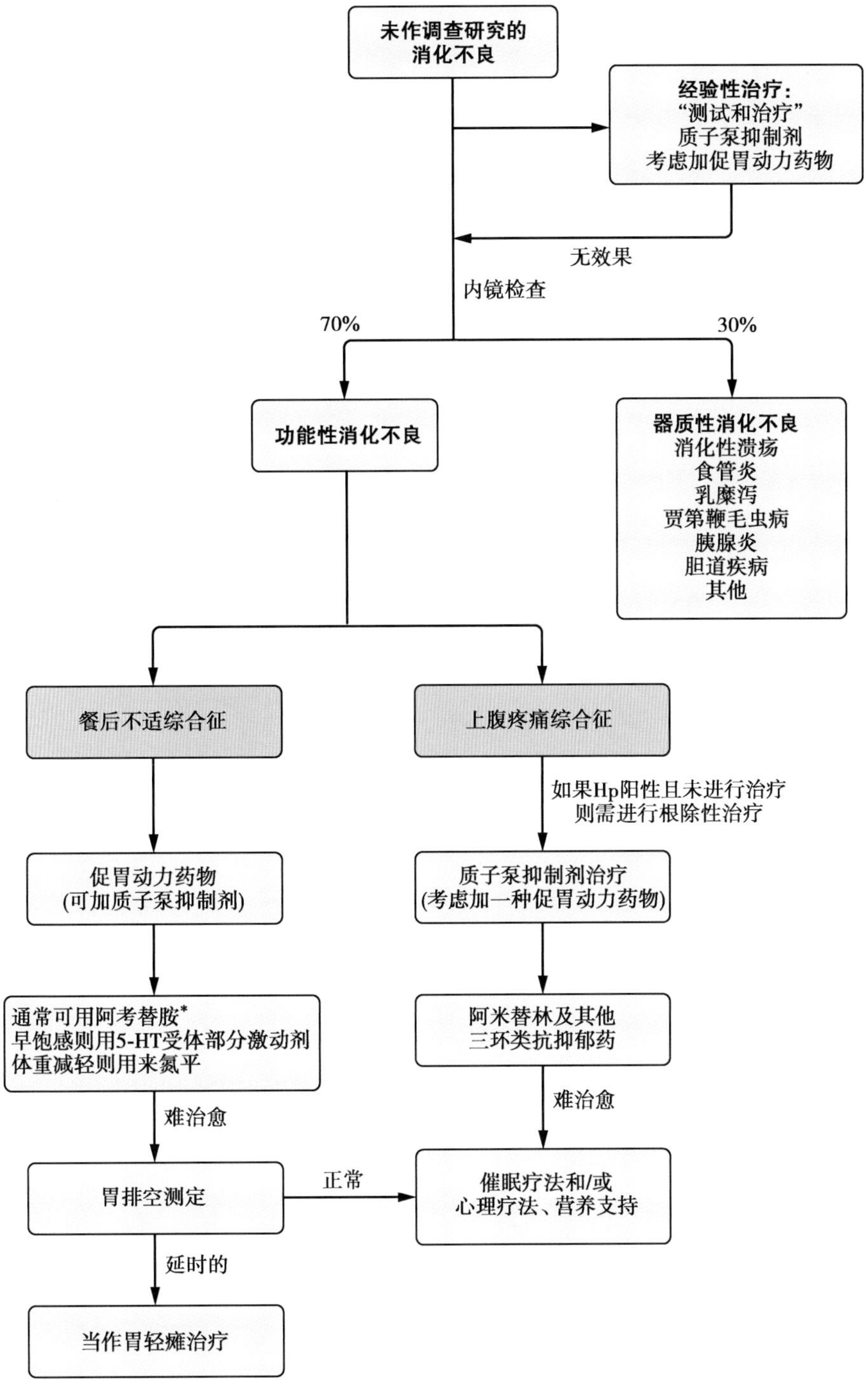

图 14.3　消化不良患者的管理算法。年龄小于 45~55 岁且无报警特征的患者可接受经验性治疗，而所有其他患者应首先通过上消化内镜检查进行评估。5-HT，5-羟色胺。* 在美国不可用

药制剂。对于难以忍受的上腹部疼痛，在排除器质性疾病后，可考虑使用止痛剂，乃至阿片类药物。

如果患者有明显的社会心理并发症、身体或性虐史，或症状严重到影响日常生活，可考虑转诊给精神科医生或心理治疗师。积极配合治疗的患者可从心理疗法、催眠疗法、认知行为疗法或放松疗法等心理疗法中获益。

（韩跃华　叶蔚 译，王立 校）

参考文献

14

第 15 章　恶心和呕吐

Arvind Rengarajan, C. Prakash Gyawali 著

章节目录

一、病理生理学 …… 182
二、临床特征 …… 183
三、病因 …… 183
（一）急性呕吐 …… 183
（二）慢性或复发性呕吐 …… 186
（三）妊娠期恶心呕吐 …… 186
（四）功能性呕吐 …… 187
（五）周期性呕吐综合征与大麻素呕吐综合征 …… 187
（六）肠系膜上动脉综合征 …… 188
（七）反刍综合征 …… 188
四、评估 …… 188
（一）急性呕吐 …… 188
（二）慢性呕吐 …… 189
五、并发症 …… 189
（一）食管和胃的呕吐损伤 …… 189
（二）声门痉挛及吸入性肺炎 …… 189
（三）水电解质代谢紊乱 …… 190
（四）营养缺乏 …… 190
六、治疗 …… 190
（一）纠正代谢并发症 …… 190
（二）药物治疗 …… 190
（三）胃电刺激 …… 193

恶心是一种即将呕吐的不愉快的主观感觉，可能与流涎、厌食、出汗、对正在进行的活动不感兴趣和焦虑有关[1]。在许多情况下，这种感觉不能准确定位，少数情况会感觉在上腹部或咽喉。恶心通常发生在呕吐之前或呕吐期间，但也可以单独出现。

干呕包括声门闭合时痉挛性呼吸运动。作为呕吐过程的一部分，干呕与强烈的恶心有关，通常（但并非总是）会以呕吐时为最终结果。

呕吐是一种通过口腔强行排出胃或肠内容物的部分自愿行为。这可能单独发生，但通常是整个呕吐序列的一部分，另外还包括恶心、干呕，呕吐需要中枢神经源性协调。

呕吐必须要与反流进行区分，反流是胃内容物毫不费力地反流到食管，有时会到达口腔，但没有呕吐典型的强烈喷射反射（见第 13 章）。反流可以从食管反流，反流物的味道完全像最近吃的食物，或从胃反流，反流物味道酸涩，且与胃灼热有关。食管流出道梗阻性疾病会出现食管反流，如贲门失弛缓症[2]。相比之下，从胃反流可能发生于胃食管反流病[3]或反刍综合征（一种行为紊乱）（见第 13 章）[4]。呕吐的鉴别诊断需要牢记，因为患者描述的呕吐症状经常没有差别，需要详细的临床病史来鉴别反流和呕吐。

一、病理生理学

呕吐的发生需要几块肌肉的同步收缩和/或舒张（包括膈肌、腹壁肌肉、咽肌和呼吸肌）以及为了适应胃内容物从口腔排出而做出姿势改变（图 15.1）[1,5-7]。虽然脑干中的神经元网络控制着呕吐反应的运动部分，但是髓质中的重要神经回路启动呕吐[8]。启动呕吐的传入神经信号来自身体的许多部位，包括咽、胃和小肠以及诸如心脏和睾丸等肠外器官。腹痛本身就可以引发恶心和呕吐。位于第四脑室底部最后在化学感受器触发区（chemoreceptor trigger zone，CTZ）的通路也可以引发呕吐。尽管 CTZ 位于中心位置，但它位于血脑屏障之外（至少部分），可以灵敏感受到循环中内源性和外源性激活呕吐的分子。来自其他中枢神经的通路，包括皮层、脑干和通过小脑的前庭系统，也可以引发症状。

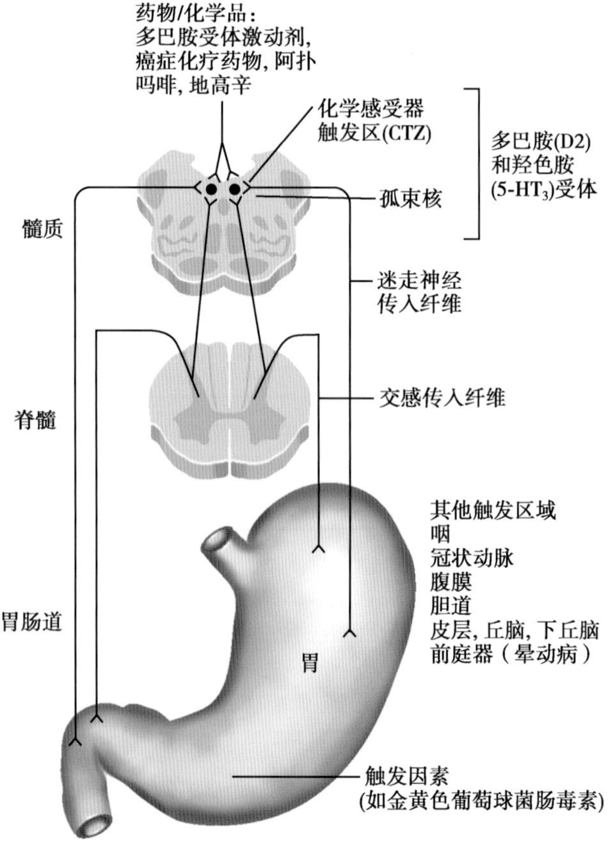

图 15.1　介导呕吐的拟定神经通路示意图。5-HT，5-羟色胺

恶心的感觉需要小脑幕上区域完整的神经回路[9,10]。介导呕吐的传入信号由迷走神经纤维传送到孤束核，但即使在双侧腹迷走神经切断术后也可能发生恶心[11]，提示存在发生恶心的替代途径。因此，恶心和呕吐仅共享用于产生这些症状的神经回路的一部分，这解释了为什么恶心和呕吐在临床上和药理学上是可分离的[11]。在一些患者中，恶心可能会持续存在，并变得相当麻烦。

呕吐反射回路涉及多个受体[7]，以下要素与临床问题最为相关：

刺激脑 5-羟色胺 3（5-HT_3）受体激发释放多巴胺，进而刺激脑干的多巴胺 D2 受体，从而激活呕吐序列。该序列是止吐药｛如昂丹司琼［一种 5-HT_3 受体抑制剂，可有效治疗急性（给药后 0~24 小时）化疗诱导的呕吐］和甲氧氯普胺（一种多巴胺 D2 受体拮抗剂）｝的药代动力学作用的基础[12]。作用于胃肠道的毒素和药物（包括化疗药物）由释放 5-HT 的肠内分泌细胞检测，进而激活迷走神经传入上的 5-HT_3 受体[11]。

组胺 H_1 受体和毒蕈碱 M1 受体在前庭中枢和孤束核中大量存在，是抑制晕动病、前庭恶心和妊娠相关呕吐的首选药物靶点[13]。

位于迷走神经背侧复合体中的大麻素 CB1 受体可抑制呕吐反射[14]。大麻素激动剂也可调节 5-HT_3 离子通道。CB 和 5-HT_3 受体系统在脑干共定位并相互作用[15]。大麻素激活中缝背核胞体树突状细胞 5-HT_{1A} 自身受体可减少致吐药物引起的恶心和呕吐[16]。

位于最后区和孤束核的神经激肽-1（NK-1）受体与 P 物质结合，是终末呕吐途径的一部分。通过 P 物质激活 NK-1 受体构成了化疗诱导呕吐的基础（即，化疗药物给药后 24~72 小时呕吐）[12]。NK-1 受体拮抗剂可减少外周和中枢作用的致吐剂引起的呕吐。5-HT_3 受体似乎在中枢诱导的呕吐中的参与程度大于外周诱导的呕吐。因此，在减少各种原因引起的呕吐方面，NK-1 受体拮抗剂似乎比 5-HT_3 受体抑制剂和其他已知的止吐药物更有效，并且可用于预防化疗药物引起的迟发性呕吐[7]。相反，它们可能具有较低的抗恶心作用。

当被激活时，脑干通过神经传出神经启动呕吐序列的各个组成部分而呕吐（见图 15.1）[7]。首先，恶心是大脑皮质激活的结果，胃同时舒张，胃窦和肠蠕动受到抑制。其次，由于膈肌和肋间肌的痉挛性收缩激活以及声门闭合而引起干呕。最后，当躯体和内脏成分同时被激活时，就会发生呕吐。这些成分包括膈肌和腹肌的快速收缩、食管下括约肌的松弛，以及空肠的强烈逆行蠕动收缩，将肠内容物推向口腔方向[17]。同时保护性反射被激活。提高软腭以防止胃内容物进入鼻咽部，暂时抑制呼吸，关闭声门以防止肺误吸，误吸是呕吐的潜在严重并发症。可能伴随恶心的其他反射现象包括多涎、心律失常以及肛门排气和排便。呕吐可以缓解恶心[7]。

二、临床特征

某些临床表现可能是恶心和呕吐的特征性病因。在早晨或空腹时出现症状，呕吐物中有吞咽的唾液或胃部分泌物，这是脑干呕吐中枢或 CTZ 直接激活的表现，最典型的是妊娠、药物、毒素（如酒精）或代谢紊乱（如糖尿病、尿毒症）。功能性呕吐也可以表现为这些特征。虽然夜间过多的鼻后滴漏也有类似表现，但是缺乏直接证据证明这种关联。餐后呕吐出残留和部分消化的食物是缓慢进展的胃出口梗阻或胃轻瘫的典型表现[18]。肠内容物逆行进入胃或胃肠吻合术后多次反复呕吐发作会出现胆汁性呕吐。伴粪便气味或味道的呕吐物提示肠梗阻、慢性胃出口梗阻或胃结肠瘘。在没有恶心或干呕的情况下突然出现的呕吐（喷射性呕吐）是颅内病变（肿瘤、脓肿）或颅内压升高对脑干直接刺激的典型表现，但不是特异性的[19]。

三、病因

确定恶心和呕吐的病因可以针对潜在的机制进行特定的治疗。明确诊断的紧迫性取决于临床表现。当出现胆汁性呕吐，神经功能障碍或呕吐急剧恶化时，需要进行积极的检查。短期（<1 周）症状需要进行紧急评估，慢性症状可在门诊选择性检查。框 15.1 列出了恶心和呕吐的原因。

（一）急性呕吐

对于急性呕吐的患者，必须首先明确以下两个问题（图 15.2）：

是否需要紧急评估或治疗？通过详细的采集病史和基本的实验室检测（全血细胞计数，全面的代谢指标，血清淀粉酶和脂肪酶）评估患者是否存在休克，脱水，低血压和严重的电解质紊乱。肠梗阻、空腔脏器穿孔、感染、急性胰腺炎、脏器梗死、脑水肿、急性肾上腺皮质危象和中毒是需要考虑的急性病因。

女性患者是否妊娠？对于育龄期妇女，在考虑其他病因之前，必须考虑和排除妊娠。

一旦这两个问题得到解决，就应该考虑一些潜在的需要紧急诊断的疾病。

1. 胃出口梗阻

在过去，消化性溃疡是胃出口梗阻的一个主要原因（见第 53 章），由活动性幽门溃疡引起的水肿或先前溃疡导致的幽门狭窄所致。呕吐可以急性发作，但也可以慢性或缓慢进展，类似胃轻瘫（见第 50 章）。虽然发病率在文献中尚未确定，但是随着消化性溃疡的早期有效治疗和复杂的消化性溃疡现在相对少见，胃出口梗阻的发病率已经减少[20]。胃扭转、食管旁疝和创伤后膈疝是其他相对少见但重要的急性呕吐原因，因间歇性梗阻和自发缓解，症状可能复发（图 15.3）（见第 27 章）[21]。脾脏过度活动（即游离脾脏）及假性息肉样胃窦肿块（如异位胰腺）阻塞出口是其他罕见但明确的急性呕吐原因[22,23]。

急性和慢性胰腺炎伴有炎性渗出、坏死、假性囊肿或继发感染，可导致十二指肠梗阻或较少见的胃窦和幽门梗阻（见第 58 和 59 章）。同样，胃、十二指肠或胰腺恶性肿瘤（腺癌、淋巴瘤、胰腺囊性肿瘤）也可引起胃出口梗阻，有时表现为急性呕吐（见第 32~34、54、60 和 125 章）。

框 15.1　恶心和呕吐的主要原因

腹部

机械性梗阻

　胃出口梗阻

　小肠梗阻

动力疾病

　慢性假性肠梗阻

　功能性消化不良

　胃轻瘫

其他腹腔内病因

　急性阑尾炎

　急性胆囊炎

　急性肝炎

　急性肠系膜缺血

　克罗恩病

　胃十二指肠溃疡

　胰腺炎和胰腺肿瘤

　腹膜炎和腹膜癌

　腹膜后和肠系膜疾病

药物

阿司匹林和其他非甾体抗炎药

抗糖尿病的药物

抗痛风药物

抗菌药物

　阿昔洛韦

　抗结核药物

　红霉素

　磺胺类药

　四环素

化疗药物

　顺铂

　阿糖胞苷

　达卡巴嗪

　依托泊苷

　5-氟尿嘧啶

　甲氨蝶呤

　氮芥

　他莫昔芬

　长春碱

心血管药物

　抗心律失常药物

　降压药

　β 受体阻滞药

　钙通道阻滞剂

　地高辛

　利尿剂

中枢神经系统药物

　抗帕金森药物(左旋多巴和其他多巴胺激动剂)

　抗惊厥药物

胃肠道药物

　硫唑嘌呤

　柳氮磺胺吡啶

　麻醉品

口服避孕药

　茶碱

感染

　急性胃肠炎

　病毒

　细菌

　非胃肠道(全身性)感染

代谢性和内分泌

　急性间歇性卟啉病

　艾迪森病

　糖尿病酮症酸中毒

　糖尿病

　甲状旁腺功能亢进和其他引起高钙血症的疾病

　甲状腺功能亢进

　低钠血症

　甲状旁腺功能减退

　妊娠

神经系统

　脱髓鞘疾病

　自主神经系统紊乱

　脑积水

　先天畸形

　颅内压增高

　低压性脑积水

脑内病变伴水肿

　脓肿

　出血

　梗死

　肿瘤

迷路疾病

　迷路炎

　梅尼埃病

　晕动病

脑膜炎

偏头痛

中耳炎

癫痫

内脏神经病变

其他原因

焦虑和抑郁

大麻素剧吐综合征

心脏疾病

　心脏衰竭

　心肌梗死缺血

　治疗心律失常的射频消融术

胶原血管疾病

　硬皮病

　系统性红斑狼疮

周期性呕吐综合征

进食障碍

酒精滥用

功能性疾病

维生素 A 过多

剧烈疼痛

副肿瘤综合征

术后状态

迷走神经切断术后

放射治疗

饥饿

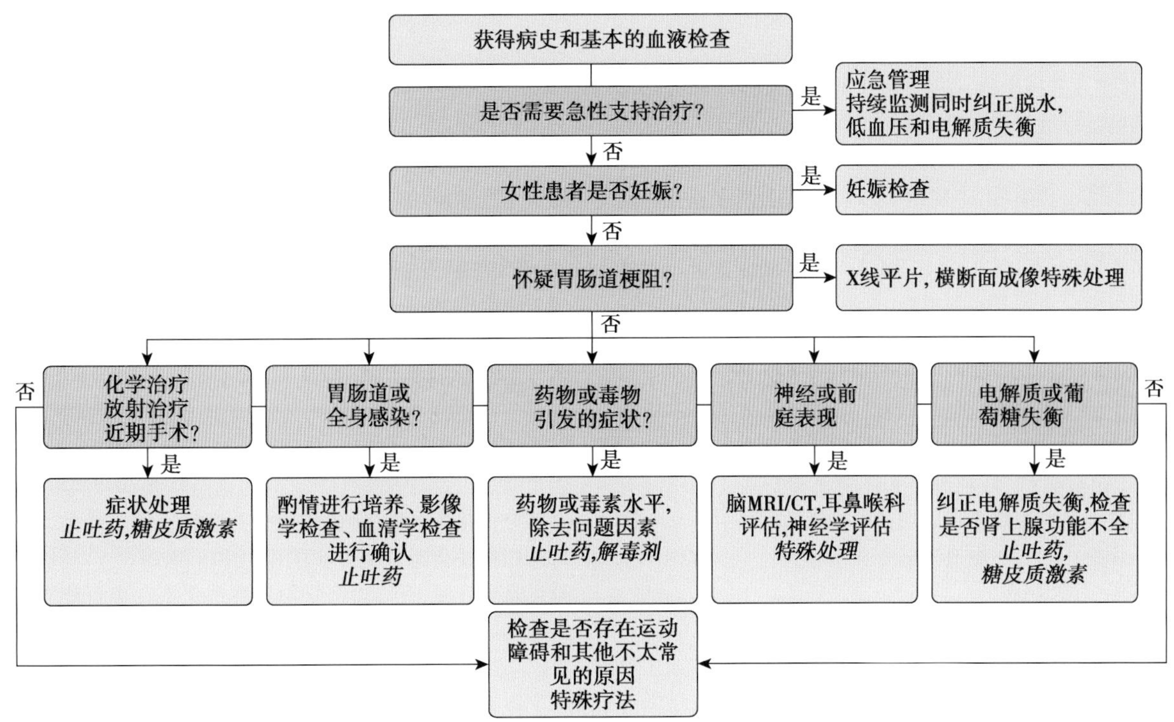

图 15.2　急性呕吐患者的诊治流程。潜在的治疗以斜体字显示

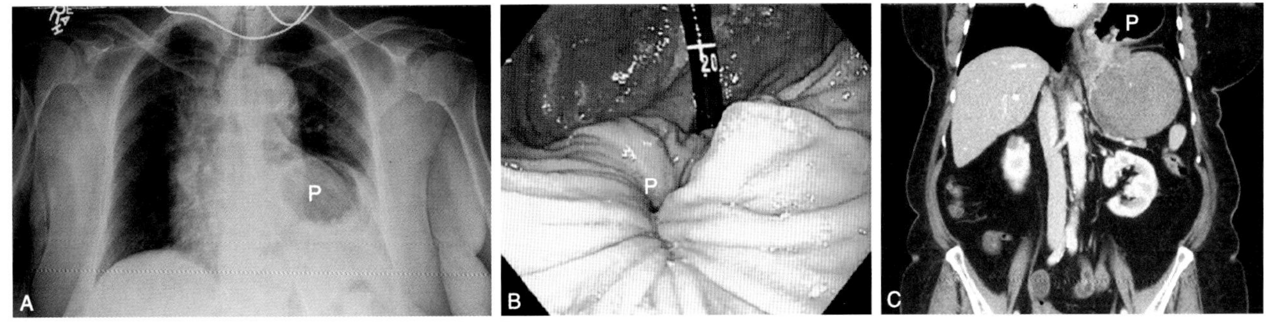

图 15.3　表现为恶心和呕吐的梗阻性食管旁疝(P)患者的腹部 X 线片(A)、内镜图像(B)和 CT 扫描(C)。成像学研究中可见左侧胸腔中存在含气的内脏。胃镜检查时翻转镜身可见开口进入食管旁疝。行急诊手术修补食管旁疝

2. 急性肠梗阻

呕吐可能是肠梗阻的主要症状。发病和严重程度取决于肠腔受损的程度和梗阻发展的速度。近端肠梗阻特别难以诊断,因为常规的上消化道内窥镜检查可能忽视或无法达到梗阻病变,在腹部平片上也可能没有典型的小肠充满液体的扩张袢(气-液平面)的典型图像(见第 123 章)。十二指肠远端和空肠近端肿瘤(腺癌、淋巴瘤、平滑肌肉瘤、类癌)可引起胃出口或肠梗阻,表现为急性或慢性呕吐。

3. 肠梗死

肠梗死可能缺乏体征,但需要迅速处理,尤其是急性动脉性肠系膜梗死,因为院内死亡率大于 60%[24]。这一诊断需要结合有相关高危因素的临床背景,[25]尤其是既往有血管疾病和血栓性疾病的患者以及老年患者(见第 118 章)。

4. 感染和炎症原因

呕吐在急性传染病中很常见。诸如病毒引起的胃肠炎是散发性或传染性病毒性疾病的常见病因之一[26]。产生毒素的细菌(如金黄色葡萄球菌等)会刺激肠嗜铬细胞释放 5-HT,激活迷走神经传入通路,从而引起呕吐[27]。在疾病初期,恶心和呕吐可能是主要甚至唯一的临床表现(见第 110 和 111 章)。全身性感染(败血症,尿毒症,肺炎,脑膜炎)也可导致恶心和呕吐。

腹腔内或腹膜后的炎症(如急性阑尾炎、急性胆囊炎、腹膜炎、急性胰腺炎,一般来说,任何引起急性腹痛的原因)都可能与呕吐有关。有时呕吐十分剧烈(但很少是唯一的症状)以至于会混淆诊断(见第 11、58 和 120 章)。

5. 肠外原因

肠外疾病可能导致恶心和呕吐。心肌梗死最初可能表现为急性呕吐,因为心脏和脑干之间的传入连接。同样,肾绞痛,胆道疼痛,卵巢或睾丸扭转可能表现为剧烈呕吐,疼痛的定位和其他特征表现可以明确诊断(见第 65 章)。

6. 药物及毒素

可引起恶心和呕吐的药物列表很长,而且恶心和呕吐都

是常用药物的常见副作用(见框 15.1)。常见的致病药物包括非甾体抗炎药、心血管药物(洋地黄、抗心律失常药)、抗生素、左旋多巴及其衍生物、茶碱、阿片类药物和硫唑嘌呤。接受多种药物治疗的患者在确定致病药物时会有困难。酒精滥用,药物过量和急性中毒也可能导致恶心和呕吐。癌症化疗经常会出现恶心和呕吐,常规给予预防性止吐治疗。化疗药物组合引起恶心和呕吐的可能性各不相同,与患者有关的因素也有所不同(见框 15.1)[28]。多达 50%~80% 接受放射治疗的患者可能会出现恶心和呕吐,这取决于放射治疗的部位、患者的易感性和放射治疗方案[29]。

7. 代谢原因

任何电解质紊乱都可能导致恶心和呕吐,包括但不限于尿毒症,高钙血症,低钠血症以及低血糖和高血糖。糖尿病酮症酸中毒、Addison 病、低钠血症和高钙血症与恶心和呕吐有特殊的相关性。糖尿病也可以通过胃轻瘫的进展引起恶心和呕吐。治疗潜在的疾病会改善恶心和呕吐。

8. 神经病学原因

与晕动病相关的恶心和呕吐涉及刺激前庭器官中的 5-HT_{1B} 和 5-HT_{1D} 受体[30]。恶心和呕吐可为脑膜炎唯一或主要的表现。前庭或小脑疾病患者的恶心和呕吐可能与眩晕有关。颅内压升高,颅内液体流动受阻或脑干直接受压等颅内病变可以表现为恶心和呕吐,有时会为喷射性。偏头痛可能伴有恶心和呕吐,轻微头痛或不存在头痛往往使诊断变得困难。发作性呕吐是一种罕见的表现,通常与右颞叶癫痫症有关[31]。一种罕见的自身免疫性疾病存在脑水通道抗体,可引起严重的恶心和呕吐[32]。运动引起的恶心和呕吐可能为嗜铬细胞瘤或副神经节瘤的诊断提供线索。

9. 术后恶心呕吐

高达 43% 的手术患者如果没有接受预防性止吐药物治疗,手术后会出现恶心和呕吐,这是与手术相关的最常见的并发症之一。许多因素与之相关,包括年龄、性别、最后用餐的时间、麻醉类型和手术类型。腹部、妇科、斜视和中耳手术风险最高,女性是男性的 3 倍[33]。全身麻醉和硬膜外麻醉有类似的风险性,而静脉麻醉的风险要低得多[34,35]。术后恶心呕吐的鉴别诊断包括手术并发症(肠穿孔、腹膜炎)、电解质紊乱和心脏病(无症状性心肌梗死、心力衰竭)。

(二) 慢性或复发性呕吐

慢性呕吐患者也必须要考虑到前面讨论的急性呕吐的相同原因,但具有特异性特征,如后面所讨论的。复发性呕吐的其他病因包括妊娠、功能性呕吐、周期性呕吐综合征(cyclic vomiting syndrome,CVS)、间歇性部分性肠梗阻和遗传性血管性水肿。

1. 部分性肠梗阻

尽管完全性肠梗阻表现为腹部症状急性发作,需要紧急评估,但部分性肠梗阻可能表现为反复呕吐,随着肠道传输的间歇性中断和自发恢复而消长。狭窄性克罗恩病、肠道肿瘤、放射性肠炎和缺血性肠狭窄是部分机械性肠梗阻可识别的主要原因(见第 41、115、118 和 123 章)。以前消化性溃疡引起的间歇性或慢性胃出口梗阻是另一个潜在的原因,但在现代该诊断相对少见。手术或盆腔炎引起的粘连可导致间歇性肠梗阻,但确立其致病作用有时比较困难。晚期腹腔内癌是肠梗阻的另一个原因。长期存在的部分性肠梗阻与慢性假性肠梗阻相似,事实上,在诊断假性肠梗阻之前需要排除隐匿性部分性肠梗阻(见第 123 和 124 章)。在老年体弱个体中,特别是伴有精神疾病合并症的患者中,便秘和顽固性便秘可能导致类似肠梗阻的表现。此时结肠受到粪便的影响,回肠流出部分受阻[36](见第 19 章)。

2. 胃肠动力障碍

胃轻瘫和慢性肠道假性梗阻可引起慢性呕吐(见第 50 章)[37,38]。反复或慢性呕吐是胃轻瘫的表现,但功能性消化不良、慢性功能性恶心呕吐和 CVS 也有类似的表现(在典型症状发作之间穿插明显的无症状期,见后文)[37,39,40]。胃轻瘫和功能性疾病的呕吐可导致厌食、进食不足、微量元素和维生素缺乏以及营养不良[41]。胃可能会扩张,呕吐物中可能含有部分消化的食物,但这些现象并不是一成不变的。明显的胃淤积往往会造成更严重的呕吐和早饱腹[42]。虽然胃排空延迟是胃轻瘫的标志,但是功能性消化不良也可能导致胃排空延迟,排空延迟的程度不一定预示着预后不良或治疗困难[43-45]。近端胃的调节减弱可以解释胃轻瘫的一些症状[46],减少胃淤积可以改善症状[47]。糖尿病是胃轻瘫的主要病因[48],胃轻瘫病因包括 Cajal 间质细胞(产生起搏活动)生长因子缺失、肠神经异常、免疫细胞增多等[42,49-51]。使用肠促胰素(普兰林肽或艾塞那肽)治疗的糖尿病患者可能发生医源性胃轻瘫[48]。特发性胃轻瘫可能在急性病毒(如巨细胞病毒、埃博拉病毒)感染后发生,其中腹痛可能是一个突出的特征[42,52-54]。可以观察到类似于吉兰-巴雷综合征的脱髓鞘表现[55],病毒性胃轻瘫往往是自限性[53]。

治疗胃食管反流病(GERD)的胃底折叠术后或减肥手术后可以短暂或长期出现慢性胃轻瘫伴复发性恶心和呕吐,这主要是因为胃适应性变化所致,迷走神经损伤也可能造成类似表现(见第 8 和 46 章)。胃轻瘫也可继发于肺移植或心肺移植手术[57,58]。

慢性恶心和呕吐,临床上与特发性胃轻瘫无法区分,但胃排空正常[51,59]。肠道假性梗阻除了腹痛和腹胀外,还可表现为恶心和呕吐,特征是在没有局限性或闭塞性肠管病变的情况下,出现部分或完全的肠梗阻[60]。胃轻瘫和慢性肠道假性梗阻之间的区别往往需要特异性的诊断试验(第 50 和 124 章)。

3. 神经系统疾病

神经系统疾病是慢性恶心和呕吐的一个重要原因,有时难以诊断。偏头痛,特别是没有先兆或家族史以及延迟或无头痛的非典型形式,是慢性或复发性呕吐的重要神经性病因。CVS 和腹型偏头痛也是偏头痛类疾病的表现形式(见后文)。脑积水压迫或刺激大脑底部的病变也可能导致慢性呕吐。

(三) 妊娠期恶心呕吐

妊娠期间会有 50%~80% 的概率出现恶性和呕吐[61]。这些症状往往在妊娠早期出现,在妊娠 6~12 周达到高峰,很少持续超过 22 周。虽然恶心和孕吐往往发生在早晨(称为"晨吐"),但症状也可以在一天中的任何时间出现。症状可能在妇女意识到自己妊娠之前就开始出现,因此对于任何孕龄期妇女有新发恶心和呕吐症状的都应该进行妊娠测试。虽然早晨的恶心和呕吐可能是妊娠的正常表现，但过度或严重的症状需要药物治疗。妊娠期间恶心和呕吐的发病机制尚不完全清楚，激素和心理影响可能是主要因素。危险因素包括多次妊娠，潜在的胃食管反流病，年龄更小和首次妊娠。尽管雌激素和孕激素可以减缓胃排空，但妊娠早期 HCG 水平升高可能会刺激胃 CCK 受体并引发症状。较高的 HCG 水平(如葡萄胎和多胎妊娠)会造成更频繁的恶心和呕吐[62,63]。

妊娠剧吐

妊娠剧烈呕吐是指严重和持续的呕吐并且诱发并发症，发生在 0.3%~3% 的孕妇。母亲的并发症包括体重减轻超过孕前体重的 5%、电解质失衡、脱水、酮症和 Mallory-Weiss 综合征。妊娠剧烈呕吐在年轻的初产妇中更为常见，特别是在亚洲和中东地区[64]。严重的呕吐会导致各种营养缺乏，包括 B 族维生素和脂溶性维生素缺乏。血清电解质紊乱可导致严重的低钾血症。剧烈呕吐还会造成畏惧再次妊娠的心理负担[65]。胎儿结局的描述较少，但剧烈呕吐常常会导致胎儿早产或者出生低体重[66]。

在美国，妊娠剧烈呕吐是妊娠前半期住院的最常见原因，仅次于早产[67]。在诊断妊娠剧烈呕吐之前，排除恶心和呕吐的其他病因(如消化性溃疡、胆囊炎、阑尾炎、肾盂肾炎)是必不可少的。初步实验室检测包括全血细胞计数、全面的代谢检测、甲状腺功能检查、血清脂肪酶水平、尿酮体检查，以及血清 β-HCG 水平用于评估可能的葡萄胎和多胎妊娠。妊娠剧烈呕吐在门诊治疗往往无效，通常需要住院进行液体和电解质补充和肠外止吐药。

简单的生活方式改变，包括多吃少餐，避免已知的饮食诱因和强烈的气味，利用非处方药如生姜、吡哆醇(维生素 B_6)，指压腕带或针灸是一线疗法。随机对照试验显示，无论生姜的剂量或制剂如何，生姜提取物比安慰剂有益[68-71]。吡哆醇和穴位按压(P6 压力点)可以改善症状[72-74]。二线治疗包括止吐药物、静脉输液和补充电解质。多巴胺拮抗剂和 5-羟色胺拮抗剂一样可以改善症状，但不良反应的可能性更大，尤其是甲氧氯普胺[75,76]。对于难治性病例的升级治疗包括在症状严重和危及生命时使用糖皮质激素和肠内营养[77,78]。

(四) 功能性呕吐

流行病学调查显示 2%~3% 的普通人群中一个月至少出现一次呕吐，罗马Ⅳ共识中功能性呕吐的标准包括每周一次或多次呕吐，持续 3 个月，症状出现至少在诊断前 6 个月，症状并非周期性的[40,79]。首先需要排除进食障碍、反刍、自我引起的呕吐、主要精神障碍、长期使用大麻素以及其他呕吐的结构性或器质性原因。社会心理压力因素和潜在的抑郁或焦虑通常起重要作用，应该加以解决[40,80]。

关于功能性呕吐的病理生理学假说主要涉及内脏高敏感、肠-脑相互作用改变、运动障碍、肠道微生物群或黏膜免疫功能紊乱以及社会心理应激。缺乏生化标志物和解剖异常对诊断造成了困难。

评估包括全面的病史和诊断性检查，以排除器质性呕吐的原因。食管胃十二指肠内镜(EGD)、造影检查[上消化道系列检查(UGIS)和小肠造影]和横断面成像(如 CT、MRI)可以排除结构性或梗阻性病变。动力检查(如放射性核素胃排空测试、十二指肠测压)可能显示胃轻瘫或肠道假性梗阻，不过胃排空延迟也见于功能性消化不良(也会造成恶心和呕吐)和其他引起恶心和呕吐的原因(如 CVS、药物)。胃窦十二指肠测压可以鉴别机械性和功能性梗阻，但是诊断的特异性较低。如果对呕吐患者进行测压，在禁食和餐后期间若能检测到强胃窦相位波和正常的肠道压力模式，则基本排除肠道假性梗阻的诊断[81,82]。经皮胃电图测量胃的起搏能力，可以识别胃的节律失常[81]，但不能确定胃的节律失常是恶心呕吐的原因还是后果[82]。

除了避免引起症状加重的食物之外，特定的饮食疗法效果甚微。同时需要纠正并存的营养不良和代谢紊乱。即使没有充分可信的证据，临床仍然使用心理疗法，行为疗法和精神药物。安慰和支持性医患关系对于功能性呕吐的治疗至关重要[83]。

(五) 周期性呕吐综合征与大麻素呕吐综合征

1. 周期性呕吐

周期性呕吐综合征(CVS)的特征为在排除其他病因的情况下，集中反复发作的呕吐。最初见于儿童，目前也见于成年人，发病率估计在 1.9%~2.3%，最常见于白人男性[84]。罗马Ⅳ标准将 CVS 定义为出现典型的呕吐发作(急性发作，持续时间少于 1 周)，在前一年出现 3 次或 3 次以上的间断发作，或者过去 6 个月出现 2 次或 2 次以上的间断发作(每次发作间隔至少 1 周)，发作间期无呕吐[40,84,85]。偏头痛的个人史或家族史支持 CVS 的诊断，特别是对于儿童患者[84,86]。经常使用大麻素可能出现一种与 CVS 无法鉴别的综合征——大麻素剧吐综合征，其解决办法是停止使用大麻素(见后文)。

典型的临床表现包括急性发作的恶心和/或呕吐伴腹痛、厌食和疲劳。发作可持续数小时至数天，间歇期无症状。体格检查无特异性，但可能反映脱水。随着时间的推移，患者经常寻求各种诊疗帮助及进行过度的实验室和诊断检查，包括血液化验，内镜检查，横断面成像，甚至手术探查[87]。鉴别诊断包括胃肠炎、消化性溃疡、胆囊疾病、胰腺炎、女性患者妊娠或潜在的代谢或精神病疾病。在儿科患者中，各种线粒体、离子通道和自主神经障碍也与间歇性呕吐发作有关，需要进一步排除。类似地，食物过敏(对牛奶、大豆或蛋清蛋白质过敏)或食物不耐受(巧克力、奶酪、坚果或味精)可能表现为呕吐，也需要排除(见第 10 章)[87,88]。

如果出现前驱症状，可以在前驱期开始流产治疗。抗偏头痛药物，特别是 5-HT_1 激动剂(例如舒马曲坦)，已经可以通过皮下，经鼻或口服给药。静脉注射常规止吐剂和苯二氮䓬类药物(例如劳拉西泮)在急性期可以发挥作用[87]。脱水和代谢并发症需要住院治疗并通过静脉治疗纠正。

三环类抗抑郁药(如阿米替林、去甲替林、丙米嗪、地西帕明)对约三分之二的成人和儿童都有预防作用[85,89]。β-肾上腺素受体拮抗剂(如普萘洛尔)也用于预防。其他有助于改善症状的药物包括 5-羟色胺再摄取抑制剂、赛庚啶、纳洛酮、肉碱、丙戊酸和红霉素。需要特别考虑 CVS 的心理因素。20% 的成人 CVS 患者有明显的焦虑障碍或其他精神疾病，发作前的预期性焦虑是常见的，并可能诱发发作。因此，管理并发的焦虑或抑郁具有治疗价值[85,90]。

2. 大麻素剧吐综合征

在部分周期性呕吐综合征患者中，长期使用大麻会激发或恶化症状，停止使用可以使症状得到缓解，这种情况称为大麻素剧吐综合征[91,92]。大麻素 CB1 受体分布在大脑和胃肠系统，而 CB2 受体分布在调节免疫功能的淋巴组织[93,94]。内源性大麻素刺激 CB1 受体可抑制下丘脑-垂体-肾上腺轴和对应激刺激的交感反应，调节胃的运动和感觉[93]。脂肪酸酰胺水解酶和单酰甘油脂肪酶负责降解内源性大麻素。假设之一是经常使用大麻导致 CB1 受体下调和脱敏，进而导致腹痛和难治性呕吐。戒除大麻素后受体恢复至原来的敏感性，这些症状就会消失[95]。大麻素受体的基因多态性也可能存在一定作用，仍需要进一步研究证实[96]。

大麻素呕吐综合征的表现与 CVS 的表现难以区分，它们有着相似的发作时间，持续时间和发作频率。长期吸食大麻及停用大麻后症状得到缓解是该综合征重要的特征[40]。许多大麻素呕吐综合征的患者需要惯例性的热水浴，但这并不是特征性表现，CVS 患者一般也存在这种情况[95]。完全戒除大麻会持续改善或缓解症状。美国大麻政策的自由化导致与大麻相关的综合征（包括大麻素呕吐综合征）的急诊患者增加，特别是在科罗拉多州，州外访客中患者的增加高于本州居民[97]。

除戒断以外，类似 CVS 的顿挫治疗和预防性措施是有效的[98]。此外，有个案报道腹壁局部应用辣椒素乳膏和静脉注射氟哌啶醇可终止症状发作[98,99]。

（六）肠系膜上动脉综合征

虽然肠系膜上动脉（superior mesenteric artery，SMA）综合征存在一些客观依据，但是该诊断不适用于功能性呕吐或 CVS 患者，否则会接受不必要的手术[100]。SMA 以锐角从主动脉分支，沿着肠系膜根部跨过十二指肠，通常位于中线右侧（见第 118 章）。在某些情况下，主动脉和 SMA 之间的夹角会变得更加锐利（身体前凸增加、肌肉张力或体重下降、卧床时间延长），导致十二指肠远端部分梗阻[101]。症状包括餐后上腹饱胀和压迫感、恶心和呕吐（通常是胆汁），以及中腹痛（俯卧或膝胸位可缓解）。影像学检查（UGIS 或 CT）显示十二指肠水平段靠近 SMA 位置的近端扩张和瘀滞。然而这种表现可能具有误导性，因为十二指肠扩张可能是由动力弛缓而非机械性梗阻引起的[100]。应在矫正手术前通过对比研究和/或闪烁显像检查证实十二指肠梗阻近端的淤滞，避免过度诊断。十二指肠和小肠测压会显示出机械性梗阻和运动障碍的不同特征性模式。将小肠营养管通过梗阻部位放置于近端空肠进行肠内营养，若能缓解呕吐，则支持诊断。

应尽可能首先纠正诱发因素。急性症状可以通过胃肠减压和静脉补液解决。只有经过充分检查的慢性复发型 SMA 综合征才应进行手术矫正。最常用的手术是腹腔镜近端十二指肠空肠吻合术，胃空肠造口术可能无效，因为近端十二指肠不能用此方法减压[102]。

（七）反刍综合征

反刍综合征是一种独特的功能性胃十二指肠疾病，其特征是反复轻松地将最近摄入的少量食物反刍到口中，然后重新咀嚼、重新吞咽或排出（见第 13 章）[103]。尽管反刍类似于呕吐，但它并不涉及由呕吐中枢协调的完整的躯体内脏反应。通常不会出现伴随恶心和自主神经表现（如唾液过多、皮肤血管收缩、出汗）。反刍通常在餐中或餐后立即开始，当反刍物变得明显酸性时停止。反刍在婴儿中相对常见，通常在 3~6 个月的时候。反刍一般没有明显的痛苦，可能会随着分心或睡眠而停止。反刍发生在成人任何年龄段，无明显性别差异[79]。

反刍的临床意义各不相同。一些健康的个体可能也经常反刍，自我认为这没有异常，另外一些在家人或朋友的压力下会咨询医生，他们可能误以为是习惯性呕吐、胃食管反流病或胃轻瘫，从而延误诊断和治疗。还有一些反刍患者会主动寻求医治，因为担心自己无法控制这个过程。另外，反刍可能与胃灼热、上腹部不适和伴有胃食管反流病、功能性消化不良或肠易激综合征患者的肠道功能紊乱有关。可能出现体重下降，这表明存在进食障碍。

在仔细询问患者病史后才可能得出反刍的临床诊断，需要排除贲门失弛缓症，其他食管动力障碍，胃出口梗阻和胃轻瘫。胃镜检测到食管炎表现并不能排除反刍。结合上消化道测压和 pH-阻抗测试可以在测压时发现胃窦和十二指肠尖锐的相位压力峰值（r 波），对应于患者将膈下的胃内容物通过松弛的食管下括约肌推向食管时突然增加的腹腔内压力。高分辨率食管测压和餐后阻抗测试有助于区分反刍与其他嗳气和反流障碍[104,105]。反刍是一种行为障碍，也需要考虑反刍与其他功能性疾病共存的可能（见第 44 章）。

反刍综合征的病理生理机制尚未完全阐明。反刍可能反映出对呃逆反射的适应（见第 17 章）。在胃内容物的突然逆行运动期间，胃食管交界部可能进入胸腔，形成一个“假性疝”，促进食管下括约肌的开放[106]。反刍综合征的一个亚组表现为反流相关的反刍，类似于反流发作，表现为腹腔内胃部张力的增加与短暂的食管下括约肌松弛同步发生[107]。

反刍综合征的治疗包括几个步骤。安慰和仔细解释这种现象会让一些患者自行控制反刍。行为矫正是最有效的治疗方法，反刍和膈肌收缩不能同时进行，所以可以教育患者掌握特殊的膈肌呼吸技术或借助生物反馈治疗[108]。借助观看监视器上显示的肌电图以训练控制腹胸肌的患者在经过仅仅 3 个疗程后，反刍发作的频率就减少了。胃灼热和内镜下有食管炎证据的患者应接受质子泵抑制剂（PPI）治疗。进一步的药物治疗包括巴氯芬（10mg，口服，每天 3 次），这是一种 γ-氨基丁酸激动剂，能增加食管下括约肌压力和降低吞咽率[109]。

四、评估

（一）急性呕吐

对急性呕吐患者的评估需从详细记录病史和仔细的体格检查开始，重点关注患者的容量状态和急性呕吐的病因。图 15.2 是急性呕吐患者的处理流程。所有育龄期妇女都应该进行妊娠测试。常规血液检查应包括全血细胞计数、肾功能、甲状腺功能、肝功能、电解质、葡萄糖、血清淀粉酶和脂肪酶水平检查，在某些情况下，还应包括动脉血气分析以评估患者的酸碱平衡状态。如有相关线索时还应进行药物和毒素水平的检测。

1. 影像学

应进行仰卧位和站立位腹部平片检查,如果影像提示为小肠梗阻,则应行进一步检查以确定梗阻原因(包括横断面影像学检查和适时的紧急手术探查)(见第 123 章)。

如果腹部平片未有明显异常,则考虑进行其他检查。胃镜检查可以评估黏膜病变、溃疡、肿瘤和胃出口或十二指肠梗阻。腹部 CT 或 MRI 可显示腹腔内炎症或感染过程(如阑尾炎、憩室炎)、急性肠缺血、梗阻或假性梗阻。这种情况下,腹部超声的敏感性较差。也可使用脑部磁共振成像以寻找肿块或呕吐的其他神经机制。

2. 其他检测

进一步的检测可以包括血液中药物和毒素水平(特别是地高辛、阿片类药物、茶碱、乙醇和卡马西平),若怀疑感染应进行血液或体液培养,腰椎穿刺后的脑脊液检测分析以及病毒性肝炎的血清学检测(如果有必要)。也可以测定血液中皮质醇,促肾上腺皮质激素释放因子和儿茶酚胺的水平。

(二) 慢性呕吐

详细的临床病史采集和仔细的体格检查是诊断功能性消化不良、功能性呕吐、CVS 和反刍综合征的关键。EGD 和/或 UGIS 是胃出口部分梗阻和十二指肠部分梗阻的首选检查。钡剂造影对贲门失弛缓症,胃轻瘫或肿瘤的诊断有帮助。腹部 CT 对于鉴别肠梗阻、腹腔内肿块和腹膜后病变特别有用,也能明确肠腔扩张程度、肠壁厚度以及通过探及肠腔直径转折点从而有助于定位肠梗阻[110]。相比之下,腹部平片往往不可靠,特别是肠袢内充满液体时。磁共振肠造影是 CT 肠造影的一种替代方法,优点是不暴露于射线[111]。脑部磁共振成像有助于诊断引起呕吐的中枢神经系统病变,包括生长缓慢的肿瘤、脑积水、炎症、血管和缺血性病变。动力学研究有助于评估运动障碍,包括胃轻瘫和慢性假性肠梗阻,这些因素相对少见但也是引起恶心和呕吐的重要原因(见第 50、99 和 124 章)。

1. 食管测压

食管测压法,最好是高分辨率测压,用于评估食管运动活动。食管运动障碍患者,如贲门失弛缓症和其他痉挛性疾病,偶尔可能出现呕吐或反流(见第 44 章)。

2. 胃排空测量

放射性核素显像是评估胃排空的首选和最准确的方法,应在 4 小时内进行,以准确评估胃排空。理想情况下,应使用双重标记(将固体和液体分开),并使用双头伽马相机进行测试。胃轻瘫的症状主要与延迟的固相胃排空有关[112]。其他可选但不太精确评估胃排空的方法包括三维胃超声评估液体餐的排空和辛酸盐 ^{13}C 呼气试验,加入测试餐中的辛酸盐是一种具有稳定的同位素标记脂肪酸[22,113]。$^{13}CO_2$ 的呼出速率反映了胃排空的速率以及随后十二指肠吸收脂质标志物的速率,但呼气试验的诊断可靠性尚未明确(见第 50 章)[114]。其他潜在的诊断方式包括无线动力胶囊、MRI 和单光子发射 CT[113,115]。

3. 皮肤胃电图

皮下放置电极的胃电图可以识别胃起搏的节律失常(如胃动过缓或胃动过速),以及进食后起搏活动频率的变化。尽管胃电图的优点在于无创和相对简单,但检查结果与临床症状不一定相关[54,81],并且某些胃电图异常可能是由恶心引起的,而不是恶心的原因(见第 50 章)。

4. 胃十二指肠测压

胃十二指肠测压是评估食管远端前肠运动障碍最具特异性的生理学检查。使用压力敏感导管记录胃窦和近端小肠管腔内压力变化。此检查烦琐昂贵,且在操作技术上具有挑战性,并且仅在少数专门研究胃肠动力障碍的中心才能实施。测压可以区分肌源性和神经源性的假性梗阻,并可以在波形分析的基础上帮助检测部分 SBO(见第 50、123 和 124 章)。如果胃十二指肠测压异常,可以考虑行腹腔镜小肠全层活检以诊断遗传性和获得性肌源性或神经源性原因的慢性假性肠梗阻。

5. 自主神经功能测试

自主神经功能测试可以评估交感神经功能,包括倾斜试验(对血压和心率调节的直立性挑战)和冷手试验(将手浸入冷水中以产生血管收缩和显著增加动脉收缩压的疼痛反射试验)。副交感神经功能可以通过测量深呼吸引起的心动过缓(通过血管迷走反射)和自发 Valsalva 动作引起的心电图 RR 间期的变化来评估。这些测试的结果可以帮助区分内脏自主神经病变(如淀粉样变或糖尿病)和中枢自主神经紊乱(如 Shy-Drager 综合征、全自主神经障碍)。

6. 组织病理学研究

在一些患者中,进一步的诊断步骤可能涉及黏膜活检的组织病理学检查,以量化神经密度和形态,作为自主神经病变的证据[116]。

五、并发症

呕吐,特别是迁延不愈或反复发作时,可导致许多潜在的可能危及生命的并发症。

(一) 食管和胃的呕吐损伤

慢性迁延性呕吐常产生食管炎,从轻度红斑到内镜下的糜烂和溃疡。与 GERD 相关的远端食管炎相反,呕吐引起的食管炎的特征是在整个食管体内均匀延伸。患者在急性呕吐后,可能会出现胃灼热或胸骨后疼痛。相反,慢性呕吐患者很少出现胸部症状,与长期呕吐相关的食管炎通常无症状。

突然的干呕或呕吐发作也可引起胃食管交界处水平的纵向黏膜撕裂和罕见的透壁撕裂。与胃食管交界处黏膜撕裂相关的急性出血和呕血构成 Mallory-Weiss 综合征(见第 20 和 45 章)。Boerhaave 综合征是指食管壁自发性破裂,伴有游离穿孔和继发性纵隔炎,死亡率较高[117]。尽管在呕吐时任何人都可能发生食管破裂,但多见于酗酒者(见第 45 章)。

长时间呕吐后,面部和上颈部可出现多发性紫癜性病变,可能是由于胸腔内压反复升高和血管破裂所致。慢性呕吐可能导致龋齿和糜烂。

(二) 声门痉挛及吸入性肺炎

由于咽部受到酸性或胆汁性物质的刺激,在呕吐过程中可能发生声门痉挛和短暂窒息。同样,在插入鼻胃管期间、镇静内窥镜检查期间、老年人或咳嗽反射抑制时发生的呕吐，可能导致胃容物吸入支气管，从而导致急性窒息和吸入性肺炎的后续风险。当胃中含有食物、液体或肠道分泌物时，更容易发生误吸，应在内镜检查期间从胃中抽出。

（三）水电解质代谢紊乱

长期呕吐后液体、电解质和代谢异常可迅速发展。可导致脱水、低血压、血液浓缩、少尿、肌无力和心律失常。低氯性碱中毒通常是首先发生的代谢异常，是由于液体以及氢离子和氯离子的丢失所致。低钾血症是由于呕吐物中钾离子丢失和碱中毒引起的肾性钾消耗所致。由于钠的丢失和抗利尿激素的释放，试图维持血容量，严重病例可发生低钠血症。代谢紊乱，尤其是代谢性碱中毒伴低尿钠排泄，可能是慢性功能性或自身诱发性呕吐的体征。

（四）营养缺乏

营养缺乏可能是由于热量摄入减少或呕吐物中营养物质的丢失所致。无论何种原因，慢性恶心和呕吐都可导致营养不良、体重减轻和需要补充营养的虚弱状态（见第 5 章和第 6 章）。

六、治疗

有效治疗恶心呕吐的患者需要纠正临床相关的代谢并发症以及进行药物治疗和根本原因治疗。

（一）纠正代谢并发症

急性、严重或反复呕吐的患者可能会迅速脱水，发展为代谢失衡、继发性循环衰竭和肾衰竭。如果口服摄入液体作用不足，应及时给予静脉输液及补充电解质。适当的替代治疗包括同时补充钾（60～80mmol/24h）和足够的生理盐水溶液（除外维持性补液）。生理盐水中也可以加入葡萄糖（例如生理盐水中加入 5% 葡萄糖），在某些情况下可能需要 10% 的葡萄糖溶液。当恢复至口服摄入时，首选含葡萄糖的液体，因为它们容易被肠道吸收。可以逐渐进行多餐、低脂、进食低纤维固体食物。

长期慢性呕吐的患者有营养不良的风险，因此当患者在 5～8 天后仍然无法通过进食获得充足的营养时，应考虑肠内或肠外营养。尽管肠内营养是一个不错的选择，但在呕吐发作期间，即使配置有导丝的口胃空肠导管也可能移位。对于长期治疗，可能需要放置经皮肠内营养管或进行肠外营养（见第 6 章）。

（二）药物治疗

用于治疗恶心和呕吐的药物主要分两大类：中枢作用止吐药和外周作用促动力药。一些药物具有两种作用机制，其中一种或另一种的优势各不相同［适用于成年患者的剂量（表 15.1）］。

表 15.1 用于治疗恶心呕吐的中枢和外周作用的药物

	药物	分类	适应证	使用方法[†]	副作用
中枢性止吐药	氯波必利	苯甲酰胺（多巴胺 D2 拮抗剂）	孕吐	10mg 口服，每日 4 次	焦虑；肌张力异常及震颤
	苯甲酰胺	外周 5-HT_4 受体激动剂	术后呕吐	25mg 口服，每日 3 次	迟发性运动障碍
			化疗及放疗后呕吐		QT 延长
			胃轻瘫相关恶心呕吐		
	氯丙嗪	吩噻嗪（多巴胺 D2 拮抗剂）	头晕	10～25mg 口服，间隔 4～6 小时一次	锥体外系反应
	奋乃静	毒蕈碱（M1 拮抗剂）	偏头痛	8～16mg 口服，每天 1 次	
	丙氯拉嗪	组胺（H1 拮抗剂）	晕动病	2.5～10mg 静推，间隔 4 小时	
	异丙嗪		化疗或术后恶心呕吐	12.5～25mg 静推，间隔 4～6 小时	
	噻乙基哌嗪			10mg 静推，间隔 8 小时	
	氟哌利多	丁酰苯（多巴胺 D2 拮抗剂）		2.5mg 静推，每日 1 次	
	氟哌啶醇	毒蕈碱（M1 拮抗剂）		1mg 静推，间隔 6 小时	
	苯海拉明	组胺（H_1 拮抗剂）	晕动病	25～50mg 口服，间隔 6～8 小时	嗜睡
	桂利嗪		前庭病	25～75mg 口服，间隔 8 小时	抗胆碱能反应
	美克洛嗪		过敏性瘙痒	25～50mg 口服，间隔 24 小时	
	羟嗪			25～100mg，间隔 24 小时	
	昂丹司琼	5-HT_3 受体拮抗剂	术后呕吐	0.15mg/kg 静推，间隔 8 小时	头痛

表 15.1 用于治疗恶心呕吐的中枢和外周作用的药物(续)

	药物	分类	适应证	使用方法†	副作用
	格雷司琼		化疗或放疗后呕吐	12~24mg 口服,间隔 8 小时	
	多拉司琼			化疗前 1 小时 100mg 口服或终止麻醉前 15 分钟 12.5mg 静推	
	托烷司琼			化疗前 5mg 静推,且连续 5 天,5mg/d 口服	
	地塞米松	糖皮质激素	术后呕吐	8~20mg 静推,间隔 6 小时	高血压
			化疗或放疗后呕吐	4mg 口服,间隔 6 小时	消化性溃疡
	大麻隆	大麻素	化疗引起的难治性呕吐	1~2mg 口服,间隔 12 小时	低血压
	屈大麻酚			2.5~10mg 口服,间隔 6~8 小时	精神症状
	阿瑞吡坦	NK-1 拮抗剂	化疗后呕吐	40mg 口服,麻醉 3 小时内	乏力;中性粒细胞减少症
	福沙吡坦		术后呕吐	130mg 静推,化疗前 30 分钟	
外周促动力制剂	普卢卡必利	外周性 $5\text{-}HT_4$ 受体激动剂	胃轻瘫相关恶心呕吐	2mg 口服,间隔 24 小时	心律不齐
	西尼必利			1mg 口服,间隔 8 小时	
	红霉素	胃动素受体激动剂	胃轻瘫相关恶心呕吐	3mg/kg 静推,间隔 8 小时	QT 延长

*临床中常用的药物;其他药物在正文中讨论。
†成人剂量。HT,羟色胺。

1. 中枢止吐药

中枢止吐剂根据药物作用的主要受体进行分类,这些药物可口服、胃肠外给药(单次推注、重复推注或连续静脉输注)或经皮给药(如可用)[118]。

(1) 多巴胺 D2 受体拮抗剂

苯甲酰胺类

苯甲酰胺类(如甲氧氯普胺、克来必利)的主要止吐作用是通过拮抗脑干的多巴胺 D2 受体。这些药物还可刺激外周 $5\text{-}HT_4$ 受体,从而促进乙酰胆碱释放,促进胃十二指肠动力活性。

副作用限制了这些药物的使用。当通过静脉途径快速给药时,甲氧氯普胺可能引起急性躁动和焦虑。重复口服给药可能会导致部分患者嗜睡。在约 1% 的治疗患者中,可能出现令人十分痛苦的锥体外系反应,包括肌张力障碍反应和震颤,并限制其使用,尤其是在高剂量时。老年患者有发生迟发性运动障碍的特殊风险[119]。甲氧氯普胺可能延长 QT 间期,因此具有致心律失常的潜在风险。该药物具有快速抗药反应性,继续使用可能会失去疗效。

这些药物最常见的适应证是妊娠恶心和呕吐、术后恶心和呕吐以及化疗和放疗引起的恶心和呕吐。由于其相关的胃促动力作用,这些药物可用于与糖尿病相关的胃轻瘫、既往迷走神经切断术和既往胃部分切除术。甲氧氯普胺的标准剂量为 10~20mg,每日 3~4 次,口服或静脉注射。

苯并咪唑衍生物

多潘立酮是苯并咪唑的主要衍生物,但在美国不可用该种药物[120]。该药物通过血脑屏障的能力较差,主要作为外周多巴胺 D2 受体拮抗剂发挥作用。它阻断最后区(部分在血脑屏障外)和胃中心的受体,其中 D2 受体抑制降低了近端胃舒张并促进了胃排空。尽管多潘立酮的止吐作用弱于甲氧氯普胺,但它可能对帕金森病患者左旋多巴治疗相关的恶心和呕吐的治疗特别有用,因为它拮抗左旋多巴的催吐副作用,而不干扰受血脑屏障保护的脑中枢的抗帕金森病作用。标准剂量为 10~20mg,每日 3~4 次口服。多潘立酮用于治疗糖尿病性胃轻瘫的综述得出结论,该药可能是有用的,但没有被设计良好的对照试验正确地评价。反应可能受到遗传特征的影响[121]。多潘立酮(以及苯甲酰胺类)可能增加催乳素的释放,偶尔伴有乳房触痛和溢乳。还观察到多潘立酮可延长 QT 间期,因此具有致心律失常的潜在影响。

(2) 吩噻嗪类和丁酰苯类

吩噻嗪类(氯丙嗪、奋乃静、丙氯拉嗪、异丙嗪和硫乙哌嗪)和丁酰苯类(氟哌利多和氟哌啶醇)除阻断毒蕈碱 M1 受体外,还阻断多巴胺 D2 受体;吩噻嗪类也阻断组胺 H1 受体。这些药物易引起松弛和嗜睡,通常用于胃肠外给药或栓剂治疗急性剧烈的中枢性呕吐,如眩晕、偏头痛和晕动病。它们也可用于毒性药物、化疗和手术后呕吐的患者[122,123],但出于安全考虑,特别是锥体外系效应,在一定程度上限制了这些药物的使用[124]。为此,氟哌利多的剂量不应超过 1mg。

奥氮平是第二代神经阻滞剂,由于其具有较强的抗呕、止吐作用,且无锥体外系副作用[125,126],是一种有吸引力的替代药物。使用奥氮平的副作用包括轻度镇静、体重增加和糖尿病风险增加。一项比较奥氮平(10mg)与安慰剂联合地塞米松、口服阿瑞匹坦或静脉注射福沙匹坦和 $5\text{-}HT_3$ 受体拮抗剂的双盲试验表明，可在临床上显著减少化疗引起的恶心和呕吐，并且获益可持续至给药后 120 小时。接受奥氮平治疗的患者的镇静程度显著增加，其中 5% 的病例尤为明显，特别是在第 2 天与基线相比时。尽管继续口服奥氮平，但这些症状会在第 3 天至第 5 天有所改善。因此，奥氮平也可以与其他药物联合使用，如地塞米松或 NK-1 拮抗剂。

（3）抗组胺药和抗毒蕈碱药

抗组胺药和抗毒蕈碱药物主要通过阻断组胺 H_1 受体（赛克力嗪、苯海拉明、桂利嗪、美克洛嗪、羟嗪）和毒蕈碱 M1 受体（东莨菪碱，可经皮给药）发挥作用[127]。东莨菪碱可引起令人烦恼的视觉适应障碍[128]。尽管异丙嗪属吩噻嗪类，但它们也可作为抗组胺 H_1 和具有强镇静作用的抗毒蕈碱药物发挥作用。赛克力嗪和苯海拉明常用于治疗晕动病，已被证明可降低胃节律障碍，因此其止吐作用可能部分通过其外周作用介导。赛克力嗪的标准止吐剂量为 50mg，每日 3 次口服或 100mg 栓剂。主要适应证是与晕动病和前庭疾病有关的恶心和呕吐。赛克力嗪可用于术后和其他形式的急性呕吐。其中一些药物也用作止痒剂。嗜睡是主要的限制性副作用，特别是在一些较老的药物中，但这种作用在急性呕吐的治疗中可能是有利的。抗胆碱能作用在青光眼、前列腺增生和哮喘患者中可能很麻烦。

（4）5-羟色胺拮抗剂

$5\text{-}HT_3$ 受体拮抗药（昂丹司琼、格雷司琼、多拉司琼、托烷司琼）是选择性阻断脑干和胃壁 $5\text{-}HT_3$ 受体的强效止吐药，通过迷走神经传递传入的呕吐冲动。除止吐作用外，它们还具有适度的促胃动力作用。这类药物的主要适应证是与化疗和放疗或手术后相关的恶心和呕吐。通常与氟哌啶醇和地塞米松联合治疗，伴或不伴使用 NK-1 拮抗剂[129]。头痛是一种常见的副作用。昂丹司琼在妊娠期间使用似乎是安全的，可以单次给药 8~32mg，静脉给药 0.15mg/kg，每 8 小时 1 次，或口服给药 12~24mg，每 24 小时，分 3 次服用。高剂量昂丹司琼存在 QT 间期延长的风险[130]。格雷司琼有透皮贴剂形式[131]。

帕洛诺司琼是第二代药物，表现出与 $5\text{-}HT_3$ 受体的独特相互作用，似乎比第一代 $5\text{-}HT_3$ 受体拮抗剂更有效。它是预防迟发性恶心和呕吐的唯一有效药物[132-136]。

（5）糖皮质激素

糖皮质激素的止吐机制尚不十分清楚，可能与抑制中枢前列腺素合成、释放内啡肽或改变 5-羟色胺的合成或释放有关。主要适应证是治疗术后或化疗或放疗引起的恶心和呕吐。糖皮质激素也可用于减轻脑水肿和减轻颅内压增高引起的呕吐。地塞米松是急性使用的制剂，剂量范围为 8~20mg 静脉注射和 4mg 口服，每 6 小时一次。因为治疗通常是短期给药，副作用并不常见。然而，在糖尿病患者中，需要密切监测血糖水平。在有消化性溃疡病史或胃肠吻合术的患者中，建议同时给予胃酸分泌抑制剂十分必要。在实践中，地塞米松常与另一种止吐药联合使用，如氟哌啶醇、奥氮平、甲氧氯普胺或 $5\text{-}HT_3$ 受体拮抗剂[137]。

（6）大麻素

尽管大麻素可引起或加剧恶心和呕吐（如 CVS、大麻素剧吐综合征），但已证实大麻素药物可用于治疗某些形式的慢性恶心和呕吐。大麻素的益处仅限于慢性恶心和呕吐的患者；相反，使用大麻素可引起间歇性刻板性恶心和呕吐，极有可能是偏头痛的一部分，继续使用大麻素可使症状加重。两种口服合成大麻素是标准治疗药物的一部分：萘哌隆和屈大麻酚。美国食品药品管理局（FDA）批准这两种药物用于常规止吐治疗无效的化疗引起的恶心和呕吐。多巴胺拮抗药和大麻素的联合应用可特别有效地预防对患者生活质量有严重负面影响的恶心症状[138,139]。情绪增强的特性使大麻素对患者具有吸引力，但这些药物的毒性可能比传统止吐药更大。低血压和精神药物反应是比较常见的副作用。老年人和有精神疾病史的患者应慎用这些药物。大麻素不再是治疗化疗引起的呕吐的一线药物，因为其副作用和更有吸引力的替代药物的可用性，尽管它们仍然对突发性恶心和呕吐有用[140]。

（7）神经激肽-1 受体拮抗剂（NK-1 受体拮抗剂）

NK-1 受体拮抗剂可抑制 P 物质和 NK-1，是强效止吐药物。有两种剂型可供选择，阿瑞匹坦（口服）和福沙匹坦（注射用）；其他制剂（如罗拉吡坦）正在评估中[141,142]。与 $5\text{-}HT_3$ 拮抗剂相比，这些药物对术后呕吐的保护作用更好，但对恶心的保护作用不佳。当 NK-1 受体拮抗剂与其他药物（如 $5\text{-}HT_3$ 拮抗剂和地塞米松）联合使用时可能特别有用，也被 FDA 批准用于预防接受癌症化疗患者的呕吐[129]。

（8）辅助药物和治疗

与化疗、放疗和手术相关的急性恶心和呕吐的患者，通常存在可能加重其症状的焦虑。苯二氮䓬类药物（如劳拉西泮、阿普唑仑）的抗焦虑作用可增强 $5\text{-}HT_3$ 受体拮抗剂和糖皮质激素等无精神作用的药物的止吐作用。加巴喷丁可能有助于预防化疗后迟发性恶心和呕吐[143]。生姜已显示出一些有效的抗恶心作用[144]。针灸、针刺、芳香疗法和穴位按摩也被证明，可以减少由虚幻的自我运动引起的晕动病相关的恶心和癌症放疗和化疗相关的恶心，但证据存在一定的争议[145,146]。

2. 胃促动力药

（1）5-羟色胺$_4$ 受体激动剂

苯甲酰胺类药物具有甲氧氯普胺（也是苯甲酰胺）的外周 $5\text{-}HT_4$ 受体激动剂作用，但不具有多巴胺 D2 拮抗剂作用，这是甲氧氯普胺的潜在中枢副作用的主要原因。普鲁卡必利是一种主要用于治疗便秘的药物，但对上消化道也有一些促动力作用，可用于这方面（见第 19 章）[147]。辛那普利是另一种药效学特性与西沙必利相似药物，西沙必利是一种与心律失常相关并已撤市的老药。在 1mg 口服，每日 3 次的剂量下，辛那普利似乎无心脏副作用，但在美国尚不可用。$5\text{-}HT_4$ 受体激动剂药物的主要适应证是治疗与胃轻瘫、假性肠梗阻和功能性消化不良相关的恶心和呕吐。

（2）胃动素受体激动剂

胃动素受体激动剂包括抗生素红霉素和其他作为平滑肌细胞和肠神经上胃动素受体配体的药物（均不常见）。在人体中的药效学作用具有剂量依赖性。在低剂量（0.5~1mg/kg，静脉推注）下，红霉素可诱导广泛的胃和肠蠕动活动，类似于消化间期移行性运动复合体Ⅲ期，但可能会使胃无效排空（见第 50 和 99 章）。在较高剂量（3mg/kg，每 8 小时 1 次，缓慢静脉输注）下，胃窦活动变得强烈，胃迅速排空，但运动爆发并不总是沿着小肠迁移。小肠收缩同时增加可引起腹部绞痛和腹泻。在临床上作为抗生素使用时,通常在较高剂量下,红霉素可能会引起恶心和呕吐。

在临床实践中,红霉素可用于治疗与胃轻瘫相关的急性恶心和呕吐(糖尿病、术后或特发性),并在 EGD 前清除胃内潴留的食物、分泌物和血液(见第 20 章)。虽然促动力作用已经很明确,但其缓解症状的作用受到质疑;有证据表明红霉素可以阻断迷走神经的交通,这是一种潜在的抗恶心机制[148,149]。

红霉素可静脉推注 200~400mg,每 4~5 小时 1 次。较低剂量更适用于假性梗阻患者,假性梗阻与小肠消化间期清除活动减少相关。红霉素不适合长期治疗,首先因为快速出现抗药反应,其次是因为口服给药的疗效不确定,而且其固有的抗生素制剂特性具有并发症的潜在风险,包括伪膜性结肠炎和 QT 间期延长。阿奇霉素是一种与红霉素结构相似的药物,已被拟定用于治疗胃轻瘫,静脉缓慢推注 250 或 500mg,但 FDA 警告提醒公众注意阿奇霉素用于心脏病患者的潜在危险[150]。无抗生素活性的新型合成胃动素激动剂目前正在研发中。

胃饥饿素是一种在结构和功能上与胃动素相关的肽,作用是加速餐后胃排空。胃饥饿素受体激动剂(如 ulimorelin, atilmolin, mitemcinal)具有促动力作用,未来可能作为促动力药治疗胃轻瘫患者的恶心和呕吐[151,152]。

(三) 胃电刺激

胃电刺激主要有两种技术方法。第一种是低频/高能量刺激("胃起搏"),涉及应用高能电流夹带胃慢波并产生相位收缩。该技术可实现胃轻瘫的纠正和恶心呕吐的改善,但需要限制患者自主性的外部能量来源。这项技术的改进—双通道胃起搏,在使胃节律障碍和排空延迟正常化方面取得了一些成功[153]。第二种方法是胃神经刺激疗法,与用于控制慢性疼痛的器械相似,使用植入式神经刺激器(Enterra 系统)向胃输送高频/低能脉冲。胃神经刺激器不引起慢波活动,也不能持续加速排空,但它能使近端胃张力松弛,减少与胃膨胀有关的不适感,并能产生明显的胃收缩,改善恶心和呕吐以及患者的营养状况和生活质量[154-156],即使是胃排空正常的患者。在应答者中,症状平均可改善至少 5 年[157]。有人提出增加幽门成形术,可提高神经刺激疗法对胃轻瘫相关恶心和呕吐患者的有效性[158]。

胃神经刺激疗法并非没有风险,常见的并发症包括电极脱位、感染和肠梗阻[155]。该器械也很昂贵,可能仅慎用于长期(至少持续 1 年)难治性胃轻瘫。可通过内镜放置的电极进行临时性神经刺激试验是可行的[159]。

(韩跃华 译,鲁晓岚　袁农 校)

参考文献

第 16 章　腹泻

Lawrence R. Schiller, Joseph H. Sellin 著

章节目录

一、定义 …… 194
二、病理生理学 …… 194
(一) 渗透性腹泻 …… 195
(二) 分泌性腹泻 …… 196
(三) 复合性腹泻 …… 196
三、临床分类 …… 198
(一) 急性腹泻与慢性腹泻 …… 198
(二) 大容量腹泻与小容量腹泻 …… 198
(三) 渗透性腹泻与分泌性腹泻 …… 198
(四) 水样泻、脂肪泻与炎性腹泻 …… 198
(五) 流行病学特征 …… 198
四、鉴别诊断 …… 199
五、评估 …… 200
(一) 病史 …… 200
(二) 体格检查 …… 201
(三) 急性腹泻 …… 201
(四) 慢性腹泻 …… 202
六、治疗 …… 206
(一) 急性腹泻 …… 207
(二) 慢性腹泻 …… 207
七、选择性腹泻综合征 …… 208
(一) 肠易激综合征和功能性腹泻 …… 208
(二) 食物性腹泻 …… 208
(三) 显微镜下结肠炎 …… 208
(四) 手术后腹泻 …… 209
(五) 胆汁酸性腹泻 …… 209
(六) 住院患者腹泻 …… 210
(七) 人为性腹泻 …… 211
(八) 特发性分泌性腹泻 …… 211
(九) 不明原因腹泻 …… 211

腹泻是人类普遍会有的经历。美国每月约有 7.5% 的人出现急性胃肠炎的症状[1]。对于大多数人来说，腹泻发作仅持续 1～2 天，无需医疗干预即可迅速好转。对另一些人来说，腹泻持续数天以上或伴有发热、虚脱或直肠出血。这些人很可能去寻求医疗保健者帮助。在美国，每年因腹泻就诊的门诊量超过 350 万次[2]。大多数可作为门诊患者成功治疗，但每年仍有 18 万多例住院和 3 000 多例死亡归因于胃肠炎[3]。在 1 年之中，约 6.6% 的人群可能发生慢性腹泻（水样便≥4 周），因此是美国人残疾的主要原因[4]。在发展中国家，急性感染性腹泻仍然是发病和死亡的重要原因，特别是在儿童中。

一、定义

腹泻是一种症状，不是一种疾病，因此在很多情况下都可能发生。大多数患者认为粪便流动性增加是腹泻的基本特征[5]。粪便的性状很难进行定量，视觉量表可能有助于患者描述其腹泻情况[6]。研究者还将大便次数或重量作为判定腹泻的替代衡量标志。每日 3 次或 3 次以上的排便被认为是异常的，西方国家普遍认为粪便重量的上限是每日 200g[7]。虽然粪便重量常被引用为腹泻的一个客观指标，但腹泻不应仅以粪便重量来定义。有些人因摄入纤维而使粪便重量增加，但因其粪便稠度正常而不主诉腹泻。当摄入高纤维膳食时，粪便排出量可高达 300g。这在一些发展中国家是惯例。相反，由于排出的是少量稀便或成形粪便排出次数增加，约 20% 腹泻患者的粪便重量可能是正常的[8]。

大便失禁在一些患者，尤其是老年人中，被诊断为严重或棘手的腹泻[9]。虽然许多失禁患者有稀便，但其主要问题是控便机制，而不是肠液或电解质吸收问题。因此，应询问所有主诉腹泻的患者是否存在大便失禁。如果大便失禁频繁，特别是在没有直肠急迫感或稀便的情况下，应评估患者是否有大便失禁，而不是诊断为腹泻（见第 18 章）。

二、病理生理学

腹泻是一种应对肠道各种损伤和攻击的保护性反应。当肠道中存在感染因子、毒素或其他有毒物质时，刺激肠道液体分泌和运动，排出不需要的物质，从而产生腹泻。这种保护性反应是有价值的急性反应，当慢性时，它是不适当的，不再起适应的目的。

腹泻是由于肠道净水和电解质转运异常导致的粪便水过多所致[5]。正常情况下，小肠和结肠通过 Treitz 韧带吸收 99% 的液体负荷，每天经口摄入和从唾液腺、胃、肝和胰腺内源性分泌的两者组成，每日总量约为 9～10L（图 16.1）。腹泻是由于这种正常微调机制的破坏所致，净吸水率降低 1% 可导致腹泻。当小肠或结肠中黏膜水和电解质转运速率改变时，可能会发生这种情况。快速转运也可以导致吸水率降低和腹泻，从而缩短了可用于吸水的时间，尤其是当液体快速通过结肠时。第三种导致腹泻的机制是粪便固体组成的变化，这可能会改变粪便的黏稠度。粪便黏稠度取决于粪便含水量与不溶性粪便固体（如纤维残渣和细菌成分）结合水的能力之间的平衡[5]。水结合减少（如脂肪泻所见）可产生稀便，甚至腹泻。

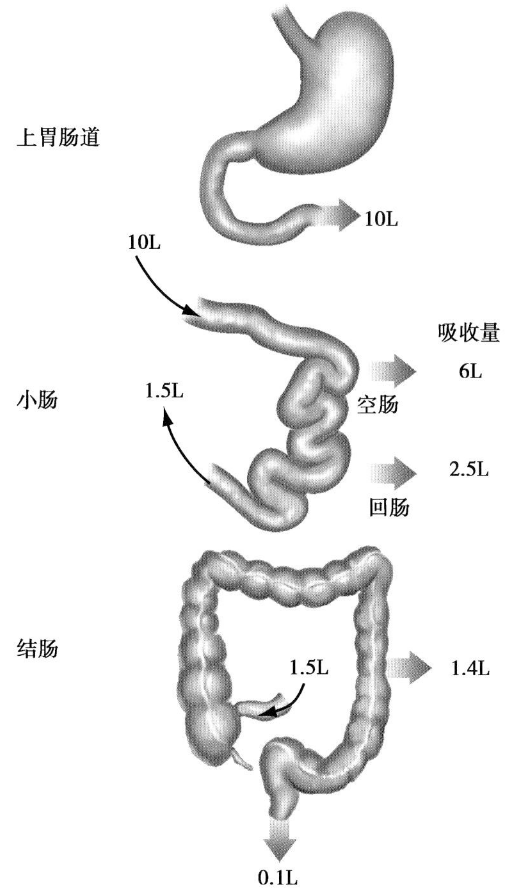

图 16.1 胃肠道的液体负荷。每天由摄入的食物和饮料以及唾液腺、食管、胃、胰腺、胆管和十二指肠的分泌物组成的接近 10L 的液体通过 Treitz 韧带。每天空肠吸收约 6L 液体，回肠吸收约 2.5L，留下约 1.5L 进入结肠。结肠吸收该负荷的 90% 以上，在粪便中仅留下约 0.1L。吸水的总有效率为 99%。这种效率降低至 1% 可能导致腹泻。（From Schiller LR. Chronic diarrhea. In：McNally P，editor. GI/Liver secrets. 2nd ed. Philadelphia：Hanley & Belfus；2001. p 411.）

在许多情况下，腹泻是许多因素相互作用的结果，由上皮功能、运动功能和管腔组成[10]。水本身不是主动运输的，相反，它通过借助电解质、营养物质等溶质转运产生的渗透压力，经细胞旁途径和跨细胞途径穿过肠黏膜（见第 101 和 102 章）。离子和营养物质跨膜转运的分子途径已得充分表征，并由细胞外和细胞内信使的复杂通信系统调节，在大多数生理条件下维持液体平衡。正常情况下，吸收与分泌同时发生，但吸收在数量上更大。吸收减少或分泌增加导致肠腔内液体增加，从而导致腹泻。毒素、药物、激素和细胞因子破坏肠上皮电解质转运或其调节系统是腹泻的主要原因。

由电解质转运紊乱引起的腹泻被称为分泌性腹泻，尽管它更常因电解质吸收减少而不是净分泌引起[11]。腹泻的另一个原因是摄入一些吸收不良的渗透性活性物质（如镁离子、乳果糖），使液体保留在肠腔内，以维持与体液的渗透平衡，从而减少吸水性。这种机制引起的腹泻被称为渗透性腹泻（表 16.1）。临床上很少出现单纯的分泌性或渗透性腹泻，但在考虑联合致病作用前，应考虑哪种机制占主导地位是有用的。

表 16.1 分泌性与渗透性腹泻

腹泻类型	病因	病种
分泌性腹泻	离子转运体缺失	先天性氯化物腹泻
	内源性分泌性腹泻	神经内分泌肿瘤（如类癌综合征）
	外源性分泌性腹泻	肠毒素（如霍乱）
	小肠缺血	弥漫性肠系膜动脉粥样硬化
	肠黏膜表面积减少	小肠切除术，弥漫性小肠黏膜病变
	小肠快速转运	迷走神经切断术后肠蠕动加速
渗透性腹泻	摄入吸收不良的物质	摄入镁离子
	营养物质输送减少	乳糖酶缺乏

（一）渗透性腹泻

摄入吸收不良的阳离子和阴离子或吸收不良的糖或糖醇（如甘露醇、山梨糖醇）是大多数渗透性腹泻的原因[12]。吸收较差的离子包括镁、硫酸盐和磷酸盐，这些离子通过在低管腔内离子浓度下达到饱和的机制主动转运，并通过容量受限的机制被动转运。总之这些过程将总吸收限制在摄入量的一小部分。由于小肠和结肠均不能维持血浆的渗透梯度，因此未被吸收的离子（及其反离子）保留在肠腔内，并强制保留水以维持与体液相同的腔内渗透压（约 290mOsm/kg）。因此，每 1mOsm 保留离子或分子保留约 3.5mL 水（1 000mL/kg÷290mOsm/kg）（见第 101 章）[12-15]。

糖和糖醇是引起渗透性腹泻的另一类主要物质[15]。单糖，而不是双糖，可以通过肠顶膜被完整吸收。当摄入蔗糖和乳糖等双糖时，缺乏适当的双糖酶将妨碍双糖的水解及其组分单糖的吸收（见第 102 和 104 章）。双糖酶缺乏症最常见的临床综合征是获得性乳糖酶缺乏症，这在许多成年人中解释了乳糖不耐受的原因[16]。乳糖酶存在于大多数未成年哺乳动物的小肠刷状缘，但在成年哺乳动物中下调，包括 70% 的成年人类[17]。主要的例外是来自北欧基因库和非洲一些地区的人，由于基因启动子区的突变[18,19]，他们通常会将乳糖酶活性维持到成年。然而，即使在这些群体中，乳糖酶活性也经常随着年龄的增长而下降。先天性乳糖酶缺乏症罕见，似乎是乳糖酶-根皮苷水解酶（成人乳糖酶缺乏症中受影响的基因）不同的基因突变的结果[20]。获得性缺陷也可能与小肠上段黏膜疾病有关，如乳糜泻。先天性蔗糖酶和海藻糖酶缺乏罕见，分别妨碍蔗糖（食用糖）和海藻糖（在蘑菇和龙虾中发现的双糖，在加工食品中用作添加剂）的充分消化。乳果糖是一种合成的双糖，不能被人双糖酶水解，当给予足量时，可引起渗透性腹泻[21]。随着人们对渗透性腹泻的认识，可能导致渗透性腹泻的食物谱已经扩大，含有吸收不良的可发酵寡糖、双糖、单糖和多元醇（fermentable oligosaccharides，disaccharides，monosaccharides，and polyols，FODMAP）的食物组（见后文）。

渗透性腹泻的基本特征是在禁食或停止摄入致病物质后消退。这一特征已在临床上用于区分渗透性腹泻和分泌性腹泻，后者通常在空腹时持续存在。渗透性腹泻时电解质吸收不受影响，大便中电解质浓度通常较低[13-15]。

（二）分泌性腹泻

分泌性腹泻有很多原因。这类腹泻的机制是阴离子（氯化物或碳酸氢盐）的净分泌、钾的净分泌或钠吸收的净抑制[22,23]。电解质转运改变的刺激来自肠腔、上皮下间隙或体循环，并显著改变调节离子转运途径的信使系统。在极少数情况下，先天性缺乏特异性转运分子限制了钠或氯化物的吸收，导致腹泻。在其他情况下，缺乏足够的吸收表面积严重限制了电解质，尤其是钠的吸收。

分泌性腹泻最常见的原因是感染[22]。来自各种感染性因子（主要是细菌，也包括寄生虫和病毒）的肠毒素与调节肠道转运并引起阴离子分泌增加的受体相互作用。例如，大肠埃希菌热稳定肠毒素与肠细胞内腔表面的鸟苷酸环化酶C受体相互作用，后者通常介导鸟苷酸的作用，鸟苷酸是一种内腔释放的肽类激素，通过囊性纤维化跨膜转导调节因子（CFTR）刺激氯化物分泌[24]。除刺激分泌外，肠毒素还可能阻断特定的吸收途径。许多肠毒素抑制小肠和结肠的 Na^+-H^+ 交换，从而是阻断电解质和液体吸收的重要驱动力之一[22]。

内分泌肿瘤产生的肽（如，血管活性肠肽）通过刺激上皮细胞分泌引起分泌性腹泻，上皮下神经元和炎性细胞释放的肽也是如此（见第4和34章）[25,26]。神经递质如乙酰胆碱或5-羟色胺（5-HT）和其他调节剂如组胺和炎性细胞因子，也是强效的分泌刺激物[27,28]。这些肠道转运的内源性调节因子大多通过改变细胞内信使引起腹泻，如控制特定转运途径的环磷酸腺苷（cAMP）、环磷酸鸟苷（cGMP）和钙[22,28]。肽和其他调节因子也可能影响单个转运蛋白的合成、定位和降解。外源性因子如药物和一些毒物可导致分泌性腹泻，可能是通过与肠细胞的细胞内调节因子或细胞内信使相互作用所致。

基因突变可能导致特定吸收途径的缺失或破坏，并可能引起腹泻。例如，罕见的先天综合征（如先天性氯腹泻和先天性钠腹泻），是由缺乏特异性转运分子引起的[29-33]。在先天性氯性腹泻中，腺瘤（DRA）蛋白中的下调和回肠和结肠中的 Cl^-/HCO_3^- 交换存在缺陷，从而将氯化物转化为吸收较差的离子。通过限制口服氯化物摄入量或氯化物分泌或通过增强短链脂肪酸吸收刺激结肠对氯化物的吸收，可减少氯化物-腹泻[31]。钠-质子交换体3活性降低是导致先天性钠腹泻的原因[32]。另一种家族性腹泻综合征是由于鸟苷酸环化酶C受体的突变，显著增加了肠细胞中环磷酸鸟苷的生成[33]。

为了使肠液和电解吸收完全，肠道必须具有足够的表面积和与肠腔内容物足够的接触时间。大量表面积损失，如乳糜泻、炎症性肠病（IBD）或切除手术后，可能影响吸水性。尽管小肠和结肠的储备吸收能力较大，但足够长的手术切除不可避免地会引起腹泻。在某些情况下，问题是暂时的，因为随着时间的推移，肠道可通过适应过程提高其吸收能力[34,35]。但在切除具有高度特异性吸收功能的某些肠段后，这种代偿是不可能的，而其他肠段根本不能替代这种功能。例如，回盲部切除术后，在浓度梯度下无法吸收氯化钠，结肠更远端部分无法克服这种情况[36]。回肠切除也可能导致胆汁酸吸收不良，可抑制结肠水和电解质吸收（见后文）。

肠运动异常可能导致同时具有分泌和渗透成分的腹泻[10,11]。为了使液体和电解质完全吸收，管腔内容物与上皮之间的接触时间必须足以允许吸收。在一些患者中，肠运动异常会产生"肠急促"[37,38]。由于快速转运阻止了足够的吸收时间，尽管黏膜吸收能力完整，但仍会引起腹泻[11]。在一些"肠急促"的患者中，口-盲肠通过时间可短至10分钟。在这种情况下，由于对腹泻产生渗透成分的营养物质吸收不良，腹泻加剧。在糖尿病和迷走神经切断术后的腹泻中，"肠急促"与肠神经系统功能异常有关[39]。在其他疾病（如淀粉样变性、餐后腹泻、IBS）中，怀疑存在肠神经系统功能障碍，但未得到证实[10,37,40,41]。许多内分泌性腹泻，如由肽分泌性肿瘤或甲状腺功能亢进引起的腹泻，可能不仅通过影响肠道电解质转运，还可能通过加速肠道运动而导致腹泻[42]。

肠道转运缓慢可能通过促进小肠细菌过度生长（SIBO）导致分泌性腹泻[43-45]。小肠中过量的细菌破坏消化，并可能改变电解质的转运。与该机制相关的腹泻的最佳记录示例是硬皮病（系统性硬化症）。虽然糖尿病常被怀疑是通过慢传输和淤滞引起腹泻，如硬皮病，但这种病理生理机制并不总是成立的（见第105章）[46,47]。结肠假性肠梗阻患者由于结肠钾的主动分泌，有时会出现分泌性腹泻，可能与自主神经或肠神经功能障碍有关（见第124章）[48]。

由于缺乏必要的工具来测量肠运动、推动力和转运时间之间的相互作用，对肠运动在腹泻病原体发生中的作用的评价受到限制。除肠道灌流研究消除了运动对电解质转运的影响外，尚无方法可以分离肠道转运和运动对净吸收的影响[11]。因此，对于运动过多或过少是否会引起腹泻，以及管腔因素如何改变肠平滑肌功能，尚未达成共识。

肠道血流量减少在腹泻中具有重要但尚不明确的作用。目前尚不清楚肠系膜缺血是否对吸收有直接影响，或者低血流量是否会引起继发性反应（例如，通过细胞因子或神经递质）从而影响液体转运并产生分泌性腹泻。放射性肠炎也会产生与持续性腹泻相关的肠道微循环异常，可能难以治疗（见第41和118章）。

（三）复合性腹泻

虽然将腹泻分为渗透性或分泌性可能对考虑腹泻的病理生理学有指导意义，但单纯分泌性或纯粹渗透性腹泻的病例并不常见。临床上大多数重要的腹泻在病理生理机制方面是复杂的，涉及多种发病机制。原因可能包括肠内分泌细胞释放的物质、局部和远程免疫反应细胞释放的细胞因子、肠神经系统的活性以及外周释放的肽和激素［自分泌、肠腔、旁分泌、免疫、神经和内分泌系统（见第4章）］的影响。上皮细胞和管腔内容物（包括细菌、营养物质和矿物质）之间发生显著的串扰越来越明显[49,50]。

对腹泻的进一步理解是认识到某些介质不仅影响上皮或肌肉功能，而且相互影响。肠神经可刺激肥大细胞，肥大细胞释放的产物（特别是组胺）可改变肠神经元功能[51]。像前列腺素这样的单一激动剂可能对上皮功能、肌肉收缩和细胞旁途径有多重同时作用，从而导致对离子转运、肠运动和黏膜通透性的影响[52]。因此，许多调节剂和效应器有助于最终的临床表现。充分了解腹泻的病理生理学，需要考虑一个被称为ALPINES（autocrine，luminal，paracrine，immune，neural，and endocrine systems，自分泌、肠腔、旁分泌、免疫、神经和内分泌系统）的调节系统（图16.2）。

体现腹泻综合征病理生理学复杂性的例子是霍乱，经常被引用为单纯分泌性腹泻的范例。霍乱毒素以肠上皮细胞为靶点，增加第二信使cAMP，cAMP开放顶端氯通道，刺激氯化物分泌，导致腹泻。然而，霍乱诱发腹泻的实际机制要复杂得多[53]。霍乱毒素刺激内分泌细胞和神经成分，加强其对肠细胞的直接分泌作用[54]。此外，霍乱毒素引起肠道运动的明显变化。霍乱弧菌产生的其他毒素靶向紧密连接，从而改变黏膜通透性（图16.3）（见第110章）[55]。

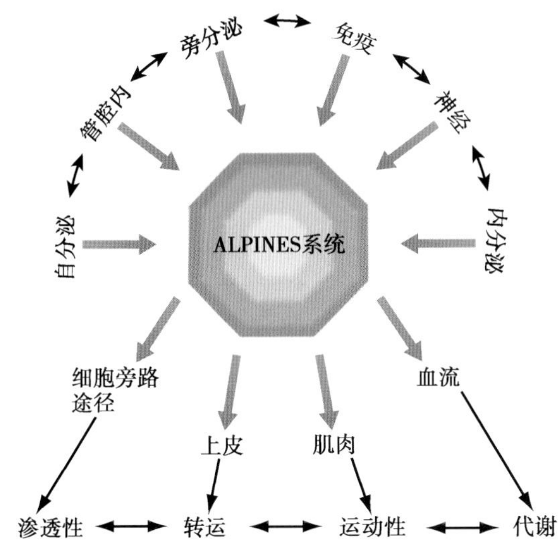

图16.2　肠道ALPINES调节系统。肠道的调节系统整合了自分泌、肠腔、旁分泌、免疫、神经和内分泌系统（ALPINES），并产生黏膜和肌肉功能的协调变化，允许对不断变化的条件作出适应性反应。调节系统可扩大或者缩小细胞旁途径，以控制电解质的被动跨膜转运，通过影响膜通道和泵加速或延缓营养物质和电解质的经上皮转运，通过松弛或收缩肠道中的各种肌肉层来改变肠运动，并增加或减少黏膜血流量，从而影响肠道代谢。腹泻可能是对急性感染的适当反应。不适应性反应可能是慢性腹泻的原因。（Modified from Sellin JH. Functional anatomy, fluid and electrolyte absorption. In: Feldman M, Schiller LR, editors. Gastroenterology and hepatology. The comprehensive visual reference, vol 7: Small intestine. Philadelphia: Current medicine; 1997. p 1. 11.）

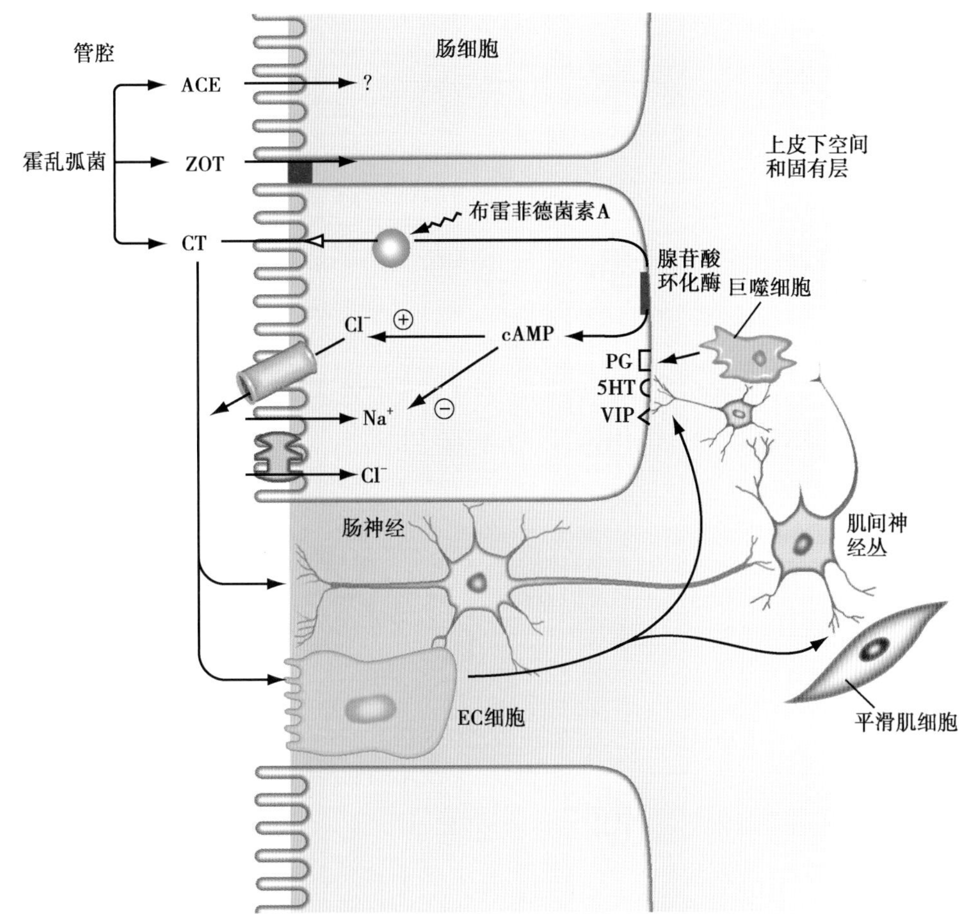

图16.3　霍乱的病理生理学。霍乱弧菌产生几种毒素，这些毒素与肠上细胞中的腺苷酸环化酶和肠道调节系统的几种成分相互作用，包括肠神经和肠嗜铬（EC）细胞，产生分泌状态和大量腹泻。除经典的肠毒素——霍乱毒素（CT）外，该菌还产生闭锁带毒素（ZOT），使肠细胞与副霍乱肠毒素（ACE）紧密连接的通透性增加，后者对肠细胞的作用尚不清楚。除CT反应下腺苷酸环化酶产生的环磷酸腺苷（cAMP）外，分泌刺激包括巨噬细胞、EC细胞和肠神经元释放的前列腺素（PG）、5-羟色胺（5-HT）和血管活性肠多肽（VIP）。在布雷菲德菌素A抑制CT跨细胞转运至基底侧膜的实验中，CT显示可激活细胞基底侧膜上的腺苷酸环化酶（锯齿状箭头）。（From Sellin JH. Functional anatomy, fluid and electrolyte absorption. In: Feldman M, Schiller LR, editors. Gastroenterology and hepatology. The comprehensive visual reference, vol 7: Small intestine. Philadelphia: Current medicine; 1997. p 1. 14.）

ALPINES 失调的另一个例子是 IBD[56]。IBD 患者的腹泻不仅仅涉及黏膜破坏导致的腔内渗出。完整的肠细胞被肠道中免疫细胞释放的多种促分泌素和可能影响肠细胞功能的细菌毒素所阻断。尽管 IBD 中腹泻的初始模型表明，氯化物分泌驱动的体液转运改变，但随后的研究表明，IBD 中的腹泻是由钠通道和泵下调相关的抗吸收作用介导的[57-59]。如果我们考虑管腔细菌的作用，IBD 腹泻的病理生理学机制更加复杂。细菌蛋白(如，鞭毛蛋白)可刺激细胞因子如白细胞介素8(IL-8)的产生，从而进一步吸引炎性细胞[60]。细胞因子和免疫细胞也可能直接影响紧密连接屏障功能和肠细胞分泌和吸收途径[61-64]。相反，上皮细胞可分泌细胞因子，如 IL-6，增强多形核白细胞(中性粒细胞)的功能[65]。炎症也可以引起肠运动的显著变化(见第 115 章)。

肠易激综合征(IBS)是病理生理学复杂的疾病的又一个例子。一系列因素，如运动改变[10]、胆汁酸吸收不良[66]、直肠储备能力受损[67]，可能加重 IBS 患者的症状。在更基础的水平上，肥大细胞或肠嗜铬细胞数量、5-羟色胺含量以及 5-羟色胺再摄取和转运的改变可能导致腹泻的发生(见第 122 章)[68-70]。

在吸收不良综合征和功能性疾病中也可观察到复杂的病理生理学，尤其是通过快速转运为特征的疾病。不吸收碳水化合物可能导致渗透性腹泻，但不吸收长链脂肪酸可能通过损害结肠对电解质的吸收而使问题复杂化[15,71]。常见的餐后功能性腹泻可能涉及运动和转运功能之间的相互作用。食物过敏引起的腹泻还涉及调节血管通透性、电解质转运和运动的免疫、旁分泌和神经机制的激活[72](见第 10 和 104 章)。

三、临床分类

腹泻可通过以下几种方式分类：时程(急性和慢性)、容量(大量和小量)、病理生理学(分泌性和渗透性)、粪便特征(水样和脂肪性和炎症性)和流行病学[7]。对于临床医生来说，分类只有在描述特定患者的诊断和管理方法时才有用。就这方面而言，没有一种分类方案是完美的，有经验的医生使用所有这些分类来帮助患者的治疗。

(一) 急性腹泻与慢性腹泻

腹泻的时间进程有助于指导治疗。急性腹泻(<4 周)通常由感染引起，通常是自限性的或容易治疗的[73]。最常见的细菌和病毒引起的腹泻在 7 天内走完其历程。如果急性腹泻发作持续超过 7 天，则原虫引起的可能性更大，如贾第鞭毛虫病或隐孢子虫病[74]。尽管很少有感染因子(如气单胞菌、耶尔森菌属)引起免疫功能低下者发生长期腹泻，但慢性腹泻通常不是由感染因子引起的。因此，当面对慢性腹泻患者时，临床医生必须首先考虑非感染性原因。

(二) 大容量腹泻与小容量腹泻

通过个体粪便量(而不是每日总排便量)来区分腹泻原因的前提是，正常的直肠、乙状结肠作为储存库发挥作用。当累及左半结肠的炎症或运动障碍损害了储存的容量时，即会出现频繁的小容量排便。如果腹泻源在右半结肠或小肠，如果直肠、乙状结肠储存库功能完整，则个体排便频率更低且量更大。频繁的、小的、疼痛性粪便可能指向结肠远端病理部位，而无痛性大容量粪便提示右侧结肠或小肠来源。尽管患者难以准确定量粪便容量，但区别小容量和大容量粪便可以指导进一步的诊断研究。

每日总排便量也可提示有关病因。肠易激综合征患者 24 小时粪便重量正常或略有增加，而其他原因的腹泻可能产生更大的粪便重量。粪便重量有时可以通过患者的病史来估计，腹泻导致脱水(在没有呕吐或口服摄入有限的情况下)的患者通常粪便重量超过 1 000g，并且不太可能患有 IBS。

(三) 渗透性腹泻与分泌性腹泻

区分因肠道吸收不良摄入的非电解质引起的腹泻(渗透性腹泻)与因吸收不良或分泌电解质引起的腹泻(分泌性腹泻)，有助于区分少量渗透性腹泻和大量分泌性腹泻。这种区分基于粪便电解质浓度的测量和粪便渗透间隙的计算[13]。在分泌性腹泻中，粪便渗透压几乎完全由钠、钾和伴随的阴离子维持，在渗透性腹泻中，肠腔内吸收不良的溶质占粪便水渗透活性的大部分(见下文)。虽然在合理的病理生理学基础上，这种区分的临床价值尚未得到前瞻性证实。

(四) 水样泻、脂肪泻与炎性腹泻

通过简单的粪便检查，将粪便特征定性为水样、脂肪性或炎性。可以通过限制鉴别诊断中必须考虑的疾病数量来加速对慢性腹泻患者的评估[7]。水样腹泻意味着分泌性或渗透性腹泻。脂肪性腹泻意味着小肠对脂肪和其他营养物质的吸收缺陷。炎性腹泻意味着存在累及胃肠道的有限数量的炎性或肿瘤性疾病之一。

(五) 流行病学特征

缩小鉴别诊断范围最有用的临床方法之一是将腹泻与其环境联系起来。例如，来自尼泊尔的"足球妈妈"和背包客可能有相同的腹泻原因，但更可能有不同的病因。应该考虑的一些常见临床情况和诊断见框 16.1。

框 16.1　定义明确的患者组或环境引起腹泻的可能原因
旅行者
细菌感染(大部分是急性的)
原虫感染(如阿米巴、贾第鞭毛虫)
热带口炎性腹泻
流行性和爆发性
细菌感染
流行性特发性分泌性腹泻(如 Brainerd 腹泻)
寄生虫感染(如隐孢子虫病)
病毒感染(如轮状病毒、COVID-19*)
糖尿病患者
动力障碍(增强或者减弱)
伴随疾病
乳糜泻
胰腺外分泌功能不全
SIBO
药物副作用(尤其是阿卡波糖和二甲双胍)
艾滋病患者
药物副作用
淋巴瘤
机会性感染(如隐孢子虫病、巨细胞病毒、单疱病毒、结核分枝杆菌)
住院患者和院内感染
艰难梭状菌介导肠炎
药物副作用
粪块嵌塞所致流水样腹泻
缺血性结肠炎
管饲
*新型冠状病毒。 SIBO，小肠细菌过度生长。

四、鉴别诊断

许多胃肠道和全身性疾病都可表现为腹泻。为了便于鉴别诊断，临床医生应首先应将腹泻病分为急性腹泻或慢性腹泻，然后根据粪便特征水样腹泻、炎性腹泻和脂肪性腹泻进行亚分类（框 16.2）。

框 16.2 腹泻的鉴别诊断

急性腹泻
- 感染（见框 16.3）
  - 细菌
  - 寄生虫
  - 原虫
  - 病毒
- 食物过敏
- 食物中毒
- 药物
- 慢性腹泻的起始阶段

慢性腹泻

水样泻
- 渗透性腹泻
  - 吸收不良综合征
  - 渗透性泻药（如 Mg^{2+}、PO_4^{3-}、SO_4^{2-}）
- 分泌性腹泻
  - 细菌毒素
  - 先天性综合征（先天性氯化物性腹泻）
  - 动力障碍、调控失调
    - 糖尿病自主神经病变
    - 肠易激综合征
    - 交感神经切除术后腹泻
    - 迷走神经切断术后腹泻
  - 憩室炎
  - 内分泌性疾病
    - 艾迪生病
    - 类癌综合征
    - 胃泌素瘤
    - 甲状腺功能亢进
    - 肥大细胞增多症
    - 甲状腺髓样癌
    - 嗜铬细胞瘤
    - 生长激素瘤
    - 血管活性肠肽瘤
  - 特发性分泌性腹泻
    - 流行性特发性分泌性腹泻
    - 散发性特发性分泌性腹泻
  - 回肠胆汁酸吸收不良
  - 炎症性肠病
    - 克罗恩病
    - 溃疡性结肠炎
  - 泻药滥用（刺激性泻药）
  - 药物和毒物（见框 16.4）
  - 显微镜下结肠炎
    - 胶原性结肠炎
    - 淋巴细胞性结肠炎
  - 肿瘤
    - 结肠癌
    - 淋巴瘤
    - 直肠绒毛状腺瘤
  - 血管炎

脂肪泻
- 吸收不良综合征
  - 肠系膜缺血
  - 肠黏膜疾病（如乳糜泻、惠普尔病）
  - 短肠综合征
  - SIBO
- 消化不良
  - 胆汁酸浓度不足
  - 胰腺外分泌功能不全

炎症性腹泻
- 憩室炎
- 感染性疾病
  - 侵入性细菌感染（如结核病、耶尔森菌病）
  - 侵入性寄生虫感染（如阿米巴虫病、圆线虫病）
  - 伪膜性结肠炎（艰难梭菌感染）
  - 溃疡性病毒感染（如巨细胞病毒、HSV）
- 炎症性肠病
  - 克罗恩病
  - 溃疡性结肠炎
  - 溃疡性空肠回肠炎
- 缺血性结肠炎
- 肿瘤
  - 结肠癌
  - 淋巴瘤
- 放射性结肠炎

SIBO，小肠细菌过度生长。

急性腹泻定义为持续时间少于 4 周，尽管许多病例持续少于 4 天[73]。常见的病因是细菌、病毒、原虫或多细胞寄生虫的感染（框 16.3）。急性腹泻也可由食物中毒、食物过敏和药物引起。导致慢性腹泻的疾病也可能表现为急性发作，因此当急性腹泻变得持续时，应考虑到慢性腹泻的急性发作。

慢性水样腹泻可能是由于摄入吸收不良的渗透活性物质（渗透性腹泻）引起的，或者更常见的是引起分泌性腹泻的情况。摄入有限数量的渗透剂中的任何一种，如镁盐、磷酸盐、硫酸盐泻药或吸收不良的碳水化合物，均可引起渗透性腹泻。相反，慢性分泌性腹泻，电解质吸收不良导致液体潴留在肠腔内，与许多临床状况相关（见框 16.2）。

尽管 IBD 通常产生以脓血便为特征的腹泻，但其他无溃疡的炎症性疾病（例如，显微镜下结肠炎）可引起具有慢性分泌性腹泻特征的腹泻。在这种情况下，腹泻是由细胞因子分泌和其他炎症介质的分泌介导的（见第 128 章）。

药物或毒物的摄入也可引起慢性水样泻（框 16.4）[75-79]。将药物确定为腹泻的原因，有赖于认识到开始摄入药物和腹泻的发作是同时发生的，但这样的时间相关性并不总是容易识别的，需要详细、仔细地询问病史。药物性腹泻的病理生理机制复杂，尚未得到很好的研究。一些药物可能激活特异性

框 16.3 引起腹泻的感染源
细菌
气单胞菌属
弯曲菌属
艰难梭菌
大肠埃希菌(产毒素的、侵入性的、出血性的)
邻单胞菌属
沙门菌属
志贺杆菌
耶尔森菌
病毒
腺病毒
诺如病毒
轮状病毒
寄生虫、原虫和真菌
隐孢子虫
环孢子虫
溶组织内阿米巴
贾第鞭毛虫
小孢子虫

框 16.4 与腹泻相关的药物和毒素
降酸剂(如 H_2 受体阻滞剂、质子泵抑制剂)
抗酸剂(如含镁的药物)
抗心律失常药(如奎尼丁)
抗生素(大部分)
抗炎药(如 5-氨基水杨酸、金盐、依克珠单抗、非甾体抗炎药)
降压药(如 β 肾上腺素受体阻滞剂、奥美沙坦)
抗肿瘤药物(许多)免疫检查点抑制剂(如纳武单抗、派姆单抗)
抗逆转录病毒药物
秋水仙碱
重金属
草药
前列腺素类似物(如米索前列醇)
茶碱
维生素和矿物质补充剂

受体和转运蛋白,例如,咖啡因与茶碱一样,可能增加细胞内 cAMP 活性和液体分泌,临床上可见所谓的“星巴克腹泻”病例。红霉素与胃动素受体相互作用,从而刺激胃肠道的推进性运动活动。其他抗生素可能改变结肠中的菌群,导致吸收不良的碳水化合物的结肠补救受损或产毒素艰难梭菌的过度生长。一些药物(如可卡因)可能会干扰肠道的血流。化疗药物与高频率的腹泻相关,这可能是由于肠上皮细胞增殖和凋亡之间的微妙平衡被破坏,导致所谓的凋亡性肠病(见第 36 章)。一组不同的药物(如阿司匹林、吗替麦考酚酯、金制剂)可激发肠道的炎症过程,也可能引起腹泻。奥美沙坦可引起口炎性腹泻样肠病(见第 107 章)[79]。在秘密滥用泻药的患者中,检测药物性腹泻的问题更加困难,这些患者故意隐瞒关于其问题原因的重要信息(见下文)[75]。

另一类慢性水样腹泻涉及肠动力障碍或肠道功能失调。迷走神经切断术后腹泻、交感神经切除术后腹泻、糖尿病自主神经病变、淀粉样变性和以腹泻为主的 IBS 等问题均属于这一类。在这些情况下,腹泻具有继发于原发性电解质转运失调或动力改变的分泌性腹泻的特征,动力可加速肠腔液体通过肠道的吸收部位(见第 37、53 和 122 章)。

水样腹泻的另一大类是内分泌功能失调引起的腹泻。相对常见的内分泌紊乱,如甲状腺功能亢进和艾迪生病(Addison 病),可并发慢性分泌性腹泻。更罕见的内分泌肿瘤也会引起腹泻,通常是通过改变电解质吸收或加速肠道转运。这些肿瘤的罕见性使得发现这些疾病的预测试概率低,尤其是在没有肝转移的情况下,因此筛查结果通常为假阳性(见后文及第 34 和 37 章)。

其他肿瘤通过阻塞肠管、阻断淋巴引流、干扰吸收或引起电解质分泌而引起水样腹泻。这种情况的例子包括结肠癌(肠梗阻)、淋巴瘤(小肠和肠系膜淋巴管阻塞)和直肠绒毛状腺瘤(大量富含钾的胶状液体分泌到肠腔内)。而在结肠近端发现的绒毛状腺瘤很少引起这种类型的腹泻(见第 32、126 和 127 章)。

慢性水样腹泻的最后一类是特发性分泌性腹泻,该规则包括两种情况:流行性分泌性腹泻(也称为 Brainerd 腹泻)和散发性特发性分泌性腹泻。这两种疾病都是长期的,但是自限性的[80,81]。

慢性炎症性腹泻是一组不同的感染性或特发性炎症和肿瘤过程。粪便特征是存在黏液和脓液,通常与黏膜溃疡有关。特发性 IBD,包括溃疡性结肠炎(UC)和克罗恩病,通常会产生此类粪便。较少见的是其他炎症性疾病,如憩室炎或溃疡性空肠炎可能与便血或脓液相关,侵袭性或溃疡性感染性疾病也是如此。引起慢性炎症性腹泻的感染包括细菌感染(如结核、耶尔森氏菌病、艰难梭菌相关性结肠炎),溃疡型病毒感染(如巨细胞病毒、单纯疱疹病毒)和侵袭性寄生虫感染(如类圆线虫病)。在免疫功能低下者中,应考虑更广泛的感染原[82]。引起慢性炎症性腹泻的非感染性疾病包括缺血性结肠炎和并发黏膜溃疡的肿瘤(如结肠癌、淋巴瘤)(见第 32、110~115、118、119、121 和 127 章)。

慢性脂肪性腹泻是由吸收不良或消化障碍引起的。由黏膜疾病引起的吸收不良综合征——最常见的是乳糜泻,但也有罕见的疾病,如惠普尔病(Whipple 病)——通常会引起脂肪性腹泻。短肠综合征或切除术后腹泻也可出现这种模式,但如果切除相对有限,腹泻可能是继发于营养或胆汁酸吸收不良的水样泻。SIBO 通过胆汁酸早期解离引起脂肪泻。肠系膜缺血可损害肠道对脂肪的吸收,但体重减轻主要是由于继发于餐后疼痛的畏食(“进食恐惧”)。胰腺外分泌功能不全或十二指肠胆汁酸浓度不足所致的消化不良可产生脂肪泻。虽然有脂肪,但在消化不良的情况下,粪便可能不是很松散的,因为在没有脂肪消化的情况下,甘油三酯保持完整,对结肠电解质的吸收影响不大。相比之下,正常消化情况下的吸收不良可能会导致大量腹泻,因为结肠中的游离脂肪酸具有导泻作用(见第 59、104~109 和 118 章)[83]。

五、评估

(一)病史

仔细采集病史对于评价腹泻患者至关重要。框 16.5 中提供了病史检查表。一个基本特征是症状持续时间。急性腹泻患者(病程<4 周)应与慢性腹泻患者相区别,后者的鉴别诊断要广泛得多。应确定腹泻的严重程度。排便频率是患者腹泻最容易定义的特征,但不一定与粪便重量相关。一些人经常排出少量粪便,但另一些人排便频率较低,量却较多。患者对粪便量的概念较差,但口干、口渴加剧、尿量减少和无力等症状提示大量排便导致脱水。急性体重减重也是严重程度的良好标志。慢性体重减轻可能提示肠道吸收不良或严重的疾病过程,如恶性肿瘤、IBD 或甲状腺功能亢进症。

框 16.5 腹泻患者的病史特征
持续时间:急性期小于 4 周、慢性期大于 4 周
起病情况:先天性、突发性、渐进性
类型:持续性,间歇性
流行病学特征(见框 16.1)
诱发因素:药物(见框 16.4)、放疗、手术
人为性腹泻(见表 16.7)
系统性疾病:内分泌,胶原血管病,肿瘤性,自身免疫性
粪便性状:水样便,血便,脂肪便
粪便失禁:有,无
腹痛:部位,与进食和排便的关系,加重及缓解的因素
体重下降
加重因素:饮食,应激
缓解因素:饮食,非处方药,处方药
既往评估情况

粪便特征也很重要。粪便中的血液提示恶性肿瘤或 IBD 的可能性,尽管这通常是由频繁排便患者的痔疮引起的。在急性感染性腹泻患者中,粪便中可见的血液对诊断侵袭性微生物感染具有高度特异性[84]。水样便提示存在渗透或分泌过程,油脂或食物颗粒的存在提示吸收不良、消化障碍或肠急促。漂浮粪便的现象通常代表气体含量的增加,而不是粪便的脂肪含量增加。医生还应询问排便与进餐或禁食的关系、白天与夜间的排便情况以及是否存在排便紧迫感或失禁。急迫性和大便失禁并不提示大量腹泻,但提示直肠顺应性或调节控便的肌肉存在问题。唤醒患者睡眠的夜间腹泻强烈提示器质性而非功能性疾病,如 IBS。还应注意其他共存症状,如腹痛、胃肠胀气、腹胀或气胀、痉挛、发热和体重减轻。过度胃肠胀气或腹胀表明,由于摄入吸收不良的碳水化合物或小肠对碳水化合物吸收不良,结肠细菌增加对碳水化合物的发酵所致。

由于腹泻的医源性原因(如药物、既往手术史、放疗治疗)很常见,医疗保健提供者应了解既往腹部手术史以及处方药和非处方药摄入史,包括营养和草药治疗。

特定的食物和饮食通常被认为是腹泻的原因,一些有很好的证据,另一些则较少[85,86]。因此,详细的饮食史非常重要,尤其是在慢性腹泻患者中。患者经常担心饮食是否会促发或加重症状[87]。在评估这些与食物的相关性时,必须考虑以下因素:①摄入过量的能引起正常肠道发生腹泻的物质(例如果糖);②由于基础疾病引起腹泻的食物(如乳糖酶缺乏的乳制品);③限制营养物质消化或吸收的胃肠道疾病(如短肠综合征,胰腺外分泌功能不全);④特异性食物不耐受;⑤真正的食物过敏。

记录摄入食物的时间、数量以及症状发作的饮食日记,可有助于确定腹泻的饮食原因。症状通常在摄入后数小时出现,可因食物类型和同时摄入的吸收不良的碳水化合物总量而异(见后文)。还应寻找流行病学线索(见框 16.1)。最近的国外旅行,特别是去不发达国家的旅行,有助于诊断旅行者腹泻。商业全球化增加了那些没有明显暴露的人群中曾经外来感染的频率[88]。医生还应考虑患者是否生活在农村或城市环境中,患者饮用水的来源,以及患者的职业、性取向和酒精或违禁药物的使用情况。从疾病中获得的间接收益或尝试减肥和注视身体形象的病史,应多考虑滥用泻药的可能性(见后文)。

患者的病史对于鉴别 IBS 患者与其他引起腹泻的功能性疾病或器质性疾病至关重要。目前 IBS 的定义强调了与排便变化(频率或一致性)相关的腹痛的存在[89],罗马Ⅳ共识委员会不再将腹部不适作为 IBS 的诊断标准,IBS 患者必须报告实际的疼痛。提示诊断 IBS 的其他附加因素包括长期病史,通常可追溯到青春期或青年期、黏液排出和应激导致的症状加重。这些特征可识别不太可能患有结构性胃肠道疾病的患者,如克罗恩病或癌症。反对 IBS 诊断和支持进一步诊断测试的因素包括:最近发生的腹泻,尤其是在老年患者中,使患者从睡眠中醒来的腹泻,体重减轻,大便中有血,粪便重量每日超过 400~500g。异常的实验室检查结果,如低血红蛋白水平、低血清白蛋白浓度、高红细胞沉降率或高粪便钙卫蛋白浓度也不支持 IBS 的诊断(见第 122 章)。并非所有“腹痛和腹泻”患者均患有 IBS,细致入微的病史有助于识别食物或碳水化合物不耐受(饮食和症状日记,显著腹胀和胀气)、SIBO(腹胀或胀气)、胆汁酸腹泻(可能主要在早晨引起腹泻)和医源性腹泻(潜在致病药物的使用、手术或放射治疗史)患者。在已发表的研究文献或临床中并不总是考虑这些细微的差别。

(二) 体格检查

体格检查结果通常在确定腹泻的严重程度方面比确定其病因更有用。可以通过观察血压和脉搏的立位变化来评估患者的容量状态。应记录发热和其他中毒性体征。仔细的腹部检查很重要,特别注意有无肠鸣音变化、腹胀、局部或全身压痛、肿块和肝脏肿大。在罕见情况下,体格检查可提供腹泻原因的更直接证据。表 16.2 列出了应寻找的特征性体格检查结果。

(三) 急性腹泻

大多数急性腹泻病例是由感染性疾病引起,病程有限(数天至数周),不需要医生干预,除非患者免疫系统受损或出现血容量不足并发症或其他重度中毒性证据,包括无法摄入液体、频繁呕吐、衰弱、肌肉或关节痛[73]。当出现这些并发症或腹泻持续数天以上时,需要进行更全面的评估。应进行全血细胞计数(CBC),以检查贫血、血液浓缩或白细胞计数异常。病毒性腹泻患者通常 WBC 和分类计数正常或淋巴细胞增多,但细菌感染患者——尤其是由侵入肠黏膜的微生物引起的感染——白细胞增多、伴过多的不成熟的 WBC。然而,沙门菌感染患者可发中性粒细胞减少。血清电解质浓度、血

表 16.2 体检结果对慢性腹泻患者的潜在影响

发现	潜在意义
直立性低血压	脱水,神经病变
肌肉萎缩,水肿	营养不良
色素性荨麻疹,皮肤划痕症	肥大细胞性疾病(肥大细胞增多症)
紫癜,巨舌	淀粉样变
色素沉着	艾迪生病
迁徙坏死性红斑	胰高血糖素瘤
面色潮红	类癌综合征
恶性萎缩性丘疹病	德戈斯综合征
疱疹样皮炎	乳糜泻
甲状腺结节,淋巴结病	甲状腺髓样癌
震颤,眼睑下垂	甲状腺功能亢进症
眼肌痉挛,心律失常	惠普尔病
右侧心脏杂音,喘息	类癌综合征
肝脏肿大	内分泌肿瘤,淀粉样变
腹部杂音	慢性肠系膜缺血
关节炎	炎症性肠病,耶尔森菌病,惠普尔病
淋巴结病	HIV 感染,淋巴瘤,癌
肛门括约肌功能不良	大便失禁

From Schiller LR, Pardi DS, Spiller R, et al. Gastro 2013 APDW/WCOG Shanghai Working Party Report. Chronic diarrhea: defnition, classifcation, diagnosis. J Gastroenterol Hepatol. 2014;29:6-25.

尿素氮和血清肌酐水平测量,可用于评估液体和电解质耗竭的程度及其对肾功能的影响。

应检查粪便样本的 WBC,以识别炎性腹泻[90]。检测粪便中 WBC 的传统方法是瑞氏染色显微镜检查。检测的准确性取决于样本的新鲜度以及检测者的经验和技能,假阳性和假阴性结果很常见。中性粒细胞的产物——钙卫蛋白和乳铁蛋白检测,对于检测粪便中的中性粒细胞具有敏感性和特异性,是显微镜检查的有用替代方法[91-93]。传统的腹泻微生物学检测方法包括常规细菌培养、粪便虫卵和寄生虫显微镜检查以及(罕见)病毒培养。这些补充了贾第鞭毛虫病和隐孢子虫病的酶联免疫吸附试验,比显微镜更准确[94]。这种诊断策略正被用于常见腹泻病原体的非培养多重聚合酶链反应(PCR)检测所取代,该技术比传统方法更快捷、更全面,而且更经济[95,96]。应在有中毒症状的患者、因腹泻入院的患者和持续性急性腹泻(持续超过 7 天)的患者中进行病原体检测(见第 110 和 113 章)。

在医院发生腹泻的患者不太可能发生常规细菌或原虫的感染,但与门诊患者相比,更可能发生艰难梭菌感染。随着社区获得性艰难梭菌感染的增加,即使无既往抗生素使用史,也应始终考虑这种可治疗的急性腹泻原因(见第 112 章)。

应对出现中毒症状的患者进行腹部 X 线检查,以评估是否存在结肠炎和肠梗阻或巨结肠。对于有明显中毒症状、大便带血或持续急性腹泻的患者,也应考虑直肠镜或软式乙状结肠镜检查。乙状结肠镜检查可能足以作为此类重度急性腹泻患者的早期检查。在 AIDS 相关性腹泻患者中,首选结肠镜检查,因为相当大比例的感染和淋巴瘤可能仅存在于右半结肠[97],尽管这种方法受到质疑(见第 35 章)[98]。如果做乙状结肠镜检查或结肠镜检查,即使黏膜没有明显的炎症,也应获得黏膜活检标本,病理检查可以提供重要线索,以助于特异性诊断[99]。相比之下,对外观正常的回肠末端进行活检通常没有帮助。评估急性腹泻患者的检查表见表 16.3。

表 16.3 基于急性腹泻患者表现的临床处理

临床表现	对症处理
无中毒症状	对症治疗,补液疗法
中毒症状	补充液体和电解质 全血细胞计数 血清电解质、血清尿素氮、血清肌酐 粪便检查:培养(如果粪便白细胞阳性),寄生虫卵检查,贾第鞭毛虫和隐孢子虫抗原,艰难梭菌检测和(或)多重 PCR 检测 结肠镜或乙状结肠镜

PCR,聚合酶链反应。

(四) 慢性腹泻

由于慢性腹泻的鉴别诊断比急性腹泻更广泛,因此评估更复杂[3,7,28,100-102]。临床医师首先应重新评估组织学和任何以前的评估,然后考虑 5 种可能性:①伪装成慢性腹泻的大便失禁;②药物、手术或放射治疗引起的医源性腹泻;③慢性感染;④肠易激综合征伴腹泻;⑤功能性腹泻(无疼痛的粪便松散、无证实的结构或生化异常)。应通过仔细的病史采集和直肠指诊排除第一种可能性。第二种可能性可以通过审查患者的用药物列表和病史来评估。第三种可能性需要通过传统检测或多重 PCR 检测来寻找粪便病原体(见前文)。第四种和第五种可能性——IBS 伴腹泻和功能性腹泻——由已发表的标准定义。如果患者符合标准且无报警特征,则不太可能患有结构性疾病,但可能存在以下 3 种可治疗疾病之一:食物不耐受、胆汁酸腹泻或 SIBO[102]。通过消除饮食、胆汁酸结合剂(如考来烯胺)或抗生素的新兴诊断试验或治疗试验可确定这些问题(见下文)。

如果诊断不能确定,或者腹泻严重、复杂、持续或难以治疗,则下一级评价包括基本的实验室检查、影像学和结肠镜检查。此时评价中推荐的实验室检查见框 16.6。这些检查侧重于鉴别并发的特征,如贫血或低蛋白血症、全身性疾病、乳糜泻、炎症性疾病和脂肪泻。炎症性腹泻的检测包括血清 C 反应蛋白、粪便钙卫蛋白或乳铁蛋白。一项系统性综述表明,炎性相关腹泻的检测包括 C 反应蛋白水平和粪便钙卫蛋白或乳铁蛋白水平。一项系统性综述报道,C 反应蛋白检测炎症相关腹泻的总敏感性为 49%,特异性为 73%,而粪便钙卫蛋白鉴定这种疾病的总敏感性为 92%,特异性为 82%[103]。粪便乳铁蛋白检测鉴定出炎症相关腹泻,总敏感性为 88%,特异性为 79%[103]。脂肪泻可通过使用苏丹红染色显微镜下估计粪便脂肪来检测，该染色可识别脂肪性腹泻患者，敏感性为 76%，特异性为 99%[103]。通过脂肪球的计数和大小的测量，可将检测的敏感性提高到 94%，特异度提高到 95%，与定量脂肪排泄量有很好的相关性[104]。

框 16.6 慢性腹泻患者需要考虑的基本实验室检查
血液检查
全血细胞计数
代谢功能检查
IgA 抗组织转谷氨酰胺酶抗体和总 IgA 测定
c-反应蛋白
粪便检查
粪便潜血试验
粪便白细胞（瑞氏染色）或粪便钙卫蛋白或乳铁蛋白
细菌培养、寄生虫卵检查、贾第鞭毛虫和隐孢子虫抗原或多重 PCR 检测
粪便脂肪定性或定量检测
PCR，聚合酶链反应。

大多数在评价中达到这一点而未确诊的慢性腹泻患者，将需要结肠镜检查（和回肠镜检查）加活检和腹部成像加 CT 或 MRI 加肠造影。这些检查可以识别或排除 IBD、缺血性肠病、胃肠道癌症、胰腺疾病或肿瘤。结肠镜检查的诊断率最高，在高达 30% 因慢性腹泻转诊的患者中得到诊断[105]。即使未见黏膜病变，也应在结肠的几个位置进行随机活检，使病理学家有最佳的机会作出诊断[106,107]。结肠黏膜在内镜下表现正常但在组织学上可以诊断的疾病包括，显微镜下结肠炎［淋巴细胞性和胶原性结肠炎（见后文）］、淀粉样变性、肉芽肿性感染和血吸虫病（见第 37、114 和 128 章）。

尽管食管胃十二指肠内镜（EGD）通常作为慢性腹泻评估的一部分进行，但在缺乏乳糜泻或脂肪泻标志物的情况下，尚无研究记录其诊断率。通过 EGD 或肠镜检查对小肠黏膜进行可视化和活检可能很有价值，但推进式肠镜检查在评价弥漫性小肠疾病的标准 EGD 中是否增加了很多尚不确定[108]。小肠活检可检出的疾病包括乳糜泻、克罗恩病、贾第鞭毛虫病、肠道淋巴瘤、嗜酸细胞性胃肠炎、热带口炎性腹泻、惠普尔病、淋巴管扩张、无 β 脂蛋白血症、淀粉样变性、肥大细胞增多症和各种感染过程（见第 30～32、37、104、107～110 和 112～115 章）。无线胶囊式内镜对小肠疾病引起的腹泻在诊断中的作用存在争议。一个回顾性综述显示胶囊内镜阳性诊断率为 42.9%，但大多数结果的重要性尚不确定[109]。便血和低白蛋白血症与较高的诊断率有关[109]，可通过深肠镜检查和活检评价结果（见第 20 章）。除非怀疑克罗恩病，否则胶囊式内镜使用指南不建议使用该技术评价慢性腹泻[110]。

如果此时评价中还没有明显诊断，则可进一步使用粪便的化学分析，将腹泻分类为水样、炎性或脂肪性，从而限制鉴别诊断中考虑的疾病数量。可对随机样本或定时（即 24、48 或 72 小时）采集的粪便进行粪便分析。分析定时采集的价值在于可以准确测量粪便重量，以及粪便组分（如脂肪）的排出量。每日粪便重量可能是腹泻对水合作用潜在影响的最佳线索。然而，在没有定时采集的情况下，随机或“点”采集的其他粪便特征评估，仍为正确诊断提供了许多线索[8]。这些评估包括粪便钠和钾的浓度、粪便 pH、粪便潜血试验和粪便白细胞检查或是否存在替代标志物如粪便钙卫蛋白或乳铁蛋白的检测[90-93]。在适当情况下，还可分析粪便样本中的脂肪含量和泻药，包括镁、磷酸盐、硫酸盐、比沙可啶和蒽醌类（见后文）。

尽管患者和医生通常认为粪便采集混乱且令人厌恶，但如果患者接受充分的指导，通常可以在家中或医院轻松地完成。也许最大的障碍是与缺乏经验或对粪便分析不感兴趣的实验室打交道。市售的采集装置可装入便池，并可以很好地分离粪便和尿液，便于采集，使用预先称重的塑料或金属容器和小冰箱或野餐冷藏器，可使标本保持低温。采集标本期间，患者应继续进行日常活动和摄入常规饮食，包括每日摄入 80～100g 脂肪。记录摄入的食物和液体日志（供营养师审查）有助于估计患者的脂肪和卡路里的摄入量，应通过计算排出量占摄入量的百分比（脂肪吸收系数）来调整粪便脂肪排出量。在采集过程中，应避免进行可能改变粪便排出量或组成的诊断性检查，如钡剂 X 线检查，仅给予基本药物。应停用任何止泻药。对于大多数腹泻患者，收集 48 小时就足够了。如果在此期间排便量不具有代表性，则可延长采集时间。必要时在禁食期间测量排便量，如果腹泻是由摄入物质引起的，禁食后腹泻应消除。禁食期间腹泻持续存在是分泌性腹泻的诊断标准。

测量粪便钠和钾浓度可计算粪便水的渗透间隙。通过从 290mOsm/kg 中减去两倍的钠和钾浓度总合（体内粪便的渗透压）计算粪便渗透间隙（考虑到这些阳离子伴随的阴离子，浓度总和加倍）。小的渗透间隙（<50mOsm/kg），这意味着粪便水的渗透压多是由于电解质吸收不全所致，是分泌性腹泻的特征（图 16.4）。较大间隙（>100mOsm/kg）是渗透性腹泻

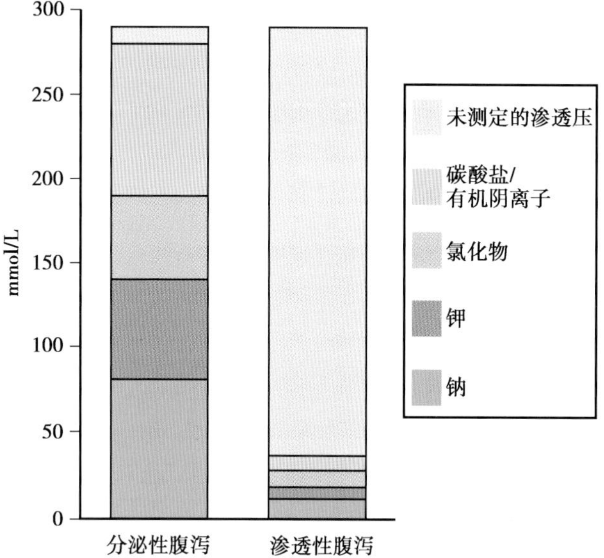

图 16.4 粪便电解质与粪便渗透间隙。结肠液和体液的渗透压处于平衡状态，大约为 290mOsm/kg。因此，电解质的总浓度不能超过 290mmol/L。在分泌性腹泻中，几乎所有结肠内容物的渗透活性均由电解质引起的，因此公式 $2\times([Na^+]+[K^+])$ 对电解质含量的估计约为 290mmo/L。在渗透性腹泻中，电解质仅占渗透活性的一小部分；摄入吸收不良物质导致的未测量渗透压占渗透活性的大部分，计算的渗透间隙将较高。（From Schiller LR. Chronic diarrhea. In：McNally P，editor. GI/liver secrets. 2nd ed. Philadelphia：Hanley & Belfus；2001. p 411.）

的特征，通常是由于摄入了一些吸收较差的物质，如镁盐或非电解质所致。当钠和钾浓度加倍的总和高于 290mOsm/kg 时，可能摄入吸收较差的多价阴离子（如磷酸盐、硫酸盐）[13]。负渗透间隙是由多价阴离子必须承担过量的阳离子造成的。粪便一旦被收集，体外持续的细菌发酵倾向于在收集后引起粪便渗透压升高[15]。因此，不应使用测定的渗透压来计算粪便渗透间隙。粪便渗透压的实际测量仅在检测被添加水或低渗尿液污染的标本时才有价值。这些样品的渗透压低于 290mOsm/kg。

粪便水的 pH 提供了关于碳水化合物吸收不良可能性的有价值信息[13,15]。到达结肠的碳水化合物迅速被细菌发酵，释放出 CO_2、H_2 气和短链脂肪酸（见第 17 章）。由于发酵 pH 呈酸性，通常降至 6 以下，这一发现间接表明结肠中碳水化合物发酵过度。

粪便隐血试验和粪便白细胞检查可识别结肠炎或恶性肿瘤导致的炎性腹泻。引起隐匿性出血的其他腹泻疾病包括小肠淋巴瘤、乳糜泻（50% 的病例粪便隐血）和难治性口炎性腹泻（70% 的病例粪便隐血）[111]。

粪便脂肪排泄量，可通过化学方法在定时（48~72 小时）采集的一次量中进行定量测量，或通过在随机标本上使用苏丹红染色进行定性估计。脂肪泻是指粪便中脂肪丢失过多（>7g/24h 或>9%/24h 的摄入量），但该定义可能不适用于所有慢性腹泻患者脂肪吸收不良或消化障碍的诊断。在一项研究中，用泻药诱发的腹泻在 35% 的正常受试者中产生了轻度脂肪泻[112]。在腹泻患者中，脂肪排泄量在 7~14g/24h 诊断脂肪吸收缺陷的特异性较低，但脂肪排泄量超过 14g/24h 强烈提示脂肪吸收的问题[112]。

在怀疑秘密摄入泻药的患者中，可通过化学或色谱法分析粪便中的泻药。这些测试容易出错，如果结果为阳性，应在另一份粪便样本中重复进行泻药测试，以核实结果，然后再让患者面对这一发现（见第 23 章）[113]。

还可通过化学试验分析粪便样本中的碳水化合物（蒽酮试剂）[15] 和 α_1-抗胰蛋白酶清除率，以检测蛋白丢失性肠病（见第 30 章）[114]。这些检测仅在特定情况下有用，不应常规用于慢性腹泻患者的初步评估。

一旦粪便分析完成，慢性腹泻可分为水样（分泌性或渗透性腹泻亚型）、炎性或脂肪性，以帮助进一步鉴别其病因。在三级转诊中心进行的一系列粪便分析的回顾性审查显示，研究结果分为 10 组，具有诊断意义，详见表 16.4[8]。

表 16.4 慢性腹泻患者粪便特征的意义

粪便特征	意义
粪便重量≤200g/24h	
没有腹泻的客观证据	排便频率改变、间隔性、大便失禁，粪便采集期间使用止泻药物治疗
排便增加（频率增加但排便量正常）	肠易激综合征、直肠炎、直肠储存功能下降可疑
粪便性状改变（大便不成形或稀变）	肠易激综合征可疑
粪便渗透压差升高	碳水化合物吸收不良或镁离子摄入过量可疑
脂肪泻	吸收不良或消化不良
粪便重量>200g/24h	
没有脂肪泻的分泌性腹泻	显微镜下结肠炎或其他分泌性腹泻
没有脂肪泻的碳水化合物吸收不良	摄入吸收不良的碳水化合物，吸收不良
脂肪泻和（或）无碳水化合物吸收不良	小肠黏膜病变，SIBO，胆汁酸分泌不足，胰腺功能不全
渗透性腹泻	摄入吸收不良的离子（如镁、磷酸盐、硫酸盐）或渗透活性聚合物（如聚乙二醇）
未分类的腹泻	血便或脓样便，提示炎症性腹泻

SIBO，肠细菌过度生长。

From Steffer KJ, Santa Ana CA, Cole JA, et al. The practical value of comprehensive stool analysis in detecting the cause of idiopathic chronic diarrhea. Gastroenterol Clin North Am. 2012; 41: 539-60.

1. 慢性分泌性腹泻

分泌性腹泻有广泛的鉴别诊断（见框 16.2），必须建立广泛的调查网络，以确定特定的原因（框 16.7）。应通过粪便细菌培养和其他微生物的特殊检测或多重 PCR 检测排除感染。此时应明确患者的 HIV 状态，因为 AIDS 患者比其他患者更有可能感染慢性腹泻（见第 35 章）[115]。虽然大多数引起腹泻的细菌在 4 周内自动清除，但一些微生物（如气单胞菌、邻单胞菌）可能引起慢性腹泻[116,117]。寻找其他病原体如球虫和微孢子虫需要特殊的微生物学检测技术[118]。酶联免疫吸附试验检测贾第鞭毛虫和隐孢子虫抗原比显微镜检查更有效[94]。可能需要用 PCR 技术、特殊染色或电子显微镜检查黏膜活检标本，以发现病原体，如 CMV 或惠普尔养障体（惠普尔病的病原体）。

SIBO 可能导致分泌性腹泻（可能由细菌毒素引起），以及胆盐解离引起的脂肪性腹泻（见后文）。葡萄糖-氢呼气试验（见后文）可用于筛查这种疾病，但 SIBO 诊断的金标准仍然是小肠抽吸物的定量培养（如可用）（见第 105 章）[119]。结构性疾病，如短肠综合征、胃结肠瘘或肠瘘、黏膜疾病、IBD 和包括淋巴瘤在内的肿瘤，应通过成像和结肠镜技术加以证实。

由肽分泌肿瘤引起的腹泻是一种有意思的慢性水样泻，相当罕见。在慢性腹泻患者中，肽分泌肿瘤检查的预测试概率极低，因此用一组血清肽水平筛查这些患者，更可能产生假

框 16.7 慢性分泌性腹泻患者的诊断方法

排除感染

细菌培养（“标准”肠道病原菌，气单胞菌，邻单胞菌）

其他病原体检测（寄生虫卵的显微镜检，贾第鞭毛虫和隐孢子虫抗原，环孢子虫、球虫和小孢子虫的特殊检测技术）和（或）多重 PCR 检测

排除器质性疾病

腹部和盆腔的 CT 或 MRI 检查

乙状结肠镜或结肠镜下黏膜活检

小肠黏膜活检及抽吸物定量培养

胶囊内镜

选择性检测

血清肽：降钙素、嗜铬粒蛋白 A、胃泌素、生长抑素、血管活性肠肽

尿液激素及代谢产物：组胺、5-羟基吲哚乙酸，甲氧基肾上腺素

其他检测：促肾上腺皮质激素刺激试验、免疫球蛋白、血清蛋白电泳、促甲状腺激素

试验性治疗

饮食排除法，如低 FODMAP 饮食

胆汁酸螯合剂

SIBO 抗生素治疗

FODMAP，可发酵的低聚糖、二糖、单糖和多元醇；SIBO，肠细菌过度生长；PCR，聚合酶链反应。

阳性结果，而不是真阳性结果[120]。内分泌介质（如 5-羟基吲哚乙酸、甲氧基肾上腺素和组胺）的血清肽水平或尿液代谢物升高的检测，应仅限于：慢性腹泻且症状和体征与肿瘤综合征（例如类癌综合征中的潮红或大的、硬的肝脏）一致；卓-艾综合征（ZES）的溃疡病；肥大细胞增生症中的头痛、潮红和色素性荨麻疹，或 CT 显示的肿瘤[25,26]。使用放射性标记奥曲肽进行闪烁显像，特别是联合正电子发射断层扫描（PET）或 CT 技术，可识别肽分泌肿瘤（见第 33 章）。

更常见的引起腹泻的内分泌疾病是糖尿病、甲状腺功能亢进症和艾迪生病（Addsion 病）。在许多情况下，其他症状和体征，如艾迪生病特有的甲状腺肿大或皮肤色素沉着，提示存在这些情况[42]。在这些疾病患者中，应选择性测量注射促肾上腺皮质激素（ACTH）类似物前后的血糖、促甲状腺激素和血清皮质醇水平。

可能与评估分泌性腹泻相关的其他血液检查包括血清蛋白电泳和免疫球蛋白电泳。选择性免疫球蛋白 A（IgA）缺乏可能表现为反复出现的肠道感染，如贾第鞭毛虫病，而联合变异性免疫缺陷可能与多种令人费解的肠道结果相关，有时酷似乳糜泻[121]。

2. 慢性渗透性腹泻

与分泌性腹泻相比，渗透性腹泻的鉴别诊断更为有限，且评估也较为简单（见框 16.8）[12]。实际上，渗透性腹泻由以下 3 种情况中的一种引起：①摄入渗透性泻药，如镁盐、磷酸盐、硫酸盐或聚乙二醇；②摄入吸收性差的碳水化合物；③全身吸收不良。摄入其他渗透活性物质是不常见的。幸运的是，通过仔细询问病史和简单的粪便检测可加以鉴别这些疾病。

渗透性泻药可通过化学试验直接在粪便中测量[14]。每日排泄镁超过 15mmol（30mEq）或粪水中浓度超过 44mmol/L（90mEq/L），强烈提示腹泻是由镁引起的。磷酸盐排泄超过

框 16.8 渗透性腹泻患者的诊断方法

粪便渗透压差升高超过 50mOsm/kg：
- 粪便镁离子浓度测定
- 粪便聚乙二醇浓度测定

粪便渗透压差降低小于 0mOsm/kg：
- 粪便磷酸盐、硫酸盐浓度检测

粪便 pH 小于 6，符合碳水化合物吸收不良：
- 饮食评估
- 乳糖氢呼气试验；黏膜乳糖酶测定（如果可能的话）
- 粪便还原性物质检测；蒽酮反应

15mmol/d 或粪水中浓度超过 33mmol/L，疑似为磷酸盐诱导的腹泻[122]。泻药的摄入可能是故意的，如秘密摄入泻药的患者，也可能是无意外的，如服用了含镁的抗酸剂或矿物质补充剂的患者。

由于结肠细菌发酵，摄入吸收不良的碳水化合物或碳水化合物吸收不良通常导致粪便 pH 较低。粪便 pH 低于 6 时，高度提示碳水化合物吸收不良[13,14]。此外，更普遍的吸收不良，除碳水化合物外，还涉及粪便中氨基酸和脂肪酸的损失，可能产生略高的 pH（如 pH=6~7.5）。单纯的碳水化合物吸收不良通常是由于摄入了难以吸收的碳水化合物，如乳糖酶缺乏者摄入乳糖。其他原因包括摄入吸收不良的糖醇（用作人工甜味剂，如山梨糖醇、甘露醇）或过量摄入吸收能力有限的糖（如果糖）[123]。治疗性使用碳水化合物吸收抑制剂（如阿卡波糖）也可能导致碳水化合物吸收不良[124]。由于发酵不仅产生酸化粪便的短链脂肪酸，还产生二氧化碳和氢气。因此，患者主诉胀气和腹胀，但存在碳水化合物吸收不良的临床线索，尽管这些症状相当无特异性（见第 17、102 和 104 章）[125]。

一旦临床表现或粪便分析提示碳水化合物吸收不良，仔细审查患者的饮食可能找到可能的来源。FODMAP，包括果糖、乳糖、果聚糖和多元醇，存在于很多食物中，许多人吸收不完全，与许多 IBS 患者引起症状有关[126]。氢呼气试验检测可用于暗示特定的碳水化合物[127,128]。在这些测试中，之前禁食的患者摄入溶于水中的固定剂量的碳水化合物，并在基线及间隔时间内对呼出的气体进行氢含量分析。由于氢不是人体代谢的正常产物，因此呼气中氢气浓度的任何增加都是细菌发酵的结果，表明未吸收的碳水化合物已到达腔内具有高浓度细菌的区域，通常是结肠段。呼吸氢检测已被用于使用葡萄糖检测 SIBO，葡萄糖是一种通常在到达结肠前应完全吸收的底物[127,128]。乳果糖是一种不可吸收但易于发酵的双糖，也被用于检测 SIBO，但由于肠道传输时间的广泛变化，为此目的使用乳果糖是有问题的[128]。乳果糖可用作测定口-盲肠通过时间的底物。在大多数情况下，当特定性诊断的试验可能性很高时，呼吸氢检测仅提供支持性证据（见第 104 章）。一旦明确了渗透性腹泻的特定原因，消除饮食的治疗性试验即可确认诊断。

3. 慢性炎性腹泻

伴有慢性腹泻和粪便中有白细胞或大便带血的患者被归类为炎性腹泻。这些特征表明黏膜被破坏和炎症。诊断考虑包括 IBD、感染、伪膜性小肠结肠炎、肠系膜缺血、放射性肠炎和肿瘤。由于这些情况可能产生分泌性腹泻，而粪便中无炎

症标志物,因此在鉴别分泌性腹泻时,也必须考虑到这种情况(见第41、110~115、118、119和125~127章)。

最初应进行结肠镜检查,以观察结构和组织学变化(框16.9)。必须从结肠获得活检标本,以帮助作出正确的诊断。CT或MRI小肠造影、胶囊式内镜和深肠镜检查,可在慢性炎性腹泻患者的评估中发挥作用。

框16.9 慢性炎性腹泻患者的诊断方法
排除器质性疾病
腹部和盆腔的CT或MRI检查
乙状结肠镜或结肠镜下黏膜活检
小肠镜下黏膜活检
排除结核、寄生虫和病毒

感染可引起慢性炎性腹泻或加重UC或克罗恩病引起的现有炎性腹泻。最可能引起慢性炎性腹泻的病原体是艰难梭菌、巨细胞病毒、溶组织内阿米巴原虫、耶尔森菌属和结核分枝杆菌,众所周知,艰难梭菌和巨细胞病毒可导致IBD加重(见第110~115章)[129]。除活检外,应获得适当的培养或非培养依赖性检测,以排除这些感染。

4. 慢性脂肪性腹泻

脂肪泻意味着小肠脂肪溶解、消化或吸收的破坏。慢性脂肪性腹泻的评价旨在区分消化不良(甘油三酯管腔内分解不充分)和吸收不良(消化产物的黏膜转运不足)(见第104章)。

消化不良的主要原因是胰腺外分泌功能不全(如慢性胰腺炎)和胆汁缺乏(如晚期原发性胆汁性肝硬化)。黏膜疾病(如乳糜泻)是吸收不良的常见原因。脂肪泻的绝对量和粪便脂肪浓度(脂肪克数/100g粪便)为脂肪泻的病因提供了线索[130]。由于脂肪同化的破坏更大,消化不良(如胰腺功能不全)的脂肪泻程度往往高于(通常>30g脂肪/d)黏膜疾病。消化障碍的粪便脂肪浓度也往往高于黏膜疾病,因为黏膜疾病可能存在液体和电解质吸收缺陷,粪便脂肪含量被未吸收的水稀释。此外,在黏膜疾病中脂肪消化通常是完整的,因此甘油三酯被水解为脂肪酸,可能会抑制结肠电解质和水分吸收,进一步稀释粪便中的脂肪含量[71]。相比之下,在消化障碍中甘油三酯水解减少,不会导致脂肪酸介导的结肠液体和电解质转运抑制,因此在消化障碍中,未吸收的脂肪分散在较小的粪便体积中,因此更集中。疑似消化不良患者的粪便脂肪浓度超过9.5g/100g,强烈提示脂肪泻是由胰腺或胆道原因引起的。

对慢性脂肪性腹泻患者的进一步评估相对简单(框16.10)。第一步是寻找涉及小肠或胰腺的结构问题。评价包括小肠影像学检查或内镜检查联合小肠活检、CT和MRCP。进行小肠活检时,应抽吸肠腔内容物,并送样本进行定量培养以排除SIBO。由于乳糜泻是导致吸收不良的黏膜疾病的最常见原因,因此应测定组织转谷氨酰胺酶抗体和肌内膜抗体(见第104、105和107章)[131,132]。

如果未发现肠道异常或检测到慢性胰腺炎的影像学证据,应考虑胰腺外分泌功能不全[133]。现有的胰腺功能检查均有局限性(见第56和59章)。胰泌素刺激试验使用外源性胰泌素刺激胰腺,并通过抽吸十二指肠内容物来测量碳酸氢盐排出量,是这些试验中历史最悠久的,但由于其复杂性很少进行[134]。已尝试将胰泌素刺激试验与内镜逆行胰胆管造影相结合,但这种改良尚未被广泛采用[135]。粪便中胰酶浓度的测定,被认为是胰腺外分泌功能不全的一种更简单的筛查试验。在慢性腹泻患者中,直接测定粪便糜蛋白酶活性的敏感性和特异性较差[136]。粪便弹性蛋白酶测定的可靠性稍好一些[137]。实际上,确定胰腺外分泌功能不全的最佳方法可能是补充胰酶的治疗性试验。如果进行此类试验,应预先设定高剂量的酶,并应监测一些如粪便脂肪排泄量或体重增加等客观指标,以评估疗效(见第59章)[133,138]。

框16.10 慢性脂肪性腹泻患者的诊断方法
排除器质性疾病
腹部和盆腔的CT或MRI检查
小肠活检和抽吸物定量培养
排除胰腺外分泌功能不全
胰酶替代试验性治疗
粪弹力蛋白酶或粪乳糜蛋白酶浓度检测
促胰液素试验
排除十二指肠胆汁酸缺乏
胆汁酸替代试验性治疗
餐后十二指肠抽吸胆汁酸浓度检测

通常可根据患者病史或体格检查推断膳食脂肪的胆盐溶解不足(如胆汁淤积性黄疸、回肠切除术、已知的小肠结肠瘘)。如果需要证明其致病机制,餐后十二指肠抽吸物分析可证明结合胆汁酸浓度降低。该检测可能无法在专业中心以外进行,外源性结合胆汁酸(牛胆汁)的治疗性试验,可能是确定诊断的最佳方法。补充胆汁酸可减轻脂肪泻,常可改善患者的营养状况,而不加重腹泻[139]。

六、治疗

腹泻最重要的治疗是确保通过静脉输液或口服补液治疗,补充液体和电解质缺乏。虽然口服补液治疗在工业化国家是一种传统的、廉价的治疗选择,但其主要影响是降低霍乱和其他传染性腹泻在欠发达国家的发病率和死亡率[140]。因为即使其他形式的钠吸收受损,营养吸收也会增强空肠对钠和液体的吸收,所以口服含有葡萄糖、氨基酸的盐水溶液或更复杂的营养物质(可在刷状缘或腔内水解)将很容易被吸收。虽然最早的口服补液用葡萄糖加速空肠对钠的吸收,但现在认为低渗高直链玉米淀粉口服补液(HAMS-ORS)也能增强短链脂肪酸的产生和结肠对液体的吸收是更优的[140]。

虽然口服补液可增加液体和电解质的吸收,但并不减少粪便排出量,使用这些溶液实际上可能会增加粪便重量。频繁呕吐的患者禁止使用口服补液溶液。大多数运动饮料(如Gatorade)旨在补充汗液中适度的电解质损失,不含足够的钠来补充替代腹泻的损失。如果同时摄入其他来源的钠和可吸收的营养物质(例如椒盐卷饼或饼干),则可使用这些溶液。Pedialyte产品(电解质水)的钠含量增加了2~3倍(45或60mmol/L),但仍然低于经典口服补液溶液(90mmol/L)。市售溶液更接近 WHO 口服补液溶液或基于谷物的补液溶液(如 Rehydralyte 和 Ceralyte 90)。

(一) 急性腹泻

由于感染是急性腹泻的常见原因,医生常经验性选择抗生素治疗[141]。如果社区或特定情况下,细菌或原虫感染的流行率较高,经验性使用抗生素是合乎逻辑的,就像用氟喹诺酮或利福昔明治疗旅行者腹泻一样,即使没有感染的细菌学证据[88]。经验性抗生素治疗通常用于病情更严重的患者,而细菌培养结果待定,但这种方法受到质疑。大肠埃希菌感染后发生溶血尿毒症综合征的患者比无溶血尿毒症综合征的患者,更可能接受经验性抗生素治疗,尽管该综合征的发生可能与特定抗生素和处方剂量相关。专家还建议不要对沙门菌病进行经验性抗生素治疗,除非存在肠伤寒[129]。对于持续性腹泻(持续>1 周)的患者,考虑潜在性原虫感染时,可使用甲硝唑或硝唑尼特的经验性治疗(见第 110 和 113 章)。多重 PCR 检测能够在数小时内(而不是数天内)鉴定出特定的病原体。因此可以避免盲目的抗微生物治疗。

非特异性止泻药可减少大便次数、大便重量和共存症状,如腹部绞痛(表 16.5)。通常处方阿片类药物,如洛哌丁胺或地芬诺酯与阿托品[142]。关于这些抗蠕动药物在很大程度上会减缓肠道病原体清除的担忧,尚未得到证实。阿片类抗腹泻药已被一些人滥用,缓解急性腹泻只需少量供给即可。肠腔内制剂如次水杨酸铋(Pepto-Bismol)和吸附剂(如高岭土)也可能有助于降低大便的流动性。消旋卡多曲是一种抑制脑啡肽酶从而增加内源性阿片类药物对 μ 阿片受体影响的药物,在一些国家可用于治疗急性腹泻[143]。

表 16.5　慢性腹泻的非特异性药物治疗

药物分类	药物	剂量*
阿片类(选择 μ 阿片受体)	可待因	15~60mg,每天 4 次
	地芬诺酯	2.5~5mg,每天 4 次
	洛哌丁胺	2~4mg,每天 4 次
	吗啡	2~20mg,每天 4 次
	阿片酊	2~20 滴,每天 4 次
脑啡肽酶抑制剂(δ-阿片受体效应)	消旋卡多曲† Racecadotril (acetorphan)	1.5mg/kg,每天 3 次
α_2-肾上腺素受体激动剂	可乐定	0.1~0.3mg,每天 3 次
生长抑素抑制剂	奥曲肽	50~250μg,每天 3 次(皮下注射)
胆汁酸螯合剂	考来烯胺	4g,每天 1~4 次
	考来维仑	1.875g,每天 2 次
	考来替泊	4g,每天 1~4 次
纤维素添加剂	多羧钙	5~10g,每天 1 次
	车前草	10~20g,每天 1 次

*口服,除非另有说明。
†未在美国获批。

(二) 慢性腹泻

慢性腹泻的经验性治疗适用于以下 3 种情况:①作为诊断试验前的暂时性或初期治疗;②诊断试验未能确诊后;③已作出诊断但没有特异性治疗可用或特异性治疗失败时。一般来说,经验性抗生素治疗对慢性腹泻的作用不如急性腹泻,因为感染是不太可能的原因。虽然一些临床医生在对患者进行广泛的诊断检测之前,尝试甲硝唑或氟喹诺酮的经验性治疗,但这种方法没有数据支持,也不推荐使用。

在适当的临床环境中,在不明原因脂肪泻患者中进行胰腺酶替代和结合胆汁酸补充的治疗性试验可能具有诊断和治疗性(见前文)。相反,当胰酶补充剂或胆汁酸结合树脂经验性试用于治疗所谓的特发性慢性腹泻时,其很少有令人满意的效果(见后文)。

慢性腹泻患者通常需要阿片类药物对症治疗,因为可能无法获得特定治疗[142]。常使用洛哌丁胺(最多 4mg,每日 4 次),但对某些患者可能不够有效。更强效的阿片类药物如可卡因、鸦片制剂或吗啡,在这些患者的治疗中剂量使用不足,主要是因为担心药物滥用。事实上,这些药物很少被慢性腹泻患者滥用,尤其是如果采取一些简单的措施。首先,需要告知患者该药物滥用的潜在风险,并应告诫患者在未咨询医生的情况下不要增加剂量。其次,初始剂量应较低,并逐渐增加剂量达到疗效。最后,应密切监测阿片类药物的使用情况,在达到预期的使用量之前,不应重新填写处方。因为对阿片类药物胃肠道效应的耐受性并未形成,因此控制腹泻所需的剂量应随时间推移保持稳定,频繁要求增加剂量可能意味着滥用。

有时用作非特异性止泻药的其他药物包括奥曲肽和可乐定。奥曲肽是一种生长抑素类似物,已被证明可以改善类癌综合征和其他内分泌疾病、倾倒综合征、化疗诱导的腹泻和艾滋病患者的腹泻[144]。对其他腹泻病的益处尚不清楚。可乐定是一种 α-肾上腺素能药物,对肠运动和转运有影响,可能对糖尿病性腹泻有特殊的作用,但其降压作用限制了其在许多腹泻患者中的作用。Crofelemer 是 FDA 批准用于接受抗逆转录病毒治疗的艾滋病患者非感染性腹泻的药物,可抑制 2 种肠上皮细胞氯离子通道——CFTR 通道和钙激活的氯离子通道——从而减少氯离子分泌(见第 35 章)[145]。Crofelemer 是否对其他形式的分泌性腹泻有作用仍有待观察。

使用益生菌作为腹泻非特异性治疗的兴趣越来越大,但有效性的证据仍然有限[146]。当应用于特殊情况时,如旅行者腹泻、抗生素相关性腹泻和婴儿腹泻。这些药物可改变肠道微生物群,刺激局部免疫,加快腹泻的康复[147,148]。治疗腹泻的草药包括那些含有小檗碱(金印草、黄连)(似乎具有刺激液体和电解质吸收的作用)和葛根(其机制尚不清楚)的草药[149,150]。

大便调节剂如车前子可,改变大便性状,但不能减轻大便重量[151,152]。其对同时存在大便失禁的患者和一些粪便重量较轻的患者有帮助(见前文)。从水样便变为半成形便可能足以缓解症状。此外,果胶可能延缓通过近端肠道的转运,增加肠腔黏度,从而作为辅助经验性治疗。每日补充 1~2g 元素钙对某些患者可能是简单有效的疗法,这种作用机制尚不明确。

七、选择性腹泻综合征

（一）肠易激综合征和功能性腹泻

在慢性腹泻患者中最常见的诊断是肠易激综合征（IBS），但实际上只有一部分慢性腹泻患者符合 IBS 的诊断标准，其中腹痛是其核心特征（见第 122 章）[89]。这些标准确定了不太可能有结构性症状（如 IBD 或癌症）的患者。动物和人体研究表明，产毒素细菌性肠炎诱导的自身免疫可能在某些个体中触发 IBS 伴腹泻的发生，并导致创建了诊断试验，以提供这种暴露的证据[153-155]。随着诊断试验的改进，引起 IBS 患者腹泻的基本问题越来越明显，从而使医生能够更精准地针对腹泻的机制（表 16.6）[102]。当 IBS 患者对非特异性治疗和生活方式改变无反应时，临床医生应该考虑这些诊断，并进一步进行针对这些机制的诊断检测或经验性治疗试验。

表 16.6　肠易激综合征（IBS）伴腹泻（IBS-D）的鉴别诊断

诊断	IBS-D 预计发病率/%	诊断策略
食物不耐受	20～67	饮食与症状日记→排查饮食
感染后并发 IBS	28～58	细胞致死性肿胀毒素 B 抗体和血管球蛋白抗体检测
SIBO	23～45	小肠抽吸物定量培养、氢呼气试验；抗生素试验性治疗
胆汁酸吸收不良	10～40	^{75}SeHCAT 残余量、C4 或 FGF19 测定；胆汁酸螯合剂试验性治疗
显微镜下结肠炎	5～10	结肠活检（直肠上端）
乳糜泻	0.4～4	IgA 抗组织转谷氨酰胺酶抗体和总 IgA 测定；十二指肠活检
胰腺外分泌功能不全	未知	粪便弹性蛋白酶-1 浓度检测；胰酶替代试验性治疗
肠道转运过快或过慢	未知	闪烁成像或基于胶囊内镜技术的肠道运动检查

C4，7-羟基-4-胆甾烯-3-酮；FGF19，成纤维细胞生长因子 19；IgA，免疫球蛋白 A；^{75}SeHCAT，硒-75-同型胆酸牛磺酸；SIBO，肠细菌过度生长。

From Schiller LR. Evaluation of chronic diarrhea and irritable bowel syndrome with diarrhea in adults in the era of precision medicine. Am J Gastroenterol. 2018；113：660-9.

无痛性腹泻不应再被认为是 IBS 的一种。罗马Ⅳ共识委员会将功能性腹泻定义为：过去 3 个月内出现"稀便或水样便，无明显的腹痛或令人烦恼的腹胀，发生在超过 25% 的大便中"，症状在诊断前至少 6 个月发作[89]。许多慢性腹泻患者在首次就诊时无法确定腹泻的明确原因，可描述为"功能性腹泻"。医生不应在没有探讨慢性腹泻的整个鉴别诊断的情况下作出这种诊断，尤其是那些能产生发作性和可变的非结构性疾病，如食物不耐受、SIBO 和胆汁酸腹泻。在大多数情况下，可以对这些患者进行特定的诊断[102]。功能性腹泻还必须与特发性分泌性腹泻相区别，后者起病急骤（见后文）。

（二）食物性腹泻

吸收不良的碳水化合物通常与腹泻有关，最有可能是由于肠道内液体的渗透潴留和细菌发酵产生的气体。因此，胃肠胀气或腹胀是提示碳水化合物吸收不良的重要线索（见第 17 章）。由于获得性乳糖酶缺乏发生率频繁，因此乳糖是饮食引起腹泻的常见原因[15,18]。果糖通过限制容量促进扩散吸收[156]。虽然很难超过天然食物的吸收能力，但食用含有高果糖玉米糖浆的加工食品更容易压倒肠道的吸收能力[157,158]。糖醇吸收障碍也可能引起腹泻：山梨醇、甘露醇和木糖醇是"无糖"口香糖和糖果等食品中吸收较差的非营养甜味剂，过量摄入可能引起腹泻[159]。各种天然食物中存在吸收不良的碳水化合物。澳大利亚的研究人员测量了食物中吸收较差的碳水化合物水平，并开发了低 FODMAP 饮食（见前文），以尽量减少这些物质的摄入[126]。在一项随机试验中，饮食学家实施的低 FODMAP 饮食减轻了 75% IBS 患者的肠道症状（见第 122 章）[160]。一旦实现获益，饮食可能会简化。一些慢性腹泻但没有乳糜泻症状的患者，似乎在无麸质饮食中病情有所改善[161]。这些患者的腹泻机制尚不确定，需要额外的研究。无麸质饮食后症状的改善，可能是由于去除了小麦相关变应原或果聚糖摄入量的偶然减少（果聚糖是小麦中吸收较差的碳水化合物）[162]。不伴有乳糜泻的腹泻患者何时应尝试无麸质饮食尚不清楚（见第 107 章）[163]。计算咖啡和能量饮料中咖啡因的摄入量也很重要，这可能是饮食引起腹泻的常见原因[164]。

脂肪和油炸食品与一些患者水样腹泻的发病有关[86]。矛盾的是，一些脂肪含量超高的食物，如冰激凌，很少暗示为脂肪食物不耐受。尽管脂肪吸收不良可刺激结肠分泌引起腹泻，但脂肪似乎可能会在无明显脂肪泻的情况下引发症状，这可能是由于刺激胃结肠反射所致。

食物过敏是免疫介导的反应，可能引起腹泻和其他症状，并且发生率似乎低于非过敏性食物不耐受（见第 10 章）[165]。流行病学研究表明，1%～2% 的成年人有真正的食物过敏，儿童的发生率更高。某些食物更容易引起过敏反应：牛奶、鸡蛋、豌豆、坚果、大豆、小麦、鱼和贝类。研究表明，香蕉，鳄梨，核桃和猕猴桃与乳胶-食物过敏综合征有关。蜱虫叮咬与哺乳动物肉类中发现的碳水化合物过敏的发生有关。虽然真正的食物过敏在成年人中并不常见，但当存在其他过敏特征如荨麻疹时，应考虑食物过敏。

（三）显微镜下结肠炎

显微镜下结肠炎包括 2 个亚型——胶原性结肠炎和淋巴细胞性结肠炎。这些疾病被定义为综合征。水样腹泻的特征是结肠镜检查正常，固有层淋巴细胞和浆细胞炎症以及上皮内淋巴细胞增多的组织学改变，伴或不伴上皮下胶原层增厚(见第 128 章)[165,166]。瑞典一项基于人群的流行病学研究表明，显微镜下结肠炎的年发病率与克罗恩病相似，10% 表现为慢性非血性腹泻的患者被诊断为该疾病[167]。在表现为慢性水样腹泻的患者中，获得足够数量(6~10 份)外观正常的结肠黏膜活检样本，对诊断至关重要。

显微镜下结肠炎的病因(或原因)至今仍未知。该病最常见于中年女性，通常与自身免疫性疾病(如关节炎和甲状腺功能减退)相关。有吸烟史和非甾体抗炎药使用史的较为常见[168,169]。许多其他药物与显微镜下结肠炎相关，包括质子泵抑制剂类药物，他汀类药物和选择性五羟色胺再摄取抑制剂，但这些相关性存在争议[169]。最令人感兴趣的是，淋巴细胞性和胶原性结肠炎与人白细胞抗原(HLA)-DQ2 和 HLA-DQ1,3(包括 HLA-DQ1,3 亚型 HLA-DQ1,7、HLA-DQ1,8 和 HLA-DQ1,9)的紧密连锁，与乳糜泻相同，提示参与显微镜下结肠炎和乳糜泻发病的免疫机制可能相似[170]。事实上，显微镜下结肠炎与乳糜泻相关，可能是接受无麸质饮食治疗的乳糜泻患者持续性腹泻的原因[171]。然而，由于许多乳糜泻患者尽管接受了无麸质饮食治疗，仍持续存在淋巴细胞性结肠炎的组织学证据，且从饮食中消除麸质对其他显微镜下结肠炎患者没有效果[172]，因此几乎可以肯定，麸质不是显微镜下结肠炎的致病抗原。结肠腔内的细菌抗原，而不是饮食抗原，可能在显微镜下结肠炎中起重要的致病作用。黏膜淋巴细胞的免疫学研究显示淋巴细胞性和胶原性结肠炎之间的异同，可能与不同的触发机制有关[173]。

无论何种原因，黏膜炎症在很大程度上对显微镜下结肠炎的腹泻有反应。结肠灌注研究表明，淋巴细胞性结肠炎和胶原性结肠炎的水盐吸收受损[174]。使用人结肠标本的体外研究表明，氯化钠吸收减少，伴随着扩散和紧密连接功能的变化[175]。结肠吸水性与固有层的细胞构成呈负相关，但与胶原层的厚度无关。尽管结肠的水和盐净分泌并不常见。典型的粪便重量为 500~1 000g/24h，与结肠很少或没有液体吸收一致。胆汁酸吸收不良也可能在这种情况下腹泻的发病机制中起一定作用[176]。

关于显微镜下结肠炎药物治疗的指南得出结论，布地奈德具有最佳的疗效证据[177]。治疗显微镜下结肠炎的不太完善的药物包括次水杨酸铋、美沙拉秦和泼尼松。难治性病例推荐使用免疫抑制剂如硫唑嘌呤[178]。大多数患者的显微镜下结肠炎随时间缓解，但通常复发。对于某些患者，止泻药对症治疗可能是适当的选择。胆汁酸螯合剂也可改善这种疾病患者的腹泻[176]。

(四) 手术后腹泻

胃肠道和胆道外科手术引起肠功能变化，可导致腹泻。尽管消化性溃疡(PUD)手术的实施频率远低于过去，但对胃肠道和胆道进行的其他手术仍并发腹泻。

1. 胃部术后腹泻

多年来，采用迷走神经切断术联合幽门成形术或胃窦切除术治疗 PUD(见第 53 章)。20 世纪 80 年代高选择性迷走神经切断术的引入，使术后腹泻的发生率下降。对于梗阻性或恶性溃疡病，仍采用传统的治疗方法。此外，用于治疗肥胖症的胃旁路手术的显著增加(见第 8 章)。该手术和其他减肥手术(如胃袖状手术和带十二指肠开关的胆胰分流术)通常与消化系统症状相关，包括腹泻[179]。腹泻也可作为腹腔镜抗反流手术的并发症，推测是由于意外的迷走神经切断术所致(见第 46 章)[180]。

胃手术后最常见的综合征是倾倒综合征，这种疾病的特征是餐后潮红、低血压、腹泻和低血糖(见第 53 章)。该综合征是由胃排空不受调节、渗透转移和肽类激素从肠道快速释放所致[181]，可以通过改良饮食、止泻药和生长抑素类似物奥曲肽成功治疗[182]。胃部手术也可能使患者易患 SIBO、肠道转运异常快、胆汁酸吸收不良和胰酶外分泌功能不全，这是由于胰腺分泌刺激不良和(或)胰酶与肠内容物混合不充分所致。

2. 肠切除术后腹泻

肠表面积的损失会促进液体、电解质或营养物质的吸收不良，取决于肠切除的部分。肠道具有大量的吸收表面积，以满足正常的营养负荷。当小肠切除后没有足够的表面积进行正常吸收时，就会发生腹泻，即所谓的短肠综合征(见第 106 章)[183]。随着时间的推移，肠道适应可能导致肠道电解质吸收改善，但不能克服特殊功能的缺陷，如对抗电化学梯度吸收钠的能力(见第 101 章)[34-36]。通过使用上皮生长因子，如替度鲁肽，可以加速适应[184]。回肠切除也可能损害结合胆汁酸的吸收，并导致胆汁酸介导的液体和结肠电解质分泌[185]。各种方法可用于纠正短肠综合征患者的营养缺乏和肠功能障碍(见第 106 章)。

3. 回肠造口术后腹泻

正常情况下，每天有 1~1.5L 液体从小肠进入结肠；回肠造口将这种液体从体内转移。如果患者有足够长度的功能性小肠，适应最终导致小肠流量减少到每日平均 750mL。这种每日过多的液体丢失，通常很容易通过增加经口服摄入量来克服，但回肠造口术患者对异常增加的液体丢失耐受性差，在这种情况下有脱水的风险。当液体丢失量超过每日 1 000mL 时，就会出现回肠造口腹泻(见第 117 章)[186]。

回肠造口腹泻的原因包括造口狭窄、部分 SBO、SIBO、复发性 IBD、造口近端复发性肿瘤、药物相关腹泻和腹腔内感染。在大多数情况下，未确定具体原因。在 UC 结肠切除术后形成回肠袋(以创建可控性回肠造口术或回肠肛管吻合术)的患者中，会发生一种特殊的情况，即由细菌过度生长或复发性 IBD 引起的袋炎症，即所谓储袋炎[187]。这种情况可用抗生素如甲硝唑、益生菌或抗炎药如美沙拉秦治疗。

特发性回肠造口腹泻用止泻药治疗，可能需要大剂量的强效阿片类药物。如果强效阿片类药物控制不佳，则使用奥曲肽。如果回肠造口每日排出量超过 2 000mL，可能必须补充口服补液或静脉补液，以防止脱水和维持正常的尿量。

(五) 胆汁酸性腹泻

二羟基胆汁酸，如鹅去氧胆酸和脱氧胆酸，可引起结肠分泌液体和电解质，如果到达结肠的浓度足够(3~5mmol/L)，则可能刺激结肠转运[188]。胆汁酸性腹泻(Bile acid-induced diarrhea，BAD)有 4 种情况，如框 16.11 所示。

框 16.11 胆汁酸性腹泻

1 型

回肠功能障碍/回肠切除(继发性胆汁酸吸收不良)

2 型

特发性(原发性胆汁酸吸收不良)

3 型

其他疾病

- 慢性胰腺炎
- 显微镜下结肠炎
- 胆囊切除术后
- 放射性肠炎
- SIBO
- 迷走神经切断术后,胃手术后

4 型

先天性转运体缺陷

- 回肠胆汁酸转运蛋白/顶端钠依赖性胆盐转运蛋白

SIBO,小肠细菌过度生长。

(1) 1 型 BAD:是定义和理解最清楚的病因学。继发于手术切除或回肠炎症性疾病(如克罗恩病)的回肠功能障碍可中断肝肠循环,从而导致肝脏合成胆汁酸增加,过量的胆汁酸进入结肠,反过来又导致结肠液体分泌增加,并更快速通过结肠[185]。

(2) 2 型 BAD:是特发性的。研究表明,在高达 30% 的腹泻型 IBS 和(或)功能性腹泻患者中,它可能是腹泻的原因(见前文和第 122 章)。这似乎与由于成纤维细胞生长因子 19(FGF19)水平降低导致的胆汁酸合成调节缺陷有关,FGF19 是一种肝脏胆汁酸合成抑制因子,通常由回肠上皮细胞响应胆汁酸吸收分泌。这导致胆汁酸池扩大,超过回肠的吸收能力,从而导致过量的胆汁酸进入结肠,增加结肠的分泌和转运[189]。

(3) 3 型 BAD:是由胆汁酸吸收不良引起的腹泻疾病的一种大杂烩,尽管其机制尚不清楚。其中最具临床意义的是胆囊切除术后腹泻,可能发生在胆囊手术后 20% 的患者中(见第 66 章)[190,191]。腹泻通常在胆囊切除术后不久开始,也可能延迟。胆囊切除术后腹泻归因于胆汁酸肝肠循环的变化,但支持该机制的证据有限。切除胆囊后,胆汁酸失去了贮存库,并且大部分胆汁酸池始终保持在小肠内。禁食期间,每 90 分钟,移行的肌电复合体通过小肠并迅速清扫肠内容物,包括固有的胆汁酸池,通过回肠末端进入结肠,从而刺激结肠分泌并加速转运(见第 64 章)。部分研究已经证实,胆囊切除术后腹泻患者的粪便胆汁酸排泄量增加。胆囊切除术后腹泻患者最好在睡前服用胆汁酸结合剂(或螯合剂)(如考来烯胺)治疗,也可以在白天的其他时间使用。阿片类止泻药对难治性病例有帮助。

(4) 4 型 BAD:是回肠顶端胆盐转运蛋白的先天性缺陷,是新生儿腹泻的一种极为罕见的原因[192]。

BAD 的临床诊断存在问题。在英国和其他一些国家,可通过全身扫描测量口服放射性标记胆汁酸(硒-75 标记的同型胆酸牛磺酸或^{75}SeHCAT)的潴留,以检测胆汁酸吸收不良[193]。如果采用严格的诊断标准(1 周时保留<5%),该检测可以预测对胆汁酸结合药物的反应性[7]。当采用不太严格的诊断标准时,检测不太可靠,腹泻本身可能使检测异常[194]。该检测在美国不可用。

在有限数量的研究中心进行了 48~72 小时定时粪便采集中粪便胆汁酸排出量的直接测量,但通常不可用。有趣的是,在 BAD 中初级胆汁酸似乎增加,这表明内源性胆汁酸的细菌解离减少,可能与结肠中的快速转运有关[195]。目前尚不清楚粪便胆汁酸排泄量的增加是否能准确预测慢性腹泻患者对胆汁酸结合剂的反应性[196]。

通过测定血清中 C4(7α-羟基-4-胆甾烯-3-酮)的浓度可以获得诊断 BAD 的支持性证据[197]。C4 是胆汁酸合成的中间体,其在血清中的浓度与总体胆汁酸合成率相关。如果由于过量的胆汁酸损失到结肠中或胆汁酸合成去抑制导致胆汁酸合成增加,则血清 C4 水平较高。该检测已上市销售,但尚不清楚其对胆汁酸结合剂反应性的预测能力。FGF19 的测量(在 BAD 患者中较低)可能会在未来可供临床医生使用。

在大多数临床情况下,胆汁酸螯合树脂的经验性试验可能是确定 BAD 诊断的最佳方法。给药剂量和时间可能至关重要,但需要科学评估。考来烯胺、考来替泊和考来维仑可用,有效性和耐受性各不相同,可能需要序贯试用[198-200]。与胆汁酸螯合剂在高胆固醇血症中的应用不同,在高胆固醇血症中,当胆汁酸在餐后存在时,胆汁酸的螯合需要发生在小肠近端,在 BAD 中,胆汁酸需要在结肠中螯合。因此,在睡前和远离食物时给予胆汁酸螯合剂是有意义的。临床反应表明 BAD 可能起了一定作用。然而,由于此类药物也可能结合毒素或具有其他作用,因此必须考虑非特异性效应的可能性。

(六) 住院患者腹泻

患者在住院期间经常发生腹泻,特别是长期住院的重症患者[201]。在这种情况下腹泻的常见原因包括药物(尤其是抗生素)、管饲、肠缺血和粪块嵌塞。

腹泻是许多药物的副作用,包括住院患者常用的药物(见框 16.4)[75,76]。抗生素治疗尤其可能通过至少两种机制引起腹泻:①损害结肠菌群的碳水化合物代谢,从而产生渗透性腹泻[202];②促进艰难梭菌过度生长并产生其毒素,从而产生炎性和/或分泌性腹泻[203]。在某些情况下,红霉素可能通过其胃动素样作用于胃肠道转运而引起腹泻。

细菌代谢受损可使碳水化合物和相关水留在肠腔内而引起腹泻[202]。通常,所有的膳食纤维和大约 20% 的小麦淀粉逃避消化和肠道吸收,到达结肠。结肠细菌将这些碳水化合物发酵为短链脂肪酸、氢和二氧化碳。这些发酵产物和相关的水被结肠迅速吸收,因此不会出现腹泻。相比之下,当抗生素杀死一些正常的结肠菌群时,发酵减少,未消化的纤维和碳水化合物以及水被保留在肠腔内,从而导致渗透性腹泻。在某些人中,疾病或伴随给予的其他药物可能改变肠道转运,导致碳水化合物更多地输送至结肠,进一步加重了腹泻。此类腹泻应在患者禁食时消退。

艰难梭菌相关腹泻是一个更严重的问题[203]。住院患者和养老院居民可能被该微生物定植,约 20% 的住院患者定植艰难梭菌。身体接触和手卫生差是其在机构内传播的主要因素。在这种情况下,诱发腹泻的因素包括抗生素治疗、化疗和免疫改变,以及质子泵抑制剂给药导致的胃液酸度降低[204]。

艰难梭菌相关疾病的严重程度范围,从轻微腹泻到危及生命的结肠炎不等,尤其是当患者定植艰难梭菌强毒株或患有基础 IBD 时(见第112章)。

腹泻可能是肠内营养的一种并发症,但通常是共存问题的结果(见第6章)[205]。管饲虽然比肠外营养更符合生理,但仍与经口摄入食物向肠道提供营养物质的正常方式不同,胃肠道的调节系统可能无法适应。一些管饲配方奶粉是高渗的,可能通过类似于倾倒综合征的机制诱发腹泻(见前文)。在这种情况下,将配方更改为等渗配方或包含纤维混合物可能是有益的。在其他情况下,减慢输注速度从而减少营养物质向肠道的输送可能是有帮助的,但如果在较慢的输注速率下不能满足患者的营养需求,这种方法的价值可能有限。在某些情况下,特定的益生菌可能有益,但尚未制定明确的指南(见第130章)[205]。在管饲中添加止泻药,如洛哌丁胺或鸦片酊可能是必要的,尽管这种方法有局限性,尤其是对于有肠梗阻风险的患者(见第124章)。

部分住院患者可能发生肠缺血,尤其是低血压或休克患者[206]。这些患者有发生缺血性结肠炎引起的血性腹泻或发生小肠缺血引起的更严重腹泻的风险(见第118章)。

老年人、长期肠道休息的患者和服用泻药的患者发生粪便嵌塞的风险增加。反常或溢出性腹泻伴大便失禁可能是嵌塞的第一个线索。发生腹泻的住院患者应接受直肠指检,以排除粪便嵌塞(见第18和19章)[207]。

(七) 人为性腹泻

对于腹泻仍未确诊的患者,特别是符合以下四类之一的患者,应考虑秘密滥用泻药(表16.7):①使用泻药调整体重的神经性厌食症或贪食症患者(见第9章);②Munchausen综合征患者,假装患病,混淆医生;③被看护者用泻药下毒的患者;④使用泻药诱导的疾病以获得二次收益(如残疾收入)或引发他人担忧的患者(见第23章)[75,208,209]。

表16.7 易滥用泻药患者的情况

状况	特征
贪食症	通常为青春期至年轻女性;担心体重或表现出进食障碍;可能暴饮暴食、呕吐或过度运动,以抵消过量的食物摄入
Munchausen综合征	患者喜欢接受诊断检查;可能反复接受各种检查
Polle综合征(代理型孟 Munchausen综合征)	受抚养儿童或成人被父母或看护者使用泻药致其中毒,以自证照顾能力;可能有兄弟姐妹死于慢性腹泻亡
继发性获益	患者可能有伤残索赔待定;疾病可能引起他人关注或照顾行为

检测泻药滥用需要高怀疑指数。医生通常认为患者是诚实的,但高达4%的普通人群或15%贪食症患者可能秘密滥用泻药[210]。在慢性腹泻评估期间,可能会发现滥用泻药的线索。例如,低钾血症可能提示摄入刺激性泻药,如番泻叶。检出结肠假性黑色素病,一种结肠黏膜的褐色色素沉着,提示长期摄入蒽醌类泻药,如番泻叶或药鼠李皮(见第128章)。存在较大的粪便渗透间隙提示镁摄入。负渗透压间隙可能表明摄入了吸收不良的多价阴离子,如磷酸盐或硫酸盐(见前文)。

对属于表16.7所列组之一的患者以及评估后未确诊的腹泻患者,应采用标准化方法对粪便样本进行通便剂分析。大多数泻药可通过分光光度法或色谱法检测,但商业分析的准确性受到质疑(见第23章)[113]。由于一些患者通过添加尿液或水而夸大粪便量,因此也应测量粪便渗透压,低于290mOsm/kg的值表明使用水或低渗尿液稀释了粪便。粪便与高渗尿液的混合通常会导致不可能的高粪便渗透压(通常>600mOsm/kg),和阴性粪便渗透间隙,因为尿液中钠和钾的浓度较高。应遵守法律法规,不应在未经授权的房间中搜查泻药。

如果诊断为泻药滥用,应在与患者或其家属讨论病情前,通过重复粪便分析确诊。患者应面对研究结果,但不是在制定善后计划之前。精神科会诊应遵循与患者讨论,一些滥用泻药的人在被发现后会有自杀倾向,因此所有滥用泻药的患者都需咨询。在由家长或看护者进行泻药给药的情况下,应提起法律程序,将患者与滥用者分开(见第23章)。

发现泻药滥用影响的结局研究很少。在一项包含11例患者的小型研究中,6例患者表示有所改善,5例声称无获益,5例未改善患者中的4例因慢性腹泻在其他地方寻求进一步医疗护理[211]。

(八) 特发性分泌性腹泻

当详尽的评估未能揭示慢性腹泻的原因,且粪便分析提示分泌性腹泻时,诊断为特发性分泌性腹泻。这种情况通常在平素健康的人中突发,通过持续超过4周与许多类似的急性腹泻疾病相鉴别。该病以两种形式发生:流行性和散发性[80,81]。

分泌性腹泻的流行形式,发生在似乎与受污染的食物或饮料有关的暴发中[80,212-216]。最先暴发这种流行性分泌性腹泻的地方是明尼苏达州布雷纳德,故常被称为布雷纳德腹泻。文献记载了几种不同社区的暴发。尽管流行病学提示感染原因,但在这些暴发中尚未确定病原体。

散发性特发性分泌性腹泻以与流行形式相同的方式影响个体,但似乎不容易被患者的家庭成员或其他人获得[81]。许多受影响的人有旅行史,但去通常与旅行者腹泻无关的目的地。腹泻突然开始,发病后很快达到最大强度。体重减轻高达9kg是其特征,几乎总是发生在患病的前几个月内,而不是患病后。抗生素和胆汁酸结合树脂的经验性试验无效。非特异性阿片类止泻药可改善症状。

两种形式的特发性分泌性腹泻均有自限性病程,通常在发病2年内消退。特发性分泌性腹泻在2~3个月内逐渐消退。了解这一自然史可以安慰患者,否则他们可能会觉得陷入无休止的疾病中。特发性分泌性腹泻可能具有与功能性腹泻相同的几个临床特征,但通常发病更离散,并与较多的大便量相关。

(九) 不明原因腹泻

尽管进行了详细的评估,医生有时还是不能对慢性腹泻患者作出特定的诊断，并可能将这些患者转诊到更专业的医疗中心。这些患者重新评估后得到的常见诊断见框 16.12。

框 16.12 不明原因腹泻患者的常见诊断
胆汁酸性腹泻
碳水化合物吸收不良性腹泻
慢性特发性分泌性腹泻
大便失禁
功能性腹泻
医源性腹泻(药物、放疗、手术)
肠易激综合征
显微镜下结肠炎
胰腺外分泌功能不全
多肽分泌性肿瘤
SIBO
隐匿性摄入泻药
SIBO，小肠细菌过度生长。

尽管在这组患者中需要特殊检查的不寻常或不明原因的疾病占主导地位，但大多数患者最终诊断是直截了当的，可能很早就作出诊断[120]。通过仔细的病史采集可以识别大便失禁和医源性腹泻。隐匿性泻药摄入和显微镜下结肠炎，可通过适当的怀疑指数和检测(分别为泻药筛检和结肠活检)进行诊断。BAD、SIBO、胰腺外分泌不足和碳水化合物吸收不良均可通过详细的病史和正确进行的试验性治疗作出诊断。肽分泌肿瘤罕见，但血清肽测定和影像学技术(如 CT、奥曲肽扫描)是广泛可用的。未能作出诊断通常是由于没有充分了解手头的证据和思考慢性腹泻的鉴别诊断。

(韩跃华 译，鲁晓岚 刘军 校)

参考文献

第 17 章　肠道气体

Fernando Azpiroz 著

章节目录

一、胃肠道气体的组成和体积 ………………………… 213
二、气体代谢与排泄 ……………………………………… 214
（一）气体在肠腔和血液之间的扩散 …………… 214
（二）从口到胃 ……………………………………… 214
（三）小肠 …………………………………………… 215
（四）结肠 …………………………………………… 215
（五）肛门排气 ……………………………………… 216
三、肠道推进、调节和对气体的耐受性 ………………… 216
四、临床气体问题 ………………………………………… 217
（一）反复嗳气 ……………………………………… 217
（二）胃肠胀气 ……………………………………… 217
（三）排气障碍 ……………………………………… 218
（四）腹胀 …………………………………………… 218
（五）肠壁囊样积气症 ……………………………… 219

尽管临床实践中遇到许多患者主诉出现肠道气体，但直到 20 世纪 60 年代，医学博士 Michael Levitt 及其同事的研究开始阐明肠道气体的病理生理学，才开始对这一主题进行系统研究[1]。

一、胃肠道气体的组成和体积

正常情况下，胃肠道含有相对少量的气体。肠腔内气体的体积取决于气体输入和输出之间的平衡，这是一个高度动态的过程。气体输入可能来自吞咽、化学反应、细菌发酵和血液扩散，而输出涉及呃逆、细菌消耗、血液吸收和肛门排泄。尽管有各种各样的因素，但在健康人群中，胃肠道内的气体量是相当稳定的，并且成分相似[2]，这说明它受到严密的自我平衡控制。可以使用专门设计的 CT 技术测量肠道气体体积[2-4]。数据采集过程相对简单，但分析相当复杂且经过仔细验证，这项技术证实了先前其他方法获得的测量结果，即空腹状态下大约有 100~200mL 的气体，进餐后的体积更大（增加 65%）（图 17.1 和图 17.2）。

气体成分分析不仅在技术上具有挑战性，而且可获得的数据比较少，也相对比较陈旧。在一项针对 10 名健康空腹受试者的研究中，研究人员采用冲洗技术评估了胃肠道内气体的组成，通过消化道置管将氩气快速注入空肠中以排出肠道气体，通过直肠管收集排出的气体，然后进行分析。99% 以上的肠道气体为 N_2、O_2、CO_2、H_2 和甲烷（CH_4），其他气体含量极微。禁食期间，肠道气体以 N_2 为主，O_2 浓度较低，CO_2、H_2、CH_4 浓度变化较大。后 3 种气体与食物残渣发酵相关，可能为餐后肠道气体的主要成分（见下文）。

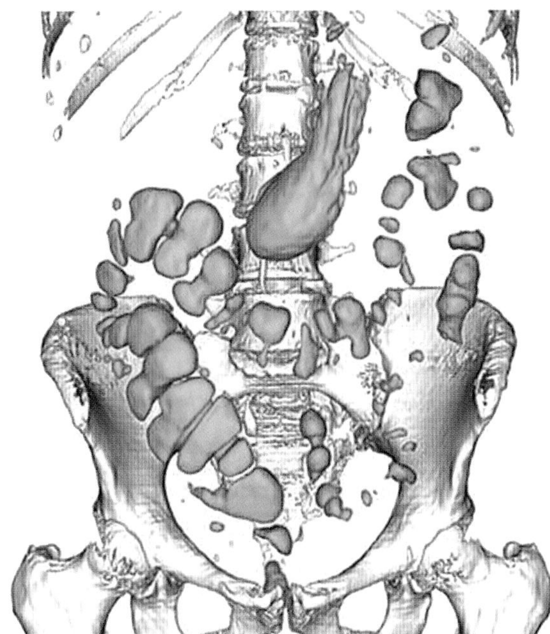
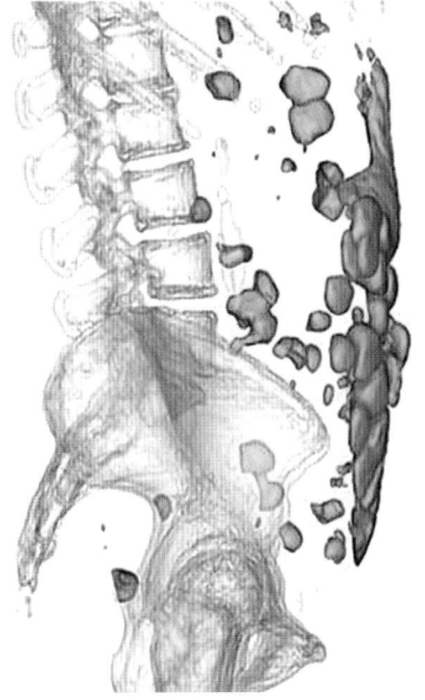

图 17.1　健康受试者仰卧位腹部气体含量（绿色）的 CT 图像分析。左图显示前视图。侧位（右）注意仰卧位时，大多数管腔气体位于近前腹壁附近。（From Accarino A，Perez F，Azpiroz F，et al. Intestinal gas and bloating：effect of prokinetic stimulation. Am J Gastroenterol 2008；103：2036-42.）

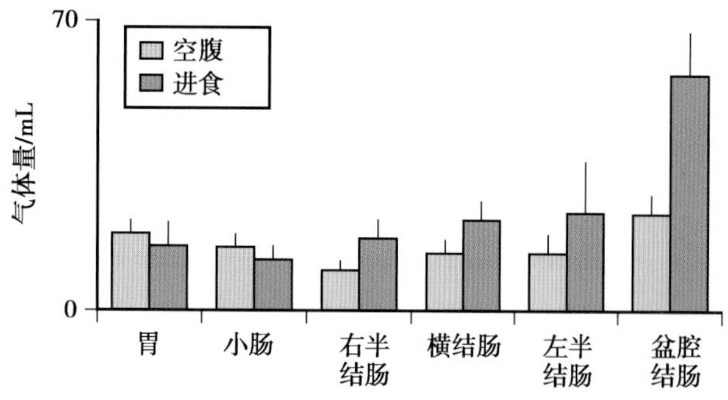

图 17.2　通过 CT 容量分析确定空腹和进食状态下胃肠道不同节段的腹部气体体积。餐后肠道气体增加主要位于结肠的盆腔部分。(From Perez F, Accarino A, Azpiroz F, et al. Gas distribution within the human gut: effect of meals. Am J Gastroenterol 2007;102:842-9.)

二、气体代谢与排泄

胃肠道气体分布在 3 个部位：胃、小肠和结肠。在每个部分，气体的体积和组成取决于气体的代谢和气体在消化道管腔内和血液之间的扩散。消化道一个部位的部分气体被推动至下一个部位，最终从肛门排出。图 17.3 示意性地描述了气体在胃肠道各分段的稳态平衡。

（一）气体在肠腔和血液之间的扩散

每种气体的扩散速度和方向与扩散率，管腔与血液之间的分压差以及气体在黏膜表面的暴露面积有关。气体在胃肠道黏膜上的扩散率取决于它在水中的溶解度。在给定的分压差下，CO_2 的扩散速度远远快于 H_2、CH_4、N_2 和 O_2。若腔内气体的分压(浓度)高于静脉血液，气体进入循环，反之亦然。气体的吸收也取决于气体在黏膜表面的暴露面积及时间。从肠道吸收的 H_2 和 CH_4 不会被人体代谢，而是通过呼出空气排出。呼吸分析提供了一种简单的方法来评估这些气体在消化道的产生过程。呼出的 H_2 和 CH_4 量是肺泡通气率和肺泡中浓度的乘积。由于静止状态下肺泡通气相对稳定，肺泡呼气末 H_2 和 CH_4 浓度可作为其总呼吸 H_2 排泄量的简单指标。

（二）从口到胃

胃通常含有相对少量的气体(约 10~20mL)[2]。它在胃中的位置是由浮力和重力决定的。在直立时，气体在胃底形成一个气泡。相反，仰卧位时，气体在靠近腹壁的胃体和胃窦

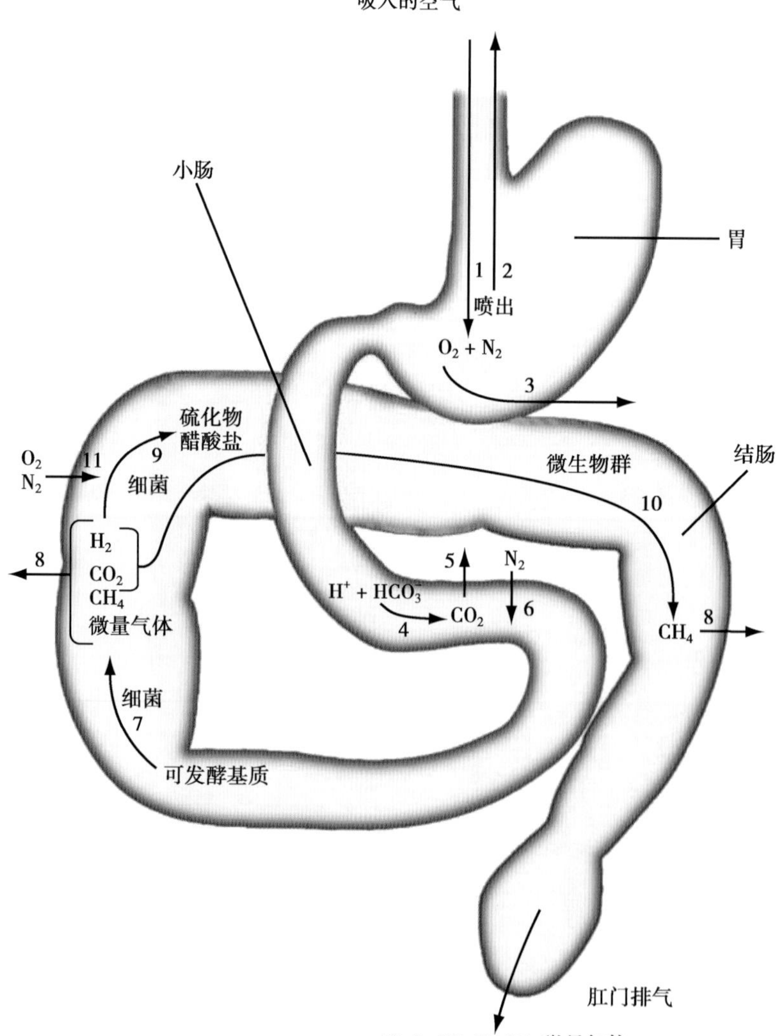

图 17.3　肠道气体的进入和消除机制。吞咽空气(1)，并被吸收入相当一部分(2)。吞咽空气中的部分氧气扩散到胃黏膜(3)。十二指肠中反应产生大量气体的 CO_2(4)，这些 CO_2 扩散到血液中(5)，而 N_2 沿着 CO_2 产生建立梯度向下融合到管腔中(6)。在结肠中，产气微生物发酵未被吸收的残留物(7)，从而释放 CO_2、H_2 和 CH_4，以及各种微量气体(8)。很大一部分 H_2 被其他微生物消耗，使硫酸盐还原为硫化物，将 CO_2 还原为醋酸盐(9)，将 CO_2 还原为 CH_4(10)，从而减少细菌代谢产生的气体净体积。N_2 和 O_2 从血液扩散到结肠腔，沿着细菌产气产生的梯度扩散(11)。气体通常沿胃肠道向下不断推进，并经肛门排出。所有这些过程的最终结果决定了不同胃肠道中气体的体积和组成

前壁形成一层薄膜(见图 17.1)。吞咽的空气(而不是管腔内产生)是胃内空气的主要来源,这也是晚期失弛缓症患者没有胃泡的原因(见第 44 章),但正常吞咽的空气量尚不明确。空气通过嗳气、吸收或排空进入十二指肠而离开胃。嗳气的过程已有很明确的记录,但是几乎没有任何气体通过胃黏膜或进入十二指肠过程的相关信息。与血液相比,吞咽的空气中 CO_2 的比例较低,O_2 的比例较高,理论上 CO_2 应从血液中扩散到胃,O_2 从胃腔中扩散到血液。由于 N_2 在黏膜中的扩散性很差,整个胃肠道中的 N_2 可能来自吞咽的空气。

(三) 小肠

小肠内通常存在 10~20mL 的气体,一般以小气泡的形式分布在肠腔内[2,5]。腹部立位平片中的气液平提示液体位于气泡下方,这是存在异常液体潴留的表现,如肠梗阻和狭窄(见第 123 和 124 章)。理论上,在小肠上部,碳酸氢盐和酸的相互作用释放大量二氧化碳。然而,基于 CT 容积分析的研究未发现餐后小肠气体体积的变化[2]。产生的气体应该扩散到血液中(这对二氧化碳来说是合理的)或者被输送到结肠。因此在餐后可以观察到结肠气体体积是微量增加的。在正常情况下,小肠微生物产生的气体微不足道,但这一结论缺乏直接证据。肠梗阻或假性梗阻(运动障碍)患者的小肠内产生大量气体,但这种积聚的来源和机制尚不清楚。

(四) 结肠

结肠通常含有 50~100mL 的气体(见图 17.2)[2,6]。一项基于 CT 图像比较禁食期间和餐后 99±22 分钟气体含量的研究显示盆腔结肠中气体含量的增加(见图 17.2)比预期食物残渣在结肠中发酵产生的气体要早。因此,胃肠道近端产生的气体(N_2 或 CO_2)可能是在进食后通过胃回肠反射被推进至结肠。然而,结肠气体主要来源于微生物群的代谢活动,并通过黏膜吸收、微生物群气体消耗和肛门排泄来消除。随着人们对肠道菌群的日益关注,对肠道气体产生和排出的研究变得尤为重要,因为它反映了肠道微生物群的代谢活动。

1. 结肠腔内微环境和气体代谢

消化道的上部主要具有营养功能:通过消化吸收过程从摄取的物质中提取出有用的成分,如营养素、水和矿物质。未吸收的残留物进入结肠后作为结肠微生物群的底物。这些微生物群有与宿主发育和体内稳态相关的关键作用(见第 3 章)。因此,结肠是一种"袋状结构",它为体内最大比例的微生物群提供了合适的环境,从而成为一个复杂的代谢器官。

微生物群对可发酵食物残渣的代谢产生一系列代谢物(包括气体)的释放,这些代谢物又作为微生物群其他亚群的底物。因此,结肠含有大量的活性物质,包括微生物群、食物残渣和动态代谢反应链中的次级代谢产物。研究表明,结肠含有 500~800mL 的生物量,这取决于每日动态周转量为 100~200mL 的饮食残渣,即粪便输出量(图 17.4)[6,7]。随着可发酵残留物进入结肠,气体生成量就会增加,但是代谢活性逐渐下降,在底物可用的情况下可持续数小时,连续进餐后的残渣有助于产气(图 17.5)[8]。因此,禁食期间的基础气体生成量取决于结肠内容物,而结肠内容物来源于前几天的饮食。产生的气体量取决于饮食中未被吸收的可发酵残留物的数量。目前对饮食中促进肠道气体生成的特定食物和产品的了解很有限,且大多是经验性的。

一些结肠微生物消耗腔内气体(H_2、CO_2 和 O_2),这种分解代谢可能占腔内气体消耗的一部分。下列 3 种微生物消耗 H_2:产乙酸菌、硫酸盐还原菌和产甲烷菌[9]。产乙酸菌消耗 H_2 和 CO_2 合成短链脂肪酸。硫酸盐还原菌利用 H_2 将硫酸盐还原为硫化物。产甲烷菌利用 H_2 将二氧化碳还原为 CH_4[10]。只有约 40% 的成年人有足够浓度的产甲烷菌能产生可检测到的呼吸 CH_4 浓度。

产甲烷菌比其他耗 H_2 微生物更快地氧化 H_2。一些人无法增加 H_2 呼出量可能反映了产甲烷菌对 H_2 的高消耗,而并非不能产生 H_2。据报道,便秘患者的产甲烷程度很高,相关的解释是便秘患者的结肠运输缓慢会促进产甲烷菌的增殖,CH_4 反过来会减缓肠道运输[10]。

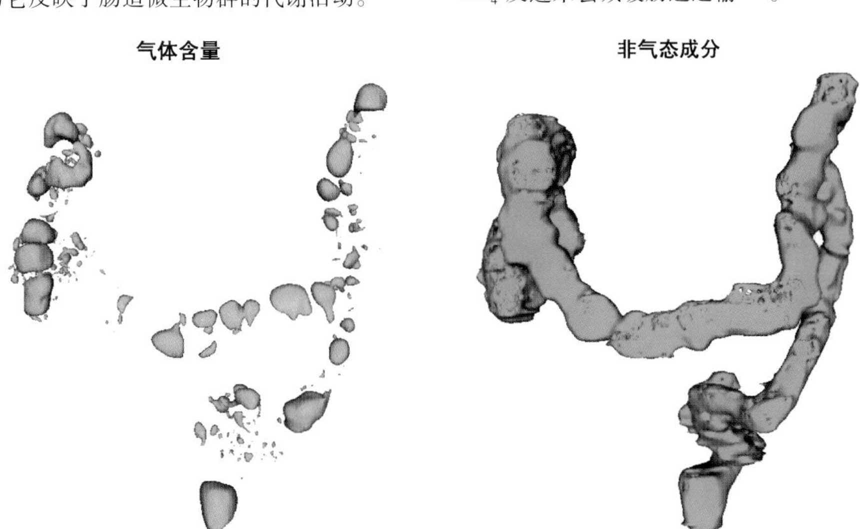

图 17.4 健康受试者 CT 上结肠内容物的气体和非气体成分的独立表现。(From Bendezu RA, Mego M, Monclus E, et al. Colonic content: effect of diet, meals, and defecation Neurogastroenterol Motil 2017;29(2)).

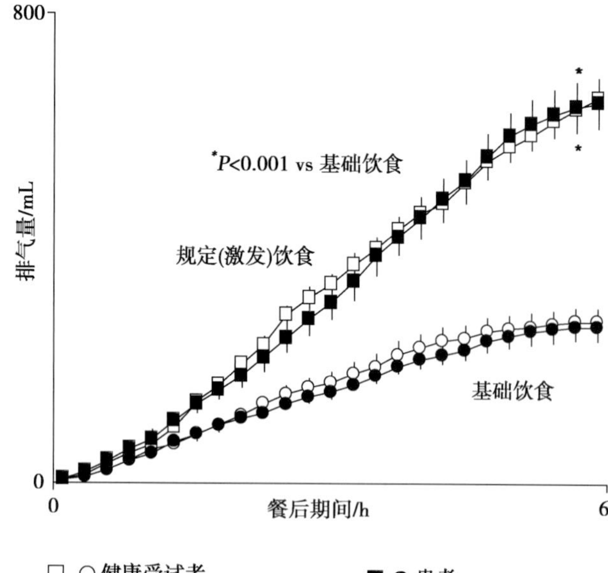

图 17.5　餐后直肠气体采集。高胀气激发餐后排气增加，但健康受试者和主诉胀气的患者相似。显示了探针餐后的累积数据(平均值±SE)。(From Manichanh C, Eck A, Varela E, et al. Anal gas evacuation and colonic microbiota in patients with flatulence: effect of diet. Gut 2014;63:401-8.)

2. 微生物群的可塑性和气体代谢

结肠菌群的组成(包括在特定饮食中产生的气体量)在个体之间有很大的差异，这取决于早期的环境条件以及后期生活中遇到的因素，如饮食和抗生素暴露[11]。即使是在同一个体中，饮食习惯也会影响微生物群的组成：富含纤维的饮食增加了多样性，而低发酵残留物的饮食则会产生相反的效果[12-14]。一项在健康受试者中进行的研究表明，进食 3 天富含促胃肠道胀气的残留物饮食会增加产甲烷菌的相对丰度。例如，长期摄入高剂量肠道吸收不良的双糖(如便秘患者的乳果糖，或肠道乳糖酶缺乏者摄入乳糖)之后，在相同双糖剂量时 H_2 的呼出量会减少[15]。这一现象可能是由诸如双歧杆菌等微生物在结肠增殖的结果，这些微生物通过非 H_2 释放途径或耗 H_2 途径发酵乳糖或乳果糖。

同样，口服具有益生元性质的低聚半乳糖可增加肠道内产生的气体量；在随后的 3 周给药期间，气体容量下降至基线水平[5]。可以想象，最初气体产量的增加是由于益生元的发酵，随后的下降是由于微生物群的适应。在给药期结束时，确实可以检测到微生物群的组成变化[16]。另一项研究表明，微生物群对益生元消耗的规律性适应涉及微生物群代谢向低产气途径的转变，而气体消耗活性无明显上调[17]。

3. 有气味的气体

肠道中容积较大的气体都没有气味；粪便的难闻气味是由微量气体引起的。肛门排气中有害气味的强度与硫化氢和甲硫醇的浓度有关[18]。有气味的气体很难研究，因为它们会穿过橡胶或塑料薄膜，而其他气体无法通透。例如，这些气体从结肠内环境扩散到用空气充气的直肠内乳胶球囊中，通过放气球囊回收的空气具有这些气体特有的气味。

(五) 肛门排气

未被吸收或代谢的肠道气体通过肛门排出。因此，肛门排气是整个胃肠道气体动力学的净结果，但事实上，肛门排气在很大程度上是由结肠气体稳态决定的。一项针对 20 名健康受试者的研究表明，在正常饮食情况下，早餐后 6 小时的气体排出量约为 40mL/h 时；在高胃肠道产气的饮食结构中，多渣饮食后的气体排出率增加到 120mL/h 左右(见图 17.5)[12]。这些数据证实了之前用不同饮食进行的观察实验结果。正常饮食的健康受试者在一天中肛门排气的平均次数约为 10 次，最高上限约为 20 次[12,16]。在高胃肠道产气的饮食结构中，排泄量要高出 2~3 倍。年龄和性别与肛门排气频率均无显著相关性。

每人每天肛门排出约 200mL 氮气，与饮食无关。排出的氧气体积要小得多，而且不受饮食的影响[19,20]。目前尚不清楚肛门排气中具体多少 N_2 和 O_2 来自吞咽的空气或者血液的扩散。从肛门(产甲烷菌群的受试者)排出的 H_2、CO_2 和 CH_4 的体积变化很大，这取决于结肠中的发酵活性。在结肠中存在可发酵残留物时，这些气体的体积增加。反之，在 48 小时流质无渣饮食后，肛门排气中的 H_2、CO_2 和 CH_4 几乎消失[20]。

研究使用冲洗技术测量了肠道内产生的内源性气体的体积。直接将标记的外源性气体高速输注到空肠中，将内源性气体从肠道中冲洗出来，从而阻止其吸收和消耗[16,21]。为了确定从管腔排出的内源性气体的比例，在配对研究中，比较了有和没有气体冲洗的肛门收集的内源性气体体积；在冲洗实验中测量的内源性气体体积近似于产生的气体的总体积，而通过肛门排出的气体在基础实验(无冲洗)中反映的是腔内消除与气体产生之间的净过量。这些研究一致表明，大部分餐后产生的气体是吸收入血液并通过呼吸排出或通过消耗气体的微生物从肠腔中迅速排出，只有小部分(约 20%~25%)从肛门被排出；然而，在这些实验中，吸收与消耗的气体清除比例没有进行区分。

在一项经典研究中，对密闭环境中的成年受试者进行了直肠和呼吸 H_2 排泄的长期同步测量[22]，发现通过肠道吸收和肛门排空排出的气体(尤其是 H_2、CO_2 和 CH_4)的比例取决于产气量。当 H_2 生成较低时，呼出量占总 H_2 排出量的 65%，肛门排出量占总 H_2 排出量的 35%；然而，当 H_2 产生较多时，只有 20% 通过呼吸排出，大部分(80%)通过肛门排出。由于 H_2 在肠道的吸收过程是不饱和的，因此呼出 H_2 比例的下降可能是由于气体更快地推进至肛门的结果。同样的，在高产气量和肛门快速排空期间，肛门排气中的二氧化碳浓度往往最高。

三、肠道推进、调节和对气体的耐受性

肠道气体的推进是决定胃肠道各节段气体体积和总体积的关键因素。气体的传输决定了其在肠腔内的停留时间，气体的吸收、细菌的消耗和从肛门排出的气体成分都受传输时间影响。在某些情况下，肛门气体排出量的增加可能与肠道气体推进力的增加有关，而不是与产气的增加有关。气体在肠道内的运动可以通过肠道气体输注的实验模型研究，但目前尚不清楚在正常情况下有多少气体从一个胃肠管腔流动至下一个管腔。与胃贲门可出现嗳气相反，正常的回盲瓣

即使在结肠的充气实验中也不允许气体回流至回肠[23]。

肠道气体输送和耐受性可通过气体激发试验进行测量，在该试验中，将混合气体持续注入空肠，并量化肛门排出的气体。一项使用高达 30mL/min（1.8L/h）输注速率的剂量-反应研究显示，大多数健康受试者在输注气体的同时迅速排出气体，几乎没有或根本没有任何不适[24]。气体的传输，就像固体和液体的传输一样，受到一系列反射机制的调节。肠内营养物质，尤其是脂质，可以延缓气体传输[25]，而机械刺激（如轻度直肠扩张）则具有很强的促动力作用[26]。气体在胃肠道内的移动速度远远快于固体和液体，但决定气体传输的胃肠道运动类型尚不清楚。可以想象，大量低阻力气体的运动和置换是由肠道的强直运动和容量的细微变化引起的，而这些变化不影响固体和液体的运动[27]。这种活动可以通过恒压器[26,27]而不是传统的压力测量法检测。传输到左结肠的气体会引起强烈的蠕动收缩，导致小部分气体排出[28]，但是直肠在持续输注气体期间没有观察到这种类型的阵发性收缩。这些阵发性收缩可能是肠腔内气体突然释放引起的局部膨胀反应。

气体传输通常是有效的，但当一定数量的气体滞留在胃肠道内时，受试者可能会出现腹胀和其他症状。不同的气体滞留实验模型表明，虽然腹胀与胃肠道内的气体量有关，但对腹部症状的感知取决于肠道运动和肠腔内气体的分布[29,30]。肠道气体滞留刺激腹部调节反射，使前腹壁和膈肌的肌肉活动适应容量负荷。在健康人群中，大量结肠气体滞留在并不会使腹围大幅度增加，因为前腹壁收缩和膈肌松弛，从而使腹腔向头侧方向扩大[31]。胸腔也参与调节反射：膈肌向头侧移动引起肋间收缩和胸壁代偿性扩张，以减少对肺容积和肺功能的影响[32]。因此，这种腹-膈-胸廓的协调限制了由于肠道内气体滞留而导致的腹围增加。

四、临床气体问题

患者经常诉说有关于气体的问题，临床医生的第一步是确定患者是指慢性嗳气、排出过多气体、有气味的排气或呼吸、肛门排气障碍，还是腹部胀气和可见的腹胀。这些诉说中的每一种都具有不同的病理生理学和治疗。已经开发了用于评价气体相关症状的特定问卷[33]。

（一）反复嗳气

1. 病理生理学

偶尔的嗳气会从胃里排出与摄入的固体或液体一起吞咽的空气。反复嗳气是由于无意或强迫性地将空气吸入下咽和食管，其中大部分空气在到达胃之前立即排出[34]；空气吸入食管可能是通过咽部注入、胸腔抽吸或两者兼而有之产生的[34,35]。Bredenoord 和 Smout 提出了吞气症（吞咽空气）和胃嗳气（从胃中排出空气）这两个术语，与"胃上嗳气"（反复嗳气吸入食管的空气）相反，尽管尚不清楚吸入的空气是否能到达胃。事实上，"胃上嗳气"可引起反流发作的反流[34,35]。

重复嗳气经常由情绪压力触发，持续嗳气经常在进食后发生；在一部分病例中，详细询问病史能发现潜在的餐后消化不良症状，而患者误认为胃内气体过多。如果吞入的空气进入胃，可能会加重不适感。嗳气可缓解部分症状，并强化患者的错误印象，从而形成恶性循环。因此，慢性嗳气是一种行为障碍，对于有相关症状或体征提示胸部或腹部病变的患者，应进行放射学检查和内镜评估。目前尚不清楚这些患者为什么以及如何学会这个动作并养成这种习惯。在一些吞气症患者中，吞咽的空气可能会进入肠道，主诉可能变为腹胀而不是持续嗳气[34,36]。胃食管反流病患者在胃底折叠术后因嗳气困难可能会导致"胀气综合征"（见第 46 章）。

2. 治疗

治疗反复嗳气首先应向患者提供明确的病理生理学解释：问题在于吞咽空气，而不是胃肠道内产生的气体。通过了解慢性嗳气的良性特质可以减少痛苦。可通过行为指导患者避免嗳气；在反复嗳气发作期间，用牙齿咬住铅笔可以有助于患者意识到吞咽并停止周期循环。如果有潜在的消化不良症状也应进行治疗（见第 14 章）。只有严重的难治性病例才建议进行精神科会诊。

（二）胃肠胀气

1. 病理生理学

少数人的过度胃肠胀气可能是由于碳水化合物吸收不良（例如乳糖吸收不良、乳糜泻）所致。吞咽空气引起的严重胃肠胀气有个案报道[37]，但是罕见。一项对 30 名主诉为肛门排气过多的患者的研究显示，部分患者的主观感受并没有完全得到客观测量的证实，用事件标记测量的日间排气量在正常范围内[12]。另一方面，当具体细致地询问时，大多数情况下胃肠胀气多与其他胃肠道症状相关，尤其是腹部胀气。有趣的是，无论是正常测量还是多通道测量，胃肠胀气患者在餐后收集的气体体积与健康受试者相似（见图 17.5）。有功能性胃肠道症状的患者结肠和直肠感觉有所增强（内脏高敏感性）（见第 122 章）[13,38]，这一发现可以解释为何直肠对气体的耐受性更低且排空更有效[39]。更频繁的少量排气可能是对直肠气体感觉的一种行为反应。基于 CT 的肠道气体容量分析，排除了在试验餐后气体仍保留在结肠内的可能性[12]。内源性黏液可能是一种可发酵的底物[40]；这一发现可以解释在小肠细菌过度生长（见第 105 章）和未经治疗的乳糜泻（见第 107 章）中观察到的空腹高 H_2 排泄。

2. 治疗

对有明确病因导致肠道碳水化合物吸收不良的患者（例如乳糖吸收不良，乳糜泻），治疗基础疾病可减少气体的产生。功能性胃肠胀气（即没有明显的肠吸收缺陷）的患者，低产气饮食可以有效地减少气体产生。虽然这些患者的基础产气量在正常范围内，但是减少这些患者的气体产生可显著改善主观的胃肠胀气与腹部症状。对气体排泄过多或正常的基础饮食的患者来说，情况也有类似改善，这表明可能与低产气饮食的膨化效应有关[12]。

虽然有许多关于食物产生气体的观点，但是关于饮食影响肛门排气的科学数据很少[41]。为结肠细菌提供少量底物的食物包括蛋白质（如肉、禽、鱼、蛋）和某些碳水化合物（如无麸质面包、大米、大米面包）。增加产气的食物包括豆类、包心菜、洋葱、芹菜、胡萝卜、葡萄干、香蕉、可发酵纤维以及小麦和马铃薯等复杂淀粉。水果和蔬菜（尤其是豆类）含有不易消化的低聚糖，如水苏糖和棉子糖，很容易被结肠细菌发酵[42]。大豆中的胰淀粉酶抑制剂减缓淀粉的消化和吸收[43]。虽然一项研究表明标准剂量的车前草可使 H_2 排泄量略有增加，但是可发酵纤维也为气体产生提供了基质[44]。软饮料和山梨醇（一种低热量的糖替代品）中的果糖可能无法被小肠吸收，但它们对结肠产气的实际作用尚不确定。选择性限制某些特定的食物，如洋葱和大蒜，可以减少气味气体，但缺乏实验证据。一般来说，经过一周的低产气饮食，患者通常会出现症状缓解[45]。通过有序地重新摄入被淘汰的食物，患者可以学会识别出有问题的膳食成分。

低发酵寡糖、双糖、单糖和多元醇（FODMAP）的饮食概念开始流行，这些饮食设计复杂，操作烦琐，相比简单的低渣饮食，似乎没有明显的优势[40,46-49]。一些数据表明，限制型FODMAP 对肠道益生菌有害[50]，尚不清楚其他低渣饮食是否也是如此（见第 122 章）。同样，在没有乳糜泻或小麦不耐受的情况下，几乎没有实验支持无麸质饮食（见第 107 章）。

β-半乳糖苷酶商业制剂（如 Beano）可以增强对豆类和其他蔬菜中的难消化的低聚糖的分解[51]，但仅在液体制剂中证实有效，而含有这种酶的片剂可能无效。二甲硅油具有消泡性能，可以消除气泡[52]，但不会减少气体体积。据报道，活性炭可减少呼出的 H_2[53]，但另一项研究显示，木炭并不能与 H_2（包括其他肠道主要气体）结合，也不会减少呼出的 H_2[54]。高剂量的水杨酸铋可以减少臭气，但是潜在毒性限制了其使用[55]。几种商用设备（床垫、护垫、内衣）用活性炭吸附异味气体；事实证明，床垫的效果不如护垫或内衣[56]。

抗生素，尤其是利福昔明，已证实可减少肠道气体产生[57]，但尚不明确是否可减少直肠排气。鉴于长期抗生素治疗带来的问题以及缺乏明确的疗效，使用抗生素控制胃肠胀气患者的肠道菌群是不可取的。益生元和益生菌调节结肠菌群的组成，从而减少肛门排气。如前所述，低聚半乳糖类益生元诱导结肠微生物群适应，从而降低产气代谢[16,17]。一项研究表明，持续 4 周摄入益生元的获益类似于低 FODMAP 饮食；这种改善在停服益生元后持续了 2 周，但在停止低 FODMAP 饮食后观察到反弹效应[58]。是否只有这种低聚半乳糖类益生元具有这种益处尚不明确。

（三）排气障碍

与胃肠胀气过多的患者相比，一些患者的气体滞留与排便障碍有关。正常情况下，气体的排出由腹内压力的轻微增加和肛门的放松共同完成[65]。这一过程的不协调会导致功能性出口梗阻，可能与排气困难和便秘有关（见第 19 章）。粪便滞留延长结肠发酵过程，增加产气量。肛门排气功能受损导致气体滞留的患者会受益于生物反馈治疗，可以改善排气和排便功能，也可能改善相关的腹部症状，尤其是腹胀。

（四）腹胀

1. 病理生理学

由过多气体引起的症状（如腹胀、腹部胀气）是胃肠道疾病中最常见的症状之一[59]。腹胀是指腹部压力增加的感觉。腹部扩张是指腹围客观增大，事实上，“可见性腹胀”这个词似乎更准确。腹胀通常发生在餐后或睡前，经过一夜的休息后会缓解。电感容积描记法和 CT 的测量可客观地证明腹胀发作时腹围明显增加（图 17.6）[3,60-63]。一些肠易激综合征的患者，特别是直肠高敏患者，在没有客观扩张的情况下也会有腹胀（见 122 章）[60]。

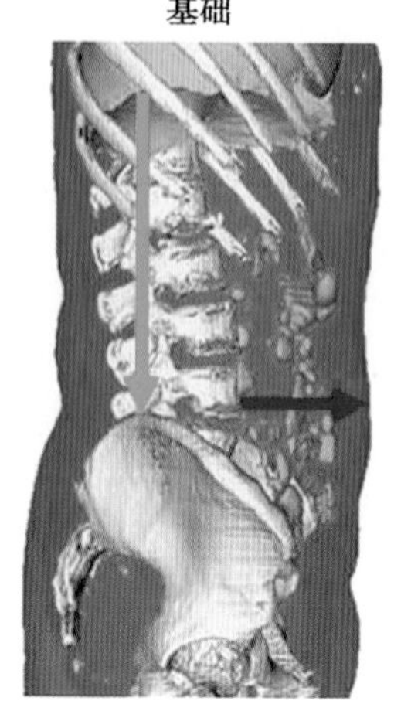

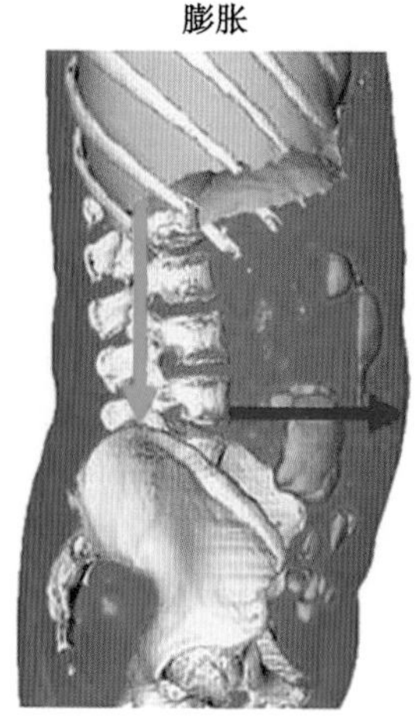

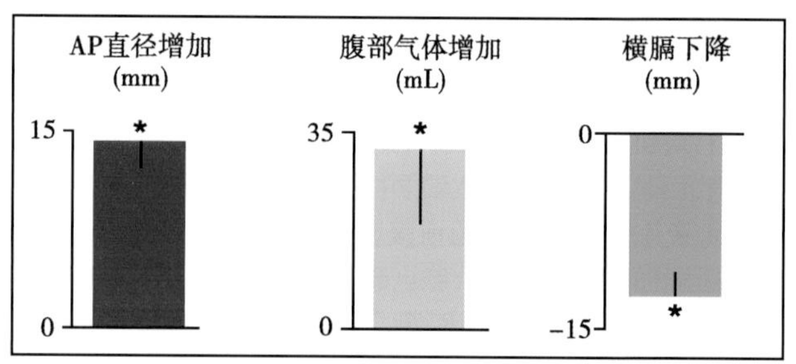

图 17.6　功能性腹胀的机制。上图，同一患者在基础状态（无腹胀）和腹胀发作期间的 CT 图像。下图，膨胀期间与基础条件的差异（$n=47$）。注意前后位（AP）腹部直径增加（红色）、腹部气体增加（蓝色）和膈肌下降（绿色）；所有变化均具有统计学意义（*）。（Adapted from Accarino A，Perez F，Azpiroz F，et al. Abdominal distension results from caudo-ventral redistribution of contents. Gastroenterology 2009；136：1544-51.）

频繁腹胀的肠易激综合征患者由于小肠细菌过度生长或肠道吸收不良而产生了更多的气体（见第 105 和 122 章）。然而，这一发现没有得到其他设计严密的研究支持[64,65]。研究表明，腹胀患者的肠道气体净产生量和腹部气体的含量与健康受试者相似[63,66]。然而，在严重运动障碍的患者中能观察到过量的气体，如慢性假性肠梗阻（见第 124 章）[67]；这种肠道神经病变或肌肉病变罕见，常见于转诊中心（图 17.7）。

多项肠内输注气体的研究均表明腹胀患者对输注气体的处理能力下降。在应对外源性气体负荷时，这些患者出现气体滞留、腹部症状或两者兼而有之[66,68-71]。这些异常明显反映了肠易激综合征患者对气体传输的反射控制受损[25,72-75]，以及对肠道扩张的高敏性[38]。因此，气体传输研究似乎提供了一种敏感的方法，可以识别传统诊断方法无法检测到的细微肠道运动障碍。

虽然前面描述了气体推进异常，但是没有发现与症状相关的肠道气体体积和分布异常[5,6]。一项针对肠易激综合征

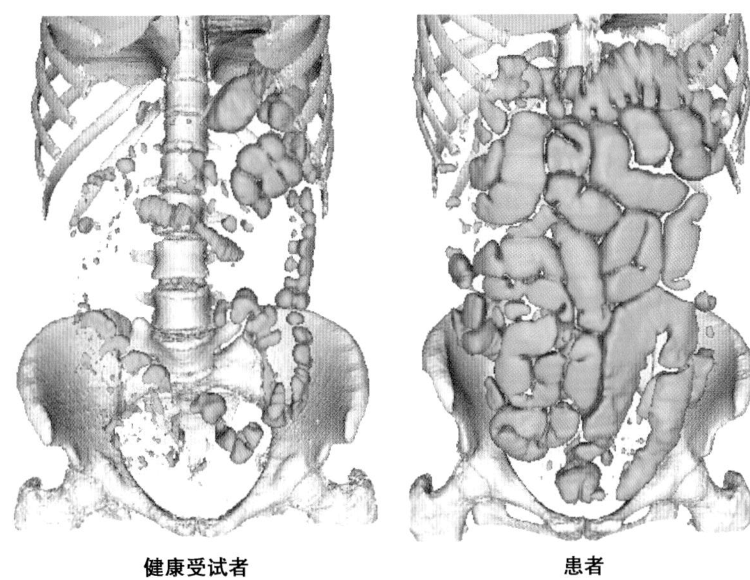

图 17.7 健康受试者和肠动力障碍患者 CT 图像的三维重建。与健康受试者相比，肠动力障碍患者存在大量气体汇聚（蓝色），尤其是小肠。（From Barba E, Quiroga S, Accarino A, et al. Mechanisms of abdominal distension in severe intestinal dysmotility: abdomino-thoracic response to gut retention. Neurogastroenterol Motil 2013;25:e389-94.）

（IBS）患者的研究比较了基础条件下和腹胀发作期间的腹部 CT 图像，证明腹胀的感觉与腹部前后径的增加和膈肌明显下降相关，肠道气体含量仅略有增加（见图 17.6）[63]。对大量患者肠道气体分布的分析未能发现异常情况，例如，在大多数有症状的患者中仅有局部气体积聚[5]；同样，结肠生物量也未检测到异常[6]。肌电图研究表明，腹部通过协调的腹部膈肌运动适应腹内容物的增加[31]。伴有腹胀的 IBS 患者有矛盾的膈肌收缩和前壁松弛，无法协调该反应[76,77]。虽然对腹部内容物的正常调节似乎是反射反应，但是一些数据表明腹胀患者的异常调节是一种行为反应，因为它可以通过生物反馈技术逆转[63,78,79]。触发这种条件反射的因素尚不清楚，对于健康受试者来说耐受良好的肠道内容物轻微增加据推测可能会导致高敏患者产生胀气感，并引发躯体条件反射，导致明显腹胀。

2. 治疗

因为腹胀的患者似乎是 IBS 的一种常见变异亚型，治疗的基本方法与 IBS 相似（见第 122 章）。

（1）非药物疗法

轻度运动和直立的姿势可以增加肠道对灌注气体的清除能力，这可以解释为什么活动相对于仰卧休息，更能改善部分患者的腹胀[80-82]。虽然腹胀患者的肠道气体量几乎是正常的，但是他们的肠道对肠道内容物的高敏感性表明将气体的产生限制在最低限度是有益的。因此，饮食控制以减少气体产生（如前所述）可能是有益的。治疗便秘可减少腹部扩张并改善腹胀。一些证据表明，使用益生菌能减轻 IBS 的症状，特别是腹胀[83,84]。但是益生菌的效果差异较大，取决于使用的细菌种类、剂量、治疗持续时间和评估终点。催眠也可以减轻 IBS 的症状，包括腹胀[85]。使用基于肌电图的生物反馈技术可以帮助“可见性腹胀”患者矫正膈肌和前腹壁的活动[21,26]。

（2）药物疗法

虽然研究表明抗生素，特别是利福昔明，可以减轻 IBS 的症状[57]，但是抗生素治疗后最先出现的副作用可能也是肠易激综合征[79]。利福昔明治疗腹部气体症状方面的有效性仍存在争议。

据报道，新斯的明是一种有效的促动力药物剂，可减轻肠内输注气体引起的腹部症状[69]。长期服用溴吡斯的明可改善腹胀患者的症状，但对肠道气体的影响微乎其微[4]。其他促动力药也可能有效。抑制肠道运动活性可增强对气体的耐受性[30]。一项关于平滑肌松弛剂治疗 IBS 的 meta 分析的结论，这些药物在治疗症状方面优于安慰剂，特别是腹痛和腹胀[86]。薄荷油的有效成分薄荷醇具有钙离子通道阻滞剂活性，对胃肠道有抑制痉挛的作用，但对 IBS 中的疗效尚不明确[87]。具有镇痛作用的药物也可能有用（见第 122 章）。

（五）肠壁囊样积气症

肠壁囊样积气症和结肠囊样积气症是小肠壁、结肠或两者同时存在的充气囊肿的特征（见第 128 章）。囊肿可无症状，也可伴有腹泻、腹胀或腹痛[88,89]。据报道，有囊样积气是结缔组织疾病的一种并发症[90]。许多积气患者的呼吸 H_2 气体浓度极高，提示 H_2 的肠腔浓度较高[91,92]。3 例结肠积气患者的粪便中的 H_2 消耗微生物浓度异常低。因此，这些受试者的高管腔 H_2 似乎反映了 H_2 的产生相对不受 H_2 消耗的阻挠。已报告肠壁内气囊肿与长期服用 α-葡萄糖苷酶抑制剂有关[89]。

高管腔 H_2 张力如何导致积气是有争议的。一种说法是，小的壁内气体收集通常以一定的频率发生，但很快被吸收到循环中。在高 H_2 产生的情况下，肠腔 H_2 快速扩散到囊肿内可稀释其他囊肿气体（如 N_2）。因此，囊肿 N_2 张力保持低于或等于血液中的张力。结果囊肿内的 N_2 不能被吸收，囊肿持续存在。消除囊肿最有效的治疗方法是通过吸入高浓度 O_2。这样可将血液 N_2 张力降低至低于囊肿的值，使 N_2 从囊肿扩散到血液中，从而囊肿消退。其他可能有效的治疗形式包括氦氧混合气（一种低密度气体混合物）、抑制 H_2 产生的抗生素（环丙沙星已成功用于小肠细菌过度生长和肠壁囊样积气患者），以及减少可发酵底物向结肠细菌输送的饮食控制，如限制乳糖摄入。

（叶蔚 译，孙明瑜 校）

参考文献

第 18 章 大便失禁

Satish S. C. Rao 著

章节目录

一、流行病学 …… 221
二、病理生理学 …… 221
（一）肛门直肠的功能解剖学和生理学 …… 221
（二）发病机制 …… 222
三、评估 …… 225
（一）病史 …… 225
（二）体格检查 …… 225
（三）诊断试验 …… 226
四、治疗 …… 231
（一）支持措施 …… 231
（二）特异性疗法 …… 232
（三）新疗法 …… 236
（四）特定患者的治疗 …… 236

大便失禁定义为粪便经肛门不自主泄漏或无法控制肠道内容物排出。其严重程度可从偶尔无意的排气丧失到液体粪质渗出或肠道内容物完全排空。因此，这个问题很难从流行病学和病理生理学角度来描述其特征，但它会造成相当大的尴尬，丧失自尊、社会孤立和生活质量（quality of life，QOL）的下降[1]。

一、流行病学

大便失禁影响各年龄段的人群，但其患病率在中年女性、老年人和养老院居民中不成比例地增高。对其患病率的估计差异很大，取决于临床环境、对大便失禁定义的界定、发生频率、社会耻辱心理的影响以及其他因素[2]。大便失禁带来的尴尬和社会耻辱心理使患者难以求医，治疗往往延误数年。这不仅造成发展率显著上升，而且也会消耗大量的医疗资源。

在一项美国住户邮件调查报告中，有 7.1% 和 0.7% 的人群报告，有频繁漏便和内裤粪便污渍现象超过 1 个月[3]。在英国，有 0.8% 的到初级保健诊所就诊的患者，报告每月发生 2 次或以上大便失禁[4]。在年龄大于 65 岁生活能自理的老年人群中，有 3.7% 的患者每周至少发生一次大便失禁，男性多于女性（比例为 1.5∶1）[5]。大便失禁发生的频率随年龄增长而增加，从 30 岁以下女性的 7% 增加到 70 岁女性的 22%[6,7]。相比之下，25% ~ 35% 生活不能自理的患者和 10% ~ 25% 的住院老年患者有大便失禁[1]。在美国，大便失禁是安置养老院的第二大原因。

在美国一项对 2 570 个家庭的 6 959 人进行的调查中，前一年至少发生 1 次大便失禁的频率为 2.2%，在受影响的人群中，63% 为女性，30% 的年龄大于 65 岁，36% 为固体大便失禁，54% 为液体大便失禁，60% 为不自主排气失禁（排气失禁）[1]。美国国家糖尿病、消化和肾脏疾病研究所（National Institute of Diabetes and Digestive and Kidney Diseases，NIDDK）专家讨论会认为，社区居住的女性和男性大便失禁的频率平均为 7% ~ 15%[8]。在另一项对参加胃肠病或初级保健诊所的患者进行的前瞻性调查中，超过 18% 的患者每周至少报告 1 次大便失禁[9]。只有三分之一的人曾经与医生讨论过该问题，因此提示大便失禁的报道不足。当按发作频率分层时，2.7% 的患者报告每日有尿失禁，4.5% 每周有尿失禁，7.1% 每月有尿失禁[9]。在另外一项调查中，在泌尿科-妇科诊所就诊的女性中，26% 的人大便失禁与尿失禁相关[10]。在疗养院的居民中也报告了高频率的混合性大小便失禁。

大便失禁对生活质量有显著影响，包括丧失自尊、信心和谦逊[8,11]。它还对心理领域有影响，包括应对策略、焦虑、恐惧、尴尬、个人卫生/气味问题和大便习惯的不可预测性[8]。其症状严重程度和生活质量之间存在显著相关性[12]。此外，与无失禁或其他功能性胃肠道症状的患者相比，大便失禁患者每年误工或误学的可能性为 6.8 倍，平均误工或误学 50 天[3]。

与大便失禁相关的医疗保健费用组成包括评估、诊断检测和失禁治疗等可衡量的部分，以及使用一次性护垫和其他辅助设备的使用、皮肤护理和护理等。仅在美国，每年用于成人尿布的费用约为 18 亿美元，在全球为 107 亿美元[13]，每年用于护理生活不能自理的住院老年失禁患者的费用，介于 15 亿至 70 亿美元之间[1,2,14]。按 2012 年的美元计算，美国每位患者每年的总费用（84.111 美元）略高于荷兰（83.521 美元）[15]。在英国，非手术治疗大便失禁的潜在经济影响，例如骶神经刺激估计每年耗资超过 35 000 美元[16]，但尚无前瞻性成本效益对照试验。在长期的医疗服务中，大便失禁和尿失禁混合患者的门诊年费用为 9 711.17 美元，每位患者的平均估计费用（包括评估）为 17.166 美元[18]。这些人的生活质量受损和社会功能障碍也会导致难以衡量的成本[7]。大便失禁造成巨大的经济负担，包括增加医疗资源的使用，并对生活质量产生大的影响。

二、病理生理学

（一）肛门直肠的功能解剖学和生理学

结构和功能完整的肛门直肠单元，对维持肠内容物有节制地排便至关重要（见第 100 和 129 章）[19]。直肠是由一层连续的纵行肌组成的肌肉管道，与下面的环形肌交错。这种独特的肌肉排列使直肠既能作为粪便的储存器，又能作为排空粪便的泵。肛门是一长约 2~4cm 的肌形管道，静息时与直肠轴线形成夹角（图 18.1）。静息状态下，肛门直肠角约为 90°，随意挤压时，肛门直肠角变得锐利，约为 70°；在排便时，肛门直肠角变为钝角，约为 110°~130°（见第 19 章）。

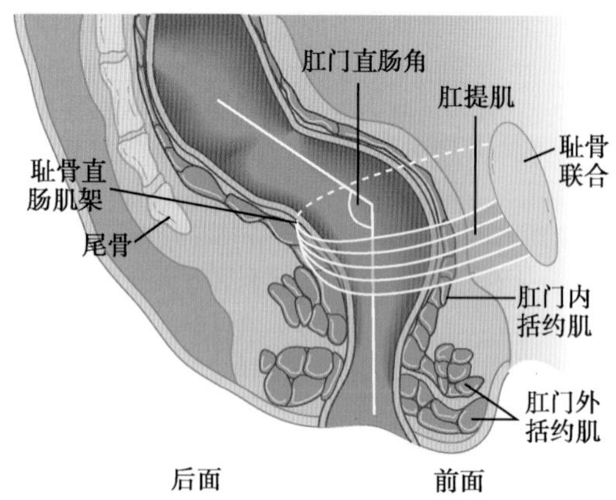

图 18.1　肛门直肠矢状位示意图。（From Rao SSC. Pathophysiology of adult fecal incontinence. Gastroenterology 2004; 126:S14-22.）

肛门括约肌由两部分肌肉组成：肛门内括约肌（internal anal sphincter，IAS），为直肠环形平滑肌层 0.3~0.5cm 厚的扩张，肛门外括约肌（external anal sphincter，EAS），为肛提肌 0.6~1.0cm 厚的扩张。在形态上，两个括约肌均是分离和异质的[20]。IAS 主要由慢收缩、抗疲劳平滑肌组成，产生频率为 15~35 周/min 的机械活动，以及 1.5~3 周/min 的超低波[19]。IAS 占静息肛门括约肌压力的 70%~85%，但在直肠突然膨胀时仅有 40% 的压力，在直肠持续膨胀期间仅有 65% 的压力，其余的压力由 EAS 或耻骨直肠肌或两者共同提供[21]。因此，IAS 主要负责维持静息时的肛门控便能力。

肛门通常由 IAS 的强直活动闭合。EAS 在自动挤压过程中加强了这一屏障。EAS 虽然在其内层呈圆周状，但其外层的前部也可能有荷包样结构，纤维插入对侧横向的会阴、尿道海绵体肌和耻骨肌支[22]。这种独特的结构可能对会阴切开术和肛门括约肌重建有意义。肛门黏膜皱襞和扩张的肛门血管垫（见后文）可提供紧密的封闭[23]。耻骨直肠肌增强了这些屏障，形成了一个类似瓣状样瓣膜，产生向前拉力加强肛门直肠角[19]。使用高清晰度三维（3D）测压法的研究显示，耻骨直肠肌对压力曲线的分布有显著影响，并在维持自控力、感觉运动反应和直肠肛门抑制反射中起着不可或缺的作用（见下文）[24]。

肛门直肠受感觉神经、运动神经、自主神经以及肠神经系统支配。肛门直肠的主要神经是阴部神经，它起源于第二、第三和第四骶神经（S2、S3、S4），支配 EAS 并辅助感觉和运动功能[25]。阴部神经阻滞可导致肛周和生殖器皮肤感觉丧失，肛门括约肌无力，但不影响直肠感觉[21]。阴部神经阻滞还能消除直肠肛门收缩反射（见下文），这一观察表明会阴神经病变可能影响直肠肛门收缩反射。直肠扩张的感觉很可能沿 S2、S3 和 S4 副交感神经传递。这些神经纤维沿着盆腔内脏神经走行，与阴部神经无关[19]。

人类如何感知肛门直肠中的粪便内容物尚不完全清楚。早期的研究未能证明直肠感觉意识[19]。随后的研究证实，直肠可感觉到气囊扩张，这种感觉在保持排便自控能力中发挥作用[23,26]。此外，感觉训练可改善直肠的低敏感性[27,28]和高敏感性[29]。对直肠的机械刺激可产生脑诱发反应[30]，证实直肠是一个感觉器官。同样，无论是健康人[31]还是大便失禁患者，电刺激肛门和直肠也可引起皮层诱发电位[32]。

虽然在直肠黏膜或肌间神经丛中不存在系统的神经末梢，但存在有髓鞘和无髓鞘的神经纤维[19]。这些神经最有可能介导扩张或伸展诱导的感觉反应，以及内脏-内脏[30]、直肠肛门抑制和直肠肛门收缩反射。直肠扩张的感觉很可能通过副交感神经沿 S2、S3 和 S4 内脏神经传递。切除生殖神经可完全消除直肠感觉和排便能力[33]。如果没有副交感神支配，直肠充盈仅被视为一种模糊的不适感觉。即使是下肢瘫痪或骶神经元病变的患者也可能保留一定程度的感觉功能，但如果脊髓损伤病变发生在较高部位，则感觉几乎丧失[16,20,34]。使用新型无创磁刺激腰骶丛神经并记录肛门和直肠运动诱发电位（motor evoked potential，MEP）的研究表明，脊髓损伤和大便失禁患者表现出明显的腰骶神经病变[35,36]。因此，骶神经与保持控制排便密切相关。

有人建议，通过肛门直肠定期取样感知肠内容物[37]，该过程使 IAS 的短暂松弛允许直肠中的粪便内容物与上肛管中的特殊感觉器接触。可能存在专门的传入神经，可感知触觉、温度、张力和摩擦，但其机制尚不完全清楚[19]。大便失禁者似乎比对照者采集直肠内容物更少。肛门感觉的可能作用是区分排气和粪便，并微调自控能力，但其确切作用尚未得到很好的证实。

直肠扩张与肛门静息压反射性降低有关，称为直肠肛门抑制反射。这种松弛的幅度和持续时间随着直肠扩张体积的增加而增加，最大可达 100~150mL，然后达到平台期[38]。这种反射由肠肌层的神经丛介导，由一氧化氮和血管活性肠肽释放引起[39]，存在下腹神经被切断的患者及脊髓病变的患者中。直肠横断后反射消失，但可恢复[26]。直肠肛门的抑制反射可能有利于排气和粪便的排出。直肠扩张也与直肠肛门收缩反应相关，这是一种防止直肠内容物释放（如排气）的潜意识反射[40,41]。这种反应涉及 EAS 的收缩，由盆腔内脏神经和阴部神经介导。直肠肛门收缩反射的幅度和持续时间的长短随着直肠的扩张而增加，最大体积可达 30mL。由咳嗽或大笑引起的腹内压突然升高与肛门括约肌压力升高有关。许多机制包括耻骨直肠肌反射性收缩也参与其中。最近，直肠肛门感觉运动反射已经描述了这种反应，即有意识地感觉到排便欲望（由球囊扩张引起）引起肛管的收缩反应[42]。这种反应主要由耻骨直肠肌的收缩介导[38]，在直肠敏感性低下的患者中明显受损。

肛门黏膜充满血液的血管组织在实现肛门最佳闭合方面也起着重要作用。一项体外研究表明，即使在最大限度的不自主收缩期间，内括约肌环也无法完全闭合肛门口，仍存有大约 7mm 的间隙。该间隙由肛门垫填充，其可施加高达 9mmHg 的压力，从而使静息肛门压力增加 10%~20%[40]。

（二）发病机制

当一种或多种维持控便的机制被破坏到其他机制无法代

偿的程度时,就会发生大便失禁。因此,发生大便失禁往往是多因素的[2,41]。在一项前瞻性研究中发现,80% 的大便失禁患者有一种以上的致病机制(图 18.2)[19]。虽然病理生理机制经常重叠,但可分为 4 大类(表 18.1)。

表 18.1　大便失禁的机制、病因和病理生理

机制	病因	病理生理学
肛门直肠或盆底结构异常		
肛门括约肌	痔切除术,神经病变,产科损伤	括约肌无力,取样反射丧失
耻骨直肠肌	老化,会阴过度下降,创伤	肛门直肠角变钝,括约肌无力
阴部神经	过度紧张,产科或外科手术损伤,会阴膨出	反射减弱,括约肌无力感觉丧失
神经系统,脊髓,自主神经系统	撕裂损伤,糖尿病,头颅损伤,多发性硬化症,脊髓损伤,脊柱手术,卒中	反射减弱,协调丧失,感觉丧失,继发性肌病
直肠	老化,炎症性肠病,肠易激综合征,脱垂,放射线损伤	超过敏反应,协调丧失,感觉丧失
肛门直肠或盆底功能异常		
肛门直肠感觉减低	自主神经系统病变,中枢神经系统病变,产科损伤	大便意识丧失,直肠肛门认知障碍
粪便嵌塞	排便协同失调	粪便潴留伴溢出,感觉障碍
粪便特征改变		
体积增加稠度松散	胆盐吸收障碍,药物,感染,炎症性肠病,肠易激综合征,泻药,代谢性病变	腹泻和急迫感,协调性障碍,粪便快速排出
粪便坚硬,滞留	药物,协同失调	粪便潴留伴溢出
其他机制		
身体活动性,认知功能	老化,痴呆,残疾	多因素变化
精神病	故意弄脏	多因素变化
药物*	抗胆碱能药物 抗抑郁药 咖啡因 泻药 肌肉松弛剂	便秘 感觉改变,便秘 括约肌紧张度松弛 腹泻 括约肌松弛
食物不耐受	果糖、乳糖或山梨醇吸收不良	腹泻,排气增多

*每一类药物都有其病理生理学特点。

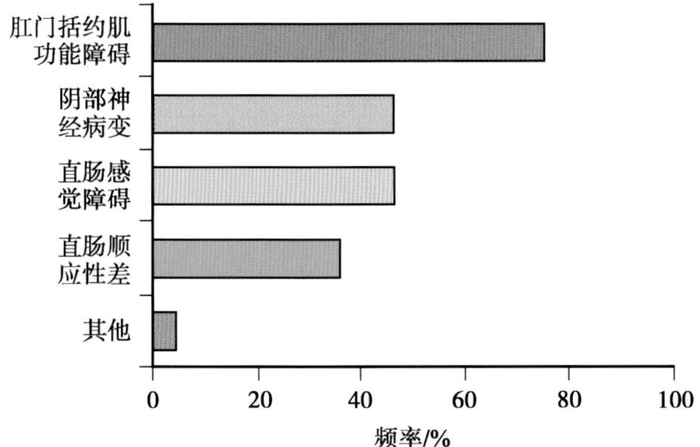

图 18.2　导致大便失禁的常见机制的相对频率。在许多患者中,涉及多种机制

1. 肛门直肠和盆底结构异常

(1) 肛门括约肌

EAS 肌肉的破坏或无力引起紧急或腹泻相关的大便失禁。相比之下,IAS 肌肉或肛门血管内垫损伤可导致密封不良和取样反射受损。这些改变可引起被动性尿失禁或粪便渗漏(见下文),通常在静息状态下发生。许多患者的两个括约肌都可能存在缺陷。肌肉损伤的程度会影响失禁的严重程度[19]。

肛门括约肌破坏的最常见原因是产科创伤,可能涉及 EAS、IAS 和阴部神经。然而,为什么大多数在 20~30 多岁时遭受产科损伤的女性,在 50 多岁之前通常不会出现大便失禁,其原因尚不清楚。在一项前瞻性研究中,35% 的初产妇(产前正常)显示在阴道分娩后有肛门括约肌的破坏[44,45]。其他重要危险因素包括产钳辅助分娩、第二产程延长、胎儿体重过大和枕后先露[19]。一项对 921 例初产妇的前瞻性研究表明,阴道分娩和括约肌撕裂的妇女产后 6 周和 6 个月大便失禁的发生率分别为 27% 和 17%,阴道分娩但无撕裂的妇女分别 11% 和 8%,在剖宫产妇女中分别为 10% 和 7.6%[46]。这项研究清楚地表明:大便失禁的发生和严重程度是由于阴道分娩时发生肛门括约肌撕裂所致。

会阴切开术被认为是肛门括约肌破坏的危险因素。一项研究表明,会阴内侧切开术与肛门括约肌功能障碍发生风险增高 9 倍相关[47]。然而,相对于分娩类型而言,仍有相当大比例的中年妇女发生大便或排气失禁,这提示与年龄相关的

盆底结构变化可能会导致大便失禁。

衰老影响肛门括约肌功能[48]。与年轻人相比，70 岁以上的男性和女性括约肌压力下降了 30%～40%[49]。在各年龄组中，女性的肛门挤压压力都低于男性[49]，在绝经期后会迅速下降[50]。在人类肛门括约肌的横纹肌中已证实有雌激素受体，切除大鼠卵巢导致肛门括约肌横纹肌萎缩[19,51]。这些观察表明，盆底肌肉的强度与活力是受激素影响的。老年女性会阴神经终末运动潜伏期（pudendal nerve terminal motor latency，PNTML）延长，用力时盆底下降过度（见后文）[52]。这些机制可能导致肛门括约肌横纹肌进行性损伤。IAS 厚度和回声增强也与衰老有关[53]。

导致解剖破坏的其他原因包括因治疗痔疮、瘘管和肛裂的肛门直肠手术。肛管扩张或括约肌外侧切开术可引起肛门括约肌破裂继发大便失禁[54]。痔疮切除术因无意中损伤 IAS 或失去血管内垫而引起大便失禁[55]。意外发生的会阴创伤或骨盆骨折也可直接引起括约肌创伤导致大便失禁[56]，但肛交与肛门括约肌功能障碍无关[57]。最后，IAS 功能障碍也可能因患肌病、变性或放射治疗而发生。

（2）耻骨直肠肌

耻骨直肠肌通过形成瓣阀机制对保持节制排便是十分重要的[58]。使用 3D 超声的研究表明，40% 的大便失禁女性有耻骨直肠肌严重异常，32% 的女性有轻微的耻骨直肠肌异常。无症状的经产妇对照组分别为 21% 和 32%[59]。应用会阴测压计评估耻骨直肠肌功能发现大便失禁患者耻骨直肠肌（肛提肌）收缩功能受损，这一发现是大便失禁的独立危险因素，并与大便失禁的严重程度相关[60]。此外，生物反馈治疗后耻骨直肠肌强度的改善与临床状态好转相关。部分原因是耻骨直肠肌上部接受的神经支配来自骶神经 S3 和 S4 分支而非阴部神经。由于耻骨直肠肌和 EAS 具有单独的神经支配，阴部阻滞并不能消除盆底的随意收缩[61]，但可完全消除 EAS 功能[21]。

（3）神经系统

盆底的完整神经支配对保持节制排便是及其重要的。由于阴部神经病变和产科损伤所致的括约肌退化可引起女性大便失禁[44]。神经性损伤通常在分娩期间持续存在，可能是由于产道拉伸过程中神经过度伸展或胎头通过时的直接创伤。当胎头过大、第二产程延长或使用产钳时，尤其是高位产钳或产程延长时，更容易发生神经损伤。

外源性自主神经支配的作用是有争论的。动物研究表明，盆腔神经传递纤维可使直肠松弛[62]，这些神经可能在调节和储存粪便和气体方面发挥作用。盆腔神经损伤可导致调节功能降低和通过直肠乙状结肠区域的快速传递受损，从而压倒排便节制屏障机制。通过刺激骶前交感神经研究的交感神经传出活动倾向于松弛 IAS，而刺激副交感神经可引起肛门括约肌收缩。随意括约肌的上运动神经元位于矢状窦旁运动皮层中支配下肢肌肉的神经元附近，并与感觉皮层中表示的生殖器和会阴邻近[19]。中枢神经系统病变对运动皮层的损伤可能导致失禁。在一些神经源性失禁的患者中，感觉神经纤维和运动神经纤维可能受损，导致感觉障碍[63]。这种损伤可损害直肠充盈的知觉意识以及盆底括约肌横纹肌的相关反射反应。

大约 10% 的大便失禁患者的病变可能比骨盆内或肛门周围神经更近。这些患者的主要异常是马尾神经损伤[64]，病变可能是隐匿性的，临床评估不明显。这些患者沿马尾神经根的神经传导延长，而 PNTML 无异常[65]。然而在少数患者中，会同时存在外周和中枢病变。其他疾病，如多发性硬化症、糖尿病和脱髓鞘损伤（或来自酒精中毒性神经病变或创伤性神经病变）也可能导致大便失禁[19]。

（4）直肠

直肠是个顺应性粪便储存器，当条件有利于粪便排出时它才排出储存的粪便[2]。如果直肠壁顺应性受损，少量粪便即可产生直肠内高压，压倒肛门阻力导致大便失禁[66]。造成直肠顺应性损伤的原因包括放射性直肠炎、溃疡性结肠炎或克罗恩病、肿瘤直肠浸润和根治性子宫切除术[67]。同样，直肠手术，特别是结肠袋手术[68]和脊髓损伤[69]也与直肠顺应性丧失相关。

2. 肛门直肠和盆底功能异常

（1）肛门直肠感觉受损

完整的感觉不仅提供了即将排便的警告，而且有助于区分成形粪便、液体粪便和排气。老年人、身体有残疾和精神上有缺陷的人以及大便失禁的儿童[70]常表现直肠感觉迟钝。直肠感觉受损可引起粪便过度堆积，从而导致粪便嵌塞、巨直肠（直肠极度扩张）和粪便溢出。感觉受损的原因包括多发性硬化症、糖尿病和脊髓病变引起的神经损伤[69]。鲜为人知的是镇痛药（尤其是阿片类药物）和抗抑郁药也可能损害直肠感觉而导致大便失禁。直肠在保持排便节制的重要性已通过手术研究得到确证，其中保留直肠远端 6～8cm 及其随同的副交感神经，有助于避免发生大便失禁[71]。相反，切除勃起神经可使直肠感觉和排便节制能力消失（见上文）[33]。

完整的采样反射允许个体选择是排泄还是保留直肠内容物。相反，采样反射受损可使受试者易发生大便失禁[37]。然而，采样反射在维持大便失禁中的作用尚不清楚。在接受结肠贯通手术的儿童中（见第 117 章），仍保留了一定程度的感觉辨别[72]。但由于这些儿童肛门黏膜感觉区缺失，因此有人推测感觉受体可能位于耻骨直肠肌，可能在促进感觉辨别方面发挥作用；对肌肉的牵引是一种强有力的刺激物，可触发排便和直肠扩张的感觉。通过局部应用 5% 利多卡因能消减肛门感觉，但不会降低括约肌静息压力（可影响自愿挤压的压力，但不影响保留注入直肠生理盐水的能力），因此，肛门感觉在维持节制排便方面的作用受到质疑[19]。

（2）排便协同失调和排空不全

在一些患者中，特别是老年人，粪便长时间滞留在直肠内或排空不完全，会导致粪便渗漏或内衣污渍[73]。大多数患者出现排便障碍或协同失调[74]，其中许多患者还表现为直肠感觉受损。虽然肛门括约肌和阴部神经功能完好，但模拟排空粪便的能力受损。同样在老年人和患有功能性大便失禁的儿童中，粪便在直肠中长期滞留会引起粪便嵌塞，久之会导致 IAS 的长期松弛，从而使液态粪便在嵌塞的粪便周围流动，并通过肛管逸出（见第 19 章）[70]。

（3）会阴下降综合征

对于长期便秘且有多年过度用力排便的女性（即使以前没有分娩史），可能导致盆底肌肉进行性去神经支配[75]。大多数患者证实有会阴过度下降和括约肌无力，可能导致直肠脱垂。但是大便失禁并不是不可避免的。大便失禁是否发生和发展取决于盆底的状态和括约肌的力量强度。

3. 粪便特征的改变

粪便的黏稠度、体积和排便频率，以及粪便中是否存在刺激物也可能是大便失禁的发病机制[2]。在大量液态粪便存在的情况下，通常迅速通过直肠，只有通过完整的感觉和强力的括约肌屏障才能维持控便能力。胆盐吸收不良、乳糖或果糖不耐受或渗透性物质快速倾倒至结肠的患者中，结肠内气体和粪便内容物转运过快，可能压倒控便机制（见第 16 和 104 章）[2]。

4. 其他混杂机制

各种不同的疾病和残疾可能易患大便失禁，尤其是老年人。无法移动和无法使用如厕设施是该人群大便失禁的主要原因[76]。几种药物可能抑制括约肌张力，有些药物用于治疗尿失禁和逼尿肌不稳定，包括抗胆碱能药物，如酒石酸托特罗定和奥昔布宁（如以及肌肉松弛剂，如巴氯芬和环苯扎必林。兴奋剂（如咖啡因产品、纤维补充剂、泻药）因引起腹泻而导致大便失禁[19]。

三、评估

（一）病史

评估大便失禁患者的第一步是建立信任关系，评估症状的持续时间和性质，特别要注意：①是否包括不能自主排气，液状粪便或固体粪便的渗漏；②症状对生活质量的影响（框 18.1）。由于许多人将大便失禁误认为是腹泻或粪便急迫[77]，因此详细描述主诉的特征很重要，临床医生应询问衬垫或其他器具的使用情况，以及患者区分成形或未成形粪便和气体的能力（缺乏这种区分能力被称为直肠失认症）[2]。询问产科史、饮食史、合并尿失禁病史以及糖尿病、盆腔放疗、神经系统问题或脊髓损伤等病史也非常重要。前瞻性排便日记，尤其是智能手机应用程序的电子粪便日记，对准确了解排便习惯、粪便性状是十分有用的。

框 18.1　大便失禁患者的病史特征
发作和诱发事件
持续时间
严重程度
粪便黏稠度和直肠急迫感
粪便嵌塞
共存问题（如腹泻、炎性肠病）
药物、咖啡因、饮食
既往病史：脊柱手术、尿失禁、背部损伤、糖尿病、神经系统疾病
临床类型：被动型、或急迫型或渗漏型大便失禁
产科病史：使用产钳、撕裂、婴儿情况、修补手术

还应确定发生大便失禁的客观环境，这种详细的查询有助于认识以下类型的大便失禁：

（1）**被动型大便失禁**：在无意识的情况下不自觉地排出粪便或排气。该类型提示知觉丧失或直肠肛门反射受损，伴有或不伴有括约肌功能障碍。

（2）**急迫型大便失禁**：尽管患者积极尝试保留肠内容物，但仍排出粪便或气体。这种类型的主要原因是括约肌功能破坏和直肠保留粪便能力下降。

（3）**粪便渗漏型**：常发生在排便之后出现的不希望有的粪便渗漏，其他情况下控便和排气正常。这种情况主要是由于粪便排空不完全或直肠感觉受损所致[73,74]。括约肌功能和阴部神经功能大多完好无损。

虽然这 3 种类型之间存在重叠，但通过确定主要类型，可获得对相关潜在机制的认识和首选处理的方法。症状评估可能与测压结果相关性不佳（见下文）。在一项研究中，应用测压计检测发现静息肛门括约肌压力较低时，渗漏发生敏感性为 98.9%。特异性为 11%，阳性预测值为 51%[78]。检测肛门括约肌挤压压力低的阳性预测值为 80%。因此，对大便失禁的个体患者而言，仅凭病史和临床特征不足以阐明病理生理学，而客观检测是至关重要的（见下文）[79,80]。

有许多自我报告的生活质量（QOL）和大便失禁严重程度量表可用，已得到验证的包括 FI-QOL（Fecal Incontinence-QOL，大便失禁的生活质量）、St. MarK/Vaizey 评分[81]、FISI（Fecal Incontinence Severity Index，大便失禁严重程度指数）[82]、FISS（Fecal Incontinence Severity Score，大便失禁严重程度评分）[12,83] 和 ICIQ-B（International Consultation on Incontinence Questionnaire-Bowels，国际大便失禁咨询委员会问卷）[84]。根据临床特征，提出了以下几种分级系统。克利夫兰诊所分级系统的修改已由圣马克医院的研究人员验证[85]，并提供了一种量化大便失禁程度的客观方法，也可以用以评估治疗效果。该分级系统基于以下 7 个参数，肛门排泄物的特征为：①固体；②液体；③排气；④生活方式的改变程度；⑤需佩戴护垫；⑥需服用止泻药物；⑦推迟排便的能力。总积分范围从 0（可节制排便）到 24 分（重度大便失禁）。如前所述，仅凭临床特征不足以确定病理生理学改变。使用问卷调查，如症状自评量表 90-R（symptom checklist 90-R，SCL-90-R）、简明健康调查量表（short form 36，SF-36）和 FI-QOL 调查，可提供有关心理社会问题和大便失禁对患者生活质量影响的附加信息。然而，前瞻性记录与大便失禁相关关键症状的粪便日记，可提供有关问题的有用观点，也可用于评估与大便失禁相关的排便百分比，这是评估治疗成功的一个关键参数[86]。使用智能手机应用程序的电子粪便日记用于记录肠道症状，可能非常有用。

（二）体格检查

大便失禁患者均应进行详细的体格检查，包括神经系统检查，因为大便失禁可能继发于全身性或神经系统疾病。已经描述了对疑似大便失禁的患者进行直肠指检的逐步方法，以及异常检查结果的记录和评分[87]。检查的重点是会阴和肛门直肠。病人应左侧卧位，光线要良好。检查时可注意有无粪质、脱出痔、皮炎、瘢痕、皮肤表皮剥脱、肛裂和有无肛周皱褶。这些特征提示存在括约肌无力或慢性皮肤刺激，并能提供了潜在病因的线索[2]。要求患者尝试排便，可证明有无会阴部过度下降或直肠脱垂。向外凸出超过 3cm 通常被定义为会阴过度下降（见第 19 章）[88]。

首先应检查肛周感觉。肛门皮肤反射检查可以了解感觉神经与皮肤间连接的完整性,脊髓S2、S3和S4段的中间神经元,以及肛门外括约肌的运动神经支配。这种反射可以通过用棉签轻轻抚摸肛周各象限的皮肤来评估。正常反应为肛门外括约肌的肛周出现快速收缩,(称肛门眨眼或瞬目反射)。肛门皮肤反射受损或消失提示传入或传出神经元损伤[2]。

临床医师将戴着润滑手套的示指插入肛门和直肠后,应评估静息括约肌张力、肛管长度、耻骨直肠肌吊带的强度、肛门直肠锐角的大小、肛门括约肌挤压的强度和主动挤压时会阴抬高的程度。可观察到是否存在直肠膨出或粪便嵌塞。

直肠指检的准确性已在几项研究中进行了评估。在一项对66例患者的研究中,由经验丰富的外科医生进行的直肠指检,在一定程度上与静息括约肌压力($r=0.56$;$P<0.001$)或最大挤压压力($r=0.72$;$P<0.001$)相关[89]。在一项280例有各种肛门直肠疾病患者的研究中,发现直肠指检与测压结果之间存在合理的相关性,但指检的敏感性、特异性和阳性预测值较低[90]。在另一项对64例患者的研究中,发现直肠指检与静息压和挤压压力之间的相关性分别为0.41和0.52[91]。这些数值表明,直肠指检仅能提供了括约肌强度的近似值,检查结果受许多因素的影响,包括检查者手指的大小、使用的技术和患者合作的程度。另外,检查者在直肠指检中缺乏足够的技能来识别大便失禁的特征[92]。尽管直肠指检能识别粪便嵌塞和漏粪的患者,但对括约肌功能障碍的诊断并不准确,不应作为有关治疗决策的依据[2]。

(三)诊断试验

评估大便失禁患者的一个重要步骤是确定该失禁是继发于腹泻还是与粪便黏稠度无关。如果腹泻与大便失禁同时存在,应进行适当的检测以确定腹泻的原因(见第16章)。此类检测包括可屈式乙状结肠镜或结肠镜检查,以排除结肠黏膜炎症、直肠肿块或狭窄以及检查粪便了解有无感染、容积、渗透压、电解质、脂肪含量以及胰腺功能障碍。应进行生化检查以寻找有无甲状腺功能异常、糖尿病和其他代谢紊乱疾病。呼吸试验用于诊断乳糖或果糖不耐受或小肠细菌生长过度[2]。有胆囊切除术史可能存在胆盐吸收不良,提示进行胆盐结合剂治疗试验。

特异性检测可用于确定大便失禁的潜在机制,通常以互补的方式使用。最常用的检查包括肛门直肠测压、肛门超声内镜检查、气囊排出试验(balloon expulsion test,BET)、特殊的神经生理学检查,包括经腰骶肛门直肠磁刺激(translumbosacral anorectal magnetic stimulation,TAMS)和PNTML[2,93-96],以及更新的测试,如用于定义肛门括约肌区域的肛门直肠腔内功能管腔成像探头(endoluminal functional lumen imaging probe,EndoFLIP)等。

1. 肛门直肠测压

肛门直肠测压是评估IAS和EAS压力(图18.3)以及直肠感觉、直肠肛门反射和直肠顺应性的有用方法。有几种类型的探头和压力记录装置可用,每种装置各有优缺点。然而,一项国际专家的调查显示,在试验方法、性能特征和试验解释方面存在显著差异[98]。尽管传统上使用的是带有密集传感器的水灌注探头[2],但目前越来越多的是,在全球范围内使

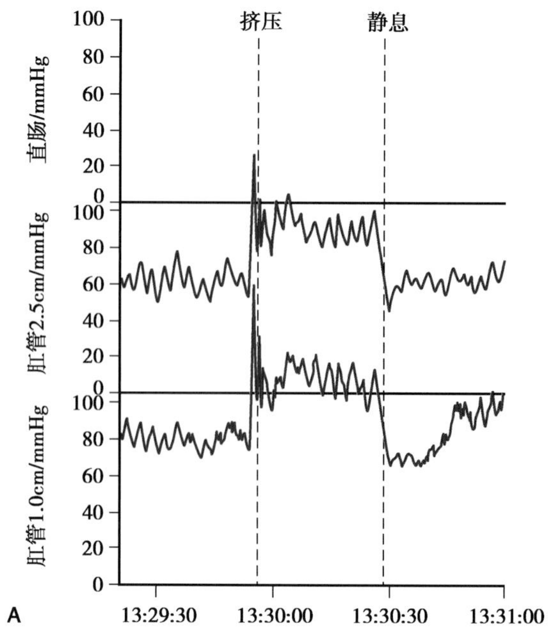

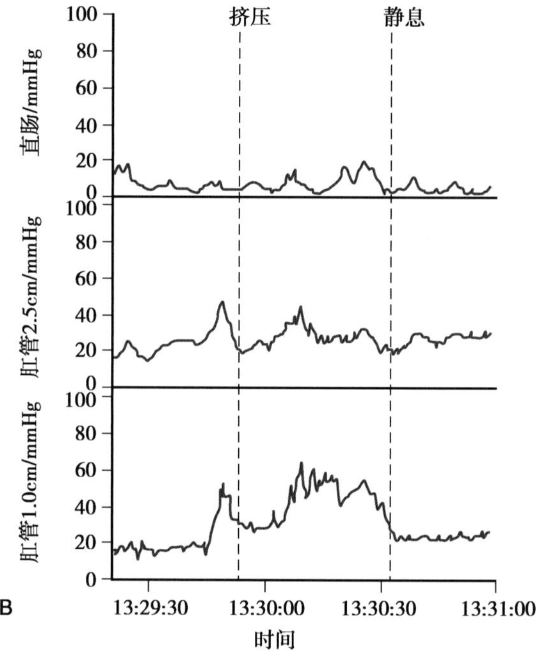

图18.3　肛门直肠测压曲线。A,挤压(肛门外括约肌)和静息(肛门内括约肌)压力正常的健康受试者。B,挤压和静息压力较弱的大便失禁者的肛门直肠测压特征。上描记图,直肠压力活动;中描记图,肛门压力活动在2.5cm;下描记图,肛门压力活动距肛缘1cm

用具有微传感器或充气小型化球囊的固态探头。固态探头具有12个圆周传感器,间隔为1cm,外径为4.2mm,气囊长度为4cm(特定成像)提供高分辨率[99]。该设备使用了一种新的压力传导技术(TactArray),能使每个压力传感元件检测长度超过2.5mm的压力,以及12个径向放射状分散的扇区中的每个扇区的压力。尽管肛门括约肌压力高于水灌注测压法记录的压力,但数据可在等压等值线图中显示,该等压等值线可以提供压力变化的连续动态表示。一个5cm探头中有256个圆周排列传感器的高清3D测压系统,正在许多实验室使用,并提供肛门括约肌压力分布和地形图(图18.4)。肛门

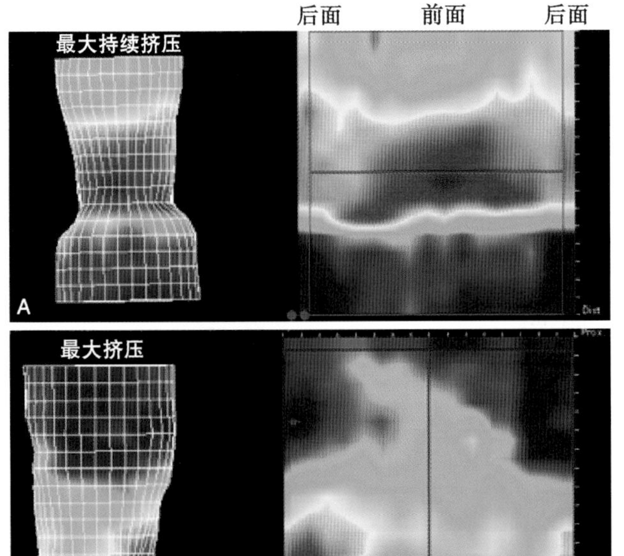

图 18.4 高清度肛门括约肌向量地形图。显示三维矢状位(左)和二维展开位(右)最大挤压期间的压力变化。A,健康对照受试者的变化。B,大便失禁受试者的变化。大便失禁受试者有明显的括约肌无力,有不对称的挤压和一些向量的变化(主要为黄色和绿色)。而健康受试者表现出强有力的挤压(橙色和红色)和括约肌直径的对称性减少

EndoFLIP(腔内功能性管腔成像探头)是一种新的系统,由一个带有球囊的探头组成,球囊内装有多个阻抗传感器,并提供肛门高压区的三维剖面,定量分析肛门括约肌扩张性指数及肛门阻力、开口力和顺应性评估(图 18.5)[97]。但仍需进一步研究评估其临床效用。

肛门括约肌压力可通过静态或定点牵拉检测技术测量[85,94],肛门括约肌静息压主要代表 IAS 功能,随意肛门挤压压力代表 EAS 和耻骨直肠肌功能。大便失禁患者静息压和挤压压降低(见图 18.3 和图 18.4),分别表明 IAS 和 EAS 疲软无力[2,90]。挤压的持续时间可提供括约肌疲劳指数。EAS 反射性收缩的能力可以在腹内压突然升高时进行评估,像患者咳嗽时。这种反射反应使肛门括约肌压力高于直肠压力,以保持控便能力。这种反应可能由盆底的受体触发,并通过脊髓反射弧介导。在脊髓圆锥以上的脊髓损伤患者中,即使随意挤压不存在,这种反射反应也得以保留,而在马尾神经或骶丛损伤的患者中,反射和随意挤压反应均不存在[2,100,101]。

肛门直肠测压可提供有关肛门直肠功能相关的有用信息[93,95,102]。美国运动协会推荐了测压测试的指南和最低标准[95],尽管有关正常值的数据不足,健康受试者与大便失禁患者之间的结果重叠[90]。试验重现性的置信区间较大[103]。然而,测压试验对大便失禁患者个体来说是很有用的[95]。肛门直肠功能测压试验也可用于评估药物治疗、生物反馈治疗和手术治疗后的客观效果[104-106]。国际上努力在专家之间就测试方法和测试解释方面达成共识,可为标准化测试铺平道

健康受试者

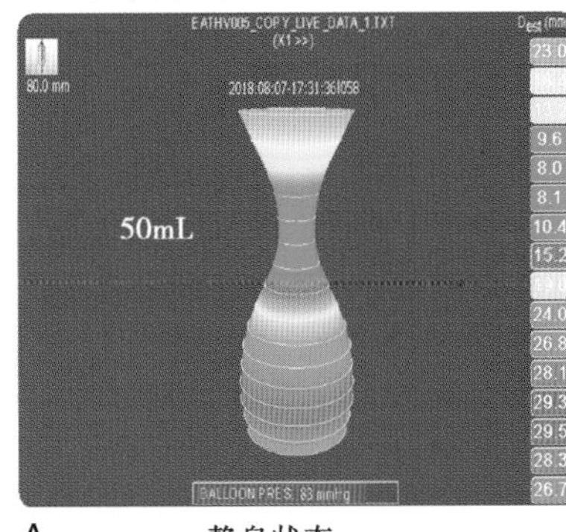

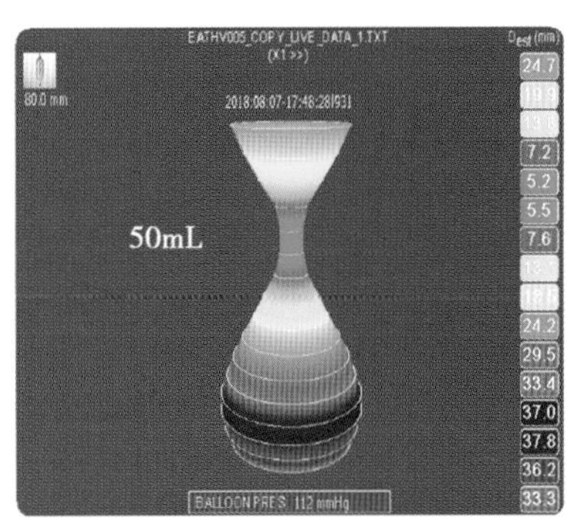

A 静息状态 挤压期间

大便失禁患者

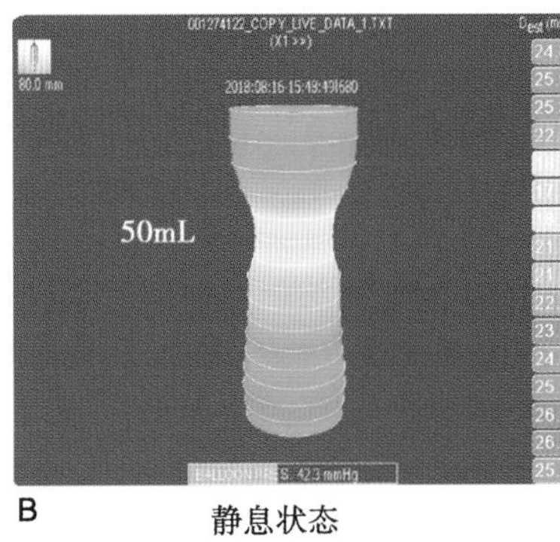

B 静息状态 挤压期间

图 18.5 肛门直肠腔内功能性管腔成像探头(EndoFLIP)地形图。(A)健康受试者,显示静息时(左图)和挤压时(右图)正常高压区剖面、横截面积和可扩张指数。(B)大便失禁患者,当在 50mL 球囊膨胀时测量,静息时大便失禁患者的肛门扩张指数(5.5mm^2/mmHg)显著高于健康受试者(0.6mm^2/mmHg),表明肛门括约肌无力且容易扩张。同样在挤压过程中,大便失禁患者的扩张指数(2.5mm^2/mmHg)显著高于健康受试者(0.2mm^2/mmHg)

路,改善临床诊断和患者的处理[95]。

2. 直肠感觉测试

用注入空气或水扩张直肠球囊,可用于评估直肠壁的感觉反应和顺应性。在直肠中放置容积递增的扩张球囊,可评估首次感知阈值、首次排便阈值和急迫排便阈值。感觉阈值越高,表明直肠敏感性越低[2,100,107]。也可评估部分或完全抑制肛门括约肌张力所需的球囊容积。大便失禁患者诱发反射性肛门松弛所需的容量低于对照组[108]。

由于肛门黏膜对直肠内容物的取样可能在维持正常节制排便中起重要作用[37],因此,提倡使用电刺激或热刺激对肛门知觉进行定量评估,但目前临床尚未使用[2]。直肠顺应性可通过评估气囊扩张时直肠压力随空气或液体的变化来计算[94,109]。结肠炎患者[66]、低位脊髓损伤患者和伴有大便失禁的糖尿病患者的直肠顺应性降低,但高位脊髓病变患者的直肠顺应性是增加的。

3. 肛管成像检查

(1) 肛管超声内镜检查

肛管超声内镜检查使用7~15mHz的旋转式超声探头,焦距为1~4cm[110]。该检查可评估EAS和IAS厚度及结构完整性,并可检测瘢痕、肌肉组织损失和其他局部病理改变(图18.6)[111]。高频(10~15mHz)探头和肛门括约肌的3D重建可改善括约肌复合体的勾画,使成像更加清晰[111]。

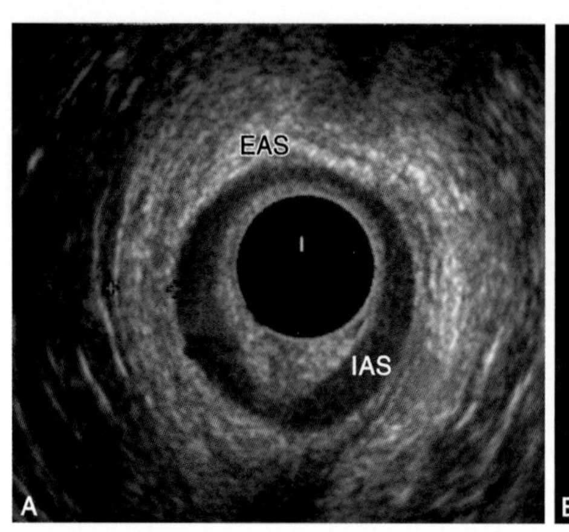

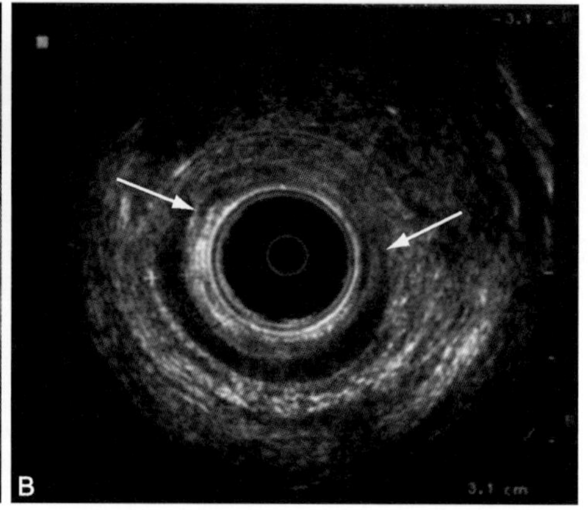

图18.6　肛管超声内镜检查。A,正常健康受试者,肛门内括约肌(IAS)呈完整的低回声,肛门外括约肌(EAS)呈完整增厚高回声。B,继发于产科损伤的大便失禁受试者,导致累及IAS和EAS的较大前括约肌缺损,跨越10点和2点位置之间的圆周(箭)

经阴道分娩后,肛管超声内镜检查发现有35%的初产妇存在隐匿性括约肌损伤,这些病变大多在临床上难以发现。在另一项研究中,85%会阴三度撕裂的女性检测到括约肌缺损,而无撕裂的患者检测到括约肌缺损的比例为33%[112]。在比较肌电图(EMG)(见后文)与肛管超声内镜检查的研究中,确诊括约肌缺损的符合率较高[113,114],但该项技术取决于操作者,需要经过培训且有一定的经验[94]。尽管超声内镜检查可以区分肛门内括约肌和外括约肌损伤,但对于确定大便失禁原因的特异性较低[2]。由于肛门超声内镜检查比EMG应用更广泛、费用更低,比需要插入针头的EMG检查疼痛更轻,因此它成为检查肛门括约肌形态和发现其缺损的首选技术[98]。

(2) 磁共振成像(MRI)

肛管内MRI可提供优质的成像,具有极好的空间分辨率,特别是在确定EAS的解剖结构方面[115,116]。在一项研究[117],而非另一项研究[115]表明,MRI比肛管内超声内镜检查的准确性低。肛管内MRI检查有助于检出外括约肌萎缩,这可能对括约肌修复产生不利影响(见后文)[118],萎缩可能存在,而无阴部神经病变[119]。增加使用快速成像序列的动态盆腔MRI或MRI阴道-膀胱造影术,包括使用超声凝胶作为接触剂填充直肠,并让患者躺在磁体内排空,可以更精确地确认肛门直肠的解剖结构[120]。使用MRI肛管内置线圈可提高分辨率并更精确地定义括约肌。然而,需要对其成本、可用性、技术因素、临床效果以及在治疗决策中的价值进行对比研究。

4. 排粪造影

排粪造影使用放射透视技术,以提供直肠和肛管的形态学信息[121]。排粪造影用于评估肛门直肠角、测量盆底下降和肛管长度,并检测是否存在直肠前突、直肠脱垂和肠黏膜套叠。将大约150mL的造影剂注入直肠,要求受试者挤压或咳嗽排出造影剂。虽然排粪造影可以检测到一些异常,但这些异常也可见于其他无症状的人[94,122]。它们的存在与直肠排空受损的相关性很差。检查者之间对测量肛门直肠角的认识也不一致。在测量肛门直肠角时,是否应该使用直肠中心轴或直肠后壁尚不清楚,从而使识别形态学缺陷的功能性意义受到质疑。尽管排粪造影可以确认在静息时或咳嗽时发生大便失禁,但它最有助于显示直肠脱垂[2,123]或直肠排空不良(见第19章)。在选定的大便失禁患者中,磁共振排粪造影可用于评估排空和识别共存的疾病,如直肠膨出、肠疝、膀胱膨出和肠黏膜套叠[111]。

5. 球囊排出实验(BET)

正常受试者可在1分钟内将50mL充满水的球囊[124]或充满硅胶的人造粪便从直肠排出[2]。一些研究使用了Foley球囊进行该实验[125],但是一项研究表明,使用Foley球囊是一种不适当的方法,高达50%的正常受试者可能会出现难以排出该装置的情况[126]。大多数大便失禁患者在很少或几乎没有便困难,但粪便渗漏的患者[74]和许多因粪便嵌塞继发大便失禁的老年人[73]证明排便受损。在这些患者中,BET有助于识别排便期间腹部、盆底和肛门括约肌之间共存的协同失调或缺乏协调能力。一项研究表明，养老院居民中协同失调的发生频率很高（见第 19 章）[127]。

6. 神经生理学检测

肛门括约肌肌肉活动的肌电图（EMG）是识别括约肌损伤以及显示神经病变的去神经-再支配电位的有用技术[30]。EMG 可采用细丝针状电极或表面电极（如肛门塞）进行。异常的肌电活动，如纤颤电位和高频自发放电，提供了慢性去神经支配的证据，常见于继发阴部神经损伤或马尾综合征的大便失禁患者[128]。PNTML 测量阴部神经终末端与肛门括约肌之间的神经肌肉完整性。阴部神经损伤导致肛门括约肌去神经支配和肌无力。因此，测量神经潜伏期时间有助于区分是肌肉损伤还是神经损伤引起的括约肌无力。使用一次性电极（St. Mark 电极测量潜伏期时间[129]。神经潜伏期时间延长提示阴部神经病变。与剖宫产或自然分娩的女性相比，经阴道分娩第二产程延长或使用产钳辅助分娩的女性 PNTML 是延长的[130,131]。美国胃肠病协会（AGA）技术评论不推荐 PNTML[94]，尽管专家评论指出，阴部神经病变患者的手术结果通常较差[132]。正常的 PNTML 并不排除阴部神经病变，因为存在少量完整的神经纤维可导致正常结果，而异常的潜伏期时间则非常显著。PNTML 可能有助于评估肛门括约肌修复前的患者，特别有助于预测手术效果。

控制肛门直肠功能的传出运动通路的外周成分的完整性，也可以通过记录和肛门括约肌对腰部和骶部神经根磁刺激的反应的 MEP 来评估。使用一种新的非侵入性方式——双侧 TAMS[25,35,36]。该技术基于法拉第原理，该原理指出，在电场不断变化的情况下，会产生磁场。因此，当电流通过导电线圈快速放电时，线圈周围会产生磁通量。磁通量会刺激神经组织。TAMS 可以更精确地定位脊髓和肛门括约肌之间的神经通路，并对传出周围神经系统、直肠和肛门括约肌进行亚成分分析。电刺激或磁刺激腰骶部神经根有利于测量马尾神经内的传导时间，可诊断骶运动神经根病为大便失禁的可能原因[133,134]。一项研究表明，记录直肠和肛门的经腰 MEP 和经骶 MEP 提供了大便失禁患者外周围神经肌肉损伤的轮廓图（图 18.7）[36]，可以揭示背部损伤患者迄今未检测到的变化。另一项研究评估了大便失禁患者的传出位点，结果表明，尽管与健康对照组相比，大便失禁患者的经颅-肛门直肠 MEP 延长，神经功能障碍的主要部位在脊神经根与肛门直肠之间，而脑与脊髓之间的部位基本完好[32]。

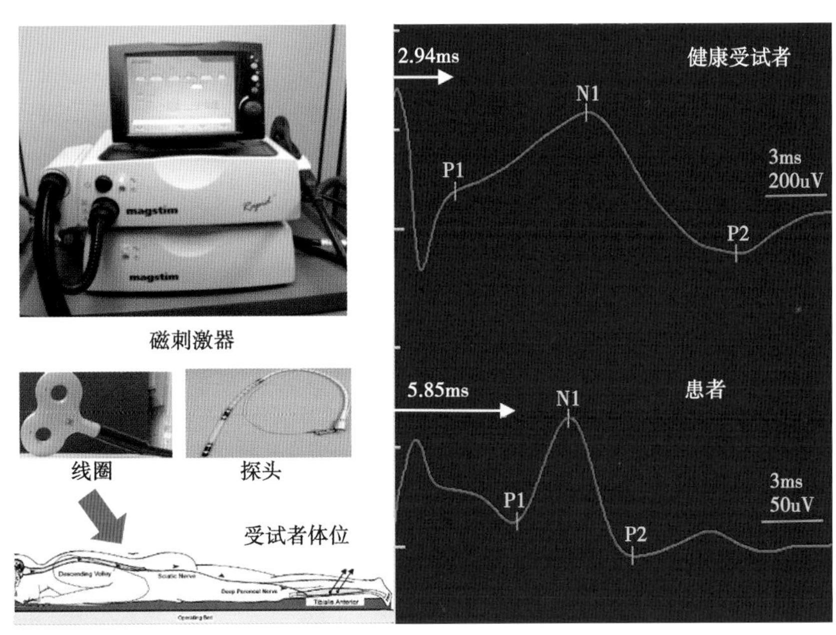

图 18.7　经腰骶部肛门直肠磁刺激（TAMS）试验（左），以及经腰磁刺激后的肛门运动诱发电位（MEP）反应（右）试验的设备。该设备由磁刺激装置、磁线圈和肛门直肠 MEP 探头组成。受试者的体位如图左下角所示。来自健康受试者（右上）的 MEP 反应显示正常的 MEP 潜伏期为 2.94ms。来自大便失禁患者（右下）的图显示 MEP 反应的潜伏期延长及振幅较小，提示肛门直肠神经病变

7. 大便失禁试验的临床应用

在一项前瞻性研究中，单独病史采集 80 例大便失禁患者中仅有 9 例可检测到潜在原因（占 11%），而 44 例患者（占 55%）的生理学试验显示异常[135]。在一项对 302 例大便失禁患者的大型回顾性研究中，仅进行肛门直肠测压、肌电图和直肠感觉测试后，确定了潜在的病理生理学异常[136]。大多数患者有一种以上的病理生理异常。在另一项 350 例患者的大型研究中发现，大便失禁患者肛门括约肌静息压和挤压压力降低，直肠容量较小，且在直肠输注生理盐水后出现泄漏较早[102]。然而单个试验或 3 种不同试验结合（肛门测压、直肠容量、生理盐水节制实验）的结果，在无失禁患者与失禁患者之间区分价值较低。这一发现说明正常值范围较广，机体有补偿大便失禁中任何一种机制丧失的能力。

在一项前瞻性研究中，肛门直肠测压和感觉试验不仅验证了临床现象，而且提供了临床上未能发现的新信息[93]。从这些研究中获取的诊断信息，可以影响大便失禁患者的治疗和预后。在 20% 的患者中发现了单一异常，而在 80% 的患者中发现了一种以上异常。在另一项研究中，40 例患者（71%）发现括约肌压力异常，42 例患者（75%）存在直肠感觉改变和直肠顺应性差[135]。这些发现得到了另一项研究的证实，该

研究表明，生理学检查对66%的大便失禁患者提供了明确的诊断[136]，而仅根据检测结果是无法预测个体患者是否患有大便失禁，异常检测结果必须与患者症状以及其他补充检测结果相互联系起来进行综合解释。肛门直肠功能检查提供了客观数据并确定了潜在的病理生理学。表18.2总结了关键试验，从中获得的信息支持其临床应用的证据。

表18.2 大便失禁的诊断试验*

试验	临床使用		质量	评论
	优点	缺点		
生理学				
肛门直肠测压(高分辨率和3D高清晰度)	量化正常或弱的EAS、IAS和耻骨直肠肌压力;识别直肠低敏感性和高敏感性、直肠顺应性受损、排便协同失调	缺乏标准化	良好	用于检测括约肌无力、直肠感觉和调节改变以及协同失调
肛门直肠内镜下功能性腔内成像探头(EndoFLIP)	测量肛门括约肌的横截面积、扩张指数和括约肌顺应性	缺乏规范的数据和可用性	合理	主要用于实验室研究;临床应用尚不完全清楚
针刺肌电图(EMG)	量化尖峰电位和再神经支配模式，提示神经病变或肌病	侵袭性，疼痛 未广泛应用	合理	有用，但主要用于实验室研究
表面肌电图(EMG)	显示EMG活动能力;可提供肌肉张力正常或减弱的信息	不精确，频发的伪影	合理	主要用于神经肌肉测试
阴部神经终末运动潜伏期(PNTML)	测量阴部神经终末部分的运动潜伏期，操作简单	微创、灵敏度低，检查者之间认识有差异	合理	数据有时相互矛盾，与其他测试和手术结果的相关性尚不清楚
经腰骶肛门直肠磁刺激(TAMS)测试	量化整个脊髓、肛门和脊髓-直肠通路的神经传导时间，微创	缺少标准化试验对照研究和实用性	良好	无创检查，更客观，比PNTML效益高;量化肛门和直肠神经病变
用不透放射线标志物进行结肠传输研究	评估有无粪便潴留，廉价且广泛可用	方法学不一致，有效性受到质疑	良好	对识别粪便渗漏和老年患者粪便嵌塞有用
球囊排出实验(BET)	简单、廉价、可在床边评估排出模拟粪便的能力，识别排便不协调	缺乏标准化	良好	BET正常也不能完全排除协同失调，应结合其他肛门直肠检查结果进行解释
影像				
肛门直肠超声检查	可视化IAS和EAS缺损、增厚、萎缩以及耻骨直肠肌	观察者间的偏倚，瘢痕难以识别	良好	使用最广泛的测试
排粪造影	检测直肠肛门脱垂、肠套叠、肛门直肠角、盆底无力、直肠前突和巨直肠	辐射暴露、令人尴尬、可利用性、观察者间的偏倚、方法学不一致	合理	实用，与其他测试互补
磁共振成像(MRI)	评估整体盆底解剖结构及动态运动;显示肛门直肠外括约肌形态和病理改变	价格昂贵、缺乏标准化和可用性	合理	用于其他检查的附加手段
腹部平片	识别结肠中的过多粪便、简单、廉价、广泛可用	缺乏标准化的解读和对照研究	差	不推荐作为常规评估，但适用于大便失禁和粪便嵌塞的老年人和儿童
钡剂灌肠	识别巨结肠、巨直肠、狭窄、憩室病、外源性压迫和腔内肿块	缺乏标准化、令人尴尬、辐射暴露、缺乏对照研究	差	不推荐作为常规评估的方法
内镜检查				
可屈式乙状结肠镜和结肠镜检查	直接观察结肠，以排除结肠黏膜病变(如孤立性直肠溃疡综合征、炎症、恶性肿瘤)	侵入性、有操作相关风险(如穿孔、出血)需用镇静剂	差	适用于不明原因的腹泻和渗漏的患者，以及年龄大于50岁的患者

3D，三维;EAS，肛门外括约肌;EndoFLIP，腔内功能性管腔成像探头;IAS，肛门内括约肌。

*循证总结。

四、治疗

大便失禁患者的治疗目标是恢复控便能力和提高生活质量。可以使用支持性和具体措施的策略。图 18.8 列出了评估和处理大便失禁的治疗流程。

（一）支持措施

一般性支持措施如避免不当食物、养成定时排便习惯、改善皮肤卫生和改变生活方式，可作为管理大便失禁患者的有用辅助措施。对于大便失禁的老年人或住院患者，可用有大便失禁治疗经验的人员，及时发现污物并立即清洁肛周皮肤是至关重要的[76]。采取卫生措施，如更换内衣、污染表皮后立即清洁肛周皮肤、使用湿巾而不是干燥的卫生纸，并使用氧化锌和炉甘石洗剂等。皮疹药膏可能有助于预防或治愈皮肤溃疡。肛周真菌感染应外用抗真菌药物治疗。更为重要的是，需在床边放置坐便桶，并采取支持措施以改善患者的总体健康和营养状况可能是有效的。使用粪便除臭剂（例如，床边护理会阴清洗液），可帮助掩盖粪便的气味。在住院患者中培养排便习惯和进行认知训练可能是有益的。使用这些措施的系列病例中报告的短期（3~6 个月）成功率高达 60%[137]。以证实使用这些措施失败的患者，死亡率高于无大便失禁和对这些措施反应差的大便失禁患者[138]。

其他支持性措施包括调整饮食习惯、如减少咖啡因或纤维食品的摄入。因为含咖啡因的饮食可增强胃结肠反射（或胃回肠反射），增加结肠运动[139]，并诱发小肠分泌[140]。减少咖啡因的摄入量，尤其是餐后，可能有助于减轻餐后急迫排便感或腹泻。剧烈的体力活动，特别是餐后或睡醒后，可能会引起大便失禁，因为这些生理反射与结肠运动增加[141]和结肠转运增强有关[142]。在一项对 2 565 名监测运动活动和大便失禁的成人的研究中，调整后，大便失禁与中度至剧烈运动呈正相关，但与轻度体力活动无关[143]。食物和症状日记可确定引起腹泻和大便失禁的饮食因素，乳糖和果糖是常见的因素，可能引起吸收不良[144]。消除含有这些成分的食品可能是有益的[2]。通常提倡使用欧车前等纤维补充剂，以增加粪便体积，减少水样便。有一项单一病例对照研究中，欧车前可使症状适度改善[145]，但纤维补充剂可通过增加不吸收纤维的结肠发酵而加重腹泻。

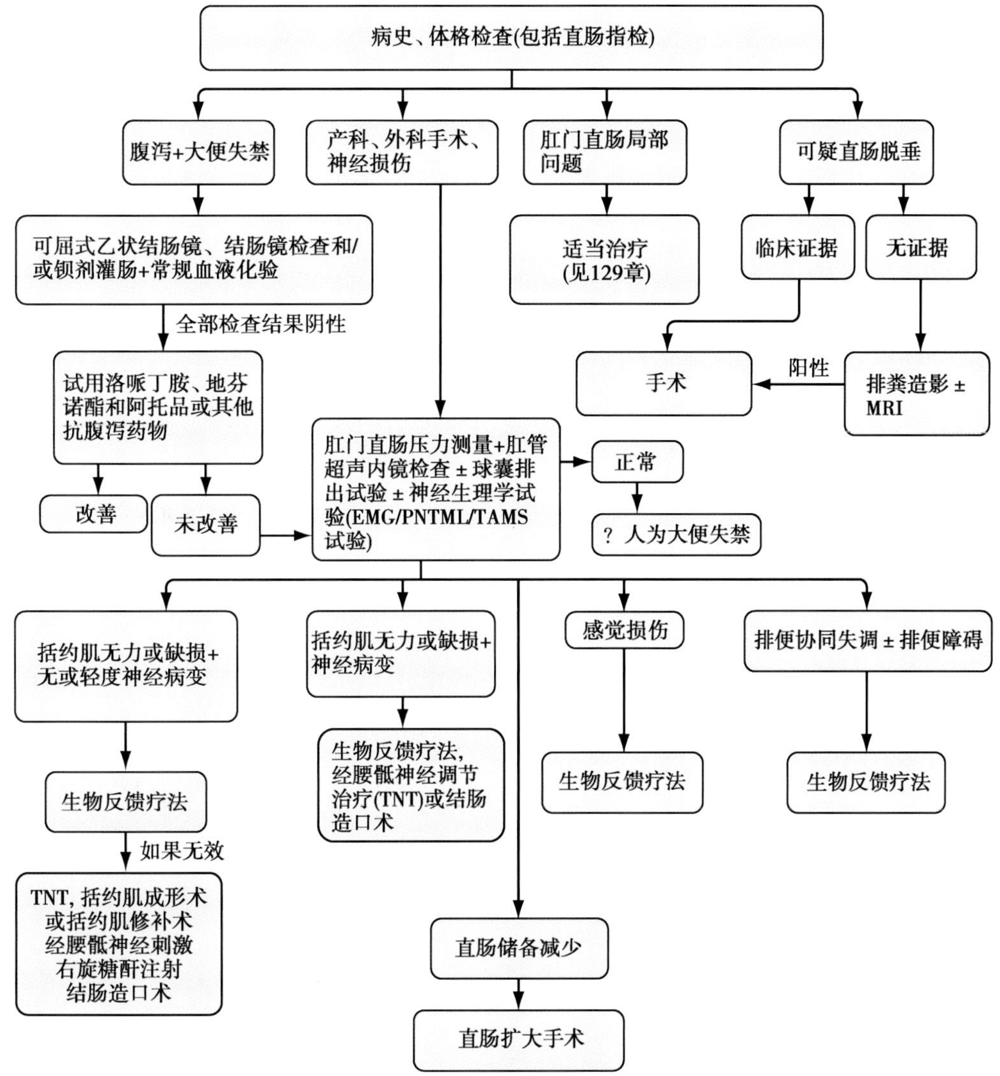

图 18.8　大便失禁患者评估和处理流程。PNTML，阴部神经终末运动潜伏期；TAMS，经腰骶肛门直肠磁刺激；EMG，肌电图

（二）特异性疗法

1. 药物治疗

尽管已经提出了其他药物治疗[2,146]，止泻药盐酸洛哌丁胺、地芬诺酯和硫酸阿托品仍然是治疗大便失禁的主要药物。在安慰剂对照研究中，洛派丁胺每次 4mg、每天 3 次，可以减少大便失禁的频率，改善排便的急迫性，增加结肠传输时间[104]，以及增加肛门括约肌静息压[147]和减轻粪便重量。一项对 80 例大便失禁患者进行的为期 8 周的随机交叉研究显示，洛哌丁胺和欧车前均可使大便失禁次数减少约 40%，但两种治疗方法之间无差异[148]。地芬诺酯和阿托品也有临床改善的报道[149]，但客观测试显示患者在直肠中保留盐水或球囊的能力没有改善。虽然大多数患者暂时受益于止泻药，但几天后发生下腹部痉挛性疼痛或排便困难，需要仔细调整剂量以获得预期效果。另一项随机对照研究在大便失禁患者中进行可乐定治疗（一种 α_2-肾上腺素能激动剂）每次 0. 1mg、每日 2 次，发现尽管腹泻减少，但大便失禁发作的次数并没有改变[150]。

特发性胆盐吸收不良可能是腹泻和大便失禁的重要潜在原因（见第 16 和 64 章）[151]。存在该问题的患者可应用滴定剂量的离子交换树脂，如考来烯胺（考来烯胺、每日 2～6g）和考来替泊或考来维伦可能受益。阿洛司琼是一种 5-羟色胺$_3$受体拮抗剂，已批准用于治疗腹泻型肠易激综合征，可作为大便失禁的辅助治疗用药，但该药的副作用限制了它的使用（见第 122 章）[152]。绝经后大便失禁的女性可从雌激素替代疗法中获益[153]。一项开放性研究表明，每天口服阿米替林 20mg，可用于治疗无结构性缺陷或神经病变的尿失禁或大便失禁患者[154]。栓剂或灌肠剂也可用于治疗直肠排空不全或排便后渗漏的失禁患者。在一些患者中，便秘药物与定期灌肠交替使用，可更有效地控制肠道内容物的排出，但这些干预措施尚未进行前瞻性研究。

2. 生物反馈疗法

神经肌肉和感觉训练，通常称为生物反馈疗法（或简称生物反馈），可改善大便失禁症状，恢复生活质量，改善肛门直肠功能的客观参数。生物反馈疗法对括约肌无力或直肠感觉受损的患者非常有用。该方法基于操作性反应训练技术，通过反复强化和即时反馈的学习过程个体获得新的行为[2,155]。生物反馈治疗大便失禁患者的目标是：①提高肛门括约肌肌力；②在自主挤压和直肠感知期间，改善腹部、臀部和肛门括约肌之间的协调性；③增强肛门直肠感官知觉。

由于每个目标都需要特定的训练方法，因此应根据潜在的病理生理机制，为每例患者量身定制治疗方案。生物反馈疗法通常采用视觉、听觉或语言反馈技术进行，通过放置在肛门直肠内的测压或肌电图探头提供反馈[2,155]。当要求患者挤压时，肛门括约肌收缩显示为肛门压力或肌电图活动的增加。该视觉提示为患者提供即时反馈。

直肠肛门协调训练的目的是，在直肠气囊充气后，在不到 2 秒的时间内达到最大程度的自主挤压。实际上这种动作模拟粪便进入直肠，并通过收缩正确的肌肉群使患者做好适当的反应准备[2,155]。指导患者学习如何选择性地挤压肛门肌肉，而不增加腹内压或不适当的收缩臀肌或大腿肌肉。该动作还可以识别感觉延迟，训练个体使用视觉线索来改善感觉运动协调性[156,157]。直肠感觉训练指导患者感知到较小体积的球囊扩张，但强度与先前感觉到的体积较大的球囊扩张强度相同，这一目标是通过在直肠内反复充盈和回缩气囊实现的。

这些神经肌肉训练技术必须与骨盆肌肉强化训练（改良 Kegel 运动）和其他支持措施一起使用，以实现肠道功能的持续改善。组成成分分析——肌肉训练、感觉训练或两者同时训练都是最有效的，单独的 Kegel 运动训练是否比多种方法更有效尚未确定。

预测需要多少次生物反馈治疗疗程往往是困难的。大多数患者似乎需要 4～6 次疗程（图 18. 9）[2,105,155]。一项使用固

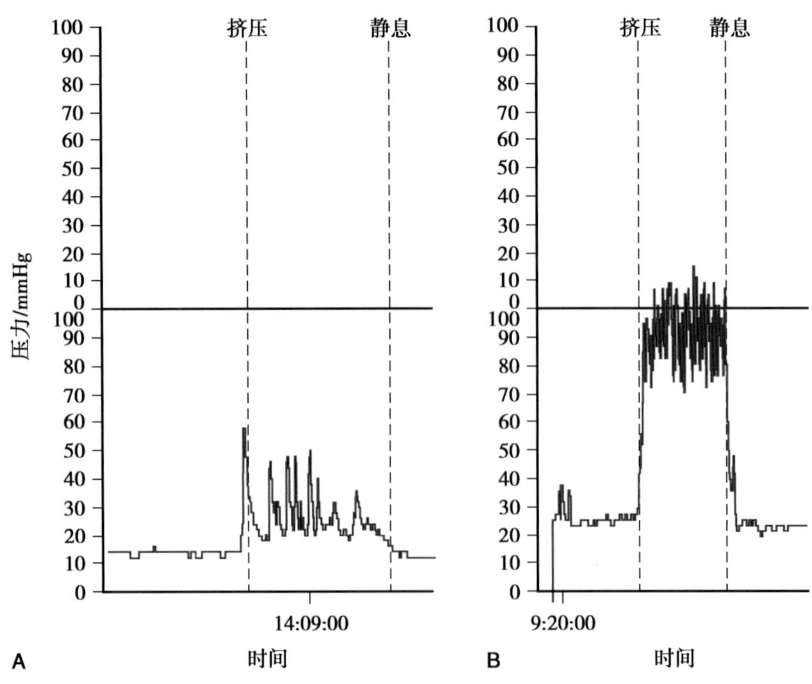

图 18. 9　大便失禁患者在挤压和静息时神经肌肉训练（生物反馈）前（A）和（B）后的肛门测压描记图。神经肌肉训练前，患者挤压乏力且持续时间较短，多次尝试挤压无效。经过 6 次训练后，患者产生和维持挤压的能力显著提高

定治疗疗程（通常少于 3 疗程）的研究显示，改善效果不如根据患者表现调整治疗疗程的效果好[158,159]。在一项研究中认为，在 6 周、3 个月和 6 个月时，通过生物反馈疗法进行定期强化，会带来额外的益处[105]和长期改善[160]。

在关于大便失禁的文献中[161-171]"改善""成功"和"治愈"的 3 个术语可互换使用，每个术语的定义都不一致。在非对照研究中，40%～85%的患者报告了主观改善[2,158]。表 18.3 总结了大便失禁患者生物反馈治疗的随机对照试验[155,156,162,163,167-170]。对 11 项随机对照试验的 Cochrane 评价得出结论，没有任何一种训练方法是最好的[172]。生物反馈疗法是否优于保守治疗也不清楚。在一项随机对照试验中[163]，108 名患者随机分配接受 6 次肌电生物反馈（$N=44$）或 Kegel 运动训练（$N=64$）加支持治疗。治疗后接受生物反馈治疗的患者中有 77% 报告症状得到充分缓解，而接受 Kegel 运动训练的患者中有 41% 报告症状得到充分缓解（$P<0.001$）。在意向性治疗分析中，两组之间大便失禁发作次数并无差异，但在按方案分析中观察到改善趋势（$P=0.042$）[163]。该研究表明，生物反馈疗法优于 Kegel 运动训练。另一项随机对照试验，将持续挤压与快速持续挤压进行比较，发现 86%的患者在控便方面有所改善，但两组之间无差异[173]。另一项研究将生物反馈和中频电刺激与低频电刺激进行了比较（见下文），显示生物反馈加电刺激与单纯电刺激相比，54%的患者明显改善[174]。一项研究将盆底锻炼加直肠球囊训练与单独盆底锻炼进行对比，结果显示大便失禁患者改善分别为 51%和 48%，但两组治疗之间无差异[175]。

生物反馈疗法尚未标准化，这种治疗方法的使用在很大程度上仅限于专科中心。基线检查时获得的测压参数似乎不能预测生物反馈治疗的临床反应[176]。同样，患者的年龄、是否存在括约肌缺陷或神经病变并不能预测结果[177]。用于选择的标准、患者个人的动机、治疗师的热情以及大便失禁的严重程度均可能影响结果[2,155,158,159,169]。

尽管缺乏统一的方法和随机对照试验的报告结果不一致，但生物反馈疗法似乎带来益处（表 18.3）。美国胃肠病学协会（ACG）[178]及美国和欧洲神经胃肠病学和运动学会推荐生物反馈疗法用于治疗大便失禁[179]。因此，应向所有使用支持性治疗失败的大便失禁患者提供神经肌肉训练，尤其是老年患者、有并发症的患者和考虑重建手术的患者。严重的大便失禁、阴部神经病变和存在潜在的神经系统疾病与生物反馈治疗的反应不佳相关[180-182]。一项研究表明，生物反馈疗法可能对急迫性大便失禁患者最有益[183]。生物反馈似乎也适用于接受肛门括约肌成形术[184]、肛门后修复术（见下文）[185]或低位前切除术的患者[186]以及接受先天性肛门直肠畸形矫正术的儿童[187]。

表 18.3　成人大便失禁的生物反馈治疗和/或训练的结果*

参考文献	受试者 F/M	治疗	对照	结果
156	17/8	测压、BFB+直肠感觉训练+协调训练（每周 1 次，共 4 周）	Sham 训练（交叉设计）	治疗症状改善
162	40/0	BFB+电刺激（增强）（每周 1 次，共 12 周）	阴道测压生物反馈	治疗组症状改善程度大于对照组（$P<0.001$）
163	83/25	BFB+PFMT+感觉训练（两周 1 次，共 12 周）	PFMT	治疗组症状改善程度大于单用 PFMT 组（77% vs 41%；$P=0.001$）
167	60/0	BFB（每周 1 次，共 12 周）+电刺激	BFB	组间 NSD
168	49/0	BFB+家庭锻炼	电刺激	两组均改善。症状和 QOL 组间 NSD
169	159/12	4 组： （1）教育+劝告 （2）组 1+PMFT （3）组 2+测压+BFB （4）组 3+家庭 BFB （两周 1 次，共 3 个月）	N/A	约 54%出现改善。症状和 QOL 组间 NSD
170	107/13	3 组： （1）PFMT （2）PFMT+肛门超声 BFB （3）PFMT+测压 BFB（每月 1 次，5 次）	N/A	症状、QOL 和测压变化组间 NSD
173	53/19	持续挤压（5 次，8 周）	快速持续挤压（5 次，8 周）	86%控便能力改善，组间 NSD
174	65/15	生物反馈和中频电刺激（每日 2 次，6 个月）	低频电刺激（每日 2 次，6 个月）	治疗组 54%肛门控便能力改善，而对照组为 0%
175	72/8	PFMT 和 RBT（每周 2 次，共 3 周，然后每周 1 次，共 12 次）	PFMT（每周 2 次，共 3 周，然后每周 1 次，共 12 次）	两组大便失禁均有改善，治疗组 51%、对照组 48%。组间 NSD
249、250	26/4	家庭生物反馈用新型电刺激和阻抗训练（每日 1 次，共 6 周）	用 ARM 探头进行诊室生物反馈（每周 1 次，共 6 周）	两组大便失禁均有改善，家庭组缓解率为 65%（大便失禁事件减少≥50%）而诊室组为 60

*选定的随机对照试验。

ARM，肛门直肠测压；BFB，生物反馈疗法（使用肌电图探头，除非另有说明）；F，女性；M，男性；N/A，不适用；NSD，无显著差异；PFMT，盆底肌肉训练；QOL，生活质量；RBT，直肠球囊试验。

Adapted from Norton C. Fecal incontinence and biofeedback therapy. Gastroenterol Clin North Am 2008；37：587-604.

3. 肛管塞、括约肌填充剂和电刺激

一次性肛管塞用于暂时堵塞肛管防止粪便渗漏[188]。遗憾的是许多患者无法忍受持久插入该器具[189,190]。肛管塞可能对肛管感觉受损的患者、神经系统疾病患者[191]、长期生活在社会福利机构缺乏自理能力以及不能正常行动的患者有用。在一些粪便渗漏的患者中,插入由手术棉制成的肛管塞可能是有益的[192]。一项多中心、前瞻性、单组、非随机对照研究,评估了91例大便失禁患者使用硅胶衬垫的疗效,其中62%接受治疗的患者大便失禁发作减少≥50%,这些患者大便失禁严重程度评分也有所降低。在完成12周治疗的患者中,约78%的患者对该器具预防粪便泄漏的效果非常满意[193]。阴道排便控制系统[Eclipse System(Pevalon,Sunnyvale,CA)]使用类似于子宫颈托的可充气、自行保持球囊,通过对肛门直肠进行外部压迫操作[194]。在一项为期4周的开放性标记试验中,110例患者中有61例成功安装了该器具,其中79%报告大便失禁发作次数减少≥50%[194],生活质量改善。主要的不良反应有盆腔不适或疼痛、阴道点滴出血、红斑和尿漏,需要等待长期对照试验进行评估。

许多大便失禁的患者选择不戴衬垫。小的肛门敷料可能对臀部间的轻微污染有用,但如果每天需要多次更换敷料,成本可能昂贵。通常认为尿布在提供安全舒适性、皮肤保护或掩盖气味方面不令人满意。然而,全球销量的不断上升和尿布技术的改进表明,尿布可能比以前更容易被接受。

尝试使用多种括约肌填充剂包括自体脂肪[195]、戊二醛处理的胶原蛋白[196]和合成大分子微粒[197]填充扩张肛门括约肌以增加其表面积,从而为肛管提供更好的密封。这些材料通常注射在括约肌缺损处的黏膜下,如果整个肌肉退化或断裂时则注射在周围黏膜下。研究表明被动性大便失禁患者在短期内有明显的改善。在一项对206例患者的随机对照试验中,在齿状线上方注射右旋糖酐微球效果优于安慰剂,其疗效与基线相比,大便失禁发作次数减少50%或更多,注射右旋糖酐微球的反应率与安慰剂的反应率分别为52%和31%[198]。一项为期36个月的长期疗效评估显示,52.2%的患者报告持续获益(发作次数减少≥50%),13.25%的患者报告完全获益[199]。另一种可注射填充剂聚苯烯酸酯聚醇,也在58名患者的前瞻性、非对照试验中进行了评估。通过肛周皮肤皮下注射到齿状线上方的肛门直肠黏膜下层。根据Cleveland诊所临床大便失禁评分标准,大便失禁改善率为50%,约60%的患者被判定为治疗成功[200],但缺乏对照组和选择偏倚是本研究的显著局限性。

用足以产生强直性不自主收缩的频率(通常30~40Hz)电刺激横纹肌,可以增加肌肉力量、阴部神经的传导速率和运动单位的大小,以及促进神经元生长和局部血流[201,202]。低频刺激(5~10Hz)可调节自主神经功能包括感觉和过度活动。电刺激治疗大便失禁的研究规模较小、无法控制、且易受运动、生物反馈或其他干预措施的影响。Cochrane对260名受试者进行的4项随机对照试验的回顾分析得出结论,电刺激可能有一定的效果[203]。一项研究发现,使用肛门生物反馈加肛门电刺激比单独使用生物反馈疗法的患者产生的短期效益更大[162],而另一项研究却发现,电刺激与单独运动和生物反馈相比没有额外的效益[167]。患者在1Hz和35Hz的刺激下显示改善程度相同[155]。两项随机对照试验报告,生物反馈和电刺激同样有效[168,204]。电刺激本身是否有帮助仍不清楚。

我们理解大便失禁治疗方法的一个关键障碍是,缺乏涉及两种或更多治疗方法的比较有效性试验。因此,目前尚不清楚用哪种治疗对哪种类型的患者最有效,谁可能受益最大。

4. 外科治疗

对于采取保守措施或生物反馈治疗失败的患者应考虑手术治疗[205]。手术方式的选择必须根据患者的需要而定,可分为4种临床类型:①肛门括约肌的简单结构缺陷;②肛门括约肌薄弱、但结构完整;③肛门括约肌复合体的复杂破坏;④括约肌外异常。表18.4总结了各种外科手术的成功率[206]。

表18.4　微创手术治疗大便失禁的成功率

操作项目	效果衡量	成功率/%	质量评价
目前使用			
左旋糖酐微球注射	与基线相比,大便失禁改善>50%	52:31(左旋糖酐:安慰剂)	合理
肛门括约肌修复术	临床、生理学	50~66*	合理†
骶神经刺激	完全控制排便 排便自制力改善≥50%	40~75 75~100	良好
动态股薄肌新括约肌	恢复控便能力	42~85	差‡
人工肠括约肌	能完全控便	50~100§	差
正在研究中			
射频治疗(Secca程序)	改善控便≥50%	84	差
直肠扩大术	避免造口	64	差

注:*5年成功率降至50%。†来自Cochrane系统评价,但一些资料仅来自一项研究的推断。‡基于对病例系列的系统回顾,无对照研究。§病例系列中的移出率约为50%

Adapted from Gladman MA. Surgical treatment of patients with constipation and fecal incontinence. Gastroenterol Clin North Am 2008;37:605-25,With permission.

在大多数患者中，特别是产科创伤患者，括约肌重叠修复通常是足够的。将括约肌的撕裂端折叠在一起，并与耻骨直肠肌相连。正如 Parks 和 McPartlin[207] 所描述的，重叠括约肌修复术涉及肛管前方的弯曲切口，游离外括约肌在瘢痕处分开，保留瘢痕组织以固定缝合线，并使用两排缝合线进行重叠修复。如果发现肛门内括约肌缺损，可对肛门内括约肌进行单独重叠修复。据报道症状改善率为 70%~80%，但有一项研究报告的改善率仅为 50% 左右[207-211]。有些患者术后可能会出现排气问题。括约肌成形术的长期疗效（超过 5~10 年）令人失望，只有 30% 的患者表现出良好的疗效[212]。在肛门括约肌薄弱无力但结构完整的大便失禁患者中，已尝试应用肛门后修补术[213]，通过括约肌间入路使肛门直肠角更加尖锐，从而改善控便能力。该方法的长期成功率在 20%~58% 之间[214]。

对于肛门括约肌严重结构损伤和重度大便失禁的患者，尝试用两种方法构建新的括约肌：①使用自体骨骼肌，通常是股薄肌，少数用臀肌[132,215]；②使用人造肠括约肌[216]。刺激股薄肌转位技术（动态股薄肌成形术），已经在许多医疗中心进行了测试，但结果却令人失望[217,218]。人造肠括约肌的植入包括一个可充气套囊装置，该装置充满植入的球囊储液器中的液体，由皮下泵控制。将袖带放气以允许排便[219,220]。一项随机对照试验证明，人造肠括约肌在改善控便方面优于保守治疗[221]。然而一项长期研究（中位随访期约为 7 年）记录的成功率低于 50%，移出率高达 49%，感染率高达 33%[156,222]。50% 的患者发生了排泄问题。

直肠扩大术是纠正继发于储液囊或直肠感觉运动障碍的难治性大便失禁患者亚组中，生理异常的一种新方法[223]。

患者表现为直肠顺应性降低、直肠感觉增强、直肠超敏。目前尚无与手术治疗、药物或生物反馈治疗相比较的对照研究，也无发表不同手术方式的对照研究资料，由于大多数手术的结局都是从最初显著改善到长期不令人满意的结果，因此目前没有一种手术被普遍接受。未来需要更好地了解潜在的病理生理学和开发更安全更优的技术，随后进行前瞻性对照试验，选择具有明确的括约肌缺损的年轻患者进行适当的手术。

5. 其他治疗措施

使用特殊设计的探头［Secca 系统（Rayfield Technology, Houston, Tex.）］将射频能量通过多个针状电极递送到肛管黏膜深处，插入大便失禁患者的肛管[224]。其作用机制是热诱导引起的肛管和远端直肠的组织收缩和重塑。在一项研究中，症状在治疗后 2~5 年持续改善[225]。一项多中心试验证实，至少在短期内（6 个月）控便和生活质量有所改善。并发症包括黏膜溃疡和延迟出血[226]。有趣的是，肛门直肠测压、PNTML 测量或肛门超声内镜检查的结果均没有变化。一项为期 6 个月的欧洲对照研究显示，射频优于安慰治疗组，但临床影响可忽略不计，生活质量不变[227]。该方法在美国完成的一项随机对照试验的结果目前尚未公布。

顺行可控性灌肠术[228]，包括形成盲肠造口按钮或阑尾造口[229]，可以定期顺行冲洗结肠，这种方法适用于儿童和神经系统疾病的患者[229-231]。

6. 结肠造口术

如果上述技术均不适用或全部失败，结肠造口术仍然是许多患者的一种安全选择，尽管在美学上不太可取[132,232-234]。它特别适用于脊髓损伤患者、瘫痪患者以及有严重皮肤问题或其他并发症的患者。结肠造口术不应被视为是药物或外科治疗的失败[206]。对于许多大便失禁患者来说，恢复正常生活质量和改善症状是有益的。使用腹腔镜辅助的方法（即环钻结肠造口术）可能有助于形成造口，并将患者的并发症降至最低[235]。在一项研究中，动态股薄肌成形术估计的直接总费用为 31 733 美元，包括造口护理的结肠造口术为 71 576 美元，以及大便失禁的常规治疗为 12 180 美元[236]。

7. 骶神经刺激

骶神经刺激（sacral nerve stimulation, SNS）已成为患者的一种有效治疗选择，虽然 SNS 改善大便失禁的机制尚不完全清楚[237]，其获益可能与结直肠感觉或运动功能的直接外周效应或与脊髓或脑水平的中枢效应有关[238]。早期研究是在肛门括约肌形态完整的患者中进行的，但随后的报告也可用于 EAS 缺损[239]、IAS 缺损[240]、马尾综合征[241] 和脊髓损伤患者的治疗[242]。

SNS 技术包括两个阶段。第一阶段是为期两周的临时试验阶段，在此期间，将电极植入第二或第三骶神经根，并用神经刺激装置刺激神经。如果患者报告症状得到满意改善，则第二阶段放置一个永久性神经刺激装置（图 18.10）。SNS 的初步报告描述了临床症状和生活质量的显著改善和对生理参数的边际效应[211,243]。SNS 多中心研究的结果报告了大便失禁和生活质量的显著和持续的改善[244-246]。一项随机对照试验发现 SNS 优于支持疗法（盆底锻炼、填充剂和饮食管理措施）[247]，但长期结果尚未提供。形态完整的肛门括约肌可能不是 SNS 成功的先决条件，EAS 缺损<33% 的患者，可用该种方法得到有效的治疗[239]。已经发表的 SNS 试验结果的系统性回顾显示，40%~75% 的患者实现了完全控便，75%~100% 的患者出现改善，不良事件发生频率低于 10%[237]。

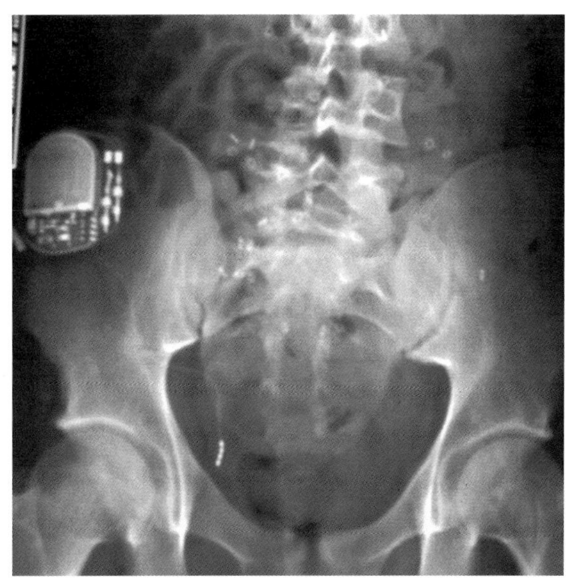

图 18.10 腹部平片显示神经刺激器装置（RLQ）以及永久植入骶神经的电极（不透射线）。该患者因大便失禁而接受结肠转运试验研究，结果显示位于结肠远端有大部分不透射线标志物保留，提示肛门直肠出口功能障碍

8. 经皮胫神经刺激

经皮胫神经刺激(percutaneous tibial nerve stimulation,PTNS)使用34号针头刺激胫后神经,并通过此刺激L4~S3神经根改善大便失禁[248]。在一项227例患者的大型多中心随机对照试验中,PTNS组与假手术组的疗效(大便失禁降低≥50%)无差异(38% vs 31%),表明对所有大便失禁患者均无益处[248]。PTNS的另一种方法是使用皮肤垫,但数据有限。

(三) 新疗法

正在探索几种创新方法来缓解大便失禁。一种新的家庭生物反馈系统,结合了肛门括约肌的机械阻力训练与自滴定充气气囊和逐渐升级的电刺激肛门括约肌与语音引导程序,已经在随机对照试验中进行了测试[249,250]。家庭生物反馈似乎与诊室生物反馈一样有效,在一项为期6周的随机对照验中,家庭组的临床有效率为65%,诊室组为60%[249,250]。另一种方法是用磁性电极导线环绕肛门括约肌以增强肛门括约肌。一项有35例患者的非对照前瞻性研究报告了23例患者(65%)的5年随访数据,1年治疗成功率为63%,3年为66%,5年为53%。不良事件包括7例器具植入、排便功能障碍(20%)、疼痛(14%)和感染(11%)[251]。另一种新方法是从肌肉活检中获得的成人干细胞,尤其是成肌细胞,有可能修复和再生受损的肛门括约肌组织[252]。在一项随机对照试验中,向括约肌内注射自体成肌细胞或安慰剂,在6个月时显示与Cleveland诊所临床大便失禁评分的改善程度相似(主要结果指标),但在12个月时成肌细胞组继续改善,而安慰剂组恢复至基线水平。随后安慰剂组接受开放标记的成肌细胞治疗,大便失禁症状改善60%[253]。而另一项使用来自脂肪组织的干细胞的研究显示,大便失禁没有改善[254]。一项初试性随机对照试验,评估了使用重复频率磁刺激腰神经和骶神经的经腰骶神经调节疗法的有效性和安全性[32]。频率为1Hz的磁刺激在改善大便失禁方面表现出明显的优势,与5Hz组(25%有效率)和15Hz组(42%有效率)相比,有效率为88%。这种无创性神经调节疗法在未来可能会被证明是有益的。

总之保守疗法和生物反馈是一线治疗方法[255],如果不成功,可以先考虑使用右旋糖酐,后再使用SNS扩张括约肌。不推荐PTNS,但术后大便失禁应考虑括约肌成形术。目前大便失禁治疗的循证总结见表18.5。

(四) 特定患者的治疗

1. 脊髓损伤患者

脊髓损伤患者证实有结肠动力延迟或肛门直肠功能障碍,可表现为大便失禁、渗漏、排便困难或直肠低敏感性[256]。这些患者的肛门括约肌压力和直肠顺应性较低,但测压结果与肠功能障碍之间的相关性较差。经腰和骶MEP的研究显示,影响整个脊髓肛门和脊髓直肠通路的神经肌肉功能严重障碍[35]。脊髓损伤患者可能因上脊髓病变或马尾病变而出现大便失禁[100,101]。在前一组中,骶神经元反射弧是完好无损的,咳嗽反射被保留下来,因此,可通过数字仿真或用栓剂出现反射性排便。对于低位脊髓或马尾神经病变的患者,数字仿真可能无效,因为排便反射常受损。在这些病例中,治疗包括使用止泻药以防止粪便持续污染,然后通过定期灌肠或使用泻药或在方便的间隙使用灌洗液[2]。盲肠造口术也可能是适宜的[257]。在一些患者中,结肠造口术可能是最佳的选择[232]。

表18.5 大便失禁的治疗方案*

治疗方案	质量评价
药物	
地芬诺酯和阿托品	适宜
洛哌丁胺	适宜
阿米替林	差
考来烯胺(考来烯胺)	差
生物反馈疗法	良好
肛管塞装置	差
外科手术	
骶神经刺激	良好
扩张括约肌	良好
人工肠括约肌	适宜
动态股薄肌成形术	适宜
括约肌成形术	适宜
结肠造口术	差
射频治疗(Secca程序)	差
新疗法	
自体成肌细胞/干细胞疗法	适宜
电气/机械阻力训练	适宜
经腰骶神经调节	适宜

*循证总结。

2. 粪便渗漏患者

有粪便渗漏的患者,表现出与直肠感觉受损相关的排便不协调,因此通过生物反馈疗法进行神经肌肉训练,以改善协同失调是有用的(见19章)[74,258]。包括感觉训练和盆底肌肉直肠协调组成的治疗,使粪便完全排空。已证明通过客观措施,能够大幅减少粪便渗漏事件的数量,改善了肠道功能和肛门直肠功能[74]。

3. 老年患者

大便失禁是老年人的常见问题,可能是养老院患者健康状况下降和死亡率增加的标志[76]。在一项研究中,20%的养老院居民在入住后10个月内出现大便失禁,长期大便失禁与生存率降低有关[138]。在一份研究报告中,长期不活动、痴呆和限制患者及时如厕是发生大便失禁的最重要风险因素[17]。

大便失禁的常见机制包括:肛门直肠感觉受损、肛门括约肌和盆底肌肉无力。活动能力下降和感觉降低也是大便失禁的常见原因[259]。这些患者中的许多人有粪便嵌塞和溢出[73,260]。粪便嵌塞是住院老年人大便失禁的主要原因,主要是由于患者对直肠中粪便无感觉和反应能力。对245例长期住院的老年患者[261]进行回顾性筛查发现,粪便嵌塞(55%)和通便剂(20%)是最常见的腹泻原因,而长期静止不动和大便失禁与粪便嵌塞或腹泻密切相关。一项研究表明，在患有大便失禁的养老院居民中，高达 75% 的人出现肛门括约肌功能受损（大便失禁的危险因素）、直肠感觉下降和协同失调[52,262]。

粪便软化剂、盐水泻药和刺激性泻药经常作为预防性治疗使用，以防止便秘和嵌塞。在一项针对住院老年患者的研究中，使用单一渗透剂和直肠刺激剂及每周一次灌肠，以达到直肠完全排空，可将大便失禁的频率降低 35%，粪便污染的频率降低 42%[263]。如果粪便嵌塞不能通过服用泻药或及时如厕缓解，应考虑采用人工手法碎裂嵌塞粪便、每周 2~3 次自来水灌肠或使用直肠栓剂等治疗方法[264]。然而，在肛门括约肌功能受损和直肠感觉减退的情况下，液状粪便可能适得其反。同样神经肌肉训练改善老年人的协同失调、程式化的排便习惯、改善提高活动能力和认知训练也可能有用[76]。

4. 儿童患者

在其他方面健康的 7 岁儿童中，有 1%~2% 的儿童出现大便失禁[265]。其原因是功能性粪便滞留（以前描述为大便失禁），功能性非潴留性大便失禁[266]是先天性异常、发育障碍或智力低下所致。

功能性粪便潴留的儿童，排便不规律，粪便体积大而且疼痛不适。因此，当儿童出现排便冲动时，他们会采取一种直立姿势，将双腿并拢，并用力收缩骨盆和臀肌。随着时间的推移，这种有意识的排便抑制会导致直肠过度调节、直肠敏感性丧失，失去正常的排便冲动。滞留的粪便逐渐变得更难以排出，从而导致恶性循环，最终结果形成溢出性大便失禁，在嵌塞的粪块周围有黏液或液体样粪便渗出。这种异常行为可能导致排便时肛门外括约肌无意识收缩，引起排便协同失调[260,267]。

相比之下，功能性非潴留性大便失禁，是指 4 岁以上无粪便潴留证据的儿童在厕所以外的地方反复和不适当的排便，而无任何粪便潴留的迹象。根据罗马Ⅲ共识委员会制定的标准[266]，功能性非潴留性大便失禁儿童通常每天在厕所排便，除此之外他们几乎每周都会有一次以上的内裤排便。在腹部或直肠部位没有触及粪便肿块，腹部 X 线平片也未发现粪便潴留的证据，结肠不透性放射线标志物检测也是正常的[268]。功能性非潴留性大便失禁儿童，白天和夜间遗尿发生频率高于功能性潴留性大便失禁儿童（40%~50%）。与对照组受试者相比，功能性非潴留性大便失禁儿童有更多的行为问题，心理社会问题外在化和内在化程度高于对照组。

治疗目标是清除任何粪便嵌塞，恢复正常的排便习惯（包括排软便、无不适感），并确保在适当的地方自行如厕和排便[268]。最好通过口服药物或灌肠解除粪便嵌塞。高剂量聚乙二醇 3350 按照 1~1.5g/kg/d，连用 3 天，已被证明是有效的[269]。一旦达到治疗目的，后续治疗应侧重于通过饮食干预、行为矫正和适当的通便剂预防复发。功能性非潴留性大便失禁的治疗是基于教育、非指责的方法、鼓励定时如厕，必要时转诊心理医生。症状的成功缓解和消退可能需要长期治疗和随访[270,271]。此外要解决与父母冲突的问题和心理社会应激源，消除对排便疼痛的恐惧，可能也是取得成功的关键[258,272]。

最常见的先天性异常是神经管畸形（如脊髓脊膜膨出、脊柱裂）和肛门闭锁（见第 98 章）。患有神经缺陷或畸形的儿童可能从行为治疗中获益，包括刺激性排便计划（见前文）[273]。肛门闭锁最好直接通过手术治疗，但约 20% 可能治疗效果不满意[274]。令人惊讶的是，患肛门直肠畸形的儿童似乎能较好地应对他们的疾病[274]，智力障碍或发育迟缓的儿童可能难以实现（永远无法）完全的控制排便，需要终生支持治疗。

（曹红燕　谢咚 译，袁农　刘军 校）

参考文献

18

第 19 章　便秘

Johanna C. Iturrino, Anthony j. Lembo 著

章节目录

一、定义和症状表现 …… 238
二、流行病学 …… 239
（一）患病率 …… 239
（二）发病率 …… 239
（三）公共卫生观点 …… 239
三、危险因素 …… 239
（一）性别 …… 239
（二）年龄 …… 240
（三）种族和国籍 …… 240
（四）社会经济地位与教育水平 …… 240
（五）饮食和体力活动 …… 240
（六）药物 …… 240
四、结肠功能 …… 241
（一）肠腔内容物 …… 241
（二）水和钠的吸收 …… 241
（三）直径和长度 …… 241
（四）运动功能 …… 241
（五）神经支配和 Cajal 间质细胞 …… 241
（六）排便功能 …… 242
（七）粪便大小及黏稠度 …… 242
五、分类 …… 242
六、病理生理学 …… 243
（一）正常传输型便秘 …… 243
（二）慢传输型便秘 …… 243
（三）排便障碍 …… 243
七、病因 …… 243
（一）肛门直肠和盆底疾病 …… 243
（二）系统性疾病 …… 245
（三）神经系统疾病 …… 245
（四）结肠、直肠和肛门结构性病变 …… 246
（五）药物 …… 247
（六）精神心理障碍 …… 247
（七）粪便嵌塞 …… 247
八、临床评估 …… 248
（一）病史 …… 248
（二）体格检查 …… 248
九、诊断试验 …… 248
（一）系统性疾病试验 …… 248
（二）结构性疾病试验 …… 249
（三）生理学测量 …… 249
十、治疗 …… 251
（一）一般措施 …… 251
（二）特效治疗制剂 …… 253
（三）其他形式的治疗 …… 259

便秘是描述一个人对排便改变的感觉，包括硬便、排便困难和排便不尽感等。当一个人自述便秘症状至少连续 3 个月时，诊断为慢性便秘。慢性便秘通常由结肠推进和/或直肠排空障碍所致[1]，可分为 3 类：慢传输型便秘、正常传输型便秘和直肠排空障碍。这 3 种类型之间可能存在明显的重叠[1,2]。慢性便秘的继发性原因不常见，包括机械性、神经性、激素和代谢疾病，以及药物治疗的反应。

慢性便秘影响了很大一部分西方人群，在女性、儿童和老年人中尤其普遍。大多数人不就医，但由于便秘影响了 3%~31% 的人群，2010 年美国仍有近 300 万人次就诊[3]。对于大多数受影响的人来说，只需最低限度干预或根本不需要干预，而对另一些人来说，便秘的治疗具有挑战性，对生活质量产生负面影响。在这种情况下，必须排除便秘的继发性原因。

一、定义和症状表现

当患者说"我便秘"时，询问他们"我便秘"是什么意思很重要。大多数患者将便秘描述为感觉排便困难或与排便有关的不适。年轻健康成年人用于定义便秘的最常见术语是排便过度用力（52%）、硬便（44%）和无能力排便（34%）[4]。国家健康访问调查（NHIS）数据分析发现，在 10 875 名 60 岁以上的受试者中，排便过度用力和硬便与自我主诉的便秘相关性最强[5]。

便秘的定义也因医护人员而异[6]。便秘的传统医学定义，是根据美国健康成年人 95% 的置信区间下限，即每周排便 3 次或更少[7]。然而，排便频率的报告通常不准确，并且与便秘的主诉相关性较差[8]。而患有便秘的人经常伴有各种各样的症状，包括排便困难、硬便、排便不尽感、腹部不适、腹胀满、过度用力、排便时堵塞感和腹胀等[2]。

为了使便秘的定义标准化，国际专家于 1992 年首次制定了共识标准（罗马 Ⅰ 共识委员会标准，简称罗马 Ⅰ 标准）[9]，并于 1999 年、2006 年和 2016 年[10]进行了修订［分别为罗马 Ⅱ、Ⅲ 和 Ⅳ 标准（框 19.1）］[11,12]。

罗马标准纳入了便秘的多种症状，其中大便次数仅为几种症状之一，并要求至少 25% 的排便中出现至少两种症状。罗马标准包括盆底肌协同失调或出口梗阻的症状（例如，感

觉到肛门直肠堵塞或梗阻,以及使用手法辅助排便),患者在不使用泻药的情况下出现罕见的稀便。罗马标准强调近3个月的症状符合标准,在诊断前症状出现至少6个月。罗马Ⅳ标准认识到功能性肠道疾病,如肠易激综合征(IBS)伴便秘和慢性便秘,存在于一个疾病谱上,并可能存在重叠症状[10]。

框19.1 功能性便秘罗马Ⅳ标准

1. 必须包括下列2项或2项以上*:
   a. 超过25%的排便过程感到费力
   b. 超过25%的排便过程出现结块状便或硬便†
   c. 超过25%的排便过程出现排便不尽感
   d. 超过25%的排便过程出现肛门直肠梗阻/堵塞感
   e. 超过25%的排便需手法辅助(如手指辅助排便、盆底支撑排便)
   f. 每周排便少于3次
2. 不使用泻药时,很少出现稀便
3. 不符合肠易激综合征(IBS)诊断标准

*诊断前症状出现至少6个月,近3个月符合以上标准。
†Bristol粪便形态量表1型或2型(见图19.2)。
From Lacy BE, Mearin F, Chang L, et al. Bowel disorders. Gastroenterology. 2016;150:1393-1407. e5.

美国胃肠病学会(ACG)将便秘定义为排便不满意,表现为排便次数减少、排便困难或两者兼有[14]。排便困难包括排便费力、排便困难感、排便不完全、硬便/块状便、排便时间过长或需要手法辅助才能排便。

二、流行病学

(一) 患病率

基于对全球超过261 000名受试者的41项研究的meta分析,便秘的患病率估计为14%[95%置信区间(CI)12~17][15]。在西方国家,便秘的患病率从3%~31%不等[16-31],具体取决于人口统计学、便秘的定义(例如,自我叙述的症状、每周排便少于3次、罗马标准)和提问方法(例如邮寄问卷、访谈)。一般而言,便秘自我叙述时患病率最高[16],采用罗马便秘标准时患病率最低[16]。女性、老年人和社会经济地位较低者便秘发生频率较高。而使用国家健康和营养检查调查(NHANES),当以粪便黏稠度定义时,美国普通人群中便秘的患病率较高[33](即Bristol粪便形态量表上的1型或2型[32],见图19.2),而不是按排便频率(即每周排便少于3次)来定义便秘时(7.2%,95% CI 7~8 vs 3.1%,95% CI 3~4)[33]。

(二) 发病率

Talley及其同事在首次和12~20个月后对明尼苏达州奥姆斯特德县的690名非老年居民进行了调查[34]。便秘定义为经常用力排便和排出硬便,每周排便频率少于3次,或两者兼有,在首次调查中17%的调查对象和第二次调查中15%的调查对象均存在便秘。本研究中新发便秘的发生率为50/1 000人/年,而消失率为31/1 000人/年。在一项类似的研究中,在首次和约12年后对居民进行调查。12年期间便秘的累积发生率为17.4%,在年龄小于50岁的受试者中,女性(18.3%)高于男性(9.2%)[35,36]。

(三) 公共卫生观点

便秘是医疗保健就诊的常见原因,就诊频率和相关费用似乎呈上升的趋势。2007—2012年,便秘在美国的门诊就诊人数接近约300万[3]。根据国家急诊部的样本数据,2006—2011年,美国便秘急诊的就诊频率增加了41.5%,相关费用增加了121.4%[37]。约85%的便秘患者需要医生开具泻药处方[38]。在健康维护理机构中,便秘的年平均直接医疗费用估计为7 522美元,在15年期间,年度自付费用为390.39美元。便秘女性的直接医疗费用63 591美元,是无便秘女性(24 529美元)的两倍多[40]。2004年,便秘的直接费用接近16亿美元,间接费用为1.4亿美元,使便秘成为直接费用排名前十的消化系统疾病之首[41]。便秘由多种医生治疗,在一项2001—2004年美国因便秘就诊的医生分析中,有33%需要治疗的患者就诊于内科医生和家庭医生,其次为儿科医生(21%)和胃肠病科医生(14.1%)[42]。然而,并非所有患者都因便秘寻求医疗帮助。加拿大一项全国性调查显示,只有34%的便秘患者因其症状曾看过医生[16]。

三、危险因素

尽管便秘的危险因素尚未进行系统评估,但女性、高龄、多种族、低收入、教育水平低以及体力活动少与慢性便秘相关[8,15,30,43]。其他危险因素包括使用某些药物[如对乙酰氨基酚(每周>7片)、阿司匹林、其他非甾体抗炎药][20]和存在某些基础疾病(稍后讨论)。饮食和生活方式也可能在便秘的发生中起作用(框19.2)。

框19.2 便秘的危险因素

高龄
女性
教育水平低
体力活动少
社会经济地位低
多种族
使用某些药物(见框19.3)

(一) 性别

女性自我叙述的便秘患病率是男性的2~3倍[18,26,30,44],尤其是育龄期女性,几乎完全由女性自述排便很少(例如每周一次)[32]。在26项研究的meta分析中,女性便秘的总患病率为17.4%(95% CI为13.4~21.8),几乎是男性9.2%的两倍(比值比为2.2,95% CI为1.87~2.62)[15]。女性占优势的原因尚不清楚。与雌激素水平相对较低的卵泡期相比,女性在月经周期黄体期结肠的转运明显延迟[45]。在患有严重特发性便秘的女性中观察到体内类固醇激素水平降低,尽管这一发现的临床意义尚不明确[46]。据报道,结肠平滑肌细胞上孕酮受体的过度表达可下调收缩性G蛋白,上调抑制性G蛋白[47]。结肠上皮细胞中孕酮受体的过度表达也与血清素转运体减少、5-羟色胺(5-HT)升高和色氨酸羟化酶水平正常有关[48]。此外,结肠肌细胞上孕酮受体 B 的过度表达,使其对生理浓度的孕酮更敏感,这为一些女性患严重慢传输型便秘提出了一种解释[49]。

(二) 年龄

老年人自我报告的便秘患病率为 15% ~ 30%,许多研究[18,43,50,51]但并非全部研究[15,16,18,20,30,52]显示患病率随年龄增长而增加。老年人便秘最常见的特征是排便费力和硬便[53],而不是排便次数减少。在一个由 209 名年龄在 65~93 岁的人组成的社区样本中,描述便秘的主要症状是排便时需要用力;只有 3% 的男性和 2% 的女性报告他们的平均排便频率每周少于 3 次[54]。老年人排便用力频率增加的可能原因包括摄食量减少、活动减少、腹壁和骨盆壁肌肉减弱(会阴下降综合征)、慢性疾病、心理因素以及使用某些药物,特别是止痛药[55]。老年人比年轻人更容易因便秘寻求医疗援助。在 1958—1986 年间美国因便秘就诊的患者进行的分析中,60 岁以下人群的便秘就诊频率约为 1%,60~65 岁人群约为 1%~2%,65 岁以上人群约为 3%~5%[38]。

在疗养院入住的居民中,便秘问题尤为严重,其中几乎近半数的人报告有便秘,50% ~ 74% 的居民需每天使用泻药[55]。同样,住院的老年患者发生便秘的风险也较高。一项针对英国老年病房患者的研究显示,高达 42% 的老年患者在住院期间出现粪便嵌塞[56]。一项针对美国 34 家养老院的研究发现,慢性便秘的发生率为 71%(95% CI 为 67~74),自我报告的粪便嵌塞发生率为 47%(95% CI 为 44~51)[57]。来自芬兰的一项研究显示,养老院中 79% 的女性和 81% 的男性报告慢性便秘或直肠排空障碍[58-61]。

便秘在 4 岁以下的儿童中也很常见[62]。在英国,0~4 岁儿童因便秘就诊的频率为 2% ~ 3%,15 ~ 64 岁的女性约为 1%,65~74 岁的男女均为 2% ~3%,75 岁或以上的人群中为 5%~6%。粪便滞留伴粪便污染是儿童生活质量受损和需要医疗护理的常见原因。

(三) 种族和国籍

在北美,有色人种比白种人更容易患便秘。在一项对 15 014 人的调查中,有色人种便秘的发生率为 17.3%,白种人便秘的发病率为 12.2%[8,30,63]。两组中均发现患病率的年龄特异性增加[8]。关于发展中国家的便秘数据有限。一项 meta 分析主要纳入了来自北美和北欧的研究,少数来自南美和中东的研究发现,所有国家慢性便秘的患病率相似,在 14%~16%之间[15]。一项比较南美洲和亚洲患病率的研究发现,便秘的发生率具有可比性,哥伦比亚为 21.7%,韩国为 16.7%[51]。在亚洲国家,包括中国、韩国和印度,便秘的患病率为 8.2%~16.8%[64-66]。在斯里兰卡有 15.4% 的 10~16 岁儿童报告了便秘(使用自填调查,依据罗马Ⅲ标准定义)。有便秘家族史的儿童(49% vs 14.8%)、生活在受战争影响地区的儿童(18.1% vs 13.7%)和上都市学校的儿童(16.7% vs 13.3%),便秘的患病率显著增加[67]。

(四) 社会经济地位与教育水平

较低的社会经济地位和教育水平是慢性便秘的危险因素。在以人口为基础的调查中,收入较低的人比收入较高的人便秘的发生率更高[8,12,28,30]。同样,受教育程度较低的人往往比受教育程度较高的人便秘的患病率更高[8,16,30,63]。一项 meta 分析的汇总数据显示,与社会经济地位较高的人相比,社会经济地位较低的人慢性便秘的患病率适度增加[15]。这些结果已在其他国家重现,如巴西、德国和克罗地亚[68-70]。

(五) 饮食和体力活动

横断面研究没有将纤维摄入量低与便秘联系起来[33,71]。然而数据表明,纤维摄入量增加会降低结肠转运,增加粪便重量和排便频率[72]。护士健康研究的一项分析,评估了 62 036 名 36 岁~61 岁女性自我报告的排便习惯,结果表明纤维摄入量最高的五分之一(中位摄入量,20g/d)且每天运动的女性,与纤维摄入量最低的五分之一(中位摄入量,7g/d)且每周运动少于一次的女性相比,报告便秘(每周排便次数少于 3 次)的可能性降低 68%[43]。尽管其他观察性研究支持体力活动对便秘的保护作用,但旨在检验这一假设的试验结果却相互矛盾。在一项试验中,经过 4 周的运动后,便秘症状没有改善[73]。同样,在退伍军人事务部的雇员中,有便秘或无便秘的人的体力活动水平没有差异[74]。

脱水被认为是便秘的潜在危险因素。一些观察性研究(但非全部)发现结肠传输缓慢与脱水之间存在关联[75,76]。然而,在日本女性低热量饮食研究中,总摄水量与发生便秘无关[71]。对于便秘患者通常建议他们增加液体摄入量,但其益处尚未得到研究的证实。

(六) 药物

一项来自全科医学数据库的 7 251 例慢性便秘患者(和非便秘对照组)的回顾中,与便秘显著相关的药物有阿片类药物、利尿剂、抗抑郁药、抗组胺药、解痉药、抗惊厥药和铝抗酸剂(框 19.3)[52]。对乙酰氨基酚(>每周 7 片)、阿司匹林和其他非甾体抗炎药的使用也发现与便秘风险增加相关[20]。

框 19.3 便秘的继发原因

机械性梗阻

肛门狭窄
结直肠癌
外源性压迫
直肠膨出或乙状结肠膨出
狭窄

药物

对乙酰氨基酚(>每周 7 片)
抗酸药(含铝制剂)
抗胆碱能药物(如抗帕金森病药、抗精神病药、解痉药、三环类抗抑郁药)
抗惊厥药(如卡马西平、苯巴比妥、苯妥英钠)
抗肿瘤药物(如长春花衍生物)
钙通道阻滞剂(如维拉帕米)
钙补充剂
利尿剂(如呋塞米)
5-羟色胺 3 拮抗剂(如阿洛司琼)
铁补充剂
非甾体抗炎药(如布洛芬)

框 19.3 便秘的继发原因(续)
阿片类药物激动剂(如芬太尼、洛哌丁胺、吗啡)
代谢及内分泌疾病
糖尿病
重金属中毒(如砷、铅、汞)
高钙血症
甲状腺功能亢进
低血钾症
甲状腺功能减退
垂体功能减退
嗜铬细胞瘤
卟啉病
妊娠
神经与肌病类疾病
淀粉样变性
自主神经病变
Chagas 病
皮肌炎
假性肠梗阻
多发性硬化症
帕金森病
Shy-Drager 综合征(直立性低血压综合征)
脊髓损伤
卒中
系统性硬化

四、结肠功能

(一) 肠腔内容物

结肠腔的主要内容物是食物残渣、水和电解质、细菌和气体。未被吸收的碳水化合物,如进入盲肠的淀粉和非淀粉多糖,作为细菌增殖和发酵的底物,产生短链脂肪酸和气体(见第 17 章)。平均而言细菌约占粪便重量的 50%[77]。在对 9 名接受代谢控制的英国饮食的健康受试者粪便的分析中,细菌占粪便总固体的55%,纤维约占粪便重量的 17%[78]。肠道微生物菌群在便秘中的作用才刚开始探索(见第 3 章)[79,80]。

一项 meta 分析表明,麦麸增加了健康志愿者粪便的重量并减少了平均结肠运输[78]。麸皮的作用主要是增加了结肠腔内体积,刺激推进性运动。一些纤维的微颗粒性质也可能刺激结肠。摄入粗麸皮(每次 10g,每天两次)可使结肠转运减少约三分之一,而摄入等量的细麸皮并未使结肠转运显著减少[77]。同样,摄入大小与粗麸皮相当的惰性塑胶颗粒可使粪便排出量增加几乎是自身重量的 3 倍,并减少结肠转运时间[81]。

(二) 水和钠的吸收

结肠大量吸收水和钠(见第 101 章)。结肠可提取 1 000~1 500mL 液体中的大部分,这些液体可穿过回盲瓣,每天只排出 100~200mL 粪水。氯化钠交换和短链脂肪酸转运是刺激结肠吸收水分的主要机制。水在结肠中的吸收还依赖于完整的上皮屏障功能,以防止电解质和其他溶质一旦被上皮细胞吸收后的反向扩散[1]。便秘的病理生理学机制之一是,延迟转运使细菌降解固体粪便有更多的时间,钠和水的吸收增加,从而降低粪便重量和频率,并增加其硬度[82,83]。

(三) 直径和长度

结肠较宽或较长可导致结肠传输速度变慢(见第 100 章)。虽然只有一小部分便秘患者有巨结肠或巨直肠,但大多数结肠或直肠扩张的患者主诉有便秘。在钡剂灌肠检查的 X 片中,盆腔边缘结肠宽度超过 6.5cm 为异常,与慢性便秘有关[84]。

(四) 运动功能

结肠肌肉有 4 个主要功能(见第 100 章):①延迟肠腔内容物通过,留出吸收水分的时间;②混合内容物并使其与黏膜充分接触;③使结肠在两次排便之间储存粪便;④将肠腔内容物推向肛门。肌肉活动受睡眠和清醒、进食、情绪、结肠内容物和药物的影响。神经控制部分是内在的、部分是外在的,由交感神经和副交感神经骶部传出神经控制。

健康志愿者的平均结肠转运时间为 34~35 小时,正常值上限为 72 小时[85,86]。在一些患者中,缓慢的结肠转运是由升结肠和横结肠(近端结肠)中物质通过延迟引起的,而不是左半结肠[87-89]。其他患者表现为结肠右侧和左侧均传输缓慢[90]。

蠕动是肠道固有的,由节段性收缩和远端松弛组成。由乙酰胆碱激活的兴奋性运动神经元引起肠平滑肌收缩,而 ATP 和一氧化氮激活的抑制性神经元可引起肠平滑肌松弛[1]。肠蠕动可通过肠神经节中的肠嗜铬细胞和机械感受器感受到的化学或机械刺激激活引起。一旦启动,肠蠕动可以长距离传播,从而使物质通过肠道移动[1]。肠嗜铬细胞在营养物质、短链脂肪酸、胆盐和机械刺激下合成 5-羟色胺(5-HT)。5-HT 激活上游兴奋性运动神经元和下游抑制性运动神经元,从而导致蠕动。

结肠推进性收缩有两种基本类型:低振幅推进性收缩(low-amplitude propagated contraction,LAPC)和高振幅推进性收缩(high-amplitude propagated contraction,HAPC)[91]。在一些便秘患者中,HAPC 的频率和持续时间降低。在一项包括 14 例慢传输型便秘患者的研究中,在 24 小时内 4 例患者没有蠕动,而在其余的 10 例患者中,与健康对照组相比,蠕动运动的次数较少,持续时间较短[92]。直肠乙状结肠重复逆行收缩 2~6 次/min 可作为一种"制动"机制。

(五) 神经支配和 Cajal 间质细胞

便秘,尤其是慢传输型便秘,可能与自主神经功能障碍有关[93,94]。组织学研究表明,参与结肠运动兴奋性或抑制性控制的肌间神经丛神经元数量异常,从而导致兴奋性递质 P 物质[95]的数量减少和抑制性递质血管活性肠肽或一氧化氮的数量增加(见第 4 章)[96]。

Cajal 间质细胞(interstitial cell of Cajal,ICC)是肠起搏细胞,在调节肠神经系统和平滑肌细胞之间的兴奋性和抑制性信号中发挥作用(见第 99 和 100 章)[1]。ICC 在整个胃肠道中启动慢波。慢传输型便秘患者的 ICC 共聚焦图像不仅显示 ICC 数量减少,而且显示形态异常,表面标记不规则,树突数量减少。在慢传输型便秘患者中,已证实乙状结肠[97]或整个结肠中的 ICC 数量减少[98,99]。对 14 例严重顽固性便秘患者的结肠切除标本进行病理检查，发现整个结肠的 ICC 和肌间神经节细胞数量减少[100]。

（六）排便功能

健康人的排便过程从排便前期开始，在此期间传播序列（3 个或更多连续压力波）的频率和振幅增加。诸如清醒和进餐等刺激（胃回肠反射，也称为胃结肠反射或反应）可刺激这一过程。在慢传输型便秘患者中，这种排便前期迟钝，甚至消失[91]。慢传输型便秘患者的胃回肠反射也减弱。粪便在直肠内出现时才产生排便冲动。排便冲动通常是在粪便与肛管上部的感受器接触时产生。当排便冲动被抑制时，可发生粪便逆行运动，整个结肠的通过时间增加（见第 100 章）[101]。

虽然坐姿或蹲姿似乎有助于排便，但蹲姿的益处在便秘患者中尚未得到深入的研究[102]。充分屈曲髋关节使肛管沿前后方向伸展，使肛门直肠角变直，从而促进直肠的排空[103]。膈肌和腹肌的收缩增加了盆腔内压力，盆底同时放松，横纹肌活动排出直肠内容物。结肠或直肠推进波的作用很小。在直肠内压力增加时，耻骨直肠肌（维持肛门直肠角）和肛门外括约肌协调松弛，导致粪便排出（图 19.1）。

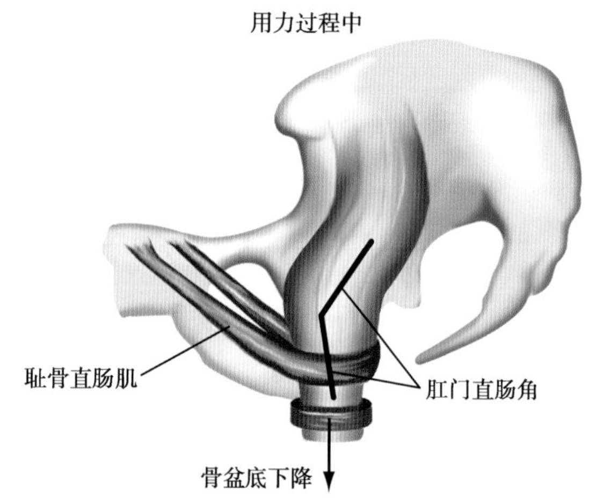

图 19.1　排便生理学。排便需要放松耻骨直肠肌，盆底下降，用力时拉直肛门直肠角，同时肛门内括约肌松弛。（From Lembo A, Camilleri M. Chronic constipation. N Engl J Med 2003;349:1360-8.）

在自发排便时，结肠排空的长度通常从降结肠延伸到直肠[104]。当平滑肌的推进作用正常时，排便通常需要最小的自主用力。如果结肠和直肠推动波很少或没有，则可能不会出现正常的排便冲动[105]。

（七）粪便大小及黏稠度

在一项对健康人的研究中，要求受试者从直肠壶腹排出不同大小的单个硬球，通过这些物体所需的直肠内压力和时间与其直径成反比。小而硬的粪便比大而软的粪便更难排出。当测试更大的刺激性粪便时，硬粪便比形状和体积大致相同的软硅胶物体排出所需的时间更长。类似的，更多的受试者能够排出充满 50ml 水的可压缩球囊[106]，而不是一个 1.8cm 的硬球体。

人类粪便的黏稠度从小的硬块到液体不等，粪便的含水量决定其黏稠度。粪便残留物的快速结肠传输导致水分吸收减少和（可能与直觉相反）粪便中的细菌含量增加。Bristol 粪便形态量表[32]用于便秘的评估，被认为是粪便形态和黏稠度的最佳描述（图 19.2）。粪便黏稠度似乎比排便频率或排便量，能更好地预测整个肠道的传输时间[107]。

全肠道传输时间	粪便类型	描述	图示
长传输（如100小时）			
	类型 1	分散的干球硬块，如同坚果，很难排出	
	类型 2	腊肠形状，但呈块状	
	类型 3	腊肠形状，表面有裂缝	
	类型 4	腊肠形状或蛇形，光滑而柔软	
	类型 5	软柔的团块，边缘清晰（容易排出）	
	类型 6	软片状，边缘毛糙	
	类型 7	水状，无固体碎片	完全水样便
短传输（如10小时）			

图 19.2　Bristol 粪便形态量表。显示常见粪便形态及其与全肠道传输时间相关的一致性。（From Heaton KW, Radvan J, Cripps H, et al. Defecation frequency and timing, and stool form in the general population: a prospective study. Gut 1992;33:818-24.）

五、分类

必须排除便秘的继发性原因（如小肠或大肠梗阻、药物、系统性疾病），尤其是新发便秘的患者（见框 19.3）。慢性便秘最常见的原因是结肠或直肠功能紊乱（有时称为功能性便秘）。慢性便秘可分为 3 大类：正常传输型便秘、慢传输型便秘和排便或直肠排空障碍（表 19.1）。梅奥诊所对 1 000 多例慢性便秘患者进行评估的一项研究中，59% 的患者存在正常传输型便秘，25% 的患者存在排便障碍，13% 的患者存在慢传输型便秘，3% 的患者同时存在排便障碍和慢传输型便秘[108]。

表 19.1　功能性便秘的临床分类

类别	特征	生理学测试结果
正常传输型便秘	排便不完全、腹痛可能存在，但不是主要特征	正常
慢传输型便秘	排便次数减少（如 ≤1 次/周），缺乏排便冲动、对纤维饮食和泻药反应差，全身症状（如不适、疲乏），在年轻女性中更为常见	结肠传输延迟（如摄入 5 天后，滞留结肠的不透射线标志物>20%）
排便障碍疾病*	频繁用力、排便不完全，需要手法辅助排便	球囊排出试验和/或肛门直肠测压异常

*盆底功能障碍、肛门痉挛、会阴下降综合征和直肠脱垂。

六、病理生理学

（一）正常传输型便秘

在正常传输型便秘中，粪便以正常速率沿结肠传输[109]。正常传输型便秘患者可能对自己的排便频率有误解，并经常表现出心理社会困扰[110]。一些患者的肛门直肠感觉和运动功能异常，与慢传输型便秘患者难以区分[111]。直肠顺应性增加和直肠感觉减弱是否影响慢性便秘，或者是导致这些患者无法排便的原因目前尚不清楚，但大多数患者的生理测试结果是正常的（见下文）。

（二）慢传输型便秘

慢传输型便秘最常见于年轻女性，其特征为排便次数少（每周<1 次排便）。相关症状包括腹痛、腹胀和腹部不适。症状往往难以控制，纤维补充剂和渗透性泻药等保守措施通常无效[112,113]。便秘症状的出现是逐渐的，通常发生在青春期前后。慢传输型便秘源于结肠运动功能紊乱。结肠传输轻度延迟的患者症状与肠易激综合征患者相似（见第 122 章）[114]。在症状更严重的患者中，其病理生理学包括近端结肠排空延迟和餐后 HAPC 减少。结肠乏力是用于描述患者症状处于疾病谱中最严重的术语。在这种情况下，餐后[115]、摄入比沙可啶[116]或服用胆碱酯酶抑制剂如新斯的明后[117]，结肠运动没有增加。

（三）排便障碍

直肠排空障碍是由于不能协调腹部、直肠肛门和盆底肌肉，从而导致无法有效排空直肠引起的。许多排便障碍的患者也合并有慢传输型便秘[118]。排便障碍也称为协同失调、盆底协同失调、痉挛性盆底综合征、梗阻性排便或出口梗阻。这些疾病似乎是后天获得的，可能始于儿童时期。它们可能是一种习得性行为，以避免在排出大量硬便或在活动性肛裂或痔疮发炎的情况下试图排便时引起不适感和疼痛。排便障碍的患者通常在用力下压时出现肛门括约肌不适当收缩（图 19.3）。这种现象可能发生于无症状者，但在抱怨排便困难的人群中更常见[119]。一些排便障碍患者，不能将直肠内压力提高到足以排出粪便的水平，这种障碍在临床上表现为用力时盆底不能下降[120]。

直肠排空障碍在患有慢性便秘和过度用力的老年人中尤为常见，其中许多人对标准医疗无反应[121]。偶尔，直肠排空障碍与结构异常有关（如直肠肠套叠、梗阻性直肠膨出、巨直肠、会阴过度下降）[122]。

直肠排便障碍患者可能会主诉排便不规律、无效和过度用力，以及需要手法解除嵌塞粪便，在盆底功能障碍的情况下症状特别严重，但无可靠的相关性生理学发现[123]。对于直肠排空障碍的诊断，罗马工作组规定了框 19.4[124]中列出的标准。患者必须符合罗马便秘标准，并通过生理学测试确定有盆底肌肉功能障碍的证据（见下文）。盆底协同失调影响到这些患者中的一部分，尽管直肠内存在足够的推进力，但在尝试排便期间肛门括约肌不能放松超过 20% 的基础静息压力。与其他类型的便秘相比，直肠排空障碍患者的直肠气量更大，因此直肠成像（即通过 CT）可提供一种敏感（>70%）和特异性（>60%）的方法来区分直肠排空障碍与其他类型便秘[125]。

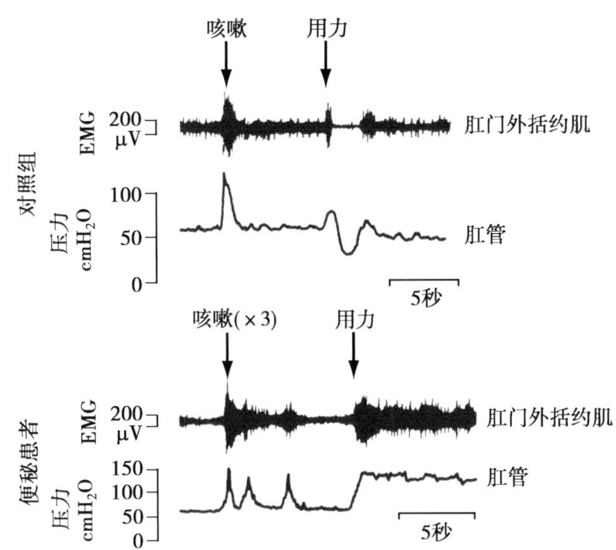

图 19.3　正常（对照）受试者和排便障碍的便秘患者排便期间的肌电图（EMG）和压力描记图。在对照组和便秘患者中，咳嗽均导致压力升高。当正常受试者用力时（上描记图），肛门外括约肌的肌电图活动受到抑制，肛管内的压力下降。在排便障碍的便秘患者中，用力时肛门外括约肌的肌电图活动不受抑制，肛管内的压力增加（下描记图）。这种自相矛盾的收缩被称为肛门痉挛、肛门协同失调和会阴痉挛。（From Preston DM, Lennard-Jones JE. Anismus in chronic constipation. Dig Dis Sci 1985; 30: 413-8.）

框 19.4　功能性排便障碍罗马Ⅳ标准*

1. 患者必须符合功能性便秘和/或伴有便秘的肠易激综合征的诊断标准
2. 在反复尝试排便过程中，必须有排空障碍的特征，如以下 3 个测试结果中的 2 个证明：
   a. 球囊排出试验异常
   b. 测压或肛门表面肌电图显示肛门直肠排空异常
   c. 影像学检查显示直肠排空障碍

*诊断前症状出现至少 6 个月，近 3 个月符合以上诊断标准。

From Rao SSC, Bharucha AE, Chiarioni G, et al. Anorectal disorders. Gastroenterology. 2016; 150(6): 1430-42.

功能性粪便潴留（FFR）是儿童最常见的排便障碍。这是一种习得性行为，由排便受阻导致，通常是因为害怕排便疼痛或社会原因所致[126]。这些症状很常见，并可能因粪便嵌塞周围的液体粪便渗漏而导致继发性大便失禁。功能性粪便潴留是儿童大便失禁最常见的原因（见第 18 章）[127]。

七、病因

（一）肛门直肠和盆底疾病

1. 直肠膨出（直肠前突）

直肠膨出是指直肠因直肠前壁的缺损而膨出或移位。在女性，会阴体支持肛门直肠交界处上方的直肠前壁（阴道后壁），从道格拉斯的直肠阴道袋延伸至会阴体有一层筋膜，并黏附于阴道后壁。直肠前壁在会阴体水平以上无支撑，直肠阴道隔可向前突起形成直肠膨出（图 19.4）。阴道分娩时，直肠膨出可由直肠阴道隔或其支撑结构受损引起。这些损伤因腹内压的反复增加和重力的长期影响而加剧。也可能存在其他盆腔器官脱垂。与排便困难但无明显直肠膨出的患者相比，尿失禁和既往子宫切除术在直肠膨出患者中更常见[128]。

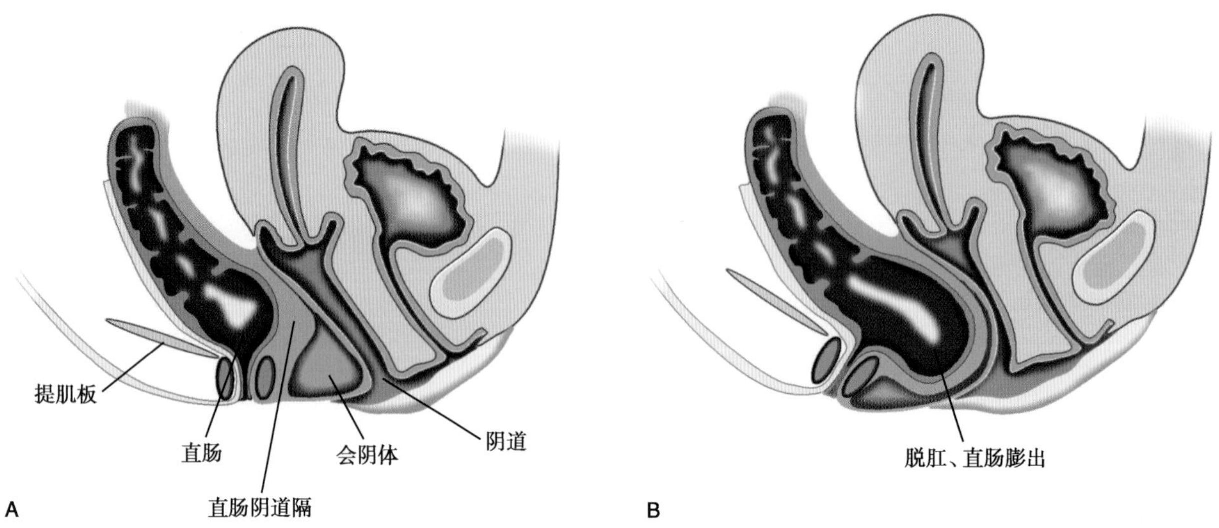

图 19.4　直肠膨出的形成。A，女性骨盆的正常解剖。提肌板几乎是水平的，支撑着直肠和阴道。会阴体为阴道后壁下部提供支撑；其上方是直肠阴道隔。B，盆底无力导致提肌板更加垂直。会阴体变薄，有利于形成直肠膨出。盆底松弛也有利于直肠黏膜脱垂。（From Loder PB，Phillips RKS. Rectocele and pelvic floor weakness. In：Kamm MA，Lennard-Jones JE，editors. Constipation. Peterfield：Wrightson Biomedical；1994. p 281.）

排便直肠造影的研究（见下文）表明，直肠膨出常见于无症状的健康女性，可从直肠前壁连线突出 4cm 以上，而不引起肠道症状。一般认为直肠膨出公认的下限是 2cm 具有临床意义[129]。有症状的女性患者常主诉无法完成排便、会阴疼痛、局部压迫感和用力时阴道口出现凸起。女性可能描述需要用拇指或手指支撑阴道后壁完成排便[128]。女性也可能描述必须要用手指辅助排空直肠。

排便直肠造影可用于显示直肠膨出，测量其大小，并确定钡剂是否滞留在直肠膨出内。在一项研究中，钡剂在直肠膨出中的潴留随直肠排空的程度而变化，并与直肠膨出的大小有关[130]。然而，直肠膨出的大小或排便时的排空程度尚未被证明与手术修复的结果相关[131,132]。

无症状的直肠膨出女性不需要手术治疗。Kegel 训练（旨在加强支撑尿道、膀胱、子宫和直肠的盆底肌肉）和指导避免腹内压反复增加，可能有助于防止直肠膨出的进展[133]。手术仅考虑用于排便造影时有潴留造影剂的患者和需用阴道指压缓解便秘以利排便的患者[134]。手术修复可经直肠、经阴道或经会阴途径进行。其他类型的生殖器脱垂也可能存在，外科和妇科医生间的合作可能是适宜的。在仔细选择患者中，手术修复使 75% 的患者受益。在对 89 名因梗阻性排便症状接受经阴道和经肛门行直肠膨出联合修复术的女性进行的综述中，根据一年后症状消失的情况评估，71% 的患者修复成功[135]。随后的一项研究[136]发现，50% 的患者肠道症状有所改善，夹板固定时间较长是术后症状持续存在的危险因素。通过排便直肠造影术判断的直肠膨出尺寸的缩小似乎与症状改善无明显相关性[132]。

2. 会阴下降综合征

在会阴下降综合征中，当患者用力排便时，盆底下降的程度比正常大 1~4cm，直肠排出困难。由于盆底无力导致肛门直肠角增宽，直肠比正常更垂直。会阴体薄弱（有利于直肠膨出形成）肌肉支持松懈，有利于直肠内黏膜套叠或直肠脱垂。盆底不能提供固体粪便通过肛管排出所需的阻力。盆底无力的常见原因是分娩过程中的创伤或过度拉伸。在某些情况下，反复和长时间排便似乎是损伤的有害因素。症状包括便秘、直肠排空不全、过度用力和需用手指辅助排空直肠[137]。电生理学研究显示横纹肌部分失去神经支配和阴部神经损伤（见下文）。盆底肌肉手术标本的组织学检查证实肌纤维丢失。

3. 直肠感觉减弱

排便冲动部分取决于直肠壁内的张力（由直肠壁环形肌肉的张力决定）、直肠扩张的速度、容积以及直肠的大小。一些便秘患者在直肠扩张至最大可耐受容积时似乎感觉不到疼痛，但在中等容量时，未出现排便冲动[138]。在一项对患有严重特发性便秘的女性研究中，需要对直肠黏膜施加高于正常的电刺激才能引起疼痛，提示可能存在直肠感觉神经病变[139]。

直肠低敏感性（rectal hyposensitivity，RH）是指直肠对肛门直肠生理学检查中的球囊扩张不敏感，尽管 RH 的病理生理学尚不完全清楚。便秘是 RH 最常见的症状。在一项对 261 例 RH 患者的调查中，38% 有盆腔手术史，22% 有肛门手术史，13% 有脊柱创伤史[140]。

4. 直肠脱垂和孤立性直肠溃疡综合征

全层直肠脱垂和孤立性直肠溃疡综合征是由盆底功能减弱引起的一系列缺陷的一部分。一些患者主诉多次去卫生间无排便，对持续排便冲动的反应是长时间用力。患者有排便不尽感，每天要用1小时或更长的时间上卫生间。小而硬的粪便不易排出的情况很常见，功能性肠病的其他特征如腹痛和腹胀也是常见的。

直肠脱垂是指直肠通过肛门完全突出（见第129章）。在33%的临床确诊为直肠膨出和排便功能障碍的患者中发现了隐匿性（无症状）直肠脱垂[141]，通过要求患者像排便一样用力，很容易在体检中发现。推荐采用腹腔镜直肠固定术——将脱垂的直肠提起并用缝线固定到邻近的筋膜上[142]的治疗方法。

孤立性直肠溃疡综合征是一种罕见的疾病，其特征为红斑或溃疡，通常发生在直肠前壁，是慢性损伤的结果（见第119章）。当患者在排便过程中用力时，可排出黏液和血液[143,144]。内镜检查结果包括红斑、充血、黏膜溃疡和息肉样病变。该综合征的异质性表现和误导性名称（溃疡无须存在）可能导致误诊。在一项对98例孤立性直肠溃疡综合征患者的研究中，26%的患者最初被误诊。在直肠溃疡或黏膜充血的患者中，最常误诊为克罗恩病和溃疡性结肠炎。在息肉样病变患者中，最常误诊为肿瘤性息肉[145]。病变全层标本的组织学检查显示，黏膜肌层在隐窝之间延伸，固有肌层组织紊乱。排便造影、经直肠超声和肛门直肠测压有助于诊断。

不同程度的直肠脱垂与孤立性直肠溃疡综合征有关。直肠脱垂和耻骨直肠肌的反常收缩可导致直肠创伤，继发于直肠内产生的高压。此外，直肠黏膜血流量减少[146]。

药物治疗可能很困难。应建议患者克制排便过度用力的冲动。大量的泻药和膳食纤维可能有一些益处[147]。有些患者可能需要手术治疗，最常见的是直肠固定术。孤立性直肠溃疡综合伴有直肠脱垂手术后，55%～60%的患者表示长期满意，尽管约三分之一的患者最终需要施行结肠造口术[148]。据报道，应用氩气等离子凝固治疗可减少出血并改善愈合[149]。直肠脱垂的修复可能会加重便秘。生物反馈治疗似乎是孤立性直肠溃疡综合征患者的一种很有前途的治疗方式[150,151]。

（二）系统性疾病

1. 甲状腺功能减退

便秘是甲状腺功能减退患者最常见的胃肠道症状。其病理生理是由于肠道运动功能的改变和黏液水肿样组织浸润肠道所致。甲状腺功能减退患者十二指肠产生蠕动波的基本电节律降低，小肠转运时间增加[152]。黏液性水肿在巨结肠是罕见的，但可由结肠肌肉层的黏液水肿浸润引起。症状包括腹痛、胃肠胀气和便秘（见第37章）[153]。

2. 糖尿病

糖尿病患者的结肠平均转运时间比健康对照组长。在一项研究中，28例糖尿病患者的平均结肠传输时间（34.9±29.6小时；平均值±SD）明显长于28例健康受试者（20.4±15.6小时；$P<0.05$）[154]。在28名糖尿病患者中，有9名（32%）符合罗马Ⅱ便秘标准，有14名（50%）患有心血管自主神经病变。糖尿病合并有或无合并心血管自主神经病变患者的平均结肠传输时间相似。相比之下，先前的一项研究报告，无症状糖尿病患者合并心血管自主神经病变的患者的全肠道传输时间（尽管仍在正常范围内）明显长于无神经病变的对照组[155]。在另一项研究中，轻度便秘的糖尿病患者，在摄入标准膳食后表现出结肠肌电和运动反应延迟，而重度便秘的糖尿病患者在进食后这些反应没有增加。新斯的明可增加所有糖尿病患者的结肠运动，表明这种缺陷是神经性的而不是肌性的（见第37章）[156]。

3. 高钙血症

便秘是由甲状旁腺功能亢进引起的高钙血症的常见症状[157]。它也可能是其他疾病引起的高钙血症的主要表现。如结节病、累及骨骼的恶性肿瘤（见第37章）。

（三）神经系统疾病

1. 意识控制丧失

大脑残疾或痴呆伴身体知觉下降或完全丧失可导致排便失败，可能是由于注意力不集中。

2. 帕金森病

便秘多发生于帕金森病（Parkinson disease，PD）患者[158]，通常早于PD的诊断[159]。便秘严重损害患者的日常生活活动和生活质量。在一项对12例PD患者与正常对照组相比较的研究中，结肠传输缓慢、直肠时相性收缩减少、腹壁肌肉收缩无力以及排便时肛门括约肌反常收缩和频繁便秘均为PD患者的特征[160]。与PD患者便秘发生的相关因素包括发病年龄较大、病程较长、疾病分期为晚期、以及严重的运动和非运动症状[158]。中枢神经系统中含多巴胺神经元的缺失是PD的潜在缺陷，肠神经系统中的多巴胺能神经元也可能存在缺陷。对11例PD伴便秘患者升结肠肌间神经丛的组织病理学研究显示，9例患者的多巴胺阳性神经元数量为对照组的十分之一或更少。PD患者外肌层多巴胺浓度显著低于对照组（$P<0.01$）[161]。

导致便秘的另一个可能因素是一些PD患者在排便时不能放松骨盆横纹肌。这一发现是锥体外系运动障碍影响骨骼肌的局部表现。临床观察表明，在耻骨直肠肌内注射肉毒毒素是治疗这种类型便秘有潜力的方法（见第37章）[162,163]。

3. 多发性硬化症

便秘在多发性硬化症（multiple sclerosis，MS）患者中很常见[164]。在未经选择的280例MS患者中，便秘（定义为排便频率减少、使用手指促进排便或使用泻药）发生的频率为43%。几乎25%的受试者每周排便少于3次，18%的受试者每周使用泻药超过一次。便秘与MS病程相关，45%的患者便秘早于MS诊断。在这项研究中，便秘与静止不动或使用药物无关[165]。在另一项对221例MS患者的问卷调查研究中，便秘的发生频率高达54%[166]。MS患者便秘的原因可能是多因素的，与餐后结肠运动减少、有限的体力活动和药物治疗有关。

晚期MS伴便秘的患者有内脏神经病变的证据。在一组晚期MS和重度便秘的患者中，所有患者均有腰骶部脊髓疾病和结肠顺应性降低的证据。通常餐后结肠运动没有增加。在受影响程度较轻的患者中，结肠传输缓慢、盆底肌肉测压证据和肛门括约肌功能障碍已被证实。患者可有大便失禁[167,168]。据报道，生物反馈疗法可缓解便秘和大便失禁，但在一项13例伴有便秘或失禁的MS患者的研究中，仅有38%

的患者通过生物反馈疗法得到改善(见第18和37章)[169]。

4. 脊髓病变

(1) 骶段以上脊髓病变

脊髓病变或骶段以上的脊髓损伤可导致上运动神经元障碍伴有严重便秘。由此导致的结肠传输延迟主要影响直肠乙状结肠[170,171]。在一项对重度胸脊髓损伤患者的研究中,结肠顺应性异常,在滴注相对少量的液体后结肠压力迅速升高。餐后运动没有增加,但结肠对新斯的明反应正常,从而排除了肌肉病变。

对严重脊髓损伤患者的肛门直肠功能的研究表明,直肠对膨胀的感觉消失,尽管一些患者在直肠球囊扩张达最大程度时体验到隐匿的盆腔迟钝感。直肠扩张时肛门松弛被夸大,发生在球囊容积低于正常人时。直肠扩张导致直肠压力呈线性增加,在正常受试者的中间值处于无平台期,在滴注相对较小容积(100mL)后以高压性直肠收缩结束。正如预期的那样,患者应变产生的直肠压力低于对照组,高于下脊髓病变的直肠压力较少。患者表现出丧失有意识的肛门外括约肌控制,用力时括约肌不松弛,表明在正常受试者中,存在下行抑制途径[172]。这些发现解释了为什么一些脊髓病变患者不仅会出现便秘,还会突然出现无法控的直肠排便和大便失禁。其他患者对泻药或灌肠的反应不能排空直肠,可能是因为肛门外括约肌不能松弛,需要人工手动排出。

通过植入电极对截瘫患者的骶前神经根S2、S3和S4进行电刺激以控制尿漏,导致乙状结肠和直肠内压力升高,肛门外括约肌收缩。刺激停止后,直肠收缩和肛门内括约肌松弛会持续很短时间。通过适当调整刺激,12例截瘫患者中有5例可完全排空粪便,其他大多数患者能够增加排便频率,并缩短排空直肠的时间[173]。在另一个系列中,常规骶神经刺激后左侧结肠传输时间缩短[174]。

(2) 骶髓、脊髓圆锥、马尾神经、勃起神经病变(S2~S4)

肛门括约肌控制和直肠乙状结肠推进的神经整合发生在脊髓的骶段。供给横纹肌括约肌的运动神经元在S2水平的Onuf神经核中分组。有证据表明,从骶段发出的副交感神经传出神经在直肠乙状结肠交界处进入结肠,并在肌间平面向远端延伸到达肛门内括约肌水平,并通过升结肠神经向近端延伸至结肠中部,以保留周围神经结构(见第100章)[175]。

损伤脊髓骶段或传出神经导致严重的便秘。X线透视检查显示,左半结肠收缩进程丧失。当结肠充满液体时,产生的腔内压力低于正常,这与脊髓较高病变的情况相反。远端结肠和直肠扩张,粪便积聚在远端结肠,可发生肛管痉挛。会阴部皮肤感觉丧失可扩展至肛管,直肠感觉减弱。直肠壁张力取决于脊髓病变的水平。在一项对25例脊髓损伤患者的研究中,急性和慢性脊髓圆锥以上病变患者的直肠张力明显高于正常,而急性和慢性圆锥或马尾病变患者的直肠张力明显低于正常[176]。

(四) 结肠、直肠和肛门结构性病变

1. 梗阻

婴儿期肛门闭锁、晚年肛门狭窄或结肠梗阻可表现为便秘。小肠梗阻一般表现为腹疼和腹胀,但便秘和不能排气也可能是其特征(见第98和123章)。

2. 平滑肌疾病

(1) 影响结肠平滑肌的肌病

先天性或后天性结肠肌病通常表现为假性肠梗阻。结肠低张力和惰性(见第124章)。

(2) 遗传性肛门内括约肌肌病

遗传性肛门内括约肌肌病是一种罕见的疾病,其特征为便秘伴直肠排出困难和严重的一过性直肠痉挛性疼痛。定义为肛门直肠区域突然出现短暂的疼痛发作[177-179]。已报道了3个发病家系。常染色体显性遗传伴不完全性外显率是遗传的表现方式。有症状的人,肛门内括约肌增厚,静息肛门压力大大增加。2例患者用钙通道阻滞剂治疗改善了疼痛,但对便秘没有影响。在另一个家族中,2例患者接受了肛门内括约肌条状肌切除术治疗,1例显示全部症状明显改善,另1例便秘症状有所改善,但疼痛仅有轻微的改善。肌条检查显示肌病性改变,平滑肌纤维中有多聚糖体(葡萄糖聚合物)肌内膜纤维化增加。

(3) 系统性硬化症

系统性硬化症(硬皮病)可能导致便秘[180]。在系统性硬化症伴便秘的患者中,10例中有9例在摄入1 000kacl膳食后结肠运动没有增加。这些受试者结肠标本的组织学检查显示结肠壁平滑肌萎缩(见第37章)[181]。

(4) 肌营养不良

肌营养不良通常被认为是横纹肌疾病,但内脏平滑肌也可能是异常的。在强直性肌营养不良症中,骨骼肌不能正常松弛,可发现巨结肠,并证实肛门括约肌功能异常[182]。已报告了与假性肠梗阻相关的病例(见第124章)[183]。

3. 肠神经疾病

(1) 先天性无神经节细胞症或神经节细胞减少症

先天性结肠神经节缺失或数量减少导致功能性结肠梗阻伴近端扩张,如先天性巨结肠病(Hirschsprung病)和相关疾病(见第98章)。在先天性巨结肠中,由于胚胎发育期间肠内神经嵴细胞的尾部迁移停滞,远端结肠中的神经节细胞缺失。虽然大多数患者在婴儿早期出现,常伴有胎粪排出延迟,但有些受累结肠段相对较短的患者在以后的生活中出现[184]。通常,结肠在缺乏神经节细胞的区域变窄,变窄近端的肠管通常扩张。在先天性巨结肠患者中发现了两种遗传缺陷——一种是在转染原癌基因过程中发生重排突变,它参与神经嵴细胞的发育,另一种是编码内皮素B受体的基因突变,它影响细胞内钙离子水平[185,186]。

当观察到小而稀疏的肌间神经节时,可能报告为神经节细胞减少症。可对全层组织标本进行神经元计数,并与已发表的尸检材料获得的参考值进行比较。由于神经元正常密度的变化,确定神经节细胞减少症的诊断并不容易[187]。肠神经系统中神经元数量定量的下降也见于严重慢传输型便秘患者,其形态学特征为寡神经元神经节细胞减少症[188]。

(2) 先天性高神经节细胞增多症(肠神经元发育不良)

先天性高神经节细胞增多症即肠神经元发育不良,是一种以黏膜下神经丛增生为特征的发育缺陷。该病的临床表现与先天性巨结肠相似,包括发病年龄小,有肠梗阻症状(见第98章)。与功能性便秘相反,受累儿童没有脏污的症状或粪结的证据[189]。一项多中心研究表明,观察者之间对肠神经

系统异常引起便秘儿童的组织学解释的差异，在先天性巨结肠的诊断中完全一致，但在结肠运动障碍（无神经节细胞增多症除外）患儿中仅有 14% 诊断一致。先前与先天性高神经节细胞增多症有关的一些临床特征和组织学改变，可能随着儿童年龄的增长而演变为正常[187]。先天性高神经节细胞增多症的诊断，可根据黏膜下神经丛的巨大神经节和直肠活检标本中至少有下列特征之一作出：①异位的神经节细胞；②固有层中乙酰胆碱酯酶活性增加；③黏膜下血管周围乙酰胆碱酯酶神经纤维增加。大多数先天性高神经节细胞增多症患者对保守治疗有反应，如使用泻药。如保守治疗失败可行肛门内括约肌切除术[190]。

（3）获得性神经病变

Chagas 病是唯一已知的传染性神经病变，由克鲁兹锥虫（*Trypanosoma cruzi*）感染引起。这种疾病中神经元变性的原因尚不清楚，但可能有免疫基础[191]。Chagas 病患者表现为进行性加重的便秘症状和节段性巨结肠引起的腹胀，可能并发乙状结肠扭转（见第 113 章）。

副肿瘤性内脏神经病变可能与胃肠道外的恶性肿瘤有关，尤其是肺小细胞癌和类癌。受累肠道的病理检查显示神经元变性或肌间神经丛炎症[192]。在一些患有这种疾病的患者中发现了一种抗肌间神经元成分的抗体（见第 124 章）[193]。结肠 ICC 的破坏与小细胞肺癌相关的副肿瘤性结肠运动障碍有关[194]。

（4）不明原因的神经病变

重度急性神经病变，主要表现为梗阻症状而不是便秘。如前所述，一些严重的特发性便秘患者可能出现影响结肠神经的病变特征。

（五）药物

便秘可能是长期服用药物或某些制剂的副作用。通常涉及的药物列于框 19.3（见上文）。可引起便秘的常见药物包括：用于治疗慢性疼痛的阿片类药物、抗胆碱能药物（包括解痉药）、钙补充剂、一些三环类抗抑郁药、非甾体抗炎药、用作长期抗精神病药的吩噻嗪类药物和用于 PD 的抗毒蕈碱药物。

（六）精神心理障碍

便秘可能是精神疾病的症状或是其治疗的副作用（见第 22 章）。具有社交能力、性格外向、精力充沛、乐观而不焦虑的健康男性，比没有这些性格特征的男性排便更容易而规律[195]。便秘患者结肠传输时间延长的相关心理因素，包括高度抑郁的情绪状态和经常控制愤怒[196]。在一项研究中，便秘女性的躯体化障碍和焦虑评分高于健康对照组。心理评分与直肠黏膜血流量（作为远端结肠神经支配的指标）呈负相关[197]。在一项评估老年人便秘心理特征的研究中，结肠传输时间延迟与躯体化障碍、强迫症、抑郁和焦虑症状显著相关[75]。在一项对 28 例女性患者连续进行难治性便秘心理评估的研究中，60% 的患者有当前情感障碍的证据。三分之一的人对食物的态度扭曲。在评定量表上，慢传输型便秘患者比正常传输型便秘患者出现更多的心理社会困扰[198]。

1. 抑郁症

对一些患者来说，便秘可能是一种情感障碍的躯体表现。在一项针对抑郁症患者的研究中，27% 的患者表示便秘在抑郁症发作时发生或恶化[199]。便秘可能发生在没有其他严重抑郁症典型特征的情况下，如厌食或伴缺乏体力活动的精神运动发育迟滞。心理因素很可能通过自主传出神经通路影响肠道功能[197]。在对 400 万美国退伍军人出院记录的分析中，重度抑郁症与便秘有关，精神分裂症与便秘和巨结肠均有关[200]。

2. 进食障碍

有神经性厌食症或贪食症的患者常主诉便秘，这些疾病患者的全肠道转运时间延长[201]。大多数神经性厌食症患者一旦摄入均衡饮食，体重增加至少 3 周后，结肠转运时间恢复正常[202]。在一些进食障碍的患者中发现盆底功能障碍，随着体重增加和均衡饮食盆底功能障碍没有改善[203]。

神经性厌食症应被认为是低体重年轻女性出现便秘的一种可能诊断。进食障碍患者经常需要定期服用泻药来治疗便秘或减少暴饮暴食促进体重减轻。此类患者的治疗是针对潜在的进食障碍（见第 9 章）。

3. 拒绝承认（否认）排便

通过影像学检查证实固体惰性标志物从腹部消失，证明粪便已经排出（见下文），但患者否认排便或报告未排便。这类患者需要有经验的精神科医生帮助。

（七）粪便嵌塞

粪便嵌塞是指直肠或结肠内有大量粪便无法排出[204]，通常表现为慢性或严重便秘患者的并发症（而不是原因）。粪便嵌塞在老年人中更常见[205]，但也可见于儿童和脊髓损伤或神经肌肉疾病的患者中[56,206]。住院老年人发生粪便嵌塞的风险特别高[57,207,208]。

多种因素可导致粪便嵌塞。这些因素通常包括慢性便秘、纤维和水摄入不足、结肠阻塞性病变、或因年老导致的缺乏活动、脊髓损伤或神经肌肉疾病、减缓胃肠运动的药物（如阿片类药物、抗胆碱能药物、钙通道阻滞剂、抗酸剂、抗精神病药、抗高血压药、铁剂、滥用泻药）均可能对一些患者产生影响[205,206,209]。

粪便嵌塞常表现出与肠梗阻相类似的症状，包括恶心、呕吐、腹痛、腹胀和厌食[209]。粪便嵌塞的其他症状包括直肠不适、反常性腹泻、大便失禁、尿频和溢出性尿失禁[205]。粪便嵌塞可伴有严重的并发症和高死亡率。并发症包括肠穿孔、肠梗阻、粪石性结肠炎或溃疡、直肠阴道瘘和巨直肠或巨结肠[205,210-212]。高龄（即>85 岁）老人因粪便嵌塞而急诊就诊很常见[213]。在高达 30% 的住院病例中，死亡可能继发于粪便嵌塞并发症[211]。

解除粪便嵌塞的常用方法包括手指解除、使用灌肠剂和口服泻药。在成功解除嵌塞后，应进行结肠检查，包括结肠镜或钡灌肠检查，以评估患者是否存在狭窄或恶性肿瘤[209]。还应进行内分泌和代谢筛查，以排除便秘和粪便嵌塞的肠外原因[205]。如果未发现解剖结构异常，应采取措施降低复发的可能性。与预防便秘一样，增加纤维摄入、补水和适当使用泻药（但不是过度使用）可能有助于降低再嵌塞的风险[209]。如果适用，应解决其他危险因素，包括便秘用药方案和缺乏活动能力的问题。

八、临床评估

（一）病史

评估病史对准确判断患者便秘的病情是很重要的。应获得详细的病史，包括症状持续时间、排便频率以及相关症状，如腹部不适和腹胀等。病史还应包括粪便硬度和大小以及排便用力程度。应提示报警症状和体征的存在，如意外的体重减轻、直肠出血、粪便粗细改变、严重腹痛或有结肠癌家族史。保守治疗无效的长期症状提示功能性结直肠疾病。相反，新发生的便秘可能提示器质性的疾病。

应获得饮食史，评估每日纤维和液体消耗量。许多患者不吃早餐[214]，这种做法可能会加重便秘，因为早餐对餐后结肠运动的增加是最大的[215,216]。虽然咖啡中的咖啡因（150mg咖啡因）也会刺激结肠运动，但进餐对结肠运动的影响更大[217]。

必须回顾患者的既往病史，产科和外科手术史尤为重要。神经系统疾病也可以解释一些便秘病例。仔细询问用药史，包括非处方泻药和草药的使用及其服用频率非常重要。

详细的社会史可以提供有用的信息，如患者此时为什么寻求便秘治疗，也可以获得潜在的相关行为背景信息。在IBS患者中，与健康对照组相比，有性虐待史的发生频率增加[218]。在对120例排便协同失调患者的调查中，22%的患者有性虐待史，32%的患者有身体虐待史。肠功能障碍对56%患者的性生活和76%患者的社交生活产生不利影响[219]。医生应警惕抑郁症的各种表现，如失眠、精神不振、对生活失去兴趣、丧失信心和绝望感。初次就诊期间可能不会发现患者有身体或性虐待史。但是如果医生指出有肠道症状的患者通常有虐待史，同时保持敏感、鼓励的态度，那么在随后的就诊中，如果有隐私、保密和足够的时间，逐渐会获得完整的病史（见第22章）。

（二）体格检查

患者的一般外观或声音可能为甲状腺功能降低、帕金森病或抑郁症提供临床诊断的依据。体格检查应排除主要的中枢神经系统疾病，特别是脊髓病变。如果怀疑有脊髓疾病，应检查骶骨皮区有无感觉丧失。检查腹部有无腹胀、触及结肠内有无硬便、炎症或肿块。如果腹部膨胀，应在患者仰卧时将手置于腰椎下方，以排除腰椎前拱引起的体位性腹胀（见第17章）。

直肠检查对评估便秘患者至关重要。患者取左侧卧位方便进行彻底的直肠检查。应排除肛周疼痛和直肠黏膜疾病，并评估排便功能。应在患者静息和像排便一样用力后观察会阴。正常情况下，会阴在用力时下降1~4cm。患者取左侧卧位，会阴下降到坐骨结节平面以下（即>4cm）通常提示会阴过度下降。如下降不足可能表明排便时盆底肌肉不能松弛，而会阴过度下降可能提示会阴下降综合征。会阴下降综合征患者因肛门直肠角未伸直而过度劳损，只能达到直肠排空不全。最终，会阴过度下降可能导致骶神经因拉伸而受损，直肠感觉降低，因无神经支配而导致大便失禁[137]。另外，当要求患者用力时可发现直肠脱垂。

应检查肛周区域是否有瘢痕、瘘管、裂隙和外痔。进行直肠指检，以发现患者是否存在粪便嵌顿、肛门狭窄或直肠肿块。肛门括约肌扩张可能提示既往肛门括约肌受创伤或神经系统疾病损害括约肌功能。直肠指检时应评估的其他重要功能总结见框19.5。具体讲，检查手指不能插入肛管可能表明肛门括约肌压力升高，当盆底横过直肠后部时触诊盆底有触痛可能提示盆底痉挛。在试图用力和排出检查手指时，会阴下降的程度提供了另一种评估会阴下降程度的方法。与高分辨率测压法和球囊排出法相比（见下文），直肠指检在诊断排便协同失调中的敏感性、特异性和阳性预测值分别为93.2%、58.7%和91.0%，两种诊断方式之间中度一致（κ系数=0.542，$P<0.001$）[220]。详细的病史和体格检查可以排除大多数继发性便秘的原因（见框19.3）。

框19.5 排便障碍的临床诊断线索

病史
需要长时间用力排出粪便
在马桶上摆出特定姿势，以促进粪便排出
需支持会阴，手指辅助直肠，或需要对阴道后壁施加压力以促进直肠排空
无法排出灌肠液
结肠次全切除术后便秘
直肠检查（患者左侧卧位）
望诊
在试图模拟排便用力时，肛门被“拉”向前方
在尝试模拟排便用力时，肛门边缘下降<1cm或>4cm（或超过坐骨结节）
在用力时会阴向下膨胀，直肠黏膜经肛管部分脱垂
触诊
静息状态时肛门括约肌张力高，检查手指不易进入［在无疼痛的肛周疾病情况下（如肛裂）］
随意挤压时肛门括约肌压力仅略高于静息时肛门压力
模拟用力排便时会阴及检查手指下降<1cm或>4cm
通过直肠壁向后触诊耻骨直肠肌有触痛，或触诊重现疼痛
用力时可触及的黏膜脱垂
直肠前壁“缺损”，提示直肠膨出
肛门直肠测压及球囊排出试验（患者处于左侧卧位）
静息时肛门括约肌压力升高
球囊排出试验延迟（<50岁女性的正常值为4~75秒；≥50岁女性的正常值为3~15秒）[246]

九、诊断试验

对于大多数主诉症状较轻的患者，尤其是青少年、青壮年和无报警症状的患者，不需要进一步的诊断检测。检查目的可能有以下两种原因之一：①排除导致便秘的系统性疾病或胃肠道结构病变；②当症状对简单治疗无反应时，需阐明潜在的病理生理机制。

（一）系统性疾病试验

如果临床症状提示是由炎症、肿瘤、代谢或其他系统性疾病所致的便秘，则需测定血红蛋白水平、血沉和生化筛查试验（如甲状腺功能、血钙、血糖及其他适当的检查项目）。

（二）结构性疾病试验

通过 CT、MRI 或钡灌肠造影对结肠进行成像，可显示结肠的宽度和长度，可用于排除足以引起便秘的严重梗阻性病变。当存在粪便嵌塞时，应用水溶性造影剂灌肠研究可以显示出结肠和粪便团块的轮廓，而不会加重病情。只有当怀疑肠梗阻或假性肠梗阻累及小肠时，才需要进行小肠成像（见第 123 和 124 章）。内窥镜检查可直接观察结肠黏膜。慢性便秘患者在无"警报"症状的情况下进行结肠镜检查的阳性率较低，与接受结肠镜检查进行结肠癌筛查的无症状患者相当[221]。786 例因便秘接受结肠镜检查的患者中，仅 5.5% 患有息肉，未发现癌症[222]。只有在近期排便习惯改变、粪便带血或其他警报症状（如体重减轻、发热）出现时，才建议进行结肠镜检查[223]。应推荐所有 50 岁及以上（或者 45 岁）的成年人接受结直肠癌筛选检查[224]。

（三）生理学测量

生理学测试仅适用于有难治性症状的患者。可以测量结肠传输时间，评估排便期间盆底功能，排除可能引起便秘的解剖异常。

1. 结肠传输时间

测量结肠传输时间的研究，对于确认和量化患者的便秘症状以及识别慢传输和区域延迟非常重要。美国和欧洲神经胃肠病学和运动学会推荐了 3 种评估结肠传输时间的方法：不透射线标志物、无线运动胶囊和闪烁扫描显像[225]。

（1）不透射线标志物

不透射线标志物试验用于区分正常结肠传输和缓慢结肠传输，评估节段传输时间，并评价对新治疗的反应[225]。在患者摄入塑料珠或塑料环后，通过在预定时间进行腹部 X 线摄像，并计算保留标志物的数量来测量结肠传输时间（图 19.5）。在研究开始之前，患者应保持高纤维饮食，避免使用泻药、灌肠剂或可能影响肠道功能的药物。由于标志物仅在排便时被清除，因此测量结肠传输的过程是不连续的，应谨慎考虑传输测量的结果，同时还要考虑最近的排便情况。如果标志物仅保留在乙状结肠和直肠中，患者可能有排便障碍。然而，标志物在整个结肠中的存在并不排除排便障碍的可能性。因此，在进行不透射线标志物试验之前，应该对适当的患者进行肛门直肠生理试验（见下文）[225]。对结肠不同节段的传输时间测量在计划治疗中的价值值得怀疑，但巨直肠除外，在巨直肠中，所有标志物都迅速移动到直肠并潴留在那里。

在非受试者中，使用不透射线标记测试的结肠平均传输时间为 30~40 小时，正常上限为 72 小时（见上文）[226]。女性结肠最大传输时间通常比男性更长（70~106 小时 vs 50 小时）。

（2）无线动力胶囊

无线记录胶囊是一种一次性使用的胶囊，可在没有放射线照射的情况下评估结肠传输。它用于区分正常的和缓慢的结肠传输，也可用于疑似上消化道动力障碍的患者，因为它可测量胃排空、小肠传输和结肠传输时间（图 19.6）。在进食标准餐和 50mL 水后摄入无线动力胶囊。当胶囊沿着胃肠道移动时，持续向数据接收器发送温度、pH 和压力测量值。患者

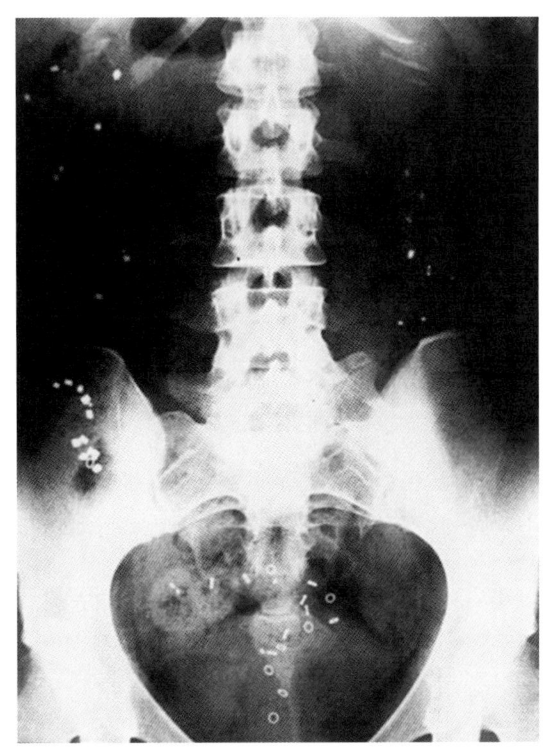

图 19.5　结肠传输研究的腹部 X 线平片。该便秘患者 120 小时前摄入了 20 个惰性环状标志物，72 小时前摄入了 20 个立方形标志物。平片显示大多数标志物仍然存在，表明整个肠道传输缓慢

在腰部佩戴数据接收器 5 天直到胶囊排出体外，并记录日常活动，如进餐、睡眠和排便状态。

大多数将无线动力胶囊与传统不透射线标志物试验进行比较的研究发现，两种方法之间存在一致性（无线动力胶囊识别异常通过时间的特异性为 0.95，灵敏度为 0.46。而不透射线标志物试验的特异性为 0.95，灵敏度为 0.40）[227-229]。然而，在一项回顾性研究中，无线动力胶囊与不透射线标志物试验的阳性试验一致性仅为 86%，阴性试验一致性为 43%[230]。还发现无线动力胶囊与胃排空闪烁扫描显像和全肠道闪烁扫描显像相当、具有可比性[231,232]。

使用无线动力胶囊测量的正常结肠传输时间为 10~59 小时，男性结肠传输时间超过 44 小时，女性结肠传输时间超过 59 小时[228]。鉴于结肠传输时间量化的方法不同，以及与不透射线标志物试验中使用的较小塑料珠相比，无线动力胶囊的尺寸较大，因此两种检查方法得出的结肠传输时间有差异并不意外[228,229]。当评估上消化道传输时，无线动力胶囊试验对结肠切除术治疗重度便秘的患者特别有用（见下文）[233]。尽管无线动力胶囊耐受性良好，允许门诊进行动态检测，但有报道，约 3% 的病例报告了装备器械失效[225]，因此，不建议在植入心脏起搏器或除颤器、吞咽障碍、疑似狭窄或瘘管风险较高的患者中使用。

（3）结肠传输闪烁扫描显像

结肠传输闪烁扫描显像用于测量累及胃或小肠的弥漫性疾病、或疑似结肠运动障碍患者的全肠道或局部结肠的传输疾病[234]。通过摄入标记食物后（^{111}In 二乙烯三胺五乙酸盐标记的水，胶囊中含有标准的^{99m}Tc 鸡蛋三明治[235]或^{111}In 标

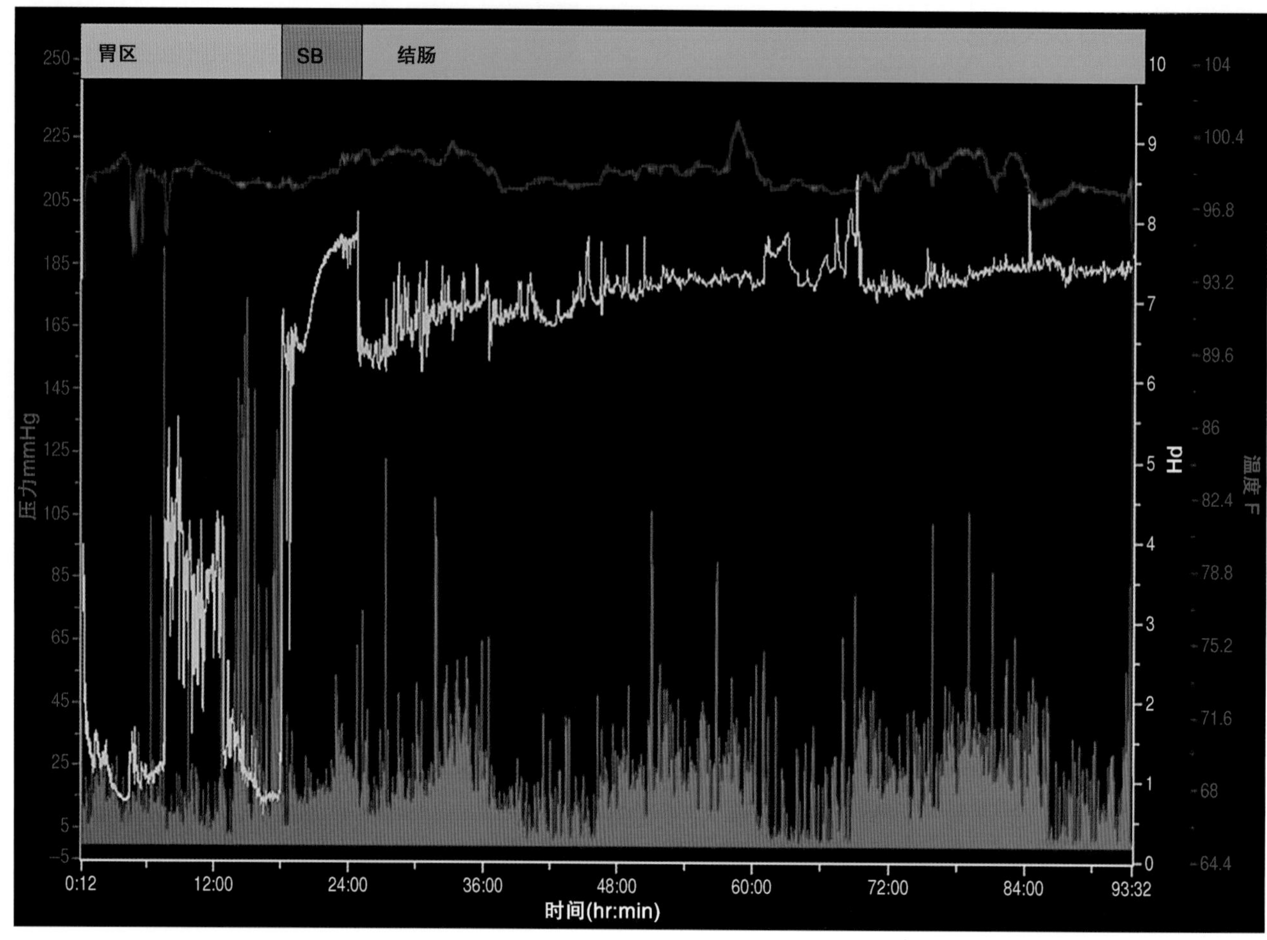

图 19.6 在便秘患者中进行的无线动力胶囊研究的追踪。吞咽无线动力胶囊后，记录温度（蓝线）、压力（红线）和 pH（绿线）。胃排空时间由 pH 的升高决定，表明胶囊已经进入十二指肠。当胶囊进入结肠时，pH 下降（约 24 小时）。胶囊通过直肠排出的时间取决于温度下降。在该患者中，结肠传输时间延长。注：SB，小肠

记的活性炭颗粒）在指定时间使用伽马照相机连续采集腹部图像来测量通过时间[236,237]。在进食后 2~3 天指定的时间内获得结肠前部和后部的图像。在同一项研究中，使用 ^{111}In 二乙烯三胺五乙酸盐标记的水与标准的 ^{99m}Tc 鸡蛋三明治，可以获得胃、小肠和结肠的传输时间[235]。含 ^{111}In 标记的活性炭颗粒的胶囊在到达回肠末端之前不会溶解，在回肠末端将标记的颗粒释放到结肠中，从而只能测量结肠传输时间[236]。结果报告为升结肠排空（表示 50% 排空的时间），或用几何中心表示的整体结肠传输（结肠和粪便内放射性分布的加权平均值）[225]。

使用闪烁扫描显像，以几何中心表示的 24 小时平均结肠传输时间为 2.7±1.05。24 小时结肠传输时间小于 1.7 被认为是慢速传输[236]。低几何中心被认为是缓慢传输，因为大部分放射性物质位于近端结肠，而高几何中心被认为是加速传输，因为大部分放射性物质已经移动到结肠左侧或随粪便排出。已证明结肠传输闪烁扫描显像与不透射线标志物试验相当，除降结肠外[238]。但仅在数量有限的专科中心应用。

2. 评估排便生理学试验

评估患者排便障碍的临床试验包括排粪造影、球囊排出试验、肛门直肠测压和肌电图。为了诊断排便不协调，罗马标准要求在尝试排便时出现以下 3 项盆底检查异常中的任何 2 项：①球囊排出或排粪造影时显示排空障碍；②测压、成像或肌电图显示盆底肌肉异常收缩；③通过肛门测压或成像评估的推进力不足[124]。

一项对 79 项慢性便秘患者研究的 meta 分析发现，慢性便秘患者普遍存在协同排便障碍。异常结果的汇总频率因检查方法而异：肛门直肠测压，48%；球囊排出，43%（根据任一标准）；排粪造影，15%（肛门直肠角无开口）和 37%（会阴过度下降）；肌电图，44%（耻骨直肠肌活动增加）[239]。

（1）排粪造影

排粪造影评价直肠排空率和完整性、肛门直肠角和会阴下降程度，并识别结构异常（如直肠膨出较大、内部黏膜脱垂、肠套叠）。将浓稠的钡剂注入直肠，在透视过程中拍摄 X 线胶片或视频，患者坐在透视的马桶上休息、延迟排便和用力排便。重要的是，确定的解剖结构异常并不总是与功能相关。例如，只有在直肠膨出首先充盈（即代替直肠壶腹部）且在模拟排便后未能排空时才与直肠膨出相关。排粪造影的局限性包括放射科医生解释结果时的差异，有时由于患者的尴尬而抑制正常直肠排空，以及钡糊与粪便的质地不同。磁共振排粪造影可能比标准钡剂排粪造影更具优势，例如无辐射暴露和增加异常检出率[240,241]。此外，磁共振排粪造影以动态方

式检测盆腔器官异常可能更灵敏，包括膀胱膨出和阴道脱垂[242,243]，但目前尚未广泛使用，且很少能在患者坐位时进行检测。

(2) 球囊排出试验

球囊排出试验可提示患者排便障碍，直肠未排空或延迟排空充满 50mL 水的球囊，试验一般是患者坐在便桶上进行[244]。在一项对 359 例便秘患者的研究中，24 例盆底协同障碍患者中（通过测压和排粪造影确定）有 21 例患者球囊排出试验异常。相比之下，在 106 例没有盆底协同障碍的患者中，有 12 例患者出现球囊排出试验异常[245]。因此，球囊排出试验通常与肛门直肠测压联合使用。在健康女性中，球囊排出时间随年龄增长而减少，50 岁以下的正常值为 4~75 秒，50 岁及 50 岁以上的正常值为 3~15 秒[246]。

(3) 肛门直肠测压

肛门直肠测压可以评估肛门括约肌的静息压力和最大挤压压力、直肠球囊扩张期间肛门括约肌是否松弛（直肠肛门抑制反射）、直肠感觉，以及在用力期间肛门括约肌松弛的能力[221,247]。静息肛门压力增高提示存在肛裂或肛门痉挛（肛管内用力或压力引起的肛门外括约肌反常收缩）。直肠低敏感性（RH）提示神经系统疾病，但在粪便潴留患者中，诱发直肠急迫感所需的直肠内容物体积可能增加，因此必须谨慎解释直肠敏感性试验的结果。直肠肛门抑制反射的缺失增加了先天性巨结肠发生的可能性。

排便障碍患者通常在用力下压时肛门括约肌有不适当的收缩。通常认为正常排便需要直肠肛门压力梯度为正值（即直肠压力高于肛门压力），直肠肛门压力梯度为负值（即直肠压力低于肛门压力）与排便障碍相关；然而，无症状患者在肛门直肠测压时常有肛门括约肌收缩异常。在一项对健康受试者的研究中，36% 的受试者在左侧卧位时有协同障碍，但协同障碍的存在与否并不能预测是否有排出球囊的能力[248]。在随后的一项使用高分辨率肛门直肠测压的研究中，大多数无症状女性的直肠肛门压力梯度为负值[246]。尽管直肠肛门压力梯度为负值，可能支持排便障碍的诊断，但其本身并不具有决定性，应与其他生理检测结合使用。

(4) 横纹肌活动肌电图

一般来说，使用同心针或表面电极记录对肛门外括约肌和耻骨直肠肌的肌电图研究并不是必需的，很少有指征。一个例外是在疑似脊髓或马尾神经病变的患者中使用肌电图，可证实双侧或单侧肛门外括约肌功能障碍。

(5) 直肠敏感性和感觉测试

直肠对膨胀的敏感性可以通过向直肠球囊中连续注入一定量的空气并记录其变化来测量。第一次感觉到刺激的体积、产生排便冲动的体积，以及由于不适而无法再忍受进一步增加空气的体积，来评价直肠的敏感度和感觉异常。

十、治疗

便秘的初始治疗是非药物干预。如果这些措施失败，可以使用药物。如果存在排便障碍，初始治疗应包括生物反馈。许多排便障碍患者对纤维补充剂或口服泻药反应不佳，而高达 75% 的患者对生物反馈有反应。否则，治疗应该包括增加体力活动、改变饮食习惯、使用膳食纤维补充剂、增加水分和纤维的摄入。补充纤维剂治疗后无改善的患者应给予渗透性泻药，如镁乳或聚乙二醇。应调整剂量，直至出现软便。刺激剂（如比沙可啶、番泻叶衍生物）应给予对纤维剂或渗透性泻药无反应的患者。对初始治疗无效的患者应考虑使用处方药物，如鲁比前列酮、利那洛肽和普立卡那肽。图 19.7 提供了评估和治疗重度便秘患者的流程。

（一）一般措施

1. 安慰（消除疑虑）

可告知患者，有一些不规则排便习惯和其他轻微的排便症状在健康的普通人群中很常见，这些症状是无大碍的。如果患者担心症状可能预示疾病，可通过适当的检查让其消除疑虑。

2. 生活方式改变

生活方式和饮食习惯的改变常作为慢性便秘患者的一线治疗。应该强调需要留出从容的、有规律的排便时间定期排便，并且始终对排便冲动作出反应。如果患者出现排便困难，建议他们坐在马桶上时，脚下放置一个大约 15cm 高的支撑物，使髋关节呈下蹲姿势屈曲。对于活动较少的人，应该鼓励体力锻炼。应避免随意使用便秘药物，包括非处方药（见框 19.3）。

3. 心理支持

便秘可能因压力而加重，也可能是情绪障碍的表现［如既往性虐待史（见第 22 章）］。对于此类患者，评估患者的情况、个性、背景以及支持性建议可能比任何药物或物理治疗措施更有帮助。行为治疗（见下文）提供了一种具有心理成分的物理方法，通常是可接受和有益的。

4. 液体摄入

脱水或盐耗竭可能导致结肠对盐和水的吸收增加，导致排出小而坚硬的粪便。然而，在无临床脱水的情况下，没有数据支持增加液体摄入量可缓解便秘[249,250]。将每日饮水量增加到 1.5~2 升，可提高便秘患者摄入纤维的治疗效果[251]。

5. 膳食变化和纤维补充

根据 20 世纪 70 年代初非洲农村的饮食和粪便模式，Denis Burkitt 博士推测，在西方社会，膳食纤维的缺乏是导致便秘和其他结肠疾病的原因[252]。此后研究表明，当非便秘人群增加膳食纤维的摄入量时，粪便重量与粪便基线重量和排便频率成比例增加，并与结肠传输时间减少相关[253]。每摄入 1g 小麦纤维，可产生约 2.7g 粪便。由此可见，当膳食纤维摄入量增加导致便秘受试者排出粪便重量增加时，产生的粪便重量仍可能低于正常。因此，高纤维膳食作为便秘的治疗方法，其治疗结果往往令人失望。在一项对 10 例便秘女性的研究中，在她们的饮食中添加了麦麸（20g/d），平均每日粪便重量从大约 30g/d 增加到 60g/d，只有一半的患者达到了正常的平均粪便重量。排便频率从平均每周 2 次增加到 3 次[254]。在一项对照交叉试验中，24 例患者每日接受 20g 麸皮或安慰剂，共 4 周。虽然麦麸在改善排便频率和口肛传输率方面比安慰剂更有效，但患者便秘发生率和严重程度在 2 个治疗期之间无差异[255]，可能是由于排便困难，而不是排便频率降低。

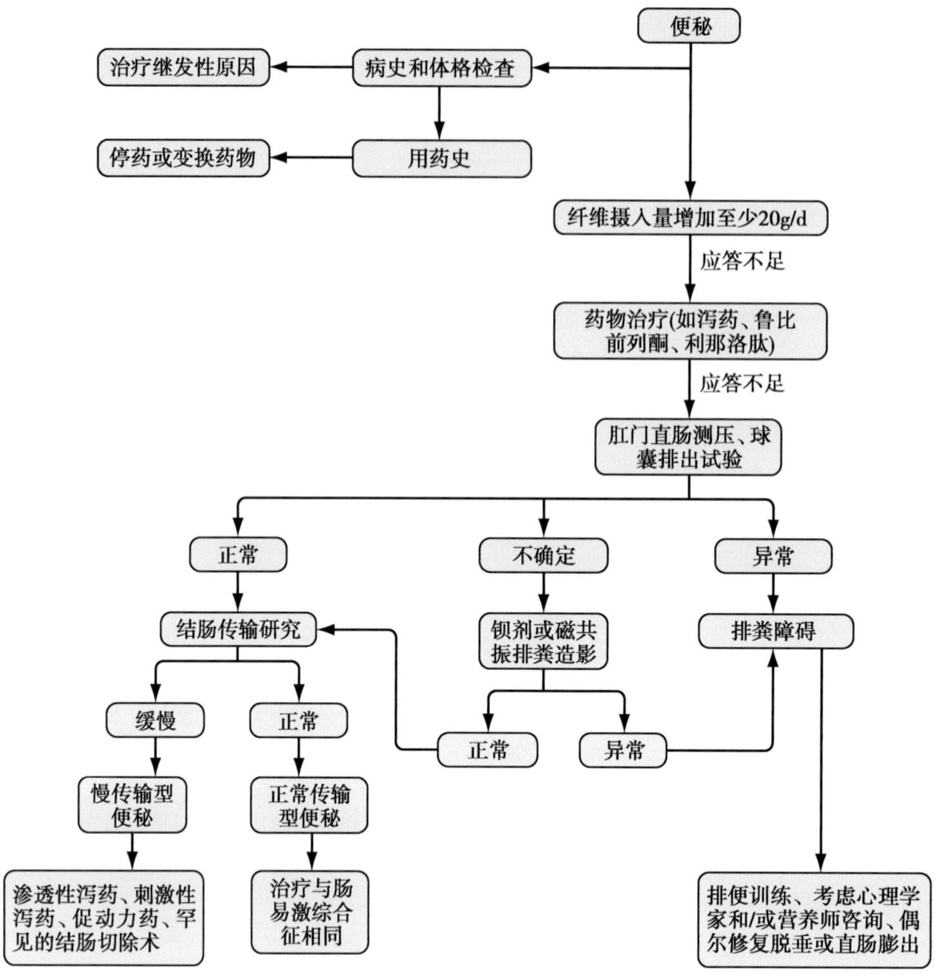

图 19.7　中重度便秘的评估和治疗流程

膳食纤维似乎可有效缓解轻度至中度便秘[81]，但不能缓解重度便秘[112]，尤其是重度便秘与结肠传输缓慢、排空障碍或与药物治疗相关时。虽然饮食调整可能不会成功，仍建议初始治疗的大多数便秘患者增加膳食纤维的摄入量，是一种最简单、最符合生理和最便宜的治疗形式。便秘治疗指南建议纤维摄入量至少为 25~30g/d 的可溶性纤维[14,256,257]，因为关于不溶性纤维作用的数据相互矛盾。对 6 项随机对照试验(4 项使用可溶性纤维，2 项使用不溶性纤维)的系统综述发现，可溶性纤维可改善便秘症状，支持不溶性纤维相互矛盾的数据[258]。可溶性纤维对慢性便秘和便秘型肠易激综合征患者的耐受性似乎更好[259]。因此，应考虑增加可溶性纤维的摄入量，如燕麦麸、坚果、大麦、种子、豆类、扁豆、豌豆、一些水果和蔬菜以及补充车前草纤维。不溶性纤维如麦麸、全谷物和一些蔬菜似乎耐受性较差，有可能加重症状，尤其是便秘型肠易激综合征患者[14,258-260]。不溶性纤维颗粒可能粗大(如麸皮)，对结肠和黏液分泌造成机械刺激。相比之下，可溶性纤维(如车前草)具有较高的保水能力，有助于将水分吸入结肠，避免脱水，从而改善粪便的稠度[1,261]。应鼓励患者每日摄入约 25g 非淀粉多糖，包括食用全麦面包、未精制的谷物食品、水果和蔬菜，必要时，可在早餐谷物食品或熟食中补充麸皮。往往需要具体的饮食咨询。

纤维补充剂的副作用包括腹部不适、腹胀和胃肠胀气，以及口味不佳，可导致患者依从性差，尤其是前几周。大多数关于纤维作用的对照研究表明，持续和显著改变肠道功能或结肠传输时间所需的最小剂量为 12g/d。为改善依从性，应指导患者在数周内逐渐增加膳食纤维的摄入量至约 20~25g/d。如果治疗效果不佳，应尝试使用市场出售的纤维补充剂(表 19.2)。纤维和膨松剂是基于小麦、植物种子黏质(卵叶车前子)、植物胶(梧桐子)或合成的甲基纤维素衍生物[甲基纤维素、羧甲基纤维素(见下文)]的浓缩形式的非淀粉多糖。

一些患者，特别是结肠传输明显延迟的女性，发现纤维加重腹胀。如果患者对膳食纤维试验没有反应，可能怀疑慢传输型便秘和/或排便障碍[112]。麸皮对患有巨结肠的年轻人和老年人可能没有帮助，在他们中可能会导致大便失禁。对于这些患者，减少纤维摄入量可能会缓解症状。

6. 低 FODMAP 食谱

限制吸收不良的可发酵碳水化合物[可发酵低聚糖、二糖、单糖和多元醇(FODMAP)]已证明对一些便秘型肠易激综合征患者有益，尽管证据不充分，需要进一步试验(见第 122 章)[259]。而目前尚未在与肠易激综合征无关的慢性便秘患者中，进行低 FODMAP 饮食的临床试验。

表19.2 市场出售的纤维剂

制剂	起始日剂量/g	注释
甲基纤维素	4~6	半合成纤维素纤维,相对抵抗结肠细菌降解,比车前草更少引起腹胀
车前草	4~6	由卵叶车前草植物磨碎的种子壳制成,与水混合时形成凝胶,因此与车前草同服时应服用足量的水,以避免发生肠梗阻 经细菌降解,可能导致腹胀和胃肠胀气的副作用 过敏反应(如过敏反应、哮喘)已有报道,但很少见
聚卡波菲	4~6	由丙烯酸聚合物制成的合成纤维,可抵抗细菌降解
瓜尔胶	3~6	从豆科灌木瓜尔豆种子中提取的可溶性纤维

(二)特效治疗制剂

1. 市售纤维产品

(1)甲基纤维素

甲基纤维素是一种半合成的非淀粉多糖,具有不同的链长和甲基化程度。甲基化可减少结肠中的细菌降解。一项对每日平均粪便重量仅为35g的便秘患者进行的研究显示,给予1、2和4g/d甲基纤维素后,可增加粪便固体,但在仅服4g剂量时可增加粪便水分。该组患者的排便频率从平均每周2次增加至4次,但患者未报告粪便硬度或排便难易程度是否改善(见表19.2)[262]。

(2)卵叶车前子(车前草、Ispaghula)

卵叶车前子是源自生长在印度的一种植物果壳,具有较高的水结合力,在结肠中适度发酵,并增加细菌细胞数量。它可制成泡腾悬浮液、颗粒和粉剂。受欢迎的悬浮液必须在果壳吸水之前迅速消耗掉。可在半杯水中快速搅拌颗粒,并立即吞服,最好是碳酸水。有些人喜欢吞下固体颗粒,然后喝一杯水。

研究显示,在便秘受试者中,卵叶车前子(3.4g Metamucil)增加粪便量的程度与1~4g/d甲基纤维素相同。尽管粪便干、湿重量均增加了,但每周粪便总重量仍低于未经治疗的健康对照组。在一项观察性研究中,149例患者接受了为期至少6周的卵叶车前子形式的治疗(15~30g/d)。结肠传输缓慢或排便障碍的患者对治疗的反应较差,而在无异常生理测试结果的患者中有85%症状改善或消失。然而,作者建议在进行诊断检测之前进行膳食纤维试验[112]。

卵叶车前子可引起免疫球蛋白E介导的急性过敏性反应,包括面部肿胀、荨麻疹、咽喉发紧、咳嗽和哮喘[263]。在生产或制备过程中吸入该化合物的工人也可能会有类似反应(见表19.2)[264]。

(3)聚碳酸钙

聚碳酸钙是一种亲水性聚丙烯酸树脂,可抵抗细菌降解,因此不可能产气引起腹胀。在肠易激综合征患者中,聚碳酸钙似乎能改善全身症状和易于排便,但不能缓解腹痛(见表19.2)[265]。

(4)瓜尔胶

瓜尔胶是一种天然高分子量多糖,从豆科灌木瓜尔豆的种子中提取的。它迅速水化形成高黏性溶液。瓜尔豆胶被批准用于许多食品和化妆品中,并作为一种补充剂。据报道,高剂量使用瓜尔豆胶会引起肠梗阻。

(5)亚麻籽

亚麻籽用于便秘患者尚未得到很好的研究,在对肠易激综合征患者的小型研究中也报告了相互矛盾的结果[266,267]。

(6)可溶性和不溶性混合纤维

可溶性纤维和不溶性纤维的组合被认为与单独使用可溶性纤维对便秘同样有效,可能耐受性稍好,因此对希望在饮食中增加纤维的患者来说是一个合理的选择[268]。在一项为期4周的试验中,梅子衍生的混合纤维补充剂(10g/d)与相同剂量的车前草在改善便秘和生活质量方面同样有效,而且在缓解胃肠胀气和腹胀方面更有效,溶解效果更好。

2. 其他泻药

除纤维外的泻药主要是渗透性和刺激性泻药。粪便软化剂和润滑剂是附加的治疗药物(见下文)(表19.3和表19.4)。

(1)渗透性泻药

渗透性泻药通过产生肠腔内渗透梯度,驱动水和电解质分泌到肠腔中,从而增加粪便量并降低粪便硬度。

(2)离子吸收不良

吸收较差的镁离子、硫酸盐和磷酸盐离子在肠道内吸收较差,从而形成腔内高渗性环境。它们的主要作用方式似乎是渗透作用,但它们可能还具有其他作用,后果尚不清楚,如增加粪便中前列腺素的浓度[269]。每增加排出1mmol可溶性镁,粪便重量增加7.3g[270]。服用标准剂量的氢氧化镁(见表19.3)通常在6小时内排便。硫酸镁是一种更有效的泻药,往往会产生大量的液体粪便,通常导致腹胀和突然排出恶臭的液体粪便。

镁的使用,尤其是在老年人中,可能受到不良反应的限制,如胃肠胀气、腹部绞痛和血容量变化等。一小部分镁在小肠中被主动吸收,其余镁通过渗透梯度将水吸入肠道[271]。肾衰竭患者和儿童特别容易发生高镁血症。高镁血症引起的麻痹性肠梗阻是一种罕见的并发症[272],儿童每天服用18g氢氧化镁7天后,发生了高镁血症伴昏迷,需要血液透析[273]。肾功能不全或心功能不全的患者可因镁的吸收而出现电解质紊乱和血容量超负荷。过量使用,即使是其他方面健康的患者,除脱水之外,也会发生这些并发症。

由于磷酸盐被小肠吸收,因此必须摄入大剂量才能产生渗透性通便作用,日常使用并不理想。一种罕见但严重的急性肾功能损伤与结肠镜检查前使用的磷酸钠溶液有关,即使在基线肾功能正常的患者中也是如此(见第42章)。磷酸盐所致肾功能损伤的危险因素包括高血压、高龄、血容量不足和使用血管紧张素转换酶抑制剂或非甾体抗炎药[274,275]。

表 19.3 便秘常用的泻药

泻药类型	通用名称	剂量	评论
渗透性泻药			
离子吸收不良			
镁	氢氧化镁	15~30ml/次 1次或2次/d	肾衰竭和儿童患者易发生高镁血症
	柠檬酸镁	75~150ml/次或2~4片/次(1次/d)	常用于肠道准备,长期使用超过1 650g的镁,可发生高镁血症
	硫酸镁	5~10g/次(1次/d)	
硫酸盐	硫酸钠(芒硝)	5~10g/次(1次/d)	硫酸钠一般不用作泻药单独使用
磷酸盐	磷酸钠	0.5~10ml/次加12盎司水	高磷酸血症,特别易发生于肾功能衰竭患者
吸收差的糖类			
二糖	乳果糖	15~30ml/次,1次或2次/d	产气和腹胀是常见的副作用
糖醇	山梨醇	15~30ml/次,1次或2次/d	通常用作无糖产品的甜味剂。在老年人中,山梨醇作用与乳果糖相似,但成本较低
	甘露醇	15~30ml/次,1次或2次/d	很少用作泻药
聚乙二醇	聚乙二醇电解质	17~34g/次 1次或2次/d	与其他药物相比,较少引起腹胀和痉挛;无味、可与非碳酸饮料混合。通常用于结肠镜检和手术前准备;也可定期使用不含电解质的粉末
刺激性泻药			
蒽醌类	鼠李皮 番泻叶	325mg(或5ml)睡前服用 1~2片/d(7.5mg/片)	引起巨噬细胞吞噬凋亡的结肠上皮细胞;导致脂褐素样色素沉着,称为假黑色素沉着症;尚未确定蒽醌类化合物与结肠癌或肌间质神经损伤(泻剂性结肠)之间无明确关联性
蓖麻油酸	蓖麻油	15~30ml睡前	常见副作用为抽筋
二苯甲烷衍生物	比沙可啶	5~10mg睡前	对小肠和结肠有作用
	酚酞	30~200mg睡前	因对动物的致畸性,已从美国和其他市场撤出
	匹可硫酸钠	5~15mg睡前	可能只对结肠有效。尽管在欧洲广泛使用,在美国只是在结肠镜检准备时使用
粪便软化剂	多库酯钠	100mg/次,2次/d	对便秘的疗效尚未完全确定
润滑剂	矿物油	5~15ml睡前	长期使用可引起脂溶性维生素吸收不良,肛门渗漏和容易误吸液体的患者发生类脂质性肺炎
灌肠剂、栓剂	磷酸盐灌肠 矿物油保留灌肠 自来水灌肠 肥皂水灌肠 甘油栓剂 比沙可啶栓剂	120ml 100ml 500ml 1 500ml 60g 10mg	直肠黏膜的严重损伤可能是由于灌肠液进入黏膜下层;高渗磷酸盐灌肠和大容量自来水或肥皂水灌肠,可导致高磷血症和其他电解质异常。如果保留灌肠,肥皂水灌肠可引起结肠炎
氯离子通道激活剂	鲁比前列酮	8~24μg/次,2次/d	增加肠分泌,其机制认为是通过氯离子2通道
鸟苷酸环化酶C激动剂	利那洛肽 普莱卡肽德	72~145μg/次 1次/d 3mg/次 1次/d	通过环磷酸鸟苷增加肠道分泌
5-HT$_4$激动剂	普鲁卡必利	2mg/次 1次/d	通过刺激5-羟色胺4受体增加肠道推动力
钠-氢化合物	特纳帕诺	50μg/次 2次/d	抑制小肠钠吸收
钠氢交换抑制剂3	导致结肠内液体分泌增加和加速		肠道转运,被批准用于治疗便秘型IBS

IBS,肠易激综合征。

表 19.4 美国胃肠病学会(ACG)关于慢性特发性便秘干预措施的总结

评论	试验的次数	患者数	症状 RR (95%CI)	NNT (95%CI)	推荐	质量证据
一些纤维补充剂可增加慢性特发性便秘(CIC)患者排便频率	3	293	0.25(0.16~0.37)	2(1.6~3)	强烈	低
PEG 能有效提高患者排便次数,改善粪便硬度	4	573	0.52(0.41~0.65)	3(2~4)	强烈	高
乳果糖能有效增加 CIC 患者的排便次数和改善粪便硬度	2	148	0.48(0.27~0.86)	4(2~7)	强烈	低
匹可硫酸钠和比沙可啶对 CIC 患者有效	2	735	0.54(0.42~0.69)	3(2~3.5)	强烈	中
普卢卡必利在改善 CIC 症状方面比安慰剂更有效	8	3 140	0.81(0.75~0.86)	5(4~8)	强烈	中
利那洛肽治疗 CIC 有效	3	1 582	0.84(0.80~0.87)	6(5~8)	强烈	高
鲁比前列酮治疗 CIC 有效	4	651	0.67(0.58~0.77)	4(3~6)	强烈	高
生物反馈对 CIC 患者有效,并证明存在盆底协同失调	3	216	0.33(0.22~0.50)	2(1.6~4)	弱	低

CI,置信区间;NNT,需要治疗的数量;PEG,聚乙二醇;RR,相对风险。

From Ford AC, Moayyedi P, Lacy BE, et al. American College of Gastroenterology monograph on the management of irritable bowel syndrome and chronic idiopathic constipation. Am J Gastroenterol 2014;109(Suppl 1):S2-26.

(3) 吸收较差的糖

乳果糖。乳果糖(lactulose)是一种不可吸收的合成二糖,由半乳糖和果糖通过耐乳糖酶键连接组成。乳果糖不被小肠吸收,但在结肠中发酵产生短链脂肪酸、氢和二氧化碳,从而降低粪便 pH。健康志愿者每日摄入乳果糖 20g(30mL)时,在粪便中检测不到糖。在较大剂量时,一些乳果糖可以原型通过结肠。

乳果糖在成人中的推荐 19. 剂量为 15~30mL,每日 1 次或 2 次。其起效时间比其他渗透性泻药长,大约 2~3 日才能起效。一些患者报告,使用乳果糖最初有效,但随后会失去作用,可能是由于药物引起肠道菌群的改变[276]。乳果糖的不良反应包括腹胀和不适,可能是结肠产气所致。已经报告了因服用乳果糖诱发巨结肠的病例[276]。

在一组每周排便少于 3 次的年轻慢性便秘志愿者中,与仅含蔗糖糖浆的对照组相比,乳果糖增加了排便频率和粪便水分百分比以及软便。乳果糖的有效性呈剂量依赖性的[277]。乳果糖对老年患者的作用,已在两项双盲安慰剂对照试验中进行了研究。在一项研究中,只有大约一半的患者被发现是真正的便秘,在这些患者中,乳果糖的有效率为 80%,而接受安慰剂(葡萄糖)的患者为 33%($P<0.01$)[278]。第二次试验在一家疗养院对 42 例老年便秘患者进行了为期 8~12 周的治疗[279]。乳果糖的初始剂量为 30ml/d,以后根据排便频率,暂时或永久减少剂量至 15mL。乳果糖在增加每日平均排便次数、明显减少粪便嵌塞($P<0.015$)和需要灌肠治疗方面优于安慰剂(50% 葡萄糖糖浆)。

山梨醇(sorbitol)和甘露醇(mannitol)。山梨醇作为人工甜味剂广泛应用于食品工业,而临床很少应用。摄入少至 5g 就会引起呼吸氢的上升,摄入 20g 会使约一半的正常受试者发生腹泻[280]。山梨醇与乳果糖一样有效且价格更便宜。一项应用乳果糖(20g/d)和山梨醇(21g/d)治疗门诊老年男性慢性便秘的随机双盲交叉试验显示,两种化合物在排便频率正常或患者偏好方面无差异[281]。除乳果糖组恶心更常见外,副作用的频率相似。甘露醇是另一种可用作泻药的糖醇。与山梨醇一样,临床上很少用于治疗便秘。

(4) 聚乙二醇

聚乙二醇(polyethylene glycol,PEG)是一种等渗性泻药,具有代谢惰性,能结合水分子,从而增加管腔内的水分潴留[282]。PEG 不被结肠细菌代谢。摄入 PEG 导致粪便量增加和粪便变软,根据 PEG 的消耗量,粪便可能变成液体。PEG 主要以原型经粪便排泄。在结肠镜检查前,将电解质添加到用于结肠灌洗的 PEG 溶液中,以避免发生与腹泻相关的潜在不良反应,如脱水和电解质失衡。在美国不含电解质的 PEG-3350 是以非处方粉末的形式提供,以小剂量与水混合,常规用于治疗便秘。

多项高质量研究已证明 PEG 治疗慢性便秘的疗效[283]。一项针对 304 例慢性便秘患者的随机对照试验显示,在使用 PEG 溶液治疗组的患者中,52.0% 的患者症状改善了 6 个月,而安慰剂组为 11%。在 75 例老年受试者亚组中也观察到相似的疗效。未观察到电解质异常或肠道吸收不良[283]。

在另一项试验中,70 例门诊患者接受了 14.6g PEG 电解质溶液治疗 4 周,每日 2 次,4 周结束时对 PEG 有反应的患者(每周排便少于 3 次)随机分配继续接受 PEG 或安慰剂治疗 20 周,剂量为每日 17g 或 34g。与安慰剂相比,PEG 改善了排便频率和粪便硬度。随访结束时,77% 随机接受 PEG 治疗的患者便秘完全缓解,而随机接受安慰剂治疗的患者仅有 20% 便秘完全缓解。安慰剂组的退出率为 46%,主要是由于治疗失败所致[284]。

另一项随机多中心试验在 266 例门诊患者中比较了 2 种不同分子量 PEG 制剂(PEG-3350 和 PEG-4000)的标准剂量和最大剂量,大多数患者在开始 PEG 治疗后 1 天内首次排便,两个治疗组的粪便硬度均有改善。最低剂量的 PEG 可产生软硬度最正常的粪便,而较高剂量则产生了更多的液体粪便[285]。低剂量 PEG 在治疗慢性便秘方面似乎比乳果糖更有效[286]并且似乎不差于普鲁卡必利(5-HT_4 受体激动剂,见下文)具有更好的耐受性[287]。

PEG 溶液可用于短期治疗粪便嵌塞。在一项研究中[288],16 例 26~87 岁的重症患者,尽管接受了各种泻药治疗,但在医院的 5~23 天内没有排便,临床检查时均有粪便嵌塞,接受 PEG 溶液治疗,1L 分为 2 份 500ml 的溶液,每份在 4~6 小时服完。如有必要,在第 2 天和第 3 天重复该方案。12 例患者在第 1 天服用全剂量,其余患者至少服用推荐剂量的一半,仅 8 例患者在第 2 天需要治疗,2 例患者在第 3 天需要治疗,治疗效果显著。最后一次给药后,大多数患者排出中等或大量的软便,嵌塞消失。除发生腹部隆隆声外,无不良副作用发生,仅有一例截瘫患者出现大便失禁。已有通过口服或鼻胃管用 PEG 成功治疗门诊难治性便秘和老年人便秘的报道[289]。

PEG 治疗的最常见不良反应包括腹胀和痉挛[282]。结肠镜检查前准备肠道应用的 PEG 最常见的副作用包括电解质失平衡、过敏反应和食管贲门黏膜撕裂(Mallory-Weiss 撕裂)[290]。有报告经鼻胃管给予 PEG 溶液后发生暴发性肺水肿的病例,其中 1 例死亡[291,292]。在每例患者中均有呕吐,提示吸入 PEG。PEG 也可能延迟胃排空[293]。

(5) 刺激性泻药

当患者对渗透性泻药无反应时,通常使用刺激性泻药。刺激性泻药可增加肠动力、增加水和电解质向肠腔分泌和前列腺素分泌[294]并加速结肠转运[1,295],它们在数小时内开始起作用,常伴有腹部绞痛。刺激性泻药包括蒽醌类(例如卡巴拉汀、芦荟、番泻叶)和二苯基甲烷类(例如比沙可啶、匹可硫酸钠、酚酞)。蓖麻油因其副作用而较少使用。刺激性泻药的作用具有剂量依赖性,低剂量可阻止水和钠的吸收,而高剂量可刺激钠的分泌,随后通过水进入结肠腔。

刺激性泻药有时会被滥用,尤其是在饮食失调的患者中(见第 9 章)[296]。即使高剂量,它们对卡路里吸收的影响很小。尽管泻药性结肠(即运动力降低的结肠)已被证实可长期使用刺激性泻药,但没有动物或人类数据支持该作用。相反,泻药性结肠如钡剂灌肠检查所见,可能是一种原发性运动障碍。

刺激性泻药在一些患者中可产生正常、柔软、成形的粪便,但即使在标准剂量下,也常伴有腹部痉挛和腹泻。它们作用迅速,特别适用于一过性便秘的单次给药。对于慢性便秘,大多数临床医生对建议无限期每日服用刺激性泻药应持谨慎态度。刺激性泻药的临床疗效差异很大,一些严重便秘患者并没有得到有益的效果。

(6) 蒽醌类

蒽醌类化合物(如药鼠李、番泻叶、芦荟、鼠李皮)是由多种植物产生的。这些化合物是无活性的糖苷,摄入时,它们以未吸收和原形通过小肠,被结肠细菌糖苷酶水解,产生活性代谢物,增加电解质向结肠腔内的转运,刺激肌间神经丛增加肠动力。蒽醌经口服给药后 6~8 小时诱导排便。

蒽醌类化合物可引起结肠上皮细胞凋亡,然后被巨噬细胞吞噬,表现为脂褐素样色素,使结肠黏膜变黑,这种情况称为结肠假性黑色素沉着症(见第 128 章)[297]。蒽醌类泻药似乎不会引起肠道功能障碍或结构的改变。动物研究表明,长期给予番泻苷后,既不会损伤肌间神经丛[298],也不会导致运动功能缺陷[299]。一项病例对照研究中,对多个结肠黏膜活检标本进行电子显微镜检查,结果显示定期服用蒽醌类泻药 1 年的患者与未服用蒽醌类泻药的患者之间黏膜下神经丛无差异[300]。使用蒽醌类泻药与发生结肠癌或肌间神经损伤和所谓的泻药性结肠之间的关系尚未确定[301]。

番泻叶在对照试验中显示可软化粪便[302],增加排便的频率和粪便重量(无论是湿的或干的粪便)。番泻叶可供临床使用的制剂,从粗糙的植物制剂、到纯化和标准化提取物、再到合成化合物不等。

(7) 蓖麻油

蓖麻油是从蓖麻豆中提取的。口服后,在小肠被脂肪酶水解为蓖麻油酸,蓖麻油酸抑制肠道水的吸收,并通过损伤黏膜细胞和释放神经递质刺激肠运动功能[303]。腹部痉挛较为常见,因此蓖麻油在临床上并不常用。

(8) 二苯基甲烷衍生物

二苯基甲烷化合物包括比沙可啶、匹可硫酸钠和酚酞。口服后,比沙可啶和匹可硫酸钠水解为相同的活性代谢物,但水解方式不同。比沙可啶可被肠酶水解,因此可在小肠和大肠中发挥作用。匹可硫酸钠被结肠细菌水解。与蒽醌类一样,匹可硫酸钠的作用局限于结肠,其活性可能无法预测,因其活性取决于菌群水解。

比沙可啶以及匹可硫酸钠对结肠的影响类似于蒽醌类泻药。当作用于结肠黏膜时,比沙可定在健康和便秘受试者中可诱导立即的、强效的推进性运动,尽管后者的效果有时会减弱[304]。这些泻药也刺激结肠分泌。

与蒽醌类泻药一样,比沙可啶可导致结肠上皮细胞凋亡,其残余物蓄积在吞噬性巨噬细胞中,但这些细胞残余物未着色[305]。除这些变化外,长期使用比沙可啶不会引起不良反应[306]。

比沙可啶是一种有效且可预测的泻药,尤其适用于一过性便秘患者的单次给药。与蒽醌类和匹可硫酸钠相比,其对小肠的不利影响是其不足之处。慢性重度便秘患者有时需要长期使用比沙可啶或相关药物。在使用的剂量中,易发生水样便和肠痉挛,而且很难调整剂量以产生柔软、成形便。在一项多中心、随机、双盲、安慰剂对照研究中,247 例慢性便秘患者被随机分为两组,接受比沙可啶治疗每次 10mg,每日 1 次,连续 4 周。与安慰剂组相比,在治疗期间比沙可啶组患者每周完全自发性排便(complete spontaneous bowel movement, CSBM)次数更多(比沙可啶组基线时 1.1±0.1 增加到 5.2±0.1,安慰剂组基线时 1.1±0.1 增加到 1.9±0.1)。与安慰剂组相比,接受比沙可啶治疗的患者在排便费力、肛门阻塞感和粪便形状方面均有所改善,并且生活质量评分比安慰剂组增加。然而,比沙可啶组中 72% 的患者至少有 1 例报告不良反应(腹泻和腹痛常见),开始治疗 1 周后,不良反应的发生频率下降。虽然可将比沙可啶剂量从 10mg/d 减少至 5mg/d,但不良反应导致比沙可啶组 18% 的患者退出研究,而安慰剂组只有 5% 的患者退出研究[307]。

匹可硫酸钠在美国以外地区常用,在美国作为部分结肠镜检查前准备使用。德国进行的一项随机、双盲、安慰剂对照研究中,233 例慢性便秘患者被随机分为匹可硫酸钠组(10mg 滴剂)或安慰剂组,每日 1 次,共 4 周。与安慰剂组相比,匹可硫酸钠组患者在治疗期间每周报告的 CSBM 次数更多(匹可硫酸钠组基线时 0.9±0.1 增加至 3.4±0.2,安慰剂组基线时 1.1±0.1 增加至 1.7±0.1)。与接受安慰剂的患者相比,接受匹可硫酸钠治疗的患者排便费力、排便不尽感、肛门阻塞感以及粪便形状方面均有改善,并且生活质量评分有所增加。32%接受匹可硫酸钠治疗的患者出现腹泻[308]。

对慢性便秘药物治疗的一项系统综述和meta分析表明,比沙可啶和匹可硫酸钠符合应答者分析的主要终点,即每周有大于或等于3次CSBM,而且比基线水平每周增加大于或等于1次CSBM[309]。然而,比沙可啶在次要终点可能优于其他处方药,包括每周自发排便次数(SBM)和每周CSBM次数较基线增加。

酚酞通过作用于类花生酸和存在于肠上皮细胞表面的 Na^+/K^+-ATP酶泵,抑制小肠和结肠的水分吸收(见第101章)。药物经过肝肠循环(见第64章)可延长其作用。尽管有效,一项为期2年的啮齿动物喂养研究发现,在接受治疗的动物中卵巢、肾上腺、肾脏和造血系统肿瘤的发病率增加[310],和1997年美国食品药品管理局(FDA)提出的,将酚酞重新归类为"一般认为不安全和有效"。从此后,大多数含酚酞的泻药已从美国和其他市场自愿退出。随后的研究未能显示酚酞类泻药与癌症之间的联系[311]。

3. 粪便软化剂和润滑剂

(1) 多库酯钠

尽管洗涤剂磺基琥珀酸二辛酯钠(多库酯钠)可用作粪便软化剂,但其功效仍需进一步研究。该化合物刺激小肠和大肠的液体分泌,但不会增加正常人的回肠造口排出量或粪便重量[312,313]。一项双盲交叉试验显示,根据患者及其护理者的判断,15例老年便秘受试者中有5例获益,排便频率显著增加[314]。然而,在一项成年人多中心双盲随机试验中,多库酯钠治疗慢性特发性便秘的疗效不如车前子[315]。

(2) 矿物油

矿物油通过乳化进入粪便团块,并为粪便通道提供润滑来改变粪便。长期使用可引起易误吸液体的患者出现脂溶性维生素吸收不良、肛周渗漏和类脂性肺炎。

4. 灌肠和栓剂

灌肠剂和栓剂化合物可被引入直肠,通过膨胀或化学作用刺激收缩,软化硬便或两者兼而有之。灌肠液外渗到黏膜下层可导致直肠黏膜严重损伤。直肠前黏膜是通过后向成角肛管插入的导管尖端最容易受到创伤的部位(见第129章)。灌肠喷嘴应在肛管通过后朝向后方。

(1) 磷酸盐灌肠剂

高渗磷酸盐灌肠通常是有效的。可以引起直肠扩张和刺激。对正常受试者的组织学研究表明,单次高渗磷酸盐灌肠后引起21例活检标本中有17例表面上皮破坏。扫描电镜显示表面上皮斑片状剥蚀,固有层暴露,杯状细胞缺失。结肠镜下观察到每个病例的黏膜外观均异常,但可在1周内恢复正常[316],表面受损的黏膜几乎迅速愈合。磷酸盐灌肠剂被广泛使用,尽管缺乏证明其疗效的研究。

磷酸盐灌肠如果对不能及时排空的患者进行,可能会导致危险的高磷血症和低钙性手足搐搦;1例患者(年龄91岁)在单次磷酸盐灌肠后死亡[317];1例成年人在未排空的情况下,每小时给予磷酸盐灌肠共6次后,出现昏迷[318]。1例肾功能正常的4岁儿童,在2次磷酸盐保留灌肠后,发生了重度高磷血症、低钙血症和癫痫发作[319]。因此不建议对3岁及以下儿童使用磷酸盐灌剂[320,321]。

(2) 盐水、自来水和肥皂水灌肠

盐水、自来水或肥皂水灌肠主要通过扩张直肠、软化粪便而见效。粪便排空通常发生在灌肠后2~5分钟。盐水灌肠不会损伤直肠黏膜是有效的[316]。也可以使用自来水和肥皂水灌肠,但若灌肠量大而且保留灌肠,有可能会发生危险的水中毒。如果大容量的水或肥皂水灌肠,也会导致高磷血症和其他电解质紊乱。肥皂水灌肠也可引起直肠黏膜损伤和坏死。

(3) 刺激性栓剂和灌肠剂

甘油可作为栓剂给药,通常是具有临床疗效的。直肠受到渗透作用的刺激,但甘油对直肠黏膜的不良影响尚不清楚。比沙可啶10mg可作为一种栓剂,它通过刺激肠神经元发挥局部作用[306]。在正常受试者中,单次给予比沙可啶栓剂或灌肠剂(将19mg比沙可啶溶于100mL或200mL水中),可使23/25份直肠黏膜活检标本发生显著变化。表面和隐窝内的上皮发生改变,使用灌肠剂时,表面上皮缺失[322]。因此,常规使用比沙可啶栓剂似乎是不明智的。奥芬那丁(Veripaque)是一种刺激灌肠剂,在美国不再上市,过去主要在诊断程序之前使用。当口服给药时,该化合物可能会有导致慢性的病例肝炎。

(4) 促分泌泻药

氯离子通道激活剂

鲁比前列酮(lubiprostone)是一种双环脂肪酸,来源于前列腺素E1,据报道主要通过在肠上皮细胞水平激活肠氯化物2通道发挥作用,从而增加肠腔中的氯化物分泌,其次是钠和水,在不改变血清电解质水平的情况下,引起肠液分泌和加速转运[323]。2006年美国批准鲁比前列酮用于治疗男性和女性慢性特发性便秘。在2项3期随机安慰剂对照试验中,鲁比前列酮(24μg/次,每日2次)增加了根据罗马Ⅱ标准定义的慢性便秘患者的SBM数量(即在过去24小时内未使用泻药而发生的排便)(鲁比前列酮治疗组患者第1周时为5.89,安慰剂治疗组患者第1周时为3.99)[324]。鲁比前列酮还可显著降低男性和女性以及老年患者的排便费力,改善粪便稠度,减轻症状的总体严重程度,同时增加SBM的数量。停药后的反弹作用不明显[325]。恶心是最常见的不良反应,发生率高达31.7%,导致5%的患者停药[318]。鲁比前列酮在美国还获批用于治疗阿片类药物引起的便秘,以及治疗伴有便秘的IBS女性,剂量为8μg/次,2次/d。

(5) 鸟苷酸环化酶C激动剂

A. 利那洛肽

利那洛肽(linaclotide)是一种吸收最少的14-氨基酸肽,可激活肠上皮管腔表面的鸟苷酸环化酶C受体,导致环磷酸鸟苷(cGMP)水平升高,增加氯化物和碳酸氢盐向肠腔的分泌。在动物模型中,环磷酸鸟苷似乎也可减少肠内传入神经的放电[326]。在涉及1 276例慢性便秘患者的2项3期研究中,利那洛肽显著增加了每周报告3次或更多次CSBM的患者百分比(即与完全排空感觉相关),在12周中至少9周,与基线水平相比增加了1次或多次(20%为接受利那洛肽145μg或290μg治疗的患者,5%为接受安慰剂的患者)。与安慰剂相比,利那洛肽还可增加大便频率,改善粪便稠度,减少排便费力、腹胀和不适。腹泻是最常见的不良反应,导致约

4%的患者停止治疗[327]。利那洛肽还可改善伴有中重度腹胀的慢性便秘患者的肠道和腹部症状[328]。于2012年FDA批准利那洛肽145μg/次、每日1次，随后改为72μg/次、每日1次，用于治疗男性和女性慢性便秘患者，对伴有便秘的IBS患者剂量为290μg/次，每日1次。6岁以下儿童禁用利那洛肽，因为实验显示3周龄以下的幼年小鼠死亡，在6周龄以上的小鼠中未发现类似结果。不推荐利那洛肽用于6~18岁的儿童。

B. 普卡那肽

普卡那肽(plecanatide)是一种鸟苷酸环化酶C激动剂，其机制与利那洛肽相似。在慢性便秘患者中进行的两项3期普卡那肽试验(每日1次，持续12周)显示CSBM应答者的总体百分比增加(在试验的12周中有9周和最后4周中的3周，每周CSBM>3个，超过基线水平>1个)[329]。在剂量为3mg和6mg时，19.5%~20.1%和20.0%~21.0%的患者为应答者，而安慰剂组为10.2%~12.8%的应答。普卡那肽还显著改善了粪便的硬度和排便频率。据报道5.1%的患者出现腹泻，2.7%的患者停药[330]。普卡那肽获得FDA批准剂量为3mg/次，每日1次。

C. 5-羟色胺能通便剂

5-羟色胺能通便剂刺激胃肠壁传入神经上的5-HT_4受体可诱导肠道蠕动收缩。已经对几种5-HT_4激动剂治疗便秘进行了检测。西沙必利是一种苯二氮䓬类药物，在治疗便秘方面效果各不相同[331]。由于发生潜在的致死性心律失常导致其于2000年7月退出美国市场。2007年从美国市场上撤出的替加色罗，由于之前在治疗便秘方面的丰富经验而重新对其进行讨论评估。无心脏效应的新型5-HT_4激动剂(例如普鲁卡必利，在美国之外地区可用)似乎对慢性便秘有效。

(a) 替加色罗

替加色罗(tegaserod)是5-HT_4部分激动剂，是5-HT的氨基胍吲哚衍生物，在结构上与西沙必利不同。由于心血管安全性问题，替加色罗于2007年4月撤出市场。既往临床试验中，心血管事件的发生率为13/13 614(0.11%)，而对照组受试者为1/7 031(0.01%)。报告的心血管事件为心肌梗死(n=3)、心源性猝死(n=1)、不稳定型心绞痛(n=6)和卒中(n=3)。FDA撤销该药的决定一直是争议的话题[332]。在一项为期12周的随机双盲、安慰剂对照试验中，1 348例慢性便秘受试者的应答率为：替加色罗2mg/次、每日两次、替加色罗6mg/次、每日2次和安慰剂组分别为41.4%、43.2%和25.1%[333]。替加色罗2mg/次和6mg/次、每日2次的腹泻发生率分别为(4.5%和7.3%)比安慰剂组(3.8%)更常见[333]。替加色罗还用于伴有便秘的IBS女性患者(见第122章)，并已被FDA重新批准用于65岁以下无心血管风险因素的患者[334]。

(b) 普鲁卡必利

普鲁卡必利(prucalopride)是一种完全5-HT_4激动剂，是苯并呋喃衍生物，可加速健康人和慢性便秘患者的结肠转运[335]。已发表了3项设计相似的大型12周随机安慰剂对照3期试验，评估了普鲁卡必利2mg/次或4mg/次、每日1次与安慰剂相比在慢性便秘患者中的疗效和安全性[336-338]。在其中一项研究中，接受普鲁卡必利2mg/次和4mg/次的患者每周达到3次以上CSBM的患者百分比分别为30.9%和28.4%，而接受安慰剂的患者为12.0%(两项比较均P<0.001)。与安慰剂组相比，使用2mg/次和4mg/次普鲁卡必利在第12周时，所有其他次要疗效均显著改善，包括患者对其肠道功能和治疗的满意度以及对其便秘症状严重程度的感觉。对2 639例便秘患者进行的7项随机对照试验的meta分析发现，必须要治疗的人数为6例，对普鲁卡必利有应答的患者百分比为28.3%，而安慰剂组为13.3%[339]。最常见的不良反应是头痛、恶心和腹泻。尽管在接受替加色罗和西沙必利(两者均为部分5-HT_4激动剂)治疗的患者中已报告了心脏副作用，但迄今为止，未观察到普鲁卡必利有心血管副作用，也未报告有任何心电图异常。此外，在一项对疗养院老年便秘患者的研究中，未发现接受普鲁卡必利和安慰剂的患者在生命体征、心电图参数或动态心电图监测结果方面存在差异。大约88%的患者有心血管疾病史[340]。目前，普鲁卡必利已被获准在欧盟、加拿大、美国和其他地区使用。

5. 其他药物(制剂)

秋水仙碱(一种治疗痛风的药物)和米索前列醇(一种前列腺素类似物)已被用于治疗严重慢性便秘患者。在一项随机、安慰剂对照、双盲交叉试验中，与安慰剂相比，秋水仙碱增加了排便频率(基线时为3次/周，而秋水仙碱0.6mg/次，每日3次时为10次/周)。然而，在秋水仙碱给药期间腹痛的发生率高于安慰剂[341]。米索前列醇的数据有限，该药的副作用很常见[342]。特纳帕诺(tenapanor)是FDA于2019年批准的第一种钠-氢交换体3抑制剂，用于治疗伴有便秘IBS，剂量为50mg/次，每日2次。它抑制小肠和结肠的钠吸收，从而增加肠液分泌，加速肠道转运。

(1) 胆碱能药物

胆碱能药物也用于治疗便秘。氯贝胆碱(bethanechol)是一种胆碱能受体激动剂，对三环类抗抑郁药治疗引起的便秘患者似乎有益，但支持氯贝胆碱用于其他原因引起的便秘的数据有限。单次静脉给予胆碱酯酶抑制剂新斯的明对急性结肠假性梗阻患者的结肠减压效果显著[343](见第124章)，但这类药物在正常传输型或慢传输型便秘患者中的对照研究尚未完成。一项新斯的明皮下给药治疗术后肠梗阻、急性结肠假性梗阻或难治性便秘患者的研究表明，难治性便秘患者(n=10)排便的中位时间为39.23小时(四分位距，19.95~57.56)。大多数患者(>75%)需要重复给药，近一半的队列患者在排便前需要5次或5次以上给药[344]。常见副作用如心动过缓、流涎增多、呕吐和腹部痉挛。

口服胆碱能药物(如溴吡斯的明)，在大多数患者以360mg/d或部分患者以180mg/d剂量给药时，显示对糖尿病慢性便秘的患者有加速结肠传输的效果。与安慰剂相比，溴吡斯的明在24小时内可加速全结肠传输[1.96±0.18(基线)，2.45±0.2U(治疗)，P<0.01]，但不加速胃排空或小肠传输。排便频率、粪便硬度和排便通畅程度有所改善。与安慰剂组相比，溴吡斯的明的胆碱能副作用更为常见[345]。

在一项对31例系统性硬化症患者接受溴吡斯的明治疗至少4周的研究中，51.6%的患者便秘得到改善。31例患者中有15例报告了不良反应，最常见的是腹泻。81.3%症状获益的患者和58.1%的患者继续使用溴吡斯的明[346]。

(2) **肉毒毒素**

A 型肉毒梭菌毒素是一种抑制乙酰胆碱突触前释放的强效神经毒素,通过肌内注射到耻骨直肠肌内治疗排便障碍。初步数据表明,肉毒毒素可能对痉挛性盆底功能障碍导致排便出口延迟的患者有效[347],包括同时患有 PD 的患者[162,163](指精神心理障碍疾病)。在一项研究中,24 例患者中有 19 例在 2 个月时症状和盆底功能生理测量值改善[348]。然而,尚未进行对照试验,因此不建议使用该方法替代生物反馈,因为生物反馈疗法的临床经验更多(见后文)。

(3) **未来制剂(未来药物)**

A. 鹅去氧胆酸

鹅去氧胆酸(chenodeoxycholic acid)是一种胆汁酸,既往用于治疗胆结石患者(见第 65 章)。在接受 750~1 000mg/d 治疗的患者中,40% 患者报告有腹泻[349]。一项双盲安慰剂对照研究纳入了 36 例便秘型 IBS 女性患者,随机接受缓释鹅去氧胆酸钠(500 或 1 000mg)或安慰剂治疗 4 天。与安慰剂组相比,2 个鹅去氧胆酸钠组的结肠传输时间、粪便硬度和排便频率均有改善。最常见的副作用是腹部痉挛或疼痛[350]。目前尚未在慢性便秘患者中进行研究。

B. 艾洛比昔巴特

艾洛比昔巴特(elobixibat)是一种新型研究的、吸收极少的回肠胆汁酸转运蛋白的抑制剂,可增加胆汁流入结肠(见第 64 章)。在一项 2 期研究中,190 例慢性便秘患者(使用改良罗马Ⅲ标准定义)随机接受艾洛比昔巴特(5、10 或 15mg)或安慰剂,每日一次治疗,持续 8 周。在接受 5、10 和 15mg 艾洛比昔巴特的患者,在第 1 周的排便频率分别增加了 2.5、4.0 和 5.4 次 SBM(自发性排便次数),而接受安慰剂的患者为 1.7 次 SBM,改善持续了 8 周以上。与安慰剂相比,艾洛比昔巴特还使腹胀和排便费力得到改善。最常报告的不良反应为腹痛和腹泻[351]。

C. 雷拉莫林

雷拉莫林(relamorelin)是生长激素受体 1a 的五肽选择性抑制剂,已知对胃有作用。在 48 例女性慢性便秘患者的随机、双盲临床试验中,雷拉莫林增进结肠传输 32 小时($P=0.040$)和 48 小时($P=0.017$),与安慰剂相比,第一次给药后 SBM 增加,首次排便时间加快。雷拉莫林不影响粪便形状。而最常见的不良影响为增加食欲、疲乏和头痛[352]。

D. 韦卢斯特拉格

韦卢斯特拉格(velusetrag)是一种完全的 5-HT_4 激动剂。在一项为期 4 周的 2 期试验中,401 例慢性便秘患者随机接受韦卢斯特拉格 15、30 或 50mg 或安慰剂,每日一次。接受韦卢斯特拉格的患者 SBM 每周增加 3.6(15mg)、3.3(30mg)和 3.5(50mg),而安慰剂组每周增加为 1.4[353]。韦卢斯特拉格改善的相对风险为 4.86,95% CI 为 2.02~11.71 较宽,表明与普鲁卡必利相比,药物疗效可能较低[309]。

(三) 其他形式的治疗

1. 排便训练

排便训练通常涉及 3~5 次治疗,每次至少持续 30 分钟。在这些课程中,讲授正常的排便过程,消除错误观念。鼓励患者详细叙述其肠道症状,由熟悉排便功能障碍经历的各种问题的同情的倾听者提示。这一过程本身就是治疗性质的,因为它使患者能够讨论可能被视为私密负担的症状。通常会给出关于纤维摄入量的建议。对于排便不频繁的患者,强调要养成有规律的排便习惯和不忽视排便冲动的重要性。对于那些由于用力排便无效而在卫生间花费过多时间的人,建议少去卫生间,多练习有效的排便方法。讲述最佳排便姿势,包括使用西式马桶时将脚抬高到地板以上的好处。每次就诊后,鼓励患者练习所讲授的技术。每次就诊时,鼓励患者减少对泻药、灌肠剂和栓剂的依赖。进步者受到赞扬。

2. 肛门直肠生物反馈

在肛门直肠生物反馈过程中,通常在排便训练后,患者接受有关其肛门括约肌和盆底肌肉功能的视觉和听觉反馈。生物反馈可用于训练患者在用力时放松盆底肌肉,并将这种放松与腹部动作协调,以促进粪便进入直肠。生物反馈可通过肌电图或肛门直肠测压导管进行。通常向患者传授使用球囊或硅胶填充的人造粪便进行模拟排便,以强调成功排便的正常协调[354]。患者教育和治疗师与患者之间的融洽关系也是生物反馈成功的组成部分[355]。患者一般在 6 周内完成 6 次治疗,每天治疗 3 次,连续 10 天。

对截至 1993 年进行的生物反馈研究的系统性综述显示,总体成功率为 67%,但缺乏对照研究[356]。生物反馈对会阴下降综合征患者的疗效可能低于痉挛性盆底疾病患者[137]。在对 38 项生物反馈研究的回顾中,发现心理因素影响对生物反馈的反应[357]。成功的生物反馈训练界定为整体排便满意度的改善,与粪便硬度增加、排便意愿增强、静息肛门压升高和球囊排出时间延长有关;而与年龄、症状持续时间、排便频率、治疗依从性、用力直肠压力或用力时肛门括约肌松弛无关[358]。

最近几项对照试验发现,生物反馈比假反馈或标准治疗[359,360]、地西泮[361]或泻药更有效[362,363]。纤维(20g/d)加灌肠剂或栓剂治疗失败的盆底协同失调患者,被随机分配到每周 5 次生物反馈治疗组($n=54$)或 PEG 治疗组(14.6~29.2g/d)加每周 5 次咨询治疗组($n=55$)。在 6 个月时,80% 接受生物反馈治疗的患者出现了显著的改善,相比之下,接受泻药治疗的患者只有 22%($P<0.001$)。生物反馈治疗的益处在 12 个月和 24 个月时持续存在,并在排便费力、排便不尽感、肛门直肠阻塞感、灌肠剂和栓剂的使用和腹痛方面均有显著减轻(全部 $P<0.01$)。两组排便频率均增加。所有接受生物反馈治疗有显著改善的患者,在 6 个月和 12 个月时均能够松弛盆底并排出一个 50mL 的球囊[362]。在另一项对照试验中,77 例排便协同障碍的患者随机接受生物反馈、虚假治疗和标准治疗 3 个月。接受生物反馈的患者更能显著纠正排便协同障碍,改善排便次数,缩短球囊排出时间,增加每周 CSBM 次数,减少使用手指辅助排便;总体肠功能满意度更高[359]。每组选择 13 例患者参与长期随访试验。1 年后生物反馈组每周 CSBM 次数显著增加(基线时为 1.91,1 年后为 4.85),但标准治疗对照组无显著增加(基线时为 1.66,1 年后为 1.43)。生物反馈组在 3 个月内出现的排便协同障碍、排便次数和球囊排出时间减少的改善,一年后得以维持,结肠传输时间恢复正常[360]。

最初,生物反馈训练是在入院时开始强化训练[364],但随后的经验表明,作为门诊患者的训练也是令人满意的。一项小型对比试验表明,使用或不使用直肠内球囊或家庭训练的结果两者没有差异[365]。当进行训练时,无论有无肌肉活动的视觉显示,结果是相似的。在没有视觉显示的情况下,指导人员向患者提供持续的信息和鼓励,并通过观察患者如何拉紧和通过在直肠球囊上轻微张力感受拉紧的有效性来评估指导的效果。

大多数完成排便训练的患者在长达2年后继续报告症状改善[364,365]。改善的症状包括排便频率、排便费力、腹痛、腹胀和需要泻药[366]。治疗前后的生理学测量表明,训练可使耻骨直肠肌和肛门外括约肌适当松弛[367-369],直肠内压力增加[118],排便用力时直肠肛门角变宽,直肠排空率、结肠转运率及直肠黏膜血流量均增加。

大多数已发表的系列研究,将排便训练和肛门直肠生物反馈限制在排便障碍患者(即盆底肌肉反常收缩)。然而,在一个研究中心,无论结肠传输或盆底功能障碍(包括结肠传输缓慢的患者)的研究结果如何,这种训练似乎有益于绝大部分未经选择的慢性便秘患者[368,370]。在另一个系列中,治疗结果并不取决于是否存在直肠前突、肠套叠或会阴下降[366]。然而,其他研究者已经表明,对排便训练和生物反馈无反应的患者比有反应的患者会阴下降的程度更大[137]。排便训练使一些在子宫切除术后发生便秘的患者和一些孤立性直肠溃疡综合征患者受益[371,372]。

3. 补充和替代医学疗法

许多补充疗法和替代疗法可用来治疗便秘患者[373],但临床研究有限且质量普遍较差(见第131章),无法就其在便秘中的使用作出明确建议。中国生物医学数据库中确定的针灸治疗慢性便秘的系统综述正在进行中[374]。益生菌普及的程度持续增长,但迄今为止进行研究的数据很少。一项前瞻性研究显示,在患有慢性便秘的女性中,动物双歧杆菌和低聚果糖(寡果糖)可改善排便频率和粪便稠度、排便费力和排便疼痛($P<0.010$)[375]。传统中药在治疗便秘中的作用仍不清楚。麻仁丸在一项小型安慰剂对照试验中对便秘显示出一定的疗效[376]。

4. 骶神经刺激

有资料表明,骶神经刺激可能对严重便秘患者有帮助[377]。对62例经使用泻药、栓剂、灌肠剂和生物反馈治疗失败的慢性便秘患者,用临时刺激导线连接到体外脉冲发生器,进行了为期21天的试验。治疗成功界定为以下任何一项改善:①排便频率从每周2次或2次以下增加至每周3次以上;②与费力排便相关的排便发生比例减少50%以上;③与排便不尽感相关的排便发生比例减少50%以上。45例患者符合成功治疗的标准,并植入了永久性神经刺激器。在接受永久性神经刺激器的患者中,87%符合成功治疗的标准。在1~55个月(中位时间为28个月)的随访期间,每周排便次数从2.3次增加至6.6次[378]。虽然前景良好,但尚不清楚获益的幅度和哪些患者最有可能从骶神经刺激中获益[379]。

5. 手术

重度便秘患者手术治疗的目标是增加排便频率和排便的通畅性,可能的额外获益是缓解腹痛和腹胀。手术方式可分为3组:部分或全部结肠切除术、造口构建和改善排便功能的肛门直肠手术[380]。

(1) 结肠切除术

结肠切除术治疗便秘会产生不同的结果。对32项已发表的慢性便秘手术研究的综述发现,患者满意度存在相当大的差异性(39%~100%)[381]。手术后最常见的并发症是小肠梗阻、腹泻和大便失禁,但术后一年腹泻和大便失禁往往会有所改善。

患者选择

术前心理评估至关重要,因为在有心理障碍的患者中,效果不佳是很常见的[382]。因为手术的目的是增加肠运动频率,所以必须通过客观的方法证实结肠慢传输。此外还必须评估排便功能。最后,应通过小肠的放射学研究、胃排空和小肠传输研究(尽可能多地)应尽可能排除全身性肠运动障碍或假性梗阻综合征。

采取这些步骤选择一组同类患者的系列研究显示了最佳结果,尽管需更长的时间随访。在一所研究中心,1 009例有可能接受手术治疗的慢性便秘患者中仅有74例接受了手术。肠道传输测量和盆底功能检测显示,597例患者没有可量化的异常,249例患者有盆底功能障碍,没有结肠缓慢传输。对52例结肠缓慢传输且排便功能正常的患者进行了结肠切除术联合回肠直肠吻合术。同时对22例结肠缓慢传输伴盆底功能障碍的患者在接受训练治疗后也进行了手术。在74例接受手术治疗的患者中,97%的患者对治疗结果满意,90%的患者在平均随访56个月后生活质量良好或有所改善。没有手术死亡病例,但有7例患者随后发生了继发性小肠梗阻[383]。

手术类型

结肠切除术联合盲肠直肠或回肠乙状结肠吻合术的效果劣于结肠次全切除术联合回肠直肠吻合术的效果[384]。偶尔有描述直肠结肠切除术联合回肠肛管吻合术和回肠袋建立的报道,通常在结肠切除术和回肠直肠吻合术失败之后实施[385]。有1例患者,由于直肠容量大于正常,发生回肠直肠吻合失败[386]。腹腔镜结肠次全切除术似乎与常规手术一样有效[387,388]。

(2) 结肠造口术

结肠造口术偶尔用于慢传输型便秘,因为它是可逆的,且结肠切除术的结果尚不确定。大多数患者报告结肠造口术后主观症状得到改善,其作为慢传输型便秘或神经系统疾病的主要手术[381]。然而,许多患者仍需要使用泻药或定期结肠灌洗。

由于便秘持续存在或发生严重腹泻和大便失禁,在结肠切除术和回肠直肠吻合术治疗慢传输型便秘失败后,偶尔会进行回肠造口术。不能从结肠切除术和回肠直肠吻合术中获益的患者,可能是患有全身性肠运动障碍或心理障碍的患者。

创建一种插入可控性导管的阑尾造口术或盲肠造口术,通过该造口术可进行顺行灌肠,有时可使截瘫患者或那些无法或不愿意接受结肠切除术的患者获益。一项对32例接受该手术并中位随访36个月(范围为13~140个月)的患者进行的回顾性研究报告称,约半数患者的长期结果令人满意。经常需要进行修订[389]。这种程序可以减少肠道护理所需的时间和药物,大部分经验是来自儿童[390]。

（3）排便障碍手术

使用吻合器经肛门直肠切除术（stapled transanal rectal resection，STARR）已取得一些成功，尤其是对同时患有直肠膨出和肠套叠的患者[391-393]。耻骨直肠肌或肛门内括约肌离断术对慢传输型便秘患者是难以成功的[394]。直肠膨出矫正术，仅适用于在排粪直肠造影过程中有造影剂滞留证据的患者或通过阴道指压缓解便秘的女性才考虑[134]。

（胡伟玲 译，袁农　刘军 校）

参考文献

第 20 章　胃肠道出血

Thomas J. Savides，Dennis M. Jensen 著

章节目录

一、急性胃肠道出血的初始评估和管理 …… 263
（一）病史 …… 263
（二）体格检查 …… 263
（三）实验室检查 …… 264
（四）临床确定出血部位 …… 264
（五）住院治疗 …… 264
（六）复苏 …… 265
（七）初始药物治疗 …… 265
（八）内镜检查 …… 265
（九）内镜下止血 …… 268
（十）影像学检查 …… 268
（十一）外科手术 …… 269
二、上胃肠道出血 …… 269
（一）流行病学 …… 269
（二）风险因素与风险分层 …… 269
（三）上胃肠道内镜技术 …… 269
（四）消化性溃疡 …… 270
（五）其他非静脉曲张原因 …… 279
三、下胃肠道出血 …… 283
（一）风险因素和风险分层 …… 284
（二）死亡率 …… 284
（三）诊断和治疗方法 …… 284
（四）病因和管理 …… 286
四、不明原因显性胃肠道出血 …… 289
（一）病因 …… 290
（二）诊断性检查 …… 292
五、隐性胃肠道出血和缺铁性贫血 …… 294
（一）粪便潜血试验 …… 294
（二）缺铁性贫血 …… 295

美国，各种类型胃肠道出血的年住院率估计为 350 次住院/10 万人，每年超过 100 万次住院[1]。大约 50% 因胃肠道出血入院的患者是由于上胃肠道出血（来自食管、胃和十二指肠），40% 是由于下胃肠道出血（来自结肠和肛门直肠），10% 是不明原因出血（来自小肠）。

重度胃肠道出血定义为记录的胃肠道出血（呕血、黑便、便血或鼻胃管灌洗液阳性）伴有休克或直立性低血压、血细胞比容值降低至少 6%（或血红蛋白水平降低至少 2g/dL），或至少输血 2 个单位的浓缩红细胞（RBC）。大多数严重胃肠道出血患者入院接受复苏和治疗。明显出血意味着胃肠道有明显的失血迹象。呕血定义为呕吐血液，提示鼻咽、食管、胃或十二指肠出血。呕血包括呕吐鲜红色血液，提示近期或持续出血，呕吐暗红色物质（咖啡样呕吐物）提示出血在前段时间已经停止。黑便是指黑色柏油样便，是由肠道细菌将血液降解为血红素或其他血色素所致。黑便可表示出血来源于上胃肠道、小肠或近端结肠，一般在 50~100mL 或更多的血液进入胃肠道时发生（通常是上胃肠道），出血事件发生后数小时便有特征性粪便排出[2,3]。便血是指从直肠流出鲜红色血液，常提示结肠或肛门直肠出血或活动性上胃肠道或小肠出血。隐匿性胃肠道出血是指无症状的亚急性出血。不明原因胃肠道出血是在食管胃十二指肠内镜（EGD）（上胃肠道内镜检查）、结肠镜和可能的推进式小肠镜检查常规内镜评价后，不明显的部位出血。严重急性上胃肠道出血的初步管理流程如图 20.1 所示。

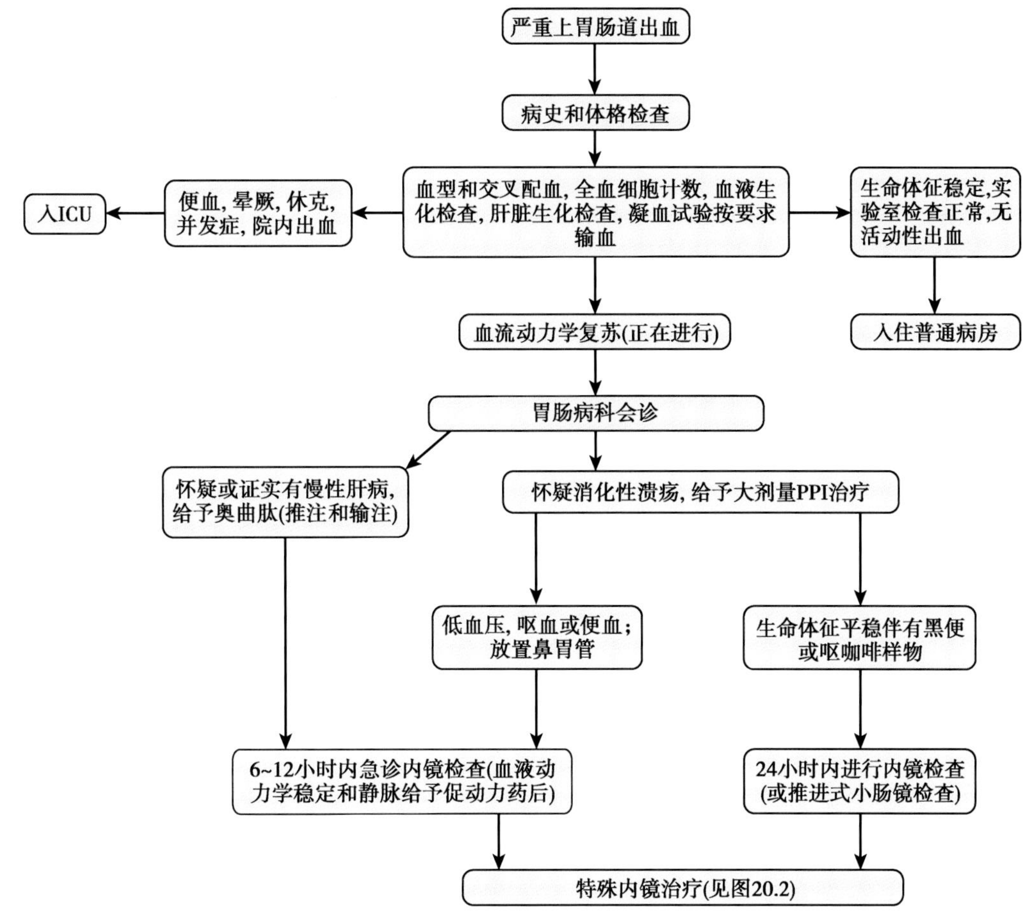

图 20.1　严重上胃肠道出血的初始处理流程。根据临床情况，一些步骤可同时进行或以不同的顺序在急诊科实施。ICU，重症监护室；PPI，质子泵抑制剂

一、急性胃肠道出血的初始评估和管理

（一）病史

急性胃肠道出血患者的初步评估包括病史采集，获取生命体征，进行体格检查（包括直肠检查）和鼻胃管灌洗。应询问患者有关风险因素，如可能引起溃疡或出血的药物、既往胃肠道手术病史和有助于确定出血部位诊断的病史性特征（表 20.1）。

（二）体格检查

在初步评估时，体格检查应侧重于患者的生命体征，注意低血压、心动过速、体位性等血容量不足的体征。应检查腹部有无手术瘢痕、压痛和肿块。慢性肝病的体征包括蜘蛛痣、肝掌、男性乳腺发育、腹水、脾大、脐周静脉曲张海蛇头样表现和掌腱膜挛缩。应检查皮肤、嘴唇和颊黏膜是否存在提示遗传性出血性毛细血管扩张症（HHT）或 Osler-Weber-Rendu 病的毛细血管扩张。指甲下毛细血管扩张和手指皮肤的特征性变化可能提示硬皮病（系统性硬化症），这与胃窦血管扩张（GAVE）或上胃肠道毛细血管扩张相关。色素口唇病变可能提示 Peutz-Jeghers 综合征。紫癜性皮肤病变可能提示过敏性紫癜。黑棘皮病可能提示潜在的恶性肿瘤，尤其是胃癌。应观察患者粪便，以识别黑便或褐红色粪便，然而，患者和医生对粪便颜色的主观描述差异很大[4]。

表 20.1　根据患者病史提示的疑似胃肠道出血的来源

疑似出血来源	病史
鼻咽部	鼻咽放射史
	既往鼻咽恶性肿瘤
	复发性鼻出血
肺部	咯血
食管溃疡	GERD
	胃灼热
	大量饮酒
	咽痛
	药物摄入
	创伤性鼻胃管放置术
食管癌	吞咽困难
	Barrett 食管病史
	体重下降
食管黏膜撕裂症	酗酒
	呕吐
Cameron 病变	大裂孔疝
食管或胃底静脉曲张或门静脉高压性胃病	肝硬化
	病态肥胖
胃血管发育不良	主动脉瓣狭窄
	慢性肾病
	系统性硬化
消化性溃疡	幽门螺杆菌感染

表 20.1 根据患者病史提示的疑似胃肠道出血的来源(续)

疑似出血来源	病史
	上腹部不适 经常服用阿司匹林或其他非甾体抗炎药 消化性溃疡病史
胃癌	早饱 体重下降
原发性主动脉肠瘘	既往严重急性不明原因出血和腹主动脉瘤未经手术治疗
继发性主动脉肠瘘	人工血管移植修复腹主动脉瘤的术前
Vater 壶腹	近期内镜下括约肌切开术
胆道	近期肝活检、胆管造影或 TIPS
胰管	胰腺炎 假性囊肿 近期胰腺造影
小肠恶性肿瘤	遗传性非息肉病性结直肠癌 腹腔内转移癌病史 间歇小肠梗阻 反复出现的不明原因胃肠道出血 体重下降
Meckel 憩室	40 岁以下不明原因胃肠道出血
小肠或结肠溃疡	炎症性肠病 阿司匹林或其他非甾体抗炎药的使用
小肠毛细血管扩张	经常鼻出血 HHT(Osler-Weber-Rendu 综合征)
小肠血管发育不良	年龄>60 岁 慢性胃肠道出血 缺铁性贫血
结肠憩室病	无腹痛的便血 憩室病史
结肠肿瘤	排便习惯的改变 慢性出血 结肠肿瘤个人或家族史 体重下降
缺血性结肠炎	心血管疾病 便血伴或不伴腹痛
溃疡性结肠炎	血性腹泻 IBD 家族史 溃疡性结肠炎病史
克罗恩病	慢性腹部不适 IBD 家族史 克罗恩病史
肛裂	便血伴肛门疼痛 严重便秘
痔疮	大便滴血 正常排便的便血
息肉切除术后出血	近期结肠镜检查伴息肉切除术 抗凝剂或抗血小板药物的使用
结肠或小肠血管扩张	年龄>70 岁 心血管疾病 慢性下胃肠道出血/缺铁性贫血 不同程度反复出血
吻合口溃疡	肠外科吻合术
放射性肠炎或直肠炎	腹部放射治疗史

GERD,胃食管反流病;IBD,炎症性肠病;TIPS,经颈静脉肝内门体分流术。

放置经鼻或口胃管,抽吸和目测视觉特征胃内容物,可用于确定是否存在大量血液、咖啡样物或非血性液体,对于有黑便而无呕血的患者特别有用。然而,鼻胃管抽吸物的隐血检测是无用的,因为插鼻胃管的创伤可能引起极少量的出血,使其隐血实验出现假阳性结果。观察到的咖啡样或新鲜血性呕吐物的患者,不需要放置鼻胃管进行诊断,但可能需要放置鼻胃管来帮助清除胃内积血,以便更好地实现内镜可视化,并将误吸风险降至最低。

(三) 实验室检查

急性胃肠道出血患者的血液应进行标准血液学、血生化、肝功能、凝血功能检查,并进行血型和交叉匹配。出血发生后,即刻的血细胞比容或血红蛋白值可能无法准确反映失血量,因为血管间隙需要 24~72 小时以上才能与血管外液体平衡,并且静脉输注生理盐水会导致血液稀释[5]。平均红细胞体积(mean corpuscular volume,MCV)低于 80fL 提示存在慢性胃肠道失血和铁缺乏,可通过发现血清铁降低,高总铁结合力(total iron-binding capacity,TIBC)和低铁蛋白水平来证实。MCV 较低和粪便潜血试验(fecal occult blood test,FOBT)阴性结果增加了腹腔出血疾病的可能性。MCV 升高(>100fL)提示慢性肝病或叶酸或维生素 B_{12} 缺乏。超过一半的上胃肠道出血患者可能发生白细胞计数升高,并且与更严重的出血相关[6]。血小板计数低有助于出血严重程度,并提示慢性肝病或血液系统疾病。在上胃肠道出血患者中,由于血液中蛋白被肠道细菌分解后,肠道对尿素的吸收增加,血尿素氮水平的升高程度通常大于血清肌酐水平[7]。凝血酶原时间(prothrombin time,PT)和国际标准化比值(INR)评估患者是否存在外源性凝血途径的损伤。在慢性肝病或使用华法林时数值可能升高。

(四) 临床确定出血部位

表现为呕血、咖啡样呕吐物或鼻胃管灌洗伴大量血液回流或咖啡样呕吐物,表明是上胃肠道来源的出血。容易清除的少量咖啡样物质或粉红色液体,可能代表鼻胃管的黏膜损伤,而不是活动性上胃肠道出血。清净的(非血性)鼻胃管抽吸物并不一定表明更远端胃肠道来源出血,因为在活动性上胃肠道出血患者中,至少有 16% 的患者是清净的鼻胃管抽吸物[8]。鼻胃管抽吸物中存在胆汁提示不太可能是急性上胃肠道出血,但可见于间歇性出血的上胃肠道来源。

黑便通常提示出血来自上胃肠道,但也可见小肠或近端结肠出血。便血意味着结肠或肛门直肠出血,除非患者存在低血压,否则可能提示重度、快速的上胃肠道出血伴血液快速通过胃肠道所致[4,9]。褐红色粪便可见于活动性出血的上胃肠道或小肠或近端结肠来源。

(五) 住院治疗

重度胃肠道出血患者需要住院治疗,而仅表现为轻度急性出血(自限性便血或罕见黑便)和血流动力学稳定(不怀疑血容量不足)的患者血液检查结果正常,如果症状复发,可以返回医院,可能是半紧急门诊内镜检查的候选者,而不是直接入住医院[10,11]。如果患者鼻胃管或经直肠有大量红色血液,生命体征不稳定,或有可能加重其他基础疾病的严重急性失血,应在重症监护室(ICU)住院。发生急性胃肠道出血,但血流动力学稳定的患者,视其临床情况,可入住监护床(观察病房)或标准病床。在急诊科对疑似上胃肠道出血的患者进行紧急内镜检查,有助于确定最佳的医院安置[12,13]。

(六) 复苏

复苏工作应在急诊科进行评估病情的同时开始,并在患者住院期间持续进行。至少应静脉置入 1 根大口径(14 号或 16 号规格)输液导管,有持续性出血的患者应置入 2 根。根据需要尽快输注生理盐水,以保持患者的收缩压高于 100mmHg 和脉搏低于 100 次/min。患者应根据需要输注浓缩红细胞,血小板和新鲜冷冻血浆,以保持血红蛋白水平大于 70g/dL、血小板计数高于 50 000/mm^3 和 PT 超过 15 秒。在巴塞罗那的一项大型研究中,重度上胃肠道出血患者随机接受血红蛋白水平低于 7g/dL 或低于 9g/dL 的输血[14]。前者("限制性")输血策略与消化性溃疡出血患者和 Child-Pugh 分级 A 级或 B 级的肝硬化患者的生存率较高和再出血率较低相关,但与 Child-Pugh 分级 C 级肝硬化患者的生存率较低和再出血率较高相关(见 92 章)。关于输血时机的决策,需根据患者的临床状况、合并症以及失血的速度进行个体化处理。

应尽快咨询内镜医师,以加快对患者的评估并确定内镜检查的最佳时机。在具有肝移植资质的医院,如果已知患者有肝硬化且是潜在的移植候选者,也应通知肝移植服务机构(见第 97 章)。

应根据住院情况,密切监测患者的生命体征。应每 4~8 小时检测血细胞比容和血红蛋白值(而不是手指针刺检测的血细胞比容值,其可靠性较低),直至血细胞比容和血红蛋白值稳定。在活动性出血患者中,应留置导尿管以监测患者的尿量。

活动性持续呕血或精神状态改变的患者,应考虑气管插管,以预防吸入性肺炎。年龄超过 60 岁、有胸痛或有心脏病史病的患者,应通过心电图和系列肌钙蛋白测定评估是否合并心肌梗死。还应考虑胸部 X 线检查。

(七) 初始药物治疗

消化性溃疡(PUD)患者使用质子泵抑制剂(PPI)有助于降低再出血率(见后文)。在对严重上胃肠道出血的患者进行内镜检查之前,在急诊科或 ICU 开始 PPI 治疗已成为一种常规,但仍存在争议[15]。几项临床研究和 meta 分析显示,在内镜检查前高剂量输注 PPI,可加速溃疡近期出血(stigmata of recent hemorrhage,SRH)的内镜下病灶消退(见后文),并减少内镜治疗的需求,但不会改善临床总的结局[16-19]。对高度怀疑门静脉高压和食管胃底静脉曲张出血的患者,应开始静脉给予奥曲肽(先静脉推注后输注)(见后文及第 92 章),可将再出血率的风险降低至类似于内镜治疗相似的速率(图 20.2;也见图 20.1)[20,21]。

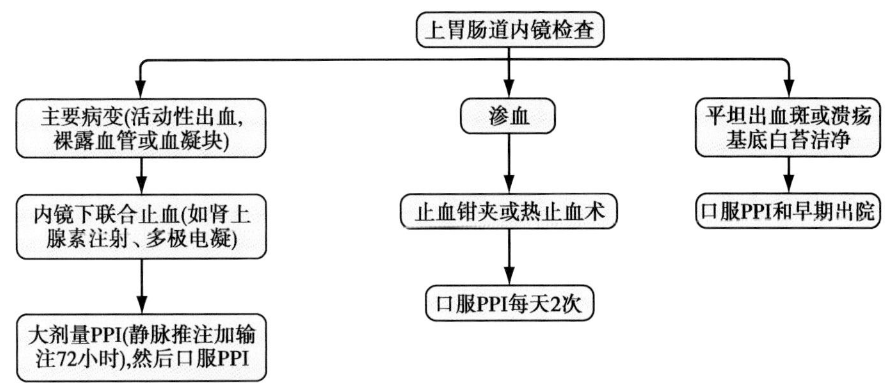

图 20.2 血流动力学稳定后重度消化性溃疡出血的内镜和药物治疗流程。PPI,质子泵抑制剂

(八) 内镜检查

胃肠道内镜检查可确定出血部位,可对大多数胃肠道出血患者进行止血治疗[22]。关于严重上胃肠道出血患者的内镜检查时机存在争议。共识意见是,对于严重共病患者(如美国麻醉医师协会体能状况分类 3~4 级)(见第 42 章),进行 EGD 的最佳时期(与死亡率最低相关)是在患者血流动力学恢复后,但在就诊后 12~20 个小时内。在此时段之前或之后进行紧急内镜检查均会导致较高的死亡率。对于合并症较轻的血流动力学稳定的患者(美国麻醉医师学会体能状况分类 1~2 级),在 24 小时内进行 EGD 的死亡率较低。内镜检查应仅在安全的情况下进行,从操作过程中获得的临床信息将会影响患者的治疗。理想情况下,患者的血流动力学应稳定,心率低于 100 次/min,收缩压高于 100mmHg。如果呼吸功能不全,精神状态改变或持续的呕血表明在紧急 EGD 前需要进行气管插管以稳定患者并保护气道。适当的医疗复苏不仅可以实现更安全的内镜检查,还可确保对容积依赖性病变(如静脉曲张)进行更好的诊断检查,并且由于凝血功能障碍的纠正,可以实现更有效的止血(图 20.3 和图 20.4;也见图 20.1 和图 20.2)。

活动性出血患者(即高容量血性鼻胃灌洗或持续便血),在药物复苏后不久接受紧急内镜检查。一般而言,急诊内镜检查最好在患者到达 ICU 病床后进行,而不是在急诊科进行,因为资源(人员、药物和空间)在 ICU 更易获得。疑似肝硬化或主动脉肠道瘘或在医院期间再出血的患者,一旦血流动力学恢复,应尽快接受紧急内镜检查。通常在入院后 6 小时内

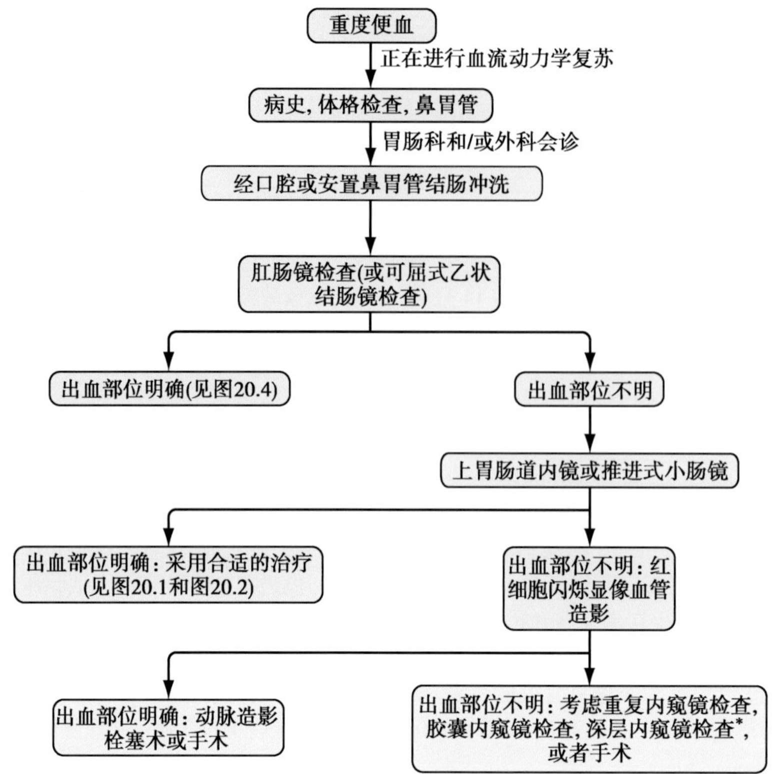

图 20.3 严重便血的处理流程。* 小肠镜检查包括双气囊肠镜检查、单气囊肠镜检查和螺旋肠镜检查

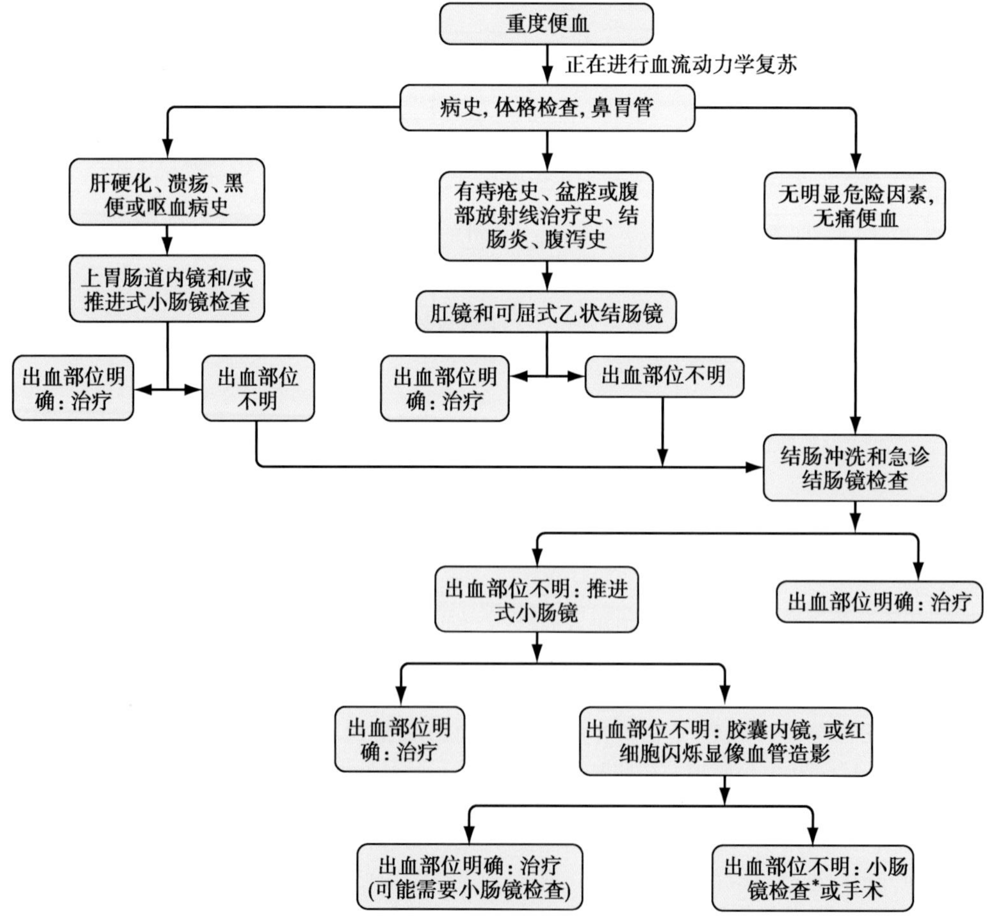

图 20.4 根据患者病史改良的严重便血的管理流程。* 小肠镜检查包括双气囊肠镜检查、单气囊肠镜检查和螺旋肠镜检查

或再出血时，血流动力学稳定且无持续出血证据的患者可接受紧急内镜检查(24 小时内)，通常在胃肠内镜检查室而不是在 ICU。除最严重出血或高风险的患者外，应该避免进行夜间内镜检查，因为经过良好培训的内镜检查护士、最佳内镜设备和血管造影备有设备可能在夜间不可用。在罕见的大出血和难治性低血压患者中，可以在手术室进行内镜检查，必要时可立即进行手术治疗。

在患有重度上胃肠道出血的患者中，使用大号(34Fr)口胃管灌洗可能有助于排空胃中的血液和血凝块，以防止误吸，并保证充分的内镜可视化(另见第 42 章)。特殊的灌洗系统有助于快速清除血液。胃促动力药物静脉给药(如红霉素或甲氧氯普胺)在 EGD 检查前 30~90 分钟用药，以诱导胃收缩并将血液从胃排空入小肠，有助于内镜可视化，减少重复内镜检查的需求，但不会减少输血需求、住院时间或手术需求[23-25]。应使用大直径单通道或双通道治疗性内镜，以便在内镜检查过程中快速清除胃肠道中的新鲜血液。此外，水泵可经辅助通道冲洗病变，并稀释胃腔内血液便于抽吸，从而促进可视化。用冰盐水灌洗对治疗上胃肠道出血没有临床价值，反而可能会损害凝血并导致体温过低。使用温自来水进行胃灌洗与使用无菌生理盐水灌洗一样安全，并且成本更低。放置在内镜头端上的透明塑料帽，可以帮助清晰观察黏膜褶皱后面的出血部位，通过调整内镜入路的角度来释放内镜夹(见后文)，避免在角落处出现黏膜"变白"，并清除血凝块[26]。

在严重便血和怀疑有活动性结肠出血的患者中，可在快速清除后可进行紧急结肠镜检查(见第 42 章、图 20.3 和图 20.4)[27,28]。患者应在 4~6 小时内口服或通过鼻胃管接受 6~8L 聚乙二醇(polyethylene glycol,PEG)冲洗，直至直肠流出液中没有粪便、血液和血凝块。一些患者可能需要额外的 PEG 清除，尤其是活动性出血、严重便秘或在医院发生便血的患者。可在清洗前静脉内给予 10mg 甲氧氯普胺，每 4~6 小时重复一次，可促进胃排空，减少恶心。有重度或持续活动性便血的患者中，应在 12~14 小时内进行紧急结肠镜检查，但必须在彻底清洁结肠后进行。轻度或中度自限性便血患者，应在入院 24 小时内进行结肠清洗后接受结肠镜检查。对于预先无法确定出血来源的褐红色粪便的患者，也应考虑紧急使用聚乙二醇制剂肠道准备。如果推进式肠镜检查不能提供诊断，在患者仍处于镇静状态的情况下，推进式肠镜检查后立即进行结肠镜检查(见后文)，将加快患者的治疗(图 20.5)。

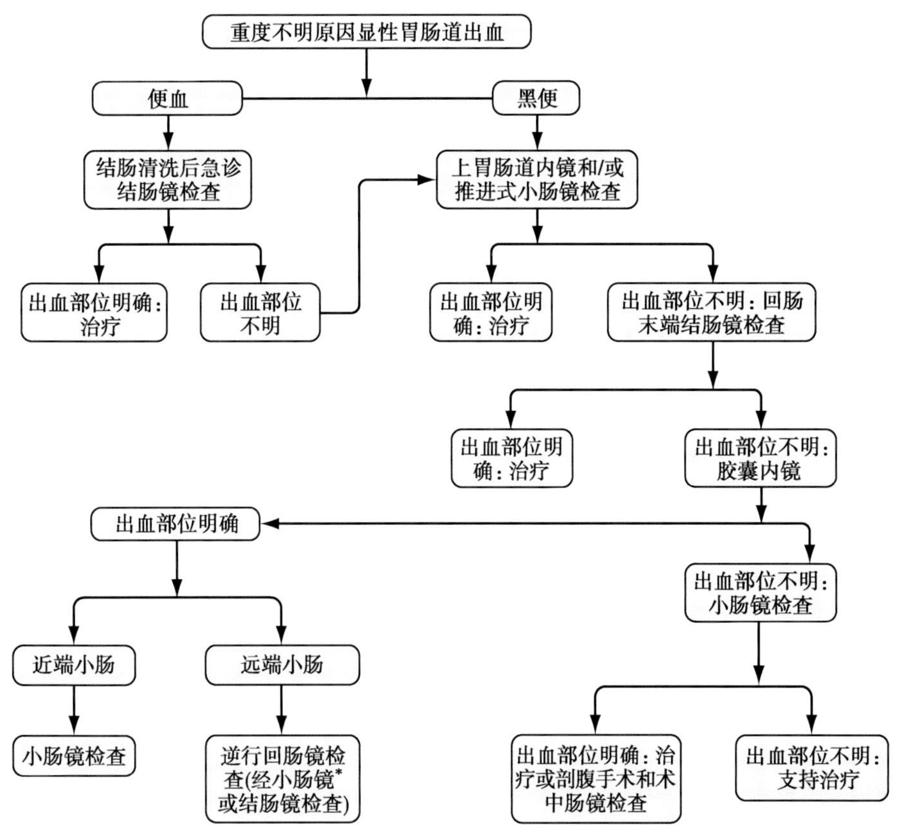

图 20.5 重度不明原因显性胃肠道出血的处理流程。* 小肠镜包括双气囊肠镜检查、单气囊肠镜检查和螺旋肠镜检查

无线视频胶囊式内镜[或胶囊内镜检查(见后文)]可用于推进式小肠镜检查和结肠镜检查正常，且怀疑小肠出血来源的明显胃肠道出血患者[29]。胶囊式内镜的优点是可直接清晰观察小肠，以识别潜在出血来源或活动性出血。缺点是该程序需要 8 小时才能完成，并且需要额外的时间来下载和审查图像，不能进行止血治疗，并且由于接受过培训的人员在休息时间放置胶囊的可用性有限，在住院患者中可能难以进行。如果胶囊式内镜检查中发现局灶性出血部位，则可为后续内镜检查，例如单气囊或双气囊肠镜检查或逆行回肠镜检查，提供最终明确的诊断和治疗。

急诊内镜检查及内镜下止血可能有1%的并发症，这取决于内镜检查和治疗的类型[30,31]。最常见的并发症包括吸入性肺炎、诱发出血、药物不良反应、低血压、低氧血症和胃肠道穿孔（见第42章）。

（九）内镜下止血

自20世纪70年代以来，热接触探头一直是内镜止血治疗的主要方法。这些探针的直径为7Fr和10Fr，长度可以适合全内镜、肠镜或结肠镜。接触探头可以物理性压塞血管以阻断血流，然后应用热能凝闭下层血管（凝血）。最常用的探头是多极电凝（multipolar electrocoagulation，MPEC）探头，也称为双极电凝探头，探头尖端交织电极之间的电流流动产生热量。在动物研究中，已经证实在对出血部位施加中等压力、中等时间（8~10秒）、应用低功率设置（12~16W）、可以获得最佳凝血效果[32]。加热探头可提供预定能量焦耳，不随组织电阻而变化，可以有效凝固直径不超过2mm的动脉，该直径远大于在切除的出血性人消化性溃疡中发现的大多数二级或三级动脉分支（通常为1mm）[33,34]。使用热探头的主要风险是过度应用凝固或压力导致的穿孔，特别是在急性或非纤维化病变中。热探针也可引起凝血损伤，使病变更大、更深，并可能在凝血功能障碍患者中诱发迟发性出血。氩等离子体凝固是一种非接触式热疗法（见后文）。

注射治疗最常使用硬化治疗针和黏膜下注射肾上腺素，将稀释至浓度为1∶10 000或1∶20 000的肾上腺素注入出血部位或有出血征象部位或其周围（见后文）。与热探头技术相比，该技术的优势在于其广泛的可用性、相对较低的成本和在凝血功能障碍的患者中使用的安全性，以及较低的穿孔风险（无热烧伤损伤）。然而，对于明确的出血来说，肾上腺素注射不如热凝固、放置止血管夹［血管夹（见后文）］或联合治疗有效[35,36]。注射治疗也可以使用硬化剂，如乙醇胺或酒精，但这些药物与组织损伤增加和其他风险相关。

自1974年以来，内镜止血夹（或称止血夹）开始应用，并在技术改进后逐渐普及[37]。血管夹对出血部位施加机械压力。第一代止血夹不能止住直径大于1mm的血管出血[38]，但后期的止血夹更大、更强，并具有抓取和释放机制，可改善内镜处理和止血。止血夹特别适用于营养不良或凝血功能障碍的患者[39]，但根据出血部位的位置、基础病变的纤维化程度和内镜进入的限制，也使其难以开展。与标准溃疡止血技术相比，新型、大号、经内窥镜止血夹可抓取更多组织，更好地固定在纤维化溃疡上，因此能够更好地控制严重溃疡出血[40]。

套扎治疗时，将黏膜（包括或不包括黏膜下层）组织吸入置于内镜末端的透明帽中，橡皮环从透明帽上释放脱落至病灶基底部并压迫之。该技术广泛应用于治疗食管静脉曲张（见第92章），偶尔也可用于其他出血性疾病。操作相对容易，但必须将足够充分的黏膜吸入到透明帽内，套扎治疗才能成功。由于制造商的不同，一些套扎器械只能安装在诊断性内镜上，因此操作时必须从较大的治疗性内镜切换到较小的诊断性内镜。

止血喷雾剂是一种具有凝血功能的无机粉剂，可以产生机械屏障，黏附和覆盖在出血部位[41-44]。该技术可用于暂时控制消化性溃疡、肿瘤和弥漫性出血病灶的出血。但是，对于严重的非静脉曲张性出血［如溃疡或Dieulafoy病变（见下文）］或静脉曲张（食管或胃）的患者，通常需要通过重复内镜检查进行后续确定性止血，血管造影或外科手术。

（十）影像学检查

血管造影可以用来诊断和治疗重度出血，尤其是上、下胃肠道内镜无法确定病因时。血管造影通常仅在动脉出血率至少达到0.5mL/min时诊断外渗进入肠腔[45]。肠系膜血管造影术的灵敏度为30%~50%（活动性胃肠道出血的灵敏度高于复发性急性或慢性隐匿性出血），特异性为100%[46]。血管造影允许治疗性动脉内输注加压素或经导管栓塞止血，如发现活动性出血，不需要肠道清洁。血管造影主要并发症的发生率为3%，包括血肿形成、股动脉血栓形成、造影剂反应、急性肾损伤、肠缺血和短暂性脑缺血发作[47]。而且，血管造影通常不能确定出血的具体原因，只能确定其出血部位。

放射性核素成像偶尔对不明原因胃肠道出血的患者有帮助，但由于内镜的广泛使用和缺少用于紧急情况的核医学服务，特别是在晚间和周末，目前使用频率低于过去。放射性核素成像可以相对快速地进行，可有助于定位出血的一般区域，从而指导后续的内镜检查、血管造影和手术。这项技术包括将放射性标记物质静脉注射到患者血液中，然后通过连续闪烁显像检测放射性标记物质的局灶性聚集区域。据报道，放射性核素成像检测出血的速率为0.04mL/min[48]。红细胞通常用高锝酸盐标记，因为它们可在血液循环中保留24小时，因此在活动性或间歇性胃肠道出血患者中，可以进行重复扫描[49]。

标记红细胞扫描诊断便血的总体发生率较低（<30%），高达25%的扫描表明出血部位是不正确的[50-52]。活动性出血与血流动力学不稳定时的真实阳性扫描率高于出血不严重时的真实阳性扫描率[53]。假阳性结果最常见的原因是管腔内血液的快速转运，因此在结肠中检测到标记的血液，即使起源于更近端的胃肠道出血。因此建议谨慎使用延迟扫描的结果来定位和确定手术切除病灶[54]。

高锝酸盐闪烁显像可以识别Meckel憩室中的异位胃黏膜。对于未明确胃肠道出血的儿童或青年人，应考虑该诊断。据报道，所谓Meckel憩室扫描的阳性预测值、阴性预测值和总体准确性在年轻患者中高于90%[55,56]。然而，在25岁以上的患者中，Meckol憩室扫描的敏感性要低的得多（小于50%）[57]。

在既往接受过腹主动脉瘤修复术和植入物的患者中，CT静脉造影可识别移植物与十二指肠之间的炎症，并提示植入物瘘管形成进入十二指肠[58]。在选定的患者中，腹部CT还可以确定占位病变，如腹腔内肿瘤或可能提示出血原因的小肠异常。随着CT和MRI技术的进步使CT和MRI小肠造影和血管造影获得了可喜的结果[59,60]。

(十一) 外科手术

在未通过紧急内镜或结肠镜检查做出诊断的选定重度、持续性胃肠道出血患者中,建议进行外科会诊。大出血、且血流动力学不稳定的患者应接受紧急血管造影或紧急手术探查[既往未进行内镜检查或手术室进行紧急内镜检查(见后文)]。内镜检查治疗或血管造影无法控制的出血患者或重度复发性不明原因胃肠道出血患者,也可能从术中肠镜检查手术中获益(见后文)。

二、上胃肠道出血

(一) 流行病学

在重度上胃肠道出血的潜在病因中,消化性溃疡是最常见的,约占 40%[61,62](表 20.2)。尽管药物治疗、ICU 护理、内镜检查和外科手术方面取得了进展,但自 20 世纪 70 年代以来,严重的上胃肠道出血的死亡率并没有改变,仍在 5%~10%之间[1,61-65]。部分原因是老年胃肠道出血患者死于重度合并症而非出血的比例增加,以及肝硬化和静脉曲张出血患者数量的增加。

表 20.2 UCLA CURE 数据库中重度上胃肠道出血的原因(N=968)

病因	发生率/%
消化性溃疡	35.2
食管或胃静脉曲张	21.9
门静脉高压相关病变*	4.6
食管炎	4.6
血管扩张+	4.0
食管黏膜撕裂症	4.0
Dieulafoy 病	3.2
胃肠道肿瘤	3.1
鼻出血	2.2
糜烂	1.2
其他	8.8
不明原因	7.3

*食管或胃静脉曲张除外;+血管扩张和毛细血管扩张。
CURE,溃疡研究和教育中心;UCLA,加州大学洛杉矶分校。

80%的上胃肠道出血患者的出血是自限性的,即使没有特殊治疗[63,66]。在剩余的 20%继续出血或再出血的患者中,死亡率为 30%~40%[8]。持续性出血或再出血风险高的患者,可能从急诊救治、内镜、血管造影或外科手术治疗中获益最大。

(二) 风险因素与风险分层

已经开发了风险因素和风险分层评分工具,以尝试识别死亡率和再出血风险最高的非静脉曲张性上胃肠道出血患者,并将患者分流到更高水平的医院诊治或进行更紧急的内镜检查。非静脉曲张出血的内镜检查前的评分系统包括 Blatchford 评分、临床 Rockall 评分、人工神经网络评分和 AIMS65 评分。Blatchford 评分采用内镜检查前变量,包括血压、血尿素氮水平、血红蛋白水平、心率、晕厥、黑便、肝病和心力衰竭,以评估患者需要临床干预以控制出血的风险(如输血、内镜治疗,手术)[67]。临床 Rockall 评分是基于患者的年龄、休克和共存疾病来进行评估[68]。人工神经网络仪器使用 21 个临床变量来帮助预测内镜检查时 SRH 的存在(见后文)和内镜治疗的需求[69]。AIMS65 是 5 个内镜检查前变量的总评分(血清白蛋白<3.0g/dL、INR>1.5、精神状态改变、收缩压≤90mmHg 和年龄>65 岁);AIMS65 评分小于 2 分与死亡率、住院时间和住院费用低于 2 分或以上相关[70]。

最常用的内镜检查后评分系统是完整 Rockall 评分(表 20.3)[68]。完整 Rockall 评分包括临床 Rockall 评分(内镜检查前变量-患者年龄、休克和共存疾病)和内镜检查结果,包括内镜 SRH(见后文)。内镜治疗后的 Rockall 评分与死亡率密切相关,但与再出血风险无关[71-73]。Rockall 风险分层方案也可用于识别临床预后较差的低风险患者(即 Rockall 评分为 0~2),这些患者可考虑提前出院[74]。

预测内镜检查后上胃肠道出血结局的其他评分系统,包括 Baylor 评分系统和 Cedars-Sinai 出血指数[75-78]。一般来说,所有这些评分系统在确定死亡率方面都优于评估再出血[79]。

(三) 上胃肠道内镜技术

治疗性内镜有助于抽吸胃腔内血液和使用大型配件。应使用脚踏泵将水经过单独的分离管道喷射冲洗靶目标获得清晰视野。在内镜检查前,应对患者进行血流动力学医药复苏(见前文),如果活动性出血严重,应考虑预防性气管插管,以尽量减少呼吸道吸入的风险。

内镜插入后,首先要寻找的是胃肠道腔内的血液。快速检查所有非血性黏膜通常最好记录这些区域没有任何病变。然后,应清除任何可抽吸的血性液体。可通过水冲洗稀释血液来帮助抽吸血液。清除血液和血凝块的其他选择是使用带有非常大(6mm)抽吸通道的内镜或使用治疗性内镜上的附件,通过抽吸口直接抽吸。如果无法通过抽吸清除大的血凝块,可以将患者翻转向背部或右侧,前提是对患者进行气管插管以防止误吸。抬高床头也有助于将血凝块从胃底向远端移动。应跟踪任何可见的黏附新鲜血液或血凝块,以查找其来源。如果胃内存在过多的血液而无法检测到出血性病灶时,应考虑再次给予(或初始剂量)促动力药(如红霉素、甲氧氯普胺),使用大口径胃管重复灌洗,或者如果患者病情稳定,应在接下来的 24 小时内重复内镜检查。如果怀疑十二指肠出血,但前视内镜未发现时,应使用侧视十二指肠镜检查十二指肠壁和壶腹部。

表 20.3　上胃肠道出血的 Rockall 评分系统

变量	评分			
	0	1	2	3
年龄	<60 岁	60~79 岁	≥80 岁	—
心率	<100 次/min	≥100 次/min	—	—
收缩压	正常	≥100mmHg	<100mmHg	—
伴随疾病	无	—	缺血性心脏病，心力衰竭，其他重要伴随疾病	肾衰竭、肝衰竭癌肿播散
诊断	食管黏膜撕裂症或未观察到病变	所有其他良性诊断	恶性病变	—
内镜下新近出血性病灶	无或仅见溃疡基底黑斑	—	上胃肠道出血、黏附血凝块、裸露血管、活动性出血	—

总分	频率/%	再出血发生率/%	死亡率/%
0	4.9	4.9	0
1	9.5	3.4	0
2	11.4	5.3	0.2
3	15	11.2	2.9
4	17.9	14.1	5.3
5	15.3	24.1	10.8
6	10.6	32.9	17.3
7	9	43.8	27
≥8	6.4	41.8	41.1

Modified from Rockall TA、Logan RF、Devlin HB、Northfield TC. Selection of patients for early discharge or outpatient care after acute upper gastrointestinal Haemorrhage. National Audit of Acute Upper Gastrointestinal Haemorrhage. Lancet 1996;347:1138-40.

（四）消化性溃疡

过去消化性溃疡主要是指胃溃疡或十二指肠溃疡，占上胃肠道出血的 50% 以上，在美国每年约有 100 000 例住院[80,81]。一些数据表明，1993 年至 2002 年间消化性溃疡出血的发生率下降，而非甾体抗炎药（NSAID）引起的溃疡比例增加[82]。然而，其他数据发现 1990 年至 2000 年间出血性溃疡的总发生率没有变化，但服用 NSAID 的老年患者亚组比率增加（图 20.6）[83]。与消化性溃疡出血相关的死亡率为 5%~10%[61,62]。在美国，消化性溃疡出血的住院费用估计每年超过 20 亿美元（见第 53 章）[84]。消化性溃疡出血患者的临床和内镜因素与发病率和死亡率增加相关，见框 20.1。

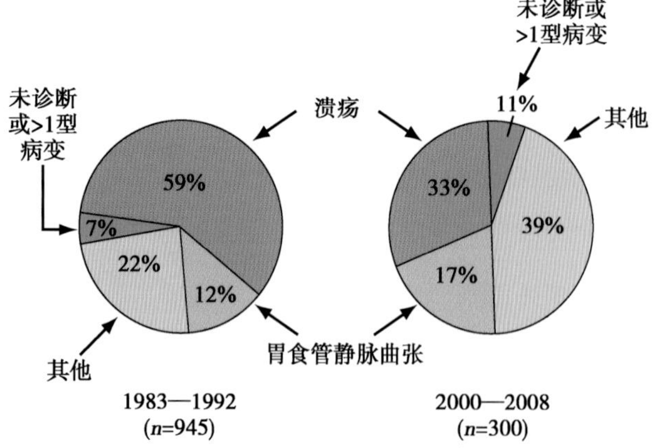

图 20.6　在 UCLA CURE 就诊的患者中，2 个时间段内重度上胃肠道出血的主要原因发生频率（两个时间段之间的所有差异均具有统计学显著性；$P<0.05$）。请注意，在最近的时期内，重度上胃肠道出血的病例总数和消化性溃疡引起的病例百分比均下降。CURE，溃疡研究和教育中心；UCLA，加州大学洛杉矶分校

框 20.1　消化性溃疡出血预后不良的预测因素
年龄>60 岁
院内出血
严重共病
休克或直立性低血压
鼻胃管存在新鲜血液
凝血功能障碍
需要多次输血
高位小弯侧胃溃疡（胃左动脉旁）
十二指肠球部后溃疡（邻近胃十二指肠动脉）
内镜发现动脉出血或裸露血管
内镜治疗后残端动脉血流

1. 发病机制

消化性溃疡最常由阿司匹林或其他 NSAID、Hp 感染或两者导致的黏膜防御机制降低引起的（见第 52 章和第 53 章）[85,86]。在一项针对重症消化性溃疡出血患者的大型多中心研究中，57% 的胃溃疡出血患者（$n=2\ 057$）服用阿司匹林或另一种 NSAID，45% 感染 Hp，而 53% 的十二指肠溃疡出血患者（$n=033$）服用过阿司匹林或另一种 NSAID 或两者兼

有，且 50% 感染 Hp[87]。在本研究的消化性溃疡出血的患者中，10% 无明显溃疡原因(Hp 阴性、未使用阿司匹林或其他 NSAID、无癌症、无胃泌素瘤)。

在许多发展中国家，Hp 感染率超过人口的 80%，而在发达国家为 20%～50%[88]。Hp 相关胃炎最常累及胃窦，使患者易罹患十二指肠溃疡，而以胃体为主的胃炎与胃溃疡有关。Hp 感染引起的消化性溃疡的终生风险范围为美国的 3% 至日本的 25%(见第 52 章)。

NSAID 是美国使用最广泛的药物，11% 的成年人群每天使用 NSAID[89]。许多是在药店柜台上购买的，并无医生的处方[87]。NSAID(包括阿司匹林)主要通过抑制环氧合酶(COX)介导的前列腺素合成引起溃疡，从而损害黏膜保护功能，而不是通过引起直接局部损伤[86]。在定期服用 NSAID 的患者中，15%～45% 在内镜检查时发现胃十二指肠溃疡[90,91]。在服用 NSAID 的患者中，胃溃疡的发生率约为十二指肠溃疡的 4 倍[92]。然而，在一项对上胃肠道出血和 NSAID 相关溃疡患者的大型研究中，胃和十二指肠溃疡的发生频率相同(见第 53 章)[87]。

2. 组织病理学

Swain 及其同事的一项具有里程碑意义的研究中，对 27 例内镜下裸露血管的手术切除出血性胃溃疡的病理学检查，在 96% 标本中显示了潜在的动脉[33]。大约 50% 的血管突出于溃疡表面上方，而另外 50% 的血管有连续的黏附血凝块，动脉壁有破口。出血动脉的平均直径 0.7mm，范围为 0.1～1.18mm。

3. 内镜风险分层

在英国、亚洲和其他一些国家，Forrest 分类用于对消化性溃疡出血内镜评估期间的结果分类包括：活动性喷射性出血(Forrest ⅠA)、活动性渗血(Forrest ⅠB)、黑色突起或裸露血管(nonbleeding visible vessel，NBVV)(Forrest ⅡA)、黏附血凝块(Forrest ⅡB)、平坦黑色出血斑(Forrest ⅡC)和基底洁净溃疡(Forrest Ⅲ)[93]。在美国和其他国家使用描述性术语略有不同。对 SRH 依据 Forrest 分级进行分类，专家之间总体观察的共识意见一致性为中等程度，而对 NBVV 的一致性较差[94,95]。

溃疡内镜下 SRH 见图 20.7，再出血相关风险的每个征象如图 20.8 所示。未经治疗的再出血高危患者是活动性动脉出血(90%)、裸露血管(50%)或黏附血凝块(33%)[96,97]。这些患者受益于内镜下止血(见后文)。内镜下确定的半透明(珍珠色或发白)NBVV 比深色突起(血凝块)具有更高的再出血风险，因为半透明突起可能代表动脉壁[98,99]。非静脉曲张性上胃肠道出血患者持续或复发出血预测因子的多变量数据分析见表 20.4。严重 SRH(喷血，NBVV 或黏附血凝块)患者从内镜下止血中获益最大，而基底洁净溃疡的患者则没有。有渗出性出血或平坦黑色出血斑且无其他病灶(如血凝块或 NBVV)的患者可能从内镜止血中获益，但不能从输注高剂量 PPI 中获益(见后文)。

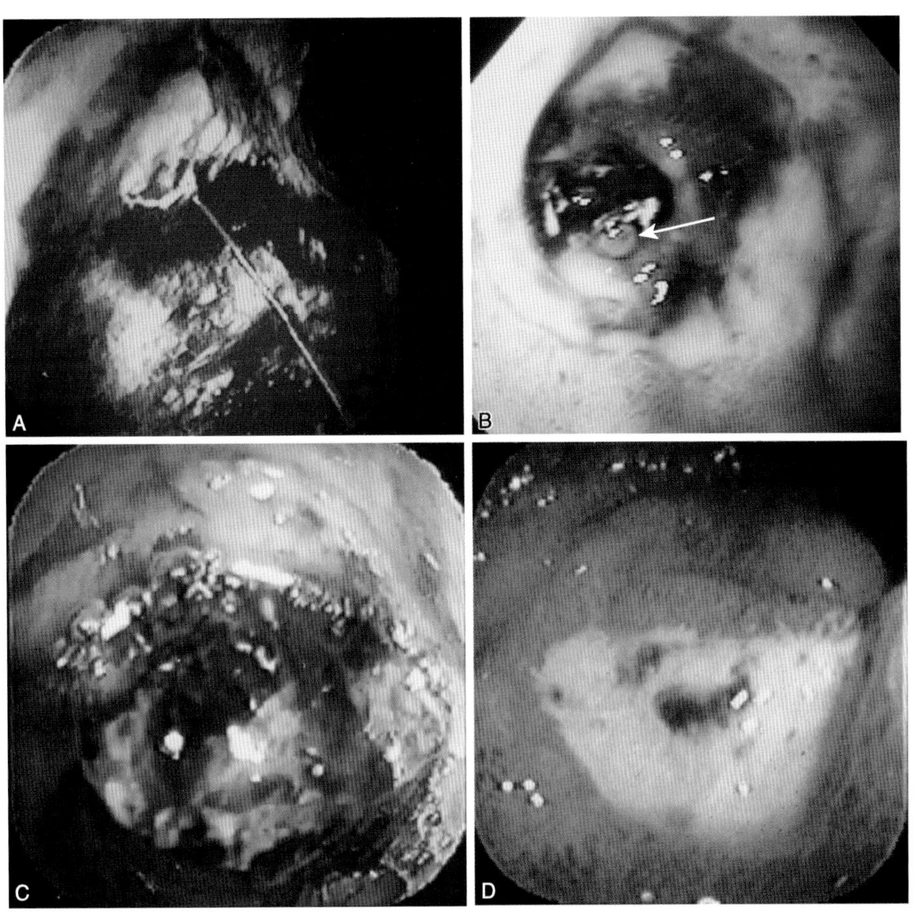

图 20.7 近期消化性溃疡出血的内镜下特征。A，活动性喷射性出血。B，有邻近血凝块的裸露血管(箭)。C，黏附血凝块。D，溃疡中央冲洗后有轻微渗血，无血块及裸露血管

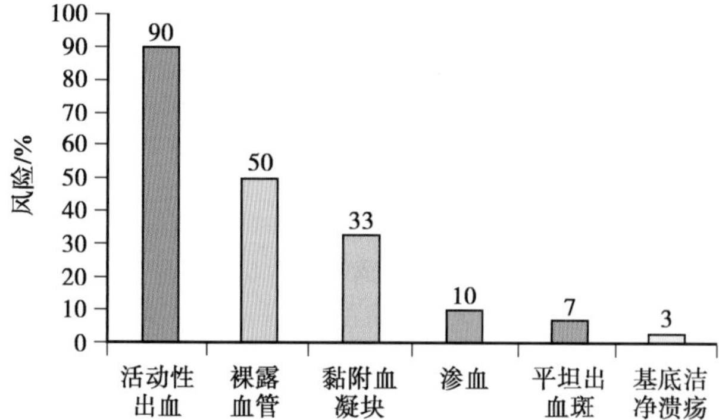

图 20.8　在加州大学洛杉矶分校 CURE 研究中，溃疡患者在未接受内镜治疗或 PPI 给药的情况下的再出血率。CURE，溃疡研究和教育中心；UCLA，加州大学洛杉矶分校

表 20.4　持续性或复发性胃肠道出血的独立危险因素

危险因素	风险增加的范围
临床因素	
健康状态（ASA 1 级 vs 2~5 级）	1.94~7.63
伴随疾病	1.6~7.63
休克（收缩压<100mmHg）	1.2~3.65
精神状态不稳定	3.21
持续出血	3.14
年龄≥70 岁	2.23
年龄>65 岁	1.3
输血需求	N/A
出血表现	
呕血	1.2~5.7
直肠检查见红色鲜血	3.76
黑便	1.6
实验室因素	
初始血红蛋白≤10g/dL	0.8~2.99
凝血功能障碍	1.96
内镜因素	
十二指肠前壁溃疡	13.9
十二指肠后壁溃疡	9.2
活动性出血	2.5~6.48
高风险出血征象	1.91~4.81
溃疡大小≥2cm	2.29~3.54
小弯侧溃疡	2.79
胃或十二指肠溃疡	2.7
溃疡覆盖血凝块	1.72~1.9

ASA，美国麻醉医师学会；N/A，不适用。

Data from Barkun A, Bardou M, Marshall JK. Consensus recommendations for managing patients with nonvariceal upper gastrointestinal bleeding. Ann Intern Med 2003;139:843-57.

首次出血发作后 72 小时，消化性溃疡再出血的风险显著降低。该结论是基于仅通过内镜治疗活动性出血的研究，观察到所有其他病灶，所有患者均接受静脉注射 H_2RA 并停用阿司匹林和其他 NSAID[98-102]。对未经治疗的 NBVV 的自然史研究发现，这些病变可在 4 天内消退，黏附的血凝块倾向于在 2 天内消退[103]。

多普勒内镜探头

便携式多普勒内镜探头（Doppler endoscopic probes，DEP）可通过内镜的工作通道，应用于溃疡检查，以确定溃疡基底部病灶下是否存在血流（图 20.9）[104,105]。DEP 已被用于将 SRH 患者风险分层为：再出血高风险（活动性动脉出血（Forrest ⅠA）、NBVV（Forrest ⅡA）和黏附血凝块（Forrest ⅠB）]；中等风险[渗出性出血（Forrest ⅠA）和平坦黑色出血斑（Forrest ⅡC）]；低风险[基底洁净溃疡（Forrest Ⅲ）][106,107]。血流信号的存在与内镜治疗前后再出血的风险相关。多普勒探头也被用来反映病变下方的动脉血流方向，对再出血的风险进行分层，并确认完成非静脉曲张止血和基础动脉血流闭塞。然而，关于使用 DEP 是否可改善急性消化性溃疡出血患者内镜下止血的结局，之前报告了相互矛盾的结果[108,109]。一项决策性分析研究发现，在急性消化性溃疡出血患者中，与单独

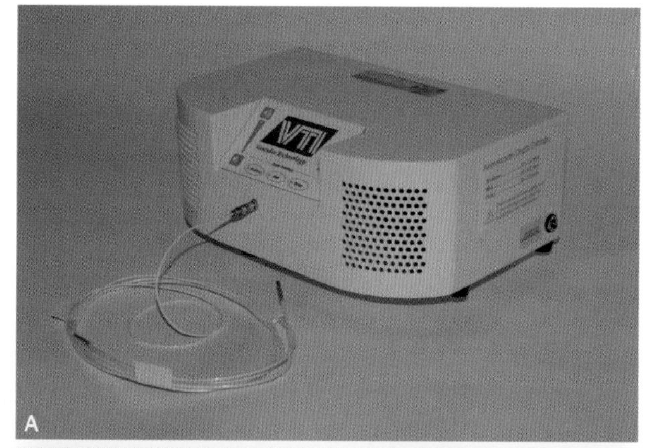

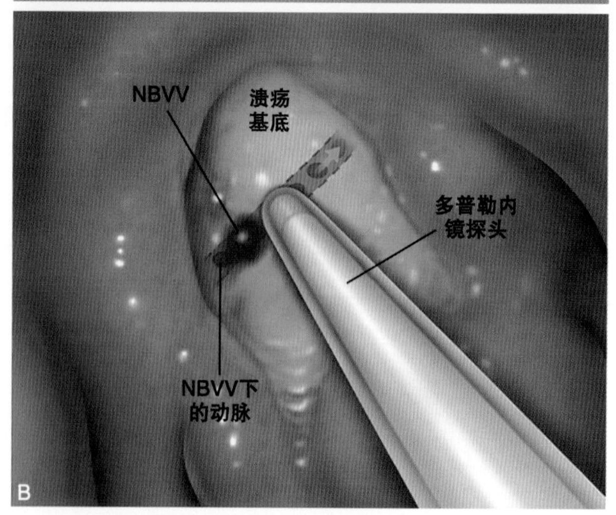

图 20.9　A，多普勒内镜探头和控制单元。B，在内镜治疗前后，通过多普勒内镜探头检测出血病灶下方的动脉血流和动脉血流的标测方向，有助于进行风险分层、内镜止血和降低再出血率（如果动脉血流闭塞）。NBVV，裸露血管

的传统内镜治疗相比，DEP 是首选的成本最小化策略[110]，加州大学洛杉矶分校（University of California，Los Angeles，UCLA）溃疡研究和教育中心（Center for Ulcer Research and Education，CURE）止血小组，在一项随机对照试验中报告，与随机分配至标准目视引导止血组相比，随机分配至 DEP 组的再出血率显著降低，且治疗安全有效[111]。内镜止血后再出血率与残余动脉血流高度相关。在另一项研究中，UCLA CURE 小组用 DEP 治疗的重度非静脉曲张性上胃肠道出血患者与匹配的既往对照进行了比较，DEP 治疗的患者再出血率和手术率也显著降低，而标准视觉引导内镜治疗的患者，则没有显著降低（见图 20.7A）[112]。

4. 内镜下止血

（1）活动性出血和裸露血管

许多实施良好的随机对照研究、meta 分析和共识建议得出结论是，使用肾上腺素注射或热探头疗法进行内镜下止血，可显著降低溃疡再出血、急诊手术率以及活动性动脉出血和 NBVV 等高风险病灶患者的死亡率[22,113-116]。不同内镜下消化性溃疡的再出血率如图 20.8 所示。这些再出血率是基于在广泛使用大剂量 PPI 输注之前进行的研究，主要使用注射治疗、MPEC 治疗、或注射和热探头联合治疗。一般而言，对于持续出血或再出血风险最高的病变，包括活动性出血（持续出血风险为 90%）或 NBVV（持续出血风险为 50%），单独内镜止血可将再出血率降低至约 15%～30%（表 20.5）。如下一节所述，大剂量 PPI 的辅助静脉用药（如泮托拉唑，80mg 推注和 8mg/h，持续 72 小时），进一步降低了再出血率。泮托拉唑、兰索拉唑和埃索奥美拉唑的静脉制剂在美国可用。

表 20.5　近期溃疡出血与再出血风险的内镜下征象

内镜下出血征象（Forrest 分级）	发生率/%	再出血风险/%	内镜止血后再出血的风险*/%
活动性动脉出血（ⅠA）	12	90	15～30
裸露血管（ⅡA）	22	50	15～30
黏附血凝块（ⅡB）	10	33	0～5
活动性渗血（ⅠB）	14	10～14†	0～5
平坦黑色出血斑（ⅡC）	10	10～25†	0
基底洁净溃疡（Ⅲ）	32	3	N/A

*出血风险的降低无须使用 PPI。
†风险取决于在内镜止血前是否检测到动脉血流[111,112]。
N/A，不适用。

全球最常用的溃疡出血治疗方法是肾上腺素注射治疗，它应用广泛，操作简便，安全、价廉。高剂量（13～20mL）肾上腺素单药注射治疗比低剂量（5～10mL）更有效[117]。注射肾上腺素可以导致循环血中肾上腺素水平升高 5 倍，但很少认为可导致具有临床意义的心血管事件[118]。大量研究和 meta 分析显示，联合热探针止血或机械止血方式可进一步降低再出血率，手术率和死亡率[35,119,120]。一些研究表明，在热探头治疗的基础上加用肾上腺素注射的唯一益处是对活动性出血患者，对 NBVV 没有益处[121,122]。

尚未对内镜止血夹以及注射治疗和热探头技术进行研究，但比单独注射肾上腺素更有效，并且与热探头疗法相比显示出协同的结果[123-126]。在一项溃疡出血结局的 meta 分析中，应用止血夹的效果优于单独注射肾上腺素，但与热凝治疗疗效相当[36]。

（2）黏附血凝块

黏附血凝块通常定义为溃疡上的血凝块，对几分钟剧烈的目标喷射水冲洗具有抵抗性。单独药物治疗的溃疡伴黏附血凝块的再出血率为 8%～35%，大多数大型研究报告再出血率为 30%～35%[127-130]。随机对照研究表明，内镜下治疗黏附血凝块，可将再出血率降低至 5% 以下（见表 20.5）。在 DEP 研究中（见前文），约有 69% 的溃疡患者报告了黏附血凝块具有潜在的动脉血流。表明如果不进行内镜治疗，其再出血的风险增加[106,111]。一项 meta 分析发现，内镜治疗在预防有黏附血凝块的消化性溃疡复发性出血方面优于药物治疗，但在手术需要、住院时间、输血次数或死亡率方面无差异[131]。这些研究是在内镜治疗前广泛使用 PPI 之前进行的，也可降低再出血率（见前文）。

（3）基底洁净溃疡

目标冲洗后内镜检查时有基底洁净溃疡的患者，其再出血率低于 5%。Laine 及其同事发现，这类患者立即恢复进食，与上胃肠道出血后恢复进食前等待天数的患者的结局没有差异[132]。Longstreth 和 Feitelberg 表明，经筛选的临床上轻度上胃肠道出血和基底洁净溃疡的低风险患者可以安全地出院回家，大大节省了医疗成本[10,11]。

5. 内镜下止血

内镜下止血目的是控制活动性出血和预防再出血。自 20 世纪 80 年代以来，标准方法一直以治疗 SRH 为基础。然而，一些研究者对于 DEP 提出了另一个治疗目标，即消除潜在的动脉血流，从而显著降低溃疡和其他非静脉曲张性上胃肠道病变的再出血率[106,107,111,112]。

（1）活动性动脉出血

在 UCLA CURE 用于活动性喷射性溃疡出血（Forrest ⅠA）的标准视觉引导技术，是通过硬化疗法针将 0.5～1mL 等份的肾上腺素（1∶20 000）注射到出血部位 1～2mm 内的溃疡 4 个象限中（表 20.6）。当进行联合治疗时，用大的 10Fr 多极探头进行凝固。注射肾上腺素后，将热探头直接放在出血部位以填塞并止血，在低（12～15W）功率设置下，以长（10 秒）脉冲和牢固的压力进行凝固（图 20.10）。然后从溃疡处缓慢取出探头（有时轻轻冲洗以防止牵拉凝固的组织），并根据需要重复热凝固以止血并使下面的任何潜在肉眼裸露血管变平。如果出血持续，可重复注射肾上腺素。内镜下成功止血后，再出血率可在单药治疗时降至 30%，联合治疗时可降至 15%（见表 20.5）。或者，注射肾上腺素后直接在活动性出血部位放置血管夹也可能是有效的。一些研究者建议在注射肾上腺素之前放置止血夹，以便将夹子直接放置在血管上，而不是放置在肾上腺素注射后肿胀的黏膜上。DEP 诱导的最初目标是跟踪动脉的血流方向。CURE 止血组首先探寻到溃疡基底部，以确定下方动脉的走行方向和位置，注射肾上腺素以减少动脉血流，然后在出血点顶部凝固止血或放置止血夹止血，并沿动脉两侧封闭，防止再出血（见图 20.7B）。DEP 引导和潜在动脉血流闭塞进一步降低了再出血率[106,107]。

表 20.6　使用多极电凝术治疗出血性病变的内镜技术参数

	消化性溃疡			食管黏膜撕裂症	Dieulafoy病	胃血管扩张	结肠憩室可见血管	结肠血管扩张
	活动性出血	裸露血管	黏附血凝块					
肾上腺素注射	是*	否	是†	可能	是	否	可能‡	否
探头大小§	大	大	大	大或小	大	大	大或小	大或小
压力//	坚固	坚固	坚固	适度	坚固	轻	轻	轻
功率设定¶/W	12~15	12~15	12~15	10~15	10~15	10~15	10~15	10~15
脉冲持续时间/s	8~10	8~10	8~10	4	8~10	2	2	2
终点	出血停止	血管扁平	扁平出血斑	出血停止	血管扁平	黏膜变白色	血管扁平	黏膜变白色

*应使用肾上腺素（1∶20 000）以 1mL 等分试样注射到 4 个象限中的每个象限，以最初控制出血，随后进行凝血。

†肾上腺素（1∶20 000）以 1mL 等分注射到 4 个象限中的每个象限，最初应在血凝块周围注射，然后分块圈套切除血凝块并治疗潜在的血管柱头。

‡伴有活动性出血的结肠憩室可通过在颈部或底部注射肾上腺素（1∶20 000）进行治疗。如果在颈部观察到裸露血管，可采用多极电凝进行治疗。

§大探头为 10Fr（直径 3.2mm），适合 3.8mm 内镜通道。小探头为 7Fr（2.4mm），适合通过 2.8mm 内镜通道。

//压力是直接通过接触探头施加在病变表面或切线上的填塞压力。

¶使用 BICAP Ⅱ发生器进行功率设置。功率设置是通用指南，可能因使用的发生器而异。

UCLA CURE 的这些指南来自实验性和随机内镜研究。对于较小、急性或较深的出血病灶，必须降低功率、压力和缩短持续时间设置。

CURE，溃疡研究和教育中心；UCLA，加州大学洛杉矶分校。

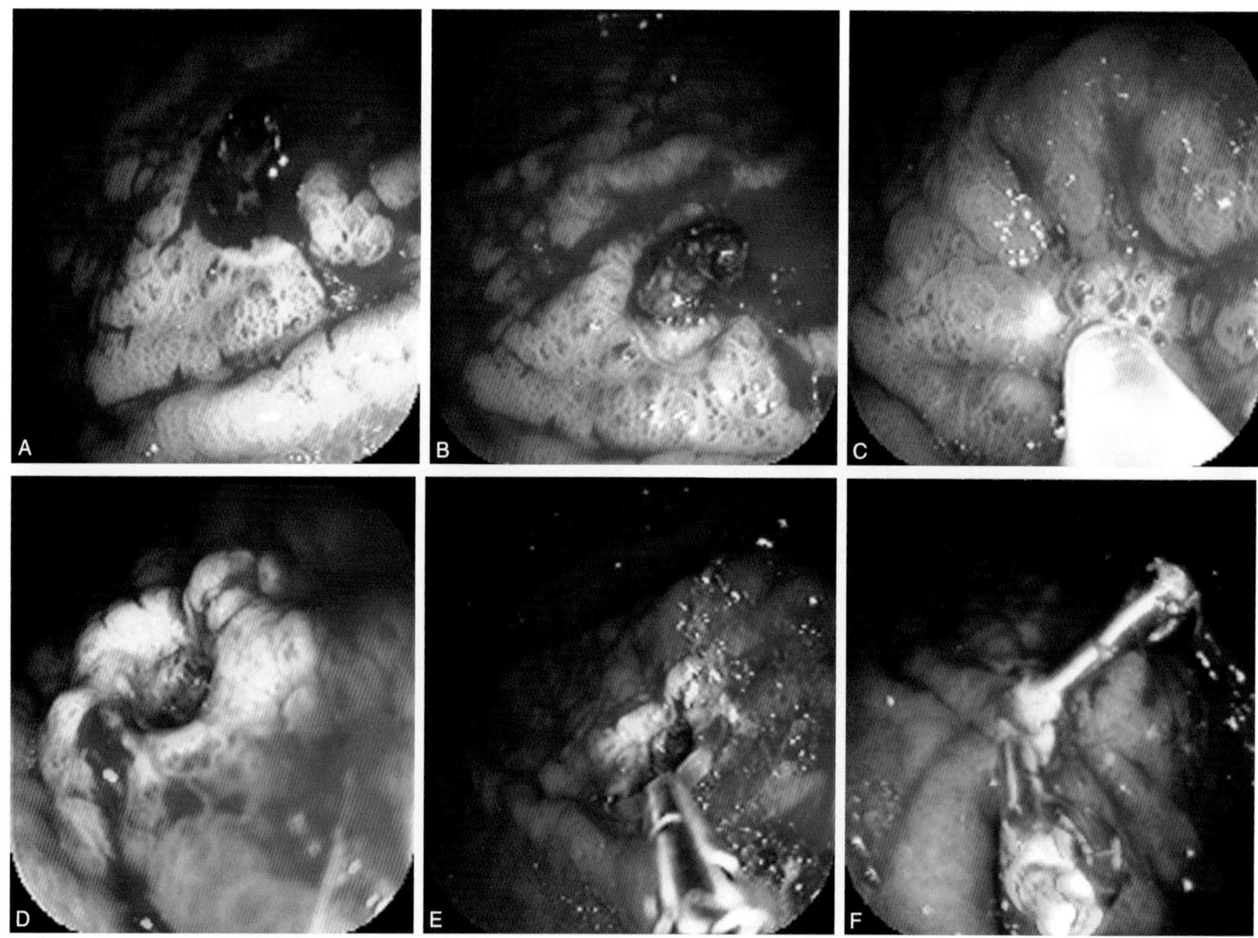

图 20.10　联合使用肾上腺素注射、多极电凝和放置止血夹治疗活动性出血性胃溃疡。A，可见血凝块伴渗血。B，注射肾上腺素后，渗血已消退，溃疡边缘可见于凝血块下方。C，用探头进行多极电凝。D，电凝后溃疡外观；在火山口边缘 7 点钟位置观察到一些渗血。E，使用单个止血夹，出血已完全停止。F，使用了第二个止血夹

(2) **非出血性裸露血管**

与活动性动脉出血相比，使用 NBVV（Forrest ⅡA），单独热凝与热凝和肾上腺素联合注射治疗的结果无显著差异。我们使用与用于停止活动性出血相同的技术，使用大探头、牢固的压力和低功率设置，使内镜下裸露血管变平（图 20.11）。如果将止血夹跨过 NBVV 放置，并静脉给予高剂量 PPI 72 小时，则止血夹也可有效预防 NBVV 再出血（图 20.12）[87,133]。内镜下成功进行止血后，单独注射的再出血率可降至 30%，热凝固、止血夹或联合治疗的再出血率可降至 10% 至 15%（见表 20.5）。

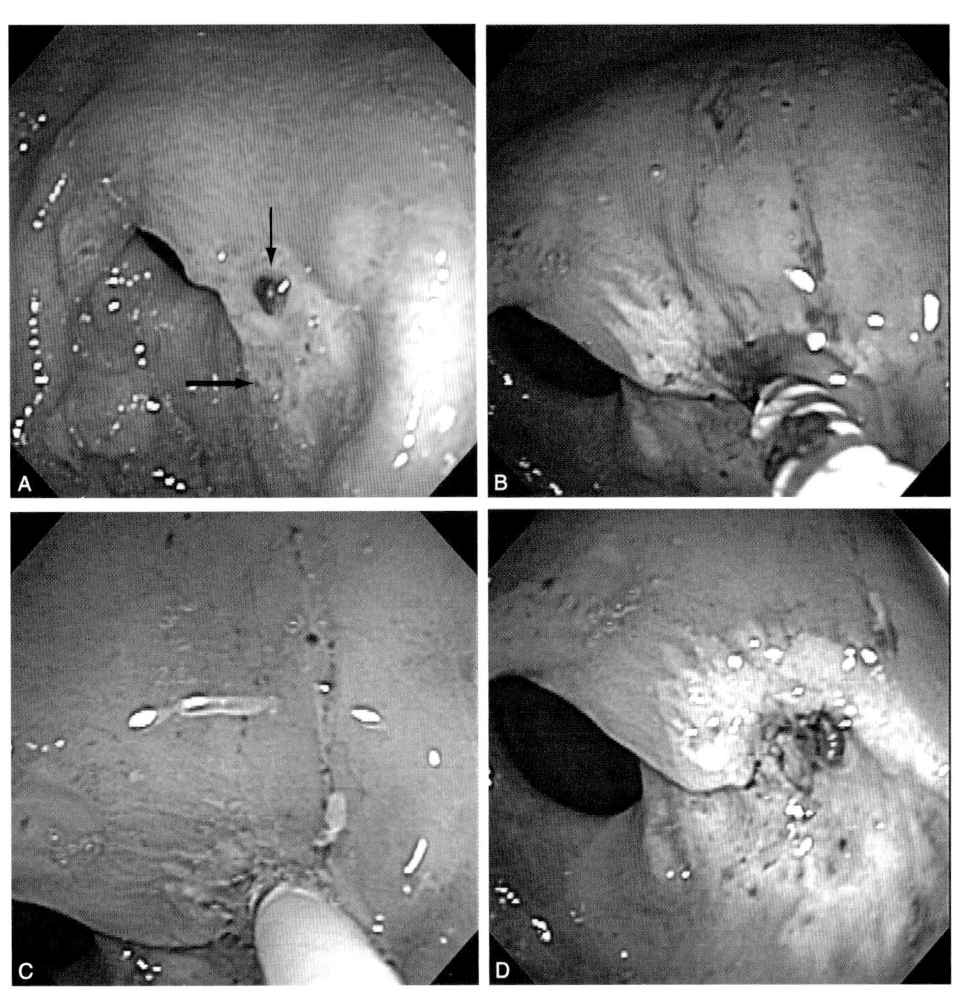

图 20.11　A，肾上腺素注射和多极电凝止血，用于无出血裸露血管（细箭）的慢性胃溃疡（粗箭）。B，对无出血的裸露血管注射肾上腺素之后，周围黏膜发白、肿胀（注意，表 20.6 中不建议对不出血的裸露血管注射肾上腺素）。C，应用多极电凝探头，施加压力和电凝牢固。D，治疗完成后，裸露血管已凝固变平

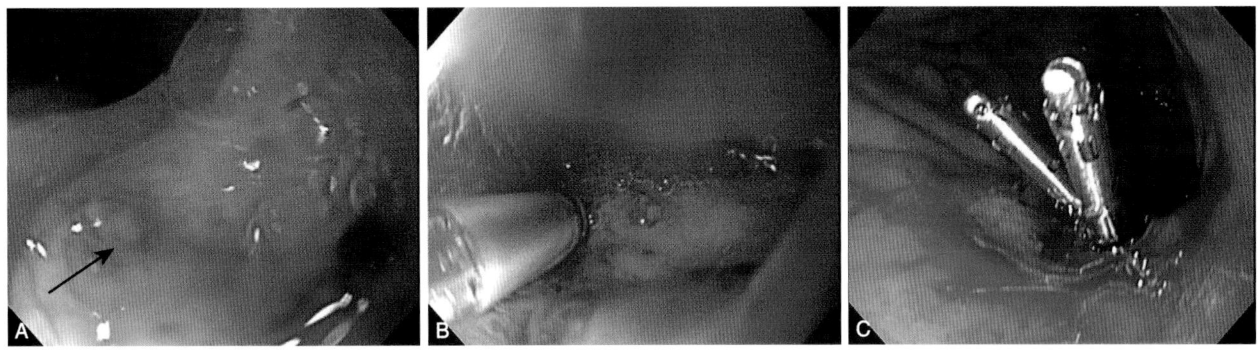

图 20.12　A，通过内镜注射肾上腺素（B）和放置止血夹（C）治疗裸露血管（箭）不出血的胃溃疡（注意，表 20.6 不建议对不出血的裸露血管注射肾上腺素）

(3) **黏附血凝块**

对于标准的、目视引导的内镜止血，对于溃疡上黏附血凝块(Forrest ⅡB)病变的治疗，建议是在血凝块蒂部周围4个象限中，以1mL剂量注射肾上腺素(1∶20 000)，然后使用可旋转的冷圈套器将血凝块碎片断开，而不是将其从基底剥离，直到在溃疡底部发现出血的潜在征象或留下3mm或更小的血凝块。如果见活动性出血、裸露血管或血管残蒂，则进行凝血或止血夹止血(图20.13)。联合治疗技术将再出血率从高达35%(仅用药物治疗)降至5%。黏附血凝块被认为是一种高风险的征象，建议在内镜止血后给予高剂量PPI治疗[130,131]。最近，建议在注射肾上腺素之前，对蒂附近的血凝块进行DEP检查——69%具有潜在的动脉血流[106,111]。止血后应重复DEP检查，以确保无动脉血流和再出血风险较低。

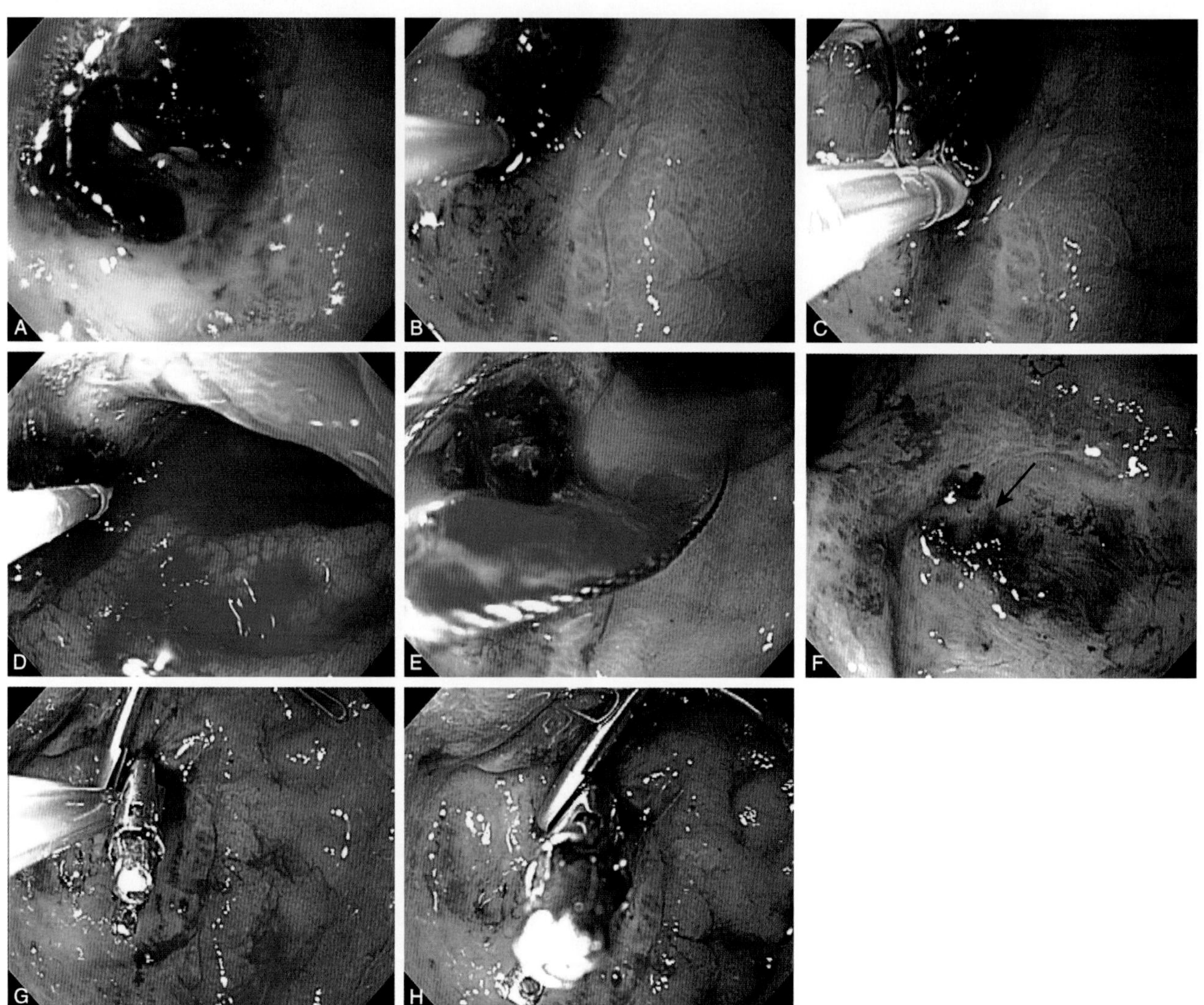

图20.13　A，十二指肠溃疡伴黏附血凝块的内镜治疗。B，血凝块注射肾上腺素，然后分块圈套切除术去除血凝块(C～E)，之后显露下方血管(F中箭)。G和H，在可见血管上放置了两个内镜止血夹

(4) **无其他出血征象的溃疡渗血**

尽管进行了水冲洗和观察(Forrest ⅠB)，溃疡边缘或基底部轻微出血(无其他出血征象)仍持续存在，这表明需要进行内镜治疗。内镜治疗的持续渗血溃疡的再出血率从10%(UCLA CURE)到27%(中国香港)不等。使用热探头或肾上腺素注射进行单药治疗可将再出血率降至5%以下。在渗血患者中，出血动脉可能较小，临床结局优于活动性动脉出血患者[106,134]。渗血和没有其他出血征象的患者(如黏附血凝块或NBVV)，可以单独使用肾上腺素注射进行有效治疗，因为联合治疗没有额外获益[134]。内镜下止血成功后，有渗血且没有其他出血征象的患者并不能从大剂量PPI给药中获益[135]。在DEP引导下，在46%的渗血性溃疡中检测到了潜在的动脉血流，使用MPEC探头或止血夹实现了止血，均无残余血流，并且在每日两次口服PPI治疗后，没有再出血[106]。渗血性溃疡应被认为具有中期再出血风险[106,107,111,112,135]。

(5) **平坦黑色出血斑**

以往认为溃疡内有平坦黑色出血斑的患者(Forrest ⅡC)再出血风险低，不推荐内镜下止血。但在DEP的研究中，40%至49%的平坦黑色出血斑溃疡具有潜在的动脉血流。当血流DEP阳性的患者未接受内镜治疗和药物治疗时，一半患者会再次出血[111]。与活动性渗血(Forrest ⅠA)相似，我们现在将平坦黑色出血斑(Forrest ⅡC)患者归类为具有中度再

出血风险[106,111,135]。单独注射肾上腺素治疗仅能短暂减少动脉血流。当 DEP 为阳性时，建议使用 MPEC 或止血夹闭塞潜在的动脉血流，以防止再出血[111]。

(6) 基底洁净溃疡

在内镜检查中，基底洁净溃疡(Forrest Ⅲ)的患者再出血率低于 5%，且不需要内镜治疗。如果患者有基底洁净型胃溃疡，应考虑对溃疡边缘和胃黏膜进行活检，以排除潜在的恶性肿瘤(见第 53 章)。这些患者可在内镜检查后进食，并接受口服抑酸药物治疗，除非合并有其他医疗问题，否则他们不需要继续住院。

6. 新的内镜技术

(1) 血液喷雾剂

据报道，血液喷雾剂可阻止非静脉曲张性上胃肠道病变、静脉曲张和肿瘤引起的活动性出血，但血液喷雾剂不能治疗潜在的动脉或静脉曲张性血流。因此，再出血的风险较高，对于患有静脉曲张或溃疡伴严重出血的患者，通常需要使用标准技术进行确定性止血。现行指南建议使用血液喷雾剂作为临时替代或辅助技术[116]。需要等进一步的研究，包括随机对照试验，以确定血液喷雾剂在胃肠道出血临床治疗中的疗效和作用。

(2) OTSC 血管夹

在一项随机对照试验中报告了一种 OTSC(large over-the-scope)止血夹(OVESCO Endoscopy AG，Tübingen，Germany)，在复发性溃疡出血患者中与标准内镜止血相比，它显著降低了再出血率。病例系列也报告了使用 OTSC 止血夹作为主要治疗的良好效果，但没有报告溃疡性出血的随机对照试验，来证明 OTSC 止血夹作为初始治疗是否优于标准止血治疗。我们已经证明，当成功应用时，OTSC 止血夹与通过内镜止血夹或 MPEC 的标准止血相比，可更有效地闭塞高危 SRH 消化性溃疡基底的潜在动脉血流。

7. Hp 感染检测

在胃或十二指肠溃疡出血的患者中，应获得外观正常的胃窦和胃体大弯中段的内镜黏膜活检标本，以评估是否存在 Hp 感染。内镜止血成功后可安全获取活检标本，但出血降低了快速尿素酶检测的敏感性。因此，建议进行粪便抗原和其他 Hp 感染检测(见第 52 章)。

8. 药物治疗

(1) 抑酸药物

体外研究表明，正常凝血功能(血小板聚集和纤维蛋白形成)，需要胃内 pH 大于 6.8，pH 小于 5.4 几乎可消除血小板聚集和血浆凝固的作用[136]。血小板聚集物在酸性 pH 下可溶解，这种作用因胃蛋白酶的存在而增强，因此，通过维持胃内 pH 高于 6，理论上可以降低急性出血和消化性溃疡再出血的风险。静脉注射 H_2RA 可急性升高胃内 pH，但对这些药物的耐受性迅速发展，pH 通常在 24 小时内恢复到 3~5。几项研究表明，在正常受试者中，PPI 静脉给药可在 72 小时输注期间持续保持胃 pH 高于 4(并且通常高于 6)[137,138]。而静脉给予 H_2RA 预防复发性溃疡出血的试验未显示明确的效果[139,140]。

多项研究表明，PPI 可有效降低消化性溃疡的再出血率。在一项来自印度的研究中，未接受内镜止血的内镜下高风险消化性溃疡出血病变(如活动性出血、NBVV、血凝块或渗血)的患者被随机接受奥美拉唑 40mg 口服、每日 2 次或安慰剂治疗。奥美拉唑治疗组再出血率为 11%，安慰剂治疗组为 36%($P<0.001$)[141]。来自同一组研究者的另一项研究表明，奥美拉唑 40mg 口服、每日 2 次，持续 5 天，可降低活动性出血、NBVV 或血凝块溃疡内镜止血注射治疗后的再出血率，从安慰剂治疗组的 21% 降至口服奥美拉唑治疗组的 7%($P=0.02$)[142]。在中国香港的一项研究中，因活动性出血或 NBVV 成功接受内镜止血的患者，被随机分配接受大剂量静脉注射奥美拉唑、80mg 推注、随后 8mg/h 或安慰剂治疗。奥美拉唑治疗组 30 天再出血率为 6.7%，而安慰剂治疗组为 22.5%($P<0.05$)[143]。来自香港的同一位研究者发现，单独接受静脉注射奥美拉唑的黏附血凝块或 NBVV 患者的 30 天再出血率为 12%，而接受静脉注射奥美拉唑并接受内镜下止血的患者为 1%($P<0.05$)[144]。另一项来自香港的研究发现，上胃肠道出血患者在上胃肠道内镜检查前开始静脉给予奥美拉唑，可减少发现高危出血征象的数量和内镜治疗的需求，但临床结局无差异，如输血单位数、复发性出血的频率、手术率和死亡率[145]。

Leontiadis 及其同事对 PPI 治疗急性上胃肠道出血的临床有效性和成本效益进行的系统和 Cochrane 综述发现，与安慰剂或 H_2RA 相比，在内镜诊断为消化性溃疡出血后即开始 PPI 治疗，可显著降低再出血率和手术率，亚裔人群的获益比非亚裔人群更为明显[146-148]。在亚洲的研究以及高危内镜下征象患者中，PPI 治疗与死亡率降低相关。与安慰剂或 H_2RA 相比，内镜检查前开始 PPI 治疗显著降低了首次内镜检查时发生 SRH 的患者比例，但未降低死亡率、再出血率或手术率。

建议谨慎将亚洲消化性溃疡出血患者的 PPI 试验结果推广至异质性非亚洲人群。亚洲患者对 PPI 的反应通常高于异质性人群或白人[149]。亚洲患者平均壁细胞量较小，PPI 代谢较慢、并且常合并 Hp 感染，所有这些均增加了 PPI 的有效性。这些因素可以解释在 PPI 治疗消化性溃疡出血试验的 meta 分析中，亚裔的死亡率低于非亚裔的原因。

是否应在 EGD 之前或之后给予 PPI 治疗尚不清楚。尽管一些小型随机研究未显示内镜检查前给予 PPI 可改善临床结局(尽管需要治疗的高危征象数量减少)，但大多数建模研究已表明内镜检查前给予 PPI 治疗具有成本效益[16,18,19,145,148]。内镜止血治疗后的最佳有效 PPI 剂量尚不确定，一项 meta 分析发现，高剂量静脉连续输注 PPI(80mg 推注，随后 8mg/h，3 天)与非高剂量间歇或口服给药(3 天)之间无差异[150]。口服给药与 PPI 静脉给药是否同样有效尚不清楚，但研究表明，高剂量口服给药(如奥美拉唑，40mg，每日 2 次)可将再出血降低至内镜止血的预期发生率。事实上，高剂量口服 PPI 给药时胃内 pH 值的增加与静脉 PPI 给药时几乎相同(尽管延迟了 1 小时)[141,151]。在近期发生上胃肠道出血和某 SRH(如 NBVV、渗血或黏附血凝块)的患者中，单独静脉给予 PPI 是否足以治疗(无内镜止血)仍存在争议。在一项亚洲研究中，Sung 及其同事报告，单独静脉 PPI 给药的 30 天再出血率(12%)与既往的内镜止血研究相似，但他们也发现内镜治疗联合静脉 PPI 给药的再出血率更低(1%)[152]。由于几乎所有PPI治疗急性消化性溃疡出血的主要研究均在亚洲人群中进行,因此需要在非亚洲人群中进行研究来证实亚洲数据。一项大型国际研究证实了高剂量静脉PPI给药,在活动性动脉出血、NBVV或黏附血凝块但无渗出的高危患者中的获益[135,153]。

(2) 生长抑素和奥曲肽

一项meta分析表明,与安慰剂或H_2RA相比,生长抑素或其长效类形式奥曲肽静脉给药,可降低消化性溃疡再出血的风险[154]。拟定的作用机制包括减少内脏和胃十二指肠黏膜血流量、降低胃肠动力、抑制胃酸分泌、抑制胃蛋白酶分泌和胃黏膜细胞保护作用。然而,在内镜或PPI治疗的时代,尚未对这些药物进行研究,因此,不能考虑常规使用[155]。生长抑素或奥曲肽可考虑用于对内镜治疗、静脉注射PPI或两者均无反应的重度持续出血的患者,且不是手术候选者。尽管其在这些患者中的有效性尚不确定。作为内镜下止血和PPI的辅助治疗,静脉注射奥曲肽也可用于门静脉高压和消化性溃疡出血患者(见第92章)。

9. 二次内镜检查

在初次内镜止血后24小时进行常规重复或第二次内镜检查,如果发现持续性高危内镜下出血的征兆,应进行二次内镜止血,已被建议作为一种改善患者预后的方法。对PUD和高危内镜下出血征兆患者的4项前瞻性随机试验的meta分析显示,二次内镜检查可降低再出血和手术率,但并不会降低死亡率。然而,给予患者高剂量PPI治疗的唯一试验显示,二次内镜检查没有任何益处,大多数试验没有采用已成标准治疗的内镜止血技术[156]。因此,不建议大多数消化性溃疡出血患者进行常规的二次内镜检查[114],除了由于胃内血液过多导致初次内镜检查不理想的患者,因为视野模糊,发生了止血的技术问题、复发了临床上显著的出血或使用了如单独注射肾上腺素效果较差的内镜技术。

10. 内镜治疗后再出血

在门诊开始出血并需要内镜止血的消化性溃疡再出血的风险,在诊断和治疗后的前72小时内最大。内镜止血后,患者应保持高剂量PPI治疗至少72小时,之后可将转换为标准剂量。在广泛使用静脉PPI之前,活动性出血性溃疡或NBVV溃疡内镜止血后的再出血率高达30%,随着PPI的使用和内镜技术的改进,大多数研究中的再出血率低于10%。

门诊开始的溃疡出血与住院后开始的出血之间的差异很大(表20.7)。由于住院患者(比门诊患者)溃疡出血至再出血时间可能更长,再出血的风险高,因此应考虑联合内镜止血和高剂量静脉PPI给药治疗超过72小时。需要在该高危人群中进行进一步的研究,以确定最佳治疗方案。

如果消化性溃疡再出血严重,应紧急重复EGD(而不是立即手术)。来自中国香港的一项大型、设计良好的随机试验发现,初次内镜止血后血流动力学稳定再出血的患者,重复进行内镜止血时,73%的患者可实现持续止血,不需要手术[157]。达到和未达到止血者的总死亡率相同,但后者(需手术者)严重并发症的发生率明显增高。预测内镜再治疗失败的因素包括溃疡大小至少2cm和初次就诊时有低血压。

表20.7 门诊与住院患者的消化性溃疡出血发作的比较

参数	发病	
	门诊	住院
频率/%	80~90	10~20
美国麻醉师学会身体状况评分*	≤3	>3
再出血时间/%		
≤72h	70~80h	40~50h
4~7天	10~15天	15~20天
8~30天	1~5天	15~20
>30天	0天	5~10天

*1分表示健康人;5分表示24小时内死亡的可能性很高。
数据引自UCLA CURE数据库。
CURE,溃疡研究和教育中心;UCLA,加州大学洛杉矶分校。

11. 血管造影、外科手术和OTSC血管夹

尽管进行了两次内镜下止血,但仍复发出血的患者可考虑进行血管造影栓塞或手术治疗。几个回顾性系列报告称,血管造影栓塞治疗与外科手术治疗在再出血率和死亡率方面不存在任何显著差异,尽管血管造影治疗的患者年龄较大、医疗问题也更严重[158,159]。这些研究表明,内镜治疗失败后可以考虑血管造影。如果栓塞治疗无法控制出血,手术仍然是一种选择。

一项随机对照试验表明,OTSC止血夹治疗复发性消化性溃疡出血比标准内镜止血(主要是通过止血夹)更有效。这种新的治疗方法有可能减少复发性溃疡出血对手术或血管造影术需求。OTSC止血夹在消除潜在动脉血流方面也比标准止血治疗更有效,后者存在再出血的风险[106,111]。对于大量持续性出血和无法进行医学复苏的患者,应立即进行急诊手术干预。如果内镜医师在治疗较大的或搏动的裸露血管时,感觉无把握(例如,在可能代表侵及十二指肠动脉的深在十二指肠后壁溃疡中的血管),或者如果内镜检查发现出血性恶性溃疡肿块时,也应考虑手术治疗。

12. 内镜治疗后的即时处理

(1) 高风险内镜下出血病灶

对于活动性动脉出血、NBVV或黏附血凝块的内镜下治疗后,高风险内镜下出血病灶的患者,应在医院观察72小时,同时接受高剂量PPI静脉输注。在成功的内镜治疗和镇静恢复后,患者可以开始进食流质饮食,随后推进饮食。对于已经使用并需要继续使用抗血小板药物或抗凝药物的患者,应咨询心脏病专家或血管内科医师,以帮助确定这些药物是否可以继续使用,以及使用多长时间可以停用。但是,对于需要阿司匹林治疗的严重动脉粥样硬化性心血管疾病患者,应在7天内开始81mg/d剂量的阿司匹林。

(2) 中风险内镜下出血病灶

患者内镜下有平坦出血斑并在病灶下方检测到动脉血流、溃疡渗血和无其他出血征象(例如喷血、NBVV、血凝块)的患者,以及有严重共病或休克的患者均应接受内镜下止血。建议开始每日两次口服PPI,并在内镜下成功止血后在医院观察24至48小时。此类患者在内镜止血后成功后,不能从高剂量静脉PPI治疗中获益[106,135]。

（3）低风险内镜下出血病灶

基底洁净溃疡或溃疡基底未检测到动脉血流的平坦出血斑的患者，通常可立即恢复正常饮食，开始口服 PPI，每日 1 次，并在内镜检查稳定后早期出院[132]。这些患者通常可以完全避免住院或提前出院[10,11,74,161]。一般来说，如果患者年轻且血流动力学指标稳定，无严重共存疾病，血红蛋白水平高于 10mg/dL，凝血参数正常，如果在家中出血复发，具有良好的社会支持系统。

13. 预防复发性溃疡出血

（1）Hp 感染

所有消化性溃疡出血患者均应进行 Hp 感染检测（见前文），如果结果为阳性，应接受 Hp 感染的标准治疗（见第 52 章）[88]。需要注意的是，出血可导致快速尿素酶检测结果假阴性，在这种情况下，患者可能需要接受另一种检测 Hp 的方法。抗生素治疗不必立即开始，当患者恢复正常饮食时，可在门诊开始治疗。在 Hp 感染诱导的溃疡患者中，建议在治疗后确认 Hp 根除（见第 52 章）。

（2）阿司匹林、其他非甾体抗炎药和抗血小板药物

由阿司匹林或其他非选择性 NSAID 引起的溃疡出血患者，在病情允许情况下应该停药。如果患者的 Hp 检测结果也呈阳性，则应采用标准疗法根除 Hp（见第 52 章）[162]。在有溃疡出血史、Hp 阳性且需要继续服用低剂量阿司匹林（每日 81mg）的患者中，单纯根除 Hp 导致的溃疡再出血率与每日 PPI 治疗相似（如果 Hp 未根除）[163]。相比之下，在有溃疡出血史、Hp 阳性且需要继续全剂量 NSAID 治疗的患者中，单纯根除 Hp 而不使用 PPI 治疗导致再出血率显著高于每日 PPI 联合 NSAID。在没有 Hp 感染但需要继续每日服用阿司匹林的溃疡出血患者中，与安慰剂相比，每日服用 PPI 联合治疗可显著降低再出血率[164]。与单用氯吡格雷相比，需要抗血小板药物（如氯吡格雷）且有溃疡出血史的患者，如果每日服用阿司匹林（81mg）和一次 PPI，复发出血的概率较低[165]。

溃疡出血后需要 NSAID 治疗的患者，可考虑使用选择性 COX-2 抑制剂。选择性 COX-2 抑制剂引起的溃疡少于非选择性 NSAID，但与心血管并发症发生率更高相关。由于选择性 COX-2 抑制剂导致的再出血率与非选择性 NSAID 和 PPI 联合治疗相关的再出血率相似，所以不值得考虑使用选择性 COX-2 抑制剂增加心血管的风险[166]。

14. 重复内镜检查以确认胃溃疡愈合

胃溃疡患者在抑酸治疗 6～10 周后，应考虑重复进行 EGD 检查，以确认溃疡愈合且无恶性肿瘤（见第 53 和 54 章）。在世界上胃癌中等风险人群的地区，2%～4% 用于确认溃疡愈合的重复上胃肠道内镜检查报告显示胃癌[167-169]。一些专家认为，当首次内镜检查和活检显示恶性肿瘤阴性，且溃疡在内镜下显示为良性时，无须进行随访内镜检查[170]。一项小型回顾性研究发现，当重复内镜检查中以评估胃溃疡愈合时观察到胃癌，其生存率并不优于未接受推荐的随访内镜检查的患者[171]。

（五）其他非静脉曲张原因

1. 食管炎

严重糜烂性食管炎的患者可表现为呕血或黑便。来自法国一个中心的多变量分析发现，其中 8% 的上胃肠道出血是由糜烂性食管炎引起的。出血性食管炎的独立危险因素为：根据 Savary-Miller 分级系统的 3 级或 4 级（中度至重度）食管炎（见第 46 章）、肝硬化、体能状态差以及抗凝治疗[171]。仅有 38% 的患者有胃灼热病史。胃食管反流性食管炎引起的严重出血需采用 PPI 进行药物治疗（见第 46 章）。EGD 检查对于诊断严重糜烂性食管炎至关重要，但内镜治疗一般没有任何作用，除非发现局灶性溃疡伴 SRH。这些患者应每日接受 PPI 治疗 8 至 12 周，并接受重复内镜检查以排除潜在的 Barrett 食管（见第 47 章）。

患者有时可表现与 GERD 无关的食管炎引起的轻度上胃肠道出血，但与感染（如念珠菌，单纯疱疹病毒，巨细胞病毒）或药物诱导的食管炎有关。内镜活检和刷检对于做这些诊断和选择适当的药物治疗至关重要（见第 45 章）。

2. 住院患者溃疡出血

住院患者的溃疡出血或糜烂出血通常分为两类。典型的原因是与应激相关的黏膜损伤（stress-related mucosal injury，SRMI，或应激性溃疡），以糜烂和浅表溃疡弥漫性出血为特征。第二类是住院溃疡，是大的、局灶性、慢性溃疡，无痛，表现为严重上胃肠道出血，出现便血、黑便或呕血。在急诊内镜检查中，局灶性住院溃疡通常是活动性出血或显示裸露血管或黏附血凝块，尽管联合内镜治疗，但再出血率较高，并且在高剂量 PPI 治疗时延迟愈合。

SRMI 发生在 ICU 重症住院患者的上胃肠道，可能是由于黏膜保护作用下降和黏膜缺血共同引起的。SRMI 通常发生于胃，但也可见于十二指肠、食管，甚至直肠。弥漫性渗血常见，患者预后差，再出血率高，常与伤口愈合障碍和多器官功能衰竭有关。

SRMI 出血现在并不常见，在 ICU 患者中的发生频率约为 1.5%。严重的凝血功能障碍和机械通气超过 48 小时是其 2 种主要危险因素[172]。具有这些风险因素之 1 或 2 种时，临床上显著 GI 出血频率为 3.7%，而不存在风险因素时为 0.1%。其他促发风险因素包括上胃肠道出血史、败血症、入住 ICU 超过 7 天、隐性 GI 出血超过 5 天和大剂量糖皮质激素治疗。

有出血危险因素的 ICU 患者是药物预防出血 SRMI 的主要目标人群。使用 H_2RA 治疗已被证明可降低 SRMI 高风险 ICU 患者的临床显著出血率[173]。一项大型多中心研究发现，口服奥美拉唑或静脉输注西咪替丁预防性治疗的出血率相似，但奥美拉唑比西咪替丁更能有效地维持胃腔 pH 在 4[174]。胃酸抑制预防应激性溃疡的潜在有害作用是继发于胃 pH 升高的胃内细菌增殖，以及吸入性肺炎和呼吸机相关性肺炎的相关风险，然而，比较抑酸治疗（用 H_2RA 或抗酸剂）和硫糖铝（不降低胃 pH）的随机试验并没有令人信服地表明，升高胃 pH 会增加罹患肺炎的风险[175,176]。

一般情况下，如果对 SRMI 患者或住院溃疡患者进行血流动力学和医学支持治疗，随着患者总体医学状况的改善，病变将会愈合。由于 SRMI 是弥漫性的，通常不采用内镜治疗。相比之下，局灶性住院溃疡出血的患者往往需要内镜下止血治疗严重出血（见图 20.9）。但是，与住院前开始出血的患者相比，其再出血率更高，愈合速度更慢（见表 20.7）[177,178]。一

项研究在院内溃疡发生率较高的患者队列中，比较了肾上腺素注射加止血夹放置与肾上腺素注射联合 MPEC 治疗，发现注射加止血夹放置组的再出血率显著较低[133]。

3. Dieulafoy 病变（恒径小动脉畸形）

Dieulafoy 病变是突出于黏膜下的一支较大的（1～3mm）黏膜下动脉，与消化性溃疡无关，可引起大出血。通常位于胃底，胃食管交界处 6cm 以内，尽管有十二指肠、小肠和结肠病变的报道。病因不明，认为是先天性和获得性（与黏膜萎缩或小动脉动脉瘤有关）原因所致（见第 38 章）。

由于其出血的间歇性，Dieulafoy 病变在内镜检查时可能很难识别；如果病变没有出血，覆盖的黏膜可能显示正常。内镜检查可见 NBVV 或无溃疡的黏附血凝块。如果大量上胃肠道出血似乎从胃发出，应仔细检查近端胃部，以寻找可能是 Dieulafoy 病变的突起。DEP 已被用于帮助识别内镜检查未可视化的 Dieulafoy 病变[179]。由于很难确定出血部位，并且再出血并不少见，我们建议，如果发现并治疗 Dieulafoy 病变，应在该部位黏膜下注射墨水标记，以便在再出血和需要再治疗的情况下，能尽快找到病变部位。

Dieulafoy 病变的内镜下止血可以采用注射治疗、热探头、止血夹夹闭或橡皮圈套扎[111,179-185]。大型病例系列报告的初始止血率约为 90%，4%～16% 的病例需要手术[182]。联合治疗或 OTSC 止血夹闭术的再出血率可能较低，因为基础动脉血流的根除比注射或单药治疗更有效[111]。虽然所有的内镜止血技术似乎都是有效的，但有报道在套扎止血术后发生穿孔和迟发性再出血（见第 42 章）。

4. Mallory-Weiss 综合征（食管黏膜撕裂症）

Mallory-Weiss 综合征是发生在胃食管交界处的黏膜或黏膜下撕裂伤，通常向远端延伸成食管裂孔疝（图 20.14）。患者一般表现为呕血或咖啡样呕吐物，有非血性呕吐后呕血的病史，尽管部分患者不记得呕吐。该综合征被认为是腹内压力升高所致，结合膈肌上方的胸内负压引起的剪切效应，通常与呕吐有关。在结肠镜检查前服用肠道清洗剂时呕吐的患者中也有报道[186]。内镜检查通常发现始于胃食管交界处的单个撕裂，并向远端延伸数毫米进入食管裂孔疝囊。偶尔可见 1 处以上的撕裂。胃镜返转观察比前视观察能提供更好可视效果。Mallory-Weiss 综合征的出血征象可能包括干净的基底、黏附性血凝块、NBVV、渗血或罕见的活动性喷血。通常出血是自限性和轻度的，但偶尔可能是严重的，尤其是食管静脉曲张或凝血功能异常疾病的患者。黏膜（浅表）Mallory-Weiss 综合征可在数小时内开始愈合，并可在 48 小时内完全愈合。

虽然大约 50% 的 Mallory-Weiss 综合征导致上胃肠道出血的住院患者接受了输血，但在大多数未就医的患者中，撕裂表现为轻度、自限性呕血[187]。Mallory-Weiss 综合征住院患者的再出血率约为 10%，再出血的风险因素包括就诊时休克和内镜检查时有活动性出血[188]。由于存在持续和复发性出血的风险，Mallory-Weiss 综合征活动性出血的患者应接受内镜治疗，可通过注射肾上腺素、MPEC、放置止血夹或套扎治疗。比较 MPEC 止血和药物治疗与 H_2RA 的随机试验发现，内镜治疗可降低再出血、输血和急诊手术的发生率[189]。

目前治疗无门静脉高压或食管静脉曲张患者活动性出血 Mallory-Weiss 综合征的内镜技术，是应用内镜下止血夹止血和闭合撕裂口。如果止血夹不可用，建议在低功率设置（12～14W）下使用 MPEC 止血并施加 1～2 秒的轻微压力，注射肾上腺素，以减缓出血并对出血部位进行局灶性止血。对于门静脉高压引起的食管静脉曲张患者，如果还存在 Mallory-Weiss 综合征，应针对食管静脉曲进行食管套扎或静脉曲张硬化治疗（见后文和第 92 章）。

Mallory-Weiss 综合征患者如果出现恶心或呕吐，也可使用止吐药物治疗，并使用 PPI 加速黏膜愈合。不需要 PPI 长期治疗。

5. Cameron 病变

Cameron 病变为大裂孔疝末端靠近横膈夹角近端胃的线状糜烂或溃疡（图 20.15）[190]。Cameron 病变被认为是由机械创伤和局部缺血引起的，因为疝向膈肌移动，仅继发于酸和胃蛋白酶。它们可能是急性上胃肠道出血的来源，但更常见的可能表现为慢性胃肠道出血和缺铁性贫血。Cameron 病变是不明原因胃肠道出血的常见原因（见下文），并不罕见，经

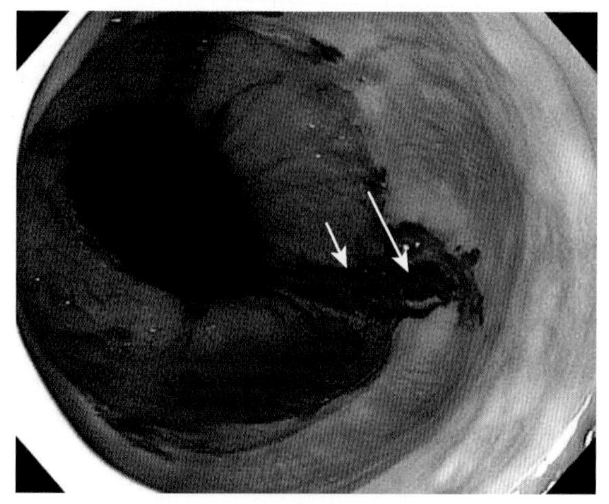

图 20.14　内镜下 Mallory-Weiss 综合征伴轻度渗血。注意，撕裂开始于胃食管交界处（长箭），并向远端延伸至食管裂孔疝（短箭）

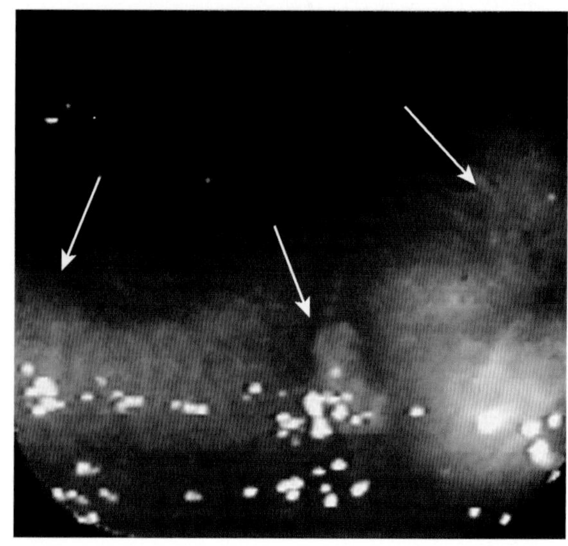

图 20.15　Cameron 病变的内镜表现。注意这些线状溃疡（箭）位于食管裂孔疝的远端

常被不知情的内镜医师遗漏。其内镜下治疗已有报道[191]。通常是补充铁剂和口服 PPI 进行长期治疗[192,193]。对于严重急性或慢性胃肠道出血和药物治疗失败的患者,可能需要手术修补食管裂孔疝(见第 27 章)[192]。

6. 上胃肠道恶性肿瘤

恶性肿瘤占严重上胃肠道出血的 1%。肿瘤通常是食管、胃或十二指肠大的溃疡性肿块。使用 MPEC、激光、注射治疗或止血夹进行内镜下止血可暂时控制大多数患者的急性出血,并有时间选择适当的长期治疗方案[194,195]。溃疡型上皮下肿块(通常为胃肠间质瘤或平滑肌瘤)患者应手术切除肿块,以防止再次出血,在胃肠间质瘤的情况下,则应考虑转移的风险。对于内镜治疗无效的恶性肿瘤引起的严重上胃肠道出血患者,应考虑血管造影与栓塞治疗。外照射放疗可为晚期胃癌或十二指肠癌出血患者,提供姑息性止血(见第 54 章)。在一项小的病例系列中,使用血液喷雾剂治疗上胃肠道肿瘤的渗出出血[42]。

7. 胃窦血管扩张症

胃窦血管扩张症(GAVE),也被称为"西瓜胃",是胃血管扩张症的一种变异(见第 92 章),其特征是扩张的黏膜血管成排或条状,从幽门发出,并向近端延伸至胃窦(图 20.16)。病因尚不清楚,病变可能代表胃窦收缩波对黏膜创伤的反应。GAVE 与肝硬化和系统性硬化症(硬皮病)相关(见第 37 章、第 38 章和第 92 章)。无门静脉高压的 GAVE 患者表现出血管瘤的线性排列(经典 GAVE),而门静脉高压患者有更弥散的胃窦血管瘤[196]。弥漫性胃窦血管瘤和偶尔的经典 GAVE 有时被不知情的内镜医师误认为是胃炎。这些病例是医学转诊中心不明原因胃肠道出血的常见原因(见后文)[57]。

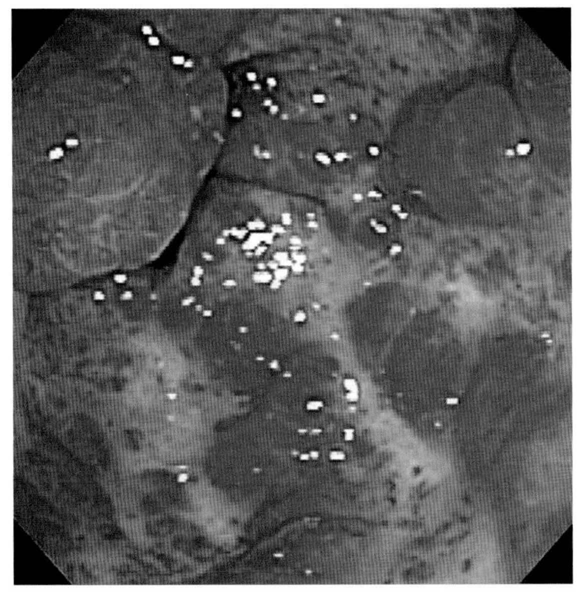

图 20.16　内镜下表现为 GAVE 或西瓜胃。该视图中观察到的模式被认为是典型的,幽门发出成排扩张的黏膜血管

患者通常表现为缺铁性贫血或黑便,血细胞比容值轻度降低提示缓慢上胃肠道出血。GAVE 最常见于老年女性[196],似乎也更常见于终末期肾病患者。

使用热模式(如激光、MPEC 或氩等离子体凝固)的内镜止血已经成功使用。使用热模式的内镜止血和热消融治疗可使病情得到良好的缓解,血细胞比容值增加,输血和住院需求降低[196,197]。通常需要几个疗程来根除病变和减少胃窦扩张的出血,每次间隔约 4~8 周。已证明氩等离子体凝固内镜治疗对伴有 GAVE 的肝硬化和非肝硬化患者同样有效(80%)[198]。初步研究证明,黏膜套扎、射频消融和冷冻治疗也可使选定患者根除 GAVE[199-201]。

在门静脉高压症和肝硬化患者中,经颈静脉肝内门体分流术(TIPS)不会减少 GAVE 或弥漫性胃窦血管瘤造成的出血。由 GAVE 引起的持续严重慢性出血的患者,很少需要手术胃切除来控制症状(见第 38 和 92 章)[202]。

8. 门静脉高压性胃病

门静脉高压性胃病(portal hypertensive gastropathy,PHG)是由于门静脉压力增高和严重的黏膜充血,导致近端胃体和贲门血管扩张、血液渗出所致。不严重的 PHG 内镜下表现为镶嵌或蛇皮样模式,与出血无关[203]。通常严重 PHG 患者表现为慢性失血,但偶可表现为急性出血。

严重 PHG 伴弥漫性出血可通过降低门静脉压的措施进行治疗,通常使用 β-肾上腺素能受体阻滞剂,或可能使用 TIPS 或施行门腔静脉分流术治疗。除非发现明显的局灶性出血部位,否则内镜治疗无效。其最佳的治疗方法是肝移植(见第 92 章)。

9. 胆道出血

胆道出血可能发生在肝创伤、肝活检或肝胆系统操作的患者中(如 ERCP、经皮肝穿刺胆管造影术或 TIPS 发生的情况),或患有 HCC 或胆道寄生虫感染的患者中[204]。患者可能同时出现胃肠道出血和肝脏生化检测水平升高。使用十二指肠侧视镜识别壶腹部出血可明确诊断(图 20.17)。持续或复发性出血可通过动脉造影进行动脉栓塞治疗。

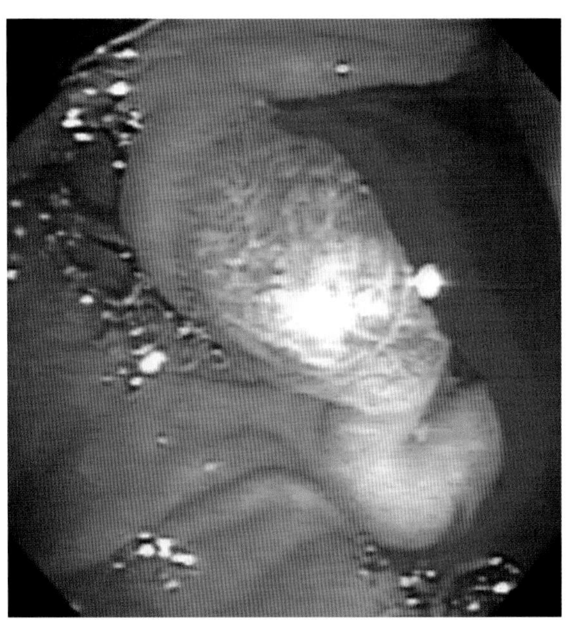

图 20.17　Vater 壶腹部和胆道出血的内镜下表现。注意当天早些时候接受经皮肝活检的患者,可见壶腹部右侧有新鲜的红色血液渗出

10. 胰源性出血

胰源性出血是一种罕见的上胃肠道出血形式，最常见于急性胰腺炎、慢性胰腺炎、胰腺假性囊肿或胰腺癌患者或ERCP联合胰管操作后的患者（见第42和58~61章）。也可由于脾动脉瘤破裂入胰管所致[205]。CT可显示以前未被疑诊的胰腺病变。十二指肠侧视镜内镜检查显示壶腹部有血液流出。严重出血的治疗通常采用血管造影栓塞或手术。

11. 括约肌切开术后出血

内镜下括约肌切开术后出血的发生率约为2%（见第42章）[206]。潜在的风险因素包括凝血功能障碍、使用抗凝剂、门静脉高压症、肾功能衰竭以及括约肌切开术的类型和长度。括约肌切开术后出血的成功止血，通常是通过内镜方法实现的，如注射肾上腺素、止血夹或MPEC（见第42章）。

12. 主动脉肠瘘

主动脉肠瘘出血通常是急性和大量的，死亡率高[207]。原发性主动脉肠瘘是自体腹主动脉（通常是动脉硬化性腹主动脉瘤）与十二指肠第三部分之间的交通[208]。往往在发生严重出血前有数小时至数月发生自限性先兆出血。偶尔通过腹主动脉瘤病史或搏动性腹部肿块触诊怀疑主动脉肠道瘘的诊断。在无活动性出血的情况下，内镜检查很难做出诊断。腹部CT或MRI（使用静脉造影剂）显示主动脉瘤提示主动脉肠瘘的诊断[58]。继发性主动脉肠瘘更常见，通常发生在小肠和感染的腹主动脉外科移植物之间。瘘管通常发生在十二指肠的第三部分和移植物的近端之间，但也可以发生在胃肠道的其他部位。瘘管通常在移植物植入后3~5年形成。在大出血发生之前，患者通常会出现轻度和自限性的预兆性出血，以及偶尔的间歇性出血[209]。十二指肠第三部分和血管内支架之间也可发生第二瘘，在这种情况下，瘘可能是由于支架对十二指肠的压力、支架感染或自体动脉瘤扩张引起的[210]。

有急性上胃肠道出血和动脉瘤修复病史的患者应首先接受紧急CT或MRI血管造影（使用静脉造影剂）。CT或MRI可显示血管支架周围炎症，并可显示瘘管。如果这些不能诊断，应考虑推进式小肠镜检查，以评价十二指肠第三部分是否有压迫、血液或移植材料，以及排除其他出血来源。还应请血管外科医师会诊。需要手术治疗清除感染的移植物。治疗性内镜检查对治疗主动脉肠道瘘出血没有作用（见第38章）。

13. 静脉曲张出血

静脉曲张出血是上胃肠道出血的重要原因，将在第92章中详细讨论。与门静脉高压相关的食管静脉曲张出血是严重上胃肠道出血的第二大常见原因（仅次于PUD）。每次出血的急性死亡率约为30%，单纯内科治疗1年后的长期存活率低于40%[211]。尽管药物治疗、内镜止血、血管造影和TIPS方面取得了进展，但静脉曲张出血患者的总体长期生存率并没有改善。未行肝移植的静脉曲张出血患者的生存率，受潜在肝脏疾病严重程度的明显影响，MELD评分较高或Child-Pugh C级肝硬化患者的生存率低于Child-Pugh A级或B级肝硬化患者（见第74、92和97章）。肝移植可提高所选患者的生存率。

出血性胃底静脉曲张是一个很难治疗的问题，因为与出血性食管静脉曲张相比，大多数可行的非手术治疗是无效的，除非发现孤立的胃底静脉曲张而不伴有食管静脉曲张时，与脾静脉血栓形成时相同，往往与胰腺炎或胰腺癌有关。采用多普勒超声、MRI或常规血管造影可诊断脾静脉血栓形成。脾静脉血栓形成引起的胃底静脉曲张出血采用脾切除术治疗。局灶性胃底静脉曲张伴出血，可通过注射氰基丙烯酸酯胶水或放射学手术治疗，如球囊闭塞逆行经静脉闭塞术来治疗（见第92章）。

（1）急性静脉曲张出血的药物治疗

生长抑素及其长效类似物奥曲肽可引起选择性内脏血管收缩和门静脉压力降低，而不会引起血管升压素所致的心脏并发症（即使与硝酸甘油联合使用）。研究显示，在治疗静脉曲张出血方面，生长抑素是否比安慰剂更有效，结果好坏参半，但它似乎至少与血管升压素一样有效，而且更安全。一项meta分析显示，血管活性药物［如奥曲肽、生长抑素、特利加压素（一种长效血管升压素类似物）］在控制静脉曲张出血方面与硬化疗法同样有效，且不良事件更少[21]。尚无研究显示，血管升压素或生长抑素对静脉曲张出血患者有生存益处。鉴于奥曲肽控制急性静脉曲张出血的潜在能力、其低毒性以及在美国的可用性，奥曲肽一直是作为内镜治疗静脉曲张出血辅助治疗的首选药物。奥曲肽治疗急性静脉曲张出血的剂量为50μg推注，然后以50μg/h速度连续静脉输注持续5天。

PT延长但未用新鲜冷冻血浆纠正的患者，可能从人重组因子Ⅶa输注中获益，但PT延长与出血风险无关（见第92章和第94章）。在一项非对照试验中，单次给予80μg/kg剂量的重组因子Ⅶa，所有10例患者的PT均在30分钟内恢复正常，所有患者的出血均立即得到控制[212]。在一项大型随机、安慰剂对照研究中，在内镜止血的基础上加用重组因子Ⅶa可降低Child-Pugh B级和C级肝硬化静脉曲张出血患者的再出血率[213]。由于重组因子Ⅶa价格昂贵，且有血栓形成的危险，因此在等待其他临床和成本效益研究结果的情况下，应将其用于严重的持续出血和不可逆的凝血病患者。

因胃肠道出血住院的肝硬化患者中，高达20%的患者在入院时有细菌感染，高达50%的患者在住院期间发生感染（见第93章）。Meta分析表明，肝硬化静脉曲张出血患者给予抗生素与死亡率和细菌感染率降低相关[214,215]。常用处方抗生素为氟喹诺酮类药物，如口服诺氟沙星（400mg，每日两次）（在美国不可用）、静脉输注环丙沙星（400mg，每12小时一次）、静脉输注左氧氟沙星（500mg，每24小时一次），以及最常见的静脉输注头孢曲松（1g，每24小时一次，给药7天）。

（2）球囊压塞止血

尽管现在很少使用球囊压塞来控制胃食管静脉曲张出血，但它可以在确定性治疗前，用于治疗大出血患者（见第92章）。有3种类型的压塞球囊可供选择。Sengstaken-Blakemore导管有胃和食管球囊，胃内有一个抽吸端口。Minnesota导管具有胃和食管球囊，并在食管和胃中各有一抽吸端口。Linton-Nachlas导管在胃和食管中有一个大的胃球囊和抽吸端口。大多数报告表明，球囊压塞可在85%~98%的病例中初步控制出血，但21%~60%的患者在球囊回缩后不久再次发生静脉曲张再出血[216]。球囊压塞的主要问题是30%的严重并发症，如吸入性肺炎、食管破裂和气道阻塞。在放置球囊导管之前应对患者进行插管，以将肺部并发症的风险降至最低。临床研究未显示血管升压素给药与球囊压塞止血之间存在显著差异。

(3) 内镜下硬化剂治疗

内镜下静脉曲张硬化治疗包括在食管曲张静脉内或附近注射硬化剂。最常用的硬化剂是油酸乙醇胺、十四烷基硫酸钠、鱼肝油酸钠和乙醇。氰基丙烯酸酯是一种注射到食管或胃静脉曲张处时能有效止血的胶水,但该药使用困难,也未获得美国食品药品管理局(FDA)的批准。各种技术的使用,其共同目标是通过按计划进行硬化治疗,达到初步止血并降低再出血风险,直至静脉曲张闭塞。食管静脉曲张比胃底静脉曲张更适合通过内镜治疗根除。

前瞻性随机试验表明,与单纯药物治疗出血性食管静脉曲张相比,硬化治疗可改善即刻止血,降低急性再出血风险[217-220]。85%~95%的病例可达到止血,再出血率为 25%~30%[221]。内镜下静脉曲张硬化治疗的并发症包括:食管溃疡伴出血或穿孔、食管狭、纵隔炎、胸腔积液、吸入性肺炎、急性呼吸窘迫综合征、胸痛、发热和菌血症,部分原因是,使用食管静脉曲张套扎术作为静脉曲张出血的首选内镜治疗方法。

(4) 内镜下套扎术治疗

内镜下套扎技术与内痔套扎术相似(见第 129 章)。在静脉曲张上放置橡皮筋,随后形成血栓,纤维化和脱落。前瞻性随机对照试验表明,内镜下套扎术与硬化治疗在实现初始止血和降低食管静脉曲张再出血率方面同样有效。一般 80%~85%的病例可达到急止血,再出血率为 25%~30%。套扎术与较少的局部并发症相关,尤其是食管狭窄。在一项研究中,与硬化疗法相比,需要较少的内镜治疗疗程[222]。一项 meta 分析报道,与硬化治疗相比,静脉曲张套扎术可降低再出血率、总死亡率和出血死亡率[223]。然而,在活动性静脉曲张出血期间,套扎术在技术上可能比硬化疗法更难以进行。用于套扎的器械最多允许放置 10 个条带,而不需要取出内镜来重新加载捆扎器。推荐的策略是先控制活动性出血,然后在每个食管静脉曲张上放置 2 个束带,一个在胃食管交界处附近的远端,另一个在近端 4~6cm 处[224-246]。

(5) 经颈静脉肝内门体分流术(TIPS)

TIPS 是一种介入性放射学手术,通过经皮插入肝静脉和门静脉之间置入可扩张的金属支架,从而形成肝内门体分流。TIPS 可有效短期控制出血性胃食管静脉曲张,尤其是内镜治疗失败的静脉曲张[226,227]。最初被设想为肝移植的过渡治疗,在非移植情况下使用频率也增加。将 TIPS 与内镜硬化疗法进行比较的随机试验表明,TIPS 在长期预防再出血方面更有效[228]。TIPS 的主要问题是分流系统在 1 年内的闭塞率高达 80%(使用聚四氟乙烯涂层支架的闭塞率较少),以及约 20%的患者出现新的肝性脑病或肝性脑病恶化[229]。大多数相关研究表明,与内镜治疗相比,TIPS 并不能延长静脉曲张出血患者的生存期。在急性静脉曲张出血的治疗中,TIPS 通常适用于内镜治疗失败的患者。在一项对以酒精性肝硬化和酗酒为主的患者进行的研究中,在初始稳定后 72 小时内接受血管活性药物和内镜治疗稳定的 Child-Pugh B 级肝硬化患者,被随机分配接受紧急 TIPS 或 β-肾上腺素能受体阻滞剂和内镜下套扎术作为维持治疗,接受 TIPS 治疗的患者再出血率较低,1 年生存率提高[230]。该研究结果可能不适用于非酒精性肝硬化患者(另见第 92 章)。

(6) 门体分流手术

为降低门静脉压力,已经进行了多种门静脉分流术的尝试。与硬化治疗相比,分流手术可显著降低再出血率,但不能改善生存率[221,231-234]。分流手术可能与肝性脑病相关,并且可能使未来的肝移植在技术上更加困难,但在降低门静脉高压和治疗胃静脉曲张破裂出血方面,它们比内镜下静脉曲张治疗具有优势。目前很少进行分流手术,但是对于内镜治疗失败并且预期不会成为肝移植候选者的患者,可以考虑分流手术(见第 92 和 97 章)。

三、下胃肠道出血

下胃肠道出血通常是指结肠或肛门直肠的出血。下胃肠道出血的年发生率约为 20 例/100 000 人,老年人中的风险增加[235]。下胃肠道出血的住院率低于上胃肠道出血。大多数患者年龄超过 70 岁。患者通常表现为无痛性便血和血细胞比容值降低。如果临床出现直立性低血压与便血有关,应排除快速出血的上胃肠道来源(见前文)。大约 15%非肝硬化患者出现的严重无痛性便血是由上胃肠道病变出血引起的[236]。UCLA CURE 关于严重便血胃肠道内起源部位见图 20.18。

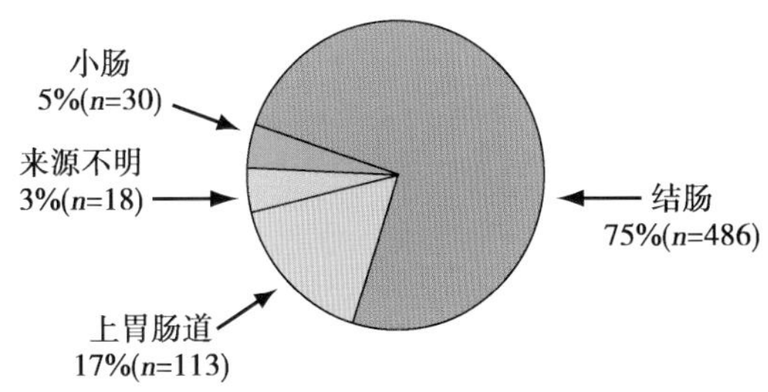

图 20.18 在 UCLA CURE 就诊的患者中,严重便血来源的频率。注意,在大多数(75%)病例中严重便血来自结肠;17% 来自上胃肠道(食管、胃或十二指肠);5% 来自小肠。CURE,溃疡研究和教育中心;UCLA,加州大学洛杉矶分校

下胃肠道出血患者最初应进行药物复苏。在病情稳定后,通常应在聚乙二醇清除后接受紧急结肠镜检查[27]。对于肝硬化、近期有黑便或呕血病史或 PUD 病史的患者,建议首先进行"泛内镜检查"(上、下胃肠道内镜检查)[236,237]。在早期报道中,大约 70% 的病例是通过紧急结肠镜检查得到了诊断[238,239];然而在随后的报告中,紧急结肠镜检查以及必要时的推进式小肠镜检查、肛门镜检查和胶囊式内镜检查的合,在 95% 的病例中得到了诊断(见图 20.4)[236,237]。

下胃肠道出血的最常见原因见表 20.8。憩室病通常是急性下胃肠道出血的最常见原因,其发生率约为 30%[2]。结肠息肉或癌症、结肠炎和肛门直肠疾病各约占病例的 20% 的[240]。

在大多数情况下,急性下胃肠道出血会自行停止,从而无需紧急诊断和诊治。对于持续或复发性便血的患者,需要紧急诊断和治疗以控制出血。在加州大学洛杉矶分校医疗中心和沃兹沃思退伍军人管理医院的大量患者中,64% 的严重便血患者需要治疗干预以控制持续出血或再出血[27]。其中 39% 接受内镜止血,1% 接受血管造影栓塞治疗,24% 行手术治疗。

表 20.8　重度便血的结肠原因(%)

病变	研究		
	239 例	240 例	UCLA CURE* (2018)
憩室病	30	33	33
结肠癌或息肉	18	21	5.2
结肠炎	17	17	N/A
缺血性结肠炎	N/A	7	11.9
IBD	N/A	4	3.6
非感染性结肠炎	N/A	5	2.7
感染性结肠炎	N/A	1	1.2
血管扩张症	7	6	5
息肉切除术后溃疡	6	N/A	7.8
直肠溃疡	N/A	1	8.4
痔疮	N/A	20	10.3
肛门、直肠源(其他)	4	3	1.8†
放射性结肠炎	0	0.5	2.2
结肠吻合口溃疡	N/A	N/A	2.1
其他	8	3	4.1
未知	16	0	0

*N=823。

†橡皮筋结扎后的肛裂、溃疡、直肠癌或其他肛门直肠病变。

CURE,溃疡研究和教育中心;IBD,炎症性肠病;UCLA,加州大学洛杉矶分校。

N/A,无相关资料。

(一) 风险因素和风险分层

与安慰剂相比,非选择性 NSAID 增加了下胃肠道出血的风险[241,242]。NSAID 相关下胃肠道出血的主要危险因素似乎是年龄≥65 岁,以及既往合并下胃肠道出血病史[243]。与长期服用非选择性 NSAID 相比,长期服用选择性 COX-2 抑制剂是否具有较低的下胃肠道出血风险,目前尚不确定。

表 20.9 显示了预测严重下胃肠道出血的临床因素(定义为住院前 24 小时内持续出血,需要至少输血 2 个单位的浓缩红细胞或血细胞比容值降低 20% 或以上)[232,233];或稳定 24 小时后复发性出血(定义为需要额外输血,血细胞比容值进一步降低至少 20%,或出院 1 周内因下胃肠道出血再次入院)。预测因素包括心动过速、低血压、晕厥、腹部无触痛、就诊时有直肠出血、使用阿司匹林和 2 种以上共病[244,245]。这些风险因素用于预后评分系统,确定严重下胃肠道出血风险最高的患者,占下胃肠道出血患者的 19%,可从紧急结肠镜检查中获益最大。

由 94 例因下胃肠道出血入院的患者组成的单中心病例系列[246]发现,在所有需要住院的下胃肠道出血病例中,39% 为重度,定义为患者离开急诊科后排出鲜血,并伴有低血压或心动过速,或住院期间需要输血超过 2 个单位浓缩红细胞。严重下胃肠道出血的独立风险因素为初始血细胞比容值≤35%、入院时生命体征异常(收缩压<100mmHg 或心率>100 次/min)和初始直肠检查时肉眼可见血液。

表 20.9　重度急性下胃肠道出血的临床预测评分和预后

总危险评分*	发生率	严重出血的危险	外科	死亡率	住院日	平均输血单位数(红细胞)
0	6	6	0	0	2.8	0
1~3	75	43	1.5	2.9	3.1	1
≥4	19	79	7.7	9.6	4.6	3

*风险因素(各 1 分):使用阿司匹林;2 种以上共病;心率≥100/min;腹部检查无压痛;评估的前 4 小时内直肠出血;晕厥;收缩压≤115mmHg。

严重下胃肠道出血定义为:住院前 24 小时内持续出血(输注≥2 个单位浓缩红细胞和/或血细胞比容值降低≥20%);和/或稳定 24 小时后复发性出血(需要额外输血,血细胞比容值进一步降低≥20%;或出院后 1 周内因下胃肠道出血再次入院)。

Data from Strate LL, Saltzman JR, Ookubo R, et al. Validation of a clinical prediction rule for severe acute lower intestinal bleeding. Am J Gastroenterol 2005;100:1821-7.

人工神经网络也被用于开发严重下胃肠道出血的预测模型[247,248]。但是从临床角度来看,必须输入计算机程序进行分析的大量变量限制了它们的广泛应用。

(二) 死亡率

一项美国大型数据库研究纳入了 227 000 例出院诊断为下胃肠道出血的患者,研究报告 2008 年的总死亡率为 3.9%[240]。多变量分析发现,住院死亡率的独立预测因素为年龄大于 70 岁、肠道缺血、至少 2 种共病、因不相关疾病、凝血功能障碍、血容量不足、输注浓缩红细胞和男性性别。结肠直肠息肉和痔疮与较低的死亡风险相关。本研究中确定的下胃肠道出血死亡风险较低,与来自 Kaiser San Diego(2.4%)和加州大学旧金山分校(3.2%)的小系列数据一致[235,246]。Kaiser 研究还发现院内下胃肠道出血的死亡风险增加。

(三) 诊断和治疗方法

便血患者应接受与急性胃肠道出血患者一般方法相同的病史采集、体格检查和实验室检查(见表 20.1)。病史应特别关注确定下胃肠道出血的来源。对于无痛性、严重、急性便血和有憩室病史的患者,应怀疑憩室出血,尽管缺血性结肠炎也可能是无痛性的[249]。

患者应接受医学复苏。由于下胃肠道出血的严重程度通常低于上胃肠道出血,因此可能不需要输血。大多数患者应在肠道准备后接受结肠镜检查的初步评价,尽管在选定的病例中,可进行肛门镜检查或可屈式乙状结肠镜检查,无需任何肠道清洁或在灌肠后进行。其他诊断检查包括:放射性核素出血扫描或血管造影,可用于选定病例或结肠镜检查未能发现出血源时。

1. 肛门镜检查

肛门镜检查可用于病史中怀疑有内痔出血或其他肛门直肠疾病(如肛裂、瘘管、直肠炎)的患者。对于内痔,可立即用橡皮筋结扎治疗(见第 129 章)。然而,大多数患者,特别是年龄超过 50 岁的患者,也需要进行结肠镜检查,至少是择期检查,以评价结肠的其余部分。

2. 可屈式乙状结肠镜检查

可屈式乙状结肠镜检查可评价直肠和结肠左侧的出血部

位，无需标准结肠镜肠道准备即可进行。尽管不足以评价肛管情况，但单独可屈式乙状结肠镜检查将在约 9% 的病例中得出诊断[250]。如果远端结肠可以用灌肠剂充分清洁，那么紧急可屈式乙状结肠镜检查可用于疑似患有孤立性直肠溃疡、溃疡性结肠炎、放射性直肠炎、息肉切除术后出血（直肠乙状结肠）或内痔的患者（见第 41、116、119、126、128 和 129 章）。治疗性止血可以通过注射治疗、放置止血夹、套扎或 MPEC 提供。如果未进行肠道准备，则不应使用单极电烙器（如氩等离子体凝固、圈套息肉切除术、热活检钳），以避免点燃易燃结肠气体的风险（见第 17 章）。

3. 放射性核素成像

放射性核素成像包括将放射性标记物注入患者血液中，并进行连续闪烁显像以检测放射性标记物质的局灶性聚集（见前文）。据报告，该技术检测出血的速率低至 0.04mL/min[48]，总体阳性诊断率约为 45%，定位真实出血部位的准确率为 78%[238]。放射性核素成像的缺点是延迟扫描可能会产生误导，确定出血的具体原因通常取决于内镜检查或手术。当肠腔内血液快速转运时，最有可能出现假阳性结果。因此，即使放射性标记血液起源于上胃肠道，也可在结肠中检测到。放射性核素显像可能对不明原因的胃肠道出血（见后文）或在血管造影之前有助于定位病灶，特别是在早期扫描（如注射放射性标记物后 30 分钟至 4 小时）显示红细胞外渗阳性。

4. 血管造影术

当动脉出血率至少为 0.5mL/min 时，血管造影术最有可能检测到出血部位[45]。诊断率取决于患者的选择、手术时机和血管造影医师的技能，12% 至 69% 的病例为阳性结果。血管造影术的一个优点是可以进行栓塞以控制一些出血性病变。然而，3% 的病例会发生严重并发症，包括肠缺血、血肿形成、股动脉血栓形成、造影剂过敏反应、急性肾损伤和短暂性脑缺血发作[47]。

血管造影的其他缺点是大多数患者在进行血管造影术时没有活动性出血，无法检测非出血性 SRH（NBVV，血凝块或出血斑），而且检测费用昂贵，导致在许多情况下无法确定出血部位[236,237]。

一项 11 例接受血管造影栓塞的结肠出血患者的小型回顾性病例系列报告称，10 例出血停止，7 例发生肠系膜缺血，6 例死亡[251]。另外一项研究纳入了 65 例急性下胃肠道出血患者，这些患者未接受结肠镜检查作为第一诊断步骤，发现诊断性血管造影提供的额外临床信息很少，因为大多数患者的出血自发停止。此外，血管造影术无助于指导随后的手术治疗，并且与 11% 的并发症发生率相关[252]。

5. CT 和 CT 结肠成像术

多排螺旋 CT 可以识别结肠中可能是出血来源的异常，如憩室病、结肠炎、肿块和静脉曲张。如果患者有便血伴腹痛，则常行 CT 检查。法国的一项研究报告称，CT 检查准确识别了 19 例下胃肠道出血患者中的 17 例，包括憩室、肿瘤、血管瘤和静脉曲张[253]。对于下胃肠道出血患者，多排螺旋 CT 已被证明比锝标记的红细胞扫描更准确[254]。

CT 结肠成像术越来越多地用于筛查结肠息肉和结肠癌患者，并且可能对下胃肠道出血患者有一定的辅助诊断作用（见第 127 章）。CT 结肠成像术检测大息肉（>1cm）或结肠癌，敏感性为 90%[255]。快速多排探测扫描仪还可以进行 CT 血管造影以及小肠评价。这种功能可以检测到肿块和血管病变，是 CT 血管造影术相对于其他放射成像技术的潜在优势。

多排螺旋 CT 已被推荐作为疑似结肠出血患者的早期诊断步骤，以帮助结肠镜评价[256]。由于这种方法可能使患者暴露于不必要的辐射中，并且几乎所有患者无论如何都会接受急诊或择期结肠镜检查，因此，CT 结肠成像不太可能在下胃肠道出血患者的急诊评价中发挥重要作用。而且，CT 血管造影使用的静脉造影剂可引起肾功能不全患者的急性肾损伤。

6. 结肠镜检查

快速肠道清洁后的紧急结肠镜检查已被证明是安全的，可以提供重要的诊断信息，并可同时进行治疗干预[236,237]。患者通常在 4~6 小时内口服或通过鼻胃管摄入 6~8L 聚乙二醇溶液，直至直肠排泄物中无粪便，血液和凝块。可以在肠道准备前静脉内给予 10mg 甲氧氯普胺，并每 3~4 小时重复给药一次，以促进排空并减轻恶心症状。由于高钠和磷酸盐负荷的潜在风险，对疑似下胃肠道出血的患者应避免使用磷酸钠进行肠道准备。

下胃肠道出血的紧急结肠镜检查通常在患者入院后 6~24 小时进行。大多数出血可自行停止，因而，结肠镜检查通常选择在初次住院后的第二天进行，使患者在住院第一天接受输血和肠道准备。

基于对 13 项研究的回顾性分析，通过结肠镜检查推测或明确原因的下胃肠道出血的总体发生率范围为 48%~90%，平均为 68%[238]。然而，除非发现有活动性出血、裸露血管、黏附血凝块、平坦黑色出血斑、黏膜脆性增加或溃疡等出血性征象，或可见仅限于结肠特定节段的新鲜血液存在，否则通常不可能明确诊断出血原因。

进行急诊肠道准备和结肠镜检查的最佳时间尚不清楚。理论上，越早进行内镜检查，发现可能适合内镜止血的病变（如出血性憩室、息肉出血）伴出血征象的可能性越高。然而，梅奥诊所的一项回顾性研究表明，在憩室出血患者中，内镜检查的时间（入院后 0~12 小时、12~24 小时或超过 24 小时）与发现活动性出血或其他可能提示结肠镜止血的征象无显著相关性[257]。一项前瞻性研究显示，紧急（入院后≤12 小时）和择期（入院后 36~60 小时）结肠镜检查在进一步出血、输血、住院天数或住院费用方面无差异[9]。早期结肠镜检查（入院后不久）与较短的住院时间相关，主要是因为诊断率提高而不是治疗干预[258]。

尚未对严重便血患者采用的单一治疗方法达成共识，采用的方法取决于当地的医疗资源和专业知识。在大型医疗中心，建议采用图 20.4 中详述的方法。使用急诊内镜方法进行诊断和治疗，明确和假定出血部位的诊断率超过 90%，估计直接费用明显低于择期评估相关费用[28]。

7. 钡剂灌肠

急诊钡剂灌肠检查对下胃肠道出血患者没有诊断价值。该检查很少是诊断性的，因为它不能显示血管病变，如果只看到憩室可能会产生误导。它不能检测到 50% 大于 10mm 的息肉[259]。此外，钡剂造影液可影响紧急结肠镜检查时的观察视野，使诊断更加困难，或延误其他检查如血管造影术。需要对钡灌肠中观察到的任何可疑病变或需要治疗的病变，进行结肠镜检查。

8. 外科手术的作用

下胃肠道出血患者很少需要进行外科手术治疗，因为大多数出血是自限性的，或通过药物或内镜治疗很容易得到控制。手术的主要适应证是恶性肿瘤、通过药物治疗未能停止的弥漫性出血（如缺血性结肠炎或溃疡性结肠炎），以及憩室复发性出血。目前，绝大多数患者是通过内科治疗而不是外科手术治疗。

（四）病因和管理

结肠镜检查期间可视化活动性出血的原因和处理并非总是可能的，但结肠镜检查可以识别近期出血征象（可见裸露的血管，黏附血凝块，平坦黑色出血斑），并提供有关病变部位和风险分层的信息。结肠镜检查越早进行，发现活动性出血病灶或 SRH 的概率越高。如果观察到活动性出血、裸露血管或黏附血凝块，通常可明确诊断为出血性病变。如果观察到潜在出血原因的病变，并且通过肛门镜检查和回肠末端插管的全结肠镜检查，以及在某些情况下的推进式小肠镜检查，未发现其他可能的来源时，则可以对出血原因进行推定性诊断[28]。

1. 憩室病

结肠憩室是结肠黏膜和黏膜下层通过结肠肌层形成的疝（见第 121 章）。组织病理学上，结肠憩室实际上是假性憩室，因为它们不包含结肠壁的所有结构层。当结肠组织在小动脉（直血管）的进入点被腔内压力推出时形成憩室，在那里它们穿透结肠壁的环形肌肉层。直肠血管的入口点是相对薄弱的区域，当腔内压力增加时，黏膜和黏膜下层可通过该区域疝出[261]。憩室直径从几毫米到几厘米不等，最常见于左半结肠。大多数结肠憩室无症状且并不复杂。憩室颈部或基部血管可能发生出血[261]。根据我们对确诊憩室出血病例的诊断经验（见后文），52% 的憩室出血来自基底部，48% 的憩室出血来自颈部[262]。

憩室在西方国家很常见，老年人的发病率为 50%[263]。相比之下，在非洲大陆和亚洲人群中发现憩室的比例不到 1%[264]。据推测，患病率的地区差异可能是因为西方饮食中膳食纤维含量较少（见第 121 章）。估计有 3%～5% 的憩室病患者发生憩室出血[265]。尽管大多数憩室位于左半结肠，但有一些系列研究表明，右半结肠憩室更容易出血[265,267,268]。三分之二的明确憩室出血（伴有 SRH）来自结肠脾曲区域或近端区域[262]。

应根据结肠镜检查、血管造影或外科手术的结果，对憩室出血进行仔细分类[28]。特别是对可能患有结肠憩室病的老年严重便血的患者。在结肠镜检查时发现 SRH（如活动性出血、裸露血管、黏附血凝块），或在血管造影或放射性核素成像时证实活动性出血时诊断为明确的憩室出血，随后通过结肠镜检查或手术证实该部位的憩室为出血源。当结肠检查发现无出血征象的憩室病，结肠及肛门镜检查、回肠末端检查和推进式肠镜检查均未见其他明显病变时，可诊断为假定憩室出血。当另一种病变被确定为便血的原因，并且有明显的结肠憩室病时，诊断为偶发憩室病。在一项大型前瞻性队列研究中，我们机构使用图 20.4 所示的管理方法对便血患者进行分类，52% 的病例为偶发结肠憩室，31% 的病例发生假定憩室出血，17% 的病例确定为憩室出血[237]。

憩室出血患者通常年龄较大，一直服用阿司匹林或其他 NSAID 药，表现为无痛性便血[269,270]。至少 75% 的憩室出血患者中，出血自发停止，这些患者需要输注少于 4 个单位的浓缩红细胞。在一个手术系列中，60% 的患者进行了节段性结肠切除术，尽管输注了 4 单位的血液，但大多数患者仍持续出血[267]。因出血性憩室接受切除术的患者的再出血率为 4%。在自发停止出血的患者中，结肠憩室病的再出血率在未来 4 年内报告为 25%～38%，大多数患者有轻度再出血[235,267]。然而，这些数据并非基于结肠镜下记录的憩室出血，再出血的实际发生率似乎更低。在我们小组对结肠憩室出血记录的患者进行的一项大型前瞻性队列研究中，（确定或推定）4 年内再出血的总发生率为 18%。9% 来自复发性憩室出血，9% 来自其他胃肠道来源[262]。

（1）内镜下出血征象

大约三分之一的真正的憩室出血（假定的或明确的）患者，在充分清洁肠道后进行紧急结肠镜检查时发现有近期出血征象，如活动性出血、裸露血管、黏附血凝块或单个憩室中的平坦出血斑[237,262]。如上所述，下胃肠道出血的早期结肠镜检查可能更容易发现近期出血征象，尽管梅奥诊所的一项小型病例系列研究未发现这些病灶的检出率存在任何差异，无论结肠镜检查是在 0～12 小时和 12～24 小时之间进行，或距住院时间超过 24 小时[257]。

有人主张通过应用与高危消化性溃疡出血（活动性出血、NBVV 和黏附血凝块）相同的内镜下出血征象，对憩室再出血的风险进行分层。例如，在对裸露血管的出血性溃疡切除标本进行组织病理学检查时，在一些憩室边缘发现的黑色突起是组织病理学上潜在破裂血管上的机化血凝块（图 20.19）[271]。据

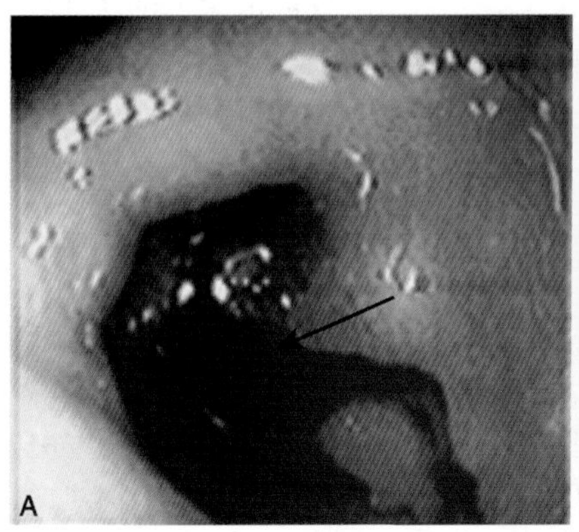

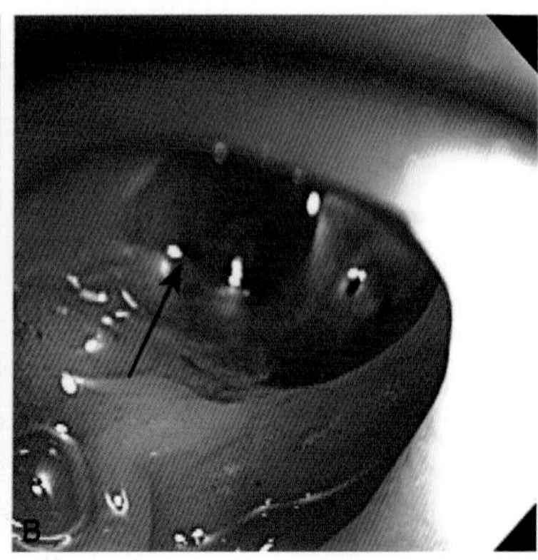

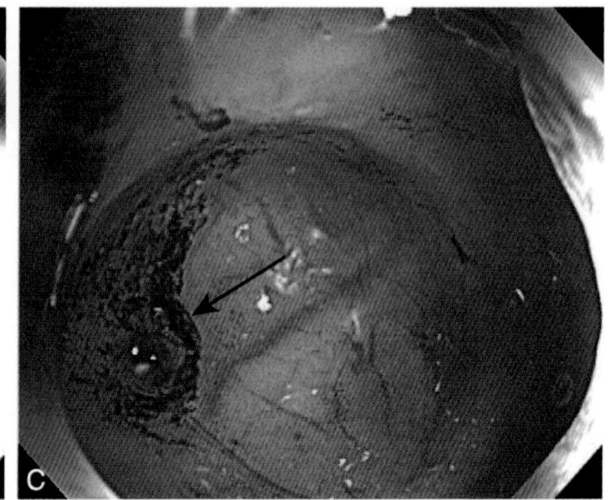

图 20.19　近期结肠憩室出血的内镜下特征。A，活动性出血（箭）。B，黏附血凝块（箭）。C，可见裸露血管（箭）

报道，与这些出血征象相关的短期自然史与消化性溃疡出血相关的征象相似[272]。憩室活动性出血的药物治疗患者中，83%(15/18)再次出血，56% 需要介入(手术或血管造影栓塞)止血。在单腔憩室 NBVV 患者中，再出血率为 60%，止血干预率为 40%。在药物治疗的黏附血凝块患者中，再出血率为 43%，介入率为 29%。对于具有这些高危风险因素的 37 例患者，药物治疗的再出血率为 65%，干预率为 43%。这些再出血和干预率比消化性溃疡出血更差，因为没有类似于 PPI 的药物可用于降低高危 SRH 患者的再出血风险。

UCLA CURE 使用 DEP 止血研究在 91% 的严重 SRH(活动性出血、NBVV 或黏附血凝块)的患者中检测到潜在血流，但在没有这些征象的患者中没有检测到。DEP 还用于紧急结肠镜检查出血期间，憩室平坦黑色出血斑患者的风险分层，并作为 SRH 患者止血完整性的指南[273]。在 DEP 引导下闭塞血流，30 天内再出血率低于 5%[272,273]。

(2) 内镜下止血

据报道，可使用 MPEC、肾上腺素注射液、止血夹、纤维蛋白胶、橡皮筋结扎、圈套器或联合肾上腺素注射和 MPEC 或止血夹进行结肠镜下止血[28,271,274-278]。如果在结肠局灶节段观察到新鲜血液，应用水大力冲洗该段肠管，以清除血液并识别潜在的出血部位。如果出血来自憩室边缘或在边缘观察到黑色突起，可使用硬化治疗针在出血周围的 4 个象限内，黏膜下注射 1mL 等份的肾上腺素(在盐水中以 1∶20 000 稀释)。随后，可在低功率设置(10~15W)和轻压下进行 1 秒脉冲持续时间的 MPEC，以烧灼憩室边缘并止血或使裸露血管变平，或者可以应用止血夹。非出血性黏附血凝块可在 4 个象限内注射 1∶20 000 肾上腺素，每象限 1mL，之后用冷息肉圈套器将血凝块剪碎，直至延伸到憩室上方 3mm。潜在的出血征象可以用 MPEC 或止血夹治疗(见前文)。

在内镜下完成出血憩室的止血后，应在病灶周围放置永久性黏膜下标记，以便在复查结肠镜或手术治疗复发出血时进行部位识别。结肠镜止血后，应告知患者避免服用阿司匹林和其他 NSAID 药物，并长期服用纤维素补充剂。

2000 年，Jensen 和 UCLA CURE 小组公布了他们在紧急结肠镜检查中，对严重憩室出血的诊断和治疗的结果[28]，报告称 20% 的严重便血患者有内镜下病灶，疑似明确的憩室出血。这组患者，接受结肠镜下止血，再出血率为 0%，急诊部分结肠切除率为 0%。而有高风险征象但未接受结肠镜下止血的历史对照组患者，再出血率分别为 53% 和 35%。结肠镜下止血患者随访 3 年未再出血。

在 UCLA CURE 研究组的另一份报告中，63 例确诊憩室出血的患者接受了内镜止血治疗，再出血率为 4.8%，再出血的手术或血管造影栓塞率仅为 3.2%[273]。研究人员注射肾上腺素和使用止血夹治疗憩室底部 SRH(在出血征象两侧阻断潜在的动脉血流)，或憩室颈部注射肾上腺素及 MPEC 治疗。憩室 SRH 约 50% 位于颈部，50% 位于底部；超过 55% 的憩室伴 SRH 见于在脾曲或脾曲近端。通过治疗后无血流的 DEP 记录完全止血，无血流与无再出血相关。2012 年日本的一项研究中，87 例因急性出血在憩室口放置止血夹的患者，早期再出血率为 34%，大部分再出血事件发生在位于升结肠的憩室[279]。该研究中的高再出血率可以用结肠憩室的血管解剖结构和远离位于憩室底部的 SRH 放置止血夹来解释。由于憩室内存在双向动脉血流和 2 条不同动脉的拱形结构，当 SRH 位于底部时，在憩室颈部使用止血夹进行治疗，不会在出血征象下方封闭动脉，因此，预计再出血率较高。该研究中的急性再出血率[279]与 UCLA CURE 自然史报告中药物治疗患者的急性再出血率相似，其中 65% 的患者再次出血，43% 的患者需要手术或介入放射学治疗[272]。

内镜下套扎术也有治疗结肠憩室出血的报道。2012 年来自日本的一项 29 例患者的研究显示，套扎术是成功和安全的，早期再出血率为 11%，仅一例升结肠憩室出血的患者需要手术切除[280]。然而，由于右侧结肠存在厚壁完全被套入的潜在风险，可能会增加穿孔的风险[281]。套扎术后也有憩室炎的报道。在一项日本的研究中报告，套扎术的再出血率低于止血夹[282]，但是许多患者接受了远程止血夹治疗，即当出血点在憩室底部时，在颈部放置止血夹以闭合憩室。

(3) 血管造影和外科手术

血管造影可在选定的憩室出血病例中进行，但存在肠道血管阻塞、造影剂反应和急性肾损伤的风险。一项研究发现，手术切除前常规血管造影无助于降低并发症的总体风险[252]。

憩室出血很少需要手术治疗，反复出现的憩室出血可以考虑手术。手术决策最好在结肠镜检查、血管造影或放射性核素成像的指导下进行，探明出血可能来自的结肠段，以及相关合并症。在无严重 SRH 的患者憩室出血通常较轻。老年患者手术并发症的风险增加。如果可能，应避免盲法结肠次全切除术，通常是在过去无法确定明确的出血部位时。

2. 结肠炎

结肠炎是指任何形式的结肠炎症。严重下胃肠道出血可能由缺血性结肠炎、IBD 或感染性结肠炎引起。

缺血性结肠炎可表现为无痛或疼痛性的便血，伴有轻度左侧腹部不适(见第 118 章)。无痛亚型通常由黏膜缺氧所致，被认为是肠壁壁内血管灌注不足引起的，而不是由大血管闭塞或栓塞所致。后者常有腹部疼痛，临床上症状更严重，预后更差。估计缺血性结肠炎的发病率为(4.5~44 例)/(100 000 人·年)[283]。大多数病例没有明确的原因。

据报道，与缺血性结肠炎相关的风险因素包括高龄、休克、心血管手术、心力衰竭、慢性阻塞性肺疾病、回肠造口术、结肠癌、腹部手术、肠易激综合征、便秘、使用泻药、口服避孕药和使用 H_2RA[283-286]。肠系膜上动脉向右半结肠(盲肠、升结肠、肝曲、近端横结肠和中段横结肠)供血，而肠系膜下动脉向左半结肠供血(远端横结肠、脾曲、降结肠、乙状结肠和直肠)。结肠血供丰富，但肠系膜上、下动脉之间的分水岭区域侧支血管最少，发生缺血的风险最大。结肠正常接受心输出量的 10%~35%，如果血流量减少 50% 以上可发生缺血。虽然缺血最易发生在脾曲分水岭区，但也可发生在结肠的任何部位[287]。

缺血的诊断通常是通过结肠镜检查作出的，但在大血管缺血的严重病例中，X 线平片上可注意到“拇指印征”或 CT 片上结肠壁增厚。结肠镜下黏膜外观包括红斑、脆性和渗液。黏膜活检标本可能提示缺血性改变，但通常用于排除感染性或克罗恩结肠病。缺血性结肠炎通常在几天内消退，一般不需要结肠镜下止血或抗生素治疗。在 UCLA CURE 经验中，约10%的缺血性结肠炎和严重便血患者发生局灶性溃疡，在紧急结肠镜检查时主要提示出血征象的溃疡[288]。经DEP探测动脉血流后，这种病例推荐的治疗方法与其他溃疡治疗相似，用肾上腺素黏膜下注射治疗和血管夹夹闭。Kaiser的一个大型回顾性临床研究显示，4年随访期内未发生缺血性结肠炎再出血事件[235]。另一方面，肠系膜大血管缺血患者预后通常较差，包括更高的再出血、穿孔、手术和死亡的发生率。

累及结肠的IBD很少引起重度急性下胃肠道出血(见第115章)。在梅奥(Mayo)诊所的一个病例系列中，这些患者中的大多数患有克罗恩病，并且大多数得到了成功的药物治疗[289]。该系列31例患者中的3例，接受了单独肾上腺素注射或MPEC内镜治疗黏附血凝块或渗血性溃疡。这3例患者无再出血，但其他28例患者中有23%在初次出血后中位时间3天(1~75天)发生再出血，39%的严重出血患者最终需要手术治疗。

任何患有严重下胃肠道出血和结肠炎的患者都应排除感染性结肠炎(见第110和112章)。由空肠弯曲杆菌、沙门氏菌、志贺氏菌、肠出血性大肠埃希菌(O157:H7)、巨细胞病毒或艰难梭菌引起的感染可发生下胃肠道出血。除严重凝血功能障碍患者外，严重失血罕见。通过粪便培养和可屈式乙状结肠镜检查或结肠镜检查进行诊断。治疗采用药物治疗，抗生素的使用取决于致病微生物。内镜治疗一般对感染性结肠炎无作用。

3. 息肉切除术

大约1%的结肠镜息肉切除术后发生无痛性出血。最常见于息肉切除术后5~7天，但可发生于术后1~14天的任何时间。一般为自限性，轻度至中度出血，50%~75%的患者需要输血[290-293]。报告的息肉切除术后出血的风险因素包括大息肉(>2cm)、粗蒂、无蒂类型、位于右半结肠、使用抗凝剂和使用阿司匹林或另一种NSAID药物。在息肉切除术后严重迟发性出血患者的紧急结肠镜检查过程中，通常在息肉切除部位发现具有出血征象的溃疡(图20.20)。在溃疡中发现SRH的严重出血患者中[294,295]，可使用DEP检测潜在的动脉血流和内镜止血需求。息肉切除术后迟发性出血的内镜治疗技术取决于发现的出血征象，与用于消化性溃疡出血的内镜治疗方法相似，包括肾上腺素注射、热凝固、放置止血夹和联合治疗。息肉切除术后溃疡中的大多数主要SRH均采用止血夹治疗(注射或不注射肾上腺素)，因为止血夹不会造成如热凝固所见的组织损伤。

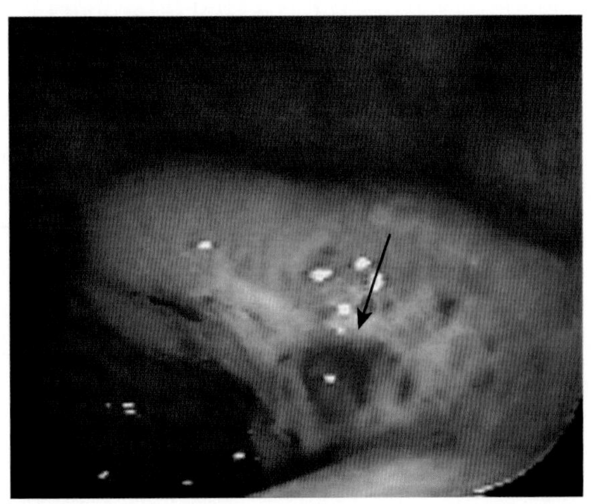

图20.20　结肠息肉切除术后出血的内镜表现。大的带蒂息肉圈套切除术后7天发生出血。注意溃疡息肉切除部位的未出血的裸露血管(箭)

4. 结肠肿瘤

结肠息肉和癌症患者可出现急性便血。通常，这些患者在发生更明显的出血之前，有与缓慢胃肠失血一致的小细胞低色素性缺铁性贫血(见后文)。在大型CURE系列研究中，结肠肿瘤是严重便血的第八大常见原因[296]。结肠镜检查时，可将肾上腺素注射到病变中以减缓活动性出血，可应用止血夹治疗内镜下无法切除的溃疡病变上的SRH。在确定性治疗前，止血粉可能对减少急性出血具有姑息治疗作用(见前文)[43]。如有可能，可切除结肠息肉止血。通常需要手术切除以防止大的、溃疡型无蒂病灶再出血(见第126和127章)。然而，大多数结肠息肉或癌症和严重便血患者的疾病分期较晚，早期死亡率较高，应考虑非手术治疗[296]。

5. 放射性直肠炎

放射性直肠炎通常引起轻度慢性便血，但偶尔可引起急性严重的下胃肠道出血。当用于治疗妇科盆腔肿瘤、前列腺、膀胱或直肠肿瘤时，电离辐射可对正常结肠和直肠黏膜造成急性和慢性损伤(见第41章)。在接受4 000cGy放射剂量的患者中，大约75%的患者发生急性自限性腹泻、里急后重、腹部绞痛和罕见的出血，持续数周。慢性辐射效应发生在治疗完成后6~18个月，表现为鲜红色血液样排便。慢性辐射引起的肠道损伤与血管损伤有关，随后出现黏膜缺血、增厚和溃疡。这种损伤大部分被认为是由慢性缺血缺氧和氧化应激导致的。

可屈式乙状结肠镜检查或结肠镜检查可发现直肠内毛细血管扩张、质脆、有时有溃疡(图20.21)。常见渗血，也常见其他非出血性直肠毛细血管扩张症。内痔也经常被看到，并经常被那些不熟悉放射性毛细血管扩张的人误诊为直肠出血的原因。

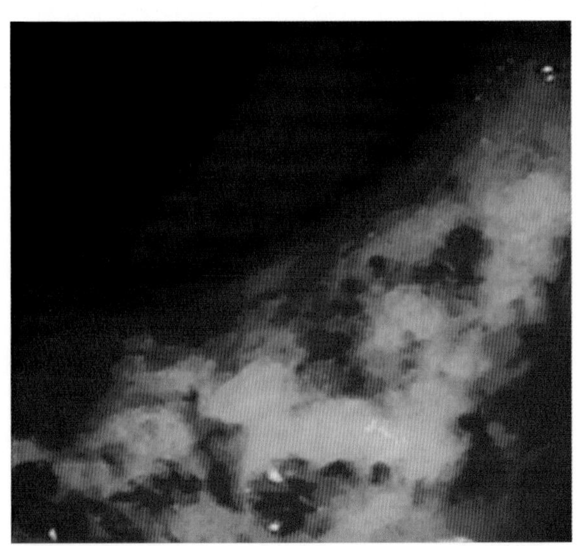

图20.21　放射性直肠炎的内镜表现。可见弥漫性渗出和毛细血管扩张

最初的治疗重点是避免使用阿司匹林和其他 NSAID 药物,食用高纤维饮食,如果患者贫血,应补充铁剂治疗。可以局部使用或口服 5-氨基水杨酸(美沙拉秦)、硫糖铝或糖皮质激素的药物治疗,但通常无效[297]。热凝通常是有效的,但可能需要重复应用 MPEC 或氩等离子体凝固治疗以获得良好疗效[289]。局部福尔马林直接用于直肠黏膜可以减少出血[299],使用高压氧治疗也可以减少出血[300]。也有报道使用抗氧化维生素,如维生素 E 和 C,可以减少慢性放射性直肠炎的出血(见第 41 章)[301]。

6. 结肠血管扩张

结肠血管扩张出血,是老年人下胃肠道出血的一个重要原因,在小肠和不明原因出血章节中讨论。当血管扩张是结肠出血的原因时,病变通常是多发的,使得内镜止血成为一个挑战(见第 38 章)。

7. 内痔

痔疮出血是无痛的,其特征是经直肠排出鲜红色血液,可附着在粪便的表面,滴入马桶内,擦拭后可见在纸巾上,常在马桶内出现大量的新鲜血液。通常出血是轻度的、间歇性和自限性的,但偶尔也会出现需要输血的重度出血[302]。在一项对便血出院患者的大型研究中,20% 被认为是痔疮出血[240]。在因重度便血(见前文)住院的 UCLA CURE 系列患者中,内痔是第二大常见的原因(见表 20.8)[237]。在结肠清洁准备后,通过紧急肛门镜检查和结肠镜检查记录了 237 例痔疮。可通过肛门镜、乙状结肠镜或结肠镜检查进行诊断。

内痔的治疗通常从补充纤维剂、大便软化剂、润滑直肠栓剂(含或不含糖皮质激素)和温热坐浴等药物治疗开始。也可以使用肛门镜治疗,包括注射硬化治疗、橡皮筋结扎、冷冻手术、红外光凝固术、MPEC 和直流电凝等。虽然大多数轻度痔疮出血患者对药物治疗有反应,但严重或复发性出血患者可能需要橡皮筋结扎或其他一些内镜治疗,或如果这些措施失败,则需要手术治疗(见第 129 章)。

8. 肛裂

肛裂患者通常表现为便秘,随后排便疼痛伴或不伴便血。便血通常为轻度,擦拭时可观察到。罕见情况下,便血为中度至重度。治疗的重点是愈合肛裂,而不是采用特异性止血技术。外用钙通道阻滞剂(如 2% 地尔硫䓬乳膏)和纤维补充剂、大便软化剂加坐浴控制便秘,可治愈大多数肛裂(见第 129 章)。

9. 直肠静脉曲张

门静脉高压症患者直肠黏膜在痔上静脉(门静脉循环)和痔中下静脉(体循环)之间可发生异位静脉曲张。在乙状结肠镜检查中,反转镜身可见直肠静脉曲张,静脉结构位于齿状线上方几厘米处并延伸至直肠。它们与内痔不同。直肠静脉曲张的发生概率随门静脉高压程度的增加而增加。大约 60% 有食管静脉曲张出血史的患者有直肠静脉曲张,但它们是严重便血的罕见原因[27,230,294]。直肠静脉曲张出血的治疗与食管静脉曲张相似,可采用硬化疗法、套扎术或门体分流术(见第 92 章)[303-305]。

10. 直肠 Dieulafoy 病变

Dieulafoy 病变是黏膜下大的动脉,其上无覆盖的黏膜溃疡,可引起大出血。它们可发生在胃肠道的任何部位,但通常发生在前肠(见前文)。直肠出血性 Dieulafoy 病变,已通过内镜止血成功治疗,已在几份报告中描述[179,306]。

11. 直肠溃疡

几个病例系列描述了位于齿状线上 3~10cm 的孤立或多发性直肠溃疡,突发无痛性严重便血的重症住院患者。在来自台湾的 19 例病例系列中,2.7% 评估为严重便血的患者,被诊断为急性出血性直肠溃疡综合征[307]。患者的平均年龄为 71 岁。在出血发生前 3 至 14 天(平均 7.5 天)因其他医学问题住院。所有患者均出现低血压,需要转入 ICU 并输血。结肠镜检查发现位于距齿状线 1~7cm 的多发性和孤立性溃疡病例数相等,溃疡多较大(1cm 以上),外观呈圆周状或地图状。患者接受了热凝固、注射治疗和缝合结扎的联合治疗,由于多器官衰竭,死亡率为 26%。病变的病理学显示坏死提示存在黏膜缺血,如胃应激性溃疡所见(见前文)。这种疾病似乎与直肠溃疡综合征、深囊性结肠炎、感染性溃疡、放射性溃疡、NSAID 溃疡或便秘引起的粪石性溃疡不同,可被认为是直肠应激性溃疡的一种类型,与住院病情严重患者的十二指肠溃疡相类似(见第 128 章)。

在 UCLA CURE 研究中,孤立性或多发性无痛性直肠溃疡,是住院患者发生严重便血的第三大常见原因(见表 20.8)。与孤立性直肠溃疡综合征相反,它们发生在严重便秘老年患者、ICU 患者和卧床不起的人中。结肠镜检查,溃疡呈慢性、大的、单发或多发。他们往往患有 SRH,可以在内镜下进行治疗(图 20.22)[308]。住院患者直肠溃疡所致便血的再出血率高于在家中治疗出血者。对于大的质硬有红斑的溃疡急性止血,推荐使用 OTSC 血管夹治疗。

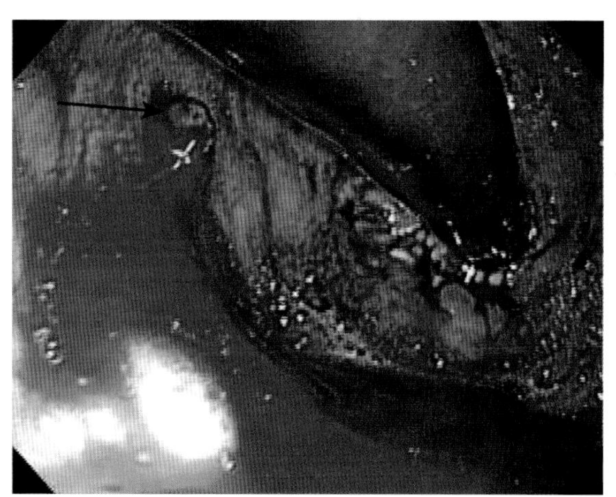

图 20.22 内镜下见直肠孤立性溃疡出血,反转镜身可见血管(箭)

四、不明原因显性胃肠道出血

不明原因胃肠道出血传统上定义为非诊断性 EGD、结肠镜检查断和钡剂小肠随访后原因不明的胃肠道出血[309]。不明原因胃肠道出血可能有显性或隐匿性表现。不明原因的显性胃肠道出血是指在非诊断性 EGD、结肠镜检查和小肠检查的患者中,可见的急性胃肠道出血(如黑便、褐红色便、便血),不明原因的隐匿性胃肠道出血是指粪便潜血试验阳性,通常与不明原因的缺铁性贫血有关。在大多数大型系列中，5%的显性胃肠道出血住院患者在EGD和结肠镜检查未发现出血原因。在这些患者中，75%的出血部位位于小肠。

在不明原因胃肠道出血患者中，存在以下可能性：①病变在标准内镜和结肠镜可触及范围内，但未被识别为出血部位（如Cameron病变、血管扩张、内痔）；②病变在内镜和结肠镜可及范围内，但难以显示（例如，血凝块遮挡病变的可视化；低血容量患者静脉曲张变得不明显；病变隐藏在黏膜皱褶后面）或表现为间歇性出血（如Dieulafoy病变、血管扩张）；③病变位于标准内镜无法触及的小肠（如肿瘤、血管扩张、Meckel憩室）。在几个系列中，发现转诊至三级医疗中心进行不明原因出血评估的50%或更多患者的病变在标准内镜可触及范围内（即造成出血的遗漏病变或难以看见的病变）[310]。

在无低血压的复发性严重不明原因的便血患者中，应怀疑结肠来源，有经验的内镜医师有必要进行重复结肠镜检查，并进行良好的结肠准备。应考虑可先出血后停止的结肠病变，如憩室病或痔疮。在复发性重度黑便的患者中，应考虑使用推进式肠镜检查，重新检查食管、胃和十二指肠以及近端空肠是否存在遗漏或未识别的病变。十二指肠镜检查可用于十二指肠第二至第四部分的出血或病变。

一旦确定上胃肠道或下胃肠道道的出血性病变没有遗漏，则应将评价重点集中在小肠。过去，小肠的主要成像模式是钡剂造影，但该技术受到小肠长度、移动性、运动性以及肠袢覆盖的限制。由于小肠出血常为间歇性，放射性核素显像或血管造影在诊断评价中的价值有限。自20世纪90年代末以来，用于评估小肠的选项已经大大扩展了，并且由于新的小肠成像技术的发展而发生了革命性变化，包括无线视频胶囊内镜、深部小肠镜检查和CT小肠成像，与过去相比，现在可以实现更大的可视化和更多的治疗选择（见后文）[311]。

（一）病因

许多病变可引起不明原因的胃肠道出血（框20.2）。在年龄小于40岁的人群中，出血更可能是由于肿瘤、Meckel憩室或克罗恩病引起。血管扩张症或NSAID诱导的溃疡是40岁及以上人群患者的常见原因。

框20.2 不明原因的胃肠道出血*

上胃肠道	Meckel憩室
Cameron病变	肿瘤
Dieulafoy病变	胰腺或胆道疾病
胃窦血管扩张症（GAVE）	溃疡
小肠	**结肠**
血管扩张	血管扩张
主动脉肠瘘	憩室病
Dieulafoy病变	痔疮
憩室病	

*排除上胃肠道出血常见原因后。

1. 血管扩张

多种血管病变可能引起胃肠道出血（见第38章）。血管扩张，也称血管发育不良，是随着年龄增长在整个胃肠道中发现的异常血管形成。病变与先天性动静脉畸形（arteriovenous malformation，AVM）和肿瘤性血管瘤不同。毛细血管扩张是由于血管终末端扩张所致的病变。任何血管病变都可导致成人显性或隐性胃肠道出血，尤其是老年人和服用抗血小板和抗凝药物的患者。获得性血管病变（血管扩张和毛细血管扩张）与各种疾病有关，如慢性肾病、肝硬化、风湿病和重度心脏病[57]。虽然血管扩张可表现为显性出血，但常表现为隐匿性出血或缺铁性贫血。最常见的出血部位是结肠和小肠。

结肠血管扩张的组织病理学表现为扩张的黏膜下静脉[312,313]。血管扩张在结肠中的形成机制是，在肌肉收缩和盲肠膨胀过程中，黏膜下静脉的部分、间歇性、轻度阻塞导致黏膜下静脉扩张和迂曲。随着时间的推移，压力的增加还会导致黏膜血管的小静脉、毛细血管和动脉扩张。最后，毛细血管前括约肌可能出现功能不全，从而导致动静脉交通发展，并可能导致局部黏膜缺血。由于血管扩张可发生在胃肠道的其他部位，因此推测了其他形成机制，包对黏膜刺激或局部缺血的反应，如放疗后发生的反应。

大多数血管扩张发生在60岁以上的患者中，可累及胃肠道的任何节段。通常，病变在特定肠段多发。大约20%（可能更多）的患者在胃肠道的至少2个部位有血管扩张[314,315]。

在接受结肠镜检查的无症状者的研究中，发现血管扩张占1%～3%[316,317]。在这些人中，血管扩张主要发生在右半结肠，分布如下：盲肠，37%；升结肠，17%；横结肠，7%；降结肠，7%；乙状结肠，18%；直肠，14%。在偶然发现结肠血管扩张的无症状患者中，3年随访期间未发生出血。

几种情况似乎与血管扩张频率增加有关。慢性肾病和尿毒症患者肠道血管扩张的发生率增加。一项在患有和未患有慢性肾病的不明原因胃肠道出血患者中进行的研究发现，血管扩张是47%的假定来源，与之相比，在未患有肾病的胃肠道出血患者中为18%[318]。慢性肾脏病患者血管扩张出血的风险增加可能与尿毒症诱导的血小板功能障碍有关。

血管性血友病（Von Willebrand病）（先天性或后天性）也与出血性血管扩张相关[319]。血管性血友病因子是血小板有效聚集所必需的。一项对照良好的前瞻性研究发现，几乎所有上胃肠道出血和结肠血管扩张患者，相对于非出血性血管扩张或出血性憩室病，都患有获得性血管假性血友病。与最大形式的血管假性血友病因子选择性丢失以及主动脉瓣狭窄相关[320]。由于大的血管假性血友病多聚体促进以高剪切力为特征的微循环中的初次止血，如发生在血管扩张中，大多聚体的缺失可解释为什么一些血管扩张患者会发生出血。

主动脉瓣狭窄与血管扩张引起的胃肠道出血相关（Heyde综合征）[321]。这种关联是存在争议的，因为这两种情况都很常见，关联可能并不意味着因果关系[322]。然而，67%～92%的患者由于机械因素，主动脉瓣狭窄与获得性血管性血友病相关。在通过狭窄主动脉瓣的过程中，破坏血管性血友病蛋白，而获得性血管性血友病又增加了血管扩张出血的风险[323,324]。Sev-eral系列报告了主动脉瓣置换术后血管扩张导致的出血停止，尽管血管扩张持续存在。但该观察结果与假设一致，即出血是血管假性血友病因子受损的结果，在主动脉瓣置换术后恢复正常[325]。

使用左心室辅助装置的患者中大约 20% 发生显性或不明原因的胃肠道出血，特别是老年患者，血管扩张是最常见的出血原因之一[326-328]。血管扩张形成和出血的可能病理生理机制包括与剪切应力相关的血管性血友病因子的丢失（导致血小板聚集受损），以及与管腔压力增加和脉压降低相关的肠灌注不足[328]。由于许多老年人因肠血管扩张出血而有心血管疾病，但没有严重的主动脉瓣狭窄，其他心血管疾病如轻至中度主动脉瓣狭窄、主动脉硬化、肥厚型心肌病和外周血管疾病可能导致足够高的剪切应力来破坏血管性血友病因子，并导致出血性血管扩张[325]。

在内镜下，血管扩张症表现为 2~10mm 的红色病变，有分枝扩张的血管从中央血管（图 20.23）。使用内镜探头对血管扩张施加压力可能导致病变变白。一项研究表明，在内镜检查过程中使用麻醉剂对患者进行镇静，会因为一过性黏膜或黏膜下灌注不足而使血管扩张可视化变得困难，这会导致充盈减少或引起血管收缩，而使用阿片类拮抗剂纳洛酮逆转会使血管扩张更加明显[329]。然而在实践中，这种手法在临床上不太可能有用，可能使患者更加不舒服。

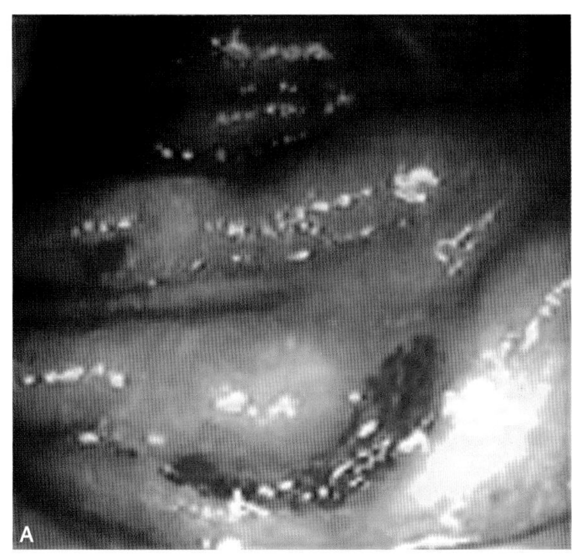

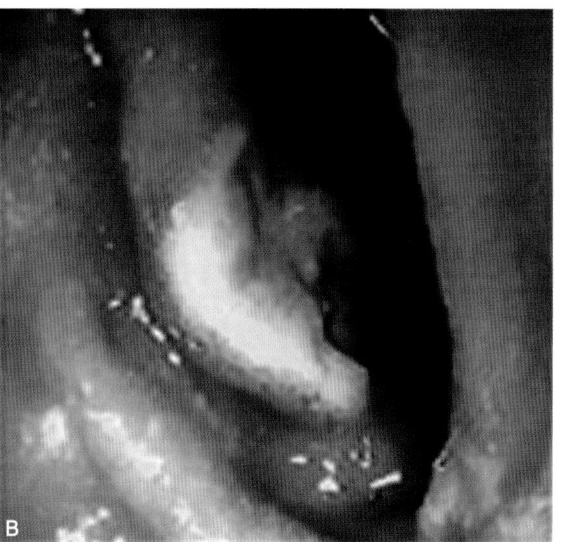

图 20.23　多极探头电凝之前（A）和之后（B）的空肠血管扩张的内镜表现

血管扩张可以通过各种方式进行内镜治疗，包括肾上腺素注射、热探头凝固、氩等离子体凝固、止血夹和套扎术。考虑到受影响患者的异质性和出血的间歇性性质，评估疗效可能很困难。在一个 16 例因血管扩张而需要输血的患者的系列研究发现，无论是手术治疗、内镜治疗还是单纯输血治疗，持续出血的频率（50%）没有差异，推测是因为弥漫性血管扩张[330]。在另一项研究中，33 例缺铁性贫血和推进式小肠镜检查可见小肠血管扩张的患者在内镜治疗后 1 年，在大多数患者中未发现临床或内镜检查结果的变化[331]。相比之下，在另一项对疑似小肠血管扩张引起胃肠道出血的患者进行的研究中，与单独观察相比，电凝治疗使其输血需求显著降低（但未消除）[332]。在一项双气囊小肠镜的初探性研究中，对大约一半的血管扩张患者进行了内镜治疗，治疗和未治疗患者在随访期间的再出血率相似[333]。

在一个小的病例系列中，雌激素治疗被认为对控制慢性肾病患者毛细血管扩张症出血有益[334]。病例报告表明，雌激素也可减少遗传性出血性毛细血管扩张症（HHT）[Osler-Weber-Rendu 病）（见后文）]和血管性血友病患者的出血。然而，一项涉及 72 例患者的多中心随机对照试验发现，雌激素-孕酮联合治疗组与安慰剂组的再出血率无差异，分别为 39% 和 46%[335]。因此，不推荐常规使用激素治疗血管扩张出血。

沙利度胺是一种血管生成抑制剂，可能对选定的血管畸形患者有效。一项在血管发育不良或 GAVE 患者中，比较沙利度胺与口服铁剂治疗的随机试验显示，沙利度胺治疗患者的出血事件、输血次数和住院次数以及血管内皮生长因子水平显著降低[336]。然而在这些数据得到证实之前，考虑到沙利度胺可能发生严重的副作用（包括出生缺陷），使用沙利度胺需要谨慎。

大多数间歇性出血的胃肠道血管扩张患者除了内镜止血外还需要药物治疗。应避免或至少尽量减少可加重慢性低水平出血的药物（特别是阿司匹林、其他非甾体抗炎药、华法林、其他抗血小板药物如氯吡格雷和直接作用的口服抗凝剂）。许多患者可通过长期服用铁剂（口服或静脉注射）进行治疗，偶尔尽管持续出血，但肾功能不全患者也可能需要注射促红细胞生成素以维持足够的红细胞计数。

2. 遗传性出血性毛细血管扩张症

遗传性出血性毛细血管扩张症（HHT），也称为 Osler-Weber-Rendu 病，是一种以弥漫性毛细血管扩张和大的 AVM 为特征的遗传性疾病（另见第 38 和 85 章）。最显著的临床特征是嘴唇、口腔黏膜和指尖的毛细血管扩张。此外，高达三分之一的患者患有肺、肝或脑动静脉畸形（见第 85 章）。患者通常表现为复发性严重鼻出血、胃肠道出血和缺铁性贫血。通常因鼻出血，而不是胃肠道出血，会引起更严重的失血和贫血。由于栓塞性卒中或与肺和脑 AVM 相关的脑脓肿，HHT 常可危及生命。HHT 症状一般在儿童期或成年早期出现。

HHT 为常染色体显性遗传，表型表达不一。至少 4 个基因[*ENG*（编码内皮糖蛋白、1 型 HHT 或 HHT1）、*ALK-1*（编码激活素受体样激酶 1、2 型 HHT 或 HHT2）、*SMAD4* 和 *HHT3*]

发生突变,编码维持血管内皮完整性所需的蛋白质,这些蛋白质的缺陷允许 AVM 的形成。

HHT 的诊断基于 4 个标准:①自发性和复发性鼻出血;②多发性皮肤黏膜毛细血管扩张;③内脏动静脉畸形(胃肠道、肺、脑、肝);④一级亲属患有 HHT[337]。检测 *ENG*、*ALK-1* 或 *SMAD4* 基因突变的基因检测可能对选定的病例有帮助。疑似 HHT 的患者应接受脑和肺动静脉畸形筛查,患者的家庭成员应考虑基因检测。

毛细血管扩张可发生于 HHT 患者小肠中的任何部位。在一个病例系列中,对 32 例 HHT 患者和 48 例非 HHT 患者进行了胶囊内镜检查,对小肠出血进行了评价,发现 81% 的 HHT 患者出现小肠毛细血管扩张,而非 HHT 的患者为 29%[338]。毛细血管扩张症在整个小肠中均匀分布,但所有活动性出血病变均见于十二指肠或近端空肠,且在标准推进式肠镜可触及的范围内。5 支或 5 支以上毛细血管扩张的检出诊断 HHT 的敏感性为 75%,阳性预测值为 86%。

HHT 的治疗通常注重控制急性出血(鼻出血和胃肠道出血)、预防再出血和治疗贫血(补充铁剂)。胃肠道出血患者应接受内镜检查(或推进式肠镜检查)和结肠镜检查,以发现可能出血的任何胃肠道病变。局灶性胃肠道出血可通过内镜下凝固治疗。激素治疗也被报告为 HHT 小肠出血的治疗方法[339]。对于症状性或大的脑或肺动静脉畸形患者,应考虑对这些病变进行放射学栓塞治疗(见第 38 章)。

3. 蓝色橡皮疱痣综合征

蓝色橡皮疱痣综合征是一种罕见的综合征,以于皮肤、软组织和胃肠道静脉畸形为特征[340,341]。出血通常发生在儿童期,并持续到成年期,导致需要补充铁剂和输血的慢性铁缺乏。在内镜检查时,病变表现为大的隆起性息肉样蓝色静脉泡,可发生在胃肠道的任何部位,尤其是小肠和结肠,可以通过内镜下套扎术或手术切除治疗(见第 38 章)。

4. Meckel 憩室

Meckel 憩室(梅克尔憩室)是一种先天性、盲性肠袋,由妊娠期间卵黄管不完全闭塞所致(见第 98 章)[342]。Meckel 憩室的特征已被"2 的规则"描述:它们发生在 2% 的人群中,在回盲瓣的 2 英尺(约 0.61m)内发现,长 2 英寸(约 5.1cm),导致 2% 的病例出现并发症,憩室内有 2 种类型的异位组织(胃和胰腺),临床上最常见于 2 岁(与肠梗阻有关),且男女之比超过 2∶1。Meckel 憩室最常见的并发症是出血、梗阻和憩室炎,可发生于儿童或成人。出血性憩室的组织病理学评价显示异位胃黏膜,可导致高达 75% 的患者出现酸分泌和溃疡。Meckel 憩室的诊断试验是 ^{99m}Tc-高锝酸盐扫描(Meckel 扫描),因为高锝酸盐对胃黏膜具有亲和力。Meckel 扫描具有较高的特异性(几乎 100%)和阳性预测价值,但在憩室不含异位胃黏膜的患者中,25%~50% 可为阴性[343]。在试验前给予 H_2RA 24~48 小时,可提高 Meckel 扫描的准确性。Meckel 憩室也可通过 CT 肠造影、胶囊式内镜和双气囊肠镜检查(通过口腔或直肠途径)确诊。

5. NSAID 诱导的小肠糜烂和溃疡

在使用全剂量非选择性 NSAID 的患者中,25%~55% 的患者在胶囊式内镜检查中观察到黏膜糜烂或溃疡[344-348]。服用选择性 COX-2 抑制剂的患者,在胶囊式内镜检查中黏膜溃疡发生率较低(见第 119 章)。

6. 小肠肿瘤

小肠肿瘤仅占所有胃肠道肿瘤的 5%~7%,是 50 岁以下患者不明原因胃肠道出血的最常见原因[349]。最常见的小肠肿瘤是腺瘤(通常是十二指肠)、腺癌(图 20.24)、类癌(通常是回肠)、胃肠道间质瘤(GIST)\淋巴瘤\错构瘤性息肉(黑斑息肉综合征)和幼年性息肉(见第 32~34、125 和 126 章)。

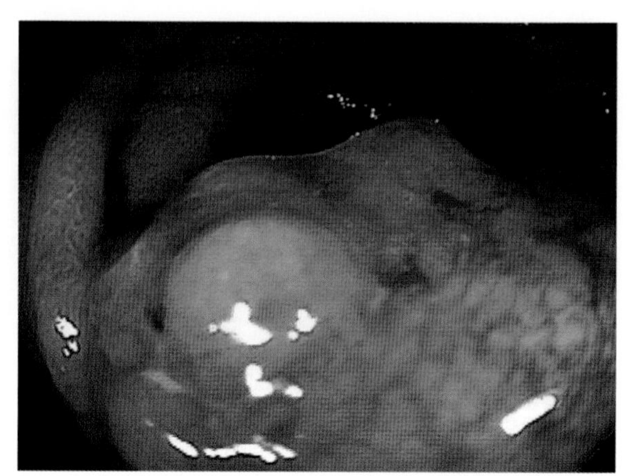

图 20.24　在一例有遗传性非息肉性结直肠癌病史并有不明原因显性胃肠道出血的患者中,通过深部肠镜检查发现了回肠腺癌。该病变最初在胶囊式内镜研究中可视化

7. 小肠憩室

十二指肠是小肠憩室最常见的部位。在一个大型系列中[350] 79% 的小肠憩室发生在十二指肠,18% 发生在空肠或回肠,只有 3% 发生在所有节段——十二指肠、空肠和回肠。在高达 20% 的人群中观察到十二指肠憩室,发生频率随年龄增长而增加[350-353]。它们通常位于 Vater 壶腹部 1~2cm 内沿十二指肠第二部分内侧壁。十二指肠憩室出血罕见。一些报告描述了通过内镜治疗的十二指肠憩室出血[353,354]。空肠和回肠憩室在人群中的发生率为 1%~2%,最常与硬皮病、其他运动障碍或小肠细菌过度生长(SIBO)相关,并且很少与出血相关(见第 26、37 和 105 章)。

8. 小肠 Dieulafoy 病变

一些报告描述了在十二指肠、空肠和回肠的 Dieulafoy 病变(见第 38 章)[355]。大多数患者年龄小于 40 岁,与那些有胃 Dieulafoy 病变的人相比,他们往往年龄较大(见前文)。病变发现往往具有挑战性,过去通过血管造影和术中内镜检查发现。胶囊式内镜还可以定位和诊断些病变,可以通过单气囊或双气囊小肠镜进行治疗。

(二)诊断性检查

1. 影像学

钡剂小肠造影随访已不再使用,因为其确定不明原因胃肠道出血的诊断率低(扩张肠和可视化黏膜病变如血管发育不良的能力有限)。不建议对急性出血患者进行钡剂检查,胃肠道中残留的钡剂造影剂可能使紧急内镜检查、结肠镜检查或血管造影更难进行。

腹部 CT 的优势在于成像小肠腔外结构以及黏膜和壁内病变。高质量的腹部 CT(有和无口服造影剂)可显示小肠增厚,提示克罗恩病或恶性肿瘤。标准 CT 对低位肠梗阻、黏膜溃疡和瘘管的诊断不如钡剂小肠造影准确。与标准 CT 相比,使用多排 CT 小肠造影提供了更好的小肠视图。由于通常需要放置鼻十二指肠管,患者有时会接受中度镇静进行 CT 小肠造影[356]。使用大量口服造影剂扩张小肠的 CT 小肠造影可能具有与 CT 小肠造影相似的诊断率,且不需要鼻十二指肠管。MRI 小肠造影和小肠成像也有描述,但初步研究表明,迄今为止的结果劣于多排螺旋 CT。MRI 技术的优点在于无辐射。

核医学研究和血管造影可用于评价不明原因的胃肠道出血。如前所述,Meckel(^{99m}Tc-高锝酸盐)扫描可用于 Meckel 憩室的诊断评估,尤其是在年轻患者中。用锝标记的红细胞进行放射性核素扫描的效用有限,因为其定位小肠出血部位的能力较差。由于治疗性栓塞的可能性,血管造影术可用于活动性、急性小肠出血患者。小型病例系列描述了诱导性血管造影,其中给予肝素或另一种抗凝剂以引起间歇性胃肠道出血。该技术提高了检测出血性病变的诊断率,但存在可引起危及生命的并发症的风险[357]。

2. 内镜

(1) 推进式肠镜检查

可以使用结肠镜(长度为 160~180cm)或专用推进式肠镜(长度为 220~250cm)进行推进式肠镜检查[358]。这些内镜可用于评价 Treitz 韧带外约 50~150cm 的食管,胃,十二指肠和近端空肠。内镜在胃内成环通常会限制插入。推进式肠镜检查可识别约 50%或更多患者的潜在出血部位,发现的病变大约 50%均在标准胃肠道内镜可触及的范围内,表明初次检查时病变被遗漏或未被识别[309,310,358]。推进式肠镜的总体诊断率约为 40%,各种研究中的诊断范围为 3%至 80%,最常检测到的病变是血管扩张[309]。在 UCLA CURE 研究中,对反复发生的严重、不明原因的、明显胃肠道出血(表现为黑便)患者的止血经验显示,诊断率为 80%[57]。漏诊的病变可分类为上胃肠道遗漏的病变、十二指肠遗漏的病变(第一至第四部分)和空肠遗漏病变,大多数病变都在推进式小肠镜可触及的范围内。对局灶性病变可进行内镜下治疗、活检或标记。推进式肠镜检查未做出诊断的患者需接受进一步检查(见图 20.5)。

(2) 术中内镜检查和手术探查

当其他检查无诊断价值时,可以进行小肠手术探查。手术时,应连续触诊小肠("走行肠管")以发现占位病变。一般而言,首先进行标准的剖腹探查或腹腔镜检查以解除任何粘连并寻找明显的肿瘤、Meckel 憩室或大血管病变。通常通过腹部切口取出小肠,以便外科医生协助推进内窥镜到胃肠道腔内,从而实现黏膜可视化及透照。可以使用各种内镜(标准上内窥镜和结肠镜、儿科结肠镜或推进式小肠镜),具体取决于进入途径。内镜可以经口通过,以便进行自然腔道检查,也可以使用无菌内窥镜通过肠切开术进行检查[359]。由于注气将使整个小肠膨胀,从而使腹腔镜或开放性可视化变得困难,外科医生应手动或用无创夹钳夹住内镜头远端的肠道,以捕获足够的空气进行可视化。另外,肠道注入二氧化碳气体而不是空气,可以使气体更快地从肠道扩散出去。外科医生通过在内镜上打褶小肠来帮助推进内镜。任何已识别的病变都可以通过手术或内镜治疗解决,这取决于病变的性质。大多数系列报告了 50%~75%的病例的整个小肠的完整肠镜检查[360,361]。术中肠镜检查的诊断率为 58%~88%,但也有 13%~60%的患者报告术中肠镜检查后再出血[309]。中等性能特征以及手术探查的风险限制了该手术作为检查诊断工具,但在选定的患者中,内镜和手术联合评价可能是有用和明确的。

已经报告了在引入胶囊式内镜和深部肠镜检查之前和之后,术中内镜在严重不明原因胃肠道出血处理中的作用[361]。在胶囊式内镜前时代的手术前,36%的患者实现了出血部位的推定诊断或定位,与之相比,胶囊式内镜后时代为 63%。在胶囊式内镜前时代,100%的患者在术中作出了明确诊断,而在胶囊式内镜后时代为 76%。对于手术可切除的病变——小肠肿瘤、Meckel 憩室、主动脉肠瘘和局灶性缺血性溃疡——在长期随访期间没有患者发生术后出血,但是,其他患者的再出血率较高——血管病变为 67%、小肠溃疡为 44%、克罗恩病为 50%和 63%无明确诊断。胶囊式内镜或深部肠镜的术前诊断变得更为重要,尤其是在可能有明显并发症或手术死亡的老年患者中。需要仔细选择患者[363]。

(3) 胶囊式内镜检查

患者摄入可传输小肠图像 8 小时或更长时间的胶囊型照相机,行胶囊内镜检查。在严重复发性胃肠道出血患者中,该技术可识别小肠中出现新鲜血液的转变点,从而定位出血部位,有时可识别特定来源的病变[363]。胶囊式内镜不允许应用于治疗,只能根据通过小肠的时间来定位小肠中的病变,由腹部上的传感器和遥测确定。但是,该信息可用于指导后续治疗程序,如深部肠镜检查、血管造影或外科手术。尽管胶囊式内镜偶尔可检测胃、十二指肠或结肠病变,但它不能替代 EGD 和结肠镜检查。

与小肠钡剂研究相比,胶囊式内镜显著改善了小肠病变的检出率(67% vs 8%)和影响临床治疗的结果(42% vs 6%)[363,364]。一个小系列发现,对于不明原因胃肠道出血的诊断,胶囊式内镜优于 CT 小肠造影,因为其能够识别血管扩张[365]。

对已发表的在不明原因出血患者中,比较推进式小肠镜检查与胶囊式内镜检查的研究(显性 79%,隐性 21%)进行评价,发现推进式小肠镜检查的平均阳性率为 23%,胶囊式内镜检查为 63%[309]。在已发表试验和摘要的 meta 分析中发现了相似的结果,推进式小肠镜检查的诊断率为 28%,胶囊式内镜检查为 63%[364]。一项比较推进式小肠镜检查与胶囊式内镜检查作为不明原因胃肠道出血一线治疗方法的随机试验报告,在 24%的推进式小肠镜检查和 50%的胶囊式内镜研究中确定了出血源($P=0.02$)[366]。在这项研究中,胶囊式内镜在 8%的患者中遗漏了病变,所有遗漏的病变均在标准上胃肠道内镜可触及的范围内。

一项针对急性、明显、不明原因胃肠道出血(非诊断性EGD和结肠镜的黑粪症或便血)患者的研究随机分为胶囊式内镜或血管造影,报告称胶囊式内镜检查的诊断率明显高于血管造影(53% vs 20%),但长期结局无差异,包括输血、住院和死亡率[367],在一项47例患者的研究中,比较了胶囊式内镜与术中内镜检查,这些患者接受了两种方法,主要用于治疗不明原因的显性胃肠道出血[368]。以术中内镜检查作为金标准,胶囊式内镜检查的敏感性为95%,特异性为75%,阳性预测值为95%,阴性预测值为85%。大多数出血病变为血管扩张。

一些研究发现,在持续或近期(<2周)明显胃肠道出血或严重慢性胃肠道出血(血红蛋白<10g/dL、缺铁性贫血或一次以上明显出血)的情况下,胶囊式内镜的诊断率会有所增加[368-370]。在一项来自希腊的研究中,34名患者有活动性轻度至中度显性胃肠道出血,EGD和结肠镜检查结果均为阴性,并且在住院期间接受了紧急胶囊式内镜检查,其诊断率为92%,根据出血病变(18例血管扩张、3例溃疡、2例肿瘤)或肠段出血(11例患者)的确定[29]。相比之下,来自希腊的同一组发现胶囊式内镜对隐匿性出血和缺铁性贫血患者的诊断率为57%(血管扩张24%、多发性空肠或回肠溃疡12%、多发糜烂8%、孤立性溃疡6%、息肉4%和其他肿瘤4%)[371]。

(4)空肠和回肠的深部肠镜检查

特别设计的超柔性、200cm长的肠镜与外套管结合使用,通过在其上对小肠进行打褶来推进内镜。可用系统包括双气囊内镜(内镜头端有一个气囊,外套管上有另一个气囊)、单气囊内镜(仅在外套管上有一个气囊)和螺旋外套管(未使用气囊)。所有肠镜均通过在内镜上对小肠进行折叠推进内镜来工作。这些肠镜可以经口插入(顺行)并推进至回肠中段的近端,或经直肠插入(逆行)并推进至回中段的远端。在罕见情况下,可以使用双气囊肠镜通过顺行方法进行小肠到盲肠的完整肠镜检查,而在发表研究的大型综述中,44%的病例使用顺行和逆行相结合的方法进行了全肠镜检查(整个小肠完全可视化)[372]。深部肠镜检查不仅可以可视化,还可以对病变进行活检、止血和标记等干预。用于深部肠镜检查的内镜具有标准工作通道,允许通过适合的附件,如活检钳、MPEC探头、止血夹和注射针。双气囊小肠镜检查的主要并发症风险约为1%,并发症包括穿孔、胰腺炎、出血和吸入性肺炎(第42章)[373]。

对双气囊小肠镜治疗723例患者的不明原因出血的12个病例系列进行汇编,发现总体诊断率为65%(表20.10)[309]。胶囊式内镜和双气囊小肠镜的比较研究显示,胶囊式内镜的诊断率略高。在一项115例患者的大型多中心研究中,这些方法的一致性:血管扩张为74%、溃疡为96%、息肉为94%和其他大型肿瘤为96%[374]。另一项研究发现,对于不明原因出血患者,一致性为92%,但对于息肉病患者,胶囊式内镜在特定肠段的诊断率仅为33%,而双气囊小肠镜为67%,然而,胶囊式内镜可能检测到双气囊小肠镜无法到达的息肉[374]。

表20.10 488例患者在双气囊小肠镜检查不明原因胃肠道出血期间发现的小肠病变

病变	频率(范围)/%
无	40(0~57)
血管扩张	31(6~55)
溃疡	13(2~35)
恶性肿瘤	8(3~26)
其他	6(2~22)

Data from Raju GS, Gerson L, Das A, Lewis B. American Gastroenterological Association(AGA) Institute technical review on obscure gastrointestinal bleeding. Gastroenterology 2007;133:1697-717

3. 总体方法

对于不明原因的显性胃肠道出血和上胃肠道内镜及结肠镜检查阴性结果的患者,通常建议将胶囊式内镜检查作为下一步方案。如果胶囊式内镜检查发现近端空肠有病变,可进行推进式小肠镜检查。如果在小肠中段发现病变,根据病变的性质,可考虑深部小肠镜检查或手术。回肠末端病变可提示经结肠途径进行深部小肠镜检查。如果胶囊式内镜未检测到病变,但高度怀疑病变仍然存在,则应重复进行胶囊式内镜检查或进行深部小肠镜检查。随着深部小肠镜和附件可用性的增加,深部小肠镜检查可能成为首选的初始诊断步骤(在胶囊式内镜检查之前)。建模研究表明,这种方法可能是一个具有成本效益的策略[375,376]。但理想情况下,该问题应在一项随机研究中解决。

UCLA CURE小组用于管理发生不明原因严重显性胃肠道出血患者的,且有黑便病史,同时需要输血的患者,其临床处理方法如图20.5所示。对于这类患者,诊断率在80%以上[57]。

五、隐性胃肠道出血和缺铁性贫血

(一)粪便潜血试验

隐匿性胃肠道出血通常通过常规基于愈创木脂的FOBT或粪便免疫化学试验(fecal immunochemical test,FIT)检测,发生(根据定义)粪便中无可见血液,伴有或不伴有铁缺乏。正常粪便失血量为0.5~1.5mL/d[377]。许多FOBT可用于检测粪便中的血液量增加,详见第127章。

对FOBT阳性患者的治疗方法取决于为何要进行这项检测。如果FOBT或FIT用于50岁或以上患者的结肠癌筛查,患者应接受结肠镜检查和可能的上胃肠道内镜检查(EGD),即使无缺铁性贫血。该建议是基于248例粪便潜血患者的研究结果,EGD在上胃肠道发现的病变(主要是食管炎、胃病和溃疡)多于结肠镜检查在结肠发现的病变(主要是大腺瘤和癌症)[378]。FIT结果阳性(仅检测下胃肠道的人血红蛋白)和结肠镜检查结果正常的患者,是否需要EGD尚不确定(且不太可能)[379]。如果因缺铁性贫血进行了FOBT,应通过EGD和结肠镜检查对患者进行评估。如果两次检查的结果均为阴性,小肠应如前所述用胶囊式内镜成像,如果在胶囊式内镜检查中检测到病变,则可能随后进行深部小肠镜检查。

尽管使用 FOBT 进行结肠癌筛查通常基于 6 份自发排便样本，但当在直肠指检期间获得粪便时，可能发现阳性 FOBT 结果（并不罕见）。尽管直肠指检可能导致肛管创伤，但几项研究发现，当通过直肠指检获得粪便时，FOBT 的假阳性率没有增加[380,381]。因此，无论采用何种方法获得粪便样本，均应以相同的方式接近阳性 FOBT 结果。此外，直肠指检的单一阴性 FOBT 结果不被视为充分的结肠癌筛查，也不会降低患者发生晚期肿瘤的概率[382]。

（二）缺铁性贫血

缺铁性贫血很常见，在成年男性和绝经后妇女中发生率为 2%～5%[383]。缺铁性贫血占所有门诊胃肠病会诊、转诊患者的 4%～13%[384]。

缺铁性贫血的治疗方法取决于患者的性别和是否存在具有临床意义的明显非胃肠道失血[385]。应考虑缺铁性贫血年轻女性的贫血原因为月经失血，根据临床情况，可能不需要进行胃肠道评估。相比之下，男性和绝经后女性缺铁性贫血患者，应始终评价铁缺乏的胃肠道原因。对低 MCV 和贫血患者应考虑缺铁性贫血。

在缺铁性贫血时，血清铁浓度降低，转铁蛋白（TIBC）水平升高。转铁蛋白饱和度指数（血清铁除以 TIBC）低于 15% 是缺铁性贫血的敏感指标。血清铁蛋白水平低于 15ng/mL 对铁缺乏的敏感性为 59%，特异性为 99%，而铁蛋白水平为 41ng/mL 的临界值敏感性和特异性为 98%[386]。骨髓穿刺可提供有关身体贮存铁的信息，但很少需要。

缺铁性贫血可由于显性或隐性失血（胃肠道病变、月经、鼻出血、肺部病变或泌尿道病变）、肠道铁吸收不良（如腹腔疾病或胃萎缩或胃旁路手术后）、促红细胞生成素治疗（因铁需求过多）和红细胞破坏（溶血）。对铁缺乏患者的胃肠道评价应侧重于内镜检查（上和下），以检测可治疗的病变，尤其是恶性肿瘤。重新确认胃肠道铁吸收不良对铁缺乏尤其重要。十二指肠是小肠吸收铁的部位。大多数膳食中铁以三价铁形式存在，但只有亚铁形式的铁才能被十二指肠吸收。需要低 pH 的抗坏血酸释放非血红素铁，并将其转化为亚铁形式在小肠内吸收[387]。多项研究表明，20% 至 30% 的缺铁性贫血患者有胃萎缩，因此不产生有利于铁吸收的酸性环境[383,388,389]。缺铁性贫血也与 Hp 感染有关[390]。因此，不明原因的缺铁性贫血患者应在上胃肠道内镜检查时应进行胃活检（见第 52、53 和 103 章）。

乳糜泻通常表现为缺铁性贫血，主要是由于十二指肠绒毛变钝导致的铁吸收不良。据报道，乳糜泻患者的 FOBT 阳性率高于健康对照组，但随后使用放射性标记红细胞的研究未发现失血量真正增加[391,392]。事实上，乳糜泻患者缺铁性贫血的原因可能是多因素的。任何接受缺铁性贫血评价和上胃肠道内镜检查的患者都应该采集十二指肠活检样本，以检查乳糜泻（见第 107 章）。

接受过 Roux-en-Y 胃旁路手术的患者发生铁吸收不良的风险较高，因为十二指肠旁路术，（大部分铁在十二指肠被吸收）。这些患者可表现为严重的不明原因的铁缺乏，而无隐匿性粪便出血。它们通常具有极低的体内铁储，需要静脉补铁（见第 8 章）。

缺铁性贫血的鉴别诊断包括慢性病贫血和地中海贫血。在慢性疾病性贫血中，血清铁水平和 TIBC 均较低，血清铁蛋白水平正常。地中海贫血患者有贫血、脾大家族史，外周血涂片有靶细胞，血清铁蛋白水平正常。

不明原因的缺铁性贫血患者应接受上胃肠道内镜和结肠镜检查，以排除可能导致慢性失血的胃肠道病变。在 100 例缺铁性贫血患者的前瞻性研究中，在 62 例患者中发现胃肠道病变，其中 36 例病变位于上胃肠道（多为溃疡），25 例位于结肠（主要是癌症），1 例位于上胃肠道和结肠[393]。在接受 EGD 的不明原因缺铁性贫血患者中，应获得十二指肠活检标本，以排除乳糜泻是铁吸收不良的原因。还应获取胃活检样本，以排除胃病和 Hp 感染。根据缺铁性贫血的严重程度，即使没有阳性 FOBT 结果，也应考虑如前所述评价小肠的出血性病变。如果未发现贫血的特定原因，应建议患者避免使用抗血小板和抗凝药物，并补充铁剂。

（陈立刚 译，王立　袁农 校）

参考文献

第21章 黄疸

Steven D. Lidofsky 著

章节目录

一、胆红素的代谢及检测 …… 296
(一) 胆红素的代谢 …… 296
(二) 胆红素的检测 …… 297
二、高胆红素血症的鉴别诊断 …… 297
(一) 胆红素代谢紊乱 …… 298
(二) 肝脏疾病 …… 299
(三) 胆管梗阻 …… 301
三、黄疸的诊断方法 …… 301
(一) 病史与体格检查 …… 301
(二) 基本实验室检查 …… 302
(三) 综合方法 …… 303
(四) 影像学检查 …… 303
(五) 其他检查 …… 304
四、治疗方法 …… 305
(一) 梗阻性黄疸 …… 305
(二) 非梗阻性黄疸 …… 305

黄疸为胆红素在组织广泛沉积所致,临床表现为人体皮肤、眼结膜以及黏膜明显的黄染。虽然黄疸通常是肝脏和胆管疾病的征兆,但鉴别诊断范围广泛,确定黄疸的原因和如何进行最好的治疗已经困扰了临床医生数千年。

黄疸的诊断分型具有悠久的历史演变。早在希波克拉底的论著中就曾描写与黄疸有关的疾病的临床表现。到19世纪晚期,正如Osler的《医学原理与实践》所述,胆管梗阻与非梗阻引起的黄疸之间已经有了重要的区分。到20世纪后半叶,分子生物学和临床影像的革命分别阐明了胆红素代谢和转运的基本机制,并通过技术手段使查明大部分黄疸病因成为可能。虽然有这些进展,但是仍然需要在评估潜在病因可能性的基础上仔细选择适当的诊断和治疗工具,以便为此类患者提供有效的治疗策略。

一、胆红素的代谢及检测

(一) 胆红素的代谢

胆红素是一种由血红素降解产生的四吡咯化合物。图21.1简要概述了胆红素代谢过程。20世纪后半叶,有大量文献描述了胆红素这种疏水性和潜在毒性物质的代谢过程,并进行了详细的综述[1,2]。一个健康成年人每天平均产生4mg/kg胆红素(如70kg约为0.5mmol)。大多数胆红素(70%~80%)是由衰老的红细胞释放的血红蛋白分解代谢产生的。

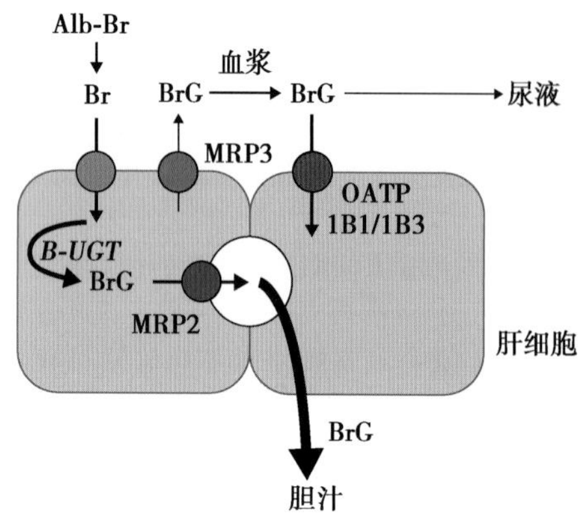

图21.1 胆红素形成、代谢和转运的示意图。来源于血红蛋白及其他血红素蛋白中的血红素主要在骨髓和脾脏中的巨噬细胞中转化为胆绿素,然后转化为胆红素(Br)。Br被释放到血浆中(以非结合形式),在血浆中与白蛋白(Alb)紧密但可逆地结合。随后Br可能通过有机阴离子转运蛋白(OATP)家族成员在肝细胞的窦状隙膜上被摄取。Br通过胆红素-尿苷二磷酸葡萄糖醛酸转移酶(B-UGT)的活性结合,形成胆红素单葡萄苷酸和双葡萄糖苷酸(BrG)。BrG的胆汁分泌是通过多特异性有机阴离子转运蛋白MRP2在小管膜上进行的。在生理条件下,绝大多数BrG经胆汁被消除。少量BrG通过多特异性有机阴离子转运蛋白MRP3从肝窦侧膜转运回血浆,并主要通过OATP(OATP1B1和OATP1B3)摄取重新捕获。剩余的血浆BrG进入肾循环,在肾循环中经过肾小球滤过并消除到尿液中。因此,在正常情况下,血浆中至少95%的胆红素是以非结合形式存在的。如果长期保留异常高浓度的BrG,就会形成不解离、不能通过肾小球滤过的BrG-Alb复合物。MRP,多药耐药相关蛋白

剩下的20%~30%的胆红素主要来自肝细胞中其他含血红素的蛋白质(如过氧化氢酶、细胞色素氧化酶)的分解。肝外组织中肌红蛋白等其他血红蛋白也可分解为胆红素,但转换率较低。因此,在健康个体中,这些血红蛋白分解产生的胆红素极少。

血红素转化为胆红素的过程包括血红素加氧酶(heme oxygenase,HO)和胆绿素还原酶的先后作用。HO有两种酶活性亚型:(a)HO-1,一种可诱导蛋白,它是一种位于内质网并广泛表达的蛋白;(b)HO-2,位于线粒体,在特定的组织中(包括肝细胞)表达[3]。这些蛋白质催化了血红素环的打开从而产生胆绿素(biliverdin,BV)(一种水溶性化合物)。异构体选择性胆绿素还原酶(biliverdin reductase,BVRA)[4]是一种广泛表达的细胞表面膜蛋白,它将BV Ⅸα转化为这种分子的主要成体形式胆红素Ⅸα。胆红素产生的主要部位取决于血液蛋白前体的组织来源。红细胞源性血红蛋白转化为胆红素主要发生在脾、骨髓和肝脏的巨噬细胞(Kupffer细胞)。游离血红蛋白、触珠蛋白结合的血红蛋白和正铁白蛋白主要在肝细

胞中分解为胆红素。

疏水性的非结合胆红素在血浆中循环并与白蛋白非共价结合。在肝细胞内,非结合的胆红素转换成水溶性结合物随胆汁排泄。胆红素的代谢和排泄是一个多步骤的过程,目前已经明确一些胆红素相关的遗传性疾病,详见后文。

肝细胞的肝窦侧膜(基底侧)可以摄取非结合胆红素。虽然对非结合胆红素被动扩散和载体转运的相对作用进行了大量的研究和讨论,但是肝细胞胆红素摄取的机制尚未完全阐明。磺溴酞钠、吲哚菁等一些有机阴离子可以竞争性地抑制非结合胆红素的摄取,根据对转染细胞的研究推测,推测有机阴离子转运蛋白(organic anion transport protein,OATP)家族成员参与了这一过程(见第64章)。OATPB1在肝窦侧膜吸收结合胆红素的过程中发挥明显的作用(见后文),但是对于肝细胞吸收非结合胆红素的重要性仍存在争议[1,5]。相比之下,胆红素代谢的后续步骤更为明确。

非结合胆红素被肝细胞摄取后,与谷胱甘肽S转移酶B、脂肪酸结合蛋白等特定的具有高亲和力的细胞质蛋白相互结合,通过扩散作用运输到内质网。由胆红素-尿苷二磷酸葡萄糖醛酸基转移酶(bilirubin UDP-glucuronyl transferase,B-UGT)介导,胆红素与尿苷二磷酸(uridine diphosphate,UDP)-葡萄糖醛酸结合。然后亲水性胆红素葡萄糖醛酸酯产物(结合胆红素)扩散到细胞质膜上。在顶端小管区域,结合胆红素通过多耐药相关蛋白-2(MRP-2,基因符号*ABCC2*,一种ATP依赖的输出泵)转运到胆小管。MRP2还可以转运多种其他有机阴离子,包括磺溴酞钠、谷胱甘肽和结合胆盐[1,6]。在肝窦侧膜(基底外侧)区域,结合胆红素通过独特的多特异性有机离子输出泵即多耐药相关蛋白-3(MRP-3,基因符号*ABCC3*)被转运到血浆中[1,6]。一旦跨过肝窦侧膜,结合胆红素可以被肝窦转运蛋白OATP1B1(基因符号*SLCO1B1*)和OATP1B3(基因符号*SLCO1B3*)重新摄取,这可能是由下游肝细胞介导的[1,5]。结合胆红素排泄的另一种途径是通过肾脏排泄到尿液中(见图21.1)。在胆汁淤积(胆汁流动减少)性疾病中,MRP3介导的结合胆红素输出可以上调[6],导致结合胆红素的血清浓度不成比例地升高(见下文)。慢性胆汁淤积(或结合高胆红素血症代谢紊乱[见下文])时,血浆中过量的结合胆红素会与白蛋白共价结合,这种形式的胆红素不能排泄到尿液中。

在生理条件下,胆汁中几乎都是结合胆红素,只有微量非结合胆红素。人类胆汁中约80%的胆红素都以二葡糖醛酸酯形式存在,其余的胆红素几乎均以单葡糖醛酸的形式存在。胆囊和肠道对结合胆红素的吸收微不足道;从胆管释放的大部分胆红素以结合形式进入肠道,随粪便排出。但是胆红素可以在回肠末端和结肠被细菌分解,转化为无色的四吡咯化合物,称为尿胆素原[7]。多达20%的尿胆素原在肠道内吸收,最终随胆汁和尿液排出。

(二) 胆红素的检测

正常成年人血清胆红素浓度低于1~1.5mg/dL。轻度高胆红素血症无法通过肉眼观察,血清胆红素浓度超过3mg/dL时才出现黄疸。在健康个体中,大部分胆红素以未结合形式在血液中循环;血浆中仅有不到5%的胆红素以结合形式存在。在胆汁淤积的条件下,由于胆小管输出受损和MRP3表达代偿性上调导致的肝窦侧输出增加,血浆中结合胆红素的比例会增加。因此血浆中胆红素的浓度和组成在健康和疾病之间有很大差异。

从新生儿黄疸到确定肝移植优先次序,准确测量血清胆红素具有重要临床意义[9]。临床实验室检测血清胆红素的常用技术基于20世纪初提出的重氮反应。在这项技术中,重氮试剂作为化合物可以裂解胆红素,例如重氮化的磺胺酸裂解,形成可以通过分光技术定量的偶氮二吡咯。结合胆红素被重氮试剂快速或直接裂解。相比之下,非结合胆红素内部氢键减少了重氮试剂对化学裂解位点的可及性,形成偶氮二吡咯的过程更缓慢。所以可靠测量总胆红素浓度需要加入另一种促进剂(如乙醇、尿素),以破坏氢键并促进重氮试剂裂解非结合胆红素。利用该技术,在不添加促进剂的情况下测定的胆红素浓度为"直接"胆红素浓度,而在添加促进剂化合物的情况下测定的为总胆红素浓度。总胆红素浓度与直接胆红素浓度之间的数值差就是间接胆红素浓度。

关于直接胆红素和间接胆红素的临床意义出现了一定的混乱。虽然直接血清胆红素浓度受结合胆红素水平变化的影响,但是直接胆红素和结合胆红素彼此并不等同。同样,间接血清胆红素浓度不等于非结合胆红素浓度。依赖直接和间接胆红素测量会引起对孤立性胆红素代谢紊乱的诊断错误[如疑似Gilbert综合征(见后文)]。因此,许多临床实验室改为使用自动反射光谱法,可以更准确地估算血清中结合和非结合胆红素浓度。这些测定可为新生儿黄疸的治疗提供有用的信息,其中非结合高胆红素血症的治疗与其他疾病的治疗有所不同(请参阅后面的讨论)。然而,在慢性胆汁淤积性疾病中,此类测定法可能会低估结合胆红素的浓度,因为它们不能准确检测结合白蛋白的结合胆红素(所谓的δ胆红素)。对于成年人来说,准确测定结合胆红素浓度通常不是关键,所以这可能不是很重要。但是在某些特殊情况下,确定胆红素代谢异常的诊断是有必要的。在这种情况下,诊断可能需要更复杂的色谱技术,以精确测量非结合胆红素、单葡萄糖醛酸胆红素、二葡萄糖醛酸胆红素和结合胆红素-白蛋白复合物的浓度[10]。实际上,这些技术并未得到广泛使用。即使采用这种精确的方法,结合和非结合胆红素浓度的测定也不能区分由肝病引起的高胆红素血症和由胆管阻塞引起的高胆红素血症。因此,在大多数情况下,对血清中结合和非结合胆红素浓度的精确测量用途有限。

二、高胆红素血症的鉴别诊断

血清胆红素水平反映了胆红素的产生与清除之间的平衡。这些过程之间的不平衡会导致黄疸。从实践的角度来看,与高胆红素血症(黄疸)相关的疾病可以归类为胆红素代谢紊乱、肝病和胆管梗阻(表21.1)。

表 21.1 黄疸和高胆红素血症的鉴别诊断

病症	举例
胆红素代谢紊乱	
孤立性非结合高胆红素血症	
产量增加	溶血,无效的红细胞生成,输血,血肿的吸收
肝细胞摄取减少	药物(如利福平、环孢霉素)
结合减少	Gilbert 综合征,Crigler-Najjar 综合征,新生儿生理性黄疸,药物(如茚地那韦、阿扎那韦)
孤立性结合或混合性高胆红素血症	
Dubin-Johnson 综合征	-
Rotor 综合征	-
肝脏疾病	
肝细胞功能障碍	
急性或亚急性肝细胞损伤	病毒性肝炎,肝毒素(如乙醇、对乙酰氨基酚、鹅膏菌);药物(如异烟肼、苯妥英钠);缺血性肝炎,血管流出受阻;代谢紊乱(如 Wilson 病);妊娠相关疾病(如妊娠急性脂肪肝、先兆子痫)
慢性肝细胞性疾病	病毒性肝炎;肝毒素(如乙醇、氯乙烯、维生素 A);自身免疫性肝炎;乳糜泻;代谢异常(如非酒精脂肪性肝病、血色素沉着病、Wilson 病、α_1-抗胰蛋白酶缺乏症)
肝病伴明显胆汁淤积	
浸润性疾病	肉芽肿疾病,如分枝杆菌感染,结节病,淋巴瘤,肉芽肿性多血管炎;淀粉样变;恶性肿瘤
胆管细胞损伤	原发性胆汁性肝硬化;移植物抗宿主病;药物(如红霉素、甲氧苄啶/磺胺甲噁唑);囊性纤维化
其他状况	良性复发性肝内胆汁淤积;药物(如雌激素/合成类固醇);全肠外营养;细菌感染;副肿瘤综合征;妊娠肝内胆汁淤积
胆管梗阻	
胆总管结石	-
胆管疾病	
炎症,感染	原发性硬化性胆管炎,AIDS 相关性胆管病,肝动脉化疗或化学栓塞引起的损伤,术后狭窄
肿瘤	胆管癌
外源性压迫	
肿瘤	胰腺癌,转移性淋巴结肿大,肝细胞癌,壶腹腺瘤或癌,淋巴瘤
胰腺炎	-
血管扩张	动脉瘤,门静脉海绵样变性(门静脉海绵状瘤)

AIDS,获得性免疫缺陷综合征。

(一) 胆红素代谢紊乱

1. 孤立性非结合高胆红素血症

3 种机制导致孤立性非结合高胆红素血症:①胆红素产量增加;②肝细胞对非结合胆红素的摄取减少;③肝细胞结合胆红素减少。在每种情况下,血清胆红素都会单独升高,而总体肝功能以及肝细胞损伤和胆汁淤积的生化指标正常(见第 73 章)。

(1) 胆红素生成增加

各种肝外过程均可产生过多的胆红素。包括溶血、无效的红细胞生成和血肿的吸收。出现这些疾病时,胆红素浓度通常不超过 4~5mg/dL。大量输血也会出现黄疸,因为储存的红细胞脆性增加,导致过多的血红蛋白释放,这可能是严重创伤患者出现高胆红素血症的主要原因[11]。

(2) 肝细胞对胆红素的摄取减少

有些药物可能会干扰肝细胞摄取胆红素。例如,抗生素利福平和免疫抑制剂环孢菌素 A 可以竞争性地抑制肝窦转运蛋白 OATP1B1,会造成高非结合胆红素血症[12],但是这种机制对非结合高胆红素血症的临床重要性仍有疑问[1]。

(3) 肝细胞结合胆红素结合减少

3 种非结合高胆红素血症的常染色体遗传性疾病是由于肝细胞中胆红素结合受损(表 21.2)。最常见的是 Gilbert 综合征,在美国的发病率约为 3%~7%,并且不同种族之间的发病情况也不同(中东最高、东亚最低)。Gilbert 综合征患者通常是在常规生化检测中偶然发现孤立性高胆红素血症;临床上黄疸少见。禁食或脱水可使血清胆红素水平升高 2~3 倍,但低于 4mg/dL。Gilbert 综合征的分子基础是启动子区和编码区(少见)突变导致的 B-UGT 基因 *UGT1A1* 转录减少[1,2]。虽然 Gilbert 综合征是良性疾病,但是可能会增加胆结石风险以及某些药物的毒性(如伊立替康),这些药物的代谢需要葡萄糖醛酸化过程[13]。另一方面,一些(但不是全部)研究表明 Gilbert 综合征患心血管疾病的风险降低[2]。这在生物学上是合理的,因为非结合胆红素是一种抗氧化剂,可抵消脂质过氧化和血管张力的改变[14]。

UGT1A1 编码区的突变与 Crigler-Najjar 综合征有关[1,15]。在Ⅰ型 Crigler-Najjar 综合征中,B-UGT 活性缺失,出生后不久就出现明显的非结合高胆红素血症。非结合胆红素可穿过血脑屏障,所以Ⅰ型 Crigler-Najjar 综合征胆红素会在脑中积聚(核黄疸),产生的神经毒性作用可导致新生儿死亡(见表 21.2)。需使用光疗法来预防核黄疸(见后文),行肝移植可以挽救生命。相比之下,Ⅱ型 Crigler-Najjar 综合征的 B-UGT 活性降低,并且血清胆红素水平低于Ⅰ型(见表 21.2)。Ⅱ型 Crigler-Najjar 综合征在新生儿期不发病,可能直到幼儿期才确诊。大多数Ⅱ型 Crigler-Najjar 综合征可以使用苯巴比妥治疗,苯巴比妥是一种合成的雄甾烷受体(CAR)的激动剂,可以增加 *UGT1A1* 的表达。[15]。苯巴比妥治疗后血清胆红素水平通常降至 2~5mg/dL。

一种与胆红素代谢相关的疾病是新生儿生理性黄疸,这是由于 B-UGT 迟缓表达所致,黄疸通常在新生儿期迅速消退[16]。需要一个短疗程的光疗预防核黄疸(见后文)。

表 21.2 胆红素代谢和转运的遗传性疾病

特征	综合征				
	Gilbert	Ⅰ型 Crigler-Najjar	Ⅱ型 Crigler-Najjar	Dubin-Johnson	Rotor
发病率	6%~12%	很少	罕见	罕见	稀少
受影响基因	*UGT1A1*	*UGT1A1*	*UGT1A1*	*MRP2*	*OATP1B1* 和 *OATP1B3*
代谢缺陷	↓胆红素结合	无胆红素结合	↓↓胆红素结合	结合胆红素的小管输出受损	结合胆红素的肝窦摄取受损
血浆胆红素/(mg/dL)	≤3,无空腹或溶血,几乎均为未结合	通常>20(范围 17~50)全部非结合	通常<20(范围 6~45)几乎均为非结合	通常<7,约一半为结合	通常<7,约一半为结合
肝组织学	通常正常,偶发性脂褐素	正常	正常	中心小叶肝细胞中的粗色素	正常
其他区分特征	↓胆红素浓度与苯巴比妥	对苯巴比妥无反应	↓胆红素浓度与苯巴比妥	↑胆红素与雌激素的浓度;↑↑尿原卟啉Ⅰ/Ⅲ比	轻度的↑尿原卟啉Ⅰ/Ⅲ比
预后	正常(所选药物毒性的理论风险)	未经治疗导致的婴儿死亡	通常正常	正常(所选药物毒性的理论风险)	正常(所选药物毒性的理论风险)
治疗	无	光疗作为肝移植的桥接治疗	苯巴比妥用于↑↑胆红素浓度	避免雌激素	无法获取

MRP2,与多药耐药相关的 protein-2 基因;*OATP*,有机阴离子转运蛋白;*UGT1A1*,胆红素尿苷二磷酸-葡萄糖醛酸转移酶基因。

逆转录病毒蛋白酶抑制剂阿扎那韦和茚地那韦竞争性抑制 B-UGT,在接受这些药物的患者中超过 25% 会产生高胆红素血症。Gilbert 综合征出现这种并发症的风险更高[17,18]。

2. 孤立性结合胆红素或混合性高胆红素血症

两种常染色体遗传性疾病,Dubin-Johnson 综合征和 Rotor 综合征,与结合性或混合性高胆红素血症相关(即结合性和非结合性胆红素的血清浓度升高)。在每个病例中,血清胆红素的浓度均会升高,而肝功能和肝细胞损伤和胆汁淤积的生化指标均正常(见第 73 章)。但是 Dubin-Johnson 综合征和 Rotor 综合征的潜在机制是不同的。在 Dubin-Johnson 综合征中,缺乏 MRP2 的表达或靶向性缺陷会损害结合胆红素向胆管分泌[1]。MRP3 的代偿性上调允许 MRP2 正常分泌的潜在毒性有机阴离子的肝窦侧输出(这可以防止肝细胞中这些化合物过载),从而放大该疾病中高胆红素血症的程度。Rotor 综合征的分子基础更加复杂。转基因小鼠的研究表明,MRP3 分泌到血浆中的结合胆红素被肝窦运输蛋白 OATP1B1 和 OATP1B3 所吸收[19],而 OATP1B1 和 OATP1B3 的联合缺乏会削弱结合胆红素的再摄取并导致 Rotor 综合征。

如表 21.2 所示,我们可以从生化和组织学上区分 Dubin-Johnson 综合征和 Rotor 综合征。在 Dubin-Johnson 综合征中,肝细胞在溶酶体中含有有特征的黑色素,这是由 MRP2 底物的芳香族氨基酸代谢产物形成的[1]。需要强调的是,在怀疑 Dubin-Johnson 综合征或 Rotor 综合征的患者的诊断评估中,肝活检是不必要的,因为没有一种疾病与肝损伤加重相关。然而,通过 OATP1B 介导的肝脏摄取进行代谢处置的某些药物(如他汀诱导的肌病)对 Rotor 综合征患者产生的毒性可能会增加[1]。

(二) 肝脏疾病

黄疸是肝实质疾病的一个常见特征,高胆红素血症通常与其他肝脏生化检查异常有关(见第 73 章)。以高胆红素血症和黄疸为表现的急性或慢性肝细胞功能不全的疾病与以胆汁淤积为主要问题的疾病不同。

1. 急性或亚急性肝细胞损伤

多种疾病可引起急性或慢性肝细胞损伤导致肝功能损伤,包括病毒性肝炎、暴露于肝毒性物质或环境、缺血和某些代谢紊乱。血清转氨酶水平会有特征地升高(见下文)。急性病毒性肝炎的先兆症状有厌食、乏力和肌痛,多早于黄疸出现(见第 78~83 章)。5 种嗜肝病毒中的甲型肝炎病毒和戊型肝炎病毒,它们是通过肠道传播的,一般是自限性的;乙型肝炎病毒、丙型肝炎病毒和丁型肝炎病毒是通过肠外传播的,可能导致慢性疾病。每一种疾病的诊断都有特异性血清学抗体可检测(见下文)。

中毒性肝损伤最常见的原因之一是摄入大量的止痛剂对乙酰氨基酚(见第 88 章),服药几天后可能导致黄疸和肝衰竭。在存活的患者中,既往没有肝病的患者黄疸可消退,肝功能可完全恢复。产生特异性(即与剂量无关的)肝细胞损伤和黄疸的药物和其他化学制剂将在本文其他部分讨论(见第 88 和 89 章)。酗酒可引起酒精性肝炎而导致黄疸(见第 86 章)。

缺血性肝炎和其他导致肝血流障碍的病因也可以引起黄疸。其中包括低血压、缺氧、高热、肝静脉流出道阻塞(Budd-Chiari 综合征)和肝窦阻塞综合征(见第 85 章)。

肝豆状核变性(Wilson disease)是一种肝胆的铜代谢异常的遗传性疾病,其临床特征与急性病毒性肝炎无明显区别(见第 76 章)。多见于年轻人的黄疸,中年人的病例也有报道。溶血性贫血是肝豆状核变性的一部分,并导致这些患者出现高胆红素血症。临床上通过生化检查、裂隙灯检查角膜铜沉积(K-F 环)和肝脏铜含量分析能诊断肝豆状核变性。

2. 慢性肝细胞疾病

慢性肝细胞疾病与急性肝细胞损伤不同,除非出现肝硬化,否则不会出现黄疸。慢性病毒性肝炎应作为疑似肝硬化患者的诊断依据,特别是存在肠外接触病原体的危险因素(见第79~81章)。血清学特异性抗体检测也有助于诊断(见下文)。肝硬化是脂肪性肝病的一部分,无论是在慢性饮酒的背景下(见第86章),还是作为代谢综合征(非酒精脂肪性肝病)的组成部分(见第87章)。某些遗传性代谢疾病也可能发展为肝硬化。血色病是一种由于过度铁吸收引起的肝细胞损伤性疾病,是最常见的一种遗传性代谢疾病(见第75章)。一般需要几十年的肝脏铁超载才会出现临床症状,然而血色素沉着症往往直到中年才被诊断出来。也可以通过检测HFE基因的特征性突变或肝脏铁含量分析来诊断血色素沉着症。肝豆状核变性患者中肝脏内铜代谢异常引起的肝损伤也可能发展为肝硬化。在患有慢性肺部疾病的黄疸患者中,应怀疑α_1-抗胰蛋白酶缺乏症(见第77章)。在这种疾病中,错误折叠的突变α_1-抗胰蛋白酶(ZZ表型)在肝细胞内质网中积聚可引发肝损伤。需要通过血清学分型和肝脏活检来辅助诊断α1-抗胰蛋白酶缺乏症。自身免疫性肝炎可能伴有全身症状,如疲劳、关节痛和皮疹,但黄疸可能是自身免疫性肝硬化的唯一表现(见第90章)。血清学检测和肝脏活检有助于诊断此类疾病(见下文)。虽然乳糜泻的特点是在小肠中引起免疫介导性疾病(见107章),但偶尔也会表现为无法解释的慢性肝病,但很少以肝硬化伴黄疸出现。

3. 伴有显著胆汁淤积的肝脏疾病

肝内胆汁淤积性疾病的特点是在没有广泛肝细胞损伤或胆管梗阻的情况下,胆汁形成受损。这些疾病和相关生化异常的表现可能与胆管梗阻相似,并可能导致诊断混乱。肝内胆汁淤积性疾病在组织学上可分为浸润性损伤,肝内胆管细胞损伤和组织学无明显改变。

(1) 肝脏浸润性疾病

肝脏浸润性疾病破坏了肝内胆管网络,常伴有明显的胆汁淤积,最终导致黄疸。最常见的原因是肉芽肿性疾病、淀粉样变和恶性肿瘤(见第37章)。包括传染病、毒素、淋巴瘤和其他系统性疾病(如结节病)等各种各样的疾病均可导致累及肝脏的肉芽肿性疾病[20]。这些导致黄疸的疾病中最常见的是结核病和结节病[21,22]。当黄疸伴不明原因发热时,应尤其怀疑肉芽肿性疾病。体格检查会发现患者肝脾肿大伴有淋巴结肿大。胸片异常为结节病或分枝杆菌感染的诊断提供线索。如果没有其他组织病理,诊断可能需要肝脏活检。黄疸也是淀粉样变性的一种不寻常表现,当淀粉样变性合并黄疸时会伴随着明显的肝脏肿大[23]。如果黄疸合并如巨舌、吸收不良、心力衰竭、周围神经病变、蛋白尿等其他相关器官的迹象,应怀疑是淀粉样变性。在没有其他线索的情况下,肝脏活检可能是诊断淀粉样变性的必要条件。由肝脏实质广泛的肿瘤性病变而引起的黄疸通常以厌食和体重减轻为先兆。无创性影像学检查可以诊断(见下文)。

(2) 与胆管细胞损伤相关的疾病

许多疾病会导致胆管细胞损伤。在其中许多病例中,以原发性胆汁性肝硬化(PBC)为例(见第91章),胆管细胞是免疫介导的炎症反应的靶标。PBC主要发生在女性群体中。随着黄疸发展,肝硬化一直存在,早期诊断及积极治疗可获得良好预后。生化和血清学检查[抗线粒体抗体(AMA)]通常足以诊断PBC,如果不确定,则可能需要进行肝活检。胆管细胞也是移植物抗宿主病的靶标(见第36章),这是造血细胞移植后黄疸的常见原因[24]。某些药物也会由于胆管细胞损伤而产生胆汁淤积(见第88章)[25],如红霉素、甲氧苄啶/磺胺甲噁唑和阿莫西林-克拉维酸[26]。一般来说,胆汁淤积在停用致病药物几个月内就会消失。约30%的成人囊性纤维化(CF)患者因胆管细胞损伤引起胆汁淤积(见第62章),CF是由于编码囊性纤维化跨膜转录调节因子(CFTR)的第7号常染色体基因突变导致的一种遗传性疾病。

(3) 伴细微组织学异常的胆汁淤积

在没有肝浸润病变或肝细胞或胆管细胞损伤的情况下,黄疸可能伴有胆汁淤积。可能有几个机制与此有关,包括编码与胆汁形成有关的转运蛋白的基因突变和干扰这些蛋白功能或表达的条件。

良性复发性胆汁淤积症是一种常染色体遗传性疾病,与编码肝细胞小管膜上的2种转运蛋白的基因突变有关,这些转运蛋白调节胆汁的形成:(a)家族性肝内胆汁淤积1蛋白(familial intrahepatic cholestasis 1 protein, FIC1, 基因符号*ATP8B1*);(b)胆盐输出泵[bile salt export pump, BSEP, 基因符号*ABCB11*(见第64和77章)][27]。FIC1是一种P型ATP酶,在肝细胞膜中作为氨基磷脂"转位酶"发挥作用,FIC1功能障碍通过增加疏水性胆汁酸对小管膜损伤的易感性和/或干扰调节BSEP表达或功能蛋白质的位点而引起胆汁淤积[28]。BSEP是一种依赖ATP的胆盐输出泵,胆盐排泌减少致使BSEP活性受损从而出现胆汁淤积[29]。良性复发性胆汁淤积代表是FIC1和BSEP突变相关疾病谱系的一端;另一端是进行性家族性肝内胆汁淤积症1型和2型,这些疾病可导致儿童肝功能衰竭,需要进行肝移植。

良性复发性胆汁淤积症患者通常在二十岁前出现反复发作的乏力和瘙痒伴黄疸;其中,发热和腹痛症状比较少见。在黄疸发作期间进行肝活检时,结果是局限于小叶中央的胆汁淤积,少见门脉的炎症细胞浸润。胆汁淤积发作可能持续数月,并由临床缓解期分隔开。虽然该病可能会影响生活质量,但是不会导致进行性肝损伤,而且(不同于进行性家族性肝内胆汁淤积症)也不会发生肝衰竭。

许多药物会引起组织学上无刺激性的肝内胆汁淤积(见第88章)。雌激素主要通过抑制胆盐分泌来减少胆汁形成[30]。多种机制导致了这种情况的发生,包括肝窦胆汁盐摄取蛋白钠离子-牛磺胆酸盐共转运肽(Na^+-taurocholate cotransporting peptide, NTCP, 基因符号*SLC10A1*)的下调,BSEP的竞争性抑制以及对MRP2功能的干扰。口服避孕药诱发的黄疸通常在开始治疗后2个月内出现,且伴有瘙痒,停药后,这些症状迅速消失。合成代谢类固醇可以产生一种临床上与雌激素诱导的胆汁淤积症难以区分的综合征。全胃肠外营养相关的胆汁淤积的临床特征,可能与肠肝循环改变和胆汁分泌的神经内分泌刺激减少有关,也可能类似于与雌激素和合成代谢类固醇相关的临床特征,但也有进展性肝纤维化的报道[31]。

在细菌感染过程中也可能出现胆汁淤积和黄疸,可能是因为细胞因子依赖地下调转运蛋白 NTCP、MRP2 和 BSEP 的下调所致[32]。与其他胆汁淤积性疾病一样，其临床特征可能难以与胆管梗阻区分，需要影像学研究来解决这个问题。

由肝内胆汁淤积引起的黄疸也是淋巴瘤患者和特定的非血液病恶性肿瘤（称为 Stauffer 综合征）的副肿瘤现象（即无肝脏恶性浸润）[33]。后者最初见于肾细胞癌，成功治疗原发肿瘤可消除胆汁淤积。对原发性肿瘤的成功治疗会使胆汁淤积得到解决。虽然发病机制尚不清楚，但是研究提示可能与肿瘤衍生的细胞因子分泌有关，而这些细胞因子干扰 NTCP、MRP2 和 BSEP 功能。

（4）胆汁淤积的非典型表现

病毒性肝炎很少会引起严重的伴有瘙痒和黄疸的胆汁淤积[34]。除非患者有病毒性肝炎的危险因素，否则没有明显的临床特征能可靠地将这种疾病与其他胆汁淤积综合征或胆管梗阻区分开来。在高度怀疑时结合适当的实验室检测将有助于确定诊断。表现为发热、黄疸、腹痛和白细胞增多的酒精性肝炎也很难与胆管梗阻相区别[35]。因此，可能需要肝活检来确认诊断。

4. 妊娠期黄疸

在妊娠过程中出现几种特有的胆汁淤积性疾病（请参阅第 40 章）。妊娠剧吐是妊娠早期的一种自限性疾病，黄疸是少见的并发症，而肝衰竭不是这种疾病的特征[36]。在妊娠晚期会发生肝内胆汁淤积症，并伴有瘙痒和偶尔的黄疸[37]。胆汁淤积症通常在分娩后 2 周内消退，并经常在随后的妊娠中复发。编码小管转运蛋白 BSEP、FIC1、MRP2 和 MDR3（基因符号 *ABCB4*）和紧密连接蛋白 2（TJP2）的基因多态性与这种疾病有关[37,38]。这些转运蛋白的功能改变可能增强它们对雌激素抑制胆汁形成作用的敏感性。更严重的综合征是妊娠期急性脂肪肝，通常发生在妊娠晚期，并与肝细胞损伤有关。黄疸出现时，通常伴有恶心、腹痛和肝功能衰竭的迹象。如果进行肝活检可以看到肝内微泡性脂肪变性。除非及时进行产科分娩，否则这种疾病是致命的。子痫前期是妊娠晚期的一种微血管疾病，以高血压和蛋白尿为先兆，约 10% 的病例中观察到肝脏损伤。还有一种特别严重的情况，即 HELLP 综合征，需要通过在产科及时分娩进行治疗。

5. 危重患者的黄疸

确定危重患者黄疸的病因对重症监护室医师和会诊医师来说是一个挑战。鉴别诊断相当广泛。诱发因素包括肝缺血、输血、肝毒性药物、胃肠外营养和隐匿性败血症[39,40]。肾损伤可能减少结合胆红素的肝外清除。持续黄疸可能会使患者的亲属感到惊慌沮丧，他们可能将黄疸视为病因，而不是危重病的表现。如果在没有胆管梗阻证据的情况下紧急胆管引流（见下文）会加剧病情恶化。值得注意的是，即使其他临床参数有所改善，黄疸的缓解可能也会有所滞后。因此，在重症监护条件下治疗黄疸不仅需要仔细寻找可逆的原因，而且需要很大的耐心。

（三）胆管梗阻

胆管梗阻性疾病包括胆道管腔阻塞、胆管内在疾病和胆管外源性压迫。

1. 胆总管结石

胆管梗阻的最常见原因是结石引起的管腔阻塞（胆总管结石）。胆总管结石按成分常分为 3 种，最多见也是最常见的是在第 65 章会讲到的胆固醇结石。胆固醇结石通常起源于胆囊，可迁移至胆管。胆红素钙结石，也就是所谓的黑色素结石，在非结合高胆红素血症患者胆囊内形成，也可能在胆管的任何部位形成原位结石。而棕色素结石是胆红素结石的一种独特类型，可导致反复发作的胆管炎，即复发性化脓性胆管炎，多见于东亚某些地区和既往接受过胆管手术或内镜介入手术的患者（见第 68 章）。

2. 胆管疾病

在炎症性、感染性或肿瘤性胆管疾病中会出现胆管的内源性狭窄。先天性胆管疾病，包括囊肿和胆管闭锁，将在第 62 章中讨论。原发性硬化性胆管炎（PSC）是一种进行性胆管炎症性疾病，其特征是局灶性和节段性胆管狭窄，会在第 68 章中讨论。第 35 章会看到类似的胆管离散狭窄和局限性梗阻综合征，它是艾滋病的一种罕见并发症，即所谓的艾滋病相关性胆管病变。胆管狭窄也可能是由肝动脉灌注或栓塞某些化疗化合物引起的[41]，或由胆管或肝动脉的外科损伤引起的（见第 68 章），而第 69 章会详细讨论胆管肿瘤。

3. 外源性胆管压迫

胆管的外源性压迫可能是由肿瘤累及或周围脏器的炎症引起的。动脉瘤、门静脉海绵样变（门静脉海绵状瘤）等周围脉管系统的显著增大几乎不会压迫胆管（见第 85 章）。

无痛性黄疸是胰头癌的典型特征（见第 60 章）。肝细胞癌或因转移性肿瘤或淋巴瘤而增大的门脉周围淋巴结可压迫肝外胆管（见第 32 章）。胰腺炎可因水肿或假性囊肿形成而导致胆管压迫（见第 58 和 59 章）。胆囊管或胆囊漏斗部的结石压迫肝总管（Mirizzi 综合征）引起黄疸的情况少见[42]。

三、黄疸的诊断方法

图 21.2 描述了诊断黄疸的一般方法。一个有逻辑的方法包括 4 个基本步骤：①仔细记录的病史，全面的体格检查和筛选实验室研究；②制订有效的鉴别诊断；③选择专门的测试来缩小诊断的可能性；④如果出现非预期的诊断可能性，制订治疗或进一步测试的策略。

（一）病史与体格检查

病史采集和体格检查会提供关于黄疸病因的重要线索（表 21.3）。一方面，有胆管手术史，发热和腹痛，特别是右上腹，表明胆管梗阻伴胆管炎。另一方面，与病毒前驱症状相似的症状（如厌食、乏力、肌痛），使急性病毒性肝炎诊断可能性明显增加，尤其是在存在潜在感染风险因素的情况下。仔细记录的病史可能提示环境毒素、乙醇或药物（包括非处方药或草药补充剂）是黄疸的基础。黄疸或肝病家族史增加了遗传性高胆红素血症或遗传性肝病的可能性。所有线索必须谨慎解读；例如，发热和腹痛伴有除胆管梗阻以外的疾病，病毒性肝炎可能在有胆管手术史的患者中同时发生。此外，厌食和乏力并不是病毒性肝炎特有的，有些慢性肝病患者可能会出现胆结石。当根据体格检查和常规实验室检查结果对患者病史的细节进行评估时，约 75% 的病例可以准确地定性黄疸为梗阻性或非梗阻性黄疸，该比率尚未被计算机模拟所超越[43]。

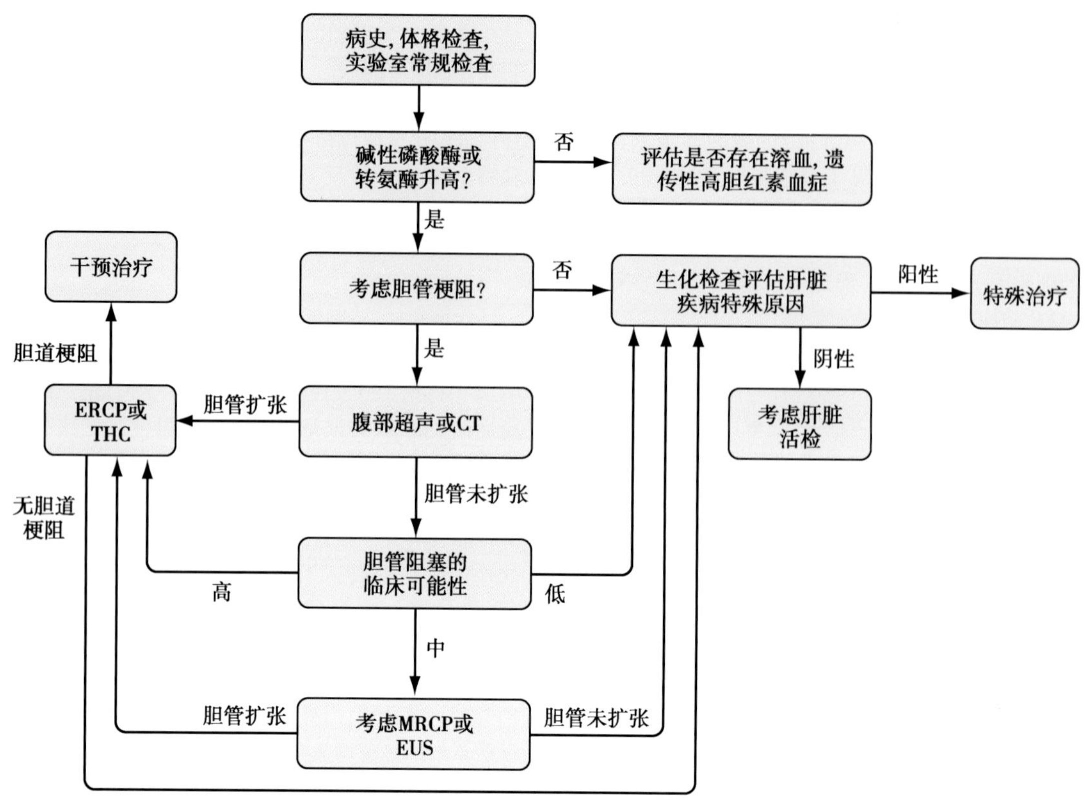

图 21.2　黄疸及高胆红素血症的评估与处理方法。CT，计算机断层扫描；ERCP，内镜逆行胰胆管造影；EUS，超声内镜检查；MRCP，磁共振胰胆管造影；THC，经肝胆管造影术

表 21.3　黄疸的鉴别诊断：胆管梗阻与肝病

特征	胆管梗阻	肝病
病史	腹痛	厌食、不适、肌痛（病毒性前驱症状）
	发热、寒战	
	高龄	暴露于已知的肝性毒素
	既往胆管手术	肝病家族史
		接受血液制品或注射药物史、肝病家族史
		已知的病毒暴露
实验室研究	血清淀粉酶或脂肪酶水平升高	相对于碱性磷酸酶而言，血清氨基转移酶水平显著升高
	白细胞增多	
	相对于氨基转移酶而言，血清碱性磷酸酶显著升高*	凝血酶原时间延长，不能正常使用维生素 K
		血清学显示特定肝病
	凝血酶原时间（INR）正常或服用维生素 K 后恢复正常	血小板减少症
体检	腹部手术瘢痕	扑翼样震颤
	腹部压痛	蜘蛛状毛细血管扩张
	发热	门静脉高压的特征（如腹静脉曲张、脾大、腹水）
	可触及腹部肿块	

*除了急性梗阻后的早期，此时可以短暂看到相反的情况。

体格检查提供的线索对于黄疸的诊断也很重要。发热或腹部压痛（特别是在右上腹）提示胆管炎，可触及的腹部肿块提示肿瘤引起梗阻性黄疸。肝硬化可由门静脉高压（如腹水、脾大、腹部静脉显露）、蜘蛛状毛细血管扩张症、男性乳房发育和扑翼样震颤。我们有时在肝豆状核变性患者中可看到角膜色素环，一些特殊体征可能是特定肝胆疾病的表现。

（二）基本实验室检查

黄疸患者的基本实验室检查包括血清总胆红素、碱性磷酸酶、氨基转移酶、全血细胞计数和凝血酶原时间（见第 73 章）。血清碱性磷酸酶活性来源于多种类型细胞膜上表达的相关同工酶；肝胆（“肝”）碱性磷酸酶同工酶是一种主要位于肝细胞和胆管细胞顶端的膜连接蛋白。在肝细胞和胆管细胞中，生理条件下的酶促裂解将碱性磷酸酶从细胞顶膜释放到胆汁中；少量从基底外侧膜释放到血浆中。胆管梗阻和肝内胆汁淤积增加碱性磷酸酶的基底外侧释放，在这些条件下血清碱性磷酸酶活性增加。因此，在黄疸患者中血清碱性磷酸酶（相对于转氨酶）活性的显著增加表明存在胆管梗阻或肝内胆汁淤积。然而，血清碱性磷酸酶活性增加（尤其是转氨酶活性正常时）可能反映肝外组织中碱性磷酸酶同工酶的释放。如果存在诊断不确定性，如 γ-谷氨酰转肽酶（GGTP）、5'-核苷酸酶、碱性磷酸酶同工酶等血清其他蛋白质的活性升高可证实肝胆疾病的存在（见第 73 章）。

通常在血清中可检测到低浓度氨基转移酶——丙氨酸转

氨酶(ALT)和天门冬氨酸转氨酶(AST),ALT为一种主要存在于肝细胞中的胞浆酶,AST是一种在肝细胞和其他组织细胞中共同存在的同工酶。如病毒性肝炎、中毒性肝损伤、缺血性肝炎(见上文)等因素导致肝细胞损伤同时会增加质膜通透性,并向血浆中释放氨基转移酶。相对于碱性磷酸酶,血清转氨酶水平的显著升高表明黄疸是由肝细胞损伤引起的。然而,也有例外。如胆总管结石引起的暂时性胆管梗阻可能导致血清转氨酶活性短暂性显著的升高(>正常的10~20倍)[44]。

全血细胞计数提供的信息补充了前面描述的生化测试的结果。白细胞增多提示胆管梗阻或其他与胆汁淤积有关的炎症性疾病的线索。贫血的存在增加了溶血性疾病引起黄疸的可能性,尤其是孤立性高胆红素血症的存在(即在肝脏生化测试中没有其他异常)。而血小板减少症是肝硬化的一个特征性发现,是由血小板生成调节剂血小板生成素合成减少或与门静脉高压相关的脾亢增加引起的。

凝血酶原时间反映了凝血因子Ⅰ、Ⅲ、Ⅴ、Ⅶ和Ⅹ的活性(见第94章)。当这些凝血因子肝脏合成受损时,凝血酶原时间延长,通常报告为INR增加,但这一发现并不特定于与肝细胞损伤的疾病相关。凝血酶原时间延长也可见于肝内胆汁淤积或胆管梗阻,因为维生素K(它是合成因子Ⅱ、Ⅶ、Ⅸ和Ⅹ所需的脂溶性因子)吸收受损。外源性补充维生素K可使由于肝内胆汁淤积或长期胆管梗阻而延长的凝血酶原时间恢复正常,但是不能纠正肝细胞损伤。

(三) 综合方法

综合患者的病史、体格检查和实验室结果,可估计黄疸是胆红素生成或代谢异常、内源性肝病还是胆管梗阻所引起。一种极端情况是除黄疸外体格检查无异常的无症状患者。这时如果ALP和转氨酶活性、血小板计数和凝血酶原时间正常,那么肝病或胆管梗阻的可能性很小。此时需要进一步检测特定的疾病,如孤立性胆红素代谢缺陷或溶血(见图21.2)。另外,如果病史、体格检查和实验室检查结果提示了胆管梗阻的可能性,需要进一步进行肝胆影像学检查。选择合适的影像学检查取决于胆管梗阻的情况、诊断准确性、成本、并发症发生率和每项检查的可用性(见下文),尤其是急诊。下面内容概述了科学家们早在20世纪至今对黄疸评估中影像学的探索。

(四) 影像学检查

1. 腹部超声

对疑似患有肝胆疾病的黄疸患者进行的首选影像学检查是腹部超声(US)[45,46]。US可显示胆石症(虽然胆管结石可能无法被很好地观察到)和直径超过1cm的肝内病变。与其他影像学研究相比,US具有无创,便携且价格低廉的优势(表21.4)。缺点包括检查结果依赖于操作者的技能水平、肥胖患者技术操作困难或肠道气体过多覆盖胰腺等某些器官。

表21.4 评估黄疸病因的各种影像学检查

检查	敏感性/%	特异性/%	致病率/%	死亡率/%	优点和缺点
腹部US	55~91	82~95	0	0	优点:无创,便携 缺点:肠内气体可能会阻塞胆管;对于肥胖者有困难,依赖操作者
腹部CT	63~96	93~100	见缺点	0	优点:无创,比US分辨率更高,不依赖操作者 缺点:有电离辐射,造影剂可能引起过敏反应
MRCP	82~100	94~98	见缺点		优点:无创,胆管造影优于US和CT 缺点:需要屏气,可能会漏诊小口径胆管疾病
ERCP	89~98	89~100	5	0.2	优点:提供胆管的直接成像,允许直接显示壶腹周围区域和获取肝管分叉远端的组织;允许同时进行治疗干预,尤其适用于肝管分叉远端的病变 缺点:需要镇静,如果解剖结构改变可能使内镜无法进入壶腹部(如Roux-en-Y),则不能进行手术;可能导致并发症(如胰腺炎)
经皮THC	98~100	89~100	3.5	0.2	优点:提供胆管的直接成像,允许同时进行治疗干预,特别适用于肝总管近端病变 缺点:未扩张的肝内胆管更困难;可能引起并发症
EUS	89~97	67~98	见缺点	0	优点:胆管成像优于超声和CT;允许对疑似肿瘤进行针吸活检 缺点:需要镇静

CT,计算机断层扫描;ERCP,内镜逆行胰胆管造影;EUS,超声内镜检查;MRCP,磁共振胰胆管造影;THC,经肝胆管造影术;US,超声。

2. 计算机断层扫描

腹部增强计算机断层扫描(CT)是评估肝胆疾病的另一种无创手段[47]。腹部CT可以精确测量胆管的直径,灵敏度和特异性与US相当[45]。腹部CT可以检测小到5mm的肝内占位性病变,不依赖于操作者,并且在肥胖人群中提供技术上更好的图像。然而它缺乏便携性,使患者暴露在电离辐射下,并且比US贵(见表21.4)。

3. 磁共振胰胆管造影

磁共振胰胆管造影(MRCP)是标准磁共振成像的技术改进,能够快速清晰地描绘胆管。在胆管梗阻方面MRCP优于传统的US或CT[48,49],在这种情况下为黄疸诊断发挥重要作用(见表21.4)。此外,如果有肝胆肿块的问题,或者如果造影剂过敏，可以在MRCP检查中进行标准的MRI。但是，MRCP比US或CT贵。

4. 内镜逆行胰胆管造影

内镜逆行胰胆管造影（ERCP）能够直接观察胆管[50]。比US、CT和MRCP（见表21.4）更具侵入性，费用与MRCP相当。内镜下识别壶腹乳头后，插入导管可将造影剂注入胆管；术中镇静和止痛是必要的。ERCP对胆管梗阻的诊断非常准确。如果确定了病灶原因（如胆总管结石、胆管狭窄），可在检查同时采取如括约肌切开术、取石术、狭窄扩张术、支架植入术等措施缓解梗阻（见第70章）。同样，如果怀疑肿瘤，可以进行活检和细胞学刷检。通过ERCP获取活检标本和治疗干预主要局限于左右肝管分叉处远端的病变。然而，胆管镜等附件的改进已经允许对常规ERCP不能清楚观察的病变进行光学可视化检查，并且在适当的情况下可进行靶向光动力治疗[51]。诊断性ERCP的技术成功率高于90%；当壶腹部乳头插管不成功，提示ERCP失败，这可能是由于患者先前进行过胃旁路术、胆总管空肠吻合术等腹部手术并改变了解剖结构。ERCP的主要并发症是胰腺炎，至少发生在5%的ERCP患者中，死亡率约为0.2%。这些比率在一定程度上受患者的基本特征和手术过程中对治疗器械需求的影响[52]。

5. 经皮肝穿刺胆管造影

经皮肝穿刺胆管造影（percutaneous transhepatic cholangiography，THC）是对ERCP的补充。THC需要穿刺针穿过皮肤和皮下组织进入肝脏，并进入周围胆管。当抽吸出胆汁时，通过针道引入导管，还可以注射造影剂了解肝胆管情况。经皮THC的敏感性和特异性与ERCP相当[53]。与ERCP一样，可在经皮THC检查同时进行球囊扩张和支架植入等介入手术，以解除胆管的局灶性梗阻，也可通过这种途径进行胆管镜（见第70章）。对于胆管梗阻位于肝总管近端或解剖结构的改变不能行ERCP的情况，经皮THC有显著优势（见上文）。在没有肝内胆管扩张的情况下，经皮THC技术上有一定挑战性；在这种情况下，可能需要多次穿刺，至少有10%的尝试失败[54]。约2%经皮THC患者会出现并发症，包括出血、穿孔和感染；死亡是罕见的。经皮THC比US和CT贵（见表21.4）。

6. 超声内镜检查

超声内镜检查（EUS）可以检测胆管和肝内胆管的梗阻情况，敏感性和特异性与MRCP相当[55-57]。EUS的潜在优势是允许对疑似恶性的病变进行活检，在适当的情况下，术者可以在EUS后直接通过ERCP行胆管减压（见表21.4）。诊断性EUS的风险与诊断性上消化道内镜检查的风险相当；使用细针穿刺活检时，死亡率仅仅约为0.1%。若不能确定患者是否存在胆管梗阻，且ERCP或THC的并发症的风险较高时，EUS可能是最有效的方法。

7. 核素显像技术

胆管核素显像[58]，如前所述具有可行性，可以使肝胆成像具有更高的空间分辨率，有助于胆囊炎的诊断，但其并不常用于成人黄疸的诊断评估。然而有两个潜在的例外情况。在胆管梗阻的早期阶段，胆管的扩张可能是不可见的，行核素成像是更加有利的[59]。核素显像在诊断肝胆外科手术或钝性腹部创伤后发生的罕见的潜在的胆漏性黄疸时也有重要作用（见第66章）[60,61]。

8. 影像学检查策略

影像学检查的顺序主要取决于梗阻性黄疸的临床可能性（见图21.2）。在MRCP和EUS之前的时代，通过临床决策分析比较了几种诊断策略；这一比较的后续改进尚未公布[62]。根据分析，如果胆管梗阻的概率约为20%，以US为首选策略的阳性和阴性预测值分别估计为96%和98%。如果胆管梗阻的概率为60%，采用US为首选检查的阳性预测值为99%，而阴性预测值将降至89%。这意味着，如果高度怀疑胆管梗阻，但是US显示胆管无明显扩张时，应进一步研究胆管的可视化检查。

因此，对于有可能出现胆管梗阻的黄疸患者，腹部US或CT是一种合适的首选影像检查方法。如果胆管扩张，应直接用ERCP或经皮THC对胆管进行成像；如果发现胆管梗阻，应采取适当的治疗措施。如果腹部US或CT提示胆管无明显扩张，应取决于临床上胆管梗阻的可能性而制订下一步检查策略。如果胆管梗阻的可能性较低，应评估患者的肝脏疾病情况（见下文）。如果胆管梗阻的可能性是中等的，建议EUS或MRCP评估肝胆情况，以决定下一步是否进行胆管干预或评估肝脏疾病。若很有可能是胆管梗阻引起的黄疸，下一步就可考虑ERCP（或经皮THC）。如果ERCP或经皮THC未显示胆管梗阻，应评估患者是否患有胆汁淤积性肝病。选择ERCP还是经皮THC受到多种因素的影响（见表21.4），包括医疗机构每种手术的可用性、初始影像学检查胆管是否扩张（这将阻碍经皮THC）、既往是否有阻碍内镜检查的胃肠道手术史（如胃旁路术、胆肠吻合术等）及胆管梗阻的可疑程度。在大多数胆管梗阻情况下，ERCP应该是首选的手术方法，因为它在准确性、技术成功率和主要并发症的发生频率方面与经皮THC相当，利于更广泛地使用，能提供更好的术后耐受性（如不需要外置胆管引流管）。

（五）其他检查

1. 血清学检测

对有肝细胞功能障碍或胆汁淤积生化证据的黄疸患者，影像学检查未发现胆管梗阻，应针对潜在肝病进行评估。根据疑似疾病，筛查实验室研究包括病毒血清学；针对血色素沉着症的血清铁、转铁蛋白和铁蛋白检测；针对肝豆状核变性的血浆铜蓝蛋白检测；针对PBC的血清AMA和抗核抗体（ANA）检测、对于自身免疫性肝炎检查血清平滑肌抗体和免疫球蛋白；对于乳糜泻的组织转谷氨酰胺酶抗体检测。若这些血清学分析未查明黄疸的病因，可以通过肝脏活组织检查（或乳糜泻情况下的小肠活组织检查）协助诊断。

2. 肝脏活组织检查

肝脏活组织检查提供了关于小叶结构以及肝脏炎症和纤维化的程度和模式的精确信息，这对持续且未确诊的黄疸患者最有帮助。通过特殊的组织学染色（以及是当时对铁或铜含量的定量检查），肝脏活组织检查有助诊断脂肪性肝病（根据患者的病史评估酒精相关或非酒精相关）、血色病、肝豆状核变性、自身免疫性肝炎、PBC、肉芽肿性肝炎和肿瘤。偶尔肝活检标本还意外地提供胆管梗阻的线索，其组织学特征如图21.3所示。然而，急性胆管梗阻的肝脏组织学可能完全正常。肝活检并发症发生率低但较为明确，主要是出血和穿孔，1%的病例需要住院治疗，死亡率约为0.01%[63]。

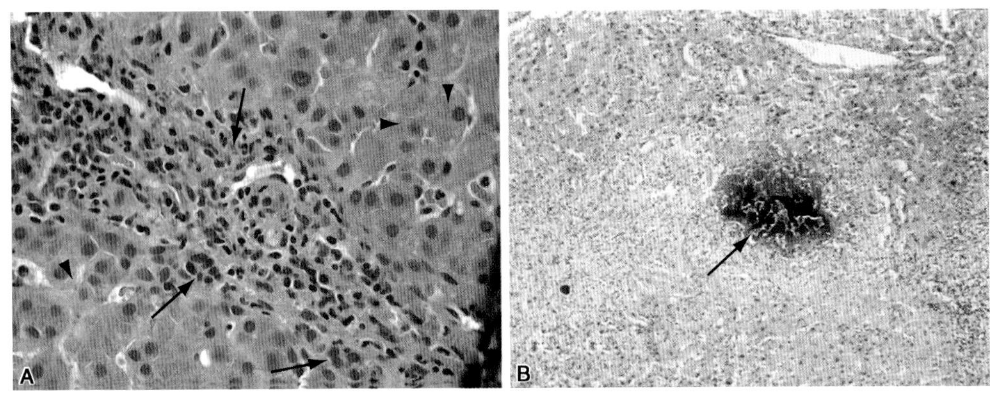

图 21.3 胆管梗阻的肝组织学。A,可见明显的胆管增生(箭头)和基于肝门的混合性炎性浸润。门静脉周围肝细胞呈羽毛状变性(箭头),表明胆酸盐淤积,长期胆汁淤积引起的细胞学变化(HE 染色,×200)。B,坏死细胞包围的门静脉周围胆红素染色区域(箭头)代表胆汁梗死(HE 染色,×40)

四、治疗方法

(一) 梗阻性黄疸

对于胆管梗阻的患者,治疗旨在解除梗阻。内镜或介入治疗方法包括括约肌切开术、局灶性狭窄的球囊扩张术和放置引流管或支架(见第 70 章);另一种方法是外科手术。对治疗策略的选择部分取决于梗阻病变的位置和可能的原因。介入放射学方法可以治疗局灶性肝内狭窄,而肝管分叉处远端的病变则更适合内镜治疗(如括约肌切开术治疗胆总管结石);如果可行,肝胆肿瘤引起的梗阻性黄疸的应考虑手术。

(二) 非梗阻性黄疸

当黄疸是由肝病引起时,最佳治疗是针对基础的疾病的治疗(例如,戒酒、停止使用违规药物、感染乙型或丙型肝炎病毒后进行抗病毒治疗、对自身免疫性肝炎使用免疫抑制剂)。在某些情况下,肝移植可能是唯一可行的选择(见第 97 章)。高胆红素血症本身的治疗在成人中通常是不必要的,因为胆红素的神经毒性仅限于以新生儿和婴儿中以非结合胆红素极度升高为特征的疾病(例如,新生儿的生理性黄疸,Ⅰ型 Crigler-Najjar 综合征)。在这些疾病中,光疗可以降低神经毒性的风险,即暴露于波长范围 460~490nm 的蓝绿色光中会使胆红素光异构化为水溶性更强的对映异构体,而这些对映异构体不需要结合即可在胆汁中排泄[1,64]。

熊脱氧胆酸(UDCA)是一种口服胆汁酸,可有效刺激胆汁流动,成功用于治疗多种胆汁淤积性疾病。在 PBC 患者中,UDCA 改善了大多数患者的生化指标并减缓了疾病进展(见第 91 章)[65]。研究还显示 UDCA 改善了妊娠期肝内胆汁淤积症患者的生化指标和临床结果[66,67],还能预防造血细胞移植后的高胆红素血症(见第 36 章)[24,68]。胆汁淤积症的其他治疗,主要是针对与高胆红素血症无关的并发症的治疗,如脂溶性维生素(A、D、E 及 K)吸收不良和瘙痒(见第 68 和 91 章)。

(王萍 译,鲁晓岚 校)

参考文献

第 22 章　胃肠病学的生物心理社会问题

Douglas A. Drossman, Laurie Keefer 著

章节目录

一、胃肠疾病的概念 …… 306
（一）生物医学模式 …… 306
（二）生物心理社会模式 …… 307
二、早期生活 …… 308
（一）学习 …… 308
（二）文化、家庭和社会 …… 308
三、社会心理环境 …… 309
（一）生活压力与虐待 …… 309
（二）心理因素 …… 310
（三）应对和社会支持 …… 310
四、脑-肠轴 …… 310
（一）应激与胃肠道功能 …… 311
（二）神经递质的作用 …… 311
（三）下丘脑-垂体-肾上腺轴 …… 312
（四）内脏疼痛的调节 …… 312
（五）细胞因子和脑 …… 315
五、症状体验和行为 …… 315
六、临床应用 …… 315
（一）病史采集 …… 315
（二）数据评估 …… 317
（三）诊断决策 …… 317
七、治疗方法 …… 317
（一）建立治疗关系 …… 317
（二）精神药理学治疗 …… 318
（三）行为治疗 …… 319
（四）临床医生相关的问题 …… 319

本章概述了心理社会因素与胃肠功能、疾病易感性、临床疾病和临床疗效的关系，并提供了胃肠疾病诊治的综合方法。

一、胃肠疾病的概念

（一）生物医学模式

在医学实践中，当观察到的与我们所期望的不一致时，会感到迷惑、困顿，这样的情况并不少见。当患者的症状与我们考虑诊断的疾病症状不相符时，则这种情况时有发生。在西方，对有症状或不适（由当前或以前的疾病、心理社会、家庭、文化等因素引起的健康状况不佳或身体功能障碍）和疾病（器官和组织的结构或功能异常）[1]的传统理解被称为生物医学模式[2,3]。该模式有两个特征。首先，任何不适症状都归于一个病因（还原论），因此确定病因是必须的，这足以解释疾病并最终治愈。这种方法似乎对急性传染病有效，但对结核病和 HIV 感染等慢性感染并不适用，因为宿主因素亦在临床表现中发挥作用。此外，生物医学模式不适用于慢性疾病，如炎症性肠病受遗传、环境、社会心理因素等多因素影响。其次，有症状或不适（illness）可分为疾病（disease）或器质性障碍，其具有客观定义的病理生理学或没有病理生理学改变的功能性紊乱（二元论）。这种二分法假定将医学（器质性）疾病与心理（功能性）疾病区分开来，或将功能性疾病降至没有病因或无治疗的状态。然而，近年来我们已经看到功能性胃肠疾病的“器质化”[4]以及疾病的功能化[5]。

以下病例很好地说明了生物医学模式[6]的局限性。

病例 1

42 岁女性，主诉中下腹疼痛伴恶心、间歇性呕吐 20 年。她说，“我再也忍受不了这种痛苦了。”经检查她的肠道功能正常，体重稳定。她觉得这些症状严重影响了她的生活和工作，没有任何能缓解这种症状的治疗。她有严重的精神创伤和抑郁史，童年时经历过性虐待和肉体摧残。她要求医生使用麻醉剂来帮她缓解疼痛，因为“这是唯一有效的方法。”她要求医生尽快“找出疼痛的原因并将其治愈”。就诊记录显示其频繁地急诊就诊，多次住院，各种诊断性检查（上消化道检查、胃镜、结肠镜、胶囊内镜、腹部和盆腔的 CT、盆腔超声、腹腔镜检查）均为阴性，以及用于止痛的持续加量的麻醉剂使用。她曾行胆囊切除术，但没有胆囊结石；因子宫内膜异位症行子宫切除术，手术均没有减轻她的疼痛。胃镜检查只显示幽门螺杆菌（Hp）阳性，为期 2 周的 Hp 根除治疗并没有减轻她的疼痛。鉴于她童年时的受虐史，她被转诊精神科，诊断为严重抑郁症和创伤后应激障碍（PTSD），同时精神科医生建议她排除其他可能的疾病。当她再次门诊就诊时，要求使用麻醉剂止痛，但医生建议其进行心理治疗。为此，患者要求转诊到上级医院进行其他的医学检查和治疗。

该患者患有严重功能性胃肠病（functional gastrointestinal disorder，FGID）[7,8]，从生物医学模式角度来看，这是一个挑战。除了诊断和治疗方面的困难外，多种原因可能会导致医患关系紧张[9]。首先，医生和患者从二元论的角度来处理这个问题。20 多年来，由于没有结构性（或器质性疾病的）诊断来解释她的疼痛，患者反复被要求进一步检查以“找到并解决”问题，如上消化道内镜检查。在门诊诊治中，经常找不到病因是一种普遍现象。一项涉及 1 000 名内科门诊就诊患者的研究显示，在 3 年内就诊的 567 例患者中[10]，16%（11% 是腹痛）最终被发现有器质性病因，只有 10% 的患者被诊断患有精神性疾病。这位患者有中枢介导的腹痛综合征[11]，每 37 个成人中有一个功能性胃肠病[12]，占消化科就诊者中的 40% 以上（见第 12 章）。相互接受这个诊断是开始一个适当治疗的关键。由于功能性胃肠病不符合生物医学模式，通常不被认为是一种疾病[6]，增加了不必要的检查和高昂检查（例如，

再次行上消化道内镜检查）的风险。Linedale 等的一项研究显示，当把功能性胃肠病与“器质性”胃肠道疾病作对比时，消化科医生在诊断时使用了更具限定性（不确定，不太自信）的语言；正是这种对诊断的不确定，往往导致不必要的检查和对疾病生物心理社会模式的拒绝[13]。更重要的是，可能进一步发展成麻醉性肠综合征，会进一步对临床结果产生不利影响，但可以经过适当的治疗缓解（见第 12 章）[11]。

这个患者出现了特征性的心理社会表现，其原因显而易见——如重大损失、抑郁、虐待史相关的创伤后应激障碍、灾难化的思维——然而这些特征被忽视了。患者认为社会心理因素与特定的医学疾病是分开的，两者的关系并不重要，而医生觉得不能或不愿意解决这些问题，故将患者转诊到精神科。反之，精神科医生注意到了心理特征，但是因为关注了是否有疾病漏诊而忽视了这些特征性的心理社会表现。就是因为这样的观点使患者继续不停地检查直到有诊断为止，而忽略了相关诊断和适当的治疗。

在这个病例中出现了医患互动障碍，因为他们对治疗的目标和期望产生了分歧。当患者需要的是快速缓解疼痛症状，而医生认为她的病情是慢性的，最终需要心理干预。作为回应，患者要求转诊到另一所医院，如果医生注重宣教的沟通技巧和患者协商制订治疗方案，那么这种分歧是可以避免的[1]。

这种无效治疗的“恶性循环”（图 22.1）源于生物医学模式的局限性。这种情况不仅发生在功能性胃肠病患者，也发生于器质性病变，如炎症性肠病，这些患者的疼痛和腹泻不能用实验室检查或内镜检查中看到的炎症程度来解释[5]。实际上，40%～60% 的炎症性肠病患者在疾病缓解期表现为肠易激综合征的临床表现[14]。实际情况是：①患者的症状不完全由机体结构异常解释；②社会心理因素诱发疾病，使患者有疾病的感受，并严重影响临床疗效；③对患者的体谅和适当的治疗有助于缓解医患关系。

（二）生物心理社会模式

生物心理社会模式[15]认为疾病不是由单一原因引起的，而是同时在细胞、组织、机体、人际关系和环境水平上相互作用的体系造成的。此外，心理社会因素有直接的生理和病理后果，反之亦然。例如，亚细胞水平的变化（如 HIV 感染、对炎症性肠病的易感性）有可能影响器官功能、个人、家庭和社会。同样，在人际层面上的变化，如配偶的死亡影响心理状况、细胞免疫，最终使疾病易感性增加[16]。该模式还解释了为什么生物学机体的临床表现（例如原癌基因的改变）和对治疗效果在不同患者之间存在差异。

图 22.2 解释了在疾病的临床表现中社会心理因素和生物

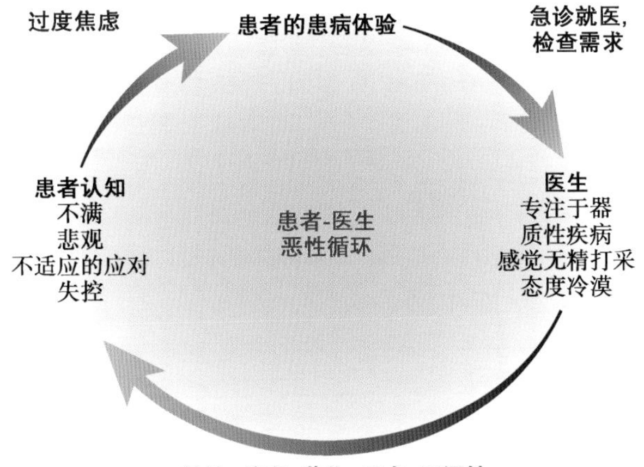

图 22.1　患者-医生恶性循环。恶性循环涉及 3 个组成部分：①功能性与器质性疾病二分法，其中未识别功能性胃肠疾病的诊断，并努力尝试进一步检测以确定器质性疾病；②识别和解决导致该疾病的潜在心理社会因素的能力有限；③患者-医生关系受损，缺乏关于诊断和治疗的共同决策。如本图所示，恶性循环的风险在于检测增加、医疗费用高、转诊次数多和护理中的相互不满，直至周期被打破。（Adapted from Longstreth GF, Drossman DA. Severe irritable bowel and functional abdominal pain syndromes: managing the patient and health care costs. Clin Gastroenterol Hepatol 2005; 3: 397-400.）

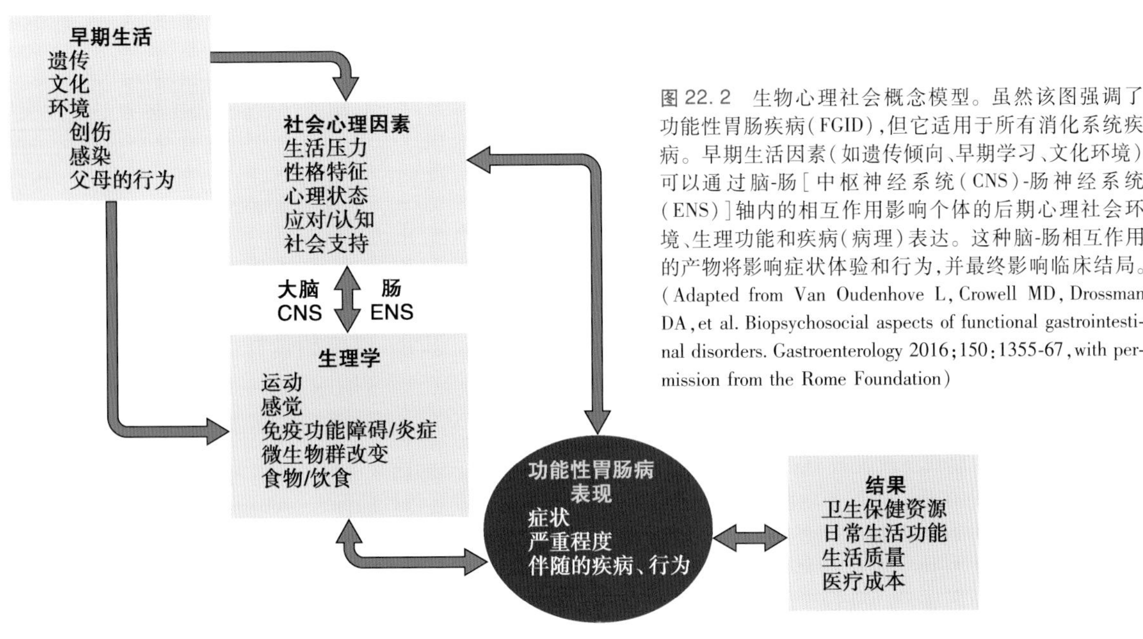

图 22.2　生物心理社会概念模型。虽然该图强调了功能性胃肠疾病（FGID），但它适用于所有消化系统疾病。早期生活因素（如遗传倾向、早期学习、文化环境）可以通过脑-肠［中枢神经系统（CNS）-肠神经系统（ENS）］轴内的相互作用影响个体的后期心理社会环境、生理功能和疾病（病理）表达。这种脑-肠相互作用的产物将影响症状体验和行为，并最终影响临床结局。（Adapted from Van Oudenhove L, Crowell MD, Drossman DA, et al. Biopsychosocial aspects of functional gastrointestinal disorders. Gastroenterology 2016; 150: 1355-67, with permission from the Rome Foundation）

因素之间的相互作用关系。早期生活因素(如遗传易感性、早期学习、文化环境)可以通过脑-肠轴(中枢神经系统-肠道神经系统)之间的相互作用,影响一个人后来的社会心理环境、生理功能和疾病的病理表现。这种脑-肠相互作用的产物将影响症状体验和行为,最终影响临床疗效。图 22.2 将作为以下大纲和讨论的模板。

二、早期生活

(一) 学习

胃肠道问题的早期学习涉及发育方面和生理条件反射。

1. 发育方面

从出生或出生前,一个人的基因组成与环境的相互作用就开始影响机体后天的行为和对疾病的易感性。这种作用最早的体现包括进食和排便。根据精神分析理论,当儿童的早期先天冲动(如进食或排便)面对外部环境(即父母)的限制时,就会出现冲突;正常的人格发展依赖这些冲突的成功解决。复杂的喂养和排便行为——给婴儿带来强烈满足感的源泉——根据普遍的家庭和社会习俗,儿童在成长过程中逐步学会妥协。在成长过程中,这些妥协在不同程度上与可立即获得的满足感相互冲突。儿童可以通过选择进食、拒绝进食、咬人、排便或拒绝排便来违抗或遵守环境限制,从而增加对这些功能的控制。这些行为何时以及如何显现,将取决于儿童的需求以及环境对他们的影响。在此期间养成的行为是孩子个性和后天与环境互动的关键,包括自主性的发展、是非分辨以及以一种社会认可的方式约束冲动,更不用说肠道功能了。相反,如果不能解决这些早期冲突,可能会影响成年后的性格,遇到困难变得脆弱。

某些胃肠疾病可能会受到早期学习困难或情感冲突的影响。肛门直肠功能紊乱(如排便失调、便秘)可能是由于排便疼痛、排便困难、排便训练[17]、滥用药物[18]所致,可以通过肛门直肠生物反馈进行康复治疗[19]。排便异常的儿童可能会因害怕上厕所、掌控或为得到父母关注而不解大便[20]。

一项设计严谨的研究揭示了症状体验与行为的早期构建模式在胃肠道症状和疾病的临床表现中的作用[21]。尤其是儿童期性虐待和身体虐待可带来生理性伤害,从而影响功能性肠病的产生或严重程度[22]。早期家庭对胃肠症状和其他疾病的关注可能会影响后来的症状主诉、健康行为及健康医疗保健费用的支出[23]。

2. 生理调节

早期条件反射经验也可能影响生理功能和心理生理疾病的发展。心理生理反应包括由心理引起的靶器官的功能性改变,而非器质性改变。这种生理心理反应通常被认为是愤怒或恐惧等情绪的生理反应,但是人们往往意识不到这种反应。一些学者认为,持续的生理状态改变或对心理刺激的生理反应强化也是一种心理生理疾病。内脏的功能,如消化液分泌、胆囊、胃和肠的运动,甚至可以通过家庭交互进行经典途径的调控[24]。经典条件作用,如巴甫洛夫所描述的,是将非条件刺激(钟声)与条件刺激(食物)联系起来,从而引起条件反应(流涎)。经过几次试验,无条件刺激可以产生条件性反应。已经证明,对良性胃肠道感觉的恐惧可以通过经典条件作用获得,这一发现对采用基于暴露技术的新型行为疗法有影响意义(见下文)[25]。此类研究中的第一项研究,将 52 名无胃肠道症状病史的健康受试者随机分为两组,一组是先行无痛性食管球囊扩张再行疼痛性食管球囊扩张(试验组),另一组仅行疼痛性食管球囊扩张(对照组)。试验组表现出较高的预期疼痛,增强的皮肤电导反应和对良性球囊扩张的恐惧反射增强,幸运的是,试验完成后该组受试者能够通过消除模式恢复[26]。

相反,操作性条件反射是通过动机和强化来发展期望的反应。打篮球就是一个例子,通过练习提高投篮精准度而得分,来看以下这个病例。

病例 2

一位叫约翰尼的儿童,学校有考试,当天早晨当他醒来时出现焦虑和“战斗或逃跑”症状,包括心动过速、出汗、腹部痉挛和腹泻。由于“肚子痛”,父母让孩子待在家里,并允许他躺在床上看电视。几天后,当孩子被鼓励回学校上课时,症状再次出现。

在这个病例中,父母把注意力集中在腹部不适上,认为是一种需要停课休息的疾病,而不是对痛苦情绪的生理反应。待在家里可以使儿童避免产生恐惧情绪,而不必考虑引起恐惧的原因。这种恐惧情绪的重复可能会导致条件性地强化心理生理症状反应,也可能改变儿童对这些症状作为一种疾病的认知,导致在以后的生活中寻求治疗的行为(疾病模式)[27]。与其他孩子相比,母亲强化疾病行为的孩子会出现更严重的胃痛和更多的学校缺勤[23]。

两项研究显示[24,28],寻求诊疗的肠易激综合征(IBS)患者比那些不寻求诊疗的 IBS 患者更能唤起父母对他们疾病的关注;他们休学在家,经常去看医生,并获得了更多的礼物和特权。采用经过验证的症状激发试验[29]来评估父母对腹痛主诉的关心程度,要求父母对孩子的疼痛主诉表现出积极或同情的反应。当他们这样做时,孩子对疼痛的主诉要比那些父母无视或分散注意力的孩子对疼痛的主诉频率要高[30]。

纠正父母这样的行为可能会防止胃肠道疾病的发展或恶化。在一项针对患有功能性腹痛(现在称为中枢性腹痛)儿童的大型临床试验中,200 名儿童及其父母被随机分配到认知行为疗法(CBT)组,该疗法针对的是父母对孩子疼痛主诉的反应和应对策略,或者是教育控制状态。父母对孩子疼痛主诉的认知改变会改善儿童的临床疗效,从而证明父母的认知会影响孩子的功能性胃肠病[31]。

(二) 文化、家庭和社会

社会和文化信仰体系改变了患者的患病体验以及与医疗保健体系的相互影响[32]。随着医学教育和医疗保健体系的全球化,这一问题变得越来越重要[33,34]。

对于没有很好的标志物的器质性或生理性疾病,诊断受到文化因素的影响,必须理解这些因素以便适当治疗。全球 70%~90% 的自我识别的疾病是在传统医疗机构之外进行治疗的,通常是由自助团体或宗教信徒提供大部分的治疗[35]。据居住在美国边境的墨西哥农民所述,即使可以免费享受标准医疗服务，他们还是会找民间治疗师（如巫医）治疗胃肠道症状[36]。

对身体感觉的认知过程受文化因素影响，取决于人们对机体运作的认知；某些症状在某些群体中，可能会被认为比其他群体更具有危险性和威胁性。在某些文盲群体中，个人可以任意自由地描述某种幻觉，而这些幻觉可能被这个群体中的其他人完全接受[37]。事实上，幻觉的意义并不在于它们是否存在，而是人们关注的焦点，尤其是在被那些掌权者说出来时，就越是如此。相反，在西方社会，人们强调的是理性和控制，幻觉会产生恐惧。除非有其他原因，否则幻觉可能被视为精神疾病的一种表现。

个体间的文化差异（如社会阶层结构）可能会影响医患之间的诊疗过程。在西方国家，以患者为中心的医疗模式正在成为主导模式，而在社会阶层差异很大的非洲国家，医患都不接受这种模式。患者常常认为，在诊疗过程中，医生要求患者的参与是一种软弱或无知的表现。

文化因素同样影响症状的表达。在 20 世纪中叶，在纽约进行的一项种族地域研究显示[37,38]，第一代、第二代犹太人和意大利患者比其他白种人移民主诉更多的身体部位症状、功能障碍和情感表达。相比之下，爱尔兰人倾向于尽量减少对痛苦的描述，而“老美国人”（新教徒）则是坚忍的。这些行为表现与家人态度与合并疾病相关，可以加强或减少主诉症状。意大利人因听到“疼痛不是一个严重的问题”而感到满意，而犹太人需要了解疼痛的原因及其可能导致的后果，这也许就是由于文化差异导致的。在欧洲，一项对炎症性肠病患者的调查中，南欧患者（即来自意大利和葡萄牙）与北欧患者相比，他们对炎症性肠病的担忧和关注度更高[39]。

文化差异也体现在医生和患者的解释模式上，这种差异可能会扭曲交流，产生误解或负面见解。例如，西班牙语中没有词汇来定义“腹胀”的概念，但在英语国家它是常见的症状[33]。在中国，表达心理压力常常受非议[35]，因此，当一个人处于痛苦状态时，主诉身体症状（躯体化）容易被别人接受[40]。但是在南欧，情感表达不仅会被接受，而且会稳固家庭关系[38]。美国南部农村，医疗保健服务者需要熟悉“root working”，这是一些非裔美国农民使用的一种巫术[41]。

食物和饮食是症状的主要决定因素，可能因文化和地理区域而异，因此，它们可能会影响肠道菌群、宿主免疫功能和治疗建议。

文化差异影响症状的处理，有的认为是需要治疗的疾病、有的自我治疗、有的被忽视。在墨西哥人中腹泻很常见，所以通常认为腹泻不是一种需要治疗的疾病[37]。据玛格丽特米德报道，阿拉佩什的孕妇不存在孕吐现象，她们有可能否认受孕直到孩子出生[42]。

是否坚持处方治疗受文化影响。如果有选择，罗马人（吉卜赛人）将只挑选最好的医生（ganzos）来照顾家庭成员，而不会听从其他人的建议[43]。在波多黎各人中，疾病的类型与基于“热-冷”理论的治疗相匹配。如果医生为“热症”患者开了一种“热药”（与体温无关），患者可能不会服用该药，因为它会破坏机体平衡[44]。

这些影响的类型表明询问患者对发病的理解、对病因的想法、临床病程以及希望或预期的治疗方法的重要性。它们可能会影响患者的依从性和治疗反应[33]。

三、社会心理环境

随着儿童步入成年期，遗传、文化、早期学习和其他环境影响都会融入个体独特的个性和行为方式中。生活压力、当前的心理状态（包括是否有精神疾病的诊断）、应对方式和社会支持程度等因素结合起来，将共同确定肠道生理功能对压力刺激的反应、疾病的易感性和活动性、疾病的认知和表现以及临床疗效。

（一）生活压力与虐待

未解决的生活压力，如失去父母、流产、重大个人灾难事件或周年纪念，或日常生活压力（包括患有慢性疾病）可能通过以下几种方式影响一个人的疾病：①产生心理-生理反应（如运动、血流、体液分泌或身体感觉的变化，加重症状）；②提高对症状（称为躯体或内脏焦虑）的警惕性；③导致个体适应不良、更严重疾病行为、寻求医疗服务[11,21,45,46]。虽然已有科学证据显示社会心理因素在病理性疾病的发展中起着因果作用，但是基于目前回顾性研究和相关数据还不足以证明其因果关系。然而生活事件压力对一个人的心理状态和疾病行为的负面影响，需要医生在对所有患者的日常诊疗中加以解决。

身体或性虐待史会严重影响症状的严重程度和临床疗效[46]。最新研究表明适应性低或无法恢复和适应压力生活事件（压力高反应性）可能是一个潜在的原因，通过早期生活的逆境增加肠易激综合征的风险[47]。与无虐待史的患者相比，有性虐待或身体虐待史的胃肠病转诊患者的疼痛程度比对照组增加 70%（$P<0.0001$），心理压力增加 40%（$P<0.0001$），在过去 3 个月内卧床时间是对照组的 2.5 倍（11.9 天 vs 4.5 天，$P<0.0007$），日常生活功能比对照组几乎差 2 倍（$P<0.0001$），6 个月内就诊的次数更多（8.7 次 vs 6.7 次；$P<0.03$），甚至接受了更多与胃肠道疾病诊断无关的手术（4.9 次 vs 3.8 次；$P<0.04$）[48]。因此，生活压力和虐待史具有生理和行为方面的影响，会放大所经历的病情的严重程度。这些影响导致寻求更多的医疗服务，并解释了与初步诊治相比，在转诊中心和专科诊治的胃肠道疾病患者有更高比例的虐待史[45,46,49]。

有几种可能的机制解释了虐待史与预后不良之间的关系[22,46]。这些机制包括：①易患心理疾病，这些状况会增加对内脏信号或其有害性的感知（中枢高敏性和躯体化）；②发生心理生理（如自主性、体液性、免疫性）反应，表现为肠道功能改变、感觉功能异常、促进炎症[50]；③由于运动增加或身体创伤（内脏痛觉过敏或异位性痛觉）引起的外周或中枢敏感；④对感知威胁的身体感觉的异常评价和行为反应（反应偏差）；⑤采用不当应对方式的反应加强，导致更多的疾病症状和就医诊治（如小题大做）。从生理上讲，与无虐待史的肠易激综合征患者相比，直肠扩张使有虐待史的肠易激综合征患者产生更多的疼痛，伴有背侧前扣带回皮层（anterior cingulate cortex，ACC）的敏感性更高（见下文）[7]，经治疗后疼痛和大脑活跃度减弱[51]。

(二) 心理因素

如图 22.2 所示,伴随着生活压力和虐待,并发的心理社会因素可以影响胃肠道的生理变化、发生病理状态的易感性以及其症状和行为表现,所有这些都会影响预后。心理因素与长期存在的或特质的特征(如性格、精神病诊断)和更易改变的或状态特征(如心理困扰、情绪)有关,后者适用于心理和精神药物的干预。此外,应对方式和社会支持均能提供调节(缓冲)效果[52,53]。

1. 人格

人格特征(轴Ⅱ障碍)是指成年早期明显的、终生稳定的持久行为。病理特征的例子包括边缘型、强迫型或偏执型人格障碍;它们不适合特定的药物或心理治疗。

在精神分析主导的心身医学时代(1920—1955 年),某些心理冲突被认为是表达特定的心身疾病(如哮喘、溃疡性结肠炎、原发性高血压、十二指肠溃疡)的人格发展的基础[54]。然而,人格特征与医学疾病的因果关系特别相关(尽管是在生物学上易感的宿主中)的观点过于简单。研究者现在将人格和其他心理特征视为疾病的驱动因素或调节因素。

2. 精神疾病诊断

精神疾病诊断是可定义的精神症状和行为的集合(轴Ⅰ)。消化科医生通常把这些症状看作是胃肠道疾病的一个伴随因素。比起专科诊治,患有内科疾病(合并症)的精神病患者在转诊中更常见,并且精神疾病加重了疾病的临床表现和预后。焦虑症是最常见的精神病,全球 30% ~50% 的功能性胃肠病患者有焦虑症[55]。抑郁症也很常见;在社区医院中,抑郁症和胃肠道疾病重叠的患者约占 30%,而在三级医院中略多[56]。据估计,15% ~38% 的肠易激综合征患者有过自杀的想法,当症状严重影响生活、治疗无效时更感绝望[57]。抑郁和焦虑适合精神药物或心理治疗[21,45,57]。

某些精神障碍和人格特征会对疾病的表现产生不利影响,甚至会干扰家庭互动、社交、与医生的互动。《精神疾病诊断与统计手册》(DSM-5)摒弃了"躯体化"的概念,取而代之的是躯体症状障碍(somatic symptom disorder, SSD; DSM5 300.82)。在这一诊断类别中,躯体症状可能或可能不是医学上能解释的,但是它令人痛苦、致残,并伴随着超过 6 个月的过度的、与症状不相符的想法、感觉和行为[58,59]。这一类别中的其他疾病包括人为障碍(DSM5 300.19),其特征是伪造症状和与这些症状相关的欺骗行为,也可能是孟乔森综合病症,患者伪装或制造自身疾病(例如,服用泻药引起胃肠道出血,假装有疾病症状)以赢得某种效果(例如得到麻醉药、手术、就医)(见第 23 章)。边缘型人格障碍(DSM5 301.83)也包括在内,患者表现强烈又极不稳定的(如过度依赖)人际关系模式,有难以控制的情绪,并表现出冲动行为(如自杀、自残、性行为)[60]。对于患有这些疾病的患者,医护人员必须建立清楚明晰的诊疗界限(例如不要仅根据患者的要求来安排治疗),明确时间限制,并避免不必要的情感互动。

3. 心理困扰

即使是以前体健的人,患病也会引起心理困扰,这被理解为短暂的和可改变的焦虑、抑郁和其他情绪障碍(心理状态)。在转诊实践中,42% ~61% 的患者会出现心理困扰,并具有放大效应:降低疼痛阈值[61],是感染后肠易激综合征和消化不良发生的共病因素[62],并影响症状严重程度、医疗保健寻求、服务利用和临床结局[21]。患者可能不清楚心理困扰与疾病之间的关联。当就诊的 IBS 患者与未就诊的 IBS 患者进行比较时,前者报告了更大的心理困扰,但也否认了这些困扰在其疾病中的作用[60]。这种模式可能是在生命早期通过家庭的调节而形成的。来自病例 2 中的 Johnny 在抑郁时报告了躯体症状,他可能没有认识到或传达症状均与应激前因的关系,因为这些前因在家庭中没有被承认或照顾。有意识地意识到自己感觉的能力被认为是一种认知技能,经历了一个类似于 Piaget 描述的其他认知功能的发展过程[16]。然而,这种认知发展可能在压抑的家庭环境中受到抑制,似乎与躯体化有关。

(三) 应对和社会支持

应对和社会支持通过缓冲(拒绝)或能(增加和放大)调节生活压力、虐待和共病心理因素对疾病及其结局的影响。应对被定义为"以行动为导向和内在精神的努力",以管理(即掌握、容忍、最小化)环境和内部需求以及对个人资源征税或超出个人资源的冲突[63]。基于应激源的应对策略的灵活性(当问题有解决方案时,以问题为中心进行应对;当问题没有解决方案时,以情绪为中心进行应对)是适应疾病的一个关键方面[64]。有一些证据表明,功能性胃肠道疾病患者可能在应对方式上缺乏灵活性,导致负性情感和强烈的症状主诉[65-67]。基于回避的应对策略(分散注意力、麻木、转移)评分较低的克罗恩病患者最不可能复发[68]。对于所有类型的胃肠道诊断,不适应的情绪应对方式,特别是灾难性的,以及无法减轻症状的感知,与随后 1 年期间较高的疼痛评分、较多的医生访视和较差的功能相关[69]。灾难性情绪应对也与更困难的人际关系有关[70],预示着术后疼痛[71],并导致肠易激综合征(IBS)患者更大的担忧和痛苦[72]。通过心理治疗努力改善人们对疾病压力及其管理能力的评估,会改善健康状况和预后[45]。

通过家庭、宗教和社区组织及其他社会网络提供的社会支持,在减少心理困扰对身心疾病的影响方面也有类似的好处,从而提高应对疾病的能力[73,74]。消极的社会关系尤其与不良的健康结果密切相关[75]。从医务人员获得社会支持的患者也有可能得到症状改善和生活质量的提高[76]。

四、脑-肠轴

脑-肠轴是神经解剖的基础,如上描述的社会心理因素影响胃肠道的神经解剖基础,反之亦然。脑肠轴"硬接线"类似于一种复杂的集成电路,它将中枢神经系统和肌间神经丛[77]之间的信息传递至末端器官结构。它是一个双向系统,思想、感觉和记忆引起神经递质释放(软件),进而影响感觉、运动、内分泌、自主神经、免疫和炎症功能[78,79]。肠道菌群还通过神经、内分泌和免疫途径与大脑进行双向交流,从而对包括焦虑,抑郁和认知障碍以及慢性内脏疼痛在内的行为障碍产生重大影响[80]。该系统的失调解释了运动障碍、疼痛和其他胃肠道症状以及功能性胃肠病。实际上,脑-肠轴是生物心理社会模式临床应用的神经解剖学和神经生理学基础。

（一）应激与胃肠道功能

1. 应激的定义

任何需要调整或适应的对稳定状态的影响都可以认为是应激,但这个术语是非特异性的,包括刺激及其影响。刺激可以是像感染这样的生物事件,也可以是像搬家这样的社会事件,甚至是一个令人不安的想法。应激可以是预期的,也可以是不想要的。某些刺激,如疼痛、性或受伤的威胁,往往会在动物和人身上引起一种可预测的反应。相比之下,生活事件有更多不同的影响,取决于个人对事件的个人解释。离婚对一个人来说可能是积极的体验,对另一个人来说则是失望。刺激可以让不同的人或同一个人在不同的时间产生不同的反应。这种影响可能是观察不到的,也可能是心理反应(焦虑、抑郁)、生理变化(腹泻、出汗)、疾病发作(哮喘、结肠炎)或以上反应的任何组合。一个人对事件的解释是否有压力以及他或她对压力的反应取决于先前的经验、态度、应对机制、性格、文化和生物因素,包括对疾病的易感性。

有前瞻性的研究表明,应激性生活事件的经历与肠易激综合征患者的症状恶化[70]、频繁就诊有关[81]。据报道,即使控制了肠易激综合征的严重程度、焦虑、人口学特征后,慢性生活压力仍然是肠易激综合征患者 16 个月内症状强度的主要预测因素[69]。最后,应激会影响治疗结果。一项肠易激综合征治疗的研究中,治疗前 6 个月内存在单一应激源的患者,与没有应激源的患者相比,前者在 16 个月随访时的不良预后、症状更严重[82]。

2. 应激对胃肠道功能的影响

健康人通常也会在沮丧或不安时出现腹部不适或肠道功能改变[83]。当这些症状足够严重时(例如导致寻医就诊),医生会考虑到这些症状,评估应激的类型、程度,予以相应的治疗[84]。

Cannon 注意到当猫对一只咆哮的狗作出反应时,猫的肠道活动停止运作[85]。Pavlov 首次报道精神因素通过迷走神经影响狗的胃酸分泌[86]。Beaumont[87]、Wolf[88]和 Engel[89]观察到人们在心理和生理应激作用下,胃袋或瘘管分泌功能、黏膜颜色改变。当人们出现愤怒、强烈的快感或对他人的攻击行为时,胃充血、胃动力增加和分泌增加。相反,当人们出现恐惧或抑郁、退缩状态(即放弃行为)或脱离他人时,胃黏膜苍白、分泌减少、动力减弱。复杂的认知活动使食管高振幅、高速地收缩[90],导致第二阶段肠道运动减少[91],小肠移行性肌电复合体(MMC)[92]第三阶段活动延长(见第 99 章)。实验引发的愤怒会增加结肠的运动电位和尖峰电位活动,这在功能性肠病患者中更明显[93]。生理或心理压力也会降低痛阈,肠易激综合征患者的痛阈比其他患者更低[61]。

在动物模型和人类研究中,应激促使促炎细胞因子的产生和肥大细胞的激活、脱颗粒,从而影响黏膜的改变,特别是在肠神经元附近,从而导致内脏致敏[94]。应激还会削弱紧密连接,从而增强黏膜通透性,增加细菌向肠壁的移位[95-97]。急性应激触发下丘脑-垂体轴,导致皮质醇水平升高,自主神经系统激活,促炎细胞因子如肿瘤坏死因子-α、白细胞介素-6和干扰素-γ 升高[98,99]。应激可改变肠道菌群组成,使“好”菌变为“坏”菌。这些变化伴随着免疫应答的改变,可导致炎症的发生和肠易激综合征(特别是感染后的肠易激综合征)、炎症性肠病易感性增加[100]。相反,肠道菌群的改变可以通过脑-肠轴反过来影响中枢神经系统的功能,包括情绪、学习和记忆[101]。

一个有效的模型验证应激和免疫改变之间的相互关系,即被称为感染后肠易激综合征,约有 10% 的患者在一次感染性肠炎后会出现这种情况[102]。据 2018 年罗马基金会工作组报告中的报道,感染后肠易激综合征会出现肠道微生物的改变以及肠道上皮、5-羟色胺、免疫因子变化[102],这些观点支持人们早期对于感染后肠易激综合征发病机制的认识,即炎症诱导的黏膜免疫反应改变,在情绪困扰的情况下使内脏传入神经敏感[103]。对于有心理困扰的人,当感染后或黏膜损伤(如炎症性肠病和肠易激综合征患者中)发生时,其内脏信号的中枢神经系统被放大来引起意识感知,从而导致对症状的感知增强[104]。肠嗜铬细胞增生(伴随 5-羟色胺的增加)、抑郁症都是感染后肠易激综合征进展的重要预测因素(风险比分别为 3.8 和 3.2)[105]。

（二）神经递质的作用

如前所述,中枢神经系统和神经内分泌系统丰富的神经丛与神经内分泌的联系为脑-肠轴提供了固有链接的基础。介导这些活动的神经递质和神经肽在中枢神经系统和肠道神经系统中可见。由于这些物质存在的位置,故对胃肠功能和人类行为都有综合作用。这一研究结果并不令人惊讶,因为大脑和肠道之间的固有链接是从一个神经元(神经管)开始,然后以不同的形式随着机体生长分化为肠道中的“大脑”和“小脑”。如图 22.3 所示,胚胎神经系统的发育始于神经嵴。随着时间的推移,神经嵴分化为前脑、中脑和脊髓。脊髓神经节从未来的脊髓迁移到早期的肠道成为未来的肠道神经系统,因此,肠道神经系统、脊髓、中枢神经系统是“固有链接”的。没有其他器官系统像胃肠道系统那样与大脑联系如此紧密。这有助于解释临床观察到的社会心理特征与肠道功能(脑-肠轴)之间的密切关系。

例如,应激激素促肾上腺皮质激素释放因子(CRF)具有中枢应激调节作用,但对肠道有不同的生理作用。在心理厌恶刺激作用下,CRF 促使胃潴留、结肠转运率增加[106],内脏超敏性增加[107]、免疫功能改变[78];因此,CRF 可能在应激诱导的肠易激综合征[108](见第 122 章)、循环呕吐综合征[109](见第 15 章)和其他应激介导的疾病中发挥作用。

肽类可作为神经递质在神经末梢分泌,也可以直接从细胞壁分泌,因此具有局部或旁分泌作用。一些关键的神经递质作用于脑-肠轴[77,110]。乙酰胆碱是副交感神经系统的主要介质,驱动肠道系统的运动;功能紊乱会导致便秘和胃轻瘫。5-羟色胺、去甲肾上腺素和多巴胺等生物胺在周围发挥调节交感神经系统的作用,调节便秘和腹泻之间的平衡,并集中调节情绪、情绪行为和疼痛。降钙素基因相关肽(CGRP)、缓激肽和速激肽(如 P 物质)参与内脏痛觉过敏和疼痛综合征。阿片类物质系统可提高疼痛阈值,减弱蠕动和减少分泌;它可能会引起痛觉过敏[111]。

这些联系在治疗方面具有相关性。慢性胃肠道引起的疼

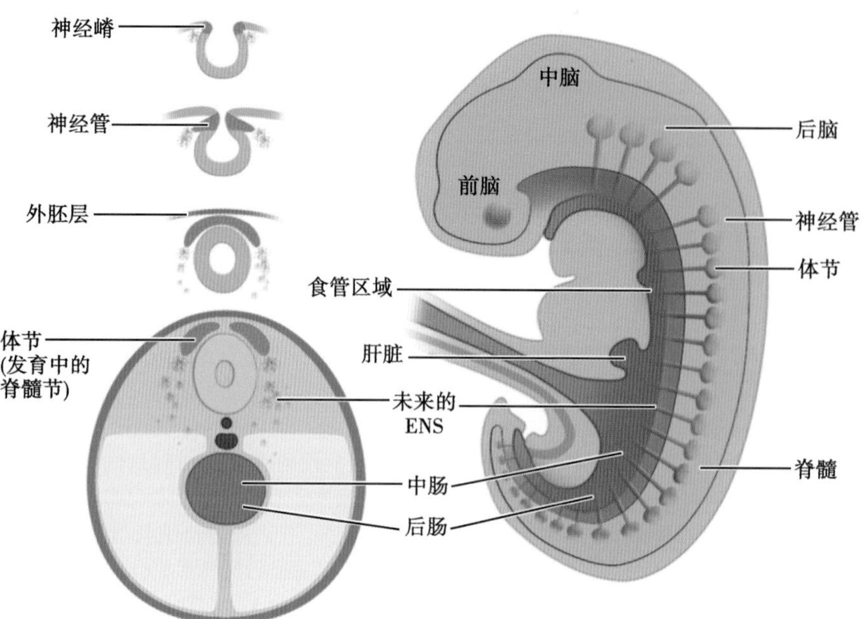

图 22.3　大脑与胃肠神经系统之间的联系。这张图显示了从神经嵴开始的胚胎中神经系统的发育。随着时间的推移,神经嵴生长并分化为前脑、中脑和脊髓。从未来的脊髓,脊髓神经节迁移到早期肠道,成为未来的肠神经系统(ENS)。因此,肠神经系统、脊髓和中枢神经系统是"固有连接"的。没有其他器官系统像胃肠系统那样与大脑紧密相连。这有助于解释心理社会特征与肠道功能(脑-肠轴)之间密切关系的临床观察结果。(From Van Oudenhove L, Crowell MD, Drossman DA, et al. Biopsychosocial aspects of functional gastrointestinal disorders. Gastroenterology 2016;150:1355-67, with permission from the Rome Foundation.)

痛是由脑-肠轴的门控系统调节的(参见第 12 章)。由于大脑的某些区域具有上调或下调传入内脏信号的功能,因此可以通过大脑和肠道共有的神经递质(例如去甲肾上腺素能和 5-羟色胺能神经递质)来尝试减少疼痛体验。罗马基金会工作小组报告[112]中推荐使用中枢神经调节剂(以前称为抗抑郁药、抗精神病药和其他精神药物)用于治疗慢性胃肠道疼痛或其他胃肠道功能紊乱,这是基于脑-肠轴疼痛控制机制及其可能对神经发生的中枢作用[112](见下文)。

(三) 下丘脑-垂体-肾上腺轴

应激免疫反应的主要介质包括 CRF 和中枢神经系统中的蓝斑-去甲肾上腺素(LC-NE)系统。这些系统受到许多正反馈和负反馈系统的影响,这些系统允许行为和外部环境适应应激[113]。CRF 系统的外周延伸是下丘脑-垂体-肾上腺(HPA)轴,一种参与心理神经免疫调节的负反馈系统。在 HPA 系统中,炎症细胞因子(主要是 TNF-α、IL-1、IL-6)在炎症过程中释放,以及来自下丘脑其他区域和包括杏仁核和内侧前额叶皮质在内的其他大脑区域的多个神经输入,刺激下丘脑室旁核的 CRF 分泌。CRF 刺激垂体释放促肾上腺皮质激素(ACTH,或促肾上腺皮质激素),进而刺激肾上腺释放糖皮质激素。最后,糖皮质激素抑制炎症和细胞因子的产生,从而完成负反馈循环[114]。儿茶酚胺能增加促炎细胞因子释放。副交感神经系统具有抗炎作用。HPA 的激活也可能是由于负反馈的减少(例如,海马糖皮质激素受体下调在早期生活压力的动物模型中所示)[115,116]。

CRF 通过中枢和外周神经系统在应激相关的胃肠道运动和感觉功能中起调节作用,并发挥重要作用[106],并可能参与对心理应激调节敏感的疼痛相关症状的产生或维持[99]。由于 HPA 轴反应性的增加(如库欣综合征、抑郁、感染易感性)或降低(如肾上腺功能不全、类风湿关节炎、慢性疲劳综合征、创伤后应激障碍),HPA 系统的紊乱可导致行为异常和全身性疾病[113]。

IBD 可能通过这种应激介导的系统受到影响[117]。疾病的激活不仅具有遗传和感染作用,而且表型表达也可能受到脑-肠通路的影响,包括自主神经系统和 HPA 轴、促炎的胃肠道 CRF、肠道屏障和肠内菌群,所有这些都是由中枢神经系统介导的。越来越多的证据表明,疾病的激活受到心理脆弱性的影响,包括感知压力、适应不良的应对方式和精神疾病[117-119]。

(四) 内脏疼痛的调节

1. 内脏信号放大

各种类型的刺激都能放大上行的内脏通路信号。值得注意的是,内脏痛觉不一定直接映射到外周传入输入的程度或强度,而是通过大脑水平的认知和情感回路以及下行调节通路放大。例如,消极情感,包括神经质和躯体化,会影响各种健康状况下的内脏疼痛的处理和调节[120]。在认知上,注意力分散和期待都可以减轻内脏疼痛的感知体验[121]。这种内脏疼痛神经基质的功能障碍会使生理(非伤害性)刺激被感知为疼痛或不愉快的,这种现象被称为内脏超敏反应。随着时间的推移,这种疼痛的持续形成了 FGID 作为肠脑疾病模型的基础。此外,随着疼痛变得更加严重,中枢机制开始在症状体验中发挥更大的作用[8]。

在通过脑-肠轴上行之前，内脏信号可以通过多种方式被放大。这些过程是相互关联的，在不同的患者中可能有所不同。感染、创伤和其他引起炎症的因素，以及由于反复扩张引起的运动障碍可能会导致初级传入通路的敏感化[122]。肠易激综合征患者的黏膜活检显示神经可塑性重塑以及蛋白酶的释放影响初级传入神经的反应特性，从而导致超敏反应[123]。如前所述，肠道感染和心理困扰反映了导致感染后 IBS 和消化不良的脑-肠机制[124]。上皮细胞免疫激活与黏膜炎性细胞因子的表达增加和初级感觉神经末梢神经肽（如 P 物质、CGRP）的释放增强有关（见上文[125]）。应激介导的肥大细胞脱颗粒，尤其是靠近肠道的神经元，与传入神经元的致敏有关[84]。最后，上皮细胞的通透性随应激反应而增加是通过肥大细胞脱颗粒产物（包括 CRF 和蛋白酶）介导的[126,127]。

2. 传输至中枢神经系统

图 22.4 显示了结肠的上行传入通路。在一级内脏神经元受到刺激后，它们投射到脊髓，与二级神经元突触上升到丘脑和中脑。在一些脊髓上行通路（脊髓丘脑、脊髓网状结构和脊髓中脑束）中，图 22.4 右侧所示的脊髓丘脑束终止于内侧丘脑，并作为三级神经元投射到初级躯体感觉皮层。这条通路对内脏和躯体刺激的感觉辨别和定位（即确定疼痛的位置和强度）很重要。脊髓节束（中间通路）将感觉信息从脊髓传导到脑干（网状结构）。这个区域主要涉及内脏刺激的情感和动机特性，即疼痛的情感成分。丘脑束从网状结构投射到左侧丘脑内侧，然后投射到扣带回皮层。扣带回皮层（见图 22.3）分为以下部分，参与情感的膝周前扣带回皮质（pACC）、参与行为反应修饰的中扣带皮层（MCC）、与接收传入的内脏信号相关的脑岛叶。这些区域参与处理有害的内脏和躯体信息。这种多成分的伤害性信息整合，分散到躯体型强度区域（外侧感觉皮层）和内侧皮层的情绪或动机-情感区

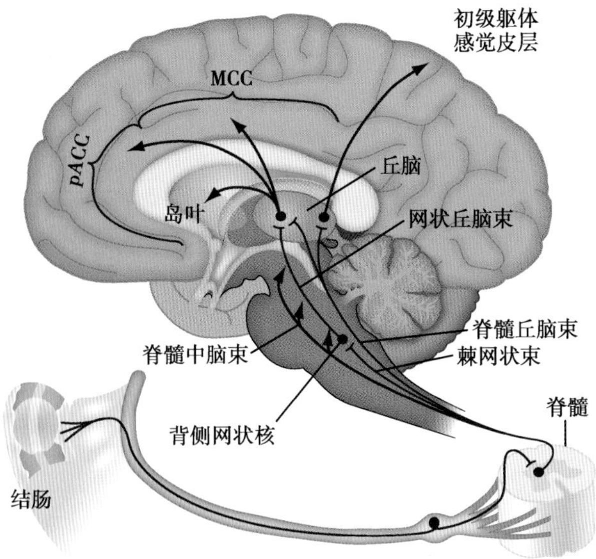

图 22.4　内脏疼痛传递至中枢神经系统。该图显示了通过脊髓和中脑通路从肠道到大脑躯体感觉和边缘结构的上行内脏通路。MCC，中扣带回皮层；pACC，前扣带回周围皮层。（From Drossman DA. Functional abdominal pain syndrome. Clin Gastroenterol Hepatol 2004；2：353-65）。

域，这解释了疼痛体验和主诉的变异性。

这种通过感觉和动机-情感成分进行疼痛调节的概念方案得到了使用放射性标记氧进行正电子发射断层成像（PET）研究的支持[128]。健康受试者将手浸入热（47℃）水中，催眠暗示可使其体验痛苦或愉悦。值得注意的是，两组在躯体感觉皮层激活方面没有观察到差异，但在经历手浸入疼痛的催眠受试者中，前扣带皮层（ACC）的激活更高。催眠暗示区可分为两种疼痛系统的功能。不愉快的暗示特异性地编码在 ACC 的前中扣带回部分，该区域涉及恐惧和不愉快的负面认知，并与功能性疼痛综合征相关（见下文）。

3. 中枢性放大

参与疼痛调节和情绪状态的回路涉及重叠的大脑区域（前岛叶皮质、ACC、内侧前额叶区域和杏仁核），这种重叠可能是胃肠道疾病患者疼痛情绪特征的基础[51,129,130]。在焦虑症患者中，大脑回路与其过度警觉、对威胁的关注度增加和适应不良的应对方式有关[131]。与高度警戒有关的大脑网络活动增加，导致对感觉输入的调节；因此，这些网络代表了疼痛回路失调的可能途径[132]。

有数据支持以下假设：共病精神诊断、重大生活压力、性虐待或身体虐待史、社会支持不佳和适应不良与更严重、更慢性的腹痛和更差的健康结果相关[21,48]。图 22.5 说明了这种与功能性和结构性胃肠道疾病的关系。对于大多数轻、中度症状的患者，环境和肠道相关因素（如肠道感染、炎症或损伤、饮食、激素因素）可导致传入兴奋和传入神经元活动上调。由于各种社会心理因素的影响，中、重度症状的患者的疼痛中枢调节功能受损，脊髓水平的传入信号中枢抑制作用减弱（去抑制）。实际上，疼痛越严重，持续时间越久，与其他合并症症状越相关，疼痛就越有可能是中枢介导的[8]。图 22.6 展示了中枢致敏的概念。内脏致敏与肠黏膜水平上发生的 ENS 一阶神经元内神经信号的上调有关（如黏膜免疫激活改变、肥大细胞脱颗粒、肠黏膜下层细胞因子释放）。中枢敏化与中枢神经系统的上调有关。反复刺激一阶神经元导致脊髓回路敏感化，从而增加来自背角突触发出的信号，然后通过二阶神经元传递到大脑。中枢敏化也可能在大脑水平上通过来自包含应激相关激活的中枢的连接而增强。其结果是疼痛加剧或其他类型的胃肠道功能障碍，通过这些上传增强途径从肠道传递到大脑。

了解疾病的严重程度和作用部位（如肠、脑或两者）有助于选择治疗方法（见下文）。当外周影响因素对严重程度占主导地位时，药物、手术或其他作用于肠道的方法是主要的治疗考虑因素。然而，随着疼痛变得更加严重，必须增加行为和精神药理治疗[11]。药理学建议稍后讨论。有 4 种心理疗法最有希望治疗中枢介导的疼痛，包括认知行为疗法、心理动力-人际疗法、正念接受疗法及肠道催眠疗法。这些通常是由健康心理学家或其他熟悉胃肠道生理学的心理医生单独治疗的，需要始终与药物治疗及良好的医患关系相结合[133,134]。

4. 应激介导的效应

脑成像研究显示，与对照组相比，大脑边缘系统的各个部位对心理困扰、直肠扩张和其他刺激有优先激活作用。ACC 参与了边缘（内侧）疼痛系统的动机和情感成分，在 IBS 和其他慢性疼痛如纤维肌痛患者中功能失调[135,136]。pACC 是一

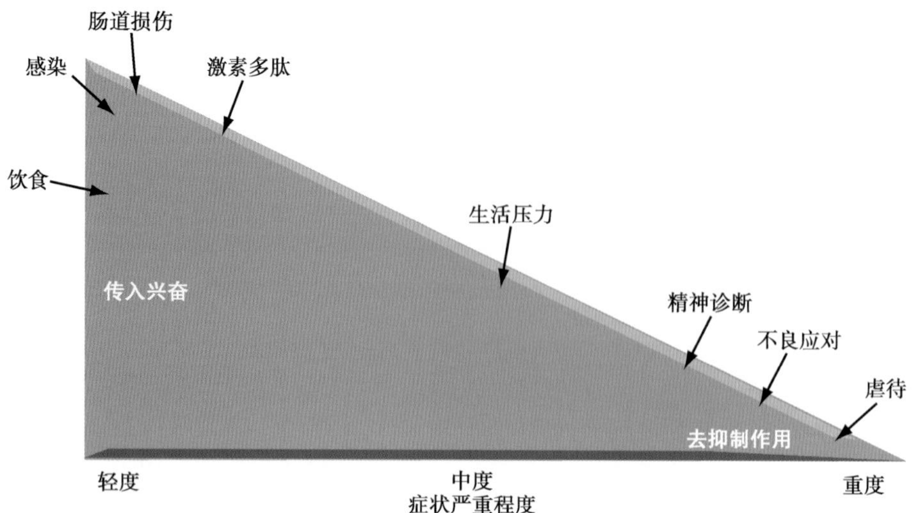

图 22.5　脑-肠轴对症状严重程度的影响。该图概念化了脑-肠轴对症状严重程度(水平轴)的影响。对于轻度至中度症状,肠道相关因素(如感染、炎症、肠道损伤、激素、肽)导致传入兴奋和传入神经元活动上调。对于具有中度至重度症状的较小患者组,痛觉的中枢调节受损,导致脊髓水平传入信号的中枢抑制作用降低(去抑制)。导致这种影响的因素可能包括生活压力和虐待、共病精神病诊断和应对不良。了解据称的作用部位(肠,脑,或两者)有帮助于确定治疗方法,例如是否使用靶向肠或脑的药物。(Adapted from Drossman DA. The biopsychosocial continuum in visceral pain. In: Pasricha PJ, Willis D, Gehhart GF, editors. Chronic abdominal and visceral pain: theory and practice. New York: Informa Healthcare; 2006.)。

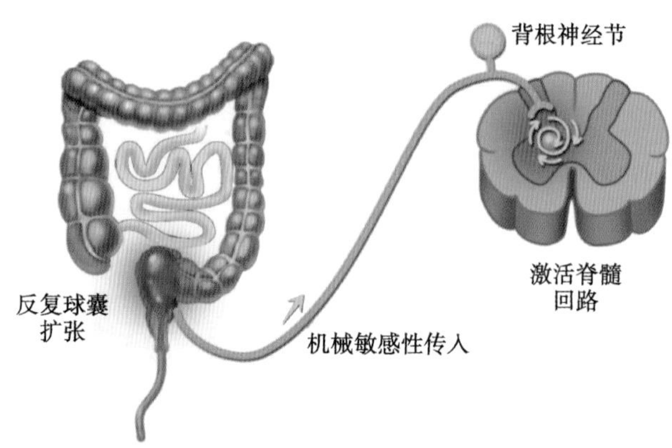

图 22.6　中枢敏化。中枢敏化与中枢神经系统上调有关。一阶神经元的重复刺激导致脊髓回路的敏化,从而增加源于背角突触的信号,然后通过二阶神经元传递到大脑。中枢敏化也可能通过来自包括应激相关激活的中枢的连接在大脑水平增强。其结果是疼痛加剧或其他类型的胃肠道功能障碍,通过这些上行增强途径从肠道传递到大脑。(From Van Oudenhove L, Crowell MD, Drossman DA, et al. Biopsychosocial aspects of functional gastrointestinal disorders. Gastroenterology 2016; 150: 1355-67, with permission from the Rome Foundation。)

个富含阿片类物质的区域,与情绪编码和疼痛下调有关,背侧 ACC(也称为头侧或前 MCC)对疼痛刺激的反应可能被不同程度地激活。背侧 ACC 和杏仁核一起与不愉快、恐惧和对运动疼痛反应的增加有关[137]。当 PET 和功能性磁共振成像(fMRI)用于评估 ACC 对直肠扩张或预期扩张的反应时,与对照组相比,IBS 患者表现出 MCC 的优先激活和对 pACC 的较少激活[135,138]。在 IBS 中,源于富含阿片类物质的 pACC 的下行抑制性疼痛通路的激活可能被 MCC 的激活所取代,MCC 是与恐惧和不愉快相关的区域。

与单独的任何一种情况相比,肠易激综合征患者的虐待史导致更大的背侧 ACC 的激活和直肠扩张引起的疼痛[7]。早期生活逆境还与情绪调节和显著相关的核心大脑网络的改变有关[139]。随着临床康复,中枢神经系统的活动恢复正常(即 MCC 降低和岛叶激活增加)[51,138]。类似地,其他情感创伤,如社交痛苦(由于重大损失和社交混乱)会激活大脑的相同区域(背侧 ACC 和脑岛),再次表明患者的社会心理状态与疼痛密切相关[140]。

医学研究所的一项关于波斯湾战争退伍军人的研究报告[141]显示了将士兵部署到战区(遭受外伤、肢解和尸体的创伤)与随后出现的医学和心理症状和综合征之间的密切关系。事实上,除了创伤后应激障碍和认知障碍,研究者还注意到了多种医学症状的集合,如所谓的“海湾战争综合征”,包括肠易激综合征、慢性疲劳、化学敏感性综合征。虐待或战时暴露的心理影响可能会破坏中枢疼痛调节系统以及情感和疼痛交界的大脑回路[7]。这些变化导致感觉阈值降低,导致大脑失去过滤身体感觉的能力。其结果是身体和心理症状的增加,以及更剧烈的疼痛和综合征(如 IBS、纤维肌痛、头痛、全身疼痛),这种情况被可变地描述为躯体化、合并症或肠外功能性胃肠道症状[141]。这些数据表明,心理和抗抑郁治疗对更严重的慢性疼痛有益,而中枢神经系统的作用是最重要的[112](见下文)。

5. 脊髓胶质细胞激活

有证据表明,神经胶质细胞(小胶质细胞、星形胶质细胞)的激活也可能增强心理应激、外周炎症和其他因素引起的疼痛放大[142-144]。胶质细胞活化与促炎细胞因子的产生有关,促炎细胞因子可上调 N-甲基-D-天冬氨酸受体信号传导系统,从而促进中枢致敏和慢性疼痛的发生。这一机制还没有在慢性胃肠道疼痛方面进行研究,但被认为是与麻醉肠道综合征有关的中枢性痛觉致敏机制[111](见第 12 章)。

6. 结构变化

越来越多的证据表明,严重的压力、精神疾病和慢性疼痛——单独或结合——都是神经退行性疾病,类似阿尔茨海默症和帕金森病一样;使用基于体素的形态测量学的功能性 MRI 研究显示,与这些疾病相关的大脑关键区域的皮质神经元密度显著下降。据报道,这些变化涉及重度抑郁和双相情感障碍中的 ACC 和眶额皮质[145],创伤后应激障碍和性虐待、身体虐待史患者的海马体[146],慢性躯体疼痛中的 ACC,后扣带皮层和腹内侧前额叶皮层[147],以及 IBS[141] 和疼痛性慢性胰腺炎中的背侧 ACC[148]。一种假设是,这些结构变化是应激介质对中枢神经系统退行性作用的结果,中枢神经系统的疲劳中枢控制机制并产生中枢致敏。这些变化可能在间歇性内脏疼痛(如 IBS)多年后转变为慢性持续的疼痛中发挥作用,如中枢介导的腹痛综合征[11]。值得注意的是,有证据表明中枢靶向治疗(如抗抑郁药)可能会导致神经元再生(神经形成),长期使用这些药物可能有助于预防复发[112]。

7. 下行调制

图 22.7 显示的是起源于富含阿片类物质的 pACC 的中枢下行抑制系统[149]。内脏传入活动可能通过降低皮质激素抑制通路下调传入信号激活这一区域。从 ACC 和杏仁核到脑桥延髓网络的下行连接——包括导水管灰质、头侧腹侧延髓和中缝核——通过阿片能、5-羟色胺能和去甲肾上腺素能系统激活抑制通路,到达脊髓背角[150]。背角就像一扇门,可以增加或减少从外周痛觉部位产生的传入冲动向中枢神经系统的投射。心理治疗和抗抑郁药可以激活这些下行通路。

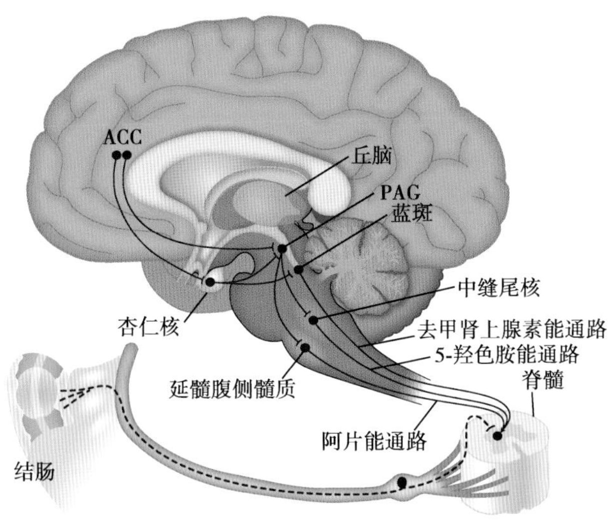

图 22.7　疼痛调节信号下行传递。该图显示了从中枢神经系统到脊髓的离皮层下行抑制通路。下行通路与疼痛调制的门控理论相一致。ACC,前扣带回皮质;PAG,中脑导水管周围灰质。(From Drossman DA. Functional abdominal pain syndrome. Clin Gastroenterol Hepatol 2004;2:353-65)。

(五) 细胞因子和脑

应激有促炎作用,肠道炎症也可能通过激活细胞因子相互影响行为。即使在大脑中,炎症也可能是一种常见的致病机制。炎症可影响神经递质代谢、神经内分泌功能和大脑神经可塑性,越来越多的证据表明,抑郁症和其他精神疾病可能是由炎症因子介导的[151]。从背角神经胶质细胞释放炎性细胞因子可上调疼痛通路,并可产生麻醉性痛觉过敏和麻醉肠道综合征[111]。

慢性炎症性疾病(包括 IBD、癌症、感染和其他分解代谢疾病)的许多行为特征(如发热、疲劳、厌食、抑郁)会产生所谓的“疾病行为”,而这个过程与产生中枢效应的外周细胞因子活化有关[152,153]。研究表明,炎症生物标志物升高的抑郁症患者对治疗反应差,在一些研究中,抗抑郁药治疗与体内炎症反应减少有关。来自炎症性疾病患者及无器质性病变的抑郁症患者的初步数据表明,抑制促炎细胞因子或其信号通路可能改善患者的抑郁情绪,并增加对传统抗抑郁药物治疗的反应[112]。

五、症状体验和行为

脑和胃肠道相互作用的产物与疾病和疾病的临床表现有关,即症状体验和随后的疾病相关行为。疾病的含义、身体形象改变的可感知效果(如行结肠造口术)、社会可接受性、功能损害的程度及其在工作和家庭中的影响、手术或过早死亡的可能性都必须由患者自己处理。除了医生参与的质量外,患者适应能力如何,对患者的心理健康和临床进程至关重要。有些慢性病患者病情恶化,变得依赖他人。他们持续的症状、活动受限以及健康保健负担,使得家人、朋友和医生都可能感到无助,无法提供足够的情感或医疗援助。有些患者拒绝接受帮助,以避免被迫产生依赖性。然后家人不得不来面对其内疚和愤怒的情绪,虽然这种情绪的表达是不可避免的,但是在社会层面上通常是不被接受的。医生肩负着患者和家属的感情负担,必须调和两者之间的矛盾。在大多数情况下问题可以得到解决,患者能建立一种应对模式。如果患者在心理上对疾病的应对能力有限,或疾病使人丧失能力,或家庭关系不稳定,就需要医生和相关人员(例如心理咨询师、社会工作者、同伴支持小组)做出额外的努力。

六、临床应用

医生应获取、组织和整合社会心理信息,以实现最佳的治疗。这里提出的建议对患有慢性疾病或重大心理社会问题的患者特别有用[1,154]。

(一) 病史采集

医生与患者的对话对增进医患关系、作出诊断和制订治疗方案具有最重要价值,但往往没有得到充分利用。考虑以下医患对话中获得的信息:

医生(看着图表):“我能为您做些什么?”

患者(停顿了一下,看上去在沉思):“我的克罗恩病突然发作了……自从我度假回来后,我感到疼痛、恶心和呕吐。”

医生(打断了他的话):“这种疼痛和以前一样吗?”

患者:“是的,我觉得差不多。”

医生(抬起头):“进食后疼痛会加重吗?”

患者:“是的。”

医生(身体前倾):“有发热吗? 有腹泻吗?”

患者(低下头):“嗯,是的,我想是的。我没有量体温。”

医生:“所以你发热和腹泻?”

患者:“呃,不,我觉得大便有些稀烂。”

在这次交流中,部分信息没有引出,并且由于打断和引导性的提问,第一个问题之后的信息准确性不确定。此外,非语言沟通并没有促进有效的医患互动。

应通过以患者为中心的非指导性访谈获取病史,在此期间鼓励患者以自己的方式讲述自己的经历,从而使导致疾病的事件自然展开。开放式问题最初是用来产生假设的,通过促进表达——“什么?”“你能告诉我更多吗?”重复患者之前的陈述,点头,甚至带着期待的表情沉默,都可以帮助采集病史。一开始要避免使用封闭式(是-否)的问题,尽管这些问题稍后可以用来进一步描述症状。避免使用多项选择题或诱导性提问,因为患者想要遵从医生的愿望可能会使回答产生偏差。

传统的医学史和社会史不应该分割开来,而应该结合起来,这样医学问题就可以在围绕疾病的社会心理事件背景下进行描述。应始终了解症状的发作或加重情况。在任何时候,这些问题都应该传达出医生对疾病的生理和心理方面的意愿:

医生(关切地看着患者):“我能帮你什么忙?”

患者(停顿):“当我度假回来时,我的克罗恩病突然发作了……疼痛、恶心和呕吐。”

医生:“是吗?”

患者:“我找了一份楼层主管的新工作,我想我应该放个假准备一下,然后就发生了这一切。”

医生(停顿):“哦,我明白了。”

患者(接着说):“我开始觉得这里抽搐(指下腹),然后吃完东西就更厉害了。所以我觉得我如果不来看病,我又会很困扰的。”

医生:“嗯。有其他症状吗?”

患者:“嗯,我觉得有些发热,但没有量体温。”

医生:“大便情况如何?”

患者:“在我度假的时候就开始有些稀烂。然后慢慢在好转。我今天没有排便。”

口头交流的次数是一样的,但是患者提供了更多的信息。临床特征更加清晰,并且获得了有关症状与开始新工作情况之间的额外信息。这种面谈方式不仅鼓励了患者的自我意识,而且考虑到了可能的行为治疗(如减压、换工作、咨询),这些治疗可能会改善患者以后的症状。应从患者对疾病的认识角度获取病史信息。问诊应包括:

“你认为是什么引起了这种不适?”

“你为什么今天来看病?”

“你认为你应该接受什么样的治疗?”

“你最担心你得了什么病?”

关于提高病史采集和沟通技巧的方法,更多信息见表22.1[1,155]。

表22.1　非语言和语言促进或抑制交流的因素

影响因素	促进	抑制
非语言		
诊室环境	私密,舒适	嘈杂,物理屏障
眼神交流	频繁	不频繁或持续
倾听	积极倾听,提问与患者所述有关	分心或只顾于他事(如打字)
身体姿势	直接,敞开,放松	转身,双臂交叉
点头	适时	极少或过度
身体距离	足以接触的距离	太近或太远
面部表情	表示感兴趣和理解	出神、无聊、不赞同
声音	温柔	刺耳,急促
身体接触	适时的接触有助于表达共情	不适当的接触显得不真诚
同步(胳膊,腿)	协调	不协调
语言		
问题形式	开放式的以产生假设	死板的,老套的
	封闭式的以测试假设	多选项或诱导性的(你没有……是吗?)
	使用患者熟悉的单词	使用患者不熟悉的单词或术语
	通过“回应”和肯定的手势促进患者谈论	打断,过度控制对话
	使用总结性的陈述	不使用
问题/面谈方式	非评判性的	评判性的
	遵循患者先前评论的引导(以患者为中心)	遵循自己预设的风格或议程

表 22.1　非语言和语言促进或抑制交流的因素(续)

影响因素	促进	抑制
	使用叙事线索	无组织性的
	适当沉默	打断或过度沉默
	适当安慰和鼓励	过早地或无端地安慰或鼓励
	表达共情	不提供或不真诚
建议	得到反馈并协商	未得到反馈或直接表达观点
提问/提供医学信息	适合临床问题	问了太多的生物医学问题,提供了太多的详细信息
提问/提供社会心理学信息	以一种敏感且不具威胁性的方式引出	忽视社会心理学信息或询问侵入性或探究性的问题
幽默	在适当和方便的时候使用幽默	不使用或不适当的幽默

(二) 数据评估

医生必须评估生物、心理和社会因素对疾病的相关影响。没有必要确定是心理社会还是生物过程在疾病中起作用,而且可能起到相反治疗效果。通常,两者都很重要,治疗基于确定哪些是可识别和可补救的。负面的医学评估不足以作出社会心理诊断。框 22.1 列出了在评估和评估患者时需要考虑的几个问题。

框 22.1　患者临床评价中需要考虑的问题
患者是否患有急性或慢性疾病?
患者的疾病生活史是什么?
患者为什么现在来就医?
患者的看法和期望是什么?
患者是否表现出异常的疾病行为?
疾病对患者有什么影响?
是否有并发精神病诊断?
是否存在文化或种族影响?
家庭是如何围绕疾病进行互动的?
患者的其他心理社会资源是什么?
评价的范围应该有多大?
患者是否应转诊至精神科吗?

(三) 诊断决策

决定安排哪些检查取决于其临床实用性。有几个问题需要考虑:检测是否安全且具有成本效益?结果会对治疗产生影响吗?持续要求进一步研究或挑战医生能力的患者可能会出于不确定性或出于自己需要做某事的感觉而诱使医生安排不必要的研究或手术。这种诱导可以通过基于数据客观评价(例如,粪便中的血液、发热、异常血清生化值),而不仅仅是根据患者的疾病行为作出决定来避免。

L 女士的病例(病例 1)是一名患有持续性和不明原因腹痛的患者,是胃肠病学家熟悉的示例。对慢性腹痛患者进行检查的冲动必须通过充分的初步评估大大降低以后发现被忽视原因的可能性的证据来缓和。在这里,临床方法不是医学诊断,而是心理社会评估和慢性疼痛治疗[11]。与慢性疼痛症状相关或加重的因素包括:①近期家庭或社会环境受到破坏(例如,孩子离家出走、争吵);②重大损失或损失周年(例如,家庭成员或朋友死亡、子宫切除术、干扰妊娠结局);③有性虐待或身体虐待史的;④抑郁或者其他精神病诊断的发作或恶化;⑤隐藏的事件(例如,寻求麻醉品的行为,泻药滥用,未决诉讼,残疾)。尽管会诊和治疗可能需要精神健康提供者,重要的是医生应继续参与患者的治疗,并对新发现的进展保持警惕[156]。

有时必须在信息不完整或不明确的情况下作出决定。特别是对于慢性症状,当诊断未明确且患者临床稳定时,明智的做法是容许诊断的不确定性,并在一段时间内观察患者的新发展。有经验的医生通常根据病情在数周或数个月内的变化程度作出诊断和治疗决策,而不是根据 1 次或 2 次的就诊。

当额外的心理数据可以澄清疾病或改善患者治疗时,应考虑咨询精神病学家或健康心理学家[156],例如:①确定可能对特定治疗(如精神药理学药物)有益的精神病诊断;②患者心理社会功能水平严重受损(如无法工作);③在客观医学数据无明确指征的情况下,根据患者主诉考虑侵入性诊断或治疗策略。

七、治疗方法

(一) 建立治疗关系

医生可以通过使用特定指南实施良好的沟通技巧与患者建立治疗关系:①允许患者完成他或她的开场白;②引起关注并建立融洽关系;③采用开放式和封闭式问题的组合来收集和澄清信息;④识别并回应患者的个人情况、信仰和价值观;⑤使用患者能够理解的语言解释诊断和治疗计划;⑥评估患者的理解程度;⑦鼓励患者参与决策,并探索患者遵循治疗计划的意愿和能力;⑧询问患者可能存在的其他问题;⑨在结束访视前讨论患者预期的随访活动[157]。该策略必须个体化,因为患者需要的协商和参与程度不同。总的来说,医生必须不做任何判断,对患者的健康表现出兴趣,并学会运用有效的沟通技巧[1,158]。

1. 激发、评估和沟通心理社会因素的作用

对不赞成的恐惧和缺乏信任往往会阻止患者分享亲密的

想法和感受，这一障碍可以通过良好的医患关系来克服。当患者不愿意或不能接受心理社会因素在疾病中的作用时，医生仍然可以通过推断间接地获得这些信息，不应试图为患者提供预见。如果患者询问问题是否只是“在我的头脑中”，医生应该解释疾病很少是精神或身体上的；理解所有因素，包括患者的感觉，是很重要的；许多慢性疾病与抑郁或不现实的恐惧相关。与疾病的生物心理社会模式一致，在因果关系（例如，通过陈述“压力引起你的问题很常见”）或排除（例如，通过陈述“检查结果为阴性；必须为压力”）方面讨论心理社会和生物学因素没有帮助。

2. 提供保障

患者的恐惧和担忧需要安抚。如果安抚过早、不充分或不恰当，医生会认为这是不真诚的，或不够彻底的。医生应该真诚地回应患者的需求和请求，而不要屈服于压力去做任何不符合患者最佳利益的事情。例如，残疾可能不利于帮助患者重建健康并重返有酬工作岗位。如果患者不符合残疾资格，医生应该明确说明这一点。

3. 患者对慢性病的适应能力的识别

疾病与患者的某些“获益”有关，如关注和支持的增加，日常职责的减轻，以及可能的社会和经济补偿。对一些患者来说，放弃疾病状态所失去的可能比健康所获得的更多，而且改善可能是缓慢的。可以通过改善患者对疾病的心理社会适应（例如改善应对策略）来帮助他或她。

4. 强化健康行为

有时，对身体不适的抱怨是一种表达情绪困扰或引起关注的不良适应的表现。医生可能在不经意间通过多种方式强化这种行为：①对患者的抱怨给予极大的重视，其他方面不予考虑；②根据每一项主诉进行诊断性检查或给予处方药物；③对患者的健康负全部责任。患者不是试图改善症状，而是通过主诉症状来保持医生对其关注度，从而使症状反复和被动循环地延续下去。

为了鼓励患者对自己的治疗承担更多的责任，并有更强的掌控感，医生可能会在多种治疗方法中提供一个选择，或帮助提供一个治疗方案。医生应该将关于症状的讨论限制在满足医学关注的所需内容上，重点放在对疾病的适应能力，而不是治疗上。我的经验是最好不要问患者的症状（例如“你的疼痛怎么样?”），因为这个问题会让我注意到患者有症状这一事实上。相反，我是在询问患者在康复治疗过程中的促进恢复健康的行为背景下的症状（例如“你是怎么控制疼痛的?”）。

（二）精神药理学治疗

精神药物作用于脑-肠调节通路中的神经递质受体，这些通路针对5-羟色胺能、去甲肾上腺素能、多巴胺能和阿片能受体位点，并产生各种效应，包括：①减少胃肠道疼痛引起的内脏传入信号；②通过促进中枢下调通路治疗胃肠道疼痛；③取决于药物，改善腹泻或便秘；④减轻焦虑、抑郁、恶心、食欲不振；⑤大剂量用于治疗重度抑郁症或其他精神疾病[112,142]。

随着罗马Ⅳ诊断标准的出版，罗马基金制定了新的指南[159]，将同时作用于大脑和肠道的药物重新定义为“肠-脑神经调节剂”。该术语[112]主要包括中枢神经调节药物（如抗抑郁药、抗精神病药、阿扎哌隆类等中枢神经调节药物）以及主要的外周神经调节剂，包括5-羟色胺、氯离子通道、δ配体制剂等（本节未讨论）。相信这个新的术语将提高人们对其药理价值的理解，当治疗胃肠道疾病患者时使其减少羞耻感，并可能提高治疗依从性。

用于治疗胃肠道疾病的中枢型抗抑郁神经调节剂的主要种类包括三环类抗抑郁药（TCA）（如阿米替林、丙咪嗪、地西帕明、去甲替林），选择性5-羟色胺再吸收抑制剂（SSRI）（如氟西汀，舍曲林，西酞普兰，艾司西酞普兰，帕罗西汀），5-羟色胺和去甲肾上腺素再摄取抑制剂（SNRI）（如度洛西汀、文拉法辛、去甲文拉法辛、米那普仑）和去甲肾上腺素能和特异性的5-羟色胺药物（四环类）（如米氮平、米安色林）。抗焦虑药物包括苯二氮䓬类（如劳拉西泮、氯硝西泮）和氮杂环类（如丁螺环酮）。新型非典型抗精神病药（如喹硫平、奥氮平、阿立哌唑）除了抗焦虑作用外还用作增强剂。关于这些药物治疗胃肠道疾病的药理学、临床作用和副作用的内容可以在其他文献中找到[112,142]。

1. 三环类抗抑郁药

TCA可通过外周和中枢机制减轻慢性疼痛[160,161]，包括通过去甲肾上腺素能和5-羟色胺能激活肾上腺皮质的疼痛抑制通路，减少肠道内的传入信号，并在较大剂量下治疗兼有焦虑和抑郁症状的患者。这类药物的去甲肾上腺素能和抗胆碱能作用也能降低肠道转运率，因此对腹泻患者有用。起始剂量通常是25~50mg，根据需要剂量可加至100mg。当用到抗抑郁药最大剂量（≥150mg/d）时，TCA还可以治疗内因性和反应性抑郁症状。抗组胺和抗胆碱能副作用包括便秘、直立性低血压、口干和眼干，这些副作用可能导致患者依从性差。然而与三胺类药物（TCA：阿米替林，丙米嗪）相比，二胺类抗抑郁药物（去西帕明、去甲替林）对胆碱能和组胺受体的激活程度低，产生的副作用少。

2. 选择性5-羟色胺再摄取抑制剂

由于缺乏去甲肾上腺素能作用，SSRI类药物对缓解胃肠道疼痛无效。通常使用全剂量来减少并发的焦虑、重度抑郁、恐慌症和其他高度焦虑的特征（例如强迫症、创伤后应激障碍、社交恐惧症）。由于其主要的5-羟色胺作用，SSRI在治疗开始时可以产生腹泻甚至焦虑。

3. 5-羟色胺和去甲肾上腺素再摄取抑制剂

SNRI对治疗疼痛症状特别有效，因其与TCA一样，具有显著的去甲肾上腺素能和5-羟色胺能作用，并且批准用于治疗糖尿病周围神经痛、纤维肌痛和其他躯体疼痛综合征。也可以用于标签说明以外的内脏疼痛，并且没有TCA或SSRI的抗组胺或抗胆碱能副作用。恶心是其主要的副作用，如果随餐服用可以改善。度洛西汀通常起始剂量为30mg/d，如果需要，几周后增加到60mg，甚至90mg。由于低剂量的文拉法辛没有去甲肾上腺素能作用，因此需要较高剂量（超过150mg/d）用于治疗疼痛症状。米那普仑（50~100mg，每日两次）不是作为抗抑郁药销售，而是用于治疗躯体疼痛。

4. 四环类药物

除了治疗抑郁症外，米氮平还具有复杂的5-羟色胺能和去甲肾上腺素能特性，产生多种作用。5-羟色胺3（5-HT_3）拮抗作用与止吐、止泻作用有关，抗组胺作用有助于镇静。它也是一种食欲刺激剂（体重增加是副作用之一），可以用于治疗焦虑症。由于镇静作用，通常在夜间服用，剂量为 7.5~30mg。

5. 抗焦虑药物

苯二氮䓬类药物常用于缓解急性焦虑，尤其是当焦虑与应激性肠道紊乱有关时。潜在益处应与镇静、药物相互作用、依赖性和停药后反弹等的长期风险权衡，不建议长期使用。丁螺环酮是一种非苯二氮䓬类药物，用于广泛性焦虑症，由于其 5-HT_1 作用引起胃底松弛，已被推荐用于功能性消化不良（推荐剂量：15~30mg，每日两次）。

6. 非典型抗精神病药物

非典型抗精神病药物最初是用于精神分裂症和双相情感障碍，在低剂量时，具有较明显的抗焦虑作用，一些药物（如喹硫平、奥氮平）具有镇静作用，有些（如阿立哌唑、依匹哌唑）更具活性，但可能产生静坐困难。可以用于胃肠道疾病患者以增强抗抑郁药对慢性疼痛的作用，就像用于抑郁症的辅助治疗一样（见下文）。剂量是精神分裂症的三分之一到一半。

7. 阿片类药物

由于阿片类药物有滥用、依赖性和引起麻醉肠道综合征的可能，因此不用于治疗慢性疼痛或心理社会障碍患者[162,163]。需要识别出有麻醉肠道综合征的患者，可以通过戒毒治疗治愈[164]（见第 12 章）。

8. 强化治疗

当单一药物治疗不成功时，可采用小剂量联合用药，达到协同效应。强化的概念涉及激活大脑中不同的受体位点以增强治疗效果[112,142]。当使用单一药物时增至更大剂量，这种方法还可以最大限度地减少副作用。可通过增加抗抑郁药、外周神经调节剂（如加巴喷丁）或肠道症状调节剂（如阿洛司琼、鲁比前列酮）来实现增强效应（见第 16 和 19 章）。另一种可以添加的中枢神经调节剂是丁螺环酮[165,166]。低剂量的非典型抗精神病药（如喹硫平）可与 TCA 或 SNRI 一起使用，以增强疼痛控制、减少焦虑和改善睡眠[167]。

9. 预防复发

预防复发涉及这样一个概念，即在达到临床治愈后继续使用神经调节剂治疗将减少复发或复发的可能性[168]。有证据表明，持续的抗抑郁药治疗与通过神经发生逆转临床疾病有关[169,170]。为了减少治疗 FGID 复发的可能性，我们根据经验建议在治疗应答后继续治疗 6~12 个月。

10. 药物基因组学检测

药物基因组学可以在细胞、组织、个体或群体水平上检测与疾病易感性以及药物反应相关的单个基因表达的变异性。基因多态性也可能通过对药物代谢的影响来影响其对药物的反应[171]。几乎所有中枢神经调节剂都可以通过药物基因组学检测，并且使用度逐渐增加，特别是在慢性疼痛的治疗中[172]。因此，药物基因组学检测对于选择最佳神经调节剂、优化效益、降低毒性，或通过几种药物来强化治疗同时避免药物相互作用等方面可能具有价值[173]。

（三）行为治疗

诱导积极生理效应的对症治疗，尤其适用于不想服药或对药物敏感的患者。然而与药物联合使用，这些方法可以产生增强获益[11]。所有的行为方式都有助于患者处理不适应的疾病信念和行为，以及压力、生活事件和症状之间的关系。

认知行为疗法（CBT）是一种简短的、以有技能为基础的协作治疗，旨在纠正已知可放大胃肠道症状的不适应想法和应对方式[174]。CBT 治疗 IBS 的最常见靶点包括过度觉醒、内脏焦虑/症状特异性恐惧和疼痛灾难化[175]。CBT 可通过互联网[177,178]对个人或群体进行治疗[133,176]，已证明在少至 4 次治疗中有效[179]。CBT 已被证明对一系列消化系统疾病有效，包括青少年[180,181]和成人的 IBD[182]。

人际动态心理治疗也是一种短期心理治疗，重点是识别导致症状加重的人际状况。当通过治疗师-患者关系解决冲突时，症状改善。该技术已被证明可改善 IBS 患者的症状，减少残疾和医疗费用[183]，尤其是在有虐待史的情况下[184]。

减轻压力（放松训练）的目的是对抗压力产生的生理效应。骨骼肌张力降低可降低自主觉醒和主观紧张和焦虑，并可改善肠动力。减压和放松训练包括引导意象、放松反应冥想、瑜伽和生物反馈等方式。正念冥想是一种放松形式，涉及对身体感觉和情绪的主动非评判性意识。团体正念冥想可减轻 IBS 女性患者症状和改善与健康相关的生活质量，以及降低压力水平[185]。

肠道定向催眠疗法是一种意识和精神集中的增强状态，通常由深度放松引起，允许肠道特异性治疗建议无阻力地进入大脑。来自不同中心的研究数据支持催眠术作为 IBS 的一种有效、可行的治疗选择，可改善症状和生活质量，减轻压力和焦虑[186,187]；长期随访表明催眠的有益作用持续存在[188]。催眠术也成功地减少了乙状结肠镜检查时获得的粪便中的炎性标志物[189]，延长了 IBD 患者的临床缓解期[190]。

行为治疗有利结果的预测因素包括对治疗成功的信心、对症状的控制感、与治疗医生的良好关系和早期疗效反应[191,192]。患者必须将心理治疗视为与个人需求相关，而不是"证明我不是疯子"。干预措施的选择取决于当地的专业知识和可用性以及患者的偏好。

（四）临床医生相关的问题

患者的心理社会问题可能会影响医生的态度和行为[9]。医生如果没有意识到这点，会对患者的治疗产生不利影响。在诊断不确定的情况下，医生不愿意作出决定[193]，因为他们认为对疾病了解越多，就越容易治疗。然而许多临床治疗是针对他们关心的症状或社会心理问题治疗的，并非针对以这一症状或社会心理问题表现的疾病，尤其是对于那些需要诊断又不明原因的抱怨者或那些被认为会投诉的患者。医生冒着对这些患者进行过度检查、不必要的检查或有害性治疗的风险（有时被称为"狂怒的医学"）[194]。另一种情况是，医生可能认为这些主诉是不合理的并有所行动（例如将患者转给精神科），而患者会排斥这种做法。

一些患者和医生之间会发生人际关系冲突。患者感到无助和失控，医生可能会将其行为解释为依赖和苛求，这些感觉可能会被医生指责或谴责。医生必须明白，这些行为是患者不适应沟通方式的一部分，不应该被视为个人行为。有些患者对慢性病产生了心理社会适应（如家人的关注、通过疾病行为控制、残疾），从而导致疾病治愈延迟，这些患者可能不认可医生的治疗。在这种情况下，虽然症状持续，但是治疗的重点最好从治疗转向改善日常生活功能。医生可以从个人努力中获得满足感，而不是从患者的感激之情中获得。最后，每个医生都必须在时间和精力上对那些特别有挑战性的患者设定个人限制。限制就诊时间，将患者的部分治疗分配给其他医生，必要时要对患者说"不"，这些都是在医生的个人需要和患者利益之间取得平衡的重要方法。

（陈立刚 译，孙明瑜 校）

参考文献

第 23 章 人为胃肠疾病

John S. Fordtran，Anahit A. Zeynalyan 著

章节目录

一、人为疾病及其隐匿形式 …… 321
（一）病因和动机 …… 321
（二）医源性疾病的风险 …… 321
（三）诊断和检测 …… 322
（四）管理 …… 323
（五）与隐私和保密有关的伦理问题 …… 324
（六）法律问题 …… 324
二、相关异常疾病行为 …… 324
（一）躯体症状障碍 …… 324
（二）诈病 …… 325
（三）贪食症患者的人为行为 …… 325
三、与胃肠病学相关的特殊问题 …… 326
（一）秘密服用泻药 …… 326
（二）人为腹泻 …… 326
（三）隐匿性呕吐 …… 327
（四）人为贫血和人为胃肠道出血 …… 327
（五）人为癌症 …… 327
（六）来自病例报告的经验教训 …… 328
四、异常疾病行为诊断和处理的隐患 …… 329

医患关系中一个公认的原则是，患者应尽一切努力恢复健康，包括诚实、毫无保留地与他的医生沟通疾病的假定病因[1-3]。在至少 4 种公认的疾病中，患者通常或有时会通过自我诱导疾病、装病、隐瞒有关病因的信息、夸大症状的严重程度或提供虚假的病史或病历等方式而背离这一原则。这些疾病包括人为疾病、躯体症状障碍、诈病和进食障碍。在这 4 种疾病中，偏离正常疾病行为的假定动机各不相同，但不管动机如何，结果均为医生被欺骗了。

本章的目的是讨论这些异常疾病行为的可能原因，提供如何识别它们的建议，并指出处理此类患者的医生面临的一些伦理冲突。我们强调在肠胃病诊疗中最可能遇到的欺骗行为类型，和最可能因此而发生的医源性疾病。我们不讨论这些患者中出现精神症状或人为障碍的极端表现，如 Munchausen 综合征或代理型 Munchausen 综合征。

一、人为疾病及其隐匿形式

1864 年，Hector Gavin 首次描述了人为疾病（factitious disorder，FD）的隐匿形式[4]。他主要在“放纵女性”中观察到 FD，她们“模仿或伪造疾病，以满足自己的愿望，或激发兴趣，或以欺骗为乐。”。这种行为的动机被认为是通过假定“病态的角色”来缓解情绪上的困扰。这些患者通常是 30 多岁的女性。通常她们会过上外在的正常生活，有工作和医疗保险，并与其护理人员高度合作。FD 被认为是一种精神疾病[5]，但患者向非精神科医生寻求医疗护理。病例 1 说明了隐匿的 FD，也称为“社会顺应”型 FD[6-8]。

（一）病因和动机

按照普遍能接受的说法，具有 FD 隐匿形式的患者有意识地、有意假装或自我诱导身体症状，以承担“病态角色”，从而获得情绪抑郁的缓解。他们表现为属于医生职权范围内的残疾和障碍[9]。

对 FD 的行为有几种可能的解释，可以借鉴各种理论框架。学习理论认为，在早年学习到的过度或欺骗性疾病行为是人们所知道的最佳反应。心理动力学理论利用了一些可能的冲突——特别是在儿童-父母关系中——导致需要得到照顾、需要欺骗、需要报复、需要感到处于控制之中、需要控制父母的虐待以及需要受到惩罚或伤害[10]。通过关注身体疾病，患者可以避免引发这些需求的潜在痛苦感觉，对养育的渴望和需求分散对真实生活问题的注意力[11]也是可能的动机。行为理论指出暴露与加强病态角色活动。自我增强模型[10,12]表明，个人渴望自己疾病的特殊性以及他们与高地位专业人员（尤其是医生）的关系。

对诱发或假装的疾病的选择，通常没有明显的象征意义[13]。FD 患者几乎可以模拟所有器官系统的真实疾病（表 23.1）。事实上，一个患者可能在不同的时间模仿出不同的症状和疾病。一般认为 FD 患者知道自己在做什么，在大多数情况下仔细计划就证明了这一点。他们知道对不对，他们的智商通常是正常的或高的（即使他们的受教育程度相对有限），只有极少数是精神病患者。有些患有抑郁症，可能会有自杀的想法。他们有时被描述为不成熟和缺乏人际交往能力的一个群体[14]。

（二）医源性疾病的风险

FD 患者通常愿意，有时似乎渴望接受危险的诊断程序，以便维持患病的角色。由于他们的欺骗，医生会开出不必要的、侵入性和有潜在风险的诊断试验、程序和治疗，反过来这些可能导致医源性疾病。在大多数情况下，对这些患者最大的伤害是医生导致的，而非患者自己[15]。表现为胃肠道症状或体征的 FD 患者可能接受不必要的剖腹手术、胃或肠切除术、胰腺切除术、肾活检、肾上腺切除术或长期应用糖皮质激素治疗。病例 2 说明了其中的一些要点。

病例 1　一位 37 岁女性腹泻患者

患者在接受颌骨重建手术后数天开始出现腹泻，全身检查未能发现腹泻原因，患者被转到我们的医疗中心，在那里她被评价为门诊患者。通过粪便定量采集，她的平均粪便重量为 1 008g/d（女性的正常粪便重量为 87±8g/d）。根据电解质分析，腹泻为分泌性。粪便脂肪排出量在正常范围内。血清胃泌素和血管活性肠多肽（VIP）浓度正常，粪便培养未发现病原菌。

由于我们无法找到患者慢性分泌性腹泻的原因，并且在腹泻发作前（见后文）还患有多种其他内科和外科疾病，因此我们怀疑患者秘密摄入泻剂比沙可啶或番泻叶。但是，该患者否认摄入泻药，尿液和粪便泻药筛查（Toxi-lab 法）结果均为阴性，且患者的结肠活检标本未发现结肠假性黑色素病（见第 128 章）。我们没有搜查她的私人物品（这些物品存放在酒店房间里），我们也没有与她直面我们的怀疑，患者出院建议进行液体和电解质替换补充和对症治疗，并建议如有不适随时复诊。

在贝勒（Baylor）大学医学中心接受评估后约 1 年，患者前往另一个医学中心重复进行了内镜检查，但没有得到诊断。结肠镜活检合并大出血，她需要大量输血。由于体重持续下降，开始进行肠外营养。腹泻出现约 4 年后，她返回 Baylor 大学医学中心。当时，我们已经证明泻药的 Toxi-lab 法检测不可靠，因此，我们通过薄层色谱法对她的尿液进行了分析，显示比沙可啶检测结果呈阳性。

我们决定以一种支持的方式面对患者（见下文），并在她丈夫在场的情况下这样做，在她门诊评估期间，他一直陪伴着她。她流着泪平静地说，她"绝对没有"服用泻药，并补充说"我不知道比沙可啶是什么"。出院后，她的丈夫在家中搜查她的衣柜，发现了一个空的女性专用盒子，里面装有比沙可啶。她的丈夫和当地的医生同意为患者寻求精神科的帮助。

随后，我们与患者家属交谈，试图深入了解她秘密摄入泻药的动机。据她的家人说，她没有进食障碍或性虐待史。在过去的 6 年里，她曾在医生办公室工作，在那里她的医学知识有所增加。"她一直都坚信医学，而且不认为有风险"。她在没有明确需要的情况下接受了多次整形手术，而颌骨手术的适应证也值得怀疑。这些手术使她成为了关注的焦点。她嫁给了一个充满爱心的丈夫。在她被诊断为不孕症后约 3 个月开始腹泻疾病。（有人观察到 FD 的发病通常在应激事件后不久开始）[6,7]。

在诊断为 FD 3 年后，我们再次联系了患者的家人和她的一些当地医生以了解最新情况。总的来说，患者的情况要好得多。尽管与患者直面的决定可能是明智的，但这让患者感觉到了背叛。她从不接受这个诊断，也拒绝看精神科医生。她仍然有各种医疗问题，经常预约专科医生。她对疾病仍然着迷，但不那么戏剧性，因此受到的关注也较少。在这次交谈的前两周，患者接受了髋关节手术，几个月前接受了胆囊切除术。年初她曾做过手术，矫正磨牙造成的损伤。"她可能不再服用泻药了，但每年中几次她的血钾水平很低，一次在她的尿检中发现了利尿剂。"基于这些信息，很明显她对药物的迷恋和她的"多手术成瘾"[8]仍然存在。

表 23.1　机械机制引起的人为疾病的表现*

机制	临床表现
自身诱导感染	脓肿，菌血症，发热，败血症，伤口感染
秘密摄入药物、维生素、矿物质	Bartter 综合征，凝血功能障碍导致的出血或紫癜（双香豆素、肝素），骨髓抑制，腹泻，甲状腺功能亢进，低血糖，低钾血症（泻药和/或利尿剂），低镁血症，肝脏疾病，嗜铬细胞瘤（肾上腺素注射液），肾功能衰竭，盐中毒，呕吐
自残	瘀伤，复杂区域疼痛综合征（反射性交感神经营养不良），畸形，皮肤病（也可能因摄入某些药物诱发），未愈合的伤口
静脉切开术（自身或动物）	贫血，呕血，便血，血尿，黑便
温度计操作或温度计的替代	发热
模拟特定疾病或综合征的临床表现（有时使用伪造的病历或体液污染）	艾滋病，癌症，囊性纤维变性疾病（CF），抑郁症，多发性硬化症，疼痛综合征，胰腺炎，蛋白尿，癫痫发作，精神病，肾结石

*改编自参考文献[14]

病例 2　一位 33 岁女性的医源性疾病

患者平素体健，直到 8 年前出现便秘，需要使用通便剂，同年晚些时候出现腹泻。结肠镜检查提示轻度结肠炎，X 线提示为回肠炎。在接下来的 2 年里，尽管调整了饮食、服用了多种药物（包括泼尼松），腹泻仍然持续存在。经常因低钠血症多次住院治疗。患者出现双髋关节无菌性坏死，可能是泼尼松治疗的结果，接受了左侧全髋关节置换术。重度腹泻持续存在，她接受了几次外科手术：剖腹探查术、无肠切除的回肠袢造口术和随后的全结肠切除术与标准回肠造口术。病理报告显示非特异性慢性炎症。术后患者出现严重回肠造口腹泻，怀疑为神经内分泌肿瘤综合征，将她转诊进一步研究。

平衡研究显示，回肠造口排泄量为 2 561mL/d（正常 600mL），腹泻为分泌型，肠道对膳食脂肪的吸收正常。肠灌注检查显示小肠对水和电解质的吸收正常。患者自腹泻发作后否认使用泻药，然而，她的房间被秘密搜索，发现了一盒卡特（Carter）的小药丸，其中含有包括鬼臼草和芦荟在内的几种蒽醌类物质（见第 19 章）。回顾性分析了她行结肠切除术时的病历，发现直肠活检标本的病理报告描述了结肠假黑色素病。

（三）诊断和检测

早期识别 FD 患者是预防医源性疾病的最佳方法，但大多数内科医生和胃肠病专科医生在对特发性躯体症状患者的鉴别诊断中从未考虑 FD。在传统医学的背景下，造成身体症状的人为病因根本没有意义。因此，真实疾病的阴性检测结果被视为假阴性结果，从而重复检查，咨询新的医生，还可能对极为罕见的真实疾病进行低特异性检测，造成的假阳性结果导致更多的检测。

即使在鉴别诊断中考虑了 FD，但有几个因素也使医生难以识别 FD 的隐匿形式。第一，这些患者似乎与其他由真实疾病引起的症状相似的患者没有区别[16-17]。第二，他们所患的精神疾病不容易被识别[18]，而且这些患者通常没有明显的过度二次收益。第三，患者如果被问到，他们会令人信服地否认自己诱发引起的疾病[17,19]。第四，是当前和之前的医生之间缺乏沟通，也没有对既往病历进行研究。第五，医生不敢与患者讨论 FD 的可能性。

一些线索（如果存在）会增加特定患者诊断 FD 的可能性（框 23.1）。然而，FD 的诊断不能仅根据这些线索，因此必须获得某种形式的证实。框 23.2 提供了一些用于支持或证实自我诱发疾病的方法。

框 23.1 增加隐匿形式的人为疾病可能性的线索

- 主要为女性
- 既往在医学领域的经验，提供了对术语和获取医疗用品的不同寻常的理解
- 多次手术，多次检查操作
- 无法解释的实验室检查结果
- 病史上某些方面不一致性和不可靠性
- 之前因相同症状到 3 个或更多的医疗中心就诊，或到全国知名的医疗中心就诊，尽管居住在很远的地方
- 药物滥用史或既往有精神疾病史
- 对既往病史的细节不清楚和/或不愿意公开既往病历

框 23.2 用于支持或确认自我诱导或人为疾病的方法

- 审阅旧病历，如果适用的话，与既往医生和家属讨论该病例，识别差异和不一致，并评估从患病角色中获得的影响。询问患者的心身疾病、既往精神病治疗、自杀企图、患者生活压力、童年期虐待、婚姻/性问题、进食障碍等。互联网可以用来促进这样的调查。一个可以访问多个记录的法医顾问可以独特地帮助识别相互矛盾的事件
- 审查之前的活检组织切片，根据患者的症状寻找伤口中的异物[22]结肠假黑色素病[23]和其他线索
- 获得精神病学评估，以帮助确定患者是否患有人格障碍或精神疾病，如果没有人格障碍或精神疾病，将反驳人为疾病
- 如果症状和体征可以通过秘密摄入药物和毒物来解释，则获得适当的药物和毒理学筛查。即使无肾功能异常或电解质异常，也要考虑进行利尿剂尿检。根据所用试验的灵敏度和特异性来评价此类筛选的结果
- 检测直接观察下采集的生物体液，并将结果与患者私下采集的体液结果进行比较。例如，将在“未准备”乙状结肠镜检查时获得的粪便标本与患者提交的粪便标本进行比较
- 让护理人员观察患者以发现篡改行为
- 搜索患者的个人物品（见正文）

如果主治医生考虑 FD 并进行精神科会诊，重要的是要认识到，即使是经验丰富的精神科医生，也不能通过从疑似 FD 但否认 FD 存在的患者中采集精神病史来可靠地做出或排除 FD 的诊断。

（四）管理

两个主要假设构成了拟议管理建议的基础。首先是 FD 代表患者试图应对情绪困扰。其次是医疗团队的支持态度，将使患者有可能度过 FD 诊断可能导致的羞耻感和破坏的自我形象。不幸的是，几乎所有报告的管理建议均基于住院患者的经验。据我们所知，没有针对门诊患者的建议。

用于治疗 FD 的方法包括患者对峙、心理治疗、药物治疗、行为治疗和多学科联合方法。Eastwood 和 Bisson[24] 试图通过回顾 32 例病例报告和 13 例病例系列来评价这些管理方法的有效性。根据他们的综述，这些作者得出结论，文献中的证据不足以评价任何管理技术的有效性。

然而，文献中似乎就框 23.3 中所列的 FD 治疗的几个方面达成了普遍的共识。尽管这些建议可能被大多数专家接受，但在面对诊断为 FD 的患者的价值和智慧方面存在意见分歧。结合 3 项研究作者的建议[14,25,26]，似乎达成共识，即当存在重大医源性疾病的风险时，应对“确诊的 FD”患者进行对峙。所有人都同意，如框 23.4 所列，对峙应该是支持性的。当怀疑 FD 但“未被证实”或判断医源性疾病的风险较小时，是否应该进行对峙目前尚未达成共识。

框 23.3 关于治疗人为疾病的共识意见*

- 实现洞察力不应成为治疗的主要早期目标，因为它会削弱患者的防御能力
- 一个人应对患者管理负主要责任
- 应该对患者进行全面的精神病学评估，包括自杀风险的评估
- 多学科综合治疗组的所有成员都应了解评估和治疗计划
- 治疗方案应个体化
- 应对共病进行适当治疗
- 如果使用对峙技术，它们应该是非惩罚性的和支持性的

*来源于文献。

框 23.4 支持性对峙的特征

- 告诉患者你所怀疑的是什么，完全没有直接指责
- 用事实支持人为疾病的诊断
- 提供富有同情心和保留情面的意见*
- 避免探究以揭示患者的潜在感受和动机†
- 除非法律要求，否则未经患者许可，不得向他人披露诊断结果‡
- 确保工作人员继续接受患者
- 鼓励接受精神科医生的帮助，但不要强迫

*“也许你不知道你在服用什么药物，这种药物可能会让你生病”“也许你是在睡梦中服用的”“你所做的是求助，我们理解”“我们意识到你一定处于非常痛苦的境地”“我们想继续照顾你。”

†“这样做是为了尽量减少对基本情绪防御的破坏”。

‡之后，可能会决定在患有潜在致命性人为疾病的患者中打破这一希望，例如通过将污染物质注射到体内而导致败血症的患者。只有在伦理道德委员会、法律人员和其他人员进行协商并达成共识意见后，才能打破这一承诺。如文中所述。

没有对峙的管理有时被称为“保全面子的技术”[27,28]。在这里，向患者委婉地传达的信息是，医生对欺骗是明智的，给他或她提供一个机会，在疾病暴露前放弃这种人为的疾病。可能会告知患者，“如果下一次治疗无效，我们将被迫得出您是自身疾病来源的结论。”。然后应用下一种治疗（几乎是任何治疗），将有惊人数量的患者得到奇迹般的改善，而不是冒着被揭露为欺诈的风险。一份报告得出结论，在采用这种非

对峙方法后，约有三分之一的患者结束了他们的恶作剧，他们可能极力地否认自己在做什么，但如果医生以某种方式让他们挽回了面子，这种行为就会停止一段时间。因此，在相当一部分患者中避免了发现造成的尴尬。然而，即使患者承认了部分或全部的欺骗，大多数仍会继续诱发或假装疾病。这种权衡是可以接受的，前提是医源性疾病的风险被判定为很小，并认识到没有一种治疗技术是持续有效的[27]。尽管这种保全面子的技术受到一些专家的青睐，但是这种方法在一些具有隐匿形式的 FD 患者中是否有效尚不明确。

一般来说，FD 的治疗很少能够"治愈"。一些患者暂时停止寻求疾病的行为，但大多数患者不愿意接受转入精神科治疗，可能会继续自我诱导或假装疾病。在可能的情况下，精神科医生应评估患者是否存在可能使患者易患或导致表达人为疾病行为的共病精神疾病（如重度抑郁症或人格障碍）。如果能识别和治疗潜在的精神疾病，驱动 FD 的心理力量可能会减轻。还应评估患者的自杀倾向，并在适当时候转移到更安全的环境中。当患者有自杀意念或自杀企图、社会状况恶化或表现出严重的行为时[25,29]，表明需要住精神病院。当康复发生时，通常是由于患者生活状况的变化，而不是医疗的干预[30]。

（五）与隐私和保密有关的伦理问题

在一些 FD 患者中，秘密搜索患者的个人物品可以挽救生命[14]。它还可以预防毁灭性的医源性疾病[31]。此外，患者可能会否认自残，但当他们面对从房间搜索到的证据时，他们往往会停止这种做法。

由于两个原因很难在医院里秘密搜索患者的私人物品，即使怀疑是自我诱发的疾病可能是致命的。首先，对秘密搜索患者的私人财产存在伦理和法律上的反对意见[32]。其次，一些综合医院基本上都承诺不会进行秘密搜索（大多数精神病院并非如此）。这一"承诺"是给予我院收治的每一位患者[33,34]。如果严重的自我诱发或医源性疾病对患者的风险极小或仅为中等，那么遵守承诺就不是一个主要问题。但当怀疑患有危及生命的 FD 患者或认为严重医源性疾病的风险很高时，应采取什么措施呢？一种可能是医生将对他或她的怀疑告诉患者，并要求知情同意对患者的私人物品进行搜查。这种方法需要制定计划，包括撰写一份具体的知情同意书。在进行进一步侵入性诊断检查之前，将告知患者有必要进行搜索。如果患者同意搜索，并且发现 FD 的证据，则怀疑将得到确认。如果患者不允许进行搜索，就可告知转诊医生（可能还有患者家属）说明可能的影响，希望这些知识能够降低疑似自我诱发疾病未来产生有害影响的可能性。如果搜索结果为阴性，或者如果患者拒绝进行搜索，医生可能会被迫退出这个病例，但前提是应找到另一位医生来承担患者的责任。就像任何其他医疗程序一样处理对患者私人物品的搜索听起来很简单，并且已经被推荐[32]，但据我们所知，没有报告描述要求患者同意搜索其私人物品的结果和影响。

一些 FD 患者禁止医生将 FD 诊断告知家人。这可能会造成了一个两难的困境，因为根据《健康保险可携带性和责任法案》（HIPAA 法案），医生可能会因违反保密规定而受到制裁。正如 Charles Ford 博士（医学博士 Feldman 个人交流 2000）报告的病例说明了这一点。一名医学生的妻子巧妙地模拟了肺出血肾炎综合征（Goodpasture 综合征）。面对照顾她的需要，这个医学生有可能不及格。如果顾问（作出正确诊断的顾问）违反保密原则并将其疾病的真实情况告知她的丈夫或她的初级保健医生，则其妻子威胁他将提起诉讼。

解决这类困境的最佳方法是咨询风险管理部门和其他医生，比如院长以及该机构的伦理和法律委员会。这些问题最好在团队中进行彻底讨论，以便达成共识。

（六）法律问题

医生可以假设，他们永远不会受到 FD 患者的医疗事故诉讼。毕竟患者伪造了自己的疾病，没有提供真实的病史。然而，有可能人为疾病的原告提起诉讼的人数不断增加[35]。这类诉讼可能是由患者的愤怒引起的，也可能是为了将注意力从医院转移到法庭[36]。同样，医生未能认识 FD 可作为诉讼的依据。在一个这样的案例中，一名前医科学生起诉了 35 名医生，指控他们疏忽大意，因为他们对她进行了化疗，治疗她并没有的癌症。这起案件已经庭外和解[37]。另一个例子涉及假装反射性交感神经营养不良患者的腿部截肢。

原告针对其医生提出的一个论点是，医疗记录中存在其疾病的人为病因的有力证据，但医生未阅读这些记录。因此可以得出结论，人为疾病并不能可靠地防御不良结局[38]，患者的欺诈行为并不能消除医患关系的法律和伦理方面的问题[39]。

同时必须认识到，揭露欺骗行为并不能否定真实疾病或伤害的风险。例如，故意夸大症状可能反映了患者对实际存在的医疗问题的绝望[10]。

我们没有发现与侵犯隐私、违反保密协议或未获得知情同意有关的诉讼。显然，任何违反保密规定的行为都应该符合维护患者健康或显著减少对他人利益的损害[40]。在有争议的案件中，详细和完整的同期文件将提供一些保护。支持所采取行动的第二种意见也将降低提起诉讼或证明诉讼成功的可能性。

二、相关异常疾病行为

（一）躯体症状障碍

躯体症状障碍（somatic symptom disorder，SSD）可定义为在 30 岁之前开始的特发性身体症状，随着时间的推移，这些症状位于身体的不同部位，并导致不成比例的重度残疾和功能受损。主要症状是疼痛，没有证据表明 SSD 患者的疼痛是故意假装或夸大的，但也没有办法证明不是（另见第 12 和 22 章）。

身体症状通常紧随创伤事件后发生，且身体症状可能与其他精神疾病如抑郁症共存。绝大多数患者为女性，患者因其症状就医，但找不到真实的医学解释。从"病态角色"的假设中获得的二次收益往往是显而易见的。在一些患者中，症状和疾病成为一种沟通的手段[41]，也是控制其环境的一种方式。症状导致的功能障碍和残疾往往与症状的严重程度不成比例。SSD 的病程通常是慢性的，一旦在年轻时建立，它可以一直持续到老年[42]。病例 3 介绍了 SSD 的一个例子。

病例 3 一位 20 岁腹痛的女性

一名大学生出现了与恶心相关的左侧脐周疼痛,她因疼痛而致残,不得不辍学。患者接受了阿片类药物治疗,但疼痛持续存在。CT 检查显示空肠套叠。患者计划接受腹部手术,但其家属决定征求第二意见。

在我们医疗中心,患者将疼痛描述为持续性疼痛伴灼烧感(严重程度为 10/10),位于左中腹部。疼痛与进餐、排便或月经周期无关。患者未出现便秘或腹泻。既往病史有腹股沟疝、右膝关节镜手术、慢性背痛、慢性盆腔痛、抑郁、疲乏和月经失调。体格检查期间,患者表现很被动、出现抑郁,未出现重度疼痛。触诊时有轻微的压痛。

放射科医生检查 CT 图像,证实为间歇性空肠套叠无梗阻。由于已知 CT 扫描偶然发现的大多数小肠套叠是无症状的、短暂的,且不需要手术治疗[43]。我们怀疑空肠套叠是否是她腹痛的原因。内镜检查回肠中段未发现异常。外科会诊同意患者的疼痛不是由 CT 扫描观察到的空肠套叠引起的。胃肠病学家和外科医生诊断为 SSD 的,患者被转诊到精神科,以评价其抑郁和自杀风险。

几年后,她的病情基本上没有变化。她仍然感到疼痛,但疼痛位于胸部而不是腹部。她没有返回学校或就业,她似乎身体功能严重失调,然而,在愉快的环境下,如在聚会上,她有时显得很快乐、很有活力。

SSD 的潜在病因尚不清楚,但已经提出了几种机制。一种假设是 SSD 患者经历的心理痛苦以身体症状的形式表现出来[44]。另一种理论是,患者了解到表现出他或她对假定痛苦信念的行为,由此产生的"疾病"有助于患者应对困难[45]。SSD 的边界明显不清晰,一边与疾病焦虑症不易察觉地融合,另一边与 FD 融合[45]。

SSD 的诊断依赖识别患者该疾病的两个特征。首先,与不同器官系统相关的多种特发性症状存在疾病寻求行为;其次是症状导致的残疾和功能障碍比例较高。在一份报告中,SSD 患者每月卧床 7 天,而一般人群为 0.48 天[46]。SSD 患者并不像 FD 患者那样被医生关注。

不幸的是,即使是高技能的医生也反复多次不能识别 SSD[42]。因此这些患者获得了少见或罕见疾病的诊断检测。这些患者极易受到这种做法的影响,因为重复的诊断检查往往会发现可疑的异常,这些异常可能导致药物治疗(如糖皮质激素或麻醉药)、侵入性操作或手术的并发症。

对于 SSD 患者的管理,建议采用"关怀"而不是"治愈"的方法[47]。最好由一位医生实行,应建立同情的、情感移入的长期关系。应安排定期随访,简短的体格检查优于广泛的诊断检查和程序[48]。处方药物应保持在最低限度,并避免使用阿片类药物[47]。由于抑郁症很常见,应该评估这些患者自杀的风险[5]。避免对峙,因为 SSD 中的动机被认为是无意识的,但可以实现对情感成分的一些意识[47]。在一项随机对照临床试验中,发现认知行为治疗与自我报告功能和躯体症状的显著改善以及医疗费用的降低相关[49]。然而,这些改善可能是由于在实验性认知行为治疗中投入了更多的注意力和额外的时间[47]。

(二) 诈病

与 FD 的隐匿形式一样,Gavin 是第一个描述诈病的人[4]。诈病是指为物质利益,如金钱、住宿、食物、麻醉品等,有意识地、有目的地制造或夸大疾病的症状和体征,逃避刑事起诉。诈病并不总是贪婪的反映。相反,这可能是经济拮据或试图逃避身体或情感虐待的结果[50]。我们的一位秘密服用泻药的患者说 为了不让丈夫离开她,她诱发了她的疾病。显然需要详细的病史和社会史,将这种医疗欺骗置于适当的背景下[50]。

与 FD 一样,诈病者因其假装或产生的症状和体征而就医,他们向医生隐瞒其症状的真实病因。诈病者通常不像 FD 患者那样愿意接受危险的诊断或治疗程序,他们试图尽量减少与医护人员的接触,以避免检测[50]。

诈病与 FD 之间的区别是基于对动机的感知:诈病的物质收益和 FD 生病角色的情感收益。然而,对动机的感知并不总是正确的,而且存在偏见[50]。临床医生还应意识到,个人的目标,无论是内部的还是外部的,有意识的还是无意识的,都会随着时间的推移而变化或共存[51]。此外,《精神疾病诊断与统计手册》第五版认识到,动机可以在个别病例中合并,并允许同时诊断 FD 和诈病。与 FD 和 SSD 不同,诈病不被认为是一种精神障碍。

(三) 贪食症患者的人为行为

伴有进食障碍的患者常发生胃肠道症状,其中大多是由于滥用泻药或自我诱发的呕吐所致(见第 9 章)[52]。当他们因这些症状而就医时,他们往往不会告知医生他们的饮食紊乱或他们的净化活动。内科住院医师 Michael Carmichael 博士进行了一次录像采访[33],探讨了这些异常疾病行为的动机。该采访的部分内容如下:

患者:当我第一次去医院做检查时,他们什么也没发现。

医生:好吧。你当时在吃什么药吗?

患者:没有吃药。

医生:那时你服用泻药了吗?

患者:是的。

医生:好吧。你离开医院之后发生了什么?

患者:我的症状改善了一段时间,但几个月后变得更严重了,我又去了另一家医院,做了同样的检查。他们只发现我得了胃炎。

医生:可是,这些医院的医生给你做了不少检查,我相信有些检查对你来说既痛苦又昂贵,还很麻烦。你想过这个问题吗?我很好奇你是怎么想的。

患者:我真的试着告诉自己,一定是哪里出了问题。

医生:那时候医生有没有问过你泻药的事,你有没有在吃泻药?

患者:没有。

医生:如果医生告诉你,你需要做手术,看看出了什么问题,你认为你会有什么反应?

患者:我相信我会按照他们说的去做。

医生:为什么?

患者:我真的不知道。

医生:你能告诉我们更多关于服用泻药的事吗?以及你为什么选择泻药而不是其他药?

患者:我觉得我可以想吃什么就吃什么,而且不用担心吃了什么,体重也不会增加。

医生:原来是为了减肥。

患者:是的。

医生:好吧。我想你吃的是 Correctol,对吗?

患者:是的。

医生:您平均一天吃几片?

患者:最严重的时候,大约 40 片。

医生:一天 40 片,那很多啊。

患者:是的。

医生:当我们告诉你体重减轻是因为你服用了泻药时,你是什么感觉?当我们提起这件事的时候你是怎么想的?

患者:我松了一口气。我这辈子从没这么轻松过。我想让别人知道,但我不能告诉任何人。

与其他患者的非录像采访揭示了性质上相似的动机,只有一些人认识到了他们胃肠道症状的原因,仅因为他们的家人坚持这样做而就医。没有证据表明寻求病态角色是为了缓解情绪困扰。所有的人都为他们的净化行为和向医生隐瞒而感到羞愧。其中两例患者因胃肠道症状接受了腹部手术。

为了评估泻药减少暴食后热量吸收的程度,在代谢研究实验室对正常受试者和 2 名贪食症患者进行了研究。结果发现,泻药对热量吸收的影响相对较小[53]。例如,在摄入 1 726kcal 的食物后,再服用 50 片 Correctol,其中 1 例患者的腹泻液量为 6.1L,重 6.2kg。与对照试验日相比,当患者摄入不含 Correctol 的相似食物时,这种高容量腹泻仅使热量吸收降低了 188kcal 的。

三、与胃肠病学相关的特殊问题

(一) 秘密服用泻药

秘密服用泻药引起的腹泻通常与腹痛、体重减轻、电解质紊乱和/或直立性低血压相关。根据这些表现中的哪一种向医生揭示,哪种被隐藏,临床表现可能具有高度变异性。与低钾血症、腹痛、体重减轻或直立性低血压相关的腹泻具有不同的众所周知的内涵,可引发特定的诊断研究。如果存在腹泻被隐藏,患者可能有一种外来的疾病,这种疾病会引起肾病学家和内分泌科医生的兴趣[54,55]。在任何情况下,胃肠病学常用的诊断工具都不会揭示正确的诊断,往往会被误导。只有掌握了框 23.1 和框 23.2 中信息的胃肠病学家才有可能作出正确的诊断。

(二) 人为腹泻

当胃肠病学家将慢性特发性腹泻患者转诊到对腹泻疾病有特殊兴趣的医疗中心时,最常见的特异性诊断是摄入泻药(见第 16 章)[56]。在很大程度上,对拒绝摄入泻药的患者,摄入泻药的诊断取决于通过分析方法检测粪便或尿液中泻药或其代谢产物的能力。然而,重要的是要认识到,在确定泻药摄入量时出现的任何错误都可能造成严重的有害后果。假阴性结果使人为疾病的诊断延迟数年,并导致不必要或不适当的医疗或手术治疗的并发症。相反,假阳性结果会过早地停止对真实疾病的诊断评价,并可能导致患者被错误地指责为自我诱导疾病,这可能造成严重的心理伤害。

比沙可啶和番泻叶是秘密摄入的最常见的泻药,可导致人为腹泻[57]。实验室研究报告通过尿液薄层色谱法(thin layer chromatography,TLC)鉴别这些药物的敏感性和特异性为 100%,建议特发性腹泻患者在进行侵入性或昂贵的诊断和治疗程序之前,常规检测这些泻药的摄入[17,18]。在 2007 年以前,美国的一家参考实验室提供了尿液和粪便的薄层色谱法分析,以检测这些药物的摄入情况。为了评估该程序的准确性,我们通过让健康志愿者摄入比沙可定、番泻叶或对照泻药来诱导腹泻。以设盲方式将尿液和腹泻粪便样本送至临床参考实验室进行比沙可啶和番泻叶分析。结果显示,该实验室对番泻叶的 TLC 检测方法灵敏度为 0%;换句话说,所有因番泻叶引起腹泻的受试者均有假阴性结果。公司的比沙可啶检测在 18% 提交的尿液和粪便样本中产生假阴性结果,在 7% 的样本中产生了假阳性结果。尿液中比沙可啶阳性试验的计算预测值,是不同人群中比沙可啶诱导性腹泻发生率的函数。如图 23.1 所示。在接受全科医生管理的隐源性腹泻患者中,比沙可啶诱发腹泻的报告发生率约为 2.4%[57]。在这种频率下,绝大多数比沙可啶尿液检测阳性结果将显示假阳性结果。除检测程序中的分析错误外,TLC 的部分问题可能是结果报告为"未检出"或"阳性",而不是以每升重量或每天重量进行定量。理论上,摄入物质或内源性代谢产生的少量物质(太小而不足以引起腹泻)可能会产生假阳性结果。

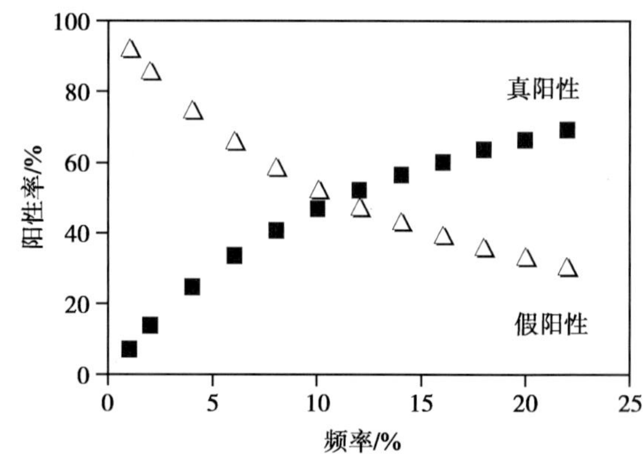

图 23.1　薄层色谱法测得的比沙可啶阳性尿液检测结果为真阳性或假阳性结果的可能性,与检测人群中比沙可啶诱导腹泻的频率之间的相关性

该相同的参考实验室目前通过高效液相色谱/串联质谱法提供比沙可啶和蒽醌类药物的尿液检测,但不提供粪便检测。这些结果也在阳性或未检测的基础上报告的,无需量化,我们尚不清楚当正常研究受试者摄入不同泻药的尿液样本被提交进行盲法检测时,这些程序的敏感性和特异性研究。根据我们在 2019 年获得的所有信息,我们认为,除非判断为人为疾病的可能性很高(见框 23.1 和框 23.2),并且除非粪便分析显示为分泌性腹泻,否则不应进行这些检查。在渗透性腹泻患者中获得的任何阳性结果几乎肯定是假阳性,因为比沙可啶和番泻叶不会引起渗透性腹泻。如果商业实验室能够证明他们的尿液比沙可啶和蒽醌的检测在腹泻患者中具有高度特异性和敏感性,则这种情况将会改变。

在慢性特发性腹泻患者中，分析粪液中的单价电解质（钠、钾和氯）、pH 和渗透压可确定是否存在渗透性或分泌性腹泻（见第 16 章）。当摄入吸收不良的溶质如镁、硫酸盐、磷酸盐或聚乙二醇引起渗透性腹泻时，化学方法可以定量测定这些溶质在粪液中的百分比含量[58]。已在正常受试者中研究了这些渗透性泻药的作用，并确定了正常人群和泻药诱导腹泻的正常人群中每种溶质的粪便浓度。当在 158 例慢性特发性腹泻患者中评估这种检测方法时，发现 8%（12/158）的患者的粪液中存在一种渗透性泻药的致腹泻浓度[58]。（乳果糖也引起渗透性腹泻，但通过粪便分析来看，它与碳水化合物吸收不良的“合法”原因难以区分。）这些结果表明，在特发性慢性渗透性腹泻患者早期使用简单的化学检查，可显著减少使用昂贵且有时危险的诊断程序，这些程序无法检测泻药摄入。

在特发性慢性腹泻患者中发现泻药摄入的真阳性检查结果，并不是秘密摄入泻药或人为腹泻的决定性证据，因为患者可能是在不知情的情况下摄入了泻药（例如，抗酸剂中的镁）或保健品中（可能含有蒽醌类）。当获得泻药摄入试验阳性结果时，需要仔细考虑此类无害解释[59]。未知泻药摄入，是医生可能在慢性特发性腹泻患者中作出的最令人满意的诊断之一，因为停止意外摄入泻药可以治愈慢性腹泻。

可以用水稀释粪便来假装腹泻。这种稀释可在粪便采集后在体外进行，也可以在体内给予自来水灌肠，然后收集直肠流出物。这种类型的人为腹泻可以通过测量粪便表面的上清液渗透压摩尔浓度来鉴别，发现其数值远低于平均生理水平 290mOsm/kg。在我们医院就诊的一例患者，提交的 48 小时粪便采集物的粪液渗透压为 83mOsm/kg。如果用生理盐水稀释粪便，通过测量粪液渗透压将无法检测到这种稀释形式的人为腹泻。

如第 128 章所讨论的，超过 70% 使用蒽醌类泻药（如药鼠李、芦荟、番泻叶等）的患者平均在定期摄入这些药物的 9 个月内发生结肠假性黑色素病。据说这种影响在停止服用蒽醌类药物后一年内是可逆的。在结肠镜检查或活检标本中发现这种色素（脂褐素）只提示但不能诊断近期摄入蒽醌类泻药。这种情况的其他明显原因包括摄入非甾体抗炎药[60]。

（三）隐匿性呕吐

在 20 世纪早期，胃肠病学家和外科医生认识到，由于胃出口梗阻引起的持续性呕吐可能导致严重的毒血症，伴有血容量不足、低氯性代谢性碱中毒、低钾血症、尿毒症和手足搐搦[61]。基于随后的临床研究发现，呕吐引起的电解质异常的发病机制如下：呕吐→氯化氢（HCl）损失和容积收缩→代谢性碱中毒→碳酸氢盐肾脏排泄增加→钾和钠肾脏排泄增加→低钾血症和血液浓缩。碱中毒还导致钾从细胞外液进入细胞内间隙，进一步降低血清钾浓度。

在 20 世纪 60 年代报道了原发性肾性钾消耗所致的低钾血症和低氯性碱中毒（Bartter 综合征）[62]。此后不久，研究表明，隐匿性呕吐或秘密摄入噻嗪类利尿剂几乎可以模拟 Bartter 综合征的所有特征，包括血浆肾素和醛固酮浓度升高以及肾小球旁器增生[63-66]。突然间，隐秘呕吐的代谢影响成为医学病例研讨中令人热议的话题，这重新唤起了学者对慢性呕吐其他原因的兴趣。

当患者秘密地自我诱导呕吐，然后到医生那里寻求呕吐的原因时，这时识别呕吐的人为性质可能是困难的。当患者隐瞒诱发呕吐发作，并出现低氯性碱中毒和低钾血症时，将对其进行提示 Bartter 综合征或其他具有相似特征的罕见疾病的诊断研究。隐蔽性呕吐是引起低钾血症和碱中毒的一个有用的线索是尿氯排泄率极低，即使患者摄入了含有正常量氯的饮食，这在 Bartter 综合征或秘密摄入噻嗪类利尿剂中并不存在[63]。

我们回顾了吐根糖浆的有趣历史[67]。1965 年，FDA 批准了这种化合物作为催吐剂的非处方药。2003 年取消了这个批准[68]，由于中毒儿童缺乏临床获益、药物不良事件和贪食症患者的滥用[69]。

（四）人为贫血和人为胃肠道出血

当反复出现不明原因的血红蛋白浓度急剧下降，并对输血有适当但不能维持的反应时，应考虑人为贫血[70]。FD 患者通常采用静脉切开术和/或放置静脉导管进行自我放血，以造成人为贫血。他们还会口服采集的血液来模拟呕血和黑便，或者将血液添加到尿液或粪便样本中，造成血尿和便血。一名患者用长编织针撕破了其远端结肠，从而导致血性腹泻[71]。一名肝硬化伴急性上、下胃肠道出血患者接受了结肠镜检查，发现直肠有线性溃疡，并在盲肠处发现了 2 个直刃剃须刀片[72]。一份报告[73]一例 23 岁患者，曾因胃肠道反复出血入院，多次内镜检查未发现真实的出血部位。因此进行了多种治疗，进行了手术包括胃血管栓塞。后来，她的医生注意到 FD 的行为特征，包括对她长期住院缺乏关注以及她愿意在最低的镇静下接受多次内镜手术。在与患者沟通后，她承认将从其经外周静脉置入的中心静脉导管管路采集的血液与注射器一起储存在她床头柜中的塑料瓶中。另一例患者通过使用针头自己从腋窝静脉切开，插入导管，然后通过吸管吸食血液，造成贫血和明显的胃肠道出血[74]。如果患者在注射同位素标记的红细胞后自行抽血，然后将血液饮用或注入腹腔，则出血扫描可能显示异常，并可能导致不适当的治疗[75,76]。

（五）人为癌症

假装癌症的患者经常会进入一个新的医院，寻求继续治疗他们的“癌症”，并声称他们是被另一个城市或州的医生转诊的。他们提供了令人信服的病史，瘢痕与以前的癌症手术治疗相容，并且经常提供（假的）病理报告。他们声称他们的其他医疗记录将很快发送过来。另外，也有一些患者假装癌症，并进入了癌症互助小组。一名这样的患者参加了关于死亡的课程。这个班级被她的勇气所感动，甚至为她募集了资金，让她骑上热气球——这是她的“最后的愿望”之一[77]。

一些动机显然导致人们假装癌症。一种是次要物质获得

(诈病,也许是为了获得麻醉剂)。另一个是无意识的需要欺骗医疗系统,并接受诊断测试和治疗过程。有些人可能寻求与癌症的诊断相关的社会地位(例如,被称赞为“幸存者”),以便得到朋友、同事和其他人的同情和礼物[77]。一些人显然是假装患有癌症,因为他们爱的人患了癌症。一名女性后来表示,她希望死于免疫抑制[78]。这些动机可能同时存在。无论动机如何,假装癌症的发作似乎通常发生在被亲人拒绝后或其他类型的损失后。孤独和孤立似乎是许多假装癌症的人的促发因素。

在患者接受癌症化疗或接受癌症手术之前,几乎总是需要相关的病历。希望假装癌症的患者可能会从其他患者的病历中窃取和篡改真实的记录,并将其作为自己的病历传递出去。在一种情况下,一名患者扫描并修改了记录,这使得识别他们的欺诈行为变得更加困难[78]。对于医院员工来说,获得医学术语、症状学、病理报告以及诊断和治疗计划是最容易的,这可能解释了为什么最好和最完整的伪造品是来自医院的工作人员。尽管肿瘤学家努力地仔细审查病历,但在某些情况下,病例伪造得足够好,使FD患者能够获得化疗[78]。

人为癌症的诊断通常是通过检测病史中的不一致性、伪造病历的证据、患者讲述自己的医疗保险或个人病史的谎言或医生提出的对患者故事的偶然怀疑来进行的。关于通常致命的癌症延长生存期的说法,有助于在某些情况下揭示人为癌症。

(六) 来自病例报告的经验教训

表23.2列出了所选病例报告的简要摘要,以进一步说明在消化病学实践中可能发生的各种各样的做作性障碍。

表23.2　胃肠病学中的人为疾病(FD)病例

表现	评估
造瘘性克罗恩病伴造口出血[79]	组织学仅显示非特异性异常,浆膜层炎症比黏膜层更严重,提示外源性创伤。本病是采用经阴道、直肠造口进针自伤感染所致
难治性乳糜泻[80]	患者患有乳糜泻,最初对无麸质饮食有反应。患者随后发生重度腹泻,认为是由于难治性乳糜泻所致。通过粪便分析确定诊断,发现腹泻是由于摄入含有镁的牛奶引起的。如果FD的正确诊断尚未确立,患者将接受免疫抑制治疗
卟啉病[81]	腹痛、尿红患者。新鲜的尿液呈红色,但在卟啉病中,新鲜排出的尿液颜色正常,暴露在日光下时变为红色或棕色。搜查患者房间发现了一种含有芦巴膦酸的药物,一种酸性红色溶液
死于肝衰竭[82]	一名29岁女性死于肝衰竭。鼻出血、贫血、脱发、肝肿大和肝脏生化检查水平升高。死亡前18个月进行的肝活检提示维生素A过多症的变化(包括富含脂肪的星状细胞)。虽然她的血清维生素A水平很高,但她否认过量摄入维生素A。临死前,她承认自己秘密地摄入了过量的鱼肝油
假性肠梗阻[83]	一名18岁男性经胃肠道及泌尿系检查后,被诊断为假性肠梗阻。患者卧床不起,需要接受全肠外营养(TPN)和留置导尿,但生理检查未发现胃肠道和膀胱运动障碍的证据。怀疑患者的母亲患有代理型Munchausen综合征。患者的粪便和尿液中吐根的一种成分依米丁检测为阳性。经法院裁定与母亲分离1周后,患者完全恢复良好,最终诊断为代理型Munchausen综合征
导致Bartter综合征诊断的双重欺骗[84,85]	该患者发生与低钾血症和代谢性碱中毒相关的发作性瘫痪。血浆肾素和醛固酮浓度较高,肾活检标本显示肾小球旁器增生,诊断为Bartter综合征[84]。随后,发现患者在秘密摄入酚酞,但一直隐瞒她腹泻的事实[85]
一例近期捐献部分肝脏进行移植的女性患者发生复发性伤口感染[86]	捐献肝脏5周后,发生术后伤口感染伴感染性休克。捐赠者的医院账单巨大,被送到接受者的保险公司,从而威胁到接受者的终身福利。她被怀疑FD,因为培养出抗生素敏感的多种微生物细菌。既往病历显示既往FD的证据
诱导呕吐以产生难治性高血压[87]	一位25岁女性高血压患者,通过消除抗高血压药物的作用,使用自我诱发呕吐来升高血压。她的动机是延长住院时间,以避免紧张的家庭环境
致死性非血栓性肺栓塞[88]	一例32岁女性在Roux-en-Y胃旁路术和胰腺自身胰岛细胞移植并发症后接受TPN治疗。患者表现为非典型病原体菌血症反复发作。心搏骤停伴右心衰竭导致她死亡。尸检时的死亡原因归因于肺微晶纤维素栓子引起的并发症,这可能是由于通过中心静脉导管自行注射口服药物所致
克罗恩病女性患者中的复发性全血细胞减少症[89]	一例50岁女性患者,有瘘管性克罗恩病病史,既往接受过6-巯基嘌呤(6-MP)治疗,但因药物性胰腺炎而停药。两个月后,患者出现复发性全血细胞减少症。重复骨髓活检的结果无诊断价值。硫代嘌呤代谢物检测显示,即使6-MP已在数月前停用,6-MP的水平也易引起毒性。该患者否认重新填写旧处方和服用6-MP,但她的社区药师证实最近分发了再填写的6-MP。全血细胞减少归因于秘密摄入6-MP

四、异常疾病行为诊断和处理的隐患

在病例 4 中，未发现可解释其剧烈腹痛和体重减轻的器质性原因，这导致胃肠病学家怀疑患者症状的精神病学的原因，并请了精神科会诊。在采集精神病史并查看患者后，精神科医生诊断为“精神性疼痛”，这一术语意味着疼痛主要是由情绪抑郁引起并维持的。胃肠病学家完全接受了这个诊断，并将患者转诊到医院精神病科。

病例 4　一位 31 岁男性腹痛

该患者因 6 周前剧烈腹痛入住我院，疼痛部位为中腹部，主要发生在餐后[33]。他的体重减轻了约 5.5kg，体格检查显示无腹膜炎的体征，除小的良性胃溃疡外，食管胃十二指肠内镜、结肠镜检查、CT、超声和内镜逆行胰胆管造影检查结果均正常。他的疼痛对强效抗溃疡药物无反应，因此认为溃疡不是他疼痛的原因。

一位精神科医生检查了该患者，发现他患有重度抑郁症伴忧郁症，复发型伴躯体化，并开了安非他明。药物最初似乎有帮助，第二天患者感觉好转；然而在第二天，他再次在餐后出现了严重腹痛，查体腹部柔软、无压痛，肠鸣音正常。给予哌替啶止痛。病程记录指出，“患者的申诉模式和他对抗抑郁药的反应表明，精神性疼痛问题与依赖性/对立人格障碍相结合”和“患者病情继续严重恶化，他从每个躯体问题中取得了最大的次要收益。”

住院第 10 天，患者以胎儿式卧位，持续剧烈腹痛。出现脐周压痛，但无反跳痛。一份病程上记录：“他的妈妈和朋友们一直在他身边徘徊。他看起来确实很抑郁，但疼痛综合征似乎是源于心因性的（不是抑郁的等价物），其次是他的依赖性自恋人格结构”。2 天后患者放置了营养管，患者转入精神科，后来发现他反应迟钝。腹部 X 线片显示图表下方有空气。患者不久后死亡。尸检显示，粥样硬化斑块完全阻塞了患者的肠系膜上动脉，导致其在过去 6 周内的疼痛、小肠坏死和穿孔[33]。

这种思维过程是错误的，原因有两个。首先，不能确切排除躯体（或器质性）疾病，未能发现严重腹痛的器质性疾病，并不构成该病例精神病病因的证据。此外，没有任何线索表明异常疾病行为的积极证据。尽管请精神科医生会诊以帮助管理任何相关的抑郁症可能是明智的，但胃肠内科医生应该知道，精神科医生无法通过进行精神学评估来准确地将情绪困扰诊断为严重腹痛的主要原因。其次，精神科医生应该知道，二次获得是正常疾病行为的一部分，他应该认识到，没有支持异常疾病行为的证据，就不应该作出“精神性疼痛”的诊断，这就为进一步寻找该患者严重腹痛的医学原因关上了大门[90]，这是典型的腹部心绞痛。

在这方面，Nadelson 的建议是正确的：“精神科医生必须鼓励转诊医生根据临床证据面对患者，认识到精神科医生自己的诊断能力可能无法预测隐藏的真相”[91]。根据我们对这一建议的解释，作为身体症状主要原因的异常疾病行为的诊断应基于临床证据（如框 23.1 和框 23.2 中所讨论的），而不是根据从精神病学评估中获得的信息。在这种情况下，阴性的临床证据可以由胃肠病学家或精神科医生进行汇编。不幸的是，没有人这样做。

（郭晓燕　译，鲁晓岚　孙明瑜　校）

参考文献

第四部分 多器官相关问题

第 24 章 口腔疾病及胃肠道和肝脏疾病的口腔表现

Kimberly L. Pham, Ginat W. Mirowski 著

章节目录

一、唇部疾病 ········· 331
（一）唇炎 ········· 331
（二）唇部肿瘤 ········· 331
二、唾液腺疾病 ········· 332
（一）口干症 ········· 332
（二）干燥综合征 ········· 332
三、舌部疾病 ········· 332
（一）舌炎、舌痛和口腔感觉障碍 ········· 332
（二）味觉减退和味觉障碍 ········· 333
（三）地图舌 ········· 333
（四）裂纹舌 ········· 333
（五）黑毛舌 ········· 333
（六）草莓舌 ········· 333
（七）萎缩性舌 ········· 334
（八）肥大舌 ········· 334
（九）白斑 ········· 334
（十）疱疹性几何学舌炎 ········· 334
四、牙龈疾病 ········· 335
（一）牙龈肿大 ········· 335
（二）牙龈口炎 ········· 335
（三）急性坏死性溃疡性牙龈炎 ········· 335
（四）铅中毒 ········· 335
五、感染、肿瘤和其他选定疾病的口腔表现 ········· 335
（一）念珠菌病 ········· 335
（二）疱疹病毒感染 ········· 335
（三）人乳头瘤病毒感染 ········· 336
（四）卡波西肉瘤 ········· 336
（五）其他 HIV 相关疾病 ········· 336
（六）鳞状细胞癌 ········· 336
（七）炎症性肠病 ········· 336
六、胃食管反流病 ········· 337
七、肝脏疾病 ········· 337
八、复发性阿弗他口腔溃疡 ········· 337
九、白塞病 ········· 338
十、伴有口腔表现的皮肤疾病 ········· 338
十一、淀粉样变性 ········· 338
十二、营养缺乏 ········· 338

一、唇部疾病

唇部是成对的结构，在中面部高度可见，功能是促进咀嚼、语言和许多习惯。嘴唇左右是对称的。将唇的皮肤与唇红分开是一个略微隆起的边缘，其被称为唇红缘。

（一）唇炎

唇炎即口唇的炎症，可涉及唇红、黏膜和口周皮肤，包括唇联合。其治疗包括针对或终止导致炎症的根本原因。

口角炎（口角干裂，口角炎）表现为唇联合处炎症和发红引起的疼痛性水肿和皲裂。维生素 B_2（核黄素）或铁缺失均可引起口角炎。感染可能会刺激嘴唇。舔唇和咬唇等口腔习惯也可能使患者易患口角炎[1]。

剥脱性唇炎（慢性唇裂）是一种唇红的慢性炎症。患者在一些疾病（如特应性皮炎、银屑病、慢性刺激和过敏）的背景下出现口唇的干燥或瘙痒，局部外用糖皮质激素或钙调磷酸酶抑制剂可能对对症治疗有效。

接触性唇炎是由接触刺激物或过敏反应引起，表现为唇部和口周水肿、红斑和鳞屑。在个人卫生用品和化妆品、食品、个人习惯和外用药物（如庆大霉素）中使用的香精、羊毛脂、没食子酸十二烷基酯和过氧化苯甲酰已被证实是导致过敏性接触性唇炎的病因。最常见的过敏原包括秘鲁的香料混合物和香脂[2]。

肉芽肿性唇炎是一种少见的病症，表现为反复发作的口唇肿胀伴有口唇慢性肿大和坚硬[3]。唇活检示非干酪样肉芽肿。肉芽肿性唇炎与克罗恩病和结核病相关，并且是 Melkersson-Rosenthal 综合征（一种以裂纹舌和肉芽肿性唇炎为特征的罕见疾病，伴或不伴面瘫和偏头痛）的组成部分[3-5]。

（二）唇部肿瘤

光化性唇炎（光化性唇角化病，日光性唇炎）是一种与长期日光或紫外线辐射有关的唇上皮细胞异型增生的癌前病变。肤色浅的人，特别是职业暴露者、老年人和有实体器官移植史（随后的免疫抑制治疗）的个体发生光化性唇炎的风险更高[6,7]。虽然本病的表现多种多样，但唇红缘消失，伴弥漫性红斑、片状白斑、干燥和唇红部脱屑是最典型的症状。由于唇部异型增生的部位和程度不能仅凭临床表现来推断，因此需行多点活检帮助诊断。虽然目前尚无美国食品药品管理局（FDA）批准的治疗本病的方法，但应针对整个唇部进行治疗，

因为光化性唇炎可能进展为鳞状细胞癌。

鳞状细胞癌是最常见的口腔肿瘤,最常累及下唇[8]。白种人、男性和 HPV 16 或 18 感染易导致患者发生唇上皮细胞的恶变。因为鳞状细胞癌具有高度转移风险,因此在初始评估时诊断应包括肿瘤分期。治疗方法包括手术切除和放射治疗。

二、唾液腺疾病

口腔健康的前提是唾液充足。唾液有利于进食、吞咽、说话等正常功能。唾液还具有防龋齿作用,启动消化过程,以及抗细菌,抗真菌和免疫作用[9,10]。

(一) 口干症

口干症是一种常见的主诉,由唾液腺破坏或萎缩所致。自身免疫性疾病(如干燥综合征、系统性红斑狼疮、原发性胆汁性胆管炎)、放射治疗、糖尿病、感染、肉芽肿性疾病(如结节病和结核病)、慢性移植物抗宿主病、终末期肾病、血色病、淀粉样变性、帕金森病以及多种药物:抗胆碱能药物、H_1 抗组胺药、三环类抗抑郁药、选择性 5-羟色胺再摄取抑制剂(selective serotonin reuptakes inhibitor,SSRI)、催眠药、镇静剂、抗高血压药、抗精神病药、抗帕金森病药和利尿剂都可引起口干[11,12],口干可易患口腔念珠菌病[13]。随着患者年龄的增长,药物数量的增加和相关的诱发条件可能进一步导致口干症的发生并不奇怪[14]。

除体格检查外,测量唾液流率或刺激唾液产生的唾液测量试验和唾液腺闪烁照相可能有助于口干症的诊断和治疗管理[12]。吸吮无糖薄荷糖和咀嚼口香糖有助于刺激唾液流量增加,进而帮助清除食物残渣,而不增加发生龋齿的风险。口干症患者应避免甜食、酸性食物或饮料,以限制诱发龋齿。应鼓励患者经常小口喝水和含冰屑。也可含 1% 羧甲基纤维素钠的制剂用于湿润口腔。唾液兴奋剂如西维美林(Evoxac)30mg,每日 3 次,或毛果芸香碱(Salagen)5mg,每日 3 至 4 次,可有效刺激唾液分泌[15]。在放射治疗期间预防性使用毛果芸香碱可能会降低放射性口干的程度[16]。使用针刺、口内电刺激、高压氧疗或氨磷汀用于放射治疗患者,是目前一些新兴的治疗手段[12]。

(二) 干燥综合征

干燥综合征是一种慢性自身免疫性疾病,根据口干症、干燥性角膜结膜炎(干眼症)和关节炎三联征分类,但其他全身性作用(腺外)也被认识到(见第 37 章)[15]。超过 400 万美国人受到影响,女性比男性多 9∶1。干燥综合征的特征是没有其他疾病时为原发性,当存在其他全身性疾病时为继发性。干燥综合征的口腔表现是由于淋巴细胞浸润破坏唾液腺,导致唾液减少或缺失,导致咀嚼困难、吞咽痛、味觉和嗅觉减弱、黏膜红斑、龋齿、口腔念珠菌病以及唾液腺结石的发生率增加。边缘带淋巴瘤是一种非霍奇金淋巴瘤,是干燥综合征中最严重的并发症。本病的诊断通常是基于临床表现,尽管实验室检查证明相关的抗 SSA 抗体、抗 SSB 抗体和/或类风湿因子,Schirmer 口腔和眼部干燥试验或唾液测定法可能有用[15]。唾液腺闪烁显像用于客观评估唾液腺受累的严重程度和范围,可能有助于干燥综合征的诊断和治疗[17]。一般性口干症的治疗策略也有助于治疗干燥引起的口干症。

三、舌部疾病

舌部是口腔中的一种肌肉器官,对味觉、咀嚼、吞咽和言语至关重要。舌背面的特征是广泛的 1~2mm 丝状或角化性乳头,以及较少的红斑性 1mm 的光滑、圆顶状丘疹。在有色个体中,可能存在单个蕈状乳头的良性色素沉着。

(一) 舌炎、舌痛和口腔感觉障碍

舌炎,即舌头的炎症和刺激,是一组异质性疾病(框 24.1)。患者可能主诉舌部疼痛(舌痛)或烧灼感(舌头灼热)。

框 24.1 原发性和继发性舌痛及相关病因
原发性(特发性)
舌部表现正常,通过病史或体格检查未发现其他病因
继发性
口腔疾病
感染(念珠菌病、梭菌螺旋体性、病毒性)
过敏/接触性超敏反应(假牙、汞合金、添加剂)
机械性损伤(异常用舌习惯、假牙)
口干症
地图舌
裂纹舌
囊泡性疾病
颞下颌关节功能紊乱
牙齿或扁桃体引起的牵涉性疼痛
系统性疾病
贫血(缺铁性,恶性)
营养缺不良(叶酸、锌、维生素 B_{12}、复合 B 族维生素)
糖尿病
胃食管反流病
干燥综合征
甲状腺功能减退
获得性免疫缺陷综合征
围绝经期(尚有争议)
药物相关的
抗生素、精神类药物、化疗药物等
任何可能导致口干症的药物
神经系统
周围神经病变
糖尿病性神经病
三叉神经痛
听神经瘤
精神疾病
抑郁症
焦虑症
恐癌症
躯体化障碍
强迫症
Modified from Gick CL, Mirowski GW, Kennedy JS, et al. Treatment of glossodynia with olanzapine. J Am Acad Dermatol 2004;51:463-465.

丝状乳头的缺失会导致一系列的改变,从伴或不伴有糜烂性改变的片状红斑到表面完全光滑、萎缩、红斑(图 24.1)。正中菱形舌炎表现为舌背中后部无症状、边界限清楚的红斑斑片。念珠菌感染,主要是白色念珠菌[18],可表现为丝状乳头的缺失。

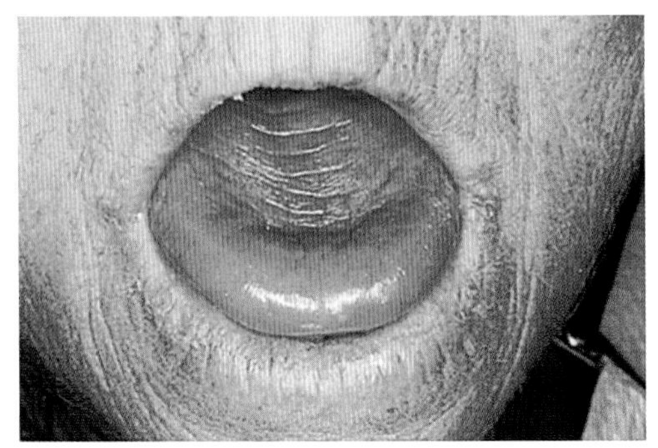

图 24.1　糖尿病和吸收不良患者的舌炎,舌部光滑(无舌乳头)且为红色,同时也存在口角炎

舌痛是指在没有炎症或刺激的临床或组织学证据的情况下出现疼痛,可能与焦虑或抑郁有关。舌痛常见于绝经后妇女,但激素替代治疗价值不大[19]。低镁血症,维生素 B_2、维生素 B_9(叶酸)或维生素 B_{12}(钴胺素)缺乏症的血清学评价,以及完整的用药史,偶尔可能提示可纠正的病因[20]。框 24.2 可作为治疗舌痛的原发性和继发性原因时考虑的指南。奥氮平可能是一种治疗选择[21]。

框 24.2　舌痛和舌灼痛的治疗方法
消除舌痛的病因(见框 24.1)
避免刺激物,包括食物和牙科设备
营养和维生素替代治疗
外用抗真菌药物
外用糖皮质激素
利多卡因凝胶(可暂时缓解)
催涎剂(如西维美林,毛果芸香碱)
苯二氮䓬类药物(如氯硝西泮、氯重氮环氧化物)
三环类抗抑郁药物(如阿米替林、多塞平)
抗精神病药物(如奥氮平)
Modified from Gick CL, Mirowski GW, Kennedy JS, et al. Treatment of glossodynia with olanzapine. J Am Acad Dermatol 2004;51:463-465.

口腔感觉迟钝,又称灼口综合征,以舌和口腔烧灼感为特征,最常见于绝经后妇女[22]。这种情况的病理生理学目前尚不十分清楚。然而,口腔感觉迟钝与维生素 B_3(烟酸)、维生素 B_{12} 和锌缺乏、糖尿病、甲状腺功能亢进及干燥综合征相关[20,23]。虽然口腔感觉迟钝可见于多种口腔黏膜疾病的患者,但它与较高的念珠菌感染率并无特定相关[24]。治疗包括纠正任何潜在的营养缺乏或使用三环类抗抑郁药、α-硫辛酸、外用氯硝西泮或认知行为治疗[22]。

(二) 味觉减退和味觉障碍

味觉减退(味觉减退)和味觉障碍(正常味觉失真)是另一类口腔疾病,有时与舌炎相关。味觉减退和味觉障碍归因于各种神经、营养和代谢疾病,包括嗜酸性肉芽肿伴多血管炎、大量药物和衰老[25-27]。然而在其他方面健康的儿童中也发现了味觉减退[28]。吸烟者、假牙佩戴者、焦虑或其他精神疾病的患者通常主诉味觉减退和味觉障碍。头颈部放射治疗可能导致味觉改变。尽管味蕾及其受体如何受到衰老、药物或疾病状态的影响尚不十分清楚,但味蕾变化可能与味觉相关基因表达的变化相关(见第 4 章)[29]。本病的治疗是经验性的,包括识别和纠正任何相关疾病。患者可接受补锌、低剂量抗焦虑药或抗抑郁药物治疗,如 SSRI 等药物。矛盾的是,三环类抗抑郁药物可阻断对广泛味觉刺激的反应,并可能导致味觉减退和味觉障碍[21,30]。

(三) 地图舌

地图舌(良性游走性舌炎、游走性红斑、游走性斑疹性舌炎)是以丝状乳头缺失为特征,形成不规则的片状构型,类似地图上的地理标志。地图舌与舌微生物群生态学的变化有关[31],或作为银屑病患者与裂纹舌相关的口腔症状[32]。患者可主诉疼痛或进食酸性、辛辣或咸味食物困难。反复发作常见。组织学上,在上皮中发现海绵样的中性粒细胞微脓肿,且无念珠菌病的证据。治疗包括局部麻醉剂、氢氧化镁铝(Maalox)保护涂层和局部应用糖皮质激素,以及控制基础皮肤病(如银屑病存在的话)。苯佐卡因(Orabase)与高铁血红蛋白血症的罕见风险相关,FDA 未推荐用于治疗该疾病的。地图舌是良性的,与恶性肿瘤无已知相关性。

(四) 裂纹舌

裂纹舌(皱襞舌、沟纹舌、阴囊舌)表现为舌背侧的良性中央沟槽,常见于高龄人群,但也与地图样舌、干燥综合征和 Melkersson-Rosenthal 综合征(以裂纹舌、肉芽肿性唇炎和偏头痛为特征,伴或不伴面瘫)有关。食物和细菌可能会积存在裂缝中,导致口臭和炎症,饭后和睡前轻刷舌部可获得症状缓解[33]。

(五) 黑毛舌

在患黑毛舌,舌背表面呈黄色、绿色、棕色或黑色,这是由于外源性色素积存于丝状乳头的细长角蛋白丝内所致。这种良性疾病最常见于长期吸烟者,通常遵循一个疗程的全身使用抗生素、使用过氧化氢或喝咖啡或茶出现[34]。超说明书的治疗包括使用 25% 足叶草或局部应用维甲酸(全反维生素 A 酸)凝胶[34]。通过刮舌器进行慢性清创术也可能有帮助。

(六) 草莓舌

草莓舌是舌炎的一种,以舌面的菌状乳头肿胀、肥大为特征。这些增大的蕈状乳头最常与猩红热和川崎病有关。由化脓性链球菌(A 群链球菌)感染引起的猩红热,除咽炎、砂纸样皮疹和口周苍白外,常表现为草莓舌。本病可应用青霉素治疗。

川崎病,也称为皮肤黏膜淋巴结综合征,是一种中到大血管炎(见第37章)。它一般影响5岁以下的儿童,在美国已取代风湿热成为儿童心脏病的首要原因,多见于东亚和东亚后裔的儿童。诊断标准包括以下至少4项:①急性颈部淋巴结肿大;②肢体末端水肿、红斑或脱屑;③双侧无痛性结膜充血;④多形性皮疹;⑤口腔黏膜红斑或草莓舌。川崎病也可引起结肠水肿。静脉用免疫球蛋白和口服阿司匹林是常用的治疗方法。

(七) 萎缩性舌

萎缩性舌(萎缩性舌炎)以无丝状乳头和舌痛为特征。它与许多营养物质缺乏有关,如蛋白质热量营养不良导致的丝状乳突萎缩,长期缺铁性贫血、维生素 B_2(舌部通常呈品红色)、维生素 B_6(吡哆醇)、维生素 B_9(伴有舌红斑和肿胀),和维生素 B_{12} 等缺乏[20]。萎缩性舌炎也见于 Plummer-Vinson 综合征(以缺铁性贫血、食管上蹼和萎缩性舌炎三联征为特征),同时其也与导致口干症的疾病有关[35]。它也是念珠菌感染的口腔表现,主要来自白色念珠菌,尽管从萎缩性念珠菌性舌炎患者中也培养出了平滑念珠菌、热带念珠菌、克柔念珠菌和近平滑念珠菌[18,36]。高龄及营养不良与舌厚度下降有关,也可使患者易发生萎缩性舌炎[35]。治疗涉及针对基础的营养缺乏或状况,可建议柔软、清淡的饮食有助于缓解症状。

(八) 肥大舌

肥大舌(巨舌)是舌超出口腔和颌骨的肿大,可影响咀嚼、吞咽和语言功能。其与许多疾病有关,包括先天性甲状腺功能减退、肢端肥大症、唐氏综合征、Beckwith-Wiedemann 综合征和原发性淀粉样变性[37]。

先天性甲状腺功能减退症可表现为舌体肥厚和黄疸,如果不及时治疗可进展为智力残疾。肢端肥大症是生长激素(如垂体腺瘤)过量产生的结果,除口腔软组织肥大和代谢变化进展为骨骼增大和糖尿病外,还可表现为舌肥大、裂纹舌[38]。Beckwith-Wiedemann 综合征是一种先天性过度生长综合征,其以舌体肥厚为特征,伴有脐膨出和器官肿大。

虽然巨舌症的治疗取决于基础疾病的治疗,但重度巨舌症的手术治疗包括舌前部楔形或锁孔切除术[39]。

(九) 白斑

毛状白斑(hairy leukoplakia,HL)是一种无症状的 EB 病毒感染表现,其表现为舌侧缘和背面的波纹状白色斑块(图24.2)。尽管 HL 主要发生在人免疫缺陷病毒(HIV)感染患者中,但肾和其他器官移植受者也易感(见第36章)。HIV 感染者中出现 HL 的提示预后不良。在198例 HL 病例中,至获得性免疫缺陷综合征发病的中位时间为24个月,至死亡的中位时间[在未接受高效抗逆转录病毒治疗(highly active antiretroviral therapy,HAART)的情况下]为41个月[40]。大约一半的 HL 病例合并念珠菌病,也必须进行治疗。治疗的第一步是进行抗念珠菌治疗。由于 HL 通常无症状,可选择超说明书使用阿昔洛韦、局部外用维甲酸和足叶草[33]。然而当停止此类治疗时,HL 通常会复发。HAART 的引入降低了 HL 的发生率。

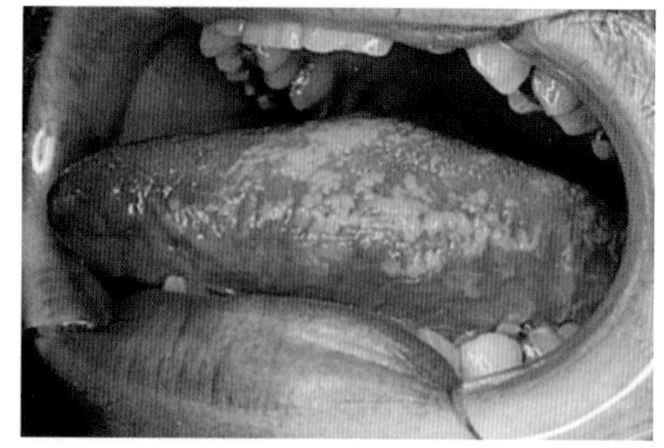

图24.2 艾滋病患者累及舌部的毛状白斑。(Courtesy Dr. Sol Silverman,Jr.,DDS,and Dr. Victor Newcomer.)

其他白色黏膜病变,如口腔白斑(图24.3),可类似于 HL 病变;如果考虑 HL 的诊断,需要行进行活检证实和 HIV 血清学检测。

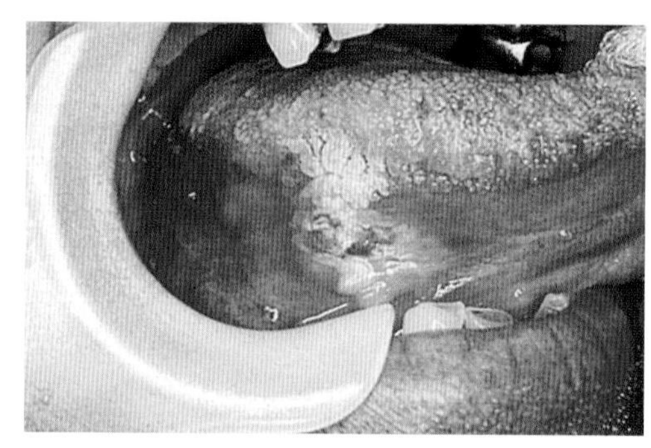

图24.3 口腔白斑及相关鳞状细胞癌

口腔白斑是口腔临床上的白色斑块,与可识别的病因无关。诊断需排除其他原因的白色口腔病变,包括念珠菌感染和 HL。在诊断口腔白斑之前,应排除和消除这些情况。口腔白斑最常见于老年人,73%至81%的受累者有吸烟史[41]。虽然口腔白斑本身通常是无症状的,但由于其与口腔鳞状细胞癌相关,因此该病变具有临床相关性[41]。如果消除其他可能的原因(例如念珠菌病)后仍不能使病变消退,则有必要对病变进行活检,以检查口腔上皮细胞是否存在异型增生或癌变。虽然目前还没有随机对照试验数据支持该治疗,但回顾性数据表明,切除的高风险口腔白斑病变不太可能发生恶变,尽管它不能完全消除复发或恶变的风险[41]。

增殖性疣状白斑(proliferative verrucous leukoplakia,PVL)是一种多发性、持续性、通常反复发作的口腔白斑,可类似于疣状癌[41]。由于其发生异型增生和恶变的风险极高,所以在临床上具有高度特异性,70%至87%的 PVL 患者在病变部位进展为鳞状细胞癌[42]。然而,在那些发生恶变的患者中,只有31%的患者有吸烟史[42]。PVL 的其他风险因素尚不清楚。

(十) 疱疹性几何学舌炎

疱疹性几何学舌炎(herpetic geometric glossitis,HGG)的特征是舌背面出现疼痛性、几何性线状裂隙,使患者进食困难。HGG 倾向于在免疫抑制患者中表现为慢性口腔单纯疱疹病毒感染的再激活,但也可出现在免疫功能正常的个体中[43]。口服抗病毒药物如阿昔洛韦治疗有效。

四、牙龈疾病

（一）牙龈肿大

牙龈肿大（牙龈增生、草莓样牙龈炎、牙龈肥大）的特征是牙龈细胞数量或大小增加。牙龈肿大是肉芽肿性多血管炎的常见表现（见第 37 章）[44]。在罕见的溶酶体贮积症、I 细胞病中也观察到这种情况，并与一些药物有关，包括环孢素、苯妥英钠及非二氢吡啶类钙通道阻滞剂如维拉帕米。

（二）牙龈口炎

牙龈口炎表现为牙龈和口腔黏膜的疼痛性炎症，是原发性疱疹病毒感染的常见表现（讨论如下）。

（三）急性坏死性溃疡性牙龈炎

急性坏死性溃疡性牙龈炎（acute necrotizing ulcerative gingivitis，ANUG）是一种累及牙间乳头的急性炎症和坏死性感染。治疗包括手术清创、口腔冲洗和全身性抗生素[45]。

（四）铅中毒

慢性铅中毒可表现为无症状的牙龈铅线（Burton 线），是沿牙龈边缘沉积的硫化铅的一种蓝黑色细线，受累者还可有腹痛和铁粒幼细胞性贫血。

五、感染、肿瘤和其他选定疾病的口腔表现

（一）念珠菌病

念珠菌（主要是白色念珠菌）是几乎半数人群中的正常口腔共生微生物[18]。口腔念珠菌病（鹅口疮、念珠菌感染、念珠菌病）的诊断需要有念珠菌感染或临床过度生长的临床和细胞学证据。其症状包括疼痛、口干、嘴唇肿胀和味觉改变。当吞咽困难和/或上消化道出血伴发鹅口疮时，很可能并发念珠菌性食管炎（见第 45 章）。口腔念珠菌病表现为白色凝乳样斑块（假膜性）或任何黏膜表面呈红色（萎缩性）或白色、红色的易碎皮损（图 24.4）。所有新生儿均出现与念珠菌定植相关的念珠菌初始过度生长，这与其消化道有关。

口腔念珠菌病，尤其是白色念珠菌[13]，可发生于 11%～15%的儿童出生后的第 1 年，特别是环境暴露于宠物和兄弟姐妹的儿童[46]。使用氢氧化钾（KOH）制剂涂片上出现假菌丝和芽殖酵母是感染白色念珠菌的证据，然而 KOH 涂片阴性并不排除活动性感染。念珠菌病可发生于抗生素或口服糖皮质激素治疗期间或之后，也可发生于义齿佩戴者、妊娠期以及口干症、萎缩性舌炎、糖尿病、桥本氏甲状腺炎、库欣病或家族性甲状旁腺功能减退患者[13,18,47]。全身和环境风险因素包括吸烟、饮食、极端年龄或营养缺乏[13]。艾滋病、其他使人衰弱的疾病或癌症化疗所致的免疫抑制也可能导致念珠菌病。当失去正常的感染屏障时，可能导致全身性念珠菌病。白念珠菌是培养的主要菌种。然而在耐药病例中必须考虑平滑念珠菌、克柔念珠菌、热带念珠菌、近平滑念珠菌和其他唑类药物耐药菌种[48]。平滑念珠菌和近平滑念珠菌的发病率因地区、患者易感条件和当地医院流行病学而异[48]。需要通过培养来确定种属和测定耐药性。

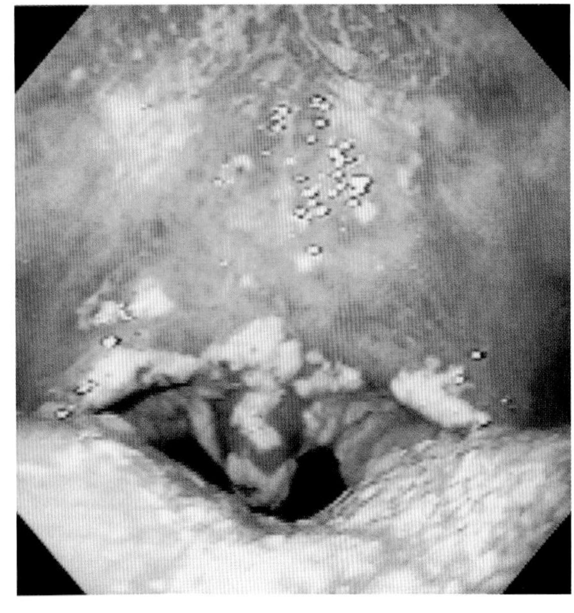

图 24.4　口腔念珠菌病。软硬腭、悬雍垂、舌可见多个白色、黄色斑块

口腔念珠菌病的早期治疗可缓解症状并防止局部疾病的全身扩散（常见于晚期 HIV 感染患者或免疫功能低下的移植患者，如第 35 和 36 章所述）。虽然白色念珠菌是念珠菌血症的最常见原因，但念珠菌病的治疗选择包括外用混悬剂、乳膏、软膏、含片以及口服胶囊和片剂。当风险因素被消除时，局部治疗对健康患者是有效的。在义齿佩戴患者中，通过将义齿浸泡在稀释的漂白剂溶液中并过夜取出，定期清洁义齿对于清除感染非常重要。然而给药方案、难吃的味道和伴随使用口腔矫治器都可能导致不依从和治疗失败。有多种全身疗法可用于治疗难治性疾病、免疫功能低下的宿主、或由于器具或其他因素而无法进行局部治疗时（见第 35、36 和 45 章）[13]。全身抗真菌药物（酮康唑和伊曲康唑），由于对细胞色素 P450 3A4 肝脏代谢途径的强抑制作用，体外耐药性增加[49]，因此在需要长期预防性治疗的患者中较少使用。最常见的 HIV 相关口腔感染是念珠菌病（见第 35 和 45 章）。

（二）疱疹病毒感染

原发性疱疹性龈口炎是由单纯疱疹病毒（HSV）1 型（偶尔为 2 型）引起的。高达 90%的人群在青春期前发生初次感染。该病通常症状较轻，常被误认为是常规的上呼吸道感染；其表现可能包括不同程度的发热、不适、淋巴结肿大以及口腔和牙龈溃疡。皮损可出现于口唇。一般 1～2 周愈合。治疗是姑息性的，但应用阿昔洛韦 400mg，每日 3 次，可缩短病程，减轻严重程度。本病继发细菌感染常见，可局部药物治疗。

复发性口唇 HSV 是由休眠在局部神经节内的病毒再激活引起的，与 HSV 抗体滴度无关。发热性疾病、日光照射、身体或精神压力都可能促发本病。复发的频率和严重程度各不相同。通常病变累及唇部（唇疱疹），并在数小时前出现前驱

症状,如烧灼感、刺痛或瘙痒。然后出现小水泡,但很快会破裂,留下小的不规则的疼痛性溃疡。溃疡相互融合、结痂和病变的渗出是常见的。口内复发性疱疹性溃疡发生在角质化的黏膜上(即硬腭或牙龈,见表 24.1),其表现为浅的、不规则的小溃疡、而且可融合。唇部和口腔疱疹性溃疡通常在两周内愈合。复发性 HSV 是复发性多形性红斑最常见的原因。HGG(前面讨论过)是 HSV 再激活的附加表现。

表 24.1 口疮和疱疹性口腔溃疡的区别

疾病	黏膜	部位
阿弗他溃疡	非角化性	舌侧部,口底部,唇和颊部黏膜,软腭,咽
疱疹性溃疡	角化性	牙龈,硬腭,舌背

在免疫功能低下的患者中,HSV 可累及任何皮肤-黏膜表面,可表现为大的、不规则的、有假膜覆盖的溃疡。在 HIV 感染者中尤其如此,所有会阴部和口腔唇部溃疡均应视为是 HSV 的表现,直至有证据可以除外(见第 35 章)。应注意避免眼部的自体接种。

HSV 感染或再激活通常根据病史和临床表现进行诊断。有前驱症状或小水泡病史,病变部位和同一部位病变的再次出现,有助于鉴别 HSV 与其他溃疡性疾病。显示多核巨细胞的细胞学涂片(Tzanck 涂片)具有提示性,尽管病毒培养和涂片单克隆抗体染色是诊断 HSV 感染更敏感和特异性的试验。外用阿昔洛韦对复发性唇疱疹的疗效甚微,对复发性生殖器 HSV 的疗效也是有限的。全身性阿昔洛韦定期用于治疗免疫抑制患者的原发性或复发性 HSV 发作的治疗(2g,分次口服,或 5mg/kg 静脉注射,每日 3 次,直至病变愈合)。泛昔洛韦(125mg,每日两次),或伐昔洛韦(500mg,每日两次)也有效。口服治疗最好在前驱症状的最初几个小时内开始。对于每年复发超过 4 次的患者,可以使用阿昔洛韦进行长期的抑制治疗,口服 200mg、每日 3 次或口服 400mg、每日 2 次。阿昔洛韦用于预防与骨髓移植相关的复发性口腔和生殖器 HSV(见第 36 章)。抗病毒药物也用于预防其他免疫功能低下患者的复发性疱疹感染,如白血病或 HIV 感染或实体器官移植后的患者。

带状疱疹(缠腰龙)是由水痘-带状疱疹病毒(VZV,HHV-3)再激活导致的。可出现类似于阿弗他溃疡的口腔损害,除下列特征外,溃疡为单侧;唇和/或皮肤损害可同时存在;起病突然,急性疼痛,通常沿皮节分布且常伴发热。发病 72 小时内给予大剂量阿昔洛韦(4g/d 口服)、泛昔洛韦 500mg 每 8 小时 1 次或伐昔洛韦 1g 每 8 小时 1 次,可能有助于加速愈合和减轻带状疱疹后神经痛。接种疫苗可降低老年人发生带状疱疹的风险,即使是那些已经康复的人。

(三) 人乳头瘤病毒感染

口腔 HPV 感染表现为口唇部疣状丘疹[1]。在婴儿和儿童中,感染 HPV 6 和 11 最常见的表现是口腔乳头状瘤或罕见的喉部乳头状瘤[50]。据报道,3%~5% 的病例可恶变为疣状癌,但几乎所有恶变的病例都与乳头状瘤的放射治疗有关。虽然目前的证据支持 HPV 可以通过母婴垂直传播的观点,但剖宫产并不适合预防 HPV 传播。HPV 疫苗接种可降低 HPV 感染的发生率。

(四) 卡波西肉瘤

卡波西肉瘤(Kaposi sarcoma,KS)是 HIV 感染的常见后果,是由人类疱疹病毒 8 感染引起的。在 1996 年和 1997 年 KS 的发病率显著下降,这与 HAART 的引入有关。虽然 KS 通常见于皮肤,但半数以上的患者也有口腔内病变(图 24.5)。22% 的患者 KS 的首发体征发生在口腔,另有 45% 的患者 KS 同时发生在口腔和皮肤[40]。口腔损害的外观可从轻微的无症状、扁平的、紫色或红色的斑疹到大结节不等。硬腭是最多发的部位,其次是牙龈和舌(见图 24.5)。

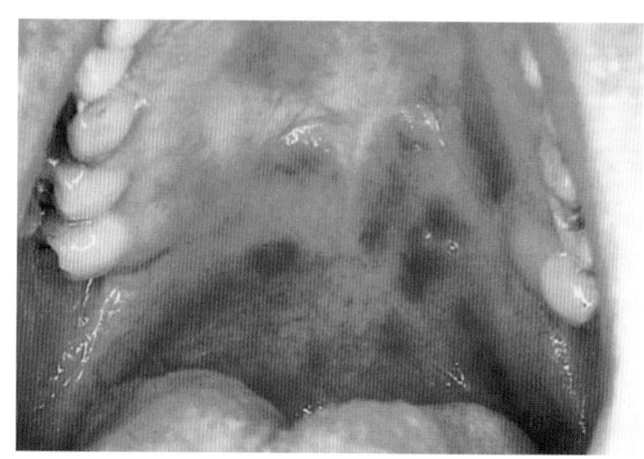

图 24.5 累及腭部的卡波西肉瘤。(Courtesy Dr. Sol Silverman,Jr.,DDS,and Dr. Victor Newcomer.)

(五) 其他 HIV 相关疾病

与 HIV 感染相关的其他口腔疾病包括淋巴瘤;广泛的口腔、生殖器或皮肤疣;复发性口疮;慢性皮肤黏膜 HSV 感染;大唾液腺淋巴细胞浸润导致继发性干燥综合征;药物反应包括药物诱发的 Stevens-Johnson 综合征和急性坏死性溃疡性牙龈炎。

(六) 鳞状细胞癌

白斑作为前驱病变占口腔鳞状细胞癌病例的 15%,但口腔鳞状细胞癌(squamous cell carcinoma,SCC)的临床表现变化很大,从无症状的红斑到白色疣状斑块,更常见的是无症状或偶尔伴有疼痛的红色和白色变化的组合(红白斑)[41]。需通过临床记录任何相关的同侧和/或对侧颈部淋巴结病变、活检和成像对 SCC 进行分期。治疗包括手术切除受累区域并辅助放疗或放化疗[41]。

(七) 炎症性肠病

克罗恩病是一种炎症性疾病,可累及整个胃肠道,伴有透壁性炎症和非干酪样肉芽肿(见第 115 和 116 章)。4%~14% 的患者出现克罗恩病的口腔表现,包括口疮(图 24.6)、唇裂、鹅卵石样斑块、唇炎、黏膜赘和口周红斑。患者也可能主诉金属味觉障碍。大约 5% 的克罗恩病患者发生口疮,病变在临床和组织学上均不属于典型口疮。相比之下,在溃疡性结肠炎中未观察到口疮和肛管周-瘘管周溃疡。在极少数情况下，克罗恩病可能与肉芽肿性唇炎相关（上文讨论）。增殖性化脓性口炎（见图 25.4）是炎症性肠病（IBD）的特异性标志物，包括克罗恩病和溃疡性结肠炎，它可能会先于胃肠道症状出现前数月至数年[51]。增殖性化脓性口炎表现为脓疱、糜烂和赘生物，累及上下唇的唇黏膜、颊黏膜、牙龈黏膜，以及腋窝、生殖器、躯干和头皮的皮肤。组织学上，上皮内和上皮下嗜酸性粟粒性脓肿具有特征性。浅表脓疱覆盖口腔脆弱、红斑和糜烂的黏膜，最不常见的是口底和舌。症状可能为重度或极轻度。嗜酸性粒细胞增多和贫血常见。根据活检结果进行诊断。治疗采用局部或全身糖皮质激素、氨苯砜或柳氮磺吡啶[52]。

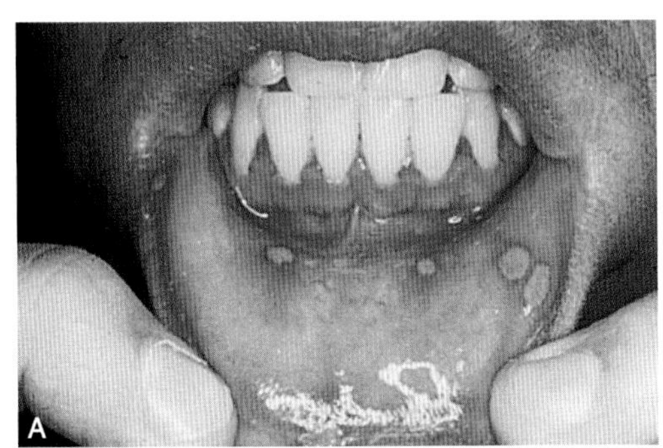

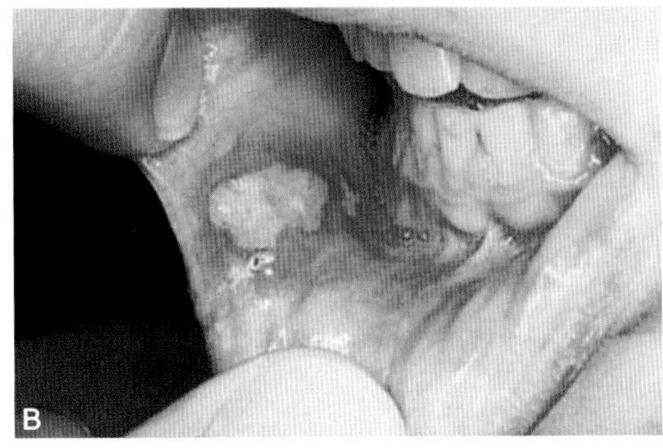

图 24.6　(A)多发性轻微阿弗他口腔溃疡。(B)大的阿弗他口腔溃疡

六、胃食管反流病

长期暴露于口腔中的酸性液体导致牙齿表面溶解（牙釉质侵蚀），最常见于上颌牙的腭表面，下面暴露牙本质，这是一种更软和更不透明的黄色物质。由于牙釉质被侵蚀，牙齿对温度的变化极为敏感。胃食管反流病患者的龋齿患病率并没有增加，可能是因为酸性环境干扰了牙科细菌生物膜的形成。牙釉质的侵蚀是不可逆的。成人最有效的药物治疗是质子泵抑制剂，尽管 H_2 受体拮抗剂可能有益。患者也可能从减少酸性食物和饮料的摄入中获益。

七、肝脏疾病

黄疸可见于慢性肝病患者的口腔内，这是由于胆红素沉积于黏膜下层，口腔黏膜可呈现黄色。由于舌下和软腭黏膜非常薄，它们往往首先出现这种黄色色调。对这些区域的检查可能为深色皮肤或生理性结膜色素沉着的患者提供有用的诊断线索。

八、复发性阿弗他口腔溃疡

复发性阿弗他口腔溃疡（recurrent aphthous ulcer，RAU，复发性口疮，口坏疽病）是一种疼痛性浅溃疡，常被灰白色或黄色渗出物覆盖，周围有红斑边缘环绕。在免疫功能正常的个体中，它们几乎只出现在未角化的口腔黏膜表面（见表 24.1）。罕见情况下，RAU 可能发生在食管、上消化道和下消化道以及肛门直肠上皮。RAU 是口腔溃疡最常见的原因，一般人群中 25% 的个体在某个时间发生，并以不规律的间隔复发。

阿弗他口腔溃疡有 3 种临床形式：轻型阿弗他口腔溃疡（最常见）、重型阿弗他口腔溃疡（较少见）和疱疹型阿弗他口腔溃疡（最不常见）。轻型口腔溃疡通常直径小于 5mm，1~3 周即可愈合（见图 24.6A）。重度口腔溃疡直径可超过 6mm（见图 24.6B），需要数月才能愈合，且常留下瘢痕。疱疹样口腔溃疡直径一般为 1~3mm，成群发生 10 个至数百个溃疡，且很快消退[53]。

RAU 的发生机制被认为是多因素的，其促发因素包括：①免疫异常，如乳糜泻和由组成性口腔屏障受损（推测来自牙科产品中使用的十二烷基硫酸钠）引起的变应原表达增加；②慢性创伤，如佩戴不合适的义齿[54]；③铁、叶酸和/或钴胺素缺乏[20]；④遗传易感性；⑤压力和焦虑；⑥对食物或药物过敏，如环氧化酶 2（COX-2）抑制剂或舍曲林；⑦口干症[20,53]。幽门螺杆菌感染可能与 RAU 有关，因为从胃中根除幽门螺杆菌似乎与减少溃疡复发以及减少溃疡数量和症状天数有关[53]。

形态相同的口疮病变（阿弗他溃疡；口疮病）可见于 IBD 患者和白塞综合征（讨论如下）。根据病史和系统回顾的指导，RAU 的检查可能包括全血血细胞计数、红细胞沉降率、血清铁和铁蛋白、血清叶酸和维生素 B_{12} 水平、KOH 染色、Tzanck 涂片、病毒培养，共存皮肤病变活检以排除 HSV 感染，以及结肠镜检查以解决 IBD 的可能性。组织学上，病变组织显示黏膜溃疡伴慢性混合炎性细胞。

RAU 的治疗包括姑息性和治愈性措施。首先，如发现缺乏维生素，应予以补充。同时应建议患者使用富含铁的多种维生素，并避免食用硬的、咸的或辛辣的食物，以尽量减少对口腔病变的刺激。应使用软牙刷、修复牙列等措施来避免不必要的口腔创伤。镇痛药和局部麻醉剂，如 2% 黏性利多卡因可能有帮助，同时局部外用次水杨酸铋（高岭土果胶）和硫糖铝保护病变并加速愈合。阿弗他溃疡可局部外用糖皮质激素有效治疗，如氟轻松醋酸酯或氯倍他索凝胶或软膏。二线治疗包括秋水仙碱 0.6mg，每日 3 次；四环素 250mg，每日 4 次；西咪替丁 400~800mg/d；硫唑嘌呤 50mg/d；或沙利度胺 200mg/d。当更保守的方法不能令人满意时，短疗程的全身泼尼松（20~60mg/d）治疗可重复有效。消除饮食可能有助于对某些食物或药物有过敏反应的患者，包括不含十二烷基硫酸钠的牙科产品试验[55]，麸质敏感性肠病患者需要无麸质饮食（见第 107 章）。应用 0.5mg/5mL 地塞米松剂、100mg/100mL 多西环素冲洗液或 0.12mg/15mL 葡萄糖酸氯己定口腔冲洗液，也可能有一定帮助。

九、白塞病

白塞病(Behçet 病、贝赫切特病)是一种小血管炎,其特征为 RAU、生殖器溃疡、葡萄膜炎和结节性红斑(见第 37 章)。复发性口腔阿弗他溃疡是该疾病最常见的症状,通常伴有生殖器阿弗他溃疡,这些生殖器阿弗他溃疡往往比口腔溃疡更大、疼痛更剧烈,瘢痕形成的风险更高[56]。罕见的胃肠道表现包括黏膜炎症和溃疡,通常局限于回盲部,肝脏受累继发于 Budd-Chiari 综合征[56]。因为白塞病可能被误认为复杂的 RAU,特别是在非流行区,因此必须采集详细的病史。临床上通过注意到口腔溃疡和同时存在以下至少两种情况进行诊断:生殖器溃疡、皮肤损害、眼部受累和针刺试验(过敏反应性试验)阳性[56]。治疗在第 37 章中讨论。

十、伴有口腔表现的皮肤疾病

许多皮肤病都有重要的口腔和消化道表现,包括类天疱疮、天疱疮、大疱性表皮松解症、多形性红斑、扁平苔藓和 Stevens-Johnson 综合征/中毒性表皮坏死松解症(见第 25 章)。

十一、淀粉样变性

淀粉样变性通常有明显的口腔表现(见第 37 章)。巨舌伴舌硬度增加,讨论较早,除颌下结构扩大外,20% ~ 50% 的患者出现舌侧压痕。巨舌症可能干扰进食和闭口,并可能引起气道阻塞伴睡眠呼吸暂停,尤其是在平卧位时。增大的舌头因血管丰富,可导致出血。口腔内复发性出血性大疱很常见。有时可通过皮下脂肪抽吸或通过牙龈或舌头活检诊断淀粉样变性。

十二、营养缺乏

营养缺乏见表 24.2(另见第 5、25 和 104 章)[20]。

表 24.2　选定的营养异常和相关的口腔表现

营养异常	病因	临床表现
核黄素缺乏(维生素 B_2)	酗酒 胃肠疾病 氯丙嗪	咽部及口腔黏膜红斑 酒红色萎缩性舌炎 舌痛症 唇干裂 口角炎
烟酸缺乏(维生素 B_3)	摄入不足 药物(如异烟肼) 先天性肠道和/或肾脏色氨酸转运缺陷 类癌综合征	黏膜水肿 唇干裂 口角炎 鲜红色舌炎 口灼感 牙龈红斑 龋齿 皮炎、腹泻、痴呆、死亡
吡哆醇缺乏(维生素 B_6)	高龄 酗酒 慢性肾功能衰竭 肝病 营养不良	萎缩性舌炎 唇干裂 口角炎 牙龈红斑
叶酸缺乏(维生素 B_9)	营养不良 吸收障碍性疾病(如乳糜泻、炎症性肠病) 药物(如甲氨蝶呤、丙戊酸)	萎缩性舌炎伴红斑及舌体肿胀 口角炎 舌疼痛或烧灼感 吞咽困难
钴胺素缺乏(维生素 B_{12})	恶性贫血 摄入不足	广泛性口炎 味觉障碍 红色,萎缩性,牛肉样舌伴烧灼感和丝状乳头消失
视黄醇缺乏(维生素 A)	营养不良 吸收不良 酗酒	口干症 牙周病 增加口腔内感染风险 损害牙齿发育(儿童)
维生素 K 缺乏	完全母乳喂养的婴幼儿 吸收障碍 药物(如华法林)	黏膜下出血 牙龈出血

表 24.2　选定的营养异常和相关的口腔表现(续)

营养异常	病因	临床表现
铁缺乏		口角炎 萎缩性舌炎 舌痛症 复发性阿弗他口炎
锌缺乏(若为遗传性则表现为肠病性肢端皮炎) 必需脂肪酸缺乏 生物素缺乏	先天性代谢异常 肝硬化酗酒患者 静脉营养 克罗恩病	灼口综合征 复发性阿弗他口炎 口周或口内糜烂 味觉障碍(味觉改变)
维生素 C 缺乏(坏血病)	酗酒 克罗恩病 Whipple 病	黏膜瘀点 出血性牙龈炎 牙龈出血 牙龈肥厚 牙间梗死

(郭晓燕　译,袁农　刘军　校)

参考文献

第 25 章　胃肠道和肝脏疾病的皮肤表现

Lawrence A. Mark 著

章节目录

一、水疱样大疱性皮肤病 …… 340
（一）类天疱疮 …… 340
（二）天疱疮 …… 340
（三）大疱性表皮松解症 …… 340
（四）多形性红斑 …… 341
（五）Stevens-Johnson 综合征/中毒性表皮坏死松解症谱 …… 341
二、扁平苔藓 …… 341
三、炎症性肠病的皮肤表现 …… 342
四、血管和结缔组织疾病 …… 343
五、胃肠道恶性肿瘤的皮肤表现 …… 345
（一）息肉病综合征 …… 345
（二）内部恶性肿瘤及相关疾病 …… 346
（三）皮肤转移瘤 …… 348
六、肝脏疾病的皮肤表现 …… 348
七、皮肤病患者的药物性肝病 …… 349
八、皮肤和胃肠道的寄生虫病 …… 350
九、疱疹样皮炎和乳糜泻 …… 350
十、维生素和矿物质缺乏 …… 351

一、水疱样大疱性皮肤病

水疱性皮肤病包括类天疱疮、天疱疮、大疱性表皮松解症（epidermolysis bullosa，EB）、多形性红斑（erythema multiforme，EM）以及 Stevens-Johnson 综合征/中毒性表皮坏死松解症疾病谱，他们可能有以下所讨论的口腔和胃肠的表现。

（一）类天疱疮

类天疱疮是多种水疱性疾病的总称，特征为存在血清免疫球蛋白（immunoglobulin，Ig）G 或者 IgA 自身免疫抗体，这是针对鳞状上皮基底膜的 230kD 和 180kD 的半桥粒蛋白（以及其他角质形成细胞抗原）而产生的。这种抗原-抗体反应导致上皮与其支持基底膜基质之间丧失黏附。类天疱疮的临床表现为影响口腔黏膜、咽、食管、肛门、结膜和皮肤的张力性大疱和溃疡。口腔表现为颊和牙龈黏膜的高度黏膜炎症（红斑）。

有两种类型已被确定的类天疱疮：大疱性类天疱疮（自身免疫和药物诱导的变种）和瘢痕性（黏膜）类天疱疮。大疱性类天疱疮的患者通常患有皮肤病变，约有三分之一的患者也患有黏膜病变。自身免疫亚型最常出现在老年人中，他们先前可能患有非大疱性的强烈瘙痒的“荨麻疹”的阶段性疾病。药物诱导的大疱性类天疱疮与噻嗪类利尿剂、抗生素（如青霉素、万古霉素）、非甾体抗炎药、血管紧张素转换酶（angiotensin-converting enzyme，ACE）抑制剂（如卡托普利）以及可能的血管紧张素受体阻滞剂（angiotensin receptor blocker，ARB；如缬沙坦），以及许多其他少有文献支持它们因果关系的药物有关[1]。停用疑似有损害作用的药物是主要的治疗方法。与大疱性类天疱疮相比，所有瘢痕性类天疱疮患者均有黏膜病变，约 1/3 的患者也有皮肤病变。睑球粘连（即睑板与球结膜之间的粘连）常与瘢痕性天疱疮合并发生。据报道，食管受累的天疱疮所致上消化道出血可能会致命[2]。

对于所有类型的类天疱疮，受累黏膜和皮肤的免疫荧光染色是诊断性的，表现出抗体和补体在基底膜区线性沉积。血清 IgG 和 IgA 自身抗体升高的患者更有可能对系统性药物有反应。治疗范围为从低剂量到高剂量的泼尼松。对于糖皮质激素使用禁忌或有全身毒性的患者，可选择的治疗包括氨苯砜、四环素和烟酰胺联合用药、硫唑嘌呤、氯丁二烯、血浆置换、IVIG、环孢素、环磷酰胺、甲氨蝶呤、利妥昔单抗和英夫利西单抗[3]。

（二）天疱疮

寻常型天疱疮不同于类天疱疮，前者的血清自身抗体直接针对细胞间角质形成细胞蛋白，导致细胞间黏附丧失，这种抗原-抗体反应会导致大疱性皮肤损伤，通常是缓慢的，如果不治疗可能会危及生命。口腔黏膜的受累可能是广泛的。黏膜受累可造成营养不良和剧烈疼痛。一半的寻常型天疱疮患者存在口腔病变，而口腔病变几乎会 100% 发生于天疱疮患者的疾病过程中。活检材料直接免疫荧光是具有诊断性的，表现为鳞状上皮细胞表面有 IgG 抗体和补体。间接免疫荧光检测到大多数寻常型天疱疮患者循环中的 IgG 抗体。治疗包括各种局部或全身泼尼松治疗方案，有时辅助用细胞毒性或免疫抑制药物。

副肿瘤性天疱疮与寻常型天疱疮和 EM 具有共同特征。它与胃肠道恶性肿瘤、淋巴瘤、白血病、胸腺瘤和软组织肉瘤有关。副肿瘤性天疱疮的特征包括：①疼痛性黏膜糜烂和多形性皮疹；②表皮内棘皮松解、角质细胞坏死、空泡界面反应；③IgG 和 C3 在细胞间和沿表皮基底膜区沉积；④血清自身抗体以天疱疮的模式特征结合皮肤和黏膜上皮，并以同样的方式结合单层、柱状和移行上皮；⑤通过自身抗体从角质形成细胞免疫沉淀形成 4 个蛋白复合物（250、230、210 和 190kD）[4]。副肿瘤性天疱疮的预后通常较差，因为症状的改善取决于潜在的恶性肿瘤的成功治疗。

（三）大疱性表皮松解症

大疱性表皮松解症（EB）是一组异质性罕见的遗传性皮

肤脆性疾病(图 25.1),其特征是形成水疱,创伤极小,分为营养不良型(瘢痕)、交接型和单纯型。口腔糜烂、前驱龋齿和牙龈受累,以及胃肠道疾病,以营养不良形式常见,但也见于一些交接型患者。除口腔糜烂外,食管狭窄是营养不良型 EB 最常见的胃肠道并发症[5]。最常发生于食管的上三分之一,但也可见于下三分之一处。食管狭窄可能是由食物和/或反流的胃内容物反复创伤所致;因此,严格遵守软食饮食仍然是主要的管理方法。尽管既往曾因长期食管狭窄增加的风险不可接受而对探条扩张术进行分流,但证据支持使用球囊扩张是缓解食管狭窄的一种安全有效的方法,并且不存在这种风险。食管切除、胃造口术喂养、结肠间置术已有效地用于伴有严重食管狭窄的营养不良型 EB 患者。环状肌后区域的食管网也有相关描述。肛管狭窄和便秘(有或没有狭窄)在营养不良型 EB 患者中很常见。连接型 EB 与幽门闭锁有独特的联系。贫血和生长迟缓经常发生在重度营养不良和连接型 EB 患者中,部分是因为胃肠道和口腔并发症。

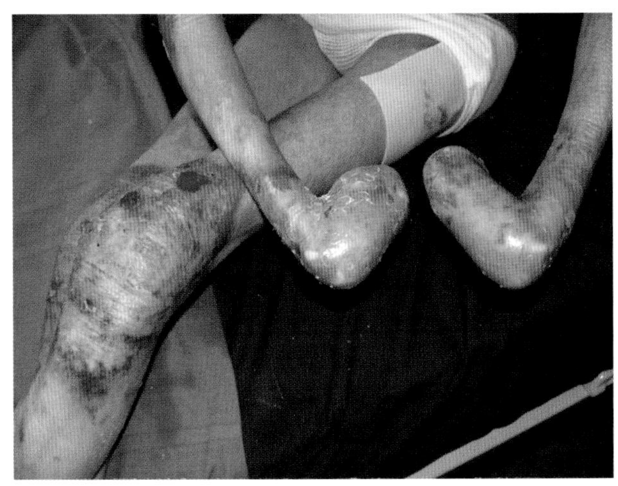

图 25.1　重度隐性营养不良型大疱性表皮松解症引起的皮肤脆性导致的特征性病变。(Courtesy Dr. Benjamin Lockshin, Silver Spring, MD.)

临床病变患者与营养不良型 EB 相同,但前者已被证实没有家族史和成人发病的患者;他们的情况被称为获得性 EB 或后天性 EB(EB acquisita, EBA)。EBA,像天疱疮和类天疱疮一样,是一种自身免疫性疾病。EBA 中的自身抗体直接针对Ⅶ型胶原。EBA 的诊断是建立在皮肤活检标本的常规组织学和直接免疫荧光检查。与瘢痕性类天疱疮患者一样,EBA 患者可能有显著的黏膜受累,特别是口腔和食管疾病。据报道,在一些 EBA 患者中存在克罗恩病。治疗方法是使用免疫抑制剂。

(四) 多形性红斑

多形性红斑(EM)是一种与潜在感染(特别是 HSV)相关的急性皮肤黏膜皮疹。通常在发病前或伴随出现低热、乏力以及提示上呼吸道感染的症状。这些皮疹包括在肘部、膝盖、手掌和脚掌交替出现的粉红色和红色病变,以及表浅宽大的口腔糜烂。EM 患者可能只有口腔受累,可发现不同程度的非特异性红斑,伴或不伴溃疡,可能出现结痂、出血和潮湿的嘴唇溃疡。严重的口腔和咽部疼痛,继发性细菌和真菌感染,以及出血是常见的并发症。诊断是根据临床特征,排除其他明确诊断的疾病,并根据对治疗的反应而得出的。活检显示非特异性界面反应。口腔 EM 可以是自限性的,也可以是慢性的,而且通常刺激过程是不清楚的。治疗包括对症缓和措施和消除任何有害因素,通常需要糖皮质激素和/或其他免疫抑制药物。复发和耀斑有不同的模式。疱疹相关的 EM 病变治疗用暂时的或抑制性抗病毒治疗包括阿昔洛韦,伐昔洛韦,泛昔洛韦,或膦甲酸[6]。

(五) Stevens-Johnson 综合征/中毒性表皮坏死松解症谱

Stevens-Johnson 综合征(Stevens-Johnson syndrome, SJS;存在 10%~30% 的皮肤蜕皮)和中毒性表皮坏死松解症(toxic epidermal necrolysis, TEN;存在超过 30% 的皮肤蜕皮),在发生严重急性疼痛的靶样病变和皮肤蜕皮并累及眼睛、皮肤和黏膜时可诊断。与 EM 不同,EM 通常与感染相关,而 SJS 和 TEN 几乎总是由药物引起的反应,如抗生素(尤其是磺胺类)或抗惊厥药。弥漫性口腔和咽部溃疡可抑制经口进食。内镜检查中,食管可表现为弥漫性红斑、脆性和白色斑块,可能误诊为念珠菌病。胃和十二指肠可能出现弥漫性红斑和脆性,而食管不受累。结肠镜表现类似于严重的溃疡性结肠炎或伪膜性肠炎。然而,结肠活检显示广泛的坏死和淋巴细胞浸润,没有隐窝脓肿或中性粒细胞。这种模式使人想起移植物抗宿主病(见第 36 章)。SJS 的大部分肠黏膜可能蜕皮,导致呕血、黑便和肠穿孔的报道。治疗主要包括停止使用刺激性药物(通常是抗惊厥药或抗生素),在可能的情况下住进烧伤病房,并通过多团队方法进行支持性护理。没有可靠的证据证明使用全身糖皮质激素、静脉注射免疫球蛋白或血浆置换治疗 SJS/TEN 有效,但有微弱的证据表明,在病程早期使用环孢素可能减少疾病进展和死亡率[7]。

二、扁平苔藓

扁平苔藓(lichen planus, LP)是一种常见的累及黏膜和皮肤的慢性炎症性疾病。该病通常开始于成年期,三分之二的患者是女性。口腔病变的表现是多样的,可以在任何黏膜表面表现为白色、花边状和/或点状图案(图 25.2),黏膜红斑或溃疡是常见的。口腔病变可表现为无症状的颊黏膜花边样斑块,或累及舌头、颊黏膜或牙龈的疼痛性红斑或糜烂性斑块。局部和/或全身使用糖皮质激素可以有效地减少几乎所有口腔和皮肤 LP 的症状和体征。外用他克莫司是一种有效的类固醇节制治疗选择。食管 LP 可能表现为进行性吞咽困难和吞咽痛、上消化道出血、狭窄和鳞状细胞癌[8]。内镜检查结果包括红斑、溃疡、近端食管的蹼和整个食管的糜烂。据报道,在 LP 患者中慢性肝病(包括慢性丙型肝炎和原发性胆汁性胆管炎)的患病率增加。无论何种治疗方法,口腔 LP 可能与萎缩或糜烂区域发生鳞状细胞癌的风险增加相关,与治疗无关[9,10]。使用抑制程序性死亡-1(inhibit programmed death-1, 抗 PD)的癌症免疫治疗药物可能发生大疱性 LP[11]。

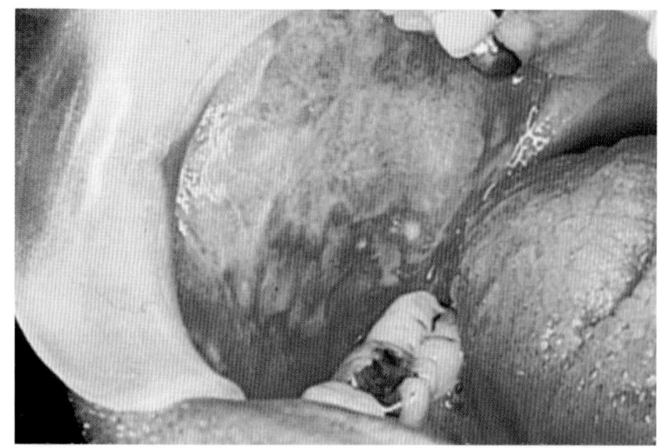

图 25.2 口腔扁平苔藓的糜烂型,累及颊黏膜。可见花边样角化、红斑和溃疡

三、炎症性肠病的皮肤表现

克罗恩病和溃疡性结肠炎(ulcerative colitis,UC)都可以伴有皮肤表现(见第 115 和 116 章)。皮肤病变在克罗恩病中更常见(高达 44%),而且通常比 UC 更典型。在有症状的肠道疾病出现之前,克罗恩病累及皮肤是罕见的,最常见的克罗恩病皮肤并发症是肛周或瘘管周围皮肤的肉芽肿性炎症,它是由下层的肠道病变直接延伸而发生的。转移性克罗恩病是指罕见的发生在远离肠道部位的溃疡性病变、斑块或结节。这种病变多见于间擦区,如耳后和乳腺下区。在组织学方面,局部皮肤扩展和转移性克罗恩病表现为结节样肉芽肿性炎症,两者在克罗恩病累及结肠的患者中发生的频率更高[12]。

在克罗恩病中口腔病变表现发生在 4%~14% 的患者,包括阿弗他溃疡、嘴唇干裂、鹅卵石斑块、唇炎、黏膜赘生物和口周红斑。患者也可自诉金属性味觉障碍。约 5% 的克罗恩病患者发生阿弗他溃疡,且临床上和组织学上无法与典型的口疮区分。溃疡性结肠炎中未见口疮和肛周-瘘管周围溃疡。肉芽肿性唇炎是一种罕见的情况,反复的嘴唇肿胀导致嘴唇的肿大和坚韧,唇活检显示非干酪样肉芽肿。在与克罗恩病相关的罕见病例中[13],这种情况可能是 Melkersson-Rosenthal 综合征(裂缝舌、嘴唇肿胀、伴或不伴面神经麻痹和偏头痛)的组成部分,或者也可能是特发性的。

增殖性脓性口炎(图 25.3)和与之对应的皮肤部分——增殖性脓皮病,其特征是脓疱、糜烂和疣状赘生物,累及上唇和下唇的唇黏膜、颊黏膜和牙龈黏膜,以及腋窝、生殖器、躯干和头皮的皮肤。增殖性脓性口炎和增殖性脓皮病都是炎症性肠病(克罗恩病和溃疡性结肠炎)的特异性标志物,并且可能发生先于胃肠道症状数月至数年。组织学上,上皮内和上皮下具有特征性嗜酸性粟粒脓肿。嗜酸性粟粒脓肿具有特征性。浅表脓疱覆盖易碎、红斑状和被破坏的口腔黏膜,最不常见于口腔底和舌部。症状可能很严重或者很轻微。嗜酸性粒细胞增多和贫血很常见。诊断是依据活检的结果,治疗是局部或全身糖皮质激素、氨苯砜或柳氮磺吡啶。

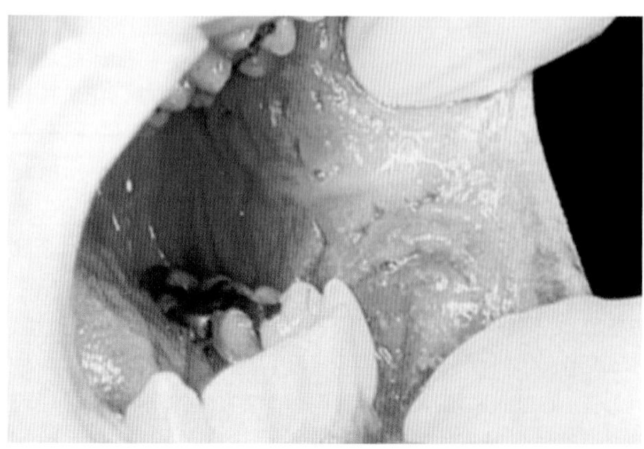

图 25.3 溃疡性结肠炎患者的化脓性口腔黏膜炎。活检标本显示微脓肿

结节性红斑是一种常见的皮下脂肪炎症性疾病,好发于女性。病变的特征性表现为胫前 1cm 或更大有光泽的痛性深红色结节,发病机制尚不清楚。结节性红斑的病因是感染(特别是链球菌、系统性真菌和结核),药物(特别是口服避孕药)和白血病。7% 的克罗恩病患者和 4% 的溃疡性结肠炎患者有结节性红斑,另外,小肠结肠炎耶尔森菌、福氏志贺菌和空肠弯曲菌的胃肠道感染也与结节性红斑有关。治疗基础疾病,严格卧床休息,抬高腿部,以及使用消炎药或碘化钾都是有效的。

坏疽性脓皮病是一种发病机制不明的非感染性溃疡性皮肤病(图 25.4),典型的病变是触痛或者痛性、边界升高、暗紫色且被广泛破坏的溃疡,可能出现一个或多个病变。病变开始时是小丘疹脓疱,破裂迅速。过敏反应性,经常表现为在轻微创伤或手术部位出现新的溃疡。这个诊断是必须排除包括人为皮炎在内的感染性和其他原因的溃疡。大多数坏疽性脓皮病发生在没有基础疾病的患者。坏疽性脓皮病发生在大约 5% 的 UC 患者和 1% 的克罗恩病患者中。当皮肤病变出现时,肠道疾病可能是亚临床的,因此在坏疽性脓皮病病例中,肠道评估——特别是直肠和远端结肠的评估是很有必要的。如果疾病与潜在的肠道疾病相关,肠道疾病的治疗可能导致

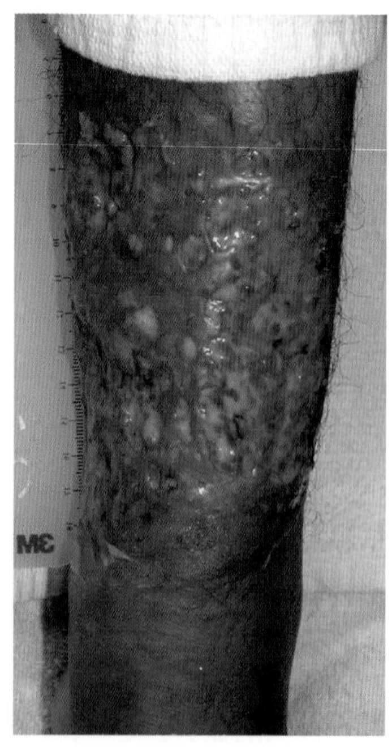

图 25.4 一例溃疡性结肠炎(UC)患者发生坏疽性脓皮病。(Courtesy Dr. Benjamin Lockshin,Silver Spring,MD.)

皮肤病变的改善。坏疽性脓皮病的一般治疗包括局部伤口护理、大剂量全身糖皮质激素或类固醇的免疫抑制剂，如硫唑嘌呤、吗替麦考酚酯、甲氨蝶呤和环孢霉素[12]。

四、血管和结缔组织疾病

结缔组织疾病如系统性红斑狼疮（SLE）、皮肌炎（见下文）和进行性系统性硬化症（progressive systemic sclerosis，PSS）都具有特征性的皮肤和胃肠道表现（见第 37 章）。典型的 SLE 患者有光敏性的蝶形红斑，常伴有滤泡堵塞的红斑隆起斑（盘状狼疮）。SLE 患者可有口腔溃疡。PSS 患者通常表现为全身硬化皮肤，或者少数情况下表现为硬斑病（带有象牙色中心的硬化斑块），席纹状的毛细血管扩张和雷诺现象。

小血管的免疫复合性血管炎（白细胞碎屑性血管炎）出现在依赖部位的皮肤上，表现为可触及的紫癜，是由免疫复合物沉积在毛细血管后小静脉介导的（图 25.5；见第 38 和 80 章）。尽管任何小血管血管炎都可累及胃肠道，但却发生在 50%～75% 过敏性紫癜患者中（图 25.6）[14]。血管性出血、肠壁水肿和肠套叠最常影响空肠和回肠。直接免疫荧光检测早期皮肤病变在大多数小血管炎病例中显示 IgG 沉积，以及在过敏性紫癜中显示 IgA 沉积。

结节性多动脉炎，有时与乙型肝炎相关，是一种中动脉及小动脉的血管炎。腹部脏器的动脉病变可导致肠道、肝脏和胆囊梗死，缺血性胰腺坏死，以及胃肠道梗死或穿孔。累及阑尾、胆囊或胰腺时可类似急性阑尾炎、胆囊炎或胰腺炎。25% 的病例有皮肤受累，最典型的表现为分布于沿浅动脉走行的 5～10mm 结节。网状青斑也很常见。

恶性萎缩性丘疹病（Degos 病、Köhlmeier-Degos 综合征、进行性动脉肠系膜血管闭塞病或播散性肠和皮肤血栓性血管炎）是一种血管疾病，其有可能是家族性的，已报道了约 200 例。这是一种纯粹的皮肤形式，但多系统亚型是重要的，因为它意味着近乎一致的致命结果由于胃肠道穿孔造成的（见第 37 章）。皮肤病变是最初的表现，最常表现于成年早期。它们表现为无症状的 2～15mm 粉红色丘疹，迅速变成脐状形，并发展为特征性的萎缩、凹陷、瓷白色中心（图 25.7）。这些病变代表皮肤梗死。相似的病变可发生在高达 60% 的病例可发生在胃肠道，但也可累及神经系统、心脏、肺、肝脏和肾脏。虽然胃肠道受累最初可能是无症状或非特异性的，但急性腹部疾病最终会发生，通常有必要进行腹腔镜检查或剖腹手术。小肠经常会出现穿孔，小肠内常出现完整的绒毛膜下多发白色、淡黄色或玫瑰色扁平或轻微凹陷的斑块。约 20% 的患者出现脑和周围神经梗死，导致神经系统并发症，包括偏瘫、失语、脑神经病变、单瘫、感觉障碍和癫痫。显微镜检查显示梗死是非炎性血栓形成的结果。Degos 病的发病机制尚不清楚，但在 SLE 和有抗心磷脂抗体和狼疮抗凝物的无 SLE 患者中有相同的病变报道。已经尝试用抗血栓药物如阿司匹林、噻氯匹定和双嘧达莫来治疗，然而所看到的疗效是有限的[15]。

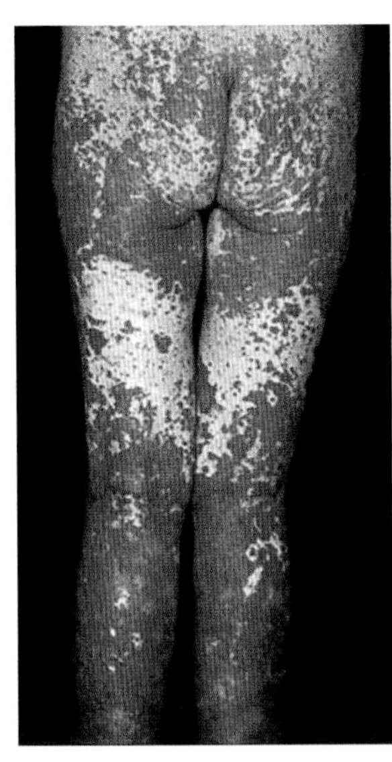

图 25.5　药物引起的冷球蛋白血症性血管炎。这种类型的血管炎也可见于慢性丙型肝炎患者，尽管通常不像图中所示的那么严重

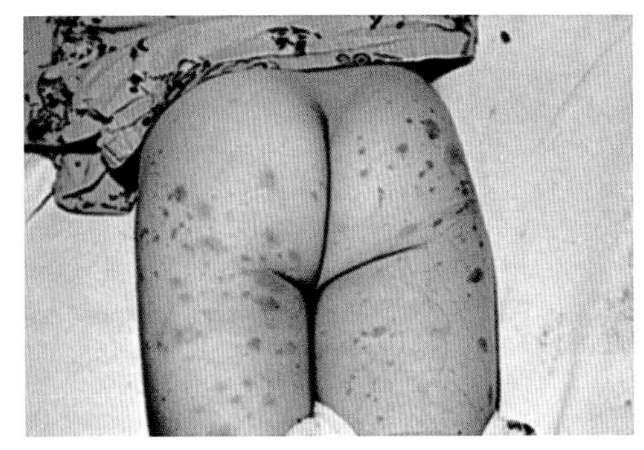

图 25.6　过敏性紫癜的皮肤病

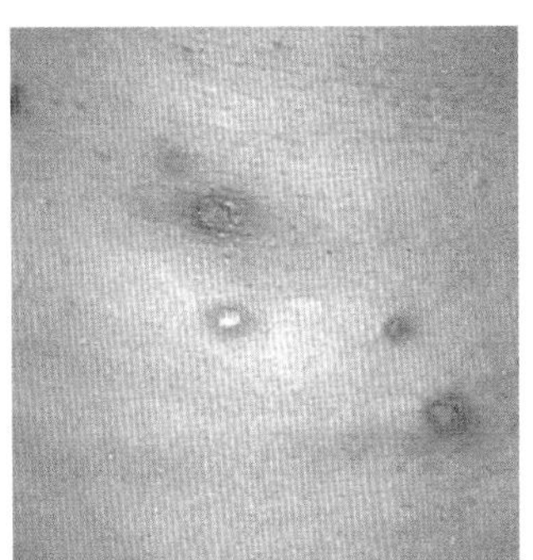

图 25.7　恶性萎缩性丘疹病（Degos 病）伴不同阶段的皮肤损害

遗传性出血性毛细血管扩张症（HHT），又称 Osler-Weber-Rendu 病，是一组常染色体显性遗传疾病，其特征是血管病变，包括毛细血管扩张、动静脉畸形和累及皮肤和内部器官（肺、脑和胃肠道）的动脉瘤性血管，鼻衄（80%～90%）和消化道出血是最常见的并发症（见第 38 章）。皮肤病变为面部、嘴唇、舌头、结膜、手指、胸部和足部的 1～3mm 黄斑毛细血管扩张（图 25.8）。皮病变出现晚于鼻衄，通常在生命的第二或第三个 10 年。在第五至第六个 10 年，可能发生反复的上、下消化道出血。血管畸形在胃肠道、肝脏、肺、中枢神经系统、泌尿生殖道和几乎所有其他器官系统都有报道。消化道出血的

处理可能是困难的，但双极电凝或激光技术的使用是有益的（见第 20 章）。可能缺乏相关的血管性血友病因子，去氨加压素治疗消化道大出血是成功的，长期使用雌激素和孕酮治疗也许可以减少消化道毛细血管扩张所致出血。尽管前没有美国食品药品管理局批准的治疗方法来抑制 HHT 患者毛细血管扩张病变的发展，目前的研究专注于所提出的相关遗传途径。转化生长因子 β 信号通路的突变，包括 *ENG*、*ACVRL1* 和 *SMAD4*，可能是抗血管生成药物的靶点，如贝伐珠单抗和沙利度胺[16]。

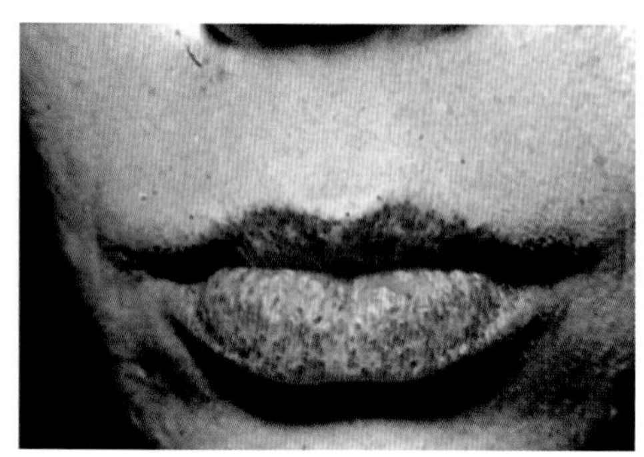

图 25.8 遗传性出血性毛细血管扩张症（Osler-Weber-Rendu 病）患者的嘴唇扁平毛细血管扩张症和唇红边缘。

蓝色橡皮泡痣综合征是一种罕见的皮肤和胃肠道疾病包括各种多发性皮肤和胃肠道静脉畸形，大多数病例是散发性的。在受累患者中，皮肤出现蓝色的皮下可压缩性结节（图 25.9）。胃肠道血管畸形是常见的，特别是在小肠或结肠，而且出血几乎是一个普遍的特征。急性消化道出血、肠套叠、肠扭转、肠梗死和直肠脱垂已被描述。手术或光凝是主要的治疗方法。

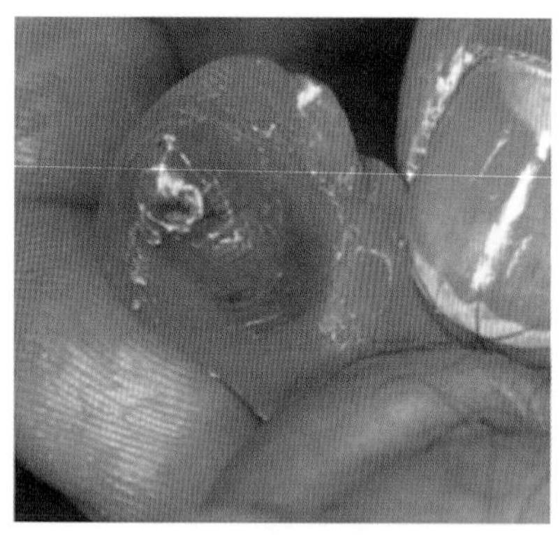

图 25.9 蓝色橡皮泡痣综合征患者的指尖病变

淀粉样变通常有明显的皮肤和口腔表现（见第 37 章），眼睛、鼻子和面部中央周围的蜡状丘疹，以及累及面部、颈部和上眼睑的紫癜，都是常见的。如果蜡质丘疹被挤压，就会出现出血（挤压性紫癜）。内镜检查后的眼窝紫癜、呕吐或咳嗽几乎可以诊断。20% ~ 50% 的患者会出现巨舌症，舌头硬度增加，颌下腺结构扩大以及牙齿的舌侧凹陷。巨舌症可干扰进食和闭口，尤其在仰卧位时，可在气道阻塞时出现呼吸暂停。增大的舌头可能有大量血管，最终出现出血，口腔中反复出现出血性大疱是很常见的。患者可能有腕管综合征、水肿、肩垫征（肩周软组织淀粉样沉积物）、胃肠道出血、周围神经病变、小关节类风湿性关节炎沉积物和心脏受累。充血性心力衰竭或心律失常造成了 40% 系统性淀粉样变性患者的死亡。淀粉样变性可以通过皮下脂肪抽吸或骨髓、直肠、皮肤或舌的活检来诊断。

弹性假黄瘤是一种罕见的 *ABCC6* 基因突变的常染色体隐性遗传病，其特征是成熟弹性组织的异常钙化。皮肤病变通常是最初的表现，在第二个十年出现在颈部侧方的黄色到橙色丘疹（“拔毛鸡皮”）（图 25.10）。皮肤病变可向尾部进展，累及其他弯曲部位（如腋窝、腹股沟、肘前和腘窝）。动脉弹性组织的钙化导致视网膜出血、间歇性跛行、过早冠状动脉疾病和消化道出血等主要并发症。高达 13% 的患者会经历胃肠道出血，通常是胃出血，而且往往并未发现特定的出血点。与弹性假黄瘤的其他并发症不同，消化道出血往往发生在较年轻的患者（平均年龄 26 岁）中，常发生在孕期，而且可能复发。皮肤病变在出血时可能无法见到。由于明显正常的弯曲或瘢痕皮肤可能产生诊断结果，而无其他解释的消化道出血的年轻人可能需要盲性皮肤活检。那些在皮肤上看到的病变同样也可能存在于下唇和直肠黏膜[17]。

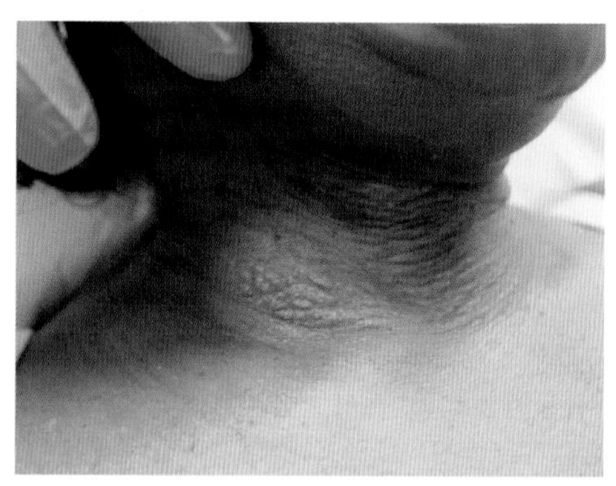

图 25.10 弹性假黄瘤患者的特征性“拔毛鸡皮”外观。（Courtesy Dr. Benjamin Lockshin, Silver Spring, MD.）

神经纤维瘤病 1 型（neuroffbromatosis type 1, NF1; von Recklinghausen 病）的定义是其皮肤表现为 6 个或更多的咖啡牛乳色斑（处于青春期前的人中每个直径大于 5mm 和处于青春期后的人中每个直径大于 15mm）。

多发软丘疹［神经纤维瘤（图 25.11）］或单发丛状神经纤维瘤以及腋窝或腹股沟区域的斑点。10% ~ 15% 的 NF1 患者胃肠道受累，肠道神经纤维瘤可以发生在胃肠道的任何部位，然而小肠受累是最为常见的。这些肿瘤一般位于黏膜下，但也可延伸至浆膜。肠系膜或腹膜后间隙密集生长的丛状神经纤维瘤可能导致动脉受压或神经损伤。其他肿瘤可能发生于神经纤维瘤病。嗜铬细胞瘤的发病率增加，伴或不伴有多发性内分泌腺瘤综合征 Ⅱ B 型[18]。十二指肠和壶腹类癌（有时产生梗阻性黄疸；见第 34 章）、恶性神经鞘瘤、肉瘤和胰腺腺癌的发生率增加。NF1 的胃肠道表现包括腹痛、便秘、贫血、黑便和腹部包块。已被报道的严重并发症包括肠或胆道梗阻、肠缺血、穿孔和肠套叠，累及肌间丛导致巨结肠。

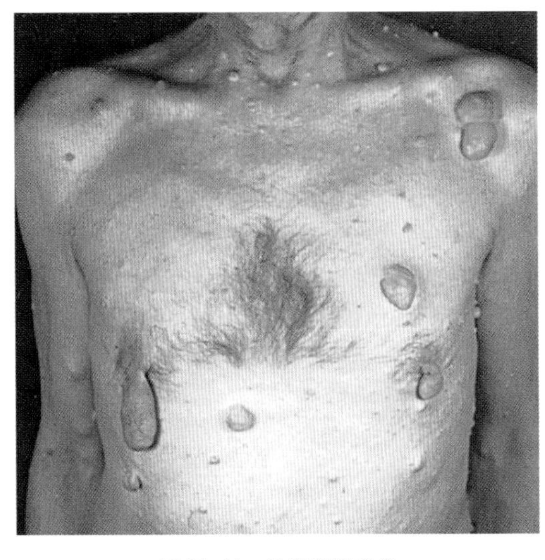

图 25.11　神经纤维瘤病

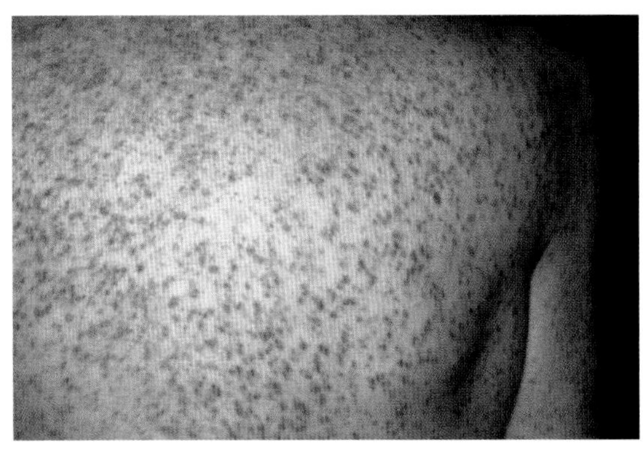

图 25.12　成人色素性荨麻疹。红棕色雀斑样皮损是本病成人型的特征。术语“荨麻疹”用词不当，因为这些病变与荨麻疹不相似

肥大细胞增多症的特征是肥大细胞浸润骨髓、皮肤、肝脏、脾脏、淋巴结和胃肠道，它发生在成人和儿童中（见第 37 章）。在儿童中，最常见的病变包括大的红棕色斑块（孤立性肥大细胞瘤），多发的红棕色丘疹或斑块（色素性荨麻疹），或弥漫性皮肤受累，伴或不伴发红或起泡。在成人患者中，大多数有色素荨麻疹型病变（图 25.12），有时有明显的毛细血管扩张。病变常位于躯干，由于肥大细胞浸润器官或肥大细胞释放介质（如组胺、前列腺素），导致头痛、晕厥、潮红、出汗、呼吸短促、气喘，或甚至是过敏反应等临床症状谱。最常见的胃肠症状是消化不良和组胺诱导的胃酸分泌过多引起的消化性溃疡（见 51 章）。腹泻和腹痛也是常见的问题，并可伴有吸收不良[19]。在儿童，病变通常是逐渐自发的，而且全身性疾病是不常见的。在成人，皮肤病变也可以治疗，但没有改善全身症状。在孤立性肥大细胞瘤伴有明显的全身症状的罕见的儿科病例，切除皮肤病变可能解决全身并发症。肥大细胞增多症的成人患者应考虑皮肤外受累，因为该症状很容易处理。

五、胃肠道恶性肿瘤的皮肤表现

皮肤表现可能是识别个人是癌或是遗传自亲属有癌发生的高风险的重要因素。这些皮肤标志物分 3 个部分讨论：胃肠道息肉和皮肤表现的综合征、内部恶性肿瘤的皮肤标志物、转移性胃肠道癌的皮肤表现。

（一）息肉病综合征

在第 126 章中讨论的息肉病综合征，有许多皮肤表现，是临床鉴别和独特鉴别的关键。表 25.1 回顾了相关的黏膜与皮肤的临床表现，以及遗传性息肉病综合征、遗传性非息肉病性结直肠癌（hereditary non-polyposis colorectal cancer，HNPCC；Lynch 综合征）和 Muir-Torre 综合征（图 25.13）。最近有一篇关于这一主题的全面综述[20]。

表 25.1　息肉综合征的相关皮肤表现和遗传学

综合征（遗传）	皮肤/黏膜表现	其他发现	基因缺陷
Gardner 综合征 家族性腺瘤息肉病变异（常染色体显性遗传）	青春期前表皮样（包含）囊肿 脂肪瘤 硬纤维瘤 牙齿异常发育： 骨瘤 牙瘤 多余的牙齿 多个未露出的牙齿 长而尖的后牙根	100~1 000 个腺瘤性结肠息肉 先天性视网膜色素上皮肥大 恶性肿瘤： 结肠/直肠 十二指肠 壶腹部 甲状腺 髓母细胞瘤 肾上腺 肝母细胞瘤	*APC*（肿瘤抑制基因缺陷） OMIM#175100
Muir-Torre 综合征 Lynch 综合征变异（常染色体显性遗传）	皮脂腺瘤和癌 上皮瘤 角化棘皮瘤	恶性肿瘤： 结直肠黏液腺癌 （通常为近端结肠） 胃 小肠 壶腹部 子宫内膜 泌尿道 卵巢 肝/胆道	*MLH1*，*MSH2*，*MSH6*，*PMS2* 错配修复基因缺陷 OMIM#158320

表 25.1　息肉综合征的相关皮肤表现和遗传学(续)

综合征(遗传)	皮肤/黏膜表现	其他发现	基因缺陷
Peutz-Jeghers 综合征(常染色体显性遗传)	早发性皮肤黏膜黑素细胞斑: 口周 唇/唇红缘 颊黏膜 舌黏膜 手指 眼周 肛周	胃肠道错构瘤性息肉(胃肠道的任何部分) 恶性肿瘤: 小肠和大肠 胰腺 乳房 子宫 子宫颈 睾丸	*STK11*(丝氨酸/苏氨酸激酶种系突变) OMIM#175200
Cowden 综合征 多发性错构瘤综合征 (常染色体显性遗传)	毛膜瘤 面部丘疹 脂肪瘤 肢端角化病 阴茎小痣 口腔表现: 乳头瘤病 裂缝舌/舌裂 颊/舌鹅卵样变	息肉病: 食管 胃 结肠/直肠 错构瘤: 骨 中枢神经系统 眼 泌尿生殖道 漏斗胸 脊柱侧凸 巨头畸形 恶性肿瘤: 结肠/直肠 乳腺 甲状腺 子宫内膜	*PTEN* 肿瘤抑制基因缺陷 OMIM#158350
Cronkhite-Canada 综合征(散发的)	斑秃(斑片状) 色素沉着(弥漫性) 指甲营养不良: 变薄 开裂 甲脱离 脱甲病(周期性甲脱落)	遍布胃肠道的弥漫性息肉病,保留食管,导致腹泻、体重减轻、厌食、消化道出血、肠套叠和蛋白质丢失肠病	OMIM#175500

OMIM,人类孟德尔遗传在线研究。

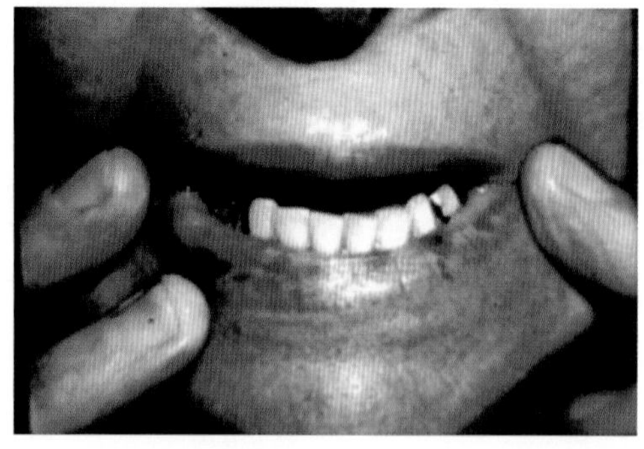

图 25.13　黑斑息肉综合征(Peutz-Jeghers 综合征)患者的皮肤黏膜色素沉着

(二)内部恶性肿瘤及相关疾病

皮肌炎(dermatomyositis,DM)表现为眼睑呈紫罗兰色,常伴有水肿(淡紫色);指节的角化性丘疹[Gottron 丘疹(图 25.14)];广泛的红斑,通常在肘部和膝盖处加重(Gottron 征),类似银屑病;光敏性;指甲角质层异常,包括毛细血管扩张、增厚、粗糙、生长过度和不规则。约 25% 的 DM 患者有内部恶性肿瘤,特别是 40 岁以上的患者[21]。最常与 DM 相关的癌症是胃癌、结直肠癌、胰腺癌、卵巢癌、肺癌和非霍奇金淋巴瘤,这在性别中没有区别。为检测相关的癌症,需要一个完整的病史、体格检查(包括直肠、骨盆和乳腺检查)、全血细胞计数(complete blood count,CBC)、常规血清化学分析、血清蛋白电泳、粪便隐血试验、尿液分析、胸部 X 线片、(女性)乳房 X 线检查和阴道超声检查,每年都推荐检查,以及在 DM 的发病后的前 3 年,出现的新症状,任何异常应作进一步的调查[22,23]。

掌跖角化病(Howell-Evans 综合征;胼胝症和食管癌)是一种成年期起病的手掌和脚掌弥漫性角化过度症,在英格兰利物浦的几个家族中被描述为与食管癌的高发病率相关。这是一种常染色体显性表型,是由位于染色体 17q 上的胼胝症

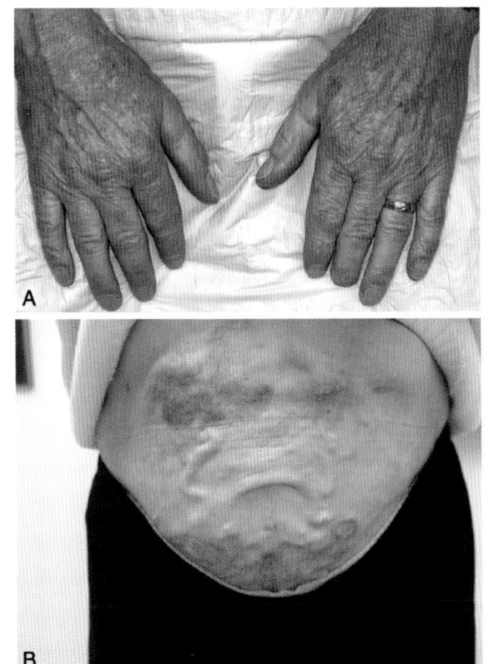

图 25.14　A，皮肌炎伴红斑性斑块，尤其是指关节（Gottron 丘疹）。B，皮肌炎伴海蛇头的皮肤钙质沉着症。（Courtesy Dr. Benjamin Lockshin，Silver Spring，MD.）

食管癌基因 *RHBDF2* 杂合缺失引起的[24]。皮肤病变出现在青春期或成年早期，而癌肿平均出现年龄在 45 岁。食管癌发生在几乎所有的有家族性胼胝症的患者中。

黑棘皮病是一种皮肤症状，表现为颈部和腋窝皮肤呈绒毛状增生和色素沉着（图 25.15），常伴多个皮赘，这是胰岛素抵抗的最常见表现。然而，一些黑棘皮病患者有内部恶性肿瘤，即所谓的恶性黑棘皮病。在这些患者中，受累程度可能很严重，包括双手、生殖器和口腔黏膜。当黑棘皮病影响到手时，称为牛肚掌（手掌棘皮病、厚皮纹、手掌角化过度和手掌角化病），牛肚掌表现为苔藓状或天鹅绒般的质地，有明显的皮肤纹，手掌和手指表面呈鹅卵石状或蜂窝状。相关的癌症通常与黑棘皮病同时出现，但可能临床表现不明显。腹内腺癌占相关恶性肿瘤的 85% 以上，其中胃癌占 60% 以上。患者的生存期很短，超过 50% 的患者在 1 年内死亡[25]。

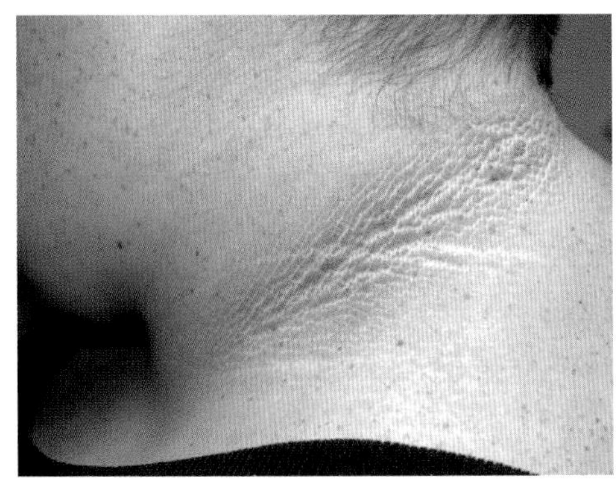

图 25.15　颈部黑棘皮病。（Courtesy Dr. Benjamin Lockshin，Silver Spring，MD.）

副肿瘤性肢端角化病（Bazex 综合征）是一种罕见但独特的综合征，与原发性恶性肿瘤有关的上呼吸消化道或转移到颈部淋巴结的癌。到目前为止报道的超过 50 例患者有恶性肿瘤，包括食管癌和 1 例伴有颈部淋巴结转移的胃癌。皮疹开始时集中于趾甲周围皮肤增厚和明显的指甲营养不良，皮疹向近端发展，也累及鼻尖和耳尖。手掌和脚掌先开始增厚，伴有中央保留完好，这使行走会很痛，最终脸部和头皮也受累。潜在癌症的治疗通常与改善或解决皮肤病变相关。

皮疹开始时集中于趾甲周围皮肤增厚和明显的指甲营养不良，皮疹向近端发展，也累及鼻尖和耳尖。手掌和脚掌先开始增厚，伴有中央保留完好，这使行走会很痛，最终脸部和头皮也受累。潜在癌症的治疗通常与改善或解决皮肤病变相关。

胎儿性多毛症是另一种罕见的副肿瘤综合征，包括细小、绒毛样、无色素的胎毛型毛发，典型表现在面部、前额、耳朵、鼻子、腋窝、四肢和躯干。相关表现包括舌痛、舌乳头肥大、味觉和嗅觉障碍、腹泻、硬皮病、黑棘皮病、脂溢性角化、淋巴结肿大和体重减轻。结直肠癌的发病率仅次于肺癌。

类癌产生大量血管活性物质，可导致皮肤潮红（见第 34 章）。最常见的类癌（阑尾和小肠）直到血管活性物质到达系统循环时才出现潮红，因此，潮红通常表示转移到肝脏或不同的原发肿瘤部位（如肺或卵巢）。胰高血糖素瘤是一种罕见的胰脏 α 细胞的神经内分泌肿瘤，可导致皮肤出现坏死游走性红斑，这些皮疹常见于孔口、弯曲部位和手指。病变为典型的丘疹，继发糜烂、结痂和裂隙呈环状分布（图 25.16）。患者也可能出现体重减轻、腹泻、贫血、精神障碍、低氨基酸血症和糖尿病。成功切除肿瘤后，皮疹通常会消失（详细讨论在第 34 章）。

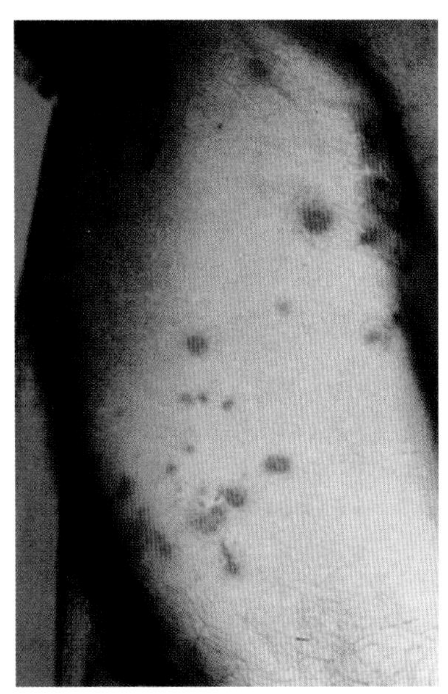

图 25.16　一例胰高血糖素瘤患者的坏死性游走性红斑，表现为迅速侵蚀的浅表水疱。皮损通常局限在臀部、腹股沟、会阴、肘部、手、足和口周。（Courtesy Dr. Carl Grunfeld，San Francisco，CA.）

皮下脂肪坏死和多关节痛与胰腺腺泡细胞癌、胰腺炎和胰腺假性囊肿有关，这种集合现在越来越被称为 PPP 综合征（pancreatitis，panniculitis，polyarthritis syndrome，胰腺炎、脂膜炎、多发性关节炎综合征)[26],多数受影响的是男性。腿部常出现深皮下、直径1至数厘米的红斑性结节。罕见的病例中,结节可破裂,渗出奶油状物质。关节炎,常累及多个关节,尤其是踝和膝关节,也许伴有结节或不出现皮肤损害(图25.17)。当皮肤病变或关节炎发生时,腹痛可能消失。除了预期的血清脂肪酶(和淀粉酶)升高外,嗜酸性粒细胞升高也很常见。皮肤病变的组织病理学检查通常显示诊断性发现——苍白染色的坏死脂肪细胞(鬼影细胞)和坏死脂肪中的钙沉积。与癌症无关的病例死亡率可接近50%。在PPP综合征中,皮下结节通常表现在胫前。

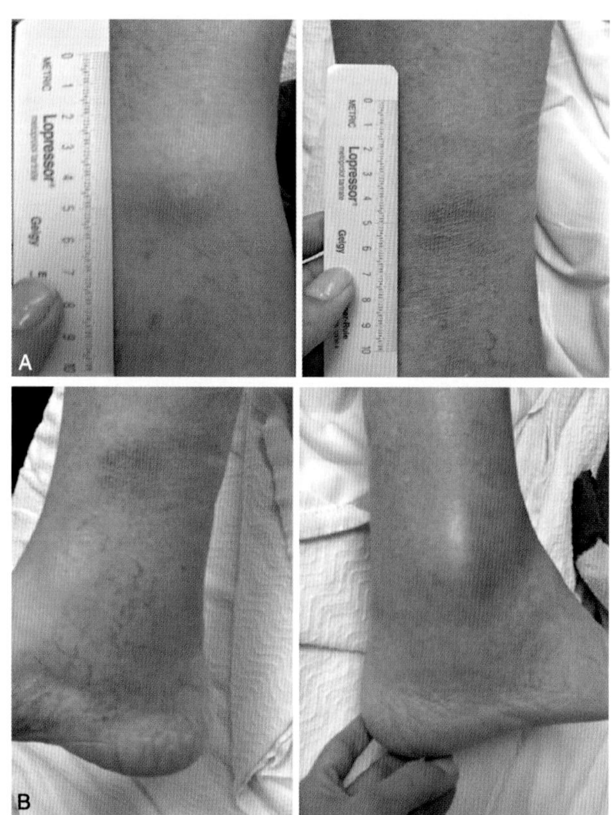

图25.17　A和B,胰腺炎、脂膜炎、多关节炎综合征。一例69岁酒精性男性患者,患有慢性钙化性胰腺炎、假性囊肿和明显的高脂血症(>6 000U/L),发生急性双侧踝关节疼痛伴发红和肿胀。3天后,患者注意到右前臂后部及右踝关节区域出现疼痛性红色肿块,随后扩散至右踝关节。掌指关节、数个指间关节疼痛、肿胀,双侧跟腱肿胀。其中一个皮下结节活检显示脂肪坏死。病变和关节炎在数周内逐渐消退。且无瘢痕。(Courtesy Ann Malbas,MD.)

脐周围皮肤呈蓝色(瘀斑),有时与出血性胰腺炎相关,称为Cullen征;当一个类似的过程发生在胁腹部,则被称为Grey-Turner征(见第58章)。

一些过去被认为与内部恶性肿瘤相关的皮肤特征,最近越来越被忽视且认为没有直接关系。这些疾病包括Bowen病(皮肤原位鳞状细胞癌)和皮赘。Leser-Trelat征(突然出现的多发性脂溢性角化)仍有争议,但当伴有其他副肿瘤性发现时,如恶性黑棘皮病,可能对胃肠道或肺腺癌更有特异性[25]。Sweet综合征(急性热性中性粒细胞性皮肤病)可能与淋巴组织增生性肿瘤有关。

(三)皮肤转移瘤

胃肠道腺癌很少发生皮肤转移,它们可能出现在皮肤的任何部位,通常是非特异性的、非常硬的真皮或皮下结节。当转移到脐部时,超过一半的病例发现腹腔内胃肠癌转移灶,胃癌占20%。这种病变称为Sister Mary Joseph结节。免疫过氧化物酶标记可以帮助病理学家预测转移性结节活检标本的原发灶。

六、肝脏疾病的皮肤表现

肝病可导致多种皮肤表现,尤其与乙型和丙型肝炎有关时(框25.1和框25.2)。

框25.1　特定的肝脏疾病的皮肤表现
肝脏疾病的一般表现
黄疸
蜘蛛痣
螺旋形巩膜血管
肝掌
条纹
脐周静脉曲张
血色病
通常的古铜色皮肤,在日晒部位有加重
原发性胆汁性胆管炎
躯干、面部或四肢的黄色瘤,包括掌痕上的明显黄色瘤
乙型及丙型肝炎
见框25.2

框25.2　乙型和丙型肝炎的皮肤表现
乙型肝炎多于丙型肝炎
结节性多动脉炎
荨麻疹
血清病
婴幼儿丘疹性肢端皮炎(Gianoti-Crosti综合征)
结节性红斑
乙型和丙型肝炎均有
小血管炎
荨麻疹性血管炎
瘙痒
多形性红斑
丙型肝炎多于乙型肝炎
白细胞破裂性血管炎伴冷球蛋白血症
迟发性皮肤卟啉症
丙型肝炎
扁平苔藓
网状青斑
坏死松解性肢端红斑

瘙痒是胆汁淤积性、炎症性和恶性肝病的一种令人苦恼的并发症。肝病的瘙痒不能通过抓挠或局部外用糖皮质激素减轻，可能尤其在手掌和脚掌症状特别突出，很难处理。紫外线 B 光治疗、考来烯胺或利福平对瘙痒的改善对说明这种令人痛苦的疾病的发病机制没有帮助。阿片拮抗剂可以缓解肝脏疾病的瘙痒，而与肝脏转移性疾病相关的瘙痒已成功被 5-HT_3 受体拮抗剂昂丹西酮治疗。密集的研究正在应用于瘙痒领域，并提出了多种潜在的瘙痒通路，包括 TRPV1 受体激活、阿片受体、5-HT、组胺受体、GABA 受体、神经激肽-1、TRPA1 等其他通路[27]。

维生素 K 经常用于肝病和低凝血酶原血症患者，尽管少见，但皮下、肌内注射或静脉注射后可能发生皮肤反应。大的红斑、质硬的瘙痒斑块会在几天到几周内出现，这些反应可能是迟发型过敏反应，因为皮肤试验可以重现这些反应。当检测时，患者被发现对维生素 K 过敏，而不是苯甲醇过敏。然而，维生素 K_3 是水溶性的，并没有报道引起类似的反应。如果在臀部注射维生素 K 后发生反应，这些斑块有一种诊断倾向，因为其扩散到腰部并下至大腿，复制所谓的“牛仔枪带和枪套”模式。这些反应位点会在几天到几周内消失，但也可能会存在几个月到几年。在注射后数月至数年会出现红斑反应，或无先前反应，会发生扩大的与局限性硬皮病类似的紫罗兰色边界的硬化斑块。后一种情况通常发生在注射大剂量维生素 K 后。除了这些局部反应外，静脉注射后的过敏反应也可能是致死性的。

结节性多动脉炎与乙型肝炎之间的联系是有充分证据的，荨麻疹和血清病以经典方式发生在乙型肝炎患者身上，尽管这两种病都曾被报道与丙型肝炎相关（见第 79 和 80 章）。慢性丙型肝炎病毒与白细胞破裂性血管炎伴冷球蛋白血症有关，皮肤上有瘀点和明显的紫癜。

迟发性皮肤卟啉症（porphyria cutanea tarda，PCT）是一种卟啉代谢障碍，其特征是暴露在阳光下的皮肤是脆弱、水疱、多毛和色素沉着的（图 25.18）。PCT 是最常见的卟啉症，其特征是缺乏尿卟啉原脱羧酶，诊断通常通过 24 小时尿液显示尿卟啉水平升高。酒精摄入、雌激素、铁和阳光都是使 PCT 恶化的因素。PCT 和丙型肝炎之间存在明显和实质性的联系[28]。PCT 患者中丙型肝炎的患病率表现出地区差别，从欧洲南部和北美洲的 65% 到欧洲北部和澳大利亚的 20%[29] 不等。治疗包括静脉放血和抗疟疾药物。

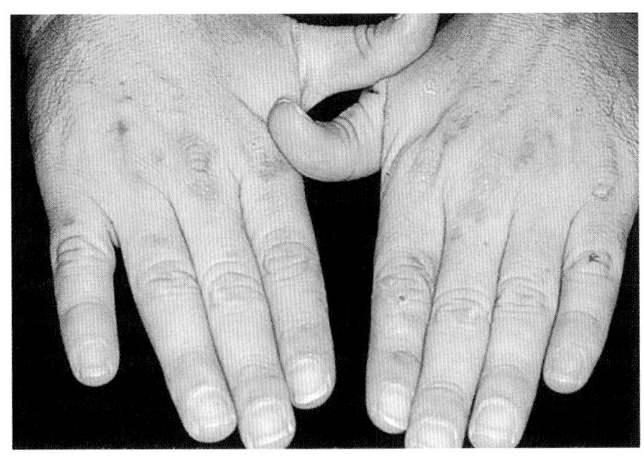

图 25.18　迟发性皮肤卟啉症，其特征为手背非炎性水疱和糜烂。受累患者经常感染丙肝病毒。（Courtesy Dr. Timothy Berger，San Francisco，CA.）

LP 是一种常见的特发性炎症，其可影响皮肤、头发、黏膜和指甲（见前面）。LP 的典型表现是手腕、手臂和腿部弯曲区域的紫罗兰色多边形扁平丘疹，丘疹通常覆盖白色网状鳞片被称为 Wickham 纹。LP 和丙型肝炎之间存在相关性，但不如 PCT 和丙型肝炎之间的相关性显著[30]。

七、皮肤病患者的药物性肝病

皮肤科医生经常咨询消化科医生来评估正在接受甲氨蝶呤或类维甲酸治疗的患者，因为这些药物可导致急性和慢性肝病（见第 88 章）。甲氨蝶呤常用于治疗严重银屑病和银屑病关节炎，但也用于皮肤 T 细胞淋巴瘤、结缔组织疾病（如风湿性关节炎）和其他炎症性疾病。甲氨蝶呤剂量通常是每周给药 10～25mg，但也可给特定的患者增加剂量。皮肤科医生通常遵循已经建立的肝脏活检的分级系统，根据这些活检的结果决定是否继续治疗（表 25.2）[26]。美国皮肤病学会最新的共识指南建议肝活检相比以前减少频率并且不再建议在无附加肝毒性危险因素（如慢性酒精使用、肥胖、糖尿病、活动性或慢性肝炎）的患者中进行预处理肝活检。值得注意的是，肝活检仍然建议用于银屑病的监测（每 3.5～4g 总累积剂量）[32]，是因为严重的银屑病伴随的固有代谢紊乱引起的慢性肝损伤，但越来越多的工作表明现在肝脏弹性成像或其他非侵入性的检查可能取代目前许多需要活检[33]。

表 25.2　服用甲氨蝶呤患者的肝活检结果分级系统和继续/停止甲氨蝶呤治疗的指南

分级	标准	指南
Ⅰ	正常的；轻度脂肪浸润；核变异，门脉炎症	可继续接受甲氨蝶呤
Ⅱ	中度至重度脂肪浸润；核变化；门静脉扩张、门静脉炎症、坏死	可继续接受甲氨蝶呤
ⅢA	轻度纤维化（形成纤维化性间隔并延伸至小叶）	可以继续接受甲氨蝶呤治疗，但在使用甲氨蝶呤约 6 个月后应再次进行肝活检。替代疗法应该被考虑
ⅢB	中度至重度纤维化	不应再使用甲氨蝶呤。然而在特殊情况下，可能需要继续服用甲氨蝶呤并随访肝活检
Ⅳ	肝硬化（再生结节和门静脉桥接）	不应再使用甲氨蝶呤。然而，在特殊情况下，可能需要继续服用甲氨蝶呤并随访肝活检

Modified from Roenigk HH Jr，Auerbach R，Maibach H，Weinstein GD. Methotrexate in psoriasis：revised guidelines. J Am Acad Dermatol 1988；19：145-56.

类维生素 A(如异维 A 酸、阿维 A、贝沙罗汀)是维生素 A 的衍生物,目前用于治疗某些类型的严重银屑病、囊性痤疮和其他角化疾病。在治疗过程中需要进行定期的肝化学检查,血清甘油三酯、胆固醇、谷丙转氨酶(ALT)和谷草转氨酶(AST)水平轻度升高是常见的(20%~30%的患者被治疗),这通常是短暂的,或可以很容易通过减少剂量而控制水。然而,严重或甚至致命的肝炎也有报道。类维生素 A 可用于曾接受甲氨蝶呤治疗的银屑病患者或既往有肝脏疾病而不可使用甲氨蝶呤的患者。有限的经验表明,这些患者在使用类维生素 A 治疗后不会出现肝脏疾病的进展。与甲氨蝶呤一样,在类维生素 A 治疗期间,肝脏化学检查结果与肝脏组织学之间的相关性较差。因此,某些长期口服维甲酸治疗的高风险患者可能需要预处理和间断进行肝活检。

八、皮肤和胃肠道的寄生虫病

人和动物线虫的幼虫形式可能引起游走性红斑性皮肤损害,称为匐行性皮疹(见第 114 章),最常见的模式是由狗和猫钩虫引起的皮肤幼虫移行症(图 25.19)。瘙痒性线性丘疹以每天 1~2cm 的速度在与粪便污染土壤接触的皮肤部位移动,通常是在脚、臀部或背部,病变会在几周到几个月后自行消退。幼虫移行是由于粪类圆线虫的幼虫在皮肤中迁移,它以两种形式发生,一种局限于有免疫能力的宿主直肠周围皮肤,另一种播散形式发生于免疫抑制宿主。粪类圆线虫在线虫中具有独特的能力,可以在肠道内发育成具有感染性的幼虫。这些感染性幼虫可侵入具有免疫能力的感染者的直肠周围皮肤,引起荨麻疹、红斑、线状病变,每天移位长达 10cm,通常在肛门 30cm 以内的范围。皮肤损害可间歇性发生,这使诊断变得困难。在免疫抑制宿主中,反复的自体感染通过肠道导致巨大的寄生虫负担(重度感染),最常见的表现为肺部疾病。与重度感染相关,播散的幼虫移行型病变可能出现在全身,躯干较为显著,点状或紫癜性蛇形病变也可发生在脐周。

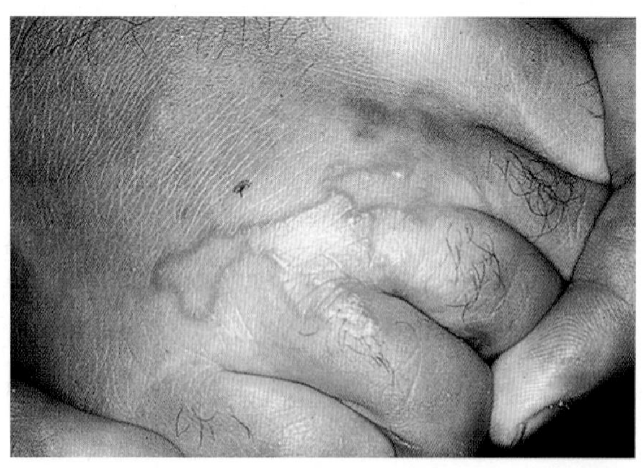

图 25.19　皮肤幼虫移行症,其特征是感染大钩虫引起的匐行性红斑移性病变。(Courtesy Dr. Timothy Berger, San Francisco, CA.)

寄生虫感染通常被认为是荨麻疹中经典的鉴别诊断,然而除了肝片吸虫病和包虫病外,与荨麻疹的直接关系很少被证实。如果血液嗜酸性粒细胞增多和胃肠道症状消失,大便检查寄生虫作用不大。

九、疱疹样皮炎和乳糜泻

疱疹样皮炎(dermatitis herpetiformis, DH)是一种特别瘙痒的皮肤病,常见于成年早期(见第 107 章)。皮疹由荨麻疹、水疱或大疱性病变组成,特征性分布于头皮、肩膀、肘部、膝盖和臀部[34]。这种疾病瘙痒极其严重,常常所有的皮损都被抓破了,而且诊断必须基于此症状和皮损分布(图 25.20)。

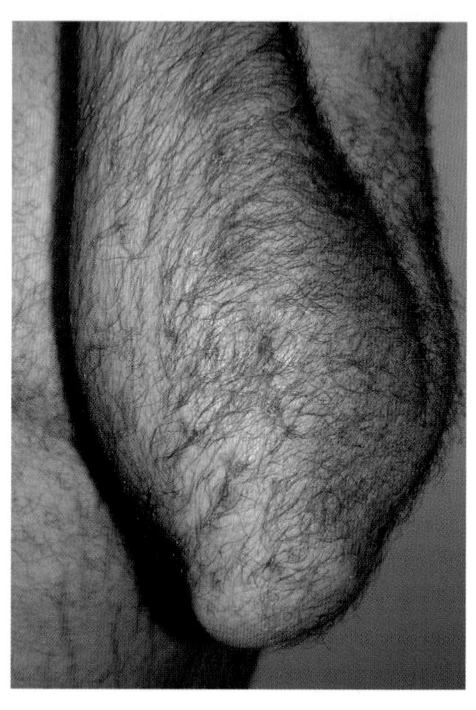

图 25.20　疱疹样皮炎表现为瘙痒、荨麻疹性丘疹和集中在肘、膝和臀部的小水疱。(Courtesy Dr. Benjamin Lockshin, Silver Spring, MD.)

DH 的诊断是由皮肤活检和皮肤直接免疫荧光检查得出的,在皮肤乳头瘙痒处和囊泡形成处发现 IgA 沉积。DH 患者通常患有与乳糜泻(celiac disease, CD)无法区分的肠病。其人白细胞抗原(HLA)模式包括单倍型 B8、DR3 和 DQw2,肠道吸收不良,出现肌内膜抗体,醇溶蛋白,组织型转谷氨酰胺酶(transglutaminase, TG),以及小肠活检结果,均类似于 CD 患者。尽管有这些相似之处,只有不到 5%的患者 DH 有胃肠道疾病症状。已证实谷蛋白是 DH 的食物诱因。即使是肠道活检结果正常的微小肠道疾病患者,无麸质饮食也能改善病情。无谷蛋白饮食的无症状患者再次摄入谷蛋白会导致瘙痒和皮肤病变的再次出现。

一个致病机制可以说明 DH 和 CD 的关系。在 CD 患者中,IgA 抗体产生于与脱氨基麦胶蛋白肽交联的 TG2 组织(来源于饮食中的小麦、大麦或黑麦,由抗原提呈细胞上的 HLA-DQ2 或 HLA-DQ8 分子呈现)。表皮形式的 TG、TG3 的 IgA 抗体被认为是表位扩散的结果,这些抗体最终在真皮乳头状区与 TG3 形成抗原-抗体复合物,导致 DH 的临床和病理结果。这个模型可以解释为什么 DH 通常比有症状的 CD 出现在较晚的年龄,而且较轻的肠道疾病,因为在该表位中传播可能需要时间以及持续暴露于谷蛋白[35]。

因为有时很难将 DH 与其他水疱性皮肤病区分开来，因此可将严重瘙痒性皮疹患者转诊进行内镜检查。在瘙痒患者中发现与乳糜泻一致的小肠异常，高度提示 DH（见第 107 章）。DH 的皮损对磺胺类药物（氨苯砜或磺胺吡啶）有显著的反应，但磺胺类药物对肠道病理和皮肤免疫荧光无影响。无麸质饮食治疗可逐渐清除皮肤病变，改善肠道异常，消失皮肤中 IgA，并降低对氨苯砜控制皮疹的依赖性[36]。

十、维生素和矿物质缺乏

虽然许多维生素缺乏会导致不同的皮肤表现（图 25.21 和图 25.22），但表 25.3 总结了所有与胃肠道和肝脏疾病最相关的结果，以及治疗剂量[31]（另见第 6 和 104 章）。

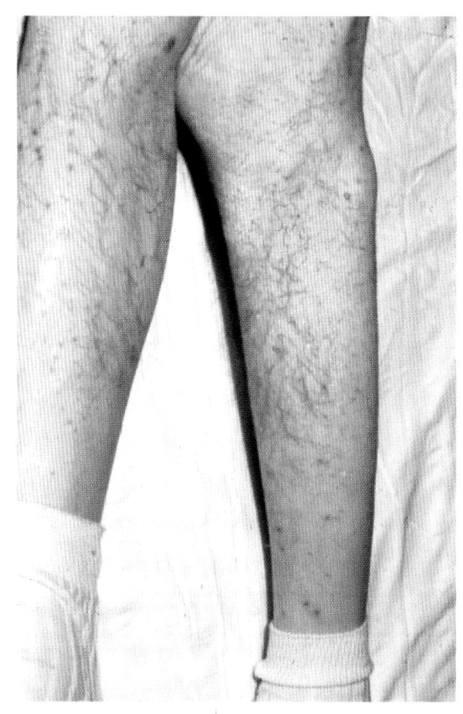

图 25.21　患有惠普尔病的老年男性的下肢，毛囊周围出血明显。血浆维生素 C 水平降低。补充维生素 C 后，皮损迅速消失。（Courtesy Dr. Mark Feldman，Dallas，TX.）

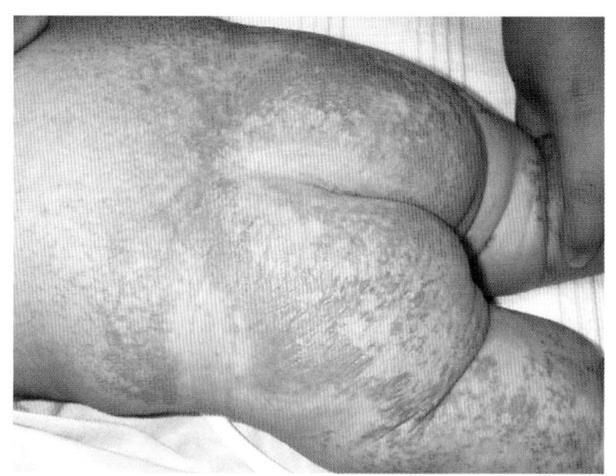

图 25.22　营养锌缺乏继发肠病性肢端皮炎女婴。她以米饭和水为食。（Courtesy Dr. Genevieve Wallace，Dallas，TX.）

表 25.3　营养异常和相关皮肤表现

营养异常	原因	临床特征	治疗
烟酸缺乏症（糙皮病）	饮食不当	暴露在阳光下的对称红棕色水疱或者鳞样斑块	烟酸：
	用药（异烟肼）	舌痛、萎缩性舌炎	轻度：50mg 口服 每日 3 次
	类癌综合征	4Ds：皮炎，腹泻，痴呆，死亡	有症状：25mg 静脉或肌内注射 每日 3 次
			进展：50～100mg 静脉或肌内注射 每日 3 次×3～4 天，口服治疗维持
缺锌	先天性代谢异常	浅表鳞屑疹，突出于腹股沟及口周	锌：获得型口服 1～2mg/kg/d；先天型和肠病性肢端皮炎口服 3mg/kg/d
（遗传性肠病性肢端皮炎）	酒精性肝硬化	脱发	生物素：口服或者肌内注射，10～40mg/d
必需脂肪酸缺乏	无充分补充的高营养		
生物素缺乏	克罗恩病		
维生素 C 缺乏（坏血病）	酗酒	滤泡角化过度及滤泡周出血	抗坏血酸，口服，800mg/d
	克罗恩病	瘀斑	
	Whipple 病	干燥病	
		伤口愈合不良	
		螺旋状体毛	
		牙龈炎伴牙龈出血	
胰高血糖素瘤综合征（坏死性迁移性红斑）	胰腺分泌胰高血糖素的神经内分泌肿瘤	张力大的红斑进展为松弛大疱和结痂并破裂	手术切除肿瘤
	肝硬化和空肠黏膜绒毛萎缩时亦会出现	最常见于面部中央、间擦区域、大腿、臀部和四肢远端	生长抑素类似物或补充锌有时在等待手术时可获益
		常有疼痛或瘙痒	

Modified from Nieves D，Goldsmith L. Cutaneous changes in nutritional disease. In：Freedberg I，Eisen A，Wolff F，editors. Fitzpatrick's dermatology in general medicine. New York：McGraw-Hill；2003. pp 1399-1412.

（郭晓燕　译，鲁晓岚　校）

参考文献

第 26 章 咽、食管、胃和小肠憩室

Kerry B. dunbar, D. Rohan Jeyarajah 著

章节目录

一、Zenker 憩室 …… 352
(一) 流行病学、病因学和病理生理学 …… 352
(二) 临床特征和诊断 …… 352
(三) 并发症 …… 353
(四) 治疗和预后 …… 353
二、食管体部憩室 …… 354
(一) 流行病学、病因学和病理生理学 …… 354
(二) 临床特征和诊断 …… 354
(三) 并发症 …… 354
(四) 治疗和预后 …… 355
三、食管壁内假性憩室 …… 355
(一) 流行病学、病因学和病理生理学 …… 355
(二) 临床特征和诊断 …… 356
(三) 并发症 …… 356
(四) 治疗和预后 …… 356
四、胃憩室 …… 356
(一) 流行病学、病因学和病理生理学 …… 356
(二) 临床特征和诊断 …… 356
(三) 并发症 …… 356
(四) 治疗和预后 …… 357
五、十二指肠憩室 …… 357
(一) 腔外憩室 …… 357
(二) 腔内憩室 …… 358
六、空肠憩室 …… 359
(一) 流行病学、病因学和病理生理学 …… 359
(二) 临床特征和诊断 …… 359
(三) 并发症 …… 359
(四) 治疗和预后 …… 359

憩室是管状结构向外突出而形成。真性憩室累及肠壁的各个层面，而假性憩室是由于黏膜和黏膜下层通过肌层形成的疝。许多憩室含有变薄的肌层，因此很难定义为真或假。真性憩室常被认为是先天性病变，假性憩室常被认为是后天获得的，但并非总是如此。一些作者保留了"假性憩室"这一术语，是基于假性憩室系炎症过程所致的。本章讨论胃肠道各部分的憩室，但 Meckel 憩室和结肠憩室除外，这两部分在第 98 和 121 章中都有涉及。

一、Zenker 憩室

Ludlow 于 1767 年首次描述了一位下咽憩室患者，在 1877 年 Zenker 和 Von Ziemssen 报道了 23 个这样的患者[1,2]。

(一) 流行病学、病因学和病理生理学

据统计，Zenker 憩室的患病率在 0.1% ~ 0.01%，发病年龄通常在 70 ~ 80 岁。患 Zenker 憩室的男性是女性的两倍[3,4]。Zenker 憩室。当吞咽过程中出现异常高压，通过咽部解剖薄弱的 Killian 三角，导致黏膜突出（见第 43 章）。Killian 三角位于食管上括约肌（upper esophageal sphincter，UES）环咽肌横纤维与咽下缩肌斜纤维相交的后方。这一薄弱点的大小因人而异。相对较大的三角可能易导致 Zenker 憩室的发生[4]。

在 Zenker 憩室中，食管 UES 开放受损，吞咽时产生高压。在 Zenker 憩室患者中，环咽部有多种病理生理改变，包括炎症和纤维化，导致环咽部顺应性差和异常松弛[5,6]。这些改变导致食管 UES 顺应性降低和开放减少[3]。其他与 Zenker 憩表现相似的憩室已被报告为颈椎前路手术的并发症[7,8]。Killian-Jamieson 憩室位于环咽肌下方，与 Zenker 憩室相似[9]。

(二) 临床特征和诊断

常见症状见框 26.1，吞咽困难和反流是最常见的症状。小憩室患者可能无症状。在一些患者中，可以发现 Boyce 征，即左前颈部可触及的结节或肿块，触诊时可能发出咯咯声[10]。

框 26.1 Zenker 憩室患者的常见症状
误吸
窒息
吞咽困难
口臭
反流
声音改变
体重减轻

通过仔细询问病史发现高度怀疑 Zenker 憩室的患者。吞钡是最有用的诊断方法。应事先通知放射科医生，以提供适当的意见（图 26.1B；参见第 44 章）。小憩室只能短暂可见。钡剂吞入侧位透视有助于小憩室的检出。大的 Zenker 憩室的开口常常与食管的轴线对齐。口服造影剂将优先填满憩室，并逐渐从憩室中清空。因此，大憩室即使在延迟图像中也很明显。Zenker 憩室几乎总是发生在颈部左侧。

Zenker 憩室可能是在吞钡或上胃肠道内镜检查不相关问题中偶然发现的（见图 26.1A）。当评估有可疑症状的患者是否存在 Zenker 憩室时，考虑在内镜检查前先进行钡餐检查。

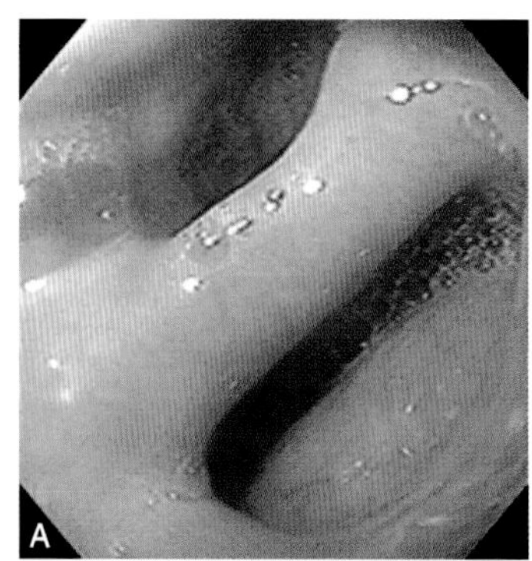

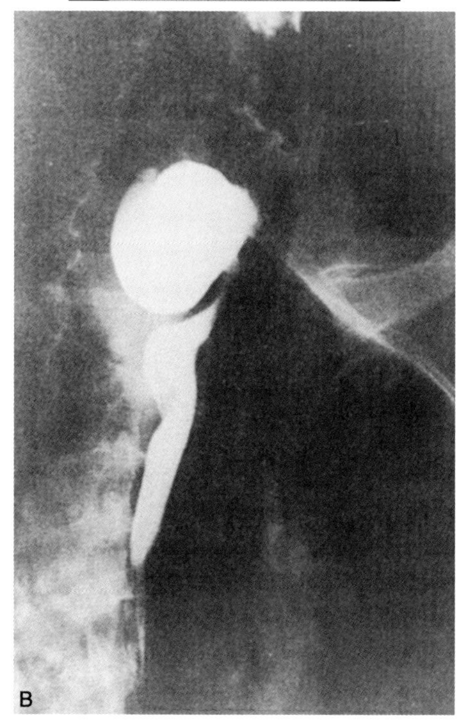

图 26.1　Zenker 憩室。A,内镜视图。食管腔与憩室腔往往难以区分。B,钡餐食管造影显示憩室大到足以充盈时,引起食管梗阻。(A,Courtesy of the late Dr. David Langdon;B,Courtesy Dr. Charles E. Pope,Seattle,WA.)

在内镜检查中,如果在进入咽部时无法定位 UES,应怀疑 Zenker 憩室。在这种情况下,应停止内镜检查,并将患者送往钡餐检查。

(三) 并发症

Zenker 憩室可发展为鳞状细胞癌;其发病率大约为 0.4%~1.5%[3,11]。如果在没有憩室切除术计划的情况下行肌切开术,应仔细检查憩室内壁有无癌变迹象。

溃疡性 Zenker 憩室可出血[12]。吸入残留食物可能导致吸入性肺炎[13,14]。药物可能卡在 Zenker 憩室,引起溃疡和疼痛,也会导致药物疗效降低[15,16]。由于 Zenker 憩室在体检中偶尔可触及,因此很难与甲状腺结节区分开来,而且 Zenker 憩室中放射性碘示踪剂的积累也被报道是转移性甲状腺癌的误诊[17]。用于胶囊内镜检查的视频胶囊也可能滞留在 Zenker 憩室中,当需要进行此类研究时,应通过内镜将其送入胃中[18]。

Zenker 憩室的存在导致气管或食管插管困难。大憩室使食管腔移位。插管器械的尖端往往优先导向憩室。在内镜下,很难将憩室腔与食管的真腔区分开(见图 26.1A)。气管插管、放置鼻胃管、食管插管用于上胃肠道内镜检查、内镜逆行胆管胰造影术或经食管超声心动图可能都很困难,会发生穿孔。Zenker 憩室患者食管插管应在直视下进行。当较大的 Zenker 憩室引起明显的解剖畸形或需要侧视内镜插管时,直接插管是不谨慎的。在这种情况下,可以使用前视内镜将导丝穿过食管腔[19]。然后将导丝反装入内镜中,内镜通过导丝进入食管。另一种技术是通过一个装载了外套管前视内镜。当内镜进入食管后,外套管推进,前视内镜被撤回,侧视或超声内镜通过外套管[20]。

(四) 治疗和预后

小的无症状或轻微症状的憩室患者可以随访,因为进展性扩大是不常见的[21,22]。大憩室且有症状的 Zenker 憩室患者应予以治疗[22,23]。

Zenker 憩室可采用开放式手术或使用硬性或软性经口内镜技术治疗。通过左侧颈部的开放手术方式是向胸腔延伸的大 Zenker 憩室(>5cm)患者典型的选择[24]。年轻患者和小憩室患者也可能是开放手术的候选对象[25]。大憩室可切除、内翻或悬吊(憩室固定术)。环咽肌切开术用于治疗高张力环咽肌,是治疗这种疾病的关键;切开高张力环咽肌以解除远端梗阻。如果憩室在不做肌切开术的情况下被切除,术后瘘和复发的风险也会增加[25,26]。开放式手术并发症包括吻合口瘘、纵隔炎、食管皮肤瘘、喉返神经损伤引起的声带麻痹(喉返神经位于气管食管沟内)。一项对 22 项研究的回顾,包括 1 793 名因 Zenker 憩室接受开放式手术的患者,发现在 36 个月的中位随访中,初始成功率为 96%,发病率为 11%,穿孔或瘘发生率为 5%,症状复发率为 3.5%[23]。

Zenker 憩室的内镜治疗可以使用硬性或软性内镜,在食管和憩室之间分隔纤维间隔[25,27]。与开放手术相比,内镜手术具有麻醉时间更短,并发症发生率更低,住院时间更短的三大优势。内镜技术适用于中等大小(2~5cm)憩室患者。已采用硬性憩室镜和软性内镜。憩室镜用于提供最佳的食管管腔、憩室及其间隔的显示(图 26.2)。这个隔膜是由食管后壁和憩室前壁组成的,包括食管上括约肌。切开隔膜和食管上括约肌的肌层,从而恢复单腔。

切口可以通过许多技术来完成。在硬性憩室镜下,可以使用二氧化碳激光、外科吻合器、氩等离子体凝固、电灼术或超声刀进行手术[22,25]。内镜下吻合器的技术依赖于将吻合器的一条腿置入食管,另一条腿置入憩室。然后将隔膜分开,在分隔线的每一边用两行吻合器钉住。Zenker 憩室必须至少 3cm 的长度,才能容纳一个足够长度的吻合器。吻合器和其他技术的改进可以改善短憩室的疗效[28]。内镜手术的并发症包括出血、穿孔和瘘,但如果使用吻合器辅助技术,这些是不常见的。在对 Zenker 憩室进行硬性内镜治疗的综述中,结合 494 例患者的 11 项研究,中位初始成功率为 95%,中转开放手术率为 4%,主要发病率为 3%,中位随访 16 个月后症状复发率为 5%[23]。软性内镜技术在治疗 Zenker 憩室方面也有一定作用,因为硬性内镜不能用于颈部伸展受限或张口能力受限的患者[26]。在内镜上连接透明帽或软性憩室镜可以

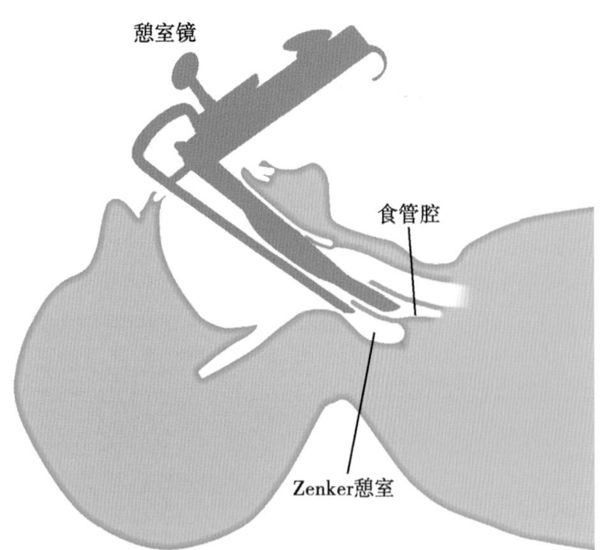

图 26.2　憩室镜。该器械的定位旨在暴露食管腔与 Zenker 憩室之间的共同壁

改善视觉效果[29-31]。多种技术可用于实施内镜肌切开术，包括针刀、氩等离子凝固、单极钳和超声刀[22,29]。软性内镜技术的并发症包括常见的颈部和纵隔气肿，以及穿孔和纵隔炎。在对 813 例接受软性内镜治疗的 Zenker 憩室患者的 20 项研究中，初始成功率 91%，不良事件发生率 11%，中位随访 23 个月后复发率 11%[32]。软性内视镜治疗 Zenker 憩室通常由外科医生进行，但一些内镜专家已经开始实施这些手术[4]。

二、食管体部憩室

食管体部憩室最常位于食管中下三分之一处(图 26.3)。

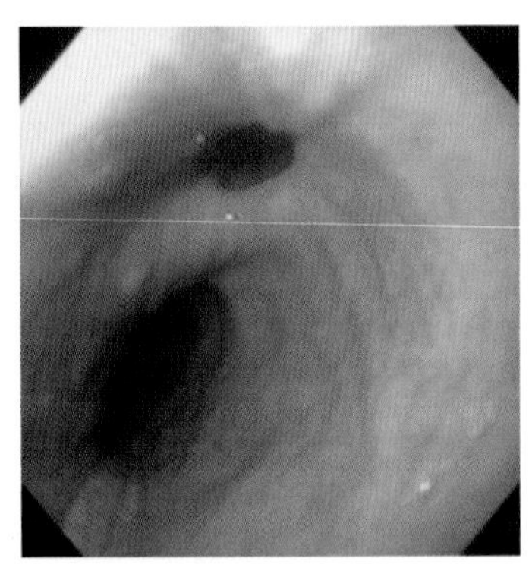

图 26.3　食管中段憩室的内镜视图。当食管充气良好时，这些憩室最明显

(一) 流行病学、病因学和病理生理学

食管体部憩室的发生率从尸检的 0.015% 到吞咽障碍放射学评估的患者的 2% 不等[33,34]。这些憩室可分为两类：牵引型和膨出型憩室。牵引型憩室是由食管外的炎性、纤维化或肿瘤过程引起的。牵引型憩室常与结核或组织胞浆菌病引起的纵隔炎有关[35]。肺恶性肿瘤引起的纵隔淋巴结肿大也可能导致牵引型憩室。膨出型憩室是由运动障碍引起的典型症状。

膨出型最常见的类型是位于膈肌裂孔附近的憩室，称之为膈上憩室(图 26.4)。大约 80% 的膈上憩室与食管运动障碍有关，如贲门失弛缓症或食管远端痉挛，这将在第 43 章讨论[36,37]。膈上憩室已被报道为束带式肥胖手术的并发症，其原因在于束带阻塞食管和胃的上段(见第 8 章)[38,39]。先天性支气管肺-前肠畸形也可合并食管憩室[40]。

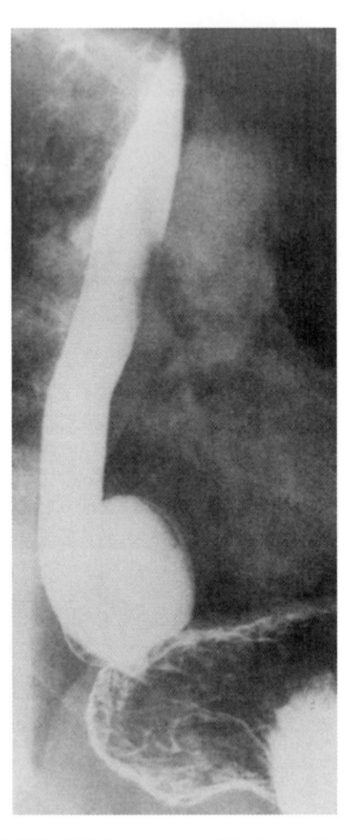

图 26.4　食管钡剂造影显示胃上方有膈上憩室。在这种投影中，憩室可能与食管裂孔疝相混淆。(Courtesy Dr. Charles A. Rohrmann and Dr. Charles E. Pope, Seattle, WA.)

(二) 临床特征和诊断

先天性和牵引性食管憩室通常无症状，特别是在食管中下段。如果诊断时没有出现症状，则在随访期间很少发生。当症状出现时，最常见的是吞咽困难、食物反流、反流、体重减轻和胸部不适[41]。吞咽困难可能是由潜在的动力障碍或由大的憩室压迫食管，使憩室优先充盈而引起的[36,37,42]。然而，支气管肺-前肠瘘可以发展，导致咳嗽、肺炎和反复的支气管肺部感染[43]。膈上憩室的诊断在内镜或钡剂造影时可以得出。膈上憩室在胸片上可能被误认为膈疝或重复囊肿。内镜检查可显示空憩室或食物残渣的存在(图 26.5A)。最好的诊断方法是吞钡，这样可以比内镜检查更精确地观察憩室并定位(图 26.5B)。放射科医生必须警惕这种诊断的可能性，因为需要斜位视图来显示憩室。CT 也应该考虑，以确保没有可能导致膨出型憩室的相关病理性淋巴结肿大或肿块病变。

(三) 并发症

鳞状细胞癌已被报道发生在膈上憩室中[44,45]。与 Zenker

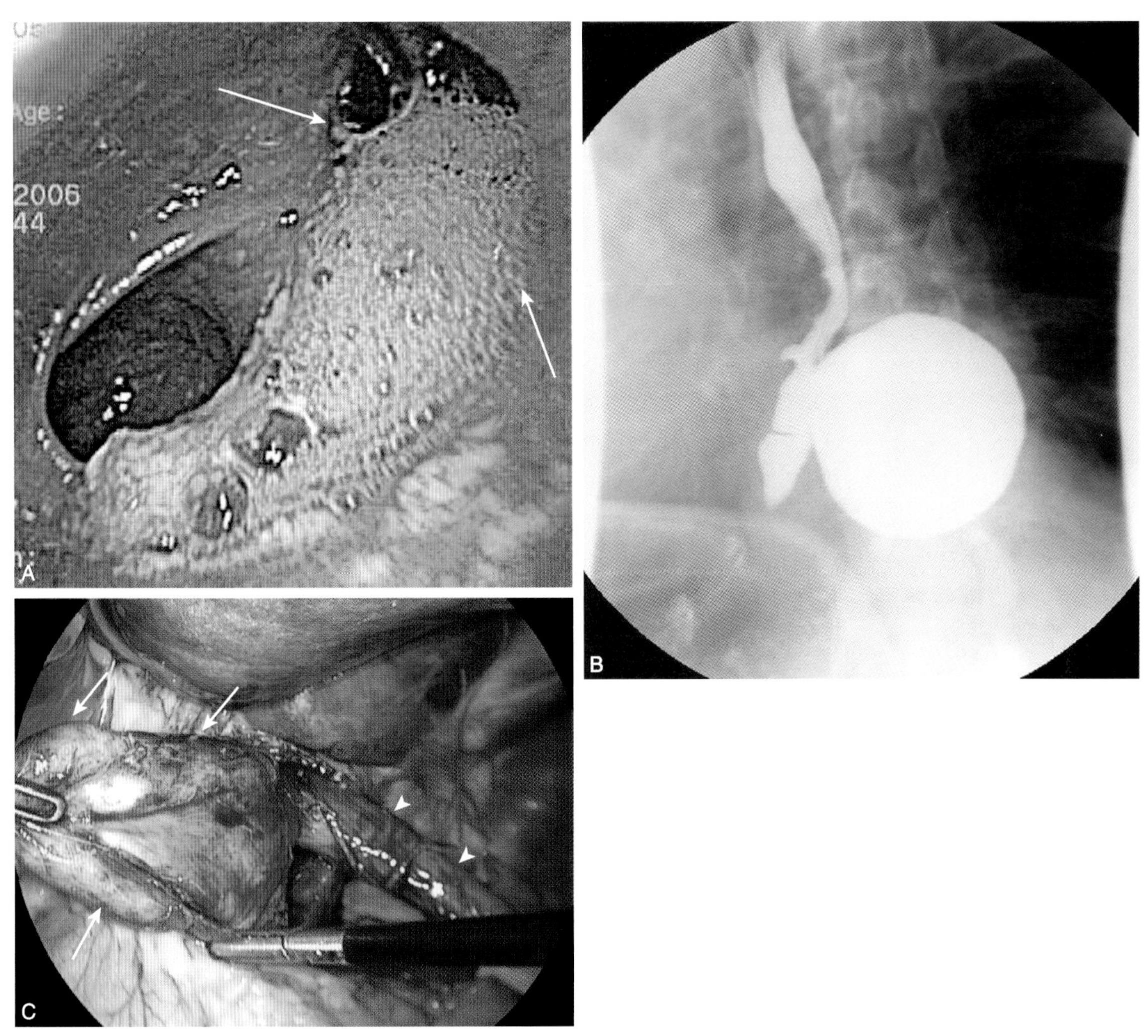

图 26.5　巨大食管憩室。A,含食物和液体(箭)的巨大食管憩室的内镜视图。B,食管钡餐造影显示食管憩室较大。C,腹腔镜下切除食管(箭头)大憩室(箭)。(B 和 C,Courtesy Dr,Thai Pham,Dallas,TX.)

憩室一样,放射性碘示踪剂在食管憩室积聚被误认为转移性甲状腺癌[46]。食管憩室溃疡出血同样会出现[47]。憩室内容物的反流和误吸可能使麻醉的诱导复杂化。在鼻胃管插管或上胃肠道(upper gastrointestinal,UGI)内镜检查时可能发生穿孔。

(四) 治疗和预后

无症状的食管憩室不需要治疗。只有与憩室症状明显相关的患者才应治疗。术前内镜检查和测压是可取的。将测压导管通过憩室进入胃是困难的,但贲门失弛缓症或远端食管痉挛的证明有助于指导治疗[48]。食管憩室的手术治疗可采用开放式、腹腔镜、腹腔镜-胸腔镜联合手术或机器人技术[49,50]。膈上憩室通常适合腹腔镜手术,其优点是住院时间较短,恢复正常活动较快(见图 26.5C)。大憩室可内翻或切除。考虑到贲门失弛缓症等相关运动障碍的高发病率,食管肌切开术可在大多数情况下进行[41,49]。小憩室可以不切除而行肌切开术。放弃憩室切除术的好处是没有要愈合的缝合线,降低了渗漏的风险。必须认识到,这些症状通常与潜在的运动障碍有关,而与憩室本身无关。因此,治疗潜在疾病,通常用肌切开术,是手术的关键组成部分。这可以在没有做过多次手术的健康人腹腔镜下完成。为了防止胃食管反流,通常要进行部分后(Toupet)或前(Dor)的胃底折叠术[41,49]。

食管憩室手术患者预后良好,症状改善率为 88.5%,实施憩室切除术后症状缓解率较好[49]。

三、食管壁内假性憩室

食管壁内假性憩室(esophageal intramural pseudodiverticul,EIP)最早于 1960 年被发现[51]。假性憩室是大小 1~4mm、来自食管腔的烧瓶状外袋物。

(一) 流行病学、病因学和病理生理学

EIP 比少量已发表病例报告中更为常见。0.09%~0.15%的吞钡研究证实了 EIP[52,53]。EIP 患者好发于 60~70 岁。这种情况男性略多于女性[54]。

EIP 是黏膜下腺体异常扩张的导管。它们被认为是后天获得的,通常与引起慢性食管炎症的条件有关。导管因周围炎症或纤维化而扩张[55]。食管狭窄通常与 EIP 有关,但胃食

管反流病、慢性念珠菌病、腐蚀性摄入、食管癌和嗜酸性食管炎也与 EIP 有关[52-54,56,57]。在一些病例中，CT 或超声内镜检查显示食管壁明显增厚[58,59]。

（二）临床特征和诊断

EIP 可在因吞咽困难或胃灼热做吞钡时发现（图 26.6A）。EIP 也可能是无相关症状患者的偶然结果。在大多数病例中，食管假性憩室是局部的，但在 40% 的病例中弥漫性分散在整个食管中[54]。狭窄是常见的，也可能发生相邻假性憩室之间的跟踪或交通[60,61]。吞钡检查的鉴别诊断包括食管溃疡。虽然 EIP 的内镜表现具有特征性（图 26.6B），EIP 的开口很小，经常被遗漏。位于狭窄区域内的 EIP 在内镜检查时特别难以看到。当出现症状时，一般与相关疾病（如狭窄或念珠菌病）有关，而不是与 EIP 相关。

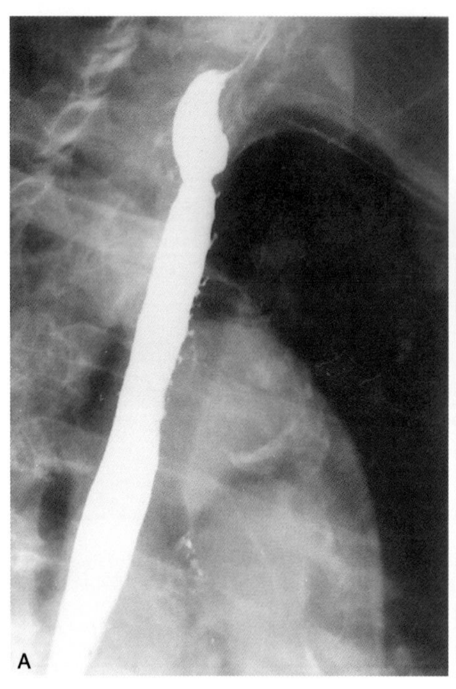

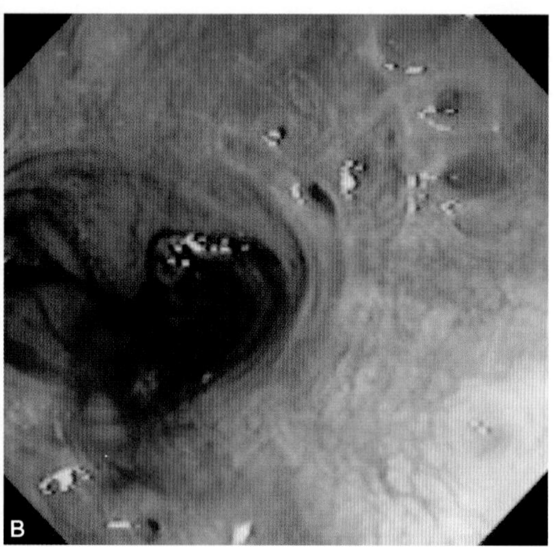

图 26.6　食管壁内假性憩室。A，钡餐食管造影显示有小的突出。B，内镜视图。在该患者中观察到假性憩室的微小开口，该患者还存在远端食管消化性狭窄

（三）并发症

EIP 引起的并发症很少。如果存在狭窄，必须通过上胃肠道内镜排除癌症；食管癌在 EIP 患者中发病率增加[52]。EPI 穿孔导致纵隔炎的病例报道罕见[62,63]。

（四）治疗和预后

EIP 的治疗应针对潜在的情况，如狭窄、酸反流或念珠菌病。据报道，食管扩张可以改善 EIP 患者吞咽困难的症状。在一系列 22 例 EIP 患者中，吞咽困难的患者经食管探条治疗后症状均有改善，常常需要多次扩张。另外，57% 的患者因复发性吞咽困难而需要再次行扩张术[61]。即使治疗后患者的症状能缓解，EIP 也可能持续存在[54]。

四、胃憩室

胃憩室并不常见，通常是内镜或影像学检查中偶然发现的。

（一）流行病学、病因学和病理生理学

胃憩室仅在 0.04% 的上胃肠道造影和 0.02% 的尸检中发现[64]。近贲门憩室占所有胃憩室的 75%。它们最常位于胃食管交界处的小弯侧后壁（图 26.7A）[65]。尽管在儿童和青少年中也有报告，但最常见于中年患者[66]。它们的直径一般在 1~3cm，但偶尔也会更大。胃憩室或部分憩室是由胃黏膜通过肌层凸出而形成的。这些憩室在大弯侧最常见[67,68]。消化性溃疡或其他炎症过程引起的畸形类似于钡餐检查或内镜检查时的幽门前憩室（图 26.7B）。虽然胃憩室也可以在 Roux-en-Y 胃旁路术后见到，但是胃憩室已被报道为肥胖手术的并发症，尤其是垂直捆绑胃成形术[69,70]。

（二）临床特征和诊断

近贲门憩室几乎总是无症状的。患者偶尔会因憩室引起的疼痛或消化不良。内镜检查时，近贲门憩室最好反转镜身观察。除非采用侧位观察，否则钡餐检查就可能错过它们。CT 表现为充满空气或造影剂的肾上肿块，可误认为肾上腺肿块或囊肿[71]。憩室如果只有液体填充，会导致诊断困难；这可能被误认为是胰腺囊性病变。空气和液体的结合使放射科医生考虑与胰腺脓肿的鉴别。壁内憩室通常不会引起症状。在钡餐检查中，它们经常被误认为是溃疡。

（三）并发症

胃憩室的并发症是罕见的。癌症很少发生[72,73]。出血很少发生，可能需要联合治疗止血，如止血夹和注射肾上腺

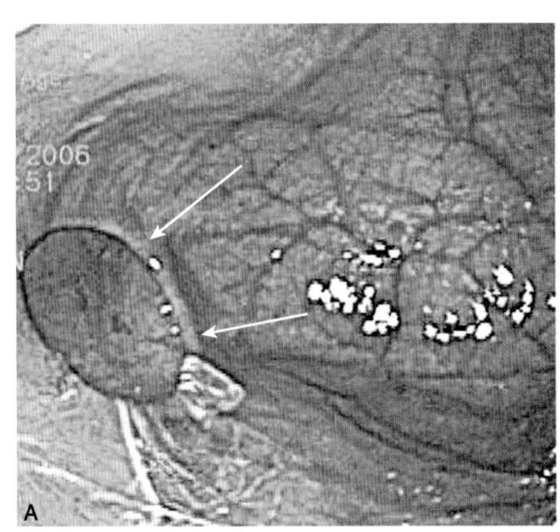

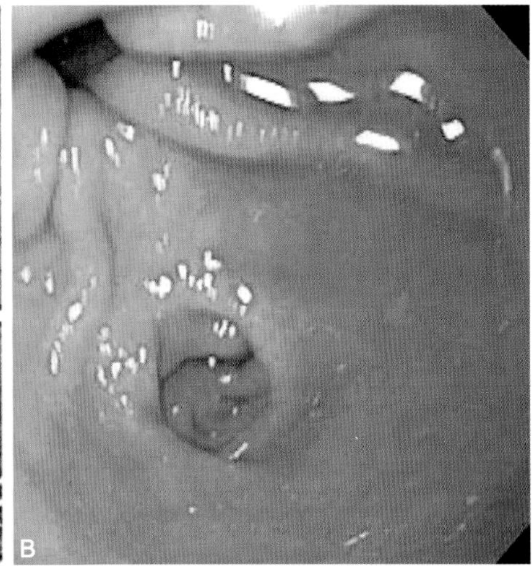

图 26.7　A，近贲门憩室。在反转镜身观察到该宽口憩室（箭）。憩室内黏膜正常。B，幽门前胃憩室

素[74,75]。穿孔也很罕见[75]。内镜技术不能控制的出血，可能需要中转手术。

（四）治疗和预后

壁内憩室无需干预。近贲门憩室几乎不需要治疗。在考虑切除术前，应明确特定症状之间的关联，因为更常见的诊断（如消化不良、反流）可能导致不明原因的上胃肠道症状。如果近贲门憩室患者被转诊接受手术，应谨慎在憩室附近放置内镜标记，以在手术过程中辅助定位。腹腔镜憩室切除术可用于症状或穿孔的简单切除[76]。在这些病例中，在腹腔镜下游离胃，吻合憩室，使大部分胃保持完整。小心处理食管胃交界处附近的近端憩室，避免吻合器造成该区域狭窄。在胃食管交界处放置探条，有助于避免憩室手术引起的狭窄。

五、十二指肠憩室

十二指肠憩室可以是腔外的，也可以是腔内的。

（一）腔外憩室

1. 流行病学、病因学和病理生理学

在大约 5% 的上胃肠道 X 线检查中可观察到腔外十二指肠憩室，在大约 20% ~ 30% 的 ERCP 研究中观察到[77,78]。它们被认为是获得性的，通常见于年龄超过 50 岁的患者[78]。它们发生在十二指肠壁的一个区域，在该区域中血管穿透肌层或背侧和腹侧胰腺在胚胎发育中融合。约 75% 位于壶腹部 2cm 以内，十二指肠内侧壁上，称为乳头旁憩室（juxtapapillary diverticula，JPD）（图 26.8A）。

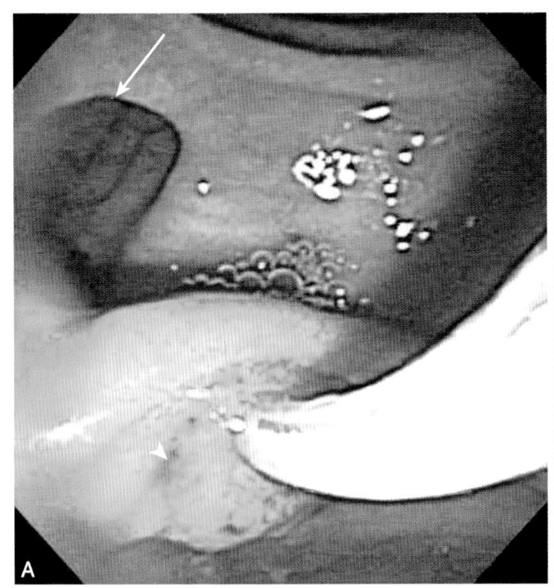

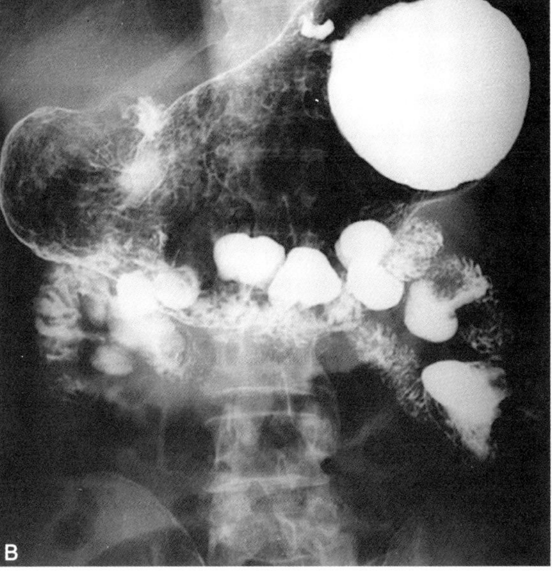

图 26.8　A，ERCP 中发现的乳头旁憩室（箭）。将括约肌刀插入附近的壶腹部（箭头）。B，上胃肠道造影显示多发性十二指肠大憩室。（A，Courtesy Dr. Zeeshan Ramzan，Dallas，TX.）

2. 临床特征和诊断

十二指肠憩室有时可通过上胃肠道 X 线诊断。除非使用侧视内镜,否则很容易在内镜检查中遗漏。十二指肠憩室在各种影像学检查(超声、CT、MRI 或 PET-CT)中可能被误认为是胰腺假性囊肿、胰周积液、胰腺脓肿、胰腺囊性肿瘤、高代谢肿块或远端胆管结石[79-83]。

如果在 CT 或 MRI 上怀疑憩室,可以通过让患者饮水并重复扫描,或者在 MRI 过程中使用阴性造影剂来明确诊断[84,85]。

3. 并发症

虽然十二指肠腔外憩室较为常见,但并发症少见。十二指肠腔外憩室的并发症包括穿孔或憩室炎、出血、急性胰腺炎和胆管结石[77,86-88]。十二指肠憩室炎可表现为游离或包裹性穿孔。患者表现为上腹部疼痛,常向背部放射,可能有脓毒症的症状和体征。腹部 CT 扫描可显示十二指肠增厚、腹膜后积气、蜂窝织炎或脓肿。

十二指肠憩室内的 Dieulafoy 样病变或溃疡曾报告出血[89,90]。十二指肠憩室出血可能很难诊断,需要用侧视内镜或血管造影检查。在一些患者中,只有手术时才能发现出血部位。

多发性十二指肠憩室患者可能出现细菌过度生长和吸收不良(图 26.8B)(见第 104 和 105 章)[91]。JPD 与胆管结石、胆管炎、奥迪括约肌功能障碍(sphincter of Oddi dysfunction, SOD)(见第 63 章)和复发性胰腺炎有关,被认为是由于胰管异常进入憩室引起的[77,92-95]。即使在括约肌切开术后,也可能发生胆管延迟排空。憩室内淤积可导致细菌过度生长,加快胆盐解离,从而增加原发性胆管结石的危险[77,96]。

由经验丰富的内镜医生进行 ERCP 时,JPD 不会明显增加插管的难度或并发症的风险[78,97]。有几种方法可以克服位于憩室深处的壶腹相关的困难[78,97]。

4. 治疗和预后

十二指肠腔外憩室很少需要治疗干预。对于腹部症状不明确的患者绝不能实施十二指肠憩室切除术。

出血、憩室炎和穿孔是与十二指肠憩室相关的最常见的并发症。憩室出血已能通过内镜下各种技术(包括双极电灼术、肾上腺素注射和止血夹)控制[89,90,98]。如果术前无法确定诊断,可以通过十二指肠切开术来止血。

如果可行的话,许多十二指肠穿孔或憩室炎患者接受诊断性和治疗性的手术,包括引流和切除所涉及的憩室。在切除憩室时,可损伤胰管和胆管,导致胆胰瘘和胰腺炎。如果十二指肠憩室炎在术前明确诊断,经皮穿刺引流和抗生素保守治疗是首选[88]。胰十二指肠切除术(Whipple 手术)是最后的治疗手段,对于在憩室切除术时意外横断胆管和胰管的患者可能需要。

(二) 腔内憩室

1. 流行病学、病因学和发病机制

十二指肠腔内憩室罕见。大多数患者的年龄在 30~60 岁,男女发病率相同[99]。十二指肠腔内憩室(袋状憩室)是起源于十二指肠第二部分的单个囊状结构。它们与整个圆周相连或仅与十二指肠壁的一部分相连,可向远端突出至十二指肠壁的第四部分。通常在囊内有一个偏心的第二开口(图 26.9)。憩室两侧衬有十二指肠黏膜。

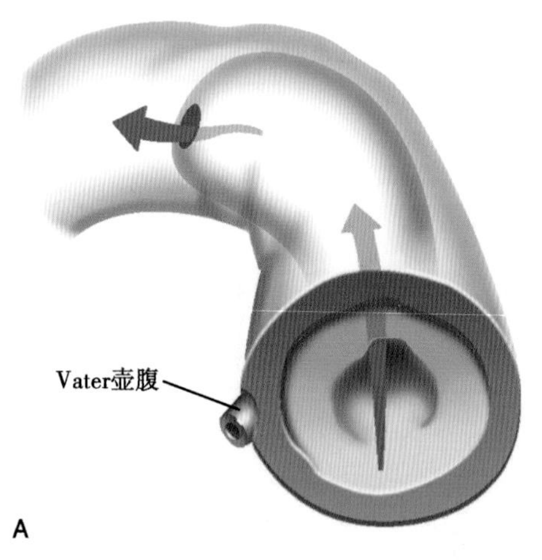

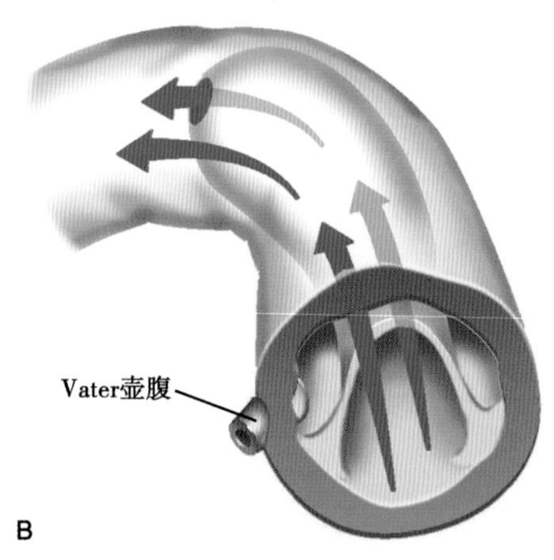

图 26.9　壁内十二指肠憩室[风向袋憩室(windsock diverticulum)]。A,憩室附着于整个十二指肠周。B,憩室仅附着于十二指肠周的一部分

在胎儿发育早期过程中,十二指肠管腔被增生的上皮细胞堵塞,随后再通(见第 49 章)。异常再通可能导致十二指肠隔膜或十二指肠蹼。随着时间的推移,蠕动拉伸可将隔膜转变为腔内憩室。

2. 临床特征和诊断

腔内憩室通常无症状,但可能在任何年龄出现症状。最常见的症状是十二指肠不完全梗阻,包括恶心、呕吐和腹痛[99]。典型的 X 线表现为长度不一的、充满钡剂的球状结构,起源于十二指肠的第二部分,其底部延伸至第三部分,并由较细的放射透线勾勒出来。CT 表现报告为十二指肠第二部分管腔内环形软组织密度影,轮廓为口服造影剂,含口服造影剂和少量空气(晕轮征)[100]。

在内镜检查时,腔内憩室是呈偏心性囊状结构,如为内翻性口,表现为一个大的、柔软的息肉样肿块[101,102]。内镜诊断可能很困难。长囊可能被误认为十二指肠腔,而内翻的憩室可能被误认为大息肉。

3. 并发症

由于植物性物质或异物滞留在憩室内可引起梗阻,通常

包括食物和较少见的硬币或大理石[103-105]。还报告了胰腺炎和出血[92,101]。憩室引起的慢性部分梗阻,可能导致胃潴留或十二指肠球部扩张。

4. 治疗和预后

治疗可能包括对有阻塞或出血症状的患者进行切除,可在腹腔镜下进行[99]。同时也有内镜下成功切除十二指肠腔内憩室的报道[106]。

六、空肠憩室

1881 年,William Osler 爵士写了一篇关于一位空肠憩室患者的文章。多年来,这位患者"一直饱受腹部里巨大隆隆作响的痛苦,尤其是每顿饭后。声音太大了,以至于在进餐后不久习惯出去散步以远离人群,因为在一定距离内都可以听到噪声"[107]。

(一) 流行病学、病因学和病理生理学

小肠憩室(十二指肠和 Meckel 憩室除外)最常见于近端空肠,见于约 1% 的人群[108]。大约 80% 的空回肠憩室发生在空肠,15% 发生于回肠,5% 两者均有,约 0.5% ~5% 通过小肠 X 线检查和尸检发现小肠憩室[109,110]。它们通常是多发性的,大小从几毫米到几厘米不等。它们通常位于小肠的肠系膜缘。小肠憩室通常缺乏真正的肌肉壁,被认为是获得性的。

空回肠憩室的病因尚不清楚。许多患者有潜在的肠动力障碍。周期性腔内压力升高可通过血管穿透肌层的肠系膜缘薄弱区导致疝的形成。内脏神经病变和肌病,包括进行性系统性硬化症,可导致肠壁慢性萎缩和纤维化,从而导致疝和憩室的形成(见第 37 章)[111]。

(二) 临床特征和诊断

空肠憩室最好通过上胃肠道 X 线摄影联合小肠随访或 CT 联合口服造影剂进行诊断,也能通过小肠镜检查或胶囊内镜检查进行识别[112-115]。空肠憩室最常发生在肠管肠系膜缘,而 Meckel 憩室则发生在肠系膜对侧肠壁。

许多空回肠憩室病病例无症状或伴有非特异性症状,患者可能不会就医。大约 40% 的病例是偶然发现的[110]。空肠憩室可出现各种症状和临床问题。最常见的临床特征是反复腹痛、早饱和胃胀。可能出现响亮的肠鸣和间歇性腹泻,这些症状可能是由潜在的运动障碍引起的[116]。

(三) 并发症

与结肠憩室相似,空肠憩室的并发症包括出血、憩室炎和穿孔。空肠憩室出血在双气囊小肠镜检查中得到了治疗,尽管存在一定的穿孔危险[117-119]。相关的小肠细菌过度生长可能导致吸收不良(见第 104 和 105 章)[110,120]。空肠憩室病且伴有严重运动障碍的患者可发展为肠假性梗阻(见第 124 章)。假性肠梗阻患者可能会周期性地有少量腹腔内游离空气(气腹),而没有明显的穿孔[121]。如果这些患者在其他方面都很好,就应该仔细观察。外科手术通常是不必要的。

小肠憩室出血可能难以定位[117,122]。如果在血管造影术中发现小肠出血源,在患者被送至手术室时,在供养血管内留下小导管可能是有用的。当对患者进行探查时,可以通过导管注射少量染料,对受累的肠道进行染色。这可以帮助外科医生定位其他不明确的病灶。憩室炎可导致肠系膜内游离穿孔或脓肿[123]。肠系膜炎性肿物的发现增加小肠憩室穿孔的概率[124]。由于空肠憩室通常向外突入肠系膜内,即使在手术中也很难发现。

空肠憩室可形成大的小肠结石,引起黏膜糜烂、出血、憩室炎、穿孔或肠梗阻[123,125,126]。空肠憩室病被发现与小肠扭转有一定联系[127]。

(四) 治疗和预后

在小肠憩室病和疑似动力障碍的患者中,可使用口服抗生素治疗相关的细菌过度生长,可能会改善腹胀和腹泻以及吸收不良(见第 104 和 105 章)[128]。

在出血、穿孔或憩室炎的患者中,应进行有限的手术切除受影响的肠段,但这可能难以精确定位[123,129]。对于有慢性假性肠梗阻症状的患者,一般应避免手术,尽管仔细挑选的患者可能会获益[130]。如果为了切除所有憩室而切除了一段较长的肠段,患者有可能遗留短肠综合征,这可能会导致严重的残疾(见 106 章)。

(张烁 译,鲁晓岚 校)

参考文献

第 27 章　腹部疝和胃扭转

D. Rohan Jeyarajah，Kerry B. Dunbar 著

章节目录

一、横膈膜疝（膈疝） …… 360
（一）食管裂孔疝和食管旁疝 …… 360
（二）先天性膈疝 …… 363
（三）创伤性和创伤后膈疝 …… 365
二、胃扭转 …… 365
（一）病因学和病理生理 …… 365
（二）流行病学 …… 365
（三）临床特点、诊断和并发症 …… 365
（四）治疗和预后 …… 366
三、腹股沟疝和股疝 …… 367
（一）病因学和病理生理学 …… 367
（二）流行病学 …… 367
（三）临床特点、诊断和并发症 …… 367
（四）治疗和预后 …… 368
（五）术后并发症及复发 …… 369
（六）腹股沟疝和结直肠癌筛查 …… 369
（七）腹股沟疝和良性前列腺增生 …… 369
四、其他腹壁疝 …… 369
（一）切口疝 …… 369
（二）上腹壁疝和脐疝 …… 371
（三）腹侧壁疝（半月线疝） …… 371
五、骨盆疝和会阴疝 …… 372
（一）病因学和病理生理学 …… 372
（二）流行病学 …… 372
（三）临床特征、诊断和并发症 …… 372
（四）治疗和预后 …… 372
六、腰疝 …… 372
（一）病因学和病理生理学 …… 372
（二）流行病学 …… 373
（三）临床特征、诊断和并发症 …… 373
（四）治疗和预后 …… 373
七、内疝 …… 373
（一）病因学和病理生理学 …… 373
（二）流行病学 …… 374
（三）临床特征与诊断 …… 374
（四）治疗和预后 …… 375

疝是器官或结构突入开口或囊袋中。腹壁疝通过腹部的肌层和筋膜壁突出形成，分为两个部分：①腹壁腱膜壁的孔口或缺损；②疝囊，由腹膜和腹部内容物组成。如果疝囊突出于腹壁或壁间疝（疝囊位于腹壁内），则腹壁疝为腹壁外疝；如果疝囊包含在腹腔内，则为腹内疝，腹内疝不一定有疝囊。

当突出的疝内容物可以回纳腹部时为可复性疝，如疝内容物不能回纳或不能完全回纳时为不可复性疝或嵌顿疝。当突出器官的血供应受损、器官缺血或坏死时为绞窄性疝。嵌顿疝通常是需要矫正复位的，因为存在绞窄的危险，可导致肠的损失。由于有时很难确定疝是嵌顿性还是绞窄性，嵌顿疝被认为是紧急，需要手术干预治疗。另一种类型的疝是肠管壁疝（Richter 疝），只有一侧肠管（最常见的是反肠系膜侧）突出于疝孔。与其他疝不同，Richter 疝可发生绞窄而无肠梗阻，因而使这类疝难以诊断。

一、横膈膜疝（膈疝）

膈疝主要有 3 种类型：食管裂孔疝和食管旁疝（均累及食管裂孔）、先天性膈疝和创伤性膈疝。

（一）食管裂孔疝和食管旁疝

最常见的膈疝是胃经食管裂孔的滑动疝，包括食管裂孔疝和食管旁疝。严格来说，所有这些疝都是裂孔疝，均通过横膈膜的食管裂孔，是位于中央的疝。

1. 病因学和病理生理学

滑动性食管裂孔疝（Ⅰ型）发生在胃食管交界处和部分胃移位至膈肌上方，但胃轴的方位不变。滑动性食管裂孔疝的发生率随着年龄的增长而增加，膈食管膜将胃食管交界处锚定在横膈膜上（见第 43 和 46 章）。食管裂孔疝可能是由于膈食管膜的年龄相关性恶化，再加上正常的腹内正压和吞咽过程中食管缩短时食管对胃的向上牵拉引起的[1]。

食管旁疝（Ⅱ型）发生于胃沿食管向前穿过食管裂孔时（见图 27.1A），由于保留了膈食管后韧带和胃食管交界处的正常锚定，胃食管交界处在膈肌水平保持正常位置，只有胃向近端移动[2]，有时甚至整个胃都可进入胸腔（见图 27.1B）。大多数食管旁疝除含有食管旁疝成分外，还含有滑动裂孔疝成分，因此是混合性膈疝[Ⅲ型（见图 27.1C）][3]。食管旁疝，其他腹内结构（如网膜、结肠、脾脏）也可疝出为Ⅳ型。通常通过钡餐检查来诊断这些缺陷。然而，CT 扫描的横断面成像将是证实Ⅳ型缺陷的首选测试，因为钡餐检查可能无法通过裂孔显示邻近的结肠或胰腺。在诊断食管裂孔疝或食管旁疝时，放射科医师需要解决的重要问题包括：①胃食管交界处是否位于食管裂孔处或食管裂孔上方？②胃或任何其他内脏结构是否位于胃食管交界处上方？例如，如果胃食管交界处位于裂孔上方，且在裂孔上方有胃，则该患者为Ⅲ型（混合型）食管裂孔疝。

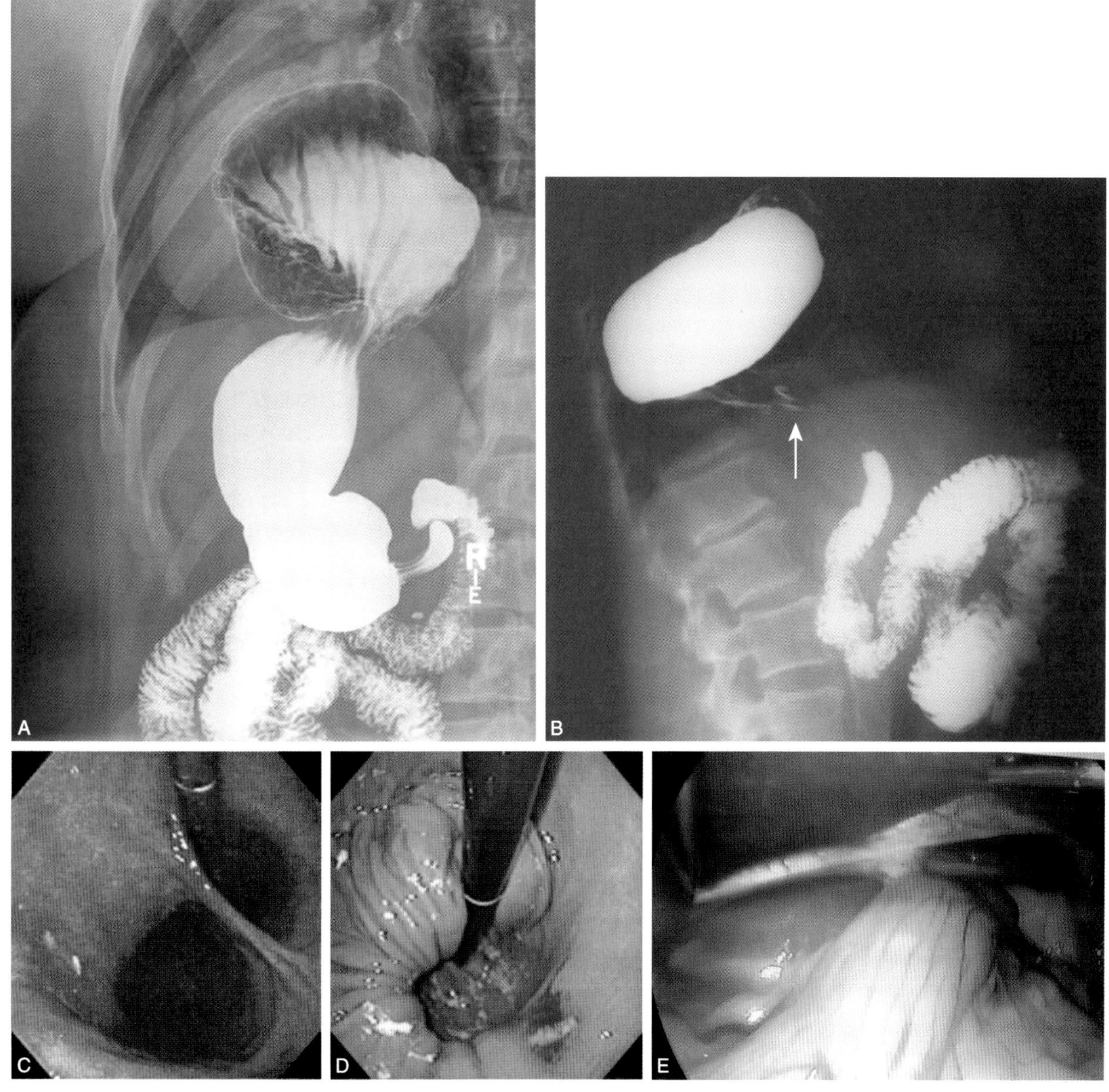

图 27.1　A,食管旁疝(Ⅱ型)。钡剂检查显示食管旁疝,部分胃位于横膈膜上方。B,本钡餐检查显示食管旁疝并发胃器官轴性扭转(见图 27.5)。胃食管交界处在横膈膜下方保持相对正常的位置(箭)。C,近端胃的反折内镜视图显示,内镜穿过邻近大食管旁疝的滑动性食管裂孔疝。D,肠管壁疝(Cameron 疝)病变,内镜下后屈位可见巨大食管裂孔疝,5 点钟位横膈膜裂孔水平可见 Cameron 病变。E,食管旁疝的腹腔镜视图。(B,Courtesy Dr. Herbert J. Smith,Dallas,Tex.)

2. 流行病学

食管裂孔疝患病率的估计值差异很大,根据患者人群、诊断方法和存在的症状,检查的患者范围为 14%~84%[4-8]。一般而言,食管裂孔疝在 GERD 患者中更常见[8]。X 线片发现约 90%~95% 的食管裂孔疝为滑动性食管裂孔疝(Ⅰ型),其余为食管旁疝[3,7]。大多数滑动性裂孔疝较小,临床意义不大。有症状的食管旁疝患者多为中老年人。

3. 临床特征、诊断和并发症

许多小的单纯性滑动性食管裂孔疝患者无症状。滑动性裂孔疝的主要的临床意义是它对胃食管反流的作用(见第 44 章)。大的滑动性食管裂孔疝患者除反酸、胃灼热外,可诉吞咽困难或胸部或上腹部不适。胸部 X 线检查时,食管裂孔疝可表现为心脏后区的软组织密度影或气液平面。食管裂孔疝有时在钡餐检查中也可诊断,CT 可显示膈肌裂孔上方的近端胃。在内镜检查时,注意到胃食管交界处在膈肌压迹的近端。

食管旁疝或混合性食管裂孔疝患者如果受到密切质疑,很少完全无症状。许多食管旁疝患者合并胃食管反流,特别是伴有较大食管旁疝的患者[3,9]。其他症状包括吞咽困难、胸痛、餐后不适和呼吸短促,一些患者会因慢性胃肠道失血而出现缺铁性贫血[9,10]。

食管旁疝或混合性食管裂孔疝在胸部 X 线片上可见到纵隔或左胸部出现异常软组织密度影(常伴有气泡)。上胃肠道放射成像是最佳的诊断检查(见图 27.1A)。CT 扫描可显示部分胃在胸部。有时可以看到上胃肠放射成像和CT扫描之间的差异，因为后者在仰卧位进行，此时胃可能会进一步移动到胸部。通常在内镜检查往往很容易发现食管旁疝（见图27.1B），但巨大混合疝的食管旁成分可能被漏诊。

滑动性食管裂孔疝患者，尤其是大型疝患者，可出现Cameron病变或线状糜烂（见第20章）。这些黏膜病变通常见于膈肌裂孔水平的胃小弯处（见图27.1D），这是膈肌中央腱形成的裂孔坚硬前缘的位置。机械损伤、缺血、药物刺激和消化性损伤被认为是这些病变的原因。据报道，在接受内镜检查的食管裂孔疝患者中，Cameron病变的患者约为5%，在最大的疝中患病率最高，在转诊接受手术修复的食管旁疝中的患病率约30%[11-13]。Cameron病变可引起急性或慢性上胃肠道出血，对抑酸治疗反应不佳[14]。慢性出血引起的缺铁性贫血见于30%～40%的食管旁疝患者[9,13]。Cameron病变和隐匿性胃肠道出血的存在是影响外科医生修复明显无症状的食管旁疝决定的一个因素。

胃扭转是食管旁疝的一种危及生命的并发症。症状包括急性腹痛和干呕，并可迅速进展为外科急症（见“胃扭转”）。在使用上胃肠道（UGI）X线摄影或CT检查中，胃腔缺乏造影剂充盈或胃壁增厚伴积气时，可增加对胃扭转和相关胃坏死的怀疑[15]。胃扭转的诊断主要是临床诊断，临床医生必须有较低的阈值才能对已知有食管旁疝和出现新症状的患者进行该诊断。如果疝合并胃扭转，内镜检查可能会很困难，而且由于胃的定位，到达幽门可能是一个挑战[16]。

4. 治疗和预后

单纯性滑动性食管裂孔疝通常不需要治疗，除非有反流症状（见第46章）。症状性巨大滑动性食管裂孔疝、食管旁疝或混合性食管裂孔疝患者应接受手术治疗。当仔细询问时，大多数Ⅱ、Ⅲ或Ⅳ型疝患者都会有症状[9,10]。过去，认为所有食管旁疝都是外科急症，但现在很明显，进展为胃坏死的风险比最初认为的要低[17]。择期食管旁疝修补术常常提供给症状性食管旁疝患者，但一些专家建议所有食管旁疝的患者均应手术治疗，因为未来存在并发症的风险[3,9,18,19]。一般而言，有选择地治疗大型食管旁疝患者是必要的，那些症状可能是由于疝引起的患者应根据其他合并症考虑手术治疗。仔细的病史对于确定症状是否存在至关重要。应仔细关注胸痛和餐后呼吸短促，这些症状可能与食管旁疝有关。事实上，存在肺部疾病的患者可能受益于其食管旁疝的修复，以在胸部创造空间并减少误吸事件。

食管旁疝修补术所需的术前评价范围存在争议。患者通常已经接受过食管钡剂造影或其他食管研究来描述食管旁疝的特征。许多外科医生建议术前常规进行食管测压和动态食管pH监测，因为相关胃食管反流和食管动力障碍的患病率高。而其他外科医师则可能放弃pH检测，并使用反流症状作为所选修复类型的指南[20]。放弃pH检测背后的想法是，pH检测结果不会改变患者的手术治疗，无论如何患者都会接受疝复位和某种形式的包裹。食管pH评估的选项包括24小时阻抗/pH检测和48小时无线胶囊pH监测。测压评价的目的是确定患者是否有明显的动力障碍（如贲门失弛缓症、无蠕动症），以及有反流症状的患者需要何种类型的胃底折叠术（完全包裹与部分包裹）。然而在这些患者中，食管测压具有挑战性，解剖结构的扭曲可能使其难以识别食管下括约肌，从而使得这种测量结果不可靠[21-24]。应研究吞咽困难患者，以确保不存在明显的动力异常。许多外科医师常规在疝修补术中增加胃底折叠术，以防止术后反流性食管炎，并将胃固定在腹部。然而，在动力障碍的患者中，外科医生可以选择进行松散的前包裹（Dor胃底折叠术）或使用胃造口管或胃固定术将胃固定在腹内。作者的实践是放弃动力和pH测试，因为偏好进行某种类型的不完整包裹，而不是依赖于良好动力的360度包裹。增加胃固定术可降低疝修补术后的复发率[25,26]。

食管裂孔疝或食管旁疝修补术的手术原则包括4个主要要素：①纵隔或胸部疝复位，疝囊切除；②重建膈肌裂孔，用或不用假体补片加固单纯后闭合；③通过胃底折叠术在裂孔处提供体积以防止脱垂到胸部，从而减少术后反流；④增加胃固定术或胃造瘘管，为腹内胃提供额外的固定机制。这些要素可以通过微创（腹腔镜或机器人）或通过腹部或胸部的开放式手术完成[3,18,27,28]。大多数患者是通过腹部进行微创手术的，从而缩短了住院时间，减轻术后疼痛，但复发风险相当（见图27.1E）[27,28]。慢性食管旁疝从胸部复位可能很困难，可通过胸腔镜和腹部联合手术进行。术中用力牵引可发生肺损伤，然而，由于膈肌缺损位于中央（内侧）而不是外周（外侧），如创伤性缺损，通常不存在强烈的肺粘连。疝囊切除可能会累及左胸，需要放置胸管引流。横膈膜重建可通过在食管后方放置不可吸收的缝线进行[22,23]。在一些研究中，使用假体补片减少了复发[29-31]，但使用补片仍存在争议，因为尚无明确的长期结果证明疝复发风险降低。然而，大多数外科医生对靠近食管使用合成补片持谨慎态度，因此“生物”产品受到青睐。补片的形状也是一个有争议的领域。可使用锁孔补片，在这种情况下，食管被补片完全环绕，担忧的是吞咽困难[30,32]。或者可使用U形补片，其中前部保持开放，仅在后部加固（复发的主要区域）。通常通过蕈状折叠术将胃固定在腹部，在裂孔处提供一些支撑作用，使胃保持在腹部，并可减少术后胃食管反流。额外使用胃固定术，将胃缝合到腹壁或放置胃造瘘管2周，使胃成熟到腹壁，可能会减少复发[25]。作者倾向于行Dor胃底折叠术，用锁孔生物补片闭合横膈膜，并放置临时胃造瘘管，用于所有大型食管旁疝患者。

滑动性食管裂孔疝或食管旁疝患者可有食管短缩，这使得在没有张力的情况下很难恢复横膈膜下方的胃食管连接，而这是降低术后复发的关键因素。在这种情况下，可以从近端胃构建额外长度的新食管（全胃底折叠胃成形术——Collis-Nissen术）[33]。在这种情况下，沿着穿过胃的探条平行于食管轴线击发吻合器，形成延长的食管。或者经纵隔剥离至进入胸腔超过5cm食管，通常可获得足够的腹内食管长度，而不需要额外的吻合[34]。根据作者的经验，如果通过切除疝囊进行充分的经纵隔分离，则很少需要食管延长术。潜在的手术并发症包括食管和胃穿孔、气胸和肝撕裂伤。潜在的长期并发症可能包括吞咽困难（如果包裹太紧）或因胃底折叠术分解或移入胸部出现的胃食管反流。如果仔细检查，食管旁疝修补术后的影像学复发率为 15%～25%[28,35]。然而，复发的临床影响可能极小，因为这些患者中的大多数保持无症状，不需要进一步治疗[36]。食管旁疝修补术后同时发生反流和吞咽困难患者应进行症状复发评估，最好通过 UGI 钡剂进行研究。上消化道内镜检查也可能有帮助，可提供动态信息。胃的后屈视图将显示是否存在食管旁疝。

肥胖患者的复发率更高，许多人倾向于 BMI 大于 35kg/m² 的患者接受 Roux-en-Y 胃旁路（Roux-en-Y gastric bypass，RYGB）手术[37,38]。

（二）先天性膈疝

先天性膈疝（congenital diaphragmatic hernia，CDH）罕见，但可有明显的并发症，大多数在出生时被诊断。

1. 病因学和病理生理学

先天性膈疝是由于膈肌多个发育成分融合失败所致（图 27.2）。在胚胎学上，膈肌来源于横膈，横膈分隔腹膜和心包间隙、食管的隔膜、胸膜腹膜和胸壁的肌肉。先天性胸骨旁疝（Morgagni 疝）在膈肌胸肋交界处向前形成，先天性胸腹膜裂孔疝（Bochdalek 裂孔疝）在膈肌腰肋交界处后外侧形成[39]，Bochdalek 裂孔疝最常在出生后立即表现，通常与肺发育不全有关。

2. 流行病学

先天性膈疝的发生率约为 1/10 000～1/2 000 出生儿，部分类型多见于男性[40-43,44]。表现在新生儿中的疝最常见的是 Bochdalek 疝。随着产前超声的常规使用，先天性膈疝可以在产前发现。在胎儿发育过程中由于胸部腹腔内容物的存在，导致胎儿肺明显发育不全。决定患儿预后的是肺功能障碍的程度，而不是疝本身的存在。然后采取产前措施，为始终伴随大的先天性膈疝的肺发育不全做好准备。只有少数 Bochdalek 疝是在成年后首次发现的[45]，约 80% 的 Bochdalek 疝发生于左侧胸部（图 27.3）[46-48]。右侧 Bochdalek 疝通常在右侧胸部包含肝脏。Morgagni 疝约占手术治疗膈疝的 2%～3%（图 27.4）[49,50]，虽然被认为是先天性的，但通常在成人中表现出来，且 80%～90% 的病例发生在右侧[49]。

3. 临床特征、诊断和并发症

先天性膈疝的临床表现差异很大，从新生儿期死亡到成人无症状意外发现。患有 Bochdalek 疝的新生儿有呼吸窘迫、一侧胸部呼呼吸音消失或舟状腹[51]。在约 30% 的病例中发现了严重的染色体异常，但在大多数病例中无法确定确切的突变（或突变）[52]。肺发育不全好发于疝侧，但对侧肺也可发生一定程度的发育不全。肺动脉高压很常见。导致 Bochdalek 疝婴儿死亡的主要原因是呼吸衰竭和相关异常，可能包括心脏异常和肌肉骨骼缺陷[51]。这些新生儿大多是在子宫内通过常规使用产前超声作出诊断的，产前超声可显示胸部内的胃或肠襻。当产前诊断出先天性膈疝时，妊娠被认为是高风险的。这些婴儿是择期分娩的，应为分娩后立即进行体外膜氧合（ECMO）做好准备。

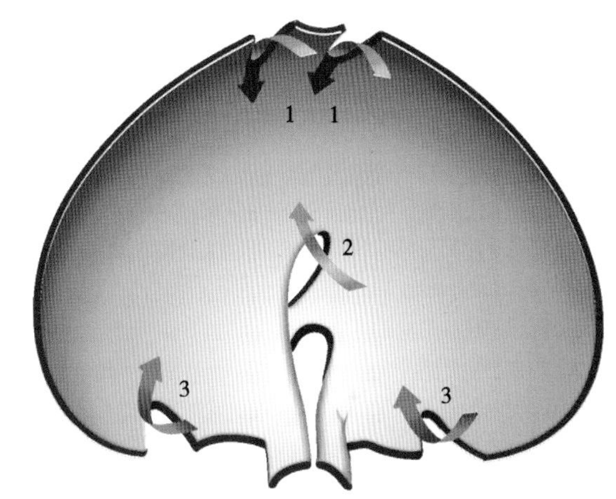

图 27.2 先天性膈疝。从下方观察的横膈膜示意图，显示了潜在的疝形成区域。1，前方为 Morgagni 的胸肋孔。2，食管裂孔。3，Bochdalek 腰肋孔后方。箭头表示疝形成的方向

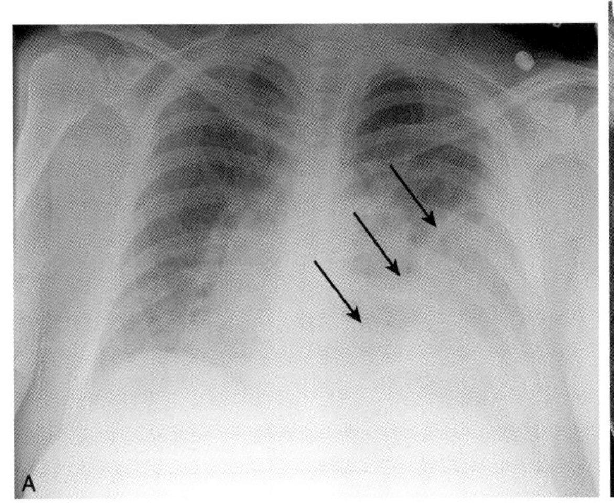

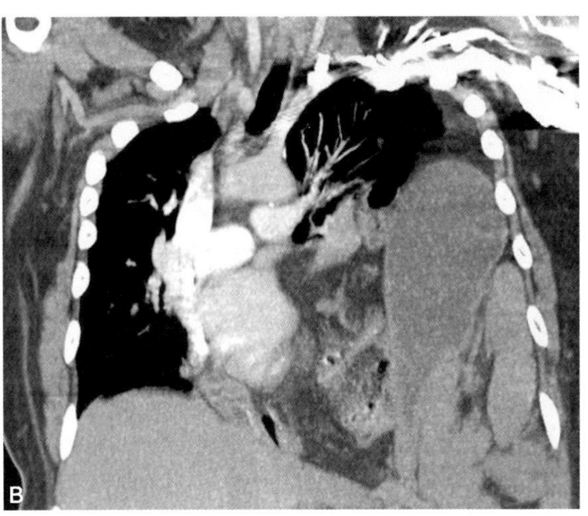

图 27.3 Bochdalek 疝。A，胸部平片显示 Bochdalek 疝为胸部横膈水平后的小阴影，左侧胸内有肠管（箭）。B，同一患者的 CT 显示肠管位于横膈膜上方并引起纵隔移位

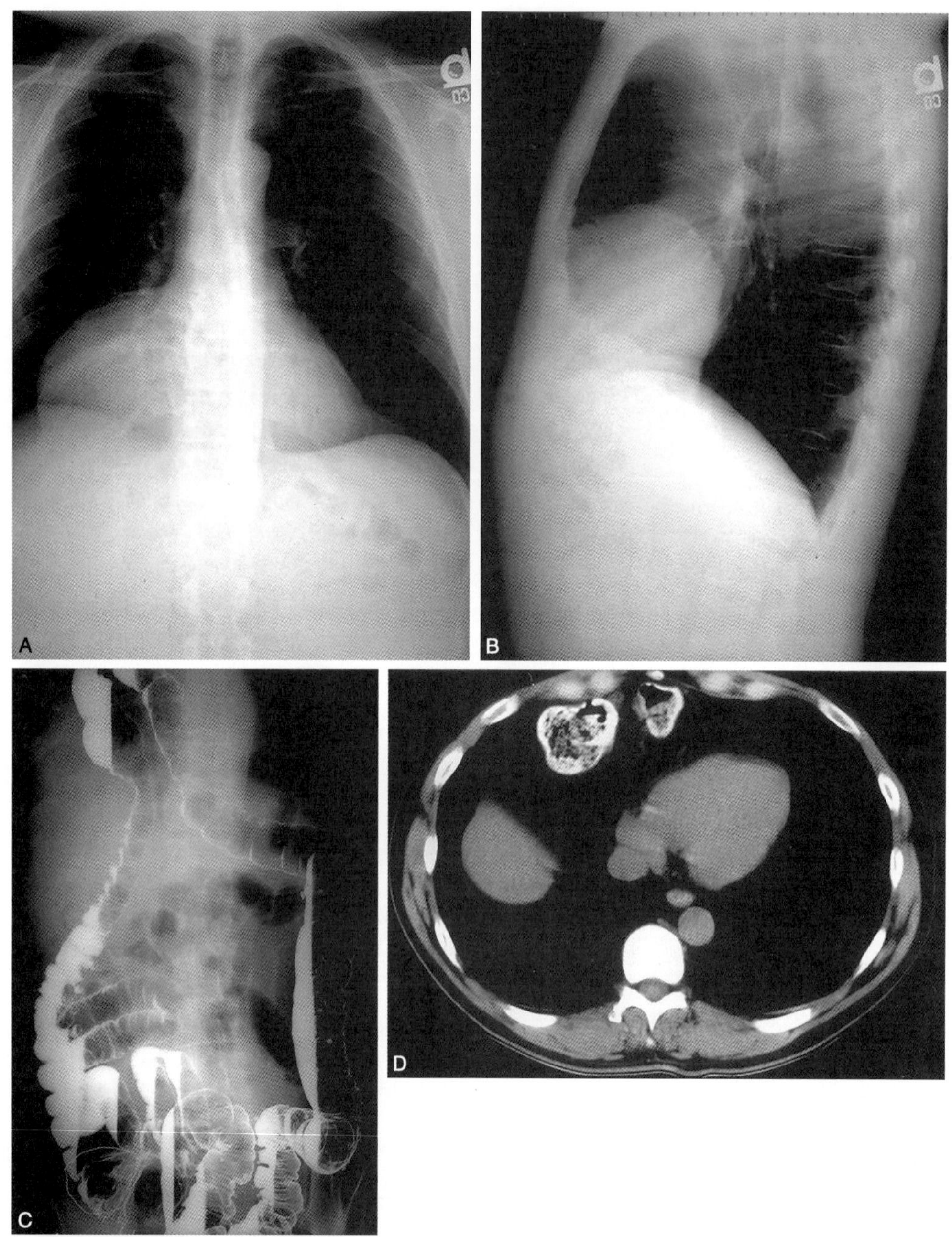

图 27.4　Morgagni 疝。A,胸片(后前位)右胸部可见肿块。B,侧位胸片显示肿块位于前胸。C,钡灌肠见横结肠的一部分为疝(左上)。D,CT 显示右前胸部(11 点钟位置)造影剂充盈的结肠

在大龄儿童和成人中,Bochdalek 疝可能是无症状的胸部肿块,需要与纵隔或肺囊肿或肿瘤、胸腔积液或脓胸相鉴别。当 Bochdalek 疝出现症状时,可能包括疼痛、肺部症状和梗阻症状,是由于胃、网膜、结肠或小肠疝所致。约 30% 的成人患者表现为绞窄引起的急性急症,可发生胃扭转[48]。其他患者可能有慢性间歇性症状,包括胸部不适、呼吸短促、吞咽困难、恶心、呕吐和便秘。在胸片上,尤其是侧位片上可能怀疑该诊断。关键发现是胸部后肿块,因为 Bochdalek 疝的缺损位于后部。可通过钡剂 UGI 造影(仅累及胃时有用)、CT 或 MRI 确诊[40,48]。

Morgagni 疝最有可能在成年后出现,它们可能含有网膜、胃、结肠或肝脏。如果肠道已通过缺损处疝出,可在胸部听到肠鸣音。与 Bochdalek 疝一样,通常是通过胸片诊断,特别是侧位片,因为 Morgagni 疝位于前部,将这种疝与 Bochdalek 缺损相鉴别(图 27.4)。用钡剂造影或 CT 可证实疝内容物(见图 27.3A 和 B 及图 27.4C 和 D)。鉴别诊断与 Bochdalek 疝相似。许多患者无胸部不适、咳嗽、呼吸困难、上腹不适等症状或非特异性症状。胃、网膜或肠嵌顿伴梗阻和缺血则可引起急性症状[49,50]。

4. 治疗和预后

对患有 Bochdalek 疝的新生儿,出生时通常需气管插管和机械通气。体外膜氧合(ECMO)对某些心功能不全和肺动脉

高压病例是有用的[51]。一旦婴儿的肺部问题稳定后,需要尽快使用补片假体进行开放或腹腔镜下手术修复。尽管重症监护和手术技术不断进步,但死亡率仍在 60% 左右,尽管一些中心报告了较高的存活率[51]。当疝内容物还纳后,腹部可能无法承受增加压力,因此也可以使用渐进式腹腔闭合(Silo 技术)[53]。

腹腔镜和胸腔镜修补 Bochdalek 疝已有报道[48,54]。已使用开放式、胸腔镜和/或腹腔镜技术通过胸部或腹部修补了 Morgagni 疝[49,50]。对小的膈疝倾向于采用腹腔镜手术。必须注意 Morgagni 疝位置存在的腹壁下血管。这种前部缺损可以用合成补片桥接。较大的 Bochdalek 缺陷需要使用假体补片进行开放式手术。

(三) 创伤性和创伤后膈疝

1. 病因和发病机制

创伤性膈疝是由钝性创伤引起的,约 75% 的病例发生机动车事故,其余病例由穿透性创伤所致,如刀刺伤或枪伤[55]。在钝性创伤期间,由于腹内压的突然变化可能导致膈肌的巨大撕裂。往往需要巨大的冲击才能造成膈肌损伤。因此,在钝性膈肌损伤的情况下,相关损伤通常会危及生命。穿透性损伤通常仅造成小的撕裂伤。钝性创伤比穿透性创伤更容易最终导致腹部内容物疝入胸部,因为钝性创伤导致的缺损较大。钝性创伤时,右侧膈肌在一定程度上受到肝脏的保护。因此,在一个系列中,68% 的钝性创伤膈肌损伤发生在左侧,24% 发生在右侧,1.5% 发生在双侧,1% 发生在心包,5% 未分类[55]。膈肌损伤可能不会即刻导致疝形成,但随着时间的推移,正常胸内相对负压可能会导致小的膈肌缺损逐渐扩大,腹部内容物通过缺损突出,导致约 15% 的病例延误诊断[56]。胃、网膜、结肠、小肠、脾脏甚至肾脏都可能见于创伤后膈疝。

2. 流行病学

创伤后膈疝的发生率尚无确切数据,大约 5% 的接受剖腹手术的多发创伤患者发生膈肌损伤,在大型创伤数据库中大约 1% 的患者发现膈肌损伤[57,58]。

3. 临床特征、诊断和并发症

创伤后膈疝可能引起呼吸道或腹部症状。严重创伤后,膈肌破裂常被其他损伤所掩盖[59]。第 4 肋间与脐部之间的穿透性损伤应提高对膈肌损伤的怀疑程度。创伤后数天至数周内出现的呼吸道或腹部症状应表明可能遗漏了膈肌损伤。因此,在剖腹探查或腹腔镜检查时必须仔细检查膈肌以发现损伤,因为这些损伤很容易被忽略。仔细阅读胸片或 CT 很重要,但根据所做的 CT 类型,仅有 40% ~ 80% 的病例具有诊断意义[60],冠状位和矢状位重建可显示膈肌的缺损。在创伤后接受机械通气支持的患者中,胸腔内正压可防止膈肌撕裂疝的形成。然而,在尝试脱机时,可能发生疝形成,导致呼吸功能受损。这些症状也可能在受伤后很长时间内才表现出来。据报告,延迟时间超过 10 年[56],在这种情况下,患者可能不会将急性疾病与远程创伤联系起来。因此,当膈肌缺损不是裂孔性的,并且不位于先天性缺损的通常位置时,主治医生应考虑创伤性原因。

4. 治疗和预后

急性膈肌破裂在剖腹探查或腹腔镜检查时最常从腹部入路。在这些病例中,必须排除可能危及生命的相关腹内损伤。但是也可采用胸部入路。诊断性腹腔镜检查已用于被认为有膈肌损伤高风险但似乎没有其他内脏损伤(例如,下胸部刺伤后)的患者[61]。慢性创伤后膈疝的特征是缺乏腹膜内衬或疝囊。因此,这些疝通常与邻近肺的广泛粘连相关,粘连减少可引起大出血。在这种情况下,最好通过胸部或胸腔镜-腹部联合入路进行修复,尽管有腹腔镜或胸腔镜修复的报道[61]。如果粘连和无腹膜疝囊使腹部入路复杂化,胸腔镜-腹部联合入路可降低撕裂肺的风险。

二、胃扭转

胃扭转是胃自身扭转的结果,但很少发生,除非伴有膈疝。Paré 描述了 1579 年首例剑伤导致膈肌损伤患者发生胃扭转的病例。胃扭转可能是一过性,产生的症状很少,也可能导致梗阻或缺血。

(一) 病因学和病理生理

胃通常通过与脾、肝和膈肌的韧带附着物固定在适当位置。当肠旋转正常时,十二指肠固定在腹膜后,从而导致远端胃固定。这些韧带附着点松弛、左侧膈肌抬高或将可移动的胃固定在特定点可导致胃扭转。局灶性粘连、胃肿瘤或邻近器官的肿块可能易发生胃扭转。在三分之二的病例中,胃扭转发生在膈肌上方,与食管旁疝或混合性膈疝相关,另外三分之一的病例,胃扭转发生在膈肌下方。

胃扭转可为肠系膜轴性或器官轴性[62](图 27.5)。在肠系膜轴扭转中,胃在其短轴上折叠,短轴从胃小弯沿伸至胃大弯穿过胃(见图 27.5,1A 和 1B),胃窦向前上扭转。在极少数情况下,胃窦和幽门向后旋转。肠系膜轴扭转常为不完全性和间歇性的,表现为慢性症状。在器官轴扭转中,胃沿其长轴扭转,长轴通过食管胃交界处区域至幽门。在大多数情况下,胃窦向前上旋转,胃底向后下旋转,沿其长度的某一点扭转大弯(见图 27.5,3A 和 3B)。较少见的是长轴通过胃体本身,在这种情况下胃窦和胃底的大弯侧向前上旋转(见图 27.5,2A 和 2B)。这种类型的胃扭转通常与膈疝有关。器官轴扭转通常是一种急性事件。混合肠系膜轴向和器官轴向扭转也有报道[63]。

(二) 流行病学

胃扭转的发病率和患病率尚不清楚。很难估计有多少病例是间歇性的和未确诊的。大约 15% ~ 20% 的病例发生于 1 岁以下儿童,通常与先天性膈肌缺损相关。成人发病高峰在 40 ~ 50 岁,男性和女性受到的影响相同[64,65]。

(三) 临床特点、诊断和并发症

急性胃扭转引起上腹部或下胸部突发性剧痛,与不能吞咽有关,常见持续性干呕。在完全扭转的情况下,不可能将鼻胃管插入胃内。呕血罕见,可能是由于食管撕裂或胃黏膜缺血所致[65]。可能发生血管损害和胃梗死。疼痛、干呕和无法通过鼻胃管的组合称为博尔夏特三联征(Borchardt 三联征)[66]。如果胃扭转合并膈疝,胸部或腹部平片将显示胸部

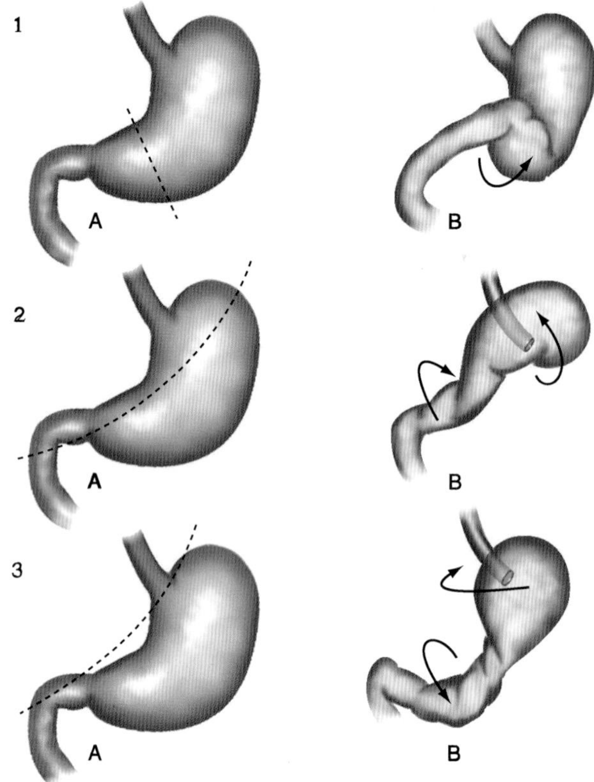

图 27.5　胃扭转的发病机制。1A,轴为将小曲率和大曲率一分为二的潜在肠系膜轴扭转。1B,胃窦沿该轴前旋导致的肠系膜轴扭转。2A,通过胃体的潜在器官轴扭转的轴。2B,胃窦沿该轴前上旋转导致的器官轴扭转。3A,通过胃食管交界处和幽门的潜在器官轴扭转的轴。3B,胃窦前上旋转和胃底沿该轴后下旋转导致的器官轴扭转。(Adapted from Carter R, Brewer LA 3rd, Hinshaw DB. Acute gastric volvulus. A study of 25 cases. Am J Surg 1980; 140:101-6.)

内有较大的充气结构[15]。CT 通常在急诊科获得,可显示胸部的胃。钡剂 UGI 放射照片可确诊,但对于有典型三联征和诊断性 CT 的情况下通常是不必要的。上消化道内镜可显示胃皱襞扭曲(图 27.6C)。急性胃扭转是外科急症。外科医生必须有一个较低的阈值,才能对出现这种综合征的患者进行诊断。手术延迟可导致胃坏死,其死亡率很高。

慢性胃扭转与轻度和非特异性症状相关,如吞咽困难、上腹部不适或饱胀、腹胀和胃灼热等症状,尤其是餐后。症状可呈间歇性,持续数月至数年[65]。有相当数量的病例可能未被识别。如果 UGI X 线片或 CT 显示巨大膈疝,即使在 X 线检查时胃没有扭转[15],也应在适当的临床环境中怀疑诊断。

(四) 治疗和预后

急性胃扭转是一种急症,死亡率在 30%左右[62]。如有可能应进行鼻胃管减压,如果不存在胃梗死体征,可考虑急性内镜下解除扭转。使用 X 线透视,推进内镜在近端胃内形成 α 环[67],如果可能,将内镜头端穿过扭转区域进入胃窦或十二指肠,避免压力过大。扭矩可使胃扭转还原。该技术最常用于无缺血迹象的慢性胃扭转[67,68]。内镜检查不应延迟确定的手术干预。胃扭转手术可采用开放或微创技术进行。近年来,微创修复术已成为修复慢性胃扭转的金标准。对于重症

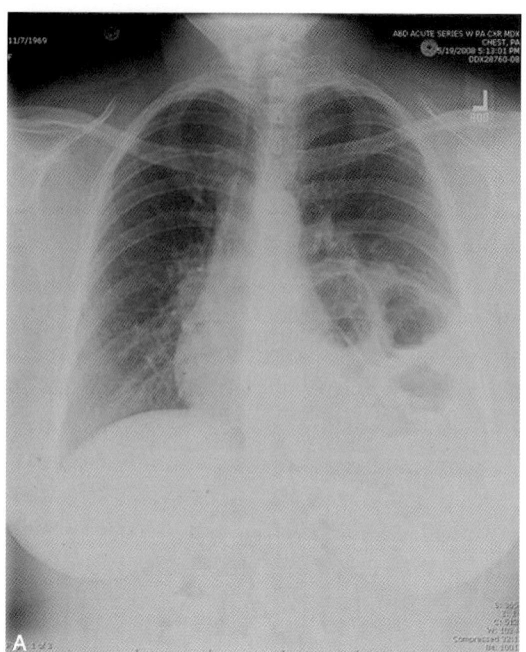

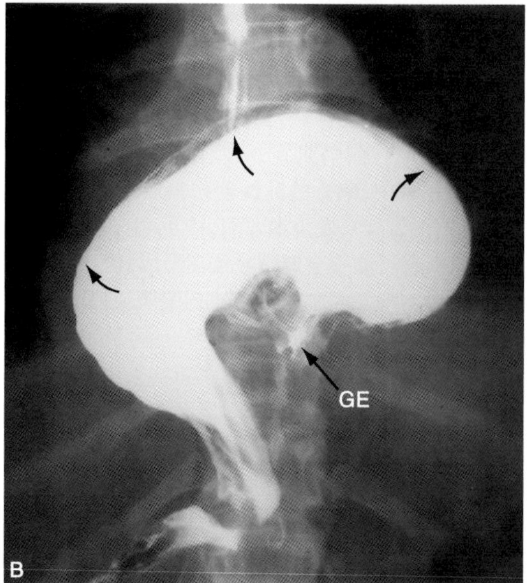

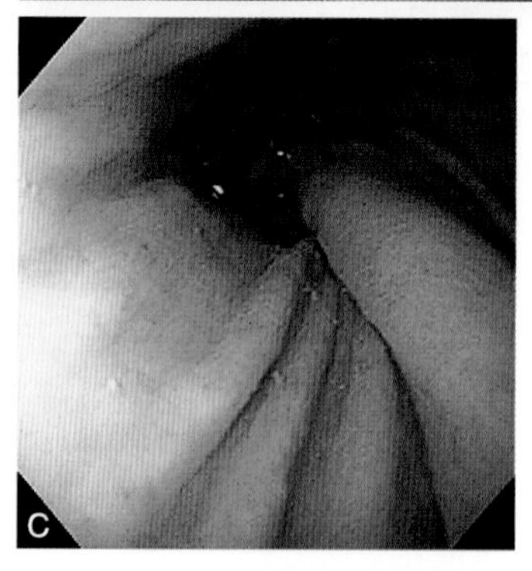

图 27.6　胃扭转伴食管旁疝。A,胸片显示充气纵隔肿块。B,钡剂检查显示胃大弯和胃小弯位置颠倒(胃倒置)。C,在胃的内镜视图中观察到在扭转点胃皱襞扭曲。(A, Courtesy Dr. Mark Feldman, Dallas, Tex.)

患者,腹部注气在血流动力学上可能无法耐受,在这种情况下,急性胃扭转应开放修复[64,65]。扭转复位后,通过胃固定

术或胃造瘘术固定胃。合并的膈疝必须修补[65,69]。但是，对于危重患者，外科医生可以选择放置胃造瘘管，随后返回手术室完成其他部分的修补，如前所述。有报道通过放置经皮胃造瘘管进行内镜和腹腔镜联合修补或单纯内镜下胃固定术[69-71,72]。

慢性胃扭转的治疗方式与急性胃扭转相同。如果患者的临床状况稳定，外科医师可选择以常规方式治疗胃扭转的根本原因（如相关的食管旁疝），以及修复膈肌或胃底折叠术。在没有相关食管旁疝的情况下，胃扭转是不常见的。

三、腹股沟疝和股疝

（一）病因学和病理生理学

有多种机制保护腹壁不形成疝。在外侧腹壁，有数层肌肉连同中间的筋膜提供支持。这些肌肉以相互倾斜的角度行进。因此在不同的平面上处理作用力，比彼此平行时提供了更大的支撑。在腹部中央，粗大的腹直肌为疝形成提供了屏障。腹壁疝发生在这些肌肉和筋膜层变薄的区域，疝可以是先天的，也可以是后天性的。在腹股沟，易发生疝的区域内侧为腹直肌，外侧为腹股沟韧带，下方为耻骨支，最深层是腹横肌腱膜。在该区域，腹外斜肌和腹内斜肌薄至筋膜腱膜，因此腹横筋膜和腹膜没有肌肉支撑。直立姿势导致腹内压持续不断地指向该区域。在腹压一过性增加时（咳嗽、用力、举重物），反射性腹壁肌肉收缩使耻骨肌孔变窄，并拉紧覆盖的筋膜（快门机制）[73]。因此，慢性咳嗽、吸烟、年龄增长和男性性别与疝风险增加相关[74,75]。

在胚胎发育过程中，男性的精索和睾丸（女性的圆韧带）从腹膜后通过前腹壁迁移到腹股沟管，同时形成腹膜突起（鞘状突）。与该过程相关的腹壁（腹股沟内环）缺损代表了可能形成腹股沟斜疝的潜在薄弱区域（图 27.7）。12%～20% 的成人鞘状突可持续存在，进一步易形成疝[76]。腹股沟直疝不通过腹股沟内环口，而是通过腹股沟三角（Hesselbach 三角）区的缺损突出，该三角区的内侧为腹直肌，外侧为腹壁下动脉，下方为腹股沟韧带（见图 27.7）。因此，腹股沟斜疝随精索（或圆韧带）一起行进，位于腹壁下动脉外侧，而腹股沟直疝位于腹股沟管底部，该区域仅由薄弱的腹横筋膜支撑，且位于腹壁下动脉内侧。

股疝穿过与股动脉和静脉相关的开口，位于腹股沟韧带下方，股动脉内侧（见图 27.7）[73]。临床检查不容易区分腹股沟斜疝和腹股沟直疝。术前区分这两种情况的重要性并不关键，因为手术入路和修复方法是相同的。然而，准确诊断股疝很重要，因为它们很容易被误认为是腹股沟淋巴结。如将股骨疝缺损中的肠袢嵌顿误判为淋巴结可导致肿块的细针穿刺和肠损伤。因此，应评估位于股动脉搏动内侧和腹股沟韧带下方的任何肿块是否存在股疝。

网膜、结肠、小肠和膀胱是腹股沟疝最常见的疝内容物，尽管阑尾、Meckel 憩室、输卵管和卵巢均有疝形成的报道[77-82]。在肠管壁疝（Richter 疝）中，只有系膜小肠游离部突入，在这种情况下，患者可能会在没有肠梗阻迹象的情况下发生肠绞窄，通常在肠嵌顿于疝中时出现。外科医生必须警惕 Richter 疝，

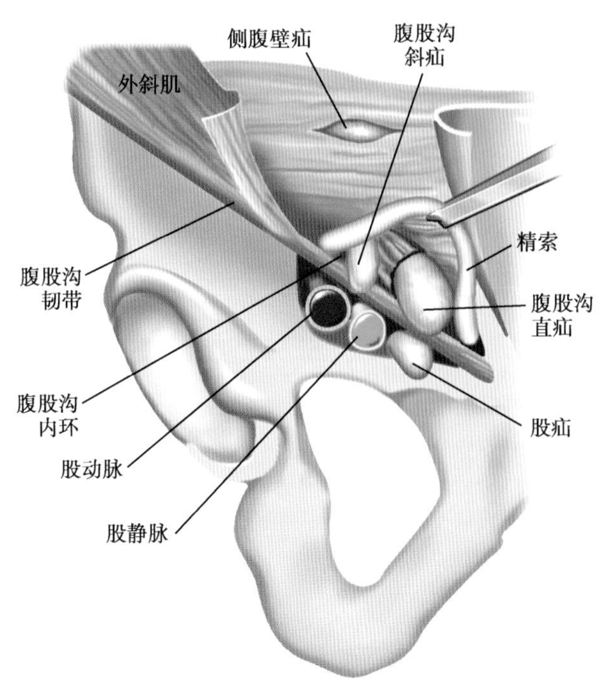

图 27.7　侧腹壁疝、腹股沟斜疝、腹股沟直疝和股疝的解剖图。腹外斜肌已被省略，精索（女性为圆韧带）被牵开。腹内斜肌和腹横肌融合性腱膜坏死的缺损可发生侧腹壁疝（又称半月线疝）。腹股沟斜疝通过腹股沟内环口发生。腹股沟直疝是通过腹股沟三角（Hesselbach 三角）腹横筋膜的缺损发生的。股疝好发于腹股沟韧带下方及股静脉、股动脉内侧

因为这可能导致肠坏死，尽管缺乏与肠梗阻的典型相关性。

（二）流行病学

需要修补的腹股沟疝的终生风险男性为 27%，女性为 3%，修补最常见于 5 岁以下儿童和 70 岁以上老年人[83,84]。发生率随年龄增长而增加，从 45 岁以下男性的 1% 增加至 45 岁以上的 3%～5%。在美国每年约进行 80 万例腹股沟疝修补术[85]，其中 80%～90% 为男性[83,86]。腹股沟斜疝约占男女腹股沟疝的 65%～70%。在男性中，腹股沟直疝约占 30%，股疝约占 1%。在女性中，约 25% 需要修补的腹股沟疝为股疝，且发生率随年龄增长增加[83,86]。腹股沟疝似乎右侧比左侧更常见。

先天性疝多见于男性，因为其代表了腹膜鞘状突未闭合。这些小儿疝通常是双侧，因此教导小儿外科医生始终注意评估对侧。

（三）临床特点、诊断和并发症

许多腹股沟疝无症状。最常见的症状是腹股沟或股部区域的肿块，当患者站立或用力时肿块增大。嵌顿时可能产生持续的不适，若有绞窄则疼痛加剧，可能出现肠梗阻或肠缺血症状。Richter 型疝可发生肠绞窄引起的疼痛但没有肠梗阻症状，因为疝仅累及一侧肠壁。应详细询问患者疝形成的风险因素（例如，患有慢性咳嗽、前列腺疾病、便秘的吸烟者），这些因素若在疝修补术前不予纠正，可能会导致复发[87,88]。

体格检查时，腹股沟疝表现为腹股沟部软包块，站立或用力时肿块可能变大。可有轻微压痛，甚至可触及与疝相关的

筋膜缺损。应在直立位检查患者,检查者的手指应插入腹股沟管,并开始长时间的瓦氏动作(Valsavla 动作),咳嗽时感觉到有轻微冲动碰到检查者的手指是正常的。然而当存在疝时,长时间的 Valsalva 动作将导致疝囊突出,对检查者的手指有压痛。直疝和斜疝有时难以区分,腹股沟疝也可在腹平片(图 27.8)、钡剂放射照片、超声、CT 上发现,MRI 可能有助于确定腹股沟疼痛的其他原因[89]。

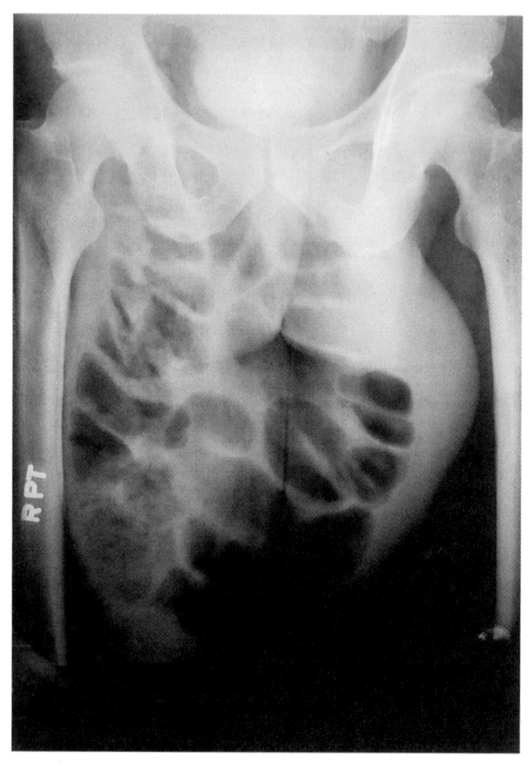

图 27.8　平片:一例 28 岁男性巨大嵌顿性腹股沟疝。(Courtesy Dr. Michael J. Smerud, Dallas, Tex.)

股疝比其他腹股沟疝更难诊断,30%～40% 的股疝表现为因绞窄引起的外科急症[74,86],手术前往往不能作出正确的诊断。股疝的颈部通常很小,即使是难以扪及的小股疝也可能引起梗阻或绞窄。Richter 疝最常见于股骨区,使诊断更加复杂化。股疝最常见于女性,临床医师对女性疝的怀疑程度低于男性。股疝也可发生于儿童[90]。诊断延误、绞窄和需要急诊手术是常见的[86,91]。位于腹股沟韧带下方和股动脉内侧的任何肿块均应怀疑为股疝。股疝常被误认为是股淋巴结病或腹股沟脓肿[91]。显然,嵌顿性股疝的床旁切开和引流是必须避免的,因此,应广泛使用超声或 CT 有助于区别股疝和腹股沟淋巴结病、脓肿或其他肿块[89]。放射科医师应在进行和不进行长时间 Valsalva 动作的情况下进行这些检查,以便发现小的缺陷。

(四)治疗和预后

很多外科医师建议即使无症状,也应修补腹股沟直疝和斜疝,然而这也是有争议的。美国外科医师协会的一项研究,表明有轻微症状腹股沟疝的男性可以安全地观察[92]。该研究将 720 例男性患者随机发配至择期疝修补术组或观察等待组。在研究的观察等待组的 364 例患者中,仅有 2 例在 4.5 年内发生了与其疝相关的并发症。这表明症状轻微的患者可以安全地观察,并在症状增加时再修复疝[93]。股疝因为绞窄的风险较高,必须及时修补[79,84]。

当患者出现嵌顿疝,并且没有明确的肠缺血体征和症状时,应注意尝试手法复位疝,这将使急诊手术转为半择期手术。可对患者进行镇静并取头低脚高位,必须用两只手通过疝缺损处将疝复位,必须密切观察患者,以确保坏死的肠管未被缩入腹腔内,这种情况可能导致腹膜炎和死亡。作者的经验是,缺血性肠水肿如此严重,通常不可能进行手法复位。疝修补应在同一医院内进行,除非有医学问题证明延迟是合理的(如近期急性心肌梗死)。

腹股沟疝可以使用各种技术进行修复,包括开放或微创手术、使用或不使用补片,是外科医生持续争论的来源。历史上,一直使用自身组织修复。然而,几项研究显示,使用补片进行无张力修补(无论是开放修补或腹腔镜修补)的复发率降低[94-97]。使用补片被认为是当前疝修补时代的标准治疗。

在 20 世纪 90 年代之前,传统的组织修复一直是独一无二的。成功的疝修补有 2 个关键组成部分:①治疗直接缺损的疝囊高位结扎;②治疗间接缺损的管底修补。即使没有直接的组织部件,也要常规对其底部进行修补。这些修复涉及通过平行于腹股沟韧带并以腹股沟内环为中心的小切口进入腹股沟管。通过腹外斜肌继续分离,暴露腹股沟内环。然后分离并彻底探查精索结构,以识别斜疝囊,对其进行结扎和横断。然后通过腹直肌腱膜外侧缘与腹股沟韧带(Bassini 或 Shouldice 法修复)或 Cooper 韧带(McVay 法修复)对合,加固 Hesselbach 三角底部[98-100]。组织修补本身不是无张力修补,与无张力补片修补相比,复发风险更大。使用补片被认为是择期疝修补术的金标准[85],然而,在可能存在污染的情况下(如在绞窄性疝中),重要的是进行初次组织修补,而不是补片修补,因为补片感染的风险很高。

开放补片修补最常按照 Lichtenstein 的描述进行[97,101]。这些可以在局部、区域或全身麻醉下进行[102,103]。成功修复的主要组成是从高位结扎疝囊开始,使用合成补片修复底部,以桥接联合肌腱(腹直肌腱膜的边缘)和腹股沟韧带之间的间隙,从而重建腹股沟管底。补片可缝合或钉合到位。还开发了网塞(疝环充填式补片)修复术,其结果似乎与其他修复相似[104]。在这些情况下,进行最小剥离,将看起来像羽毛球梭子的网塞放入缺损处,并用几根缝线固定在适当位置。补片导致成纤维细胞长入和瘢痕形成,从而导致腹股沟管底部加强。补片修补的优点是比组织修补更简单,张力更小,急性疼痛更轻,复发率更低[94,95,96]。双侧、非常大或复杂的腹壁疝可以用加强整个腹侧腹壁的大补片修补。这被称为内脏囊巨大假体加固术或 Stoppa 手术[105]。

几个系列比较了开放式疝修补术与腹腔镜疝修补术。最大规模和最近的研究是由退伍军人协作组织进行的[106],对近 1 700 例患者随机分配接受开放式手术与腹腔镜腹股沟疝修补术后进行 2 年随访。腹腔镜下疝修补的患者最初疼痛较轻,比开腹疝修补者早 1 天恢复工作。但腹腔镜组的复发率较高(10% vs 开放组的 4%),腹腔镜组并发症的发生率高于开腹修补组且更严重。开放式与腹腔镜修补术的荟萃分析表明,腹腔镜修补术引起的疼痛较轻,但复发率较高,并发症风险也较高[107,108,109]。对原发性腹股沟疝患者采用开放补片修补治疗,除非他们强烈偏好腹腔镜方法。对复发或双侧疝的患者可考虑采用腹腔镜修补术。这可由经验丰富的医生有效进行,微创疝修补术可经完全腹膜外(totally extraperitoneal,TEP)入路或经腹膜前入路(transabdominal preperitoneal approach,TAPP)进行[110-112]。在前一种情况下,使用球囊在腹膜正上方进行分离,然后将补片放置在该平面上。在 TAPP 手术中,进入腹部并抬起腹膜皮瓣,放置补片并重新连接皮瓣,以防止补片与肠管接触。TAPP 入路可引起腹腔内粘连和未来粘连性肠梗阻的风险,这是该入路的不利方面。机器人方法使用了 TAPP 技术。

(五) 术后并发症及复发

择期腹股沟疝修补术是安全的,严重的并发症少见[106-108]。可能发生肠、膀胱或血管的撕裂伤,特别是在 TAPP 修复过程中,如果不能及早发现,可能会造成严重后果。在嵌顿疝复位过程中也可能发生肠管损伤。

轻微的急性并发症包括急性尿潴留、血清肿、血肿和感染[92,104,113],严重感染的发生率低于 1%。精索的损伤可能导致缺血性睾丸炎[92]。组织剥离易致睾丸静脉血栓形成,其症状是精索和睾丸肿胀和疼痛,病情持续 6 至 12 周,可导致睾丸萎缩。幸运的是,这是一种罕见的并发症,发生在约 0.04% 的组织修复后[114,115]。鞘膜积液或输精管损伤的发生率不到 1%[115]。在腹股沟疝手术期间,感觉神经的损伤并不常见,这可能与髂腹股沟神经穿过腹股沟管时的分离或保留有关[116-118]。约 10% 的患者报告阴囊内侧慢性感觉异常和疼痛,这或是由感觉神经损伤或神经瘤引起,可以通过局部神经阻滞、脱敏治疗和神经切除术进行治疗[118-120]。

有些复发疝实际上是首次疝修补时遗漏的斜疝。复发风险与导致组织恶化的疾病有关,如营养不良、肝或肾衰竭、糖皮质激素治疗和恶性肿瘤[121]。阴囊疝和复发疝患者分别有较高的复发或再复发风险[88]。吸烟者中复发疝也比不吸烟者更常见[75]。据报道,在无腹水或有中度腹水的肝硬化患者中,腹股沟疝修补是安全的,尽管在某些系列中复发率增加[122,123]。理想情况下,在择期疝修补术前积极控制腹水,应考虑经颈静脉肝内门体分流术(TIPS)或肝移植。

如上所述,腹腔镜疝修补术的复发率高于开放式疝修补术[106-108]。常规使用补片可减少复发,因为开放补片修补的学习曲线比腹腔镜或组织修补更快。总的来说,组织修补后的复发率高于无张力补片修补[95,108]。对于腹股沟疝,据报道加拿大和库珀韧带(Cooper 韧带)修复术复发率最低:初次修复约为 1.5%~2%,复发疝修复约为 3%[98,100]。报道的初次补片修补的复发率从 0% 到 4% 不等,使用补片似乎可减少复发[94,106,108]。

(六) 腹股沟疝和结直肠癌筛查

一些执业医生建议 50 岁或 50 岁以上的腹股沟疝患者在疝修补术前应筛查结直肠肿瘤。一项使用软式乙状结肠镜筛查主要患有腹股沟疝的中年或老年男性的老年前瞻性研究报告称,结直肠息肉的患病率为 26%,结直肠癌的患病率为 3.6%[124]。然而,最近的数据清楚地表明,腹股沟疝患者患结直肠癌的风险没有增加。在一项结肠镜筛查无症状美国退伍军人的前瞻性研究中,息肉的患病率为 37.5%,结直肠癌的患病率为 1%[125]。因此,结直肠肿瘤的患病率在有或无腹股沟疝的中年或老年男性中相当高。在最近的几项研究中,发现疝患者的结直肠癌的风险(5%)与没有疝的对照组(4%)相似[126]。巨大的腹股沟疝,特别是嵌顿疝,在乙状结肠镜检查或结肠镜检查时可能造成困难,对于这类患者,建议将检查推迟到疝修补术后进行。有报道,结肠镜会嵌顿在疝囊内[127]。

(七) 腹股沟疝和良性前列腺增生

腹股沟疝和症状性良性前列腺增生常见于老年男性[128],用力排尿可导致腹股沟疝恶化。相反,前列腺增生会增加疝修补术后尿潴留的风险,应告知有任何前列腺疾病症状的老年男性患者疝修补术后尿潴留的风险[128]。随着良性前列腺增生药物治疗的改进,大多数患者可以在疝修补术前接受药物治疗。在择期疝修补术前对前列腺疾病进行医学处理是非常重要的,这将避免术后尿潴留引起的痛苦和延长住院时间。如果需要进行择期腹股沟疝修补术和经尿道前列腺切除术,一些外科医生会考虑同时进行这些手术[129,130],但更多担心补片感染会导致连续的手术。

四、其他腹壁疝

真正的腹壁疝包括切口疝、上腹壁疝、脐疝和侧腹壁疝(Spigelian 疝,又称半月线疝)。患者常将直肠分离误认为是腹壁疝。直肠分离是指直肠和腹部肌肉的分离,腹部筋膜没有缺损,可以通过 Valsalva 手法显示为中线缺损,不能扪及筋膜环,缺损常很宽很长。这种情况不需要修复,仅为外观问题。

(一) 切口疝

切口疝,顾名思义,是术后切口发生的疝。切口疝包括剖腹术后疝、造口旁疝和穿刺部位疝。

1. 病因学与病理生理学

切口疝是由患者和手术相关因素引起的。前者包括可能增加腹内压的情况(如肥胖、胶原血管疾病、手术修复主动脉史、营养因素、腹水)[123,131-133]。损害伤口愈合的情况,如在接受糖皮质激素治疗和吸烟患者中的胶原血管疾病,也会增加术后疝的形成[134]。手术相关因素包括切口的类型和位置,垂直正中切口后发生疝比横向切口后更多见[135],这导致一些外科医生对易患疝的患者使用横向切口,如正在接受糖皮质激素或其他免疫抑制剂治疗的克罗恩病患者。术后伤口感染的发生可导致疝形成的发生率升高[135]。

放置造口导致有意识地产生肠道通过的疝。通过将这些切口疝置于腹直肌内而不是腹直肌外侧,或使用补片加固该区域,可降低发生腹壁旁疝的风险[136]。

穿刺部位疝随着微创手术应用的增多已成为一种较常见的事件。疝形成率与所用套管针的大小(套管针直径>10mm 更常与疝形成相关)、手术时长、肥胖和年龄增长有关[137]。

与中线放置相比，外侧放置套管针形成疝的概率较低。

2. 流行病学

剖腹手术后切口疝很常见。当长期仔细随访时，可发现高达20%的患者发生切口疝，当伤口感染或伤口裂开时，该发生率增加到35%~50%[138,139]。高达50%的此类疝在术后1年以上出现[138]。垂直切口(与横向切口相比)、肥胖、高龄、糖尿病、败血症、术后肺部并发症、免疫抑制和糖皮质激素的使用增加了切口疝的风险[135]。

据报道，造口旁疝在造口放置后发生的病例高达50%[136]。在手术时采取具体措施以降低疝形成的发生率。例如，在腹直肌鞘内而不是在其外侧创建最小的筋膜缺损。在初次造口放置中使用生物补片可降低疝形成的发生率，但这种常规使用补片是有争议的，计划进行一项多中心随机对照试验来解决这一问题[136,140]。在放置造口之前导致肠管扩张的疾病(例如梗阻)可导致造口放置后的肠收缩，这种皱缩可增加肠壁与筋膜之间的间隙，有利于疝的形成。

穿刺部位疝估计发生在0.5%的腹腔镜胆囊切除术后[137]。它们通常发生在最大套管针的位置，套管针的直径通常大于10mm，位于脐部。

3. 临床特征、诊断和并发症

切口疝可引起慢性腹部不适。由于切口疝的筋膜缺损通常较大，即使嵌顿也不常见绞窄。自愿增加腹内压的能力降低会干扰排便和排尿，由于平衡“核心”的减少，可能会发生脊柱前凸和背痛[139]，大切口疝可能导致“膨出病”。随着腹壁完整性的消失，膈肌在吸气时不能与腹腔脏器收缩，而是迫使内脏进入疝内。因此，膈肌变得薄弱，疝有扩大的趋势。内脏可能会失去腹腔内所谓的右侧区域。外科医生需要小心缩小和修复这些大型疝，因为腹压的急剧升高可能导致肺呼吸衰竭和静脉回流减少，从而导致有效的腹腔间隔室综合征[141]。

造口旁疝常干扰造口功能和器械的安装，这可能导致大便泄漏，从而造成失能。通过造口可发生肠管脱出，这有时导致造口处突出为长鼻状。患者可能会带来造口溢出和突出的图片，即脱垂的肠道。肠嵌顿和绞窄可发生在造口旁缺损内，表现为肠梗阻[136]。

套管针部位疝通常会引起套管针部位疼痛和凸起。由于开口很小，腹腔内容物更有可能在缺损处发生绞窄。Richter疝已有报道，其他器官(如胃)也可疝入套管针疝[142,143]。

如果切口疝很小、很柔软或是肥胖患者，则诊断切口疝可能很困难。超声或CT是诊断的有用辅助手段。要求进行超声或CT的医生应仔细地将自己的怀疑传达给放射科医生，因为放射医生可以进行特定操作来证实缺损。例如，可以在患者处于直立位或CT处于俯卧位时进行超声检查[144]。造口旁疝也可通过造口内超声识别[145]，尽管CT是首选的诊断方式。穿刺部位疝的诊断尤其具有挑战性，因为筋膜进入的部位可能与皮肤切口部位相切。这是因为在放置套管针时向腹部注入二氧化碳，导致筋膜进入点与腹部充气时不同。在靠近套管针部位的部位发现局部疼痛，应进行CT扫描评估。

4. 治疗和预后

切口疝最好用假体补片修补，术后复发率明显低于传统组织修补[135]。合成补片和生物补片(可提供组织基质，重塑时向内生长)可供使用。疝修补术的关键要素是实现无张力修补。一般来说，应尽一切努力将筋膜与筋膜下方的补片结合在一起，以加强修复。事实上，“腹壁重建”一词是对这类手术的最好描述。这个术语强调了通过腹壁成分的内侧化来恢复解剖结构的尝试，趋势是尽可能恢复解剖结构。尽可能在腹腔内容物和补片之间放置一层腹膜或疝囊，但是，如果无法做到这一点，则可以使用特殊的双面补片，其一面有某种屏障材料，以防止内脏粘连。这种物质不会黏附在肠道上，因此不太可能侵蚀到肠道中[141]。在伤口愈合不良高风险的患者中存在使用生物补片的趋势，例如肥胖症、糖尿病或有吸烟史的患者。如果怀疑膈肌功能障碍(膨出病)，在修复前，腹壁可能必须通过反复进行性气腹来拉伸。2%~60%的病例报告了切口疝复发[146]，这取决于修复方法和随访持续时间[139,147,148]。可以对腹侧缺损进行微创修复。有一些证据表明，微创修复术可降低复发率和发病率[135,147]。

微创疝修补术是通过向腹部注入气体，并通过仔细分离粘连逐渐创造工作空间来进行的。然后将双面补片置于腹膜后位置，并使用固定钉和缝线进行固定，这种方法有效地桥接了间隙，而不是内侧化疝边缘。这可能产生残留疝的感觉，是由于补片和皮肤之间的疝囊内液体潴留引起，这可能使临床医生和患者感到沮丧。与开放式修补术相比，在微创疝修补术中筋膜不会聚集在一起，因此患者的疝区域会持续凸起。这是由于疝缺损本身缺乏腹部肌肉组织，仅含有补片。一些外科医生进行微创部件分离，将外侧部件切开并滑动至中线处相接。这种微创手术，不会导致与补片桥接，因此不会出现凸起。缝合或固定部位的慢性疼痛似乎是腹腔镜疝修补术比开放式疝修补术更严重的问题[149,150]。

小而症状轻微的造口旁疝可用改良的造口带进行治疗。如果必须手术，有几种治疗方式。最好的治疗方法是彻底消除造口。这需要重建患者的能力，而对于接受经腹会阴联合切除术的患者来说，这是一种不可能的选择。造口可重新定位在腹部的另一侧或另一象限。造口旁缺损的一期修复不再被认为是充分适当的治疗，提倡放置补片。可以使用带有锁孔缺损的补片，通过该补片可将造口外置[136]。或者，可以采用“腹腔镜下造口旁疝修补术”技术(“Sugarbaker”技术)，即在肠段退出离开造口时，将一块扁平的补片放置在肠段上，这改变了平行于肠壁的角度，并产生了防止未来疝形成的生理效应。在这种情况下，胃肠内科医生了解的重要信息是潜入腹部之前腹腔镜将与腹壁平行行进移动。这些修复术均可微创手术进行[151,152]。

为了降低套管针部位疝的发生率，建议在直视下取出穿刺器端口并闭合缺损，尤其是与直径大于10mm的穿刺器相关的缺损。

具有生物成分的新型修复材料现已上市。这些生物补片可用于污染患者，如有必要进行肠切除术时，代替补片。生物补片基质可随时间降解，植入后，它们会引起成纤维细胞内流，从而形成有力的瘢痕，可以提供与补片相似的强度。随着时间的推移，生物补片降解，只留下自体组织，这被称为组织长入和重塑。但疝复发仍然是一个重大的问题，发生率高达21%[153]。由于复发率高，在使用生物补片时应避免桥接缺损。

（二）上腹壁疝和脐疝

1. 病因和病理生理学

上腹壁疝是通过剑突和脐之间的腹直肌鞘（白线）腱膜坏死的中线缺损发生的。这些缺陷通常较小，并且经常是多个缺陷。由于位于腹壁上部，肠管嵌顿于上腹疝是很少见的。镰状韧带位于此位置，为肠管嵌顿提供保护。更常见的是，腹膜前脂肪或大网膜通过这些疝突出[154]。

婴儿脐疝是先天性的（见第 98 章），它们常自行闭合。非洲人后裔儿童先天性脐疝的发病率增加[155]。一般情况下，这些缺陷会在 4 岁时自行闭合[156]。如果在这个年龄后仍然明显，则是手术修复的指征。在成人中，由于腹水、妊娠或肥胖，腹内压升高可导致脐疝。

2. 流行病学

在 0.5%～10% 的尸检中发现上腹壁疝[154]。很多人在一生中无症状或未确诊。一般发生在 30～50 岁。上腹壁疝的危险因素包括肥胖、吸烟、提重物等[154]。在腹壁下动脉穿支皮瓣乳房重建术后也有上腹壁疝的报告[157]。

在出生时大约 30% 的非裔美国婴儿和 4% 的白人婴儿发生脐疝，到 1 岁时分别有 13% 和 2% 存在[158]。脐疝在低出生体重儿中较正常体重儿多见。其他风险因素包括肥胖和妊娠，大约 20% 的肝硬化和腹水患者会发生脐疝[159]。

3. 临床特征、诊断和并发症

上腹壁疝的主要症状是上腹疼痛，通常局限于腹壁，而不是伴随肠道病理性深部内脏痛。非肥胖患者可触及特定的结节或压痛点。临床诊断可能很困难，尤其是肥胖患者。然而，症状有时被误认为是消化性溃疡或胆道疾病。确定不适在腹壁，而不是腹膜深处，有助于区分嵌顿的肠管和疝中的脂肪组织。超声和 CT 检查可能有助于诊断[160,161]。上腹壁疝的并发症罕见，据报道，胰头嵌顿、疝内胃十二指肠溃疡穿孔和疝内肠绞窄均可导致急性胰腺炎[162-164]。

儿童脐疝通常无症状。成年人可无症状或报告疝在触诊时有一些不适。嵌顿和绞窄可发生于儿童和成人。自发性脐疝破裂多发生于腹水患者，罕见于妊娠妇女[165,166]。通常在脐疝明显破裂之前发生浸润和溃疡的皮肤变化。因此，如发现脐疝患者的皮肤改变时应保证紧急修补。对脐疝患者进行治疗性腹腔穿刺术时必须小心，在腹腔穿刺过程中必须使疝复位并保持复位，因为快速清除腹水有时会导致脐疝绞窄[159,167]。

4. 治疗和预后

如果手术治疗上腹壁疝，应广泛暴露腹白线，因为可能发现称为“瑞士奶酪”缺损的多个缺损。在这种情况下，首选微创入路，只需几个 5mm 的孔即可实现中线的极佳可视化。单个缺损可以很容易地修复，“瑞士奶酪型”情况（筛孔样缺损）也可以在不打开腹部整个中线的情况下微创修复。将补片置于腹内以覆盖所有这些缺损。手术修复通常是成功的，复发率很低。

脐疝在儿童中通常不予治疗，并发症很少见，如果直径小于 1.5cm，通常可自行闭合。如果脐疝大于 2cm 或在 4 岁后仍然存在者应考虑修复[158]。对于难以复位或有症状的成人应建议修补脐疝。所有腹壁缺损的修复技术均依赖于无张力修补来降低复发风险，为此可使用开放式或微创技术[168]。数据支持常规使用补片修补这些缺损，因为可以降低复发率[169]。补片始终用于微创修复。

当脐疝患者出现并发症时，预后明显恶化。脐疝修补术时需要肠切除或伴有腹水和肝硬化的患者死亡率增加[167,170]，肝硬化腹水患者脐疝的修补是临床上的一大难题。一般而言，应积极控制腹水。如果不可能，应考虑 TIPS 或肝移植（见第 93 和 97 章）。腹水患者脐疝缺损自发性破裂预示预后不良，据报道死亡率可高达 60%[159,165,171]。对肝硬化患者应考虑采用微创技术和早期疝修补术，尽管即使是套管针穿刺部位的腹水渗漏也可能是致命的。择期修复的发病率似乎并没有人们想象得那么高，最近的一项试验报告称择期修复的死亡率为 3.7%，终末期肝病模型评分小于 15 分的患者的死亡率更低（1.3%）[172]。手术修复后的结果直接取决于营养状况和腹水控制。控制腹水可能需要频繁穿刺，以保持腹部平坦以便于愈合。局部纤维蛋白封闭剂已被成功用于治疗腹水患者的脐疝渗漏[173]。一般情况下，肝硬化腹水患者应慎行脐疝修补术。在这种情况下，疝修补术前的肝移植评估是谨慎的。

（三）腹侧壁疝（半月线疝）

1. 病因学和病理生理学

半月线疝是通过腹横肌和腹直肌鞘外侧的腹内斜肌融合腱膜的缺损处发生的，最常发生在脐水平正下方（见图 27.7）。这个区域被称为 Spigelian 筋膜，以比利时解剖学家 Adriaan vanden Spiegel 的名字命名。该筋膜是半月线与 Douglas 半圆线相交的地方。半月线是腹横肌成为筋膜而非肌肉的水平。上腹部血管穿透该区域的直肌鞘。所有这些解剖特征的组合可导致潜在的缺损和半月线疝。Spigelian 筋膜被外斜肌覆盖，因此半月线疝确实不能穿透腹壁的所有层，使得疝的诊断具有挑战性[156]。

2. 流行病学

半月线疝罕见，仅报告了约 1 000 例[174]。最大的患者系列包括 81 例患者[175]，半月线疝在女性中的发生率是男性的两倍，在某种程度上更常见于左侧腹部[176,177]，通常发生在 60 岁左右的患者中[175-177]。

3. 临床特征、诊断和并发症

由于腹外斜肌覆盖了深层筋膜的缺损，因此半月线疝可能很难诊断，只有 75%～80% 的半月线疝患者在术前被正确诊断[175,177]。当患者主诉腹直肌外侧缘、脐下疼痛时，检查者必须高度怀疑。仔细检查会提示疼痛起源于腹壁，而不是腹腔。这种确定是至关重要的，因为半月线疝可能被误认为急性阑尾炎和憩室炎等疾病[178-180]。通常疝中只有网膜，但大肠或小肠、卵巢、阑尾或输卵管也可能疝出[175,179,181]，可能发生 Richter 疝或小肠嵌顿引起的肠梗阻[182]。鉴别诊断包括腹直肌鞘血管瘤、脂肪瘤或肉瘤。超声检查和 CT 是诊断半月线疝最有用的辅助手段[175,177,183]。放射科医生将使用各种技术（如 Valsalva 动作）进行这些研究，以增加即使是很小的半月线疝的检测。在正确位置发现脏器结构穿透腹壁的两个内层，则可诊断为半月线疝。

4. 治疗和预后

半月线疝可通过开放或微创技术进行处理[184,185]。腹腔镜检查可作为疑似半月线疝患者的诊断工具,即使预期进行开放修复[186]。疝可以从腹腔中找到。可采用腹膜前腹腔镜技术,其优点是腹腔镜留在腹膜腔外,从而避免粘连[185]。腹膜内腹腔镜修补术可以使用一侧覆盖涂层的补片进行,以避免粘连到下面的肠管上[185,187]。与开放技术相比,微创方法可以减少疼痛并缩短住院时间[188]。然而,这些疝罕见,外科医生应该根据个人经验选择手术方式。作者倾向于从腹腔镜方法开始,因为这可以确认诊断并帮助定位疝本身。和其他疝一样,大多数半月线疝是使用补片修补进行闭合的,这种技术的复发率似乎低于一期修复的技术[175,185]。

五、骨盆疝和会阴疝

骨盆和会阴疝的 3 种主要类型是闭孔疝、坐骨疝和会阴疝。

(一) 病因学和病理生理学

闭孔疝罕见,好发于老年女性,因此有时被称为“小老太太疝”[189]。闭孔疝发生在闭孔的大孔和小孔。女性的闭孔比男性大,通常充满脂肪。明显的体重减轻易导致疝[190]。

坐骨疝是通过坐骨切迹和骶棘韧带或骶结节韧带形成的孔发生。梨状肌发育异常或萎缩可能易患坐骨疝。坐骨疝可包含卵巢、输尿管、膀胱或大肠或小肠[191]。

会阴疝罕见,好发于会阴的软组织。其可是原发性的或术后的。原发性会阴疝发生在泌尿生殖膈前方或肛提肌后方或肛提肌与尾骨肌之间。继发性会阴疝最常发生在手术后,如经腹会阴联合切除术、盆腔脏器切除术或子宫切除术[192-194]。放射治疗、伤口感染和肥胖易导致继发性会阴疝的发生[195,196]。

(二) 流行病学

闭孔疝通常发生在年龄较大、恶病质、经产妇中,已报道约 800 例[197]。在亚洲,闭孔疝约占所有疝修补术的 1%,但在西方,闭孔疝占所有疝修补术的 0.07%[198,199]。

坐骨疝比闭孔疝更少见,报道的病例不足 100 例[191],最常见于老年妇女,但偶尔也见于儿童[200]。

会阴疝也很少见。原发性会阴疝最常见于中年妇女。继发性会阴疝发生在不到 3% 的乙状结肠直肠癌盆腔脏器切除术的患者和不到 1% 的经腹会阴联合切除术的患者[196,201]。

(三) 临床特征、诊断和并发症

闭孔疝几乎只发生在老年女性中,更常见于右侧[197,202]。通常会引起痉挛性下腹疼痛、恶心和呕吐。几乎所有患者均出现小肠梗阻的症状[202]。由于疝孔较小,常见 Richter 疝和绞窄,肠坏死并不少见[202,203]。嵌顿闭孔疝有 3 种特异性体征[202]:①闭孔神经痛,表现为沿大腿内侧延伸的感觉异常;②Howship-Romberg 征,由闭孔神经受压引起,导致臀部和大腿内侧感觉异常和疼痛,髋关节屈曲时疼痛减轻,髋关节伸展、内收或内旋时疼痛增加,这一征象见于 25%~50% 的闭孔疝患者,被认为是特异病症;③Hannington-Kiff 征,通过叩击膝上内收肌引出,无正常内收肌反射收缩是闭孔疝引起闭孔神经受侵犯的有力指征。在骨盆或直肠检查时,偶尔可在大腿内侧上部或骨盆内触及包块。该病诊断困难,常常被延误,术前通常不能作出诊断。治疗医生必须对患有骨盆肠梗阻的老年恶病质女性患者,进行低阈值的诊断。术前诊断有时在超声或 CT 上很明显[202,204,205]。

坐骨孔疝可表现为臀部或臀下区肿块或肿胀,但因发生在臀肌深部,一般难以触及。可发生输卵管和/或卵巢嵌顿引起的慢性盆腔疼痛[206],侵犯坐骨神经也可能产生臀部深部疼痛或放射至大腿处[207]。可能发生肠梗阻或输尿管梗阻。鉴别诊断包括脂肪瘤或其他软组织肿瘤、囊肿、脓肿和动脉瘤[208]。诊断往往很困难,只有 37% 的患者通过体格检查结果确诊[191]。CT 和 MRI 可能对明确诊断有帮助,但许多患者是在开腹手术或腹腔镜检查时被诊断的。

在女性中,原发性会阴疝发生于大阴唇前方(阴部疝)或阴道后方[195]。在男性中,其发生于坐骨直肠窝。原发性和术后会阴疝通常柔软且可复位。大多数患者主诉坐位时产生不适肿的肿块。由于疝孔通常很宽,因此嵌顿少见。如累及膀胱,可能会出现泌尿系统症状[209]。术后会阴疝可能会并发皮肤溃疡。鉴别诊断包括坐骨疝、肿瘤、血肿、囊肿、脓肿和直肠或膀胱脱垂[210]。

(四) 治疗和预后

骨盆疝的治疗通常是手术。腹腔镜下修补闭孔疝、坐骨孔疝和会阴疝已有报道[192,211,212]。然而,大多数盆腔疝患者表现为急性外科疾病,通常是肠梗阻,因此经常有必要进行开放式手术来处理该问题。会阴疝的修复可能很复杂。当需要切除肠管时,由于发生感染的风险较高,通常不使用补片。生物制品的出现使这些材料可以用于受污染领域[191]。腹膜瓣或肌肉推进瓣可用于这些缺损的组织修复[213]。当患者表现为急性疾病时预后很差,并且更多地与基础疾病有关,而与疝本身无关。营养耗竭、高龄和医疗健康状况不佳都是混杂的变量。

六、腰疝

(一) 病因学和病理生理学

腰疝可以发生于肋部两个单独的三角形区域。上三角(Grynfeltt 腰三角)上方以第 12 肋骨为界,下方以内斜肌为下界,内侧以骶棘肌为界。下三角(Petit 小腰三角)后方以背阔肌为界,前方以腹外斜肌为界,下方以髂嵴为界(图 27.9)[214]。上腰三角疝比下腰三角疝更常见,左侧腰疝多于右侧。这可能是因为肝脏在发育过程中将右肾推向下方,形成对腰三角的保护。由于胸背神经轻瘫,腰区可能发生假性疝[215,216],这是由于肌肉控制和张力丧失引起的,但没有相关的筋膜缺损。假性疝的原因包括糖尿病神经病变、带状疱疹感染、神经损伤和脊髓空洞症[217]。

在后天性腰疝中,大约半数为自发性的,其余为切口疝或创伤后疝。侧腹部切口用于进入腹膜后进行肾切除术等手

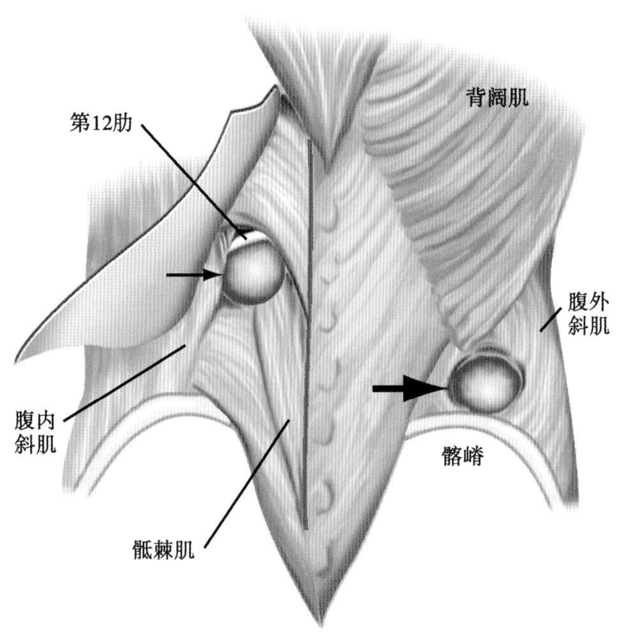

图 27.9　腰疝解剖图。下三角疝即 Petit 疝(粗箭头),以背阔肌、腹外斜肌、髂嵴为界。上三角疝 Grynfeltt 疝(细箭头)以第 12 肋骨、内斜肌和骶棘肌为界

术,可能导致后天性腰疝形成,也可能是术后肌肉麻痹引起的真正疝或假性疝[218,219]。从髂嵴采集骨后也有腰疝的报告[220]。机动车事故是创伤后腰疝的最常见原因。如果在机动车事故后发现腰疝,则必须假定患者有其他腹内损伤。这些患者大多会接受紧急开腹手术,其中 60% 以上会有严重的腹腔内损伤[221,222]。

(二) 流行病学

腰疝很少见,据报道约有 300 例[215]。大约 20% 为先天性的,很少为双侧性[223,224]。

(三) 临床特征、诊断和并发症

腰部切口疝一般表现为较大的隆起,可能引起不适。当患者负重或处于直立位时,这一点尤为明显。由于缺陷面积较大,嵌顿并不常见。此外,腹膜后的位置使得腹腔内结构的嵌顿罕见。腰上、下三角疝可通过小缺损发生,可表现为嵌顿(24%)和绞窄(18%)[225]。鉴别诊断包括脂肪瘤、肾肿瘤、脓肿和血管瘤。据报道,肠、肠系膜、脾脏、卵巢和肾脏都可疝出[223]。偶尔小的腰疝可能会侵犯腰骶神经的皮支,引起腹股沟或大腿的疼痛。CT 可能有助于诊断[226]。

(四) 治疗和预后

大型腰疝以及上、下腰三角疝的闭合,通常需要使用假体补片或腱膜瓣,这些可能是具有挑战性的案例。识别具有良好抗拉强度的筋膜,并使用补片以无张力方式修复缺损,对于预防复发至关重要[223,227]。需要将补片固定到骨性结构上(如肋骨、髂嵴)。已有报道腹膜前和经腹膜腹腔镜修补术,可以减轻疼痛并更快地恢复活动[215,219,228,229]。大的有症状的假性腰疝应该通过处理潜在的疾病进行治疗,据报道,带状疱疹治疗后症状消退[217]。

七、内疝

腹内疝是指腹腔内脏器突入到腹腔内间隙或囊袋内,而不是通过腹壁。内疝可能是发育异常的结果,也可能是后天获得的[230]。通常,腹内疝发生在早期腹部手术后,如 RYGB 手术后。

(一) 病因学和病理生理学

发育异常引起的内疝包括十二指肠旁疝、小网膜囊孔疝(Winslow 孔疝)、肠系膜疝和膀胱上疝。在妊娠期间,肠在腹腔外。在胎儿发育过程中,十二指肠、升结肠和降结肠的肠系膜固定在后腹膜上,这些肠段重新排列并附着于腹膜后。肠系膜固定异常可能导致发生内疝的异常开口。这方面的极端例子是完全性肠旋转不良,其中十二指肠悬韧带(Treitz 韧带)没有位于其在脊柱左侧的适当位置,这种情况易引起中肠扭转,并可导致广泛的肠系膜缺血(见第 98 章)[231,232]。较小的固定异常导致缺陷,如十二指肠旁疝和膀胱上疝。肠系膜固定异常可能导致小肠和右半结肠活动异常,从而有利于内疝的形成。在胎儿发育过程中,盲肠周围、小肠、横结肠或乙状结肠系膜以及网膜可发生异常开口,导致肠系膜疝[230]。不寻常的疝可能发生在阔韧带等结构上[233]。

降结肠或升结肠肠系膜固定异常可能导致十二指肠旁疝。75% 的病例十二指肠旁疝发生于左侧,男女比例为 3∶1[234,235-237]。患者最常见于 40 岁。在左侧十二指肠旁疝的病例中,异常孔,即十二指肠旁隐窝(Landzert 隐窝),通过靠近 Treitz 韧带的肠系膜发生,在肠系膜上动脉后方的远端横结肠和降结肠下方。小肠可通过 Landzert 隐窝突出,并固定在左上腹。因此,结肠的肠系膜形成囊的前壁,包绕小肠的一部分。右十二指肠旁疝通过另一个异常孔——即十二指肠结肠系膜隐窝(Waldeyer 窝)以相同的方式发生,位于升结肠下方[230,238]。

当该孔异常大时,特别是小肠和右半结肠肠系膜固定异常时,可发生 Winslow 孔疝。最常见的是,右半结肠异常固定在腹膜后,导致 Winslow 孔扩张。异常活动的小肠和结肠可经 Winslow 孔疝入小囊内,可能会出现小肠或结肠梗阻的症状。这些症状可能是间歇性的。因为疝会自行缩小。可能发生门静脉结构撞击,但很少导致胆道阻塞或门静脉受压[239,240]。如果疝出的肠管膨胀,也可能出现胃部症状,因为疝出的肠袢位于胃后方的小囊内。

当肠袢突入小肠或结肠肠系膜的异常开口时,就会发生肠系膜疝。这些肠系膜缺陷被认为是先天性的,尽管它们也可能是由于手术、创伤或感染而获得的。这种开口最常见的区域是小肠的肠系膜,最常在回结肠交界处附近。据报道,在阑尾、乙状结肠和梅克尔憩室(Meckel 憩室)的肠系膜中存在缺陷[241-243],肠管通过正常的蠕动活动可通过这些缺陷,不同长度的肠管可向后疝入右半结肠旁沟(图 27.10)。肠袢受压可能导致疝入的肠管梗阻,疝段受压或扭转时可发生绞窄。梗阻可为急性、慢性或间歇性的。疝入的肠管也可能压迫肠系膜缺损边缘的动脉,引起非疝入的肠缺血。小肠系膜、横结肠系膜、网膜和乙状结肠系膜可出现类似的缺陷。

累及乙状结肠的肠系膜疝有 3 种类型。经乙状结肠疝没

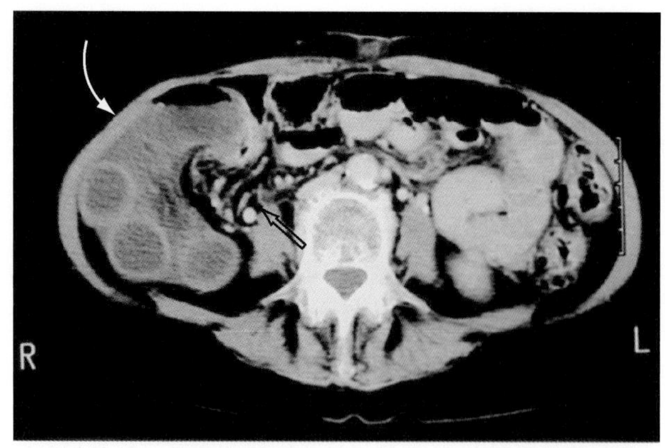

图 27.10　内疝（盲肠周围）伴绞窄的 CT。在腹部右侧可见一团梗死的小肠（白色箭）。疝形成区域（脊柱右侧的开放箭）显示小肠穿过肠系膜时扭曲。（Courtesy Dr. Michael J. Smerud, Dallas, Tex.）

有真正的疝囊，它们通过结肠系膜的两层发生。一般情况下，肠管陷入左结肠旁沟，乙状结肠外侧。乙状结肠系膜间疝是发生在乙状结肠系膜内的疝。这导致疝内容物包含在乙状结肠肠系膜内，通常在乙状结肠后方。乙状结肠间疝发生在腹膜后融合平面之间、乙状结肠肠系膜与腹膜后之间。这些疝位于腹膜后，一伴将其肠系膜上的乙状结肠提起剥离出左侧沟[236]。

膀胱上疝突入膀胱周围的异常隐窝内，分为膀胱内疝或膀胱外疝。膀胱上内疝发生在腹部，因此是内疝，它们可延伸至膀胱的前方、外侧或后方。膀胱外疝发生在腹壁外，其表现很像腹股沟斜疝，它们通常包含小肠，但也可能包含网膜、结肠、卵巢或输卵管[244-246]。

如果出现异常间隙和肠系膜缺损，获得性内疝可能作为手术或创伤的并发症发生。粘连可形成肠疝入的空间。分离肠系膜以形成管道。如 Roux-en-Y 分支，可能导致肠系膜内或重建周围的缺损，从而导致疝形成。随着 RYGB 手术治疗病态肥胖症的普及，与该手术相关的异常疝的发生率也在增加（稍后讨论）[247,248,249]。

吻合后疝可发生在胃空肠吻合术、结肠造口术或回肠造口术、回肠旁路术或血管旁路术后，此时可能会形成异常间隙，小肠、结肠或网膜可能疝入其中。胃空肠吻合术后可发生吻合口后疝，通常发生在胃切除 Billroth Ⅱ式重建术后，输入袢、输出袢或两者均向前进入吻合口后方的间隙。输出袢疝的发生率约为输入袢疝的 3 倍，可能是由于输入袢长度有限和参与输入袢的固定结构的栓系作用所致。例如，Billroth Ⅱ式吻合术后，输入袢与十二指肠连接固定，输出袢与小肠其余部分相连，因此，输出回路更易移动，并可疝入潜在的间隙中[236,250]。结肠造口术、回肠造口术、回肠旁路术或血管旁路术也可能导致形成器官可突入的空间，从而形成疝。据报道，肝移植术后出现吻合口后疝继发的梗阻[251]。肾移植手术为腹膜外手术，但腹膜意外撕裂可能导致肾旁肠疝[252]。

RYGB 手术后疝随着该手术需求的增加而变得越来越常见。这些可以是通过切口或端口部位的内疝或外疝。RYGB 术后与内疝相关的小肠梗阻发生率为 2%～3%[247,248,253]。在 RYGB 手术期间形成了 3 个可能导致内疝的潜在间隙。Peterson 缺损发生在空肠右侧，因为它穿过横结肠的肠系膜到达吻合胃的囊袋。根据定义，Roux 支必须在结肠后位置移动才能发生这种情况。内镜器械遇到这种情况时，Roux 分支假体在距离胃袋-空肠吻合口远端约 40～60cm 处发生狭窄。空肠空肠吻合肠系膜缺损发生在小肠肠系膜离断叶之间，分离肠系膜以形成 Roux 支，该支被提起至胃袋。然后将横断肠系膜的两个边缘缝合在一起，以防止这种缺损。然而，尽管采取了这些措施，但仍可能发生缺损，导致腹腔内容物疝形成。横结肠系膜缺损是通过横结肠系膜层的缺损发生的，空肠支通过横结肠系膜缺损到达胃袋。将空肠支置于结肠前位置可避免 Peterson 和横结肠系膜缺损。在这种情况下，空肠不是穿过横结肠系膜的裂隙放置的，而是带到横结肠的前面。尽管这具有直觉意义，但并不总是能够达到足够长度的小肠系膜，以确保无张力的结肠前吻合。由于大多数 RYGB 手术是在腹腔镜下进行的，术后形成的粘连较少，这实际上允许小肠有更大的移动性和通过疝缺损脱垂的能力更大。开放式手术的术后粘连实际上可以降低这种类型内疝的风险，然而，肠梗阻的粘连性原因，在开放式胃旁路手术中更常见。

疝可罕见发生在结肠镜检查后的结肠系膜[254,255]。这可能是由于结肠注气时导致乙状结肠系膜发生裂隙。疝可能通过子宫阔韧带发生，最常见的是妊娠期间发生的撕裂，因为这些疝大多数发生在经产妇。其他病例可能是先天性的，也可能是由手术引起的[233,256]。

（二）流行病学

内疝罕见，最常见于成人。在 0.2%～0.9% 的尸检中发现，但其中相当一部分患者仍无症状[236]。约 5% 的肠梗阻是由内疝引起的。

虽然一半的先天性内疝是十二指肠旁疝，但在所有肠梗阻病例中，1% 或更少的是由十二指肠旁疝引起[230,237,257]。男性多于女性。可发生于儿童或成人，但通常出现在 30～60 岁之间，大多数（75%）十二指肠旁疝发生在左侧[234-237]。

Winslow 孔疝非常少见，占内疝的 8%[230,257]。肠系膜疝罕见，可发生于任何年龄[236,250]。膀胱上疝极为罕见，病例报告有限。男性多于女性。几乎所有报告的病例均发生在成人中，最常见于 60 岁或 70 岁[246]。同样，阔韧带疝也极为罕见[233]。胃肠吻合术后内疝已变得不太常见，因为消化性溃疡病的手术频率已经下降。其他吻合后内疝也很少见[246]。由于治疗病态肥胖的手术越来越普遍，与 RYGB 手术相关的内疝也变得更加常见。在大多数患者中，与内疝相关的小肠梗阻在 RYGB 手术后的发生率为 2%～3%[247,248,253]。

（三）临床特征与诊断

各种形式的内疝均可表现为急性或慢性间歇性肠梗阻的症状。对有慢性症状的患者诊断困难，因急性梗阻、绞窄就诊的患者术前很少做出诊断[230,236,250]。

约半数十二指肠旁疝患者发生肠梗阻，肠梗阻可为轻度、慢性和复发性或重度和急性的[236,237]。已证明 UGI 造影 X 线摄影具有极好的准确性。钡剂 X 线摄片可显示小肠成串或结块，好似被包裹在一个袋子中，并移位到结肠左侧或右侧。小肠常在骨盆内缺如，似乎存在于胃后方的小囊内。结肠可因内疝囊而偏离，疝近端肠管可扩张[236,258]。然而，如果疝在研究时缩小，则钡剂 X 线检查可能是正常的。内镜检查对十二指肠旁疝的诊断并不可靠。如果进行 CT 静脉造影或动脉造影检查，可观察到肠系膜血管移位[234,236]。然而，CT 检查可能会遗漏十二指肠旁疝，因此需要特别注意小肠与结肠和肠系膜血管的关系。

在 Winslow 孔疝中，约 2/3 的病例小肠疝入门静脉结构后方，其余病例右半结肠疝入小囊。胆囊疝已有报道[239]。患者可能有胃或近端肠梗阻的症状，即使是在结肠疝的情况下，因为疝入的肠管对胃的压力。偶尔可触及上腹包块。腹部平片可显示胃向前和向左移位。肠道，最常见的是右半结肠，将在胃后部的小囊中看到。造影剂灌肠可显示盲肠向上腹部移位。CT 对 Winlow 疝孔的诊断是准确的，疝入的肠管位于胃后方的小囊内。可伴有胆管树扩张或门静脉结构受压引起的门静脉狭窄。该结果很少有任何生理后果[236,240]。

肠系膜疝术前诊断困难。症状和体征是急性或慢性间歇性肠梗阻或急性绞窄的症状和体征[250]。腹部平片可显示肠梗阻或正常气体模式移位的证据。例如，通过乙状结肠系膜的疝，小肠气体模式位于乙状结肠气体模式的外侧[236]。这一发现与肠梗阻有关，可能会增加对内疝的怀疑。

膀胱上内疝会产生肠梗阻症状。约 30% 的病例出现膀胱压迫的相关症状。前膀胱上疝可导致耻骨上肿块或压痛。膀胱上疝患者也可有腹股沟疝。口服造影剂的钡剂造影或腹部 CT 可能有助于对本病的诊断[244,246]。

子宫阔韧带疝在约一半的病例中引起肠梗阻症状，并可引起慢性盆腔疼痛[256]。其他病例是在手术时偶然发现的。据报道，小肠、乙状结肠、阑尾、网膜和输尿管都可疝出。CT 扫描可显示小肠扩张和子宫偏离。

吻合后疝引起的症状和体征与其他内疝相似。胃空肠吻合术后疝引起胃出口梗阻症状。输出袢疝出最常见。输入袢疝是输入袢综合征的原因之一（见第 53 章）。约 50% 的胃空肠吻合术后疝发生在术后第一个月内，25% 发生在术后第一年内，其余发生得较晚[257]。体格检查无特异性。血清淀粉酶和脂肪酶水平常随传入肢体梗阻而升高，腹部平片可显示胃扩张和充满液体的袢。钡剂 UGI X 线片最有助于记录传出肢体梗阻与传入肢体梗阻。超声检查或 CT 可显示传入肢体扩张、或"漩涡征"，即肠系膜血管和小肠似乎围绕一个点扭转（图 27.11）[259]。胆道闪烁显像将显示放射性核素排泄到胆管树中，但示踪剂保留在阻塞的传入肢体中[256]。

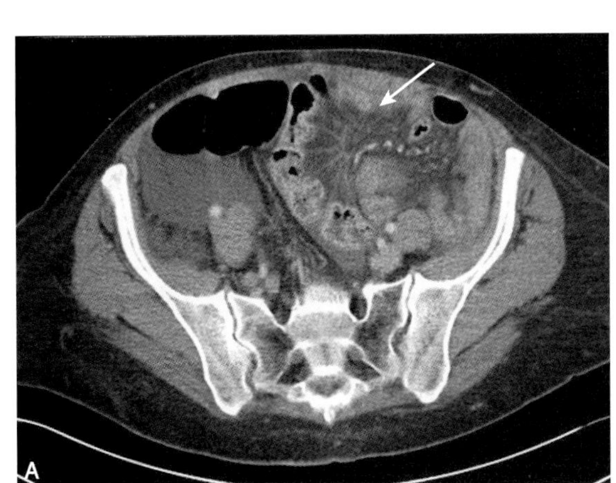

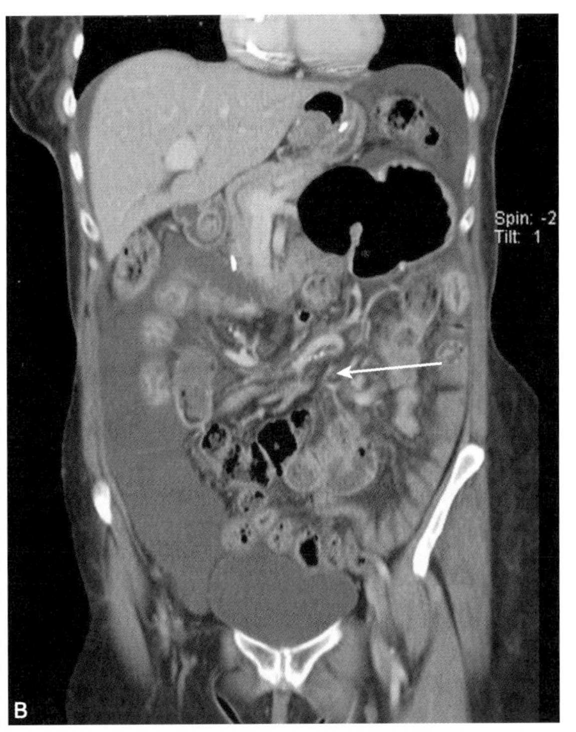

图 27.11　内疝 CT 显示"漩涡征"。A，漩涡征见于一例 Roux-en-Y 胃旁路术后内疝患者（箭）。B，同一患者直立位显示肠管和肠系膜扭曲点（箭）

RYGB 术后疝的临床表现与其他内疝相似，最常见的是肠梗阻。空肠-空肠吻合的传入支（携带胰胆管分泌物的支）的疝形成可呈现一个有趣的诊断困境，因为该袢不携带食物物质，因此，可能不会发生呕吐。传入支疝可能表现为胆道梗阻和胰腺炎，而不是典型的肠梗阻。CT 和平片将显示十二指肠扩张的证据，在胆道闪烁显像中，放射性核素从扩张的十二指肠进入小肠远端缺乏进展。远端小肠疝表现为肠梗阻的症状和体征。有症状的患者在 RYGB 术后发现"漩涡征"，应立即进行手术评估。治疗延迟可导致肠道损失和死亡。Roux 支基底部狭窄可表现为类似的梗阻综合征。然而，更远端肠梗阻的发现应增加对内疝的怀疑。

（四）治疗和预后

有症状的内疝需要手术[230,236,250,257]。如果在并发症之前检测到疝，则首选腹腔镜修补术[240,246,256]。一旦患者出现肠梗阻的体征和症状，对患者进行探查、缩小疝、确保肠存活和修补缺损是合理的。急性梗阻如治疗不及时会导致绞窄、肠缺血和死亡[243]。

十二指肠旁疝往往通过切开包绕的肠系膜来矫正。必须注意避免损伤肠系膜上动脉或肠系膜下动脉，因为它们在疝的边缘内走行异常。有时可经疝的开口还纳小肠而不需切开肠系膜[234,237]。但此后必须闭合十二指肠旁缺损。如果疝与真正的旋转不良相关，这可能涉及进行正式的 Ladd 手术(见第 98 章)[231,232]。如果十二指肠旁间隙扩张，简单切除疝囊和折叠缺损即可提供充分的修补。但是一旦发生嵌顿，死亡率可能高于 20%[237]，因此建议尽可能择期修复所有十二指肠旁疝。

阔韧带疝和膀胱上疝均可在腹腔镜下成功修补[223,246,256]。

RYGB 手术后疝是当今时代的常见事件，胃肠病学家必须具备解剖学和可能发生的缺陷的工作知识。RYGB 术后无法进食的患者，如果袋空肠吻合处无梗阻，可能会发生内疝。CT 通常会显示“漩涡征”，提醒主治医生可能存在内疝[259]。外科医生对这些患者进行手术的阈值应较低，因为遗漏内疝会导致肠坏死和短肠综合征。

(王萍 译，刘军 校)

参考文献

第 28 章　胃肠道异物、胃石和腐蚀物摄入

Patrick R. Pfau, Mark Benson 著

章节目录

一、胃肠道异物 …… 377
（一）流行病学 …… 377
（二）病理生理学 …… 378
（三）病史和体格检查 …… 378
（四）诊断 …… 379
（五）治疗 …… 379
（六）特殊异物 …… 381
（七）操作相关的并发症 …… 384
二、胃石 …… 384
（一）流行病学 …… 384
（二）临床特征 …… 385
（三）诊断 …… 385
（四）治疗 …… 385
三、腐蚀物摄入 …… 385
（一）流行病学 …… 385
（二）病理生理学 …… 386
（三）临床特征 …… 386
（四）诊断 …… 386
（五）治疗 …… 387
（六）晚期并发症 …… 387

胃肠道异物是由食物团块嵌塞和有意或无意摄入或插入的异物组成。胃石是一种在正常或异常胃中蓄积的摄入物质（食物或其他物质）。摄入酸性或碱性物质后会出现腐蚀物摄入，这可能导致食管和胃的急性和/或慢性损伤。本章将详细讨论这些主题。

一、胃肠道异物

胃肠道异物（gastrointestinal foreign body，GIFB）是胃肠外科医生经常遇到的问题。多数康复后无严重临床后遗症[1]。早期的研究表明，在美国有 1 500~2 750 人死于 GIFB[2-4]。最近的研究表明，GIFB 的死亡率明显降低，超过 850 名报告的 GIFB 成年人没有人死亡，大约 2 200 名报告的 GIFB 儿童中只有 1 人死亡[5-11]。尽管发病率和死亡率不精确，异物摄入都会导致严重并发症，甚至死亡[12-14]。由于 GIFB 的频繁发生和可能产生的不良后果，了解哪些患者处于风险之中，并知道如何诊断和治疗 GIFB 以及处理其并发症是很重要的。

（一）流行病学

GIFB 可能由意外或故意摄入导致。意外摄入异物的最常见患者群体是儿童，尤其是 6 个月到 3 岁的儿童。儿童占真正异物摄入患者的 80%[15]。儿童天生的好奇心会导致他们把物体放进嘴里，偶尔还会吞下去。硬币是儿童最常吞咽的物品，但其他经常被吞下的物品还包括弹珠、小玩具、蜡笔、钉子和大头针[6,10,16,17]。

有牙套或假牙的成年人也可能因吞咽时触觉失去而意外摄入自己的假牙[18]，这种情况并不少见[19]。精神状态或感觉中枢改变的患者，包括年纪很大、痴呆或醉酒的患者，都有意外异物摄入的风险（图 28.1）。在一个名为“Quarters”的酒馆喝啤酒游戏中，在大学生、老年人中观察到意外的硬币摄入，其中硬币会卡在食管中[20]。最后，从事某些职业的人（如屋顶工人、木匠、裁缝）在工作时，如果将钉子或大头针放在口中，就有意外误食的危险。

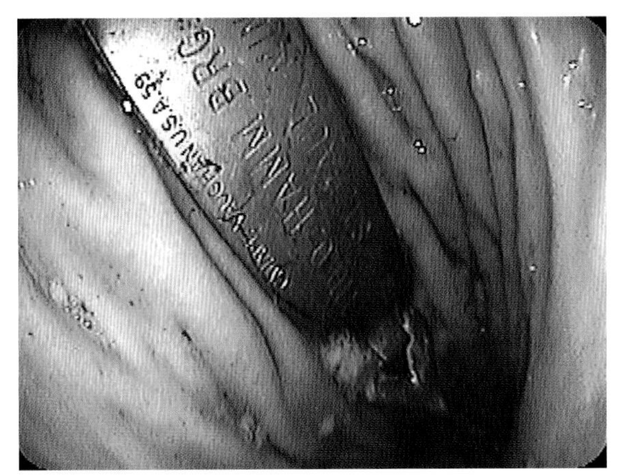

图 28.1　醉酒患者摄入开瓶器（胃内）的内镜图像

最常见的故意摄入异物的群体是精神病患者和囚犯[21]，他们往往是为了附带收获；他们经常多次摄入多种物体，而且往往是最复杂的异物。

由于胶囊内镜检查、移位支架（食管、肠道和胆道）以及移位的肠内引流管和支撑物的并发症，医源性异物的发生率越来越高[22,23]。

在美国最常见的并且需要医疗救治的 GIFE 为食管食物嵌塞，本病发病率为 16/10 万[24]。绝大多数（75% ~ 100%）的食管食物嵌塞患者都有潜在的易患食管病变[25,26]，最常见的是消化道狭窄、Schatzki 环和越来越多的嗜酸性食管炎（eosinophilic esophagitis，EoE）[27]。食管癌很少出现急性进食障碍[28]。其他导致食管食物障碍的原因包括食管切除、胃底折叠术或减肥手术后的解剖改变，以及运动障碍，如贲门失弛缓症和远端食管痉挛[29]。

食物嵌塞最常发生在 40 岁或 50 岁的成年人身上，但随

着嗜酸性食管炎发病率的上升，本病在年轻人中也变得越来越普遍。GIFB受文化和地区饮食习惯的影响。

鱼骨损伤在亚洲国家和环太平洋地区很常见，而肉类（如热狗、猪肉、牛肉、鸡肉）造成的嵌塞在美国很常见（图28.2）[30,31]。

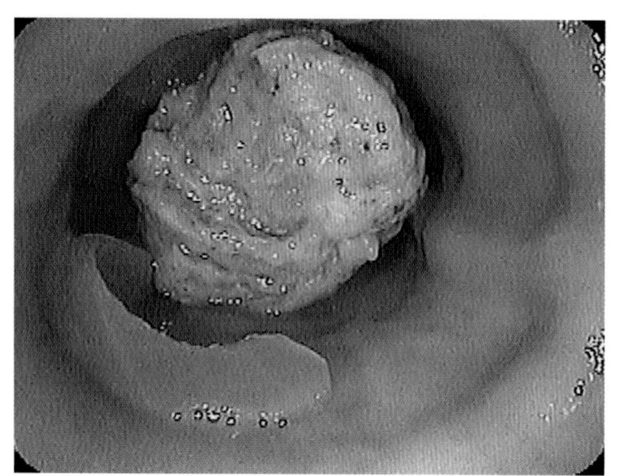

图28.2　当患者观看足球比赛时，摄入带有泡菜的烤香肠时嵌入食管的内镜图像

有症状的直肠异物更多的是通过肛门插入的结果，而不是口服和转运的结果。这在年轻的成年男性中最为常见[32]。引起医学注意的直肠异物最常带有自体性欲的意图，但也可能出现双方自愿的性行为或性侵犯[33]。不太常见但仍然普遍的直肠异物的原因包括走私期间隐藏非法药物，患者试图缓解便秘时插入的物品，甚至有报道称跌倒在物品上[34]。

（二）病理生理学

大多数（约80%～90%）的GIFB能够通过胃肠道，没有任何临床后遗症，对患者没有任何伤害[1,35]。其余10%～20%的GIFB需要内镜干预，1%的GIFB可能需要手术治疗[5,36]。最近的数据表明，在故意摄入的情况下，内镜和外科干预的需求更高，三分之二的病例需要内镜检查，超过10%的患者需要手术[37]。真正的异物和食物嵌塞可能会导致严重的发病率，最严重的并发症是肠穿孔或梗阻，很少会导致死亡[3]。为了帮助对治疗干预进行分层，重要的是要了解与GIFB相关的并发症容易发生的条件、患者和解剖位置。

GIFB穿孔和梗阻可发生在消化道的任何部位，但更容易发生在狭窄、成角、解剖括约肌或既往手术部位（图28.3）[38]。咽部是异物可能被困并引起并发症的首要部位。在下咽，像鱼骨和牙签这样的短而锋利的物体可能会撕裂黏膜或卡在里面[39,40]。

一旦进入食管，就会有4个狭窄的区域，即食管上括约肌、主动脉弓水平、主支气管水平和食管胃交界处。这些区域的腔狭窄均小于或等于23mm[41]。

然而，食物和异物更多地停留在食管的病理部位，包括环、蹼或狭窄。与嗜酸性食管炎相关的多发食管环（见第30章）导致食管食物嵌塞在年轻人中越来越普遍[27,42,43]。同样，食管运动异常（见第44章），如远端食管痉挛或贲门失弛

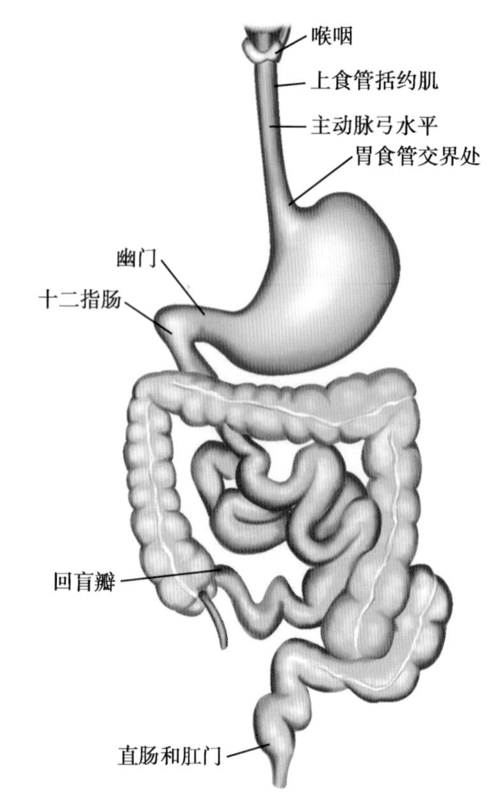

图28.3　易发生异物嵌塞和阻塞的胃肠道管腔狭窄和成角的区域

缓症，可导致食管内食物或异物嵌塞[44-47]。食管异物和食物嵌塞不良事件的总发生率最高，并发症发生率与物体在食管内停留的时间成正比。儿童食管异物的自然通过率明显低于其他GIFB，仅为12%[48]。食管异物的严重并发症包括穿孔、脓肿、纵隔炎、气胸、瘘管形成和心脏压塞[49,50]。

如果GIFB通过食管，绝大多数也能通过整个胃肠道，不会有进一步的困难或并发症。锋利、长的和大的物体例外。锋利或尖锐的物体穿孔率可达35%。较大的物体（直径>2.5cm）可能无法通过幽门。较长的物体（大于5cm），如钢笔、铅笔和餐具等，不能通过十二指肠或幽门。

物体可能在小肠的Treitz韧带或回盲瓣形成阻塞。小肠内的粘连、炎症后狭窄和外科吻合术也可能是异物滞留和阻塞的地方，然而，大多数物体，即使是锋利的物体，一旦进入小肠和结肠就很少造成损害，因为肠道通过蠕动和轴向流动自然地保护自己。这些因素往往会使异物集中在粪便残留物的中心，钝端领先，尖端拖尾[51,52]。

由于肛门括约肌痉挛和水肿，插入的直肠物体通常会顽强滞留，物体很难自发通过。直肠角度和直肠瓣也可能阻碍物体通过直肠。

（三）病史和体格检查

儿童或沟通障碍的成年人的病史往往是不可靠的。大多数儿童胃异物和高达20%～30%的食管异物是无症状的[53]。其中大多数是在父母、照顾者或年长的兄弟姐妹目击或怀疑之后发现的，但在高达40%的病例中，没有目击进食的历史[54]。因此，儿童的症状通常很轻微，表现为流口水、不想吃

东西和发育不良。

对于可以交流的成年人来说，进食时间和类型的病史通常是可靠的。患者能够准确地描述他们摄入了什么，何时摄入，以及疼痛和/或梗阻的症状。食管食物丸嵌塞的患者有症状，表现为完全性或间歇性梗阻。他们不能喝液体或保留自己的口腔分泌物。流涎很常见。摄入不受重视的小而锋利的物体，包括模糊的鱼或动物的骨头，可能会因黏膜撕裂而引起咽痛或持续的异物感。症状的类型有助于判断食管异物是否仍然存在。如果患者出现吞咽困难、吞咽疼痛或发音困难，则80%的可能性有异物存在，造成至少部分梗阻。流口水和无法处理分泌物的症状表明食管几乎完全阻塞。如果症状仅限于胸骨后胸痛或咽部不适，只有不到50%的患者仍会有异物存在[55]。患者对摄入异物的定位是不准确的，只有30%～40%的正确定位在食管，对胃内异物的准确率基本上为0%[53,56]。一旦物体到达胃、小肠或结肠，除非出现并发症（如梗阻、穿孔、出血），否则患者不会报告症状。

直肠异物患者通常无症状[33]，因尴尬可能会妨碍获得准确的病史。症状呈现通常是在患者或另一个人多次尝试移除物体之后[39]。症状可能包括肛门直肠疼痛、出血和瘙痒，少数患者出现更严重的并发症，包括梗阻、穿孔和腹膜炎。

既往病史有助于确定是否曾摄入异物；重复犯罪者可能摄入多种更复杂的异物。食管嵌塞或食管异物患者有吞咽困难的病史提示潜在食管病变的可能性很高。既往食物嵌塞或需要食管扩张使反复发作的可能性更大。过敏史（如哮喘、过敏性鼻炎、食物过敏）提示患者可能患有嗜酸性食管炎[57]。

体格检查对确定异物残留的诊断或定位几乎无济于事，但对于确定与异物摄入相关的并发症至关重要。在开始移除 GIFB 的治疗之前，评估患者的气道、通气状态和误吸风险是至关重要的。颈部和胸部检查有无皮下捻发感、红斑和肿胀可提示近端穿孔。应进行肺部检查以检测是否有吸入或喘息。应进行腹部检查，以评估是否有穿孔或梗阻的迹象。

（四）诊断

1. 影像

对于疑似吞食异物的患者，建议拍摄胸部和腹部的平片，以确定异物的存在、类型、数量和位置。无并发症的非骨性食物嵌塞患者不需要常规的放射学评估[58]。正位胸片和侧位胸片都是必要的，因为侧位片有助于确定异物是在食管还是气管[59]，并可能在正位片中详细描述被上脊椎遮挡住的异物。如果下咽或颈部食管有可疑物体或并发症，则推荐使用颈部双平面平片。平片也有助于确定并发症，如游离空气、误吸或皮下肺气肿（图 28.4）[60]。

但是射线照相不能对非放射不透明物体（如塑料、玻璃、木头）成像，可能会遗漏小骨头或金属物体。异物平片检查假阴性率高达 47%，假阳性率高达 20%。据报道，食品嵌塞的假阴性率高达 87%[61]。如果临床怀疑或症状继续存在，应对患者进行进一步的临床检查[62]。

在儿童中使用普通胶片更具争议性，因为儿童不能说出病史和相关的辐射暴露。一些人建议用口-肛门筛查片来检测儿童体内是否存在异物。在不需要放疗的情况下，床旁超声已能有效鉴别儿童食管异物[63,64]。此外，为了限制辐射，还使用了手持式金属探测器，其灵敏度从 89% 到 95% 不等，用于检测和定位金属异物[65,66]。

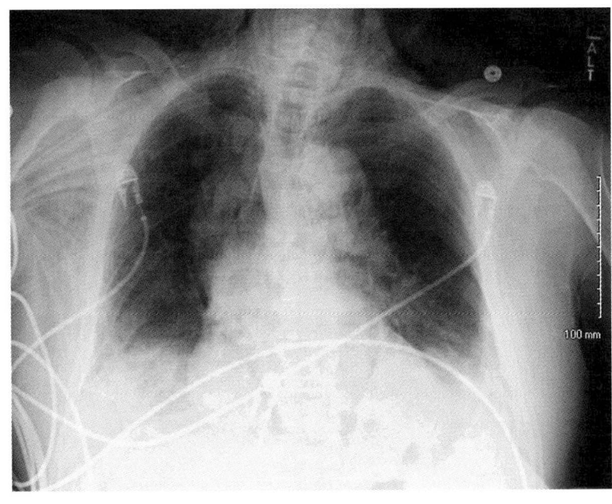

图 28.4　胸片显示患者因食物嵌塞超过 24 小时未治疗而继发食管穿孔，出现纵隔气胸和双侧气胸

在评估 GIFB 时，一般不推荐进行钡检查。完全或接近完全食管梗阻的患者吸入高渗造影剂可能导致吸入性肺炎[67]。钡剂还可能会干扰内镜显影，从而延迟或损害治疗性内镜介入治疗的效果[68]。即使钡剂检查被认为是正常的，如果症状持续存在或高度怀疑有异物，仍建议进行内镜检查[39]。

诊断 GIFB 很少需要 CT 或 MRI。但 CT 可以检测出其他方式遗漏的异物[69]，并可能有助于在使用内镜检查之前检测异物吞入的并发症，如穿孔或脓肿[70]。在内镜检查前对颈段食管或下咽部进行 CT 扫描可能有助于诊断[71]。

2. 内镜检查

内镜检查为诊断可疑异物或食物嵌塞提供了最精确的手段。这确保了内镜所能触及的物体的几乎达到 100% 的诊断准确性，包括不透射线的物体和被覆盖的骨结构遮挡的不能通过放射照相看到的物体。

内镜可以最准确地诊断基础的病理，如食管狭窄，它可能导致食物嵌塞或食管异物嵌塞。内镜检查还可以显示可能由异物引起的黏膜缺损、擦伤或溃疡。诊断性内镜检查也是 GIFB 最有效的治疗，用治疗性内镜来移除或治疗。

当有穿孔的临床或影像学征象时，上胃肠道内镜检查是相对禁忌的。一旦吞入的异物通过 Treitz 韧带，一般不进行内镜检查，因为这些异物通常会畅通无阻地通过，但有明显的例外（见后文）。同样，成人患者胃中的大多数小（<2.5cm）钝物不需要内镜取出；大多数都可以顺利通过，无并发症。

（五）治疗

1. 非内镜方法

在计划治疗 GIFB 时，应始终考虑到 80%～90% 的 GIFB 会自发通过胃肠道而不会出现并发症[5,8]。这使得一些研究者建议，所有的异物都可以通过保守的观察来处理[72,73]。虽然保守治疗在大多数 GIFB 病例中是有效的，但根据异物的位置、大小和类型进行选择性内镜治疗更为合适[21,74]。

食管异物和食物嵌塞的主要治疗方法有几种。平滑肌松弛剂胰高血糖素是目前应用最广泛、研究最多的治疗食管食物和异物嵌塞的药物。静脉注射 0.5~2mg 的胰高血糖素可以使下食管括约肌松弛高达 60%，并有可能允许阻塞的食物或异物通过[75,76]。胰高血糖素治疗食物嵌塞的成功率从 12% 到 58% 不等[77-79]。一项多中心研究表明，胰高血糖素仅对 14% 的病例有效，与未接受胰高血糖素治疗的患者无统计学差异[80]。一项小型随机研究显示，与安慰剂相比，使用胰高血糖素没有任何好处[81]。胰高血糖素可能会引起恶心、呕吐和腹胀，当存在固有梗阻时，效果甚微，从而阻止异物通过。硝苯地平和硝酸甘油不推荐使用，因为会出现与低血压相关的副作用和疗效值得怀疑。

气体形成剂如碳酸饮料或由碳酸氢钠和柠檬酸组成的制剂已被描述用于治疗食管嵌塞。它们被释放二氧化碳气体以扩张管腔，并充当活塞将物体从食管推入胃[82]。然而，这种方法的有效性值得怀疑。已有报道认为穿孔与使用造气物体有关[83]。同样，肉类嫩化剂木瓜蛋白酶不推荐用于食管肉类嵌塞的治疗，因其缺乏疗效和存在并发症（如穿孔、纵隔炎）的风险[84,85]。

放射学方法治疗食管异物通常是成功的。透视引导下，Foley 导管、抽吸导管、金属丝篮和磁铁被用来收回物体[60]。最常见的抽出装置是 Foley 导管，它的尖端穿过物体，气球膨胀，然后物体被收回到口咽部。这种方法在透视下的成功率高达 90%。然而，有的影像学检查方法都缺乏对目标的控制，特别是在上食管括约肌和下咽的水平。并发症包括鼻出血、喉痉挛、误吸、穿孔，甚至死亡[86]。一般情况下，只有当柔性内镜检查不可用时，才推荐使用放射检查方法。

2. 内镜方法

可曲式内镜因其安全、高效，已成为治疗胃肠道食物嵌塞和异物的首选方法。多个大型系列报道指出，内镜治疗 GIFB 的成功率超过 95%，并发症发生率不到 5%[5,36,66,74,87-89]。当进食尖锐或多个物体时，以及当进食是故意的而不是意外的时候，并发症的风险就会增加。

由于大多数 GIFB 会自发通过而不会引起症状，因此了解内镜干预的适应证和时机是很重要的。一般来说，所有滞留在食管内的异物都需要紧急处理。食管异物或食物嵌塞造成不良后果的风险与物体或食物在食管内停留的时间有直接关系[90]。理想情况下，任何物体在食管内停留的时间都不应超过 24 小时。

一旦进入胃内，大多数摄入的物体都会自发通过，并发症的风险也低得多，因此观察是可以接受的。也有明显的例外情况。尖锐和锋利物体的穿孔率高达 15%~35%[90]。长度超过 5cm 的物体和宽度超过 2.5cm 的圆形物体也不能通过，应在出现时或在 3~5 天内没有进展的情况下用内镜将其从胃中取出。如果更复杂或尖锐的物体已经移动到胃以外，并且无法取出，应定期拍摄 X 线片，以记录其通过胃肠道的进展情况[91]。然后随访患者是否有任何提示梗阻或穿孔的症状（如发热、心动过速、腹痛、腹胀）。此外，随着双气囊和单气囊小肠镜的使用越来越多，病例报告详细介绍了如何使用这些气囊小肠镜安全、有效地从小肠取出异物[92,93]。鉴于大多数异物到达小肠后没有后遗症，使用气囊辅助肠镜检查应考虑到异物的类型和异物摄入的患者情况。球囊肠镜的附件包括网篮、网兜和钳子已经被设计出来，以便能够取出异物。

对于食物嵌塞和异物摄入的处理，需要个体化的镇静治疗以协助内镜检查。对于成年人来说，清醒镇静对于大多数食物嵌塞和简单异物的治疗是足够的，但对于不合作的患者或吞咽多个复杂异物的患者可能需要麻醉辅助（见第 42 章）。内镜治疗小儿异物通常在麻醉和气管插管的帮助下进行的[94]。

对于喉咽水平以下的嵌塞和吞咽的处理，最好使用可曲式内镜[95]。可以使用硬性食管镜和软性鼻内镜，但效果有限，而且通常只有少数的内镜医师可以使用[7,96]。硬性和可曲式内镜治疗食管异物的比较发现，可曲式内镜治疗食管异物的穿孔明显减少[97]。在 Kelly 钳或 McGill 钳的辅助下进行喉镜检查对近端手术是有用的。

获取和熟悉多种内镜下取出异物和食物嵌塞的设备是至关重要的（框 28.1）。内镜检查套件和/或移动车应至少配备鼠嘴钳或鳄嘴钳、息肉勒除器、篮形取石器械和网形取物器[98]。内镜医生应使用长度为 45cm 和 60cm 的套管。套管可以保护气道、多次交换内镜，并保护黏膜免受尖锐物体的伤害[99]。较长的 60cm 套管可以从胃中取出尖锐而复杂的物体，并包绕下食管括约肌。另一种用于取出尖锐物体的附件是安装在内镜顶端的乳胶保护罩（稍后讨论）[100,101]。

框 28.1 胃肠道异物和食物嵌塞的治疗和清除的设备
内镜
可屈式内镜
硬式内镜
喉镜
外套管
标准食管外套管
45~60cm 异物外套管
配件设备
检索网
抓钳
网篮
息肉切除圈套器
透明真空帽
乳胶保护罩
Kelly 钳或 McGill 钳

当计划取出被摄取的复杂、尖锐或尖端物体时，以及在机会允许的情况下，在考虑取出器械和取出技术时，对类似物体进行体外演练可能是有价值的[5]。取出异物的成功和速度与内镜医师的经验直接相关[102]。当没有人员或设备来完成内镜治疗时，应考虑将患者转移到其他中心。

（六）特殊异物

1. 食物嵌塞

在美国，食物嵌塞是最常见的摄入异物[29]。在美国最常见的引起异物嵌塞的食物是肉类产品，包括牛肉、热狗和鸡肉。鱼骨嵌塞在沿海地区和亚洲国家更为常见。在吃大块肉的同时饮酒可能会增加食物阻塞的风险，并导致后院烧烤综合征和牛排餐厅综合征。

考虑到食团可能会自发排出，内镜干预的必要性是基于症状的持续。出现完全或接近完全梗阻并有流涎或过多唾液的患者应接受紧急上消化道内镜检查。最迟应在症状出现后 24 小时内完成内镜治疗，最理想的是在最初的 6～12 小时内完成。食物嵌塞时间越长，内镜成功率越低[103]。并发症风险的增加被认为与食管食物嵌塞的持续时间成正比[1,18,104]。

治疗食物嵌塞的主要方法是推法，成功率超过 90%，且并发症最少[25]。在食物嵌塞被推入胃中之前，应尝试引导内镜绕过食物进入胃内。一般来说，如果内镜能绕过食物嵌入物进入胃内，则嵌入物就可以毫无困难地安全地进入胃内。这也可以评估任何梗阻性食管病变以外的嵌顿。

即使内镜不能绕过食物嵌塞，也可以安全地尝试温和的推压。可以用内镜或附件将嵌顿的大块肉分开，然后安全地将小块肉推入胃中。

EoE 越来越多地与食管食物嵌塞有关（图 28.5）（见第 30 章）。食物嵌塞往往更频繁发生在 EoE 患者，镜下可见食管环形以及活检中可见较高的嗜酸性粒细胞密度[105]。报告表明，推法可有效安全治疗 EoE 患者的食物嵌塞[42]，但应注意尽量减少引起的黏膜撕裂[106]。虽然 EoE 的穿孔总体较低，但大多数穿孔发生在食物团长期嵌塞[107]。如果怀疑是嗜酸性食管炎，在使用硬质内镜时应特别小心。据报道，在这一患者群体中使用硬性镜的穿孔率高达 20%[108]。如果怀疑有 EoE，应在食物嵌塞治疗后进行黏膜活检。然而，只有 34% 的内镜医生在食物嵌塞时进行食管活检，这大大降低了诊断和适当治疗的机会[109]。外用糖皮质激素治疗 EoE 可降低后续食物团嵌塞的风险[110]。

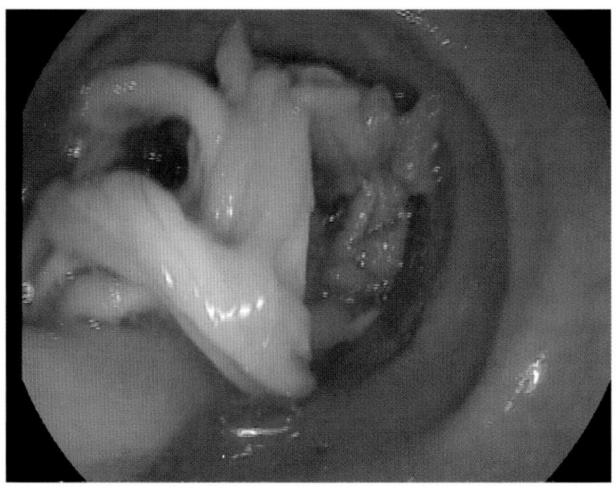

图 28.5　具有多个同心环并已知诊断为嗜酸性食管炎患者的食物嵌塞

不能轻轻推入胃内的食物嵌塞必须取出并收回。逆行摘除可以用各种取回装置来实现，包括圈套、篮、网和镊子。最初手动将食物团分成更小的碎片，通常会更容易取出。这种情况下，食管套管是有用的，因为它保护了气道，并允许在取出时多次交换内镜。专用的食物团块取回网在不使用外管的情况下可以很好地清除大块食物，因为食物可以在网内得到很好的保护，降低误食的风险[111]。所有的拔出方法也可以有效和安全地用于 EoE 患者，但放置外管时要小心，特别是对于食管管径狭窄的患者。

透明塑料兜或帽，类似用于实施静脉曲张结扎术和内镜黏膜切除术的器械，已成功地用于移除大的、紧密嵌塞的肉丸。与使用其他器械相比，使用兜帽可能是一种更有效、并发症更少的方法来取出食物嵌塞[112]。将兜帽固定在内镜的顶端，该设备可用于将食物吸入真空室，并每次取出很大剂量[113,114]。

超过 75% 的食物嵌塞患者伴有食管病变[5,26]，和大约一半的患者有 24 小时食管 pH 测定和/或食管测压异常。如果食管狭窄或沙茨基环在食物丸清除后出现，在条件允许的情况下，可以安全有效地同时扩张食管狭窄或沙茨基环。更常见的是长时间停留在食管内的食物引起的黏膜擦伤或红斑，扩张延迟 2～4 周，在此期间应给予患者质子泵抑制剂治疗。当存在多个食管环时，应进行活检以评估嗜酸性食管炎。缺乏对患者的适当随访，特别是那些有狭窄或环的患者，已被证明是预测复发性食物嵌塞的一个因素[115]。

2. 尖锐物体

尖锐物体可能导致穿孔的风险高达 15%～35%，占所有胃肠道异物穿孔的三分之一，与其他 GIFB 相比，并发症的风险高 2.5 倍[116,117]。尖锐物品，特别是牙签和动物骨，是最有可能导致穿孔的异物，需要手术治疗[118]。精神病患者和被监禁的患者更容易摄入更复杂、多个尖锐和锋利的物体。如剃须刀片（图 28.6）、大头针、别针以及书写和饮食用具（图 28.7）。

锋利和尖锐的物体留在食管被认为是一种医疗紧急情况，应该在 6～12 小时内取出。此外，如果可以安全地完成，内镜可触及范围内的任何尖锐物体也应移除（图 28.8）。取出锋利尖锐的异物时，应抓住并定位异物，使尖端在取出时尾随，以减少穿孔和黏膜撕裂的风险[119]。

对于尖锐的异物，最好使用抓取钳、圈套器或篮形取石器械取回[102]。所有这些装置都能固定异物；如前面所述，调整设备方向使锐端指向远端。在清除尖锐物体时，检索网倾向于剪切，可能影响视觉。

应考虑使用套管来保护食管和咽。可以抓住长而尖的物体并将其引导到套管中；然后将整个组件（包括锋利而尖端的物体、内镜和套管）一齐取出。

用于取出尖锐物体的套筒的另一种选择是可伸缩的乳胶罩，它可以固定在内镜的尖端（图 28.9）。当内镜通过下食管括约肌被拉回时，乳胶罩会翻转抓住的物体，并在取出时保护黏膜[100,120]。

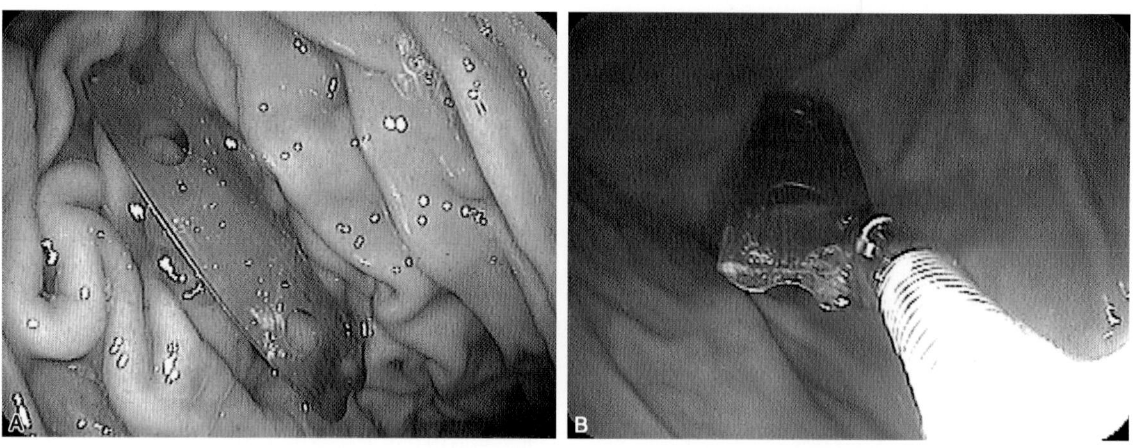

图 28.6 A,一名囚犯吞下的剃须刀片(胃内)。B,用抓钳和外套管取出刀片

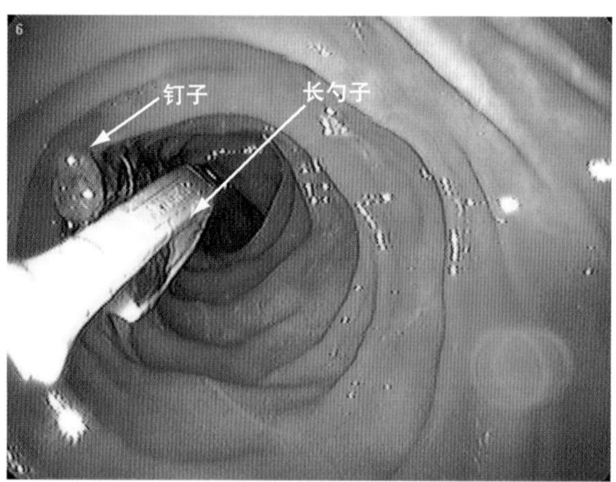

图 28.7 精神病患者吞咽后嵌塞在十二指肠清除中的钉子和长勺子的内镜图像

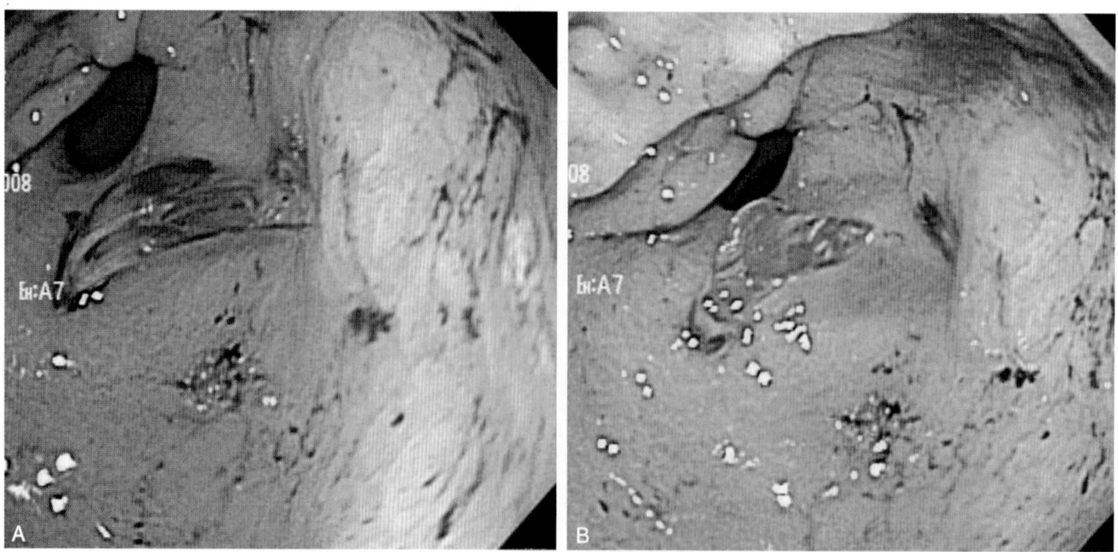

图 28.8 幽门前胃窦部玻璃碎片的内镜图像。(Courtesy Dr. Jamie Anderson and Dr. Tushar Dharia,Dallas,Tex.)

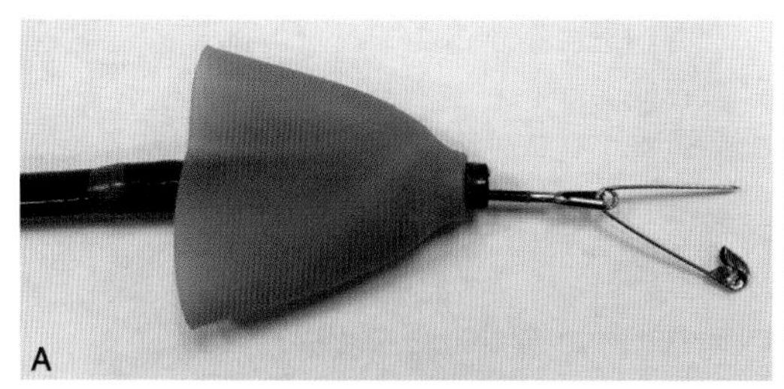

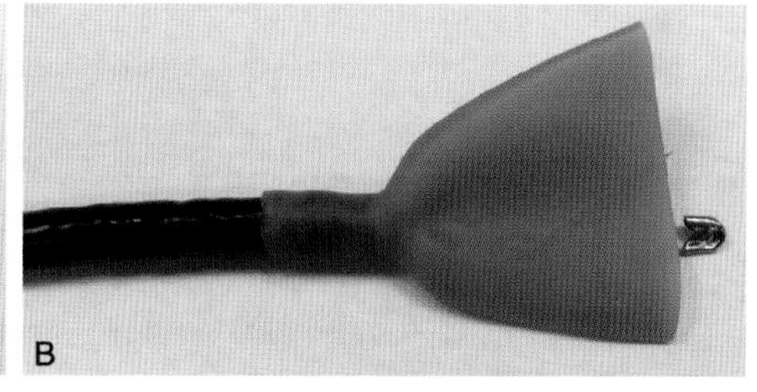

图 28.9　A,拉回乳胶保护罩。该位置能够实现完全可视化,并允许内镜医生轻松抓取锐利物体。B,当保护罩通过下食管括约肌拉回时,保护罩向前翻转,保护胃肠道黏膜免受锋利物体的损伤

虽然会增加穿孔的风险,但大多数超出内镜范围的尖锐物体都可以畅通无阻地通过胃肠道,而不会出现并发症。由于穿孔的风险增加,尖锐的物体应每天连续拍 X 线片以确保进展。如果锋利或尖锐的物体超过 3 天没有进展,应该考虑手术干预。

3. 长物体

吞食的物体超过 5cm,特别是超过 10cm 的物体,很难通过幽门和十二指肠降部,并可能被挂起,导致这些部位梗阻或穿孔(见图 28.8)。最常被摄取的长物是钢笔、铅笔、牙刷和餐具。抓取钳和息肉夹是固定和切除长物体最常用的设备。长物体应握在一端,纵向定位以便移开。对于长物体的提取,如前所述,应该考虑使用 60cm 长的套管式内镜组件。

4. 钝性物体：硬币、电池和磁铁

小型钝器,如玩具和硬币,是儿童最常吞食的物体。圆盘(按钮)电池和磁铁摄入并不常见,但会造成独特的潜在危险。食管内的钝物应立即取出。嵌顿硬币可导致食管壁压迫性坏死,引起穿孔和瘘管。任何大小的硬币都可能卡在儿童的食管里,但人们吞下的硬币,尤其是直径为 17mm 或 18mm 的一角硬币通常会穿过成人的食管。在影像学上,位于食管远端的硬币自然通过的可能性是位于食管近端硬币的两倍[121]。

息肉或专用的取石网可以捕获并安全地取出硬币和大多数小的钝物[102]。抓取钳和胆道取石篮也是有效的。不推荐使用标准的活检钳和诱捕器,因为它们在提取过程中不能可靠地固定硬币。如果难以将钝器固定在食管内,则将其推入胃内是安全的,因为胃内有更大的通过空间。

一旦小的钝器进入胃,对于许多患者来说保守的门诊治疗是合适的[122]。例外情况包括手术改变了消化道解剖结构的患者和那些摄入了大型钝器的患者。成年人的幽门,可以通过大多数直径 25mm 以下的钝物。否则,一旦进入胃内,就应定期饮食,每 1~2 周进行一次影像学检查,以确认病情进展或消除。如果钝器在 3~4 周后仍未通过,则应进行内镜取出[123]。

纽扣电池现在装在许多幼儿可接触到的小玩具和电子设备中。食用纽扣电池尤其值得关注,因为电池中含有一种碱性溶液,可能会导致食管迅速液化坏死。纽扣电池摄入最常发生在年龄较小的儿童中,大约 10% 会出现症状[124]。任何临床怀疑食管中嵌塞纽扣电池的病例都应立即进行紧急内镜检查。大多数纽扣电池将在内镜检查前在平片上发现,较大的电池(>2cm)更有可能留在食管并导致并发症[125]。镊子和诱捕器通常对取出纽扣电池无效,但使用回收网可以在几乎 100% 的情况下成功取出[126]。使用套管保护气道,或者对于儿科患者,气管插管在回收纽扣电池中至关重要。胃内纽扣电池有一半的患者有黏膜损伤,因此胃电池也应该通过内镜取出[127]。一旦进入小肠,纽扣电池很少引起临床问题,可在 X 线片上观察到,85% 的纽扣电池在 72 小时内通过胃肠道[128]。

圆柱形电池引起症状的频率较低,没有严重危及生命的损伤报告,只有 20% 的人在摄入后出现一些轻微症状,包括黏膜溃疡和很少的肠梗阻[128]。圆柱形电池应从食管取出,大于 20mm 的电池或 48 小时内没有进展的电池应通过内镜取出(图 28.10)。

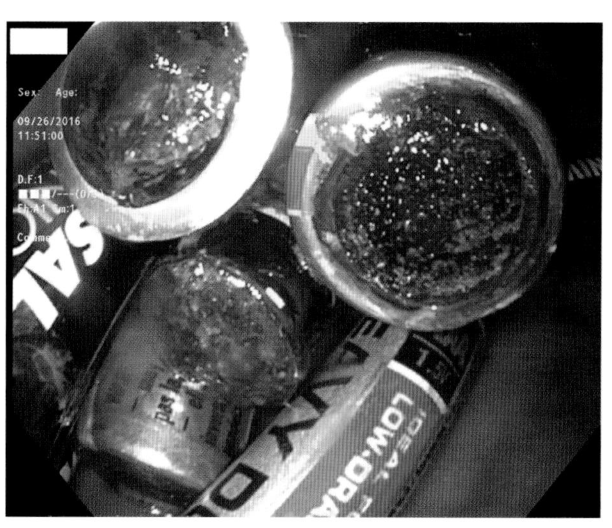

图 28.10　在胃内发现多个大于 2cm 的圆柱形电池,随后用内镜取出

小型耦合磁铁作为儿童玩具已变得流行起来。在内镜可触及范围内摄入的磁铁也应紧急取出。虽然单个磁铁很少会引起症状,但如果摄入了多个磁铁,或者磁铁与其他金属物体一起摄入,就会引起人们的担忧。这可能导致肠袢间的磁吸引和耦合,随后出现压迫性坏死、瘘管形成和肠穿孔[129,130]。当磁铁很可能在标准内镜的范围内时,应该紧急进行移除;这可以通过抓取钳、网形取物器或篮形取石器实现。对金属回收装置的磁引力可以减小取出的难度。

5. 麻醉包

胃肠道中摄入的袋装非法麻醉品通常分为两类:人体填充

者和人体包装者。"人体填充者"指的是吸毒者或毒贩,他们很快地摄入少量毒品,但包装或内含的包裹很容易泄漏。身体包装者是毒品走私者用来运输毒品的"骡子",他们摄入大量精心准备的包裹,以抵御胃肠道的蠕动转运[131,132]。这些患者可能会因为包裹而出现肠梗阻,或者出现与摄入的药物相关的症状。后者可能会导致5%的人严重中毒和死亡[133]。

疑似患者通常不合作,并由执法人员陪同。诊断始于X线平片或CT扫描,可见多个圆形或管状包。内镜手术是禁忌的,因为包装穿孔的风险很高,并导致药物过量[1]。建议连续拍X线片的同时观察清澈的流质饮食。当怀疑肠梗阻、进展失败或药物泄漏/毒性时,应进行手术干预。在一项大型研究中,高达45%的患者可能需要根据包装的位置进行胃切开术、肠切开术或结肠切开术[134]。

其他数据表明,仅凭观察就对麻醉药品包装器进行保守治疗导致手术的病例不到3%[135,136]。

6. 结直肠异物

摄入的物体很少会在结肠内滞留。更常见的情况是,结肠异物有意或无意插入直肠。在试图取出结直肠异物之前,应拍摄X线片,以便更好地观察异物的位置、方向和形态(图28.11)。为了避免医护人员受伤,应该推迟手动移除或直肠指诊的尝试,直到排除了尖锐或尖锐的物体。

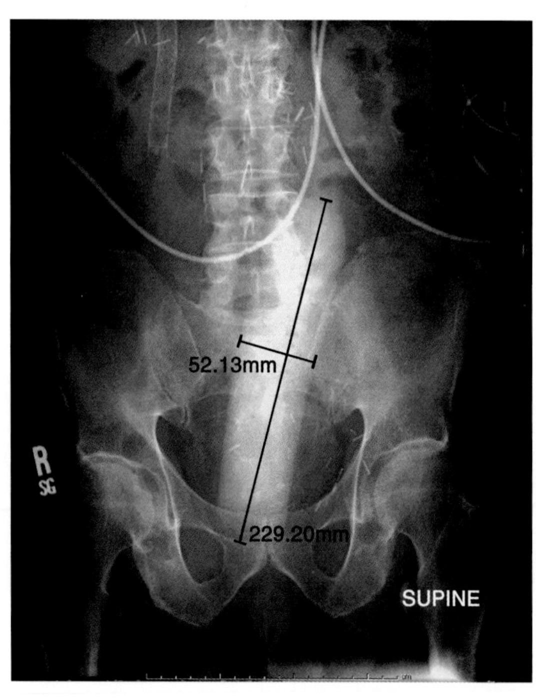

图28.11 平片显示一例73岁男性自行塞入的直肠异物,表现为下腹疼痛。(Courtesy Dr. William Beaujohn, Plano, Tex.)

对于直肠远端的小的、钝的、可触到的物体,手动拔除很有可能成功。在一些患者中,清醒镇静可能足以进行手动摘除,但在其他患者中,可能需要在全身麻醉下进行检查和摘除,以便使肛门括约肌得到更大的松弛和成功地取出物体。

不可触及的尖锐或有尖的物体应使用硬性直肠镜或可曲式性乙状结肠镜直接观察移除[137]。标准的回收装置可以像前面描述的用于上消化道的那样。乳胶罩或外管在取出长而尖的物体时特别有用,可以保护直肠黏膜免受撕裂,并克服试图移除物体时肛门括约肌收缩的趋势。虽然有清醒镇静通常会有助于切除,但全身麻醉可以最大限度地扩张肛门括约肌,以帮助取出更大、更复杂的物体[138]。

对于直肠或结肠异物继发的任何疑似并发症,包括穿孔、脓肿和梗阻,都需要手术干预。并发症多发生在靠近直肠的部位[139]。

(七) 操作相关的并发症

虽然报告的与内镜下摘除GIFB和食物嵌塞相关的并发症发生率较低(0%至1.8%),但在实践中被认为要高得多[5,9,24,25,36,68]。穿孔是最严重的并发症,尽管与误吸和镇静相关的心肺并发症也可能发生(见第41章)。增加并发症风险的因素包括:取出尖锐的物体,患者不合作,多次和/或故意摄入,以及食物嵌塞或异物摄入的时间延长[12]。

二、胃石

胃石积聚在胃肠道,最常见的是在胃的消化不良物质的集合。最常见的3种类型的胃石是:植物胃石,由植物物质组成;毛发胃石,由毛发或毛状纤维组成;以及药物胃石(药用胃石)(图28.11和框28.2)。

框28.2 与药物胃石形成相关的口服药物
不可吸收的抗酸药
容积性泻药
心血管药物
硝苯地平
维拉帕米
普鲁卡因胺
维生素和矿物质
维生素C
维生素B_{12}
硫酸亚铁
其他药物
硫糖铝
瓜尔胶
考来烯胺
肠内喂养配方
茶碱
聚磺苯乙烯(聚苯乙烯磺酸钠)树脂

(一) 流行病学

植物胃石是最常见的胃石类型。引起胃石的水果和蔬菜包括芹菜、南瓜、李子、葡萄干、韭菜、甜菜和柿子[5]。所有这些食物都含有大量的不溶性和不可消化的纤维,如纤维素、半纤维素、木质素和水果单宁[140]。当大量摄入和积累时,就会形成植物胃石。

毛球性胃石最常见于年轻妇女和儿童,因为他们摄入了大量的头发、地毯纤维或衣物纤维。动物性胃石通常与精神障碍、智力迟钝或异食癖有关[141]。

药用胃石与含有纤维的药物、树脂水产品或旨在抵抗消化的缓释药有关[142]。当活性物质被困在胃石中不能被吸收时,用药胃石的药理作用可能会降低,或者,当大量胃用药胃石的内容物一次性释放到小肠时,会产生毒性。

大多数胃石患者(除动物性胃石外)都有减少胃内容物排空的易感因素。70%~94%的胃石患者有明显的胃部手术史。在接受迷走神经切断术和幽门成形术的患者中,可观察到高达65%~80%的胃内容物残留[56]。胃手术后胃石形成的原因是胃排空延迟,胃调节功能降低,酸消化活性降低[143]。胃结石患者常可见胃排空障碍。糖尿病或终末期肾病患者以及使用机械通气的患者形成胃石的风险更大[144]。

(二) 临床特征

胃结石患者可能没有症状,但大多数(80%)有上腹部不适的模糊症状[144]。还可能出现相关的食欲减退、恶心、呕吐、体重减轻和早饱。胃石可引起继发于压迫性坏死的胃溃疡。胃石引起的胃溃疡可导致出血和胃出口梗阻[145]。

胃石也可能聚集在小肠内,通常表现为机械性梗阻。Rapunzel综合征是一个术语,主要用来描述位于胃部的毛状石,它穿过幽门进入十二指肠,甚至由于在壶腹水平的梗阻导致黄疸或胰腺炎[146,147]。

(三) 诊断

病史有助于胃石的诊断,重点是食物或药物的用量和类型。应考虑既往胃石病史、胃手术史或胃动力障碍史。虽然偶尔可以发现可触及的腹部肿块,但体格检查通常对诊断帮助不大。秃顶和散乱的头发可能出现在毛球症患者身上,他们一直在吞食自己的头发。

腹部平片可以显示胃石的轮廓。对比片显示,胃结石通常表现为胃内的充盈缺损[140]。平片和造影剂检查只能发现25%的上消化道内镜检查发现的胃石。CT扫描可以帮助识别小肠结石,并根据组成胃石的植物性物质的大小和程度预测是否会发生梗阻[148]。胃结石通过上消化道内镜检查可以更明确地诊断,植物胃石在胃内呈深棕色、绿色或黑色的无定形植物体。毛球性胃石的外观坚硬,发黑,几乎是混凝土。药物胃石将被视为物质中间的完整药片或药片碎片(图28.12)。

(四) 治疗

较小的胃石可以采用保守的药物治疗;通常包括短期的流质饮食和促进胃排空的促动力剂[140]。据报道,使用纤维素酶进行化学溶解的成功率高达85%[145]。纤维素酶可以片剂形式服用,也可以通过内镜或鼻胃管以液体形式滴入胃中。鼻胃灌洗可能有助于小胃石的物理溶解。碳酸饮料(例如可口可乐)可有效溶解超过50%的植物胃石,当与内镜方法联合使用时,可有效溶解90%以上的植物胃石[148]。其他已证明有效治疗胃结石的药物包括胰酶和熊去氧胆酸,单用或与纤维素酶和碳酸饮料联合使用[149]。

对于较大的胃石和耐药的胃石,内镜治疗可能是有效的。

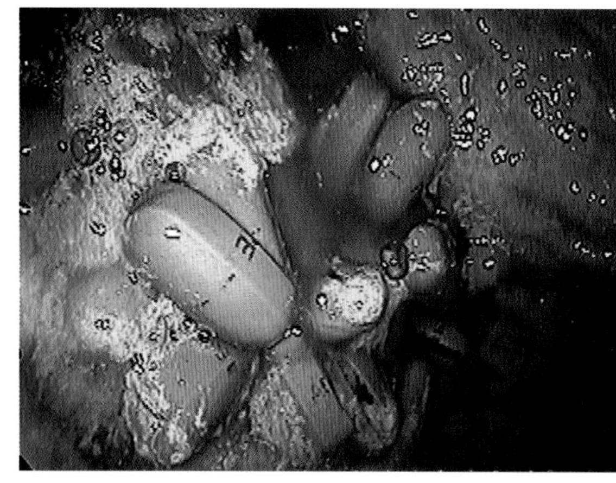

图28.12　有胰十二指肠切除术史并有梗阻症状的患者的药物胃石的内镜图像。用内镜网取出这些药丸,随后患者症状缓解

用内镜将胃石切成小块。碎片可以通过内镜本身,以及镊子或诱捕器等辅助设备进行,或者通过内镜滴注盐水或冲洗水来完成。胃石的碎片可以推入小肠或用嘴取出。如果要移除大部分胃石,建议使用外管,以方便内镜的频繁通过,并保护气道。在85%~90%的胃结石中,机械破碎和内镜取出的成功率为85%~90%。顽固性胃结石可采用机械碎石、液电碎石、Nd:YAG激光或针刀括约肌切开术治疗[150-152]。

如果内镜治疗失败或出现与结石有关的并发症(如穿孔、梗阻、出血),可能需要手术干预。与植物胃石相比,毛球性结石更需要手术治疗。胃结石通常通过小的胃造口术去除[145,147]。可以通过小肠切开术切除,也可以经黏膜挤到盲肠,在大直径结肠中很少引起梗阻的问题。在切除胃石时,可以先尝试腹腔镜切除,但一半以上的患者可能会转行开腹手术[153]。当考虑手术干预时,必须注意排除在一个以上位置的多个结石。

预防胃石复发与积极治疗同等重要。如果胃石形成的根本原因得不到纠正,就有可能复发。应避免食用高纤维和其他不易消化的食物。起始剂量的纤维素酶是一种酶溶解药物,经常复发的胃石患者可以预防性服用。促动力药物可能对潜在的运动障碍患者有用。尤其是难治性复发性胃结石患者,反复进行周期性内镜检查,并对食物材料进行物理破坏,可以防止较大的、临床上有意义的胃石形成。

三、腐蚀物摄入

(一) 流行病学

在美国,每年报告大约5 000例摄入腐蚀物[154]。大多数是6岁以下儿童意外摄入[155]。成人的腐蚀物摄入是自杀企图、有心理健康问题的患者,以及由于酒精或娱乐性药物摄入导致的醉酒者。成年人可以摄入更多的腐蚀物,所以他们往往比儿童有更严重的伤害,儿童通常会吐出或呕出他们吞下的腐蚀物。

广义上,最常被摄入的腐蚀物有两种:碱性剂或酸性剂。碱性清洁剂最常见于家用清洁剂,如排水管、马桶和烤箱清洁剂。Lye 是一种含有氢氧化钠或氢氧化钾的碱液。碱液通常是无臭、无味,这可能会导致大量的误服。最后,如上所述,圆盘电池也可能引起碱诱导损伤。

酸摄入通常来自吞咽马桶清洁剂、游泳池清洁剂或电池酸。酸摄入通常会引起即刻疼痛,从而导致摄入物被快速排出体外。家用漂白剂可能同时含有酸碱产品,但由于其浓度被稀释,很少会引起严重损伤。

(二) 病理生理学

1. 强碱

强碱摄入会导致液化坏死,并迅速蔓延至黏膜、黏膜下层、食管肌层和胃[156]。坏死后会发生血管血栓形成。最初的碱损伤可以是跨壁的,导致穿孔、纵隔炎和腹膜炎[157]。食物摄入后几天会出现表面上皮脱落和溃疡。最后,大量肉芽组织、成纤维细胞活性和胶原沉积持续数周,导致慢性狭窄形成(图 28.13)。强碱摄入对食管的影响最大,胃酸中和可限制对胃的损伤。少数患者的小肠也有损伤[158]。损伤的程度还取决于摄入的药剂、其数量以及胃肠道暴露的时间长短[159]。

2. 酸性制剂

酸性制剂可引起凝固性坏死,伴有黏膜血管血栓和更有限的浅表坏死。酸性制剂更容易损害胃,特别是胃窦,而不是食管(图 28.14)。酸性制剂由于其刺激性的味道和即刻的疼痛,往往摄入量较少,因此与碱性制剂相比,其总体损伤较小。

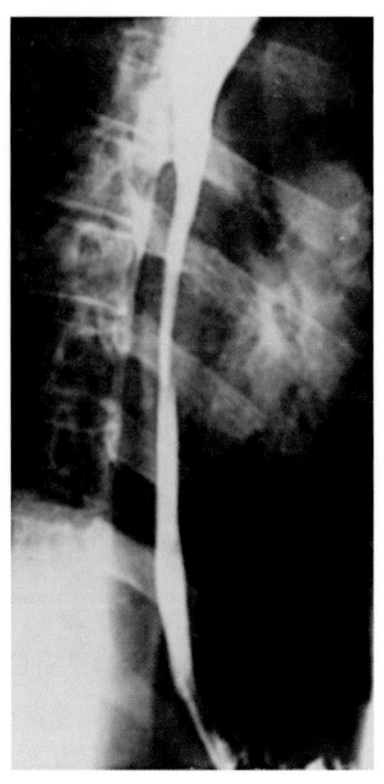

图 28.13　钡剂食管造影显示腐蚀物摄入数周后食管上段狭窄伴食管中段狭窄。(Courtesy Dr. Robert N. Berk, University of California, San Diego, Calif.)

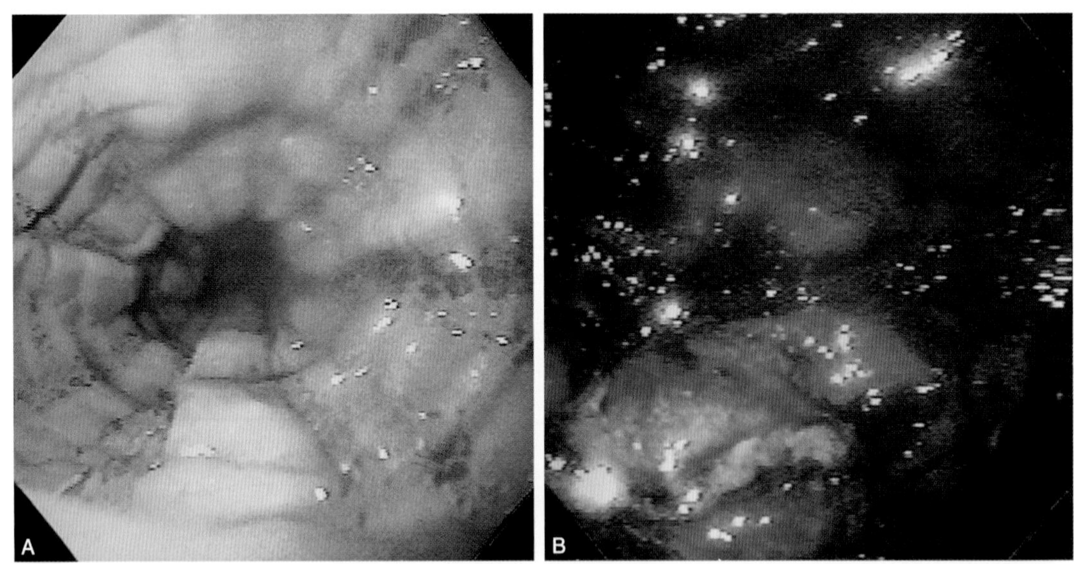

图 28.14　酸对食管和胃的腐蚀性损伤。A,食入酸后,食管鳞状黏膜呈线状脱落。食管黏膜水肿,呈蓝色变色。B,该患者胃黏膜出血水肿。(From Wilcox MC. Atlas of clinical gastrointestinal endoscopy. Philadelphia: WB Saunders; 1995. p 85.)

(三) 临床特征

患者可能出现口咽痛、上腹痛、胸痛、吞咽困难或吞咽疼痛。口咽受累可引起流涎和流口水。声音嘶哑、喘鸣和呼吸困难提示会厌、喉部和上呼吸道损伤。持续性胸痛或背痛可能提示食管穿孔和纵隔炎,而剧烈腹痛可能与胃穿孔和腹膜炎有关。重要的是,早期体征和症状并不总是与腐蚀性损伤的程度和晚期并发症的可能性相关[160]。在体检中,患者可能有口腔烧伤、水肿、溃疡和渗出的迹象,但多达 20%～45% 的患者体格检查正常[161]。

(四) 诊断

胸部 X 线和腹部平片等放射影像无助于直接诊断或对损伤严重程度进行分级。但可通过显示肺纵隔、气胸或气腹来提示穿孔的存在。当颈部、胸部和/或腹部高度怀疑有穿孔时，尽管平片呈阴性，仍应考虑 CT 检查。如果有穿孔，应紧急进行手术而不是内镜检查(图 28.15)。

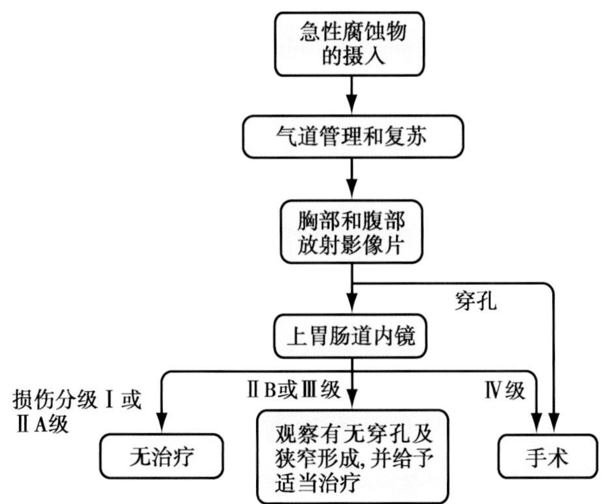

图 28.15　急性腐蚀性损伤处理的流程。有关内镜下损伤分级的定义见表 28.1

腐蚀物摄入后的症状和体格检查可能与损伤程度不匹配，因此对于没有穿孔的患者，应在摄入后的 24~48 小时内进行上消化道内镜检查[162]。上消化道内镜检查可以诊断胃肠道损伤，对损伤程度进行分级，确定预后，并指导治疗(见图 28.15)。也可以在摄入后 5 天重新检查胃镜，因为它比最初 24 小时的胃镜检查更能预测食管和胃的并发症[163]。值得注意的是，40%~80% 的有腐蚀性咽下的患者在内镜检查中没有损伤的证据[164]。急诊 CT 扫描也可以用于在腐蚀性进食时对食管损伤进行分级和预测狭窄程度[165]。

内镜检查中看到的损伤程度可以分级，并提供预后信息(表 28.1)。Ⅰ级和ⅡA 级烧伤相当于一度和二度烧伤，通常会痊愈而不会有后遗症[158]。然而，70%~100% 的ⅡB 级烧伤患者会出现狭窄，这会导致环状溃疡，而Ⅲ级烧伤患者会出现相关的坏死[166]。伴有穿孔的Ⅳ级损伤死亡率高达 65%，需要紧急手术。

表 28.1　内镜下腐蚀性损伤的分级

等级	内镜检查结果
Ⅰ	水肿和红斑
ⅡA	出血、糜烂、水疱、溃疡伴渗液
ⅡB	环周溃疡
Ⅲ	多处深溃疡，伴棕色、黑色或灰色变色
Ⅳ	穿孔

(五) 治疗

初始处理应评估复苏管理 ABC：即气道(airway)、呼吸(breathing)和循环(circulation)。与区域控制中心联系。一旦初步稳定，根据患者的临床状态和内镜所见的损伤程度进行治疗。内镜检查正常或仅有Ⅰ级或ⅡA 级损伤的无症状患者，可以在最初 24~48 小时内开始口服治疗，通常在同一时间段内出院。

临床上有低血压、呼吸窘迫、内镜检查显示ⅡB 级(周围性溃疡)或Ⅲ级坏死的患者应入院重症监护室，进行静脉输液复苏，并密切监测穿孔的证据。呼吸窘迫患者应行喉镜检查。喉咽水肿、坏死的患者不应接受气管内插管，需要气管切开以维持气道。

如果有穿孔，须行食管切除或胃切除等紧急手术。有时需要结肠代食管术。操作人员和机构的经验影响急诊食管胃切除术的死亡率和发病率，条件允许时最好在转诊中心进行[167]。

对于没有明确穿孔证据的严重溃疡或坏死患者，手术干预的必要性和时机仍然存在争议。在这样的患者群体中，比较分析是困难的。一些权威人士认为，早期手术探查可降低死亡率[168,169]，但另一些权威人士指出，在接受非手术支持治疗的患者中，死亡率较低且患者完全康复[159]。高龄、气管支气管损伤、延长切除术和急诊食管切除术是早期手术治疗患者存活的负面预测因素[169]。因此，治疗必须在个体化的基础上考虑。

由于可能会使食管、口咽和气道再次暴露于腐蚀物，所以禁止使用诱导呕吐或放置鼻胃管来清除或稀释胃肠道中的腐蚀物。诱发性干呕和呕吐可能会增加穿孔的风险。不推荐使用中和剂，因为它们没有被证明是有效的，可能会导致更多的热损伤，还可能会促进干呕和呕吐[170]。不建议常规使用糖皮质激素[156]和全身抗生素[154]，但使用质子泵抑制剂可能会减少并发症[171]。

(六) 晚期并发症

高达三分之一的腐蚀物摄入患者在初次恢复后会发生食管狭窄(见图 28.13)。狭窄形成最常见于损伤后 2 个月，但也可能发生在最初受伤后 2 周至数年的任何时间[158]。损伤越严重(ⅡB 级或Ⅲ级)，越容易形成狭窄(见表 28.1)。腐蚀物摄入继发食管狭窄的主要治疗方法是频繁扩张。腐蚀性狭窄的内镜治疗必须是谨慎的，逐渐渐进性扩张到 15mm 或直到症状缓解[172]。报道称，内镜下在狭窄处注射曲安奈德或局部使用丝裂霉素对治疗腐蚀性狭窄有益[173,174]。慢性腐蚀性狭窄的内镜下扩张的穿孔率为 0.5%，多达 10%~50% 的患者最终将需要手术干预。与需要早期手术治疗腐蚀物摄入的患者相比，需要手术干预治疗晚期并发症的患者具有更好的功能结构和生存率[169]。可以考虑食管切除联合食管胃吻合术、食管空肠吻合术或结肠间置术[175]。有病例报告描述了在摄入腐蚀物后不久，使用临时食管支架治疗的成功案例，但没有足够的证据支持常规预防性支架置入或预防性早期内镜扩张以防止腐蚀性相关狭窄[170]。

腐蚀性损伤后也可发生胃窦和幽门狭窄(图 28.16)。胃窦和幽门狭窄通常在摄入腐蚀物后 1~6 周发生，但也可能在数年后发生[154]。胃窦狭窄的风险也与损伤程度有关。内镜下扩张加抑酸在许多患者中是成功的，但也有许多患者需要行胃切除术。

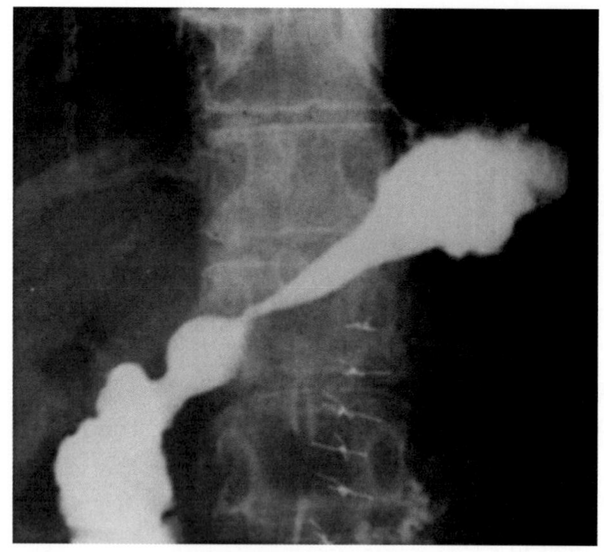

图 28.16　误食所致慢性胃窦狭窄的钡剂研究。(Courtesy Dr. Robert N. Berk, San Diego, Calif.)

尤其是碱性腐蚀物的摄入与食管鳞状细胞癌风险增加相关。有碱液摄入史的患者患食管癌的风险增加 1 000 倍,从损伤开始的滞后时间约为 40 年[176]。建议从摄入腐蚀物后 20 年开始,每 1~3 年定期进行一次内镜监测。

图 28.17 总结了本节综述的摄入腐蚀物后并发症的时间进程。

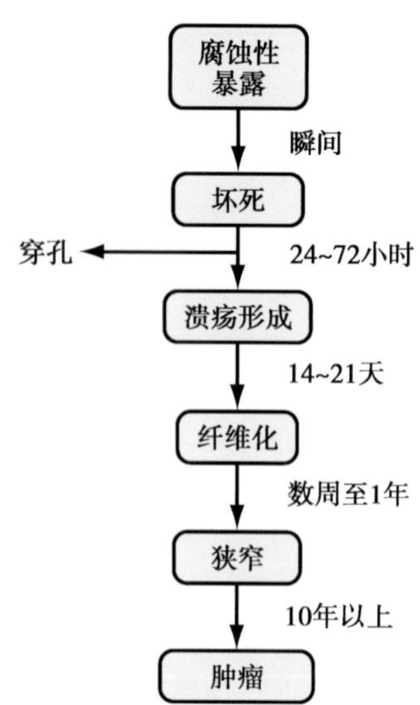

图 28.17　在摄入后,胃肠道腐蚀性损伤后果随时间变化的顺序图

(边艳琴　刘璐 译,闫秀娥 校)

参考文献

第 29 章　腹腔内脓肿和胃肠道瘘

Gregory de prisco, Scott Celinski, Cedric W. Spak 著

章节目录

一、腹腔内脓肿 …… 389
（一）病理生理学 …… 389
（二）细菌学 …… 390
（三）诊断 …… 390
（四）处理 …… 392
（五）预后 …… 396
二、胃肠瘘 …… 396
（一）分类 …… 396
（二）病理生理学 …… 396
（三）诊断 …… 396
（四）处理 …… 398
（五）结果 …… 399

一、腹腔内脓肿

腹腔内脓肿（intra-abdominal abscess，IAA）是在感染性腹膜炎背景下发生的局部腹部感染。原发性腹膜炎（自发性细菌性腹膜炎，在第 93 章中讨论）通常与脓肿的形成无关，而继发性腹膜炎，由胃肠道炎症过程引起的腹膜感染，通常与脓肿的形成有关（见第 39 章）。大多数 IAA 病例是在肠穿孔引起的继发性腹膜炎的情况下发生的（框 29.1）。第三型腹膜炎是在治疗继发性腹膜炎后 48 小时出现的持续性或复发性感染，通常发生在已有合并症的情况下，可能与 IAA 有关（见第 39 章）[1,2]。实质性器官脓肿将在第 58、61 和 84 章中讨论。

框 29.1　腹腔内脓肿的原因
腹部创伤
阑尾炎
胆囊切除术和其他手术或侵入性操作
克罗恩病
憩室炎
肿瘤性疾病
胰腺炎
空腔脏器穿孔（如十二指肠或胃溃疡）

（一）病理生理学

当机体防御能力大于细菌致病作用时，腹腔就保持无菌状态。细菌通常通过穿孔的肠壁进入腹腔。大部分的细菌通过膈肌的持续淋巴引流作用被运送到网状内皮系统后清除[2]。淋巴清除非常有效，只有当辅助物质如血红蛋白、钡或坏死组织存在时，脓肿才会形成[3]。这些辅助物质（钡、粪便颗粒）可以阻断淋巴管，为细菌提供营养物质（血红蛋白中的铁），或削弱杀灭细菌的作用，这些促进了细菌感染。细菌进入腹膜腔后，立即被巨噬细胞吞噬，同时被淋巴系统所清除。随着细菌的增殖，多核白细胞侵入污染区域并变得越来越多。腹膜炎症导致内脏血流增加，同时蛋白质和液体渗出进入腹腔。纤维蛋白原的释放、炎症过程的促凝作用及纤溶酶原激活剂水平的降低增强了纤维蛋白的沉积，导致细菌的滞留和局部的感染[4]。腹膜腔内有许多凹陷和隐窝，使得腹腔感染分隔，以防止感染的进一步扩散和脓毒症的发生[5,6]。因此，脓肿的形成可能是控制严重腹腔内感染的一种手段。

腹膜防御机制可以预防细菌感染扩散，但也会对人体产生不利影响。淋巴系统可以有效清除细菌，但也导致脓毒症。渗出液进入腹腔导致低血容量和休克，也会削弱调理素的细菌吞噬作用。此外，纤维蛋白包裹细菌会影响抗菌药物的渗透和吞噬细胞的迁移[1]。

一些宿主因素与细菌感染相互作用增加了 IAA 的风险（框 29.2）。糖尿病、营养不良、高龄、器官功能障碍、潜在的恶性肿瘤和输血都是脓肿形成的易感因素[7-9]。在这些情况下，无论是继发性腹膜炎还是三型腹膜炎，免疫系统对抗细菌污染的能力都会下降。

框 29.2　腹腔内脓肿的临床风险因素
长期使用糖皮质激素
年龄增长
营养不良
既存器官功能障碍
输血
潜在的恶性肿瘤

炎症性肠病（IBD）背景下的医源性免疫抑制治疗加深了对 IAA 发病机制的了解。长期糖皮质激素治疗增加了 IAA 的风险[10]。同样，术前应用硫唑嘌呤治疗 IBD 也增加了腹腔感染的风险[11]。相比之下，最近 2 项大型研究显示术前 12 周内使用抗 TNF-α 治疗 IBD 不增加 IAA 的发生率[12-14]。

IAA 与术后残留纱布，所谓的纱布瘤（纺织品瘤）之间的关系已广为人知[15]。虽然这些引起 IAA 的原因不常见，但仍是重要的可预防的病因。同样的，应用介入放射学技术治疗外伤性实体内脏损伤改善了对创伤患者的护理，但可能与迟发 IAA 形成有关[16]。

（二）细菌学

IAA 的微生物学取决于临床的不同阶段以及感染发生的宿主。动物研究表明腹腔感染的细菌构成随时间而变化。在 Onderdonk 等人的经典研究中，大肠杆菌在最初的腹腔脓毒症大鼠模型中占主导地位[17]。随着腹膜炎的发展，许多动物患上了大肠杆菌菌血症并且死亡。在存活的动物中，IAA 以脆弱拟杆菌为主要微生物。因此，导致腹腔感染的细菌种类具有流动性。

IAA 的形成是有益的，因为它使感染局限、防止致命的脓毒症和死亡。拟杆菌是 IAA 形成过程中重要的微生物，为了更好地了解脓肿形成过程，人类对其进行了广泛的研究。已知脆弱拟杆菌有 8 种形式的荚膜多糖[18]，其中一些具有两性结构。脆弱拟杆菌的多糖 A（polysaccharide A，PSA）可刺激消化道的促炎或抗炎反应，这取决于它们的位置[19,20]。这被称为“爱恨”关系[19]或细菌多糖的“阴阳”关系[20]。一方面，来自脆弱拟杆菌的 PSA 似乎在诱导正常 T 细胞介导的免疫应答中起重要作用，这些免疫由肠道中正常的共生菌定植引起；而另一方面，PSA 进入腹腔，与淋巴管阻塞一起诱发脓肿形成。PSA 对脓肿形成的影响是通过调控 T-辅助 17 细胞分泌白介素（interleukin，IL）-17 及促进脓肿形成[21]，以及 Forkhead Box（FOX）转录因子调节 T 细胞和 $CD4^+$ $CD45RB^{low}$ 细胞，两者共同分泌 IL-10 促进脓肿形成[22,23]。IL-10 的另一个来源是腹膜巨噬细胞，对脓肿的形成也至关重要[23]。最近的研究表明脆弱拟杆菌与纤维蛋白原的直接结合以及纤维蛋白原水解酶的活性可能会阻碍脓肿的形成，从而导致菌血症和潜在的脓毒症[24]。很明显，细菌和免疫细胞之间存在极其复杂的相互作用，可促进或防止细菌的播散。事实上，许多学者提出的理论认为，脓肿的形成可能是“细菌凋亡”的一种形式，通过牺牲肠外共生物来避免脓毒症并防止宿主微生物死亡，从而保证了更大的肠内菌群的持续生长。

经典研究表明，腹腔感染的多种微生物实际上可能来自各种细菌亚种之间的协同作用。兼性厌氧菌如大肠杆菌可以为脆弱拟杆菌的增殖提供理想的厌氧环境[25]。因此，厌氧菌（如脆弱拟杆菌）的增加使机体防御大肠杆菌变得更加困难，因为局部反应会降低吞噬作用的效果。

在接受广谱抗生素选择性压力的 ICU 患者中，与腹腔感染及脓肿的细菌与继发性细菌性腹膜炎引起脓肿的患者不同[26]。引起三级腹膜炎的细菌不再以大肠杆菌和脆弱拟杆菌为主。相反，由耐药的革兰阴性细菌、肠球菌和/或酵母菌引起的院内感染更常见[27,28]。一项对重症患者脓肿的微生物学分析[急性生理学与慢性健康评价（Acute Physiology and Chronic Health Evaluation，APACHE）Ⅱ评分>15]显示，38% 的患者有单微生物感染。最常见的微生物是念珠菌（41%）、肠球菌（31%）、肠杆菌（21%）和表皮葡萄球菌（21%），大肠杆菌和拟杆菌分别仅占 17% 和 7%[29]。

（三）诊断

IAA 的典型表现为腹痛、发热、寒战和腹部包块，但这四联征在临床中并不常见。根据脓肿位置的不同，可表现为其他症状及体征。膈下脓肿可引起胸膜炎；小网膜囊或胃周脓肿可导致恶心和早饱。肠间脓肿可出现肠麻痹或肠梗阻症状和体征，包括呕吐和腹胀。盆腔脓肿可引起里急后重或直肠刺激征。在老年人及有潜在合并症的患者中，IAA 的症状和体征更多变和隐匿，这就要求临床（对这类患者）要高度怀疑[30]。无论是急诊科就诊的患者，还是临床状态较差的住院患者，影像学都是诊断 IAA 的一线方法。

1. 计算机断层扫描（CT）

CT 是诊断 IAA 的金标准。口服及静脉造影剂的运用，使脓肿的检测得到了优化。IAA 的经典 CT 表现是边缘强化的含气液化灶[31]。多层螺旋 CT 可快速扫描，创建冠状位和矢状位图像，尽可能地描述复杂外观和影射集合（图 29.1）[32]。选择适当的 CT 成像方案可以诊断 IAA 相关的肠梗阻、门静脉炎，并可能提示或确认瘘管的存在[33]。尽管 CT 检测腹腔积液的敏感性高，但据最近报道诊断腹腔积液感染的正确率为 83%，特异性仅为 39%[34]。CT 检测到腔外气体是诊断感染最特异的指标，但仅在不到 40% 的患者中可检测到[35]。衰减大于 20 亨氏单位（Hounsfield unit，HU）的积液也提示脓肿存在[34]。血肿、浆液瘤、假性囊肿和坏死性肿瘤都可能影响 CT 诊断 IAA 的准确性。因此，抽吸物的革兰染色和细菌培养仍然是确诊脓肿的必要条件。

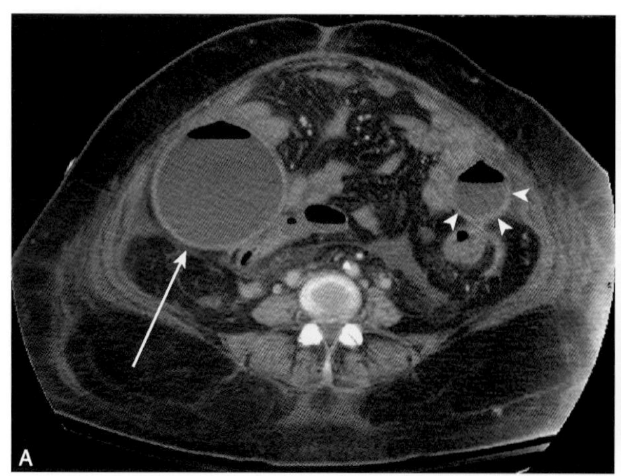

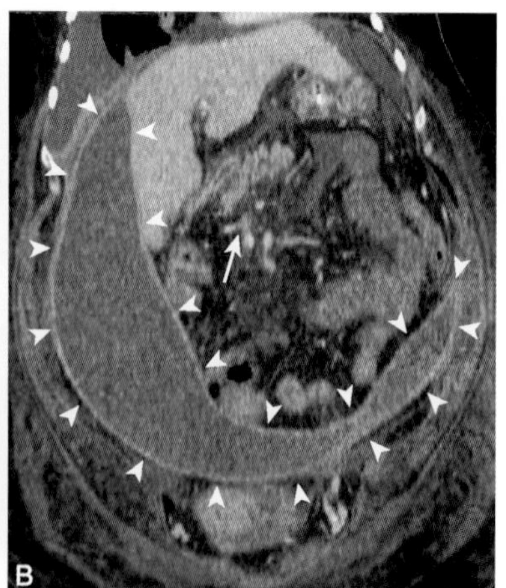

图 29.1 A，轴位 CT 图像显示，右下象限（箭）一个含有气液平的大边缘增强结构，左下象限（箭头）含有一个较小的类似结构。B，同一患者的冠状位图像显示，2 个病灶聚集形成一个大的 C 形病灶，在低位骨盆越过中线（箭头），并证明肠系膜上静脉血栓形成（箭），这是脓肿的潜在并发症之一

CT 检测 IAA 的缺陷是将充满液体的肠袢误认为脓肿。在 CT 检查前 90 分钟(或更长时间)口服造影剂是避免这种缺陷的最佳方法。口服造影剂在肠道通过缓慢偶尔会使部分肠道黏膜不被显影,部分病例需要延迟扫描及重复扫描,使口服造影剂有更多的时间向远端移动(图 29.2)。急诊科为增加患者的周转,不使用口服造影剂而直接行腹部 CT 的趋势越来越明显[36,37]。然而,部分急诊患者需要口服造影剂、重复扫描以确认疑似脓肿的诊断。

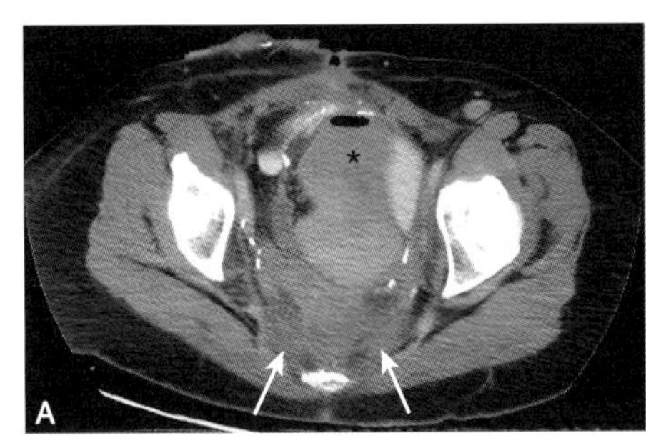

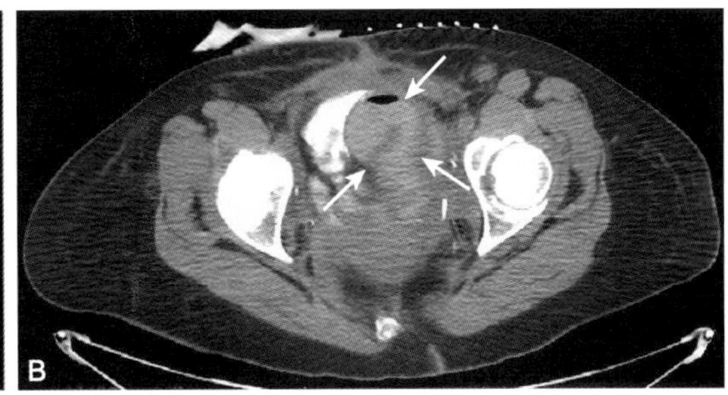

图 29.2　A,轴位 CT 图像显示,在既往接受过盆腔放疗的患者中,骨盆深部邻近栓系肠袢的边缘增强结构中含有气体(星号)。该结构可能代表脓肿或扩张的小肠袢。骶前炎症(箭)与辐射改变有关。B,2 小时后获得的 CT 图像显示该结构中摄入的口服造影剂(箭),证实这是肠袢而不是脓肿

2. 超声检查

超声是一种常规的筛查方式,它简便、快速、无辐射,特别适用于年轻和妊娠患者。脓肿的表现可以是一个相对单纯的无回声积液区,也可是一个复杂的、回声不均的积液区,反映了存在的残渣和气体的量(图 29.3)[38]。对于可疑的实性腹腔脏器 IAA 和盆腔积液,超声是一种极好的评价方法。膀胱内液体是 IAA 定位的超声窗。经阴道超声能发现大多数盆腔脓肿。气体会阻碍超声波穿透,腹部中央含气的肠腔阻碍了脓肿的发现,在最近的报道中,脓肿检出率为 43%[39]。此外,手术伤口、敷料和引流管可能妨碍或限制术后超声的使用。这些局限性在一定程度上被机器的便携性所抵消。危重患者转运到放射科做检查是不安全的,而超声检查在床旁就可以进行。

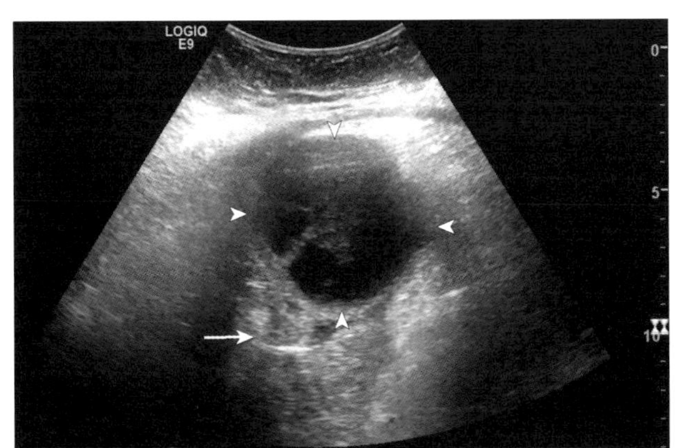

图 29.3　憩室病患者典型脓肿(箭头)的腹部超声显示中央回声减弱、壁增厚和碎屑出现在降结肠(箭)前方,与憩室脓肿一致

3. 磁共振成像(MRI)

随着 MRI 成像方案和设备的改进及对 CT 辐射剂量认识的提高,MRI 越来越多应用于急性和亚急性疾病的诊断。MRI 最初用于诊断妊娠期阑尾炎[40]。现在,MRI 在急诊科急腹症患者中的应用更常见[41,42]。此外,最近的一项多中心研究证明对于有经验的人员,MRI 在阑尾炎的诊断上优于 CT,这可能会增加 MRI 在阑尾炎患者中的应用[43]。磁共振小肠成像已成为评估克罗恩病的标准方法[44]。该技术将含钆的静脉造影剂与高分辨率磁共振成像相结合以检测肠壁的异常。在增强 MRI 小肠成像中,脓肿表现为位于肠腔外的、边缘强化的积液区,在液体敏感序列上具有异质信号升高(图 29.4)[45]。弥散加权成像可以提高鉴别脓肿和囊肿的能力[46]。MRI 诊断 IAA 的主要问题是急诊情况下 MRI 的可用性,因为放射科医生和临床医生更习惯 CT 检查,以及与 CT 相比,MRI 检查时间长、费用高[41]。

4. 放射学检查

X 线片可显示有明显占位效应的巨大脓肿。仰卧位和直立位片可显示巨大脓腔内的气液平、局部肠麻痹或肠梗阻,可支持 IAA 诊断。但总的来说,X 线片对大多数 IAA 的检测是不敏感的,大的脓肿也可能被忽略。CT 在诊断急性非创伤性腹部病变的敏感性(96%)、特异性(95%)和准确性(96%)方面远远优于 X 线片(敏感性、特异性和准确性分别为 30%、88% 和 56%)[47]。

5. 核医学检查

可用于诊断 IAA 的核医学检查包括镓扫描、标记白细胞扫描和 PET/CT 扫描等[48]。以前镓扫描是诊断 IAA 最常用的方法,但肠道以及肿瘤中的正常摄取可能会产生假阳性结果。放射性同位素标记白细胞扫描可提供高灵敏度和特异性的全身成像。不过,这些扫描也有缺点;由于合成放射性标记物需要时间长、不易获得,通常需要 18 个小时甚至 72 小时才能完成[49]。此外,肝脾中的示踪剂摄取可能会混淆上象限脓肿的检测,这可能需要增加硫胶体扫描以区分生理性摄取和感染[50]。PET/CT 扫描在 IAA 诊断中具有重大作用。参与炎症过程的细胞摄取大量葡萄糖,故使得 ^{18}F-FDG PET 扫描的使用非常有用。^{18}F-FDG 摄取,结合 CT 扫描,可对异常结构进行准确的解剖定位,这解决了一个长期困扰核医学检查的问题。在持续菌血症患者中,使用 PET/CT 获得的全身图像可能会发现隐匿的 IAA[51]。PET/CT 是不明原因发热的首选检查,它可以检测发热的感染、炎症和肿瘤来源[52]。PET/CT 和镓扫描最大的缺点是不能区分无菌性炎症和感染[48]。尽管

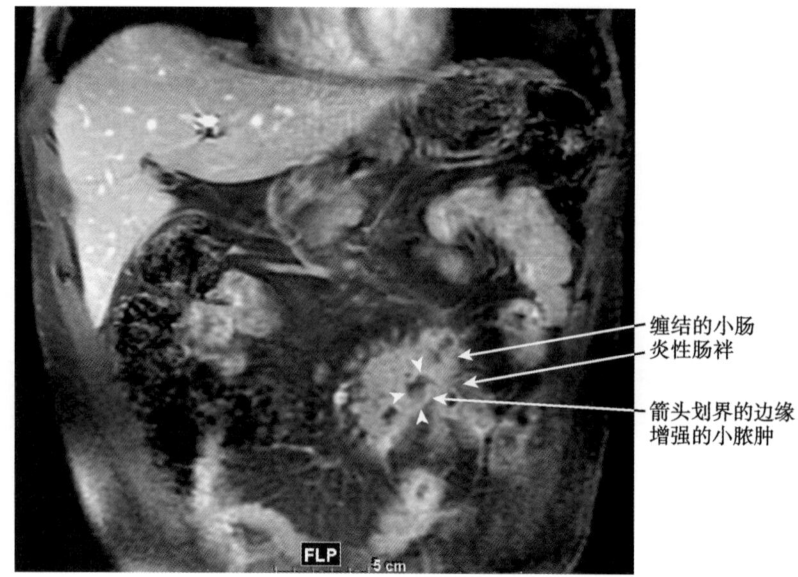

图 29.4 克罗恩病患者的与钆对比冠状面磁共振显示,在发炎肠的几个肠袢(箭)之间,有一个小的边缘增强集合(箭头),与肠袢间脓肿一致。肠袢间脓肿不适合经皮引流管置入

在可预见的未来,CT 仍将是 IAA 的一线首选检查方法,但是 PET/CT 扫描和其他核医学检查可用于疑难病例的诊断。

(四) 处理

1. 一般治疗

最初的治疗需要进行液体和电解质复苏和重要器官功能的支持,如果有脓毒症的表现上述支持治疗则尤其重要。根据脓毒症治疗指南,脓毒症休克中的液体复苏需要大量晶体液输注[33,53]。

2. 抗生素治疗

一旦作出 IAA 的推定性诊断,最好在血培养之后立即开始经验性治疗。虽然抗生素是早期治疗的重要组成部分,但由于无法渗透感染区,在脓肿引流前抗生素可能达不到理想效果。这是由宿主因素(例如:组织坏死、酸性环境、灌注不足)和致病因素(例如:菌落数多、细菌及其产物生长缓慢)共同造成的。这些因素会对某些抗生素的治疗效果造成影响:例如,β-内酰胺类抗生素在密集菌落中效果不佳,而氨基糖苷类抗生素在 pH 值较低时活性降低。

抗生素的初步选择应根据每个患者的临床情况而定。IAA 合并继发性腹膜炎选择抗生素时应该针对大肠杆菌和其他大肠菌群,包括脆弱拟杆菌。这些病例通常不复杂,也没有菌血症等肠外表现。然而,没有随机对照试验表明一种药物优于另一种。多项非劣性研究提供了多种选择(框 29.3)。需根据患者的因素选择抗生素,如肾功能和过敏史。医院抗菌谱也有帮助;例如在一些医院大肠杆菌对氟喹诺酮类抗生素有很高的耐药性。

美国传染病学会和外科感染学会发布的指南建议,单一药物(例如 β-内酰胺类/β-内酰胺酶抑制剂合剂,碳青霉烯,第二代头孢菌素头孢西丁、氟喹诺酮类莫西沙星,甘氨酰环素替加环素)适用于轻度至中度感染(见框 29.3)[26]。革兰氏染色和细菌培养可能对感染治疗的选择有帮助,但最新的指南指出还没有研究证实这一做法。临床医生也可以选择组合方案。大多数专家建议对病情较重或伴有高危并发症的病例应做到对假单胞菌的覆盖。

框 29.3 治疗腹腔内感染的抗生素选择

第二代头孢菌素
头孢西丁*

第三代和第四代头孢菌素
头孢曲松*†
头孢他啶†
头包吡肟†

碳青霉烯类
亚胺培南-西司他丁
美罗培南
厄他培南*

对耐药病原体具有广谱活性的联合抗生素
哌拉西林/他唑巴坦
头孢派酮/他唑巴坦†
头孢他啶/阿维巴坦†
美罗培南/瓦博巴坦
亚胺培南-西司他丁/瑞维巴坦

四环素衍生物
替加环素*
埃拉瓦环素*
欧马霉素*

氟喹诺酮类
环丙沙星†
左氧氟沙星†
莫西沙星*

*不覆盖假单胞菌属。
†添加甲硝唑静脉或口服覆盖厌氧菌。

选择经验性抗生素时需要考虑的要点来自最近发表的研究。某些病原菌不太可能在社区获得性腹腔内脓肿患者中发挥作用。耐甲氧西林金黄色葡萄球菌(Methicillin resistant *Staphylococcus aureus*,MRSA)在这些病例中并不常见。因此,万古霉素或其他抗耐甲氧西林金黄色葡萄球菌抗生素不建议初次使用。在感染的这个阶段,肠球菌通常不具有致病性,因此选择抗生素不需要覆盖肠球菌[26]。

不再常规推荐联合氨基糖苷或者克林霉素。最近的研究表明,氨基糖苷类具有较高的肾毒性且并不增加疗效[54];在过去的 10 年中,克林霉素的耐药率一直在上升,尤其是对脆弱拟杆菌。头孢替坦也已证明对厌氧菌如脆弱拟杆菌的疗效下降。由于大肠杆菌对氨苄西林的耐药率增加,不推荐常规使用氨苄西林/舒巴坦。

与三级腹膜炎相关的 IAA 包括处于晚期或更具侵袭性的腹腔感染阶段的病例,以及具有更强耐药性的院内感染病原体引起的“医院获得性感染”(见第 39 章)。考虑铜绿假单胞菌、肠球菌、MRSA、耐药革兰阴性杆菌,甚至念珠菌感染的可能性,这些患者的经验性抗感染治疗必须覆盖更广泛的病原菌。抗铜绿假单胞菌 β-内酰胺抗生素、碳青霉烯、抗铜绿假单胞菌头孢菌素或喹诺酮联合甲硝唑均是不错的选择。在 β-内酰胺抗生素中,哌拉西林/他唑巴坦的使用最广泛。碳青霉烯可以选择亚胺培南-西司他汀、多利培南或美罗培南;厄他培南无抗铜绿假单胞菌活性。头孢吡肟和头孢他啶对假单胞菌均有活性,但应联合甲硝唑覆盖厌氧菌。环丙沙星或左氧氟沙星可联合甲硝唑用于喹诺酮耐药不常见的患者群体(定义为在抗菌谱上,医院分离出的耐药菌株少于 10%)。由于抗生素的选择性压力改变了三级腹膜炎中 IAA 的菌群,脓肿的微生物学检查有助于指导抗生素的选择[26]。

较早的外科文献表明,覆盖肠球菌是不必要的,但现在已经知道,这些细菌能发挥致病作用[26]。哌拉西林/他唑巴坦和万古霉素对于社区获得性粪肠球菌和屎肠球菌感染均有抗菌活性。然而,青霉素的耐药性一直在增加,有时只有万古霉素才有效。迄今为止,在腹腔感染的系列报道,尚未发现耐万古霉素肠球菌(vancomycin-resistant *enterococci*,VRE),但在肝移植病例除外[55]。

MRSA 在 IAA 中并不常见。万古霉素仍然是治疗 MRSA 的首选抗生素。FDA 已经批准利奈唑胺和替加环素治疗 MRSA 引起的腹腔感染,但是很少有发表的临床研究,因此大多数专家不建议在一开始就使用上述药物。

在治疗复杂性腹腔感染时,院内耐药革兰阴性杆菌成为一个难题。在有过感染和大量使用抗生素的患者中,脓肿培养可以发现多重耐药菌。最值得注意的是产超广谱 β-内酰胺酶的大肠杆菌以及其他只对碳青霉烯敏感的肠杆菌(因此没有口服药物可用)。最近,产碳青霉烯酶的克雷伯菌甚至对碳青霉烯类产生耐药性,临床医生除了使用替加环素、氨基糖苷类或基于碳青霉烯酶抑制剂的新型抗生素,除头孢他啶/阿维巴坦外,几乎没有抗菌药物可供选择。其他更新的抗生素组合制剂即将上市,但目前缺乏临床数据。

念珠菌属可以在晚期的 IAA 病例中表现致病作用。传统上,氟康唑是首选药物,但在一些中心,对氟康唑耐药的非白色念珠菌呈上升趋势,推荐使用米卡芬净或卡泊芬净等棘白菌素。除特殊情况外,两性霉素不再推荐用于真菌性 IAA。

一旦获得培养结果后,经验性抗生素的选择应根据治疗的需要进行调整。这是一种常见的做法,但奇怪的是,很少有证据从患者预后的角度支持这一点。大多数医疗中心正在经历抗菌药物管理的复兴,这很可能继续成为进化过程中的实践。重要的是,一些研究表明不恰当的抗生素选择会导致患者病情恶化[56]。

在某些情况下,患者可能出现进一步的感染症状,如发热、腹部不适或白细胞增多。这些患者应复查腹部影像学以确保感染灶得到有效控制(下面讨论),评估是否有二重感染发生,这需要多次培养指导抗菌治疗。

一旦诊断 IAA,应该立即进行抗生素治疗,并持续至患者临床症状好转,通常为 5~7 天。在 STOP-IT 研究中,复杂腹部感染患者在与腹部感染相关的病理生理异常消失(最长治疗 10 天)后 2 天或 4±1 天接受控制原发病加抗生素治疗,结果没有显著性差异[57]。

治疗后白细胞持续增多的患者复发风险高(37%),白细胞增多和发热的患者复发的风险更高(57%)[58]。对于肠吸收不良、持续性肠麻痹、需引流的巨大脓肿、营养状况差的患者,指导抗生素选择的资料较少。随着多重耐药菌和特殊病原体的出现,一些中心更依赖于门诊静脉注射抗生素来治愈那些有多种危险因素的患者。

3. 控制原发灶和引流

(1) 经皮穿刺脓肿引流术

经皮穿刺脓肿引流术(percutaneous abscess drainage,PAD)已经成为脓肿的标准治疗[59,60],与手术引流相比,PAD 的疗效已经得到证实[61]。大多数 IAA 病例(85%~90%)可接受 PAD[59,62]。PAD 的禁忌证包括缺乏安全的引流途径、无法控制的凝血功能障碍、弥漫性腹膜炎和/或肠穿孔、大量气腹或腹腔积液[62,63]。对于不能手术的腹膜炎患者,可以选择性地进行 PAD。边界不清或蜂窝织炎聚集的脓肿不适合 PAD。直径小于 3cm 的脓肿,通常采用经皮穿刺抽吸、不放置引流管的方法治疗,尽管没有试验验证这种做法[61,64]。

介入技术的进步扩大了 PAD 在 IAA 中的应用,可以达到以前认为经皮穿刺无法到达的位置[62,65](例如将无菌生理盐水注入腹膜后间隙,可引流邻近胃、十二指肠和结肠的 IAA[65])。如果临床需要,可以用小口径导管穿过肝脏或胃,但不能用导管穿过大肠和小肠。因此,PAD 禁用于由克罗恩病或其他疾病引起的肠系膜内或肠间脓肿(见图 29.4)。然而研究表明,克罗恩病并发 IAA 的患者,如果手术前行 PAD,则较少出现术后腹腔内脓毒症,且造瘘率更低[66,67]。对于克罗恩病和肠间脓肿的患者,不留置 PAD、直接用小口径针头穿过小肠抽吸肠间脓肿在技术上是可行的,但目前没有研究证实这一做法[62,64]。有多个且独立的 IAA 患者,手术效果比 PAD 更好(图 29.5)。虽然在有多个 IAA 的患者中放置多根经皮穿刺引流管在技术上是可行的,但患者的不合规引流的复杂性限制了这种做法的应用。与血管移植物或外科补片相关的脓肿,只有在确定感染后方可行 PAD;无菌脓肿行 PAD 可能导致感染[62]。行 PAD 要考虑的技术因素包括脓肿的大小和位置。医生可以根据脓肿的位置和个人习惯,选择超声、

CT 或透视进行定位。在引流前 CT 能对脓肿涉及的脏器、血管和神经进行最全面的评估，而超声则更快，更适合于腹部浅表脓肿的引流。超声的主要局限是可能穿透中间肠管。经直肠和经阴道超声可用于诊断盆腔深部脓肿。如果在诊断时遇到多腔 IAA 或 PAD 后成像检查发现脓肿分隔，可以通过滴注溶栓剂来实现引流，成功率可高达 96%[68]。

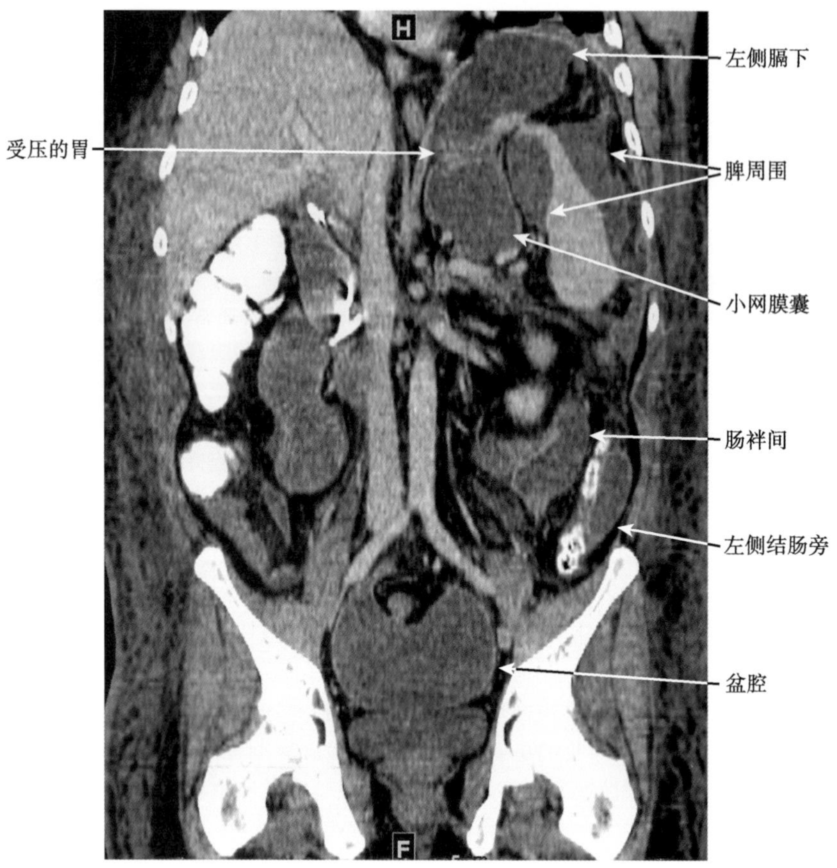

图 29.5　冠状位 CT 图像显示，肝移植受者腹部和盆腔中有大量边缘增强的积液（箭）。可见左侧膈下、脾周、小网膜囊、肠袢间、左侧结肠旁和盆腔脓肿。此类病例最好采用手术治疗

确定安全的经皮穿刺路径后，采用套管针法或针、导丝法进入脓腔（图 29.6）。将管道扩张至接近计划导管的直径，并将导管推进到空腔中。初始 8Fr 或 10Fr 导管尺寸可能是适当的，尽管经常需要增大或更换尺寸[69]。导管一旦放置，应通过复查影像确认其位置，确保所有导管侧孔都在脓肿内。

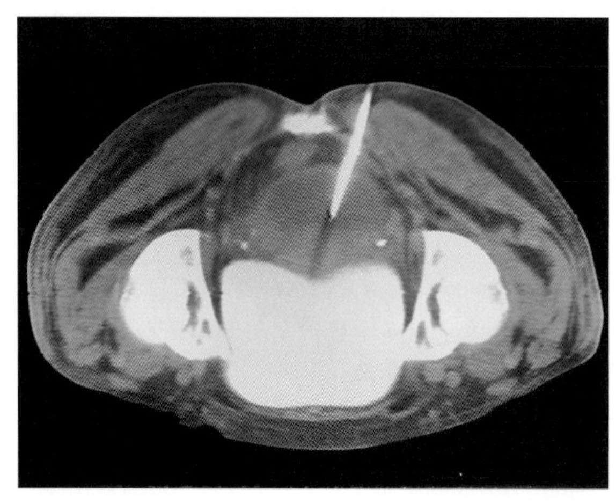

图 29.6　俯卧位 CT 图像显示，使用针经臀肌穿刺通过沿坐骨切迹进入盆腔脓肿，产生脓性物质。随后放置了引流管

通常先将脓腔抽吸干净，然后用无菌盐水冲洗清除残留物质。将引流管放置在便于吸引或通过重力作用引流的部位，并固定在皮肤上。脓液送到实验室进行革兰氏染色和培养。每天用无菌生理盐水冲洗导管以保持通畅。应每日记录引流量和引流物特征。应通过评估体温和白细胞计数来监测临床状态以获得充分的治疗效果。

PAD 的治疗终点和后续影像学检查取决于临床效果、引流量和引流物性质以及是否存在疑似肠内瘘。如果临床效果满意，引流量减少到每天 20mL 以下，则可以安全地取出导管。如果临床效果不理想，需要重复影像学检查。持续大量的引流量应怀疑瘘。在透视下通过导管注入水溶性对比剂进行造影，是评估瘘存在的最佳方法（图 29.7）。如果瘘管被定位，导管可以重新放置在靠近瘘管开口的位置，以更好地控制肠道流出物。PAD 临床效果差可能是由于导管滑脱、脓肿分隔、多个脓肿或形成新的脓肿。重复 CT 检查可以评估这些可能的原因，并适时指导其他的经皮介入治疗。较大的碎片可能堵塞导管、影响冲洗。在这种情况下，可以更换更粗的导管[69]。

PAD 的成功率取决于 IAA 的基础病因和患者的并发症。穿孔性阑尾炎和术后 IAA 的成功率为 64% 至 90% 或更高，这

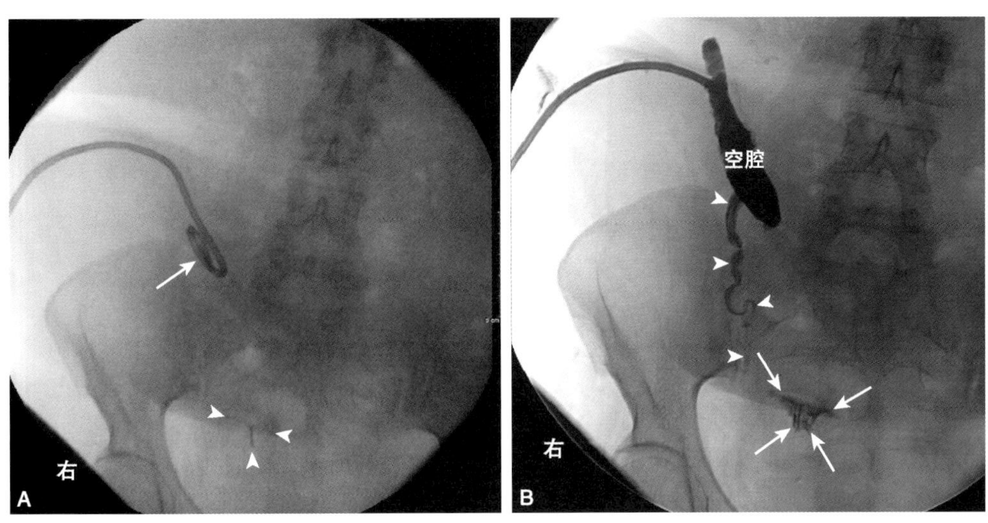

图 29.7　A,包含经皮引流管的右下腹脓肿患者的点透视图像(箭)。注意盆腔内的宫内节育器(IUD)(箭头)。B,同一患者在将造影剂滴入引流导管后显示造影剂充盈脓腔(箭),脓腔与输卵管相通(箭头)表明有瘘管,造影剂充盈节育器周围的宫腔

与术后 IAA 引流比非术后 IAA 引流成功率更高的说法相矛盾[70-74]。术后 IAA 引流成功率高的相关因素为单个脓肿、低级别脓肿、无残留物集聚以及脓肿形成于术后 8 天内[71,73,74]。克罗恩病 IAA 引流成功率约为 80%[71]。

PAD 并发症的发生率为 4% ~ 15%[61,75-77]。并发症包括脓毒症、器官损伤、出血、气胸、腹膜炎、脓胸和疼痛。IAA 复发率从 1% 到 9% 不等[61,76,78,79]。即使脓肿复发,也应考虑再次行 PAD 以达到治愈目标。尽管成功引流所需的时间更长,但复发性脓肿的二次 PAD 成功率高达 91%[78]。

(2) 特殊类型脓肿的引流

A. 膈下脓肿

只要注意技术,膈下脓肿可以经皮引流。避开胸膜腔是防止气胸和感染扩散到胸部的最佳方法。胸膜腔通常向前延伸到第八胸椎(T8)水平,向外侧延伸至 T10 水平,向后延伸至 T12 水平。这些标志可用于防止穿入胸膜腔。一些膈下积液的采集可能无法通过胸膜外入路,在这种情况下,应权衡手术引流的风险与经胸膜 PAD 引起气胸和脓胸的风险[80]。有报道称内镜下膈下脓肿的引流可以降低气胸和脓胸的风险[81]。

B. 盆腔脓肿

如果盆腔脓肿的前路受到肠、膀胱、子宫和/或血管结构的干扰,可以采用俯卧位、经坐骨切迹的臀后入路穿刺,以引流盆腔深处脓肿(见图 29.6)[82]。必须小心操作以避开臀部血管和坐骨神经。超声引导下经阴道和经直肠引流技术越来越多地用于盆腔深处脓肿的引流。经直肠和经阴道技术的比较表明,患者对经直肠引流耐受性较好;经阴道引流疼痛更明显[83]。

C. 阑尾周围脓肿

阑尾周围脓肿可以通过 CT 表现来判断(见第 120 章)。PAD 逐渐成为阑尾周围脓肿合并脓毒症的初始治疗,这使得外科医生可以择期进行随后的阑尾切除术,通常是腹腔镜手术[84,85]。研究表明,存在与腔外阑尾结石相关的一个或多个边界不清的脓肿预示 PAD 临床治疗失败(图 29.8)[70]。低级别脓肿定义为阑尾周围蜂窝织炎或小于 3cm 的脓肿,CT 引导和经臀部入路是治疗成功的相关因素[73]。

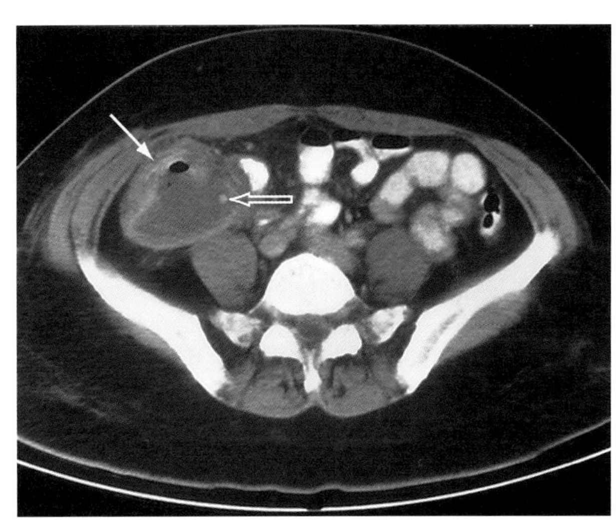

图 29.8　轴位 CT 显示右下腹脓肿(实心箭)伴阑尾结石(空心箭)。这种腔外阑尾结石可能预示经皮引流术的临床失败

D. 憩室周围脓肿

经皮穿刺引流憩室周围脓肿已逐渐得到临床应用(见第 121 章)。对于最终需要行结肠手术的憩室脓肿患者,引流可以使症状得到初步控制,有利于实现一期手术,避免二期手术所需的肠道造瘘(见图 29.3)[86]。

4. 内镜治疗

随着胰腺假性囊肿和胰腺脓肿治疗的成功(见第 58、59 和 61 章)及超声内镜检查(EUS)技术的进步,内镜引导下的 IAA 引流成为一种新的治疗模式[81,87,88]。虽然还没有大型的随机对照试验证实这一方法,但病例系列报道显示经胃和经结肠引流 IAA 效果良好,可引流膈下、肝周、小网膜囊、结肠周围和盆腔脓肿[81,88,89]。如果脓肿距内镜传感器 20mm 以上、中间有血管或腹水,IAA 引流是不可行的[89]。

如果横断面成像(CT、MRI、超声)发现有可引流的脓肿,则用 EUS 定位脓腔,用 19 号 EUS 细针穿刺针穿刺。将坚硬的导丝置入脓腔中。脓肿壁用线针刀导管或者 ERCP 导管穿刺。然后扩张管道、放置双猪尾塑料支架(7~10Fr)。将 IAA 的标本做革兰氏染色和培养。术后 2~3 天 CT 随访。如果脓肿明显缩小,且患者的临床症状改善,则可以在患者出院前取出支架。如果脓肿持续存在,则支架保持原位,并在 6 至 8 周内复查 CT。如果脓肿仍然存在,可以进行额外的支架置入、PAD 或外科手术治疗[88]。只有少数病例有支架移位[89]。

病例系列研究表明内镜引流术后积液的成功率和并发症与经皮引流术相当[90]。

5. 手术治疗

IAA 的手术治疗适用于弥漫性腹膜炎、未控制的胃肠道穿孔、PAD 或内镜引流不安全的患者、PAD 或内镜引流失败的患者。需要外科治疗的主要是肠系膜内或肠间脓肿及多个独立脓肿(见图 29.5)。由于持续存在感染源而导致 PAD 治疗失败的患者需要手术清除污染物(如腔外阑尾结石、脱落的胆结石,大块碎片)[70,91]。

有复杂腹部外伤、腹部脓毒症休克、腹部出血性休克或腹腔间隔室综合征的患者越来越多地采用损伤控制剖腹手术(damage control laparotomy,DCL)进行治疗,如腹腔造口术或“腹腔开窗术”(open abdomen,OA)[92],一种先将筋膜和皮肤打开并计划在后期关闭的手术。DCL 为急腹症患者提供简单的治疗,目的是防止这些患者出现凝血功能障碍、酸中毒和体温过低等并发症。首次 DCL 治疗失败或严重感染可导致腹部脓毒症休克和继发性腹膜炎的患者进展为三级腹膜炎,从而需要多次清创和冲洗。这类 IAA 患者面临特殊挑战,主要是如何选择抗生素以覆盖医院感染。在这些患者中,IAA 和肠瘘的进展与筋膜闭合失败有关,并导致与 OA 相关的高死亡率,通常超过 20%[92]。负压设备,如封闭负压引流技术(vacuum-assisted closure,VAC)仍然是 OA 治疗的基础,但提高 OA 闭合率的技术仍在不断研究中,包括将肉毒杆菌毒素注射到腹壁肌肉组织以实现闭合的新方法。

(五) 预后

IAA 治疗后的效果取决于许多因素。单纯性继发性细菌性腹膜炎的死亡率低于 5%,复杂的三级腹膜炎的死亡率为 65%或更高[27,28,93-95]。穿孔性阑尾炎引起的单纯脓肿,手术引流和抗生素治疗效果好,死亡率较低。较高的死亡率出现在老年患者、男性患者、复杂脓肿、高 APACHE Ⅱ评分、多脏器功能障碍、治疗延迟、使用糖皮质激素或其他免疫抑制的患者[1,96]。其他导致高死亡率的危险因素包括多次手术以控制腹腔脓毒症、营养不良、生理储备不足、心功能不全和多脏器功能障碍综合征。有研究者认为持续的腹腔感染是器官衰竭的另一种表现,而不是病因[97]。换言之,患者死亡时存在感染,而不是死于感染。这类患者需要积极的手术、抗生素和支持治疗,他们可以从明确的临床路径中受益,最大限度地减少实践中的变异性[98]。

二、胃肠瘘

瘘管是两个上皮表面之间任何异常的解剖连接,该定义包括多种临床表现。发生在腹部的瘘管可以起源于胃肠道或泌尿生殖道、肝脏或胰腺中空腔脏器或导管的任何上皮表面。

(一) 分类

一般来说,瘘管是根据其解剖学和生理学来分类的。解剖分类基于瘘管的起源和引流点。这种解剖学分类特点是瘘管是位于内部还是外部,内瘘管在两个上皮表面之间引流,而外瘘管则是引流到身体外表面。生理或体积分类是根据瘘管在 24 小时内的引流量,一般分为高流量瘘和低流量瘘(框 29.4)。临床上经常使用这两种瘘管分类法对瘘管进行描述(例如高流量的胃皮瘘管)。一个特殊例子是肠空气瘘,定义为肠道和大气之间的瘘管(稍后讨论)。本章主要集中在肠皮瘘。关于胆瘘和胰瘘的具体讨论见第 58、59、61 和 70 章。

框 29.4 瘘管的分类
解剖学分类
内瘘(如回结肠瘘、结肠膀胱瘘)
外瘘(如肠皮肤的瘘)
生理学分类
高流量瘘(>500mL/d)
低流量瘘(<200mL/d)

(二) 病理生理学

胃肠道瘘可自发产生或医源性产生。自发性瘘占 15%~25%,与炎症/感染、癌症和放疗有关[99-107]。炎症有助于自发性瘘的形成,包括结肠憩室炎、IBD、IAA、消化性溃疡病和阑尾炎。这些瘘管可以是内瘘也可以是外瘘,在特殊情况下,它们有不同的自发闭合率。其余 75%~85%的瘘管是由于手术或其他因素造成的[108-113];其中大部分为术后发生的,提示吻合口裂开或肠损伤。术后瘘形成的危险因素包括营养不良、脓毒症、休克、低血压或需要加压素治疗、糖皮质激素治疗、相关的合并症以及手术吻合的难度[114]。

确定瘘管形成的原因很重要,因为这会影响后续治疗。IBD 的瘘管可能对抗炎治疗有反应,而由恶性肿瘤引起的瘘管则不太可能自发闭合,通常需要手术干预。因吻合口裂开引起的术后低流量瘘可通过保守治疗闭合。与瘘自发性闭合失败相关的情况列于框 29.5。

框 29.5 与无法愈合的自发性胃肠道瘘相关的疾病
瘘管内异物(见第 28 章)
累及受累肠道的放射性肠炎(见第 41 章)
瘘管起源处的感染或炎症
瘘管上皮化
瘘管起源处的肿瘤
远端肠梗阻

(三) 诊断

准确诊断瘘管在很大程度上取决于解剖因素。肠皮瘘通常是通过观察到肠液引流到体外从而诊断。通过检测引流液中胆红素和淀粉酶的水平，以确认液体是肠源性的。另一种确认外瘘的简单方法是给患者口服活性炭。如果引流物中含有木炭，则证实为肠瘘。在尿液中发现摄入的罂粟籽则可证实存在肠尿道瘘。外引流的瘘管比内引流的瘘管更明显，内瘘的诊断难度较大。例如，在胆囊十二指肠瘘中，除非形成胆石性肠梗阻，否则可能不会被发现（见第 65 章）。在结肠膀胱瘘中，主要表现为尿路感染、粪尿和气尿。

特别是在合并感染的情况下，在体格检查中确认瘘的存在更加困难。在怀疑有瘘的情况下，稳定患者内环境是最重要的。影像学检查有助于确定瘘管的诊断、病因和来源，确定适当的引流路径。这些检查包括口服或经直肠（取决于可疑病灶的位置）使用造影剂后的透视检查。将造影剂注入一个空脏器（如膀胱）导致另一个脏器［如直肠乙状结肠（图 29.9）］显影时，可诊断为内瘘。也可逆行注射造影剂到引流部位（瘘管造影术），追踪原发部位（图 29.10；也可参见图 29.7 所示）。增强 CT 或 MRI，尤其是使用肠显像方案，可显示瘘管（图 29.11）。这种横断面成像还有额外的优点，可以确定是否存在未引流的脓肿。最后，内镜检查有助于观察瘘管的腔内起源。

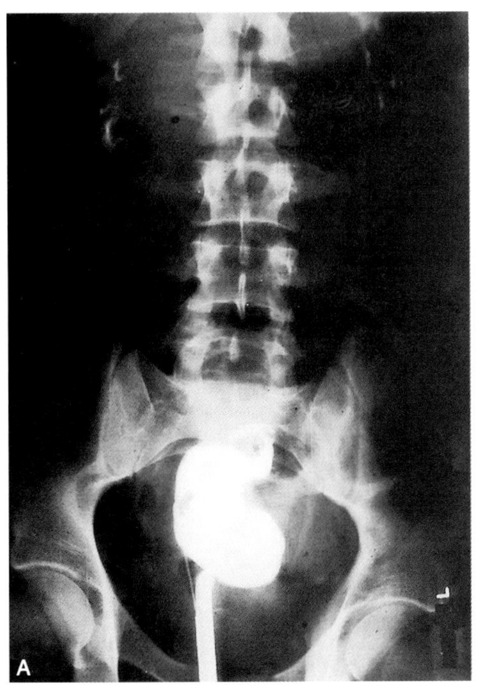

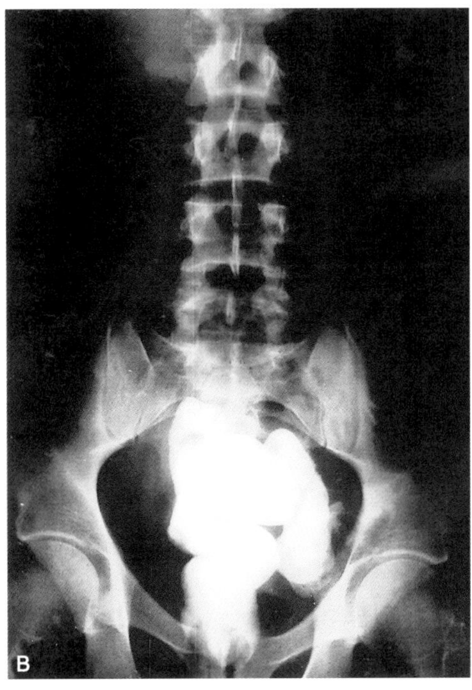

图 29.9 腹部 X 线片显示 1 例克罗恩病、气尿症和尿路感染患者的直肠膀胱瘘。A，导管在膀胱内，造影剂开始充盈肠道。B，造影剂通过瘘管充满乙状结肠和直肠。（Courtesy Dr. Mark Feldman, Dallas, TX.）

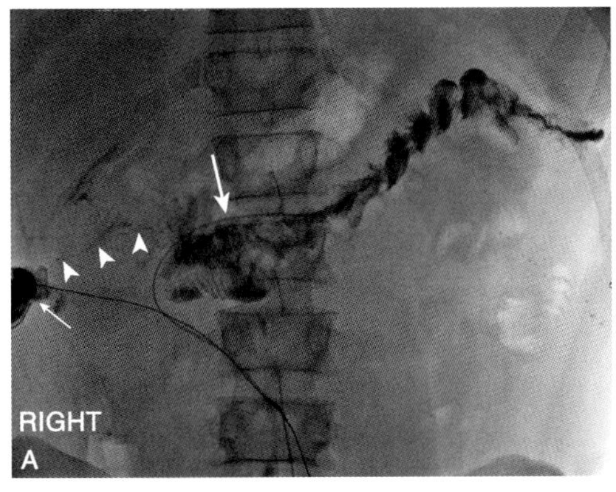

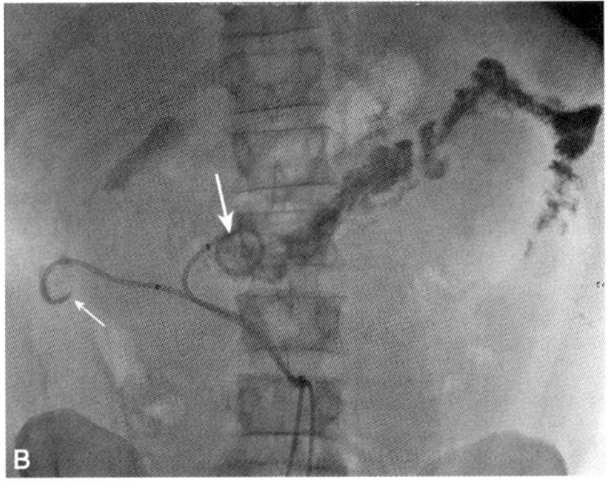

图 29.10 A，克罗恩病患者的 X 线透视图像，有 2 个引流腹部伤口，在每个引流腔内放置导丝，一个在横结肠内（大箭），另一个在空肠袢内（小箭）。注意另外一个连接空肠和横结肠的薄肠结肠瘘（箭头）。B，将引流导管置入该复杂瘘的横结肠（大箭）和空肠（小箭）组件后的患者相同

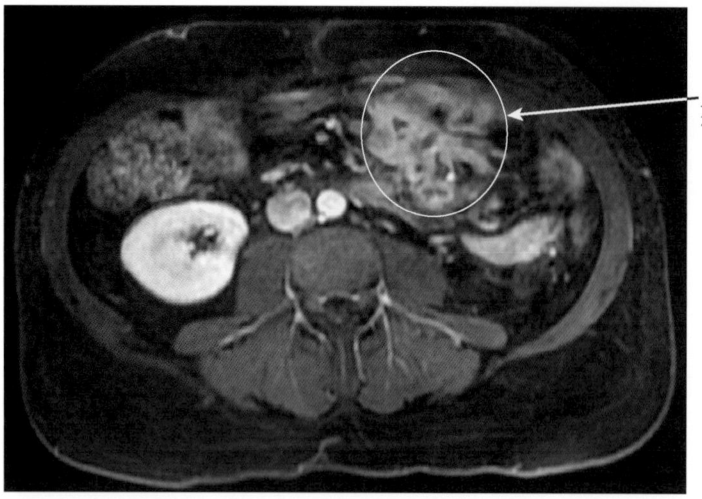

图 29.11 克罗恩病患者使用钆-林造影剂造影后的轴向 MRI，显示栓系星状结构中的暗淡小肠袢（圆圈），典型的肠-肠瘘（箭）

（四）处理

1. 一般治疗

胃肠瘘的初步治疗是稳定患者内环境，控制脓毒症，以及纠正水电解质紊乱。如果患者有严重脓毒症或瘘管输出量大（>500mL/d；见框 29.4），治疗会变得困难。如果瘘管起源于近端小肠，那么输出量多大于 1 000mL/d。为了防止血容量减少和电解质失衡，在进行更详细的诊断性检查之前，必须优先考虑液体和电解质的替代治疗。液体替代治疗应考虑瘘管丢失的液体量和电解质含量。一般来说，瘘液是等渗的富含钾的液体。最初，瘘管输出量应该用添加了钾的平衡盐将瘘管排出量替换为毫升/毫升。如果在处理电解质失衡时遇到困难，瘘液样本可送实验室进行电解质测定，然后根据实验室结果进行后续的电解质补充。

2. 建立充分的引流

肠皮瘘治疗的基础是建立充分的引流。因为如果未建立充分的引流，瘘内容物聚集可导致感染，形成脓肿和脓毒症。通常需要微创的手术操作，例如打开最近的手术切口以获得充分的引流。可能需要放置经皮导管以排出脓液并控制瘘管流出物。一些弥漫性腹膜炎患者，不能仅经皮引流，可能需要剖腹探查和冲洗。在腹膜炎手术时对这样的瘘管进行彻底修复很少成功。在这种情况下，手术的目的是清除污染物并建立引流，通常在手术过程中放置引流管。

在适当的情况下，需要进行改道肠造口术和放置外科喂养管[115]。一旦持续的腹膜污染得到解决，并建立外部引流，从瘘管排出的污物就必须加以控制。大多数肠皮瘘发生在术后，所以需要一些技巧保护皮肤免受瘘管输出物腐蚀。大多数急性术后肠皮瘘通过手术切口减压。由于切口有感染和液化的迹象，所以必须切开。重新切开、引流肠内容物的切口不适合简单地放置一个造口袋来收集引流物。有多种可供选择的容器，应咨询经验丰富的肠造瘘口治疗师来处理这个难题[116]。最近肠皮瘘的辅助治疗是使用前面所述的 VAC 系统进行局部伤口护理。VAC 装置可以同时处理排泄物和开放伤口从而简化了这些复杂伤口的处理[108,117-119]。

随着 DCL 和 OA 的日益普及，肠空气瘘也越来越常见[120-122]。这些“暴露的瘘管”往往很难处理，并导致引流困难。许多创新的策略已经被用来治疗这些复杂的瘘管[123-126]。

3. 营养支持

营养状况良好且无感染并发症的患者更容易实现瘘口自发性闭合，如果需要手术修复，发生手术并发症的风险更低[103,127-130]。因此，必须积极进行营养评价和营养支持（见第 5 和 6 章）。胃肠道瘘患者营养不良的原因是多方面的，包括潜在的疾病状态、缺乏蛋白质摄入、通过瘘管丢失蛋白质以及潜在的伴有高分解代谢的脓毒症[114]。在胃肠瘘确诊后不久，必须给予积极的热量支持。一旦确定了瘘的解剖来源，就要考虑喂养途径。全肠外营养（total parenteral nutrition，TPN）是肠皮瘘患者的首选，但并非所有患者都必须使用 TPN。在一项对 335 例肠外瘘患者的研究中，85% 的患者仅给予了肠内营养[131]。在本研究的一组非复杂瘘患者中，50% 的患者仅通过这种营养治疗模式自行愈合。在另一项研究中，胃肠瘘合并严重脓毒症患者入院后 2 周内开始肠内营养较 2 周后开始肠内营养的患者，腹部伤口更快愈合，死亡率降低[132]。肠内营养通过直接和间接机制促进黏膜增殖和绒毛生长。与肠黏膜接触的营养物质可直接刺激肠细胞，喂食谷氨酰胺含量高的食物特别有益，因为谷氨酰胺是肠细胞的主要能量来源[133]。此外，肠腔内的营养物质会导致肠激素的释放，这些激素对肠黏膜有间接的营养作用（见第 4 章）。相反，TPN 会导致肠黏膜萎缩，一部分原因可能是标准 TPN 溶液中不含有谷氨酰胺，谷氨酰胺会从溶液中结晶出来。在一项对 TPN 患者的小型研究中，补充口服谷氨酰胺的患者更可能出现瘘管的自发闭合[134]。尽管最近胃肠瘘患者的肠内营养治疗取得了进展，TPN 仍然是大多数患者营养支持治疗的主体，因为他们无法通过肠内营养吸收足够的热量[135]。积极的营养支持对于改善胃肠瘘患者的预后至关重要[136]。

决定胃肠瘘患者采取肠内营养或 TPN 是基于解剖学和生理学考虑的。在大多数患者中,病情稳定后应开始肠内营养。通常情况下,肠内营养并不会显著增加瘘管输出量。如果输出量明显增加,应该考虑减少或停止肠内喂养。如果瘘管位于小肠近端,同时肠远端通路已建立(如在许多术后瘘管中,在手术时已放置空肠造瘘口),应在肠远端开始肠内喂养。随着肠内营养的开始,将近端瘘管引流物输入到远端肠管,可以使液体和电解质管理更容易,以及减少近端瘘的输出量[106,137]。此外,瘘管灌流或直接将管饲喂入瘘管的传出段对特定患者也是有效的[138]。并非一定要通过全肠内途径以获得肠内营养的益处,TPN 也可以补充蛋白质和热量需求。

4. 药物治疗

生长抑素类似物

生长抑素类似物,如奥曲肽或兰曲肽,可以辅助 TPN 治疗胃肠道瘘患者。奥曲肽通过几种机制减少瘘管输出。首先,它抑制胃泌素、胆囊收缩素、胰泌素和许多其他胃肠道激素的释放。该抑制作用减少了进入肠道的电解质、水和胰酶,从而减少肠液分泌量。其次,奥曲肽能松弛肠平滑肌,使肠腔容量更大。最后,奥曲肽增加肠道水分和电解质的吸收[139]。

随机研究评价生长抑素类似物治疗肠皮瘘的 Meta 分析显示瘘管愈合率增加,瘘管输出量减少,愈合时间缩短,住院时间缩短,而对死亡率没有影响[140,141]。奥曲肽通过将高输出的瘘管转变为低输出的瘘管,提高了瘘管愈合率[142]。主张进行有时限的试验以评估添加奥曲肽是否会减少瘘管输出。如果在奥曲肽治疗开始后 72 小时内,瘘输出量没有下降,则应停止使用。

5. 克罗恩病的治疗

曾经,保守治疗克罗恩病相关的瘘管价值不大,因为大多数腹部和肛周瘘管需要手术矫正。克罗恩病患者肠黏膜产生 TNF-α 增加[143],从而开发了针对 TNF-α 的嵌合单克隆抗体(英夫利西单抗)以及其他抗炎单克隆抗体(乌司奴单抗和维得利珠单抗),用于治疗克罗恩病(见第 116 章)。对于克罗恩病瘘管的最初治疗,应考虑抗 TNF-α 抗体疗法,该疗法得到 Cochrane 数据库支持[144]。一些小的病例系列研究主张当其他非手术治疗失败时,对克罗恩病患者的瘘管使用甲氨蝶呤或他克莫司进行积极的免疫抑制治疗[145,146]。

用于治疗瘘管型克罗恩病的药物数据主要偏向于肛周疾病的治疗,而专门针对肠皮瘘的数据很少。Meta 分析表明 TNF 拮抗剂、间充质干细胞治疗、免疫抑制剂以及 TNF 拮抗剂联合抗生素治疗在瘘管型克罗恩病中的作用存在不同等级的证据支持[147,148]。在内科治疗无效的情况下,可以考虑外科手术治疗。

6. 非手术干预

治疗顽固性瘘管的非外科手术干预包括使用带膜支架、组织夹、腔内真空(endoluminal vacuum,E-vac)治疗、经内镜缝合、闭塞及经皮或内镜下放置纤维蛋白胶。虽然目前仅限于病例系列研究,但已经有各种非外科手术技术,包括瘘管镜、荧光透视和内镜[149-152]。内镜下夹闭内瘘口也取得了成功。现有的夹闭器可以用于内镜下夹闭较大的缺损[153-158]。

E-vac 治疗在上消化道和下消化道瘘管和漏的治疗中具有广阔的应用前景。与其他技术相比,该项技术具有理论上的优势,通过应用负压吸引改善了感染和肠道流出物的引流,同时也可以增加血流量以促进黏膜愈合。这项技术包括内镜评估管腔缺损,冲洗和抽吸任何相关的脓腔或瘘管,然后插入一个开孔大小合适的聚氨酯海绵,且连接到鼻胃管的末端(目前在美国没有可用的商品化 E-vac 产品)。一旦海绵到位,将其置于 100~125mmHg 的连续负压下。海绵每 3~5 天更换一次,直到空腔和缺损闭合。一些小规模研究的评估结果令人鼓舞[159-162]。

内镜和非手术技术作为保守治疗难治性瘘管的有用辅助手段,越来越成为一线治疗的选择。最初尝试非手术干预并不妨碍手术的可能性,可能使一些患者免于接受高危的手术。

7. 手术干预

手术治疗仍然是肠-皮肤瘘的主要治疗方法,其中保守治疗和内镜治疗未能解决瘘管输出[103,106]。早期手术的适应证包括在不进行手术引流的情况下无法控制瘘管、脓毒症、脓肿形成、瘘管远端的肠梗阻和出血。早期手术干预往往采取临时措施,以消除脓毒症的来源和建立瘘管控制,如冲洗和引流和/或造口形成。更复杂的瘘管可能需要手术取出补片或其他异物,然后瘘管才能自行闭合或进行确定性手术。手术治疗的目标是解决感染和恢复肠道的连续性——通常需要切除[163]。直接闭合瘘管的尝试很少成功,一般应避免。微创手术是特定患者的一种选择[149,164]。

目前没有明确的数据来确定最终手术的时机,但手术时机应考虑当前患者的临床情况。对于术后肠皮瘘,应于开腹手术后 7~12 天的有利"窗口期"或推迟至少 6 周后进行再次手术,以改善腹腔内炎症和粘连[165]。等待的基本原理是避免手术,直到腹部严重的炎症反应消退,相关的致密血管粘连减少。如果手术干预超过了窗口期,往往注定会失败。此外,这些患者进行额外肠切开术的可能性增加。在败血症的情况下,文献中的普遍共识是在败血症稳定和消退后等待至少 6 周,许多人主张等待更长时间[165,166]。

手术治疗的主要方法是切除受累的肠段,进行并吻合。在瘘管的外科治疗中使用了不同的技术,并且在创新技术中取得了一些成功,如带蒂皮瓣[167]。

(五) 结果

外瘘的早期患病和死亡是由于最初的液体和电解质紊乱没有得到控制。然而,胃肠瘘患者死亡的主要原因是脓毒症和多器官衰竭。出现脓毒症的典型情况是引流不充分或不受控制的复杂瘘管。在这种情况下,肠内容物聚集在腹腔内,形成感染灶。如前所述,必须进行积极的治疗,以确保瘘管引流良好。瘘管患者的全因死亡率在 10% ~ 30%[100,101,103,106,108,128,129,165,168]。存在并发症、年龄大于 55

岁、脓毒症、营养不良、以前接受过放射治疗、或术后腹壁裂开并发复杂瘘的患者死亡率更高[109,129,165]。胃肠道瘘患者死亡的第二个主要原因是严重的潜在疾病，最常见的是癌症。通常继发于恶性肿瘤的终末期患者会放弃进一步的手术治疗[169]。

5%～38%的术后患者出现瘘管复发。与术后瘘管复发相关的因素包括IBD、营养不良、复杂性瘘管、筋膜延迟闭合、补片植入、感染、严重的基础疾病以及缝合瘘管而不是切除和再吻合[100-102,108,128,163,165]。研究表明，高输出瘘管患者的复发率是低输出瘘管患者的4倍[167]。在单因素分析中，与瘘管闭合术后复发相关性最大的因素包括高输出量、肠空气瘘和/或OA史。专家们建议将所有的复发性瘘视作是新出现的瘘并且遵循标准的治疗流程[167]。

除了预防发病率和死亡率，闭合瘘管是治疗的最终目标。通常这是通过支持治疗自发完成的。文献中瘘口自然愈合率为15%～71%。在自然愈合的瘘管中，大约90%会在脓毒症稳定和控制后30天内闭合。脓毒症的控制、瘘管输出量的控制和营养支持是治愈的重要因素。表29.1列出了一些在决定自发性瘘愈合率方面重要的预测因素[170]。最终需要手术闭合的瘘管往往与高输出量，短通路及持续脓毒症相关。

表29.1 非手术治疗自发性瘘管闭合的预后指标

有利因素	不利因素
外科病因	回肠、空肠、非手术病因
阑尾炎，憩室炎	炎症性肠病，癌症，辐射
转铁蛋白>200mg/dL	转铁蛋白<200mg/dL
无梗阻，无感染，无肠炎，无肠发炎	远端梗阻、肠不连续、邻近感染，邻近活动性炎症
长度>2cm，末端瘘管	长度<2cm，外侧瘘，多发性瘘
输出量<200mL/24h	输出量>200mL/24h
无败血症，血清电解质平衡	败血症，电解质紊乱
初步转诊至三级医疗中心和亚专科治疗	延迟转诊到三级医疗中心和亚专科治疗

Adapted from Gribovskaja-Rupp I, Melton GB. Enterocutaneous fistula: proven strategies and updates. Clin Colon Rectal Surg 2016;29:130-7.

虽然创新疗法和支持治疗提高了瘘的自发闭合率，但这些难题的处理需要多学科参与，包括营养支持治疗、肠造口治疗师、外科医生、介入放射科医生和胃肠科医生[171]。图29.12给出了胃肠道瘘的治疗流程。

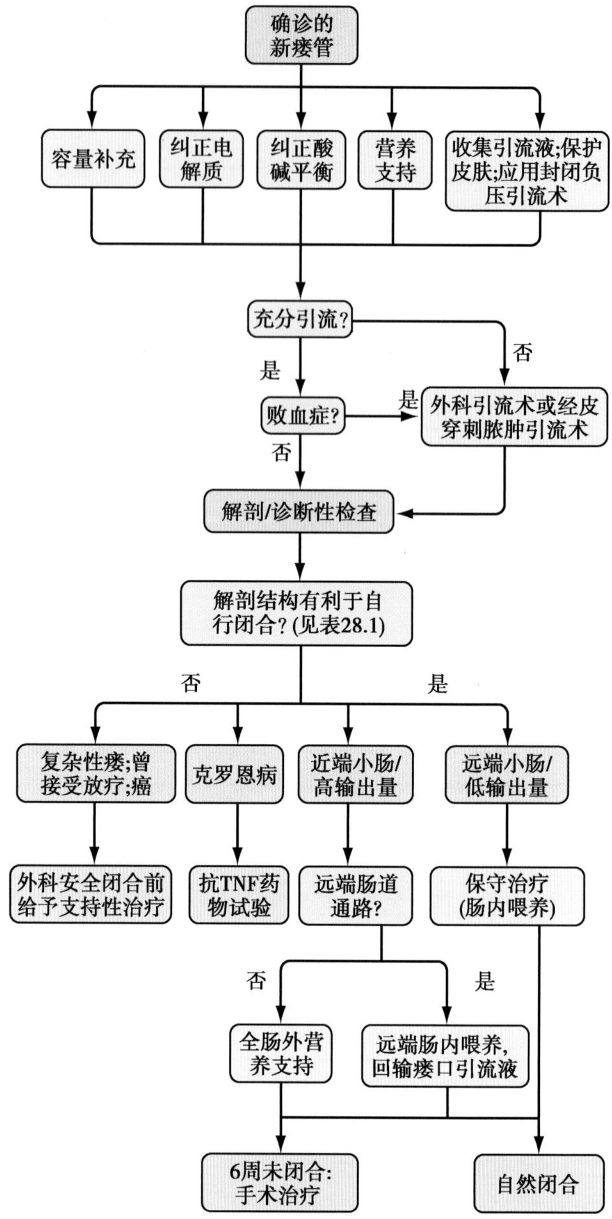

图29.12 胃肠道瘘的治疗流程。详见正文

（丁静 田文广 译，施海韵 李鹏 校）

参考文献

30

第 30 章　胃肠道嗜酸性粒细胞性疾病

Marc E. Rothenberg, Vidhya Kunnathur 著

章节目录

一、嗜酸性粒细胞生物学、潜在诊断和治疗目标 ……… 401
二、健康状态的胃肠道嗜酸性粒细胞 ………………… 402
三、嗜酸性粒细胞相关胃肠道疾病 …………………… 403
（一）嗜酸性粒细胞性食管炎 ……………………… 404
（二）嗜酸性粒细胞性胃炎、肠炎、胃肠炎 ……… 408
（三）嗜酸性粒细胞性结肠炎 ……………………… 409
四、资源 ……………………………………………… 410

嗜酸性粒细胞增多性胃肠疾病（eosinophilic gastrointestinal disorder, EGID）定义为在没有已知的嗜酸性粒细胞增多原因（例如药物反应、寄生虫感染、恶性肿瘤）的情况下，沿胃肠道发生的选择性嗜酸性粒细胞富集性炎症，并与胃肠道相关症状有关。EGID 包括一系列疾病，根据相关嗜酸性粒细胞浸润的解剖位置命名：嗜酸性粒细胞性食管炎（eosinophilic esophagitis, EoE）、嗜酸性粒细胞性胃炎（eosinophilic gastritis, EG）、嗜酸性粒细胞性肠炎和嗜酸性粒细胞性结肠炎（eosinophilic colitis, EC）。我们保留术语嗜酸性粒细胞性胃肠炎，用于描述超过一段胃肠道受累的情况。越来越多的证据表明，嗜酸性粒细胞在许多胃肠道疾病的发病机制中起着关键作用。我们对肠道嗜酸性粒细胞病理生理学的理解主要来自 EoE 更普遍和研究的实体，对于这一实体，关于临床诊断和管理也有公认的共识。越来越多的数据支持这一概念，即 EGID 的发生与以下因素之间的相互作用有关：遗传因素（家族中患病率较高[1,2]和 EoE 遗传风险因素，包括常见的单核苷酸多态性[3]和罕见的损伤性变体[4]、环境因素（如饮食[5-7]）及宿主免疫系统因素。EGID 的免疫系统特征介于免疫球蛋白 E（immunoglobulin E, IgE）介导和延迟的 2 型辅助性 T 细胞（T-helper type 2, Th2）应答之间[8-11]。研究已确定了变应原[5-7]、细胞因子［如白细胞介素（interleukin, IL）-5, IL-13］、微小核糖核酸（microRNA, 如 miR21）[12]、趋化因子［如嗜酸性粒细胞趋化因子（eotaxin）］[12]、Th2 免疫极化［如胸腺基质淋巴细胞生成素（thymic stromal lymphopoietin, TSLP）］[12]、屏障功能丧失[13]和蛋白酶/蛋白酶抑制剂失衡的促进作用，在疾病病理生理学中有利于蛋白酶激活[14]。因此，这些因素可作为未来潜在的疾病生物标志物以及治疗靶标。

一、嗜酸性粒细胞生物学、潜在诊断和治疗目标

嗜酸性粒细胞含有调节固有及适应性免疫应答所必需的全部介质（细胞因子和趋化因子）。它们可以作为抗原递呈细胞发挥作用，它们表达 Th2 细胞因子（IL-4、IL-5、IL-13）、Th1 细胞因子（干扰素-γ）、促炎性细胞症因子（TNF、IL-6、IL-8）、抑制性细胞因子［转化生长因子（transforming growth factor, TGF）-β 和 IL-10］，以及其中许多细胞因子的受体[15]。嗜酸性粒细胞来源于骨髓的多能干细胞，其产生受球蛋白转录因子-1[16]、细胞因子 IL-3、IL-5 和粒细胞-巨噬细胞集落刺激因子的调节[17]。嗜酸性粒细胞含有特殊的次级颗粒，其蛋白含量对包括肠上皮在内的多种组织有毒性[18]。嗜酸性粒细胞颗粒含有由主要碱性蛋白（major basic protein, MBP）-1 和 MBP-2 组成的晶体核心以及由嗜酸性粒细胞阳离子蛋白（eosinophil cationic protein, ECP）、嗜酸性粒细胞衍生的神经毒素和嗜酸性粒细胞过氧化物酶组成的基质[19]。临床调查证明 MBP 和 ECP 在嗜酸性胃肠炎患者小肠细胞外沉积[20-24]，EoE 患者循环中嗜酸性粒细胞来源的神经毒素水平也升高，因此可以区分活动期和非活动期患者[25]。

IL-5 是嗜酸性粒细胞谱系中最特异的，负责嗜酸性粒细胞的选择性分化[26]，它们从骨髓释放到外周循环中[27]并存活[28]。小鼠中的研究表明，IL-5 表达水平与血液嗜酸性粒细胞增多呈正相关，IL-5 水平降低导致变应源激发后血液、肺和胃肠道中的嗜酸性粒细胞显著减少[29-32]。这些结果导致了瑞利珠单抗和美泊珠单抗等 IL-5 调节剂的开发[33,34]。在一项双盲随机安慰剂对照试验中[34]抗 IL-5 的中和抗体瑞利珠单抗显著降低了 EoE 儿童和青少年的食管上皮内嗜酸性粒细胞计数[34]。然而，在所有治疗组中均观察到症状改善，与食管嗜酸性粒细胞计数变化无关。这两种抗 IL-5 药物，以及一种直接针对 IL-5 受体的嗜酸性粒细胞耗竭单克隆抗体，现在美国食品药品管理局（FDA）批准用于治疗嗜酸性粒细胞性哮喘，很可能会有更多的应用[35]。这些结果也可能提示参与组织嗜酸性粒细胞相关炎症变化的其他分子的重要性，这是 EoE 发病机制的特征。事实上，Th2 细胞的其他产物（如 IL-4 和 IL-13）可影响嗜酸性粒细胞[36]。IL-4 和 IL-13 通过几种协同机制间接诱导嗜酸性粒细胞的募集和存活。它们通过诱导与嗜酸性粒细胞上的 β1 和 β2 整合蛋白结合的关键黏附分子（如细胞间黏附分子-1、血管细胞黏附分子-1）以及趋化因子（如嗜酸性细胞趋化因子）和影响嗜酸性粒细胞的其他分子（如几丁质酶）的内皮表达来介导其功能[36,37]。IL-4 和 IL-13 通过使用 Janus 激酶/信号转导和转录激活因子（STAT）-6 通路的共同受体亚基 IL-4Rα 转导信号[38]，嗜酸性粒细胞表达由 IL-4Rα 和普通 γ 链组成的主要 IL-4R 受体。STAT-6 靶向缺失的小鼠胃肠道 Th2 相关反应的发展受损[39,40]。此外，活化的 STAT-6 二聚体与一系列炎症基因中的特异性启动子基序结合，如嗜酸性细胞趋化因子-1、嗜酸性细胞趋化因子-2 和嗜酸性细胞趋化因子-3 启动子[41-45]。事实上，几项研究中发

现IL-13与食管组织的疾病活动以及IL5和嗜酸性细胞趋化因子-3信使RNA表达呈正相关[46]。此外,小鼠模型中IL-13过表达诱导EoE样变化,包括与EoE转录组部分重叠的食管转录组[47]。抗IL-13和抗IL-4受体抗体的早期临床试验证明,食管嗜酸性粒细胞增多和组织学、内镜和临床症状的改善,进一步的研究将有望确定这些基于机制的EoE和可能的其他EGID治疗的定位[48,49]。嗜酸性粒细胞在胃肠道固有层的定位,受到嗜酸性粒细胞趋化因子的调节,嗜酸性粒细胞趋化因子在整个胃肠道组成性表达[50]。嗜酸性粒细胞趋化因子受体、趋化因子(C-C基序)受体(CCR)-3在表达[51],3种嗜酸性粒细胞趋化因子中,嗜酸性粒细胞趋化因子-3与EoE的发病的相关性最强[52]。对288例食管活检组织的分析发现,单独的嗜酸性细胞趋化因子-3信使RNA水平对区分有和无EoE个体的敏感性为89%[46]。总的来说,这些研究表明IL-5、IL-13和嗜酸性粒细胞趋化因子-3可作为诊断疾病和疾病是否活动的替代标志物。此外,这些研究为开发旨在阻断嗜酸性粒细胞趋化因子和/或CCR3作用的治疗药物提供了动力。事实上,已经开发了CCR3的小分子抑制剂和人源化抗人嗜酸性粒细胞趋化因子-1抗体[36,53,54]。在过敏性鼻炎患者中进行的人源化抗嗜酸性粒细胞趋化因子-1的一期试验结果显示,当该药物通过静脉或鼻内途径给药时,没有出现严重的不良反应[53,55]。值得注意的是,抗嗜酸性粒细胞趋化因子-1可以降低鼻腔冲洗液和鼻黏膜活检中嗜酸性粒细胞的水平,并可改善鼻腔通畅性[53,55]。抗嗜酸性粒细胞趋化因子-1可能对嗜酸性粒细胞占优势的哮喘和/或嗜酸性粒细胞趋化因子-1明显增加的严重哮喘患者特别有帮助,但这尚未经临床证实[56]。此外,抗嗜酸性粒细胞趋化因子-1可能对其他以嗜酸性粒细胞为特征的胃肠道疾病(如炎症性肠病)有获益[57]。然而,从抗IL-5抗体临床试验中得到的结果提示,研究人员应该同时关注组织学和临床研究终点,并注意研究应针对高嗜酸性粒细胞和嗜酸性粒细胞趋化因子-1水平的患者。

最近引入了EoE诊断组合(EoE diagnostic panel,EDP)(表30.1)。EDP是一组96个基因,在EoE患者的食管中不一致表达,除了识别那些吞咽糖皮质激素暴露的患者外,在确定成人和儿童患者中EOE的敏感性为96%,特异性为98%。EDP也有助于作为亚临床组织学患者的预测工具[<15个嗜酸性粒细胞/高倍视野(high power field HPF)][58]。

表30.1 嗜酸性粒细胞性食管炎诊断小组:6个主要类别,每个类别有5个代表性基因

细胞黏附	上皮	炎症	重构	嗜酸性粒细胞/肥大细胞	趋化因子/细胞因子
CDH26	*FLG*	*TNFAIP6*	*POSTN*	*CLC*	*CCL26*
DSG1	*UPK1A*	*ALOX15*	*KRT23*	*CCR3*	*CXCL1*
CLDN10	*SPINK7*	*ARG1*	*COL8A2*	*TPSB2/AB1*	*IL4*
CTNNAL1	*CRISP3*	*MMP12*	*CTSC*	*CPA3*	*IL5*
CHL1	*MUC4*	*IGJ*	*ACTG2*	*CMA1*	*IL13*

Modified from Rothenberg ME, Stucke EM, Grotjan TM, et al. Molecular diagnosis of eosinophilic esophagitis by gene expression profiling. Gastroenterology 2013;145(6):1289-99.

二、健康状态的胃肠道嗜酸性粒细胞

在健康状态下嗜酸性粒细胞在许多组织中含量较低,但在胃肠道、脾脏、淋巴结、胸腺和脂肪组织中含量较高[59,60]。有趣的是,嗜酸性粒细胞浸润仅与胃肠道中的嗜酸性粒细胞脱颗粒相关;然而,以前认为形态学脱颗粒可能在胃肠道中正常观察到,可能与组织处理有关[59,60]。在健康的儿童胃肠道中,嗜酸性粒细胞水平从近端到远端逐渐增加[61],食管通常无嗜酸性粒细胞(表30.2列出了明显正常内镜活检胃肠道中嗜酸性粒细胞水平)。在常规健康小鼠(如未处理的野生型

表30.2 正常小儿内镜黏膜活检标本中的胃肠道嗜酸性粒细胞水平

部位	固有层		绒毛膜固有层		表面上皮		隐窝/腺上皮	
	Mean±SD	Max	Mean±SD	Max	Mean±SD	Max	Mean±SD	Max
食管	N/A	N/A	N/A	N/A	0.03±0.10	1	N/A	N/A
胃(胃窦)	1.9±1.3	8	N/A	N/A	0	0	0.02±0.04	1
胃(胃底)	2.1±2.4	11	N/A	N/A	0	0	0.008±0.03	1
十二指肠	9.6±5.3	26	2.1±1.4	9	0.06±0.09	2	0.26±0.36	6
回肠	12.4±5.4	28	4.8±2.8	15	0.47±0.25	4	0.80±0.51	4
升结肠	20.3±8.2	50	N/A	N/A	0.29±0.25	3	1.4±1.2	11
降结肠	16.3±5.6	42	N/A	N/A	0.22±0.39	4	0.77±0.61	4
直肠	8.3±5.9	32	N/A	N/A	0.15±0.13	2	1.2±1.1	9

注:嗜酸性嗜酸剂/HPF的平均数±胃肠区和黏膜区域指示的解剖区域的平均值的标准差。HPF,高倍镜视野;Max,最大值;Mean,平均值;N/A,不适用。

Reproduced from Debrosse CW, Case JW, Putnam PE, et al. Quantity and distribution of eosinophils in the gastrointestinal tract of children. Pediatr Dev Pathol 2006;9:210-8.

小鼠,在无病原体条件下饲养)的胃肠道中,嗜酸性粒细胞通常存在于胃、小肠、盲肠和结肠的固有层中[62],而通常不存在于派尔集合淋巴结或上皮内部位,但在 EGID 小鼠模型中嗜酸性粒细胞通常会浸润这些区域[63]。有趣的是,胎鼠的嗜酸性粒细胞位于和成年小鼠相似的区域且浓度相似[62],证明嗜酸性粒细胞归巢至胃肠道独立于内源性菌群。组织中嗜酸性粒细胞在炎症或非炎症条件下具有不同的细胞因子表达模式,EoE 患者的食管嗜酸性粒细胞 Th2 细胞因子表达水平相对较高[64,65]。

三、嗜酸性粒细胞相关胃肠道疾病

胃肠道嗜酸性粒细胞聚集是许多胃肠道疾病的共同特性,包括典型的 IgE 介导的食物过敏[11,66,67]、嗜酸性粒细胞性胃肠炎[23,68]、过敏性结肠炎[69-71]、EoE[72-74]、炎症性肠病(IBD)[24,75,76]和胃食管反流病(GERD)(表 30.3)[77-79]。在 IBD 中,嗜酸性粒细胞通常仅占浸润白细胞的一小部分[76,80],但其水平被认为是不良预后指标[80,81]。同样,在 GERD 中,通常仅有低水平的食管嗜酸性粒细胞[77,82],但已描述了质子泵抑制剂反应性食管嗜酸性粒细胞增多(proton pump inhibitor-responsive esophageal eosinophilia, PPI-REE)的实体[83]。PPI-REE 与 EoE 具有重叠的内镜、遗传学和组织学特征,目前被认为是相同疾病谱的一部分[84,85]。EGID(即 EoE、嗜酸性粒细胞性胃炎、嗜酸性粒细胞性肠炎和嗜酸性粒细胞性结肠炎)定义为在没有已知嗜酸性粒细胞增多症原因(例如,药物反应、寄生虫感染、恶性肿瘤等)的情况下,主要累及胃肠道的嗜酸性粒细胞增多性炎症疾病[8]。此外,EoE 和遗传性结缔组织疾病(connective tissue disorder, CTD)共同产生过多的 TGF-β,EoE 使 CTD 的风险增加 8 倍。这种相关性在过度活动综合征中尤其明显,如勒斯-迪茨综合征(Loeys-Dietz 综合征)、马方综合征(Marfan 综合征)Ⅱ型和先天性结缔组织发育不全综合征(Ehlers-Danlos 综合征),称为嗜酸性粒细胞性食管炎-遗传性结缔组织病(EoE-CTD)[86,87]。EGID 患者存在多种问题,包括发育停滞、腹痛、易怒、胃动力障碍、呕吐、腹泻和吞咽困难[88-90]。

越来越多的证据支持 EGID 继发于遗传和环境因素相互作用的概念。值得注意的是,很大比例(约 10%)的 EGID 患者,尤其是 EoE 患者,有一个与 EGID 直接相关的家庭成员[1,2]。此外,几项证据支持过敏性病因:包括组织标本中发现肥大细胞脱颗粒[91,92];约 75% 的 EGID 患者为特应性[5,7,93-99];疾病的严重程度通常可通过无变应原饮食逆转[5-7];重要的是,疾病通常在食物重新引入后复发[100]。此外,EGID 的小鼠模型支持这些疾病的潜在过敏性病因[101,102]。有趣的是,尽管在 EGID 患者中常见食物特异性 IgE,但食物诱导的过敏反应仅发生在少数患者中[8]。因此,EGID 具有介于纯 IgE 介导的食物过敏和细胞介导的超敏反应疾病(如乳糜泻)之间的特性[8-11]。

尽管尚未严格计算原发性 EGID 的发病率,但在过去 10 年中已注意到这些疾病(尤其 EoE)的小规模流行[73]。例如 EoE 是目前在澳大利亚[103]、巴西[104]、英国[105]、意大利[106]、以色列[107]、日本[108]、西班牙[109]和瑞士报告的全球健康问题[110]。Liacouras 和他在费城儿童医院的研究小组发现,约 10% 对酸阻断无反应的 GERD 样症状儿童患者患有 EoE[79]。Furuta 和他在波士顿儿童医院的同事们报道,他们的食管炎患者中有 6% 患有 EoE[111]。最后,Noel 等据报道,在 10 年期间,辛辛那提大都市地区的儿童患病率约为 1∶1 000[2]。随着这些疾病的 ICD-9/10-CM 编码的引入,嗜酸性粒细胞性胃肠疾病研究者联盟(Consortium of Eosinophilic Gastrointestinal Disease Researchers, CEGIR)的研究人员最近的研究能够准确估计 EGID 的患病率。使用高度特异性的病例定义[112],在美国 EoE 的患病率估计为 39.0/100 000~56.7/100 000[113],与早期研究结果一致[2],外推全国患病率约为 105 000~150 000 例[113,114]。尽管在过去 20 年中 EoE 的患病率有所增加,但它仍然是一种罕见的疾病。最近的一项荟萃分析估计汇总患病

表 30.3　胃肠道嗜酸性粒细胞增多的鉴别诊断

GERD
胃肠道嗜酸性粒细胞性疾病
嗜酸性食管炎(EOE)
孟德尔和遗传性结缔组织病(CTD),包括过度活动综合征相关的 EoE(EoE-CTD)
高 IgE 综合征——常染色体显性和隐性遗传
Ehlers-Danlos 综合征,过度活动型
ERBIN 基因缺陷
Loeys-Dietz 综合征(LDS)
Netherton 综合征
PTEN 错构瘤综合征(PHTS)
与代谢消耗(SAM)综合征相关的重度特应性综合征
嗜酸性粒细胞性胃炎
嗜酸性粒细胞性肠炎
嗜酸性粒细胞性胃肠炎
嗜酸性粒细胞性结肠炎
感染
血吸虫病
异尖线虫病
胃肠道蛙粪霉病
弓蛔虫病
十二指肠钩虫病
Hp 感染
乳糜泻
嗜酸性粒细胞增多综合征
药物超敏反应
炎症性肠病
移植相关性嗜酸性肠炎
嗜酸性肉芽肿性多血管炎(Churg-Strauss 综合征)
中毒性损伤
移植物抗宿主病
血管炎
胶原血管性疾病

率仅为22.7/100 000[115],这表明美国存在的病例甚至少于10万。在CEGIR进行的一项单独研究中,发现EG的患病率为6.4/100 000,外推至美国约17 000例病例,EC的患病率估计为3.5/100 000,外推至约9 000例病例[116]。在一项独立研究中也证实了这种罕见的患病率[117,118]。

EGID通常与外周血嗜酸性粒细胞增多无关(>50%的时间),表明胃肠道特异性调节嗜酸性粒细胞水平机制的潜在意义,事实上,已证实嗜酸性粒细胞趋化因子途径在该过程中的重要性[119,120]。然而,一些EGID患者(通常是EG患者)外周血嗜酸性粒细胞水平显著升高,并符合高嗜酸性粒细胞综合征(hypereosinophilic syndrome,HES)的诊断标准[121]。该综合征的定义为持续性、严重的外周血嗜酸性粒细胞增多(>1 500个细胞/mm^3)以及在无已知嗜酸性粒细胞增多原因的情况下存在终末器官受累[122]。值得注意的是,虽然HES通常涉及胃肠道,但通常与HEB相关的其他终末器官(如心脏和皮肤)很少累及EGID。已经认识到HES患者的一个子集在4号染色体上有微缺失,该微缺失可产生对甲磺酸伊马替尼治疗敏感的活化酪氨酸激酶(*FIP1L1-PDGFRA*融合基因)[123]。目前正在研究EGID患者中的该事件和其他遗传事件,尤其是具有显著循环嗜酸性粒细胞增多的患者。

(一)嗜酸性粒细胞性食管炎

由于食管通常无嗜酸性粒细胞,如发现食管嗜酸性粒细胞则表示病理改变[8,73]。现已认识到许多疾病伴有食管嗜酸性粒细胞浸润,如EoE、嗜酸性粒细胞性胃肠炎、GERD、寄生虫和真菌感染、IBD、HES、食管平滑肌瘤病、骨髓增生性疾病、癌症、结节性多动脉炎、过敏性血管炎、胶原血管疾病(如硬皮病)、增生型天疱疮和药物损伤[63]。嗜酸性粒细胞相关食管疾病分为原发性和继发性。主要亚型被称为EoE,包括特应性、非特应性和综合征性疾病,尤其是与CTD相关的疾病,如过度活动综合征[124]和家族性EoE变体[125]。家族性EoE见于5%~10%的患者[1],其同胞复发风险比估计超过50倍[126]。此外,还有其他几种与EoE相关的孟德尔疾病:ERBIN基因缺陷、Netherton综合征、PTEN错构瘤综合征和与代谢消耗综合征相关的严重特应性综合征(见表30.3)[86]。次要亚型分为2组,一组由系统性嗜酸性粒细胞疾病(即HES)组成,另一组基本为非嗜酸性粒细胞疾病(即HES)组成。

1. 病因

EoE是一种临床病理状态,在世界过敏和胃肠病门诊就诊的儿童和成人患者中普遍公认。在多项研究中,EoE的年发病率在0.1/10 000~1.2/10 000之间变化,EoE是慢性食管炎的第二大常见原因[2,103]。EoE的病因知之甚少,但食物过敏被认为是主要原因。事实上,根据皮肤点刺试验和/或过敏原特异性IgE检测的定义,大多数患者有食物过敏原和空气过敏原致敏的证据,然而,其中只有少数患者有食物过敏反应史[73]。尽管被认为是食物过敏原驱动的过敏性疾病,但已积累的证据表明,阳性皮试验和过敏原特异性IgE是相关免疫应答的标志物,而不是主要机制的反映[86]。也有人提出食管嗜酸性粒细胞性炎症在机制上与肺部炎症有关。这一理论是基于以下发现:向小鼠肺重复递送特异性变应原或Th2细胞因子IL-13,以及在小鼠肺中转基因过表达IL-13,均可诱导出实验性EoE[47,127,128],以及对草过敏的季节性变应性鼻炎患者食管中存在嗜酸性粒细胞聚集增加的观察结果[129]。其他研究也表明特应性和EoE之间有很强的关系[130]。事实上,EoE患者报告了其食管症状的季节性变化。食管黏膜活检除嗜酸性粒细胞外,T细胞和肥大细胞增多,提示慢性Th2相关性炎症[131,132]。嗜酸性粒细胞和肥大细胞产生的TGF-β升高,已被证明有助于组织重塑和平滑肌功能障碍[133]。此外,表皮抗原暴露使食管在单次气道抗原激发后发生明显的嗜酸性粒细胞炎症[134]。

食管组织全基因组微阵列表达谱分析是EoE研究的一个里程碑[3]。研究人员比较了EoE或慢性食管炎(典型的GERD)患者和正常个体食管组织中的基因转录表达。值得注意的是,大约1%的整个人类基因组的表达失调构成了EoE遗传特征。有趣的是,嗜酸性细胞趋化因子-3是EoE患者中过度表达最多的基因,其表达水平与疾病严重程度相关,事实上,单独过表达嗜酸性粒细胞趋化因子-3对单次食管活检诊断EoE的预测价值为89%[46]。同一研究者证明,嗜酸性粒细胞趋化因子受体(CCR3)基因消融的小鼠受到保护,免于发生实验性EoE。总的来说,这些结果强烈提示嗜酸性粒细胞趋化因子-3在EoE的病理生理学中起作用,并提供了Th2炎症与EoE发生之间的分子联系。第一项全基因组关联研究将EoE与含有*TSLP*基因的基因位点区域5q22相关联。值得注意的是,TSLP在与EoE相关的过程中具有已知的作用,包括Th2免疫的极化和嗜酸性粒细胞趋化因子的诱导[135]。随后的全基因组关联研究验证了*TSLP*位点,还在2p23的*CAPN14*基因位点鉴定出一个很强的遗传易感位点[136]。*CAPN14*编码钙蛋白酶-14,钙蛋白酶-14是一种食管特异性细胞内半胱氨酸蛋白酶,可调节上皮细胞屏障功能。有趣的是,钙蛋白酶-14是由IL-13诱导的,将过敏性2型适应性免疫反应与先天性上皮细胞反应联系起来。因此,这种食管特异性途径有助于解释过敏个体会发生EoE的原因,将2型免疫(过敏性)与食管特异性反应联系起来[136]。为了支持这一点,*CAPN14*遗传变异与特应性易感变异的遗传相互作用(上位性)已被证实[137]。此外,使用广泛的候选基因方法,证实*TSLP*及其受体的遗传变异体与EoE易感性相关[138]。

2. 临床特征和诊断研究

EoE代表一种慢性、抗原驱动、免疫介导的疾病,临床表现为与食管功能障碍相关的症状,组织学特征为以嗜酸性粒细胞为主的炎症[83]。EoE应由临床医生诊断,同时考虑所有临床和病理学信息,这些参数均不应单独解释。2011年EoE的诊断标准[83]强调EoE需要在食管中发现15个或更多的嗜酸性粒细胞/HPF(峰值)。该定义是基于2017年的共识建议,即在EoE的诊断中不考虑PPI反应性,因为PPI-REE具有与PPI耐药性食管嗜酸性粒细胞增多重叠的表型、遗传和分子特征[84,85]。除少数例外的情况,15个嗜酸性粒细胞/HPF(峰值)被认为是EoE诊断的最小阈值。这种以嗜酸性粒细胞为主的食管炎症的后果会对患者及家属产生深远的全身和情绪影响[124,139]。

关于EoE的病史,该疾病在儿童和成人患者人群中已被确定,通常是有特应性证据的男性患者,并且该病通常对局部糖皮质激素治疗或饮食限制有反应。目前,EoE的治疗是长期的,在停止限制饮食或药物治疗后,疾病活动迅速复发[140]。这种疾病的主要症状因患者年龄而异,这些症状包括进食困难、发育停滞、胸部和/或腹部疼痛、吞咽困难和食物嵌塞[105]。这些症状通常根据患者年龄按时间顺序发生，为儿童 EoE 的自然史进展为成人 EoE 提供了支持性证据[141]。在婴儿和幼儿经常表现为喂养困难，而学龄儿童则表现为呕吐或疼痛。吞咽困难是青少年的主要症状。儿童 EoE 最常与其他特应性体质表现相关(如食物过敏、哮喘、湿疹、慢性鼻炎和环境过敏)，这些表现也遵循时间顺序以类似于“过敏(或特应性)”的进展流程。成人 EoE 患者的症状则比较固定，包括吞咽困难、非吞咽相关胸痛、食物嵌塞和上腹痛。其中固体食物吞咽困难仍然是最常见的症状[142]，33%~54% 的 EoE 成人发生需要内镜下取出导致食物嵌塞的团块[143]。

考虑到 EoE 与特应性进展的相关性，EoE 的评估包括寻找共存过敏性疾病的过敏评价。不再认为有必要通过皮肤点刺试验或测定血清中变应原特异性 IgE 来寻找食物变应原和空气变应原致敏，因为与经验性避免最常见变应原相比，这对成功的饮食治疗几乎没有影响[144]。然而，这些检测在决定哪些食物添加回饮食时，可能是有用的，特别是当 EoE 患者有食物急性反应史(过敏反应)时。临床适当时应考虑排除 GERD 是食管嗜酸性粒细胞增多的主要原因。一项研究表明，与单独皮肤点刺试验相比，通过延迟皮肤斑贴试验来评价食物蛋白致敏可增加食物过敏的识别[5]，但这些结果主要限于一个部位，通常不推荐使用。

EoE 患者的体格检查有助于识别儿童的正常生长模式，并识别儿童和成人的共病过敏性疾病。然而，体格检查在诊断 EoE 方面并无特异性。此外，虽然一些患有 EoE 的儿童可能出现喉部症状，但尚未发现 EoE 的口腔或咽部表现。EoE 患者通过内镜检查可识别的食管异常的疾病包括：固定食管环/气管化(又名纤维狭窄并发症)、一过性食管环、白色渗出物、长纵沟(图 30.1 显示沟纹和渗出物)、水肿、弥漫性食管狭窄、窄口径食管及内镜通过时引起的食管撕裂(为黏膜脆性的表现，严重时食管出现皱褶纸样外观)。然而，由于所有这些内镜特征在其他食管疾病中均有描述，因此均不能被视为 EoE 的特征性病症。2013 年 ACG 的临床指南建议，胃肠病学家评价时可以使用 EoE 内镜参考评分对 EoE 进行分类和分级，该系统在表 30.4[145] 中进行了描述。此外，已经评价了内镜参考评分的准确性，分类系统可以成功识别 EoE 患者，也可用于评价治疗反应[146]。内镜检查与食管黏膜活检仍然是

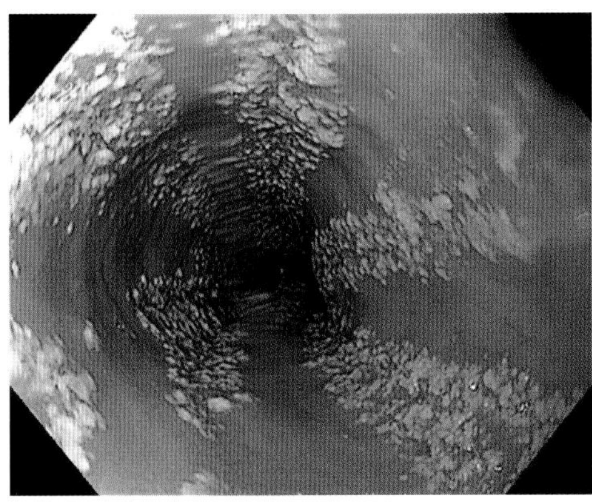

图 30.1 嗜酸性食管炎，食管有沟纹和渗出物

EoE 唯一可靠的诊断试验(图 30.2)，典型的组织学表现包括存在 15 个或更多的嗜酸性粒细胞/HPF、细胞间隙扩张，在某些情况下还包括乳头变长及固有层炎症和纤维化(见图 30.2)。2017 年，对新开发的 EoE 组织学评分系统(histologic scoring system，HSS)进行了验证。除了确定 15 个或更多的嗜酸性粒细胞/HPF 外，8 个其他组织学特征显示可区分治疗和未治疗患者，HSS 在疾病诊断和监测方面优于食管嗜酸性粒细胞水平。8 个 HSS 特征包括嗜酸性粒细胞密度、基底区域增生、嗜酸性粒细胞脓肿、嗜酸性粒细胞表面分层、细胞间隙扩张、表面上皮改变、角化不良上皮细胞和固有层纤维化。使用 4 分量表对严重程度和范围进行评分，0 表示正常值，3 表示最大变化[147]。然而，在不确定确证症状和排除食管嗜酸性粒细胞增多的其他原因的情况下，孤立性食管嗜酸性粒细胞增多的发现不足以作出 EoE 的诊断[83]。

表 30.4 内镜下嗜酸性粒细胞性食管炎的评分参考

主要特征
水肿
(也称为血管纹理减少、黏膜苍白)
0 级：无存在明显的血管分布
1 级：血管纹理清晰度丧失或缺失
固定环
(也称为同心环、波纹环、环形食管、气管环)
0 级：无
1 级：轻度-轻微圆周嵴
2 级：中度-明显的环，不影响标准诊断性成人内镜通过(外径 8~9.5mm)
3 级：重度-明显的环，诊断性成人内镜不能通过
渗出液
(也称为白斑、斑块)
0 级：无
1 级：累及食管表面积小于 10% 的轻度病变
2 级：累及食管表面积大于 10% 的严重病变
沟纹
(也称为垂直线、纵向沟纹)
0 级：无
1 级：存在垂直线
狭窄
0 级：无
1 级：存在(请说明估计的管腔直径)
次要特征
皱纹纸样食管(牛皮纸样食管)
(诊断性内镜通过时，而不是食管扩张后的黏膜脆性或撕裂)
0 级：无
1 级：存在
狭窄口径食管
(大多数管状食管的管腔直径缩小)
0 级：无
1 级：存在

Adapted from Hirano I，Moy N，Heckamn MG，et al. Endoscopic assessment of the oesophageal features of eosinophilic oesophagitis validation of a novel classification and grading system. Gut 2013；62：489-95.

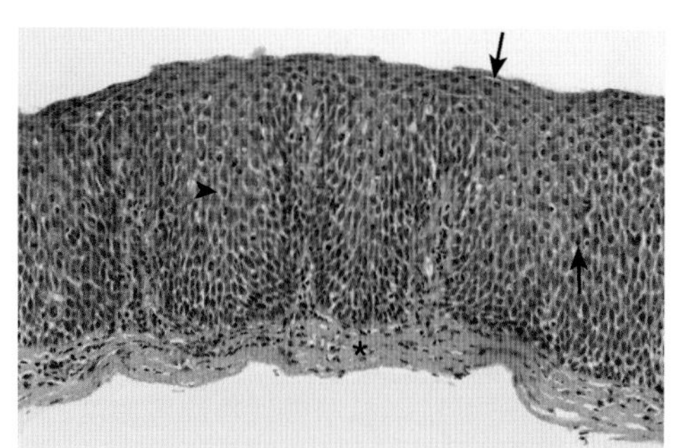

图 30.2 嗜酸性食管炎患者食管苏木精和伊红染色。箭指向嗜酸性粒细胞，包括表面，箭头指向扩张的细胞间隙。星号标记固有层显示炎症和纤维化，绿色箭指向细长的乳突。也有明显的基底层增生，基底层几乎达到表面

具体来说，其中一些表现症状不容易区分 EoE 和 GERD。表 30.5 总结了 GERD 和 EoE 之间的区别特征。嗜酸性粒细胞的数量和位置助于鉴别 EoE 和 GERD。高达 7 个嗜酸性粒细胞/HPF(放大倍数 400×)最有可能为 GERD，7~15 个嗜酸性粒细胞/HPF 可能代表 GERD 和食物过敏的组合，至少 15 个嗜酸性粒细胞/HPF 是 EoE 的特征[63,148]。嗜酸性粒细胞在食管近端和远端的解剖位置均表示 EoE，而主要在食管远端的嗜酸性粒细胞蓄积是 GERD 的特征[73]。一些研究也发现，与 GERD 患者相比，EoE 患者活检标本中肥大细胞增加[149,150]。与 GERD 患者相比，EoE 患者活检标本中携带 IgE 的细胞更常见，在对照样本中未检测出[151]。食管 pH 监测(和 pH 阻抗，如可用)是评价食管嗜酸性粒细胞增多患者 GERD 的有用诊断试验。此外，共识指南表明，钡剂造影可识别 EoE 的许多解剖和黏膜异常，但 X 线造影作为该疾病诊断试验的灵敏度似乎较低。因此，不建议将放射学作为 EoE 的常规诊断试验，但在选择的病例中可能有助于描述难以通过内镜定义的解剖异常，并收集更多关于复杂性食管狭窄长度和直径的信息。使用腔内功能性管腔成像探针(EndoFLIP)的新技术提供了与 EoE 相关的食管功能的独特评估。研究显示，EoE 患者的食管扩张性降低，伴有食物嵌塞或需要治疗性扩张的相关风险。一项研究甚至证实了药物和饮食治疗(无扩张)可改善食管体部的扩张性，这种扩张性改善与症状改善的相关性大于食管黏膜嗜酸性粒细胞计数的降低。在将 EndoFLIP 最终用作结果测量标准之前，还需要完成更多的研究[152,153]。

表 30.5 嗜酸性粒细胞性食管炎和胃食管反流病的比较

特点	嗜酸性粒细胞性食管炎	胃食管反流病
临床		
发病率	约 1/1 000	约 1/10
特应性发生率	非常高	正常
食物过敏发生率	非常高	正常
性别偏好	男性	女性
腹痛和呕吐	常见	常见
食物嵌塞	常见	不常见
检查所见		
pH 监测及阻抗	正常	不正常
内镜下沟槽样改变	非常常见	偶尔可见
组织病理/发病机制		
近端食管受累	有	无
远端食管受累	有	有
上皮增生	增生明显	有增生
食管嗜酸性粒细胞水平	>15/HPF	0~7/HPF
嗜酸性粒细胞趋化因子-3 水平升高	是	否
EoE 诊断面板阳性	是	否
治疗		
H_2 受体拮抗剂	无效	有效
PPI	有时有效(但嗜酸性粒细胞仍>15/HPF)	有效
糖皮质激素	有效	无效
食物抗原剔除	有时有效	无效
要素饮食	有效	无效
抗 IL-13 和抗 IL-4Rα	有效	无效

注：HPF，高倍镜视野；IL，白细胞介素；PPI，质子泵抑制剂。

Modified from Rothenberg ME. Eosinophilic gastrointestinal disorders (EGID). J Allergy Clin Immunol 2004;113:11-8. © 2004, with permission from the American Academy of Allergy, Asthma, and Immunology.

3. 治疗

EoE 有几种一线治疗方法，包括：饮食疗法、局部糖皮质激素和 PPI。有研究表明，对于原发性 EoE(过敏或非过敏亚型)患者，饮食疗法常常可以改善症状并减少食管活检标本中的嗜酸性粒细胞的数量[6,154]。一项特定食物过敏原和避免空气中过敏原的试验，通常适用于特应性 EoE 患者。如果该方法不令人满意或实际上很难(即，当患者对许多过敏原过敏时)，则建议采用基于氨基酸的配方组成的饮食，称为要素饮食，或避免最常见的过敏食物(牛奶、大豆、小麦、鸡蛋、花生/树坚果和海鲜/贝类)，被称为 6 种食物的消除饮食(6-food elimination diet，SFED)是提倡的[155]。接受要素饮食的患者有时需要放置胃造瘘管，以获得足够的热量支持。观察不同饮食方案有效性的研究重点是经验性 SFED、改良 SFED(SFED 加通过皮肤试验确定或作为病原体的食物消除)和要素饮食之间的比较[100,144,156]。在这些研究中，表明要素饮食优于经验性 SFED 和皮肤试验导向饮食(改良 SFED)。此外，已有研究表明，经验性 SFED 是成人 EoE 的有效治疗方法，经验性 SFED 的应答率与皮肤试验导向饮食治疗的应答率相似(应答率为 74%~81%)，此类应答率与成人和儿童 EoE 人群中报告的对吞服糖皮质激素的应答率相似[157-160]。低限制性饮食，如 2-食物消除饮食(乳制品和麸质)和 4-食物消除饮食(乳制品、麸质、鸡蛋和豆类)已被用于儿科人群，体面有效率分别为 43% 和 54%。已经提出了将消除饮食从 2-食物消除饮食升级为 4-食物消除饮食，然后进行 SFED 的方法，因为其避免了不必要的饮食限制[161,162]。初步研究结果表明，1-食物消除饮食(1-food elimination diet，OFED)可能在 EoE 的治中发挥作用[163,164]。Kagalwalla 等提出使用牛奶乳的 OFED，结果显示 65% 的儿科患者表现临床和组织学缓解[164]。此外，消除牛奶的 OFED 组与吞服氟替卡松组患者相比，发现 64% 的 OFED 患者食管嗜酸性粒细胞计数低于 15 个嗜酸性粒细胞/

HPF,症状评分显著改善,而氟替卡松组为 80%[163]。

Gonsalves 团队[100]和 Spergel 团队[156]的研究只确定了 34%~40%的 EoE 的相关致病食物(基于皮肤试验和内镜检查对食物消除或再引入的反应),这意味着 EoE 是由非食物相关刺激触发的,或者更可能是,识别食物超敏反应的方法目前不充分,因此未常规用于 EoE 患者的评估。成人队列中最常见的食物触发因素为小麦(60%)、牛奶(50%)、大豆(10%)、坚果(10%)和鸡蛋(5%),而儿童队列中最常见的触发因素为牛奶(35%)、鸡蛋(13%)、小麦(12%)和大豆(9%)。基于这些描述的频率,以及重新引入最不可能首先是诱因的食物原理,建议儿童患者重新引入食物的顺序首先是海鲜/坚果,然后依次是大豆、小麦、鸡蛋,最后是牛奶。成人患者首先是海鲜,然后依次是鸡蛋、坚果/大豆、牛奶,最后是小麦。

全身性[79]或局部糖皮质激素[165]也被用于治疗 EoE,疗效满意。急性加重使用全身性糖皮质激素,而局部糖皮质激素可提供长期控制。一项对 EoE 患者随访 10 年的研究支持继续糖皮质激素和食物消除治疗 EoE 的疗效[166]。当使用氟替卡松形式的局部糖皮质激素时,建议使用不含储雾罐的定量吸入器[83],或者也推荐使用布地奈德(以雾化器形式使用)与蔗糖[三氯蔗糖(Splenda)]的浆液[83,159]。指导患者吞服剂量,以促进其沉积在食管黏膜上。虽然建议将定量吸入器与局部氟替卡松一起使用,但其他研究表明,对于无法使用吸入器的 EoE 患者,使用布地奈德口服混悬液也是有效的方法[158,167]。在 EoE 的第一项安慰剂对照、双盲临床试验中,发现吞服局部氟替卡松可有效诱导疾病缓解,包括嗜酸性粒细胞、肥大细胞和 CD8 T 细胞水平降低以及上皮增生的程度[157]。然而,重要的是要指出,糖皮质激素抵抗也会发生。吞服氟替卡松或布地奈德不太可能出现与糖皮质激素相关的显著毒性(如肾上腺抑制),因为这些药物经胃肠道吸收后首次通过肝脏代谢[168]。然而,在 Cincinnati 儿童中心,10%接受氟替卡松每日使用大于 440μg 治疗的 EoE 儿童显示有肾上腺抑制的证据[169]。此外,患者可发生食管念珠菌病,可通过抗真菌治疗(见第 45 章)[170]。尽管局部糖皮质激素被认为是 EoE 的一线治疗药物,但迄今为止,在美国尚无局部用剂型获批用于 EoE,布地奈德崩解膜剂(口崩片)已在欧洲获批[171]。目前正在进行一些关于口服布地奈德黏性制剂以及布地奈德泡腾片的临床试验。

PPI 治疗可分别使 50% 和 60% 的 EoE 患者获得组织学缓解和症状改善[85,117]。2017 年欧洲指南在 EoE 治疗方案中使用高剂量 PPI 治疗 8 周作为一线治疗。此外,一些系统综述和荟萃分析证实了支持 PPI 作为一线治疗的证据,尤其是在高剂量下。

食管扩张联合或不联合药物或饮食疗法均可缓解部分 EoE 患者的吞咽困难。然而,在没有严重食管狭窄的情况下,在扩张前进行药物或饮食疗法的试验是合理的。然而食管扩张作为一种主要治疗,而不伴随药物或饮食疗法并不能解决潜在的炎症过程。描述的 EoE 患者食管扩张技术包括使用内镜和探条扩张器。虽然穿孔的风险较低,但与其他良性疾病患者相比,建议 EoE 患者采用更保守和谨慎的食管扩张技术[172]。逐步扩张食管的实践目标是 15~18mm,如果遇到阻力,将每次治疗的扩张直径限制在 3mm 或更小是合理的,但尚未在 EoE 患者中得到专门解决。已证实并发症与患者年龄较小和扩张次数较多、食管上三分之一狭窄以及在扩张前内镜无法穿过狭窄有关[173]。扩张后胸痛的风险是显著的,应在扩张前与患者讨论。

针对嗜酸性粒细胞生长因子 IL-5 的治疗在动物研究中证实有效[174],最近已在临床试验中进行了测试[33,34]。已经开发了两种不同的人源化 IL-5 特异性抗体美泊利单抗(mepolizumab)和瑞利珠单抗(reslizumab),并在 EoE 的临床试验中进行了测试[33,34,175]。美泊利单抗治疗导致 EoE 患者血液嗜酸性粒细胞增多急剧下降,食管嗜酸性粒细胞浸润减少,但对症状的影响各不相同[33]。其他减少 EoE 患者中嗜酸性粒细胞组织聚集的治疗可能靶向 IL-13。动物模型表明,IL-13 是调节炎症部位嗜酸性粒细胞募集的关键细胞因子,其主要是通过诱导趋化因子表达来实现[176,177]。最近在轻度哮喘患者中研究了人源化 IL-13 特异性抗体 Lebrikuzumab 单抗,然而,这种治疗似乎对组织嗜酸性细胞增多有不同的影响,并可能引起外周嗜酸性细胞计数增加[178]。临床前数据证实抗 IL-13 药物可能对 EoE 特别有效,已经进行了临床试验,一些有希望的结果证明平均嗜酸性粒细胞计数减少 60%[179]。评价人抗 IL-13 抗体(RPC 4046)以及抗 IL-4 受体 α 链的人抗体(dupilumab)(其阻断 IL-13 和相关细胞因子 IL-4)的多中心研究已显示可改善 EoE 的组织病理学(包括食管嗜酸性粒细胞增多)、内镜和临床特征[86]。FDA 批准 Dupilumab 用于治疗特应性皮炎,而 RPC4046 正在开发中。靶向 EoE 治疗的另一种候选药物是 Th2 细胞的趋化受体[CRTH2,也称为前列腺素 D2 受体 2(PTGD2R2)],被认为是 Th2 应答的效应因子。CRTH2 表达于 Th2 细胞、嗜酸性粒细胞和嗜碱性粒细胞表面[180],是一种 G 蛋白偶联受体[181]。低分子量 CRTH2 拮抗剂可部分减弱不同模型中的肺嗜酸性粒细胞增多[182]。此外,在一项Ⅱ期临床试验中,中度持续性哮喘患者的痰嗜酸性粒细胞计数显著降低[183],哮喘控制得到改善[184]。来自活动性 EoE 患者临床试验的初步数据显示,CRTH2 拮抗剂治疗可使组织嗜酸性粒细胞增多中度减少[185]。然而,还需要更多的临床数据来评估这种 G 蛋白偶联受体拮抗剂的有效性。

4. 预后

EoE 需要长期治疗,类似于过敏性哮喘。EoE 的自然史尚未充分阐明,然而,从儿童期至成年期食管嗜酸性粒细胞增多的 15 年随访显示,绝大多数患者的症状持续存在[186]。因此,慢性 EoE 如果不及时治疗,很可能发展为进行性食管瘢痕和功能障碍。EoE 的并发症包括食物嵌塞、食管狭窄、窄口径食管和食管穿孔。未经治疗 EoE 的持续时间是狭窄风险的良好预测因素[187]。成人中"食物嵌塞"(定义为需要内镜取出的食物潴留)的患病率范围为 30%~55%[188,189]。狭窄定义存在问题,因为"食管环"是成人疾病状态的常见表现,并且环的存在意味着一定程度的食管狭窄。共识指南指出,在这方面影像学定义可能优于内镜评估,因为影像学定义可能提供关于狭窄长度的补充信息,这可能影响可能的治疗选择及扩张。EoE 成人狭窄患病率为 11%~31%[172,188,190,191]。全层撕裂定义为食管或胃内容物进入胸腔,需要手术治疗。局部破裂定义为有限的空气或造影剂渗入纵隔,并可通过保守治疗愈合。食管壁内撕裂在内镜下被确定为延伸至食管黏膜下层的深部撕裂,或通过造影剂延伸至食管腔外但仍包含在食管壁内的影像学撕裂。尤其是在同时存在 EoE 和 GERD 的患者中,尚未确定发生巴雷特食管的风险,但似乎不是问题(见第 47 章)。此外,EoE 患者发生其他形式 EGID6 的风险增加,因此,可能需要通过内镜对整个胃肠道进行常规监测。

(二) 嗜酸性粒细胞性胃炎、肠炎、胃肠炎

与食管相反,健康条件下胃和肠易于检测到嗜酸性粒细胞的基线水平。因此做出嗜酸性粒细胞性胃炎(EG)、嗜酸性粒细胞性肠炎或嗜酸性粒细胞性胃肠炎(eosinophilic gastroenteritis,EGE)的诊断比作出 EoE 的诊断更为复杂。由于嗜酸性粒细胞性胃炎、肠炎和胃肠炎在临床上相似,并且关于其发病机制的可用信息很少,因此将一起讨论。然而,在大多数患者中,这些情况可能确实是不同的。在一项基于人群的研究中,EGE 和 EC 的患病率分别为 5. 1/100 000 人和 2. 1/100 000 人[118]。EGE 是 EGID 的第二种常见形式,但尚无关于临床或病理诊断的共识建议。Lwin 等提出,当在胃中至少 5 个不同的高倍镜视野中鉴定出至少 30 个嗜酸性粒细胞/HPF 时,就可以诊断 EG[192],而 Chehade 等建议在 3 个 HPF 中鉴定出至少 70 个嗜酸性粒细胞/HPF[193]。EG、EGE 和 EC 的发病率和患病率正在增加,其背后的原因尚不清楚[116]。这些疾病的特征是嗜酸性粒细胞选择性浸润胃和/或小肠,食管和/或大肠受累程度不一[23,194,195]。胃嗜酸性粒细胞浸润的继发性病因包括寄生虫和细菌感染(例如幽门螺杆菌)、IBD、HES、骨髓增生性疾病、结节性多动脉炎、过敏性血管炎、硬皮病、药物损伤和药物超敏反应。主要亚型包括特应性、非特应性和家族性变异型,次要亚型分为两组,一组由系统性嗜酸性粒细胞疾病(HES)组成,另一组由非嗜酸性粒细胞疾病组成(见表 30. 3)。原发性嗜酸性粒细胞胃炎、肠炎和胃肠炎也被称为特发性或过敏性胃肠炎。家族性尚未得到很好的表征,但在这些作者自己的患者中约 10% 可见(未发表的结果)[1]。原发性嗜酸性粒细胞性胃肠炎包括多种疾病实体,根据组织学受累程度细分为 3 种类型:黏膜、肌层和浆膜形式[196]。值得注意的是,胃肠道的任何一层均可受累,因此,在肌层和/或浆膜亚型患者中,内镜下黏膜活检可能是正常的。

1. 病因学

虽然嗜酸性粒细胞性胃炎、肠炎和胃肠炎在本质上是特发性的,但在至少一个患者亚组中提示了过敏机制[197]。事实上,已检测到总 IgE 和食物特异性 IgE 升高。另一方面,伴有局灶性糜烂性胃炎、肠炎和偶见的伴有明显嗜酸性粒细胞增多的食管炎的综合征,如饮食(食物)蛋白诱导的小肠结肠炎和饮食蛋白性肠病,以皮肤试验阴性且无特异性 IgE 为特征[198]。大多数患者对多种食物抗原的皮肤试验呈阳性,但没有典型的免疫反应,这符合迟发型食物超敏综合征。在一项研究中,23% 的 EGE 患者缺乏外周血嗜酸性粒细胞增多,但高达 50% 的黏膜型患者有食物过敏或不耐受史[20,196]。在另一项关于 EG 的研究中,接近 90% 的患者血嗜酸性粒细胞水平升高,并显示与胃嗜酸性粒细胞水平密切相关,表明血嗜酸性粒细胞水平可作为一种非侵入性的生物标志物,与 EoE 不同[199]。事实上,小鼠嗜酸性粒细胞性胃肠炎(累及食管、胃和肠)的实验性诱导,可以通过对致敏小鼠经口给予变应原(以肠溶变应原珠的形式)来完成[102]。值得注意的是,小鼠出现嗜酸性粒细胞相关的胃肠道功能障碍,包括胃胀、食物转运延迟和体重减轻,所有这些都强烈依赖于趋化因子嗜酸性细胞趋化因子-1[200]。肠组织的超微结构分析表明,嗜酸性粒细胞介导了轴突坏死,这一发现在 IBD 相关的肠嗜酸性粒细胞增多患者中已有报道[201]。值得注意的是,肥大细胞在 EGID 中也增加,一种口服过敏原诱导腹泻的小鼠模型已证实,IL-9 驱动的肥大细胞在 EGID 这种特定主要特征(过敏性腹泻)的发病机制中起着关键作用[202,203]。

在 EGE 患者中报告了外周血 T 细胞分泌 IL-4 和 IL-5 增加[197]。此外,当用牛奶蛋白刺激时,来源于 EGID 患者十二指肠固有层的 T 细胞优先分泌 Th2 细胞因子,尤其是 IL-13[204]。与包括感染幽门螺杆菌的患者在内的对照个体相比,胃活检显示出独特的转录组。EG 转录组表达高水平的嗜酸性细胞趋化因子-3 以及与 Th2 相关免疫相关的其他基因,但仅与 5% 的 EoE 转录组重叠[199]。IgA 缺乏也与 EGE 相关,有趣的是,推测这可能与这些患者中特应性或隐匿性胃肠道感染的相关发生率增加有关[205]。重要的是要记住,EGE 和膳食蛋白诱导的综合征(小肠结肠炎、小肠病和结肠炎)可能代表具有相似潜在免疫病理机制的 EGID 的连续统一体。此外,EGE 常与蛋白质丢失性肠病相关(见第 31 章)[193]。值得注意的是,已有嗜酸性粒细胞性肠炎伴系统性红斑狼疮的报告,具体病理相关性未知[206,207]。

2. 临床特征和诊断研究

一般来说,这些疾病表现为与胃肠道受累程度和面积相关的一系列症状。然而,即使是患孤立性嗜酸性粒细胞性肠炎(如十二指肠炎)的患者也可能有一系列的胃肠道症状。EGE 的黏膜型是最常见的变异型,其特征为呕吐、腹痛(甚至可以酷似急性阑尾炎)、腹泻、便血、缺铁性贫血、吸收不良、蛋白丢失性肠病和发育停滞[193,208]。肌层型的特征是嗜酸性粒细胞主要在肌层中浸润,导致肠壁增厚,这可能导致酷似幽门狭窄的胃肠道梗阻症状或胃出口梗阻的其他原因。浆膜型发生在少数 EGE 患者中,其特征为渗出性腹水,与其他形式相比,外周血嗜酸性粒细胞计数更高[20]。

对 EGID 的评估从全面的病史采集和体格检查开始,然后进行诊断检测(框 30. 1)。应通过检查粪便样本、结肠镜检期间获得的肠抽吸物或特异性血液抗体滴度来评价肠道寄生虫,特别是当患者有高风险暴露时(如出国旅行、居住在农场、饮用井水)(见第 114 章)。作为预防措施,在使用全身性免疫抑制治疗 EGID 之前,应排除粪类圆线虫感染,因为在全身性免疫抑制的情况下,这种感染可能危及生命[209]。总 IgE 水平的评价,在对 EGID 特应性变体患者进行分层或建议进一步考虑隐匿性寄生虫感染方面具有重要意义。值得注意的是,对一组食物过敏原和空气过敏原进行皮肤点刺试验,有助于识别对特定过敏原的致敏作用。针对特定食物抗原的皮肤超敏反应试验(皮肤斑贴试验)可能有助于进一步识别 EoE 的变异型变应原[5]。事实上,有证据表明 EGID 特应性变异型患者对平均 14 种不同食物的 IgE 致敏[1]。目前尚无诊断 EG、肠炎或 EGE 的标准[20,208]。支持诊断的一些发现是:胃肠道壁活检标本中嗜酸性粒细胞升高(与表 30. 2 所示的正常水

平相比）；肠隐窝和胃腺内嗜酸性粒细胞浸润；其他器官未受累；并排除引起嗜酸性粒细胞增多的其他原因（如感染、IBD）。这些疾病患者的小肠组织学分析显示嗜酸性粒细胞颗粒成分在细胞外沉积，免疫组化检测到细胞外 MBP 和 ECP 沉积[20,23,24,68]。EG 患者内镜下可观察到微结节（和/或息肉病），这些病变常含有明显的淋巴细胞和嗜酸性粒细胞聚集。

框 30.1 嗜酸性粒细胞增多性胃肠道疾病的诊断检查注意项目

一般检查

全血细胞计数及分类计数

总 IgE 水平

红细胞沉降率和 C 反应蛋白（EGID 中正常）

皮肤针刺试验和特异性 IgE 检测（作为综合检查的一部分）

感染检查（粪便和结肠抽吸物分析）

上、下消化道内镜检查及活检

pH 探针阻抗研究

内镜下功能性腔内成像探针技术（食管顺应性测量）

EoE 诊断组合

存在嗜酸性粒细胞增多

骨髓检查

血清类胰蛋白酶

血清维生素 B_{12}

超声心动图

染色体和细胞遗传学筛查

基于染色体研究的 FIP1L1-PDGFRA 融合基因和其他基因异常的遗传分析

任何其他潜在受累组织的评估和活检

EGID，嗜酸性粒细胞性胃肠道疾病；EoE，嗜酸性粒细胞性食管炎；IgE，免疫球蛋白 E。

Reproduced from Rothenberg ME. Eosinophilic gastrointestinal disorders (EGID). J Allergy Clin Immunol 2004; 113: 11-28. © 2004, with permission from the American Academy of Allergy, Asthma, and Immunology.

3. 治疗

消除皮肤点刺试验（或测量变应原特异性 IgE 水平）涉及的食物的饮食摄入具有不同的影响，但通常使用基于氨基酸的要素饮食实现完全消退[193,210]。通过饮食调整获得疾病缓解后，缓慢重新引入特定食物组（每个食物组约间隔 3 周），每 3 个月进行一次内镜检查，以确定疾病是持续缓解或疾病复发。值得注意的是，作者所在机构使用嗜酸性粒细胞耗竭抗体（抗 IL-5 受体-α）贝那利珠单抗（benralizumab）（目前 FDA 批准用于嗜酸性粒细胞性哮喘）治疗 EG 和 EGE 的临床试验正在进行中。有人主张使用色苷酸钠、孟鲁斯特、酮替芬、甲磺司特、吗替麦考酚酯（也称霉酚酸酯）和“替代中药”等药物[1,90]，但根据作者的经验，这些药物一般都不成功。然而，有报道孟鲁司特治疗后 EGE 成功获得长期缓解[211]。在作者所在机构，适当的治疗方法包括通过皮肤点刺试验和/或特异性 IgE 水平测定，发现食物致敏时进行食物消除试验。如果未发现致敏作用或特定的食物回避不可行时，则采用要素配方喂养。

除上述要素饮食外，EGID 的管理包括：全身和局部应用糖皮质激素、非糖皮质激素抗炎治疗、EGID 并发症（如缺铁性贫血）管理以及治疗毒性的管理[212]。如果饮食限制不可行的或未能改善疾病，则以抗炎药物（全身或局部糖皮质激素）为主。对于全身性类固醇治疗，相对低剂量的 2 到 6 周疗程似乎比 7 天疗程的冲击性糖皮质激素效果更好。有几种局部糖皮质激素可以保证药物在胃肠道的特定部位释放［如布地奈德片（Entocort EC）］，在回肠和结肠近端释放）。与哮喘治疗一样，与全身性应用糖皮质激素相比，局部应用糖皮质激素具有更好的获益-风险效应。在糖皮质激素无效或依赖的严重病例中，可选择静脉营养或硫唑嘌呤或 6-巯基嘌呤免疫抑制抗代谢治疗。最后，即使不存在 GERD，用 PPI 中和胃液酸度也可以改善症状以及食管和胃部病理的程度。

4. 预后

嗜酸性粒细胞性胃炎、肠炎和 EGE 的自然史尚未得到很好的证实。然而，这些疾病会长期反复消长（时好时坏）。在明确食物抗原诱导疾病的患者中，循环 IgE 水平和嗜酸性粒细胞水平异常通常作为组织受累的标志物。由于这些疾病常常是另一种原发性疾病过程的表现，因此建议对心肺系统进行常规监测。嗜酸性粒细胞的受累情况。当疾病在婴儿期出现并可确定特异性食物致敏时，到儿童晚期疾病获得缓解的可能性很高。

（三）嗜酸性粒细胞性结肠炎

嗜酸性粒细胞聚集在各种疾病患者的结肠中，包括嗜酸性粒细胞性胃肠炎、婴儿期过敏性结肠炎、感染（如蛲虫、犬钩虫）、药物反应、血管炎（如嗜酸性肉芽肿伴多发性血管炎）和 IBD[213,214]。婴儿期过敏性结肠炎又称饮食蛋白引起的婴儿期直肠结肠炎综合征，是出生后第一年血便最常见的原因[215,216]。与其他 EGID 相似，这些疾病可分为原发性和继发性。

1. 病因学

嗜酸性粒细胞性结肠炎通常是一种非 IgE 相关性疾病。一些研究指出 T 淋巴细胞介导的过程，但造成这种情况的确切免疫学机制尚未确定[217]。在口服抗原诱导的与结肠炎症相关的腹泻小鼠模型中，结肠 T 细胞已被证明通过 STAT-6 依赖机制将疾病转移到幼稚小鼠[40]。据报道，婴儿过敏性结肠炎可能是蛋白诱导的肠病或蛋白诱导的小肠结肠炎综合征的早期表达。牛奶和大豆蛋白是婴儿期过敏性结肠炎最常涉及的食物，但其他食物蛋白也可激发这种疾病。一般而言，虽然缺乏数据，但认为 EC 与自身免疫过程（包括 IBD）比 EoE 和胃炎更一致，后者更符合过敏性疾病。

2. 临床特征和诊断研究

根据组织受累的程度和部位，观察到与嗜酸性结肠炎相关的各种症状。虽然腹泻是一种典型的症状，但可独立于腹泻发生的其他症状通常包括腹痛、体重减轻和厌食。该病存在双峰年龄分布，婴儿型在诊断时的平均年龄约为 60 天[71]，另一种形式在青春期和成年早期出现[1]。在婴儿中，血样腹泻先于诊断前数周出现，因失血引起的贫血并不少见。大多数婴儿没有全身症状,其他方面健康。内镜检查时,斑片状红斑、血管分布缺失和淋巴结增生多局限在直肠但可扩展至整个结肠(图 30.3.A)[217]。组织学检查常显示黏膜的整体结构保存完好,然而,在黏膜固有层、隐窝上皮和肌层中均有嗜酸性粒细胞的局灶性聚集,偶尔在黏膜下层中存在多核巨细胞(见图 30.3.B)。没有单一的检查是诊断的金标准,但外周血嗜酸性粒细胞增多或粪便中出现嗜酸性粒细胞提示嗜酸性粒细胞性结肠炎。

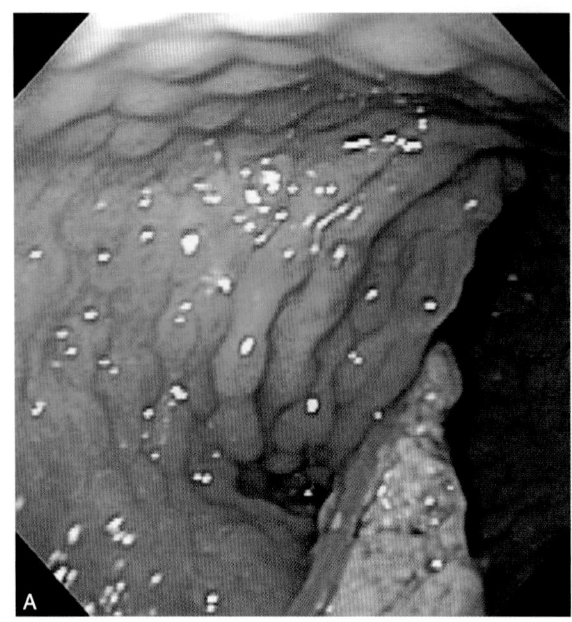

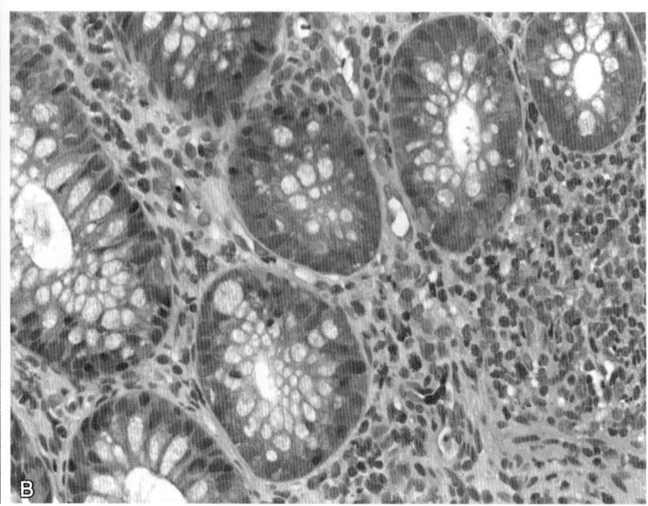

图 30.3 表现为血红素阳性大便和贫血的婴儿嗜酸性结肠炎。A,直肠的内镜图像显示黏膜结节,中央脐状凹陷,是结节性淋巴样增生的特征,这种所见通常与食物过敏有关;B,直肠黏膜活检的显微照片显示固有层中嗜酸性粒细胞数量增加,形成聚集体,偶尔侵入上皮和隐窝。(苏木精和伊红染色×40)

3. 治疗

嗜酸性粒细胞性结肠炎的治疗主要取决于疾病亚型。例如,婴儿期嗜酸性粒细胞性结肠炎通常是一种良性疾病。在撤除饮食中的致病蛋白触发物后,粪便中的肉眼血液通常在72 小时内消退,但显性和隐匿性失血可能会持续更长时间[70,218]。老年嗜酸性粒细胞性结肠炎通常需要药物治疗,抗炎药物包括 5-氨基水杨酸盐和全身或局部糖皮质激素是常用的,似乎有效,但尚未进行仔细的临床试验。有几种形式的局部糖皮质激素,旨在将药物递送至远端结肠和直肠,但嗜酸性粒细胞性结肠炎通常也累及近端结肠。在对全身性糖皮质激素治疗抵抗或依赖的严重病例中,替代方案包括静脉营养或硫唑嘌呤或 6-巯基嘌呤免疫抑制性抗代谢治疗。

4. 预后

当嗜酸性粒细胞性结肠炎在出生后第一年出现时,预后良好,绝大多数患者到 1~3 岁时就能够耐受致病食物。生命后期发生的嗜酸性粒细胞性结肠炎的预后比婴儿亚型更保守。与嗜酸性粒细胞性胃肠炎相似,自然史尚未见记载,本病被认为是一种慢性消长性(时好时坏)疾病。由于嗜酸性粒细胞性结肠炎通常可能是其他原发性疾病过程的表现,因此心肺系统的常规临床监测很重要,可能需要定期进行上消化道和下消化道的内镜检查。

四、资源

最近 EoE 的小规模流行促成建立了以患者为基础的支持/倡导团体,如美国嗜酸性粒细胞疾病合作伙伴(American Partnership for Eosinophilic Disorders,APFED)和敦促研究嗜酸性粒细胞疾病运动(Campaign Urging Research for Eosinophilic Disease,CURED)。此外,最近形成的 CEGIR 这是美国国立卫生研究院罕见病临床研究网络的一部分,将使人们更好地了解和治疗 EGID[219]。虽然在胃肠道嗜酸性粒细胞和 EGID 方面取得了很大进展,但与其他细胞类型和可能更不常见的胃肠道疾病相比,知识仍然很少。可以预见,通过结合过敏、胃肠病学、营养学和病理学领域专家参与的综合临床和研究方法,将会更好地了解 EGID 的发病机制和治疗方法。

(王萍 张莉 译,闫秀娥 袁农 校)

参考文献

第 31 章　蛋白丢失性胃肠病

David A. Greenwald 著

章节目录

一、定义与正常生理学 …… 411
二、病理生理学 …… 412
三、临床特征 …… 413
四、与蛋白质丢失性胃肠病相关的疾病 …… 414
（一）无黏膜糜烂或溃疡的疾病 …… 414
（二）伴有黏膜糜烂或溃疡的疾病 …… 415
（三）伴有淋巴管阻塞或淋巴管压力升高的疾病 …… 415
五、诊断 …… 415
（一）实验室检查 …… 415
（二）疑似蛋白丢失性胃肠病患者的处理方法 …… 416
六、治疗和预后 …… 416

一、定义与正常生理学

蛋白质丢失性胃肠病是指各种原因所致的血清蛋白质过量丢失入胃肠道所致低蛋白血症的一组疾病[1-16]。血清蛋白质过量丢失引发低蛋白血症，可表现为水肿、腹水和营养不良。框 31.1 列出了与蛋白质丢失性胃肠病相关的疾病[17-76]。

1947 年，Maimon 等推测 Ménétrier 病患者胃内巨大皱襞中流出的液体富含蛋白质。1949 年，Albright 等通过静脉注射白蛋白发现，导致低蛋白血症的原因是白蛋白的分解代谢过度，而不是白蛋白的合成下降[1]。直到 1956 年，Kimbel 等发现，慢性胃炎患者胃内白蛋白的生成增加。一年后，Citrin 等[2]证明在 Ménétrier 症患者中消化道是蛋白质过量流失的实际部位，因为他们在这类患者的胃液中发现了静脉内注射标记放射性碘的蛋白质。

框 31.1　与蛋白丢失性胃肠病相关的疾病

无黏膜糜烂或溃疡的疾病

AIDS 相关胃肠病[17]
急性病毒性胃肠炎[18]
过敏性胃肠病[19]
乳糜泻[20]
维生素 B_{12} 缺乏[21]
胶原性结肠炎[22]
巨细胞病毒感染[23]
嗜酸粒细胞性胃肠炎[24]
巨大肥厚性胃病（Ménétrier 病）[25,26]
贾第虫病、血吸虫病、线虫病（毛细线虫病）、圆线虫病
移植物抗宿主病
幽门螺杆菌相关性胃炎
过敏性紫癜[27]
肥大高分泌胃病[28-30]
肠道寄生虫[22]
淋巴细胞性结肠炎
淋巴细胞性胃炎
混合结缔组织病[31]
副球孢子菌病
麻疹后腹泻
小肠细菌过度生长（SIBO）[32]
干燥综合征[33]
系统红斑狼疮（SLE）[34-40]
热带性口炎性腹泻[41]
血管扩张（胃、肠）[43]
肠源性脂肪代谢障碍（Whipple 病）[43]

有黏膜糜烂或溃疡的疾病

α 链病[44]
淀粉样变性[45]
白塞病[460]
类癌综合征
克罗恩病[47,48]
十二指肠炎[49]
糜烂性胃炎[49]
消化道肿瘤
移植物抗宿主病[50]
幽门螺杆菌相关性胃炎[51-53]
特发性溃疡性空肠回肠炎[54]
感染性腹泻（如艰难梭菌[55]，志贺菌属[56]）
缺血性结肠炎
卡波西肉瘤[57]
白血病/淋巴瘤
黑色素瘤
多发性骨髓瘤
神经纤维瘤[582]
NSAID 肠病[59]
结节病[60]
脓毒症休克综合征（溶血性链球菌）
华氏巨球蛋白血[62]

伴淋巴管阻塞或淋巴管内压力增高的疾病

布-加综合征[68]
心脏病[63,64]
CD55 缺乏症[69]
缩窄性心包炎，心力衰竭，三尖瓣反流，Fonton 手术[70,71]
克罗恩病[47,48]
肠道子宫内膜异位症[65]
肠道淋巴管扩张症（先天性、获得性）[66,67]
淋巴-小肠瘘[28]
淋巴瘤，包括蕈样真菌病
肠系膜结核及结节病[60]
肠系膜静脉血栓形成[73]
累及肠系膜淋巴管的肿瘤性疾病
门静脉高压性胃肠病[74]
移植后淋巴增生性疾病[75]
腹膜后纤维化
硬化性肠系膜炎[76]
上腔静脉血栓形成
系统性红斑狼疮[35-40]
结核性腹膜炎
Whipple 病[43]

之后的研究都采用放射性标记的聚乙烯吡咯烷酮、白蛋白和其他蛋白质以及免疫学方法进行测定肠道内 α_1-抗胰蛋白酶(α_1-antitrypsin,α_1-AT)的丢失,进一步阐明了胃肠道在血清蛋白质代谢中的作用特点。正常情况下,胃肠道丢失的白蛋白占机体白蛋白降解总量的 2%~5%,但在严重蛋白质丢失性胃肠道疾病患者中,这种胃肠道蛋白丢失可达到白蛋白总量的 60%[3-6]。

在生理条件下,大多数在胃肠腔内发现的内源性蛋白来源于脱落的肠细胞以及胰腺和胆道的分泌物[7,8]。大量研究通过各种方法(如 ^{67} 铜-铜蓝蛋白、^{51} 铬-白蛋白和 α_1-AT 清除率)检测血清白蛋白在胃肠道内的丢失,结果显示健康成人每日肠道丢失的血清蛋白不多,估计这些蛋白质不到血清蛋白总量的 1%~2%,而肠道丢失的白蛋白不到白蛋白每天分解率的 10%。正常女性和男性的白蛋白总量分别约为 3.9g/kg 和 4.7g/kg,白蛋白半衰期为 15~33 天,肝白蛋白合成速率为 0.15g/(kg·d),与降解速率相等[9-10]。上消化道内多余的蛋白质会像其他肽类一样,被上消化道内的蛋白酶代谢分解为氨基酸后被重吸收。在健康成人中,消化道丢失的蛋白在总蛋白代谢中只起很小的作用,血清蛋白水平反映了蛋白质合成与总蛋白代谢之间的平衡。然而,在蛋白丢失性胃肠病患者中,这种平衡出现显著改变[5,11]。

二、病理生理学

大量的血浆蛋白通过胃肠道上皮细胞丢失,可由多种黏膜病理过程引起。黏膜损伤可导致血浆蛋白通透性增加;黏膜糜烂和溃疡可导致富含炎性蛋白的渗出液渗出,淋巴管阻塞或淋巴管静水压增高可导致含有血浆蛋白的淋巴液直接漏出。血管通透性的改变可影响间质液中血清蛋白的浓度,进而影响肠黏膜蛋白的丢失[12,16]。

在研究蛋白质丢失性胃肠病的发病机制中,Bode 等认为可能与肠上皮细胞表面的硫酸乙酰肝素蛋白的丢失有关[11,13,14]。硫酸乙酰肝素蛋白聚糖通过具有与质膜结合的大细胞外结构域(称为多配体蛋白聚糖)或附着在称为蛋白聚糖的膜糖脂上来影响肠道屏障[15]。这些多配体蛋白聚糖在维持细胞间紧密连接中起到了重要作用。

被基因改造为缺乏多配体蛋白聚糖或其他硫酸乙酰肝素蛋白的小鼠,其细胞间紧密屏障发生改变,蛋白质通过细胞旁通路漏至肠腔(图 31.1)。此外,用促炎细胞因子(如肿瘤坏死因子-α 或干扰素-γ)治疗此类小鼠会导致细胞间连接的显著缺陷,甚至更多的蛋白质漏入肠腔[13]。多配体蛋白聚糖缺乏状态和暴露于促炎细胞因子的同时存在,会加重蛋白质的漏出和蛋白质的流失。最后,重新引入硫酸肝素或其他多配体蛋白聚糖可消除蛋白质漏入肠腔[13]。

蛋白丢失性胃肠病患者血清蛋白的丢失与其分子量无关,因此循环血内每日各种蛋白质的降解比例保持不变,包括白蛋白、免疫球蛋白(IgG、IgA、IgM)和铜蓝蛋白[5,11,16]。相反,肾病综合征患者选择性地漏出分子量较低的蛋白质,如白蛋白。当蛋白质进入胃肠道时,蛋白质的合成代偿性地增加。进入胃肠道的蛋白质被胃、胰腺和小肠的酶代谢分解成氨基酸,再被特定的转运体吸收,然后再循环。当胃或肠的蛋白质丢失率,或两者都超过身体合成新蛋白质的能力时,就会发生低蛋白血症[7,8]。例如,低白蛋白血症在蛋白丢失性胃肠病中很常见,当肝白蛋白合成(其能力有限,只能增加 25%)和白蛋白丢失不平衡时,就会导致血液循环中白蛋白总量减少和白蛋白半衰期缩短。

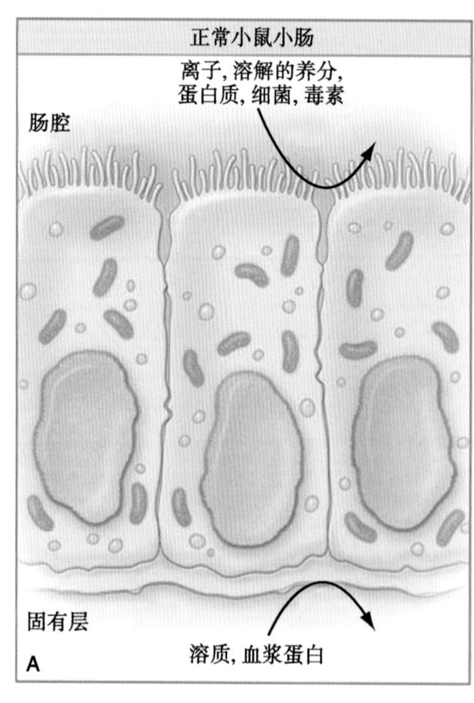

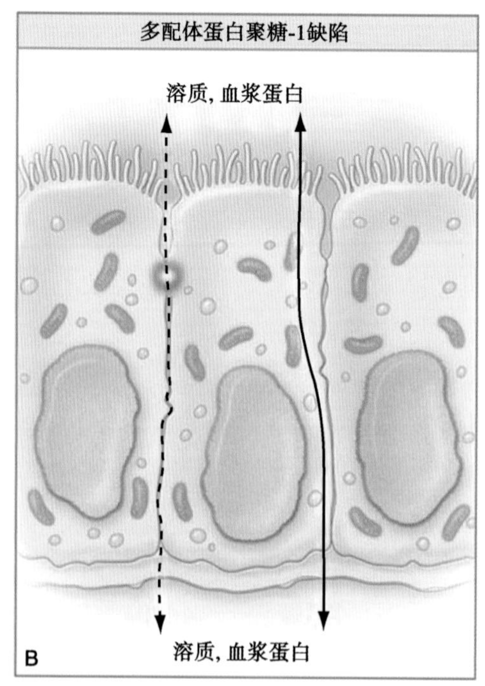

图 31.1　影响小鼠肠道完整性因素的示意图:A,正常小鼠肠道是抵御某些离子、营养溶质、蛋白质、细菌和毒素自由扩散的有效屏障,将肠腔(外)与固有层(内)有效分离。B,多配体蛋白聚糖-1 缺陷小鼠,由于细胞间连接缺陷和细胞旁渗漏增加(虚线)或跨细胞蛋白转运增加(实线),导致肠道屏障功能下降[13]。

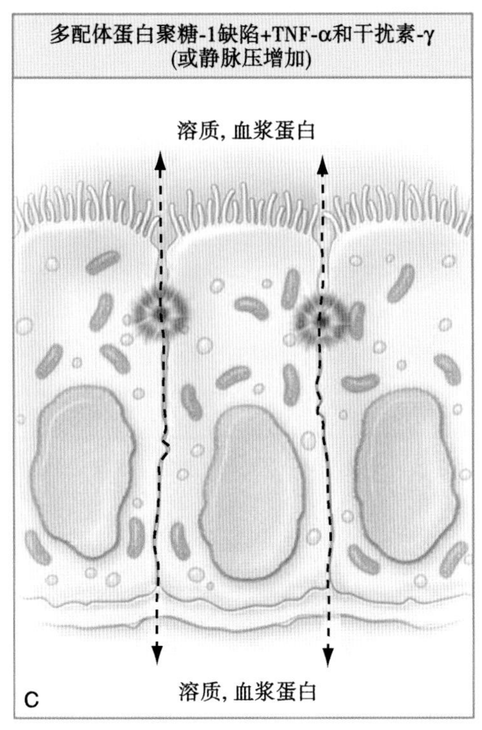

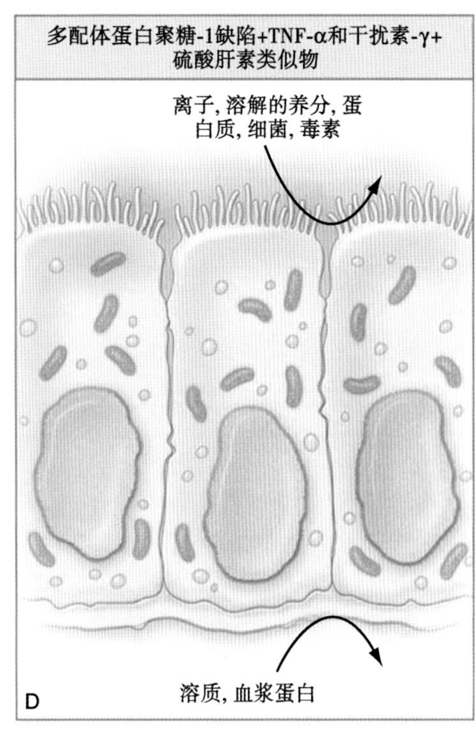

图 31.1(续)　C,给予炎性细胞因子(TNF-α 和干扰素-γ)或手术增加其门静脉压力的多配体蛋白聚糖-1 缺陷小鼠,有大量缺陷的细胞间连接和大量的细胞间蛋白渗漏(虚线),与蛋白质丢失性肠病一致。D,输注硫酸肝素类似物可完全逆转给予炎症细胞因子的多配体蛋白聚糖-1 缺陷小鼠中观察到的肠道屏障功能障碍。更多详情请参见正文。TNF-α,肿瘤坏死因子-α。(From Lencer WI. Patching a leaky intestine. N Engl J Med 2008;359:526-8, with permission.)

内源性蛋白质分解代谢的适应性变化可能弥补肠道蛋白质的过度丢失,导致特定蛋白质的丢失不平衡。像胰岛素、一些凝血因子和 IgE 等蛋白质分解代谢周转率快(短半衰期),因此相对不受胃肠道丢失的影响,因为这些蛋白质的合成随之而来。另一方面,除了 IgE 外,白蛋白和大多数免疫球蛋白的加速合成是有限的,因此从肠道中丢失这些蛋白会表现为低蛋白血症(低白蛋白血症和低球蛋白血症)[11]。其他因素促发的肠内蛋白的过度丢失见于各种疾病,如肝脏蛋白质合成受损和血浆蛋白质内源性降解增加。

除了引起低蛋白血症外,蛋白质丢失性胃肠病还可能与其他血清成分(如脂类、铁、微量金属)浓度降低有关[11]。淋巴管阻塞可导致淋巴细胞减少,从而引起细胞免疫功能降低。

三、临床特征

低蛋白血症和水肿是蛋白质丢失性胃肠病的主要临床表现,胸腔积液、心包积液以及营养不良也很常见。大多数其他临床表现反映了潜在疾病,因此,蛋白质丢失性胃肠病的临床表现多种多样(框 31.2)[17-76]。蛋白质丢失性胃肠病在儿童和成人中均可见[77],临床上常见的是低蛋白血症,表现为血清白蛋白降低,免疫球蛋白(IgG、IgA、IgM,除了 IgE)、纤维蛋白原、脂蛋白,α1-AT、转铁蛋白、血浆铜蓝蛋白降低[11]。尽管存在低蛋白血症,但视磺醛结合蛋白、前白蛋白等周转较快的蛋白则维持正常水平[78]。因为血浆胶体渗透压降低,临床上常出现严重的坠积性水肿,但全身水肿在蛋白丢失性胃肠病中罕见。单侧水肿、上肢水肿、面部水肿、黄斑水肿(伴有可逆性失明)和双侧视网膜脱离多认为是肠道淋巴管扩张的结果[79]。虽然血清丙种球蛋白降低,但感染的易感性增加并不常见。虽然凝血因子在胃肠道中丢失,但合成较快,因此凝血功能常不受影响。另外,某些情况下有血管病性血栓形成(见

框 31.2　蛋白丢失性胃肠病的临床表现

症状和体征

水肿(依赖性,上肢,面部,黄斑;单侧淋巴管扩张症)

腹泻

视网膜脱离(见于淋巴管扩张症)[79]

实验室检查异常

低蛋白血症

低白蛋白血症

血清 γ 球蛋白下降(IgG,IgA,IgM)

血清蛋白—铜蓝蛋白、α1-抗胰蛋白、纤维蛋白原、转铁蛋白、激素结合蛋白降低

血清脂蛋白降低

有证据的脂肪吸收不良

有证据的碳水化合物吸收不良

有证据的脂溶性维生素吸收不良或缺乏

细胞免疫功能改变[80]

淋巴细胞减少症

Ig,免疫球蛋白。

后面讨论）[69]。循环中结合激素的蛋白尿（如皮质醇结合球蛋白和甲状腺结合球蛋白）的浓度可能会显著降低，但血液循环中游离激素浓度没有显著改变。

大多数蛋白丢失性胃肠病患者的临床表现是其潜在疾病本身的表现，而非蛋白质丢失本身造成的。例如，以蛋白质丢失为特征的小肠疾病（如乳糜泻、热带性口炎性腹泻）临床症状与吸收不良有关，继而引起腹泻、脂溶性维生素缺乏和贫血。由淋巴管扩张导致的淋巴管阻塞，可引起淋巴细胞减少或细胞免疫功能的异常[80]。

四、与蛋白质丢失性胃肠病相关的疾病

蛋白质丢失性胃病相关的疾病可分为 3 大类：①无胃肠道黏膜糜烂或溃疡的疾病；②有胃肠道黏膜糜烂或溃疡的疾病；③导致淋巴管阻塞和间质压力升高的疾病（见框 31.1）。在某些疾病状态下，这些机制中不止一种可起作用，某些感染性疾病的情况也是如此。

（一）无黏膜糜烂或溃疡的疾病

虽然有些疾病胃肠道上皮层损伤而没有造成糜烂或溃疡，但仍可能导致表面上皮细胞脱落，从而引起蛋白质的过量丢失。小肠病变引起的吸收不良往往与肠内血浆蛋白的渗漏有关。蛋白质丢失可由血管损伤引起的血管通透性改变引起，如狼疮性血管炎、IgE 介导的 1 型超敏反应、感染（寄生虫、病毒、细菌过度生长），也可由细胞间通透性增加或毛细血管通透性增加引起[28-38,36]。

1. Ménétrier 病

巨大肥厚性胃病（Ménétrier 病，见第 52 章）是引起严重蛋白质丢失的最常见的胃部病变[25,26]。患者通常有消化不良、恶心、呕吐、水肿、体重减轻和低蛋白血症。可见胃皱襞突出、肥厚，表面有大量黏液及富含蛋白质的渗出物，正常的胃腺体被黏液分泌细胞取代，壁细胞数量减少，进而引起胃酸减少或胃酸缺乏。细胞间通透性的增加导致蛋白质丢失。该病患者细胞间的紧密连接比健康人宽，由此证明蛋白质的转运由这些增宽的间隙通过胃黏膜漏出。组胺-2 受体拮抗剂（H_2RAs）、抗胆碱能药物和奥曲肽可改善该病患者症状，但持续性腹痛或严重持续蛋白质丢失的患者需要接受胃大部或全胃切除术缓解[26]。如第 52 章所说，幽门螺杆菌（Hp）感染、Ménétrier 病与蛋白质丢失性胃肠病之间可能存在因果关系，在清除 Hp 后，低蛋白血症得以纠正，胃皱襞也可能恢复到正常的形态[51-53]。

2. 幽门螺杆菌相关性胃炎

没有梅尼埃病（Ménétrier 病）的幽门螺杆菌相关性胃炎（见第 52 章）与蛋白质丢失性胃病有关，并对根除 Hp 感染有反应[51-53]。其中一些患者可能有胃糜烂，从而导致蛋白质的丢失。

3. 过敏性胃肠病

虽然过敏性胃肠病（见第 10、30 和 52 章）是儿童多见的疾病，但是也发生在成年人。临床表现为腹痛、呕吐和阵发性腹泻。实验室检查可见低蛋白血症、缺铁性贫血和外周血嗜酸性粒细胞增多，血清总蛋白、白蛋白、IgA 和 IgG 水平显著降低，而 IgM 和转铁蛋白轻度降低。小肠的组织学特征性表现为固有层嗜酸性细胞数量的显著增加，粪便检查可发现夏科-莱登结晶（Charcot-Leyden 结晶）[19]。

4. 系统性红斑狼疮

系统红斑狼疮（systemic lupus erythematosus，SLE）是一种全身性自身免疫性疾病，通常与蛋白丢失性胃肠病相关，该病被称为狼疮蛋白丢失性肠病（图 31.2）[34-39]。SLE 引起的肠系膜血管炎可导致肠缺血、水肿和肠道血管通透性改变。此外，SLE 患者可发生胃炎和黏膜溃疡，这两种情况都可以引起蛋白质的过度丢失。蛋白丢失性胃肠病可以视为 SLE 的首发临床表现。全身应用糖皮质激素以及其他免疫调节剂（如硫唑嘌呤、环磷酰胺和他克莫司等）可以缓解临床症状，包括蛋白质丢失性胃肠病导致的临床症状[38-40]。

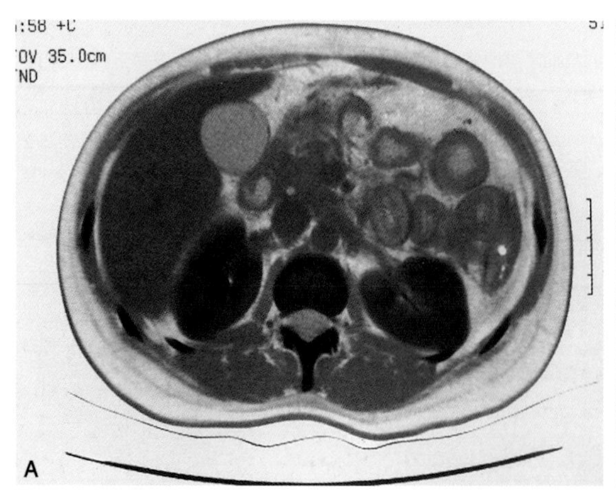

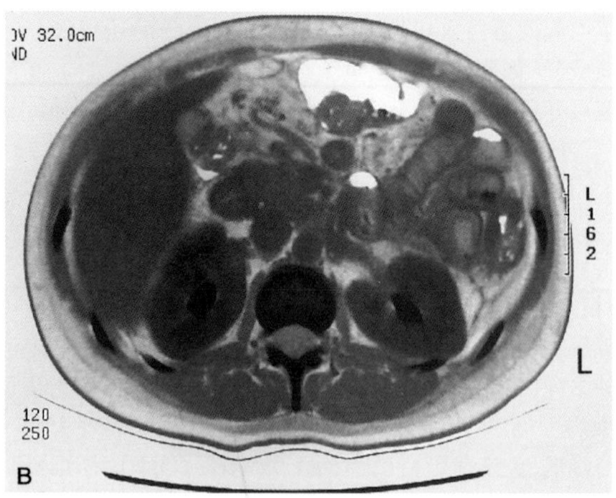

图 31.2　A，腹部 CT。一例 29 岁女性患者，有严重的水样腹泻和弥漫性非放射性腹痛。血清白蛋白水平为 2.9g/dL，肌酐水平为 0.6mg/dL。粪便检查显示病原体阴性。CT 显示弥漫性小肠壁增厚。抗核抗体滴度为 1∶1 280，该患者接受甲基泼尼松龙治疗后，症状迅速改善，腹泻和腹痛缓解。B，5 天后复查 CT 显示肠壁增厚明显改善，此时血清白蛋白水平为 3.4g/dL，肾活检符合狼疮性肾炎

（二）伴有黏膜糜烂或溃疡的疾病

导致蛋白质丢失性胃肠病中伴有胃肠黏膜糜烂或溃疡的疾病可由良性或恶性疾病引起，可以是局灶性或弥漫性的（见框 31.1）。蛋白质丢失的严重程度取决于细胞损伤以及相关的炎症和淋巴管阻塞的程度。弥漫性小肠或结肠溃疡（如克罗恩病、溃疡性结肠炎和伪膜性结肠炎）可导致严重的蛋白质丢失[47,48,61]。低白蛋白血症在胃肠道恶性肿瘤患者中常见，虽然这通常是白蛋白合成下降导致的，但也有肠道蛋白质过度丢失导致的相关报道。蛋白质丢失性胃肠病也与肿瘤治疗有关，包括化疗、放疗和骨髓移植。

（三）伴有淋巴管阻塞或淋巴管压力升高的疾病

淋巴管阻塞可导致肠道淋巴管扩张，并可导致富含血浆蛋白、乳糜微粒和淋巴细胞的乳糜管破裂。当中心静脉压升高时（如心力衰竭或缩窄性心包炎），肠壁淋巴管充血，导致富含蛋白质的淋巴液渗入胃肠道[8,63,64]。黏膜和黏膜下淋巴管弯曲、扩张可见于原发性肠淋巴管扩张症（图 31.3）。该病患者一般在 30 岁时出现水肿、低蛋白血症、腹泻和淋巴细胞减少（由于淋巴液渗漏和淋巴管破裂所致）[66,67]。常染色体显性纯合子患者存在编码 CD55 的基因突变，该病患者表现为腹痛、腹泻、伴有肠淋巴管扩张的蛋白质丢失性胃肠病、水肿、消化不良、反复感染和血管病性血栓栓塞疾病[69]。腹膜后病变如腺病、纤维化和胰腺炎也可影响淋巴液引流。肝移植术后的布-加综合征（Budd-Chiari 综合征）与蛋白质丢失性胃肠病有关[68]。肺动脉下心室旷置术（Fontan 手术）是先天性单心室心脏或严重左心室发育不良的外科矫正手术，在右心房和肺动脉之间建立了一个大吻合口，使静脉血绕过右心室。Fontan 手术后 10 年内，有高达 15% 的患者出现了蛋白质丢失性胃肠病[8,70,71,72]。血流动力学研究提示这些患者的中心静脉压升高。

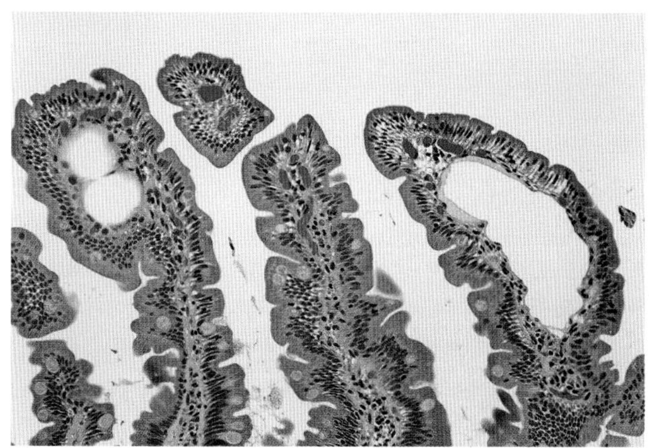

图 31.3　肠淋巴管扩张症。该小肠活检标本获自蛋白质丢失性肠病患者。显示局灶性淋巴管扩张（即 2 个绒毛受累，2 个未受累），与获得性（继发性）淋巴管扩张一致。先天性淋巴管扩张症可表现为弥漫性的淋巴管扩张。（Courtesy Dr. Edward Lee, Washington, D. C.）

五、诊断

（一）实验室检查

除了蛋白丢失性胃肠病，低蛋白血症和水肿还可出现于许多其他疾病，因此确定蛋白质是否从胃肠道过度丢失是非常重要的。对于没有蛋白尿、肝病、营养不良等不明原因的低蛋白血症患者，应注意是否存在蛋白质丢失性胃肠病。以往诊断蛋白质丢失性胃肠病的金标准是将放射性标记的大分子（如 ^{51}Cr-白蛋白）静脉给药后，测量在粪便中排出量。这种方法的使用有很大的局限性，比如需暴露于放射性物质，有 6～10 天的标本收集期，因此不具有临床实用性[81]。

α_1-AT 是一个有用的肠道蛋白质丢失的标志物。α_1-AT 是一种 50kD 的糖蛋白，其大小与白蛋白（67kD）相似；与白蛋白一样，其在肝脏内合成，但在肠道既不吸收也不分泌，且可以抵御肠腔内的蛋白水解。在粪便可检出低浓度的 α_1-AT[81-83]。通过定量测定粪便中的 α_1-AT 浓度或血浆中 α_1-AT 的清除率，可以判断是否存在肠道蛋白质的丢失，其中，后者更加准确。因此，最佳方法是通过收集 72 小时粪便和血浆 α_1-AT 的浓度，计算 α_1-AT 血浆清除率（单位：mL/d），计算公式为：

$$\alpha_1\text{-AT 血浆清除率} = (\text{每天粪便的体积} \times \text{粪便 } \alpha_1\text{-AT 浓度}) / \text{血浆 } \alpha_1\text{-AT 浓度}$$

α_1-AT 的血浆清除率也可以用来监测治疗反应。

α_1-AT 的血浆清除率正常情况下不超过 24mL/d。腹泻本身可以增加 α_1-AT 的血浆清除率；对于腹泻患者，α_1-AT 的血浆清除率超过 56mL/d 认为是异常。此外，α_1-AT 的血浆清除率和血清白蛋白浓度呈负相关，当血清白蛋白低于 3g/dL，α_1-AT 的血浆清除率可超过 180mL/d。在婴儿中，胎粪会干扰 α_1-AT 结果（假阳性）。由于胎粪中的 α_1-AT 浓度更高，因此本试验不适用于怀疑患有蛋白质丢失性肠病的婴儿[81-84]。肠道出血也会导致 α_1-AT 的血浆清除率呈假阳性；当粪便隐血试验阳性时，α_1-AT 的血浆清除率的结果不可靠[81-84]。在胃内 pH<3 时，α_1-AT 被胃蛋白酶降解，因此可能在胃蛋白丢失患者中出现假阴性；应用 PPI 防止 α_1-AT 在胃内被消化降解，可用来检测蛋白质丢失性胃病[84]。

核医学研究有助于诊断蛋白质丢失性胃肠病，常用的有 ^{99m}Tc 标记的人血清白蛋白（^{99m}Tc-HSA）、^{99m}Tc 标记的亚甲基二膦酸盐（^{99m}Tc-MDP）、^{99m}Tc 标记的葡聚糖显像、^{99m}Tc 标记的人免疫球蛋白和铟-111（^{111}In）标记的转铁蛋白[85-89]。当 α_1-AT 的血浆清除率结果不明确时，核素显像有助于蛋白质丢失的定量和定位，有助于确定诊断。在这些检测中，^{99m}Tc 标记的葡聚糖显像比 ^{99m}Tc-HSA 更敏感，但这两种检测都还没有广泛使用。^{99m}Tc-HAS 检测已应用于儿童和成人，用于检测胃或肠道蛋白丢失的定位和监测治疗反应。^{99m}Tc 标记的人免疫球蛋白和 ^{111}In 标记的转铁蛋白也有助于胃肠道蛋白质丢失的定量和定位[85-89]。磁共振成像（MRI）可以诊断原发性蛋白质丢失性胃肠病，可以明确病变，如腹部肠系膜淋巴管扩张、四肢皮下淋巴管扩张[90]。据报道，肠道磁共振成像可确诊放射性核素显像疑似的蛋白丢失性肠病，同时定位结肠和小肠中蛋白丢失的炎症区域[91]。胶囊内镜可观察到蛋白丢失性胃肠病的特征性改变，但需要通过小肠镜进行活检样本[92]。

（二）疑似蛋白丢失性胃肠病患者的处理方法

在没有上述讨论的混杂因素下，根据 α_1-AT 的血浆清除率增加，即可作出蛋白质丢失性胃肠病的诊断，^{99m}Tc-HSA 等放射性核素显像有助于蛋白质丢失的定量和定位（具体到器官）（图 31.4）[85,86]。能确认蛋白质从胃肠道丢失的检测对于诊断蛋白质丢失性胃肠病至关重要，因为许多其他疾病也可以出现水肿和低蛋白血症而没有肠内蛋白质丢失，例如肾病综合征、肝硬化、恶性肿瘤、饮食失调（包括贪食症和厌食症）、营养不良、利尿剂或泻药滥用。

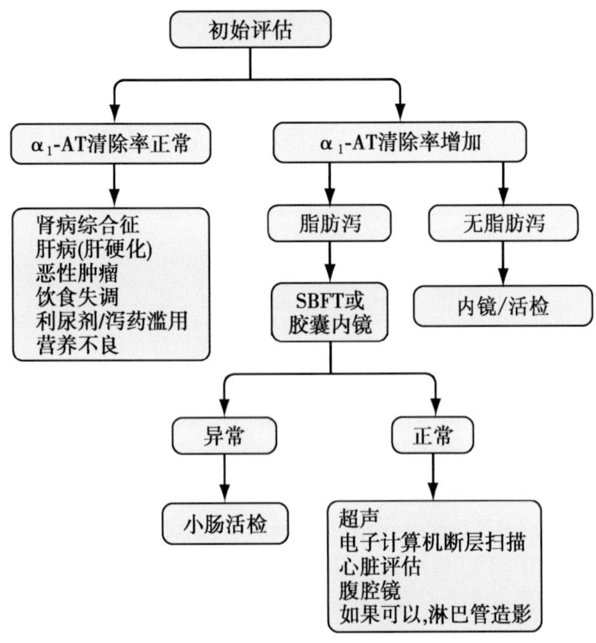

图 31.4　蛋白丢失性胃肠病患者的治疗方法。初步评估包括完整的病史和体格检查，实验室评价（见正文）和测定 α_1-抗胰蛋白酶（α_1-AT）血浆清除率。SBFT，小肠钡餐造影

在确认存在胃肠内蛋白丢失后，需要进一步评估确认潜在的病因。初步评估应包括详细的病史采集和体格检查。血液检测通常包括全血细胞计数、分类（特别是嗜酸性粒细胞）、血红蛋白、电解质、钙、镁、血清蛋白电泳和免疫电泳、c反应蛋白、血沉、抗核抗体（antinuclear antibody，ANA）和类风湿因子、凝血指标、HIV 检测、铁和铁结合力和甲状腺功能。对于腹泻患者，收集 72 小时粪便脂肪测定也是有用的，包括虫卵、寄生虫、贾第虫抗原、艰难梭菌毒素和 Charcot-Leyden 结晶（如果有外周血嗜酸细胞增多症）的检测。

胸片可显示肉芽肿疾病或心脏扩大。如怀疑静脉压增高，可进行心电图或超声心动图检查。脂肪肝患者应该集中检测上消化道，并对小肠进行影像学和内镜检查（包括胶囊内镜和小肠镜）[91,92]。

食管胃十二指肠检查和结肠镜检查有助于发现黏膜炎症、溃疡、肿瘤或其他异常，异常部位应进行活检，随机活检也是有意义的。有些疾病如胶原病或淋巴细胞性结肠炎内镜下正常，但随机活检可能有阳性发现。研究发现小肠和大肠可表现为溃疡和黏膜异常。可能导致淋巴管阻塞的疾病（如腹膜后纤维化、胰腺疾病、恶性肿瘤）可进行腹部和骨盆的 CT 或 MRI 检测。胶囊内镜检查有助于判断蛋白质丢失性胃病是否存在肠淋巴管病[93]。可以对一些患者进行淋巴管造影，但大多数中心很少进行这项检查。当诊断不明确时，有时需剖腹探查以排除隐匿的恶性肿瘤。

六、治疗和预后

由于蛋白质丢失性胃肠病是一种综合征，而不是一种特定的疾病，治疗的目的是纠正基础疾病，还包括支持性治疗和饮食调整。高蛋白饮食可以弥补部分蛋白质的丢失，低脂饮食有益于白蛋白代谢[94]。此外，奥曲肽可减少肠道液体分泌和蛋白质渗出，可能对某些蛋白质丢失性胃病患者有用[95]。在小鼠实验中，输注肝素类似物有助恢复肠黏膜紧密连接，防止肠表面蛋白丢失，疗效尚需进一步的临床研究验证[15]。

累及胃部的疾病，如巨大肥厚性胃病（Ménétrier 病），胃切除可以逆转蛋白质丢失，须在术前明确是否有 Hp 感染，如有应先根除治疗（见第 52 章）。累及小肠的疾病应根据具体情况治疗，例如涉及致病菌的疾病（如小肠细菌过度生长症和 Whipple 病），应采用适当的抗生素治疗；炎症性疾病（如克罗恩病或系统性红斑狼疮），可能需要免疫抑制治疗[38,40,96,97]。累及结肠的疾病，如溃疡性结肠炎、胶原性结肠炎等可能需要长期的免疫调节剂治疗或手术治疗；而感染性结肠炎需要抗生素治疗。恶性肿瘤引起的肠内蛋白丢失需要针对癌症治疗。心脏疾病（如心力衰竭、缩窄性心包炎）引起的肠内蛋白质丢失和淋巴细胞减少可通过针对心脏病的药物治疗、外科治疗而得到改善[8,64,97]。布地奈德和大剂量的螺内酯推荐用于 Fontan 术后导致的蛋白丢失性胃肠病患者[98,99]。

获得性肠淋巴管扩张症应纠正原发疾病，而先天性肠淋巴管扩张症可通过饮食限制得到控制。先天性肠淋巴管扩张症患者可以通过低脂饮食（富含中链甘油三酯）来减少肠道蛋白质的丢失，因为中链甘油三酯不通过淋巴管转运，不会刺激淋巴液流动[100,101]。

支持性治疗可以减少并发症的发生率。水肿是因血浆胶体渗透压低引起的，通常不用利尿剂；但利尿剂可以减少低白蛋白血症的坠积性水肿，提高患者的舒适度。弹力袜可以促进淋巴回流，减轻水肿。应鼓励适当的运动和走动，以减少静脉血栓形成的风险。皮肤护理是防止皮肤破损和蜂窝组织炎发生的关键。虽然这些治疗没有减少肠蛋白质的丢失，但可以最大程度减少并发症的发生。

大多数引起胃肠道蛋白质丢失的病因很容易发现和治

疗，而且很多都可以治愈。因此，蛋白丢失性胃肠病的治疗目标就是明确病因，饮食控制、药物治疗、外科干预或各种治疗联用[5,11]。随着原发病的控制或好转，大多数患者的肠内蛋白丢失、水肿和其他相关症状将得到部分或完全缓解。

（张莉　译，孙明瑜　校）

参考文献

第 32 章　胃肠道淋巴瘤

Praveen Ramakrishnan Geethakumari, Syed Mujtaba Rizv 著

章节目录

一、淋巴瘤管理的一般原则 ………… 419
（一）诊断 ………… 419
（二）分期和预后 ………… 419
（三）治疗 ………… 420
二、胃淋巴瘤 ………… 420
（一）胃边缘区黏膜相关淋巴组织 B 细胞淋巴瘤 ………… 420
（二）胃弥漫性大 B 细胞淋巴瘤 ………… 423
三、小肠淋巴瘤 ………… 425
（一）MALT 型边缘区 B 细胞淋巴瘤 ………… 425
（二）弥漫性大 B 细胞淋巴瘤 ………… 425
（三）套细胞淋巴瘤 ………… 425
（四）滤泡性淋巴瘤 ………… 426
（五）Burkitt 淋巴瘤 ………… 427
（六）免疫增殖性小肠疾病 ………… 427
（七）肠病相关性 T 细胞淋巴瘤 ………… 429
（八）不常见的小肠淋巴瘤 ………… 430
四、消化道其他部位淋巴瘤 ………… 430
（一）Waldeyer 环淋巴瘤 ………… 430
（二）原发性肝淋巴瘤 ………… 430
（三）胰腺淋巴瘤 ………… 430
（四）原发性结直肠淋巴瘤 ………… 430
五、免疫缺陷性相关淋巴瘤 ………… 431
移植后淋巴增殖性疾病 ………… 431
六、医源性淋巴增殖性疾病 ………… 431
七、HIV 相关性非霍奇金淋巴瘤 ………… 432

淋巴瘤是淋巴系统的恶性实体肿瘤，分为霍奇金淋巴瘤和非霍奇金淋巴瘤（non-Hodgkin lymphoma，NHL）。2017 年，预计美国将有 8 260 例新发霍奇金淋巴瘤和 72 240 例新发非霍奇金淋巴瘤患者[1]。霍奇金淋巴瘤很少累及胃肠道，本章将不再讨论。

本章讨论原发性胃肠道淋巴瘤（primary gastrointestina lymphoma，PGIL），其主要病变位于胃肠道，伴或不伴邻近淋巴结受累。PGIL 占所有胃肠道恶性肿瘤的 1%～4%，占所有 NHL 的 10%～15%，占所有结外 NHL 的 30%～40%[2]，使胃肠道成为结外 NHL 最常见的部位。不同国家 PGIL 的发病率为 0.58/10 万人～1.31/10 万人不等，好发于 50～70 岁。累及胃肠道，但大部分病变位于淋巴结内的淋巴瘤，其治疗方式与不累及胃肠道的淋巴瘤相似。

广义上讲，免疫系统可以被认为是淋巴组织和非淋巴组织之间高度结构化和严格调控的相互作用，旨在保护宿主免受有害物质的侵害（见第 2 章）[3]。淋巴细胞在骨髓和胸腺中产生，然后进入淋巴组织中，包括淋巴结、脾、咽淋巴环和黏膜相关淋巴组织（mucosa-associated lymphoid tissue，MALT）。胃肠道淋巴组织是 MALT，以末端回肠的派尔斑（Peyer patches）为代表。MALT 含有处于不同分化阶段的 B 细胞，组成不同的区域（图 32.1A）。受到抗原刺激的 B 细胞穿过黏膜弥散进入 MALT 的生发中心，并经历反复的免疫球蛋白基因突变（体细胞突变）[4]，形成一种能分泌高度抗原特异性免疫球蛋白的 B 细胞亚克隆，它比分泌低特异性免疫球蛋白的 B 细胞更具生存优势。这些抗原特异性 B 细胞随后离开生发中心，进入血液循环，分化成记忆 B 细胞或可产生抗体的浆细胞，并返回到肠黏膜。记忆 B 细胞位于 MALT 的边缘区。一些边缘区 B 细胞位于派尔斑表面的上皮组织，被称为上皮内边缘区 B 细胞。没有遇到抗原的 B 细胞构成 MALT 的套区。T 细胞在免疫系统的调节和呈递中起作用，因此在 MALT 中也能够见到（见图 32.1A）。因此，MALT 由处于多个分化阶段的 B 和 T 细胞组成；在特定分化阶段的免疫细胞具有特征性的组织学、免疫表型和遗传学特征。每个分化阶段的细胞都可能发生恶性转化，导致具有不同临床病理特征的恶性肿瘤（图 32.1B）。这就可以理解世界卫生组织（WHO）淋巴瘤系统中，NHL 有 60 多种不同的临床病理类型[5]。

胃肠道淋巴瘤大多数是 B 细胞淋巴瘤，其中大部分是由边缘区 B 细胞转化引起的，WHO 将其分类为结外边缘区 B 细胞淋巴瘤。然而，B 细胞淋巴瘤也可以来自 MALT 的其他细胞，例如生发中心的中心细胞[滤泡性淋巴瘤（follicular lymphoma）]或套区的细胞[套细胞淋巴瘤（mantle cell lymphoma MCL）]。不同个体大 B 细胞淋巴瘤的确切组织起源不同。胃肠道 T 细胞淋巴瘤较少见，通常与乳糜泻患者上皮内 T 细胞恶性转化有关（见第 107 章）。

PGIL 最常累及胃或小肠，口咽、食管、结肠或直肠受累并不多见。在发达国家，胃是最常见的受累部位（大约 60% 的病例），但在中东地区，小肠是最常见的胃肠道受累部位。PGIL 首次定义是由 Dawson 等于 1961 年提出的，诊断标准严格，即以胃肠道病变为主，伴或不伴区域淋巴结受累，不累及远处淋巴结，并排除有白血病表现或骨髓、脾脏、肝脏受累的患者[6]。该定义后来扩展到包括邻近肝脏和脾脏受累，允许有远处淋巴结受累，前提是结外胃肠道受累并是肿瘤负荷的主要部位（占 >75% 的肿瘤总体积），作为治疗的主要靶点[7-9]。

临床医生在处理胃肠道淋巴瘤时，面对的是发生在特定部位具有特定病理诊断的淋巴瘤，在某些情况下，还需要根据

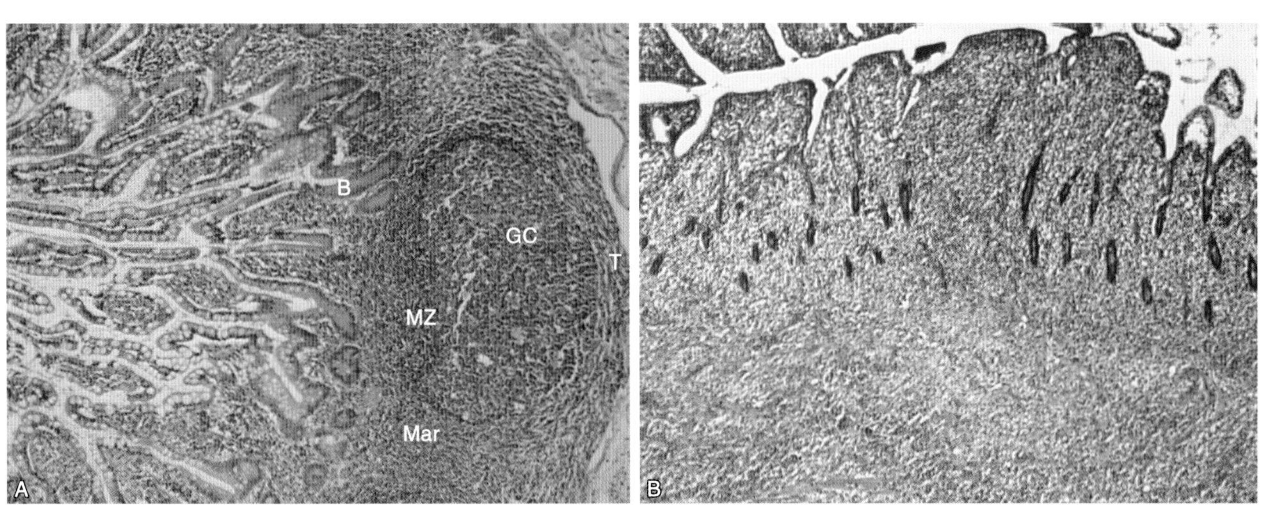

图 32.1 A,小肠正常黏膜相关淋巴组织。T 区位于浆膜面(T),还存在上皮内 B 细胞(B)。B,小肠大 B 细胞淋巴瘤。可见肿瘤细胞对黏膜的浸润和扩张,固有上皮结构的萎缩。GC,生发中心;Mar,苍白的外部边缘区,MZ,黑暗的外套膜区。(Courtesy Dr. Pamela Jensen, Dallas,TX.)

重要的患者特征[如人免疫缺陷病毒(HIV)感染]而调整方案。本章讨论临床医生可能遇到的主要临床病理类型。

一、淋巴瘤管理的一般原则

(一)诊断

由于 NHL 的亚型众多,因此需要专家对其进行准确的诊断和分类。准确的诊断需要足够的组织供病理检查。在胃肠道中,这通常意味着要有多个内镜活检。由于标本小,只能分析单个细胞形态,而不能深入观察这些细胞所处的背景环境,细针穿刺活检不能满足诊断需要。最基本的病理检查包括光学显微镜检查和通过流式细胞术或免疫组织化学(immunohistochemistry,IHC)进行的免疫表型分析。当存在明确轻链限制性(κ/λ 比值或 λ/κ 比率≥10:1)时,免疫球蛋白轻链染色有助于证实其单克隆性,高度提示为 B 细胞淋巴瘤。有时,分子遗传学分析如 Southern 印迹试验、聚合酶链反应(PCR)可证实单克隆免疫球蛋白或 T 细胞受体基因重排,或评估特征性的原癌基因重排。但有一点必须要重视,克隆性标志物在各种炎症条件下也可能是阳性的,并不一定是恶性肿瘤。因此,由专业的血液病理学医生对活检样本进行评估对于准确的诊断极为重要。

(二)分期和预后

NHL 的累及范围可以通过仔细的病史采集和体格检查,颈部、胸部、腹部和盆腔的 CT 检查,高度恶性 NHL 行正电子发射断层摄影(PET)检查,骨髓检查以及对于 PGIL 行超声内镜检查(EUS)来评估[10]。胃肠道淋巴瘤常累及 Waldeyer 环,因此需要检查咽部。在开始治疗之前,还应该进行血清 HIV、乙型肝炎病毒(HBV)和丙型肝炎病毒(HCV)的检测,胃淋巴瘤须行幽门螺杆菌(Hp)筛查。Ann Arbor 分期系统[11]最初用于霍奇金淋巴瘤,也可用于非霍奇金淋巴瘤,但许多人认为其用于 PGIL 分期并不充分。因此提出了替代的分期系统(表 32.1)。[12]

表 32.1 原发性胃肠道淋巴瘤的分期系统

分期	改良的巴黎分期系统*	TNM 分期系统(针对胃淋巴瘤修订)	Ann Arbor 分期系统	肿瘤累及
Ⅰ	T1 N0	T1 N0 M0	$Ⅰ_E$	黏膜,黏膜下
	T2 N0	T2 N0 M0	$Ⅰ_E$	固有肌
		T3 N0 M0	$Ⅰ_E$	浆膜
Ⅱ	累及腹部			
	$Ⅱ_1$=局部淋巴结受累	T1~3 N1 M0	$Ⅱ_E$	胃周或肠周淋巴结
	$Ⅱ_2$=远处淋巴结受累	T1~3 N2 M0	$Ⅱ_E$	远处区域淋巴结
$Ⅱ_E$	穿透浆膜累及邻近器官或组织	T4 N0 M0	$Ⅱ_E$	侵犯邻近器官组织
Ⅳ	广泛结外受累或伴膈上淋巴结受累	T1~4 N3 M0	$Ⅲ_E$	膈两侧淋巴结
		T1~4 N0~3 M1	$Ⅳ_E$	远处转移(如骨髓或其他结外部位)

*Modified from Ruskoné-Fourmestraux A, Dragosics B, Morgner A, et al. Paris Staging System for primary gastrointestinal lymphomas. Gut 2003;52:912-3.
TNM,肿瘤淋巴结转移。

通过确定淋巴瘤亚型和临床特征,包括肿瘤分期、患者年龄、一般状况和血清乳酸脱氢酶(LDH)水平来评估预后。国际预后指数(International Prognostic Index,IPI)是用于预测侵袭性NHL患者预后的模型[13]。该模型已被修订为R-IPI,以反映针对CD20的单克隆抗体靶向药利妥昔单抗的疗效[14],并已得到前瞻性验证,在应用利妥昔单抗时具预测价值。

(三) 治疗

治疗方法因淋巴瘤亚型和分期的不同而异,但应该注意的是,许多胃肠道淋巴瘤的最佳治疗方法仍然存在争议。虽然许多大型对照试验已经确定了多种淋巴结淋巴瘤的最佳治疗方法,但胃肠道淋巴瘤的情况并非如此。因此,许多治疗建议都是基于小样本的病例研究和淋巴结淋巴瘤的治疗经验。在开始全身化疗之前,除了所用药物的副作用外,对有需求的患者还应给予有关保留生育能力的咨询[15]。MALT淋巴瘤时,我们还常规筛查相关的慢性感染,如HIV、HBV、HCV和Hp。我们认为这一点很重要,因为相当大比例的低度恶性淋巴瘤在慢性感染充分治疗后会自发消退。

二、胃淋巴瘤

原发性胃淋巴瘤占胃肿瘤的5%,在世界范围内呈上升趋势[16]。胃是淋巴瘤最常见的结外受累部位,占PGIL的68%~75%[17]。这些胃淋巴瘤多数为MALT型边缘区B细胞淋巴瘤或弥漫性大B细胞淋巴瘤(diffuse large B cell lymphom,DLBCL)[2]。

(一) 胃边缘区黏膜相关淋巴组织B细胞淋巴瘤

黏膜相关淋巴组织(MALT)结外边缘区B细胞淋巴瘤又称MALT淋巴瘤,由Isaacson和Spencer于1983年[18]首次报道,约占所有NHL的8%[19]。这些淋巴瘤来源于MALT边缘区B细胞的恶性转化[20]。它们可能来自正常生理环境下的MALT(如胃肠道中的派尔斑),或来自感染、自身免疫过程相关的MALT。例如,胃组织通常不含MALT,但在慢性Hp感染时可能会获得MALT(见第52章)[21]。"淋巴细胞归巢"现象,涉及淋巴细胞整合素和组织特异性地址素介导的循环淋巴细胞和内皮微静脉之间的相互作用,是结外淋巴瘤发生的关键[22]。

恶性转化发生在一小部分获得性胃MALT患者中,并导致惰性淋巴瘤。恶性转化过程似乎在很大程度上是由慢性幽门螺杆菌感染引起的,因为根除Hp可使50%~80%的淋巴瘤消退[23,24]。

1. 流行病学

胃MALT边缘区B细胞淋巴瘤占胃淋巴瘤的38%~48%[25]。其发病率根据人群中Hp发病率的不同而存在差异。因此,在Hp感染率非常高的意大利东北部,发病率大约是英国的13倍[26]。胃MALT淋巴瘤的年龄范围很广,中位年龄约为60岁,男女比例相等[27]。

2. 病因和发病机制

(1) 幽门螺杆菌感染

很多证据支持幽门螺杆菌(Hp)在胃MALT淋巴瘤发展中具有关键作用(见第52章)。胃MALT淋巴瘤的绝大多数病例都存在Hp感染[28]。早期流行病学研究表明,在特定人群中,Hp感染率与胃淋巴瘤的患病率密切相关[29,30]。同时,病例对照研究显示,既往Hp感染与胃淋巴瘤发生具有相关性[31]。体外研究表明,胃MALT淋巴瘤组织中含有可以与Hp发生特异性反应的T细胞,这些Hp反应性T细胞促进肿瘤性B细胞的增殖[32]。慢性幽门螺杆菌感染可诱导小鼠胃MALT淋巴瘤[33]。多项研究证实根除Hp后胃MALT淋巴瘤消退[23,24,34]。有趣的是,尽管Hp在非胃器官中的作用尚不清楚,小肠和直肠淋巴瘤在Hp根除后改善也有报道[34,36]。海耳曼螺杆菌感染患者中也有淋巴瘤的报道,在感染根除后肿瘤消退[37]。

(2) 抗原驱动的B细胞增殖的证据

如前所述,B细胞免疫球蛋白可变区(V)基因在T细胞依赖性B细胞对抗原的反应过程中发生体细胞超突变[4],产生抗原亲和力改变的新的抗原受体。与含有低亲和力抗原受体的B细胞克隆相比,新产生的表达高亲和力抗原受体的B细胞克隆具有生存优势。因此,体细胞突变是抗原驱动性B细胞克隆筛选的标记。胃MALT淋巴瘤恶性B细胞序列分析显示,免疫球蛋白基因发生了体细胞突变[38]。

(3) 遗传学研究

结外边缘区淋巴瘤主要有4种染色体易位:t(11;18)(q21;q21)、t(14;18)(q32;q21)、t(1;14)(p22;q32)和t(3;14)(p14.1;q32)。最常见的易位t(11;18)(q21;q21)见于30%的病例中,其发生率因患病部位而异:在胃(和肺)中较为常见,但其他部位很少见[39,40]。t(11;18)(q21;q21)易位导致*API-2*和*MALT-1*基因的相互融合。API-2是一种凋亡抑制因子,MALT-1参与核因子κB(NFκB)的激活。这种易位的MALT淋巴瘤对根除Hp感染的抗生素治疗,治疗反应不如没有易位的淋巴瘤好[23]。然而,他们也不太可能发生其他染色体易位,或转化为更具侵袭性的大细胞淋巴瘤[39,41]。

t(14;18)(q32;q21)易位使染色体18q21上的*MALT-1*基因易位到免疫球蛋白基因重链增强子区域,导致其过度表达,不同于*bcl-2*基因相关的滤泡性淋巴瘤t(14;18)易位。t(14;18)(q32;q21)易位发生在大约20%的MALT淋巴瘤中,发病率因患病部位而异,常见于唾液腺和眼附属器的MALT淋巴瘤,胃肠道中少见[39]。

大约5%的胃MALT淋巴瘤存在t(1;14)(p22;q32)易位[42]。这种易位使得*bcl-10*基因处于免疫球蛋白重链基因增强子的控制之下,从而导致表达失控。该易位只在MALT淋巴瘤患者中发现,通常同时具有3、12和18号染色体的三体突变,且更常见于晚期病例,对根除Hp治疗反应较差。

最后,t(3;14)(p14.1;q32)易位导致转录因子*FOXP1*出现在3p14.1上,与免疫球蛋白基因重链增强子区域并列,导致B细胞发育所必需的*FOXP1*表达失控[43,44]。

(4) MALT淋巴瘤染色体易位的共同分子通路

前面列出的3种染色体易位都激活了促进细胞激活、增殖和存活的转录因子(参见第1章和第2章)-核因子κB(NF-κB)[45,46]。在未被刺激的B和T淋巴细胞中,NF-κB由于与抑制蛋白IκB结合而被隔离在细胞质中。IκB磷酸化后发生泛素化和降解,从而释放NF-κB,后者转位到细胞核,发挥转录因子的作用。IκB 磷酸化通路受到严格调控，涉及 BCL-10 和 MALT-1。t(11;18)、t(14;18)或 t(1;14)引起的 *BCL-10* 或 *MALT-1* 过度活化可导致 NF-κB 的持续激活[39]。

(5) 胃 MALT 淋巴瘤发病机制模型

胃 MALT 淋巴瘤是一个多阶段的演变过程，包括从 Hp 胃炎、低度恶性 B 细胞淋巴瘤到高度恶性 B 细胞淋巴瘤的顺序发展[42]。这一模型得到了慢性胃炎患者活检标本的支持，这些活检组织在淋巴瘤发病前几年，就显示出 B 淋巴细胞克隆，最终发展为具有明显临床证据的淋巴瘤。在这个模型中，Hp 感染引起免疫反应，T 细胞和 B 细胞被趋化到胃黏膜，并形成 MALT。Hp 特异性 T 细胞辅助异常 B 细胞克隆的生长。异常的 B 细胞可能不是 Hp 特异性的，甚至可能是自身反应性的。然而，它们最初的持续增殖依赖于 T 细胞的辅助。Hp 特异性 T 细胞在促进 B 细胞增殖中的关键作用，或许可以解释为什么肿瘤倾向于保持局限，以及为什么在根除 Hp 后肿瘤会消退。然而，持续 B 细胞增殖最终会引起更多异常基因的累积，导致自主生长和更具侵袭性的临床行为。

由于只有小部分 Hp 感染者会患上淋巴瘤，因此其他目前未知的环境、微生物或遗传因素也必然起一定作用。炎症反应和抗氧化能力相关基因 *IL1RN* 和 *GSTT1* 的基因多态性，可能是 MALT 淋巴瘤遗传背景的一部分[47]。有研究表明，表达某些蛋白质如 CagA 的 Hp 菌株，和氧化损伤在胃淋巴瘤的发病中发挥作用[48]。

3. 病理学

(1) 大体外观和部位

低度恶性胃 MALT 淋巴瘤可表现为单一或多发病灶。单发病灶通常表现为溃疡、隆起或浸润性肿块，也可表现为糜烂或单纯红斑，最常见于胃窦。

(2) 组织学

低度恶性 MALT 淋巴瘤的主要组织学特征是存在“淋巴上皮病变”(图 32.2)[18,49]，即肿瘤细胞聚集对胃腺体或小凹的明确侵袭和部分破坏。然而，需要注意的是，这些病变有时也可见于慢性胃炎。肿瘤细胞是小到中等大小的淋巴细胞，核形态不规则，胞质量中等。这些细胞的形态多样，从小的淋巴浆细胞样细胞到具有丰富的苍白细胞质和明确边界的单核细胞样细胞[50]。也可以看到散在的较大的细胞或转化的淋巴母细胞。淋巴瘤细胞弥漫性地浸润固有层并在反应性滤泡的周围生长；甚至侵入生发中心，这一现象称为滤泡定植。由于从胃炎到淋巴瘤的转变过程是连续的，因此对临界病例的诊断可能很困难。各一些参数可能有助于鉴别，如淋巴上皮病变的严重程度，细胞异型性的程度，以及是否存在含有 Dutcher 小体(过碘酸希夫染色阳性的核内假包涵体)的浆细胞。

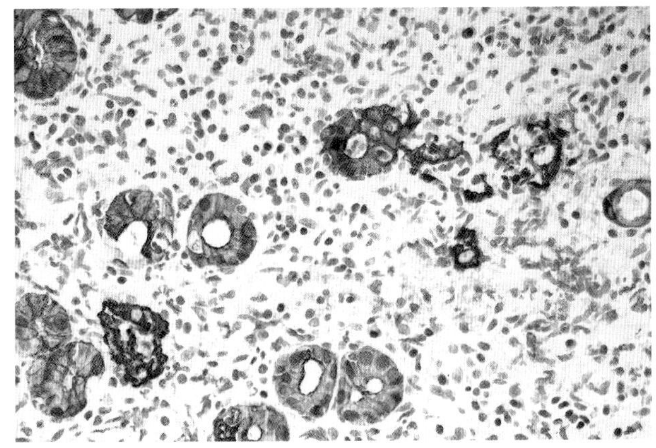

图 32.2　显微镜下照片显示胃黏膜相关淋巴组织淋巴瘤的“淋巴上皮病变”特征。细胞角蛋白染色显示单形态淋巴细胞群侵袭和破坏一些胃腺体。注意与照片底部中间未受累的正常腺体相比较。特殊染色(未显示)显示幽门螺杆菌感染。(Courtesy Dr. Edward Lee, Washington, DC.)

大细胞的存在会进一步增加诊断的难度[16]。低度恶性 MALT 淋巴瘤可能有散在的大细胞，但肿瘤主要由小细胞组成。另一方面，仅包含大细胞或仅局灶可见 MALT 样淋巴瘤小细胞的胃淋巴瘤应归类为 DLBCL(见后文)[5]。在这两种情况之间是低度恶性淋巴瘤向侵袭性更强淋巴瘤转变的过程，可观察到逐渐增多的大细胞。

(3) 免疫表型

胃 MALT 淋巴瘤细胞具有边缘区 B 细胞的典型免疫表型，表达泛 B 细胞抗原(CD19、CD20 和 CD79a)，不表达 CD5、CD10、CD23，和 cyclin D1[2]。经验丰富的病理医生可以通过进一步免疫染色识别淋巴上皮病变(见图 32-2)，并鉴别滤泡定植与滤泡性淋巴瘤(胃部罕见，见后文)。

(4) 单克隆性的分子测试

免疫球蛋白重链重排的 Southern 印迹试验或 PCR 检测有助于确定细胞的单克隆性。然而，值得注意的是，在 Hp 相关性胃炎中也可以检测到 B 细胞的单克隆性增殖(见第 52 章)。虽然单克隆性可以预测后期有可能进展为淋巴瘤，但仅凭单克隆性增殖不能诊断淋巴瘤。因此应始终在组织学所见的背景下进行分子检测。

4. 临床特征

(1) 症状、体征和实验室检查

最常见的症状是消化不良和上腹痛。其他不常见症状包括厌食、体重减轻、恶心和/或呕吐以及早饱[42]。胃出血和 B 症状(发热，盗汗，体重下降)很少见。血清 LDH 和 β_2-微球蛋白水平通常正常[51]。

(2) 诊断与分期

MALT 淋巴瘤患者可采用食管胃十二指肠内镜(EGD)进行评估。内镜检查前最好停用 PPI 至少 2 周，以避免 Hp 检测的假阴性结果。内镜表现包括红斑、糜烂和/或溃疡。弥漫性浅表浸润是 MALT 淋巴瘤的典型表现，而肿块更常见于侵袭性非霍奇金淋巴瘤 DLBCL(图 32.3)。胃最常见的受累部位是胃窦，但由于病变通常是多灶性的，所有异常部位均需取活检，胃内各个区域以及十二指肠和胃食管交界处也要随机活检。由于一些淋巴瘤仅侵犯黏膜下层而不累及黏膜层，活检组织需要足够深、足够大，以进行组织病理学和免疫组织化学分析。Hp 感染可通过组织学检查、呼气试验或粪便抗原检测来确定(见第 52 章)[52]。EUS 可以确定浸润深度并评估是否存在胃周淋巴结肿大[10]。此外，肿瘤分期还需完善上呼吸道检查，胸部、腹部和盆腔 CT，骨髓穿刺和活检，以及血清 LDH 水平的测定。由于胃 MALT 淋巴瘤对氟脱氧葡萄糖(FDG)的摄取率低，PET 通常不用于分期[53,54]。

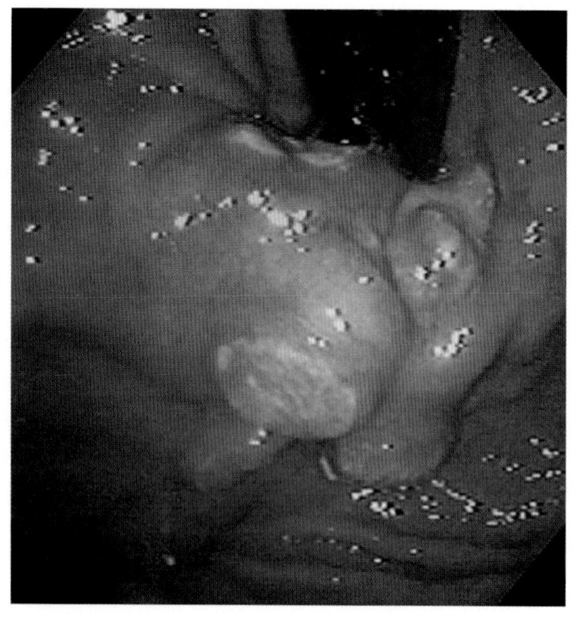

图 32.3　胃弥漫性大 B 细胞淋巴瘤的内镜表现，胃食管交界处邻近有多个脐样病变。在鳞柱交界处稍远处可见一个大的溃疡

(3) 分期系统和预后分析

1994 年，一个关于胃肠道淋巴瘤分期的国际研讨会提出了 Lugano 分期系统[55]，改良自 Blackledge 分期。Paris 分期（见表 32.1）改良自 TNM 分期，纳入了 EUS 对浸润深度和淋巴结受累的判断[56]。约 75% 的胃 MALT 淋巴瘤在诊断时局限于胃内（Ⅰ期）[42]，表现为惰性淋巴瘤；因此，大多数患者预后良好，整体 5 年生存率为 80% 至 95%，少数进展期的患者预后差。胃壁浸润深也提示预后不良，因其常伴有区域淋巴结受累[57]和组织学见高比例大细胞。

已研发并验证的 MALT 淋巴瘤特异性预后指数（MALT-IPI）包含以下 3 个关键参数：年龄≥70 岁、Ⅲ期或Ⅳ期以及血清 LDH 水平升高。队列研究显示，MALT-IPI 低危、中危和高危组 5 年无事件生存率分别为 70%、56% 和 29%。该预后判断工具重复性好，适用于胃和非胃 MALT 淋巴瘤，以及不同的治疗方案[58]。

5. 治疗

由于 MALT 淋巴瘤较少见，尚未进行大规模的随机临床试验。因此，治疗建议基于病例报道和专家意见。Wotherspoon 及其同事首次报道了胃 MALT 淋巴瘤在根除 Hp 后达到了内镜、组织学和分子水平的完全消退[24]。大量研究证实了上述发现[59-62]，根除 Hp（见第 52 章）已成为治疗低度恶性胃 MALT 淋巴瘤的主要方法。即使晚期患者也可以通过根除 Hp 使病情得到消退。然而，现有文献仍存在以下几个方面的不足：很早之前的研究分期不充分，分类系统过时。此外，这些报道都不是对照或随机试验，缺乏长期随访。但是，现有的文献足以表明，早期的胃 MALT 淋巴瘤首选根除 Hp 治疗（第 52 章），对不伴 Hp 感染或抗生素应答不佳的病例给予毒性较大的治疗方法，如放疗、化疗或手术治疗。需要强调的是，从治疗到缓解可能需要几个月的时间。

表 32.2 显示了依据 Lugano 分期系统的分期治疗方案。

表 32.2　MALT 型胃边缘区 B 细胞淋巴瘤的治疗*

Lugano 分期	治疗†‡
Ⅰ期，病变局限于黏膜和黏膜下层	单独使用抗生素
Ⅱ期，累及固有肌或浆膜	目前最佳治疗方法尚不清楚。放疗或化疗可能优于手术（见正文）
Ⅳ期，累及胃壁以外	对有症状的患者给予化疗 在某些情况下选择局部放疗或手术治疗

*根据 Lugano 分期系统。

†Hp 感染的患者均应使用抗生素以清除感染，与疾病分期无关（见第 52 章）。

‡大细胞百分比高且疾病仅限于黏膜的患者可能对抗生素单药治疗有效，有必要对该问题进行进一步研究。

大细胞比例高且疾病分期较晚的患者应按表 32.4 中弥漫性大 B 细胞淋巴瘤的方案进行治疗。

MALT，黏膜相关淋巴组织。

(1) Ⅰ期病变

大多数患者属于这一期，可以用根除 Hp 的抗生素治疗。第 52 章中讨论的任何治疗方案都可以使用。治疗结束后 3 至 6 个月应进行内镜随访和多点活检，以确定感染的清除情况及淋巴瘤的消退[57]。首次治疗后复查时，淋巴瘤的消退（但不一定是完全消退）通常会很明显。持续 Hp 感染的患者应接受二线抗生素根除方案（见第 52 章）[63]。首次治疗后的组织病理学检查可以预测最终疗效。若活检显示只有小灶性淋巴瘤提示随后可能完全缓解，活检显示弥漫性持续性病灶提示随后完全缓解的可能性较低。1993 年，Wotherspoon 指数最初是作为一种评估疗效的组织学工具，但它实际上更多地被用于初始诊断。2003 年成人淋巴瘤治疗小组提出的治疗后组织学评估系统[64]是一个有效、可重复胃淋巴瘤治疗过程监测标准（表 32.3）。治疗后 2 年内患者每 6 个月进行一次内镜检查，之后每年一次内镜随访。总的来说，大约 75% 局限于黏膜和黏膜下层的Ⅰ期患者达到了完全缓解[30]。中位缓解时间为 5 个月，通常在 12 个月内实现。然而，也有缓解时间长达 45 个月的报道[23,65]。在临床缓解的患者中，大多数 PCR 仍能检测到肿瘤性克隆[59]。对这些患者持续随访，恶性克隆逐渐减少；目前的研究表明，组织学缓解时，PCR 阳性并不能预测疾病复发，但必须进行更长时间的随访。大约 90% 根除 Hp 治疗后获得临床完全缓解的患者会持续处于缓解期[30]，但仍可能发生晚期复发。复发可能与 Hp 再感染有关，可以通过再次根除 Hp 来治愈。在没有 Hp 再感染的情况下，复发通常是短暂的[66]。一项根除 Hp 治疗有效患者的随机试验表明，与对照组相比，苯丁酸氮芥治疗并没有显示出益处[67]。

大约 25% 的患者对根除 Hp 治疗无应答[68]。t(11;18)(q21;q21) 易位的患者中，无应答比例高；一项研究显示，67% 的无应答患者存在这种变异，而在应答患者中只有 4% 存在这种变异[69,70]。对根除 Hp 治疗的抗生素无应答还见于 Hp 阴性的胃 MALT 淋巴瘤[71]和确诊时有淋巴结受累的患者[57]。

表 32.3 拟定用于评价抗生素治疗后 MALT 胃淋巴瘤的组织学评价系统(根据成人淋巴瘤研究小组提出)

治疗结果	定义	组织学特征
CR	组织学完全缓解	固有层正常、疏松和(或)纤维化,固有层中浆细胞和淋巴样细胞缺失或稀疏,无淋巴上皮病变
pMRD	可能的微小残留	固有层疏松和(或)纤维化伴病灶聚集,或固有层、黏膜肌层和/或黏膜下层见淋巴细胞结节
rRD	消退中的残留病变	固有层部分疏松和/或纤维化;致密、弥漫或结节状浸润的淋巴细胞在固有层的腺体周围延伸。无或局灶性淋巴上皮病变
NC	无改变	致密、弥漫或结节状淋巴细胞浸润,+/-淋巴上皮病变

Hp 根除治疗无效的患者,最佳治方案尚不确定。可选择手术切除、化疗和放疗,具体将在 $Ⅱ_E$ 期治疗中讨论(见后)。

病变局限,但大细胞比例较高的患者,其治疗方案亦不明确。最近的研究显示根除 Hp 后可使病情缓解,与早期的研究结果相反。例如,1 项包含 34 名组织学为高度恶性淋巴瘤患者的研究中,18 名患者在根除 Hp 后出现疾病消退,并且在中位随访 7.7 年期间无复发[72]。如果采用这种方法,需对患者进行密切随访,如果应答不佳,则采用下一节讨论的方法进行治疗。

如前所述,偶有胃 MALT 淋巴瘤病例是 Hp 阴性的,这些患者对抗生素治疗应答的可能性较小,但仍应尝试根除 Hp 治疗,因为 Hp 检测可能会出现假阴性结果,或者可能存在其他螺旋杆菌(如海耳曼螺旋杆菌)引起的淋巴瘤[57]。

局部进展期:Ⅰ期但肌层或浆膜受累或对 Hp 根除治疗反应差($Ⅱ_E$ 期)。Hp 阳性的进展期患者也应接受抗生素治疗,但仅用抗生素治疗通常不足以根除淋巴瘤。目前对该类患者的最佳治疗方案尚未达成共识。全胃切除术可以治愈 80% 以上的 $Ⅱ_E$ 期患者,但降低患者的生活质量,且与更保守的方法相比,未显示出更好的效果[73]。受累区域放射治疗(胃及胃周淋巴结累积照射剂量 30~40Gy,分为 15~20 次)疗效显著,完全缓解率为 90% ~ 100%,5 年无病生存率约为 80%[74,75]。放射治疗通常耐受性好,且能保留胃功能。因此,放疗已成为进展期患者的首选治疗方案,包括 Hp 阴性、根除 Hp 治疗无效的持续性胃 MALT 淋巴瘤患者[76]。这些患者的其他治疗选择包括化疗、免疫治疗、化学免疫联合治疗或较新的靶向化疗,如依鲁替尼(ibrutinib)。较早的研究表明,口服化疗药物如环磷酰胺[23]或苯丁酸氮芥,以及嘌呤类似物如克拉屈滨(cladriine,2 CdA)单药治疗都有效,对 t(11;18)(q21;q21)易位患者可能更有效[77]。抗 CD20 的单克隆抗体利妥昔单抗联合苯丁酸氮芥[78,79]、氟达拉滨[80]、克拉屈滨[81]和苯达莫司汀[42]进行化疗免疫联合治疗,类似于其他低度恶性 B-NHL 的治疗方案,显示出 80% ~100% 的治疗应答率,且毒副作用尚可接受。

(2) Ⅱ期或Ⅳ期病变

已扩散到远处淋巴结或结外部位的低度恶性胃 MALT 淋巴瘤,应按进展期低度恶性 B 细胞 NHL 治疗。可使用多种治疗方案,多数包含利妥昔单抗[82,83]。这种疾病通常被认为是不可治愈的,但基本上都是惰性的,对化疗有短暂的应答[84]。无症状患者可以随访等待观察。

(二) 胃弥漫性大 B 细胞淋巴瘤

1. 流行病学

大约 50% 的胃淋巴瘤是 DLBCL。发展中国家的发病率可能高于发达国家,但临床特征相似。中位年龄约为 60 岁,男性略多见[17]。

2. 病因和发病机制

胃 DLBCL 的发病机制尚不清楚。许多大细胞肿瘤含有低度恶性 MALT 的成分,并被认为是由低度恶性病变转化而来。通常,这些细胞具有相同的免疫球蛋白重排基因。根据 WHO 的分类,此类疾病现在被称为"弥漫性大 B 细胞淋巴瘤,伴边缘区 MALT 型淋巴瘤区域"[5]。然而其他 DLBCL 没有与低度恶性 MALT 相关的证据。新发胃 DLBCL 是否比伴边缘区 MALT 型淋巴瘤区域的 DLBCL 预后差尚不清楚[85]。

如果大细胞病变通常由低度恶性病变进展而来,那么可以想象 Hp 可能在最初的发病机制中发挥作用。一项研究表明,Hp 感染在具有低度恶性成分的大细胞病变患者中更为常见[86]。此外,对早期大细胞淋巴瘤行 Hp 根除治疗的应答观察表明 Hp 参与其中,至少在某些患者中,Hp 发挥了一定的作用[72,87]。如先前在关于 Hp 诱发淋巴瘤模型的讨论中所述,大细胞转化来源于遗传突变,包括 p53 和 p16 缺失,导致肿瘤细胞生长失去对 Hp 的依赖[2]。在一项对胃 DLBCL 的研究中,免疫球蛋白重链可变区基因重排的体细胞突变发生率很高,提示抗原选择与淋巴瘤的发生有关。

3. 病理学

DLBCL 病变明显,可表现为大溃疡、隆起性肿瘤(见图 32.3)或多发浅表溃疡[88,89]。最常见的受累部位是胃体和胃窦。有低度恶性成分的肿瘤比没有低度恶性成分的肿瘤更有可能是多灶性的。大细胞淋巴瘤通常侵犯固有肌层,甚至更深。

显微镜检查可见大细胞呈紧密的团簇状、汇合聚集或大片状,类似于免疫母细胞或中心母细胞,最常见的是两者混合存在(图 32.4)[2]。25% 至 40% 的病例显示出来源于 MALT 的证据,包括固有层中密集的中心细胞样细胞浸润和典型的淋巴上皮病变[86]。

免疫表型分析显示,肿瘤细胞表达一种或多种 B 细胞抗原(CD19、CD20、CD22、CD79a)和 CD45。有低度恶性 MALT 证据的病变不表达 CD10,这与它们是从 CD10 阴性边缘区低度恶性病变演变而来是一致的。没有 MALT 证据的病变可能表达,也可能不表达 CD10。基因分析显示单克隆免疫球蛋白基因重排。*BCL6* 经常发生突变或重排[90];如果与涉及 myc 的易位一起出现,则该淋巴瘤被称为"双重打击"DLBCL,或者根据 WHO2016 年的分类,为具有 MYC 和 BCL2 和/或 BCL6 重排的高度恶性 B 细胞淋巴瘤[5]。

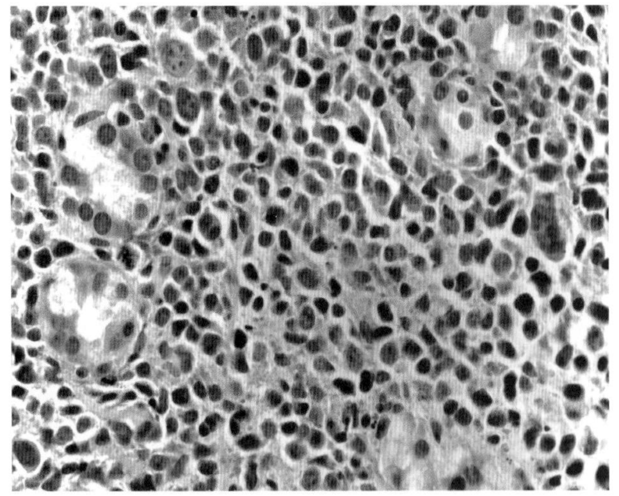

图 32.4 显微镜下照片显示胃弥漫性大 B 细胞淋巴瘤。胃黏膜内有中等大小至大 B 淋巴细胞的致密浸润。(Courtesy Dr. Weina Chen, UT Southwestern Medical Center, Dallas, TX.)

MYC 易位伴随 BCL2 和/或 BCL6 重排越来越被认为是预后不良的特征,基于此,大多数专家采用更激进的化疗免疫治疗方案。同样,IHC 染色 myc 和 bcl2 的表达越高,预后越差;虽然俗称为"双表达",但这一分类尚未得到 WHO 的正式认可,除临床试验外,大多数专家仍使用标准的 R-CHOP 治疗方案。

关于胃 DLBCL 术语的演变值得讨论。许多病理学医生将起源于 MALT 的具有高度恶性特征(有或无低度恶性病变成分)的淋巴瘤称为高度恶性胃 MALT 淋巴瘤。然而,参与制定 WHO 分类的专家们担心,许多临床医生已经将胃 MALT 淋巴瘤这一术语看作等同于对抗生素治疗有效的病变。MALT 起源的高度恶性淋巴瘤通常不是这种情况。因此,参与制定 WHO 分类[5]的专家们同意将 MALT 型结外边缘区 B 细胞淋巴瘤用于低度恶性病变,将弥漫性大 B 细胞淋巴瘤用于高度恶性病变,省略 MALT 一词。包含 MALT 的低度恶性病变通常含有不同比例的大细胞,大细胞的比例越高,预后越差。然而,在这一点上,尚未设计出针对这种情况的精确分级系统,仍然是正在进行的研究目标。

4. 临床特征

患者表现为上腹痛(70%)或消化不良(30%),症状与胃腺癌患者相似[88,91]。较大的肿瘤可引起梗阻。溃疡性病变可引起消化道出血。B 症状(发热、盗汗、体重下降)和血清 LDH 升高不常见。

准确分期需完善 EGD(见图 32.3),上呼吸道检查,胸部、腹部和盆腔 CT 或 PET 扫描,骨髓穿刺涂片及活检和血清 LDH 水平的测定。此外,EUS 在评估胃壁受累深度方面具有重要作用。应评估 Hp 感染情况。35%的胃 DLBCL 患者存在 Hp 感染,伴有胃 MALT 的患者更常见[88]。大多数患者按 Ann Arbor 分期系统属于Ⅰ期或Ⅱ期[92]。然而,随着其他分期系统的出现,多种系统的使用使得不同研究间结果很难比较。

5. 治疗

胃 DLBCL 的最佳治疗方法尚有争议,但目前的共识推荐化疗免疫疗法联合或不联合放疗以代替手术治疗(表 32.4)[88]。传统上,对具有预后不良特征的患者,采用单纯手术或术后联合放疗和/或化疗的方法治疗局部病变[93]。这种方法的优势在于可提供诊断和分期信息,且可避免因化疗或放疗导致的穿孔或出血风险。Ⅰ期患者术后 5 年的无病生存率约 70%[94]。然而,一些研究者质疑手术在局部胃 DLBCL 治疗中的作用。他们注意到,随着内镜的应用,手术不再是诊断所必需,并且随着 CT 和 EUS 的发展,手术也不再是分期所必需。此外,化疗期间出血或穿孔的风险低于 5%,只有少数出血者需要行紧急胃切除术[95]。而手术的死亡率为 5%至 10%,且会显著增加并发症的发生率。

表 32.4 胃弥漫性大 B 细胞淋巴瘤的治疗*

Lugano 分期	治疗
Ⅰ	CHOP†×3~4 周期+RT‡+利妥昔单抗§
Ⅱ, $Ⅱ_1$, $Ⅱ_2$, $Ⅱ_E$	CHOP×3~4 周期+RT+利妥昔单抗
Ⅳ	CHOP×6~8 周期+RT+利妥昔单抗

*根据 Lugano 分期系统,该病的最佳治疗尚存争议。然而,正在形成的共识似乎倾向于联合化疗和放疗,避免手术(见正文)。

†环磷酰胺、多柔比星(羟基柔红霉素)、长春新碱(安可平)、泼尼松。

‡RT(放疗);通常为 30~40Gy,分为 20~30 次。

§在这种情况下加用利妥昔单抗的建议包括外推淋巴结弥漫性大 B 细胞淋巴瘤的随机数据。

因此,有研究对化疗和放疗作为手术的替代方案进行了分析。回顾性研究显示,单纯手术与单纯化疗患者的预后相似[17]。一项对胃 DLBCL 患者的前瞻性研究,将患者随机分为单纯手术、手术联合放疗、手术联合化疗,或单独化疗四组,结果显示,与单纯手术或手术联合放疗的患者相比,手术联合化疗和单纯化疗的患者的完全应答率和整体生存率较高[96]。德国多中心研究 GIT NHL 01/92 是一项前瞻性的非随机研究,比较手术联合化疗和放疗与单纯化疗和放疗对局部原发性胃淋巴瘤治疗效果。是否行手术治疗由每个参与中心自行决定。手术后再接受放化疗的患者和单纯接受放化疗患者生存率没有差别[97]。这些结果在随后的一项更大规模的前瞻性非随机试验(GIT NHL 02/96)中得到了证实[98]。

对于进展期淋巴结 DLBCL 患者,在 CHOP[环磷酰胺、多柔比星(羟基柔红霉素)、长春新碱(安可平)、泼尼松]化疗方案的基础上加用抗 CD20 的单克隆抗体利妥昔单抗,较单纯 CHOP 方案治疗的整体生存率提高[99-102]。这种联合疗法也已用于胃 DLBCL 患者,被认为是安全有效的[103,104]。

放疗在胃 DLBCL 的治疗中的必要性还存在争议。一项小规模的回顾性研究对接受了化疗的Ⅰ期或Ⅱ期原发性胃高度恶性 DLBCL 患者进行了分析,结果显示同时接受了巩固放疗的患者比未接受放疗患者的复发率低[95]。但是,该研究仅纳入了 21 例患者,其中 3 例复发,其结论还有待前瞻性随机试验证实。

因此,胃大 B 细胞淋巴瘤的标准治疗参照淋巴结大 B 细胞淋巴瘤的标准治疗方案。局部(Ⅰ期或Ⅱ期)淋巴结大 B 细胞淋巴瘤的治疗包括 3 到 6 个周期的联合化疗(通常为 CHOP 方案)联合利妥昔单抗,如果使用简化的化疗方案(3 个周期,而不是 6 个周期)则通常联合放疗[105,106]。专家正越来越多地使用更激进的 DA-R-EPOCH 方案[利妥昔单抗、依托泊苷、泼尼松、长春新碱(安可平)、环磷酰胺、多柔比星(羟基柔红霉素)]治疗具有“双重打击”特征的 *DLBCL* 或 *myc/bcl2/bcl6* 重排的高度恶性 B 细胞淋巴瘤。该方案主要基于回顾性研究,数据显示,使用该方案获得完全缓解的人数增加,且获得完全缓解的患者长期无病生存机会最大。目前还没有前瞻性研究对“双重打击”DLBCL 进行两种治疗方案的比较。然而,根据 2016 年美国血液病学年会上公布的一项前瞻性试验(CALGB/Alliance 50303)的数据,DA-R-EPOCH 对于很多 DLBCL 并不带来更好的治疗效果,反而增加副作用风险[107]。同样,IHC 染色 myc 和 bcl2 表达增加与预后不良相关。尽管俗称“双表达”,但这一类别尚未得到 WHO 的正式认可,在临床试验之外,大多数专家仍继续使用标准的 R-CHOP 方案。有 Hp 感染证据的 DLBCL 患者应接受根除 Hp 治疗,因为有报道显示根除 Hp 对治疗大细胞淋巴瘤有效[108,109]。然而,这些研究有明显的局限性,大多数单独使用抗生素治疗的患者病变仅限于黏膜层;而多数胃 DLBCL 患者的病变处于进展期,单独使用抗生素治疗是不够的。

对于两种治疗方案(包括基于蒽环类药物的方案)失败的复发/难治性 DLBCL 患者,嵌合抗原受体 T 细胞疗法是 FDA 最近批准的一种新的治疗方案。虽然这种治疗可以使病情得到持久缓解,但仍有待长期疗效数据观察[110,111]。

6. 罕见的胃淋巴瘤

除边缘区 MALT 淋巴瘤或 DLBCL 外,其他 B 细胞淋巴瘤很少累及胃[如 MCL(1%)、FL(0.5%~2%)],T 细胞来源的胃淋巴瘤也少有报道(1.5%~4%)[112-114]。

三、小肠淋巴瘤

小肠淋巴瘤可分为 B 细胞和 T 细胞肿瘤,占 PGIL 的 20%~30%[115]。B 细胞肿瘤包括免疫增殖性小肠疾病(immunoproliferative small intestinal disease,IPSID)和各种非 IPSID 亚型,包括 MALT 边缘区 B 细胞淋巴瘤、DLBCL、MCL、FL 和 Burkitt 淋巴瘤。有关非 IPSID 小肠淋巴瘤各亚型的描述报道相对较少,较大宗的病例研究在归纳其临床表现和治疗结果时,倾向将所有亚型归为一类[116-118]。由于对这些疾病在肠道中的生物学行为不甚了解,最好参考其对应的淋巴结病变来考虑。因此,边缘区和 FL_S 被认为是惰性的,虽不可治愈,但可以通过化疗控制,并且通常有相对长的生存期。DLBCL、MCL 和 Burkitt 淋巴瘤更具侵袭性,通常需要化疗作为其治疗的一部分。小肠 T 细胞淋巴瘤通常是肠病型肠道 T 细胞淋巴瘤,其他形式的 T 细胞淋巴瘤罕有报道。最近有自然杀伤(natural killer,NK)细胞或 NK 型 T 细胞肠道淋巴瘤的报道[119-122]。

(一) MALT 型边缘区 B 细胞淋巴瘤

发生在小肠的淋巴瘤可具有边缘区 B 细胞淋巴瘤的特点,与前面描述的胃边缘区 B 细胞淋巴瘤具有相同的组织学和免疫表型特征[121,123]。然而,目前尚无小肠边缘区 B 细胞淋巴瘤与 Hp 感染相关的证据,尽管有研究显示对抗生素治疗有一定反应。大多数发生在老年患者,表现为黑便。该病通常表现为单个环状或外生性肿物[124],可发生于小肠的任何部位,常局限于肠道或局部淋巴结。治疗一般是外科手术。部分患者接受了化疗,但有关治疗方案和预后的数据很少。值得注意的是,在淋巴结边缘区淋巴瘤中,化疗通常只用于有症状的患者,因为该肿瘤生长缓慢,对化疗敏感,但化疗不能使其治愈。5 年生存率在 75% 左右。与胃边缘区 B 细胞淋巴瘤一样,小肠淋巴瘤可能出现不同的大细胞转化成分。这一特征可能会使预后变差,但数据较少。

(二) 弥漫性大 B 细胞淋巴瘤

小肠 DLBCL 在组织学和临床行为上与胃 DLBCL 相似。患者可能出现腹痛、体重减轻、肠梗阻、腹部肿块、出血和/或穿孔。肿瘤通常呈外生性或环状。组织学表现与前述胃 DLBCL 相似,部分患者可有低度恶性成分,部分患者只有大细胞成分。约半数患者仅为局部病变,另有半数患者疾病可扩散到区域或远处淋巴结。梗阻或穿孔时需要手术治疗[125],附加治疗包括含蒽环类药物的化疗和抗 CD20 单克隆抗体利妥昔单抗[126]。此外,有时还需要放射治疗。预后取决于疾病分期和患者因素,如年龄和身体状况。

(三) 套细胞淋巴瘤

套细胞淋巴瘤(mantal cell lymphoma)MCL 是 B 细胞 NHL 的亚型[127]。就临床行为而言,是一种异质性淋巴瘤,有的患者表现为类似低度恶性 B-NHL 的惰性病程,有的患者病程极具侵袭性,类似于高度恶性 B 细胞淋巴瘤。患者通常表现为广泛的淋巴结肿大,多有骨髓和结外受累。超过 80% 的患者有胃肠道受累(图 32.5),但并不是所有胃肠道受累的患者都有症状[128]。胃肠道受累最常见的表现是多发性“淋巴瘤样息肉病”,即胃肠道中存在多发的淋巴样息肉[129,130]。最常见的受累部位是回盲部,但从胃到直肠的任何其他部位都可能受累;偶尔有患者会累及上述所有部位(图 32.6;另见图 32.5)。胃肠道受累也可不表现为多发性息肉,亦有单纯累及胃肠道的报道。当患者出现胃肠道受累相关症状时,通常表现为腹痛、梗阻、腹泻或便血。值得注意的是,多发性淋巴瘤样息肉病也可见于其他淋巴瘤,特别是 MALT 边缘区 B 细胞淋巴瘤和滤泡性淋巴瘤。显微镜下,MCL 累及黏膜和黏膜下层,肿瘤细胞形态上呈非典型小淋巴细胞,包绕良性生发中心或破坏淋巴组织。肿瘤细胞表达泛 B 细胞标志物和 T 细胞标志物 CD5。本病的特点是 t(11;14)(q13;q32)易位,导致编码原癌基因 cyclin D1 的 *bcl-1* 基因重排和过度表达[131]。治疗的主要方法是化学免疫治疗,有梗阻性肿块的患者需要外科手术治疗。有侵袭性表现的 MCL,通常在化疗后首次缓解期续贯利妥昔单抗维持治疗的基础上,给予自体干细胞移植巩固治疗[132]。虽然 MCL 最初对化疗有反应,但最终会变为难治性;中位生存期为 3~5 年。Bruton 酪氨酸激酶抑制剂依鲁替尼(ibrutinib)已被批准用于难治性或复发性 MCL[133,134]。

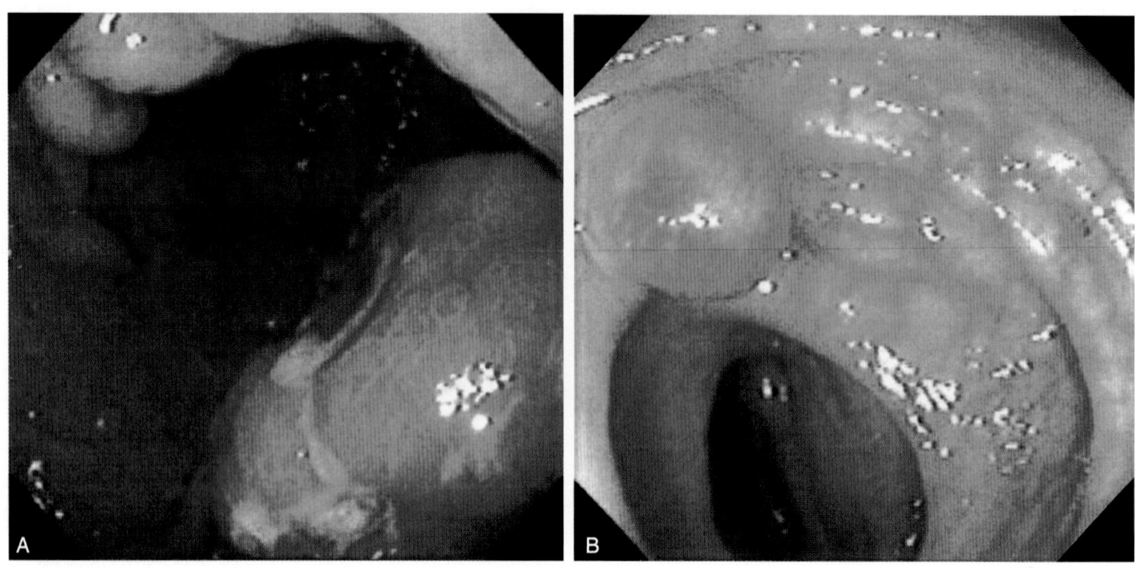

图 32.5　套细胞淋巴瘤的内镜表现为胃内(A)和结肠内(B)多发性淋巴瘤样息肉病

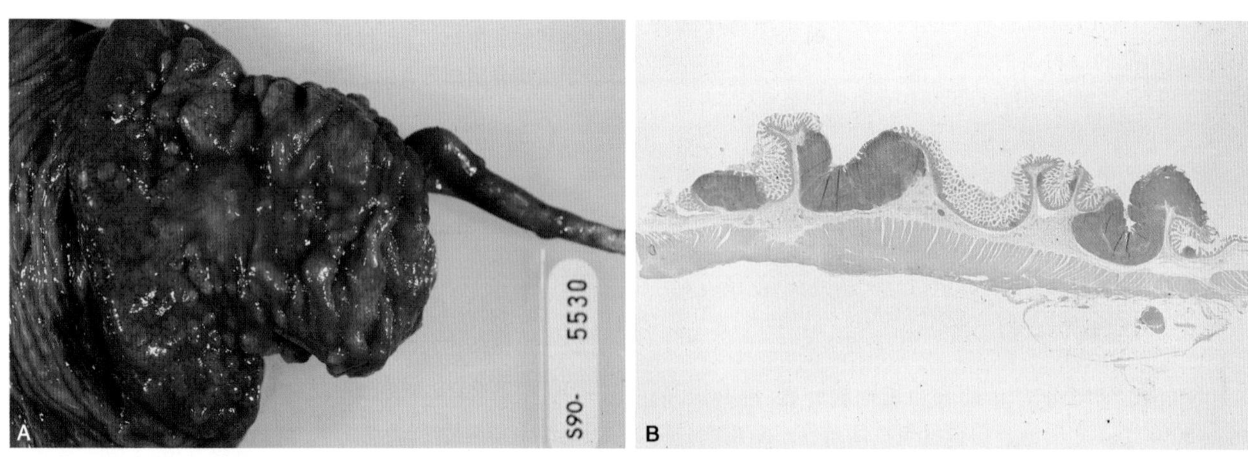

图 32.6　多发性淋巴瘤样息肉病(套细胞淋巴瘤)。A,大体标本显示盲肠内有多发小息肉样病变。在回肠、十二指肠以及直肠和乙状结肠中存在或随后发生的其他同步或异时性病变。B,回肠低倍显微镜照片显示淋巴瘤样息肉病累及黏膜和黏膜下的多个离散部位。(Courtesy Dr. Edward Lee,Washington,DC.)

(四) 滤泡性淋巴瘤

胃肠道的滤泡性 B 细胞淋巴瘤很少见[135]。最常见的表现是末端回肠的梗阻性病变,如前所述,也可呈多发性淋巴瘤样息肉病的大体表现。显微镜下,大多数 FL 由小的裂隙淋巴细胞或中心细胞组成(图 32.7),与大细胞不同程度地混合在一起。t(14;18)(q24;q32)易位是本病的特征,导致 *bcl-2* 基因过度表达[136]。梗阻性病变需要手术治疗。有时需要化疗和放疗,虽呈惰性但无法治愈。

十二指肠型 FL(duodenal-type FL,D-FL)是 2016 年 WHO 更新分类中新确认的类型。与其他 FL 不同,D-FL 几乎都是在内镜检查中偶然发现(单发或多发结节,或息肉样病变,直径在 1~5 毫米之间),诊断时级别和分期都较低,并且大多局限于十二指肠降部。从基因表达谱和发病机制来看,它与 MALT 淋巴瘤的关系比 FL 更密切。由于该病的预后极好(中位生存期>12 年),大多数专家建议对其采取"等待和观察"策略[137,138]。

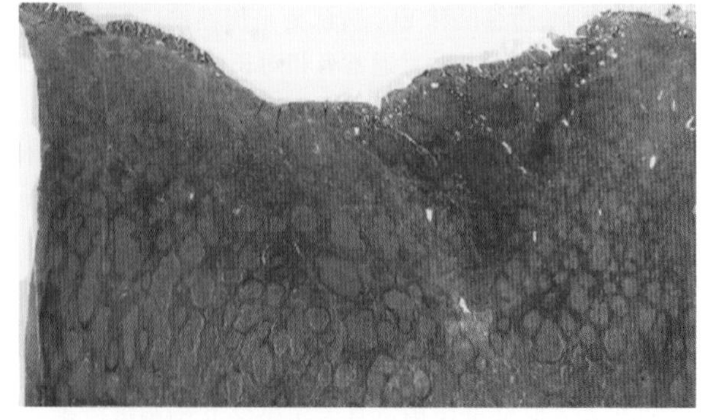

图 32.7　显微镜照片显示滤泡性淋巴瘤,世界卫生组织Ⅱ级。肿瘤性淋巴滤泡明显,累及小肠壁,正常结构消失(HE 染色,低倍镜)。(Courtesy Dr. Imran Shahab and Dr. Pamela Jensen,Dallas,TX.)

（五）Burkitt 淋巴瘤

Burkitt 淋巴瘤是一种高度侵袭性的恶性肿瘤，在 HIV 阴性的患者中，呈地方性分布于非洲或其他地区散发[139]。在散发病例中，患者通常表现为累及远端回肠、盲肠和/或肠系膜的腹部病变。Burkitt 淋巴瘤细胞形态单一、中等大小，核圆、多核仁，胞质嗜碱性（图 32.8）。受累的淋巴组织在显微镜下呈星空样，这是由大量吞噬了凋亡肿瘤细胞的良性巨噬细胞所致[140]。肿瘤细胞表达 B 细胞相关抗原和表面免疫球蛋白。大多数病例有 8 号染色体上的 *c-myc* 基因易位，或易位到 14 号染色体上的免疫球蛋白重链区，或易位到 2 号或 22 号染色体上的免疫球蛋白轻链区，导致 t(8;14)、t(2;8) 或 t(8;22) 易位[141]。Burkitt 淋巴瘤在未治疗的情况下可迅速致死，但会立即对积极的化疗有反应。治疗易导致溶瘤综合征。治愈率为 50% 至 90%，具体取决于疾病的严重程度[142,143]。

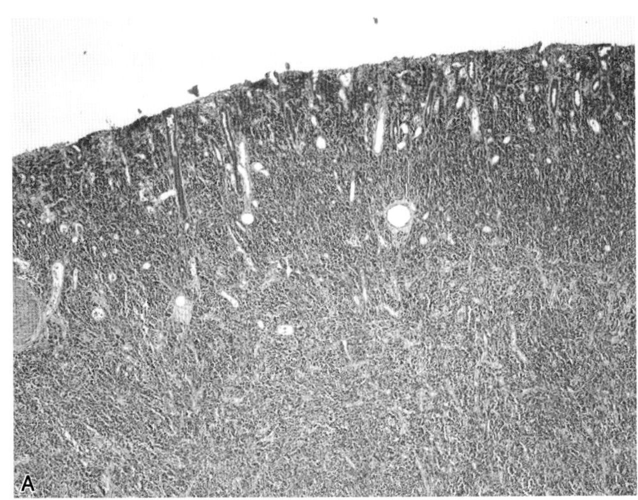

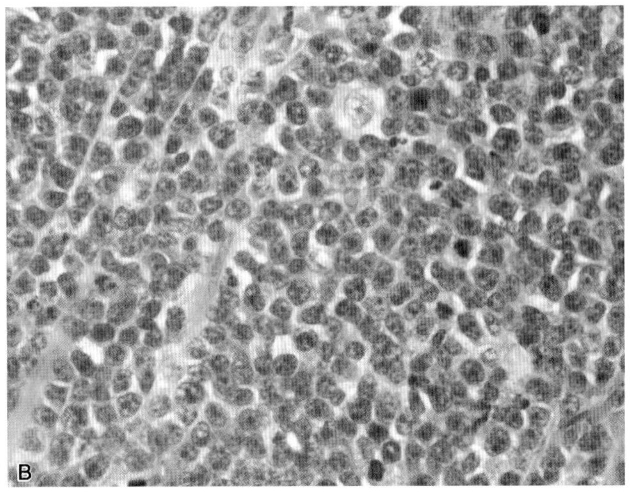

图 32.8　Burkitt 淋巴瘤。A，Burkitt 淋巴瘤弥漫性累及小肠。注意原腺体结构周围的浸润。B，高倍视图显示活跃的有丝分裂活动和背景有巨噬细胞。CD20 免疫染色（未显示）在肿瘤细胞群中呈强阳性。（A，HE 染色，×20；B，HE 染色，×600）（Courtesy Dr. Pamela Jensen，Dallas，TX.）

（六）免疫增殖性小肠疾病

1. 流行病学

免疫增殖性小肠疾病（IPSID）（也称为 α 重链疾病或地中海淋巴瘤）仅限于世界某些地区，特别是北非，以色列以及中东和地中海周边国家[144]。IPSID 在其他地区较少见，包括中非、南非、印度、东亚以及南美洲和中美洲。在北美或欧洲诊断该病要谨慎，除非患者曾有流行地区生活史。该疾病发生在社会经济地位较低及个人和环境卫生条件差的人群中[145]。尽管该病常见于 20~30 岁人群，但老年人也可患病。男女发病率相等。

2. 病因和发病机制

一些观察结果表明，IPSID 可能是由一种或多种传染性病原体引发的：①该病与较低的社会经济地位和卫生条件差有关；②肠道细菌过度生长和寄生虫病的患病率高；③当流行地区的生活条件改善时，发病率降低；④早期病变抗生素治疗有效。此外，众所周知，肠道微生物刺激分泌免疫球蛋白（Ig）A 的细胞，来自流行区的正常个体的肠黏膜活检显示固有层淋巴细胞和浆细胞数量增加，类似于 IPSID 患者的表现。已证实 IPSID 与空肠弯曲杆菌感染有关[147,148]。

正如稍后将讨论的，IPSID 与一种异常的 IgA 重链蛋白（称为 α 重链）有关，该蛋白由浆细胞分泌，可以在各种体液中检测到[149,150]。浆细胞是浅表黏膜中的主要组织学特征，细胞表面和胞质均含有 α 链蛋白。在黏膜深层增殖的中心细胞样细胞主要具有胞质 α 链蛋白。这些中心细胞样细胞很可能在微生物抗原刺激下分化为浆细胞，分泌该病特有的 α 链蛋白。基因分析表明，即使在早期病变中，细胞增殖也是单克隆性的[151,152]。

因此，可以认为，在某种程度上类似于 Hp 感染相关的胃 MALT，肠道 MALT 中的淋巴细胞可能会受感染原，尤其是空肠弯曲杆菌[153]的刺激而出现增殖反应。淋巴细胞的反应为单克隆性，最初依赖于抗原的存在。然而，随着时间的推移，恶性细胞获得了额外的基因变化，导致它们失去对抗原的持久依赖性。这种抗原依赖性的丢失，使其侵袭性进一步增高。

3. 病理学

大体病变通常局限于近端小肠，伴周围肠系膜淋巴结肿大[154]。有些患者只表现为黏膜皱襞增厚，其他患者可见肠壁广泛增厚、不连续的肿块、结节或息肉样病变。尽管大体上仅累及近端小肠壁，但组织学上整个小肠均可见该病的特征性表现，黏膜和黏膜下层致密细胞浸润。目前有多种病理分期系统（表 32.5）[154,155]。在早期病变中，浸润细胞由外观良性的浆细胞或淋巴浆细胞组成。然而，如前所述，各种评估免疫球蛋白基因重排或轻链限制的研究表明，即使是最早期的浸润肿瘤细胞也是单克隆的。这种早期浸润使绒毛变宽，隐窝缩短和分离，但上皮细胞仍完整。已经发现在一些患者中有一种组织学变异型，即滤泡性淋巴型（见图 32.7），其特征是伴淋巴滤泡样结构的黏膜弥漫浸润。随着疾病进展到中晚期，绒毛进一步变宽并可能完全消失，隐窝减少，免疫增殖延伸至更深层。非典型淋巴细胞浸润良性外观的浆细胞和淋巴浆细胞。随着时间的推移，逐渐演变成典型的淋巴瘤。病变早期，肠系膜淋巴结肿大，结构正常，尽管淋巴滤泡可能被组织学上看起来良性的淋巴细胞或浆细胞浸润。随着疾病进展，淋巴结外观的异型性可能会愈加明显。

表 32.5　免疫增殖性小肠疾病病理分期系统

世界卫生组织(WHO)

(a) 弥漫、密集、致密、明显良性的淋巴增殖性黏膜浸润
　ⅰ. 单纯浆细胞性
　ⅱ. 混合淋巴浆细胞性
(b) 加上小肠和/或肠系膜淋巴结内局限的"免疫母细胞"淋巴瘤
(c) 弥漫性"免疫母细胞"淋巴瘤,伴或不伴明显良性的淋巴浆细胞浸润

Salem 等[146]

0 期:良性外观的淋巴浆细胞黏膜浸润(LPI),无恶性迹象
Ⅰ期:LPI 和恶性淋巴瘤累及肠道(Ii)或肠系膜淋巴结(In),但不是两者都有
Ⅱ期:LPI 和恶性淋巴瘤累及肠和肠系膜淋巴结
Ⅲ期:累及腹膜后和/或腹腔外淋巴结
Ⅳ期:不连续的非淋巴组织受累
未知或不充分分期

Galian 等[147]

分期	部位Ⅰ:小肠	部位Ⅱ A:肠系膜淋巴结	部位Ⅱ B:其他腹部及腹膜后淋巴结	部位Ⅲ:其他淋巴结	部位Ⅳ:其他部位
A	固有层† 成熟的* 浆细胞浸润,淋巴结结构无紊乱或轻微紊乱;多样且不同程度的绒毛萎缩	所有部位浸润细胞与部位Ⅰ相似			
B	不典型浆细胞或淋巴浆细胞浸润,伴或多或少的不典型免疫母细胞样细胞,至少延伸至黏膜下层;大部分或完全绒毛萎缩	不典型浆细胞或淋巴浆细胞浸润,伴多少不等的不典型免疫母细胞样细胞;淋巴结结构全部或部分消失			浸润细胞与部位Ⅰ相似
C	淋巴瘤样增生浸润肠壁全层	淋巴瘤样增生伴淋巴结结构完全破坏†			淋巴瘤样增生与部位Ⅰ相似

*罕见细胞可能呈现不成熟模式。
†可观察到局限的和浅表的黏膜下层扩散。
Modified from Fine KD, Stone MJ. Alpha-heavy chain disease, Mediterranean lymphoma, and immunoproliferative small intestinal disease: a review of clinicopathological features, pathogenesis, and differential diagnosis. Am J Gastroenterol 1999;94:1139-52.

4. 临床特征

患者通常表现为腹泻、腹部绞痛、厌食和显著的体重下降;症状持续数月至数年。腹泻最初可能是间歇性的,但随着吸收不良的进展,腹泻量逐渐增大并伴恶臭。约半数患者有发热。体格检查显示营养不良、杵状指和外周水肿。疾病晚期表现为腹水、肝脾肿大、腹部包块和外周淋巴结肿大。内镜检查可见黏膜皱襞增厚、结节、溃疡或黏膜下浸润征象,肠道蠕动减弱、僵硬和扩张不良。小肠钡餐造影显示十二指肠、空肠及回肠近端弥漫性扩张,黏膜皱襞增厚。患者通常因维生素缺乏而贫血,1/3 的患者血沉增快。外周血淋巴细胞计数低,体液和细胞免疫受损。粪便检查常发现贾第鞭毛虫感染。正如前述,通过对肠道活检样本的 PCR、DNA 测序、荧光原位杂交和免疫组化检查,发现大部分患者存在空肠弯曲杆菌[153]。血清 IgG 和 IgM 水平可升高或降低;IgA 水平通常降低或检测不到。

该病特征和特异性的实验室检查是检测到 α 链蛋白[156]。这种 32~34kD 的蛋白质是一条可变(V_H)区和 C_H1 区内缺失的游离 α1 重链。它没有轻链,因此对应 $IgA\alpha_1$ 亚单位的 Fc 段。α 链蛋白氨基末端包含不与任何已知的免疫球蛋白序列同源的序列。这些变化通常是由于插入或缺失导致的,常涉及 V_H-J_H 和 C_H2 区域[147],但这些插入的遗传物质的来源尚不清楚。

血清蛋白电泳显示,α 链以宽带形式位于 α_2 和 β 区之间。除了血清电泳,还可以通过免疫电泳或免疫选择(最灵敏和特异的方法)[147]检测血清、尿液、唾液或肠道分泌物中的 α 链蛋白。这些样本中的 α 链蛋白在早期患者中比晚期患者中更容易检测到,但不论分期如何,在大多数 IPSID 病例的组织切片中可以通过免疫荧光或免疫过氧化物酶染色浆细胞或淋巴瘤细胞检测到 α 链蛋白[156]。

据推测,抗原对肠道 IgA 分泌细胞的慢性刺激会导致数个浆细胞克隆的扩增。最终,在某个特定克隆中发生结构突变,导致 α 重链内缺失。从而无法形成完整的轻链并分泌 IgA,代之以分泌 α 链蛋白[144,147]。

5. 诊断和分期

由于更恶性的组织学形态表现可能仅出现在深层肠壁,所以通常认为仅用内镜活检评估分期是不充分的;有些研究者强烈建议手术分期,以便进行肠壁全层活检和肠系膜淋巴结活检[157]。然而,有的研究者并不常规行腹腔镜或开腹手术,而是进行上、下消化道的内镜检查、小肠系列检查、骨髓活检和肿大淋巴结的针吸活检[158],然后可以应用其中一个分期系统(见表 32.5)进行分期。病情晚期、一般情况差及出现并发症,提示预后差。

6. 治疗

由于这种淋巴瘤相对罕见，目前还没有大规模的试验来研究其治疗方法[158,159]。患者通常需要加强营养支持[160]。早期患者［如 Salem 0 期（见表 32.5）］一般给予抗生素治疗 6 个月或更长时间。两种最常用的治疗方案是单独使用四环素或甲硝唑和氨苄西林联合，应答率为 33%～71%[161]。在一项研究中，完全应答率为 71%，5 年无病生存率为 43%[158]。对于 6 个月没有明显好转或 12 个月仍未完全缓解的患者，或发现时已是晚期的患者，应给予化疗。大多数研究者推荐含蒽环类药物的方案，如 CHOP[162,163]。例如，一位研究者报道了，在接受抗生素、全肠外营养和基于蒽环类药物联合化疗的患者中，完全缓解率为 67%，3.5 年生存率为 58%[163]。然而，也有报道称非蒽环类方案亦可获得良好的治疗效果；一份报告显示晚期患者 5 年无病生存率为 56%[158]。最后，由于全腹放疗仅用于少数患者，目前难以评估其疗效[164]。

（七）肠病相关性 T 细胞淋巴瘤

肠病相关性 T 细胞淋巴瘤（enteropathy-associated T cell lymphoma，EATL）是乳糜泻的并发症（见第 107 章）[165]。上皮内 T 细胞的恶性转化导致侵袭性恶性肿瘤，大多数患者在确诊后几个月内死亡[166,167]。用无麸质饮食治疗乳糜泻可能会降低患这种恶性肿瘤的风险[168]。

1. 流行病学

EATL 是一种罕见的恶性肿瘤，发病率仅为 0.016/10 万，但经年龄校正后的总体发病率呈上升趋势[169]。乳糜泻在美国和欧洲的患病率为 0.5% 至 1%[170,171]，与非裔美国人和亚洲人相比，白人更常见。在有症状的乳糜泻患者中，最常见的死亡原因是 NHL[172]。淋巴瘤的诊断通常是在诊断乳糜泻的同时或之后不久，尽管这两种情况通常是同时诊断的，特别是在有长期吸收不良病史的患者中。坚持严格的无麸质饮食似乎可以降低死亡率[173]。EATL 的确诊中位年龄为 60 岁，男性和女性的发病率相等[174]。

2. 病因和发病机制

EATL 发生在成人乳糜泻患者[175]。如第 107 章所述，乳糜泻的特点是对麸质具有遗传敏感性[176]。麸质肽由乳糜泻特异性 HLA-DQ2 和 HLA-DQ8 阳性的抗原递呈细胞呈递，从而引发免疫反应，其中麸质特异性上皮内淋巴细胞损伤肠上皮。乳糜泻患者的上皮内 T 细胞具有正常的免疫表型（$CD3^+/CD8^+$），并且是多克隆的[177,178]。这些 T 细胞的恶性转化导致具有异常表型的上皮内 T 细胞的单克隆增殖[179-182]。乳糜泻患者黏膜上皮内的单克隆 T 淋巴细胞可能导致以下几种相互关联的疾病过程中的任何一种[182,183]。一是难治性乳糜泻，无麦胶饮食治疗无效[184]。二是溃疡性空肠炎，其特征是炎性空肠溃疡和无麦胶饮食治疗无效[185]。三是 EATL，一种侵袭性的小肠恶性肿瘤[180,181]。以上 3 种情况的患者，其病变附近未受累肠黏膜内都可有含有相同重排 T 淋巴细胞受体基因的单克隆 T 细胞[186]。此外，溃疡性空肠炎患者可发展为 EATL，在空肠和随后的淋巴瘤中可以分离到相同的 T 淋巴细胞克隆。因此，这三种情况被认为是代表了由单克隆上皮内 T 细胞介导的一系列疾病。

比较基因组杂交研究显示，在 EATL 中染色体 9q，7q，5q 和 1q 反复增加，以及染色体 8p，13q 和 9p 反复丢失。最常见的是 9q 增加，在 58% 的检测病例中可见[187]。另一项研究显示，9q21 杂合性丢失也常见[188]。此外，一项研究表明 1q 染色体的增加可能是淋巴瘤发生的早期事件[189]。

3. 病理学

肿瘤通常发生在空肠，但也可能发生在小肠的其他部位。淋巴瘤可以单发或多发。大体上，淋巴瘤通常表现为小肠全周受累的溃疡性病变。也可表现为结节，斑块或狭窄，但大的肿块并不常见。由于肿瘤累及，水肿或反应性改变，肠系膜淋巴结通常肿大。远隔部位，尤其是骨髓或肝脏，有时也会受累。

组织学上，淋巴瘤的一般特征是炎症背景下，可见大的、高度多形性（大量、异形、多核）的细胞。少数患者（10%～20%）可能表现为单一形态的中等大小的细胞（图 32.9），曾经被称为Ⅱ型 EATL，现在命名为单形性嗜上皮性肠道 T 细胞淋巴瘤（monomorphic epitheliotropic intestinal T cell lymphoma，MEITL）[5]，并且可能发生于没有乳糜泻的患者。MEITL 在亚洲和西班牙裔人群中的发病率增加。未受累的黏膜通常可见典型的乳糜泻表现，包括绒毛萎缩、隐窝增生、固有层浆细胞增多，以及上皮内淋巴细胞增多（见第 107 章）。然而，在某些情况下，肠病可能是轻微的，只有上皮内淋巴细胞的增加。

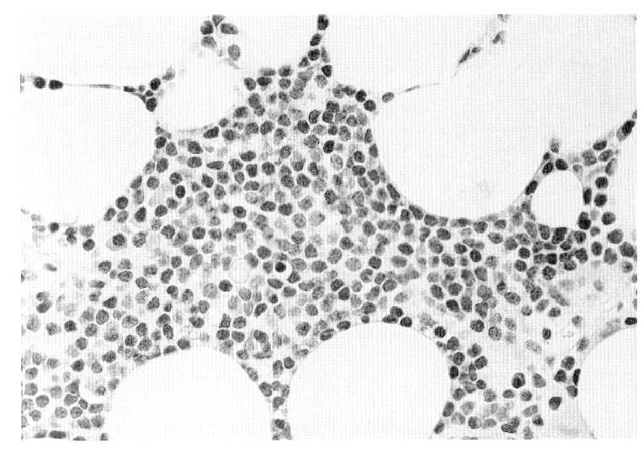

图 32.9　乳糜泻患者肠病型肠道 T 细胞淋巴瘤的显微镜照片。可见小肠壁的肠系膜脂肪与小到中等大小的不规则 T 淋巴细胞的单一形态群。T 淋巴细胞 CD2、CD3、CD7 呈阳性，CD5 呈阴性。T 细胞基因重排研究呈阳性（即显示克隆条带，表明克隆 T 细胞过程）。（Courtesy Dr. Edward Lee，Washington，DC.）

根据对国际外周 T 细胞淋巴瘤项目中 62 例 EATL 患者的研究显示，典型的恶性细胞免疫表型为 $CD3^+$、$CD2^+$、$CD5^-$、$CD4^-$、$CD8^+$、$CD30^+$、$CD103^+$，并含有被抗体 TIA-1 识别的细胞毒性颗粒[190]。在无淋巴瘤累及的黏膜中也可检测到单克隆 T 细胞群。全基因组分析和 HLA 基因分型已鉴定出 2 个 EATL 亚型[191]。Ⅰ型为 CD56 阴性，发病机制与乳糜泻有关，和难治性乳糜泻具有相同的 *HLA-DQB1* 基因型。MEITL（曾经的 EATL Ⅱ型）为 $CD56^+$ 和 MYC^+，与正常白种人群有相似的 *HLA-DQB1* 基因型。

4. 临床特征

患者可能有乳糜泻病史，发展为淋巴瘤的时间差异很大。然而，至少有一半的患者在诊断淋巴瘤的同时诊断乳糜泻。最常见症状是腹痛，体重减轻，腹泻或呕吐。其他症状可能包括发热、盗汗、小肠梗阻或穿孔。患者很少有可触及的腹部肿块或外周淋巴结肿大，但肠外受累部位可能包括肝脏、脾脏、甲状腺、皮肤、鼻窦和脑[165]。有研究显示，β_2 微球蛋白和血清 LDH 水平升高分别见于 85.7% 和 62% 的患者，贫血和低白蛋白血症分别见于 91% 和 88% 的患者[192]。

确诊通常是通过内镜活检或腹腔镜全层小肠活检。传统上，患者通过 CT 和骨髓活检进行分期，但在鉴别 EATL 和难治性乳糜泻方面，^{18}F-FDG PET-CT 比 CT 更敏感和特异[193]。Lugano 系统被提出作为分期系统，但其在评估预后方面的作用尚不清楚[55]。

5. 治疗

目前尚无关于 EATL 治疗的大型对照试验的报道，因此，标准治疗尚不明确。通常，给予患者手术和化疗的联合治疗[192]。手术需尽可能多地切除肿瘤，术后再进行强化的化疗，最常见的方案是含有蒽环类药物的方案，如在老年患者应用 CHOP，在年轻的成年患者应用 CHOEP（CHOP 加依托泊苷）[174]。单纯应用蒽环类药物为基础的化疗，其 5 年总体生存率约为 10%~20%。基于这个原因和回顾性数据，大多数专家建议，在首次缓解期，对没有或较少合并症的健壮患者进行自体干细胞移植。患者的营养状况普遍较差，需要肠外营养支持。由于营养不良和一般情况差，只有不到 50% 的患者适合全身化疗，其中能够完成规定治疗方案的患者不到 50%。大约 80% 的患者在确诊后的 6 个月（中位时间）内复发，部位通常在小肠。虽然对于复发的患者已经尝试了各种挽救治疗方案，但复发患者很少能存活下来[194]。由于常规化疗效果不佳，于是在少数一般情况良好的患者中开展了大剂量化疗后进行自体干细胞移植的研究。欧洲血液和骨髓移植组织进行了一项回顾性研究，纳入了 2000 年至 2010 年间自体干细胞移植的 44 名患者，结果显示 4 年复发率、无进展生存率和总体生存率分别为 39%、54% 和 59%[195]。还尝试了新药治疗，如阿仑单抗（Alemtuzumab，Campath），一种抗 CD52 单克隆抗体，已用于治疗难治性乳糜泻[196]，以及本妥昔单抗（Brentuximab vedotin），一种抗 CD30 单克隆抗体与抗有丝分裂剂-单甲基奥瑞他汀 E（monomethyl auristatin E）的耦联产物[197]。可想而知，早期诊断可能改善预后。对于中年乳糜泻患者和无麸质饮食治疗使病情稳定后又出现临床恶化的患者，应考虑该诊断。

（八）不常见的小肠淋巴瘤

自然杀伤 T 细胞肠道淋巴瘤

鼻型结外 NK/T 细胞淋巴瘤，是 WHO 血液淋巴系统恶性肿瘤分类中的一种独特病理类型[5]。肠道 NK 细胞淋巴瘤罕见[198]。已报道的大多数病例与乳糜泻或麸质敏感无关[120,121]。尚未确定这种罕见疾病的最佳治疗方案。大多数数据来自东亚国家，传统化疗方案如 CHOP 和 CHOEP 治疗的失败率高。激进的治疗方案，如 DeVIC（地塞米松、依托泊苷、异环磷酰胺、卡铂）和 SMILE（地塞米松、甲氨蝶呤、异环磷酰胺、L-门冬酰胺酶、依托泊苷），联合或不联合放射治疗，都取得了一定程度的成功。抗 PD1 检查点抑制剂（如帕博利珠单抗）的免疫疗法，在一些复发/难治性患者群体中显示出可期的疗效[199]。

四、消化道其他部位淋巴瘤

NHL 很少发生在消化系统胃、小肠以外的其他部位，包括口咽、食管、肝脏、胰腺、胆道、阑尾、结肠和直肠。患者的体征和症状与病变部位有关。由于这些疾病相对罕见，文献相当有限。因此，无法就这些罕见的消化系统淋巴瘤的最佳诊疗方案给出明确的结论。淋巴瘤诊疗规范规定了诊断程序、分期、预后评估和治疗。与所有淋巴瘤一样，组织学和分期指导治疗。

（一）Waldeyer 环淋巴瘤

通常是弥漫性大细胞淋巴瘤，但也可能存在其他组织学类型[200,201]。分期检查必须包含胃肠道其他部分的内镜检查和影像学检查，因为淋巴瘤累及其他部位时可能同时出现 Waldeyer 环受累。Ann Arbor Ⅰ期或Ⅱ期弥漫性大细胞淋巴瘤建议采用蒽环类药物为基础的联合化疗和/或局部放疗[106]。

（二）原发性肝淋巴瘤

多见于男性，中位发病年龄约为 50 岁[202,203]。原发性肝淋巴瘤可表现为单发、大的、多分叶状肿物，也可表现为单个或多个结节。组织学通常是弥漫性大 B 细胞，而 MALT 淋巴瘤（结外边缘区 B 细胞淋巴瘤）也有报道。肝 T 细胞淋巴瘤罕见。诊断主要通过穿刺活检。由于该病罕见，最佳治疗方案尚不确定。已有报道，肿物切除后可获得长期无病生存，但肝 DLBCL 可能更适合多药联合的化学免疫疗法。温和的化学免疫疗法或利妥昔单抗单药可能适用于边缘区淋巴瘤。已经证明肝脾边缘区淋巴瘤与 HCV 有关，且丙型肝炎治疗对其有效[204,205]。其他肝炎病毒是否与肝淋巴瘤相关尚不清楚。

（三）胰腺淋巴瘤

很少见（占所有胰腺肿瘤的 0.5% 以下）[206]。患者的临床表现与胰腺腺癌相似，可有腹痛和梗阻性黄疸；乳糜性腹水也有报道。组织学上 80% 以上为弥漫性大 B 细胞淋巴瘤，已发表的文献支持含蒽环类化疗（如 CHOP）与利妥昔单抗和放疗的联合治疗。胆道梗阻患者在接受化疗前需要进行胆汁引流，以避免严重的化疗毒性。

（四）原发性结直肠淋巴瘤

最常见于盲肠[207,208]，组织学表现为中-高度恶性。大多数结直肠淋巴瘤处于 Ann Arbor $Ⅰ_E$ 期或 $Ⅱ_E$ 期。治疗由组织学类型和疾病分期决定。首选手术切除，对组织学为侵袭性的病变患者应给予辅助化疗。

五、免疫缺陷性相关淋巴瘤

移植后淋巴增殖性疾病

移植后淋巴增殖性疾病(posttransplantation lymphoproliferative disorder,PTLD)[209-211]并发于0.8%~20%的实体器官移植患者(见第36章),其中接受心肺移植患者的发病率最高。PTLD也见于接受了骨髓移植的患者,尤其是在接受T细胞耗竭的同种异体移植患者。PTLD由EBV转化的B细胞克隆性增殖所致,其部分归因于免疫抑制[212]。PTLD的组织学表现差异很大,病变呈多形性或单形性(类似淋巴瘤);组织学可能类似于传染性单核细胞增多症、侵袭性NHL或浆细胞瘤。病变可以是多克隆,寡克隆或单克隆的。单克隆病变在外观上类似于低度恶性淋巴瘤,如FL、边缘区淋巴瘤、小淋巴细胞性淋巴瘤,按惯例不被认为是PTLD。临床表现也有很大差异,部分患者呈类似传染性单核细胞增多症的临床表现,部分患者有淋巴瘤样表现,伴淋巴结或结外病变。PTLD累及淋巴结外部位很常见,胃肠道是常见受累部位。有关治疗的文献尚缺乏前瞻性研究和标准化的组织学分类。

治疗方法各不相同,但对于多形性PTLD通常首先是停止或调整免疫抑制方案[213]。对于$CD20^+$的单形性PTLD,除了尽量减少免疫抑制外,首选的治疗方法是使用抗CD20抗体利妥昔单抗进行免疫治疗,对于单独免疫治疗无效的患者可以联合以蒽环类药物为基础的化疗。这种序贯疗法主要基于欧洲的数据,利妥昔单抗治疗的早期应答者可获得长期无病生存,从而避免了CD20阳性PTLD患者使用有毒性的化疗[214]。

外科或放射疗法可以治愈那些经严格筛选的病变局限的患者。其他治疗方法包括针对EBV的阿昔洛韦或更昔洛韦,同种异体细胞毒性EBV特异性T细胞或EBV-CTL和干扰素-α。供体白细胞输注常用于同种异体骨髓移植后发生的PTLD患者[215]。

六、医源性淋巴增殖性疾病

因非移植原因使用免疫抑制药物[其他医源性免疫缺陷相关淋巴增殖性疾病(other iatrogenic immunodeffciency-associated lymphoproliferative disorder,OIIA-LPD)]引起的淋巴增殖性疾病,越来越多地被认识和描述[216]。甲氨蝶呤引起的淋巴瘤已经得到公认。我们越来越多地发现,正在接受免疫抑制剂治疗或有免疫抑制剂治疗史(包括TNF抑制剂在内的生物制剂)的炎症性肠病患者,出现了淋巴增殖性疾病。EBV是这类疾病的核心驱动因子,其诊疗参考PTLD文献(参见移植后淋巴增殖性疾病一节)。

多形性淋巴增殖被认为是反应性的,主要通过停用免疫抑制来治疗。单形性淋巴增殖类似于各型的非霍奇金淋巴瘤或霍奇金淋巴瘤,治疗主要根据发病时淋巴瘤的分期、分型和累及范围。

在我们中心,情况允许时,我们倾向于对低度恶性病变和低肿瘤负荷患者停用免疫抑制剂,并进行密切观察。这些患者中多达40%可以出现肿瘤自发性消退。在广泛器官受累或脏器危象情况下,通常对高度恶性淋巴瘤的患者给予辅助化疗。

WHO 2016年的分类中有一临时条目,这是一种特殊的疾病,通常影响老年人,称为EBV阳性黏膜皮肤溃疡,具有霍奇金淋巴瘤的一些病理特征(图32.10)。本病常见于免疫抑制状态下,主要表现为边界清楚的口咽部病变,但可累及皮肤和胃肠道的任何部位。病变大多呈惰性病程(45%自发缓解,15%复发/缓解),临床病理相关性是其区分霍奇金淋巴瘤的重要特征,后者很少出现结外受累[217]。

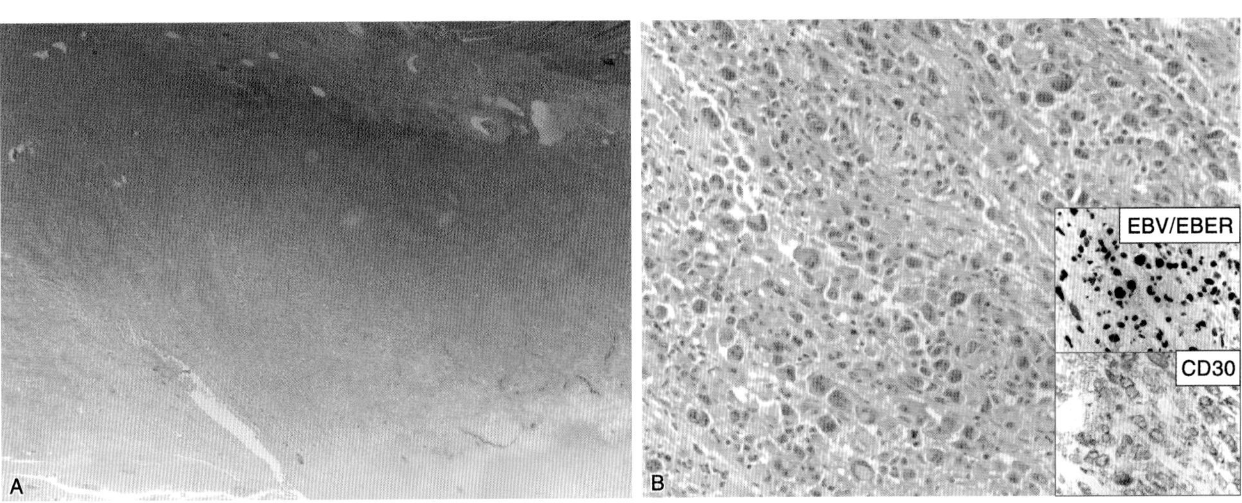

图32.10 显微镜下照片显示小肠EBV阳性黏膜皮肤溃疡。A,显示小肠黏膜多形性浸润,包括小淋巴细胞、组织细胞和大的非典型淋巴细胞伴溃疡。B,显示大的淋巴样细胞,细胞核不规则、核仁明显、细胞质丰富,与表达EBV/EBER和CD30(插图)易变的霍奇金细胞类似。(Courtesy Dr. Weina Chen, UT Southwestern Medical Center, Dallas, TX.)

七、HIV 相关性非霍奇金淋巴瘤

HIV 患者发生非霍奇金淋巴瘤的风险显著增加(见第 35 章),进展至淋巴瘤是获得性免疫缺陷综合征诊断的必要条件。这类恶性肿瘤是 B 细胞肿瘤[218],组织学上大多数具有小的无裂细胞或弥漫性大细胞。EBV 与约半数的非中枢神经系统 HIV 相关淋巴瘤有关。HIV 相关性非霍奇金淋巴瘤通常表现为侵袭性,疾病发展迅速,B 症状突出。胃肠道是常见受累部位,包括肛门和直肠等不常见部位。从既往研究看,患者对化疗的耐受性差,多使用低剂量的化疗方案。然而,CD4$^+$T 细胞计数较高的患者(常见于使用标准 HAART 治疗的患者)可能更能耐受全剂量化疗方案,并且预后好于既往研究[219]。

浆母细胞性淋巴瘤(plasmablastic lymphoma,PBL)是 DLBCL 的一种侵袭性变异,最初在 HIV 患者的口腔中被发现。大多数 HIV 感染胃肠道 PBL 病例存在肛管受累。PBL 不表达 CD20、CD45 和 PAX5,表达浆细胞相关蛋白,包括 CD38、CD138 和 VS38c。多数病例 EBV 阳性,HHV-8 阴性。多数存在 *MYC* 重排(图 32.11)。采用激进的化疗免疫治疗联合策略,如 V-EPOCH[硼替佐米(Velcade)+EPOCH]在这种难治性疾病中显示出了良好的疗效[220]。

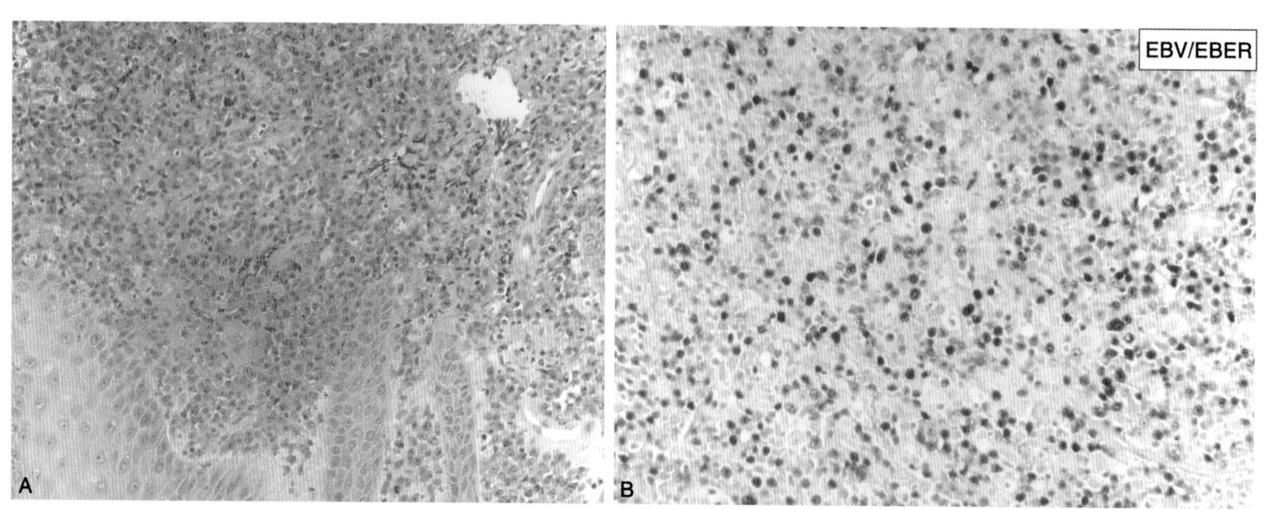

图 32.11 显微镜下照片显示累及直肠的浆母细胞淋巴瘤。A,显示大淋巴瘤细胞浸润直肠黏膜(鳞状上皮下方)。B,显示 EBV/EBER 表达的淋巴瘤细胞。(Courtesy Dr. Weina Chen,UT Southwestern Medical Center,Dallas,TX.)

*原发性渗出性淋巴瘤*是与疱疹病毒 HHV-8(卡波西肉瘤相关病毒)相关的临床病理学类型[221,222]。组织学表现出独特的形态,介于大细胞免疫母细胞淋巴瘤和间变性大细胞淋巴瘤之间[223]。肿瘤细胞显示单克隆免疫球蛋白基因重排,常丢失 B 细胞相关抗原。通过 PCR 方法可以检测到 HHV-8。患者通常为 HIV 阳性,但也有 HIV 阴性的病例报道。患者存在恶性胸腔积液或腹腔积液,这些积液局限于原发性体腔。疾病进展迅速,生存期仅为数周至数月。最佳治疗方案尚不明确。

(王欣欣 胡伟玲 译,李鹏 校)

参考文献

第 33 章　胃肠道间质瘤

Margaret von Mehren 著

章节目录

一、病理学 …… 433
二、分子发病机制 …… 434
三、分子药理学 …… 436
四、流行病学 …… 436
五、临床特征 …… 436
（一）食管肿瘤 …… 436
（二）胃肿瘤 …… 437
（三）十二指肠和空回肠肿瘤 …… 437
（四）结肠和肛门直肠肿瘤 …… 437
六、诊断 …… 438
（一）影像学 …… 438
（二）活检 …… 438
（三）鉴别诊断 …… 438
七、治疗 …… 440
（一）原发性局部疾病（早期疾病）…… 440
（二）进展期疾病（晚期疾病）…… 441
八、特殊状况 …… 444
（一）克隆进展的影像 …… 444
（二）Carney 三联征和 Carney-Streatakis 综合征 …… 444
（三）家族性胃肠道间质瘤 …… 445
（四）其他与胃肠道间质瘤相关的遗传肿瘤综合征 …… 445
（五）儿童胃肠间质瘤 …… 445

胃肠道间质瘤（GIST）占所有胃肠道恶性肿瘤的 1%～3%，是最常见的胃肠道间叶组织肿瘤。20 多年前，一项开创性的发现开始在分子水平上阐明大多数 GIST 的发病机制[1]。此外，这一新的认识已转化为高效的分子靶向治疗，如甲磺酸伊马替尼和相关药物，适用于大多数 GIST 患者[1]。

一、病理学

胃肠道间质瘤一词最初是由 Mazur 和 Clark 在 1983 年提出的纯粹描述性术语，用于定义非癌性（即非上皮性肿瘤）但具有平滑肌和神经成分组织学特征的腹腔内肿瘤[2]。当时，肿瘤细胞的形态是诊断的主要依据。在胃肠道间质病变中，用于标记肌细胞（如平滑肌肌动蛋白）和神经细胞（如 S100）的分化抗原存在很大差异，从而推测，认为不同患者的 GIST 病变是否可以体现不同的肌源性或神经分化程序。为了解释观察到的这些现象，有人提出，大约三分之一的 GIST 病变沿平滑肌谱系分化，另外三分之一是神经源性分化，最后三分之一缺乏通过免疫组化分析可检测到的谱系特异性标志物（无效表型）[3-5]。

1999 年以前，对于胃肠道间质瘤的诊断和分类，缺乏客观的、可重复的和明确的诊断标准。它们经常被误诊为平滑肌瘤或平滑肌肉瘤，因为它们在组织学上与这些平滑肌肿瘤相似。其他经常用于 GIST 的术语还包括良性平滑肌母细胞瘤[6]，以及具有某些神经特征的，如神经丛肉瘤[7]或胃肠道自主神经肿瘤[8]。几个病理学小组的深入研究表明，这些被归类为胃肠道平滑肌肿瘤的肿瘤可能不仅仅是平滑肌肉瘤或良性平滑肌瘤；一些起源于肠壁的肿瘤的具有几个独特的组织学特征，可能属于完全不同的诊断类型[9,10]。由于胃肠道间质瘤这一诊断术语所体现出的异质性，以及在特异性激酶指导诊断和分子标志物被广泛使用之前，对该肿瘤的诊断不足，因此对 2000 年之前发表的 GIST 的解读是困难的。

20 世纪 90 年代初，GIST 的免疫组织化学分析试图找到特定的标志物来区分 GIST 与其他胃肠道梭形细胞瘤，如神经鞘瘤和肉瘤样癌。最初 CD34 作为这样一种抗原标志物一度成为研究的热点，然而，这种抗原也可表达于造血干细胞、血管和肌成纤维细胞。并且，CD34 的敏感性和特异性较低，因为只有约半数的 GIST 病例表达 CD34，以及其他平滑肌，肌成纤维细胞（如硬纤维瘤）或施万细胞肿瘤也可表达 CD34[11,12]。

20 世纪 90 年代后期，人们在分子水平上对 GIST 的认识取得了重大进展，认识到这些肿瘤的细胞在组织病理学上与肠道起搏细胞 Cajal 间质细胞（ICC）有相似之处[13]。ICC 通常存在于肠道肌间神经丛，通过协助肠壁平滑肌细胞与自主神经系统的联系来协调肠蠕动（见第 98～100 章）。GIST 细胞和 ICC 具有某些共同的超微结构特征，如神经表型和肌肉表型联合。此外即使不是大多数，全身也有许多胃肠外组织也有类似于 ICC 的间质细胞；最初被称为 ICC 样细胞，现在被称为特络细胞（telocytes）。特络细胞具有能够影响其他细胞的细长突起[14]。特络细胞可能是 GIST 和胃肠道外间质肿瘤的前驱细胞，如胰腺 GIST[15,16]。

免疫组织化学染色显示，GIST 特征性地（>95%）表达 CD117（肥大/干细胞因子受体）[1]。该受体的其他名称包括原癌基因 c-KIT、酪氨酸激酶受体 KIT 或简称 KIT。CD117 由 *KIT* 基因编码。CD117 蛋白在梭形细胞 GIST 亚型中呈弥漫强阳性表达（图 33.1）。相反，在上皮样 GIST 亚型中，CD117 的表达通常是局灶性的，呈点状弱阳性（图 33.2）。正如后面讨论的，CD117 阴性的 GIST 很少见。

真性平滑肌肉瘤表达两种平滑肌标志物，平滑肌肌动蛋白和结蛋白（desmin），但不表达 CD117。神经鞘瘤通常神经

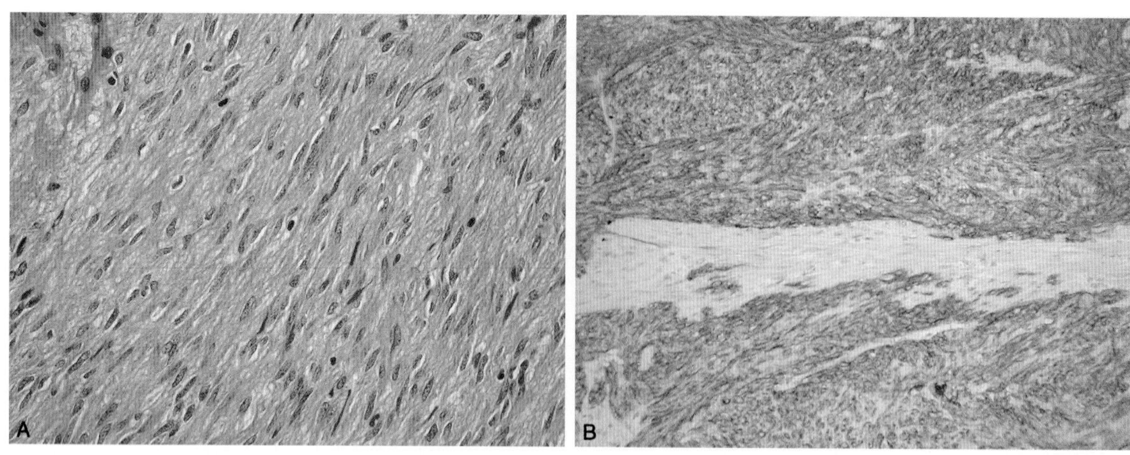

图 33.1　A,典型梭形细胞 GIST 的显微照片。细胞呈单形性,胞质丰富苍白、嗜酸性、纤维性,缺乏有丝分裂活性(HE 染色,×100)。B,KIT(CD117)免疫组化染色。这种梭形细胞 GIST 的中倍显微照片显示 KIT 具有弥散和强烈的细胞质免疫反应性。来自肠壁的残留肌纤维 KIT 的 CD117 免疫组化染色呈阴性(CD117 免疫染色,×100)。(Courtesy Dr. Brian P. Rubin,Cleveland,OH.)

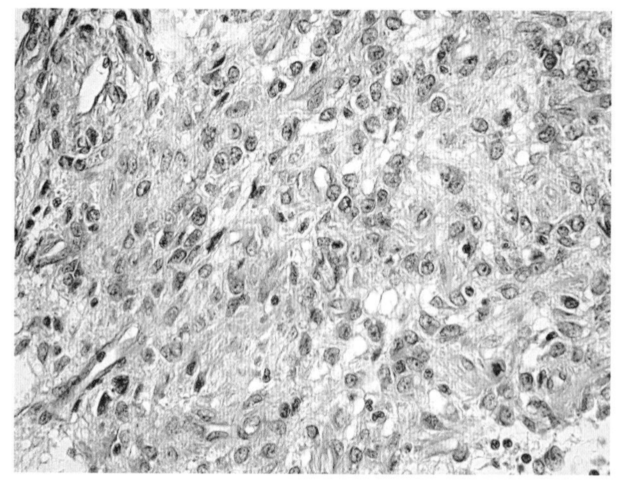

图 33.2　胃肠道间质瘤的显微照片显示上皮样细胞形态,纤维状细胞质和缺乏有丝分裂活性(HE 染色,×200)。(Courtesy Dr. Brian P. Rubin Cleveland)

抗原 S100 呈阳性,但 CD117 也是阴性。周围间质组织中的正常肥大细胞和 ICC 是理想的阳性对照,因为这些正常细胞强烈表达 CD117。

GIST 病变在 CD117 的表达上是存在异质性的,即使在单个肿瘤内也是如此。因此,仅由于取样偏差,就可以导致针刺活检取到了组织学上与 GIST 一致的细胞,但 CD117 表达阴性。有一些罕见的 GIST 亚群(不到总病例的 5%)没有 CD117 表达;这些亚群很可能依赖于另一种激酶,如突变的血小板衍生生长因子受体-α(PDGFRA)(见分子发病机制部分)[17]。少见的 CD117 阴性 GIST 的明确诊断需要借助于 DOG-1 鉴定[18]。DOG-1 是代表了在 GIST 发现的蛋白质,TMEM16A 或 anoctamin 1 蛋白,其功能是 Ca^{2+} 激活的氯离子通道蛋白[19]。DOG-1 已被发现在 98% 的 GIST 中呈阳性,特别是在那些 *PDGFRA* 突变且不表达 KIT 的人群中;它已成为许多病理科 GIST 诊断的标准。另一个有助于诊断 KIT 阴性的胃肠道间质瘤的标志物是 PKC-θ[20];在 KIT 阴性的胃肠道间质瘤中,96% 表达 PKC-θ。需要注意的是,在 KIT 阳性的胃肠道间质瘤中,DOG-1 和 PKC-θ 也有表达。因此,GIST 的诊断应基于形态学、临床病理学和免疫组织化学数据,如果其他病理学评估有任何歧义,也可进行分子检测(见分子发病机制部分)。CD117 阳性的 GIST 也有可能去分化,发生间变,并失去表达 CD117 的能力[21]。

评估 GIST 恶性行为的标准最初是基于 GIST 专科病理学家在美国国立癌症研究所(National Cancer Institute)会议上达成的共识[22]。这次共识会确定了原发性 GIST 的两个最可靠的预后因素:①原发肿瘤的大小;②反映细胞增殖活性的核分裂数[22]。现在认为其他因素对预后也非常重要,如肿瘤发生部位,胃的原发肿瘤比其他部位来源的预后好。此外,在切除前或切除过程中原发肿瘤发生穿孔的,预后很差[23,24]。除大小和有丝分裂外,还有一些因素,例如特殊的组织亚型[上皮样细胞和梭形细胞(见图 33.1 和图 33.2)]、细胞多形性程度和患者年龄,可能对预后有一些影响,但在决定临床结果方面的作用较小。

列线图(nomogram)和分期系统已发表用于评估初次切除后复发的风险[25,26]。由 Memorial Sloan Kettering 癌症中心的研究人员开发的 GIST 列线图,可以在线获得[25]。虽然很简单,但有人担心,与其他风险标准相比,分配给胃来源肿瘤的权重太高。Joensuu 及其同事开发的基于人群的疾病复发预测模型提供了最大的清晰度,因为肿瘤大小和有丝分裂计数是作为连续变量测量的;该模型还考虑了破裂的证据[26]。提倡使用简化的"5s 原则",其中,中-高风险胃 GIST 指肿瘤大于 5cm 且每 50 个高倍视野(high-power field,HPF)含 5 个以上的有丝分裂象,而中高风险非胃 GIST 指肿瘤直径大于 5cm 或每 50 个 HPF 有 5 个以上有丝分裂象[27]。

二、分子发病机制

1998 年,Hirota 及其同事的重要发现推动了 GIST 的分子发病机制的提出[28]。该小组研究 KIT 蛋白(CD117)在细胞生长和发育中的作用。在正常细胞信号转导中,KIT 与其配体肥大/干细胞因子(SCF)结合,导致 2 个 KIT 分子二聚化。形成的同源二聚体复合物导致 KIT 胞内结构域关键酪氨酸残基的交叉磷酸化,从而激活 KIT 下游的信号转导通路。正常情况下配体诱导的 KIT 活化产生的生理净效应是控制细胞增殖和提高细胞存活率,因此,失去调控的 KIT 激活理论上可能导致肿瘤生长和细胞的恶性转化。

Hirota 及其同事在细胞和分子水平上证实了 GIST 中存在 *KIT* 突变,并可导致小鼠模型中 GIST 的发生[28]。同一团队,在 Nishida 领导的一个项目中,也观察到家族性 GIST 患者中,存在 *KIT* 种系突变[29]。这项出色的工作证实 GIST 和 ICC 细胞之间的一些关键性生物相似性[30,31],因为这两种细胞都表达 CD117。GIST 和正常的 ICC 可能具有共同的前体细胞,可能是一种干细胞[13,30,31]。KIT 及其配体 SCF 在正常 ICC 以及其他细胞(包括黑素细胞、红细胞、生殖细胞和肥大细胞)的发育和维持中发挥重要作用。KIT 在绝大多数(>95%)的 GIST 中都有表达,但在胃肠道真正的平滑肌肿瘤(即平滑肌瘤和平滑肌肉瘤)或其他解剖位置的间质肿瘤(如子宫内膜间质瘤)中不表达。尽管 GIST 肿瘤细胞的起源仍在进一步研究中,一些数据表明 GIST 起源于位于肠壁内的 CD34 阳性干细胞,这些干细胞随后可向 ICC 表型不完全分化[30,31]。

最初由 Hirota 及其同事分析的 6 例人类 GIST 中,有 5 例存在 *KIT* 的活化突变[28],有证据表明这些突变导致不受调控的配体非依赖性 KIT 活化,或者 KIT 的组成型激活,导致受体在没有配体的情况下磷酸化。携带有突变过度活性 KIT 蛋白的基因工程细胞在裸鼠中具有致瘤性,这证明了 GIST 的恶性表型是由不受调控的配体非依赖性 KIT 活化相关的异常信号转导通路直接诱导的。

具有常染色体显性遗传模式和异常高的 GIST 发生率的家族性综合征(见家族性 GIST 部分)的鉴定也支持了突变体组成型激活 KIT 在人类 GIST 发病机制中的潜在致癌性,患病个体通常表现为多发病灶[29,32,33]。对这类患者亲属的遗传分析表明,它们具有种系激活的 *KIT* 突变,这与首次在散发性 GIST 病例中描述类似。

重要的是,大多数 GIST 最初表现为 *KIT* 基因单一位点的突变;还发现了其他多种基因和细胞遗传学改变,其中一些与侵袭性恶性行为有关[34,35]。最常见的功能突变是在 *KIT* 外显子 11,该外显子编码 KIT 的胞内膜旁结构域[36-41]。外显子 11 的某些突变导致出现终止密码子或缺失,预示着预后较差[41]。突变也可见于 *KIT* 外显子 9[38],激酶的胞外区,以及较少见的外显子 13 和 17(激酶结构域)[35-39],很少发生在外显子 8[40]。与那些寻求晚期疾病治疗的患者相比,原发肿瘤患者的突变分布有所不同(表 33.1)。

结构生物学研究揭示,正常(野生型)KIT 保持自身抑制构象,直到与它的配体 SCF 结合并导致 2 个 KIT 激酶二聚化。突变引起的蛋白质构象改变会干扰这种自抑制作用,并成为 KIT 激酶异常活化的结构基础[44,45]。正如后面将讨论的,甲磺酸伊马替尼[和其他一些酪氨酸激酶抑制剂(tyrosine kinase inhibitor,TKI)]可以阻止这些突变肿瘤中的这种异常激活和激酶活性。

表 33.1 新诊断的胃肠道间质瘤与转移性胃肠道间质瘤中特定 *KIT* 和 *PDGFRA* 突变频率的比较

	新诊断 GIST[42]	转移性 GIST[43]
GIST(*N*)	106	414
KIT 突变	67%	81%
外显子 8	未报道	<1%
外显子 11	53%	71%
外显子 9	9%	8%
外显子 13	4%	1%
外显子 17	1%	1%
PDGFRA 突变	16%	2%
外显子 12	2%	<1%
外显子 14	0%	0%
外显子 18	15%	2%
野生型 *KIT* 和 *PDGFRA*	17%	17%

GIST,胃肠道间质瘤;PDGFRA,血小板衍生生长因子受体-α。

对 GIST 的认识的另一个关键进展是发现是除 KIT 之外的其他不受调控的激酶信号也可以驱动 GIST 细胞的肿瘤表型。具体地说,现在已经认识到至少 10% 的 GIST 细胞具有相关激酶(称为 *PDGFRA*)的突变,最常见于外显子 18,但也出现在外显子 12(见表 33.1)[17,43]。家族性 GIST 病例中已鉴定出种系 *PDGFRA* 突变,在稍后讨论[46-48]。

即使在小的 GIST(最大径小于 1cm)中,也存在 *KIT* 和 *PDGFRA* 突变[49,50]。此类病变通常是被偶然发现(例如,因反流症状行胃镜检查时发现的胃或食管 GIST),并且可能在形态上表现为良性。这些发现支持以下假说:*KIT* 或 *PDGFRA* 原癌基因的活化突变代表了从正常前体细胞向 GIST 病变转化的早期事件。由于具有种系 *KIT* 或 *PDGFRA* 突变的家族性 GIST(见家族性 GIST 部分)可能要到 20~30 岁甚至更晚才出现临床表现,因此有可能需要二次打击才能获得更具侵袭性的恶性肿瘤表型。赋予 GIST 细胞更恶性表型的其他关键信号步骤仍然不清楚。然而目前人们正努力研究 GIST 特有的信号级联特征,它似乎不同于血液肿瘤中的 KIT 信号转导。例如,白血病细胞的 STAT5 途径通常不在 GIST 中被激活,而 STAT1 和 STAT3 则被高水平激活[36]。现在的共识是,KIT 基因型本身不能解释可能表现为惰性的 GIST(肿瘤小,仅通过切除即可治愈)与那些根据所有功能定义明显具有侵袭性和恶性的 GIST 之间的差异。仅凭分化好的良性细胞形态不能保证病变持续为良性。然而,小于 2cm 的胃 GIST 被认为是良性的,如果切除,则无需随访[51]。

大约 5%~10% 的 GIST 是野生型 *KIT* 和 *PDGFRA*(即这两个关键基因没有突变)[1]。许多这样的 GIST 被认为具有琥珀酸脱氢酶(SDH)蛋白的表达和功能缺失。SDH 蛋白是一个酶家族(SDH A、B、C 和 D),它们在线粒体壁上形成一个复合体,对细胞呼吸至关重要。有些患者存在 SDH 基因突变,有些患者存在SDHC启动子在内的基因高度甲基化,导致该蛋白表达和活性丧失。这些肿瘤可以通过肿瘤细胞中SDHB染色的缺失来识别;这些肿瘤也表达高水平的胰岛素样生长因子-1受体[52-57]。这类肿瘤现在被称为SDH缺陷型GIST;Carney三联征和Carney-Stratakis二联体(在家族性GIST一节中讨论)综合征的GIST就是具有这种肿瘤机制。这种形式的胃肠道间质瘤发生在胃,可能是多灶性的,并有淋巴结转移。肿瘤在女性中更常见,而且往往比典型的突变型GIST更早被诊断出来;儿童年龄组中的GIST大多数是SDH缺陷型。

在没有*KIT*和*PDGFRA*突变的患者中,一种罕见的突变涉及*BRAF*(编码丝氨酸/苏氨酸蛋白激酶B-raf)[35,58]。最近,还报道了包括成纤维细胞生长因子受体1和嗜神经酪氨酸受体激酶(NTRK)的其他可塑性突变[59]。

除了已经讨论过的基因和蛋白质外,其他基因、转录因子、microRNAs和通路也被报道在GIST的发病机制、生物行为、诊断和预后中发挥作用[60-77]。其中一些将无疑是重要的预后预测因素或未来的治疗靶点。对这些因素的详细讨论超出了本章的范畴。

三、分子药理学

*KIT*突变的发现提供了对GIST病理生物学的重要理解,并提供了一个有吸引力的治疗靶点。偶然的是,一种为完全不同的用途而研发的药物对KIT活性具有显著的抑制作用。这种分子靶向药物的最初概念来自针对BCR-ABL研发的小分子,BCR-ABL是慢性粒细胞白血病(chronic myeloid leukemia,CML)发病中重要的肿瘤蛋白靶点。诺华公司的Druker及其同事发现了一种2-苯基氨基嘧啶类小分子,该分子在体外对ABL和失调的BCR-ABL具有有效的抑制作用[78,79]。Druker和Buchdunger及其同时实验室的其他筛选研究表明,这种药物[信号转导抑制剂-571(signal transduction inhibitor-571,STI-571)]后来被称为甲磺酸伊马替尼(在美国为Gleevec,在其他地方为Glivec),也能有效抑制KIT和PDGFRA的酪氨酸激酶活性[80]。随后在具有与GIST相似的*KIT*突变的人类肥大细胞白血病细胞系中进行的研究发现,伊马替尼对野生型和突变KIT蛋白均有抑制作用[81]。在具有*KIT*激活突变的人类胃肠道间质瘤细胞系中测试伊马替尼的实验揭示了该药抗胃肠道间质瘤活性的明显证据。在培养的人类胃肠道间质瘤细胞中加入伊马替尼可迅速抑制KIT的活性,抑制细胞增殖,并诱导肿瘤细胞凋亡[82]。因此,从所有标准来看,伊马替尼的临床研发有望作为靶向GIST的基本分子发病机制的治疗药物。甲磺酸伊马替尼和其他酪氨酸受体激酶抑制剂治疗胃肠道间质瘤将在后面讨论。

四、流行病学

很难获得胃肠道间质瘤发病率的准确数据。这是因为转诊偏倚,即将预后更差、生物行为更恶性的GIST病例集中到学术癌症中心,以及在1998年及以后GIST分子定义出现之前缺乏明确的诊断技术。2000年以前,新发GIST病例数量是被低估和报道不全的。随着对GIST分子基础的了解和分子靶向药物的获得,该病的诊断准确性有所提高[83]。最近一项使用监测、流行病学和最终结果(Surveillance,Epidemiology,and End Result,SEER)数据库对2001年至2011年间诊断病例的研究发现,年龄调整后的发病率从2001年的0.55/100 000增加到了2011年的0.78/100 000。发病率随年龄增长而增加,在70~79岁年龄组最高,为3.06/100 000[84]。

据报道,男性的发病率略高于女性[84]。对因非肿瘤性疾病行胃切除术的手术标本的研究和尸检研究表明,隐匿性显微镜下胃肠道间质瘤病变的发病率很高,达20%~35%[85,86]。

五、临床特征

大多数胃肠道间质瘤(60%~70%)发生在胃部;20%~30%源于小肠,不到10%源于食管、结肠和直肠。胃肠道外的腹部或盆腔,如网膜、肠系膜或腹膜后,包括胰腺,也可发生胃肠道间质瘤[87-100];胃肠外间质瘤被称为E-GIST[16]。

胃肠道间质瘤患者的临床表现取决于原发病灶的解剖位置,以及其他因素,如肿瘤大小和有无症状性转移。对于许多胃肠道间质瘤患者来说,胃肠道间质瘤的最初发现可能是偶然的或在对非特异性症状的评估时发现。胃肠道间质瘤本身的症状通常仅在肿瘤大于5cm或累及特定解剖区域(例如,胃GIST导致胃出口梗阻)后出现。出现的症状可能包括可触及的腹部肿块或腹部肿胀、腹痛、恶心、呕吐、厌食和早饱。据报道,高达40%的GIST患者因肿瘤破裂出现急性出血进入胃肠道或腹腔;然而,这样的报告可能存在对大病灶或多发病灶患者的转诊偏倚。有些患者因长期失血而出现贫血。由于胃肠道间质瘤可能无法通过常规内镜检查进行识别,因此对消化内镜检查阴性的缺铁性贫血患者,应考虑腹盆腔影像学检查以确定出血来源(见第20章)。

绝大多数胃肠道间质瘤的转移,在出现症状或疾病复发时,都是在腹腔内的,转移到肝脏、大网膜或腹膜[88]。转移到淋巴结和其他区域很少见;影像学检查认为的淋巴结转移大多数仅代表大网膜或腹膜中肿瘤结节的转移性沉积,而不是真正的淋巴转移。晚期疾病的转移部位也包括肺和骨。胃肠道间质瘤可表达一种甲状腺激素失活酶(3型碘甲状腺原氨酸脱碘酶),可导致"消耗性"甲状腺功能减退,需要超正常剂量的甲状腺激素治疗[91]。

(一)食管肿瘤

GIST可以出现在食管,尽管少见较大病变[92-94]。大多数食管GIST病变都是因为一些不相关的症状或疾病,如反流性食管炎而行上消化道内镜检查时偶然发现的。食管GIST可能很小(只有几毫米大小),并且可以通过内镜切除[95]。如果病变未被怀疑为GIST并被认为是良性的,行内镜切除可能会有病变残留。目前尚不清楚等待观察和定期内镜随访是否适合所有病灶较小(最大径<1cm)的GIST患者。较大的食管

GIST 可能会穿孔[96]。在影像学上，与其他部位的 GIST 一样[92]；它们往往边界清晰，^{18}F-FDG 亲和力强，衰减低，呈局部扩散（如胸膜）或血液扩散（如肝脏）[94]。

如上所述，由于组织学不能完全预测 GIST 的恶性行为，因此组织病理学即使表现为良性的 GIST 细胞形态也不能令人放心。仔细的风险评估还包括肿瘤的其他方面，以及患者特异性因素（如年龄、合并症和患者偏好）。通过前瞻性研究积累与患者预后相关的大量客观数据库是很重要的，这样医学决策就可以建立在可靠证据的基础上。虽然小的食管 GIST 病变可能是单一的原发病变，但最好仔细记录家族史，并进行腹部和盆腔的 CT 检查，以确保不存在其他病变，特别是在年轻人首次发现这种疾病时。一些研究试图区分 GIST 患者和平滑肌肉瘤或其他间叶性肿瘤（如平滑肌瘤）患者的临床预后[92]。

（二）胃肿瘤

胃肠道间质瘤最常见的原发部位是胃（图 33.3 和图 33.4）。患者可以无症状，也可以表现为出血、疼痛或梗阻。内镜下观察到的大多数胃肠道间质瘤病变是黏膜下的，而不是黏膜的，表面没有溃疡。这就解释了为什么许多 GIST 肿块在内镜下只显示为细微、光滑的突起，表面黏膜正常[97]。同时，位于黏膜下层的病变难以通过内镜活检诊断。浅表活检常常只能取到正常黏膜，而深层活检或明确切除的组织病理学检查可以观察到真正的 GIST 细胞。超声内镜检查（EUS）的使用通常可以获得合适的采样和足够用于诊断的活检样本。

（三）十二指肠和空回肠肿瘤

GIST 的第二大常见部位是小肠[98,99]。在一项研究中，通过小肠胶囊内镜检查发现的小肠肿瘤约半数是 GIST[100,101]。

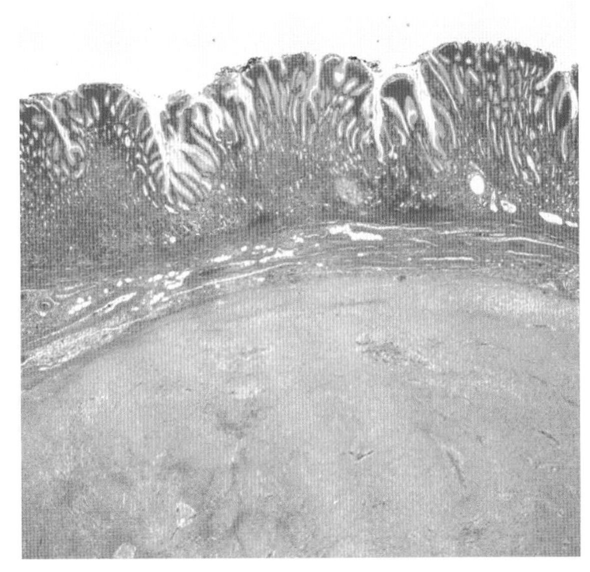

图 33.3　显微照片显示胃黏膜下胃肠道间质瘤的梭形细胞。病变界限清楚，不侵犯被覆的黏膜肌层。如黏膜肌层浸润被认为是不良预后的因素（HE 染色，×50）。（Courtesy Dr. Brian P. Rubin，Cleveland，OH.）

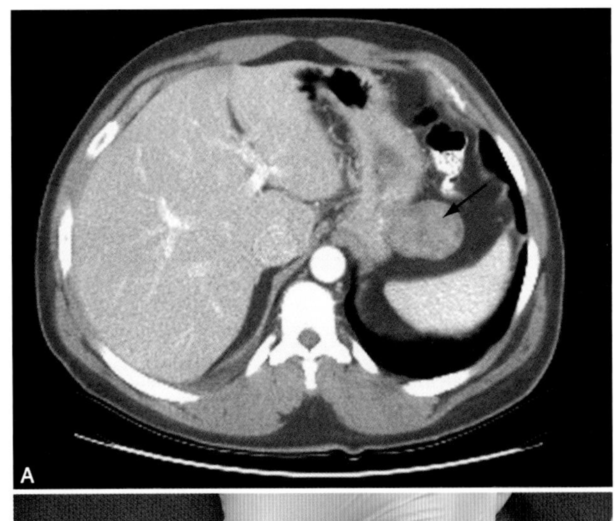

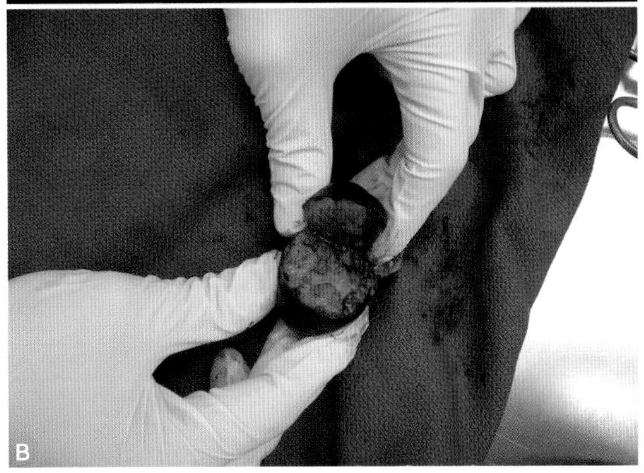

图 33.4　胃 GIST。A，CT 显示起源于胃大弯的 4～5cm 外生性胃肠间质瘤（箭头）。B，3.5cm×4.5cm×4cm 肿瘤切除切开后的大体照片。组织学显示梭形细胞胃 GIST，KIT（CD117）免疫反应阳性。（Courtesy Dr. Jay N. Yepuri and Dr. Christopher Bell，Dallas，TX）

小肠中的 GIST 主要发生在空肠，其次是回肠和十二指肠。由于临床表现和生物学行为的差异，更多的研究者现在将十二指肠 GIST 与其他小肠 GIST 分开。十二指肠 GIST 似乎比空肠 GIST 的预后好，即使切除更保守和有限（即不进行胰十二指肠切除术）[102-106]。小肠 GIST 病变通常明显大于原发于其他部位的 GIST。大的病变血管丰富，即使仅进行活检也存在显著的出血风险。由于完整的手术切除是 GIST 的首选治疗方法，因此对于是否需要进行术前活检或活检是否会给患者带来额外风险尚存在争议（下文将进一步讨论）。这是极具挑战性的问题，因为小肠 GIST 需要和其他伴小肠和肠系膜受累的腹部肿瘤相鉴别。指南建议，如果强烈怀疑胃肠道间质瘤，并且手术可以完成且没有显著的并发症风险，则可以在没有预先活检的情况下进行手术切除。如果只有导致严重功能障碍的根治性手术才能切除病变，那么考虑术前活检以确定胃肠道间质瘤的诊断并允许新辅助治疗（见下文）可能对患者最有益（见下文）。

（四）结肠和肛门直肠肿瘤

直肠和结肠 GIST 很少见，约占 GIST 病例的 5%，并且其诊疗独具挑战性[107-112]。与其他部位一样，直肠的小的 GIST

病变可能表现为直径小于 1cm 的小而硬的结节,在直肠指检或直肠镜检查中被偶然发现。然而,大的肿瘤表面可有溃疡,表现为急性或慢性出血,类似直肠腺癌。诊断可能具有挑战性,GIST 的上皮样细胞或混合细胞变异可能被误诊为腺癌,特别是小的活检可能受到严重的炎性变化或相关脓肿形成的影响而出现混淆。

六、诊断

一些专业组织已经制定了基于共识(并尽可能以证据为基础)的临床实践指南。国家综合癌症网络(National Comprehensive Cancer Network,NCCN)已经制定了广泛的可公开获取的指南,以帮助临床医生诊断和治疗胃肠道间质瘤患者。欧洲医学肿瘤学会(European Society of Medical Oncology,ESMO)也发布了专家主导的临床实践指南[113]。

疑似或确诊 GIST 病例的诊断评估与其他 GI 肿瘤的诊断评估相似。最重要的是要与其他消化道肿瘤以及位于腹盆腔的胃肠外肿瘤进行鉴别诊断。对于 GI 病变的评估,病变部位决定了使用哪种诊断工具最合适。内镜检查在胃、十二指肠、食管、结肠和肛门直肠 GIST 的诊断中起主要作用。胶囊内镜检查对于空肠和回肠 GIST 的诊断具有重要价值[100,101];双气囊小肠镜也可用于诊断小肠 GIST,尤其是伴出血的小肠 GIST[114]。

(一) 影像学

1. EUS

由于肿瘤位于黏膜下层,因此 EUS 是评估 GIST 的有用技术。EUS 显示 GIST 为邻近正常肠壁第四层(固有肌层)或第二层(黏膜肌层)的低回声肿块。一项研究显示,预测所谓良性胃肠道 GIST 的 EUS 特征为边缘规则,肿瘤大小≤3cm,回声均匀[115]。多因素分析显示囊性腔隙和不规则边缘的存在是恶性潜能的独立预测因素。另一项研究显示肿瘤大小超过 4cm、腔外边缘不规则、强回声灶大于 3mm,囊性腔隙大于 4mm 是 GIST 恶性行为表现的相关因素[116]。

2. CT 和 MRI

CT 是对胃部原发病灶进行成像的最有效方法,因为口服造影会勾勒出肿块和胃增厚(见图 33.4)。对胃扩张不足的鉴别诊断有一定难度,尤其是在监测术后复发时。CT 对疾病的分期也很重要。对于可测量的胃肠道间质瘤,采集 CT 平扫图像,以及在静脉注射造影剂后评估早期和晚期图像特别有用。由于胃壁和周围组织的运动无法控制,常规 MRI 对胃 GIST 的显示不如 CT。然而,MRI 的弥散加权成像可能与 PET/CT 相当[117]。MRI 可用于评估肝转移,因为一些 GIST 病灶与正常组织完全等密度,在 CT 上与周围的肝实质无法分辨,因此观察不到。

基线 CT 成像对于 GIST 患者很重要,因为内镜检测可能只显示了肿瘤的一小部分。此外,可以定性地解释成像模式,以用肿瘤大小以外的指标评估靶向治疗的影响[118,119]。激酶抑制剂的治疗效果可表现为 CT 上肿瘤密度的降低,即使病灶大小没有变化(CHOI 标准);CT 上的低密度病变与 FDG-PET 成像上的代谢活性的丧失相关[119]。

3. PET/CT

GIST 影像诊断中最有效的方法之一是使用^{18}F-氟脱氧葡萄糖(^{18}F-FDG)PET 扫描,对常规解剖成像作信息补充(图 33.5)。虽然 CT 或 MRI 可以准确评估 GIST 病变的大小,但^{18}F-FDG PET 对 GIST 的功能成像可以提供有效的附加信息,帮助临床医生处理 GIST 患者。引起 GIST 对^{18}F-FDG 示踪剂高水平亲和力的机制可能是通过过度活化的 KIT、RTK 和葡萄糖转运蛋白(如 GLUT4)信号通路[120]。在治疗过程中,细胞活力和葡萄糖摄取减少与 GLUT4 表达减少相关,因此解释了与药物抑制 KIT 信号通路有关的 PET 成像的快速变化[121,122]。体积较大的 GIST 在 CT 或 MRI 上主要表现为中央囊性或低衰减特征。通过^{18}F-FDGPET 扫描可以清楚地看出,大的 GIST 肿块的内部表现为代谢静止,这可能是由于肿瘤中心部位的坏死所致。尽管 GIST 病变是血供丰富的,但肿瘤内部仍然可以表现为坏死物质的混合肿块,而 GIST 更有活力的部分向病变边缘推出。^{18}F-FDG PET 系列成像中的许多附加信息也可以通过 CT 对肿瘤密度的定性评估来获得[119]。然而,有时大网膜中的转移性 GIST 病灶可能很细微,在 CT 上很容易被忽略,因为小的病灶可能会混入肠壁的褶皱中,即使是最有经验的放射科医生也很难发现。^{18}F-FDG PET 成像可以毫无困难地检测到约 1cm 或更大的病变,因为正常的肠和大网膜都不会过度吸收^{18}F-FDG 示踪剂。然而,国家指南并不鼓励常规使用 FGD-PET 成像。

4. 生长抑素受体显像

生长抑素受体显像对胃肠道和胰腺神经内分泌肿瘤的诊断很有价值(见下一章)。最近的研究显示生长抑素受体(SSTR1 和 SSTR2)在大多数 GIST 中表达,在使用生长抑素受体显像检测的患者中,有一半可以观察到肿瘤(参见第 34 章)[123]。这一发现可能允许肽受体介导的放射治疗在未来用于部分 GIST 患者,但到目前为止还没有进行评估。

(二) 活检

如前所述,GIST 具有丰富的血供,这可能给内镜活检带来不可接受的风险。另外,即使仅使用 FNA 技术,经皮活检也可能会增加肿瘤破裂和肿瘤细胞沿活检孔道播散或通过腹膜或肠系膜播散的风险。为了最大限度地降低患者的风险,许多外科医生建议,如果计划手术切除,则不要进行术前活检。但对无法切除的 GIST,必须进行活检以明确诊断,并为术前(新辅助)给予伊马替尼治疗提供证据(后面讨论)。此外,对胃 GIST 患者行超声引导下的 FNA 活检[124],或者黏膜切口辅助活检[125],都可以进行确诊,并且是安全的。对于出现转移性病灶的患者,活检有利于确定诊断并开始全身治疗。

(三) 鉴别诊断

GIST 最初被描述为单一形态的梭形细胞肿瘤。然而,现已明确,GIST 可以表现出多种组织学形态,从具有大圆细胞的上皮样形态(见图 33.2)到梭形细胞形态(见图 33.1),以及具有混合组织学形态的病变。梭形细胞 GIST 最为常见,约占 70%。上皮样细胞或圆形细胞 GIST 占其余 30% 中的大部分,并且可能含有梭形细胞的混合成分。上皮样 GIST 以前被诊断为平滑肌母细胞瘤,有些可能被误诊为低分化癌。

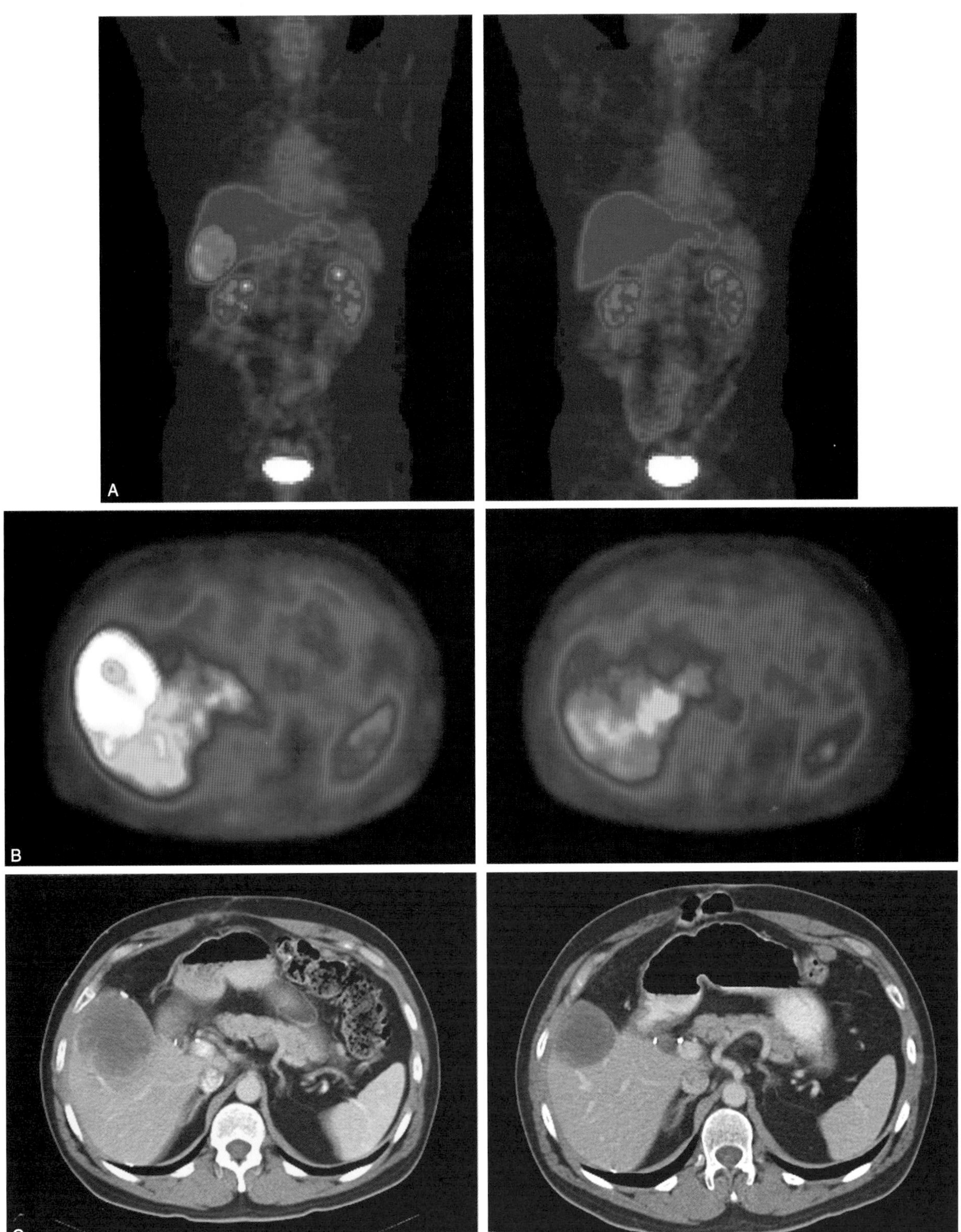

图 33.5　转移性 GIST。甲磺酸伊马替尼治疗前（左）和治疗后（右）。1 例胃肠间质瘤肝转移患者的 PET（A，B）和 CT（C）检查。治疗后可见肿瘤部分消退，^{18}F-FDG 摄取减少。（Courtesy Dr. A. Van den Abbeele, Boston, MA; and modified from Demetri GD, Benjamin RS, Blanke CD, et al. NCCN Task Force report: management of patients with gastrointestinal stromal tumor［GIST］—update of the NCCN clinical practice guidelines. J Natl Compr Canc Netw. 2007; 5［Suppl 2］: S1-S29.）

起源于间叶细胞的胃肠道肿瘤的鉴别诊断包括胃肠道间质瘤（80%），但也有真正的胃肠道平滑肌肿瘤，包括真正的平滑肌瘤和平滑肌肉瘤（约 15%）以及神经鞘瘤（约 5%）。CT 表现有助于帮助鉴别小的胃 GIST 和胃神经鞘瘤；而且，在连续 CT 随访时，胃 GIST 的生长速度往往比神经鞘瘤更快[126]。如上所述，KIT 的表达不限于 GIST 细胞。正常 ICC 和肥大细胞均表达 CD117，其正常生长和发育有赖于 KIT 进行。数量相对有限的其他一些肿瘤，也可能表达 CD117 且免疫组化可检测得到。这些肿瘤包括软组织肉瘤的某些亚群，包括尤因肉瘤和血管肉瘤，以及其他肿瘤，如偶发的小细胞肺癌、黑素瘤、硬纤维瘤、精原细胞瘤、卵巢癌、肥大细胞瘤、神经母细胞瘤、腺样囊性癌以及一些罕见的淋巴瘤和急性髓性白血病亚型[127-130]。需要注意的是，CD117 抗原的表达并不意味着 KIT 靶点的激活，也不一定与任何 *KIT* 基因突变相关。具有正常（野生型）*KIT* 基因的细胞与 *KIT* 突变活化细胞表达相同的 CD117 抗原。此外，KIT 蛋白的表达并不一定意味着该蛋白参与了某特定肿瘤的发生。

七、治疗

（一）原发性局部疾病（早期疾病）

1. 外科手术

专业的外科手术仍然是原发性局限性 GIST（早期 GIST）患者的主要治疗手段。原发灶手术切除时应当考虑到疾病本身的生长和行为特征。GIST 很少侵犯区域淋巴结，也很少有广泛的淋巴结探查或切除的指征。GIST 病变血管丰富且常有易破的假包膜，因此，外科医生应尽量减少肿瘤破裂的风险，否则可能会使腹膜播散的风险增加。外科病理学医生对肿瘤标本的切缘应仔细定位和检查，并对肿瘤不同部位进行取材和评估。腹腔镜[131-135]和内镜[136,137]切除术越来越多地被采用，且效果良好。

一些转诊机构对早期原发性 GIST 的自然病程进行了单中心的研究。这些研究必然存在选择偏倚，并且在这个不断发展的领域中，显然许多早期 GIST 患者可能由包括消化科和普外科在内的多个专科医生进行了诊疗。Memorial Sloan-Kettering 癌症中心对 200 名患者进行了前瞻性的随访[88]；其中 80 名（40%）原发性 GIST 患者接受了完整手术切除。结果显示 5 年疾病特异性生存率仅为 54%，这证明了这样一个事实，即使在这样的学术性转诊中心，GIST 可能有很高的复发风险，并最终危及生命。多因素分析显示，肿瘤大（>10cm）是降低疾病特异性生存率的唯一因素。原发肿瘤的解剖学部位似乎也是原发性局限性 GIST 的重要预后因素[90]。如前所述，小肠 GIST 的预后比胃 GIST 差；结肠/直肠 GIST 和 E-GIST 罕见，预后最差。

小肠 GIST 的预后与切除是否充分有关[88,138]。多数局限性或局部进展期的病灶可以完全切除，这些患者的中位总生存期超过 5 年。接受完整切除的患者的 5 年整体生存率远高于不能完整切除病变的患者。

直肠和直肠周围部位的 GIST 与小肠 GIST 类似；应选择创伤小且能使微小 GIST（<1cm）获得阴性切缘的手术方式。然而，许多直肠 GIST 的手术切除难度大，特别是如果没有事先行新辅助治疗，手术可能仅在有明显功能异常的情况下进行。

由于现在对晚期 GIST 有有效的治疗方法（伊马替尼，后面讨论），因此对所有术后 GIST 患者进行定期随访监测是非常必要的。通过这种方式，任何复发性疾病都可以在第一时间被发现并给予治疗，从而有望避免由于肿瘤复发体积增大而引起的并发症（如肿瘤出血）。

2. 辅助放射治疗

只有少数病例报告和小规模研究探讨使用常规方案进行辅助治疗的作用，例如早期 GIST 手术切除后的放疗。放射治疗在 GIST 的辅助治疗中似乎作用不大，部分原因是考虑到对小肠和其他腹腔脏器的毒性，放射治疗无法给予有效剂量。还有一小部分患者接受了全身或腹腔内辅助化疗，这些数据尚未发现任何明显的益处。因此，在使用伊马替尼之前，对原发 GIST 完整切除术后的标准治疗仅仅是观察随访。

3. 伊马替尼辅助治疗

现已明确，在 GIST 切除术后（辅助）给予伊马替尼治疗可延迟肿瘤复发，尤其是对于肿瘤体积大且有很高复发和转移风险的患者[139-144]。辅助治疗患者的风险分层通常不使用 AJCC 分期系统，利用前面讨论过的 GIST 列线图、基于人群的疾病复发预测模型或 5s 原则来评估具有中高复发风险的肿瘤[25-27]。

几个大型多中心试验研究了辅助应用伊马替尼在胃肠道间质瘤患者中的效果[139-144]。在美国外科肿瘤学会（American College of Surgical Oncology Group，ACOSOG）开展的第一个随机辅助试验 Z9001 中，伊马替尼（或安慰剂）的使用时间为 1 年。与安慰剂相比，在原发性局限性胃肠道间质瘤切除后应用伊马替尼显著延长了无复发生存期（1 年无复发的比率分别为 98% 和 83%；风险比为 0.35），尽管没有发现总体的生存益处[139]。ACOSOG 试验招募了任何大小的胃肠道间质瘤患者。根据肿瘤的大小（即 3~6cm、6~10cm 和 10cm 或更大）对治疗受益程度进行分析发现，虽然在所有组中都有数值上的改善，但仅在大于 10cm 的肿瘤中才有统计学意义。欧洲癌症研究和治疗组织（European Organization for the Research and Treatment of Cancer，EORTC）比较了 2 年的辅助治疗与没有辅助治疗的结果，最初以总生存期作为主要研究终点[141]。后来发现，这项试验可能需要十多年才能得到结果，因此将研究终点改为出现伊马替尼耐药的时间。服用伊马替尼 2 年并出现疾病进展的患者被允许重新开始伊马替尼治疗，而安慰剂组中出现进展的患者则开始治疗。两组对伊马替尼耐药的时间无统计学差异。在斯堪的纳维亚试验中[142,143]，免疫染色检测 KIT 阳性，由于其大小、有丝分裂比例和/或出现肿瘤破裂而术后复发风险高的 GIST 患者，随机接受甲磺酸伊马替尼（400mg/d）辅助治疗 1 年或 3 年，从术后 1~12 周开始。伊马替尼治疗 3 年的总体生存率明显优于仅治疗 1 年的患者（91.9% vs 85.3%，HR，0.6，$P=0.036$），但常由于不良反应或患者偏好，3 年组的伊马替尼停药率较高。该试验证明了接受辅助治疗的患者有生存优势[142,143]。PERSIST-5 研究是一项Ⅱ期单臂研究，纳入了高危胃肠间质瘤患者，其定义为原发性胃肠间质瘤（任意部位）≥2cm 且有丝分裂计数≥5/50HPF 或非胃原发性胃肠间质瘤≥5cm[144]。伊马替尼在 5 年的试验期内保持了其有效性。伊马替尼的辅助治疗效果是显而易见的，值得对所有的 GIST 切除术后，根据目前的风险分类系统评估存在中重度复发的风险的患者的用药风险和益处进行充分的讨论[22,25,26]。指南建议至少治疗 3 年。目前正在进行研究，以评估更长期治疗的益处。

4. 新辅助治疗

随着高效药物治疗的出现，目前的指南建议，只有当手术引起的功能障碍或并发症风险较小的情况下，才首选外科手术治疗。对于较大的GIST，且有围手术期并发症的风险，应考虑新辅助（术前）伊马替尼治疗。在这种情况下，在开始治疗之前需要行组织活检；这种诊断性活检可能因组织太小而不能用于详细的风险评估，但应该可以满足分子检测所需。试验表明，这种新辅助用药可以有效缩小肿瘤体积，从而提高手术疗效[145-147]。在这种情况下，^{18}F-FDG PET扫描可以对治疗效果进行早期评估，从而将疾病进展的风险降至最低，否则可能会使患者面临无法切除的风险。在伊马替尼的效果达到最大后（中位时间为6个月或更长），可以进行手术治疗。对于这类患者，也建议术后伊马替尼辅助治疗，总疗程至少3年。

（二）进展期疾病（晚期疾病）

1. 全身和局部化疗、放疗和减瘤手术

医学肿瘤学家曾经指出，胃肠道的"平滑肌肉瘤"比发生在身体其他部位（如子宫）的平滑肌肉瘤预后更差。胃肠道的"平滑肌肉瘤"对标准化疗方案的耐药性更强；这些"平滑肌肉瘤"被证明主要代表胃肠道间质瘤。对接受常规细胞毒性化疗的晚期GIST患者的研究显示，各种化疗药物的客观抗肿瘤反应率一般为0~4%，益处甚微[1,148]。一些研究者试图通过腹腔给药途径来改善化疗的这些令人沮丧的结果[149]。然而，由于GIST很少局限于腹膜表面，可以通过血行转移到肝脏和其他腹腔内部位，而且GIST的大多数危及生命的并发症都来自肝脏受累或累及大网膜的巨大肿块，因此这种腹膜内给药方法并不特别有希望。基于这些令人失望的结果，传统的细胞毒性化疗被认为对GIST患者无效。GIST对化疗表现出高度耐药性，部分原因可能是P-糖蛋白（*MDR*-1的产物）表达增加。研究表明，GIST的P-糖蛋白表达水平高于平滑肌肉瘤[150]。这些细胞外排泵阻止某些类型的化疗药在靶向GIST肿瘤细胞中达到有效的细胞内浓度。

单中心的数据显示转移性GIST可以通过局部外科或介入放射技术在有限时间内得到控制，如肝切除[151]、肝动脉栓塞/化疗栓塞[152]、或射频消融[153]。尽管有一部分累及肝脏的转移性GIST患者在化疗栓塞后表现出抗肿瘤反应和有限的无进展生存期（progression-free survival，PFS），但获益通常以月而非年计算。这些手段现在被用作其他系统治疗的辅助方法[154,155]。

减瘤手术在某些转移性GIST患者中具有有限的作用。如果患者出现累及肝脏和腹膜表面的转移性疾病，一线治疗是TKI。一旦疾病对TKI有反应，减瘤手术的作用就是通过消除含有耐药克隆的肿瘤，可能延长疾病控制时间，而伊马替尼的PFS与肿瘤大小相关[156]。EORTC开展了一项试验来验证这一假设，在该试验中，患者被随机分为持续伊马替尼治疗组和持续伊马替尼治疗的肿瘤切除组，主要研究终点为PFS。可惜这项研究进展不佳，提前终止。

来自几个机构的大规模研究报道了疾病进展期患者接受TKI治疗时给予有限肿瘤切除的益处[157-161]。大多数报道了接受伊马替尼治疗的患者的结果。尽管使用舒尼替尼进行手术是可行的，但由于舒尼替尼以血管内皮生长因子受体为靶点，导致出血和伤口并发症的风险增加，手术前需要停药2周或更长时间[158]。在伊马替尼治疗进展性疾病的情况下，切除的孤立进展性疾病的患者在接受伊马替尼治疗后可以多活大约1年。对于弥漫进展的病变，手术作用有限，调整全身治疗可能对患者更有利。

放射治疗在转移性GIST患者的治疗中作用有限。在一定程度上是因为将治疗剂量的射线照射到肝脏或胃肠道时通常是弊大于利。然而，在晚期疾病伴有疼痛性骨转移或肿瘤出血的情况下，放射治疗可以起到姑息治疗的作用[162]。

显然，对于转移性或不可切除的GIST患者，在分子靶向治疗出现之前，预后是很差的。对于转移性或复发性GIST或GI肉瘤患者（其中大多数可能是真正的GIST），在采用激酶抑制靶向治疗之前的大多数研究都记录了生存率低，疾病进展导致的致命结果通常发生在首次复发或转移后1~2年[88]。

2. 甲磺酸伊马替尼

伊马替尼作为GIST的分子靶向治疗在全球范围内的合作临床开发进展迅速。2000年，对一名晚期、接受过大量的前期治疗和广泛转移的胃肠道间质瘤患者进行了单患者试点研究。该患者对伊马替尼的反应迅速，持续临床受益近3年[163]。基于该患者的显著而持久的受益，以及惊人的科学依据和强大的临床前数据，开始了伊马替尼治疗胃肠道间质瘤的其他研究。由EORTC肉瘤小组发起的一项剂量探索研究主要招募了GIST患者[164]。据报道，伊马替尼的最大耐受剂量为800mg/d（每天两次给药400mg）；在每天给药1 000mg（每天两次给药500mg）的高剂量水平下，出现了不可接受的严重的剂量限制性毒性，如恶心、呕吐和严重水肿。一项多中心的美国-芬兰合作研究将147名转移性胃肠间质瘤患者随机分为两种剂量水平（每天400mg或每天两次300mg）[121]。两种剂量水平之间的应答率或疾病控制持续时间似乎没有差异，但该研究没有足够的统计学效力证实有无差异。EORTC小组继续在GIST和其他形式的肉瘤中扩大对伊马替尼的研究。在该试验中，再次证实了对GIST的高水平抗肿瘤效果，而对于其他形式的软组织肉瘤患者则没有明显的益处[165]。这些完全独立的试验，其结果非常一致（表33.2）。这些数据支持以下假说：对GIST细胞生长和存活的关键分子驱动因素的*KIT*和*PDGFRA*突变的靶向治疗，可以带来有意义的治疗益处。如果没有这种抑制靶点（如在肉瘤中），伊马替尼治疗就没有明显的抗癌活性。

表33.2 转移性或不可切除的胃肠道间质瘤患者对伊马替尼的抗肿瘤反应

参考文献	GIST/*N*	伊马替尼剂量/（mg/d）	CR/%	PR/%	DSD
164	36	400~1 000	0	53	17
121	147	400或600	0	54	28
167	946	400 vs 800	5	47	32
166	746	400 vs 800	4	41	23

在这些研究中，不同剂量的抗肿瘤反应无显著差异。CR，完全缓解；DSD，持久稳定疾病；GIST，胃肠道间质瘤；PR，部分缓解。

在由西南癌症组织(SWOG)和EORTC同时设计和开展的两项大型试验中,进一步评估了伊马替尼对晚期不可切除GIST的最佳剂量[166,167]。这些研究纳入了1 700名患者,足以明确每天两次400mg(与每天一次400mg相比)是否会带来显著的临床益处,从改善应答率、PFS(SWOG试验)或生存率(EORTC试验)方面进行评估。此外,低剂量组的进展期患者允许转到高剂量组。两项研究均没有证实这两个剂量水平的生存差异。尽管SWOG研究仅显示了高剂量伊马替尼组患者在疾病控制持续时间方面呈现有利趋势,欧洲的研究显示高剂量组在PFS方面具有一些统计学意义上的受益。在一项联合荟萃分析中,高剂量伊马替尼的受益仅限于相对较少的GIST患者,这些患者的肿瘤含有*KIT*外显子9的突变,该突变编码促进激酶分子二聚化的细胞外KIT结构域[166]。因此一些专家建议,对存在*KIT*外显子9突变的患者,使用较高剂量伊马替尼作为晚期胃肠道间质瘤患者的一线治疗。然而,由此带来的获益应该与额外的药物毒性进行权衡,因为更高剂量的伊马替尼与更大的不良反应发生率相关,并导致更多因毒性导致的药物减量。可以通过以400mg/d开始治疗,1~2个月后增加至每天两次来缓解药物毒性的增加;在由低剂量转换到较高剂量400mg每天两次的患者中,药物毒性副作用的发生率较低[167]。

美国和欧洲的这些试验结果证实了伊马替尼在控制转移性胃肠道间质瘤方面的有效性,客观应答率为45%~53%,与历史对照相比,可以控制症状并延长生存期。客观应答的中位时间是3个月以上,也有一些患者在开始口服伊马替尼后的一周内就出现了显著的疾病消退。在两项研究中,伊马替尼总体耐受性良好。基于这些试验,美国食品药品管理局(FDA)于2002年批准使用伊马替尼治疗转移性或不可切除的胃肠道间质瘤。此后,欧洲和世界其他地区也很快批准了该药物。

相关的分子研究是与美国-芬兰试验以及SWOG和EORTC进行的Ⅲ期试验一起进行的[43,168]。这些研究根据胃肠道间质瘤的基因型记录了伊马替尼治疗效果的差异。具体地说,GIST含有外显子11(最常见的分子亚型)*KIT*突变的患者比具有*KIT*外显子9突变或没有检测到*KIT*突变的患者有更高的客观应答率和更持久的疾病控制率。对Ⅲ期SWOG和EORTC研究的荟萃分析显示,在*KIT*外显子9突变患者中,起始给予400mg每日两次治疗对PFS有益,尽管总体生存没有差异,也可能支持在疾病进展的情况下,将药物剂量从400mg增加到每日两次400mg[169]。伊马替尼敏感的*PDGFRA*突变患者也可以受益,除了那些存在D842V突变且对已批准的激酶无效的患者[17,43,168]。

伊马替尼在晚期胃肠道间质瘤中的研究一致报道了伊马替尼的总体耐受性[121,164,166,167]。幸运的是,当KIT功能被伊马替尼治疗阻断时,依赖于KIT受体的正常受体-配体信号的正常生理过程(如造血)不会因此而受影响并导致致命后果。伊马替尼的副作用通常较轻(1级或2级),包括水肿,尤其是在面部眶周区域的疏松皮下组织,以及腹泻、肌痛或肌肉骨骼疼痛、皮疹和头痛。与使用伊马替尼治疗的慢性粒细胞白血病患者相比,GIST患者的骨髓毒性要少得多。尽管如此,接受伊马替尼治疗的胃肠道间质瘤患者偶尔会出现严重的血细胞减少;对于这种风险,应该对患者进行严密监测。在伊马替尼治疗晚期胃肠道间质瘤患者中,最令人担忧的不良事件是腹部或胃肠道出血,见于约5%的患者,主要与巨大肿块出血有关;出血被认为是由伊马替尼的强效快速抗肿瘤作用引起的。对于伊马替尼产生毒性的患者,减少剂量可以降低毒性并可以继续治疗。

伊马替尼治疗的大多数副作用会随着时间的推移而减轻,这表明可能存在某种快速防御机制[170]。例如,与伊马替尼治疗GIST相关的水肿通常会随着用药时间延长而改善,尽管合理使用利尿剂通常能有效地控制这种副作用。建议GIST患者使用低盐饮食也有助于控制这种副作用。伊马替尼引起的恶心通常是轻微的,并且是自限性的。应建议患者坚持低脂饮食,并且每天喝一大杯水;如果症状严重,可以使用止吐药。腹泻通常根据需要用止泻药治疗。肌肉痉挛,经常发生在小腿,一般是短时性和自限性的,通常通过增加液体和电解质的摄入量来缓解。

在功能性PET成像中,伊马替尼能够迅速而显著地导致肿瘤的^{18}F-FDG示踪剂摄取减少(见图33.5)[120]。单剂伊马替尼治疗后24小时就可以检测到肿瘤中^{18}F-FDG的减少。在反映伊马替尼的有效应答和记录在少数对于伊马替尼原发耐药的患者中的疾病进展方面,PET的结果都是高度可靠的。这些数据表明,GIST的^{18}F-FDG PET扫描功能成像是评估伊马替尼治疗早期应答的一种有效诊断方法。然而,鉴于辐射暴露的增加以及与使用PET相关的更高成本,并不建议将PET作为监测治疗效果的标准影像学方法。

根据现有证据,伊马替尼治疗转移性胃肠道间质瘤的最佳疗程为终身治疗[171,172]。法国肉瘤组织的一项随机研究测试了在病情稳定或在治疗1年、3年或5年后有应答的GIST患者中停止伊马替尼治疗的影响。发现停用伊马替尼与疾病快速复发有关。转移性疾病的最佳管理方案需要肿瘤内科医生、外科医生、放射科医生和核医学影像专家密切合作,以确定适合这些患者的最佳诊疗方案[173]。

对伊马替尼的耐药性可以是原发性的,表现为使用伊马替尼期间疾病的快速进展;然而,原发性伊马替尼耐药相对少见,已发现主要与PDGFRA D842V和其他非伊马替尼敏感的肿瘤驱动因子有关(见表33.2)[43]。此外,由于GIST的克隆进化,伊马替尼耐药性可能在持续应答1年或2年后出现[174]。这种继发性伊马替尼耐药机制在GIST中与在伊马替尼耐药的CML中大致相似[175]。

3. 苹果酸舒尼替尼

舒尼替尼可抑制多种受体酪氨酸激酶,包括:KIT、血小板衍生生长因子受体α和β;VEGF受体1、2和3;FMS样酪氨酸激酶-3受体(FLT 3);巨噬细胞集落刺激因子受体(CSF-1R)和胶质细胞源性神经营养因子受体(RET,在转染过程中重排)[176]。在Ⅰ期临床试验中,舒尼替尼显示了在胃肠道间质瘤中的抗肿瘤活性[176]。该项研究测试了几种剂量和方案,选择了50mg口服,为期28天,停药14天的疗程方案。纳入舒尼替尼Ⅰ期及后续Ⅱ期临床试验的患者大部分是伊马替尼难治性患者,并伴广泛转移。PET扫描显示舒尼替尼治疗4周期间出现了代谢降低,但在2周停药(洗脱)期间代谢活性重新激活。与伊马替尼相似,CT扫描反应发展更慢。早期试验和关键的安慰剂对照的Ⅲ期试验的应答数据非常相似，没有完全应答，部分应答率为 7%～13%[176-178]。早期研究中，肿瘤进展的中位时间为 7.8 个月，中位生存期为 19.8 个月。

在使舒尼替尼获得监管机构批准的Ⅲ期试验中，312 名因耐药或药物不耐受而导致伊马替尼治疗失败的转移性或手术无法切除的 GIST 患者被随机分为两组，接受舒尼替尼 50mg/d（$n=207$）或安慰剂（$n=105$），方案为 4 周给药，然后停药 2 周[177,178]。该研究的主要终点是通过进展时间（TTP）评估疾病的控制情况。由于计划内的中期疗效分析显示舒尼替尼与安慰剂相比中位 TTP 显著改善 4 倍以上时，该试验提前揭盲。接受舒尼替尼治疗患者的 PFS 明显高于接受安慰剂治疗的患者（舒尼替尼 24.1 周，安慰剂 6.0 周，危险比为 0.335，$P=0.0001$）。在最初的分析中，舒尼替尼还显著提高了总体生存率（风险比，0.49）；在中期分析时，接受舒尼替尼治疗组尚未达到中位总体生存期。在最终分析中，TTP 与中期分析的结果相似（6.7 个月 vs 1.6 个月）。尽管研究采用了交叉设计（18.2 个月 vs 16.2 个月），87% 被分配到安慰剂组的患者接受了开放标签的舒尼替尼治疗，初始接受舒尼替尼治疗组患者的总体生存期也是延长的。

对来自Ⅰ期和Ⅱ期临床试验的 GIST 样本的分子分析表明，在伊马替尼耐药的 GIST 患者中，KIT 的原发性和继发性突变影响舒尼替尼的治疗结果；PDGFRA 突变患者数量不足限制了对该部分患者的评估[179]。与外显子 11 突变患者相比，对伊马替尼不太敏感的突变患者（如 *KIT* 外显子 9 和野生型 KIT）更常出现应答和临床获益。TTP 时间最长的是肿瘤中含有 *KIT* 外显子 9 突变的患者，其次是野生型 *KIT*，外显子 11 突变，最差的是同时含有外显子 11 突变和新突变的肿瘤。*KIT* 外显子 9 突变和野生型的患者总体存活期最长。这并不表明舒尼替尼在外显子 11 肿瘤中是无活性的；相反，它代表了这样一个事实，即外显子 11 突变的患者在伊马替尼治疗期间产生了耐药性出现疾病进展，通常会有其他的突变克隆。进一步的研究表明，涉及 *KIT* 外显子 13 或 14 的继发性突变对舒尼替尼敏感，而外显子 17 和 18 的继发性突变往往对舒尼替尼耐药[179,180]。对这些突变激酶的结构生物学分析解释了当突变编码某些氨基酸变化导致对伊马替尼的结合和抑制作用产生空间位阻时，舒尼替尼如何抑制激酶功能[181]。

对于一些患者来说，中断 2 周治疗的方案伴随着疾病相关症状的复燃。然而，舒尼替尼治疗需要通过中断剂量来控制副作用。胃肠道间质瘤患者最常见的 3 级和 4 级舒尼替尼毒性包括疲劳、无症状血清脂肪酶和淀粉酶升高以及高血压[176-178]。其他副作用包括恶心、腹泻、口腔炎、手足综合征、贫血和皮肤变色。当患者使用该药物时，肿瘤活检部位也可能出血。服用舒尼替尼的患者皮肤异常的发生率也更高，包括掌足红斑感觉异常（手足综合征）和口腔黏膜刺激。此外，一些有冠状动脉疾病史的患者出现了无症状的心肌酶升高。某些患者也可能出现心功能异常，通常在舒尼替尼停药后逆转[182]。甲状腺功能减退症也有报道，须在治疗过程中监测甲状腺功能[183]。

在 GIST 患者中进行了一项舒尼替尼的Ⅱ期临床试验，连续每日低剂量给药[184]。该方案旨在减轻药物相关的副作用，控制在 2 周停药间期出现疾病相关症状。该研究证明了以每日 37.5mg 舒尼替尼起始剂量治疗的其安全性和耐受性。毒性类型与其他治疗方案相似，但低剂量的毒力更小，可以连续给药。有人建议用每日给药方案来长期控制疾病。大多数医生都倾向于这种方案。

因此，作为二线治疗，舒尼替尼对伊马替尼耐药的 GIST 似乎具有独特的治疗活性，但对其他激酶信号通路的强大抑制可导致更多的不良反应，需要密切监测并适当调整剂量。

4. 瑞戈非尼

最近批准的药物是瑞戈非尼。它有多个靶点，包括 KIT、血小板衍生生长因子受体、血管内皮生长因子受体 1-R3、TIE2、RET、成纤维细胞生长因子受体 1、RAF 和 p38 丝裂原激活蛋白激酶[185,186]。GIST 的初期Ⅱ期临床试验显示应答率为 17.6%，临床受益率为 76%，定义为≥16 周有客观应答或病情稳定。此外，中位 PFS 为 13.2 个月[185,186]。

这些引人注目的Ⅱ期临床研究数据带动了 GRID 研究，这是一项国际双盲Ⅲ期临床试验，使用与Ⅱ期临床研究中相同的入组标准，对瑞戈非尼和安慰剂进行比较[187]。该试验以 2∶1的方式将 199 名患者随机分为瑞戈非尼治疗组和安慰剂对照组，允许任一组患者在病情进展时接受瑞戈非尼的揭盲治疗。总体应答率（overall response rate，ORR）非常低，瑞戈非尼组为 4.5%，安慰剂组为 1.5%（一例部分应答）。瑞戈非尼组的中位 PFS 为 4.8 个月，安慰剂组为 0.9 个月。鉴于 85% 的安慰剂组患者转为接受瑞戈非尼治疗，两组患者的总体生存期没有统计学差异。

与伊马替尼相比，该药的毒性更接近于舒尼替尼。Ⅱ期临床试验中最常见的毒性是手足综合征、疲劳、腹泻和高血压，分别出现于 91%、85%、79% 和 76% 的患者，最常见于第一个治疗周期[185]。总体而言，67% 的患者在研究期间经历了至少一种或多种 3/4 级毒性。在Ⅲ期临床试验中，与药物相关的不良事件在瑞戈非尼组患者中比安慰剂组更常见（分别为 98.5% 和 68.2%），3 级或更高级别的不良反应发生率分别为 61.4% 和 13.6%。瑞戈非尼组中最常见的 3 级或更高级别的不良反应是高血压（23.5%）、手足皮肤反应（19.7%）和腹泻（5.3%）[185]。

对Ⅲ期临床研究中，瑞戈非尼改善 PFS 的相关因素分析表明，无论作为几线治疗方案，瑞戈非尼对 *KIT* 外显子 11 和 9 的原发突变的肿瘤都是有效的[187]。倾向于安慰剂的唯一因素是之前的伊马替尼治疗的时间少于 6 个月。一项Ⅱ期临床研究的临床获益分析显示，76% 的患者获益，其中 SDH 缺陷肿瘤（100%）、外显子 11 突变肿瘤（79%）和外显子 9 突变肿瘤（67%）的获益最大[187]。有一名 *BRAF* 外显子 15 突变的患者没有获益。3 例基因型未知，其中 2 例有临床获益。

5. 替代药物

其他一些药物也在 GIST 治疗中进行了评估，在有限的Ⅱ期临床试验中显示了一定程度的有效性，但尚未获得 FDA 的批准；对这些药物的情况不在此阐述。一些被批准用于其他适应证的药物可能在身体状况良好，足以继续治疗，并且没有合适的临床试验选择的晚期患者中发挥作用。表 33.3 列出了这些药物以及支持其使用的相关研究。

表 33.3　FDA 未批准的胃肠道间质瘤治疗药物

药物	疾病状态	研究阶段	参考文献
尼罗替尼		Ⅰ/Ⅰb	188
	转移一线 与伊马替尼比较	Ⅲ	189
	转移三线 伊马替尼和舒尼替尼治疗后进展，与最佳支持治疗和持续激酶治疗相比	Ⅲ	190
索拉非尼	二线或以上	Ⅱ	191-193
帕唑帕尼	三线和四线	Ⅱ	194，195
达沙替尼	三线和四线	Ⅱ	196
依维莫司	二线和三线	Ⅰ/Ⅱ	197
达拉非尼	不适用	病例报道	58
拉罗曲替尼	不适用	Ⅰ	203

尼罗替尼是研究最深入的药物。初始Ⅰ期临床数据显示，无论尼罗替尼单独使用或与伊马替尼合用，都证实了其安全性和耐受性，并具有一定的治疗效果[188]。后续研究，包括 2 项Ⅲ期临床研究，均不支持该药在 GIST 中适用[189,190]。在转移性 GIST 患者的一线治疗中，与伊马替尼相比，尼罗替尼不如伊马替尼有效，特别是对于有外显子 9 突变的肿瘤[189]。关于Ⅲ期临床试验，在伊马替尼和舒尼替尼治疗失败的晚期 GIST 患者中，允许对照组患者接受激酶治疗有很多讨论。如果该研究是安慰剂对照的，可推测其将对 PFS 的改善产生积极影响[190]。

其他可用的激酶抑制剂单药（FDA 批准用于其他适应症）在胃肠道间质瘤中的益处有限，包括索拉非尼、帕唑帕尼和达沙替尼（主要用于 *PDGFRA* D842V 突变胃肠道间质瘤）（见表 33.3）[58,191-200]。

已经根据抑制 KIT 通路以及同一通路或替代通路的其他分子的基本原理对联合治疗进行了评估。伊马替尼加依维莫司，一种丝氨酸-苏氨酸激酶 mTOR 抑制剂，在伊马替尼和至少另一种 TKI 治疗后进展的患者中进行了评估[197]。研究者发现，有 37%的患者，在接受每日伊马替尼 600mg 和依维莫斯 2.5mg 治疗时，疾病没有进展。已证实在伊马替尼治疗中加入 MEK 抑制剂比美替尼（binimetinib）是安全的。一项正在进行的研究评估了其对转移性疾病的一线治疗效果[198]。由于突变的激酶蛋白对热休克蛋白 90（Hsp90）的保护性伴侣功能的依赖性[199]，已有一些研究使用多种 HSP-90 抑制剂[200,201]或与伊马替尼联合使用[202]。Hsp90 抑制剂 IPI-504 的早期Ⅰ和Ⅱ期临床试验结果令人鼓舞，但该药已不再开发[200]，Hsp90 抑制剂 B11B021 对少数难治性疾病患者也有部分缓解作用[201]。然而，HSP-90 药物是否会被批准用于 GIST 治疗尚存疑虑。

对于罕见的 *BRAF* 突变患者，达拉非尼已显示出治疗活性[58]。最近，有报道称伴有 NTRK 易位的胃肠道间质瘤对拉罗曲替尼治疗有反应[203]。

6. 未来的制剂

BLU-285，也被称为阿法利替尼，已经在Ⅰ期临床试验条件下，在各种 GIST 亚型的扩展队列中进行了测试[204]。该药经过优化，可以抑制涉及远端激酶结构域的激酶突变，该结构域通常会发生继发性突变[205]。该区域也是 *PDGFRA* D842V 突变的位点，这种突变对标准疗法耐药。到目前为止，GIST Ⅰ期临床试验的疗效仅以摘要形式报道（NCT02508532），但值得注意的是，该药对具有 *PDGFRA* D842V 突变的 GIST 患者有显著疗效，而这些突变对已批准的激酶类药物通常耐药[204]。在Ⅰ期临床研究的首次报道中，对 17 例 *PDGFRA* D842V 患者应用一项或多项疾病应答评估，7 例确认部分应答（ORR 为 41%），10 例病情稳定。鉴于已获批药物对该基因型的治疗有效性不足，这些结果还是相当有意义的。除了对 *PDGFRA* D842V 型 GIST 的显著疗效外，该药对标准治疗耐药的其他 *KIT* 和 *PDGFRA* 突变也有效，并可延长疾病控制时间。比较阿法利替尼和瑞戈非尼作为三线治疗的Ⅲ期临床试验 Voyager 研究正在进行中（NCT03465722）。

DCC-2618 采用了一种新的方法来治疗 GIST[206,207]。KIT 有一个内部开关袋，激酶的 2 个部分作为抑制开关（外显子 11 近膜结构域）或激活开关（外显子 17 激活环）。外显子 11 的突变使激酶具有了组成型活性，幸运的是，它可以被批准的激酶抑制剂抑制，这些抑制剂具有 ATP 竞争性抑制剂的作用。然而，外显子 17 的突变并不被抑制。DCC-2618 的设计目的是在激活环路阻止进入开关袋，使激酶处于非激活状态。鉴于 PDGFRA 与 KIT 的结构相似，预计可能会观察到类似的疗效。该药的Ⅰ期临床试验（NCT02571036）报告显示，在 99 名接受一项或多项研究中肿瘤评估的 GIST 患者中，ORR 为 16%[208]。对该药物的进一步测试正在进行，InVictus 试验评估 DCC-2618 与安慰剂在对所有计划治疗失败患者中的疗效（NCT03353753）。

八、特殊状况

（一）克隆进展的影像

当监测恶性肿瘤对治疗的反应时，疾病进展与肿瘤增大相关。在临床研究中，随着 RECIST 标准的使用，这一点已经标准化。RECIST 标准将疾病进展定义为可测量的病变增加 20%或更多，以及新病灶的出现[209]。如上所述（见 CT 和 MRI），随着 TKI 治疗在 GIST 中的使用，也可以使用 CHOI 标准通过肿瘤密度的降低来评估治疗的获益。在有应答的转移病灶中，可以通过出现密度增加或强化的新结节来判断疾病进展[210]。对这些新病变的基因组研究已经发现了新的突变，可以解释对治疗的耐药性和疾病进展的原因[211]。必须仔细观察 CT 和 MRI 影像以识别这些病变。

（二）Carney 三联征和 Carney-Streatakis 综合征

Carney 三联征在 20 世纪 70 年代被首次描述[212]。据报道，年轻患者，通常为女性，出现胃平滑肌肉瘤、副神经节瘤和肺软骨瘤[213]。我们现在认识到该胃肿瘤是 GIST，通常是多灶性的，伴淋巴结侵犯[213]。对该三联征的描述已经演变，现在可能包括肾上腺腺瘤和食管平滑肌瘤[214]。Carney-Stratakis 二联体（Carney-Stratakis 综合征）被描述为有副神经节瘤和胃肠道间质瘤家族史的患者[215,216]。这两种综合征的 GIST 没有 *KIT* 或 *PDGFRA* 突变；它们的特征是免疫组织化学染色显示 SDHB 表达缺失。对这些肿瘤的评估和基因检测发现，作为二联体一部分的肿瘤携带 SDH 基因家族突变，而与三联征相关的肿瘤没有这种突变[57]。对于临床医生和患者来说，区分这些是非常重要的。通过免疫组织化学染色发现缺乏 SDHB 表达的胃 GIST 患者需要转诊进行遗传咨询，以确定患者是否有种系突变的二联体；二联体患者需要持续筛查可能发生在颈部、胸部和腹部的副神经节瘤，以及考虑遗传咨询和其他家庭成员的筛查。

SDH 缺陷型 GIST 患者的治疗有其特殊性。这些肿瘤通常是多灶性的，可能发生出血。就诊时，淋巴结转移并不少见，并且可以转移到肝脏。然而，其临床病程可能相当缓慢，因此治疗这些患者必须在控制症状和这些症状是否具有治疗意义之间取得平衡。不推荐通过激进的胃切除来根除疾病；相反，这些患者最好通过选择性外科手术来处理引起症状的病变[217]。

对于转移性和进展性疾病患者，激酶抑制剂的临床获益并不完全清楚。这在一定程度上是因为肿瘤突变检测的发展。早期研究使用的检测方法遗漏了对 *KIT* 或 *PDGFRA* 突变的检测，甚至不做基因检测。虽然有报道称伊马替尼是有效的[44,168,169]，但现在认为它对大多数患者无效。有报道称舒尼替尼和瑞戈非尼对 SDH 缺陷的 GIST 患者有效[186,218]。

（三）家族性胃肠道间质瘤

除了 Carney-Stratakis 综合征，GIST 很少与家族遗传模式相关[29,32,33,46-48,216]。在一些家族中报道了 *KIT* 突变。这些家族性病例往往有常染色体显性种系突变，而受累成员中的 GIST 往往是多灶性的。患病家庭成员的其他临床特征包括皮肤病变，如色素沉着过多或类似于色素性荨麻疹临床表现的皮肤病变。这些皮肤色素沉着异常可能是由于突变激活了 KIT 激酶对黑素细胞生长和发育的影响。这种色素沉着障碍保持局灶性而不是播散性的机制，可能会为解释为什么 GIST 病变需要数十年才出现在这些罕见的家族性病例中提供线索。

应该注意的是，也有家族性 *PDGFRA* 相关突变的报道。家族性 GIST 病例也被发现具有种系 *PDGFRA* 突变[46-48]；与未受影响的家族成员相比，具有该突变的家族成员的手和胃肠道间质瘤更大。另一个种系 *PDGFRA* 突变的病例具有肠多发性纤维性息肉和脂肪瘤[47]。最近，*PDGFRA* 突变综合征被描述为包括 GIST、炎性纤维性息肉和纤维瘤[48]。该综合征与 *PDGFRA* 外显子 14 的突变有关，是 GIST 中的一种不常见的突变。

（四）其他与胃肠道间质瘤相关的遗传肿瘤综合征

Ⅰ型神经纤维瘤病（NF1）患者罹患 GIST 以及其他恶性肿瘤的风险增加[220-223]。对 NF1 患者胃肠道间质瘤的分子分析表明，这些胃肠道间质瘤通常没有可检测到的 KIT 或 PDGFRA 基因突变，但这些突变也可能存在，因此应该进行分子检测[220,221]。正如预期的那样，标准治疗对具有经典突变的肿瘤有效。对于那些没有经典基因突变的患者，使用标准方案进行全身治疗的获益似乎有限，尽管关于这一小部分肿瘤结果的文献非常有限。通常不会预期基于靶向 KIT 和 PDFRA 治疗的疗效，但抗血管生成药物可能有一些效果。NF1 驱动的肿瘤可能表现为腹腔多灶性病变，长期呈惰性病程。对于这些患者，观察等待是非常合理的选择。

（五）儿童胃肠间质瘤

GIST 很少出现在儿童[224-226]。儿童 GIST 通常是我们以前所说的野生型 GIST，现在被认为是 SDH 缺陷的 GIST。对这些肿瘤的初步评估发现很少有分子改变[225,226]。儿童和年轻人的 GIST 指南已经发表[227]。

（王欣欣　郭雪燕 译，闫秀娥 校）

参考文献

第 34 章　神经内分泌肿瘤

Jonathan R. Strosberg, Taymeyah Al-Toubah 著

章节目录

一、历史由来 …… 447
二、流行病学 …… 447
三、起源和组织化学特征 …… 448
四、分类 …… 449
五、分子发病机制 …… 449
六、多发性内分泌瘤和其他遗传综合征 …… 450
（一）多发性内分泌肿瘤综合征 1 型（MEN-1） …… 450
（二）Von Hippel-Lindau 病 …… 451
（三）神经纤维瘤病 1 型 …… 451
（四）结节性硬化症 …… 451
七、功能性肿瘤 …… 451
胰岛素瘤 …… 451
八、胃泌素瘤 …… 453
（一）病理生理学与病理学 …… 453
（二）临床特征 …… 455
九、胰高血糖素瘤 …… 457
病理生理学与病理学 …… 457
十、血管活性肠肽瘤 …… 458
病理生理学与病理学 …… 458
十一、其他功能性胰腺神经内分泌肿瘤 …… 459
十二、无功能性胰腺神经内分泌肿瘤 …… 459
（一）临床特征 …… 459
（二）治疗 …… 459
十三、胃肠道神经内分泌肿瘤（类癌）（GI-NET） …… 459
（一）胃神经内分泌肿瘤（胃 NET） …… 460
（二）小肠神经内分泌肿瘤（空肠/回肠类癌）（SI-NET） …… 462
（三）阑尾神经内分泌肿瘤（类癌） …… 463
（四）直肠神经内分泌肿瘤（类癌） …… 463
（五）十二指肠及壶腹神经内分泌肿瘤（类癌） …… 464
（六）结肠神经内分泌肿瘤（类癌）（结肠 NET） …… 464
十四、类癌综合征 …… 465
（一）病理生理学 …… 465
（二）临床特征与诊断 …… 465
（三）治疗 …… 466
十五、肿瘤定位 …… 467
（一）内镜检查 …… 467
（二）超声内镜检查（EUS） …… 467
（三）计算机断层扫描（CT）和磁共振成像（MRI） …… 467
（四）生长抑素受体成像 …… 467
十六、转移性疾病的治疗 …… 467
（一）减瘤手术 …… 468
（二）肝导向的非手术治疗 …… 468
（三）肝移植 …… 468
（四）生长抑素类似物（SSA） …… 469
（五）α-干扰素 …… 469
（六）依维莫司 …… 469
（七）舒尼替尼 …… 469
（八）肽受体放射性核素放射治疗 …… 469
（九）细胞毒性化疗 …… 470
（十）低分化肿瘤的治疗 …… 470

神经内分泌肿瘤（neuroendocrine tumor, NET）起源于第 4 章中讨论的弥漫性神经内分泌系统[1,2]。胃肠胰腺神经内分泌肿瘤（gastroenteropancreatic NET, GEP-NET）可起源于胃肠道［即胃肠道神经内分泌肿瘤（GI tract NET, GI-NET，也称为类癌）和胰腺［即胰腺神经内分泌肿瘤（pancreas NET, pNET）］。GEP-NET 的特征是倾向于产生激素和其他血管活性物质。分泌激素导致临床综合征的肿瘤也称为“功能性肿瘤”（表 34.1）[3-18]，而非分泌性或分泌无活性蛋白的肿瘤称为“无功能性肿瘤”。GI-NET 和 pNET 有许多相似之处，因而两者常被一起探讨。如果存在重要差异时，则对其进行单独讨论。

表 34.1　胰腺神经内分泌瘤相关综合征[a]

综合征	年发病率/每 100 万	症状/体征	恶性肿瘤率/%	分泌的激素
胰岛素瘤	1~2	见表 34.5	<10	胰岛素
胃泌素瘤(ZES)	0.5~1.5	见表 34.6	60~90	胃泌素
血管活性肠肽瘤(Verner-Morrison 综合征,WDHA,胰性霍乱)	0.05~0.2	见表 34.7	>60	血管活性肠肽
胰高血糖素瘤	0.01~0.1	见表 34.7	50~80	胰高血糖素
生长激素释放因子瘤	未知	肢端肥大症	>30	生长激素释放因子
促肾上腺皮质激素瘤	不常见	异位库欣综合征	>95%	促肾上腺皮质激素
分泌甲状旁腺激素相关蛋白的 pNET	罕见	高钙血症引起的症状	84%	甲状旁腺激素相关蛋白
胰腺类癌	罕见(<1% 的类癌)	类癌综合征(见表 34.11)	77%	5-羟色胺,速激肽
分泌肾素的 pNET	罕见	高血压	未知	肾素
分泌促红细胞生成素的 pNET	罕见	红细胞增多症	未知	促红细胞生成素
分泌黄体生成素的 pNET	罕见	男性化(女性) 性欲丧失(男性)	未知	黄体生成素
分泌胆囊收缩素的 pNET(胆囊收缩素瘤)	罕见	腹泻、胆结石、消化性溃疡、体重减轻	未知	胆囊收缩素

[a] 这些综合征也可能由胃肠道神经内分泌瘤(GI-NET)(类癌)引起。
pNET,胰腺神经内分泌肿瘤;WDHA,水样腹泻、低血钾、胃酸缺乏。

一、历史由来

1869 年 Langerhans 描述了类癌的组织学。Lubarsch 于 1888 年在尸检时描述了回肠类癌。类癌(karzinoide)一词是由 Oberndorfer 提出来描述一种侵袭性低于腺癌的肿瘤[19]。Scholte 于 1931 年描述了 1 例患者发生的类癌综合征,该患者出现了水肿、出汗、面部潮红和腹泻症状,且发现 1cm 大小的回肠类癌以及增厚的三尖瓣。Lembeck 在 1952 年再次证明了 Kulchitsky 于 1897 年描述的肠嗜铬细胞(enterochromafffn cell,EC)是假定的类癌起源细胞,且合成并分泌 5-羟色胺[19]。1927 年(发现胰岛素后 5 年),在 1 例伴有转移性胰岛细胞瘤的低血糖患者中描述了第一例胰腺激素生成肿瘤综合征;该肿瘤提取物有降血糖作用[20]。此后,描述或提出了许多其他产生激素的 pNET(见表 34.1)。

二、流行病学

具有临床意义的 GEP-NET 的年发病率正在显著上升(图 34.1)。来自监测、流行病学和最终结果(SEER)18 数据库(2000—2012 年)的数据显示,原发部位未知的 GEPNET 年发病率为 3.56/10 万,NET 的年发病率为 0.84/10 万[21]。尸检时 GI-NET 的发生率甚至更高,为 8.4/10 000,这意味着许多患者无临床症状[22-24]。NET 发病率升高的主要原因尚不清楚,因为尚无已知的环境风险因素。这种增加很可能与内镜操作的广泛使用、成像的增加和病理学家对 NET 的识别提高有关[22-24]。

pNET 占胰腺肿瘤的 1%~10%[25-27]。功能性 pNET 的总患病率很低,据报道约为 1/10 万[5]。相比之下,尸检研究中 pNET 的患病率为 0.5%~1.5%[28]。pNET 的年发病率约为 0.8/10 万[24]。pNET 的总发病率随着年龄的增长而增加,60 岁和 70 岁达到高峰。在最近的研究中,无功能性 pNET 占所有 pNET 的 60%~80%[12,29,30]。功能性 pNET 的发病率各不相同,其中胰岛素瘤和胃泌素瘤是最常见的亚型,每年的发病率为(0.5~30)/100 万[12,31-34](见表 34.1)。

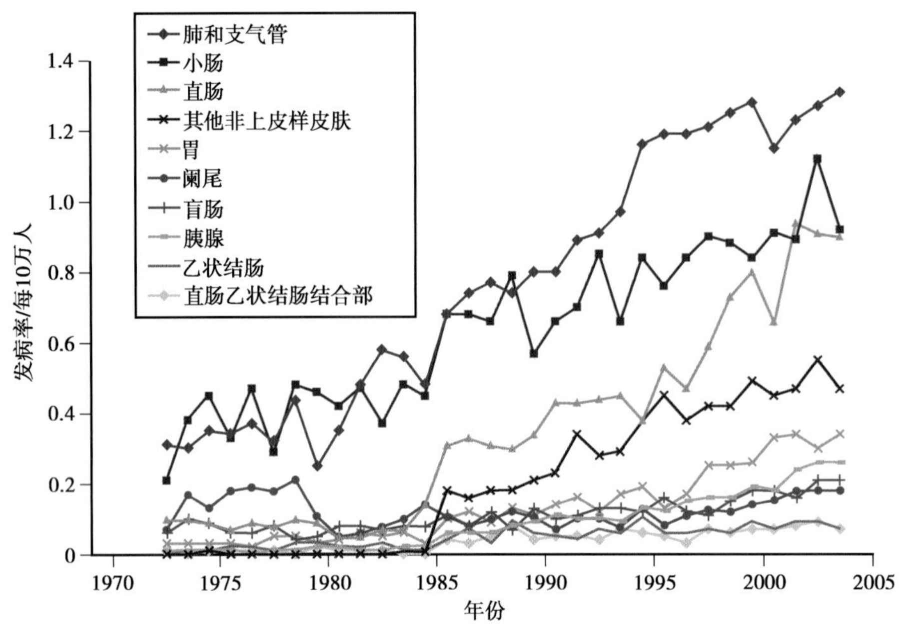

图 34.1　1970—2005 年不同亚型神经内分泌肿瘤的发病率。(From Modlin IM, Oberg K, Chung DC, et al. Gastroenteropancreatic neuroendocrine tumours. Lancet Oncol. 2008;9:61-72.)

三、起源和组织化学特征

GI-NET 起源于肠嗜铬细胞,它们形成分散在胃肠道、呼吸道和其他组织中的弥漫性神经内分泌细胞系统的一部分[22,35];pNET 可能起源于朗格罕岛,它也是弥漫性神经内分泌系统的组成部分[12,36,37]。该系统的细胞具有一定的细胞化学性质,最初被认为具有神经嵴细胞的共同胚胎起源,尽管目前更多的研究支持神经嵴和内胚层起源[35]。在超微结构上,神经内分泌细胞通常含有多种调节激素和胺类、神经元特异性烯醇化酶、突触素和嗜铬粒蛋白的电子致密颗粒。

GI-NET 和 pNET 具有明显的组织学相似性[38]。分化良好的肿瘤由相对均一的小圆形细胞组成,细胞核和细胞质均匀,常排列在胰岛或骨小梁中(图 34.2)。核有丝分裂象的特征性是不常见的(<2 个有丝分裂/高倍视野),坏死亦不常见[39]。恶性肿瘤只能通过转移灶或组织侵袭来确定,不能通过显微镜或超微结构研究来预测[40]。围绕 pNET 起源的确切细胞存在争议[36,41]。pNET 常被称为“胰岛细胞瘤”,但尚不确定它们起源于胰岛[11,34,36]。这些肿瘤经常含有导管结构,并往往产生成人胰腺中正常情况下不存在的激素,如胃泌素和血管活性肠肽(vasoactive intestinal polypeptide, VIP)[42]。在许多 pNET 中发现的导管结构,以及在胰腺个体发育过程中内分泌细胞从导管出芽(见第 55 章),导致人们推测这些肿瘤起源于导管[41]。GI-NET 和 pNET 可产生多种胃肠激素,可通过免疫细胞化学方法定位[38,39]。在许多研究中,大多数功能性和无功能性的 GI-NET(类癌)和 pNET 具有含有不引起临床症状的多肽细胞[39,42]。尽管肿瘤中存在多种激素,但尚不清楚为什么通常仅观察到一种综合征或无临床综合征。[40,42]。因此,功能性 pNET 综合征或类癌综合征只有在出现适当的临床症状时才能诊断,而不仅仅是基于免疫细胞化学。

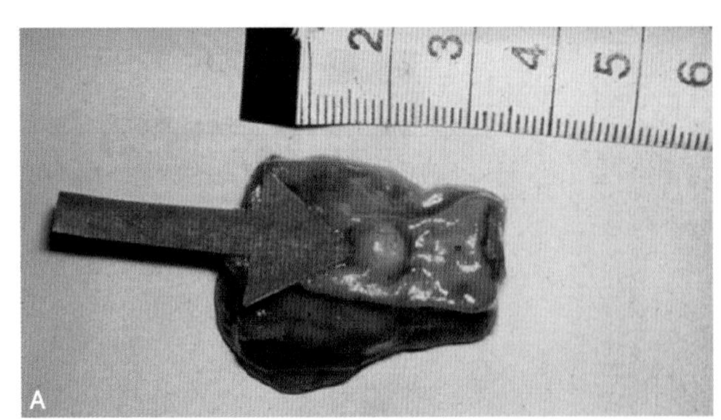

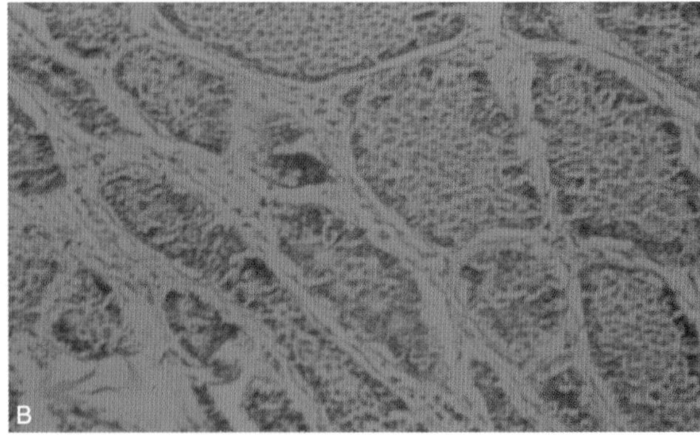

图 34.2　GI-NET(类癌)和 pNET 的大体和组织切片。A,小肠类癌的大体切片。这种大小是原发性小肠类癌的典型特征,肿瘤位于上皮下。B,小肠类癌的组织病理学及其特征性的岛叶状生长方式(HE 染色,×80)

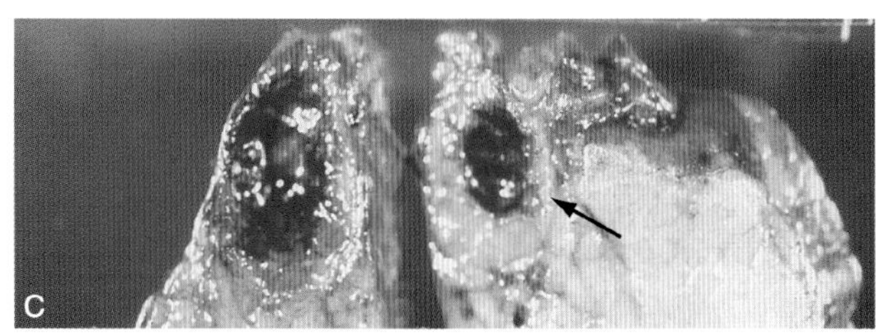

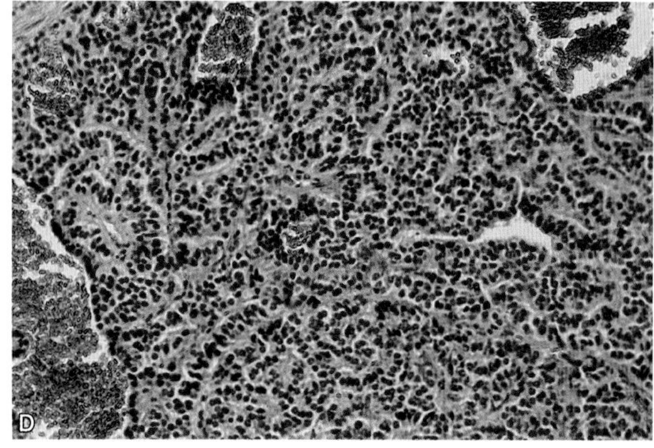

图 34.2(续)　C,胰腺尾部出血性和囊性 2cm pNET(胃泌素瘤)(箭头)。D,胃泌素瘤的组织病理学,与其他 pNET 相似。这种血管丰富的肿瘤由清一色的内分泌细胞的小管组成

分化良好的 GI-NET、pNET 和呼吸道神经内分泌肿瘤在组织学上似乎相似。因此,预测转移患者原发性神经内分泌肿瘤的部位是困难的。最近的研究报道,来自不同位点的 NET 可能差异表达转录因子,包括 CDX-2、胰腺和十二指肠同源核因子 1(pancreatic and duodenal homeobox factor-1,PDX-1)、TTF、PAX-1 和 ISL-1。一组这些因素可用于从转移灶定位原发性 NET 的来源[43,44]。

四、分类

肿瘤按其分级和分化程度进行分类,肿瘤的分级和分化是非常重要的预后标志物。等级是指使用核有分裂率和 Ki-67 指数测量的肿瘤的增殖活性。分化是指肿瘤形态与起源的内分泌细胞相似的程度。低分化肿瘤常表现为成片的多形性细胞,有坏死区[45]。低分化神经内分泌癌倾向于具有高增殖活性的高度侵袭性恶性肿瘤;几乎所有低分化肿瘤均为高级别肿瘤。在 2010 年世界卫生组织(WHO)GI-NET 分类中,低分级肿瘤定义为每 10 个高倍视野(high powered field,HPF)有 0~1 个有丝分裂,Ki-67 指数为 0%~3%,中分级肿瘤的核有分裂率为每 10 个 HPF 有 2~20 个或 Ki-67 指数为 3%~20%,高级别肿瘤,即核有丝分裂率>20 个/10HPF 或 Ki-67 指数>20%。高分化 NET 被细分为低级别和中级别肿瘤,而低分化癌被认为等同于高级别的肿瘤(见表 34.2a)[46]。该分类的一个缺陷是它否定了分化良好的高级别肿瘤的可能性,这是一个逐渐被认识的实体,特别是在胰腺 pNET。因此,2017 年 WHO pNET 分类将高分化分类扩展为包括低、中、高级别肿瘤(表 34.2b)[47]。值得注意的是,目前的分类使用术语“神经内分泌肿瘤”一词来描述高分化 NET,而“神经内分泌癌或 NEC”来表示低分化形态。

在过去的 10 年里,美国癌症联合委员会(American Joint Committee on Cancer,AJCC)和欧洲神经内分泌肿瘤学会(European Neuroendocrine Tumor Society,ENETS)已经为 GEPNET 引入了正式 TNM 分期分类。在人群和机构数据库上对这两种分期系统进行了验证。

表 34.2A　WHO 2010 年胃肠道 NET 分类

分化程度	分级	WHO 分级	WHO 命名
高分化	低级别(G1)	<2 个有丝分裂/10HPF 和<3% Ki67 指数	NET 1 级
	中级别(G2)	2~20 个有丝分裂/10HPF 或 3%~20% Ki67 指数	NET 2 级
低分化	高级别	>20 个有丝分裂/10HPF 或>20% Ki67 指数	神经内分泌癌,3 级(大细胞或小细胞型)

HPF,高倍视野;NET,神经内分泌肿瘤;WHO,世界卫生组织。

表 34.2B　WHO 2017 年胰腺 NET 分类

分化程度	分级	WHO 分级	WHO 命名
高分化	低级别(G1)	<2 个有丝分裂/10HPF 和<3% Ki67 指数	NET 1 级
	中级别(G2)	2~20 个有丝分裂/10HPF 或 3%~20% Ki67 指数	NET 2 级
	高级别(G3)	>20 个有丝分裂/10HPF 或>20% Ki67 指数	NET 3 级
低分化	高级别	>20 个有丝分裂/10HPF 或>20% Ki67 指数	神经内分泌癌,3 级(大细胞或小细胞型)

HPF,高倍视野;NET,神经内分泌肿瘤;WHO,世界卫生组织。

五、分子发病机制

迄今为止,NET 的发病分子机制仍知之甚少[48-51]。与许多非内分泌胃肠肿瘤(如结肠或胰腺腺癌)相比,常见癌基因(如 *ras*、*fos*、*myc*、*src*、*jun*)和抑癌基因(如 *p53*、*rb*)突变在高分化 NET 中是罕见的[12,28]。

最近对 pNET 的基因组分析为这些肿瘤的遗传背景提供了重要的见解。在一项对 68 例散发性 pNET 的里程碑式的全外显子组研究中,44% 的病例观察到 *MEN1* 的体细胞突变,而 44% 的病例观察到死亡结构域相关蛋白(death-domain-associated protein, DAXX）或 α-地中海贫血/X 连锁精神发育迟缓综合征蛋白（α-thalassemia/mental retardation syndrome X-linked, ATRX）突变[50]。

这 3 个基因都与染色质重塑有关。此外，14%的样本存在哺乳动物西罗莫司靶蛋白（mTOR）通路基因的突变，包括 *PTEN*、*TSC2* 和 *PIK3CA*。在对 102 例原发性 pNET 的全基因组测序研究中也报道了类似的结果。4 种失调的信号通路如下：①DNA 损伤修复；②染色质重塑；③端粒的维护；④mTOR 激活。临床上散发的 pNET 中发现种系突变的比例高于预期，其中 11%的患者发生 *MUTYH*、*CHEK2* 和 *BRCA2* 突变[52]。

驱动 pNET 发展和进展的基因突变的精确序列目前尚不清楚。DAXX/ATRX 表达缺失与端粒选择性延长和染色体不稳定性的激活有关。额外的突变会随着时间累积，并与临床进展相关。低分化 pNEC 的遗传背景与高分化 pNET 明显不同。据报道，55%和 49%的 pNEC 患者存在 *KRAS* 突变和 Rb 丢失。总而言之，NEC 的突变频率明显高于 NET[53]。

与 pNET 相比，GI-NET 的分子结构更不为人所知。超过 60%的小肠神经内分泌肿瘤（SI-NET）存在 18 号染色体的缺失，但这种改变的生物学意义尚不明确[54]。总的来说，在 SI-NET 中观察到低突变率（0.1 个体细胞单核苷酸变异/10^5 个核苷酸），8%的患者中观察到细胞周期蛋白依赖性激酶抑制剂基因 *CDKN1B* 的突变或缺失[55]。表观遗传变化似乎在 SI-NET 的发展中起着基础性作用。全 DNA 低甲基化是 SI-NET 的一个特征，而高甲基化指数的肿瘤往往具有临床侵袭性。DNA 甲基化在原发肿瘤和转移瘤之间已被检测到渐进式的变化[56,57]。

在许多 GEP-NET 中，mTOR 通路似乎明显失调，即使在通路成分中没有可识别的突变。mTOR 是一种丝氨酸/苏氨酸激酶，可调节细胞存活和增殖、血管生成和代谢。mTOR 和/或其下游目标的过表达在 NET 中经常被检测到，并与较差的预后相关[58]。结节性硬化症-2（tuberous sclerosis-2, TSC-2）和 mTOR 通路抑制剂磷酸酶和张力蛋白同源物（phosphatase and tensin homolog, PTEN）的表达在大多数 pNET 中降低。此外，TSC-2 和 PTEN 的表达降低与存活率降低相关[59]。

NET 是富含血管的肿瘤，血管生成已被确认为 NET 进展的关键事件。促血管生成因子，包括成纤维细胞生长因子（fibroblast growth factor, FGF）、血小板衍生生长因子（platelet-derived growth factor, PDGF）和血管内皮生长因子（vascular endothelial growth factor, VEGF）及其受体的过表达已被报道[60]。

六、多发性内分泌瘤和其他遗传综合征

（一）多发性内分泌肿瘤综合征 1 型（MEN-1）

MEN-1（Wermer 综合征）主要表现为甲状旁腺功能亢进、多灶性胰十二指肠 NET 和垂体腺瘤。MEN-1 基因缺陷位于染色体 11q13 上，是由编码 610 个氨基酸蛋白 menin 的第 10 外显子基因的种系突变引起的（表 34.3）[61,62]。Menin 是一种可与许多蛋白相互作用的核蛋白，包括 AP1 转录因子、核因子（NF）-κβ、RPA2（一种 DNA 加工因子）、FAN CD2（一种 DNA 修复因子）以及各种细胞骨架相关蛋白和组织修饰酶[61-63]。Menin 在转录调节、基因组稳定性、细胞分裂、细胞周期控制等方面具有重要作用[61,63,64]。致癌的确切机制尚不清楚[65,66]。

表 34.3 遗传性胃肠道神经内分泌肿瘤综合征

综合征	患病率/10^5	遗传缺陷：蛋白改变	NET 频率	pNET 的类型
多发性内分泌肿瘤 1 型（MEN-1）	1~10	11q13：menin，一种由 610 个氨基酸组成的核蛋白，与参与细胞生长、细胞周期调控、基因组稳定性和凋亡相关的通路相互作用	pNET：80%~100%（显微镜下）、20%~80%（临床） 类癌：胃（15%~35%）、肺（0%~8%）、胸腺（0%~8%）	NF-pNET： 80%~100%（显微镜下）、0%~20%（大的） 功能性 pNET： 胃泌素瘤（54%） 胰岛素瘤（18%） 胰高血糖素瘤（3%） 血管活性肠肽瘤（3%） 生长激素释放因子瘤（<1%） 生长抑素瘤（<1%）
von Hipper-Lindau 病（VHL）	2~3	3p25：pVHL，一种由 232 个氨基酸组成的蛋白，与下调 HIF 和 VEGF 的转录因子相互作用	10%~17%（pNET）	NF-pNET：98% 功能性 pNET：2%
神经纤维瘤病 1 型（NF-1, Von Recklinghausen disease）	20~25	17q11.2：神经纤维蛋白，一种 2484 氨基酸蛋白，具有 Ras-GTP 酶活性，结合微管，调节 mTOR 生长，诱导细胞骨架改变	0%~10%（十二指肠类癌） 罕见 pNET	生长抑素瘤
结节性硬化症（Bourneville）	10	9q34（TSC1）和 16p13（TSC2）：Hamartin（1164-氨基酸蛋白）和 tuberin（1807-氨基酸蛋白），与调节 mTOR 生长的 PI3K 信号级联，影响细胞生长的 GTP 酶活性、能量调节、对缺氧反应和营养	不常见	NF-pNET>功能性 pNET

GTP，三磷酸鸟苷；HIF，缺氧诱导因子；mTOR，哺乳动物西罗莫司靶蛋白；pNET，胰腺神经内分泌肿瘤；NF，无功能；VEGF，血管内皮生长因子。

MEN-1 患者内分泌肿瘤的发生符合 Knudsen[11,61]“二次打击”肿瘤模型理论，一条染色体的遗传（种系）突变被另一条正常染色体的体细胞缺失或突变所掩盖，从而消除了正常基因产物的肿瘤抑制作用[61,62]。在 *MEN1* 中已经描述了许多（>1 300）种不同的突变，超过 75% 的突变是无活性的[62]。

甲状旁腺功能亢进是 MEN-1 患者最常见的异常临床表现（表 34.4）[61,67-69]。典型的甲状旁腺功能亢进是 MEN-1 的

表 34.4 多发性内分泌腺瘤 1 型患者的临床特征

特征	频率/%[范围]
甲状旁腺功能亢进	97[78~100]
胰腺内分泌肿瘤（任何种类）	
任何种类，包括胰多肽瘤或无功能性	80~100
胃泌素瘤	54[20~61]
胰岛素瘤	18[7~13]
胰高血糖素瘤	3[1~6]
血管活性肠肽瘤	1[1~12]
生长抑素瘤	0~1
生长激素释放因子瘤	<1
垂体瘤	
任何种类	60[15~100]
分泌催乳素	[15~46]
分泌生长激素	[6~20]
分泌促肾上腺皮质激素（库欣综合征）	16
肾上腺皮质肿瘤	[27~36；有症状者<2]
类癌	
胃（1 型胃肠道类癌）	[7~35；有症状者<5]
肺	[0~8]
胸腺	[0~8]
皮肤异常[a]	
血管纤维瘤	88
胶原瘤	72
咖啡牛奶斑	38
脂肪瘤	34
中枢神经系统肿瘤[a]	
脑膜瘤	[0~8]
室管膜瘤和神经鞘瘤	
平滑肌瘤、平滑肌肉瘤[a]	[1~7]
甲状腺腺瘤[a]	5[0~30]

[a] 有症状者<1%。

Data modified from Jensen RT GJ. Gastrinoma. In: Go VLW DE, Gardner JD, et al, eds. The pancreas: biology, pathobiology and disease. 2nd ed. New York: Raven Press; 1993, pp 931-78; Jensen RT, Berna MJ, Bingham DB, et al. Inherited pancreatic endocrine tumor syndromes: advances in molecular pathogenesis, diagnosis, management, and controversies. Cancer 2008; 113: 1807-43; Thakker RV. Multiple endocrine neoplasia type 1. Endocrinol Metab Clin North Am. 2000; 29: 541-67; Gibril F, Schumann M, Pace A, et al. Multiple endocrine neoplasia type 1 and Zollinger-Ellison syndrome: a prospective study of 107 cases and comparison with 1009 cases from the literature. Medicine (Baltimore) 2004; 83: 43-83; Gibril F, Jensen RT. Advances in evaluation and management of gastrinoma in patients with Zollinger-Ellison syndrome. Curr Gastroenterol Rep 2005; 7: 114-21.

最初表现，通常在 30 岁时出现，然后在 40~50 岁时发展为 pNET[61]。大约 20% 的患者患有垂体腺瘤。无功能性 pNET 在 MEN-1 患者中几乎普遍存在，病理学研究表明[12,61,68,70]，在几乎所有 MEN-1 患者中，胰腺表现为弥漫性微腺瘤、伴或不伴较大的肿瘤。在功能性肿瘤中，胃泌素瘤最常见（通常发生在十二指肠）。重要的是要认识到 pNET 患者何时患有 MEN-1，因为有和无 MEN-1 的患者在临床表现、是否需要家族筛查、手术治愈的可能性以及临床和诊断方法方面存在差异[61,71-73]。

（二）Von Hippel-Lindau 病

von Hipper-Lindau 病（von Hipper-Lindau disease，VHL）是由染色体 3p25 编码 232 个氨基酸蛋白 pVHL 的缺陷引起的，pVHL 与许多蛋白质形成复合物，调节大细胞蛋白的泛素依赖性蛋白水解，并以缺氧诱导因子（HIF）α 为靶点[74]。VHL 突变导致转录调节的改变，导致血管生成、生长和有丝分裂因子的病理改变。胰腺病变（主要是囊肿）发生在 60% 的 VHL 患者。10% ~ 17% 的 VHL 患者存在 pNET。pNET 通常（>98%）无症状和无功能。VHL 诊断为 pNET 的平均年龄为 29~38 岁。大多数患者有单一并可能是恶性的 pNET[75]。伴有 pNET 的 VHL 患者中有 9%~37% 发生肝转移。

（三）神经纤维瘤病 1 型

神经纤维瘤病 1 型（NF1）是由染色体 17q11.2 编码 2 845 个氨基酸蛋白神经纤维瘤蛋白的缺陷引起的，该蛋白是 Ras 信号级联抑制剂（见表 34.3）[61,76]。0%~10% 的 NF1 患者通常在十二指肠壶腹周围区域[61,77,78]发生 GI-NET（类癌）。虽然生长抑素瘤综合征很少出现，但这些肿瘤通常含有生长抑素瘤的典型圆形钙结核（砂粒体）。转移到肝脏或淋巴结的 NF1 占 30%[61,78]。

（四）结节性硬化症

结节性硬化症是由 1 164 个氨基酸蛋白，即 hamartin（TSC-1）或 1 807 个氨基酸蛋白 tuberin（TSC-2）突变引起的（见表 34.3）[61]。这两种蛋白调节 PI3K 信号级联和小鸟苷三磷酸酶（GTP）结合蛋白 RHEB（大脑中富集的 Ras 同源物），其在蛋白质翻译和合成、生长和增殖的调节中以及维持细胞能量水平方面发挥重要作用。4% 的 TSC-2 患者存在 pNET。

七、功能性肿瘤

胰岛素瘤

胰岛素瘤是分泌胰岛素的 pNET，主要起源于胰腺，引起低血糖症状（表 34.5）。

1. 病理生理学与病理学

胰岛素瘤几乎都位于胰腺[12,28,31,39,79-81]。胰岛素瘤均匀分布于胰腺，通常相当小[12,28,31,39,79-82]。在一个系列研究中，39% 的病灶小于 1cm，只有 8% 大于 5cm[82]。胰岛素瘤在 2%~13% 的患者中以多发性肿瘤的形式出现[28,82]，在这种情

表 34.5　胰岛素瘤患者的症状、体征和实验室检查异常

	频率/%
临床过程期间的任何时间[a]	
神经精神症状(意识丧失、意识模糊、头晕、复视)	92
意识模糊或行为异常	80
肥胖	52
失忆症或昏迷	47
癫痫发作(癫痫大发作)	12
心血管症状、心悸、心动过速	17
胃肠道症状(饥饿、呕吐、腹痛)	9
第一次发作[b]	
神经性低血糖症状	
视觉障碍(复视、视物模糊)	59
意识模糊	51
意识改变	38
虚弱无力	32
短暂性运动缺陷,偏瘫	29
头晕	28
疲劳	27
不当行为	27
言语困难	24
头痛	23
癫痫发作	23
晕厥	21
注意力不集中或思考困难	19
感觉异常	17
记忆丧失	15
嗜睡	12
健忘症	8
昏迷	12
共济失调	4
定向障碍	4
精神改变	4
肾上腺素能症状	
出汗	43
震颤	23
饥饿、恶心	12
心悸	10

[a]Data from Refs Service FJ, Dale AJ, Elveback LR, et al. Insulinoma: clinical and diagnostic features of 60 consecutive cases. Mayo Clin Proc 1976; 51: 417-29; Stefanini P, Carboni M, Patrassi N, et al. Betaislet cell tumors of the pancreas: results of a study on 1,067 cases. Surgery 1974; 75: 597-609.

[b]Data modified from Hirshberg B, Cochran C, Skarulis MC, et al. Malignant insulinoma: spectrum of unusual clinical features. Cancer 2005; 104: 264-72.

况下应该怀疑是 MEN-1[61]。胰岛素瘤通常有完整的包膜,比正常胰腺更硬,且血管密度高。只有 5%~16% 的胰岛素瘤是恶性的[83]。恶性胰岛素瘤一般体积比较大(平均 6cm[84]),最常转移到肝脏和/或局部淋巴结。

胰岛素是由胰岛 β 细胞中粗面内质网以前胰岛素原的形式合成的。胰岛素原从前胰岛素原中释放并转移到高尔基体中[32]。胰岛素原,包括 21 个氨基酸的 α 链和 30 个氨基酸的 β 链、再由一条 33 个氨基酸连接肽(C 肽)连接在一起,储存在 β 细胞分泌颗粒中。在这些颗粒中,蛋白酶切除 C 肽,C 肽和双链胰岛素分子以等摩尔量分泌[32]。在正常受试者中也检测到一些胰岛素原,但不到总免疫反应性血浆胰岛素的 25%,而在几乎所有(>90%)胰岛素瘤患者中,胰岛素原相对于总胰岛素的比例升高[85]。

2. 临床特征

胰岛素瘤通常发生在 20~75 岁之间的患者,60% 为女性[10,12,28,31,39,79-81]。低血糖症状特征性表现与禁食相关[10,28,79-81]。低血糖症状在运动中也可能出现。空腹或运动引起的低血糖症与饭后低血糖症(餐后低血糖症)在时间上有所不同,后者可由多种不相关的原因引起[86-91]。空腹低血糖和餐后(反应性)低血糖的区别通常可以通过仔细的病史来确定。

除胰岛素瘤外,胰岛细胞病引起的空腹低血糖伴高胰岛素血症的其他不常见原因包括胰岛素瘤病、胰岛增生[92]和胰岛细胞增殖症[93]。在胰岛素瘤病中,许多表达胰岛素的大腺瘤和微腺瘤伴有多个表达增生性单激素的小内分泌细胞簇。

胰岛素瘤的大多数症状[12,28,31,39,82]是由神经性低血糖引起的,因为葡萄糖是大脑能量的主要来源。儿茶酚胺释放也可引起低血糖症状(肾上腺素能症状)。患者经常通过频繁进食来避免症状,并可能导致肥胖[83]。神经性低血糖症状可在胰岛素瘤确诊数年前出现[85]。

3. 诊断

胰岛素瘤确诊的关键是根据临床病史怀疑患者的症状可能是由低血糖引起的,并确定其症状与空腹的关系[10,12,28,31,39,79-81,90]。Whipple 三联征,即低血糖症状、低血糖(血糖<50mg/dL)和摄取葡萄糖后症状缓解,这对胰岛素瘤并不是特异性的[83]。经过一夜的禁食,只有不到 40% 的胰岛素瘤患者的血糖水平低于 50mg/dL。然而,如果空腹血糖测定同时伴有空腹血浆胰岛素水平升高,65% 的胰岛素瘤患者的胰岛素水平会不成比例的升高[12]。

对于缺乏明确的疾病影像学证据的患者,可以延长禁食时间,每隔 3~6 小时测量血糖、血浆胰岛素和 C 肽水平[10,12,28,31,39,79-81,90]。传统上,根据计划一般禁食 72 小时,但如果禁食期间患者出现症状,应在静脉注射葡萄糖和停止试验前确定血浆胰岛素和血糖值。75%~80% 的胰岛素瘤患者在禁食后 24 小时内出现症状、血糖低于 40mg/dL,72 小时内几乎 100% 出现症状[10,12,28,31,39,90]。在健康、非肥胖的禁食受试者中,当血糖水平降至低于 40mg/dL 时,血浆胰岛素浓度降至 6μU/mL 以下,而血浆胰岛素(以 μU/mL 计算)与葡萄糖(以 mg/dL 计算)的比值仍小于 0.3。因此,血浆胰岛素与血糖之比超过 0.3 被认为是胰岛素瘤阳性。在一项研究中[85],72 小时禁食试验诊断胰岛素瘤最敏感和最特异的标准

是空腹血糖水平低于 45mg/dL 联合胰岛素原水平升高。

多重影像学检查有助于胰岛素瘤的定位。这些包括多相 CT 扫描和超声内镜检查(EUS)。生长抑素受体显像,通常采用与生长抑素受体-2 类似物^{68}Ga-dotatate PET 扫描[68];临床上除非怀疑有转移,或除非怀疑胰岛素瘤不能用其他方法检测到,否则常规检查下该检查是不必要的。侵入性影像学检查(如动脉钙刺激后肝静脉采样)很少有必要用于定位隐匿性胰岛素瘤。

4. 治疗

胰岛素瘤的治疗包括控制低血糖症状,其次是肿瘤定位和切除。所有 pNET 的肿瘤定位以及 5%~13% 的转移性胰岛素瘤患者的化疗或其他针对肿瘤本身的治疗将在后面进行讨论[84,94-97]。

5. 药物治疗

大多数胰岛素瘤患者的低血糖可通过饮食和药物治疗相结合来控制的[10,12,28,31,39,83,97]。零食的摄入不应局限于快速吸收的碳水化合物,因为它们的摄入偶尔会刺激肿瘤分泌胰岛素。吸收缓慢的碳水化合物(如淀粉、面包、马铃薯、大米)更可取。然而,在低血糖发作期间,快速吸收的碳水化合物,如含葡萄糖或蔗糖的果汁更为可取。偶尔,严重低血糖的患者可能需要持续静脉输注葡萄糖,同时增加膳食碳水化合物[12]。

二氮嗪是一种非利尿噻嗪类似物,具有显著的高血糖作用[10,12,96,98,99]。它通过刺激 α 肾上腺素能受体,直接抑制 β 细胞释放胰岛素,还具有促进糖原分解的胰外高血糖效应[83]。随餐服用二氮嗪来减少胃肠道副作用。二氮嗪的起始剂量应为每天 3~8mg/kg,分为 2 或 3 次/d;如果无效,可将二氮嗪增加至每日最大剂量 15mg/kg。不良反应与剂量有关,可能限制使用至最大剂量。不良反应包括钠潴留/水肿、胃肠道症状如恶心和多毛。添加噻嗪类利尿剂可以纠正水肿,并增强二氮嗪的高血糖效应。生长抑素类似物可控制 40%~60% 的胰岛素瘤患者的低血糖症状。生长抑素类似物被认为主要是通过与肿瘤上的生长抑素受体相互作用,特别是亚型 2 和 5[100]。因为胰岛素瘤通常生长抑素受体水平较低,所以胰岛素瘤对奥曲肽的症状反应率低于其他功能性 pNET[101]。由于生长抑素类似物还会降低胰高血糖素和生长激素的分泌,有时给药可能会加重低血糖[94]。因此,在给药长效奥曲肽或兰瑞肽之前,通常建议对短效奥曲肽进行密切监测。依维莫司(everolimus)是一种 mTOR 抑制剂,其副作用是导致高血糖,已被证明能有效控制其他疗法难以治愈的转移性胰岛素瘤患者的低血糖。其他的细胞毒性全身和肝靶向治疗(稍后讨论)也能控制转移性胰岛素瘤患者的低血糖[10,102]。

6. 手术治疗

由于绝大多数胰岛素瘤是局限性的[103-105],70%~97% 的患者可通过手术切除治愈[12,98,106,107]。因为胰岛素瘤几乎都是胰腺内的,通常是良性的,所以术前影像学上发现的胰岛素瘤越来越多地被腹腔镜手术成功切除[98,108,109]。

八、胃泌素瘤

胃泌素瘤(gastrinoma),又称为 Zollinger-Ellison 综合征(Zollinger-Ellison syndrome,ZES),是由神经内分泌肿瘤(胃泌素瘤)异位分泌引起的,可导致胃酸分泌过多,特点是引起消化性疾病(通常是严重的)和/或胃食管反流病(GERD)[110]。1955 年,Zollinger 和 Ellison 首次报道了 2 例胰腺非 β 细胞肿瘤引起的极度酸分泌过多和难治性消化性溃疡(PUD)的患者。

(一) 病理生理学与病理学

几乎所有的 ZES 症状都是由胃酸分泌过多引起的(表 34.6)。当胃酸分泌亢进得到控制后,PUD、GERD 和腹泻会消

表 34.6 NIH(Zollinger-Ellison 综合征胃泌素瘤)的临床和实验室特征

	NIH	文献中的范围
临床特征		
发病平均年龄/岁	41	41~53
症状平均持续时间/年	5.2	3.2~8.7
男性/%	56	44~70
腹痛/%	75	26~98
腹泻/%	73	17~73
确诊 PUD 病史/%	71	71~93
胃灼热/%	44	0~56
恶心/%	30	8~37
呕吐/%	25	26~51
出血/%	24	8~75
MEN-1/%	22	10~48
食管狭窄/%	4	4~6
胃肠穿孔/%	5	5~18
实验室特征/%		
空腹高胃泌素血症/%	99	96~100
胃泌素试验阳性(增加>120pg/mL)/%	94	94
BAO>15mEq/h(无既往胃部手术史)或>5mEq/h(有既往胃部手术史)/%	93	43~100

BAO,基础胃酸输出;MEN-1,多发性内分泌腺瘤 1 型;NIH,美国国立卫生研究院。

Data from Gibril F, Schumann M, Pace A, et al. Multiple endocrine neoplasia type 1 and Zollinger-Ellison syndrome: a prospective study of 107 cases and comparison with 1009 cases from the literature. Medicine (Baltimore) 2004; 83: 43-83; Osefo N, Ito T, Jensen RT. Gastric acid hypersecretory states: recent insights and advances. Curr Gastroenterol Rep 2009; 11: 434-41; Berna MJ, Hoffmann KM, Serrano J, et al. Serum gastrin in Zollinger-Ellison syndrome: I. Prospective study of fasting serum gastrin in 309 patients from the National Institutes of Health and comparison with 2229 cases from the literature. Medicine (Baltimore) 2006; 85: 295-340; Berna MJ, Hoffmann KM, Long SH, et al. Serum gastrin in Zollinger-Ellison syndrome: II. Prospective study of gastrin provocative testing in 293 patients from the National Institutes of Health and comparison with 537 cases from the literature. evaluation of diagnostic criteria, proposal of new criteria, and correlations with clinical and tumoral features. Medicine (Baltimore) 2006; 85: 341-64; Gibril F, Jensen RT. Advances in evaluation and management of gastrinoma in patients with Zollinger-Ellison syndrome. Curr Gastroenterol Rep 2005; 7: 114-21; Rogers A, Wang LM, Karavitaki N, et al. Neurofibromatosis Type 1 and pancreatic islet cell tumours: an association which should be recognized. QJM 2015; 108: 573-6.

失[10,16,111,112]。高胃泌素血症引起的壁细胞增生增加了胃最大酸分泌能力，慢性高胃酸血症也增加了基础酸分泌，这是ZES的特征性表现[112]。高血清胃泌素水平对胃黏膜有营养作用，导致胃皱襞增大（图34.3），不仅有壁细胞增生，还有胃嗜铬样细胞（gastric enterochromaffinlike cell，ECL）增生[11,112-115]。超过99%的ZES患者表现出一定程度的ECL增生[114-116]，而MEN-1/ZES患者的ECL增生更为明显。此外，2型胃类癌（稍后进一步阐述）很少见于散发性（非MEN-1）ZES病例，而23%的MEN-1/ZES患者发展为2型胃类癌[116]。

胃酸分泌增加直接导致小肠酸损伤，从而引起腹泻。此外，低pH会使胰脂肪酶失活，并能沉淀胆汁酸[16]。半数以上的胃泌素瘤发生在十二指肠，其中56%发生在十二指肠的第一部分，大约32%、6%和4%分别发生在十二指肠的第二、三和第四部分[71-73,81,111,117,118]。目前，60%～90%的胃泌素瘤位于"胃泌素三角"，即由后方胆囊管与胆总管的交界处、下方十二指肠的第二和第三部分交界处以及胰腺颈部与胰体内侧交界处形成的区域[119]。胃泌素瘤很少起源于非十二指肠/非胰腺腹部部位[120]。

淋巴结原发性胃泌素瘤在散发的ZES病例中有高达11%的报道[81,111,121,122]。一些散发性ZES的患者在仅切除含有胃泌素瘤的淋巴结后随访20年，仍能保持正常的胃泌素水平，几近治愈。根据淋巴结或肝转移情况，60%～90%的胃泌素瘤为恶性[40,123]。几乎三分之一的肝转移患者也发生骨转移，最常见的是转移到骨盆、肩胛骨和肋骨[124]。

胃泌素瘤有两种常见的生长模式：侵袭性疾病（占25%）和非侵袭性疾病（占75%）[27,110,125,126]。在一项研究中，预测肝转移的因素是胰腺（相对于非胰腺）胃泌素瘤和原发性肿瘤大于3cm。即使在转移到肝脏的胃泌素瘤患者中，肿瘤生长速度差异也很大[127]。超过90%的十二指肠胃泌素瘤是小的（<1cm），而只有8%的胰腺胃泌素瘤很小。十二指肠和胰腺胃泌素瘤生物学行为和预后的差异被用来支持它们有不同起源的假说[128]。

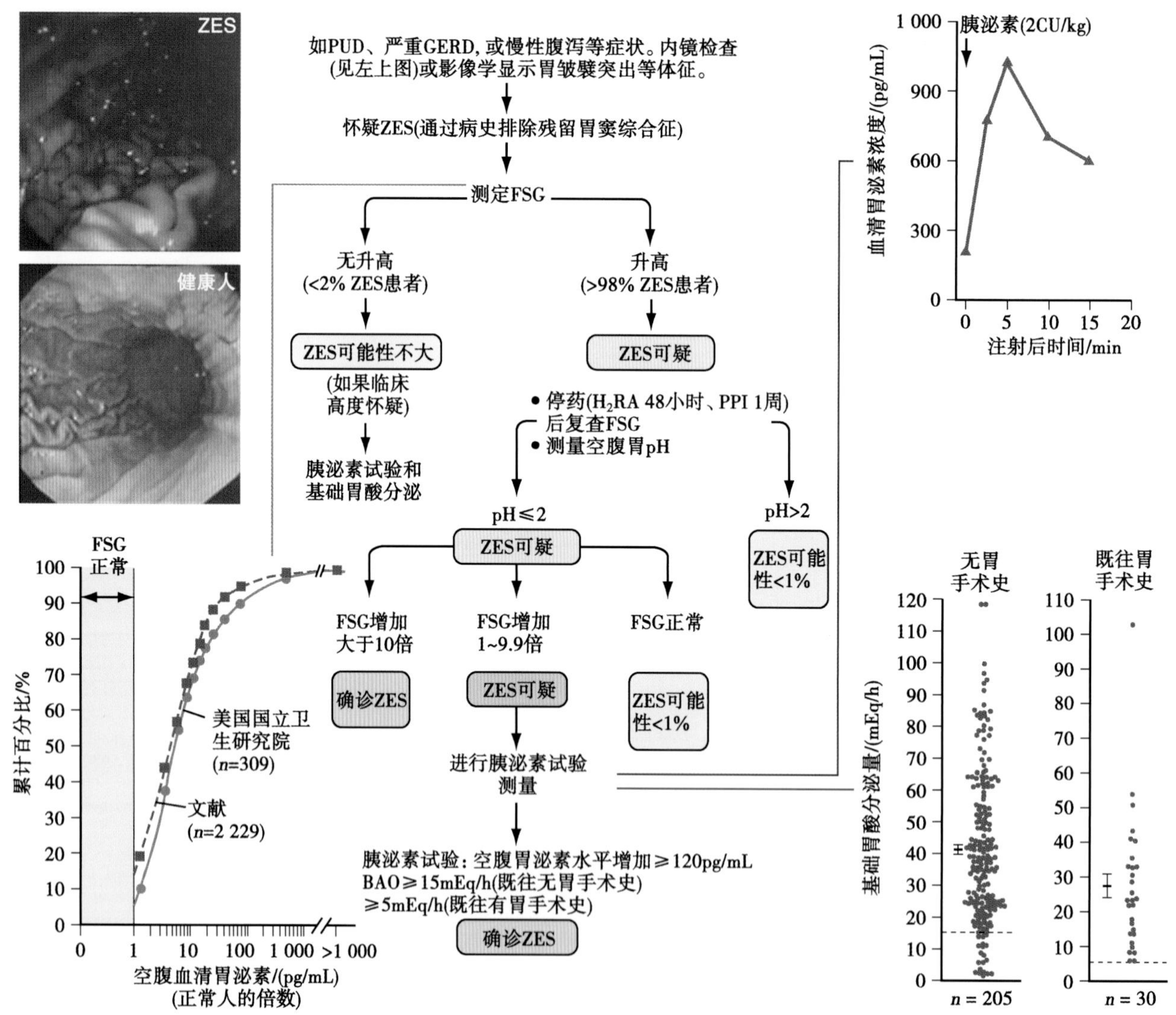

图34.3　胃泌素瘤（ZES）的诊断流程。右上图：典型ZES患者，促胰液素试验结果阳性（即，空腹胃泌素水平升高≥120pg/mL）。右下图：平均基础胃酸排出量（BAO）显著升高，既往接受过或未接受过胃酸减少手术。水平虚线表示拟用于区分ZE患者与非ZES患者的>15mEq/h或>5mEq/h标准。与正常受试者相比，ZES患者内镜检查发现左上胃皱襞明显。左下图：ZES患者中空腹血清胃泌素水平表示为水平轴上正常上限的倍数。极少数患者具有正常值，60%的患者血清胃泌素升高小于10倍[40,73,130,142,150]。CU，临床单位；FSG，空腹血清胃泌素

（二）临床特征

表 34.6 总结了 ZES 的临床特征[129]。主要由 PUD 引起的腹痛仍然是最常见的早期症状。溃疡疼痛在临床上与其他形式的 PUD 患者难以区分[40,111,129]。当溃疡样症状持续、药物治疗难治或伴有并发症时，提示 ZES 的诊断（见图 34.3）[10,130]。大多数 ZES 患者诊断时都有典型的十二指肠溃疡。这与以往研究的一个重要区别，在过去的研究中，90%以上的患者出现 PUD，通常伴有多发性溃疡或在非典型部位出现[112,123,131]。在较早的研究中，高达 100%的患者出现或发展为消化性疾病并发症（如出血、穿孔、梗阻、穿透、食管狭窄）。目前，只有不到 30%的患者出现这些并发症，即使大多数患者有 PUD 的确诊史[129]。

腹泻伴腹痛在 28%～56%的病例中发生，可能是 10%患者唯一的初始症状[10,129]。近 1/3 的患者以 GERD 为首发症状，约半数患者在初步评估时有 GERD 症状和/或食管病变[129,132]。

1/4 ZES 患者合并 MEN-1，但临床表现与散发性 ZES 患者相似[61,68,73,133]。提示 MEN-1/ZES 而非散发性 ZES 的线索包括：①有肾结石和/或肾绞痛史（47% vs 4%）；②症状出现时较年轻（平均 34 岁 vs 43 岁）；③某些内分泌疾病的个人或家族史（见表 34.4）。在对 MEN-1/ZES 患者的回顾中[68]，68%～90%的患者患有甲状旁腺功能亢进，31%～60%存在垂体疾病，6%～30%合并其他 NET（典型为肺），6%～16%的患者有其他功能性 pNET[61,68]。

1. 诊断

尽管广泛使用血清胃泌素测定法，但对 ZES 的诊断仍然可能推迟到症状出现后 4～6 年[68,129,134]。出现这种延迟诊断存在诸多原因。第一，由于 ZES 罕见（见表 34.1），因此通常不被考虑。第二，ZES 通常与其他 PUD 和 GERD 患者难以区分[40,112,133]。第三，最近广泛使用的质子泵抑制剂（PPI）既会使诊断复杂化，又会延迟诊断[130,134-137]。PPI 的使用降低了可能发生 ZES 的转诊人数，减少了被诊断为 ZES 的病例数，还与误诊 ZES 患者的增加有关[137]。由于长期 PPI 治疗导致 80%～100%的 PUD 或 GERD 患者出现高胃泌素血症，血清胃泌素水平经常达到正常水平的 5 倍，60%的 ZES 患者出现这种水平，因而可能导致误诊[130,134-136]。在过去，当 H2 受体拮抗剂（H2RAs）被广泛使用时，当常规剂量的 H2RAs 不能控制酸分泌过多和溃疡病时，常常建议诊断 ZES[7]。目前，常规剂量的强效 PPI 可能掩盖了 ZES 的诊断，因为它们控制了大多数患者的症状，PPI 治疗失败的情况并不常见[10,129,134,138]。

另一个使 ZES 诊断复杂化、有时会延迟的因素是当前血浆胃泌素测定的可靠性[134,139,140]。一项检查了 12 种不同的商用血浆胃泌素试剂盒（7 种放射免疫测定法和 5 种 ELISA 测定法）的研究[139]，结果表明 7 种分析法测定血浆胃泌素浓度不准确，既有高估亦有低估。因此，可靠的胃泌素测定法很有必要[134,139]。

胃酸性疾病或腹泻患者具有这些临床和实验室特征应提示诊断为 ZES（见图 34.3 和表 34.6）。第一，73%的 ZES 患者出现腹泻，但在常规的 PUD 或 GERD 患者中并不常见。高达 27%的 ZES 患者以腹泻为主要症状[40,112,129]。第二，由于 MEN-1 导致了 20%～25%的 ZES（见表 34.4）[61,68]，任何患有酸性消化性疾病且有 MEN-1 相容性内分泌病的个人史、家族史或实验室证据的患者都应被怀疑患有 MEN-1/ZES[68,134]。第三，50%～90%的 ZES 患者 Hp 阴性，显著高于其他 PU 人群，因此 Hp 阴性、NSAID 阴性的溃疡应怀疑是 ZES[10,141]。胃影像学检查中 EGD 上显著的胃皱襞提示了这种诊断。（见图 34.3 和表 34.6）[129]。胃镜下发现 ZES 患者的胃皱襞增大，与许多胃酸过少患者的胃皱襞消失形成对比，低胃酸血症可导致空腹高胃素血症（如慢性萎缩性胃炎，见第 52 章）。

ZES 的诊断需要在高胃泌素血症同时存在胃酸分泌不当（见图 34.3）[10,40,118,131,134,136]。空腹高胃泌素血症出现在 97%～99%的 ZES 患者中[142]。因此，如果空腹血清胃泌素水平正常，尤其是反复测定，则不太可能诊断 ZES。所以，当怀疑是 ZES 时，应首先测定空腹血清胃泌素[10,98,134,136,139,140]。由于 PPI 可提高大部分 ZES 患者的空腹血清胃泌素水平，且与血浆胃泌素水平重叠，因此当患者服用 PPI 时很难诊断 ZES[12,73,134-137,143,144]。如果患者服用 PPI 时空腹胃泌素水平升高，一般建议停止 PPI 至少一周后重复测定（见图 34.3）[12,134-136,143,144]。然而，如果患者有 ZES，突然停止 PPI 可导致消化性并发症的迅速发展。基于这个原因，一项研究建议不应停止 PPI，而应通过寻找胃泌素瘤的其他征象（如影像学上的 pNET）或尝试以某种方式降低 PPI 剂量来进行 ZES 的诊断[145]。在极少数情况下，转诊至有 PPI 停药经验的特殊中心，以保障停药带来的潜在危险[98,134,136,146]。

无论是由于疾病（如慢性萎缩性胃炎）或 PPI 使用所致的胃酸缺乏，都是比 ZES 更常见的空腹高胃泌素血症的原因，并可导致胰泌素试验假阳性[147]。在一项针对 ZES 患者的研究中[131]，99%的患者空腹时胃 pH 低于 2。因此，如果发现空腹胃泌素水平升高并怀疑有 ZES，下一步应该检测空腹胃 pH 排除生理性、"适当"高胃泌素血症（如胃酸减少或胃酸缺乏引起）（见图 34.3）。另一个生理性高胃泌素血症的原因（除慢性萎缩性胃炎和 PPI 的使用外）是减少胃酸的手术，如迷走神经切断术[10,40,98,130,134,136]。慢性肾脏病也会由于胃泌素清除率降低而导致空腹高胃泌素血症。

慢性萎缩性胃炎患者空腹血清胃泌素水平可升高 70 倍以上，在服用 PPI 患者中，超过 25%的患者胃泌素水平升高 4 倍以上[134]。相比之下，大多数 ZES 患者空腹胃泌素水平升高不到 10 倍（图 34.3）。因此，血清胃泌素水平的升高并不能单独将 ZES 与生理性高胃泌素血症区分开来[134]。

空腹血清胃泌素水平升高小于 10 倍（如<1 000pg/mL）且空腹胃 pH 值低于 2 的患者可能患有除了 ZES 外的其他疾病，如幽门梗阻、Hp 感染、肾功能衰竭、短肠综合征、胃窦 G 细胞功能亢进或增生、残窦综合征。在这类患者中，如果怀疑为隐匿性胃泌素瘤，则应考虑进行分泌素试验和基础胃酸分泌（basal acid output，BAO）测定[134,142,148]。胰泌素试验的基础是胃泌素瘤在静脉注射分泌素后会释放出过量的胃泌素，这可能是由肿瘤细胞分泌素的特定受体引起的[149]。静脉注射 2U/kg 分泌素后，血清胃泌素增加≥120pg/mL，敏感性高（94%），特异性接近 100%[150]。在胃 pH 低于 2 的高胃泌素血症患者中，未见胰泌素试验假阳性的报道[131,148,150-152]。90%以上的 ZES 患者 BAO 升高，未经胃手术的患者 BAO 水平高于 15mEq/h，而存在减少胃酸的手术史的患者 BAO 高于 5mEq/h（见图 34.3）[40,131,152]。胃酸分泌现在不是常见的测量方法，但如果需要，EGD 期间可以测量胃酸分泌量[153]。

2. 治疗

同其他恶性功能性 pNET 一样，ZES 患者有两个治疗问题[10,73,94,146,152]。第一,必须控制胃酸高分泌;第二,必须处理胃泌素瘤[10,40,71,73,96,98,117,118,152]。如果胃酸分泌亢进得不到控制,几乎一定会发生危及生命的消化性疾病并发症,有时发生得很快[10,40,123,130,134,152,154]。尽管大多数患者在 ZES 确诊之前接受了某种形式的抗胃酸分泌治疗,但仍有近 25% 的患者出现出血,6% ~ 7% 出现溃疡穿孔,8% ~ 10% 出现食管狭窄[12,129]。随着医学上控制胃高分泌能力的提高,肿瘤的自然病史正成为长期生存的主要决定因素(图 34.4)[110,126]。

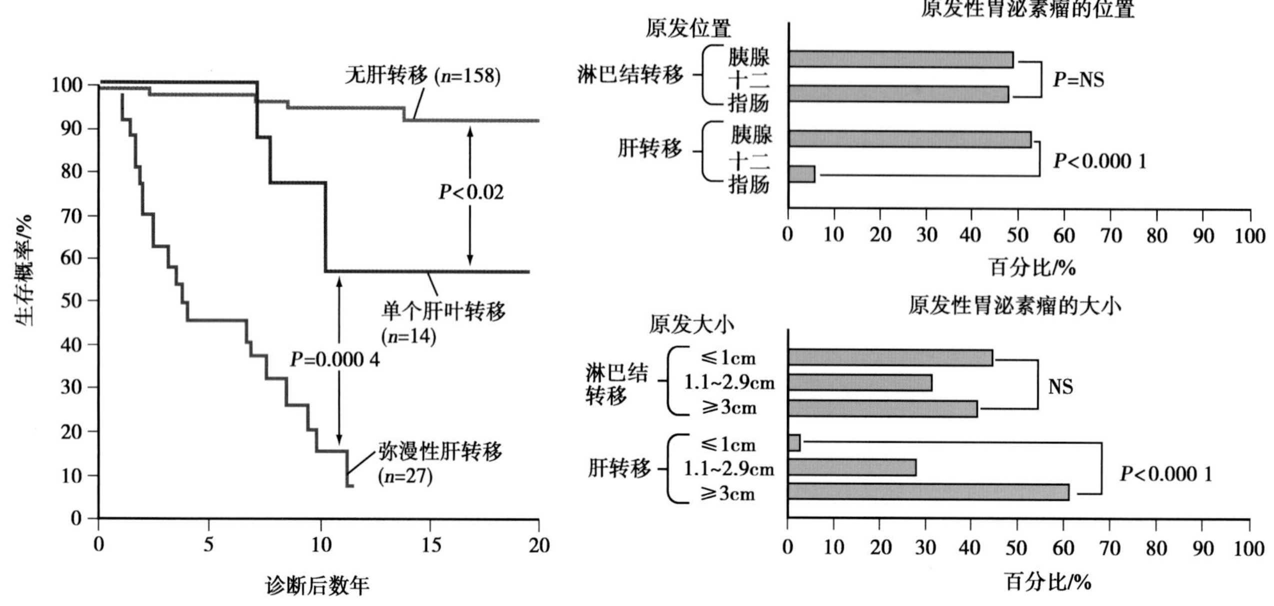

图 34.4 胃泌素瘤的范围对生存期以及原发性胃泌素瘤位置和大小对淋巴结或肝转移发展的影响。左图,伴或不伴肝转移的胃泌素瘤患者的生存期。右上部分显示了 83 例原发性胰腺或十二指肠胃泌素瘤患者发生淋巴结或肝转移的百分比。右下部分显示 118 例不同直径的原发性胃泌素瘤患者发生淋巴结或肝转移的百分比。(左,adapted from Yu F, Venzon DJ, Serrano J, et al. Prospective study of the clinical course, prognostic factors, causes of death, and survival in patients with long-standing Zollinger-Ellison syndrome. J Clin Oncol 1999;17:615-30。右,adapted from Weber HC, Venzon DJ, Lin JT, et al. Determinants of metastatic rate and survival in patients with Zollinger-Ellison syndrome: a prospective long-term study. Gastroenterology 1995;108:1637-49.)

3. 控制胃酸高分泌

由于其作用和效力持续时间较长,PPI 允许在大多数 ZES 患者(>95%)中每日给药 1~2 次,是首选药物[10,40,73,152,155-157]。所有的 PPI(奥美拉唑、兰索拉唑、泮托拉唑、埃索美拉唑和雷贝拉唑)均有效[10,152,155,156]。H2RAs 也有效,但通常需要高于常规剂量[10,111,152]。

对于大多数 ZES 患者,PPI 的起始剂量通常为 60mg/d 的奥美拉唑。需要给予足够的抗分泌药物,以将下一次给药前一小时内测得的酸高分泌量降低至 10mEq/h 以下(无胃酸减少手术史)或小于 5mEq/h(有胃酸减少手术史)。这种程度的酸抑制可使消化道病变愈合并防止其复发。尽管 PPI 的初始剂量较低,但由于需要快速控制 ZES 患者的酸分泌过多,因此建议使用较高剂量的 PPI[158]。

对于某些患者,如那些 MEN-1/ZES、严重 GERD 或既往存在 Billroth II 切除术的患者,推荐更高的 PPI 初始剂量,相当于每日两次、每次 60mg 奥美拉唑[98,132,152]。这类患者需要更强的酸抑制,应增加抗分泌药物,以控制症状和治愈所有黏膜病变,这通常需要酸抑制到 1~2mEq/h 甚至更低[159]。MEN-1/ZES 和甲状旁腺功能亢进患者进行甲状旁腺切除术,可降低空腹胃泌素水平,降低 BAO,并增加了对抗分泌药物的敏感性[40,134,160,161]。这种干预尤其重要,因为,如前所述,甲状旁腺功能亢进的 MEN-1/ZES 患者对 PPI 相对耐药[152,156,157]。

长期口服抗分泌药治疗 10 多年来一直有效,没有发展快速耐药性[40,111,130,152,155,157]。PPI 的安全性已经引起了人们的关注[162-167],但诸如铁吸收不良导致的铁缺乏和 GI-NET(类癌)风险增加等问题在临床上并不显著。PPI 治疗可导致维生素 B_{12} 缺乏,应每年进行监测。

4. 局限性胃泌素瘤的治疗

大多数权威人士建议对 ZES 患者进行手术探查,只要肝脏没有弥漫性扩散转移灶,且患者没有 MEN-1[72,73,98,117,146,168,169] 便可能根治性切除。在散发性(非 MEN-1)ZES 患者中,92% 的患者发现胃泌素瘤,51% 的患者肿瘤切除后立刻缓解,34% 的患者 10 年后无病[72]。手术治愈率远高于许多早期研究报道的治愈率,这在很大程度上取决于更多小的十二指肠胃泌素瘤的发现。在手术中进行常规的十二指肠切除术比其他常用方法可发现更多的肿瘤[111,117,170-172]。治疗性手术在 MEN-1/ZES 患者中的作用是有争议的,因为如果不采用更积极的切除(如胰十二指肠切除术),这类患者的无病治愈率低于 5%[61,71,73,98,169,173,174]。这种不利的手术结果是因为 MEN-1/ZES 患者常常为多发十二指肠胃泌素瘤,并经常在手术时已出现淋巴结转移[175]。手术的作用存在争议,其中部分原因在于尚不清楚早期手术切除能否提高 MEN-1/ZES 患者的生存率。有人建议对 MEN-1/ZES 患者进行常规探查,也有人建议仅进行药物治疗而不探查,还有人建议仅在发现较大的病变(≥2~3cm)时才进行探查[98,146,173,176]。虽然胰十二指肠切除术可以治愈较高比例的 MEN-1/ZES 患者[177],但由于手术的不良影响和未手术的小 pNET(<2cm)患者的长期预后良好,因此一般不推荐行胰十二指肠切除术[198,146,178]。

九、胰高血糖素瘤

胰高血糖素瘤是一种罕见的 NET(几乎都是 pNET),它分泌过多的胰高血糖素,并引起一种以体重减轻、葡萄糖不耐受、贫血和一种称为坏死溶解性移行性红斑(NME)的特殊性皮炎为特征的独特综合征(表 34.7)。Becker 等在 1942 年描述了一个合并皮疹的 pNET 患者[179],McGarvan 等 1966 年报道了一例高胰高血糖素水平、皮炎、糖尿病和 pNET 患者[180],Wilkinson 等 1973 年描述了 NME[181]。最后,Mallinson 等[5]于 1974 年建立了 NME 与产生胰高血糖素肿瘤的关联。

表 34.7　胰高血糖素瘤或血管活性肠肽瘤综合征患者的临床和实验室特征

胰高血糖素瘤	血管活性肠肽瘤
临床特征(%)	
皮炎(54~90)	分泌性腹泻(89~100)
糖尿病/葡萄糖不耐受(22~90)	血容量不足(44~100)
体重减轻(56~96)	体重减轻(36~100)
舌炎/口腔炎/唇炎(29~40)	腹部绞痛、肠绞痛(10~63)
腹泻(14~15)	潮红(14~34)
腹痛(12)	
静脉血栓栓塞(12~35)	
精神障碍(不常见)	
实验室特征(%)	
贫血(34~85)	低钾血症(67~100)
低氨基酸血症(26~100)	胃酸过少(34~72)
低胆固醇血症(80)	高钙血症(41~50)
肾性糖尿病(不详)	高血糖症(18~100)

胰高血糖素瘤数据来自:Mallinson CN, Bloom SR, Warin AP, et al. A glucagonoma syndrome. Lancet 1974; 2: 1-5; Jensen RT, Norton JA. Endocrine tumors of the pancreas and gastrointestinal tract. In: Feldman MFL, Brandt LJ, ed. Sleisenger and Fordtran's Gastrointestinal and Liver Disease. 8th ed. Philadelphia: Saunders; 2006. pp 625-66; Eldor R, Glaser B, Fraenkel M, et al. Glucagonoma and the glucagonoma syndrome—cumulative experience with an elusive endocrine tumour. Clin Endocrinol (Oxf) 2011; 74: 593-8; Kindmark H, Sundin A, Granberg D, et al. Endocrine pancreatic tumors with glucagon hypersecretion: a retrospective study of 23 cases during 20years. Med Oncol 2007; 24: 340-7; Soga J, Yakuwa Y. Glucagonomas/diabetico-dermatogenic syndrome (DDS): a statistical evaluation of 407 reported cases. J Hepatobiliary Pancreat Surg 1998; 5: 312-9; Guillausseau PJ G-SC. Glucagonomas: clinical presentation, diagnosis, and advances in management. In: Mignon M, Jensen RT, eds. Endocrine tumors of the pancreas: recent advances in research and management. Frontiers in GI Research Basel, Switzerland, S. Karger, 1995; Chastain MA. The glucagonoma syndrome: a review of its features and discussion of new perspectives. Am J Med Sci 2001; 321: 302-306; van Beek AP, de Haas ER, van Vloten WA, et al. The glucagonoma syndrome and necrolytic migratory erythema: a clinical review. Eur J Endocrinol 2004; 151: 531-7.

血管活性肠肽瘤数据来自:Jensen RT, Norton JA. Endocrine tumors of the pancreas and gastrointestinal tract. In: Feldman MFL, Brandt LJ, ed. Sleisenger and Fordtran's gastrointestinal and liver disease. 9th ed. Philadelphia: Saunders; 2010, pp 491-522; Matuchansky CR, JC. VIPomas and endocrine cholera: clinical presentation, diagnosis, and advances in management. In: Mignon MJR, ed. Endocrine tumors of the pancreas: recent advances in research and management Frontiers in GI Research. Basel, Switzerland, S. Krager; 1995, pp 166-82; Song S, Shi R, Li B, et al. Diagnosis and treatment of pancreatic vasoactive intestinal peptide endocrine tumors. Pancreas 2009; 38: 811-4; Adam N, Lim SS, Ananda V, et al. VIPoma syndrome: challenges in management. Singapore Med J 2010; 51: e129-32; Soga J, Yakuwa Y. Vipoma/diarrheogenic syndrome: a statistical evaluation of 241reported cases. J Exp Clin Cancer Res 1998; 17: 389-400; Jensen RD, GM. Carcinoid tumors and the carcinoid syndrome. In DeVita VT Jr HS, Rosenberg SA, ed. Cancer: principles and practice of oncology. 7th ed. Philadelphia: Lippincott Williams and Wilkins; 2005, pp 1559-74.

病理生理学与病理学

与胰岛素瘤相比,大多数胰高血糖素瘤在诊断时体积较大,平均大小为 5~10cm(范围为 0.4~35cm)[12,182-187]。与胰岛素瘤以外的其他 pNET 类似,胰高糖瘤通常是恶性的[12,182,183,188]。最常见的转移部位是肝和淋巴结,骨和肠系膜较少见[11,182]。大部分胰高血糖素瘤(>97%)发生在胰腺,通常(88%~90%的病例)为孤立性肿瘤[185]。

胰高血糖素瘤综合征的病理生理学与已知的胰高血糖素的作用有关(见第 4 章)[189]。高血糖是由肝糖原分解和糖异生作用增加引起的。减肥被归因于胰高血糖素的已知分解代谢作用[185],尽管胰高血糖素样肽-1(GLP-1)(7~36 个酰胺)介导的味觉厌恶效应可能是原因之一[190]。特征性皮疹(NME)是否由高胰高血糖素血症引起尚存争议。长期服用胰高血糖素引起的高胰高血糖素血症确实会引起典型的皮疹[12,191,192]。低氨基酸血症(80%~90%)或必需脂肪酸缺乏可能与皮炎的发生有关,因为如果这些缺陷得到纠正,NME 可以在不改变血浆胰高血糖素水平的情况下得到改善。皮肤损伤与锌缺乏症的相似性导致了锌的试验,并取得了一些效果。皮疹甚至会随着容量的增加而消退。因此,不同的患者可能有不同的影响因素。高胰高血糖素血症可能导致贫血,因为用胰高血糖素治疗会降低动物中红细胞生成。胰高血糖素在引起静脉血栓栓塞和精神疾病中的作用尚不确定[193]。

胰高血糖素细胞腺瘤病[194]可模拟胰高血糖素瘤综合征[12,195,196]。胰高血糖素细胞腺瘤病中有许多微腺瘤和染色为胰高血糖的增生性胰岛素。此外,在单一病例中,人胰高血糖素受体的纯合 P86S 突变与 α 细胞增生、高血糖素血症和 NF-pNET 有关。这种疾病,即 Mahvash 病,可以在缺乏胰高血糖素受体的小鼠身上重现[196,197]。

1. 临床特征

胰高血糖素瘤通常发生在 50~70 岁的人中[12,90,182,184-186]。NME 是一种常见的表现(图 34.5,另见表 34.7)[12,90,183-185,198,199]。皮炎往往先于该综合征的诊断数年[12,198]。在 70%的患者中,皮肤损伤是该病的主要症状,并且在确诊 pNET 前 3 年就被发现[200]。皮肤病变可能会时轻时重,常被误诊[200,201]。特征性的病变开始是红斑,通常出现在口周或擦烂区域,如腹股沟、臀部、大腿或会阴部,然后向侧面扩散。随后病灶升高,并出现中央表浅水疱。大疱的顶部经常脱落或破裂,留下形成硬痂的侵蚀区域。病灶往往在中心趋于愈合,而边缘继续扩散,边缘有明显的痂皮。愈合与色素沉着的发展有关。整个过程通常需要 1~2 周。组织病理学可随临床表现而变化[11]。典型的早期病变表现为浅表性海绵样变和坏死,伴有角膜下和中表皮大疱。镜下可见梭形角化细胞的核固缩,也可见单核细胞炎性浸润[5,12,198,199]。

葡萄糖不耐受或糖尿病可能先于诊断胰高血糖素瘤很多年[90,183-186]。严重的低氨基酸血症(通常低于正常值的 25%,尤其是糖原性氨基酸)很常见[5,11,90,184,186],而且有时也会出现必需脂肪酸缺乏症。大多数患者,即使是小的、非转移性肿瘤[5,11,182],也会出现严重的、与厌食症相关的体重减轻[11,90,183-186]。

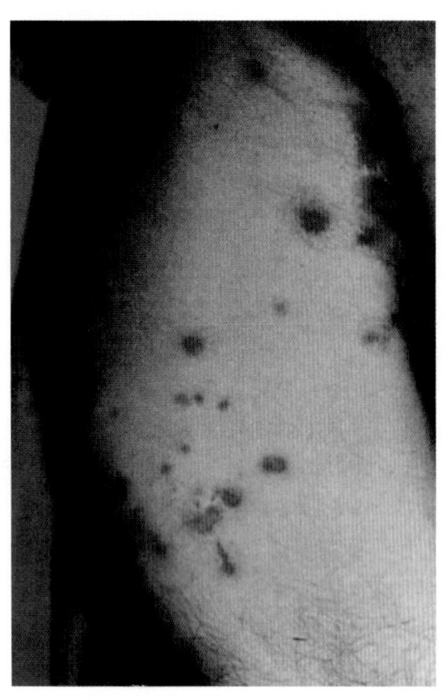

图 34.5　一例胰高血糖素瘤患者的坏死溶解性移行性红斑(NME)。NME 的特征是快速侵蚀浅表水疱。病变通常局限于臀部、腹股沟、会阴、肘部、手、足和口周区域。(Courtesy Dr. Carl Grunfeld, San Francisco, Calif.)

静脉血栓栓塞在胰高血糖素瘤综合征中比在其他 pNET 中更常见。出现的轻度贫血通常为正细胞性正色素性的,血清铁、叶酸和维生素 B_{12} 水平是正常的,对成功的肿瘤治疗有反应。

2. 诊断

常因皮疹、NME(见图 34.5)而怀疑胰高血糖素瘤[90,176,177,179-187,195,198,202-205]。胰高血糖素瘤的诊断可以通过证明空腹血浆胰高血糖素浓度的增加而得到证实(正常值低于 200pg/mL)。大多数胰高血糖素瘤患者的血浆胰高血糖素水平显著升高[11,12,90,182,183,186,206],平均血浆胰高血糖素浓度为 2 110pg/mL(范围 550~6 600pg/mL)[11]。轻度高胰高血糖素血症(200~500pg/mL)也发生在许多其他情况下,如肝硬化、慢性肾脏病、糖尿病酮症酸中毒、长期饥饿、急性胰腺炎、肢端肥大症、库欣综合征、败血症、严重烧伤、严重应激(创伤、运动)、腹腔疾病、达那唑治疗和家族性高血糖素血症[10,11,181,185]。胰高血糖素瘤激发试验已有报道,但没有一种足够可靠。

3. 治疗

(1) 药物治疗

随着肿瘤定位研究(稍后讨论)的进行,最初的药物治疗旨在缓解症状、恢复营养状况和控制高血糖。胰高血糖素瘤患者手术风险一般较低。胰高血糖素的分解代谢作用联合葡萄糖不耐受和糖尿病可显著影响患者的营养状况。静脉血栓栓塞的风险增加了术后发病率。

生长抑素类似物(somatostatin analog, SSA)在控制胰高血糖素瘤患者的症状方面很有用[182,183,185,207]。大多数患者经 SSA 治疗后皮疹好转,消失率高达 30%。80%~90% 患者的血浆胰高血糖素水平降低了,但仅 10%~20% 患者的血浆胰高血糖素水平恢复至正常范围。

(2) 手术治疗

所有局限性肿瘤患者都应考虑手术切除[208]。不幸的是,50%~90% 的胰高血糖素瘤患者在诊断时已经转移[182-184,209]。

十、血管活性肠肽瘤

血管活性肠肽瘤综合征是一种由过量分泌的血管活性肠肽(VIP)引起的 NET。该综合征的特征是严重的水样腹泻、胃酸过少、胃酸缺乏和低钾血症(见表 34.1 和表 34.7)[4,210]。由于腹泻液与霍乱的相似之处,人们提出了"胰性霍乱"一词,并创建了首字母缩略词 WDHA(水样腹泻、低钾血症和胃酸缺乏)这一简称[211]。VIP 被怀疑为该综合征的介质,并证实了输注 VIP 能够在人体内产生与血管活性肠肽瘤患者血液水平相同的分泌性腹泻[212]。

病理生理学与病理学

大多数(80%~90%)的成人血管活性肠肽瘤是 pNET,42%~75% 发生在胰腺尾部[12,213,214];分泌 VIP 的 SI-NET、肺癌或嗜铬细胞瘤是罕见的[12,211,213-217]。血管活性肠肽瘤几乎总是巨大的孤立性肿瘤,通常在诊断或手术时已经转移,类似于胃泌素瘤和胰高血糖素瘤。在幼儿(<10 岁)和很少的成人(5% 的成人病例)中,血管活性肠肽瘤综合征是由胰腺外神经节瘤或神经节神经母细胞瘤引起的,只有 10% 是恶性肿瘤[11,211]。

几乎一半的血管活性肠肽瘤分泌多种激素,包括胰高血糖素、生长抑素、胰岛素和胃泌素[11,16]。

VIP 是该综合征的主要介质[11,16,211,218];血浆 VIP 水平通常升高[219],正常人连续静脉输注 VIP,达到与血管活性肠肽瘤综合征患者相似的血浆水平,在 6~7 小时内产生水样腹泻[212]。VIP 与肠上皮细胞上的特定受体相互作用,导致肠电解质和液体分泌(见第 101 章)[11]。

血管活性肠肽瘤患者的面部潮红被归因于 VIP 强大的血管舒张作用[11]。尽管血浆 VIP 水平很高,但只有少数的血管活性肠肽瘤综合征患者出现潮红,这一发现被认为是由于 VIP 灌注时间过长导致潮红逐渐消失,即快速耐受。严重的低钾血症可能主要是由粪便 K^+ 丢失引起的,继发性醛固酮增多症是由于肾 K^+ 损失和肾素释放的 VIP 刺激所致[11]。胃酸缺乏或胃酸减少的发病机制尚不完全清楚,但已归因于 VIP 对胃酸分泌的抑制作用。高钙血症的机制也不清楚。高血糖被认为是 VIP 对肝脏的糖原分解作用。

1. 临床特征

成人血管活性肠肽瘤的平均发病年龄为 42~51 岁(范围为 32~81 岁)[10,211,219-221]。儿童平均发病年龄为 2~4 岁(范围为 10 个月~9 岁)。血管活性肠肽瘤综合征的主要特征是伴有低钾血症和血容量不足的严重分泌性腹泻(见表 34.7)[10,211,219-221]。腹泻可间歇性发作[211,222],超过 1L/d(通常为超过 3L/d)[11,16,213,214]。腹泻液呈淡茶状,并且在禁食期间仍有发作[11,16,218]。大多数(90%)患者每天有 5 次或更多的大便。

血管活性肠肽瘤患者的实验室异常见表 34.7[10,211,219-221]。在超过 90% 的患者中,低钾血症在病程的某个阶段往往是严重的(<2.5mmol/L)[12,211,222]。可能发生手足搐搦症,并归因于由

腹泻引起的低镁血症[11]。如果测量,在许多情况下都会发生胃酸减少。

2. 诊断

血管活性肠肽瘤综合征的诊断需要在禁食时持续的大量分泌性腹泻和血浆 VIP 浓度升高[10,16,213,214,216,218]。在被确诊前腹泻可能会持续长期存在。腹泻具有分泌性腹泻的特征(见第 16 章)。

其他疾病可引起慢性、大量分泌性腹泻,具有血管活性肠肽瘤综合征除血浆 VIP 水平升高(假性血管活性肠肽瘤综合征)外的大部分临床特征。这样的疾病包括胃泌素瘤[16,40,129]、慢性泻药滥用[223]、腹腔疾病[224]、艾滋病肠病[225]或特发性分泌性腹泻[12,16,223,226-228]。仅血浆 VIP 水平升高不能作为诊断腹泻患者血管活性肠肽瘤的唯一依据,因为其他情况(如长期禁食、IBD、小肠切除术、放射性肠炎、慢性肾脏病、胰岛细胞增殖症[229])偶尔也会升高 VIP 水平[11,16,230]。

3. 治疗

(1) 药物治疗

首要目标是补充液体和电解质的损失,以纠正严重的容量不足、低钾血症和高氯性代谢性酸中毒(见表 34.7)。患者可能需要每天 5L 或更多的液体[11] 和超过 350mEq 的钾[11,16,211,231]。可发生低钾性肾病伴严重肾功能衰竭[4]。应仔细监控液体和电解质的需要量。使用 SSA 可控制腹泻的量[10,12,16,98,146,207,232]。奥曲肽可控制 78% ~ 100% 患者的腹泻[10,207,220,232]。奥曲肽在 6 个月后仍对 56% ~ 100% 的患者有效,但 22% 的患者需要增加剂量[11,12]。服用奥曲肽的患者血浆 VIP 浓度下降了 80% ~ 89%。奥曲肽治疗后血浆 VIP 浓度的降低并不总是反映临床治疗反应[11,16,233]。转移性血管活性肠肽瘤的治疗稍后讨论。

(2) 手术治疗

一旦纠正了液体和电解质不足,患者应该进行影像学检查(稍后讨论),以评估肿瘤能否切除。完成这些影像学研究后,所有没有转移性病灶的患者都应考虑手术治疗[10,98,105,208,214,222]。手术切除胰腺血管活性肠肽瘤可减轻三分之一患者的所有症状,其中 30% 的患者可治愈[12,211,234]。在儿童(和罕见的成人)中[12],78% 的患者可以手术切除并控制所有症状。

十一、其他功能性胰腺神经内分泌肿瘤

表 34.1 总结了不常见的 pNET。分泌促肾上腺皮质激素(ACTH)的 pNET 可导致库欣综合征。这些肿瘤往往是转移性、侵袭性的,并且对包括 SSA 治疗在内的治疗无效[10,11,235,236]。

分泌甲状旁腺激素(PTH)相关肽的 pNET,可导致高钙血症,通常在诊断时体积较大和/或转移到肝脏。除了抗肿瘤治疗,双膦酸盐可用于控制高钙血症[237]。产生 5-羟色胺的 pNET 会导致类癌综合征,是一种罕见、体积巨大、主要是恶性的肿瘤[12,13,188]。

"生长抑素瘤"一词有时用于描述罕见的胰腺或十二指肠肿瘤,这些肿瘤分泌大量的生长抑素,导致相对非特异性的症状,如糖尿病、胆结石、腹泻/脂肪泻和体重减轻。该词有时也用于描述十二指肠 NET,其生长抑素染色呈阳性,也以砂粒体为表征,但不一定分泌生长抑素。这种肿瘤在 NF1 患者中出现频率较高。由于生长抑素瘤综合征的临床表现相对隐匿,这种诊断罕见[238]。

十二、无功能性胰腺神经内分泌肿瘤

无功能性胰腺神经内分泌肿瘤(NF-pNET)是一种与引起功能综合征的肽/胺分泌无关的 pNET,其症状完全是由肿瘤本身的局部效应引起[12]。

(一) 临床特征

典型的高分化 NF-pNET 患者发病年龄为 40~60 岁。从最初症状到确诊的中位时间从 6 个月到近 3 年不等。越来越多的小 NF-pNET 患者因不相关的原因进行扫描时被偶然诊断出来。肿瘤的症状/体征包括腹痛、黄疸和体重减轻[10,25,29,67,239-241]。

(二) 治疗

对于局部可切除的 NF-pNET 患者,一般建议手术切除。未来的复发取决于肿瘤大小、分级和淋巴结阳性。对于小的(≤2cm)、散发性、偶然诊断为低级别 NF-PETs 患者的治疗存在争议[67]。一些研究表明,接受监测的患者的疾病稳定性很高[242]。某些提示肿瘤惰性的影像学特征包括清晰的肿瘤边界和肿瘤的均质性[243]。最终,手术和监测的决定需要考虑患者的年龄、合并症和接受长期监测的意愿[67,244,245]。

十三、胃肠道神经内分泌肿瘤(类癌)(GI-NET)

GI-NET(类癌)几乎占所有类癌的 70%。其他大部分(近 25%)存在于呼吸道。GI-NET 最常发生在小肠、直肠、阑尾或胃(表 34.8)[246]。在小肠内,回肠是最常见的部位,其次是十二指肠和空肠[246]。GI-NET 的发病率在增加,但并不一致(见图 34.1)[23]。GI-NET 生存率高度依赖于肿瘤分期[247],如表 34.9 所示。

表 34.8 选定类癌的相对频率及其转移和类癌综合征的患病率

	所有类癌中[a] 的百分比/%	有转移的百分比/%	伴类癌综合征的百分比/%
胃	2~6	22~31	10
小肠[b]	10~28	14~71	3~13
阑尾	2~38	2~35	<1
结肠	4~10	60~71	5
直肠	10~19	3~14	<1

[a] 此处不包括的其他较少见的类癌部位包括食管、肝脏、胆囊、胆道、喉、子宫颈、卵巢和睾丸。

[b]小肠包括十二指肠、壶腹、空肠、回肠和 Meckel 憩室。

Data from Yao JC, Hassan M, Phan A, et al. One hundred years after "carcinoid": epidemiology of and prognostic factors for neuroendocrine tumors in 35,825 cases in the USA. J Clin Oncol 2008;26:3063-72; Modlin IM, Lye KD, Kidd M. A 5-decade analysis of 13,715 carcinoid tumors. Cancer 2003;97:934-59; Modlin IM, Sandor A. An analysis of 8305 cases of carcinoid tumors. Cancer 1997;79:13-29; Godwin JD. 2nd: Carcinoid tumors. An analysis of 2,837 cases. Cancer 1975;36:560-9.

其他研究可能有所不同(见正文)。

表 34.9 所选类癌分期的中位生存期(月)

	局部阶段	区域阶段	远处转移阶段
胃	154	71	29
小肠	111	105	103
阑尾	>360	>360	NA
结肠	261	36	14
直肠	290	90	34

Data from Dasari A, Shen C, Halperin D, et al. Trends in the incidence, prevalence, and survival outcomes in patients with neuroendocrine tumors in the USA. JAMA Oncol 2017;3:1335-42; Yao JC, Hassan M, Phan A, et al. One hundred years after "carcinoid": epidemiology of and prognostic factors for neuroendocrine tumors in 35,825 cases in the USA. J Clin Oncol 2008;26:3063-72.

NA,不可用。

(一) 胃神经内分泌肿瘤(胃 NET)

在美国,胃 NET 占了所有胃肿瘤的 0.3% 和所有类癌的 2%~6%。它们的发病率在过去 30 年里显著增加(见图 34.1)[247-260]。目前尚不清楚这是否是疾病发病率的真正增加,还是由于上消化道内窥镜检查(EGD)使用的增加导致检测率的提高[248]。因此,在 EGD 过程中,由于其他原因,经常会偶然发现胃 NET[118,250,251,253,257,258,260]。

胃 NET 分为 3 种类型(表 34.10)。为了将胃类癌正确分类,除了病灶切除或活检外,还应采集胃窦、胃体/底的黏膜[146,248,250,260]。

(1) 1 型胃 NET:是最常见的类型,一般较小且多发,多见于伴或不伴恶性贫血的慢性萎缩性胃炎患者(多为女性)[248-250,260]。1 型胃 NET 出现在 1%~2% 的慢性萎缩性胃炎患者中(见第 52 章)[253]。在 EGD 时,1 型胃 NET 通常表现为息肉样病变,并伴有黏膜萎缩(图 34.6A)[253]。尽管在内镜下看不到、但如果随机黏膜活检,会发现额外的黏膜内 NET[253]。组织学上,1 型胃 NET 分化良好,常伴有不同程度的胃 ECL 细胞增生。ECL 增生是由胃酸对胃泌素(G)细胞反馈抑制缺失引起的高胃泌素血症引起的(见第 51 章)[249]。通常严重的慢性高胃泌素血症,导致 ECL 细胞的增生(弥漫性、线性、小结节),在某些情况下,会出现异常增生和瘤变[249]。1 型胃 NET 一般侵袭性较弱,27% 局限于黏膜层,64% 局限于黏膜下层,只有 9% 侵犯固有肌层[257,260]。转移到淋巴结或肝脏罕见[22,248,261]。

表 34.10 胃类癌的分类

	1 型	2 型	3 型
相对频率/%	65~80	5~6	14~25
性别	女性>男性	女性=男性	男性>女性
肿瘤特征			
肿瘤大小/cm	<1(80%) 1~2(15%~20%) >2(<1%)	<1(35%) 1~2(45%) >2(20%)	2~5
肿瘤数目	多发	多发	单发
组织学,等级(G)	高分化,G1	高分化,G1	高分化,G1 或 G2
ECL 细胞增生/%	100	100	0
胃黏膜	萎缩	增生	正常
相关因素	胃萎缩	MEN-1/ZES	无
胃 pH,酸度水平	高 pH,酸缺乏	低 pH,酸过多	正常 pH 和酸度
空腹血清胃泌素	高	高	正常
转移			
淋巴结/%	2~9	15~30	75~100
远处/%	0~2	<10	50~100
肿瘤相关性死亡/%	无	<10	25~30
5 年生存率(疾病相关)/%	100	60~90	50
治疗	<1cm:EndoR 1~2cm:EndoR 或手术 >2cm:手术	<1cm:EndoR 1~2cm:EndoR 或手术 >2cm:手术	手术,切除局部淋巴结(如果无晚期疾病)

EndoR,内镜下切除术;MEN-I/ZES,多发性内分泌腺瘤 1 型/胃泌素瘤。

数据来自 Delle Fave G, Kwekkeboom DJ, Van Cutsem E, et al. ENETS Consensus Guidelines for the management of patients with gastroduodenal neoplasms. Neuroendocrinology 2012;95:74-87; Lawrence B, Kidd M, Svejda B, et al. A clinical perspective on gastric neuroendocrine neoplasia. Curr Gastroenterol Rep 2011;13:101-9; Delle Fave G, Capurso G, Milione M, et al. Endocrine tumours of the stomach. Best Pract Res Clin Gastroenterol 2005;19:659-73; Scherubl H, Cadiot G, Jensen RT, et al.: Neuroendocrine tumors of the stomach(gastric carcinoids) are on the rise: small tumors, small problems? Endoscopy 2010;42:664-71; Rindi G, Azzoni C, La Rosa S, et al. ECL cell tumor and poorly differentiated endocrine carcinoma of the stomach: prognostic evaluation by pathological analysis. Gastroenterology 1999;116:532-42; Rindi G, Bordi C, Rappel S, et al. Gastric carcinoids and neuroendocrine carcinomas: pathogenesis, pathology, and behavior. World J Surg 1996;20:168-72; Ruszniewski P, Delle Fave G, Cadiot G, et al. Welldifferentiated gastric tumors/carcinomas. Neuroendocrinology 2006;84:158-64.

(2) 2 **型胃 NET**：是最不常见的类型，几乎只发生在 MEN-1/ZES 患者中[61,68,114,116,250,258]。它们发生在 23%～33% 的 MEN-1/ZES 患者中，通常伴有甲状旁腺功能亢进[61,68,116,160]。2 型胃 NET 仅在散发型 ZES 患者中很少被提及[68,114,116]。2 型胃 NET 与 1 型胃 NET 一样，一般是多发的，但往往更大，小于 1cm 的只有 35%，大于 2cm 的有 20%（图 34.6B）。2 型胃 NET 通常表现为息肉样病变，尽管它们也可以通过盲活检发现为黏膜内肿瘤[116,250]。它们分化良好，常伴有 ECL 细胞和胃黏膜增生[114,116,250,258]。2 型胃 NET 比 1 型更有侵袭性，15% 侵袭限于黏膜，60% 侵袭至黏膜下层，10% 至固有肌层。2 型胃 NET 的转移比 1 型更常见[116,250,257,260]，2 型胃类癌患者的 5 年生存率低于 1 型（见表 34.10）。然而，目前还不清楚这种低存活率是否是由于胃 NET 本身[61,68,250]。

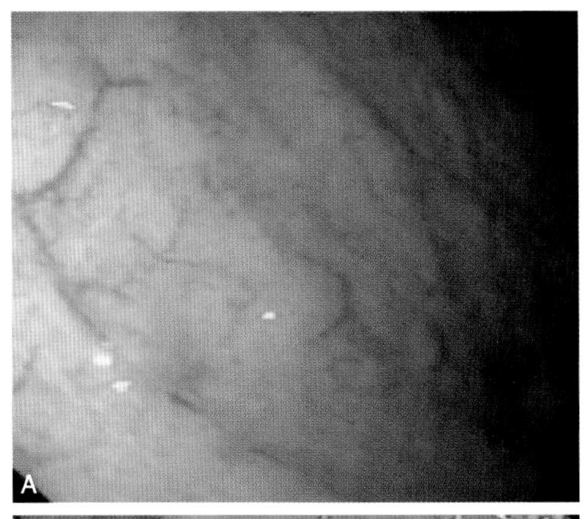

1 型胃类癌
(PA, CAG)

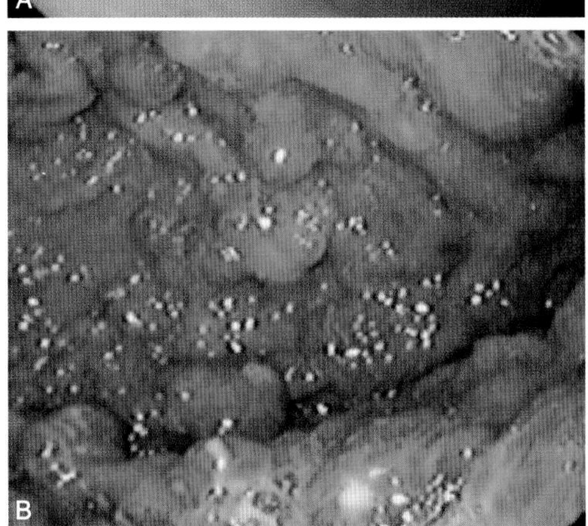

2 型胃类癌
(MEN1/ZES)

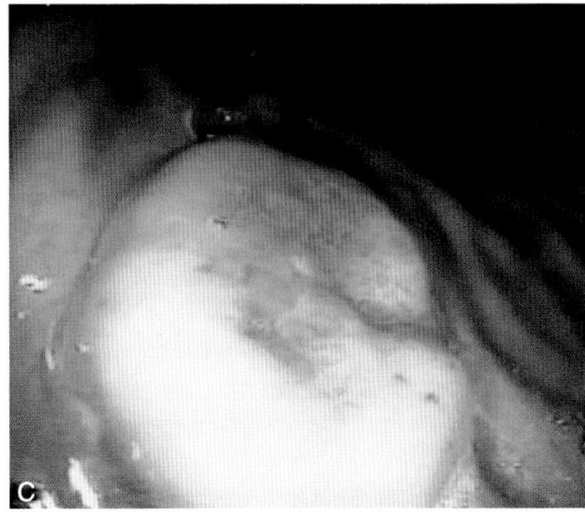

3 型胃类癌
(散发性)

图 34.6　3 种胃类癌的内镜图像。A，1 型胃类癌，慢性萎缩性胃炎（CAG）和恶性贫血（PA）患者。注意苍白萎缩的黏膜和多个小类癌。B，2 型胃类癌，MEN-1/ZES 的患者。注意病变的多样性和突出的胃皱襞。C，3 型胃类癌，特征性孤立，且通常较大。Modified from Scherubl H, Cadiot G, Jensen RT, et al. Neuroendocrine tumors of the stomach[gastric carcinoids]are on the rise: small tumors, small problems? Endoscopy 2010;42:664-71.

(3) 3 **型胃 NET**：不同于其他 2 种类型，它们与高胃泌素症或胃酸分泌的改变无关。它们是孤立、散在的 NET，与胃的其他疾病无关（见图 34.6C）[248,257,258,260]。内镜下，3 型胃 NET 通常是单一、大的、浸润性病变，有时可形成溃疡（见图 34.6C）。组织学上，它们通常是分化良好的 NET（见表 34.2a）。3 型胃 NET 的患者 EGD 检查时可能存在胃肠道出血或晚期恶性肿瘤的迹象[260]。大多数 3 型胃类癌确诊时已经是侵袭性的。5 年生存率接近 50%，3 型患者中出现 25%～30% 肿瘤相关性死亡[248,257,258,260]。

类癌综合征（稍后讨论）发生在一小部分 2 型和 3 型胃 NET 患者中[248,251,255]。这些患者可能出现不典型的红晕，因为这些胃 NET 可能缺乏 L-氨基酸脱羧酶，所以它们不会产生 5-羟色胺，而是分泌未经加工的前体 5-羟色氨酸（5-HTP；图 34.7）[248,251,256]。不典型的红晕是累及躯干和四肢的长时间的红紫色红晕[248,256]。更典型的类癌性红晕如图 34.8 所示。罕见的胃 NET 也能释放组胺，导致支气管痉挛、瘙痒、皮肤潮红和泪流满面[259]。

1 型和 2 型胃类癌的最基本实验室评估是血清胃泌素的评估。对于怀疑 1 型胃 NET 伴慢性萎缩性胃炎的患者，临床医生应考虑进行全血细胞计数、壁细胞抗体、血清 B_{12}（见第 51 和 52 章）和甲状腺功能检查（以检查可能相关的自身免疫性甲状腺炎）[250]。对于可能存在 MEN-1/ZES 的患者，应全面评估 MEN-1 的特征。对于所有大于 1cm 的胃 NET 和局限性的 3 型胃 NET，在内镜切除前应进行 EUS 检查，以评估浸润深度[248,250]。

在美国 SEER 数据库中，所有类型胃类癌的 5 年生存率为 49%（见表 34.10），但这些数据仅包括主要的恶性肿瘤；因此，许多 1 型类胃癌（具有更好生存率）可能没有被包括在内。

与 3 型类癌的处理方法有显著不同，1 型和 2 型胃 NET 有许多相似的处理方法（见表 34.10）：

- 小的（<1cm）1 型和 2 型类癌在大多数情况下应采用内镜治疗[248]。对于浸润至黏膜下层的 1 型或 2 型胃类癌，尽管许多仍采用传统的息肉切除术，但建议考虑内镜下黏膜切除（EMR）。至少每年进行一次 EGD 监测[248,254]。在一项对经内镜治疗的 1 型胃类癌患者的研究[253]中，在 46 个月的随访中生存率为 100%；没有发生转移，一名患者发生了需要手术治疗的低分化肿瘤；在接受内镜治疗后中位时间 8 个月的复发率为 64%。因此，内镜治疗是安全有效的。
- 对于大小为 1～2cm 的 1 型和 2 型胃类癌，目前还没有完全一致的最佳治疗方案[248,254]。最常见的是，在 EUS 评估深度后，通过内镜切除这些病变[248,250,252,253,260]，尽管一些作者建议手术治疗[248,249,260]。对于有高危肿瘤（如大小>2cm、Ki-67 指数较高）的患者，可以考虑手术楔形切除[248]。长期使用 SSA 可能导致小（<1cm）胃类癌的消失[248,250,250]。对于大量 1 型类胃癌的患者，胃窦切除术消除了驱动 ECL 细胞生长的高胃泌素血症，对 80% 以上的患者有效[260]。

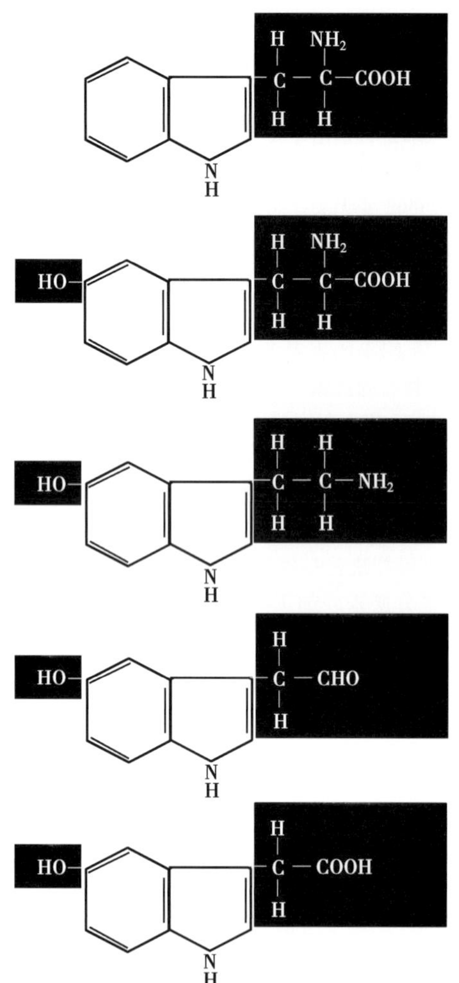

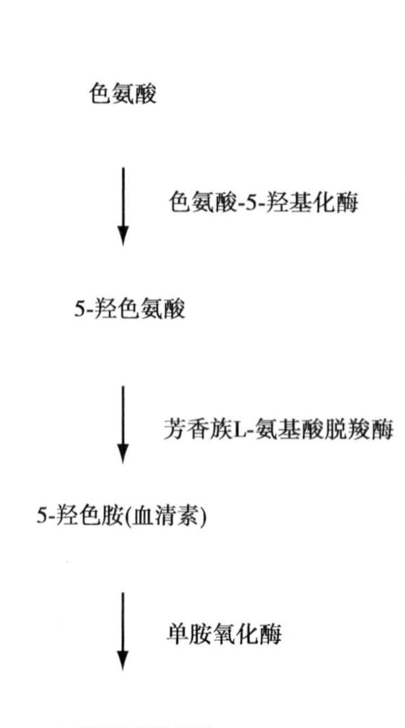

图 34.7 5-羟色胺(5-HT)的合成与降解。图中所示的是在色氨酸合成 5-羟色胺及其降解为 5-羟基吲哚乙酸(5-HIAA)(经尿液排泄)过程中发挥重要作用的各种酶

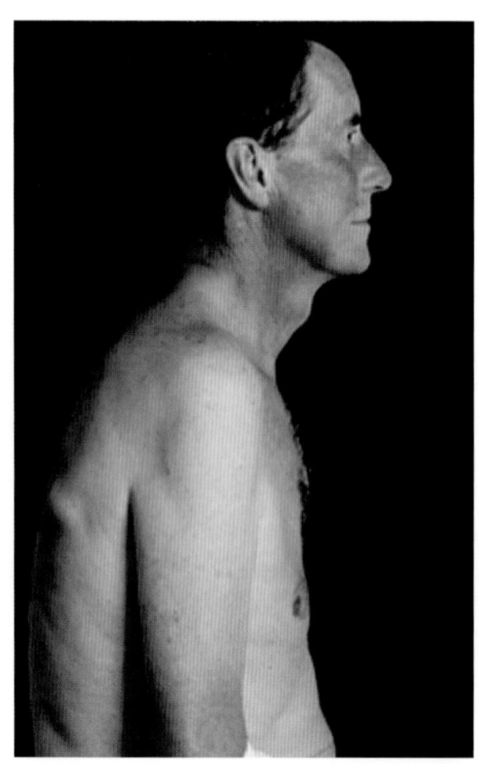

图 34.8 类癌性潮红。小肠类癌和类癌综合征患者累及面部和颈部的典型类癌性潮红

- 3 型胃 NET 的患者需要进行影像学检查以进行疾病分期(稍后讨论)。如果不存在远处转移,这些患者应该接受手术治疗[248,250,260]。有人建议对没有任何危险因素的、罕见的小(<1cm)3 型胃类癌,可以采用内镜下黏膜切除术进行保守治疗[262]。

晚期转移性胃癌 1 型(罕见)、2 型(不常见)或 3 型如后文所述,需要全身抗肿瘤治疗。

低分化胃 NET 占所有胃类癌的 3%~8%[248]。它们通常为单发较大的肿瘤(>2cm);80%~100%的病例与转移有关,超过 50%的患者出现肿瘤相关性死亡[248]。这些肿瘤的治疗方法和其他部位的低分化 GI-NET 一样(见下文)[263,264]。

(二) 小肠神经内分泌肿瘤(空肠/回肠类癌)(SI-NET)

在美国,SI-NET 的发病率正在升高(见图 34.1)。SI-NET 占所有小肠肿瘤的一半以上[265]。在本章中,我们使用术语 SI-NET 指空肠和回肠 NET(也称为中肠 NET);稍后将讨论十二指肠 NET。

SI-NET 患者平均发病年龄为 60 岁[266]。这些肿瘤在亚洲人中发病率较低,在非裔美国人中发病率较高[24]。罕见的家族性回肠 NET 似乎有常染色体显性遗传。肿瘤在临床上与散发性病例相似,并且在 18 号染色体上常见突变[267]。

空肠 NET(9%~18%)比回肠(70%~87%)少得多,后者

的 40%～70% 发生在距回盲瓣约 60cm 范围内[246,266]。SI-NET 通常很小，1/3 小于 1cm，另外 1/3 为 1～2cm，最后 1/3 大于 2cm（其中 8%＞5cm）[22,266]。约 25% 为多灶性[233,268,269]。尽管典型的 SI-NET 病灶分化良好，但通常具有侵袭性：只有 28% 是局限于黏膜或黏膜下，52% 延伸到固有肌层或呈透壁生长。转移发生在大多数 SI-NET 患者（范围为 20%～100%）[22,233,266,268]，通常转移到肝脏、淋巴结、肠系膜/大网膜/腹膜、肺或骨[22,30,266,270-278]。大的肠系膜中央淋巴结，通常伴有周围的结缔组织增生，是 SI-NET 的特征，通常表明小肠的起源，即使原发肿瘤在扫描时是隐匿的。

SI-NET 被认为来自肠嗜铬细胞（EC）。它们主要是高分化（G1）肿瘤，其中 9%～19% 为 G2，2% 为 G3[271]。许多遗传/表观遗传变化已经在 SI-NET 中被报道，包括 3p13 的缺失（与更好的生存有关）和 14 号染色体的增加（与较差的生存相关）[279]。

虽然典型小肠类癌在 60 岁时被确诊[266]，但确诊时间往往比症状出现的时间推迟 4～5 年，甚至有报道说推迟时间更长[22,272]。大多数（＞90%）患者出现与肿瘤或类癌综合征相关的症状（稍后讨论）。与肿瘤相关的症状包括腹痛，常为间歇性痉挛。由于原发性肠道肿瘤或肠系膜转移，也可能反复发作肠梗阻。体重减轻和肝大是与这些肿瘤相关的其他体征/症状。类癌性心脏病的症状（呼吸困难、水肿）通常是疾病的晚期表现[22,265,266,280,281]。

SI-NET 患者的治疗首先需要通过影像学研究对疾病的程度进行分期，同时也需要确定是否存在类癌综合征（两者稍后讨论）[105,265,282]。根治性切除原发性 NET 和邻近淋巴结可提高局部或限于局部 SI-NET 患者的 5 年生存率[277]。肠系膜上动脉周围淋巴结受累可能需要淋巴结清扫[265,282]。即使存在远处转移，也常建议手术切除原发性 NET（稍后讨论）。手术时，通常会进行胆囊切除术，因为许多患者随后会接受 SSA 治疗，而 SSA 通常会导致胆汁淤积和胆结石[265,282]。

转移性 SI-NET 患者的 5 年总生存率约为 70%[283]，中位生存期为 8～9 年[270,272,273]。生存率在很大程度上取决于疾病的分期（见表 34.9）。SI-NET 患者生存率降低的预后因素包括男性、高龄、转移、类癌综合征（尤其是类癌性心脏病）和尿 5-HIAA 水平明显升高[22,270,272,274-276,278,284]。与许多其他 NET 不同，原发性 SI-NET 的大小与生物活性没有很好的相关性。例如，约 46% 小于 1cm 的肿瘤与肝转移有关[22,272,278]。

（三）阑尾神经内分泌肿瘤（类癌）

阑尾 NET 占阑尾肿瘤的 32%～80%，在不同分类中，占 GI-NET（类癌）的 2%～38%（见表 34.8）。阑尾 NET 患者多为中年人（平均年龄 38～51 岁）[265,285,286]。这些肿瘤在男性中不太常见，在亚洲人中也比其他种族少。每 1 000 例阑尾切除术可发现 3～9 个阑尾 NET[22,24,233,246,265,285,287]。大多数（95%）是典型的类癌。腺癌（也称为杯状细胞类癌），作为一种独立的阑尾恶性肿瘤，在临床行为和治疗上完全不同。

大多数的阑尾 NET 出现在阑尾的顶端（60%～75%），5%～20% 在体部，7%～10% 在阑尾基部[265,287]。他们中的大多数（60%～80%）直径小于 1cm，5%～25% 是 1～2cm，2%～17% 是大于 2cm[265,287]。阑尾 NET 通常为高分化（G1）肿瘤（87%），其余为高分化 G2 肿瘤（13%）[288]。低分化 G3 阑尾神经内分泌癌不常见（＜1%）[288]。

几乎所有的阑尾 NET 都是在阑尾切除术或其他原因偶然发现的。阑尾类癌很少引起阑尾炎[265]。与 SI-NET 相比，阑尾 NET 极少引起类癌综合征（见表 34.8）[265]。

阑尾顶端小于 2cm 的低级别 NET 几乎与恶性行为无关[289]。局部或远处转移的主要危险因素是肿瘤直径大于 2cm。其他不良预后因素包括肿瘤位于阑尾基部、阑尾系膜浸润超过 3mm、高级别肿瘤和切缘阳性[265,282]。局部发病患者的 5 年生存率为 88%～100%；区域性受累患者的 5 年生存率为 78%～100%；远处转移患者的 5 年生存率为 12%～34%（见表 34.9）[24,265,282,288]。由于阑尾 NET 的诊断通常是阑尾切除术后手术标本中的偶然发现，所以在术前可能需要进行横断面成像研究来评估腹痛[105,265]。然而，如果横断面成像（如 CT、MRI）术前未行，术后若阑尾 NET 直径小于 1cm，则不推荐术后行横断面成像。对于直径 1～2cm 肿瘤的患者，即使已经完成了切除，影像学检查也需完善、以排除其他局部疾病或远处转移的可能性[265]。阑尾 NET 直径大于 2cm，有明显的阑尾系膜浸润和/或血管浸润，需要进行影像学分期研究[265,290]。同样的方法也适用于切除不完全或有转移的病例[265]。阑尾 NET 的治疗以手术为主，但手术的选择取决于以下几个因素：

对于 1cm 或更小且无明显转移的典型肿瘤，肿瘤浸润深度不超过浆膜下，阑尾系膜浸润极少（＜3mm），且手术切缘清晰，简单的阑尾切除术就足够了[265,282,287]。幸运的是，这些严格的标准适用于大多数典型的阑尾的 NET[285]。103 例患者接受简单阑尾切除术并随访至少 5 年（其中 83 例随访 10～35 年），没有患者出现局部复发或转移[291]。在位于阑尾基部的阑尾 NET 罕见病例中，如果阑尾系膜侵犯超过 3mm，或者切除不完全，则应考虑右半结肠切除术[265]。

对于直径 1～2cm 的阑尾类癌，T2（ENETS）或 T1B（UICC/AJCC）病变，目前还没有完全一致的最佳治疗方案[265]。有些人建议右半结肠切除术，而另一些人则推荐简单的阑尾切除术[22,265,287,291]。ENETS 指南建议使用额外的标准，即肿瘤的位置和局部浸润[265]。如果肿瘤位于阑尾基部或阑尾系膜浸润超过 3mm，建议右半结肠切除术[265]。

对于直径超过 2cm 的阑尾类癌，T3/T4（ENETS）或 T2b 或以上（UICC/AJCC），大多数但非全部[292] 权威人士[265,287,291] 建议行右半结肠切除术。

稍后讨论远处转移患者的治疗。

（四）直肠神经内分泌肿瘤（类癌）

直肠 NET 的发病率正在增加（见图 34.1）[24,293-296]。目前尚不清楚该病的发病率是否真的增加，或者仅仅是由于广泛使用下消化道内镜进行癌症筛查和其他适应证而更好地发现[295]。直肠类癌早期发现是过去几十年来典型直肠 NET 变小的原因[295]。每 1 500～2 500 例直肠镜/结肠镜检查中就发现 1 例直肠类癌[233,295]。在美国，直肠 NET 在亚裔美国人尤其常见，在高加索美国人少见，非裔美国人发病率居中[246]。在日本和其他亚洲国家的研究中，直肠 NET 占所有 GI-NET 的 60%～90%[297,298]。

直肠 NET 通常在 60 岁时被确诊，一般没有症状[246,294,295,298-302]。类癌综合征在直肠 NET 患者中非常少见(0.7%)(见表 34.8)[293,302]。

直肠 NET 是典型的小(平均直径 0.6cm)息肉样病变，发生在齿状线以上 4~13cm 的直肠前壁或外壁[302]。大部分(98%)的直肠类癌为 ENETS/WHO G1 级(72%)或 G2 级(28%)的高分化 NET[293,300,302]。近 80% 的肿瘤侵袭深度不超过黏膜下层，有些肿瘤侵袭至肌层(10%)，穿透性生长(7%)，或累及邻近结构(5%)[302]。直肠 NET 的转移与大小有关，大多数直径小于 1cm 的病灶很少转移(2%~5%)[302]。相比之下，1~2cm 肿瘤的转移率为 5%~30%，15% 的超过 2cm 肿瘤转移率为 60%~80%[246,302]。在美国，直肠 NET 转移的发生率为 22.6%，主要部位为淋巴结、肝、骨、肠系膜/大网膜/腹膜和肺。采用 AJCC-TNM 分期，81% 的直肠类癌为Ⅰ期，5% 为Ⅱ期，11.5% 为Ⅲ期，2.5% 为Ⅳ期[301]。直肠 NET 的 5 年生存率为 88%，生存率很大程度上取决于疾病的分期(见表 34.9)[246,293,299,300]。更晚期疾病和更差生存的危险因素包括原发肿瘤较大(尤其是>2cm)，浸润深度增加，分化不良，Ki 增殖指数升高，浸润至神经、淋巴或血管，以及淋巴结、肝脏或远处转移[293,299,300]。

如果直肠 NET 相对较大(>2cm)，则可能为晚期，可通过横断面成像(CT 或 MRI)和生长抑素受体成像进行分期[293]。直肠 EUS 对评估肿瘤大小、浸润深度和淋巴结也很重要[293,303]。

直肠 NET 的治疗取决于其大小、浸润深度和分期[293,295,299]：

对于直径小于 1cm 且未浸润固有肌层或有淋巴血管浸润或淋巴结转移的肿瘤，建议内镜下切除。通常可以进行标准的息肉切除术，但如果存在局部的黏膜/黏膜下浸润，则可能需要更广泛的内镜治疗(如 EMR 或黏膜下剥离)[293,295,299]。

对于直径 1~2cm 的直肠类癌，首选的治疗方法存在争议，有人建议内镜下切除，而有些人则建议更积极地治疗[293,295,304]。这些肿瘤的转移率为 10%~15%，相比之下，直肠类癌小于 1cm 的转移率为 3%[246,293]。由于一些研究表明更积极的治疗没有额外的好处，指南建议对核分裂象低且 EUS 未发现病灶浸润至固有肌层的直径 1~2cm 直肠 NET 患者进行内镜下局部切除[118,250,293]。

对于直径大于 2cm 的直肠 NET，其转移风险高达 60%~80%[246,293]，通常建议患者像直肠腺癌患者一样治疗，尤其是当肿瘤为 T3 或 T4 病变，分级为 G3 级，或局部区域淋巴结受累时，依据取决于肿瘤与肛缘的距离，行全直肠系膜切除术或腹会阴联合切除术(见第 127 章)[293,299]。

转移瘤患者的治疗将在后面的章节讨论。

(五) 十二指肠及壶腹神经内分泌肿瘤(类癌)

十二指肠 NET 在美国每年的发病率为 0.19/10 万[24]。它们占了所有 GI-NET 的 5%[24,250]。它们的发病率在英国较低[296]，在日本较高、占所有胃肠 GI-NET 的 10%，在近 10% 的尸检中发现[118,305]。

大部分(>90%)十二指肠 NET 位于十二指肠的第一或第二部分，18%~20% 位于壶腹周围区域[305,306]。十二指肠生长抑素瘤和节细胞性副神经节瘤偏爱壶腹区域，前者可能与 NF1 有关(见表 34.3)[61,118]。事实上，25% 的壶腹 NET 与 NF1 有关[307]。十二指肠 NET 一般较小，平均直径 1.2~1.5cm；其中 75% 小于 2cm[305]。大多数病例(63%)局限于黏膜或黏膜下层，但仍可转移至淋巴结(19%~60%)，尽管肝转移发生率不到 10%[118,250,295,299,305]。大多数十二指肠类癌是单发的，但在 MEN-1 患者中多发率为 9%~13%，MEN-1 患者占所有十二指肠 NET 患者的 6%[118,250,306]。例如，在 MEN-1/ZES 患者中，80%~90% 的胃泌素瘤发生在十二指肠，且通常是多发的[61,68]。

十二指肠 NET 可分为 5 种亚型：十二指肠胃泌素瘤(48%~66%)、生长抑素瘤(15%~43%)、无功能 NET(即与临床综合征无关、19%~27%)、节细胞性副神经节瘤(<2%)和低分化神经内分泌癌(<3%)[40,118,247]。许多研究也将壶腹部或壶腹周围区域的 NET 与其他十二指肠 NET 区分开来[118,250,306]。十二指肠 NET 几乎从未见过类癌综合征[12]。

十二指肠生长抑素瘤可能含有砂粒瘤体[118,305]。十二指肠节细胞性副神经节瘤包含上皮细胞、神经节和梭形细胞，S-100 蛋白免疫反应性 Schwann 细胞染色[118]。

发病的平均年龄为 60 岁，男性稍多[118,250,305,306,308]。由于绝大多数十二指肠 NET 与临床综合征无关，通常因非特异性症状行 EGD 时被确诊[118,250,305,306,309]。最常见的功能综合征是 ZES(10%)和类癌综合征(4%)；其他综合征(见表 34.1)罕见(<1%)[250]。壶腹周围 NET 通常(50%~60%)伴有黄疸，也可引起疼痛、恶心/呕吐和腹泻[118,250,307]。

高分化十二指肠 NET 患者的 5 年生存率为 80%~95%。十二指肠胃泌素瘤患者 5 年生存率超过 90%[72,126]。预后不良的因素包括远处转移、晚期、原发肿瘤较大、浸润黏膜肌层或更深、有丝分裂活性增加和分化较差[247,305,306]。由于壶腹 NET 的大小与肝转移瘤的发生无关，所以 Vater 壶腹 NET 的生长特征可能与其他十二指肠 NET 不同[247,305,306]。

EGD 联合活检是诊断十二指肠 NET 最常见的方法，其次应进行 EUS 检查以评估浸润深度[250]。对于怀疑或确诊为晚期疾病的患者，应进行 CT(或 MRI)和生长抑素受体成像。

依据 NET 的大小、位置和类型进行治疗：

——如果没有转移，且肿瘤侵犯局限于黏膜或黏膜下层，内镜下可摘除小的(≤1cm)十二指肠非壶腹 NET[118,247]。但若十二指肠 NET 位于壶腹区，则建议手术切除及淋巴结切除术。

——对于中等大小(1~2cm)的十二指肠 NET，一般建议手术治疗[118,310-313]。

——大的(>2cm)十二指肠 NET，或任何大小的淋巴结受累者，都应手术切除[247]。

——对于散发的(非 MEN-1)ZES 和十二指肠胃泌素瘤的患者，推荐十二指肠切开探查、切除，而不是内镜治疗，因为十二指肠胃泌素瘤几乎都位于黏膜下，而且至少有一半的病例存在淋巴结转移[71,118,172]。

对于少数十二指肠 NET 功能性激素综合征患者，如前所述，应给予特定的治疗以控制症状。

(六) 结肠神经内分泌肿瘤(类癌)(结肠 NET)

结肠 NET(不包括直肠和阑尾)的年发病率为 0.06~0.19/100 万[24,293,296]。结肠 NET 占所有 GI-NET 的 11%[246]。

结肠 NET 大部分出现在盲肠,其余出现在升结肠、横结肠、降结肠和乙状结肠(分别为 11%、8%、4% 和 9%)[314]。盲肠 NET 属于"中肠 NET"范畴,转移时常与类癌综合征相关。结肠 NET 往往较大,一半以上大于 5cm[314]。这些肿瘤通常是恶性的,诊断时已转移至淋巴结(55%)、肝脏(53%)、肠系膜/网膜/腹膜(24%)、肺(8%)和骨(4%)[293,299,314]。只有 14% 局限于黏膜/黏膜下层;另外 10% 浸润至固有肌层。其余 76% 为透壁浸润或累及邻近结构[314]。

结肠 NET 的患者的 5 年生存率为 33% ~ 70%,生存率随分期的不同而变化很大(见表 34.9)[293,314]。预后差与年龄较大、淋巴结和/或远处转移、肿瘤分化差、肿瘤体积大、组织浸润深度和组织学异型有关[293,314,315]。

结肠 NET 平均发病年龄 55 ~ 65 岁,男性居多[293,314]。越来越多的结肠 NET 是无症状的,因癌症筛查结肠镜检查中发现。类癌综合征发生在 5% ~ 12% 的结肠 NET 患者中,主要起源于盲肠[314,315]。

大多数局限性结肠 NET 应通过适当的淋巴结切除术进行手术治疗,但非常小、浅表的和低级别的肿瘤除外[293,315]。远处转移患者的治疗将在后面讨论。

十四、类癌综合征

类癌综合征发生在大约 8% 的 GI-NET 患者中(范围为 2% ~ 18%)[233,316-335]。表 34.11 总结了其症状,主要发生在转移性 SI-NET(中肠)患者。

表 34.11 类癌综合征患者的临床特征

特征	就诊时/%(范围)	病程中/%(范围)
面部潮红	70(23~100)	78(45~96)
腹泻	69(32~93)	78(58~100)
类癌性心脏病	26(11~40)	30(14~41)
喘息/哮喘	11(4~14)	12(3~18)
糙皮病(烟酸缺乏症)	2(0~7)	1(0~5)

发病时特征的数据:from Davis Z, Moertel CG, McIlrath DC. The malignant carcinoid syndrome. Surg Gynecol Obstet 1973; 137: 637-44; Norheim I, Oberg K, Theodorsson-Norheim E, et al. Malignant carcinoid tumors. An analysis of 103 patients with regard to tumor localization, hormone production, and survival. Ann Surg 1987; 206: 115-25; Garland J, Buscombe JR, Bouvier C, et al. Sandostatin LAR(long-acting octreotide acetate) for malignant carcinoid syndrome: a 3-year experience. Aliment Pharmacol Ther 2003; 17: 437-44.

病程中特征的数据:from Feldman JM. Carcinoid tumors and syndrome. Semin Oncol 1987; 14: 237-46; Soga J, Yakuwa Y, Osaka M. Carcinoid syndrome: a statistical evaluation of 748 reported cases. J Exp Clin Cancer Res 1999; 18: 134-41; Norheim I, Oberg K, Theodorsson-Norheim E, et al. Malignant carcinoid tumors. An analysis of 103 patients with regard to tumor localization, hormone production, and survival. Ann Surg 1987; 206: 115-25; Kvols LK, Moertel CG, O'Connell MJ, et al. Treatment of the malignant carcinoid syndrome. Evaluation of a long-acting somatostatin analogue. N Engl J Med 1986; 315: 663-6; Garland J, Buscombe JR, Bouvier C, et al. Sandostatin LAR(long-acting octreotide acetate) for malignant carcinoid syndrome: a 3-year experience. Aliment Pharmacol Ther 2003; 17: 437-44; Ruszniewski P, Ish-Shalom S, Wymenga M, et al. Rapid and sustained relief from the symptoms of carcinoid syndrome: results from an open 6-month study of the 28-day prolonged-release formulation of lanreotide. Neuroendocrinology 2004; 80: 244-51; Khan MS, El-Khouly F, Davies P, et al. Long-term results of treatment of malignant carcinoid syndrome with prolonged release Lanreotide(Somatuline Autogel). Aliment Pharmacol Ther 2011; 34: 235-42; Moertel CG, Rubin J, Kvols LK. Therapy of metastatic carcinoid tumor and the malignant carcinoid syndrome with recombinant leukocyte A interferon. J Clin Oncol 1989; 7: 865-8.

(一) 病理生理学

当肿瘤释放足够浓度的激素产物进入体循环时,就会发生类癌综合征。它的发生和严重程度与进入体循环的肿瘤大小有关。在 90% 以上的病例中,该综合征伴有转移性疾病,特别是转移到肝脏[22,233,335-338]。

患者发展为典型或不典型类癌综合征[233,321,339]。在典型的综合征中,色氨酸羟基化为 5-羟色氨酸(5-HTP)是限速步骤(见图 34.7)。5-HTP 一旦形成,就迅速由芳香族 L-氨基酸脱羧酶转化为 5-羟色胺或血清素(5-HT)。5-HT 要么储存在肿瘤的神经分泌颗粒中,要么释放到循环系统中,其中大部分被血小板吸收和储存。循环中仍有少量的 5-HT,其中大部分通过单胺氧化酶和乙醛脱氢酶转化为 5-羟基吲哚乙酸(5-HIAA)。这样产生的 5-HIAA 随后通过尿液排出[233,321,340]。在不典型类癌综合征中,肿瘤被认为缺乏芳香族 L-氨基酸脱羧酶。因此,该 NET 不能将 5-HTP 转化为 5-HT,5-HTP 就被分泌到循环中[256,321,340]。这种情况下血浆 5-HT 水平正常,但尿 5-HT 水平通常升高,因为一些循环中的 5-HTP 在肾脏中脱羧为 5-HT,并以 5-HT(或 5-HIAA)的形式排出体外。前肠 NET 的患者更有可能在尿液中排泄高水平的 5-HTP,并出现不典型类癌综合征。然而,5-HTP、5-HT 和 5-HIAA 在类癌综合征患者之间的尿排泄量有相当大的重叠[340]。

最初,类癌综合征的症状归因于 5-HT[22,233,321]。然而,5-HT 在面部潮红中的作用仍不清楚[233,325]。引起面部潮红的原因可能因肿瘤类型而异。在胃 NET 患者中,红斑瘙痒性潮红被认为是由组胺引起的,因为这种类型的潮红可以通过 H1 和 H2 抗组胺药来预防[233,259,340]。其他候选的面部潮红介质包括速激肽(P 物质、神经激肽)和其他胃肠肽[12,325,341-343]。

类癌综合征患者腹泻的发病机制也很复杂。类癌综合征患者的 5-HT 介导的结肠运动增加,肠道转运时间缩短,而且可能改变肠分泌/吸收[343,344]。5-羟色胺分泌过量可能导致大多数患者腹泻[16,233,325,343,344]。

5-羟色胺(与组胺结合)可能导致支气管痉挛。关于类癌性心脏病的发病机制[317,331,345],心脏病患者比非心脏病患者有更高的尿 5-HIAA 排泄量和血浆速激肽及其他多肽[12,316,318,328,346,347]。5-羟色胺可能是最重要的致病因素[323,331,345,348]。长期接受 5-羟色胺的动物以及 5-羟色胺转运体基因缺乏的动物,会发生类癌性瓣膜斑块/纤维化[331]。此外,5-羟色胺刺激培养的心内膜下细胞和心脏瓣膜间质细胞合成胶原[317,331]。由食欲抑制药物(如 5-羟色胺激动剂右芬氟拉明)引起的心脏瓣膜病与类癌性心脏病难以区分。5-羟色胺也可能参与其他纤维化反应,有时可见于类癌综合征,如腹膜后纤维化[233,320,327]。

(二) 临床特征与诊断

类癌综合征主要与中肠 SI-NET 有关。最常见的症状是自发性皮肤潮红(见图 34.8)和腹泻,其次是支气管痉挛,伴有喘息和哮喘症状,在病程后期出现类癌性心脏病,以右心衰为主(见表 34.11)。

典型的类癌性潮红是身体上部突然出现深红色红斑,主要位于面部和颈部(见图 34.8)[349,350]。潮红常伴有不愉快的温暖感，偶尔伴有流泪、瘙痒、心悸、面部或结膜水肿和腹泻。面部潮红可能是自发的，也可能是由压力、酒精、某些食物（如奶酪）或运动引起的，也可能是由注射儿茶酚胺、钙或五肽胃泌素引起的[22,233]。面部潮红可能是短暂的，特别是开始时、持续2~5分钟，之后也可能延长数小时。呼吸道NET患者潮红的时间往往会延长（持续数小时至数天），而且颜色会变红，伴有流涎、流泪、出汗、面部肿胀、心悸、额头较深的皱纹、腹泻和低血压。呼吸道类癌的面部潮红更容易引起全身弥漫性病变，反复这种类型的脸红后，患者可能会出现持续的红色或紫绀色。与胃NET相关的不典型潮红也呈红色，但在颈部和面部呈斑片状分布。它经常由食物摄入引起，红斑伴有斑点和中央褪色的风团，经常发生在颈部和手臂上，病变常与瘙痒有关[22,233]。

腹泻通常（85%的病例）与潮红一起发生，但15%的病例可能单独发生[16,321,345]。腹泻通常是水样的，较少见的是泡沫状或苍白的脂肪性大便，每天大便2~30次。大多数病人（60%）每日粪便排出量小于1L[16]。腹痛可伴腹泻或单独出现[16]。

类癌性心脏病可以是类癌综合征的晚期表现（图34.9；见表34.11）[316,323,328]。纤维沉淀物呈弥漫性，最常见于三尖瓣及其相关索部，较少见于肺动脉瓣尖部[233,317,323,331]。在30%的尸检病例中，左心瓣膜病变发生在二尖瓣，且比右心范围小[233]。三尖瓣反流是最常见的结果（90%~100%），其次是三尖瓣狭窄（43%~59%）、肺动脉瓣反流（50%~81%）和肺动脉瓣狭窄（25%~59%）[318,323,333]。在诊断时，27%~43%的类癌性心脏病患者为功能性Ⅰ级，30%~40%为Ⅱ级，13%~31%为Ⅲ级，3%~12%为Ⅳ级[318,329]。类癌性心脏病的发生频率和严重程度似乎在降低[22,318,331]。这种减少归因于SSA的广泛使用，它控制了5-羟色胺、速激肽和其他生物活性物质的释放，这些物质被认为在类癌性心脏病的发病机制中很重要[22,318,331]。

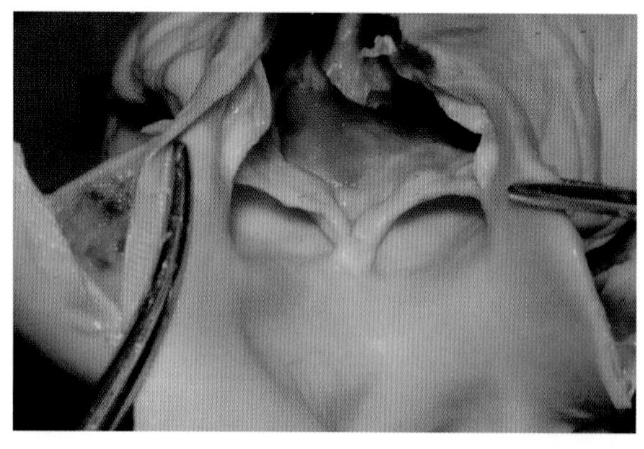

图34.9 类癌性心脏病。小肠类癌伴肝转移患者的肺动脉瓣尖部和心内膜呈纤维化增厚

喘息或哮喘样症状、伴有角化过度和色素沉着的糙皮病样皮损、关节炎/关节病、精神状态或意识混乱的改变、面部潮红伴眼睛变化、认知障碍也可能发生[233,332]。此外，在类癌综合征患者中，由于纤维组织增多而导致的各种非心脏问题已经被报道，包括腹膜后纤维化、阴茎Peyronie病（阴茎硬结症）[351]、腹腔内纤维化（尤其是SI-NET）、胸膜和肺纤维化、皮肤纤维化、肠系膜动或静脉栓塞[320,327]。

类癌综合征的一个严重并发症是类癌危象[22,325]。类癌危象通常是在手术、麻醉、化疗、内镜检查或介入放射治疗（如活检、肝肿瘤栓塞术）等过程中发生的[22,322,324,326,334]。危象的症状包括血压的剧烈变化（通常是低血压，但有时是高血压）、神志不清、昏迷、面色呈深红色、腹泻、支气管痉挛、体温过高和心律失常[22,325]。

如果类癌患者出现任何典型症状，应怀疑为类癌综合征（见表34.11）。为了确认该综合征，通常测量5-羟色胺或其分解产物之一（见图34.7）。在一项对类癌患者的研究中[352]，前肠、中肠和后肠的5-HIAA/5-羟色胺水平分别升高了14%/18%、76%/46%和0%[352]。24小时尿5-HIAA检测通常比血清5-羟色胺检测更具特异性。单次血浆5-HIAA测定与24小时尿5-HIAA排泄量之间有非常密切的相关性[353]，提高了血浆测量可以取代目前金标准的但更不方便的尿路采集的可能性，这是由于尿液的采集不完整和不当导致这种方法并不总能产生可靠的结果[353]。

如果患者食用富含5-羟色胺的食物，如香蕉、芭蕉、菠萝、猕猴桃、核桃、山胡桃、山核桃和鳄梨，则可能出现假阳性尿5-HIAA[354-356]。愈创甘油醚、对乙酰氨基酚、水杨酸盐和左旋多巴也可能影响尿液5-HIAA水平[233,355,356]。尿5-HIAA水平的升高也可发生在肠道吸收不良和其他情况下[355]。在产生不典型类癌综合征的前肠NET中，血浆5-HTP水平升高（见图34.7），尿5-HIAA可能不会显著升高。如果适当控制饮食和药物摄入，尿中5-HIAA的正常排泄范围为2~8mg/d，尽管使用更高的临界值（15mg/d）可能会减少假阳性结果[355]。许多分泌5-羟色胺的NET患者尿液中的5-HIAA分泌量为8~30mg/d。在一项研究中，尿5-HIAA检测对类癌综合征的敏感性为73%，特异性为100%[342]。

诊断困难常见于因类癌综合征以外的原因而面部潮红的患者，有该综合征但没有面部潮红的患者，有如5-HIAA可能正常或轻微升高的前肠类癌的肿瘤患者，或少数面部潮红而无转移性疾病的患者[338,357]。面部潮红的鉴别诊断很广泛，包括更年期潮热、对酒精和谷氨酸盐的反应、药物的不良反应（如氯磺丙脲、钙通道阻滞剂、烟酸）、慢性粒细胞白血病和全身性肥大细胞增多症[357]。上述这些面部潮红的情况都不会导致尿液5-HIAA排泄增加。

（三）治疗

生长抑素类似物（SSA）是治疗类癌综合征的首选一线药物[233,358,359]。生长抑素本身的使用由于其半衰期短（2.5~3分钟）而受到限制[233,360]。随着合成SSA如奥曲肽的发展，皮下治疗可以每6~12小时进行一次[233,360,361]。缓释制剂（奥曲肽LAR和兰瑞肽注射）每4周给药一次，可以控制大部分患者的类癌症状[362,363]。奥曲肽LAR是肌内注射，而兰瑞肽是深层皮下注射。奥曲肽和兰瑞肽具有相似的作用机制，与生长抑素受体2亚型结合，与5亚型结合程度较低[364,365]。个体的反应各不相同，一些患者需要更高或更频繁的剂量[366-368]。为预防类癌危象，接受手术的类癌综合征患者应接受额外的生长抑素类似物[207,369]。术前1~2小时内，应补充皮下注射奥曲肽250~500μg[207]。对于初诊患者的急诊手术,目前的指南建议在手术前 1~2 小时静脉注射 500~1 000μg 奥曲肽或皮下注射 500μg 奥曲肽[207],尽管有些人使用更高的剂量[334],其他人则建议持续输注奥曲肽[207]。

SSA 的短期不良反应是常见、轻微和短暂的,最常见的是注射部位疼痛、恶心和腹泻。长期的副作用通常是轻微的,很少会导致停药[94,232,233,359,370]。长期副作用包括胆汁淤积/结石、脂肪泻和葡萄糖耐量异常[94,233,366]。长期使用奥曲肽治疗的患者胆道疾病的发生率约为 30%,大多数患者出现淤积,1%~10% 出现有症状的胆囊疾病[94,232,233,367]。

对于严重的难治类癌综合征和肝脏显性疾病患者,肝动脉栓塞(稍后讨论)在大多数情况下是姑息性治疗[233,371-373]。

使用标准剂量的 SSA 治疗后出现难治性腹泻的患者可以通过口服色氨酸羟化酶抑制剂——telotristat——进行治疗。在三期 TELESTAR 试验中,135 例难治性腹泻(定义为每天排便次数≥4 次)患者随机分为 2 种剂量 telotristat(每天 3 次、每次 250mg 和每天 3 次、每次 500mg)与安慰剂(同时继续服用稳定剂量的 SSA)[374]。主要终点是每日排便次数减少。经过 12 周的双盲试验后,250mg 剂量组的每日排便量次数平均减少值为 0.81,500mg 剂量组为 0.69。两种剂量的 telotristat 可使尿液 5-HIAA 水平降低约 50%。本试验结果表明,每天 3 次、每次服用 250mg telotristat 被批准用于治疗难治性腹泻。该药耐受性较好,伴有轻度恶心和无症状的血清 GGPT 增加。便秘是一种罕见的副作用。

随着术前和围手术期控制类癌综合征的能力的提高,心脏瓣膜手术相关的死亡率已经下降到 10%,手术后的中位生存期可以长达 11 年[317,375]。瓣膜手术的主要适应证是右心衰。心脏手术可以降低死亡率[329,345]。

十五、肿瘤定位

NET(pNET 和 GI-NET)患者的治疗需要确定肿瘤的范围(分期),如果可能的话,还需要确定原发肿瘤的部位[12,22,98,369,376,377]。多种肿瘤定位方法可供选择[12,22,98,369,377]。

(一) 内镜检查

如前所述,内镜对于发现原发性胃十二指肠和结直肠 NET 以及起源于回盲瓣附近的末端回肠 NET 是必不可少的[378]。隐匿性原发性 SI-NET 有时可以通过胶囊内镜或双气囊小肠镜检查发现,尽管常规使用这些方法是不必要的或不推荐的。横断面影像上出现典型的肠系膜肿块提示为原发性小肠肿瘤。

(二) 超声内镜检查(EUS)

EUS 有助于胃和直肠 NET 的 T 分期(可能还有 N 分期)[12,247,250,260,379-381]。EUS 在检测 pNET[98,178,382] 和通过 FNA 提供疾病组织学确认方面也相当敏感。EUS 可检测到约 80% 的胰岛素瘤(范围为 57%~92%),这优于传统的影像学检查[12,71]。EUS 还可检测大约 70% 的胃泌素瘤(范围为 40%~100%)[12,379]。在 MEN-1 患者中,EUS 可以检测到其他诊断方法无法检测到的 pNET,对诊断时未切除的小病变的大小进行连续评估尤其有用[12,381]。

(三) 计算机断层扫描(CT)和磁共振成像(MRI)

腹部 CT 和 MRI 被广泛用于评估原发性肿瘤的位置和肿瘤分期[22,376,377,382-385]。许多 SI-NET 太小,在 CT 或 MRI 上看不到。胰岛素瘤和十二指肠胃泌素瘤通常也很小(<1cm),而大多数非胰岛素瘤 pNET 出现在病程晚期,体积较大(>4cm),更容易成像[12,101]。

为了增强肝转移病灶的显著性,建议采用动脉期(造影剂注射后约 20 秒)、静脉期(大约 70 秒后)和非造影剂期的 CT 三期成像。多相成像还可以提高 CT 扫描检测小胰腺 NET 的敏感性。MRI 对肝转移瘤的检测比 CT 扫描更为敏感。对于接受基于钆的 MRI 扫描的患者,钆塞酸二钠(Eovist)与肝胆期成像对比可提高小肝转移瘤的显著性[386]。

(四) 生长抑素受体成像

生长抑素受体成像可用于疾病的最佳全身分期以及评估生长抑素受体的表达。后一个功能对于评估 SSA 和放射性标记 SSA 治疗的潜在获益非常重要(稍后讨论)。过去,使用^{111}Indium-喷曲肽(OctreoScan)的生长抑制素受体闪烁显像(SRS)是生长抑制素受体成像的主要方法。最近,基于^{68}镓的 PET 成像使用依多曲肽(dotatoc,dotanoc 或 dotatate,后者通常获得批准),和 CT 融合的镓成像提供了更高的灵敏度和更高的空间分辨率[387]。对于生长抑素受体表达的肿瘤,与 CT 或 MRI 扫描相比,^{68}Ga-dotatate PET 可提高检测转移灶及小原发性肿瘤的灵敏度。研究表明,适当有序的^{68}Ga-dotatate 扫描可以影响相当大比例病例的临床决策[388]。尽管生长抑素受体成像并不能常规用于疾病监测,但应在基线时对大多数高分化肿瘤患者进行生长抑素受体成像检查,并在考虑使用放射性标记的 SSA 治疗之前,以及在手术或肝栓塞等手术之前,肿瘤的光学定位可能是有益的。

其他定位 GI-NET 患者肿瘤的扫描方法最近已被描述,但尚未广泛使用。胰岛素瘤过表达 GLP-1 的受体,一项研究[389]表明,放射性标记的 GLP-1 类似物可以检测到其他成像模式未定位的隐匿性胰岛素瘤。^{11}C-和^{18}F-标记的左旋多巴已被用于使用 PET 可视化 NET[22,377];^{11}C-5-HTP 也被使用[22,382]。使用^{18}F-脱氧葡萄糖(FDG)的 PET 也可能有助于高增殖率和低细胞分化的 NET 亚群的显像(稍后讨论)[377,390,391]。

十六、转移性疾病的治疗

由于类癌综合征和功能性 pNET 患者的药物治疗(如长效 SSA)的有效性,这些患者的生存时间越来越取决于肿瘤的生物学和生长模式[2,27,94,100,110,207,215-220,222-225,232,261,274,361,364,392-502]。NET 在不同的患者中生长速度不同,生长速度是一个预后因素。一般来说,虽然低分化神经内分泌癌具有高侵袭性,但与常见的腺癌相比,转移 NET 生长相对缓慢[24,126,443,503]。治疗的基本类型包括肝减瘤手术、肝动脉栓塞治疗和全身治疗。

（一）减瘤手术

切除可切除的转移性肿瘤（减瘤手术、去瘤和转移切除术）经常被考虑，尽管没有对照研究来确定其价值[12,67,94,98,146,204,265,369,394,411,504]。如果90%以上的肝转移瘤可以切除，5年生存率在75%～80%之间、偶尔也能治愈[12,67,94,146,204,265,369,394,411,467,504]，但只有5%～15%的患者可以进行这样的切除。当其他疗法不能充分降低血浆激素水平以控制症状时，可能还需要对功能性NET患者进行肝减瘤手术[12]。

一些SI-NET患者的肠系膜淋巴结肿大和/或纤维化可能在肠系膜根部发展，导致肠梗阻、腹痛和其他症状[282,433,498]。有些人建议对这样的患者，即使他们有肝转移，也应该消除肠系膜疾病[94,265,282,433,468,498,502]，这一方法可以减轻或预防症状，并可能延长生存时间[94,265,433,468,498,502]。在减瘤手术时，有时联合预防性胆囊切除术是由于未来长期使用SSA治疗可导致胆汁淤积或结石[265,433,478]。

（二）肝导向的非手术治疗

有几种肝靶向治疗针对NET肝转移。尽管它们在管理指南中被广泛使用和提及，但还没有完整的随机试验来比较它们[282,369,402,502]。这些以肝脏为导向的非手术方法主要用于不能切除的转移NET患者，这些转移仅限于肝或以肝为主，特别是对于激素过量状态不能通过其他方式很好地控制的功能综合征患者[369,372,502]。

1. 射频消融（RFA）和其他消融方法

NET肝转移瘤的局部消融技术、射频消融、乙醇注射和冷冻治疗可以在手术时或者经皮介入性放射治疗时[94,203,371,438,458,480,482,497]。RFA是应用最广泛的技术，并越来越多地与其他技术如减瘤手术相结合[203,371,438,458,480,482,497]。RFA的相对禁忌证包括大病灶(>3.5cm)、大量病灶(>5个)和邻近重要结构的转移瘤[51,369,371,438,458,480,482]。有效率为80%～95%，有些反应长达3年[203,371,438,497]。与减瘤手术或肝栓塞术（下一章讨论）相比，射频消融的并发症发生率更低（<15%），并且射频消融可缩短住院时间。RFA的严重并发症包括出血或脓肿形成[203,371,497]。虽然RFA的价值尚未在对照试验中确立，但一些指南认可RFA是一种有效的治疗方法[94,146,369]。

2. 肝动脉栓塞和化疗栓塞

大多数NET是富血管性的，阻断NET的动脉供应可以选择性地损毁肿瘤；未受累的肝脏不太容易受影响，因为它接受的大部分血液来自门静脉（见第71章）[94,371,435]。选择包括单独经动脉栓塞（TAE）或联合动脉内化疗药物（TACE）。TACE最常用的化疗药物是阿霉素、5-氟尿嘧啶（5-FU）、顺铂、丝裂霉素C或链脲佐菌素[94,371,435,440]。栓塞颗粒包括微栓子、聚乙烯醇颗粒或凝胶泡沫粉末[396,425,451]。

TAE或TACE的完全或相对禁忌证包括门静脉阻塞、明显的肝功能障碍、肿瘤累及超过50%～75%的肝脏、胆道重建术和体力状态不佳[94,203,371,396,399,435]。60%～100%接受TAE或TACE治疗的患者症状改善，25%～86%的患者在高度变化的时间内有客观的肿瘤反应[371,399,435,451]。在类癌综合征患者中，TAE或TACE可减少64%～75%的症状，5-HIAA排泄/肿瘤标志物可减少50%～70%[486,505]。

转移性GI-NET患者栓塞后5年生存率为30%～50%，在转移性pNET患者中为20%～35%[94,371,440]。TAE和TACE均可导致死亡（<6%）和病态并发症（10%～80%），包括腹痛、发热、恶心/呕吐的栓塞后综合征[203,371,396,399,442,451]。严重的并发症并不常见，包括胆囊坏死、肝衰竭、肝脓肿和肾功能衰竭[94,203,371,396,399,442,451]。最近的指南总结道，在有手术经验的中心，对于局限于肝、不能切除的肝转移瘤NET患者，应考虑采用TAE或TACE作为姑息性治疗[146,369]。目前还没有完整的比较TAE和TACE的前瞻性随机研究[356]。

3. 肝放射性栓塞

对不可切除的肝非转移性NET患者的另一种栓塞选择是使用^{90}钇（^{90}Y）微球进行放射性栓塞，称为选择性内放射治疗（SIRT）。可使用两种类型的^{90}Y微球：树脂（SIR-spheres，Sirtex Medical，Australia）和玻璃（Thera Spheres，Nordion，Canada）[94,395,488]。在动脉内注射^{90}Y微球之前，进行肝血管造影，以确定导管头端是否处于恰当的位置，并避免将微球注射到十二指肠动脉或胆囊动脉中，以免导致十二指肠溃疡或胆囊炎[94,488]。另一个需要避免的严重并发症是^{90}Y微球分流到肺导致的放射性肺炎[94,488]。后一种并发症可以通过确认闪烁扫描上的肺分流程度为10%或更低以及通过调整^{90}Y剂量在很大程度上避免[94,444,456,488]。SIRT后栓塞后综合征很常见[356]。43%的患者发生2级体质性副作用（如体重减轻、疲乏、发热），胃肠道副作用很常见。3级短期不良反应罕见。然而，长期辐射诱导的肝病是一个重要问题，特别是在广泛双叶转移的患者中。这种并发症的表现包括黄疸、腹水和由以下原因引起的肝脏假性肝硬化表现[506]。对SIRT的有效率为55%（范围为12%～89%），另有32%（范围为10%～60%）的患者病情稳定[94,395]。半数患者症状改善，包括生活质量改善，平均生存30个月[94,422,447,455]。

（三）肝移植

肝移植用于少数转移性GI-NET患者，尽管其使用存在争议[94,369,421,439,445,446,465,472,507]。在一篇综述中，移植后5年总生存率为52%，无病生存率为30%。手术死亡率为10%～14%[445,446]。在UNOS数据库中，移植后1年、3年和5年生存率分别为81%、65%和49%[472]。预测预后不良的因素包括伴有肝移植术的大部切除手术、肿瘤分化差和肝大。随着对这些不良预后因素的认识，2000年后的5年生存率提高到59%。再分析后发现年龄大于45岁、肝大、肝移植同时进行大或小的切除手术是预后不良的其他预测因素[445]。其他不良危险因素[94,439,446,465,472]包括：十二指肠或胰腺的原发性NET[446]、移植时肝外转移、广泛（>50%）肝受累、Ki67指数超过10%[94,465]。一般来说，指南将肝移植限制在只有肝脏疾病的患者，或极小且可切除的肝外肿瘤（即未切除的原发部位）的患者。

（四）生长抑素类似物（SSA）

SSA 不仅控制功能性 NET 释放激素，还能抑制肿瘤生长[12,22,94,100,365,401,405,424,508]，尽管客观反应率微不足道。这种抗增殖作用的确切机制尚不清楚。除了胰岛素瘤，超过 90% 的高分化的 GEP-NET 具有生长抑素受体，可以激活细胞内抑制细胞增殖的级联反应。生长抑素还可以抑制生长因子从 NET 或邻近细胞的释放，并对其他可能促进癌症生长的细胞（如血管、基质及免疫细胞）具有抑制作用[360,401,508]。

两个关键的Ⅲ期试验已经证实了 SSA 对肿瘤生长的抑制作用。PROMID 将 85 名高分化、低级别转移性中肠 NET 患者随机分为两组：奥曲肽 LAR 30mg、每 4 周一次与安慰剂组。中位进展时间（主要终点）从安慰剂组的 6 个月改善到奥曲肽 LAR 组的 14.3 个月（$P<0.001$）[365]。对总生存率没有显著的影响，可能是因为在研究期间患者的死亡人数很少，以及接受安慰剂的患者在疾病进展后能够过渡到活性药物治疗。在 CLARINET 试验中，204 例肠胰 NET 患者（生长抑素受体阳性、ki-67 指数 ≤ 10%）随机分为每 4 周服用一次兰瑞肽 120mg 组与安慰剂组[364]。绝大多数患者（96%）在随机分组前病情稳定。在数据分析时，安慰剂组的中位无进展生存期（PFS）为 18 个月，而兰瑞肽组的 PFS 尚未达到（风险比 0.47；$P<0.001$）。兰瑞肽的副作用包括腹泻、腹痛和胆石症。

根据 PROMID 和 CLARINET 研究的结果，奥曲肽和兰瑞肽被各种指南推荐用于治疗生长抑素受体阳性的 GEP-NET。由于相似的作用机制和结果，很少有数据支持使用一种 SSA 而不是另一种，也没有任何数据支持在另一个 SSA 进展后换用别的 SSA。

（五）α-干扰素

与 SSA 相似，干扰素-α 能有效地控制功能性 GI-NET 激素过量状态的症状，并具有抗增殖作用，其主要作用是使疾病稳定（30% ~ 80%）、而不是缩小肿瘤（<15%）[94,407,430,509]。干扰素的抗增殖作用被认为由以下机制介导：抑制 DNA 合成，阻断细胞周期进展到 G_1 期，刺激 bcl-2 增加，抑制蛋白合成，通过降低 VEGF/VEGFR 表达抑制血管生成，诱导细胞凋亡[94,430,501,509]。干扰素的副作用包括流感样症状、厌食、疲劳、骨髓抑制和肝毒性。由于这些副作用和缺乏有力的随机试验证实疗效，干扰素-α 很少用于 GEP-NET 的管理，并且在指南中被认为是具有争议性（NCCN 类别 3）[369]。

（六）依维莫司

mTOR 是一种丝氨酸-苏氨酸激酶，在细胞生长、增殖和凋亡中发挥重要作用[94,477,492,510]。mTOR 级联激活在 NET 尤其是 pNET 的生长中发挥重要的作用[94,151,392,413,464,466,487,490,492,510]。口服 mTOR 抑制剂依维莫司已经在 3 个关键的Ⅲ期试验中进行了研究，所有试验均以 PFS 为主要终点。

在 RADIANT-3 研究中，410 名晚期进展期 pNET 随机接受依维莫司（10mg/d）或安慰剂，安慰剂治疗进展后允许交叉。依维莫司使中位 PFS 从 4.6 个月延长到 11 个月（风险比 0.35，$P<0.0001$）[151]。客观有效率为 5%。最常见的 3 级或 4 级副作用是骨髓抑制、腹泻、口腔炎或高血糖，发病率从 3% ~ 7% 不等；这些副作用一般可以通过减少剂量或中断药物来控制。肺炎和感染是临床上其他重要的副作用。总生存率（OS）无明显改善趋势。

RADIANT-2 研究将进展期、不可切除、高分化的非胰腺 NET 和有类癌综合征病史（主要是中肠 NET）的患者随机分为奥曲肽 LAR（每月 30mg）和依维莫司（10mg/d）或安慰剂。这项研究的结果是模棱两可的：依维莫司/LAR 患者的中位 PFS 为 16.4 个月，而 LAR/安慰剂组为 11.3 个月（风险比 0.77；$P=0.026$），这一差异没有达到预先规定的显著性水平。尽管结果没有统计学意义，OS 分析在数值上支持安慰剂组。RADIANT-2 研究并没有在这类患者中批准依维莫司[511]。

最后一项Ⅲ期研究——RADIANT-4 评估了依维莫司与安慰剂在 302 例无功能胃肠道和肺 NET 患者中的疗效。作为合格标准的结果，不同类型的肺、胃十二指肠和结直肠 NET 被纳入，与 RADIANT-2 相比，中肠 NET 相对较少。本研究不允许交叉。这项研究达到了其主要终点，证明了中位 PFS 从安慰剂组的 3.9 个月改善到使用依维莫司的 11.0 个月（风险比 0.48，$P<0.001$）。由于 RADIANT-4 的研究，依维莫司被批准用于治疗无功能胃肠道和肺 NET[512]。

目前尚不清楚肿瘤功能状态（类癌综合征史）是否应是进展期 GEP-NET 选择依维莫司的决定因素。总的来说，依维莫司适用于临床有显著进展的患者，并且可能更适用于非中肠 NET 而不是中肠 NET。风险与收益需要仔细权衡，尤其是年长的、虚弱或合并临床重大疾病如肺部疾病或糖尿病的患者。

（七）舒尼替尼

GEP-NET 是富血管性肿瘤，同时表达 VEGF 及其受体（VEGFR）。一些抗血管生成药物在单臂和小型随机研究中显示出活性，但只有舒尼替尼被批准用于晚期 pNET 患者[369,494,513]。舒尼替尼是一种口服活性小分子抑制剂，可抑制多种酪氨酸激酶受体，包括 PDGFR、VEGFR-1、VEGFR-2、c-KIT 和 FLT-3[479,513]。在安慰剂对照试验中[513]，进展期、不可切除、转移性、高分化的 pNET 患者被随机分为口服舒尼替尼（37.5mg/d）或安慰剂组。舒尼替尼使中位 PFS 从 4.5 个月增加到 11.4 个月（风险比 0.42；$P=0.001$），与 OS 获益趋势相关，其结果与 RADIANT-3 试验中与依维莫司相关的结果非常相似[513]。主要不良事件包括高血压、骨髓抑制和掌跖红肿疼痛（手足综合征）[513]。通过减少剂量或停药，不良反应通常是可控的[513]。与依维莫司一样，尚不清楚舒尼替尼与其他治疗方法相比何时应用于晚期进展期 pNET 患者[94,356]。

（八）肽受体放射性核素放射治疗

生长抑素受体在大多数高分化的 GEP-NET 中高表达，用放射性标记的 SSA 治疗可使靶向细胞毒性的放射性标记生长抑素受体配体与肿瘤结合[397,398,449,495]。这种治疗方式也被称为肽受体放射性核素治疗（PRRT）。对一些与SSA耦合的放射性同位素进行了评估，包括^{90}钇（^{90}yttrium，^{90}Y）和^{177}镥（^{177}lutetium，^{177}Lu）[397,398,449,495]。最常用的SSA是奥曲肽或奥曲酸，这是一种与生长抑素受体亚型2有较高亲和力的SSA；常见的螯合剂是DTPA或DOTA[94,397,398,495]。^{90}Y是一种发射β的同位素，组织穿透范围相对较长、约12mm。在一项对87名患者的研究中，用^{90}Y-dotatoac观察到的客观影像学反应为28%。另一项仅评估难治性类癌综合征患者的研究显示，客观缓解率仅为4%，但病情稳定率较高（70%）[514,515]。以^{90}Y为基础的PRRT的主要毒副作用之一是肾功能不全，这种副作用可以通过同时输注氨基酸来部分改善，它可以抑制肾小球对放射性肽的再吸收[516]。在1 109例接受以^{90}Y为基础的PRRT治疗的患者中，102例（9%）出现了严重的肾毒性。大约2%的患者出现长期骨髓毒性（骨髓增生异常综合征或急性白血病）[517]。

基于^{177}Lu的PRRT代表了新一代放射性标记的SSA，其粒子范围更短、约为2mm。使用^{177}Lu-dotatate的研究表明，客观缓解率在18%～44%之间，中位PFS持续时间约为30个月。预防性使用氨基酸输液，3级或4级肾毒性的发生率小于1%。骨髓增生异常综合征或急性白血病的长期发病率约为2%[518,519]。

NETTER-1研究是放射性标记生长抑素类似物的第一个前瞻性Ⅲ期研究，231例高分化、标准剂量奥曲肽LAR治疗进展和奥曲肽扫描有生长抑素受体表达的中肠NET患者，被随机分配，接受4周期^{177}Lu-dotatate（200mCi每8周）和30mg奥曲肽，对照组接受高剂量奥曲肽（每4周60mg）治疗。主要终点是通过盲态中心放射学检查评估的PFS。这项研究显示PFS在临床和统计学上有显著改善，研究中高剂量奥曲肽组的中位PFS为8.4个月，而^{177}Lu-dotatate组的中位PFS未达到（风险比0.21；$P<0.001$）。^{177}Lu-dotatate的客观缓解率为18%，而高剂量奥曲肽组为3%。也有初步证据表明^{177}Lu-dotatate可以改善OS（风险比0.4；$P=0.004$），这需要在计划的最终OS分析中得到确认[520]。

基于NETTER-1研究的结果以及单臂机构注册数据，^{177}Lu-dotatate被批准用于治疗晚期进展期的GEP-NET。适当选择患者需要在影像学研究中确认生长抑素受体的表达（奥曲肽扫描或^{68}Ga-dotatate PET）。有证据表明，生长抑素受体的表达程度与肿瘤反应相关[521]。一个标准治疗过程包括4个周期的^{177}Lu-dotatate，尽管关于剂量测定在改善治疗剂量和周期数方面的潜在作用存在一些争议。对于在PRRT初始疗程后病情稳定或有反应的患者来说，随后的再治疗是一种选择[522]。在某些机构，8个个体治疗周期（1 600mCi）被认为是终生最大剂量，尽管有些患者可能能够耐受更高的终生剂量。总治疗剂量与不可逆性骨髓毒性风险之间没有明确的相关性。

（九）细胞毒性化疗

细胞毒性化疗在GEP-NET中的作用正在逐渐发生演变。显而易见，与中肠NET相比，pNET对烷基化剂为主的化疗更加敏感。化疗在胃、十二指肠和结直肠NET中的作用尚不清楚[481]。

基于链脲佐菌素的治疗方案在20世纪70年代和80年代在NET中进行了广泛试验，发现在pNET中是有效的。两项关键性研究予以开展。据报道，链脲佐菌素联合5-氟尿嘧啶（5-fluorouracil，5-FU）治疗的客观缓解率为63%，而链脲佐菌素单药治疗组为36%[523]。另一项研究报道链脲佐菌素联合阿霉素治疗的有效率为69%，而链脲佐菌素和5-FU治疗的有效率为45%[524]。这两项研究都没有使用严格的放射两项研究都没有采用严格的放射学反应标准，使得数据难以应用于现代治疗结果学反应标准。最近的一项回顾性分析显示，使用客观的放射学参数，由链脲佐菌素、阿霉素和5-FU组成的三联用药方案的有效率为39%[454]。

替莫唑胺是一种口服烷基化剂，与链脲佐菌素相比，其副作用更为耐受。一些小规模Ⅱ期研究评估了替莫唑胺与其他药物的联合作用[400,483,525-529]。一项关于替莫唑胺和沙利度胺的小型研究报告了11例pNET患者的客观缓解率为45%（而胃肠道NET没有应答）[529]。另一项关于替莫唑胺和贝伐珠单抗的研究报告有效率为33%，中位PFS为14.3个月[526]。

卡培他滨（一种口服氟嘧啶）和替莫唑胺的联合应用已在多个回顾性系列研究和最近的前瞻性随机临床试验中进行了研究。在一个由30名初试化疗的pNET患者组成的研究机构中，观察到70%的影像学有效率和18个月的中位PFS[400]。另一个主要由pNET患者组成的研究应答率为61%[530]。基于这些数据，一项旨在比较卡培他滨联合替莫唑胺与替莫唑胺单药治疗进展性高分化pNET患者疗效的随机Ⅱ期研究得以启动。他们的结果显示，卡培他滨/替莫唑胺联合用药后的PFS和OS均出现了统计学上的显著改善：联合用药组的中位PFS为22.7个月，而替莫唑胺单药组的中位PFS为14.4个月（风险比0.58；$P=0.02$）。与替莫唑胺中位OS 38个月相比，联合用药组未达到中位OS（风险比0.41；$P=0.01$）。该方案耐受性良好，3～4级中性粒细胞减少率为13%，3～4级血小板减少率为8%[531]。在替莫唑胺之前预防性使用昂丹司琼，严重恶心的发生率相当低。目前指南推荐卡培他滨/替莫唑胺用于转移性pNET的治疗。关于甲基鸟嘌呤甲基转移酶（MGMT）表达的潜在预测价值存在相互矛盾的数据[532]。迄今为止，在进展期pNET的治疗中，还没有完整的比较细胞毒性药物和非细胞毒性药物（依维莫司或舒尼替尼）的研究。

（十）低分化肿瘤的治疗

低分化癌占GEP-NET的5%以下[94,261,263,264,404,409]。识别它们很重要，因为在于它们的侵袭性过程，以及与前面讨论的高分化肿瘤的独特治疗[263,264,404,499]。低分化GI-NET的组织学特征为侵袭性生长（3级，Ki67指数>20%、通常为50%～90%）、坏死、核异型性、快速生长和临床预后不良[94,261,263,264,404,499]。组织学上可分为小细胞和大细胞。这些癌症通常含有少量的生长抑素受体；因此很少有未标记或放射性标记的SSA的指征。^{18}FDG PET、CT和MRI经常用于这些低分化NET进行成像[264]。由于大多数低分化的 NET 患者表现为局部或远处转移，手术很少能治愈，尽管在偶有有限病变的患者中仍应考虑手术治疗[94,263,264,404,499]。

在不能手术的典型患者中，建议使用顺铂（或卡铂）联合依托泊苷进行化疗。这些药物可在 14%～80% 的患者中诱导缓解，平均缓解持续时间小于 12 个月[263,264,369,404,462,463,481,499]。治疗的中位生存期为 4～16 个月，平均 5 年生存率仅为 11%（范围为 0%～31%）[404]。化疗方案可能与显著毒性相关，尤其是胃肠道（恶心/呕吐）、骨髓抑制和肾损害[264,369,404,462,463,481]。

尽管缺乏前瞻性数据，但接受手术切除的局部未分化肿瘤患者通常应接受顺铂（或卡铂）加依托泊苷的辅助化疗。放化疗是局部或局部低分化神经内分泌癌患者的另一选择，也是食管局部小细胞癌的首选治疗方法[533]。

对于铂类药物耐药患者（定义为一线或辅助铂类药物化疗后 3～6 个月内病情进展），有效的治疗选择很少。与小细胞肺癌的结局相比，PD-1 抑制剂帕博利珠单抗（pembrolizumab）的免疫治疗显示出相对较低的缓解率[534]。评价联合免疫治疗的研究正在进行中。

（鲁晓岚　王俊雄 译　李鹏 校）

参考文献

第 35 章　人类免疫缺陷病毒感染的胃肠道后果

C. Mel Wilcox 著

章节目录

一、吞咽疼痛和吞咽困难 …… 473
二、腹泻 …… 474
三、腹痛 …… 478
四、肛管直肠疾病 …… 478
五、消化道出血 …… 479
六、肝胆疾病 …… 479

1981 年,有人描述了现在被认为是艾滋病的第一批病例。随后,世界上暴发了以机会性感染(opportunistic infection,OI)为典型表现的疾病,如肺孢子虫肺炎和人疱疹病毒 8(human herpesvirus 8,HHV-8)感染所致的卡波西肉瘤等肿瘤。超过 3 500 万人死于艾滋病,据估计全世界目前有超过 3 600 万人感染艾滋病毒,每天约 5 000 人感染,这使其成为我们这个时代最重要的全球健康问题。在该病流行的初期,人们关注的焦点在明确病原(HIV-1 及 HIV-2)、发现这些疾病的特点及有效的使用预防性病原菌疗法上。1995 年,高效抗逆转录病毒治疗(HAART)概念的诞生,使艾滋病的流行形式迅速改变。HAART 能减少病毒复制,从而减少 HIV 病毒的传播。在一些患者的血液中检测不到 HIV 病毒。免疫功能的实质性改善与病毒载量减少具有相关性,这可通过如 CD4 淋巴细胞计数增加和临床上 OI 发病率降低,以及生存率的升高等客观方法进行评估[2,3]。在发达国家,目前的重点是病毒控制,而在资源匮乏的国家,像结核病这样的 OI 比比皆是,它们和发达国家流行病中疾病早期阶段最先出现的情况相似[4,5]。尽管流行病的规模很大,但仍有许多值得乐观的地方,包括数据显示预暴露预防能降低传播风险;夫妻中有一方感染 HIV,使用 HAART 治疗后可降低未感染一方感染的风险;抗逆转录病毒疗法能减少母婴传播;男性包皮环切能有效减少传播;较早使用 HAART 可能会提高完全免疫恢复率;在全球范围内增加 HAART 的使用;最后,早期试验提示开发一种有效疫苗的可能性[6]。

随着与 HAART 有关的免疫的重建,人们关注的重心也已经转变为慢性疾病的治疗以及药物副作用。现在已经认识到,使用 HAART 的 HIV 感染患者的死亡率通常与非艾滋病事件有关,例如由于 HCV 感染引起的慢性肝病[7,8]。同样,对 HAART 治疗有应答的同时存在胃肠道症状的 HIV 感染患者,更有可能出现药物引起的副作用或非机会性胃肠道感染,治疗策略应转回到免疫功能正常者普遍存在的疾病上[9]。

因为患者通常出现临床表现后来就诊,因此,本章主要围绕症状诊断进行阐述。特定的 HIV 相关疾病(仅限于最常见和毒力最强的 HIV-1)及其治疗是在其最常见的相关症状和体征的背景下提出的。此外,还要讨论 HAART 对这些综合征和疾病的相关作用。在本章当提到艾滋病患者中,我们特指那些 CD4 计数低于 200/mm³ 且存在机会感染风险或已发生机会感染疾病的患者。通常这些患者是尚未接受 HAART、无法接受 HAART 或对 HAART 治疗无效的患者。

虽然 HAART 显著改变了胃肠道并发症的发生,但在应用 HAART 治疗之前建立的许多相同管理原则仍然适用。一般而言,调查艾滋病患者胃肠道症状的方法与非艾滋病毒感染患者相似。在评估艾滋病的胃肠道症状时必须考虑一些普遍的因素:

1. 临床症状和体征很少能给出明确的诊断。

2. 在接受 HAART 的患者中,胃肠道症状在病因学上通常是药物诱导的或非机会性的。

3. 机会性疾病的危险分层可根据免疫功能低下的程度预测[即 CD4 计数>200/mm³ 多见于常见细菌和其他非机会性疾病;CD4 计数<100/mm³ 多见于巨细胞病毒(CMV)、真菌、分枝杆菌复合体(MAC)和不常见的原生动物)(图 35.1)。

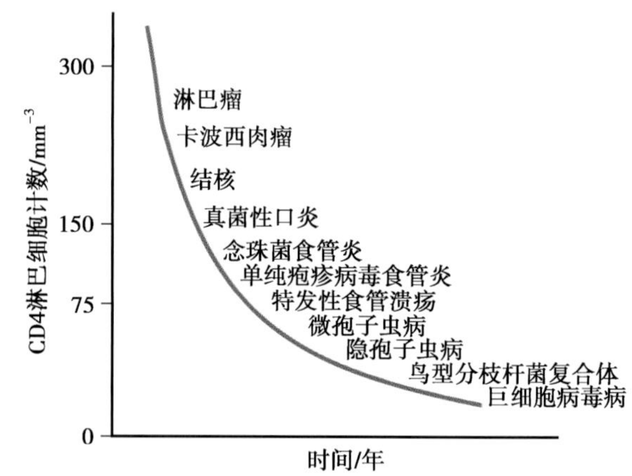

图 35.1　基于淋巴细胞 CD4 计数的机会性疾病时间表。(From Wilcox CM, Saag MS. Gastrointestinal complica-tions of HIV lnfection: Changing priorities in the HAART era. Gut 2008;57:861-70.)

4. 在艾滋病中,胃肠道常涉及机会性感染过程,且常常是多个机会性感染过程(图 35.2)。胃肠道病原体常为全身性感染的一部分(如 CMV、MAC)而且通常是多重感染。因此,在临床实践中,发现了肠道外的病原体有可能会取消对胃肠道的评估。

5. 评估应从侵入性由小到大进行,并且应根据症状和体征的严重程度和特异性来决定。

6. 应寻求组织侵入的证据作为致病性的标志。

7. 在没有改善免疫功能的情况下(通过 HAART),OI 的

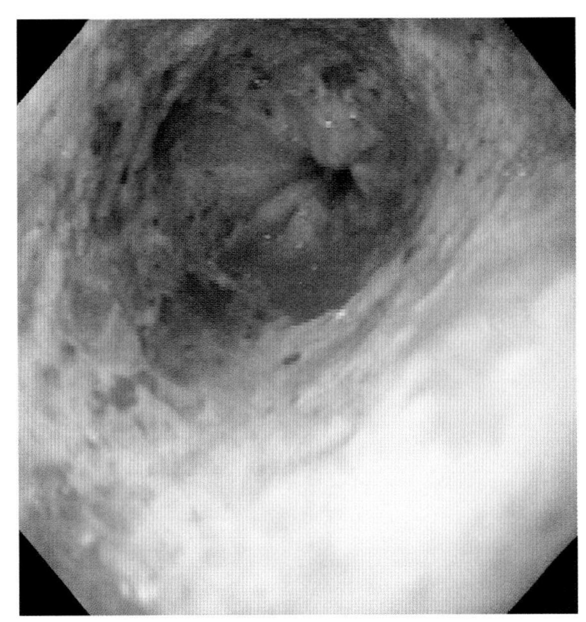

图 35.2　巨细胞病毒和 HSV 食管炎。在该内镜视图上观察到弥漫性环周溃疡，在远处观察到食管胃交界处。在艾滋病患者中，经常发现多种病原体。(From Wilcox CM. Atlas of clinical gastrointestinal endoscopy. Philadelphia：Saunders；1995. p 28.)

复发几乎是一致的，需要维持抗病原体治疗。

8. 所有机会性疾病的治疗应包括 HAART。

一、吞咽疼痛和吞咽困难

在 HAART 时代来临之前，HIV 疾病过程中至少 1/3 的患者发生食管不适（吞咽困难和吞咽疼痛）。由于 HAART 的使用，食管疾病的发病率明显下降，非艾滋病患者特异性疾病（如胃食管反流）的人数有所增加[10]。

白色念珠菌，艾滋病中最常见的食管感染，在这种情况下常常与其他疾病共存。虽然大多数病例发生在艾滋病的情况下，但由于短暂的免疫抑制，念珠菌性食管炎可能发生在 HIV 感染初期[11]。口腔鹅口疮常预示食管不适的患者合并食管炎（见图 24.2）。然而，没有鹅口疮并不排除这类患者食管念珠菌病的可能性[12]。

食管念珠菌病患者通常会主诉胸骨后吞咽困难[13]。吞咽疼痛通常并不严重。通过上消化道内镜检查能明确诊断，表现为与黏膜充血和脆性相关的局灶性或弥漫性斑片。一个界限清晰的溃疡或多个溃疡表明疾病有所进展。活检显示脱落的上皮细胞具有典型的酵母样外观；真菌侵犯通常仅存在于浅表上皮[14]。

尽管 CMV 是艾滋病中最常发现的病原体，但其与食管疾病的相关性不如念珠菌常见。CMV 引起特征性的黏膜溃疡。因此，CMV 食管炎患者可表现为躯干痛或胸骨后胸痛，症状十分严重[15]。吞咽困难比念珠菌性食管炎患者少得多，并且极少是最初主诉。发热罕见。尽管内镜下的表现有多种，但是一般表现为大而深的大面积溃疡（图 35.2）[16]。念珠菌合并感染较为常见。黏膜活检应能证实肉芽组织内间质细胞和（或）内皮细胞的病毒细胞病变效应。可能缺乏特征性包涵体，这就需要通过免疫组织化学染色来确认。溃疡底部肉芽组织的活检结果为病毒致细胞病变效应提供了最有力的依据，而病毒培养则不那么敏感，细胞刷片也无太大的作用[17]。

非特异性（特发性，口疮）食管溃疡综合征很常见（图 35.3）[15]。临床和内镜表现无法和 CMV 感染区分。诊断特发性溃疡的标准包括：①通过组织病理学证实的内镜溃疡；②通过常规组织学和免疫组化染色，没有病毒致细胞病变效应的证据；③没有 GERD 或药物诱导的食管炎的临床或内镜证据。与 CMV 溃疡一样，非特异性溃疡发生在疾病晚期，大多数患者的 CD4 计数小于 50/mm^3。然而，它们也可以出现在急性 HIV 感染患者中[11]。这些溃疡的发病机制尚不清楚。

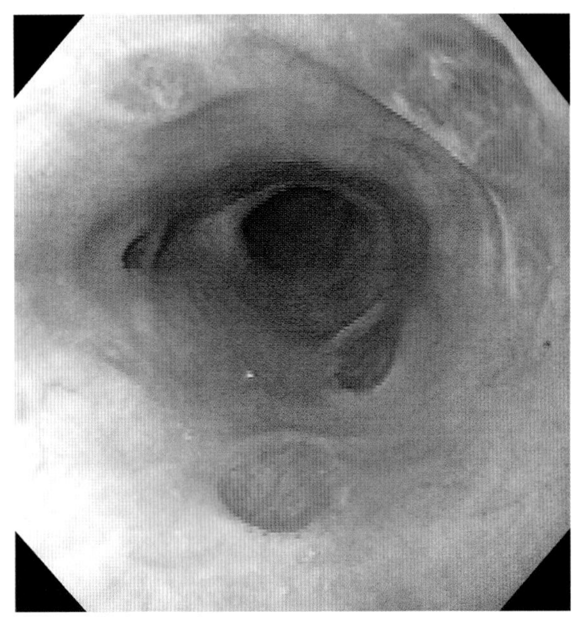

图 35.3　HIV 相关特发性溃疡。在该内镜视图中，可见整个食管内多处界限清晰的溃疡。溃疡呈穿凿样外观，中间黏膜外观正常，似乎隆起，造成火山口样堆叠的外观。(From Wilcox CM. Atlas of clinical gastrointestinal endoscopy. Philadelphia：Saunders；1995. p 75.)

与其他免疫功能低下的宿主相比，HSV 食管炎在艾滋病中并不常见[15]。在免疫功能正常的患者中，疱疹性食管炎通常归因于 1 型 HSV。然而，艾滋病患者可能患有感染 1 型或 2 型 HSV 导致的食管炎。该疾病类似于其他黏膜的疱疹感染，其特征遵循可预测的方式发展，先形成分散的囊泡，然后出现浅溃疡，最终聚集成弥漫性浅溃疡区域。与 CMV 食管炎和非特异性溃疡相比，这些溃疡常较浅；罕见大而深的溃疡（图 35.4）。从溃疡边缘（活跃的病毒复制位点）活检和细胞刷检最有可能显示上皮细胞受侵和疱疹感染典型的核变化。活检标本的病毒培养通常是阳性的[17]。

由各种感染及药物（齐多夫定、去羟肌苷）引起的孤立性食管炎/溃疡病例，已有报道。

艾滋病患者患食管肿瘤的风险可能增加。报告的肿瘤包括霍奇金和各种非霍奇金淋巴瘤、卡波西肉瘤、鳞状细胞癌和腺癌。

艾滋病患者食管症状的具体原因不能仅根据症状或体格检查确定（框 35.1）。但是可以适当进行一些概括。与不伴吞咽疼痛的轻度至中度吞咽困难相关的口腔鹅口疮可能是由念珠菌性食管炎引起的。相反，患有严重的吞咽痛而无吞咽困难或鹅口疮的患者更可能患有溃疡性食管炎（病毒性，特发性）。胸骨后烧灼感和反流者最有可能患有GERD，特别是在HAART治疗中。

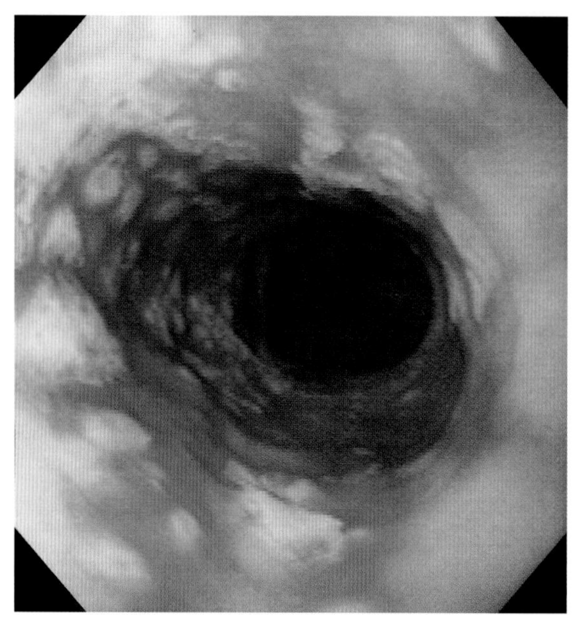

图35.4　单纯疱疹病毒食管炎（HSV食管炎）。该内镜视图显示围绕多个发白斑块的弥漫性红斑，代表浅溃疡。外观正常的食管黏膜岛仍然存在

框35.1　艾滋病患者吞咽困难和吞咽疼痛的鉴别诊断

感染	特发性溃疡*
白色念珠菌*	胃食管反流病（GERD）*
巨细胞病毒（CMV）*	**肿瘤**
单纯疱疹病毒（HSV）	卡波西肉瘤
荚膜组织胞浆菌	淋巴瘤
鸟分枝杆菌复合体	鳞状细胞癌
隐孢子虫属	腺癌
刚地弓形虫	**药物诱发的食管炎**

*更常见的原因。

内镜下活检是明确吞咽困难和吞咽疼痛病因的唯一方法。对于溃疡性病变，多次黏膜活检优于细胞刷检[17]。然而，当怀疑有运动功能障碍时，钡餐造影对免疫功能尚好的HIV感染者可能有用。

鉴于念珠菌感染占优势，大多数艾滋病患者采用经验性方法治疗食管症状是合理的。吞咽困难和（或）吞咽疼痛，且合并口腔鹅口疮的患者应在氟康唑200mg负荷剂量后给予100mg/天进行经验治疗[18]。伊曲康唑或氟康唑悬浮液是有效的替代品。经过1周的经验治疗后如果症状仍持续存在，则应进行内镜下活检，而不是开始其他经验性治疗或加大氟康唑剂量。除非用HAART改善了免疫功能，否则念珠菌性食管炎可反反复复。此外，尽管进行了慢性预防，但因抗真菌药耐药引起食管炎的复发仍频繁发生。

CMV和HSV感染的治疗应与这些病毒感染其他肠道部位相似（见下文）。90%以上特发性溃疡患者对口服糖皮质激素应答（例如，最初每天40mg泼尼松，4周内逐渐减少）。糖皮质激素有效的依据尚不清楚；在此情况下使用糖皮质激素前应该谨慎排除感染的原因。沙利度胺也非常有效，当泼尼松治疗失败时也可能有治疗效果[19]。其致畸作用极其强大，要求仅限于男性使用。HAART本身显示可使溃疡愈合。

二、腹泻

HAART问世之前，在HIV疾病过程中，高达90%的患者出现腹泻，尤其是来自发展中国家的患者[20]。在HAART时代，腹泻并不常见，现在最常见的病因是药物诱导（HAART）或由与HIV感染无关的疾病引起[21,22]。

HIV感染导致整个胃肠道中CD4 T细胞快速消耗，及出现以固有层炎症加重并损伤胃肠上皮细胞层为特征的肠病，这与微生物易位和免疫激活有关[23]。这些艾滋病患者黏膜免疫的改变易患肠道感染，健康人感染后呈自限性病程的微生物（如隐孢子虫）可能会导致AIDS患者无法治愈的慢性感染，也可能导致其他常见肠道感染（如沙门菌、志贺菌、弯曲杆菌属）的更为致命的临床过程。临床和社会环境因素与肠道OI相关，包括低CD4淋巴细胞计数及不使用HAART、社会经济状况差、缺乏安全饮用水以及接触农场动物[20]。尽管有多种原虫，病毒，细菌和真菌生物可引起艾滋病患者腹泻，可以根据临床表现和免疫缺陷程度进行鉴别诊断（框35.2）。

框35.2　艾滋病患者腹泻的鉴别诊断

感染	腺病毒
原生动物	轮状病毒属
微孢子虫*	诺如病毒
隐孢子虫属*	人类免疫缺陷病毒（HIV）?
贝氏囊等孢球虫属	**真菌类**
环孢子虫属	组织胞浆菌病
蓝氏贾第鞭毛虫	球孢子菌病
溶组织内阿米巴	隐球菌病
杜氏利什曼原虫	念珠菌病
耶氏肺孢子虫	马尔尼菲篮状菌
弓形虫属	**肿瘤**
细菌	淋巴瘤
艰难梭菌	卡波西肉瘤
沙门菌*	**特发性**
志贺菌*	“获得性免疫缺陷肠病”
空肠弯曲杆菌*	**药物诱导**
鸟分枝杆菌复合体	HIV蛋白酶抑制剂
结核分枝杆菌	**胰腺疾病**
小肠细菌过度生长（SIBO）	胰腺功能不全
病毒	慢性胰腺炎
巨细胞病毒（CMV）*	感染性胰腺炎（CMV，MAC）
单纯疱疹病毒（HSV）	药物性胰腺炎（如喷他脒）

*更常见的病因。

原生动物是绝大多数腹泻病原体中最常见的[24-26]。很大程度上是因为一部分感染可导致慢性腹泻并且难以治疗。能引起健康人自限性腹泻的隐孢子虫仍然是世界范围内HIV

患者感染的最常见的原生动物。临床表现和转归与免疫功能低下的程度和微生物的亚型有关[26]。尽管这些病原体可以在肠道的所有区域以及胆道和呼吸道上皮中找到,但是小肠是最常见的感染部位。腹泻通常很严重,每天几升的粪便量并不少见。腹鸣,恶心和体重减轻是常见的相关症状;右上腹疼痛表明胆道受累(见后文)。这种感染的发病机制尚不确定。肠隐孢子虫病最常通过粪便抗酸染色诊断,微生物表现为与红细胞大小相似的鲜红色球体。粪便检测的敏感性各不相同,取决于病原体的载量,粪便的特征(成形还是水样)以及感染的原始部位。粪便抗原检测和 PCR 技术能明显增加粪便检测的敏感性。即使粪便检查结果为阴性,也可在小肠或直肠活组织检查中发现隐孢子虫[27]。

隐孢子虫感染的特异性的抗菌治疗仍不尽如人意。当前已经测试了许多抗微生物试剂,但是大多数没有明显效果(表 35.1)[28]。目前针对隐孢子虫最有效的疗法是 HAART,与安慰剂相比,硝唑沙奈有部分疗效。其中免疫功能的改善可致腹泻临床缓解,并且粪便和小肠活检发现隐孢子虫已清除[29]。对于 HAART 治疗失败和(或)抗菌治疗无效的患者,对症治疗应包括液体支持和止泻药,偶尔可使用阿片类药物来控制腹泻。

表 35.1　艾滋病患者腹泻感染原因的治疗

病因	治疗	持续时间/d
原虫		
隐孢子虫属	巴龙霉素,阿奇霉素,硝唑尼特	14~28
环孢子虫属	甲氧苄啶/磺胺甲基异噁唑或环丙沙星	14~28
贝氏囊等孢球虫属	甲氧苄啶/磺胺甲基异噁唑或环丙沙星	14~28
微孢子虫	阿苯达唑(脑胞内原虫)	14~28
	甲硝唑,阿托伐醌,福尔马林(在美国不可用)	
病毒		
巨细胞病毒(CMV)	更昔洛韦	14~28*
	膦甲酸钠	14~28*
	西多福韦	14~28*
单纯疱疹病毒(HSV)	阿昔洛韦或代昔洛韦	5~10*
细菌		
沙门菌,志贺菌,弯曲杆菌属。	氟喹诺酮类(例如,环丙沙星)	10~14*
艰难梭菌	甲硝唑,万古霉素	10~14
小肠细菌过度生长(SIBO)	甲硝唑,环丙沙星	10~14
结核分枝杆菌	利福平,异烟肼,吡嗪酰胺,乙胺丁醇	270~365
鸟分枝杆菌复合体	症状性感染的多种药物治疗方案(见文)	270~365
真菌		
组织胞浆菌病	两性霉素 B,然后是伊曲康唑	28
球孢子菌病	两性霉素 B,然后是氟康唑	28
隐球菌病	两性霉素 B,然后是氟康唑	28

* 治疗持续时间取决于 HAART 的免疫重建。

贝氏囊尾蚴是一种孢子虫,与微小隐孢子虫一样,是未经治疗的 AIDS 患者的慢性腹泻的原因。这种疾病在美国很少见,但在发展中国家更为常见和流行。微生物可通过粪便或十二指肠分泌物的抗酸染色或黏膜活检来明确。与隐孢子虫病不同,抗生素对贝氏囊尾蚴感染治疗有效,特别是甲氧苄啶/磺胺甲噁唑和环丙沙星[30]。

环孢子虫菌属是一种球虫寄生虫,很少引起免疫功能正常和免疫缺陷的人急性或慢性腹泻。它在艾滋病中的流行率很低。粪便检查可检测到该菌,可用甲氧苄啶/磺胺甲基异噁唑或环丙沙星治疗。

微孢子虫是艾滋病患者常见的肠道感染,但在 HAART 时代,其患病率明显下降[31]。肠道和肝胆疾病可能由 2 种微孢子虫引起:比氏肠微孢子虫(最常见)及肠脑炎微孢子虫。报道的未经 HAART 治疗的微孢子虫患病率从 15% 到 39% 不等[32]。典型症状包括轻度至中度的水样、非血性腹泻,通常不伴相关的痉挛性腹痛。感染与严重的免疫缺陷有关,感染者的 CD4 计数中位数小于 100/mm^3[27]。与隐孢子虫感染一样,其发病机制仍未明。在塑料或石蜡包埋的组织中,可以用光学显微镜识别微孢子虫(图 35.5)。使用 Brown-Brenn(革兰氏菌染色试剂盒),Gram 染色或改良的 Masson(马松染色)三色染色法对包埋的黏膜活检组织进行染色,优于常规 H&E 染色[28]。肠脑微孢子虫(*E. intestinalis*)通常体积较大且可感染固有层巨噬细胞,由此可将其与比氏肠微孢子虫(*E. bieneusi*)区分开来;电子显微镜可以明确诊断。粪便染色技术仅中度敏感,而小肠活检一般为阳性。尽管阿苯达唑治疗 E 肠脑微孢子虫有效[33],但是尚无广泛的针对比氏肠微孢子虫的有效治疗。与隐孢子虫病的治疗一样,HAART 是最好的治疗方法,可在清除这种病原体的同时消除腹泻[29]。

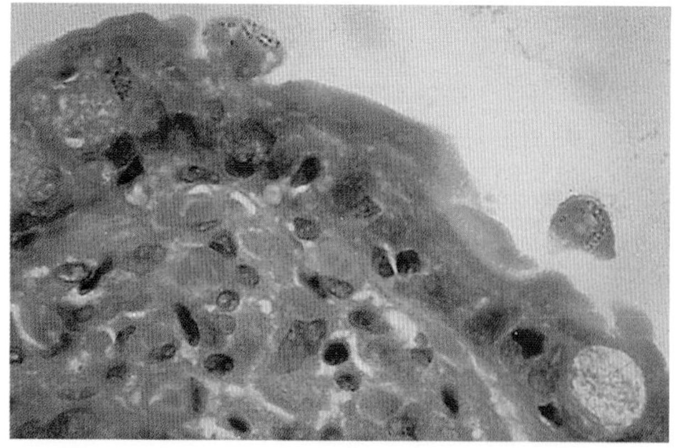

图 35.5　小肠微孢子虫病的内镜活检标本。该薄塑料切片显示含有微孢子虫卵囊的上皮细胞脱落。(From Gazzard BG. Diarrhea in human immunodeficiency virus antibody-positive patients. Semin Gastroenterol 1991;2:3.)

由于原因未明,原虫蓝氏贾第鞭毛虫和溶组织内阿米巴感染并未在艾滋病中频繁出现或毒力增加。然而,在溶组织内阿米巴流行的东亚地区,阿米巴结肠炎被确定为腹泻的常见原因[34]。非致病性阿米巴在形态上与溶组织内阿米巴相似,只能通过更特异性的粪便或酶联免疫吸附试验来区分[35]。人芽囊原虫、结肠内阿米巴原虫和内阿米巴是非致病性原生动物,在男男性接触者(MSM)中更常见,常与其他原虫寄生虫有关。肠道利什曼病(地方性),肺孢子虫感染和弓形虫病鲜有报道。

蠕虫,特别是粪类圆线虫和蛔虫,在 AIDS 中并不常见[36]。患者可能出现腹痛,腹泻和嗜酸性粒细胞增多。在 HIV 感染的情况下,与这些寄生虫相关的临床综合征和复发率似乎没有改变。

大肠的病毒感染,罕见于小肠,是 HIV 患者腹泻的重要原因。CMV 是引起腹泻最常见的病毒,也是 AIDS 和多次粪检阴性的患者慢性腹泻的最常见原因[37]。这种感染特征性地发生在 HIV 感染过程的晚期,即当 CD4 淋巴细胞计数低于 100 个/L 时(见图 35.1)。感染在结肠中最常见,但可见伴随食管、胃或小肠的疾病(见图 35.2)。孤立的胃或小肠疾病通常导致腹痛而非腹泻。

肠道 CMV 感染的临床表现差别很大,包括无症状携带,非特异性症状如体重减轻和发热,局灶性肠炎/结肠炎—包括阑尾炎或弥漫性溃疡出血或穿孔。因此,患者可出现几种症状中的一种,包括腹痛、腹膜炎、非血性水样腹泻或便血[38]。然而,最常见的表现是与慢性腹泻相关的腹痛。虽然内镜表现多样,但 CMV 肠炎/结肠炎的特征是上皮下出血和黏膜溃疡(图 35.6)[38]。

如前所述,诊断胃肠道 CMV 感染最好通过组织样本中的病毒致细胞病变效应来确定。如果包涵体的数量很少并且肉眼观察组织正常,则应该认为患者是 CMV 定植而不是真正的 CMV 感染。

许多治疗方法可用于有效治疗 CMV(见表 35.1)。更昔洛韦,一种经静脉给药的阿昔洛韦衍生物,在约 75% 的病例中有效[39]。缬更昔洛韦是更昔洛韦的前体口服药物,具有良好的胃肠道吸收和治疗巨细胞病毒视网膜炎的疗效,但在胃肠道疾病的诱导治疗方面尚未得到充分研究。HAART 的免疫重建将减少长期抑制治疗的需要。在诊断胃肠道 CMV 感染时,所有患者都应进行眼科检查以排除 CMV 视网膜炎,因为这个部位感染需要密切随访以确保缓解,以防止失明。虽然广泛用于移植领域,但 CMV 抗原血症或通过 PCR 检测 DNA 浓度来预测随后的疾病并指导使用优先治疗的作用仍然不太明确[40]。

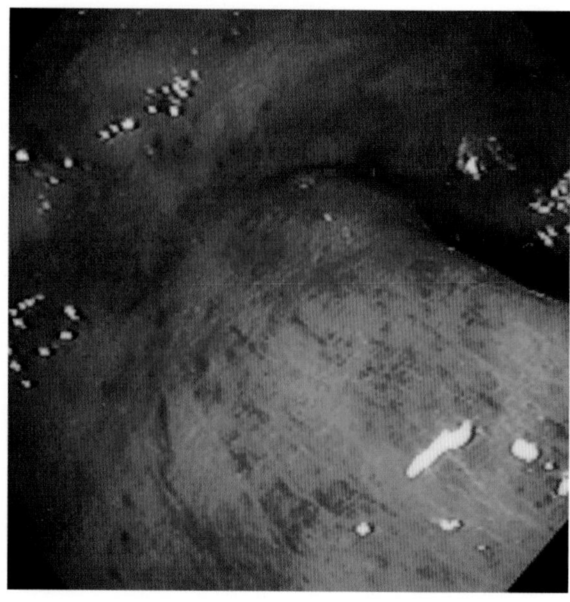

图 35.6　巨细胞病毒(CMV)结肠炎。乙状结肠的内镜照片显示 CMV 典型的水肿和弥漫性上皮下出血。这种内镜下表现与特发性溃疡性结肠炎相似

已经在有症状和无症状的患者中发现了许多其他病毒(例如诺沃克,腺病毒,轮状病毒)以及新型诺如病毒,但它们对艾滋病患者腹泻的总体作用很小。

HIV 本身作为腹泻病原体的作用很有限。已经有人提出用特发性艾滋病肠病来解释缺乏可识别病原体的艾滋病患者的腹泻,并且可能反映艾滋病毒对肠道内环境稳态的间接影响。随着诊断技术的改进、对艾滋病腹泻病原体谱认识的提高、对药物作为腹泻额外原因重要性的认识,以及对粪便检测结果阴性的患者进行全结肠镜检查并活检,真正患有“特发性腹泻”的患者的比例越来越少。蛋白酶抑制剂的研究已被证明可以改善慢性不明原因的腹泻[41]。

与健康宿主相比,肠道细菌感染在艾滋病个体中更频繁且更具毒性。沙门菌,志贺菌和弯曲杆菌出现菌血症和抗生素耐药的概率较高。诊断较为简单,因为这些病原体常可从粪便样本中培养出来(见第 110 章)。这些肠道感染通常表现为伴有高热,腹痛和可能带血的腹泻。腹痛可能很严重,类似于急腹症。如上所述,菌血症常见在怀疑重症感染患者中,应该根据经验给予重症患者肠外抗生素,直到获得粪便和血培养及敏感性的结果,之后可针对分离出的病原体使用相应的抗生素。

艰难梭菌已成为引起腹泻的一个常见的细菌病原体,不是因为它是一种 OI,而是因为抗生素的使用和住院频率在这

一人群中比健康宿主更高[42]。临床表现、对治疗的反应、复发率与免疫功能正常的患者相比没有差异[43]。诊断依赖于对粪便中艰难梭菌肠毒素的标准测定(见第 112 章)。

小肠细菌过度生长(见第 105 章)在艾滋病患者中并不常见[44],其在腹泻中发挥的作用似乎有限。

在晚期艾滋病患者中,细胞内分枝杆菌(MAC)或结核分枝杆菌累及肠道,可导致腹泻、腹痛,很少出现梗阻或出血。大多数 MAC 患者出现的是无症状胃肠道感染,而结核分枝杆菌感染似乎在所有病例中都有症状。十二指肠受累是最常见的,内镜下可见黄色黏膜结节,常伴有吸收不良、菌血症和全身性感染。胃镜活检是诊断胃肠道 MAC 感染的最佳方法;粪便抗酸涂片的敏感性远低于培养。在抗酸染色的活组织切片标本中上很容易看到这种微生物,而且数量往往惊人(图 35.7),血培养阳性可能提示诊断。受累患者具有严重的吸收不良和体重减轻,伴有绒毛低平和巨噬细胞内充满分枝杆菌。尽管与 MAC 相反,已经提出伴 PAS 阳性巨噬细胞的假 Whipple 综合征,它是抗酸染色阳性而非 PAS 阳性的巨噬细胞;电镜可以鉴别 Whipple 和假 Whipple 病。艾滋病患者 MAC 感染的典型表现是炎症反应不明显,且很少出现肉芽肿。对多种抗生素治疗的反应不一,部分取决于免疫低下的程度。然而,很少能实现根除。与其他 OI 一样,在这些患者中采用 HAART 疗法可以提高免疫功能,加快临床清除感染,防止复发,从而不再需要长期抗菌治疗,并提高生存率。

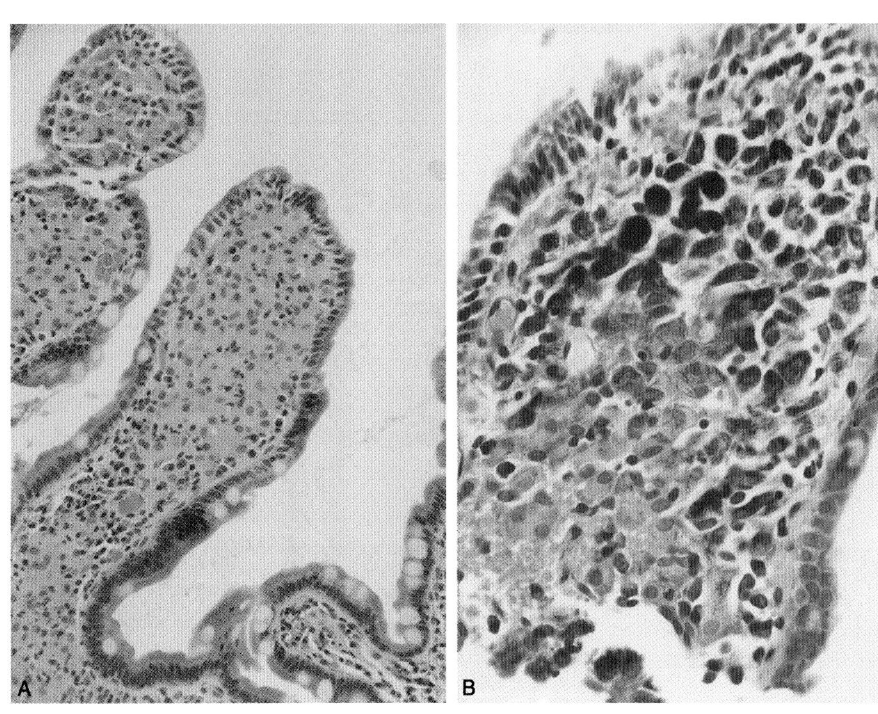

图 35.7　肠道鸟分枝杆菌复合体。A,小肠活检标本的 H&E 染色显示绒毛明显增厚,伴细胞浸润。B,抗酸染色高倍视野显示大量巨噬细胞充满分枝杆菌

尽管肺外结核是艾滋病的特征性表现,但胃肠道腔内受累并不常见,通常累及回盲部或结肠。[42] 也有报道发现瘘管形成、肠套叠和穿孔,以及腹膜和直肠受累。HIV 感染者的肠结核最常见于发展中国家。与 MAC 相比,艾滋病患者的结核感染一般会对多药抗结核治疗产生应答[如 RIPE(见表 35.1)][39]。

已有发现,HAART 治疗后分枝杆菌(如 MAC 淋巴结炎)和病毒(如 CMV 葡萄膜炎)引起的感染。这种免疫重建炎症综合征(immune reconstitution inflammatory syndrome,IRIS)引起针对先前静止或潜伏状态病原体的强烈的炎症反应[45]。此外,随着诊断出 OI 和使用 HAART 后,这些感染的反常恶化可能导致更糟糕的结局。

艾滋病肠道真菌感染中,描述最多的是组织胞浆菌病,并且发生在播散性感染的情况下,通常与肺和肝组织胞浆菌病有关。组织胞浆菌病可能表现为伴有大溃疡和腹泻的弥漫性结肠炎、肿块或与腹膜炎相关的浆膜性疾病[46]。在高热且血清 LDH 明显升高的患者中,可怀疑播散性组织胞浆菌病的诊断[46]。通过真菌涂片和尿液、感染组织或血液培养可以建立诊断;尿液组织胞浆菌病抗原检测可提供支持性证据。一些罕见病例还描述了肠道受累的全身性隐球菌病、球孢子菌病和马尔尼菲篮状菌(主要在东南亚)的感染。

随着 HAART 的出现,药物引起的腹泻变得越来越重要。尽管几乎每一种治疗方案都与腹泻有关,但与腹泻相关的最常见药物是蛋白酶抑制剂,奈非纳韦的发生概率最高[47]。一般来说,腹泻的严重程度为轻度至中度,不伴体重减轻。这些药物导致腹泻的机制尚不清楚。对症治疗通常有效。一种新的药物 crofelemer 可能对这种情况下的腹泻有用[48]。框 35.3 概括了评估腹泻的方法。

框 35.3　艾滋病患者腹泻的评估
所有患者
用于细菌培养的粪便标本;艰难梭菌毒素
用于粪便白细胞,虫卵和寄生虫检测以及抗酸染色的粪便涂片
直肠出血、里急后重、或粪便白细胞增多的患者
软式乙状结肠镜检查或结肠镜检查及黏膜活检,用于组织病理学、病毒、原虫检查
在某些情况下,对直肠组织进行细菌(尤其是弯曲杆菌属)和病毒培养
持续性腹泻和体重减轻且高于评估结果为阴性的患者
上消化道内镜检查及小肠黏膜活检

三、腹痛

艾滋病患者腹痛的发生频率尚不清楚,但如同艾滋病其他胃肠道并发症,其患病率和病因已被 HAART 改变。大多数艾滋病患者较为严重的腹痛与 HIV 及其后果直接相关。然而,医生不仅要考虑 OI 和肿瘤的表现,还要考虑一般人群腹痛的常见原因。

表 35.2 中列出了艾滋病腹痛的鉴别诊断。此表格不包括在 HAART 时代认为更为重要的非艾滋病相关诊断。表 35.3 根据 4 种最常见的疼痛综合征、可疑诊断、最可能的原因和所示的诊断方法来描述腹痛。通常,症状的持续时间和严重程度决定了评估的紧迫性。

表 35.2　艾滋病患者腹部疼痛的鉴别诊断*

器官	病因
胃	
胃炎	CMV†,隐孢子虫(见第 52 章)
胃溃疡	CMV†,PUD
胃出口梗阻	隐孢子虫,CMV,淋巴瘤,PUD
肿块	淋巴瘤,KS,CMV
小肠	
肠炎	隐孢子虫†,CMV,MAC
梗阻	淋巴瘤†,KS
穿孔	CMV†,淋巴瘤
结肠	
结肠炎	肠道细菌†,CMV,HSV
梗阻	淋巴瘤†,KS,肠套叠
穿孔	CMV†,淋巴瘤,HSV
阑尾炎	KS†,隐孢子虫,CMV
肝、脾	
浸润性疾病	淋巴瘤†,CMV,MAC
胆道	
胆囊炎	CMV†,隐孢子虫†,微孢子虫
乳头狭窄	CMV†,隐孢子虫†,KS
胆管炎	CMV†
胰腺	
胰腺炎	CMV†,KS,药物诱导
肿瘤	淋巴瘤,KS
肠系膜,腹膜	
浸润性疾病	MAC†,隐球菌属,KS,淋巴瘤,组织胞浆菌病,结核,球孢子菌病,弓形体病

CMV,巨细胞病毒;HSV,单纯疱疹病毒;KS,卡波西肉瘤;MAC,鸟分枝杆菌复合体;PUD,消化性溃疡病。

*鉴别诊断不包括许多非艾滋病特异性疾病。

†更常见的诊断。

表 35.3　艾滋病患者腹痛综合征的评估

症状	疑似诊断	诊断方法
钝痛,腹泻,轻度恶心,呕吐	感染性肠炎	粪便培养,粪便虫卵和寄生虫检测、乙状结肠镜检查
急性剧烈疼痛伴腹膜刺激征	穿孔,感染性腹膜炎	腹部平片和直立位胸部平片,外科会诊,US 或 CT,腹腔穿刺(如果有腹水),腹腔镜检查
右上腹疼痛,肝脏生化检查水平升高	胆囊炎,胆管炎,肝脏浸润,胆管病	US 或 CT,MRCP,ERCP,肝活检
亚急性疼痛,严重恶心和呕吐	肠道梗阻	腹部平片,CT,小肠系列,内窥镜检查,钡灌肠

ERCP,内镜逆行胰胆管造影;MRCP,磁共振胰胆管造影;US,超声。

病史有助于确定腹痛的原因。相关症状和体征提示受累的特定器官,腹痛的性质和持续时间可能涉及特定的疾病。一般来说,对非艾滋病患者也应该进行相同的检查。腹部 CT 扫描在评估早期腹痛特别有用。急性胰腺炎患者必须考虑药物引起的原因[49]。腹痛的治疗主要涉及手术与非手术治疗。艾滋病患者手术干预的指征和没有患艾滋病的患者相同。所有组织标本必须进行病毒和真菌培养以及病理检查,肿大的肠系膜淋巴结也应进行活检。

四、肛管直肠疾病

艾滋病男男性接触患者肛门直肠疾病的发病率高于其他性传播感染的艾滋病患者。HIV 感染患者的常见表现包括直肠周围脓肿、肛瘘、肛周 HSV、特发性溃疡和感染性直肠炎,但也可见淋巴瘤,以及由 CMV、TB 和组织胞浆菌病引起的溃疡(框 35.4)。MSM 中肛门直肠鳞状细胞癌的发生率明显高于其他组。而且随着 HIV 病变的进展,这种风险会增加。尽管使用了 HAART,但这些肿瘤的发病率仍然在上升[49]。这些肿瘤是通过性接触获得的 HPV 感染,特别是 HPV16 和 18 型。形态学研究记录了组织学进展,通常在同一病变中,可见从良性病变、尖锐湿疣,进展至高级别上皮内瘤变或鳞状细胞癌;但是,对进展的发生率和危险因素了解甚少。高级别上皮内瘤变与 HPV16 或 HPV18 和低水平的 CD4 细胞计数有关,并可能迅速发展为癌症[50]。尽管未做常规推荐,与巴氏涂片相似的肛管的细胞学标本,可用于筛查病变,对异型增生具有很高的预测价值[51]。

框 35.4　艾滋病患者肛门直肠疾病的鉴别诊断

感染	真菌
细菌	白色念珠菌
沙眼衣原体*	荚膜组织胞浆菌
性病淋巴肉芽肿	**肿瘤**
淋病奈瑟菌*	淋巴瘤*
福氏志贺菌	卡波西肉瘤
结核分枝杆菌	鳞状细胞癌
原虫	泄殖腔源性癌
溶组织内阿米巴	尖锐湿疣
利什曼原虫	**其他**
病毒	特发性溃疡*
HSV*	直肠周围脓肿，瘘*
巨细胞病毒*	

*更常见的诊断。

有症状的 HIV 感染者和艾滋病患者，体格检查应包括仔细检查皮肤和黏膜，以及淋巴结的触诊。在直肠指诊之前，应先观察肛门是否有溃疡、裂隙和肿块。应行肛周区域和臀部触诊以检查是否有脓肿。直肠检查中出现剧烈疼痛高度提示有溃疡性疾病、痔疮或肿瘤。触诊肛管可能会发现肿块或裂隙，但其他情况并不明显。所有伴肛门直肠症状的患者都应进行肛门直肠镜检和乙状结肠镜检查（硬式或软式）并行黏膜活检。高分辨率的肛门镜检查可能对肛门细胞学筛查起辅助作用。疼痛严重时，可能需要在全身麻醉下进行。应评估标本有无肿瘤或感染的证据；适当时候应行细菌（包括淋球菌和衣原体）、病毒和真菌培养或核酸扩增试验。如果发现肿瘤，CT 扫描可确定病变的范围。肛肠疾病在手术或药物治疗后的恢复情况将主要取决于 HIV 感染的阶段。在 HAART 时代，鳞状细胞癌患者的存活率有所提高[52]。

五、消化道出血

艾滋病机会性感染和肿瘤很少引起消化道出血（框 35.5）。然而，这些患者上消化道出血的原因大多是与艾滋病无关的疾病，包括消化性溃疡疾病，相反，艾滋病患者下消化道出血的最常见原因是机会性感染，即 CMV 结肠炎[53]。引起黏膜溃疡的感染（如 CMV、HSV、侵袭性肠细菌）是出血最常见的原因。尽管大多数肠道卡波西肉瘤无症状，肠道淋巴瘤（如 Burkitt 淋巴瘤）、卡波西肉瘤或腺癌可能会自发溃疡形成和出血。

艾滋病患者消化道出血的初步评估与其他健康患者采用的方法相似（见第 20 章）。所有患者优先选择内镜检查，特别是那些具有严重免疫缺陷的患者，考虑到机会性疾病的可能性，需要黏膜活检来诊断，因为内镜下可以进行止血治疗。

框 35.5　艾滋病患者胃肠道出血的鉴别诊断（排除非艾滋病特异性诊断）

食管	巨细胞病毒
念珠菌属*	沙门菌属
巨细胞病毒*	隐孢子虫属
HSV	**结肠**
特发性溃疡	巨细胞病毒*
胃	卡波西肉瘤*
巨细胞病毒*	溶组织内阿米巴
卡波西肉瘤*	空肠弯曲杆菌
隐孢子虫病	艰难梭菌
淋巴瘤	志贺菌属
小肠	特发性溃疡
卡波西肉瘤*	淋巴瘤
淋巴瘤	

*更常见的诊断。

六、肝胆疾病

HAART 的出现显著改变了 HIV 患者的肝病和肝脏生化检查异常的原因、方法和结局（框 35.6）。肝胆疾病可大致分为肝实质异常、胆道异常或两者均有。如前所述，肝病已成为最常见的非艾滋病相关死因之一；1/3 或更多接受 HAART 治疗的患者死于肝病并发症[54,55]。在 HAART 时代，实质性肝病的最常见原因是与病毒性肝炎（最重要的是慢性丙型肝炎），药物相关性肝毒性，脂肪性肝病，以及酒精性肝病相关。

框 35.6　艾滋病患者肝脏肿大和肝脏生化试验水平升高的鉴别诊断

肝实质疾病	肿瘤
感染	淋巴瘤
丙型肝炎*	卡波西肉瘤
鸟分枝杆菌复合体*	**胆道疾病**
结核分枝杆菌*	**胆管炎**
巨细胞病毒	巨细胞病毒*
杆菌性肝紫癜症	隐孢子虫*
隐球菌属	微孢子虫
乙型、丁型肝炎	**肿瘤**
耶氏肺孢子虫	淋巴瘤*
微孢子虫	卡波西肉瘤
药物†	

*更常见的诊断。
†特别是磺胺类药物、蛋白酶抑制剂。

药物性肝损伤是肝脏检查异常的最常见原因，常与抗逆转录病毒药物使用增多有关。在 HAART 之前，磺胺类药物最常引起肝毒性，并且这些药物不良反应发生率的增加在艾滋病中得到了充分认识。其他处方(或非处方)药以及中草药的使用也必须考虑肝生化异常的原因,或是药物单独作用,或是潜在的药物之间的相互作用。

药物性肝损伤的危险因素与慢性病毒性肝炎具有高度的相关性,最明显的是 HBV 或 HCV,风险增加了 3 倍或者更高。其他报告的危险因素包括既往肝纤维化、治疗前肝生化指标升高、年龄较大,酗酒以及同时进行抗结核药物的治疗[56,57]。

HAART 导致肝损伤的机制包括药物诱导的毒性和(或)代谢、直接超敏反应、线粒体毒性、IRIS 和脂肪变性[58]。超敏反应具有特质性、免疫相关,通常发生在药物开始使用的前 4 到 6 周。

乳酸酸中毒综合征,通常由核苷逆转录酶抑制剂(即齐多夫定、地丹宁或司坦夫定)引起,以明显肝大、脂肪变性和代谢性乳酸性酸中毒为特征,最终导致肝衰竭。鉴于这些药物在目前的 HAART 疗法中很少使用,因此这种综合征也很少见[59]。

在启动 HAART 治疗并随后的 CD4 细胞恢复后,特别是在那些合并慢性 HBV 感染的患者中,会发生 IRIS 相关性肝损伤,该综合征通常在药物治疗开始的前 2 个月内表现出来,并伴随着 HIV RNA 的急剧下降和 CD4 计数的上升。转氨酶升高和 HBV DNA 高水平是诱发因素[60]。肝损伤程度的变化范围从轻微肝功异常到致命的急性肝功能衰竭。

鉴于病毒性肝炎感染的共同风险因素,包括使用静脉注射药物和性传播,在这一人群中病毒性肝炎的高流行率和发病率并不意外。HBV(+/-HDV)、HCV 和 HAV 感染的临床表现和组织学特征在合并 HIV 感染的情况下发生改变,但每种病毒的感染方式截然不同。

性感染,但全球差异显著[61]。在非洲和亚洲,垂直传播是最常见的 HBV 感染途径,而在西方,吸毒和性传播占主导地位。最近的研究表明,乙肝病毒感染率降低,可能部分归因于乙肝疫苗的使用[62]。同时感染 HIV 和 HBV 导致 HBV 抗原-抗体表达,病毒复制和临床结局的改变。HIV 感染者 HBeAg 自发清除率较低、HBV 复制增加、抗 HBs 阴性率更高、HBV 再激活,而且在急性暴露于该病毒后更有可能发展为慢性 HBV 感染。与 HCV 一样,与不伴 HIV 感染的 HBV 患者相比,HBV/HIV 合并感染的患者肝硬化进展速度更快,死亡率也更高。HBsAg 的再次出现可能是再感染或因免疫缺陷的进展而再次激活。随着对 HBV 免疫力的丧失或降低,乙型肝炎 e 抗原(HBeAg)表达增加,DNA 聚合酶的平均水平升高,乙型肝炎核心抗体滴度增加。血清 HBV DNA 病毒载量的增加提高了肝细胞癌(HCC)发生的风险。在艾滋病毒感染的患者中获得慢性携带者状态的可能性也更大,特别是在免疫缺陷更严重时发生了感染。因此,与 HIV 阴性的患者相比,HIV/HBV 合并感染患者有更大比例的慢性 HBV 携带者状态,具有高度传染性的血清和体液。

尽管 HIV 感染导致出现更多的慢性 HBV 携带者,但它似乎减轻了肝生化和组织学的严重程度。HIV 感染后 HBV 相关的肝损伤降低的机制尚不确定,但已被认为是由于 HIV 对淋巴细胞的损伤作用减少了淋巴细胞介导的肝细胞损伤。在既往或目前无 HBV 和 HIV 感染血清学证据的患者中,乙肝疫苗接种的效果与免疫受损阶段和 HIV 病毒血症程度有关[63]。对 HBV 疫苗接种的免疫应答可通过 HAART 治疗后接种、提高免疫功能、使用高剂量疫苗接种和重复接种疫苗来提高[64]。

相反,慢性 HBV 携带者应用 HAART 治疗可能会在免疫重建后产生灾难性后果(IRIS)。患者可能出现重度病毒性肝炎急性发作,导致暴发性肝衰竭。然而,使用 HAART 后发生急性乙型肝炎发作的共感染患者的比例似乎较低[65]。值得信赖的说法是,如同正常宿主一样,应用 HAART 重建免疫功能会产生针对被感染的肝细胞的抗体,也可能产生抗-HBe 和(或)抗-HBs。在 HAART 方案中包含的对 HBV 具有效抗病毒作用的拉米夫定可以降低乙型肝炎急性发作的可能性。长期拉米夫定单药治疗可能导致逃逸突变并突发急性肝炎。HIV 或 HBV 的治疗必须考虑到每一种感染,因为许多抗逆转录病毒药物对两种病毒都具有双重活性。如果对某一感染进行治疗,应使用替诺福韦和恩曲他滨或替诺福韦和拉米夫定加上第三种药物联合启动治疗 HIV。目前建议使用包括 2 种对 HBV 有活性的药物,以防止出现耐药株。对于晚期免疫抑制的患者,治愈 HBV 不太可能;因此,目标应该是尽可能降低 HBV DNA。这种治疗可以减少疾病进展并且可能降低 HCC 的风险。这些观察结果表明,所有接受 HAART 治疗的患者都应接受活动性或既往 HBV 感染的筛查。所有符合条件的患者都应考虑接种疫苗。目前已经总结出来 HIV 感染者 HBV 感染的治疗方案[66]。HIV、HBV 和 HDV 三联感染很少见。尽管一些数据表明 HDV 相关肝脏疾病进展性可能更强,但 HIV 合并 HDV 感染结局似乎与 HBV 感染相似。HDV 感染 HIV 的后果似乎与 HBV 相似,尽管一些数据表明 HDV 肝病可能更具侵袭性[67]。

与这一人群密切相关的 HAV 感染的主要风险因素包括旅行和高危性行为。在 MSM 中已经发现了 HAV 的暴发[68]。虽然在 HIV 感染者中发生 HAV 感染可能导致 HAV RNA 血清滴度更高以及迁延的病毒血症,但并没有证据表明病程会更为严重。与乙型肝炎一样,在免疫功能低下的人群中,对 HAV 疫苗的免疫应答更弱,但是当免疫功能得以保留时,应答率很高且持续时间也会延长,特别是当接种 3 剂而不是 2 剂疫苗时[69]。鉴于粪-口传播途径,应考虑在所有非免疫 MSM 中接种疫苗。

艾滋病患者感染 HCV 的患病率是不同的,与异性恋者和男男性接触者(1% 至 10%)相比,静脉注射吸毒者和血友病患者的发病率较高(约 50% 至 90%)[70]。HIV 明显改变了 HCV 合并感染的自然史。肝脏疾病现在是导致 HIV 感染者死亡的重要原因,其中大部分与 HCV 合并感染有关。与 HBV 不同,HCV 的临床过程随着 HIV 相关免疫功能的降低而恶化。急性感染 HCV 的 HIV 患者不太可能清除 HCV 病毒血症,HCV RNA 水平也高很多,纤维化的进展速度也增快,失代偿性肝硬化和致命性肝病发生的时间比 HIV 阴性患者早发生 10 年或更久[71]。合并感染者的纤维化进展更迅速,首次是在血友病人群中观察到。发生肝硬化的风险增加 2 倍,发生失代偿期肝病的相对风险增加 6 倍,发展为肝癌的风险也增加。预测合并感染的患者纤维化和进展为肝硬化的因素包括感染年龄较大、血清 ALT 水平较高、炎症活动较高、饮酒量超过 50 克/天、CD4 计数低于 500 细胞/mm^3[72]。脂肪性肝炎也可能发挥一定的作用[73]。这种快速发展为纤维化的机制是多因素的，但在其他免疫功能低下的患者中也有类似情况。共感染者出现失代偿期肝硬化，生存率较低，中位生存期约为 1 年。持续的病毒学应答者不太可能出现肝脏相关事件以及死亡，这支持了对有效治疗的迫切需求[74,75]。虽然在这些患者中，与肝病相关的大部分死亡率是 HCV 感染造成的，但 HCC 的发病率正在上升，艾滋病患者的发病率比一般人群高 4 倍[76]。与乙型肝炎一样，HCV 不会引起艾滋病的进展。三联感染（HCV，HBV，HIV）甚至四联感染（HCV，HBV，HDV 和 HIV）极少见，这与注射毒品有关，可能预后更差，包括较高的肝硬化发生率。

随着新的治疗丙型肝炎的简化口服药物的出现（第 80 章），对合并感染患者的治疗、应答和自然史都发生了改变。对许多患者来说，随着新的 DAA 治疗的应用，丙肝治愈已成为现实。以往的以干扰素为基础的治疗存在副作用且效果差。DAA 通常与 HAART 联合使用可产生与 HCV+/HCV-患者相同的持续病毒应答（SVR）（>95%）[77,78]。此外，早期治疗可降低肝纤维化和 HCC 的发生率。已观察到再感染。

戊型肝炎合并感染似乎很少见，呈地方性，对孕妇的任何其他影响尚不确定[79]。

非酒精性脂肪性肝病（NAFLD）在世界范围内逐渐被认识，这与肥胖有关。这种疾病 HIV 感染者中逐渐增多，它在肝功异常、肝纤维化和肝硬化的发展中尤其是在代谢综合征的发展中起着重要作用[80]。此外，可能有多种原因，包括 HCV 感染，饮酒，以及 HAART 本身或其对脂肪生成的影响。

虽然罕见，但结节再生性增生和非肝硬化门静脉高压症在这一人群中的报道越来越多。相关的风险因素是使用去羟肌苷和血栓形成的倾向[81]。

细胞内分枝杆菌（MAC）感染是 HIV 感染后期肝脏最容易出现的特异性表现[82]。这种感染的病理特征是在泡沫状组织细胞中存在含有抗酸杆菌的形态不佳的肉芽肿。在发展中国家，结核病是 HIV 感染者最常见的累及肝脏的机会性感染。与 MAC 相反，结核病可能在 HIV 感染患者严重免疫功能低下之前发生。在感染 HIV 的患者中，肺外结核病很常见（≈80%）[83]。已有报道部分粟粒性结核累及肝脏。结核性脓肿和胆管结核瘤等症状比较罕见[84]。通过经皮或腹腔镜活检获得的肝组织培养出结核杆菌来诊断肝结核。PCR 可以更早诊断。与 MAC 一样，通过对活检标本进行适当染色可以观察到典型的分枝杆菌。

CMV 是一种罕见的肝脏病原体，最常见于 HIV 患者的尸检中。然而，它很少是临床肝炎的原因或其他肝脏症状的原因。典型的病毒包涵体通常出现在库普弗细胞中，但有时可在肝细胞或窦内皮细胞中或与肉芽肿相关。

当免疫功能低下较严重时，肝脏的真菌感染在 HIV 感染中并不罕见。在播散性真菌疾病患者中可观察到肝组织胞浆菌病，隐球菌病和球孢子菌病，主要但不仅限于该病原体高流行区域[84]。与其他黏膜部位的高发率相比，肝脏的念珠菌感染很少见。

卡波西肉瘤最常见于尸检或肝脏活检时意外发现，但有时可能导致转氨酶升高或黄疸。

非霍奇金淋巴瘤肝脏受累可能是艾滋病的特征性表现和肿瘤的原发部位。艾滋病患者的这种肿瘤往往在组织学和临床上更具侵袭性，迅速扩散到结节外部位，使肝脏更容易受累[85]。病变通常是局灶性的，也可能很大。预后在很大程度上取决于潜在的免疫损伤程度和表现评分，而不是淋巴瘤本身。已证实接受 HAART 的患者存活率有所提高[86]。

已有报道许多多种病原体感染累及肝脏的单发病例，包括吉罗韦氏疟原虫、隐孢子虫、微孢子虫、双色瓢虫和利什曼原虫[87]。

由亨氏巴尔通体或昆氏巴尔通体引起的细菌性肝球囊病是一种全身性感染，可能伴有发热、皮肤病变、腹痛和溶骨性损害[88]。肝生化结果通常显示血清碱性磷酸酶不成比例地升高。肝脏活检证实黏液样基质区域与紫色颗粒状物质关系密切，Warthin-Starry 染色或电子显微镜显示微生物团块。

目前与胆道疾病最可能相关的是胆石症、胆总管结石或慢性胰腺炎。一个类似于硬化性胆管炎伴乳头状狭窄的综合征已被公认且被称为 AIDS 胆管病[89]。患者特征性地出现明显的上腹痛，伴有血清碱性磷酸酶显著升高，以及胆红素、AST 和 ALT 的轻微升高。目前，非 HIV 相关的胆道疾病（如胆管结石）与 AIDS 相关的疾病一样很常见。

胆管改变包括单纯的乳头狭窄，硬化性胆管炎样病变，或者两者合并出现，或较长时间的肝外狭窄。大多数案例发现乳头狭窄伴肝内疾病最常见（图 35.8）。在大多数经胆管造影证实为胆管病变的患者中，超声或 CT 可见胆管异常，以扩张为主，这意味着影像学阴性并不能完全排除诊断。在大多数情况下，病因是由于隐孢子虫、CMV、微孢子虫或囊尾蚴感染十二指肠及胆道上皮所致。对于以乳头狭窄为主的患者，括约肌切开术可改善大多数患者症状[89]。然而，血清碱性磷酸酶可能继续升高，这可能反映了相关肝内疾病的进展。HAART 可能使部分影像学异常的患者得到改善[89]。艾滋病胆管病患者的存活与免疫缺陷的严重程度有关[90]。

艾滋病中胆道疾病的其他不常见原因包括原发性胆管淋巴瘤、肝门部淋巴瘤样淋巴结阻塞胆管树、卡波西肉瘤和肝外胆汁聚积（胆汁瘤）。

在艾滋病患者中也描述了非结石性胆囊炎，表现为严重的腹痛和偶发性腹膜炎。这种综合征通常由特定感染引起，最常见的是 CMV，也可是微孢子虫，隐孢子虫和贝氏囊尾蚴[91]。可能发生胆石症。腹腔镜胆囊切除术是首选治疗方法。

临床病史和有症状的肝大或肝生化检查异常非特异性，需要进一步评估。但是可以得出一些概括性结论。血清转氨酶的显著升高倾向于药物诱导或病毒原因。相比之下，若无肝外阻塞，血清碱性磷酸酶的显著升高与 AIDS 中肝脏 MAC 感染存在统计学相关性。应尽早使用超声（US）、CT 和 MR 胆管造影（MRC），因为它们在识别胆管扩张，胆囊病理和局灶性肝脏病变方面特别有用。

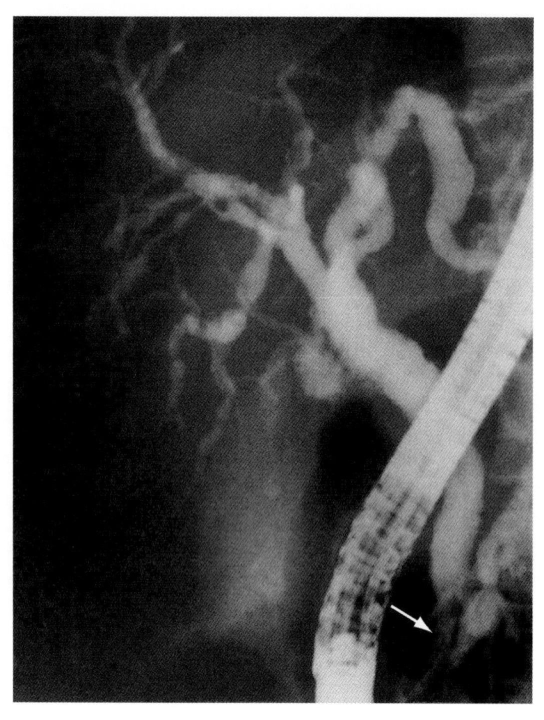

图 35.8　艾滋病胆管病患者的内镜逆行胰胆管造影(ERCP)图像。存在乳头狭窄(箭)

对疑有肝内疾病的患者,肝活检的适应证有限。虽然在大多数患者中都有可能出现特殊诊断,但肝活检很少发现以前未确诊的机会性感染,这表明不易出现在别处的疾病也极少累及肝脏。这一观察结果强调了在血液培养和骨髓检查等微创诊断方法尚未得出结论的情况下肝活检的重要性[92]。肝活检和肝弹性可能在 HCV 的治疗决策中发挥作用,如同对正常人一样。腹部影像发现的局灶性肝脏病变可以在 US 或 CT 引导下取样。在特殊情况下,例如血友病,经颈静脉肝活检可能优于经皮活检。活检组织切片的恰当染色常可证实特殊感染或肿瘤。

CT 或 US 显示胆管扩张,则提示黄疸为肝外原因,也可能显示其他胆道和(或)胰腺异常。一旦发现肝外阻塞,必须考虑与艾滋病胆管病相关的乳头狭窄的可能性,以及胆总管结石或其他疾病的可能性,这取决于影像表现和临床情况。额外的检查如 CT、磁共振胰胆管造影(MRCP)或内镜 US 可以更好地显示背后的病因,计划内镜治疗的患者可行内镜逆行胰胆管造影(ERCP)。在 ERCP 期间收集的胆管、壶腹和十二指肠活检标本或胆汁和(或)胆汁细胞学(适当染色)可以检测是否存在病毒、原生动物或肿瘤细胞。

(刘晖 译,孙明瑜　闫秀娥 校)

参考文献

第 36 章　实体器官和造血细胞移植的胃肠道和肝脏并发症

Anne M. Larson, Rachel B. Issaka, David M. Hockenbery 著

章节目录

一、实体器官移植的并发症 …… 483
二、肾脏和肾脏/胰腺移植 …… 485
三、肝移植 …… 486
四、心脏移植、肺移植和心-肺移植 …… 487
五、肠移植 …… 487
六、实体器官移植受者以问题为导向的诊断方法 …… 487
（一）上消化道症状和体征 …… 487
（二）腹泻和便秘 …… 488
（三）腹痛 …… 488
（四）胃肠道出血 …… 489
（五）胃肠道恶性病变 …… 489
（六）肝胆并发症 …… 489
七、造血细胞移植并发症 …… 489
（一）造血细胞移植前肠道和肝脏疾病的评估 …… 490
（二）移植术后 1 年内发生的问题 …… 491
（三）移植后长期存活的问题 …… 500

实体器官移植是同种异体造血细胞移植的免疫学镜像：移植受体可以排斥移植的实体器官，而同种异体造血细胞可以损伤或“排斥”其受体的器官。这些移植手术的肠道和肝脏并发症有相似之处，特别是在感染和免疫抑制药物的副作用方面。然而，移植患者群体、移植准备以及免疫抑制程度和时间长短方面存在极大差异。因此，本章针对实体器官和造血细胞移植的并发症提出了基于问题为导向的处理方法。

一、实体器官移植的并发症

据报道，实体器官移植（solid organ transplan，SOT）后胃肠道并发症发生于 20%～35% 的受体中，而印度报道其概率高达 60%。大多数问题与机会性感染、移植后功能紊乱，药物不良反应或恶性肿瘤有关（表 36.1）[1-3]。感染仍然是 SOT 后高发病率和死亡率的主要原因，尤其是在最初 6 个月内[4]。然而，SOT 受体在最初 6 个月后发生感染的概率也多达 16%[5]。SOT 术后第一个月内，感染包括移植前的感染（如尿路感染），与手术过程本身相关的并发症（如胆道败血症）有关的感染，或与同种异体移植物一起传播的感染。机会性病毒、真菌和寄生虫感染在第一个月后更有可能发生，疱疹病毒感染是最常见的（图 36.1）[4]。普遍预防—预防性抗菌药、抗病毒药物和抗真菌药物可能减少这些感染的发生[6]。也有一些与感染类似的非感染并发症（见表 36.1）。

巨细胞病毒（CMV）感染是一种普遍存在的病毒感染，感染率从美国约一半的成年人到全球超过 95% 的人不等[7,8]。CMV 是 SOT 后第一年内发生的感染的主要病毒病原体，如果没有抗病毒预防措施，40%～60% 的血清阳性受者会出现病毒血症[9]。CMV 感染会大幅增加移植物排斥的概率，同时降低移植物存活率和增加受者死亡率[10-13]。CMV 的几种易感因素[10,11]：①免疫抑制增加，如除了常规免疫抑制或高剂量吗替麦考酚酯（MMF）维持治疗外的抗淋巴细胞抗体[4]；②CMV 供体和受体错配[10,11,14]；③同种异体移植物排斥或与免疫调节病毒［即人疱疹病毒（HHV）-6，HHV-7］、细菌、真菌共感染[4,15]。CMV 感染的发病高峰期通常在停止预防抗病毒感染，移植后 4～6 个月内。表现包括无症状的病毒血症、CMV 综合征（发热、不适，白细胞减少，中性粒细胞减少，非典型淋巴细胞增多，肝转氨酶升高）以及侵袭性疾病（如胃肠道和肝胆感染，肺炎，视网膜炎）（见图 36.1）[7,16]。SOT 受者器官侵袭性疾病的病例中约 70%～80% 继发于胃肠道 CMV 感染[17,18]。疾病活动度可通过多种方式确诊，包括 CMV DNA

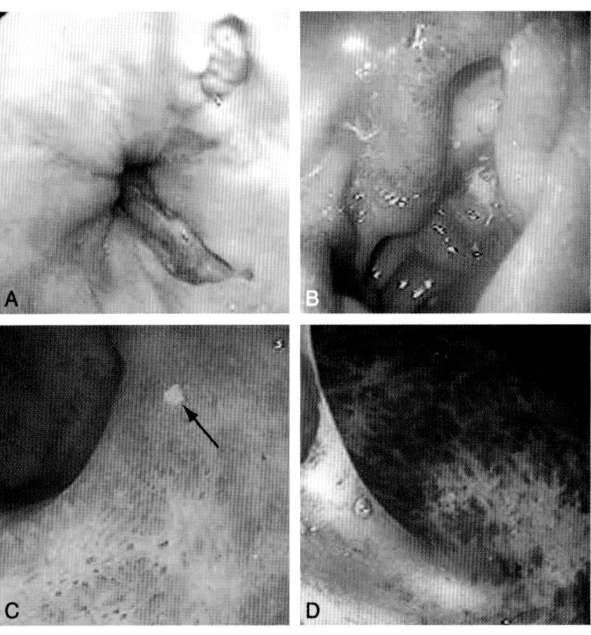

图 36.1　实体器官移植后肠道感染的内镜照片。A，巨细胞病毒（CMV）引起的远端食管溃疡。B，HSV 引起的十二指肠溃疡，溃疡较深，不规则，周围黏膜水肿。C，CMV 感染的结肠黏膜，表现为局灶性溃疡（箭头），和周围黏膜苍白溃疡及黏膜内出血。D，CMV 感染的结肠黏膜，有弥漫性脆性黏膜及溃疡

表 36.1 实体器官移植受者肠道和肝胆系统疾病的原因*

	食管症状	恶心、呕吐、厌食	腹痛	胃肠道出血	腹泻	恶性肿瘤	肝胆管疾病
感染性原因	白色念珠菌 其他真菌种属 CMV 单纯疱疹病毒(VZV) (结核分枝杆菌) (寄生虫)	CMV 单纯疱疹病毒 幽门螺杆菌相关的溃疡(VZV) (贾第鞭毛虫) (隐孢子虫) (诺瓦克病毒) (轮状病毒) (EBV-PTLD)	CMV 艰难梭状芽孢杆菌 幽门螺杆菌相关的溃疡 脓肿穿孔,腹膜炎、急性胆囊炎、(病毒性胰腺炎) (VZV) (真菌感染)	CMV 真菌(念珠菌,霉菌)感染 幽门螺杆菌-相关的溃疡(EBV-PTLD) 梭状芽孢杆菌(单纯疱疹病毒食管炎)	CMV 其他病毒 梭状芽孢杆菌 (寄生虫) (EB 病毒-PTLD) (肠道细菌致病菌)	EBV-PTLD MALT 淋巴瘤 (幽门螺杆菌相关) (卡波西肉瘤)	败血症相关的胆汁淤积 慢性感染性胆囊炎 疱疹病毒(CMV、单纯疱疹病毒、VZV、EBV) HBV HCV 脓肿(真菌、细菌)
非感染性原因	胃酸反流±消化道狭窄 药物性食管炎 胸腔导管术	药物 阻塞 尿毒症 透析 胰腺炎 肝炎 胆囊炎 胃肠动力不足 GVHD	肠梗阻 假性肠梗阻 麻醉肠道综合征 免疫抑制药物 憩室炎 缺血性结肠炎 阑尾炎 急性胰腺炎、(急性 GVHD) 肠动力障碍(肠移植) 胆汁泄漏(LT)	非甾体抗炎药胃溃疡 消化性食管炎 憩室炎(特别是 KT) 缺血性结肠炎(特别是 KT) 胆道或 Roux-en-Y 吻合口出血(原位肝移植) 肝活检(肝活检致胆道出血) 静脉曲张出血(急性 GVHD)	促胃肠动力药 免疫抑制剂(山梨醇结肠炎) 缺血性结肠炎 Mg^{2+} 盐类 抗生素相关腹泻	淋巴瘤 皮肤癌 结肠癌 复发肝细胞癌 肺癌	药物毒性 血管损伤(原位肝移植) 结节性再生性增生 胆道疾病 复发性肝细胞癌

*括号中为文献中描述过但很少见到的情况。
CMV,巨细胞病毒;EBV,EB 病毒;GVHD,移植物抗宿主病;KT,肾移植;LT,肝脏移植;MALT,黏膜相关淋巴组织;PTLD,移植后淋巴增生性疾病;VZV,水痘-带状疱疹病毒。

定量检测、抗原血清学、培养、组织病理学和免疫学检测，这些检测反映了对 CMV 的细胞免疫应答[16,19]。然而，在器官终末期疾病的情况下，血液中可能检测不到病毒，必须从肠道或肝脏活检组织中检测 CMV[20]。疾病预防的两种主要方法是移植后普遍采用的预防性抗病毒或先行治疗（如果发生 CMV 病毒血症，则进行治疗）[21,22]。这两种方法都能有效降低 CMV 相关疾病的发病率[23,24]。更昔洛韦或缬更昔洛韦可显著降低移植受者中 CMV 疾病的发病率；使用的药物取决于移植的器官。然而，因为临床试验中组织侵袭性疾病的发病率较高，所以缬更昔洛韦未被美国食品药品管理局（FDA）批准用于肝移植。更昔洛韦耐药的 CMV 已有报道，是一个在治疗 CMV 疾病中新出现的问题[25]。

单纯疱疹病毒（HSV1/HHV-1 和 HSV2/HHV-2）和水痘-带状疱疹病毒（VZV/HHV-3）是第二常见的病毒感染，是受体内潜伏病毒再激活的典型表现[25-27]。如果不使用抗病毒预防，多达 70% 的移植受体中均可发生 HSV 或 VZV 感染[26]。HSV 对于鳞状上皮（鼻、口、食管、生殖器）具有趋向性，但如果患者没有接受预防性阿昔洛韦（见图 35.1B）治疗，则可能累及肠、肺和肝。原发性 HSV 感染并不常见，但在 SOT 受者中通常更严重且持续时间更长。HSV 再激活常见且通常无症状。症状与原发感染相似。罕见情况下，HSV 可发生播散，表现为发热、白细胞减少和肝炎[26]。原发性 VZV 感染也可能导致终末器官损害。幸运的是，很少有成年 SOT 受者易感，因为只有约 2%～4% 的成人为 VZV 血清阴性[28]。尽管可能出现严重的播散性疾病，再激活的病变可能只表现为局部带状疱疹[28]。高达 20% 的 SOT 受者会出现有症状的感染[25]。肺移植受体风险最大，其次是心脏、肾脏和肝脏[28-30]。阿昔洛韦、伐昔洛韦、缬更昔洛韦或泛昔洛韦的预防可减少 SOT 后 HSV 和 VZV 的复发[31]。据报道，高达 11% 的免疫功能低下的宿主出现了 HSV 抗病毒耐药，但在 SOT 研究中几乎没有数据[25]。

EB 病毒（EBV）和其他人类疱疹病毒引起的感染（HHV-6、HHV-7 和 HHV-8）不太常见。与其他疱疹病毒一样，EBV 感染可以是原发性或继发性的。临床表现从无症状的病毒血症到症状性疾病，包括传染性单核细胞增多症和移植后淋巴组织增生性疾病（post-transplant lymphoproliferative disorder，PTLD）[32]。原发感染通常有症状，并且与更严重的疾病相关[33]。根据移植的器官以及受者是成人或儿童，EBV 相关的 PTLD 的发生率不等（0.6%～16%）[34]。对于需要持续高水平免疫抑制的 SOT 受者，PTLD 总是个问题，B 细胞和 T 细胞淋巴瘤均可见（图 36.2）。HHV-6 在不到 1%～2% 的 SOT 受者中可引起临床疾病[25,35-37]。原发感染很少见，并且再激活主要导致亚临床、短期感染。已有引起胃肠道疾病的报道[38]。缺乏 HHV-7 作为病原体的结论性证据[25,39]。HHV-6 和 HHV-7 均使 SOT 受体易患其他机会性感染。预防性抗病毒在这种情况下的作用尚未得到证实，目前不建议进行预防。HHV-8 可致癌，能导致卡波西肉瘤、巨大淋巴结病和原发性渗出性淋巴瘤（一种非霍奇金淋巴瘤）。HHV-8 也可能导致发热、骨髓抑制和多器官衰竭[38]。

真菌感染通常在移植后第一个月后发生，特别是那些停止预防性抗真菌治疗的患者。SOT 受者真菌感染的发生率估计不到 5%[40,41]。最常见的真菌是念珠菌种（白色念珠菌，热带念珠菌），但曲霉菌和接合菌等真菌的发病率正在增加[42,43]。SOT 超过 6 个月后，机会性感染的发生频率降低，但移植受者仍然面临社区获得性感染的风险。有些不太常见的感染［组织胞浆菌病（<1%）、球孢子菌感染（1.5%～8.7%）、诺卡菌感染、肺孢子虫感染、弓形虫感染和类圆线虫感染］也可能发生于移植第一个月后[38,44-46]。

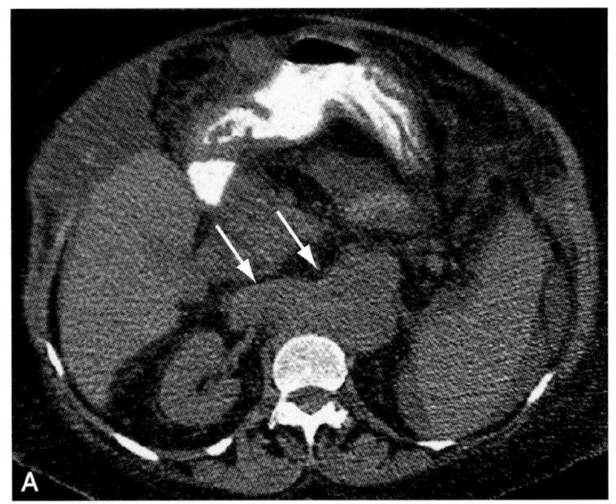

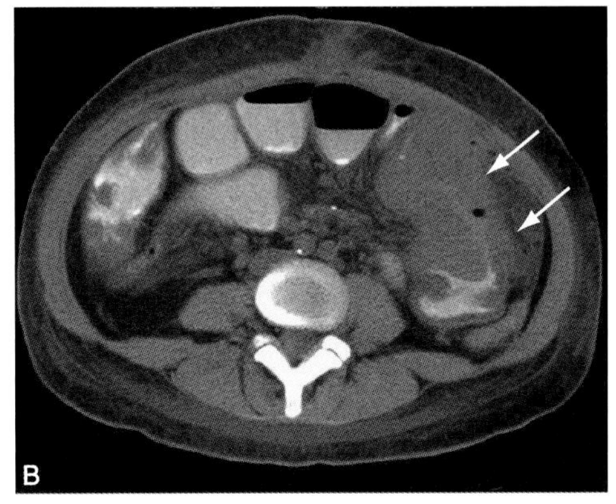

图 36.2　实体器官移植后淋巴组织增生性疾病的计算机断层扫描结果。A，肝移植后由 EBV 阳性 B 细胞淋巴瘤引起的腹膜后肿块（箭）。B，T 细胞淋巴瘤引起的肾移植后远端小肠肿块（箭）。肿块引起肠梗阻，肿块近端可见扩张的小肠袢

二、肾脏和肾脏/胰腺移植

胃肠道并发症是肾移植（kidney transplant，KT）最常见的并发症之一，可见于多达 50% 的患者中，与患者的长期生存相关[47-49]。据报道，经历 GERD 或消化不良的 KT 患者移植物失去功能和死亡的风险增加，其机制尚不清楚[50]。移植物胰腺炎和移植物十二指肠炎通常发生在肾/胰腺移植（kidney/pancreas transplant，KPT）后早期，并可能导致腹腔内感染[51,52]。依据其出生国家不同，KT 和 KPT 受者 HCV 或 HBV 感染的发生率为 5%～66%[53,54]。HCV 对患者和移植结局的影响仍存在争议[55]。许多结果表明长期感染 HCV 或 HBV 的患者预后较差[56-59]。接受 KT 的肝硬化患者 10 年生存率明显低于非肝硬化患者，HCV 肝硬化比 HBV 肝硬化严重。在这种情况下，肝肾联合移植仍然存在争议。HBV 和 HCV 抗病毒治疗都显著改善了 KT 和 KPT 受者的临床转归[60]。

由于更严密的监测、预防性抗感染治疗以及对病毒和真

菌感染的预先治疗，所报道的 KT 受者中许多严重感染现在都不太常见。但是，如果发生无法治愈的危及生命的感染，需要停止使用免疫抑制剂，必要的话，患者可以维持透析。其他器官的受者无法使用此选项。CMV 感染是一种相当常见的感染，报道高达 100%，其中很大一部分患者会出现症状[61-63]。胃肠道 CMV 感染可见于约 50% 的 KT 和 KPT 受者，胰腺受者由于接受更高水平的免疫抑制而有更大的风险[17,54,64]。据报道，成人中约 3.5% KT 受者及 15.5% KPT 受者会发生艰难梭菌感染[65]。约 4% 发生肠道真菌感染，最常见的是念珠菌，还必须考虑寄生虫感染（微孢子虫、粪类圆线虫）[66]。KT 后的 HSV 感染通常无症状，可自限，但可能表现为口腔炎、单核细胞增多症、肝炎或肺炎[67]。KT 受者可发生胆囊炎，在糖尿病患者的发病率较高[68]。

在过去几年中，高达 20% KT 受者发生胃肠道出血。尽管发病率已下降至约 5%，但胃肠道出血仍然有较高的发病率和死亡率[69,70]。手术预后与过去相比有所改善[71,72]。许多患有胃十二指肠溃疡的 KT 受者将不会有胃十二指肠疾病的病史。然而，无症状者高达 40%，大约 50% 的患者会出现消化不良的症状，约 30%～40% 的患者 HP 感染[66,73,74]。随着糖皮质激素的使用减少和质子泵抑制剂（PPI）或 H_2RA 的使用，溃疡形成和出血已不太常见[3]。许多胃肠道症状（如腹泻、恶心、呕吐、腹痛）与 MMF（吗替麦考酚酯）的使用有关，MMF 已基本上被肠溶性霉酚酸（麦考酚酸）代替，肠道副作用较少[75,76]。急腹症见于 10% 左右的患者，可能与胰腺炎、胆囊炎、憩室炎、阑尾炎和肠梗阻有关[77]。与其他 SOT 受者相比，肾脏受者特别容易发生肠缺血。然而，发病率低（<5%）且病因多样[78]。患有多囊肾的受者更常发生肠缺血和梗阻[79]。这一组也有较高比例的病人患憩室疾病及并发症[66,79,80]。在这种情况下，肠缺血具有很高的死亡率。有腹痛的 KT 受者应考虑缺血，特别是接受尸体供肾的老年患者（>40 岁）[78]。

三、肝移植

如第 97 章所述，原位肝移植（orthotopic liver transplantation，OLT）特有的胃肠道并发症通常与手术本身有关，包括腹腔内出血、肝动脉狭窄或血栓形成、胆道功能障碍、肠穿孔、肠梗阻和胃肠道出血[81]。大约 5%～9% 的成人受者发展成肝动脉血栓，并呈现一系列的后果，从伴或不伴发热的转氨酶轻度升高到需要紧急再次移植的急性肝功能衰竭[82]。而且，胆道系统接受来自肝动脉的全部血供，而动脉血流的丧失导致胆管坏死和渗漏，伴肝内胆汁瘤和脓肿形成（图 36.3A 和 B）[83,84]。肝动脉血流的逐渐丧失也可导致肝内胆管消失，这难以与胆管消失性排异反应区分。

高达 12% 的移植物出现门静脉血栓，如果发生在移植后早期，则可导致肝脏缺血和严重的肝功能障碍；后期可出现门静脉高压表现。罕见情况下，肝静脉血栓和下腔静脉血栓或狭窄，可以产生类似 Budd-Chiari 综合征的表现。

胆道并发症是 OLT 后死亡的最常见的原因，占 5%～30%[85]。胆汁渗漏伴胆汁瘤以及狭窄形成一般在吻合口部位，是最常见的胆道异常（见图 36.3A 和 B）[85,86]。吻合口狭

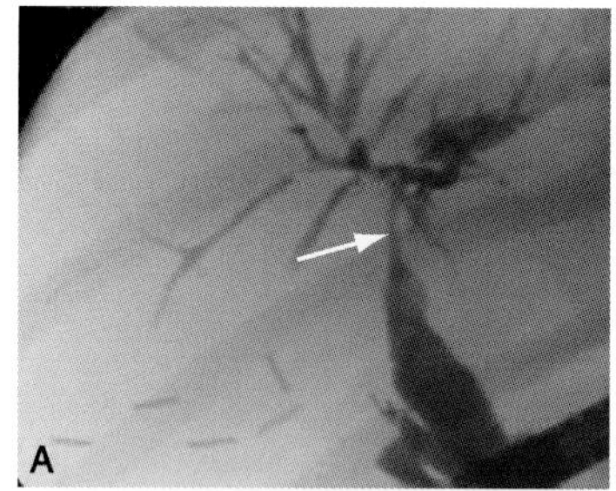

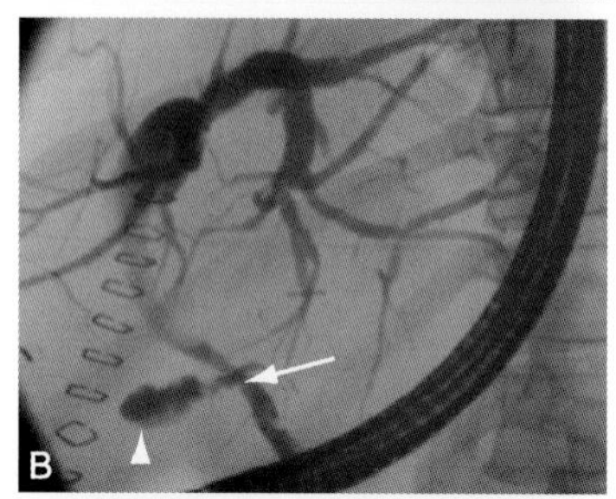

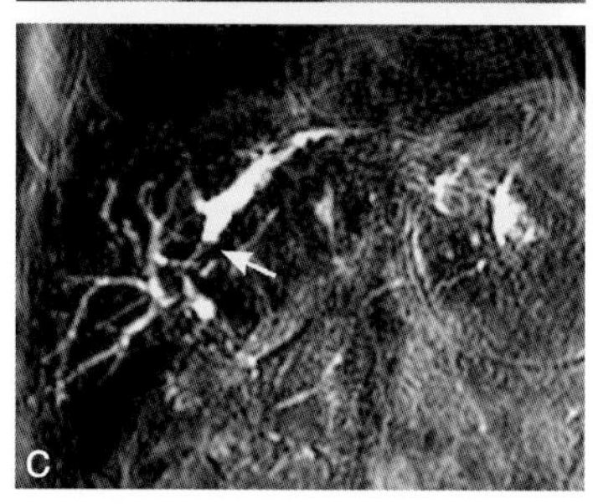

图 36.3　肝移植后的肝胆成像。A，内镜逆行胆管造影显示移植后胆管缺血性狭窄（箭）。B，内镜逆行胆管造影显示移植后胆道吻合口（箭）胆漏（箭）。C，肝内胆道系统磁共振胆管成像显示移植肝复发性硬化性胆管炎。箭头指向狭窄，伴上游胆管扩张

窄占狭窄性疾病的 80%，通常发生在 OLT 后 2～6 个月内，但也可能发生于新近移植的患者。行胆管-胆管吻合术患者的狭窄和渗漏常适用于内镜治疗，而行胆管空肠吻合术的患者可能需要经皮或手术矫正。非吻合口狭窄引起肝动脉供血不足[87]。胆汁铸型可能发生在高达 18% 的受者中，通常发生在 OLT 后第一年中[39,88]。与胆管铸型发生相关的临床因素包括肝缺血和胆道狭窄。内镜和经皮治疗成功率高达 70%，但也可能需要手术治疗，据报道死亡率为 10%～30%[39,89]。

肝移植术后发病率和死亡率的最高是感染，见于 75% 的受者[90]。移植后紧接着可见医院获得性感染和伤口感染。据报道，胃肠道 CMV 感染在高达 40% 的肝脏受者中发生[17]。CMV 肝炎是 OLT 后 CMV 最常见的表现，并且在 OLT 受者中比在其他器官的受者中更严重[91,92]。患者通常血清转氨酶升高，可能与排斥反应相混淆，因此肝脏活检对于诊断十分必要。血中 CMV DNA 检测常可明确诊断[93]。无症状的低水平 CMV 病毒血症通常不需要抗病毒治疗[94]。LT 受者比其他 SOT 受者更常发生侵袭性真菌感染，死亡率高。在没有预防性抗真菌的情况下，多达 42% 的受者发生侵袭性感染，念珠菌属占大多数[95,96]。血清半乳甘露聚糖测定可用于检测真菌感染，特别是侵袭性曲霉菌[97,98]。这些真菌对抗真菌治疗越来越耐药。急性胰腺炎罕见，但据报道可发生于高达

5.7% 的 OLT 受者中，且死亡率高(64%)[39,99]。

OLT 后存在潜在肝病复发的风险，包括 HCV、HBV、自身免疫性肝炎、NASH、PBC 和 PSC(见图 36.3C)[100-103]。肝脏同种异体移植物 HCV 几乎全部复发(见第 80 和 97 章)。以前，这会导致移植物失功显著增加[104-107]。然而，随着多种高效直接作用抗病毒药物的发展，这已不再是一个问题。使用乙肝免疫球蛋白(hepatitis B immune globulin，HBIG)和抗病毒药可预防 HBV 复发。OLT 后，约 26% 的患者 PBC 复发(见第 97 章)[101]。

四、心脏移植、肺移植和心-肺移植

多达一半的心脏移植(heart transplantation，HT)、肺移植(lung transplantation，LT)和心-肺移植(heart-lung transplantation，HLT)受者会出现胃肠道并发症，多达 20% 的受者需要手术[108,109]。最常见的并发症包括腹泻、GERD、消化不良、恶心呕吐、腹痛、胰腺炎、疱疹病毒感染(尤其是巨细胞病毒感染)、胆石症、溃疡和肝胆疾病[108-110]。据报道，高达 40% 的患者患有胆道疾病，外科治疗的死亡率很高[111]。肺移植或心肺移植后 GERD 和胃动力不足问题尤其严重，可能与药物和术中迷走神经损伤有关[109,112-115]。在 25% 的肺移植受者和高达 80% 的心肺移植受者中有胃动力不足症状[116-118]。病程常起伏，提示神经病理性、感染性(CMV)或药物引起[117,119]。有 GERD 和/或胃动力不足的受者特别容易发展为支气管炎闭塞综合征，严重威胁 LT 患者的寿命[115-117]。质子泵抑制剂可用于治疗反流；然而，如果反流疾病不能被控制，可能要采用腹腔镜胃底折叠术[120-122]。

尽管常规使用抑酸剂，但 LT 受体也可能发展为巨大的胃溃疡(直径>3cm)。这些溃疡具有显著的发病率和死亡率，通常与双侧肺移植、移植后大剂量非甾体抗炎药的使用、急性排斥反应时大剂量糖皮质激素的使用和环孢素免疫抑制有关[123]。基于这个原因，一些作者认为非甾体抗炎药不应该在移植后使用。LT 和 HT 受体比其他 SOT 受体更容易发生巨细胞病毒感染(15%~25%)。巨细胞病毒感染一般表现为肺炎，但胃肠道巨细胞病毒感染仍是其发病的主要原因(见图 36.1)[14]。LT 和 HLT 受体在 SOT 环境中真菌感染发生率最高，以非念珠菌属为主[124,125]。

接受 LT 的心力衰竭患者胃肠道并发症较为独特[126]。胰腺功能不全——严重心力衰竭的一个标志——相当常见。心力衰竭诱导的继发性胆汁性肝硬化可使免疫抑制剂的吸收复杂化，如环孢素等药物。如果在肺移植之前检测到严重的肝脏疾病，可以考虑进行肺-肝移植。远端肠梗阻综合征发生率高达 10%，与非移植的心力衰竭中发生率相似[127]。CF 患者也可能出现胆囊炎，PUD 和 GERD[128]。

HT 后的原发性 HCV 感染导致移植后 1~3 年死亡率显著增加。现在，随着新的抗 HCV 药物出现，过一段时间这可能就会改变。然而，HT 后获得 HBV 似乎不会影响生存，至少可达 5 年[129,130]。

五、肠移植

大多数并发症与潜在疾病、移植物排斥反应、肠缺血和吻合口漏有关。细菌和真菌感染常见，通常与手术后黏膜破坏有关，但来源可能无法确定。有两种恶性肿瘤与强烈的免疫抑制有关：EBV 淋巴组织增生性疾病(lymphoproliferative disease，LPD)和非淋巴瘤起源的新发癌[131,132]。EBV DNA 监测和通过减少免疫抑制或使用利妥昔单抗的先行治疗减少 LPD 的发生率。肠动力改变和厌食症已被报道。高达 9% 的肠移植受者出现 SOT 移植物抗宿主病。

六、实体器官移植受者以问题为导向的诊断方法

(一) 上消化道症状和体征

有食管或胃症状的 SOT 患者的治疗方法受高发的非特异性症状的影响，这些症状是严重感染的先兆(如 CMV 感染，表现为恶心和呕吐)，也受疾病快速发展的影响。GERD 是引起胃灼烧和胸痛的最常见原因，尤其是在肺移植后，但病毒性和真菌性食管炎可能是这些症状的基础，尤其是在停止预防性抗菌之后。糖尿病患者念珠菌性食管炎发生率较高；其他危险因素包括使用广谱抗生素、大剂量免疫抑制剂以及肝移植受体中存在胆管空肠吻合术(Roux-en-Y 吻合术)。严重的坏死性真菌性食管炎可导致穿孔，穿孔可导致多达三分之一病例死亡。吞咽痛、吞咽困难或呕血应考虑到食管感染；疱疹病毒(CMV，HSV)和真菌类(念珠菌)占的比例最大，但也可以看到不常见的病原体[133]。吞咽困难可能继发于 SOD 受体的药物性食管炎，因口服抗生素、抗病毒药物、氯化钾、双膦酸盐、非甾体抗炎药和铁制剂所致。曾报道过严重食管感染后的食管狭窄，并且可能在根除病原体很久后才出现。

SOT 后常见厌食，恶心和/或呕吐，特别是在移植后的早期阶段[48,108,109]。这些症状通常与疱疹病毒感染或药物(包括免疫抑制药物)有关，因此，内镜评估对大多数患者的诊断是必要的。他克莫司是大环内酯类，可引起恶心、腹痛和腹泻，常导致厌食和体重减轻。这些副作用是剂量依赖性的，可以通过减少剂量来控制，很少选择停药。西罗莫司是一种较新的大环内酯类免疫抑制剂，具有类似于他克莫司的胃肠道副作用。MMF 是一种核酸合成的抑制剂，胃肠道副作用明确，包括恶心、呕吐和腹泻，通常需要剂量调整。霉酚酸缓释片配方的胃肠道副作用显著减少，但疗效相似[75,76,134]。厌食和恶心偶见于胰腺炎、胆囊炎或膀胱炎。

SOT 后，移植物抗宿主病(graft-versus-host disease，GVHD)很少(约 1%)在 SOT 后和移植后 2~6 周内表现为发热、皮疹和胃肠道症状，特别是恶心、呕吐和腹泻[135,136]。如果怀疑患有 GVHD 并且没有皮肤病变，则必须进行内镜活检，确认其他病症，如病毒感染和药物反应可能具有类似 GVHD 的组织学模式[137]。症状性胃动力不足常见于肺移植情况下，但在其他 SOT 中报告较少[117]。CMV 和 VZV 可能很少累及肠道神经丛，导致肠扩张或胃肠动力不足。Hp 感染可能与症状性消化不良、胃炎和胃十二指肠溃疡有关，但免疫抑制的应用或免疫抑制的程度与 Hp 定植之间没有关系；其发病率与非移植者相似[2]。Hp 感染在透析和 KT 患者中很常见[66]。

（二）腹泻和便秘

据报道，所有类型的SOT后都会出现结肠和小肠并发症（憩室炎、缺血性结肠炎、恶性肿瘤和感染）。移植后早期，以感染为主。腹泻通常是感染性的，并伴有发热（37%）、腹痛（46%）、恶心（32%）和呕吐（22%）[138,139]。病原主要是CMV和艰难梭菌，但文献中所描述的SOT受者中的致病原较为广泛，特别是当他们在感染流行地区就医时[例如，腺病毒，诺如病毒，轮状病毒，柯萨奇病毒，细菌肠道病原体，肠出血性大肠杆菌，耶尔森菌小肠结肠炎，蓝氏贾第鞭毛虫，念珠菌属，隐孢子虫，小孢子虫目（微孢子虫），贝氏等孢球虫和粪类圆线虫][139,140]。如果患者同时伴有系统性CMV感染，则更易发生细菌性肠道感染[65]。除了CMV、某些寄生虫和EBV相关淋巴组织增生性疾病（EBV-associated lymphoproliferative disorders，EBV-LPD），几乎在所有病例中都可以通过检查粪便标本进行诊断。尤其是如果诊断延误，CMV累及小肠，常常导致伴有蛋白质丢失的大量水样泻。结肠受累可以表现为炎性结肠炎，导致血性腹泻，并且通常伴发热、腹胀和疼痛[141,142]。CMV的诊断可能需要进行黏膜活检，特别是如果血液标本中CMV DNA或抗原呈阴性。2%～30%住院的SOT受者发生艰难梭菌感染，其发病率高于一般住院人群（1%～2%）[143]。艰难梭菌感染可能在SOT后出现更严重的病情；暴发性结肠炎和中毒性巨结肠患者需要及时进行外科手术以防止穿孔和腹膜炎[139,140]。结肠炎的体征可能很轻微，是因为同时使用了免疫抑制剂。治疗将在第112章讨论。高达20%的病例可能复发[144]。

在SOT受者中使用某些益生菌（如布拉德酵母菌）仍然存在争议，因为有报道称免疫低下的宿主中有酵母菌传播和感染[145,146]。但是，似乎使用细菌益生菌可能有助于预防感染[147]，并且正常结肠细菌菌群移植可用于治疗复发性艰难梭菌结肠炎。多达25%的SOT受者可见肠道真菌感染。在没有预防的情况下，肠道真菌过度生长和腹泻可能由使用抗生素或肠道运动障碍所致。在免疫功能低下的宿主中也必须考虑常见的寄生虫感染，特别是在高度流行的地区。原生动物和多细胞动物寄生虫是一种不太常见的SOT后急性腹泻的病因，但必须要考虑到。小孢子虫（*E. bieneusi*）在慢性腹泻病因中很少报道，也许确实在SOT后几乎没有找到[148]。临床上，这种感染患者会出现疲劳、间歇性腹泻和体重减轻。对小孢子虫没有明确有效的治疗方法。结肠炎或中毒性巨结肠的症状通常与感染有关，但在多达20%的病例中，未发现明确的病因[139,149]。早期识别、诊断和治疗结肠炎可降低与疾病相关的死亡率。有供体传播的粪链球菌感染的报道，其死亡率很高，当供体来自流行地区时，应考虑这种病原体。已有伴腹泻的嗜酸性粒细胞性结肠炎应用他克莫司和环孢素治疗的报道。组织学特征是嗜酸性粒细胞结肠浸润和外周血嗜酸性粒细胞增多；一些患者可能血清免疫球蛋白（Ig）E升高。通常只有在非侵袭性检测未能查明感染原因时才需要进行结肠镜检查。如果未找到感染的病原体，必须要考虑到下消化道的GVHD。

多达三分之一的SOT患者出现与药物相关的腹泻，最常见的是他克莫司或西罗莫司[139,150,151]。30%的使用MMF的患者中会出现水样泻，可能需要减少剂量或停药。MMF引起的腹泻的机制尚不清楚，它是剂量依赖性的，可能抑制肠上皮细胞内新的嘌呤合成。组织学显示类似于GVHD的局灶性炎症病变，伴十二指肠绒毛结构的丧失[152]。使用肠溶麦考酚酸可以减少这种副作用。抗胸腺细胞球蛋白（ATG）和抗T细胞抗体（OKT3）治疗都可致腹泻，腹泻可预测持续3～4天并自发消退。大多数免疫抑制剂引起的腹泻都可以通过剂量调整来控制，但是一些病例非常严重，以至于需要停用免疫抑制剂。腹泻也可以由于应用纠正肾脏镁消耗的含镁制剂和预防性或治疗性使用抗生素引起，导致结肠的常驻菌群不能重吸收碳水化合物。据报道，非感染性腹泻会增加移植器官失去功能和死亡的风险[150]。

在接受某些药物（例如，麻醉剂，含钙和铝的抗酸剂，抗胆碱能药）的活动较少的SOT患者中可出现便秘。增加患者活动、降低使用麻醉剂、在接受麻醉剂的人中使用甲基纳曲酮[153]、应用聚乙二醇泻药和番泻叶治疗后通常会得到改善。

（三）腹痛

SOT后腹部并发症很常见，多达30%的患者可发生[153]。尽管存在危及生命的并发症，但症状可能很轻微。应对所有腹痛患者进行积极评估，特别注意患者是否需要紧急手术或特别的药物治疗。大多数腹痛患者不需要手术治疗。

需要紧急手术的腹内情况是脓肿、穿孔、严重结肠炎、阑尾炎、肠梗阻、肠缺血和急性胆囊炎，表现为疼痛。这些疾病可能出现在移植后早期。免疫抑制可掩盖症状并抑制宿主反应，导致诊断延迟及死亡率增加。大多数移植患者急性阑尾炎时会出现典型的右下腹疼痛，但并发症的发生率更高[154]。总体而言，低于5%的SOT患者发生肠穿孔，尽管肺移植手术的发生率可能略高[47,155]。穿孔可自发而没有明确的病因，但在多达三分之二的病例（特别是肾脏受者）和15%的缺血中，它与结肠憩室有关。穿孔，尤其是憩室，具有很高的死亡率[78,142]。结肠穿孔发展的危险因素包括憩室疾病、免疫抑制（尤其是糖皮质激素）、巨细胞病毒感染、真菌感染（如毛霉菌病）、未被确认的淋巴瘤（EBV-LPD）、结肠癌和缺血[2,142]。腹部X线和CT可以明确穿孔的存在，但在手术前可能无法确定其来源。肾移植术后憩室穿孔较为常见，常形成脓肿及瘘管，有时无严重疼痛及腹膜炎表现。50岁以下患者在移植前结肠筛查并不能预测移植后结肠穿孔。SOT受者罹患胆石症的风险也有所增加[156]，与胆结石相关的因素包括环孢素、肥胖和作为潜在疾病的心力衰竭。腹痛常因组织浸润性CMV疾病所致。CMV一般造成黏膜弥漫性水肿，但也可引起局灶性溃疡、灌注障碍、高度狭窄和肠梗阻（见图36.1）。VZV播散性感染的首次表现往往是与假性梗阻和内脏神经病变有关的严重腹痛。CMV和VZV感染的早期治疗可提高生存率。

腹痛也可能是移植相关并发症的一种表现，这些并发症通常不会有可怕的后果。据报道疼痛往往与口服他克莫司、西罗莫司和MMF伴随出现。接受MMF治疗的患者中，高达19%的患者出现了继发于MMF的腹痛，使MMF的使用明显受限[157]。所提出的假定的MMF导致疼痛的病因包括炎性溃疡（内镜所见）及肠道细胞快速分裂受到干扰，有一个假说研究表明和MMF相比，缓释霉酚酸的胃肠道并发症较少[75,76,134]。麻醉或抗胆碱能药常导致手术后假性梗阻。必须注意排除感染性病因，如巨细胞病毒或 VZV，两者都可能累及肠神经丛[2]。非感染性假性梗阻往往可保守处理，采用鼻胃管减压、努力纠正电解质失衡、停用阿片类药物。阿片类药物引起的肠道症状也可以通过使用甲基纳曲酮来阻断，同时不会干扰中枢疼痛的缓解[153]。新斯的明可安全用于移植情况下假性梗阻的治疗[142]。明显结肠扩张时可能需要手术干预。据报道，1%～2% 肾移植受者、6% 的 LT 受者以及 18% 的 HT 受者患有急性胰腺炎，这可能会有致命的后果[158]。急性胰腺炎的发生与 CMV 感染、高钙血症、胆石症、胆道处理、恶性肿瘤、近期饮酒和药物（如阿扎硫普林、环孢素，他克莫司和糖皮质激素）有关。除了需要排除 CMV 感染和一些免疫抑制剂的使用，移植后胰腺炎与非移植状况下治疗相同（见第 58 章）。

肠道积气可能在 SOT 后的腹部影像学检查中偶然发现，但也可能是危及生命的肠道缺血或产气病原体感染的表现[159]。肠道积气与 CMV 感染、艰难梭菌结肠炎和脓毒症有关，并可见于接受糖皮质激素治疗的患者。大多数患者不需要特殊干预，除非是由于缺血或梭状芽孢杆菌感染，否则聚集的气体会自行消散[159]。

（四）胃肠道出血

胃肠道出血通常继发于感染性溃疡。非感染因素导致出血的原因包括非甾体抗炎药导致的胃十二指肠溃疡、憩室出血、吻合口出血、缺血性结肠炎。目前移植人群胃十二指肠溃疡的发病率约为 5%，穿孔率不足 1%[3]。H_2RA 或 PPI 预防可减少该人群中溃疡的发生，这两种疗效相同[3]。移植前感染 Hp 的患者移植后更容易发生 PUD[160]。在缺乏有效的抗病毒预防治疗的情况下，病毒性溃疡是肠出血最常见的病因。与 HSV 相关的食管溃疡可出现严重出血，甚至没有食管症状。巨细胞病毒可导致整个肠道溃疡。CMV 食管溃疡通常较浅（见图 36.1A），而其他地方的溃疡可能较深，侵蚀血管，导致严重出血。CMV 还可引起与 IBD 相似的弥漫性炎症（见图 36.1C 和 D）。VZV 和 EBV 感染很少出现胃肠道出血。虽然 EBV 本身不会引起黏膜溃疡，但与 EBV 相关的 LPD 可形成导致溃疡和出血的黏膜肿瘤（见图 36.2）。已有侵袭性真菌感染所致大量出血的报道[161]。

（五）胃肠道恶性病变

多达 20% 的移植受者可发生 PTLD、淋巴样增生或与 EBV 感染相关的淋巴瘤[32,162]。虽然大多数 PTLD 起源于 B 细胞，但也有 T 细胞淋巴瘤的报道[163]。移植后早期，EBV 再活化通常表现为单核细胞增多症样综合征，伴有弥漫性腺病和发热；血液中检测到 EBV DNA，可能允许使用低剂量的免疫抑制或利妥昔单抗进行预先治疗[164]。PTLD 在移植 1 年后的表现更具隐匿性，常表现为结外病变或内脏受累。胃肠道 PTLD 可表现为腹泻、肠梗阻（见图 36.2B）、出血或穿孔。移植后的黏膜相关性淋巴瘤也有报道[165]。幸运的是，它们对免疫抑制、抗生素（如果与 Hp 有关）、手术或化疗都有反应（见第 32 章）。

长期存活的移植受者罹患癌症的风险高于一般人群，尤其是淋巴瘤、皮肤癌、结肠癌和肛门癌、头颈部癌及卡波西肉瘤[166,167]。因继发于 PSC 的肝硬化而接受肝移植的患者发生与原有溃疡性结肠炎相关的结肠异型增生和弥漫性结肠癌的风险明显增高[168]。如果有重度异型增生，在移植后 10～12 周内行结肠切除术比较安全。

（六）肝胆并发症

药物引起的肝毒性在移植后可能会是个问题，因为这通常是排他性诊断。多达 10% 的受者会出现硫唑嘌呤肝毒性，表现为血清转氨酶升高；常为胆汁淤积性损伤，并伴有小叶中心肝细胞坏死。较少见的表现是缓慢而隐匿出现的肝窦阻塞综合征（sinusoidal obstruction syndrome，SOS；以前称为小静脉闭塞病），常表现为门静脉高压症，通常在停药后消退。现在，硫唑嘌呤在器官移植后已很少使用，已被霉酚酸所取代。血药浓度较高时，环孢素或他克莫司可致胆汁淤积。西罗莫司已被报道引起剂量依赖性的血清转氨酶升高。移植受者还应用许多其他药物，这些药物单独或联合使用，可产生胆汁淤积、脂肪肝、肝炎或多种组织学表现。

细菌性脓毒症对肝功能影响较大（见第 37 章），严重的胆汁淤积是最常见的表现（有时称为感染性胆管炎或高胆红素脓毒症综合征）[169]。CMV 感染可导致转氨酶升高，或表现为胆汁淤积或表现为肝细胞损伤。CMV 肝炎在肝移植受者中较其他器官受者更为常见和严重[91]。VZV 和 HSV 感染可导致肝炎和暴发性肝功能衰竭[26,67]。SOT 后 2%～3% 可见 EBV 肝炎，但一般较轻。原发性或复发性 HCV 或 HBV 可导致移植后肝病。这些病毒可以通过任何实体器官传播。幸运的是，对这两种抗病毒治疗效果都有明显改善[104]，随着直接作用抗病毒药的发展，移植后丙型肝炎的治疗有了很大改善，高达 98%～99% 的受者被治愈[170]。在事实上，在撰写本文时，由于这些药物的成功，已经考虑对 HCV 阴性受体使用 HCV 病毒血症供体[171,172]。慢性 HBV 携带者（乙型肝炎表面抗原阳性受者）可能在移植后突然加剧，但通常对抗病毒药物反应良好（见第 79 章）。

与 OLT 相关的血管损伤可能导致肝功能障碍。已有报道肾移植后出现结节性再生性增生，之后会出现门静脉高压及紫癜性肝炎。

器官移植受者，特别是肝移植者，患胆道疾病的风险很高。包括非结石性胆囊炎、胆囊泥沙样结石、胆囊壁增厚、胆管扩张或胆石症[111]。需要胆囊切除术的胆囊和胆道疾病的移植后发生率约为 1%～6%。移植后紧急胆囊切除术的死亡率很高（29%）[111]。然而，移植前胆道筛查和预防性胆囊切除仍存在争议。胆道疾病的病因很多，包括肥胖、使用全肠外营养（TPN）、禁食、胆管狭窄和药物。环孢素可能从胆汁中排出，可能会增加胆石症和胆管炎的发生率[68,173]。一些中心建议胆道结石应在移植前或移植后一旦发现立即清除。

因肝细胞癌行肝移植的患者在移植器官中有复发风险，特别是如果移植前病变大或多发。PTLD 也可能累及肝脏。

七、造血细胞移植并发症

造血细胞移植（hematopoietic cell transplantation，HCT）使

用以下 3 种造血和免疫细胞来源之一：骨髓、外周血造血细胞或脐带血[174]。移植的细胞可以是自己的（自体 HCT）、来自同卵双胞胎的（同源 HCT）或者来自另一个人的（异体 HCT）。异体细胞可以来自 HLA 与受体匹配的兄弟姐妹、另一个家庭成员、HLA 匹配不相关的供者，或来自 HLA 不匹配不相关的供者（如脐带血供者）。HCT 与 SOT 有 3 个重要的区别：①HCT 的适应证往往包括潜在的致命性恶性肿瘤、骨髓衰竭（再生障碍性贫血）、先天性免疫缺陷或遗传性血液病，如地中海贫血或镰状细胞病；②HCT 的准备需要大剂量的骨髓抑制治疗或强烈的免疫抑制，极易感染，使用预防性治疗，对肝、肾、肺、心脏也造成损害；③使用异体供体细胞的受者常发生急性和慢性 GVHD。HCT 患者面临化疗药物毒性、感染、急性和慢性 GVHD、复发性恶性肿瘤等多种并发症[174]。HCT 的胃肠道和肝脏并发症现在已大大减少，过去所见的一些问题已经消失[174,175]。有时晦涩难懂的关于 HCT 术语和缩写的指南对那些不熟悉 HCT 的人是有用的[176]。

（一）造血细胞移植前肠道和肝脏疾病的评估

1. 肠道溃疡和肿瘤

对于可能接受 HCT 治疗的免疫缺陷患者，黏膜溃疡可能具有感染性病因（如 CMV、HSV 或真菌感染），需要特殊的抗菌治疗[177]。CMV、溶组织阿米巴及艰难梭菌是结肠溃疡的原因，可能似 IBD。应在开始预处理前治愈肠溃疡，避免 HCT 后血小板减少时大出血。已行异体和自体 HCT 的溃疡性结肠炎和克罗恩病患者，未出现出血、穿孔或异常微生物播散等并发症[178,179]。异体 HCT 清髓治疗后，克罗恩病得到了的长期缓解，自体 HCT 也得到了改善。单基因自身免疫综合征，包括许多有极早期 IBD 的患者，可以通过同种异体 HCT 治愈[180]。任何近期有胃肠道出血史的患者，都应在 HCT 前做结肠镜和上消化道内镜检查。可能需要内镜活检对某些容易累及肠道的恶性疾病（如套细胞淋巴瘤；见第 32 章）进行分期。

2. 腹泻

腹泻患者应检查 HCT 后可能引起发病的病原体（溶组织内阿米巴，粪链球菌，鞭毛虫，隐孢子虫，微孢子虫，梭状芽孢杆菌，CMV，轮状病毒，诺如病毒，腺病毒）[181,182]。这些病原体的多数，而非全部，已包含在目前可使用的多重分子队列中，并且针对梭菌、巨细胞病毒、腺病毒、阿米巴病、贾第鞭毛虫病、圆线虫病等寄生虫及微孢子虫有了特效治疗[183]。隐孢子虫病可能对免疫抑制患者的治疗产生耐药性，但异体 HCT 术后，正常的免疫功能恢复可以清除隐孢子虫[184]。盲肠炎是在中性粒细胞减少症患者中表现为盲肠水肿、黏膜屏障受损和溃疡形成的一种综合征，常与多菌性脓毒症有关。其病因通常是肠梭菌感染，尤其是脓毒梭菌感染[185]。经过治疗，HCT 后盲肠炎的风险与其他患者相似。

3. 肛周疼痛

粒细胞减少症患者肛管附近的疼痛都源于细菌感染，除非证明有其他感染。在大多数情况下，给予覆盖厌氧的广谱抗生素的治疗足够了，手术切开引流用于进行性感染[186]。外部的体格检查观察不到广泛的骨盆直肠间隙和括约肌内的脓肿，但可以通过 CT，MRI 或经会阴超声检查来诊断[187]。由 HSV 感染引起的直肠炎和生殖器溃疡、肛周 CMV 溃疡以及罕见的真菌感染也可能导致肛周疼痛[188]。

4. 肝脏真菌感染

诊断依赖于肝脏影像（高分辨率 CT 或 MRI），并结合真菌的生物标志物（半乳甘露聚糖和葡聚糖测定）、PCR 或肝脏活检物培养[189]。真菌性肝脏感染应使用棘白菌素治疗，与原先的药相比，它能降低毒性、减少药物相互作用，并且覆盖范围更广[190]。完全移植的患者也可以清除 HCT 后难治性真菌性肝脓肿。

5. 同种异体造血细胞移植供体中的病毒性肝炎

患有 HBV 或 HCV 病毒血症的供体将会把病毒传给受体。当有 2 个相同的 HLA 匹配的供体可用时，首选未感染的供体。如果最合适的供体患有慢性乙型肝炎，供体使用恩替卡韦或替诺福韦治疗，受体接受主动或被动免疫，可能会阻止病毒传播[191]。如果血清和外周血干细胞 HBV DNA 阴性，HBsAg 阴性、抗 HBc 阳性的供体是可以使用的，移植后，受者需每月检测血清 HBV DNA。如果受体 HBsAg 阳性或抗 HBc 阳性，那么本身为抗 HBc 阳性的供体可能是首选供体，因为免疫的过继转移可以影响病毒的清除[192]。

如果供体被 HCV 感染并且时间允许，在收获供体细胞之前对供体进行治疗可能会使它们变成非病毒血症，并且更不可能传染[193]。新的直接抗病毒药（DAA）联合是该症治疗的合适选择（见第 80 章）[194]。如果 HCV 传播，HCV 感染的急性期可能是在 HCT 恢复 T 细胞功能后 2~3 个月引起转氨酶升高；10 年后，结局与不伴 HCV 感染的移植受者无异[195,196]。然而，在接受 MMF 免疫抑制治疗的患者中，HCT 后纤维淤胆性丙型肝炎很少被描述[197]。应该给慢性丙型肝炎患者提供抗病毒治疗—特别是纤维淤胆性肝炎、失代偿性肝硬化和 HCV 相关淋巴瘤患者。初步研究表明抗病毒治疗可以降低非复发性死亡率，以及肝硬化和肝细胞癌进展的长期风险[198]。

6. 造血细胞移植候选者中的肝脏疾病

伴有炎性纤维性肝脏疾病的患者所面临的风险包括在使用清髓药物后出现的致命性 SOS[176]。Child-Pugh B 或 C 级肝硬化是大多数大剂量预处理方案的禁忌证，因为有发生致命肝窦损伤的危险；这些患者即使给予低强度的预处理方案，在接受 HCT 治疗后，也可能出现致命性脓毒症或肝功失代偿[199,200]。如果临床怀疑肝硬化或广泛纤维化是由慢性病毒感染、酒精、NASH 引起，应考虑肝活检或瞬时弹性成像。骨髓增生性肿瘤可表现为非肝硬化门静脉高压症和移植后早期肝毒性发生率增加[201,202]。Gilbert 综合征患者在接受含白消安（BU）的治疗后无复发性死亡率增加[203]。移植前几个月化疗或放疗引起的更多的新的肝损伤也会带来风险。许多化疗药物直接（胆汁淤积性损伤、肝细胞坏死或肝窦损伤）或间接（脓毒症或内毒素血症引起的胆汁淤积，如胆管炎）引起肝功能障碍[204]。虽然标准化疗本身与致命性 SOS 的风险增加并无相关性，但持续黄疸和转氨酶升高的患者行 HCT 仍可能有危险[205]。肝损伤与长期暴露于 6-硫鸟嘌呤等抗代谢物以及伊马替尼和新型酪氨酸激酶抑制剂等药物有关[206]。吉妥珠单抗奥唑米星可使患者在肝毒性骨髓抑制方案后更易发生 SOS，尤其是在患者接受大剂量吉妥珠单抗 3 个月内进行移植的情况下[207]。

7. 胆囊和胆管结石

无症状胆结石的 HCT 患者(在 CT 或 US 检查中偶然发现)不需要手术干预。有症状的胆石症或胆总管结石患者应考虑行移植前胆囊切除术或内镜下胆道手术移除结石。

8. 铁过载

患有地中海贫血、再生障碍性贫血、骨髓增生异常综合征、慢性白血病或淋巴瘤等疾病的 HCT 候选者,都有明显的肝脏铁过载。肝脏铁含量的中度升高(最好通过 T2 加权 MRI 评估)与 HCT 术后非复发死亡率增加的相关性不一致[208]。对于重型地中海贫血患者,有效的 HCT 前螯合治疗可改善 HCT 后的生存率。然而,在大多数其他患者中,组织铁储备的定量和铁清除的考虑可以推迟到 HCT 恢复后进行。

(二) 移植术后 1 年内发生的问题

1. 恶心、呕吐和厌食的问题

大剂量预处理引起的黏膜炎可导致口腔黏膜肿胀、疼痛,严重时可导致咽部和食管上皮脱落、剧烈的干呕、无法吞咽、呕吐、胸骨后疼痛和气道阻塞。一些治疗方案,特别是含有 5-氟尿嘧啶、阿糖胞苷、依托泊苷、高剂量美法仑(MEL)或多种烷化剂的方案,可能会引起异常严重的肠黏膜坏死,导致进一步延迟进食。已证明口服冷冻治疗可以降低 5-氟尿嘧啶、高剂量美法仑使用后口腔黏膜炎的严重程度和持续时间[209]。清髓性预处理治疗使大多数患者出现恶心和厌食,伴胃排空延迟[175]和经口摄食差,在移植后第 10~12 天最严重,但通常持续至第 20 天[210,211]。5-HT_3 受体拮抗药物在预处理治疗期间缓解这些急性症状非常有效,第二代 5-HT_3 受体拮抗剂帕洛诺司琼也有助于治疗迟发性恶心和呕吐(第 2~5 天)[212]。加入地塞米松和/或神经激肽受体拮抗剂,如阿瑞匹坦、奈妥匹坦和罗拉匹坦,可阻断 P 物质启动冲动到达延髓呕吐中枢的途径,并可能预防突发性恶心和呕吐[213,214]。长期厌食可能与循环中白细胞介素(IL)-1、IL-6 和 TNF-α(已知影响食欲中心的细胞因子)有关[211]。

上消化道急性 GVHD 是同种异体移植受者出现这些症状的最常见原因。早期症状包括食欲减退、进食时无快感和饱腹感,常伴有恶心和呕吐。例如,当 GVHD 发生在外周血同种异体移植后第 15 天之前时,GVHD 的组织学特征可能与由预处理产生的那些特征无法区分。第 20 天后,超过 80% 伴有难治性厌食、恶心或呕吐的同种异体移植患者,将胃和十二指肠 GVHD 作为唯一解释[215]。内镜检查显示胃窦和十二指肠黏膜水肿、斑片状红斑和胆汁性胃液(图 36.4)[216]。组织学可能显示上皮细胞凋亡和脱失,常伴有局限性淋巴细胞浸润[216,217]。当组织学模棱两可时,需要结合全部临床表现、内镜外观、无感染和组织学的范围来得出诊断[216-218]。使用 10 天诱导疗程的泼尼松 1mg/kg/d 加口服二丙酸倍氯米松 8mg/d 进行免疫抑制治疗是一种治疗上消化道 GVHD 的有效方法,可避免延长泼尼松的暴露时间[219,220]。自体移植物的受体也可能发生厌食,恶心和呕吐综合征,与弥漫性胃水肿和红斑相关[221]。

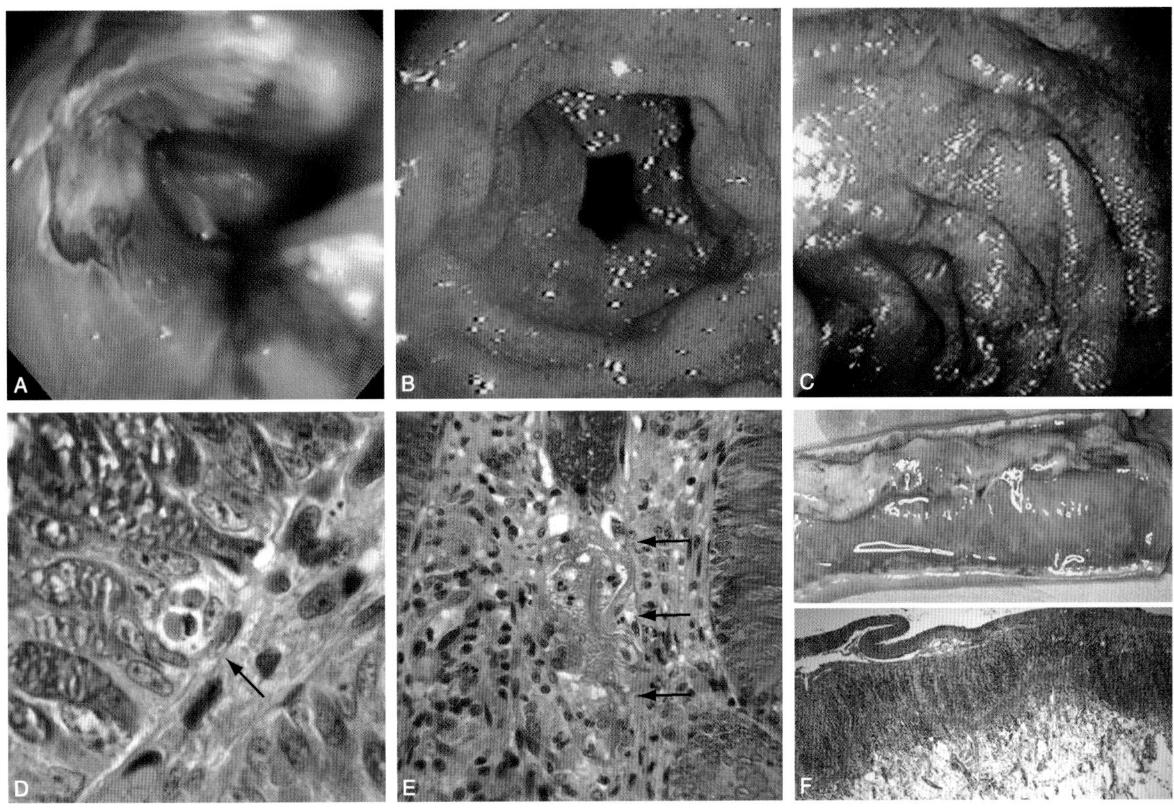

图 36.4 胃肠道急性移植物抗宿主病(GVHD)的内镜和组织病理学表现。A,食管:严重 GVHD 时食管远端鳞状上皮脱屑。B,胃:中重度 GVHD 胃窦部弥漫性黏膜水肿和红斑。C,小肠:重度 GVHD 的黏膜水肿,局灶性出血和溃疡。D,组织病理学:直肠活检隐窝上皮 GVHD 引起的局灶性细胞凋亡(箭头)(HE 染色,阿尔辛蓝染色)。E,组织病理学:结肠隐窝底部(箭头)上皮细胞缺失;隐窝底部细胞凋亡碎片与黏液混合(HE 染色,阿尔辛蓝染色)。F,致死性 GVHD 的大体和组织病理学结果:打开小肠段的尸检照片显示黏膜脱落(上图);组织病理学显示完全不存在上皮细胞、淋巴细胞浸润和黏膜下水肿(下图)(HE 染色)

内窥镜检查也有助于排除肠道疱疹病毒、细菌和真菌感染是引起上消化道症状的原因。在更昔洛韦治疗前的时代，食管、胃和上消化道的CMV感染占不明原因恶心和呕吐的患者的三分之一，但CMV感染现在是这些症状的一个不常见的原因[215]。胃肠道CMV感染通常在HCT后50～150天被诊断，但如果患者在HCT前感染CMV或接受脐带血移植，则可能诊断更早。在外周血中不存在CMV抗原或DNA的情况下，可在胃肠道中检测到CMV感染[177,222]。恶心和呕吐可能是一些寄生虫感染（如果在HCT前筛查期间遗漏）和不可培养病毒（诸如病毒、轮状病毒、星状病毒）引起的感染的突出症状[182-184]。厌食和呕吐也可能是与中枢神经系统感染、假性脑瘤或硬膜下血肿相关的颅内压升高的表现。

口服不可吸收的抗菌药物（特别是制霉菌素）、环孢霉素、MMF、甲氧苄啶/磺胺甲基异噁唑、伏立康唑、泊沙康唑、伊曲康唑、两性霉素和大剂量阿片类药物也会引起恶心，偶尔也会引起呕吐。即使在停止TPN后，食欲抑制也可能持续1～3周[223]。

2. 黄疸、肝大和肝功能检查异常（表36.2和图36.5）

HCT后发生黄疸是一种预后不良的体征，无论是否由药物毒性、GVHD、感染还是缺氧引起[224,225]。然而，最近的研究进展使几乎所有的移植肝脏并发症都是可以预防的[176,225,226]。

（1）肝窦阻塞综合征

肝窦阻塞综合征（SOS）（见图36.5A和B）是一种使用高剂量清髓性预处理方案后出现的综合征，表现为压痛性肝大、液体潴留、体重增加以及血清胆红素浓度升高[227]。由于这种形式的肝损伤是由肝窦损伤引起的，因此旧称“静脉闭塞性疾病”（veno-occlusive disease，VOD）是不准确的。SOS的发生频率和严重程度已显著下降，这是因为：①已很少使用高于14Gy的全身照射（total body irradiation，TBI）剂量；②氟达拉滨正在取代环磷酰胺（CY）；③目前对有SOS风险的患者给予不含CY或TBI超过12Gy的乙型肝炎治疗方案；④慢性丙型肝炎在移植候选者中的患病率，以前是SOS的常见风险因素，现在非常低；⑤治疗药物监测允许代谢不同的化疗药物个性化给药[176]。SOS是由某些预处理方案中的毒素引起的；SOS发病率变异性的重要促成因素为：①CY/TBI方案中患者之间CY代谢的差异；②基础纤维炎症性肝病；③多药预处理方案中的药物递送顺序[203,228]；④在预处理治疗期间和治疗后合并使用影响清髓药物代谢（如伊曲康唑）或导致伴随肝损伤的药物（如甲氨蝶呤、西罗莫司、炔诺酮）。虽然致命性SOS在大多数成人移植单位中几乎消失[175,229]，但是接受白消安（BU）/美法仑（MEL）预处理方案的儿童患者仍存在风险[230]。既往许多根据黄疸被诊断为SOS的患者，可能主要是患有胆汁淤积性肝损伤，而不是肝窦损伤，这一结论是基于熊去氧胆酸预防研究的数据[175,226,231]。

SOS的发作预示着肝脏增大、右上腹压痛、肾钠潴留和体重增加，发生在CY开始后10～20天，以及其他清髓方案治疗

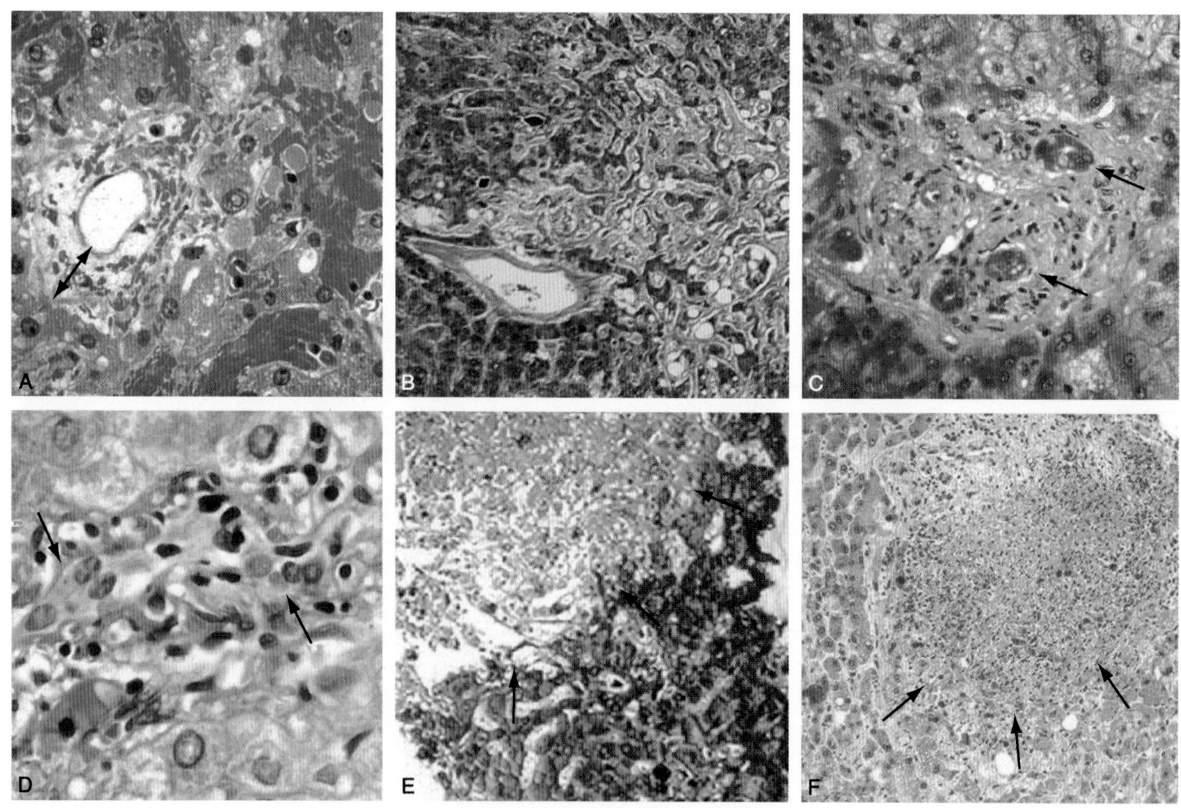

图36.5　造血细胞移植后肝脏疾病的组织病理学。A，移植后23天的肝窦阻塞综合征（也称为肝小静脉闭塞性疾病）；高倍镜可见Disse间隙出血、肝细胞坏死、肝窦破坏和中央静脉内皮下水肿（箭头）。静脉管腔通畅（HE染色）。B，由吉妥珠单抗（奥佐米星）引起的肝窦阻塞综合征；腺泡3区高倍视图，显示广泛的肝窦纤维化，肝细胞脱失和通畅的中央静脉（Masson染色）。C，移植后第82天的急性移植物抗宿主病（GVHD）；汇管区含有异常小胆管（箭头），伴上皮细胞脱落、胞浆嗜酸性变和空泡变（HE染色）。D，移植后第184天的慢性GVHD；高倍视图见淋巴细胞浸润的受损伤的汇管区小胆管（箭头）（HE染色）。E，水痘-带状疱疹病毒性肝炎；低倍视图见与正常肝细胞邻近的肝细胞融合性坏死（箭头，指向苍白区域）（过碘酸-希夫染色）。F，腺病毒性肝炎；低倍镜下见灶状肝细胞融合性坏死区域（箭头，指向嗜碱性区域），及含典型的腺病毒核内包涵体的肝细胞残余物（“破碎细胞”），最好在高倍率下观察（HE染色）

表 36.2　造血细胞移植后肝脏疾病

疾病	频率	时间	诊断	治疗	预防
肝窦阻塞综合征	<10%（方案依赖性）	在>20 天前发作	典型的临床特征，影像学，WHVPG，组织学（见图 36.5A，B），注意非典型表现（急性肝炎，全身水肿）	没有证据；去纤维蛋白核因子在严重 SOS 患者中的治疗成功率约为 40%	评估患者的风险。选择对“肝友益性”的调节方案
脓毒症型胆汁淤积（亚急性胆管炎）	常见于中性粒细胞减少症患者	继发脓毒症或中性粒细胞减少症发热（通常>30 天前）	排除胆汁淤积的其他原因；临床诊断	治疗潜在的感染	感染期预防或预期治疗；熊去氧胆酸
急性 GVHD	同种异体移植后，罕见于≈20% 的受者	15~50 天	确认皮肤和肠道中的 GVHD，排除胆汁淤积的其他原因；组织学（见图 36.5C 和 D）	糖皮质激素（2mg/kg/d）；熊去氧胆酸	选择最优供体；彻底预防 GVHD；T 细胞耗竭方案；熊去氧胆酸
急性病毒性肝炎	不常见，使用预防措施对抗疱疹病毒、HBV	单纯疱疹病毒：>20~50 天不等；腺病毒：>30~80 天 VZV：>80~250 天 HBV、HCV：免疫重建期间	移植前的血清学和 PCR 结果；从其他标本中分离病毒（粪便和尿液中的腺病毒）；对特定病毒用血清 PCR 法；肝脏组织学/PCR/免疫标记（见图 36.5E 和 F）	HSV；带状疱疹；阿昔洛韦；腺病毒；西多福韦；HBV：恩替卡韦或替诺福韦；HCV：如果肝损伤严重，考虑直接作用的抗病毒药物	HSV 和 VZV 感染：对所有患者进行阿昔洛韦预防；如果患者有感染 HBV 的风险：拉米夫定或恩替卡韦；选择 HBV 免疫了的供体血清或免疫球蛋白
真菌性脓肿	很少使用预防措施	10~60 天	肝区疼痛、发热；肝脏成像；血清真菌抗原	抗真菌药物	移植前的筛选；所有患者口服抗真菌药物预防
药物性肝损伤	常见	0~100 天	临床诊断	持续停药	无
缺血性肝脏疾病	仅限于脓毒症、失血性休克或呼吸衰竭患者	0~50 天	临床诊断	恢复心输出量、血氧饱和度	早期治疗脓毒血症、出血
胆道梗阻	短暂性胆汁淤积常见于胆石症；绿色瘤罕见	15~60 天	病史，胆道超声检查	如果梗阻持续，乳头切开±引流支架	无
特发性高氨血症	罕见	10~50 天	检测静脉血氨	未证实	未知，可能是遗传缺陷
慢性丙型肝炎	下降	80 天后	血清中 HCVRNA；免疫重建后血清 AST、ALT 升高	完全免疫重建后，抗 HCV 治疗	筛选造血细胞供体
铁过载	很常见	移植前；移植后需长期随访	铁定量检查 MRI 特异；转铁蛋白饱和度；骨髓铁定量；肝铁定量	放血疗法可能不是必需的；如果铁含量过高，可采用螯合剂治疗	避免使用铁补充剂
慢性 GVHD	常见	80 天后	GVHD 前兆；其他器官慢性移植物抗宿主病；特征性的 ALT、碱性磷酸酶水平；组织学（见图 36.5D）	免疫抑制药物治疗，熊去氧胆酸	在第 80 天筛查慢性 GVHD

GVHD，移植物抗宿主病；SOS，肝窦阻塞综合征（静脉闭塞性疾病）；VZV，水痘-带状疱疹病毒；WHVPG，楔形肝静脉压力梯度。

后较晚期[176]。高胆红素血症后4~10天。伴有肾和肺功能障碍和难治性血小板减少症则强烈提示SOS[227,232]。SOS临床发作后数周血清AST/ALT升高反映了肝窦纤维化引起的缺血性肝细胞坏死[233]。多普勒超声可用于显示肝大、腹水、门静脉周围水肿、肝脏静脉血流减弱和符合SOS的胆囊壁水肿,以及排除肝大和黄疸的其他原因。SOS病程后期的异常表现可能包括门静脉内径扩大、门静脉或其节段分支血流缓慢或反向、充血指数高、门静脉血栓形成和肝动脉血流阻力指数增加。剪切波超声弹性成像是一种新兴的技术,可帮助在儿科患者中比传统多普勒超声更早地检测出SOS[234]。经颈静脉肝活检和肝静脉压力测定是最准确的诊断方法。在这种临床环境中,高于10mmHg的肝静脉压力梯度对SOS具有高度特异性[235]。初始组织学变化为肝窦扩张、红细胞通过Disse间隙外渗、小静脉周围肝细胞坏死以及中央静脉内皮下区增宽[236,237]。SOS的后期表现为星状细胞的激活和增殖、血窦广泛胶原化、小静脉腔有不同程度的阻塞,导致血窦血流闭塞[236,237]。反映在血清ALT水平上的肝窦和中央静脉胶原化强度和肝细胞坏死程度与结局相关[233,237]。在仅接受支持治疗的患者中,超过70%的患者SOS完全恢复。严重SOS患者很少死于肝衰竭,而是死于肾和心肺衰竭[227,232]。不良预后结果包括体重增加和血清胆红素升高的速度、血清ALT水平超过1 500U/L、发生腹水、肾功能不全和低氧血症[227,232,233,239]。

预防SOS的关键在于了解其发病机制[237,239]。肝窦内皮细胞的毒性损伤、非小静脉损伤和非肝血管内血栓形成是SOS的直接原因。肝窦损伤最常见的原因是含有CY的治疗方案和使用TBI的治疗方案,CY和TBI剂量超过12Gy的组合是致死性SOS的最常见原因[232]。产生大量毒性CY代谢物的患者更有可能发生致死性SOS[228,240]。CY总剂量为100~110mg/kg,而不是120mg/kg,将降低CY/TBI方案中器官毒性的频率[240]。当与CY120mg/kg联合应用时,TBI的总剂量与严重SOS的频率有关——CY/TBI 10Gy后约为1%,CY/TBI 12~14Gy后约为4%~7%,CY/TBI 14Gy以上后约为20%。BU是SOS频率较高方案的另一个组分,但BU本身似乎没有肝毒性[241]。BU可能通过诱导氧化应激、降低肝细胞和肝窦内皮细胞中的谷胱甘肽水平以及改变CY代谢而导致肝损伤[228]。在静脉靶向BU前给予CY,尤其是在骨髓纤维化患者中[202],导致的肝毒性低于靶向BU/CY小[228]。MEL的药代动力学也因患者而异,可以通过治疗性药物监测来实现标准化[242]。当大剂量吉妥珠单抗(奥唑米星)与含有肝窦毒素的清髓方案同时给药时,发生SOS的风险增加[204]。前胶原肽和纤维溶解抑制剂一起出现在更严重的SOS患者血清中,与致命性SOS中伴随的血窦和小静脉壁的严重纤维化完全一致。SOS患者肝脏中α-肌动蛋白(α-actin)的免疫组化染色在活化的星状细胞中呈强阳性,星状细胞是胶原沉积到血窦中的来源[237]。由遗传决定的药物代谢差异或对毒性损伤的敏感性可以解释SOS频率的一些变异性,但目前没有基于基因组数据改变药物剂量或确定个体患者对肝窦损伤敏感性的方法[243]。

预防致死性SOS的唯一方法是避免损伤肝窦内皮细胞,尤其是在有风险的患者中。预防严重肝窦损伤,首先是评估基础肝病患者接受给定的清髓性预处理方案的风险。这些策略对作为HCT并发症的SOS发生频率有显著影响[175,229]。有致死性SOS风险的患者有几种选择:①不涉及HCT的基础疾病的常规治疗;②降低强度的条件治疗方案;③不含环磷酰胺的清髓性治疗方案,例如,用于同种异体移植的靶向氟达拉滨(BU-fludarabine)[243,244]或用于自体造血干细胞移植(auto-HCT)的BEAM[245];④通过改变顺序(如CY/靶向BU[228])或将CY剂量降低到100~110mg/kg,修改基于CY的治疗方案;⑤使用药理学方法预防肝窦损伤。如果必须对有致死性SOS风险的患者使用CY/TBI方案,应考虑调整CY(100~110mg/kg)和TBI(≤12Gy)剂量。如果必须对有致死性SOS风险的患者使用BU/CY方案,如果在目标BU前给予CY或如果在BU完成后延迟CY给药1或2天,则肝毒性频率较低。静脉BU的代谢是可变的,曲线下面积(AUCBU)有数倍的范围,这一问题可以通过治疗药物监测来解决[244,246]。使用治疗药物监测使MEL使用规范化也是可行的[242]。降低含BU和MEL方案毒性的另一种方法是按相反顺序给药(MEL/BU)。在窦状隙损伤动物模型中实现了药物预防SOS,但在人类中尚未实现,可能的去纤苷输注除外(稍后讨论)[230]。前瞻性研究显示,预防性使用肝素、抗凝血酶Ⅲ或N-乙酰半胱氨酸预防致死性SOS方面没有任何获益。一项荟萃分析表明,熊去氧胆酸可能预防SOS[226],但在这些研究中,SOS与胆汁淤积性肝病并无差异,一项大型随机试验显示,熊去氧胆酸对SOS的频率没有影响,但对胆汁淤积性黄疸的频率有较大的影响[231]。

对于70%以上将自行恢复的SOS患者,治疗包括管理钠和水的平衡、维持肾血流量和反复腹水穿刺,以缓解不适和/或肺损伤。预后不良的患者在发病后不久即可被识别出,表现为生血清总胆红素和体重急剧升高、血清ALT值超过1 500U/L、门静脉压力超过20mmHg、发生门静脉血栓形成,尤其是多器官衰竭需要透析、血液滤过或机械通气[227,232,233,238]。重度SOS没有令人满意的治疗方法,静脉去纤苷治疗是目前最好的结果(46%的完全缓解率,定义为总血清胆红素<2mg/dL和多器官衰竭消退)[247,248]。去纤苷在美国和欧洲获批用于重度SOS的治愈性治疗,但高昂的治疗费用对移植中心来说是一个挑战。去纤苷治疗严重SOS的成本-效益分析发现,每获得一个质量调整生命年的增量成本-效益比为47 735美元[249]。在SOS患者中实施肝内分流术,可降低门静脉压力和控制腹水,但血清胆红素水平和患者预后均未得到改善。持续性腹水和血清胆红素正常的患者已经成功进行了门-体分流术。难治性腹水的腹腔静脉分流术未成功。有报道严重SOS成功实施了OLT[250]。然而在大多数中心,有恶性肿瘤复发风险的患者是尸体肝脏的低优先级候选者。与治疗严重肝窦损伤患者相比,预防肝窦损伤已被证明是改善HCT结局更有效的策略[175]。

(2) 胆汁淤积性疾病

与安慰剂相比,预防性熊去氧胆酸可总体上降低胆汁淤积的发生,特别是GVHD相关的胆汁淤积,并改善预后[175,231]。既然SOS的发病率已经大幅下降,HCT后黄疸的主要原因则为胆汁淤积性肝损伤[176,225]。

Lenta胆管炎:高胆红素血症常见于中性粒细胞减少和发热,以及因预处理方案导致的肠黏膜损伤的患者。结合胆红素的肝细胞滞留是由内毒素、IL-6和TNF-α介导的[169]。虽然这种疾病常被称为“脓毒症的胆汁淤积”,但它发生在单纯发热和肺和软组织存在局限性感染的患者中(见第37章)。

急性移植物抗宿主病：高达70%的同种异体移植受者可发生急性GVHD(见图36.5C)。熊去氧胆酸的预防大大降低了移植后黄疸的发生率，改变了GVHD的临床表型[175,231]。回顾发现，所谓的“肝脏GVHD”是3个过程的混杂。第一个过程是在GVHD早期发生的黄疸，其中胆汁淤积是由细胞因子如IL-6引起的[209,251]。第二个过程的特征是血清胆红素、碱性磷酸酶和GGTP增加，通常在胃肠道GVHD患者中进行肝活检，可见淋巴细胞浸润小胆管，伴上皮细胞核多形性、上皮细胞脱落和肝脏腺泡3区的胆汁淤积[251]。由于免疫抑制，炎症浸润可能非常轻微。持续性肝脏GVHD和黄疸恶化与胆管消失有关。肝脏GVHD的第三个过程最常见于同种异体移植受者免疫抑制减少或供体淋巴细胞输注后，其中GVHD表现为急性肝炎，血清ALT明显升高[252,253]。患者GVHD的预后与症状和体征的峰值严重程度无关，而是疾病活动曲线下的区域，此区域中持续性黄疸是死亡率的独立预测因子[254]。

药物性肝损伤：环孢素抑制毛细胆管胆汁转运并且通常引起血清胆红素浓度的轻度升高，而不影响血清ALT或碱性磷酸酶。除了血药浓度很高，他克莫司较少引起胆汁淤积。HCT后使用的许多其他药物与肝功能障碍有关(例如，甲氧苄啶/磺胺甲噁唑，伊曲康唑，伏立康唑，氟康唑，泊沙康唑)，尽管药物通常在这种情况下不造成严重的肝损伤[203,233]。

(3) 急性肝细胞损伤

自20世纪90年代以来，HCT后严重肝细胞损伤的发生率已显著下降[175,233]。HCT后血清转氨酶(AST和ALT)突然升高通常是由于非感染性原因，如SOS中的3区肝细胞坏死(在第20天左右达到峰值)、缺氧性肝损伤(如感染性或心源性休克或呼吸衰竭)、急性胆道梗阻(胆总管结石)、药物性肝损伤(DILI)、或前面讨论的GVHD的急性肝炎的表现[176]。如果可能的原因不明显，应怀疑急性病毒性肝炎；早期诊断和治疗可预防致死性的结局。

由HSV、VZV、腺病毒和HBV引起的急性肝炎可导致HCT后致死性的暴发性肝衰竭，而CMV和HCV引起的肝脏感染则很少这么严重(参见图36.5E和F)。常规使用预防性阿昔洛韦或伐昔洛韦，由HSV和VZV引起的急性肝炎现在很少见；然而，HCT后HHV-6和HHV-8再激活以及HEV作为肝炎的原因已有报道[255,256]。当血清ALT和AST水平升高的原因尚不确定时，应进行疱疹病毒、腺病毒、HCV、HBV的血清PCR检测，以及在某些情况下，进行HEV的血清PCR检测。病毒的血液检测在很大程度上取代了获取肝活检组织进行病毒诊断的需要，但通过肝活检经静脉测量楔形肝静脉压力梯度可用于诊断疑似SOS或其他原因引起的肝细胞坏死。如果未给予阿昔洛韦，应该根据经验开始治疗，特别是当患者出现VZV感染的典型腹部症状时[257]。如果患者同时有肺、肾、膀胱或肠道症状，但可能仅表现为发热、转氨酶升高和腹部CT上显示肝脏低密度区，以及骨髓抑制的特征，应该怀疑腺病毒性肝炎[258]。最有效的治疗方法是在腺病毒感染早期给予西多福韦，但许多病例都是致命的[259,260]，新的药物制剂正在开发中。

暴发性乙型肝炎可能在高危患者的免疫重建期间发生，但可通过预防性抗病毒药物预防[261]。如果确实发生重度乙型肝炎再激活，通常是因为在HCT前未诊断为HBV，应立即开始使用可用的最强效抗HBV药物(恩替卡韦或替诺福韦)进行抗病毒治疗，然而，进展为致死性肝衰竭并不少见[262]。在停止预防性抗病毒治疗后也报道了暴发性乙型肝炎，所有患者，特别是移植前HBV DNA水平高的患者，应在抗病毒药物停药后进行监测[263,264]。

HCT受者的慢性丙型肝炎通常导致血清ALT从第60~120天无症状性升高，与免疫抑制药物逐渐减量同时发生[198]。近年来，用直接抗病毒药(DAA)治疗血液系统恶性肿瘤患者的慢性HCV感染已成为标准治疗。无DAA禁忌证且移植前未接受治疗的HCT受者，一旦患者停用所有免疫抑制药物且无活动性GVHD证据，应接受HCV治疗[198,265]。DAA对HCT后HCV引起的罕见的重度肝炎以及纤维化胆汁淤积性肝炎提供有效的治疗[197]。

(4) 真菌和细菌感染

预防性抗真菌显著降低了HCT患者肝脏真菌病的发病率[266]。有发热、轻度肝大、血清碱性磷酸酶水平升高等特征时，应怀疑有耐药的念珠菌种或霉菌[266]。高分辨率CT或MRI可能表现出多发的真菌性脓肿，真菌抗原的血清学检测有助于诊断[190]。HCT后中性粒细胞功能恢复可影响先前的难治性曲霉菌感染的缓解[267]。HCT受者中罕见细菌性肝脓肿，可能是因为系统抗生素的广泛使用；然而，潜伏的分枝杆菌感染(包括结核杆菌)可能随着长期的免疫抑制治疗在肝脏内重新激活。播散性梭菌感染和产气病原体的胆囊感染可能导致肝脏和胆道系统积气。

(5) 胆囊和胆道疾病

HCT受者中胆泥(胆红素钙和钙调神经磷酸酶抑制剂晶体)形成很常见[268]。胆泥进入胆管可能导致上腹部疼痛、恶心和血清转氨酶异常。胆泥可能是急性“非结石性”胆囊炎、急性胰腺炎和细菌性胆管炎的原因[269,270]。HCT受者不常见急性胆囊炎，它往往是由于较大的胆结石引起[270]。这种情况下的胆囊炎也可能是由于白血病复发累及胆囊所致，或是CMV、真菌感染，或其他少见的病原体比如流感嗜血杆菌感染所致。由于无症状患者US或CT检查中常常会发现胆囊异常，致使HCT后胆囊炎的诊断很困难。胆囊周围渗液、胆囊壁坏死或局限性压痛提示胆囊炎。用输注吗啡行放射性核素胆汁排泄实验，胆囊不显影，提示胆囊炎。胆道梗阻相当罕见，原因很多：胆总管结石或浓缩胆汁淤积；壶腹黏膜GVHD，EBV-LPD患者胆总管、胆囊、壶腹淋巴细胞浸润，CMV相关的胆道疾病，内镜活检所致的剥脱性十二指肠血肿，以及胰头部的白血病复发(绿色瘤)[270,271]。自体HCT的患者，胆道狭窄通常是由复发性恶性肿瘤引起的[272]。应用熊去氧胆酸刺激HCT后胆泥患者的胆汁流出无效。ERCP适用于有胆管炎临床证据和胆道梗阻影像学证据的患者，允许胆道支架植入或扩张，风险可接受[271,272]。

(6) 恶性肝脏疾病

EBV-LPD现在是罕见的HCT并发症，主要是因为EBV DNA监测和利妥昔单抗的预防治疗。发生率最高的是接受HLA不匹配、T细胞耗竭的移植物和那些因GVHD接受有效的抗T细胞治疗的患者。症状包括发热、出汗、全身不适、扁桃体增大和颈淋巴结肿大，常伴有肝、脾受累(血清碱性磷酸酶异常和肝脾肿大)和胃肠道侵犯。作为移植适应证的恶性肿瘤可作为复发的一部分出现在肝脏中。

(7) 特发性高氨血症与昏迷

已有报道，在接受大剂量化疗，包括HCT预处理的患者中描述了特发性高氨血症与高氨血症昏迷综合征[273]，患者表现为进行性嗜睡、意识模糊、无力、不协调、呕吐和过度换气伴呼吸性碱中毒。当血氨超过 200μmol/L，且无肝衰竭证据时可确诊[274]。

3. 胃肠道出血（图 36.6）

轻微的出血很常见，特别是当血小板计数低于 50×10^9/L 时。原因包括呕吐引起的食管或胃黏膜损伤、预处理引起的黏膜损伤、反流性食管炎、难治性结肠炎、肛裂、内痔、急性 GVHD。HCT 术后胃肠道大出血的发生率为 1%～2%，由于对病毒、真菌和急性 GVHD 的有效预防，发生率较过去有所下降[275]。然而，严重的肠道出血的致死率仍然是 40%[275,276]。严重出血最常见的原因是难治性急性 GVHD，出血原因为小肠和盲肠广泛溃疡[277]。出血是严重肠道 GVHD 患者死亡率的独立预测因素。在更昔洛韦预防和早期优先治疗下，CMV 溃疡出血已很罕见。胃溃疡也可由 VZV、侵袭性细菌（黏液性胃炎）或 EBV（LPD）感染引起（见第 52 章）。虽然目前 HCT 后很少发生 EBV-LPD，但 20%～25% 的病例累及胃肠道，可表现为胃肠道出血。胃窦血管扩张是 HCT 受者发生严重上消化道出血的原因之一，尤其是口服 BU 的受者[278]。胃窦内可见弥漫性出血区，偶尔可见于小肠和大肠，但其下层黏膜是完好的[278-280]。组织学为固有层异常的毛细血管扩张、血栓形成和肌纤维增生。因晚期系统性硬化症而移植的患者也可能因类似的血管病变而出血。可以选择内镜激光治疗或氩离子凝固术来控制血管扩张出血，但可能需要多种治疗来阻塞扩张性病变[278]。HCT 后出血的其他罕见原因包括真菌引起的溃疡、Dieulafoy 病变、应激性溃疡、十二指肠活检部位、霉酚酸诱导的肠炎、腺病毒肠炎和败毒梭菌感染（伤寒炎）。重度淀粉样变行自体 HCT 的患者，可因肠内多处缺血性溃疡出血[281]。

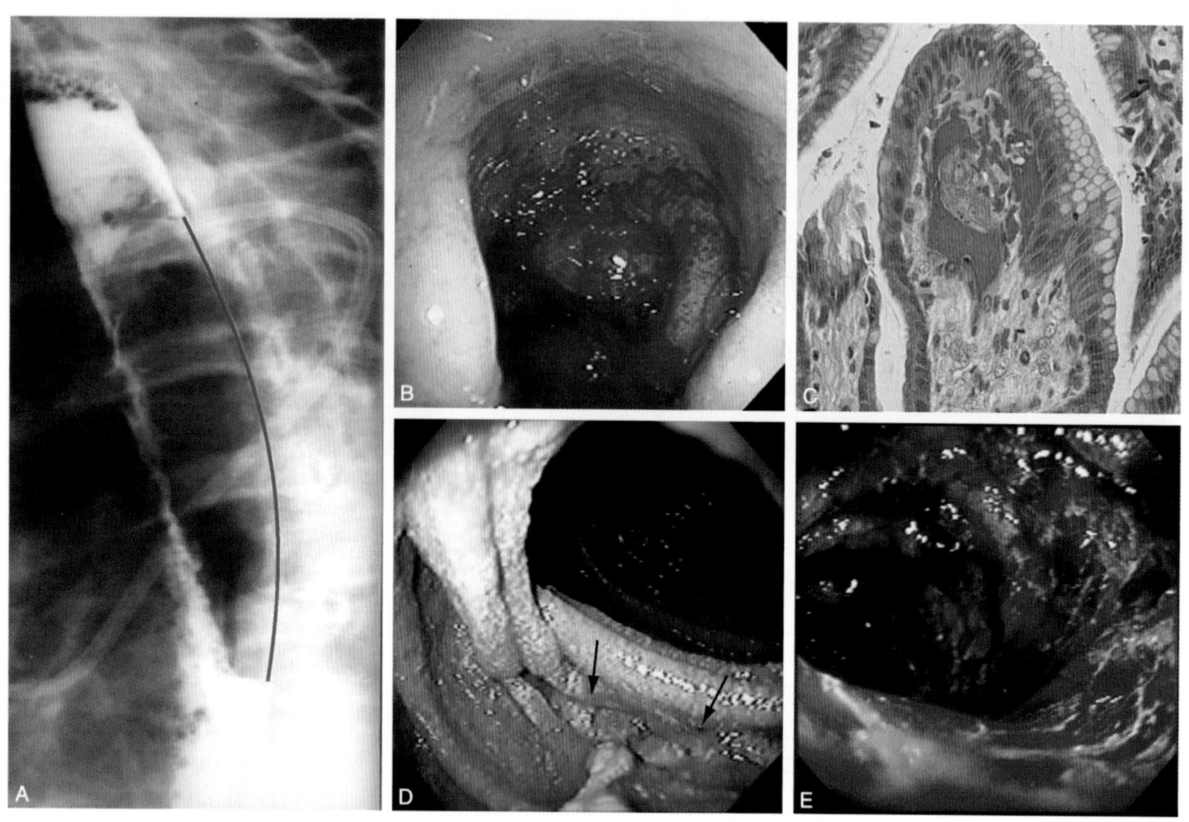

图 36.6 造血细胞移植受者不常见的胃肠道问题。A，食管：钡剂造影显示从主动脉弓到食管下段占据食管一壁的壁内血肿。红线接近正常食管轮廓。该血肿是由血小板减少症患者干呕引起的。B，胃：GAVE 中胃窦黏膜弥漫性渗血。当血液被冲洗掉时，观察到下面的黏膜没有溃疡，但是再次出现血液。C，胃组织学：胃窦活检的高倍视图，说明 GAVE 的特征—毛细血管扩张、血栓形成和肌纤维增生（HE 染色）D，十二指肠：接受免疫抑制治疗移植物抗宿主病（GVHD）的移植患者因根霉感染引起的线状十二指肠溃疡伴黄色渗出物（箭）。由于 GVHD，周围黏膜异常。E，结肠：腺病毒结肠炎中的乙状结肠，表现为弥漫性黏膜水肿、溃疡、出血

对于弥漫性血液渗出的黏膜，如果可能，除了将血小板计数提高到 50×10^9/L 以上并治疗其基础症状外，没有其他有效的治疗方法。连续输注 25μg/h 的奥曲肽，可使 GVHD 出血停止，但如果剂量减少，会再出血[282]。在 GVHD 中，溃疡性肠黏膜的上皮再生非常缓慢。局灶性病变，特别是黏膜感染，只要血小板数量足够，内镜烧灼、热探针或注射肾上腺素均可治疗，但对于弥漫性渗血的黏膜无效。除非基础的疾病被消除，否则内窥镜方法不会治愈出血问题。试图切除 GVHD 累及的大量弥漫性出血肠段没有取得成功[277]。

4. 吞咽困难、吞咽疼痛和食管疼痛

预处理引起的口腔和下咽黏膜炎、反流性食管炎和药物性食管炎是目前引起吞咽困难和食管疼痛的主要原因。由于预防性抗微生物治疗，食管感染（真菌、病毒、细菌）已很少见；当发现真菌性食管炎时，这种微生物很可能是一种具有耐药性的念珠菌种或霉菌[283]。真菌性食管炎很少会导致穿孔[284]。预处理可能很少导致难以愈合的食管溃疡、狭窄和吞咽困难[285]。与急性 GVHD 有关的胃潴留患者，胃酸和胆

汁反流引起的食管痛常见。严重急性 GVHD 患者，食管水肿、红斑和上皮细胞脱落会导致溃疡[286,287]。HCT 服用某些药物后可发生药物性食管炎，如苯妥英、福司卡托普利、口服双膦酸盐、抗坏血酸、环丙沙星、克林霉素、口服高氯酸钾等。

突然出现严重胸骨后疼痛、呕血和吞咽痛提示食管壁有血肿，这是血小板计数非常低时呕吐的结果（见第 45 章）[288]。内镜检查是相对禁忌证，因为许多壁内血肿说明包含有穿孔。CT 是可以选择的诊断方法[289]。血肿 1～2 周后逐渐消退。

5. 腹泻

（1）预处理治疗

大剂量预处理治疗所致的黏膜损伤引起的腹泻很少是严重的，通常在第 12～15 天消退。但有一些例外。含阿糖胞苷的治疗方案、大剂量美法仑（MEL）（≥200mg/m²）和含有多种烷化剂的治疗方案可能导致更严重和更持久的腹泻。静脉输注奥曲肽和口服洛哌丁胺可能对预处理治疗相关的严重腹泻有效[290]。

（2）移植物抗宿主病

急性 GVHD（表 36.3；也见图 36.4）是第 15 天后腹泻的最常见原因[291]。然而，GVHD 可能不是个体患者腹泻的唯一原因，尤其是在接受长期免疫抑制的患者中，其中重新评估腹泻原因可能检测到基线时不存在的感染[292]。对 HCT 后复发的血液系统恶性肿瘤，新兴的非标准治疗（即检查点抑制剂）也可能加重 GVHD[293]。GVHD 腹泻可突然发作，严重者每天大便量超过 2L。在降低强度预处理方案后接受移植的患者发生移植物抗宿主病的时间可能会延迟，许多患者在第 100 天后发生[294]。GVHD 的腹泻液呈水样，有黏液性物质链，反映出黏膜蛋白的丢失。这种表现几乎可诊断肠道 GVHD，尤其是伴有血清白蛋白水平降低和粪便感染检查阴性时[295]。在怀疑 GVHD 的非典型病例中，腹部影像学可发现肠水肿和黏膜增强，特别是回肠和右半结肠，尽管急性 GVHD 和 CMV 感染的表现重叠[296-299]。用 PET 可获得相似的信息。肠壁积气可能与 GVHD 或 CMV 肠炎相关，可通过 X 线平片、CT 或 MRI 观察到，在缺乏临床严重程度辅助检查证据的情况下，保守处理[300]。确诊 GVHD 需要内镜下黏膜视图、胃肠黏膜组织的组织学变化和排除感染。内镜医师所见的诊断与病理学家通过显微镜所见的诊断具有同等的诊断价值[216]。中重度 GVHD 导致整个胃肠道黏膜弥漫性水肿和红斑。重度 GVHD 可能导致胃、小肠和结肠溃疡和大面积黏膜脱落[301]。即使外观正常，直肠乙状结肠或胃窦的黏膜活检也常显示肠隐窝坏死和凋亡小体，而诊断为急性 GVHD[302]。当从远端结肠和胃或结肠和回肠进行活检时，黏膜活检的诊断率最佳[291,301,302]。应将黏膜的目视检查视为组织学结果的补充。支持 GVHD 诊断的其他组织学结果包括毛细血管周围出血、中性粒细胞或嗜酸性粒细胞浸润以及内皮损伤的证据。使用胶囊式内镜诊断 GVHD 可以提供常规内镜通常看不到的空肠和回肠的目视检查[303]。小肠胶囊式内镜检查的阴性预测值似乎较高，因此，有用于排除更严重的急性 GVHD。

表 36.3　造血细胞移植后引起腹泻的原因

原因	频率	诊断	严重性	治疗
清髓预处理治疗	常见	排除感染，超急性 GVHD	通常是轻度，在某些方案后可能为重度	自限的，奥曲肽适用于严重的病例
急性 GVHD	常见于同种异体移植后；发生在大约 10% 的自体移植物中	与皮肤和肝脏 GVHD 的相关性；排除感染。血清白蛋白突然下降是更严重 GVHD 的标志；有问题病例的黏膜组织学	范围从轻度到难治性高容量性腹泻	免疫抑制药物，通常最初使用泼尼松
巨细胞病毒感染	现在不常见	血液中巨细胞病毒抗原或 DNA；病毒培养、黏膜活检的免疫组织学	如果早期未检测到，可能会致命	更昔洛韦或磷甲酸钠
腺病毒	散发的	血液或粪便中的腺病毒 DNA；病毒培养，黏膜活检的免疫组织学	血清型依赖性；可能迅速致死	西多福韦
诺如病毒	不常见；可通过医院内传播获得	粪便标本 PCR 检测	如果免疫缺陷持续存在，可能是重度和长期的	无
星状病毒	不常见	ELISA、粪便 PCR	自限性	无
轮状病毒	罕见	ELISA、粪便 PCR	血清型依赖性；可能为重度	无
EBV（淋巴组织增生性疾病）	现在罕见	血液 EBV DNA；黏膜活检	当发生淋巴瘤性肠道受累时，通常是致命的	早期发现用利妥昔单抗；停用免疫抑制药物
细菌感染艰难梭菌	常见	粪便中的 PCR、毒素和抗原	通常为轻度至中度	口服万古霉素>非达霉素>甲硝唑

表 36.3 造血细胞移植后引起腹泻的原因(续)

原因	频率	诊断	严重性	治疗
败血梭状芽孢杆菌	散发性	伤寒临床综合征	有可能致命	亚胺培南,口服万古霉素
肠道病原体	罕见,流行区除外	粪便,血培养	有可能致命	基于微生物的敏感性
寄生虫感染:蓝氏贾第鞭毛虫	罕见	粪便 ELISA	可迁延不愈	甲硝唑
人隐孢子虫	罕见	粪便、血培养,粪便显微镜检查,PCR	常迁延不愈	恢复免疫力
溶组织阿米巴	罕见	粪便显微镜检查、抗原、PCR;血清 EIA	可能致命	甲硝唑或替硝唑,随后使用巴龙霉素
粪类圆线虫	罕见	粪便显微镜检查	潜在致命性	伊维美替尼
渗透性腹泻:口服镁盐	常见	临床诊断	剂量依赖性	降低剂量;静脉注射 Mg^{2+}
碳水化合物吸收不良	常见肠道 GVHD、感染	临床诊断	饮食依赖性	二糖饮食限制
抗生素的使用	常见	临床诊断	药物依赖性	停用抗生素
药物:他克莫司	不常见	临床诊断	剂量依赖性	减少剂量;洛派丁胺
吗替麦考酚酯	常见	临床诊断、内窥镜检查结果	剂量依赖性	减少剂量;替代肠溶麦考酚酸制剂;咯派丁胺
甲氧氯普胺(胃复安)	不常见	临床诊断	药物依赖	停药

EBV,EB 病毒;EIA,酶免疫分析法;ELISA,酶联免疫吸附试验;GVHD,移植物抗宿主病。

在 GVHD 的严重病例中,整个隐窝被破坏,然后是邻近的隐窝破坏,最后是整个肠黏膜节段。黏膜溃疡患者的腹泻常伴有出血[275]。采用免疫抑制疗法成功治疗急性 GVHD 可使大便量急剧减少,伴随的腹痛、恶心和呕吐的症状消退。在免疫抑制治疗 5 天后,腹泻及其他肠道 GVHD 症状未缓解的患者的治疗不理想,是因为二次治疗失败率较高[304]。GVHD 引起的高容量腹泻患者的死亡率,可以通过发病 14 天内的一组临床特征来预测:黄疸、年龄大于 18 岁、对泼尼松无反应和胃肠道出血[305]。预测 GVHD 患者预后的其他方法包括计算急性 GVHD 活动指数、测量血清白蛋白水平相对于基线和血清生物标志物的下降[254,295,306,307]。

(3) 感染

异体移植受者,因感染引起的腹泻远没有 GVHD 常见,仅占腹泻发作的 10%~15%[276,291,308]。常见的致病菌在 HCT 后极为罕见[308],特别是在感染流行区域以外[309]。有几种感染与肠道 GVHD 极为相似,或者更常见的是与 GVHD 共存,包括不可培养的肠道病毒(诺如病毒、轮状病毒、星形病毒)、分枝杆菌、真菌和寄生虫[283]。如果腹泻起病就被诊断,那么艰难梭菌性结肠炎通常相对温和并可治疗[291,310]。在复发或难治性艰难梭菌结肠炎的 HCT 受者中,通过仔细选择供者和受者,粪便微生物群移植似乎是安全有效的[311]。一个经常被忽视的因素是在边缘适应证中不适当地使用 PPI,这会使艰难梭菌性结肠炎的风险增加 2 倍[312]。在一项前瞻性研究中,感染性腹泻最常见的病因是星形病毒(一种与诺如病毒相似的小而圆的病毒);诊断可通过粪便标本 PCR 或小肠活检组织的电镜检查[291,313]。诺如病毒作为 HCT 患者的医院内感染也可在医院内传播,后果很严重[314]。一些血清型腺病毒会引起坏死性肠炎,并迅速导致包括肠、肝、肺和肾在内的多器官衰竭[283,315]。在确定腺病毒为肠炎成因方面,应有紧迫感;延迟治疗往往无效[316,317]。然而,并非所有在腹泻粪便中发现腺病毒的患者都感染了腺病毒。

CMV 是 HCT 后肠炎唯一常见的感染原因,需要肠道活检诊断[291]。与腺病毒一样,从未被证实黏膜 CMV 感染患者的腹泻粪便标本中可以检测到 CMV DNA。血液中 CMV 抗原或 DNA 阴性的患者黏膜活检可发现 CMV[177,318]。另外,粪便检查阴性结果对其他病毒、细菌、真菌和寄生虫的预测值很高,特别是如果使用了分子方法[319]。HCT 后继发于肠道寄生虫感染的水样泻(隐孢子虫,蓝氏贾第鞭毛虫,溶组织阿米巴,蠕虫)较为少见,但可见与 GVHD 易混淆的散发性病例[320-322]。HCT 后类圆线虫感染和高度感染综合征已被报道;应在 HCT 前对流行地区的患者进行筛查[182]。HCT 后非结核分枝杆菌小肠感染也有报道[323,324]。

(4) 腹泻的其他原因

除了感染,其他几种情况可能也与 GVHD 类似,包括刷状缘双糖酶缺乏、胆盐吸收不良、胰腺功能不全、MMF 引起的黏膜毒性和肠道血栓性微血管病变。肠道炎症常常导致乳糖酶和蔗糖酶/异构化酶的下调,如果摄入乳糖或蔗糖,就会导致腹泻。作为腹泻原因的小肠内胆盐吸收障碍可以用考来伟伦治疗[325]。胰腺炎和胰腺功能不全与钙调神经磷酸酶抑制剂治疗有关[326]。短暂性胰腺功能不全被认为是壶腹黏膜水肿所致[327]。日本研究者描述了钙调磷酸酶抑制剂相关的肠微血管病,与 GVHD 类似[328]。MMF 引起肠道溃疡和隐窝细胞凋亡类似于急性 GVHD 的组织学改变[329],转化成肠溶霉酚酸后 SOT 受者的胃肠道副作用减少[75]。腹泻也可能是由于碳水化合物吸收不良(特别是服用抗生物制剂的患者,这些药物会影响结肠菌群保留碳水化合物的能力)、口服镁盐、他克莫司(一种胃动素激动剂)和普列里沙因(一种免疫兴奋剂)引起的。“脐结肠炎”腹泻综合征已在脐带血受者中报道。内镜活检病理显示慢性活动性结肠炎伴肉芽肿,患者对抗生素有反应,但复发率高[330]。然而,其他研究中心还没有确定其结肠炎是 HCT 后腹泻的原因，大多数病例是由 GVHD 所引起的[331]。

6. 腹痛

腹痛可能是进展迅速的致命性疾病的指征，或者是一种只需要保守治疗自然病史良性的疾病（表 36.4）。可能迅速致命的疾病包括肠道穿孔、某些感染（如由败毒梭菌引起的伤寒、腺病毒肠炎、内脏 VZV 感染、曲霉菌血管炎）、胆囊坏死和细菌性肝脓肿。幸运的是，这些疾病远没有肠道假性梗阻、麻醉性肠综合征、急性 GVHD、与 SOS 相关的肝脏疼痛以及出血性膀胱炎那么常见。出血性膀胱炎当然是导致严重疼痛的原因，但不会立即死亡。第一个问题是疼痛病人是否需要紧急手术。HCT 术后疼痛的外科干预比较罕见，但适用于肠道穿孔、急性胆囊炎、脓肿引流、阑尾炎，以及一些肠道或胆道梗阻、盲肠炎和剥离性血肿的患者[332]。手术决策取决于临床情况、腹部检查和影像学的正确判断。外科医生根据目前的影像学检查和仔细体检，在入选患者时具有高度的选择性，但当患者不能排除有外科疾病，如不明原因的腹腔游离气体影或怀疑胆囊坏死，临床可能对这些疑难病例行手术探查或腹腔镜手术。预处理治疗后不久透壁性淋巴瘤或转移癌坏死或时间较久的 CMV 溃疡或憩室穿孔，可发展成肠道穿孔。穿孔可表现为只有轻-中度的腹痛和腹部 CT 上所见的气腹，尤其是粒细胞减少症患者。气腹可能是肠积气的一个表现，是一个比游离穿孔和缓得多的情况，由 CMV 感染和 GVHD 引起[333]。诊断急性胆囊炎比较困难，因为右上腹部疼痛（通常来自 SOS）和发热在 HCT 后早期常见，影像学经常显示完全无症状的患者胆囊壁增厚和腔内淤泥。一项用吗啡进行的放射性核素研究显示胆囊充盈，提示不存在外科性胆囊炎，但假阳性结果（即缺乏胆囊充盈）可以发生在全肠外营养的重症患者[334]。当疼痛局限在右下腹，盲肠炎（败毒梭菌感染）和阑尾炎可通过影像并排除其他引起右下腹痛的原因（肾脏、卵巢、腹壁）来诊断。引起中度到重度腹痛最常见的原因——肠假性梗阻伴肠胀气；在阿片类或抗胆碱能药物暴露情况下，叩诊发现胀气及鼓胀就足以做出诊断。在内脏 VZV 感染中，腹胀、剧烈疼痛、发热和血清 ALT 水平升高可先于皮肤表现 10 天，这种表现仅发生在未接受阿昔洛韦预防的患者中[257,335]。临床怀疑时应开始使用阿昔洛韦，并对血清进行 PCR 检测 VZV DNA。临床胰腺炎是 HCT 患者不常见的引起腹痛的原因；亚临床胰腺炎的确有发生，其症状被免疫抑制剂所掩盖[269]。血小板计数低或凝血时间延长的患者，可能会见到少数病例，特别是十二指肠活检后，出血进入腹膜后、腹壁或腹腔脏器，引起明显疼痛。

表 36.4　造血细胞移植后腹痛的原因分析

原因	频率	诊断	严重程度	治疗
肝窦阻塞综合征（SOS）	现在不常见	触痛性肝大、体重增加、黄疸	可能致命	见病例描述
预处理治疗引起的肠损伤	不常见	检查、成像	某些治疗后可能会延长	无
结肠假性梗阻	常见，特别是在使用 μ-阿片类药物或抗胆碱能药物的患者中，GVHD 和 VZV 或 CMV 感染也可能发生，既往长春新碱暴露会增加风险	腹胀、鼓音、腹部平片	当与药物相关时，通常可消退；当 GVHD 或病毒感染体征可能为重度时	减少阿片类药物、抗胆碱能药物的暴露；排除可治疗的基础原因；考虑使用甲基纳曲酮；如果持续或重度，则用新斯的明
出血性膀胱炎	常见于环磷酰胺治疗后和病毒性膀胱感染	耻骨弓上疼痛、血尿、病毒培养（JC/BK 病毒或腺病毒）	可因病毒感染而迁延不愈	泌尿系统治疗，抗病毒药物（如适用）
急性 GVHD	常见，尤其是更严重的 GVHD	评估皮肤、肠道症状、血清胆红素、肠道成像（CT、US、MRE、PET）、黏膜活检	可能严重，但不会立即致命	免疫抑制药物治疗
胆道疼痛	不常见	右上/上腹定位；胆囊淤泥、胆囊水肿、积气；超声显示胆管扩张	胆泥的通过通常是自限性的；坏死的胆囊需要手术	持续性胆道梗阻需要放置支架；胆囊坏死手术
胰腺炎	不常见	血清脂肪酶	通常为自限性，但可发生出血性胰腺炎	治疗胆道、感染和药物原因
血肿	罕见；可见于十二指肠活检术后	检查、腹部成像、内镜检查	可迁延不愈	恢复血小板计数；肠梗阻可能需要手术
肠道感染	不常见	梭状芽孢杆菌感染、VZV、CMV、腺病毒、诺如病毒、真菌的诊断和成像检测	如果不治疗可能致命（特别是梭状芽孢杆菌败血症、病毒或真菌感染）	治疗发现的病原体
肠穿孔（CMV 溃疡、肠肿瘤坏死、憩室）	现在罕见	腹平片、CT 检查	可能致命	手术

表 36.4 造血细胞移植后腹痛的原因分析(续)

原因	频率	诊断	严重程度	治疗
肝脏脓肿/细菌感染	罕见(通常为真菌感染)	肝脏成像(首选 MRI)、检查、血清真菌抗原检测	如果不治疗,可能致命	抗真菌治疗,抗菌治疗
肠梗死(通常由播散性曲霉菌感染引起)	罕见	肠道成像、检查、胸部 X 线、半乳甘露聚糖 ELISA	致命	抗真菌药物治疗
EBV-淋巴组织增生性疾病	罕见,监测到血清中 EBV DNA	腹部成像,内镜活检	一旦肿瘤形成,通常是致命的	早期发现用利妥昔单抗;停用免疫抑制药物

CMV,巨细胞病毒;EBV,EB 病毒;ELISA,酶联免疫吸附试验;GVHD,移植物抗宿主病;JC/BK,多瘤病毒;MRE,磁共振肠动描记法;US,超声;VZV,水痘-带状疱疹病毒。

下一个问题是疼痛是否由 GVHD 引起,因为 GVHD 的早期治疗势在必行。急性胃肠道 GVHD 可仅表现为腹痛,但更常见的是伴有疼痛的皮疹、恶心、呕吐、厌食症或腹泻。表现为腹部僵硬,反跳痛,但更常见的是腹绞痛和脐周痛。胃黏膜水肿时,疼痛局限于上腹部。如未掌握 GVHD 的确切证据,以经验治疗为主是很困难的,但 GVHD 的验前概率高,穿孔或感染率很低,应使用强的松[2mg/(kg·d)]治疗。CT 或腹部超声(尤其是超声造影)显示急性 GVHD 患者肠壁增厚,这是一种非特异性但具有高度提示的发现,尤其是在 CMV 感染不太可能发生的情况下[297,299,336]。延误治疗可能导致更广泛的黏膜坏死和发病率[337]。如果后来证明疼痛是由于 GVHD 以外的原因,强的松可以停用。

接下来要考虑的是疼痛是否由可治疗的感染引起。最近在抗病毒和抗真菌预防方面的进展使得肠道和肝脏感染成为引起腹痛的罕见原因[175]。累及内脏的播散性 VZV 在未接受阿昔洛韦或更昔洛韦治疗的患者 HCT 后 2~6 个月可能出现难以解释的腹痛。重要的是,腹痛可能比典型的 VZV 皮肤病变早几天[257]。患者应开始静脉注射阿昔洛韦,同时寻求明确的诊断(血清、胃黏膜或肝脏活检中 VZV DNA 检测)。其他肠道感染可能表现为明显疼痛,包括腺病毒、巨细胞病毒、隐孢子虫病感染和侵袭性真菌,如根霉菌、梭菌性结肠炎和败血症性结肠炎(盲肠炎)。盲肠炎症状包括发热、右下腹部疼痛、恶心呕吐、腹泻、大便隐血、休克;诊断盲肠炎通常根据影像显示盲肠水肿作出[338]。手术切除盲肠炎几乎是没有必要的,只要对脓毒杆菌进行抗生素治疗(如亚胺培南和口服万古霉素),并对发热病人的腔内细菌和真菌进行全身覆盖即可[339]。

假性肠梗阻和胀气的患者,药物治疗几乎总是有效的,并且穿孔罕见。虽然某些肠道神经元感染(VZV 和 CMV)能导致假性梗阻,但是阿片类激动剂药物和抗胆碱能药物也是常见的原因,尤其是在患者肠道炎症时。阿片类药物相关性假性梗阻的治疗方法有 3 种:①减少阿片类药物的剂量;②甲基纳曲酮阻断外周血阿片受体[153];③改用 κ-阿片类激动剂(如布托啡诺)。假性梗阻患者禁用抗胆碱能药物,有抗胆碱能副作用的药物应停止使用。新斯的明(2mg 静脉注射)已成功用于 HCT 后急性结肠假性梗阻的患者[340]。奥曲肽治疗伴液体的肠胀气相关的假性肠梗阻有效。

7. 肛周疼痛

HCT 后肛周疼痛可由肛裂、血栓性外痔、与组织浸渍相关的蜂窝织炎和感染所致。在粒细胞减少症的患者中,会阴或肛周间隙感染通常是多种微生物感染,来自肛腺或肛管撕裂。也可出现广泛的上提肌和括约肌间脓肿,但外观检查不明显[341]。CT 或 MRI 或内镜检查或经会阴超声均可清晰显示受累解剖结构,特别是存在脓液时[342]。自从对"隐窝炎"(初发肛周感染)患者使用了覆盖厌氧菌和需氧菌的抗生素后,需要手术引流的患者远少于过去。肛周疼痛的不常见原因还包括 HPV 引起的巨大尖锐湿疣(生殖器疣)、HSV 感染、真菌感染和 CMV 诱导的皮肤血管病变伴肛周会阴溃疡[343,344]。

(三) 移植后长期存活的问题

胃肠道和肝胆问题发生在同种异体 HCT 后的几年,通常是长期急性 GVHD、慢性 GVHD(chronic GVHD,cGVHD)、药物副作用和与免疫相关的感染症状的延续[345,346]。

1. 食管症状

如果存在 cGVHD,胃灼烧可能会恶化,因为唾液腺破坏会减少碳酸氢盐的产生。慢性 GVHD 可累及食管,导致动力障碍,而无法清除反流的胃酸[347]。累及胃的长期急性 GVHD,导致胃潴留以及胃酸和胆汁反流。幸存者食管炎较少见的原因包括真菌和病毒感染以及滞留药物引起的炎症(药物性食管炎)。吞咽困难的常见原因包括食管和口腔 cGVHD、感染、口干和牙列不良[345]。广泛 cGVHD 患者常诉固体食物和药物吞咽困难,儿童还表现为隐匿的体重减轻、胸骨后疼痛及误吸胃内容物,导致肺部疾病可误认为 GVHD 相关的闭塞性细支气管炎综合征。食管 cGVHD 的诊断是通过钡剂造影 X 线或内镜检查进行的,后者应谨慎进行,因为已有穿孔的报道。放射学表现包括肺大泡、蹼、同心环、缩窄、锥形狭窄和蠕动停止[348]。特征性内镜表现食管上段脱屑、独特的食管上蹼。组织学可见食管黏膜淋巴细胞、中性粒细胞和嗜酸性粒细胞浸润;基底层单个鳞状细胞坏死;浅表上皮脱屑。食管 cGVHD 患者通常需要内镜扩张,以避免进行性腔腔狭窄,但扩张必须非常小心,因为穿孔风险高于消化性狭窄。局部糖皮质激素治疗可有效。HCT 后食管鳞状细胞癌的风险是对照组的 8.5 倍;cGVHD 是主要的风险因素[349]。

2. 上消化道症状:厌食、恶心、呕吐和饱腹感

长期生存者的胃十二指肠 GVHD 被称为持续性、复发性或迟发性急性 GVHD,因为无论是在移植后第 100 天前还是数年内,症状、内镜表现和组织学均相同[350]。长期使用口腔

局部糖皮质激素对上消化道 GVHD 迁延不愈的患者可能有效[351]。然而,长期暴露于糖皮质激素引起的肾上腺抑制和的肾上腺功能不全的症状(如厌食、恶心)可能与上消化道 GVHD 相似。局灶性肠狭窄可视为肠道 GVHD 的后遗症。如果停用预防性抗病毒药物和病毒监测,疱疹病毒(HSV,CMV,VZV)可能引起幸存者出现恶心、呕吐和饱腹感。当上消化道症状同时出现腹胀和血清 ALT 水平升高时,应怀疑内脏 VZV 感染,并通过 PCR 检测血液中的 VZV DNA 证实[283,352]。HCT 后可能发生胃轻瘫,通常对促动力药物有反应[353]。

3. 中消化道和结肠症状:腹泻和腹痛

迟发性急性 GVHD 或与急性和慢性 GVHD 重叠的疾病可在移植数年后引起胃肠道症状[354]。一些既往发生过较严重症 GVHD 的患者可发生肠狭窄[354,355]。艰难梭菌、诺如病毒、巨细胞病毒以及罕见的兰氏贾第鞭毛虫和微小隐球菌可能导致散发性肠道感染病例,且可能酷似 GVHD[283,320,321]。在需要阿片类药物治疗的患者中,麻醉性肠综合征可能表现为腹痛和便秘加重[356]。在接受来那度胺治疗的患者中,回肠中胆汁酸吸收不良可能导致持续性低容量腹泻,胆汁酸螯合剂(如考来维仑)可能有用[357]。罕见的肠道疾病"传播"病例,如通过供体 T 细胞传播的乳糜泻也有报道[358]。

4. 肝脏 GVHD

HCT 的长期存活者有 3 种肝脏 GVHD 表现[176,345,346]:①在无黄疸的情况下,血清 ALT、碱性磷酸酶和 GGTP 无症状性升高;②缓慢性进展的胆汁淤积性黄疸伴血清碱性磷酸酶升高,是小胆管损伤的结果(见图 36.5D);③急性肝细胞损伤(肝炎 GVHD),血清 ALT 突然升高至 500U/L 以上,而之前无肝功能障碍。在长期存活者中,黄疸的鉴别诊断比第 100 天之前更窄。胆汁淤积性黄疸的鉴别诊断包括 GVHD、胆道梗阻、DILI 和纤维化胆汁淤积性乙型或丙型肝炎[176]。如果转氨酶升高的原因不明显,可进行肝活检以确定 GVHD 的原因。在免疫抑制方案中添加熊去氧胆酸(12~15mg/kg/d)可显著改善肝脏 GVHD 生化指标[359,360]。重度肝脏 GVHD 可进展为胆管缺失和深度黄疸,可能需要泼尼松、钙调磷酸酶抑制剂和熊去氧胆酸治疗几个月才能消退[251]。一些病例系列,并没有随机试验,却吹捧以下几种作为有效的类固醇节制治疗:环磷酰胺冲击[361]、体外光分离术[362]、改变钙调磷酸酶抑制剂或加用西罗莫司。口服二丙酸倍氯米松或布地奈德可用于治疗肝脏 GVHD,因为这些局部糖皮质激素中分别有 40% 和 90% 到达门静脉循环[363] 和肝脏,这种方法对其他炎症性肝病,如自身免疫性肝炎有效[364]。OLT,包括来自原始造血细胞供体的活体供者移植,已在难治性胆汁淤积或 GVHD 所致的终末期肝病的患者中实行[250,365,366]。在免疫抑制治疗停止或逐渐减量后或供者淋巴细胞输注后可发生肝脏 GVHD[252,253]。患者出现血清 ALT 水平急剧升高、伴或不伴黄疸,表现为病毒感染、DILI 和肝炎 GVHD 的鉴别诊断。这些患者需要紧急诊断和治疗。肝组织学表现包括肝细胞损伤、小叶炎症、小胆管内和周围淋巴细胞浸润、小胆管上皮细胞广泛损伤(和缺失)、胆汁淤积、汇管区纤维化和碎屑样坏死[252]。病毒抗原或病毒 DNA/RNA 的血液检测,将排除疱疹病毒(HSV 或 VZV)、肝炎病毒 A-E 或腺病毒引起的急性肝炎。应在等待疱疹病毒检测结果时开始阿昔洛韦治疗,如果病毒检测结果为阴性,应开始钙调磷酸酶抑制剂和泼尼松(1~2mg/kg/d)治疗,同时等待组织学检查结果,以预防 GVHD 引起的广泛胆管损伤[252]。

5. 慢性病毒性肝炎和肝硬化

在长期 HCT 存活的慢性丙型肝炎患者中,肝硬化发生的中位时间为 10~18 年,而对照组为 40 年[367,368]。采用肝活检或非侵入性方法(如瞬时弹性成像)确认肝硬化是至关重要的[369],以便监测患者的并发症,包括食管静脉曲张和肝细胞癌。慢性丙型肝炎也可能是移植后发生淋巴瘤和其他淋巴增生性疾病的风险因素[370,371]。所有慢性 HCV 幸存者,包括肝硬化患者,均应接受抗病毒治疗,除非存在禁忌证[198]。直接作用抗病毒药物组合高度有效且耐受性良好。无干扰素治疗方案在 HCT 后患者中特别有吸引力,其中干扰素诱导慢性 GVHD 激活的可能性是一个问题。

由于免疫抑制,HCT 幸存者 HBV 感染的血清学模式可能不典型。可观察到表面抗原血症的清除,如果献血者既往 HBV 感染抗-HBs 阳性或对疫苗接种产生强烈应答,则特别可能清除表面抗原血症[192,372]。HCT 后 HBsAg 仍为阳性的患者存在乙型肝炎活动复发的风险,特别是在免疫抑制减少时,如慢性 GVHD 治疗逐渐减量或停止期间,这些患者应在停止免疫抑制治疗后服用抗病毒药物如替诺福韦或恩替卡韦 12 个月[373]。应定期监测所有慢性乙型肝炎长期存活者,以评估病毒学和疾病状态以及是否需要抗病毒治疗[374,375]。由于担心 cGVHD 的发作,不推荐聚乙二醇干扰素用于同种异体 HCT 幸存者。在重新化疗前应重新评估 HBV 病毒状态[373]。生物制剂,如用于治疗 B 细胞恶性肿瘤的利妥昔单抗,具有特别高的隐匿性乙型肝炎再激活风险(HBsAg 阴性和抗 HBc 阳性),建议采用预防性抗病毒治疗[376]。与在围移植期一样,HBsAg 阳性患者在接受免疫抑制或细胞毒性治疗时应接受抗病毒药物治疗。

6. 腹水

HCT 生存者新发腹水的最常见原因是肝硬化(例如慢性丙肝患者肝硬化进展加速[367,368],而肝脏 GVHD 患者罕见),以及非肝硬化患者的结节性再生性肝增生(在特发性非肝硬化性门静脉高压范畴)[377]。因为肝脏成像和楔形肝静脉压测量均可能误导正常,致使结节性再生性增生的诊断可能具有挑战性[378]。HCT 后结节性再生性增生的预后通常良好,尽管处理并发症可能需要频繁的大量穿刺或行 TIPS[379]。HCT 后不明原因腹水的其他可能包括缩窄性心包炎、胰源性腹水、腹膜转移癌和与 cGVHD 相关的浆膜炎综合征[380]。

7. 其他肝脏疾病

接受 HCT 的患者中,发生 DILI 与抗高血压药物、降脂药、降糖药、非甾体抗炎药、抗抑郁药、抗生素、抗真菌药或中草药制剂相关[204]。虽然大多数 DILI 对停药有反应,但一些药物反应可导致慢性肝病。与一般人群相比,患者新发实体器官恶性肿瘤的发生率是预期的两倍[381]。由于慢性丙型肝炎感染率的增加,肝细胞癌的风险特别升高。根据国际指南,有肝细胞癌危险因素(HCV 肝硬化、慢性 HBV 感染或任何原因的肝硬化)的移植幸存者,应每 6 个月接受一次肝脏超声监测[382]。在 HCT 基础肝脏 MRI 的一个儿科存活者系列中,5.2% 存在偶发局灶性结节性增生病变[383]。这些病变具有特征性的中央瘢痕，可与肝细胞癌和真菌性病变相鉴别。由于它们在MRI上的表现非常具有特征性[384]，通常不需要肝脏活检。然而，当有明显局灶性结节性增生的患者血清AFP水平升高时，可能需要活检以排除肝细胞癌[385]。由真菌和细菌引起的肝脏感染是现在罕见的晚期并发症。幸存者服用被真菌受污染的非无菌中草药制剂也可能导致肝脓肿[386]。

8. 胆囊和胆道疾病

长期HCT存活者胆结石和胆结石并发症的发病率增加，这与清髓预处理治疗后与胆红素钙微粒(胆泥)的形成有关[268,387]。环孢素和可能的他克莫司，可诱发胆固醇性结石[388,389]。胆泥和胆结石可能引起胆囊管梗阻、胆管梗阻和急性胰腺炎[270]。

9. 胰腺疾病

急性胰腺炎在长期HCT存活者中罕见，大多数病例与胆道结石或(罕见)与他克莫司相关的胰腺损伤有关[390]。HCT后的胰腺萎缩导致的胰腺功能不全已被报道，胰腺萎缩可由CT或MRI检查发现[391,392]。

10. 铁过载

在红细胞生成无效的情况下，反复输血和胃肠道铁吸收增加均可引起继发性铁过载。严重铁过载的发病率主要来自心脏铁蓄积，其仅与肝脏铁含量略微相关[393]。铁特异性MRI方法不仅可以准确测量肝脏铁，还可以准确测量心脏、垂体、胰腺和甲状腺中的铁调节[394]。持续性铁过载对长期HCT结局的影响尚未得到充分研究，但因地中海贫血而接受移植的患者除外，在这些患者中，极高的铁负荷转化为心脏原因导致的死亡率增加。铁过载可能是HCT存活者发病和非复发死亡的危险因素，其铁负荷远低于地中海贫血患者，尽管铁状态的最佳指标仍有待确定[176,395]。异体HCT后第100天前死亡的患者，其肝脏铁水平在血色病范围内(1 832～13 120mg/g干重)[396]。

(刘晖 译，闫秀娥 李鹏 校)

参考文献

第37章　系统性疾病的胃肠道和肝脏表现

Frederick Weber 著

章节目录

一、胶原血管及炎性疾病 503
（一）类风湿性关节炎 503
（二）成人型 Still 病 505
（三）系统性硬化 506
（四）系统性红斑狼疮 507
（五）肌病 508
（六）干燥综合征（SjÖgren 综合征） 508
（七）混合性结缔组织病 509
（八）结节性多动脉炎 509
（九）过敏性紫癜 509
（十）嗜酸性肉芽肿性多血管炎 510
（十一）肉芽肿性血管炎 510
（十二）冷球蛋白血症 510
（十三）白塞病 510
（十四）脊柱关节病 511
（十五）家族性地中海热 511
（十六）结缔组织疾病 511
（十七）IgG4 相关性疾病 511
二、肿瘤与血液系统疾病 511
（一）胃肠道转移瘤 511
（二）副肿瘤综合征 512
（三）血液系统恶性肿瘤 512
（四）系统性肥大细胞增多症 513
（五）骨髓性和骨髓增生性疾病 514
（六）蛋白异常血症 515
（七）红细胞异常 515
（八）凝血功能障碍 517
三、内分泌疾病 517
（一）糖尿病 517
（二）甲状腺疾病 519
（三）甲状旁腺疾病 520
（四）肾上腺疾病 520
（五）脑垂体疾病 520
四、脂质代谢紊乱 520
五、肾脏疾病 521
六、神经系统疾病 522
（一）中枢神经系统疾病 522
（二）脊髓损伤 522
（三）锥体外系（运动）障碍 523
（四）自主神经系统疾病 523
（五）神经肌肉接头疾病 523
（六）肌营养不良 523
七、肺部疾病 524
八、危重症 524
九、脓毒症 524
十、心血管疾病 525
十一、浸润性疾病 525
（一）淀粉样变 525
（二）肉芽肿性肝病 527
（三）结节病 527
（四）其他 530

诸多系统性疾病都有胃肠道及肝脏表现，本章主要对常见的和近期有进展的疾病进行讨论。系统性疾病可以直接累及胃肠道/肝脏的结构、功能或两者同时受累，胃肠道和肝脏也可能受到治疗的影响间接受累。需要留意的是，一些罕见疾病如系统性硬化病（硬皮病）和淀粉样变等通常在三级医院诊治，从而可能会有倾向认为这些患者病情较重。读者也可参阅其他章节，其中对具体的系统性疾病的胃肠道和肝脏表现进行了更详细的讨论。

一、胶原血管及炎性疾病（表 37.1）

（一）类风湿性关节炎

在北美及欧洲，类风湿性关节炎（rheumatoid arthritis，RA）的患病率为 0.5%～1%[1,2]。RA 的胃肠道症状很常见，且很大程度上与药物，尤其是非甾体抗炎药（NSAIDs）的使用相关。口腔干燥和颞下颌关节、颈椎和喉部（尤其是环杓关节）受累可导致口咽部症状[3,4]。寰枢关节半脱位可导致吞咽困难以及其他脊髓受压的表现，对此类患者行内镜检查应慎重。食管运动功能障碍以食管下 2/3 段蠕动乏力以及食管下括约肌（lower esophageal sphincter，LES）压力降低为特征，患者常表现为烧心、吞咽困难和食管炎。相关的类风湿性血管炎，干燥综合征（Sjögren syndrome，SS）和淀粉样变（稍后讨论）也可能导致食管症状和运动功能障碍，并且血管炎可造成缺血而导致食管狭窄。

消化性溃疡可能与使用抗炎药物有关。在 RA 患者的活检标本中，慢性浅表性和慢性萎缩性胃炎分别占 30% 和 65%。约 1/3 的 RA 患者有低氯血症或胃酸缺乏症，易出现小肠细菌过度生长（small bowel bacterial overgrowth，SBBO）。高胃泌素血症可能与胃酸缺乏症、抗壁细胞抗体、维生素 B_{12}

表 37.1　胶原血管及炎性疾病的胃肠道表现

疾病	病变	临床表现
类风湿关节炎	颞下颌关节炎	咀嚼功能受损
	食管运动功能障碍	吞咽困难、胃灼热
	血管炎	肠道溃疡与梗死、穿孔、出血
	淀粉样变性	假性肠梗阻、吸收不良、PLGE、肠道溃疡与梗死、胃出口梗阻
	Felty 综合征	肝脾肿大、肝生化检查异常
成人型 Still 病	肝脏病变	肝脾肿大、肝生化检查异常、高铁蛋白血症
系统性硬化	食管运动功能障碍	吞咽困难、胃灼热、巴雷特食管、食管念珠菌病
	胃轻瘫	恶心、消化不良
	肠道运动功能障碍	便秘、假性肠梗阻、吸收不良、PLGE、SIBO、肠壁囊样积气、真性憩室
	胰腺病变	胰腺外分泌功能障碍、钙化性胰腺炎
	肛管功能障碍	大便失禁、直肠脱垂
	消化道出血	胃窦血管扩张、毛细血管扩张
系统性红斑狼疮	肠系膜血管炎	肠缺血、溃疡
	食管运动功能障碍	吞咽困难、胃灼热
	胰腺病变	胰腺炎
	浆膜炎	腹水、腹膜炎
	肝脏病变	肝生化检查异常、肝炎
多发性肌炎/皮肌炎	骨骼肌功能障碍	吞咽功能受损、舌无力、误吸、吞咽困难
	胃肠道运动障碍	胃灼热、吞咽困难、胃轻瘫、假性肠梗阻、肠壁囊样积气
干燥综合征	口腔干燥	口角炎、龋齿、口腔念珠菌病、声音嘶哑
	食管运动功能障碍	吞咽困难
	胰腺病变	胰腺炎
	肝脏病变	肝生化检查异常、PBC、AIH、HCV 感染
混合性结缔组织病	食管运动功能障碍	胃灼热、吞咽困难
	硬皮病样改变	吸收不良、PLGE、假性肠梗阻、肠壁囊样积气
	血管炎	肠道缺血、溃疡、穿孔
结节性多动脉炎	血管炎	肠道缺血、溃疡、穿孔，动脉瘤，非结石性胆囊炎，硬化性胆管炎，胰腺病变，HBV 感染相关
过敏性紫癜	血管炎	腹痛、消化道出血、肠套叠
嗜酸性肉芽肿性多血管炎	嗜酸细胞浸润期	嗜酸细胞性胃肠炎、嗜酸细胞性腹水
	血管炎期	腹痛、出血、肠溃疡、穿孔
肉芽肿性多血管炎	口腔病变	口腔溃疡、牙龈增生（草莓牙龈）、舌梗死
	血管炎	食管及胃溃疡，肠道缺血伴溃疡及穿孔，胰腺炎，坏疽性胆囊炎
白塞病	血管炎	口腔溃疡、回盲部溃疡及穿孔、淀粉样变
	大血管病变	门静脉或肝静脉血栓形成、动脉瘤
脊柱关节病	相关肠道炎症	急性表现类似于细菌性肠炎
		慢性表现类似于克罗恩病
家族性地中海热	浆膜炎/淀粉样变	腹膜炎、急腹症样症状
Cogan 综合征	克罗恩病	血性腹泻、腹痛、瘘管、肛裂
	肠系膜血管炎（少见）	出血、溃疡、肠梗死、肠套叠
马方综合征/Ehlers Danlos 综合征/关节过度活动综合征	胶原蛋白缺陷	巨食管、动力不足、憩室、巨结肠、吸收不良、穿孔、动脉破裂
IgG4 相关性疾病	浸润/纤维化	自身免疫性胰腺炎、硬化性胆管炎、肝炎、腹膜后纤维化、炎性假瘤、主动脉炎、硬化性肠系膜炎、小肠炎、结肠炎、储袋炎

AIH，自身免疫性肝炎；PLGE，蛋白丢失性胃肠病。

缺乏或恶性贫血有关[3,5,6]。

类风湿关节炎有时也与溃疡性结肠炎相关，且类风湿性血管炎的临床表现与炎症性肠病（IBD）相似[7-9]。与 RA 不同，IBD 相关的外周关节病变通常类风湿因子（rheumatoid factor，RF）为阴性、无关节变形且为非侵蚀性病变，RA 患者很少出现肠壁囊样积气（图 37.1）。

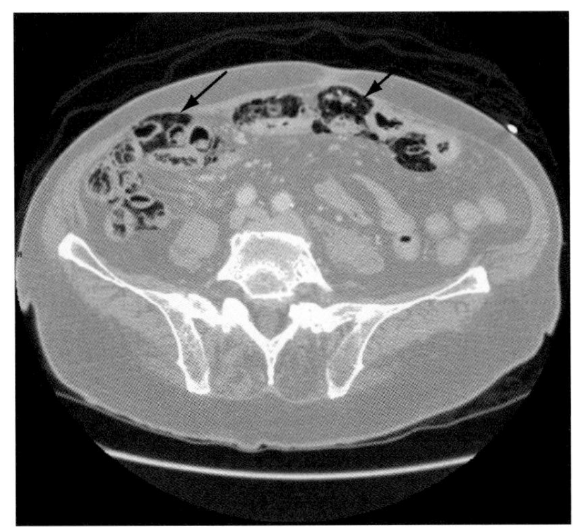

图 37.1　CT 显示一例类风湿性关节炎（RA）患者肠壁囊样积气（箭头）。（From Ebert EC，Hagspiel KD. Gastrointestinal and hepatic manifestations of rheumatoid arthritis. Dig Dis Sci 2011；56：295-302，with permission from Springer.）

1%～5% 的 RA 患者可出现类风湿性血管炎，这是一种中小血管的炎症性疾病，通常这些患者疾病程度较重且类风湿因子滴度较高[10,11]。这些患者中约 10%～38% 有肠道受累，常伴有皮肤（手指坏疽、皮肤溃疡）和周围神经系统（神经病变、多发性单神经炎）表现。肠道小血管受累可导致缺血性溃疡、疼痛和出血；当累及大血管时可导致肠梗死、狭窄形成、肠穿孔或腹腔积血。部分小样本非对照研究显示糖皮质激素和/或环磷酰胺可用于治疗血管炎。值得注意的是，使用托法替尼或托珠单抗治疗的 RA 患者下消化道穿孔的发生率也有所增加，而这种情况在使用 TNF 抑制剂治疗的患者中没有发现。

1. 肝脏受累

RA 通常无肝脏受累的临床表现。患者的血清转氨酶和胆红素水平通常正常，而血清碱性磷酸酶（肝和骨同工酶）可能升高[12-14]。包括汇管区炎症、充血、肝脂肪变、肝窦扩张、淀粉样变性、汇管周围纤维化和结节性再生性增生在内的肝脏组织学改变无特异性[15]。RA 很少与原发性胆汁性肝硬化、自身免疫性胆管病和自身免疫性肝炎（autoimmune hepatitis，AIH）相关[14,16,17]。

Felty 综合征是中性粒细胞减少、脾大和严重 RA 的三联征，其可能与肝大和肝脏生化检查异常有关。门静脉高压可能是由于肝脏微结构改变（结节性再生增生）或脾大引起的脾血流量增加所致。对于脾大所致的门静脉高压，行脾切除术可治疗静脉曲张[18]。由于 HCV 感染和 RA 均为常见疾病，故而患者可能同时罹患丙肝和 RA。HCV 感染患者常有关节痛、干燥综合征和肌痛，并且可表达 RF 和抗核抗体（ANA）[19]。因此有一部分 HCV 感染患者可出现混合性冷球蛋白血症伴有关节炎表现，与 RA 难以鉴别。HCV 感染所致的关节炎通常是累及大中型关节的非破坏性单关节炎或少关节炎。抗环瓜氨酸肽抗体很少在这些患者中出现，因此可以作为 RA 的可靠标志物[20]。用 TNF-α 拮抗剂治疗 RA 通常不会导致潜在 HCV 的再激活，但长期影响尚不明确[21]。一项对 216 名暴露于一种或多种 TNF 拮抗剂的 HCV 感染患者的研究显示，在 260 个累积患者年中，仅有 3 例因肝脏问题停药[22]。然而，抗 TNF-α 治疗和其他免疫抑制剂却可能激活乙型肝炎病毒（HBV），因此合并 HBV 感染的患者可能需要抗病毒治疗[23]。在因 RA 接受常规免疫抑制治疗的 HB 表面抗原（sAg）阳性或 HB 核心抗体（cAb）阳性的患者中，约 2% 会出现 HBV 再激活[24]。

2. 药物副作用

水杨酸类药物引起的肝毒性通常无临床症状，最常见于大剂量用药时[3,25]。血清丙氨酸氨基转移酶（ALT）升高水平与水杨酸类药物的剂量呈正相关，并且 ALT 水平可在阿司匹林停药或减量后的数天内恢复正常。肝脏活检可见汇管区单核细胞浸润，肝细胞坏死很少，很少出现严重的肝坏死。少数情况下，NSAIDs 可能出现肝毒性，特别是与其他有潜在肝毒性的药物联用时[26]。布洛芬与包括胆管消失综合征在内的肝细胞或胆汁淤积性疾病有关。

柳氮磺吡啶可引起迟发性超敏反应，偶尔会导致肝衰竭[27]。患者通常在开始用药的 6 周内出现皮疹、淋巴结肿大、恶心、呕吐、嗜酸性粒细胞增多，以及肝细胞性或混合性肝损伤。

甲氨蝶呤与肝纤维化和肝硬化有关，尤其是在银屑病而非类风湿性关节炎患者中。高达 25% 的 RA 患者可能有轻度的血清转氨酶升高，但尚不清楚转氨酶升高与肝纤维化或肝硬化的关系。尽管糖尿病、肥胖、饮酒和非酒精性脂肪性肝病（NAFLD）等因素可能起作用，但慢性乙型肝炎和丙型肝炎对其无影响[28]。硫唑嘌呤和巯基嘌呤与无症状血清转氨酶一过性升高、胆汁淤积性损伤和以紫癜性肝炎，结节性再生性增生和肝窦阻塞综合征为特征的慢性肝损伤有关，通常发生在治疗的前 5 年。也可能增加淋巴瘤和肝细胞癌的风险。很少有关于肝脾 T 细胞淋巴瘤的报道，大多出现在硫唑嘌呤和 TNF 抑制剂联合治疗的年轻男性中，其表现为发热、乏力、全血细胞减少和肝脾肿大。可通过骨髓或肝活检确诊，该病预后差。来氟米特可引起腹泻和肝毒性，通常在用药的前 6 个月内发生，并且和肝脏硬度异常升高相关，尤其当与甲氨蝶呤联用时更为显著[29]。

（二）成人型 Still 病

成人型 Still 病（成人型幼年型类风湿关节炎）是一种炎症性疾病，表现为骤起骤降的高热、咽炎、一过性斑丘疹、关节痛/关节炎和中性粒细胞增多[30-32]。患者腹痛通常较轻且短暂，但也可严重。偶尔可发现小肠扩张和气液平面。患者常有肝脾肿大和淋巴结肿大。实验室检测可见铁蛋白明显升高[33]，C 反应蛋白（CRP）和血沉（ESR）升高，而 ANA 和 RF 阴性或滴度较低[34]。50%～75% 的患者可出现肝功能异常，通常是轻微的、一过性的，与疾病活动度有关。偶可发展为重型肝炎，甚至暴发性肝衰竭，导致死亡或需肝移植。肝脏组织学可无异常，表现为汇管区单核细胞浸润或与 AIH 类似的淋巴浆细胞浸润的界面性肝炎。可有门静脉血栓形成[35]。药物治疗包括 NSAIDs、糖皮质激素、甲氨蝶呤、环孢素和阿那白滞素，阿那白滞素罕有肝毒性报道[36]。

（三）系统性硬化

超过 90% 的原发性系统性硬化病（PSS）患者有消化道症状，以食管症状为主[37]。患者常以厌食、反流、吞咽困难、早饱、恶心、腹胀、腹泻、便秘、大便失禁和社会心理健康程度下降为主诉[37,38]。常见营养不良，偶尔需要肠外营养[38]。引起营养不良的原因包括厌食、胃排空延迟、吸收不良、小肠细菌过度生长及小肠蠕动缓慢。

长期以来的理论认为首先出现神经病变过程，而后随着肌肉萎缩和纤维化的发展出现肌病过程。只有在第一阶段，促胃肠动力药才是有效的[39,40]。血清抗毒蕈碱-3 乙酰胆碱自身抗体可阻断神经传递，从而导致继发性组织/肌肉萎缩[41]。在部分 PSS 患者中也可能发现与肌炎相关的抗体[42]。

1. 食管受累

PSS 食管受累可出现胃灼热、反流和吞咽困难。引起反流的原因有：①食管蠕动减弱/缺失；②LES 压力降低；③短食管型食管裂孔疝；④胃轻瘫；⑤自主神经功能障碍；⑥伴唾液碳酸氢盐丢失的干燥综合征；⑦因咳嗽和用力而引起的腹压升高[43]。

PSS 患者可出现巴雷特食管，罹患食管腺癌的风险增加[44,45]，尽管最常见的恶性肿瘤可能是肺癌。PSS 患者因食管排空缓慢、使用免疫抑制剂和抑制胃酸而易出现念珠菌性食管炎。药物与黏膜接触时间延长可继发药物性食管炎。PSS 主要累及食管下三分之二的平滑肌。食管上段主要由横纹肌组成，通常不受累，除非出现近端反流[46]。采用食管测压判断是否具有运动障碍有助于诊断 PSS。典型表现为食管下三分之二收缩或蠕动幅度降低，以及 LES 压力降低或消失（图 37.2）。然而，这些发现在 PSS 中并非普遍可见，也不是 PSS 特有的，也可见于其他疾病：如淀粉样变性、糖尿病、慢性酒精中毒、食管念珠菌病、严重反流、甲状腺功能减退和其他结缔组织疾病[43]。200 例硬皮病患者（117 例局限性硬皮病，83 例弥漫性硬皮病）接受了高分辨率测压，并根据芝加哥分类标准对其结果进行了分类，无论是局限性还是弥漫性硬皮病，最常见的是无收缩（56%）、动力正常（26%）和无效运动（10%）。仅在 33% 的患者中观察到典型的食管硬皮病。严重的运动障碍与病程、间质性肺病和胃肠道症状评分有关[47]。此外，在 111 例系统性硬化症患者（89 名女性）中，进行了多次快速吞咽的高分辨率测压，多次快速吞咽期间的蠕动增加幅度（18%）远低于年轻健康对照组（100%）。蠕动储备异常是系统性硬化症患者最常见的测压异常[48]。食管阻抗检测显示食团清除不完全[46,49,50]。和贲门失弛缓症一样，影像学检查可能显示食管扩张，但是 PSS 不存在机械性阻塞，因此除非存在狭窄，否则观察不到气液平面。即使患者没有症状，内镜检查也经常显示异常[51]。腔内超声检查可见食管固有肌层出现高回声异常，被认为是代表纤维化[43]。反流可能通过吸入胃内容物和/或食管中的胃内容物刺激迷走神经而引起肺部疾病。相反，肺病时由于通气所需的胸腔内负压升高以及支气管扩张剂降低 LES 压力，从而导致反流。

在 PSS 患者中，胃食管反流与间质性肺疾病有关[43,52,53]；这些临床表现可能会一起演变。虽然两者的因果关系尚不明确，在腔内嗜碱性内容物与消化性坏死一致的 PSS 患者中，21% 出现了呈支气管中心性分布的小叶中心性纤维化，这提示存在胃内容物吸入的肺部反应[54]。肺部疾病是 PSS 的主要死因，且对治疗的反应不佳。防止误吸和针对反流的生活方式改善很有必要。

PPI 可以治愈食管炎，甚至可以逆转食管纤维化[55]。剂量可能需要高于标准剂量的 PPI，但可能无法阻止运动障碍的进展[56]。目前尚不明确 PPI 是否能改善 PSS 的肺部疾病

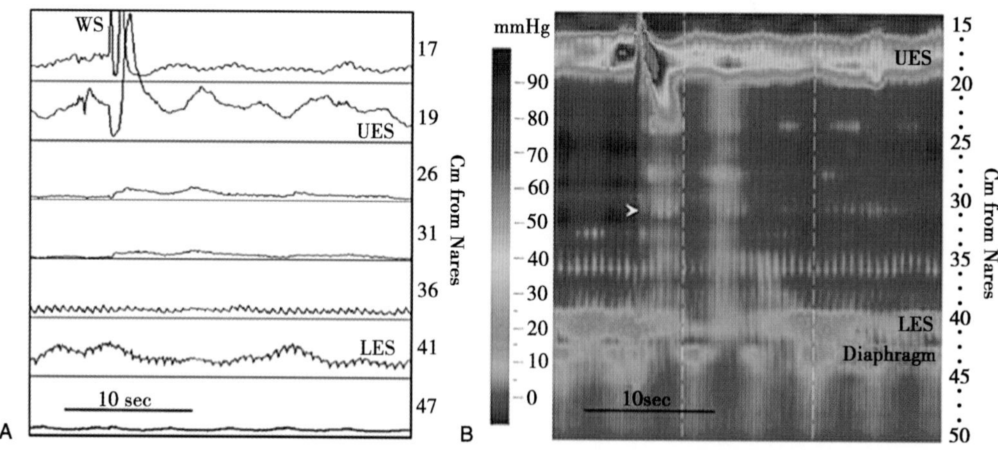

图 37.2　A，PSS 患者在线模式的高分辨率测压（HRM）。嘱患者湿吞咽（WS）可使食管上括约肌（UES）正常松弛，但无食管蠕动。很难确定食管下括约肌（LES）是否松弛。B，在 HRM 彩色轮廓图中，横纹肌食管的 UES 和蠕动是正常的。食管平滑肌未见蠕动。在胃食管交界处，有一小的食管裂孔疝，LES 适当松弛。WS 产生与 UES 开放一致的团注压力（视为同时向浅蓝色或更高压力移动）（箭头）。在没有蠕动压力波的情况下，浅蓝色仅缓慢恢复到空食管中观察到的深蓝色，表明食团未从食管中清除。（From Conklin J，Pimentel M，Soffer E. Color atlas of high resolution manometry. New York：Springer Science and Business Media；2009. Fig. 2. 23，p 38，with permission.）

情况。在疾病的早期，促动力药也许有效。丁螺环酮（一种5HT1受体激动剂）可能对改善食管蠕动和LES功能有利。一项用丁螺环酮（20mg/d）治疗30例PPI难治性PSS患者的开放标签试验结果显示，4周后静息LES压力显著增加，胃灼热和反流评分显著降低[57]。考虑到食管无蠕动时吞咽困难可能加重，胃底折叠术的治疗效果有限[43]。Roux-en-Y胃旁路术可作为一种选择[58]。

2. 胃受累

原发性系统性硬化病常表现为固体食物为主的胃排空延迟，从而可能出现早饱、腹胀、恶心和呕吐，也可无症状[59,60]。应除外胃出口梗阻和消化性溃疡，尤其在应用NSAIDs的患者中。超声内镜可能显示胃壁增厚，尤其是黏膜下层和肌层[61]。目前，对PSS胃排空延迟的治疗尚无广泛研究[62]。此外，患者可有胃窦血管扩张。

3. 小肠受累

PSS小肠功能障碍的实际患病率尚不清楚。除小肠细菌过度生长或罕见的乳糜泻外，小肠的吸收能力是正常的[63]。PSS患者小肠通透性可能增加，进而出现蛋白丢失性胃肠病（protein-losing gastroenteropathy，PLGE）或吸收不良[64]。病情严重者可出现肠衰竭，需要静脉营养且预后不良。

PSS患者常见口盲肠通过时间延长[65]以及小肠测压异常[66,67]。缺乏、异常或不协调的移行性复合运动提示PSS神经病变过程，而收缩幅度降低表明已发展到肌病过程。

小肠可能因钡剂的絮凝和淤积而扩张。肠绷紧征为弥漫性肠管扩张伴密集的小肠皱襞，后者由小肠固有肌层纵行纤维萎缩后缩短肠管而形成的[68]。空肠和结肠可出现包含肠壁全层的真憩室，其颈部宽大，不易发生憩室炎[60]。患者可无任何症状，也可表现为腹痛、呕吐、出血、穿孔或小肠细菌过度生长。少数情况可见肠壁囊样积气（见图37.1）、假性肠梗阻或气腹[69,70]。

由于存在口盲肠通过时间延长、正常的移行性复合运动缺失、憩室以及使用PPI引起胃内pH升高，PSS患者常有小肠细菌过度生长[71]。抗生素治疗可改善症状，有时联合每日小剂量的奥曲肽治疗，这可能会改善PSS患者移行性复合运动的第Ⅲ相。

4. 结肠受累

PSS患者常有结肠受累，但多数患者可无症状。部分患者可表现为大便性状改变、腹胀、排便不畅、大便失禁和直肠出血[72]。结肠造影的典型表现为肠腔积液、排空不全及结肠袋消失伴扩张[60]。

结肠受累的并发症包括假性肠梗阻、粪石慢性嵌顿所致的直肠和乙状结肠溃疡、肠扭转、穿孔、结肠狭窄、直肠脱垂、肠壁囊样积气和良性气腹[59,60]。

对于食管功能受损且有误吸风险的患者，应避免口服矿物油。渗透性泻药可能会加重假性梗阻。对于促动力药物的疗效尚缺乏研究数据。一篇报道中使用普卢卡必利（一种$5\text{-}HT_4$受体激动剂）在2名PSS患者的治疗中获得了成功，但仍需进一步研究[73]。奥曲肽可能对难治性病例有效，并可与红霉素联合使用[74,75]。

5. 肛门受累

腹泻、肛门功能障碍、直肠脱垂和长期排便用力可引起大便失禁。肛管内超声和功能性管腔成像探头可发现由平滑肌组成的肛门内括约肌（IAS）萎缩、变薄[76,77]。患者可出现肛门括约肌静息张力降低、肛门感觉阈值减低、直肠顺应性降低以及出现直肠-肛门抑制反射受损[78,79]。治疗方法包括生物反馈疗法（常不成功）和骶神经刺激，但研究数据有限[80]。类似胃窦血管扩张，患者直肠也可出现西瓜状血管条纹，伴固有层毛细血管扩张和血栓形成[81]。此外，毛细血管扩张可发生于胃肠道的任何部分，并且可能是消化道出血的原因。

6. 其他问题

有病例报告表明，特发性钙化性胰腺炎和动脉炎可导致胰腺缺血性坏死[60,82]。抗着丝粒抗体是PSS的标志性抗体，可在9%～30%的PBC患者中出现，25%的PSS患者抗线粒体抗体（AMA）呈阳性。合并PSS的PBC患者的肝病进展较单纯PBC患者缓慢[12,13,83]。

（四）系统性红斑狼疮

系统性红斑狼疮（SLE）是一种累及多个系统的自身免疫性疾病[84,85]。SLE常有胃肠道症状（如：恶心/呕吐、厌食、腹痛），但往往较轻微。这些症状在成人中病因多样，严重程度不同，有时与狼疮无关。在儿童中腹痛常与SLE相关，常见于血管炎、胰腺炎和/或腹膜炎/腹水[86,87]。

1. 血管炎

在无法留取病理时，血管炎也被称为狼疮性肠炎，累及9.7%的SLE患者，其中高达65%表现为急腹症[88]。其炎症型的特征为血管壁内免疫复合物沉积所致的白细胞破碎性血管炎，而血栓型则是由抗磷脂抗体相关的血管内血栓形成引起的，且两者可相互激活。临床表现可以从轻微症状到急腹症，几乎总是伴有全身活动性疾病[88-90]。通常有疼痛、恶心呕吐、压痛、低补体血症和白细胞减少。并发症包括有症状的肠道缺血、梗死、狭窄形成、出血和穿孔。

CT的典型表现为：肠壁增厚、靶征或双晕征、肠段扩张、齿梳征（肠系膜血管栅栏样突出）、腹水，在疾病晚期还可见肠壁囊样积气症或肠系膜静脉积气[91]。空肠和回肠是最常受累的部位，病变为节段性或多灶性，而不是像血栓栓塞性缺血那样局限于血管供血区域[89]。肠系膜血管造影可用于除外结节性多动脉炎（PAN），而由于SLE通常累及中小动脉，故肠系膜血管造影常为阴性。内镜下可见缺血和深凿样溃疡，其间黏膜正常，但结肠镜检查偶可诱发缺血性结肠炎和/或穿孔[92]。

除非对黏膜下血管取样，否则内镜活检一般不能明确诊断。其组织病理学表现为：小血管的动静脉炎及其导致的弥漫性同心性纤维化、病变血管内血栓形成及纤维蛋白样坏死、白细胞破碎和炎性浸润[88]。

患者通常对糖皮质激素反应良好[88,89]，难治性患者可考虑使用环磷酰胺。抗磷脂抗体综合征和机会性感染的患者由于免疫低下，常可出现类似胃肠道血管炎的症状，应予以鉴别[93]。

2. 食管和胃肠道受累

SLE食管受累主要表现为胃灼热，有时会因食管运动功能障碍以及出现与干燥综合征相关的唾液分泌减少而出现吞咽困难加重。虽然SLE患者食管运动功能障碍可发生在食管的任何部位，但其发生率较 PSS 或混合性结缔组织病（mixed connective tissue disease，MCTD）低[94]。患者也可出现食管上段和咽部受累，但目前尚不清楚是这由 SLE 还是其合并的多发性肌炎所致。SLE 本身或其重叠的 PSS 或 MCTD 也可引起食管下段蠕动停止伴括约肌张力减退。

胃受累则表现为消化不良。目前尚不清楚狼疮是否存在与 NSAIDs 和/或糖皮质激素的协同或额外作用而引起胃溃疡。SLE 患者可能存在血清 B_{12} 水平低下、内因子抗体阳性，少部分患者可出现恶性贫血[84,85]。

尽管 SLE 所致的低白蛋白血症常归因于肾病综合征，但也应警惕疾病加重、肝病以及肠道大量丢失。蛋白丢失性胃肠病有时是系统性红斑狼疮最初的表现，且青年女性多见，特征表现为明显的低白蛋白血症、腹水、胸腔或心包积液、外周水肿以及低血清补体水平[95-97]；而腹痛或腹泻等胃肠道症状少见。小肠是蛋白丢失的主要部位，结肠的蛋白丢失则不多见[96]。其可能的机制包括微血管/内皮细胞通透性增加，补体介导的血管损伤以及血管炎。除此以外，其他一些病因如心包积液/缩窄和小肠细菌过度生长等也可导致 SLE 患者出现蛋白丢失性胃肠病（见第 31 章）。

乳糜泻与 SLE 之间也存在一定的关系。虽然有研究表明乳糜泻患者发生 SLE 的概率升高了 3 倍，但发展为 SLE 的 10 年绝对风险较低，最多为每 1 000 人中出现 2 人[98]。SLE 可与 IBD、嗜酸性粒细胞性肠炎和胶原性结肠炎合并存在，提示其中可能存在些许关联[84,85,99]。

免疫抑制的 SLE 患者可能会感染巨细胞病毒（CMV），症状类似于以肠炎和/或胰腺炎为表现的狼疮活动[100,101]。此外，SLE 患者常可见到沙门氏菌感染[102,103]。出现发热和腹痛的菌血症较之于腹泻更为多见，并且患者的血液较粪便更容易分离出病原微生物。致病的危险因素包括：免疫抑制、低补体水平、机体病原微生物清除能力受损和脾功能减退。SLE 和沙门氏菌感染均可出现胸膜炎、滑膜炎、血细胞减少和皮疹等类似症状。与健康对照组相比，系统性红斑狼疮患者中贾第鞭毛虫病的发病率有所增加[104]。

肠壁囊样积气（见图 37.1）和气腹均为 SLE 相关的良性病变，发生率较低[105]。假性肠梗阻（见第 124 章）病因多样，常见于活动性狼疮且有时为疾病的首发表现。它与输尿管肾盂积水和间质性膀胱炎有关[84,106,107]。通常糖皮质激素治疗有效。

3. 胰腺和胆囊受累

在 SLE 患者中，SLE 相关胰腺炎的年发病率约为每 1 000 人中 0.4~1 人[108]，但可能遗漏了亚临床病例，且其他原因所致的胰腺炎在 SLE 中也很常见[109]。大约 22% 的病例以胰腺炎为首发症状。患者通常有活动性狼疮[110]。只有极少数患者会出现抗磷脂抗体相关的血管病变[108]。糖皮质激素的使用降低了疾病的死亡率[108]，也可能需要加用硫唑嘌呤。慢性胰腺炎罕见，这些患者此前通常有急性胰腺炎反复发作，且无胰腺外分泌或内分泌功能不全[111]。

SLE 患者可出现原发性硬化性胆管炎和自身免疫性胆管炎[84,112]。明显的胆总管不规则可能是由于既往亚临床的血管炎发作影响了脆弱的壁内毛细血管网。而血管炎或血栓形成可能导致急性非结石性胆囊炎[113]。外科手术治疗为常用手段，对于无胆囊扩张和败血症的患者可考虑使用糖皮质激素。

4. 腹水及腹膜炎

SLE 患者易出现腹水可因多种原因所致：如感染、心力衰竭、肠梗死、肾病综合征、蛋白丢失性胃肠病、缩窄性心包炎、胰腺炎、肠系膜血管炎、布-加综合征或浆膜炎[114]。较之于腹膜炎，浆膜炎更多为胸膜炎或心包炎[115]。急性狼疮性腹膜炎的腹水往往发展迅速，伴腹痛及狼疮活动。而慢性腹膜炎患者腹水发展缓慢且多为无痛性。无菌性腹水中可能出现补体水平低、ANA 阳性、抗 DNA 抗体水平升高以及典型的低血清腹水白蛋白梯度（<11g/L）。糖皮质激素治疗对腹膜炎可能有效，也可能需要额外的免疫抑制治疗。

5. 肝脏受累

虽然 SLE 患者肝脏生化检查常存在异常，但却很少发展为终末期肝病[13,116]。肝损害的病因多样，包括脂肪肝、肝动脉炎、PBC、AIH、结节性再生性增生、病毒性肝炎、药物反应（见 RA 部分）。有学者认为 SLE 肝炎是与抗核糖体-P 抗体相关的一种特殊类型 AIH[12,13,84,116]。HCV 感染可有与 SLE 类似的临床表现和血清学检查结果[117]，且干扰素治疗时可诱发 SLE[118]。对于 IBD 患者，使用英夫利西单抗可分别引起 53% 和 35% 的患者出现 ANA 和抗双链 DNA 阳性，但却很少导致药物性狼疮[119]。肝脏血管疾病包括布-加综合征和肝梗死，通常是由于抗磷脂综合征引起的[12,13,120]。在 SLE 患者中，肝脏供血的局灶性失衡可能可以解释 SLE 患者中局灶性结节增生和肝血管瘤发生率增加。

（五）肌病

炎性肌病包括多发性肌炎、皮肌炎和包涵体肌炎，其诊断依据为肌肉无力、肌酶水平升高、肌电图提示肌病表现和典型的肌肉组织学改变[121]。由于血清天冬氨酸氨基转移酶（AST）的释放和清除均增多，两者相互抵消，故血清 AST 水平和 ALT 水平大致相等[122]。一般情况下，ALT 约 100U/L 时肌酸磷酸激酶（CPK）约 1 000U/L[123]，但常出现例外。治疗胃肠道疾病的药物方面，可导致肌炎的为抗 TNF 药物和干扰素，质子泵抑制剂（PPI）有时也能引起肌炎[124]。肌炎也常与 IBD、乳糜泻、HBV 或 HCV 感染以及 PBC 有关[121,125]。皮肌炎也可能与胃肠道血管病变有关，这是一种严重但罕见的表现，可导致血管扩张、溃疡和肠穿孔[126]。皮肌炎和更少见的多发性肌炎可能是与胃、结肠、胰腺和其他器官的恶性肿瘤相关的副肿瘤性表现。

咽和食管上括约肌（upper esophageal sphincter，UES）均由骨骼肌组成，当其受累时，可出现鼻反流、误吸、舌肌无力和吞咽困难（固、液体）[127,128]。食管动力检查可见咽部收缩幅度降低以及 UES 压力降低。同时，平滑肌也可能受累，表现为食管和胃排空延迟[121]。LES 压力降低和低振幅非蠕动性食管收缩还可导致胃灼热。目前针对食管受累的治疗方法包括：免疫抑制治疗（如糖皮质激素）、静脉注射免疫球蛋白、环咽肌切开术和咽部扩张，但其疗效不一[127,128]。

（六）干燥综合征（SjÖgren 综合征）

干燥综合征可单独存在（原发），也可继发于自身免疫性疾病(继发性)。SS 的特征表现为:泪腺和唾液腺的淋巴细胞浸润,伴有干燥性角膜结膜炎和口干燥症。口(见第 24 章)和食管是最常受累的器官[129]。唾液的中和作用减弱可能会增加食管对酸暴露的时间,使其易出现反流症状和/或黏膜损伤。虽然可以见到食管的唾液流率减少以及运动功能障碍,但患者的吞咽困难普遍和两者无关[129,130]。干燥综合征患者常有慢性萎缩性胃炎的表现,但维生素 B_{12} 水平低下和/或恶性贫血并不多见[129]。SS 患者中 Hp 相关胃炎的患病率是否升高尚有争议;但抗幽门螺杆菌治疗后并不会减轻胃淋巴细胞浸润、萎缩或消化不良[131,132]。众所周知,SS 与黏膜相关淋巴组织淋巴瘤有关。胃淋巴瘤是 SS 中最常见的腺体外淋巴瘤。有研究提出 SS 患者中,和炎症标志物、IgA 水平和 SS-B 抗体相关的疾病严重程度可能与患胃腺癌的风险成正比。在 SS 患者中行胃癌筛查或监测的作用尚不明确。多达 15% 的 SS 患者可出现与之相关的乳糜泻[133]。

SS 患者胰腺炎的发生率高达 7%[129],常表现为自身免疫性胰腺炎或慢性胰腺炎[134]。大约 25% 的 SS 患者可能出现具有形态学改变和/或分泌试验异常的慢性胰腺炎,但通常无临床症状[135]。

10%~49% 的 SS 患者可出现肝脏生化检查异常,通常较轻且没有明确特征,临床意义有限[136,137]。11%~21% 的患者可出现肝脏肿大[129]。肝脏损害的常见原因有:非酒精性脂肪肝病、PBC、AIH 和 HCV 感染。PBC 患者中发生干燥综合征、唾液腺组织学和造影异常的情况较为常见,但抗 SS-A/B 抗体通常为阴性。此外,HCV 感染也可出现口干、唾液流率降低以及涎腺炎的表现,但抗-Ro/SS-A/B 抗体常为阴性[138]。丙型肝炎病毒相关性 SS 的发病机制包括:丙型肝炎病毒感染唾液腺、分子模拟和/或含丙型肝炎病毒的免疫复合物的形成[129]。

(七) 混合性结缔组织病

混合性结缔组织病(MCTD)是和抗核糖核蛋白抗体相关,出现 SLE、PSS 和多发性肌炎等特征的一种重叠综合征。患者可出现胃灼热和吞咽困难[139]。大多数患者表现为食管运输迟缓,24 小时 pH 检测发现病理性胃食管反流,食管蠕动幅度和协调性降低[139-141]。如果类似于多发性肌炎中的食管上段受累以及 PSS 中的食管下段受累同时存在,即全食管运动功能障碍,可提示 MCTD 的诊断。与 PSS 一样,MCTD 的食管异常通常与肺部异常相关[139,140]。糖皮质激素在食管疾病中的作用尚不明确。

患者肠道内可见与 PSS 相似的病变[142]。一些患者还可能存在血管炎、淀粉样变性或胰腺炎[143]。肝脾肿大、AIH、特发性门静脉高压或布-加综合征也可发生[144]。

(八) 结节性多动脉炎

结节性多动脉炎(polyarteritis nodosa,PAN)是一种主要累及中动脉的血管炎,可导致坏死性炎症、纤维蛋白样坏死、中性粒细胞浸润以及血管壁成纤维细胞增生[145,146]。可发生动脉瘤、血管狭窄、血栓形成、血管闭塞和动脉破裂。如果损伤局限于黏膜或黏膜下层会导致肠灌注受损、溃疡、出血,缺血,全层受累时出现肠穿孔。虽然 PAN 可累及全消化道,但小肠受累最为常见[147]。肝脏受累一般为无临床症状,可包括致肝叶萎缩的坏死性血管炎、肝脏梗死或结节性再生性增生[148]。若肝脏内动脉瘤破裂可导致胆道出血、被膜下出血或肝内出血,但发生率很低。HBV 相关的 PAN 常见于 HBV 感染的早期,较无 HBV 感染 PAN 而言,其与胃肠道疾病关系更密切、血管炎更严重并且死亡率更高[145,146]。HBV-PAN 的特征性改变为出现含有 HBs 抗原和抗 HBs 抗体的循环免疫复合物,这表明 HBV-PAN 是由病毒抗原抗体复合物的沉积所介导的。大多数病例中乙型病毒性肝炎处于静止状态,仅表现为血清转氨酶轻度升高[149]。HCV 也偶可引起 PAN,但与 HBV 暴露后的早期发病不同,HCV 引起的 PAN 通常发生在 HCV 病毒暴露后的几年,通常与 HBV-PAN 一样表现为严重的血管炎[150]。

35%~37% 的尸检病例出现胰腺受累,表现为急性胰腺炎、胰腺梗死、假性囊肿、胰腺肿块或胰腺功能不全[145]。当供应小胆管的动脉出现血管炎时可引起肝内硬化性胆管炎,胆囊动脉炎可导致非结石性坏疽性胆囊炎[147,151]。但血管炎很少引起腹水[152]。

60% 以上患者的血管造影可出现血管异常改变[153,154],表现为动脉瘤、不规则和血栓形成,这些情况都可能进一步发展为血管狭窄和闭塞。动脉瘤是局灶性和节段性的,处于不同的发展阶段,好发于血管分叉处。一般于实质器官内多发,直径可达 1 厘米。动脉瘤偶可破裂,尤其在血压升高时。RA、SLE 以及肉芽肿性多血管炎等其他疾病中有时也可出现微动脉瘤。动脉瘤可能形成血栓或愈合,故而即使内脏血管造影未见异常仍不能排除 PAN。CT 可见肠壁增厚及靶征[155]。三维 CT 血管造影可发现直径 3mm 的动脉瘤以及在常规血管造影上无法见到的早期血管病变(如血管壁增厚和钙化)。

可对皮损部位、腓肠神经和肌肉行活检。内镜活检通常过于浅表,以至于无法作出诊断,而深部活检又会增加穿孔风险[147]。

运用糖皮质激素联合免疫抑制剂,特别是环磷酰胺,可显著降低 PAN 的死亡率。HBV-PAN 或 HCV-PAN 常使用免疫抑制剂和抗病毒药物治疗,必要时可进行血浆置换(以去除免疫复合物)[145,146,149]。

(九) 过敏性紫癜

过敏性紫癜(Henoch-Schönlein purpura,HSP)是儿童最常见的系统性血管炎,偶见于青年人。过敏性紫癜的临床特征为可触及的紫癜、关节炎以及肾脏和胃肠道受累。成人通常有更严重的临床综合征,且肾脏受累较常见。该病由免疫沉积(常为 IgA)介导而造成引起小血管壁坏死的白细胞破碎性血管炎[156-158]。大多数患者都可出现胃肠道受累,而且症状有时可发生在皮疹前。腹痛常为绞痛,位于脐周或上腹,进食后可能加重。明显的便血少见,多为黑便或便潜血阳性。小肠是最常受累的部位,十二指肠降部比球部受累常见[156,158]。该病主要需与 Crohn 病相鉴别。由于存在回肠某个部位的肠壁内出血或水肿,肠套叠通常是回肠-回肠或回肠-结肠。肠套叠可自发缓解,也可通过空气或造影剂灌肠而缓解,但操作时应尽量动作轻柔以免造成肠穿孔[159]。如果肠套叠超过 24

小时,则应考虑手术治疗。患者很少发生急性非结石性胆囊炎、腹水合并浆膜炎、胰腺炎[156]。复发时症状较第一次发作的程度轻、病程短。

内镜检查可见胃肠道黏膜瘀点、糜烂和溃疡、充血和瘀斑(图 37.3)。黏膜活检可见 IgA 沉积及炎症表现。黏膜下层取样可见血管炎。胶囊内镜检查可以确定疾病的范围和出血部位[160]。CT 可见肠壁增厚伴跳跃性损伤、肠梗阻、肠扩张。为避免儿童受到辐射,有学者认为腹部超声检查是首选检查方法,并有可能帮助确定预后[161]。

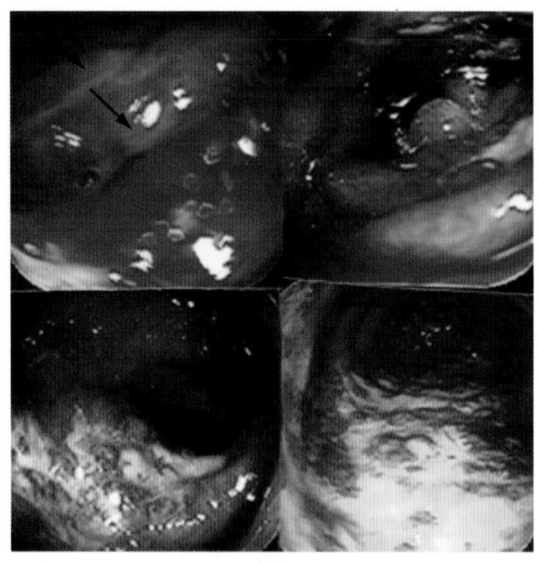

图 37.3　过敏性紫癜患者的内镜视图。上图显示空肠黏膜弥漫性增厚,呈结节状,有浅表线状溃疡(黑色箭头)。下图显示了具有鹅卵石样外观的回肠黏膜。(From Ebert EC. Gastrointestinal manifestations of Henoch-Schönlein purpura. Dig Dis Sci 2008;53:2011-19,with permission from Springer.)

对肾脏受累的高危患者可用糖皮质激素治疗;但因为超过 80% 的患者消化道症状可自发缓解,激素在消化道病变中的作用尚不明确[156,162]。必要时也可考虑使用血浆置换、氨苯砜、静脉注射免疫球蛋白等其他疗法。

(十)嗜酸性肉芽肿性多血管炎

嗜酸性肉芽肿性多血管炎(又称为 Churg-Strauss 综合征),是一种中、小血管的血管炎,高达 59% 的患者可出现胃肠道症状[163]。疾病包括前驱期、组织嗜酸性细胞浸润期及血管炎期,后两期可出现胃肠道受累。嗜酸细胞性胃肠炎主要表现为外周嗜酸性粒细胞增多以及嗜酸性粒细胞浸润胃肠道黏膜[163,164]。腹痛、腹泻、恶心/呕吐及出血是最常见的症状。血管炎可导致溃疡、穿孔,胃肠道狭窄少见[165]。溃疡以红斑样边缘为特点[166]。其他非常见并发症包括非结石性胆囊炎、胰腺炎以及腹膜受累所致的嗜酸粒细胞性腹水[164]。肠切除标本和膜下活检可见血管炎伴纤维蛋白样坏死、嗜酸性浸润和/或肉芽肿。糖皮质激素治疗的有效性约 90%,但需要密切监测肠穿孔的发生。对于糖皮质激素难治性疾病可以使用环磷酰胺、静脉注射免疫球蛋白或血浆置换治疗[167]。严重胃肠道受累者常预后不良。

(十一)肉芽肿性血管炎

肉芽肿性血管炎是一种影响中小血管的坏死性血管炎,可累及大部分消化道。由于消化道受累时常无临床症状,故其发病率尚不清楚。口腔受累时可出现溃疡、舌梗死和有病理提示意义的“草莓龈”表现为牙龈增生,并且散在如成熟草莓般的瘀点[168]。可出现食管和胃溃疡,其病理表现为坏死性肉芽肿性炎症[169]。血管炎可导致肠溃疡、缺血、梗死以及穿孔。它可能类似于 IBD,也可能与 IBD 有关[170]。动脉炎可能导致胰腺炎或胆囊坏疽[171]。肝脏受累通常是非特异性的,也有如缺血所致的不完全间隔纤维化等罕见报道[172]。表浅的肠道活检可能仅有非特异性发现,血管造影可正常。髓过氧化物酶特异性核周染色抗体 ANCA(p-ANCA)可能呈阳性,但定位于髓样溶酶体的蛋白酶 3 抗原的细胞质染色抗体 ANCA(c-ANCA)更具有特异性。环磷酰胺等免疫抑制剂对大多数病变有效。

(十二)冷球蛋白血症

冷球蛋白是指在 37℃ 以下体外沉淀的免疫球蛋白[173]。冷球蛋白血症可通过引起高黏滞状态或血管炎而造成器官损伤,后者是胃肠道受累的主要机制。虽然感染、自身免疫性疾病和癌症均可导致冷球蛋白血症,但其最常见的病因是 HCV 感染。多达 7% 的冷球蛋白血症患者有胃肠道受累症状,通常表现为肠系膜血管炎(见 RA,SLE,PAN)[174]。对于非 HCV 相关的血管炎,胃肠道严重受累是预后不良的独立因素。治疗措施主要为控制基础疾病,以及运用免疫抑制剂、血浆成分分离和/或利妥昔单抗等。

(十三)白塞病

白塞病(Behçet disease,BD)为多系统性血管炎,其临床表现包括反复发作的口腔和生殖器溃疡,关节炎以及特征性皮肤病变。也可出现中枢神经系统症状、胃肠道病变、高凝状态和内脏动脉瘤。虽然白塞病好发于古代丝绸之路沿线的国家,但其所致的胃肠道表现却最常见于其他某些国家(如日本和英国)[175,176]。小血管炎主要累及静脉和微静脉,表现为黏膜炎症并且可引起溃疡;而大血管受累则导致缺血和梗死。和克罗恩病类似,这种血管炎主要累及回盲部。口腔溃疡、葡萄膜炎、关节炎和结节性红斑等肠外表现也可能与 IBD 相似。有几个特征可以将白塞病与克罗恩病区分开来[177-179]:与克罗恩病不同,白塞病很少引起肠管狭窄、肛周疾病或直肠溃疡,并且多节段或弥漫性胃肠道受累也很少见。白塞病常导致口腔溃疡、黏膜水肿、肠穿孔和静脉炎(不伴肠道炎症、纤维化或肉芽肿),且常可自发缓解。一些感染过程可能会类似于白塞病,或与其并发[180]。由于肠溃疡通常非常深,内镜检查应考虑到穿孔的风险并谨慎操作。除此以外还可能出现淀粉样变性(稍后讨论)、动脉瘤形成或肝静脉、门静脉血栓形成[181]。由于血栓性静脉炎是由静脉炎症所引起,故而抗凝治疗可能无效。急性胰腺炎、布-加综合征、多发性无菌性肝脾脓肿[182]和硬化性胆管炎在白塞病中均有报道。针对胃肠道受累的药物治疗包括美沙拉秦、免疫调节剂和 TNF 抑制剂。目前尚不清楚糖皮质激素是否会延长溃疡愈合时间以及导致肠道穿孔[183]。一项 2 期试验发现，口服磷酸二酯酶抑制剂阿普斯特（apremilast）显著减少了 BD 患者口腔溃疡的发生，但治疗时间较短（12~24 周）且可引起腹泻、恶心呕吐。此外，阿普斯特对胃肠道症状等疾病其他方面的效果，仍有待阐明[184]。约 1/2 的患者可出现术后复发，且通常发生在吻合部位[185]。

（十四）脊柱关节病

多达 2/3 的脊柱关节病患者可有亚临床肠道炎症的表现[186-188]。回肠炎的出现可能和关节病长期迁延有关。急性脊柱关节病（如反应性关节炎）的肠炎症状与细菌性肠炎相似，伴有中性粒细胞浸润，但其肠道结构正常。慢性脊柱关节病（如强直性脊柱炎）的胃肠道表现类似于克罗恩病，为单核细胞浸润且肠道结构紊乱。虽然脊椎关节病相关回肠炎可能与克罗恩病回肠炎在组织学上难以区分，但它通常无症状，影像学表现不明显，并且患者通常 HLA-B27 呈阳性。多达 15%的 IBD 患者和约 50% HLA-B27 阳性的 IBD 患者患有强直性脊柱炎。对于中轴关节受累者，非甾体抗炎药可减缓关节疼痛和僵硬症状，但却可能加重潜在的 IBD。糖皮质激素对脊柱关节病几乎无效，而且会导致骨密度降低。柳氮磺胺吡啶和甲氨蝶呤可能对脊椎关节病有一定的疗效，特别是对阑尾受累的患者。TNF-α 阻断剂，包括不用于 IBD 治疗的依那西普，对于脊柱关节病也非常有效。

（十五）家族性地中海热

家族性地中海热（familial mediterranean fever，FMF）是一种常染色体隐性遗传疾病，其特征表现为：反复自限性发热、腹痛和关节疼痛，其在具有地中海地区血统的人中最常见[189,190]。FMF 的致病基因是 *MEFV*，其位于 16 号染色体，编码 Pyrin 蛋白。行 MEFV 基因检测有助于疾病的诊断。

患者常由于腹膜炎而出现急腹症。躺着不动且屈曲卧位可缓解剧烈腹痛。腹部查体可见板状腹、压痛、反跳痛、肠鸣音减弱、腹膨隆。辅助检查可见多个气液平，白细胞增多伴核左移，ESR 升高并出现急性期反应物升高。症状在 24 小时后开始消退。腹膜炎会导致含有纤维蛋白和中性粒细胞的富含蛋白的无菌渗出物，其机化可能导致粘连和小肠梗阻，甚至出现绞窄和坏死。虽然患者在发作之间没有症状，但是急性时相反应物可能升高，提示存在亚临床炎症。

发热过程中，血清淀粉样蛋白浓度急剧上升［请参阅淀粉样变性（浸润性疾病章节中）］。AA 淀粉样变性与疾病发作的频率、持续时间和复发强度无关。虽然最具意义的临床表现为肾脏损害，但淀粉样蛋白可以沉积在胃肠道并在多年后引起症状。FMF 还与 IBD[191]、某些血管炎以及肠易激综合征等其他疾病相关。胃肠道黏膜受累可能提示 IBD，但单独使用秋水仙碱可使黏膜愈合。

无论淀粉样变性程度如何，食管均可能出现运动障碍[192]。肝脏疾病则主要由淀粉样变性引起，且持续性炎症刺激可导致脾肿大[189,190]。尽管对于疾病急性发作暂无特别的治疗方法，但秋水仙碱降低了大多数 FMF 患者的发作频率、严重程度和持续时间。由于秋水仙碱能够预防、延缓，甚至逆转肾脏淀粉样变性，故而应该终生使用。抗 IL-1β_1 单抗卡那单抗（canakinumab）可能对难治性病例有效。

（十六）结缔组织疾病

已有多种结缔组织疾病被报告存在胃肠道表现。这些表现可被归类为结构或功能异常。

马方综合征的心血管、眼部和肌肉骨骼的临床表现通常会掩盖其胃肠道的临床表现。原纤维蛋白-1（fibrillin-1）基因突变导致糖蛋白原纤维蛋白-1 的质和/或量的改变，继而导致肌原纤维缺陷和结缔组织不稳定。在胃肠道中，这可能导致内脏疝、腹壁疝、憩室/假憩室，以及一些临床事件，如异常年轻时发作的急性阑尾炎或急性憩室炎。肝囊肿、肾囊肿和胆石症的发生率似乎也有所增加。如 IBS 等功能性胃肠病也可能比对照组更常见[193]。

在 Ehlers Danlos 综合征（EDS）中，虽然主要为功能性胃肠病，但也可能出现膈上憩室、膈膨出、巨食管症、自发性消化道穿孔和急性消化道出血。一项大型回顾性研究发现，在经典型、过度活动型和血管型的 687 例 EDS 患者中，有 378 例（56%）有相关的胃肠道表现。血管型患者都有频繁的胃肠道症状，但这些症状较过度活动型患者少见。典型症状包括腹痛（56%），恶心（42%），便秘（39%），胃灼热（38%）和 IBS 症状（28%）。胃和结肠转运分别延迟了 12% 和 28%。所有的腹部动脉瘤均发生在血管型 EDS 中[194]。

在综合三级中心的功能性胃肠病患者中，发现良性关节过度活动综合征的频率高于一般人群（10%~20%）。在 129 个（97 名女性）综合三级中心转诊至神经胃肠病诊所的患者中评估了关节过度活动的发病率，发现有 63 名（49%）患者存在关节过度活动的证据；较之于无关节过度活动的患者，不明原因的胃肠道症状在这些患者中更常见。评估的 25 名患者中，有 23 名被风湿科医生证实存在关节过度活动的临床诊断[195]。

（十七）IgG4 相关性疾病

这种罕见的多系统炎症和纤维化疾病通常会累及胰腺（Ⅰ型或Ⅱ型自身免疫性胰腺炎；请参阅第 59 章）或胆管，且可与胰腺癌、胆管癌或 PSC 类似。报告的其他腹腔内受累包括腹膜后纤维化、主动脉炎、硬化性肠系膜炎、炎性假瘤、肝炎、小肠炎、结肠炎和储袋炎。只有 60%~70% 的患者血清 IgG4 升高；通常情况下需要对病变器官进行诊断性活检，典型表现为致密的 IgG4 染色淋巴浆细胞浸润，席纹状纤维化和闭塞性静脉炎。糖皮质激素治疗通常有效，有时需要免疫调节剂维持治疗。

二、肿瘤与血液系统疾病

（一）胃肠道转移瘤

肿瘤可通过血液或淋巴扩散以及腹腔种植等方式发生肠道转移，最常见的是乳腺癌[196]。转移瘤与原发性肿瘤的区别在于正常细胞与癌细胞之间没有移行区，且原发灶与继发灶之间在组织学和免疫组化上具有相似性。

由于许多患者并无症状，故尸检时发现的胃肠道转移比临床上更多。其主要的临床表现有:腹痛、贫血、消化道出血、梗阻、体重减轻,偶可出现蛋白丢失性胃肠病[196,197]。某些肿瘤可在发现原发灶数十年后出现胃肠道转移,特别是黑色素瘤(图 37.4)、乳腺癌和肾细胞癌[198,199]。

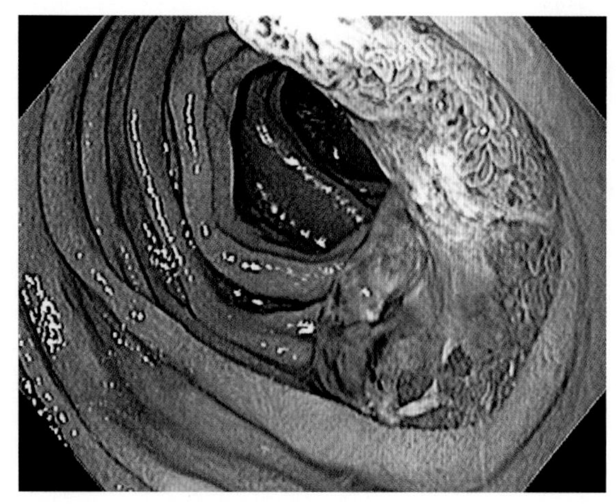

图 37.4　一名出现上消化道出血的年青男性的累及十二指肠降部的溃疡性转移性黑色素瘤病变的内镜视图

肠黏膜息肉样转移灶可引起肠套叠[200],或由于转移瘤生长迅速而其血液供应相对不足而发生溃疡或空洞出血。肿瘤的肠黏膜下转移可形成黏膜下层肿块或弥漫性浸润,而引起壁增厚和僵硬。转移灶中央出现溃疡时可出现"牛眼"征[198,201]。肿瘤破裂入腹腔时可出现癌细胞扩散及恶性腹水[198]。化疗引起肿瘤坏死时也可发生肠穿孔。

胃转移最常见于肺癌、乳腺癌、食管癌和黑色素瘤[201]。小肠转移最常见于小叶性乳腺癌或恶性黑色素瘤。胰腺转移较为少见,其中 60% 由肾癌转移所致[202]。肾癌在 CT 上表现为高密度肿块,血管造影可见血管增多[203]。切除胰腺转移灶可能可以提高患者生存率[202,203]。

有色素或无色素的黑色素瘤转移最常见于小肠[198,199]。通常因为贫血或梗阻而行手术切除转移灶,尽管术后疾病复发很常见,但可改善症状并降低发病率或死亡率。黑色素瘤是导致胆囊转移的最常见原发肿瘤[204]。

虽然最常见的乳腺癌类型是导管癌,但小叶癌最常发生胃肠道转移[205]。患者偶尔可出现假性贲门失弛缓症、口咽性吞咽困难或食管狭窄。胃转移可能与有浸润表现的皮革胃相似,而回肠末端受累的表现类似于 Crohn 病,直肠浸润可能类似于原发性直肠癌(Schnitzler 转移)。胃肠道转移性乳腺癌可由无腺体形成的印戒细胞组成,与原发性胃肠道恶性肿瘤的病理表现类似。由于肿瘤中普遍表达雌激素受体,可借此进行疾病的诊断。尽管罕见,发生胃肠道转移的肺癌通常为大细胞性肺癌[206]。

(二) 副肿瘤综合征

副肿瘤性胃肠运动功能障碍表现为假性贲门失弛缓症、胃轻瘫或假性梗阻[207,208]。副肿瘤综合征最常见的病因是小细胞肺癌,胃肠道症状通常在肿瘤诊断前数周或数月出现。其他与副肿瘤性胃肠运动功能障碍相关的原发性肿瘤包括乳腺癌、膀胱癌、前列腺癌、肾癌、睾丸癌、卵巢癌、神经母细胞瘤,以及胰腺癌等原发性胃肠道恶性肿瘤。最常见的自身抗体是 1 型抗神经元核抗体,该抗体可作用于肿瘤细胞和神经元核(包括肌间神经丛的神经元)。抗 HuD 抗体可诱导神经元凋亡[209]。若此类抗体和类似的抗神经元抗体阳性应积极寻找恶性肿瘤。1 型抗神经元抗体最常引起的是神经病变,30% 的患者可出现胃肠运动功能障碍。

患者通常会出现体重快速下降、吞咽困难、恶心和呕吐、早饱、便秘和/或腹痛,尽管存在小细胞肺癌,但胸部 X 线检查一般无异常[208]。也常可出现食管运动功能障碍、胃排空延迟、肠道排空延迟以及自主神经反射试验异常[210]。胃十二指肠测压表现为神经性胃肠运动功能障碍。胃肠运动功能障碍的鉴别诊断包括病毒感染、药物(尤其是阿片类药物)、化疗(如长春新碱)和放射性损伤。

常规治疗方法,如促胃肠动力、止吐以及导泻药物的疗效有限[208]。虽然化疗可缩小肿瘤体积,却无法缓解胃肠道症状。

副肿瘤性肝病较罕见,副肿瘤现象表现为肝内胆汁淤积,最常与肾细胞癌(Stauffer 综合征)和淋巴瘤相关。其典型表现为碱性磷酸酶水平异常,而高胆红素血症或黄疸较不常见。副肿瘤性肝病还与嗜铬细胞瘤、前列腺癌、甲状腺髓样癌、卵巢无性细胞瘤和神经内分泌肿瘤有关。在组织学上,这种胆汁淤积与非特异性肝脏炎症或肝窦扩张有关,且通常在肿瘤切除术后消退,但可能随着肿瘤复发而复发。副肿瘤性胆管损伤(继发性硬化性胆管炎)和胆管消失综合征与淋巴瘤有关[211]。

POEMS 综合征(多发性神经病变、脏器肿大、内分泌障碍、M 蛋白血症、皮肤改变)是一种罕见的累及多系统的浆细胞肿瘤疾病。其通常在 50~60 岁时隐匿起病。诊断 POEMS 的必要标准包括多发性神经病和单克隆浆细胞异常(通常为 λ 轻链)。主要标准还可能包括 Castleman 病、硬化性骨病和血管内皮生长因子(VEGF)升高;次要标准包括脏器肿大、血管外积液[水肿、低 SAAG(5%)腹水、胸腔积液]、皮肤改变、内分泌障碍、视乳头水肿和红细胞/血小板增多症。临床表现可能是由血管内皮生长因子升高使微血管通透性显著增加所引起的。大多数患者有单发或多发浆细胞瘤。骨髓检查通常显示克隆性浆细胞,并且针对潜在的浆细胞恶性增生进行治疗。肝脏肿大和腹水可能错误地提示存在潜在的慢性肝病[212]。

(三) 血液系统恶性肿瘤

肝脏属于网状内皮系统的一部分,常因播散性淋巴增生性疾病而受累,并且通常意味着疾病发展到了晚期[213]。血液系统恶性肿瘤常出现肝脏生化指标升高,但通常不会引起临床上明显的肝功能障碍。各类型的恶性肿瘤之间肝脏受累情况差异很大。此外,如药物毒性、感染、淀粉样变性以及肝门淋巴结肿大所致的肝外梗阻等一些其他原因也可能导致肝脏生化检查异常。

1. 系统性淋巴瘤所致的肝脏受累

肝脏为系统性淋巴瘤扩散的常见部位,部分罕见的原发性淋巴瘤也可能发生于肝脏。淋巴瘤与 HIV、HCV 或 EBV(移植后)感染、常见变异型免疫缺陷病、风湿性疾病、乳糜泻、IBD、硫唑嘌呤治疗以及可能的 TNF 抑制剂治疗有关。HBV 感染者患非霍奇金淋巴瘤(NHL)的风险也增加了 2~3 倍,但两者的因果关系尚不明确[214]。

NHL 占肝淋巴瘤的 90% 左右,且大多数为 B 细胞来源[213,215]。NHL 较霍奇金淋巴瘤(HL)更易出现肝脏的恶性侵犯。影像学检查通常阴性,或表现为多个或弥漫性浸润病灶。肝脏局灶性病变较少见,其超声表现为低回声,CT 显示低密度改变[216,217]。脾脏受累以及淋巴结肿大可进一步佐证淋巴瘤的诊断。NHL 和 HL 的非特异性组织学表现:汇管区淋巴细胞浸润、含铁血黄素沉着症、脂肪变性和肉芽肿(通常为非干酪性肉芽肿);较之于 NHL,肉芽肿在 HL 中更常见[213,215,218]。免疫分型可以区分这些细胞的表型。

许多患者并没有肝脏受累的临床症状或生化异常。肝脏肿大或血清碱性磷酸酶水平中度升高等肝脏化验异常,与淋巴瘤累及肝脏的关系不大[219]。少数情况下,当肿瘤大面积浸润肝脏时可引起急性肝衰竭,患者的平均存活时间为 10 天[220]。

在 NHL 中,弥漫大 B 细胞淋巴瘤是最常见的亚型。其主要表现为弥漫分布于整个肝脏的肿瘤结节,伴有致密的淋巴瘤浸润[213,215]。相比之下,富于 T 细胞的 B 细胞淋巴瘤的特征表现为汇管区散在少量的肿瘤细胞浸润,常被误诊为反应性炎症疾病或 T 细胞淋巴瘤的肝脏浸润。T 细胞淋巴瘤的发生率较低,且缺乏典型的浸润形式;若活检仅显示 T 细胞数量增加,则往往容易误诊为药物性肝炎或病毒性肝炎。需要进行 T 细胞受体或者免疫球蛋白重链位点 PCR 进行克隆分析加以鉴别。

实际上肝脏受累的 HL 患者常伴有脾受累,但脾脏受累者其肝脏却不一定受侵犯。较之于出现肿块,肝脏受累更多呈弥漫性粟粒样改变。最常见的组织学表现为显著的汇管区浸润,偶可见 Reed-Sternberg 细胞[213,215]。

胆汁淤积症最常见的原因是肝内肿瘤浸润,但应考虑淋巴结增大造成的肝外胆管梗阻。同时,特发性胆汁淤积和胆管消失综合征等罕见疾病也可引起胆汁淤积[221]。胆汁淤积常与明显的肿瘤负荷不成比例,并且可能对化疗有效,其也可能导致致命性肝损伤。

2. 白血病所致的胃肠道及肝脏受累

白血病可累及胃肠道的任何部分,约 10% 的患者可有临床症状[222]。胃肠道受累通常发生在白血病复发期间,其原因包括白血病肠壁浸润、免疫缺陷、凝血障碍以及化疗。抗白血病治疗也可阻碍正常细胞的增殖,引起骨髓抑制,并因破坏肠壁潜在的恶性肿瘤而使肠壁变薄弱。白血病累及胃肠道时一般无临床表现,但少数患者可出现腹痛、出血或腹泻症状。

白血病常见的口腔问题包括:口干、牙龈出血、黏膜炎、感染(尤其是念珠菌)和牙科疾病[223]。食管可能出现白血病浸润、感染性食管炎(最常见的念珠菌病,HSV 或 CMV)、出血性病变(如瘀点、瘀斑、糜烂、溃疡)或化疗导致的黏膜炎[222,224]。

白血病肠浸润可表现为溃疡或结节性病变,进而发生肠套叠、梗阻或类似癌症的表现[222,225,226]。病变可浸润整个肠壁并导致穿孔。少见的有蛋白丢失性胃肠病及营养吸收不良。由于淋巴组织丰富,回肠末端和阑尾是白血病最常见的浸润部位。症状与 IBD 相似,或者和肠壁囊样积气或气腹相关[222,227]。免疫缺陷可能导致粒细胞缺乏性溃疡伴细菌侵袭和出血。凝血障碍可导致肠壁血肿和出血性肠坏死。白血病浸润也可导致血栓痔、粪石和中性粒细胞减少性溃疡、瘘管以及脓肿等痛性肛直肠病变。

中性粒细胞减少性小肠结肠炎或盲肠炎(来源于希腊语“*typhlon*”,意为“盲肠”)是累及回肠末端、盲肠和升结肠的坏死性病变[222,227-230]。多出现在急性髓系白血病发作或复发期间,常见于化疗后,是导致发热的一个重要原因。其他与中性粒细胞减少相关的疾病也可能与之同时发生。盲肠扩张有时与低血压有关,可导致肠道灌注不足从而引起肠黏膜受损,随着中性粒细胞减少,微生物从破损的黏膜入血并增殖[222,231]。

患者可出现发热、右下腹疼痛、腹泻、出血、恶心、呕吐、脱水和脓毒症,偶尔还可表现为急腹症。脓毒症最常见的病原体为革兰氏阴性菌。肠壁厚度大于 10mm 时在 CT 和超声上可见,而其死亡率约为 60%[229,232]。多数患者可通过静脉补液、血及血小板输注、粒细胞集落刺激因子和广谱抗生素控制病情,但并发症需要手术治疗。

肝、脾和淋巴结的浸润在白血病中很常见,但肝活检可能导致的出血并发症,导致难以明确白血病浸润、骨髓外造血以及这些疾病的其他感染性和毒性并发症在这种情况下的作用。虽然肝脏浸润的患者一般无症状,但却可能发生急性肝衰竭[233]。白血病很少发生胰腺、胆囊或胆管浸润[234-236]。急性白血病出现脾破裂的主要原因是脾大,也可能是由于白血病浸润、脾梗死或凝血功能障碍(特别是血小板减少)所致[237]。

弥漫性非破坏性肝脏浸润常无症状且实验室检查一般无明显的异常。慢性淋巴细胞白血病浸润汇管区时,界板常不受累,但有时却可出现肝细胞坏死、桥接坏死以及少见的假小叶形成[215]。其他类型的白血病可出现肝窦受累,伴或不伴汇管区浸润。

(四) 系统性肥大细胞增多症

系统性肥大细胞增多症的特征表现为:骨髓或皮肤以外的器官及组织内肥大细胞(mast cell,MC)的多发致密浸润,存在 c-kit 基因(*CD117*)突变以及血清类胰蛋白酶浓度升高[238,239]。皮肤的典型病变为色素性荨麻疹,伴或不伴全身受累。胃肠道受累的发病率报道差异很大,但可能是除了瘙痒以外最多的表现[240]。目前认为系统性肥大细胞增多症的症状主要是由于介质释放(如组胺、白三烯、肝素、蛋白酶)引起,一般不是肥大细胞浸润肠道所致。其临床表现为腹痛、腹泻和恶心/呕吐,可因为药物、压力和进食某些食物而加重。腹痛呈胀痛或下腹绞痛。

食管受累可伴有胃灼热、食管炎或运动障碍等表现[241]。组胺介导的胃酸过度分泌可导致消化性溃疡,其可能会被漏诊。胃酸分泌过多还可能与腹泻、肠道吸收障碍、前列腺素 D_2 生成过多有关,有时也可造成肠道运动的改变[238-240,242]。

胃肠道受累的内镜表现不具有特异性(结节、红斑、溃疡、荨麻疹样病变、皱襞增厚、紫色色素沉着病变)[240]。组织学可见包括肥大细胞的混合性细胞浸润,由于肥大细胞浸润也常见于其他疾病,故组织学表现可能具有诊断意义,也可能为非特异性的(图 37.5)。然而,系统性肥大细胞增多症的组织

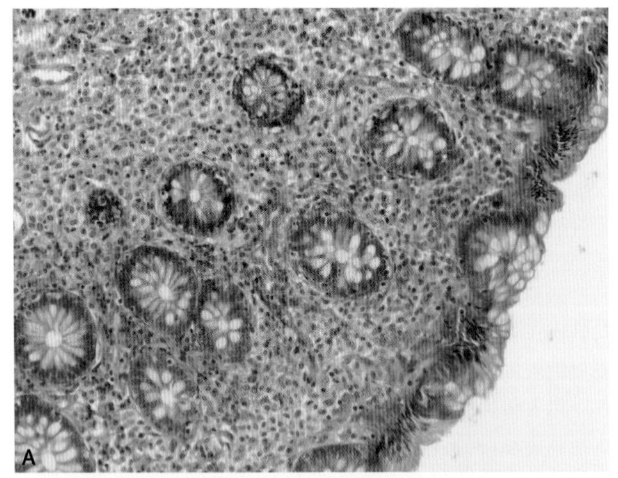

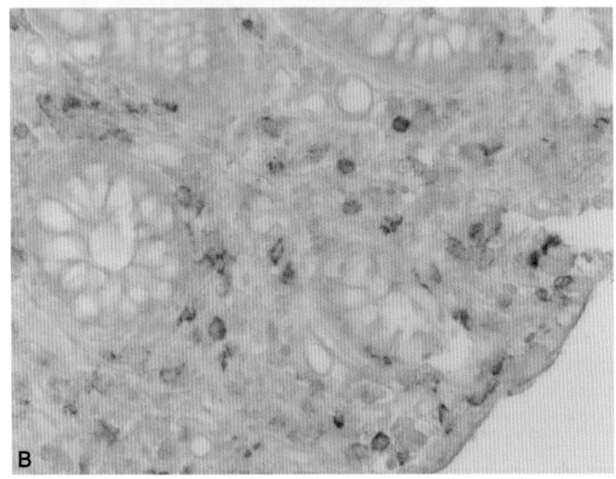

图 37.5　累及结肠的系统性肥大细胞增多症。A，可见肥大细胞间质浸润，胞质苍白（HE 染色，×100）。B，肥大细胞类胰蛋白酶免疫组化染色突出显示间质浸润（×400）。该患者还出现骨髓受累。（Courtesy Shahab I，MD，Dallas，TX.）

学表现与其他炎性疾病也有不同，主要表现为存在大量的肥大细胞，其聚集或融合成片、肥大细胞形态异常以及 CD25 染色阳性[243,244]。虽然系统性肥大细胞增多症也存在浆细胞和嗜酸性粒细胞的浸润，但嗜酸性粒细胞性胃肠炎一般无如此大量的肥大细胞浸润。同时，系统性肥大细胞增多症还可出现隐窝结构扩张及变形等与 IBD 相似的改变[245]，然而却一般不出现隐窝脓肿。此外还可表现为肠绒毛萎缩，而常无乳糜泻中典型的隐窝增生。

肝脏受累时，患者常表现为肝脏肿大及生化检查异常。肝脏生化检查可见混合性改变或单纯为碱性磷酸酶水平升高，其升高的来源常为骨质[239]。肝脏活检表现为：汇管区肥大细胞浸润、嗜酸性粒细胞浸润、髓外造血、汇管区纤维化，有时可见肝硬化表现。虽然脾大可能是由于肥大细胞浸润所致，但也可能为门静脉高压症所致。瞬时弹性成像可表现为肝脏质地坚硬[246]。

治疗的目的是限制肥大细胞脱颗粒和控制病理性肥大细胞组织浸润[238]。使用 H_1 和/或 H_2-受体拮抗剂、口服色甘酸二钠，或运用糖皮质激素可缓解胃肠道症状。对于有器官功能障碍的进展期疾病，干扰素或克拉屈滨（cladribine）的细胞减灭疗法显示出有限的应答率和持续时间。90% 的系统性肥大细胞增多症患者存在 *KIT* D816V（Asp-→Val）突变，一项对 116 名此类患者进行的多国非对照观察性研究报告称，一种多激酶抑制剂（米哚妥林[midostaurin]）对晚期肥大细胞增多症及其高致死性变体——MC 白血病都有效。目前 FDA 批准伊马替尼（格列卫）用于治疗 D816V 突变的患者[247]。

通常，惰性型和阴燃型（后者存在器官浸润但无器官功能障碍）预后较好，而侵袭型（器官浸润伴功能障碍）或转化为肥大细胞白血病的预后较差。

与系统性肥大细胞增多症不同，肥大细胞活化综合征不是由于肥大细胞数量增加导致的，而是由于高反应性 MC 产生炎症介质所驱动的多系统疾病。肥大细胞活化综合征可能与常见变异型免疫缺陷病、体位性直立性心动过速综合征、莱姆病和 EDS 有关，但也可能是特发性的。典型的症状包括：皮肤症状（荨麻疹、潮红和灼热）、心血管症状（头晕、晕厥前期/晕厥）、胃肠道症状（腹泻、腹部绞痛、恶心/呕吐和吞咽困难）、神经症状（短时记忆障碍、记忆改变和头痛）、呼吸系统症状（呼吸困难、喘息和鼻塞）和躯体症状（疲劳/不适）。实验室证据可能包括血清类胰蛋白酶基础值升高，24 小时尿中组胺以及前列腺素 D_2 或其代谢产物前列腺素 F_2 升高，或者是在出现症状时这些标志物明显高于基线。治疗包括 H_1 和 H_2 受体拮抗剂、拮抗白三烯或 MC 稳定剂[248,249]。

（五）骨髓性和骨髓增生性疾病

骨髓外造血（extramedullary hematopoiesis，EMH）是由骨髓衰竭和/或浸润或者慢性溶血性贫血引起的反应性过程[250,251]。最常见的髓外造血器官为肝和脾。因此 EMH 常表现为由于弥漫性浸润所致的肝脾肿大，而腹部症状不明确。虽然肝脏生化检查可出现异常，但临床上很少发生严重的肝功能障碍。组织学可见肝窦内、Disse 间隙和汇管系统内存在成群的红系和髓系前体细胞，并伴有巨核细胞。这种多形性可用于与白血病浸润相鉴别。EMH 通常为弥漫性浸润，但有时也表现为界限清晰的多发性结节或肿块。超声检查呈低回声或不均匀回声，CT 扫描呈低密度。磁共振成像（MRI）的影像学表现因 EMH 的活动度和铁沉积的程度而异[252,253]。胃肠道髓外造血少见，可导致肠梗阻、腹痛、出血或腹水[254,255]。腹膜、网膜、肠系膜或肠壁的髓外造血均可产生腹水。

骨髓纤维化的特征为伴有骨髓纤维化和髓外造血的克隆性骨髓增生。脾大引起的门脉血流量增加、EMH 所致的肝窦狭窄以及肝内阻力增加和/或高凝状态所致的 Budd-Chiari 综合征或门静脉血栓形成均可能导致门静脉高压[256,257]。脾切除可改善 EMH 所致的高动力循环状态，但不能降低肝内门静脉阻塞所致的门静脉高压。脾切除术的并发症包括血小板增多伴血栓事件，以及由于 EMH 转移到肝脏导致的肝大，有时是巨大的。血栓并发症与骨髓纤维化、真性红细胞增多症和原发性血小板增多症有关[258]。脾梗死可引起左上腹疼痛。多达 50% 的 Budd-Chiari 综合征患者有明显的骨髓增生综合征。

朗格汉斯细胞组织细胞增生症（也称为组织细胞增生症 X、嗜酸性肉芽肿、Letterer-Siwe 病和 Hand-Schuller-Christian 病）是一种主要涉及婴儿和儿童的罕见病[259,260]。胃肠道浸润少见（1.6%～2.6%），且多伴有严重的全身性疾病以及特征性皮疹，且通常预后不良，超过 50% 的患者在诊断后 18 个月内死亡。胃肠道受累的表现为呕吐、出血、腹泻、便秘和/或肛周疾病。还可能出现营养吸收不良、蛋白丢失性胃肠病，甚至肠穿孔。内镜下的多种表现包括结节、溃疡、息肉、管腔狭窄和结肠炎。肝脏浸润的发生率为 18%～20%；肝肿大的发生率尚不清楚。朗格汉斯细胞组织细胞增生症的病理学改变可出现在皮肤、肝脏和胃肠道。肝脏及胆管受累可出现门脉三联症、胆管增生、纤维化伴组织细胞改变、胆汁淤积、硬化性胆管炎和肝硬化[261,262]。

噬血细胞性淋巴组织细胞增多症（Hemophagocytic lymphohistiocytosis，HLH），又称噬血细胞综合征，是一种罕见的血液病，属于细胞因子风暴综合征的一种。由于 HLH 中固有免疫系统的自然杀伤细胞活性失控，导致淋巴细胞和巨噬细胞反应性升高，从而造成细胞因子大量过度产生，因此是一种致命的严重炎症疾病。原发性 HLH 是一种异质性常染色体隐性遗传疾病，亲缘关系会增加其发病率。继发性 HLH 发生在强烈的免疫激活之后，如成人型 Still 病（如前所述）等风湿性疾病、全身感染、免疫缺陷综合征或有潜在恶性肿瘤的患者。继发性 HLH 也称为巨噬细胞活化综合征。由此导致的 T 淋巴细胞和巨噬细胞的过度激活会导致临床症状和血液系统障碍，如果不治疗则最终会导致死亡。临床表现包括发热、淋巴结病、肝脾肿大和皮疹（60%）。典型的实验室检查可见全血细胞减少、低纤维蛋白原、低白蛋白血症、可伴有黄疸的肝脏化验指标升高，以及 C 反应蛋白、血沉、血清甘油三酯和铁蛋白显著升高。可以在骨髓、淋巴结和脾脏中发现噬血现象。常可见 CD25 升高。如果可能，应治疗潜在原发病，通常可能需要同时使用大剂量糖皮质激素、依托泊苷、环孢素、甲氨蝶呤或静脉注射免疫球蛋白进行治疗[263]。

脂质肉芽肿瘤样增生病（Erdheim-Chester 病）或多骨硬化性组织细胞增生症是一种罕见疾病，其特征是由于 RAS/MARK 细胞内信号通路的紊乱，导致非朗格汉斯组织细胞异常增殖。通常中年起病，表现为骨髓浸润以及淋巴细胞和组织细胞炎性浸润所致的普遍长骨硬化。骨外受累呈浸润性，胃肠道表现不常见，但肝活检可能包括黄色肉芽肿性浸润。腹膜后纤维化可能导致乳糜性腹水[264]和蛋白丢失性胃肠病。其死亡率很高，治疗可能包括大剂量糖皮质激素、长春花碱类、蒽环类药物、环孢霉素或 α 干扰素[265]。

（六）蛋白异常血症

多发性骨髓瘤可通过直接侵袭具体器官、占位效应或产生恶性渗出而累及胃肠道[266]。轻链淀粉样变性所致的胃肠道症状将在后续章节介绍。骨髓瘤侵犯最常见的部位是肝、脾和淋巴结。临床上很少出现明显的肝脏或胃肠道受累，其通常发生在疾病晚期，且预后不良。多达 58% 的患者可出现肝大，常伴脾大。肝脏以弥漫性浸润为主，也可为结节型[267]。肿瘤浸润的患者常可出现血清碱性磷酸酶水平升高。

胃、肠、胰腺和腹膜是累及部位。直接浸润胃肠可导致出血或穿孔，患者还可出现占位样改变伴有胃肠道或胆管梗阻，以及产生腹水等。患者出现腹水的常见原因有：淀粉样变性所致的门静脉高压、肝脏的恶性浸润、心力衰竭、腹腔的恶性种植以及感染性（如结核性）腹膜炎。多发性骨髓瘤可能与 IBD 有关，或者呈 IBD 样改变[268]。

无多发性骨髓瘤证据的原发性髓外浆细胞瘤占所有浆细胞性疾病的 3%～5%。虽然肠道受累较少见，但从口腔到肛门的全消化道均可受累。患者可表现为吞咽困难、出血、假性梗阻和息肉病[269]。抗幽门螺杆菌治疗后部分胃浆细胞瘤可得到改善，但这些患者可能实际上患有具有明显浆细胞分化的黏膜相关淋巴组织（MALT）淋巴瘤[270]。手术及放疗为常规治疗方法，内镜下切除病灶也是可选择的手段[271]。

Waldenström 巨球蛋白血症以产生 IgM 的 B 淋巴细胞恶性增殖为特征。患者常表现为肝脾肿大及淋巴结病变，很少出现胃肠道症状。胃肠道受累的原因可能是：①免疫球蛋白轻链片段等淀粉样蛋白的沉积；②产生单克隆 IgM（刚果红染色阴性）的淋巴浆细胞浸润肠壁；③高黏度的组织间液造成的淋巴管扩张及阻塞[272,273]。IgM 沉积物可能会被过碘酸-希夫染色，并可能导致肠绒毛增粗膨大以及淋巴管扩张。其对胃肠道功能的影响可能导致营养吸收不良、蛋白丢失性胃肠病或假性梗阻。患者也可出现门静脉高压，其原因包括淋巴浆细胞样细胞浸润汇管区和/或脾肿大继发的脾静脉血流增加[274]。腹水少见。

（七）红细胞异常

镰状细胞性贫血

镰状细胞性贫血（sickle cell disease，SCD）是血红蛋白（Hb）β-珠蛋白链异常引起的一种常染色体隐性遗传病[275,276]。HbS 在脱氧状态下聚集成多聚体，从而形成胶状网状结构，使红细胞膜变硬且黏度增加。这可进一步导致红细胞破裂以及微血管堵塞，从而引起器官缺血和梗死。约 8% 的非裔美国人为 HbS 性状杂合子，而 0.2% 为纯合子。

（1）脾脏受累

在出生后的 6 个月内脾脏充血，镰状细胞可导致功能性无脾[277]。随着出血和梗死的发生，脾脏体积逐渐缩小并最终被纤维组织取代，称作脾自截（图 37.6）。在出生后的 18 至 36 个月内，随着保护性 HbF 的消失，常出现脾梗死。脾萎缩可导致机体对荚膜细菌感染的易感性增强，并在红细胞中可出现 Howell-Jolly 小体的特征性改变。腹部影像学可见脾脏体积缩小，常伴钙化[277]。

较之于纯合子 SCD 患者，由于 SC-HbC 或 SC-地中海贫血患者同时存在 Hb 水平接近正常的脾大以及相对升高的血液黏度，故更容易出现急性脾梗死[275]。甚至可能在非缺氧条件下出现 SC 样表现。脾梗死表现为左上腹疼痛、恶心呕吐、脾区可闻及摩擦音以及白细胞增多，可能会形成脓肿或假性囊肿。患者有时还可出现脾脏破裂、脾脏的髓外造血或含铁血黄素沉着。

急性脾隔离症，或血液短期内迅速汇集到脾脏，可导致脾脏迅速肿大以及血红蛋白下降[278]。少数可表现为患者若不及时输血，可在数小时内出现低血容量性休克甚至死亡。在纯合子 SCD 中，由于继发的纤维化进展可遏制脾隔离，故而该症状仅见于婴儿和儿童。在 SC 地中海贫血患者中，急性脾隔离可发生在任何年龄且复发率很高，可通过脾切除或长期输血预防。

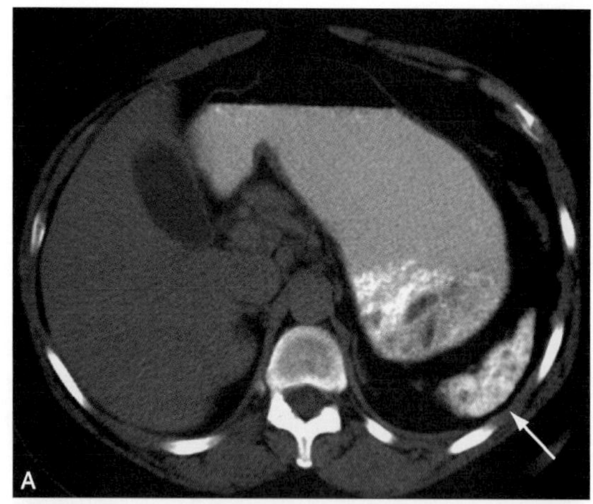

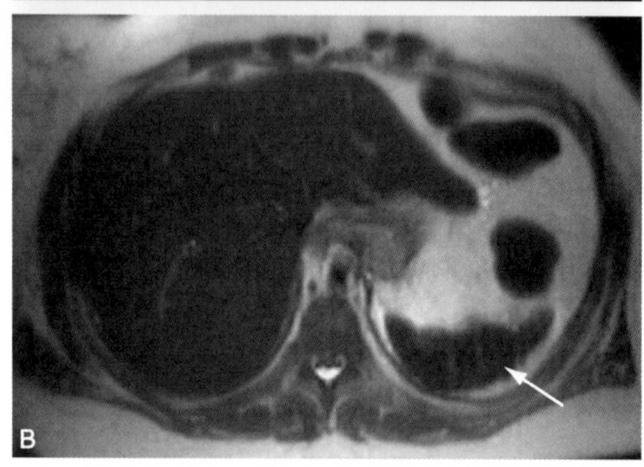

图 37.6 镰状红细胞贫血患者脾自截的影像学检查。腹部CT平扫(A)显示小脾脏密度增加(箭头)。腹部MRI(B)也显示脾脏较小,所有序列中均呈弥漫性低信号(箭头),与CT上致密钙化的发现相一致。由于钙化和脾脏体积缩小,使超声难以检测到脾脏。(From Ebert EC, Nagar M, Hagspiel KD. Gastrointestinal and hepatic complications of sickle cell disease. Clin Gastroenterol Hepatol 2010;8:483-9.)

(2) 胆道受累

约70%的患者一生中可发生胆结石,其成分为色素结石,是由慢性溶血引起的胆红素排泄增加所致[279-281]。由于射线不能透过胆红素钙结石,故X平片可显影。在SCD合并胆结石的患者中,胆总管结石的发生率在18%~30%之间,高于胆固醇结石患者。

无症状SCD患者行腹腔镜胆囊切除术尚存在争议[282,283]。患者围手术期的管理包括:监测动脉氧分压和pH的变化、补液、可能的围手术期输血、术后早期下床活动、必要时予以术后持续气道正压通气以避免肺不张以及SCD相关的术后并发症。术前或术后应考虑行磁共振胰胆管成像(MRCP)或EUS以探查胆总管结石情况[284]。

镰状红细胞性胆管病患者常表现为不伴胆总管结石的胆汁淤积性黄疸,可能是由于胆管缺血性损伤所致[285]。需要对这些患者进行随访,以确定是否有可能发生的胆管结石。

(3) 肝脏受累

由于镰状细胞在肝窦内淤积,肝血流量减少,患者可出现急性镰状细胞肝危象,约占腹痛急症入院患者的10%[275,279]。临床表现为:右上腹疼痛、恶心、疼痛性肝大、低热、白细胞增多以及血清转氨酶与结合胆红素水平升高。转氨酶水平通常为正常值的1~3倍,但也可能达到1 000IU/L以上。最主要的治疗措施为支持治疗,必要时可行血浆置换。

虽然血隔离症最常见于肺部和脾脏,但偶尔也会累及肝脏。镰状红细胞可阻塞肝窦导致胆管受压。血液在肝脏内淤积可导致急性肝肿大、红细胞比容迅速下降、网织红细胞数目增加、转氨酶和胆红素水平轻度升高。而反向隔离则可使肝脏体积缩小、红细胞比容增加,这表明并非所有的被隔离细胞都会被破坏。有时反向隔离可导致血容量增加、心力衰竭和脑出血。

镰状细胞在肝窦内广泛淤积可导致缺氧和以及小胆管内胆汁淤积,从而引起急性镰状细胞性肝内胆汁淤积症,这是一种发病率极低的致命性并发症[286]。其为肝脏危象的一种,可有严重的高胆红素血症、凝血障碍、肾功能不全/衰竭,最终导致肝功能衰竭。包括血浆置换在内的早期治疗至关重要。

急性肝衰竭少见,多在具有潜在慢性肝病的基础上发生[287]。其表现为黄疸、血清转氨酶水平升高、进行性凝血功能障碍以及肝性脑病。肝衰竭患者可行肝移植治疗。

在纯合子SCD或镰状地中海贫血的住院患者中,肝脏急性静脉闭塞的发生率约为39%。其发生与肝脏危象的严重程度无关,表现为肝细胞性、胆管性或混合性胆汁淤积,且通常为良性经过[288,289]。肝脏梗死在CT上表现为肝脏外周低密度楔形病变,是一种相对罕见的临床事件。在功能性无脾、血清中针对多糖类抗原的IgG抗体水平低等情况下,血流中清除细菌的能力减弱,可能会出现继发于感染性肝梗死的肝脓肿,伴有发热和疼痛。由于门静脉阻塞,也可见到局灶性结节增生。可卡因具有肝毒性,可使肝功能显著恶化,并且可使肝脏动脉血管收缩,引起组织缺氧、血管闭塞,并进一步加重镰状贫血[290]。除此以外,SCD患者也可能出现肝静脉或门静脉阻塞。

(4) 其他胃肠道问题

急性血管闭塞常出现腹痛症状,可能与急腹症难以区分。腹痛较为弥漫且伴有如上肢和胸部等部位的疼痛。及时补液及吸氧后,急性血管闭塞所引起的腹痛可在48小时内缓解。这种腹部危象常由于肠系膜和腹腔脏器小血管梗死引起的剧烈腹痛、腹膜刺激和广泛肠梗阻[275]。相较于胆结石的发生率,急性胰腺炎少见,可能是由于胆结石或微血管闭塞合并缺血性损伤[291]。SCD患者可出现十二指肠溃疡,但其发生并非由于胃酸分泌过多,而是缺血导致黏膜抵抗力下降所致。由于血管内镰状细胞增多以及微血管闭塞,患者有时可出现肠缺血[292]。

(5) 胃肠道受累的诊断

以非结合胆红素为主的血清胆红素升高主要是由于在急性肝脏损伤时红细胞血红素负荷增加。在这些患者中胆红素诱导的尿苷二磷酸葡萄糖醛酸转移酶水平会升高,从而增加胆红素结合水平[293]。血清胆红素与乳酸脱氢酶(LDH)水平相关表明引起高胆红素血症的原因并非肝脏疾病,而是慢性溶血和无效的红细胞生成。血清AST升高一部分可能是由于红细胞中存在AST以及肌肉损伤所致,因此血清ALT水平的升高更能反映肝细胞损伤。疼痛发作期间血清碱性磷酸酶水平往往升高,但主要为骨碱性磷酸酶,而并非肝脏同工酶。

尽管急性镰状细胞危象时常不进行,肝活检可见肝窦内镰状细胞、Kupffer 细胞增大并出现红细胞吞噬现象、含铁血黄素沉着，伴有不同程度的肝纤维化。在 SCD 患者中不常见到能在肝缺血中出现的肝细胞皱缩或静脉周围坏死等典型征象[275,279]。尤其是对于处于急性镰状细胞危象的患者而言，肝脏活检的安全性仍存在疑虑[294]。活检的并发症包括慢性静脉流出道梗阻、明显的红细胞肝隔离和肝窦扩张等。

（6）含铁血黄素沉着症

由于 SCD 患者反复输血与溶血，可出现含铁血黄素沉着，由于 Kupffer 细胞吞噬红细胞，铁最先沉积于肝窦内[295]。随着病情的进展，肝细胞内也可出现铁沉积，从而增加了肝脏损伤的风险。地中海贫血患者的肝窦和肝细胞内均可见铁沉积。与 SCD 患者相比，地中海贫血患者往往需要更频繁地输血，并且无效红细胞生成也增加了肠道对铁的吸收，因此内脏铁负荷增加[296]。CT 检查可见肝、脾随着含铁血黄素沉着而密度增加。而在 MRI 上，随着肝脏的铁浓度增加，磁性信号减弱[297,298]。MRI T2 相和肝脏铁含量相关并可用于指导治疗。由于肝脏和心脏之间铁含量缺乏相关性，故应单独评估。铁蛋白是一种急性期反应物，不能有效地反映铁超载情况。可用的铁螯合剂有：去铁胺（非胃肠道给药）以及口服制剂去铁酮（deferiprone）和地拉罗司（deferasirox）。

（八）凝血功能障碍

外伤和出血体质分别容易引起十二指肠和空肠出现肠壁内血肿[299,300]。外伤最易导致十二指肠降部和水平部受损。十二指肠降部和水平部固定在前腹壁和脊柱之间更易活动的部位可能对其造成挤压或撕裂。过度抗凝或出血体质是自发性血肿最常见的原因。患者症状不一，可出现肠梗阻以及肠套叠等并发症。平扫 CT 检查可见肠壁呈均匀对称性增厚，在最初的 10 天内，病变呈现高密度，随后演变为低密度区域。除非肠道广泛受损，通常经过保守治疗症状可迅速缓解。若病变持续超过 2 个月应考虑其他病因。

血管性血友病是最常见的遗传性出血性疾病，消化道出血通常与胃肠道血管扩张有关，或无可见病变。对于 Heyde 综合征患者，其消化道出血与主动脉瓣钙化狭窄之间的关系可能是获得性血管性假血友病因子缺乏所致，因为在剪切应力的作用下，血管性假血友病因子多聚体在尺寸上会减小[301,302]。这种异常可以通过主动脉瓣置换得到纠正或改善。在放置左心室辅助装置后也会出现类似的现象，这类患者中有 30%～40% 的患者出现血管扩张相关的消化道出血。

血友病常和以上消化道为主的消化道黏膜出血有关，尤其是使用传统的非甾体抗炎药的患者[303,304]。血友病常合并与因子获得性丙型肝炎相关的慢性肝病，并可增加消化道出血的可能性。

溶血性尿毒综合征（hemolytic-uremic syndrome，HUS）是以肾损害、微血管病变性溶血性贫血和血小板减少为表现的三联征（见第 110 章）。散发的非产毒性大肠杆菌感染造成的 HUS 的常见诱因包括非肠道感染（尤其是肺炎链球菌）、恶性肿瘤、妊娠、器官移植、抗癌药物、免疫抑制剂和抗血小板药物[305]。产志贺样毒素的大肠杆菌 0157：H7 感染为 HUS 的主要病因。主要传播载体为未煮熟的汉堡，以及苹果汁、莴苣等其他食物[306]。可通过粪-口途径（特别是幼儿园）、饮水（包括游泳池）和接触动物等其他传播途径而感染。感染人群主要为儿童，常在夏秋季发病。在平均 3 天的潜伏期后，患者可出现腹部绞痛、呕吐、发热和腹泻，其中 70% 的患者有出血。在散发性病例中，3%～7% 的患者会发生 HUS，在某些暴发病例中，高达 30% 的患者会发生 HUS。由于大肠杆菌的排泄呈间歇性且排菌量少，所以粪便培养可能为阴性。CT 可见结肠壁增厚，常伴有靶征和结肠周围索条[307]。胰腺炎、腹腔积血、结肠穿孔或狭窄的发生率低[308,309]。使用抗生素治疗大肠杆菌 0157：H7 并增加 HUS 发病风险受到一项 meta 分析的质疑[310]。抗胃肠蠕动的药物可能延缓病原体的清除，甚至增加 HUS 的发生风险，故应禁用。

血栓性血小板减少性紫癜（thrombotic thrombocytopenic purpura，TTP）包括微血管病性溶血性贫血和血小板减少，伴或不伴神经功能障碍和肾功能不全[311-313]。大多数患者中可以分解大的血管性假血友病因子的 ADAMTS13 蛋白酶活性较低，易诱发血栓性微血管病变和血小板消耗。患有严重的血小板减少症时，也可能发生出血。与 HUS 不同，TTP 的好发人群为 40 岁左右的中年人。约 70% 的患者有胃肠道症状，可能包括肠腔缺血和消化道出血。血浆置换可以使 80% 的 TTP 患者在没有永久性器官损伤的情况下存活。

三、内分泌疾病

（一）糖尿病

糖尿病患者中胃肠道症状是否更加频繁仍存在争议[314]。所研究的人群差异很大，对照组的肥胖人群造成的混杂越来越多，很可能存在发表偏倚。提示自主神经功能障碍的症状（例如姿势性头晕、无汗、勃起或射精障碍、膀胱排空困难、口干和味觉性出汗）应予以鉴别。血糖的急剧变化会影响运动功能和感知[315-317]。血糖控制不佳会延迟胃排空，进而影响血糖控制。二甲双胍是引起腹泻和大便失禁的常见原因[318]。

间质卡哈尔细胞（interstitial Cajal cell）的丢失[319]、兴奋性和抑制性肠神经元数量失衡[320]、自主神经病变、迷走神经和交感神经分布的损伤可以改变胃肠运动功能。中枢突（central processing）能以异常的方式感知胃肠道事件[321]，从而导致感觉神经肽（如 P 物质）的减少、平滑肌收缩能力受损、微血管病变引起的缺血[316]。

1. 糖尿病与癌症

糖尿病可能与某些胃肠道恶性肿瘤（如胰腺癌、肝癌、结肠癌）的风险增加有关，尽管数据并不一致[314,322-324]。这种关联可能部分归因于两者存在共同的风险因素，如老化、肥胖、饮食和缺乏运动。二甲双胍可能会降低癌症的风险，而胰岛素可能会增加癌症的风险[324,325]。

糖尿病并发癌症会增加总体死亡率和癌症相关手术[326]。继发性高胰岛素血症伴随的胰岛素抵抗可降低胰岛素样生长因子（IGF）结合蛋白的浓度，导致生物可利用的 IGF-1 浓度的增加[323,324,327]，可能会刺激肿瘤的生长。

糖尿病病程超过 5 年的患者中，胰腺癌的发病率略有增加[328,329]。相反，胰腺癌也会导致糖尿病，这一点可由某些肿瘤切除患者中新发糖尿病的发展和改善所证明。此外，伴有胰腺功能不全的慢性胰腺炎会增加糖尿病和胰腺癌的风险（见下文）。对于老年患者，出现新发且控制不佳的糖尿病，尤其伴有体重减轻者应当考虑胰腺腺癌。胰高血糖素瘤更为罕见，但也可能出现类似的唇炎、舌炎和典型的环状、结痂和大疱性皮疹——坏死松解性游走性红斑（见第 34 章）。

糖尿病是肝细胞癌的危险因素[330,331]。混杂因素包括肝硬化患者（肝细胞癌风险增加）可能存在葡萄糖不耐受，并且30%的患者可能会出现明显的糖尿病，并发 HBV、HCV、肥胖、脂肪性肝病或饮酒可能会增加 HCC 的风险。

糖尿病还与结直肠癌的风险增加有关[327,332]。高循环水平的胰岛素、C 肽或 IGF-1 以及长期使用胰岛素会增加这种风险。与 HbA_{1c} 低的糖尿病患者或非糖尿病患者相比，血糖控制不佳（HbA_{1c}>7.5%）与发病年龄较小、肿瘤较晚期和存活率较低有关[333]。

2. 食管受累

尽管高达 50%的糖尿病患者可能出现食管运动功能障碍，但只有 25%出现症状[314]。其包括 LES 压力降低、转运延迟、多峰或自发收缩以及收缩幅度降低[334]。神经传导速度测定表明，食管运动功能障碍与周围运动神经病变相关。

糖尿病患者胃食管反流的发病率不一，高达 40%的患者有内镜下食管炎[335]，并且肥胖、腮腺碳酸氢盐分泌减少和高血糖会加重胃食管反流。食管转运延迟不一定与胃排空相关，表明消化道并不总是受到糖尿病的影响，并且反流也不是胃排空延迟的主要结果。对于吞咽痛和/或吞咽困难的患者应考虑口腔和食管念珠菌病；糖尿病的易感因素包括免疫功能受损、运动障碍导致的食管淤积、高血糖性中性粒细胞功能及调理作用障碍。

3. 胃受累

糖尿病患者胃排空情况各异，并且与症状关系不大。1 型糖尿病患者可出现壁细胞抗体阳性（15%~25%），自身免疫性萎缩性胃炎（5%~10%）和恶性贫血（2.6%~4%）[336]。自身免疫性萎缩性胃炎可导致缺铁性贫血（由于酸缺乏性铁吸收不良）；这些患者患 Ⅰ 型胃类癌和胃癌的风险增加。1 型糖尿病患者应定期检测壁细胞抗体。存在该抗体的患者应进一步检查全血细胞计数、空腹血清胃泌素、血清铁和维生素 B_{12} 水平。

虽然糖尿病与消化性溃疡之间的关系存在争议，但有证据表明，糖尿病增加了溃疡出血的风险，可能是继发于糖尿病相关的微循环改变破坏了黏膜完整性[337]。从感染的流行率、症状与胃排空的关系或根除率来看，幽门螺杆菌和糖尿病之间似乎没有明确的关联[338]。

4. 小肠受累

在美国和西欧的 1 型糖尿病患者中平均有 4%的人患有乳糜泻（celiac disease），而在没有糖尿病的人群中，这一比例约为 0.5%[339,340]。共同的 HLA Ⅱ类基因和非 HLA 基因座表明了两者有共同的自身免疫起源[341]。乳糜泻患者可能没有胃肠道症状，也可能表现为如身材矮小、青春期延迟、脂溶性维生素缺乏、贫血、骨质疏松和（或）生殖障碍等非胃肠道疾病。1 型糖尿病合并乳糜泻的患者可能存在血糖控制不佳、低血糖发作和微血管并发症[342]。这些患者有发展成其他自身免疫性疾病的倾向，如恶性贫血、Addison 病和自身免疫性甲状腺疾病。目前在所有的糖尿病患者中筛查乳糜泻存在争议。

糖尿病患者的小肠转运时间变化很大且并不一定与胃或结肠的转运时间有关。多达 22%的糖尿病患者有腹泻，但便秘更为常见[314]。腹泻常常呈间歇性、无痛性、偶在夜间发生，必须与大便失禁相鉴别（见后文）。有腹泻的糖尿病患者中多达 75%可能会发生脂肪泻。即使在已经使用了数年的患者中，二甲双胍仍是最常见的导致腹泻的降糖药物[318,343]。与糖尿病相关的腹泻的病因包括：药物、肠道快速转运、自主神经病变、乳糜泻、小肠细菌过度生长、过度使用无糖甜味剂、胰腺功能不全以及激素。神经病变可通过改变液体和电解质的运输以及改变肠道运动引起腹泻。分泌激素的罕见肿瘤，例如分泌胰高血糖素或生长抑素，可诱发糖尿病和腹泻。治疗腹泻应针对特定的病因，对症治疗可使用洛哌丁胺。可乐定能刺激 α_2-肾上腺素能受体，但可能会加重直立性低血压。如果不能耐受口服剂型，可以尝试贴剂[314]。奥曲肽或者长效奥曲肽类似物兰瑞肽可能对腹泻有帮助[344,345]。也有使用选择性 5-HT_3 受体拮抗剂治疗糖尿病腹泻的报道[346]。

糖尿病性胸神经根病变可引起糖尿病性神经病变患者不明原因的上腹痛。疼痛可能与厌食和体重减轻有关，类似于腹部恶性肿瘤。体格检查可见受累的皮肤感觉丧失和肌肉萎缩/无力。腹部肌肉的肌电图显示失神经支配[347]。

5. 结肠及肛门受累

半数以上的长期糖尿病患者会出现便秘，部分原因是胃结肠反射受损和结肠转运延迟。偶尔也会出现巨结肠和假性肠梗阻（很少）。糖尿病可致结肠毛细血管基底膜增厚，黏膜下小动脉管腔狭窄，进而导致缺血性结肠炎[348]。大便失禁可能与 IAS 功能障碍和直肠对扩张的敏感性降低有关[314]。控制高血糖及生物反馈治疗可能会改善大便失禁。

6. 胰腺受累

胰腺外分泌功能不全在糖尿病中很常见，并且和 MRI 和 MRCP 显示胰腺体积缩小和慢性胰腺炎改变有关[349-351]。糖尿病引起胰腺功能不全的可能机制包括：胰腺的糖尿病性血管改变和伴有肠胰反射受损的自主神经病变。在 1 型糖尿病中，自身免疫过程可能损害内分泌 β 细胞和邻近的外分泌细胞，并且低胰岛素水平会降低其对腺泡细胞的营养作用。此外，一半的 1 型糖尿病患者的胰腺外分泌有明显的变化。

此外，胰腺疾病可能会导致糖尿病，被称作 3 型糖尿病对其诊断可能不足[352,353]。病因包括慢性胰腺炎、血色素沉积症、胰腺癌（前面已讨论）、自身免疫性胰腺炎和部分胰腺切除术。在血色素沉积症中，铁通常沉积在胰腺腺泡细胞中，但也可能影响胰岛细胞。糖尿病往往在患者诊断为自身免疫性胰腺炎之前或当时就已存在，糖皮质激素疗效并不稳定[354]。胰腺切除术的效果取决于胰腺切除的部分，因为分泌胰高血糖素的细胞主要位于胰尾，分泌胰多肽的细胞位于胰头部，分泌胰岛素的细胞则均匀的分布在整个胰腺中。不同于 1 型和 2 型糖尿病，胰源性糖尿病的特点是受营养物质刺激分泌的胰多肽和胰高血糖素释放不足，从而导致容易出现低血糖症以及糖尿病酮症酸中毒（diabetic ketoacidosis，DKA）的发生率下降。饮酒和/或肝脏糖原储存减少会加重低血糖症状。胰酶替代在血糖控制中的作用存在争议。长期来看，这些患者可能会出现许多与其他糖尿病患者相同的并发症，但他们肥胖和高脂血症发病率较低，可能是由于消化不良导致的，降低了血管并发症的风险。

囊性纤维化患者中 50% 的人在 30 岁前会发生糖尿病。其增加死亡率并使肺功能恶化[355,356]。氯通道功能异常分泌的黏稠分泌物会造成胰腺梗阻性损伤，导致胰腺纤维化和脂肪浸润以及严重的胰腺萎缩。进而出现 α、β 和胰腺多肽细胞的缺失和胰岛素抵抗。低血糖是由于胰高血糖素因刺激、肝病和营养不良而缓慢增加造成的，但患者很少有酮症倾向。当患者出现生长缓慢、体重减轻或肺功能意外下降时，建议使用胰岛素，而不是口服糖尿病药物。营养支持应采用高热量、高脂肪饮食。

糖尿病会增加急性胰腺炎的发病率，而服用降糖药物可以降低急性胰腺炎的发病率[357]。11% 的急性胰腺炎患者可并发 DKA，并且认为一过性高甘油三酯血症是一个诱发因素[358]。患者可能没有腹痛或较轻微。急性胰腺炎可加重与 DKA 相关的血容量不足和高血糖。DKA 本身也可能出现腹痛、淀粉酶和脂肪酶轻度升高，但不会出现胰腺炎症改变。

7. 胆囊受累

在糖尿病患者中，超声检查可见空腹胆囊容积正常或增加[359]。糖尿病胆囊功能障碍的可能原因包括：胆碱能通路缺陷、α-肾上腺素能紧张度减少、缩胆囊素受体缺乏[360]、微动脉疾病损害肌肉收缩、高血糖和高胰岛素血症。

因为肥胖、高甘油三酯血症、高龄和高胰岛素血症等已相当明确为胆石症的危险因素，证明糖尿病是其危险因素存在困难[314]。当控制了相关的心血管和肾脏疾病时，糖尿病患者胆石症的自然病史和手术风险可能与非糖尿病患者相似[361]。高血糖、血管疾病和宿主防御功能受损会增加糖尿病患者对感染的易感性。气肿性胆囊炎是一种罕见的疾病，通常与糖尿病有关。这可能是由于血管受损致胆囊缺血，以及产气微生物的繁殖所致。

8. 肝脏受累

肝功能异常在 2 型糖尿病中很常见，尤其是血清 ALT 异常[362]。如果 ALT 不明原因地升高且小于 3 倍正常值上限，可以开始口服降糖或调脂药物；这些治疗方案通常使血清 ALT 水平随着血糖水平的降低而降低。目前使用的降糖药物中肝毒性罕见。有研究报道称噻唑烷二酮类药物可以引起肝炎或急性肝功能衰竭，磺酰脲类药可引起胆汁淤积[363]。尚不认为二甲双胍存在肝毒性。脂肪肝在糖尿病患者中很常见，是胰岛素抵抗的表现，常伴随代谢综合征。现已证明糖尿病会增加急性肝衰竭的风险，且独立于潜在的肝脏疾病[364]。

横断面和纵向研究显示，与未感染丙肝病毒的对照组、HBV 阳性患者或其他肝病患者相比，HCV 阳性患者发生 2 型糖尿病[优势比(OR)为 1.6~2.1]的风险增加[363,365,366]。同样，HCV 也是肝移植后新发糖尿病的有力预测因子[367]。胰岛素抵抗会加速纤维化的形成，并且 HCV 中 TNF-α 的上升会促进胰岛素抵抗[368]。清除丙型肝炎病毒可改善胰岛素的敏感性，降低糖尿病发病率。

在病情控制不佳的糖尿病患者中，右上腹部疼痛、肝大和血清氨基转移酶显著升高的急性肝损伤可能与糖原累积性肝病有关，但这种情况很罕见。肝活检可以用于该疾病与肝脂肪变性的鉴别，活检结果可见前者存在广泛的肝细胞核 PAS 糖原染色阳性；而控制血糖可以逆转这种表现。

肝硬化患者中有 30%~60% 的患者存在肝源性糖尿病[369,370]。其特点是肌肉、肝脏和脂肪组织中存在胰岛素抵抗，以及高胰岛素血症和胰岛细胞反应受损。与 2 型糖尿病相比，肝源性糖尿病患者由于体重指数、血脂和血压较低，微血管和大血管病变并发症的发生率下降。同样，他们可能在糖尿病并发症出现之前就死于肝病。由于肝脏中糖原的储存量极少，肝脏摄取胰岛素受损，高分解代谢率，有时并发酒精中毒，因此存在发生低血糖的危险。这类病人因为经常出现营养不良，所以一般不限制饮食。口服降糖药物由肝脏代谢，因此可能导致低血糖。虽然双胍类药物有助于降低胰岛素抵抗，但二甲双胍具有乳酸酸中毒的风险，而且在饮酒的肝硬化患者中相对禁忌[371]。α-糖苷酶抑制剂和噻唑烷类药物可能对非酒精性脂肪性肝病有效。阿卡波糖可能会降低肝性脑病患者的血氨水平[372]。67% 的肝硬化糖尿病患者肝移植后糖尿病可以治愈[373,374]。

（二）甲状腺疾病

1. 甲状腺功能亢进

甲状腺功能亢进的临床表现多样，可表现为淡漠型甲状腺毒症到甲状腺危象(伴有发热、心动过速、激越和谵妄)。胃肠道症状包括腹痛、呕吐、体重减轻和排便习惯的改变[375]。甲状腺功能亢进症可能与其他自身免疫性疾病有关，如恶性贫血、乳糜泻和溃疡性结肠炎[375-378]。

吞咽困难是一种罕见的临床表现，可能与甲状腺肿或甲状腺结节直接压迫、过量的甲状腺激素引起的肌病(累及咽部和食管上三分之一的横纹肌)或食管收缩速度增加有关。目前已证实甲状腺功能亢进的患者的胃排空速度可能正常、延迟或加快[375]。一些研究发现甲状腺功能亢进的患者存在低胃酸分泌和高胃泌素血症。自身免疫性甲状腺疾病与萎缩性胃炎有关[379]。

多达 25% 的患者有腹泻[380]。常表现为肠道转运时间缩短和粪便中脂质排泄增多。脂肪泻的机制包括过量的脂肪摄入和肠道过度蠕动。甲状腺功能亢进患者的腹泻可能是由于溃疡性结肠炎或乳糜泻引起的[375,378]。普萘洛尔可能会减少腹泻，提示肾上腺素能的相对兴奋状态有所改善。在甲状腺功能亢进的患者中，虽然甲状腺功能本身异常，药物治疗(丙基硫氧嘧啶)或并发自身免疫性肝病(AIH 和 PBC)可以导致血清氨基转移酶或碱性磷酸酶的轻度异常，但是临床上甲状腺功能显著异常罕见。甲状腺功能亢进的患者很少出现严重的胆汁淤积性肝炎、黄疸和/或急性肝功能衰竭，但在肝脏氧耗增加与肝血流不匹配时可能出现。典型表现为以 3 区为主的肝坏死，伴或不伴有右心衰竭。药物治疗可能会对甲状腺毒症有一定的作用，但必要时可行紧急的甲状腺切除术和/或肝移植。

2. 甲状腺功能减退

甲状腺功能减退最常见的原因是桥本甲状腺炎或甲状腺功能亢进患者行甲状腺消融术后。前者是一种自身免疫性疾病，有时与其他自身免疫性疾病有关，如溃疡性结肠炎、恶性贫血、糖尿病、乳糜泻和 PBC[375,378]。甲状腺功能减退最常见的胃肠道症状是便秘、厌食、恶心/呕吐和腹痛。

食管运动功能障碍可出现吞咽困难和反流等症状，其原因可能是 LES 压力降低和收缩幅度降低[375]。患者可能有胃酸分泌减少或胃排空延迟，其病因尚不清楚。植物粪石可能存在于胃或肠内，偶尔会导致梗阻。

甲状腺功能减退症与小肠细菌过度生长有关，导致腹部不适、胃胀、腹胀；通常抗生素治疗可以改善这些症状[381]。小肠转运时间可能正常或延迟[377]。结肠动力不足可导致便秘、肠梗阻、巨结肠或肠扭转。巨结肠和假性扭转少见，通常与严重的甲状腺功能减退或黏液水肿昏迷有关，静脉注射甲状腺激素治疗可能有效[382]。可能存在结肠袋横向增厚或肠袢扩张，并伴有液气平面，这需与肠梗阻相鉴别。这些患者可能因长时间的肠梗阻而使手术变得复杂[383]。病理可见神经病变或间质组织中糖胺聚糖沉积[375]。黏液水肿患者腹水的特点是蛋白浓度高(>2.5g/dL)，伴血清-腹水白蛋白梯度变化，白细胞计数低，以淋巴细胞为主[384]。治疗方案选择甲状腺素替代治疗，不选用利尿剂。

3. 甲状腺髓样癌

甲状腺髓样癌是甲状腺中分泌降钙素的 C 细胞来源的肿瘤。它可能与 2 型多发性内分泌瘤(MEN)综合征有关。三分之一的患者会出现腹泻，尤其是那些广泛转移的患者[375]。其机制多种多样，包括降钙素、前列腺素、6-羟基吲哚乙酸或非激素机制。

(三) 甲状旁腺疾病

1. 甲状旁腺功能亢进

随着包括血清钙测定在内的多通道生化筛查的出现，严重的甲状旁腺功能亢进症现已不常见，多数病例症状较轻。胃肠道症状包括结肠动力不足引起的便秘、胃动力不足引起的恶心呕吐、厌食和体重减轻[385,386]。腹痛可能与消化性溃疡，胰腺炎或胃肠运动迟缓有关。甲状旁腺功能亢进症是否会增加消化性溃疡的发病率目前还存在争议。在一些研究中发现甲状旁腺功能亢进患者胃酸分泌过多和(或)存在高胃泌素血症，而在另外的一些研究中并没有此发现。高钙会降低神经肌肉的兴奋性，进而可能导致便秘。

甲状旁腺功能亢进症中急性胰腺炎的发病率为 1%～12%。同时患有胰腺炎和甲状旁腺功能亢进的患者中 80% 存在胰腺结石，主要是导管内结石[385]。此外，钙能促进胰蛋白酶原向胰蛋白酶的转化，从而导致胰腺泡细胞损伤。相反，急性胰腺炎(常为重症)也可以由于甲状旁腺素的相对不足导致低钙血症，而通过给予甲状旁腺素可以纠正血清钙水平。此外，液体隔离和有效动脉血容量减少会引起骨骼和肾脏出现甲状旁腺激素抵抗现象，从而导致低钙血症。甲状旁腺功能亢进和胰腺炎很少有遗传因素参与，如丝氨酸蛋白酶抑制因子 Kazal1 型和 CFTR 突变[387]。一旦甲状旁腺功能亢进引起的急性胰腺炎的诊断成立，就应该进行甲状旁腺切除术。甲状旁腺切除术后可能会出现急性胰腺炎，可能是因为对甲状旁腺的操作导致钙含量急剧上升，或者是由于导致分泌降钙素细胞疲劳而反应迟钝[385]。甲状旁腺功能亢进也可能与慢性胰腺炎有关。

2. 甲状旁腺功能减退

甲状旁腺功能减退症的主要胃肠道表现为脂肪泻。可能是由于进餐后十二指肠黏膜分泌的内源性缩胆囊素释放不足，从而减少胆囊收缩和胰酶分泌[388]。用中链甘油三酯代替膳食中的长链甘油三酯可减少粪便中脂肪的丢失，从而减少因皂化作用造成的粪便中钙丢失。甲状旁腺功能减退症有时和乳糜泻有关，无麸质饮食可缓解吸收不良[389]。即使没有腹泻，对于治疗后血清钙水平无变化的甲状旁腺功能减退症患者，应该怀疑存在潜在的乳糜泻。

甲状旁腺功能减退症可导致血清碱性磷酸酶降低，但其他原因也可导致血清碱性磷酸酶降低，如锌缺乏、镁缺乏、营养不良、肝豆状核变性和低磷血症。

(四) 肾上腺疾病

超过一半的肾上腺功能不全(Addison 病)患者有胃肠道症状，如恶心、呕吐、腹泻和腹痛[390]。8% 至 12% 的 Addison 病患者有乳糜泻，这两种疾病具有相似的 HLA 关联[391]。由于相关的乳糜泻会导致糖皮质激素吸收不良，可能会使 Addison 病的治疗变得复杂，而糖皮质激素治疗可能会减轻乳糜泻。患者还可能出现萎缩性胃炎和恶性贫血[392]。Addison 病患者可能出现血清氨基转移酶升高，而糖皮质激素替代疗法可以降低血清氨基转移酶的水平[393]。

嗜铬细胞瘤是一种罕见的分泌儿茶酚胺的肿瘤，表现为高血压、心悸、头痛和出汗。胃肠道常见症状包括恶心、呕吐、腹痛，其他少见症状包括便秘、肠梗阻、巨结肠、缺血性结肠炎和穿孔[394,395]。儿茶酚胺能够松弛肠道平滑肌而减少肠道蠕动和张力，并引起内脏小动脉血管收缩而引起缺血。酚妥拉明等 α-肾上腺素能受体阻滞剂可以拮抗这种效应。使用阿片类和其他药物(如在内镜操作中)可能出现高血压急症。

(五) 脑垂体疾病

下丘脑-垂体-肾上腺轴是大脑和肠道之间重要的联系通路[396,397]。除Ⅰ型多发性内分泌瘤(MEN-Ⅰ)综合征外，垂体疾病很少累及胃肠道。库欣病患者中促肾上腺皮质激素分泌异常可能会引起皮质醇增多症，当同时使用非甾体抗炎药时，可增加胃溃疡的发病率。肢端肥大症是一种罕见的疾病，其特征为生长激素(GH)分泌过多，使结肠的长度和周长增加并且能够延缓结肠的转运时间，因此标准肠道准备常常不够充分[398]。肢端肥大症患者罹患结直肠癌、结肠息肉和其他消化道癌症的风险增加[399]。目前认为增加的生长激素和胰岛素样生长因子-1 在其中发挥了一定的作用，因为它们能够促进上皮细胞增殖。肢端肥大症患者是否应该在 50 岁前行结肠镜检查以筛查结直肠癌目前尚存在争议。可能是由于奥曲肽抑制了缩胆囊素的释放和胆囊排空，用其治疗肢端肥大症会增加胆囊结石形成风险[400]。停用奥曲肽后可能发生有症状的胆石症[401]。

四、脂质代谢紊乱

当血清甘油三酯水平超过 10g/L 时可引起急性和复发性胰腺炎，但很少引起慢性胰腺炎[402]。通常情况下，患者存在家族性高脂蛋白血症以及其他一些危险因素,包括糖尿病控制不佳、饮酒或使用某些药物(如雌激素)。高甘油三酯血症会影响淀粉酶的测定,因此血清淀粉酶水平可能正常或轻度升高。家族性高脂蛋白血症,尤其是Ⅳ型家族性高脂蛋白血症中,胆结石的发病率较高[403]。

低 β 脂蛋白血症可继发于营养不良或严重的肝病[404]。主要病因包括:无 β 脂蛋白血症、乳糜微粒滞留症和家族性低 β 脂蛋白血症[405]。无 β 脂蛋白血症是一种表现为脂肪吸收不良、血清转氨酶升高的罕见常染色体隐性遗传疾病,与载脂肝细胞导致的肝脏肿大有关,偶尔会进展为肝硬化。由于脂质不能被转运到高尔基体内,所以能在肠细胞中发现脂滴存在,尤其是在电子显微镜下[406]。家族性低 β 脂蛋白血症患者通常是无症状的杂合子,伴有或不伴有脂肪性肝病。

Fabry 病是一种 X 染色体连锁的 α-半乳糖苷酶 A 缺乏性疾病,与胃肠道症状有关,50% 至 60% 的患者表现为腹痛和腹泻[407-409]。它可能与腹泻型肠易激综合征相混淆。患者可能出现胃轻瘫、呕吐、自主神经病变、肠扩张、憩室形成、蠕动减弱和小肠细菌过度生长。使用 α-或 β-半乳糖苷酶替代疗法可以改善症状。

Gaucher 病是一种由于缺乏葡萄糖脑苷脂酶,导致葡萄糖脑苷脂在单核细胞/巨噬细胞来源的细胞内蓄积的疾病[410,411]。典型的戈谢细胞是充满脂质的巨噬细胞,呈皱褶纸样外观,细胞核移位。肝窦内富含糖脂的网状内皮细胞引起的肝脾肿大很常见。由于肝细胞不受累,因此肝衰竭罕见。门静脉高压症可能是由于脾大引起门脉正向血流增加和(或)大量戈谢细胞沉积致肝内梗阻所致,但也较少见。前者可采取脾切除治疗,两者均可通过酶替代疗法治疗。然而,由于脾切除会导致脾储存糖脂能力丧失,可能增加肝脏糖脂沉积。胆固醇为主要成分的胆结石发病率增加,特别是在脾切除术后[411]。

B 型 Niemann-Pick 病是由于缺乏酸性鞘磷脂酶,导致鞘磷脂在以单核细胞/巨噬细胞为主的细胞溶酶体内积聚[412]。疾病早期,肝脏中鞘磷脂蓄积限于库普弗细胞,但随着疾病的进展,其他类型的细胞,特别是肝细胞,也会发生鞘磷脂蓄积。门静脉高压、肝衰竭和肝硬化罕见。

Tangier 病是一种常染色体隐性遗传病,特征是扁桃体、胸腺、淋巴结、骨髓、肝脏和肠道的巨噬细胞中出现胆固醇酯蓄积。丹吉尔病是由三磷酸腺苷结合盒蛋白 *ABCA1* 突变引起的,ABCA1 介导过量的细胞固醇流出到载脂蛋白 A-I,这是高密度脂蛋白形成的一个步骤。由于缺乏载脂蛋白 A-I,这些患者的血浆胆固醇和 HDL 水平非常低。显著的临床表现包括:80% 的病例存在橘黄色"条纹"扁桃体、肝脾肿大和外周神经病变。患者可能有腹泻但无脂肪泻。结肠镜显示整个结肠和直肠有橙褐色黏膜斑点,腹腔镜显示肝脏表面出现类似的黄色斑点,这是由于肝脏网状内皮细胞中的胆固醇酯蓄积造成的。

五、肾脏疾病

厌食、恶心、呕吐、腹痛和便秘等症状在肾功能衰竭中常见[413-415]。恶心有许多原因,包括透析失衡综合征、尿毒症毒素、低血压和渗透压的快速变化。胃食管反流在特别是接受腹膜透析的患者中也有发生。尤其在夜晚尽量减少交换量可能会减少胃食管反流的发生[416]。对胃排空的研究结果相互矛盾,且与症状不相符。胃功能障碍可能与胃肌电活动受损[417]、调节胃肠动力的胃肠激素(如缩胆囊素和胃泌素)水平升高[414]、尿毒症毒素、糖尿病、自主神经功能障碍和帕金森病引起的身体受限有关。

胃十二指肠病变(通常为炎症、红斑和糜烂)在肾衰竭患者中很常见,但与症状无关[418]。胃酸或血清胃泌素水平是否改变尚有争议。在肾衰竭患者中,幽门螺杆菌感染的发生率通常是正常的或降低的[419]。

隐匿性和显性消化道出血在肾功能衰竭患者中很常见。这类因上消化道出血入院的肾功能衰竭患者,死亡率和再出血率高于无肾功能衰竭的出血患者[420,421]。尿毒症对胃肠道黏膜的影响、血小板功能障碍和抗血小板药物、非甾体抗炎药和/或透析期间的肝素化可能加重消化道出血。肾功能衰竭患者出现上消化道或下消化道血管扩张的发生率可能增加并且可能在检查消化道出血时发现[422]。与普通人群相比,存在这些血管病变的肾功能衰竭患者出血风险更高。

急性肠系膜缺血通常是非闭塞性的,可能是由于血液透析期间出现血流动力学不稳定所致[423-425]。它倾向于累及右侧结肠或多个区域,且预后较差。危险因素包括非甾体抗炎药和积极的促红细胞生成素的使用。

便秘和粪便嵌塞是血液透析患者的重要问题,而在腹膜透析患者中较少。原因包括缺乏活动、脱水、纤维摄入减少(由于限钾饮食)、代谢异常、磷酸盐结合物、铝抗酸剂、离子交换树脂、合并症以及结肠转运时间延长[413-415,426,427]。小肠运动功能障碍[428]、胆汁酸代谢异常、胰腺外分泌功能不全或淀粉样变性(后两种情况将在后面讨论)引起的小肠细菌过度生长也可能会导致腹泻的发生。

用于肠道准备的口服磷酸钠可能会导致磷酸盐肾病、高磷血症、低钙血症、低钾血症和(或)高钠血症或低钠血症,然而研究结果的异质性使得发生风险尚不清楚[429-432]。含镁泻药可导致高镁血症。通常用于治疗高钾血症的聚苯乙烯磺酸钠(Kayexalate)联合山梨醇预防便秘时可能会导致胃肠道坏死。清洁灌肠可能降低上述风险。含铝抗酸剂或硫糖铝可导致铝毒性或粪石,进而导致梗阻和(或)穿孔。

血液透析患者在结肠镜检查中穿孔的风险增加。部分原因是 β_2-微球蛋白的沉积,导致胃肠道淀粉样变性(见下文)[433]。血液透析患者急诊腹部手术后死亡率很高[434]。

腹膜透析患者中与透析导管相关的腹膜炎最常由单一病原体引起,通常选用适当的抗生素可治愈。然而,不缓解的腹膜炎、多种病原微生物引起的腹膜炎以及渗出物中淀粉酶浓度的增加提示肠穿孔[435]。因为患者常被考虑为腹膜透析所致的腹膜炎而被给予抗生素治疗了炎症,因此穿孔的诊断可能延迟,从而导致死亡率增加。由于壁腹膜和脏腹膜接触减少,腹痛为弥漫性但强度较小。此外,连续腹腔灌洗稀释了细菌负荷,减少了脓肿形成,因此 CT 可能无法显示。腹膜透析的患者也可发生气腹,尤其是导管源性气腹,从而使情况复杂化,但随着技术进步,其发生率越来越低[436]。硬化性腹膜炎是腹膜透析中一种罕见且致命的疾病,其特征是腹膜增厚并包裹肠道，从而造成梗阻[437,438]。CT显示腹膜增厚和钙化，包裹性积液和小肠袢粘连。疝在腹膜透析患者中很常见，尤其在插管部位、腹股沟管、脐部以及先前手术部位。腹膜透析液在腹内压升高时，可通过腹膜进入前腹壁软组织，引起水肿。

腹膜透析患者存在胰腺实质改变和外分泌功能不全[439,440]。血清高甲状旁腺激素水平、高甘油三酯血症、胰腺刺激激素（如缩胆囊素）升高、胰腺刺激、透析液引起的腹内压升高和淀粉样变性均与此有关。在肾衰竭或血液透析患者中，胰腺炎的发病率是否增加尚有争议。虽然血清淀粉酶水平会因清除率降低而升高，但血清淀粉酶（或脂肪酶）高于正常上限3倍和（或）CT有阳性表现则提示胰腺炎。

六、神经系统疾病

由于神经和神经递质对胃肠道功能的重要性（见第4章），各种各样的神经疾病常常与胃肠道症状相关并不意外。

（一）中枢神经系统疾病

腹型偏头痛在儿童中发病率为1%～4%，常见于女孩，发病年龄在7～12岁，也偶尔见于成年人[441,442]。腹型偏头痛的特点是反复急性发作的脐周的强烈非绞窄样疼痛。发作持续1～72小时，可伴厌食、恶心、呕吐和（或）苍白。头痛不是必需的特征。间歇期无疼痛。常有偏头痛家族史。非药物治疗包括去除诱因（例如某些食物、压力、长时间禁食、睡眠模式改变、旅行）。抗偏头痛药物治疗（如普萘洛尔、赛庚啶、曲坦类，苯噻啶）可能有效。

腹型癫痫是一种罕见的疾病，儿童比成人更常见。其特征是：①阵发性胃肠道不适，通常为病因不明的腹痛、恶心和呕吐；②中枢神经系统功能紊乱的症状，通常为嗜睡和意识模糊；③提示癫痫的异常脑电图；④抗癫痫药物治疗后症状持续改善[443,444]。腹痛通常持续几分钟，为锐痛或绞痛。成年人的腹部和中枢神经系统的表现可能比儿童更多样化。可能存在一个范围，胃肠道症状与癫痫发作（"腹部先兆"）或更细微的神经系统症状相关。原发问题常在大脑，通常是在颞叶，尽管它可能是由与大脑相连的内脏刺激引起的。抗惊厥药物治疗有效并不是腹型癫痫的诊断标准，因为抗癫痫药物可以通过镇静或安慰剂效应减轻腹痛，并且一些腹型癫痫患者药物治疗效果不佳。

头部外伤与应激性胃病和胃排空延迟有关[445]。这些患者常不能耐受肠内营养，并出现呕吐、腹胀、胃潴留、反流、误吸和肺炎。胃排空延迟是由于颅内压升高、促肾上腺皮质激素释放因子升高、高血糖、药物（镇静剂、阿片类、儿茶酚胺类）、炎症、电解质紊乱以及肠道菌群改变而抑制迷走神经活动所致。即使有轻度肠梗阻，也可以开始肠内营养，因为它促进肠道的完整性和肠蠕动。治疗方法包括促进胃肠道蠕动和使用阿片受体拮抗剂[445,446]。

脑血管意外可能会引起吞咽困难，尤其是吞咽中枢所在的脑干损伤[447,448]。脑血管意外也可导致应激性胃病、溃疡和消化道出血。结肠转运时间延长、行动不便和饮食改变可导致患者出现便秘。

多发性硬化（multiple sclerosis，MS）是发达国家年轻人最常见的慢性神经系统病。大约40%的MS患者存在胃肠道功能障碍，特别是便秘和大便失禁[449,450]。此外，患者还会出现早饱感、恶心和呕吐，以及与胃排空延迟相关的餐后不适。患者以及一级亲属中乳糜泻的发病率增加，但是无DQ2和DQ8遗传标记[451]。便秘可能与结肠转运时间延长、盆底功能障碍、结肠顺应性降低、肠蠕动消失、肛门反常收缩以及缺乏餐后结肠运动和肌电反应有关。排粪造影可以显示盆腔出口梗阻伴有耻骨直肠肌和肛门括约肌失弛缓[452]。偶尔发生直肠内套叠，通过会阴压力减轻。MS常用的药物（例如，肌肉松弛剂、抗胆碱能药、抗抑郁药、阿片类药物）以及全身肌无力导致腹内压降低，均会造成便秘。MS中大便失禁可能是由于肛门外括约肌张力降低，肛门直肠感觉减退和自发性直肠收缩所致。应当与大便蓄积导致的充溢性失禁相鉴别。通常典型的药物治疗有效，但有时需要机械排空。尤其对于疾病程度较轻的患者，生物反馈可能有帮助[453]。

（二）脊髓损伤

脊髓损伤（spinal cord injury，SCI）患者最常见的症状包括便秘、腹胀、腹痛、大便失禁和自主神经反射亢进[454,455]。

当损伤脊髓横断平面以下所有的自主神经和反射活动都消失时，脊髓损伤后脊髓休克可达数周。患者会出现腹膨隆和腹壁松弛，且损伤平面以下的感觉缺失，由于胃扩张和麻痹性肠梗阻，可导致肠鸣音消失或减弱。溃疡和出血的发生率增加。在此期间，急腹症诊断困难。当脊髓休克结束时，损伤平面以下自主神经反射恢复而后增强。

脊髓损伤位于T6平面以上或内脏大神经传出部分的患者，自主神经反射亢进为一种有潜在危险的强烈反射性血管收缩。患者表现为高血压、出汗、膀胱痉挛和腹泻。直肠乙状结肠扩张和肛门刺激会加剧自主神经反射亢进，而麻醉性栓剂可以减轻自主神经反射亢进[456]。

在高位脊髓损伤中，患者可能不会出现腹肌紧张和压痛反跳痛，导致急腹症诊断可能延迟，从而升高了死亡率[457]。合并阑尾炎的患者阑尾穿孔超过90%[454]。早期症状包括自主神经反射亢进、肩部放射痛、腹部的钝性和定位不明确的腹痛、腹胀、痉挛加重、恶心和呕吐。

腹部手术受到畸形或痉挛的影响，使得手术在技术层面上较为困难。由于腹部痉挛而张力增加，可能需要保留缝线缝合伤口。患者可能会出现反射性高血压、肺部运动减少、持续性肠梗阻和慢性化脓性病灶，从而增加伤口感染的风险。

脊髓损伤患者由于为仰卧位、便秘引起腹内压升高以及使用腹内肌进行移动，易出现胃食管反流[458]。因为咽后壁靠近颈椎，所以颈部创伤可能撞击甚至穿透咽部。颈部脊髓损伤患者上食管括约肌失弛缓会降低口腔分泌物的清除率，并损害吞咽功能[459]。这可能是由于上食管括约肌和（或）支配神经受损以及诸如气管切开术和前路脊柱外科手术等造成。

脊髓损伤患者胃排空延迟或正常[454]。因为肠神经系统和平滑肌层完整，促胃动力药物治疗有效。肠系膜上动脉压迫综合征（Wilkie综合征）是十二指肠水平部被肠系膜上动脉间歇性压迫所致。体重快速减轻、长时间仰卧位和使用脊柱矫形器可能发生该综合征。

便秘和大便失禁在脊髓损伤患者中很常见。患者也可能出现粪便嵌塞，巨结肠，粪性溃疡和痔疮[460,461]。患者也经常出现结肠转运时间延迟。T7 以上病变可导致增加腹内压的能力丧失，从而加重便秘。肛门外括约肌紧张，导致粪便滞留。当脊髓反射消失时，更多的是出现大便失禁，而较少出现便秘。肛门外括约肌不会因腹内压增加或直肠扩张而收缩。

结肠排空应在餐后进行，以利用胃结肠反射[462]。可以先导入泻药，然后刺激肛门和直肠，扩张肛管，放松耻骨直肠肌。其他方法包括：腹部按摩、手动排空、灌肠，以及新斯的明和格隆溴铵联用（一种减少新斯的明副作用的抗胆碱能药物）[463,464]。更积极的治疗方式包括：骶神经前根刺激，有时联合 S2～S4 骶神经后根切断术，可控性顺行灌肠，以及结肠造瘘术[454,465]。

在脊髓损伤后的前 6 个月内，患者可出现胆泥而非胆结石。随后，尽管一些患者有其他胆囊结石的危险因素，病因不明的胆囊结石或胆囊切除术的比率都很高（占脊髓损伤患者的 17%～31%）[466]。这些患者通常可以被准确诊断为急性胆囊炎，并且胆囊切除术的并发症和死亡率都尚可接受[467]。

（三）锥体外系（运动）障碍

由基底神经节病变引起的运动障碍可分为运动功能减退（帕金森病）和运动功能亢进（Huntington 病）。路易小体是帕金森病的病理特点，见于食管、胃和结肠的肠神经系统[468]。肠神经系统的多巴胺能神经元缺乏和迷走神经背侧运动核受累，可减少胃肠道的副交感神经支配，可能是致病特征。

帕金森病患者唾液过多，不是因为分泌量增加，而是因为吞咽效率降低[469]，有时会导致在弯腰或持续张嘴时出现流涎的症状。局部使用抗胆碱能药物可能能够改善症状。

吞咽的各个时期——口腔、咽、食管——都可能受帕金森病的影响。舌运动受损和咽期时间延长与吞咽反射延迟有关[470]。其结果会导致食物在咽部淤积，从而导致误吸（通常是无症状的），咳嗽反射减弱可使病情恶化，并导致肺炎，肺炎是帕金森病的主要死因。在帕金森病中发现了各种食管异常，包括失蠕动和多个同时收缩[471]。

大多数帕金森病患者胃肌电活动受损，以及以固体为主的胃排空延迟[472-474]，但与症状不一定相关，可能在疾病早期出现。恶心可能是治疗药物的副作用，而不是胃排空延迟所致。胃轻瘫可减少左旋多巴的吸收：因为胃排空延迟，胃黏膜中左旋多巴被多巴脱羧酶分解为多巴胺，而多巴胺不能被肠道吸收。这种效应可以通过在两餐之间给予左旋多巴、使用可溶性左旋多巴、或其他给药途径（胃肠外、鼻、舌下、直肠或空肠）来改善[475]。甲氧氯普胺为禁忌，它能通过阻断中枢多巴胺受体而加重帕金森病。多巴胺能 D_2 受体拮抗剂多潘立酮可安全使用，因为它不会透过血脑屏障，5-HT_4 受体激动剂可以通过增加乙酰胆碱的释放改善胃排空。

幽门螺杆菌相关性胃炎可能减少左旋多巴的吸收，根除幽门螺杆菌后，左旋多巴的疗效改善[476]。小肠细菌过度生长在帕金森病患者中比对照组更普遍，可能是由于肠道运动障碍所致，并与腹胀和胃肠胀气有关[477]。

便秘很常见，甚至在一些还没有出现帕金森症状的患者中也存在便秘[478,479]。某些药物、活动减少和腹部增压能力减弱（由于肌肉强直和声门闭合不协调性）会加重便秘。少数情况下可出现巨结肠、假性梗阻、肠扭转以及穿孔。结肠转运时间延长是发生便秘的主要原因[479]。参与排便的肌肉可能出现运动不协调。肌张力障碍可阻碍肛门括约肌松弛，导致排便后残余物异常增多。使用肉毒杆菌毒素注射耻骨直肠肌和（或）肛门外括约肌可能有帮助[480]，但可能导致大便失禁。阿扑吗啡注射（阿片类药物/多巴胺激动剂）可以改善反常的肛门括约肌收缩。

Huntington 病是一种常染色体显性遗传的神经退行性疾病，其特征是不自主运动、精神障碍和认知能力下降。亨 Huntington 病的吞咽困难可发生在口腔准备期（姿势不稳定、吞咽过快、舌控制差）、口腔期、咽期[481]或食管期[482]。无症状患者的内镜检查常表现为胃炎或食管炎[483]，但胃排空正常[484]。

（四）自主神经系统疾病

自主神经系统功能障碍通常是通过心血管功能异常（呼吸对心率变异性的影响或 Valsalva 动作或立位血压的测量）来衡量，但也可以通过定量发汗试验或节后交感神经轴突的功能来评估。相关的特征可能包括：直立性低血压、口眼干燥、手足冰冷伴颜色或营养改变、出汗改变、膀胱功能及性功能障碍[485,486]。自主神经功能紊乱常先于病毒综合征。疾病谱包括全自主神经系统到选择性肾上腺素能或胆碱能衰竭。多达 85% 的患者会出现胃肠道症状（如腹痛、腹胀、恶心、呕吐、便秘、腹泻），可能伴有胃肠动力不足或收缩活动不协调。一些患者中可见到神经鞘血管周围单核细胞浸润以及与神经节乙酰胆碱受体抗体的关联，提示自主神经系统功能障碍的发生可能是由免疫介导的。

自主神经病变的继发病因包括：卟啉病、疱疹病毒感染、风疹、糖尿病、副肿瘤性自主神经病变、淀粉样变性、重症肌无力、美洲锥虫病和肉毒杆菌中毒。

（五）神经肌肉接头疾病

重症肌无力是一种神经肌肉递质障碍性疾病，导致疲劳性肌无力。患者常出现吞咽困难和误吸，并且有时可能是该病的唯一临床表现[487,488]。患者咽部通常受累，也可能发生食管异常。通常情况下，反复的吞咽动作会使肌肉收缩减弱，而用依酚氯铵可以改善收缩（腾喜龙试验）。在干扰素治疗期间，偶尔会发生重症肌无力，并可能与如恶性贫血、AIH 或 PBC 等其他自身免疫性疾病有关[489,490]。

（六）肌营养不良

杜氏肌营养不良症（Duchenne muscular dystrophy，MD）是由肌营养不良蛋白基因突变引起的，该突变导致异常的肌营养不良蛋白，而肌营养不良蛋白对肌肉结构和功能至关重要[491]。肌营养不良蛋白不仅存在于骨骼肌中，而且存在于平滑肌细胞和肌间神经元中，因此可能出现胃肠道症状。强直性肌营养不良的特征是进行性肌肉无力。大部分消化道都可受累，但其严重程度通常与骨骼肌受累程度无关[492]。

肌营养不良患者血清转氨酶升高可能与肝病混淆。虽然肌肉中 AST 的含量远大于 ALT，但由于 AST 的清除率更高，因此在肌营养不良时血清中两者大致相等（一般不超过 600IU/L）[493]。磷酸肌酸激酶通常比血清 AST 和 ALT 高至少 20 倍，表明是肌肉疾病而非肝脏疾病。另一个鉴别方法是肌营养不良患者血清 γ-谷氨酰转移酶水平正常[494]。

肌营养不良患者的口咽症状很典型，可能导致误吸。咽部收缩不对称或低振幅，且食管上括约肌压力较低[492]。患者的食管可能出现扩张，收缩幅度降低且协调性差；部分患者可能出现食管体完全弛缓。食管下括约肌压力可以正常或降低。患者尽管存在食管运动障碍，但很少出现症状或没有症状。

患者常有早饱感、恶心呕吐、上腹部疼痛等症状，也可出现与胃排空延迟及餐后促胃动素分泌水平减少有关的胃石[495]。甲氧氯普胺治疗有效表明一些平滑肌还存在功能，并提示一些患者存在潜在的神经病变。

患者常见主诉包括发作性严重腹泻、吸收不良、非特异性腹痛和大便失禁[492]。小肠转运延迟可能导致小肠细菌过度生长，70% 的患者抗生素治疗有效[496]。空肠测压在小肠运动异常检测方面的敏感性优于小肠钡剂造影。患者可出现巨结肠，并有肠扭转或有穿孔风险。

在一些研究中，肛管直肠压力测定显示肛门静息和收缩压力较低。肌电图可表现为肌强直或肛门外括约肌运动单位持续时间和振幅减少等肌病电位。病理上可表现为萎缩、纤维化的 EAS，骨骼肌被 IAS 的平滑肌取代。

七、肺部疾病

慢性阻塞性肺疾病及其治疗与胃食管反流有关。慢性阻塞性肺疾病患者易患消化性溃疡病，尤其在使用糖皮质激素时，增加了与穿孔或出血性溃疡相关的死亡率。第 53 章讨论了吸烟本身对溃疡病的影响。第 57 章和第 77 章分别讨论了囊性纤维化和 α_1-抗胰蛋白酶缺乏症的胃肠道表现。

八、危重症

重症监护室（ICU）患者是一个异质、复杂的群体，因此很难研究。常见的上消化道运动障碍[497]表现为胃潴留、腹胀、呕吐、反流及误吸[498,499]。这些情况会导致肠内营养不耐受，而伴有分解代谢大于合成代谢，造成营养不良，并增加疾病的发病率和死亡率。上呼吸道的细菌定植可能来源于留滞的胃内容物中的菌群，并可导致肺炎[500]。目前尚不清楚抑酸治疗是否会加重这种情况。喂养不耐受与肠道菌群以及有机酸的变化有关；与那些没有喂养不耐受的患者相比，这类患者的菌血症发病率和死亡率更高[501]。

在机械通气和镇静的患者中，食管下括约肌压力很低，甚至无压力，食管体收缩频率低且幅度小[498]。唾液分泌减少以及食管紧绷（通常是由于气管内吸痰引起的咳嗽），这些都易导致反流和误吸。急性应激性胃病很常见，且在机械通气和明显凝血功能障碍的患者中出血风险增加。肠梗阻[502]将在第 124 章中详细讨论。50% 的患者在进入 ICU 后 96 个小时中无肠道运动并出现便秘[503]。主要危险因素是阿片类药物的摄入和疾病严重程度。应考虑常规给予刺激性或渗透性泻药。纤维性泻药应谨慎使用，因为如果液体摄入量不足，它们可能会导致粪便嵌塞。缺血性结肠炎可在低血压发作后出现。

非结石性胆囊炎也常见于 ICU 患者，表现为急性腹痛、不明原因的白细胞增多或腹腔脓毒症。

九、脓毒症

在 ICU 患者中，脓毒症肝脏受累是引起黄疸的最常见原因。肝脏可在脓毒症的两个阶段中受累。第一是感染性休克初期的肝脏低灌注，导致肝脏合成功能低下和血清氨基转移酶升高。第二阶段的肝功能障碍是由于肝脏作为主要保护器官对脓毒症的反应而引起的。肝脏中的库普弗细胞能够清除细菌内毒素以及循环中的细菌[504-506]。它们的激活会导致中性粒细胞的募集，而中性粒细胞反过来又会损伤肝细胞。肝内皮细胞具有促凝血和促炎症反应活性[507]。内毒素介导的肝微血管系统损害可导致内皮损伤、肝窦的血流减少和纤维蛋白微血栓的形成，造成明显的肝细胞坏死。与肝脏正常的患者相比，肝硬化患者更有可能因脓毒症住院，并增加死于脓毒症的可能性，这一事实说明了肝脏在抵御全身性感染方面具有重要作用[508]。

脓毒症肝脏受累在新生儿中比在成人中更常见，通常由革兰氏阴性细菌如大肠埃希菌引起[507]。重症脓毒症患者肝脏常常受累，并且溶血、弥漫性血管内凝血、心力衰竭、缺血性肝炎、全肠外营养、药物毒性、肾功能不全或胆道梗阻等因素可能会使情况变得不明朗。相比之下，男性患者更容易在大叶性肺炎脓毒症中出现肝脏受累，并且可能因酗酒而加重[507]。大多数肺炎病例是由肺炎链球菌引起的，也有肺炎克雷伯菌和其他微生物引起肺炎的报道。脓毒症肝脏受累发生在出现菌血症后的几天内，50% 的患者有轻度肝肿大，但没有瘙痒或腹痛[504,505,507]。更多的为潜在感染的表现。随着感染的治疗，病情慢慢好转。血清胆红素峰值水平，主要是直接胆红素，通常为 5～10mg/dL，但可能更高。大约 50% 的患者血清碱性磷酸酶升高，尽管可以出现明显的升高，但很少超过正常值的 2～3 倍。血清转氨酶通常正常，也可轻度升高。血清乳酸脱氢酶通常是正常的，相反，在缺氧/缺血性肝炎中它显著升高。血清白蛋白可能较低，但可能不会低于非黄疸性脓毒症。凝血酶原时间通常正常或可用维生素 K 纠正。

黄疸的原因包括红细胞输注和溶血导致的胆红素负荷增加[504]。此外，肝细胞功能障碍导致胆红素摄取、肝内结合和肝小管排泄减少，从而导致高胆红素血症。胆管及胆管细胞可能受累。脓毒症和创伤引起的胆管损伤可导致进行性硬化性胆管炎，通常是小胆管病变。当脓毒症消退后持续性高胆红素血症及血清碱性磷酸酶水平升高时，应作鉴别诊断[504]。

虽然通常不能获得脓毒症的肝脏组织学检查，但可表现为门静脉炎症、小叶中心坏死、小叶炎症、肝细胞凋亡、胆管炎/毛细胆管炎、脂肪变性（包括大泡性和微泡性）和不伴胆管上皮损伤的胆汁淤积[507,509,510]。胆管性淤胆可增加脓毒症死亡率，它是一种与“慢性感染性胆管炎”相关的脓毒症特异性肝脏病变[511]（图 37.7）。

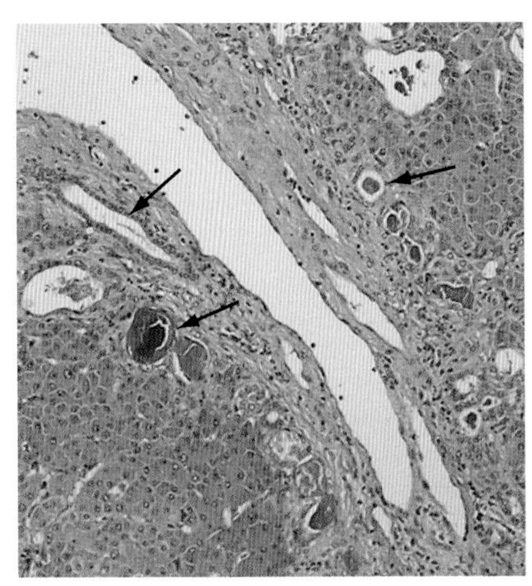

图 37.7　肝活检标本取自一例伴有明显高胆红素血症且血清碱性磷酸酶水平正常的脓毒症患者，显示"慢性感染性胆管炎"。增殖的汇管区周围胆小管内胆汁浓缩(箭头)。汇管区小叶间胆管外观正常，无胆汁淤积或损伤。(HE 染色，×25)

脓毒症肝脏受累并无特殊的治疗手段。如果需要使用经肝脏排泄到胆汁中的抗生素(如头孢曲松)时应当减量。脓毒症患者的预后与肝脏受累或高胆红素血症的程度无关，而与潜在的疾病进程有关。

十、心血管疾病

几种情况中可出现心脏和肝脏疾病相联系[512]。心脏病可继发引起充血性肝病、缺血性肝病，甚至伴有腹水的心源性肝硬化。肝脏疾病可继发影响心脏和肺，包括肝肺综合征、门静脉高压性肺动脉高压、肝硬化心包积液、肝硬化性心肌病[513]以及非肝硬化肝内动静脉瘘引起的高动力性心力衰竭(如 Osler-Weber-Rendu 即遗传性出血性毛细血管扩张症)。同时累及肝脏和心脏/循环的其他疾病包括脓毒症和浸润性疾病，如血色素沉着症、淀粉样变性和结节病。

心脏疾病(心力衰竭、缩窄性心包炎、肺源性心脏病)累及胃肠道也可以出现肠吸收不良或蛋白丢失性胃肠病。缺血性心脏病是缺血性结肠炎的危险因素[514]。纤维肌发育不良是一种非动脉粥样硬化性、非炎症性血管疾病。肾动脉和颈动脉受累最常见，但肠系膜动脉也可能受累，引起腹部绞痛和急性肠缺血[515]。主动脉瓣狭窄(Heyde 综合征)患者和多数(30%～40%)放置左心室辅助装置后的患者可能会出现有症状的消化道血管扩张(见前文"凝血障碍"疾病)。

十一、浸润性疾病

(一) 淀粉样变

淀粉样变是一组由多种血清蛋白前体、非原纤维糖蛋白血清淀粉样蛋白 P(SAP)和糖胺多糖组成的淀粉样纤维在细胞外沉积引起的浸润性疾病[516-518]。已确定超过 20 种不同的蛋白质是其致病底物。字母 A 用于表示淀粉样纤维蛋白，并用第二个字母或更多字母表示特定的原纤维蛋白。因此，对于原发性淀粉样变，最常见的表示形式为 AL，其中 L 代表在大多数患者中发现的免疫球蛋白轻链片段，无论是"原发性"还是与多发性骨髓瘤相关的。

继发性(AA)淀粉样变是由于血清淀粉样蛋白 A(SAA)沉积所致，这些血清淀粉样蛋白 A 与各种感染、炎症或(不太常见的)肿瘤性疾病有关。在过去的 40 年中，AA 淀粉样变性患者的数量有所下降，部分原因是慢性感染(如结核病)减少，慢性炎症性疾病(如 RA、IBD、家族性地中海热)得到了更好的控制，以及对 AL 淀粉样变性认识的增加。虽然过度产生的 SAA 是 AA 淀粉样变性进展的必要条件，但并不充分；SAA 是一种急性时相反应物，许多炎症性疾病也会导致 SAA 增加。

透析相关淀粉样变性($A\beta_2M$)是由于 β_2-微球蛋白沉积所致，这种蛋白存在于所有有核细胞中，通常在肾脏中代谢[519]。遗传性淀粉样变性有几种类型，最常见的是由肝脏产生的突变型甲状腺素转运蛋白(TTR)引起的。由此产生的淀粉样变(ATTR)被称为家族性淀粉样多神经病变，一种主要累及神经的常染色体显性遗传病，可通过肝移植治愈[520]。老年性系统性淀粉样变，通常累及心脏、肺和消化道，并导致野生型(非突变型)TTR 在浆膜下静脉中沉积[521]。

全身表现包括肾病综合征、周围神经病变、伴有心力衰竭和心脏传导障碍的限制型心肌病、紫癜("浣熊眼")、巨舌、关节受累、腕管综合征和体重减轻。自主功能障碍表现为直立性低血压、腹泻和阳痿。在消化道，淀粉样蛋白通常沉积在黏膜下血管壁中，使管腔变窄并最终阻塞管腔，导致血管供血区域的消化道缺血、梗死和(或)溃疡。沉积在平滑肌纤维之间淀粉样蛋白导致相邻肌纤维的压迫性萎缩，从而导致肠道运动功能障碍。沉积在消化道神经中的淀粉样蛋白也可以引起肠道运动障碍，特别是在 ATTR 淀粉样变性中。黏膜结构通常保持正常，但大量的淀粉样蛋白沉积会破坏正常的黏膜结构，导致吸收不良。

1. 口腔、食管和胃受累

巨舌最常见于 AL 淀粉样变性，通常有病理提示意义，舌体可能有干燥、皲裂、溃疡、齿痕[522,523]。它可能导致气道阻塞、构音障碍、吞咽困难和错䊀。颌下腺受累可导致口干。牙龈活检对淀粉样变性的诊断价值存在争议。

影像学发现 13% 的患者存在食管受累，而尸检发现 22% 的患者存在食管受累[516,517]。主要症状为吞咽困难、胸痛、胃灼热、呕血。可能还表现为无张力食管、溃疡、类似癌症的肿块。患者的基础食管下括约肌压力正常或降低，食管收缩幅度减小。偶尔会出现继发性贲门失弛缓症，症状发展迅速，患者体重显著减轻。

尸检发现 12% 的患者胃受累，而内镜活检中 8% 患者胃受累；但只有 1% 的患者有症状，其症状包括早饱感、恶心、腹痛、呕吐或呕血。患者可能发生胃出口梗阻。患者也可能出现胃轻瘫，尤其在影响自主神经系统的家族性淀粉样多神经病中。不规则皱襞增厚可表现为黏膜和黏膜下层低回声增厚，超声下正常壁层结构消失[524]。当平滑肌被淀粉样蛋白替代时，皱襞消失，运动能力下降。最常见的内镜表现是颗粒状外观、质脆、息肉、糜烂/溃疡和皱襞增大[525]。十二指肠病变有多种类型：扇形边缘、十二指肠炎、溃疡、肿块、低张力和扩张[516,517]。

2. 小肠及大肠受累

消化道淀粉样物质大量沉积于小肠（图 37.8），表现为腹泻、脂肪泻、蛋白丢失性胃肠病、出血、梗阻、缺血和梗死、肠壁囊样积气、肠套叠、便秘、假性梗阻、肠系膜浸润和穿孔（有时为憩室所致）[525,526]。十二指肠病变存在多种类型：扇形边缘、十二指肠炎、溃疡、肿块、低张力和扩张[516,517]。血管中淀粉样物质沉积导致的缺血性肠炎、肠壁淀粉样物质沉积或低白蛋白血症水肿可导致皱襞增厚。吸收不良、蛋白丢失性胃肠病和（或）肾病综合征可引起低白蛋白血症[527-529]。AL 淀粉样变性患者可见息肉样隆起和环状襞增厚，伴有的淀粉样物质弥漫性沉积与机械性梗阻和慢性假性肠梗阻有关[516,517]。相比之下，AA 淀粉样变性呈细颗粒状外观，沉积在黏膜可引起腹泻、吸收不良和大便潜血阳性。Aβ_2M 淀粉样变由于淀粉样蛋白沉积在固有肌层中，可导致肠道转运延迟和肠管扩张。

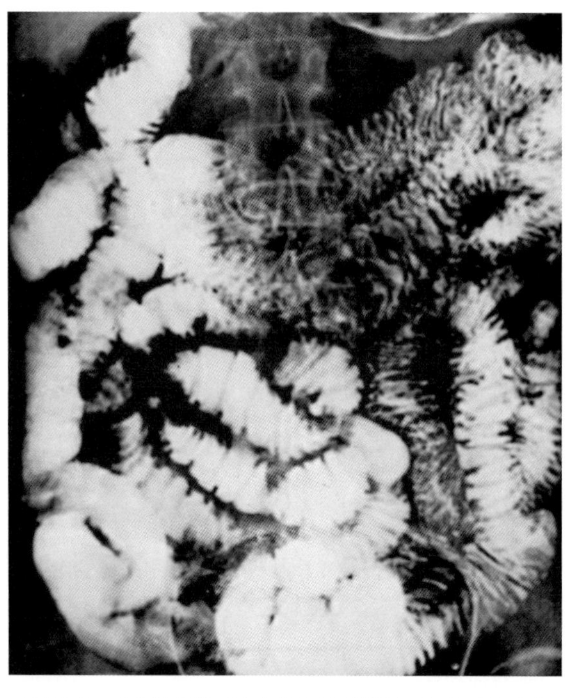

图 37.8　来自淀粉样变性患者小肠系列的胶片；显示整个小肠对称的环状皱襞边界清晰的增厚。（Courtesy Marshak RH, MD, New York.）

大肠中的淀粉样物质比小肠中的更不易辨认，常伴有管腔狭窄或扩张、结肠袋消失、皱襞增厚、结节、息肉样病变和溃疡。临床表现类似于炎症性肠病（IBD）、恶性肿瘤[530]或缺血性结肠炎。患者可出现急性假性肠梗阻，尤其是肌间神经丛有沉积物的 AA 淀粉样变性患者，病变可能是可逆的。AL 淀粉样变性和淀粉样物质浸润平滑肌引起梗阻的患者，预后较差[516]。

自主神经功能障碍所致的肠道快速转运[531]、转运延迟导致的小肠细菌过度生长、快速转运或小肠细菌过度生长引起的胆汁酸吸收不良、或血管中淀粉样物质沉积而引起胰腺腺泡组织缺血导致的胰腺功能不全均可引起腹泻。尽管常规疗法常常效果欠佳，但在个案研究中，生长抑素类似物和肠造口术可缓解腹泻[516,517,528]。脂肪泻在家族性淀粉样多神经病变中常见，在 AL 淀粉样变中不常见。体重减轻（通常严重）和营养不良影响生存质量。

出血可能是由于直接浸润了血管和组织致其脆性增加或缺血，特异性淀粉样病变，或血管脆性和血管收缩功能受损所致[532]。患者可出现如 X 因子缺乏等获得性凝血异常，特别是在 AL 淀粉样变性中。凝血酶原时间延长可能是由于肝功能障碍、吸收不良、维生素 K 摄入减少或 X 因子减少所致。

在临床上，0.9% 的克罗恩病患者和 0.7% 的溃疡性结肠炎患者会并发淀粉样变，尽管尸检结果中发生率较高。它与化脓性并发症有关，克罗恩病中多见且发展通常需要大约 15 年[533]。

3. 肝脏受累

肝淀粉样变性在大多数患者中没有临床意义，而在家族性淀粉样多神经病中，肝脏是主要受累器官。症状包括体重减轻、乏力、腹部不适和厌食[534]。在原发性淀粉样变性和活检证实肝脏受累的患者中，肝肿大（有时巨大）和血清碱性磷酸酶水平升高是最常见的表现，尽管肝脏化验异常的程度与肝脏淀粉样物质沉积的程度无关。腹水的产生多因心力衰竭而非肝病。慢性肝病的典型特征表现少见（如门静脉高压、黄疸）。通常肝大可引起脾大，偶尔会发生肝脾破裂[535]。淀粉样物质沉积可能导致肝脏硬度增加[536]。淀粉样物质可沉积于肝窦或血管。病变通常开始于汇管区周围的 Disse 间隙中，随后由于淀粉样纤维的压迫而出现肝细胞萎缩[516]。当淀粉样物质阻塞肝窦时，会促进门静脉高压症发展。有时淀粉样物质会浸润门静脉血管壁。在疑似肝淀粉样变性的患者中，皮下脂肪抽吸或骨髓活检通常为阳性（阳性率分别为 80% 和 82%），可以作为肝活检的替代诊断方法，因肝活检会增加肝淀粉样变的出血风险[534]。高胆红素血症与预后不良有关。

4. 诊断

AL 淀粉样变性中应检测血清和尿液中的单克隆轻链，免疫固定电泳可发现 89% 的患者中都存在单克隆轻链。使用免疫固定手段是用来避免遗漏小的单克隆（M）峰。患者应进行骨髓抽吸和活检，以确定浆细胞的数量和克隆性。

常见的活检部位包括肾脏、肝脏、皮下脂肪、骨髓和消化道；胃十二指肠活检结果与肾活检相当，且风险更小[537]。如果取到黏膜下血管活检，则消化道活检的阳性率会提高。在口腔活检中，88% 的患者病变部位的上皮下结缔组织中存在淀粉样物质[538]，而盲目的口腔活检几乎没有任何诊断价值。经皮肝穿刺活检由于部分研究表明会增加出血风险而存在争议[516]。出血可能是由于肝脏合成功能受损或维生素 K 依赖性凝血因子吸收不良、X 因子缺乏、淀粉样物质浸润血管所致收缩功能受损等原因导致的凝血障碍。一项研究报告指出，那些术中出血的患者凝血功能化验正常，但仍会出血[516]。

淀粉样物质 HE 染色呈粉红色（图 37.9A）。刚果红染色后，在正常光下呈红色，在偏振光下呈现苹果绿双折射（图 37.9B）。高锰酸钾预处理不影响 AL 淀粉样物质对刚果红的染色亲和力，但通常会消除 AA 淀粉样物质对刚果红的染色

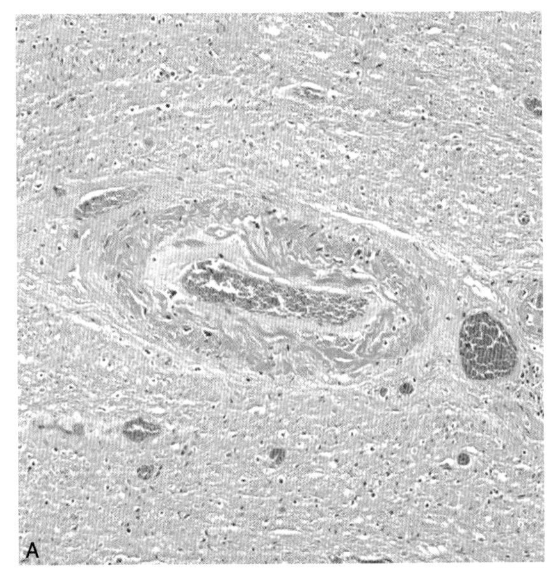

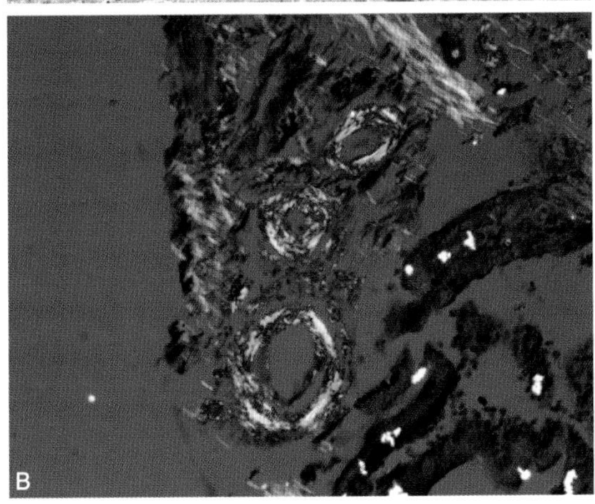

图 37.9　A，组织病理学标本显示肠系膜动脉中膜内的黏膜下血管有不规则的嗜酸性物质（淀粉样蛋白）。B，刚果红染色显示黏膜下血管呈苹果绿双折射。（From Ebert EC，Nagar M. Gastrointestinal manifestations of amyloidosis. Am J Gastroenterol 2008；103：776-87，with permission from Nature Publishing Group.）

亲和力。对活检样本进行免疫组织化学检查很重要，因为它影响治疗方法的选择[539,540]。

5. 治疗和预后

AL 淀粉样变可采用骨髓瘤化疗方案或大剂量化疗加自体造血干细胞移植治疗，以消除 B 细胞或浆细胞克隆[541,542]。虽然并发症较多，但能显著延长中位生存时间，并且淀粉样物质沉积可能消退。对于 AA 淀粉样变，控制潜在的炎性疾病可降低血清淀粉样蛋白 A 的水平和延缓疾病的进展。抗 TNF 药物可改善与克罗恩病相关的 AA 淀粉样变性患者的临床症状[543]。秋水仙碱能在家族性淀粉样多神经病患者和 FMF 患者中减轻症状并防止淀粉样物质沉积，似乎对已发生淀粉样变性的患者也有获益[516]。对于透析相关淀粉样变性，肾移植可降低血清 β_2 微球蛋白水平并使淀粉样物质沉积减慢。对于如家族性淀粉样多神经病等遗传性淀粉样变性，其前体蛋白（突变 TTR）仅由肝脏产生，可通过肝移植治愈，且大部分患者的胃肠道症状和营养状况也能够得到改善[544]。移除的肝脏除了产生淀粉样蛋白外，其他都是正常的，并且其也不是淀粉样物质沉积的部位。

奥曲肽用于治疗 AA 淀粉样变性患者的难治性腹泻[516]。有零星报道表明促动力药可能对胃肠道运动功能障碍有治疗效果。手术困难且存在许多风险：出血、伤口愈合不良、吻合口开裂（可能与切缘淀粉样物质沉积有关）、营养不良和以心脏及肾脏为主的多器官衰竭。

AL 肝脏淀粉样变性患者的中位生存期不到 1 年，尤其是那些患有心力衰竭和（或）高胆红素血症患者。大多数死亡与心脏或肾脏的并发症有关，或在多发性骨髓瘤患者中与潜在恶性肿瘤的进展有关[534]。肝脏受累程度与发病率和死亡率几乎不相关。

（二）肉芽肿性肝病

肉芽肿是一种试图将机体视为异物包裹的免疫细胞机化性积聚，作为系统性疾病的一个主要过程或表现而常在肝脏中出现[545-548]。可以在 2%～15% 肝活检中见到，常位于汇管区周围。肉芽肿性肝病存在多种病因（表 37.2），其中只有 10%～30% 为特发性。在发达国家最常见的病因可能是原发性胆汁性肝硬化，而在发展中国家（以及较早的研究）中，最常见的病因是感染性疾病，尤其是结核病。虽然患者通常无症状，但可能出现肝肿大、右上腹部疼痛、发热和（或）体重减轻。与感染相关的肉芽肿需要以巨噬细胞为基础的清除途径，因此免疫细胞聚集浸润呈混合性，并容易出现干酪样中央坏死。免疫介导的疾病通常伴有密集的淋巴细胞浸润。淀粉、硅油或矿物油等不可清除的颗粒物引起的异物性肉芽肿和脂肪肉芽肿的炎性浸润最轻。结节病、某些感染、毒物和药物相关的上皮样肉芽肿含有类似于上皮细胞的活化巨噬细胞。纤维蛋白环肉芽肿由上皮样肉芽肿和纤维蛋白环包围的中央脂质空泡组成，常见于 Q 热，但也见于其他多种疾病[548]。肉芽肿性炎症的特点是肉芽肿形态不良，边缘模糊，常伴有肝细胞和（或）导管损伤。病理医生在肝脏活检阅片时应尝试确定肉芽肿的位置、有无坏死、伴发浸润的类型、肉芽肿中有无任何生物体或异物以及相关发现。

一些罕见的并发症通常是由于肉芽肿压迫邻近结构所致，导致门静脉高压、肝内胆汁淤积、胆道狭窄、肝静脉血栓形成和肝硬化[546]。必要时应行胸部 X 线检查；细菌（包括布鲁菌）、分枝杆菌和真菌培养；血清抗线粒体抗体检测；Q 热、布鲁菌病、梅毒、乙肝和丙肝的血清学检查；感染性病原体 PCR 检测和结核病检测。

（三）结节病

结节病是一种病因不明的多系统肉芽肿性疾病[549]。本病好发于 20～40 岁的人群，与高加索人相比，非裔美国人的发病率和死亡率更高。患者可能出现全身症状、肺部疾病、淋巴结病、肉芽肿性葡萄膜炎、近端型肌病、冻疮样狼疮、脑神经麻痹、结节性红斑、高钙血症和多器官肉芽肿。肉芽肿中的上皮样细胞产生的血管紧张素转换酶（ACE）水平升高是一种较弱的诊断试验。Kveim-Siltzbach 试验是在皮内注射结节组织提取物，4 周后对该区域产生的丘疹进行活检；然而可行性和伦理准则限制了其使用。

表 37.2　肝肉芽肿的部分原因*

感染	肿瘤	药物	其他原因
细菌			
	霍奇金淋巴瘤	别嘌呤醇	自身免疫性肝炎
汉赛巴尔通体(猫抓病)	非霍奇金淋巴瘤	卡马西平	卡介苗
疏螺旋体(莱姆病)		头孢氨苄	胆道梗阻
布鲁菌	肾细胞癌	氯磺丙脲	常见变异型免疫缺陷病
土拉热弗朗西斯菌(兔热病)		氯丙嗪	
单核细胞性李斯特菌(李斯特菌病)		氨苯砜	克罗恩病
胞内鸟分枝杆菌		地西泮	异物(滑石粉,淀粉)
麻风分枝杆菌(麻风病)		双氯芬酸	蔬菜汁
结核分枝杆菌		地尔硫䓬	特发性
诺卡氏菌		依那西普	金属毒性(铍、铜)
伤寒沙门氏菌(伤寒)		格列本脲	原发性胆汁性肝硬化
梅毒螺旋体(梅毒)		黄金	原发性硬化性胆管炎
惠普尔养障体(惠普尔病)		肼屈嗪	结节病
小肠结肠炎耶尔森菌		英夫利西单抗	硅胶注射
立克次体		干扰素	系统性红斑狼疮
贝纳柯克斯体(Q 热)		异烟肼	肉芽肿性多血管炎
病毒			
		美沙拉秦	
巨细胞病毒		甲基多巴	
EB 病毒		呋喃妥英	
丙型肝炎病毒		口服避孕药	
真菌病			
		苯唑西林	
放线菌病		盘尼西林	
粗球孢子菌(球孢子菌病)		苯妥英	
新型隐球菌(隐球菌病)		普鲁卡因胺	
荚膜组织胞浆菌(组织胞浆菌病)			
寄生虫病			
		丙卡巴肼	
肝片吸虫(肝片吸虫病)		奎尼丁	
利什曼病		奎宁	
血吸虫病		罗格列酮	
犬和猫弓首蛔虫(内脏幼虫移行症)		散利痛(埃克塞德林)	
刚地弓形虫(弓形虫病)		磺胺类药	

*另见第 35、84、88 和 91 章。

1. 胃肠道受累

结节病胃肠道受累罕见[550-552]。可能会偶然发现黏膜肉芽肿,并且必须完全除外结核或克罗恩病等诊断,尤其是在进行免疫抑制治疗之前。食管很少受累,一旦累及食管可导致吞咽困难或反流。黏膜受累可引起阿弗他病变、斑块或结节[553-556]。肌肉或神经性受累导致环咽肌运动障碍,或产生糖皮质激素治疗有效的贲门失弛缓症样表现。肺门或纵隔淋巴结压迫食管可能会导致食管机械性梗阻,并且在高分辨率食管测压检测中可以看到浸润性食管胃结合部流出道梗阻。

胃肠道最常见的受累部位是胃,虽然通常无症状,但可引起疼痛、早饱感、恶心和呕吐(见第 52 章)。研究报道表明,胃受累,尤其是累及胃窦时可出现各种病变:溃疡、皱襞增厚、皮革胃样表现以及腹膜后淋巴结病引起的外源性压迫[554,557]。通常无法明确肉芽肿是偶然发现还是会引起症状。胃孤立性肉芽肿更多是由克罗恩病引起的,而非结节病。结节病很少累及十二指肠[558]。

乳糜泻和结节病之间可能存在某种联系,可能由于这两种疾病都与 HLA-DQ2 和 HLA-DR3 有关,都是由抗原加工缺陷引起的,并与Ⅱ类 HLA 分子表达增加有关[559]。

结节病很少累及肠道,主要鉴别诊断为克罗恩病。罕见的舒曼小体(细胞内同心层状包涵体)、胃肠道外肉芽肿和对糖皮质激素强烈应答是提示结节病的鉴别特征。瘘管、结构变形和急性炎症并不常见。患者可能出现肠梗阻(由于肿块、狭窄或淋巴结病的外源性压迫)、疼痛、慢性腹泻、蛋白丢失性胃肠病[560]、溃疡或结肠炎所致出血[558,561]。

胰腺的结节病相当罕见,表现为胰腺肿大、胆道梗阻、腹痛、急性胰腺炎或胰腺功能不全[562]。血清淀粉酶和脂肪酶可轻度升高[563]。淋巴结或胆囊肉芽肿性炎症压迫胆囊管可引起继发的急性胆囊炎[564]。肉芽肿累及胆管或周围淋巴结可能会引起梗阻性黄疸。因胆囊炎行胆囊切除术后可能会发现胆囊壁肉芽肿。

与淋巴瘤不同,结节病中腹部淋巴结病的特点是淋巴结直径一般小于 2cm,分离的(而非融合),且膈脚后间隙很少受累[565]。结节病必须与癌症患者淋巴结中发现的“结节样反应”相鉴别。绝大多数患者超声内镜下细针抽吸活检能够明确诊断肉芽肿[566]。

腹水是罕见的,通常是由于右心衰竭或门静脉高压所致。然而,腹膜小结节可能会引起淋巴细胞性腹水[567]。CT 可显示腹膜韧带和肠系膜浸润[568]。需要进行腹膜活检以确定诊断并排除结核、真菌感染和恶性肿瘤。腹水通常会自发吸收或经短疗程糖皮质激素治疗后消退。

干扰素治疗(通常在前 6 个月内)可能会罕见地引起结节病,通常侵犯肺和皮肤。大多数患者在停用干扰素后病情可有所好转,但也有少数患者需要糖皮质激素治疗[569,570]。然而,未经治疗的丙肝患者偶尔也可能会出现结节病。接受那他珠单抗治疗克罗恩病的患者也可能出现结节病;但目前尚不清楚维多珠单抗治疗是否也会出现这种情况[571]。

2. 肝、脾受累

肝脏受累通常无症状,且肝化验正常[550,552,572,573]。最常见的症状是腹痛。黄疸很少见,可能是由于肝内胆汁淤积、溶血、肝细胞功能障碍或肿大淋巴结阻塞肝外胆管所致。临床上,约 21% 的患者会出现肝大,超过半数的患者行腹部 CT 扫描可发现肝大。约 20% ~ 40% 的患者肝脏化验异常,通常为血清碱性磷酸酶水平较高,而血清转氨酶升高不明显[550,574]。高球蛋白血症非常常见。在一份报告中,四分之一的患者仅有肝脏受累而无肺受累[575]。

肝活检发现肉芽肿有助于结节病的诊断。肉芽肿主要位于汇管区和汇管周围区域,伴有大上皮样细胞簇集,通常伴有多核巨细胞(图 37.10A)。肉芽肿转化速度较快,大的融合性肉芽肿会导致透明瘢痕形成。肝肉芽肿内很少含有舒曼体或星形小体(星状包涵体)。虽然见不到明显的干酪样变,但也可发生肉芽肿中央坏死。

可出现多种组织学表现,可分为胆汁淤积,坏死性炎症和血管病变。胆汁淤积可能是由于肝外胆管结节病,肝门周围淋巴结肿大压迫胆管,胰腺受累,或伴发的 PBC 和 PSC 所致[572]。肝内胆汁淤积患者可能会出现肉芽肿对胆管的进行性破坏,导致小叶间胆管消失、门静脉周围纤维化和类似于 PBC 的胆汁性肝硬化[550,572]。其他患者可能有与 PSC 类似的导管周围纤维化。与 PBC 和 PSC 不同,结节病患者通常血清 IgM 水平正常,抗线粒体抗体和 ANCA 呈阴性。此外,在使用糖皮质激素治疗后结节病患者的病情可能会迅速改善,这种

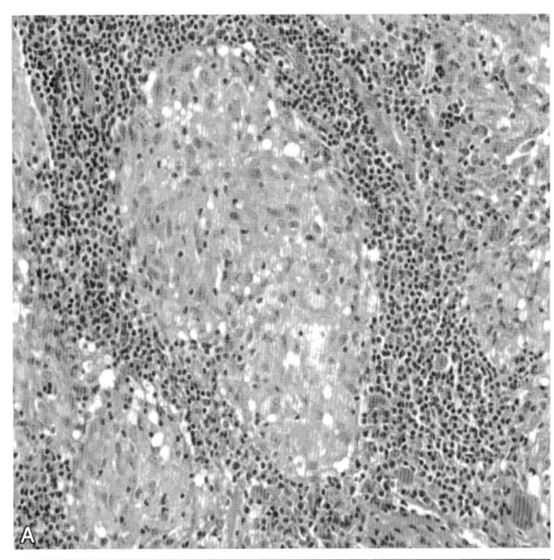

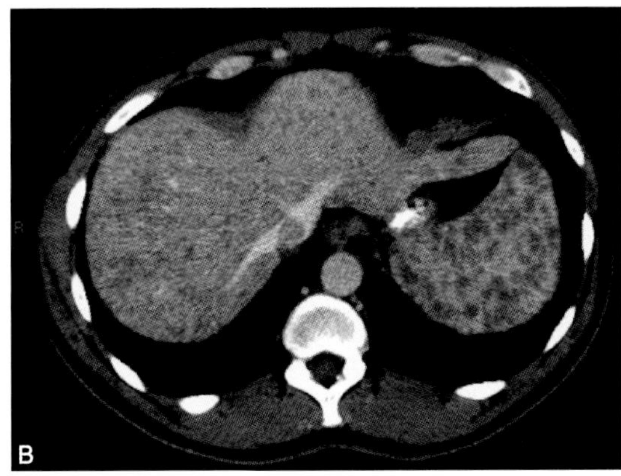

图 37.10　结节病。A,组织病理学显示淋巴结内有非干酪样肉芽肿。周围可见有上皮样组织细胞和淋巴细胞包绕的朗格汉斯型巨细胞聚集,无中心性坏死。B,腹部 CT 显示肝、脾多发低密度灶,证实 1 例结节病患者为肉芽肿。(From Ebert EC, Kierson M, Hagspiel KD. Gastrointestinal and hepatic manifestations of sarcoidosis. Am J Gastroenterol 2008;103:3184-92, with permission ffffrom Nature Publishing Group.)

情况在 PBC 和 PSC 中难以见到。PBC 和 PSC 可能与肝肉芽肿有关(见表 37.2),但在结节病中,这些疾病的典型胆管表现不明显或不存在。PBC 和 PSC 很少与结节病共存。一些患者患有急性胆管炎,提示存在机械性梗阻而无真正的导管梗阻。可能会发现坏死性炎症性疾病或类似肝炎的改变,也可发现结节性再生性增生或肝窦扩张等血管改变,主要累及中央静脉周围。外源性压迫或血管壁肉芽肿导致静脉狭窄会促使肝静脉血栓形成,但发生率很低。纤维化可能局限于汇管区及周围区域或发展成汇管区间桥接性纤维化,甚至肝硬化。少数患者中可能出现窦前阻滞或者由于门静脉和肝静脉肉芽肿性静脉炎继发引起肝脏缺血而导致的窦前和窦后阻力增加,进而发生门静脉高压[573]。由于肝硬化罕见且肝功能通常正常,因此很少发生肝性脑病和肝衰竭。在一项对 350 例结节病患者的回顾性研究中,有 19 例(6%)出现了肝脏受累。约有 16 例患者接受了肝活检,其中 88% 为非干酪性肉芽肿。大约 4 名患者(20%)在诊断出肝结节病后平均 10 年的随访中发展为肝硬化[576]。

结节性肉芽肿通常较小,不能通过影像学检查发现。然

而,如果它们聚集形成大的聚集体,可能会发生纤维化和(或)被炎症包围,在影像学上可能表现为无数的小结节(图 37.10B)。增强 CT 表现呈低密度影而无强化[572]。磁共振 T1 和 T2 加权像表现为低信号病变,注射钆后无强化。正电子发射断层扫描上表现为病变摄取氟脱氧葡萄糖,这可用于监测疾病的进展或缓解。

结节病有很高的自然缓解率,并且由于目前尚无评估治疗的大型对照试验,因此不清楚是否应该以及何时治疗肝结节病[577]。糖皮质激素治疗可能可以改善肝脏化验结果,但肝脏组织学上并不一定,并且仍可能进展为肝硬化。只有个案报道支持使用其他药物,如熊去氧胆酸、苯丁酸氮芥、硫唑嘌呤和甲氨蝶呤。肝移植术后疾病复发是一种导致移植物失功或患者死亡的罕见原因[578]。

结节病脾脏受累通常无症状,但可表现为左上腹痛、全身症状、脾功能亢进,但很少发生脾破裂。脾结节往往较小、离散、多发,但随着体积增加而出现融合(图 37.10B)[579]。多达 50% 的患者伴有肝脏病变。鉴别诊断包括感染(结核病和组织胞浆菌病)、错构瘤和血管瘤等良性病变、淋巴瘤等恶性病变。MRI 可用于这些疾病的鉴别诊断。严重的脾大患者可采用糖皮质激素治疗。

(四) 其他

嗜酸细胞性胃肠炎(见第 30 章)、嗜酸细胞增多综合征、嗜酸性肉芽肿性多血管炎、结节性多动脉炎和金中毒时可出现消化道黏膜嗜酸性粒细胞浸润。朗格汉斯细胞肉芽肿病(组织细胞增生症 X,嗜酸性肉芽肿)也可浸润胃肠道。

小血管透明变性是一种罕见的家族综合征,包括腹泻、直肠出血、吸收不良和蛋白丢失性胃肠病,并伴有皮肤异色病、头发灰白和脑血管钙化[580]。病理可见肠毛细血管、小动脉和小静脉的上皮下间隙基底膜样沉积物。

(韩跃华 译,黄永辉 袁农 校)

参考文献

第 38 章　胃肠道血管病变

Joann Kwah, Lawrence J. Brandt 著

章节目录

一、原发性血管病变 …… 531
（一）结肠血管扩张 …… 531
（二）血管发育不良 …… 537
（三）Dieulafoy 病变 …… 538
（四）血管瘤 …… 539
（五）先天性动静脉畸形 …… 540
二、动脉瘤 …… 540
（一）腹主动脉瘤 …… 540
（二）内脏动脉瘤 …… 541
三、假体旁肠瘘和主动脉肠瘘 …… 542
四、系统性病变或表现形式相关的血管病变 …… 543
（一）遗传性出血性毛细血管扩张症 …… 543
（二）蓝色橡皮疱痣综合征 …… 544
（三）进行性系统性硬化症（硬皮病）…… 544
（四）Klippel-Trénaunay 综合征和 Parkes Weber 综合征（先天性静脉畸形肢体肥大综合征） …… 544
（五）辐射诱导的黏膜损伤 …… 545
（六）胃窦血管扩张症（西瓜胃）及门静脉高压性胃病、肠病和结肠病 …… 545
五、血管的解剖异常 …… 547
（一）肠系膜上动脉综合征 …… 547
（二）腹腔干压迫（正中弓状韧带）综合征 …… 547

随着我们的诊断方法的不断精进，胃肠道的血管病变和疾病诊断也越来越准确。目前常用的诊断技术包括胃镜、结肠镜、单气囊小肠镜（SBE）和双气囊小肠镜（DBE）、胶囊内镜（video capsule endoscopy，VCE）和先进的放射成像技术，如 CT 血管成像（CTA）和核磁血管成像（MRA）。血管病变是消化道出血的常见原因，可能是单发的或多发的；良性的或恶性的；孤立的、成组的或弥漫的；综合征或全身性疾病的一部分；或者由于脉管系统的解剖异常；或因治疗导致。我们首先要了解血管病变的命名法。*Vas* 及其衍生的 *vascular* 是拉丁文，意思是“血管”；对应的希腊语是 *angeion*。*Ectasia* 是一个源自希腊语的词，指的是血管扩张或延长的过程；由此产生的病变也可称为扩张症。毛细血管扩张症是指血管末梢扩张引起的病变。血管发育不良是用来描述异常形成（*dys*，“bad”；*plasis*，“molded”）血管的病变或过程的通用术语。动静脉畸形（arteriovenous malformation，AVM）是一种先天性病变，而血管瘤是一种新生物。本章讨论了临床上重要的胃肠道血管病变，其中大部分会引起消化道出血。

一、原发性血管病变

（一）结肠血管扩张

血管扩张（angioectasia，AE）是一种独特的临床和病理改变[1~3]。它是胃肠道最常见的血管异常病变，可能是导致 60 岁以上人群复发性或慢性下消化道出血的最常见原因[4]。结肠血管扩张与年龄增长有关，与性别无明显相关。与胃肠道的先天性或肿瘤性血管病变相反，获得性血管扩张与皮肤或其他脏器病变无关，尽管约有 10% 的结肠血管扩张患者在血管造影或小肠镜检查时发现小肠中存在类似病变[3,5,6]。结肠血管扩张几乎都局限于盲肠或升结肠，通常是多发的，且直径小于 10mm。该病很少被外科医生在手术中发现，病理医生使用标准的组织学技术也很少能够识别，但它们通常可以通过血管造影（稍后讨论）、结肠镜检查（图 38.1 和图 38.2）或螺旋 CTA[7] 识别。

CT 和 MRI 在所有类型血管病变中的作用正在不断演变，但随着这些复杂诊断方法的应用更加广泛，其诊断能力会进一步提高；显而易见，目前传统血管造影对血管病变的治疗作用比诊断更重要。为了确定血管病变的确切性质，有必要进行组织学检查。例如，一篇没有进行血管病变组织学确认的文献报道，在 46% 的患者中，血管扩张发生在肝曲远端[8]；随后发现小肠或左半结肠中被认为是血管扩张的组织学表现与右半结

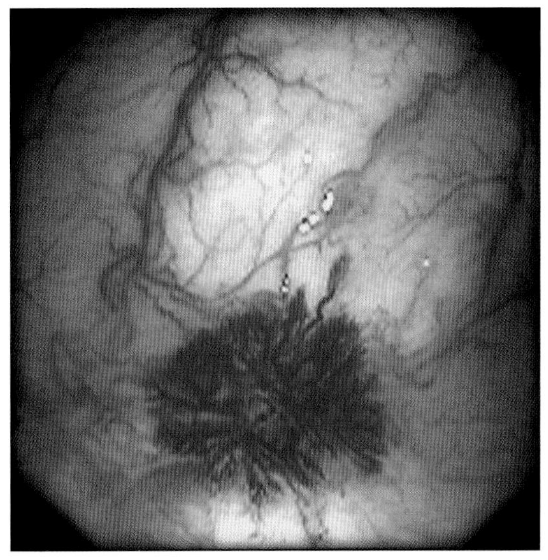

图 38.1　升结肠血管扩张（AE）的内镜图像。该 AE 具有典型的珊瑚礁样小血管模式，扭曲了黏膜层和黏膜下层。迂曲的黏膜下静脉是 AE 发生的最早阶段，可能存在于与扩张相交的线性血管中，但无法区分

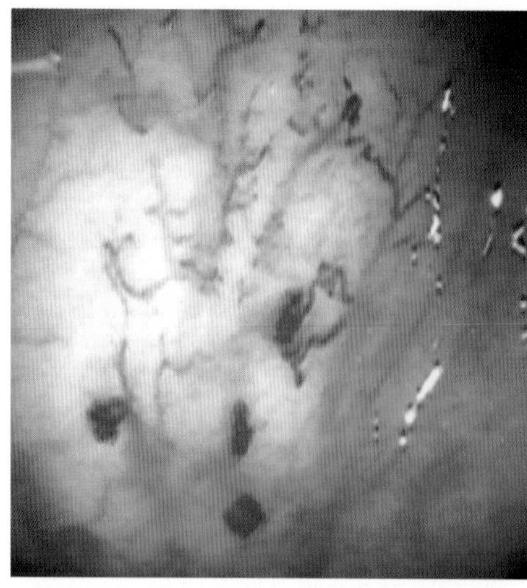
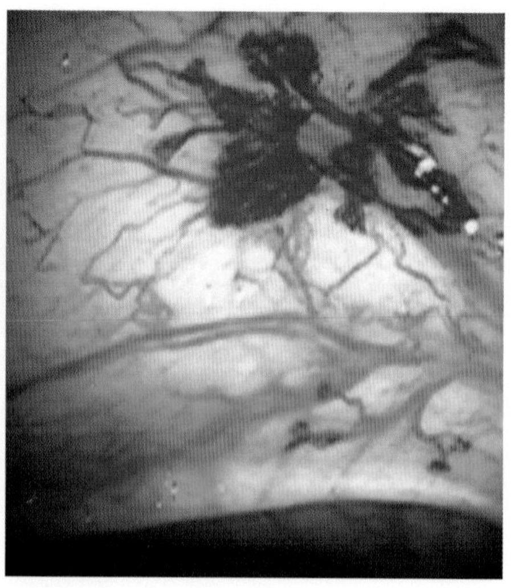

图 38.2　一例表现为反复性下消化道出血的老年患者升结肠中多发性血管扩张(AE)的内镜图像。AE 可以是单个的,也可以是多个的、形状和大小各不相同。在 AE 附近可见引流静脉

肠血管扩张存在差异(S. J. Boley 和 L. J. Brand 的综述)。

1. 病理学

除非使用特殊技术,否则很难对血管扩张进行组织学鉴定[1]。虽然通常只有不到三分之一的病变可通过常规病理检查发现,但几乎所有病变都可以通过以下方法进行鉴定:向结肠血管内注射硅橡胶,增加乙醇浓度使细胞脱水,通过将其浸入水杨酸甲酯中 24 小时来清除样本,然后通过解剖立体显微镜观察样本(图 38.3)[1]。在一项使用这些方法的研究中,我们发现手术切除的结肠具有 1 个或多个直径为 1 至 10mm 的黏膜血管扩张。血管扩张通常是多发的,并且都位于盲肠和升结肠[1]。

在显微镜下,黏膜血管扩张由扩张的、扭曲的、薄壁的小静脉、毛细血管和小动脉组成。最早期的异常是出现扩张、曲折的黏膜下静脉(图 38.4A),通常位于表面黏膜血管正常的区域。进展期病变显示越来越多的扩张和变形血管穿过黏膜肌层并累及黏膜(见图 38.4B 和 C),直到在最严重的病变中,黏膜被弯曲、扩张的血管迷宫取代(见图 38.4D)。在晚期病变中偶尔可见扩大的动脉和厚壁静脉,其中扩张的小动脉-毛细血管-小静脉单位由于动脉前括约肌功能丧失而成为小动静脉瘘。然而,大的厚壁动脉是先天性 AVM 的典型特征。

2. 发病机制

先前描述的使用注射和清除技术的研究表明,血管扩张是随着年龄的增长而发生的,它们代表了一种独特的临床和病理改变[1]。在临床上,血管扩张常在老年人的结肠镜检查和没有出血史的老年患者切除的结肠中发现[1,9]。Boley 推测血管扩张的可能形成原因是黏膜下静脉在这些血管穿透结肠

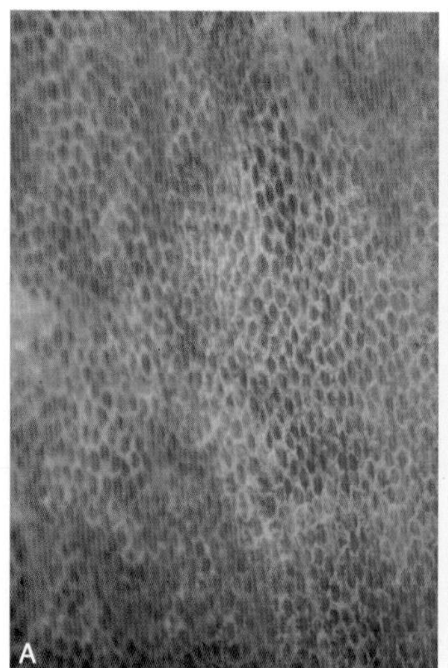

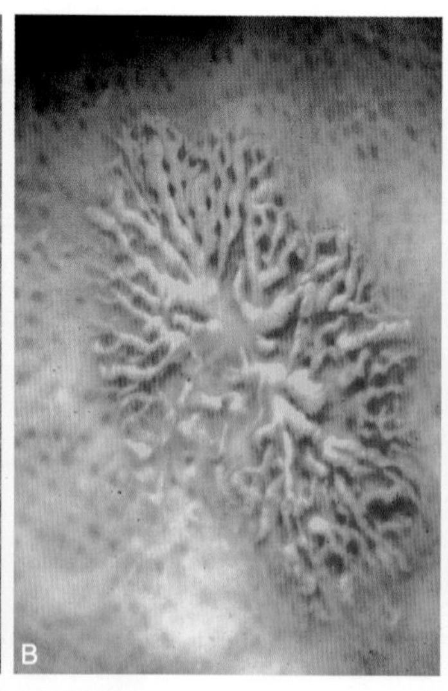

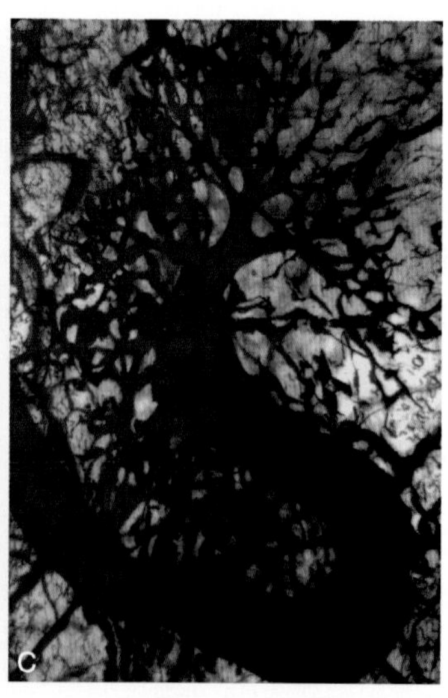

图 38.3　A,已注射硅橡胶但未清除的结肠切除标本(详见正文)。立体显微镜显示正常结肠隐窝呈蜂窝状。B,在注射但未清除的结肠中出现珊瑚礁血管扩张。在血管扩张周围可见正常隐窝。C,注射、清除和透照结肠显示黏膜扩张,周围有正常隐窝,小静脉扩张,导致黏膜下静脉变大、扩张、迂曲。(A and B, From Mitsudo S, Boley SJ, Brandt LJ, et al. Vascular ectasias of the right colon in the elderly: A distinct clinical entity. Hum Pathol 1979;10:589; C, from Boley SJ, Sammartano RJ, Adams A, et al. On the nature and etiology of vascular ectasias of the colon: Degenerative lesions of aging. Gastroenterology 1977;72:650-60, with permission.)

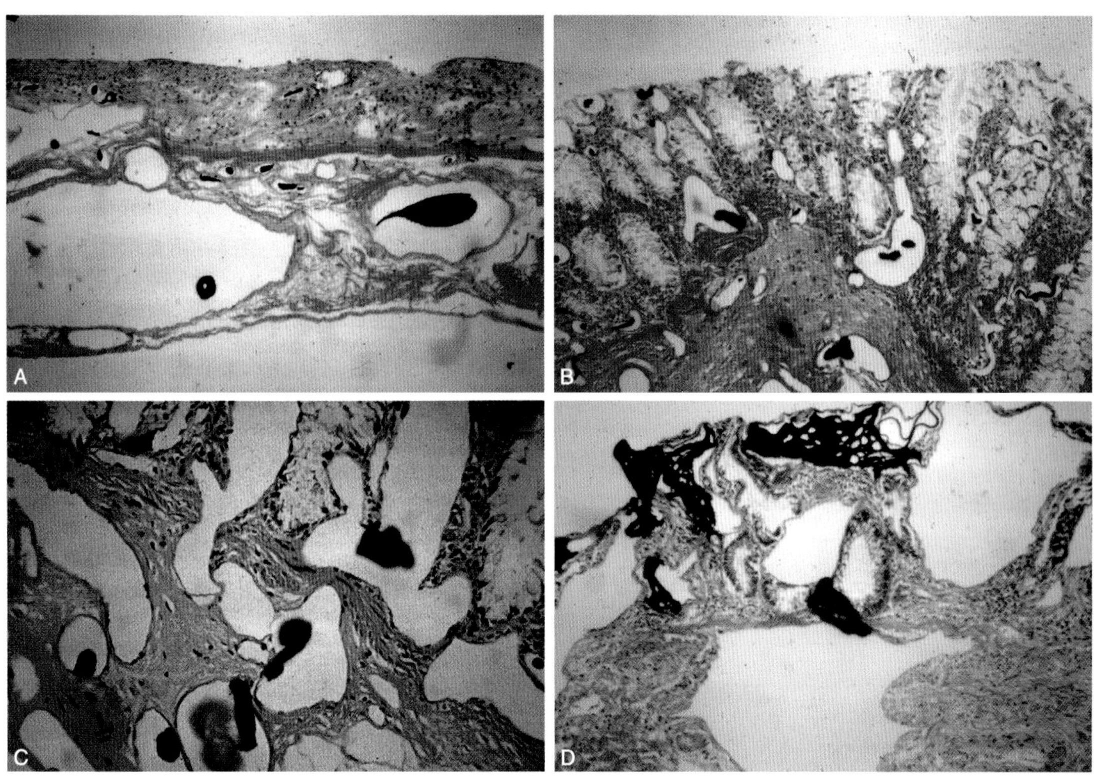

图 38.4　血管扩张(AE)的组织病理学。A,黏膜下层充满大的扩张静脉,上覆黏膜中有少数扩张的小静脉。这种表现是早期 AE 的标志。血管腔内的黑色物质是 Microfil^{R}(血管造影剂)。B,更晚期的 AE 病变,黏膜下层的扩张迂曲静脉延伸至黏膜。C,AE 病变进一步发展的阶段,其中扩张血管破坏并取代黏膜。D,晚期 AE 显示黏膜完全破坏,被扩张血管替代。只有一层内皮将盲肠腔与扩张血管腔分离。(H & E,×50)(From Boley SJ,Sammartano RJ,Adams A,et al. On the nature and etiology of vascular ectasias of the colon:Degenerative lesions of aging. Gastroenterology 1977;72:650-660,with permission.)

肌层的部位出现部分、间歇性、低度阻塞(图 38.5 和图 38.6)[1]。他进一步提出,长期在肌肉收缩和盲肠扩张时反复出现的短暂压力升高导致黏膜下静脉以及随后的小静脉和毛细血管的扩张和弯曲。他还提出,最终,毛细血管环扩张,毛细血管前括约肌功能丧失,并产生一个小的动静脉瘘;后者是“早期静脉充盈”的原因,这是该病血管造影的标志性表现(图 38.7)。动静脉瘘的血流持续增加可引起供应该区域的动脉和引流该区域的壁外静脉发生改变。血管扩张病因的这一发展概念基于以下发现:①没有任何黏膜病变,或者在由正常动脉供血的微小黏膜血管扩张之下的明显的黏膜下静脉;②从血管穿过固有肌层处开始的静脉扩张(见图 38.5);③既往的研究表明,随着结肠运动、壁内张力和腔内压力的增加,肠内的静脉血流量可能会减少[10]。按照这个逻辑,根据拉普拉斯原理:$T \propto PR$(其中 T 是张力,P 是腔内压力,R 是半径),血管扩张出现在右半结肠可归因于盲肠壁的张力大于其他部位结肠。

血管扩张发生的另一个概念是基于已证实血管扩张在因反复出血行结肠切除术的患者的手术标本中,沿其内皮层表达血管内皮生长因子(VEGF)及其受体[11];这表明血管生成的增殖期。VEGF 和 VEGF 受体 1 已被证明会因缺氧而上调[12],因此也有人认为缺氧在血管扩张的发病机制中发挥作用。进一步提出,血管性血友病因子(vWf)通过涉及 VEGF 受体 2 信号通路、血管生成素和整合素 $\alpha\nu\beta3$ 的多条“交叉通路”途径调节血管生成。在小鼠模型中,抑制内皮细胞中的

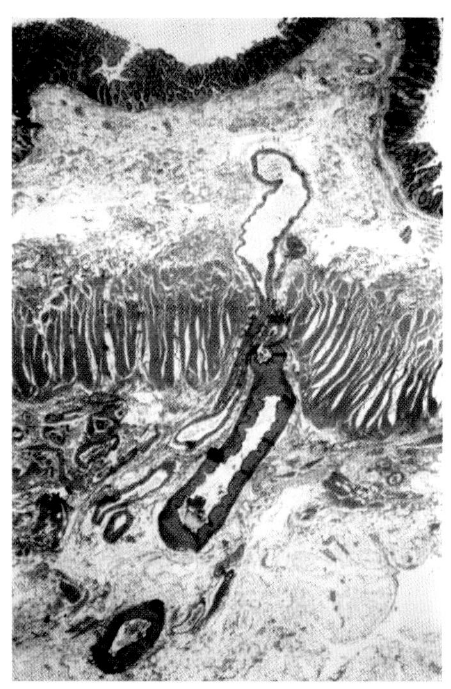

图 38.5　穿过盲肠固有肌层的直肠血管和伴随静脉。静脉压迫是其间歇性、部分低级别静脉阻塞的功能性解剖学解释。(弹力纤维染色,×50)(From Boley SJ,Sammartano RJ,Adams A,et al. On the nature and etiology of vascular ectasias of the colon:Degenerative lesions of aging. Gastroenterology 1977;72:650-60,with permission.)

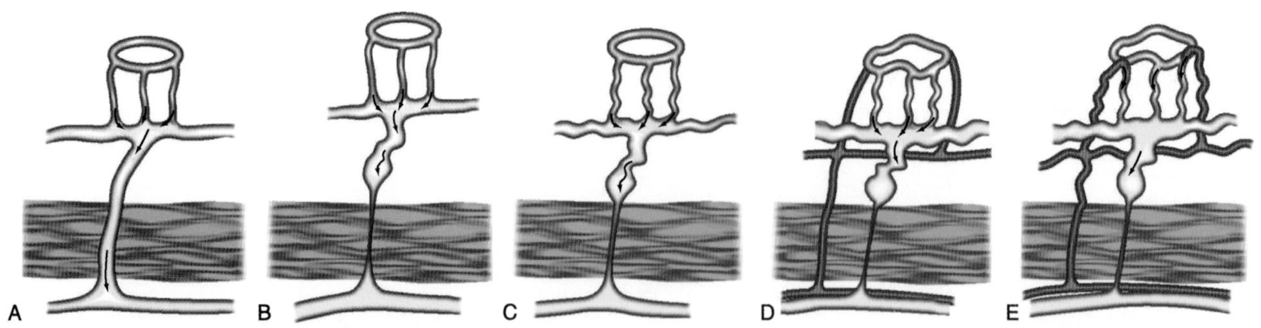

图 38.6　盲肠血管扩张发展的拟定概念。A,静脉穿过肌层的正常状态。B,随着肌肉收缩或腔内压力增高,静脉部分阻塞。C,多年反复发作后,黏膜下静脉变得扩张迂曲;肠系膜血管造影显示静脉排空缓慢。D,以后引流到异常黏膜下静脉的静脉和小静脉同样受累。E,最终,毛细血管环扩张,毛细血管前括约肌功能不全,通过血管扩张存在小的动静脉交通;这一阶段解释了肠系膜血管造影所见的早期充盈的静脉。(From Boley Sj,Sammartano RJ,Adams A,et al. On the nature and etiology of vascular ectasias of the colon:Degenerative lesions of aging. Gastroenterology 1977;72:650-60,with permission.)

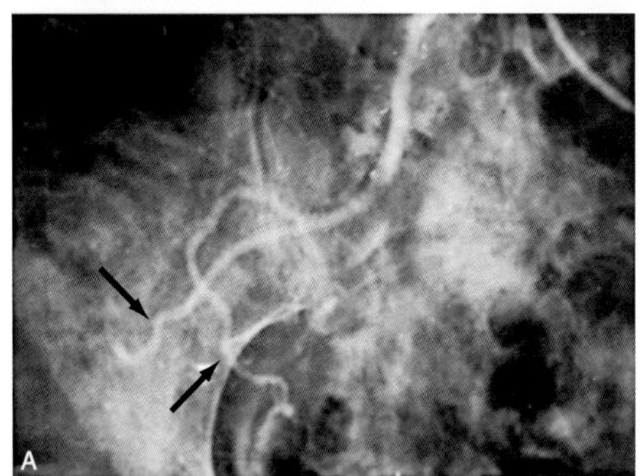

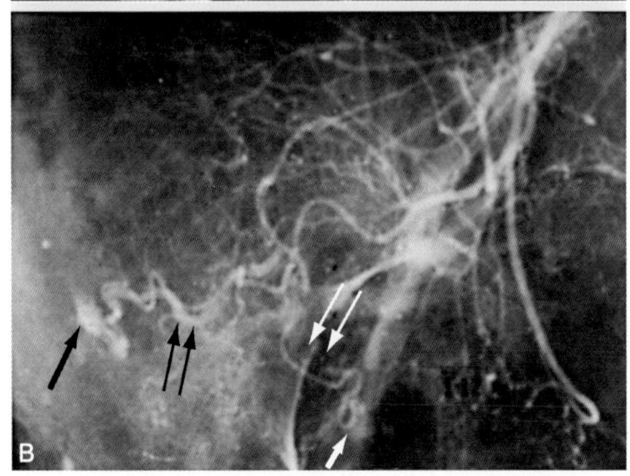

图 38.7　血管扩张(AE)的血管造影。A,发生 AE 患者的肠系膜上动脉造影显示 2 条密集不透明、缓慢排空、扩张迂曲的(箭示)盲肠静脉。注意在其他静脉清除后,晚期才显示的回结肠静脉。B,同一动脉造影的动脉期显示 2 条血管簇(粗箭示)和 2 条早期充盈静脉(各由一对细箭显示)。(From Boley SJ,Sprayregen S,Sammartano Ru,et al. The pathophysiologic basis for the angiographic signs of vascular ectasias of the colon. Radiology 1977;125:615-21,with permission.)

vWf 导致体外血管生成增加,VEGF 受体增殖和迁移增加,同时整合素 $\alpha\nu\beta3$ 水平降低,血管生成素释放增加[13]。仍需要进一步研究来阐明血管扩张的病理生理学变化。

3. 临床特征和相关情况

1961 年,Baum 及同事通过术中血管造影显示盲肠血管扩张可能会出血[8]。如今,这类疾病可以被常规的结肠镜检查很好地记录到。最近的文献指出,血管扩张和憩室病分别占急性下消化道出血的 3%～15% 和 20%～65%(参见第 20 和 121 章)[14]。当结肠镜检查或血管造影检查中的造影剂外溢未能证实病变出血时,判断出血的原因需要结合 60 岁以上人群合并这些疾病但没有出血的比例。在 60 岁以上的人群中,憩室病的患病率高达 50%。通过对手术切除的结肠进行注射检查,可以发现在该年龄段无出血征象的患者中,有超过 25% 和 50% 的患者分别存在右半结肠的黏膜和黏膜下血管扩张[1,15]。大规模的结肠镜检查结果显示,0.2%～2.9% 的非出血患者和 2.6%～6.2% 因便潜血阳性、贫血或便血行肠镜检查的患者存在血管扩张[3,9,16]。一名正在接受消化道出血检查的患者,其活动性出血部位尚未明确,确诊为结肠血管扩张或憩室所致的唯一依据是患者在消融或切除疑似病变后提供的间接证据。偶然发现出血的血管扩张是不常见的,即使是有出血史的患者也不能假定血管扩张是其原因[17]。

尽管患者可能出现大出血,但典型的结肠血管扩张出血表现为反复少量出血。同一患者不同时期的出血性质和程度往往不同:患者可能在不同情况下出现鲜血便、暗红色血便或黑便。其反映了扩张的毛细血管、小静脉和动静脉通路的不同出血速度,这取决于病变的发展阶段。在一项研究中,血管扩张出血中,20%～25% 的病例表现为柏油样便,而少数(10%～15%)患者仅表现为缺铁性贫血和间断大便隐血阳性[4]。另一项研究报道,血管扩张中有 21% 可出现血流动力学显著改变的下消化道出血,尽管 42% 的血管扩张患者没有急性出血的证据,而是表现为慢性下消化道出血或贫血[17]。目前认为大多数血管扩张患者没有临床症状或仅表现为隐匿性消化道出血。在 90% 以上的血管扩张出血可自行停止。

1958 年,Heyde 描述了至今仍然有争议的“Heyde 综合征”:血管扩张、消化道出血和主动脉狭窄(aortic stenosis,AS);当出血无法通过药物治疗控制时,建议行主动脉瓣置换术(aortic valve replacement,AVR)。许多关于 Heyde 综合征的报道出现在文献中,尽管一些分析[18]和研究[19]未能支持这种关联性表现。一项回顾性研究再次提出了 Heyde 综合征的存在[20],在这项研究中,“AVM”患者的 AS 发生率为 31.7%,而普通人群为 14%。据推测,最大形态的 vWf 多聚体缺陷(血管性血友病,2A 型)会导致止血异常,从而使已存在的血管扩张易于出血[21]。目前认为,剪切应力的增加会导致球状结构的血管性血友病聚合物展开成为细长的高度不对称蛋白,从而暴露出 A2 结构域[22]。ADAMTS13 与 A2 结构域结合,导致这种高分子量多聚体裂解成更小的聚合物,其止血能力低于其母体分子[22]。术前这些多聚体的缺陷在 AVR 后发生逆转[23],大多数接受 AVR 的 Heyde 综合征患者的出血得到解决;然而建议更换主动脉瓣以控制血管扩张引起的消化道出血是存在争议的[24]。目前,AVR 仅推荐用于重度 AS 患者,而不建议用于无症状 AS 情况下的消化道出血或缺铁性贫血患者,因为大多数血管扩张出血可以通过多种内镜技术来控制(见第 20 章)。

消化道出血是安置左心室辅助装置(left ventricular assist device,LVAD)患者的主要并发症,现在公认最常见的原因是上消化道血管发育不良(稍后讨论)。最近对 17 项病例对照和队列研究进行的 meta 分析显示,在持续血流 LVAD 患者中,消化道出血的患病率为 23%,其潜在危险因素包括年龄增长和肌酐升高[25]。LVAD 相关的消化道出血机制仍不清楚,但已被归因于 vWf 依赖性原发性止血功能受损[26]。这种损伤可能是由于 vWf 活性降低、剪切应力导致内皮细胞释放预先产生的 vWf,以及在非搏动性血流中使高分子量多聚体减少,导致获得性血管性血友病综合征[25]。脉压变大与血管性血友病多聚体增加相关[26],但是 LVAD 和 AS 患者脉压较小或为零。目前正在进行研究以确定降低这些装置的速度,是否会诱导更多的"搏动"血流从而减少消化道出血,尽管初步结果并未显示这些操作对获得性血管性血友病综合征的改善。Patel 等发表了一种新的方法,使用鼻内镜检查来确定 LVAD 患者的消化道出血风险。鼻血管增多作为胃肠道血管病变的潜在标志物,有助于确定接受 LVAD 患者的消化道出血风险。他们发现,无论是否接受 LVAD 治疗,鼻血管丰富同样常见于充血性心力衰竭患者(LVAD 组 63%,心力衰竭组 57%,对照组 20%),但 LVAD 患者的消化道出血与鼻血管增多之间存在统计学上的显著相关性,发生率为 32%。未行 LVAD 的心力衰竭患者的鼻血管增多与消化道出血之间没有显著相关性。因此,鼻内镜检查可能是胃肠道黏膜血管改变的潜在替代标志物。正在进行的进一步研究,比较 VCE 诊断的有无小肠血管病变的 LVAD 患者的鼻内窥镜检查结果,以证实这一假说[27]。

4. 诊断和治疗

结肠血管扩张的治疗从对出现急性或慢性 LGIB 的老年人怀疑患有该病开始(见第 20 章)。结肠镜是诊断和治疗的主要手段。如果找不到疑似病灶,或者因大出血无法进行结肠镜检查,则应行放射性核素闪烁扫描,然后行 CTA 检查。一项回顾性研究比较了 CTA 与 ^{99m}Tc 标记的红细胞闪烁扫描(red blood cell scintigraph,RBCS)对急性 LGIB 的总体评估和管理,发现 CTA 和 RBCS 均可用于识别活动性出血(38% 的病例),但更多的研究用 CTA 定位出血部位。在 24 名通过 CTA 准确定位 LGIB 部位的患者中,2 名患者被诊断为"AVM",而 RBCS 没有确定任何患者的出血原因[7]。

不同类型病变相似的外观限制了内镜医生诊断血管病变特定性质的能力。血管扩张、蜘蛛状血管瘤、毛细血管扩张症、血管瘤、放射性结肠炎的局灶性血管增加、溃疡性结肠炎、克罗恩病、缺血性结肠炎、某些感染、增生性和腺瘤性息肉,以及包括淋巴瘤和白血病浸润在内的恶性肿瘤,有时都可能彼此相似(框 38.1)。由于内镜创伤和吸引所致伪影可能类似于血管病变,因此必须在进镜时,而不是在退镜时评估所有病变。在内镜检查时从小的、非抬高性的血管病变获得的活检标本通常是非特异性的;因此,无须对这些病变进行活检。有时,在内镜检查时,可能会发现血管扩张的突出营养血管,血管扩张边缘的黏膜可能比远处的黏膜更显苍白,尽管在其他血管病变中也可看到这种"苍白晕"[28]。

框 38.1　内镜检查可能与血管扩张混淆的病变

结肠炎
IBD
感染性
缺血性
放射性
肿瘤
腺瘤性息肉
白血病浸润
淋巴瘤
非肿瘤性息肉
增生性
淋巴样
非血管病变
创伤
血管病变
血管瘤
动静脉畸形
静脉扩张
蜘蛛痣
毛细血管扩张
静脉曲张
静脉簇

由于血管病变的观察受患者血压和血容量的影响,在严重贫血或低血压的患者中,这种病变可能显示得不明显;因此,在红细胞和血容量不足得到纠正之前,可能无法进行准确的评估。哌替啶也可以减少细微血管异常(如血管扩张和遗传性出血性毛细血管扩张症);因此,应避免使用哌替啶,如果使用哌替啶,应使用纳洛酮进行拮抗,以便能够准确检测血管病变;而芬太尼不会产生这种掩蔽效应[29]。在接受哌替啶治疗的患者中,纳洛酮能使约 10% 的患者的正常结肠血管显示更加明显,使血管扩张显现(2.7%)或范围增大(5.4%)(图 38.8)[30]。因此,对于接受内镜检查的下消化道出血患者和接受哌替啶治疗的患者,纳洛酮是一种重要的辅助药物。在结肠镜检查中,使用冷水灌洗清理黏膜表面,也可能导致血管扩张血管收缩和暂时消失[31]。

血管造影用于确定活动性出血时血管病灶的部位和性质,甚至在出血停止后也能识别一些血管病变。血管扩张的 3 个可靠的血管造影征象是密集不透明的、排空缓慢的、扩张的、迂曲的静脉;血管簇;和早期充盈的静脉(见图 38.7)[32]。第四个征象是造影剂外溢,当出血速率至少为 0.5ml/min 时,可识别出血部位,但对血管扩张并不特异。在其他肠系膜静脉排空后,缓慢排空的静脉(见图 38.7A)持续到静脉期的晚

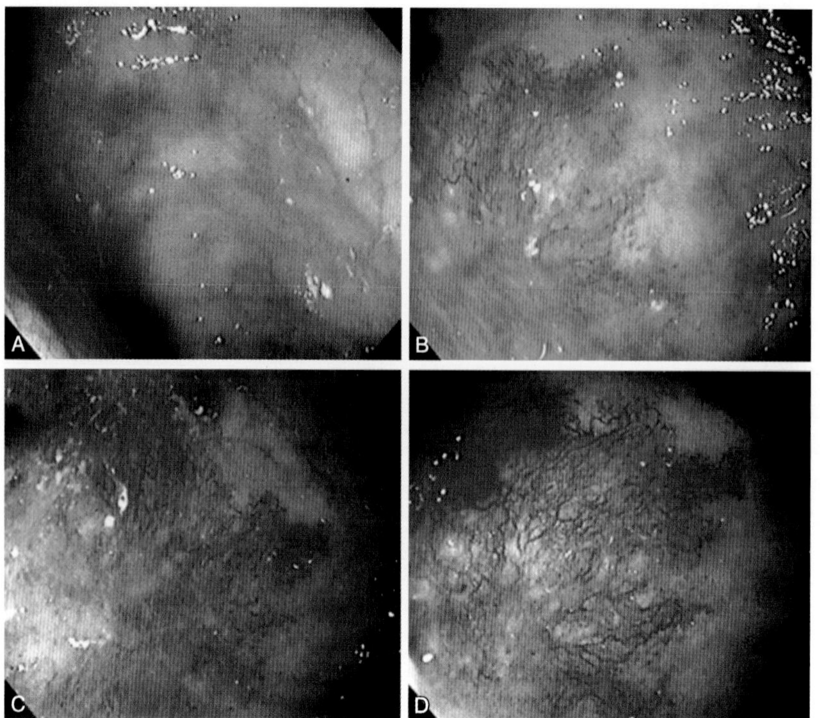

图 38.8 内镜图像显示，接受哌替啶镇静的患者在纳洛酮给药后，盲肠血管扩张（AE）外观的进行性变化。开始时不明显，AE 变为苍白，然后变为深红色扇形明显的血管病变。（From Brandt Ld，Spinnell M. Ability of naloxone to enhance the colonoscopic appearance of normal color vasculature and colon vascular ectasias. Gastrointest Endosc 1999；49：79-83.）

期。血管簇（见图 38.7B）是由扩张的小静脉形成，这些小静脉连接血管扩张黏膜成分及其黏膜下静脉。它们在动脉期表现最为明显；通常位于回结肠动脉分支的末端；呈小烛台状或椭圆形的血管簇；并且在静脉期仍可见与扩张、迂曲的壁内静脉相通。在注射后的 4 或 5 秒内，动脉期可见早期静脉充盈（见图 38.7B），但如果使用罂粟碱或妥拉唑林（Priscoline）等血管扩张剂来增强检查效果，早期静脉充盈则不是血管扩张的有效征象。当病灶出血时，造影剂的腔内外溢通常出现在动脉期，并在整个检查过程中持续存在。造影剂外溢可确定活动性出血的部位，在没有其他血管扩张征象的情况下，提示存在其他原因出血。

结肠镜检查中可能会偶然发现非出血性血管扩张。在这种情况下，不建议行内镜治疗[33]，因为一项前瞻性研究显示，无症状血管扩张患者的出血风险很低（3 年内为 0%）[31]，而结肠镜下消融术本身存在出血和穿孔风险[17,34,35]。

大多数患者的血管扩张出血可以通过内镜或血管介入得到控制，从而避免急诊手术的并发症和死亡。如今，超选择性微弹簧圈栓塞已取代动脉内血管升压素输注治疗下消化道出血。这种栓塞是非常有效和安全的，尽管并发症的发生率为 5%~9%；严重并发症（例如坏疽、血肿形成、动脉夹层、血栓形成、假性动脉瘤形成）的发生率不到 2%。然而，当肠道血管病变弥漫性分布于整个肠道或无法行超选择性导管置入时，仍建议使用血管升压素[28]。

使用雌激素与孕激素联合的激素疗法已被用于治疗胃肠道各种出血性血管病变的患者。这些药物的作用机制尚不清楚，尽管较流行的理论认为这些药物具有促凝和增强内皮完整性的作用。一项长期观察性研究[36]表明，激素联合治疗可以控制不明原因的隐匿性消化道出血（可能是由于小肠血管发育不良引起），尽管最近的一项 meta 分析详细介绍了 2 项病例对照研究，表明激素治疗对止血无效[37]。小肠血管病变对这种治疗的反应可能与结肠中出现的类似病变不同。目前，尚无对证实的结肠血管扩张进行激素治疗的研究。

生长抑素类似物是治疗胃肠道血管病变出血的另一种选择。这些药物通过抑制血管生成、减少内脏血流量、增加血管阻力和改善血小板聚集来发挥作用。在前面提到的最近的 meta 分析中，有 4 项队列研究评估了每日或每月使用奥曲肽的疗效。出血停止的总体优势比为 14.5［95% 可信区间（CI）：5.9~36］，治疗 1 年后输血需求减少，优势比为 0.55（95% CI：0.29~0.82）[37]。

抗血管生成因子是一种治疗血管扩张或胃肠道其他血管病变的新方法，包括沙利度胺、贝伐单抗和来那度胺。沙利度胺是 20 世纪 50 年代开发出来的一种镇静剂、安眠药和孕妇止吐药，但它很快因引起新生儿短肢畸形和其他畸形而臭名昭著[37]。1994 年，D'Amato 及同事报道了沙利度胺抑制 VEGF 和碱性成纤维细胞生长因子介导的血管生成[38,39]。数据表明，其抗血管生成作用的机制与整合素基因表达减少有关，导致细胞表面相互作用和对血管生成细胞因子的反应降低[40]。一些病例报告和病例系列描述了沙利度胺成功用于治疗肠道血管扩张和克罗恩病引起的危及生命的或难治性出血[41~44]。在使用沙利度胺治疗 3 个月后，VCE 记录了血管扩张的明显变化，表现为数量减少、面积减小、颜色变淡[42]。一项胃肠道血管发育不良和胃窦血管扩张（见下文）的对照研究,将患者随机分入沙利度胺治疗组和铁剂补充组,在一年的随访中,沙利度胺组 71.4% 的患者出血事件至少减少了 50%,而在铁剂补充组,这个比例只有 3.7%;然而,这些患者的病变主要局限于胃和小肠,目前还没有针对结肠血管扩张的治疗经验[45]。

贝伐单抗是一种针对 VEGF 的人源化单克隆抗体,对结肠癌和肾癌有效,并具有很强的抗血管生成活性[46]。奇怪的是,在治疗过程中,多达 59% 的患者观察到剂量依赖性的鼻腔和消化道出血,这可能是由于在血管生成活跃的高度再生黏膜组织中,贝伐单抗诱导内皮细胞脱落,从而导致血管完整性丧失所致。目前尚不清楚为什么某些抗血管生成药(如贝伐单抗)会引起黏膜出血,而其他药物(如沙利度胺)则不会;这种差异效应可能与血管生成的拮抗阶段有关,也可能反映了特别强的抗血管生成活性。

来那度胺是一种新的血管生成抑制剂,是沙利度胺的类似物,但副作用较少。来那度胺可以成为血管扩张治疗的一种新方法,尽管其作用仍有待在对照研究中进行评估[28]。虽然基于 VEGF 的抗血管生成治疗很有前景,但需要更详细地了解血管生成级联反应以及抗血管生成物质如何在其中的作用才能解决这个问题。

在过去,钕:钇铝石榴石(钕:YAG)激光[3,6,47]、内镜硬化[9]、单极电凝[48]、双极[49]电凝和加热探头[49]被用于消融胃肠道各种血管病变和控制活动性出血。然而,近年来,用止血夹与电凝烧灼术[50]、内镜套扎[51]和氩等离子凝固术(APC)[52]相结合的方式治疗(图 38.9)。对于血管扩张,最常用的是加热探头和 APC。内镜热疗法的止血成功率为 47% ~ 88%[3],并且没有一种方法明显优于其他方法[9]。热疗法后,有 5% 的结肠血管扩张患者发生了严重的迟发性出血[48]。经内镜治疗后,结肠血管扩张的复发性出血似乎有所减少,但是可能需要进行一次以上的治疗[49]。随着时间的推移,再出血率增加,在 15 ~ 36 个月的随访期内,28% ~ 52% 的患者出现了再出血[3]。

在准备内镜消融血管病变时,如有可能,应在术前几天停用阿司匹林和含阿司匹林的药物、其他非甾体抗炎药(NSAIDs)、抗凝剂和抗血小板药物,具体停药时间取决于不同药物。在热疗之前抽吸一些腔内气体增加了安全性,因为结肠壁不会因为管腔直径较小而变薄。当通过结肠镜或血管造影诊断了血管扩张,但这两种方法治疗均失败,无法进行,或不可用,并且患者有持续或复发的下消化道出血时,需要行右半结肠切除术。在这种情况下,左半结肠的憩室病并不影响结肠切除的范围;只有右半部分结肠被切除,但重要的是切除整个右半结肠,以确保无血管扩张残留。如果出血的部位(及其原因)没有确定,并且有复发或持续出血,结肠次全切除术(subtotal colectomy,STC)是合适的。当出血部位未被识别时,STC 的并发症发生率和死亡率与“盲目”半结肠切除术没有统计学差异[53,54]。在一篇外科综述中,STC、定向限制性结肠切除术和“盲目”限制性结肠切除术的死亡率分别为 0% ~ 40%、2% ~ 22% 和 20% ~ 57%;再出血率分别为 0% ~ 8%、0% ~ 15% 和 35% ~ 75%[53]。

(二) 血管发育不良

血管发育不良最常见于慢性肾病患者的胃和小肠(见第

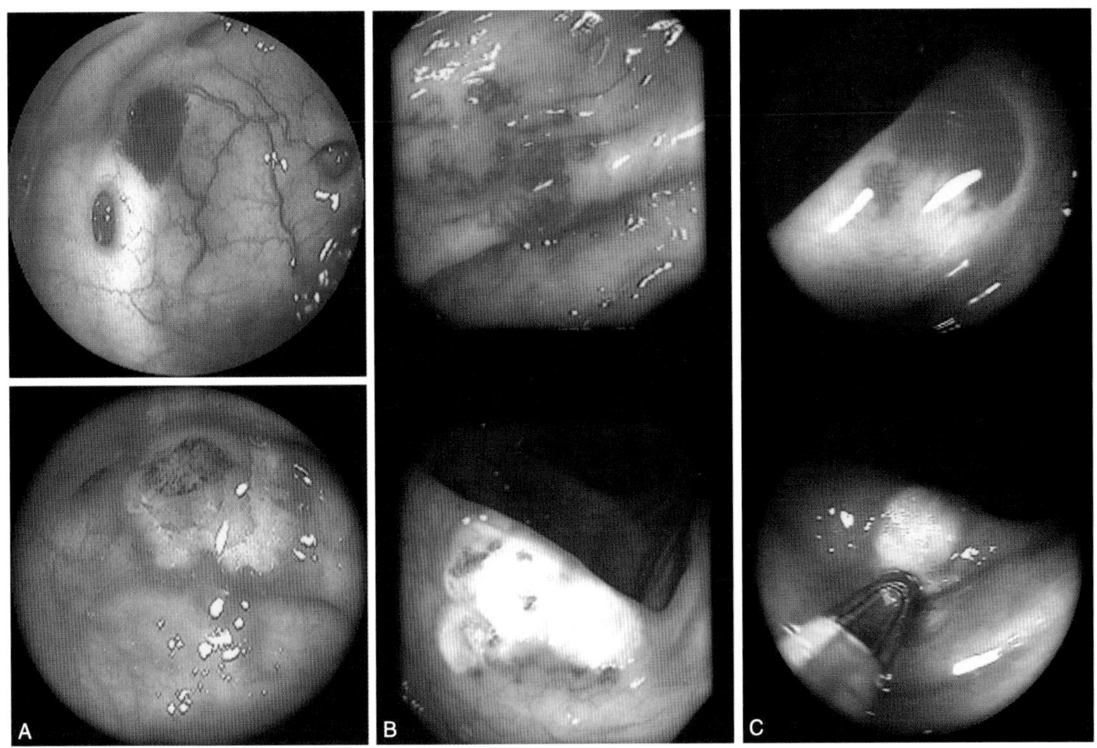

图 38.9 内镜图像显示血管扩张(AE)和结肠憩室病。A(上图),一名下消化道出血的老年男性升结肠憩室中的单个 AE。AE 和憩室是老年人严重复发性下消化道出血的两种最常见原因;因此,在同一个患者中发现它们并不罕见。A(下图),氩等离子体凝固术治疗 AE。B(上图),治疗后的 AE,升结肠中的多发 AE。B(下图),使用热探头治疗后的 AE。C(上图),单个 AE。C(下图),使用热探头消融 AE

37章)，但也见于约10%的结肠血管扩张患者。发生在小肠的其他血管病变包括蓝色橡皮泡痣综合征、血管瘤、Dieulafoy病变和门脉高压性肠病(稍后讨论)。虽然SBE和DBE(图38.10)用于诊断和治疗许多这些病变，但目前VCE(图38.11)是诊断和评估不明原因和隐匿性消化道出血患者的主要手段，因为它是无创的，易于实施，并且能够检查整个小肠。在一项前瞻性多中心研究中，VCE对明显小肠出血的总体诊断率为67%，血管扩张是最常见的诊断[55]。一项meta分析显示VCE优于推进式小肠镜和小肠钡剂造影：VCE比推进式小肠镜的诊断率增加30%，比小肠钡剂造影的诊断率高出36%[56]。在急性不明原因消化道出血患者中，VCE的诊断率也超过了血管造影(53% vs 20%)[57]。

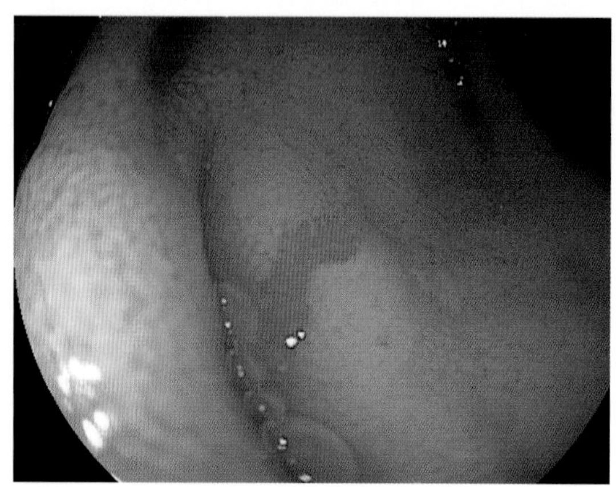

图38.10　双气囊小肠镜检查显示血管发育不良。(Courtesy Dr. Daniel Mishkin，Boston，Mass.)

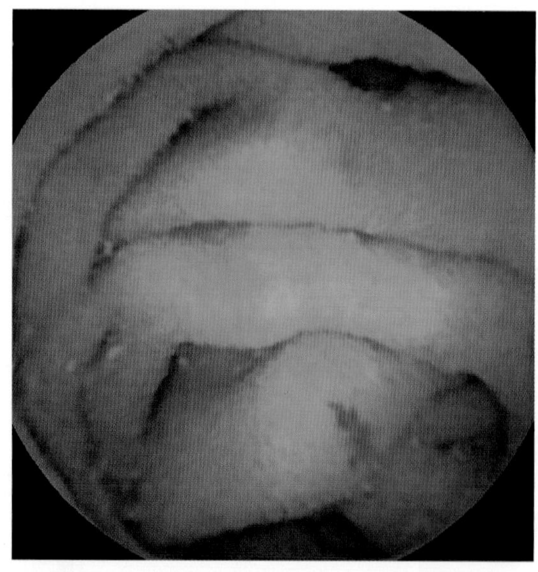

图38.11　可视胶囊内镜(VCE)显示血管发育不良。(Courtesy Dr. Daniel Mishkin，Boston，Mass.)

血管病变是因隐匿性消化道出血而行VCE检查的患者，尤其是年龄大于65岁的患者中最常见的病因[58]。而在年轻患者，贫血往往由于更严重的病变(如小肠肿瘤)[58]。

SBE和DBE可用于通过顺行或逆行的方式检查小肠，并可在诊断时实施内镜治疗。据报道，DBE的完整小肠镜检查率为57%，而SBE为0%，这证明DBE应优先使用[59]。一项对10项研究比较VCE和DBE对不明原因消化道出血患者的meta分析显示，VCE和DBE的诊断率相似，分别为60%和57%，而对VCE阳性的患者行DBE的诊断率显著高于VCE阴性患者(75% vs 27.5%；P=0.02)[60]。最近的一项研究调查了因不明原因消化道出血接受DBE患者的远期预后，研究发现51%的患者怀疑存在小肠血管病变(包括血管发育不良、毛细血管扩张、蓝色橡皮疱痣综合征和Dieulafoy病)。这些病灶在97%的患者中被APC成功治疗，36个月时累计再出血率为46%[61]。一项系统回顾和meta分析显示，约34%的血管发育不良和约45%的孤立性小肠血管发育不良病变患者在内镜治疗后再出血[25]。Meta分析还包括4项研究，观察奥曲肽类似物对内镜难治性患者再出血率的影响，显示再出血率和输血需求均显著降低。治疗1年后输血次数的标准平均减少量为0.55(95% CI：0.29~0.82)。两项研究分析了沙利度胺在难治性出血中的应用，均显示再出血率和输血需求减少[41,42]。

(三) Dieulafoy病变

这种血管病变是引起消化道大出血的一个不常见原因，可能发生在从食管到直肠的胃肠道的任何部位(图38.12)[62]。男性的患病率是女性的两倍，平均发病年龄为52岁。异常表现为持续大口径的动脉存在于黏膜下层，在一些情况下存在于黏膜层，其表面通常具有小的黏膜缺损。Dieulafoy称这种病变为“单纯性溃疡”，因为他认为这是胃溃疡的初始阶段。这种病变也被称为动脉粥样硬化性动脉瘤，这是一个不准确的术语，因为动脉壁的口径管径在整个过程中是均匀的，没有显示出异常程度的动脉硬化。据信，来自这些大“恒径”血管的局部压力使表面的黏膜变薄，导致暴露的血管壁被侵蚀，从而导致出血。大量呕血或黑便之前通常不会出现任何胃肠道症状，并且通常会在几天内出现间歇性和严重出血。最常见的出血部位是贲门食管交界处远端6cm处，那里的胃供血动脉最大，但是，如前所述，有报道Dieulafoy病灶出现在胃外，包括食管、小肠、直肠[62]，甚至在胃肠道以外的支气管出现。内镜下，Dieulafoy病变表现为被正常黏膜包围的孤立的突出血管，在上消化道出血的患者中可能难以发现，因为其上覆的黏膜缺损可能很小，并且隐藏在胃皱褶之间，而且恒径血管可能在出血后收缩和回缩。如果发现病变，一些专家提倡对病变进行标记，以便在再次出血时能快速识别病变。EUS也被用于加强对这些异常黏膜下层血管的检测，并有助于确定内镜治疗是否成功。肠系膜血管造影用于内镜无法定位出血部位时，特别适用于由于存在结直肠病变的患者，因为活动性出血和肠道准备差可导致内镜视野被遮挡[63]。

内镜技术定位和治疗Dieulafoy病变减少了手术干预的需要，并将出血死亡率从80%显著降低到8%。内镜治疗被认为是安全有效的止血方法，成功率可达75%~100%。Dieulafoy病变出血的治疗方法包括注射疗法、加热探头、APC、套扎，止血夹和内镜吻合夹(over-the scope clips，OTSC)。注射后进行热疗或机械夹闭疗法的内镜联合治疗在95%的病例中成功止血，其疗效优于单一疗法[64]。据报道，这些病变的再出血率为9%~40%[63]，并且与内镜联合治疗相比，单

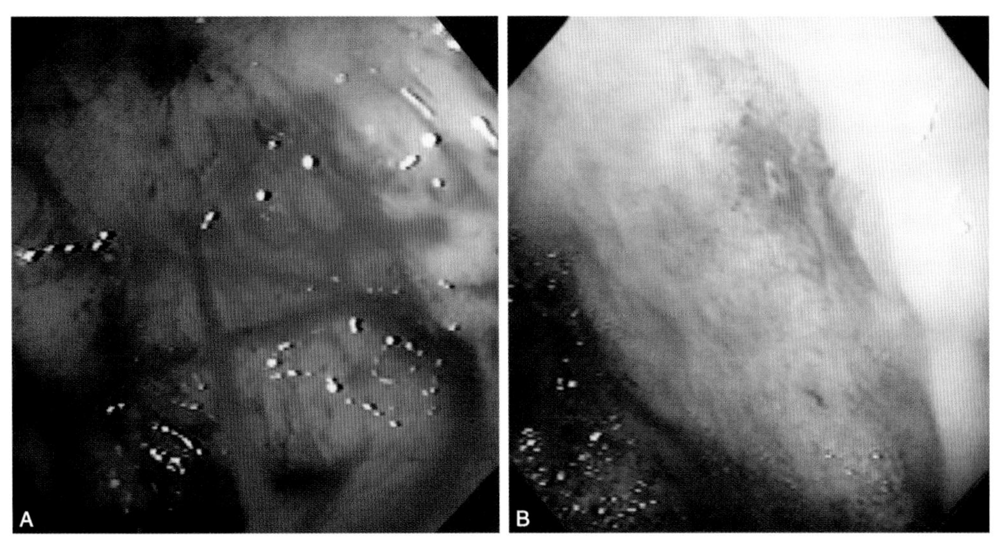

图 38.12 Dieulafoy 病变的内镜图像。A，胃食管交界处远端动脉出血（喷射状）。B，出血点为小缺损，内镜下未见溃疡病变。（From Wilcox CM. Atlas of clinical gastrointestinal endoscopy. Philadelphia：WB Saunders；1995. p 122.）

一治疗的再出血率高更[65]。

（四）血管瘤

血管瘤通常被认为是错构瘤，而另一些人认为是真正的肿瘤。血管瘤是结肠第二常见的血管病变，可表现为在结肠的单发或多发病变，或作为胃肠道弥漫性或多系统血管瘤病的一部分。血管瘤是一种结构复杂的病变，其特征是黏膜下结缔组织局部区域有过多血管，通常是静脉和毛细血管[66]。血管瘤可分为海绵状、毛细血管型或混合型；然而，胃肠道中最常见的血管瘤是毛细血管瘤[66]。

大多数血管瘤较小，从几毫米到 2cm 不等，但也有较大的病变，尤其是在直肠。结肠血管瘤出血通常较为缓慢，引起表现为贫血或黑便的隐匿性出血。便血较少见，但直肠大的海绵状血管瘤可引起大出血。最好通过内镜检查（包括小肠镜）来确诊，因为影像学检查，即便是血管造影，常表现正常。直肠海绵状血管瘤通常可以通过腹部平片上静脉石的存在和直肠气柱的移位或扭曲来帮助诊断（图 38.13）。在钡剂灌肠时，受累直肠管腔的典型表现为狭窄和僵硬，直肠壁呈扇形，骶前间隙增宽（见图 38.13）。内镜下可见隆起的梅红色结节或血管充血；也可能存在溃疡和直肠炎。CT 和 MRI 在显示海

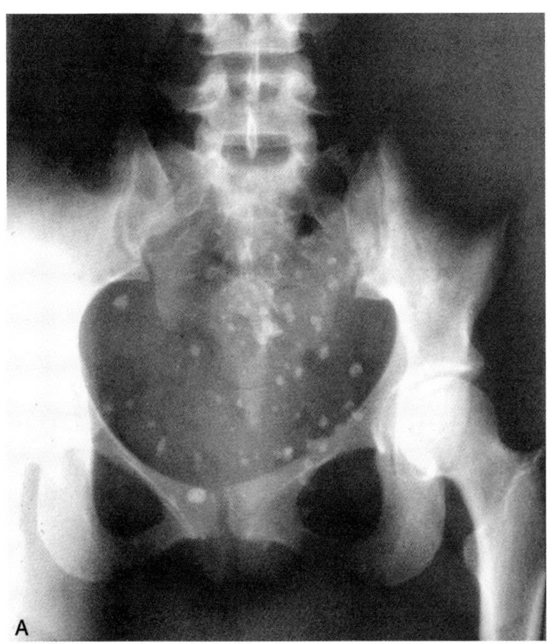

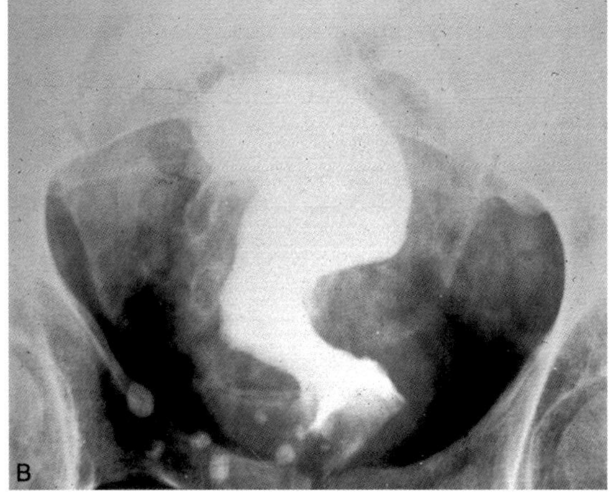

图 38.13 直肠海绵状血管瘤的两个影像学病例表现。A，骨盆平片发现软组织肿块，在异常血管通道内有钙化灶。儿童盆腔静脉石的出现是海绵状血管瘤的特征性病征。B，钡剂灌肠片显示结肠外特征性的静脉石模式，血管病变压迫引起肠腔扇贝形化

绵状血管瘤方面非常准确，EUS 也有助于确定侵入肛管和邻近结构的程度[67]。血管造影可以证实这些病变，但很少是确诊所必需的。

总体来说，海绵状血管瘤表现为息肉状或丘状红紫色黏膜病变。组织学上，在黏膜和黏膜下层可见大量扩张的、不规则的充血腔，有时会穿过肌层延伸到浆膜表面。血管腔内排列着扁平的内皮细胞，细胞核扁平或丰满。未成熟的血管瘤有饱满的内皮细胞核，经常表现出有丝分裂活性，这种特征在成熟病变中不存在；血管腔小且不规则[66]。随着病灶的成熟，内皮细胞变平且数量减少。在消退期，纤维间隔增厚，内皮细胞被脂肪细胞取代，血管结构萎缩[66]。虽然缺乏包膜，但毛细血管瘤通常界限清楚，通常有一个中心营养血管，呈放射状、小叶状延伸[66]。毛细血管瘤是斑块状或丘状红紫色病变，由被微小基质分隔的细小的、紧密堆积的、新生毛细血管增生所组成。内皮细胞大，通常是肥厚的，在某些区域可能形成实心索或结节，毛细血管间隙不清。

位于内镜可到达部位的孤立或数量少的小血管瘤可通过内镜消融治疗。大多数大的或多发的病变需要手术切除血管瘤或切除受累的结肠段。不应对大的病灶行内镜消融治疗，除非事先证实（如通过 EUS）病灶不是透壁性的。局部治疗控制直肠海绵状血管瘤大出血通常只是暂时有效。栓塞和外科结扎主要的滋养血管也用于该病治疗，但最终往往还是需要切除直肠[68]。

在一类称之为弥漫性肠血管瘤病的疾病中，许多病变，通常为海绵状，累及胃、小肠和结肠；头部和颈部皮肤或软组织的血管瘤经常存在。儿童时期出现的出血或贫血通常提示该诊断，持续、缓慢出血或肠套叠可能需要手术干预[69]。术中内镜检查有助于发现小病灶，但现今可能会首先尝试 SBE 和 DBE。VEGF 受体抑制剂（贝伐单抗）和多靶点酪氨酸激酶抑制剂，包括舒尼替尼［抑制 VEGF、血小板衍生生长因子（PDGF）］、瓦他拉尼（抑制 VEGF、PDGF、c-kit）和司马沙尼（抑制 VEGF 和 PDGF），已被用于治疗血管母细胞瘤，另一种组织来源不确定的高度血管化病变，最常见于希佩尔-林道综合征（von Hippel-Lindau disease，vHLD）患者[70]。在 vHLD 中，von Hippel-Lindau 蛋白的缺失导致缺氧诱导因子的积聚，进而导致 VEGF 的过度产生[71]。贝伐单抗是一种抗 VEGF 的人源化单克隆抗体，在 vHLD 患者中，可导致中枢神经系统血管母细胞瘤的稳定或消退，从而改善黄斑和视神经血管母细胞瘤患者的视力[70]；这些结果表明，VEGF 抑制剂可能在其他类型血管瘤的治疗中发挥一定的作用。手术是最终的治疗方式。

（五）先天性动静脉畸形

动静脉畸形（AVM）是胚胎发育缺陷，被认为是发育异常。虽然 AVM 主要见于四肢，但它们也可能发生在血管系统的任何部位。在结肠中，它们可能很小，类似于血管扩张，也可能涉及到很长一段肠道。最广泛的 AVM 通常位于直肠和乙状结肠。在组织学上，AVM 是主要位于黏膜下层的动脉和静脉之间持续存在的先天性交通。特征性表现为存在静脉的“动脉化”（即扭曲、扩张和平滑肌肥大和内膜增厚或硬化导致的管壁增厚）。在长期存在的动静脉畸形中，动脉扩张，出现萎缩和硬化变性。血管造影是主要的诊断方法（图 38.14）。小病灶的早期静脉充盈和大病灶的动脉或静脉广泛扩张是典型表现。有明显出血的大 AVM 患者应切除受累肠段；内镜治疗对较小的病灶可能是有益的。

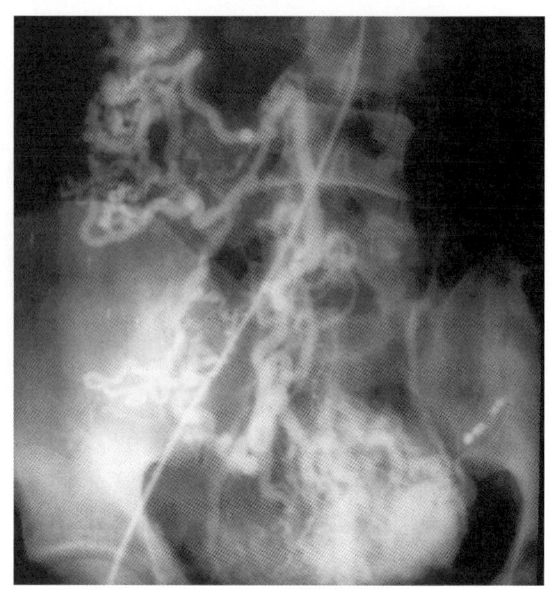

图 38.14　一例复发性 LGIB 患者的肠系膜血管造影。血管造影片显示在累及肠系膜上动脉和肠系膜下动脉循环的大型先天性血管畸形（AVM）中存在复杂的血管蔓状结构

二、动脉瘤

（一）腹主动脉瘤

约 95% 的腹主动脉瘤（abdominal aortic aneurysms，AAA）起源于动脉粥样硬化，但遗传易感性也是重要因素；不太常见的原因包括创伤、血管炎、感染和先天性异常。与腹主动脉瘤发展相关的风险因素包括年龄大于 60 岁、男性、白种人、吸烟和高血压。对 50 岁以上成年人进行的基于人群的研究发现，男性腹主动脉瘤的患病率为 3.9%～7.2%，女性为 1.0%～1.3%[72]。在 15%～20% 的病例中已经观察到腹主动脉瘤的家族聚集性，在一些家庭中，已经在 16 号染色体中发现了异常[73]；在其他家族中，Ehlers-Danlos 综合征Ⅳ型患者的前胶原蛋白Ⅲ缺陷和基因表达改变导致腹主动脉瘤的弹性蛋白和胶原蛋白异常[73]。迄今为止对腹主动脉瘤的遗传风险有最强支持证据的 2 个基因是：*CDKN2BAS* 基因，也称为 *ANRIL*，其编码一种反义 RNA 调节细胞周期蛋白依赖性激酶抑制剂 CDKN2A 和 CDKN2B 的表达；以及 *DAB2IP*，编码细胞生长和存活的抑制剂[74]。

大多数腹主动脉瘤在破裂前是无症状的，因其他症状行腹部超声、CT 或 MRI 时偶然发现，因此，目前的指南支持对年龄在 65 岁至 74 岁之间有吸烟史的男性进行“一次性”腹部超声筛查[72]。腹主动脉瘤最常见的症状是上腹痛，通常放射到背部；剧烈的疼痛可能预示着破裂。体检时，可触及搏动性上腹部肿块。在体格检查中很难区分动脉瘤和表面搏动性肿块，最好是通过影像学检查。可能存在杂音，但除非是最近才出现,否则通常对诊断没有帮助[72]。

腹部平片可能显示腹主动脉区域有软组织肿块伴周围钙化的。对于大动脉瘤,可能会出现腰椎的侵蚀或周围脏器的移位,包括肠、肾和输尿管。由于腹部平片对确定动脉瘤的存在或大小不够敏感,所以超声、CT 和 MRI 已成为评估的标准方法。超声是腹主动脉瘤的首选影像筛查手段,因为其高度敏感(95%~100%)和特异(100%)且相对便宜。此外,超声是连续监测腹主动脉瘤大小变化的首选方式[72]。术前使用 CT 和 MRI 显示主动脉和血管解剖,并帮助选择合适的支架。术前血管造影不像过去那样频繁使用,最适用于有外周血管疾病、严重高血压、慢性肠系膜缺血症状(见第 118 章)的患者,如果怀疑胸主动脉或髂动脉受累,以及用于马蹄肾或盆腔肾患者以显示肾动脉解剖结构。血管造影不用于估计动脉瘤的大小,因为腔内层状血栓限制了整个管腔的显影,更重要的原因是,现在有更简单、侵入性更小、且更便宜的成像方式可使用。

腹主动脉瘤的主要并发症是破裂,其先兆是突发或加重的腹部、两侧或背部疼痛;当"渗漏"发生在明显破裂之前时,会出现以数周疼痛为特征的隐匿性表现。平躺时疼痛可能会加重,坐位或前倾时疼痛可能会缓解。随着内脏血管受损和急性肠缺血的发展,主动脉夹层也可能出现严重的腹痛。血管外科医生的共识是,腹主动脉瘤破裂最重要的预测因素是动脉瘤的大小。直径在 3.0~3.9cm 的腹主动脉瘤的年破裂风险接近 0%,直径在 4.0~4.9cm 的腹主动脉瘤的年破裂风险为 1%,直径在 5.00~5.99cm 的腹主动脉瘤的年破裂风险为 11%[72]。其他与破裂相关的危险因素包括高血压和慢性阻塞性肺疾病。腹主动脉瘤最常破裂到主动脉周围的腹膜后组织。较少见的情况下,动脉瘤破裂至腹腔,在这种情况下,会迅速出现失血性休克。动脉瘤破裂至小肠通常发生在十二指肠的第三或第四部分,常表现为消化道大出血;如果血栓形成并从侵蚀的肠道或瘘管开口处脱落,可出现间歇性出血。事实上,大多数患者会在大出血前的几个小时或几天出现"先兆出血"[75]。内镜检查是诊断这种并发症最敏感的方法。腹主动脉瘤破裂至下腔静脉很罕见;如果发生,可以听到很大的血管杂音。

腹主动脉瘤大于 5.5cm 的无症状患者或任何大小的有症状动脉瘤患者应接受手术修复以防止破裂。腹主动脉瘤在 3.0~5.4cm 的患者应该每 3~12 个月接受一次 US 或 CT 检查[72]。腹主动脉瘤的增长速度报道不一致。一项大规模研究对小动脉瘤(平均初始大小为 4cm)患者进行了平均 3.3 年的随访,58.4% 的患者动脉瘤大小没有变化或动脉瘤缩小,25.3%的患者动脉瘤增大了 0.1~0.25cm,12.6%的患者动脉瘤增大超过 0.25cm,只有 3.7% 的患者动脉瘤增大超过 0.5cm[73]。腹主动脉瘤的平均增长速度为每年 0.35cm。

腹主动脉瘤的手术修复包括经腹膜后或经腹开放式手术,或血管内修复手术,将支架置入到血管腔内以阻挡血流进入主动脉瘤,从而将破裂风险降到最低。在择期手术病例中,术前血管造影有助于发现其他血管疾病(如内脏动脉的狭窄或闭塞),并允许有计划的血管重建,这可能有助于避免术后肠缺血。低风险患者腹主动脉瘤修复的死亡率为 1%~4%[75];而破裂或即将破裂时紧急手术的死亡率大幅度增加到 34%~85%[76]。血管内动脉瘤修复手术(endovascular aneurysm repair,EVAR)越来越多地被作为腹主动脉瘤开放修复的替代方法。与开放手术相比,EVAR 有一定优势,如避免全身麻醉、缩短手术时间、减少失血和减少术后疼痛。在 3 项比较开放手术和 EVAR 治疗大于 5.5cm 腹主动脉瘤的试验中,EVAR 的手术死亡率低于开放手术,但腹主动脉瘤特异性死亡率和全因死亡率没有差异,并且 EVAR 的再干预率较高[77]。目前的建议支持对手术并发症风险较低或中等的腹主动脉瘤患者行开放手术修复,对手术并发症风险较高的患者行 EVAR[77-79]。手术风险不高的患者也应考虑 EVAR,尽管尚缺乏支持证据[77]。

(二) 内脏动脉瘤

根据尸检报告,内脏动脉瘤的患病率估计高达 10%,尽管内脏动脉瘤的自然史尚不清楚[80,81]。内脏动脉瘤通常无症状,在影像学检查中偶然发现。耶鲁纽黑文医学中心最近的一项回顾性研究评估了自 1999 年 1 月至 2016 年 12 月的影像学检查记录的 122 名患者的 138 处 SAA 的年增长速度和破裂风险[81]。SAA 的增长速度缓慢(每年 0.064±0.18cm),最小的动脉瘤破裂发生在 2.3cm;因此建议对小于 2.5cm 的无症状患者进行观察随访。当出现症状时,SAA 可表现为腹痛或消化道出血。在体格检查中,听诊可能会听到杂音,但腹部肿块很少触及,因为动脉瘤很小。高达 25% 的 SAA 可能并发破裂,估计死亡率为 25%~70%[82]。与主动脉瘤一样,如果 SAA 侵蚀到胃肠腔内,可出现散发性消化道出血,即所谓的先兆出血。破裂至肠系膜静脉可导致动静脉瘘,并可导致门静脉高压和静脉曲张出血。如果 SAA 充分钙化,可以在腹部平片上看到,但通常通过 CT、MRI 或内脏血管造影进行诊断,这具有潜在治疗干预的额外好处。治疗取决于动脉瘤的表现、位置和大小。一般来说,如果动脉瘤的直径大于 2cm,即使没有症状,也要考虑治疗。治疗选择包括栓塞、手术修复或血管内支架植入[81]。对于难以手术处理的动脉瘤和高危患者,栓塞可能是首选。

1. 脾动脉瘤

脾动脉瘤通常呈囊状,20% 的患者有多个动脉瘤。症状是左上腹或上腹疼痛,可能会放射至左肩。常见的原因是动脉粥样硬化和门静脉高压,而不太常见的原因包括脾动脉夹层、脓毒性栓子、高血压、结节性多动脉炎、系统性红斑狼疮、Ehlers-Danlos 综合征、纤维肌发育不良和神经纤维瘤病。女性与男性的患病比例为 3:1~4:1,并且与妊娠有关[80~83]。孕妇患病率增加可能与脾血流量增加和雌激素对中膜弹性组织的影响有关,这会导致脾动脉扩张,易于形成动脉瘤。同样,脾血流量增加也是门静脉高压症患者出现脾动脉瘤的原因。动脉瘤破裂发生在不到 2% 的患者中,但孕妇动脉瘤破裂的风险明显升高。超过 95% 的孕妇动脉瘤是在破裂后诊断的,可导致 75% 的孕产妇死亡率和 95% 的胎儿死亡率[80]。如果动脉瘤破裂到小网膜囊,患者仍可以保持血流动力学稳定,但是一旦血液通过 Winslow 孔溢出到腹腔,就会出现弥漫性腹痛和低血容量性休克;这就是"双破裂"现象。据说,出血局限于小网膜囊时,约 25% 的患者有时间进行外科干预[80]。脾动脉瘤的治疗选择取决于其位置及其表现。动脉瘤破裂通常行脾切除术治疗。急诊手术后的死亡率高达40%，而择期修复术后的死亡率非常低。孕妇或计划受孕的妇女的有症状的动脉瘤或任何大小的动脉瘤都应在受孕前进行修复。如果动脉瘤的位置在近端且大于2cm，应考虑手术治疗，包括切除和端-端血管修复；如果位置在远端或涉及脾门，则建议脾切除术。1~2cm的动脉瘤应进行影像学监测。如果不能手术，可以进行栓塞。对于门静脉高压患者，倾向于栓塞治疗，因为广泛的侧支循环使手术更加困难。栓塞的并发症包括脾梗死和动脉瘤的再灌注，可发生在5%~20%的患者中。建议每年进行一次CT或MRI随访，以评估脾动脉瘤是否渗漏或生长[80,82]。

2. 腹腔动脉瘤

曾经，腹腔动脉瘤最常见的原因是梅毒或结核引起的感染，大多数病例是在动脉瘤破裂后尸检时诊断的。现在梅毒和结核病较容易识别和治疗，腹腔动脉瘤更常见的原因是动脉粥样硬化、创伤、夹层和大动脉炎[80,82]。与其他动脉瘤的关联很常见，在研究中发生在66%的患者中[83]。腹腔动脉瘤通常无症状。当出现症状时，可以类似胰腺炎。食管压迫会导致吞咽困难。动脉瘤破裂风险约为6%。大于2.5cm的腹腔动脉瘤应考虑修复，而小于2.5cm的无症状病变可通过影像学检查随访[82]。传统的开放修复可通过经腹途径或胸腰椎途径进行。可以在结扎后进行主动脉肝旁路或直接主动脉再植术。在接受血管重建术的患者中，假体移植物比隐静脉移植物闭塞的风险低，但是因为其位置而难以放置。如果动脉瘤破裂，可以行介入治疗，包括结扎或经皮导管栓塞[80]。

3. 肠系膜上动脉动脉瘤

肠系膜上动脉(superior mesenteric artery，SMA)动脉瘤很少见。它们通常累及SMA的近端5cm。可能出现动脉瘤相关的血栓或夹层，可引起肠缺血的症状。曾经，最常见的病因是感染，脓毒性栓子占所有SMA动脉瘤的三分之一。在最近的研究中，常见的原因包括动脉粥样硬化、结节性多动脉炎、胰腺炎、胆道疾病、神经纤维瘤病和创伤[83]。超过90%的SMA动脉瘤有症状，表现为腹痛和消化道出血。高达50%的SMA动脉瘤出现破裂，死亡率为30%。β-肾上腺素能受体阻滞剂对破裂有保护作用[80]。由于并发症发生率高，建议对所有有症状的患者和所有手术风险低的患者进行干预；对于小于2.5cm的无症状动脉瘤，建议进行监测[82]。外科手术方法包括动脉瘤切除术和肠系膜动脉分支的插入静脉移植或结扎以治疗动脉瘤。此外，切除任何缺血的肠段。也可行经导管栓塞和血管内支架置入术，但如果SMA的分支被支架阻塞，血管内支架置入可能会增加肠系膜缺血的风险。β-肾上腺素能受体阻滞剂可用于不愿接受介入治疗的患者[80,82]。

4. 真菌性动脉瘤

主动脉和内脏血管的真菌性动脉瘤很少见。William Osler爵士之所以如此命名，是因为它们的外观让他想起了真菌。过去，真菌性动脉瘤最常见的原因是由细菌性心内膜炎引起的脓毒性栓子。如今，主要的危险因素是静脉注射药物的使用。其他重要的危险因素包括邻近感染的连续传播、动脉操作和免疫力低下(如酒精中毒、糖尿病、化疗和糖皮质激素治疗)。沙门菌(特别是猪霍乱沙门菌)和葡萄球菌是最常见的感染微生物。受影响最大的是腹腔动脉(CA)，其次是肠系膜上动脉(SMA)和肠系膜下动脉(IMA)。在病程早期，真菌性动脉瘤的症状是非特异性的；后期出现典型表现发热、寒战和腹痛。诊断方法为血管成像；真菌性动脉瘤通常呈分叶状和囊状(图38.15)。破坏性过程会迅速发展，导致快速膨胀和破裂。治疗方法为外科手术，通常是动脉瘤切除和血管重建，然后静脉注射抗生素6周。终生抑制性口服抗生素疗法也被用于预防假体移植物感染[153,154]。

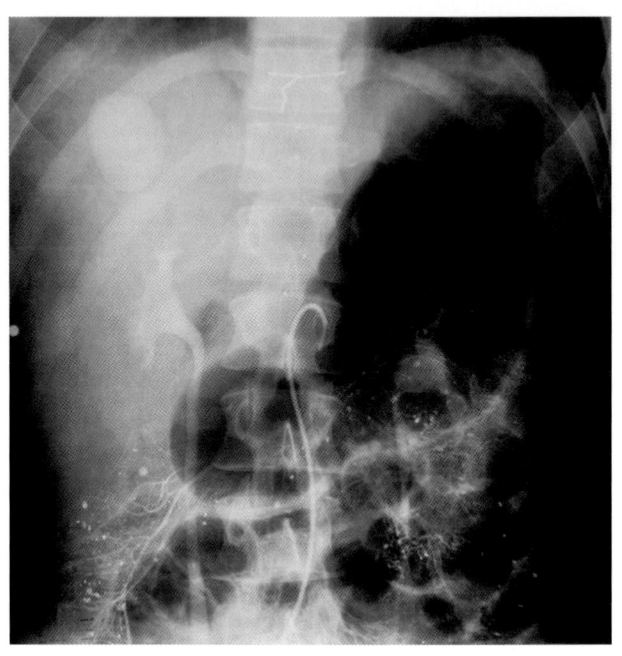

图38.15　肝动脉巨大真菌性动脉瘤患者的内脏血管造影照片。(Courtesy Dr. Lawrence J. Brandt，Bronx，NY.)

三、假体旁肠瘘和主动脉肠瘘

主动脉瘤切除术和腹膜后或腹部的血管假体置入术的一个罕见但严重的并发症是在移植物和邻近肠道之间形成瘘管，通常是十二指肠的第三或第四部分，因为它接近肾下腹主动脉(图38.16)[84]。这种并发症被称为继发性主动脉肠瘘，其发生率在0.36%~2%[85]。据报道，主动脉手术与继发主动脉肠瘘之间的平均间隔时间为44个月，但这种瘘最早可在术后21天发生，最晚可在术后14年发生；当并发腹腔内感染时，瘘可出现得更早，平均间隔时间为22个月[85]。继发性主动脉肠瘘被认为是由于移植物植入时或植入后的局部情况造成的，包括感染、解剖过程中十二指肠或其血液供应的损伤，以及随后移植物对十二指肠壁的侵蚀。较新的外科技术，包括使用血管内移植物、不可吸收缝线、抗生素、严格止血以及用腹膜后组织和腹膜覆盖缝合线，可以降低瘘形成的风险。原发性主动脉肠瘘是在没有动脉瘤修复的情况下发生，并与动脉粥样硬化、感染(最常见的是沙门菌和克雷伯菌属；其他不太常见的包括葡萄球菌属、链球菌属、大肠埃希菌、粪肠球菌、败血症梭菌和乳酸杆菌)、恶性肿瘤、放疗、创伤和异物有关。原发性主动脉肠瘘比继发性主动脉肠瘘少见，发生率为0.04%~0.07%[86]。

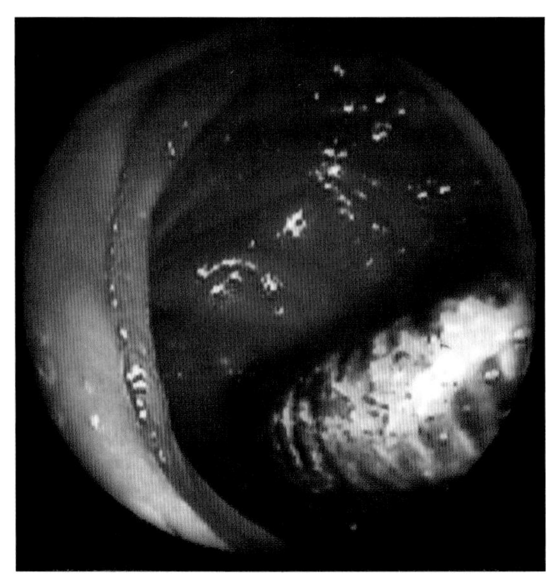

图 38.16 十二指肠第三部分的内镜视图，可见部分主动脉移植物。主动脉肠道瘘患者通常表现为胃肠道出血、腹痛和发热，因为移植物通常在侵蚀胃肠道时发生感染。（Courtesy, Dr. Lawrence J. Brandt, Bronx, New York）

主动脉肠瘘患者出现上消化道或下消化道出血，如果不及时治疗，可能会出现大出血而迅速致命。食管胃十二指肠镜（EGD）联合 CT 影像学检查用于排除其他诊断和决定治疗方案[87]。为了作出诊断，需要提高警惕，尤其是主动脉髂动脉移植术后出现消化道出血的患者，及时的诊断和迅速的外科修复对生存至关重要。

四、系统性病变或表现形式相关的血管病变

（一）遗传性出血性毛细血管扩张症

这是一种常染色体显性家族性疾病，也称为 Osler-Weber-Rendu 病，其特征是皮肤和黏膜毛细血管扩张以及反复消化道出血[88~90]。在一些患者中，其发病机制为内皮糖蛋白（*ENG*）和激活素受体样激酶-1（*ALK-1*）基因的突变，这些基因在血管生成过程中对决定内皮细胞的特性起着重要作用[91]。病变通常在出生后最初几年中被发现，儿童期反复鼻出血是其特征性表现。到 10 岁时，大约一半的患者出现消化道出血。严重出血在 40 岁之前不常见，在 60 岁时发生率最高。在大多数患者中，出血表现为黑便；BRBPR 和呕血发生率较低。HHT 患者出现便血提示出血来自毛细血管扩张以外的其他原因。出血是间歇性的、慢性的，可以很严重；患者一生中可能接受超过 60 次输血。80% 的 HHT 患者都有该病家族史，但家族史在年长才发生出血的患者中较少见。毛细血管扩张症通常出现在嘴唇、口腔和鼻咽黏膜、舌和甲周区域；如果不累及这些部位则需要对该诊断产生怀疑（图 38.17）。

目前，HHT 的诊断至少需要满足 4 项相关临床标准中的 3 项。这些所谓的 Curaçao 标准包括：鼻出血（自发性和复发性鼻出血）；毛细血管扩张（特征性部位的多处病变，如嘴唇、口腔、手指、鼻）；内脏病变（如肺、肝、脑、脊髓、胃肠道）；阳性家族史（一级亲属患 HHT）[92]；临床诊断可通过分子遗传学分析确诊。在大多数情况下，HHT 是由两个已知 HHT 基因中的一个突变引起的。*ENG* 基因突变导致 1 型 HHT[93]。*ENG* 基因位于 9 号染色体上，编码内皮糖蛋白，一种Ⅲ型转化生长因子-β（TGF-β）受体。激活素基因突变导致 2 型 HHT。患有 1 型 HHT 的人往往比患有 2 型 HHT 的人更早出现症状，并且更有可能在肺和脑中出现血管畸形；肝脏受累和门脉高压在 2 型 HHT 患者中更为常见。激活素基因位于 12 号染色体上，编码 ACVRL1 蛋白，一种Ⅰ型 TGF-β 受体[90]。这两种受体主要在血管内皮上表达，在维持血管完整性中起重要作用。已有证据表明另外 2 个基因也与 HHT 相关[94,95]。在一些 HHT 的患者中也发现了导致幼年性息肉病的 *SMAD4* 基因突变（参与 TGF-β 信号级联）[96,97]；这些患者具有幼年性息肉病和 HHT 的重叠综合征，因此罹患结直肠癌（CRC）的风险显著升高，需要进行更加积极的 CRC 筛查[96]。虽然 HHT 存在基因型异质性，但不同 HHT 基因型的临床表现相似。HHT 和非遗传性肠血管扩张均以 VEGF 生成增多为特征。在 HHT 患者中，血清高水平 VEGF 与出血的严重程度相关[98,99]。肝脏血管受累在 HHT 中很常见，尤其是 2 型，且通常无症状。在该疾病病程中，8% ~ 31% 的患者出现肝脏相关临床表现，包括由动静脉分流引起的高输出量性心力衰竭、门脉高压和胆道疾病[100,101]。肝脏受累与并发症有关，包括需要肝移植

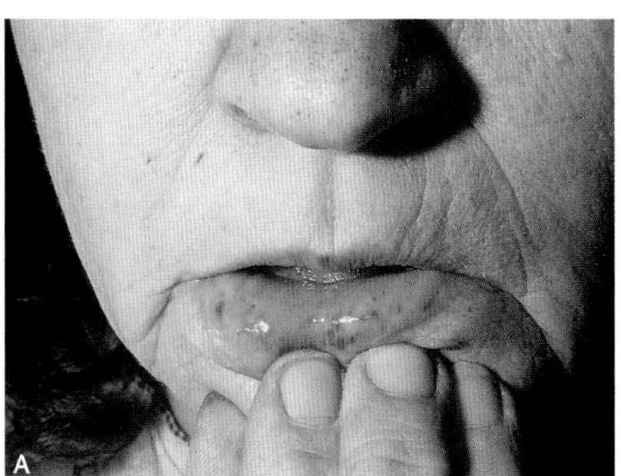

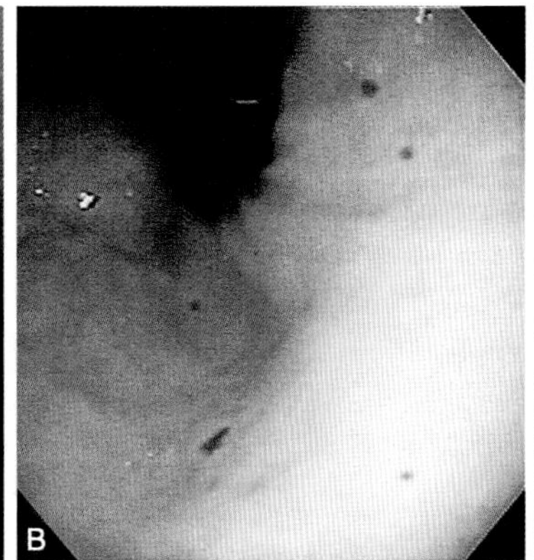

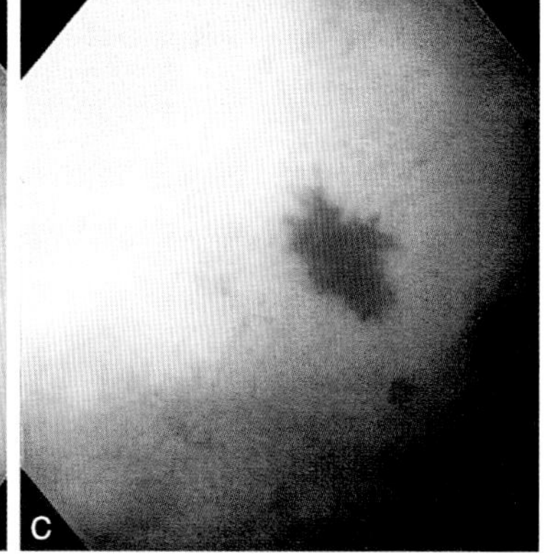

图 38.17 遗传性出血性毛细血管扩张症。A，鼻子和嘴唇上有多处毛细血管扩张。在近端胃体（B）和胃窦（C）有大小不等、形态不一的毛细血管扩张。（From Wilcox CM. Atlas of clinical gastrointestinal endoscopy. Philadelphia：WB Saunders；1995. p 123.）

的肝衰竭，以及显著升高的发病率和死亡率[102]。在一项对HHT和已知肝血管畸形患者进行的中位时间为44个月的随访研究中，5.2%的患者死亡，25.3%的患者出现并发症，包括高输出量性心力衰竭、房颤、门脉高压和消化道出血。通过多学科联合治疗，包括支持治疗、高输出量性心力衰竭和门脉高压的药物治疗、房颤的射频消融术、肝血管畸形的经动脉栓塞术和原位肝移植，完全缓解率达63%[102]。

毛细血管扩张也可发生于HHT患者的结肠，但更常见于胃和小肠，更容易导致大出血。毛细血管扩张在内镜检查中容易被发现，但在严重贫血、失血或低血压的情况下，它们可能暂时变得不那么明显甚至不可见；在纠正低血容量和低血压后，它们会再次变得明显。通过传统的血管造影或较新的技术，如螺旋CTA[103,104]和MRA进行评估可能无法显示肝实质不均匀增强、肝内动脉分支扩张和扭曲、异常血管团块、动脉瘤、动静脉交通、静脉扩张以及肝动脉和门静脉扩张[104,105]。血管造影在显示多处血管异常时可能会产生误导，因为这些病变可能位于肠系膜而不是肠道，并且不是消化道失血的潜在部位。

大体而言，HHT的毛细血管扩张相当于小米种子大小，通常表现为樱桃红色的光滑的小丘。病理上，主要改变包括毛细血管和小静脉，但小动脉也可能受到影响。病变由不规则、扩张、弯曲的血管构成，内皮细胞单层排列，并由一层细小的纤维结缔组织支撑。这些血管中没有弹力层或肌肉组织，因此无法收缩；这一特性可以解释为什么毛细血管扩张容易出血。小动脉显示内膜增生，其中常有血栓，提示血管淤滞。与血管扩张变薄的小静脉相比，HHT的小静脉异常增厚；有突出的、发达的纵向肌；并且被认为在毛细血管扩张中起着调节血流的重要作用[103]。

治疗毛细血管扩张症的方法包括雌激素[106]、氨基己酸[107]、内镜热消融[6,47]和受累肠段切除。当病灶在内镜可及范围且不是弥漫性时，内镜消融，包括APC和热接触器的使用，是最具前景的。SBE和DBE的应用将内镜治疗范围扩大到了整个胃肠道。内镜治疗可在活动性出血时或出血间期进行，减少了急诊肠切除术的需求。需要长期随访研究来评估各种治疗方法的最终疗效。

一项研究对25名HHT伴有严重肝血管畸形和高心输出量的患者使用贝伐单抗用治疗，结果显示贝伐单抗可降低心脏输出量及减少鼻出血；然而，在6个月的随访中，肝脏血管分布、肝脏体积和肝功均无明显变化[108]。这与另一例报道中观察到的相反：一位47岁女性患有HHT和严重的肝脏受累，于4年前接受了治疗，在开始治疗后3个月观察到胆汁淤积逆转、心力衰竭纠正、腹水消退，并且营养状况得到改善，在治疗6个月后肝脏的血管分布和肝脏体积明显减小[109]。关于在HHT患者中使用贝伐单抗治疗消化道出血的数据仍然有限，但是病例报告和小型研究显示该药有利于减少输血需求和提高生活质量。需要进一步研究以确定最佳治疗频率和疗程[110~112]。

（二）蓝色橡皮疱痣综合征

1860年，皮肤血管痣、肠道病变和消化道出血之间的关联被报道，近一个世纪后，这一系列发现被Bean命名为蓝色橡皮疱痣综合征（blue rubber bleb nevus syndrome，BRBNS），以区别于其他皮肤血管病变（图38.18）。除胃肠道外，其他部位也可受累，包括眼、鼻咽部、腮腺、肺、肝、脾、心脏、脑、骨骼肌、膀胱和阴茎。可能出现骨骼异常，并且在病变内可能出现钙化、血栓形成和消耗性凝血病（伴有血小板减少症）[113]。虽然有少数常染色体显性遗传的病例报道，并且一项分析确定了9号染色体上的一个易感位点，但家族史并不常见[114]。最近的一项研究假设，BRBNS可能是由于*TEK*的体细胞突变，该基因编码TIE2，TIE 2是血管生成素的内皮细胞酪氨酸激酶受体。这项研究发现，17例BRBNS患者中有15例存在*TEK*突变，支持了这些基因突变是皮肤黏膜静脉畸形原因的假设[115]。

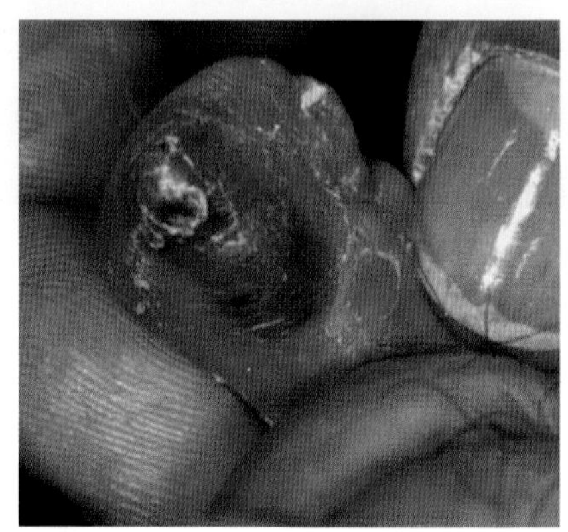

图38.18 蓝色橡皮疱痣综合征患者指尖病变

病变的表现很独特：蓝色的隆起，直径从0.1cm到5cm不等。典型表现为囊内所含血液可以被直接压空，留下一个“皱囊”，直到它再次充满。病变可能是单发或多发的，通常位于躯干，四肢和面部。可能累及胃肠道的任何部分，但最常见于小肠。在结肠中，病变在远端更常见。该病很少能通过钡剂或血管造影检查发现，CT和MRI可以较好地观察到病变。内镜检查，包括VCE，是该病最重要的诊断方法[116]。最初，这些病变被认为是血管瘤，但现在被认为是静脉畸形。对于复发性出血，建议切除受累的肠段。APC可能是危险的，因为这些病变可能累及肠壁全层；已有胃肠道病变成功硬化治疗和套扎的报道。

（三）进行性系统性硬化症（硬皮病）

毛细血管扩张是进行性系统性硬化症的一个显著特征，尤其是钙质沉着、雷诺现象、食管运动功能障碍、硬皮病和毛细血管扩张（calcinosis，Raynaud phenomenon，esophageal dysmotility，scleroderma，and telangiectasia，CREST）[117]。这些病变最常累及的部位是手、唇、舌和面部，但胃、小肠和结直肠病变也已有报道。这些微小病变可能是隐匿性或临床上显著出血的来源，如果有可能，最好通过内镜热消融术治疗[118]。

（四）Klippel-Trénaunay综合征和Parkes Weber综合征（先天性静脉畸形肢体肥大综合征）

在最初的描述中，Klippel-Trenaunay综合征（KTS）包括：①累及下肢的血管痣；②在出生或童年时出现局限于患侧的静脉曲张；③受累肢体的所有组织肥大，尤其是骨骼[119]。随后，注意到各种血管病变与肢体肥大相关，一些作者现在将该综合征分为两种不同的类型：Klippel-Trénaunay 综合征和 Parkes Weber 综合征；前者是单纯低流量状态，而后者为高流量动静脉瘘。已经在 KTS 患者中发现了血管生成因子 VG5Q 调控中的几个基因缺陷[120]。骨延长的原因是有争议的，但有一种理论认为是子宫内静脉高压和淤滞[119]。受累腿部常出现水肿，如果大腿受累（图 38.19A），通常会出现各种淋巴系统异常（例如，乳糜性肠系膜囊肿、乳糜腹、蛋白质丢失性肠病；见第 31 章）。

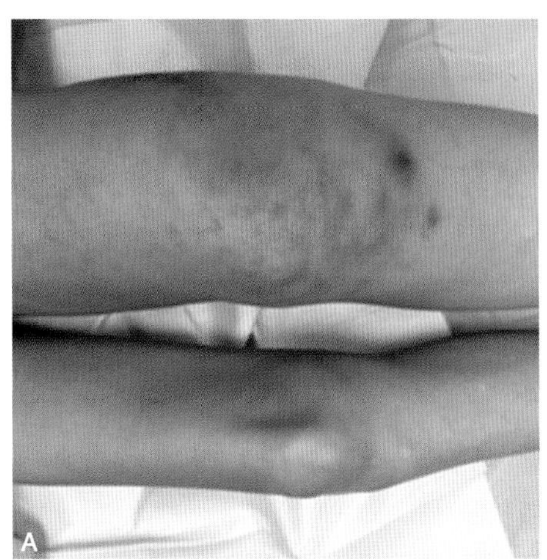

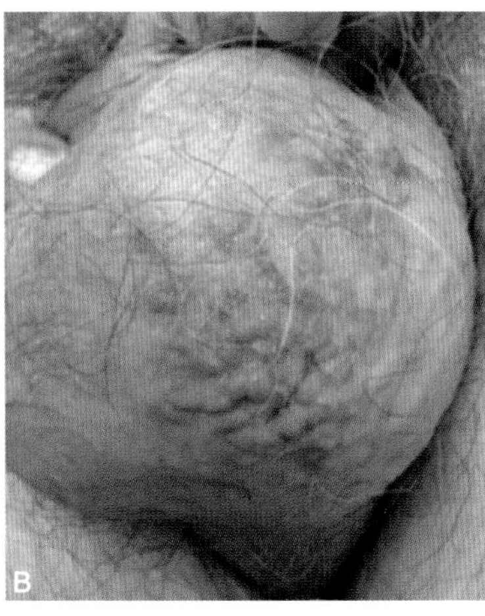

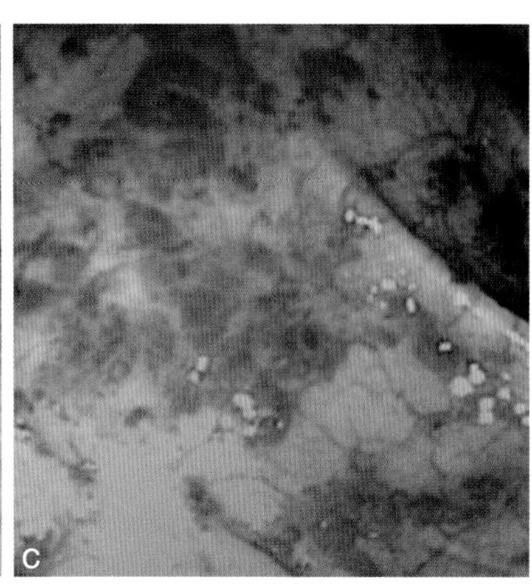

图 38.19　Klippel-Trénaunay 综合征图像。A，可见受累腿部水肿和相关血管病变。B，另一例患者阴囊受累。C，B 中同一患者的内镜图像显示广泛直肠血管病变示例，这可能是胃肠道出血的原因。（Courtesy，Dr. Lawrence J. Brandt，Bronx，NY.）

内脏病变包括胃肠道、肝脏、脾、膀胱、肾脏、肺、心脏和生殖器官（见图 38.19B）。胃肠道受累比以前认为的更常见，可能发生在多达 20% 的患者中，其中一些患者可能没有被识别内脏受累，因为他们没有症状。消化道出血是胃肠道受累的主要症状，最初是间歇性的，从生命的第一个 10 年开始；随后，KTS 引起的消化道出血可能表现为隐匿性出血，也可能为消化道大出血[121]。在最大的病例系列研究中，最常见的胃肠道症状是便血，尽管 588 例患者中仅 6 例出现[119]。消化道出血最常见部位是远端结肠和直肠，累及整个胃肠道并不常见[121]。消化道出血通常由直肠血管病变、髂内系统阻塞引起的局部直肠阴道静脉曲张或门静脉高压伴静脉曲张引起（见图 38.19C）。发生在血管病变的较小血窦内的消耗性凝血病可能会加重出血。体格检查即可诊断，各种影像学检查技术被用来定义解剖结构和计划手术修复[122]。MRI 用于诊断和发现动静脉分流[123]；血管造影仍然是金标准，并可允许介入治疗[121]。内镜热消融治疗在控制出血和预防或最大程度地减少消化道出血复发方面是有用的，特别是当病变相对局限时（L. Brandt，个人经验）；然而，临床上有明显出血的患者通常需要手术切除治疗[121]。

（五）辐射诱导的黏膜损伤

辐射损伤可诱导进行性闭塞性动脉内膜炎和内皮增生，导致新血管形成和毛细血管扩张形成，并可能出血[124]。如第 41 章所述，辐射损伤可发生在胃肠道的任何地方，但最常见的是在直肠乙状结肠，由前列腺癌和宫颈癌盆腔放疗导致[125,126]。

（六）胃窦血管扩张症（西瓜胃）及门静脉高压性胃病、肠病和结肠病

1. 胃窦血管扩张症（GAVE）

GAVE（西瓜胃）描述了胃窦的血管病变，由从幽门向外辐射的迂曲、扩张的血管组成，像轮子的辐条，类似西瓜表面的深色条纹[127]。这种病变可引起急性出血、慢性隐匿性出血或两者兼有。其原因尚不清楚，尽管有人提出胃蠕动导致松弛的胃窦黏膜脱垂，从而黏膜血管伸长（图 38.20）[127,128]。GAVE 也被假定是由于胃排空延迟以及高胃泌素血症、前列腺素 E2.5-羟色胺（血清素）和血管活性肠多肽引起的。

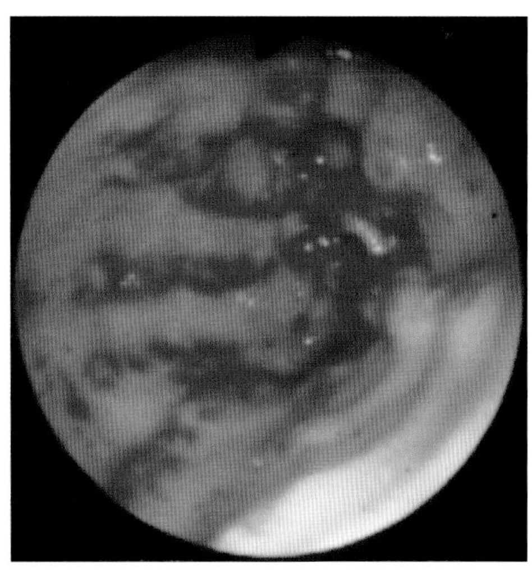

图 38.20　胃窦血管扩张（GAVE）的内镜下表现，也称为“西瓜胃”

GAVE 尤其见于中年或老年女性，并与胃酸缺乏/萎缩性胃炎、肝硬化和门静脉高压症、慢性肾病、心脏病、自身免疫性疾病和结缔组织疾病以及骨髓移植后相关[117,129,130]。约 40% 的 GAVE 病例与肝硬化和门静脉高压有关；因此，GAVE 可能由门静脉高压或肝静脉闭塞性疾病引起[131]，尽管其对旨在降低门脉压力的治疗没有反应。然而，鉴于肝移植后 GAVE 消退的病例报告，肝功能不全可能在其病理生理学中发挥作

用[132]。虽然不是病理性的，但 GAVE 的微观特征包括黏膜毛细血管扩张和充血、局灶性血栓形成、梭形细胞增殖（平滑肌细胞和肌成纤维细胞增生）和围绕固有层扩张毛细血管的纤维透明质变性[130]。一些研究者认为 GAVE 和门静脉高压性胃病是同一病理过程的不同表现，但文献表明它们是不同的两种病[133]，区分它们对给予适当的治疗干预很重要[130]。

GAVE 的药物治疗选择有限。雌孕激素已经过试验[134]，显示出一些疗效。抗纤维蛋白溶解剂氨甲环酸[135,136]和沙利度胺[137]的成功应用也有报道。在一项随机对照研究中，沙利度胺能显著减少 GAVE 和其他胃肠道血管发育不良患者的复发性出血[138]。在没有门静脉高压的情况下，TIPS 似乎对 GAVE 无效[139]。对于药物和内镜治疗失败的患者，胃窦切除是最后的选择[140]。

经内镜治疗是目前治疗 GAVE 的主要方法。多项研究表明，APC 可改善贫血并减少输血需求，尤其是在肝硬化患者中；副作用很小，尽管通常需要多次治疗。回顾性研究显示套扎治疗有效。如果 APC 不可用，可以考虑的其他治疗方法包括射频消融、冷冻疗法和使用氰基丙烯酸酯喷雾剂[141]。GAVE 伴消化道出血的患者，如果存在门静脉高压则出血更难控制，因为在这种情况下，出血量通常更大，且更难以治疗[142]。一些病例报告详细说明了肝移植后 GAVE 的逆转[143]。然而，数据不足以推荐这种治疗方法，除非患者是肝移植候选者。当 GAVE 与门静脉高压有关，或与 GAVE 伴门静脉高压胃病导致的出血不能经内镜控制时，TIPS 提供了另一种治疗方式（另见第 20 和 92 章）。

2. 门静脉高压性胃病、小肠病和结肠病

肝硬化患者中门静脉高压性胃病（portal hypertensive gastropathy，PHG）的患病率从 20% 到 98% 不等，可能是由于缺乏统一的诊断和分类标准；一般来说，这与更严重的门静脉高压有关。PHG 患者可能无症状或表现为慢性消化道出血相关的症状，据报道，后者发生率为 3% 至 60%。急性消化道出血不太常见，报告的患病率在 2% 至 12% 之间[144]。PHG 的内镜表现为 3 种形式：①黏膜的细小红斑点；②表面发红，特别是在胃皱襞的顶端；③在胃底或胃体出现带有红色斑点（蛇皮样外观）的马赛克图案（图 38.21），这种最常见。从组织学上看，PHG 发生在泌酸黏膜中，表现为扩张、弯曲、不规则的

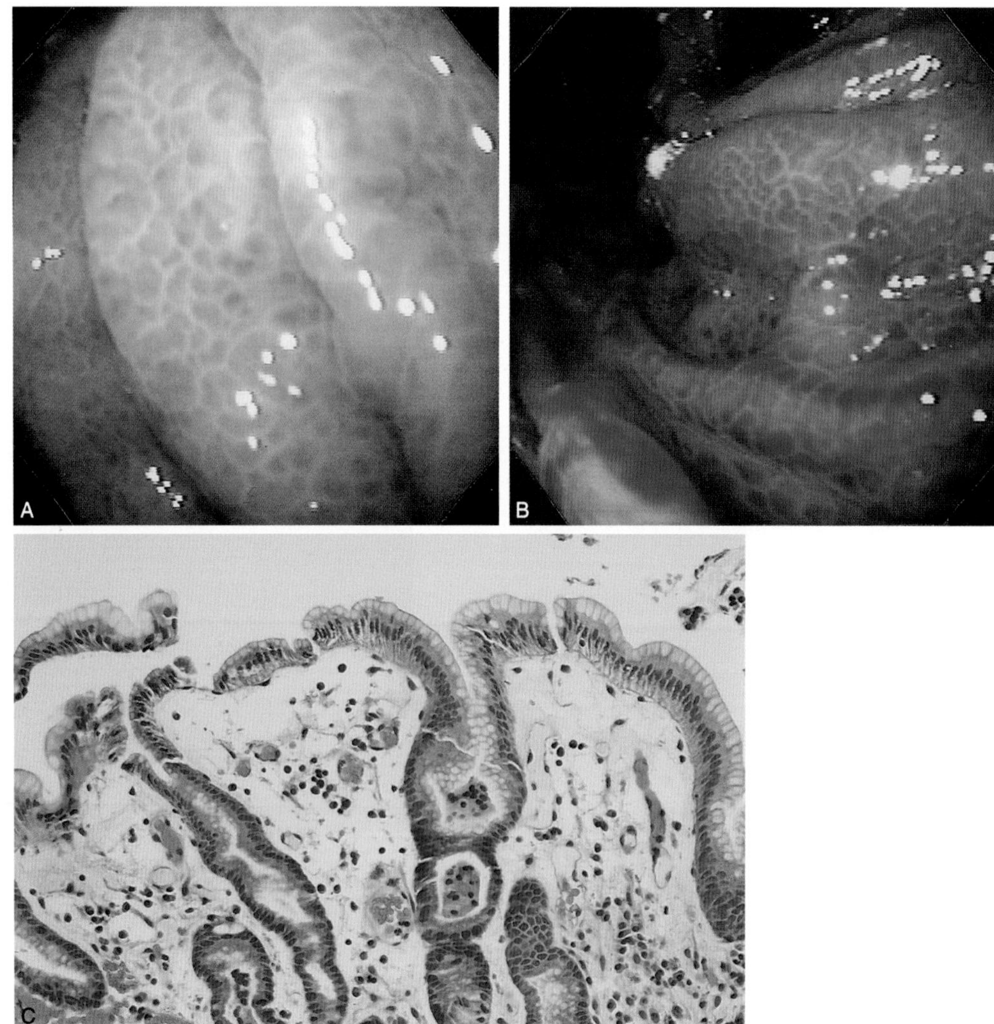

图 38.21　门静脉高压性胃病。A，轻度胃病表现为胃皱襞肥厚，有红斑和上皮下出血区。这种外观非病理学表现，可在其他引起黏膜水肿的疾病中观察到，如幽门螺杆菌胃炎。B，严重胃病伴蛇皮样弥漫性上皮下出血。C，低倍显微镜照片显示累及固有层的黏膜水肿明显，有多条充血血管。未观察到胃炎的组织学证据。（From Wilcox CM. Atlas of clinical gastrointestinal endoscopy. Philadelphia：WB Saunders；1995. p 109.）

静脉，无纤维蛋白血栓，有时伴有内膜增厚，通常无明显炎症[132]。

PHG 的管理主要集中在通过药物治疗降低门静脉压力。非选择性 β-肾上腺素能受体阻滞剂是一线治疗方法。普萘洛尔是一种非选择性 β 受体阻滞剂，在经典的随机对照试验中用于评估 β 受体阻滞剂在预防重度 PHG 复发性出血中的作用[144]。在这项研究中，与服用安慰剂的患者相比，服用普萘洛尔的患者在 12 个月（35% vs 62%）和 30 个月（48% vs 93%）的再出血率显著降低。如果患者对 β 受体阻滞剂治疗无效，则需要 TIPS 并且在大多数情况下是有效的[140,145-147]。生长抑素类似物，如奥曲肽，被认为是治疗急性静脉曲张出血的有效方法，也被证明是治疗急性 PHG 出血的有效方法。在评估这些血管活性药物对急性 PHG 出血疗效的两项研究中[148,149]，所有接受生长抑素或奥曲肽治疗的患者均成功止血。血管升压素及其类似物特利加压素也进行了试验，结果不一[148,150]。静脉曲张和蜘蛛样毛细血管扩张也可以在小肠中看到，称之为门静脉高压性小肠病。门静脉高压性结肠病是用来描述门静脉高压时结肠血管表现的术语，包括痔、静脉曲张和蜘蛛样毛细血管扩张（图 38.22A 和图 38.22B）。门静脉高压性结肠病的黏膜病变在内镜下与 PHG 相似，可能具有弥漫性结肠炎样外观，包括红斑、毛细血管扩张和脆性。门静脉高压性结肠病和小肠病的组织学变化与门静脉高压性胃病相似[151]。只要是在内镜可达范围内，对门静脉高压性肠病的病变治疗可采用与 GAVE 和 PHG 一样的热疗法[152]。

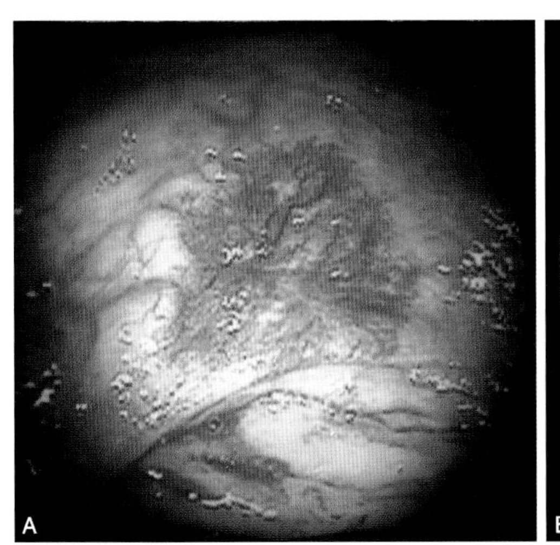

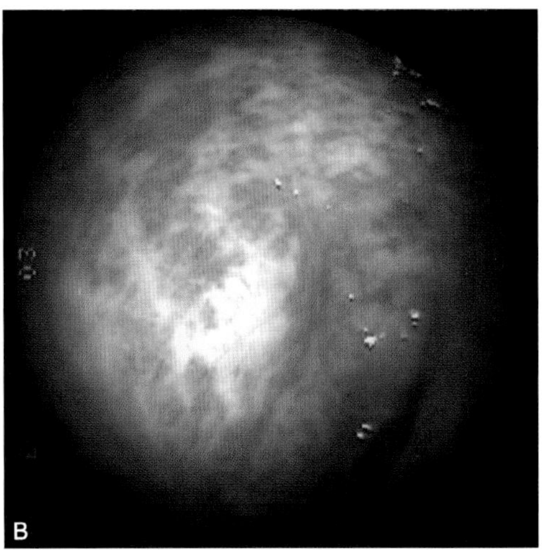

图 38.22 内镜图像显示两例门静脉高压性结肠病变。A，在直肠乙状结肠可见类似蜘蛛样毛细血管扩张或血管扩张的孤立性病变。B，肝硬化门静脉高压症患者降结肠斑片状红斑病灶。（Courtesy Dr. Lawrence J. Brandt, Bronx, New York）

五、血管的解剖异常

（一）肠系膜上动脉综合征

十二指肠的第三部分位于由肠系膜上动脉（SMA）根部和主动脉壁形成的约 45°夹角之间。当这个角度缩小到小于 25°时，SMA 压迫十二指肠，从而导致胃和肠瘀滞，这种情况被称为 Wilkie 综合征或 SMA 综合征（图 38.23）[155,156]。后一个术语可能会令人困惑，因为这种情况并不意味着血管功能不全。症状可能表现为急性或慢性，通常包括上腹痛、呕吐和早饱。该综合征与固定在身体模型中、儿童期生长迅速以及在成年人尤其是饮食障碍的年轻女性体重快速下降相关（见第 9 章）。罕见情况下，解剖异常也会导致这种情况，包括 Treitz 韧带位置过高或 SMA 起点过低。

钡剂检查可显示十二指肠第三部分突然中断，并伴有近端扩张，尤其是当患者仰卧时。CTA 和 MRA 可以提供无创和详细的解剖信息，可用于诊断和计划手术方案[157,158]。症状通常会在体重恢复或去除固定的身体模型后得到改善。很少需要手术。十二指肠空肠吻合术可以缓解症状，并且可以在腹腔镜下完成[159]。

（二）腹腔干压迫（正中弓状韧带）综合征

腹腔干压迫综合征（celiac axis compression syndrome, CACS）是否是胃肠道缺血的原因一直是一个有争议的话题，因为在一位患者中描述了餐后疼痛和上腹部杂音，该患者的血管造影显示由纤维化腹腔神经节压迫引起的 CA 变窄[160]。动脉受压解除后，杂音和餐后疼痛消失。自 1963 年 Harjola 描述以来，越来越多的人发现了膈正中弓状韧带和腹腔神经节对 CA 的压迫，但仍不太清楚。

确定 CACS 为一类疾病（有时也称为 Harjola 综合征或 Dunbar 综合征）的有效性的主要困难来自不同的研究者对它按不同的标准定义[161,162]。诊断 CACS 应具备的临床特征包括餐后上腹痛、腹泻、体重减轻和腹部杂音，当 CA 上升超过膈肌且动脉受压增加时，腹部杂音随着深呼气而加剧。

CA 受压通过侧位主动脉造影或 CA 选择性造影证实。EUS、CTA 和 MRA 是显示 CA 血管解剖结构和受压的无创手段[163]。膈脚纤维或腹腔神经节的压迫，使 CA 上段产生平滑、不对称狭窄，并将其向 SMA 方向移位（图 38.24）。这些表现最好在呼气末而不是吸气末显示。

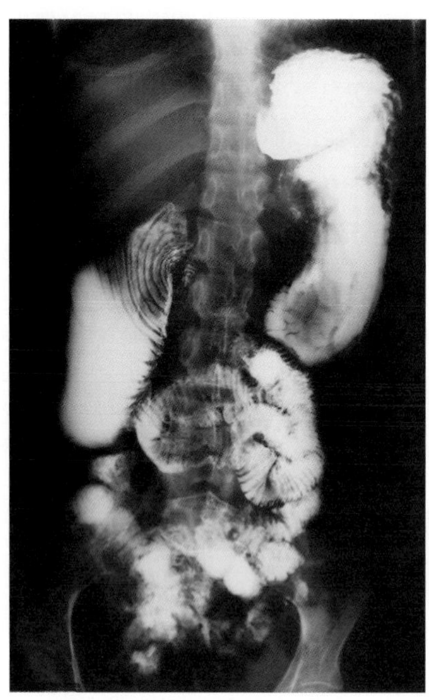

图 38.23　来自上消化道系列和小肠随访的肠系膜上动脉综合征患者的胶片。患者的症状与胃出口梗阻一致,在此胶片上,十二指肠的第二和第三部分明显扩张。(Courtesy Dr. Ellen Wolf,Bronx,NY.)

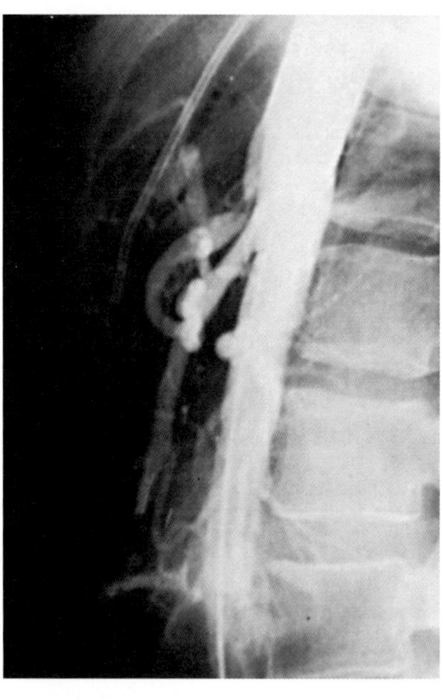

图 38.24　侧位主动脉造影片显示了腹腔干压迫综合征的结果:腹腔干起源的典型钩样压迫伴一些狭窄后扩张。该患者无胃肠道不适主诉。(From Boley SJ,Brandt Lu,Veith FJ. Ischemic disorders of the intestines. Curr Probl Surg 1978;15:1.)

血管造影 CA 狭窄的临床意义一直受到质疑,因为这一表现是非特异性的,而且在疑似肠绞痛患者,或不以疼痛为主要表现的胃肠道疾病的患者,以及胃肠道以外疾病的患者中发生的频率相同。CACS 的特征性疼痛最常见的原因是缺血,因为该综合征涉及的解剖病变是灌注上腹部内脏的主要动脉变窄。尽管临床和实验证据表明 CA 受压几乎是由 SMA 或 IMA 的侧支循环来代偿,但这一概念仍然存在。

一种流行的替代缺血的理论是,疼痛发生在腹腔神经节本身,可能继发于受压动脉的压力或搏动。进食时内脏血流量的增加和动脉的扩张可以解释疼痛与进餐的关系。

CACS 的手术方法包括分离正中弓状韧带,伴或不伴神经节切除术、动脉重建或旁路术;腹腔镜方法已成功地解除压迫[163]。CACS 的手术结果因用于诊断它们的标准而异。在对接受 CACS 治疗的患者进行的一项长期随访研究中,Evans 发现 83% 的患者在减压手术后 6 个月无症状,但只有 41% 的患者在 3~11 年后仍无症状[164]。在另一项对 400 名接受开放手术或腹腔镜下正中弓状韧带分离治疗的 CACS 患者的研究中,术后症状立即缓解的患者分别占 85% 和 96%。术后随访 6~229 个月,开放手术组和腹腔镜组分别有 6.8% 和 5.7% 的患者出现症状复发[165]。

关于 CACS 的争议仍在继续。少数其他原因不明的腹痛患者在标准方案治疗无效的情况下,通过 CACS 手术的某些方面获得了症状的缓解[166]。为了尽量减少不必要的手术,应仅对表现出上述临床特征的患者进行手术。

(汤善宏　施海韵 译,黄永辉 校)

参考文献

第 39 章　外科腹膜炎及其他腹膜、肠系膜、网膜和横膈膜疾病

Jeffrey B. Matthews, Kiran Turaga 著

章节目录

一、解剖和生理学 ………………………………… 549
（一）大体解剖 ………………………………… 549
（二）显微解剖 ………………………………… 550
（三）血液供应和神经分布 …………………… 550
（四）生理学 …………………………………… 550
二、继发性（外科）腹膜炎 ………………………… 551
（一）病因和发病机制 ………………………… 551
（二）病史和体格检查 ………………………… 552
（三）实验室检测和影像学 …………………… 552
（四）诊断 ……………………………………… 552
（五）治疗 ……………………………………… 552
（六）预后 ……………………………………… 553
三、其他原因的腹膜炎 …………………………… 553
（一）原发性腹膜炎 …………………………… 554
（二）持续性非卧床腹膜透析的腹膜炎 ……… 554
（三）结核性腹膜炎 …………………………… 554
（四）艾滋病相关腹膜炎 ……………………… 554
（五）Fitz-Hugh-Curtis 综合征或衣原体腹膜炎 …… 554
（六）真菌和寄生虫性腹膜炎 ………………… 555
（七）淀粉性腹膜炎 …………………………… 555
（八）罕见原因 ………………………………… 555
四、腹腔内粘连 …………………………………… 555
五、腹膜肿瘤 ……………………………………… 555
（一）转移到腹膜的肿瘤 ……………………… 555
（二）腹膜假黏液瘤 …………………………… 557
（三）间皮瘤 …………………………………… 557
六、盆腔脂肪增多症和腹膜囊肿 ………………… 557
七、肠系膜和网膜疾病 …………………………… 557
（一）出血 ……………………………………… 557
（二）肿瘤 ……………………………………… 557
（三）炎症性和纤维化状况 …………………… 558
（四）网膜梗死 ………………………………… 559
（五）网膜阑尾炎 ……………………………… 559
八、横膈膜疾病 …………………………………… 559
（一）疝和腹部脏器膨出 ……………………… 559
（二）肿瘤 ……………………………………… 559
（三）呃逆 ……………………………………… 559
九、腹腔镜对腹膜疾病的评估 …………………… 560
（一）一般考虑 ………………………………… 560
（二）不明原因腹水的评估 …………………… 560
（三）腹腔镜分期 ……………………………… 560

腹膜继发性炎症通常出现在需要手术干预的危急患者，一般被称为“外科腹膜炎”，原发性腹膜炎或原发性细菌性腹膜炎（SBP）具有独特的病理生理学，将在第 93 章中进行讨论。本章讨论影响腹膜、肠系膜、网膜和横膈膜的主要疾病过程。

一、解剖和生理学

（一）大体解剖

腹膜是人体最大的浆膜，估计其表面积为 1.8m^2，几乎与皮肤（或全身表面积）相同。腹膜的胚胎发育发生在原肠胚形成阶段，胚胎的 3 层——外胚层、中胚层和内胚层——进一步分化为内脏板中胚层和顶板中胚层。壁腹膜分泌浆液，而内脏腹膜包绕器官和肠系膜，使肠管悬浮于腹腔，从而为血管、神经和淋巴管提供通路。众所周知，网膜囊在男性体内是封闭的，而在女性体内则通过输卵管的开口与外界相通[1]。

完全发育的胎儿壁腹膜覆盖腹壁内表面，包括横膈膜和骨盆，而脏腹膜覆盖所有腹膜内器官（如小肠、胆囊、胃）和腹膜后器官（胰腺、肾脏、升结肠和降结肠）的前表面。我们正逐渐认识腹膜，网膜和肠系膜的解剖学。Meyers 识别了多条韧带和 2 个肠系膜，包括冠状韧带、胃肝韧带、肝十二指肠韧带、镰状韧带、胃结肠韧带、十二指肠结肠韧带、胃脾韧带、脾肾韧带、膈结肠韧带、横结肠系膜和小肠系膜。虽然这对于理解和预测在临床相关情况下表现的疾病和炎症的传播很重要，但这是对解剖学的过度简化。例如，消化性溃疡穿孔患者可能由于依赖右侧结肠旁沟的引流而出现右下腹疼痛。在影像学技术出现之前，一种常用的方法是将患者置于半卧位（Fowler 位），促进感染性液体在骨盆内聚集，以便触诊由此产生的脓肿并通过直肠进行引流。

目前对肠系膜和壁腹膜的认识表明，十二指肠空肠曲远端的肠系膜是一个连续的腹膜外器官[2]。右、左侧结肠系膜区域和乙状结肠系膜扁平地贴近腹壁，并由 Toldt 筋膜固定。有人提出，肠和肠系膜从膈肌到盆底是连续的，并且胃系膜和十二指肠系膜确实与肠系膜相连。肠系膜的这种描述被分为 6 个弯曲：十二指肠空肠，回盲部，肝脏，脾脏，降结肠和乙状结肠之间，以及乙状结肠和直肠之间。腹膜反折虽然是连续的，但也有不同的名称：Jackson 膜、前反折、Douglas 袋和腹膜侧反折（图 39.1）。这种理解被转化为“全结肠系膜或直肠系膜”用于切除肿瘤的目的。

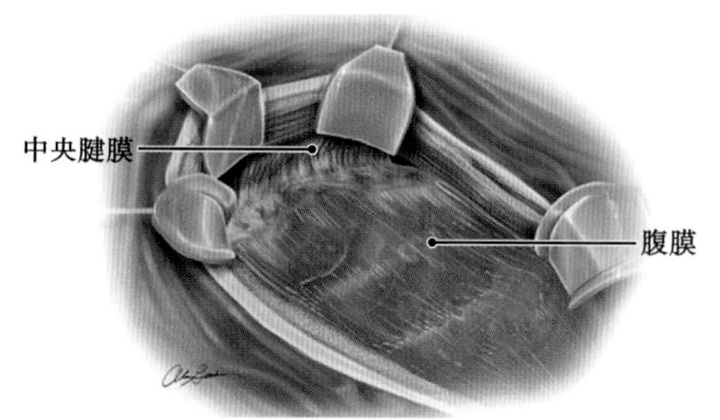

图 39.1　从前腹壁剥离后显示前壁腹膜

大网膜是一种腹腔内器官，来源于胃和脾大弯，延伸至横结肠，将腹部分隔成大小囊。小网膜连接胃小弯与肝脏，也称为胃肝网膜。小网膜的右缘也被称为肝十二指肠韧带，其后面的开口[小网膜孔(Winslow 网膜孔)]是大、小腹膜囊之间唯一的连接。

(二) 显微解剖

腹膜一词源于希腊语 peri(意为“周围”)和 tonos(意为“伸展”)，有“周围伸展”之意。壁腹膜和脏腹膜具有相似的结构，由间皮、基底层和间皮下基质 3 层构成。间皮由直径约 25μm 的单层立方间皮细胞形成。间皮细胞同时具有上皮和间充质特征，腹膜病理性改变可导致上皮-间充质转化。腹膜含有气孔，是淋巴系统的直接入口。它们大量存在于横膈膜上。在腹膜的顶端表面有许多微绒毛，偶有纤毛，其中嵌入板层小体。这些成分释放表面活性剂，营造一种无摩擦状态。在微绒毛和板层小体的顶部，存在一个糖萼，由蛋白聚糖和糖胺聚糖组成[3]。它们负责细胞间接触、炎症调节、组织重塑以及运输。间皮细胞由明确界定的细胞间连接复合物连接，包括紧密连接、黏附连接、间隙连接和桥粒，它们建立和维持了流体、溶质和微粒的半渗透屏障。

(三) 血液供应和神经分布

脏腹膜由内脏血管供应，壁腹膜由肋间、肋下、腰部和髂血管供应。来自脏腹膜的静脉血液通过门静脉回流，而壁腹膜通过下腔静脉回流。脏腹膜不由躯体神经支配，壁腹膜由躯体神经支配。因此，内脏疼痛是局限的、弥漫性的和模糊的(见第 11 章)，由伸展、扩张、扭转和旋转引起。脏腹膜受到切割或烧灼时不会产生疼痛。当中肠的内脏疼痛神经纤维受到刺激时，由于内脏疼痛纤维进入脊髓的平面与 T10 体纤维相同(见第 11 和 12 章)，因此会产生模糊的脐周不适感。这种感觉是皮区分布性不适感。同样，前肠的内脏刺激产生上腹部(T8 分布)不适，后肠内脏刺激产生耻骨上(T12)不适。壁腹膜(躯体)疼痛纤维被诸如切割、烧灼和炎症等刺激激活，这种疼痛定位明确。急性阑尾炎就是一个很好的例子。在疾病早期，患者经历继发于阑尾腔扩张的脐周不适，当炎症成为透壁性或累及壁腹膜时，会进一步表现为局限性右下腹部疼痛和压痛。

(四) 生理学

间皮细胞维持腹膜腔的稳态，并在基底面合成基质蛋白，维持腹膜的结构(图 39.2)[4]。腹膜在受伤或手术后可以再生，也可以通过上皮间充质转变引起纤维化。此外，这些细胞还可以通过将纤溶酶原转化为纤溶酶来促进纤维蛋白的降解，从而激活组织纤溶酶原激活物。在用复合网片修复腹壁疝的动物模型中，功能性新腹膜在 7 至 14 天内覆盖移植物[5,6]。

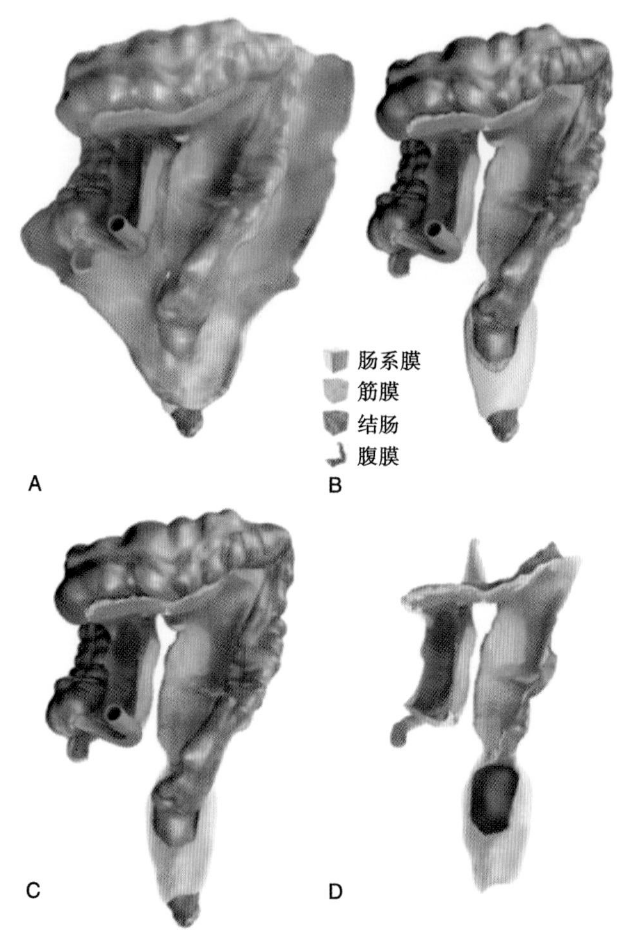

图 39.2　腹膜、肠系膜、筋膜和肠的数字表型。A，腹膜，肠系膜，筋膜和肠。B，肠系膜，筋膜和肠。C，肠系膜和肠。D，肠系膜

在炎症条件下，间皮细胞通过合成细胞因子、趋化因子和生长因子以启动和调节炎症反应。腹膜间皮细胞具有吞噬作用，也可以作为抗原呈递细胞[7]。

最后，在健康和炎症条件下，间皮细胞促进体液、溶质和颗粒物质通过腹膜进行运输。体液和溶质的运动受对流和扩散的控制[8]。颗粒通过 2 种不同的解剖途径从腹膜腔吸收。小于 2kD 的颗粒可通过腹膜静脉孔被吸收，引流至门静脉循环。大于 3kD 的颗粒通过腹膜淋巴管吸收，进入淋巴胸导管由此进入体循环。第二条吸收途径在控制腹部感染方面起着重要作用，因为它具有巨大的吸收能力。腹膜腔和膈血管之间的这些大通道的解剖结构，以及吸气时胸腔的负压使得这种机制在去除细菌和细胞方面非常有效。腹膜的巨大表面积和较好半透性的特点，使其可用作腹膜透析的治疗手段(图 39.3)。

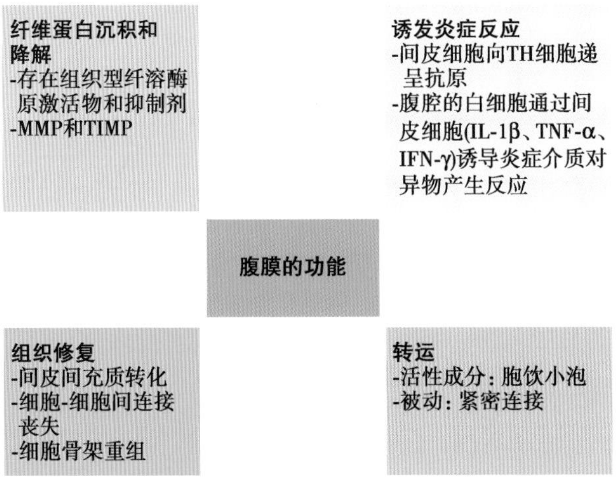

纤维蛋白沉积和降解
-存在组织型纤溶酶原激活物和抑制剂
-MMP和TIMP

诱发炎症反应
-间皮细胞向TH细胞递呈抗原
-腹腔的白细胞通过间皮细胞(IL-1β、TNF-α、IFN-γ)诱导炎症介质对异物产生反应

腹膜的功能

组织修复
-间皮间充质转化
-细胞-细胞间连接丧失
-细胞骨架重组

转运
-活性成分：胞饮小泡
-被动：紧密连接

图 39.3　腹膜的功能。IFN-γ，γ 干扰素；IL-1β，白细胞介素 1β；MMP，金属蛋白酶；TH，辅助性 T 细胞；TIMP，金属蛋白酶组织抑制剂

二、继发性(外科)腹膜炎

继发性(外科)腹膜炎是继发于腹腔内或腹膜后脏器炎症、穿孔或坏疽的腹腔炎症。通常需要手术干预治疗。然而，在某些情况下，如消化性溃疡穿孔，非手术治疗也可能成功(见第 53 章)。抗生素在严重腹腔感染中仅起辅助作用。如果不治疗，继发性腹膜炎在大多数情况下会导致感染性休克和死亡。医学上常用的说法是将非手术治疗与“保守”治疗等同起来，然而继发性腹膜炎的情况往往相反(也就是说，手术干预实际上是“保守”的方法)。

(一) 病因和发病机制

继发性腹膜炎的诊断基于病史、体格检查、影像学研究和手术探查。病史和体格检查在继发性腹膜炎中非常重要，高质量的病史和体格检查往往可以减少或避免进一步的检查。继发性腹膜炎有许多原因，常见原因包括穿孔性消化性溃疡、阑尾炎、憩室炎、急性胆囊炎、胰腺炎和术后并发症。其他炎症来源，如自身免疫性浆膜炎(如系统性红斑狼疮)，子宫内膜异位症和恶性肿瘤可引起腹膜炎症，但很少引起临床腹膜炎。

腹膜炎的其他非细菌性原因包括输卵管妊娠、卵巢囊肿或动脉瘤血管破裂导致血液渗入腹膜腔。血液对腹膜高度刺激，可能引起类似于脓毒性腹膜炎的腹痛(出血性腹膜炎)。胆汁漏入腹膜腔也可引起腹膜炎的症状和体征，特别是当胆汁内容物也有细菌污染时。然而令人惊讶的是，腹部的无菌胆汁可无症状。大的胆汁瘤可能只有轻微症状。

细菌可以通过多种病理过程进入腹膜腔：透壁性炎症伴管腔阻塞(见第 123 章)、胃肠道穿孔、细菌移位(见第 58 章)和肠缺血(见第 118 章)。细菌的初始接种量是由消化道受累部位的正常菌群决定的(见第 3 章)。

1. 菌群

虽然肠道菌群种类繁多广泛，特别是大肠杆菌，但肠道内容物漏入腹膜腔后，生物种类迅速减少[9]。以大肠杆菌、肠球菌等需氧菌和脆弱拟杆菌、梭菌等厌氧菌为主。结肠憩室炎破裂相关感染的一项研究报告发现，厌氧菌仅占 15%，需氧菌仅占 11%，混合需氧菌群和厌氧菌群占 74%；腹腔脓肿培养物仅检出厌氧菌占 18%，需氧菌占 5%，混合需氧菌群和厌氧菌群占 77%[10]。腹腔感染中除细菌外，真菌的检出率也较高，可能具有临床意义。例如，真菌培养阳性在穿孔性消化性溃疡中很常见，并可能对结果产生不利影响[11]。

基于单一微生物和多种微生物腹膜炎的动物模型，显示大肠杆菌是导致这种医源性腹膜炎死亡的最常见病原体，至少部分是由于它能够引起菌血症，厌氧菌和兼性微生物联合导致脓肿形成[12]。其他辅助物质，如失活组织、黏液、胆汁、血红蛋白和钡剂通过干扰吞噬和杀死细菌，与微生物协同增加外科性腹膜炎的死亡率。这些因素构成了外科性腹膜炎的治疗基础，后续将对此进行描述。

腹膜腔有几道防御细菌感染防线(框 39.1)[13-15]。当这些防线不堪重负时，会发生腹膜炎。

框 39.1　腹膜细菌防御机制
移除机制
通过胸导管经横膈膜腹膜清除细菌
白细胞吸引机制
间皮细胞的微绒毛
ICAM-1(CD54)和 VCAM-1(CD106)
通过网膜高内皮小静脉的中性粒细胞募集
杀灭机制
巨噬细胞(伴有谷氨酸代谢暴发)
中性粒细胞
调理素
补体 C3b
免疫球蛋白 G
纤维连接蛋白
肥大细胞衍生的白三烯
隔离机制
细菌的纤维蛋白捕获
纤维素性粘连形成
炎症病灶网膜包裹

2. 腹腔细菌清除率

一旦细菌进入腹腔，立即开始清除致病微生物。在犬腹腔内接种细菌后 6 分钟内，可以在胸淋巴导管内培养出细菌，表明微生物通过了横膈膜。12 分钟后，菌血症可能会很明显。这种清除机制在生存中可能很重要，因为在腹膜炎动物模型中阻断胸导管可以减少菌血症发作，但增加死亡率并导致肝坏死。这似乎与肝脏暴露于内毒素的量直接相关[16]。早在数十年前，横膈膜被认为是细菌清除的主要场所，Fowler 在 1900 年就建议采取头朝上、骨盆向下的姿势，以防止从受感染的腹腔吸收毒素。在没有抗生素的年代，被感染犬的试验显示，细菌清除延迟的记录证实了腹膜炎患者采取这种头低体位的明智性。

（二）病史和体格检查

临床病史和仔细的体格检查是及时诊断外科腹膜炎的关键因素。一般来说，诊断越早，预后越好。腹痛是腹膜炎的标志。疼痛发作的确切细节有助于引起对受累器官的关注（见第11章）。疼痛的性质、部位、辐射面积、随时间的变化、刺激和缓解因素是辅助诊断的关键信息。腹膜炎通常与肠梗阻有关，因此恶心和呕吐是常见症状。

在神经系统和免疫系统受损的患者中，临床医生发现出腹痛和腹膜体征的准确病史的能力是有限的。老年患者腹膜炎的疼痛可以减轻甚至消失。婴儿和儿童可能无法提供任何病史或配合体格检查。众所周知，继发性腹膜炎难以评估的患者包括酒精或违禁药物影响下的急诊室患者，中枢神经系统或脊髓损伤的创伤患者，以及镇静和通气的重症监护室（ICU）患者。镇痛药通常不会缓解体格检查时腹膜炎的表现，但可能会减轻一些不适。糖尿病患者可能在神经和免疫功能方面存在缺陷。接受免疫抑制剂和抗炎药物（如糖皮质激素和化疗药物）的患者可能会存在痛觉迟钝和轻微的腹膜刺激症状。肝硬化和腹水患者在SBP发作期间可能不会表现疼痛，除非壁腹膜参与炎症过程（见第93章）。

在检查中，外科性腹膜炎患者通常倾向于不活动，因为任何动作都会加剧疼痛。典型表现有37.8℃或更高的发热，以及心动过速，这可能是由疼痛引起的。低血压通常是脓毒症的晚期表现。发热是一种基本的内源性机制，有助于对抗感染。事实上，通常在细菌感染（包括腹膜炎）期间的体温升高，似乎在宿主抵御细菌的最佳防御中有重要作用[17]。叩诊时肝浊音区消失提示腹腔内有游离空气。由于压痛剧烈，应非常轻柔地触诊。过度用力触诊非常柔软的腹部可能会导致患者疼痛，以至于患者无法配合剩下的检查。

触诊应该从患者认为最痛的部位的最远处开始。触诊板状腹是个令人印象深刻、无法忘记的检查。其他较低的腹壁柔韧程度需要与此进行比较。如果粗暴地触诊焦虑患者，伴有轻微压痛的肌紧张可能会被缺乏经验的检查人员误认为僵硬。如果在听诊或叩诊时发现反跳触痛，一般就不需要通过触诊检查反跳痛。通常如果患者的疼痛在病床或担架震动时加重，可以推断存在反跳痛。

腹膜刺激征表明腹腔内炎症累及壁腹膜，包括反跳痛、肌紧张和触诊时极度压痛。腹膜炎可以是弥漫性的，如穿孔性消化性溃疡；或局限性的，如局限于左下腹的乙状结肠憩室炎。严重的脓毒症过程可能由于表面肠管和网膜的覆盖，而局限于盆腔，不会出现前腹壁的腹膜刺激征。因此，仔细的直肠和盆腔检查是必要的，以期发现盆腔腹膜炎。髂腰肌和闭孔征的存在（见第120章）有助于发现腹膜后或盆腔炎症和脓肿。

同一检查者的反复体检将提供进行性腹膜刺激的证据。随着时间的推移，体格检查将为诊断和对最初保守治疗的反应评估提供附加信息。连同下文所述的实验室检查和影像学检查，将提示外科干预的必要性。

（三）实验室检测和影像学

在免疫功能正常的患者中，腹膜炎最常见和广泛可用的实验室检查结果是白细胞计数增加以及核左移。血液中幼稚细胞的存在反映了对骨髓来源白细胞需求的增加。在细菌感染中，白细胞计数较低，有时与革兰氏阴性败血症相关，可能表明存在骨髓耗竭，预后较差。此外，可能存在代谢性酸中毒、血液浓缩和肾前性氮质血症。

在直立位胸片或直立或卧位腹部平片上可检出游离空气，但通过放射学检查发现气腹对肠穿孔的敏感性有限[18]。在恰当的临床环境下，缺乏游离气体不应延迟外科干预。超声检查有助于显示脓肿、胆管扩张和大量积液，但通常不是诊断成像的最佳一线选择。腹部和骨盆的CT，通常需要口服（偶尔直肠途径）和静脉注射造影剂，日益成为急性腹痛最敏感和最特异的影像学检查方法。多排螺旋CT可以在一次屏气中对整个腹部和骨盆进行成像。轴向图像具有极高的分辨率，可以在冠状面、矢状面和三维图像中重建[19]。对于游离气体的探测，CT的敏感性高于普通平片，使用多排CT可以看到穿孔的实际位置[28,29]。虽然CT越来越准确，图像也越来越有说服力，但对于可疑腹膜炎的患者，不应延迟外科会诊、复苏和手术。

（四）诊断

依据病史、体格检查、实验室检查和影像学检查可怀疑为外科性腹膜炎，当发现化脓性纤维性腹膜炎时，需开腹手术或腹腔镜检查确诊。对于病史和体格检查不可靠的患者，CT和腹腔灌洗对确诊外科性腹膜炎极具价值。CT具有较低的侵入性，但如果无法使用，或者对于血流动力学不稳定的患者，腹腔灌洗可以快速进行，是一种有效的替代方法。腹腔灌洗是在无菌条件下将导管插入腹腔，注入1L生理盐水。如果流出物中白细胞超过500个/mm^3，血清淀粉酶或胆红素水平高于正常，或革兰氏染色细菌阳性，则外科性腹膜炎的可能性约为90%，通常需要手术。最后，腹腔镜探查对外科性腹膜炎的诊断是非常准确的，许多基础疾病都可以通过腹腔镜进行治疗，避免了开腹手术[20]。

（五）治疗

外科性腹膜炎需要格外强调两个治疗原则。首先，并非所有腹膜炎患者都需要手术。例如，继发于乙状结肠憩室炎的局限性左下腹部腹膜炎患者，可以仅通过肠道休息和单独静脉注射抗生素治疗。另一名具有相同临床表现和CT扫描发现憩室脓肿的患者可以通过抗生素和经皮引流成功治疗（见第29章）。第二个原则是没有腹膜炎并不排除外科急症的可能性。典型的例子是在急性肠系膜缺血早期，腹痛与体格检查结果不成比例（见第11章）。同样，完全性机械性小肠梗阻需要在出现进展为穿孔或血管受损的腹膜体征前，进行紧急手术治疗（见第123章）。

对于大多数继发性腹膜炎，液体复苏和抗生素治疗后，急诊开腹手术或腹腔镜是治疗的主要内容。应该积极予以患者体液复苏以治疗继发于血管内液体外移而导致的血管内液体消耗。液体复苏（静推30mL/kg）是通过ICU内监测生理参数来指导的，包括血压（如果存在休克，通过动脉导管）、心率、中心静脉压、混合静脉氧饱和度和尿量。还应监测血细胞比容、白细胞、电解质、葡萄糖、肌酐和血气分析。可能会出现血容量减少、低血压、代谢性酸中毒、低氧和血浆进入腹腔导致的血液浓缩。只有在充分的容量复苏不能纠正低血压和低灌注后,才应开始加压治疗。新的脓毒症指南中包括了对血清乳酸水平的测量以指导复苏[21]。以前经验性使用的糖皮质激素仅限于对液体和血管加压药治疗无效的患者。一旦患者血流动力学稳定,应立即进行手术以控制病源。

1. 抗生素

手术前、手术中和手术后都需要抗生素治疗[22,23]。引起继发性腹膜炎的细菌种类部分取决于引起脓毒症的胃肠道的正常菌群,部分取决于临床环境。最近发布的两项关于复杂性腹腔内感染管理的指南建议,对医院获得性感染采用比社区获得性感染更广谱的抗生素治疗[22,23]。在社区获得性腹膜炎中,典型的病原菌是易感革兰氏阴性杆菌、严格的厌氧菌和肠球菌。在卫生保健相关感染中,菌群因抗生素暴露史和疾病史而改变,存在更多的抗生素耐药性菌株。一般来说,应该选择针对最有可能的病原体的抗生素。例如,结肠病变需要覆盖革兰阴性需氧菌和厌氧菌。在动物模型中,针对革兰氏阴性肠道需氧菌的抗生素可使死亡率降到最低,而针对厌氧菌的有效药物可防止脓肿的形成。在腹膜炎的实验模型中,需氧菌和厌氧菌之间存在协同作用。没有必要覆盖所有可能的病原体。外科性腹膜炎的菌群随时间而简化,甚至在开始使用抗生素之前,杀死某些关键菌群可能会改变微环境,足以抑制和杀死其他菌群。

对于感染性休克、免疫功能受损或医院获得性感染的患者,如果从腹腔培养出念珠菌,应予以相应的抗感染治疗[24]。另一方面,在社区环境中,血流动力学稳定、免疫功能强的继发性腹膜炎患者不需要治疗念珠菌。STOP-IT 试验中,抗生素短程疗程(4±1 天)的使用与抗生素持续使用直至退热或血常规正常具有相同的效果[25]。

已提出多种抗生素方案,可单独使用或联合使用以下几类抗生素:二代头孢菌素、三代头孢菌素、广谱 β-内酰胺类、氟喹诺酮类和甲硝唑、氨基糖苷类和克林霉素或甲硝唑。许多抗生素治疗方案的对照研究显示出不同方案具有同样的效果。例如,已证实广谱 β-内酰胺类单独使用和 β-内酰胺类与氨基糖苷类联合使用具有同样的效果[26]。由于研究设计不够理想和疗效标准不统一,目前还没有关于最佳抗生素治疗的指南。一项涉及 16 种不同治疗方案的 40 项随机试验的 Cochrane 综述显示,死亡率没有差异[27]。抗生素的选择应考虑到其他因素,如避免毒性、病原体的敏感性、给药的容易程度和途径、抗生素耐药性出现的风险以及成本[22]。广谱抗生素的可用性,包括 β-内酰胺类、氟喹诺酮类药物以及第三代和第四代头孢菌素,使肾功能受损的患者不需使用氨基糖苷类药物,因为它们具有潜在的肾毒性。

在适当的抗生素治疗后不能清除继发性腹膜炎或腹膜炎复发被称为三级腹膜炎。长期住院患者发生的院内感染可能包括多重耐药的假单胞菌、肠杆菌、肠球菌、葡萄球菌和念珠菌。若初次手术后出现多器官功能障碍综合征(MODS),应积极寻找未控制的感染源和脓肿,除抗菌治疗外,还包括重复 CT、经皮或手术引流脓肿、持续性体液培养[28]。

2. 手术干预

抗生素有助于治疗或预防致命性菌血症,但除非同时进行手术干预,否则不能治愈大多数外科性腹膜炎患者。在没有引流的情况下,肠内容物的漏出和大脓肿都不能通过单独使用抗生素而得到治疗。在患者病情稳定、复苏并给予抗生素后,应尽快进行手术干预。开腹手术仍然是确诊外科性腹膜炎的金标准,也是治疗腹膜炎的主要手段。然而,最近的一篇综述证实,越来越多的腹腔镜手术成功地治疗了某些形式的腹膜炎[20]。无论是腹腔镜手术还是传统的开腹手术,手术治疗的目的都是控制感染源、腹膜净化和预防复发性感染。

当初次手术无法控制感染源时,暂时关腹后再开腹手术可能有用。以下情况应该进行手术再次探查:①对感染源控制无效;②重新评估肠管活力;③引流不充分或较弱;④血流动力学不稳定;⑤初次手术时胰腺感染性坏死或弥漫性粪便性腹膜炎;⑥张力性吻合口的重新评估;⑦发生腹内高压(腹腔间隔室综合征)。这一综合征在第 11 章有更详细的描述。当腹部在筋膜或皮肤水平闭合,导致腹内压力上升到损害呼吸、肝脏和肾脏功能的程度时,就会出现腹腔间隔室综合征[29]。

术前和术后的体液和营养支持对促进伤口愈合和生存至关重要。腹膜炎的损伤与 50% 人体表面积烧伤相当,即使每天摄入 3 000~4 000kcal 的热量也不一定能达到正氮平衡。然而不能达到正氮平衡,可能是继发于蛋白降解的加速,以及病理性蛋白降解相关的负氮平衡不会因任何热量的摄入而纠正。这种蛋白降解可能只可以通过脓毒症相关治疗和患者的康复而抑制。肠内营养途径优于肠外营养途径(见第 6 章)。因此在危重患者中,初次手术时需要谨慎放置空肠造口管。

(六) 预后

尽管有了诊断和治疗继发性(外科性)腹膜炎的现代方法,但某些亚组患者的死亡率仍然很高,尤其是老年患者和腹膜炎发生前患有多器官功能衰竭的患者。总的来说,腹膜炎相关死亡率可能高达 30%[30],阑尾炎和十二指肠溃疡穿孔的死亡率最低(≈10%),术后(三级)腹膜炎的死亡率最高(高达 50%)。

三、其他原因的腹膜炎(框 39.2)

框 39.2 非外科腹膜炎的原因
SBP(见第 93 章)
长期非卧床腹膜透析
结核分枝杆菌感染
艾滋病相关因素
沙眼衣原体
淋病奈瑟菌(Fitz-Hugh-Curtis 综合征)
罕见原因
1. 结节性多动脉炎
2. 系统性红斑狼疮
3. 原发性干燥综合征
4. 家族性地中海热
SBP,原发性细菌性腹膜炎。

（一）原发性腹膜炎

SBP 或非手术来源的腹膜炎是原发性腹膜炎最常见的病因。这主要发生在肝硬化和腹水患者，并在第 93 章讨论。原发性腹膜炎也见于肾病综合征腹水患者。没有肝硬化或肾病的原发性腹膜炎要少见得多，通常发生在儿童。原发性腹膜炎的治疗无需手术干预，需要使用直接针对致病微生物的抗生素。

（二）持续性非卧床腹膜透析的腹膜炎

持续性非卧床腹膜透析（continuous ambulatory peritoneal dialysis，CAPD）是终末期肾病的一种常用治疗方法，尤其是在美国以外的地区[31]。细菌性腹膜炎的发生率因透析方案的不同而有很大差异，据报道，患者治疗年的发生率为 0.06～1.66[32]。最常见的分离株是表皮葡萄球菌和其他皮肤菌群。其他病原体，如革兰氏阴性杆菌，包括假单胞菌、真菌或结核分枝杆菌，则不那么常见。这种高感染发生率最可能的解释是留置导管的污染，但也与胃肠道、妇科和菌血症有关。因此，人们对腹膜炎提出了各种各样的预防建议[32]。这组患者中腹膜炎是主要的死亡原因，也是导致患者 CAPD 无效的最大原因。

约 80% 的患者会出现腹痛和压痛，但只有约三分之一的患者会出现发热。一致的特征是云絮样腹水，见于 84% 的病例[33]。根据体征和症状可以疑似诊断，并通过白细胞计数大于 100 中性粒细胞/mm^3 或革兰氏染色阳性而确诊。治疗应立即开始，无需等待培养结果，类似于肝硬化和中性粒细胞性腹水患者的经验治疗。疑似 CAPD 腹膜炎的初期治疗应覆盖最常见的分离细菌。如果考虑单药治疗，万古霉素或头孢菌素是很好的选择。腹腔内给药途径优于静脉给药[33]。分离出的微生物的敏感性决定了随后的抗生素选择。这些患者中的大多数在不停止透析的情况下在门诊成功治疗。及时的治疗可以确保生存；然而，复发性感染是常见的，可能导致导管移除或腹膜瘢痕形成。在腹膜炎患者透析袋中加用肝素可减少纤维蛋白的形成，从而减少感染后粘连的发生率，但尿激酶给药无任何益处。真菌感染和复发性细菌感染需要拔除导管。反复感染导致硬化性囊性腹膜炎（腹茧症）和有效透析表面积的缺失[34]。

（三）结核性腹膜炎

结核性腹膜炎是由结核分枝杆菌引起的一种罕见肺外感染部位。艾滋病、肝硬化、糖尿病和基础恶性肿瘤患者的发生风险增加[35]。非肝硬化结核性腹膜炎患者常有高蛋白含量、低葡萄糖浓度腹水和低血清腹水白蛋白梯度（<1.1g/dL）[36]。患者腹水白细胞计数几乎总是升高，淋巴细胞占优势。腹水淋巴细胞高的患者的评估流程包括腹水细胞学评估和腹腔镜检查。淋巴细胞性腹水和发热患者通常有结核病，而无发热患者通常有恶性腹水。癌症是引起淋巴细胞性腹水的原因，其发生率约为结核的 10 倍（见第 93 章）。如果存在腹膜转移癌，90% 以上的细胞学检查结果为阳性，可以避免腹腔镜检查。如果细胞学检查呈阴性，则需要进行腹腔镜检查，对结核性腹膜炎的敏感性接近 100%。然而，许多非侵入性的诊断方法可用于诊断肺外疾病。腺苷脱氨酶水平在结核性腹水中升高，这一发现有助于区分结核性腹膜炎和腹膜癌[37]。酶联免疫斑点试验（enzyme-linked immunospot assay，ELISPOT）和 PCR 试验（Xpert MTB/RIF）是一种新型、快速、无创的结核分枝杆菌检测方法。结核性腹膜炎也可在 CT 上表现为盆腔肿块，血清 CA125 水平较高，使得难以与转移性卵巢癌相鉴别。

QuantiFERON gold 等血清检测在诊断活动性结核性腹膜炎方面的检测特异性较差，特别是在仍接种卡介苗的结核病流行国家。认为由异烟肼、利福平、吡嗪酰胺和乙胺丁醇组成的 6 个月疗程（前 8 周），以及随后 4 个月异烟肼和利福平的治疗是足够的。根据当地药敏试验和耐药菌株的出现，可能需要更多的抗结核药物。肝硬化患者由于一线药物的肝毒性，可能需要改变药物治疗。抗结核治疗必须由公共卫生人员和医生仔细监督。不恰当的治疗会导致耐药菌株的出现。

（四）艾滋病相关腹膜炎（见第 35 章）

随着抗逆转录病毒治疗技术的进步，艾滋病死亡率下降了数倍，机会性胃肠道疾病的患病率下降，艾滋病相关外科疾病的手术次数显著减少。艾滋病患者可能会发生多种病原体相关腹膜炎：细菌（单一或多种病原微生物）；病毒（巨细胞病毒、疱疹病毒等）和真菌（组织胞浆菌、隐球菌和球孢子菌）；寄生虫（耶氏肺孢子虫、克氏锥虫）；以及分枝杆菌（结核分枝杆菌和鸟型结核分枝杆菌）。此外，肿瘤病变，如 Kaposi 肉瘤和非霍奇金淋巴瘤，可能累及腹膜。发生在 HIV 阳性患者中的腹膜炎，与其他形式的腹膜炎相似，常见的特征是腹痛、厌食、发热和腹水，腹水蛋白含量通常较高。除非肠道受累发生肠道穿孔，如伴发巨细胞病毒感染时，累及腹膜的这些机会性感染的治疗通常需要药物（如抗生素、两性霉素 B、更昔洛韦）。此外，开腹手术也可用于梗阻性症状，如淋巴瘤，这种情况下需要肠切除。

（五）Fitz-Hugh-Curtis 综合征或衣原体腹膜炎

Fitz-Hugh-Curtis 综合征或称肝周围炎（图 39.4）以前最常与淋病奈瑟菌感染相关。然而，近年来沙眼衣原体与肝周炎的关系日益密切[40]。由于细菌从输卵管播散到腹腔，衣原体肝周炎仅发生于妇女。这些患者的症状包括炎性腹水、右上腹痛、发热和肝脏摩擦音。如果有足够的腹水可以被临床检测到，腹水特点是白细胞计数升高、中性粒细胞为主，蛋白

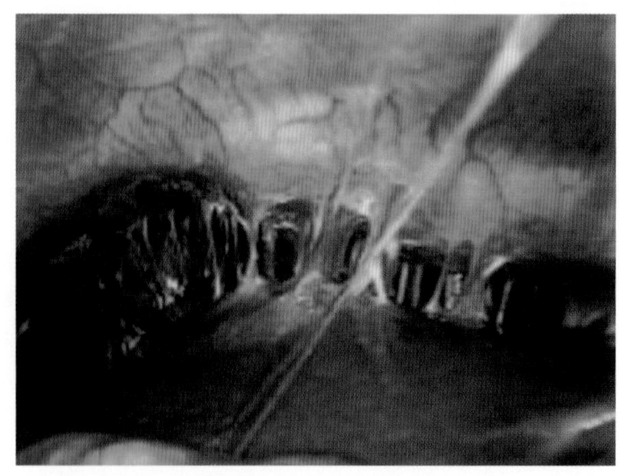

图 39.4　显示肝脏表面粘连的肝周围炎（Fitz-Hugh-Curtis 综合征）腹腔镜照片。（From Frumovitz MM，eMedicine.com，Inc.，2004）

质含量高，甚至超过 9g/dL。腹腔镜检查有助于确诊，可以发现从腹壁到肝脏的“琴弦”和“婚纱”样粘连征（见图 39.4）。多西环素常可治愈。如果粘连是在腹腔镜手术或开腹手术中偶然发现，则不需要治疗。

（六）真菌和寄生虫性腹膜炎

真菌性腹膜炎可由肠穿孔引起，尤其是上消化道穿孔，也可能是获得性免疫缺陷的并发症（见第 35 章）。妇科来源的真菌性腹膜炎可能局限于盆腔，可以用氟康唑治疗[41]。最常见的菌株是念珠菌，可能是因为常规血液培养基可以检测到念珠菌。如前所述，真菌性腹膜炎发生在慢性腹膜透析患者中。

尽管罕见，但艾滋病患者可以发生腹膜组织胞浆菌病、球孢子菌病和隐球菌感染。血吸虫病、蛲虫、蛔虫病、类圆线虫病、阿米巴病也可能累及腹腔（见章节 113 和 114）

（七）淀粉性腹膜炎

几年前，大约 1/1 000 开腹手术患者在术后 2~3 周因手套淀粉污染腹膜而出现发热和转移性腹痛。1980 年后，制造商用更多的惰性物质取代了玉米淀粉。手套玉米淀粉增加伤口感染，形成腹膜粘连，诱发肉芽肿性腹膜炎，并作为乳胶过敏原的载体[42]。手套粉性肉芽肿也可能类似于腹膜癌。如果病因不确定，或结果可能改变手术过程，则应对这些病变进行活检并行冰冻切片。淀粉性腹膜炎是一种很难诊断的疾病，需要较高的疑诊指数。治疗是非手术性的，糖皮质激素可能有益。

（八）罕见原因

约 5% 的狼疮患者[43] 和 10% 的多动脉炎和硬皮病患者可以因结缔组织疾病导致腹膜炎，并作为浆膜炎的一种表现。基础疾病的治疗通常需要控制浆膜炎（见第 37 章）。

家族性地中海热是一种常染色体隐性遗传病，可影响腹膜和其他浆膜。在犹太人、亚美尼亚人和阿拉伯血统的患者中更常见。这是一种无菌性复发性腹膜炎。患者通常表现为间歇性腹痛和发热；也可能出现滑膜炎和胸膜炎。秋水仙碱可预防发作和肾淀粉样变性（见第 37 章）。

四、腹腔内粘连

腹内粘连的形成和腹膜表面之间分隔的异常纤维条带可能是继发性腹膜炎和为纠正粘连而手术的后遗症。粘连可能是先天性的，但绝大多数是腹膜损伤所致。腹腔内异物如缝合材料、夹子和网片也有助于粘连的形成。腹腔粘连可能是发病率和死亡率的一个重要来源，是引起小肠梗阻的最常见原因（见第 123 章）。粘连是女性继发性不孕的主要原因，占 15%~20% 病例。盆腔粘连可能是慢性下腹部和盆腔疼痛的一个原因。如果需要腹膜透析或腹腔内化疗，粘连将妨碍疗效。广泛的粘连可能妨碍腹腔镜手术，并已证实可以增加失血、手术时间和再次肠切开术的风险。这些患者术后并发症的风险增加，住院时间延长。因此，需要考虑粘连性疾病的社会经济代价[44]。

在防止粘连形成方面已作出了巨大的努力。腹腔内组织损伤、出血和炎症导致纤维蛋白沉积在腹膜表面，使相邻表面黏附在这个黏稠的基质上。预防粘连形成的各种策略包括减少腹膜损伤、抑制炎症反应、预防纤维蛋白形成、促进纤维蛋白溶解、预防胶原沉积和腹膜表面屏障分离。虽然在动物实验中各种各样的实验策略已经减少了粘连的数量和严重程度，但这些策略很少转化为临床实践。在人类和动物实验中，大量的证据表明腹腔镜手术切口和手术部位的粘连比开腹手术少[45]。透明质酸为主的生物可吸收膜是一种透明质酸-羧甲基纤维素膜，已在人体试验中显示可减少一般外科手术后腹腔内粘连，但在随后的肠梗阻中没有明显的减少[46]。在妇科手术的患者中，有证据表明氧化再生纤维素（Interceed）、扩张 PTFE（Gore-Tex）和 Seprafilm 可以减少粘连，但是证据质量却相当低。

五、腹膜肿瘤

（一）转移到腹膜的肿瘤

转移性癌是目前最常见的腹膜肿瘤（图 39.5）。优先转移到腹膜的肿瘤包括卵巢癌、胃癌、结肠癌、直肠癌、阑尾癌、胰腺癌和乳腺浸润性小叶癌。腹膜的原发性肿瘤包括间皮瘤和促结缔组织增生性圆细胞肿瘤。

1. 临床特征

腹膜转移的患者往往由于影像学检查不充分而诊断较晚。腹膜转移的特征性表现是腹水、恶性肠梗阻及输尿管梗阻，都可以彼此独立发生。一些腹壁转移（包括以“Sister Mary Joseph”命名的脐带结节）患者易于检测。在腹膜转移高风险的患者中，有上述发现时应立即行腹腔镜对腹膜进行检查。

这些症状的存在通常预示预后不良，并且这个阶段的干预措施通常在其治疗效益和治疗目的方面受限。这导致许多

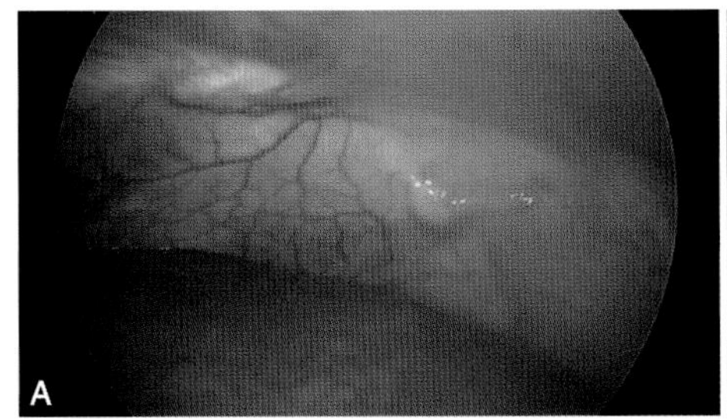

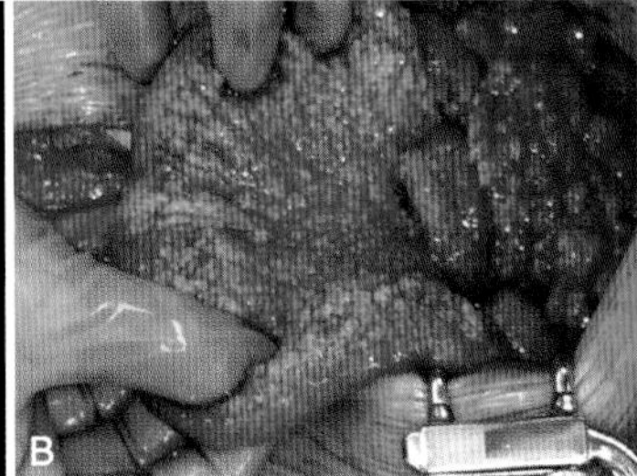

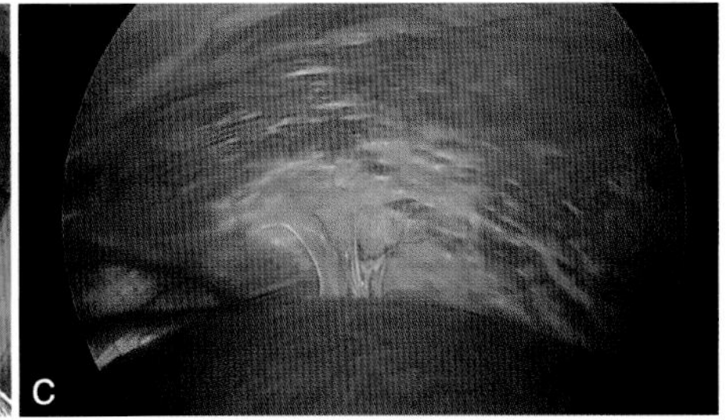

图 39.5　出现腹膜转移：A，结节型转移；B，肠系膜受累的弥漫性结节型转移；C，硬化或瘢痕样转移（最常见）

研究者尝试主动用腹腔镜诊断腹膜转移。最近的 Prophylo-CHIP 试验就是这样的一项研究，在这项研究中，接受完全切除的高危结肠癌（穿孔性肿瘤、T4 期病变、小负荷腹膜疾病/肿瘤沉积），患者如果在影像学上未见腹膜疾病，即在完成化疗后随机接受第二次剖腹手术。52%的患者诊断为腹膜转移[47]。胃和其他实体瘤恶性肿瘤正在进行类似的研究。可切除（和临界可切除）胰腺癌中可见其他无法检测的腹膜转移的发生率为 8%至 20%。

常规影像学检查一般不会发现腹腔积液。因此，在没有炎症过程的情况下出现腹水则可高度怀疑肿瘤转移。渗出性腹水的出现作为一项证据表明肿瘤患者已进入晚期，且具有较大的肿瘤负荷，而不是作为癌症的主要表现。体重减轻，腹痛和早期饱腹感较为常见。在没有腹膜转移的情况下，大量肝转移、肝细胞性肝癌伴或不伴肝硬化、恶性淋巴结梗阻如淋巴瘤、Budd-Chiari 综合征伴或不伴下腔静脉梗阻也与腹水有关。但可根据腹水的性质加以鉴别，这点非常重要，因为每种疾病所需的治疗方案不一样（详见第 93 章的发病机制和腹水分析）。细胞学检查通常可以发现腹膜转移（除了某些组织学，如间皮瘤），并且癌性腹水通常是浆液性和黏液性的，而不是血性的（见第 93 章）。

输尿管梗阻患者的影像学检查可能会提示存在肾积水。肾积水的进展可导致尿毒症，恶心和呕吐，类似肠梗阻。放置输尿管支架或经皮肾造瘘管可迅速缓解梗阻所致的肾功能恶化。

恶性肠梗阻是肿瘤腹膜转移患者的终末期表现。通常情况下有多灶性梗阻，尽管只有主要梗阻区域显现出症状。患者经常出现腹痛，闭环梗阻引起的痉挛和呕吐。乙状结肠和近端空肠是转移性疾病梗阻的常见部位。

2. 一般治疗

腹膜转移的患者需要专业的治疗管理，这类患者最好采用多学科合作下共同治疗。控制症状以及早期目标设定非常重要，可以促进决策治疗计划。

（1）手术和腹腔内化疗

并不是所有的腹膜转移预示不良的生存预后。根据疾病进展和组织学报告，有些患者可以被治愈。

低度恶性阑尾上皮肿瘤、腹膜间皮瘤（稍后讨论）、低负荷结直肠转移和卵巢癌患者通常至少可存活 5 年，其中很大一部分患者可以生存 10 年或更长时间[48]。

细胞减灭术的技术已被用于这类患者的治疗，包括腹膜切除术，其中壁腹膜系统地从腹壁内壁切除。以前，腹膜切除术被认为是一种高风险的手术，但是技术的进步使得其死亡率与其他主要肿瘤切除术不相上下。死亡率与疾病进展程度直接相关，因此积极的早期检查可使实施微创手术治疗的概率及可能性更大，完全细胞减灭技术有着非常显著的治疗效果。

在单一环境下使用腹腔内化疗［如热性腹腔化疗（hyperthermic intraperitoneal chemotherapy，HIPEC）］或随后的经导管腹腔内治疗已广泛应用于腹膜转移患者。HIPEC 在卵巢癌、阑尾上皮肿瘤、间皮瘤、胃和结直肠恶性肿瘤患者中的应用已得到很好的研究[49]。进行腹腔内治疗会增加 30 天和 90 天的发病率，且需要由经验丰富的团队进行管理。表 39.1 列出了腹膜转移性恶性肿瘤患者的管理策略。

表 39.1 腹膜表面恶性肿瘤的管理策略

组织学亚型	系统治疗	细胞减灭术	局部治疗
原发性			
原发性腹膜瘤	紫杉烷/卡铂（新辅助/辅助）	最佳细胞减灭	最佳减瘤患者腹腔内化疗（顺铂/紫杉醇）±HIPEC（顺铂/卡铂）
恶性间皮瘤	顺铂/培美曲塞	最佳细胞减灭	HIPEC（顺铂/阿霉素/丝裂霉素 C）
DSRCT（促纤维增生性小圆细胞肿瘤）	环磷酰胺，阿霉素，长春新碱与异环磷酰胺和依托泊苷交替；自体干细胞拯救；全腹放疗	最佳细胞减灭	HIPEC（顺铂）
继发性			
低级别阑尾肿瘤		最佳细胞减灭	HIPEC（丝裂霉素-C）
高级别阑尾肿瘤（包括杯状细胞类癌、印戒细胞组织学）	氟尿嘧啶，奥沙利铂，伊利替康，抗表皮生长因子抗体（西妥昔单抗/帕尼单抗）；抗血管内皮生长因子抗体（贝伐珠单抗）	最佳细胞减灭	HIPEC（丝裂霉素-C）
结直肠癌	氟嘧啶、奥沙利铂、伊立替康、抗 EGFR 抗体（西妥昔单抗/帕尼单抗），抗 VEGF 抗体（贝伐珠单抗）	最佳细胞减灭	HIPEC（丝裂霉素-C/奥沙利铂）
卵巢癌	紫杉烷/卡铂（新辅助/辅助）	最佳细胞减灭	腹腔内化疗（顺铂/紫杉醇）用于最佳减瘤者 HIPEC（顺铂）
胃癌	顺铂/氟嘧啶、多西他赛/表柔比星、曲妥珠单抗用于 HER2/neu+肿瘤 检查点抑制剂	正在研究的最佳细胞减灭术	±HIPEC（顺铂/丝裂霉素-C）；±IP 多西他赛/紫杉醇）

表 39.1　腹膜表面恶性肿瘤的管理策略(续)

组织学亚型	系统治疗	细胞减灭术	局部治疗
食管/胰腺/肝胆	氟嘧啶/奥沙利佰/伊立替康 吉西他滨/顺佰 白蛋白结合型紫杉醇 胃部治疗方案 检查点抑制剂		
肉瘤(非 GIST)	阿霉素/异环磷酰胺,艾日布林,帕唑帕尼	最佳细胞减灭术	±HIPEC(顺铂/阿霉素)
肉瘤(GIST)	酪氨酸激酶抑制剂,伊马替尼/舒尼替尼/帕唑帕尼/瑞格非尼		

HIPEC,腹腔热灌注化疗;IP,腹腔内。
From the American Cancer Society Oncology in Practice,Turaga KK(February 2018).

(2) **恶性肠梗阻**

恶性肠梗阻的治疗通常需要放置鼻胃管。软鼻胃管相比传统 Salem 管更为舒适。还可以额外采取奥曲肽,质子泵抑制剂(以减少酸分泌),抗胆碱能药物如东莨菪碱以减少痉挛和镇痛等治疗。糖皮质激素可以减少水肿和恶心,被提议可作为非手术的辅助治疗。手术咨询是适当的,以确定干预是否具有治疗性或姑息性的益处。当恶性梗阻反复发生时,则应尽早考虑放置胃造口管。40%~80%的梗阻可自发消退,且坚持低纤维饮食可能会降低复发的概率。如果是肿瘤引起的外源性压迫,该情况下放置腔内支架通常效果不佳,但可以在多学科共同商议后决定是否在特定部位实施。早期进行姑息治疗有助于帮助患者缓解症状。

(3) **治疗性穿刺术**

大多数腹膜种植转移的患者可以进行治疗性穿刺术以缓解症状,反复穿刺则会导致营养不良,发育停滞及加重身体虚弱程度。留置导管对于考虑临终关怀或临终措施的患者有很大帮助。利尿剂的使用主要基于假设而非硬数据,并且应该严格限制。

(二) 腹膜假黏液瘤

腹膜假性黏液瘤本身并不构成一种诊断,而是一种黏液性腹水综合征,主要与阑尾上皮肿瘤相关,但也可以发生在卵巢、胰腺、结直肠和胃黏液性肿瘤。腹膜假性黏液瘤的组织学起源预测着预后和结局。通常症状表现为无痛的腹胀。当在剖腹手术或腹腔镜检查中观察到特征性胶状物质时,可以作出明确的诊断。当其起源于阑尾肿瘤时,则必须区分是低度阑尾黏液性囊腺瘤(以前称为黏液性囊腺瘤,黏液囊肿)还是高度恶性肿瘤(包括腺癌)。这种情况下可以进行有效的细胞减灭手术和 HIPEC 治疗。由于淋巴结转移十分少见,进行完全细胞减灭术且无须切除结肠的患者中,内脏切除包括右半结肠切除术是不必要的。

(三) 间皮瘤

65%~70%的间皮瘤发生在胸膜,25%发生在腹膜。大多数腹膜间皮瘤是恶性的,与石棉暴露有关,并在最初暴露35~40 年后发现。石棉工人的家属也有发病风险。通常在开腹手术或腹腔镜下诊断,但偶尔在腹水分析中发现恶性间皮细胞。恶性腹膜间皮瘤患者通常存在偶发的种系 BRCA 相关蛋白-1(BAP-1)突变。多学科合作下的治疗对患者而言是最佳的。细胞减灭手术和 HIPEC 已被证明可以改善生存率,5年生存率波动于 29%到 70%之间[50]。

六、盆腔脂肪增多症和腹膜囊肿

正常情况下积聚在直肠周围和膀胱周围的脂肪可能发生非恶性过度生长,并且被认为是一个独特的临床病理过程,盆腔脂肪瘤。它主要发生在 20~60 岁非裔美国人(男∶女为18∶1),可能导致或与高血压、膀胱炎、尿路梗阻、偶与胃肠道症状相关[51]。脂肪异常增殖伴有不同程度的纤维化反应。经直肠超声和 CT 对于诊断十分重要,特别是在盆腔脂肪瘤和脂肪肉瘤的鉴别诊断中。虽然尿路梗阻可能需要改道,但大多数患者不会进展。腹膜囊肿很少见。良性囊性淋巴瘤多影响年轻男性,表现为肿块,切除后很少复发。

七、肠系膜和网膜疾病

肠系膜和网膜的疾病包括出血、肿瘤和囊肿、炎症和纤维化以及梗死(发病频率递减)。肠系膜脓肿见第 29 章。

(一) 出血

肠系膜出血、腹腔内出血和腹膜后出血及其并发症可分为外伤性出血和自发性出血。这两种类型都因抗凝而加重。外伤性血肿可能需要或不需要手术治疗,这取决于损伤的部位和创伤是钝性还是穿透性的。自发性出血可能源于妇科(如卵巢囊肿破裂)、肝脏(如肝细胞癌破裂)、脾脏(如 EB 病毒感染相关破裂)、血管(如内脏动脉瘤破裂)和凝血病[52]。

症状通常包括疼痛和血肿的占位效应,如肠梗阻症状。诊断依赖于较高的怀疑指数和超声或 CT,显示血液的集聚。超声引导 FNA 可能有助于明确诊断。治疗包括停用抗凝药物(正在接受抗凝治疗的患者)和逆转抗凝治疗。另一些治疗则取决于局部或全身出血症状。在某些情况下,血管造影栓塞可能有助于治疗腹腔出血[53]。

(二) 肿瘤

起源于肠系膜和网膜的肿瘤罕见,包括软组织肿瘤(如囊肿、纤维瘤、肉瘤、硬纤维瘤)和局部性肿瘤,如腹部弥漫性平滑肌肉瘤和卡斯特曼氏病(Castleman 病)。大多数这个部位的肿瘤在发现时都很大,因为它们生长的空间很大。当由于无关原因进行影像学检查时,它们可能被偶然发现,通常表现为非特异性症状,如腹部不适或轻度梗阻症状。

1. 肠系膜囊肿

肠系膜囊肿是一种罕见的肿瘤,可发生在各种腹内的不同部位,并有不同的表现。可以发生在儿童和成人。此类肿瘤通常较大(平均≈13cm)、充满液体(≈2 000mL),尽管其尺寸较大,但只有 3% 病例是恶性。最常见的症状是疼痛(58%),最常见的体征是腹胀(68%)[54]。一些病例可能出现发热和寒战,另一些则无症状,在开腹手术前被偶然发现和误诊。如果在开腹手术中偶然发现小的肠系膜囊肿,不需要切除。切除术是囊肿并发症(如破裂或出血)的治疗选择,可在腹腔镜下进行[94]。肠系膜囊肿通常可以因完全切除完全治愈(图 39.6)。

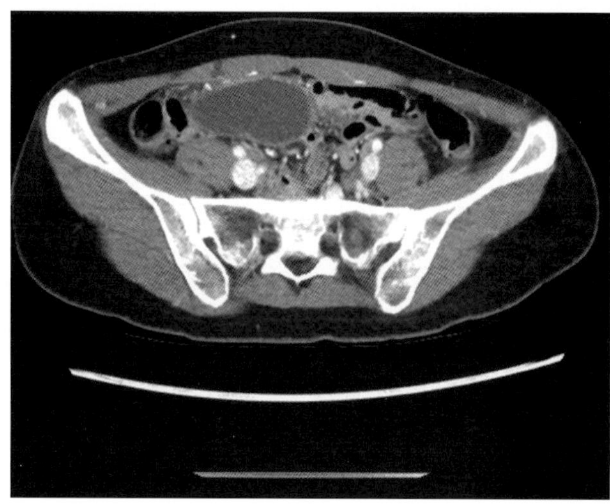

图 39.6 肠系膜囊肿的特征是解剖位置和均匀的外观,充满液体的密度

2. 实体瘤

肠系膜实体性肿瘤较肠系膜囊肿少见。大多数(67%)是良性的,包括纤维瘤、黄色肉芽肿、脂肪瘤、平滑肌瘤、毛细血管和海绵状血管瘤、神经纤维瘤和间质瘤。恶性肿瘤包括血管外皮细胞瘤、纤维肉瘤、脂肪肉瘤、平滑肌肉瘤、恶性间质瘤。网膜实体性肿瘤在组织学类型和发生率上有显著的相似性。肠系膜和网膜肿瘤的典型症状和体征包括疼痛和肿胀,并伴有较大的病灶。治疗方法是手术切除。约 18% 患者死于肿瘤,但恶性肿瘤患者的 5 年总体生存率仅为 21%[55]。尽管诊断和治疗可能需要腹腔镜或开腹手术,但对这些肿瘤可以尝试针吸活检。

3. 多灶性平滑肌瘤(腹膜分散平滑肌瘤病)

多灶性平滑肌瘤甚至比其他肿瘤更少见,可能是恶性的,可类似腹膜癌。它们可能与其他平滑肌瘤或子宫内膜异位症同时出现。这些病变由小而有弹性的结节组成,似乎对激素敏感,妊娠期间或雌激素治疗期间有时会进展,并随激素的撤退而消退。这些肿瘤可引起腹痛或胃肠道出血。这种情况必须与多灶性平滑肌肉瘤相鉴别,后者被描述为发生于子宫内膜肉瘤的子宫粉碎术后。

4. Castleman 病

Castleman 病(巨大或滤泡性淋巴结增生)罕见。该病具有相当大的异质性,可分为单中心型和多中心型。在某些情况下,Castleman 病是由人类疱疹病毒 8(HHV-8)感染引起的。肠系膜或纵隔的中央淋巴结更常以单中心形式受累。这种情况下,手术切除肿块是成功的,预后良好。多中心型采用系统性治疗,疗效不一,预后相当差,患者有转化为淋巴瘤的风险[56]。

(三)炎症性和纤维化状况

腹膜后的炎症状况是异质的,且对他们的研究正在进一步深入。这一领域的最新进展表明,这些是 IgG4 相关疾病的表现,其特点是淋巴浆细胞浸润、闭塞性静脉炎和中度嗜酸性粒细胞增多(第 37 章)。其他 IgG4 相关疾病包括自身免疫性胆管炎,自身免疫性胰腺炎和 Riedel 甲状腺炎等[37]。

腹膜后炎症在组织学上分为 3 种基本疾病:收缩性系膜炎、肠系膜脂膜炎和腹膜后纤维化。

收缩性系膜炎标志了这一疾病的纤维化部分,通常也被称为硬化性肠系膜炎、多灶性腹膜下硬化、纤维瘤病和硬纤维瘤样肿瘤(图 39.7)。炎症部分被称为肠系膜脂膜炎、肠系膜脂肪营养不良、肠系膜脂肪肉芽肿、脂肪硬化性肠系膜炎、肠系膜 Weber-Christian 病和全身性结节性脂膜炎。有人试图将这种疾病细分为弥漫性、单纯性和多发性,并提出与淋巴瘤有关[58]。

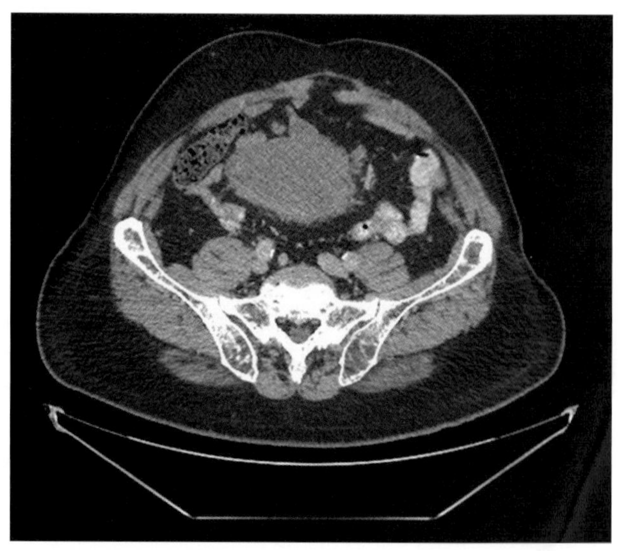

图 39.7 肠系膜硬纤维瘤患者的轴向 CT 切片

重叠性名称,如硬化性脂肪肉芽肿,在 12 年间肠系膜脂膜炎向收缩性肠系膜炎进展和转化,以及硬化性肠系膜炎和腹膜后纤维化的同时发生,表明这些只是同一基础疾病的不同阶段。

虽然肠系膜脂膜炎和收缩性肠系膜炎通常表现为腹痛、肠梗阻症状和肿块病变,但也有报道与持续高热和无腹部症状的自身免疫性溶血性贫血相关的病例。收缩性肠系膜炎和肠系膜脂膜炎通常是特发性的,但 30% 腹膜后纤维化有明确病因,包括药物、恶性肿瘤、创伤或炎症[103]。报告的病例大多数是药物引起的（二甲麦角新碱、麦角胺）。纤维化过程可导致输尿管或血管阻塞。

组织学上，收缩性肠系膜炎和肠系膜脂膜炎可伴有淋巴细胞和中性粒细胞炎症、脂肪坏死、纤维化和钙化。相反地，只有肠系膜脂膜炎具有多核巨细胞，胆固醇裂隙，脂质巨噬细胞和淋巴管扩张。腹膜后纤维化由致密结缔组织组成，伴或不伴炎症。IgG4 浆细胞，轮辐状纤维化和闭塞性静脉炎的存在应该促进开展对 IgG4 相关纤维化的评估。

诊断与治疗

这些疾病以前只有在开腹手术或尸检时才可确诊；然而，如 CT（图 39.8）或 MRI 等非侵入性技术可能有助于术前诊断。在一系列腹部 CT 扫描中，0.6% 患者放射性检查提示肠系膜脂膜炎[59]。49 例肠系膜脂膜炎患者中，以女性为主，34 例与恶性肿瘤有关。腹膜后纤维化患者常伴有肾积水。

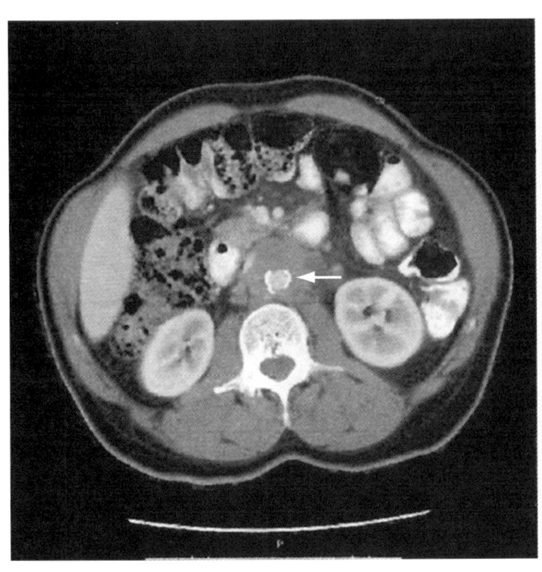

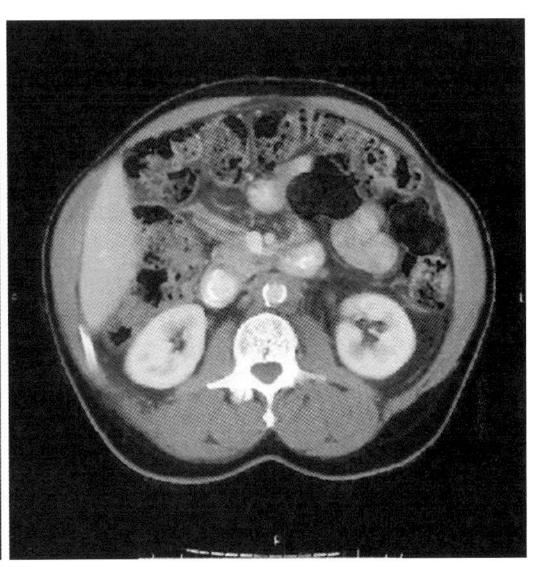

图 39.8　一名 63 岁男性因恶心、脐周疼痛和体重减轻 4.5kg 进行了腹部 CT 检查。左侧扫描显示的腹膜后软组织肿块包绕主动脉（箭）。肿块开放性活检显示炎症和纤维化，无肿瘤证据，与腹膜后纤维化一致。症状消退，糖皮质激素治疗后肿块消退。右侧扫描是在诊断和治疗后 9 个月进行的。（Courtesy Jeffrey H. Phillips，MD，Dallas，TX.）

腹膜后纤维化在男性中更为常见，其典型表现是在放射学评估中发现输尿管偏离中线。治疗通常包括去除违禁药物和糖皮质激素的试验疗程（见图 39.8）。利妥昔单抗的使用在早期Ⅱ期临床试验中显示出有一定的疗效。除非包裹的输尿管不能通过腔内支架进行管理，一般能够避免手术干预。收缩性肠系膜炎患者如果出现肠道梗阻，则必须接受治疗。据报道，给药黄体酮可以延缓纤维化的发生。腹膜后纤维化患者的预后似乎比过去更好。

（四）网膜梗死

当部分网膜在狭窄的血管处扭转时会发生网膜梗死。如果术前通过影像学技术（如 CT、超声）确诊，则可进行保守治疗。然而，诊断确有难度，往往延误，有时只有在手术时才可确诊。腹腔镜下切除坏死性肿块确有疗效。

（五）网膜阑尾炎

网膜阑尾炎（结肠网膜阑尾炎的原发性炎症）是一种偶发疾病，常与阑尾炎的诊断混淆。网膜阑尾炎的诊断需要较高的怀疑指数。典型表现为右下腹痛。然而，恶心、呕吐和厌食症等症状并不常见，而且疼痛往往是突然发作的。患者通常可以用一根手指准确指出疼痛的部位，且压痛和疼痛的部位往往比阑尾炎更局限，头侧略多。CT 可以诊断出网膜阑尾炎，确诊后采用非手术治疗。

八、横膈膜疾病

（一）疝和腹部脏器膨出

横膈疝包括腹部器官通过横膈膜进入胸腔的疝出，我们将在第 27 章详细讨论。脏器膨出并不是真正的疝，而是由导致腹部脏器向胸腔膨出的薄弱横膈顶所组成。这通常在拍胸片时偶然发现，但大的脏器膨出可引起呼吸短促，因为受累侧肺容量减少以及纵隔向健侧移位所致。有症状的患者可以通过胸腔镜下横膈折叠术治疗。

（二）肿瘤

横膈肿瘤通常起源于结缔组织，可为良性或恶性，也可由单纯囊肿组成。通常通过筛查性胸片或评估肋源性胸痛中发现。手术切除要考虑保留膈神经的胸腹入路。

（三）呃逆

呃逆是横膈膜突然有节奏的非自主收缩和声门关闭后的快速吸气所致。只持续几分钟时，被认为是一种生理肌阵挛。对于持续性呃逆（定义为>48 小时），家庭疗法包括屏住呼吸、突然惊吓、从纸袋中重新呼吸、吃干砂糖和喝冷液体。顽固性呃逆（定义为>1 个月）可以是家族性的，通常是由横膈腹受刺激、胃扩张、胸神经或中枢神经系统激惹或肿瘤、低钠血症或其他代谢紊乱引起。

治疗包括针灸、药物治疗、非侵入性膈神经刺激、膈神经挤压或植入式膈起搏器，但缺乏指导性治疗的证据。已报告治疗成功的药物包括氯丙嗪、甲氧氯普胺、奎尼丁、苯妥英、丙戊酸、巴氯酚、舍曲林、加巴喷丁和硝苯地平。腹部手术后的呃逆可能是由于膈下脓肿或其他膈肌刺激，如急性胃扩张，这应该在假定为更良性的病因前有所考虑。

九、腹腔镜对腹膜疾病的评估

（一）一般考虑

于1901年Kelling首次提出诊断性腹腔镜是一种安全有效的评估腹腔的方法。腹腔镜可以直接观察肝脏表面、腹膜表面和肠系膜，并可以直接活检，易于收集腹水。尽管像CT这样的低侵入性成像技术已经减弱腹腔镜的需要性，但它仍然在肝脏和腹腔疾病的评估中发挥着作用。在一项大型腹腔镜诊断回顾性研究中，该手术的死亡率为0%，总发病率为1.2%。可能的并发症包括长期腹痛、血管迷走神经反应、内脏穿孔、出血（活检组织或腹壁内出血）、脾脏破裂、腹水渗漏和发热。腹膜炎动物模型中显示，腹腔镜下腹腔内注气可能增加细菌易位[60]，显示了腹腔镜在脓毒性腹膜炎中的危险性。尽管存在这些问题，腹腔镜检查还是日益成为需手术治疗腹膜炎患者的一种常用方法。在大多数患者中，腹腔注气带来的不良血流动力学后果可以通过积极的复苏和细心麻醉而克服。腹腔镜手术是治疗胃十二指肠溃疡穿孔的有效方法。腹腔镜阑尾切除术是治疗急性阑尾炎和复杂性阑尾炎的首选方法。腹腔镜胆囊切除术是治疗急性胆囊炎安全有效的方法。复杂性结肠憩室炎可行腹腔镜结肠切除术[61]。已制定了腹腔镜手术在外科性腹膜炎应用的循证依据。

（二）不明原因腹水的评估

临床表现、常规实验室检查和腹水分析确定了大多数患者腹水的原因（见第93章）。然而，腹腔穿刺有时不能明确诊断。在这种情况下，诊断性腹腔镜检查成为可以获得组织进行组织学检查和培养的直接、敏感性技术。在美国，隐源性肝硬化和腹膜恶性肿瘤占大多数。亚洲国家研究显示，腹膜恶性肿瘤也是不明原因腹水最常见的原因，但结核性腹膜炎的病例越来越多。在HIV患者中，腹膜受累可能由各种机会性感染和肿瘤引起（见前面的章节和第35章）。腹腔镜检查发现的腹膜病变中，非霍奇金淋巴瘤占大多数，也有报道显示结核分枝杆菌、*M. avium-intracellulare* 和 *P. jiroveci* 感染相关。

（三）腹腔镜分期

腹腔镜在胃肠道恶性实体肿瘤分期中的应用越来越广泛（图39.9）。诊断性腹腔镜联合腹腔镜超声检查、腹腔液细胞学检查和活组织检查能够更加有效地选择患者，使得患者从更大而明确的治愈性手术治疗中获益。在胃肠道恶性肿瘤中，诊断性腹腔镜检查发现一些潜在可切除的患者有转移或局部晚期疾病，避免了不必要的开腹手术，既降低了成本，又保证生活质量[62]。在胰腺癌的腹腔镜分期中，11%～48%患者在初次CT检查阴性后会显示有转移性病灶。腹腔镜分期已被推荐用于胃癌患者，其中12%～60%患者的处理会发生变化[63]。在食管癌和胃癌分期腹腔镜检查中发现转移性疾病，可以避免进行姑息性手术。

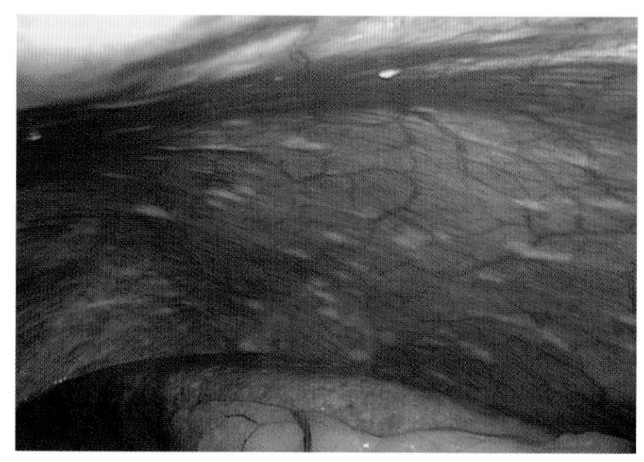

图39.9 腹腔镜检查显示术前成像未显示左侧膈肌疾病

（韩跃华 译，鲁晓岚 李鹏 校）

参考文献

第 40 章 妊娠期患者的胃肠道和肝脏疾病

Shilpa Mehra，John F. Reinus 著

章节目录

一、正常妊娠期间的胃肠道和肝脏功能 …… 561
（一）食管功能 …… 561
（二）胃肠道功能 …… 561
（三）免疫功能和肠道微生物群 …… 561
（四）胆囊功能 …… 562
（五）肝脏功能 …… 562
二、妊娠期患者的用药安全性 …… 562
三、妊娠期内镜检查 …… 562
四、妊娠期影像学和辐射暴露 …… 562
五、胃肠道疾病与妊娠 …… 563
（一）恶心、呕吐和妊娠剧吐 …… 563
（二）胃食管反流病 …… 563
（三）消化性溃疡病 …… 564
（四）炎症性肠病 …… 564
（五）阑尾炎 …… 565
六、胆囊和胰腺疾病与妊娠 …… 565
（一）胆结石病 …… 565
（二）急性胰腺炎 …… 565
七、妊娠特有的肝脏疾病 …… 565
（一）妊娠期胆汁淤积症 …… 565
（二）先兆子痫 …… 566
（三）HELLP 综合征（妊娠期高血压疾病的严重并发症，以溶血、转氨酶升高、血小板减少为特点） …… 567
（四）肝破裂、血肿和梗死 …… 568
（五）妊娠期急性脂肪肝 …… 569
八、其他肝脏疾病与妊娠 …… 570
（一）病毒性肝炎 …… 570
（二）慢性肝病及肝门静脉高压症 …… 571
（三）Wilson 病（肝豆状核变性） …… 572
（四）自身免疫性肝病 …… 572
（五）肝脏肿瘤和肿块性病变 …… 572
（六）肝静脉血栓形成（Budd-Chiari 综合征） …… 572
（七）肝脏移植后妊娠 …… 572

一、正常妊娠期间的胃肠道和肝脏功能

妊娠期间胃肠道会发生剧烈的改变，腹内器官必须移动以适应子宫生长，激素水平改变胃肠道运动能力，妊娠的免疫适应影响人体对疾病的反应。胃灼热、恶心、腹部痉挛和排便习惯的改变是妊娠期妇女最常见的胃肠道症状，这些都是由于肠道运动的正常生理变化引起的。这些症状通常是暂时的，并且很容易用保守的方法治疗。然而，要区分这种由于肠道运动的正常生理变化引起的症状和那些症状发生或恶化预示着需要立即就医的问题，可能是一项挑战。

（一）食管功能

妊娠妇女和非妊娠妇女食管肌肉收缩的幅度和持续时间相似[1]。人们发现，在妊娠期间食管下段蠕动波的速度大约减少了三分之一，但仍保持在正常范围内[2]。相反，在妊娠期间，静息状态下的食管下括约肌张力逐渐降低，这很可能是孕酮抑制食管平滑肌收缩的结果[2-4]。这种影响加上妊娠期间腹压的增加导致 70% 的孕妇出现胃食管反流症状[5]。

（二）胃肠道功能

妊娠对胃动力的影响尚不清楚。一些研究者已证实了妊娠导致的胃排空延迟，尤其是分娩期间的胃排空延迟[6]，然而，其他人没有发现妊娠对胃排空的影响[7]。孕妇胃分泌正常[8]。妊娠期间，肠道转运食糜的时间延长。小肠转运延迟在妊娠晚期最为明显，并且与消化间期移行性复合运动减弱有关[9,10]。妊娠动物结肠转运食糜的时间延长。孕酮被认为对肠道平滑肌细胞具有直接抑制作用，从而降低肠道运动能力[11]。也有人认为是内源性阿片类药物的作用[12]，通常这些变化一起导致轻度生理性便秘。妊娠期间，小肠的吸收能力增加以满足胎儿的新陈代谢需求，已经证实钙、氨基酸和维生素的吸收会增加[13-16]。动物实验表明，妊娠引起的小肠重量和绒毛高度的增加与黏膜肥厚有关[17,18]。在哺乳期间，部分小肠刷状缘肽酶活性增加，在断奶后降低[19,20]。

（三）免疫功能和肠道微生物群

在妊娠期，母体免疫系统必须适应胎儿的存在，这种适应性变化可以影响母体对感染的反应，并调节潜在的自身免疫性疾病的进程。随着 Th1 的下调和 Th2 细胞因子的上调，出现了从细胞免疫到体液免疫的转变。妊娠调节自然杀伤（NK）细胞的细胞毒性作用，并诱导影响母体免疫反应的 T 调节细胞[21,22]。不幸的是，我们仍然不能很好地了解妊娠对自身免疫性疾病（如自身免疫性肝炎和克罗恩病）的影响机制，以便让我们能够预测妊娠期间的临床结果。母体肠道菌群在妊娠期间发生变化，潜在地以有益的方式改变宿主与微生物

的相互作用[23]。母体的细菌定植在新生儿的肠道，这就建立起了具有潜在长期健康作用的微生物群[24]。虽然以前认为人类胃肠道微生物群在出生时建立，但在胎粪、胎盘和羊水中发现的细菌产物表明定植发生在子宫中[25,26]。

（四）胆囊功能

妊娠会引起胆汁成分的改变，包括胆固醇过饱和状态，鹅去氧胆酸减少和胆酸浓度增加，以及胆汁酸池大小的增加[27]。这些变化与禁食和进食状态下较大的残余胆囊体积有关。性类固醇激素可能会抑制孕妇的胆囊收缩，促进胆固醇结晶的沉淀和结石的形成[28,29]。

（五）肝脏功能

在妊娠期间，母体血容量逐渐增加，至妊娠第 30 周比正常情况高出 50%，并持续到分娩[30]。由于类固醇激素的作用以及醛固酮和肾素的血浆水平升高，这种血容量的增加导致了红细胞等一些血液成分的稀释（如生理性贫血）。因此，妊娠中期的总血清蛋白浓度下降了 20%，这主要是由于血清白蛋白水平降低所致。母体蛋白通过被动扩散方式经过胎盘到达胎儿循环[31]。同样，胎儿体内的甲胎蛋白（AFP）经过胎盘从胎儿转移到母体血液循环，从而提高了母体血清中的 AFP 水平。一些大分子的跨胎盘运动可能涉及主动转运。

尽管母体血容量增加，但在妊娠期间，许多用于评估肝脏损伤的血清蛋白的水平没有变化，甚至增加。孕酮引起滑面内质网增殖，而雌激素促进粗面内质网的形成和相关蛋白质的合成。孕妇以较快的速度合成细胞色素 P-450 基因超家族和其他蛋白质产物，包括凝血因子、结合球蛋白和铜蓝蛋白。孕妇血清碱性磷酸酶水平通常在妊娠晚期升高，主要是由于胎盘产生；因此，临床上对孕妇碱性磷酸酶的测定只在妊娠早期进行。母体血浆蛋白浓度的改变可能在产后持续数月。在正常妊娠中，轻度白细胞增多和红细胞沉降率升高也很常见。

二、妊娠期患者的用药安全性

在妊娠期间，患者和医生往往避免使用药物治疗，因为他们担心药物会伤害胎儿[32,33]。然而，拒绝医疗干预可能会对母亲的健康和妊娠结局产生不利影响，话虽如此，妊娠期间，任何药物或其他治疗干预都不能被认为是绝对安全的。事实上，胎盘并不是阻止大多数药物通过的可靠障碍，胎儿体内药物的分布情况无法准确检测，关于药物对子宫内胎儿持续影响的数据几乎无法收集。应与患者讨论推荐药物治疗的必要性，并且必须仔细评估已知和未知的治疗风险。因此，在 2014 年，美国食品药品管理局（FDA）要求变更医生说明书规则（Physician Labeling Rule，PLR）所要求的处方药说明书的内容和格式[34]。不再使用字母类别（A、B、C、D、X）。相反，FDA 现在要求标签包含对风险和支持数据的阐述。

三、妊娠期内镜检查

据估计，每年有 20 000 名孕妇接受内镜检查[35]。在这种情况下，有关内镜检查的建议主要基于专家意见和病例报告[36]。尽管妊娠期间内镜检查的安全性尚未完全确定，但如果有明确的适应证，则应常规进行检查[37]。孕妇已经安全地接受了食管、胃、十二指肠镜检查（EGD）、结肠镜检查、乙状结肠镜检查、经内镜逆行胰胆管造影（ERCP）和经皮胃镜检查[38]。尽管最近瑞典的一项大型队列研究发现，妊娠期间的内镜检查与早产或小胎龄儿的风险增加有关，但作者得出结论，这种风险很小，很可能是由于家庭内因素或疾病活动，而不是仅仅因为内镜检查[39]。除了内镜检查的一般禁忌证外，妊娠期间的特殊禁忌证还包括：临产或先兆分娩、胎膜早破、胎盘早剥和妊娠高血压综合征[40]。

在孕妇进行内镜检查时，应注意几点预防措施，以避免并发症[40]。鉴于胎儿对母体缺氧的极度敏感，孕妇应吸氧并持续进行氧饱和度监测。在妊娠 24 周左右，胎儿通常是能够在子宫外存活的，此时，建议在检查前、中和后对孕妇进行持续宫缩监测，以便在发生胎儿窘迫时能够迅速分娩。在妊娠中期和晚期，应该避免仰卧位和腹部受压，因为这会压迫腔静脉和主动脉，可能导致低血压和胎盘灌注不足。ERCP 应仅在有明确治疗目的的情况下，由内镜专家实施，并尽一切努力避免胎儿辐射（见后文）[38]。阿片类（麻醉）镇痛剂能够穿过胎盘，内镜检查时必须权衡获益以及母亲（见第 42 章）和胎儿的风险。应避免使用苯二氮䓬类药物镇静，特别是在妊娠的前 3 个月，因为有报道称地西泮会导致胎儿畸形[41,42]。缺乏广泛使用丙泊酚的经验，其高脂质溶解性是一个令人担忧的原因[43]。建议哺乳期患者避免母乳喂养，并把在使用丙泊酚后 4 小时内的母乳丢弃[40]。

四、妊娠期影像学和辐射暴露

国际辐射防护委员会建议将妊娠期间的电离辐射暴露量限制在 5cGy 以下[44,45]。美国放射学会指南和标准委员会[46]以及美国妇产科医师学会产科实践委员会[47]已经公布了参考充分的电离辐射孕妇影像指南。辐射对胎儿造成损伤的可能性取决于暴露时的剂量和孕龄（表 40.1）。CT 应仅在其潜在益处明显超过其风险的情况下进行，如果可能的话，应在胎儿的器官发育完成后进行[48]。螺旋 CT 与常规 CT 相比，对胎儿的辐射暴露较少。磁共振成像（MRI）通常是一种优于 CT 的选择；没有造影剂的 MRI 与不良妊娠结果无关，磁场也不被认为对生物体有害[49]。从理论上讲，在妊娠早期，MRI 存在对胎儿热损伤的风险，因此在妊娠前 12 周不建议进行 MRI 检查。造影剂可能会穿过胎盘，并且其对孕妇的安全性尚未得到正式评估。新生儿甲状腺功能减退症与使用某些碘化剂有关。在 MRI 检查时使用的顺磁性造影剂（如钆）尚未在孕妇中进行研究。在给药后的前 24 小时内，不到 0.04% 的钆标记造影剂在母乳中排泄，这种可以忽略不计的量婴儿胃肠道

表 40.1　妊娠期辐射对胎儿的影响*

胎龄	辐射的影响
0~9 天	死亡
13~50 天	致畸，生长受限
51~280 天	生长受限 中枢神经系统异常 可能的癌症风险

*列出的影响也与辐射剂量有关。

可以吸收[50]。因此，使用钆成像后不应中断母乳喂养。在美国，它已经被广泛、安全地使用在妊娠期间的检查。

五、胃肠道疾病与妊娠

（一）恶心、呕吐和妊娠剧吐（见第 15 章）

报道显示，在妊娠的前 3 个月，60%~70% 的孕妇有一些恶心症状，超过 40% 有呕吐症状[51,52]。这些症状的出现通常发生在妊娠的第 4~6 周，第 8~12 周达到高峰，第 20 周消失。尽管恶心和呕吐程度可能从轻微到严重不等，但大多数孕妇仍能获得足够的口服营养和（碳）水化合物。在某些情况下，通过吃少量的干淀粉类食物来获取营养。孕妇感染幽门螺杆菌可能导致呕吐[53]。

需要进行医疗干预的严重持续性呕吐或妊娠剧吐较少见，发生在 2% 或更少的孕妇中[54,55]。妊娠剧吐伴有液体、电解质和酸碱失衡、营养缺乏和体重减轻，其定义是出现酮症和较孕前体重减少 5%。它可能与胃灼热、呕血和唾液分泌过多（流涎）有关[56]。尽管妊娠剧吐的预后通常普遍良好，但严重的未经治疗的疾病可能导致（较高的）母体和胎儿发病率。症状通常在妊娠第 4~5 周开始，并在妊娠 14~16 周后有所改善。然而，在高达 20% 的有孕吐的孕妇中，呕吐持续到分娩[57]。妊娠剧吐经常在随后的妊娠中复发。据报道，导致妊娠剧吐的危险因素包括个人或家族史[58]、女性胎儿或多胎妊娠、妊娠滋养细胞疾病、胎儿 21-三体综合征、胎儿水肿和母体幽门螺杆菌（Hp）感染[59]。

妊娠剧吐的病因可能是多因素的，包括激素变化、胃肠动力障碍、Hp 感染和社会心理因素的影响。这种疾病的家族聚集性表明存在遗传倾向。与妊娠有关的激素，特别是 HCG 和雌激素，已被认为是引起剧吐的重要原因[60]。在 HCG 浓度高峰期间，症状恶化，而与血清 HCG 水平较高相关的疾病（如多胎妊娠，滋养细胞疾病和 21-三体综合征）与剧吐的发生率增加有关[61]。在肥胖患者中，血清雌激素浓度升高也与这种疾病有关[62]。雌激素和孕酮被认为通过改变胃动力和延缓胃肠道传输时间而引起恶心和呕吐[63]。与剧吐发病机制有关的其他激素包括甲状腺激素、肠源性激素、生长素释放肽和瘦素[64,65]。在三分之二的妊娠剧吐患者中发现甲状腺功能测试结果异常[66]。HCG 的 α 亚基具有促甲状腺激素（TSH）样活性，可抑制内源性 TSH 释放，并导致游离甲状腺素（T_4）水平略微升高[67]。尽管有这些发现，但这种一过性妊娠期甲状腺毒症与不良妊娠结果无关，通常不需要治疗。在两项关于妊娠期间 Hp 感染的 meta 分析中，发现 Hp 感染的孕妇妊娠剧吐的风险增加[68,69]。一些研究者记录了在 Hp 根除后，孕妇的呕吐症状得到了改善[70,71]。

妊娠剧吐患者的呕吐通常由嗅觉甚至听觉和视觉刺激引发。通过使用妊娠期间特有的恶心和呕吐量化表（PUQE 评分）来评估患病孕妇每天恶心的小时数和呕吐及干呕的次数，这有助于对症治疗[72]。当患病孕妇出现低血压、心动过速、酮症、体重减轻或肌肉萎缩时，需要住院接受静脉输液和电解质补充，有时还需要营养支持。这类患者的实验室检查结果异常，包括低钾血症、低钠血症和酮症。在 25%~40% 的病例中，妊娠剧吐与血清转氨酶和胆红素水平轻微升高有关。四分之一的患者出现高淀粉酶血症，这是由于长期呕吐刺激唾液腺过度分泌所致[73]。

严重的妊娠剧吐与不良的母婴结局有关。一项超过 150 000 例单胎妊娠的研究发现，在妊娠期间有剧吐症状且体重增加低于 7 公斤的孕妇所生的婴儿，更有可能出现低出生体重儿、早产和小于胎龄儿以及低 Apgar（新生儿）评分[54]。这些发现得到了最近荟萃分析的证实[74]。虽然罕见，但妊娠剧吐的严重并发症包括食管贲门黏膜撕裂（Mallory-Weiss 撕裂）伴上消化道出血、自发性食管破裂（Boerhaave 综合征）、脑型维生素 B_1 缺乏病（Wernicke 脑病）伴或不伴器质性遗忘综合征（Korsakoff 精神病）、脑桥中央髓鞘溶解症、视网膜出血和自发性纵隔气肿[75]。剧烈呕吐的患者在妊娠期间和产后可能患有抑郁症和创伤后应激障碍[76]。最后，有报道选择性终止妊娠后会出现严重的抑郁症[77]。

鉴于妊娠剧吐可能出现的发病率和死亡率，应对患病孕妇进行积极治疗。如果可能的话，产科治疗应由具有母胎医学资格的医生监督。治疗的目标是维持足够的母体液体摄入和营养，以及控制症状。应建议患者在可以忍受的情况下尽量少食多餐，并避免可能引发恶心的空腹。此外，应避免令人不快的气味，分别摄取固体和液体食物，以及食用高碳水化合物饮食可能会有所帮助[78]。止吐和抗反流药物是饮食调整失败的门诊患者的一线药物治疗。生姜、吩噻嗪（氯丙嗪，丙氯拉嗪）、多巴胺拮抗剂甲氧氯普胺和吡哆醇（维生素 B_6）已证明在这种情况下有益[79,80]。大量数据显示，这些药物中的大多数没有致畸性和良好的胎儿安全性[81-83]。对上述药物治疗无效的患者，应考虑使用一种 5-羟色胺-3（5-HT_3）受体拮抗剂昂丹司琼来治疗。最近的一项对照试验[84]，病例报告和广泛的临床经验都证明了妊娠期间昂丹司琼治疗的安全性。糖皮质激素可能使症状严重的个体受益。口服药物治疗的失败者可以在家庭环境中通过静脉补充液体、药物治疗和复合维生素来治疗。然而，应该指出的是，在通过中心静脉导管治疗，包括经外周插入导管的妊娠患者中，有多达 50% 的患者出现导管相关的并发症[85]，这很可能是由于孕妇的相对高凝状态和对感染的易感性增加所致。有时需要通过鼻肠管或手术放置的饲管进行肠内喂养，以维持母体营养[86]。

（二）胃食管反流病（见第 46 章）

至少有许多女性在妊娠期间会出现恶心和胃灼热。到妊娠晚期结束时,50%~80%的孕妇新发或原有的胃灼热症状恶化[87,88]。然而,胃灼热感很少伴有明显的食管炎或并发症[89]。患有胃灼热的孕妇也可能有反流,如前所述的恶心和呕吐,以及非典型反流症状,如持续性咳嗽和喘息。妊娠期间可能随时出现症状,妊娠晚期发病率最高[90],可能会持续至分娩,并可预测日后胃食管反流病复发[87]。反流的风险因素包括多胎、高龄产妇以及首次妊娠并发反流[5,87,91]。孕前体重指数和孕后体重过度增加的作用具有争议性[92]。

妊娠期胃食管反流病的发病机制与妊娠期激素对食管运动、食管下括约肌张力和胃排空的影响有关。由子宫增大引起的胃受压和腹内压增加也是导致这种疾病的发展的原因。

有胃食管反流病症状的孕妇很少需要EGD来评估[93]。在这种情况下,没有使用24小时动态pH监测评估的数据,而且使用钡餐造影是不可取的,因为它会导致胎儿辐射暴露;因此,怀疑孕妇患胃食管反流病时的诊断取决于医生的临床经验和判断,并且需要适当考虑患者病史以及解释患者目前症状的所有潜在的合理原因。

轻度反流症状通常可以通过改变饮食和生活方式来控制。液体抗酸剂和硫糖铝是一线治疗药物[94]。在妊娠晚期应避免使用含镁抗酸剂,因为在理论上它们可能会影响分娩。对于持续性胃灼热患者来说,尽管接受了液体抗酸剂治疗,但雷尼替丁仍然是首选治疗方法[95]。质子泵抑制剂(PPI)应用于难治性病例。一项大规模的人口研究和两项meta分析发现,在妊娠前3个月暴露于质子泵抑制剂的婴儿中,没有明显的胎儿畸形风险[96,97]。然而,奥美拉唑已经在动物身上造成了胎儿毒性。丹麦医疗登记处的一项调查指出,孕妇使用PPI或H_2受体拮抗剂(H_2RA)与其子代儿童哮喘的发病之间存在关联[98],但这一观察结果的意义尚不清楚。胃动力药甲氧氯普胺虽然用于产科麻醉和治疗妊娠剧吐,但在妊娠期间尚未广泛用于治疗胃食管反流病。

(三) 消化性溃疡病

病例研究和回顾性系列研究表明,妊娠消化性溃疡的发病率低于非孕妇[99,100]。如果这种情况存在,可能与谨慎的患者服用非甾体抗炎药减少有关,也可能与增加服用抗酸药物来治疗恶心或胃灼热有关。妊娠类固醇可能对胃肠道黏膜细胞有保护作用,但同样未经证实。鉴于医生不愿对孕妇进行诊断检查,消化性溃疡可能在妊娠期间未被诊断。众所周知,胃酸分泌和Hp感染的自然史不会因妊娠而改变。

通常伴随着妊娠的消化不良症状,特别是恶心、呕吐和胃灼热,可能会使消化性溃疡的诊断变得困难。由于消化性溃疡在整个人群中非常普遍,因此,诊治孕妇的医生应该警惕。经验性抑酸治疗可能对疑似消化性溃疡的孕妇有用,并认为是安全的[101-104]。在诊断不明时,通过EGD检查来明确诊断(见前面)。妊娠期消化性溃疡的一线治疗包括雷尼替丁和硫糖铝,尽管大多数PPI也有效。Hp感染的患者可以在妊娠期间或分娩后接受抗生素治疗。

(四) 炎症性肠病(见第115和116章)

治疗炎症性肠病(IBD)患者的医生有可能在孕妇中遇到这种疾病[105]。大多数女性IBD是在30岁之前,即生育高峰期出现这种疾病[106]。一些研究显示,女性患溃疡性结肠炎或克罗恩病的风险比男性高约30%。

关于IBD对生育能力的影响存在争议。IBD患者的妊娠率可能会低得离谱,因为自我形象问题导致性回避和自愿不生育[107]。对其后代患IBD的恐惧和对母体药物治疗引起胎儿畸形的恐惧经常是患病妇女无子女的主要原因[108]。然而,女性生育能力本身似乎并未因简单的炎症性肠病而受损[109,110]。一个值得注意的例外是接受全结肠切除术和回肠肛管J袋吻合术治疗的溃疡性结肠炎患者的生育能力[111,112]。一项meta分析发现,经历过这种手术的IBD患者不孕风险增加了3倍[112]。这些人的不孕症很可能是由盆腔粘连和输卵管瘢痕造成的。应该与正在考虑这种手术的育龄患者讨论潜在的不孕症。柳氮磺胺吡啶治疗会损害患有IBD的男性的生育能力,会导致精子数量减少,通常在停药后6个月内恢复正常[113]。

如果IBD的最初症状出现在妊娠期间,则通常在妊娠早期诊断出该病[114,115]。这类患者并不比非妊娠患者严重。同样,妊娠似乎不会增加原先IBD的严重程度或发病率。有证据表明,受孕前后的疾病活动会增加妊娠期间疾病复发的风险;UC患者在妊娠期复发的频率高于克罗恩病患者[116]。

治疗的目标是在受孕前将炎症性肠病的症状和发病率降至最低。大多数专家一致认为,在妊娠期间,患者应继续优化孕前治疗,以避免停药可能导致的突发问题。应积极治疗妊娠期间IBD的加重,以避免并发症,包括出血、穿孔、败血症、胎儿死亡和早产。暴发性结肠炎的治疗与非妊娠患者相同,即高剂量糖皮质激素、静脉注射抗生素、环孢菌素和抢救生物治疗。肠道手术的适应证同样与非妊娠IBD患者相同,尽管肠道手术与早产以及母婴死亡率有关[117,118]。结肠造瘘以实现结肠减压和粪便转移可能比全结肠切除术更安全[119]。对妊娠28周后的暴发性结肠炎患者,提倡同步剖宫产和结肠次全切除术[120]。IBD患者即使处于轻度活动期或非活动性期,其妊娠结局不良的风险也会增加[121]。主要并发症包括早产、出生体重低和小于胎龄儿,以及剖宫产率增加[122]。在这种情况下胎儿畸形的风险尚不清楚[123]。患有溃疡性结肠炎的孕妇发生血栓栓塞事件的风险可能会增加[124]。

大多数炎症性肠病患者需要几种药物才能保持无症状。关于最常用的炎症性肠病药物的致畸性,有一些安全性数据可参考。但目前还没有它们对孕妇后代潜在不良影响的长期研究。在妊娠前仔细评估患者治疗的风险和获益非常重要。如果可能的话,应在受孕前停用潜在的致畸药物。甲氨蝶呤和沙利度胺都是已知的致畸剂和人工流产剂,在育龄期患者中应谨慎使用。受孕前这些药物的最佳禁用期尚不清楚;但建议至少6个月。5-氨基水杨酸盐在妊娠期间被广泛用于治疗轻度炎症性肠病。一项针对接受美沙拉秦治疗的孕妇患者进行的大宗病例系列前瞻性研究,并未显示该药物有任何增加致畸风险的作用[125,126]。

硫唑嘌呤及其代谢产物 6-巯基嘌呤是孕妇中研究最多、使用最广泛的免疫抑制药物之一。它们的代谢物在脐带血中被发现,并在母乳中少量排泄。孕妇使用这些药物的有关数据未能证实动物研究中所见的致畸性[127]。许多用 6-巯基嘌呤治疗的妊娠期炎症性肠病患者的研究未能证实早产、自然流产、先天性畸形或儿童肿瘤的风险增加[128-130]。根据这些临床数据和孕妇对该药及其代谢产物的广泛经验,专家们一致认为,在妊娠前或妊娠期间停药是不可取的。相反,建议仔细监测母体内该药的代谢物水平[131]。

几十年来,糖皮质激素一直用于治疗患有中度至重度炎症性肠病的孕妇,以及其他更常见的糖皮质激素反应性疾病(例如哮喘)。早期报告显示,接受该药物治疗的母亲,其胎儿患先天性畸形的风险增加[126]。随后的前瞻性研究和使用这类药物的大量临床经验都已证实,使用该类药物继发畸形的风险极低。然而,妊娠期间的糖皮质激素治疗与其他并发症有关,包括母体葡萄糖耐受不良和高血压(先兆子痫的危险因素)、巨大胎儿和胎儿肾上腺抑制[132]。泼尼松龙比其他糖皮质激素更容易经胎盘代谢,并且肾上腺抑制的风险可能更低[133]。少数孕妇口服布地奈德后未报告不良结果[134]。

许多器官移植受者已经用环孢菌素作为免疫抑制药物来治疗,没有显著的致畸性报道。TNF-α 拮抗剂已被广泛用于治疗炎症性肠病和其他炎性疾病,妊娠期间,血清英夫利西单抗水平升高,而阿达利单抗水平稳定[135]。特别是在妊娠晚期,这些免疫球蛋白到达羊膜腔内。赛妥珠单抗可能是一个例外,它缺乏主动转运所需的 Fc 片段。这些药物集中在胎儿体内,并且在婴儿出生后的几个月内就可在其血液中检测到[114,136]。上市后的安全性数据和病例系列登记没有发现在妊娠期间使用英夫利西单抗或阿达利单抗治疗的妇女中胎儿畸形或流产的发生率增加[137]。最近公布的指南建议,除非另有说明,否则在整个妊娠期间应继续服用 TNF-α 拮抗剂[138]。一些专家对胎儿暴露于肿瘤坏死因子-α 拮抗剂对新生儿免疫系统发育的潜在有害影响表示担忧。因此,在子宫内接触这类药物的婴儿在出生后的前 6 个月内不应接种活疫苗;但是,建议接种其他疫苗[139]。在子宫内接触 TNF-α 拮抗剂的儿童感染的短期或长期发病率没有增加[140]。

关于妊娠期使用抗整合素和抗 IL-12/23 抗体[分别为维多珠单抗(vedolizumab)或那他珠单抗(natalizumab)和乌司奴单抗(ustekinumab)]的治疗效果的数据仍然有限。尽管在一项关于暴露于维多珠单抗的妇女的妊娠结局的小型研究中没有发现任何问题,但在获得更多的安全数据之前,孕妇不应该接受这些药物的治疗[141]。

在炎症性肠病患者中,阴道分娩并非禁忌,但建议活动性会阴部疾病患者进行剖宫产。建议回肠袋术后的患者避免阴道分娩以防损伤肛门括约肌。

(五) 阑尾炎(见第 120 章)

疑似急性阑尾炎是孕妇剖腹探查术中最常见的非产科指征[142,143]。1 500 例孕妇中大约有 1 例患有阑尾炎的并发症,并且可能在妊娠期间的任何时间发生[143]。阑尾炎的诊断可能很困难,因为扩大的子宫会使盲肠和阑尾头端移位,改变由阑尾炎症引起的疼痛位置,随着妊娠的周数的增加,阑尾炎的延迟诊断增加[144]。炎症性阑尾的延迟诊断是导致并发症的原因,该并发症与母体和胎儿发病率和死亡率过高有关[145]。在整个妊娠期间,右下腹疼痛是阑尾炎最常见的症状[146]。除了疼痛之外,患病孕妇经常主诉恶心,但这种症状在妊娠期间往往很难解释。超声逐步加压法检查诊断阑尾炎是疑似阑尾炎孕妇患者的首选检查方法[146]。据报道,螺旋 CT 在这种情况下也有帮助[143]。在妊娠早中晚期的任何一个时期,患有阑尾炎的孕妇都可以接受腹腔镜阑尾切除术[147],尽管在妊娠晚期妊娠子宫的潜在干扰可能是该手术的相对禁忌证[148]。孕早期妊娠期阑尾炎患者可采用腹腔镜阑尾切除术治疗[136],但在妊娠晚期,该手术对妊娠子宫的影响可能是其相对禁忌[137]。适当的支持治疗可以防止阑尾穿孔引起的胎儿死亡[149]。

六、胆囊和胰腺疾病与妊娠

(一) 胆结石病(见第 65 章)

孕妇往往会因为胆囊功能和胆汁成分的改变而形成胆结石(见前文)。在妊娠期间用超声检查评估胎儿时,经常会发现胆结石[150];据报道,孕妇的无症状胆结石患病率在 2.5% 至 12% 之间。尽管发病率很高,急性胆囊炎的发病率并没有因为妊娠而增加。必要时,胆结石相关疾病的外科干预不会增加早产或胎儿或产妇死亡的风险[73,151]。妊娠期胆总管结石在必要时可接受内镜下取石,尽量少使用透视,并进行适当的母体防护[152]。在一项研究中,相对于保守治疗,内镜治疗与较少的住院和较低的剖宫产率有关[153]。

(二) 急性胰腺炎(见第 58 章)

急性胰腺炎在妊娠期间并不常见,每 1 066~3 300 例妊娠中就会发生一例[154,155]。大多数病例是由于胆结石引起的,出现于妊娠晚期或产褥期。常见于轻度高甘油三酯血症的孕妇,在患有家族性高脂血症的人(群)中可能更严重,使其在此基础上易患胰腺炎[156]。妊娠期急性胰腺炎的临床特征与非妊娠期妇女相似,尽管大多数患有这种疾病的孕妇不会出现胰腺炎并发症[157]。

七、妊娠特有的肝脏疾病

孕妇可能患上与妊娠或妊娠并发症有关的肝脏疾病[158]。通常,这些疾病在妊娠晚期或刚分娩后临床表现明显。它们可能是严重的,甚至危及生命,但患病孕妇如果得到及时诊断和适当的处理,预计会存活下来。妊娠特有的肝脏疾病也与胎儿发病率和死亡率增加有关。

(一) 妊娠期胆汁淤积症

妊娠期胆汁淤积症是一种肝内胆汁淤积症,伴有瘙痒、血清胆汁酸水平升高,以及肝脏活检中单纯性胆汁淤积[159,160]。这种病可能有不同的病程,使其难以诊断;然而,它对胎儿健康有严重影响,必须尽快确诊[161]。

妊娠期胆汁淤积症通常出现在妊娠晚期,但也可能在更早期被发现,甚至在妊娠的前 3 个月。它的第一个也是最具特征的症状是瘙痒症，因此，患者可能会被转诊给皮肤科医生进行初步评估。与其他形式的胆汁淤积一样，妊娠期胆汁淤积症的瘙痒在手掌和足底皮肤中最严重，在夜间最强烈。只有10%～25%的患病孕妇随后出现黄疸。血清胆汁酸水平升高(>10μmol/L)证实了胆汁淤积的存在；部分孕妇患者还有胆红素尿症甚至轻度高胆红素血症[162]。血清碱性磷酸酶浓度中度升高，但γ-谷氨酸转肽酶(GGTP)水平正常或仅略微升高[162]。后者的检测结果是成人胆汁淤积症的不典型表现，但见于进行性家族性肝内胆汁淤积的儿科患者，如Byler综合征[163]。患病孕妇的血清转氨酶水平升高，有时达到1 000U/L或更高，有时难以将妊娠期胆汁淤积与病毒性肝炎区分开来。血清自体趋化素水平升高已被证明是一项敏感而特异的诊断试验，可将妊娠期胆汁淤积症与其他妊娠相关肝病区分开来[164]。孕妇患者的症状和实验室检查结果的异常可能会有波动。严重的胆汁淤积与脂肪泻有关，这通常是亚临床的，但可导致脂溶性维生素缺乏，最明显的是维生素K的缺乏。

患病孕妇分娩后母体的临床症状和实验室检查结果开始改善，虽然不是一成不变的，但这种改善通常是迅速而全面的。极少数患者出现长期的胆汁淤积症，这可能预示着潜在的胆道疾病，如原发性胆汁性胆管炎或原发性硬化性胆管炎[165,166]。患有普通胆汁淤积症的孕妇在病情缓解后不会遗留肝脏损害，但她们患胆结石、胆囊炎和胰腺炎的风险增加[167]。此外，60%～70%的患病孕妇在随后的妊娠期间或在使用口服避孕药时出现胆汁淤积(尽管反复发作可能没有最初的严重)。但在妊娠间期行胆囊切除术会增加再次妊娠时胆汁淤积复发的风险[168]。

妊娠期胆汁淤积症对胎儿健康有严重影响。许多研究表明，患有这种疾病的孕妇出现胎儿窘迫、原因不明的死产和需要早产的概率增加[169]。据报道，19%患有妊娠期胆汁淤积症的瑞典女性在分娩时出现胎儿缺氧和胎粪染色[170]。这些并发症与母体内胆汁酸水平大于40μmol/L有关[171]。虽然，通过密切监测患病母亲可以降低(胆淤)对胎儿的风险，但不能完全消除这种风险[172-175]。由于这个原因，建议一旦胎肺成熟就计划早期选择性分娩。

正如第64章所讨论的，近年来许多胆汁形成的分子机制已被阐明，从而使人们对许多胆汁淤积性疾病有了更为深入的了解[176,177]。*MDR3*(*ABCB4*)基因的突变可能导致大约15%的妊娠期胆汁淤积病例[178-181]。*MDR3*基因产物是一种磷脂翻转酶(又称磷脂转位蛋白)，它将磷脂酰胆碱从小管肝细胞膜的内小叶移位到外小叶，在那里它被胆汁酸溶解形成混合胶束。然而，妊娠期胆汁淤积症与人白细胞抗原(HLA)分型无关[182]。

环境、激素和其他因素也可能促进孕妇胆汁淤积的发展。在智利和斯堪的纳维亚半岛，妊娠期胆汁淤积症很常见，这种疾病最常发生在较冷的月份。智利的妊娠期胆汁淤积症发病率下降，可能是由于平均血浆硒水平下降所致[183]。对于在妊娠期间发生胆汁淤积的患者，其家庭成员(包括男性亲属)，已被证实对外源性雌激素的胆汁淤积作用有更高的敏感性[184]。对易感女性进行雌激素化合物的治疗性或实验性给药会加速这种疾病的发生[185,186]。类似地，妊娠期间的孕酮治疗与胆汁淤积的发展有关[187,188]。熊脱氧胆酸改变孕酮代谢可以解释其治疗效果[189,190]。可能是一些妊娠期胆汁淤积症妇女遗传了对雌激素或孕酮代谢变化的敏感性增强，从而导致胆汁淤积对各种刺激(包括一些药物和食物)的反应[191]。丙型肝炎妇女妊娠期胆汁淤积症的发生率明显高于其他孕妇[192]。

妊娠期胆汁淤积症的鉴别诊断包括其他胆汁淤积性疾病，如原发性胆汁性胆管炎、原发性硬化性胆管炎、良性复发性肝内胆汁淤积、胆汁淤积性病毒性肝炎、中毒性肝损伤和胆管梗阻。患者的肝活检标本可显示由于各种病因引起的胆汁淤积的典型变化，但通常不需要活检来作出诊断。重要的是要记住妊娠可能会加重先前存在的亚临床胆汁淤积症。例如，1997年报道了一个患有进行性肝病的姐妹家庭，她们也发生了复发的重度妊娠期胆汁淤积症[165]。

妊娠期胆汁淤积症的治疗主要是姑息治疗[193,194]。熊脱氧胆酸有助于缓解症状[190]，可能降低胎儿并发症的发生率[178]，并且母亲和胎儿对熊脱氧胆酸的耐受性很好[195,196]。对接受治疗患者的研究表明，母体血清和羊水的胆汁酸含量发生变化，胎盘胆汁酸转运增加[197-199]。大多数研究人员都已给出了治疗的常规剂量(15mg/kg/d)，尽管有一份报告表明较高的剂量(20～25mg/kg/d)更有效[186]。用胆汁酸结合剂(如考来烯胺[196]和瓜尔胶)治疗也可以缓解症状[200]，但重要的是要记住，用这些药物治疗会加重脂肪泻并导致脂溶性维生素缺乏[201]。妊娠期胆汁淤积症患者应用S-腺苷-L-甲硫氨酸(SAMe)的治疗效果好坏参半[202-204]；它与熊脱氧胆酸联合使用可以增加其益处[205]。据报道，短疗程的糖皮质激素(如口服地塞米松12mg/d，持续7天)可减轻该病患者的瘙痒症状并降低血清胆汁酸水平[206]，但也与1例患者出现的病情恶化有关[207]。镇静剂如苯巴比妥，可缓解胆汁淤积患者的瘙痒症状，但可能会对胎儿产生不良影响。在这种情况下，有人建议紫外线B段(UVB，为波长280～320nm紫外线)的光波治疗。与其他胆汁淤积综合征一样，对于妊娠期胆汁淤积症的孕妇，没有一种治疗方法是完全有效的，通常分娩除外。

(二) 先兆子痫

先兆子痫是一种多系统疾病，其特征为与内皮损伤和母体器官功能障碍相关的新发高血压，可能包括肝脏，这可能产生严重的甚至危及生命的并发症并影响妊娠结果[208]。胎盘对这种疾病的发展至关重要，并且严重的病例与胎盘缺血的病理学证据相关[209]。3%～10%的妊娠合并先兆子痫，发生在妊娠后半期或产褥期，最常见但不仅限于初产妇女或多胎妊娠妇女[210]。诊断的常用标准包括在孕前血压正常的孕妇，妊娠20周后持续血压为140/90mmHg或更高，伴有蛋白尿(≥300mg/24h)，大约相当于尿液随机试验中蛋白质浓度为30mg/dL("1+试纸")[208]。许多患者也有反射亢进和水肿。

肝病被认为是先兆子痫的常见和潜在的不祥并发症。Weinstein于1982年首次描述的HELLP综合征[211]是最常见的先兆子痫肝病形式，可能导致肝脏血肿，破裂和梗死[212-214]。有证据表明，存在不同的先兆子痫表型，并且

HELLP 综合征可能是一个不同的遗传(变异)和临床表型[215,216]。虽然,先兆子痫在妊娠期急性脂肪肝患者(acute fatty liver of pregnancy,AFLP)中很常见,并且可能在这种疾病的发病机制中发挥作用,但 AFLP 通常不属于先兆子痫肝病[217]。

(三) HELLP 综合征(妊娠期高血压疾病的严重并发症,以溶血、转氨酶升高、血小板减少为特点)

HELLP 在患有严重先兆子痫的孕妇中发生率高达 12%,在所有孕妇中发生率为 0.2% 至 0.8%[218-220]。在过去,临床医生依赖于两个主要的 HELLP 诊断分类系统:田纳西州分类和密西西比州三级分类,它根据母体血小板计数的最低点进一步对患病个体进行分类(框 40.1)。最近,HELLP 综合征的诊断标准已经由美国妇产科医师学会妊娠期高血压特别工作组标准化(框 40.2)[221]。除了溶血、血清转氨酶水平升高、血小板减少合并高血压和蛋白尿的诊断异常外,典型的 HELLP 综合征的患者经常有胸痛、上腹痛和 RUQ 腹痛的主诉(表 40.2)。这些症状常伴有恶心、呕吐、头痛和各种形式的视力模糊。然而,一些孕妇在观察先兆子痫时可能出现无症状的血小板计数下降,或这些患者最初没有高血压或蛋白尿[222]。其他女性可能会抱怨身体不适,提示诊断为病毒性综合征[223]。大多数患者在妊娠 27 周后寻求治疗,但高达 11% 的人可能会更早就诊。值得注意的是,尽管分娩时没有先兆子痫的迹象,但仍有高达 30% 的病例在分娩后出现 HELLP 综合征延迟表现的情况[218]。

框 40.1　田纳西州和密西西比州 HELLP 综合征的三级诊断分类系统

田纳西州分类

1. 微血管病性溶血性贫血伴血涂片异常、血清结合珠蛋白低和血清 LDH 水平升高
2. 血清 LDH 水平>600IU/L 或实验室正常值上限的两倍,且血清 AST 水平>70IU/L 或实验室正常值上限的两倍,或血清胆红素水平>1.2mg/dL
3. 血小板计数<100 000/μL

   不完全性 HELLP 综合征是指仅出现其中 1~2 项异常,可能较轻

密西西比州三级分类

Ⅰ类:血小板计数最低点≤50 000/mm^3

Ⅱ类:血小板计数最低值>50 000/mm^3 且≤100 000/mm^3

Ⅲ类:血小板计数最低值>100 000/mm^3 且≤150 000/mm^3

框 40.2　HELLP 综合征诊断的推荐标准(美国妇产科医师学会妊娠期高血压特别工作组)

1. 溶血和以下至少两种情况:
   a. 外周血涂片上可见裂红细胞和棘红细胞
   b. 血清胆红素水平≥1.2mg/dL
   c. 血清结合珠蛋白低
   d. 与失血无关的严重贫血
2. 转氨酶水平升高
   a. AST 或 ALT≥实验室正常值上限的两倍
   b. LDH≥实验室正常值上限的两倍
3. 血小板<100 000/mm^3

表 40.2　HELLP 综合征患者的临床特征和母体并发症

表现症状	**百分比**
腹痛(右上腹,上腹部)	65
恶心或呕吐	36
头痛	31
出血	9
黄疸	5
实验室检测值(正常值)	**中位数(范围)**
血清 AST(<40U/L))	249(70~633)
血清胆红素(<1mg/dL)	1.5(0.5~25)
血小板计数(>125×10^3/mm^3)	57(7~99)
受影响的母体并发症	**百分比**
弥散性血管内凝血	21
胎盘早剥	16
急性肾损伤	8
肝包膜下血肿	1
死亡	1

From Sibai BH, Ramadan MK, Usta l, et al. Maternal morbidity and mortality in 442 pregnancies with hemolysis, elevated liver enzymes and low platelets (HELLP) syndrome. Am J Obstet Gynecol 1993;169:100-6。

由于没有针对这一疾病的特异性诊断实验,HELLP 综合征的诊断基于出现的临床情况和疾病特征的评估,因为没有针对这一疾病的单独的特殊检测[220,224]。HELLP 患者的溶血是轻微的。涂片上可见碎片状红细胞(裂红细胞),血清 LDH 水平升高。与实验室胆汁淤积症状相关的血清氨基转移酶水平升高,但有时很低,有时高达 1 000U/L 以上[218,225]。血清胆红素水平通常可以轻度升高,与溶血的发现相一致。在患有 HELLP 综合征的孕妇中已经发现了血清中的谷胱甘肽 S-转移酶 α[226]、D-二聚体[227]、组织多肽抗原[228]和纤连蛋白[229]水平升高,而这些检测在预测肝病的存在或严重程度方面可能会有一些用处。

腹部影像,尤其是 CT 和 MRI,可能有助于诊断 HELLP 综合征和发现肝内出血和梗死(稍后讨论)。针对严重腹痛、颈部或肩部疼痛或血压突然下降患者,应进行影像学检查,一份报告显示:45% 的此类患者有异常影像学表现[212]。

HELLP 综合征患者的肝活检标本显示出门静脉周围出血,窦内纤维蛋白沉积,以及轻度反应性肝炎的不规则肝细胞坏死区,这是先兆子痫的特征(图 40.1)。如果出现肝脏脂肪变性,程度轻微,则不会出现 AFLP 患者中心周围广泛的微泡脂肪堆积(稍后讨论)。HELLP 综合征患者的肝脏活检病变严重程度与实验室检查异常之间几乎没有相关性;因此,轻度血小板减少症和血清转氨酶水平轻度升高并不一定意味着无意义的肝损伤[230]。然而,在这些患者中很少为了诊断必须进行肝活检,并且肝活检可能会导致肝实质内血肿的发展或肝破裂。

虽然大多数血小板计数减少和先兆子痫的孕妇都有 HELLP 综合征,但鉴别诊断还包括其他导致血小板减少的原

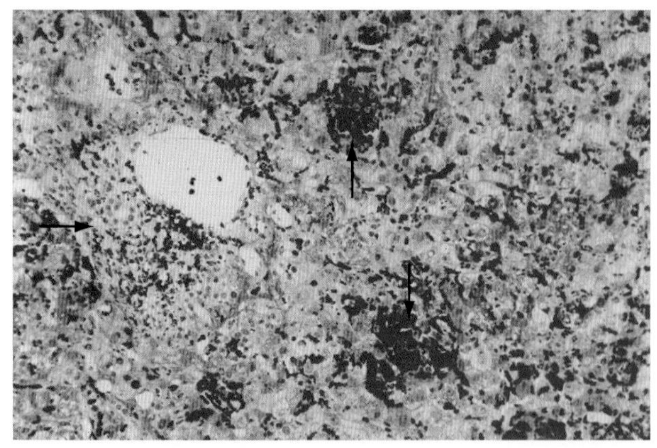

图 40.1　HELLP 综合征的组织病理学。图左侧的门脉三联征（水平箭头指向门脉三联征中的小叶间胆管）被出血囊袋（垂直箭头）和纤维蛋白沉积区域（门脉三联征左侧）包围

因，包括免疫性血小板减少性紫癜、血栓性血小板减少性紫癜[231]和抗磷脂抗体综合征，这本身可能与 HELLP 的早期发病有关[232,233]。先兆子痫患者血清氨基转移酶水平升高最常被误诊为由病毒性肝炎引起[234]。对于有 HELLP 综合征临床表现的患者，也应考虑 AFLP 的诊断，但 AFLP 通常与更严重的肝病症状和可能的肝功能衰竭有关，尽管血清氨基转移酶水平较低，并且不一定与血小板减少症有关。

现在认为先兆子痫和 HELLP 综合征是胎盘形成异常的结果，其中，滋养层细胞侵入子宫内膜和螺旋动脉扩张的失败导致生理上不能随着妊娠的进展适当地增加子宫胎盘的灌注，并伴随着胎盘产物的继发释放，从而引发临床疾病[235,236]。

女性亲属，包括先兆子痫患者的母亲，通常具有该病病史，并且一些人群中存在的证据表明，其遗传为常染色体隐性遗传或具有可变外显子的常染色体显性遗传[215,237,238]。许多母体遗传变异与患 HELLP 综合征的风险增加有关[239-242]。可以通过检测特定血清因子来预测 HELLP 或先兆子痫的早期发作，其中许多因子对血管的生成有影响[234-247]。此外，具有高凝状态的女性（例如，具有莱顿因子 V 或抗心磷脂抗体）具有发展为早期和严重先兆子痫的风险[248,249]。有令人信服的证据表明，这种疾病的发展是由可溶性 fms 样酪氨酸激酶 1（sFlt1）过量释放到循环中所介导的；sFlt1 是血管内皮生长因子（VEGF）、胎盘生长因子（PlGF）和可溶性内皮糖蛋白（sEng）的有效拮抗剂，后者是毛细血管形成的抑制剂[250,251]。过度表达 sFlt1 和 sEng 的妊娠大鼠会出现蛋白尿，严重的高血压，HELLP 综合征的实验室检查结果以及宫内生长受限[252]。患有先兆子痫的女性同样产生过量的 sFlt1 和 sEng[251]。

HELLP 综合征的临床异常通常在分娩后迅速消退[253,254]。HELLP 综合征在分娩前逐渐恶化，随后发展为产后肝功能衰竭、败血症、消耗性凝血病，极少数甚至死亡，这较为罕见[255]。如果没有适当的支持性治疗和快速分娩，患者可能发展为肾衰竭，肝血肿和肝破裂。血清转氨酶水平和血小板计数均不能预测 HELLP 综合征患者的预后[256]。这种疾病可能在随后的妊娠期间复发，但一般情况下不会[257,258]。

HELLP 综合征的治疗主要是支持性治疗[254]；患者在分娩前应在重症监护环境中接受治疗，最好由具有母胎医学执业资格的产科医生进行治疗。一些接受治疗的患者血清转氨酶水平可能下降，并且支持治疗可能导致血小板计数增加[259]。在这种情况下，在胎儿不成熟的情况下延迟分娩可能是可行的，但胎儿通常不能在先兆子痫的情况下生长。严重先兆子痫和 HELLP 综合征患者可能需要产前血小板输注和血液透析。一些权威机构提倡为一些患者进行分娩后血浆置换，预防产后血栓性微血管病变[260,261]。许多受影响的妇女在分娩前接受糖皮质激素治疗，不是作为疾病治疗，而是为了促进胎儿肺成熟；然而，糖皮质激素疗法也被用作这种情况下的治疗[262]。糖皮质激素治疗 HELLP 综合征可以改善血小板计数和血清 ALT 水平，减少住院和重症监护室时间，但与产妇发病率和死亡率的显著改善无关[263]。对于一些 HELLP 综合征患者，原位肝移植可能是适当的治疗方法[264-266]，但早期诊断和及时分娩几乎总是使这些患者没有必要采取这种和其他极端的治疗措施。绝大多数受影响的患者有望完全康复，不会有后遗症。上述支持措施也适用于近三分之一的产后 HELLP 综合征患者，通常是在分娩后的头两周内。

（四）肝破裂、血肿和梗死

自发性肝破裂可能会并发先兆子痫和 HELLP 综合征，通常在接近足月的妊娠晚期或产后早期。自发性肝破裂患者会出现腹胀和疼痛，并伴有心力衰竭[267,268]。与先兆子痫患者相比，自发性肝破裂孕妇往往年龄较大，且有多次妊娠史。肝破裂通过超声、CT 或 MRI 检查上的肝破裂征象以及腹腔穿刺术中的血液抽吸进行诊断[212,269]。影像学研究经常显示，受影响的患者有部分出现肝包膜下血肿（图 40.2）[270]。在这种情况下，肝动脉栓塞可有效控制出血并降低发病率和死亡率[271]。肝破裂必须积极治疗，由产科医生快速分娩胎儿，如果栓塞不足以控制出血，由经验丰富的肝外科医生修复肝脏[272]。术后，患者的病程很长，可能包括发生弥散性血管内凝血（DIC）和肝功能衰竭。肝破裂患者行急诊肝切除术和间

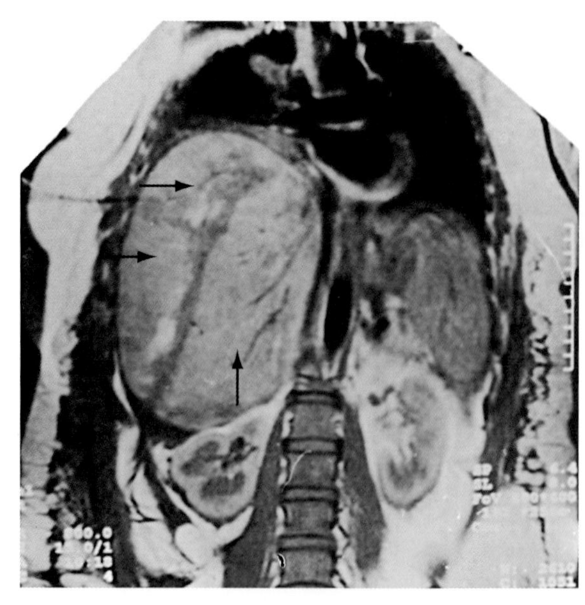

图 40.2　先兆子痫患者的肝包膜下血肿。T1 加权 MRI 扫描的冠状面显示邻近肝脏的包膜下血凝块或出血（水平箭头）（垂直箭头）。（From Barton JR, Sibai BM. Hepatic imaging in HELLP syndrome. Am J Obstet Gynecol 1996;174:1820-5.）

隔门体分流术后作为临时措施,同时寻求供体移植物进行原位肝移植[265,266,273,274]。肝破裂的幸存者可能在随后的妊娠中平安无事[275],但血肿复发和破裂也有报道[276]。

一些患有先兆子痫、HELLP 综合征和腹痛的孕妇出现肝包膜下血肿[277]。在这种情况下,可以通过连续 CT 观察并且无需手术治疗[212,276]。血管造影栓塞肝脏动脉分支,为受影响的肝脏部分供血,可能会有所帮助[271]。

肝脏血肿和破裂并发先兆子痫可能是由 Glisson 鞘下的一个或几个门静脉周围出血的微血管出血外渗引起的。门静脉周围出血是先兆子痫和 HELLP 综合征患者肝脏的典型病理表现[278]。由于不断扩大的血肿,包膜被拉伸并从肝脏表面撕开。最终,包膜可能破裂,使血液从肝脏表面自由渗入腹膜腔。

肝梗死也可能并发先兆子痫。出现发热、白细胞增多、贫血和血清氨基转移酶水平显著升高的患病孕妇[212,214,279],在最严重的情况下会发生多器官功能衰竭,包括肝功能衰竭。横断面成像显示汇合性肝脏梗死,(肝穿刺)针吸这些部位能获取血液和坏死组织;毗邻的肝实质包含先兆子痫和 HELLP 综合征的典型表现,即门静脉周围出血和纤维蛋白沉积。肝梗死有时与高凝状态的存在有关,如莱顿第五因子(即凝血因子Ⅴ莱顿突变)或抗磷脂抗体[280]。

(五) 妊娠期急性脂肪肝

妊娠期急性脂肪肝(AFLP)是一种特发于人类妊娠期间的微泡性脂肪肝,在妊娠晚期发病,常表现为暴发性肝功能衰竭,并在无肝病病史的妇女中突然出现凝血功能障碍和脑病[281,282]。基于典型的临床和病理特征,在 6 700 例妊娠晚期的妇女中大约有 1 例被诊断为 AFLP[283],但也存在亚临床病例[217]。一项使用英国产科监测系统和规范化诊断标准[Swansea 标准(框 40.3)]、调查超过 100 万例孕妇的前瞻性研究[284]仅确诊了 57 例 AFLP[285]。这种疾病发生发展的病理生理机制尚不清楚,目前已知一些 AFLP 患者具有遗传性脂肪酸氧化缺陷,这也会影响胎儿[286-290]。

框 40.3　妊娠期急性脂肪肝的诊断标准(Swansea 标准)

≥以下 6 项,在无其他可解释的情况下:
- 腹痛
- 肝脏超声检查显示腹水或明亮肝脏
- 凝血功能障碍(PT>14 秒或 aPTT>34 秒)
- 血清氨水平升高(>47μmol/L)
- 血清 AST 或 ALT 水平升高(>42IU/L)
- 血清胆红素水平升高(>14μmol/L 或 0.8mg/dL)
- 血清尿酸盐水平升高(>340μmol/L 或 5.7mg/dL)
- 脑病
- 低血糖症(<4mmol/L 或 72mg/dL)
- 白细胞增多(>11 000/mm^3)
- 肝活检显示小泡性脂肪变性
- 多饮/多尿
- 肾功能损害(肌酐>150μmol/L 或 1.7mg/dL)
- 呕吐

aPPT,活化部分凝血活酶时间;PT,凝血酶原时间。

Adapted from Ch'ng CL, Morgan M, Hainsworth I, et al. Prospective study of liver dysfunction in pregnancy in Southwest Wales. Gut 2002;51:876-80; and Knight M, Nelson-Piercy C, Kurinczuk JJ, et al. A prospective nation-al study of acute fatty liver of pregnancy in the UK. Gut 2008;57:951-6.

AFLP 在妊娠晚期,通常在妊娠第 34~37 周发病,也有在第 19~20 周发病的报道,极少发生于分娩后。早期症状通常包括恶心和呕吐,伴腹痛。瘙痒可能是早期的症状,与妊娠胆汁淤积重叠,但很少见[291]。这些症状通常误与 AFLP 孕妇伴发的其他妊娠并发症,如早产、阴道出血、胎动减少等相联系。这种疾病在初产妇女和多胎妊娠妇女中最为常见[292]。受累个体的男胎数量比预期的要多得多[293]。值得注意的是,同时也有 21%~64% 的 AFLP 患者出现先兆子痫[283,294],先兆子痫也与第一次妊娠、双胞胎妊娠和男胎有关。

实验室检查中,AFLP 孕妇通常表现出凝血酶原时间延长、血清纤维蛋白原水平降低、白细胞增多;血清氨基转移酶水平中度升高(≈750U/L),但极少数可能非常高,甚至正常。黄疸也常见于 AFLP 患者,但随着病程进展呈动态变化;AFLP 孕妇还通常存在肾功能障碍,伴血清肌酐、血尿素氮和尿酸水平升高。

AFLP 患者病情多变,可能会发生低血糖和高氨血症,当高危患者表现出中枢神经系统功能改变的迹象时,应予以警惕。肝功能衰竭的其他并发症,包括腹水、胸腔积液、急性胰腺炎、呼吸衰竭、肾功能衰竭和感染等也可能发生在 AFLP 患者身上。阴道出血或剖宫产术后出血在这些人中也很常见。有时会出现一过性尿崩症[295]。更罕见的是,受累的患者有心肌梗死[296]或肺部脂肪栓塞[297]。

AFLP 的诊断几乎总是基于患者出现的典型临床特征,包括实验室检查结果。肝脏成像可以证实疑似 AFLP 患者肝脏脂肪变性的存在[298],并在识别肝脏血肿、破裂和梗死方面起着至关重要的作用。

AFLP 的诊断通常不需要进行肝脏活组织检查,但如果确诊可能需要组织学结果,且产科医生建议继续妊娠的情况下,则有必要活检。有凝血功能障碍的患者需要经颈静脉进行肝脏组织取样。AFLP 的组织学特征是肝脏的微泡脂肪浸润,中央静脉周围的肝细胞(3 区)和汇管区周围的肝细胞最明显(图 40.3)。光学显微镜下这种类型的微泡性脂肪变性具有相对均匀的外观,在普通的 HE 染色标本检查中可能很难辨别。为了确认诊断,必须使用特殊技术;冷冻组织可以用苏丹红进行脂肪染色,或者使用电子显微镜观察经戊二醛固定的标本。必须在活体组织取样之前就将标本处理的方案制定好。AFLP 患者的其他组织学发现可能具有迷惑性,包括易误

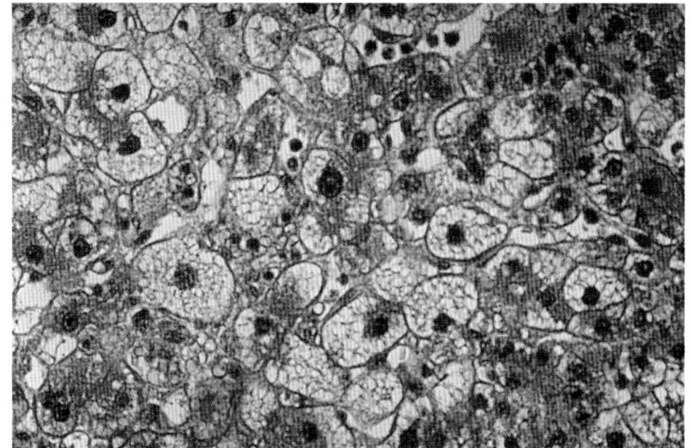

图 40.3　妊娠急性脂肪肝的组织病理学。小静脉周围肝细胞呈多形性和空泡样,并有小叶排列紊乱。未见大的脂肪滴

判为病毒性肝炎的肝小叶结构紊乱和胆管炎的炎症以及胆管增生[217,299]。AFLP 患者的肝脏中没有出现与先兆子痫和 HELLP 综合征患者相似的门静脉周围出血和(肝)窦状隙纤维蛋白沉积。

AFLP 疑似病例的鉴别诊断包括在后文讨论的非妊娠相关性急性肝功能衰竭,尤其是各型病毒性肝炎和中毒性肝损伤。罕见类型病毒性肝炎(例如戊型病毒性肝炎和单纯疱疹病毒性肝炎)妊娠患者的情况可能比普通患者更为严重[300,301]。这些病原体可以通过适当的血清学试验来鉴定。另一个难题是将 AFLP 与其他合并妊娠的肝脏疾病相鉴别,特别是先兆子痫肝病,即 HELLP 综合征伴出血性或缺血性肝损伤。如果一个 AFLP 的患者可能发展为先兆子痫、弥散性血管内凝血伴血小板减少,这就符合 HELLP 综合征的诊断标准(见框 40.1)。所幸通常不需要仔细区分这些不同的诊断,因为 AFLP、HELLP 综合征和先兆子痫都是通过加快分娩来治疗的。然而,迅速识别肝脏血肿和破裂至关重要(见前文讨论)。

AFLP 的发病机制尚未阐明。最初,AFLP 被认为是由接触特定物质引起,例如,肝脏的微泡状脂肪变性可由丙戊酸钠或静脉注射四环素治疗引起。然而,尽管进行了深入的搜索,还没有发现可能导致 AFLP 发生的毒素。由于先兆子痫和 AFLP 在许多患者中同时发作,一些专家认为 AFLP 是一种与先兆子痫相关的严重肝病[217,302,303]。胎盘氧化应激反应伴毒性介质释放,是先兆子痫的病因之一,也被认为可能与 AFLP 的发生有关[304]。然而,与此相悖的是,AFLP 患者的肝活检标本中缺乏先兆子痫常见的组织学特征,并且许多 AFLP 患者缺乏先兆子痫前期的常见临床特征。

AFLP 与脂肪酸 β 氧化的遗传缺陷之间有着较大的关联[287-289,305,306]。AFLP 患者和牙买加呕吐病患者之间相似的临床表现和组织学特征支持了这一结论。牙买加呕吐病是一种由食用未成熟的橡树果实的一种毒素引起,阻止线粒体内脂肪酸的 β 氧化失效。据报道,存在脂肪酸 β 氧化缺陷的新生儿的母亲中,有 62% 的人患有母性肝病(HELLP 综合征或 AFLP)[287]。如果胎儿缺乏长链 3-羟基酰基辅酶 A 脱氢酶(LCHAD)并且携带至少 1 个 G1528C *LCHAD* 等位基因突变,那么 AFLP 的发生与母体基因型无关[286,307]。另一种类型的脂肪酸 β 氧化缺陷,由肉毒碱棕榈酰基转移酶(CPT)-1 的缺乏引起,也与 AFLP 有关[308]。对于来自存在这种遗传缺陷家族的孕妇,通过绒毛膜取样术取出适量的绒毛组织进行产前基因诊断,已被证明有较好的可行性和准确性[309,310]。然而,并非每个研究者都能证实 AFLP 和脂肪酸 β 氧化缺陷之间的联系[311],AFLP 的发生发展也可能存在其他未知的机制。

AFLP 患者应在重症监护室进行治疗,最好是由具有母胎医学实践资质的产科医生与其他相关的专科医生合作。胎儿的早期诊断和及时分娩是将母婴发病率和死亡率降至最低的当务之急。在导致临床异常的生理缺陷解决和肝脏恢复之前,受影响的个体可能会在产后非常虚弱。支持性治疗可能包括输血产品、机械通气、血液透析和抗生素治疗。肝性脑病按照从结肠排出粪便和细菌的措施来治疗。可能需要输注浓缩葡萄糖溶液来治疗或预防低血糖。虽然,许多 AFLP 患者有 DIC 和抗凝血酶Ⅲ水平(AT Ⅲ)降低,但不推荐使用肝素或抗凝血酶Ⅲ治疗。尿崩症患者可用 1-脱氨基-8-d-精氨酸-加压素(DDAVP)治疗[295]。一些继发于 AFLP 的肝功能衰竭患者需要紧急原位肝移植作为可能挽救生命的措施[266,313,314]。然而,大多数受影响的妇女在适当的支持治疗下能够完全康复。分娩后持续或甚至增加的高胆红素血症和多种并发症并不一定意味着需要进行肝移植。

据报道,在及时诊断、分娩婴儿和重症监护的情况下,AFLP 孕妇的生存率几乎达到 100%[283,294,315,316]。受累孕妇无性婴儿围生期病死率低于 7%。幸存的婴儿可能患有长链 3-羟基酰基辅酶 A 脱氢酶(LCHAD)缺乏症并发展为非酮症性低血糖和闭塞。已有文献记载 AFLP 的复发,特别是在 LCHAD 缺乏症的妇女中[317,318]。在所有 AFLP 病例中,母亲、父亲和孩子都应接受 G1528C *LCHAD* 突变检测[286]。

八、其他肝脏疾病与妊娠

(一）病毒性肝炎

病毒性肝炎是世界范围内最常见的肝脏疾病,无论是急性或慢性感染,都常常影响育龄妇女[319,320]。甲型病毒性肝炎,除非异常严重,似乎不会改变正常的妊娠过程,妊娠似乎也不会影响甲型肝炎的自然病史。然而,其他类型的急、慢性病毒性肝炎可能会对母婴健康产生影响。

1. 戊型病毒性肝炎（HEV）(见第 82 章）

HEV 是经粪口传播的 RNA 病毒,有 4 种基因型和 1 种血清型[301,321]。其中,基因型 1 和 2 仅感染人类,通常在中亚、南亚以及印度的季风季节大规模流行;基因型 3 和 4 可以感染包括人类在内的许多物种,尤其是猪和鸡,可能还包括牛、羊和大鼠。这些 HEV 基因型是造成农民散发性肝炎的原因,还能通过食用未煮熟的肉而传播给他人[322]。与 1998 年至 1994 年相比,2009 年至 2010 年在美国采集的血液样本中戊型肝炎病毒抗体的流行率有所下降[320];最近,6 岁或以上儿童的戊型肝炎病毒抗体流行率为 6%。两种重组蛋白 HEV 疫苗已经进行了临床试验[323],其中一种已于 2011 年 12 月被中国国家食品药品监督管理总局批准于中国使用。

妊娠晚期急性 HEV 发作是导致暴发性肝功能衰竭的原因之一,病死率高达 20%[301]。母体戊型肝炎病毒感染也与胎儿宫内死亡有关[324,325]。感染的孕妇在整个孕期内发生胎儿宫内死亡和流产都较健康孕妇更大,还会导致新生儿 HEV 感染[326],目前尚无有效措施阻断其垂直传播。健康孕妇应避免在 HEV 流行季节前往疫区。

2. 单纯疱疹病毒性肝炎（HSV）(见第 83 章）

与原发性单纯疱疹病毒感染相关的亚临床肝炎很常见。在妊娠或免疫抑制的个体中,这种病毒可能导致严重的肝脏疾病[327]。妊娠期间,特别是妊娠晚期的感染可导致暴发性肝功能衰竭。患者一般无黄疸,表现为血清转氨酶水平升高、并伴有凝血功能障碍。他们可能伴有轻微的口咽部或生殖器部位疱疹病变。脑病可能是由疱疹脑炎引起的。HSV 感染可通过血清学检测和病毒 DNA 聚合酶链式反应(PCR)检测来确诊。患者的肝活检标本通常能观察到典型的胞质内包涵体和灶性出血。口服阿昔洛韦或万乃洛韦治疗疗效显著,并且似乎可以防止病毒垂直传播给胎儿[328,329]。

3. 乙型和丁型病毒性肝炎（HBV 和 HDV）（见第 79 和 81 章）

孕妇中的 HBV 感染是导致慢性 HBV 全球流行的最主要因素[330-332]。建议在孕妇中进行 HBV 普查[333]。尽管 HBV 也可以在整个妊娠期间、分娩时或出生后从母体垂直传播给婴儿，但大多数母婴传播发生在分娩过程中，这期间新生儿的免疫系统无法清除入侵的病毒。垂直传播是导致 HBV 流行地区大多数慢性 HBV 感染的主要原因，特别是在东南亚和非洲[334]。

母体的传染性与病毒载量（VL）成正比[335]。与血清乙肝 e 抗体检测阴性的母亲相比，HBV e 抗原检测阳性的母体有更高的病毒载量和围生期传播率[336,337]，尽管前者仍可能是新生儿感染源[338]。如果不进行治疗，90% HBV e 抗原阳性的母亲和 10% 的 HBV e 抗原阴性的母体所生的婴儿会出现慢性 HBV 感染。对于非活动性乙型肝炎但血清 HBV-DNA 水平高于 20 万 IU/mL 的孕妇，建议从妊娠晚期开始进行抗病毒治疗[339]。对于患有活动性乙型肝炎的孕妇，治疗应与非孕妇相同[340]。孕期适当治疗可显著降低母婴传播病毒的风险[341]。然而，如果传播的风险很低，除了推荐的婴儿预防措施外，抗病毒治疗没有任何好处[342]。妊娠期间的侵入性手术，如羊膜穿刺术，可能会引起乙肝病毒从母体传染给孩子的风险，特别是当孕妇的 HBV-DNA 水平大于或等于 7log 拷贝/mL 时[343]。

血清 HBV 表面抗原检测呈阳性的母体产下的婴儿应在分娩后 12 小时内接种乙肝免疫球蛋白和乙肝疫苗[344]。这种疗法非常有效，但即使在出生后立即进行适当的被动和（或）主动免疫预防，仍有 1% ~ 2% 接受治疗的婴儿感染 HBV[335,345]。只要婴儿接受了规范化的免疫治疗，慢性 HBV 感染的母亲进行母乳喂养就不会增加垂直传播的风险[346]。

大多数慢性 HBV 感染的育龄妇女是健康的病毒携带者，发生疾病并发症的风险非常低。然而，在围生期以前无症状的孕妇可能会出现肝炎发作，在某些情况下甚至急性肝功能衰竭[347,348]。在最近的一项研究中，大约 25% 的慢性乙型肝炎妇女在分娩后的头几个月出现了疾病发作[349]。研究人员还发现，脐带血中 HBV-DNA 的存在可能会增加自发性早产的发生率[350]。基于这些原因，应在 HBV 患者妊娠期间和产后阶段进行长达 6 个月的密切监测[351]。

曾经对孕妇进行研究的乙肝治疗方法包括拉米夫定、替比夫定和富马酸替诺福韦双丙酯（TDF）。在这些药物中，TDF 因其可靠的疗效和对出现病毒耐药性的高屏障而作为首选。对于血清 HBV-DNA 水平较高的孕妇，在妊娠晚期接受 TDF 治疗已被证明能显著降低母婴病毒传播的发生率[341,352]。接受治疗和未接受治疗的妇女在早产、先天畸形和阿普加评分方面没有差异。其他研究表明，暴露于 TDF 和未暴露于 TDF 的婴儿的不良反应发生率没有差别[353-355]。患有慢性乙型肝炎的妇女在妊娠期间不应接受干扰素治疗。对未免疫的孕妇接种乙肝疫苗安全有效[357]。加速接种计划可用于接触乙肝病毒的高危妇女[358]。当乙肝治疗的适应证是妊娠晚期血清 HBV-DNA 水平高于 200 000IU/mL 时，建议在分娩时或分娩后 4 周内停止治疗[359]。产后持续治疗长达 12 周并不能保护母亲免受疾病的侵袭[360]。

HDV 感染需要同时感染急性或慢性乙肝病毒。最有可能合并感染 HDV 的孕妇包括 HIV 携带者和来自 HDV 高流行区的移民。这些人应该接受提示 HDV 感染的抗 HDV 抗体的检测[359]。

没有证据表明妊娠会改变丁型肝炎的自然病程。预防 HDV 垂直传播的最佳方法是为母亲接种预防感染乙肝病毒的疫苗，或在妊娠前对现有的孕妇进行适当的乙肝治疗，同时接种疫苗并给婴儿注射乙肝免疫球蛋白。一份病例报告记录了通过这一管理措施预防乙肝和丁型肝炎病毒垂直传播的情况[361]。

4. 丙型病毒性肝炎（HCV）（见第 80 章）

美国肝病学会和北美传染病学会的丙型肝炎指南专家组不断更新孕妇（和其他人）丙型肝炎的诊断和治疗建议[362]，并可在互联网上查阅。虽然目前没有建议对孕妇进行丙型肝炎病毒普查，但建议对有病毒暴露风险因素（如注射吸毒史）的患者进行丙型肝炎病毒抗体检测。每一位感染 HIV 的孕妇都应该接受同时感染丙型肝炎病毒（HCV）的检测。具有反应性抗体检测的患者应该进行丙型肝炎病毒核酸确认检测[363,364]。

母婴传播是儿童丙型肝炎的主要原因[365]。据报道，HCV 垂直传播的发生率在 HCV-RNA 阳性、HIV 阴性妇女的子女中为 5. 8%，在 HCV-RNA 阳性、HIV 阳性妇女的子女中为 10. 8%[366,367]。血清中丙型肝炎病毒 RNA 水平较高，如艾滋病毒和丙型肝炎病毒混合感染中所见，会增加垂直传播的风险：在多达 36% 的病例中，血清丙型肝炎病毒 RNA 水平达到 10^6 拷贝/毫升或更高拷贝/毫升与垂直传播有关[368]，产期暴露于受感染的母亲血液、胎膜长时间破裂和胎儿内部监护也被确定为新生儿感染丙型肝炎病毒的可能危险因素[369,370]。围生期丙型肝炎病毒感染的发生率似乎与婴儿是通过阴道分娩还是剖宫产无关[368]。虽然可以在母乳中检测到丙型肝炎病毒 RNA[371]，但母乳喂养并不被认为是新生儿感染丙型肝炎病毒的风险因素[372]，也没有数据表明羊膜穿刺术显著增加了胎儿感染的风险。

基于人群和病例对照的关于母体 HCV 感染对妊娠结局影响的研究结果并不一致。慢性 HCV 可能与母体妊娠糖尿病（GDM）、早产和胎儿出生低体重、发育迟缓和妊娠胆汁淤积独立相关[373-376]。尤其是肝硬化，与产妇和胎儿发病率的增加有关[377,378]。无令人信服的数据表明妊娠可能改变 HCV 感染的自然史。尽管患有丙型肝炎的孕妇妊娠胆汁淤积症的发生率高于未感染的对照组[192]。如果可能，患有丙型肝炎的育龄妇女应该在妊娠前接受抗病毒治疗；没有批准直接作用的抗病毒药物在妊娠期间使用。没有证据表明妊娠期内或产后干预可以降低丙型肝炎病毒垂直传播的风险，包括用免疫球蛋白治疗婴儿[379]。丙型肝炎患者在妊娠期间不应接受干扰素/利巴韦林治疗；利巴韦林是一种公认的致畸剂。以前感染的人在分娩后可能会自发清除丙型肝炎病毒 RNA[380]。

（二）慢性肝病及肝门静脉高压症（见第 92 和 94 章）

患有严重慢性肝病和肝硬化的女性通常无月经周期或闭

经,因此不太可能妊娠。在2005年至2009年间,加州出生登记处数据库记录的200多万名孕妇中,只有37例使用ICD-9代码识别出肝硬化[378]。

门静脉高压、腹水以及连接门脉循环和奇静脉的食管黏膜下静脉的代偿性扩张也会发生在非肝硬化性门静脉高压症的孕妇体内,并且随着循环血量的生理性增加而恶化。即使在没有引发门静脉高压的病因的情况下,一些食管静脉侧支也可在妊娠期间由于生理性的循环血量变化而充血,包括因子宫扩大造成的血流量增加和下腔静脉受压,均可通过内镜观察到。这种由生理原因引起的静脉曲张并不会自发出血。

正常妊娠相关的母体血容量增加似乎会加重潜在门静脉高压患者静脉曲张出血的风险[381,382]。据报道,在患有肝硬化的孕妇中,有18%~32%的人发生了食管静脉曲张出血,在已知的门静脉高压症患者中,多达50%的患者和先前存在静脉曲张的患者中,有78%的患者出现了食管静脉曲张出血。根据1950年至1980年发表的报告,除了静脉曲张出血,患有慢性肝病和门静脉高压的女性妊娠后死亡、肝脏失代偿、脾动脉破裂和子宫出血的风险可能会增加[377,381]。肝硬化似乎显著增加了先兆子痫、早产、低出生体重和新生儿死亡的风险[378]。

内镜下套扎术仍被认为是孕妇静脉曲张出血的首选初始治疗方法,尽管在这种情况下还没有关于其安全性和有效性的研究。生长抑素类似物奥曲肽的输注也是根据其对非妊娠患者的有效性而使用的。理论上,注射血管升压素和奥曲肽可能导致子宫缺血和早产。尽管存在相关的放射暴露风险,但当静脉曲张出血不能通过任何其他方法控制时,可以建议行经颈静脉肝内门体分流术[383-385]。美国肝病研究学会年会(AASLD)建议每个肝硬度不低于20kPa(FibroScan)、血小板计数不超过15万/mm^3的肝硬化患者都要进行食管静脉曲张的内镜筛查[386],尽管目前还没有正式的孕妇食管静脉曲张预防性管理指南。β-肾上腺素能受体拮抗剂可以拮抗宫缩,但这些药物不会抑制长期治疗的孕妇的正常分娩。使用β受体阻滞剂作为孕妇静脉曲张出血的主要预防措施尚未得到正式评估。一些作者建议预防性套扎、门体分流术和剖宫产以降低妊娠期静脉曲张出血的风险。

慢性肝病孕妇的腹水和肝性脑病按常规方式处理。对于妊娠期严重的肝脏失代偿,唯一可用的治疗方法是肝移植。妊娠期已成功进行了原位肝移植[387,388]。MELD评分可以帮助预测妊娠期肝硬化妇女的临床失代偿情况。例如,在1项研究中,妊娠时MELD评分在10或更高时预测腹水、脑病或静脉曲张出血的敏感度和特异度分别为83%和83%[389]。

(三) Wilson病(肝豆状核变性)(见第76章)

育龄妇女的肝豆状核变性闭经和不孕有关。对患病个体进行治疗以清除多余的铜可能会导致排卵周期的恢复和随后的妊娠。孕妇必须继续服用药物来治疗威尔逊病,因为停止治疗会导致铜离子的突然释放,引起溶血、急性肝功能衰竭和死亡[390]。D-青霉胺虽然有致畸的可能[391],但其作为铜离子螯合剂时所需的剂量对于胎儿而言是安全的[392]。同样地,曲恩汀在动物身上是致畸的,但作为铜超载的治疗方法,在人类身上似乎是安全的。醋酸锌等锌盐似乎不会致畸,因此一些专家倾向于在妊娠期间使用锌作为威尔逊病的治疗方法[393]。

(四) 自身免疫性肝病(见第90和91章)

包括自身免疫性肝炎在内的大多数自身免疫性疾病,在女性中的发病率较男性更高。自身免疫性肝病有多种临床表型。在女性中,典型的(1型)自身免疫性肝炎通常出现在预期的月经初潮时间,但与闭经有关。当患有自身免疫性肝炎的妇女妊娠时,她们自然流产和早产的发生率比预期的要高[394]。患者在妊娠和产后也可能出现疾病症状[395,396]。出于这个原因,妊娠的自身免疫性肝炎患者应该在妊娠期间继续服用免疫抑制药物。作为标准治疗方案的一部分,硫唑嘌呤的剂量被认为不致畸。自身免疫性肝炎患者在孕期和产后应仔细监测。

原发性胆汁性胆管炎(PBC)在绝经后妇女中比在有生育能力的妇女中更常见。患有PBC的妇女在妊娠期间可能会出现严重的瘙痒症状[397]。瘙痒可以通过熊脱氧胆酸治疗以改善症状[398],但其安全性尚未得到正式验证。

(五) 肝脏肿瘤和肿块性病变(见第96章)

在美国,妇女妊娠期间可能会在接受超声检查时偶然观察到肝实质的类肿块病变,育龄妇女肝脏常见的良性病变包括腺瘤、局限性结节性增生和血管瘤。肝腺瘤的发生与口服避孕药有关,瘤体可能在妊娠期间增大,增大的病变可能会出血并破裂进入腹腔。已有妊娠患者的局灶性结节性增生和肝血管瘤出血的报道。已知患有肝脏良性结节性病变的女性应进行系列超声检查,以观察肿块大小、判断病灶出血的风险。

肝细胞癌几乎全部发生在慢性肝病患者中,对于慢性乙型病毒性肝炎(HBV)感染的年轻人中可能没有肝硬化。高危患者应给在妊娠期间进行肝癌的标准筛查。需要注意的是,在正常妊娠期间,孕妇血清AFP水平总是轻度升高[399],在胎儿唐氏综合征、神经管缺陷和葡萄胎的病例中,AFP水平可能进一步升高,从而限制了妊娠期间诊断肝细胞癌的阳性预测价值。

据报道,肝纤维板层癌可发生于孕妇[400]。纤维板层癌是一种生长缓慢的肝癌,通常见于年轻人(中位年龄,25岁)[401]。与典型的原发性肝癌不同,这种肿瘤与肝硬化或慢性肝病没有已知的联系,也不是血清AFP水平升高的原因。这是一种侵袭性肿瘤,5年存活率低于50%。

其他癌症引起的肝转移在育龄妇女中很少见。

(六) 肝静脉血栓形成(Budd-Chiari综合征)(见第85章)

妊娠是静脉血栓的诱发因素之一。体内含有抗磷脂抗体的孕妇,肝静脉血栓的形成可能与HELLP综合征[402]和先兆子痫有关[403]。发生肝静脉血栓形成的孕妇应检查抗磷脂抗体和其他循环促凝剂(如因子V莱顿)的存在,以及JAK-2,以及可能的其他基因突变[404]。

(七) 肝脏移植后妊娠(见第97章)

育龄妇女在原位肝移植成功后可能妊娠并产下正常胎

儿[127,405,406]。将妊娠推迟到移植后第二年可能与早产风险较低有关。移植患者必须在妊娠期间继续接受免疫抑制治疗，但治疗方案可能需要调整。吗替麦考酚酯是移植术后免疫抑制治疗方案的常见药物之一，但具有强致畸性[407]，其他免疫抑制药物的副作用，包括高血压和高血糖等，可能会增加孕妇患者发生胎儿窘迫和先兆子痫的风险。少数情况下，妊娠还会因器官排斥反应而变得棘手。

（汤善宏　译，孙明瑜　闫秀娥　校）

参考文献

第 41 章 放疗的急性和慢性胃肠道副作用

Jarred P. Tanksley, Christopher G. Willett, Brian G. Czito 著

章节目录

一、辐射引起胃肠道损伤的分子机制 …… 574
二、串联对比并联的器官功能 …… 575
三、小肠 …… 575
(一) 发病率及临床特征 …… 575
(二) 治疗和预防 …… 577
四、食管 …… 579
(一) 发病率和临床特征 …… 579
(二) 治疗与预防 …… 580
五、胃 …… 581
(一) 发病率和临床特征 …… 581
(二) 治疗与预防 …… 581
六、结肠和直肠 …… 581
(一) 发病率和临床特征 …… 581
(二) 治疗与预防 …… 583
七、肛门 …… 583
(一) 发病率及临床特征 …… 583
(二) 治疗 …… 584
八、胰腺和肝脏 …… 584
(一) 发病率及临床特征 …… 584
(二) 治疗 …… 584
九、降低毒性的治疗技术 …… 585

在胸部、腹部和盆腔胃肠道或非胃肠道恶性肿瘤的放疗(radiation therapy, RT)之后,可能会发生早期或晚期胃肠道器官损伤。与所有放疗相关的毒性反应一样,胃肠道副作用大致分为两类:早期或急性反应,如腹泻和恶心,可在治疗过程中或治疗结束后不久发生;晚期或慢性反应,如溃疡、狭窄和肠梗阻,可在几个月到几年后出现。严重的急性反应可导致放疗中断,进而不能达到理想的疗程;而对慢性放疗毒性的关注,尤其是对小肠的毒性,通常是制定放疗计划时限制放疗剂量的考虑因素。辐射引起的胃肠道疾病的发病率和严重程度取决于总剂量和分次剂量、放疗区域和放疗技术、是否存在其他治疗方式,如全身治疗和手术,以及患者的基础疾病。本章讨论放疗和联合放化疗(combined chemoradiation therapy, CRT)方案对食管、胃、小肠、结肠、直肠、肛门、胰腺和肝脏的早期和晚期毒性。

接下来的章节将重点介绍胃肠道各个器官可能发生的各种放射毒性,以及放射肿瘤科医生为降低上述毒性的可能性和严重性而采取的措施。在此之前,我们对放射损伤的细胞机制进行了简要的综合性讨论,并介绍了串联功能器官和平行功能器官的概念,这样的概念提示了要注意放疗的剂量限制。

一、辐射引起胃肠道损伤的分子机制

在细胞水平上,放疗的治疗效应和急性损伤效应都是其能够通过产生自由基诱导 DNA 双链断裂的结果。在某些类型的细胞中,这种损伤会导致程序性细胞死亡(凋亡),这是通过一系列明确的信号级联反应进行的,这种级联反应通常在肿瘤发生过程中被破坏。在快速分裂的癌细胞中,通常缺乏正常 DNA 损伤反应系统和凋亡级联反应的重要组成部分,放疗诱导的 DNA 双链断裂可导致致死性染色体畸变,当尝试分裂时引起细胞死亡,这种现象被称为有丝分裂灾难。

在动物模型中研究了正常胃肠道辐射暴露的急性效应,在暴露于低剂量辐射(1~5cGy)后,可观察到肠隐窝/干细胞凋亡率快速增加。细胞凋亡率呈剂量依赖性,在 1Gy 时达到平台期。辐射暴露可增加胃肠上皮中 *TP53* 基因产物 p53 的表达,从而诱导 PUMA(p53 上调凋亡调节因子,也称为 BBC3 或 Bcl-2 结合成分 3)的表达,PUMA 是一种通过内源性凋亡途径引起细胞死亡的促凋亡蛋白。相反,在缺乏促凋亡 bcl-2 多结构域蛋白 bax 和 bak 的动物中,辐射诱导的内皮细胞凋亡率显著降低[1,2]。因此推测 p53 在照射后促进细胞凋亡,而 bcl-2 家族的抗凋亡成员保护正常黏膜。

除了细胞凋亡和有丝分裂灾难导致的细胞急性丢失外,放射损伤是细胞间一系列复杂相互作用的结果,涉及多种细胞因子和分子通路,可导致急性黏膜水肿,慢性纤维化,并可通过细胞外基质的过度沉积及基质金属蛋白酶等重塑酶的表达减少而导致器官功能障碍。辐射诱导的纤维化本质上是伤口愈合不当,当与黏膜干细胞丢失结合时,是放疗相关的慢性毒性,如运动障碍、狭窄和瘘管形成的基础[3,4]。该过程通常在放疗疗程结束后数月至一年开始,并且可在接下来的几年内继续进展。

这一过程的最初步骤是将免疫细胞募集到放疗诱导损伤的部位,进而导致许多细胞因子的局部表达增加,包括血小板源性生长因子和转化生长因子(TGF)-β。血小板源性生长因子促进成纤维细胞向损伤区迁移,而 TGF-β 既促进成纤维细胞的增殖,又促进其转分化为促纤维化肌成纤维细胞[5,6]。研究认为活性 TGF-β 的持续局部表达是辐射诱导纤维化的主要介质。TGF-β 除了促进肌成纤维细胞的生成外,还促进细胞外基质蛋白的生成并减少基质金属蛋白酶的表达[7,8]。对接受放射性肠病患者的肠道标本进行病理学检查,发现与因其他原因接受手术的患者相比,血管硬化区域以及浆膜和固有肌层的纤维化区域的 TGF-β 增加[9]。在大鼠肝脏中,照射后长达 9 个月,发现肝细胞中 TGF-β 表达呈剂量依赖性上

调[10]。TGF-β 和小分子抑制剂的中和抗体已在临床前模型中显示出抑制或逆转纤维化的作用，但迄今为止尚未在临床实践中应用[11-13]。

纤维化组织的急性至亚急性形成和上皮的丢失，反过来可导致慢性和永久性纤维化，其风险也与患者的合并症有关，如吸烟状态、营养、糖尿病，以及某些炎症性疾病[14]。认为整体情况是最初的损伤和损伤反应的产物，导致血管变化，最终导致组织缺血和进行性纤维化[15]。

二、串联对比并联的器官功能

通过上皮干细胞的丢失和瘢痕组织的形成，放疗可导致胃肠道各器官的功能减弱。其临床表现与器官的功能排列有一定关系，器官功能排列分为串联和平行两种类型。

串联排列的器官各个节段串联组成，并且每个节段都依赖于前一节段的功能，因此任何单个节段的丢失都会使器官功能失调，甚至在受到损伤的下游并可能在上游出现功能障碍甚至功能丧失。这种排列的典型器官是脊髓，单个脊髓水平的严重损伤会导致损伤下游各个层面的功能丧失。就胃肠系统而言，大部分胃肠道管腔都是这种功能结构。

另一方面，具有平行结构的器官具有一定的功能冗余，以致各个节段丢失到某一程度可能也不会出现临床表现。肝脏有这种类型的排列方式，尽管关于肝脏到底需要保留多少才能保持整体功能的争论仍在继续，特别是在有潜在肝病的患者中。

在制定放疗计划时，考虑这些功能排列方式会提示需要使用的剂量限制类型。串联功能的器官受到最大剂量的限制，因为可以造成小面积小肠消融的高剂量可以导致整个器官的功能障碍，如小肠梗阻。具有平行功能结构的器官受到辐射体积限制，应保护相对足够的组织体积，以发挥功能。正如在肝脏，讨论关注的重点是不要让特定的肝脏体积接受超过特定剂量的辐射。

三、小肠

1897 年，第一次描述了在照射腹部皮肤的情况下，小肠放射性损伤或放射性肠病[16]。放疗在治疗几乎所有胃肠道癌症和妇科癌症的过程中都会损伤小肠，但放疗很少作为小肠癌初始治疗的一部分。大多数腹部和盆腔恶性肿瘤放疗的剂量限制因素通常是降低放射性肠炎和慢性小肠损伤的风险和严重程度。

（一）发病率及临床特征

胃肠道上皮具有较高的增殖率，每 3~5 天更新一次，使其易受放疗和化疗引起的黏膜炎的影响。肠黏膜受照射主要影响 Lieberkühn 隐窝内的克隆形成肠干细胞（通过自我复制和最终成熟提供肠绒毛中替代细胞的细胞）。由于直接辐射损伤或辐射诱导的微血管损伤导致的干细胞损伤，使肠绒毛细胞储备减少。这导致黏膜剥脱、绒毛缩短、吸收表面积减少以及相关的肠道炎症和水肿。组织学变化在照射后数小时内可见。

在 2~4 周内，可见白细胞浸润并形成隐窝脓肿（微脓肿），导致溃疡形成（图 41.1）。这种急性损伤可导致脂肪、碳水化合物、蛋白质、胆盐和维生素 B_{12} 的吸收受损，并导致水分、电解质和蛋白质的损失。回肠胆盐吸收受损会增加进入结肠的结合胆盐的负荷，这些胆盐被结肠细菌解偶联，导致管腔内盐和水的积聚以及随后的腹泻。此外，放疗照射后对乳糖的消化可能受损，导致细菌发酵增加，并因此导致胃肠胀气、腹胀和腹泻。另有证据表明放疗照射后胃肠动力也有明显改变[17]。

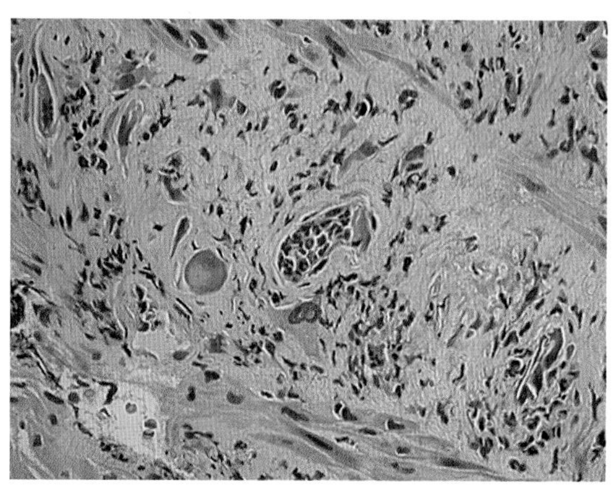

图 41.1　组织病理学显示微脓肿和放射相关成纤维细胞。黏膜下反应显示大的、奇异的放射成纤维细胞，同时有巨细胞和细胞核增大。平滑肌细胞也有反应性改变。由过量中性粒细胞组成的微脓肿浸润间质。（Courtesy Dr. Robin Amirkahn Dallas，TX.）

急性放射性肠炎患者出现腹泻、腹部绞痛或疼痛、恶心呕吐、厌食和乏力。放射诱导的腹泻常出现在分次放疗的第 3 周，据报道发病率为 20%~70%[18]。部分患者通过常规分次方式接受 18~22Gy 剂量照射后，可能会出现急性放射性肠病并腹泻，这与治疗第 3 周开始的时间相吻合，而接受 40Gy 的患者大多数可以出现以上反应。虽然有证据表明，急性小肠毒性的患者可能有更高的慢性反应风险，但症状和病理表现通常在放疗完成后 2~6 周消退[19]。

小肠慢性毒性的组织学改变包括进行性闭塞性血管病，表现为泡沫细胞侵犯动脉内膜和小动脉壁玻璃样增厚，伴有胶原沉积和纤维化。小肠变厚，出现毛细血管扩张，小动脉的血管壁破坏消失，造成组织缺血（图 41.2）[20]。随着血管病变的进展，可以看到黏膜溃疡、坏死，偶尔肠壁穿孔，导致瘘管和脓肿形成。淋巴组织损伤导致黏膜水肿和炎症。组织学上，黏膜萎缩，腺体不典型增生，肠壁纤维化（图 41.3）[21]。随着溃疡愈合，可能会出现纤维化及肠腔变窄，随后形成狭窄，甚至出现狭窄近端肠道扩张的肠梗阻。细菌过度生长可能是由狭窄近端的肠袢扩张淤滞引起的间接并发症。尽管受累的肠段和浆膜看起来有增厚，并有区域性的毛细血管扩张[22]，但应注意的是，即使肠道看起来正常，患者仍有自发性穿孔的风险[23]。

慢性放射性肠炎可导致严重的并发症。这种并发症往往是进行性的，至少在放疗后 6 个月出现。小肠的迟发放射性

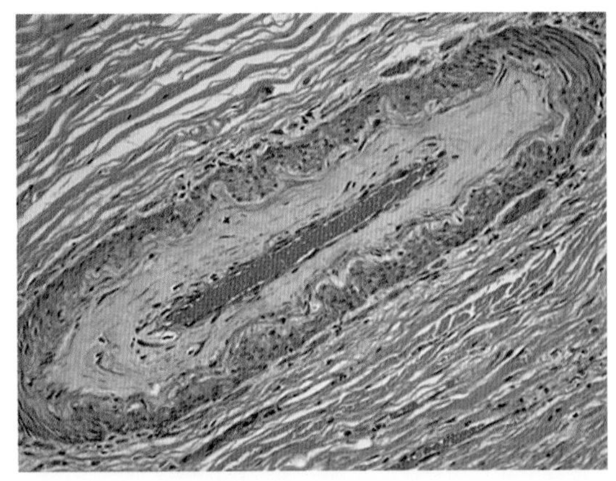

图 41.2　组织病理学显示慢性放射性肠病的黏膜下小动脉。辐射引起的变化包括血管壁增厚、血管内膜下水肿变化和纤维化，导致血管腔狭窄和闭塞，以及随后的组织缺血。（Courtesy Dr, Robin Amirkahn, Dallas, TX.）

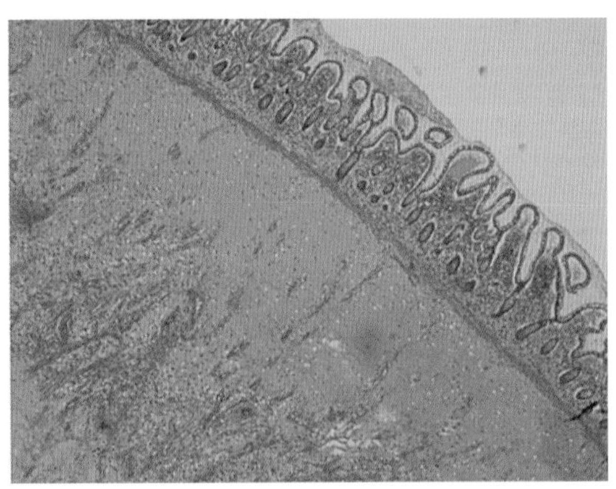

图 41.3　组织病理学显示放疗后小肠黏膜下纤维化。由于该狭窄患者出现小肠梗阻。（Courtesy Dr. Robin Amirkahn, Dallas, TX.）

损伤出现的中位时间是在放疗后的 8～12 个月，也可能出现在数年后[24]。放射性肠炎的慢性阶段有许多临床表现（表 41.1）。肠纤维化和血管炎可能导致运动障碍、狭窄形成和吸收不良[25,26]。受累肠段可以出现蠕动加快，这可能会导致慢性营养不良，并进一步导致贫血和低蛋白血症。吸收不良和其他并发症可能需要外科手术和肠外营养。严重的慢性放射性肠炎患者长期预后差，死亡率约为 10%[27-32]。

表 41.1　慢性放射性肠炎或直肠炎的临床并发症

并发症	损害	临床特征
梗阻	狭窄	便秘、恶心、呕吐、餐后腹痛
感染	脓肿	腹痛、发热、寒战、败血症、腹膜炎
瘘管形成	瘘管	粪便、阴道或膀胱分泌物；气尿
出血	溃疡	直肠疼痛、里急后重、直肠出血、贫血
吸收不良	小肠损伤	腹泻、脂肪泻、体重减轻、营养不良、恶病质

From Girvent M, Carlson GL, Anderson I, et al. Intestinal failure after surgery for complicated radiation enteritis. Ann R Coll Surg Engl 2000;82:198-201.

慢性放射性肠炎的总体发病率还没有得到准确确定。回顾性的系列研究显示发病率为 20%，但这些研究通常包括大量在放疗结束后到研究结束前失去随访或死亡的患者[33]。一篇关于直肠癌辅助放疗随机试验的综述显示，严重的长期并发症可低至 1.2%，高达 15%，这与以前的研究结果相比有了很大的改进，表明技术进步降低了慢性小肠毒性发生率[34]。

已经发现某些因素使患者易出现放疗引起的小肠毒性。女性、老年患者和体形较瘦的患者的直肠子宫陷凹（男性为直肠膀胱陷凹）中可能有大量小肠，这会增加盆腔恶性肿瘤治疗中放射性损伤的可能性[35]。有盆腔炎性疾病或子宫内膜异位症病史的患者也有较高的辐射并发症风险[36,37]。曾做过腹部手术的患者可能会出现粘连，从而降低小肠的活动度，使其持续暴露于分次的放疗[38,39]。此外，有盆腔手术的患者可能会增加骨盆内的小肠数量。在 Eifel 及其同事发表的一系列文章中，先前接受过剖腹手术的女性出现小肠并发症的风险明显升高[40]。

吸烟者、糖尿病、高血压和心血管疾病的患者，也有增加原有血管损伤或闭塞的风险[41]。慢性辐射损伤的病理变化（包括血管病变和缺血）使这些共存疾病加重，使患者易于罹患与辐射相关的小肠毒性损伤。胶原血管病和炎症性肠病患者有较高的急性和慢性放射性损伤风险。这些疾病的患者可能有病理改变，包括透壁纤维化、胶原沉积和黏膜炎症浸润。放疗对小肠的后期效应可能是对这些先前存在的变化的继续累积效应，研究表明这些患者对放疗的胃肠道耐受性较低[42,43]。炎症性肠病（IBD）或非恶性全身性疾病处于静止状态或得到良好控制的患者比疾病活动状态的患者表现出更好的耐受性。

研究还探讨了辐射剂量对小肠毒性发生的影响。治疗野体积、受照小肠体积、总剂量、分剂量、治疗时间和放疗技术均影响小肠耐受性。一小段小肠的 TD5/5（治疗 5 年时毒性风险为 5% 的剂量）估计为 50Gy。患者一般可接受 45～50Gy 的盆腔照射，每日 1.8～2Gy，无明显毒性[44]。对接受 CRT 治疗的局部晚期胰腺癌患者的回顾性分析发现，每 1mL 十二指肠最大剂量不超过 55Gy 是预防长期毒性的重要指标[45]。

对于术后患者，5 周接受 45～50Gy 的辐射量，出现需要手术的小肠梗阻的发病率约为 5%。而剂量大于 50Gy 时，发病率高达 25%～50%[35]。术后分次剂量大于 2Gy 也会增加毒性风险[46]。在放射剂量为 70Gy 或更高时，毒性发生率急剧上升[47]。

研究分析了接受基于 5-氟尿嘧啶（5-FU）的 CRT 治疗直肠癌患者的急性小肠毒性相关的剂量-体积参数，发现在每个被分析的剂量水平上，急性毒性与小肠受照射的体积之间存在强烈的相关性[48,49]。一项旨在使用不同治疗技术尽量减少盆腔辐射对小肠影响的研究表明，照射较小体积的肠道产生的毒性较小[50]。此外，对俯卧位患者辅以腹外加压和充盈膀胱，可减少副作用，可能是由于小肠的一部分被挤出照射野之外（图 41.4）[51]。

CRT 通常与 5-FU 或卡培他滨同时使用，用于治疗胃肠道恶性肿瘤，已知这可增加小肠毒性的风险。在法国癌症学联合会消化试验中，患者随机接受单纯放疗或 CRT 联合 5-FU

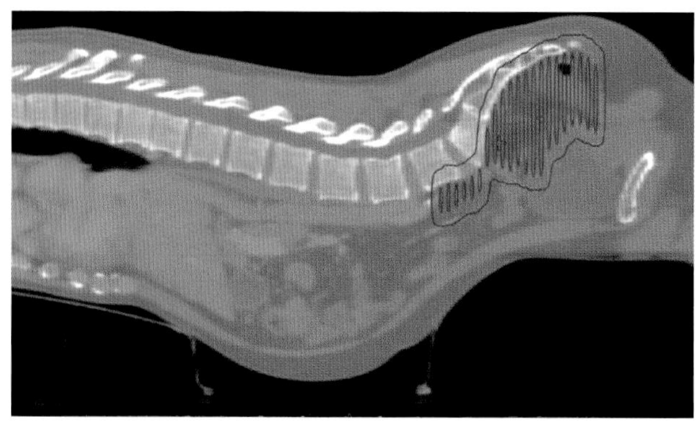

图 41.4　图像来自对直肠癌患者进行的计划扫描。患者俯卧于腹板上，这使得小肠从计划处方剂量的解剖区域脱离（用红色表示）

和甲酰四氢叶酸，放疗组的急性毒性发生率为 2.7%，在放疗基础上加用化疗组的急性毒性发生率为 14.6%[52]。由欧洲癌症研究和治疗组织进行的第二项试验，对术前放疗或 CRT 加或不加辅助化疗的晚期直肠癌患者随机进行研究。加用化疗导致 3 级急性毒性发生率更高（13.9% vs 7.4%）。在同时接受化疗的患者中，2 级腹泻的发生率更高（37.6% vs 17.3%），晚期毒性无差异[53]。

目前正在研究将新型化疗和“靶向”药物与放疗整合在胃肠道肿瘤的新辅助治疗中。将奥沙利铂纳入新辅助治疗方案的早期Ⅱ期研究取得了有希望的结果，但在随后的随机试验中则显示这样的毒性更大，而对疾病没有益处[52,54]。来自使用伊立替康、VEGF 受体和 EGF 受体抑制剂等新型药物的Ⅰ期和Ⅱ期试验的数据表明，与常规新辅助放化疗方案药物相比，添加上述药物可显著提高 3 级和 4 级胃肠道毒性，进一步强调仔细制定放疗计划的重要性，以确保最大限度地保留这些患者的正常组织。

慢性（晚期）放射性肠病的临床诊断见表 41.2。症状出现的原因可能因人而异，诊断和治疗方法也应个体化。治疗方案见表 41.3。如果出现与放射性肠炎特征符合的临床表现，应向实施治疗的放射肿瘤科医生咨询。回顾患者先前的放疗记录可了解总剂量、分次剂量、照射体积和其他放疗参数。对治疗方案的分析可能会显示高剂量区域，尤其是如果

表 41.2　慢性（晚期）放射性肠病患者的病理生理特征及其临床表现

病理生理特征	临床表现
黏膜功能障碍	乳糖不耐受 维生素 B_{12} 缺乏性 脂肪泻
伴小肠细菌过度生长的狭窄或盲袢综合征	腹泻
肠道动力障碍	腹胀 便秘 腹泻
异常胆汁酸再循环	胆汁性腹泻

From Hauer-Jensen M, Wang J, Denham J. Bowel injury: current and evolving management strategies. Semin Radiat Oncol 2003;13:357-71.

表 41.3　慢性（晚期）放射性肠病患者的治疗选择

病理生理特征	治疗选择
营养缺乏	纠正特定营养缺乏
	低脂饮食
	无乳糖饮食
	要素饮食
	全肠外营养
肠道动力障碍（增加或减少）	洛哌丁胺
	奥曲肽
	促动力药
胆汁酸吸收不良	胆盐结合剂
小肠细菌过度生长	抗生素

From Hauer-Jensen M, Wang J, Denham J. Bowel injury: current and evolving management strategies. Semin Radiat Oncol 2003;13:357-71.

患者进行了腔内植入或近距离放疗。内镜检查或影像学检查中遇到的病变通常局限于高剂量区。黏膜溃疡、空肠皱襞增厚和肠袢增厚是提示小肠受到辐射损伤的放射学征象（图 41.5）。慢性放射性肠炎患者的肠道转运速度加快，胆汁酸和乳糖吸收减少[55]。服用洛哌丁胺后，这些作用可能会得到改善。如果有小肠细菌过度生长（SIBO）综合征，则应使用抗生素（见第 105 章）[56,57]。

（二）治疗和预防

急性放射性小肠毒性的处理应根据症状的严重程度。大多数急性放射性肠炎是自限性的，只需要支持性治疗。对腹泻、恶心、呕吐和腹部绞痛行对症治疗，可以使用止泻药物，如洛哌丁胺、地芬诺酯阿托品或阿片类等。止吐药也可能有效。低脂肪、无乳糖的饮食可以改善症状。一项对接受盆腔照射的患者口服硫糖铝的研究表明，在早期和晚期两个时间点，口服硫糖铝可降低排便次数，改善大便性状[58]。考来烯胺治疗胆汁酸吸收不良引起的腹泻也显示出一些益处[59]，阿司匹林治疗也有效[60]。在 CRT 期间，顽固性腹泻可能需要住院接受肠外液体和电解质补充。对常规止泻药物无效的患者，可通过使用人工合成的生长抑素类似物（如奥曲肽）获益[61]。

考虑到病理生理的渐进发展，包括闭塞性动脉内膜炎和纤维化，慢性放射性肠炎的治疗仍然是一个重大挑战。考虑到该过程的弥漫性和与手术相关的高发病率，治疗应该是保守的；但是，对于肠梗阻、穿孔、瘘管和严重出血，手术治疗是必要的。

慢性腹泻可通过少渣饮食进行对症治疗。在一些病例中，纤维补充剂（例如，美达施纤维粉、甲基纤维素）已显示出益处。在与慢性辐射损伤有关的营养不良这样的罕见情况下，全肠外营养（TPN）可改善临床结果，甲基泼尼松龙可增强 TPN 的效果[36]。尽管采取了这些干预措施，接受 TPN 的患者的 5 年生存率在 36% 到 54% 之间[32,62]。据估计，与慢性放射性肠炎相关的总死亡率约为 10%[63]。

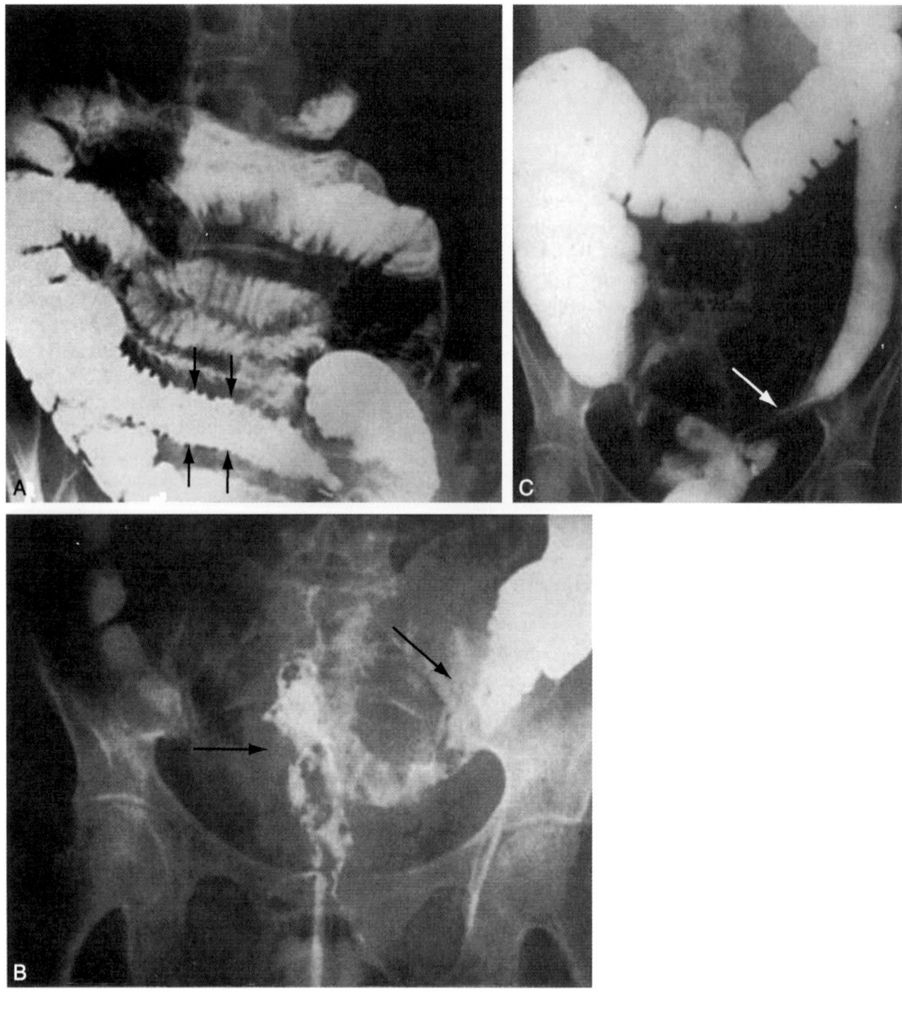

图 41.5　肠道放射性损伤的放射学证据。A,在早期损伤中,肠和肠系膜水肿可引起肠袢分离,导致黏膜皱襞增厚和变直,并使小肠黏膜呈尖峰状(箭)。B,患者接受宫颈癌放疗后 2 个月进行的钡灌肠,在该胶片上发现直肠乙状结肠明显严重异常。结肠亚急性辐射损伤可能表现为水肿,偶见黏膜溃疡合并不对称性狭窄区域,提示克罗恩病结肠炎或复发性肿瘤(箭)。C,结肠晚期放疗改变,累积剂量约 55Gy 后狭窄形成(箭)

有时需要应用内镜技术诊断出血性肠道溃疡。双气囊小肠镜和胶囊内镜检查有助于此诊断[64]。双气囊小肠镜可用于某些情况下的治疗干预,包括小肠毛细血管扩张症的凝固治疗。对内镜治疗无效的大出血可通过手术治疗。

小肠梗阻一般通过肠道休息和置管减压进行保守治疗。在极少数情况下,肠梗阻严重或呈明显慢性,可能需要肠切除术或粘连松解术。由于小肠及肠系膜发生弥漫性的纤维化和改建,慢性放射性小肠炎的手术难度大,有很高的手术并发症发病率及再次手术风险[65,66]。如果使用照射野内的肠段进行吻合术,则吻合口瘘的风险很高[63]。如果吻合口至少有一个肠段是先前未经放疗的肠段,则吻合口瘘的风险可以降低。然而,在手术时,甚至在病理评估时,可能很难区分正常组织和受照组织[67]。外科医生可以用来规避这一技术难题的另一种方法是与未经放疗的结肠进行吻合。术中内镜检查可发现放射性黏膜损伤,可提高肠损伤定位的准确性[68]。

我们的目标是有限度地切除病变的肠道,但如果病变过于弥漫,可以尝试旁路手术。如果可行的话,切除病变肠道比肠道旁路手术效果更好。然而,通过外科手术广泛切除病变的肠段可能导致短肠综合征(见第 106 章)及需要全肠外营养。在接受外科广泛小肠切除术的患者中,5 年生存率约为 65%,其中三分之二的患者脱离了肠外营养[69]。鉴于纤维化的进展,如果不进行广泛的外科切除,患者可能需要额外的手术。外科手术旁路绕开损伤的肠道可能出现盲袢综合征,由于受损伤的肠道持续存在,患者仍有穿孔、出血、脓肿和瘘管的风险。旁路手术应当在不能切除时进行,或作为在以后切除前的临时处理。手术应该由一个经验丰富的团队进行,他们熟悉放射性肠炎的处理。穿孔和瘘管最好通过手术治疗。需要注意的是,许多有慢性小肠放射毒性的患者营养缺乏,术后更容易发生吻合口瘘和裂开。这些患者的术后死亡率可能很高,在决定继续手术前必须考虑到这一点。

高压氧已被用于治疗慢性放射性肠炎,其基本原理是在缺氧组织中产生一个氧梯度将刺激新生血管生成[70,71]。在对 36 例药物治疗反应不佳的严重放射性肠炎患者的回顾性研究中,三分之二接受了高压氧治疗的患者的临床症状有改善[72]。高压氧可能有助于治疗因慢性放射性肠炎而导致的出血,这些患者不能通过诸如福尔马林和激光治疗(稍后讨论）等保守措施得以控制[73,74]。一项临床病例系列对 65 例以慢性出血为主要表现的慢性放射性肠炎（小肠和直肠）患者采用高压氧治疗。直肠和近端部位的有效率分别为 65%和 73%。对控制出血的有效率为 70%，对缓解其他症状（疼痛、腹泻、体重减轻、瘘管、梗阻）的有效率为 58%。作者的结论是，高压氧治疗使三分之二的慢性放射性肠炎患者的临床症状显著改善[75]。

其他降低慢性放射性肠炎发病率的药物也被研究过。有人认为己酮可可碱可能通过抗氧化作用和抑制 TGF-β1 来消除放射性纤维化。在一项小型研究中，用己酮可可碱和维生素 E 治疗放射性肠炎，并用主观、客观、管理、分析量表评估疗效。通过主观、客观、管理和分析量表评估，40%的患者在 6 个月时以及 80%的患者在 18 个月时出现症状消退[76]。

鉴于慢性放射性肠炎比较复杂且很难治愈，所以预防其发生是关键，使用减少其发病率的措施势在必行。胰酶可加剧急性肠道辐射毒性，使用合成生长抑素受体类似物（如奥曲肽）减少胰腺分泌可减少动物研究中的早期和迟发性放射性肠炎[77]。放射性损伤的主要危险因素之一是先前的腹盆腔手术，这会导致小肠脱垂到盆腔并暴露在照射野中。术前或术后实行放疗和化疗需要外科、放射科和肿瘤科医生密切合作。如果在手术中意外发现肿瘤残留，用金属夹标记肿瘤床有利于术后放疗计划的实施。另外，术中使用一些手术技术（例如大网膜成形术或聚乙醇补片）使小肠尽量离开盆腔，可能会显著降低并发症的发生。

正常小肠通常是活动的，术后粘连肠管活动受限，可能会增加受照射的小肠体积。如果术后预计会进行放疗，则应在手术时尝试将肠道移到照射野之外[78]。一种简单的技术是手术放置聚乙醇、可生物降解的补片，将小肠移出骨盆[79,80]。这种手术的并发症发病率很低，不会显著增加手术时间。也不需要第二次手术来移除补片，因为补片在术后 3~4 个月会被吸收。磁共振成像可以在手术后用来确认补片和小肠的位置，以及补片的最终消失。手术中放置补片可使暴露在照射野的小肠体积减小 50%，允许术后根据需要给予更高剂量的辐射[81,82]。其他技术，如骨盆重建、网膜成形术、结肠移位也可显著减少放疗时暴露的肠体积[82-84]。

放疗技术是降低并发症发生率的关键。由于照射剂量大，被辐射肠道体积大，应尽可能避免仅使用前后野进行盆腔放疗。放疗的毒性与受照小肠的体积有关[85]。在许多患者中，俯卧位治疗时应用"腹压板"可使小肠脱离照射野[86,87]。应指导患者在放疗期间保持膀胱充盈，这进一步将肠道移出骨盆[38]。三维（3D）治疗计划通过更精确的剂量分布来优化治疗技术。3D 放疗算法可通过精确地使用多个形状的多个照射野照射到目标体积，确保了正常组织免受过量辐射剂量[88]。此外，更现代的技术，如调强放疗（intensity-modulated radiotherapy，IMRT）可使用复杂的放疗技术来避免重要器官受到损害。

放射性肠炎的治疗往往只能部分成功。治疗需要个体化并应尽可能保守，因为病情是持续发展的，并可能会因该区域的进一步损伤而恶化。更好地了解纤维化的机制以及控制细胞凋亡和纤维化的分子事件之间的相互作用，可能有助于识别有辐射并发症风险的患者，并有助于开发新的治疗方法。

四、食管

（一）发病率和临床特征

食管的早期和晚期效应通常发生在胸部和上腹部恶性肿瘤（如食管/食管胃交界处癌、肺癌）放疗后。正常食管黏膜持续更新。急性食管损伤被认为主要与基底上皮层的辐射损伤有关，组织学上表现为空泡化，导致上皮变薄，随后剥脱（图 41.6）。这些变化在临床上表现为吞咽困难、吞咽疼痛和胸骨后不适，通常发生在放疗开始后 2~3 周内。患者可能会出现突然的、尖锐的、剧烈的胸痛，并放射到背部。随着治疗的推进，疼痛可能会持续，不一定与吞咽有关。这些症状可能与念珠菌性食管炎混淆，后者可能与放射性食管炎合并发生。同时化疗会加重这些毒性作用。内镜检查可能会观察到黏膜炎症和溃疡形成。急性期很少发生穿孔和出血[89]。治疗结束后不久，基底细胞增殖恢复并再生[90]。若同时给予化疗与放疗，这样的方案在肺癌和食管癌中常见，3 级或更严重的急性食管炎的发病率可增加约 5 倍[91]。

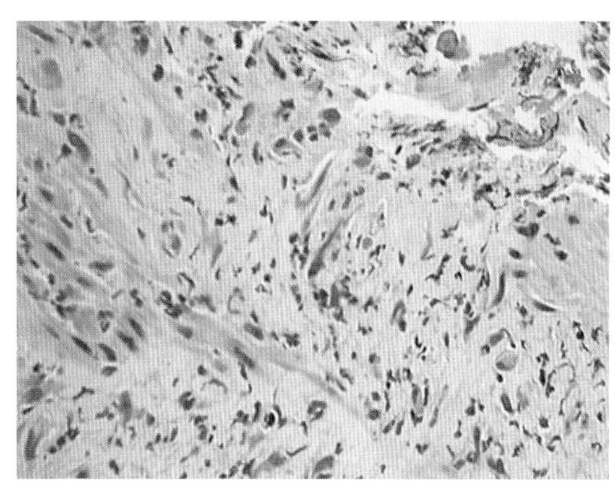

图 41.6　急性放射性食管损伤的组织病理学显示食管溃疡伴大量的成纤维细胞

急性损伤恢复后，治疗后数月至数年内可能会出现良性狭窄导致持续性吞咽困难、溃疡和瘘管形成。这些主要是由于炎症和食管肌层内瘢痕的形成所致。随着时间的推移，食管周围的结缔组织也可能表现出严重的纤维化，内镜下可以看到小血管毛细血管扩张。先前曾接受照射患者的食管组织学检查显示上皮增厚、慢性炎症、黏膜下层和固有肌层纤维化，但很少有慢性溃疡。受损上皮从辐射效应中完全恢复可能需要 3~24 个月[21]。晚期效应通常表现为狭窄引起的吞咽困难，以及纤维化或肌肉损伤导致的运动改变，还可能伴有神经损伤。瘘管形成并不常见，与辐射剂量相关。钡餐检查可显示受照射食管段的狭窄和蠕动中断，在受照区域上下有重复波和非蠕动波出现。据报道，在治疗结束后 1~3 个月出现异常蠕动，而大多数狭窄发生在治疗结束后的 4~8 个月。晚期效应通常在放疗完成后 3 个月才出现，在一些系列病例中，发病时间中位数为 6 个月[24,92,93]。

辐射相关晚期并发症的发生与剂量相关。关于急性放射性食管炎对不同剂量分割方案依赖性的许多随机数据来自肺癌试验。在局限期小细胞肺癌患者中进行的组间 0096 试验比较了 CRT 方案,即在 3 周内每日输送两次 1.5Gy 的治疗分割,与在 5 周内每日输送一次 1.8Gy 的治疗分割,与相同的总剂量 45Gy。在每日接受 2 次治疗的组中,3 级食管炎的发生率几乎是 3 倍[94]。在放疗肿瘤组(RTOG)0617 试验中,比较总剂量 60Gy 与 74Gy 治疗局部晚期非小细胞肺癌,也观察到 3 级或更高级别食管炎在 74Gy 组增加了 3 倍[95]。历史上,当食管长度的三分之一接受辐照时,TD5/5(即 5% 的患者将在 5 年时发生并发症的剂量)估计为 60Gy[96]。建议平均食管照射剂量保持在 34Gy 以下,同时将治疗的食管部分限制在不超过 60Gy[97]。

很少有食管癌的随机试验报告晚期食管毒性。在 RTOG 0113 号研究中,使用 50.4Gy 的放疗剂量联合化疗,严重晚期食管毒性的发生率为 12%(3% 出现 5 级毒性,即死亡)[98]。在 RTOG 85-01 中,这是一项随机试验,比较了剂量为 64Gy 的单纯放疗和剂量为 50Gy 的 CRT,在每个组中近 20% 的患者经历了严重的晚期食管毒性[99]。最近对采用现代计划技术治疗的患者进行的分析发现,长期性的食管并发症显著减少[100]。

近距离放疗(将放射源暂时插入肿瘤或肿瘤附近)也被用作食管癌放疗加量的技术。尽管一些机构报告了近距离放疗发生瘘的概率较低。但是 Gaspar 及其同事报告了一项Ⅰ/Ⅱ期研究的结果,该研究检查了在进行外照射放疗时加用近距离放疗在食管癌治疗中的作用。1 年的食管瘘发生率为 18%,因此作者建议谨慎使用这种方法,尤其是在同时进行化疗的情况下[101,102]。一个更加近期的对 62 名患者的病例系列的研究发现,同时接受外照射和近距离放疗可导致 16% 的严重毒性反应,包括溃疡、狭窄、食管穿孔、瘘管和急性食管出血[102]。

癌症治疗的强度增加,例如同时使用化疗和放疗,会增加急性食管炎的发生率[103]。Maguire 及其同事评估了 91 例接受放疗的非小细胞肺癌患者,发现食管放疗时受照区域接受的照射剂量大于 50Gy 时预示着晚期食管毒性增加。既往有胃食管反流病(GERD)和继发于肿瘤的食管糜烂患者发生晚期毒性的风险亦增加。超分割(每天多次放疗)也与急性毒性增加有关[104]。Singh 及其同事研究了非小细胞肺癌患者,这些患者每天接受适形放疗,同时接受或不同时接受化疗。他们发现最大食管"点"剂量 69Gy(单独放疗)和 58Gy(同时化疗)预示着显著的毒性发生。26% 同时接受放疗及化疗的患者出现 3 级或更高的食管毒性,而仅接受放疗治疗的患者仅有 1.3% 出现这种程度的毒性[105]。

Ahn 及其同事发现,在 254 例非小细胞肺癌患者中,晚期食管毒性的最有力预测因子是急性食管毒性的严重程度。严重急性毒性可通过每日两次的照射、更大的年龄、淋巴结分期增加和各种剂量学参数进行预测。总的迟发性毒性发生率为 7%,中位和最长发病时间分别为 5 个月和 40 个月[92]。Wei 和同事评估了 215 名同时接受化疗的患者,发现相对食管容积接受大于 20Gy 的照射可预测 3 级或更严重的急性毒性,第二组发现当超过 30% 的食管容积接受大于 50Gy(V50)时,这将导致 1 级或更高的急性毒性[106,107]。根据这些和其他数据,很明显,在放疗中同时进行化疗会增加急性和慢性食管毒性的发生率。

(二)治疗与预防

随着积极的联合化疗和放疗方案的应用,放射性食管炎的治疗和预防越来越受到重视。中断治疗可以缓解急性食管炎的症状,但也可能降低治疗效果,通常只适用于严重病例。急性食管炎的治疗通常包括对症治疗,如应用局部麻醉药(包括基于黏性利多卡因方案)、口服镇痛药(包括抗炎药和麻醉药)、胃抑酸药(组胺阻滞剂、质子泵抑制剂)、促动力剂(如甲氧氯普胺),以及治疗重叠感染(念珠菌病)。调整饮食,包括清淡的食物、糊状或松软的食物和汤,可以帮助患者保证摄食量。其他的调整包括避免吸烟、酒精、咖啡、辛辣或酸性食物、薯条、饼干和高脂肪食物。一项针对放射性食管炎的研究报告认为,饮食调整和药物预防可以使治疗毒性降低,使治疗中断减少。建议在两餐之间饮水,每天少食多餐吃 6 顿,主要包括半固体食物、汤、高热量补充剂、果泥、布丁、牛奶和软面包[108]。此外,如果可能,应避免摄入热的或冷的食物;相反,食物和液体应保持在室温水平。在严重情况下,可能需要放置鼻饲管。

研究认为辐射防护化学制剂可以减轻辐射引起的正常组织毒性。研究得最多的放射性保护剂阿米福汀是一种有机硫代磷酸盐。这种药物是一种自由基清除剂,可作为核酸烷基化或铂类药物的替代靶点[109]。试验结果相互矛盾,并受患者人数较少的限制[110-114]。在最大的随机试验中,接受化疗和放疗治疗的非小细胞肺癌患者被随机分为接受阿米福汀或不接受该药治疗。虽然阿米福汀不能显著降低 3 级或更高级别的食管炎,但患者自我评估表明,接受阿米福汀治疗的患者急性食管炎发病率显著降低。然而,接受阿米福汀的患者出现恶心、呕吐、感染、发热性中性粒细胞减少症和心脏事件的发生率显著增高[115]。鉴于此,不建议常规使用阿米福汀预防放射性食管炎[116]。

第二种放射性保护剂谷氨酰胺引起了大家的兴趣。在高分解代谢状态下、如癌症,谷氨酰胺缺乏可以持续进展。一项对 41 名肺癌患者的回顾性研究表明,患者对谷氨酰胺具有良好的耐受性,补充谷氨酰胺的患者 2~3 级食管炎的发病率较低,而且治疗期间体重增加[117]。来自同一机构的第二项分析评估了 104 名患者,其中 56 名患者接受谷氨酰胺治疗,谷氨酰胺组患者出现 3 级食管炎、治疗中断和体重减轻的比例较低,给药与达到终点事件时间的差异无关[118]。一项对 75 名患者的初步研究证实了回顾性数据:未出现谷氨酰胺不耐受或相关毒性。大多数(73%)接受序贯放化疗的患者,和 49% 同时接受放化疗的患者没有发生食管炎[119]。最近对 122 例晚期肺癌患者的回顾性分析表明,预防性使用谷氨酰胺治疗的患者急性食管炎明显减轻,因此,显著地防止了体重下降[120]。尽管谷氨酰胺几乎没有毒性,但在其广泛应用于临床实践之前,还需要对其疗效进行进一步评估。

晚期食管放射性狭窄的治疗包括一系列内镜扩张以改善症状。晚期狭窄扩张治疗可导致食管破裂,因此应谨慎处理。推荐长期使用抑酸药物以及甲氧氯普胺等促动力药物治疗胃食管反流。少数体重明显减轻无法维持体重的患者或只能摄入流食的患者,可能需要管饲。对于发生穿孔或瘘管的患者可能需要外科手术。最后,值得注意的是,与晚期放射性损伤相关的临床症状通常很难与复发或新的原发性恶性肿瘤所引起的症状相区分。对有狭窄或溃疡的患者也应该进行评估，以区分慢性放射性改变和癌症复发。

五、胃

（一）发病率和临床特征

上腹部癌症，包括食管-胃接合部、胃癌和胰腺癌等放疗后，胃可能会出现放射损伤。非常高的单次剂量照射动物的胃会导致糜烂性胃炎及胃溃疡。稍低的单次剂量会导致胃扩张和胃轻瘫，正常胃黏膜被角化过度的鳞状上皮替代。用更低的剂量照射后数月可以出现胃梗阻，在存活动物中可以观察到胃黏膜萎缩和肠化生[121]。

对消化性溃疡患者放疗后进行连续胃活检，发现主细胞和壁细胞坏死，以及黏膜变薄、水肿和慢性炎症浸润[24,122]。此外，相对低剂量的胃照射后，胃酸生成减少。在过去，放疗被用于减少消化性溃疡患者的胃酸量。即使是相对较低剂量 18Gy 分 10 次放疗，约 40% 的溃疡患者胃酸分泌减少 50%，持续 1 年或更长时间[123]。

临床上，放射性胃炎可能发生在放疗开始后一周内，显微镜下改变包括水肿、出血和渗出。组织学改变包括在治疗后 1 周内，壁细胞和主细胞中细胞质的细节和颗粒消失。细胞损伤和随后的细胞死亡通常首先出现在腺体的深处，随后胃黏膜变薄。其他的黏膜变化包括腺体凹陷加深和腺体颈部细胞增生。放疗第 3 周可见腺体结构丧失和黏膜增厚。组织学恢复大约从放疗结束后 3 周开始。早期胃放射性损伤恢复的征象包括上皮再生和纤维化。

急性放射性胃损伤的症状主要包括恶心呕吐、消化不良、厌食、腹痛和不适感。这些症状更常见于同时化疗的情况。辐射引起的恶心和呕吐可能发生在治疗后的最初 24 小时内。据估计，大约一半接受上腹部放疗的患者在放疗后 2~3 周内会出现呕吐[124]。

胃照射的晚期效应分为 4 类：①急性溃疡（发生在放疗完成后不久）；②胃镜下表现为黏膜皱襞平滑和黏膜萎缩的胃炎，伴有胃窦狭窄的影像学证据（照射后 1~12 个月）（见第 52 章）；③消化不良，包括模糊的胃症状，无明确的相关临床特征（放疗后 6 个月~4 年）；④迟发溃疡（放疗后平均 5 个月）[24,125]。用于整个胃的 TD5/5 剂量估计为 50Gy[96]。上腹部放疗的大型研究表明，先前的腹部手术以及分剂量每次使用更高剂量的辐射，可能会增加晚期效应的风险[126]。

沃尔特里德陆军医疗中心的研究表明，应用目前已经过时的技术对睾丸癌患者实施腹部放疗，高辐射剂量会增加迟发性胃溃疡和穿孔的风险，接受 45~50Gy 照射治疗的患者溃疡发生率约 6%，接受 50~60Gy 照射治疗的患者溃疡发生率约 10%，接受超过 60Gy 剂量的患者发生溃疡的比例为 38%。剂量小于 50Gy 和大于等于 50Gy 时，穿孔率分别为 2% 和 14%。有症状的胃炎发生在放疗完成后约 2 个月，溃疡形成的中位时间为 5 个月。在 233 例患者中，有 6 例（3%）患者因溃疡出血或溃疡疼痛需要外科手术治疗，这些患者几乎均接受大于 50Gy 的照射剂量[24,127]。另外一些关于霍奇金淋巴瘤、睾丸癌、胃癌或宫颈癌患者接受放疗的研究建立了胃承受辐射的耐受剂量[126-129]。这些研究的照射剂量分别从 40~60Gy。接受剂量大于 50Gy 的患者出现胃溃疡和胃溃疡相关穿孔的发生率分别为 15% 和 10%。需要指出的是，适形放疗对整个胃的剂量应限制在 45~50Gy，估计有 5%~7% 的严重辐射毒性风险，其中主要是发生溃疡[130]。

与食管一样，化疗与放疗联合应用可降低胃黏膜对放疗的耐受性。以 5-FU 为基础的化疗是与放疗同时进行的最常见的胃肠道肿瘤治疗药物。这种药物可以在辅助治疗或新辅助治疗环境下使用，或作为胃食管结合部癌、胃癌、胰周癌和胆管癌的“最终”治疗。5-FU 是一种辐射增敏剂，历史上曾安全地应用于 45~50Gy 剂量的放疗，毒性没有显著增加。较新的全身性药物，包括紫杉醇、吉西他滨和表皮生长因子受体抑制剂，已被证明在放疗时同时应用时会增加急性胃毒性。一项Ⅰ期研究评估了 5-FU、吉西他滨和放疗对局部晚期胰腺癌的疗效。在入选的 7 名患者中，3 名患者出现胃或十二指肠溃疡并严重出血，需要输血[131]。这些治疗方案仍然是腹部恶性肿瘤治疗研究的内容。

（二）治疗与预防

急性胃辐射中毒症状的治疗包括止吐药（5-羟色胺-3，5-HT3］拮抗剂、吩噻嗪类、甲氧氯普胺、糖皮质激素、苯二氮䓬类、抗组胺药或抗胆碱能药物），以及在接受放疗前少量进食。预防性 5-HT3 抑制剂的随机试验表明，与安慰剂相比，5-HT3 抑制剂在预防放射导致恶心呕吐方面有效[132]。一项对 211 名接受上腹部放疗的患者进行的随机试验，所有患者接受 5-HT3 抑制剂昂丹司琼每日两次，比较了在前 5 次分剂量放疗时同时每日应用或者不应用地塞米松。接受地塞米松治疗的患者在完全控制恶心上有改善的趋势（50% vs 38%），在呕吐的完全控制率上则有显著改善。作者的结论是，加入地塞米松后，对辐射引起的呕吐有适当的预防效果[133]。麻醉剂和非麻醉剂通常用于止痛。此外，建议患者使用抑酸药物，包括质子泵抑制剂。细心的营养支持加上止吐治疗对腹部放疗患者是必不可少的。急性症状一般在放疗完成后 1 至 2 周内消失。

晚期胃炎相关症状通常用抑酸药，包括组胺拮抗剂和质子泵抑制剂，和/或硫糖铝治疗。这些药物可以长期使用，以避免迟发性溃疡形成。由于出血、溃疡、胃出口梗阻、瘘管形成或穿孔等更严重的并发症，患者可能需要内镜治疗，或者极少数情况下需要进行胃部分切除手术。

六、结肠和直肠

（一）发病率和临床特征

大肠的放射敏感性比小肠低。然而，大肠的急性和慢性损伤的基本机制与小肠损伤相似。干细胞有丝分裂率降低，导致上皮细胞正常脱落并再生时所需的前体细胞减少。急性损伤可伴有浅表黏膜糜烂和固有层出血。另外，还会出现黏膜增厚及成纤维细胞增生（图 41.7）[134]。晚期变化包括血管纤维化伴缺血和毛细血管扩张的形成，这可能是出血的来源

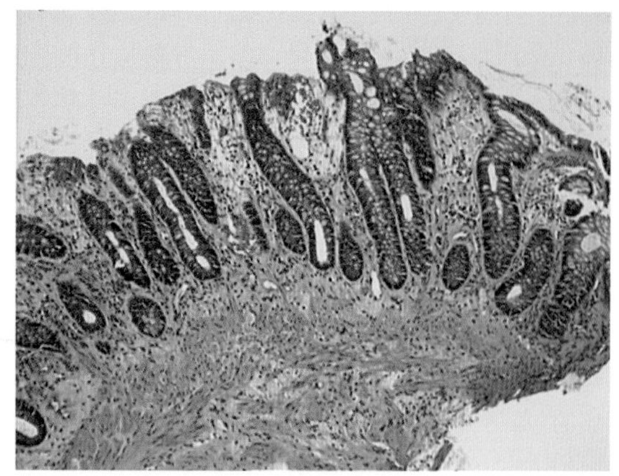

图 41.7 直肠急性放射性损伤伴浅表性直肠黏膜糜烂和局灶性固有层出血的组织病理学表现。(Courtesy Dr. Robin Amirkahn, Dallas, TX.)

(图 41.8)。晚期放射性大肠改变可导致液体和电解质吸收障碍、梗阻、慢性直肠炎和瘘管形成。缺血性改变还包括溃疡(图 41.9)、穿孔和瘘管[22]。肠壁纤维化可能会发生,导致运动性和顺应性下降,以及狭窄[135]。直肠顺应性降低可降低直肠蓄积粪便的能力,导致大便频次增加、急迫和失禁。

急性放射性结肠炎的临床表现包括腹泻、腹部绞痛、里急后重、大便急迫、大便失禁,以及少见的黏液脓血便。这些症状可由直肠炎症、水肿和痉挛引起。症状通常在治疗后 2~3 周开始,在照射完成后的数周至 3 个月内消失。急性和慢性放射性损伤的发病率之间的关系尚不确定[136,137]。慢性改变出现在放疗完成后 6 个月至 2 年或更久,症状与急性损伤相似。患者可能表现为里急后重、出血、少量的腹泻、直肠疼痛,偶尔出现轻度梗阻或瘘管(见表 41.1)[138]。患者可发展为类似 IBD 的全结肠炎症。此外,盆腔照射是直肠癌发生的一个

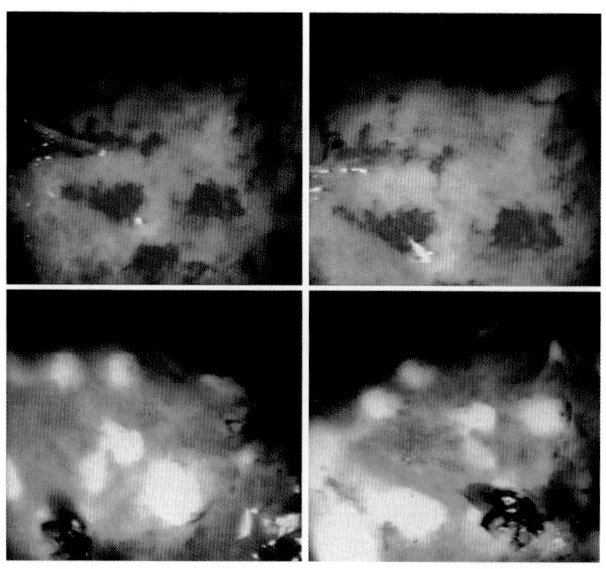

图 41.8 接受前列腺癌治疗的患者放射性直肠炎的典型结肠镜检查结果。上图,直肠内镜视图显示了新生血管的特征性细微迂曲和卷曲。下图,显示了氩等离子体凝固造成的浅表烧伤,用于该患者的止血。不需要完全消融病变,而只需造成黏膜和黏膜下纤维化,从而使血管陷入瘢痕环过程。(Courtesy Lawrence J. Brandt, MD, Bronx, New York.)

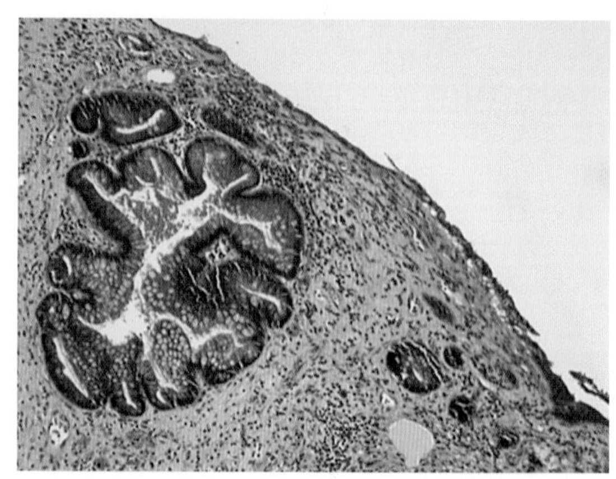

图 41.9 放疗后直肠黏膜的组织病理学,在放射性直肠溃疡区域可见残留畸形的直肠隐窝和平坦、再生的表面黏膜。注意固有层的纤维化和炎症。(Courtesy Dr. Robin Amirkahn, Dallas, TX.)

危险因素,有证据表明接受前列腺放疗的患者患直肠癌的风险与直肠癌一级亲属相似[139]。

与小肠相比,结肠和直肠的放射敏感性较低,直肠上相对较小的体积接受更高的放射剂量的事实可以部分解释这样的情况(如前列腺癌和妇科癌症治疗中的病灶"旁"直肠照射)。直肠也是一个容易通过内镜检查的器官,可以做到早期诊断和干预,这样可能会防止症状恶化。有数据表明,尽管直肠黏膜改变在治疗后 5 年时仍然存在,但在并发症和黏膜改变消失后通常会恢复[140]。

一系列报道表明,当照射剂量少于 80Gy 时,严重的晚期直肠并发症的风险为 5% 或更低[24]。大肠的辐射损伤最常见于直肠,因为它靠近前列腺、膀胱、宫颈、子宫和卵巢,因此在治疗这些疾病时,直肠受到附带的照射[21]。急性直肠损伤通常是自限性的,但慢性放射性直肠炎的发病率随着盆腔放疗次数和照射剂量的增加而增加[141,142]。

与其他部位一样,大肠毒性的发生率与放射剂量、接受放疗的体积和同期化疗的使用有关。直肠癌的治疗通常使用 45~54Gy 的剂量,而前列腺癌和宫颈癌的治疗则使用 60~80Gy 的更高剂量。宫颈癌患者严重直肠乙状结肠毒性的发生率在接受剂量小于 80Gy 的患者中为 4% 或更低,在大于 95Gy 的患者中为 13%[143]。治疗前列腺癌的剂量为 60~70Gy 时,严重直肠炎的发生率低于 8%[144]。放疗剂量为 60~70Gy 的肛管癌患者的严重直肠毒性发生率为 5% 或更少[145-147]。

总的来说,建议少于 20% 的直肠接受大于 70Gy 的剂量,相应 2 级或更高级别的直肠毒性发生率为 6%~23%[148]。使用适形放射、3 野和 4 野技术进行放疗进一步降低了直肠毒性的风险[143,149]。一项研究表明前列腺癌适形放疗与常规放疗相比放射性直肠炎更少(分别为 5% 和 15%)[150]。一项对近 1 000 例接受照射剂量高于 80Gy 的前列腺癌患者的最新分析表明,IMRT 的使用可能会进一步降低放射性直肠炎的发生率。治疗后 7 年时 2 级或更高直肠毒性的精确发生率为 4.4%,晚期 3 级毒性的发生率为 0.7%,没有患者出现 4 级毒性[151]。即使是中度及重度的小分割放疗,包括立体定向体放疗(stereotactic body radiotherapy, SBRT),已成为前列腺癌治

疗中更常用的方法，在现代放疗技术和图像引导下，晚期胃肠道毒性发生率仍保持在可接受的低水平[152,153]。

联合化疗和放疗会增加毒性发生率。5-FU、丝裂霉素 C 联合使用 40~55Gy 的辐射剂量治疗肛管癌，其严重直肠并发症的风险低于 5%[154]。多个试验联合以 5-FU 为基础的化疗和放疗作为直肠癌的新辅助和辅助治疗[155-158]。联合化疗和放疗的治疗毒性表现从不显著增加到表现为 24% 出现严重腹泻和 25% 出现慢性肠损伤[159]。考虑到使用单野或对穿野时毒性的增加，使用联合治疗时有必要使用适形和多野技术。尽管一项大型随机试验显示，接受新辅助治疗的患者的急性和慢性胃肠道毒性的发生率显著降低，但越来越多的新辅助放化疗的使用也引起了对这些患者术后并发症增加的担忧[158,160]。

与小肠损伤不同，先前的腹盆腔手术似乎并不会使直肠更倾向于受到辐射损伤，这可能是因为直肠本身不可移动。考虑到与小肠辐射损伤类似的血管变化，糖尿病、高血压、心血管疾病或外周血管疾病的患者可能更易出现大肠辐射毒性[41-43,161]。胶原血管病和 IBD 患者也有大肠辐射毒性增加的倾向。

（二）治疗与预防

大肠辐射毒性的治疗以症状控制为基础。急性毒性可用抗动力药物治疗，如洛哌丁胺或地芬诺酯与阿托品和少渣饮食。阿片类和抗胆碱能药物也可能有益。含糖皮质激素的栓剂可能有助于肛门直肠炎症患者的治疗。因为放疗期间，直肠黏膜脆弱可能导致穿孔，应尽可能避免结肠镜检查[162]。建议在前列腺近距离放疗之前进行筛查性结肠镜检查，以减少直肠并发症[163]。这也是开始外照射放疗之前的合理步骤。

对于因直肠顺应性下降引起的慢性腹泻，大便软化剂或纤维补充剂可以缓解症状。与急性直肠炎一样，糖皮质激素栓剂可能是有益的。糖皮质激素保留灌肠的益处尚不清楚[164]。短链脂肪酸和氨基酸衍生物可滋养和保护结肠黏膜，其在急性放射性直肠炎中的作用也有被研究[165]。经治疗，症状能够得到初步缓解，但停止治疗后症状很快就会复发[166]。高压氧已用于稳定毛细血管扩张相关的出血，但这种治疗方法并不广泛可行，并且需要多次治疗才能见到效果[167]。尽管如此，一项针对难治性慢性放射性直肠炎患者的随机试验报告，高压氧治疗显著促进愈合[168]。

结直肠溃疡合并出血的最初治疗是内镜下使用凝固技术，如氩离子凝固。放射性直肠炎引起的出血通常是轻微的，通常通过内镜下的保守方法控制出血，如用激光烧灼治疗毛细血管扩张症（见图 41.8）[169]。应用福尔马林或用口服抗生素进行结肠灌洗可产生长期疗效[170-174]。硫糖铝灌肠可通过与直肠黏膜形成保护复合物来减轻放射性直肠炎。它还能增加局部成纤维细胞生长因子和前列腺素水平。硫糖铝灌肠似乎有助于慢性直肠病变，但其益处在急性期尚不清楚[175-177]。短链脂肪酸灌肠也可通过抑制炎症反应（包括核因子 κB 通路）来帮助治疗慢性出血性放射性直肠病变[178,179]。

狭窄也可以通过内镜扩张。对于难治性出血、狭窄、穿孔或肠瘘的患者，可能很少需要外科手术治疗。盆腔瘘（如阴道瘘或膀胱瘘）的处理很复杂，需要在矫正手术前先进行粪便改道术。术前应进行彻底的放射学检查，包括钡灌肠、小肠示踪检查或小肠造影，以确定瘘管的范围。我们处理瘘管患者时可能会遇到额外的挑战，如电解质失衡、营养不良和感染。修复瘘管有许多外科技术，但是矫正手术最好是在患者身体稳定和改造手术后足够的时间时进行。这有助于伤口愈合以及受影响组织的炎性减轻[180,181]。

预防放射性大肠毒性的研究发现前列腺素是潜在的放射保护剂。前列腺素 E_2 和前列腺素类似物在动物实验中显示出辐射防护作用[182-185]。临床上也证明米索前列醇栓剂可以减轻前列腺癌放疗患者的急性放射性肠炎症状。然而，一项来自德国的随机安慰剂对照试验发现，在接受放疗的前列腺癌患者中，米索前列醇组出现直肠出血的患者明显增多[186,187]。

有研究应用阿米福汀预防慢性放射性肠炎，并在临床前研究中证明其对小肠和大肠有保护作用[188]。还有研究证明该药可以减少多个解剖部位的早期和迟发放疗损伤的发生率。在一项随机研究中，接受阿米福汀肠外给药组的放疗后晚期损伤显著减少[189]。然而，中位随访时间很短（24 个月），考虑到晚期肠道并发症的发生率随着时间的推移而增加，需要更长时间的随访来确认药物的益处。另一项随机试验评估了 205 例盆腔恶性肿瘤患者，他们单独接受放疗或同时静脉注射阿米福汀。接受阿米福汀治疗的患者 2 级和 3 级膀胱和下消化道毒性的发生率显著降低，两组之间在肿瘤对治疗的反应方面没有显著差异[190]。也有证据表明，直肠内应用阿米福汀可降低前列腺癌的放疗患者发生直肠炎的风险[191]。在一项Ⅱ期研究中，患者在盆腔放疗的同时接受预防性阿米福汀治疗，在放疗开始前、放疗结束后以及 6~9 个月后进行乙状结肠镜检查。接受阿米福汀治疗的患者发生组织学上可检测到的黏膜病变的比例较小。放射性结肠炎的发病率在阿米福汀放疗组为 29%，没有使用阿米福汀的放疗组为 52%[192]。

一项临床前研究表明，抗 TGF-β1 干预治疗可减少迟发性放射性纤维化和肠病[193]。许多特殊饮食和营养素，如膳食纤维、要素饮食、短链脂肪酸和氨基酸（如谷氨酰胺）可降低对肠道的辐射毒性。但是，没有观察到一致的临床结果[194-198]。预防性治疗必须具有高效、低毒、低成本的特点，并且不能保护肿瘤免受放疗的影响。不幸的是，目前还没有一种有效的治疗方法能够达到所有这些目标。如前所述，优化的照射计划和具体照射方式至关重要。

七、肛门

（一）发病率及临床特征

除了治疗肛管癌、低位直肠癌和妇科癌症外，肛管通常不会受到严重的辐射照射。肛管癌放疗的主要急性毒性是大肠暴露引起的腹泻。对于肛门自身的损伤，一般表现为黏膜剥离及溃烂，随后继续发展为溃疡、狭窄、肛门直肠瘘，以及大便失禁[199]。放疗所致肛门毒性的数据的主要来源为应用放疗或放化疗治疗肛管癌的研究。肛门毒性表现为黏膜水肿和变脆[200]。这些变化通常因直肠毒性引起的腹泻而加剧。肛门纤维化可能会慢性发展。

肛门毒性最初表现为肛周皮肤反应，从轻微的皮肤变化和红斑到湿性脱屑和腹泻。这些变化具有自限性，通常在治疗结束后的几周内就会缓解。急性毒性可导致治疗中断，尽管这在现代放疗技术中可能不太常见[200-202]。急性毒性的发生率很高，并且随着同时进行化疗或因使用较大的分割剂量而增加[146,154,203,204]。一些Ⅲ期研究和对一系列联合化疗和放疗的患者的研究发现，在使用45～60Gy照射剂量（分割剂量为1.8～2.25Gy）的患者中，26%至78%的患者出现3级或更严重的皮肤毒性[154,199,201,205-207]。与先前的随机试验结果相比较，多个机构的经验显示，在肛管癌患者接受基于IMRT的放化疗时，38%的患者出现3级皮肤毒性，没有观察到4级毒性[202]。一项比较IMRT和常规放疗的研究发现，接受常规放疗的患者经过的治疗天数更长，并且出现2级或更大毒性的概率更高，因此导致的治疗中断明显增多[208]。

迟发肛门毒性发生在治疗完成后的几个月到几年内。最常见的晚期并发症是肛门直肠溃疡。患者还可能出现肛门狭窄、大便失禁、肛门疼痛或肛瘘[154,199,206,209]。在放疗中加入化疗后，慢性肛门毒性的发生率似乎没有增加[201,209,210]。45～60Gy的剂量（分割剂量为1.8～2Gy）被认为是安全的，3级或更高级慢性毒性的发生率为0～22%[145,147,154,204,211,212]。剂量大于65Gy或分割剂量大于2Gy会导致肛门毒性的高发生率[203]。HIV和肛管癌患者在接受联合化疗和放疗时，急性和迟发肛门毒性的风险都会增加[213]。

（二）治疗

急性毒性的治疗主要是支持性治疗，包括皮肤护理、饮食调整、止痛药和局部糖皮质激素药物，毒性严重时可暂停放疗。这种副作用是自限性的，通常在治疗结束后的几周内消失。慢性毒性如肛门狭窄的治疗方法包括括约肌扩张。在非常少见的情况下，患者会因为严重症状而需要行结肠造瘘。有小型研究证明，高压氧治疗对慢性肛门直肠溃疡有效[214]。也有口服维生素A治疗肛门直肠溃疡的报告，但缺乏确证性研究[200]。

八、胰腺和肝脏

（一）发病率及临床特征

1. 胰腺

日本的一项研究将可切除胰腺癌患者随机分为手术组和放化疗组，结果显示3年生存率分别为20%和0，这表明即使是在最早期的患者中，手术也是长期生存的必要条件[215]。反过来，胰腺放疗的长期后遗症仍不明确。在动物研究中，胰腺照射对外分泌功能的影响比对内分泌功能的影响更大[216]。一项评估胰头病变切除后术中放疗早期和晚期效应的研究指出，与未接受放疗的患者相比，接受放疗的患者术后即刻出现更明显的外分泌功能暂时性降低，这种差异在较长的随访中逐渐消失[217]。

2. 肝脏

当整个肝脏辐射剂量达到30～35Gy、分割剂量为2Gy时，约5%的患者会出现放射性肝病（radiation-induced liver disease，RILD）[218]。RILD的病理损害是小叶中央静脉血栓形成（静脉闭塞性疾病），导致明显的窦性瘀血，导致小叶出血和周围肝细胞继发性损伤[219]。中央静脉纤维蛋白沉积被认为是静脉闭塞性损伤的原因。目前尚不清楚是什么刺激了纤维蛋白的沉积，但有假说认为，在暴露于辐射的组织中，TGF-β增加，这反过来又刺激成纤维细胞向损伤部位迁移，导致纤维蛋白和胶原沉积。坏死灶位于受累小叶部分[220]。严重急性肝毒性可进展为肝纤维化、肝硬化和肝衰竭。

典型的RILD是一种临床综合征，包括无黄疸的肝大、腹水和转氨酶升高。RILD通常发生在放疗完成后的2周到4个月之间。患者出现疲劳、体重增加、腹围增加，偶尔还会出现右上腹疼痛。血清碱性磷酸酶升高水平与其他转氨酶升高不成比例，最初血清总胆红素水平正常。非经典形式的RILD包括明显异常的转氨酶和胆红素水平，更可能发生在潜在肝病患者，如病毒性肝炎或肝硬化。腹部CT或MRI检查可用于诊断。RILD可发展至慢性阶段，患者可发展为日益严重的肝纤维化和肝衰竭[221]。

考虑到肝脏的平行结构，尽管未被照射的肝脏能够继续发挥肝脏功能，但在一定剂量的放疗中未被照射的肝脏体积是预测RILD可能性的一个重要因素。虽然放射性肝病可发生在整个肝脏接受35～40Gy的剂量后，但如果保留足够体积的正常肝脏，则可以给予明显更高的剂量，并且几乎没有临床并发症。Lawrence和其同事的研究报道，如果少于25%的正常肝脏接受了放疗，则可能不会有能够产生放射性肝病的剂量上限[219]。当对1/3、2/3及整个肝脏进行均匀照射放疗时，能够使5%的患者产生放射性肝病的估计剂量分别为90Gy、47Gy和31Gy。联合化疗和放疗会增加肝脏损伤，尤其是当化疗药物具有肝毒性时。苯丁酸氮芥、白消安和铂类药物联合放疗用于骨髓移植患者，是潜在的肝毒性药物。相比之下，氟嘧啶似乎不会增加辐射相关的肝毒性[218,222]。

在考虑患者肝定向治疗的适当性时，考虑基线肝功能是很重要的。目前根据Child-Pugh评分对患者进行分层。其他分级系统也存在（如MELD评分），但尚未在接受放疗的患者中得到评估。大多数对肝细胞性肝癌（HCC）放疗的研究试验都排除了肝功能最差的患者。

因为HCC患者的基线肝功能通常比非肝脏起源的癌症患者差，指南建议在原发性肝癌患者中坚持较低的平均肝脏放射剂量[223]。从使用SBRT治疗肝转移瘤的试验中推断出的结论建议保留700毫升的正常肝脏[224]。在使用3个分割剂量的SBRT方案中，这一限制要求在整个治疗过程中至少要有700毫升的肝脏体积接受小于15Gy的辐射剂量，然而要记住这是在没有潜在肝脏疾病的患者中进行的。对于潜在肝脏疾病患者，需要避免照射的容量可能是800mL[225]。

（二）治疗

1. 胰腺

胰腺外分泌功能不足是实施Whipple手术的患者胰腺体积损失和解剖结构改变的结果，然而这在接受远端胰腺切除术的患者中也常见。脂肪吸收障碍是症状发生的主要原因，首先建议调整饮食。胰酶替代疗法能够成功地增加脂肪吸收，进而降低脂肪泻的严重程度，但是还没有试验评估术后患者的酶替代疗法的具体效果[226]。尽管如此，胰酶替代治疗已被 FDA 批准用于该适应证，并且应该在该人群中使用，应密切注意给药建议，包括总剂量、与进食相关的时间，以及是否需要 PPI 或抗酸剂来优化疗效。

2. 肝脏

支持疗法是放射性肝病治疗的支柱。一项随机试验比较了间质近距离放疗治疗肝转移患者接受己酮可可碱、熊脱氧胆酸和低分子量肝素与不接受上述治疗的情况，发现治疗 6 周后放射性肝损伤显著减轻[227]。不幸的是，因为缺乏有效的治疗方法，且患者通常缺乏储备肝功能，RILD 通常是致命的。

九、降低毒性的治疗技术

胃肠道毒性是许多恶性肿瘤放疗中的一个重要障碍，它限制了患者可使用的放射剂量，导致患者发病和肿瘤控制效果差。放射肿瘤科医生的主要目标是最大限度地避免正常组织受影响，并向靶点提供足够的治疗剂量。如前所述，可实施不同的技术来减少非目标胃肠道的受照体积，包括使用多个照射野以避免“热点”、俯卧位治疗、使用腹压板，以及使治疗患者膀胱充盈以将肠道移出照射野。

在过去，放疗计划是基于二维（2D）规划，其中治疗区域是通过放射平片和已知的解剖标志来确定的。随着成像和计算能力的提高，3D 治疗规划在 20 世纪 80 年代开始出现。作为 3D 规划的一种高级形式，IMRT 现已在临床实践中得到实施[228,229]。与传统的“静态”放射野不同，IMRT 使用多个“野中野”的原理，在避开正常结构的同时，更精确地将辐射剂量聚焦到靶组织。IMRT 需要靶组织和正常器官的精确定位。限制周围正常组织的剂量，并且使治疗体积得到所需的处方剂量。然后执行“逆向规划”，即计算机搜索算法建立多个（有时是非常规的）束流或野设计，以试图满足规定的目标剂量和正常组织剂量限制。用多个小“束流”而不是一束均匀的束流来处理单个照射野，并且每个束流向靶标的不同部分传递不同的剂量强度。这使得辐射剂量与靶标的形状接近，并优先保护附近的正常组织。

总之，使用基于 IMRT 的 CRT 治疗不同癌症的早期临床结果显示治疗相关毒性显著降低，与癌症治疗相关的结果与常规放疗方法相似。例如，Mundt 及其同事发现，与常规 3D 计划相比，接受 IMRT 治疗的妇科恶性肿瘤患者的小肠放射剂量测定结果有显著改善。将 36 例接受调强全盆腔放疗的妇科恶性肿瘤患者与 30 例在同一机构接受三维适形放疗患者的结果进行比较。患者在人口统计学和治疗因素方面匹配良好。IMRT 组的慢性胃肠道毒性发生率显著降低，仅 11% 接受 IMRT 治疗的女性出现 1~3 级毒性（3 级为 0），而非 IMRT 组为 50%[230]。在另一系列研究中，Salama 及其同事报告了 53 例采用基于 IMRT 的 CRT 治疗的肛门癌患者。骨盆和原发性疾病的中位辐射剂量分别为 45Gy 和 52Gy。15% 的患者出现 3 级急性胃肠道毒性，未观察到 4 级毒性；与使用常规放疗计划的当代试验中观察到的严重胃肠道毒性发生率相比更有利[202]。IMRT 是目前肛管癌治疗的主要方法，在食管癌和胰腺癌的治疗中广泛应用。

（王萍 刘军 译，鲁晓岚 李鹏 校）

参考文献

第 42 章　胃肠内镜检查的准备及并发症

Aravind Sugumar, John J. Vargo II 著

章节目录

一、新型内镜技术的并发症 …… 586
二、内镜检查患者的准备 …… 586
（一）病史及体格检查 …… 586
（二）预防性使用抗生素 …… 586
（三）抗凝和抗血小板药物的使用 …… 587
（四）知情同意书 …… 587
三、镇静 …… 587
四、感染 …… 588
五、电外科学 …… 588
六、并发症发生的时间和严重程度 …… 588
七、食管、胃、十二指肠内镜 …… 588
（一）心肺事件 …… 588
（二）局部麻醉 …… 588
（三）穿孔 …… 588
（四）内镜下止血 …… 588
（五）肠内置管的操作程序 …… 588
（六）黏膜消融和切除术 …… 589
（七）其他治疗操作 …… 589
八、小肠镜 …… 589
（一）气囊辅助小肠镜 …… 589
（二）胶囊内镜 …… 589
九、结肠镜 …… 590
（一）穿孔 …… 590
（二）出血 …… 591
（三）息肉切除术后电凝综合征 …… 591
（四）结肠准备的相关并发症 …… 591
（五）其他并发症 …… 591
十、内镜逆行胰胆管造影 …… 591
（一）出血 …… 591
（二）穿孔 …… 591
（三）胆管炎 …… 592
（四）胰腺炎 …… 592
十一、超声内镜 …… 592
十二、新型内镜技术 …… 593

一、新型内镜技术的并发症

胃肠道内镜检查在各种胃肠道疾病的诊断和治疗中起着不可或缺的作用。风险和获益是任何手术的固有性能。近年来，胃肠道内镜检查的“范围”不断扩大，包括经口内镜下肌切开术（POEM）、肿瘤内镜黏膜下剥离术（ESD）和内镜下减重手术等。随着这种扩展，需要了解这些风险并将其与潜在获益进行权衡。这一过程的重要性不容小觑。并发症是难以避免的，但通过结合最佳的技术和认知能力，严格关注此类手术的适当适应证，可最大限度地减少并发症。

二、内镜检查患者的准备

（一）病史及体格检查

应在内镜检查前获得患者全面和相关的病史，还应仔细审查既往的内镜手术。这应包括识别任何不良事件、目标镇静水平和患者对镇静的满意度。还应获得当前药物使用情况以及相关过敏反应的列表。患者使用镇静剂、止痛剂和酒精的情况可以帮助我们预测是否需要更大剂量的镇静剂和镇痛药，或使用监测的麻醉护理。每次内镜检查前，应进行重点体格检查，包括气道、心脏、肺部和腹部。强烈建议分配美国麻醉医师学会身体状况（American Society of Anesthesiology Physical Status, ASA PS）类别（表 42.1），因为已证明该类别可预测心肺不良事件[1]。

表 42.1　用于评估胃肠道内镜手术风险的 ASA PS 分类系统

ASA PS 分类	检查前健康状况
1	健康（正常）
2	轻度全身性疾病
3	重度全身性疾病
4	重度全身性疾病，持续危及生命
5	濒死（未经内镜手术，预计不会存活）
6	脑死亡（用于器官采集）

ASA PS，美国麻醉医师学会身体状况。

（二）预防性使用抗生素

表 42.2 列出了需要预防性使用抗生素的内镜操作[2]。在经皮内镜下胃造口术（percutaneous endoscopic gastrostomy, PEG）置入前使用抗生素，可以降低造口周围蜂窝织炎的风险，这是预防性给予抗生素的最有力证据[3]。在所有接受内镜逆行胰胆管造影（ERCP）的肝移植患者中也推荐使用抗生素预防，但这类患者使用抗生素的必要性受到质疑[4]。一般来说，在 ERCP 或超声内镜（EUS）过程中对无菌胰腺坏死或胰腺假性囊肿进行有意或无意的操作，以及对胃肠道内和胃肠道周围的囊性结构进行 EUS 引导的细针穿刺（FNA）时，应接受抗生素预防[2]。接受 ERCP 的广泛 PSC 或肝门部肿瘤继发胆道树预期引流不完全的患者，也应接受抗生素预防[2]。值

表 42.2　内镜手术中需要抗生素预防的患者状况和程序

患者状况	程序	预防目标
胆管梗阻不伴胆管炎	ERCP 伴预期不完全的胆管引流	预防胆管炎
与胰管相通的无菌胰腺积液	ERCP	预防囊肿感染
无菌胰液收集	经壁引流	预防感染性囊肿
沿胃肠道(包括纵隔)的囊性病变	EUS-FNA	预防囊肿感染
肝硬化伴急性胃肠道出血	所有内镜治疗	预防感染并发症,包括 SBP
任何疾病	经皮内镜鼻饲管置入	预防造口周围感染(蜂窝织炎)

ERCP,内镜逆行胰胆管造影;EUS,超声内镜;FNA,细针穿刺;SBP,自发性细菌性腹膜炎。

得注意的是,因为没有数据证明胃肠道手术和感染性并发症之间存在明确联系,也没有数据证明抗生素预防可以预防内镜手术后的感染性并发症[5],所以并非所有心脏瓣膜疾病、合成血管移植物和人工关节患者均应接受抗生素预防。当预防性使用抗生素时,抗生素的选择取决于特定的胃肠道程序、临床情况和患者的过敏史[6]。

(三) 抗凝和抗血小板药物的使用

随着新型抗血小板药物和抗凝药物的出现,了解此类药物的作用持续时间,对于减少出血和血栓并发症非常重要。抗血栓形成和抗血小板药物的管理应基于内镜手术的紧迫性以及如果不停用药物与手术相关的出血风险[7]。需要一个良好的框架工作来将内镜手术分类为低与高出血风险,以及将基础疾病状态分类为高与低血栓并发症风险。ASGE 关于接受胃肠内镜检查的患者抗血栓药物管理的立场声明是一个有用的资源[8]。例如,胆道括约肌切开术、EUS 联合细针穿刺、经皮胃造瘘术和息肉切除术等手术增加了接受华法林治疗的患者出血的风险[7,8]。在高危择期手术中,应停用华法林,使国际标准化比值(INR)恢复正常,华法林通常可在术后 1 周内重新开始[9,10]。在具有高风险状况(如机械心脏瓣膜)的患者中,应在内镜手术前 12 小时内使用低分子量肝素“桥接”,以将血栓栓塞风险降至最低。

当抗血栓治疗是暂时性时,例如在静脉血栓栓塞的治疗中,择期胃肠手术应尽可能延迟,直至无抗凝治疗指征[7,8]。对于出血风险较低食管、胃、十二指肠镜(EGD)和结肠镜活检等手术,可继续使用阿司匹林、非甾体抗炎药和氯吡格雷。对于出血风险较高的手术,如内镜下括约肌切开术,继续使用抗血小板药物的决定将与血栓栓塞事件的风险相关。

目前关于使用较华法林半衰期更短的新药(如直接凝血酶抑制剂达比加群或直接Ⅹa 抑制剂利伐沙班)进行抗凝治疗,或使用新型 $P2Y_{12}$ ADP 受体抑制剂(如替格瑞洛)进行抗血小板治疗的患者最佳管理的数据有限。

(四) 知情同意书

在进行任何内镜手术之前,应由内镜医师获得书面知情同意书。获得知情同意的过程是一项法律要求,也是一项基本的道德义务。从而使患者全面了解拟定程序,包括涉及的潜在风险和可能的替代方法,并回答所有问题。知情同意书的内容应包括对程序本身的讨论,包括风险、获益和替代方案。并发症的发生频率和严重程度也应加以评价[11]。

三、镇静

镇静用于大多数内镜手术,以便为手术提供一个舒适和安全的环境。大多数门诊病例(包括 EGD 和结肠镜检查)需要中等水平的镇静。通常联合使用苯二氮䓬类药物和阿片类药物,尽管过去 10 年中异丙酚介导的镇静的应用有所增加。深度镇静或全身麻醉通常针对高级内镜手术,如 ERCP、EUS、ESD 和 POEM 等,以及用于中度镇静的药物可能存在问题的患者。这可能包括使用麻醉剂和/或镇静剂的患者,以及有严重合并症的患者,这些患者有发生不良心肺事件的风险。血流动力学不稳定或呼吸功能受损的患者也可能从麻醉辅助镇静中获益。

0.9%的手术会发生计划外心肺不良事件,如低血压和低氧血症[1,12]。这些事件的风险因素包括年龄、ASA PS 分级升高(见表 42.1)、住院手术,以及针对长期深度镇静或全身麻醉的手术,如 ERCP[1]。呼吸系统并发症包括低氧血症和通气不足。在行门诊内镜检查的 ASA PS 1 级和 2 级患者中,低氧血症的风险因素包括体重指数(BMI)、高龄和术中使用更高剂量的麻醉性镇痛药[13,14]。使用脉搏血氧仪可以早期识别低氧血症,在大多数情况下,常规使用吸氧可以预防低氧血症。肺泡通气不足可能是由于中枢神经系统抑制或下咽肌松弛所致。使用二氧化碳描记术(二氧化碳监测仪)测量有效的 CO_2 消除,可显著降低了接受结肠镜检查、ERCP 和 EUS(使用深度镇静)的患者呼吸暂停的发生率[15,16]。但是,目前没有数据支持在进行 EGD 或结肠镜检查的受试者中,当以中度镇静为目标时,常规使用二氧化碳监测仪。

内镜检查过程中的低血压通常是由于血容量不足患者的药物诱导静脉扩张所致。通常对静脉液体推注有反应。血管迷走神经反应是内镜检查过程中观察到的心律失常最常见的原因。这种反应通常是由于疼痛刺激引起,可通过改善内镜定位和减少肠膨胀来补救。偶尔需要静脉注射阿托品和液体推注。对于有心脏病史的患者、年龄超过 55 岁的患者以及所有以深度镇静或全身麻醉为目标的患者,应考虑使用心电图监测。内镜医生应该熟悉他们使用的所有镇静药物的药代动力学和不良反应特征,包括其逆转剂,如用于苯二氮䓬类药物的氟马西尼和用于麻醉药物的纳洛酮。在内镜检查室张贴带有该信息的标语牌是明智的。

在恢复区域，一旦去除了手术刺激，就有再镇静的风险。恢复至基线生命体征是一项重要的出院标准。需要强调的是，即使在接受丙泊酚等速效药物治疗的患者中，其精神运动恢复也可能延迟[17]。因此，建议患者在出院时由其他人陪同，并建议患者在术后第二天之前不要驾驶或操作机器。

四、感染

据估计，在美国通过胃肠道内镜的传播感染率为 1 人/180 万人[2,18,19]。感染性不良事件是未遵循内镜器械和配件的既定再处理指南、未遵循使用镇静剂（如丙泊酚）的无菌技术或手术本身导致的[2,20,21]。

短暂性菌血症在内镜手术中并不少见，但菌血症引起的感染后遗症（如心内膜炎或其他的部位播散）罕见，以致于美国心脏协会和 ASGE 的目前建议仅针对非常特殊的情况推荐抗生素预防（见前文"抗生素预防"和表 42.2）[5,22]。由于胃肠道不是无菌的，因此在两次使用之间对内镜进行高水平消毒被认为足以防止患者之间传播感染性微生物[23]。该过程包括对通道和内镜外部进行机械清洁，然后浸泡在消毒剂溶液中（如戊二醛或过乙酸），随后对器械进行彻底冲洗和干燥。最近十二指肠镜引起的耐碳青霉烯类肠球菌感染的暴发，引发了对内镜设计局限性的担忧与仔细消毒方案的思考[24]。一次丙型肝炎的暴发与不当的无菌技术和对多名患者使用同一瓶镇静剂有关[25]。需要强调的是，高水平消毒可以杀死大多数可能污染内镜的病原体，包括 HBV、HCV 和 HIV。尽管朊病毒（如 Jakob-Creutzfeldt 病原体）不能通过高水平消毒灭活，但在唾液、肠组织、粪便和血液中并未发现朊病毒，因此世卫组织判定其为非感染性[26]。

五、电外科学

心脏起搏器或植入式心脏除颤器（implantable cardiac defibrillator，ICD）的存在需要特别考虑，因为内镜手术期间进行的电烙术可能会抑制心脏起搏器功能，并可能导致除颤器不适当放电。因此，应谨慎将接地垫放置在远离起搏器的患者大腿或臀部，并使用短暂的电外科输出脉冲。此外，使用双极平台或在内镜止血的情况下，使用机械或热器械可以将风险降到最低[27]。对于 ICD，电外科器械可诱发意外激活。应使用体外除颤器对 ICD 进行临时去激活，同时对患者的心律进行连续心脏监测。了解所使用的电外科设备的操作能力是非常重要的。这应包括了解器械上的各种设置及其与所需组织效应的对应关系。此外，注意电路中如果出现错误信号或电路中断，内镜医生应能够对器械进行故障排除[28,29]。

六、并发症发生的时间和严重程度

内镜并发症可能发生在手术过程中或也可能延迟。了解潜在并发症是知情同意过程的关键要素（见前文）。同样重要的是，对患者进行教育，使其能早期识别可能提示延迟并发症的体征和症状，并提供一个简化的流程，就潜在并发症联系内镜医生进行适当治疗。从质量改善和治疗的角度来看，重要的是使用这组标准的不良结局定义，包括时间、归因、严重程度和最终结果[30]。

七、食管、胃、十二指肠内镜

（一）心肺事件

与镇静和镇痛相关的心肺不良事件占所有食管、胃、十二指肠内镜（EGD）不良事件的 30%~60%[1,31,32]。不良事件可能包括缺氧、呼吸暂停、低血压/休克、误吸、呼吸骤停、肺炎、心肌梗死和脑血管意外。心肺事件的风险与手术的复杂性增加和共病的严重程度相关[1,12]。ASA PS 分类（见表 42.1）与心肺疾病风险增加相关[12]。

（二）局部麻醉

局部麻醉剂如苯佐卡因和利多卡因与严重不良事件相关，包括高铁血红蛋白血症和严重的类过敏反应。高铁血红蛋白血症的临床表现为，尽管动脉血氧饱和度正常，但在脉搏血氧测定中显示发绀伴低血氧饱和度的临床证据。通常采用动脉血氧，使用一氧化碳血氧仪诊断这种潜在的致命性疾病。静脉注射亚甲蓝可逆转高铁血红蛋白血症[33,34]。使用局部麻醉剂也可能增加误吸的风险。

（三）穿孔

据估计，在诊断性 EGD 期间，上消化道穿孔的发生率为 1/2 500~1/11 000[35,36]。最常见的穿孔部位是口咽或颈段食管。因此，食管近端狭窄和癌症患者，以及 Zenker 憩室或较大的颈椎前路骨赘患者，存在穿孔的特殊风险。出现捻发音伴相关颈部或胸部疼痛应紧急评估。一般情况下，应考虑使用水溶性造影剂进行食管造影或使用口服造影剂进行颈部和胸部 CT 扫描。如果发现及时，大多数颈部穿孔可以保守治疗，配合适当的手术治疗，采用广谱抗生素和鼻胃管抽吸。胸内穿孔也可采用这种方式处理。在适当的环境下，可使用一系列内镜器械治疗穿孔，包括金属夹、内镜系统组织定位装置、支架和缝合平台[37-42]。

（四）内镜下止血

高达 78% 的患者在静脉曲张硬化治疗后可发生溃疡[43]。高达 6% 的患者可在硬化治疗后即刻发生显著的出血[44]。其他硬化治疗并发症包括误吸、穿孔、狭窄形成、心包积液、胸腔积液以及纵隔炎[45,46]。内镜下套扎术与内镜下静脉曲张硬化治疗的疗效相同，但其不良事件发生率和死亡率较低，已基本上取代了静脉曲张硬化治疗[45,46]。高达 15% 的患者发生套扎食管溃疡形成。内镜止血的罕见并发症包括吸入性肺炎、穿孔和腹膜炎。如果在初始治疗后 24 到 48 小时内重复使用加热器探针治疗，会增加并发症的风险[47,48]。使用聚多卡醇、乙醇等药物进行注射止血很少有引起穿孔或出血加剧的报告，现已成为临床研究的热点[49,50]。

（五）肠内置管的操作程序

内镜常用于提供肠内置管。内镜下放置螺旋形鼻肠饲管可以确保饲管进入小肠，并与轻微的自限性并发症相关[51,52]。鼻衄最常见，发生率高达 5%。也可能发生近端移位以及插管移位。

PEG 置入的不良事件可高达 10%[53,54]。2% ~ 10% 的病例发生严重不良事件，包括误吸、伤口感染、出血、穿孔、坏死性筋膜炎、肠梗阻（图 42.1）和其他器官的损伤[55,56]。术前单次给予头孢菌素或 β-内酰胺可显著降低造口周围感染[56]。PEG 置入期间或置入后的出血通常是轻微和自限性的，但偶尔可能需要内镜止血。应暂停使用抗凝剂，并在 PEG 置入前常规记录凝血参数[57]。PEG 的外部缓冲物保持过紧，引起内部缓冲物迁移到胃壁时。会发生“埋藏综合征”[58]。治疗包括取出插管并在不同部位置入另一根插管。有报道，在口咽和食管恶性肿瘤患者中描述了 PEG 插入部位发生的肿瘤转移。目前尚不清楚转移是局部扩散还是血行播散的结果。在这些癌症患者中，可考虑肠内营养的替代途径，如放射学辅助置管[59]。如果尚未形成成熟的瘘管，PEG 管在置入后一个月内意外移位可导致腹膜炎。在成熟管道和管道移位的情况下，应尽快插入替代管道[60]。注射造影剂可在 X 线透视下进行，以确定适当的定位。经皮内镜下空肠造口术的不良事件与 PEG 置入相似，尽管堵塞、移位和意外取出的发生率可能更高[61]。吸入性肺炎可能是由于口咽内容物的吸入或是由于管饲本身所致。误吸的危险因素可能包括口咽部的神经肌肉或结构问题、长时间仰卧位、有记录的误吸史、意识水平降低或呕吐/反胃[62]。

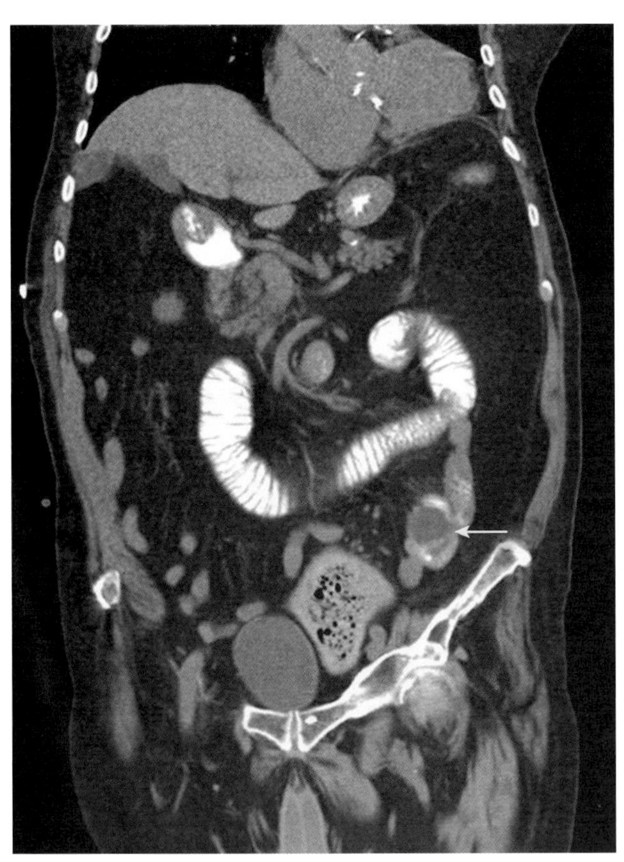

图 42.1　磁共振肠造影显示回肠近端有一个移位的、充满水的经皮内镜下胃造口术（PEG）缓冲物（黄箭头）。该患者有 7 天小肠梗阻病史。进行单气囊小肠镜检查，用注射针回缩气囊，用圈套器捕获缓冲物，经口取出，肠梗阻解除

（六）黏膜消融和切除术

在巴雷特食管（伴或不伴异型增生）和黏膜癌的患者中（见第 47 和 48 章），热电凝、射频消融、冷冻治疗和内镜下黏膜切除术（endoscopic mucosal resection，EMR）与吞咽困难/吞咽痛、胸痛、消化不良、溃疡伴出血和穿孔相关[63-66]。发生如穿孔和出血的严重事件，EMR 的发生率通常在 0.5% ~ 5% 之间[67]。在环周 EMR 的情况下，食管狭窄形成的风险升高。这些狭窄大多可以通过食管扩张进行充分治疗[68]。内镜黏膜下剥离术允许使用各种专用工具，并选择黏膜下层作为剥离平面进行整块切除。ESD 的不良事件与 EMR 相似，但出血和穿孔的发生率可能更高一点[67,69]。

（七）其他治疗操作

置入可膨胀的金属支架用于治疗恶性和良性难治性狭窄。其相关并发症发生率高达 12%，包括胸痛、误吸、定位不当、气管压迫引起的呼吸功能受损和穿孔[70]。当食管胃交界处被支架桥接时可导致 GERD，需要大剂量的 PPI 抑酸治疗。恶性肿瘤置入支架后的晚期并发症包括肿瘤过度生长、气管食管瘘和 CRT 后肿瘤收缩后支架移位[71,72]。

内镜下上消化道异物取出的并发症包括误吸、穿孔和胃肠道出血（见第 28 章）。使用外套管或气管插管可以降低异物吸入的风险。穿孔的风险因素包括内镜干预延迟超过 24 小时或存在不规则或尖锐的物体[73-75]。

八、小肠镜

（一）气囊辅助小肠镜

气囊辅助肠镜检查的出现将诊断和治疗前景的视野扩展到小肠。诊断性双气囊小肠镜并发症发生率为 0.8%，治疗性操作的并发症发生率为 4.3%[76]。一项双气囊手术的多中心调查发现出血（0.8%）、穿孔（0.3%）和胰腺炎（0.3%）是最常见的并发症[76]。几乎所有出血并发症均发生在进行息肉切除术的治疗过程中。还报告了球囊扩张后的穿孔率为 2.9%。虽然关于单气囊小肠镜检查的数据并不多，但它们似乎具有相似的并发症[77,78]。

（二）胶囊内镜

无线胶囊内镜的禁忌证包括已知或疑似肠梗阻、狭窄、瘘或扩展性克罗恩病、吞咽障碍、肠梗阻或假性肠梗阻（见第 124 章）[79]。更多的相对禁忌证包括妊娠、长期使用非甾体抗炎药、Zenker 憩室、胃轻瘫、既往盆腔或腹部手术或放射治疗以及存在心脏起搏器或 ICD 和左心室辅助装置。这些心脏装置和胶囊内镜之间存在电磁干扰的理论风险。然而，这一问题的研究并没有证明这是一个具有临床意义的问题[80-83]。

也许最可怕的并发症是胶囊滞留在小肠内，该疾病的风险患者包括有炎症性肠病（IBD）病史、既往放疗史、既往手术史和使用非甾体抗炎药的患者[79]。在大型病例系列中观察到胶囊滞留率为 1.4%。在几乎所有情况下，均识别出了需要手术干预的严重小肠病变[79]。在胶囊滞留、无梗阻症状、

无即刻手术指征且基础疾病可能通过药物或内镜治疗的患者中，使用双气囊小肠镜可成功取出胶囊并治疗非甾体抗炎药引起的膈膜狭窄等病变[84]。在进行胶囊内镜检查前需要评估管腔通畅性的患者中，使用通畅性胶囊系统是确定是否存在足够的管腔狭窄以导致胶囊滞留和后续并发症的有用工具[85-87]。

在吞咽困难的患者中，应在胶囊内镜检查之前进行适当的结构和动力评价。在某些情况下，在吞咽胶囊之前应吞咽钡剂外加13mm钡丸。曾有报告胶囊滞留在环咽肌及Zenker憩室内，并成功通过内镜取出[88]。还报告了胶囊内镜误吸并成功经支气管镜取出[89,90]。内镜置入器械可绕过胃，在胃轻瘫或可能导致胃延迟通过的术后解剖结构存在的情况下，成功对小肠进行了胶囊内镜检查[91]。

九、结肠镜

结肠镜检查并发症的整体风险率为0.28%[92]。风险因素包括患者年龄、合并症（如卒中、房颤或心力衰竭病史）和接受息肉切除术[92,93]。结肠镜检查的主要并发症是心血管和肺部事件（图42.2）、穿孔、出血和息肉切除术后电凝综合征[94]。与其他内镜检查过程一样，ASA PS级内镜手术（见表42.1）与手术相关的计划外心血管事件（如低血压和低氧血症）的风险相关[1,95,96]。

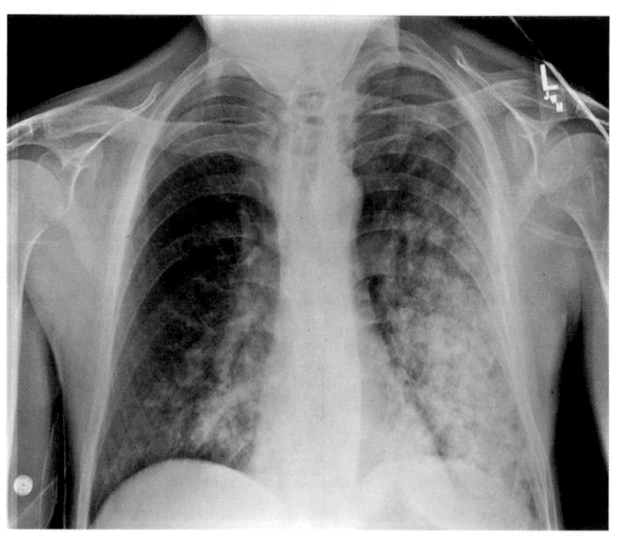

图42.2 胸片显示1例接受结肠镜检查并监测麻醉护理的患者，发生双侧吸入性肺炎。既往无胃轻瘫病史

（一）穿孔

结肠镜检查的穿孔率为0.05%～0.3%[95,97,98]。有趣的是，在接受结肠镜息肉切除术的患者中，穿孔风险并没有增加[93]。穿孔可能是由于结肠袢压力过大、空气/气体压力过大（气压伤）或电外科应用部位损伤导致结肠抗畸变边界撕裂所致。结肠撕裂主要发生在乙状结肠，结肠镜最容易在乙状结肠打弯成环。气压伤最常见于盲肠，此处结肠直径最大，因此，结肠壁上的张力最高。血管扩张（尤其是右半结肠）的消融治疗与高达2.5%的穿孔率相关[99]。假性梗阻患者放置结肠减压管发生穿孔的风险为2%[100-102]。球囊扩张治疗结肠克罗恩病的穿孔风险接近2%。腹部或肩部疼痛的患者如腹胀无改善应考虑穿孔[103]。结肠镜检查时经常可发现穿孔（图42.3A）。在许多情况下，使用内镜夹联合抗生素和密切观察进行缺损闭合是有效的（见图42.3B）[104,105]。在这种情况下，建议胃肠病医生与外科医生一起仔细观察。存在撕裂较大或明显腹膜炎的病例，应考虑手术干预。

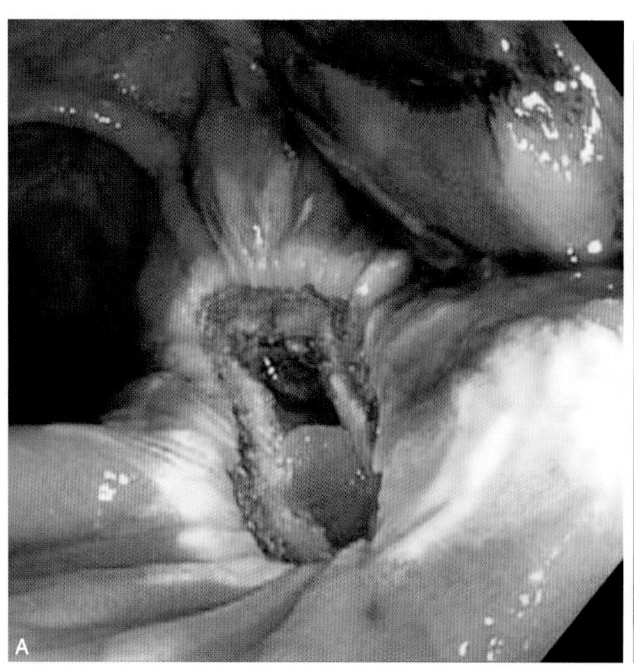

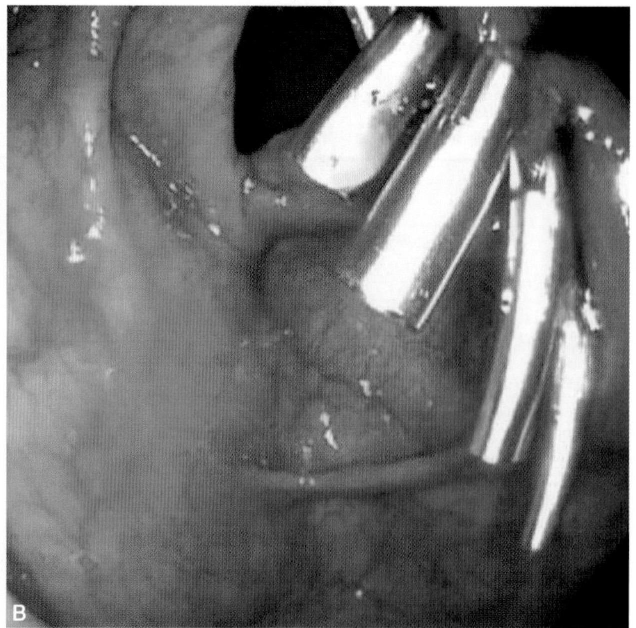

图42.3 A，2cm无蒂息肉切除术后升结肠穿孔的结肠镜视图。B，使用金属夹在内镜下闭合穿孔部位。患者接受抗生素治疗48小时，保持无症状，并出院

(二) 出血

结肠镜检查即刻或延迟出血的最常见原因是进行息肉切除术。尽管与结肠镜检查相关的总体出血发生率为 0.1% ~ 0.6%，但息肉切除术的出血风险为 0.87%[97]。患者年龄、心血管合并症和使用抗血栓和/或抗血小板药物与息肉切除术相关出血的风险增加有关[93,106-108]。息肉大小可能是息肉切除术后出血的额外风险因素[106,108,109]。内镜下切除大的(≥2cm)无蒂息肉后，在切除部位使用预防性止血夹可以降低息肉切除后迟发性出血的风险[110]。息肉切除后的急性出血通常适合多种内镜下治疗措施(图 42.4)[111,112]。在切除息肉之前，使用可拆卸圈套器可显著减少出血[113]。

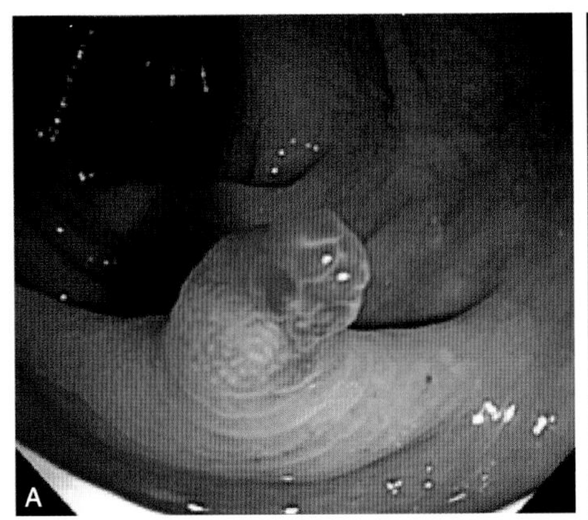

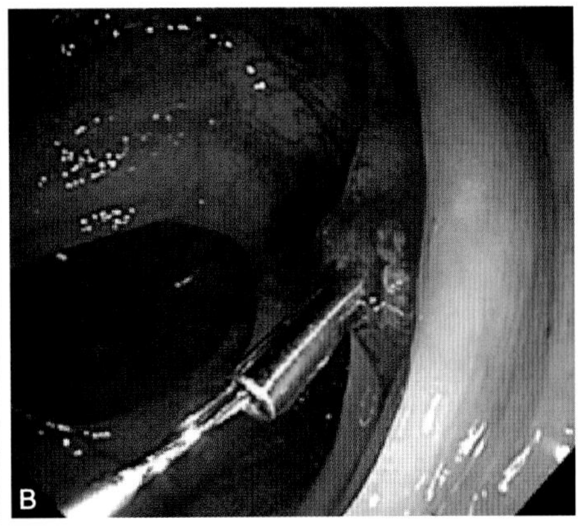

图 42.4　A，结肠息肉切除术后 5 天，便血患者息肉切除部位的结肠镜视图。该息肉被认为是出血的原因。B，虽然在第二次结肠镜检查期间未发生出血，但放置了止血夹，以降低进一步出血的风险

(三) 息肉切除术后电凝综合征

息肉切除术后电凝综合征是指一系列发热、局限性腹痛伴反跳痛和白细胞增多。该综合征通常发生在结肠镜检查联合息肉切除术后 1 ~ 5 天。该综合征的发生率为 0.003% ~ 0.1%[97]。通常患者需要接受静脉补液、广谱肠外抗生素和禁食治疗，直至症状改善[114]。还应进行腹部 CT 检查，以排除局部穿孔的可能性。如果在连续、频繁的腹部检查中观察到令人担忧的结果，也应进行 CT 检查。较轻的息肉切除术后电凝综合征病例，可在门诊接受口服抗生素治疗[115]。

(四) 结肠准备的相关并发症

在液体/电解质紊乱或慢性肾病、心力衰竭和/或肝衰竭的患者中，与结肠制剂相关的并发症，聚乙二醇通常比磷酸钠制剂更安全。血管紧张素转换酶(ACE)抑制剂、非甾体抗炎药和利尿剂等药物可能会导致即将接受结肠镜检查的此类患者出现液体/电解质问题。一般而言，有液体和电解质紊乱易感因素的患者在使用上述药物时，应逐渐地进行肠道准备，并密切监测，并测定其基线血清肌酐水平[116-119]。

(五) 其他并发症

结肠镜检查的罕见并发症包括脾破裂，阑尾炎和意外被消毒剂溶液污染后的化学性结肠炎[120-123]。结肠镜检查特异性死亡率罕见，发生率为 7/100 000 例手术。结肠支架置入的并发症包括穿孔、移位和支架闭塞。由于穿孔风险较高，不推荐在支架置入前或置入后，对恶性结肠狭窄进行狭窄扩张[124-126]。

气体爆炸罕有报道，被认为是由于使用电灼或氩等离子体凝固时，结肠腔内存在的甲烷或氢气达到可燃水平所致。风险因素可能包括结肠清洁不彻底和使用不可吸收或不完全吸收制剂，如用山梨醇、乳果糖和甘露醇[127-129]。

EMR 和 ESD 是切除结肠大息肉的技术，出血和穿孔均与任一技术相关。尽管 ESD 的并发症发生率更高(稍后讨论)，但大多数可以通过内镜治疗[105,130,131]。

十、内镜逆行胰胆管造影

随着 EUS 和 MRCP 的出现，内镜逆行胰胆管造影(ERCP)几乎完全成为一种治疗技术。幸运的是，治疗性 ERCP 的严重并发症是罕见的(图 42.5；另见第 61 和 70 章)。内镜医师有责任通过尽可能使用微创检查来尽量减少并发症，并获得适当的知情同意。

(一) 出血

ERCP 术后的大多数出血并发症与括约肌切开术有关，发生率为 1% ~ 2%[132,133]。括约肌切开术出血的风险因素包括血小板减少、凝血功能障碍、胆管炎和术后 3 天内开始抗凝治疗。此外，观察到每周进行少于 1 次胆道括约肌切开术的内镜医师，在括约肌切开术后出血率较高[132]。括约肌切开术后出血的治疗方法包括注射稀释的肾上腺素、热灼法(如使用 BICAP 探头)、机械法(如在括约肌切开术中使用充气的球囊)、使用金属夹或置入覆膜可扩张的金属支架。在出血未得到控制的情况下，可能需要进行治疗性血管造影或手术。必须注意避免损伤胰腺括约肌。

(二) 穿孔

ERCP 病例中穿孔的发生率低于 1%[132-134]。十二指肠外侧壁穿孔往往较大，通常需要手术干预。随着超范围夹闭器械的出现，内镜下闭合穿孔是可能的[135]。胆道括约肌切开术或取石术后造成的壶腹周围穿孔，如果早期发现，需要手术

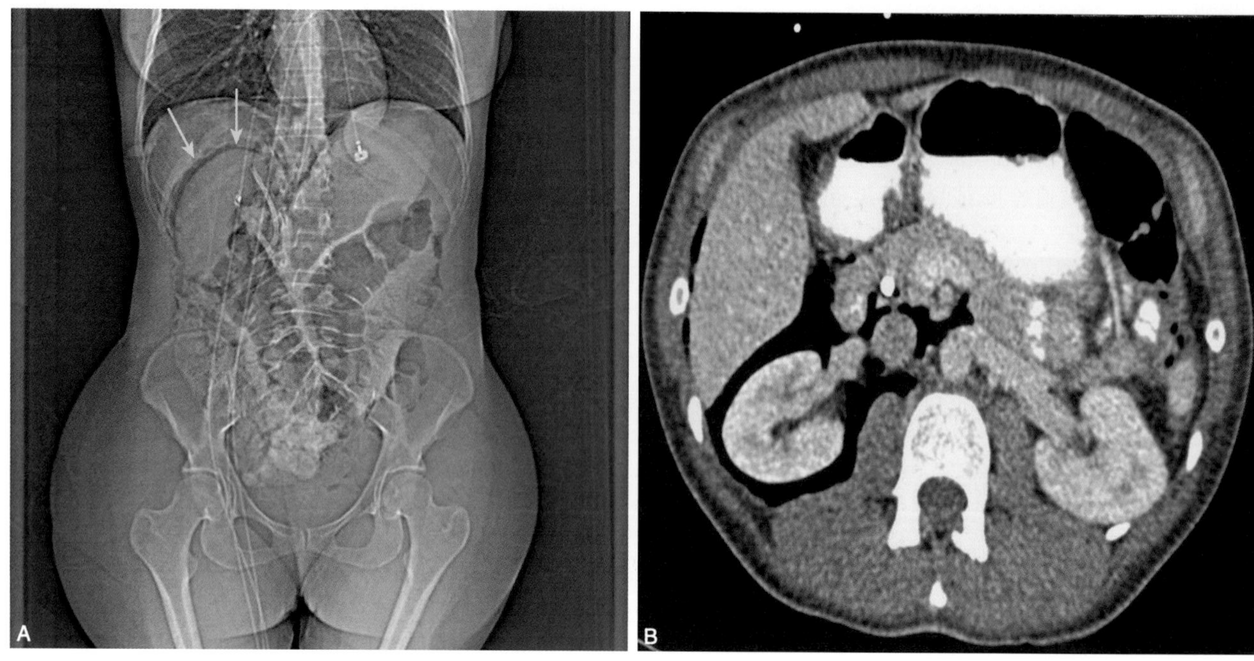

图 42.5 A,放射学图像显示胆道括约肌切开术后右肾周积气。确定穿孔,置入胆道支架(箭头)。B,CT 示腹膜后积气。患者接受抗生素治疗观察 48 小时后平安出院

干预的可能性较小(见图 42.5)。内镜治疗包括放置塑料或全覆膜金属支架[136,137]。胆管穿孔通常是在梗阻附近使用导丝或网篮进行内固定的结果。其中大多数可以通过放置塑料或全覆膜金属支架进行保守治疗。在闭合失败、延迟入路或有明确腹膜后外渗证据的患者中,应考虑手术干预。

(三)胆管炎

胆管炎和胆囊炎的发生率分别为 1% 和小于 0.5%[132]。上行性胆管炎的风险因素包括经皮/内镜联合手术、恶性肿瘤支架植入术和胆道通路阻塞或引流失败[132]。在 ERCP 之前,使用其他成像方式(如 MRCP)进一步确定复杂的胆道解剖结构可能是有用的。这些疾病的管理可能包括重新尝试内镜治疗、经皮入路或手术干预。预防性抗生素不能降低 ERCP 术后胆管炎的风险。现行指南建议仅在接受 ERCP 且预期引流不完全的患者中,进行预防性抗生素治疗[138]。

(四)胰腺炎

ERCP 术后胰腺炎的讨论见第 58 章。其发病率从 5% 到 10% 不等[132,133]。与手术和患者相关的某些风险因素,可能将该风险放大到 20% 以上。患者和手术因素均被确定为 ERCP 术后胰腺炎的危险因素(框 42.1)。胰腺炎的严重程度从轻度的短暂住院到重度的多器官衰竭和死亡不等。也许 ERCP 方案最重要的组成部分是确保遵守框 42.1 中列出的风险因素,并在知情同意的前提下使用适当的无创成像检查。随机对照试验和荟萃分析显示,预防性放置胰腺支架有助于预防 ERCP 术后胰腺炎[139,140]。特定的电烙术切割电流是否会影响风险存在争议[141,142]。最近在高风险患者中进行的一项随机对照试验报告,使用直肠吲哚美辛可显著减少 ERCP 术后胰腺炎的发生[143]。ERCP 术后胰腺炎的治疗仍然是支持性的(见第 58 章),在这种情况下重复 ERCP 是没有作用的。

框 42.1 ERCP 术后胰腺炎的风险因素(另见第 58 章)
十二指肠乳头括约肌球囊扩张
插管失败或困难
ERCP 后胰腺炎病史
血清胆红素水平正常
胰管注射
胰管导丝置入
胰管括约肌切开术
胰腺组织取样
乳头括约肌预切开术
疑似 SOD
青年人
ERCP,内镜逆行胰胆管造影;SOD,奥迪括约肌功能障碍。

如果存在假性囊肿感染,ERCP 始终是一种可能性。应结合 ERCP 考虑囊肿引流方案。在大多数情况下,可通过内镜下囊肿胃造口术或囊肿十二指肠造口术引流[144]。

十一、超声内镜

由超声内镜(EUS)通过引起的食管穿孔罕见(0.03%)[145]。食管穿孔的风险因素包括患者年龄较大、操作者缺乏经验和食管插管困难[145]。在高达三分之一的食管恶性肿瘤患者中,超声内镜难以通过或无法通过。在这些患者中,连续食管探条扩张至 16mm 是安全的,可以完成 EUS 检查[146,147]。

囊性病变的 FNA 增加了发热、靶向囊肿感染和败血症的风险。有证据支持在术前开始预防性抗生素治疗,并持续至

术后 48 小时[148,149]。此外，接受直肠周围病变 FNA 的患者应考虑预防性使用抗生素。目前的数据不支持在淋巴结或实体性肿块的 FNA 过程中使用预防性抗生素。在高达 4% 的 FNA 病例中可能发生轻度管腔内胃肠出血[150]，在 1.3% 的 FNA 病例中可能发生管腔外出血[151]。在高达 2% 的患者中报告的胰腺炎最有可能继发于细针穿刺针通过胰腺组织所形成的通道[152]。

十二、新型内镜技术

随着新的内镜技术的出现，如内镜黏膜下剥离术（endoscopic submucosal dissection，ESD）、经口内镜下食管括约肌切开术（peroral endoscopic myotomy，POEM）和内镜减重手术，必须彻底了解风险和收益。ESD 是一种技术，现在越来越多地用于整块切除大的肿瘤病变。该技术并发症的发生率取决于部位（直肠与盲肠）。POEM 是贲门失弛缓症最首选的内镜治疗方法（见第 44 章），并发症低于腹腔镜 Heller 肌切开术。内镜减重手术属于微创手术范围，如胃内球囊至内镜袖状胃成形术（见第 8 章）。此类手术的适当适应证正在演变。

使用单人操作的胆道镜观察胆管具有与 ERCP 相似的并发症特征，但胆管炎的风险增加。一项前瞻性研究表明，当有指征时直接胆道镜检查胆总管的菌血症风险似乎与 ERCP 一样安全，即使在老年患者中也是如此[153]。内镜下引流已经成为处理复杂胰腺积液和包裹性胰腺坏死的首选疗法（见第 58 章）。管腔相对的金属支架具有极好的安全性特征，需要干预的并发症包括支架移位（4.2%）、感染（3.8%）、出血（2.4%）和支架闭塞（1.9%）[154]。

（王萍　张烁 译，李鹏 校）

参考文献

第五部分　食管

第 43 章　食管解剖学、组织学、胚胎学和发育异常

Ryan D. Madanick, Vishal Kaila 著

章节目录

一、解剖和组织学 …… 595
（一）肌肉组织 …… 595
（二）神经支配 …… 596
（三）血液和淋巴循环 …… 597
（四）黏膜 …… 597
（五）黏膜下层 …… 598
二、胚胎学 …… 598
三、发育异常 …… 598
（一）食管闭锁和气管食管瘘 …… 598
（二）先天性食管狭窄 …… 601
（三）食管重复畸形 …… 602
（四）血管异常 …… 602
（五）食管环 …… 603
（六）食管蹼 …… 604
（七）异位胃黏膜（入口斑）…… 604

一、解剖和组织学

食管作为将食物从口腔输送到胃的管道。为了安全有效地实施这项任务，食管被构造成一个 18~26cm 长的中空肌肉管，内有一层复层鳞状上皮的“皮肤样”衬里（图 43.1）。吞咽之间食管塌陷，但吞咽时管腔向前后扩张达 2cm，向外侧扩张 3cm，以容纳吞咽的食块。在结构上，食管壁由 4 层组成：从内向外依次为最内层的黏膜、黏膜下层、固有肌层和最外层的外膜；与胃肠道的其余部分不同，食管没有浆膜[1,2]。这些层在解剖学上的描述，如图 43.2 中超声内镜（EUS）所示。

（一）肌肉组织

食管固有肌层负责执行食管的运动功能。其上端 5%~33% 由骨骼肌组成，远端 50% 由平滑肌组成。两者之间的中段是两种肌肉类型的混合[3]。食管近端起始于咽下缩肌与环咽肌汇合处。环咽肌是骨骼肌的一个区域，在功能上称为食管上括约肌（upper esophageal sphincter，UES）（图 43.3A）。UES 在静息时收缩，因此形成一个高压区，阻止吸入的空气进入食管。在 UES 下方，食管壁由内环肌层和外纵肌层组成（见图 43.2A）。食管体位于气管和左主支气管后方的后纵隔

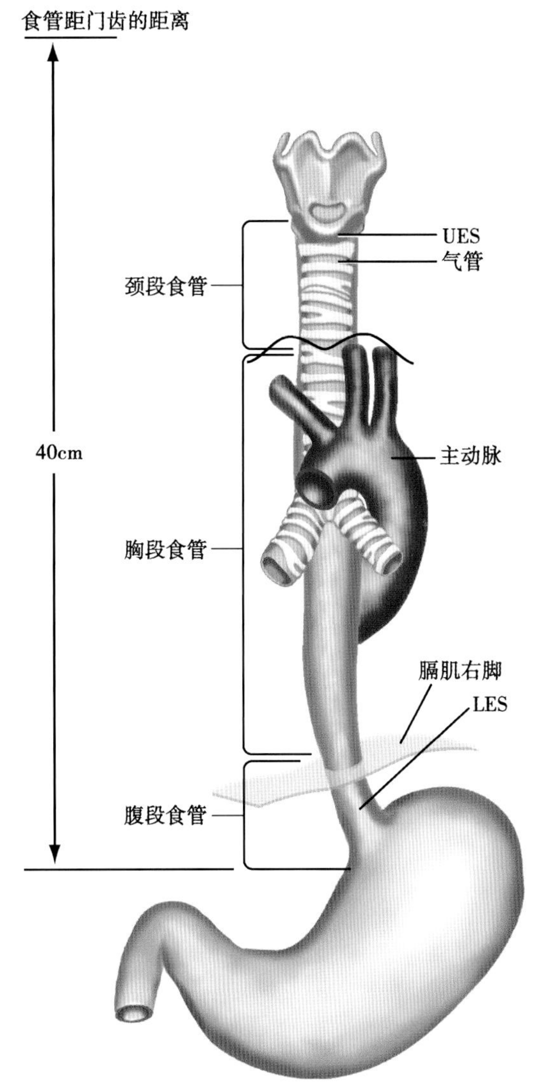

图 43.1　食管的解剖及其与邻近结构的关系。食管长约 25cm，起源于环状软骨水平的颈部，穿过胸部，通过膈肌右脚裂孔后，与下方的胃连接而结束。钡剂食管造影：邻近结构可使食管壁凹陷，包括主动脉弓、左主支气管、左心房和膈肌。LES，食管下括约肌；UES，食管上括约肌。（Modified from Liebermann-Meffert D. Anatomy, embryology, and histology. In: Pearson FG, Cooper JD, Deslauriers J, et al, editors, Esophageal surgery. 2nd ed. Philadelphia: Churchill Livingstone; 2002. P 8.）

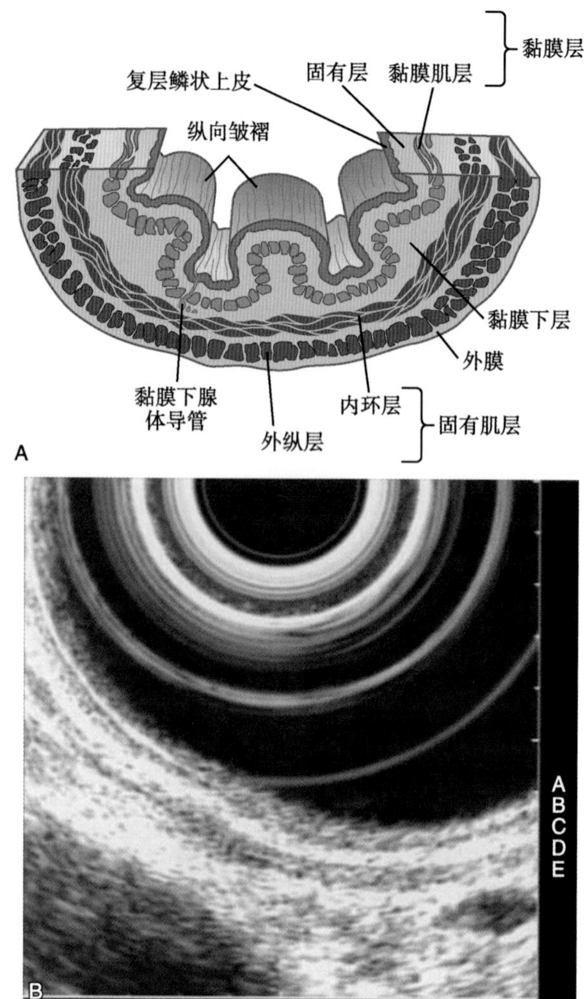

图 43.2　食管的横断面和超声内镜解剖。A,图示食管壁内的解剖层。B,一张超声内镜图像,描绘了食管不同层回声产生的亮环(高回声)和暗环(低回声)图像。(A,食管腔与黏膜之间的界面;B,黏膜;C,黏膜下层;D,固有肌层;E,外膜。)注意 A、C 和 E 为高回声,B 和 D 为低回声。(A,Modified from Neutra MR,Padykula HA. The GI tract. In:Weiss L,editor. Histology,cell and tissue biology. 5th ed. New York:Elsevier Science;1983. P 664.)。

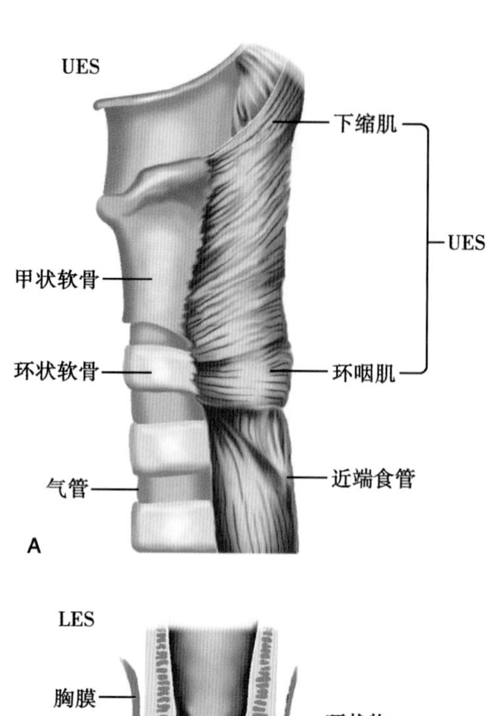

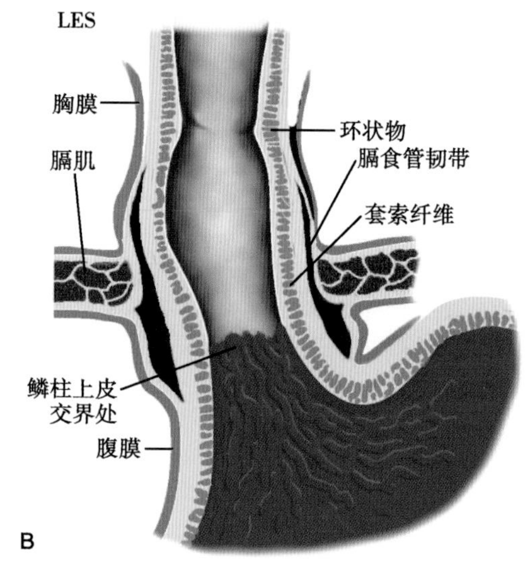

图 43.3　A,食管上括约肌(UES)的解剖细节及其与邻近结构的关系。B,食管下括约肌(LES)的解剖细节及其与膈肌、膈食管韧带和鳞状上皮与柱状上皮连接的关系。(A,Modified from AGA Clinical Teaching Project. Esophageal disorders:Upper esophageal sphincter anatomy,slide 14,American Gastroenterological Association,1995;B,modified from Kerr RM. Hiatal hernia and mucosal prolapse. In:Castell DO,editor. The esophagus. Boston:Little,Brown & Company;1992. p 763.)

内,并向左转弯通过心脏后方和主动脉前方[1]。在胸 10 椎体水平食管体通过右膈脚内的裂孔离开胸腔(见图 43.1)。在膈肌裂孔内,食管体以 2~4cm 长的不对称增厚的环形平滑肌终止,称为食管下括约肌(lower esophageal sphincter,LES)(见图 43.3B)[4]。膈食管韧带起源于膈肌的腹横筋膜,嵌入食管下段,有助于将 LES 固定在膈肌裂孔内。这种定位是有益的,因为它使膈肌收缩,以协助 LES 在运动期间维持高压区。LES 在静息时收缩形成高压区,阻止胃内容物进入食管。在吞咽过程中 LES 松弛,以通过蠕动将吞咽的食团从食管推入胃内。

(二) 神经支配

食管壁由副交感神经和交感神经支配,副交感神经通过迷走神经调节食管蠕动(图 43.4)。迷走神经的细胞体起源于延髓。位于疑核内的控制骨骼肌,而位于背侧运动核内的控制平滑肌。延髓迷走神经节后传出神经直接终止于食管上段骨骼肌的运动终板,而通向食管远端平滑肌的迷走神经节前传出神经,终止于位于环形肌层和纵行肌层之间的 Auerbach(肌间)神经丛内的神经元[3]。第二个神经感觉网络,Meissner 神经丛位于黏膜下层,是食管壁内传入冲动的部位。这些冲动通过迷走神经副交感神经和胸交感神经传递至中枢神经系统。感觉信号通过迷走神经传入通路传递到中枢神经系统内的孤束核(见图 43.4);从那里神经传递到迷走神经的疑核和背侧运动核,其信号可能影响运动功能[5]。

由食管引起的疼痛感觉通常是由食管黏膜或黏膜下层的化学感受器和/或食管肌肉组织中的机械感受器刺激触发的[6]。当这些冲动通过交感神经和迷走神经传入神经传递到大脑时,就会产生中枢感知。交感神经传入通过背根神经节到达脊髓后角,而迷走神经传入通过结状神经节到达延髓的孤束核。来自交感神经/脊髓传入的神经信息随后通过脊髓-

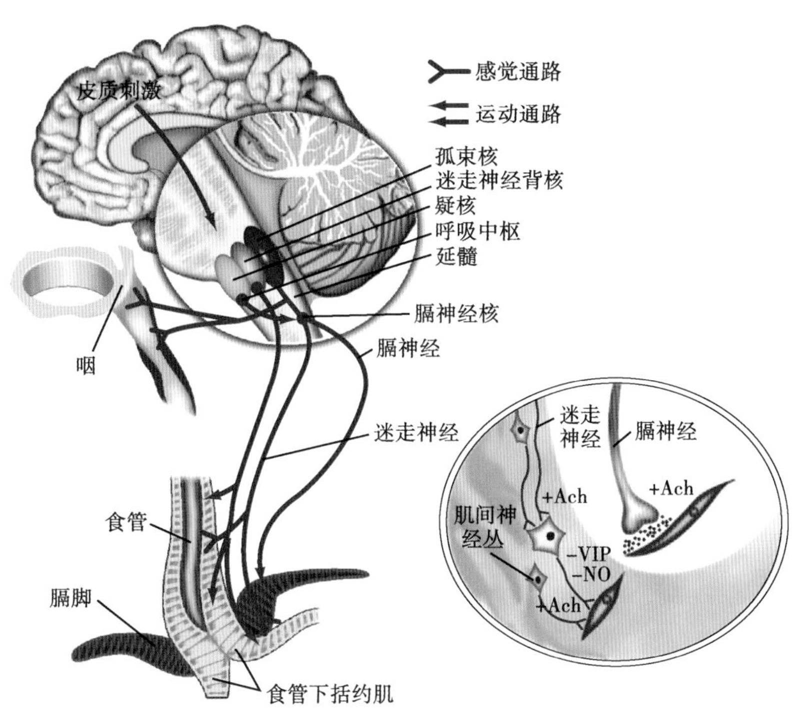

图 43.4　食管神经通路。外源性神经支配主要由迷走神经提供。迷走神经传入通路将刺激传递到孤束核，起源于迷走神经背核的传出通路介导食管蠕动和食管下括约肌松弛。Ach，乙酰胆碱；NO，一氧化氮；VIP，血管活性肠肽。（From Mittal. RK，Balaban DH. The esophagogastric junction. N Engl J Med 1997；336：924.）

丘脑和脊髓网状通路传递到丘脑和网状核，然后再传递至躯体感觉皮层进行痛觉感知，传递到边缘系统进行痛觉调节。来自延髓的迷走神经传入信息也传递至边缘系统和额叶皮质进行疼痛调节。此外，由于食管神经解剖通路与心脏和呼吸系统的神经解剖通路相互重叠，在临床实践中，可能难以辨别某些胸痛综合征的起源器官[6]。

（三）血液和淋巴循环

食管的动脉和静脉血液供应是分段的。食管上段由甲状腺上、下动脉分支供血；食管中段由支气管动脉、右肋间动脉和降主动脉分支供血；食管远端由胃左动脉、膈下左动脉和脾动脉分支供血[1-3]。这些血管吻合在黏膜下层形成致密的网状结构，被认为是食管梗死的罕见的原因。食管上段静脉经上腔静脉引流，食管中段静脉经奇静脉引流，食管远端静脉经门静脉的胃左静脉和胃短静脉引流。食管远端黏膜下静脉吻合网很重要，因为它是门静脉高压症患者形成食管静脉曲张的部位[1-3]。

食管的淋巴系统也是节段性的，食管上段引流至颈深淋巴结，食管中段引流至纵隔淋巴结，食管远端引流至腹腔和胃淋巴结。然而，这些淋巴系统也通过许多通道相互连接，这解释了大多数食管癌在发现时已扩散到该区域以外的原因。

（四）黏膜

在内镜检查时，正常食管黏膜光滑、呈粉红色。正常食管胃交界处呈不规则的白色 Z 线（锯齿状缘），这是分隔颜色较浅的食管黏膜和颜色较红的胃黏膜之间的界面。组织学上，食管黏膜为非角化的复层鳞状上皮（图 43.5）。该上皮由功能截然不同的 3 层组织组成：角质层、棘层和生发层。最面向管腔的角质层是管腔内容物与血液之间的通透性屏障，由多层薄饼状富含糖原的细胞通过紧密连接和小带黏附横向相互连接，细胞间隙内充满致密的糖复合物基质[7]。中间的棘层含有代谢活跃的棘状细胞。棘状是由于在整个层中有大量桥粒连接细胞。此外，这种相同的桥粒网络维持了组织的结构

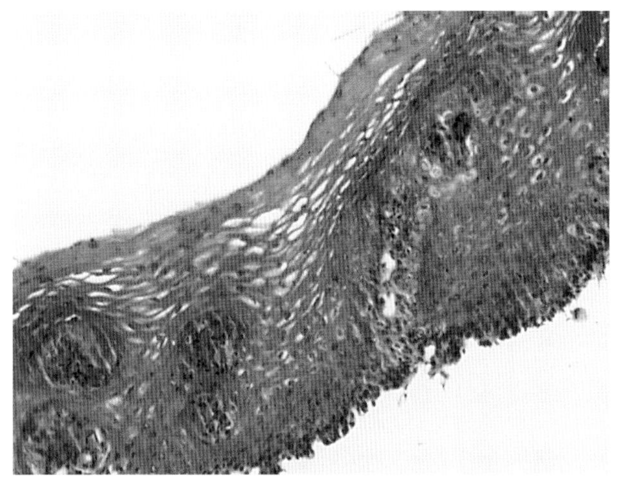

图 43.5　食管上皮。该活检标本显示人食管内衬为非角化复层鳞状上皮。表面（顶部）的细胞长而扁平，核浆比例小；而基底层（底部）的细胞，密度大、呈立方状、核浆比例大是其突出的原因。这些基底层细胞的一个亚群似乎具有食管干细胞的特性[7]。上皮钉突或真皮乳头含有固有层成分，通常延伸至上皮中，距离管腔约一半。（Courtesy Pamela Jensen，MD，Dallas，TX）

完整性。生发层的基底层含有立方细胞，占上皮厚度的10%～15%，具有独特的复制能力[2]。基底细胞增生是指基底细胞占上皮厚度的15%以上，反映了组织修复率增加。这在胃食管反流病(GERD)中常见(见第46章)。

食管上皮含有少量其他类型的细胞，包括嗜银神经内分泌细胞、黑色素细胞、淋巴细胞、朗格汉氏细胞(巨噬细胞)和嗜酸性粒细胞。在健康上皮中不存在中性粒细胞[2]。

上皮下方是固有层，为疏松的结缔组织网，其内有血管和分散的淋巴细胞、巨噬细胞和浆细胞(见图43.5)。固有层以一定间隔突入上皮，形成钉突或真皮乳头。正常情况下，这些突起不到上皮厚度的50%，当其厚度超过时，被认为是诊断GERD的标志物[8]。黏膜肌层是一层较薄的平滑肌，将上方的固有层与黏膜下层分开。其功能尚不清楚。

(五) 黏膜下层

黏膜下层由致密的结缔组织网络组成，其中包括血管、淋巴管、麦氏神经丛(Meissner)和食管腺体(见图43.2A)。这些腺体沿食管的数量及分布各不相同，由立方细胞组成的腺泡组织形成[9]。其产生并分泌润滑剂、黏液、碳酸氢盐和表皮生长因子等，对上皮防御和修复很重要。这些腺体的分泌物进入迂曲的集合管，将其输送到食管腔。

二、胚胎学

本文简要回顾上消化系统的胚胎学，以了解本章讨论的

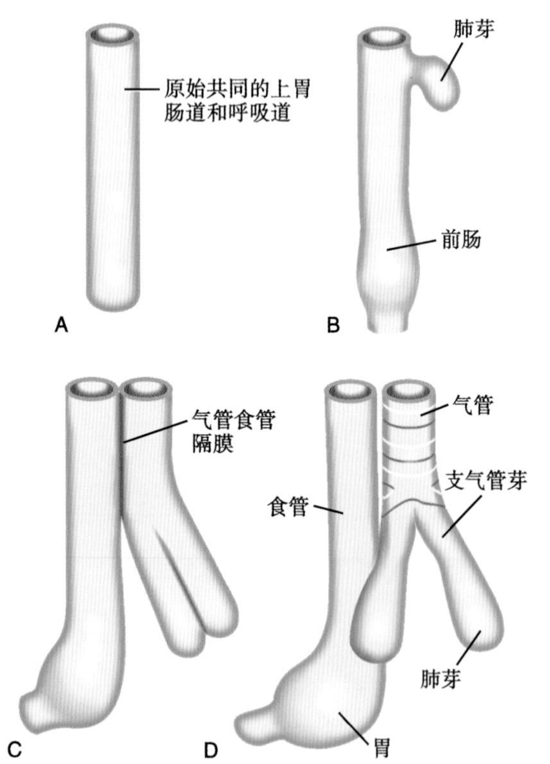

图43.6　形成单独呼吸系统和消化系统的发育阶段。这些系统起源于胚胎形成过程中的内胚层共同管。A，单个原始管。B，第4周形成肺芽。C，背管(原始前肠)和肺芽延长，4～6周形成气管食管隔。D，6周时原始前肠从气管支气管树中分离

许多发育异常的起源。在发育中的胎儿中，胃肠道的口咽和食管成分以及呼吸道的喉、气管、支气管和肺由一根共同的管道发育而来[3]。到妊娠第4周，该管道由内胚层组成，在其腹侧表面形成憩室，该憩室注定成为呼吸道的上皮和腺体(图43.6A～D)。憩室随后伸长，被内脏间充质(未来的软骨、结缔组织和平滑肌)包裹，并出芽、脱落发育成为原始呼吸道。同时，背管的管腔即原始前肠，充满增殖的纤毛柱状上皮。到第10周，空泡出现，随后在原始前肠内融合，重建管腔。到第16周，原始前肠和未来食管内衬的柱状上皮被复层鳞状上皮取代，这一过程在出生时完成。

三、发育异常

先天性食管异常相对常见。是由于遗传缺陷的传递或阻碍胎儿成熟的子宫内应激所致。食管异常见于早产儿，60%有其他异常，这可通过术语VACTERL(以前称为VATER)来反映，VACTERL是与脊椎、肛门、心脏、气管、食管、肾脏和肢体系统(vertebral, anal, cardiac, tracheal, esophageal, renal, and limb systems)异常相关疾病的简要记忆方法。常见的特异性缺陷包括动脉导管未闭、心脏间隔缺损、肛门闭锁等[10]。

(一) 食管闭锁和气管食管瘘

食管闭锁即食管上下段之间的连续性丧失，气管食管瘘是气管与食管之间的异常连接，都是食管最常见的发育异常(图43.7和图43.8)。食管闭锁和气管食管瘘的发病率约为1/4 000[11]。前者是由于原始前肠未能再通所致，后者是由于肺芽未能与前肠完全分离所致。尽管机制尚不清楚，但食管闭锁和气管食管瘘可能是由遗传缺陷引起的(表43.1)[12]。正确的音猬因子信号是实现呼吸道与原始前肠分离的关键通路之一[13]。实验研究将抗肿瘤药物阿霉素注入小鼠或大鼠胚胎，通过改变音猬因子信号通路，导致食管闭锁和气管食管瘘，以及构成VACTERL组的其他异常[14,15]。

食管闭锁仅在7%的病例中作为孤立异常发生。其余病例伴有一种形式的气管食管瘘，最常见(89%)为远端型瘘(见图43.7B)，以及少见(3%)的H型瘘(见图43.7C)[16]。在孤立性闭锁中，食管上段末端为盲袋，食管下段与胃相连(图43.7A)。这种情况在产前即表现为羊水过多(因为胎儿无法吞咽和吸收羊水)和胃泡缺如或很小[17]。产前超声检查发现近端食管扩张并伴有盲端，又称为食管袋，对食管闭锁具有高的特异性，尽管该发现的敏感性有限[18]。产前超声或MRI检查时，胎儿下咽部膨胀是食管闭锁的另一产前征象，敏感性优于食管袋。产前MRI可提供食管全长的图像，可用于辅助诊断食管闭锁[19]。此外，产前MRI显示下食管管腔则提示存在气管食管瘘(图43.9)。若出生时出现唾液反流和舟状(无气)腹则强烈提示孤立性食管闭锁，无远端气管食管瘘，因为不存在吸入或吞咽的空气进入肠道的途径。在首次喂养时，食管闭锁的高度完全性胃肠道梗阻导致快速发生窒

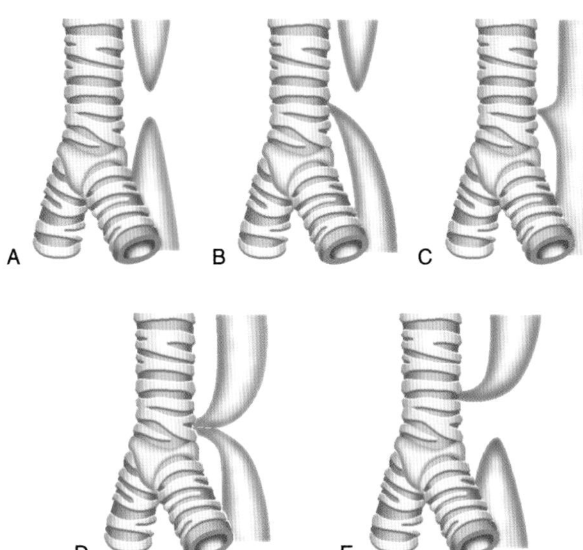

图 43.7　食管闭锁(A)和气管食管瘘(TEF)。在最常见的TEF中,气管与闭锁食管远段(B)相通。其次最常见的类型是H型TEF,在该类型中,气管与其他正常食管(C)相通。气管与闭锁食管的上下段(D)或仅与闭锁食管的上段(E)相通的TEF是罕见。(Modified from nonneoplastic esophagus. In: Fenoglio-Preiser CM, editor. GI pathology. An atlas and text. 2nd ed. Philadelphia: Lippincott-Raven; 1999. p 31.)

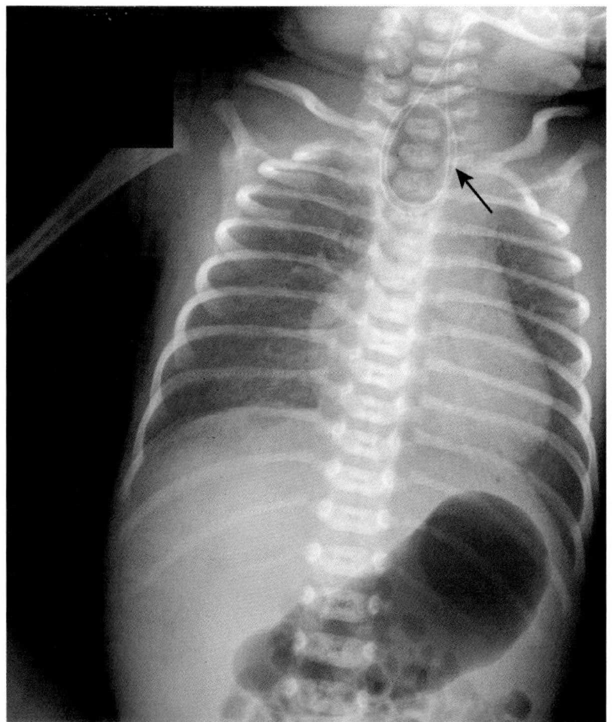

图 43.8　气管食管瘘胸片。显示导管盘绕在第二胸椎水平的食管(箭)中,胃内有空气。(From Forero Zapata L, Pappagallo M. Esophageal Atresia and Tracheoesophageal Fistula. N Engl J Med. 2018;379(7):e11.)

表 43.1　气管食管瘘和食管闭锁综合征的原因和临床特征

综合征	基因	临床特征
无眼-食管-生殖器综合征	*SOX2*	无眼症/小眼症 EA/TEF 泌尿生殖系统异常
CHARGE 综合征	*CHD7*	眼缺损 心脏异常 后鼻孔闭锁 智力障碍 生长迟缓 生殖器异常 耳部异常 听力丧失 EA/TEF
Feingold 综合征	*MYCN*	食管/十二指肠闭锁 小头畸形 学习障碍 并指/趾畸形 心脏缺陷
Fanconi 贫血	>20 基因	骨髓衰竭 恶性肿瘤 身材矮小 异常皮肤色素沉着 放射线缺陷 眼部异常 肾脏异常 心脏缺陷 耳部异常 中枢神经系统异常 听力丧失 发育延迟 胃肠道异常,包括 EA/TEF
VACTERL-H	*FANCB*	脊椎畸形 肛门闭锁 心脏畸形 TEF 肾脏异常 肢体异常 脑积水

EA,食管闭锁;TEF,气管食管瘘。

Adapted from Scott DA. Esophageal atresia/tracheoesophageal fistula overview. In: Adam MP, Ardinger HH, Pagon RA, et al., editors. GeneReviews®[Internet]. Seattle: University of Washington, Seattle; 1993.

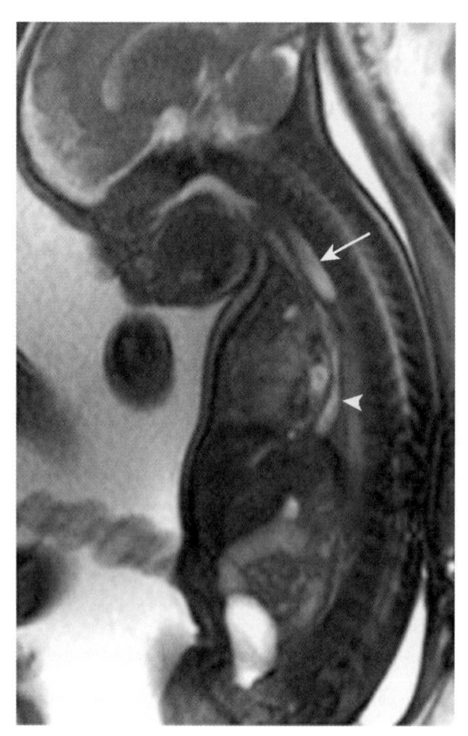

图 43.9　矢状位 T2 加权 MRI 序列显示食管闭锁。显示近端盲袋(箭)和远端长食管(箭头)。(From Cassart M. Fetal Body Imaging:When is MRI Indicated? J Belg Soc Radiol. 2017;101(S1):3.)

息、咳嗽和反流(表 43.2)。一旦怀疑,通过鼻胃管不能插入胃部,同时进行食管上段空气造影胸部 X 线检查(空气通过位于食管上段内的导管导入)即可确诊。在某些情况下,向阻塞段注射 1mL 水溶性造影剂有助于诊断。

气管食管瘘通常伴随食管闭锁。气管食管瘘最常见的类型是与食管闭锁相关的远端型(见图 43.7B)[16]。在这种类型中,闭锁的上食管末端在盲袋中,气管与远段食管段相通。这种结构的临床表现通常与孤立性食管闭锁相似。胃内容物通过瘘管反流进入气管会增加吸入性肺炎发生的风险(见表 43.2)。尽管如此,孤立性闭锁与远端气管食管瘘之间的区别是显而易见的,因为气管和食管之间的连接导致腹部充满气体,如平片所示(见图 43.8)。在某些情况下,可通过用或不用支气管镜检查的食管造影来确认构型类型。

有 3 种少见的气管食管瘘:①闭锁的上段食管与气管相通;②闭锁的食管上段和下段均与气管相通;③非闭锁食管中的 H 型瘘与气管相通(分别见图 43.7E、D 和 C),由于这些类型具有共同的上食管和气管之间的交通,它们在临床上均表现为复发性(吸入性)肺炎的症状和体征(见表 43.2)。然而,区分不同类型并不困难。伴有近端气管食管瘘的食管闭锁在婴儿期表现为反复发作的肺炎,X 线平片上有无肠内气体表明是否存在伴有远端气管食管瘘。相比之下,在没有食管闭锁的 H 型气管食管瘘患者中,诊断可延迟到儿童期甚至成年期。疑似 H 型瘘的诊断通常做食管造影,但由于一些交通口的尺寸太小,明确诊断可能很困难[20]。在这种情况下,可摄

表 43.2　食管发育异常的临床表现

异常	出现年龄	主要症状	诊断	治疗
孤立性闭锁	新生儿	喂食反流、误吸	食管造影* 腹部平片:无气腹	外科手术
闭锁+远端 TEF	新生儿	喂食反流、误吸	食管造影* 腹部平片:腹部充气	外科手术
H 型 TEF	婴儿至成人	复发性肺炎及支气管扩张	食管造影* 支气管镜检查†	外科手术
食管狭窄	婴儿至成人	吞咽困难食物嵌塞	食管造影* 内镜检查†	扩张‡ 外科手术§
食管重复囊肿	婴儿至成人	呼吸困难、喘鸣、咳嗽(婴儿)、吞咽困难、胸痛(成人)	EUS* MRI/CT†	外科手术
血管异常	婴儿至成人	呼吸困难、喘鸣、咳嗽(婴儿)、吞咽困难,胸痛(成人)	食管造影* 血管造影† MRI/CT/EUS	饮食调整‡ 外科手术§
食管环	儿童至成人	吞咽困难	食管造影* 内镜检查†	扩张‡ 内镜下切开§
食管蹼	儿童至成人	吞咽困难	食管造影* 内镜检查†	探条扩张术

*首选诊断试验。
†确诊性试验。
‡主要治疗方法。
§二级治疗方法。
CT,计算机断层扫描;EUS,超声内镜检查;MRI,磁共振成像;TEF,气管食管瘘。

入亚甲蓝和通过支气管镜寻找蓝染的瘘管部位来改善检出率。

食管闭锁和气管食管瘘的治疗首选外科手术。术前应评价患者是否存在其他 VACTERL 异常,尤其是心脏异常[21]。手术方式的选择取决于食管上段与下段之间的距离。短间隙(间隙小于 3 个椎体)可行端端吻合,通过探条扩张术或术中肌切开术延长上段后的一段间隙也允许端端吻合[16]。磁性压迫吻合术,或称磁压榨吻合术,已用于一些食管闭锁患者的修复[22]。如果无法对合两个节段,则进行食管初次重建。结肠可插入近端食管残端和胃之间,或将胃向近端牵拉并与食管残端吻合。当食管闭锁作为孤立异常存在时,其手术矫正的效果非常好,总体结局主要由伴随心脏异常的严重程度和婴儿的出生体重决定[23,24]。近年来,成功修复孤立性食管闭锁后的存活率稳步提高,在没有其他严重畸形的情况下,存活率已接近 100%[25]。

尽管在过去几十年中患者生存率显著提高,但长期并发症仍然很常见。在长期随访中,57% 的患者发生无食管炎的胃食管反流[26]。40% 的患者发生 GERD 伴食管炎,Barrett 食管的患病率为 6.4%[27]。胃食管反流病的发生可能与手术修复后食管运动异常和酸清除受损有关[28]。大约 20%~35% 的患者在其一生中的某个时间点需要胃底折叠术治疗 GERD。遗憾的是,这些患者中 20%~30% 的胃底折叠术将会失败[29]。50% 存活至成年期的患者发生吞咽困难[26]。30%~56% 的患者可发生吻合口狭窄。虽然在接受食管闭锁修复术的成年人中报告有发生食管癌的病例(腺癌和鳞状细胞癌),但芬兰和瑞典的登记研究中,这些患者的癌症风险不一定有统计学意义[28,30]。

(二) 先天性食管狭窄

食管狭窄是一种罕见的异常,每 25 000~50 000 例活产儿中仅有 1 例发生[31]。狭窄段的长度从 2cm 到 20cm 不等,通常位于食管的中 1/3 或下 1/3 段(图 43.10A)。先天性食管狭窄的确切原因尚不完全清楚。部分患者(17%~33%)有其他相关异常,最常见的是食管闭锁(见图 43.10B)和气管食管瘘[32]。根据组织学,可识别出 3 种类型的狭窄:①异位气管支气管残留部分(tracheobronchial remnant,TBR),其为隐蔽的呼吸组织(透明软骨、呼吸道上皮),表明其起源为肺芽与原始前肠的不完全分离[33];②纤维肌性肥大,与肌间神经丛损伤和丧失肌肉松弛的氮能神经成分相关;③膜性膈,仅限于黏膜,不累及肌层[34]。一项系统性综述显示,继发于纤维肌性肥厚的先天性食管狭窄占病例的 54%,30% 的病例继发于 TBR,16% 继发于膜性膈[35]。膜性膈通常见于食管上段和中段,纤维肌性肥厚见于食管中段和下段,TBR 主要见于食管下 1/3[35]。大约四分之一的病例伴有食管闭锁和气管食管瘘[36]。

尽管严密的狭窄在婴儿期有症状,但当摄入更多固体食物时,大多数狭窄在儿童期表现为吞咽困难和反流(见表 43.2)。食管造影能很好显示狭窄,可显示突然狭窄或锥形狭窄。狭窄近端的食管扩张是常见的(见图 43.10)。内镜检查可显示狭窄区域的正常黏膜,这有助于排除获得性狭窄(如 GERD)的原因。使用高频微型探头 EUS 可显示伴有声影的强回声病变,这表明 TBR 所致狭窄的患者存在软骨结构[37]。

一些患者在内镜引导下行探条或球囊扩张术后有所改善。但由于常常发生胸痛和黏膜撕裂,因此内镜医师在为这

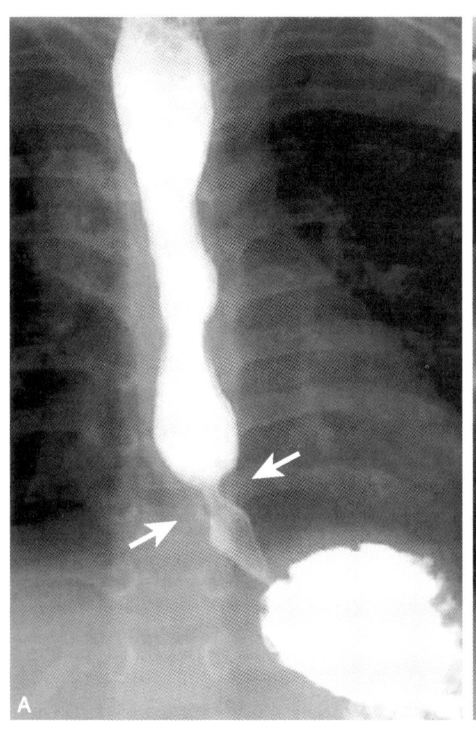

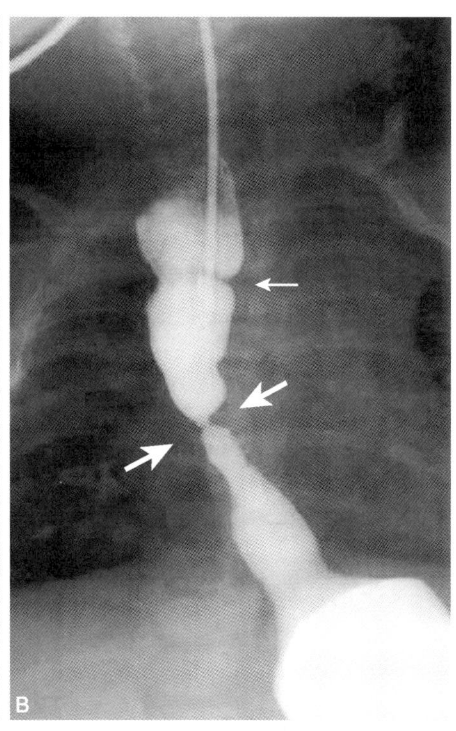

图 43.10 2 例先天性食管狭窄患者的食管钡剂造影。A,食管钡剂造影,食管远端逐渐狭窄,近端食管扩张。B,食管钡剂造影显示食管中段突然狭窄(粗箭)。细箭表示既往食管闭锁修复术的部位。(A and B, From Usui N, Kamata S, Kawahara H, et al. Usefulness of endoscopic ultrasonography in the diagnosis of congenital esophageal stenosis. J Pediatr Surg 2002;37:1744.)

些患者进行食管扩张时应该格外小心。据报告,扩张术后的食管穿孔率为10%~44%[38-40]。有问题的狭窄需要手术切除受累节段。治疗这种病变的新型手术方法是环形肌切开术,该技术涉及剥离含有TBR的食管肌层,保留黏膜层。这样做的优点是避免了一期修复和食管端-端吻合术相关的许多潜在并发症[41]。继发于纤维肌性肥厚的狭窄段可行纵向肌切开术[42]。

(三) 食管重复畸形

先天性食管重复畸形的发生率为1/8 000活产婴儿,约占胃肠道重复畸形的20%[2,43]。食管重复畸形的发病机制尚不确定,尽管它们可能是器官形成过程中异常空泡化的结果。食管重复体是由上皮内衬和发育良好的平滑肌层组成,是与食管连接的附属物。重复体在形态上可以是囊性的、管状的或是憩室性的。囊肿占重复体的80%,通常是单个充满液体的结构,不与食管相通[2]。大多数重复囊肿发生于食管下段,位于后纵隔内,尽管有腹内食管重复囊肿的报道[44]。食管重复囊肿大多数在儿童期确诊,7%的病例在成年期表现为症状性囊肿[45]。有些囊肿是在无症状时被发现的,表现为胸片上的纵隔肿块或食管造影上的黏膜下病变(图43.11A)。其他表现为气管支气管树邻近结构受压的症状(咳嗽、喘鸣、呼吸急促、发绀、哮鸣或胸痛)和食管壁邻近结构受压的症状(吞咽困难、胸痛或反流)(见表43.2)[46]。

食管重复囊肿的诊断是通过CT、MRI或EUS显示囊性肿块来支持的(见图43.11B)[47]。重复囊肿表现为食管管腔外源性压迫病变,黏膜外观正常。在EUS上,重复囊肿可表现为边缘清晰的均匀无回声或低回声肿块[48]。囊肿内可见的蠕动是食管重复囊肿非常特异的(并被认为是诊断特征)[49]。由于存在与手术相关感染的显著风险,EUS引导下的FNA对重复囊肿进行病理诊断存在争议[48]。手术切除是有症状和无症状重复囊肿确诊病例的首选治疗方法[48]。罕见的大的重复囊肿可表现为急性危及生命的呼吸道症状。在这种情况下,可通过放射学或内镜引导下的针吸术实现紧急减压。

管状食管重复畸形的发生率远低于囊性食管重复畸形(20%的病例),憩室型食管重复畸形很少见。管状型囊肿通常位于食管壁内,与食管真腔平行,与重复囊肿相反,管状囊肿在管的一端或两端与真腔相通[46]。食管重复畸形在婴儿期通常会引起胸痛、吞咽困难或反流,通过食管造影或内镜检查可确定诊断。虽然有些病例可以通过内镜进行治疗,但重建手术适用于大多数有症状的患者[46,50,51]。

(四) 血管异常

2%~3%的人群存在胸廓内血管异常。尽管食管造影显示血管明显受压,但很少出现食管梗阻症状。在婴儿期,大多数胸廓内血管异常表现为气管支气管树受压引起的呼吸道症状。然而,在儿童期或成年人后期,由于食管受压迫,这些异常也会导致吞咽困难和反流(见表43.2)。

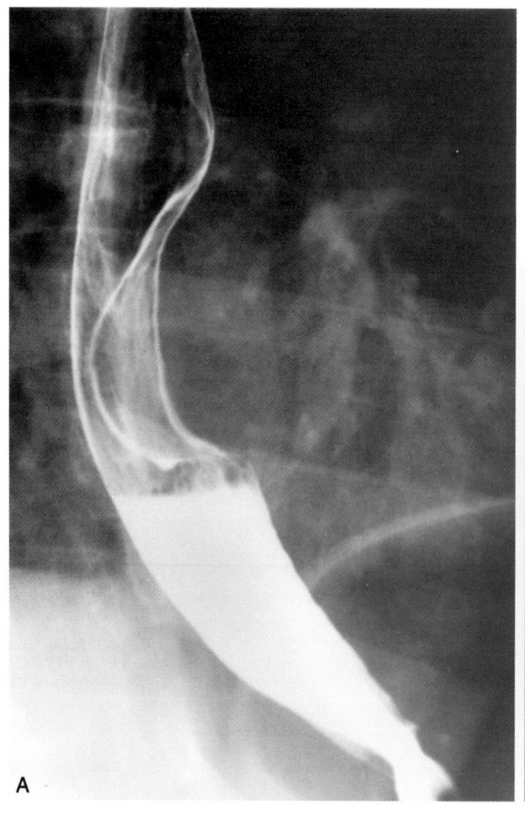

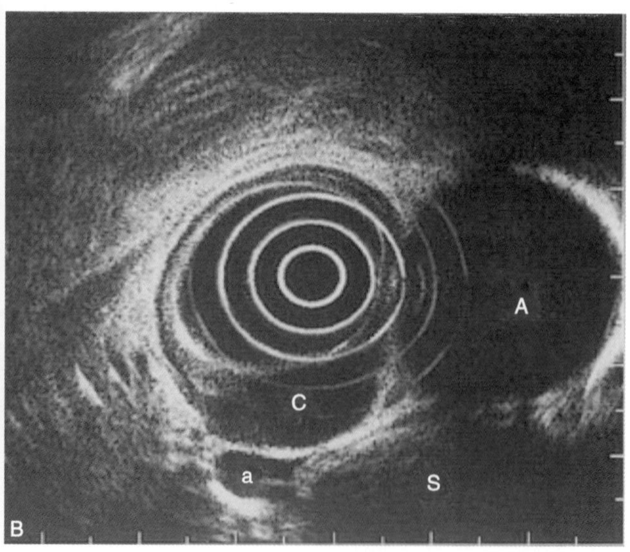

图43.11　影像学检查显示食管重复囊肿。A,钡剂食管造影显示食管壁外源性压迫。B,EUS图像显示低回声囊肿。(C)造成的食管壁扭曲,囊肿与主动脉(A)、奇静脉(a)和脊柱(S)造成的其他低回声区的关系。(A,Courtesy David Ott,MD,Winston-Salem,N. C.;B,from Kimmey MB,Vilman P. Endoscopic ultrasonography. In:Yamada T,editor. Atlas of gastroenterology. 3rd ed. Philadelphia:Lippincott Williams & Wilkins;2003. p 1044.)

Lusoria 吞咽困难是由变异的异常右锁骨下动脉压迫食管引起的症状(图 43.12)[52]。这种情况是由于右侧咽弓发育缺陷所致,在正常情况下,咽弓转变为右锁骨下动脉。右锁骨下动脉起源于主动脉弓的左侧,从食管后的左下方走行至食管的右上方。在 20% 的病例中,该动脉走行于食管前方[53]。根据尸检研究,估计 0.7% 的普通人群中存在鲁索里亚动脉。通常通过钡剂食管造影来确定诊断。钡剂食管造影显示第三和第四胸椎水平的特征性铅笔状凹痕(见图 43.12B)[52]。通过 CT、MRI、动脉造影或 EUS 检查可证实(见图 43.12C)。鉴于此类病变无症状的发生率相当高,内镜检查或食管测压可能有助于排除其他原因引起的吞咽困难。在内镜检查过程中,右桡动脉搏动可能因仪器压迫右锁骨下动脉而减弱或消失。食管测压显示在变异动脉部位有搏动性高压区[54]。该症状通常对简单地调整饮食作出反应,即食用稀软和小块食物。必要时手术,通过将异常动脉与升主动脉吻合来解除梗阻(见图 43.12A)[54]。

(五) 食管环

远端食管可包含两个"环",即 A 环和 B 环(Schatzki 环),从解剖学上划分食管前庭的近端和远端边界。A 环(肌肉)位于近端边缘(见图 43.3)。它是一条宽(4~5mm)对称的肥厚肌肉带,在其与前庭的交界处收缩食管腔。在该位置,被鳞状上皮覆盖的 A 环对应于 LES 的上端[55]。A 环是罕见的,食管造影的口径取决于食管扩张的程度,一般无症状。偶尔发现 A 环与固体和液体的食物吞咽困难有关(见表 43.2)[55]。有症状的 A 环可通过大口径水银加权食管扩张器、注射肉毒杆菌毒素或经口、内镜下肌肉切开术治疗[56,57]。

B 环,也称为黏膜环或 Schatzki 环,非常常见,在 6%~14% 常规上胃肠道序列检查的受试者中发现[58]。最近一项对 10 000 多例上消化道内镜检查的回顾性研究中发现,4% 的

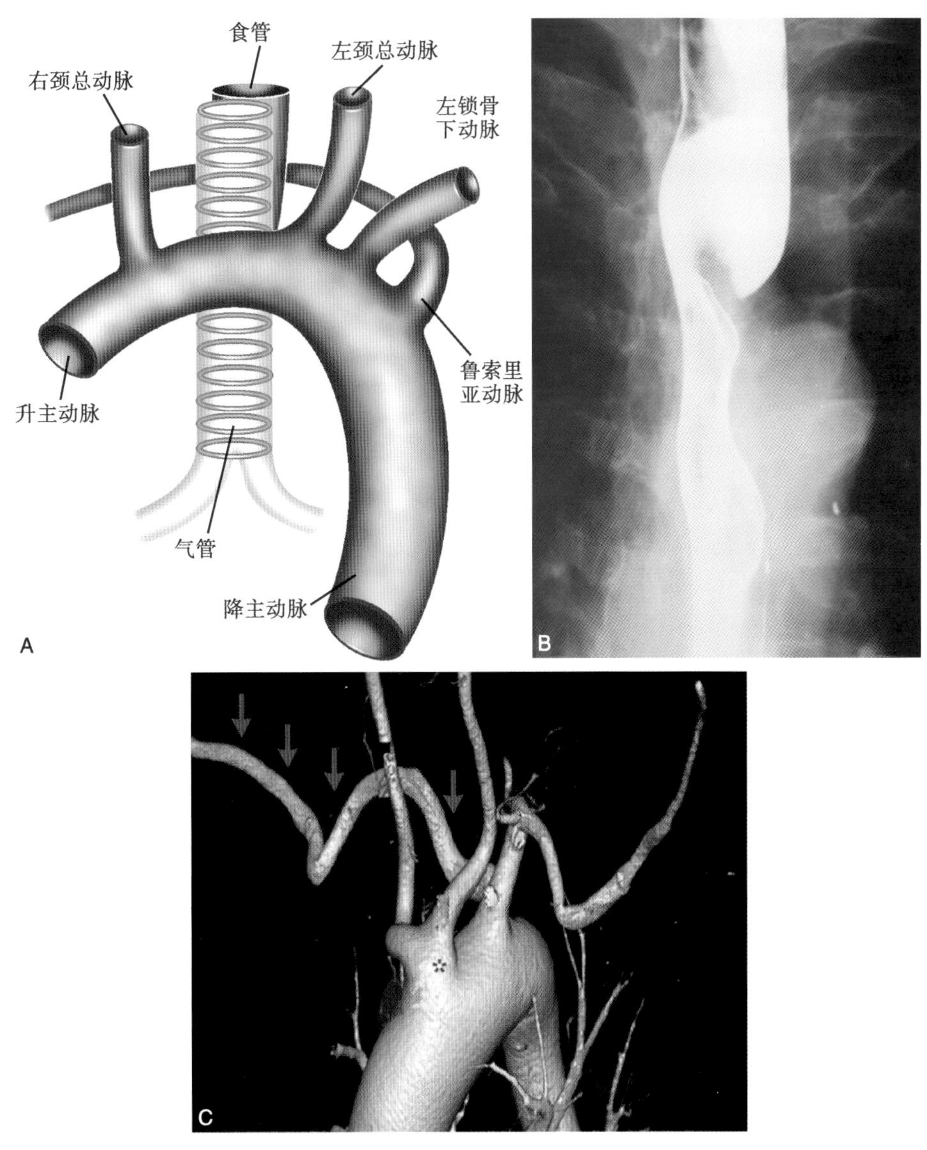

图 43.12　Lusoria 吞咽困难。A,变异的右锁骨下动脉(Lusoria 动脉)的解剖结构,从主动脉弓到右肩在食管后走行。B,食管钡剂造影显示第三、第四胸椎水平食管壁的特征性对角线压痕。C,CT 与 3D 重建。(A,From Janssen M,Baggen MG,Veen HF,et al. Dysphagia lusoria:Clinical aspects,manometric findings,diagnosis,and therapy. Am J Gastroenterol 2000;95:1411;B,courtesy David Ott,MD,Winston-Salem,NC;C,from(1)Hudzik B,Gasior M. Dysphagia Lusoria. N Engl J Med. 2016;375(4):e4.)

病例有 Schatzki 环[59]。在钡剂研究中,总是发现其与食管裂孔疝有关,被认为是一层 2mm 薄的膜,在前庭和胃贲门交界处收缩食管腔(图 43.13A)。Schatzki 环的上表面有鳞状上皮,下表面有柱状上皮,因此划分出鳞柱上皮的交界处。B 环本身仅由黏膜和黏膜下层组成,无固有肌层。Schatzki 环可以是先天性的,也可以是后天获得性的,很可能与 GERD 有关(见第 46 章)[58]。

大多数 B 环无症状,但当食管腔直径缩小至 13mm 或更小时,B 环通常是固体食物或突发急性固体食物嵌塞引起间歇性吞咽困难的原因(见表 43.2)[60]。食管造影(见图 43.13A)或内镜检查(见图 43.13B)通常不难识别有症状的环,但应注意充分扩张食管远端[58]。在某些情况下,阻塞环最好通过其捕获吞咽的棉花糖或钡片的能力进行影像学证明,该技术也可以帮助确定阻塞环的直径。无症状的 B 环不需要治疗。而产生吞咽困难的患者可通过单个、大的水银加权扩张器或一系列直径逐渐增大的此类扩张器得到有效的治疗[61]。早期研究报告,32% 的患者在 1 年后需要重复扩张[58]。最近的研究报告了更低的重复扩张率(13%),可能是由于常规地使用更大的扩张器和一个疗程扩张治疗后的抗反流治疗的原因[62]。在对 44 例有症状的 Schatzki 环患者进行的一项随机安慰剂对照研究中,平均随访 35 个月后,使用奥美拉唑维持治疗可使患者的再扩张需求减少 40%[63]。最近的一项观察性研究证明,使用四象限大型冷活检钳完全切除 Schatzki 环可安全有效地预防复发[64]。通过内镜电烙术切口方法成功治疗了 64 例难以扩张的有症状 B 环[65]。针对有症状 Schatzki 环的标准探条扩张术与电烙术切口的随机对照试验证明,这两种治疗的初始成功率相当,但内镜下切口的症状消退持续时间更长[66]。

(六) 食管蹼

食管蹼是一种发育异常,其特征是食管上段(颈部)和食管中段内有一层或多层鳞状上皮的薄层水平膜。与食管环不同,这些异常很少环绕管腔反而是从前壁突出,向外侧延伸而不向后壁延伸(图 43.14A 和 B)。食管蹼常见于颈段食管,在食管造影侧位片上最容易显示。高达 5% 的病例为无症状状态,但当其出现症状时,会导致固体食物吞咽困难(见表 43.2)[67]。食管蹼是脆弱的膜,因此对使用水银加权的食管探条扩张器反应良好。

正如第 37 章所讨论的,成人颈部食管蹼、吞咽困难和缺铁性贫血的相关性被称为 Plummer-Vinson 综合征或 Paterson-Kelly 综合征[67]。该综合征虽然不常见,但主要发生在女性。Plummer-Vinson 综合征与乳糜泻之间可能存在关联[68]。该综合征确定了一组咽和食管鳞状细胞癌风险增加的患者[67]。纠正 Plummer-Vinson 综合征中的铁缺乏,可使相关吞咽困难症状缓解以及食管蹼消失[67]。

(七) 异位胃黏膜(入口斑)

入口斑是指在食管浅粉色鳞状黏膜中,内镜下发现一个小的(0.5~2cm)独特的天鹅绒样的红色异位胃黏膜岛,一般位于 UES 正下方(图 43.15A)。当寻找时,在高达 10% 的内

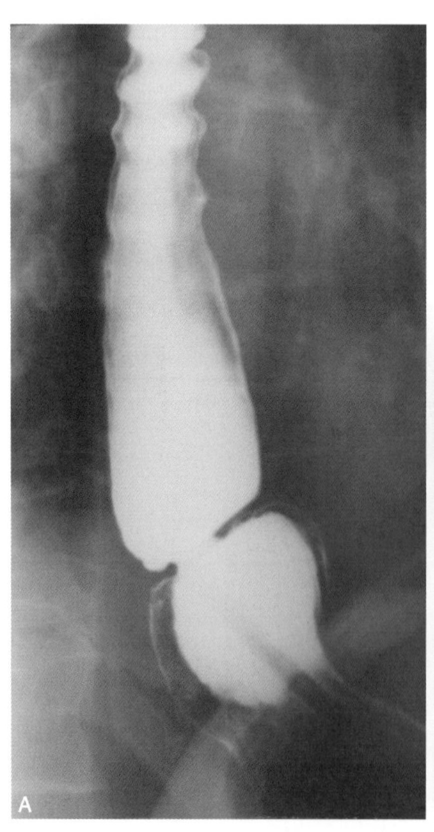

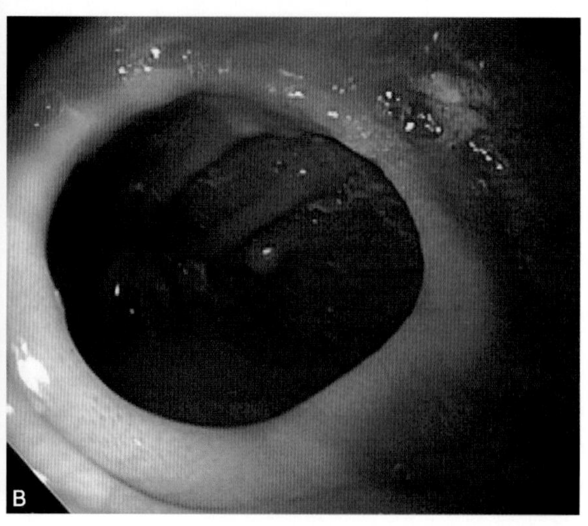

图 43.13　影像学检查显示食管 B(Schatzki)环。A,钡剂食管造影显示黏膜环局限于鳞柱交界处。B 环下方为裂孔疝,疝显示为上方 B 环与下方膈肌之间的一个小囊。B,B 环的内镜视图。(A,Courtesy David Ott,MD,and Winston-Salem,NC;B,courtesy John D. Long,MD,and Winston-Salem,NC.)

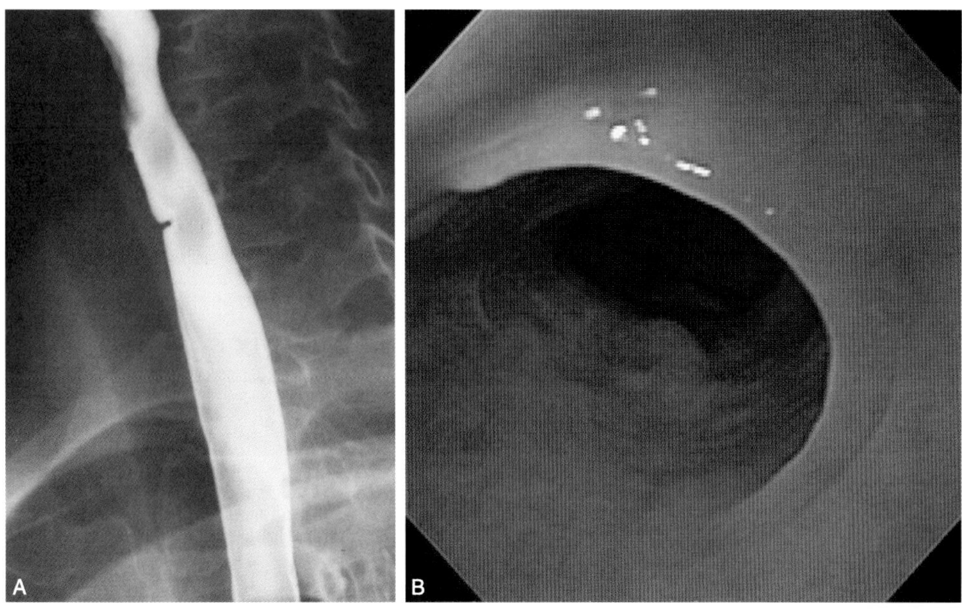

图 43.14　食管蹼的影像学研究。A，颈段食管蹼的钡剂食管造影。在侧位片上可见从食管前壁突出的薄膜。此为蹼不是环，通常不完全环绕食管腔。B，颈段食管蹼的内镜视图。（A，Courtesy David Ott，MD，and Winston-Salom，NC；B，Courtesy John D. Long，MD，and Winston-Salem，NC.）

镜检查中发现入口斑，且活检标本显示胃底或胃窦型黏膜（见图 43.15B）[69,70]。胃底型黏膜含有主细胞和壁细胞，因此，在一些标本中保留了分泌酸的能力[71]。与胃内胃黏膜相似，入口斑可感染 Hp[72]。然而，入口斑通常无症状，与疾病无关，因此不需要治疗。在一项研究中提示了其与癔球症（globus pharyngeus，即咽部异感症）可能相关，在该研究中，使用氩等离子凝固器消融入口斑后，该症状得到改善[73]。在极少数情况下，在与食管蹼、狭窄[74]或溃疡相关的部位发现入口斑，后者导致食管出血或穿孔[69]。尽管入口斑与近端食管腺癌之间存在统计学显著相关性，但发生于入口斑的腺癌仍是一种罕见并发症[69,75]。通过内镜检查监测的必要性存在争议，尚未达成正式共识。

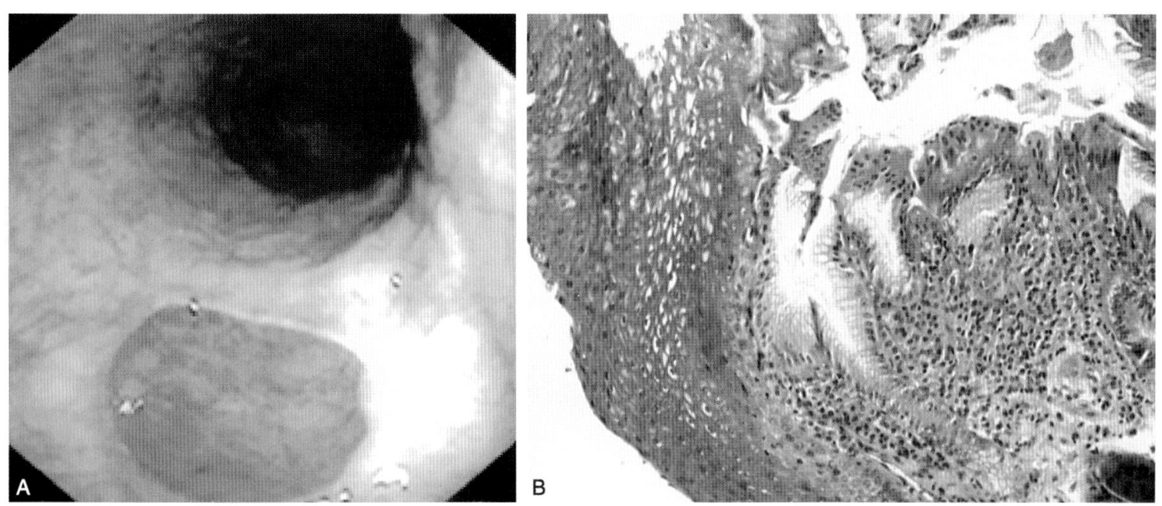

图 43.15　入口斑的内镜图像。A，颈段食管异位胃黏膜的内镜视图（“入口斑”）。B，入口斑的显微组织照片视图，显示腺上皮和壁细胞（右）与正常食管鳞状上皮相邻（左）。（A，From Avidan B，Sonnenberg A，Chejfec G，et al. Is there a link between cervical inlet patcch and Barrett's esophagus? GastrointestEndosc 2001；53：717；B，courtesy Pamela Jensen，MD，Dallas，TX.）

（程妍　刘军 译，袁农 校）

参考文献

第 44 章　食管神经肌肉功能及动力障碍疾病

John E. Pandolfino, Peter J. Kahrilas 著

章节目录

一、运动和感觉功能 …… 606
（一）口咽部和食管上括约肌 …… 606
（二）咽部吞咽 …… 608
（三）食管 …… 608
（四）食管胃交界处 …… 610
（五）食管感觉 …… 611
二、食管动力障碍 …… 613
（一）流行病学 …… 613
（二）发病机制 …… 613
（三）临床特点 …… 616
（四）鉴别诊断 …… 617
（五）诊断方法 …… 618
（六）治疗 …… 622

食管是一个长管状的肌性器官，连接下咽部和胃，两端有括约肌相连，具有运输食物、液体和气体等简单功能。因此，食管肌层存在由口咽部的横纹肌向胃肠道平滑肌的解剖和生理转变。在神经学上，口咽部横纹肌由大脑皮质和延髓控制，能够精确感知触觉；食管远端完全由平滑肌组成，受迷走神经和肠神经系统控制，感觉相对不敏感。虽然食管横纹肌和食管平滑肌之间是逐渐过渡的，但口咽和食管体部的运动功能是截然不同的，考虑到这一点，接下来的讨论包括与食管功能密不可分的咽、胃和膈肌功能的特定方面。

一、运动和感觉功能

（一）口咽部和食管上括约肌

在口腔内，口唇、牙齿、硬腭、软腭、下颌、口底和舌用于形成和容纳食物，使之成为适合转移到咽部的食团。咽部分为3个部分：鼻咽、口咽和下咽（图 44.1）。鼻咽从颅底延伸至软腭的远端边缘。鼻咽肌肉在吞咽过程中抬高软腭，封闭鼻咽部，阻止鼻咽反流。口咽从软腭延伸至舌根。口咽下缘由前方的会厌谷和后方的会厌移动尖端分界。下咽从会厌谷延伸至环状软骨下缘，包括食管上括约肌（upper esophageal sphincter, UES）。

软腭、舌和咽部的肌肉组织在吞咽过程中均会塌陷，缩短咽腔，然后将其内容物排入食管。此外，外部肌肉将咽部抬高并向前拉动，从而封闭气道并开启食管上括约肌。咽部固有肌：上、中、下咽缩肌（见图 44.1）重叠排列并插入一个胶原薄

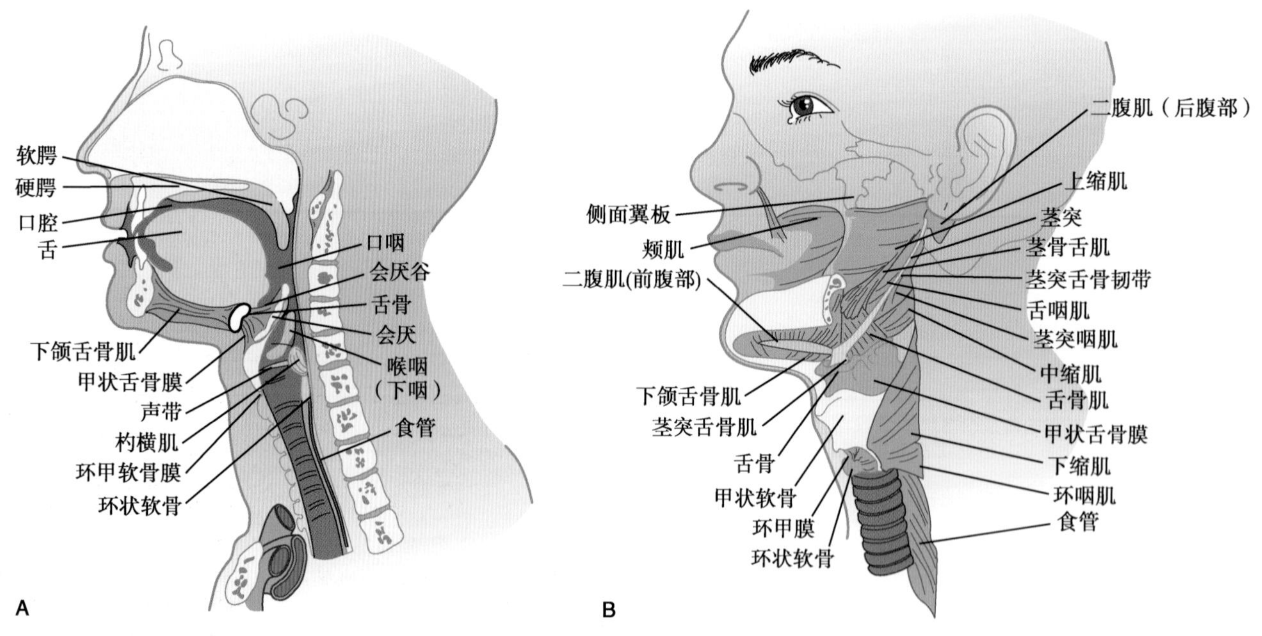

图 44.1　咽部解剖图。A，咽部矢状位图。显示参与吞咽过程中的肌肉骨骼结构。食管在静息状态时是塌陷和空虚的。在吞咽的过程中，通过高度协调的肌肉活动，封闭喉部入口，打开食管入口。B，咽部肌肉组织的剖面图。舌骨被定位为一个支点，有助于引导向前、向上的牵引力（舌骨前移），在吞咽过程中舌骨前移对封闭喉部和打开食管入口至关重要。（Reprinted from Kahrilas PJ, Frost F. Disorders of swallowing and bowel motility. In: Green D, editor. Medical problems of the chronically disabled. Rockville, MD: Aspen Publishers; 1990. p 11-37.）

层,即颊咽腱膜。下咽缩肌由甲咽肌(上部分)和环咽肌(下部分)组成。甲咽肌起自甲状软骨,经后内侧,插入中缝正中。环咽肌有上、下两部分,每部分均起自环状软骨板两侧;上部分环咽肌行走于中缝后内侧,而下部分环咽肌环绕食管入口,不经中缝。Killian 三角(环咽肌上三角)一个由薄肌肉形成的三角形区域,在这些成分之间的后方形成,是咽部搏动性憩室最常见的起源部位。

咽部还含有 5 个单个或成对的软骨(见图 44.1)。下缩肌外侧端和甲软骨外侧壁之间形成的间隙为梨状窦,其末端止于环咽肌下方,将咽与食管分开。喉和气管悬吊在舌骨上方和胸骨下方之间的颈部。许多肌肉,被归类为喉带肌,有助于这种悬吊,加之气管的固有弹性,使喉部得以上升和下降。舌依附在舌骨上,舌骨是舌活动的根基。喉部运动对吞咽反应至关重要,因为在吞咽过程中,喉入口是关闭的,并且从推注路径中物理移除食团,若未能实现这种同步喉部运动可能会导致误吸。

咽肌由来自三叉神经核、面神经核、舌咽神经核、舌下神经核以及迷走神经疑核和脊髓 C1 至 C3 段的运动纤维密集支配。疑核内的所有运动神经元均参与吞咽,其中食管横纹肌的运动神经元位于口侧,支配咽、喉的运动神经元位于尾侧[1]。食管上括约肌的肌肉成分是环咽肌、邻近食管和相邻环咽肌的下缩肌,有助于构成 1cm 的最大压力区[2]。闭合的食管上括约肌呈狭缝状结构,在环状软骨板前方,和环咽肌的侧后方。起源于疑核的迷走神经干的神经输入维持食管上括约肌的压力,若迷走神经横断则会消除这种收缩活动。

食管上括约肌功能的测压评估是很困难的,因为它是一个短而复杂的解剖区域,在吞咽过程中快速移动。此外,由于其明显的不对称性以及对咽部和食管刺激的反射性收缩,食管上括约肌压力受到记录方法的严重影响。因此,无法界定有意义的食管上括约肌压力的正常范围[3]。吞咽过程中食管上括约肌松弛也给记录带来了很大的挑战,使得技术和解释存在很大的差异。然而,利用固态技术的高分辨率测压(high-resolution manometry,HRM)可准确地跟踪吞咽过程中食管上括约肌松弛和食团内的压力变化(图 44.2)。

食管上括约肌保持食管交界处近端闭合,除非吞咽或嗳气时需要打开。它还构成了一个额外的屏障,阻止反流物质从食管进入咽部。并通过与吸气同步收缩防止空气进入食管。吸气增强在食管上括约肌处于低压期间最为明显,往往在有癔球感的个体中可能被夸大[4]。食管气囊扩张刺激食管上括约肌收缩[5],在近端气囊位置的影响更明显。然而,当使

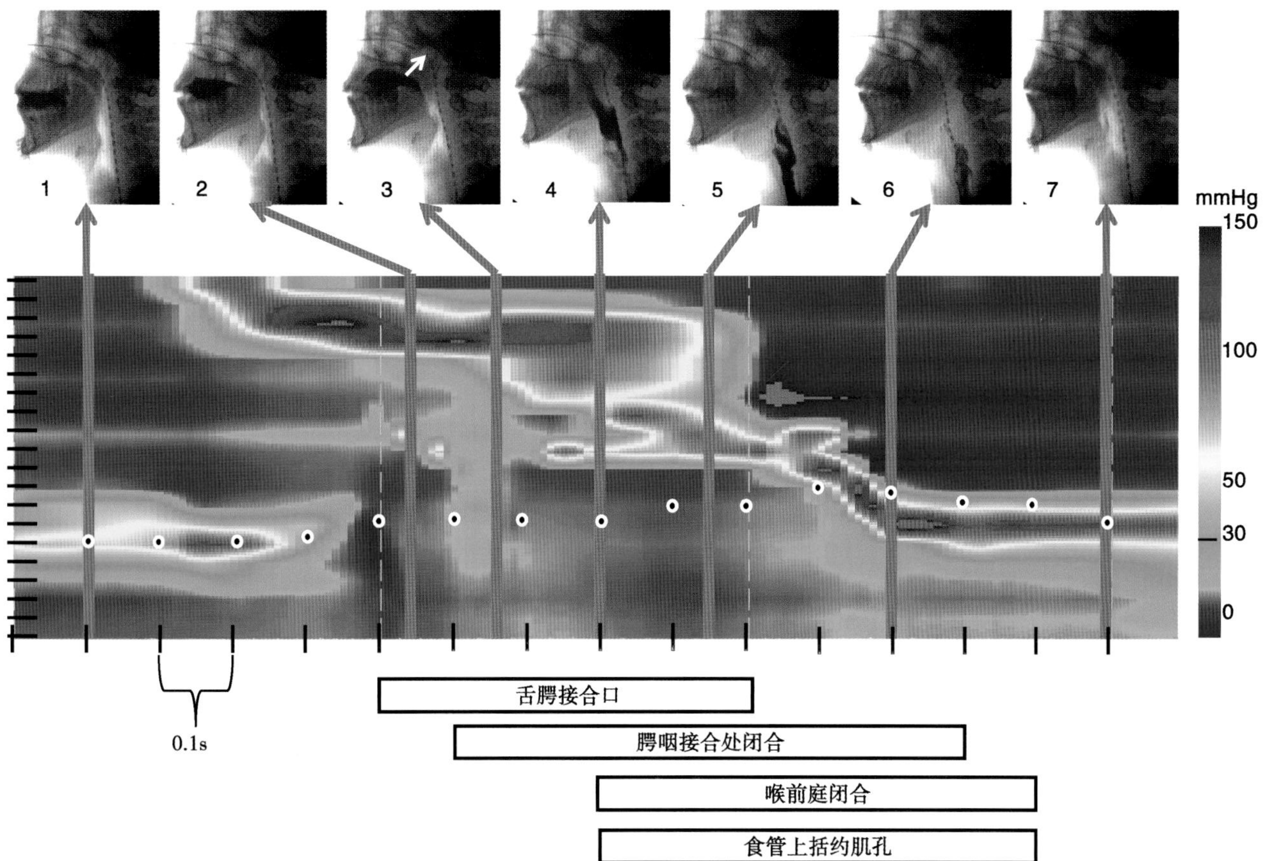

图 44.2 荧光透视结合高分辨率测压(HRM)。在 HRM(彩色面板上用粉色箭头标出)上的特定时间进行描绘的透视图像(顶部)。时间线显示了荧光透视下咽部吞咽活动的协调和时间段。每个水平线(横线)均描述了其中一个口咽瓣处于其吞咽构型的时间段,与呼吸时的构型相反,并与透视图像相关:①口腔内食团的基线解剖,②舌腭开口与食管上括约肌松弛同步发生,压力通常低于 10mmHg,③腭咽接合处闭合,封闭鼻咽以防止反流(注意白色箭头所示的抬高),④喉前庭闭合和食管上括约肌开放发生在会厌内翻时,当空气引导的食团快速通过食管上括约肌时,喉前庭关闭,⑤随着咽剥离波的开始食团持续通过,⑥当咽部剥离波穿过食管上括约肌而喉前庭始终保持闭合状态时,完成食团向食管的转移,⑦咽部恢复呼吸构型,喉前庭打开,会厌恢复直立位。地形图(HRM)上的黑点表示食管上括约肌在每个时间点的近端位置。(With permission from the Esophageal Center at Northwestern.)

用圆柱形气袋或向食管快速注入空气来模拟气体反流的扩张模式时，会发生食管上括约肌松弛而不是收缩[2]。嗳气引起的食管上括约肌松弛也与声门闭合有关。精神压力会增加食管上括约肌压力，而麻醉或睡眠[6]几乎会消除压力。无论是在正常志愿者还是在消化性食管炎患者中，无论是实验性食管酸灌注还是自发性胃食管酸反流均不会改变连续记录食管上括约肌压力。

（二）咽部吞咽

口腔吞咽期出现的吞咽紊乱可伴随着许多以整体神经功能障碍为特征的疾病，如创伤性脑损伤、脑肿瘤或舞蹈病（见第37章），这些疾病的详细讨论可在关于吞咽评估及治疗的文本中找到。吞咽主要是下意识地协调收缩，将口腔内容物转移到食管。能够触发咽部吞咽的传入感觉神经纤维通过喉上神经（来自喉）和舌咽神经（来自咽）的内侧支传输到中枢，这些感觉神经纤维在终止于延髓吞咽中枢之前汇集。

虽然在生理学上理解为运动神经元及其相应运动单位的模式化活动，但吞咽在临床上是用机械术语进行评估的，最好通过荧光透视或X线电影照相分析进行评估。咽部吞咽迅速将咽部结构从呼吸路径重构为消化路径，然后在1秒钟内恢复为呼吸路径。咽吞咽反应可分为几个密切协调的动作：①通过抬高和回缩软腭关闭鼻咽，②食管上括约肌开放，③喉部关闭，④舌负载（斜坡），⑤舌推进，⑥咽清除。这些行为的精确协调是非常必要的，在某种程度上，这些行为的相对时机既受到意识的控制，又受到食团体积大小的影响（见图44.2）。

将口咽从呼吸路径转换为吞咽路径所需的最基本的解剖重构是打开食管入口，并封闭喉的入口。这些活动以紧密同步的方式发生，通过喉抬高和舌骨轴向前牵引促进的。认识到食管上括约肌松弛和开放之间的区别是至关重要的。食管上括约肌松弛是由于喉部抬高时兴奋性神经输入停止所致。一旦喉部抬高，食管上括约肌开放是由于舌骨上、下肌肉组织收缩引起的前括约肌壁牵拉所致，也会导致舌骨移位的特征性模式。

舌和咽缩肌促进食团从口咽输送出。舌的运动适应不同的吞咽状态，并在咽部收缩开始前将大部分食团推入食管。另一方面，咽部收缩更为模式化，其功能是从咽壁上剥离最后的残留物。食管上括约肌闭合与咽部收缩的通路同时发生。

然而，括约肌的收缩活动也有一个额外的维度，在喉下降期间表现出收缩力增强，导致抓握效应，使得括约肌和喉部下降相互补充以清除下咽的残留物[8]。当呼吸恢复时，这种清除功能可能通过阻止残留物质黏附在喉部入口，从而将吞咽后吸入的风险降至最低。

（三）食管

食管是由骨骼肌和平滑肌组成的长20~22cm的管道。每种肌肉类型的比例取决于具体情况，但在人类中，食管近端5%为横纹肌，中间35%~40%为远端平滑肌比例越来越增加的混合肌肉，而远端50%~60%完全为平滑肌。外层的纵行肌，起自环状软骨，从环咽肌滑脱，经背外侧，在环状软骨远端约3cm处向后融合。这导致后三角区缺乏纵行肌，即Laimer三角（Laimer triangle）。在Laimer三角的远端，纵行肌在食管周围形成一个薄厚均匀的连续鞘。相邻的内肌层由环形肌，或更准确地说，螺旋肌构成，沿食管长度形成厚度均匀的鞘。螺旋度向远端移动的程度降低，从食管近端的60°到食管下括约肌（lower esophageal sphincter，LES）的近0°[9]。与远端胃肠道不同，食管没有浆膜层。食管的外源性神经支配通过迷走神经，迷走神经的运动神经元位于疑核（支配横纹肌部分）和迷走神经背侧运动核（支配平滑肌部分）。迷走神经传出纤维通过咽食管神经到达颈段食管，并直接在横纹肌上形成突触。

迷走神经也提供感觉神经支配，在颈段食管中，感觉纤维通过喉上神经和结状神经节中的细胞体传递，而在食管的其余部分，感觉纤维通过喉返神经传递，或者在食管最远端，通过迷走神经的食管支传递。食管扩张强烈刺激迷走神经传入纤维。

食管还包含一个自主神经网络，即肌间神经丛，位于纵行和环形肌层之间。肌间神经丛神经元在食管近端稀疏，其功能尚不清楚，因为横纹肌直接受疑核运动神经元控制。另一方面，在食管平滑肌中，迷走神经突触背侧运动核的节前神经元位于肌间神经丛神经节的中继神经元上。第二个神经网络，即黏膜下神经丛或称Meissner神经丛，位于黏膜肌层和环形肌层之间，但在人类食管中是稀少的。

1. 食管蠕动

食管通常是无张力的，其腔内压力密切反映胸膜压力，在吸气时变为负值。然而，吞咽或局部性扩张会启动蠕动。原发性蠕动由吞咽引起，并自上而下穿过食管的整个长度。继发性蠕动可在食管局部扩张时发生，从扩张部位开始，（用空气、液体或球囊扩张）。蠕动相关的机械力是一个剥离波，剥离波将食管从近端到远端挤奶式挤压干净。剥离波的传播与测压记录的收缩密切相关，因此，在每个食管位点处荧光透视观察到的管腔闭合点与在线追踪的压力波上行或食管压力地形图（esophageal pressure topography，EPT）上的收缩波前相对应（图44.3）。食管远端达到完全排空的可能性与蠕动幅度成反比。随着蠕动振幅≤30mmHg时，食管排空逐渐受损[10]。然而，通过食管胃交界处（EGJ）的压力梯度也可调整食管排空，这种相互作用会对食团的转运和蠕动收缩产生显著影响。

食管蠕动的另一个基本特征是吞咽抑制。在食管近端仍在进行早期蠕动收缩时开始第二次吞咽，可以完全抑制由第一次吞咽引起的收缩。食管远端的退行性抑制归因于环形平滑肌的超极化，并通过肌间神经丛中的抑制性神经节神经元介导。吞咽抑制可通过扩张腔内气囊刺激食管收缩的实验证实[11]。一旦高压区建立，吞咽后吞咽抑制明显，可同时记录气囊和食管壁之间的腔内压力。

食管横纹肌和平滑肌的生理控制机制各不相同。横纹肌只接受兴奋性迷走神经支配，其蠕动收缩是肌肉连续激活的结果。这些迷走神经纤维释放乙酰胆碱（ACh），并刺激横纹肌细胞上的烟碱类胆碱能受体。横纹肌蠕动是由延髓吞咽中枢编程，其方式与咽部吞咽大致相同。迷走神经在食管平滑肌中也表现出对原发性蠕动的控制，但迷走神经控制的机制比横纹肌更复杂，因为迷走神经纤维的突触连接在肌间神经

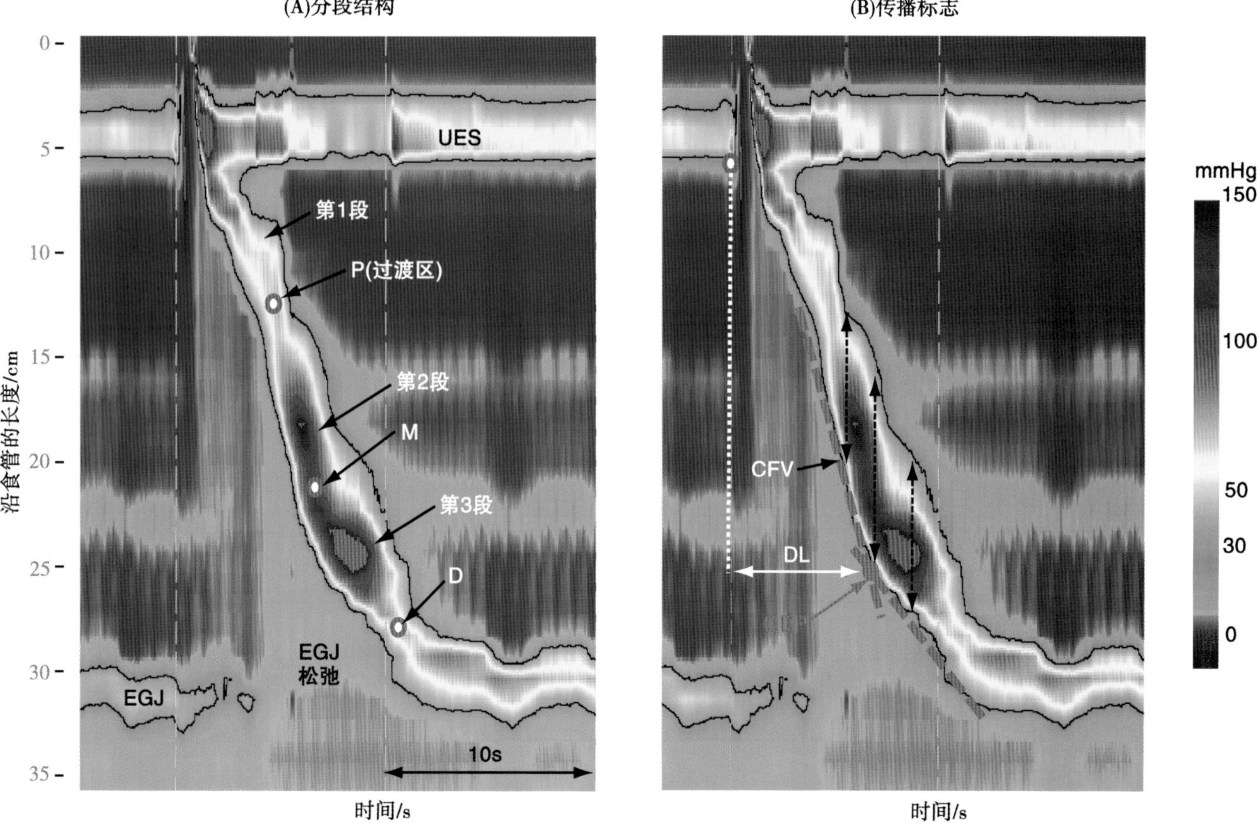

图 44.3　使用高分辨率测压(HRM)对食管蠕动进行地形图描绘,显示食管蠕动的节段性结构和收缩传播的标志。A,30mmHg 等压等值线图(黑线)显示通过食管的过程并非无缝的。近端横纹肌段 1 和远端食管平滑肌第 2 和 3 收缩段由过渡区(P)分隔。远端食管也分为 2 个不同的收缩段(第 2 和 3 段),由压力槽(M)分隔。EGJ 区域还通过一个明显收缩段来区分,该收缩段通过另一个压力槽(D)与相邻的食管分离。B,与蠕动地形图标志相同的描述。位于第 3 段内的粉红色圆圈定位 CDP,即收缩波前速度减慢点,分界从蠕动到括约肌重建的过渡。DL 是吞咽抑制的表现,从 UES 松弛到 CDP 进行测量。收缩前速度是通过从 CDP 到过渡区 P 的最佳拟合切线来测量的。有趣的是垂直虚线箭头所示的同时食管收缩的概念。从收缩前沿开始到近端收缩的偏移之间,食管同时收缩的长度平均为 10cm,并且在接近 CDP 时近似达到最大化。在 CDP 之后,同时收缩的长度随着"后部"赶上缓慢收缩的前部而缩短。P,近段;M,中段;D,远段;EGJ,食管胃交界处;CFV,收缩推进速度;DL,吞咽抑制形式;CDP,收缩减速点。(With permission from the Esophageal Center at Northwestern.)

从的神经元上,而不是直接在肌肉细胞上。然而,肌间神经丛也以独立于迷走神经激活而编排蠕动,即使存在外源性去神经支配,但沿食管平滑肌的任何部位均可诱发继发性食管蠕动。相反,横断食管横纹肌并不会抑制横断部位或远端的蠕动进程。

无论中枢或神经节控制如何,食管平滑肌收缩最终是由神经节胆碱能神经元引起的。蠕动方向和速度的控制机制尚不太清楚。神经传导的研究表明,吞咽引起的神经刺激基本上能同时到达沿食管长度的神经节神经元。然而,迷走神经刺激到达和肌肉收缩之间的潜伏期逐渐增加,运动中止。在人类中,食管近端平滑肌的潜伏期为 2 秒,而 LES 近端的潜伏期为 5~7 秒。目前的假设是,蠕动方向和速度是由沿食管分布的神经梯度导致的,其中兴奋性神经节神经元在食管近端占主导地位,而抑制性神经节神经元在食管远端占主导地位(图 44.4)。该组织与压力地形图在平滑肌节段内显示的 2 个亚节段一致,其中第一个亚节段对胆碱能药物具有强烈的反应[12]。主要的抑制性神经递质是一氧化氮,由 L-精氨酸在肌间神经元中通过一氧化氮合成酶产生[13]。也有证据表明含血管活性肠多肽(vasoactive intestinal polypeptide,VIP)的神经元介导抑制作用[14]。

高分辨率 EPT 不仅可以在时间上,而且还可以沿着食管的长度对食管收缩力进行连续成像。Clouse 及同事开创了这项技术,注意到蠕动不是无缝的加压波,而是 4 个连续收缩节段的协调序列(见图 44.3)。在第一和第二节段之间存在一个过渡区,以蠕动幅度最低、进展稍微延迟、偶尔传递失败为特征。地形图分析还显示了食管平滑肌内蠕动进展的节段性特征,两个收缩节段被一个压力低谷隔开,随后是 LES,其收缩活力和持久性与邻近的食管平滑肌完全不同[15]。最近,沿波前的一个明显的标志被识别定位于第三节段,此时收缩传播急剧减慢(见图 44.3)[16]。该标志被定义为收缩减速点(contractile deceleration point,CDP),具有病理生理学意义,因为它位于 LES 近端,并假设这代表了食管蠕动终止的位点[17]。超过这一点的收缩更符合 LES 的重建,LES 在蠕动过程中松弛、伸长和消失形成膈壶腹。

2. 纵行肌

食管的纵行肌肉在蠕动过程中也会收缩,其净效应是将食管结构短暂缩短 2~2.5cm。与环行肌肉收缩模式相似,纵行肌肉的收缩作为活跃节段以 2~4cm/秒的速度向远端传

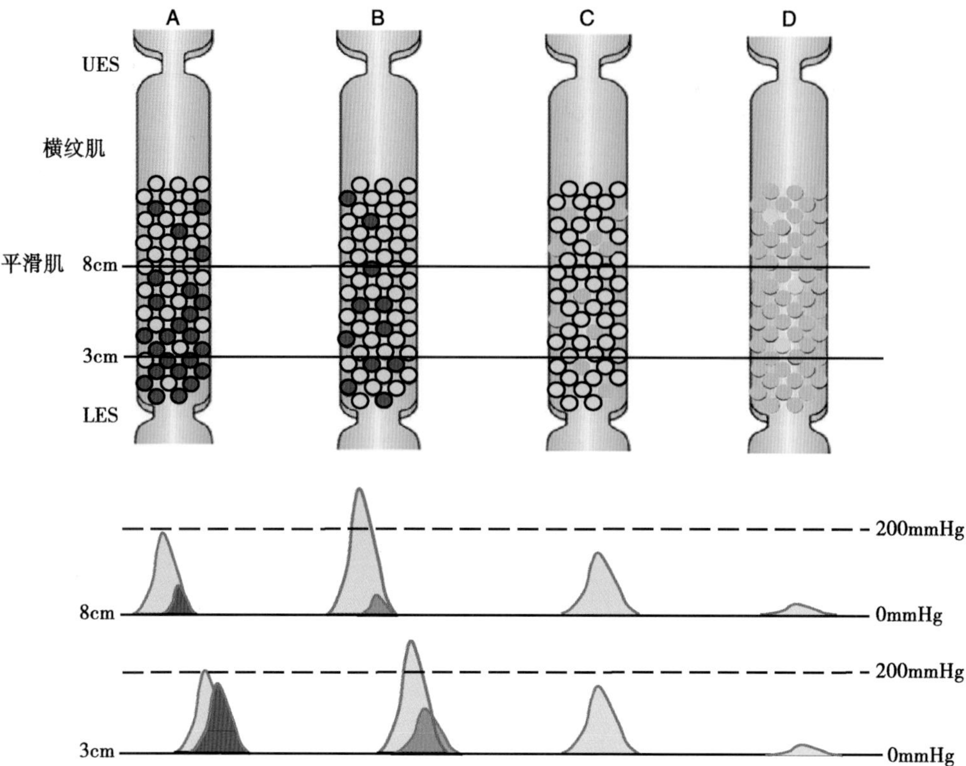

图 44.4　食管运动障碍的病理生理机制——食管远端兴奋性(胆碱能)和抑制性(硝基能)神经元平衡和梯度的改变。上图描绘了食管中的神经节成分,下图显示了 LES 上方 3cm 和 8cm 处的测压描记。蓝色圆圈代表兴奋性神经元,红色圆圈代表抑制性神经元。A,在正常受试者中,胆碱能神经元近端最密集,远端变得越来越稀疏。相反,抑制性神经元在远端更加突出,在近端相对稀疏。这种反向的神经梯度导致收缩的潜伏期随着向远端进展而逐渐增加。随着沿食管长度同时刺激迷走神经神经节,收缩首先发生在近端,只有随着越来越密集的抑制作用逐渐消失时才向远端传播。因此,药物操作可改变收缩活力和传播时间。从概念上讲,食管运动病理生理学可以通过这些神经梯度的改变来解释。B,过度收缩和正常传播(或快速)的患者兴奋性神经元可能相对增加。C,抑制性神经元丧失的患者会失去吞咽抑制,收缩会同时和过早发生。D,兴奋性和抑制性神经元均丧失的患者,可能表现为蠕动缺失或不能传播的弱蠕动。UES,食管上括约肌;LES,食管下括约肌。(Modified from Goyal R, Shaker R, GI Motility Online.)

播[18]。在蠕动过程中,中心机制控制纵行肌肉收缩,潜伏期由近及远逐渐延长,这点与环形平滑肌是相似的。然而,与环形平滑肌不同的是,神经刺激研究表明纵行肌肉不受抑制性神经控制。

(四) 食管胃交界处

食管胃交界处(EJG)的解剖结构十分复杂(另见第 43 章)。食管的远端通过膈食管韧带固定在膈肌上,膈食管韧带环向插入靠近鳞柱交界处(SCJ)的食管肌肉组织中,然后食管穿过膈肌裂孔,几乎与胃切线连接。因此,EGJ 高压区有 3 个促成因素:LES(食管下括约肌)、膈脚和构成 EJG 远端的贲门肌肉组织。LES 是位于食管远端的一段 3~4cm 的具有张力性收缩的平滑肌。在 SCJ 水平围绕 LES 的是膈脚,最常见的右膈脚束在其主要轴上形成长约 2cm 的泪滴状管(图 44.5)[19]。SCJ 远端的 EGJ 高压区的组成主要归因于胃贲门肌肉组织中层的反吊带和扣环纤维[20]。在该区域,食管的外侧壁与胃穹窿的内侧面以锐角相交,该锐角定义为 His 角。从腔内观察,该区域在胃腔内延伸,形成一个折叠,在概念上被称为"瓣阀",因为当胃内压力增加时迫使瓣阀闭合,从而封闭食管入口。

在生理学上,EGJ 高压区归因于 LES 和围绕的膈脚两者的组合,延伸至 SCJ 近端 1~1.5cm,并延伸至 SCJ 远端约 2cm[21]。相对于胃内压,静息 LES 张力范围为 10~30mmHg,并伴有相当大的时间波动。通过 HRM 将其量化为 EGJ 收缩强度,正常值范围为 28~125mmHg/cm[22]。LES 强直性收缩的机制可能是肌源性和神经源性的,这与观察到的在河豚毒素消除神经活动后括约肌内的压力持续存在一致。肌源性 LES 张力变化与导致 Ca^{2+} 内流的膜电位直接相关。除肌源性因素外,LES 压力还受腹内压、胃扩张、肽类激素、食物和许多药物的调节。移行性复合运动(MMC)使 LES 压力大幅增加,在移行性复合运动的第三阶段,LES 压力可超过 80mmHg。LES 压力全天波动较小,餐后压力下降,睡眠时压力升高[23]。

叠加在肌源性 LES 收缩上,迷走神经、肾上腺素能、激素及机械影响的输入将改变 LES 压力。迷走神经的影响与食管体部相似,迷走神经刺激同时激活兴奋性和抑制性肌间神经元。因此,任何时刻的 LES 压力瞬间都反映了兴奋性(胆碱能)和抑制性(硝基能)神经输入之间的平衡,改变迷走神经放电模式可导致 LES 松弛。膈脚也是构成 EGJ 压力的主要因素。即使在食管胃切除术后,随之切除 LES 平滑肌,在呼气

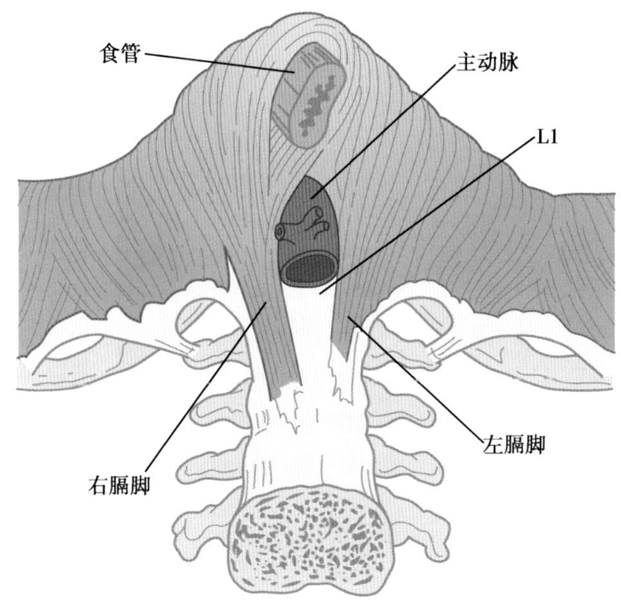

图 44.5 膈肌裂孔的解剖结构，如下图所示。图中显示了最常见的解剖结构，其中膈脚的肌肉成分来源于右侧膈脚。右膈脚起自于覆盖腰椎的前纵韧带。一旦肌腱中出现肌肉成分，就会形成两条扁平的肌肉带，它们以剪刀样的方式相互交叉，形成裂孔壁，然后在食管前方相互融合。L1，第一腰椎。（Modified from Jaffee BM. Surgery of the esophagus. In：Orlando RC，editor. Atlas of esophageal diseases. 2nd ed，Philadelphia；Current Medicine，lnc.；2002. p 221-42.）

期间仍可显示约 6mmHg 的持续 EGJ 压力。在吸气期间，由于膈脚收缩，EGJ 压力会显著增加。在腹部受压、用力或咳嗽时，膈脚收缩也会增强[24]。另一方面，在食管扩张、呕吐和嗳气期间，尽管持续呼吸，但膈脚内的电活动仍被选择性抑制，证明控制机制与肋横膈无关。这种对膈脚活动的反射性抑制可通过迷走神经切断术消除。

1. 食管下括约肌松弛

食管下括约肌（LES）松弛可由 EGJ 两侧的扩张或吞咽引起。食管扩张引起的松弛是一种壁内过程，不受迷走神经切断术的影响。然而，河豚毒素可拮抗松弛作用，证明其由节后神经介导的。吞咽性 LES 松弛是由迷走神经介导的，迷走神经与肌间神经丛中的抑制性神经元形成突触。NO 由前体氨基酸 L-精氨酸的 NO 合成酶产生，是节后神经元中使 LES 松弛的主要神经递质。NO 在食管、LES 和胃的神经刺激下释放，NO 合成酶抑制剂阻断神经介导的 LES 的松弛[13,25]。然而，NO 可能并不单独发挥作用。在黏膜下神经丛中已证实含有 VIP 的神经元，VIP 通过直接作用于肌肉来松弛 LES。目前认为，VIP 作为连接前神经递质作用于含 NO 合成酶的神经末梢，促进 NO 的释放，并作用于胃肌肉细胞，刺激肌肉产生 NO[26]。

在食团通过 LES 期间，另一个导致腔内压力的重要因素是食团本身。在吞咽的初始阶段 LES 松弛，但直到食团进入括约肌它才真正打开，由此涉及食团内压力。因此，EGJ 开口取决于打开它的力（蠕动产生的食团内压力）和抵抗打开的力（食管壁与膈脚的张力和机械特性）之间的平衡。尽管这些因素中的每一个都可能在特定的生理预测情况下占主导地位，除了传统的测压记录外难以梳理它们。HRM 和 EPT 对此有所改进，目前对吞咽过程中 EGJ 松弛的评估采用电子套管，或“E 套管”（eSleeve），在 4 秒的时间段内查明最低平均吞咽后压力，如果有必要，跳过吸气性膈脚收缩（图 44.6）。该测量提供了通过 EGJ 的压力动力学综合评估，EGJ 对抵抗开放的两种病理状态均敏感，如伴有贲门失弛缓症的 LES 松弛受损，以及与结构原因相关的 EGJ 机械性梗阻（狭窄、肿瘤、LES 肥大）。

2. 一过性食管下括约肌松弛

在静息期间，EGJ 必须防止胃食管反流，但也必须短暂松弛，以便选择性地使胃部排气。这些功能是通过延长 LES 松弛在没有吞咽或蠕动的情况下完成的。这种一过性食管下端括约松弛（transient LES relaxation，tLESR）是胃食管反流病（GERD）发病机制中的一个重要机制，也是 LES 压力正常期间最常见的反流机制（见第 46 章）。tLESR 与吞咽诱发的松弛有以下几种方式区别：①它们延长（>10 秒），与咽部吞咽无关；②它们与食管远端纵行肌收缩有关，使食管缩短；③无食管同步蠕动；④它们与膈脚抑制有关，与吞咽引起的松弛不同（图 44.7）[27,28]。tLESR 最常发生在餐后胃扩张期间。在 tLESR 期间，EGJ 完全松弛的情况下，即使在胃扩张时观察到的最小胃食管压力梯度（3~4mmHg）也足以促进胃排气。因此，tLESR 是嗳气的生理机制。

近端胃扩张是 tLESR 的主要刺激因素。扩张刺激近端胃的机械感受器（神经节内板层末梢），激活投射到孤束核的迷走神经传入纤维。吞咽和非吞咽 LES 松弛的传出支均位于 LES 的节前迷走神经抑制通路中。这两种松弛均可被双侧颈迷走神经切断术、颈迷走神经冷冻术或 NO 合成酶抑制剂阻断。胃扩张触发的 tLESR 可能使用 NO 和 CCK 作为神经递质，静脉输注 CCK 后 tLESR 频率增加，和 NO 合成酶抑制剂或 CCK-A 拮抗剂的阻断可以证明。最后，GABA-B 激动剂，如巴氯芬，抑制 tLESR，是作用于外周受体和位于迷走神经背侧运动核的受体[29,30]。

（五）食管感觉

人类的食管可以感觉到机械、电、化学和热刺激，感知为胸部压力、温暖或疼痛，这些刺激之间在感知上有很大的重叠[31]。食管感觉是通过迷走神经和脊髓传入神经传递。相关的迷走神经神经元位于结状神经节和颈静脉神经节，而相应的脊髓神经元位于胸、颈背根神经节。迷走神经传入纤维主要调节内环境稳态和分泌功能，而脊髓传入神经以脊髓节段重叠和与躯体传入神经汇集为特征的模式集中投射。因此，食管疼痛往往定位较为模糊，伴有牵涉到的躯体疼痛和内脏痛觉过敏[32]。食管的感觉通常在胸骨后，以疼痛为例，常放射到背部、肩部和下颌中线，与心脏疼痛非常相似。这些相似性可能是由于来自心脏和食管的感觉传入纤维在同一脊髓通路中汇聚，甚至在某些情况下汇聚到同一背角神经元。

食管的传入神经主要由管壁的牵张、温度以及酸度激活。当伴有黏膜损伤时，炎症介质（前列腺素、缓激肽等）可增强反应。近端食管比远端食管更敏感，这与观察到的食管近端刺激（如反流）更容易被感知一致[33]。过度的近端食管敏感性与食管超敏反应和功能性胃灼热有关[34]。

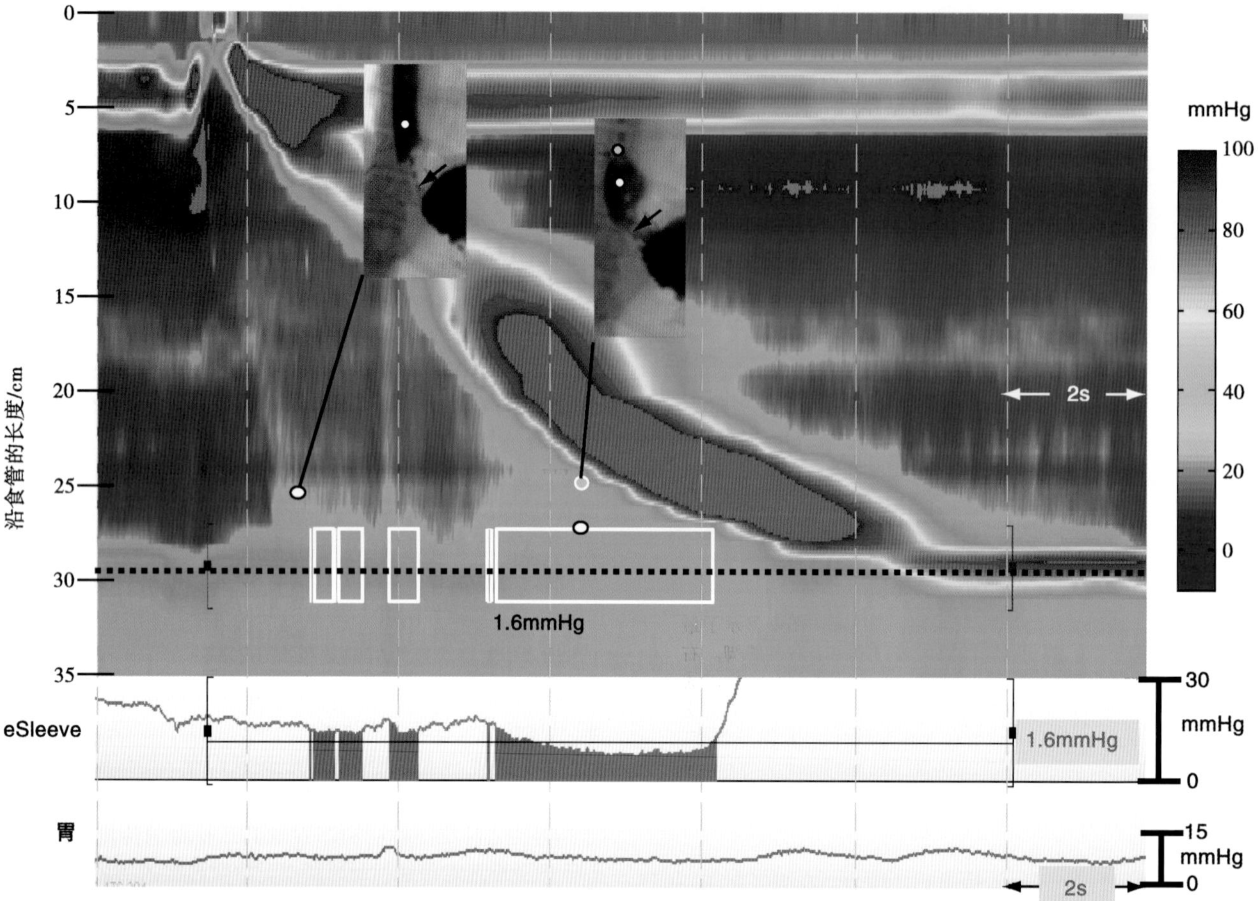

图 44.6　吞咽期间食管胃交界处(EGJ)松弛和食团转运。整体松弛压(IRP)提供了吞咽期间 EGJ 压力动态的压力地形图测量。IRP 是一个复杂的度量，因为它涉及准确定位 EGJ 的边缘，标定在吞咽时上括约肌松弛后的时间窗，在该时间窗内预测 EGJ 松弛，然后在 10 秒的时间框内应用电子套管(eSleeve)测量(用黑色括号表示)。eSleeve 指的是参考胃压力，提供了每个时间点 EGJ 轴向区域最大压力的测量值，并绘制成线条轨迹。IRP 的平均值是 4 秒，在此期间 eSleeve 值最低的。图上的白框和红线 eSleeve 轨迹描记图上的红色阴影区域表示 IRP 的时间间隔。在本例中，IRP 为 1.6mmHg，这是正常的。EGJ 关闭，吞咽开始时无流动发生，因为食团内压力不足以克服 EGJ 压力(左荧光透视图像)。当收缩波前的食团内压力克服 EGJ 处的阻力时，发生食团转运(右荧光透视图像)

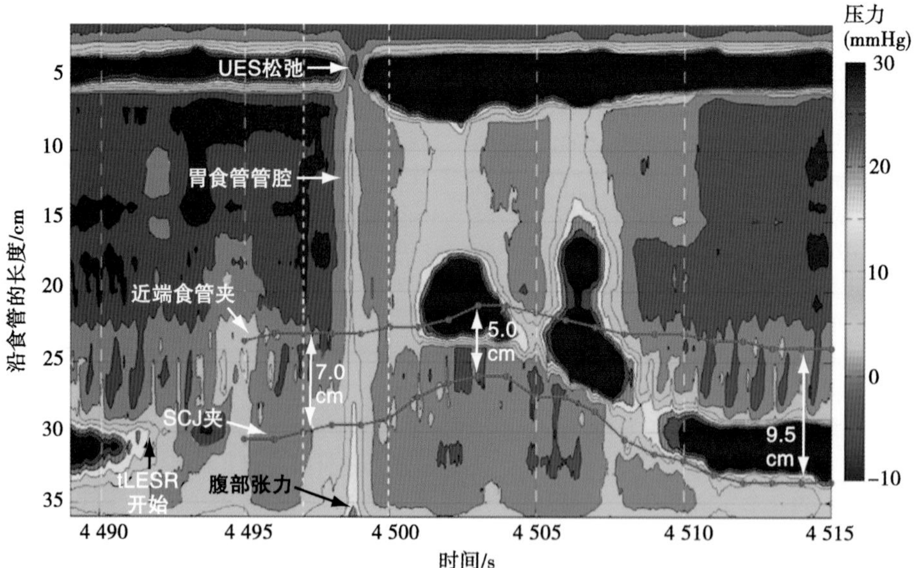

图 44.7　tLESR 期间食管缩短。以高分辨率 EPT 格式记录 tLESR 期间内镜夹移动的可视化透视图像(一个放置在 SCJ 处，一个放置在 SCJ 近端 10cm 处)。测压记录跨越咽部到胃，在这种情况下，tLESR 与腹部张力和"微打嗝"有关，通过短暂的 UES 松弛和排气食管降压突然明显。当夹子数据输入等压等高线图时，SCJ 夹数据偏移很明显反映了食管胃交界处高压带的移动。从远端 SCJ 夹约 7cm 的移动，同时近端 SCJ 夹的最小移动可以看出，食管缩短在内镜夹隔离的 10cm 段的远端最为显著。还应注意，在 tLESR 期间无膈脚收缩。SCJ，鳞柱上皮交界处；tLESR，一过性食管下括约肌松弛；UES，食管上端括约肌

由于感觉末梢集中位于较深的相对不渗透的黏膜下的固有肌层内，因此食管腔内的酸性物质似乎不太可能直接刺激到感觉末梢。然而，这些传入神经纤维很容易对黏膜分泌的胆汁或辣椒素（辣椒的一种衍生物）产生反应，表明这些化学物质诱导内源性物质的释放，进而刺激传入神经纤维。这些反应被认为是由瞬时受体电位香草酸-1（TRPV1）受体和/或酸敏感离子通道介导的[35,36]。与此一致，目前的证据表明，慢性食管炎能增加嘌呤能受体的 mRNA 表达，并伴随 TRPV1 和神经营养因子的上调，介导发炎的人食管的敏感性[37]。

鉴于 tLESR 在 GERD 发病机制中的重要性，人们对调节 tLESR 反射产生了浓厚的兴趣（见第 44 章）。目前的概念是迷走神经传入末梢终止于位于胃近端的神经节内板层末梢主要负责启动反射，然后通过髓质介导反射，并通过迷走神经传出神经和膈神经返回食管和膈肌。药理学和生理学研究表明，GABA-B 受体激动剂巴氯芬可减弱张力敏感性迷走神经传入纤维的机械传导特性，从而降低 tLESR 的频率。迷走神经和脊髓感觉传入纤维中也存在谷氨酸受体，促代谢型谷氨酸受体拮抗剂（尤其是 mGluR5 拮抗剂）也被证明能抑制 tLESR[38]。

最近的一些研究也探索了功能性脑成像，主要是功能性磁共振成像，作为对内脏感觉和疼痛的脑功能无创性评估[39]。尽管迄今为止，研究结果在研究组之间存在相当大的差异，但食管刺激最常激活的脑区域是前脑岛和后脑岛、扣带回皮质、初级感觉皮质、额叶前皮质和丘脑。初步研究还提示，GERD 患者亚组与正常对照组之间的功能性磁共振成像激活模式存在差异[40]。

二、食管动力障碍

食管动力障碍的一个有效的（尽管有限制）定义是一种由神经肌肉功能障碍引起的与食管相关的症状，最常见的症状是吞咽困难、胸痛或灼热。根据这一定义，只有 3 种确定的原发性食管动力障碍疾病：贲门失弛缓症、食管远端痉挛（distal esophageal spasm，DES）和 GERD。GERD 显然是该组中最普遍的一种疾病，在本文其他部分对其进行了详细论述（见第 46 章）。

食管动力障碍也可能是继发性的，在这种情况下，食管功能障碍是更广泛疾病的一部分，例如假性贲门失弛缓症、Chagas 病和硬皮病（PSS）。由咽部或 UES 功能障碍引起的吞咽困难也可纳入食管动力障碍的讨论中，但这通常是更全面的神经肌肉疾病过程的局部表现。本章的主要重点是原发性食管动力障碍，特别是贲门失弛缓症。然而，当存在重要的独特特征时，将提到继发性食管运动障碍和近端咽食管功能障碍。

（一）流行病学

据估计，50 岁以上人群吞咽困难的患病率为 16%～22%，其中大部分与口咽功能障碍有关。大多数口咽吞咽困难与神经肌肉疾病有关，据估计，最常见的解剖学病因 Zenker 憩室的患病率在美国人口中仅为 0.01%～0.11%，男性发病率在 20 世纪 70～90 年代达到高峰[41]。口咽吞咽困难的后果是严重的，会导致脱水、营养不良、误吸、窒息、肺炎甚至死亡。在卫生医疗保健机构内，估计有高达 13% 的住院患者和 60% 的疗养院患者存在进食问题，且与食管功能障碍相反，大多数患者都是因口咽功能障碍所致。吞咽困难和误吸的护理住院患者的死亡率在一年内可高达 45%。随着美国人口的不断老龄化，口咽吞咽困难将成为一个与复杂的医学和伦理问题相关的日益严重的问题。

贲门失弛缓症是最容易识别和最好定义的食管动力障碍性疾病。现在美国，贲门失弛缓症发病率估计约为 2.9 人/10 万人，在澳大利亚南部约为 2.6 人/10 万人[43]，男女发病率相同，通常在 25～60 岁之间[44]。由于贲门失弛缓症是一种慢性疾病，其患病率远超过其发病率。最近对芝加哥贲门失弛缓症患病率的调查显示，预期患病率可能高达 76 人/10 万人，鉴于平均诊断年龄为 56 岁，预期诊断后平均生存 26 年[42]。关于贲门失弛缓症家族聚集性的报道增加了遗传易感性的可能性。然而，与遗传决定因素相反，一项针对 159 例贲门失弛缓症患者的 1 012 名一级亲属进行的调查，尚未发现受影响的亲属。有一种罕见的遗传性贲门失弛缓综合征与肾上腺功能不全和无泪症有关。该综合征是一种常染色体隐性遗传病，表现为儿童期发作的自主神经系统功能障碍，包括贲门失弛缓症、无泪症、窦房结功能障碍、瞳孔对光反应异常和胃排空延迟[45]。它是由编码一种被称为 ALADIN 蛋白的 AAAS 基因突变引起的。

除贲门失弛缓症外，目前尚无基于人群的食管动力障碍发病率或患病率的研究。因此，估计痉挛性疾病的发病率或患病率的唯一方法是检查高危人群的数据，并参考观察到的痉挛性疾病的发生率与贲门失弛缓症的发病率，如前所述，该发病率约为 2.75 人/10 万人。这样做，DES 的患病率远低于使用现代限制性诊断标准时的患病率。有运动障碍风险的人群是胸痛和/或吞咽困难的患者，因此在这些患者中收集了大量的测压数据。测压异常在这些人群中普遍存在，但在大多数情况下，测压结果的意义尚不清楚[46]）。

（二）发病机制

1. 口咽吞咽困难

造成口腔、头部和颈部的阻塞病变都可导致吞咽困难。结构异常可能由创伤、手术、肿瘤、腐蚀性损伤、先天异常或后天畸形引起。最常见的与吞咽困难相关的下咽结构异常是下咽憩室和环咽嵴。

如果对解剖结构紊乱进行初步评估后，口咽吞咽困难的病因仍不明确，则应寻找功能异常的证据。涉及口咽部的原发性神经或肌肉疾病常伴有吞咽困难。食管吞咽困难通常由食管疾病引起，而口咽吞咽困难通常由神经或肌肉疾病引起，口咽功能障碍只是一种病理表现。虽然疾病的特征各不相同，但根据早先对吞咽的机械描述，可以分析对吞咽的净效应。表 44.1 总结了吞咽的机械因素、功能障碍的表现和后果，以及可能遇到的典型病理状态。神经系统检查可能提示脑神经功能障碍、神经肌肉疾病、小脑功能障碍或潜在的运动障碍。功能异常可由固有肌肉组织、外周神经或中枢神经系统控制机制的功能障碍所致。值得注意的是，与人们普遍认识相反，咽反射并不能预测咽部吞咽效率降低或误吸风险。有 20%～40% 的正常成年人咽反射消失[47]。

表 44.1 口咽吞咽的机械事件、功能障碍的证据和口咽吞咽困难患者的相关疾病

机械事件	功能障碍的证据	相关疾病
鼻咽闭合	鼻咽反流 鼻音	重症肌无力
喉闭合	食团转运期间的误吸	卒中 创伤性脑损伤
UES 开放	吞咽困难 吞咽后滞留物/误吸 憩室形成	环咽嵴 帕金森病
舌负载及食团推注推进缓慢	缓慢误导食团	帕金森病 手术缺陷 脑瘫
咽清除	下咽部吞咽后残留物/误吸	脊髓灰质炎及脊髓灰质炎后综合征 眼型肌营养不良 卒中

UES,食管上端括约肌。

如表 44.1 所示,口咽吞咽困难通常是神经或肌肉疾病的结果。神经系统疾病可损伤口咽吞咽传入或传出神经支所必需的神经结构。事实上,任何神经肌肉疾病都可能引起吞咽困难(见第 37 章)。由于控制吞咽的神经元没有什么独特之处,它们参与疾病过程通常是随机的。此外,在大多数情况下,相邻神经元结构介导的功能同时参与其中。下面的讨论将集中在最常遇到的神经肌肉病理学过程。

2. 卒中

据估计,并发吸入性肺炎在卒中后第一年的死亡率为 20%,此后每年造成 10%~15% 的死亡率。这通常不是吸入性肺炎的首次发作,而是随后多年的复发,甚至最终导致死亡。吸入性肺炎的最终原因是吞咽困难导致误吸,误吸可通过多种机制发生:触发吞咽的缺失或严重延迟,舌控制能力减弱或喉咽肌肉无力[7]。从概念上讲,这些病因可能涉及运动或感觉功能障碍。与脑干卒中相比,皮质梗死导致严重吞咽困难的可能性较小,且更有可能从吞咽困难中恢复。在 86 例急性脑梗死的患者中,37 例(43%)在发病后 4 天内出现吞咽困难。然而,86% 的患者能够在 2 周后正常吞咽,恢复是因为对侧区域接管丧失的功能[48]。在发生较大面积梗死的患者或既往有梗死的患者中,吞咽功能往往难以恢复。

3. 肌萎缩侧索硬化

肌萎缩侧索硬化症是一种进行性神经系统疾病,其特征是大脑、脑干和脊髓运动神经元的变性。具体症状取决于受累运动神经元的位置和受累的相对严重程度。当退行性过程涉及脑神经核时,吞咽困难随之发生。口咽功能障碍的特征是从舌开始,逐渐进展累及咽部和喉部肌肉组织。患者出现窒息发作,体力耗竭或营养不良,并导致吸入性肺炎。吞咽功能的下降是进行性的和可预测的,常需要胃造瘘喂养。患者往往因吞咽功能障碍伴呼吸抑制而死亡[49]。

4. 帕金森病

虽然只有 15%~20% 的帕金森病患者主诉吞咽问题,但通过荧光透视检查,95% 以上的患者有明显的缺陷[50]。这种差异表明,患者在疾病早期阶段进行代偿,只有在病情严重时才会主诉吞咽困难。帕金森病的异常包括咽部吞咽前舌的反复抽动、零碎吞咽和吞咽后的口腔残留。患者还可能表现出吞咽反应延迟和咽部收缩无力,造成会厌谷和梨状窦存有残留物。最近的数据表明,这与 UES 松弛不完全和咽部收缩减弱有关[50]。

5. 迷走神经病变

单侧迷走神经损伤可导致软腭、咽缩肌及喉部肌肉的轻偏瘫。喉返神经可因甲状腺手术、主动脉瘤、肺切除术、原发性纵隔恶性肿瘤或纵隔转移性病变而受损伤。由于其在胸部有更广泛的袢,左侧喉返神经比右侧喉返神经更容易受到纵隔恶性肿瘤的侵袭。单侧喉返神经损伤导致单侧声带内收肌麻痹。由于喉闭合受损,该缺陷可导致吞咽过程中的误吸。然而,喉返神经损伤导致的任何原发性咽功能障碍是罕见的。

6. 眼咽型肌营养不良

眼咽型肌营养不良是一种以上睑下垂和进行性吞咽困难为特征的综合征。过去,年满 50 岁受折磨的患者通常死于咽麻痹导致的饥饿。该病现在已知为肌营养不良的一种形式,是常染色体显性遗传疾病,发病集中在法裔-加拿大裔血统的家族中。对受累家族的遗传学研究表明,与第 14 号染色体有连锁关系,可能涉及心脏 α 或 β 肌球蛋白重链的区域编码。眼咽型肌营养不良影响咽横纹肌和上睑提肌。虽然其他形式的肌营养不良偶尔会影响咽缩肌,但这很少是显性表现。眼咽型肌营养不良的首发症状通常是上睑下垂,进展缓慢,最终影响患者的外貌。吞咽困难可在上睑下垂之后、伴随或甚至在上睑下垂之前开始。主要的功能异常为咽部收缩无力或缺失,环咽开口减少和下咽淤滞[51]。吞咽困难进展缓慢,但最终可能导致饥饿、吸入性肺炎或窒息。

7. 重症肌无力

重症肌无力是一种进行性自身免疫性疾病,其特征是血液循环中乙酰胆碱受体抗体水平升高和神经肌肉连接处乙酰胆碱受体的破坏。几乎总是累及由脑神经控制的肌肉组织,尤其是眼部肌肉。超过三分之一的重症肌无力患者有明显的吞咽困难,在不寻常的情况下,吞咽困难可能是该疾病最初的和主要的表现。在轻症病例中,吞咽困难可能在进食 15~20 分钟后才明显。经典的测压研究显示,反复吞咽时,咽部收缩幅度逐渐恶化。静息状态或给予 10mg 乙酰胆碱酯酶抑制剂依酚氯铵后,蠕动幅度恢复。在晚期的病例中,吞咽困难可能很严重,并伴有鼻咽反流和鼻音,甚至在一定程度上与延髓肌萎缩侧索硬化或脑干卒中混淆[52]。

8. 下咽憩室和环咽嵴

下咽憩室是与环咽嵴密切相关的一种疾病,因为环咽嵴可导致憩室形成。最常见的类型是 Zenker 憩室(图 44.8),它起源于 Killian 裂开处的后方中线,即咽下缩肌斜纤维与环咽横肌之间的咽壁薄弱点。获得性咽憩室的其他位置包括:①将环咽肌与食管近端纤维分离的外侧裂隙处,喉返神经及其伴行血管通过此裂隙供应喉部;②甲状腺下动脉穿入下咽处;③中下缩肌交界处。这些部位的相同特点是,它们是下咽肌层潜在的薄弱部位,黏膜通过这些部位疝出,形成"假"憩室。憩室形成的最有说服力的解释是,它们是由于环咽肌顺应性降低引起的限制性肌病所致。来自下咽憩室患者的环咽

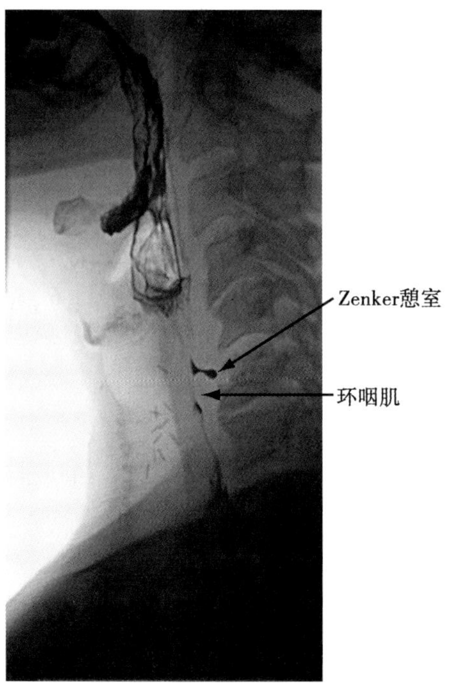

图 44.8　吞钡研究的 X 线胶片，显示小的 Zenker 憩室。虽然疝出点在 Killian 裂开处的后方中线，但随着憩室的增大，憩室在颈部向外侧迁移，因为咽后壁和脊柱之间没有潜在的间隙

肌的手术标本证实结构改变会降低 UES 的顺应性和开放[53]。这些患者的环咽肌术后样本有"纤维脂肪组织替代和（肌肉）纤维变性"。因此，虽然在吞咽过程中肌肉能正常松弛，但不能正常扩张，导致在吞钡过程中出现环咽肌凹痕或条状（图 44.9）。括约肌顺应性降低必须增加下咽食团内压力，以维持

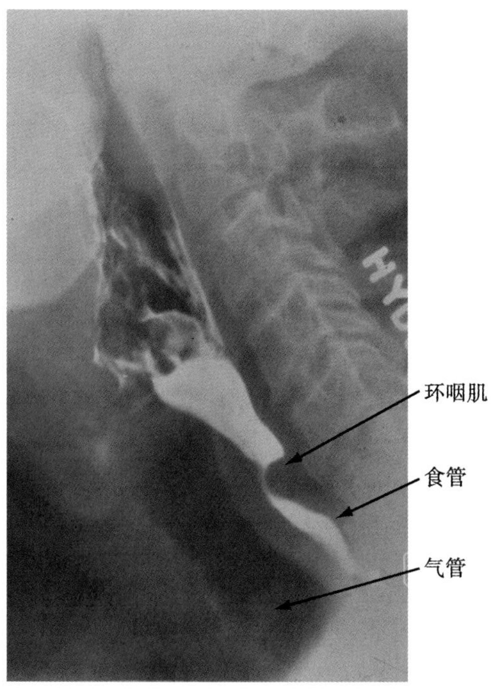

图 44.9　吞钡研究的 X 线胶片，显示口咽吞咽困难患者的环咽嵴。钡柱的后压痕是由不顺应的环咽肌引起的。（Courtesy Dr. Richard Gore，Evanston，IL.）

通过较小 UES 开口的经括约肌流量。食团内压力的增加对下咽的应力增加可能最终导致憩室的形成。

9. 贲门失弛缓症

贲门失弛缓症的特征是吞咽时 LES 松弛受损，伴有食管平滑肌蠕动停止。如果食管体部出现过早的痉挛性收缩，这种疾病称为痉挛性（Ⅲ型）贲门失弛缓症[54]。这些生理变化是由于食管平滑肌段（包括 LES）的神经支配受损伤伴肌间神经丛（Auerbach）内的神经节细胞丢失所致。一些观察者报告，在贲门失弛缓症患者的食管平滑肌中，神经节细胞和被单核炎性细胞包围的神经节细胞较少[55]。神经节细胞丢失的程度与疾病的持续时间相平行，可能从 EGJ 流出道梗阻进展到Ⅱ型贲门失弛缓症、到Ⅰ型贲门失弛缓症，再到终末期贲门失弛缓症[55,56]。Ⅲ型贲门失弛缓症似乎具有独特的发病机制，其特征是肌间神经丛炎症和功能改变，但不是破坏[55]。

贲门失弛缓症的生理学研究表明，食管平滑肌节后去神经支配的功能障碍，可能会影响兴奋性神经节神经元（胆碱能）、抑制性神经节神经元（NO±VIP）或两者兼有之（见图 44.4）。当乙酰胆碱直接刺激时，贲门失弛缓症患者食管体部环形层的肌肉条收缩，但对尼古丁刺激的神经节无反应，表明神经节后兴奋性缺陷。然而，通过观察发现，在某些情况下，在给予 AChE（乙酰胆碱酯酶）抑制剂依酚氯铵后，贲门失弛缓症患者的 LES 压力增加，而在给予毒蕈碱拮抗剂阿托品后，其 LES 压力降低，这表明保留了部分节后胆碱能通路，是了解为什么肉毒毒素可能具有一定治疗益处的关键性观察结果（见治疗章节）。不管兴奋性神经节神经元损伤如何，抑制性神经节神经元功能障碍显然是贲门失弛缓症的早期表现。这些神经元介导吞咽抑制（包括 LES 松弛）和食管蠕动的有序传播，它们的缺失为贲门失弛缓症的关键生理异常提供了一个统一的假说：LES 松弛受损和无蠕动。贲门失弛缓症缺乏一氧化氮合成酶和胃食管交界处 VIP 染色神经元显著减少。

有大量证据表明，贲门失弛缓症患者的食管节后抑制性神经支配受损。来自 LES 的肌肉条在尼古丁刺激神经节时不会像正常对照组那样松弛。此外，CCK 正常刺激抑制性神经节神经元，从而降低 LES 压力，但矛盾的是 CCK 增加了贲门失弛缓症患者的 LES 压力[57]。LES 上方的食管平滑肌抑制性神经支配受损更难确定，因为该区域缺乏静息张力。然而，在一项精确的实验中，Sifrim 和同事们使用食管内球囊在管状食管中形成一个高压区，然后随着吞咽抑制的开始而放松。在早期非扩张的贲门失弛缓症病例中，食管体部的这种吞咽松弛是不存在的[58]。

特发性贲门失弛缓症的神经节细胞变性的最终原因正在被逐渐阐明，越来越多的证据表明在遗传易感性个体中存在自身免疫过程[59]。对贲门失弛缓症患者肌间神经丛炎性细胞浸润的分析显示，大多数炎性细胞是静息状态或是活化的细胞毒性 T 细胞。在贲门失弛缓症患者的血清中，特别是在具有特异性 HLA 等位基因的患者中，已检测到抗肌间神经元的抗体。启动自身免疫反应导致贲门失弛缓症发生的触发因素仍存在争议，被怀疑是一种慢性或潜伏的人类疱疹病毒 1 型（HSV-1）感染[59]。有趣的是，在非贲门失弛缓症器官供体的 LES 组织中也检测到 HSV-1，这表明贲门失弛缓症的发生取决于病毒和遗传易感性。

10. 食管远端痉挛

虽然食管远端痉挛(DES)的诊断常被认为是食管性胸痛的原因之一,但实际上这种疾病罕见,大多数食管性胸痛可归因于反流性疾病或贲门失弛缓症。从历史上看,诊断食管远端痉挛的测压标准是非特异性的,导致对该病的过度诊断。这一点通过芝加哥高分辨率测压分类法和采用缩短蠕动远端潜伏期(DL)作为食管远端痉挛的主要异常,目前已得到一定程度的澄清[60]。

虽然DES明显是一种蠕动障碍,但大多数患者在大部分时间表现出正常的蠕动收缩。DES的神经肌肉病理学尚不清楚,也没有已知的危险因素。最显著的病理改变是食管远端弥漫性肌肉肥大或增生,增厚达2cm。然而,还有其他文献记载的病例,在开胸手术中没有发现食管肌肉增厚,还有一些病例的肌肉增厚与DES症状无关。

尽管缺乏明确的组织病理学证据,但生理学证据表明痉挛时肌间神经丛神经元功能障碍,因为沿食管平滑肌的收缩潜伏期是节后肌间神经丛神经元的功能。吞咽引起的迷走神经冲动同时到达整个食管平滑肌段,肌间神经丛内兴奋性和抑制性神经节神经元的平衡决定了每个食管位点的收缩时间。此外,实验证据表明痉挛患者之间存在异质性,例如一些患者主要表现为抑制性中间神经元功能降低,而在另一些患者缺陷表现为过度兴奋。

根据吞咽后收缩潜伏期来定义DES使其与贲门失弛缓症形成病理生理学连续体,这与患者经历这种演变的病例报告的记录相一致[61]。此外,痉挛性贲门失弛缓症和DES之间存在显著的相似性,因为两者都具有食管远端快速传播收缩的特征。强有力的贲门失弛缓症的特征鉴别是LES受累和缺乏任何正常的蠕动。

11. 高收缩性食管(jackhammer食管)

正常DL的剧烈食管收缩,在芝加哥分类中定义为高收缩性食管或jackhammer食管(即手提钻食管,又称胡桃夹食管),可同时伴有吞咽困难和胸痛。高收缩性被认为是过度兴奋性冲动或流出道阻塞的反应性代偿导致肌细胞肥大的表现[62]。与此一致的是,高收缩性患者表现出对胆碱能激动剂(如依酚氯铵)高度敏感性。支持阻塞作为高收缩性病因学的数据来自在猫远端食管周围植入充气压力袖带的生理学研究[63]。小袖带的充气体积增加了蠕动幅度,但体积较大时,蠕动完全中断。

从临床角度来看,HRM中量化食管远端收缩力的汇总指标是远端收缩积分(DCI)。DCI值大于8 000mmHg·cm·s代表一种极端的过度收缩模式,通常与重复收缩相关,在正常受试者中很少见到,几乎总是与胸痛和吞咽困难有关。当在测压研究中发生2次此类收缩时,当前版本的《芝加哥分类法》将这种情况称为"jackhammer"食管[64,65]。

12. 蠕动缺失

蠕动受损的范围从收缩无力到收缩力缺失,如在贲门失弛缓症和硬皮病中所见。虽然收缩力缺失通常是特发性的,贲门失弛缓症和硬皮病可作为阐明贲门失弛缓症神经节细胞缺乏症(见图44.4)和硬皮病中肌源性破坏发病机制的一种模型。硬皮病患者的超微结构研究报告了毛细血管基底膜增厚和食管平滑肌萎缩或纤维化。因此,蠕动无力和收缩力缺失可能与肌源性或神经源性过程有关,类似于胃肠道的其他部位。

(三)临床特点

吞咽困难是食管动力障碍的基本症状。食管(与口咽相反)吞咽困难是指不伴有误吸、咳嗽、鼻咽部反流、流涎、吞咽后咽部残留或同时发生的神经肌肉功能障碍(如无力、感觉异常、口齿不清)。另一方面,灼热、反流、胸痛、吞咽疼痛或间歇性食管梗阻等相关症状也提示食管吞咽困难。食管吞咽困难患者病史记录的一个重要限制是患者对识别梗阻位置的准确性有限。具体而言,食管环、狭窄或贲门失弛缓症引起的食管远端梗阻通常被视为颈部吞咽困难,患者仅能在60%的时间内正确定位远端食管功能障碍。由于区分食管近端和远端病变方面存在主观困难,颈部吞咽困难的评估应包括整个食管长度。

患者处理中的另一个重要考虑因素是,食管动力障碍比吞咽困难的机械性或炎症性病因(如肿瘤、狭窄、食管环或食管炎)要少见得多,可能是消化性的、药物诱导的、嗜酸性的或感染性的。提示运动障碍的病史要点是对固体和液体食物均有吞咽困难,而仅是固体食物吞咽困难则更提示机械性梗阻。然而,机械性或炎症性疾病的后果可以完全模拟原发性动力障碍性疾病。因此,与口咽吞咽困难的评估一样,只有在通过内镜、组织学检查和/或放射学检查排除了更常见的诊断后,运动障碍才应被视为食管吞咽困难的病因。

1. 贲门失弛缓症

贲门失弛缓症的临床表现包括吞咽困难、反流、胸痛、呃逆、口臭、体重减轻和吸入性肺炎。所有患者均有固体食物吞咽困难,大多数患者还存在不同程度的液体吞咽困难。吞咽困难的发作通常是渐进的,并且在陈述时通常已持续数年。吞咽困难的严重程度有波动,但最终会趋于平稳。对于久治不愈的患者,存在食管进行性扩张,卧位时反流变得频繁。反流物通常是之前数小时甚至数日内吃过的食物。它倾向于无胆汁、无酸,并与大量唾液混合。患者往往不能识别黏稠的黏液样反流物与唾液,对其所见的黏稠度不认识。大约三分之二的患者在贲门失弛缓症的早期出现胸痛。其病因尚不清楚,但被认为与食管痉挛的发生有关(最近认为是纵行肌痉挛)。贲门失弛缓症的治疗在缓解胸痛方面不如缓解吞咽困难或反流方面有效。然而,与吞咽困难或反流不同,胸痛可能会自发改善或随着时间推移而消失。

对于晚期贲门失弛缓症,高达10%的病例因反流和误吸而发生支气管肺并发症,在某些情况下,正是这些并发症而不是吞咽困难促使他们就医。贲门失弛缓症的另一个令人关注的罕见症状是,扩张的食管压迫颈部膜状气管导致的气道受损和喘鸣。据推测,这可能是因为促进LES放松的神经肌肉装置受到损害,而这部分神经肌肉同样是作为嗳气反射的一部分[66]。

值得思考的是,许多贲门失弛缓症患者甚至在出现吞咽困难后仍有胃灼热症状。虽然反流可能是贲门失弛缓症治疗的常见后遗症,但从生理学角度来看,同时存在LES松弛受损引起的吞咽困难和LES过度松弛引起的反流似乎是不一致的。为了支持这一怀疑,对贲门失弛缓症患者进行24小时食管 pH 动态研究，仅显示食管内滞留食物的细菌发酵引起的周期性食管酸化，而不是离散的胃食管反流事件[67]。此外，失弛缓症患者发生 tLESR 是罕见的。相反，贲门失弛缓症患者表现为不完全的 tLESR，伴有膈脚抑制、食管缩短和明显的松弛后收缩，但缺乏 LES 松弛的要素[68]。

2. 远端食管痉挛

端食管痉挛（DES）的主要症状是吞咽困难和胸痛，体重减轻比较少见。吞咽困难通常是间歇性的，有时与在极热或极冷的温度下吞咽特定物质如红酒或液体有关。在某些情况下，患者在进食时会出现食管梗阻，持续到呕吐才缓解。

食管性胸痛在性质上与心绞痛非常相似，常被描述为压榨性与挤压性疼痛，放射到颈部、下颌、手臂或背部正中。疼痛发作可持续数分钟至数小时，但持续吞咽并不总是受损。引起食管性胸痛的机制尚不清楚。高频腔内超声检查数据表明，这可能与食管纵行肌持续收缩有关[69]。

胸痛在随后发现测压异常的患者中也很普遍，这些异常不足以确定贲门失弛缓症或 DES 的诊断。在这些人中，反流和精神病诊断的患病率很高，尤其是焦虑和抑郁[46]。

3. 高收缩性食管

食管过度收缩性疾病也通常表现为胸痛和吞咽困难，虽然吞咽困难不太可能涉及食团转运受损。根据定义，收缩潜伏期正常，收缩力亢进，因此食管蠕动进程和食团转运是正常的。然而，jackhammer 模式与持续的、长时间的重复性收缩有关，这种收缩在食团转运后仍会持续很长时间（图 44.10）。食管过度收缩的自然史尚不清楚，但至少在某些情况下很明显，jackhammer 患者的临床病程会延长且较为困难。

4. 蠕动缺失

缺乏食管蠕动的患者可出现吞咽困难或严重胃食管反流的症状，如灼热、反流和胸痛。症状的严重程度在某种程度上取决于 EGJ 的功能，当缺乏蠕动并伴有严重的 EGJ 功能不全时，胃食管反流症状更为严重。另一方面，对于完整的 EGJ，缺乏蠕动可能难以与贲门失弛缓症区分，由于具有相似的症状学和生理学。

（四）鉴别诊断

患者病史在吞咽困难的评估中至关重要。病史的主要目的是鉴别口咽吞咽困难与食管吞咽困难、口干（唾液分泌不足）或癔球症。以上症状经常相互混淆。尤其是癔球感觉，经常与吞咽困难相混淆。与吞咽困难不同，吞咽困难只发生在吞咽过程中，而癔球感觉在吞咽之间明显。患者几乎总是感觉到咽喉有肿块或异物卡在咽喉内的感觉。在某些情况下，癔球症与反流症状相关，而在另一些情况下与严重的焦虑有关。正是与焦虑的联系导致了旧的命名为“歇斯底里癔球症”（hystericus globus）。遗憾的是，研究未能阐明癔球症的客观解剖或生理学原因，我们留下了历史上的关键数据，无论吞咽行为如何，癔球样感觉都会持续存在。

1. 贲门失弛缓症

贲门失弛缓症的鉴别诊断，包括其他食管动力障碍和与贲门失弛缓症功能性后果相同而病理生理学不同的疾病。关于其他运动障碍，DES 与贲门失弛缓症有许多相似之处，尤其是痉挛性贲门失弛缓症亚型。事实上，这些疾病之间的唯一区别是Ⅲ型贲门失弛缓症中 LES 松弛不完全的证明，并且也有 DES 演变痉挛性贲门失弛缓症的病例报告[61]。然而，鉴于这两种疾病的罕见性和如何诊断的历史异质性，似乎只有少数贲门失弛缓症病例是 DES 连续体的一部分。

与特发性贲门失弛缓症功能后果相同的其他疾病，主要考虑的是与浸润性疾病、恶性肿瘤、梗阻或手术相关的 Chagas 病和假性贲门失弛缓症。

2. Chagas 病（美洲锥虫病）

食管受累的 Chagas 病主要流行于巴西中部、委内瑞拉和阿根廷北部地区，该病与特发性贲门失弛缓症难以区分。估计有 2 000 万南美洲人受到感染。由于移民的原因，在美国大

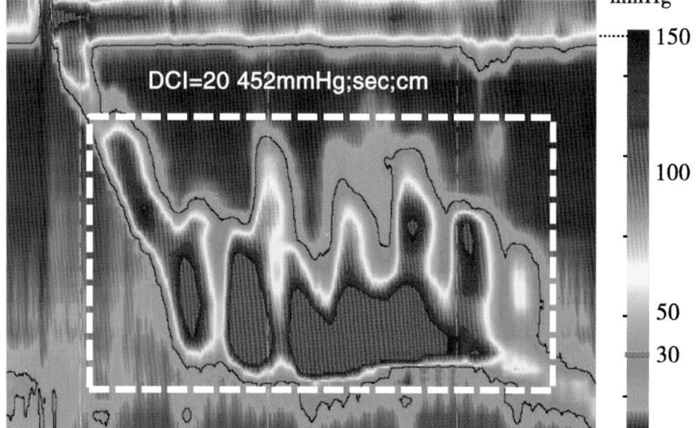

图 44.10　正常与异常的收缩活力。A，正常吞咽，远端收缩间隙（DCI）为 3 212mmHg · s · cm，正常传播，单次均匀一致收缩。B，极高的 DCI 吞咽。该吞咽表现出重复性收缩，无 EGJ 流出道梗阻的证据。这是芝加哥分类中的一种过度收缩或“jackhammer”模式（见表 44.2）。（With permission from the Esophageal Center at Northwestern.）

约有50万人被感染。Chagas病是通过一种猎蝽小昆虫叮咬(接吻)传播的,这种小昆虫能传播寄生原生动物克鲁兹锥虫。在疾病的急性败血症期之后,其严重程度从被忽视到致命不等。该病的慢性期在感染后长达20年发展,是由于全身自主神经节细胞破坏引起,包括心脏、肠道、泌尿道和呼吸道。慢性心肌病伴有传导系统紊乱和心律失常的是最常见的死亡原因。在消化道内,最常受累的器官是食管、十二指肠和结肠。食管功能障碍的严重程度与壁内神经节细胞的丢失程度成正比,50%的神经节细胞被破坏后,首先可检测到异常蠕动,90%的神经节细胞被破坏后,出现食管扩张。与此相平行的是,最初的功能障碍仅限于食管体部,LES功能障碍发生在疾病的晚期。特发性贲门失弛缓症与Chagas病食管受累之间最明显的临床区别是Chagas病中外加的管状器官受累的证据(如心肌病、巨十二指肠、巨结肠、巨直肠、巨输尿管)[70]。关于食管病理学,这两个疾病在其他方面难以区分。在急性期Chagas病的诊断是通过在血液涂片中观察到寄生虫作出的。在慢性期通过补体结合或PCR的血清学试验确诊。Chagas病相关的贲门失弛缓症的治疗与特发性贲门失弛缓症相似。感染本身的治疗在急性期效果有限,而在慢性期没有证明有效。

3. 假性贲门失弛缓症

贲门失弛缓症的放射影像学和测压特征对特发性贲门失弛缓症或与Chagas病相关的贲门失弛缓症均无特异性。肿瘤相关的假性贲门失弛缓症最常见于胃贲门,占测压定义的贲门失弛缓症病例的5%。与特发性贲门失弛缓症相比,假性贲门失弛缓症更常见于高龄(>50岁)、突然和近期出现症状(<1年)及早期体重减轻超过7kg[44]。然而,尽管这些标准使假性贲门失弛缓症的可能性更大,但它们在个体病例中的预测价值仍然较差。正是由于这一潜在的缺陷,进行全面的解剖学检查(包括内镜检查),应作为每例贲门失弛缓症新发病例诊断评价的一部分。如内镜通过EGJ的阻力最小这可能是假性贲门失弛缓症存在的线索。在特发性贲门失弛缓症中,内镜仅需轻轻按压即可突然弹出。如果高度怀疑假性贲门失弛缓症,则应根据个体情况考虑内镜活检、CT、MRI或EUS进行进一步评价。

EGJ腺癌占肿瘤相关假性贲门失弛缓症病例的一半以上,其余病例为多种肿瘤(如胰腺癌、肝细胞癌、前列腺癌、肺癌、食管癌和淋巴管瘤)[44]。这些肿瘤通过浸润EGJ处的食管壁,引起LES处的恶性梗阻,伴食管近端扩张,从而发生贲门失弛缓综合征。类似地,假性贲门失弛缓症可由浸润性疾病(如嗜酸细胞性食管炎、结节病)、血管梗阻、腹型肥胖、阿片类药物作用或手术相关梗阻(如下文所述)引起的食管壁僵硬[71]导致。尽管经常在文献中讨论,但贲门失弛缓症综合征作为副肿瘤综合征发生而不直接累及EGJ的情况要少见得多。

4. 术后功能障碍

术后吞咽困难常见于胃底折叠术后早期,劝告患者在术后的前2~4周食用软食。对于持续时间超过4周的吞咽困难,应通过上消化道内镜检查或食管钡剂造影进行评价,以评估包裹的完整性,并评价有无食管旁疝形成。对无明显机械性破坏的受试者应通过测压法评估蠕动功能、EGJ松弛和食管加压,以确定包裹是否过紧或存在潜在的运动障碍,如贲门失弛缓症。在胃底折叠术的背景下诊断贲门失弛缓症可能很困难,因为关键的测压结果(胃蠕动停止和EGJ松弛受损)可能是完全相同的。

减肥手术,特别是腹腔镜可调节胃束带术,也可能并发假性贲门失弛缓症的发生。一份手术报告检查了121例术后1年的患者,发现其中14%的患者食管扩张超过3.5cm。受累患者发生伴吞咽困难和呕吐的贲门失弛缓症[72]。这种形式的假性贲门失弛缓症通常(但不总是)在消除胃束带后可逆转[73]。

5. 远端食管痉挛

远端食管痉挛(DES)引起的疼痛与心绞痛非常相似。鉴于心肌缺血的潜在致死性后果,因此在鉴别诊断时必须始终仔细考虑这一点。提示食管而非心脏疼痛的特征包括:①长期非劳力性疼痛,②中断睡眠的疼痛,③与进餐相关的疼痛,④抗酸剂可缓解,⑤其他伴随的食管症状,如灼热、吞咽困难或反流。然而,即使是这些特征也可能与心脏疼痛重叠。此外,即使在食管疾病谱中,胸痛和吞咽困难也不是DES所特有的,这两种症状也是食管常见疾病的特征,包括消化性或感染性食管炎。因此,只有在通过适当的放射影像学评估、内镜评估和质子泵抑制剂(PPI)的治疗性试验排除了这些更常见的诊断可能性后,才应考虑DES。

(五)诊断方法

1. 内镜检查

上消化道内镜检查应是评估新发吞咽困难的首选方法,因为内镜组合了查明大多数吞咽困难结构性原因的能力和获得活检的能力。越来越多的人认识到嗜酸粒细胞性食管炎(见第30章)是一种易混淆的临床疾病,这在进行上消化道内镜检查评估吞咽困难时增加了活检的潜在价值。内镜医师在获取多个食管黏膜活检标本以评估吞咽困难患者的嗜酸粒细胞性食管炎时应具有非常低的意识阈,即使是食管黏膜外观正常的患者。此外,如果检测到狭窄或黏膜环,可在同一内镜检查过程中完成扩张。然而,尽管上消化道内镜检查是评估吞咽困难的极佳工具,但其在评估腔外结构和食管运动异常方面存在很大的局限性,它还有可能遗漏细微的梗阻性病变,如食管网和食管环。

2. 对比成像

如果内镜检查结果不确定,口咽与食管的对比成像研究可用于评估吞咽困难。电视透视对于检查后用解剖结构解释吞咽口咽期的功能评估特别有用。Logemann常被称为改良吞钡,描述了一系列吞咽活动的规程[7]。图像在侧位投影中获得,一帧内包括口咽、上颚、食管近端和气道近端。然后根据4大类口咽功能障碍评价这些图像:①咽吞咽无能力启动或过度延迟,②误吸,③鼻咽反流,④吞咽后咽腔内残留物质。此外,该程序可以评价各种补偿性饮食调整、姿势以及吞咽动作在补偿观察到的吞咽功能障碍方面的功效。

钡剂食管造影还可提供有关UES功能、蠕动和通过EGJ的钡团清除率的关键信息。伴贲门失弛缓症进展期病例(图44.11)的发现有些明显,临床上仅需区分原发性和继发性病因。然而,应用良好的技术,正常的蠕动也可以被证实。蠕动

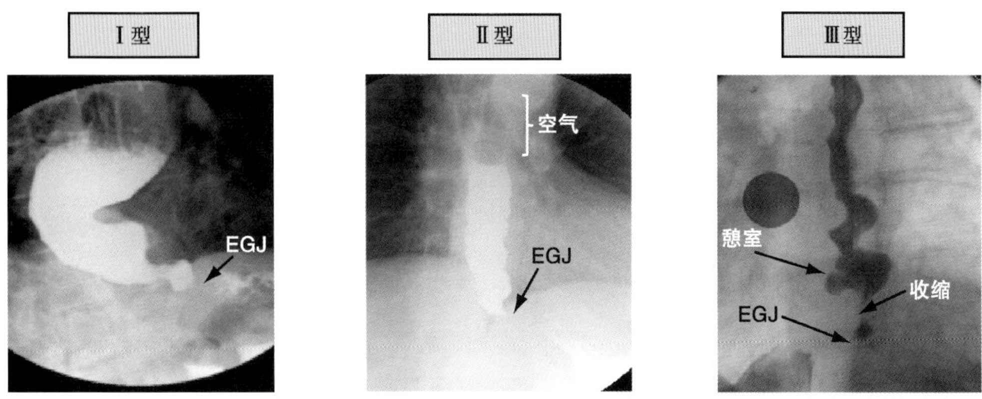

图 44.11　特发性贲门失弛缓症 3 种亚型吞钡研究的 X 胶片(见表 44.2)。注意食管扩张与气液平面(左图和中图)和 EGJ 处的逐渐变细。在疾病的早期阶段,放射学表现可能更微妙。右侧的胶片是在定时食管钡剂造影期间拍摄的,表明在 5 分钟时钡剂仍保留在扩张的食管内。EGJ,食管胃交界处

最好在俯卧位进行评估,这样在重力作用下不会出现明显的间隙[44]。蠕动异常可通过蠕动波前的钡团逆行逸出造成食管排空不全推断的。通常,当钡团到达该区域时,EGJ 会变得明显通畅,当在 EGJ 观察到平滑逐渐变细或钡团通过 EGJ 受阻时,可以推断松弛受损。另外,荧光透视偶尔会显示痉挛性收缩,表现为出现螺旋形外观而证实(图 44.12)。

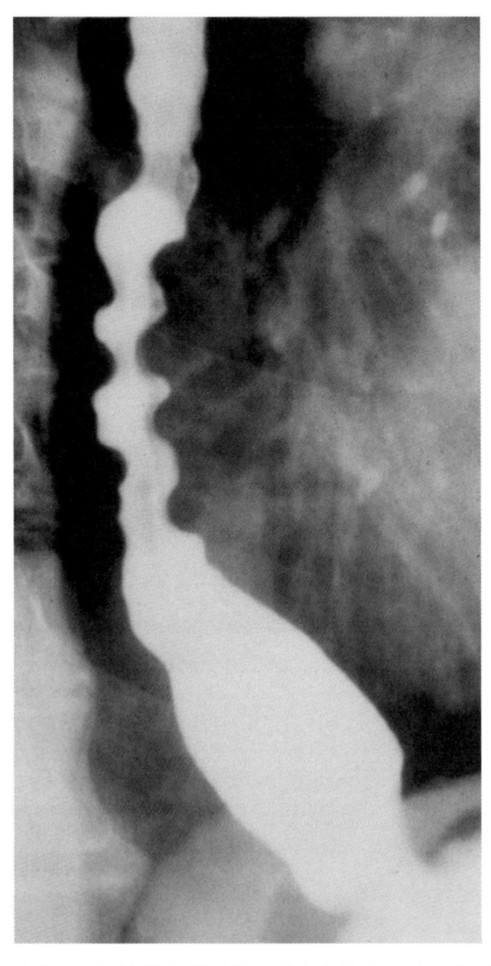

图 44.12　钡剂食管造影显示一例有症状的 DES 患者的螺旋状食管

3. 高分辨率测压(HRM)

食管测压是将腔内压力传感器定位在食管内,以测量食管的收缩特征并将其分离为功能区的一种检查。高分辨率食管测压的概念是在食管内使用足够数量的压力传感器,使腔内压力能被监测为沿食管长度的连续体,就像时间被视为常规测压线描记的连续体一样,如图 44.3 所示。当 HRM 结合复杂的算法将测压数据显示为压力地形图时,食管收缩力是可视化的,压力地形图上等色区域指示的传感器间的等压条件。图 44.3 在压力地形图中描述了包括两端括约肌和中间食管的正常吞咽,括约肌松弛和节段性收缩的相对时间以及过渡区的位置均易于证实。

鉴于我们在过去的 15 年中对 HRM 的理解取得了重大进展,利用新技术提高的准确性和细节开发了一种新的分类。芝加哥食管运动障碍分类由一组国际专家审核并定期更新,最新版本(3.0)于 2015 年发表[64]。芝加哥分类结合标准化指标量化 EGJ 松弛[即整体松弛压(integrated relaxation pressure,IRP)]和蠕动(DCI,DL)进入生成 4 大类功能的算法:①EGJ 流出道梗阻疾病;②主要蠕动障碍疾病;③蠕动轻微障碍疾病;④正常(图 44.13)[64]。

吞咽 EGJ 松弛的测压评估可能是临床食管测压期间最重要的测量。EGJ 不完全松弛是贲门失弛缓症诊断的基本特征,贲门失弛缓症是治疗最特殊的运动障碍疾病。尽管具有这一重要意义,但在芝加哥分类法之前,没有定义不完全吞咽性 EGJ 松弛的协议。芝加哥分类发展的关键是一项研究,该研究在大量患者和对照受试者中比较了检测吞咽 EGJ 松弛受损的标准,从而导致 IRP 的发展,分析中使用的测压装置的正常值为 15mmHg 或更低[74]。从概念上讲,IRP 是吞咽后 10 秒内最大松弛 4 秒的平均 EGJ 压力(见图 44.6)。这种吞咽 EGJ 松弛的单一测量方法,在区分明确定义的贲门失弛缓症患者与对照受试者和其他诊断患者方面,显示出 98% 的敏感性和 96% 的特异性[74]。

除了改善测压检测贲门失弛缓症的敏感性外,HRM 还定义了贲门失弛缓症的临床相关分类亚型[54]。贲门失弛缓症的诊断需要满足蠕动消失和吞咽 EGJ 松弛受损两种异常。在其最明显的形式中(Ⅰ型),这发生在食管扩张的情况下,食管内压可忽略不计(图 44.14)。然而,尽管没有蠕动,食管

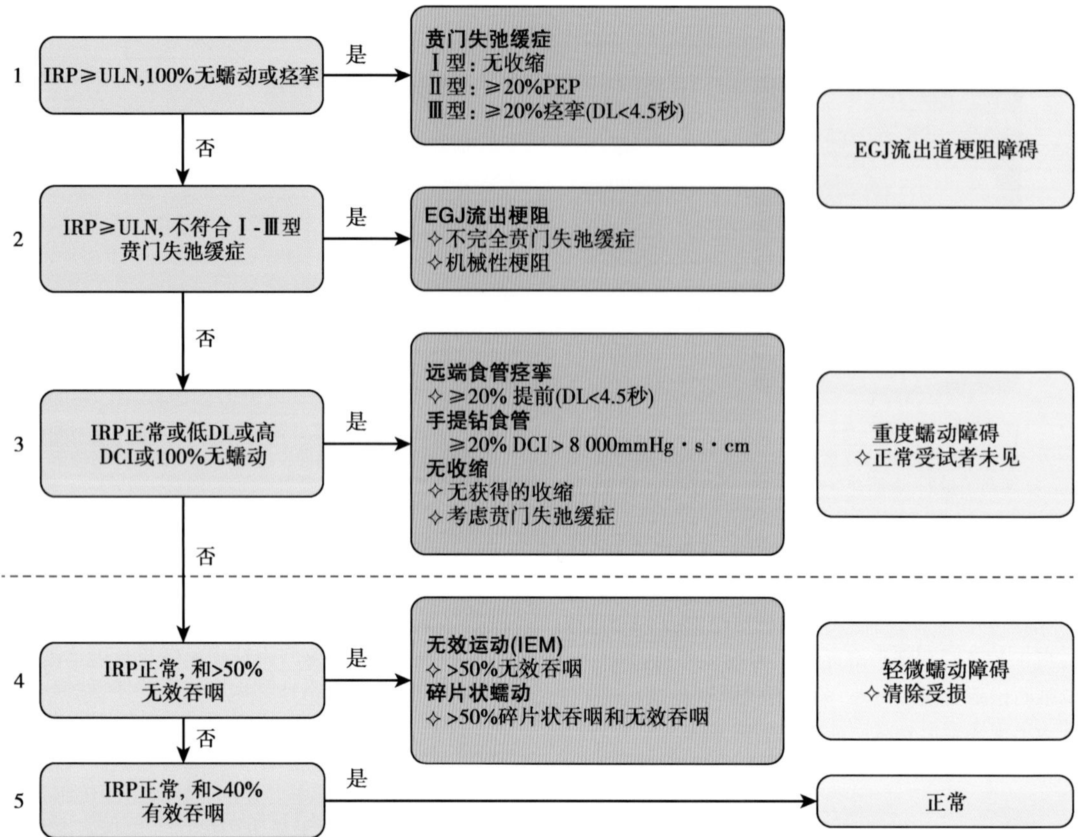

图 44.13 食管运动障碍疾病芝加哥分类的流程。DCI，远端收缩间期；DL，远端潜伏期；EGJ，食管胃交界处；IRP，整体松弛压；PEP，全食管加压；ULN，正常值上限。（更多信息参见表 44.2）

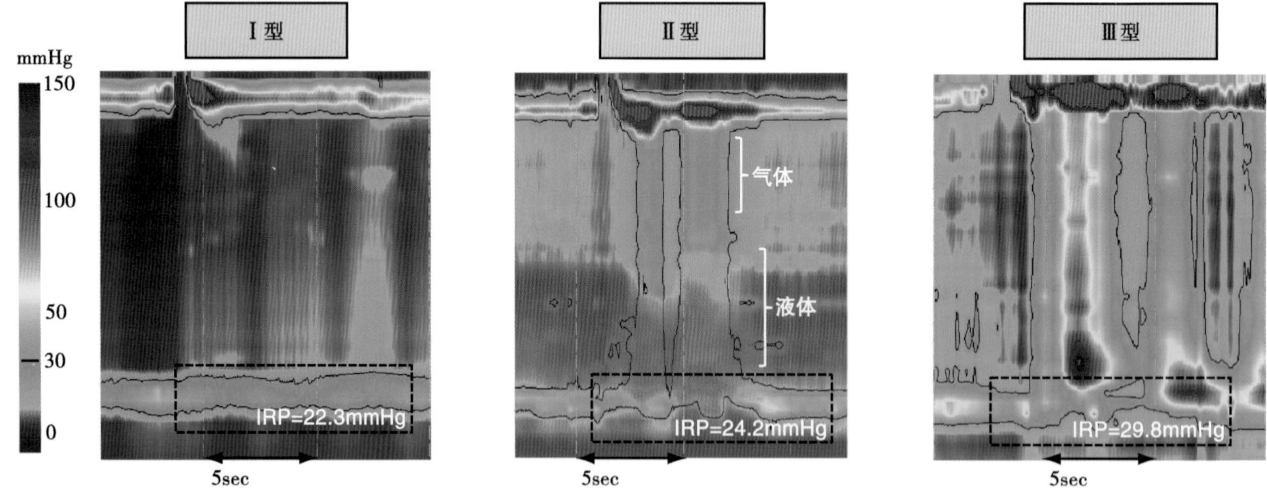

图 44.14 贲门失弛缓症亚型。这 3 种亚型通过食管体收缩力的不同测压模式进行区分。在典型贲门失弛缓症（Ⅰ型）患者中，食管体内无明显压力，EGJ 松弛受损；在本例中 IRP 为 22.3mmHg。一例Ⅱ型患者“即贲门失弛缓症伴压迫亚型”的吞咽显示，随着食管缩短，截留在括约肌之间的液柱快速全食管加压。Ⅲ型患者的压力地形图是典型的痉挛性贲门失弛缓症。虽然这种吞咽也与快速传播的加压有关，但加压可归因于异常的管腔闭塞性收缩。EGJ，食管胃交界处；IRP，整体松弛压。（Modified from Pandolfno JE，Kwiatek MA，Nealis T，et al. Achalasia：A new clinically relevant classifcation by high resolution manometry. Gastroenterology 2008；135：1526-33. With permission from the Esophageal Center at Northwestern.）

内仍有大量的压力。事实上，最常见的模式（Ⅱ型）是贲门失弛缓症伴食管压迫和全食管加压（见图 44.14B）。另一种较少见的模式（Ⅲ型）是痉挛性贲门失弛缓症，食管远端内存在痉挛性收缩（见图 44.14C）。随后的几个系列，包括比较腹腔镜 Heller 肌切开术与充气扩张术的欧洲随机对照试验的随访报告[75]，证实了该开创性研究的初步观察结果，即Ⅱ型贲门失弛缓症对治疗的反应性最强，Ⅲ型反应最低。

EGJ 松弛受损的患者，被定义为持续蠕动活动的异常 IRP 不符合贲门失弛缓症的诊断标准，在芝加哥分类中被归类为 EGJ 流出道梗阻[64]。从一开始，这些患者就被认为是一组异质性患者，其中只有一些患者从贲门失弛缓症治疗中获益[76]。图 44.15 显示了 EGJ 流出道梗阻的两个代表性示例。因此，某些情况下，如图 44.15A 所示，这可能是贲门失弛缓症的变体或早期表现。然而，最近的系列研究报道称，许多 EGJ 流出道梗阻的患者症状轻微甚至无症状，20%～40% 的病例中"病变"自行消退，只有 12%～40% 的病例最终治疗后被视为贲门失弛缓症[77,78]。

在分析 EGJ 松弛之后，分析远端收缩的定量特征，以识别蠕动障碍。该分析在很大程度上基于 DCI 和 DL，基于关键地形图标志的指标：UES 开始松弛、第一个压力谷（过渡区）和 CDP（见图 44.3）。CDP 接近 LES 的近端边缘，被确定为沿 30mmHg 等压线的拐点，在此发生减速，这表示从蠕动到壶腹排空的过渡[16]。UES 松弛和 CDP 之间的间隔定义了收缩的 DL，如图 44.3 所示。DL 值小于 4.5 秒定义为提前收缩，可能提示抑制性神经元控制受损，以定义收缩失败（DCI<100mmHg·s·cm），弱收缩（DCI<450mmHg·s·cm）和过度收缩（DCI>8 000mmHg·s·cm）。

根据上述列出的标准对个体吞咽进行分析后，根据表 44.2 中详述的标准，将组分结果综合为整体测压诊断。EGJ 松弛正常、完整性正常、DL 正常、收缩前速度正常和 DCI 小于 5 000mmHg·s·cm 的患者属于正常。所遇到的异常以特定的功能术语描述，目的是在临床背景下解释这些异常。表 44.2 详述的分类代表了当前的芝加哥分类版本，该版本由国际 HRM 工作组采用协商共识的方法进行审查。

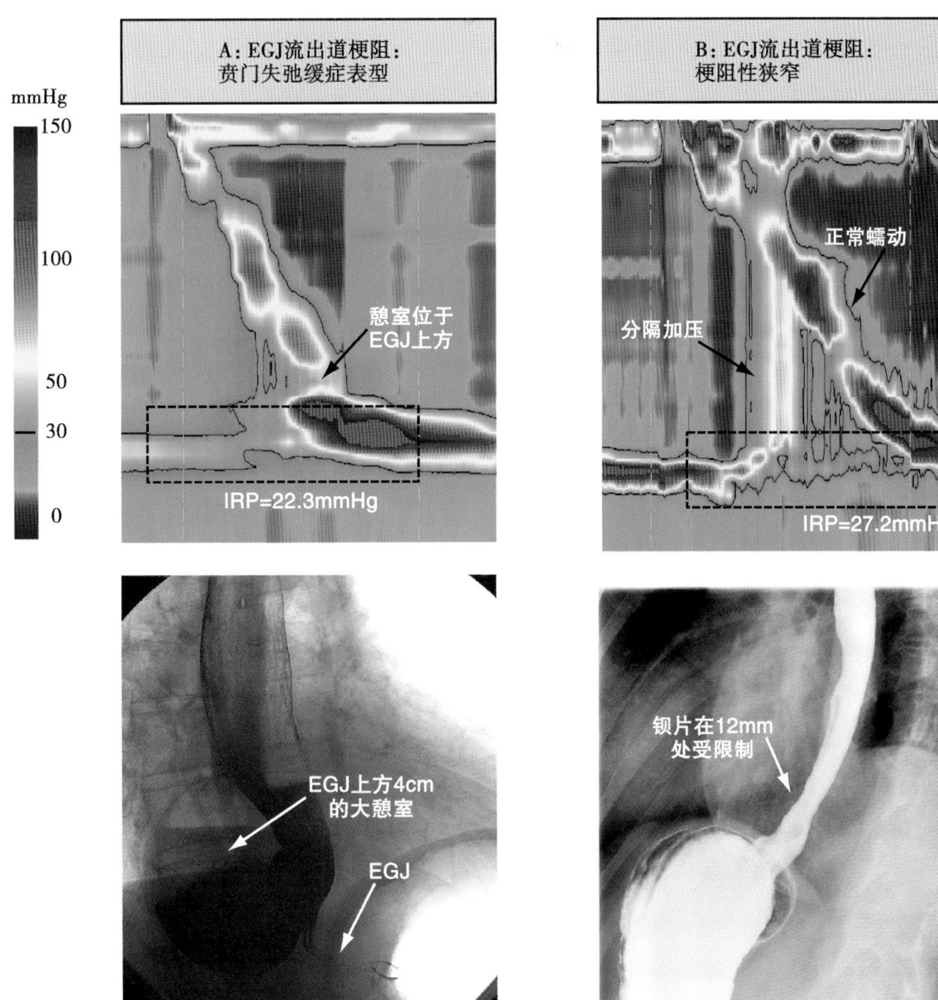

图 44.15 EGJ 流出道梗阻。EGJ 流出道梗阻的诊断标准是 IRP 升高与一些保留下来的微弱或正常蠕动相关，因此不符合Ⅰ型、Ⅱ型或Ⅲ型贲门失弛缓症的诊断标准。最终，这种模式可能被证明是贲门失弛缓症的一种表型（A，上图）。该患者还患有较大的膈上憩室（A，下图），曾接受腹腔镜肌切开术和憩室切除术治疗，效果良好。另外，EGJ 流出道阻塞模式可能与机械阻塞有关（B）。该患者的 EGJ 扩展，通过了 9mm 内镜，未遇到阻力。然而，IRP 增加，并且在保留的蠕动收缩和 EGJ 之间存在分隔加压（B，上图）。食管造影图（B，下图）显示 EGJ 近端轻微狭窄（箭头），12.5mm 处钡片通过延迟。患者对 18mm 球囊扩张和 PPI 治疗有反应。EGJ，食管胃交界处。（With permission from the Esophageal Center at Northwestern.）

表 44.2 食管运动障碍的芝加哥分类 3.0 版

诊断	诊断标准
贲门失弛缓症	
Ⅰ型(经典型)	100%蠕动消失,IRP>正常上限
Ⅱ型(伴食管受压)	100%蠕动消失,≥20%吞咽伴全食管加压,平均 IRP>正常上限
Ⅲ型(痉挛型)	无正常蠕动,≥20%吞咽提前收缩,平均 IRP>正常上限
EGJ 流出道梗阻	平均 IRP≥正常上限,有足够的蠕动证据表明不符合贲门失弛缓症的标准
主要蠕动障碍(正常人未观察到的模式)	
远端食管痉挛	平均 IRP<正常上限,≥20%提前收缩,DCI>450mmHg·s·cm,可能出现一些正常的蠕动
高收缩性(jackhammer)食管	至少有 2 个吞咽 DCI>8 000mmHg·s·cm,可能累及或局限于 LES
收缩力缺乏	平均 IRP≤10mmHg,100%无收缩力(DCI<100mmHg·s·cm)
轻微蠕动障碍(超过正常的统计极限定义)	
无效食管蠕动	≥50%无效吞咽,DCI<450mmHg·s·cm
频繁蠕动失败	>30%,但<100%吞咽蠕动失败
碎裂蠕动	≥50%碎裂蠕动,DCI>450mmHg·s·cm
正常	未达到上述任何诊断标准

DCI,远端收缩间隔;EGJ,食管胃交界处;IRP,整体松弛压(见正文)。

4. 腔内阻抗测量

在十多年前,腔内阻抗监测被描述为一种不用荧光透视评估腔内食团转运的方法。该技术需使用具有多对紧密间隔的金属环的腔内导管。在每对相邻环上施加交流电,环之间的合成电流取决于组织阻抗和环之间的管腔内容物。当电极被液体桥接时,阻抗降低,当电极被空气包围时,阻抗增加。因此,来自多个阻抗段的数据,揭示了食团转运的方向、内容和完整性。确认数据表明,阻抗下降 50%表示在电极水平的液体团注进入。阻抗描记恢复到基线的 50%与荧光透视下团注尾部通过相关,也可通过测压期间观察到的收缩性上升表明。针对荧光透视的验证研究显示,在确定团注转运方面具有极好的一致性。

最近,腔内阻抗测量也与测压相结合,以评估食管排空的效果。随着蠕动振幅的减小,排空的效果降低。目前,HRM 与阻抗联合的主要用途是评估食管转运异常,特别是反刍和嗳气,并评估贲门失弛缓症患者食管潴留的严重程度[79]。

5. 感觉测试

食管感觉神经在确定食管运动障碍症状中起着关键作用,因为食管对各种刺激都敏感,包括机械刺激(由管腔扩张或高幅度收缩引起)、化学刺激(酸和/或反流的其他成分)和温度刺激[31]。通常情况下,内脏传入不会被有意识地感知到,尽管一些患者可能会出现症状,痛觉过敏(过度疼痛感知)或痛觉超敏(对通常不痛的刺激的疼痛感知)[32]。食管症状可描述为灼热感、压迫感、刺痛感或热感觉。然而,症状并非给予特定的刺激,不同刺激之间的感知有大量重叠是很常见的。

虽然食管刺激引起疼痛或吞咽困难感知的确切机制尚不清楚,但设计通过模拟生理活动引起或刺激疼痛的方法,可用于评估持续症状和疑似原因之间的可能关系。这些试验通常使用扩张研究的形式(气囊、稳压器、阻抗平面测量或容积要求)或直接刺激黏膜(化学、电或热)。气囊扩张研究显示,食管扩张可引起胸痛,与对照组相比,食管胸痛患者的疼痛阈值往往较低[31]。

化学敏感性的标准试验是 Bernstein 试验,其中将 0.1 N HCl 灌注到食管中以重现胸痛或灼热症状。通常,酸输注与盐水灌注以设盲方式交替进行,以增加试验的客观性,但此不存在标准化方案。除了 Bernstein 试验,还设计了新的探针来测试食管对热刺激和经黏膜神经电刺激的反应性。然而,尽管这些工具无疑有助于改善我们对外周感受器和中枢痛觉之间相互作用的理解,但由于缺乏标准的方案和研究的烦琐性,目前,这些设备的使用仅限于专业中心,在提倡主流临床使用之前,还需要进一步改进。

(六) 治疗

1. 口咽吞咽困难

口咽吞咽困难的处理集中在 4 个特定问题上:①确定基础疾病;②描述适合手术或扩张的疾病特征;③确定适合吞咽治疗的吞咽困难特定模式;④评估误吸风险。

(1) 确定基础疾病

基础疾病识别评价的潜在结果是确定特定处理的基础神经肌肉、肿瘤或代谢疾病。例如吞咽困难可能是肌肉病变、肌无力、甲状腺毒症、运动神经元疾病或帕金森病患者的症状。基础疾病的治疗是否能改善吞咽功能取决于特定疾病的自然史以及是否存在有效的治疗。

(2) 适于手术的疾病

口咽吞咽困难最常见的手术治疗是环咽肌切开术,但对神经源性或肌源性吞咽困难的肌切开术疗效不一。大多数系列评价肌切开术疗效是不受控制的,并且缺乏经过验证(甚至是特定的)的结局指标。因此,尽管本文献中报告的总体有利应答率超过 60%,但尚无有效的患者选择标准。从理论上讲,神经源性或肌源性吞咽困难患者面临的功能受限是咽推进力较弱,而肌切开术的潜在益处在环咽水平梗阻的情况下不太明显。

(3) 适于吞咽治疗的口咽吞咽困难模式

识别口咽吞咽困难的潜在治疗从异常生理学的定义开始,如表 44.1 所示。这最好通过视频透视吞咽研究来完成,该研究首先描述患者的吞咽功能障碍特征,然后继续测试所选补偿或治疗策略的有效性。补偿治疗包括体位改变、改变食物输送或黏稠度或使用假体。例如,在轻偏瘫患者中,转头偏向功能性更强的一侧来消除误吸或咽部残留[7]。同样,饮食调整可以降低吞咽的难度。治疗策略的设计旨在改变吞咽的生理功能,通常通过改善口腔或咽部结构的活动范围,达到使用意志控制的可能程度。根据损伤的严重程度、推动水平、和整体神经系统的完整性,可以有选择地修复吞咽的缺陷成分。关于吞咽治疗技术和局限性的详细介绍，请读者参考该主题的论文[7,80]。

（4）评估误吸风险

口咽吞咽困难是每年成千上万人死于吸入性肺炎的原因。荧光透视被认为是检测误吸的最敏感的测试，据报道在大约 50% 的患者中检测床边评估不明显。然而，尽管吞咽性误吸与随后发生的肺炎之间存在逻辑联系，但该顺序并非不可避免。尽管如此，证据的平衡表明，误吸的检测是肺炎风险的预测因素，其检测决定了采取补偿性吞咽策略、非经口喂养或矫正手术的实施。非经口喂养是否能消除误吸的风险是有争议的，这是一个由挑衅性发现提出的问题，即在放射线检查误吸的患者中，接受饲养管的患者肺炎和死亡更常见。这表明防止口腔分泌物的吸入可能对控制肺炎风险至关重要，并导致一些人考虑诸如气管切开术等以保护呼吸道。

2. 下咽憩室和环咽嵴

下咽憩室（Zenker 憩室）的治疗方法是环咽肌切开术加或不加憩室切除术或憩室固定术。环咽肌切开术降低了静息括约肌张力和流经 UES 的阻力。据报道，有 80%～100% 的 Zenker 憩室患者，采用经颈肌切开术联合憩室切除术或憩室固定术治疗结果良好或极佳。在某些情况下，有限的手术操作是足够的，但解决牵拉性憩室的最终方法应包括憩室切除术和肌切开术。单纯憩室切除术有复发的风险，因为环咽肌水平的潜在狭窄没有得到纠正[80]。同样，单纯的肌切开术也有可能无法解决憩室内食物积聚的问题，同时伴有反流和误吸。然而，小憩室也可在肌切开术后自行消失。最近的趋势是通过硬式或软式内镜治疗 Zenker 憩室。两种技术的治疗原理都是分离憩室腔和食管腔之间的隔膜。该分离使食物和液体从环咽肌远端的憩室内流出（位于隔膜内），而不是在憩室内蓄积。该手术操作是在全身麻醉下，使用硬式内镜用吻合器完成，或在轻度镇静和软式内镜下，使用针刀、氩气等离子凝固或热活检钳完成。尚未对不同手术操作进行对照试验，但许多病例系列表明，在操作娴熟的情况下，每种手术操作都是有效的[81]。

在没有 Zenker 憩室的情况下，环咽嵴是否需要治疗目前尚不清楚。当然，如果存在吞咽困难，并且结合荧光透视/测压分析确认括约肌开口减小连同上游食团内压力升高，则为良好的治疗依据。一项非对照系列的研究表明，对于有症状的环咽嵴患者，使用大口径探条扩张可有效缓解吞咽困难，认为这是肌切开术前合理的治疗选择[82]。

3. 贲门失弛缓症

由于贲门失弛缓症的潜在神经病理学改变无法纠正，治疗的目的是补偿食管排空不良和预防并发症。实际上，这相当于降低 LES 压力，因此重力以及存在的任何残余食管收缩力都会促进食管排空。LES 压力可通过药物治疗、强制扩张或手术肌切开术来降低。总的来说，药物治疗并不是很有效，因此药物只适合作为临时的措施。

HRM 将贲门失弛缓症分为 3 种不同的亚型：①经典型贲门失弛缓症；②压迫型贲门失缓症；③痉挛型贲门失缓症（见图 44.14）。从概念特点的角度来看，Ⅰ型和Ⅱ型代表一个连续统一体，Ⅱ型是Ⅰ型食管扩张特征进展之前的早期疾病。而Ⅲ型是一种以食管远端痉挛为特征的亚型。这些疾病亚型的意义在于它们对治疗的反应有所不同。直到最近几年，贲门失弛缓症的持久治疗选择是腹腔镜 Heller 肌切开术或充气扩张术。大量文献对这些治疗方法进行了比较，最终在一项欧洲多中心随机对照试验中得出结论，这两种方法的有效率均约为 90%，两者之间不存在任何统计学显著差异[83,84]。然而，此项研究和先前所有的试验一样，在设计或治疗效果的评估时均未考虑贲门失弛缓症亚型。随后，大量回顾性数据和对欧洲贲门失弛缓症试验[85]的重新评估表明，贲门失弛缓症亚型在确定治疗效果方面具有重要的相关性。事实上，在欧洲贲门失弛缓症试验中，充气扩张术治疗Ⅱ型贲门失弛缓症的有效性为 100%，而 Heller 肌切开术的疗效仅为 93%（$P=0.03$）。相比之下，对于充气扩张和腹腔镜肌切开术治疗Ⅲ型贲门失弛缓症的成功率分别为 40% 和 86%，尽管数量较少，且该差异无统计学显著性。考虑到与腹腔镜肌切开术相比，充气扩张术的成本较低，且两种技术之间发生食管穿孔的风险相当（约 1%）[86]，这些结果证明充气扩张是Ⅱ型贲门失弛缓症的首选初始治疗方法。

大部分与贲门失弛缓症治疗相关的文献是使用各种质量终点作为疗效指标的非受控病例系列组成。如前所述，关于定义贲门失弛缓症的标准、疾病严重程度或如何进行治疗的技术细节的标准化程度很小。此外，一些系列病例的收集是前瞻性的，一些是回顾性的，一些是混合性的。考虑到所有这些局限性，对各种技术进行详细比较几乎没有价值，现存的治疗资料总结如下。

（1）药物治疗

餐前即刻舌下含服平滑肌松弛剂，如硝酸盐类或钙通道阻滞剂，可通过降低 LES 压力缓解贲门失弛缓症的吞咽困难。亚硝酸异戊酯、舌下含服硝酸甘油、茶碱和 β_2-肾上腺素能受体激动剂也曾试用。报告的最大经验是使用硝酸异山梨酯和硝苯地平。然而，硝酸盐类药物的副作用，特别是头痛很常见，疗效非常有限。安慰剂对照试验尚未报告。钙通道阻滞剂（主要是硝苯地平）的副作用是面部潮红、头晕、头痛、外周水肿和直立性低血压。对 29 例早期贲门失弛缓症患者餐前舌下含服硝苯地平（30～40mg/d）进行了研究，其疗效明显优于安慰剂，70% 的贲门失弛缓症患者在随访 6～18 个月后疗效良好[87]。然而，随后进行的硝苯地平安慰剂对照交叉试验发现其获益极小[88]。

西地那非（万艾可）是另一种平滑肌松弛剂，可通过阻断 5 型磷酸二酯酶，该酶由 NO 诱导代谢环磷酸鸟苷来降低贲门失弛缓症患者的 LES 压力。一项双盲安慰剂对照试验发现，与安慰剂相比，50mg 西地那非可显著降低 LES 压力和 LES 松弛压[89]。该效应在给药后 15～20 分钟达到峰值，持续时间不到 1 小时。虽然西地那非在概念上具有吸引力，但临床上使用西地那非的实用性受到其成本和潜在副作用的限制。

（2）肉毒毒素注射

肉毒杆菌毒素在治疗贲门失弛缓症中的初步标志性研究报道，向括约肌内注射 80 单位肉毒毒素，在 6 个月期间，66% 的患者 LES 压力下降 33%，吞咽困难症状改善[90]。肉毒毒素不可逆地抑制突触前胆碱能神经末梢释放乙酰胆碱，有效地消除 LES 压力的神经源性成分。然而，由于这种效应最终会被新轴突的生长所逆转，因此这并不是一种持久的治疗方法。该技术涉及使用硬化剂治疗导管针，将等份肉毒毒素分别注射到 LES 的 4 个象限。副作用罕见，但有可能发生数天胸部不适和偶发的皮疹。虽然许多患者最初反应良好，但 1 年后的持续疗效极小[91]。重复注射可能有效，但反复注射会导致局部炎症反应和纤维化，最终限制了这种策略。注射剂量大于 100 单位不会增加疗效[92]。因此，这种选择最好保留给老年人或确定治疗风险较低的个人。

(3) 充气扩张术

充气扩张治疗贲门失弛缓症需要将 LES 直径扩张至少 3cm，以持续降低 LES 压力，推测可能是通过部分破坏括约肌的环形肌肉实现的。只有专门设计用于治疗贲门失弛缓症的扩张器，才能达到足够的直径以获得持久的益处，扩张到较小的直径最多只能提供非常短暂的益处。Rigiflex 扩张器有 3.0cm、3.5cm 和 4.0cm 直径可供选用，这些是长的、不顺应性、带有不透射线标记的圆柱形气囊，它们被设计为沿导丝穿过并在 X 线透视下穿越 LES。定位后，使用手持式压力计将气囊充盈至全直径，注意观察气囊膨胀时括约肌在气囊表面的压痕。气囊扩张通常在门诊进行，患者处于清醒镇静状态。但是，充气扩张技术在患者准备、气囊充盈参数、和扩张后监测方面在从业医师中存在高度差异[93]。对于食管内大量潴留的患者，应在术前 1 天或更长时间采用清淡的流质饮食是有益的。尽管从业医师之间的方法一致性极小，但只有当较小直径扩张器被证明无效时，才使用小直径扩张器(3.0cm)开始，并逐步进展至较大直径(3.5cm 和 4.0cm)的谨慎做法相当普遍。至于充盈压力，这些与现代非顺应性气囊扩张器的相关性极小，因为无论充盈压力如何，其膨胀不会超过规定的直径。因此，有必要在 X 线透视下观察气囊是否正确定位以捕获 LES，观察为沙漏形气囊轮廓的“腰部”，并且随着充气的进行，腰部完全消失。

气囊扩张术的主要并发症是食管穿孔，据报道发生率为 0~5%，总体平均值为 1%[86]。由于持续或严重的胸痛、发热或皮下气肿，大多数穿孔在术后 1 小时内很明显(或至少可疑)，应在术后至少 2 小时内观察患者是否有食管漏体征。或者一些从业医师在充气扩张后常规进行 X 线透视检查，以确保未发生穿孔。通常先给予水溶性造影剂，然后再给予钡剂。如果穿孔很小且为包含型或在壁内，应进行保守治疗包括住院治疗和密切观察，同时维持患者禁食(NPO)，静脉给予抗生素。较大的穿孔可以使用内镜钛夹闭合。如果出现完全性穿孔或者如果发生胸痛和发热恶化，则应立即进行手术修复。能识别并及时手术治疗(6~8 小时内)的充气扩张穿孔患者的结局与接受择期 Heller 肌切开术的患者相当[94]。

在充气扩张后结果不满意的情况下，可在数周内使用逐渐增大的扩张器进行后续扩张是合理的。如果最初扩张的收益持续了 1 年或更长时间，通常会根据需要重复充气扩张。据报道，扩张的临床有效性范围为 32%~98%，这可能是因为技术、评估治疗结果的方法以及随时间推移进行重复扩张的可接受性存在极大差异[93]。手术肌切开术的后续反应不会受既往扩张史的影响。

(4) Heller 肌切开术

目前治疗贲门失弛缓症的外科手术是 Heller 于 1913 年描述的食管肌切开术的变体。随后，通过开胸术将该手术改良为前肌切开术。肌切开术的吸引力在于它提供了一种比充气扩张术更能预测降低 LES 压力的方法。虽然开放式 Heller 肌切开术明显有效，但与开胸术相关的发病率相当高。然而，采用腹腔镜方法进行贲门失弛缓症手术在很大程度上缓解了这种情况。

已发表的 Heller 肌切开术治疗贲门失弛缓症的疗效系列报告，62%~100% 的患者结果优良，持续性吞咽困难的患者不到 10%。与通过开胸术、剖腹术或胸腔镜行肌切开术相比，腹腔镜方法具有相似的疗效、发病率降低和住院时间缩短。在过去，肌切开术后胃食管反流可能特别严重，然而，通过使用 PPI 通常很容易控制。因此，腹腔镜 Heller 肌切开术结合部分胃底折叠术应用(Toupet 或 Dor)已成为治疗贲门失弛缓症的首选术式。Heller 肌切开术后不满意的结果可能是由于肌切开术不完全、肌切开术后瘢痕形成、手术中抗反流成分引起的功能性食管梗阻、食管旁疝形成或严重的食管扩张。

只见到 1 项多中心前瞻性随机对照试验比较了充气扩张术与腹腔镜 Heller 肌切开术[83,84]。在欧洲贲门失弛缓症试验中，200 例贲门失弛缓症患者被随机分配接受腹腔镜肌切开术结合 Dor 胃底折叠术或充气扩张术，充气扩张术组最多允许进行 3 个系列的扩张。随访 2 年后，成功率无差异：充气扩张术成功率为 92%，腹腔镜肌切开术成功率为 87%[84]。基于这一证据，腹腔镜肌切开术和充气扩张术的成功率相当，并且可以对这些成功率进行有力的论证。因此，在选择初始治疗时，应评估可用的当地资源以及患者的偏好。

(5) 经口内镜下肌肉切开术

最近，开发了一种用于治疗贲门失弛缓症的混合技术，主要是使用内镜来实现手术肌切开术，该手术称为经口内镜肌切开术(per oral endoscopic myotomy，POEM)。首先需要在食管中段做一个横向黏膜切口，然后进入该切口，并使用带有远端透明帽和三角形剥离刀的前视内镜创建一条通向胃贲门处的黏膜下隧道。一旦黏膜下隧道完成，撤回内镜，使用电灼工具对环形肌肉进行选择性肌开术，在食管上方和 EGJ 远端 2cm 至胃贲门处使用不同长度的电灼工具。然后使用内镜钛夹闭合进入切口。在接受 POEM 手术治疗的贲门失弛缓症患者的前瞻性队列中，最初报告的成功率大于 90%，与腹腔镜 Heller 肌切开术的成功率相当。最近一项系统性综述和 meta 分析比较了 POEM 术(1 958 例患者)和 LHM 术(5 834 例患者)的结果，发现 POEM 在短期(平均随访 16 个月)缓解吞咽困难方面比 LHM 更有效，但是与病理性反流的发生率极高相关(糜烂性食管炎的比值比为 9.31)[95]。2017 年以摘要形式发表的一项随机对照试验将 POEM 术与充气扩张术进行比较，发现 POEM 手术在治疗成功方面更有效，但也更有可能导致术后反流性食管炎[96]。1 年后，92% 的 POEM 患者($n=67$)获得临床缓解，而充气扩张术后为 70%($n=66$)($P<0.01$)。

(6) 治疗失败

贲门失弛缓症治疗后持续性吞咽困难提示治疗失败，应结合内镜检查、高分辨率阻抗测压[97]、功能性管腔成像探头[98]及荧光透视成像进行评估。内镜检查可发现食管炎、狭窄、食管旁疝或解剖畸形。阻抗测压法可用于量化持续性或复发性括约肌功能障碍、远端痉挛或食管潴留。功能性管腔成像探头研究可以识别括约肌扩张不良，即使在 HRM 提示充分松弛的情况下也是如此[99]。荧光透视有助于识别解剖问题，也可通过定时吞钡评估食管排空，这是一种标准化的方法，需在吞钡 1 分钟和 5 分钟后测量食管钡柱的高度[97]。在某些情况下，这些评估将导致进一步干预，这可能是重复扩张、POEM 术或 Heller 肌切开术。在已经接受肌切开术的患者中，从手术的抗反流部分检测到肌切开较短或功能性食管梗阻可能需要再次手术，但可以寻求充气扩张术作为替代方法。一般而言，对于贲门失弛缓症的任何适应证，再次手术的有效性均低于初次手术。

偶尔患者对最佳充气扩张或肌切开术无反应，需要替代治疗。在极晚期或难治性贲门失弛缓症的患者中，食管切除加胃上提或插入一段横结肠或小肠可能是唯一的选择。这种干预的适应证包括：无法解决的梗阻症状、营养不良、出血、慢性误吸、癌症和扩张期间的穿孔。虽然可以获得功能良好的长期结果，但报道的该手术的死亡率约为 4%，与针对其他适应证进行的食管切除术相同。

（7）鳞状细胞癌的风险

贲门失弛缓症食管可能发生鳞状细胞癌。肿瘤在贲门失弛缓症诊断多年后发生，通常发生在严重扩张的食管伴淤积性食管炎中。可因癌症的症状出现延迟，在检测时肿瘤往往较大且属晚期，这就提出了内镜监测检查的问题。然而，一项包含 1 062 例贲门失弛缓症患者瑞典人群的数据库分析表明，在剔除意外发生的癌症后，贲门失弛缓症患者的鳞状细胞癌总体风险是年龄匹配对照组的 17 倍，导致癌症发病率为 0.15%。作者计算出，如果每年进行一次监测内镜检查，在发现一例潜在的可治疗肿瘤之前，必须对男性进行 406 次检查，女性进行 2 220 次检查。然而，即使是这样的计算也是乐观的，但在严重扩张的食管伴食物滞留和淤积性食管炎中发现一个小癌病灶是远不能保证的。因此，最新的 ASGE 指南不提倡对贲门失弛缓症患者进行常规内镜监测。然而，他们还指出，如果考虑进行监测，在贲门失弛缓症症状出现后 15 年开始是合理的[100]。

4. 弥漫性食管痉挛

弥漫性食管痉挛（DES）尽管采用平滑肌松弛剂治疗，但关于 DES 药物治疗的对照数据极少[101]。长期研究尚不可用，这种疗法的整个基础都是轶闻。此外，大多数食管源性胸痛是由于反流而不是 DES 引起的，使用平滑肌松弛剂治疗可能使会反流症状恶化。少数 DES 患者的非对照试验报告了硝酸盐类、钙通道阻滞剂、肼屈嗪和抗焦虑药物治疗有临床反应。

肉毒杆菌毒素注射是 DES 有吸引力的治疗方法，因为它可以阻断胆碱能神经传递。在一项涉及 22 例 DES 或胡桃夹食管患者的随机对照试验中，50% 的患者对肉毒杆菌毒素有反应，而对照注射生理盐水的患者为 10%（$P=0.01$）[102]。在随后仅对用 HRM 诊断的患者进行的回顾性分析中，6 例 DES 患者在 2 个月时对肉毒杆菌毒素均呈阳性反应，其中 4 例患者的反应持续超过 6 个月[103]。然而，在接受肉毒杆菌毒素治疗的 DES 患者中报告了 1 例致死性纵隔炎，因此不能将该治疗视为无风险[104]。

直到最近，DES 治疗很少采用外科手术，因为选择是开胸术联合长肌切开术或食管切除术。但是，自 2012 年以来，明确定义的 DES 病例已通过 POEM 成功治疗[105]。POEM 术的独特优势是肌切开的长度可以延长到可能累及用 HRM 测量的整个食管平滑肌、EUS 显示的食管壁增厚或术中翻转。支持这一点的是，最近一项非对照 POEM 系列的 meta 分析报告，平均肌切开长度为 13.5cm[106]，DES 的加权汇总反应率为 88%（CI 61%～97%）。

5. 高收缩性食管（Jackhammer 食管）

对于高压（高收缩性）食管蠕动的患者，也提倡使用 DES 相同的治疗选择。平滑肌松弛剂，如钙通道阻滞剂和硝酸盐已被用于这些疾病。尽管它们能降低蠕动幅度，但在临床试验中，上述药物均不能缓解胸痛或吞咽困难。西地那非是一种很有吸引力的替代药物，因为其具有降低收缩幅度和潜在减少重复性收缩的深远影响[107]。同样，不存在支持性临床试验数据。同样，在有或无 EUS 引导下，向食管肌内注射肉毒杆菌毒素，可能是难治性症状患者的一种选择。最后，与痉挛性贲门失弛缓症和 DES 病例相似，POEM 最近被提出作为高收缩性治疗的方法。上述讨论的关于 DES 的非对照 POEM 系列的相同 meta 分析也分析了 jackhammer 食管的数据，并报告了 72% 的加权汇总反应率（CI 55%～83%），明显低于Ⅲ型贲门失弛缓症 92% 的反应[106]。

由于高收缩性食管蠕动和胃食管反流病之间可能存在重叠，并且观察到许多患者同时存在心理忧虑，因此也尝试了针对酸分泌、内脏敏感性和应激的治疗。基于 GERD 可引起胸痛和高收缩性食管蠕动的假设，提出应用 PPI。同样，使用低剂量三环类抗抑郁药治疗可能通过抗胆碱能作用减少收缩，并可能降低内脏敏感性。

6. 蠕动缺失

尽管治疗与蠕动缺失相关的潜在疾病可能改善食管动力在生物学上是有道理的，但尚未发现在蠕动缺失的背景下显著改善蠕动的药物。因此，治疗的重点是通过改变生活方式（如体位动作）尽可能减少潜在的并发症，以改善食管清除率，以及随餐大量饮水，以促进食团的通过。蠕动缺失和 EGJ 功能不全（“硬皮病模式”）的患者容易发生重度 GERD，因为一旦发生反流，由于抗反流屏障降低，食管清除功能受损（见第 46 章）。这些患者通常需要每日服用两次 PPI 治疗。此外，这些患者容易发生药物性食管炎，应注意避免使用可能具有腐蚀性的药物，并将药物转换为液体制剂、舌下制剂或更小的制剂，以预防药物性食管炎。

7. 食管超敏反应

食管运动障碍的治疗传统上以改善食管收缩力和排空为中心。然而，除了贲门失弛缓症外，这些治疗的疗效非常有限。最近，人们认识到，以前被解释为症状性高收缩状态疾病的微小测压结果通常提示是超敏反应综合征的附带现象。因此，现在人们对开发旨在降低食管超敏反应的治疗方法有着浓厚的兴趣，许多药物和行为治疗已被确定可调节食管痛觉。

（1）药物治疗

抗抑郁药是治疗调节内脏疼痛或食管源性胸痛的最常见的处方药物。在抗抑郁药中，研究最多的是三环类抗抑郁药物。这种治疗获益的作用机制尚不清楚，因为这些药物在中枢及外周都有多个受体靶点。这些药物的拟定治疗剂量低于情绪改变作用的剂量，抗抑郁药(阿米替林、去甲替林)的典型起始剂量为睡前10~25mg，以10~25mg的增量递增至50~75mg的目标剂量。然而，正如最近的一项随机对照试验所强调的，很难区分三环类药物的非特异性作用和它们对超敏反应的作用[108]。在该试验中，43例功能性胃灼热和食管超敏反应患者随机接受25mg丙米嗪治疗，40例随机接受安慰剂治疗，根据反流症状减少50%判断，应答率分别为37.2%和37.5%。然而，根据SF-36总分评估，接受丙米嗪治疗的患者更有可能体验到生活质量的改善，这毕竟是治疗功能性疾病的主要目的。

实验数据也支持选择性5-羟色胺再摄取抑制剂治疗食管超敏反应的有效性。在一项随机双盲交叉研究中，发现20mg剂量的西酞普兰静脉注射可显著降低化学性(酸灌注)和机械性(气囊扩张)食管的敏感性[109]。尽管临床试验尚未获得，但评估其他选择性5-羟色胺再摄取抑制剂的机制研究也取得了令人鼓舞的结果。与此类似的，鉴于5-羟色胺通路对肠动力的作用和作为恶心的治疗，人们对开发影响5-羟色胺通路的药物产生了很大兴趣。遗憾的是，这些药物中有几种被证明是不可接受的，有引起心律失常或肠道缺血相关的风险，导致其撤回被禁止应用。

(2) 非药物治疗

虽然食管超敏反应、心理因素和精神异常之间的联系尚不清楚，但以安慰、行为矫正和放松技术为重点的治疗可能是有帮助的。这些疗法最有可能使惊恐障碍、广泛性焦虑和抑郁症等共病患者获益。然而，使用控制呼吸、放松技术或催眠疗法的治疗，也可能通过转移精神注意力和减少对内脏刺激的高度警觉，使超敏反应患者获益。有必要进行良好的前瞻性试验来确定这些治疗的临床作用。

(程芮　孙元隆 译，袁农 校)

参考文献

45

第 45 章　药物、创伤和感染引起的食管疾病

David A. Katzka 著

章节目录

一、药物引起的食管损伤 …… 627
（一）发病机制 …… 627
（二）临床特征及诊断 …… 627
（三）预防、治疗和临床病程 …… 628
（四）特殊药物 …… 628
二、鼻胃管和其他非内镜管引起的食管损伤 …… 630
三、食管穿透性损伤或钝挫性损伤 …… 631
四、食管撕裂和血肿 …… 631
（一）Mallory-Weiss 综合征（食管黏膜撕裂症）…… 631
（二）Boerhaave 综合征（自发性食管破裂综合征）…… 631
（三）自发性食管血肿 …… 632
五、在免疫活性宿主中的食管感染 …… 632
（一）白色念珠菌 …… 632
（二）单纯疱疹病毒 …… 633
（三）巨细胞病毒 …… 633
（四）人乳头瘤病毒 …… 633
（五）其他感染 …… 634
六、急性食管坏死 …… 634

一、药物引起的食管损伤

药物引起的食管损伤发生在任何年龄以及来自各种常用的药物。尽管如此，药物引起的食管损伤在临床实践中较少被诊断出。有以下几个原因：第一，由于严重的胸痛（通常为胸膜炎性质）与药物引起的食管炎相关，最初可能考虑常见和更严重的问题，如急性冠脉综合征和肺栓塞。第二，可假定患者有严重的酸反流发作，这是一种比药物引起的食管溃疡更常见的疾病。第三，导致药物性食管炎的几种药物是非处方药（如非甾体抗炎药）或可能已安全服用多年（如四环素）而没有损伤，因此患者不认为是导致其症状的可能原因。第四，由于没有常规报告或重新认识，药物引起的食管损伤被认为是不常见的[1,2]。这种认识上的不足可能存在问题，因为未能认识到这一疾病，可能无法及时停用相关药物，并导致对其他疾病进行广泛和错误的评价与治疗。由于认识不足可能导致无法向患者提供避免损伤的正确指导。因为本章对药物引起的食管损伤进行了详细概述，特别注意的是，通过其症状和可能引起潜在损伤的药物怀疑该疾病。

（一）发病机制

药物可通过多种机制引起食管损伤。最初可分为因其腐蚀性或通过其他机制如诱导酸反流（如钙通道拮抗剂）促进损伤而导致食管黏膜直接损伤。药物通过 4 种已知机制中的一种直接损伤食管黏膜：①产生腐蚀性酸溶液（如抗坏血酸和硫酸亚铁）；②产生腐蚀性碱性溶液（如阿仑膦酸钠）；③产生与食管黏膜接触的高渗溶液（如氯化钾）；④对食管黏膜的直接毒性药物（如四环素）。对于许多药物，损伤食管的机制不属于这些已知的类别。其他因素也可能影响药物的毒性作用。特别是接触时间、涂有凝胶材料的药丸[3]、缓释制剂和药物的蜡基质形式[4]。纤维素纤维和瓜尔豆胶丸可能在食管内膨胀和滞留，因其吸水能力引起完全梗阻。最后，药物可能通过诱导影响食管的全身反应而引起食管损伤[5]。

通常认为药物引起的食管损伤的倾向是由于食管的解剖或运动功能障碍，或药物服用不当，这两种情况都会导致药物长期暴露于食管黏膜。例如，研究表明，左房扩大[6]、食管狭窄[7]、食管动力障碍[8]、食管憩室（Zenker 或膈上憩室）[9]患者发生药物性损伤的风险更大。同样，在食管功能正常的患者中，药物性损伤的部位最常发生在有正常动力不足或外源性压迫的区域，例如在食管的低压槽区（平滑肌和骨骼肌重叠处）或在食管的主动脉或左支气管压迹的水平[10,11]。这些相对容易停滞的位置，在药物服用不当时即可引起食管黏膜的损伤。然而，食管的任何部分均可能受累。不正确的服药方法易于损伤，包括没有足够水的服药、采取卧位或在服药后立即入睡，或两者兼而有之。后两个因素特别有问题，因为消除了食管运输中重力的帮助，减少了在清醒时正常的唾液分泌和频繁的吞咽。然而，重要的是，许多（如果不是大多数）药物诱导的食管损伤患者可能具有正常的食管功能、不一定以错误的方式摄入药物。药物引起的食管损伤可以在“正常”条件下发生，这一点得到了数据的支持，这些数据表明正常受试者即使在直立位用水送服时，正常人食管中胶囊的 X 线影像显示滞留时间延长[3,12]。胶囊的食管滞留时间可能长于片剂[13]。

（二）临床特征及诊断

患者通常会注意到胸痛急性发作，疼痛可能会辐射到胸部中央及背部。吸气时疼痛加重，可能伴有严重的吞咽痛，甚至啜饮一小口液体也是如此。一些患者可能主诉严重的灼热症状急性发作。这组症状与误服潜在损伤性药物有关（尤其是在睡前未饮用足够的水），则强烈提示了诊断。如果有必要客观上确认诊断，可使用内镜或 X 线摄影检查，内镜检查被认为更敏感。镜下可见从离散性溃疡到带有假膜的弥漫性重度食管炎，可见于双膦酸盐[14]或聚磺苯乙烯混悬液，酷似念珠菌性食管炎[15]。也可发现食管黏膜弥漫性脱落，也称为食管浅表剥脱[16]。偶尔会发生引起狭窄和肿瘤样外观的严重

炎症反应[17,18]。在 X 线上可见到类似的表现,特别是使用 X 线双重对比摄影时[19,20]。食管造影所描述的发现范围也可能包括孤立或多发性溃疡;小溃疡或大溃疡;溃疡呈点状、卵圆形、线形、匐行性、或钡剂星状聚集;融合性溃疡;或外观正常的黏膜区域分离性溃疡(图 45.1)[10]。也描述了多发性食管隔膜的发生[21]。药物性损伤的严重并发症较为罕见,诸如食管-气管瘘、食管穿孔、溃疡继发出血、慢性狭窄形成等。病理学上,受累区域的食管活检显示细胞间隙扩张,T 淋巴细胞和嗜酸性粒细胞占优势,其模式与其他原因引起的食管炎不同[22]。

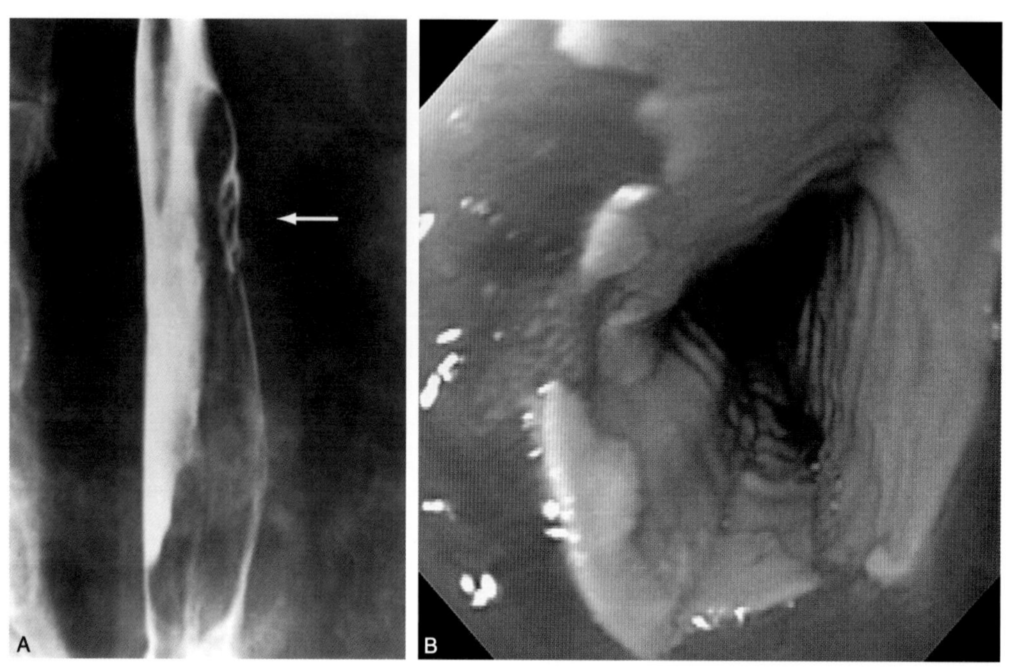

图 45.1　A,食管钡剂造影显示服用四环素继发的食管溃疡,箭指向溃疡区域。B,四环素诱发的食管灼伤的内镜图像。(A,Courtesy Dr. Marc Levine,Philadelphia.)

(三) 预防、治疗和临床病程

目前尚无特殊的治疗显示有益于改变药物诱导损伤的过程,治疗的目的是控制症状,预防酸反流引起的叠加损伤,维持充足的水分,并清除惹麻烦的药物。使用局麻药如黏性利多卡因溶液可达到控制症状。偶尔应用麻醉剂也是必要的。使用每日两次质子泵抑制剂能最好地预防叠加反流,但尚无数据显示酸反流加速药物诱导损伤的症状或病理学改善。对于有严重吞咽疼痛妨碍经口摄入的患者,需要静脉补液数天。消除损伤原因是不言而喻的,尽管这并不总是容易实现的。在临床情况下尤其如此,因为在这种情况下可能没有适当的替代品,例如阿司匹林预防心血管疾病、双膦酸盐治疗重度骨质疏松症、或大剂量非甾体抗炎药治疗慢性炎症性关节炎的疼痛。没有数据阐述如果谨慎地服用既往诱发食管炎的药物,再次服用该药物是否会增加复发性损伤的风险,但双膦酸盐可能除外。尚不清楚理论上具有潜在风险(例如食管动力障碍)的患者再激发时发生食管炎的风险是否更高。在没有狭窄形成或灾难性表现的情况下,大多数患者症状在 2~3 周内临床消退,7~10 天内放射影像学描述消退[19]。

由于目前尚无有效的治疗方法,因此希望适当给予潜在的损伤性药物将有助于避免食管损伤的发生。根据药物通过食管的速度有时较慢,尤其是明胶胶囊和较大的片剂[3],因此提出以下建议:①药物应该用至少 240mL 的澄清液体吞服;②患者应在服药后保持直立至少 30 分钟;③潜在增加药物诱导损伤风险的患者(例如无能力遵循之前的指示、食管动力差、食管腔的解剖结构受损),应寻找更安全的替代药物,或仔细权衡该药物的风险和获益,以及该药物对疾病治疗的必需性。

(四) 特殊药物

有几大类药物会引起食管损伤。这些药物包括抗生素、抗病毒药物、非甾体抗炎药、特异性抗心律失常药物、维生素和各种不同类别的其他混杂药物。

1. 抗生素类(框 45.1)

框 45.1　通常与食管炎或食管损伤相关的药物

抗生素类	达克霉素
克林霉素	柔红霉素
多西环素	5-氟尿嘧啶
青霉素	甲氨蝶呤
利福平	长春新碱
四环素	克唑替尼
氯唑西林	**非甾体抗炎药**
抗病毒药	阿司匹林
奈非那韦	布洛芬
扎西他滨	萘普生
齐多夫定	**其他药物**
双膦酸盐	抗坏血酸
阿仑膦酸钠	硫酸亚铁
依替膦酸钠	兰索拉唑
帕米膦酸二钠	复合维生素
化疗药物	氯化钾
博来霉素	奎尼丁
阿糖胞苷	茶碱

到目前为止，四环素、多西环素及其衍生物是药物诱发食管炎最常见的原因，报告的此类病例数几乎与所有其他病例的总和一样多[11]。其损伤的共性可能更多地反映了这些药物的使用频率，而不像四环素产生这种损伤的强烈倾向。在最近对 491 例接受多西环素治疗的海湾战争退伍军人进行的一项调查中，没有发现任何食管损伤病例，这表明所有使用者使用四环素后食管溃疡的发生率相对较低[2]。损伤的机制被认为是腐蚀性损伤，因为四环素溶于水可产生 pH 非常低的溶液[12]。症状可能是急性发作[23]，通常持续数天至数周。溃疡的外观各不相同，但通常较小且表浅，可具有"对吻"外观，位于主动脉弓或左支气管正上方的食管中段[10]，并具有烧伤样外观（见图 45.1）。形成狭窄并不常见。

其他抗生素引起的损伤并不常见，主要记录在病例报告中。这包括克林霉素[24,25]、利福平[26]、环丙沙星[27]、青霉素[28,29]和氯唑西林，鉴于它们经常使用，但发病率仍然极低。如果病史与药物诱导的食管损伤一致，目前使用的任何抗生素都应该被视为可能的致病因素，尽管罕见。

据报道，抗病毒药物，特别是用于治疗 HIV 的药物，也可引起药物诱导的食管损伤。如扎西他滨[30]、齐多夫定[31]和奈非那韦[32]。

2. 双膦酸盐类

最迅速出现的药物性食管炎是继发于用于治疗骨质疏松症的双膦酸盐的损伤。事实上，这类药物已成为药物诱导的食管炎的最普遍的病因。

迄今为止，据报道，损伤主要见于阿仑膦酸钠[14,33-39]，但也见于依替膦酸钠[40]和帕米膦酸二钠[41]。尽管损伤的总体发生率可能很低（报告的病例<100 例）[11]，但考虑到使用药物的数百万患者，损伤可能是严重的，甚至是致命的。遗憾的是，反流型症状很常见，很难与药物引起的黏膜损伤区分开来。如果有的话，利塞膦酸钠引起的食管损伤可能性较低[42]。解释部分原因可能是食管快速转运，随后药物与食管黏膜接触的时间极短[43]。在一项前瞻性研究中，对 255 例接受利塞膦酸钠治疗的患者进行随访，并在 8 天和 15 天后接受内镜检查，无患者发生食管溃疡。这项研究还强调了双膦酸盐的总体安全性，因为在 260 例接受阿仑膦酸钠治疗的患者中仅有 3 例发生了食管溃疡[44]。

本病最好通过内镜进行诊断，镜下可见明显的渗出物和炎症。组织活检显示严重的炎症渗出物和肉芽组织，可能含有可极化晶体和多核巨细胞[45]。狭窄形成[46]发生在高达三分之一的患者中[11]，危及生命的出血[37]，Zenker 憩室炎（由于药丸嵌顿）[47]，出现食管穿孔[35]已有报告。持续损伤的患者通常被描述为不按照指导服用双膦酸盐（即直立位饮用至少 240mL 液体送服、保持直立至少 30 分钟）。然而，与其他药物诱导的食管炎一样，正确服用药物的患者也可能会遭受食管损伤。对于有胃食管反流病史的患者是否应该避免使用双膦酸盐，这个问题经常被轶事回答，但科学上尚没有明确解决的问题。此外，如果胃食管反流是一个危险因素，那么还不清楚什么程度的反流构成风险。这个决定应权衡骨质疏松的严重程度、发生骨折的风险与并发食管炎的风险。对胃食管反流病易于淤滞的患者，如伴有食管狭窄或食管动力严重障碍的患者，应特别谨慎。

3. 非甾体抗炎药

非甾体抗炎药是诱发食管损伤的另一种常见原因。与药物引起的食管损伤的其他常见原因相似，它们发生在所有非甾体抗炎药使用者中的一小部分。阿司匹林、萘普生、吲哚美辛和布洛芬占大多数病例[11]，但在病例报告中，大多数其他非甾体抗炎药可引起食管损伤。出乎意料的是，严重的出血可能是这些食管溃疡的常见并发症[48]，尤其是与其他药物引起的食管炎相比。支气管食管瘘也有报道[49]。值得注意的是，非甾体抗炎药的非处方使用最常与损伤相关[50]，与它们更常使用的药物场地相一致。

在一项针对 1 122 例因胃肠道出血住院患者的研究中，任何剂量的阿司匹林（包括低剂量）都与发生食管炎的风险增加相关[51]。其他研究也认为非甾体抗炎药通常是糜烂性食管炎的危险因素[52]。这些研究中的食管炎是否都是由这些药物的直接作用，或者它们是否与反流引起的损伤协同作用尚不清楚，尽管一项研究表明，阿司匹林可使食管黏膜对酸和胃蛋白酶更敏感[53]。

4. 其他药物

氯化钾（KCl）药片与食管损伤相关。损伤可能是严重的，如食管狭窄形成[54,55]或穿孔进入左心房[56]、支气管动脉[57]或纵隔[58]。因使用氯化钾药片而遭受食管损伤的患者通常报告相关疾病，如心脏（包括左心房）扩大或既往心脏手术史[59-61]。目前这些过程是否真正容易因心脏外源性食管压迫，或是因使用氯化钾药片的患者心脏病患病率较高，而导致的药片淤滞和损伤尚不清楚。

奎尼丁是另一种可能导致重度食管炎的药物[18]，内镜下发现，奎尼丁可能与从轻度溃疡到明显的炎症反应伴水肿提示癌症的结果相关[17,18]。硫酸亚铁[62]、茶碱[63,64]、口服避孕药[65]、抗坏血酸[28]、麦考酚酸[66]和多种维生素[67]均可引起食管溃疡。在单个病例报告中，许多其他药物可引起食管溃疡。例如包括西地那非[68]、苯妥英钠[12]、华法林[69]、格列本脲[70]、兰索拉唑[71]、丙戊酸钠[72]、氯氮䓬[73]、卡托普利[74]、膦甲酸钠[75]、地拉罗司[76]、达比加群[77]、扑热息痛[78]和咽喉含片[79,80]。

5. 化疗诱导的食管炎

达克（更生）霉素、博来霉素、阿糖胞苷、柔红霉素、5-氟尿嘧啶、甲氨蝶呤、长春新碱和造血干细胞移植中使用的化疗方案均可能引起口咽黏膜炎导致严重的吞咽疼痛，这一过程也可累及食管黏膜[81]。在没有口腔变化的情况下，食管损伤是不常见的。虽然黏膜炎症在大多数情况下是自限性的，但一些患者发生口腔和食管损伤，会持续数周至数月。胸部 X 线照射食管后给予化疗数月，特别是多柔比星，可引起"回忆性"食管炎。长春花生物碱类药物具有神经毒性，吞咽困难可能使长春新碱治疗复杂化[82]。克唑替尼是一种酪氨酸激酶抑制剂，用于治疗非小细胞肺癌，据报道可引起重度溃疡性食管炎，与更典型的药物诱导食管炎相似[83-89]。

6. 静脉曲张硬化治疗导致的食管损伤

多年来，静脉曲张硬化治疗是内镜下控制食管静脉曲张出血的主要治疗方法。尽管它仍然是一种可接受的治疗方式，但在很大程度上已被其他几种方法所取代，包括静脉注射奥曲肽、曲张静脉套扎术和经静脉肝内门体分流术（TIPS）。

然而，一些医生仍继续使用它，由于可能持续数年的并发症的发生，迫使胃肠病学家认识到其有各种形式的潜在食管损伤。

静脉曲张硬化治疗的并发症可分为两大类：严重的结构损伤和食管动力改变。静脉曲张注射会造成大范围的重度损伤。向曲张静脉内及周围注射硬化剂会引起食管组织坏死和黏膜溃疡，风险与注射次数和硬化剂的量有关。几乎所有患者在硬化治疗后的最初几天内都会出现小溃疡，大约一半的患者会出现较大的溃疡。其他并发症包括食管壁内血肿[90]、狭窄[91]和穿孔[92]。大约15%接受硬化剂治疗的患者发生狭窄[91,93,94]，通常适合接受Savary探条扩张器或球囊扩张术治疗。深针穿刺硬化治疗的异常表现包括心包炎、食管胸膜瘘、胸腔积液和因壁内血肿压迫引起的气管阻塞[95,96]。一例食管鳞状细胞癌被认为是因5年前静脉曲张多次硬化治疗所致[97]。

几项研究已经证明，在完成硬化治疗疗程后，食管动力异常。这些异常可能与食管壁损伤或迷走神经功能障碍有关[98]，具体的动力异常包括食管传输延迟、食管收缩幅度及协调性降低[94,99]。关于这些变化是否可逆存在争议，不同的研究证明，动力异常超过4周可恶化[94]或消退[100]。这些动力变化是否反映了不可逆纤维化或可逆性炎性神经病变的影响尚不清楚。硬化治疗后动力功能障碍的一个潜在后果是发生病理性胃食管反流，可通过食管pH检测异常[101]以及通过异常闪烁显像和钡剂造影研究证实[94]。其他研究也显示硬化治疗后出现异常反流与食管动力障碍相关，在接受套扎术治疗的患者中尚未发生[99]。此外，在静脉曲张旁注射硬化剂的量似乎与酸反流增加有关[101]。

唯一被证明能有效预防硬化治疗后狭窄和愈合溃疡的药物是硫糖铝，可单独使用或与抗酸药和西咪替丁联合使用[102,103]。单独使用 H_2 受体拮抗剂或质子泵抑制剂进行抑酸治疗，未显示可有效预防或愈合硬化治疗后溃疡或狭窄[104,105]。

二、鼻胃管和其他非内镜管引起的食管损伤

长期以来，鼻胃管被认为是食管损伤和狭窄形成的潜在来源（图45.2）。推测其机制为胃食管反流。在接受择期剖腹手术的患者中，最近的数据显示，在最初24小时内有近9小时的食管pH低于4，而在未放置导管的对照组中，pH在半小时内低于1[106]。一项研究表明，即使在接受鼻胃管放置的正常志愿者中，酸暴露也会增加[107]。当发生狭窄时，其特征是长而狭窄，难以用内镜处理。尚不清楚一般使用强效抑酸治疗是否会降低这些狭窄的发生率。

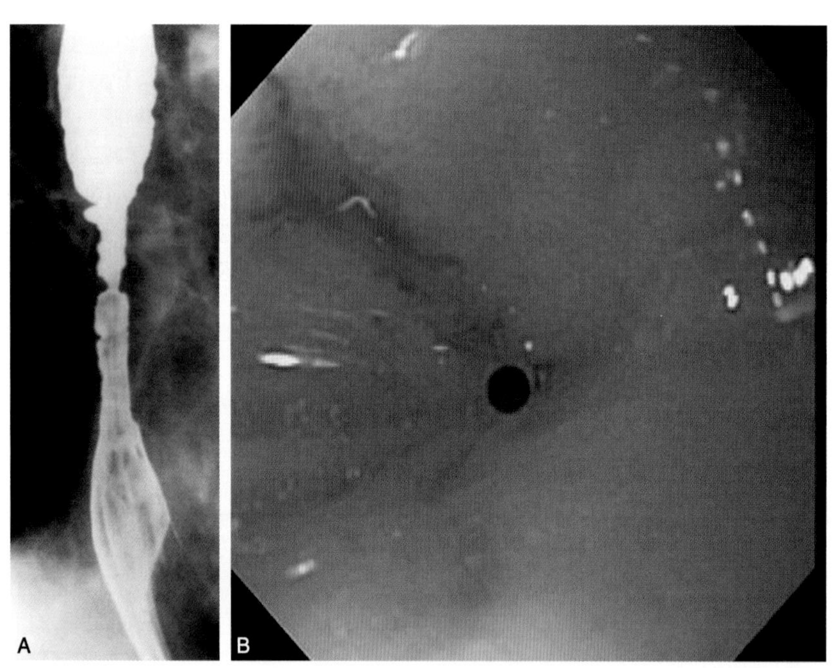

图45.2 A，食管钡剂造影证实鼻胃管诱发的狭窄。B，内镜下出现紧贴鼻胃管诱导的狭窄。
（A，Courtesy Dr. Marc Levine，Philadelphia；B，courtesy Dr. Gregory. G，Ginsberg，Philadelphia.）

呼吸道管腔器械也被报告为食管创伤的潜在来源。已报告了使用食管气管联合导管导致的食管撕裂[108]、带套囊的气管导管所致的气管食管瘘[109]及胸廓造口术导管引起的食管穿孔[110]或经食管超声心动图探针导致的食管穿孔[111]。

最近，一些作者报告了心脏射频消融术并发心房—食管瘘的发生[112-117]。据估计，房颤消融术的发生率为0.1%～0.25%。这种严重且通常致命的并发症发生在消融术后10天至5周。最初的前驱症状包括发热和神经系统异常，后者由空气栓子从食管经瘘口进入左心入脑所致。实验室检查可发现白细胞增多和血培养阳性。影像学检查可发现左心房内有气泡。尽管败血症和上消化道出血通常具有致死性，但最近的一份报告描述了一例瘘管手术修复后存活的患者[115]，表明及时识别可降低死亡率。还报告了一例经保守疗法消退的食管壁内血肿的病例[118]。

最后，用于经食管超声心动图的探头可能发生食管穿孔[119-121]，即使内镜通过没有明显阻力或明确的解剖异常（容易发生穿孔），也可能发生穿孔。

三、食管穿透性损伤或钝挫性损伤

非医源性食管创伤性损伤可能通过穿透性损伤或较少见的钝挫性损伤发生。导致食管穿孔的钝挫性创伤罕见，大多数病例发生在机动车事故引起的颈段食管[122]，有时会延迟诊断[123,124]。损伤可能由方向盘[125]、安全带[126]甚至外部车辆冲击引起[127]。还描述了因从摩托车上投掷所经历的剪切力导致的颈段食管横断[128]。食管穿透性损伤通常是由枪伤或刀伤引起的，已公认颈段食管穿孔也可继发于颈椎手术[129]。一般情况下，穿透伤的损伤分为颈段和食管下段。颈段食管穿孔可通过 X 线影像学检查，如颈部侧位片或 CT 发现壁外空气可初步诊断。泛影葡胺对比研究证实了诊断，尽管该检测并不总是适用于严重创伤损伤的患者。虽然常规内镜检查是这些患者的相对禁忌证，但术中内镜检查可能是诊断穿孔的有价值的诊断工具[130]。

颈段食管穿透伤通常与并发气管、颈动脉或脊柱损伤有关。处理这些损伤是否需要对所有患者进行手术探查，是一个有争论的领域。等待中的担忧是发生败血症、气道损伤或气管食管瘘[131]，估计发生在大约 4% 的穿透性食管损伤中[132]，尤其是那些因气管损伤而进行气管造口术的患者。谨慎等待的另一个不利因素是先前无菌区域的污染。这可能消除了一期闭合的选择，需要两步操作，首先在确定修复前进行改道颈部食管造口术。因此，一些研究者继续推荐一种积极的多模式手术方法[129]。与此相反，最近一项对 17 例因刀伤或枪伤所致的颈段食管损伤患者的研究表明，肠内营养和抗生素的保守治疗可能会达到非手术愈合[133]。形成一个共识似乎是，对那些有小管腔颈部穿孔、无败血症和无需手术探查其他损伤的患者，可尝试保守方法治疗[134]。

对于食管远端的穿透性损伤，适用相似的原则，但存在一些重要差异。第一，尽管通常通过在胸片或 CT 上发现食管外气泡(或在食管对比造影研究中发现外渗)进行诊断，但也可以进行内镜检查，特别是对于食管对比造影不真实、不稳定的患者[135]。一些研究者认为内镜应该作为首选的诊断检查[130]。第二，与紧密组织平面决定的发生在颈部的包裹性更强的穿孔相反，更远端的食管穿孔可能进一步延伸到纵隔和胸膜。同时主动脉也存在共存损伤的威胁。

第三，因食管血供的节段性且经常变化(尤其是在食管远端)，由于伤口缺血和随后的渗漏，穿孔的简单闭合通常是不够的[136]。结果这些患者常需行食管切除与食管胃吻合术[135]。第四，由于通过纵隔进入食管比通过颈部进入食管要困难得多，因此纵隔、胸膜或主动脉穿孔的后果可能更具破坏性，食管远端穿孔所需的手术可能要广泛得多。因此，决定是否手术要困难得多。尽管有这些告诫，手术并非是唯一的建议，在大多数患者中[136,137]，仍必须及时进行手术，因为当手术延迟超过 1～12 小时时，其发病率和死亡率显著增高[138]。仅在选定的患者组中，保守治疗可能发挥作用，使用抗生素和鼻胃管绕过穿孔置入。最后，尽管金属支架已成功地用于其他原因食管穿孔的非手术治疗[139]，但其在治疗创伤性食管穿孔中的作用仍在逐步发展中。

四、食管撕裂和血肿

(一) Mallory-Weiss 综合征(食管黏膜撕裂症)

Mallory-Weiss 综合征(见第 20 章)最初由 Kenneth Mallory 和 Soma Weiss 医生于 1929 年描述，他们描述了由于剧烈呕吐导致的胃贲门撕裂伤患者[140]。认为撕裂是由于胃食管交界处和胃近端受到剪切力所致，因为用力呕吐导致腹内压较高，从而使其通过膈肌疝出[141,142]。根据 Laplaces 定律(拉普拉斯定律)，当存在食管裂孔疝时，这种剪切力的作用最大，从而使相对较大体积的扩张囊壁张力增高。因此，大多数 Mallory-Weiss 撕裂的患者都有食管裂孔疝并不奇怪[143]。尽管大多数撕裂发生在胃食管交界处 2cm 内，但当存在较大的食管裂孔疝时，胃近端部分出现更远端撕裂的可能性增加。任何导致腹内压突然升高和胃疝的身体动作均可能导致贲门黏膜撕裂。这些动作包括剧烈咳嗽、过度用力、呃逆[144]、内窥镜检查、经食管超声心动图和心肺复苏期间的干呕[141,145-150]。引起撕裂的其他因素包括饮酒和服用阿司匹林[142,151,152]。

大多数患者出现呕血，但一些患者仅出现黑便。虽然典型的病史包括呕吐或干呕后的呕血，但高达三分之一的患者无呕吐的前期病史，呕血是其主要的症状[151,152]。典型的是，内镜检查时可观察到一处撕裂，最常见的是沿着贲门小弯侧，尽管高达 10% 的患者可能会发生不止一处撕裂[143]。出血通常是自限性的，但可能在高达 10% 的患者中大量出血[143]甚至是致命的[153]。内镜检查不仅对诊断撕裂很重要，而且对排除在初始内镜检查评估期间在超过三分之一的患者中发现的其他上消化道病变也很重要。这些病变包括消化性溃疡、胃炎或胃病、糜烂性食管炎、食管静脉曲张和胃出口梗阻。

Mallory-Weiss 综合征的治疗通常是支持治疗，因为出血伴随干呕和呕吐的减少可能是自限性的。最近，使用了几种内镜治疗的方法。内镜下注射肾上腺素和乙氧硬化醇可显著减少出血和输血需求，缩短住院时间[154]。内镜下结扎术也被证明是有效的[155,156]，在一项试验研究中证明效果相当于注射治疗[157]。内镜下放置止血夹、圈套器[158,159]以及内镜下圈套结扎术[160]也被用作控制 Mallory-Weiss 综合征出血的治疗替代方法[161]。对于内镜治疗后仍持续出血的患者，可通过胃左动脉进行血管造影栓塞术[162]，很少需要外科手术干预。

(二) Boerhaave 综合征(自发性食管破裂综合征)

Boerhaave 综合征是一种更为极端形式的食管撕裂，发生于腹内压急剧增加和胃内-胸内压力梯度增强的情况下。在该综合征中，会发生透壁性撕裂伴穿孔。穿孔特别发生在“卡环”和斜行食管纤维之间相接触的边缘[163]。与 Mallory-Weiss 综合征类似，先前的症状，如严重呕吐和干呕、腹部紧张用力、钝挫性创伤和咳嗽可能导致这种穿孔[143]。除了胃食管交界处的急性压力变化之外，一些研究者推测食管黏膜异常可能诱发穿孔。这些疾病包括反流性食管炎[164]、Barrett 食管炎伴溃疡[165]、感染性食管炎[166,167]和嗜酸性食管炎[168,169]。

临床表现常常是灾难性的，由于食管大穿孔引起休克和败血症。毫不奇怪，高达三分之一的患者死亡[170]。由于严重胸痛的急性表现，常与急性心脏或肺部事件、主动脉夹层动脉瘤或胰腺炎相混淆[171]，常导致诊断延误和更高的发病率和死亡率。通过皮下气肿伴捻发音以及X线影像照相发现纵隔气肿和左侧胸腔积液（可能含有唾液淀粉酶，错误地提示胰腺炎）甚至明显的脓胸提示诊断。食管穿孔可通过使用泛影葡胺食管造影得到证实。治疗通常是手术修复和引流，也可通过放置自膨式覆膜金属支架[172-175]和夹子[176,177]成功进行非手术治疗，以及2例患者使用胸腔引流胶，在早期发现的穿孔中越来越常用。

（三）自发性食管血肿

自发性食管血肿是一种罕见的疾病，在食管壁的黏膜与固有肌层之间发生突然出血，通常在食管发生较长。“自发性”一词有点用词不当，因为已经确定了几个容易形成血肿的潜在因素。这些包括使用阿司匹林[178-180]、潜在的凝血疾病[181]、使用抗凝剂（包括直接凝血酶抑制剂）[182-184]、先兆子痫[185]或突然增加腹内-胸内压力梯度（如剧烈呕吐、咳嗽和打喷嚏）[186]及异物摄入[187]。然而并非所有病例都有明显的诱发因素，本质上是自发出现的[188]。三分之一的患者典型表现为胸骨后疼痛、吞咽困难和呕血三联征，50%的患者至少表现其中两种症状[188]。与Boerhaave综合征一样，由于症状与更常见的心肺疾病重叠，常常会延误诊断[189]。有趣的是，中年女性可能有这种综合征的倾向，尽管这种相关性并不一致[190-192]。

可通过多种方法进行诊断。胸部CT检查显示食管弥漫性增厚，有时呈“双筒”状食管腔闭塞的外观[193]。MRI检查也可能是作出诊断的准确方式[194]。内镜检查可见食管腔闭塞，可见一长、深、易碎的蓝色黏膜下肿块，伴或不伴可见的撕裂[187]。有时很难区分血肿和食管恶性肿瘤[195]。保守治疗是主要的治疗方法，保持患者不经口进食，并监测血流动力学状态[187]，通常需要数周才能完全愈合。通常每隔1周，通过重复CT或内镜检查监测其进展，很少需要手术干预。

五、在免疫活性宿主中的食管感染（框45.2）

框45.2 免疫活性宿主的食管感染
通常与免疫缺陷有关
疱疹病毒（HSV）
白色念珠菌
结核分枝杆菌
与食管淤滞相关（如贲门失弛缓症、硬皮病）
白色念珠菌
与使用糖皮质激素吸入剂有关
白色念珠菌
其他食管感染
克鲁兹锥虫
梅毒螺旋体
人乳头状瘤病毒（HPV）

食管感染最常见于免疫功能低下的患者，如感染HIV的患者（见第35章）以及接受化疗或免疫抑制治疗的患者，尤其是血液恶性肿瘤或器官移植后患者（见第35章）。尽管如此，仍有一些食管感染发生在具有免疫活性的宿主（免疫功能正常的宿主）。这些感染包括：①更典型的与免疫缺陷相关，但偶尔见于免疫系统完整的患者；②发生于有基础食管疾病的患者，特别是与食管腔内容物长期淤滞相关的患者；③累及食管局部免疫受损的区域，例如使用吸入性类固醇治疗呼吸系统疾病。在这些情况下发现的微生物类型数量很少，而念珠菌是优势微生物。

（一）白色念珠菌

白色念珠菌是免疫活性宿主中最常见的食管感染。尽管有几种念珠菌与食管感染有关，包括热带念珠菌和*Guilliermondii*念珠菌[196]，但白色念珠菌占绝大多数。在印度933例吞咽困难或吞咽疼痛患者的一个大型系列研究中，发现56例患者有不同严重程度的念珠菌性食管炎[197]。有多少患者患有明确的食管动力障碍或与念珠菌相称而不是病理微生物的尚不清楚，因为据报道，健康经常活动的成年人食管念珠菌定植的流行率约为20%[198]。

尽管念珠菌性食管炎在没有明确潜在机制的情况下可能很少发生，但通常应该设定易感的诱发条件，即使在免疫活性宿主中也是如此。最常见的诱发条件是与严重淤滞相关的疾病，如贲门失弛缓症或硬皮病（见图45.3）。在贲门失弛缓症中，感染似乎与严重程度相关，那些长期患有明显食管扩张疾病的患者风险最高。在贲门失弛缓症得到有效治疗之前，这些感染可能很难进行药物治疗，因此需要进行食管引流。与贲门失弛缓症相比，硬皮病伴有食管受累的患者念珠菌性食管炎较少见，但同样，念珠菌性食管炎常见于有食管扩张和蠕动不良的患者。硬皮病患者念珠菌感染的一个危险因素可能是酸抑酸，正如一项针对系统性硬化症患者的研究所表明的，其中未接受抑酸治疗的患者念珠菌性食管炎的患病率为44%（48例患者中的21例），而接受强效抑酸治疗的患者为89%（18例中的16例）[199]。局部使用糖皮质激素（包含在治疗哮喘的吸入器中）可能会导致其他方面健康的成人发生口咽和食管念珠菌病[200]。同样，在接受口服氟替卡松治疗的嗜酸性食管炎的患者中也描述了念珠菌性食管炎[201,202]。尽管免疫机制受损，但易患真菌性食管炎的其他疾病包括糖尿病、肾上腺功能不全、酗酒和高龄[203]。此外，一种称为食管壁内假性憩室病的罕见病，可能与念珠菌感染有关[204]。念珠菌性食管炎的诊断可通过内镜下其特征性的表现作出诊断，即黏附在食管黏膜上的白色伪膜状或斑块样病变。通过刷检病灶，进行细胞学检查或活组织检查进行确认，其中可见炎症、菌丝和芽殖酵母团块（通常不单独定植）。“黑色食管”（见后文）也被描述为念珠性食管炎[205]。虽然不如内镜检查敏感，但念珠菌性食管炎可通过食管气钡双重造影确诊[206]。其特征性表现为纵向分离的斑块样病变，呈线状，或由滞留钡剂产生的边缘清晰的不规则充盈缺损。偶见肿块样病变和狭窄。

大多数真菌性食管炎且无免疫缺陷患者的治疗是口服氟康唑或局部用抗真菌剂。常使用氟康唑（100~200mg/d）口

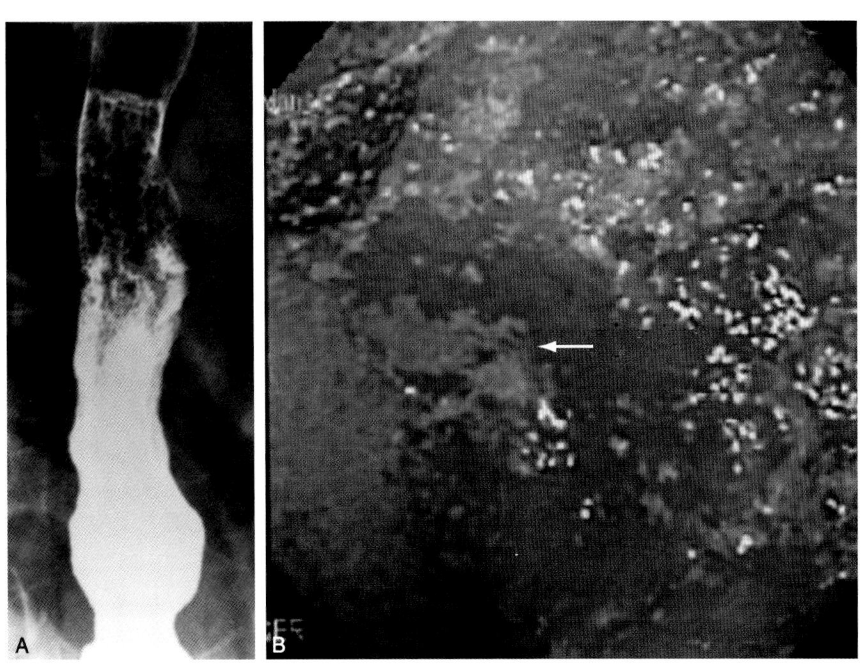

图 45.3　A，食管钡剂造影显示贲门失弛缓症伴念珠菌感染。B，贲门失弛缓症患者食管扩张伴碎片状念珠菌斑（箭）的内镜照片。（A，Courtesy Dr Marc Levine，Philadelphia.）

服，因其比局部治疗更方便。不易吸收的局部药物的优点是几乎没有不良反应和药物相互作用。克霉唑是一种不可吸收的咪唑类药物，以 10mg 口含片溶解于口腔内，每日 5 次，共 1 周，耐受性良好。制霉菌素是一种不可吸收的多烯类，作用机制与克霉唑不同，适口性也较克霉唑差，使用剂量为 1～2 片/次（每片 20 万单位），每日 4～5 次，最长使用 14 天。

（二）单纯疱疹病毒

单纯疱疹病毒（HSV）性食管炎[207-211]已在广泛年龄范围内的免疫缺陷宿主中描述了，可以代表原发感染，或更常见的是，喉神经、颈上神经和迷走神经分布中的潜伏病毒的再激活。可能由于身体密切接触或常见暴露而发生[212]，并与嗜酸性食管炎有关[213]。所有年龄段均可受累，口咽部病变仅在 5 例中发现 1 例。严重的吞咽疼、胃灼热和发热是主要症状。也可出现恶心、呕吐和胸痛。内镜下表现为弥漫性、易碎的圆形或线状溃疡和渗出物，主要发生在食管远端。典型的、最早的食管病变是位于食管中远端的 1～3mm 圆形小囊泡，其中心剥脱形成离散的边缘隆起的局限性溃疡。这些病变在 X 线影像上也可被显现。HSV 也有出现“黑色食管”外观的报道[205,214]。HSV 食管炎可通过几种方法诊断：这些包括：①特征性病毒致细胞病变效应和/或通过电子显微镜在食管刷检或活检中证实病毒颗粒；②通过培养从黏膜活检中分离的 HSV；③通过聚合酶链反应（PCR）在食管组织中检测 HSV DNA；④通过免疫组织化学技术在食管组织中显示 HSV；⑤从口腔炎和多发性食管溃疡患者的口咽分泌物中分离 HSV[215]。HSV 感染上皮细胞的组织学染色显示多核巨细胞、气球样变性、“毛玻璃”核内 Cowdry A 型包涵体和染色质边缘化。使用 HSV 抗原单克隆抗体的免疫组织学染色或原位杂交技术，可通过识别缺乏特征性形态变化的感染细胞，提高疑难病例的诊断率。

大多数患者有自限性疾病，伴有一致的鼻唇疱疹（如果存在），但上消化道出血和穿孔已有报道[207]。疱疹性食管炎的治疗与免疫活性宿主的其他单纯疱疹病毒感染相同，例如，立即开始 7～10 天疗程的阿昔洛韦或伐昔洛韦口服治疗。偶尔严重的吞咽痛，需要静脉给予阿昔洛韦 250mg/m^2，每 8 小时一次初始治疗。然后，在患者可以口服药物时改为口服治疗。然而，考虑到食管受累的相对罕见性，目前尚无治疗食管单纯疱疹感染的具体结果数据。

（三）巨细胞病毒

巨细胞病毒（CMV）是疱疹病毒家族的一员，最常见于免疫功能低下患者的食管感染（见第 35 章和第 36 章）。然而，近期一系列研究记录了 4 例明显免疫功能正常的患者 CMV 感染引起的食管溃疡[216]，经抗病毒治疗全部反应良好。

（四）人乳头瘤病毒

人乳头瘤病毒（HPV）是一种小型双链 DNA 病毒，可感染健康人的鳞状上皮，产生疣和尖锐湿疣。该病毒可通过性传播。食管感染 HPV 通常无症状，HPV 病变最常见于食管中远段，为红斑斑疹、白色斑块、结节或茂盛的叶状（菜花样）病变[217]。在一例患者中，在硬化治疗注射部位发生了乳头状瘤[218]。通过组织学证实挖空细胞（koilocytosis，一种被环包围的非典型细胞核）、巨细胞或经免疫组织化学染色作出诊断。尽管大的病变需要内镜下切除，但通常不需要治疗。其他治疗如使用全身干扰素（IFN）-α、博来霉素和依托泊苷治疗产生了不同的结果[219]。曾有一位患者食管和上呼吸道有许多病变，对所有形式的治疗均无反应，最终导致死亡[220]。

HPV 感染被认为是鳞状细胞癌，特别是宫颈癌的危险因素。在南非、中国北方和阿拉斯加的食管肿瘤标本中，通过 PCR 或原位 DNA 杂交已证实 HPV 与食管鳞状细胞癌之间的相关性[221]。相反，在美国大陆、欧洲、日本和中国香港[222,223]的食管鳞状细胞癌中未发现 HPV DNA，因此其与食管癌的相关性受到质疑[224]。

（五）其他感染

1. 克鲁兹锥虫（*Trypanosoma cruzi*）

Chagas 病（见第 113 章）是由克鲁兹锥虫（一种南美洲特有的寄生虫）进行性破坏全身间充质组织和神经神经节细胞的结果。心脏、食管、胆囊和肠道异常是临床所见的后果。食管表现可能在急性感染后 10～30 年出现，通常包括吞咽困难、胸痛、咳嗽和反流，夜间误吸很常见的。食管测压记录与贲门失弛缓症的结果相同，尽管 Chagas 病的食管下括约肌压力较低[225]，在无症状血清阳性患者中可发现食管测压异常[226]。设定疾病的发病机制是在感染后产生抗毒蕈碱受体抗体的反应[227]。锥虫病食管可能对硝酸盐、球囊扩张或最终胃食管交界处的肌切开术治疗有反应[228]。继发于巨食管的难治性症状或肺部并发症的患者，可能是食管切除术的候选者[229]。Chagas 病所致的长期淤滞患者通常有食管鳞状上皮增生，与贲门失弛缓症一样，发生食管鳞状细胞癌的风险增加。

2. 结核分枝杆菌

大多数食管结核分枝杆菌感染的报告来自地方性结核病地区。结核病的食管表现几乎完全是相邻纵隔结核直接扩散的结果，但也有充分证实的原发性食管结核病例[230,231]。继发性食管结核的临床表现与大多数其他原因引起的感染性食管炎有很大不同。具体来说，吞咽困难常伴有体重减轻、咳嗽、胸痛和发热。后续并发症包括出血、穿孔和瘘管形成[231]。吞咽时哽噎可能表明食管和呼吸道之间存在潜在的瘘管。

其他 X 线表现包括纵隔淋巴结转移和延伸至纵隔的窦道。在 CT 成像上，这种表现可能与伴有溃疡性肿块病变和气管旁腺病的癌症相似[232]。确诊活动性结核病常需内镜检查，但建议慎用，防止气溶胶结核杆菌感染医务人员。内镜检查表现包括浅溃疡、类似肿瘤形成的堆积病变和食管外源性压迫[233]。对病灶处应进行活检和彻底刷检获取标本，除常规研究外，还应留取标本进行抗酸染色、结核分枝杆菌培养和 PCR 检测。当外源性压迫是结核唯一的食管表现时，必须通过支气管镜检、纵隔镜检或经食管细针穿刺细胞学评价确诊[234]。有时需要手术修补瘘管、穿孔和出血性溃疡。

3. 梅毒螺旋体

梅毒在 20 世纪 90 年代在美国越来越流行，在免疫活性的个体中很少引起食管疾病。早期文献描述了三期梅毒的树胶样肿、弥漫性溃疡和食管狭窄[235]。当患者有炎性狭窄和其他三期梅毒证据时，应考虑梅毒性食管的诊断。组织学检查评价可显示血管周围淋巴细胞浸润，然而，如果有可能诊断，应进行特异性免疫染色。

4. 罕见的感染

病毒感染很少累及有免疫活性的成年人的食管，包括带状疱疹病毒和 EB 病毒[236,237]，两者感染均可产生溃疡。在接受糖皮质激素治疗的有免疫活性的患者中，也描述了发生巨细胞病毒性溃疡性食管炎[238]。罕见的食管真菌感染包括芽生菌病，表现为食管肿块[239]和组织胞浆菌病，通过与结核相似的纵隔腺病直接扩散[240]。

六、急性食管坏死

急性食管坏死（黑色食管）是一种罕见的知之甚少的疾病。缺血和黏膜屏障受损被认为在其发病机制中起作用[241]，尽管其他病因包括严重反流和巨细胞病毒感染[242]。已描述有黑色食管背景的疾病包括糖尿病、血液和实体器官恶性肿瘤、营养不良、肾功能不全、心血管损害、创伤和高凝状态[243]。

（程芮　译，袁农　校）

参考文献

第 46 章 胃食管反流病

Joel E. Richter, Michael F. Vaezi 著

章节目录

一、流行病学 …… 635
(一) 症状和 GERD 并发症的患病率 …… 635
(二) 人口统计的危险因素 …… 636
(三) 环境风险因素 …… 636
二、对医疗卫生的影响 …… 636
三、发病机制 …… 636
(一) 抗反流屏障 …… 636
(二) 反流机制 …… 637
(三) 裂孔疝 …… 639
(四) 食管酸清除 …… 639
(五) 胃因素 …… 640
(六) 一种新的细胞因子介导的食管损伤机制 …… 641
四、临床特征 …… 642
(一) 典型症状 …… 642
(二) 食管外表现 …… 642
(三) 睡眠障碍 …… 643
五、鉴别诊断 …… 643
六、相关条件 …… 643
七、诊断 …… 643
(一) 酸抑制试验 …… 644
(二) 内镜检查 …… 644
(三) 食管黏膜活检 …… 644
(四) 食管反流试验 …… 645
(五) 食管钡剂造影 …… 647
(六) 食管测压 …… 647
八、临床病程 …… 647
(一) 非糜烂性疾病 …… 647
(二) 糜烂性疾病 …… 647
九、并发症 …… 648
(一) 出血、溃疡和穿孔 …… 648
(二) 消化性食管狭窄 …… 648
(三) Barrett 食管 …… 648
十、无并发症疾病的治疗 …… 648
(一) 非处方药物治疗 …… 648
(二) 处方药 …… 649
(三) 维持疗法 …… 651
(四) PPI 治疗的安全性 …… 651
(五) 手术治疗 …… 652
(六) 新型内镜/外科手术治疗 …… 653
十一、消化性食管狭窄的治疗 …… 654

胃食管反流(gastroesophageal reflux, GER)是胃内容物从胃逆行移动至食管的生理过程。GER 本身不是一种疾病,每天发生多次,不会产生症状或黏膜损伤。相反,胃食管反流病(GERD)是一种疾病谱,通常产生胃灼热和反酸症状。GERD 是正常抗反流屏障无法防止频繁和异常数量的反流物质的结果。大多数患者在内镜检查时没有可见的黏膜损伤,而其他一些患者可有食管炎、消化道狭窄或 Barrett 食管。其他症状可能包括胸痛或食管之外的表现,如肺、耳、鼻或咽喉症状。GERD 是一个多因素的过程,也是人类最常见的疾病之一。2009 年,美国有 890 万人次 GERD 患者在门诊就诊,是所有胃肠道疾病的首要诊断[1]。

一、流行病学

(一) 症状和 GERD 并发症的患病率

GERD 的准确患病率很难精确确定,因为许多受影响的个体,即使是 Barrett 食管患者,也没有任何症状。此外,基于客观检查如内镜检查(即食管炎)和食管 pH 检测的数据在大量筛查人群中是不切实际的[2]。

根据症状,全球基于人群的研究报告的 GERD 每周至少出现一次症状的总患病率约为 13%,但存在相当大的地理差异[3]。研究设计的异质性使其难以获得准确的测量,但 GERD 的患病率在南亚和东南欧最高(超过 25%),在东南亚、加拿大和法国最低(低于 10%)。没有来自非洲的患病率数据。在美国,GERD 每周至少发生一次的患病率约为 20%[4],但由于使用的问卷的差异性,包括定义 GERD 所需症状的频率和持续时间,患病率估计在 6% 到 30% 之间[3]。美国每年约有 11 万例因 GERD 住院的患者[5]。重要的是,北美、欧洲和东南亚 GERD 症状的患病率与 20 世纪 90 年代早期至中期的患病率相比增加了近 50%,但此后趋于平稳[4]。

GERD 的主要并发症是反流性食管炎、消化性狭窄和食管癌。食管炎的真实患病率很难确定,因为健康受试者很少接受上消化道内镜检查。在以人群为基础的研究中[3],不管症状如何,接受内镜检查患者的糜烂性食管炎患病率在中国为 6.4%、在瑞典为 15.5%[6-8]。在无症状受试者中,糜烂性食管炎的患病率在中国为 6.1%,在瑞典为 9.5%。糜烂性食管炎可能是一种暂时现象——在基线时患有非糜烂性反流病的受试者中,25% 在 2 年后的近期内镜检查中发现了食管炎,而另一项具有相似设计的研究发现 5 年时的发病率为 10%[9,10]。需要重复内镜扩张的复发性消化性狭窄从 1992 年的 16% 下降至 2000 年的 8%,可能与质子泵抑制剂(PPI)的使用增加有关[11]。从 2003 年至 2006 年,每年约有 10 570

例因糜烂性食管炎住院,14 000 例因食管狭窄住院[5]。因糜烂性食管炎的死亡罕见,从 1988 年至 1992 年约为 2.1/100 万人[5]。

(二) 人口统计的危险因素

GERD 及其并发症有许多公认的风险因素。在北美和欧洲,性别不是一个因素,但在南美和中东,女性 GERD 症状的发生率比男性高 40%[3]。性别与消化性狭窄无明确相关性,但男性患食管炎、Barrett 食管和食管腺癌的风险大于女性[12]。年龄的增长与 GERD 症状增加的相关性不一致,但与 GRED 并发症密切相关,包括食管炎、食管狭窄和 Barrett 食管癌[3,5]。在美国,不同种族之间 GRED 症状的患病率似乎相似[12],但白人发生糜烂性食管炎、Barrett 食管和食管腺癌的风险更大。

(三) 环境风险因素

西方国家 GERD 的患病率呈上升趋势[4],可以解释这种趋势的两个主要因素是肥胖盛行和 HP 相关胃炎患病率的下降。肥胖是 GERD 症状(比值比 1.73)、糜烂性食管炎(比值比 1.59)、Barrett 食管(比值比 1.24)和食管腺癌(比值比 2.45)的主要风险因素[3,13]。通过腰臀比测量的中心型肥胖可能比 BMI 更重要,与复杂性 GERD 相关[13]。已经提出了几种机制来解释中心性肥胖与 GERD 之间的相关性:胃内压升高压倒反流屏障[14]和内脏脂肪产生多种细胞因子,包括白细胞介素 6(IL-6)和肿瘤坏死因子-α(TNF-α),其可能调节食管下括约肌(lower esophageal sphincter,LES)压力和促进胰岛素抵抗[15]。观察性研究表明,将体重指数降低至少 3.5kg/m^2,会使 GERD 症状缓解的概率增加 1.5~2.4 倍[16]。随机试验证实,体重减轻,尤其是腰围减少,可改善 GERD 症状并减少食管酸暴露[16]。

除了肥胖患病率的增加外,Hp 胃炎患病率下降可以解释 GERD 及其并发症的趋势(见"发病机制"中"胃因素")[17]。与 Hp 感染相关的胃萎缩似乎与糜烂性食管炎[18]、Barrett 食管和食管腺癌呈负相关[19,20]。然而,东亚的负相关比北美强得多,而欧洲的负相关则模棱两可。

还有其他与 GERD 相关的环境暴露,但它们相对较弱而且在人群中不可预测。某些形式的体力活动可能会增加易感个体的 GER 症状,如弯腰、骑自行车、举重和游泳[21]。另一方面,适度、有规律的有氧运动与 GERD 症状呈负相关[22]。在横断面研究中,烟草使用与 GERD 症状的相关性较弱(汇总优势比,1.26)[3]。这种关系得到了一项为期 18 年的纵向研究的支持,在该研究中,与继续吸烟的个体相比,吸烟减少与 GRED 症状减少 3 倍相关[23]。同样,在观察性研究中,饮酒与 GERD 症状无强相关性(汇总优势比,1.11)[3]。尽管患者经常报告饮红酒后的症状比饮白酒后更严重(可能与红酒中的鞣酸有关),但一项随机试验发现,红酒对 LES 压力和反酸的影响小于白酒[24]。烟草是糜烂性食管炎和食管腺癌的重要风险因素,但酒精与糜烂性食管炎或 Barrett 食管之间无关系[2]。

与环境因素一起,GERD 的流行病学可能受到遗传的影响。GERD 及其并发症的家族聚集性,尤其是 Barrett 食管,已有报道[25,26]。两项来自美国和瑞典的双胞胎进行的大型病例对照研究表明,GERD 的遗传易感性范围为 30%~45%[27,28]。遗传机制尚不清楚,但可能与食管裂孔疝、LES 压力降低和运动受损相关的平滑肌疾病有关。

二、对医疗卫生的影响

虽然 GERD 很少是引起死亡的原因,但 GERD 与相当多的其他疾病发病率和并发症有关,如食管溃疡(5%)、消化性狭窄(4%~20%)和 Barrett 食管(8%~20%)[2]。不出所料,GERD 对医疗卫生的负担很大。在 2009 年,GERD 是门诊就诊中最常见诊断的消化系疾病[1]。对于胃肠道疾病,GERD 是出院时第 13 位最常见的主要诊断,估计每年总人数为 66 000 例,平均住院时间为 2 天,中位费用为 4 366.1 美元[1]。作为次要出院诊断,它是最常见的胃肠道疾病,被列为 450 万次,比任何其他诊断高出 3 倍[1]。在美国 2005—2010 年期间,近四分之一的上消化道内镜检查的适应证是评估反流症状[29]。2005 年美国 PPI 治疗的每例患者总费用估计为 2 040 美元[30]。对疑似食管外 GERD 患者的经济负担甚至可能更高。在最初第一年,Vanderbilt 的一项研究发现,食管外 GERD 患者的直接费用(5 154 美元)是典型 GERD 患者报告的直接费用(971 美元)的 5.6 倍[31]。

来自德国的一项经济民意调查报告,6% 确诊 GERD 的个体中因该病每年至少缺勤 1 天;其中 61% 的患者在前一年至少就诊一次,2% 的患者因 GERD 住院治疗[32]。他们估计每位患者每年的直接和间接费用约为 600 美元。来自美国的数据表明,GERD 对工作损失的影响相对较小[1]。最近的一项跨国民意调查报告,患有严重 GERD 症状的工人每周平均误工 2 小时,这是直接的结果[33]。

已证实 GERD 可严重损害生活质量。毫不奇怪,对抗胃酸分泌治疗无反应的 GERD 患者生活质量较低。无论是精神上还是身体上的生活质量均低于有反应者[34]。GERD 的共病很常见,包括肠易激综合征和心理痛苦的患者分别占 36% 和 41%[35]。这些共病可加重 GERD 患者对生活质量的负面影响,并可能影响 PPI 治疗的反应。

三、发病机制

GERD 的发病机制是复杂的,其原因是保护食管的防御因素(抗反流屏障、食管酸清除、阻抗)和胃反流的攻击性因素(胃酸、胃容量和十二指肠内容物)之间的不平衡所致。

(一) 抗反流屏障

抗反流屏障是 3 层食管防御酸损伤的第一层,是一个解剖学上复杂的区域,包括固有的 LES、膈肌脚、LES 的腹内位置、膈食管韧带和 His 锐角。

LES 涉及食管远端 3~4cm,静止时呈张力性收缩[36]。它是抗反流屏障的主要组成部分,即使因裂孔疝膈肌脚完全移位,也能防止反流[37]。LES 的近端部分通常在鳞柱上皮交界处上方 1.5~2cm,而远端部分长约 2cm,位于腹腔内。解剖学研究,将这部分抗反流屏障归因于与胃贲门反吊带和卡环纤维有关的折叠样功能。该位置在腹内压波动期间保持胃食管能力。静息时 LES 的压力范围为 10~30mmHg,具有充足的储备能力[38],因为仅需要 5~10mmHg 的压力防止 GER 是必要的。LES 通过其肌肉的固有张力和胆碱能兴奋性神经元维持一个高压区[39]。基础 LES 压力有相当大的昼夜变化,餐后最低,夜间最高,并且随着移行性复合运动Ⅲ期而大幅增加。它还受循环肽类和激素、食物(特别是脂肪)和许多药物的影响(表 46.1)。

LES 位于右膈肌脚形成的裂孔内,由膈食管韧带锚定,插入鳞柱上皮交界处水平。裂孔为沿着其长轴约 2cm 的泪滴状管道。

表 46.1 LES 压力的调节

	增加 LES 压力	减少 LES 压力
激素/肽类	胃泌素	CCK
	胃动素	胰泌素
	P 物质	生长抑素
		血管活性肠肽
神经因子	α-肾上腺素能激动剂	α-肾上腺素能拮抗剂
	β-肾上腺素能拮抗剂	β-肾上腺素能激动剂
	胆碱能激动剂	胆碱能拮抗剂
食物和营养素	蛋白质	巧克力
		脂肪
		薄荷糖
其他因素	抗酸药	巴比妥类
	巴氯芬	钙通道阻滞剂
	西沙必利	地西泮
	多潘立酮	多巴胺
	组胺	哌替啶
	甲氧氯普胺	吗啡
	前列腺素 $F_{2\alpha}$	前列腺素 E_2 和 I_2
		血清素
		茶碱

LES,下食管括约肌。

在发育上,来自食管背侧系膜与来自肋膈膜的膈脚分开受神经支配。它可被食管扩张、呕吐和一过性 LES 松弛(transient LES relaxation,tLESR)所抑制,但在吞咽过程中不被抑制。膈脚为固有 LES 提供外源性挤压,有助于吸气期间增加静息压力,并在腹压增加期间增加 LES 压力,如咳嗽、打喷嚏或弯腰[39]。下肢收缩对 LES 压力记录施加约 5~10mmHg 的节律性压力增加。在深吸气和一些腹部用力增加的时期,这些变化会导致 50~150mmHg 的压力[40]。

食管斜行进入胃,在胃食管交界处大弯侧形成锐角,即 His 角。这个角已在尸体上显示出产生瓣阀效应,然而对胃食管交界处所起的功能尚不清楚[41]。

(二)反流机制

反流一般通过 4 种机制发生:tLESR、低 LES 压力、吞咽相关 LES 松弛和低 LES 压力期间的紧张[42]。

1. 一过性食管下括约肌松弛(tLESR)

在括约肌压力正常的患者中,tLESR 是最常见的反流机制(图 46.1)。tLESR 发生是独立于吞咽之外,不伴有食管蠕动,比吞咽诱导的下食管括约肌松弛(LESR)持续时间长(>10 秒),并伴有膈脚抑制[43]。tLESR 几乎可以解释健康受试者所有的反流发作。GERD 患者中有 50%~80% 的发作取决于食管裂孔疝的存在和相关食管炎发作的严重程度[44](图 46.2)。然而一项研究表明,是低基础 LES 压力,而不是 tLESR,可能是不可复性裂孔疝患者发生 GER 的主要机制[45](见图 46.2)。

tLESR 并不总是与 GER 相关。在正常受试者中,40%~60% 的 tLESR 伴有反流发作,对比 GERD 患者为 60%~70%[44,46]。确定是否发生反流的可能因素包括腹部紧张用力、食管裂孔疝、食管缩短程度以及 tLESR 的持续时间。tLESR 的明显刺激物是食物或气体引起的近端胃扩张。这并不意外,tLESR 是呃逆的机制。在触发 tLESR 方面,牵拉感受器似乎比张力感受器更相关[39]。更多不同的刺激是食物脂肪、精神压力和咽部阈下值(用于吞咽)的刺激[47]。各种不同药物可能减少 tLESR,包括 CCK A(CCK-1)受体拮抗剂、抗胆碱能药物、吗啡、生长抑素、一氧化氮抑制剂、5-羟色胺(5-HT3)拮抗剂和 γ-氨基丁酸($GABA_B$)激动剂[47]。

tLER 的主要刺激是近端胃膨胀,它激活迷走神经传入纤维神经节内板层末梢的机械感受器[48]。这些纤维最终投射到脑干和迷走神经背侧运动核。这些神经元投射到位于食管远端肌间神经丛的抑制性神经元。这导致整合运动反应,涉及 LES 松弛、纵向肌肉收缩、减少胃食管交界处(EGJ)阻塞并将 LES 重新定位在膈肌脚上、膈肌脚抑制和肋膈肌收缩[49]。几种神经递质参与 tLESR 的控制,包括 GABA、谷氨酸盐和内源性大麻素[50]。

2. 吞咽诱导的食管下括约肌松弛

在吞咽诱导的 LESR 期间约有 5%~10% 的反流发生。大多数发作与蠕动缺陷或不完全有关[46]。在正常吞咽诱发的 LESR 期间,反流并不常见,因为:①膈脚不松弛;②LESR 持续时间相对较短(5~10 秒);③反流被即将到来的蠕动波所阻止(见图 46.1 描记的右侧)。吞咽诱导的 LESR 期间的反流更常见于食管裂孔疝。这可能是由于裂孔疝患者 EGJ 的顺应性较低,使其在低于或等于胃内压的压力下打开,从而使食管裂孔疝中蓄积的胃液反流[43,51]。

3. 食管下括约肌压力低下——过度用力诱导或自由反流

GER 可发生在过度用力诱导或自由反流导致的低 LES 压力的情况下[45,52]。当相对低压的 LES 被突然增加的压力所克服时,就会发生过度用力诱导的反流,因咳嗽、用力或弯腰引起的腹内压增加。当 LES 压力大于 10mmHg 且无食管裂孔疝时,不太可能发生这种类型的反流[42]。自由反流的特征是食管内 pH 下降,胃内压没有可识别的变化,通常发生在 LES 压力小于 5mmHg 时。由于 LES 压力低或无压力引起的反流并不常见,通常见于终末期硬皮病患者或贲门失弛缓症肌切开术后[44]。多发生于严重食管炎患者,其中可占反流发作的 25%,很少发生于无食管炎的患者[44]。

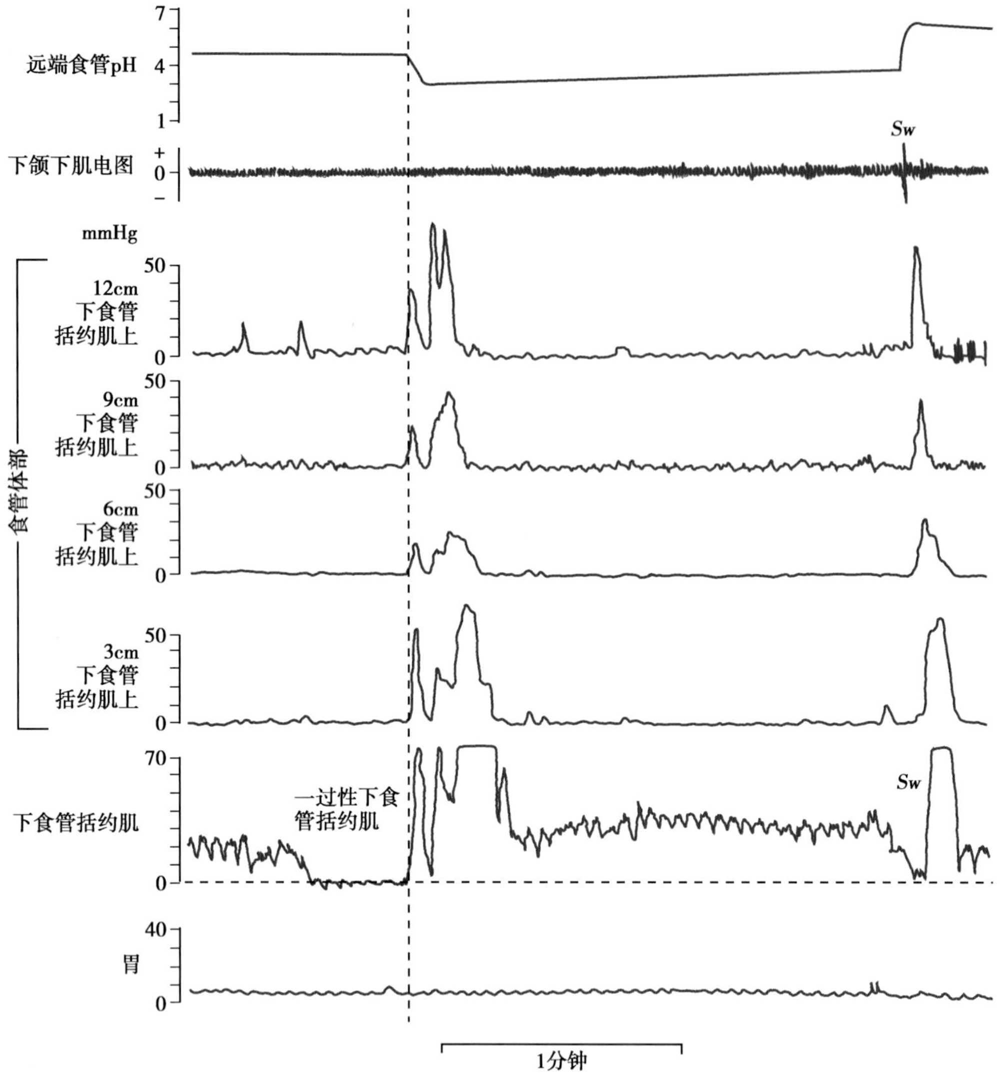

图 46.1　食管测压研究中一过性下食管括约肌松弛(tLESR)示例。LES 压力是作为胃压力的参考,用水平虚线表示。注意,tLESR 持续了近 30 秒,而吞咽诱导的 LESR 向右(Sw)仅持续了 5 秒。还应注意 tLESR 期间没有下颌下肌电图(EMG)信号,这表明缺少咽部吞咽。最后,两种类型 LESR 的相关食管运动活动不同:吞咽诱导的松弛与初级蠕动相关,而 tLESR 与整个食管体部的剧烈的、重复的"收缩停止"相关。(From Kahrilas PJ, Gupta RR. Mechanisms of reflux of acid associated with cigarette smoking. Gut 1990;31:4)

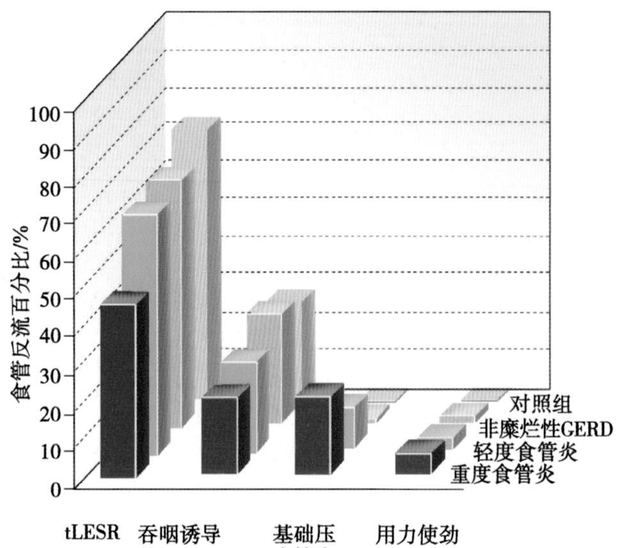

图 46.2　对照受试者和胃食管反流病(GERD)患者通过以下机制发生的反流发作百分比:一过性下食管括约肌松弛(tLESR)、吞咽诱导的下食管括约肌松弛(LESR)、下食管括约肌(LES)基础压力缺失和用力使劲 LES 压力下降。(From Holloway RH. The anti-reflux barrier and mechanisms of gastro-oesophageal reflux. Ballieres Clin Gastroenterol 2000;14:681-99.)

最后 3 种反流机制几乎总是与食管裂孔疝的存在相关。这些观察结果支持 EGJ 的功能完整性是取决于膈肌裂孔的内在 LES 和外在括约肌功能的概念。从本质上讲，GER 需要对 EGJ 进行 2 次"击打"[42]。EGJ 正常的患者需要抑制 LES 和膈脚才能发生反流（即 tLESR）。相反，当食管裂孔疝损害了膈肌脚括约肌的功能时，在 LES 低压、吞咽引起的松弛和用力期间，仅通过松弛 LES 即可发生反流[51,52]。

（三）裂孔疝

尽管存在食管裂孔疝，但许多人没有出现 GERD 的证据。其他无可识别疝的个体可因其他因素，如 tLER 过度或延长证明有 GERD。然而有 54%～94% 的反流性食管炎患者发生食管裂孔疝，该发生率显著高于健康人群[53]。研究还发现，在有反流症状的个体中，食管裂孔疝的存在使糜烂性食管损伤的风险显著增加[54]。最近的流行病学数据证实了食管裂孔疝在发生 Barrett 食管和食管腺癌患者中的重要性[55]。

食管裂孔疝通过几种机制促进反流（图 46.3）。LES 从膈脚向胸部的近端移位降低了 LES 的基础压力，并缩短了高压区的长度，这主要是由于腹腔内 LES 节段丧失所致[50]。裂孔疝消除了用力时 LES 压力的增加，增加了气体扩张胃时的 tLESR 频率[56,57]。裂孔疝可充当胃酸持久的前庭（即所谓的酸袋）。因此，在吞咽诱导的 LESR 和 tLER 过程中，疝囊发生反流的趋势增加。较大裂孔疝（≥3cm）和不可还纳（在吞咽间隔，胃皱襞仍位于膈上方的疝）的食管裂孔疝尤其容易发生反流[58]。

最后，EGJ 顺应性增加，尤其是在伴有食管裂孔疝的 GERD 患者中已被确定[51]。对于相同程度的胃内压，食管交界处以较低的压力开放，随着胃内压的增加，横截面积更大、更对称。

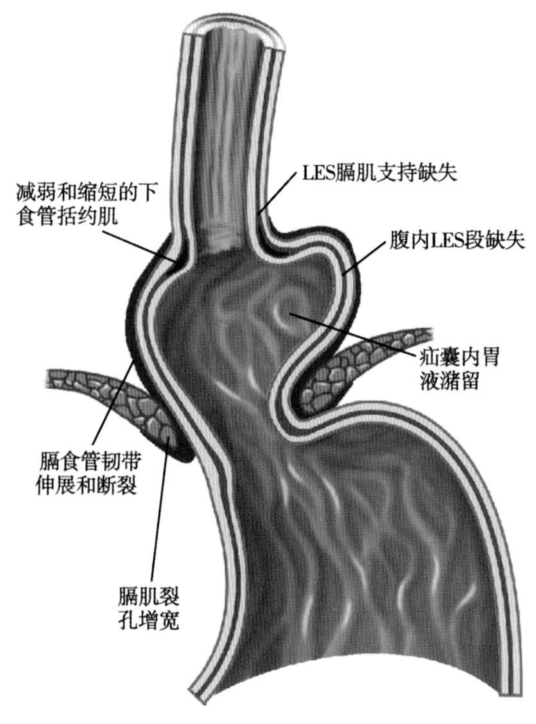

图 46.3　裂孔疝对抗反流屏障影响的示意图。LES，下食管括约肌

食管裂孔疝的病因仍不清楚。GERD 的家族聚集性提示有遗传性平滑肌疾病的可能性[27]。动物研究提出，反流本身会引起食管短缩，促进食管裂孔疝的发生[59]。其他研究发现与肥胖[60]和举重[61]也有关，随着时间的推移，慢性腹内应激源可削弱食管裂孔，可引起食管裂孔疝的发生。这一理论具有吸引力，因为它助长了随着人口老龄化食管裂孔疝患病率增加[53]。

酸袋

在空腹状态下，胃 pH 通常约为 2。在进餐期间以及此后大约 90 分钟内，由于食物的缓冲作用 pH 保持上升。在此，存在一个矛盾的情况，因为大多数酸反流发作都在餐后立即发生。这种矛盾情况的解释是，在胃贲门中发现了一个未被缓冲的区域，该区域现在被称为酸袋[62,63]。设定该囊袋是酸性反流液的来源，其 pH 远低于餐后食管远端和胃的其余部分。一项后续研究证实，在正常受试者和有症状的 GERD 患者中，该区域在进餐时缓冲作用很差[64]。在 GERD 患者中，酸袋的存在比对照组更常见，并且由于从 LES 向远端延伸而更大[65]。在伴有食管裂孔疝的 GERD 患者中，由于 LES 向近端移位，酸袋进一步扩大。此外，当酸袋位于膈肌周围时，尤其在食管裂孔疝中，超过 70% 的 tLESR 伴有酸反流。相比之下，当酸袋位于膈肌下方时，只有不到 20% 的 tLESR 伴有酸反流[58]。

（四）食管酸清除

防止反流损伤的第二层保护是食管酸清除。该现象涉及两个相关但独立的过程：容积或团块清除（即从食管中实际清除反流物质）和酸清除（即通过唾液和食管腺分泌物中的碱滴定酸暴露后恢复正常食管 pH）。尽管抗反流屏障的能力决定了 GER 的频率和体积，而食管酸清除决定了酸暴露于黏膜的持续时间，并可能决定黏膜损伤的严重程度。

1. 容量清除

食管蠕动可清除直立和仰卧位的酸容量，但在深度快速眼动睡眠期间是无效的。Helm 及其同事[66]研究显示，1 或 2 次原发性蠕动收缩可完全清除食物中的 15mL 液体团块。原发性蠕动是通过吞咽引起的，由酸反流引起的食管扩张引起的继发性蠕动，在清除反流物方面的效果要差得多，因此只能提供辅助保护作用。

蠕动功能障碍［即蠕动收缩失败、压力低或不完全排空食管的微弱（<30mmHg）蠕动收缩］的频率随着食管炎的严重程度增加。Savarino 及其同事发现，GERD 严重程度的增加与食管远端振幅降低和食管动力功能不良的患病率增加相关[67]。与非糜烂性食管炎反流病和功能性胃灼热患者相比，糜烂性食管炎患者的液体团块传输明显受损[67]。食管炎本身是否会导致蠕动功能障碍，或食管潜在的平滑肌运动障碍是否会诱发反流性疾病尚不清楚。动物研究发现，与活动性食管炎相关的食管动力障碍是可逆的。但与狭窄或广泛纤维化相关的食管动力障碍是不可逆的。临床观察结果表明，在有效的药物或手术治疗后，受损的运动功能不会恢复正常。

食管裂孔疝也会损伤食管排空。EGJ 上方的同步 pH 记录和闪烁扫描显示，清除受损是由于吞咽过程中疝囊内液体再回流所致[52]。在非复位疝患者中，这种清除率受损最严重，即使在吞咽松弛期间，疝内液体也会发生逆行流动。

当反流发生在直立位置时，重力有助于食团清除。在夜间仰卧位时，除非抬高床头，否则这种机制不起作用。这一重要的生活方式改变，显著改善了酸清除时间，对蠕动停止的患者（如硬皮病）最有益。

2. 唾液和食管腺分泌

唾液是正常食管酸清除所需的第二个重要因素。唾液分泌的刺激似乎是食管近端（LES 上方 20cm）存在酸[68]。正常每日唾液量为 1.2L，在持续的食管酸化反应中可能增加 3 倍[69]。反流酸激活食管化学受体，刺激唾液腺，并通过迷走神经介导的神经反射弧增加蠕动活动[70]。唾液为弱碱性，pH 为 6.4~7.8[71]。但在几次蠕动收缩后，易中和食管内残留的少量酸[71]。

唾液分泌的调节可能有助于 GERD。睡眠期间唾液分泌减少是夜间反流发作与酸清除时间明显延长相关的原因。口腔干燥症与长期的食管酸暴露和食管炎有关[72]。吸烟会促进 GER。最初归因于尼古丁降低 LES 压力的作用，吸烟者也有唾液分泌减少，导致食管酸清除时间延长[73]。

除唾液外，食管黏膜下腺分泌的富含碳酸氢盐的水性分泌物稀释并中和残留的食管酸[74]。酸反流到食管腔刺激这些腺体，有助中和酸，即使是不发生吞咽[75]。

3. 组织抵抗力

虽然清除机制可以缩短酸与上皮的接触时间，但即使是健康受试者，在白天、有时晚上也会有酸反流。然而，仅有少数受试者有症状性 GER，而发生 GERD 的受试者更少。这是由于食管防御的第三层被称为组织抵抗力。从概念上讲，组织抵抗阻力可细分为上皮前、上皮和上皮后因素，这些因素共同作用，使有害胃反流物对黏膜的损害降至最低[76]。

食管上皮前防御系统发育不良。表面细胞既没有明确的黏膜层，也没有缓冲能力将碳酸氢根离子分泌到未搅拌的水层中。食管分泌糖结合物（主要是黏蛋白）和前列腺素 E2 可能在上皮前防御中发挥作用[77]。

上皮防御由结构和功能成分组成。结构成分包括食管黏膜的细胞膜和细胞间连接复合体。该结构是一层 25~30 个细胞厚的非角化鳞状上皮，功能上分为增殖的基底细胞层（基底层）、代谢活跃的鳞状细胞中间层（棘层）和黏膜表面 5~10 个细胞厚的死细胞层（角质层）。食管黏膜是一个相对“紧密”的上皮，可抵抗细胞间以及细胞水平的离子运动，这是由于细胞间隙紧密连接和富含脂质的糖复合物基质形成的结果[78]。管腔内酸通过损伤细胞间连接来攻击上皮防御，使氢离子进入并酸化细胞间隙。正如透射电子显微镜所证实的，细胞间隙扩大，最终该间隙的缓冲能力被击垮，通过基底外侧膜导致相邻细胞质酸化[76]。组织抵抗力的功能成分包括食管上皮缓冲和排出氢离子的能力。细胞内的缓冲作用是由带负电荷的磷酸盐和蛋白质以及碳酸氢根离子完成的。当超过黏膜缓冲能力和细胞内 pH 下降时，上皮具有主动清除和中和 H^+ 的能力。这可能是通过两种跨膜蛋白的作用：一种是 Na^+/H^+ 交换器，另一种是 Na^+ 依赖的 Cl^-/HCO_3^- 交换器[68,79]。在反流诱导的细胞酸化后，这些转运蛋白分别通过将 H^+ 交换为细胞外 Na^+ 或将 Cl^- 交换为细胞外 HCO_3^-，使细胞内 pH 恢复到中性。此外，食管细胞在其胞膜内含有 Na^+ 非依赖性 Cl^-/HCO_3^- 交换器，当细胞内 pH 过高时，会将 HCO_3^- 从细胞质中排出[68]。当上皮细胞不再能够维持细胞内 pH 时，它们失去了容积调节能力，发生细胞肿胀，形成气球样细胞，随后细胞死亡。上皮防御的其他促成因素包括唾液表皮生长因子（EGF）、转化生长因子-α（TGF-α）和前列腺素 E2。这些因子可增强上皮细胞更新，增加食管黏蛋白的生成，并调节碳酸氢盐的分泌[78]。支持上皮细胞骨架的桥粒蛋白转录上调也会发生[80]。

数据表明，细胞间隙扩张是食管上皮细胞损伤的最早标志（图 46.4）[76]。这些改变发生在胃食管反流期间暴露于酸和胃蛋白酶时，但细胞间隙连接处受损伤的确切途径仍不清楚[81]。一种可能是调节紧密连接通透性的关键分子 E-钙黏蛋白的蛋白水解降解[82]。反流物中的其他有害成分，如胆汁酸也是有害的，急性心理应激可诱发细胞间隙扩张[83]。扩张的细胞间隙可用电子显微镜定量评估，但也可用光学显微镜识别[76]。在 Calabrese 及其同事的研究中[84]，所有对照组的细胞间隙均小于 1.69μm，有症状患者的平均细胞间隙值和最大扩张细胞间隙的平均值至少是对照组的 3 倍。在食管炎患者与非糜烂性 GERD 患者之间未观察到统计学差异。作者推测，在没有明显食管炎的情况下，细胞旁通透性增加可以部分解释了胃灼热的发生。这一假设得到了细胞间隙内浅表迷走神经和脊髓感觉传入神经元鉴别的支持[85]。重要的是，PPI 的强酸抑制可在 3~6 个月内，使几乎所有患者扩张的细胞间隙完全消失。这些变化与胃灼热的缓解密切相关[84]。

上皮后防御是由食管血液提供。血流输送氧气、营养物质和碳酸氢盐，清除 H^+ 和 CO_2，从而维持正常的组织酸碱平衡。在管腔内酸的应激下，流向食管黏膜的血流量增加[86]。

（五）胃因素

胃因素（胃反流液的容积和成分）在反流性食管炎的发生中具有潜在的重要作用。胃液酸度决定了反流液潜在的黏膜损伤程度。胃容积的增大可增加 tLESR 的发生率，使胃内容物更容易反流。

1. 胃酸分泌

胃酸和胃蛋白酶是胃反流产生食管炎的关键成分。在动物研究中，在 pH 小于 3 时，酸单独引起的损伤最小，主要是由于蛋白质变性。然而，酸即使是结合少量胃蛋白酶也会破坏黏膜屏障，导致 H^+ 通透性增加、组织学变化和出血[87]。从非糜烂性 GERD 到 Brrett 食管的食管损伤程度与酸反流（pH<4）的频率和持续时间增加相平行[88,89]。相反，用 pH 为 4~7.5 的胃蛋白酶溶液灌注动物的食管，产生的黏膜破坏或黏膜通透性变化极小[87]。这些观察结果是酸抑制治疗 GERD 相关食管炎的基础。然而，弱酸性胃内容物的反流可能是反刍的一个主要因素，由于胃内容物反流到食管，可能引起胃灼热和咳嗽[90]。

总的来说，GERD 患者的胃酸分泌是正常的[91]。另一方面，胃酸的局部分布而不是胃液分泌总量，可能与 GERD 的发病机制更相关。数据表明，胃食管交界处可能逃逸了膳食的缓冲作用，与胃体相比保持高酸性。前面讨论过的这个近端酸袋，从贲门延伸到食管远端。

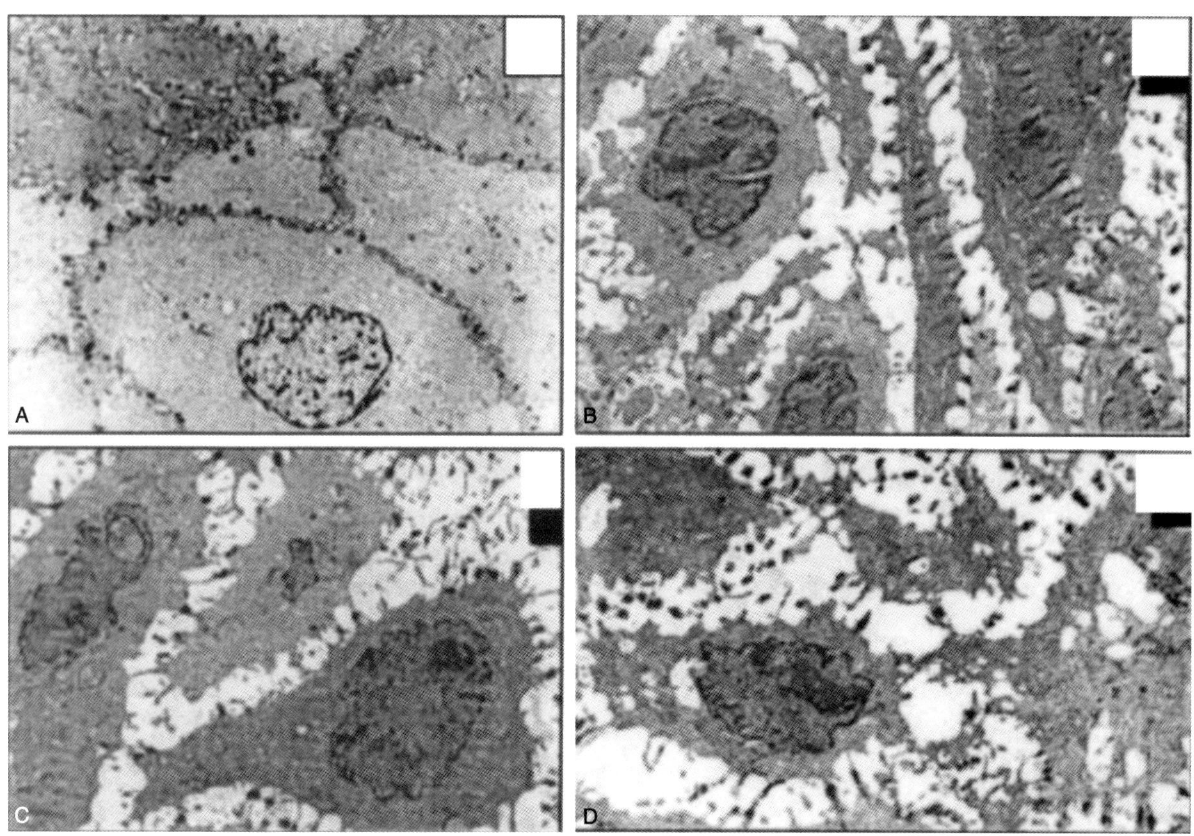

图 46.4 食管上皮的透射电子显微镜照片。正常受试者(A)没有扩张的细胞间隙。相反,"胆汁"反流(B)、非糜烂性 GERD(C)和糜烂性 GERD(D)患者的细胞间隙扩张(不规则的白色间隙)。这些扩张似乎是 GERD 最早的细胞标志物,与食管炎的程度无关。(From Calabrese C, Fabbri A, Bortolotti M, et al. Dilated intercellular spaces as a marker of oesophageal damage: Comparative results in gastro-oesophageal reflux disease with or without bile reflux. Aliment Pharmacol Ther 2003;18:525-32.)

Hp 感染,尤其是 $cagA^+$ 毒株的感染,有可能升高或降低胃液酸度,这取决于感染的部位。酸输出降低可能通过以下几种机制:①胃体感染,可进展为多灶性萎缩性胃炎;②胃碱性(碳酸氢盐)分泌增加,Hp 根除后恢复正常;③细菌本身产生氨[92]。根除 Hp 后,胃体黏膜可再生至正常,增加酸分泌。在亚洲,以胃体为主的胃炎很常见,这些患者的根除治疗可能增加发生 GERD 的风险。在一项来自日本的研究中,Hp 根除后反流性食管炎的累计患病率为 26%。有胃体萎缩性胃炎者为 33%,无胃体萎缩性胃炎者为 13%[93]。相反,以 Hp 胃窦为主的胃炎已被证明与高胃泌素血症和胃高分泌有关。以胃窦为主型胃炎的患者根除治疗后,胃灼热和反刍常明显改善[94]。

2. 十二指肠胃反流

胆汁酸可通过破坏细胞功能和损伤膜结构而改变黏膜屏障的完整性。动物研究表明,在酸和胃蛋白酶存在的情况下,结合胆汁酸产生的损伤最大,而在更中性的环境中,去结合胆汁酸和胰蛋白酶具有损伤性[95]。食管暴露于胆汁中总是与酸混合,导致更严重的食管炎。酸与胆汁反流(使用胆红素吸光度定量)与 GERD 的相关性分析支持以下假设:糜烂性食管炎的存在和严重程度主要取决于酸反流,而 Barrett 食管取决于酸和胆汁的暴露[96]。

3. 胃排空延迟

胃排空延迟在 GERD 发病机制中的重要性存在争议。早期研究提示发生率高达 50%,但最近使用标准化 4 小时胃排空试验的研究发现,有 8%~20% 的患者存在重叠[97]。从概念上讲,胃排空受损导致胃内物质容量更大,由于近端胃扩张,这些物质可直接反流至食管中。最近的阻抗-pH 测试研究发现,酸反流值没有增加,但与膳食内容物的反流相一致,增加的是在餐后液体或混合反流和非/弱酸反流[98]。女性和糖尿病患者更容易出现胃轻瘫伴继发性反流。主诉腹胀、疼痛、恶心、呕吐和便秘应是有帮助的线索,测压通常显示 LES 压力正常。

(六) 一种新的细胞因子介导的食管损伤机制

最近的动物和人类研究表明,食管损伤的一种新模式是反流的胃内容物不直接损伤食管,而是刺激食管上皮细胞分泌趋化因子介导食管组织的损伤。Souza 等人使用食管十二指肠吻合术的大鼠模型[99],在不同时间点切除食管,对炎症变化进行组织学分析。术后第 3 天开始出现反流性食管炎,黏膜下层淋巴细胞浸润,最终发展到上皮表面。基底细胞和乳头状增生先于表面糜烂的发展,这些发现与腐蚀性化学损伤预期的结果正好相反。在同一研究的另一项实验中,将人食管鳞状细胞系暴露于酸化胆汁盐中显著增加了 IL-8 和 IL-1β 的分泌,从而触发了 T 细胞和中性粒细胞的迁移。

在一项对 12 例有严重食管炎病史的患者接受 PPI 治疗愈合的初步研究中,同一组观察到,停止服用抗酸药物与 T 淋巴细胞为主的食管炎症和基底细胞以及乳头状增生有关[100]。这些变化发生在PPI停药后1~2周,活检组织中的中性粒细胞和嗜酸性粒细胞很少或缺如,没有表层细胞的丢失(即糜烂)。

四、临床特征

(一) 典型症状

胃灼热是GERD的典型症状,患者通常主诉从胃或下胸部开始出现灼热感,并向颈部、咽喉、偶尔还向背部放射[101]。它通常发生在餐后,特别是在大餐后或摄入辛辣食物、柑橘类食品、脂肪、巧克力和酒精后。仰卧位和弯腰可能会加重胃灼热。睡眠缺少,以及心理或听觉应激可能会降低症状感知的阈值[102,103]。夜间胃灼热可发生在自发意识觉醒后,导致再入睡困难。GERD通常通过每周2天或2天以上发生胃灼热症状来诊断,尽管较少频率的胃灼热症状并不排除该疾病[101]。虽然胃灼热有助于诊断,但其发生频率和严重程度并不能预测食管损伤的程度[101]。

胃灼热症状可由酸反流、弱酸性反流、胆汁反流和食管的机械性刺激引起。尽管辣椒素受体或香草醛受体1(TRPV1)是主要候选受体,但在酸灌注过程中介导胃灼热感觉的受体尚未确认。TRPV1是一种由感觉神经元表达的阳离子通道,其被热、酸性pH或乙醇激活可能引发灼痛[104]。通过pH和阻抗联合技术检测到的弱酸性反流,当反流物到达较大的近端范围、较大的反流量和延长的酸清除时间时,似乎会出现症状[105]。胆汁酸诱发食管症状的机制尚不清楚。设想胆汁酸是通过损伤脂质质膜诱导细胞内介质的释放[106]。除了酸诱导和胆汁酸诱导的食管损伤外,胃蛋白酶可对食管黏膜造成直接损伤,导致细胞间隙扩张和食管黏膜通透性增加[107]。食管扩张和持续食管收缩是解释胃灼热症状的其他机制。Balaban及其同事使用高频腔内超声证实了自发性胸痛或氯化依酚氯胺(一种抗胆碱酯酶药)诱发的胸痛与持续的食管纵向肌肉收缩之间的相关性[108]。

反刍定义为"感觉胃内容物流入或反流到口腔或咽部"[101]。在GERD的临床试验和流行病学研究中描述不一致。在每日有反刍的患者中,LES压力往往较低,许多患者伴有胃轻瘫,食管炎很常见,使这种症状比典型的胃灼热更难以药物治疗[109]。

由于缺少GERD诊断的金标准,因此很难确定GERD胃灼热和/或反刍的准确性。来自英国的Diamond研究通过仔细评估308例疑似GERD的普通内科患者,解决了这个问题[110]。经内镜下食管炎和/或24小时pH检测异常或阳性症状相关的203例患者(占66%)中明确GERD。只有49%的GERD患者记录到胃灼热或反刍是他们最烦恼的症状,其敏感性和特异性分别为63%和63%。反流问卷没有更好执行。症状对PPI治疗(埃索美拉唑40mg,持续2周)的应答也不能提高诊断的精确度——对PPI治疗应答阳性的GERD患者为69%和无GERD的患者为51%[111]。同样,一项性能良好的meta分析对PPI试验提出了质疑,发现该试验确定GERD患者的敏感性为78%,特异性为54%[112]。

超过30%的GERD患者报告有吞咽困难[113]。它通常发生在长期胃灼热的情况下,出现缓慢进展的固体食物吞咽困难。体重减轻并不常见,患者食欲良好。最常见的原因是消化性狭窄或Schatzki环,其他病因包括单纯严重的食管炎症、蠕动功能障碍和食管癌。

与GERD相关不太常见的症状包括胃灼热、吞咽痛、呃逆、恶心和呕吐[114]。胃灼热是指口腔内突然出现的一种略带酸味或咸味的液体,它不是反流液,而是唾液腺对酸反流的反应[71]。吞咽痛可见于严重的溃疡性食管炎。然而,它的存在应引起对食管炎另一种原因的怀疑,尤其是嵌塞药丸引起的感染或损伤。

部分GERD患者无症状,在老年人中尤其如此,可能是由于一些人的反流物质酸度降低或另一些人的痛觉降低。因为疾病长期存在且症状极微,许多老年患者首先表现为GERD的并发症。例如,高达40%的Barrett食管患者在就诊时对酸不敏感[2]。

(二) 食管外表现

GER可引起多种疾病,包括非心源性胸痛、哮喘、后喉炎、慢性咳嗽、复发性肺炎、牙齿腐蚀和睡眠障碍[115]。其中一些患者有典型的反流症状,但许多患者是"沉默的反流者",这导致了诊断上的问题。此外,即使可以通过检测(如pH研究)记录GER,也难以建立因果关系,因为有些个体可能仅患2种无因果关系的常见疾病。

1. 胸痛

GER相关胸痛可能与心绞痛相似,具有挤压或灼热性质,位于胸骨后,并放射到背部、颈部、下颌或手臂。常在饭后加重,情绪紧张时可能会恶化。与反流相关的胸痛可能持续数分钟至数小时,通常可自行缓解,服用抗酸剂可缓解。GERD相关胸痛的机制知之甚少,可能是多因素的,与H^+浓度、容积和酸反流持续时间、继发性食管痉挛和纵向肌肉的长时间收缩有关[116,117]。胸痛发作与pH检测记录的酸反流事件相关,通常对抗酸分泌治疗反应良好[118]。

2. 哮喘和其他肺部疾病

哮喘患者GERD的估计患病率为34%~89%,这取决于研究的患者组和GERD如何定义(例如症状或24小时pH监测)[119]。反流诱发哮喘的可能机制包括将胃内容物吸入肺内,继发支气管痉挛并激活从食管到肺部的迷走神经反射,导致支气管收缩。动物[120]和人[121]研究报告,食管酸化后支气管收缩,但反应轻微且不一致。与单纯的食管相比,酸反流进入气管,可预见引起哮喘患者呼气峰流速值发生显著变化[122]。与GERD相关的其他肺部疾病包括吸入性肺炎、间质性肺纤维化、慢性支气管炎和支气管扩张症。此外,在一部分患者中,GER可能会加重阻塞性睡眠呼吸暂停(OSA)的病程[123]。

高达30%的与GERD相关的哮喘患者无任何食管症状的主诉。因此,即使在哮喘控制不佳的无症状患者中,也热衷于对酸反流进行经验性治疗。但随机双盲试验的数据不支持这种方法。一项针对使用吸入性糖皮质激素治疗但哮喘控制不佳且GER症状轻微或无症状的成年人试验中,使用40mg埃索美拉唑2次/d或匹配的安慰剂。埃索美拉唑对哮喘控制不佳的发生频率没有显著的影响。作者还发现,埃索美拉唑对肺功能、气道反应性、夜间觉醒或生活质量无影响。即使在 pH 异常哮喘控制不佳的亚组患者中,抑酸也无获益[124]。最近一项在儿童患者中使用兰索拉唑的研究也发现了相似的结果[125]。此外报告了,接受兰索拉唑治疗的儿童有更多的呼吸道感染[126]。

3. 耳鼻咽喉疾病

喉部炎症可能与各种前驱症状有关,包括声音嘶哑、癔球症、频繁清喉、复发性咽喉痛和长时间的声音热身练习[127]。归因于 GERD 的耳鼻喉体征包括后部喉炎伴水肿和红肿、声带溃疡、肉芽肿、白斑,甚至癌[128]。这些改变通常局限于声带后 1/3 和杓间区,两者均靠近上食管括约肌(图 46.5)。动物研究发现,酸、胃蛋白酶和结合胆汁酸的组合对喉部的损伤非常大[129]。人体研究证实,与一般人群相比,有喉部症状和体征的患者食管酸暴露增加更为常见[127]。尽管抑酸治疗通常推荐作为慢性喉部症状的经验性治疗,使用 PPT 治疗的对照试验结果的 meta 分析,未能发现与安慰剂相比的客观症状改善[130]。

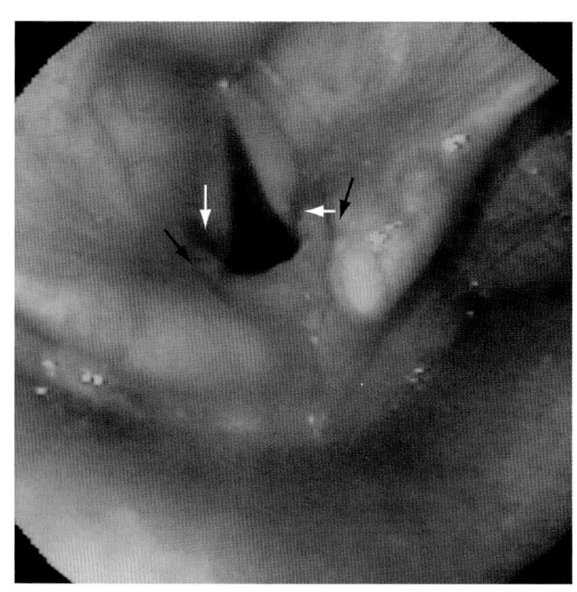

图 46.5 一例 31 岁声音嘶哑男性患者的“反流性喉炎”特征性表现,经 PPI 治疗 3 个月后症状和体征消失。黑色箭头:杓状软骨内侧壁红斑。白色箭头:真实声带上的红色条纹。喉部的反流改变通常局限于最接近食管上括约肌的后部(杓状软骨复合体后面的蓝灰色隆起)

GERD 被设定为慢性咳嗽的主要原因(鼻窦问题和哮喘之后)[131],GER 可增加慢性咳嗽患者的咳嗽敏感反射(即降低咳嗽阈值)[132]。然而,这种相关性在人类中的重要性尚未在治疗研究中得到证实。总的说来,治疗研究并未证明 PPI 优于安慰剂[133]。牙侵蚀,即非细菌化学过程导致的牙齿结构丧失,可由 GER 引起,抑酸治疗有助于对抗反流相关牙齿侵蚀的进展[134]。

(三) 睡眠障碍

夜间 GERD 可引起睡眠中断,导致高缺勤率和生活质量下降[135]。已证明 PPI 治疗在缓解夜间胃灼热和减少 GERD 相关睡眠障碍方面优于安慰剂,从而改善睡眠质量和工作效率[136]。流行病学研究也发现夜间 GERD 和 OSA(阻塞性睡眠呼吸暂停综合征)之间存在相关性[137]。在一项使用 pH 阻抗的研究中证实了这一点,发现 OSA 患者比无 OSA 的患者有更多的病理性反酸发作[125]。这种相关性的机制仍不清楚。尽管 GERD 似乎是 OSA 的结果,而不是相反。例如一项研究发现,OSA 患者在睡眠期间有更多的 tLESR 与之前的睡眠觉醒和浅睡眠相关[138]。

五、鉴别诊断

与 GERD 相关的症状可能与其他食管和食管外疾病类似,包括贲门失弛缓症、嗜酸粒细胞性食管炎(EoE)、Zenker 憩室、胃轻瘫、胆结石、消化性溃疡病、功能性消化不良和心绞痛。这些疾病通常可以通过积极的 PPI 治疗和适当的诊断试验无反应来识别。虽然 GERD 是食管炎最常见的病因,但在难以处理的病例、老年人或免疫功能低下的患者中,需要考虑食管炎的其他病因(药丸、感染或辐射损伤)。

六、相关条件

有几种内科和外科疾病易诱发 GERD。最常见的是妊娠,其中 30%~80% 的妇女主诉胃灼热,尤其是在妊娠的前 3 个月(见第 40 章)。由于雌激素和孕酮的影响,以及可能来自妊娠子宫的机械因素,妊娠通过降低 LES 压力增加了反流的风险[139]。虽然症状可能很严重,但食管炎并不常见,这类情境性 GERD 通过分娩治愈。高达 90% 的硬皮病[原发性干燥综合征(PSS)或 CREST 综合征(系统性硬皮病亚型)]患者因平滑肌纤维化导致 LES 压力较低和蠕动较弱或蠕动缺失而发生 GERD(见第 37 章)。严重疾病很常见,高达 38% 的患者有食管炎[140]。高酸分泌和胃容量增加是引起 Zollinger-Ellison 综合征(即胃泌素瘤)患者 GERD 的主要因素(见第 34 章)。在这些患者中,食管炎和并发症比溃疡病更难治疗[141]。在 Heller 肌切开术或最近的经口内镜肌切开术治疗贲门失弛缓症后(见第 44 章),10%~39% 的患者可能发生 GERD[142]。对于因病态肥胖而接受减肥手术(腹腔镜胃绕道手术)治疗的患者(见第 8 章),术后可能出现 GERD 的新发症状[143]。最后,长时间鼻胃管插管可能导致反流性食管炎,部分原因是胃酸沿着插管轨道流出,以及插管机械性干扰 LES 屏障功能有关(见第 45 章)[144]。

七、诊断

大量检测可用于评估疑似 GERD 的患者[145]。但许多情况下这些检查是不必要的,因为胃灼热和反酸的典型症状具有足够的特异性,可以识别反流疾病并开始药物治疗。然而,情况并不总是如此,临床医生必须根据所需信息决定选择哪种检测方法,以便以及时、可靠和具有成本效益的方式作出诊断(框 46.1)[145]。

框 46.1　胃食管反流病(GERD)检测
GERD 问卷(RDQ,GERD Q)
PPI 测试
测压
吞钡检查
内镜检查
组织学
pH 监测(基于导管或无线)
腔内阻抗-pH 监测
黏膜阻抗
RDQ,反流性疾病问卷;GERD Q,胃食管反流病问卷;PPI,质子泵抑制剂。

(一) 酸抑制试验

酸抑制试验是诊断 GERD 和评估其与症状关系的最简单方法。随着 PPI 的出现,它已经成为第一个用于无报警主诉的典型或非典型反流症状患者的检测方法。症状通常在 1~2 周内对 PPI 试验有反应,如果症状在治疗后消失,然后在停药后复发,则 GERD 已经确立。

在胃灼热的经验性试验中,初始 PPI 剂量较高(如奥美拉唑 40~80mg/d),通常至少给药 2 周,阳性反应定义为胃灼热症状至少改善 50%。使用这种方法,PPI 经验性试验确定 GERD 存在的敏感性为 68%~83%,但特异性较差[146,147]。然而,这些研究富含 GERD 患者,可能不代表一般人群。例如 PPI 试验在英国初级保健机构中对大量具有各种 UGI 症状的患者不那么有用[148]。在 64% 有充分证据的 GERD 患者和 51% 的无 GERD 患者中观察到阳性反应,并不比掷硬币好多少。

用于诊断 GERD 的经验性 PPI 试验具有许多优点:该试验基于办公室、易于完成、价格低廉,可供所有医师使用,并避免了许多不必要的程序。例如 Fass 及其同事研究显示[149],由于非心源性胸痛的诊断性检查次数减少,每例患者节省 570 美元以上。缺点很少,包括安慰剂反应和如果延长经验性治疗后症状未完全消退,则无法确定症状终点。然而,在一般实践中,假阳性率可能比以前预期的要高[148]。将成功 PPI 治疗的诊断试验特征与 24 小时 pH 监测作为参考标准,一项研究显示,短期 PPI 试验诊断 GERD 的敏感性和特异性的综合估计值分别为 78% 和 54%[150]。

(二) 内镜检查

上消化道内镜检查是证明食管炎存在和程度及排除引起患者症状的其他病因的标准检查。然而,经 pH 检测异常食管反流患者中,只有 20%~60% 在内镜检查时有食管炎。因此,内镜对 GERD 的敏感性较低,但其特异性高达 90%~95%[151]。

胃酸反流的最早内镜征象包括水肿和红斑,但这些表现是非特异性的,取决于内镜视觉图像的质量[151]。更为可靠的征象是易碎、颗粒感和红色条纹。易碎性(易出血)是由于在酸的作用下,黏膜表面毛细血管扩张所致。红色条纹从食管交界处沿食管黏膜皱襞嵴向上延伸[152]。糜烂伴进行性酸损伤,其特征为黏膜浅层破裂,伴有白色或黄色渗出物,周围有红斑包绕。典型的糜烂开始于胃食管交界处,沿食管黏膜皱襞顶部发生,此处最易发生酸损伤,可能是单个的,也可以是多个的。非甾体抗炎药(NSAIDs)、大量吸烟和感染性食管炎也可引起糜烂[151]。溃疡反映了更严重的食管损伤,病变深入黏膜和黏膜下层,孤立地沿着皱襞或食管交界处周围。全面评估食管炎分类是洛杉矶系统(Los Angeles,LA),目前在全世界广泛使用(图 46.6 和表 46.2)[153]。

食管胶囊内镜检查对反流症状的评估至今令人失望,该胶囊为 11mm×26mm,每秒可获取 14 帧的视频图像。吞咽后,图像通过数字射频传输到便携式接收器。在一项研究中,与标准的上消化道内镜检查相比,胶囊内镜对糜烂性食管炎诊断的敏感性仅为 50%,对食管裂孔疝的诊断敏感性为 54%,对 Barrett 食管的敏感性为 79%[154]。

大多数 GERD 患者最初接受 PPI 治疗,无需内镜检查。一个重要的例外情况是患者出现"报警"症状:吞咽困难、吞咽痛、体重减轻、呕吐和胃肠道出血。在此,应尽早进行内镜检查,以诊断 GERD 的并发症(如狭窄),并排除感染、溃疡、癌症或静脉曲张等其他疾病。美国医师学会目前的指南建议,内镜检查的主要作用是诊断和治疗 GERD 的并发症,尤其是消化性狭窄,并确定 Barrett 食管[155]。其他适应证包括尽管进行了为期 4~8 周的每日 2 次 PPI 治疗试验,但仍持续存在的典型 GERD 症状,以及经过 2 个月 PPI 疗程后的重度食管炎患者,以评估愈合情况并排除 Barrett 食管。

(三) 食管黏膜活检

与内镜检查一样,食管黏膜活检在评估 GERD 中的作用逐年不断发展[145]。即使内镜检查显示黏膜正常,也可能发生反流引起的显微镜下微观变化[156]。典型变化是基底细胞增生和表皮钉突高度增加,均代表鳞状黏膜上皮更新增加,对 GERD 是敏感的但非特异性组织学发现[157]。以中性粒细胞和嗜酸性粒细胞为特征的急性炎症(图 46.7),对食管炎诊断具有很强的特异性,但敏感性较低,在 15%~40% 范围之间[158]。因此,对外观正常的鳞状黏膜进行组织学检查以识别 GERD 的价值很小。然而,由于需要区分 EoE 和 GERD,尤其是在主诉吞咽困难的患者中,这一论断最近有所缓和[159]。在吞咽困难的年轻患者中,尤其是食物嵌塞,嗜酸性粒细胞性食管炎的临床疑诊很高,需要在食管远端和近端进行黏膜活检。对典型的反流性食管炎,除非为排除肿瘤、感染或大疱性皮肤病外,通常不进行活检。因此,目前食管黏膜活检的主要适应证是,确定 Barrett 上皮和排除嗜酸性粒细胞性食管炎[160]。当怀疑 Barrett 食管时,必须强制进行活检,最好在食管炎治愈时进行(见第 47 章)。

表 46.2　洛杉矶食管炎内镜检查分类系统

A 级	一个或多个局限于皱襞的黏膜破损≤5mm
B 级	一个或多个>5mm 的黏膜破损,局限于皱襞但在黏膜皱襞顶部之间不连续
C 级	黏膜破损在 2 个或多个黏膜皱襞顶部之间连续,但周围无环形包绕
D 级	黏膜破损呈环形包绕

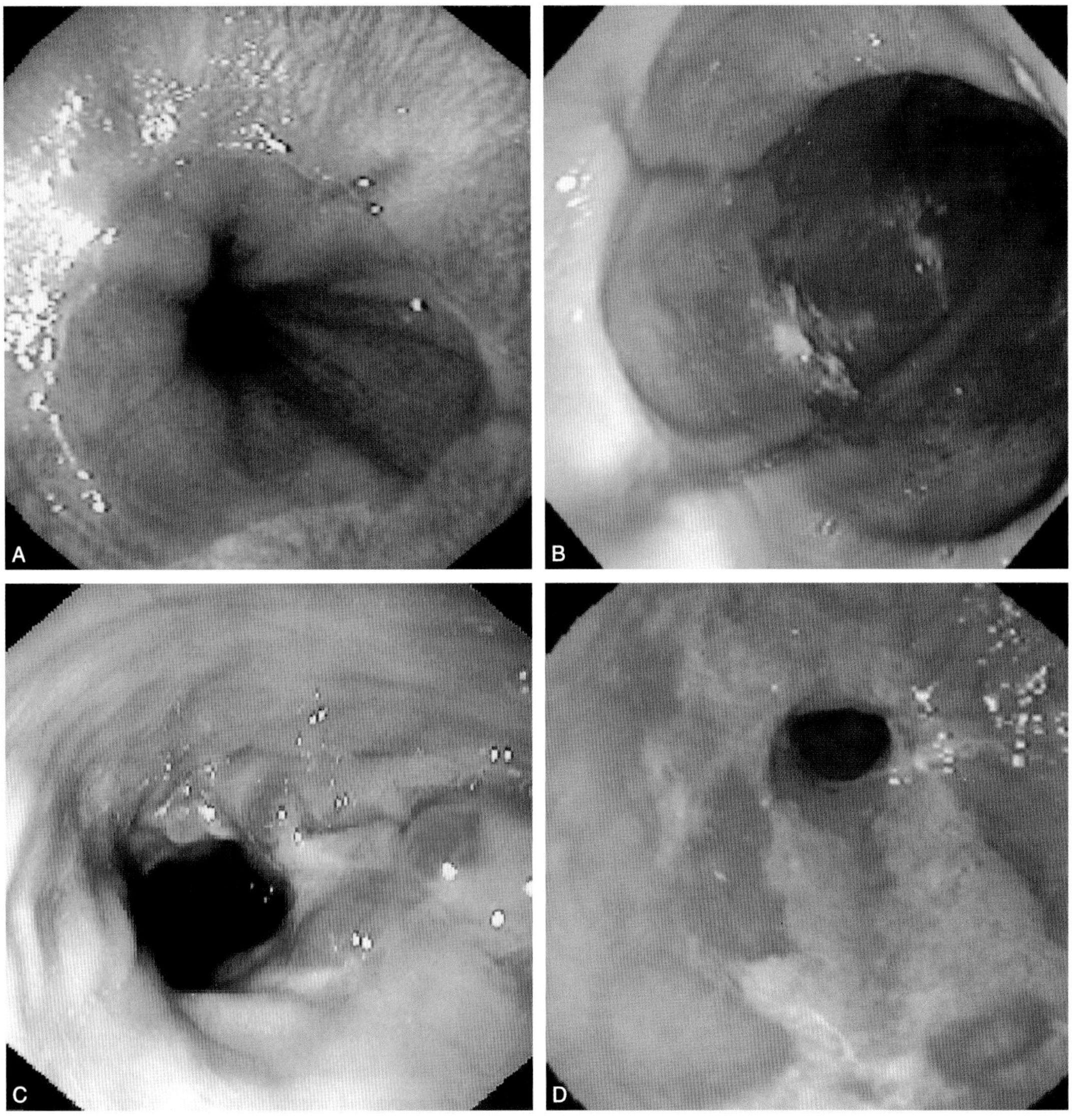

图 46.6　使用洛杉矶分类系统(见表 46.2)的 4 级食管炎(A 至 D)的内镜照片

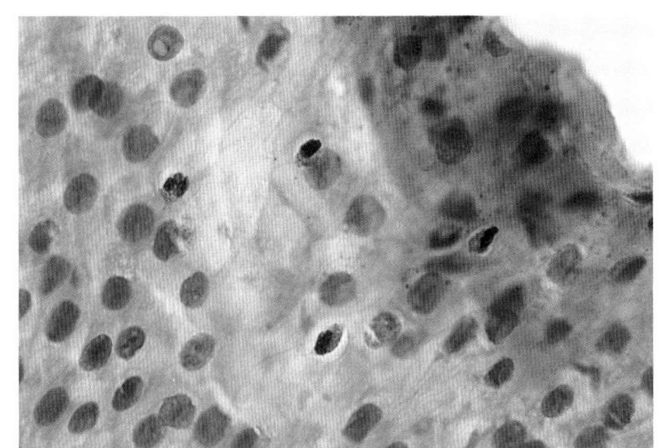

图 46.7　胃食管反流病的组织病理学。炎性细胞(嗜酸性粒细胞和中性粒细胞)散布在鳞状上皮细胞之间。(Courtesy Edward Lee, MD, Mashington, DC.)

(四) 食管反流试验

食管反流监测在过去 10 年中发生了重大变化[145]。无线 pH 胶囊和测量所有形式反流(包括酸和非酸)的能力是反流检测领域的重要进展。动态食管内 pH 监测仍然是确定病理性酸反流的标准[145,161,162]。基于导管的 pH 测试,探头通过鼻腔,处于测压 LES 上方 5cm 处,并连接到电池供电的数据记录仪上,该记录仪能够每 4~6 秒收集一次 pH。当出现症状、进饮和体位改变时,事件标记被患者激活。鼓励患者正常进食,从事日常活动,并进行 18~24 小时的监测。反流发作定义为 pH 下降小于 4。常规测量的参数包括:pH 小于 4 时的总时间百分比、pH 小于 4 时的直立和仰卧时间百分比、反流发作总数、最长反流发作持续时间以及大于 5 分钟的发作次数。总时间 pH 小于 4 的百分比是 GERD 最具重现性的测量值,报告的正常上限范围为 4%~5.5%[161]。动态 pH 检测可识别 GER、进食和睡眠相关事件的位置变化,并有助于将症状与反流事件联系起来。

反流试验 3 项新技术进展中的第一项是无导管系统(图 46.8 上图)[163]。该系统使用无线 pH 胶囊,用驱动小针进入上皮输送系统固定在食管黏膜上。然后胶囊利用射频信号将 pH 数据传输到便携式接收器。无导管检测现在是 pH 检测的首选方法,因为监测时间可以延长到 24 小时以上(通常为 48 小时),对每日正常活动和进餐的限制可以忽略不计[164]。由于胶囊只能准确测量酸反流(pH<4),因此所有研究必须停用 PPI 至少 7 天[165]。

第二项技术改进将阻抗与 pH 检测相结合,可测量酸和非酸反流(见图 46.8 下图)。后者对于 PPI 治疗后仍有持续反流的患者尤为重要,但现在大多数发作的 pH 都高于 4[160]。非酸性反流是通过检测食管内富含离子液体的逆行食团来测量的。液体和空气混合物的回流液也很容易被检测到。在不使用 PPI 的一大组正常受试者中,约 40% 的反流发作为弱酸性(pH 4~6.5)或碱性(pH>6.5)[166]。在一项联合阻抗-pH 测试的多中心研究中,37% 的患者尽管每日两次 PPI 治疗,但仍出现持续的反流症状,这是由于非酸性反流所致[167]。

在内镜检查期间检测 GERD 黏膜完整性改变的最新技术,是通过检测黏膜阻抗变化或基于腔内阻抗测试(夜间基线阻抗和吞咽后诱导的蠕动波指数)[168-171]。黏膜阻抗测量对确定 GERD 和 EoE 患者具有高度准确性。现在评估这项新技术的临床影响还为时尚早,但诊断 GERD 而不需要长时间的动态测试是有希望的。夜间基线阻抗和吞咽后诱发的蠕动波的作用预计将受到限制,因为需要以导管为基础的测试和测量这两个参数的复杂方法。最后,据称唾液胃蛋白酶检测和基于导管的经口 pH 监测有助于诊断食管外反流,然而,关于其临床获益的研究显示了混杂的不同结果[145]。

食管 pH 监测的一个关键限制是,没有可靠的绝对阈值识别 GERD 患者。对接受 pH 测试的内镜下食管炎患者进行比较的研究报告,敏感性为 77%~100%,特异性为 85%~100%[145]。然而,食管炎患者很少需要 pH 测试,相反,内镜检查正常和疑似 GERD 的患者可能从该测试中获益最大。遗憾的是,这些患者的数据不太确定,对照组与非糜烂性反流患者之间有相当大的重叠[161]。pH 检测的其他缺点包括可能

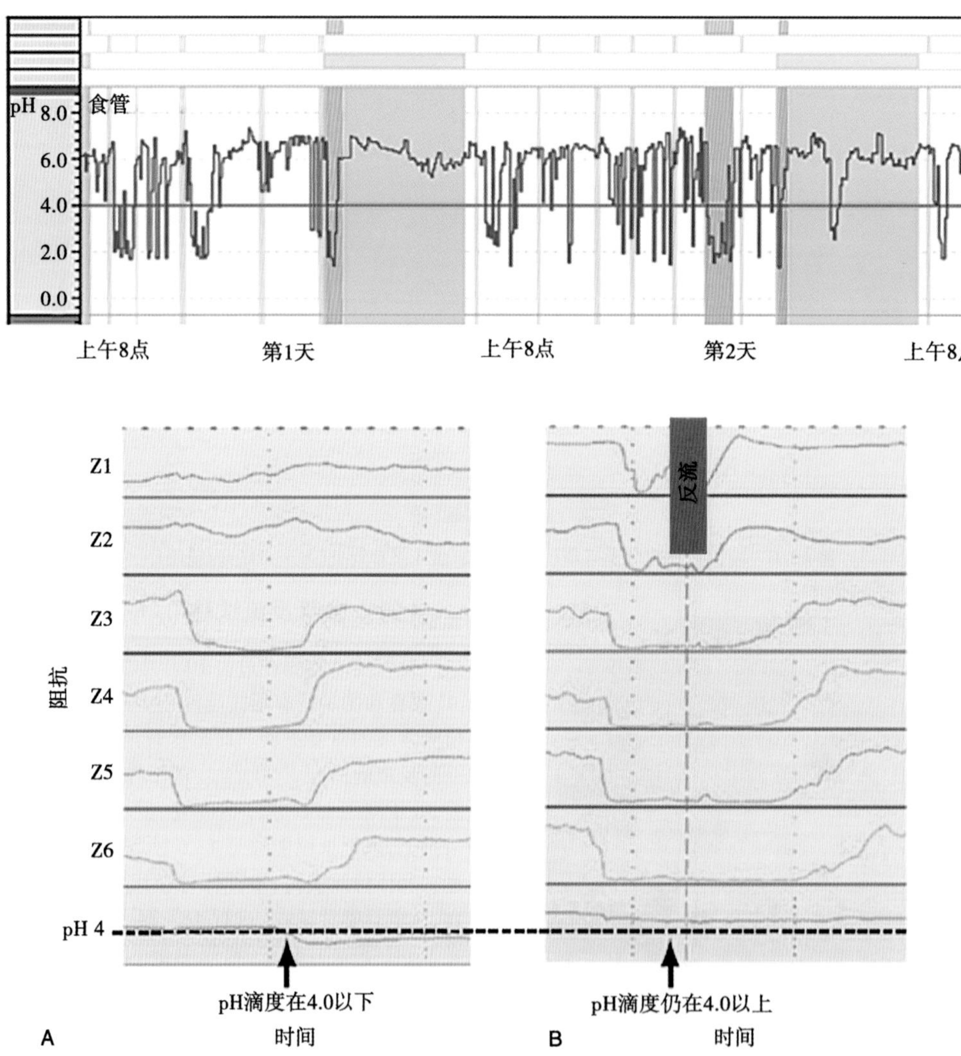

图 46.8 48 小时食管 pH 和多通道阻抗-pH 的追踪研究。上图是对 GERD 患者进行的 48 小时 pH 胶囊研究。膳食/饮料用黄线表示、仰卧位用蓝色表示、橙色条代表与酸反流相关的症状。下图是通过多通道阻抗-pH 监测检测酸和非酸反流的示例。A,胃酸反流,具有典型的顺序阻抗模式呈逆向行下降,到达第三个阻抗测量段(Z3),并伴有食管 pH 下降至 4.0 以下。B,PPI 治疗的非酸性反流患者,在反流发作期间出现典型的逆流阻抗模式,达到 Z1,尽管食管 pH 仍在 4.0 以上。Z,段

发生的设备故障、由于探头埋藏在黏膜皱襞中而遗漏反流事件，以及由于鼻探头耐受性差受到饮食或活动限制而导致的假阴性研究结果。

动态反流 pH 监测是唯一记录和关联长期反流发作症状的测试。然而，由于只有 10%～20% 的反流发作与症状相关，因此，不同的统计学分析已经逐渐形成，试图定义症状和反流发作之间的显著关联，包括症状指数、症状敏感性指数和症状关联概率[171]。遗憾的是，没有研究确定这些症状评分在预测治疗反应方面的准确性。此外，验证研究仅针对胃灼热、反流和胸痛伴酸反流进行，而未对非典型反流症状或非酸反流进行研究。最近的研究对症状关联概率的有效性提出了质疑，并警告不要使用它，尤其是在反流参数正常的患者中[172,173]。因此，pH 检测可以确定主诉和 GERD 之间的相关性，但只有治疗试验解决了因果关系的关键临床问题。

建立了动态反流监测的临床适应证[145]。胃底折叠术之前，内镜检查正常的患者应进行 pH 检测，以确认存在病理性酸反流。抗反流手术后，持续或复发症状需要重复进行 pH 检测。在这些情况下，pH 监测是在患者停用抗反流药物下进行的。食管反流试验特别有助于评估对治疗有抵抗、且内镜检查结果正常或模棱两可的 GERD 样症状患者。然而，是在 PPI 治疗期间还是停药期间仍有争议[162]。对于这种情况，可以在 PPI 治疗期间进行阻抗-pH 检测，以确定 2 种人群：有和无持续异常酸或非酸暴露时间的人群。持续性胃食管反流的患者需要强化药物治疗，而有症状且反流控制良好的患者可能有另一种病因。非 PPI 方法获得普及，因为 50%～60% 的患者症状反应差且内镜检查正常的患者没有 GERD。pH 检测阴性的治疗是有用的，因为它可指导针对其他原因的诊断检查，并可以停止不必要的 PPI 治疗。然而，最近的一项研究发现[174]，超过 42% 的胃酸反流检测阴性患者仍在继续 PPI 治疗。最后，动态 pH 检测可能有助于确定 GERD 食管外表现的患者。然而，它最重要的作用是排除反流是导致患者持续反流的原因。最初，这些研究中的大多是在停用抗反流药物的情况下进行的，以确认 GERD 的共存，然而，这并不能保证症状的因果关系。因此，一种方法是首先使用 PPI 进行积极治疗，对治疗 4～12 周后无反应的患者保留 pH 检测[160]。

（五）食管钡剂造影

食管钡剂造影是一种价廉、易获得、无创的食管检查方法[175]。它在证明食管解剖学狭窄和评估食管裂孔疝的存在和可复性方面是最有用的。Schatzki 环、蹼或轻微缩小的消化性狭窄可能仅在食管造影时才能发现，而内镜检查可能因无法充分扩张食管而漏诊。在钡液中加入 13mm 的不透射线药丸或棉花糖有助于识别这些细微的狭窄。食管钡剂造影可以很好地评估蠕动，并有助于术前识别食管泵虚弱无力。食管钡剂造影检查食管炎的能力各不相同，对中度至重度食管炎的敏感性为 79%～100%，而轻度食管炎通常被漏诊。钡剂检查在诊断 Barrett 食管时存在不足。钡剂自发反流至食管近端对反流很有特异性，但并不敏感。激发性动作（如抬腿、咳嗽、Valsalva 动作、水虹吸）可引起应激性反流，提高钡剂食管造影的敏感性，但有争论，认为这些手法可降低其特异性[176]。

（六）食管测压

与反流试验一样，多通道高分辨率测压的出现彻底改变了这种食管功能测试[177]。有 32～36 个压力传感器跨越整个食管，测压现在可以准确评估 LES 的压力和松弛，以及蠕动活动，包括收缩幅度、持续时间和速度。然而，食管测压通常不适用于无并发症的 GERD 患者的评估，因为大多数患者的静息 LES 压力正常。传统上建议在抗反流手术之前进行食管测压，以记录充分的食管蠕动，并排除贲门失弛缓症和硬皮病的变异[160]。如果研究发现无效蠕动（低振幅或频繁蠕动失败）或无蠕动，则可能禁忌进行完全胃底折叠术。然而，这一假设受到挑战，因为与部分胃底折叠术相比，完全胃底折叠术后蠕动较弱的患者的反流控制更好，吞咽困难不再常见[178]。传统测压法的改进，结合阻抗测试，有助于澄清这一争议。使用该技术研究发现，不到 50% 的蠕动无效患者通过阻抗测量的食管团注传输显著延迟[179]。因此，可能只有这些有明显运动生理缺陷的患者才需要改进胃底折叠术。

八、临床病程

GERD 的临床病程在很大程度上取决于患者是否有糜烂性或非糜烂性疾病。关于 GERD 是作为一种严重程度不同的疾病谱还是作为 3 组不同分类的疾病：糜烂性、非糜烂性和 Barrett 食管是有争议的。患者往往不会从一个组转到另一个组。在 6 个月～22 年以上的随访中，不到 25% 的非糜烂性疾病患者随着时间的推移演变为糜烂性食管炎，几乎所有患者都是 LA 分类中的 A/B 级疾病，或有 GERD 并发症[180,181]。

（一）非糜烂性疾病

来自三级转诊中心的早期研究表明，大多数 GERD 患者患有食管炎[182]。然而，最近的数据表明，高达 70% 的 GERD 患者内镜检查正常[183,184]。内镜检查阴性的 GERD 患者更可能是女性、更年轻、更瘦且无食管裂孔疝，他们的功能性胃肠道疾病患病率更高[185]。尽管只有轻微黏膜损伤，但这些患者表现出一种慢性症状模式，伴有加重和缓解期[186]。在具有典型反流症状和内镜检查正常的患者中怀疑非糜烂性 GERD，可通过患者对抗分泌治疗的反应得到证实。食管 pH 检测可识别 3 个不同的非糜烂性 GERD 患者亚群。首先是胃酸反流过多的患者，他们通常对 PPI 治疗有反应。其次是胃酸反流参数正常，但其症状与酸反流发作有良好相关性的患者。该组占非糜烂性 GERD 患者的 30%～50%，根据最近的罗马Ⅳ标准，被归类为“反流性超敏反应”[187]。这些患者食管可能对酸敏感性更高，抗反流治疗反应较小[188]。第 3 组的特点是酸暴露时间正常和症状相关性差。这一组被归类为“功能性胃灼热”[187]。

（二）糜烂性疾病

糜烂性食管炎患者多为男性、年龄较大、超重、更容易发生食管裂孔疝[185]。这些糜烂性食管炎患者的临床病程更可预测，并与 GERD 的并发症相关。纵向研究表明，高达 85% 的糜烂性 GERD 患者在停止 PPI 治疗后 6 个月内未接受维持反流治疗的将复发，重度食管炎患者的复发率更高（见表46.2）[189,190]。几项研究证实，糜烂性食管炎患者容易发生反流并发症，包括溃疡、狭窄和 Barrett 食管。在芬兰的一项研究中，20 例糜烂性 GERD 患者接受了生活方式改变、抗酸剂和促动力药物治疗，平均随访 19 年。14 例患者持续糜烂，发现 6 例新的 Barrett 食管[180]。在最近另一项欧洲研究中[181]，LA 分类为 C/D 级的食管炎患者在 2 年内发展为 Barrett 食管，发生率为 5.8%，而 LA 分类为 A/B 级的食管炎患者仅为 1.4%，非糜烂性 GERD 为 0.5%。

九、并发症

（一）出血、溃疡和穿孔

与 GERD 相关的非癌症死亡罕见（0.46/100 000 人）。最常见的致死原因是出血性食管炎、吸入性肺炎、溃疡穿孔和重度食管炎破裂[191]。大出血和食管穿孔通常与食管深部溃疡或重度食管炎有关[192]。食管穿孔在 PPI 治疗时代罕见，但可导致纵隔炎和死亡。据报道，7% ~ 18% 的 GERD 患者临床出现大出血[193]，可能导致缺铁性贫血。

（二）消化性食管狭窄

未经治疗的反流性食管炎患者中有 7% ~ 23% 发生食管狭窄。它们常见于老年男性患者[194]，与长期使用 NSAIDs 有关[195]。狭窄的形成是复杂的，从可逆性炎症开始伴水肿、细胞浸润和血管充血，进展为胶原沉积，最终导致不可逆的纤维化。随着吞咽困难的进展，胃灼热通常会减少，反映出狭窄充当进一步反流的屏障，吞咽困难通常仅限于固体食物。与恶性狭窄不同，消化性狭窄患者食欲好，饮食习惯改变，体重减轻很少。消化性狭窄是壁光滑、呈锥形的食管下段环形狭窄，通常长度不到 1cm，但偶尔可延伸至 8cm（图 46.9）。在异常的情况下，临床医师应怀疑有其他易感疾病，如 Zollinger-Ellison 综合征、药物性食管炎或长期鼻胃管插管[194]。食管中上段狭窄应引起对 Barrett 食管或恶性肿瘤的关注。虽然曾经备受争议，但如今 Schatzki 环被认为是早期消化性狭窄的一种形式[196]。所有狭窄患者均应接受内镜检查，以证实病变的良性性质，并进行活检排除 EoE、癌症和 Barrett 食管。

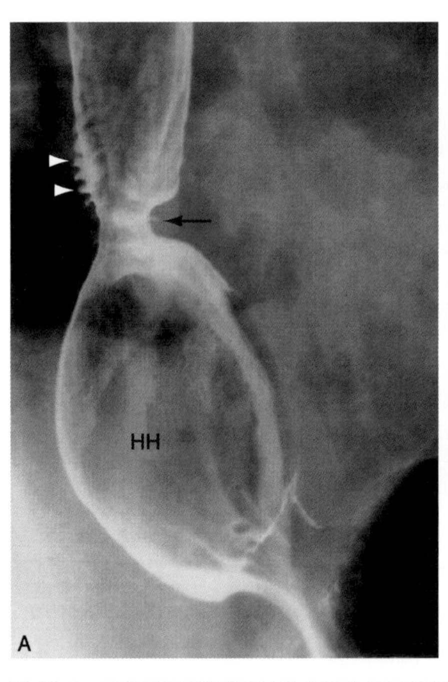

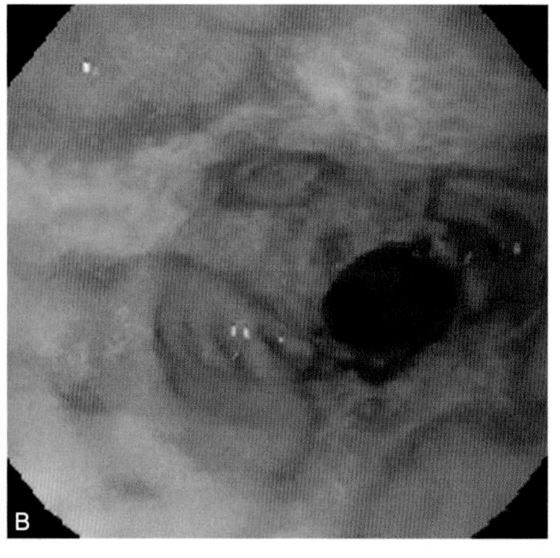

图 46.9　经食管钡剂造影（A）和内镜检查（B）证实的典型消化性食管狭窄。图片显示了所有 GERD 狭窄常见的大食管裂孔疝（HH）。黑色箭头指短而厚的纤维性狭窄，白色箭头指与其相关的多个假性憩室。虽然在钡剂检查中未观察到，但内镜视图也证实了环周状食管炎（LA 分类 D 级）。（Los Angeles grade D.）

（三）Barrett 食管

见第 47 章。

十、无并发症疾病的治疗

GERD 治疗的基本原理取决于对特定目标的仔细定义[197]。对于无食管炎的患者，治疗目标是缓解反流症状和防止频繁的症状复发。在食管炎患者中，目标是缓解症状和治愈食管炎，同时防止进一步复发和并发症。

（一）非处方药物治疗

虽然 GERD 很常见，但许多患者并不就医，而是选择改变生活方式，自行使用非处方（OCT）抗酸制剂自我治疗。这些观察结果导致了 GERD 人群的“冰山”模式，绝大多数胃灼热的痛苦是看不见的，因为他们自我治疗，不寻求专业医师帮助，只有那些处于冰山一角的人，通常是有严重症状或反流并发症的患者，才会被专业医师看到[21]。

1. 改变生活方式

有选择地改变生活方式，并仔细向患者解释，应作为最初治疗计划的一部分，特别是对轻度、间歇性主诉的患者尤其有用。这些措施包括抬高床头、超重时减肥、限制饮酒和吸烟、改变饮食习惯、避免饭后躺卧以及避免睡前吃零食。生理学研究表明，这些行为可提高食管酸清除率，减少酸反流相关事件，或缓解胃灼热症状[198]。床头抬高可以通过使用 15~20cm 的垫块或泡沫楔形物来抬高上半身。在临睡前几小时进食，避免睡前吃零食，可以使夜间保持胃排空，从而减少夜间反流发作。减肥的目的是通过"腹部应激"机制降低反流的发生率。有针对性的减肥可能是有帮助的，而不连续的体重增加期可能与反流症状的加重有关[199]。戒烟和减少饮酒是有价值的，因为这两种动因都会降低 LES 压力，降低酸清除率，并损害固有的鳞状上皮防护功能[21,73]。减少进餐量、避免脂肪、祛风剂、排出胃肠气体和巧克力通过减少 tLESR 的发作，以及降低 LES 压力来减少反流频率[21]。此外，一些患者主诉在喝柑橘类饮料、辛辣食品、番茄制品、咖啡、茶或可乐饮料后感到胃灼热。刺激胃酸分泌或食管对低 pH（或高渗溶液）的敏感性可能是这些症状的原因[200]。然而，应避免不加区分地禁用食品，而是根据个人的敏感性进行调整，以更好地促进依从性。最后，如果可能，患者应避免使用降低 LES 压力（见表 46.1）或促进局部食管炎的药物，如某些双膦酸盐类（见第 45 章）。

评估生活方式改变疗效的临床研究有多好？在一项以循证为基础的综述中[21]，关于吸烟、饮酒、巧克力、脂肪食品和柑橘类产品的研究得到了可靠的生理学数据，表明它们的摄入会对症状产生不利影响，或在食管 pH 检测中促进反流。然而，几乎没有令人信服的证据表明，停用这些产品可预料能改善反流症状。在病例对照研究中，只有抬高床头、左侧卧位和体重减轻与 GERD 改善相关[21]。

2. 非处方用药（OTC）

这些药物用于治疗因生活方式不当而引发的轻微的、不频发的胃灼热症状。抗酸剂可增加 LES 的压力，但主要是通过缓冲胃酸起作用。尽管短期内胃灼热症状迅速缓解，但患者可能需要经常服用抗酸剂，通常在餐后 1~3 小时服用。Gaviscon 含有海藻酸和抗酸剂，与唾液混合形成一种高黏性溶液，漂浮在胃池上，起到机械屏障的作用。最近的研究发现，可大量与餐后酸袋共定位，并将其移动到横膈膜下方，导致显著抑制餐后酸反流[201]。一项非处方药的 meta 分析发现，与安慰剂相比，抗酸剂显示出轻微的症状改善[绝对收益为 8%，治疗次数（NNT）为 13]，而 Gaviscon 的疗效最好（绝对收益 26%，NNT 为 4）[202]。然而，这些治疗不能治愈食管炎，长期试验表明，只有 20% 的患者症状得到缓解[203,204]。

非处方用药组胺 2 受体拮抗剂（OTC H2RAs）的剂量通常是标准处方剂量的一半。虽然开始症状缓解的速度不如抗酸剂快，但 OTC H2RAs 可能在 6~10 小时内缓解症状。基于 3 项研究的 meta 分析，在症状缓解/改善方面，激发餐前服用 H2RAs 效果则优于安慰剂（绝对收益为 11%~16%，NNT 为 9~6）[202]。因此，当存在潜在反流活动之前，服用时特别有用。与抗酸药一样，OTC H2RAs 在治愈食管炎方面无效[205]。

由于 PPI 的长期安全性和有效性使 FDA 于 2003 年批准奥美拉唑全剂量（20mg）用于非处方药。药物标签建议每日使用仅 2 周，并建议医生对持续症状进行随访。尽管最初担忧在"现实生活"中滥用这种药物，但早期实际使用数据支持消费者可准确地自我选择是否适合使用 OTC 奥美拉唑，并遵守两周的治疗方案，对频繁胃灼热的处理，需寻求医生的长期治疗[206]。

（二）处方药

经常有胃灼热、食管炎或并发症的患者通常会就诊并接受处方药治疗。促动力药物可纠正与 GERD 相关的动力障碍。然而，临床上治疗短期和长期反流最有效的药物是抑酸药物。

1. 促动力药

直到最近，美国已有 3 种治疗 GERD 的促动力药：①氯贝胆碱，一种胆碱能激动剂；②甲氧氯普胺，一种多巴胺拮抗剂；③西沙比利，一种 5-羟色胺（5-羟色胺 4）受体激动剂；可增加肌间神经丛乙酰胆碱的释放。这些药物通过增加 LES 压力、酸清除或胃排空来改善反流症状。然而，没有一种能改变 tLESR，它们的有效性随着疾病的严重程度而降低[207]。目前的促动力药物在控制胃灼热方面提供了适度的益处，特别是在胃排空延迟的患者中，但在治愈食管炎方面的疗效不可靠，除非与抑酸药物联合使用[207]。

目前促动力药物的使用受到其副作用的很大限制。氯贝胆碱通常会引起面部潮红、视力模糊、头痛、腹部绞痛和尿频。甲氧氯普胺可通过血脑屏障，其疲乏、嗜睡、焦虑和躁动不安的发生率为 20%~50%，罕见引起震颤、帕金森综合征、肌张力障碍和迟发性运动障碍，尤其是老年患者。可通过将给药方案减少到每日两次、晚餐前或睡前服用较大的单次剂量或使用缓释片剂来减少副作用。多潘立酮是另一种不能通过血脑屏障的多巴胺拮抗剂，副作用较少，主要是引起高泌乳素血症和乳头压痛/溢乳。它在美国尚未获批用于 GERD，但可以从加拿大或复合药房买到。西沙必利是治疗 GERD 的最佳促动力药物，但由于报告了严重的心律失常（室性心动过速、室颤、尖端扭转型心动过速和 Q-T 间期延长），以及与药物相关的心搏骤停和死亡报告，西沙必利于 2000 年撤出美国市场[208]。

欧洲研究人员通过对大环内酯类药物（如阿奇霉素）的研究，重新激发了人们对 GERD 促动力药物的兴趣。这类药物可增加胃排空、增加 LES 和近端胃张力，且在小裂孔疝患者中，可取代膈下的酸袋[209]。小型临床研究发现，阿奇霉素可降低 GERD 合并食管裂孔疝患者[209]和肺移植患者[210]的酸反流发作和总酸暴露。

2. tLESR 抑制剂

调节 tLESR 的频率是治疗 GERD 的一个有吸引力的靶点，因为它在所有类型的反流发作中起着关键作用。目前，唯一可降低 tLESR 的药物是巴氯芬，一种 γ-氨基丁酸（GABAB）激动剂，多年来用于治疗痉挛。巴氯芬（5~20mg，每日 3 次）可显著降低 tLESR，减少胃酸和十二指肠反流，并改善治疗 4 周至数月的 GERD 患者的症状[211,212]。巴氯芬的关键问题是耐受性。有高达 20% 的患者因嗜睡、头晕、恶心和呕吐的副作用需要停止服用[211]。已经开发出其他耐受性改善的

GABAB 激动剂[莱索加贝兰(lesogaberan)、阿巴克罗芬-普拉卡比尔(arbaclofen-placarbil)],但主要由于临床疗效有限而被放弃。例如,莱索加贝兰作为 PPI 的附加治疗药物,用于难治性 GERD 症状患者,其缓解率仍较低为 16%,但与 PPI 单药治疗缓解率为 8% 相比具有显著性[213]。在 150 例经常出现胃灼热和/或反刍的患者中,阿巴克罗芬-普拉卡比尔(20mg、40mg 和 60mg,每日 2 次)减少胃灼热事件并不比用 4 周多安慰剂好[214]。最后 mGluR5(代谢型谷氨酸受体 5)受体的负性变构调节剂(ADX 10059)作为单药治疗显示可以改善反流症状和减少反流事件,但在难治性 GERD 患者中未能显示出显著的临床疗效,该成分的进一步开发已经停止[215]。

3. 组胺 2 受体拮抗剂(H2RAs)

这些药物(西咪替丁、雷尼替丁、法莫替丁和尼扎替丁)在控制夜间酸分泌方面比膳食刺激更有效[216]。4 种 H2RAs 在使用适当剂量时同样有效,通常每日两次在餐前服用。GERD 试验发现,与安慰剂相比 H2RA 可显著降低胃灼热,尽管症状难以消除。一项全面的 meta 分析发现,H2RA 治疗长达 12 周后,即使使用更高剂量,食管炎总体的愈合率很少超过 60%(图 46.10B)[217]。但个体间试验的愈合率不同,主要取决于接受治疗的食管炎的严重程度:Ⅰ级和Ⅱ级食管炎的治愈率为 60%~90%,而Ⅲ级和Ⅳ级食管炎尽管采用了高剂量方案,治愈率仅为 30%~50%[217]。

虽然 PPI 比 H2RAs 更有效,但在 PPI 治疗期间夜间酸突破,可能会导致一些患者出现反流症状。在一项研究中,睡前给予 H2RAs 成功消除了这一问题,表明在 PPI 时代 H2RAs 有了的新适应证[218]。然而,这项研究仅使用晚上单次剂量给药,并不能解释在数周至数月内经常对 H2RAs 产生的耐受性[219]。这种耐受性损害了 H2RA 长期夜间给药消除夜间酸突破的有效性[220],但在生活方式不谨慎可能导致夜间不适的情况下,提示根据需要服用药物会起到有用的作用。

H2RA 非常安全,副作用发生率约为 4%,大多数副作用轻微且可逆[216]。服用西咪替丁和雷尼替丁后,发现苯妥英钠、普鲁卡因胺、茶碱和华法林的血清浓度较高,而其他 2 种 H2RAs(法莫替丁、尼扎替丁)未报告这些相互作用。H2RAs 不抑制氯吡格雷的抗血小板作用。

4. 质子泵抑制剂(PPI)

PPI 对膳食刺激和夜间酸分泌的抑制程度明显大于 H2RAs[221],但很少使患者胃酸缺乏。口服摄入之后,酸抑制被延迟,因为 PPI 需要在壁细胞分泌小管中蓄积,以不可逆地与主动分泌的质子泵结合[232]。因此,PPI 从血浆中清除越慢,可递送至质子泵的量就越多。PPI 应该在一天中的第一餐之前服用,此时大多数质子泵变得活跃。因为并非所有质子泵在任何给定的时间都处于活跃状态,因此单次 PPI 剂量不会抑制所有的质子泵。如有必要,可在晚餐前服用第二剂药物,然而,这是一种标签外的指示。PPI 不能"治愈"反流性疾病,而是通过减少酸反流发作次数,以间接方式治疗 GERD。作为交换,弱酸性(pH>4)发作增加,而反流发作总数和近端范围不受 PPI 治疗的影响[164]。

与 H2RAs 相比,PPI(奥美拉唑、兰索拉唑、雷贝拉唑、泮托拉唑和埃索美拉唑)的疗效优于 H2RAs,因为它们能够在每日 10~14 小时内维持胃内 pH 大于 4,而 H2RAs 每日约 6~8 小时[222,223]。PPI 通常在 1~2 周内,完全缓解重度 GERD 患者的胃灼热症状优于 H2RAs(见图 43.10A)[217]。一项 Cochrane meta 分析显示,PPI 治疗在非糜烂性 GERD 和初始治疗中未确诊的反流症状方面优于安慰剂和 H2RA,但其疗效比治疗食管炎患者低 20%~30%[224,225]。与胃灼热不同,

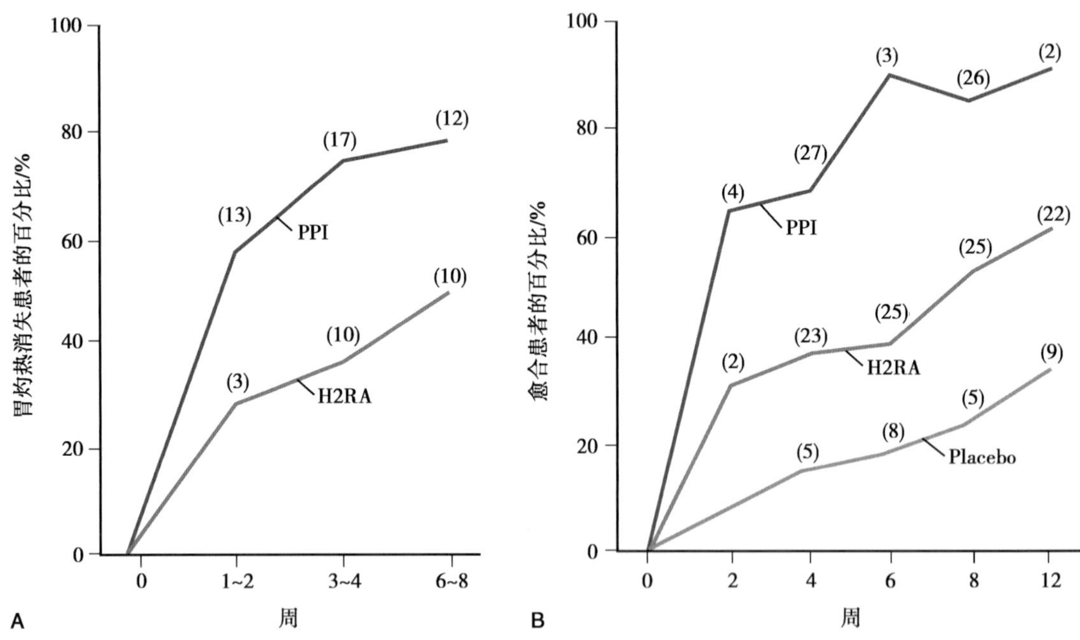

图 46.10 A,基线检查时用 PPI 或 H2RA 纠正胃灼热患者的 8 周症状缓解时间曲线图。与 H2RA 治疗的患者相比,PPI 治疗 2 周的患者中无症状的患者更多,即使在 H2RA 治疗更长时间后也是如此。B,用 PPI、H2RA 和安慰剂治疗的食管炎在 12 周内愈合时间曲线图。在 12 周内,PPI 治疗 4 周愈合食管炎的患者比其他两组多,表明治疗效果显著。每个时间点和治疗纳入的研究数量显示在括号中。PPI,质子泵抑制剂;H2RA,组胺 2 受体抑制剂。(Data based on meta-analysis from Chiba N, Gara CJ, Wilkinson JM, Hunt RH. Speed of healing and symptom relief in grade Ⅱ to Ⅳ gastroesophageal reflux disease: A meta-analysis. Gastroenterology 1997;112:1798-810.)

GERD 反刍症状对 PPI 没有强劲的反应。在最近对 7 项安慰剂对照试验的综述中,与安慰剂相比,反刍的治疗增益平均仅为 17%,比观察到的胃灼热治疗的增益至少低 20%[226]。

对照研究和一项大型 meta 分析报告,80% 以上服用 PPI 的患者在 8 周后甚至重度溃疡性食管炎也完全愈合。相比之下,H2RAs 组为 51%,安慰组为 28%(见图 43.10B)[217,227-229]。在最近的另一篇 Cochrane 综述中[230],PPI 在治疗 4~8 周食管炎愈合方面优于 H2RAs(风险比为 0.47),NNT 为 3。在最初未愈合的患者中,使用相同剂量长期治疗或增加 PPI 剂量通常会 100% 治愈[231]。直至最近,PPI 之间的治疗效果是相似的。然而大量研究发现,在治愈食管炎方面,埃索美拉唑 40mg 优于奥美拉唑 20mg 和兰索拉唑 30mg[232,233]。一项比较埃索美拉唑与所有其他 PPI 的 10 项随机临床试验[234]的 meta 分析发现,LA A/B 级食管炎的治疗优势最小(NNT 分别为 50 和 33),重度 LA C/D 级食管炎的治疗优势更大(NNT 分别为 14 和 8)。这种优势与埃索美拉唑的系统生物利用度较高和患者间变异性较小有关。尽管每日两次频繁用于治疗 GERD,但只有最近的一项日本研究[235],记录了每日两次 PPI 非说明书剂量给药在 8 周内愈合食管炎方面优于每日一次用药。雷贝拉唑 20mg 每日两次(77%)和 10mg 每日两次(78%)的愈合率相似,明显优于雷贝拉唑每日早晨 20mg(59%)。在美国有几种 PPI 可供静脉使用[236]。

最近使用 PPI 增强抑制酸作用的方法包括立即释放奥美拉唑和右旋兰索拉唑。前者含有非肠溶奥美拉唑和抗酸剂,可防止奥美拉唑在胃中不被酸降解,并使其快速吸收。立即释放奥美拉唑可在睡前空腹服用,与埃索美拉唑或兰索拉唑相比,它可更快地控制夜间胃 PH 和夜间酸突破[237]。右旋兰索拉唑 MR 是兰索拉唑的 R-对映体,有 2 个不同的药物释放期(摄入 90 分钟和 4~5 小时),可延长血浆浓度-时间曲线,从而延长酸抑制的持续时间。最佳疗效可能不需要精确的进餐时间[238,239]。在最近的一项安慰剂对照研究中,178 例接受每日两次 PPI 的患者减至每日一次 30mg 右旋兰索拉唑,88% 的患者在 6 周内保持了良好的症状缓解[240]。

PPI 耐受性良好,头痛和腹泻是最常见的副作用。所有 PPI 治疗后空腹血清胃泌素水平均升高,但升高幅度一般不超过正常范围,并在停药后 1~4 周内恢复至基线值。由于与细胞色素 P450 同工酶 P2C19[241]的竞争,奥美拉唑可降低地西泮、华法林和氯吡格雷的清除率。

(三) 维持疗法

GERD 可能是一种慢性复发性疾病,尤其是在 LES 压较低、重度食管炎和症状难以处理的患者中[204]。食管炎治愈后,80% 以上的重度食管炎患者和 15%~30% 的轻度食管炎患者在停药后 6 个月内复发[189,242]。

Cochrane 综述已经确定 PPI 在维持食管炎缓解 6~12 个月以上优于 H2RA[243]。在 10 项随机试验中,PPI 组食管炎的复发率为 22%,而 H2RAs 组为 58%(NNT 为 2.5)。美国食品药品管理局(FDA)已批准所有 PPI(有时为急性剂量的一半)作为维持治疗,但 H2RA 中仅雷尼替丁 150mg 每日两次,具有轻度食管炎维持适应证。现在许多临床医生将严重疾病患者(每日有症状、严重食管炎或并发症)无限期地接受长期 PPI 治疗。这种方法的疗效得到了主要来自荷兰和澳大利亚的公开、有同情心使用数据的支持[244]。在一项 230 例接受 40mg 奥美拉唑治愈的严重食管炎患者的研究中,所有受试者在服用奥美拉唑维持治疗后均保持缓解长达 11 年。超过 60% 的患者维持奥美拉唑 20mg/d 治疗,而仅 12% 的患者需要更高剂量 60mg 或需要更多,证实对 PPI 缺乏耐受性。复发罕见(随访 9.4 年 1 例),未发生狭窄,Barrett 食管也没有进展。

尽管 PPI 能最好地缓解症状和治愈食管炎,但许多患者在最初使用 PPI 缓解症状后,仍长期服用低剂量治疗效果良好。使用这种"降阶梯方法",美国退伍军人事务部的一项研究报告称,71 例接受长期 PPI 治疗的患者中,有 58% 可以转换为 H2RAs 和/或促动力药物或完全停药[245]。年龄较轻和严重的胃灼热症状预示需要 PPI 治疗。总的来说,这种方法为医疗保险体系节省了资金。同一研究者的一项类似研究发现,80% 使用多剂量 PPI 的患者可以减至单剂量 PPI,在 6 个月内保持无症状,并节省大量成本[246]。因此,"一旦服用 PPI,总要服用 PPI"这句格言是不真实的。尽管接受 PPI 治疗,但仍有症状的患者可能有 GERD 以外的其他病因[247]。

(四) PPI 治疗的安全性

PPI 是非常安全的一类药物。由于它的有效性和安全性,2009 年 PPI 在全球的销售额接近 140 亿美元。最初关于发生胃类癌和结肠癌的担忧尚未得到证实[248,249]。最近,文献中充斥着 PPI 长期抑酸会出现潜在不良事件的报告[250]。在美国,此类报告导致 FDA 发布了一些有广泛基础的产品警告(即黑盒子警告),包括所有可用的 PPI,无论是处方药还是非处方药。然而这些研究均来自回顾性护理对照研究,并证明了相关性,而非因果关系[250]。非前瞻性、观察性或随机试验可以证实所涉及的以下讨论的问题。

胃底腺息肉是胃镜检查中最常见的胃息肉,自从这些药物首次被描述以来,它们与长期使用 PPI 的相关性一直是一个有争论的话题。最近的一项研究评估了 599 例患者,其中 322 例使用 PPI,发现 107 例有胃底腺息肉[251]。长期使用 PPI 与胃底腺息肉风险增加高达 4 倍相关。发现 1 例胃底腺息肉伴低度异型增生。这些息肉的发生是由于壁细胞增生和酸抑制导致壁细胞凸起。

最近的研究证实,慢性酸抑制可能与社区获得性肺炎和肠道感染风险增加有关。在一项以斯堪的纳维亚人为主的大型研究中[252],与停止使用 PPI 的患者相比,当前 PPI 使用者发生肺炎的校正相对风险为 1.89。当前 H2RA 使用者患肺炎的风险是停药者的 1.63 倍。在 PPI 使用者中观察到显著的阳性剂量-反应关系。同样,系统回顾和 meta 分析发现,使用抑酸剂时,肠道感染(沙门氏菌、弯曲杆菌和艰难梭状芽孢杆菌)和自发性细菌性腹膜炎风险增加[253,254]。与社区和医院获得性艰难梭状芽孢杆菌相互作用的关系尤其令人惊慌,PPI 使用开始接近抗生素可作为这种感染的一个危险因素。

长期使用 PPI 会影响钙、维生素 B_{12}、镁和铁的吸收。一项来自英国 13 556 例患者的巢式病例对照研究发现,长期使用 PPI 超过 1 年(校正比值比,1.44),尤其是接受高剂量 PPI 的患者(校正比值比,2.65),髋部骨折的风险会增加。在长期 H2RA 使用者中观察到较少,但仍有显著风险[255]。加拿大的一项大型研究也得出了类似的结论[256]，但发现髋部骨折的风险仅在治疗5年后(校正比值比，1.62)和所有骨质疏松性骨折7年后(校正比值比，1.92)才变得明显。然而，最近的横断面、纵向和前瞻性研究(即使是由同一个加拿大研究中心进行研究[257])并不支持这些早期的观察结果，表明存在未被发现的偏倚问题，未来需要进行随机研究来解决这个问题[250,258]。研究表明，如果PPI导致骨质疏松，它们可能干扰不溶性钙的吸收，或可能抑制破骨细胞质子转运系统，从而潜在地减少骨吸收。

PPI可通过降低胃酸度，减少膳食蛋白质中钴胺素的释放或通过促进小肠细菌过度生长(SIBO)，从而增加腔内钴胺素的消耗量，延缓维生素 B_{12} 的吸收。然而队列研究和病例对照研究并未显示PPI的使用与维生素 B_{12} 缺乏之间存在令人信服的联系[250]。

最近，一系列(<50例)病例报告将低镁血症与长期使用PPI相关联[259]。出现重度症状需要住院治疗，一些患者对镁离子补充有抵抗，但所有患者均可通过停用PPI得到纠正，有几例在PPI重启后复发。镁丢失的机制尚不清楚，不能识别是胃肠道或是肾源性消耗。

膳食铁主要是非血红蛋白铁，需要酸才能吸收。动物研究表明，在低酸状态下，铁的吸收受到损害。接受长期PPI治疗的血色病患者每年必须清除的血量显著减少，以使铁保持在适当的水平[260]。另一方面，由于Zollinger-Ellison综合征引起胃酸分泌过多，需要长期高剂量PPI来减少酸分泌的患者，在4年内没有铁缺乏的证据[261]。

PPI被认为是急性间质性肾炎的病因。这似乎是一个罕见的特异质事件，可引起肾间质和肾小管超敏性炎症损伤[262]。慢性肾衰竭、痴呆和死亡也归因于PPI使用，然而，对这种相关性的压倒性担忧可能是潜在的混杂因素[250]。

2009年，FDA发布了一份关于使用PPI和氯吡格雷的患者心血管不良事件可能增加的警告，尤其是与奥美拉唑、兰索拉唑和埃索美拉唑合用。这种担忧是因为氯吡格雷的抗血小板活性需要通过CYP2C19同工酶将前体药转化为活性代谢物。这是一些PPI类药代谢所需的相同通路，但泮托拉唑或右旋兰索拉唑不需要。然而，目前的数据尚不能确凿地表明药物-药物之间的相互作用具有显著的临床意义。最近一项meta分析(27项研究)[263]，集中观察其主要结果(心肌梗死、卒中、支架阻塞或死亡)和次要结果(因心脏事件或血管重建操作的再次住院)发现，PPI和氯吡格雷之间没有一致的不良相互作用。唯一一项大型随机试验证实，与单独使用氯吡格雷相比，氯吡格雷和奥美拉唑联合治疗可显著减少胃肠道出血事件(风险比，0.34)，且无明显的心血管病发病率(风险比，0.99)[264]。

这些不断增加的有关PPI相互作用的报告可能会让公众感到震惊。尽管目前的数据相对薄弱，但它增加了所有医生的职责，即仅为有适应证的患者适当开具PPI，当每日一次治疗剂量足够时，尽量较少每天两次使用PPI，并对长期连续使用PPI保持警惕，用按需治疗替代有症状而无并发症的GERD患者。然而，同样重要的是要认识到，大多数这样的关联是微弱的，并不表明存在因果关系[250]。

(五) 手术治疗

只有外科胃底折叠术才能纠正引起GERD的生理因素，并可能消除长期用药的需要。抗反流手术通过增加基础LES压力、降低tLER和抑制LES完全松弛来减少酸性和非酸性GER[265]。这是通过减少食管裂孔疝进入腹部，重建膈肌裂孔和加固LES来实现的。最常用的两种手术是通过腹部腹腔镜进行的Nissen 360°胃底折叠术和Toupet部分胃底折叠术(图46.11)[265]。前者是一种优越的手术方式，具有较好的长期耐用性，但引起术后吞咽困难和胀气症状较多[266]。一般住院时间为1~2天，许多患者在2周内恢复正常活动。对于病情较重且食管较短的患者，提示有较大的不可复性食管裂孔

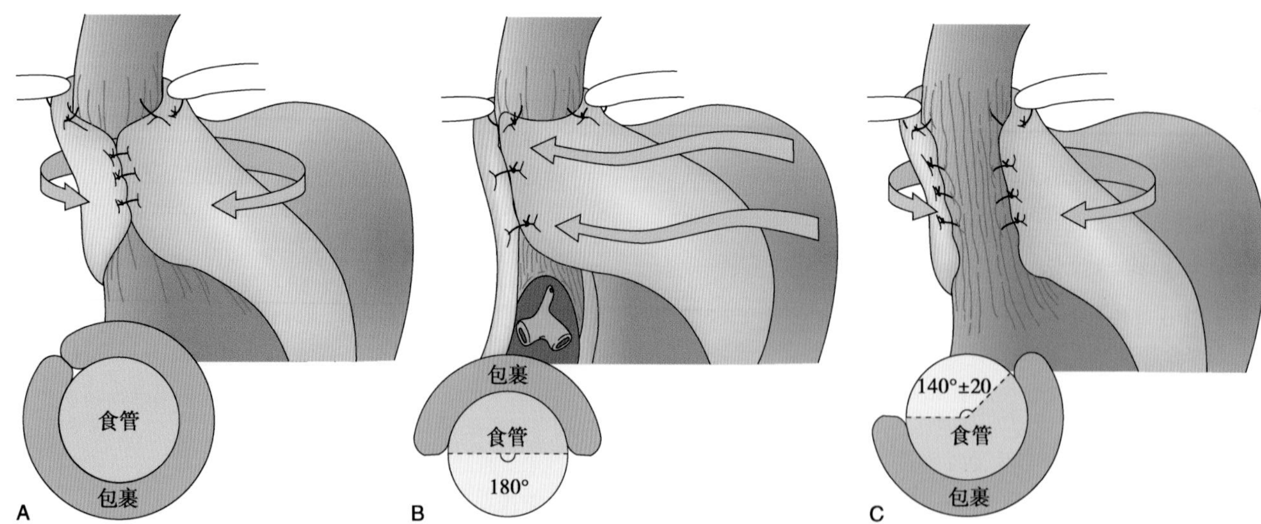

图46.11　抗反流手术中使用的胃底折叠术。A，全世界最流行的是360°折叠的Nissen胃底折叠术。B，在贲门失弛缓症行Heller切开后，为预防胃食管反流，通常使用前包裹(如Thal，Dor)。对于典型的GERD患者，这种修复的经验有限。C，在食管动力不良的患者中流行使用后包裹(Toupet)，因为术后吞咽困难的发生频率低于其他手术。Toupet手术需要220°±20°的包裹。(From Oelschlager BK, Eubanks TR, Pellegrini CA. Hiatal hernia and gastroesophageal reflux disease. In: Townsend CM, Beauchamp RD, Foshee JC, et al., editors. Sabiston textbook of surgery: The biological basis of modern surgical practice. 18th ed. Philadelphia: Saunders; 2007.)

疝、狭窄或长节段 Barrett 食管，需要进行 Collis-lenging 延长手术，以创建一个 3~5cm 长的新食管，使胃底折叠能够在最小张力下放置于腹部[267]。

自从腹腔镜手术问世以来，美国进行的抗反流手术数量几乎是以前的 3 倍。从 1985 年（开放手术）每年 11 000 例，1999 年达到高峰近 32 000 例，但 2006 年趋于平稳，每年约 20 000 例，并在继续逐渐下降[268,269]。在一项系统性综述中，确定了 6 项随机对照试验，涉及 449 例患者，对开放式和腹腔镜胃底折叠术进行了比较[266]，两种手术的复发率无显著差异，腹腔镜胃底折叠术与手术发病率较低（NNT 为 8）和较短的住院时间有关。

在 PPI 治疗时代，治疗后症状消退有助于预测典型或非典型症状的抗反流手术的成功[270]。抗反流手术是以下患者的合理选择：①PPI 控制良好的典型或非典型 GERD 症状的健康患者，由于药物费用、药物依从性差或担心长期用药的副作用而希望进行替代治疗；②PPI 治疗不能控制的反刍容量大和误吸症状的患者；③年轻患者中复发性消化性狭窄[266]。对 PPI 治疗难以控制的患者很可能有其他病因（如药物性食管炎、胃轻瘫、贲门失弛缓症、功能性胃灼热），应谨慎进行手术，尤其是那些仅有食管外主诉的患者[271]。

抗反流手术前必须进行检测。有必要进行内镜检查以排除狭窄、Barrett 食管、异型增生或癌。食管钡剂造影检查有助于确定不可复位的食管裂孔疝、食管缩短和食管动力不良。食管测压结合阻抗检查可确定食管泵功能薄弱，以及既往误诊的贲门失弛缓症或硬皮病。在非糜烂性 GERD 或对 PPI 治疗无反应的食管炎患者中，食管 pH 检测是必须的。胃酸分泌功能测定（如有）、空腹血清胃泌素测定和胃排空试验可能适用于选定的患者。经过仔细的检测可使大约 30% 的患者修改原来手术或改变原来的诊断[272]。

抗反流手术可缓解 90% 以上患者的反流症状，减少食管狭窄扩张的需求，但 Barrett 食管很少消退，发生显性食管癌的风险没有变化[273]。在两项大型随机研究中[274,275]，开放式和腹腔镜抗反流手术未发现优于 PPI 治疗，尤其是在允许剂量滴定时。例如，在欧洲 LOTUS 随机研究中，埃索美拉唑组 5 年症状缓解率为 92%（95% 可信区间为 89%~96%），腹腔镜手术组为 85%（95% 可信区间为 81%~90%）[275]。抗反流手术后死亡率罕见（<1%），但高达 25% 的患者术后出现新的症状，包括吞咽困难、胀气、腹泻和排气增加[276]。大多数症状在 1 年内有所改善，但持续主诉表明包裹过紧、胃底折叠术移位或迷走神经意外损伤。而成功的抗反流手术并不能保证永久治愈，但长期研究表明症状可持续缓解 20~30 年[277,278]。最佳手术结果是由经验丰富的外科医生在高手术量中心获得，他们报告只有 10%~17% 的患者出现长期症状复发[265,276,279]。然而，许多手术是在低手术量社区医院进行的，手术效果差异很大[278]。根据长期随访研究，25%~62% 的患者在抗反流手术后 5~15 年重新恢复使用某种类型的抑酸药物[269,276,280]。然而，通过 pH 检测发现 GERD 复发的证据并不常见。

三级专科中心医院的胃底折叠术失败率增加。失败最常见的原因是完整的胃底折叠疝入胸腔、“滑脱”的胃底折叠伴复发性食管裂孔疝（可能是由于食管过短）、通过完整胃底折叠的食管旁疝、胃底折叠过紧和胃底折叠错位（通常发生在胃贲门）。胃底折叠术的彻底失败现在很少见[281]。修正抗反流手术必须由经验丰富的外科医师在进行彻底的食管测试后进行，因为与初次手术相比，再次手术增加了发病率和死亡率。

（六）新型内镜/外科手术治疗

自 20 世纪 90 年代末推出以来，一系列内镜治疗[射频治疗（Stretca）、非手术内视镜疗法（Endocinch）、液态化学聚合物注射治疗（Enteryx）等]GERD 都未能显示长期疗效。此外，副作用和并发症（有些是致命的）在广泛使用中很常见[282]。因此，2006 年美国胃肠病学会声明建议“现有的数据表明，目前尚无 GERD 内镜治疗的明确适应证”[283]，这一点最近得到了美国胃肠病学会指南的支持[284]。尽管射频治疗（Streta）在第二次弃用前有一个短暂的重现，但这些设备中的大多数已经被拆除。尽管如此，通过内镜重建正常食管裂孔和有效 LES 的新尝试仍在继续。最新的方法是经口无切口胃底折叠术，使用内镜下放置的聚丙烯紧扣件重新折叠 200°~270°[285]。初步研究显示症状改善，尤其是反刍症状和 PPI 的使用减少。但是，随着时间的推移，紧扣件往往会脱落，一项系统性综述报告称，60% 的患者 GERD 症状复发率与 PPI 的复发率相似，尽管剂量通常低于治疗前[286]。

在不改变贲门解剖结构的情况下，一些新型的手术创新可以缓解反流症状，副作用极小甚至没有。第一种是磁性括约肌，它是一条钛珠项链，在贲门周围放置磁芯，对食管裂孔剥离最小。当食管处于静止状态时，磁力会充分增强 LES 足以防止反流，但足够弱，允许蠕动伴吞咽打开装置。在一项对 100 例 GERD 患者进行的为期 3 年的前瞻性研究中[287]，64% 的患者酸反流值恢复正常，93% 的患者 PPI 使用量减少了 50%，92% 的患者生活质量显著改善。68% 的患者术后经常出现吞咽困难，1 年时为 11%，3 年时为 4%。6 例患者移除了该设置，3 例因严重吞咽困难。这种长期疗效可维持长达 5 年，仅 15% 的患者恢复使用 PPI[288]。目前有报告称设置侵蚀食管或胃，但似乎很少见。

第二项手术创新是在不干扰 LES 松弛的情况下，对 LES 进行电刺激以改善 LES 压力[289]。该手术是通过腹腔镜在 LES 固有肌层中放置双极缝合电极，该电极与前腹部皮下囊袋中的植入式脉冲发生器连接[290]。来自智利的对 24 例 GERD 和小食管裂孔疝（<2cm）患者进行的一项研究报告显示，在 6 个月内，电刺激使症状评分提高了 75%，91% 的患者停用 PPI，24 小时内食管 pH 低于 4 的中位时间从基线时的 10.1% 改善至 6 个月时的 5.1%。无患者主诉吞咽困难、腹部胀气或无法嗳气。美国正在进行一项 FDA 为期 1 年的随机随访研究。

这些新疗法的潜力令人兴奋，但为了避免重蹈 GERD 内镜治疗时代的覆辙，需要进行至少随访 5 年的仔细随机研究，并对社区使用这些设备的经验进行细致的监测。此外，到目前为止，在随机研究中尚未将新设置与金标准 Nissen 胃底折叠术进行比较。出于这些原因，许多私营保险公司对这些新业务一直迟迟不采取补偿措施[285]。

十一、消化性食管狭窄的治疗

食管狭窄和食管环患者的吞咽困难与狭窄直径和食管炎的严重程度有关[291]。当食管管腔直径小于13mm时，吞咽困难是常见的，需要进行食管扩张。简单的短狭窄可以通过橡胶Hurst(圆形末端)或Maloney(锥形末端)尺寸递增的充汞扩张器(16~60Fr;3Fr=1mm)盲法经口进行扩张。复杂的、更长的、更紧的或更不规则的狭窄需要使用中心中空、Savary、塑料覆盖的聚乙烯扩张器或球囊(Gruentzig)扩张器沿导丝进行探条扩张[292]。PPI的广泛使用显著影响了我们对消化性狭窄和食管环的治疗。PPI在缓解狭窄患者的胃灼热和吞咽困难症状方面优于H2RAs，同时降低了重复扩张的频率和治疗这些患者的成本[293]。社区和退伍军人医院的几项研究表明，复发性狭窄的发生率下降了约33%。这种减少的时间线与1995年以来PPI使用的显著增加相平行[294]。另一项随机研究令人信服地表明，在有症状的Schatzki环患者中，探条扩张术后维持PPI治疗可显著降低环的未来复发[196]。对更多PPI和扩张治疗无效的顽固性狭窄，可能需要在病灶内注射类固醇或用自膨式塑料支架[295]。病灶内注射类固醇可阻止胶原沉积并促进其分解，这种疗法有可能减少瘢痕形成。通常剂量为40mg/mL，用生理盐水以1:1稀释，然后在最狭窄部位的所有4个象限中以0.5mL等份注射[296]。自膨式塑料支架是可以取出的，比金属支架具有更高的膨胀力，从而减少了移位。在其他治疗失败的患者中，在手术干预之前，大系列样本显示正确放置的成功率为100%，短期缓解率为80%[297]。支架通常在3个月后取出。支架移位是最常见的并发症，发生率为1%。对于选定的患者，食管自扩张可能是一种替代方法，避免了手术并显著降低了医疗卫生服务[298]。

（程妍　曹红燕 译，袁农 校）

参考文献

第 47 章　Barrett 食管

Stuart Jon Spechler, Rhonda F. Souza 著

章节目录

一、诊断 …… 655
二、流行病学 …… 655
三、发病机制 …… 656
四、肿瘤的分子生物学 …… 656
五、异型增生 …… 658
六、治疗 …… 659
（一）胃食管反流病的治疗 …… 659
（二）阿司匹林和其他非甾体抗炎药 …… 659
（三）异常增生的内镜监测 …… 659
（四）黏膜肿瘤的治疗 …… 660
（五）建议 …… 662

Barrett 食管是一种具有胃和肠特征且易发生恶性肿瘤的异常柱状上皮取代了通常位于食管远端的复层鳞状上皮的病变[1]。该病症以澳大利亚外科医生 Norman Barrett 的名字命名，他于 1950 年提出的引起人们对柱状上皮内衬食管的关注[2]。Barrett 食管是慢性胃食管反流病（GERD）的结果，损伤的食管鳞状上皮通过化生过程而愈合，在化生过程中柱状上皮取代了反流受损的鳞状上皮。柱状上皮内衬的食管不会引起症状，这种情况之所以具有临床意义，只因为它是食管腺癌发生的危险因素，食管腺癌在过去的几十年中发生频率增加了 7 倍以上[3]。

一、诊断

Barrett 食管通过内镜检查确诊，必须满足 2 个标准。第一，内镜医生必须确定柱状上皮内衬在食管远端 1cm 或以上。第二，柱状上皮的活检标本必须显示有肠化生的证据，即从一种成熟的组织类型转变为另一种成熟的组织类型。为了确定柱状上皮内衬在食管远端，内镜医师首先必须定位食管胃交界处（EGJ），它被认为是 EGJ 胃皱襞的最近端范围，然后确定柱状上皮从 EGJ 上方延伸 1cm 或以上进入食管（图 47.1）。内镜下，柱状上皮呈淡红色、质地呈丝绒样，很容易与正常的食管鳞状上皮区分，后者苍白而有光泽。专家们对确认食管中是否存在化生所需的上皮组织类型存在分歧[1]。几乎所有人都同意，发现有杯状细胞的肠型上皮（被称为肠化生、特异肠化生或特异柱状上皮）是化生的明确证据。大多数已发表的关于 Barrett 食管的研究都已将肠化生作为必要的诊断标准。然而，一些权威人士认为，胃贲门型黏膜几乎完全由黏液分泌细胞组成，也是化生的，具有恶性倾向[4]，可考虑 Barrett 食管的诊断[5]。尽管这一争论仍未解决，但美国胃肠病

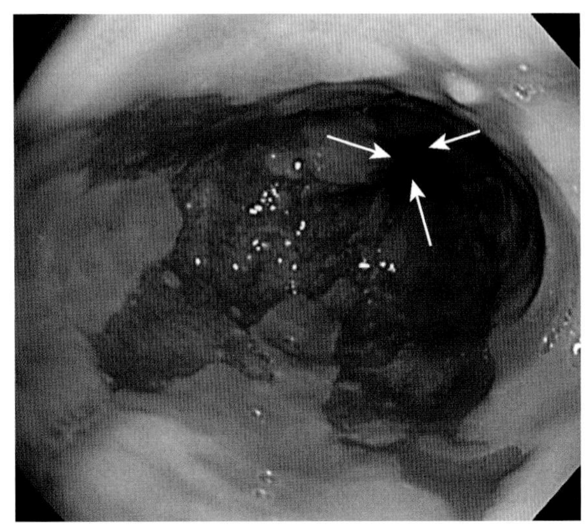

图 47.1　Barrett 食管的内镜照片。箭头标记食管胃交界处（EGJ），内镜下确定为胃皱襞的最近端范围。Barrett 上皮为淡红色和丝绒样质地与食管鳞状上皮的灰白色有光泽外观形成鲜明对比。注意，Barrett 柱状上皮延伸到 EGJ 上方至食管远端

学会要求具有杯状细胞的肠化生，作为 Barrett 食管的诊断标准。

Barrett 食管可进一步分类为长节段（当化生上皮延伸至 EGJ 上方至少 3cm 时）或短节段（当化生上皮沿食管远端延伸<3cm 时）[6]。短节段 Barrett 食管是目前最常见的疾病形式，直到 1994 年 Spechler 等对其进行了描述，才被广泛认识[7]。另一个 Barrett 食管分类系统，即 Prague C 和 M 标准，确定了 Barrett 化生的圆周（C）和最大范围（M）[8]。数据表明 Barrett 食管的癌变风险随内衬的化生黏膜范围而变化。

二、流行病学

典型的 Barrett 食管通常是在中老年人为评估 GERD 症状而进行的内镜检查中发现的[9]。诊断时的平均年龄约为 55 岁。这种情况在 10 岁以下的儿童中罕见，在 5 岁以下的儿童中几乎不存在[10]。在大系列检查中，白种人男性占主导地位，由于未知的原因，Barrett 食管在黑人和亚洲人群中并不常见[11]，尽管最近在亚洲国家的患病率有所增加[12]。吸烟也与 Barrett 食管相关[13]。在因 GERD 症状而接受内镜检查的成年患者中，长节段 Barrett 食管占 3%～5%，而短节段 Barrett 食管占 10%～20%。在西方国家的一般成年人中，Barrett 食管（主要是短节段）的患病率为 1.6%～6.8%[14,15]。

已发表的关于长节段 Barrett 食管患者癌症年发病率估计高达 2.9%，但 2000 年发表的一份报告显示，其中许多估计

被夸大了,因为它们是基于存在发表偏倚的较老的小型研究[16]。在新千年的前十年,人们普遍认为非异型增生 Barrett 食管患者的癌症风险约为每年 0.5%。然而,最近的研究表明,此类患者的癌症风险更低,每年仅为 0.12%~0.33%的范围内[17-20]。

食管腺癌的流行病学与 Barrett 食管相似[21-24]。GERD 与这两种疾病密切相关,与 Barrett 食管一样,食管腺癌主要影响白种人男性。肥胖,尤其是中心性肥胖,易患 Barrett 食管和食管腺癌[25],美国肥胖率的急剧上升与 Barrtt 食管癌患病率的类似上升相平行。这些与肥胖相关的机制尚不清楚,但可能与中心性肥胖易患 GERD 有关。这可能是由于腹内压增加而诱发 GERD(另见第 46 和 48 章)。肥胖还与血清促增殖激素[如胰岛素样生长因子 I(IGF-1)和瘦素(leptin)],水平升高相关,并与抗增殖激素脂联素水平降低相关,这些因素可能是导致 Barrett 食管癌变的原因。

有人提出,在西方人群中 Hp 感染频率的下降也可能是食管腺癌发病率上升的原因之一(见第 48 章)。许多研究表明,Hp 感染可预防 Barrett 食管的发生和肿瘤发展,这可能是因为在一部分患者中,这种感染可通过减少胃酸的分泌来预防 GERD[21]。似乎可预防食管腺癌发生的其他因素包括使用阿司匹林和其他非甾体抗炎药,以及摄入富含水果和蔬菜的饮食[22-24]。虽然吸烟和饮酒是食管鳞状细胞癌非常强的风险因素,但吸烟仅适度增加食管腺癌的风险,而饮酒似乎根本不会影响该风险。最后,有人提出,食管腺癌发病率的上升可能是由于第二次世界大战后西方国家广泛使用硝酸盐肥料,导致绿叶蔬菜中膳食硝酸盐的摄入量增加有关[26]。

三、发病机制

Barrett 食管的发病机制始于 GERD 引起的食管损伤,长节段 Barrett 食管患者通常伴有重度 GERD(见第 46 章)。表 47.1 列出了在 Barrett 食管患者中报告的一些生理异常,并提示了这些异常如何造成 GERD 严重程度。个体患者可能表现出任何、全部或无这些异常,其在 Barrett 食管中的患病率存在争议。例如,一些研究者描述了长节段 Barrett 食管患者的胃酸分泌正常[27]。此外,许多短节段 Barrett 食管患者无 GERD 症状,且无食管炎的内镜征象。事实上,一项大型研究表明,无论是否存在 GERD 症状,短节段 Barrett 食管可能影响大约 5% 的成年人[14]。研究表明,即使是健康志愿者中,食管最远端在一日中也有 10% 以上的时间暴露在酸液中[28]。当亚硝酸盐(由膳食硝酸盐产生)与酸反应生成一氧化氮时,此类酸暴露可直接或间接损害食管。在摄入硝酸盐的 GERD 患者中,观察到食管远端存在高浓度的一氧化氮[26]。

表 47.1 在 Barrett 食管患者中导致 GERD 的生理学异常*

异常	潜在后果
食管下括约肌极度低压	胃食管反流
食管动力无效	反流物质的清除缺陷
胃酸分泌过多	高酸性胃液反流
十二指肠胃反流	胆汁酸和胰酶反流引起的反流性食管损伤
唾液分泌 EGF 减少	反流损伤的食管黏膜愈合延迟
食管对反流腐蚀性物质引起的疼痛敏感性降低	未能开始治疗

*这些异常的详细讨论见第 46 章。
EGF,表皮生长因子;GERD,慢性胃食管反流病。

在 Barrett 食管中,反流受损的鳞状上皮被肠型上皮所取代,推测这种上皮对 GERD 损伤更具抵抗力。由于在食管中正常发现不了肠型细胞,这一过程必须涉及 GERD 诱导的祖细胞中关键发育转录因子的分子重新编程,从而引起化生[29]。然而,这些祖细胞的身份特征尚不明确,有几种候选细胞。有人认为,当 GERD 导致成熟的食管鳞状细胞转分化为柱状细胞,或当 GERD 引起未成熟的祖细胞异常分化时,就会发生 Barrett 化生[30]。这些祖细胞的潜在食管来源包括鳞状上皮的基底细胞,或食管黏膜下腺导管内衬的细胞[30,31]。另外,如第 46 章所述,Barrett 祖细胞可能从胃贲门迁移到反流损伤的食管[32],从胃食管交接处发现的残留胚胎型细胞巢[33],或来自最近描述的位于鳞柱交界处的移行基底细胞群[34]。最后,在反流性食管炎大鼠模型中,显示 Barrett 化生是由循环骨髓干细胞发展而来[35]。反流性食管炎导致 Barrett 食管的鳞状到柱状上皮化生的上调基因,包括 *CDX* 基因,已知其介导肠上皮细胞分化和刺猬靶基因 *BMP4*(骨形态发生蛋白-4)和 *FOXA2*,也参与柱状细胞分化[36-38]。

Barrett 上皮细胞似乎比天然鳞状上皮细胞更能抵抗反流诱导的食管损伤。例如,与鳞状细胞不同的是,Barrett 细胞分泌黏蛋白并表达紧密连接蛋白 18(claudin 18),这些特征使上皮更能抵抗酸消化性攻击[39,40]。遗憾的是,Barrett 上皮也容易发生肿瘤。

四、肿瘤的分子生物学

在癌变过程中,Barrett 上皮细胞积累了一系列遗传和表观遗传学改变,这一改变赋予细胞恶性肿瘤的核心生理属性(2000 年由 Hanahan 和 Weinberg 提出的)(见第 1 章)[41]。这些属性包括生长信号的自给自足、对抗生长信号不敏感、逃避细胞凋亡、无限的复制潜能、持续的血管生成以及侵入邻近结构和转移的能力(图 47.2)。最近,Hanahan 和 Weinberg 增加了恶性肿瘤的另外两个生理标志:重新编程能量代谢以支持持续增殖的能力,以及逃避免疫细胞(T 和 B 淋巴细胞、巨噬细胞和自然杀伤细胞)破坏的能力[42]。

在 Barrett 食管肿瘤进展的过程中描述了许多基因改变。尽管单一的这种改变可能有多种不同的效应,但从概念上讲,根据其赋予的主要生理性癌症属性对改变进行分类是有用的[43]。例如,癌基因[如细胞周期蛋白 D1(cyclin D1)、K-ras]、生长因子(如转化生长因子-α)和生长因子受体(如 EGF 受体)的表达使 Barrett 细胞能够获得生长信号的自给自足。对抗生长信号的不敏感主要通过肿瘤抑制基因(如 TP53 和 p16)的失活而发生。TP53 的失活也能使细胞逃避凋亡。端粒酶的重新激活,使细胞能够取代细胞分裂所需的端粒,从而可赋予细胞无限的复制潜能。肿瘤可通过分泌血管生成因子,如血管内皮生长因子(VEGF)增加其血管供应。最后,为了使肿瘤细胞侵袭和转移,它们必须通过破坏细胞黏附蛋白(如钙黏蛋白和连环蛋白)和通过分泌酶(如基质金属蛋白酶)降解细胞外基质,使自身与周围细胞分离。

在 Barrett 食管中,基因组不稳定性和促肿瘤微环境促进了恶性肿瘤核心生理属性的获得[44]。Barrett 上皮细胞通过改变细胞 DNA 含量的染色体片段的得失来显示基因组的不稳定性。非整倍体是细胞 DNA 含量异常的状态,非整倍体细胞发生肿瘤进展的风险增加[45]。非整倍体可通过流式细胞仪、荧光原位杂交和自动图像细胞仪检测,后两种技术用于常规临床实践更可行[46,47]。在一些肿瘤中,具有促肿瘤作用的免疫细胞浸润也有助于获得恶性属性,但对免疫细胞在 Barrett 食管中的促肿瘤作用知之甚少[45,48]。非整倍体被认为是 Barrett 食管肿瘤进展的生物标志物,上一段讨论的许多基因改变也是如此。尽管已经有一些有前途的研究,尤其是那些使用生物标志物的研究[49],胃肠病学协会目前不赞同临床常规使用生物标志物对 Barrett 食管患者进行临床管理。

全基因组测序和全外显子测序(仅限于基因编码区)等基因组技术的最新进展,对了解 Barrett 细胞如何成为肿瘤细胞有很大贡献。对从 Barrett 腺癌相关的 Barrett 化生区域提取的 DNA 进行全外显子测序,结果发现非肿瘤化生的体细胞突变频率高于前列腺癌或乳腺癌,突变模式表明氧化应激引起的基因组织损伤(可能是由于 GERD 引起的)(见图 47.2)[50]。非异型增生的 Barrett 化生和相关的腺癌都表现出 p53 肿瘤抑制基因的突变,这证明 *p53* 突变发生在 Barrett 癌变的早期。致癌基因激活似乎发生较晚,因为它们只在异型增生和癌组织中发现[50]。

有趣的是,新的基因组技术揭示了 Barrett 癌变的两条一般途径:"传统途径"(涉及肿瘤抑制基因改变的逐步积累,随后是癌基因激活、基因组不稳定和恶性转化)和 *p53* 突变后全基因组加倍,导致基因组不稳定、癌基因扩增和恶性转化的"基因组加倍途径"(图 47.3)。Barrett 化生中的大多数肿瘤(62.5%)似乎是通过基因组加倍途径发展的,这可能是比传统途径更快的恶性肿瘤途径[50]。通过基因组加倍的快速癌症发展,可能解释了内镜监测在 Barrett 食管中检测癌症进展的频繁失败。

与上述通过组织样本基因组分析确定体细胞突变的研究不同,全基因组关联研究(GWAS)确定了种系变异,通常使用全血标本中的 DNA 进行。GWAS 表明,不相关的 Barrett 食管和食管腺癌受试者在基因组特定位置的单核苷酸多态性(SNPs)有大量重叠,提示 Barrett 食管及其癌症具有共同的遗传易感性[51]。最近的 GWAS 分析了炎症通路中选择的 SNPs,发现环氧合酶通路(特别是抗氧化微粒体谷胱甘肽 s-转移酶 1 基因)的种系变异与 Barrett 食管和食管腺癌的发生显著相关[52]。另一项 GWAS 探索了 7 个 SNP(作为 Barrett 食管的风险因素)与几种众所周知的 Barrett 食管流行病学风险因素(GERD、吸烟和 BMI)之间的相关性[53]。只有 FOXP1 基因中的一个 SNP(它调节食管发育)和至少每周出现反流症状被发现可改变发生 Barrett 食管和食管腺癌的风险。通过这些新的"生物组学"方法鉴定新的基因环境相互作用,很可能彻底改变我们对 Barrett 食管如何发展和进展为食管癌的认识。

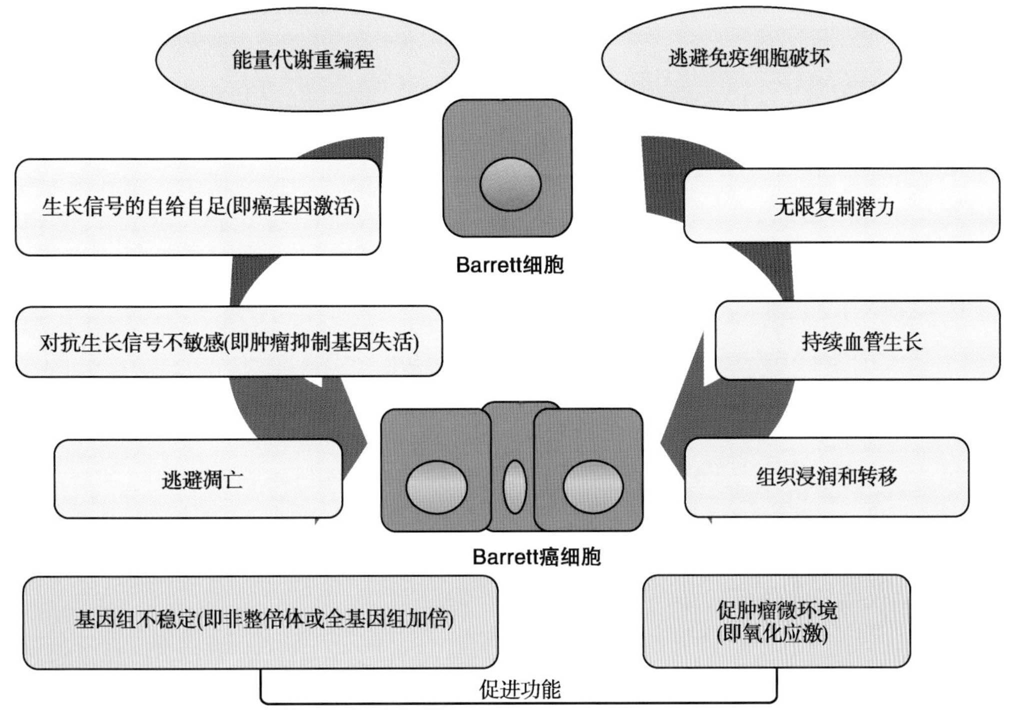

图 47.2　Barrett 食管肿瘤的分子生物学。癌细胞的核心生理属性显示为蓝色。2011 年提出的 2 个额外病理生理学特征以绿色显示。橙色的方框是促进的特征,如基因组不稳定和促肿瘤的微环境,可能允许 Barrett 细胞快速获得癌细胞的生理属性

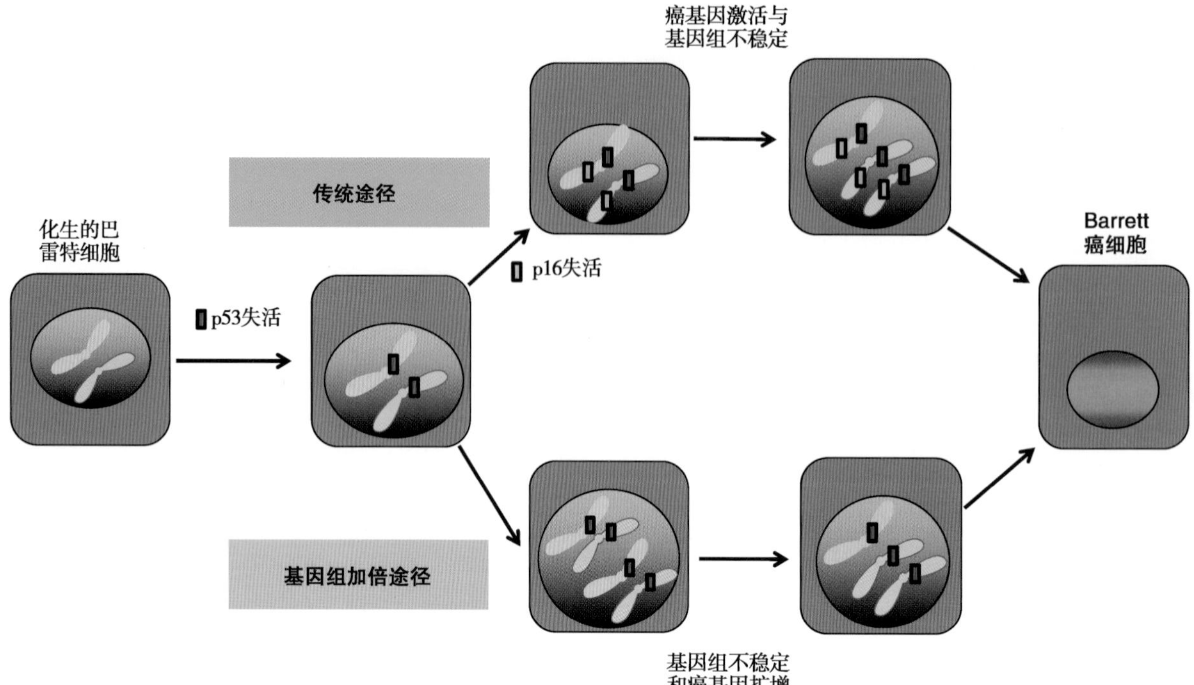

图 47.3　Barrett 食管癌发生的途径。化生性 Barrett 细胞首先获得导致 p53 失活的突变。在传统途径中，抑癌基因 *p16* 的改变逐步累积，随后癌基因激活，基因组不稳定最终导致癌形成。在基因组加倍途径中，*p53* 突变的 Barrett 细胞发生全基因组加倍，随后基因组不稳定和癌基因扩增，导致癌形成。基因组加倍途径已被认为是一种癌形成的更快途径，可能解释了内镜监测无法检测 Barrett 食管癌进展的原因

五、异型增生

在肿瘤性 Barrett 细胞恶性变之前，赋予恶性肿瘤生理属性的一些相同的遗传和表观遗传学改变，也会引起病理学家认为是异型增生的组织形态学改变（图 47.4）。异型增生（也称为上皮内瘤变）可被视为不受调控的细胞生长的遗传和表观遗传学改变的组织学表达[54,55]。通过食管活检标本的细胞学和结构异常可识别异型增生，包括：①细胞核变化，如增大、多形性、深染、分层和非典型有丝分裂；②细胞质成熟丧失；③小管和绒毛状表面拥挤。根据组织学异常的程度，将异型增生分为低级别或高级别，更明显的异常反映了更严重的

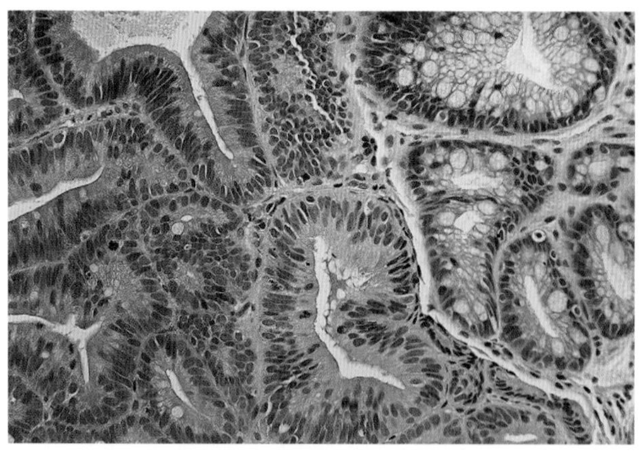

图 47.4　Barrett 食管异型增生的组织病理学。在内镜监测期间采集的活检标本病理检查显示，显微照片 11 点位的低级别异型增生和中心的高级别异型增生

基因损伤和更大的致癌可能性。病理学家很难区分 Barrett 食管的低级别异型增生和反流性食管炎引起的反应性改变，对低级别异型增生的诊断观察者之间一致性可能低于 50%。而对高级别异型增生的诊断观察者之间一致性更好（约 85%），但病理学家在区分高级别异型增生和黏膜内癌方面存在很大分歧（见第 48 章）。

Barrett 食管中的异型增生通常与可见的黏膜不规则性相关，但这些不规则性通常不易观察到，很容易遗漏，特别是经验不多的医师[56]。此外，异型增生的范围和严重程度可能是片状、分布不均的。这些因素导致了识别异型增生的活检取样误差的实质性问题。为了发现 Barrett 食管中的异型增生，内镜医师传统上使用“西雅图活检方案”，这是一种随机活检取样系统，在整个 Barrett 化生长度上，以 1～2cm 的间隔进行 4 象限活检[57]。然而，最近对 2 项射频消融（RFA）试验的分析发现，异型增生最有可能出现在 Barrett 化生节段的近端一半，这提示未来的活检方案可能会被修改为优先对近端节段进行活检[58]。很明显，西雅图活检方案经常遗漏异型增生区域，甚至癌区域。最近一项系统性综述和 meta 分析发现，在初次内镜检查诊断为非异型增生或低度异型增生 Barrett 食管并随访 3 年或以上的患者中，25% 后来诊断为食管腺癌的患者在初次内镜检查 1 年内发现癌症[59]。这表明在首次检查时已存在和遗漏了癌。在因内镜活检显示 Barrett 食管高度异型增生而接受食管切除术的老年患者系列中，在多达 30%～40% 的切除食管中发现了侵袭性癌[60]。然而，对那些早期研究的评论性综述表明，13% 是对这种情况下侵袭性癌频率的更准确估计[61]。随着现代高清内镜和较新的诊断技

术，如内镜黏膜切除术（见后文），发现异型增生患者侵袭性癌的误诊率应非常低。

许多先进的成像技术已被用于提高 Barrett 食管异型增生和早期癌症的检测，包括色素内镜、自发荧光内镜、放大内镜、窄带成像、光学相干断层扫描、拉曼（Raman）检测方法、共聚焦激光显微内镜和容积激光显微内镜（见第 48 章）[52,62-64]。在经过适当培训和专业技能的内镜医生手中，这些先进技术可以识别常规白光内镜检查可能不明显的肿瘤性病变。然而，胃肠病学协会并不强制要求在常规临床实践中使用这些先进的成像技术，使用高清晰度白光内镜检查和随机四象限活检进行仔细的内镜检查仍然是标准方法。

非异型增生 Barrett 食管患者发展为癌的总发生率约为每年 0.25%。一项研究表明，非肿瘤性 Barrett 食管患者每年发生 4.3% 的低级别异型增生，每年发生 0.9% 的高级别异型增生[65]。由于难以确诊和研究结果的相互矛盾，Barrett 食管低级别异型增生的自然史仍存在争议。在一项研究中，两位病理学专家复查了在荷兰社区医院诊断为低级别异型增生的 147 例患者的病理切片，专家们仅在 15% 的病例中证实了这一诊断[66]。然而，在这些确诊病例中，9 年后进展为肿瘤的累积风险为 85%。相反，美国一项 210 例低级别异型增生患者平均随访 6.2 年的研究发现，每年的进展率仅为 0.4% 和病理学家的诊断共识与肿瘤进展无关[67]。对于高级别异型增生的患者，癌的年发展率约为 6%[54]。

六、治疗

（一）胃食管反流病的治疗

Barrett 食管患者 GERD 治疗的一般方法与无 Barrett 食管的 GERD 患者推荐的方法非常相似（见第 46 章）。然而，一个重要的区别是，许多权威人士提倡对 Barrett 食管患者进行质子泵抑制剂（PPI）维持治疗，而不考虑 GERD 的症状和内镜体征如何。这种做法是基于间接证据表明酸反流促进 Barrett 化生的癌变，积极控制酸反流可能会阻止癌变[68-72]。然而，这个问题仍然存在很大的争议，因为对它的研究已经得出了相反的结果。对 7 项研究的 meta 分析发现（包括 2 813 例 Barrett 化生患者和 317 例 Barrett 肿瘤患者），PPI 的使用与高级别异型增生和/或食管腺癌风险显著降低相关[校正比值比 0.29；95% 可信区间（CI）0.12～0.79][73]。然而，随后对 5 712 例 Barrett 患者进行的 9 项观察性研究的 meta 分析发现，与 PPI 使用相关的食管肿瘤风险降低并不具有统计学意义（未校正的比值比 0.43，95% 可信区间 0.17～1.08）[74]，一项基于人群的 796 例患者的队列研究，492 例接受 PPI 维持治疗的瑞典成人甚至描述了 PPI 使用者食管腺癌的总体 SIR 升高为 3.93（95% 可信区间 3.63～4.24）[75]。然而，大多数研究表明 PPI 可降低 Barrett 食管恶性进展的风险[76]，ACG 关于 Barrett 食管治疗的最新指南建议 Barrett 患者应接受每日一次 PPI 治疗进行化学预防[77]。

使用食管 pH 监测的研究表明，PPI 给药剂量未能使食管酸暴露正常化时，Barrett 患者可能会无症状。在一项 48 例 Barrett 食管患者的此类研究中，24 例在 PPI 治疗期间出现持续性异常酸反流，从而消除了 GERD 症状[78]。有人提出，长节段 Barrett 食管患者可能对 PPI 特别耐药，但一项研究表明，该问题并非由于胃对 PPI 的抗分泌作用产生耐药所致[79]。在该研究中，接受高剂量埃索美拉唑治疗的长节段 Barrett 食管患者表现出正常程度的胃酸抑制，但高达 23% 的患者仍有异常的食管酸暴露。这表明 Barrett 食管患者所谓的 PPI 抵抗是其具有严重的反流素质的结果。

有人提出，在预防 Barrett 食管癌方面，胃底折叠术可能比 PPI 药物治疗更有效，但关于该问题的高质量研究通常驳斥了这一论点[80-83]。在最近对 10 项比较手术或药物治疗 GERD 患者癌风险的研究进行的系统综述和 meta 分析中，总体固定效应模型显示，两种治疗对癌风险的影响相似（IRR 0.76，95% 可信区间 0.42～1.39）[84]。然而，仅限于 4 项最现代研究（2000 年后发表）的亚组分析表明，手术在降低 Barrett 食管癌风险方面显著优于药物治疗（IRR 0.26，95% 可信区间 0.09～0.79）。这些分析的结果是不确定的，如果胃底折叠术比药物治疗有任何预防癌的益处，那么对个体患者的潜在优势是很小的，并且不能清楚地证明抗反流手术的风险。我们不认为在 Barrett 食管患者中，抗反流手术仅用于癌症预防。

（二）阿司匹林和其他非甾体抗炎药

许多间接证据表明，阿司匹林和其他非甾体抗炎药通过抑制 COX-2 和通过独立于 COX-2 抑制的机制预防食管腺癌[85-87]。体外实验证明，非甾体抗炎药（NSAIDs）可降低细胞增殖、增加细胞凋亡和减少血管生成[88-91]。在 GERD 和 Barrett 食管动物实验模型中，已证实 NSAIDs 可减少 Barrett 化生的发生及其进展为癌[92-94]。在 Barrett 食管患者中，NSAIDs 已显示可降低 Barrett 化生的增殖[91]，阿司匹林每日 325mg 剂量（与埃索美拉唑联合使用）可降低 Barrett 食管黏膜中前列腺素 E_2 的水平[95]。使用 NSAIDs 似乎可减少 Barrett 化生中体细胞外显子突变的积累[96]。许多流行病学和观察性研究也表明，使用 NSAIDs 与降低食管腺癌风险相关[97-99]，尽管有一些相反的数据报告[100]。医学会目前不推荐常规应用阿司匹林或其他 NSAIDs 处方药用于 Barrett 食管患者的化学预防，因为尚不清楚 NSAIDs 的潜在获益是否超过其严重的胃肠道和心血管副作用的风险。然而，Barrett 食管患者通常伴有心血管疾病和/或心血管风险因素，适用阿司匹林治疗[101]。

（三）异常增生的内镜监测

尽管在临床实践中推荐常规内镜监测来预防 Barrett 食管患者死于食管腺癌，但权威人士对这种监测的明智性提出了质疑，其论点可概括如下[102]：①内镜检查费用昂贵；②内镜检查有风险，以及产生不良情绪和财务负担；③Barrett 食管患者患癌症的绝对风险很小，因此大多数患者不能从内镜监测中获益；④没有随机对照试验的证据表明，内镜监测 Barrett 食管可预防食管癌死亡或延长患者生存期。而内镜监测的支持者反驳了这些论点：①Barrett 食管监测可以预防食管腺癌死亡的概念是合理的；②在可预见的未来，不太可能获得随机对照试验形式的有效证据；③许多观察性研究表明监测是有益的；④几乎所有已发表的关于该问题的计算机模型都表明监测是有益的；⑤对于其他方面健康的 Barrett 食管患者个体来说，内镜检查的风险非常小；⑥没有研究表明监测项目对患者的总体生存是不利的。对确立 Barrett 食管诊断所产生的潜在不良情绪和经济负担令人遗憾，但不如未能预防食管癌那么严重。因此，支持者认为，医生在等待可能永远不会出现的最终研究结果的同时，放弃对 Barrett 食管进行内镜监测这一可能挽救生命的做法，在伦理上是错误的。目前，胃肠病学会倾向于支持者的论点，并通常推荐具有一定资质的支持者监测[103]。

由于对大量个体进行 Barrett 食管筛查主要是为了将其纳入未经证实的监测项目，因此这种筛查尤其存在争议并不奇怪（见第 48 章）。美国胃肠病学会（AGA）最新指南[101]、美国消化内镜学会（ASGE）[104]、美国胃肠病学会（ACG）[77]、美国医师学会[105]、英国胃肠病学会[106]和欧洲胃肠内镜学会[107]建议仅考虑对具有食管腺癌多种风险因素的患者进行 Barrett 食管内镜筛查，包括慢性 GERD、年龄≥50 岁、男性、白人、食管裂孔疝、腹内脂肪分布（中心性肥胖）、吸烟史，以及一级亲属中有 Barrett 食管或食管腺癌病史。由于女性患食管腺癌的风险很低，ACG 特别指出，不建议对女性进行 Barrett 食管筛查，但在具有多种风险因素的女性个体病例中可考虑进行筛查[77]。

（四）黏膜肿瘤的治疗

黏膜肿瘤，如 Barrett 食管高级别异型增生和黏膜内癌，传统上采用食管切除术治疗。目前，大多数黏膜肿瘤的患者接受内镜根除治疗（endoscopic eradication therapy，EET），尽管食管切除术仍然是高度选择病例的有效选择。低级别异型增生的治疗是有争议的，因为诊断和疾病自然史存在不确定性。然而，最近的指南认为 EET 是低级别异型增生患者的首选治疗[77,107,108]。

内镜治疗

Barrett 食管有两种常见的内镜治疗方法：①内镜消融治疗，使用热（通过激光、电凝、氩离子凝固或射频能量输送）、冷（冷冻治疗，通过喷射冷二氧化碳或一氧化二氮气体或光化学能量[光动力疗法（PDT）]破坏 Barrett 上皮；②内镜切除术，包括内镜黏膜切除术（EMR）和内镜黏膜下剥离术，即使用透热圈套器或内镜刀切除一大段 Barrett 上皮黏膜和黏膜下层。在这些内镜治疗后，患者接受 PPI 治疗，使得消融或切除的黏膜可以随着正常食管鳞状上皮的再生长而愈合，而不是随着更多 Barrett 黏膜的再生而愈合。消融治疗可破坏化生组织，但不能提供病理学标本来判断肿瘤浸润的深度和消融的完整性。相反，EMR 和内镜黏膜下剥离术提供了大的组织标本，可由病理学家进行检查，以确定黏膜异常的特征和范围，以及肿瘤性病变浸润的深度和切除的彻底性。虽然，早期的研究主要集中在使用消融术或 EMR 治疗 Barrett 食管肿瘤，但现在这两种技术通常被联合使用。EET 用于描述使用任何一种或多种内镜联合治疗方式，其目的是完全根除 Barrett 化生。

EET 可以消除局限于食管黏膜的肿瘤，但不能治愈已转移到淋巴结的癌灶。对于累及黏膜下层的食管腺癌患者，淋巴结转移的频率超过 10%，因此，通常不建议进行 EET[109,110]。然而，即使是黏膜肿瘤也有可能转移到淋巴结。对 Barrett 食管黏膜肿瘤患者的淋巴结转移频率进行了系统性回顾，确定了 70 份相关报告，其中包括 1 874 例因 Barrett 食管合并高级别异型增生或黏膜内癌进行食管切除术的患者[111]。仅 26 例患者发现淋巴结转移（1.39%，95% 可信区间，86%～1.92%）。这种低风险使得 EET 可行。

（1）内镜消融治疗（另见第 48 章）

理想的消融技术会造成足够深的损伤，破坏所有的异常上皮，但深度不足以造成严重的并发症，如食管出血、穿孔或狭窄形成。到目前为止，没有一种消融治疗能达到这一理想效果，并且都与严重的并发症有关。已经实施了 PDT 和 RFA 治疗异型增生的随机对照试验。

对于 PDT，给予患者全身剂量的光激活化学物质，被食管细胞摄取。然后，使用激活化学物质的低功率激光对食管进行照射，化学物质将获得的能量传递给分子氧。这种转移导致形成单线态氧，这是一种破坏异常细胞及其血管系统的毒性分子。在一项使用卟吩姆钠 PDT 治疗 Barrett 食管高级别异型增生的多中心随机试验中，138 例患者接受 PDT 联合奥美拉唑 20mg，每日 2 次治疗，70 例患者接受奥美拉唑 20mg，每日 2 次单独治疗[112,113]。在 77% 接受 PDT 治疗的患者和 39% 接受奥美拉唑单药治疗的患者中，重复内镜检查和活检未发现异型增生（$P<0.0001$）。在长达 5 年的随访中，15% 的 PDT 患者发生癌症，而单独用奥美拉唑治疗的患者为 29%（$P=0.027$），无手术相关死亡。但接受 PDT 治疗的患者中有 69% 发生光敏反应，36% 发生食管狭窄，这通常很难治疗。由于并发症的高发生率和手术难度大，PDT 在很大程度上已被放弃作为 Barrett 食管异型增生的治疗，而倾向于 RFA。

RFA 使用基于球囊的紧密间隔电极阵列输送射频（微波）能量以消融食管黏膜。该系统旨在造成均匀的圆周热损伤，其深度由发生器控制，发生器可以改变应用能量的功率、密度和持续时间。还有一些更小的射频导管消融装置，用于消融短节段 Barrett 化生或使用基于球囊的系统治疗后持续存在的残余化生病灶。在一项 RFA 的多中心随机假性对照试验中（肠上皮化生消融异型增生试验），127 例 Barrett 食管异型增生的患者（64 例低级别、63 例高级别）被随机分配接受 RFA 或假内镜手术[114]。1 年时的意向性治疗分析显示，消融组中 90.5% 的低级别异型增生患者的异型增生完全根除，而对照组为 22.7%（$P<0.001$）。同样，消融组中 81.0% 的高级别异型增生患者完全根除，对照组为 19.0%（$P<0.001$）。消融组 77.4% 的患者肠化生完全根除（complete eradication of intestinal metaplasia，CE-IM），而对照组为 2.3%（$P<0.001$）。此外，消融组患者进展为肿瘤的程度更低（3.6% vs 16.3%，$P=0.03$），1 年时发现的癌更少（1.2% vs 9.3%，$P=0.045$）。在接受消融的 84 例患者中有 6 例（7%）出现严重并发症，包括 1 例上消化道出血和 5 例食管狭窄，均对治疗反应良好。在欧洲监测与射频消融（European Surveillance versus Radiofrequency Ablation，SURF）试验中，136 例经病理专家证实的低级别异型增生患者被随机分配接受 RFA 或内镜监测，RFA 使进展为高级别异型增生或腺癌的风险降低 25.0%（消融为 1.5% vs 对照组 26.5%；95% 可信区间，14.1%～35.9%；$P<0.001$），进展为腺癌的风险为 7.4%（消融为 1.5% vs 对照组 8.8%；95% 可信区间，0～14.7%；$P=0.03$）[115]。RFA 目前被广泛认为是消融 Barrett 食管伴异型增生的首选手术，包括高级别和低级别[116,117]。

在内镜冷冻治疗中，在内镜下将压缩二氧化碳或液态一氧化二氮等冷冻剂应用于 Barrett 食管，引起组织快速冻融，破坏细胞膜,诱导细胞凋亡,并导致局部血管血栓形成[118]。与 RFA 不同,冷冻疗法不会引起蛋白质结构的永久性变化,因此,保留了细胞外胶原基质结构。理论上,这可能会限制狭窄的形成,但冷冻治疗在这方面的临床优势尚未确立。对于体积较大的病变治疗,冷冻疗法也可能优于 RFA。观察性研究表明,冷冻疗法在根除 Barrett 化生和异型增生方面的有效性与 RFA 相似[119-121]。但是,可用的长期数据很少,RFA 仍然是目前最常用的消融技术。

(2) 内镜黏膜切除术(EMR)(另见第 48 章)

EMR 可采用"抽吸和切割"的方法进行,其中内镜医师通过向黏膜下层注射液体来抬高异型增生区域,然后将抬高的黏膜抽吸到装在内镜顶端的透明帽中[122]。之后在抽吸区域周边放置息肉切除圈套器将其通电摘除。EMR 也可以通过使用结扎装置的"束带和圈套器"方法操作,该装置类似于内镜下静脉曲张结扎术,其在抽吸的黏膜段周围放置弹性束带,而不需要预先向黏膜下注射液体[123]。使用息肉切除圈套器去除束带结扎段(见第 48 章)。有限(非环周)EMR 可获得的报告描述了很少的严重并发症,几乎没有与手术相关的死亡率。但是,如果在单次内镜治疗中使用 EMR 去除 Barrett 上皮的整个圆周范围,则食管狭窄经常发生[124]。

尽管 EMR 最初是作为一种治疗手段发展起来的,但临床医生最终认识到 EMR 作为 Barrett 食管早期肿瘤 T 分期的价值。由于 Barrett 肿瘤累及黏膜下层时淋巴结转移的风险很高,准确的肿瘤 T 分期对于确定内镜治疗是否可行至关重要。EUS 被认为是 T 分期最准确的诊断方式,但许多研究表明,EUS 对 Barrett 食管早期肿瘤 T 分期的准确性非常有限[125]。相反,有报告描述了早期 Barrett 肿瘤 EMR 术前 T 分期[125]与术后食管切除标本检查 T 分期之间有良好相关性[126]。因此,胃肠病学会现在建议,在进行内镜消融术前,应通过 EMR 对 Barrett 食管中的结节性病变和其他可见的不规则性病变进行 T 分期。如果 EMR 标本显示黏膜下浸润,则不建议进一步的内镜治疗。

关于 EMR 作为 Barrett 食管早期癌主要治疗方法获取的长期有效数据有限,但令人印象深刻。Ell 及其同事对 100 例 Barrett 食管早期腺癌患者进行了 EMR(肿瘤直径<20mm,组织学分化良好,无淋巴管或血管浸润,无转移、黏膜下浸润或淋巴结受累的证据)[127]。无严重并发症,计算出的 5 年生存率意想不到高达 98%。然而,在平均 37 个月的随访期间,11%的患者发现复发或出现异时性癌。复发的肿瘤经更多的内镜治疗获得成功,但这种高复发率表明 EMR 治疗往往会留下具有肿瘤潜能的细胞。

梅奥(Mayo)诊所的一项研究比较了接受食管切除术或 EMR 和 PDT 联合治疗的高级别异型增生患者的长期生存率[128]。尽管在随访期间发现 6.2%接受 PDT 和 EMR 治疗的患者患有异时性食管癌,但接受这两种治疗中任何一种治疗的患者的生存率无统计学显著差异。

另一份报告描述了 349 例 Barrett 食管高级别异型增生或黏膜腺癌患者内镜治疗的长期结果[129]。内镜治疗包括单纯 EMR 治疗 279 例,单纯 PDT 治疗 55 例,EMR 和 PDT 联合治疗 13 例,单纯氩等离子凝固治疗 2 例。5%的病例发生内镜治疗的严重并发症(2 例患者严重出血,15 例患者食管狭窄)。在平均 64 个月的随访期间,97%的患者获得完全缓解(定义为肿瘤病变完全消除,至少一次随访内镜检查显示无肿瘤)。计算出的 5 年生存率为 84%,无一例死于食管癌。然而,在随访期间发现异时性肿瘤的比例占 21%。研究者指出,这些异时性病变的一个主要风险因素是未能根除残留的非肿瘤性 Barrett 上皮。在切除原发性肿瘤后进行 Barrett 上皮消融的 200 例患者中,17%发生了异时性肿瘤,但在未进行 Barrett 上皮消融的 137 例患者中,30%发生了异时性肿瘤。主要基于这一经验,专家们现在建议对 Barrett 食管黏膜肿瘤进行 EET 应包括尝试根除所有 Barrett 黏膜,而不仅仅是明显的肿瘤病灶。

(3) Barrett 食管异型增生的 EET 进展状况

EET 目前被广泛认为是治疗 Barrett 食管黏膜肿瘤的首选方法,包括低级别异型增生、高级别异型增生和黏膜内癌。但是,在进行 EET 以发现黏膜肿瘤之前,应仔细检查 Barrett 食管,在整个 Barrett 化生节段以 1cm 的间隔按照西雅图活检方案采取标本,并应通过 EMR 去除任何可见的黏膜不规则,EMR 提供了关键的分期信息。EMR 现在被认为是如此重要,以至于最近的 ACG 指南特别指出,"计划实施内镜消融手术的内镜医师应额外提供 EMR"[77]。内镜下夹取活检或 EMR 标本中任何级别的异型增生的诊断,应由具有胃肠病理学专业知识的病理学家确认。如果确认为黏膜肿瘤,应消融所有剩余的 Barrett 化生(通常使用 RFA),以尽可能减少异时性肿瘤的发生。

当 EMR 显示黏膜下浸润时,通常不建议进行 EET,因为在这种情况下淋巴结转移的频率较高。然而,在专家中心使用 EET 治疗组织学特征良好的肿瘤的经验有限和仅能对穿透黏膜下层最表层产生了极好的长期生存效果[130]。目前,EET 治疗 Barrett 食管黏膜下肿瘤存在很大争议,应仅在专家中心考虑作为一种选择。

EET 的并发症比传统的食管切除术治疗异型增生的并发症要少得多,但 EET 并非无风险。最近对 37 篇文献(包括 9 200 位既往接受或未接受 EMR 的 RFA 患者)进行的系统性综述和 meta 分析发现严重不良事件的汇总发生率为 8.8%(95% CI,6.5%~11.9%),包括食管狭窄(5.6%,95% CI 4.2%~7.4%)、出血(1%,95% CI 0.8%~1.3%)和穿孔(0.6%,95% CI,0.4%~0.9%)[131]。此外,当 RFA 联合 EMR 时,不良事件的风险显著高于单独使用 RFA 时(相对风险 4.4,$P=0.015$)。尽管食管切除术的不良反应远远多于 EET,但食管切除术在选定的 Barrett 食管黏膜肿瘤患者中仍有一定作用。在少数 EET 未能根除肿瘤黏膜的患者中可能需要食管切除术,尤其是分散在长节段 Barrett 食管中的多发性异型增生病灶。对于不愿意或无法坚持多次内镜治疗和确保治疗效果所需的监测程序的患者,也可考虑食管切除术(见下文)。

早期报告表明,一种称为鳞状肠上皮化生(subsquamous intestinal metaplasia,SSIM;也称"埋藏腺体")的疾病是 EET 的并发症,但似乎并非如此[132]。SSIM 是一种可能具有恶性潜能的化生腺体,存在于食管固有层鳞状上皮下方的疾病,内镜医师在此处观察不到这些腺体。SSIM 被认为是内镜消融手术不完全的结果,该程序根除了 Barrett 化生的浅层,但留下了更深的腺体层,被覆盖在消融伤口上的新鳞状上皮"掩埋"。然而,最近的报告表明,绝大多数从未接受过消融治疗的 Barrett 食管患者在其与 Barrett 化生交界处附近的食管鳞状上皮下有 SSIM[132,133]。SSIM 的发病机制和临床重要性尚不清楚。

在考虑 EET 时，患者和医生均应认识到随访的重要性，因此化生和肿瘤复发均很常见。在一项回顾性队列研究中，有 218 例患者使用射频消融治疗 Barrett 食管异型增生并达到 CE-IM 的患者，有 52 例（24%）的化生或肿瘤复发率超过 540.6 人/年，总复发率为 9.6%/年[134]。其中 30 例（58%）实现了第二次 CE-IM，4 例（占总数的 1.8%，复发的 7.7%）进展为侵袭性腺癌，癌症发病率为 0.65%/年。在 39 项 EET 研究的系统综述和 meta 分析中，任何复发的汇总发生率为 7.5（95% CI 6.1~9.0）/（100 患者·年）[135]，化生复发率的汇总发生率为 4.8（95% CI 3.8~5.9）/（100 患者·年），而异型增生复发率为 2.0（95% CI，1.5~2.5）/（100 患者·年）。这些令人担忧的复发率表明，即使在达到 CE-IM 后，所有接受 EET 治疗的患者均应接受内镜监测。

经过 EET 治疗达到 CE-IM 后的第一年，Barrett 化生和异型增生的复发最常见[136]。复发的风险因素包括基线异型增生、长节段 Barrett 食管和在低手术量中心治疗[137]。Barrett 食管高级别异型增生或黏膜内癌患者达到 CE-IM 后，当前基于指南的意见要求第一年每 3 个月进行一次内镜监测，第二年每 6 个月一次，此后每年 1 次[77]。对于低级别异型增生 EET 后 CE-IM 的患者，基于指南的意见要求内镜监测，第一年每 6 个月监测一次，之后每年监测一次[77]。最近一项旨在建立 Barrett 食管 RFA 后循证监测间隔的研究表明，基于患者风险因素的内镜监测计划大大减少，将提供相似的癌症保护，但提出的循证监测项目尚未得到胃肠病学协会的认可[138]。

EET 后，复发似乎主要累及新的鳞状-柱状交界区域。在 RFA 达到 CE-IM 后进行 2 次或更多次内镜检查的 198 例患者的研究中，研究者在现在被新鳞状上皮覆盖的整个消融区域以 1cm 间隔进行 4 象限活检，活检在新的鳞-柱上皮交界处进行[139]。在平均随访 3 年期间，32 例患者（16%）有化生或肿瘤复发。32 例复发中有 29 例发生在鳞-柱交界处或其上方 1cm 处，3 例更近端食管复发均在内镜下可见。基于这些发现，作者推荐了一种活检方案，涉及 Z 线周围 8 个均匀分布的活检，Z 线上 1 和 2cm 处的 4 象限活检以及仅针对可见异常的更近端活检。

（4）非异型增生 Barrett 化生的 EET 治疗

一些权威专家提出，EET 应该提供给所有 Barrett 食管患者，而不仅仅是那些异型增生和早期癌患者[140]。这些权威专家认为 Barrett 化生即使未表现出异型增生的组织学特征，也可能是肿瘤性的，而内镜监测作为癌预防策略的有效性是值得怀疑的，在治疗异型增生的高质量研究中已经确定了 RFA 的安全性和有效性。El-Serag 和 Graham 甚至认为，在结肠镜检查过程中发现的结直肠息肉常规进行息肉切除术的做法在认知上等同于消融治疗非异型增生的 Barrett 食管[141]。

尽管存在这些有趣的论点，但一些尚未解决的问题限制了对非异型增生 Barrett 食管患者 EET 治疗的支持。早期讨论的化生频繁复发表明，EET 不排除内镜监测的需要。应缓和使用 EET 治疗非异型增生 Barrett 食管热情的其他考虑因素包括，EET 通常需要几种内镜手术才能完全根除 Barrett 化生，导致大量费用和患者不便。EET 具有相当高的并发症发生率，其降低非异型增生 Barrett 食管本来较低的癌发生率的疗效尚未确立。目前，不推荐将 EET 用于一般无异型增生的 Barrett 食管患者[77]。

（五）建议

Barrett 食管患者的治疗策略目前尚未得到确定性研究的证实，这些研究证明可延长患者的生命或预防因食管癌死亡。我们支持美国胃肠病学协会、ACG 和 ASGE 提出的总体管理策略，并稍做修改如下：

- Barrett 食管患者应使用任何剂量的 PPI 治疗，以控制 GERD 症状和消除反流性食管炎的内镜表现。无症状的非反流性食管炎患者可采用每日一次 PPI 治疗进行化学预防。对于担心 PPI 不良反应的患者，可以考虑将抗反流手术作为长期 PPI 治疗的替代方案，但在癌症预防方面，抗反流手术并不明显优于 PPI。
- 对于非异型增生 Barrett 食管患者，应在详细讨论中介绍内镜监测的风险和益处。选择监测的患者应每 3~5 年进行一次。
- 应使用高分辨率白光内镜进行监测。接受过先进成像技术培训的内镜医生可能会发现它们是有用的，但常规监测不需要先进的成像技术。内镜医师应仔细检查 Barrett 化生。对于出现不规则或疑似肿瘤的区域，内镜医师应进行靶向活检，或最好通过 EMR 去除可疑区域。除了这些靶向标本外，内镜医师还应在整个 Barrett 化生长度上每隔 2cm 采取 4 象限活检标本。对于已知异型增生的患者，应在 Barrett 化生长度上每隔 1cm 取一次 4 象限活检标本。
- 如果活检被解读为"不确定异型增生"，应优化 PPI 治疗，并在大约 8 周内重复内镜检查，每隔 1cm 采集活检标本。如果"不确定异型增生"的诊断持续存在，治疗选择包括每 12 个月进行一次内镜监测或转诊到具有管理 Barrett 食管专业知识的中心治疗。
- 当首次发现任何级别的异型增生时，如果对初始检查的充分性有任何疑问，应尽快进行其他内镜检查，并进行广泛的活检取样，以寻找浸润性癌。应在黏膜不规则的区域进行 EMR。应由病理学专家（最好不止 1 名专家）判读组织学切片。
- 在广泛活检采样和黏膜不规则 EMR 后，建议对证实为黏膜各种新生物形成（低级别异型增生、高级别异常增生、黏膜内癌）的患者进行 EET。
- Barrett 食管高级别异型增生或黏膜内癌患者实现 CE-IM 后，第一年每 3 个月进行一次内镜监视，第二年每 6 个月进行一次，此后每年进行一次。
- 对低级别异型增生患者实现 CE-IM 后，第一年每 6 个月进行一次内镜监视，此后每年进行一次。

（程妍 译，袁农 校）

参考文献

第 48 章 食管肿瘤

Hazem Hammad,Sachin Wumo 著

章节目录

一、癌 …… 663
（一）食管鳞状细胞癌 …… 663
（二）食管腺癌 …… 664
（三）发病机制 …… 665
（四）临床特征 …… 666
（五）诊断 …… 666
（六）筛查和监测 …… 668
（七）分期 …… 669
（八）治疗 …… 673
（九）预后 …… 678
二、其他恶性上皮性肿瘤 …… 678
（一）鳞状细胞癌变异体 …… 678
（二）小细胞癌 …… 678
（三）恶性黑色素瘤 …… 679
三、良性上皮性肿瘤 …… 679
（一）鳞状细胞乳头状瘤 …… 679
（二）腺瘤 …… 679
（三）炎性纤维性息肉 …… 679
四、恶性非上皮肿瘤 …… 679
（一）淋巴瘤 …… 679
（二）肉瘤 …… 679
（三）胃肠间质瘤 …… 680
（四）转移瘤 …… 680
五、良性非上皮性肿瘤 …… 680
（一）平滑肌瘤 …… 680
（二）颗粒细胞瘤 …… 680
（三）纤维血管息肉 …… 680
（四）错构瘤 …… 681
（五）血管瘤 …… 681
（六）脂肪瘤 …… 681

食管癌是全球第八大常见癌症，估计发病有 45.6 万例，占每年诊断的所有癌症病例的 3.2%。它也是全球癌症死亡的第六大原因，每年约占所有癌症死亡的 40 万人（5%）[1,2]。2018 年，估计美国有 17 290 例新发病例和 15 850 例死于食管癌[3]。美国食管癌的终生风险约为每 125 名男性中就有 1 例，每 400 名女性中就有 1 例[4]。食管癌通常表现为进展期，因此治愈有限，预后差，死亡率与发病率之比为 0.88（总的 5 年生存率低于 20%）[2,5]。最近的数据表明其 5 年生存率有所改善，特别是早期和局部进展期癌[4,6]。食管癌有两种亚型——食管鳞状细胞癌和食管腺癌，这两种亚型都与不同的地理分布、时间趋势和风险因素有关[6,7]。

一、癌

（一）食管鳞状细胞癌

食管鳞状细胞癌（esophageal squamous cell carcinoma，ESCC）是全球最常见的一种食管癌。尽管在西方社会中 ESCC 不再是最常见的食管癌类型，但在东方，ESCC 仍然是最普遍的食管癌类型，在大多数亚洲、非洲和东欧国家，ESCC 占所有癌症的 90%[8]。ESCC 风险最高的区域有两个地理带，从里海到中国北部横跨中亚的亚洲食管癌带和从埃塞俄比亚到南非的非洲东部海岸带[9,10]。

1999 年至 2008 年美国 ESCC 发病率趋势的最新数据表明，存在显著的地区差异。所调查的数据覆盖了 85% 的美国人口，发现全国年龄标准化的发病率男性为 4.93/10 万，女性为 2.30/10 万。65 岁以上的患者发病率最高。在研究期间，美国男性和女性的 ESCC 发病率每年分别下降 3.41% 和 3.13%。在研究期间诊断的食管癌中大多数（70.8%）为食管腺癌（esophageal adenocarcinoma，EAC），而不是 ESCC[11]。

虽然 ESCC 在男性中比女性更常见，但在低风险地区如美国（4∶1）和中国及伊朗的高发地区中，（这些地区的比率较低，接近甚至或超过 1∶1），该比率存在差异[12]。环境因素可能在解释 ESCC 发病率的地理变异方面很重要。在低发病率和高发病率地区，病因和风险因素各不相同[13]。在美国的一项研究中报告，89% 的人群归因于吸烟、饮用酒精饮料和低水果、蔬菜消费的风险[14]。相反，在中国进行的一项大型队列研究发现，吸烟在 ESCC 风险中的作用很小[15]。

在工业化国家，两个最重要的风险因素是吸烟和过量饮酒（框 48.1）[16-19]。此外，这两个独立的风险因素对癌症发病

框 48.1 ESCC 和 EAC 的风险因素
ESCC
烟草
酒精类饮料
水果和蔬菜摄入量低
社会经济地位低
微量营养素缺乏
高温食物
贲门失弛缓症
摄入碱性液体
罕见疾病（Plummer-Vinson 综合征、Fanconi 贫血和胼胝症）
EAC
烟草
胃食管反流病
肥胖
EAC，食管腺癌；ESCC，食管鳞状细胞癌。

率具有协同作用[20]。主动吸烟发生ESCC的风险增加了3~9倍[21,22]。虽然吸烟的风险最高,但使用其他形式的烟草,如烟斗、雪茄、水烟、咀嚼烟草和亚洲槟榔也与ESCC有关[23]。据报道,接触强度和持续时间较长与ESCC风险有关[24,25]。烟草特有的亚硝胺和多环芳烃被认为是烟草中主要的致癌物质。据报道,与烟草相比,使用酒精的风险略低,ESCC的风险增加3~5倍[21]。如果酒精摄入量超过美国饮食指南建议的每周140g的上限,风险会显著增加[18]。乙醛是乙醇代谢的第一个代谢产物,是一类致癌物。

在发展中地区,营养缺乏等因素似乎与ESCC发病率有更密切的关系[19,26]。尽管确切的机制尚不清楚,但低社会经济状态本身就是ESCC的一个风险因素,即使在调整了烟草、酒精、年龄和许多潜在的风险因素之后也是如此[7,27,28]。微量营养素的缺乏(例如维生素A、C和E)也是危险因素[29,30],这些维生素被认为具有重要的抗氧化作用,可防止自由基和亚硝胺的形成。然而,在中国进行的一项为期6年的随机对照试验(随访20年)表明,补充多种维生素并不能降低ESCC高危人群的风险[31]。其他营养素缺乏,如叶酸、锌和硒,也被报告为ESCC的风险因素。叶酸摄入量减少和代谢受损(主要由于基因多态性)已被认为是几种胃肠道恶性肿瘤(包括ESCC)的风险因素[32]。在一项病例对照系列中,ESCC患者的血清叶酸水平较低[29]。微量元素锌和硒对抗ESCC有保护作用[33-35]。锌缺乏被认为可增强亚硝胺的致癌作用。补充硒也被认为对ESCC具有化学预防作用。经过10年的随访,一项研究表明,硒补充剂(以及β-胡萝卜素和维生素E)可使55岁以下年轻参与者的食管癌死亡风险降低17%[33,36]。一项以病例对照研究为主的系统性综述表明,水果和蔬菜摄入量增加可能会降低食管癌的风险,生蔬菜和水果每增加50g/d,食管癌的风险分别降低31%和22%[14]。其他饮食因素也被推理为增加ESCC的风险。在多项研究中证实,饮用高温饮料与ESCC风险增加相关,可能是由于慢性热损伤所致[37]。Yerba mate,一种在南美洲普遍饮用的热香草茶,已被发现是ESCC的风险因素[38]。以前报告的其他风险因素,如摄入N-亚硝基化合物(在腌肉制品和腌菜中发现的动物致癌物)和轮状镰刀菌(在玉米上发现的一种真菌)有混杂证据表明,它们也是发生ESCC的风险因素[39,40]。

多项研究显示ESCC与人乳头状瘤病毒(HPV)感染可能有关[41]。最近,一家大型国际联盟对ESCC病例和对照受试者的多种HPV血清型进行了复杂的血清学分析,发现HPV与ESCC相关性的证据非常有限[42]。目前还不能证明两者之间存在明确的相关性,有必要进一步调查研究[43]。

一些食管疾病增加了ESCC的风险。如第44章所述,估计贲门失弛缓症患者中ESCC的患病率约为5%[44]。在贲门失弛缓症确诊后的1~24年间,风险增加了16倍,尤其是男性[45]。事实上,来自瑞典的一个大型贲门失弛缓症队列研究显示,ESCC和EAC的风险均增加[46]。其机制很可能是由于食物等物质在食管内淤积,导致慢性炎症。同样,如第28章所述,因摄入碱液而导致食管狭窄的患者在初次摄入后数十年发生ESCC的风险增加[47]。食管蹼患者,如患Plummer-Vinson综合征(缺铁性贫血、吞咽困难和环状软骨后蹼)患者和Fanconi贫血(与多种癌症有关的遗传性骨髓衰竭)患者,发生ESCC的风险也增加(见第43章)[7,48]。

与ESCC相关的另一种罕见疾病是胼胝症(tylosis),这是一种常染色体显性遗传病,以手掌/足底角化过度和白斑为特征(见第25章)。胼胝症的食管癌基因TOC(*RHBDF2*)已定位于染色体17q25[49]。最近的报告认为,该基因可能是表观遗传沉默而不是突变[50]。在一项报告中,携带该基因的人到65岁时发生ESCC的风险为95%[51]。某些因素对ESCC具有保护作用,其中包括肥胖症和经常使用阿司匹林和非甾体抗炎药(NSAIDs)[52-55]。

(二) 食管腺癌

食管腺癌(EAC)是全球第二常见的食管癌。EAC的患病率和发病率不仅随着时间的推移发生了变化,而且在地理上也发生了变化。ESCC曾经是西方和东方国家最常见的食管癌类型。根据外科手术资料,食管腺癌在1978年以前并不常见[56]。在西方国家,其发病率显著增加,以至于在1994年,EAC在美国的患病率超过了ESCC。如今,EAC是西方食管癌的主要类型。在美国,其在白人男性中的发病率从20世纪70年代的0.5/10万~0.9/10万,上升至随后20年的3.2/10万~4.0/10万[57]。这种转变代表白人男性和白人女性发病率分别增加了463%和335%[58]。最近开展基于人群的研究,从2003年至2007年估计EAC的发病率为5.3/10万[59]。EAC在男性中的发病率是女性的8倍,在高加索人中的发病率是非裔美国人的5倍。此外,EAC发病率的快速增长并不局限于美国,在其他西方国家如英国、冰岛和澳大利亚也出现了类似的趋势[60-64]。此外,基于数学预测模型,预计EAC的发病率将持续升高到2030年,届时EAC的预测发病率将为(8.4~10.1)/10万人/年[65]。EAC的总体5年观察生存率强烈依赖于诊断时的分期,是所有癌中最低的。最近一项使用美国国家癌症研究所监测、流行病学和最终结果(Surveillance,Epidemiology,and End Results,SEER)注册的分析显示,患有局限性、区域性或远期疾病的EAC比例保持相对稳定(40%的EAC患者被诊断为远期疾病)。最近的数据还表明,5年生存率总体改善,局限性疾病患者的改善最大,这反映了治愈性治疗方式的改善[4]。远端食管EAC与食管胃交界处腺癌和胃贲门腺癌之间的关系在第47和54章中讨论。

EAC发病率随时间的地理变化被认为与GERD的显著增加有关(见第46章),更重要的是,与西方社会的肥胖有关。西方和东欧国家的流行病学梯度可能部分与社会经济状态有关,因为高社会经济状态在EAC中更常见,而低社会经济状态在ESCC中更常见[27,58]。然而,社会经济状况改善的其他指标,包括人均国内生产总值和教育水平,与在世界不同地区观察到的食管癌梯度无关[58]。

由于EAC发病率的上升是如此引人注目,因此提出了错误分类和/或过度诊断的可能性也随之增加。一项基于人群的研究使用了SEER的数据[9],该数据代表了1973年至2001年间约10%的美国人口,发现将EAC重新分类为ESCC和邻近贲门癌不太可能改变EAC的发病率。食管癌的解剖分布已经从食管的上1/3转移到下1/3。食管下1/3是腺癌通常发生的部位,是食管发病率增加的唯一部位。由于原位和局部疾病的发病率变化极小,并且事实上EAC的死亡率也显著增加(7 倍,从 2 例死亡/100 万增加到 15 例死亡/100 万),过度诊断不太可能解释 EAC 发病率的显著增加[66]。此外,EGD 作为观察到的 EAC 发病率急剧增加的潜在原因而加强监测的可能性被否定,因为显示在所有阶段和年龄组的白人男性和女性中,EAC 的发病率均增加[67]。

一般来说,影响 EAC 发病率的风险因素常见于经济发达国家[5]。与 ESCC 相似,烟草是 EAC 的一个风险因素(见框 48.1)[13,17,18]。国际 Barrett 和食管腺癌联合会(Barrett and Esophageal Adenocarcinoma Consortium,BEACON)的汇总数据证实了吸烟与 EAC 之间的相关性(OR 1.96,95% CI 1.64~2.34)。还观察到剂量-反应关系,重度吸烟者患癌症的风险最高。此外,戒烟已被证明与癌症风险降低相关(戒烟≥10 年与 EAC 风险降低 30% 有关)[68]。与 ESCC 相比较,酒精似乎不是 EAC 或 Barrett 食管的强风险因素[69]。与 ESCC 不同,BEACON 从事的 11 项研究的综合分析显示,饮酒与 EAC 风险之间无关联性[70]。

GERD 是发生 EAC 最重要的风险因素(见第 46 和 47 章)[71]。尽管大多数大型研究在风险增加方面认识是一致的,但报告的风险从 4 倍到 8 倍不等[72-74]。瑞典的一项研究表明,GERD 症状复发(至少每周出现胃灼热和/或反流症状)的个体发生 EAC 的风险比症状不太频繁的个体高 8 倍(OR 7.7,95% CI 5.3~11.4)[72]。这项研究还表明,在 GERD 症状更严重和持续时间更长的个体中,EAC 的风险尤其高(OR 43.5,95% CI 18.3~103.5)。最近对 BEACON 中 5 项基于人群的大型病例对照研究的个体水平数据进行了汇总分析,结果显示 GERD 症状频率与 EAC 之间存在强烈的剂量依赖关系(至少每周;OR 4.81,95% CI 3.4~6.8;每日症状:OR 7.96,95% CI 4.51~14)[75]。尽管 GERD 是 EAC 的公认风险因素,但大多数 GERD 患者从未发生 EAC。事实上,大多数 EAC 患者否认既往 GERD 的任何实质性症状[76]。据认为,在易感个体中,GERD 引起远端食管损伤,导致异常愈合过程,从而引起 Barrett 食管(BE)。BE 是 EAC 唯一确定的癌前状态,定义为远端食管正常复层鳞状上皮被柱状上皮排列伴肠化生所替代(见第 47 章)。在约 7%~15% 的 GERD 个体中观察到 BE,估计存在于 1%~2% 的一般成年人群中[77]。BE 患者发生 EAC 的风险高达 10~55 倍,然而,据报道从 BE 进展为 EAC 的比例较小(每年 0.12%~3%)[77-79]。

同样,肥胖是 EAC 的另一个强风险因素,这种风险随着 BMI 的升高而增加[80-82]。据估计,肥胖患者发生 EAC 的风险增加了 2~5 倍[83]。此外,腹型肥胖(独立于 BMI)已被证明与 EAC 风险增加相关[84,85]。高热量和高脂肪摄入本身也是 EAC 的风险因素[86]。肥胖可能通过增加腹内压增加食管裂孔疝和 GERD 的风险[71]。然而,即使在调整 GERD 后,腹型肥胖也与 BE 相关,即使在没有 GERD 症状的情况下,肥胖也与 EAC 相关[83]。除其机械效应外,腹型肥胖还与 BE 和 EAC 相关的肽类循环水平的改变有关[10,87]。代谢综合征与 BE 和 EAC 有关[88,89]。此外,研究还发现胰岛素样生长因子、瘦素和脂联素与 BE 进展为 EAC 相关[10]。

男性在食管癌中的显著优势提出了性激素是否可能起作用的问题。当计算 1992 年至 2006 年间确诊的 EAC 和 ESCC 的男女比例时,西班牙裔的男女比例最高(20.5),其次是白种人(10.8)和非洲裔美国人(7.0)。相比之下,ESCC 的男女发病率比率要低得多。这些发现支持了女性性激素暴露可能在 EAC 发生中起保护作用的假设[90]。男性患 EAC 风险的差异也可能与吸烟或肥胖类型的不同有关。

据报道,有几个因素对发展中的 EAC 具有保护作用。幽门螺杆菌感染(胃癌的已知风险因素)的患病率与 EAC 呈负相关[91-93]。这种风险降低估计为 50%。感染似乎通过降低胃液酸度来降低 EAC 的风险。此外,与 ESCC 一样,使用阿司匹林和 NSAIDs 似乎对发生 EAC 具有保护作用[94-96]。如系统综述和荟萃分析所示,观察性研究也表明,使用质子泵抑制剂可将 BE 患者的肿瘤进展风险降低 71%[97]。同样,他汀类药物已被证明可以降低发生 EAC 的风险,尤其是 BE 患者[98]。最后,水果和蔬菜的摄入量与 EAC 呈负相关[71]。

(三) 发病机制

由于表观遗传学变化和基因改变的积累,人类癌症以多步骤方式发生(见第 1 章)[99,100]。环境因素、遗传因素和获得性基因改变的组合很可能是食管癌发生的重要风险因素。在 EAC 中,食管上皮化生—异型增生—癌序列期间发生的体细胞遗传异常逐渐积累(见第 1 和 47 章)。干细胞群中的炎症微环境和体细胞基因组改变被认为介导了从 BE 到 EAC 的进展[101]。了解这些异常的序列,可能会导致根据患者的个体癌症风险对其进行更准确的分层[102]。因为有一些证据表明,只有对新辅助治疗有完全病理反应的患者才有生存获益(稍后讨论),所以正在寻找预后和预测性遗传标志物,以定制更有效的多模式治疗[103-105]。另一方面,ESCC 被认为是起源于过度增殖的上皮细胞,这些上皮细胞发展为低、中和高级别异型增生(high-grade dysplasia,HGD),最终成为侵袭性癌[106,107]。同时发生的基因变化和表观遗传修饰,以肿瘤抑制基因的高甲基化形式,在 EAC 和 ESCC 中都经常发生[108-110]。

虽然大多数 BE 和 EAC 病例都是散发的,也没有明确的家族史,有几项发现表明存在遗传成分。这些发现包括家族聚集性,事实上,只有一部分 GERD 患者发生 BE,反流量不是 BE 发生的准确预测因素[111-113]。在这些情况下,发生 BE 的风险受到基因-基因和基因-环境相互作用的强烈影响(见第 47 章)。

基于对人类致癌过程中 6 个基本成分的描述[114],食管癌的这 6 个步骤中的每一步都描述了分子因素,概括如下[115]。

1. **生长信号的自给自足**。癌细胞既可以产生自身的生长因子(自分泌效应,见第 4 章),也可以改变其生长因子受体和信号通路,使其解脱外源性生长限制信号。例如,EGF 受体 2(*HER2/neu*)的基因表达是食管癌的预后因素[116-118]。*HER2/neu* 基因扩增与患者生存期缩短相关,并可独立预测 EAC 患者的不良结局[119]。相反,与 *HER2/neu* 高表达的肿瘤相比,*HER2/neu* 低表达与新辅助放化疗反应的改善相关[120]。ESCC 也有类似的效应[121,122]。此外在 ESCC 中,与细胞周期蛋白 D1(cyclin D1)阴性患者相比,细胞周期蛋白 D1 的表达(一种关键的细胞周期调节因子)(见第 1 章)与患者生存期缩短相关[123]。

2. **对抗生长信号不敏感**。肿瘤抑制基因的失活是肿瘤细胞对抗生长信号脱敏的重要机制。这可能通过突变、杂合性缺失或启动子超甲基化发生[115]。肿瘤抑制基因 *TP53* 在 ESCC 中的表达是一个独立的预后因素。p53 蛋白低表达的肿瘤比 p53 蛋白高表达的肿瘤生存期显著延长[124,125]。此外,ESCC 中的 p21 染色与生存率的改善相关[126,127],以及肿瘤中 p16 水平高的 ESCC 患者的生存期更长[128]。

3. **避免细胞凋亡**。细胞凋亡(程序性细胞死亡)阻碍了细胞池的扩张。肿瘤的扩增能力不仅取决于其细胞的增殖速度,还取决于其避免凋亡的能力。凋亡的一些重要调节因子包括 Bax、Bcl-2 和 Bcl-X 蛋白。这些蛋白单独或联合应用与预后和对新辅助放化疗的反应相关[129,130]。存活素(survivin)是凋亡抑制基因家族的另一个成员[129,130],已被发现是食管癌新辅助治疗中一个有用的预测因素。具体而言,新辅助化疗的部分应答者其存活素的表达低于无应答者[131]。因此,未来减少存活素表达或阻断存活素信号通路的治疗策略,可能会提高组织病理学应答率和预后[132]。

4. **不受控制的复制潜能**。恶性肿瘤细胞通过端粒酶的过度表达,破坏了限制其增殖能力的机制,从而对细胞衰老和死亡产生抵抗力。尽管在 EAC 的发病机制中人端粒酶逆转录酶催化亚基的表达似乎有所增加,但尚无研究表明这一发现有任何预后意义[133-135]。

5. **持续血管生成**。持续的血管生成对于癌症的发生、进展和最终转移是至关重要的。血管生成因子如血管内皮生长因子(vascular endothelial growth factor, VEGF)、环氧化酶-2(COX-2)和成纤维细胞生长因子受体 1 被认为是食管癌的潜在预后因素。其中,VEGF 似乎是最重要的[132]。VEGF 的高表达在 ESCC 中是一个独立的负面预后因素,尽管在 EAC 中的相关性尚未得到证实[136]。已知 COX-2 随着组织通过 Barrett 化生、异型增生和直接成为 EAC 的进展而进行性增加[132]。在 ESCC 中,COX-2 过度表达与肿瘤浸润深度、肿瘤分期和生存率降低相关[137]。成纤维细胞生长因子受体 1 的扩增显示是 ESCC 的一个独立的不良预后因素[138]。胸苷磷酸化酶(另一种血管生成因子)的表达可预测 ESCC 患者对放化疗仅有部分应应[139]。

6. **侵袭和转移**。细胞间黏附分子(即 e-钙黏蛋白糖蛋白、连环蛋白和基质金属蛋白)及其抑制剂的异常与组织学分化不良、肿瘤侵袭和淋巴结转移增加相关[140-142]。

(四) 临床特征

尽管在人口统计学和风险因素方面存在差异,但 EAC 和 ESCC 患者的临床表现相似。在早期大多数患者并无症状。但随着疾病进展,进行性吞咽困难和体重减轻是最常见的症状。由于出现吞咽困难的患者倾向于避免摄入引起症状的食物和调整饮食摄入量,因此诊断常被延误。吞咽困难最初表现为固体食物,但在疾病后期发展为液体食物。固体食物的吞咽困难通常发生在食管腔直径≤13mm 时。吞咽困难的严重程度和因经口摄入量减少而伴随的体重减轻与管腔阻塞的程度成正比。患者定位的吞咽困难点不能很好地预测肿块的实际位置。吞咽痛是一种较少见的症状,通常提示存在溃疡性病变。

其他不太常见的临床表现包括缺铁性贫血、可触及的颈部淋巴结肿大和/或胸痛。胸痛常放射到背部,提示可能侵入食管周围结构。肿瘤侵蚀可导致食管-气管瘘,表现为顽固性咳嗽、复发性肺炎或胸腔积液。一种罕见的并发症是食管-主动脉瘘,可引起上消化道大出血和失血。由于喉返神经损伤,声音嘶哑是另一种罕见的临床表现,来自肿瘤本身或相关淋巴结肿大。转移病灶不仅可见于淋巴结,也可见于肺、肝、脑和骨。

(五) 诊断

实验室检查是非特异性的,可以显示贫血(缺铁性或慢性疾病型)、低蛋白血症和/或高钙血症(通常与溶骨性转移有关)。尽管食管癌的副肿瘤综合征很少见,但由于肿瘤产生的循环甲状旁腺激素相关蛋白,ESCC 很少引起高钙血症[143]。目前食管癌没有特异性血清学标志物。

食管癌的诊断主要是通过内镜活检对表现为固体食物进行性吞咽困难的患者作出的(图 48.1)。晚期 ESCC 与 EAC 的内镜表现相似,然而,约 3/4 的 EAC 病变发生在食管远端,而 ESCC 更常见于在食管近端至中端。食管癌内镜下可表现为黏膜的肿块、隆起的结节、溃疡、凹陷、狭窄或黏膜细微不规则病变。重要的是,内镜医师必须花费足够的时间检查食管并记录标志,如胃食管交界处、使用 Prague C(环周)和 M(最大范围)标准的 BE 范围、是否延伸到胃,以及肿瘤的确切位置[144]。这些数据点确定了使用治疗食管癌患者的手术技术。清晰描述肿瘤的形态学特征也有助于确定内镜根除治疗的候选资格,内镜根除治疗已成为早期食管癌(ESCC 和 EAC)标准的治疗方法。

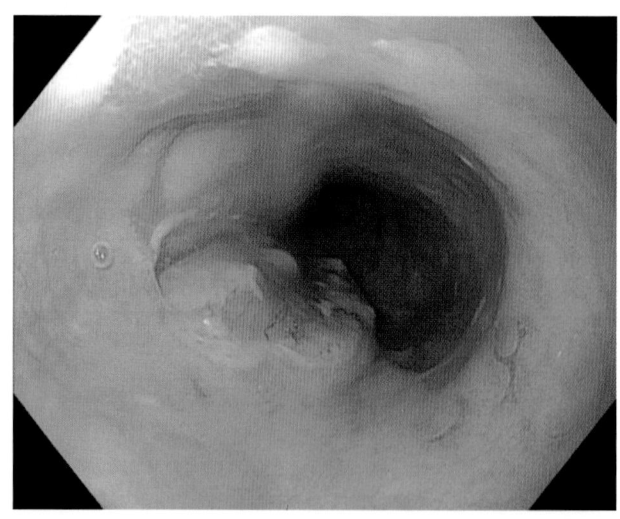

图 48.1 Barrett 食管背景下食管远端肿块的内镜图像,符合腺癌

其他各种成像方式可以帮助诊断。常规胸片可显示非特异性表现,如吸入性肺炎、食管扩张伴气液平面(假性贲门失弛缓症)、肺实质转移性病变、胸腔积液或瘘征象。食管钡剂造影有助于食管癌的诊断。这种检查模式的早期癌征象是食管黏膜内衬异常,可表现为斑块、息肉样病变、溃疡或非特异性局灶性不规则病变。进展期肿瘤可表现为明显肿块、肩胛样明显狭窄或管腔狭窄。由于内镜的广泛应用,食管钡剂造影通常已不受青睐,但在疑似食管-呼吸瘘的内镜检查之前,

食管钡剂造影是非常有用的。当涉及此问题时，内镜医师可在内镜支架置入术前获得解剖学的“路线图”。应特别注意使用钡作为对比剂，而不能使用高渗剂（泛影葡胺和泛影葡胺钠），后者有引起严重肺水肿和吸入性肺炎的风险。

CT 检查可显示食管壁增厚/不规则、局灶性食管狭窄伴近端扩张或可见腔内肿块。可见到吸入性肺炎、转移病灶、淋巴结肿大和食管-气管瘘的征象。

如上所述，内镜检查和活检对食管癌的诊断率最高，是确定诊断的标准（图 48.2 和图 48.3）。在 3 个主要临床应用中已经使用了几种成像方式：(a) 在内镜筛查和监测期间检测和识别早期癌症患者；(b) 预测内镜检查期间的组织学和实时诊断；(c) 指导内镜根除治疗。技术进步使得能够生产出更小的电荷耦合器件芯片，这些芯片能够产生高分辨率的图像（超过 85 万~210 万像素），并以 16∶9的纵横比显示在显示器上，与标准清晰度白光内镜（WLE）相比，成像质量更优。高分辨率放大内镜可将图像放大 150 倍（虽然在美国并非常用）。一些研究表明，高分辨率内镜无论是否使用放大内镜，均可提高异型增生和早期癌的检出率[145-149]。总体而言，在早期 ESCC 的检测中，白光内镜检查总体灵敏度较低，为 55%~63%[150]。在可行的情况下，使用高分辨率 WLE 应是评估接受监测或考虑内镜根除治疗（EET）的 BE 患者和食管中其他细微病变（食管鳞状上皮异型增生和早期 ESCC）的最低标准，这一做法得到了胃肠协会指南的认可[151,152]。内镜检查结果可以从相对正常的黏膜（黏膜下浸润型）到溃疡、结节和明显的肿块不同。其他几种内镜技术也可以帮助识别异型增生和恶性肿瘤区域，包括窄带成像、色素内镜（常规或电子）、自发荧光成像（autoffuorescence imaging，AFI）和共聚焦激光内镜（confocal laser endomicroscopy，CLE）。关于 Barrett 食管的章节将进一步详细讨论这些成像方式（见第 47 章）。

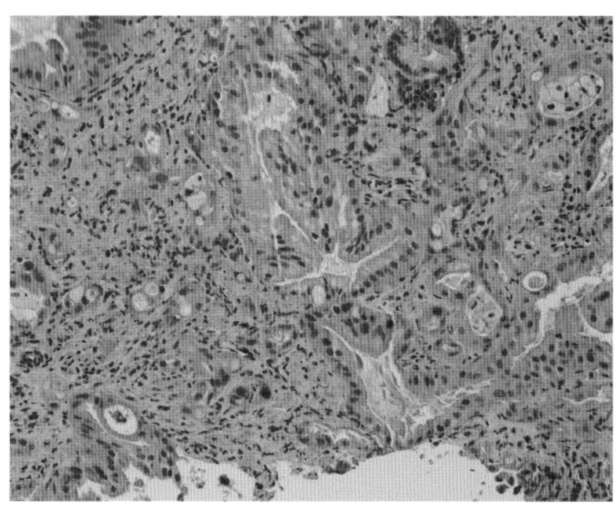

图 48.2　食管腺癌标本的组织病理学显示不规则的恶性腺体，管腔内黏蛋白产生，累及食管黏膜，并伴有炎症性基质反应。在图左侧中心可见一部分“印戒”细胞，胞浆内见大的空泡和偏心的细胞核。×200。（Courtesy Dr. Michael Argyres，Denver，Colo.）

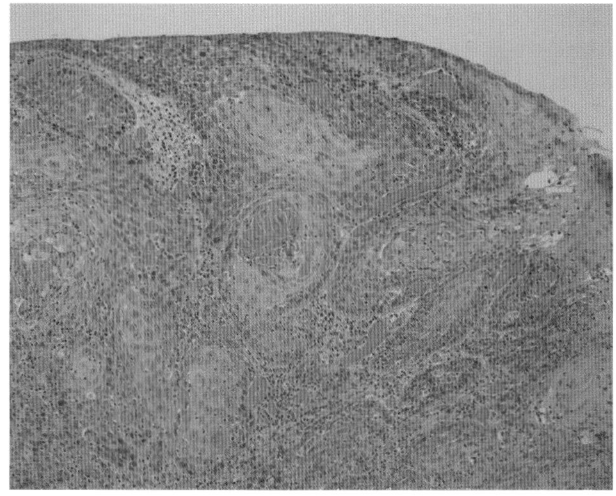

图 48.3　食管鳞状细胞癌的组织病理学显示，恶性角质形成细胞巢，细胞质、核仁和角蛋白呈玻璃样，累及食管黏膜，并伴有炎性基质反应。图像中心可见角化珠。×100。（Courtesy Dr. Michael Argyres，Denver，Colo.）

传统染色内镜涉及使用特殊染色剂来突出细微的结构变化，以帮助指导活检和预测组织学改变。卢戈式碘、亚甲蓝、乙酸、结晶紫和靛胭脂红是最常用的染色剂[153,154]。卢戈式碘液由 0.5%~3.0% 的碘化钾水溶液组成。正常食管上皮含糖原的细胞碘染色正常，异型增生或恶性细胞糖原耗竭碘染色不被吸收（呈“粉红色征”）。卢戈式碘染色的染色内镜检查已成为高危人群中 ESCC 筛查的标准方法，具有 89%~100% 的高敏感性，由于存在假阳性病变，其特异性具有高度变异性[150,155]。相比之下，亚甲蓝、乙酸和靛胭脂红染色在检测腺体异常方面更有用，如 EAC 所示。将这些染色剂喷洒在食管内，以改善黏膜的特征，从而黏膜选择性摄取（活体染色—亚甲蓝）或增强黏膜表面模式（对比染色法——靛胭脂红、乙酸）。重要的是，传统的染色内镜有许多局限性，包括：(a) 异型增生和炎症（食管炎）染色彼此无法区分；(b) 这些技术通常烦琐、耗时，且需要染料喷洒设备；(c) 难以用染料在黏膜表面实现完全且均匀的涂层；(d) 无法检测血管模式；(e) 与已发表的数据矛盾；(f) 需要放大内镜检查；(g) 缺乏标准化分类。在评估 Barrett 食管和 EAC 患者时，传统的染色内镜已基本被光学染色内镜检查所取代（见下文）。

光学染色内镜检查是另一种检测异型增生和癌的方式，它使用选择性滤光片来突出黏膜的细微结构和血管变化。这种方法避免了上述传统染色内镜检查相关的一些问题。不同的制造商提供了几种不同的电子染色内镜，但大部分已发表的研究都描述了在 BE 病变中使用窄带成像技术（narrow band imaging，NBI）。NBI 是一种基于光穿透组织深度的光学现象的成像技术，光穿透组织的深度取决于波长，波长越短，穿透越浅。使用带窄带滤光器的蓝光，能够以高分辨率和对比度对黏膜和血管表面模式进行精细成像，而无需染色内镜检查[156]。NBI 是研究最广泛的电子染色内镜技术，可在监测期间预测组织学变化，提高异型增生的检出率，并指导内镜根除治疗。一个国际专家工作组最近使用 NBI 建立了 BE 的分类系统[157]。一项系统性综述和 meta 分析表明，先进的成像技术（传统和光学染色内镜检查）使异型增生或癌的检出率增加了 34%（95% CI 20%~56%）[158]。

已在 ESCC 和鳞状上皮异型增生的检测中评价了无放大

的 NBI。早期 ESCC 内镜可疑病变在无放大的 NBI 上表现为边界清晰的褐色区域(图 48.4)。一项前瞻性比较研究表明,NBI 检查对早期 ESCC 的诊断是可靠的,敏感性为 88%,特异性为 75%[150,159]。

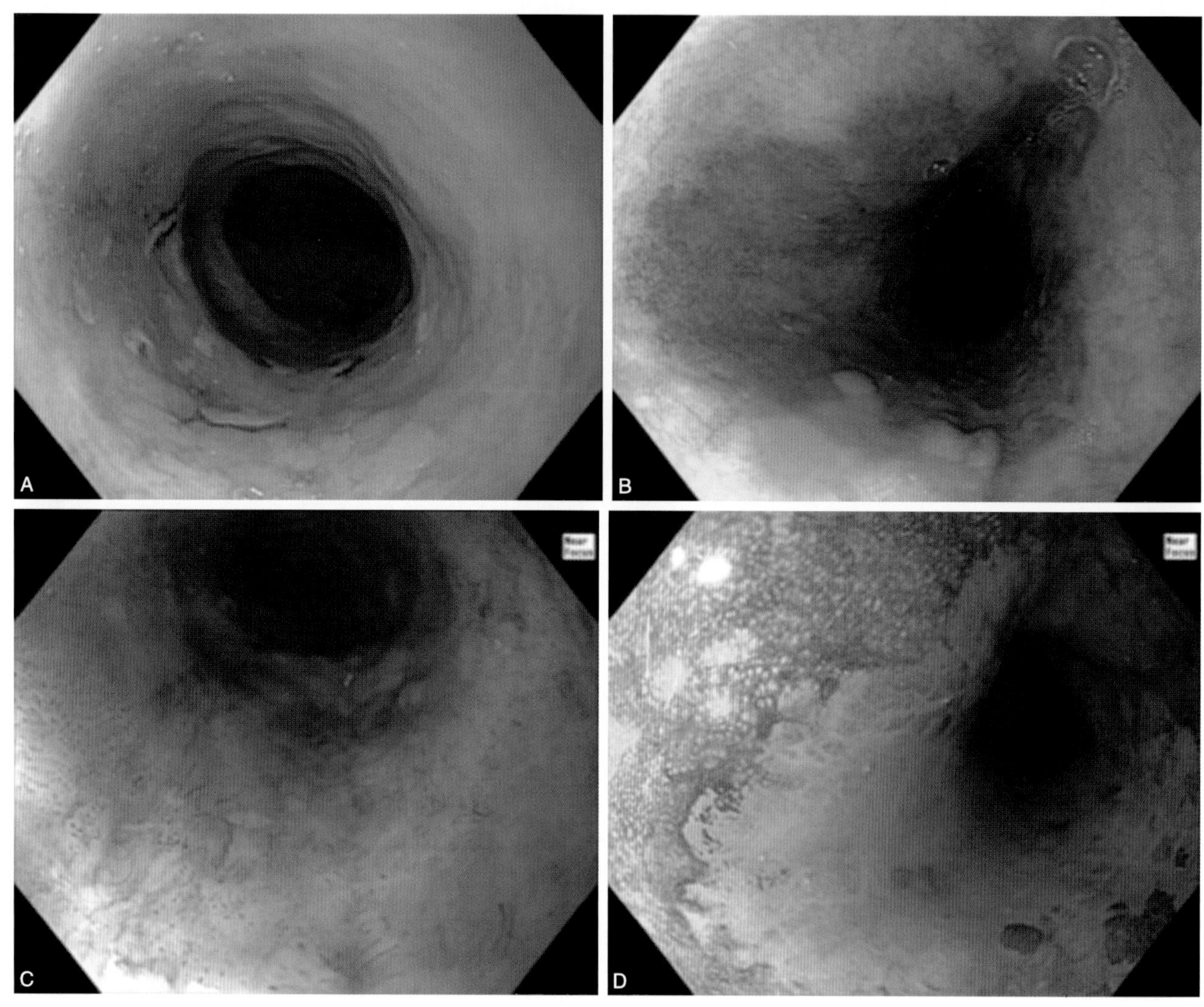

图 48.4 A,食管鳞状细胞癌的高清晰度白光内镜图像,显示食管内细微的不规则。B,同一区域窄带成像显示边界清晰的深褐色区域。C,放大 NBI 图像显示上皮内异常乳头状毛细血管袢模式。D,Lugo 染色内镜检查可见周围环绕的未染色病变

自发荧光成像(AFI)是一种使用短波蓝光或紫外线光刺激食管中生物荧光团(如胶原蛋白、卟啉、黄素、芳香族氨基酸)的技术。该技术主要用于检测 BE 相关肿瘤的临床试验。来自 5 项前瞻性试验的汇总分析表明,AFI 对肿瘤诊断几乎无效应,与 WLE 相比,附加诊断值为 2%,假阳性率高(78%)[160]。鉴于这种有限的附加诊断治疗值,AFI 在临床上未被广泛应用。

共聚焦激光内镜(CLE)是对食管黏膜进行实时活体显微成像的技术。它涉及静脉注射能被正常黏膜细胞吸收的荧光染料(最常见的是荧光素钠)。在异型增生的细胞中看不到摄取的荧光染料,因此显示黑暗。该方法可产生 1 000 倍的放大倍数。目前 CLE 的唯一市售方法是基于探针的仪器,该仪器可以通过标准上消化道内镜的附件通道。几项前瞻性随机对照研究报告,在高清晰度 WLE 中增加 CLE 可显著提高 BE 相关肿瘤的阳性诊断率[161,162]。

*光学相干断层扫描术*通过发射近红外光,提供组织的横断面图像,这在识别黏膜下病变方面也具有潜在优势。初步的研究显示检测异型增生的结果令人鼓舞,但其使用的局限性包括视野小和成像处理缓慢[163]。

容积激光显微内镜(VLE)是第二代光学相干断层扫描技术,可产生食管大面积的实时横断面图像。Nvision-VLE 已获得美国食品药品监督管理局的批准,目前已上市销售。该设备能够对可疑区域进行激光标记,以便进行后续治疗。在前瞻性队列中使用诊断算法,显示 VLE 检测 BE 相关异型增生的敏感性为 86%(95% CI 69% ~ 96%),特异性为 88%(95% CI 60% ~ 99%),诊断准确性为 87%(95% CI 86% ~ 88%)[164]。但目前这项新技术尚未广泛应用。

(六) 筛查和监测

EAC 筛查和监测包括在 Barrett 食管下进行(见第 47 章)。ESCC 的组织学前身包括异型增生和原位癌(图 48.5)[165]。鉴于异型增生发展为恶性肿瘤所需的时间,筛查

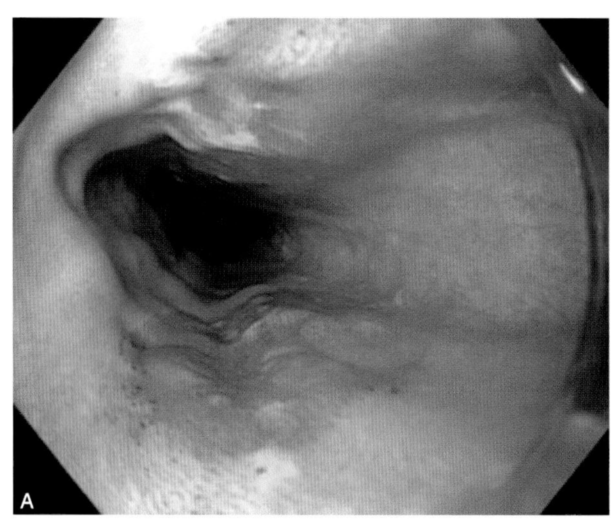

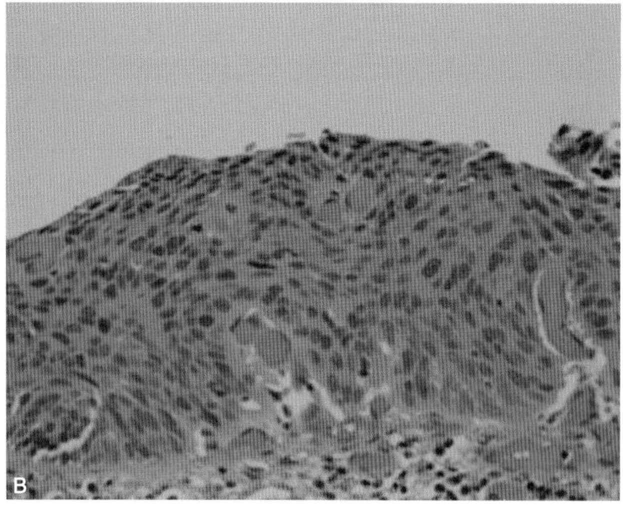

图 48.5 A,食管上段 6 点钟位置见边界清晰的微小结节,与早期肿瘤有关。B,活检病理证实为高级别鳞状上皮异型增生。(Courtesy Dr. Jeffrey Kaplan, Denver, Colo.)

和监测程序旨在检测这些早期组织学前身,以提高生存率。通过手术治疗,早期癌与显著改善的生存期相关(5 年生存率高达 86%)[166]。

ESCC 高发病率地区的主要筛查策略涉及 Lugo 染色内镜检查,从未染色区域获得活检标本。Lugo 活体染色是基于正常上皮细胞中碘和糖原之间的可逆化学反应。异型增生、癌性细胞和炎性细胞通常不被染色(因为糖原含量较少),可以进行靶向活检以确认异型增生/恶性肿瘤[167]。如上所述,Lugo 染色内镜检查的敏感性和特异性均大于 90%[155]。一些研究表明,Lugo 染液检测早期 ESCC 的特异性较低,这可能是由于难以区分异型增生/肿瘤和炎症,但靶向活检在这种原位中应该是有帮助的[168]。Lugo 溶液活体染色虽然简单且价格低廉,但存在一些局限性,包括可能的碘过敏、误吸风险或食管痉挛引起的胸痛。

NBI 可以更清晰地描述毛细血管网和浅表黏膜模式。在鳞状细胞异型增生和早期 ESCC 的鉴别和分期中,已提出并验证了这些异常的详细分类(见图 48.4)[169]。最近对 18 项研究进行的荟萃分析(包括超过 1 900 例患者)表明,与染色内镜相比,NBI 的特异性显著提高,但敏感性没有差异[168]。

已经开展了一项成本效益研究,以评估食管癌筛查策略[170]。一项研究发现,在不发达的高危地区,50 岁时进行一次分层筛查的策略是最好的方法,而在医疗卫生资源较好的地区,从 40 岁开始(间隔 10 年)进行 3 次筛查的策略是更为可取的[171]。

在中国一项随访 10 年的社区分配研究显示,在 40~69 岁成年人接受一次 Lugo 染色内镜检查的社区中,与未接受筛查的社区相比,与 ESCC 相关的累积死亡率降低了 1/3[172]。

头颈癌患者也建议进行 ESCC 常规筛查。来自台湾的一项回顾性研究发现,接受常规内镜检查的头颈部癌患者继发 ESCC 的患病率高于未筛查组(4.5% vs 3%, P=0.04),而且是早期诊断(P=0.03)[173]。

目前的筛查指南包括[9]:

1. 对高风险的亚洲和非洲人群从 40 岁开始进行一次 Lugo 染色内镜检查。

2. 头颈部鳞状细胞癌治疗完成后,每 6 个月至 1 年进行一次 Lugo 或 NBI 内镜检查,持续 10 年。

3. 也可以考虑对高危患者(胼胝症、贲门失弛缓症和食管腐蚀性损伤)进行筛查。

早期涉及的其他内镜技术,如 NBI 和 AFI,也已被评价为筛查工具。多项研究显示,NBI 可以基于浅表血管系统和表面模式检测早期食管病变,具有良好的敏感性和特异性,但仍需与 Lugo 染色内镜联合使用[168]。AFI 对小于 10mm 的病变不够敏感,因此作为筛查是不太有用的[174]。

使用经鼻非镇静的超薄内镜检查(TNE)已被证明是安全的,且耐受性良好[175]。一项对高危患者的研究表明,TNE(无论是否使用光学染色内镜)对早期 ESCC 具有极好的特异性和敏感性[176]。TNE 仍未广泛使用,但可作为 ESCC 筛查的重要工具。

其他内镜技术包括细胞内镜和高分辨率显微内镜,可对组织进行实时病理检查。有限的初始数据表明它们很有前景,但这些技术并不广泛使用[177,178]。

与内镜检查相比,用于筛查的非内镜方法(如使用经口气囊和海绵擦)具有成本低、侵入性小的优势。然而,由于对异型增生甚至浸润性癌检查的敏感性差,这些技术显然是不够的[179]。将非内镜细胞学样本与生物标志物(如 P53)相结合可能提高检测的敏感性[180]。正在研究的其他非侵入性筛查方法包括呼吸标志物(挥发性有机化合物)、肿瘤相关抗原抗体、循环微小 RNA 和甲基 DNA 标志物。

(七) 分期

食管癌的分期采用美国癌症联合委员会分期系统进行(图 48.6),该系统 2017 年最后一次更新(第 8 版)[181]。该系统不仅将 EAC 和 ESSC 的分期分开,还分别为 EAC 和 ESCC 提供了 3 种分类系统:经典参考病理学分期组(pTNM)(图 48.7)、新引入的新辅助后病理学分期组(ypTNM)(图 48.8)和临床分期组(cTNM)(图 48.9)。该分期系统最近修订了食

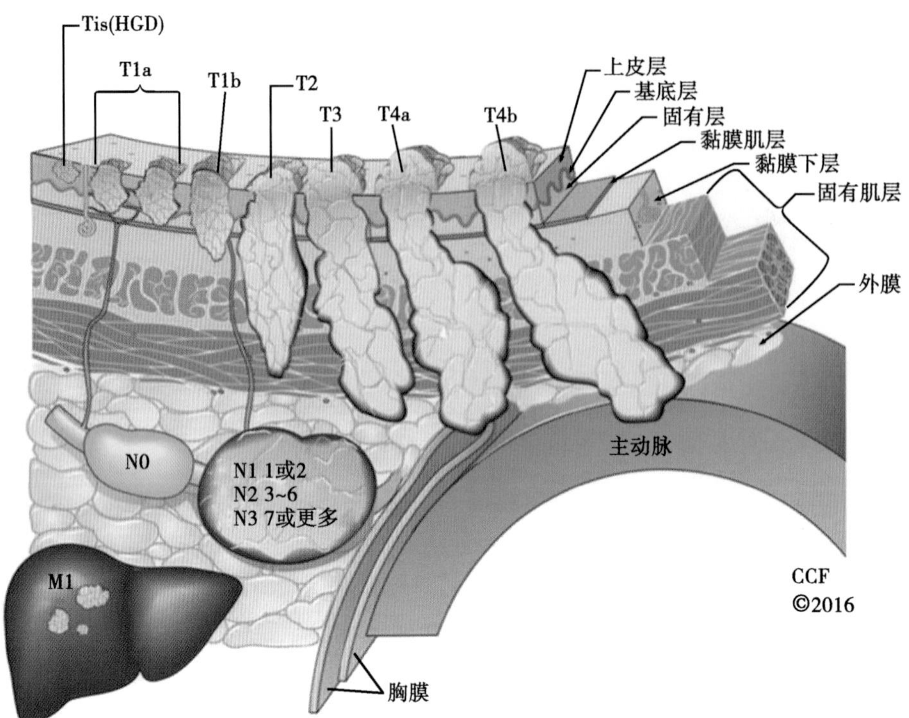

图 48.6　美国癌症联合委员会（AJCC）对食管-胃交界处癌 TNM 分期分类。T 分类为：Tis（高级别异型增生）；T1 癌侵犯固有层、黏膜肌层和黏膜下层，并细分为 T1a（侵犯固有层或黏膜肌层的癌）和 T1b（侵犯黏膜下层的癌）；T2 癌侵犯固有肌层；T3 癌侵犯外膜；T4 癌侵犯局部结构，被细分为 T4a（癌侵犯邻近结构如胸膜、心包、奇静脉、膈膜或腹膜）和 T4b（癌侵犯主要的邻近结构，如主动脉、椎体或气管）。N 分类为：N0（无局部淋巴结转移），N1（局部淋巴结转移侵犯 1 或 2 个淋巴结），N2（局部淋巴结转移侵犯 3 至 6 个淋巴结）和 N3（局部淋巴结转移侵犯 7 个或更多淋巴结）。M 分类为 M0（无远处转移）和 M1（远处转移）。（From Rice TW，Ishwaran H，Ferguson MK，Blackstone EH，Goldstraw P. Cancer of the esophagus and esophagogastric junction：an eighth edition staging primer. J Thorac Oncol 2017；12：36-42.）

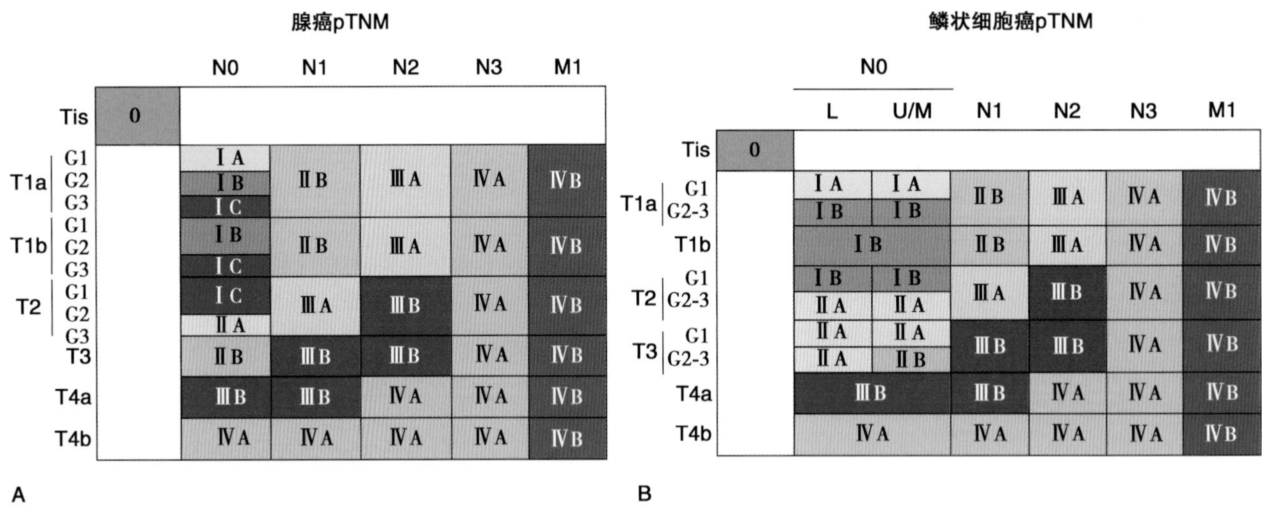

腺癌pTNM

		N0	N1	N2	N3	M1
Tis		0				
T1a	G1	ⅠA	ⅡB	ⅢA	ⅣA	ⅣB
	G2	ⅠB				
	G3	ⅠC				
T1b	G1	ⅠB	ⅡB	ⅢA	ⅣA	ⅣB
	G2					
	G3	ⅠC				
T2	G1	ⅠC	ⅢA	ⅢB	ⅣA	ⅣB
	G2					
	G3	ⅡA				
T3		ⅡB	ⅢB	ⅢB	ⅣA	ⅣB
T4a		ⅢB	ⅢB	ⅣA	ⅣA	ⅣB
T4b		ⅣA	ⅣA	ⅣA	ⅣA	ⅣB

A

鳞状细胞癌pTNM

		N0 L	N0 U/M	N1	N2	N3	M1
Tis		0					
T1a	G1	ⅠA	ⅠA	ⅡB	ⅢA	ⅣA	ⅣB
	G2-3	ⅠB	ⅠB				
T1b		ⅠB		ⅡB	ⅢA	ⅣA	ⅣB
T2	G1	ⅠB	ⅠB	ⅢA	ⅢB	ⅣA	ⅣB
	G2-3	ⅡA	ⅡA				
T3	G1	ⅡA	ⅡA	ⅢB	ⅢB	ⅣA	ⅣB
	G2-3	ⅡA	ⅡB				
T4a		ⅢB		ⅢB	ⅣA	ⅣA	ⅣB
T4b		ⅣA		ⅣA	ⅣA	ⅣA	ⅣB

B

图 48.7　食管腺癌（A）和鳞状细胞癌（B）的病理学分期组（pTNM）。（Redrawn from Rice TW，Ishwaran H，Ferguson MK，Blackstone EH，Goldstraw P. Cancer of the esophagus and esophagogastric junction：an eighth edition staging primer. J Thorac Oncol 2017；12[1]：36-42.）

ypTNM

	N0	N1	N2	N3	M1
T0	Ⅰ	ⅢA	ⅢB	ⅣA	ⅣB
Tis	Ⅰ	ⅢA	ⅢB	ⅣA	ⅣB
T1	Ⅰ	ⅢA	ⅢB	ⅣA	ⅣB
T2	Ⅰ	ⅢA	ⅢB	ⅣA	ⅣB
T3	Ⅱ	ⅢB	ⅢB	ⅣA	ⅣB
T4a	ⅢB	ⅣA	ⅣA	ⅣA	ⅣB
T4b	ⅣA	ⅣA	ⅣA	ⅣA	ⅣB

图 48.8 食管腺癌和鳞状细胞癌的新辅助治疗后病理学分期组(ypTNM)。(Redrawn from Rice TW, Ishwaran H, Ferguson MK, Blackstone EH, Goldstraw P. Cancer of the esophagus and esophagogastric junction: an eighth edition staging primer. J Thorac Oncol 2017;12[1]:36-42.)

腺癌cTNM

	N0	N1	N2	N3	M1
Tis	0				
T1	Ⅰ	ⅡA	ⅣA	ⅣA	ⅣB
T2	ⅡB	Ⅲ	ⅣA	ⅣA	ⅣB
T3	Ⅲ	Ⅲ	ⅣA	ⅣA	ⅣB
T4a	Ⅲ	Ⅲ	ⅣA	ⅣA	ⅣB
T4b	ⅣA	ⅣA	ⅣA	ⅣA	ⅣB

A

鳞状细胞癌cTNM

	N0	N1	N2	N3	M1
Tis	0				
T1	Ⅰ	Ⅰ	Ⅲ	ⅣA	ⅣB
T2	Ⅱ	Ⅱ	Ⅲ	ⅣA	ⅣB
T3	Ⅱ	Ⅱ	Ⅲ	ⅣA	ⅣB
T4a	ⅣA	ⅣA	ⅣA	ⅣA	ⅣB
T4b	ⅣA	ⅣA	ⅣA	ⅣA	ⅣB

B

图 48.9 食管腺癌(A)和鳞状细胞癌(B)的临床分期组(cTNM)。(Redrawn from Rice TW, Ishwaran H, Ferguson MK, Blackstone EH, Goldstraw P. Cancer of the esophagus and esophagogastric junction: an eighth edition staging primer. J Thorac Oncol. 2017;12(1):36-42.)

管-胃交界处的定义,将累及食管-胃交界处的中心距胃贲门不超过 2cm 的癌分期为 EAC,受累距胃贲门>2cm 者分期为胃癌。

肿瘤浸润深度(T 分期)是一个重要因素,由于食管有丰富的淋巴供应可以提供转移途径。浅表性癌定义为原位癌(Tis)或 T1 期肿瘤。根据黏膜下层是否受累,T1 分为 T1a 和 T1b。T1a 的进一步分类包括 M1(上皮内癌)、M2(侵犯固有层)和 M3(侵犯黏膜肌层)。T1b 病变还可细分为 SM1(侵犯黏膜下层的上 1/3)、SM2(侵犯中 1/3)和 SM3(侵犯下 1/3)。与 T1b 病灶相比,Tis 和 T1a 病灶预测的淋巴结转移率高达 8%,T1b 病灶的淋巴结转移率高达 56%[182-184]。除纵隔淋巴结外,颈部和上腹部也可能发生淋巴结转移[185]。淋巴结受累的风险与以下几个因素有关(按频率递减顺序排列):Ⅲ级组织学、SM3 侵袭、淋巴管浸润、血管浸润、SM2 浸润和 SM1 浸润。在 ESCC 中,淋巴结浸润的最佳预测因素是 SM3 浸润和血管浸润,而在 EAC 中,最重要的预测因素是淋巴浸润[186]。图 48.10 显示了生存期与 T 分期的相关性。

分期可通过几种方法进行:内镜下黏膜活检、内镜下切除、多排螺旋 CT(MDCT)和 ^{18}F-氟-2-脱氧-d-葡萄糖 PET(^{18}F-FDG-PET,正电子发射计算机断层显像),以及超声内镜-细针穿刺(EUS-FNA)进行细胞学检查[187,188]。

1. 内镜下黏膜活检

内镜下黏膜活检在分期中的作用是描述肿瘤的腔内黏膜范围(位置特征),并确定组织学类型(ESCC 或 EAC)和组织学分级(分化程度)[189]。当进行多次活检时(通常为 6~8 次),黏膜活检的敏感性可达到 96%[190]。如前所述,NBI 和其他先进的成像技术可更精确的评估肿瘤范围。

2. 多排螺旋 CT 和 ^{18}F-FDG-PET 扫描

多排螺旋 CT 和 ^{18}F-FDG-PET 扫描常用于食管癌分期(图 48.11)。ESCC 和 EAC 对 ^{18}F-FDG 均具有高亲和力,这使得 PET 扫描在食管癌评估中非常有帮助。^{18}F-FDG-PET 检测食管癌远处转移的敏感性和特异性分别为 71%(95% CI 62~79)和 93%(95% CI 89~97),而 CT 的敏感性和特异性分别为 52%(95% CI 33~72)和 91%(95% CI 86~96)[191,192]。研究表明,CT-PET 可以识别 5%~28% 的转移性疾病,尤其是在单用 CT 未检测到的部位。此外,与单独使用 EUS-FNA 或 MDCT 相比,使用 FDG-PET/CT 在新辅助治疗后再分期似乎完成得更好[193]。

3. 超声内镜(EUS)

EUS 越来越多地用于评估肿瘤浸润的深度,并将 T1 病变与较深的浸润区分开。这种区别有助于选择适当阶段治疗的候选者。EUS 是唯一可以清晰显示不同食管壁层次的成像

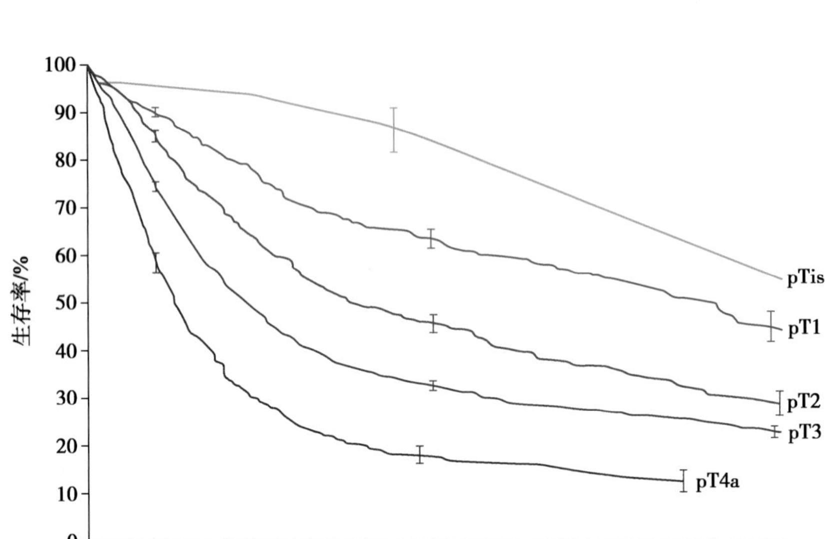

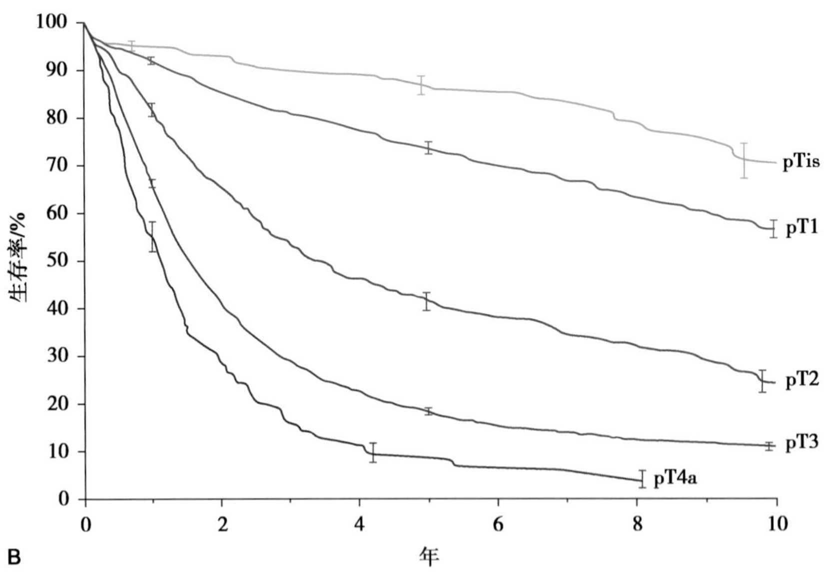

图 48.10　按 pT 类别分层的生存率。Kaplan-Meier(生存曲线分析法)估计值通过 68% 置信限的竖线代表,相当于±1 个标准误。A,食管鳞状细胞癌。B,食管腺癌。(Data from Rice TW, Chen LQ, Hofstetter WL, et al. Worldwide Esophageal Cancer Collaboration: pathologic staging data. Dis Esophagus 2016;29[7]:724-33.)

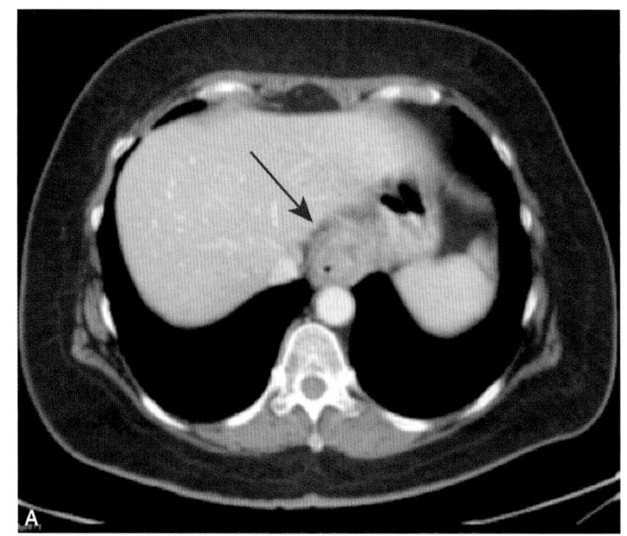

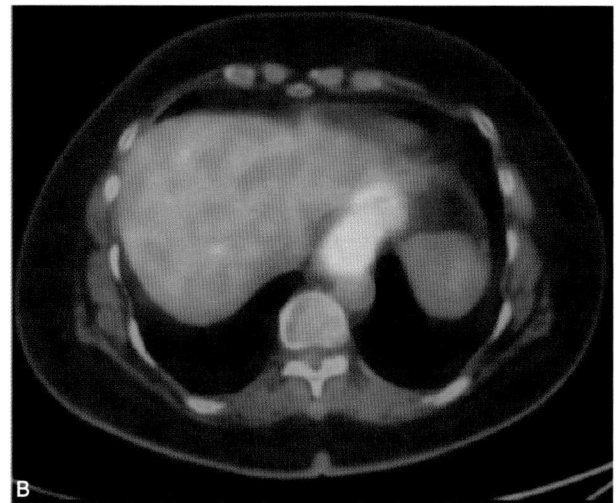

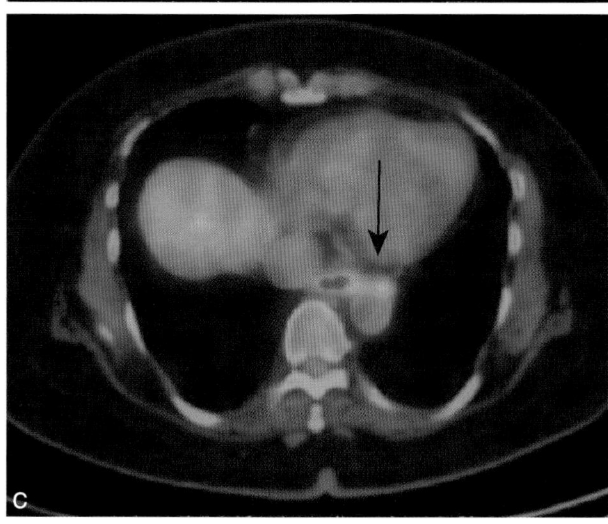

图 48.11　A，CT 扫描所见食管远端增厚的食管癌部位（箭）。B 和 C，FDG-PET 图像显示食管远端（B）和左侧食管旁淋巴结（C，箭）出现相应的强烈高代谢

方式。大多数专家认为它是 T 分期和局部区域淋巴结（N）分期的最佳分期方式。在荟萃分析中，EUS 对 T 分期的总体敏感性为 80%～90%，特异性超过 90%。对于更晚期的 T 分期，准确性更高。EUS 对 N 分期的总体敏感性为 85%（95% CI 82%～86%）。对难以解释的淋巴结进行细针穿刺（FNA）可将淋巴结分期的敏感性提高到 97%（95% CI 92%～99%）[194]。恶性淋巴结的超声内镜特征包括表面圆形光滑的低回声病变，病变>10mm，病变位于肿瘤附近[195]。

EUS 在食管癌初始分期中的作用受到质疑，尤其是在浅表性肿瘤中[196,197]。最近的一项综述和荟萃分析发现，EUS 对浅表性食管癌分期总体来说具有良好的准确性[198]。病变的位置、组织学类型、使用的 EUS 方法以及超声内镜医师的经验等因素可能会影响诊断的准确性。一项系统综述和荟萃分析的最新数据评估了 EUS 检查在肿瘤水平上的进展期疾病的假阳性率（区分 T1a 和 T1b 疾病），结果显示在 BE 伴异型增生和早期癌症患者中使用 EUS 导致高比例的患者出现虚假的过度分期和分期不足[199]。因此，诸如内镜下黏膜切除术（EMR）和内镜下黏膜剥离术（ESD）等先进技术在确定侵袭的真实程度方面起着关键作用。

与 CT 相比，EUS 对局部转移的诊断具有更好的敏感性和特异性[195,200]。一项荟萃分析比较了 EUS、CT 和 FDG-PET 结果显示，三种方式检测区域淋巴结转移的汇集敏感性分别为 80%、50% 和 57%[191]。最近一项使用 SEER 医疗保险相关数据库的食管癌近期病例研究显示，与未接受 EUS 或 CT-PET 组相比，接受 EUS 分期组的食管癌患者队列的生存率有所提高，0 期疾病除外。接受 EUS 增加了接受内镜治疗、食管切除术和放化疗的可能性。多变量 Cox 比例风险模型表明，接受 EUS 是 1 年［风险比（HR）0.49，95% CI 0.39～0.59］、3 年（HR 0.57，95% CI 0.48～0.66）和 5 年（HR 0.59，95% CI 0.5～0.68）生存率改善的重要预测因素。这种生存率的提高很可能与食管癌患者的准确分期有关，从而产生适当的分期特异性治疗[201]。

4. 先进技术

在选定中心进行的其他分期方式包括 EMR、ESD 和使用腹腔镜进行的微创分期[202]。如何选择以及选择的顺序取决于医疗机构的专业知识和偏好。关于 EUS 在浅表性肿瘤中准确性的相互矛盾的报道，使一些人认为 EMR 和 ESD 可能是更准确的诊断和分期方法[196,197,203]。这两种方法不仅为评估肿瘤浸润深度（T 期）和可能的无瘤边缘提供了组织，还提供了肿瘤分化程度和淋巴血管浸润分级的信息。EMR 和 ESD 将在后面进行更详细的讨论。对于食管远端及食管-胃交界处的肿瘤，腹腔镜分期检查被认为是可选的方式，因为它可以检测到其他放射学隐匿性转移的病变[204,205]。

（八）治疗

食管癌治疗的多学科综合方法至关重要，需要肿瘤外科学、放射肿瘤学、内科肿瘤学、胃肠病学、放射学、病理学和姑息治疗专家的共同参与[206]。肿瘤定位、分期、组织学类型、医学合并症和患者的意愿是选择适当治疗时必须考虑的因素。一般原则总结如下[207]：

- 手术是患有局部、非浅表肿瘤的医学优化手术候选者的标准治疗方法。
- 对于不能手术治疗的局部肿瘤患者，可考虑具有治疗目的的确定性放化疗。
- 对于所有其他疾病（转移性疾病），建议姑息治疗。

食管癌的治疗方案谱广泛，准确的分期对选择合适的治疗方式至关重要[208]。主要目的是确定哪些患者可能受益于新辅助治疗，哪些患者有广泛转移性疾病更适合姑息治疗。选择患者是食管癌治疗的另一个非常重要的组成部分。评估应包括医学合并症和患者目前体能状态、营养和心肺功能。肺部并发症，尤其是肺炎，是术后早期预后的重要决定因素，与死亡率增加4倍以上有关[209-211]。有趣的是，发现术前放化疗是术后肺炎的危险因素[211]。涉及肺活量测定结果、年龄和体能状态的评分系统可用于预测心肺并发症[210]。基于数学评分的选择可能并不优于医生的临床评估，这两种方法是互补的[212]。重要的是，获得的评分可能并不适用于所有机构或人群。例如，与西方国家的EAC患者（如心脏风险因素或合并症）相比，来自亚洲的ESCC患者（如吸烟和饮酒导致的肺部和肝脏合并症）具有不同的风险特征[213]。

颈段或颈胸段食管肿瘤患者（距环咽肌小于5cm），由于手术技术的限制，通常是手术的不良候选者，不适合手术[214]。这些患者通常接受确定性放化疗，在最近的一项研究中有令人鼓舞的应答率[215]。

1. 外科手术

切除食管加整体淋巴结切除术是局部进展期食管癌患者治愈性治疗的基石[216]。此外，根据美国国家综合癌症网络（National Comprehensive Cancer Network，NCCN）指南，对于无淋巴结受累或远处转移的T1b和T2食管癌，选择单独手术被认为是标准治疗。对伴有淋巴结转移的T1～T4a肿瘤，需采用手术联合多模式方法[204]。接受食管切除术的患者的最终结局不仅取决于患者的分期、合并症和体能状态，还取决于手术团队的专业技术和中心手术容量。食管切除术有可能导致较高的围手术期发病率（40%～50%）和死亡率（3%～13%）[217-221]。在外科文献中反复出现的一个主题是食管切除术的中心手术容量是决定预后的关键因素[216,220,222]。30天死亡率与在该中心进行的食管切除术数量呈负相关。在高容量手术中心由经验丰富的外科医生进行治疗，以及ICU提供的有效管理和并发症的早期发现，在不同的结局中起着显著重要的作用。

在低手术容量中心（每年<5例食管切除术），死亡率可能增加到20%[223-225]。高容量中心的手术死亡率（每年>20例）估计低于2%[226-228]。在对护理质量指标的回顾中，选择患者和多学科团队管理是影响食管癌手术结果的最重要因素[229]。

（1）技术

对食管癌患者的食管切除术，已经描述了几种不同的外科技术。使用的技术可能受到手术入路部位（经胸与经膈）、淋巴结病变的范围、所需吻合方式、食管导管的类型和制备方法、幽门引流程序和重建路径等的影响。大多数争议是基于手术入路的类型和淋巴结清扫的范围[230]。手术入路的类型不仅可能影响围手术期的发病率和死亡率，还可能影响进行广泛淋巴结清扫的能力[212]。

经胸入路包括Ivor-Lewis食管胃切除术（右开胸和剖腹手术）和McKeown食管胃切除术（开胸、剖腹手术和颈部吻合术）。经膈裂孔入路包括剖腹手术和颈部吻合术[231-236]。据报道，经胸入路的优势在于更好地显示纵隔，从而降低了邻近器官损伤的风险，更完整地切除癌和淋巴结，以及更准确地分期[234]。相反，那些赞成经膈裂孔入路的人注意到，食管癌的治愈是一种罕见的现象，只有在极早期肿瘤中才能实现，这使得食管切除术通常是一种姑息性手术。在这点上，经膈裂孔入路的手术时间较短，术后发病率较低[232]。一项基于人群的大型研究比较了经胸和经膈裂孔入路的手术方式，发现经膈裂孔入路食管切除术与较低的手术死亡率相关（6.7% vs 13.1%，$P=0.009$），但两种方法的长期生存率没有差异[221]。

微创食管切除术（minimally invasive esophagectomy，MIE）包括微创Ivor-Lewis食管胃切除术（腹腔镜和有限的开胸术或胸腔镜）和微创McKeown食管胃切除术（胸腔镜、有限剖腹术或腹腔镜和颈部切口），最近获得人们的欢迎[237]。其目的是最大限度地减少手术创伤及围手术期发病率和死亡率。这项技术需要特殊的培训和专业知识[238]。与传统手术方法相比，微创手术具有相似的肿瘤治疗效果[239]。微创手术的优点包括术后疼痛较轻、住院时间缩短、术中输血需求较少，以及总体成本较低[240-242]。最近一项前瞻性多中心试验表明，MIE是安全可行的，围手术期发病率和死亡率较低（2.1%）[243]。尽管MIE的结果令人鼓舞，但最近基于人群的研究未能证明MIE优于传统手术方法[244]。

（2）淋巴结清扫术

淋巴结状态是食管癌生存的独立预测因素[245]。因此，积极的淋巴结切除术被认为对减少局部区域复发、提高生存率和获得更准确的病理分期极其重要[246,247]。食管切除术中切除的淋巴结数量已被证明是生存的独立预测因素[248]。在未接受新辅助放化疗的食管切除术的患者中，NCCN指南建议切除15个或更多淋巴结以进行充分分期[204]。然而，在接受新辅助放化疗的患者中，淋巴结切除的数量似乎与生存率的增加无关[249]。

（3）结果

食管癌食管切除术后测量短期临床结果是难以与已发表的报告进行比较，由于缺乏标准方法学和其他不一致[250]。此外，在美国最大的胸外科数据库中纳入的食管切除术后的结果远远好于其他国家临床和管理数据库所报告的结果[251]。最常报告的并发症是吻合口瘘和术后肺炎。

最近一项更新的基于人群的无新辅助治疗食管癌手术后生存率的研究表明，自2000年以来，长期生存率没有改善。更确切地说，5年后仍保持在30.5%。尽管术后30天死亡率从近5%下降至2%，但手术患者的生存率保持不变[252]。术后死亡率的改善可能反映了ICU对并发症的更好管理和治疗[252,253]。因此，手术技术的改进并没有转化为更好的长期生存结果。

在具有潜在可切除肿瘤的患者中，有相当一部分在接受新辅助放化疗后达到病理学完全应答（EAC中23%，ESCC中49%）[254]。此外，最近一项在可切除ESCC患者中比较手术与确定性放化疗的研究显示，Ⅰ期（80% vs 75.8%）和Ⅱ期（78.2% vs 74.6%）患者的5年总生存率并无差异[255]。另一项研究显示，Ⅰ期疾病手术与放化疗的结果相似，但放化疗组局部复发（包括异时病变）的风险明显增高。放化疗组大多数复发为黏膜内癌，经挽救治疗（主要是内镜）后治愈，如下所讨论的[256]。目前正在进行研究，以确定哪些患者有可能避免手术。

2. 内镜治疗

EET彻底改变了与BE相关的异型增生和早期EAC（见第47章）以及食管鳞状细胞异型增生和早期ESCC的治疗。

内镜治疗食管癌的作用可以是治愈目的或缓解症状。前者仅限定于黏膜(M1 或上皮内)、固有层(M2)或黏膜肌层(M3)的黏膜肿瘤(T1a)。这些肿瘤发生淋巴结转移的概率极低。黏膜下肿瘤(T1b)进一步分为 SM1(黏膜下浅层浸润)、SM2(黏膜下层中心浸润)或 SM3(黏膜下层深部浸润)。与 T1a 肿瘤相比,累及黏膜下层的 T1b 肿瘤发生淋巴结转移的风险更高,在 SM3 肿瘤中高达 56%[183,184]。

(1) 以治愈为目的的内镜治疗

内镜切除术和内镜消融治疗已被广泛用于浅表性食管癌的治疗。内镜切除术具有获取大组织标本用于病理诊断和准确的癌症分期的额外优势(图 48.12)[257,258]。EMR 和 ESD 均可靶向切除组织,如结节状或扁平状 Barrett 上皮伴 HGD 以及 T1a 期癌(图 48.13)。EET 在根除 Barrett 相关肿瘤、维持缓解和防止进展为侵袭性 EAC(EET 的主要目标)方面的有效性和安全性已在多项研究中得到证实[259,260]。关于 barrett 相关异型增生和早期 EAC 处理的 EET 基本原则如下:(a)切除所有可见病变(具有隐藏最高级别肿瘤的病变);(b)根除剩余的 BE,以降低异时性肿瘤的风险;(c)即刻处理不良事件,如出血、穿孔以及长期不良事件,如狭窄和复发,(d)在实现彻底根除后注册登记参加监测项目[261]。

EET 目前已取代食管切除术成为 Barrett 相关 HGD 和早期黏膜内 EAC 患者的标准治疗[262]。尽管没有比较食管切除术与 EET 的随机对照试验,但基于人群和观察性研究的结果已报告 EET 与食管切除术后的结果相当(2 年和 5 年 EAC 生存率),为 BE 相关肿瘤患者用 EET 现代治疗提供了信心[259]。

关于 EET 作用的最新 ACGE 指南文件建议,在伴有 HGD 和黏膜内癌的 BE 患者中不进行手术而使用 EET 治疗[259]。EMR 在 BE 相关肿瘤治疗中作为一种分期和治疗工具的作用已得到充分描述。与活检标本相比较,EMR 的分期优势与提供更大、更深、且变形程度有限的组织标本有关,提供了浸入深度的最终证据,以及改善了使用 EMR 标本的病理学观察者之间的一致性[258,263]。一项对 1 000 例 T1a 食管癌患者跟踪 5 年左右的研究表明,EMR 非常有效,完全缓解率为 94%[264]。对 1998 年至 2008 年间 1 458 例 T1N0 食管癌(ESCC 和 EAC)患者的 SEER 数据库分析显示,接受手术治疗的患者(64.1%)和接受内镜治疗(包括 EMR 伴或不伴消融)的患者(55.5%)的总生存率相似[265]。EMR 的高效率似乎也是 BE 高根除率的重要预测因素[266,267]。

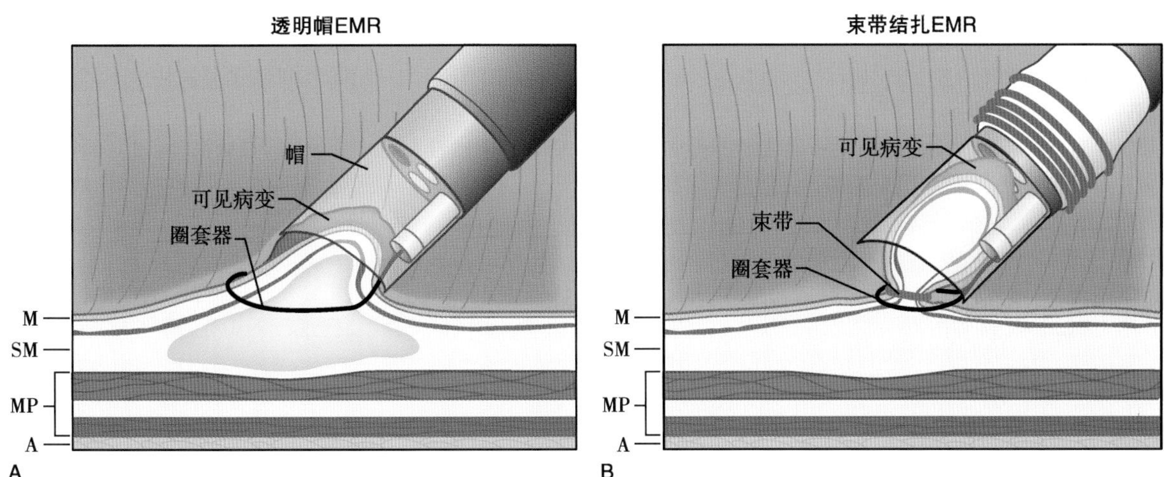

图 48.12 内镜黏膜切除术(EMR)。A,透明帽 EMR。B,束带结扎 EMR。A,外膜;M,黏膜;MP,固有肌层;SM,黏膜下层

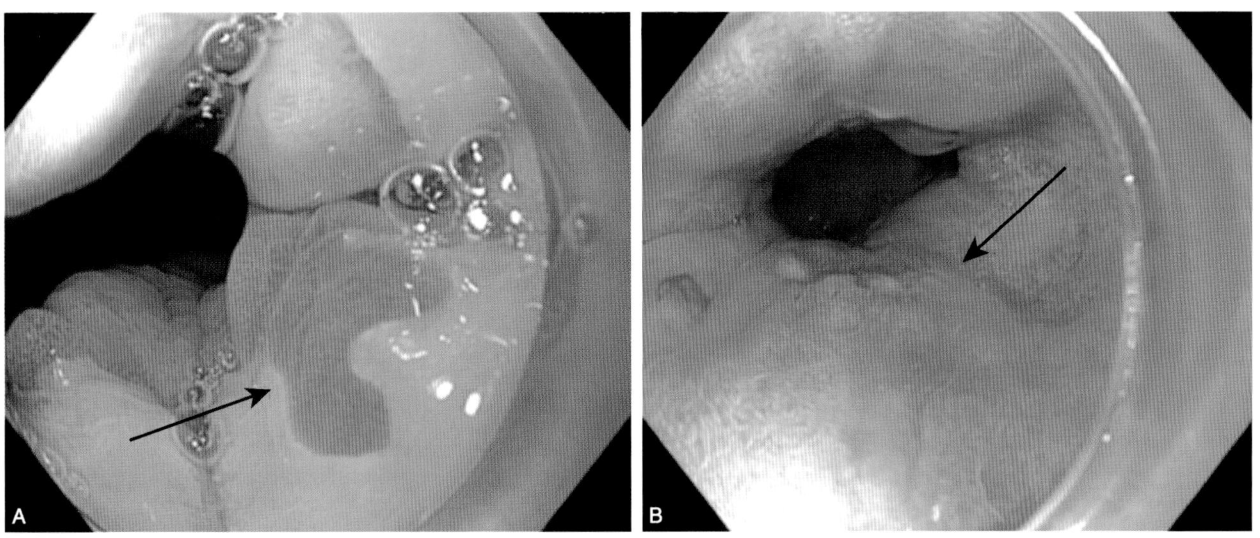

图 48.13 A~D,Barrett 食管患者在高分辨率内镜下检查到的可见病变示例(箭)

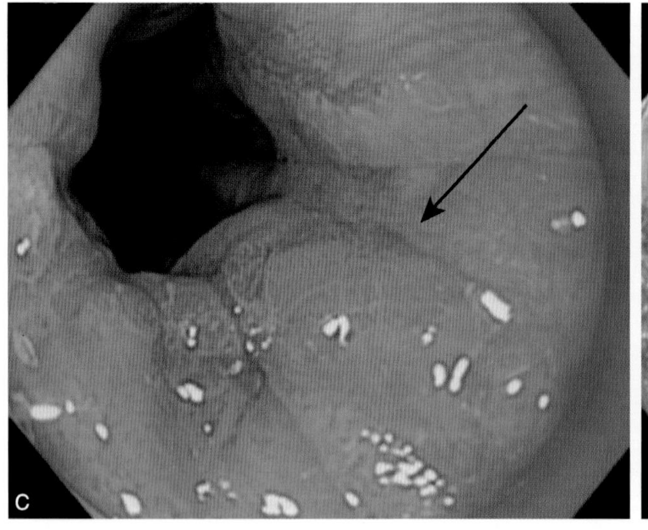

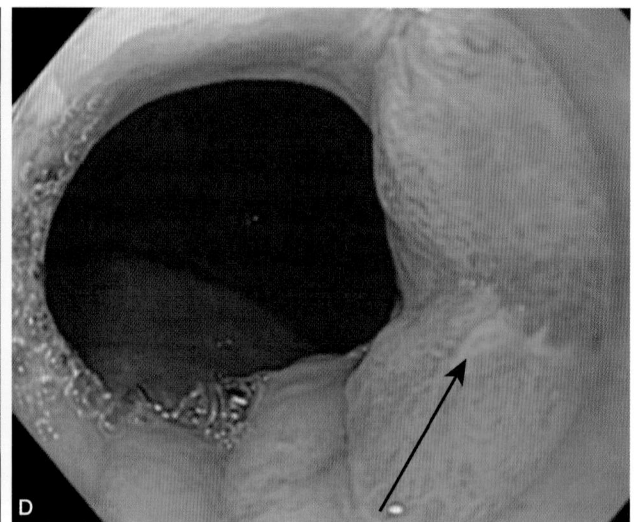

图 48.13(续)

EMR 的并发症包括出血(高达 10%)、穿孔(<3%)和狭窄[257,268]。EMR 术后狭窄大部分对内镜球囊扩张有反应,并与黏膜切除术的周长和长度有关[269]。

鉴于 EMR 在早期食管癌治疗中令人鼓舞的报道,选择患者是至关重要的。EMR 的主要限制因素是淋巴结受累、存在淋巴血管浸润和多灶性疾病[270,271]。最终,据报道,EMR 的最佳无病结果是直径小于 20mm 的非溃疡性或结节性黏膜病变,尤其是分化良好或中等分化、且黏膜内无淋巴血管浸润的病变[272,273]。

早期对内镜治疗的热情为延伸到黏膜下层的病变带来了新的技术。ESD 可以有效地增加局部整块大小的切除,并切除黏膜下肿瘤(图 48.14 和图 48.15)[274]。然而,这些病变有淋巴结受累的显著风险,因此在这种情况下,ESD 只是诊断性的,而不是治愈性的。大多数 ESD 经验来自日本,据报道 ESCC 的整体切除率为 100%,根治性切除率为 80%[275,276]。当比较 ESD 与 EMR 在治疗 20mm 或更小的食管黏膜癌中的效果时,发现 ESD 提供了 100%的整块切除率,而 EMR 的整块切除率为 87%(透明帽辅助)和 71%(需用双通道技术)。ESD 的根治性切除率为 97%,显著高于任何一种 EMR 技术(透明帽为 71%,双通道为 46%)。ESD 的并发症包括 2%～5%的穿孔和 5%～17%的狭窄[275-277]。

欧洲胃肠内窥镜学会建议,ESD 是内镜下切除 ESCC 的首选方法,因为它整块切除率较高,且具有更优越的组织学评估。如果可以确保整块切除,EMR 可用于<10mm 的病变。对

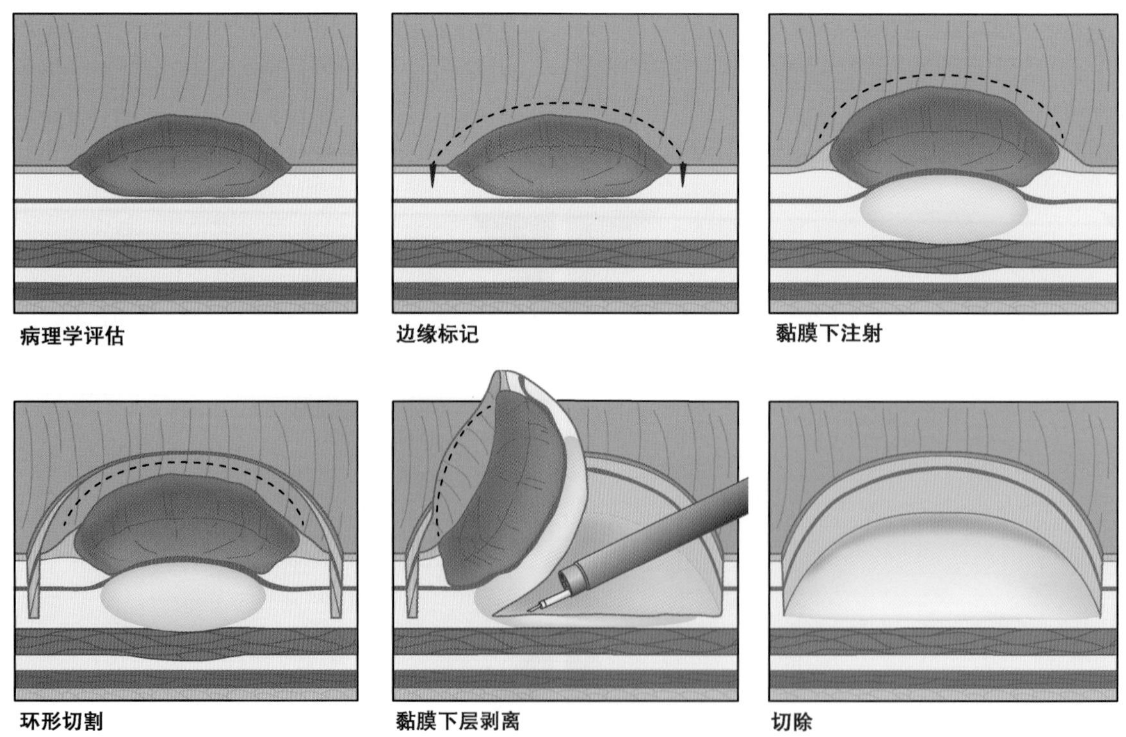

图 48.14　内镜黏膜剥离术的示意图。(Redrawn from Current Gastroenterology Reports 2014;16[5].)

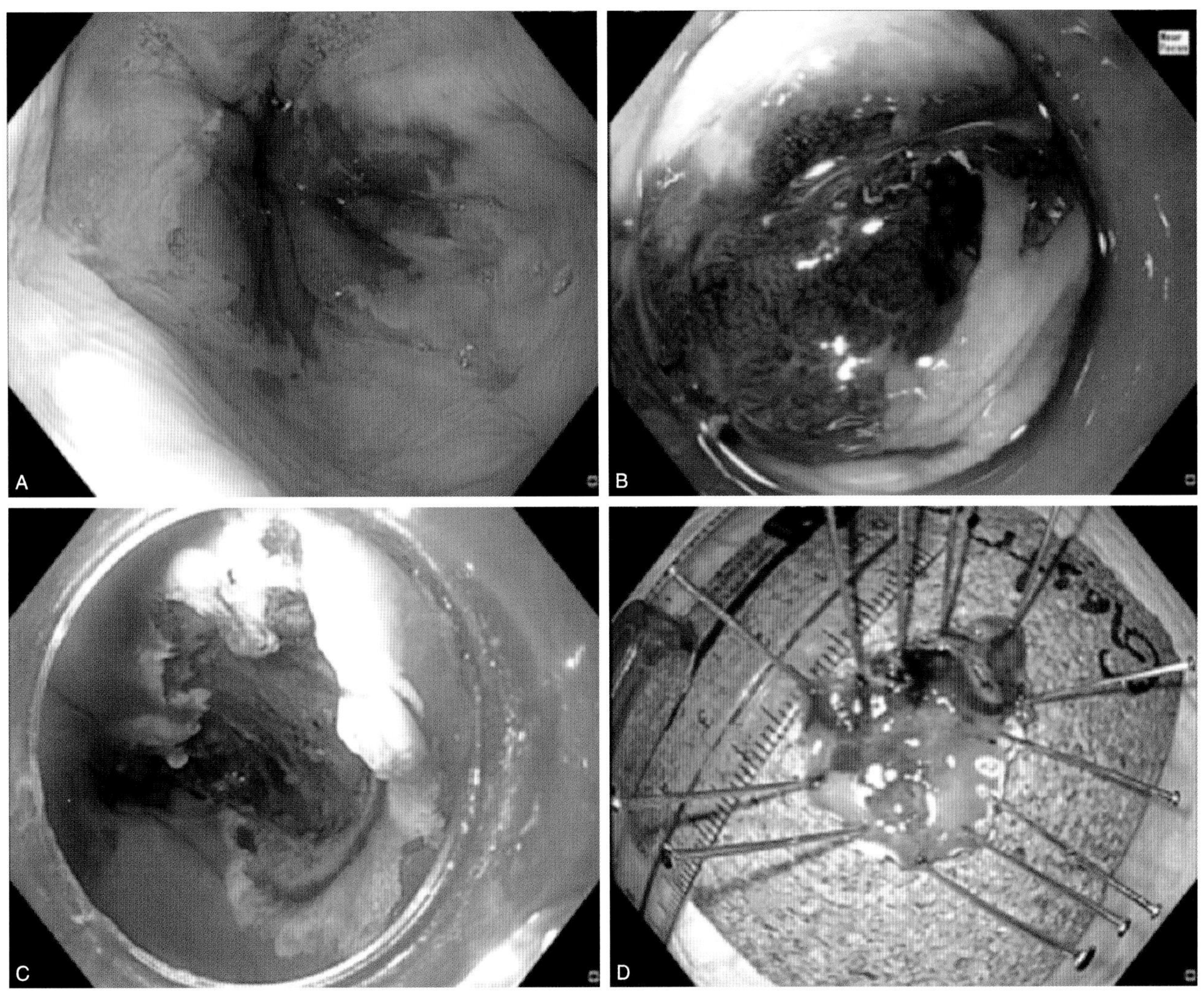

图 48.15　A，食管远端 1~3 点位的结节病变，活检符合腺癌。B，窄带成像检查的同一区域，见不规则凹陷和血管模式图像。C，结节区域行内镜黏膜剥离术（ESD）后的黏膜缺损区域。D，固定在软木板上的 ESD 切除标本

于早期的 EAC 和 HGD，EMR 仍然是内镜切除的主要方法，但对于>15mm 的病变、抬举不良的肿瘤以及具有黏膜下浸润高风险特征的病变可以考虑 ESD[278]。

消融术可通过射频消融（RFA）或冷冻疗法实现。每种方法都可以单独使用，或者更常用于 EMR 或 ESD 之后的可见结节。由于不良反应（狭窄和光敏性）风险较高及其他消融技术的可用性，目前光动力疗法很少在临床实践中使用[279]。RFA 正越来越多地用于 BE 相关 HGD 和低级别异型增生（low-grade dysplasia，LGD）和黏膜 EAC 患者，以及 EMR 后的任何可见病变（见第 47 章）和原位腺癌。与光动力疗法相比，RFA 的并发症更少，并且食管功能保存更好[280-282]。基于随机对照试验和大型观察性研究的数据，RFA 是 BE 相关肿瘤患者治疗中使用最广泛的技术。RFA 在早期 ESCC 中并不常用，但近期的一些报道证实了 RFA 治疗早期鳞状细胞肿瘤的有效性和安全性[283]。虽然证据较少，但冷冻治疗似乎对早期食管癌也有效[284]。

消融治疗的一个最大局限性是不能提供组织进行进一步的病理学评估和分期。

（2）姑息性内镜治疗

内镜扩张术可用于治疗吞咽困难。然而，这种效果通常是短暂的，并且会增加穿孔的风险[285]。还可以考虑在内镜下放置自膨式金属支架，对缓解吞咽困难有极佳的效果。目前使用的支架多为覆膜支架，因为其疗效更好，再介入率更低（图 48.16）[286]。较小直径（18mm）和大直径（23mm）支架似乎具有相同的效果[287]。支架也可以与其他治疗方式（如化疗、放疗或近距离放射疗法）联合使用以缓解吞咽困难[288]。

内镜下放置胃造瘘或空肠造瘘饲管有助于缓解吞咽困难和体重减轻。考虑到胃造瘘管可能会干扰胃作为管道的使用，因此不建议在手术候选者中放置胃造瘘管，此外，使用牵拉技术放置胃造瘘管，有报告插管部位发生转移性种植。为了避免这种风险，倾向直接放置胃造瘘管[289]。覆膜自膨式金属支架可成功封堵高达 86% 的食管癌患者的气管-食管瘘[290]。当将支架放置在食管的中 1/3 位置时，必须特别谨慎，因为可能存在从外部压迫位于正前方的气管[291]。ASGE 建议放置食管支架治疗瘘管，因为它们可提供持久和即刻的症状缓解[292]。

3. 化疗和放疗

（1）新辅助化疗

术前接受化疗后进行手术且无癌残留的患者，比那些有

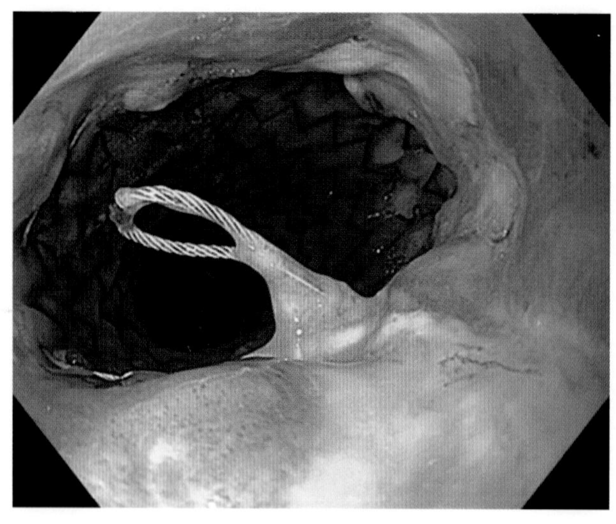

图 48.16 全覆盖食管金属支架

癌残留或持续癌的患者有更好的生存率[293-296]。北美和欧洲的一项研究显示，与单纯手术相比，术前（和围手术期）化疗具有显著的3年和5年生存优势[297-299]，在ESCC和EAC中均观察到这些结果。一项大型荟萃分析也显示，新辅助化疗与生存率的改善和较高的完全切除率（R0）相关[300]。尽管新辅助放化疗是局部进展期食管癌最常见的治疗方法，但围手术期化疗可作为食管远端及胃食管交界处（GEJ）腺癌的一种治疗选择[301]。

（2）新辅助放化疗

基于前瞻性试验和荟萃分析的数据，新辅助放化疗已成为许多国家局部进展期食管癌的标准治疗[302,303]。CROSS研究（手术后食管癌的放化疗研究）纳入了食管癌患者（75%的EAC患者和23%的ESCC患者），将患者随机分为新辅助放化疗组和单纯手术组。这项研究发现，联合治疗模式组的中位生存期更长（49.4个月 vs 24.0个月）。放化疗组患者在围手术期每周接受卡铂、紫杉醇和41.4Gy的放疗，随后接受手术。与单纯手术组相比，围手术期治疗组的局部复发患者比例较低（14% vs 34%）。组织学肿瘤类型不影响生存率，EAC和ESCC均从新辅助放化疗中获益[103,304]。

（3）新辅助放疗

与刚才讨论的新辅助化疗和新辅助放化疗相比，研究表明术前单纯放疗没有任何益处[305]。NCCN建议单独放疗应仅用于姑息治疗目的或者不适合化疗的患者[204]。新的放疗技术旨在增加对靶组织的剂量输送，同时减少对周围器官（心脏、肺、皮肤）的毒性。这些技术，如调强放疗和质子束治疗，对食管癌患者的疗效仍在评估[306,307]。

（4）辅助性放化疗

与新辅助放化疗相比，辅助性放化疗似乎无效，最近的一项网络荟萃分析显示，与单纯手术相比，辅助性放化疗无生存获益[303]。一项回顾性研究表明，新辅助放化疗和手术后的辅助性化疗对无残留病变或有残留非结节性病变的患者无效，但与残留结节性病变患者的生存率改善有关[308]。

4. 靶向治疗

EAC患者应在肿瘤组织活检中检测人表皮生长因子受体2（HER2）。如果观察到高水平表达，可以将HER2抗体［如曲妥珠单抗（Trastuzumab）和帕妥珠单抗（Pertuzumab）］添加到不适合局部治疗的转移性腺癌或局部进展期癌患者的化疗方案中[309]。

在最近的一项试验中，VEGF受体2抗体［雷莫芦单抗（Ramucirumab）］对于标准化疗方案难以治疗的进展期GEJ腺癌患者显示出了有希望的结果，并被FDA批准用于该适应证[310]。

5. 免疫治疗

最近FDA批准的另一种治疗方法是帕博利珠单抗（pembrolizumab），是一种程序性死亡配体-1（PD-L1）的抗体。帕博利珠单抗获批用于治疗PD-L1阳性的难治性腺癌或微卫星不稳定性肿瘤或DNA错配修复基因缺陷的肿瘤[311]。

（九）预后

食管癌生存的最佳预测因素是侵袭深度（T分期）和淋巴结受累（N分期）[312,313]。一项回顾性研究发现，食管癌的N分期是影响总生存期和无病生存期的独立因素（N1无病生存期为13.6%）[314]。局部、区域和远处转移病变的5年生存率分别为41%、23%和5%[315]。当诊断为高级别异型增生（原位癌）或T1a期癌时，其5年生存率可提高到90%以上[264]。然而，对于出现局部区域性进展期疾病的患者（>50%的患者），他们的预后很差，大多数在确诊后3~5年内复发并死亡[315]。此外，除侵袭深度和累及淋巴结转移的数目外，组织学类型、分化程度和肿瘤部位也会影响患者的生存率[247]。尽管最近在治疗上取得了进展，但最新报道的5年总生存率仅为19%[3]。

最近对食管癌脑转移的报告引起关注。转移性脑病变在食管癌中罕见，最近的报告显示其发病率为3.8%[316]。大多数报告的病例与EAC相关，而不是ESCC[316,317]。

二、其他恶性上皮性肿瘤

（一）鳞状细胞癌变异体

疣状癌是ESCC的一种罕见变异体，报告的病例不足30例[318]。最常见于中年人，三分之二的患者为男性。内镜下表现为乳头状或疣状外观。诊断需要高怀疑指数和多次活检，因为组织学显示分化良好的角化过度和棘皮病表现，而仅有一小柱肿瘤细胞[318]。尽管这些病变通常分化良好且生长缓慢，但由于诊断延迟，它们的预后往往很差。

ESCC的另一种变异体是癌肉瘤（又称为假肉瘤、梭形细胞癌和息肉样癌）。该肿瘤表现为息肉样外观，可为单发或多发。由于肿瘤的外生性，许多患者会出现吞咽困难或上腹部不适。组织学上，肿瘤有梭形细胞成分，在诊断时，它们往往已侵犯食管壁并扩散到局部淋巴结，并可能转移。因此，这些肿瘤预后不良（2年生存率为25%）[319]。

（二）小细胞癌

食管小细胞癌是一种罕见的疾病，约占所有食管恶性肿瘤的0.8%~3.1%。该肿瘤具有高度侵袭性，预后极差。诊断时的平均年龄为65岁，2/3的患者为男性。吞咽困难、体重减轻和上腹痛是其主要表现症状。通常有吸烟史(90%)和饮酒史(70%)。肿瘤通常位于食管的中 1/3 段(52%)或下 1/3 段(35%)。半数以上的患者在诊断时已有广泛的转移[320]。这些患者的最佳治疗尚不明确,但化疗应始终是多模式治疗的一部分[321]。对于经过精心挑选的病情有限的一组患者,切除术后化疗可提供较长的生存期[321]。中位总生存期仅为 11 个月,2 年生存率仅为 25%[320]。

(三) 恶性黑色素瘤

原发性食管黑色素瘤罕见,仅发现了 300 多例[322,323]。黑色素瘤占所有食管恶性肿瘤的 0.1%~0.5%[324]。原发性食管黑色素瘤转移早,预后极差。基底增生或慢性食管炎引起的上皮基底层黑素细胞增多被认为在其发病机制中起重要作用[325,326]。黑色素瘤男性发病率是女性的两倍,平均发病年龄接近 60 岁[324]。吞咽困难是最常见的症状。然而,由于肿瘤的柔软性质,症状可能会延迟,在超过 90% 的病例中,就诊时肿瘤的大小大于 2cm。最常见的部位是食管的中段和远端 1/3[323]。内镜特征包括非溃疡性色素性肿瘤,颜色可能因黑色素的数量而异,但也有"无色素"变异的描述[327]。"卫星"病变发生在距原发病灶几厘米处,可看到较大病变,被认为是壁内转移所致。组织学上,由于缺乏黑色素颗粒黑色素瘤可被误诊为低分化癌,免疫组化可能是确定正确诊断的必要条件[324]。这是一种侵袭性疾病,局部淋巴结和远处转移的发生率很高(40%~80%)[328]。FDG-PET 是目前检测转移最被接受的方式。区分原发性和转移性黑色素瘤很重要,因为在 4% 的病例中转移性黑色素瘤(稍后讨论)可累及食管[329]。根治性切除联合淋巴结清扫术是主要的治疗方法。经计算,原发性食管黑色素瘤的 5 年生存率为 37%[330]。年龄、分期、肿瘤部位、淋巴结受累是预后的独立预测因素[331]。

三、良性上皮性肿瘤

(一) 鳞状细胞乳头状瘤

食管乳头状瘤是一种无症状的良性上皮性肿瘤,内镜下以食管下 1/3 孤立的外生性病变为特征(图 48.17)。它们往往是白色或粉红色,质地柔软,表面光滑或略微粗糙。组织学上,显示为结缔组织的指状突起,内衬数量增多的鳞状细胞。内镜检查的鉴别诊断包括糖原性棘皮病、鳞状细胞癌的疣状边缘和疣状癌[332]。鳞状乳头状瘤罕见,据报道患病率为 0.01%~0.43%[332]。其发病机制尚不确定,但推测与潜在的炎症(例如 GERD)有关[332]。另一种发病机制理论是感染 HPV[333]。乳头状瘤通常适合内镜切除,鉴于其体积小大多使用钳子或采用黏膜切除术。切除后复发并不常见。据报道,在少数多发性乳头状瘤(食管乳头状瘤病)病例中有恶变的报道,但在单发的病变中恶变是罕见的[334,335]。

局灶性真皮发育不全综合征(Goltz 综合征)是一种罕见的疾病,多见于女性,其特征是外胚层和中胚层结构的多种异常。虽然皮肤、眼部和肌肉骨骼的临床表现占主导地位,但也可能存在食管乳头状瘤病[336,337]。由 X 染色体上 *PORCN* 的突变引起,Goltz 综合征具有一个显性 X 连锁遗传,通常对受累的男性是致命的。Goltz 综合征可以是遗传性的,也可以是新生的。

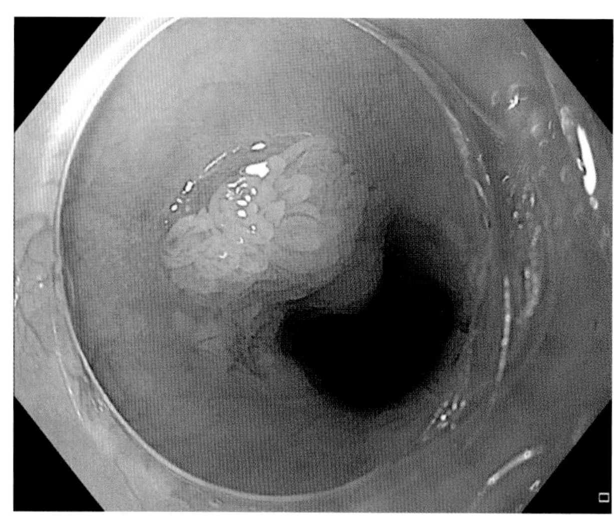

图 48.17　食管镜下所见的食管乳头状瘤

(二) 腺瘤

食管腺瘤罕见,几乎完全与 Barrett 化生有关。虽然腺癌是一种更常见的与 Barrett 相关的病变,也报告了一些腺瘤病例[338-340]。其特征表现为食管下 1/3Barrett 段内的息肉样病变。组织病理学显示异型增生的管状腺体被特殊的肠上皮覆盖。与结肠腺瘤相似,这些被认为是恶性前病变,建议内镜下切除进行诊断和治疗。

(三) 炎性纤维性息肉

炎性纤维性息肉(也称为炎性假性息肉或嗜酸性肉芽肿)具有独特的组织学特征。这包括黏膜下息肉样病变伴血管周围同心成纤维细胞增生伴嗜酸性粒细胞增多。大多数息肉表达 CD34,而 CD117 阴性。最常见于胃和大肠,其次是小肠。食管是一个不太可能发生的部位(约 2% 病例)[341]。它们是非肿瘤性息肉,呈良性病程。

四、恶性非上皮肿瘤

(一) 淋巴瘤

食管淋巴瘤可以是原发性的,也可以是继发性的,其中原发性淋巴瘤较少见。原发性食管淋巴瘤是指:以食管受累为主,仅累及局部淋巴结的淋巴瘤,而外周或纵隔淋巴结、脾或肝不存在疾病,且胸片和 WBC 计数正常[342]。淋巴瘤占食管恶性肿瘤的 1% 以下[343]。临床上,食管淋巴瘤可表现为吞咽困难、体重减轻、胃肠道出血、食管瘘和其他非特异性全身症状(如发热、盗汗、乏力)。内镜检查,报告的少数病例描述了一系列发现,包括黏膜下结节、肿块、溃疡和息肉样病变。食管淋巴瘤可以是霍奇金型或非霍奇金淋巴瘤(NHL)。弥漫性大 B 细胞性淋巴瘤(DLBCL)是 NHL 最常见的亚型,与免疫抑制状态相关,如 AIDS(艾滋病)(见第 32 章)[344]。

(二) 肉瘤

食管肉瘤是一种罕见的间叶源性肿瘤,包括平滑肌肉瘤、胃肠道间质瘤(见下文和第 33 章)、横纹肌肉瘤、纤维肉瘤、脂肪肉瘤、纤维组织细胞瘤、卡波西肉瘤和绒毛膜癌。平滑肌肉瘤是最常见的亚型,很难与良性平滑肌瘤区分。肿瘤可以是腔内、息肉样或呈浸润性/侵袭性。组织学上,由纺锤形细胞螺纹交错组成,有丝分裂相增多,多形性明显。在大多数情况下,黏膜活检不是有用的诊断工具,因为这些病变是黏膜下病变。另一方面,EUS 结合 FNA 已被证明有助于诊断。1/3 的病例发生淋巴结受累。食管切除术加淋巴结清扫术是主要的治疗方法。预后差,5 年总生存率为 35%[345]。

(三) 胃肠间质瘤

胃肠间质瘤(gastrointestinal stromal tumor,GIST)是胃肠道最常见的间叶性细胞肿瘤,在第 33 章中有详细讨论。GIST 发生于食管的病例仅占 1%~3%[346,347]。通常起源于固有肌层,更确切地说,起源于 Cajal 间质细胞。通常在 40 岁以后出现,症状包括吞咽困难、溃疡出血、消化不良和体重减轻。内镜下最常出现在食管远端 1/3 的黏膜下孤立性肿块。GIST 在 CT 扫描中表现为边界清楚的低衰减肿块[348]。EUS 是最准确的成像方式,甚至可以帮助预测恶性的可能性[349,350]。在组织学上,GIST 大多表现为特征性的梭形细胞,细胞核细长,表达 *KIT* 基因编码的 CD117。CD117 和 DOG1 阳性是一个重要的鉴别特征,因为类似的病变,例如平滑肌瘤或其他梭形细胞肿瘤,通常为 CD117 和 DOG1 阴性。

如第 33 章所述,GIST 恶变的风险取决于 GIST 的大小及其有丝分裂率。具有低度恶性潜能的 GIST 的特征包括<2cm 和有丝分裂率<5/50 高倍视野[351]。GIST 的治疗取决于病变的大小和分期。最近的报告表明,ESD 可以成为切除小的、非进展期病变的更常用的技术[352]。否则,手术切除是传统的首选治疗方法。酪氨酸激酶抑制剂,如甲磺酸伊马替尼也可作为新辅助治疗或用于不可切除的 GIST 的一种选择(见第 33 章)。CT 和 PET 扫描已显示对治疗后患者的监测是有用的[353]。

(四) 转移瘤

食管的转移瘤发生是罕见的。转移至食管的两种最常见的癌是黑色素瘤和乳腺癌。通常转移性病变会引起外源性压迫,吞咽困难是常见的症状。EUS 结合 FNA 细胞学检查可有助于诊断。治疗通常包括姑息性内镜支架植入术。

五、良性非上皮性肿瘤

(一) 平滑肌瘤

平滑肌瘤是最常见的食管良性肿瘤。它们影响男性的频率是女性的两倍[354]。内镜下可见病变为食管中段或远端 1/3 黏膜下孤立性肿块或许多肿块。活检通常无诊断价值,因为平滑肌瘤有正常的黏膜覆盖。EUS 是首选的诊断方法,平滑肌瘤通常起源于固有肌层。只有大的(>5cm)有症状的病变需要切除,对于较小的肿瘤可以在内镜下切除(使用 ESD 技术)或手术[355]。

(二) 颗粒细胞瘤

颗粒细胞瘤最常见于头颈部(包括口咽部),胃肠道较少见。胃肠道受累最常见的部位是食管,占病例的 33%。内镜表现、食管内的位置和病变的数量各不相同[356,357]。典型的颗粒细胞瘤是一种孤立的黏膜下病变,外观呈淡黄色,通常位于食管远端。由于大多数患者无症状,它们多在上消化道内镜检查中被偶然发现。组织学上,颗粒细胞瘤由圆形或多边形细胞组成,具有丰富的嗜酸性细胞质。细胞呈过碘酸-希夫和抗淀粉酶阳性。免疫组化表达 S-100 蛋白证明,它们可能起源于神经嵴。尽管报告了一些恶性转化病例,但大多数病例是良性的[358]。推荐内镜下切除,已被证明是安全的,并且在需要时可获取更准确的组织学诊断[356]。

(三) 纤维血管息肉

纤维血管息肉是食管良性病变(图 48.18)。它们几乎仅

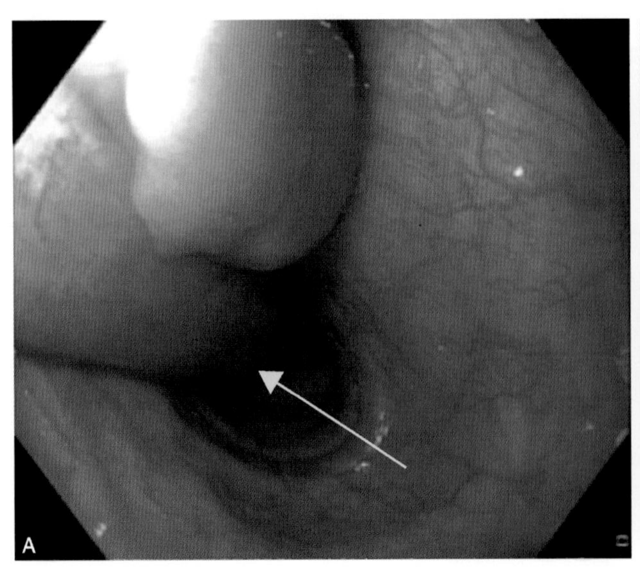

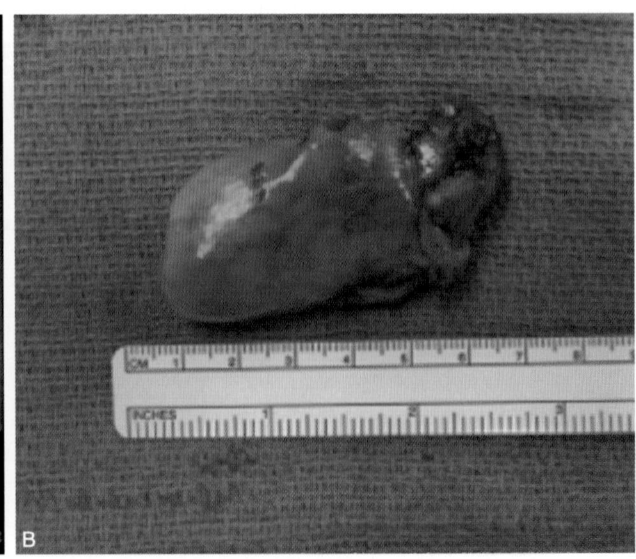

图 48.18　A,食管内巨大的纤维血管息肉内镜图像(箭头)。B,切除后的息肉。(Courtesy Dr. Julie Goddard,Denver,Colo.)

见于颈段食管，可能是由于该解剖区域黏膜下组织相对疏松，黏膜冗余所致[359,360]。它们通常是由血管、脂肪细胞和被正常鳞状上皮覆盖的基质组成的有蒂息肉。尽管大多数病例是偶然诊断的，但大的息肉可引起吞咽困难和癔球症。特殊的是，纤维血管息肉在呕吐或干呕后脱出口腔，为可见的肉质组织。罕见情况下，这些息肉可引起致命性窒息，因此建议内镜或手术切除。一些人建议在切除前对较大的息肉进行 EUS 检查，以确定是否存在大血管。

（四）错构瘤

错构瘤是食管最罕见的病变。它们是典型的有蒂息肉，可引起与纤维血管息肉相似的症状（如吞咽困难、癔球症、息肉脱垂、窒息）。在内镜下，这两个病变是无法区分的。然而，错构瘤息肉并不常见，具有不同的组织学表现。它们通常包含多种组织类型，包括软骨、骨、脂肪组织、平滑肌和骨骼肌。建议内镜或手术切除治疗[361]。

（五）血管瘤

食管血管瘤是一种罕见的血管畸形，偶尔会出现胃肠道出血或吞咽困难。食管血管瘤有两种组织学类型：海绵状血管瘤和毛细血管瘤。大多数病变为海绵状血管瘤。内镜下可见蓝色至红色的黏膜下结节，常随压迫而发白[362]。有趣的是，在报告中活检与出血无关[363]。以前，手术切除是最常见的治疗方法，而内镜治疗也是可行的[364]。

（六）脂肪瘤

脂肪瘤是一种罕见的胃肠道良性肿瘤。脂肪瘤在结肠、小肠和胃中比在食管中更常见。几乎所有患者均无症状，内镜检查偶然发现食管近端有轻微的淡黄色隆起结节。大的、有蒂的食管病变可引起吞咽困难和窒息。通常食管脂肪瘤表现为“枕头”征——有凹痕或用“触诊”松软。浅表黏膜活检通常无诊断价值。来自黏膜下层的深层标本显示分化良好的脂肪细胞。EUS 可见均匀的、高回声的黏膜下病变，外缘光滑。有症状的脂肪瘤治疗是内镜或手术切除[365]。

（程妍　译，袁农　校）

参考文献

第六部分 胃和十二指肠

第 49 章 胃和十二指肠解剖学、组织学及发育异常

M. Gaith Semrin 著

章节目录

一、胃胚胎学和解剖学 …… 683
（一）血管供应和引流以及淋巴引流 …… 683
（二）胃神经支配 …… 685
（三）胃组织的各层 …… 685
（四）显微解剖学 …… 685
二、十二指肠胚胎学与解剖学 …… 688
（一）血管供应和引流以及淋巴引流 …… 688
（二）十二指肠神经支配 …… 688
（三）显微解剖学 …… 688
三、胃与十二指肠先天性异常 …… 688
（一）胃闭锁 …… 688
（二）小胃 …… 690
（三）胃憩室 …… 690
（四）胃重复畸形 …… 690
（五）胃畸胎瘤 …… 691
（六）胃扭转 …… 691
（七）婴儿肥厚性幽门狭窄 …… 691
（八）成人肥厚性幽门狭窄 …… 693
（九）先天性幽门缺失 …… 693
（十）十二指肠闭锁和狭窄 …… 693
（十一）环型胰腺 …… 694
（十二）十二指肠重复囊肿 …… 695
（十三）肠旋转不良与中肠扭转 …… 695

一、胃胚胎学和解剖学

胃是一个 J 形的消化道扩张体，近端与食管相连，远端与十二指肠相连。它的主要功能是储存大量摄取的食物，启动消化过程，并以受控的方式向下游释放其内容物，以适应容量小得多的十二指肠。胃容量从新生儿约 30mL 到成年 1.5~2L 不等。

在妊娠第四周，由远端前肠扩张的胃就可以辨认出来了（图 49.1）[1]。随着胃的增大，胃背侧比腹侧生长得更快，因此形成大弯。此外，在发育的过程中，胃绕其纵轴旋转 90°，使其大弯（背侧）转至左侧，小弯（腹侧）转至右侧。旋转和持续差异生长导致胃横向位于中上腹和左上腹。旋转事件也可以解释胃的迷走神经支配：右边的迷走神经支配胃后壁（原始神经右侧）和左迷走神经支配前壁（原始神经左侧）。

胃解剖位置是可变的，因为胃的两点固定，即食管胃和胃十二指肠，允许相当大的灵活性。食管胃交界处一般位于 T10 椎体左侧，横膈膜裂孔下方 1~2cm。胃十二指肠连接处位于 L1，一般在横卧禁食者中线的右侧。成人直立的扩张的胃十二指肠连接处可能要低得多。左侧和尾部大弯可延伸至脐以下，这取决于胃的扩张程度、位置和胃蠕动期。

胃大弯形成了左下胃边缘，而小弯形成右上胃缘。胃后方紧邻部分胰腺、横结肠、横膈膜、脾脏、左肾顶部和肾上腺。胃的后壁实际上包括大网膜囊的前壁或小网膜囊。胃前壁与肝比邻，而前腹壁的内部边界是胃前左下侧。

胃完全被腹膜包裹，除了食管胃交界处有一小块裸露区域。腹膜呈双层结构，从小弯到肝脏，即小网膜的胃肝部分，然后从胃底部及胃大弯侧的大网膜向下延伸至横结肠（如胃结肠韧带）、脾（即胃脾韧带）和膈肌（称为腹膈韧带）。

胃分为 4 个区域，可以通过解剖学或组织学标志来确定（图 49.2）[2]。从解剖学上讲，贲门是胃的一个界限不清的小区域，紧挨着食管。胃的这个部位一直是研究的重点。对于贲门黏膜的性质、位置、范围，甚至是否存在等相关问题都存在争议。胃底向上突出，位于贲门和食管胃交界处上方。胃的穹隆区域是它的最上部，在上部与左半侧膈接触，胃左侧与脾脏紧邻。胃的最大部分是胃体，它位于胃底的下方与胃底连续。胃角切迹是一个固定的、尖锐的凹痕，在小弯向下延伸三分之二的距离，标志着胃体的尾部（图 49.3）。胃窦从其与胃体的模糊边界处，延伸到幽门与十二指肠的交界处。这些大体的解剖标志与黏膜的组织学基本一致，因为胃窦黏膜（幽门腺黏膜）实际上是从胃角切迹上方的小弯处延伸出来的。幽门（幽门管）是连接十二指肠和胃的管状结构，包含明显的环形肌肉，即幽门括约肌。由于幽门位于大网膜和小网膜的腹膜之间，故幽门位置可以出现有限的移动，但通常位于 L1 中线右侧 2cm 处。相应的胃这些区域的运动和分泌功能将在第 50 和 51 章详细讨论。

（一）血管供应和引流以及淋巴引流

胃的动脉供血来自腹腔干动脉的分支，即肝总动脉、胃左动脉和脾动脉，它们形成了沿着小弯和大弯的下三分之二处的 2 个动脉弓。胃小弯上方由胃左动脉供血，下方是由胃右

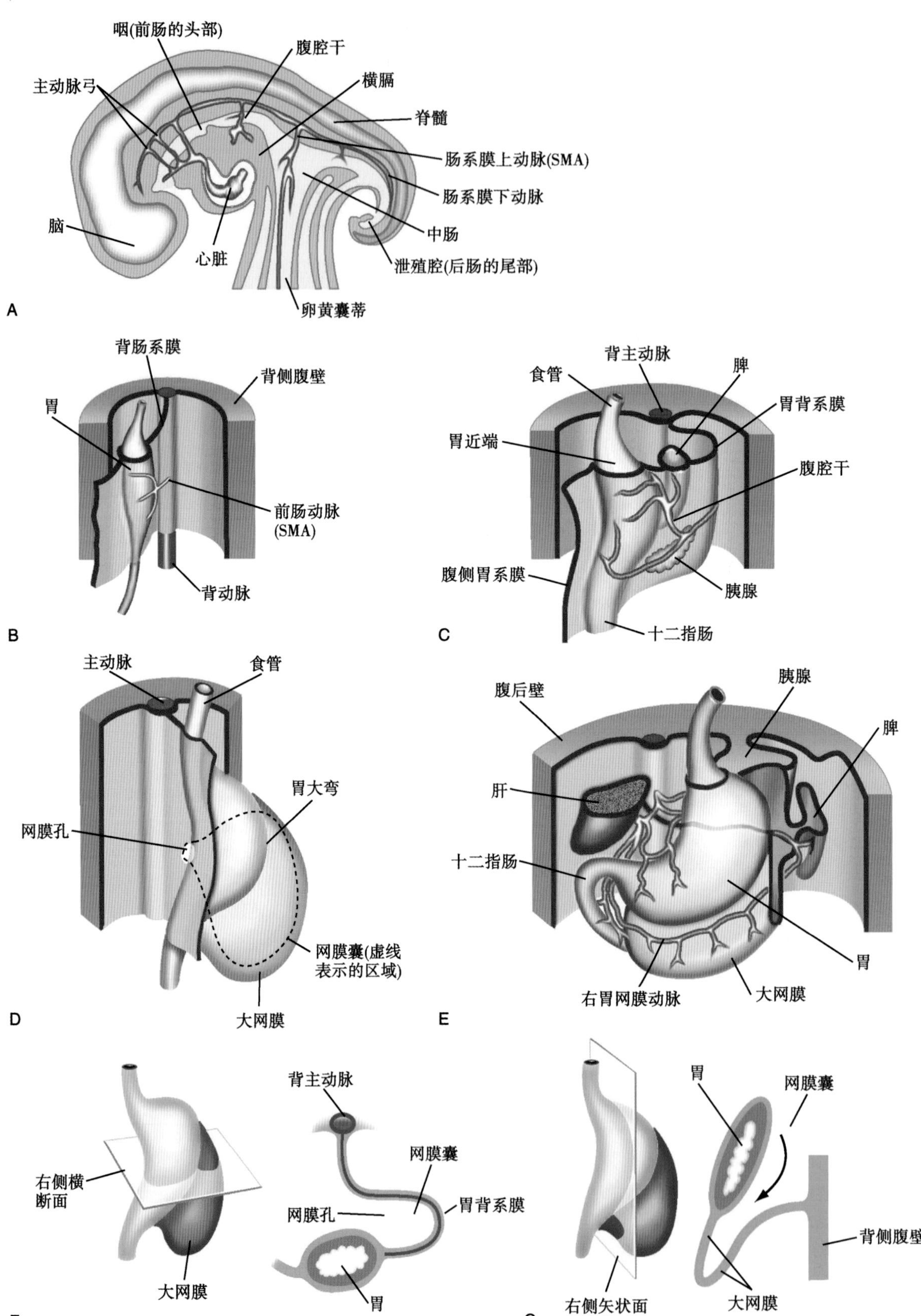

图 49.1　胃和十二指肠的发育以及网膜囊(小囊)和大网膜的形成。A,28 天胚胎的中位切片。B,28 天胚胎的前外侧视图。C,胚胎约 35 日龄。D,胚胎约为 40 日龄。E. 胚胎约 48 日龄。F,约 52 天时胚胎胃和大网膜的侧位视图。横断面显示网膜孔和网膜囊。G,矢状面显示网膜囊和大网膜。十二指肠的胚胎学在第 55 和 96 章中进一步讨论。(From Moore KL, Persaud TVN. The developing human. 7th ed. Philadelphia: WB Saunders; 2003. p 258.)

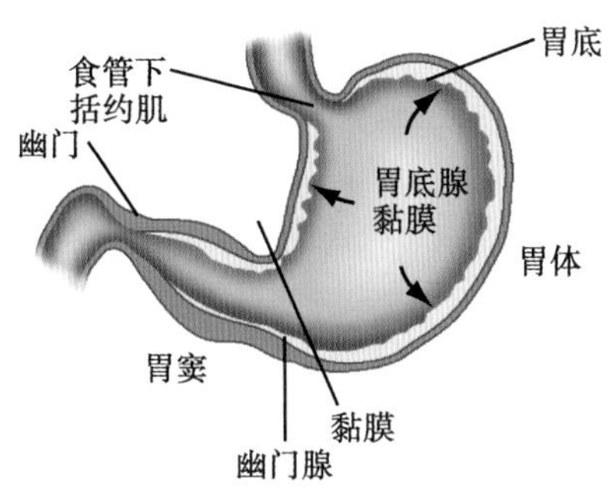

图 49.2　胃的解剖区域。该线从角切迹沿胃小弯至不清晰边界的连线沿胃大弯位于胃体和胃窦之间。(From Johnson LR. Gastrointestinal physiology. 6th ed. St Louis:Mosby;2001. p 76.)

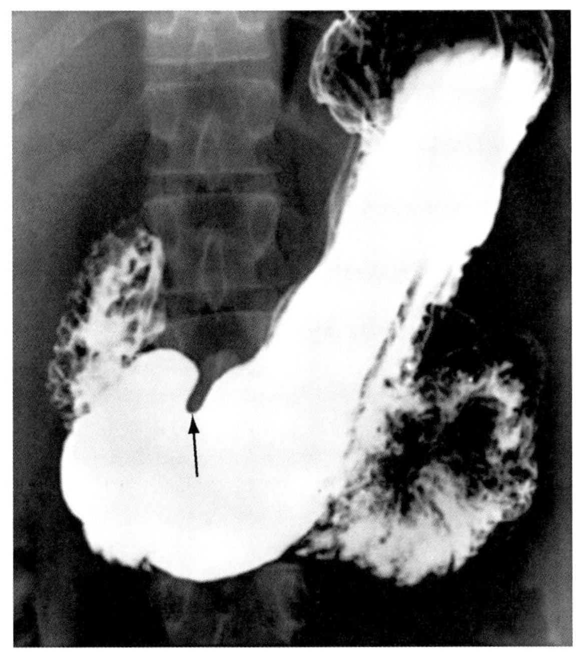

图 49.3　来自上胃肠道系列检查(UGIS)的 X 线片显示了胃小弯远端的角切迹(箭头)。(Courtesy James W. Weaver,MD.)

动脉供血。而胃右动脉属于肝总动脉,或胃十二指肠动脉(肝总动脉的分支)的分支。胃底以下的大弯由胃左网膜动脉(脾动脉的一个分支)和胃右网膜动脉(胃十二指肠动脉的一个分支)共同支配。左右胃网膜动脉吻合,形成大弯侧动脉弓;有时左右胃网膜动脉没有吻合。胃底和胃大弯左上部的动脉是由胃短动脉供应的,它起源于脾动脉。

胃的静脉引流通常伴随动脉供应,流入门静脉或其支流,即脾静脉或肠系膜上静脉。左右胃静脉引流胃小弯。胃左静脉也被称为冠状静脉。左右胃网膜静脉引流胃远端和胃大弯的一部分。右胃网膜静脉和若干远端静脉成为胃结肠静脉,最终回流于肠系膜上静脉。没有胃十二指肠静脉。胃网膜左静脉汇入脾静脉,随后接受胃短静脉,引流胃底和胃近端大弯的血流。

胃的大部分淋巴引流最终通过中间淋巴结到达腹腔淋巴结。淋巴管在胃壁自由吻合,淋巴管通过单向阀流入 4 组淋巴结中的 1 组。胃下区流入幽门下淋巴结和大网膜淋巴结,然后是肝淋巴结,最后流入腹腔淋巴结。脾或胃大弯的近端淋巴最初流入胰脾淋巴结,然后进入腹腔淋巴结。胃近端或胃小弯区域淋巴流入左右胃淋巴结,这些淋巴结紧邻左右胃的血管,并终止在腹腔淋巴结。小弯的肝或幽门部分淋巴流入幽门上淋巴结,然后进入肝淋巴结,最后进入腹腔淋巴结。

(二) 胃神经支配

胃的自主神经支配来自交感神经和副交感神经系统,通过沿内脏动脉行走的复杂神经束传递。

胃交感神经起源于 T6~T8 脊神经的神经节前神经纤维,双侧腹腔神经节的突触与神经元节后纤维,沿胃的血管走向穿过腹腔神经丛。伴随这些交感神经的是,从胃和支配幽门括约肌的运动纤维传入痛觉神经。

副交感神经通过左右迷走神经,形成食管远端神经丛,并在靠近胃贲门处形成前后迷走神经干。主干包含节前副交感神经纤维,以及来自内脏的传入纤维。两个主干分别起源于腹腔和肝分支,然后在小网膜内继续延伸至小弯右侧,作为 Latarjet 前神经和 Latarjet 后神经。这些神经在胃壁上产生多个胃分支,神经节前纤维在此与黏膜下神经(Meissner 神经)和肠肌神经丛(Auerbach 神经丛)中的神经节细胞通过突触进行信息交流,从这些神经丛的节后纤维分布到细胞、腺体和平滑肌。

(三) 胃组织的各层

胃壁管腔表面形成厚的、纵向的褶皱或皱襞,随着扩张而变平。胃壁由 4 层组成:黏膜层、黏膜下层、固有肌层和浆膜。胃腔内的黏膜,呈光滑、柔软、血供丰富的黏膜层。贲门、胃窦和幽门的黏膜色泽比胃底和胃体的稍浅。胃的大部分功能性分泌成分都位于胃底和胃体黏膜内(见第 51 章)。黏膜下层在黏膜层的下方,是由胶原蛋白和弹性蛋白纤维构成的紧密结缔组织骨架。黏膜下层还包含淋巴细胞、浆细胞、小动脉、小静脉、淋巴管和黏膜下神经丛,第三个组织层是固有肌层,由内斜肌层、中环肌层和外纵肌层组成。内斜肌纤维穿过胃底,覆盖胃壁的前后面;中间的环状纤维环绕胃体,向远端增厚形成幽门括约肌;外纵肌纤维主要沿着胃的大弯和小弯行走。胃的最后一层是透明的浆膜,是内脏腹膜的延续。

(四) 显微解剖学

胃黏膜表面主要由一层简单的柱状上皮细胞组成,柱状上皮细胞高度为 20~40μm。这些表面黏液细胞(图 49.4)在整个胃中都很相似,细胞核位于基部,高尔基体突出,细胞质致密,特别是位于顶端致密的含有黏蛋白的膜结合颗粒。细胞分泌颗粒状黏液,通过胞吐、顶端排出和细胞脱落释放。黏液和碳酸氢盐的主要作用是保护细胞免受酸、胃蛋白酶、摄入食物和病原体的侵害。胃表面黏液细胞的更新时间约为 3 天。

胃上皮由一系列胃小凹构成,这使胃腺分布在胃腔面积更大,胃小凹与胃腺的比例为 1∶4~1∶5。不同解剖区域胃腺排列着不同类型的特异上皮细胞,使这些区域可以根据胃腺类型进行分化(见图 49.2)。第一个区域是贲门,是食管鳞状上皮到胃柱状上皮的小过渡区。贲门一直是一个有争议的组织学领域,理论认为它的存在是病理的。然而,最近的观察表明,贲门黏膜在妊娠期发育,并在出生时存在[3]。贲门腺呈分

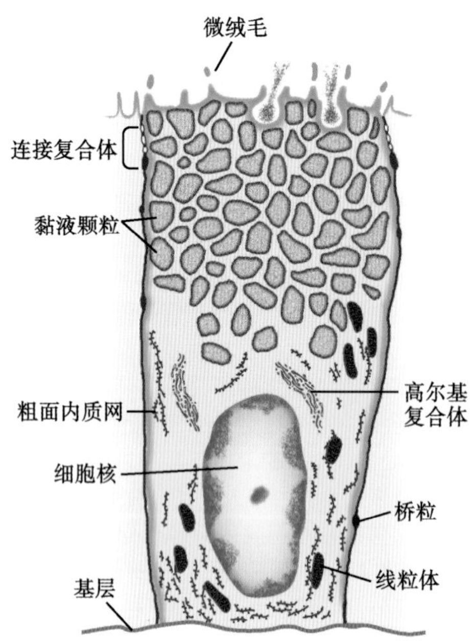

图 49.4 黏膜表面细胞的示意图

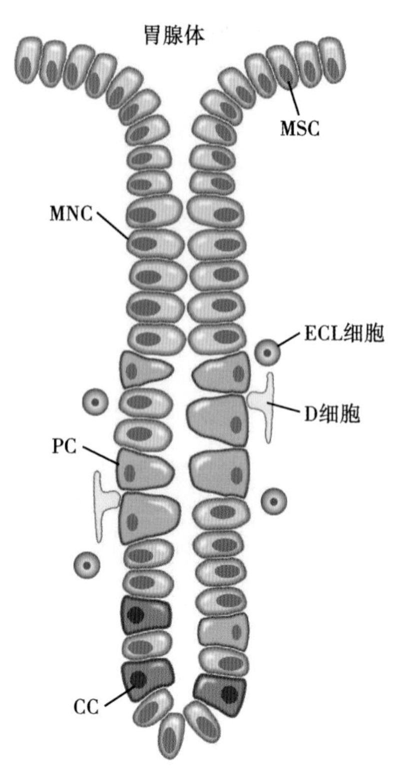

图 49.5 胃底腺的示意图。含黏液表面细胞(MSC)、黏液颈部细胞(MNC)、肠嗜铬样(ECL)细胞、含生长抑制素的 D 细胞、壁细胞(PC)和主细胞(CC)。(From Lloyd KCK, Debas T. The peripheral regulation of gastric acid secretion. In: Johnson LR, et al, editors. Physiology of the gastrointestinal tract, vol 2. 3rd ed. New York: Lippincott-Raven; 1994.)

支状,结构迂曲,并有黏液细胞、内分泌细胞和未分化细胞。从贲门腺体逐渐过渡到第二段,即胃的泌酸段,这个区域包括胃底和胃体,含壁细胞(或泌酸区或胃底部)腺体。这部分腺体由壁细胞、主细胞(又称为消化性细胞)、内分泌细胞、黏液细胞及未分化细胞组成。最后一个区域是胃窦和幽门,包含幽门腺,由内分泌细胞组成,包括产生胃泌素的 G 细胞和黏液细胞。

到目前为止,数量最多、最独特的胃腺是胃酸分泌腺(图 49.5),负责分泌酸、内因子和大多数胃酶。这些相当直而简单的管状腺体位于胃底和胃体区。一个典型的腺体可细分为 3 个区域:峡部(以表面黏液细胞为主),颈部(以壁细胞和黏液细胞为主)和基底部(以主细胞为主,以及一些壁细胞和黏液细胞)。内分泌细胞,含生长抑素 D 细胞和分泌组胺的肠嗜铬样(ECL)细胞(在其他细胞中)散布在泌酸上皮细胞中(见第 4 章)。

胃底腺的主要细胞类型是壁细胞(图 49.6),每秒可分泌 3×10^4 个氢离子,最终盐酸(HCl)浓度约为 150mmol/L。壁细胞凸向胃底腺体的管腔里,作为主要氢离子分泌细胞,具有不同于其他胃细胞的超微结构:大线粒体,多糖-蛋白质缺乏的微绒毛,以及与管腔接触的细胞质小管系统。在不分泌的壁细胞中,细胞质小管泡系统占优势,微绒毛排列在小管顶部。在分泌状态下,小管泡系统消失,只留下一个广泛的细胞内小管系统,包含长微绒毛。线粒体约占分泌壁细胞体积的 30%~40%,通过顶端微绒毛提供酸分泌所需的能量(见图 49.6)。与碳酸酐酶一样,H^+、K^+-ATP 酶也存在于顶端的微绒毛膜中,称为质子泵。顶端的 H^+,K^+-ATP 酶在胃酸分泌中起质子转位器的作用(见第 51 章)。酸分泌始于受刺激后 5~10 分钟。此外,壁细胞是分泌内因子的部位,通过膜相关囊泡运输。

与壁细胞密切相关的是颈部黏液细胞,它们单独出现在壁细胞附近,或以 2 或 3 组出现在分泌腺的颈部或峡部。颈部黏液细胞与表面黏液细胞的不同之处在于,它们合成的是酸性、硫酸盐化黏液,而不是中性黏液。此外,颈部黏液细胞有基底核,细胞核周围有较大的黏液颗粒,而不是位于顶端的颗粒。这两种细胞类型的功能表现出不同,表面黏液细胞具有细胞保护作用,而颈部黏液细胞的功能是作为表面黏液细胞、壁细胞、主细胞和内分泌细胞的干细胞前体。

主细胞,也被称为酶原细胞,主要存在于胃底腺的深层。这些金字塔形的细胞在胃蛋白酶原Ⅰ和Ⅱ的合成和分泌中发挥作用。由于核糖体丰富,主细胞的细胞质具有明显的嗜碱性染色,这些核糖体要么游离于细胞质中,要么与广泛的内质网系统有关。酶原颗粒位于细胞质的顶端;当含有酶原的颗粒与胃腔膜融合后,其颗粒内的酶原就释放入胃腔内。一旦进入胃腔内,胃蛋白酶原就被转化为胃蛋白酶。

各种内分泌,或肠内分泌细胞分散在泌酸腺的细胞中(见第 4 章),其位置不同,可以是对胃腔开放式的,也可以是封闭式的。开放的内分泌细胞有包含受体的顶膜,这些开放的细胞通过基底部细胞的胞吐方式将其内容物排入血液中,而产生内分泌的效果。封闭的内分泌细胞包含几个过程,分布在其靶细胞附近,构成所谓的旁分泌效应。D 细胞就是胃底腺的封闭内分泌细胞的形式,通过漫长过程分泌生长抑素,到达 ECL、壁细胞和主细胞。

肠内分泌细胞类型也可根据其嗜银或嗜铬染色颗粒进行分类。那些含有不经预处理就能还原银的颗粒细胞,称为嗜银细胞。能重铬酸钾染色的嗜银细胞为肠嗜铬细胞(EC);大

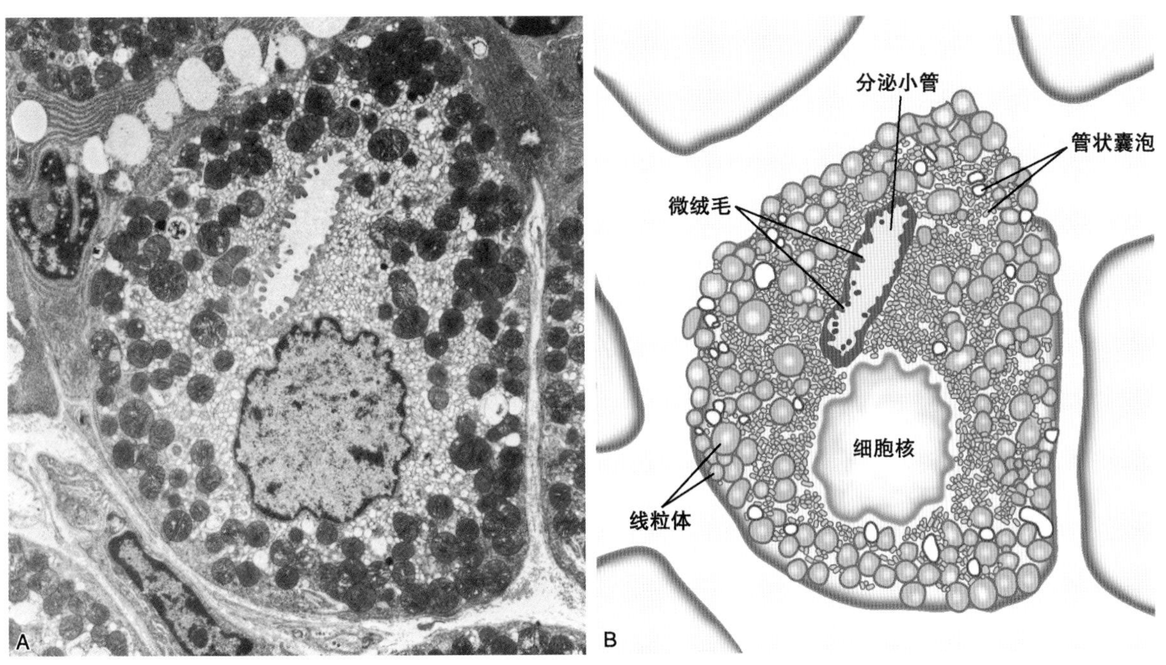

图 49.6　壁细胞。A,电子显微照片。B,示意图。(Form Johnson LR. Gastrointestinal physiology. 6th ed. St Louis: Mosby; 2001. pp 78-9.)

多数肠嗜铬细胞含有血清素。在有还原剂存在的情况下,其颗粒被银染色的细胞称为亲银细胞或 ECL 细胞。ECL 细胞主要位于泌酸腺内,是唯一含有组胺的肠内分泌细胞。

远端胃包括胃窦和幽门,其内有广泛盘绕的内分泌细胞和上皮细胞组成的胃窦腺体。上皮细胞以黏液细胞为主,也有分泌胃蛋白酶原Ⅱ的颈部黏液细胞。胃泌素分泌(G)细胞虽然数量不多,但起着重要的生理作用,是开放式肠内分泌细胞的原型。这些细胞单发或小簇分布于胃窦腺体中部至深部(图 49.7A),细胞质的基底部密集填充着含有胃泌素的分泌颗粒(图 49.7B)。胃泌素的释放受到胃舒张、迷走神经刺激、膳食氨基酸和多肽的刺激,在餐后阶段,激素迅速进入血液(见第 51 章)。G 细胞的顶端或管腔表面被缩小成小的微绒毛,被认为含有负责刺激胃泌素释放的氨基酸和肽的受体。胃腔内含有大量的胃泌素,胃泌素是一种已知的胃生长和分化因子,通过上调胃壁细胞中肝素结合表皮样生长因子(HB-EGF)来介导[4,5]。

胃窦肠内分泌 D 细胞与 G 细胞紧密相邻,可产生生长抑素,生长抑素是胃泌素分泌的有效抑制剂。D 细胞在胃底腺中也少量存在。生长抑素通过旁分泌(对肠 ECL 和壁细胞的直接作用或对 G 细胞的间接作用)或内分泌作用(对壁细胞的直接作用)抑制酸分泌(更多请参阅第 51 章)。

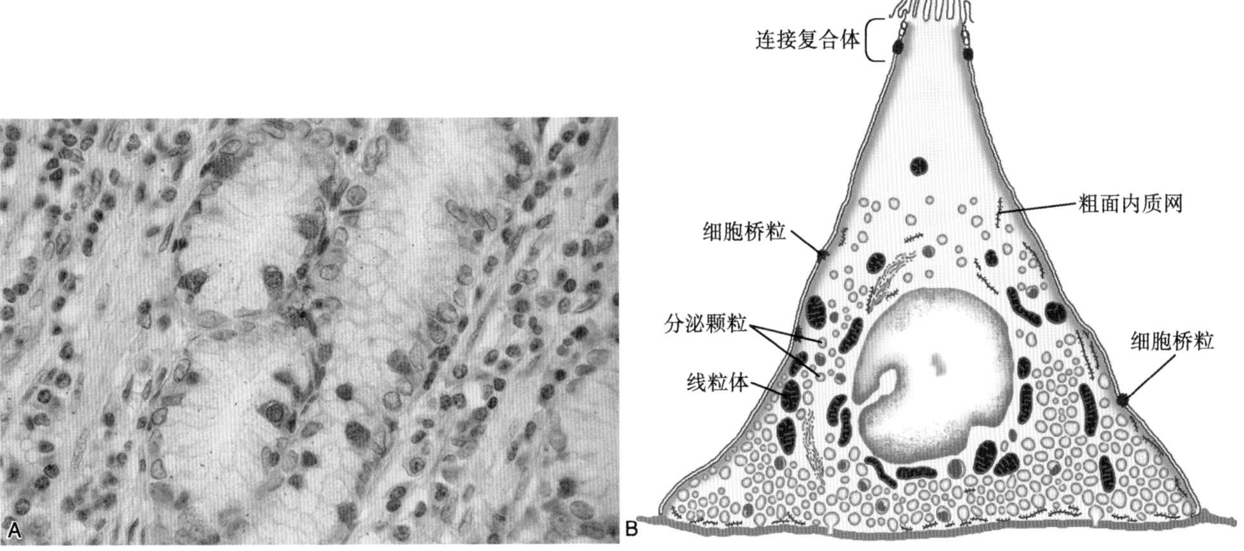

图 49.7　胃泌素(G)细胞。A,在该显微照片的幽门腺体中,可见散在的 G 细胞(粉红色)(免疫过氧化物酶染色)。B,示意图

固有层紧邻胃黏膜上皮基底膜深处,其中含有多种白细胞(多形核白细胞,浆细胞,淋巴细胞,嗜酸性粒细胞)、肥大细胞、成纤维细胞和内分泌样细胞。还有一些淋巴管穿过固有层。另外,黏膜毛细血管在固有层形成静脉丛,与黏膜肌层的小静脉相通。这些小静脉最终汇入黏膜下层静脉。

二、十二指肠胚胎学与解剖学

在妊娠第四周十二指肠由远端前肠、近端中肠和邻近内脏间充质发育而来。前肠与中肠的连接处位于十二指肠第二部,主乳头略远端。当胃旋转时,十二指肠也旋转,因此呈C形。在胚胎发育的第五和第六周,由于其黏膜层的增生,十二指肠腔短暂消失。在接下来的几周中,管腔空泡化和部分增殖细胞的变性导致十二指肠腔再通。上皮和腺体从胚胎内胚层发育而来,而结缔组织,肌肉和浆膜则来自中胚层。

十二指肠是小肠的最近端部分,在近端与幽门相连,在远端与空肠相连。它在胰头周围形成一个C形环。成人的十二指肠大约是30cm长(12英寸,因此称为十二指肠),分为4段(通常称为第一段、第二段、第三段和第四段),各段以角度改变处为界限。

十二指肠的第一段长约5cm,从幽门向右、向上和向后延伸。十二指肠第一部分的近端部分也称为十二指肠球或十二指肠帽。第一段通过小网膜的肝十二指肠部分松散地附着在肝脏上。十二指肠球部随着幽门的运动而运动。胃十二指肠动脉,胆管和门静脉位于十二指肠球部后方,而胆囊位于十二指肠球部前方。十二指肠的第二段长为7至10cm,向下走行于右肾门的前方,向右与胰头比邻。十二指肠乳头位于十二指肠后内侧壁,大约在第二段中点的远端,十二指肠乳头是Vater壶腹的位置,胰腺胆管通过该壶腹进入十二指肠。同在后内侧壁上,离主乳头约2cm处,有十二指肠小乳头,为副胰管开口处。十二指肠的第三段长约10cm,从右向左横向延伸,在下腔静脉、脊柱和主动脉的前方越过中线。肠系膜上动脉和静脉位于十二指肠第三段的前方,通常位于中线的右侧。十二指肠的第四段和最后部分长约5cm,由主动脉的左侧向上走行至胰腺下缘。十二指肠和空肠(十二指肠空肠曲)之间的连接点由Treitz韧带向后固定。

十二指肠肠壁由外纵肌层和内环肌层组成。与小肠的其余部分一样,肠腔表面衬有黏膜层,形成环形皱襞(plicae circulares)或褶皱(valvulae conniventes)。然而影像学和内镜检查显示,十二指肠球部内壁并不形成特征性的黏膜皱褶。

十二指肠起始部的几厘米被前后腹膜所覆盖。其余部分位于腹膜后方。

(一)血管供应和引流以及淋巴引流

十二指肠动脉形成起始于胚胎发育,且供应丰富,腹腔干动脉的分支(源自前肠)供应十二指肠近端,而十二指肠远端(源自中肠)则由肠系膜上动脉供应。腹腔干动脉分出肝总动脉,胃十二指肠动脉起自肝总动脉。胃十二指肠动脉分支为胰十二指肠上动脉,后者分支为十二指肠前支和后支。这些分支与胰十二指肠下动脉(肠系膜上动脉的分支)的前后分支相吻合。

静脉伴行于相应的动脉,胰十二指肠上静脉在十二指肠和胰头之间,汇入门静脉。同样,胰十二指肠下静脉汇入空肠静脉或直接汇入肠系膜上静脉。

十二指肠淋巴引流也与血管相伴行。十二指肠前部和后部小淋巴管汇入胰十二指肠淋巴结,淋巴液向上进入肝脏淋巴结,或者向下流入位于肠系膜上动脉起源处的肠系膜上淋巴结。

(二)十二指肠神经支配

与胃相似,十二指肠受到交感神经和副交感神经支配。神经节前交感神经穿过腹腔和肠系膜上神经节,神经节后神经元进入十二指肠壁内神经丛。交感神经元与传入纤维,主导内脏痛觉。副交感神经纤维由前迷走神经和肠系膜神经的肝支构成,与十二指肠壁的Meissner和Auerbach神经丛形成突触连接。

(三)显微解剖学

十二指肠的黏膜与胃黏膜有显著的差异,不同于胃黏膜的胃腺和胃小凹,十二指肠黏膜富有Lieberkühn隐窝内衬绒毛,黏膜下层具有特征性的Brunner腺。单层上皮细胞在绒毛和隐窝区域为十二指肠腔和黏膜之间提供了界面。上皮层中含有吸收细胞、Paneth细胞(分泌溶菌酶和其他宿主防御因子)、黏液细胞和内分泌细胞。

十二指肠近端绒毛外观扭曲,认为其暴露与胃酸有关。相反,十二指肠远端的绒毛又长又细,而且非常规则,类似于空肠绒毛。十二指肠远端的绒毛与隐窝的长度之比为4∶1或5∶1,也类似于空肠中之比。十二指肠黏膜下层有Brunner腺,它们分泌碱性和透明的黏液,其中含有碳酸氢盐、表皮生长因子(EGF)和胃蛋白酶原Ⅱ。Brunner腺在十二指肠近端最多,在远端较少。它们不是通过自有导管系统排入十二指肠,而是通过相邻的肠腺排出。

三、胃与十二指肠先天性异常

表49.1总结了胃和十二指肠先天性异常。先天性胃畸形在胃肠道畸形中并不常见。根据胃出口梗阻的程度,临床表现可能在新生儿期或之后出现。

(一)胃闭锁

胃闭锁通常发生在胃窦或幽门,3种形式中胃闭锁类型之一:完全的节段性缺损,由纤维索或膜(也称为蹼、膈或间隔)的残余物桥接的节段性缺损。这些病变并不常见,报告的发生率为(1~3)/100 000,其中膜型节段性缺损占大多数。膜由胃黏膜,黏膜肌层和黏膜下层组成。相反,纤维束通常缺乏黏膜成分,但含有正常的浆膜层和肌肉层。膜可以是完整的(完全阻塞),或不完整的(穿孔)。为了清楚起见,不完整的胃黏膜,根据定义不属于闭锁,也在这里一并讲述。

表 49.1　胃和十二指肠异常

异常	发病率	发病年龄	症状和体征	治疗
胃				
胃、胃窦或幽门闭锁	3/10 万(与蹼结合时)	婴儿	非胆汁性呕吐	胃十二指肠吻合术、胃空肠吻合术
幽门或胃窦膜(蹼)	同上	任何年龄	发育异常、呕吐	切开术或切除术,幽门成形术
小胃	罕见	婴儿	呕吐、营养不良	连续滴入喂养或空肠储备造口
胃憩室	罕见	任何年龄	通常无症状	通常无需治疗
胃重复畸形	罕见;男:女=1:2	任何年龄	腹部包块、呕吐、呕血、破裂引起腹膜炎	切除或部分胃切除
胃畸胎瘤	罕见	任何年龄	上腹部肿块	手术切除
胃扭转	罕见	任何年龄	呕吐、拒食	扭转复位,前胃固定术
幽门狭窄(婴儿肥厚性或成人肥厚性)	美国 3/1 000(不同地区范围 1/1 000~8/1 000);男:女=4:1	婴儿	非胆汁性呕吐	幽门成形术
先天性幽门缺失	罕见	儿童、青少年	消化不良(如有症状)	通常无需治疗
十二指肠				
十二指肠闭锁或狭窄	1/20 000	新生儿	胆汁性呕吐、上腹扩张	十二指肠空肠吻合术或胃空肠吻合术
环型胰腺(见第 55 章)	1/10 000	任何年龄	胆汁性呕吐、生长发育不良	十二指肠空肠吻合术
十二指肠重复囊肿	罕见	任何年龄	胃肠出血、疼痛	手术切除
肠旋转不良或中肠扭转(参见第 27 和 98 章)	罕见	任何年龄	胆汁性呕吐、上腹扩张	削减或可能的话切除

1. 发病机制

这些病变发生的原因仍然不清楚,但是各个发育阶段的异常可导致不同的闭锁类型。例如,如果在妊娠 8 周之前(肌层发育之前)融合了多余的内胚层,则胃壁肌肉组织的不连续会导致有或无纤维索的节段性缺损。另一方面,如果在妊娠 8 周之后,肌肉层完整发育成熟时,才出现过长内胚层融合,就仅形成简单的膜。另一种机制是在发育的关键时期发生局部缺血将导致先天畸形。最后,也有人提出了因黏膜增生造成暂时性阻塞,而胃腔再通失败的假说,但这不太可能成立,因为与食管和十二指肠不同,胃在发育过程中不会发生阻塞和再通现象[6]。在患有幽门闭锁的患儿中发现,胃黏膜上皮完全剥离,与上皮细胞和固有层的交界处的 $\alpha_6\beta_4$ 整合素表达不足有关[7]。

遗传也是一个重要的影响因素。除家族遗传(常染色体隐性遗传)外,胃闭锁还与唐氏综合征和结合性大疱性表皮松解(junctional epidermolysis bullosa,JEB)有关。在合并大疱性表皮松解症-幽门闭锁-阻塞性尿路病变的病例中,已发现半桥粒整联蛋白亚基 α_6 和 β_4 的突变[8,9]。JEB(在第 25 章中讨论)也被称为 JEB 幽门闭锁综合征[10]。

其他相关异常包括:肠旋转不良,房间隔缺损,胆囊缺失,气管食管瘘,阴道闭锁和肝外门静脉缺失[11]。此外,胃闭锁可能与多发性肠闭锁和免疫缺陷相关[12]。

2. 临床特征与诊断

在胃肠道近端梗阻中常伴有妊娠期羊水过多。各型胃闭锁的新生儿都有胃出口梗阻的现象,如初次喂奶后出现强烈的无胆汁性呕吐。临床表现可有流口水和呼吸困难。在不伴有胃部扩张时,常有舟状腹。若未及时明确诊断,可能发生严重的代谢性碱中毒,血容量减少和休克,长期胃胀可能导致胃穿孔。腹部 X 线片显示为胃扩张和肠道无气体影。上消化道造影的显示胃完全梗阻,通常发生在胃窦或幽门水平。病变的类型(例如膜)只能通过手术探查来确定。

当胃窦和幽门膜不完整时,出现临床症状的时间通常取决于阻塞的程度。从婴儿到成年期的任何年龄段都可能出现症状。除了膜穿孔之外,这些病变与膜型胃闭锁的临床表现相同。畸形本身、局部炎症和水肿是导致管腔变窄的原因。主要症状是呕吐,婴儿或幼儿体重可能因此无法达到正常范围。在儿童和成年人中,症状可能类似于消化性溃疡疾病,伴有恶心,上腹痛和体重减轻。也可出现腹泻症状,但其生理机制尚不清楚。腹部 X 线片通常是正常的,但也可能显示有胃扩张。产前超声检查偶尔发现不伴有羊水过多的胃扩张。需要进行造影、超声检查(US)或食管胃十二指肠镜检查(EGD)明确诊断。造影显示在胃窦或幽门的膜表现为薄的环周充盈缺损,造影剂在穿过膜中央缺陷时会延迟通过。胃排空时间延迟。US 显示胃窦腔分隔,而 EGD 检查,胃窦或幽门处可见一个小的固定开口,周围是无皱折的黏膜。

3. 治疗

患者经过补液和胃减压治疗,病情稳定后,最终需要外科手术治疗。完整或不完整的胃窦膜可通过简单切除来治疗。幽门膜需要进行幽门成形术。前面已经描述过十二指肠共闭锁[也称为风向袋隔膜(见第 26 章)],术中将导管由近向远端穿入十二指肠来可验证是否存在梗阻。使用圈套器,乳头切开刀,激光或球囊扩张的内镜治疗也有报道。在涉及间隔闭锁时,可使用胃十二指肠造口术达到治愈。另一种方法是通过纵向幽门肌切开术进行幽门括约肌重建,然后进行端--端吻合胃和十二指肠黏膜的末端囊[13]。不建议儿童进行胃空肠造口术,因为存在吻合口溃疡的风险。并且一项回顾性研究显示,由于存在有多种微生物(克雷伯菌,假单胞菌和念珠菌以及耐甲氧西林的金黄色葡萄球菌)感染的可能性,可导致胎儿异常和败血症,其死亡率可超过 50%。另外,如前所述部分患者还可伴有免疫缺陷[14]。

(二) 小胃

小胃是尾部前肠部分的一种极为罕见的先天性畸形。小胃、管状或囊状胃、不全扭转胃与巨食管症有关。胚胎发育第 5 周应出现胃大弯的分化,此时如果出现发育受阻,胃既没有旋转也没有扩张,便可导致各种小胃畸形[15]。局部缺血被认为是妊娠 8 周以后小胃畸形的原因[16],而局部缺血的病因不明。

幸运的是胃组织是正常的。小胃可单独发生,但更常见的是与其他畸形合并发生,如十二指肠闭锁、中肠不旋转、回肠重叠、食管裂孔疝、无脾、部分内脏异位,或肾、上肢(微胃-肢体减少异常)、心脏、肺、骨骼和脊柱等畸形。小胃单独发生是不致命的,但其他关联发生的畸形可能是致命的。有人提出,小胃与肢体减少缺陷和中枢神经系统异常有关,且具有遗传倾向,为常染色体隐性遗传[17],但染色体分析是正常的。

1. 临床特征与诊断

患儿常出现餐后呕吐和营养不良。也可有腹泻(胃排空过快导致)和倾倒综合征。也有出现呼吸系统症状的报告,如出生时喘鸣和呼吸窘迫,反复肺部感染。胃酸分泌的减少可能会影响铁的充分吸收,从而引起缺铁性贫血。内因子分泌不足可导致钴胺素(维生素 B_{12})缺乏。产前超声检查可发现小胃和羊水过多。造影可显示巨食管和管状胃或小胃,食管下端括约肌显示不清,食管胃反流严重。

2. 治疗

小胃的治疗包括少量多次的喂养,小剂量持续的滴入喂营养。另一种方法是通过空肠造口术进行夜间滴喂营养,以补充口服摄入。外科手术可行与胃大弯吻合的双腔 Roux-en-Y 袋。Hunt-Lawrence 空肠袋能够促进正常生长和发育,并能预防反流和倾倒综合征[18]。一病例报告描述了胃分离术治疗先天性小胃食管裂孔疝的案例[19]。

(三) 胃憩室

胃憩室是消化道憩室最罕见的类型。真正的先天性憩室位于贲门后壁,包含所有胃组织层。壁内(或部分)憩室通常于胃窦大弯处,伸入但不穿过肌层。假性憩室是由黏膜和黏膜下层通过肌壁缺损形成的,缺乏固有肌层。胃憩室未发现有家族聚集性。

1. 临床特征与诊断

先天性胃憩室通常无症状,大多在 X 线或内镜检查或尸检时发现(见第 26 章)。大小从 1cm 到 11cm 不等。造影显示为圆形,轮廓清晰的可移动袋,通常有气液平。憩室的排空可能会延迟。在内镜检查中,憩室表现为轮廓分明的开口;内镜扩张可能会引发症状。但是,上消化道造影检查和内镜检查常漏诊位于食管胃交界的憩室。临床表现可为上腹或下胸痛,消化不良,出血或无胆汁性呕吐。需要与胰腺炎、胃出口梗阻、创伤,溃疡病或恶性肿瘤相关的获得性胃憩室进行鉴别诊断。在造影检查中,食管裂孔疝和肥大的胃皱襞可表现为憩室。影像学无法区分先天性憩室和后天性憩室。

2. 治疗

偶发的胃近端憩室无需治疗。如果认为症状与憩室相关,则可以手术切除或封闭憩室开口。而由于远端胃憩室存在诱发恶性肿瘤的风险,因此建议通过手术治疗切除,套叠或节段切除。已有报道胃镜定位后进行腹腔镜切除的报告。

(四) 胃重复畸形

大约有 20% 的胃肠道重复是胃重复。胃重复可单独发生,如三重复(1 名患者中发生 2 次胃重叠),或与其他胃肠道重复同时发生,如食管或十二指肠。通常发生于胃大弯和胃后壁中相邻的部位,且保留所有胃壁层。胃黏膜和胰腺组织可出现在重复胃组织中,继发潜在的并发症[如消化性溃疡病(PUD)和胰腺炎],因此在临床上最为重要。重复胃一般与正常胃不相通,因此常形成管状、梭形或球形的囊性肿块。胃重复偶尔与结肠,胰腺或重复胰腺连通。可能是由于重复胃中穿透性消化性溃疡的获得性瘘导致的。胃重复的病因可能源于一些胚胎发育缺陷,包括脊索和内胚层分离错误、胚胎憩室持续存在和原始前肠上皮细胞内液泡持续存在[20]。大多数胃重复发生在女性(65%),并且在婴儿或儿童时期(80%)发现,没有家族遗传倾向。除并发其他重复外,椎骨异常是第二常见的合并症[21]。也有先天性胃重复的成人患者发生癌变报道。

1. 临床特征与诊断

胃重复的临床表现取决于大小,位置和是否有与其他脏器交通结构等因素。症状和体征各不相同,可有绞痛、腹部包块、上腹部疼痛、体重减轻、呕吐、继发于消化性溃疡的隐匿或显性上消化道或下消化道出血(通过侵蚀结肠发生),与肝内胆管连通导致胆道出血、呼吸窘迫或咯血(囊肿穿孔与肺形成瘘)[22]、幽门梗阻、破裂继发性腹膜炎,胰腺炎、胰腺假性囊肿和急腹症。在婴儿早期,症状可能类似于肥大性幽门狭窄。腹部 X 线片显示胃移位和胃腔受压可提示诊断。造影可通过胃部的占位效应显示重复(见图 49.8A)或与正常消化道连通时可以直接对重复胃进行成像。超声(见图 49.8B),包括产前超声[22],以及 CT(见图 49.8C)、磁共振胰胆管成像(MRCP)、Tc-99m 扫描和内镜超声(EUS)也可显示病变部位。EUS 检查发现在肠旁的囊状物有蠕动表现,是胃重复的诊断特征[23]。

2. 治疗

手术切除是最佳治疗方法(见图 49.8D)。已有腹腔镜切除的报道[24]。当无法完全切除时,如重复胃和内脏具有共同的肌肉层,则可能需要进行减负荷手术、胃造口术或部分胃切除术。此外,应考虑进行黏膜切除术或黏膜表面消融术,因为已有在成人肠道重复中发生恶性肿瘤的记录[25]。

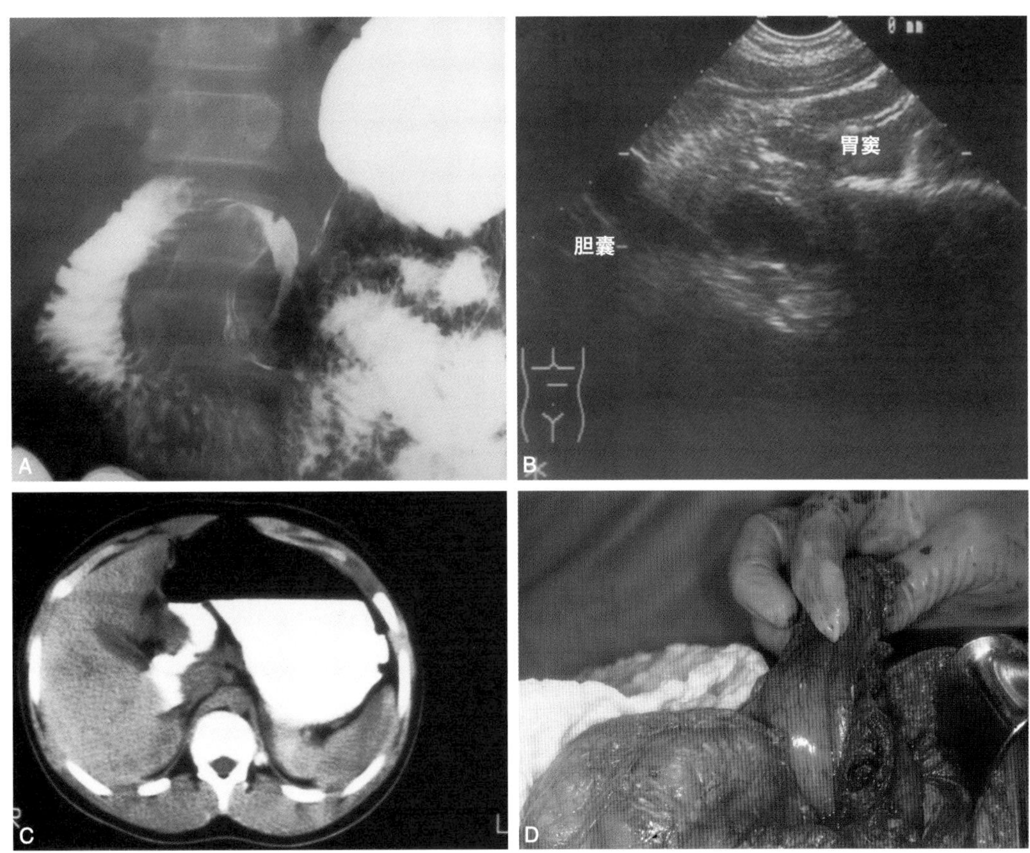

图 49.8　胃重复畸形。一例 12 岁男孩，有 1 年呕吐和间歇性腹痛史。体格检查和实验室检查均正常。A，来自 UGIS 的胶片显示外源性肿块移位并压迫胃窦和十二指肠 C 环。B，超声（US）图像显示胃窦后方和胆囊（GB）内侧低回声团块。C，CT 显示周向软组织增厚，使胃窦移位变窄。D. 解剖胃后和切除前胃重复畸形的术中图片

（五）胃畸胎瘤

胃畸胎瘤是胃的良性肿瘤，几乎只发生在男性中。胃畸胎瘤很罕见，仅占所有儿童畸胎瘤的 1%。胃畸胎瘤可能起源于多功能干细胞，且内含所有 3 胚层细胞。胃畸胎瘤体积较大，通常在婴儿期被诊断出来。尽管报道有向壁内延伸的报道[26]，多数位于胃大弯且存在位于胃外。未成熟畸胎瘤（包括卵黄细胞瘤、生殖器瘤和胚胎瘤）可能发生局部浸润，例如网膜、区域淋巴结以及肝脏的左叶，而成熟畸胎瘤则不发生局部浸润。胃畸胎瘤几乎都是单独发生而与其他肿瘤或畸形无关[27]。

1. 临床特征与诊断

典型的表现是有腹部肿块的男婴，平均年龄为 3.2 个月[28]。透壁生长引起的内在压迫和胃肠道出血可能引起呕吐，可破坏胃黏膜。产前可因羊水过多而发现胃梗阻。畸胎瘤新生患儿可因腹部压力升高而提前分娩或出现呼吸窘迫。可能出现分娩困难，使婴儿面临肩难产等伤害。已有胃畸胎瘤与胃穿孔、胎粪性腹膜炎的相关报告[29]。X 线平片显示特征性钙化。US 显示实性和囊性区域，CT 或 MRI 可证实诊断并评估区域浸润[28]。

2. 治疗

肿瘤切除和一期胃修补是治愈该病的首选方法。若肿瘤浸润壁内则需要进行部分或全部胃切除。已有癌前病变转化或直接恶变为腺癌的报告[30,31]，和腹膜性胶质瘤病的病例。幸运的是，即使有恶性组织学特征或有邻近组织浸润，患者预后也较好[27]。对于未成熟的胃畸胎瘤，血清 AFP 水平可能具有临床意义，可以提示复发或转移风险和辅助指导化疗[32]。胃畸胎瘤可在 20 年后复发，因此需要长期随访[33]。

（六）胃扭转

见表 49.1 和第 27 章。

（七）婴儿肥厚性幽门狭窄

婴儿肥厚性幽门狭窄（infantile hypertrophic pyloric stenosis，IHPS）是一种由幽门通道周围环行肌肥大引起的胃出口梗阻。IHPS 的矫治是 6 个月以内儿童最常见的腹部手术。由于幽门环形肌的肥大和梗阻往往是在婴儿出生后才出现的一个渐变过程，因此 IHPS 不属于真正意义上的先天性缺陷[34]。IHPS 的病因仍在探索中。一氧化氮合成酶（一种与平滑肌松弛有关的酶）的局部缺乏，或与肌肉神经纤维板减少，或神经末梢、突触小泡蛋白和神经细胞黏附分子减少有关的神经支配异常[35]已被证实与 IHPS 有关；然而，解剖学研究不能确定一氧化氮合成酶缺乏是原发性还是继发性因素[36]，并且一氧化氮合成酶缺乏仅在一部分病例中发现[37]。调节胃肠运动的起搏细胞，即 Cajal 间质细胞（下一章讨论）仅在 IHPS 黏膜下层附近观察到，而不是整个幽门[38,39]。在 IHPS 的平滑肌细胞中，EGF、EGF 受体以及肝素结合 EGF 样生长因子显著增加[40]，但其触发因素尚不清楚。

在美国,IHPS 的发病率约为3‰,但不同种族和地区的发病率从1‰~8‰不等。白人(尤其是北欧人)的发病率最高,而非裔美国人和非洲人的发病率较低,亚洲人的发病率最低。男性与女性的发病率比例为4∶1或5∶1。

IHPS 呈家族性聚集,有报道表明 IHPS 为常染色体显性遗传[41]。大约50%的同卵双胞胎患 IHPS,这使人们相信遗传因素和环境因素的共同作用。患病女性的男性亲属更有可能患上 IHPS,因此患病女性的兄弟姐妹和后代比患病男性的亲属更有可能患上 IHPS。此外,第一胎的男婴,特别是那些出生体重较高或由患病父母生下的男婴,患 IHPS 风险更高。IHPS 还与 Turner 综合征、18-三体综合征、Cornelia de Lange 综合征、食管闭锁、先天性巨结肠、苯丙酮尿症和先天性风疹综合征相关。多份报告已经描述了婴儿早期接触过大环内酯类药物,包括通过母乳接触[42],这可能与 IHPS 的发生有关[43-45]。此外,最近观察到 IHPS 发病率下降,与婴儿猝死综合征的发病率相一致,这与建议婴儿仰卧睡眠姿势相关;然而,德国的一项研究表明,IHPS 的地区分布与婴儿猝死综合征的地区分布不同[46,47]。

通过对具有2个或2个以上患病个体的家系进行全基因组连锁分析,研究人员确定出 IHPS 的5个遗传位点:位于染色体12q24.2-24.31位点上的一氧化氮合成酶基因 *NOS1*;与常染色体显性遗传相关的2个位点 *IHPS2*(16p12-p13)和 *IHPS5*(16q24.3);*IHPS3*(11q14-q22);以及 *IHPS4*(Xq23-q24)[48]。对1 001名丹麦 IHPS 患者和2 401名健康对照进行了全基因组相关研究。发现两个基因 *MBNL1* 和 *NKX2-5* 与该病有关,然后在其他队列研究中也重复发现[49]。

1. 临床特征与诊断

患有 IHPS 的婴儿通常在出生后3~4周内没有症状,但也有一小部分婴儿可能在出生第一周就会出现症状。最初婴儿会出现轻微吐口水,随着疾病的进展,喂食后会出现喷射性呕吐。强烈的呕吐可能会使呕吐物经口排出的同时也从鼻孔排出。呕吐物可能含有"咖啡渣"样物质或少量鲜血,但很少有胆汁。在这个过程的早期,婴儿在呕吐后仍然感到饥饿,但随着时间的推移,婴儿会不想进食,随之可能会出现虚弱和严重的脱水。脱水表现为尿量和粪便排出量减少。明显的代谢性碱中毒继发于呕吐物中的氯化物丢失。婴儿可能被误诊为配方奶过敏或胃食管反流。

体格检查时,IHPS 患儿可表现为虚弱和脱水,但其程度与症状的严重程度和持续时间有关。典型的体征是可触及幽门肿块和可见胃蠕动波。消瘦的病人在呕吐或胃内容物吸出后,最容易感觉到明显的"橄榄"形幽门肿块。幽门肿块的位置从脐部水平到上腹部都可以出现。根据检查人员的经验和耐心,在70%~90%的患病婴儿中可以触摸到幽门肿块。通过放置鼻胃管排空胃,并在婴儿俯卧时触诊胃,可以提高检测率。母亲用左臂将裸体婴儿抱在怀中喂养时最容易观察到胃蠕动波。许多婴儿出现黄疸是由于间接高胆红素血症,与脱水有关,或许还与营养不良有关。当症状典型且可触及橄榄状包块时,就可以确诊 IHPS。然而,有少数表现为喷射性呕吐的婴儿需要放射学检查来明确诊断。X 线显示胃扩张伴胃外气体不足。幽门超声已取代 X 线检查,成为确诊 IHPS 的首选方法。由于脱水可能会影响幽门超声的测量,在超声评估之前,需确保胃内有足够的液体[50]。幽门管肥厚的长度从14mm到20mm不等。幽门肌厚度下限的数值在文献中有不同的报道,范围为3~4.5mm。超声表现为典型的透声"甜甜圈"(图49.9)。许多人认为这个数值不如管道的整体形态和实时观测那么重要。美国的一项阴性对照研究显示,明确诊断的依据是有正常幽门环和扩张胃窦部[51]。

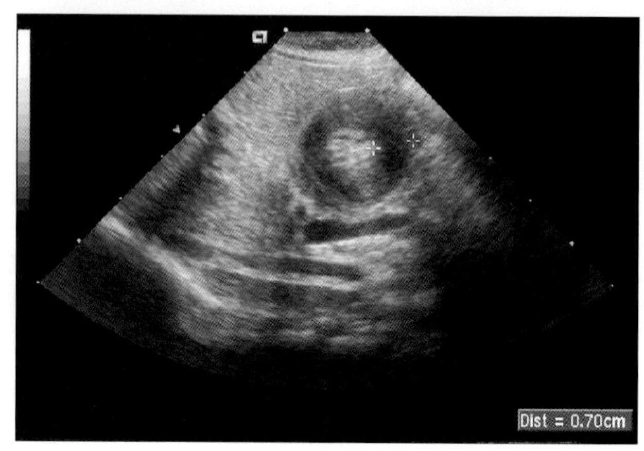

图49.9 1个月婴儿特发性肥厚性幽门狭窄的腹部超声图像,横断面显示幽门肥厚的透声"环状"。横线测量异常(7mm)肌肉厚度。(Courtesy Jeanne Joglar, MD.)

当鉴别 IHPS、胃食管反流或其他上消化道疾病时,上消化道造影检查可能是合适的首选检查手段。行上消化道造影前应排空胃内容物。婴儿通过乳头获得钡剂,并在半俯卧位成像。典型的影像学结果为一个细长狭窄的幽门,呈"双轨征"。幽门肿物还会使邻近的胃窦和十二指肠受压,形成所谓的肩部(图49.10)。类似于 IHPS 异常改变的疾病,最常见的是幽门痉挛。EGD 对 IHPS 的诊断描述为幽门呈菜花状变窄,7.8mm(外径)内镜无法通过[52];然而,另一份关于内镜诊

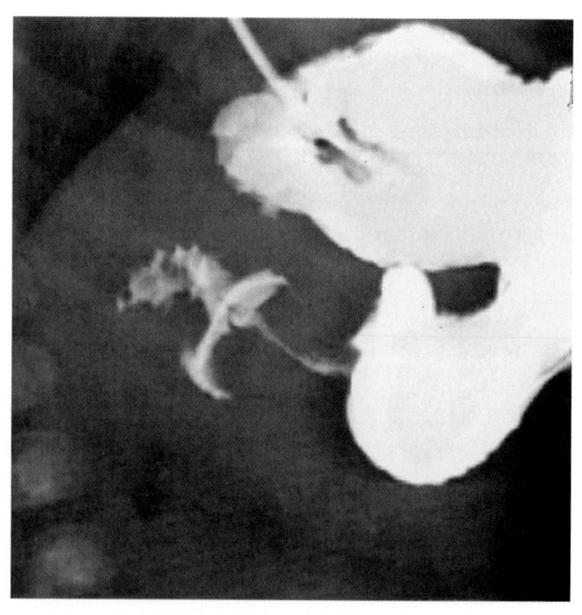
图49.10 来自 UGIS 的1个月大的特发性肥厚性幽门狭窄婴儿的胶片,显示继发于占位效应的幽门、胃窦及十二指肠"肩部"延长。(Courtesy Marcia Pritchard, MD.)

断的报告驳斥了这些说法[53]。EGD 还可能有助于评估与幽门狭窄相关的嗜酸性胃肠炎[54](见第 30 章)。

2. 治疗

IHPS 的早期治疗是补充液体和电解质,以纠正脱水和低氯性代谢性碱中毒。根据严重程度,液体和电解质的补充通常可以在 24 小时内完成。最终的治疗方法是 Ramstedt 幽门肌切开术,需纵向切开肥厚的幽门肌,直至幽门前面的黏膜下层。肌肉展开后,完整的黏膜通过切口隆起到切开的肌肉水平。另一种手术是幽门创伤成形术,用 Babcock 钳夹住幽门,在两点破坏肥大的环状肌[55,56]。腹腔镜下幽门肌切开术伤口更美观,对止痛药的需求少,在临床中应用越来越多[57,58]。虽然在术后前几天婴儿可能仍有呕吐的症状,但持续呕吐则提示幽门环肌切开不足。

非手术治疗包括使用抗胆碱能药物[59]和糊状食物喂养,直到肌肉肥大消失[60]。由于失败率高、恢复期长(与手术相比)、幽门肌切开术风险低,非手术方法在美国已很少使用。

手术预后良好,婴儿可恢复正常生长发育。虽然在 IHPS 治疗后的许多年中观察到了不同的胃排空率,但在接受手术治疗或保守治疗的患者中,使用放射性标记液体或固体进行核素扫描的胃排空功能与对照组相似[52]。

(八) 成人肥厚性幽门狭窄

肥厚性幽门狭窄(hypertrophic pyloric stenosis,HPS)很少发生于成人,文献中描述了大约 200 例。成人 HPS 具有与婴儿型相同的解剖学特征。在成人中,幽门增厚通常与 PUD、肥厚性胃病[61]或癌症有关。在少数病例中,没有确定病因;因此,尚不清楚这些病例是被遗漏的婴儿期病例,还是肥大就发生在成人期。在一些成人 HPS 病例中有 IHPS 的家族史,再次提示遗传易感性或遗漏婴儿病例的可能性。此外,80% 的成人 HPS 病例发生在男性。切除的幽门表现为黏膜正常,固有肌环周明显增厚[62]。显微镜下可见不同程度的炎症改变或水肿,以及肌间神经丛的神经节细胞退行性改变[61]。

1. 临床特征与诊断

成人 HPS 的症状与婴儿期观察到的症状相似:恶心、轻度呕吐、早饱和上腹痛,尤其是在进食后。与婴儿期相比,体格检查可能没有帮助,因为成年人很难触及幽门肿块。造影显示幽门狭长,胃排空延迟,胃扩张。超声是首选的筛查程序;如果幽门厚度大于或等于 1cm,且持续伸长超过 2cm,则通常认为是异常的[61]。EGD 用于区分成人 HPS 与癌症或慢性消化性溃疡疾病。

2. 治疗

传统上,幽门环肌切开术或切除受累区域被认为是首选治疗方法。鉴于小病灶癌变的风险,建议手术切除幽门。内镜球囊扩张术在治疗成人 HPS 病中也是有效的,但据报道扩张术后 6 个月内复发率为 80%[63]。内镜下放置支架对由胃癌引起的幽门狭窄的姑息治疗也已有文献报道[64]。

(九) 先天性幽门缺失

这是一种罕见的异常畸形,幽门像一个囊一样闭合,胃出口的开口沿着胃小弯的切迹位于一个异常的位置(见表 49.1)。

(十) 十二指肠闭锁和狭窄

十二指肠闭锁和狭窄分别是以十二指肠完全和部分梗阻为特征的先天性缺陷。闭锁有不同的解剖形态,包括与远端十二指肠无连接的盲端袋(最不常见),与远端十二指肠有纤维索带连接的盲端袋,或由隔膜完全阻塞管腔(最常见)。穿孔隔膜也是十二指肠狭窄的原因之一。所有这些病变在 Vater 壶腹附近发生的频率最高,大多数病变(80%)发生在 Vater 壶腹的远端。这 3 种异常的总发病率在新生儿中约占 1/200 000,略倾向发生于女孩。这些病变的病因可能与妊娠 8~10 周时十二指肠肠腔空泡化再通失败有关。这与子宫内血管意外引起的空肠和回肠闭锁或狭窄不同[65]。在 sonic hedgehog(shh)突变小鼠中观察到十二指肠狭窄,这一现象加深了我们对信号通路突变在这种畸形中可能起作用的理解[66]。

在 2 个系列的 100 多例患者中[67,68],超过 50% 的患者合并其他先天性缺陷,包括胰腺缺损、先天性肠索带肠旋转不良、食管闭锁、梅克尔憩室、肛门闭锁、先天性心脏病、中枢神经系统病变、肾脏畸形,极少数还有胆道畸形。小儿唐氏综合征与十二指肠闭锁/十二指肠狭窄/十二指肠蹼相关,因为 25%~50% 以上的病例发生在患有这种染色体异常的婴儿和儿童身上。家族性关联很少见,尽管个别病例报告显示可能存在遗传关联[41,69]。文献报道一对父子,因十二指肠狭窄和环状胰腺(父亲)和节段性十二指肠闭锁(儿子)导致壶腹周围梗阻,这个案例提醒人们,随着患病婴儿存活率的提高,未来可能应多关注遗传背景[70]。

1. 临床特征与诊断

当孕妇产前超声检查提示胃和十二指肠近端扩张以及羊水过多时,需考虑胎儿有无十二指肠闭锁。羊水过多出现在 33%~50% 的十二指肠闭锁病例中。羊水过多时胃和十二指肠近端无扩张不能排除此诊断,因为宫内呕吐可能会限制阻塞部位上游的扩张。在美国使用的高频经阴探头可能会过度诊断肠扩张,因此一旦怀疑梗阻,建议进行更长时间的扫描[71]。

患有十二指肠闭锁的婴儿通常早产,并有早期喂养不耐受的特点,主要表现为呕吐和上腹胀。呕吐通常是胆汁性的,因为大多数病变发生在胆管进入十二指肠的远端。非胆汁性呕吐见于 15%~20% 的继发于近端梗阻的病例。任何有小儿唐氏综合征和呕吐表现(特别是呕吐物含有胆汁的)的儿童都需要进一步评估是否有十二指肠狭窄。根据梗阻程度的不同,十二指肠狭窄或部分隔膜可在任何年龄出现。婴儿和儿童表现为呕吐、体重不能充分增加和/或误吸。呕吐可能是间歇性的,并且病情轻重不等,因此对有症状患者的诊断可能需要几个月甚至几年。更有甚者,直到成年才明确诊断。

婴儿十二指肠梗阻的 X 线造影典型表现为胃和十二指肠第一段有空气存在——“双泡”征(图 49.11)。第二个气泡以外的空气缺失应被解释为十二指肠闭锁可能。造影通常能有效显示十二指肠闭锁、狭窄、隔膜和其他导致十二指肠外压的异常(图 49.12)。此外,造影还可以评估肠道的正常或异常旋转和固定。已有某些案例观察到壶腹括约肌功能不全。

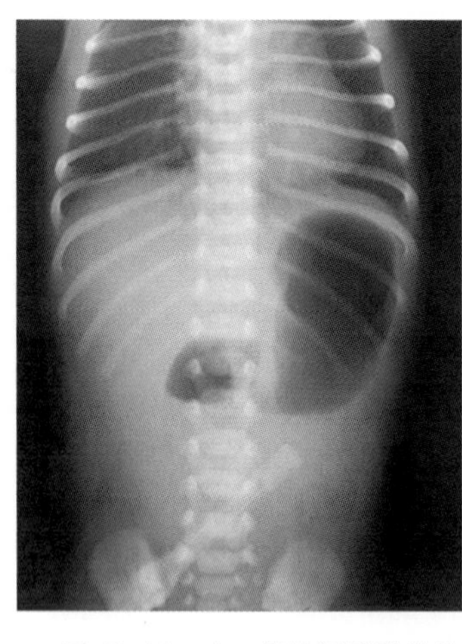
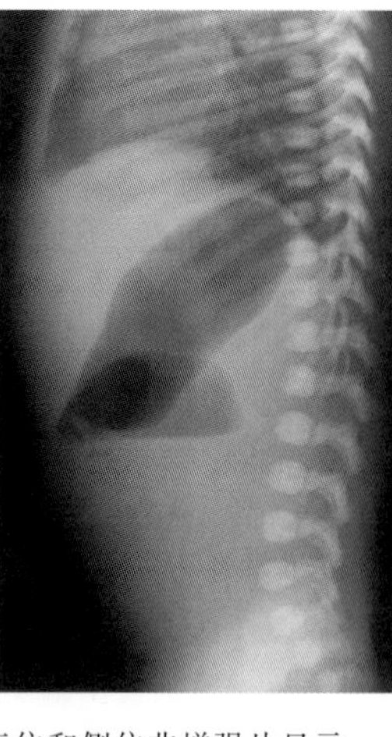

图 49.11　十二指肠闭锁婴儿的正位和侧位非增强片显示“双泡”征。(Courtesy Marcia Pritchard, MD.)

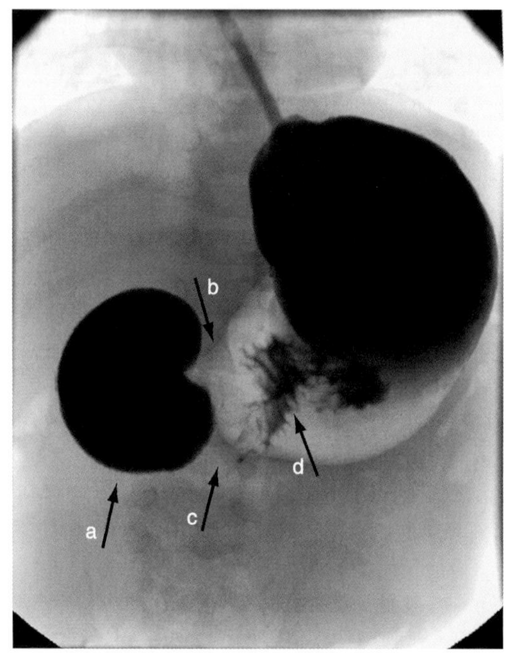

图 49.12　患有十二指肠膜/十二指肠蹼的婴儿的 UGIS 胶片显示,(a)从幽门(b)至十二指肠蹼段近端的十二指肠第三部分(无造影剂)(c)和十二指肠口径正常的第四部分(d)。(Courtesy Korgun Koral, MD.)

造影剂通过壶腹回流有发生胆管炎和胰腺炎的风险。有时,上消化道内镜检查有助于诊断或确定十二指肠狭窄或十二指肠隔膜。

2. 治疗

怀疑十二指肠梗阻的新生儿应放置鼻胃管减压,并纠正液体和电解质异常。过去的手术方式是十二指肠空肠吻合术,但现在首选十二指肠十二指肠吻合术[68]。手术方式由侧侧吻合演变为近端横向至远端纵向(“菱形”)吻合。相关的旋转不良可通过 Ladd 程序进行纠正。导管进入十二指肠远端以检查二次梗阻,大约 3% 的病例会发生二次梗阻。如果只是隔膜导致梗阻,可以切除隔膜而不行吻合术。球囊扩张已被应用于治疗膜性十二指肠狭窄[72,73]。已有内镜激光切割隔膜的报道;但随后的瘢痕形成会导致再狭窄和二次手术[74]。初次修复后可困扰患者数月至数年的并发症包括胃肠动力问题、巨十二指肠、药物治疗无效的胃食管反流、胃病、肠粘连和 PUD[68]。最近的一项研究表明,十二指肠闭锁的近段和远段在神经细胞、肌肉结构和 Cajal 间质细胞的分布上存在差异,这可能是十二指肠术后运动障碍发生的原因[75]。

在 30 年的随访期内,大约 12% 的患者需要再次修复或再次行腹腔内手术[76]。两名青少年出现胆总管囊肿[67]。梗阻近端的巨十二指肠蠕动异常是一个常见的长期问题,但大多数患者没有症状。对于有症状的巨十二指肠患者,可能需要进行肠道折叠术[77]。

(十一) 环型胰腺

环型胰腺是一种罕见的先天性畸形,其特征是胰腺组织呈薄环状,最常环绕在十二指肠的第二部分,导致不同程度的梗阻(见第 55 章)。病变可能出现在新生儿期、儿童期或成年期。这是儿童最常见的先天性胰腺异常。有些病例没有临床症状表现,直到行内镜逆行胰胆管造影(ERCP)或尸检时才被偶然发现。环型胰腺在组织学上是正常的,包含一个中等大小的胰管。胰腺组织可穿透十二指肠壁肌层,或与十二指肠保持分离。

关于环型胰腺的胚胎起源有几种假说。证据似乎支持 Lecco 1910 年的假说,即在妊娠第五周,腹侧胰腺原基在旋转之前就固定在十二指肠壁上。随着背侧和腹侧原基的生长和融合,形成了部分(75%)或完整(25%)的胰腺组织环[6]。

这种疾病的发病率约为每 10 万名活产儿中就有 1 例,但这一数字不包括成年期间通过 ERCP(通常被认为是偶然发现)或尸检中发现的病例。真正的发病率可能高达每 250 名活产儿中就有 1 名。在婴儿期,男婴和女婴的发病率相同,而成年后,男性与女性的比例为 2∶1。据估计,婴儿和儿童病例中有 40%~70% 与其他先天性畸形有关,包括小儿唐氏综合征、十二指肠闭锁、心脏缺陷、肛门直肠畸形、梅克尔憩室、气管食管瘘、肠管旋转不良、泌尿生殖系统畸形和内脏反位[78]。与儿童相比,成人更常见肠管旋转不良、十二指肠蹼、Shatzki 环(下食管括约肌环)、十二指肠闭锁、气管食管瘘和泌尿生殖系统异常。此外,成年人患胰胆管肿瘤的风险也会增加。在 13 名患有环型胰腺的成人中,6 名患有胰胆管肿瘤,包括 2 名胰腺腺癌,2 名壶腹腺瘤和 1 名胆囊腺癌[78]。在一名妇女和她的孩子以及连续两代人中发现环型胰腺,这表明可能存在遗传联系[79]。最近的一份病例报告显示,utrophin 基因的 6q24.2 微复制是环型胰腺发生的潜在危险因素[80]。

1. 临床特征与诊断

当环型胰腺组织阻塞十二指肠或胆道时会产生相应的症状。环型胰腺是否真的在梗阻中起作用还存在争议。胰腺组织位置异常提示潜在的十二指肠异常,可表现为十二指肠狭窄甚至闭锁[81]。婴儿可能出现严重的梗阻症状和体征,如胆汁呕吐和上腹胀,与十二指肠闭锁或肠管旋转不良伴中肠扭转难以区分。在儿童时期,间歇性胆汁呕吐和发育不良是常见的表现症状,而在成年期间,最常见的症状是腹痛。成人的其他症状和体征包括恶心、呕吐、胃出口梗阻、胰腺炎、胰腺结石、胰腺分裂、胰腺肿块、胃或十二指肠溃疡,或导致黄疸的胆道梗阻。在成人中,症状在 30~50 年达到顶峰。

婴儿的 X 线片检查可能显示与十二指肠闭锁相同的双泡征（见图 49.10）。为确保梗阻不是由中肠扭转引起的，应行造影检查，因为中肠扭转是外科紧急情况。在成人中，经腹 US、EUS、CT 或 MRCP 可诊断环状胰腺。ERCP 可以显示与环型胰腺一致的导管结构，但在某些情况下，由于主壶腹部近端的十二指肠梗阻，ERCP 技术就无法实施。当既往有胃切除或十二指肠梗阻无法行 ERCP 检查时，EUS 尤其适用；此外，在行 EUS 检查的同时还可对肿块进行分期或行 FNA 检查。考虑到壶腹癌与环状胰腺相关的报道，评估肿块的能力是一个新的考虑因素；因此，在排除肿瘤之前，黄疸不应完全归因于环型胰腺[82]。MRCP 可以显示整个胰胆管的空间分布，可以识别十二指肠周围的环状物和导管。此外，还可通过开腹手术在术中诊断环型胰腺。

2. 治疗

环型胰腺的首选手术疗法包括十二指肠与十二指肠吻合术或十二指肠空肠吻合术。无论哪种术式，术后预后都很好，婴儿的术后死亡通常是由于相关其他异常引起的。由于并发症风险较高，不建议对胰腺组织进行分割或剥离。这些并发症包括胰腺炎，胰瘘和因十二指肠狭窄引起不能完全缓解的症状。在器官摘取时发现环型胰腺，连同一段较长的十二指肠被移植，其移植效果良好，因此认为环型胰腺可以适合移植[83]。

（十二）十二指肠重复囊肿

十二指肠重复囊肿是一种罕见的临床异常，仅占胃肠道重复畸形的 7%。最常位于十二指肠第一或第二部分的后方，这些球形或管状囊肿通常不与十二指肠腔相通，但与十二指肠共享血液供应系统。十二指肠重复囊肿的组织学包括胃肠道黏膜，壁内有平滑肌层，与十二指肠壁有联系。典型的黏膜是十二指肠黏膜，但在 15% 的病例中有胃黏膜，很少发现胰腺组织。男性和女性患病率是一样的。人们提出了几种胚胎学理论，但没有一种理论能解释解剖变异的多样性[84]。

1. 临床特征与诊断

重复畸形在临床上可能会在数年后才出现临床表现。这些囊肿引起的典型症状和体征是胃出口部分梗阻，包括呕吐、进食减少、脐周压痛和腹胀。然而，无症状肿块可能首先通过体格检查或放射学检查被发现。如果十二指肠重复畸形存在异位的胃黏膜，出血或穿孔可能是最初的症状。已有巨大的重复囊肿引起新生儿十二指肠梗阻的报道。感染的十二指肠重复畸形囊肿也已被发现[85]。如果囊肿压迫胰管或与胰管相通，则可能发生胰腺炎。最后还可以出现黄疸和导致小肠梗阻的十二指肠空肠套叠[86]。

造影或不造影的 X 线检查都可显示梗阻或压迫征象，但一般而言，所见不具特异性，仅提示诊断。超声可见单房囊性结构，周围有薄薄的肌层低回声晕环绕的黏膜回声[85]。超声可见囊肿有蠕动波。产前超声可以识别疑似囊肿。CT 可显示十二指肠后方的包裹性、非交通性囊肿。ERCP 上可见压缩的壶腹周围肿块。

2. 治疗

手术治疗应根据囊肿的解剖学特点进行个体化治疗。由于潜在的并发症，提倡在新生儿早期切除，甚至对无症状的囊肿也是如此[87]。已开展的手术包括局部切除和囊肿空肠吻合术。黏膜剥离共同肌壁和切除游离壁已被推荐[88]。然而，这可能是复杂的，因为囊肿靠近壶腹和胆胰汇合部。内镜引流和取出术在成人和儿科病例中都取得了成功。由于浸润性癌可能发生在患有十二指肠重复畸形囊肿的成年人身上，不切除组织而只行内镜引流的方法可能需要重新考虑。

（十三）肠旋转不良与中肠扭转

参见表 49.1 和第 98 章。

（程芮 译，王立 刘军 校）

参考文献

第 50 章　胃神经肌肉功能与神经肌肉病变

Kenneth L. Koch 著

章节目录

一、正常胃神经肌肉功能的电生理学基础 ………… 696
（一）细胞外慢波、平台期电位和动作电位 …… 696
（二）胃平滑肌细胞内电记录 …………………… 696
（三）Cajal 间质细胞 ………………………… 698
（四）神经系统支配 …………………………… 700
（五）禁食期间的胃神经肌肉活动 …………… 700
（六）餐后胃神经肌肉活动 …………………… 700
二、餐后胃神经肌肉活动 ……………………… 705
三、胃感觉活动 ………………………………… 706
四、胃与摄食、饥饿和饱腹感的调节 ………… 708
五、胃神经肌肉功能的发育 …………………… 709
六、胃神经肌肉功能的评估 …………………… 709
（一）胃排空率 ………………………………… 709
（二）胃收缩 …………………………………… 709
（三）胃肌电活动 ……………………………… 710
（四）胃舒张、容纳和容积 …………………… 710
（五）胃和幽门神经肌肉病变的组织病理学研究 ………………………………………… 711
七、胃神经肌肉疾病 …………………………… 711
（一）胃轻瘫 …………………………………… 713
（二）与其他胃肠道疾病相关的胃神经肌肉功能障碍 ………………………………… 716
（三）倾倒综合征和胃快速排空 ……………… 717
八、胃神经肌肉病变的诊断 …………………… 717
（一）病史 ……………………………………… 717
（二）体格检查 ………………………………… 718
（三）标准检查 ………………………………… 718
（四）非侵入性检查 …………………………… 718
九、治疗 ………………………………………… 718
（一）药物治疗 ………………………………… 720
（二）电疗 ……………………………………… 721
（三）内镜治疗 ………………………………… 721
（四）饮食治疗 ………………………………… 721

胃神经肌肉功能是指胃的收缩、舒张和蠕动活动过程。

胃的 3 种主要神经肌肉活动是：①胃底容受性舒张；②胃体和胃窦周期性蠕动波；③胃窦蠕动与胃窦、幽门和十二指肠相互协调作用。胃的这些主要神经肌肉活动实现 3 个关键功能：①接受摄入食物（容受性舒张）；②将摄入的食物碾磨成一种名为食糜的营养悬浮液；③以高度调节的方式将食糜从胃通过幽门括约肌排入至十二指肠。这一复杂过程对于之后小肠最大限度地消化吸收食物营养成分是必要的。胃神经肌肉功能障碍会导致恶心、早饱、呕吐咀嚼过的食物以及胃内固体和液体食物排空失调。

这些重要的胃神经肌肉活动和相关功能受到中枢神经系统（central nervous system，CNS）、副交感神经系统（parasympathetic nervous system，PNS）、交感神经系统（sympathetic nervous system，SNS）、中枢神经系统与肠神经系统（enteric nervous system，ENS）的相互作用，以及 Cajal 间质细胞（interstitial cell of Cajal，ICC）的复杂调节。ICC 调节胃平滑肌收缩频率和组织蠕动波，以及最终调节胃平滑肌的收缩及舒张的神经递质的宿主。

一、正常胃神经肌肉功能的电生理学基础

（一）细胞外慢波、平台期电位和动作电位

胃是一个复杂的平滑肌球体，由环形、纵行和斜行肌组成。胃肌电活动（gastric myoelectrical activity，GMA），称为慢波或起搏电位，调节、控制和起搏胃平滑肌收缩[1,2]。在正常人胃中，慢波以大约 3cpm（每分钟周期数）或 2.5~3.7cpm 之间的速度出现[3,4]。从胃大弯处的起搏区（在胃底和近端胃体部之间），慢波每隔 20 秒向远端传播一次，以环周的形式到达幽门，在胃窦远端 2~4cm 处达最大的振幅和速度（约 7mm/s）（图 50.1）[5]。胃慢波起源于 ICC[2,6]。

慢波的去极化上行波降低了环形平滑肌收缩的电阈值，在适当的情况下，环形平滑肌收缩的幅度随着平台电位和动作电位的开始而增加[7,8]。与平台电位（有或无动作电位）相关的慢波的远向传播是胃蠕动波电生理基础（图 50.2）。与平台或动作电位相关的慢波通过胃体和胃窦传播，产生运动的“环状收缩”，最终在胃窦或幽门以胃窦收缩的形式结束。幽门在远端胃窦的 3cpm 慢波和十二指肠的 12~13cpm 慢波之间提供了电荷屏障。

（二）胃平滑肌细胞内电记录

来自不同区域（从胃底到胃体，最终达末端胃窦）胃平滑肌细胞的细胞内记录显示了区分这些区域的电生理特征（图 50.3）[1]。主要特征是：①静息电位的区域差异，范围从 −48mV 到 −75mV；②收缩阈值的区域差异，范围从 −52mV 到 −40mV；③伴有或不伴有峰电位的平台电位[1]。胃底平滑肌细胞的独特之处在于它们的静息膜电位位于或高于收缩阈值（−50mV），这种情况促进持续平滑肌收缩和持续胃底张力。吞咽过程中，胃底的抑制性迷走神经在吞咽过程中输入增加，导致与胃底“容受性舒张”和吞咽食物相关的肌张力下降[9,10]。胃底肌张力随着抑制性神经放电强度和持续时间的增加而降低。

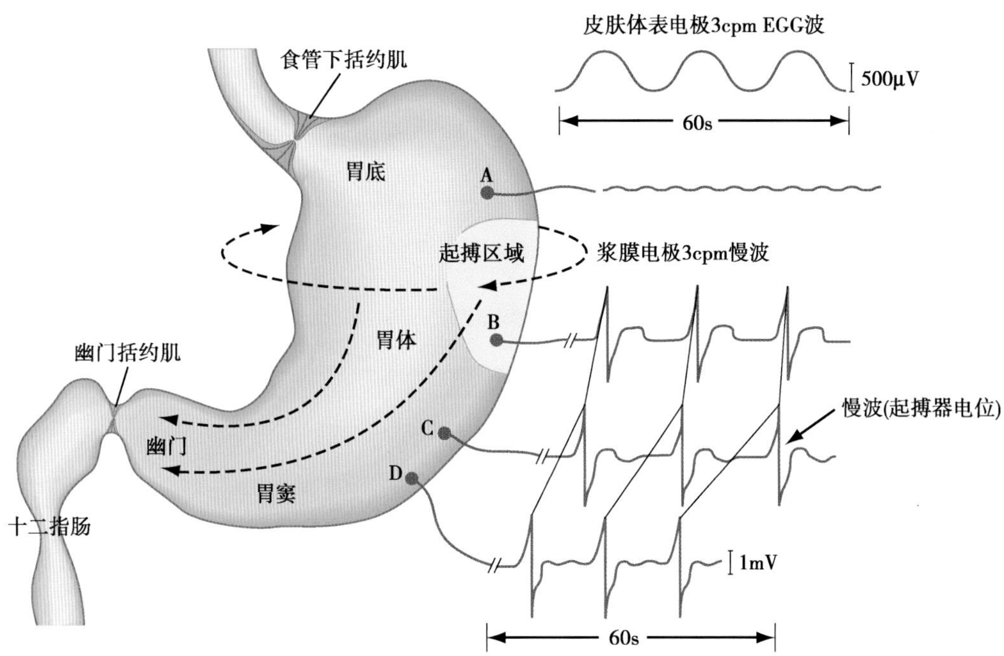

图 50.1　从胃底至胃窦在胃浆膜上放置电极(A~D),记录胃电活动。慢波起源于位于胃底与胃大弯体交界处的起搏区。注意胃底没有慢波活动(电极 A)。慢波向圆周传播,约每 20 秒或 3cpm 向远端移至幽门(箭头虚线)。可使用皮肤体表电极记录 3cpm 时的 GMA。从位于上腹部表面的电极记录的 GMA 总和被称为胃电图(EGG),正常节律为 3cpm。cpm,每分钟周期数。(Modified from Koch KL. Electrogastrography. In:Schuster M,Crowel M,Koch,KL,editors. Atlas of gastrointestinal motility. Hamilton,Ontario:BC Decker;2002. pp 185-201.)

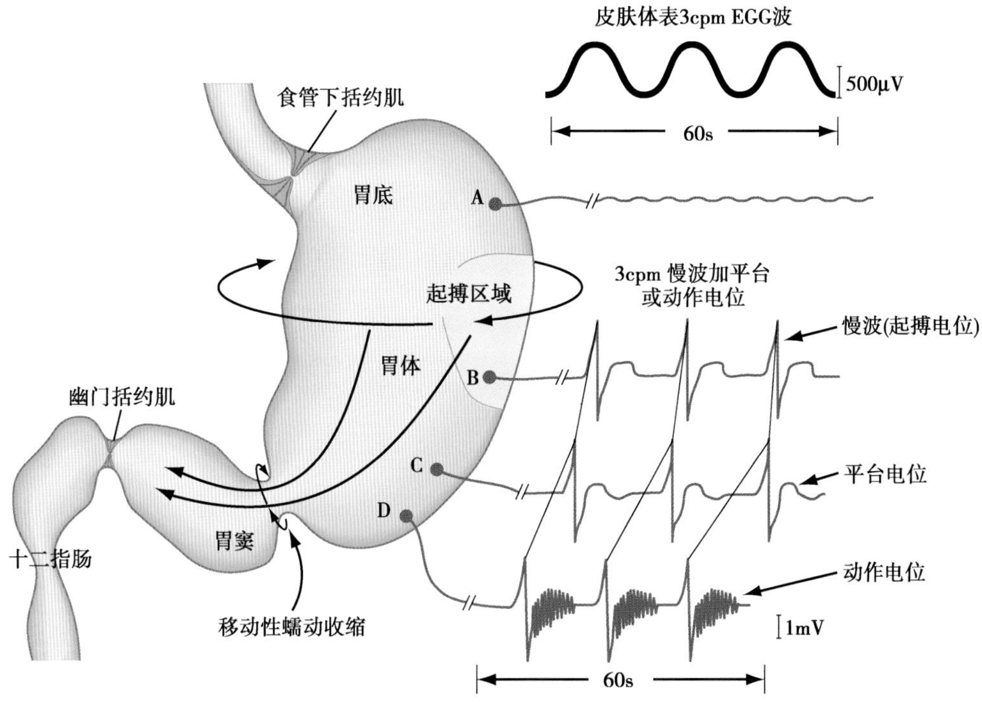

图 50.2　与平台电位(或动作电位)相关的胃慢波,是胃蠕动波的电生理基础。平台期电位和动作电位发生在环形肌肉收缩过程中。蠕动波起源于起搏区。胃蠕动波的频率(3cpm)和传播速度(≈14mm/s)由慢波控制,慢波导致胃体近端至胃窦远端收缩,如电极 A 至 D 所示。黑色实线和箭表示蠕动波的圆周向远端传播,其形成环形收缩(小箭),表明蠕动收缩移动。蠕动收缩每分钟发生 3 次,这是胃慢波的频率。与慢波相关的平台电位和动作电位的 GMA 增加,导致胃电图(EGG)信号(粗黑线)中记录的 3cpm 波振幅增加。胃底不参与胃蠕动收缩。cpm,每分钟周期数。(摘自 Koch KL. Electrogastrography. In:Schuster M,Crowel M,Koch,KL,editors. Atlas of gastrointestinal motility. Hamilton,Ontario BC Decker;2002. pp 185-201.)

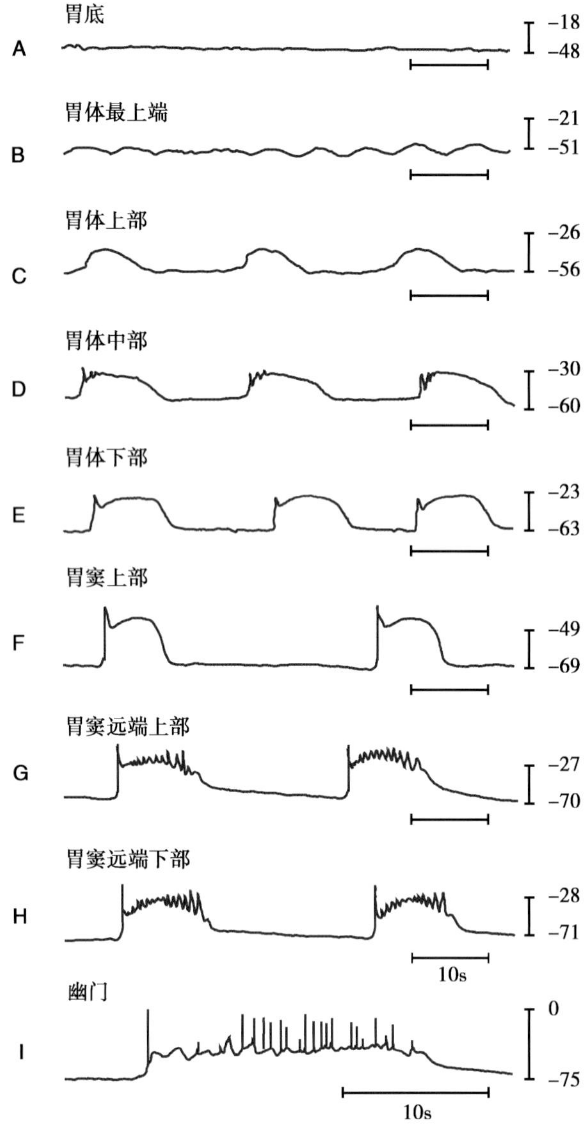

图 50.3　从胃底至幽门平滑肌的细胞内电记录(A 至 I)。静息膜电位(mV)显示在垂直轴上,时间显示在水平轴上。显示了每个区域的独特电特征:A,胃底平滑肌无自发电活动。B 至 E,与胃窦相比,胃体平滑肌的静息膜电位阴性较少(F 至 H)。平台电位部(F 到 H)的负值要小。在胃体和胃窦,以及幽门也记录到自发性上升去极化(I)。平滑肌的上升去极化由 Cajal 间质细胞启动(见正文)。上升去极化之后是平台电位和复极化(D 至 I)。上升去极化和平台电位与平滑肌收缩有关。动作电位叠加在胃窦和幽门末端的平台电位上(G 至 I),与平滑肌收缩幅度增加有关(From Szurszewski JH. Electrophysiological basis of gastrointestinal tract. 2nd ed. New York:Raven Press;1986. p 383.

与胃底相反,来自胃体的细胞内记录显示静息电位较低,为-60mV。这些细胞快速上行去极化之后就进入平台电位,然后慢慢恢复到基线的静息电位。平台电位与胃体和胃窦环形肌的收缩活动有关[1]。平台电位可伴随着胃体和胃窦的动作电位。外在的刺激,如乙酰胆碱的释放或胃壁的拉伸,可增加平台电位的幅度和持续时间,以及促使动作电位的发生,导致不同力度的收缩,如同在末端胃窦的肌肉中所见一样。根据兴奋性神经刺激、平台电位的幅度和动作电位数量的不同,环形肌层的蠕动收缩波可以从极低幅度的收缩到高幅度的闭腔收缩。在幽门平台电位持续时间较长,叠加的动作电位导致幽门括约肌关闭,同时伴有末端胃窦收缩[1]。

膜电位和平滑肌收缩力也能区分胃底、体部和窦部(图 50.4)。胃底的静息电位约为-50mV,产生胃底的持续收缩和静息张力[1]。这种张力确保胃底对兴奋或抑制刺激的敏感反应,使胃底进一步舒张或收缩。摄取食物时的容受性舒张是由胃底平滑肌的这些电生理属性完成的。胃体和胃窦的静息电位分别为-60 和-70mV。在平台电位或动作电位的作用下,膜电位可达-45mV 或以下,平滑肌发生收缩。如果平台电位的幅度较大,则会发生幅度或力度较大的收缩。当平台电位和动作电位与胃窦内传播的慢波接触后(图 50.5),胃蠕动"波"的移动收缩环就形成了。

伴随着末端胃窦收缩,幽门括约肌收缩阻止胃内容物排空进入十二指肠,并使固体食物滞留在胃中。因此,与末端胃窦和幽门括约肌收缩相关的蠕动波不会将胃内容物从胃排空到十二指肠。相反,如果幽门在胃蠕动波期间保持开放,那么部分营养食糜就会被排入十二指肠。

(三) Cajal 间质细胞

Cajal 间质细胞(ICC)是胃肠道平滑肌的起搏细胞[6,11,12]。ICC 来源于 c-Kit 表达阳性的间叶细胞前体[13]。胃内的 ICC 位于胃壁的肌下、肌内、肌间和浆膜下[14-16]。图 50.6 显示了肌间神经丛中的 ICC(MY-ICC)、肌内 ICC(IM-ICC)、肠神经元和环形胃壁平滑肌细胞之间的解剖关系。MY-ICC 位于胃的环形肌和纵行肌之间,是负责产生慢波的 ICC。这些 ICC 自发地产生慢波,传导到相邻的平滑肌细胞,通过激活电压依赖的二氢吡啶敏感(L 型)钙通道,引起平滑肌的去极化和收缩[16,17]。平台电位的幅度增加与平滑肌收

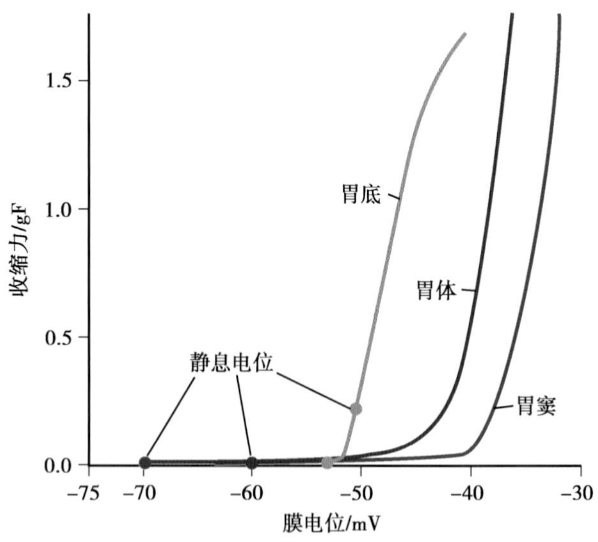

图 50.4　胃底、胃体和胃窦平滑肌膜电位(mV)与收缩力(g)之间的关系。胃底平滑肌的静息膜电位约为-50mV,该电位产生胃底的肌肉收缩和"静息张力"。胃窦平滑肌静息电位为-70mV,低于平滑肌收缩阈值近 30mV。当静息膜电位达到-40mV 或-35mV 时,在胃体和胃窦部观察到电压收缩曲线的陡峭斜率。(From Szurszewski JH. Electrophysiological basis of gastrointestinal motility. In:Johnson LR,editor. Physiology of the gastrointestinal tract. 2nd ed. New York:Raven Press;1986. p 383.)

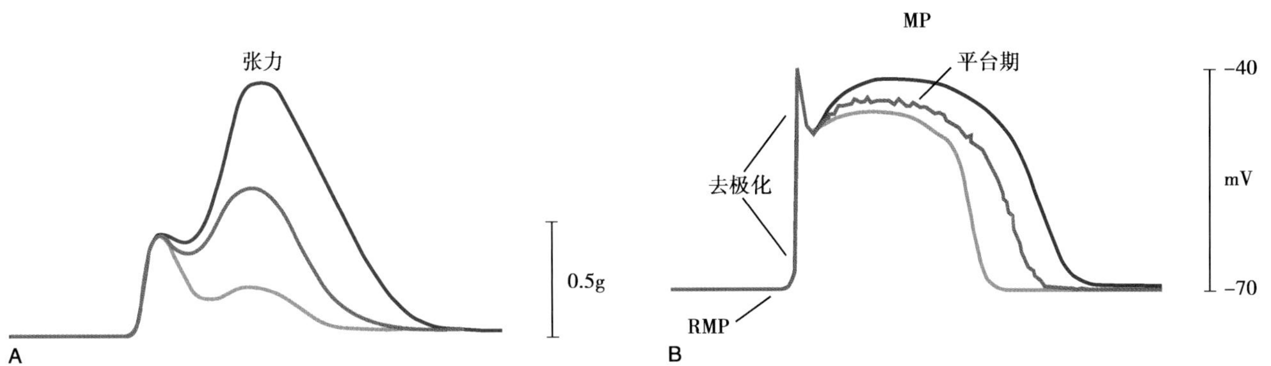

图 50.5　平滑肌收缩(张力)和膜电位(MP)的关系。在这些胃窦平滑肌的细胞内记录中,上升电位是快速去极化(上升)事件,随后是平台期。平台电位与平滑肌细胞的收缩相关,如图 A 所示,注意,平台电位振幅增加(图 B 中的红线)与更大的收缩性(张力)相关。在复极化至静息膜电位(RMP)期间,收缩消退。(Modified from Sanders KM, Ordog T, Koh SD, Ward SM. Properties of electrical rhythmicity in the stomach. In: Koch KL, Stern RM, editors. Handbook of electrogastrography. New York: Oxford Press; 2004. pp 13-36.)

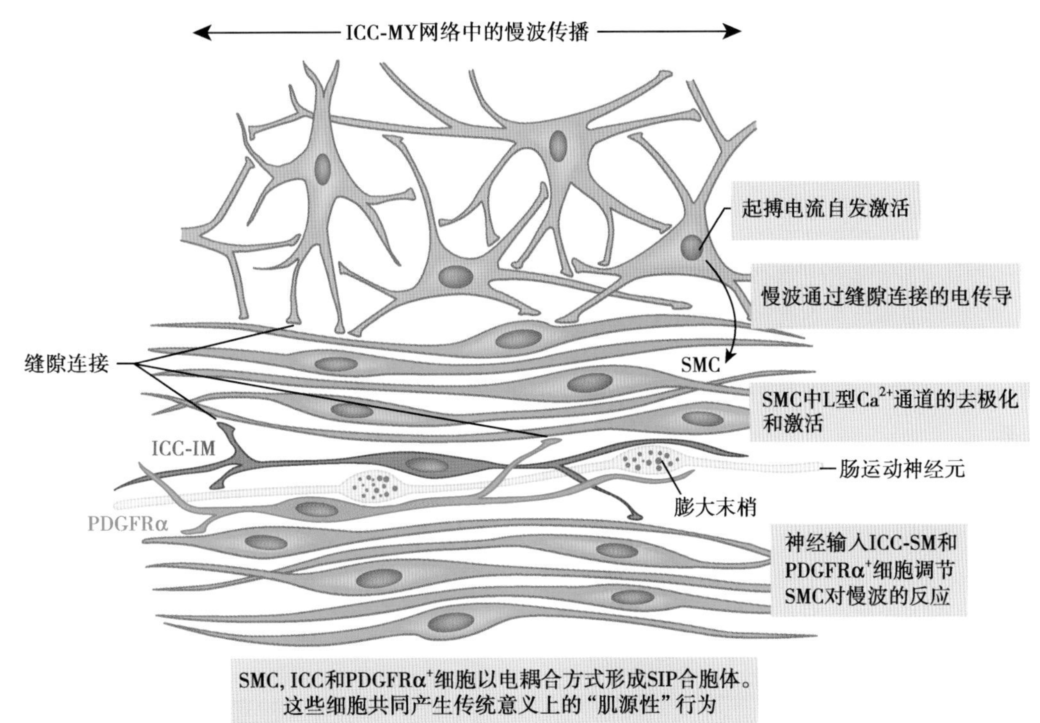

图 50.6　Cajal 间质细胞(ICC)血小板源性生长因子受体 α 阳性(PDGFRα⁺)细胞、环形肌层平滑肌细胞(SMC)和肠神经系统运动神经元之间的关系。肌间神经丛区域的 ICC(ICC-MY)是起搏细胞,可自发产生慢波去极化。慢波通过低电阻连接(缝隙连接)传导到相邻的平滑肌细胞(SMC),如弯曲箭头所示。平滑肌细胞去极化导致 L 型钙通道激活、Ca^{2+}进入和由 ICC 肌内网络(ICC-IM)协调的平滑肌细胞收缩。因此,慢波将胃平滑肌的收缩模式组织成一系列位相性和传播性收缩。平滑肌细胞不具有再生慢波所需的离子机制,因此,随着慢波在肌束中从平滑肌细胞传导到平滑肌细胞,慢波的振幅降低。慢波从主导(即最高频率)起搏点沿胃体大弯主动传播到幽门括约肌需要 ICC-MY、ICC-IM 和 SMC 的连续耦合网络。ICC-IM 是位于平滑肌束环形肌层内的 ICC。ICC-IM 似乎在介导神经传递中很重要,因为它们与肠运动神经元的膨大末梢(短箭头)形成非常紧密的突触连接(缝隙连接)。连接后神经反应可以从 ICC-IM 传导到肌肉束。因此,兴奋性肠神经元的刺激导致 ICC-IM 去极化,增加 SMC 对 ICC-MY 启动的慢波去极化的收缩反应。抑制性肠神经元的刺激引起膜电位的超极化和稳定,并倾向于抑制对慢波去极化的收缩反应。PDGFRα⁺细胞是另一类 ICC,其分布与 ICC 相似,似乎介导嘌呤能神经传递和 SMC 反应。因此,这些细胞——SMC、ICC 和 PDGFRα⁺——形成 SIP 的合胞体,产生胃的节律性、静止性和传播性收缩(肌源性)事件

缩幅度的增加相关。慢波通过缝隙连接沿 ICC 网络向四周和远端传播,并以较低的固有频率将更多的远端 ICC 同步到较高的慢波频率(正常的 3cpm 起搏频率)。

ICC 也位于环形平滑肌(IM-ICC)的各个层中,它们整合并协调慢波的传播和 MY-ICC 引发的平滑肌收缩[8]。慢波不会在平滑肌中再生,因为胃平滑肌细胞不能表达产生和传播慢波所需的离子通道。

在胃体和胃窦部,MY-ICC 和 IM-ICC 形成一个连续网格状相互连接的网络,从起搏区一直延伸到幽门。MY-ICC 建立了主要的起搏频率,IM-ICC 将慢波携带到环形平滑肌束中,

以协调收缩波的环向和远向传播。

ICC具有天然的节律性，这是基于其独特代谢和钙离子在细胞内外流动[17,18]。ICC的去极化和复极化最活跃的区域位于胃底和近端胃体之间的起搏区域。ICC的去极化和复极化是在ICC网络中再生和传播的，该波从胃大弯的起搏区通过胃体和胃窦移动到幽门，阻断了胃蠕动收缩的通路。当兴奋性因素（如胆碱能刺激、牵张）刺激MY-ICC时，可使钙通道开放，通过激活IM-ICC使平滑肌细胞去极化，以协调环形肌细胞在时间和空间上的收缩。因此，ICC网络可控制环形肌的收缩频率和传播速度，包括胃蠕动波的频率及速度。

胃底缺乏慢波。胃底的IM-ICC在机械感受中起作用，并作为感觉细胞与支配胃底的迷走神经传入神经元相互连接[19]。胃底IM-ICC还受抑制性迷走神经元支配，调节胃底张力[19]。因此，ICC还参与调节过程中胃底张力的松弛。

正常人胃体和胃窦部有5个以上的ICC/高倍视野（High-power field，HPF）[20,21]。在糖尿病和特发性胃轻瘫（idiopathic gastroparesis，IGP）患者中，胃体ICC的耗竭和CD206巨噬细胞的丢失与胃瘫（IGP）有关[20-22]。ICC的严重耗竭还与各种胃节律紊乱有关，包括胃动力过缓、胃动力过速和传导障碍[21,23]。糖尿病胃轻瘫（Diabetic gastroparesis，DGP）伴ICC缺失的患者与ICC数目正常的患者相比，胃电节律失常（快速性胃速）更明显，上消化道症状更多，对胃电刺激（GES）的反应更差[23]。非糖尿病机制阻断ICC通路也会导致胃电节律失常和异位起搏，类似于糖尿病患者的胃电节律失常[24]。DGP中ICC的丢失与M1巨噬细胞的炎性浸润和IL-6等炎性介质的产生增加有关，而M2巨噬细胞似乎对ICC具有保护作用[25,26]。

（四）神经系统支配

如第4章前面所述，神经元分布于从胃底到幽门的胃壁上[27]。这些神经元不仅位于环形肌和纵行肌之间的肌间神经丛中，也定位于黏膜下和浆膜下神经丛中。肠神经系统（ENS）在胃壁内提供如下局部反射回路：位于黏膜中的①感觉传入神经元与肌间神经丛中的②中间神经元相连，这些中间神经元与支配平滑肌和腺体的③传出神经元相连，以执行胃分泌功能[27]。兴奋性神经递质（如乙酰胆碱和P物质）的释放刺激平滑肌收缩，而抑制性神经递质（如一氧化氮和血管活性肠肽）则抑制平滑肌收缩。胃壁内的这些肠神经回路，通过相继抑制胃壁远端平滑肌节段和近端节段的收缩来调节蠕动收缩（结合前面描述的ICC活动）[28,29]。肠壁中的5-羟色胺在启动和控制胃蠕动中起主要作用[27,28]。

ENS的神经元位于MY-ICC和IM-ICC附近[30]。ENS神经元通过胆碱能兴奋性和氮能抑制性神经传递为胃平滑肌的收缩和舒张提供额外的控制和调节。ENS的神经元与MY-ICC和IM-ICC形成缝隙连接，提供整合慢波活动和平滑肌活动的关键神经控制。因此，节后兴奋性和抑制性神经元支配MY-ICC来调节胃神经肌肉的收缩和舒张，并对慢波提供变时性作用。IGP和DGP患者胃神经元体和神经末梢超微结构异常[31]。

PNS和SNS对胃神经肌肉活动有调节作用。迷走神经为胃提供PNS输入，尽管大约80%的迷走神经纤维是传入神经元。传入神经元对胃壁每时每刻的收缩和松弛（张力）作出反应[32]。迷走神经的传出活动可增加乙酰胆碱的释放，从而增加胃收缩的幅度，刺激胃酸和胃蛋白酶的分泌。SNS支配胃平滑肌，其神经元与内脏血管系统一起走行。SNS一般通过作用于ENS的肌间神经元而对平滑肌产生抑制作用[33]。

各种激素的释放，从CCK到胃泌素，都会影响胃的神经肌肉活动。胃肠激素对平滑肌、ICC和ENS以及迷走神经传出或传入功能产生影响。这些效应将在禁食和进食条件下描述，并在后面更详细地讨论。

（五）禁食期间的胃神经肌肉活动

在禁食状态下，胃体或胃窦的电活动和收缩以高度规则的模式发生，称为移行性复合肌电活动（migrating myoelectrical complex，mmC）[34]。MMC的3个时期，与管腔内收缩的变化相似，大约每90~120分钟发生一次。第1期是一个平静的时期，很少或基本没有记录到收缩活动。在第2期，出现随机、不规则的收缩。MMC的第3期是一个有规律的，高振幅的阶段性收缩，持续5~10分钟（图50.7A）。第3期的收缩也被称为“活动峰”。活动峰从胃窦向回肠迁移，持续90~120分钟。尽管约50%的第3期活动峰起源于胃，然后通过小肠迁移，但MMC的第3期通常发生在小肠[35]。起源于胃或十二指肠的MMC移行通过小肠，终止于回肠远端。如果继续禁食，那么下一个第3期的活动峰在胃窦或十二指肠以90~120分钟的间隔重新出现。胃窦远端发生的高振幅、每分钟3次的第3期收缩可排空胃内不易消化的纤维性食物。

在食管下段括约肌、Oddi括约肌和胆囊中也发现了与第3期发生相关的周期性收缩活动。第3期收缩与快速眼动睡眠相关，并与更大的生物钟系统有关[36,37]。迷走神经切断术后出现MMC，提示非迷走神经机制启动并维持MMC的神经肌肉活动。胃动素在十二指肠近端发生第3期强烈收缩时释放。

（六）餐后胃神经肌肉活动

摄取固体食物期间和之后发生的3种基本的胃神经肌肉活动：①容受性舒张以容纳摄取的食物；②反复的胃体-胃窦蠕动波将摄取的固体食物磨碎以产生食糜；③胃窦蠕动和胃-十二指肠协调运动以可控方式将食糜分次排入十二指肠，以实现最佳的食物消化和营养吸收。

1. 对摄入固体食物的反应

胃在混合、研磨和排空食物中的神经肌肉活动取决于所摄入食物的物理特性、体积及脂肪、蛋白质和碳水化合物的含量。例如，正常情况下，胃需要240分钟的神经肌肉活动才能排空255kcal固体食物的90%[38]。相比之下，胃只需要35分钟的神经肌肉工作就可以清空在4分钟内摄入的20kcal 500mL流食的70%[39]。图50.8说明了摄入、混合和清空固体食物所需胃的神经肌肉活动。胃的工作包括胃底舒张、胃蠕动及胃窦十二指肠的协调运动，在这一过程中产生食糜并

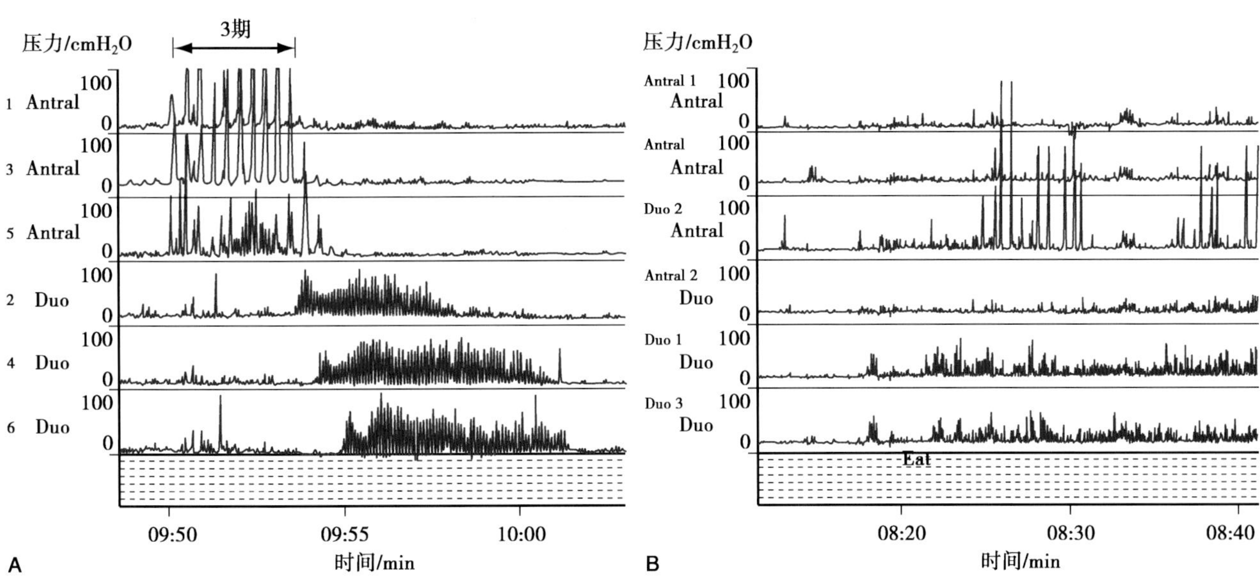

图 50.7　健康受试者的胃十二指肠运动活动。A，空腹状态：胃窦和十二指肠的 3 期收缩。该图显示了胃窦（通道 1、3 和 5）和十二指肠（通道 2、4 和 6）的腔内收缩。在通道 1、3 和 5 中观察到 3 期活动前沿，每分钟 3 次胃窦蠕动收缩，持续近 6 分钟。3 期活动前沿向远端传播，并通过十二指肠记录端口迁移。十二指肠的收缩频率约每分钟 11 或 12 次，与十二指肠慢波的频率相同。3 期收缩完成后，在胃窦部可见 1 期静止和无收缩。B，进食状态：确保受试者摄入标准流质饮食。在胃窦中观察到不同幅度的收缩，在十二指肠中观察到一系列相对低振幅的不规则收缩，所有这些收缩均代表进食状态，并且与 A 所示的空腹状态下的 3 期活动形成鲜明显对比。Antral，胃窦；Duo，十二指肠。（Modified from Koch KL. The stomach. Manometry. In：Schuster M，Crowell M，Koch KL，editors. Atlas of gastrointestinal motility. Hamilton，Ontario：BC Decker；2002. pp 135-150.）

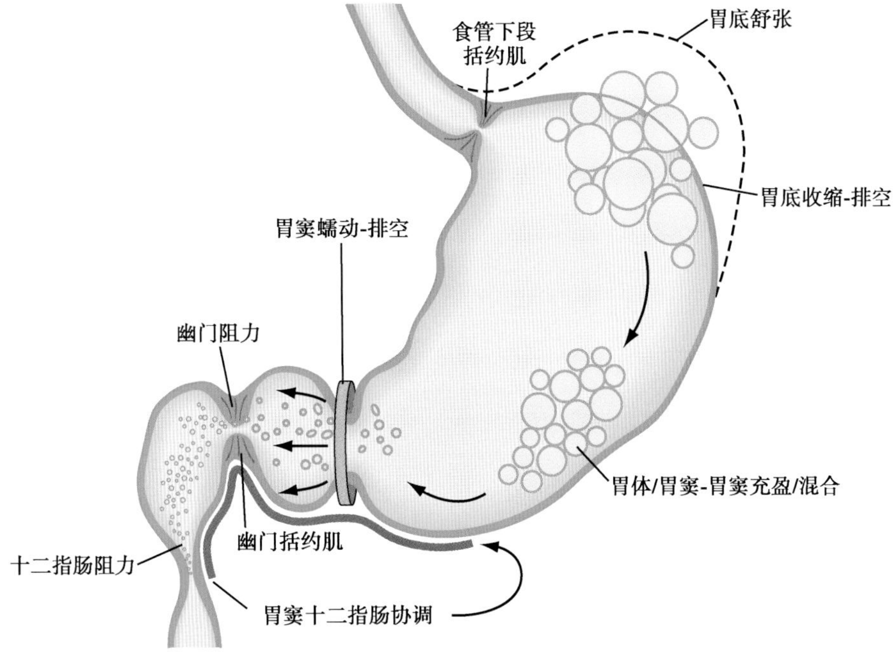

图 50.8　摄入固体食物后胃神经肌肉的活动谱。为了接受摄入的固体食物，并在不增加胃内压的情况下容纳食物体积，胃底平滑肌松弛（接受性松弛）。然后胃底收缩，将摄入的固体食物排空到胃体和胃窦，进行研磨和排空。反复出现的胃体-胃窦蠕动波将固体研磨成食糜，食糜是由悬浮在胃液中的 1～2mm 的固体颗粒组成。胃窦蠕动波，表现为胃窦内的环形凹陷，通过幽门排空 2～4mL 的食糜，并以每分钟 3 次蠕动收缩的慢波频率进入十二指肠球部。胃-幽门-十二指肠的协调作用，表明了食糜通过幽门的有效排空，它通过改变括约肌阻力来调节食糜的流动。十二指肠收缩也提供了排空阻力。（Modified from Koch KL. Physiological basis of electrogastrography. In：Koch KL，Stern RM，editors. Handbook of electrogastrography. New York：Oxford Press；2004. pp 37-67.）

将其排入十二指肠。食物摄入中断了禁食状态,在胃体和胃窦开始了每3分钟一次的规律胃蠕动来混合食物;在摄入状态下,连续小肠收缩产生2~4cm的短距离蠕动,可优化营养物的消化和吸收(见图50.7B)。

从食管进入胃底的固体食物与胃底的接受性松弛有关,即胃底肌肉的松弛。随着胃底平滑肌的松弛,胃底和近端胃体中容纳了大量的固体或液体食物,而腔内压力几乎没有增加。相反,液体立即分布在整个胃体和胃窦(下一节将讨论液体的排空)。胃底的舒张发生在胃体和胃窦的充盈之前,是迷走神经介导的事件,需要一氧化氮[40]。图50.9显示了由于进食使胃底和近端胃体松弛期间胃内容积的变化[41]。通过胃底IM-ICC介导的胃底松弛和机械感受器的刺激(牵张),激活迷走传入神经元和迷走神经反射,这些反射涉及孤束核和迷走神经背核的传出神经元,兴奋性迷走神经元被抑制,抑制性迷走神经的神经递质一氧化氮和血管活性肠肽被释放,以实现接受性舒张。

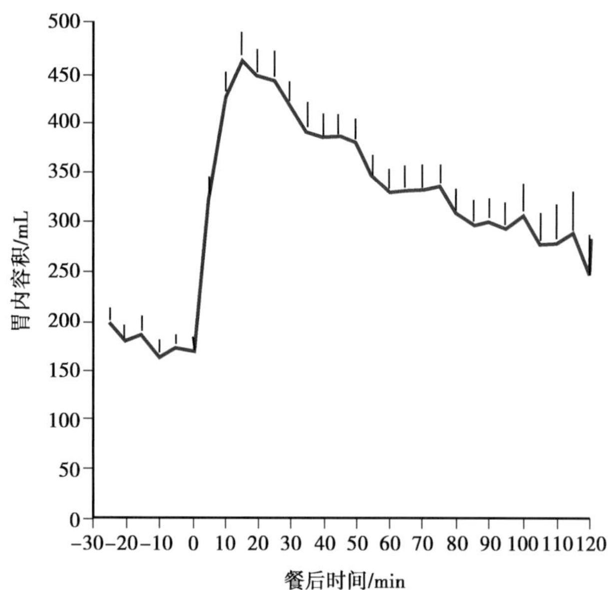

图50.9　健康受试者在试验餐后胃底和近端胃的胃调节。在餐后20分钟内,用气压调节器测量的胃内容积从约200mL增加到约450mL。当食物排空时,胃的容积在餐后2小时内缓慢减少。近端胃的松弛和餐量的调节反映了迷走神经介导的接受性松弛。(From Tack J, Piessevuax H, Coulie B, et al. Role of impaired gastric accommodation to a meal in functional dyspepsia. Gastroenterology 1998;115:1346-52.)

其他因素也会影响胃底的肌肉张力。胃窦扩张、十二指肠扩张、十二指肠酸度过高[42]、十二指肠腔内富含脂质或蛋白质以及结肠扩张,都会通过各种反射降低胃底张力。这种反射是通过辣椒素敏感的传入迷走神经引发,并由5-羟基色胺3($5\text{-}HT_3$),胃泌素释放肽和CCK_A受体介导[43]。

用锝标记的固体食物最初容纳在胃底和近端胃体中,并且通过获取频闪显像图像,可以追踪被标记固体食物的分布长达4小时以上[38]。图50.10显示,在摄入这种固体食物后,大部分食物保留在胃底和近端胃体中。随后,胃底收缩将食物按比例排入胃体和胃窦中进行研磨。胃排空食物之前的这种餐后早期的适应和研磨时间称为滞后期。对于固体食品,滞后期可能会持续45~60分钟,但是具体的持续时间取决于咀嚼食物的彻底程度,摄取食物所用时间以及食物成分组成。对于在10分钟内摄入的255kcal鸡蛋代餐,滞后期为30~45分钟。

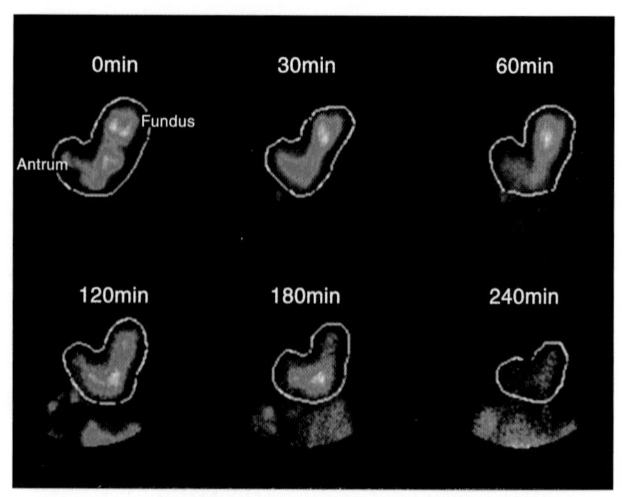

图50.10　进食鸡蛋三明治后的胃排空。该图显示了摄入后0、30、60、120、180和240分钟放射性标记255kcal鸡蛋代餐的1分钟胃内闪烁图像。黄色和粉红色区域表示胃中同位素计数较高于的区域比其他区域的食物更多。注意,摄入后120分钟,进餐从胃底缓慢地重新分布到胃窦,进行研磨和排空。到240分钟时只有少量的食物留在胃中,大部分标记的替代蛋餐都在小肠中

一旦将食物研磨成悬浮在胃液中的1~2mm颗粒,便开始胃排空食糜的阶段。反复发生的胃蠕动波将唾液,胃酸和胃蛋白酶与咀嚼的食物混合,然后将食物磨碎以产生食糜。正常胃蠕动波每20秒发生一次,这是平台期和动作电位相关的3cpm慢波产生的。在健康受试者中,大约60%的鸡蛋代餐已在2小时内排空,超过90%鸡蛋代餐在4小时内已完全排空(图50.11)[38]。

在胃排空的线性期,每个蠕动波都会使3~4mL的食糜通过开放的幽门进入十二指肠[44]。由于胃窦蠕动波的收缩期效应,食糜进入十二指肠的运动并不全是脉冲性的[44]。每次蠕动波送入十二指肠食糜的体积受很多因素影响,包括蠕动波形态(例如收缩深度、蠕动波的长度),胃内压力以及幽门括约肌和十二指肠收缩提供的阻力[45,46]。当幽门和十二指肠舒张以接受食糜时,胃蠕动波会产生较大的“搏出量”,但向十二指肠传递的总体热量比率为3~4kcal/min[43]。

进餐后,随着时间推移,咀嚼、吞咽的食物会不断从胃底重新分配到胃窦,以便进行研磨。一些胃蠕动波终止于胃窦的各点,而另一些胃蠕动波终止于与幽门关闭相关的末端胃窦收缩,从而阻止了较大的食物颗粒或难消化的固体物的排空。这些末端胃窦和幽门的收缩导致胃体和胃窦中固体颗粒的排空延迟。末端胃窦,即靠近幽门3~4cm的胃窦,也是慢波具有最大振幅和速度的地方。以这种方式,保留了需要进一步研磨的固体食物颗粒,使其进一步经受周期性蠕动波的研磨作用。

健康受试者摄取鸡蛋代餐后记录的胃内压力和管腔内pH如图50.12所示。摄入固体食物后约3.5小时,随着无线

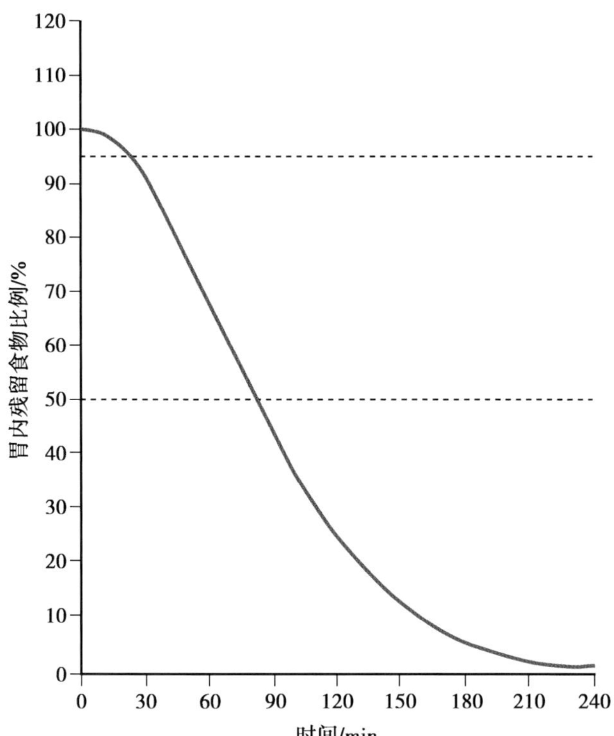

图 50.11　123 位受试者摄入 255kcal 鸡蛋代餐后(相同膳食)的固相胃排空曲线，见图 48.10。注意，仅有大约 15% 的鸡蛋代餐在前 45 分钟内排空，即进餐后胃排空的滞后期。在 90 分钟时，大约 50% 的食物已被排空，50% 被保留。到 240 分钟时，超过 91% 的膳食已被排空。(Modified from Tougas G, Eaker EY, Abell TL, et al. Assessment of gastric emptying using a low fat meal: Establishment of international control values. Am J Gastroenterol 2000;95:1456-62.)

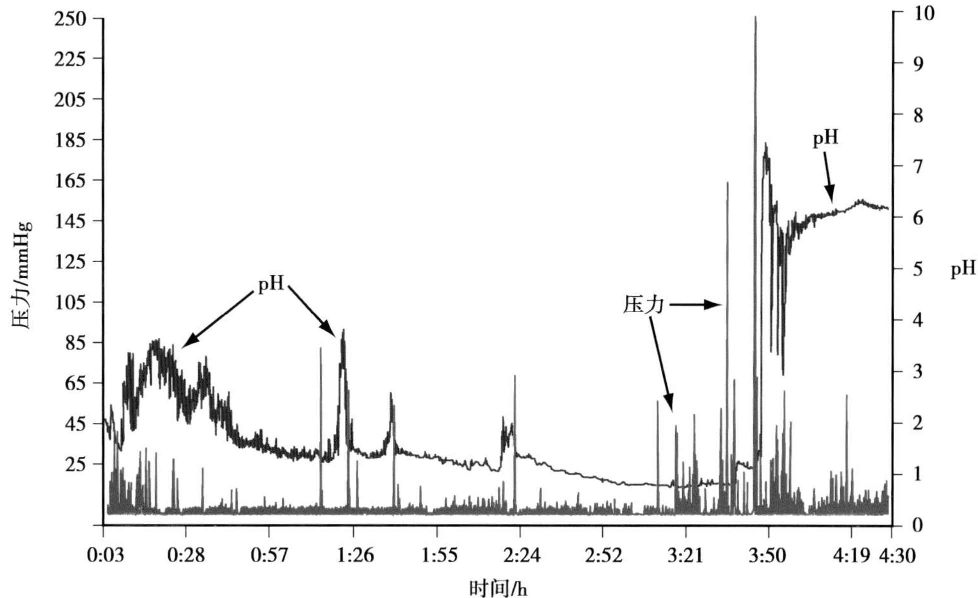

图 50.12　排空 255kcal 鸡蛋代餐期间的胃收缩和腔内胃 pH 记录，与图 50.10 所示食物相同，用动态记录 pH 胶囊和运动装置记录；pH 显示在右垂直轴上，压力(mmHg)显示在左垂直轴上。当胃酸被食物稀释时，在前 45 分钟内 pH 升高至约 3。然后 pH 逐渐降至 1，并在进餐后的 3 小时保持在 1 左右。胃收缩幅度一般较低，进餐后小于 10mmHg。在餐后约 3 小时 40 分钟，记录的 pH 突然升高至 7，然后降低并保持稳定在 6 左右。在 pH 突然升高之前，出现了一系列聚集的高幅度胃窦收缩(压力)。这些胃窦收缩使胶囊从胃窦(pH 为 1)排空进入十二指肠，其中 pH 为 6 或更高。在健康受试者中，排空食物所需的 3 小时 50 分钟内发生的收缩记录了研磨和排空食物所需的神经肌肉工作

运动装置/pH 记录胶囊从酸性窦腔排空到十二指肠较碱性的环境中，在 pH 突然从 1 升高到 6 之前，胃窦发生了高振幅收缩(>65mmHg)。排空食物的易消化成分后，强烈的胃窦收缩(类似于 3 期收缩)将胶囊从胃排空到十二指肠[47]。因此，高振幅的胃窦收缩将纤维性和难消化的物质排空，而在线性排空期，食糜中易消化的营养成分通过低振幅的蠕动波较早排空[48]。

幽门通过几种机制调节胃排空的速度。幽门张力增加和孤立的幽门压力波可阻止胃排空，促进食物保留以备进一步研磨。与胃窦终末收缩相关的幽门收缩常见于发生研磨食物的滞后期。一旦固体物排空的线性阶段开始，由于食糜可通过胃蠕动波排空，孤立的幽门收缩波的数量减少。幽门括约肌的神经肌肉功能障碍与胃轻瘫有关，较以往所重视的更为普遍，现综述于后。

2. 对摄入液体食物的反应

混合和排空液体食物所需胃的神经肌肉活动与固体食物明显不同[39,49,50]。图 50.13 显示了健康受试者在空腹状态下和摄入 500mL 液体餐后 10 分钟的胃三维超声图像[39]。禁食时胃内容积约为 40mL，摄入液体餐后 10 分钟增加至 350mL，表明除了胃底舒张外，胃窦和胃体平滑肌显著舒张，这是适应该液体餐容积所必需的(相比之下，固体餐最初是适应的，主要保留在胃底和近端胃)。与需要研磨的固体食物相比，液体食物一旦进入胃内，会以受控但更快的速度排空至十二指肠中。在描述为单指数排空的曲线中，无滞后期的零热量液体食物排空(图 50.14)[50,51]。另一方面，与零热量的液体食物相比，高热量的液体食物在胃窦中保留的时间更长，排空速度比零热量的液体食物慢。液体通过以下方式从胃中排空：①胃和十二指肠之间的压力梯度使液体食物流入十二指肠；②胃窦蠕动收缩，使液体食物以脉冲模式从胃窦排入十二指肠；③通过十二指肠胃反流机制调节胃排空速度[43,44]。从 GMA 的角度来看，摄入水直至饱腹会引起短暂的胃蠕动频率的下降，然后恢复无创胃电图(electrogastrogram，EGG)中记录的正常 3cpm 活动(图 50.15)[52]。液体食物的排空速度受摄入液体的体积、营养成分、黏度和渗透压的影响[39,45,46,51]。这些因素影响胃的神经肌肉活动，进而影响排空速度，将在后面进行讨论。

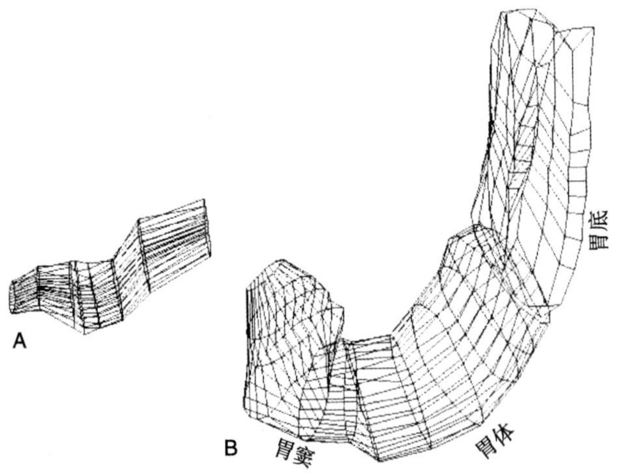

图 50.13　健康受试者摄入 500mL 液体餐前后胃的三维超声重建图像。A，在空腹状态下，胃内容积约为 38mL。B，进餐后 10 分钟，胃容量为 350mL。注意，此时胃窦、胃体和胃底明显膨胀，表明调节该液体体积所需的平滑肌明显松弛。(Modified from Gilja OH，Detmer PR，Jong JM，et al. Intragastric distribution and gastric emptying assessed by 3-dimensional ultrasonography. Gastroenterology 1997；113：38-49.)

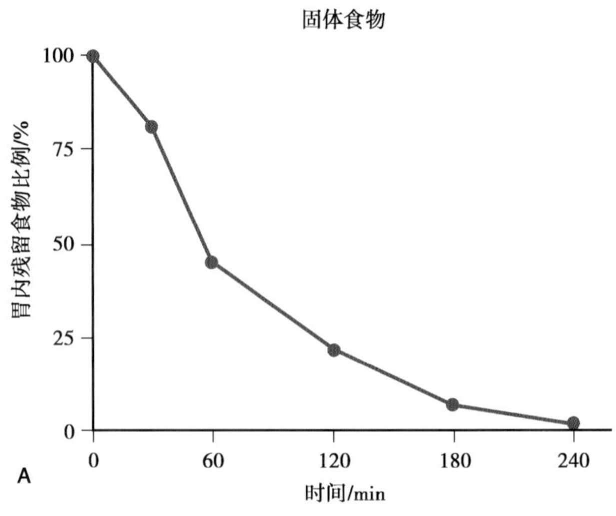

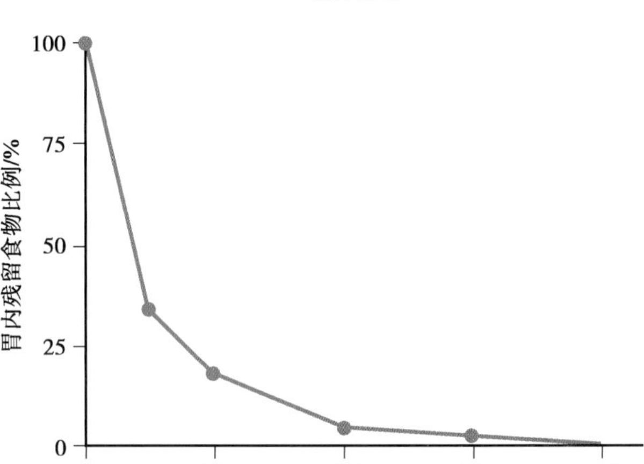

图 50.14　健康受试者摄入 300mL 放射性标记水、2 个放射性标记鸡蛋和吐司后，混合液体和固体食物的胃排空。A，固体食物的排空率。在排空的线性阶段之前观察到短暂的滞后期，到餐后 60 分钟时，大约 55% 的食物被排空(45% 被保留)。如果受试者进食时间相对较长或固体食物几乎不需要研磨，即可缩短滞后期。B，液体食物的排空速度。大约 80% 的水在 60 分钟时被排空(20% 保留)，因为液体迅速分布在整个胃窦和胃体。这被认为是单指数液体排空曲线。(Modified from Maurer AH，Parkman HP，Knight LC，Fisher RS. Scintigraphy. In：Schuster M，Crowel M，Koch，KL，editors. Atlas of gastrointestinalmotility. Hamilton，Ontario：BC Decker；2002. pp 171-84.)

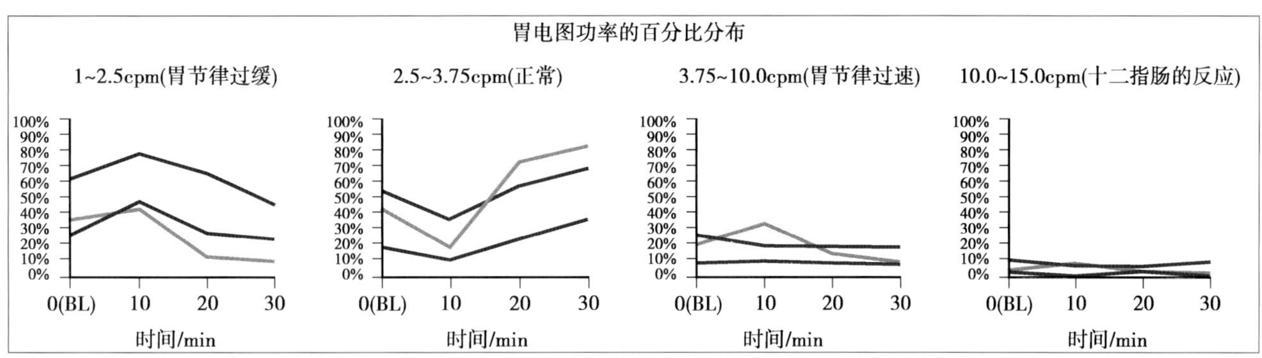

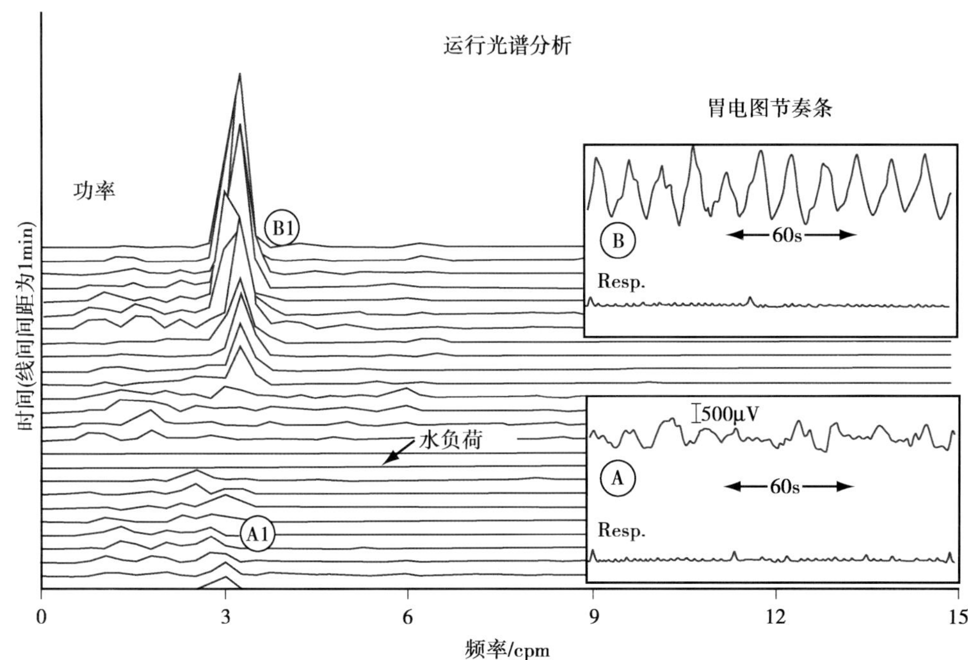

图 50.15 健康受试者中摄入水负荷前后的胃电图(EGG)信号和 EGG 节律进行运行频谱分析。X 轴显示 EGG 信号中的频率,单位为每分钟周期数(cpm)。Y 轴表示时间,峰值(或 Z 轴)表示 EGG 信号所含频率的功率。基线 EGG 节律条带(A)显示 3cpm 活动。受试者在 5 分钟内摄入 750mL 水(水负荷箭头)后,3cpm EGG 信号的规律性和振幅增加(B)。运行频谱分析显示基线(A1)时的功率相对较低的 3cpm 峰值。摄入水负荷后,峰值最消失(频率"下降"),然后出现 3cpm 峰值,并突出至 30 分钟记录结束(B1)。这是对胃充满水和随后排空水的正常胃肌电反应。插图中的 4 张图显示了基线(BL)和受试者饮水后 10、20 和 30 分钟,4 个相关频率范围内 EGG 功率的百分比分布(绿色线)。正常范围以蓝色线表示。注意摄入水后 10 分钟,正常 EGG 活动百分比的初始降低(2.5~3.75cpm)(频率下降),随后在摄入水后 20 分钟和 30 分钟 3cpm 正常范围的百分比增加。Resp.,呼吸活动。(Modified from Koch KL. Physiological basis of electrogastrography. In:Koch KL,Stern RM,editors. Handbook of electrogastrography. New York:Oxford Press;2004. pp 37-67.)

二、餐后胃神经肌肉活动

调节胃排空速率,使食糜形式的热量以一致、规律的方式进入十二指肠,以优化胰蛋白酶和胆汁的分泌,使其适合食糜内容物的消化。通过胃神经肌肉装置的变化实现各种胃排空率:胃底舒张和收缩、胃蠕动收缩特征、3cpm 慢波的暂时性暂停和胃节律障碍的发生;胃窦-幽门-十二指肠收缩和十二指肠收缩的协调;幽门括约肌收缩和舒张;以及促进十二指肠胃反流的十二指肠收缩。特定食物的属性刺激相应的胃神经肌肉反应,从而影响胃排空的速率。表 50.1 列出了影响胃神经肌肉活动的因素,食物相关因素以及其他调节胃排空速率的因素。胃节律障碍的暂时发生、胃窦收缩幅度和传播距离的调节、幽门收缩增强和胃窦-幽门-十二指肠协调减少可降低胃排空率。

影响胃排空的食物相关因素包括:固体和液体食物的易消化成分、脂肪含量(营养密度)、黏度、酸含量、体积、渗透压和不易消化的食物成分。例如,脂肪含量高的食物比蛋白质或碳水化合物含量高的食物排空慢。在胃内消化的初始阶段,甘油三酯(TG)与胃脂肪酶混合(见第 102 章),并在排入十二指肠之前分解为脂肪酸,甘油单酯或甘油二酯[53]。十二指肠对源自饮食的脂肪酸非常敏感。接触十二指肠黏膜的长链脂肪酸(>C12)导致 CCK 释放。CCK 可使胃底舒张,减少胃窦收缩,并增加幽门张力,进而导致胃排空延迟。相反,短链和中链脂肪酸(<C12)对胃排空速度没有这些神经肌肉作用[46,54]。从十二指肠释放的 CCK 还会激活迷走神经传入神经元的 CCKA 受体,而迷走神经传入神经元的突触位于孤束核[55]。来自孤束核的神经元上升到下丘脑的脑室周围核,参与饱食机制,迷走神经背核发出迷走神经传出神经元下降至胃,抑制胃排空并保持胃底舒张。十二指肠黏膜对脂肪和其他营养物质的敏感性引出了十二指肠味觉和十二指肠制动的概念,是调节胃内营养物质排空的感觉运动事件[56,57]。

表 50.1 调节胃排空率的因素

因素	对胃排空率的影响
胃的神经肌肉因素	
胃动过速	延迟
胃底调节功能减低	加速
胃底调节功能增加	延迟
胃窦动力不足	延迟
幽门痉挛	延迟
胃窦十二指肠协调功能障碍	延迟
食物相关因素	
容积	与进食容量成比例
酸度增加	延迟
渗透压增加	延迟
营养物密度:脂肪>蛋白质>碳水化合物	延迟
色氨酸	延迟
不易消化的纤维	延迟
小肠因素	
十二指肠内的脂肪酸	延迟(十二指肠试验、十二指肠障碍)
回肠内的脂肪酸	延迟(回肠障碍)
结肠因素	
便秘,IBS	延迟
其他因素	
高血糖	延迟
低血糖	加速
非真实的自我运动(矢量)	延迟

IBS,肠易激综合征。

十二指肠中的单糖刺激肠促胰岛素例如胰高血糖素样多肽-1 的释放,进而促进胰岛素分泌以控制餐后血糖水平的升高并减少胃窦收缩[58,59]。为了平衡葡萄糖吸收,血糖和胰岛素分泌之间的关系,胃排空碳水化合物是受到严格调控的[60,61]。Hasler 及其同事发现,高血糖会减少胃窦收缩并增加胃节律失常,这是一种"生理性"胃节律失常,可降低胃排空速度(图 50.16)[62,63]。高血糖还会增加胃底顺应性并减少与胃底舒张相关的感觉传入[64,65]。血糖水平高于 220mg/dL 会导致胃窦收缩减少,胃排空减少并诱发胃节律失常[62],这些胃神经肌肉活动可减少胃排空及减少十二指肠对营养成分的进一步暴露。低血糖发作与 1 型糖尿病患者的排空延迟有关[65]。

在餐后的后期,随着小肠内营养物质的消化和吸收,肠腔内营养物质间的相互作用和胃排空速度的调节持续进行。例如,如果食物中的脂肪酸或碳水化合物到达回肠腔,则所谓的回肠静息被启动,胃排空被延迟。研究证明,向回肠腔内注入营养物质会延迟胃排空[66]。

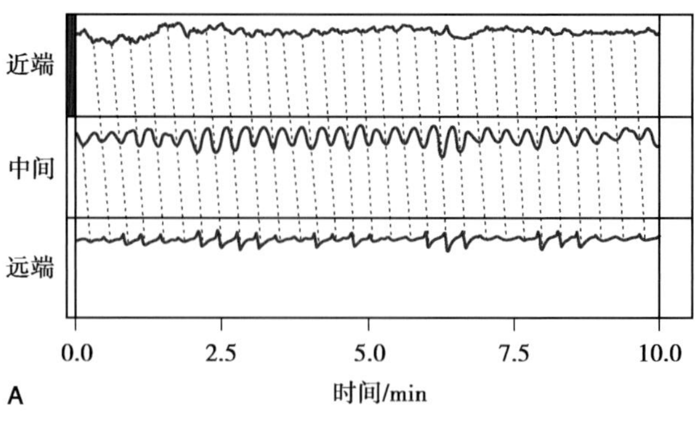

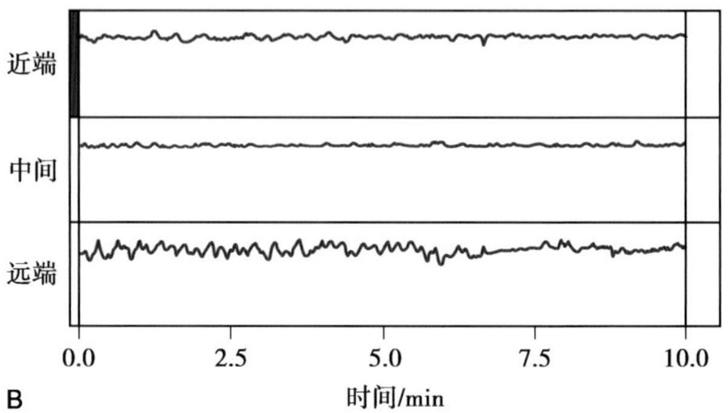

图 50.16 固定在健康受试者胃窦近端、中间和远端黏膜上的电极的电记录。A,近端、中间和远端电极导线中的 3cpm 的电慢波。慢波以虚线所示的向外终止方向传播。B,在高血糖(血糖水平为 240mg/dL)时传播中断,远端导联出现 5~6cpm 胃动过速。cpm,每分钟周期数。(Modified from Coleski R, Hasler WL. Coupling and propagation of normal dysrhythmic gastric slow waves during acute hyperglycemia in healthy humans. Neurogastroenterol Motil 2009;21:492-99.)

迷走神经和内脏神经活动通过调节胃神经肌肉活动来进一步调节胃排空。迷走传入神经时刻监视着胃神经肌肉功能,迷走传入神经、孤束核和迷走神经背核传出神经突触之间的相互作用对胃产生了持续的中枢神经系统兴奋性和抑制性作用。应激状态下胃排空会延迟。促肾上腺皮质激素释放因子在应激调节中发挥作用,并通过中枢多巴胺 1 以及脑室周围核中的多巴胺 2 和血管升压素途径抑制胃排空[67]。其他尚未提及的影响胃排空速度的因素包括直肠结肠扩张,妊娠恶心、呕吐以及矢量变化诱发的晕车病[68]。中枢神经系统各个区域的刺激影响胃神经肌肉功能。非真实的自身运动(矢量变化)导致胃窦动力不足,胃节律频率和胃排空减少[68,69]。利用非真实的自身运动的经验进行的一系列研究(一种独特的中枢神经系统感觉刺激)表明,恶心的发作与胃节律频率和血浆血管升压素水平升高有关[69,70]。

性别会影响标准餐的胃排空速度。与男性相比,健康女性的胃排空速度明显减慢[71]。胃排空速度的性别差异可能与性激素的波动有关,但是月经周期的各个阶段(雌二醇和孕酮浓度的变化)与胃排空没有显示出一致的关系[72]。胃排空速度随着体重指数的升高而增加,这可能与肥胖的发生和维持有关。

三、胃感觉活动

胃游离神经末梢具有多种模式的感受器,对轻触、压力、酸和其他化学刺激均能作出反应。胃内传入神经元被称为内源性初级传入神经元(IPAN)[73]。IPAN 的胞体位于胃壁的黏膜下层或肌间神经丛区域。从局部肠嗜铬细胞释放 5-羟色胺可以激活 IPAN[27,74]。IPAN 中的传入信息用于局部反射,分别为迷走反射和脊柱反射提供迷走和内脏传入神经元的输入信号,以帮助将内脏感觉信息传递到 CNS。迷走神经传入神经元,其胞体位于结状神经节,与孤束核相连,其二级神经元与下丘脑较高中枢相连,其中一些输入信号到达皮层,皮层会将其视为内脏感觉(胃空虚或饱腹感)或恶心或腹痛等症状(图 50.17)。

通过 SNS,胃壁的内脏或脊柱初级传入神经元介导疼痛感觉。这些神经元的胞体位于脊髓后角,其二级神经元通过后脊柱中的脊髓丘脑束和脊髓网状束上升。感觉神经元是细的、有髓的 A-δ 或无髓的 C 纤维。脊髓传入神经包括大量无髓的 C 纤维。辣椒素敏感的无髓纤维含有神经肽,例如降钙素基因相关肽,血管活性肠肽,生长抑素,P 物质和神经激肽 A。这些纤维被认为是从胃肠道到中枢神经系统各种疼痛刺激的主要传播途径。这些神经纤维可能会对炎症介质作出反应,从而唤醒"沉默的"伤害性神经纤维[75]。

除了与 IPAN 相互作用外,迷走传入神经的轴突还与肠神经元有多种连接,并通过与 ICC 的连接来支配环行肌纤维束[74]。迷走神经传入神经元还通过黏膜神经元和机械敏感神经元以及肌层中的 ICC 对化学趋化分子敏感。在禁食和进食期间,迷走神经传入神经元上的 CCK 受体主要被胃生理机械和化学刺激激活。这些迷走神经传入介导对腔内酸和脂肪的感觉反应。酸可能对神经末梢本身有直接作用[42]。

恶心是一种常见感觉,通常归因于胃神经肌肉功能障碍[76]。在非真实的自身运动中,随着健康个体出现恶心,胃节律失常会加重[77]。出现恶心受试者的血浆血管升压素水平升高,而没有恶心受试者的血浆血管升压素水平没有升高[78]。非真实的自身运动过程中的这种脑-肠、肠-脑相互作用,说明了外周胃节律失常的发作与受试者的急性、严重的恶心经历之间存有时间关系。另一方面,用气囊扩张胃窦,而不扩张胃底,会诱发健康个体的恶心感和胃节律失常[79]。这些研究表明,胃节律失常起源于人的胃窦,而胃窦壁的伸展是引起胃节律失常和胃部恶心感的另一种机制。通过水负荷试验(而不是气囊)对胃窦和胃体进行扩张,也会引起易感人群的胃节律失常和恶心[52]。

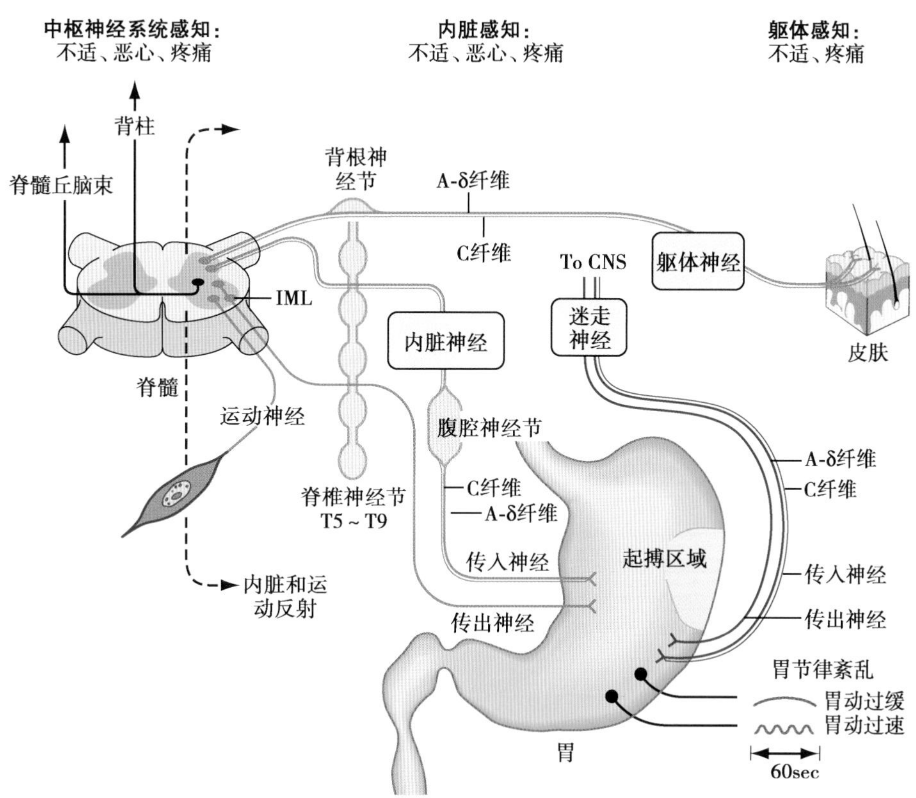

图 50.17 胃和中枢神经系统之间的传入和传出神经连接。迷走神经含有传入神经与 A-δ 和 C 类疼痛纤维,其胞体位于结状神经节,并与孤束核相连(未显示)。低阈值机械感受器和化学感受器刺激内脏感觉,如胃排空或饱胀以及症状,如恶心和不适。这些刺激是通过迷走神经通路介导的,如果感觉输入到达大脑皮质,则会成为对内脏感觉的有意识(自我)感知。内脏神经还含有传入神经与 A-δ 和 C 类纤维,在腹腔神经节与脊神经节(T5～T9)中的一些细胞体形成突触。脊髓后角白支的中间神经元与背柱和脊髓丘脑束交叉,并上升至延髓的感觉区。这些内脏传入纤维被认为介导了内脏疼痛的高阈值刺激。与内脏感觉相反,来自皮肤的躯体神经,通过背根神经节的 A-δ 和 C 类纤维传递感觉信息,并进入后角,然后通过背柱和脊髓丘脑束传递至躯体表征的皮质区域。胃电节律变化、过度收缩幅度或胃壁伸展是引起传入神经活动变化(通过迷走神经和/或内脏神经)的外周机制,可能达到有意识的程度,被视为来自胃的内脏感觉(症状)。IML,中间外侧核

四、胃与摄食、饥饿和饱腹感的调节

饥饿是人类的基本动力，可以通过摄入食物消除或减轻。饥饿也被描述为引起不适的胃“空虚”感。食物的摄入会引起胃部肌肉的舒张（容受性舒张）容纳摄入食物的体积。随着这些胃部神经肌肉事件的发生，饥饿感消失，餐后会出现饱腹感。

摄入的食物量比食物中的卡路里含量更多地抑制了饥饿并刺激饱腹感的产生[80,81]。与将相同营养成分注入十二指肠相比，将其注入胃内会引起更强的饱腹感。经口摄取营养成分时，对饥饿的抑制作用会更强，这表明中枢神经系统、口咽和胃神经肌肉因素综合在一起，产生正常的餐后饱腹感[82]。

健康个体通常会进食至吃饱为止。餐后饱腹感的生理特性尚不完全清楚，但食物摄入和胃液分泌引起的胃壁机械舒张（以及胃内压的变化）是部分原因[80,81]。受试者持续摄入水长达5分钟后，经历了从基线胃空虚感到饱腹感的巨大变化。为达到饱腹感所摄取的平均水量为600mL；相比之下，功能性消化不良患者平均摄取350mL即出现饱腹感，表明胃壁舒张和/或胃壁张力存在障碍[52]。同样，通过摄取营养饮料也可以实现饱腹感[83]。十二指肠中存在酸或营养成分或血糖水平升高会降低胃壁张力[84,85]。

摄入固体食物最初会引起胃底舒张，并且在滞后期几乎没有食物排空。在滞后期食物被研磨时，饱腹感仍然存在。一旦胃排空的线性阶段开始，随着时间的推移，会逐渐感觉到胃充盈度降低和胃空虚度增加。进餐后4~5个小时，胃完全排空，健康个体会再次感到饥饿。

饥饿和饱腹感的生理机制正在深入研究中。在禁食状态下，血浆胃动素水平在MMC的第3期增加，但饥饿感与增加的胃动素或MMC第3期启动的相关性尚不清楚。如第4章和第7章所述，胃促生长素（ghrelin）是一种28个氨基酸构成的肽，由胃底腺内分泌细胞分泌的[86]。禁食（饥饿）期间血浆中胃促生长素的水平也会升高，并刺激食物摄入，可能是通过迷走神经传入引起的[87]。食欲素或刺激食欲的肽类是由下丘脑外侧的神经元合成的，通过作用于迷走神经背核，并投射到胃底和胃体，促进食物摄入并刺激胃收缩（在大鼠中）[88]。摄入食物后，胃促生长素的水平降低[89]。在胃旁路手术后胃促生长素被显著抑制[90]。胃促生长素对胃动力也有促进作用，目前正在评估其对胃轻瘫的治疗效果[91,92]。

其他激素也在实现饱腹感中扮演重要角色，这些激素在进食后释放。从脂肪酸接触到十二指肠黏膜CCK就被释放。CCK受体参与十二指肠内脂质和胃扩张引起的饱腹感和恶心感[93,94]。瘦素在胃中合成并在食物摄入后释放，循环中的瘦素通过中枢神经系统对弓状核的调节减少食物摄入量[95]。胰高血糖素样多肽-1可以在进食标准餐后增强饱腹感，减少幽门运动并增加胃容量[59,96]。载脂蛋白A-Ⅳ在吸收TG的过程中从小肠中释放出来，部分通过CCK和迷走神经传入途径减少食物摄入并降低胃动力[97]。进食后回结肠区域释放的多肽-YY，是“回肠静息”效应[98]和食欲抑制的重要调节因素[99,100]。

大脑和这些胃肠激素与食物摄入的调节和引起胃排空的胃神经肌肉活动的调节有着明显的联系[59,100]。胃生理学的头期是众所周知的，但是多年没有被再研究。食物的外观，气味和味道刺激迷走神经中枢传出活动，从而增加胃酸分泌，提高胃收缩力并增加3cpm GMA[100-102]。假装进食过程中，受试者咀嚼并吐出测试餐而不是将其吞咽，会引起头-迷走神经反射。假装进食一个热狗面包会增强EGG记录的3cpm活动，而假装进食一种令人恶心的食物会使3cpm肌电活动没有变化或减弱（图50.18）[103]。因此，在进食的头期，食物的感官和情绪属性也影响胃神经肌肉活动。

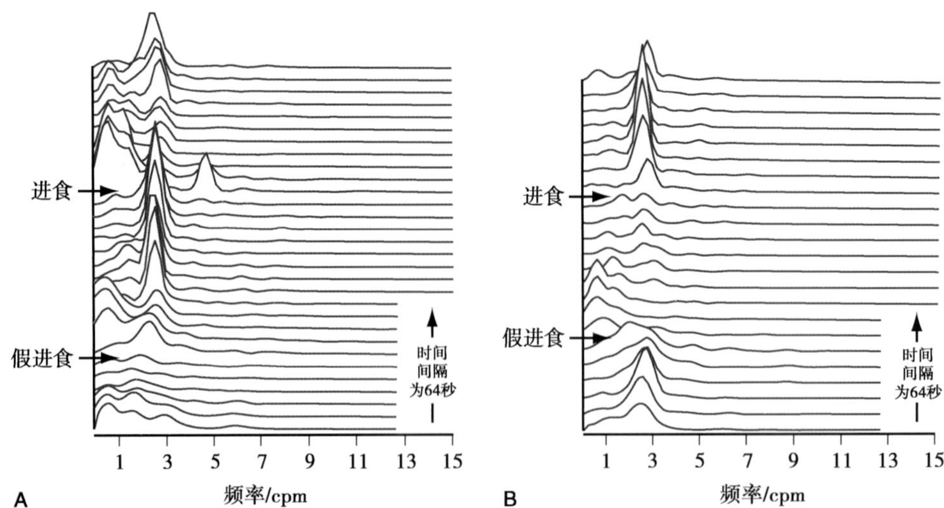

图50.18 用美味食物（A）和“恶心”食物（B）假喂养的胃肌电反应。A，健康受试者咀嚼温热的热狗并将其吐入纸袋时（假喂养），记录的胃电图（EGG）信号的运行频谱分析（RSA）。假喂养时正常3cpm范围内的峰值振幅的增加是正常反应。“用餐”表示实际摄入热狗。B，健康受试者咀嚼冷素豆腐热狗并吐出（假饲喂）时记录EGG的RSA。受试者在假喂食期间感到“厌恶”。注意与（A）相比，在假饲喂素豆腐热狗期间未出现3cpm峰值增加。在这两天，受试者在“用餐”时吃了一个热的热狗。注意随后在3cpm时峰值增加。cpm，每分钟周期数。（Modified from Stern RM，Crawford HE，Stewart WR，et al. Sham feeding. Cephalic-vagal influences on gastric myoelectric activity. Dig Dis Sci 1989；34：521-7.）

五、胃神经肌肉功能的发育

胃蠕动出现在妊娠 14~23 周之间。到妊娠 24 周时，蠕动波会成组或成簇地出现[104]。妊娠 30 周左右，负责胃排空中胃窦十二指肠协调运动的神经调节机制已经发展成熟[105]。EGG 记录显示，在 35 周分娩的早产儿中正常的 3cpm 活动与足月儿中记录的 EGG 信号相似[106,107]。另一方面，早产儿(妊娠<35 周)的 EGG 记录中有相当多的胃节律过速[106]。GMA 在出生后的 6~24 个月内会进一步成熟，并在第十年末达到成人水平[108]。

由于对胃的电节律，平滑肌收缩和胃节律不齐的关注，学者们对 ICC 的发育进行了深入研究。对酪氨酸激酶受体(c-Kit)进行标记和敲除 c-Kit 基因小鼠的研究，使人们对 ICC 的发展有了更多的了解[109]。ICC 有不同的发育过程，MY-ICC 在出生前就有 c-Kit 表达的 ICC，而 IM-ICC 在出生后发育[110]。出生时 ENS 和 ICC 网络尚未完全发育，耦合性较差，但在围生期发育期间，胃的节律性和收缩力逐渐成熟[106,107]。ENS 和深层肌丛中的 ICC 密切相关，而在没有 ENS 的情况下，肌间神经丛中的 ICC 可以正常发育[110]。幽门 ICC 的缺失与抑制性神经活动的丧失有关，而后者可导致婴儿幽门狭窄的发生(见第 49 章)[111]。

六、胃神经肌肉功能的评估

(一) 胃排空率

美国食品药品管理局(FDA)目前批准的评估胃神经肌肉功能的临床试验是闪烁显像试验，以测量胃排空速度，胶囊运动装置评估胃排空，以及 EGG 装置在进食前后测量 GMA。这些测试提供了健康和疾病状态下不同胃神经肌肉活动的客观评估。胃排空和 GMA 试验的结果为胃轻瘫和胃节律不齐的客观诊断提供了依据，并为治疗提供了合理的基础。

1. 闪烁扫描法

放射性同位素标记的试验餐可用于评估胃排空速率。固体胃排空方案是一项用锝-99m(^{99m}Tc)标记的 255kcal 包括面包和果酱的鸡蛋代餐作为标准试验餐的多国研究[38]。123 名健康个体在摄入膳食 1 分钟后立即进行扫描，并在 30 分钟、60 分钟、120 分钟、180 分钟和 240 分钟再次进行扫描。在 120 分钟时大于 60% 的食物滞留和在 240 分钟时大于 9% 的食物滞留被定义为胃排空延迟。4 小时排空试验优于 2 小时试验，因为几乎 20% 的疑似胃轻瘫患者在 2 小时排空正常，而在 4 小时排空异常[112]。

固体胃排空试验显像法存在的缺陷，包括同位素与试验餐结合不当，导致排空过快或正常，以及某些药物可干扰此试验，如长期服用一些药物可能刺激(如甲氧氯普胺)或抑制(如麻醉剂、抗胆碱能药物)胃平滑肌收缩。如果可能的话，这些药物应该在所有胃神经肌肉试验检查前 5 至 7 天停用。

受试者在闪烁扫描中会发生辐射暴露，因此不建议在同一受试者中进行多次闪烁扫描。液体胃排空试验(gastric emptying test，GET)可以用 111 二乙烯三胺、^{99m}Tc 标记的水或其他液体进行。有不明原因恶心症状的患者可能改变了液体食物胃排空，但固体食物胃排空是正常的[113,114]。

2. 胶囊技术

通过能测定管腔内 pH 和收缩的胶囊可以测得试验餐的胃排空时间。胶囊与标准试验餐一起吞咽，在餐后阶段，测得的管腔 pH 和收缩数据被传输到受试者佩戴的接收器。在健康受试者中，胶囊在摄入鸡蛋代餐后约 5 小时从胃排空至十二指肠。胶囊的排空结果与锝标记的鸡蛋固体试验餐的排空结果一致性达 90%。该试验在检测胃轻瘫方面具有良好的敏感性和特异性[115]。

3. 呼气试验

呼气试验间接反映固体和液体试验餐的胃排空情况。固体食物用^{13}C 标记，包括^{13}C 辛酸、^{13}C 乙酸盐或^{13}C 螺旋藻。^{13}C 辛酸呼气试验已经被应用在许多实验方案中，并在欧洲广泛用于实验室和临床研究[116]。^{13}C 标记的食物从胃中排出并在小肠中吸收，标记的营养物质在肝脏中代谢为$^{13}CO_2$，在肺部释出，并在呼吸样本中测得。在^{13}C 螺旋藻试验中，呼吸样本在餐后 45、90、120、150 和 180 分钟收集。^{13}C 是一种稳定的同位素，没有辐射风险。^{13}C 呼气试验通常可以取代闪烁显像[117]。其缺点在于吸收不良、肝病或肺病患者因为这些疾病可能影响^{13}C 标记食物的正常氧化和排泄，而导致出现错误结果。

4. 超声检查

经腹超声技术用于测量胃窦直径和胃窦幽门十二指肠功能[118]。三维超声可以显示试验餐的胃内分布和胃容积的区域变化[39]。超声检查技术对于液体食物的检查结果比较理想。但临床应用因为超声检查者需要高水平的专业知识而受到限制。

5. CT 和 MRI

CT 和 MRI 这两种技术已被用于测量胃排空和显示试验餐的胃内分布。CT 和 MRI 可提供空腹胃和餐后时期独特的解剖和功能视图[119]，可以观察到连续的胃窦收缩。由于费用和实用性，这些技术并没有在临床实践中使用。

(二) 胃收缩

1. 胃窦十二指肠测压

胃窦十二指肠测压是一种有创检查技术，将灌注水的多腔导管经鼻或嘴插入，使导管近端端口位于远端胃窦，远端端口位于十二指肠的位置[36]，导管的放置需要依靠内镜或透视设备的帮助。通常需要持续记录数小时，以记录消化间期 MMC 的第 1、2 和 3 期。在受试者摄入试验餐后，需再持续数小时以记录餐后收缩。胃窦十二指肠测压试验不仅是有创检查，而且需要时间集中，同时还需要耗费助手或医生大量时间来完成试验和分析数据。管腔内测压导管仅能检测闭塞管腔收缩[120]。因为大多数餐后蠕动波不是闭塞管腔收缩，所以管腔内压力传感器装置无法记录近 50% 的胃体和胃窦收缩。位于十二指肠的测压导管可以检测出神经性或肌源性功能障碍形式。

2. 胶囊技术

先前描述的无线可摄入胶囊可以测量胃壁的收缩。在摄入标准试验餐及胶囊后，每分钟出现 1~3 次不规则收缩，与胃窦测压记录一致[121]。在将胶囊排空至十二指肠之前，会出现持续几分钟的高振幅胃窦收缩，一些形式与胃窦十二指肠测压记录的 3 期收缩一致。研究显示，在胃轻瘫患者中，胶囊排空前的 20~30 分钟内，胶囊的动力指数降低，但在胶囊排空至十二指肠前的 10 分钟内，动力指数正常。这些研究表明，即使在胃轻瘫患者中,也可以维持正常的末端胃窦收缩,而将食物研磨至可消化状态,所需的胃窦收缩力是异常的[122]。

(三) 胃肌电活动

使用放置在腹部表面的电极可以无创记录胃肌电活动(GMA)[4,123]。胃电图信号总结了正在进行的 GMA:包括禁食期间的慢波活动,餐后期间与静息和动作电位活动相关的慢波活动的总和[124]。有关胃对水负荷或营养负荷的反应,可通过视觉和计算机分析来确定,胃电图信号的振幅在正常的 2.5~3.7cpm 范围内增加(例如,在正常频率范围内胃电图功率百分比,或餐后功率百分比的增加)[52,125,126]。记录和分析胃电图的缺陷包括在计算机分析中无法识别信号中的伪影和计算机分析中的谐波[127]。

胃电图频率和振幅的变化是关键的衡量指标。在摄入大多数固体或液体食物后,在进餐后的前 10~15 分钟会出现所谓的频率下降。频率下降反映了与食物体积或温度相关试验餐引起的显著胃舒张和容纳变化[128,129]。进食数分钟后,EGG 信号的频率回到正常的 2.5~3.7cpm 范围。

胃节律障碍与患有晕动病[78]、妊娠恶心和呕吐[130,131]、功能性消化不良[52,132]和胃轻瘫[133-135]受试者的恶心症状有关。胃节律障碍包括 0.5~2.5cpm 的胃动过缓信号和 3.7~10cpm 的胃动过快信号(图 50.19),同时有胃动过速和胃动过缓记录者被称为非特异性或混合性胃节律障碍[124,136]。GMA 也可以通过手术过程中放置的浆膜电极或内镜检查期间放置的黏膜电极来记录[5,21,63,137],使用多达 128 个通道的多通道浆膜记录显示了 3cpm 肌电信号,以及与心脏节律障碍相似的各种胃节律障碍[138,139]。人体慢波振幅和速度在末端胃窦处最大,即紧邻幽门 3~4cm 的胃窦处[5]。这些相同的研究进一步证实正常人的慢波频率范围为 2.5~3.7cpm。在伴有或不伴有胃轻瘫有恶心症状患者中,慢波频率在 1~2cpm(胃动过缓)和 4~9cpm(胃动过速)间[21,139,140]。

(四) 胃舒张、容纳和容积

1. 球形气压调节器(恒压器)试验

由于胃底和近端胃的球形形状,标准测压导管在记录餐后腔内压力方面没有用处。球形气压调节器的设计是为了测量近端胃球形区域的张力(或胃舒张)和容积变化[41]。在基线或禁食期间,通过注入空气维持球囊内压力,球囊略微扩张。由于摄入试验餐后胃底和近端胃舒张,同时向球囊内注入更多的空气,以维持既定的基线球囊内压力[141]。用于维持基线压力的注入气量,即是近端胃舒张时胃容量增加的估计值。

球形气压调节器(恒压器)试验研究显示,几乎 30% 的功能性消化不良患者存在胃底舒张异常[41]。胃底舒张失败与早饱相关。在胃轻瘫患者中也记录了胃底舒张失败[41,142,143]。由于恒压器方法对患者来说是有创的且有不适感,故此试验仅限于实验室研究。

2. 闪烁显像和其他试验

对液体和固体物质引起的胃底舒张过度或不良,可以通过闪烁显像、超声和 MRI 来证明。单光子发射 CT 是一种在进餐前后描记胃壁轮廓以确定胃容积变化的方法。这种方法需要静脉注射^{99m}Tc-高锝酸盐来描记胃壁。容纳反应可以通过单光子发射 CT 来识别[144]。

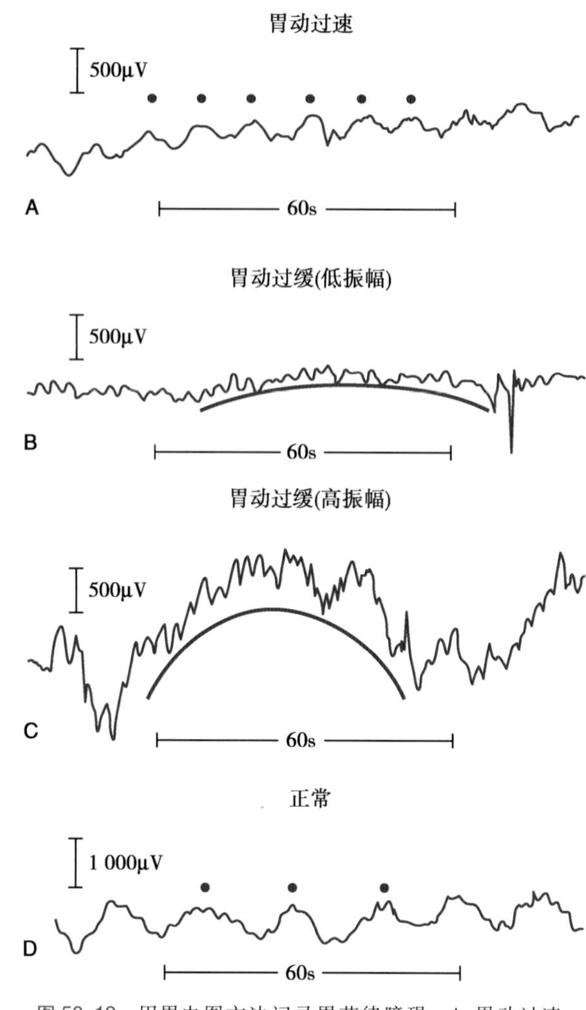

图 50.19 用胃电图方法记录胃节律障碍。A,胃动过速,6cpm 的异常快速信号,用圆点表示。B 和 C,分别在低或高振幅 1cpm 波下的胃动过缓。每分钟 1 个波用实线表示,胃电图(EGG)信号中较小的波代表呼吸活动。D,正常的 3cpm EGG 信号由圆点表示。cpm,每分钟周期数

3. 非营养液体和营养液体饱腹感测试

非营养液体(水负荷饱腹感测试)和营养液体测试用于评估总胃容积或胃容量及内脏感觉,如摄入这些液体后的恶心、饱胀不适或饱腹感[52,83,145,146],通常与 GMA、胃容纳或胃排空的检测结合使用。在水负荷饱腹感测试中,水在 5 分钟内被摄入,直到受试者感到饱腹[52,146]。在典型的热量液体测试中,受试者每 5 分钟喝 150mL 液体(如安素),直到达到最大耐受饱腹感。在健康受试者中达到这一终点需要花费近 30 分钟,并消耗 800~1 000mL 营养液体[146]。在许多健康受试者中,液体饱腹感测试会引起恶心和胃节律障碍。患有功能性消化不良或胃轻瘫的受试者摄入的水或营养液体量要少得多,并出现饱胀不适,表明胃的舒张和容纳受损[52,83]。

4. 幽门括约肌测试

幽门括约肌是胃排空的关键调节器,就像食管下括约肌是食管排空的关键调节器一样。在清醒受试者中,很难研究其空腹和餐后幽门的功能。内镜下功能性腔道成像探针或内镜功能成像探头(EndoFLIP, Medtronic, Minneapolis, MN)在内镜检查期间定位在幽门上,以测量幽门括约肌压力、直径和扩张性[147]。与胃排空正常的患者相比,几乎 30% 的胃轻瘫患

者幽门扩张性降低[148]。

5. 胃窦十二指肠测压

胃窦十二指肠测压已应用了多年，但是由于难以将导管固定在幽门括约肌同一个区域内，因此很难保持压力传感器的一致性和可靠性。

（五）胃和幽门神经肌肉病变的组织病理学研究

对胃神经肌肉疾病组织病理学基础的研究，为神经胃肠病学的发展领域提供了基础知识。大部分胃壁全层标本是在放置 GES 装置或为严重胃轻瘫患者放置空肠造口饲管时采集的。提供包含环形肌、ENS 神经元和 ICC 的全层标本的内镜活检技术已被探索了多年[149,150]。平滑肌、ENS 的神经元、ICC 的数量或位置，以及关键神经或肌肉受体分布的组织学异常，可能是胃平滑肌舒张、蠕动收缩和胃慢波活动异常的潜在机制。

据报道，糖尿病和 IGP 患者会出现 ICC（MY-ICC 和 IM-ICC）丢失[20,21,31]。有趣的是，糖尿病小鼠中也出现了类似的 ICC 丢失，并且在强化胰岛素治疗下 ICC 得以恢复，这表明 ICC 在糖尿病中并未完全破坏，而是在长期高血糖状态下去分化为未成熟的成肌细胞[151]。在炎性和肿瘤性疾病中也可以看到对 ICC，ENS，和平滑肌的损伤[152-155]。其他对人类的研究显示，在 DGP 患者中，平滑肌层纤维化但肌间神经丛和迷走神经完好，ICC 丢失但平滑肌纤维化很少，肌间神经元中有炎性 T 淋巴细胞浸润[156,157]。

来自 IGP 和 DGP 患者的全层活检显示，ICC 明显减少，肠神经细胞体和末梢大量损伤，平滑肌尚存[20-23,31]。有趣的是，与糖尿病患者相比，IGP 患者的标本中可见更严重的 ICC 减少和肠神经损伤[20,31]。这些标本中的胃平滑肌通常是正常的。因此，这些疾病可能被认为是 Cajal 细胞病变或胃肠神经病变，或在大多数情况下，更有可能是两者均同时存在。

进一步的研究表明，CD204 巨噬细胞的免疫浸润与 IGP 和 DGP 患者胃窦处 ICC 的减少有关[22]。与胃体相比，胃窦 ICC 的损失似乎更严重。CD204 巨噬细胞的增加也与血红素氧化酶缺乏和 ICC 丢失有关，而血红素氧化酶的替代物改善了小鼠的胃排空[158]。然而，在 DGP 患者中进行的一项血红素输注试验中并没有改善症状或胃排空[159]。在胃轻瘫动物体内 M2 巨噬细胞的恢复导致 ICC 数量增加和胃排空改善[160]，这提供了一条治疗胃轻瘫的新途径。

最后，组织化学研究表明，与正常幽门组织对照组相比，胃轻瘫患者的幽门组织 ICC 数量减少和纤维化增加[161]。这些研究以及关于胃轻瘫患者幽门舒张性降低的生理学研究[147,148,162]，表明幽门在调节胃排空速率，从而调节胃轻瘫的发展中起着重要作用。胃和幽门组织的全层组织化学研究结果也为理解胃神经肌肉功能障碍提供了新的方向，并激发了新的治疗方法的想法。

七、胃神经肌肉疾病

胃神经肌肉疾病包括一系列的电和收缩功能障碍。在轻度范围内的是胃节律障碍，这是一种与轻度至重度恶心症状相关的细微电干扰（图 50.20）。研究表明，这些患者的 ICC 轻度减少，约为 3~5 个 ICC/高倍镜视野（HPF）[140]。胃底舒

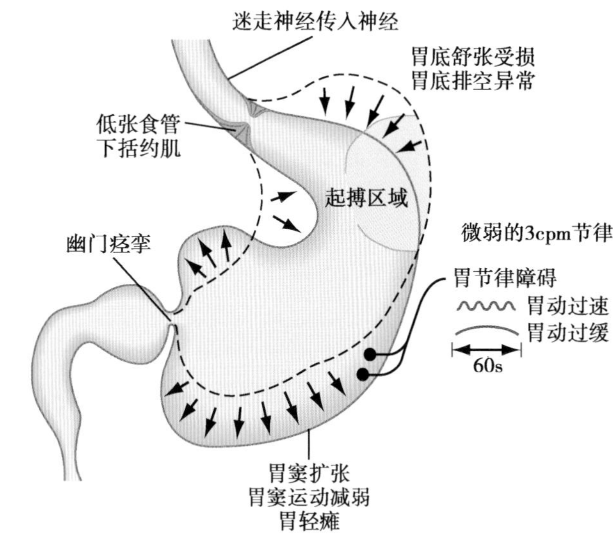

图 50.20　胃神经肌肉疾病谱。胃神经肌肉疾病从胃底松弛和排空异常到胃节律障碍、胃窦动力不足和胃轻瘫。部分胃神经肌肉疾病患者可出现幽门括约肌功能障碍、十二指肠功能障碍、胃窦十二指肠协调障碍和迷走神经超敏反应。cpm，每分钟周期数。详见正文。（Modified from Koch KL, Stern RM. Functional disorders of the stomach. Semin Gastrointest Dis 1996;7:185-95.）

张异常与早饱感有关。在严重情况下，胃窦运动减弱和严重的胃轻瘫，与长期餐后饱胀、呕吐、腹胀、体重减轻和可能需要肠内或胃肠外营养支持的营养不良相关。这些患者的 ICC 显著减少（0~2 个 ICC/HPF）[20-23]。胃轻瘫患者还可能有多种神经肌肉异常：胃节律障碍、胃窦扩张不良、胃底舒张差，以及由于迷走神经或内脏神经功能障碍引起的胃超敏反应或低敏反应[163,164]。表 50.2 总结了与胃神经肌肉障碍相关的症状。

在 20% 以上的胃轻瘫患者中，幽门括约肌是一个关键病理生理因素[165]。在这些患者中，GMA 值为 3cpm，表明在胃体和胃窦处的 ICC 数量正常。幽门固定性梗阻[134]和幽门神经肌肉功能障碍见于胃轻瘫和正常或高于 3cpm GMA 的患者[147,148,166,167]。因此，胃神经肌肉障碍反映了持续的 ICC 损耗，但也包括梗阻性胃轻瘫。

在正常的胃组织中，存在 5 个及以上 ICC/HPF，正常 GMA 为 3cpm，试验餐以正常速率排空[20-24,140]。患有慢性原因不明的恶心且胃排空正常的受试者具有 3~4 个 ICC/HPF，同时存在各种胃节律障碍，范围从胃动过速到胃动过缓和各种传导缺陷（例如，折返性节律，传导阻滞）[140]。患有恶心、呕吐且有胃轻瘫的受试者具有更严重的 ICC 减少（0~2 个 ICC/HPF），同时有从胃动过速到胃动过缓的各种胃节律障碍[20-24]。最后，有一部分胃轻瘫但具有正常 3cpm GMA 的患者[134,166,167]，这些不一致的发现（正常或高于 3cpm GMA 和胃轻瘫）表明在胃体/胃窦中具有正常数量的 ICC，这种情况与幽门功能障碍有关[134,147,148,168]。因此，幽门功能障碍引起的“IGP”可能是由于：（a）持续性的、机械性的疾病，如由消化性溃疡疾病引起的狭窄[134]或癌症[166]；或（b）神经肌肉功能障碍，如幽门痉挛[167]、幽门舒张性差[147,148]或胃窦部协调性差[168]。因此，持续的 ICC 减少似乎与胃节律障碍和胃排空速率及相关症状有关（图 50.21）。

表 50.2　基于胃电和胃排空测试结果的胃神经肌肉疾病分类和治疗方法

类别 1	类别 2	类别 3	类别 4
检查结果	检查结果	检查结果	检查结果
胃节律紊乱和胃轻瘫	正常 3cpm 胃节律和胃轻瘫	胃节律紊乱和正常胃排空	正常 3cpm 胃节律和正常胃排空
诊断	诊断	诊断	诊断
重度胃肌电收缩障碍	幽门痉挛,幽门或十二指肠的固定性梗阻 电机械收缩失耦联	胃肌电障碍	内脏高敏感性 非胃病原因
治疗	治疗	治疗	治疗
恶心和呕吐饮食* 促动力疗法 抗焦虑疗法 胃造口/空肠造口管 全胃肠外营养 针灸 内镜治疗† 胃电刺激 胃起搏器	肉毒杆菌/球囊扩张术 手术治疗固定性梗阻 恶心和呕吐饮食* 促动力疗法 抗焦虑疗法	恶心和呕吐饮食* 促动力疗法 抗焦虑疗法	恶心和呕吐饮食* 抗焦虑疗法 抗抑郁疗法 胃底/胃窦舒张药物(对非胃病原因的进一步检查,如非典型 GERD、胆囊炎、肠易激综合征或中枢或自主神经系统疾病)

*参见表 50.6。
†参见表 50.5。
cpm,每分钟周期数。
FromKoch KL, Hasler WL, Editors. Nausea and vomiting: diagnosis and treatment. Switzerland: Springer International Publishing; 2017.

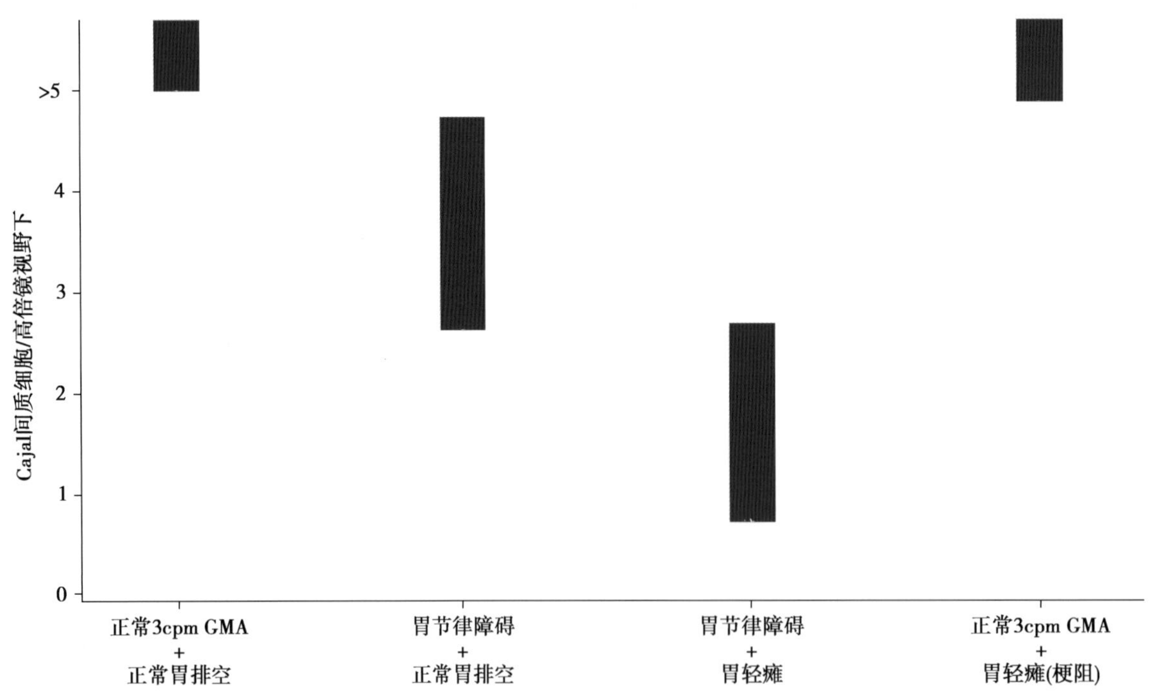

图 50.21　显示了 ICC、GMA、胃排空之间关系的示意图。正常数量的 Cajal 间质细胞[>5 个/高倍镜视野(HPF)]与正常的 3cpm GMA 和正常的胃排空相关。ICC 中度耗竭(3~4 个 ICC/HPF)与胃节律障碍和胃排空正常相关,而重度 ICC 耗竭(1~2 个 ICC/HPF)与胃节律障碍和胃轻瘫相关。相反,在梗阻性胃轻瘫亚型中,存在正常的 3cpm GMA,并反映了正常数量的 ICC 和幽门功能障碍。cpm,每分钟周期数

（一）胃轻瘫

胃轻瘫是指胃的“麻痹”，定义为在没有机械性梗阻的情况下，标准试验餐从胃中排空的速率延迟。大约 90% 的胃轻瘫患者是糖尿病、手术后或 IGP，但明确是否存在持续性梗阻性或功能性阻塞性胃轻瘫很重要，因为它们是可逆的。表 50. 3 列出了胃轻瘫的鉴别诊断。

表 50. 3　胃轻瘫的原因

诊断	发病率/%
特发性胃轻瘫* （20% 有梗阻性胃轻瘫）	40
糖尿病性胃轻瘫（1 型和 2 型糖尿病） （20% 有梗阻性胃轻瘫）	35
手术后胃轻瘫（胃窦切除术、迷走神经切断术、胃底切除术、胃底折叠术）	20
缺血性胃轻瘫	<1
其他原因	4

*可能是病毒感染后、药物诱导、肠神经、Cajal 间质细胞或平滑肌的退行性或炎症过程。

胃轻瘫的流行病学才刚刚开始被研究。来自明尼苏达州奥姆斯特德地区的数据表明年龄调整后胃轻瘫的患病率，男性为 9. 6/10 万，女性为 37. 8/10 万。男性发病率为 2. 4/10 万，女性为 9. 8/10 万。胃轻瘫病例组是根据标准胃闪烁显像结果诊断的[169]。在糖尿病患者中，2 型糖尿病患者胃轻瘫的发生率为 1%，1 型糖尿病患者胃轻瘫的发生率接近 5%，而在奥姆斯特德的人群中，非糖尿病受试者胃轻瘫的发生率为 0. 1%[169]。糖尿病患者的胃轻瘫随着时间的推移而演变，通常在 10 年或更长时间后出现。在明尼苏达州奥姆斯特德的一系列研究中，5. 2% 的 1 型糖尿病患者和 1. 0% 的 2 型糖尿病患者在 10 年内出现胃轻瘫，而在对照受试者出现胃轻瘫只有 0. 2%[170]。在以社区为基础的 2 型糖尿病患者人群中，6% 的白人和 7% 的非洲裔美国人出现中度胃轻瘫相关的症状[171]。相比之下，在转诊中心，几乎 50% 的 1 型糖尿病患者和 30% 的 2 型糖尿病患者出现胃轻瘫[172,173]。

自 2000 年以来，与胃轻瘫相关住院人数显著增加。许多因胃轻瘫入院的患者是血糖控制不佳或存在感染问题的 DGP 患者[174]。这些入院患者中的一部分也是为了行外科手术置入胃刺激器治疗糖尿病或特发性胃轻瘫[175]。

1. 糖尿病性胃轻瘫

许多长期 1 型糖尿病患者会发展为 DGP。这些患者通常糖尿病病史超过 10 年，血糖水平不稳定且过高，合并周围神经病变、肾脏病变和心血管疾病[164,175-177]。与无胃轻瘫的糖尿病患者相比，DGP 患者的 5 年死亡率有所增加[172,178]。在少数患者中，胃轻瘫是其糖尿病的初始并发症。

1 型糖尿病患者胃排空障碍的一个重要表现是血糖控制不稳定，尤其是如果在餐前使用常规剂量的胰岛素，在餐后可能会出现意外的低血糖发作。当注射胰岛素后餐后胰岛素水平增加但胃排空延迟时，进入十二指肠和小肠的营养物质葡萄糖吸收被延迟。因此，经胰岛素治疗后，患者血糖水平下降，并意外出现低血糖症状[177]。

在健康受试者和糖尿病患者中，急性高血糖症（>220mg/dL）与胃动过速和胃排空延迟有关[63,179,180]。高血糖症还与 ICC 减少[151]、胃窦运动减弱[181]、孤立性幽门收缩[182]、胃节律障碍[63,179]和促动力药物如红霉素的促动力作用受损有关[183]。在正常受试者和糖尿病患者中，血糖水平相对轻微升高，甚至在生理范围内升高，都会延迟胃排空[180]。葡萄糖钳夹法导致的急性高血糖会引起饱胀、胃窦收缩力降低、胃节律障碍，减弱幽门对十二指肠内传输脂质的收缩反应，并改变上消化道感觉[63,179,180]。

1 型糖尿病患者记录的胃神经肌肉异常包括食物在胃内的异常分布[184]、容受性舒张和调节减少[185]、胃窦部 MMC 发生率降低、胃窦扩张、餐后胃窦运动功能减弱[181]和电节律障碍[133,173,186]。在 DGP 患者中，ICC 耗尽及肠神经末梢异常[20,21]，有助于解释在试验餐试验中出现胃节律障碍和胃收缩反应差的病理机制。胃窦 3 期收缩的减少导致胃内纤维碎片排空不良，并且是形成胃石的神经肌肉基础（参见第 28 章）。因此，糖尿病患者胃的进行性神经肌肉功能障碍反映了慢性高血糖和叠加间歇性高血糖发作对胃 ENS 和 ICC 的影响。胃平滑肌功能障碍是一些糖尿病患者胃排空延迟的另一种机制。糖尿病大鼠电刺激的胃平滑肌收缩性对电刺激的反应降低[187]。高血糖可抑制对干细胞因子的抑制作用，从而能减少 ICC 数量及降低平滑肌收缩力[188]。在 DGP 患者中，胃平滑肌是完整的，但基底膜增厚[20,21]。胃轻瘫糖尿病患者接受胰岛素泵治疗并连续监测 48 周血糖水平，与基线相比，糖化血红蛋白显著降低（降低 1. 1%），根据胃轻瘫主要症状指数（Gastroparesis Cardinal Symptoms Index）的记录，与胃轻瘫相关的症状降低了 23%[189]。因此，对这些患者进行积极的胰岛素治疗有助于控制血糖和改善胃轻瘫症状[189]。

幽门痉挛可能导致一种梗阻性糖尿病性胃轻瘫[167,190]。在这些情况下，胃体和胃窦神经肌肉功能是完整的，但是由于幽门痉挛或幽门不完全舒张引起幽门功能性梗阻会导致胃排空延迟。这些患者的 3cpm GMA 正常或增加，这与胃轻瘫患者的表现不一致，这表明胃出口梗阻可能是由于幽门功能性或机械性原因（图 50. 22A；见后文关于梗阻性胃轻瘫的部分）[134,190]。

美国有近 2 500 万人患有 2 型糖尿病，许多人有可疑或亚临床胃轻瘫[191]。在三级中心，2 型糖尿病胃轻瘫发病率在 30% 至近 50% 之间[191]。2 型糖尿病患者与 1 型糖尿病患者的显著不同之处在于，2 型糖尿病患者具有胰岛素抵抗，糖尿病多发生在晚年，常伴有肥胖，易出现早饱感，胃轻瘫不太严重，与 1 型糖尿病患者相比，高血糖症在诊断前存在的时间更长[191-194]。在 2 型糖尿病早期阶段，胃排空速率可能会加快[195]。美国国立卫生研究院胃轻瘫协会的一项研究表明，与 2 型糖尿病合并胃轻瘫患者相比，1 型糖尿病患者更年轻，胃排空延迟更严重，住院次数更多。2 型糖尿病胃轻瘫患者年龄较大，胃排空延迟较轻，早饱感较明显[193,194]。

非肥胖糖尿病小鼠和 2 型糖尿病 db/db 小鼠（肥胖症、糖尿病、脂肪代谢障碍的模型小鼠）的实验性糖尿病会导致胃轻瘫。糖尿病小鼠胃中的神经元型一氧化氮合成酶（nNOS）

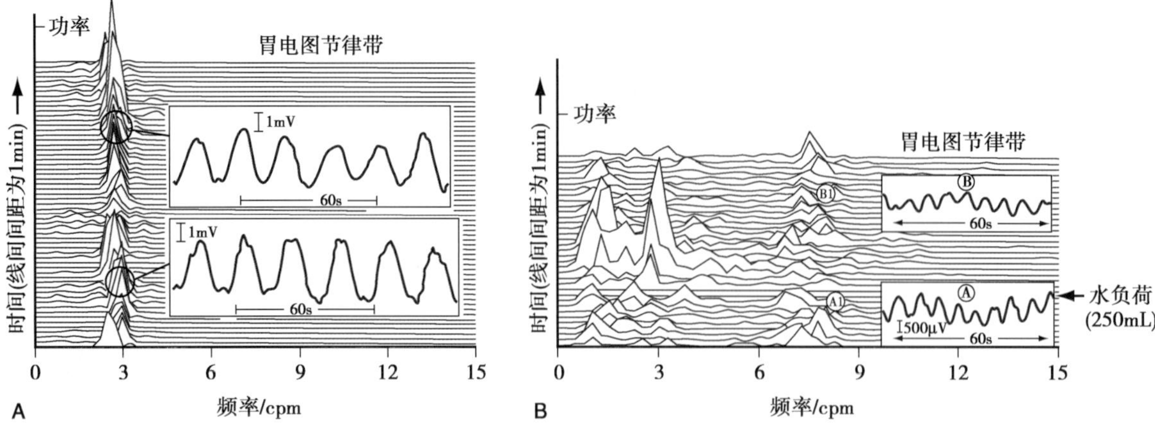

图 50.22　梗阻性和特发性胃轻瘫患者胃电图的频谱分析。A，继发于慢性消化性溃疡病的幽门机械性梗阻导致胃轻瘫患者的RSA 记录。注意胃电图节律条带中持续的高振幅 3cpm 波和 RSA 中 3cpm 的均匀且无变化的峰值，这些发现在胃轻瘫患者中是由于电和收缩功能障碍而无法预期的。B，RSA 和胃电图(EGG)节律条带。一例特发性胃轻瘫患者的记录。注意胃电图节律条带在水负荷试验前(B)和之后(A)显示 7~8cpm 的胃动过速。RSA 在 7~8cpm 的胃动过速范围显示多个峰值，在正常 3cpm 范围内显示很少的峰值。该患者有胃电和收缩异常，表现为胃动过速和胃轻瘫。cpm，每分钟周期数。(Modified from Brzana RJ，Koch KL，Bingaman S. Gastric myoelectrical activity in patients with gastric outlet obstruction and idiopathic gastroparesis. Am J Gastroenterol 1998；93：1803-9.)

减少，其减少与胃窦扩张和胃轻瘫相关[196]。值得注意的是，与对照组相比，DGP 患者胃组织中的 nNOS 减少了 40%[20]。胰岛素或西地那非治疗能恢复胃组织内一氧化氮合成酶的含量，并与糖尿病小鼠胃排空延迟逆转相关。在 db/db 小鼠中发现胃底运动减弱和幽门过度收缩[197]。在对糖尿病小鼠的其他研究中，ICC 的减少与电节律障碍、胃排空延迟和胃平滑肌神经传导减少有关[198]。

2. 手术后胃轻瘫

胃轻瘫可以发生在接受包括从迷走神经切断术到胃底折叠术再到胃窦切除术的精细或根治性胃手术的患者中。迷走神经干切断术对胃神经肌肉功能造成复杂的影响。迷走神经切断术后，饭后胃底不能正常舒张，导致胃窦快速充盈[199]。迷走神经切断术还与胃节律障碍[3]、胃窦收缩减弱和胃窦十二指肠协调性差相关[200]。由于胃窦收缩变弱，蠕动中断，胃溃疡手术中进行的迷走神经切断术需要进行幽门成形术，以减少括约肌对胃窦流出的阻力。大多数病人可以从迷走神经切断术的影响中恢复过来。但是在接受胃窦和胃体广泛切除术的患者中，可能会出现长期症状和慢性胃神经肌肉功能障碍。

食管癌的食管下段切除术包括胃底切除术，迷走神经被切断，胃底储备丧失。进行幽门成形术是为了促进胃排空，但胃底和数量不定胃体(可能包括起搏区域)的缺失通常会导致慢性恶心、胃节律障碍和胃轻瘫。采用 Billroth Ⅰ式、Billroth Ⅱ式、Roux-en-Y 式胃空肠吻合术治疗胃肿瘤或消化性溃疡时，切除胃窦可能会导致严重的胃神经肌肉功能障碍[201,202]。正常胃神经肌肉活动所需的胃体-胃窦临界数量(包括含有起搏区域胃壁的未知数量)可能会被切除，胃体和胃窦的研磨效果可能会显著降低。摄入的食物保留在残胃的胃底，无法排空到胃体内[203]；尽管吻合术已经被广泛采用，但胃体不能混合和排空胃内容物。Roux-en-Y 式胃肠造口术可能会导致 Roux 综合征，即餐后疼痛、腹胀和恶心。胃排空延迟是由于 Roux 残胃的"功能性梗阻"，因为 Roux 残胃内的神经肌肉不同步阻止了胃的排空[204,205]。在迷走神经切断术和胃窦切除术后，患者可能会出现下文所述的倾倒综合征。在肥胖症的胃"袖状"切除术中，胃的三分之二被切除，包括胃底、胃体和胃窦的部分，幽门被保留。袖状切除术后，液体和固体试验餐的胃排空速率加快，但可供查阅的研究很少[206,207]。

胃底折叠术通常用于药物治疗无效的胃食管反流病(见第 46 章)。胃底折叠术后可能出现胃轻瘫和早饱感、腹胀、长期饱胀和恶心。这些患者的胃底舒张改变、胃排空延迟和胃节律障碍，可能是由于胃底折叠术中或术后迷走神经损伤[208,209]。由于胃排空研究很少在此项手术前进行，因此不能确定有多少患者在胃底折叠术前就已经有胃轻瘫[209]。

3. 缺血性胃轻瘫

慢性肠系膜缺血是胃轻瘫的一个罕见但可逆的原因[210]。这些患者会出现与胃轻瘫相关的症状。缺血性胃轻瘫不同于急性肠系膜缺血，急性肠系膜缺血表现为急腹症和坏疽性小肠的腹部症状(见第 118 章)。慢性肠系膜缺血通常是由于进行性动脉粥样硬化，或腹主动脉、肠系膜上动脉或肠系膜下动脉内膜增生引起的。这些阻塞动脉的侧支循环随着时间推移而逐渐形成，从而至少在一段时间内可以保持胃神经肌肉功能正常。动脉搭桥手术或狭窄动脉扩张术可以缓解症状、根除胃节律障碍和逆转胃轻瘫[210]。因此，缺血性胃轻瘫是潜在的可逆性胃轻瘫，当患者有胃轻瘫、体重减轻和外周血管疾病、脑血管疾病或心肌梗死病史时应考虑缺血性胃轻瘫可能。大约 50% 的缺血性胃轻瘫患者会出现腹部杂音。

肠系膜血管损伤还有其他不常见的形式(如正中弓状韧带综合征)，可导致流向胃的血流减少[211]。弓状韧带的解除和血流的恢复与胃排空的改善相关。而肠系膜上动脉压迫综合征不是引起胃轻瘫、恶心和呕吐等症状的机械性梗阻的原因。

特发性(如下所述)、糖尿病性或手术后胃轻瘫患者，可出现因幽门功能障碍而致的胃轻瘫——梗阻性胃轻瘫亚型。由于内镜和外科治疗是针对幽门的，因此这种亚型非常重要。

(1) 固定性幽门梗阻

固定性梗阻性胃轻瘫是指由于肿瘤、慢性消化性溃疡或炎症、环状或蹼状幽门或十二指肠球部或球后区域的机械性梗阻而导致的胃排空延迟[134,166]，阻塞也可以在十二指肠球部远端的十二指肠降部和水平部。这些患者有胃轻瘫及正常或异常的 3cpm GMA[134]。图 50.22A 显示了一个在 EGG 测试中记录的高振幅 3cpm GMA 波的例子，该患者因慢性消化性溃疡和幽门持续性狭窄而患有幽门出口梗阻。在这些患者中，胃体窦的平滑肌、ENS 和 ICC 是完整的，但是正常周期性的胃蠕动波在阻塞点(幽门)遇到持续的阻力，固体食物的排空延迟。相比之下，大多数 IGP 患者出现胃动过缓、胃动过速或混合性胃节律障碍，表明存在电和收缩功能障碍(见图 50.22B)。然而，如果 IGP 或 DGP 患者有 3cpm GMA，则应考虑胃轻瘫的原因。胃轻瘫实际上可能是由于幽门狭窄或十二指肠球后部癌引起的梗阻性胃轻瘫[134,166]。尽管一些患者可能对狭窄球囊扩张术有反应，采取外科手术解除持续性幽门梗阻及采用 Billroth Ⅰ式或 Billroth Ⅱ式胃空肠吻合术改善梗阻性胃轻瘫是非常必要的(见第 53 章)。在长期机械性幽门梗阻的患者中，胃可能会扩张，平滑肌收缩减弱，但 3cpm GMA 存在，所有这些都可能代表一种由于电机械收缩失耦联引起的胃轻瘫。

(2) 功能性幽门梗阻

幽门痉挛可引起一种相对较轻的胃出口梗阻。在胃轻瘫样症状的情况下，幽门“痉挛”可能导致餐后右上腹部疼痛。幽门痉挛可阻止正常胃蠕动波将食糜排入十二指肠。Fischer 等人描述了幽门失弛缓症，表明幽门过早关闭并抑制排空时，胃窦与幽门协调性差[168]。因此，胃排空速率延迟，在幽门功能障碍的情况下诊断为胃轻瘫。然而，这些胃轻瘫患者在胃电图中记录的 3cpm GMA 是正常的，因为胃体窦神经肌肉组织是完整的(图 50.23)。

在这些患者中，用 20mm 球囊扩张幽门 2 分钟或向幽门注射肉毒杆菌毒素 A 可减少餐后症状[167]。在成功完成超过 3 次内镜下幽门治疗的患者中，建议并完成幽门成形术。所有患者的症状都有所改善，胃排空速率也有所提高[212]。最后，一些阻塞性胃轻瘫患者可能有正常的 3cpm EGG 信号，及由于“电机械失耦联”导致的胃排空差。在这些情况下，产生慢波的 MY-ICC 或 IM-ICC 可能是正常的，但是存在肠神经元和/或平滑肌功能障碍。

4. 特发性胃轻瘫

超过三分之一的胃轻瘫患者是特发性胃轻瘫(IGP)[213]。

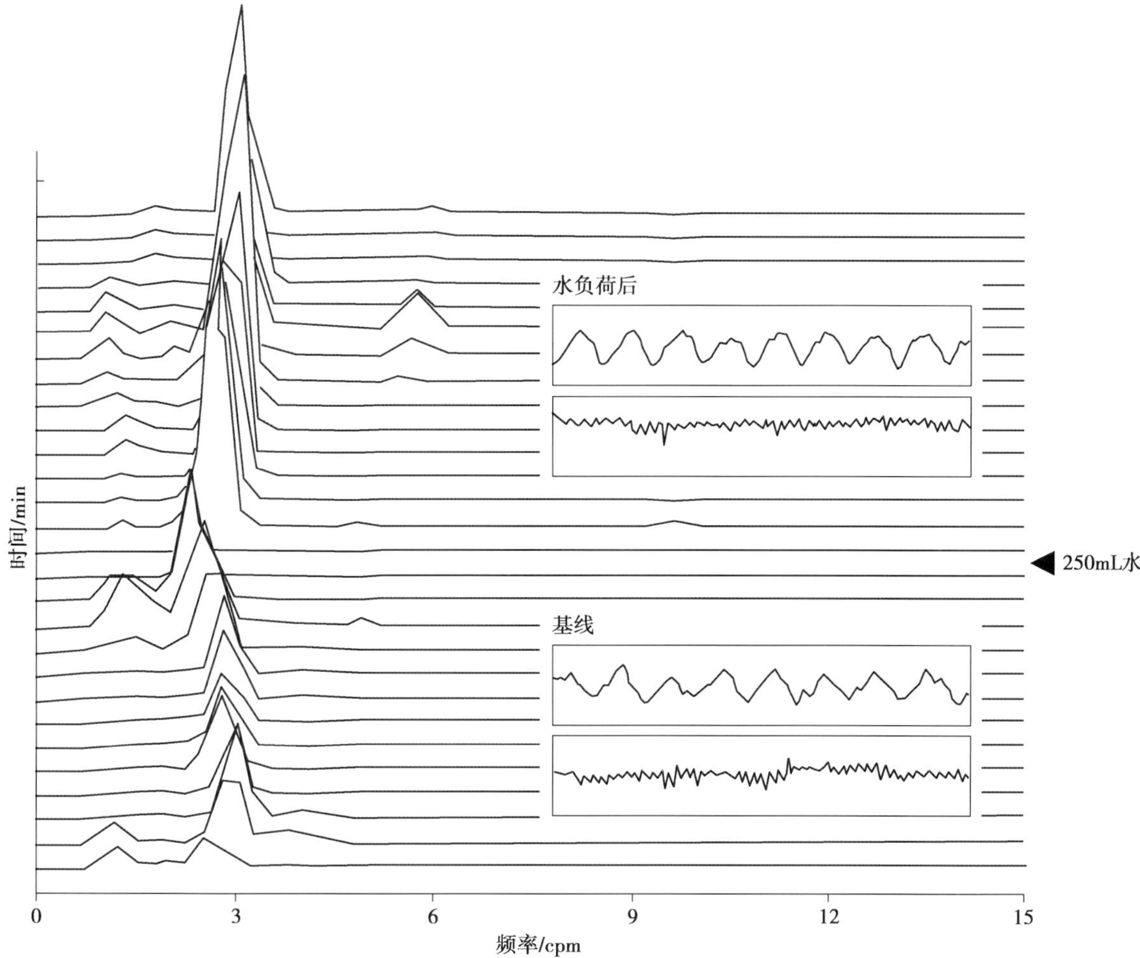

图 50.23　IGP 患者的胃电图(EGG)节律从基线和水负荷试验后 30 分钟开始条带。X 轴表示 EGG 信号中的频率，Y 轴表示时间，Z 轴表示峰值中所代表频率的功率。在节律带(右)中观察到清晰的 3cpm 波，反映了正常的慢波和 ICC 数量。EGG 记录的计算机分析(左)显示在频谱分析中有规律的 3cpm 峰值。这是胃轻瘫和正常 3cpm GMA 的胃轻瘫梗阻亚型。内镜检查排除了幽门处机械性梗阻。cpm，每分钟周期数

与DGP患者相比,IGP患者往往更易出现腹痛,但恶心和呕吐才是驱使患者去看胃肠科医生的主要症状[214]。在这些患者中,15%的患者在诊断为胃轻瘫之前数月出现急性发热性疾病[215]。这些“先兆”疾病通常被描述为伴有发热、恶心和呕吐的流感样疾病。患者通常从那时开始确定他们恶心的发作日期。有报道诺沃克病毒、单纯疱疹病毒和EB病毒感染在突发胃轻瘫的免疫系统正常的患者和免疫功能低下的患者中出现[216]。病毒后胃轻瘫可能在1~2年内完全缓解。美国国立卫生研究院胃轻瘫协会的一项新的组织学研究表明,与糖尿病性胃轻瘫患者相比,特发性胃轻瘫患者的ICC减少和肠神经末梢丢失更严重[20,31]。基因敲除小鼠中的ICC减少与胃节律障碍有关[217]。胃节律障碍在特发性胃轻瘫患者中很常见(见图50.22B),提示其胃体/胃窦的ICC严重减少[20-22]。其他IGP患者发病的病史线索是暴露于:①多疗程的抗生素(如慢性耳部或鼻窦感染的治疗);②各种常见手术的麻醉剂;③食物中毒样不明原因的疾病。然而,如前所述,近20%的IGP患者是正常的3cpm GMA,功能性梗阻性胃轻瘫亚型。

IGP诊断依据:具有消化不良样症状、胃排空延迟和胃节律障碍,排除了有胃轻瘫的主要原因,如糖尿病、缺血或胃部手术。许多其他疾病和异常,包括假性肠梗阻(稍后讨论)、副肿瘤疾病、自主神经系统异常、甲状腺和肾上腺疾病或中枢神经系统疾病等,可能导致胃轻瘫或与胃轻瘫相关。如果这些疾病能被确定,那么胃轻瘫可能是继发于这些特定的疾病。

(二)与其他胃肠道疾病相关的胃神经肌肉功能障碍

1. 功能性消化不良

功能性消化不良(functional dyspepsia,FD)症状包括上腹部不适或疼痛、早饱、腹胀、恶心和呕吐,其上消化道内镜检查和常规实验室检查结果均正常。功能性消化不良分为上腹痛综合征和餐后窘迫综合征(postprandial distress syndrome,PDS),后者占功能性消化不良患者的80%[218]。功能性消化不良患者的主要症状之一是原因不明的反复恶心和呕吐。这是一种具有较多需鉴别诊断的可使人衰弱的症状(框50.1),在评估有恶心和呕吐症状的患者时应排除这些疾病。如果患者患有这些疾病中的一种,那么不能诊断功能性消化不良。重要的是,餐后窘迫综合征也与胃轻瘫相关的症状相似[219]。

框50.1 慢性恶心和呕吐的鉴别诊断
机械性胃肠道梗阻(幽门、胆管、小肠、结肠)
黏膜炎症
腹膜刺激
恶性肿瘤(如胃、卵巢、肾、支气管源性)
代谢/内分泌紊乱(糖尿病、甲状腺功能减退、甲状腺功能亢进、肾上腺功能不全、尿毒症)
药物(抗胆碱能药、麻醉药、左旋多巴、孕酮、钙通道阻滞剂、洋地黄、非甾体抗炎药、抗心律失常药、鲁比前列酮、大麻素、二甲双胍、胰淀素类似物)
胃轻瘫(见表50.2)
胃节律紊乱(胃动过速、胃动过缓、混合性)
中枢神经系统疾病(肿瘤、偏头痛、癫痫、卒中、直立不耐受)
精神性疾病(神经性厌食症、神经性贪食症)

引起功能性消化不良症状的胃病理生理学机制仍然是一个需要深入研究的领域(见第14章)。如果内镜检查正常,那么功能性消化不良症状可能是由胃的数种神经肌肉疾病引起的。例如,胃轻瘫与功能性消化不良症状相关。81% IGP患者的症状与PDS患者的症状相似[214],这些患者的诊断是伴有相关症状的IGP。17%至40%的功能性消化不良患者有胃轻瘫,40%至62%的患者有胃节律障碍[52,132],可以设计治疗方案来解决胃轻瘫的几种病理生理学异常。如果排除了胃轻瘫的主要原因,如功能性或持续性幽门出口梗阻、糖尿病或胃部手术,则这些功能性消化不良患者可以认为患有IGP。

研究表明,功能性消化不良或胃轻瘫样症状患者与胃轻瘫患者具有相同的症状和相同的严重程度[219]。据报道,使用西沙必利治疗的患者胃节律障碍和功能性消化不良症状得到改善[220-222]。因此,胃节律障碍本身是功能性消化不良症状的潜在病理生理学机制,也是治疗目标[223]。在胃排空正常或延迟的慢性恶心患者中,与安慰剂相比,使用阿瑞匹坦治疗后,恶心症状和胃动过速显著减少[224]。

在其他功能性消化不良患者中,胃排空和GMA都是正常的。胃容纳(舒张)异常或胃对扩张的高敏感性可能是这些患者出现功能性消化不良症状的原因[225-227]。因此,在功能性消化不良症状患者中,胃的不同区域可能存在各种神经肌肉功能障碍。

2. 胃食管反流病

许多典型的胃食管反流病(GERD)患者还有早饱感、餐后饱胀和恶心等伴随症状(见第46章)。大约30%的GERD病患者也患有功能性消化不良[218]。20%~30%的GERD病患者有胃排空延迟[228,229]。在对食管下括约肌行射频消融术(RFA)治疗后,与胃轻瘫相关的症状得到改善,胃节律障碍恢复到正常的3cpm GMA[230]。在一些患者中,恶心是胃食管反流的一种轻微的非典型症状,在积极的抑酸治疗后,恶心症状得到改善[231]。

食管下括约肌异常,包括暂时性食管下括约肌松弛次数增加,可能导致这些患者出现胃排空不良和胃节律障碍[232,233]。与对照组相比,GERD患者也倾向于在近端胃迟留固体和液体[234],这种异常可能刺激引起过度的暂时性食管下括约肌松弛。胃灼热和消化不良患者经食管下括约肌区域的射频消融治疗可改善胃灼热、胃排空速率和胃节律障碍[230]。这些数据表明,在一些GERD和胃轻瘫患者中,通过射频消融或胃底折叠术治疗GERD可改善胃电节律和胃排空速率。

3. 便秘、肠易激综合征和假性肠梗阻

在一些患者中同时存在胃轻瘫、胃节律障碍、GERD和肠易激综合征,提示这些患者有弥漫性或广泛胃肠神经肌肉功能障碍[235]。胃轻瘫发生在60%的便秘型肠易激综合征患者中。在一项对350名IGP患者的研究中,89%的患者服用了质子泵抑制剂,64%的患者患有肠易激综合征[214],这些患者代表了另一种胃肠道神经肌肉异常的重叠综合征(见第122章)。

假性肠梗阻综合征患者通常有GERD、胃轻瘫、小肠运动障碍和结肠无力,反映了最严重的全身性胃肠神经肌肉疾病[235,236]。继发于进行性系统性硬化症(硬皮病)的假性肠梗

阻通常可累及食管和胃，但也可导致小肠运动障碍和随之引起的细菌过度生长[237]。假性肠梗阻可能是由于特发性退行性病变或炎症病变，累及平滑肌或 ENS，如第 37 章和第 124 章所述。胃肠道神经肌肉疾病（神经病、肌病和 ICC 异常）的病理分类正在研究中[238]。

各种神经系统疾病也可能涉及胃或消化道的其他区域，并引起假性梗阻样症状。这些神经系统疾病包括 Ehlers-Danlos 综合征[239]、体位性直立性心动过速综合征[240]、脊髓和头部损伤、肌萎缩性侧索硬化、重症肌无力、各种肌肉营养不良和帕金森病（见第 37 章）。

4. 其他情况

有胃轻瘫样症状的肝硬化伴门静脉高压症[241]、慢性肾病[242]、慢性胰腺炎[243]、晚期艾滋病病毒感染[244]患者可能有潜在的胃轻瘫。Rett 综合征是一种好发于年幼女性的疾病，其常见的临床表现包括发育不良、自闭症行为、共济失调及痴呆。此病患者常有发育不良并且有严重的胃轻瘫和食管收缩异常[245]。一些肿瘤可能也会对胃的神经肌肉产生局部或系统的作用从而导致胃轻瘫[246,247]。肿瘤性和副肿瘤性神经病变综合征，以及细胞毒性化疗和放疗均可致胃轻瘫，并影响患者的营养和血管内容量状态。

幽门螺杆菌的感染不会影响胃排空速度。然而，有报道幽门螺杆菌性胃炎患者的 GMA 异常，而这种节律紊乱在根除 Hp 后完全消失[248]。神经性厌食症的患者常有胃排空延迟[249]，而暴食症患者的胃排空时间则正常[250]。周期性呕吐综合征是一种罕见的疾病，临床表现为持续数天剧烈的恶心和呕吐（通常需要住院治疗），随后数天或数月几乎无胃肠症状[251]。成人和婴儿均会患此病[252,253]。一些立位不耐症的患者也会出现恶心和胃轻瘫的症状，并有自主神经紊乱和胃神经肌肉功能障碍的表现[240,253]。

（三）倾倒综合征和胃快速排空

倾倒综合征可见于一些迷走神经切断术、幽门成形术和 Billroth Ⅰ式或Ⅱ式胃空肠吻合术后的患者[254]。这些患者由于胃底松弛，因此摄入的食物不能被容纳并停留在胃底。此外，如果幽门被切开，食物也不能随蠕动波而被研磨。因此液态和固态的营养物质被迅速地排空或者“倾倒”至十二指肠或者空肠。

倾倒综合征也可见于一些无胃手术史的患者，因此这种疾病可能会被一些医生漏诊。倾倒综合征的症状可与一些胃轻瘫和功能性消化不良相似，包括非特异性的腹部不适、腹胀、恶心和呕吐，这些症状通常会在进食后 1 小时内出现。然而，出汗和头昏眼花等症状则可能出现在饭后 2~4 小时，随后可出现腹部绞痛和腹泻等表现，这些表现可以提示倾倒综合征。早期症状的产生是由于胃快速排空固体和液体所导致的小肠扩张，而较晚发生的症状则是由于碳水化合物的快速吸收和相应的高血糖不能与胰岛素的分泌相匹配，这种血糖和胰岛素的不匹配可以导致症状性低血糖。此外，迅速的小肠蠕动和摄入营养物质吸收不良会导致渗透性腹泻[255]。

无胃手术史的患者也可能有胃快速排空（特发性倾倒综合征）[254]，包括功能性消化不良的患者[255]。在 30 分钟内排空 30% 以上的测试餐（低脂鸡蛋代餐）或 60 分钟内排空 70% 以上的测试餐即为快速胃排空[38]。快速胃排空与早期 2 型糖尿病（见前）、Zollinger-Ellison 综合征以及之前描述过的各种胃部手术相关。没有胃手术史或其他原因的患者被诊断为特发性胃快速排空。

八、胃神经肌肉病变的诊断

（一）病史

胃神经肌肉功能障碍的患者，包括容纳缺陷、胃节律异常以及胃轻瘫等都有类似消化不良的症状。大多数胃神经肌肉失调患者在禁食时几乎没有上消化道症状。但是，进餐会刺激胃神经肌肉功能紊乱，然后会出现易饱、长期的上腹饱胀、上腹不适或疼痛，以及随之而来的轻度至重度的恶心及呕吐[218]（表 50.4）。餐后饱胀、恶心、腹胀和呕吐的症状类似于功能性消化不良，餐后恶心或胃轻瘫。

表 50.4 胃神经肌肉活动障碍疾病：生理学、病理生理学和症状

神经肌肉活动	生理学效应	病理生理学结果	病理生理学异常	症状
容受性舒张	胃底容纳	过度或不足容纳	nNOS 减少 迷走神经阻断术	ES
胃窦蠕动	胃研磨排空	蠕动减弱 胃轻瘫	ICC 减少 肠神经元减少 迷走神经阻断术	PF
正常 3cpm 慢波	正常胃蠕动排空	胃节律紊乱（例如胃动过速）	ICC 减少 迷走神经阻断术	恶心
胃窦幽门-十二指肠协调	正常胃研磨排空	幽门痉挛 幽门狭窄	nNOS 减少 PUD	ES，PF，恶心，呕吐
正常迷走神经、ANS 和 CNS 功能	正常胃神经肌肉功能	胃底功能紊乱，胃节律紊乱 蠕动停止	迷走神经功能下降 ANS 失衡	ES，PF，恶心，呕吐

ANS，自主神经系统；CNS，中枢神经系统；cpm，每分钟周期数；ES，早饱；ICC，Cajal 间质细胞；nNOS，神经一氧化氮合成酶；PF，长期饱胀；PUD，消化性溃疡病。

与糖尿病性胃轻瘫患者相比,特发性胃轻瘫患者更容易发生腹痛[214]。与2型糖尿病合并胃轻瘫的患者比1型糖尿病合并胃轻瘫的患者更容易发生腹胀。疼痛是IGP患者的主要症状,约占20%~30%[214,256]。恶心和呕吐是导致超过85%胃轻瘫患者就诊的症状。呕吐物含有咀嚼但未消化的食物是胃轻瘫的有力证据。餐后长时间饱胀,体重减轻和女性是胃轻瘫的预测因素[257]。腹胀也是与胃轻瘫相关的重要症状,但也可能是由于小肠或结肠运动障碍所致[258]。患者可以通过调整饮食来减轻餐后症状,因此可在数月或数年后才就诊或被医生所关注。

胃轻瘫主要症状指数用于量化胃轻瘫症状[259]。持续性恶心是胃神经肌肉失调最有害的症状之一,需要彻底检查恶心和呕吐的原因(请参阅第15章),并应考虑进行适当的鉴别诊断(请参见框50.1)[76,260]。胃神经肌肉失调引起的无法解释的恶心和呕吐必须与非典型胃食管反流病、反胃和反刍综合征相鉴别。非典型胃食管反流病可表现为无法解释的恶心,这些患者几乎没有胃灼热[231]。反胃是将胃内含物轻柔地输送到食管和咽中(有时会重新吞咽内含物),而呕吐是将胃内容物有力地从嘴中喷出。反刍是指使摄入的液体和固体食物毫不费力地返回口腔,而没有灼热或苦涩的恶心感觉反刍患者的胃部容纳能力受损,并且食管下端括约肌的压力更容易因胃扩张而降低[261,262]。反刍可发生在健康的青少年和年轻人中,也见于患有神经和发育障碍的儿童。

与腹胀、恶心和腹部不适相反,腹痛仅发生于约20%的胃轻瘫患者[263,264]。由于恶心和呕吐可能是继发于一些已知原因所致疼痛(例如,与恶心和呕吐相关的上腹痛可能是糜烂性食管炎引起的),因此必须对所有反复腹痛症状的患者进行全面的检查。一旦诊断并治疗了疾病如食管炎,疼痛和恶心就会消失。特定的疼痛综合征可能提示胆囊炎、胰腺炎或Oddi括约肌功能障碍(sphincter of Oddi dysfunction,SOD)等疾病。而某些胃轻瘫患者的上腹不适或疼痛可能源于胃:胃底肌肉过度紧张,胃窦高幅收缩,幽门痉挛或胃超敏反应均是引起疼痛的潜在原因[265]。干呕和呕吐通常会导致腹部疼痛,这可能是由于腹部肌肉和肋骨压痛或腹壁综合征所引起的[266-268]。

(二) 体格检查

常规检查可能是正常的,或有容量不足,体重减轻和营养不良的迹象。体位性改变可能提示体位性直立性心动过速综合征[269]。胃轻瘫患者中有近40%是超重或肥胖[213,270]。牙齿检查可能显示出与慢性反流性食管炎或贪食症相关的牙釉质侵蚀。腹部检查可发现肿块,器官肿大和部分区域压痛。胃轻瘫很少出现腹胀和振水音。上腹部听诊可能会发现腹腔或肠系膜上动脉狭窄的体征。疼痛和压痛精确地定位在愈合的腹部切口上,并且当头部弯曲和腹肌收缩时疼痛加重(Carnett征阳性),提示疼痛是由腹壁综合征而不是胃引起的[266-268]。关节松弛可能反映了Ehlers-Danlos综合征的存在[239]。神经系统检查可能发现眼球震颤,面部无力,共济失调或其他异常,提示原发性神经系统疾病。

(三) 标准检查

通过内镜检查,常规实验室检查以及腹部和头部CT排除了恶心、呕吐和餐后不适症状的常见原因[260]。在接受内镜检查的这些患者中,胃癌的检出率不到1%[271]。如果这些常规检查结果正常且仍有症状,则应考虑胃神经肌肉失调。

(四) 非侵入性检查

胃神经肌肉失调的客观诊断可通过水负荷饱腹感测试的GET和EGG结果确定。GET和EGG在界定胃神经肌肉失调的不同方面是互补的(见表50.3)[52,132,260]。通过结合GET和EGG的结果,可以定义4种病理生理学类型的胃神经肌肉功能异常,并设计合理的治疗方法,分别为:①胃轻瘫伴有胃节律异常;②胃轻瘫伴有胃电节律正常;③正常胃排空伴有胃节律异常;④正常胃排空伴有胃电节律正常。这4个类别提供了一个概念框架,用于理解胃神经肌肉失调的范围并提供一种治疗方法(见表50.2)。

胃轻瘫患者可归为两种亚型。一类患者患有严重的神经肌肉功能障碍,并伴有GET胃轻瘫和胃节律异常,如胃动过速等。这些患者可能患有糖尿病,特发性或术后胃轻瘫。在功能性消化不良患者中,有17%到32%的患者出现胃节律异常和胃轻瘫[52,132,136]。这一类患者症状通常更严重,需要多种药物,并且可能需要进行胃造口术,肠内进食和胃起搏等治疗,在下文中会有讨论。

第二类患者有胃轻瘫和正常或高振幅的3次/min EGG信号。这些患者的幽门和十二指肠可能存在有能通过外科手术逆转的持续性机械梗阻[134]。胃壁正常幅度3次/min EGG信号和胃轻瘫的患者,内镜检查通常是正常的,而有幽门神经肌肉功能障碍的患者可能会被内镜检查出来有异常疾病[167]。机电分离也是一种病理生理可能性。

关于患者的功能性消化不良或胃轻瘫样症状和正常胃排空,归为另两种亚型:第三类患者有胃轻瘫相关的症状,但具有正常的胃排空和胃节律异常[52]。这些患者有胃轻瘫样症状[219]或功能性消化不良-餐后不适综合征[218]。第三类患者对促动力药西沙必利的反应比具有正常EGG患者的效果明显更好[220]。

第四类患者的症状与胃轻瘫相关,但胃排空正常且胃肌电活动正常。胃轻瘫样症状可能是由于水负荷膨胀或热量饱腹试验引起的胃松弛不良或胃内脏超敏反应所致。非胃病也应考虑该患者组。不典型的GERD可能引起恶心,24小时食管pH测定可证实[231]。缩胆囊素(CCK)刺激的胆囊排空研究可以证明在没有胆石症的情况下胆囊功能可出现障碍。如果存在餐后腹部不适/疼痛和肠功能障碍,则应考虑肠易激综合征(IBS)。如因引起恶心的中枢神经系统疾病和体位不耐受而就诊者,还应按照如表50.1进行评估。

九、治疗

如果确认胃排空延迟,则应检查胃轻瘫的原因(见表50.3)。必须排除持续性幽门狭窄或功能性幽门痉挛引起胃轻瘫的其他可逆性阻塞原因,和由于慢性肠系膜缺血引起的缺血性胃轻瘫,因为这些疾病是可逆的。如果胃排空正常,胃节律异常和胃调节障碍可能是由神经肌肉失调导致胃的相应症状。但应考虑非胃部疾病。通过依据GET和EGG测试结果对患者进行分组,病理生理结果有助于了解症状和制定治疗方法(请参见表50.2)。表50.5和表50.6中列出的治疗方法其范围包括促动力剂、内镜、电疗法及饮食咨询等。

表 50.5　用于治疗胃神经肌肉疾病患者症状的药物和非药物治疗

治疗	机制和作用部位	剂量	不良反应
促动力药			
大环内酯类			
红霉素	胃动素受体激动剂	125~250mg 每日 4 次	恶心，腹泻，腹部痉挛，皮疹
苯甲酰胺替代物			
甲氧氯普胺（胃复安）	D_2 受体拮抗剂；5-HT_3 受体拮抗剂；5-HT_4 受体激动剂	饭前和睡前 5~20mg	锥体外系症状，肌张力反应障碍，焦虑，抑郁，高泌乳素血症，迟发性运动障碍
多潘立酮（吗丁啉）	外周 D_2 受体拮抗剂	饭前和睡前 10~20mg	高泌乳素血症、乳房胀痛、溢乳
5-HT 激动剂（血清素激动剂）			
西沙必利*	5-HT_4 受体激动剂	饭前 5~20mg	心律失常，腹泻，腹部不适
替加色罗*	部分 5-HT_4 受体激动剂	2~6mg 每日 3 次	腹泻，腹痛
促生长素激动剂			
雷拉瑞林	促生长素激动剂	待定	影响血糖
前促松弛剂			
双环胺	毒蕈碱拮抗剂	饭前 10~20mg	嗜睡，口干
丁螺环酮	5-HT_{1a} 受体激动剂	7.5~15mg 每日 2 次	头晕，头痛，恶心
肉毒杆菌毒素	见内镜治疗		
抗恶心药物			
5-HT 拮抗剂			
昂丹司琼	5-HT_3 受体拮抗剂	4~8mg 每日 2~4 次，口服或静脉注射	头痛，肝酶升高
格拉司琼	5-HT_3 受体拮抗剂	2mg 每日 1 次或 3.1mg/24 小时贴剂	头痛，肝酶升高
酚噻嗪类			
氯丙嗪	中枢神经系统	5~10mg 每日 3 次	低血压，锥体外系症状
抗组胺药			
异丙嗪	中枢神经系统，H_1 受体拮抗剂	25mg 每日 2 次	嗜睡
茶苯海明	H_1 受体拮抗剂	50mg 每日 4 次	嗜睡
苯甲嗪	H_1 受体拮抗剂	50mg 每日 4 次	嗜睡
苯丁酮类			
氟哌利多	中枢多巴胺受体拮抗剂	2.5~5mg 静脉滴注，2 小时 1 次	镇静，低血压
抗抑郁药	中枢神经系统		
阿米替林		睡前 25~100mg	便秘
去甲替林		睡前 10~75mg	便秘
米氮平		睡前 15mg	体重增加
苯二氮草/大麻素	中枢神经系统		
劳拉西泮		0.5~1mg 每日 4 次	嗜睡，头昏
阿普唑仑		0.25~0.5mg 每日 3 次	嗜睡，头昏
屈大麻酚		5~10mg 每日 2 次	镇静
P 物质拮抗剂			
阿瑞匹坦	P 物质拮抗剂	15mg 每天 1 次	疲乏，呃逆

表 50.5 用于治疗胃神经肌肉疾病患者症状的药物和非药物治疗(续)

治疗	机制和作用部位	剂量	不良反应
电疗法			
指压和针刺疗法/针灸	脊柱/迷走神经传入?/内啡肽	不适用	局部压痛
胃电刺激	迷走神经传入?	12cpm,330ms,5mÅ	囊袋感染
胃起搏	控制异常节律,改善胃排空	3cpm,300μsec,4mÅ	囊袋感染
内镜疗法			
幽门内注射肉毒毒素	松弛幽门肌肉	每象限 25~50 单位	无
幽门球囊扩张	扩张幽门肌	20mm 球囊,2 分钟	扩张后腹痛
食管下括约肌射频消融术	减少胃食管反流,改善胃肌电活动	不适用	短暂性吞咽困难
饮食疗法			
胃轻瘫饮食	基于胃排空生理的饮食	见表 50.6	无
高蛋白饮食	减少胃异常节律	未知	无
胃造口术	排气缓解胃轻瘫	不适用	见第 6 章
空肠造口术	肠内营养支持	不适用	见第 6 章
全肠外营养	旁路绕过轻瘫胃	按需	脓毒症,中央静脉血栓形成

*仅供同情许可使用。
cpm,每分钟周期数;D_2,多巴胺-2 型;5-HT,5-羟色胺;H_1,组织胺-1。

表 50.6 针对胃神经肌肉紊乱患者恶心呕吐症状的分步饮食疗法

饮食	目标	需避免食物
第一步:运动饮料和肉汤		
对于严重的恶心和呕吐:小剂量的含有一定热量的盐水,避免血容量不足 可咀嚼的多种维生素	通过多种方式每天 1 000~1 500mL(如 120mL/h 持续 12~14 小时) 患者一次可进食 30~60mL 来达到约 120mL/h	各种柑橘饮料,高甜度饮料
第二步:汤和沙冰		
如果可以耐受第一步: 带汤的面条或者米饭以及饼干 含低脂乳制品的沙冰 花生酱,奶酪和小块饼干 奶糖或其他耐嚼的糖果 摄入上述食物少量多餐,至少每天 6 次 可咀嚼的多种维生素	每天约 1 500cal 避免血容量不足,维持体重(通常比增重更现实)	含乳制品、基于牛奶的液体
第三步:淀粉,鸡肉,鱼		
如果可以耐受第二步: 面条,意大利面食,马铃薯(马铃薯泥或是烤马铃薯),米饭,烤鸡胸肉,鱼(所有胃容易混合和排空的食物) 摄入固体食物少量多餐,至少每天 6 次 多种维生素(液体或可溶解的)	患者感兴趣并喜欢的,并且最小限度导致恶心和呕吐的普通食物	延迟胃排空的脂肪类食物;需要大量胃研磨的红肉或者新鲜蔬菜;促进胃石形成的浆状纤维食物

From Koch KL, Hasler WL, Editors. Nausea and vomiting: diagnosis and treatment. Switzerland: Springer International Publishing; 2017.

(一) 药物治疗

1. 胃体和胃窦促动力剂

对于第一类和第三类患者开具促进胃收缩和对抗胃节律异常的药物(见表 50.5)。胃轻瘫和胃动过速的患者常有严重的胃电和收缩异常。治疗方法包括动力学,抗恶心治疗和饮食咨询[164,260]。

红霉素是一种大环内酯类抗生素和胃动素样分子,可通过刺激强烈的 3 相样胃窦收缩来增加胃排空[272,273]。红霉素通常会增加恶心和呕吐症状。甲氧氯普胺是一种与普鲁卡因酰胺有关的取代苯甲酰胺,是一种有用的促动力止吐药,但有“黑框”警告(“black box” warning)。该药物在美国仅获准在胃轻瘫中使用 2~8 周,并且需要进行细致的随访,因为甲氧氯普胺可能会导致抑郁,锥体外系副作用和不可逆的迟发性运动障碍[274,275]。多潘立酮是一种多巴胺拮抗剂,可减轻恶心,纠正胃节律异常,增加胃排空率[276,277]。多潘立酮可以通过 FDA 的同情用药申请流程获得。西沙必利未被批准用于胃排空障碍,但在某些患者中可提高胃排空率并减少消化不良症状[278]。西沙必利已退出市场,但可通过 FDA 同情用药流程获得。生长激素释放肽促进剂,雷拉瑞林(relamorelin)可以促进胃排空并缓解 DGP 患者的症状[279]。

2. 胃底和幽门松弛剂

很少有药物可使胃底松弛。5-HT_1 拮抗剂舒马曲坦(sumitriptan)在降低功能性消化不良患者的症状方面可降低胃底张力,但不优于安慰剂[280]。丁螺环酮可松弛胃底并可能改善餐后饱胀感[281]。尚未有使用二环胺或钙通道阻滞剂降低胃底张力的报道。肉毒杆菌毒素可减轻幽门括约肌压力,稍后在内镜治疗中进行描述。

3. 抗恶心、呕吐疗法

非特异性的治疗胃神经肌肉失调引起的恶心和呕吐方法包括 5-羟色胺(5-HT_3)受体拮抗剂,如昂丹司琼和格雷司琼(参见表 50.5)。这些药物以及吩噻嗪和抗组胺药(如异丙嗪,苯海拉明和环丙嗪)通常用于应对这些症状,但尚无针对胃神经肌肉失调患者的对照试验。劳拉西泮或阿普唑仑或其他抗焦虑药可减轻某些患者的恶心[175,176,282]。屈大麻酚和米氮平也是用于治疗恶心的药物,但尚无针对胃轻瘫的对照试验数据。一项三环类抗抑郁药的非对照试验缓解了约 70% 不明原因恶心患者的恶心症状[283],但一项近期的安慰剂对照试验表明,一种三环类化合物去甲替林在减轻胃轻瘫症状方面并不比安慰剂好[284]。阿瑞匹坦(aprepitant)是一种神经激肽-1 拮抗剂,可在正常或延迟性胃排空和慢性恶心的患者中显著减少恶心的症状,并减少胃动过速[224]。

(二) 电疗

1. 针刺疗法

穴疗电刺激(轻度电刺激穴位点)可减少妊娠恶心,化疗药物引起的恶心,术后恶心和晕动病的恶心[285,286]以及一些与胃轻瘫相关的症状[287]。

2. 胃电疗法

正在研究 3 种不同的方法来治疗胃轻瘫:①高频(如 12cpm)和短时(300 微秒)的胃电刺激(gastric electrical stimulation, *GES*);②低频(如 3cpm)和长时(300 毫秒)进行胃起搏刺激;③用位于胃体-胃窦上的多对电极进行顺序神经电刺激。

(1) 胃电刺激器

顽固性特发性糖尿病或术后胃轻瘫患者的恶心和呕吐症状在连续进行 12 个月 12cpm GES 治疗后得到显著缓解[288-291]。以 12cpm(正常慢波频率的 4 倍)刺激胃,可改善胃轻瘫患者的恶心和呕吐情况[292]。一项为期 12 周的安慰剂对照交叉研究显示,胃电刺激对 DGP 患者与安慰剂对照相比未显示获益,但在与基线相比,开放标签的接受胃电刺激的患者在 12 个月时症状明显减轻,胃排空率也在治疗 1 年后得到改善[293]。来自多个中心的非对照研究表明,接受 GES 治疗的患者中有 50%~70% 报告有慢性恶心和呕吐症状的缓解。与胃动过速和 ICC 较少的患者相比,3cpm EGG 正常和胃活检中 ICC 较多的胃轻瘫患者对 GES 的症状改善明显更好[23]。DGP 患者的症状改善比 IGP 患者更好[288,291]。短暂胃刺激可能有助于识别胃电刺激应答者[293]。术中胃慢波测量显示,12 例胃轻瘫患者中有 11 例出现胃动过速、胃动过缓、起搏和传导异常,提示 GES 可能有助于直接起搏和刺激治疗[21]。GES 并发症包括 10% 的感染发生率,主要发生于放置设备的皮下囊袋中。也有一些偶发电极线的断裂。

(2) 胃起搏

胃轻瘫患者采用 3cpm 刺激来加快或带动正常慢波节律的低频胃刺激,旨在每分钟刺激 3 次胃蠕动收缩并改善胃排空[294]。在 13 例患者中,以 4mÅ 的振幅和 300 毫秒的脉冲宽度以及比正常 3cpm 高 10% 的频率进行电刺激,来起搏慢波。可根除一些患者的胃节律异常。在另外一项类似的纳入 9 位患者的研究中,有 2 位患者成功使用电刺激形成慢波,从胃动过速转换为正常的 3cpm 节律[295]。胃起搏治疗 1 个月后,胃排空明显改善,胃轻瘫症状明显减轻。胃起搏装置引起的不良事件为电刺激部位的不适以及电极断裂或移位。

(3) 顺序神经电刺激

顺序神经电刺激是一种胃起搏,它使用微处理器顺序激活一系列围绕胃远端三分之二的电极。刺激序列会引起播散性的收缩,从而促使胃内容物强制排空[296]。

(三) 内镜治疗

内镜疗法是指通过内镜将药物或治疗器械传递到胃部相关区域的方法。向胃幽门扩约肌注射肉毒杆菌毒素 A,以降低括约肌压力并改善胃排空,恶心和呕吐的症状,但其效果与安慰剂注射相似[297-299]。然而,一项研究对 33 例有正常的 3cpm 节律以及胃肌电活动(功能性胃流出道梗阻)的胃轻瘫患者,进行了幽门球囊扩张术或肉毒杆菌毒素注射,症状改善者占 78%[167]。内镜下幽门疗法成功治疗 2 次或以上的患者,接受了幽门成形术以获得更持久的治疗效果,所有患者的症状均有所改善,6 例患者胃排空恢复正常[212]。接受胃电刺激的患者进行幽门成形术改善了 GE 和症状[300]。胃经口内镜下幽门环肌切开术(gastric-perioral endoscopic myotomy, G-POEM)是一种先进的内镜手术方法,在此过程中进行了幽门切开术治疗胃轻瘫。

近期进行的 G-POEM 研究表明,治疗后胃排空得到改善,症状也有所减轻[301,302]。正常的 3cpm 胃肌电活动合并胃轻瘫似乎可以定义为由于幽门痉挛或失弛缓所致的功能性胃流出道梗阻这一亚型[168,302]。评估幽门扩张性可能有助于进一步确定其分型[148]。RFA 治疗在 GERD 和消化不良患者的食管下括约肌区域应用可以改善 GERD,但也可以改善胃节律异常和胃排空[230]。

(四) 饮食治疗

1. 饮食咨询

很多因为胃神经肌肉失调而有急性或慢性恶心呕吐症状的患者不知应如何进行饮食,对这类患者进行膳食指导可以使其获益[260,303]。只有 1/3 的胃轻瘫患者曾接受过膳食指导[269]。在针对胃轻瘫所致恶心和呕吐的饮食方案中，会开具一些易于胃混合和排空的液体和固体食物[260,303]。这种饮食基于胃排空原理，是一种3步饮食，随着饮食的发展，其需要胃的神经肌肉活动最少（见表50.6）。

第一步主要是为了避免血容量不足而在24小时内少量消耗的电解质溶液。与固体食物相比，液体需要较少的胃神经肌肉工作来排空。如果患者可以忍受第一步，则接下来可以尝试第二步。第二步的饮食包括含有面条或米饭的汤。避免以牛奶为基础的奶油汤。第三步强调淀粉以及鸡肉和鸡胸肉。与新鲜蔬菜或红肉相比，这些固体食物需要较少的胃功进行混合和排空。避免油炸和油腻食物，因为脂肪会延迟胃排空。每天在所有3个步骤中均服用可咀嚼的多种维生素。

2. 营养品

含或不含生姜的液态蛋白质餐可减少与晕动病和胃节律异常相关的恶心、妊娠恶心和化疗后延迟的恶心[304-308]。这些基于蛋白质的餐食疗法尚未在胃轻瘫或胃节律异常患者中得到正式评估。

3. 其他方法

对于慢性恶心和呕吐患者，可放置经皮内镜下胃造口术（percutaneous endoscopic gastrostomy，PEG）管以定期排空胃内容物，以避免频繁的呕吐发作而改善生活质量[309]。PEG引流不能治疗潜在的胃神经肌肉失调，但它可以让患者排空胃，避免反复呕吐和不适。从而减少了住院治疗[175]。当通过胃造口术导管给药时，可以耐受一些药物和营养液体。有时可能需要用于肠内营养的空肠饲管，为患有胃神经肌肉失调而严重恶心和呕吐的患者提供基本的热量支持。连接有J管延长管的PEG通常会失败，因为一次呕吐就可能会将延长管推入胃中。需要通过内镜或手术方式来放置J管（参见第6章）[309]。由于肠外营养易出现脓毒症和偶发的静脉血栓形成，故应尽可能避免通过中心静脉内导管进行全胃肠外营养。

（程芮 译，王立 校）

参考文献

第 51 章　胃分泌

Mitchell L. Schubert, Jonathan D. Kaunitz 著

章节目录

一、功能解剖学 …… 724
二、胃酸分泌的旁分泌、激素、神经和细胞内调节 …… 726
（一）组胺 …… 727
（二）胃泌素 …… 727
（三）乙酰胆碱 …… 728
（四）生长抑素 …… 728
（五）混杂的肽类 …… 730
（六）壁细胞胞内途径 …… 730
（七）质子泵抑制剂和阻断剂 …… 731
（八）对一次进食的综合反应 …… 732
（九）幽门螺杆菌诱发的胃酸分泌紊乱 …… 733
三、胃酸分泌的测定 …… 734
（一）适应证 …… 734
（二）方法 …… 734
（三）基础胃酸排出量 …… 734
（四）最大胃酸排出量和胃酸峰值排出量 …… 734
（五）假喂食刺激酸排出 …… 735
（六）膳食刺激胃酸排出 …… 735
四、胃酸分泌增加的相关疾病 …… 735
五、胃蛋白酶原分泌 …… 736
六、胃脂肪酶分泌 …… 736
七、内因子分泌 …… 737
八、碳酸氢盐分泌 …… 737
九、黏液分泌 …… 737
十、胃液中的胃癌生物标志物 …… 738

如上一章所讨论的，胃是一个活跃的储存库，储存、研磨和缓慢地将部分消化的食物推送到肠道中，以进一步消化和吸收。其主要分泌功能是产生盐酸[1]。胃酸分泌从出生后第一天即开始，分泌量随着婴儿的成熟而增加[2]。到 2 岁时，按体重校正后酸分泌量与成年人相似[3]。大多数研究表明，除非有胃底腺黏膜的并存疾病（如感染 Hp 或萎缩性胃炎等），否则 20 岁以后酸的分泌速度变化不大[4-7]。

胃酸通过将酶原（胃蛋白酶原）转化为活性蛋白水解酶（胃蛋白酶），以促进蛋白质的消化。它还促进非血红素铁、维生素 B_{12}、某些药物（如甲状腺素）和钙的吸收，并防止细菌过度生长、肠道感染和可能的自发性细菌性腹膜炎（SBP）[8-22]。

胃除了分泌多种神经分泌、旁分泌和激素外，还分泌脂肪酶、内因子（IF）、电解质［如碳酸氢盐（HCO_3^-）、K^+ 和 Cl^-］和黏蛋白（图 51.1）。神经内分泌因子［如乙酰胆碱（ACh）、

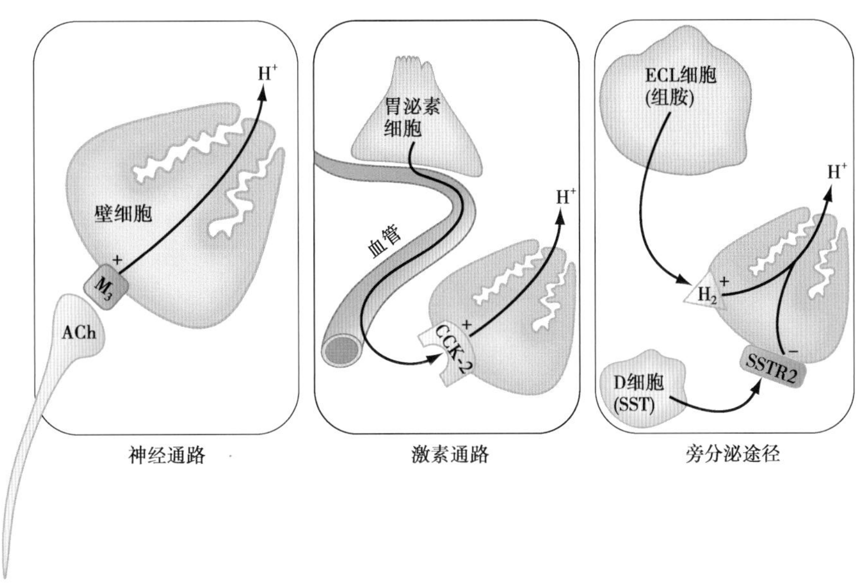

图 51.1　直接调节壁细胞酸（H^+）分泌的神经、激素和旁分泌途径。左图，乙酰胆碱（ACh）从泌酸黏膜内的节后肠神经元释放，直接通过 M_3 受体偶联细胞内钙释放刺激壁细胞分泌胃酸。中间图，胃窦 G 细胞释放的胃泌素，经血液循环到达壁细胞，并直接激活与细胞内钙释放偶联的胆囊收缩素 2 型（CCK-2）受体。右图，泌酸肠嗜铬样（ECL）细胞释放的组胺，扩散到壁细胞并直接激活组胺 H_2 受体，这些受体与环磷酸腺苷（cAMP）的生成偶联。从泌酸 D 细胞释放的生长抑素（SST）扩散到壁细胞，并直接激活生长抑素受体 2（SSTR2），与酸分泌的抑制偶联。乙酰胆碱、胃泌素和生长抑素也具有影响胃酸分泌的重要间接作用，此处未显示。+，促进；−，抑制

胃泌素释放肽（GRP）、血管活性肠肽（VIP）、一氧化氮（NO）和垂体腺苷酸环化酶激活多肽（PACAP）］从神经末梢释放并通过突触扩散达其靶细胞。旁分泌因子在其靶标附近释放，并通过扩散到达靶标（如组胺和生长抑素）。激素被释放到循环中，并通过血流到达其靶细胞（如胃泌素）（见第 4 章）。

胃黏膜的完整性取决于侵袭性物质（如酸和胃蛋白酶）和防御性物质（如碳酸氢盐和黏蛋白）分泌之间的微妙平衡（图 51.2）[23]。当黏膜防御机制不堪重负时，可能会发生溃疡。为了在没有不良反应的情况下获得胃酸的益处，精确地调节胃外分泌和内分泌，这是通过多种神经分泌、旁分泌和激素途径之间高度协调的相互作用来完成的。

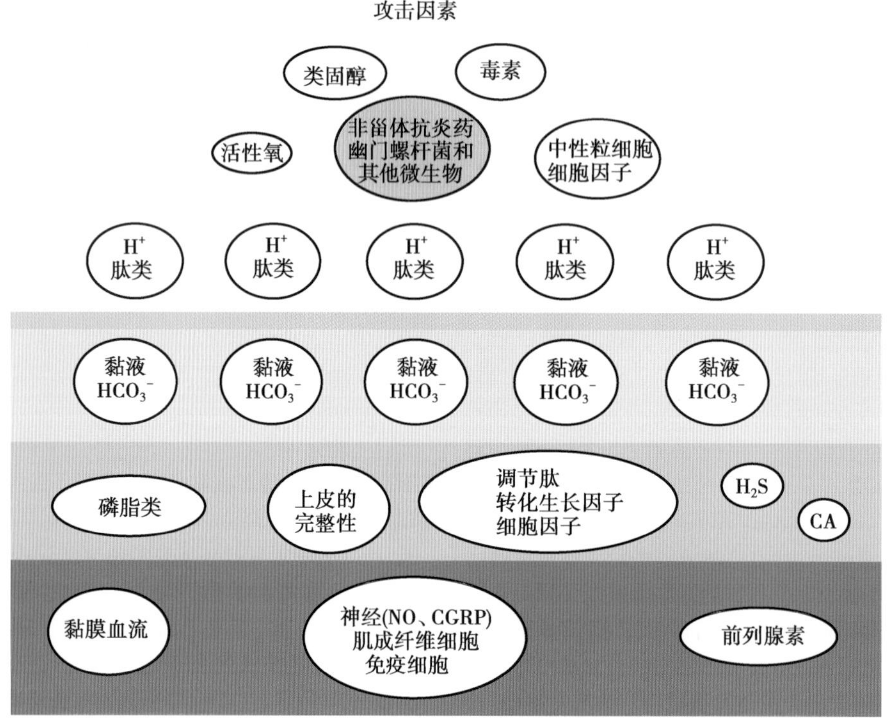

图 51.2　胃十二指肠黏膜的攻击和防御因素。黏膜完整性取决于攻击性和防御性因素之间的微妙平衡。当黏膜防御机制不堪重负时，可发生溃疡。CA，碳酸酐酶；CGRP，降钙素基因相关肽；H_2S，硫化氢；HCO_3^-，碳酸氢盐；NO，一氧化氮

一、功能解剖学

如第 49 章所述，胃由 3 个解剖区域（胃底、胃体和胃窦）和 2 个功能区域（胃底腺和幽门腺）组成（图 51.3）。胃底腺区的标志是泌酸细胞或壁细胞占器官（胃底和胃体）的 80%。幽门腺区的标志是 G 细胞或胃泌素细胞占器官（胃窦）的 20%。人胃中大约含有 1×10^9 个壁细胞和 9×10^6 个胃泌素细胞[24]。贲门是食管的鳞状黏膜和胃的泌酸黏膜之间 0~9mm 的移行过渡带，是以正常的解剖结构存在还是由于异常的反流而发展，这是有争议的（见第 44、46 和 47 章）。尸检和内镜研究提示，一般人群中 50% 以上不存在贲门黏膜[25]。

胃腺体区组织成垂直管状单位，其由顶端凹陷区、峡部和形成单位下部的实际腺体区组成；后者由颈部和基低部组成（图 51.4）。位于峡部的胃单位祖细胞产生所有胃上皮细胞。在胃底腺区，产生黏液的 pit 细胞从祖细胞向上迁移到胃腔。每个月在 1 个峡部产生 6 个产酸的壁细胞，并向下迁移至腺体的中下区域[26]。随着细胞向下迁移，它们变得更衰老，缺乏分泌酸的活性。小鼠壁细胞的周转时间为 54 天，大鼠为 164 天[24]。除盐酸外，壁细胞还产生内因子（IF）、转化生长因子-α（TGF-α）、双调蛋白、肝素结合表皮生长因子（EGF），音猬因子、铁调素和瘦素[27-29]。主细胞（酶原细胞）在腺体基底部占优势，分泌胃蛋白酶原和瘦素[30]。腺体中含有几种不同的神经内分泌型细胞，但只有其中一些细胞具有生理功能（见第 4 章）。这些细胞包括 D 细胞（分泌生长抑素和胰淀素）、肠嗜铬样（ECL）细胞（分泌组胺和甲状旁腺激素样激素）、肠嗜铬（EC）细胞（心钠素［ANP］、5-羟色胺和肾上腺髓质素）以及 A 样细胞或 Gr 细胞（生长激素释放肽和肥胖抑制素）[31-37]。含有生长抑素的 D 细胞是具有终止于壁细胞及 ECL 细胞附近的神经样胞质突起（见图 51.4）。这种解剖耦联的功能相关性是生长抑素通过抑制组胺分泌直接或间接对酸分泌施加的强烈的旁分泌抑制（图 51.5）[38-40]。肠嗜铬样细胞是胃底胃底腺黏膜中主要的神经内分泌型细胞。它们占大鼠神经内分泌细胞群的 66%，占人类的 30%。和含生长抑素的 D 细胞一样，ECL 细胞也可能具有终止于壁细胞附近的胞质突起[41]。

幽门腺区也存在含生长抑素的 D 细胞（见图 51.4 和图 51.5），它们对 G 细胞分泌胃泌素产生强烈的旁分泌抑制[42,43]。幽门腺还含有嗜铬细胞（分泌心钠素和 5-羟色胺）、

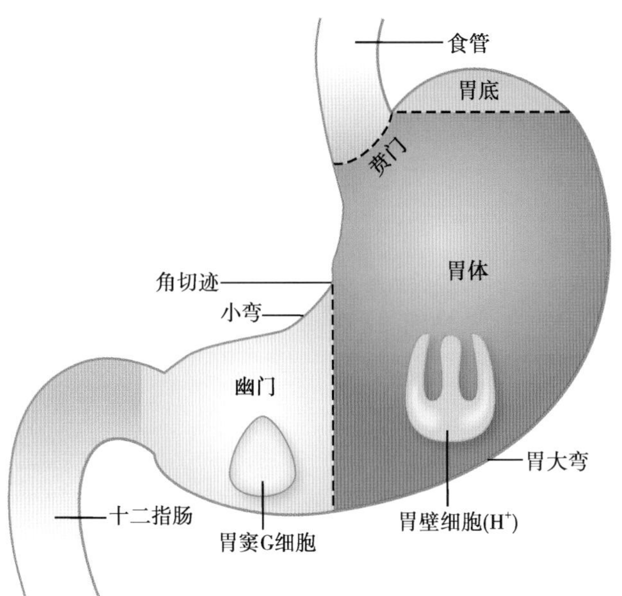

图 51.3　胃功能性解剖。胃由 3 个解剖区域(胃底、胃体和胃窦)和 2 个功能区域(胃底腺区和幽门腺)组成。胃底腺区的标志是壁细胞,幽门腺区的标志是 G 细胞或胃泌素细胞

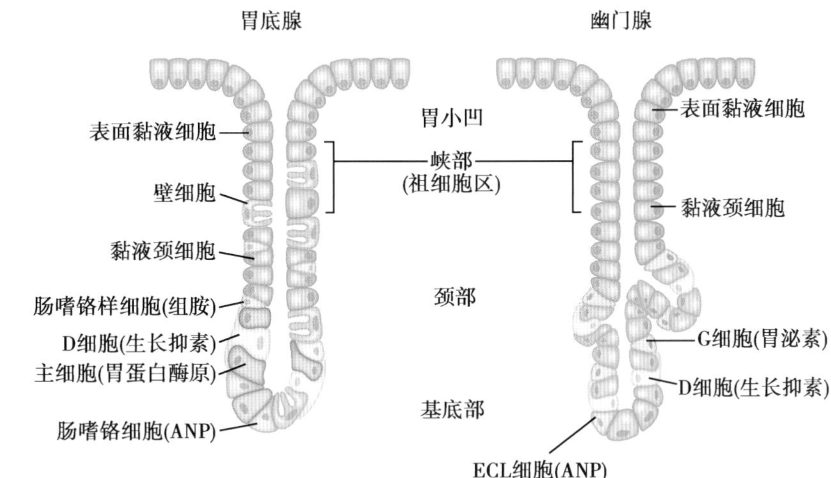

图 51.4　胃腺解剖图。含生长抑素的 D 细胞含有胞质突起,终止于胃底腺区域(胃底和胃体)分泌胃酸的壁细胞和分泌组胺的肠嗜铬样(ECL)细胞以及幽门腺区域(胃窦)分泌胃泌素的 G 细胞附近。这种解剖偶联的功能相关性是生长抑素对酸分泌强烈的旁分泌抑制,生长抑素直接作用于壁细胞,并通过抑制组胺和胃泌素分泌间接发挥作用。ANP,心钠素。(From Schubert ML, Peura DA. Control of gastric acid secretion in health and disease. Gastroenterology 2008;134:1842-60.)

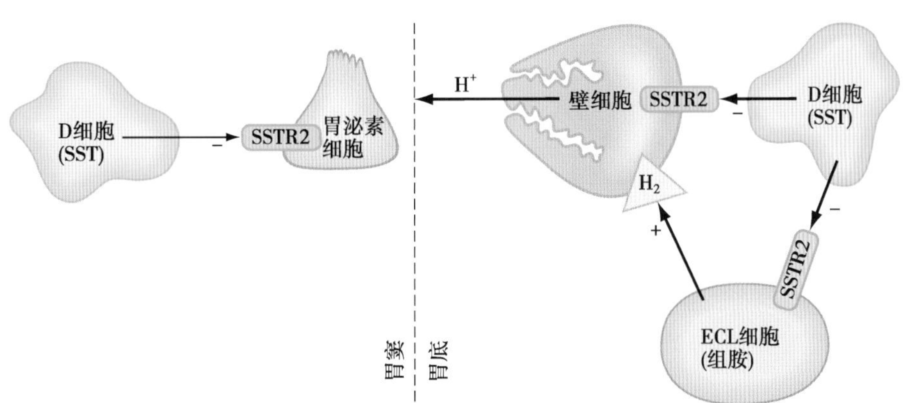

图 51.5　说明生长抑素(SST)对胃底腺区(胃底和胃体)和幽门腺区(胃窦)胃酸分泌抑制作用的模型。含 SST 的 D 细胞在结构和功能上与其靶细胞偶联:壁细胞、肠嗜铬样(ECL)细胞和胃泌素细胞。SST 通过生长抑素受体 2(SSTR2)受体发挥作用,可抑制胃酸分泌。这种抑制作用直接作用于壁细胞,也通过抑制 ECL 细胞分泌组胺和 G 细胞分泌胃泌素间接发挥作用

A 样或 Gr 细胞（分泌生长激素释放肽和肥胖抑制素），以及含有食欲肽的内分泌细胞[33,44,45]。

嗜铬粒蛋白 A（CgA）是一种酸性糖蛋白，存在于神经内分泌细胞中，如第 34 章所述，血清 CgA 已用作诊断神经内分泌肿瘤（NET，如类癌和胃泌素瘤）的敏感标志物[46]。大部分“正常”血液 CgA 来自胃 ECL 细胞。因此，在萎缩性胃炎引起的高胃泌素血症或质子泵抑制剂（PPI）治疗短至 5 天所致的 ECL 增生患者中，也观察到循环 CgA 浓度升高[47]。在停止 PPI 治疗后，血清 CgA 逐渐下降，半衰期为 4~5 天[48]。

胃由肠神经系统（ENS）的神经网络支配，ENS 含有内在神经元（即细胞体位于胃壁内的神经元）（图 51.6~图 51.8）。ENS 是自主神经系统的第三分支（另外两个是交感神经和副交感神经），通常被称为“小大脑”，因为它包含与脊髓一样多的神经元（$\approx 10^6$），可以自主进行中枢输入（见图 51.6）[49]。然而，ENS 接受来自交感神经和副交感神经元的输入，并通过交感神经和副交感神经向中枢神经系统发送输入。在大鼠和豚鼠中，胃的大部分内在神经支配起源于位于环形和纵形肌层之间的肌间神经丛，这些物种的黏膜下神经丛仅含有少量神经元。相反，人类有一个明确的黏膜下神经丛，可调节胃液分泌，并含有多种神经递质（见图 51.7 和图 51.8）。

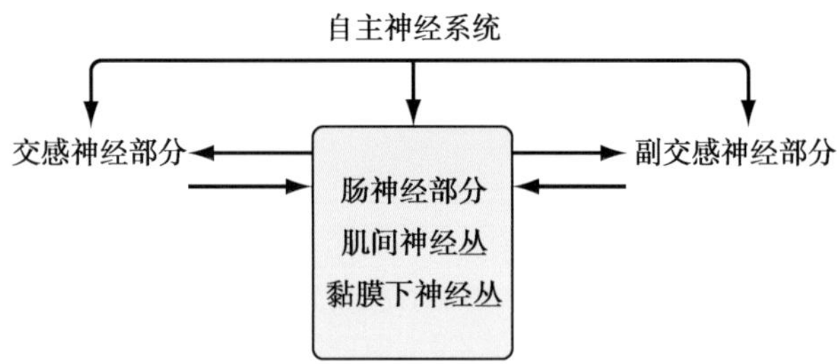

图 51.6　自主神经系统由交感神经、副交感神经和肠分支神经组成。肠分支神经由主要调节运动的肌间神经丛和主要调节分泌的黏膜下神经丛组成。虽然肠分支神经可以自主运作，但它可接受来自其他神经分支的输入并向其他分支发送投射

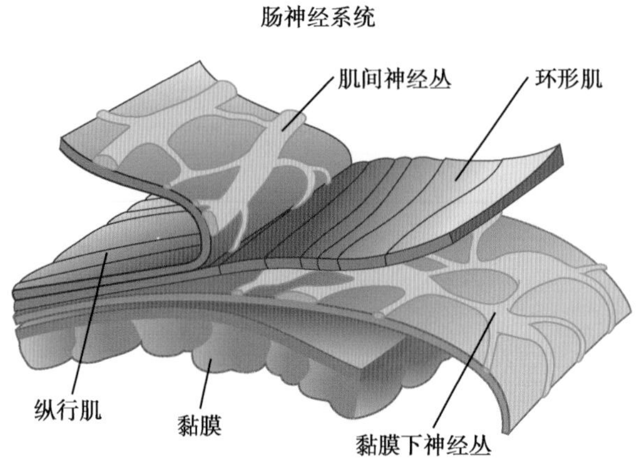

肠神经系统
肌间神经丛
环形肌
纵行肌
黏膜
黏膜下神经丛

图 51.7　肠神经系统含有内在神经元，其细胞体包含在胃壁内。肌间神经丛支配环形和纵向肌肉层，调节运动。黏膜下神经丛支配黏膜层，调节分泌

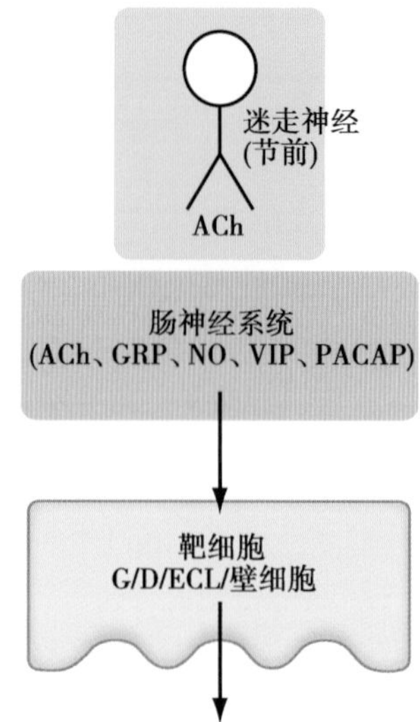

图 51.8　神经功能解剖学。迷走神经含有与肠神经形成突触的节前神经元（即作为肠神经系统一部分的胃壁内神经元）。肠神经元含有多种递质，包括 ACh、GRP（或哺乳动物蛙皮素）、NO、VIP 和 PACAP，通过调节 G 细胞的胃泌素、D 细胞的生长抑素和肠嗜铬样（ECL）细胞的组胺（可能）的分泌，来直接和/或间接调节壁细胞的酸分泌。ACh，乙酰胆碱；GRP，胃泌素释放肽；NO，一氧化氮；VIP，血管活性肠肽；PACAP，垂体腺苷酸环化酶激活多肽

迷走神经以传入神经为主，含 80%~90% 的传入纤维和 10%~20% 的传出纤维。传出纤维来自延髓中的背侧运动核。迷走神经是节前神经，不直接支配壁细胞或神经内分泌细胞，而是与 ENS 神经元突触相连。肠神经元含有多种递质，包括 ACh、GRP、NO、VIP 和 PACAP（见图 51.8）[50]。在胃中含有降钙素基因相关肽的传入神经纤维（CGRP）是外源性的，细胞体位于胃壁外[51]。ENS 神经元通过乙酰胆碱直接调节胃酸的分泌，和/或间接调节 G 细胞的胃泌素、D 细胞的生长抑素和可能的 ECL 细胞的组胺的分泌（见图 51.8）。

二、胃酸分泌的旁分泌、激素、神经和细胞内调节

壁细胞分泌浓度约为 160mmol/L 或 pH 为 0.8 的盐酸。盐酸被认为是通过黏液层通道进入腔内的，分泌过程中产生相对较高的腺内静水压力（约 17mmHg）形成了这个通道[52]。

胃酸可以促进蛋白质的消化和非血红素铁、钙和维生素 B_{12} 的吸收，还可以防止细菌过度生长、肠道感染和可能的自发性细菌性腹膜炎[8-14,18-22]。然而，当胃酸（和胃蛋白酶）的水平超过黏膜防御机制时，就会发生溃疡。为了防止溃疡形成，必须根据需要通过许多神经、激素和旁分泌通路的高度协调及相互作用来实现精确地调节及生成胃酸。这些通路可以被来自大脑的刺激直接激活，也可以被进食后来自胃部的反射性刺激激活，如机械刺激（如腹胀）或化学刺激（如蛋白质和酸）。

胃酸分泌的主要刺激物是胃肠神经元释放的乙酰胆碱、胃窦 G 细胞释放的胃泌素和泌酸区 ECL 细胞（旁分泌）释放的组胺（图 51.9；见图 51.1）。这些物质分别与特异性 G 蛋白结合受体（M_3、CCK-2 和 H_2）相互作用，与 2 条主要信号转导途径耦合：ACh 和胃泌素与细胞内钙信号通路，以及组胺与腺

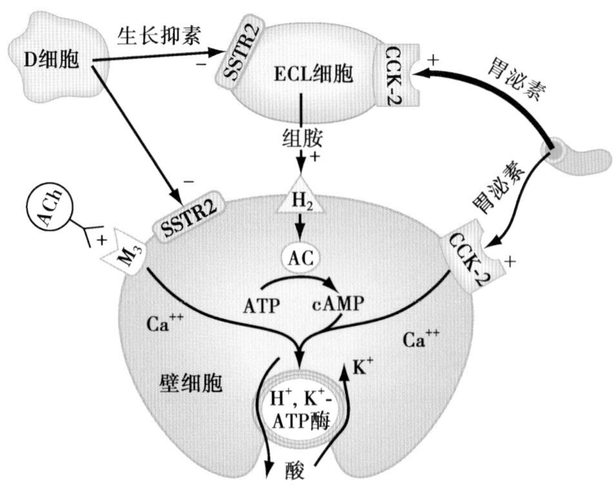

图 51.9　壁细胞受体和转导通路的模式图。壁细胞酸分泌的主要刺激物是组胺（旁分泌）、胃泌素（激素）和乙酰胆碱（ACh）（神经内分泌）。肠嗜铬样（ECL）细胞释放的组胺与 H_2 受体结合，激活腺苷酸环化酶（AC），生成腺苷 3′,5′-环磷酸腺苷（3′,5′-cAMP）。G 细胞释放的胃泌素与胆囊收缩素 2 型（CCK-2）受体结合，激活磷脂酶 C（未显示），诱导胞质钙（Ca^{2+}）释放。胃泌素通过从 ECL 细胞释放组胺直接刺激壁细胞，更重要的是间接刺激壁细胞分泌胃酸。乙酰胆碱从壁内肠神经元释放，与毒蕈碱 3 型（M_3）受体结合，后者与细胞内钙增加偶联。细胞内环磷酸腺苷（c-AMP）和钙依赖信号系统激活下游蛋白激酶，最终导致 H^+，K^+-ATP 酶（质子泵）的融合和激活。从泌酸 D 细胞释放的生长抑素是胃酸分泌的主要抑制剂。生长抑素通过 SSTR2 受体发挥作用，通过抑制 ECL 细胞释放组胺直接和间接抑制壁细胞。+，刺激，-抑制。ATP，三磷酸腺苷；SSTR2，生长抑素受体 2

苷酸环化酶或 3′,5′-环单磷酸腺苷（cAMP）途径（见图 51.9）。有证据表明组胺与乙酰胆碱或胃泌素之间存在增强作用（或协同作用），这可能是两种信号通路在受体结合后有相互作用[53]。咖啡因通过苦味感受器（2 型苦味感受器；TAS2Rs）定位于壁细胞[54]。胃酸分泌的主要抑制剂是由泌酸区的和胃窦的 D 细胞（旁分泌）释放的生长抑素（见图 51.1、图 51.5 和图 51.9）。这些分泌因子都可直接作用于壁细胞，也可通过调节神经内分泌细胞间接产生作用（图 51.10）。

（一）组胺

在 ECL 细胞中，L-组氨酸通过组氨酸脱羧酶（histidine decarboxylase，HDC）脱羧产生组胺，组胺结合 H_2 受体，偶联腺苷酸环化酶的激活和 cAMP 的产生（见图 51.9）[55]。组胺还通过与 H_3 受体结合抑制泌酸区 D 细胞释放生长抑素，从而间接刺激酸的分泌（见图 51.10）[56,57]。胃泌素、PACAP、VIP 和胃促生长素促进组胺分泌，而生长抑素、CGRP、前列腺素、肽 YY（PYY）和甘丙肽抑制组胺的分泌[58,59]。如后面讨论的，胃泌素也对 ECL 细胞有直接的增殖作用。乙酰胆碱对组胺分泌无直接影响[60-62]。

（二）胃泌素

胃泌素是在进食过程中促进胃酸分泌的主要物质，它产生于胃窦的 G 细胞，在近端小肠、结肠和胰腺中产生的量非常少且变化不定。胃泌素的合成是由 101 个氨基酸组成的前体分子，通过 N 端信号肽的裂解转化为胃泌素前体（80 个氨

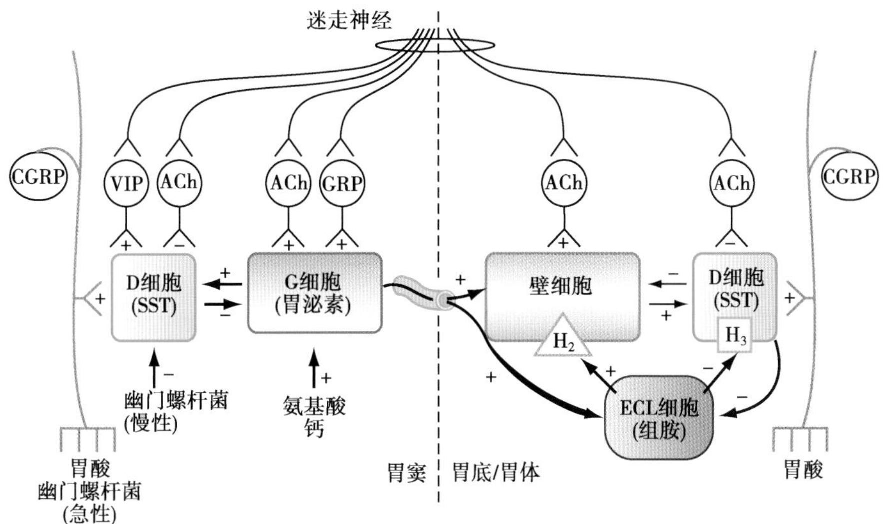

图 51.10　健康和疾病中胃酸分泌的神经、激素和旁分泌调节的模式图。迷走神经传出纤维与肠壁内胆碱能（ACh）和肽能（GRP 和 VIP）神经元形成突触。在胃底（泌酸黏膜），ACh 神经元通过抑制生长抑素（SST）分泌，直接和间接刺激胃酸分泌，从而消除其对壁细胞和含组胺的肠嗜铬样（ECL）细胞的抑制作用。在胃窦（幽门黏膜），ACh 神经元通过抑制 SST 分泌直接以及间接刺激胃泌素分泌，从而消除其对含胃泌素 G 细胞的抑制。由管腔蛋白激活的 GRP 神经元也刺激胃泌素分泌。氨基酸和钙可能直接刺激胃泌素分泌。由轻度胃膨胀激活的 VIP 神经元刺激 SST，从而抑制胃泌素分泌。双重旁分泌途径将含 SST 的 D 细胞与壁细胞和胃底/体的 ECL 细胞联系起来。ECL 细胞释放的组胺通过 H_3 受体抑制 SST 分泌。这有助于加强胆碱能刺激诱导的 SST 分泌减少，从而增加胃酸分泌。在胃窦，双重旁分泌途径将含 SST 的 D 细胞与胃泌素细胞联系起来。胃酸释放到胃腔内可激活外源性 CGRP 感觉神经元，其作用是恢复胃底和胃窦的 SST 分泌。Hp 急性感染还可激活 CGRP 神经元刺激 SST 分泌，从而抑制胃泌素（和胃酸）的分泌，抑制酸分泌有利于 Hp 的定值及感染。在慢性感染 Hp 的十二指肠溃疡患者中，炎性浸润释放的生物体或细胞因子可抑制 SST 分泌，从而刺激胃泌素（和胃酸）的分泌。+，刺激；-，抑制。CGRP，降钙素基因相关肽；VIP，血管活性肠肽；ACh，乙酰胆碱；GRP，胃泌素释放多肽

基酸）。胃泌素前体被进一步加工得到含有C端甘氨酸的多肽（即G34gly和G17gly）。最后的加工步骤包括酰胺化以产生酰胺化胃泌素34（G34amide）和酰胺化胃泌素17（G17amide）。人类分泌的胃泌素中，超过95%是胺化的，大约一半是酪氨酸硫酸化的[63]。其中，大约85%为G17，5%~10%为G34，其余为较大和较小的肽（G71、G52、G14和G6）的混合物。G34amide的血浆半衰期为30分钟，G17amide的血浆半衰期为3~7分钟。它们主要由肾脏代谢，少量由肠道和肝脏代谢[64-66]。由于G17的代谢比G34快得多，所以空腹时循环中的胃泌素大部分是G34，而餐后是G17。在肾功能不全或大量小肠切除术的患者中，空腹血G17和G34水平升高[67,68]。用于试验研究的五肽胃泌素并不是一种自然产生的肽，而是一种人工合成的类似物，它包含有生物活性的C端序列Trp-Met-Asp-Phe-NH_2。

胃泌素和CCK属于同一个多肽家族，具有相同的羧基端五肽序列（-Gly-Trp-Met-Asp-Phe-NH_2）。两类主要的胃泌素/CCK受体：CCK-1（原CCK_A）和CCK-2（原CCK_B或CCK_B/胃泌素）。CCK-1受体对CCK具有特异性，而CCK-2受体对CCK和胃泌素具有高亲和力。硫酸化和未硫酸化的G17和G34与经典的G蛋白偶联受体CCK-2具有相似的亲和力。胃泌素与受体结合可激活磷脂酶C，磷脂酶C将磷脂酰肌醇4,5二磷酸水解成肌醇1,4,5-三磷酸（IP_3）和二酰基甘油[69]。IP_3从细胞内储存中调动钙，二酰基甘油激活蛋白激酶C亚型。胃泌素通过CCK-2受体直接刺激壁细胞，更重要的是通过ECL细胞释放组胺间接刺激壁细胞（见图51.9~图51.11）[70,71]。胃泌素双相调节组胺的分泌和合成，第一阶段包括释放储存的组胺。第二阶段涉及补充组胺储存，增加HDC活性，随后增加HDC基因转录[72]。H_2受体、HDC和CCK-2受体敲除小鼠的胃酸分泌明显减少，特别是对于胃泌素的反应明显降低[73-75]。

虽然酰胺化胃泌素被认为是唯一具有生物活性的形式，但甘氨酸延伸的胃泌素可能调节壁细胞对促分泌剂的反应能力，ECL细胞释放组胺，可刺激结肠黏膜和结直肠癌细胞的增殖[76,77]。已报道N端胃泌素前体片段（如胃泌素前体片段1-35和1-19）可抑制人类胃酸分泌。ACh、GRP、PACAP、肠促胰液素、β_2/β_3肾上腺素能激动剂、5-羟色胺、钙、蛋白质、氨基酸、胺、辣椒素和发酵产生的酒精饮料刺激胃泌素的分泌；而生长抑素、甘丙肽、缓激肽和腺苷抑制胃泌素的分泌。另外，至少有2种负反馈通路通过生长抑素的释放来调节胃泌素的分泌。第一种负反馈由胃腔内酸度激活并涉及感觉CGRP神经元（见图51.10）。低胃内pH（高胃酸）激活CGRP神经元后，通过轴突反射刺激生长抑素细胞，从而抑制胃泌素分泌（见图51.10）[78-80]。相反，当胃内pH升高（胃内酸度降低）时，例如，通过使用PPI等抗胃酸分泌药物或者发生胃萎缩，生长抑素分泌不受到刺激，患者出现高胃泌素血症（见图51.11）[81]。有证据表明，胃酸过低所引起的细菌过度生长也可导致高胃泌素血症[82]。第二种负反馈途径涉及一种旁分泌作用，即胃泌素直接刺激生长抑素，从而减少其自身的分泌（见图51.10）[83]。

胃泌素也可作为一种营养激素来刺激黏膜增生。CCK-2受体定位于胃底腺的祖细胞区，慢性高胃泌素血症可直接及间接地通过自分泌或旁分泌的生长因子，如肝素结合EGF、双调蛋白、TGF-α、金属蛋白酶（见图51.11）[84,85]，促进ECL和壁细胞的增殖。给予PPI药物治疗的大鼠胃泌素升高，ECL细胞数量增加了5倍，壁细胞数量增加了1.5倍[86]。胃泌素直接作用于啮齿动物的ECL细胞，诱导其增生、异型增生，最终导致肿瘤（如，类癌）（见图51.11）[87]。与啮齿动物相反，人类很少见高胃泌素血症导致的肿瘤，除非存在其他因素，如慢性萎缩性胃炎或与多发性内分泌肿瘤Ⅰ型相关的胃腺瘤［MEN-Ⅰ（见第34章）］[88]。这可能是因为胃泌素升高的程度较低，可能需要数十年的轻度高胃泌素血症才可能诱发人类肿瘤。因为ECL细胞含有生长抑素2受体（SSTR2），^{111}铟-二乙三胺五乙酸奥曲肽生长抑素闪烁显像是检测类癌肿瘤的首选成像方法（见第34章）[89,90]。

最近的研究表明胃泌素与癌的发生有关[91,92]。胃泌素及其受体在多种人类胃肠道腺癌中表达，包括食管癌、胃癌、胰腺癌和结肠癌[93-96]。

（三）乙酰胆碱

乙酰胆碱（ACh）由节后肠内神经元释放，既可直接刺激壁细胞，也可以通过抑制生长抑素的分泌间接刺激壁细胞（见图51.10）。壁细胞毒蕈碱受体属于M_3亚型[97-99]。与CCK-2受体一样，M_3受体偶联激活磷脂酶C，生成肌醇三磷酸，释放细胞内钙（见图51.9）[97-99]。发酵酒精饮料刺激胃酸分泌，这一作用可能通过激活M_3受体来介导[100]。ACh还通过激活D细胞上的M_2和M_4受体，与抑制生长抑素分泌相结合，间接刺激酸的分泌，从而消除了该肽对胃泌素、ECL细胞和壁细胞的张力性抑制（见图51.10）。

（四）生长抑素

胃酸分泌的主要抑制剂是生长抑素。生长抑素由含有92个氨基酸的生长抑素前体分子衍生而来，该分子经处理可产生生长抑素14和生长抑素28。生长抑素14主要存在于胃、胰腺和肠道神经元中，而生长抑素28主要存在于小肠中。生长抑素14的半衰期为1~3分钟，生长抑素28的半衰期约为15分钟。

在胃中生长抑素几乎只存在于黏膜D细胞中，D细胞与其靶细胞（胃窦部胃泌素细胞、胃底/胃体的壁细胞和ECL细胞）直接通过细胞质或间接通过局部血液循环实现紧密耦合[39,101]。这种解剖耦合的功能便于生长抑素对壁细胞分泌胃酸、ECL细胞分泌组胺和G细胞分泌胃泌素的强力性抑制（见图51.5和51.10）[39-43,102,103]。通过激活胆碱能神经元来解除这种抑制（如解除抑制或消除抑制剂的影响）是刺激酸分泌的重要生理机制（见图51.10）。生长抑素的生物活性是通过6个G蛋白偶联受体介导的，称为SSTR1-SSTR5。SSTR2受体有两种剪接变体，称为SSTR2A和SSTR2B。在胃内生长抑素的作用主要通过SSTR2介导[104-106]。胃泌素、GRP、VIP、PACAP、β_2/β_3-肾上腺素能受体激动剂、促胰液素、CCK、ANP、肾上腺髓质素、抑胃肽、高浓度的腺苷、CGRP、苯丙氨酸、色氨酸和急性Hp感染刺激D细胞分泌生长抑素，而ACh、γ-干扰素、低浓度腺苷、葡萄糖、谷氨酰胺、慢性胃窦Hp感染可抑制生长抑素分泌[107-109]。如上所述，胃腔内酸度的增加通过涉及CGRP感觉神经元在胃窦和胃底释放生长抑素的途径来减弱酸的分泌。胃生长抑素分泌的变化可以在pH 3~5范围内表现出来，这是一次进食后观察到的范围变化（图51.12）[110]。

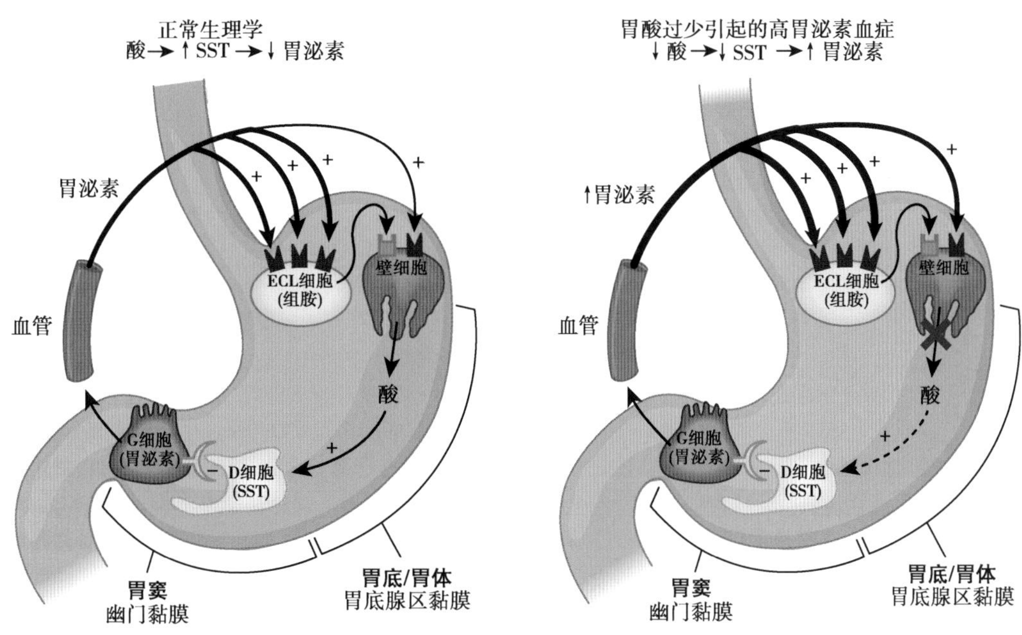

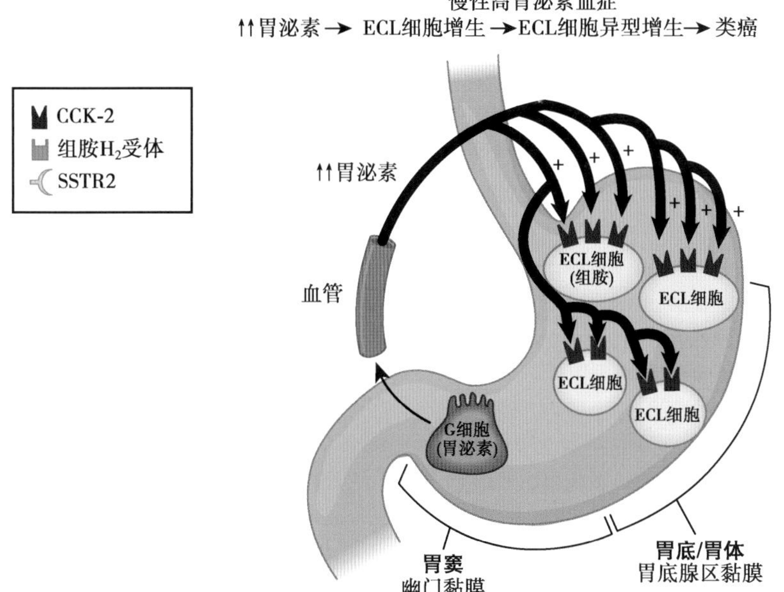

图 51.11　胃泌素作为胃内促分泌和营养激素的功能和机制的示意图。左图(正常分泌生理学):胃泌素由胃窦(幽门黏膜)的 G 细胞分泌到局部循环中,是酸分泌的主要激素刺激物。胃泌素通过胆囊收缩素 2 型(CCK-2)受体直接刺激壁细胞,更重要的是通过从肠嗜铬样(ECL)细胞释放组胺间接刺激壁细胞。组胺扩散到邻近的壁细胞(旁分泌途径),与组胺 H_2 受体结合,偶联生成环磷酸腺苷,随后激活酸性质子泵 H^+/K^+-ATP 酶。胃窦部 D 细胞分泌的生长抑素(SST)与 G 细胞上的 SST2 受体结合,对抑制胃泌素分泌发挥强烈的旁分泌抑制作用。在消化间期,局部反馈通路被激活,由此未缓冲的胃腔内酸[通过从感觉神经元释放 CGRP 发挥作用(见图 51.10)]刺激生长抑素释放,从而抑制胃泌素分泌,将酸分泌维持在较低的水平。中间图(胃酸过多诱导的高胃泌素血症):当胃酸分泌受到抑制时(例如,通过强效抗分泌药物或胃泌酸黏膜萎缩),对生长抑素分泌的刺激较小,胃泌素分泌相应增加,患者发生高胃泌素血症。右图(慢性高胃泌素血症):由于胃泌素也是一种营养激素,特别是对泌酸黏膜,慢性高胃泌素血症通过 CCK-2 受体发挥作用,诱导 ECL 细胞增生。分泌组胺的 ECL 细胞数量增加是 PPI 突然停药后观察到的反射性胃酸分泌的原因。在易感个体中,慢性高胃泌素血症诱导的 ECL 增生可进展为异型增生,并最终进展为类癌肿瘤

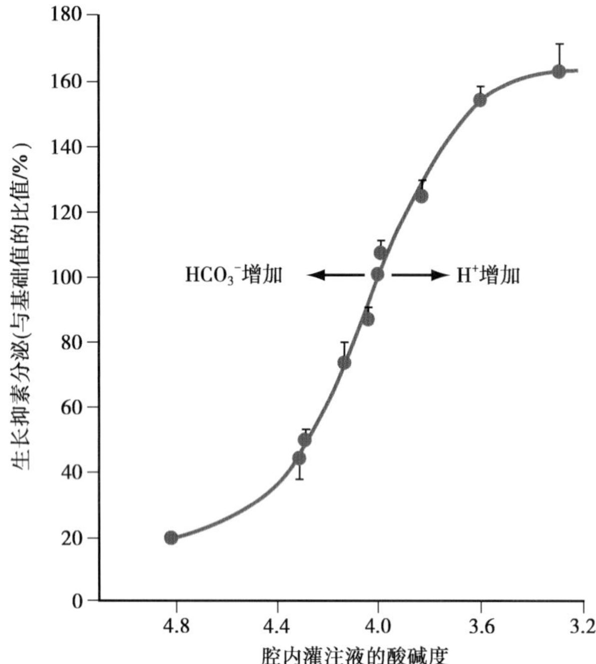

图 51.12 胃腔 pH 与胃生长抑素分泌的关系。在离体小鼠胃内,加入碳酸氢盐(HCO_3^-)中和基础酸分泌,或加入盐酸增加胃腔中的酸度,引起生长抑素分泌的相应变化。(From Schubert ML, Edwards NF, Makhlouf GM. Regulation of gastric somatostatin secretion in the mouse by luminal acid: A local feedback mechanism. Gastroenterology 1988; 94:317-22).

(五) 混杂的肽类

垂体腺苷酸环化酶激活肽(PACAP)是 VIP 肽家族的一员,存在于胃肠神经元中。PACAP 通过与一种称为 PACAP1 型受体(PAC1)的 PACAP 受体和两种 VIP 受体 VPAC1 和 VPAC2 结合而起作用。PACAP 通过结合在含组胺的 ECL 细胞上的 PAC1 受体刺激酸分泌,而通过结合在含生长抑素的 D 细胞上的 VPAC1 受体发挥抑制酸分泌的作用[111,112]。基于以上途径,已报道 PACAP 既可刺激亦可抑制胃酸的分泌[113]。

胃促生长素是生长激素促分泌受体的天然配体,以最大浓度存在于胃泌酸黏膜内,定位于 A 样(或 Gr)细胞[114,115]。少量存在于胃窦、小肠和结肠(见第四章)。哺乳动物胃黏膜产生 60% 至 80% 的胃促生长素,胃切除术后血浆胃促生长素立即减少 75%[116]。血浆胃促生长素浓度在餐前升高,餐后降低[116]。据推测,胃促生长素会引发餐前饥饿感并促进进食。Roux-en-Y 胃分流术后对它的抑制可能部分导致体重减轻[117]。此外,促胰液素、内皮素和大麻素刺激其分泌,而 Hp 感染、GRP、CCK、胰岛素、谷氨酰胺、生长抑素和干扰素-γ 降低其分泌[118-120]。大多数研究报道外源性胃促生长素刺激胃酸的分泌[121-123]。刺激作用似乎涉及迷走神经和组胺,因为在迷走神经切断术后胃促生长素的作用被消除,并且与 HDC 信使 RNA(mRNA)的增加有关[123,124]。

食欲素-A,通过从前食欲素翻译后加工衍生而来,与胃泌素共同定位于人幽门黏膜中[122,125]。侧脑室内的和外周给予食欲素-A 可刺激胃酸分泌[125,126]。在有胃瘘的大鼠中,食欲素受体 1 拮抗剂可抑制基础和五肽胃泌素刺激的胃酸分泌,这意味着内源性食欲素-A 刺激胃酸分泌[125,126]。

心钠素、胆囊收缩素、促胰液素、神经降压素、胰高血糖素样肽 1(GLP-1)、胰高血糖素、胃泌酸调节素、肾上腺髓质素、肽 YY(PYY)、胰淀素、葡萄糖依赖性促胰岛素多肽、瘦素、表皮生长因子和白细胞介素 1β 均可抑制胃酸的分泌。除了白细胞介素-1β 之外,它们的作用都是通过释放生长抑素来调节胃酸的分泌[33,38,127]。

肠胃素一词曾被用来描述一种或多种肠道因子,这些因子负责抑制胃酸的分泌,以调节肠道中的营养物质。主要包括 CCK、促胰液素、神经降压素、GLP-1、肠高血糖素和胃泌酸调节素,它们存在于肠黏膜中,由于肠腔营养物的刺激而释放到循环中,并能够在"生理"浓度下抑制胃酸分泌[128-132]。虽然这些肠胃激素的活性可能受这些多肽综合作用的影响,但最具影响的因子是 CCK(通过生长抑素起作用)。近端小肠 I 细胞产生的 CCK 由肠腔蛋白和脂肪的刺激而释放。在狗身上,通过用 CCK-1 受体拮抗剂预处理,来消除十二指肠内脂肪对胃酸的抑制作用,而在小鼠中通过敲除 CCK-1 受体来达到此目的[133-136]。

(六) 壁细胞胞内途径

在壁细胞中,胃酸分泌通过激活细胞内环磷酸腺苷和钙依赖性信号通路而增加,这些信号通路激活下游蛋白激酶,最终导致 H^+,K^+-ATP 酶(质子泵)的融合和激活,伴随着 K^+ 和 Cl^- 腔膜电导的激活(图 51.13;另参见图 51.9)[137]。质子泵以水合氢离子的形式主动泵出氢离子,对抗巨大的浓度梯度(细胞内部的 pH 为 7.4 或 40nmol/L;在 pH0.8 或 1.6 亿 nM 时分泌酸)来交换腔内钾离子。所需的能量来自壁细胞广泛的线粒体网络产生的 ATP。H^+,K^+-ATP 酶由一个 α-亚单位和另一个高度糖基化的 β-亚单位组成,α-亚单位执行酶的催化和运输功能[138],β-亚单位保护酶不被降解[139]。两个亚单位都是运输 H^+ 到顶膜所必需的,任何一个亚单位的靶向敲除都会导致胃酸缺乏[140]。

在非刺激的静止状态下,H^+,K^+-ATP 酶活性被隔离在细胞质小管泡内。当有刺激时,囊泡移位于顶端质膜并与之融合,会发生显著的形态学变化,导致膜增加 6~10 倍,并形成小管系统(图 51.14)。H^+,K^+-ATP 酶移位到小管膜,同时腔内 K^+ 激活该酶[141]。在分泌停止时,H^+,K^+-ATP 酶从顶端膜中被回收,并且小管泡室被重建。调节 H^+、K^+-ATP 酶转运的精确机制尚不清楚,但数据表明它涉及囊泡蛋白(如网格蛋白)、基于肌动蛋白的微丝、肌动蛋白结合蛋白(如 ezrin)、Rab 家族的小 G 蛋白(如 Rab10、Rab11、Rab25 和 Rab27b)、可溶性 N-乙基马来酰亚胺敏感因子附着蛋白受体(SNARE)蛋白(如 VAMP-2 和突触融合蛋白 1、2、3 和 4)和分泌载体膜蛋白(SCAMPs)[142-145]。

胃酸的分泌不仅需要有活性的 H^+、K^+-ATP 酶,还需要顶端的 K^+ 和 Cl^- 通道以及基底外侧的 HCO_3^- 和 Cl^- 交换器[146]。酸是由 CO_2 水合形成 H^+ 和 HCO_3^- 产生的,这是一种由细胞质碳酸酐酶催化的反应(见图 51.13)。因为在没有平行摄取 K^+ 的情况下,质子泵不能将 H^+ 泵入胃腔内,所以必须向胃腔输送足够量的钾离子,才能激活质子泵分泌胃酸。这种钾离

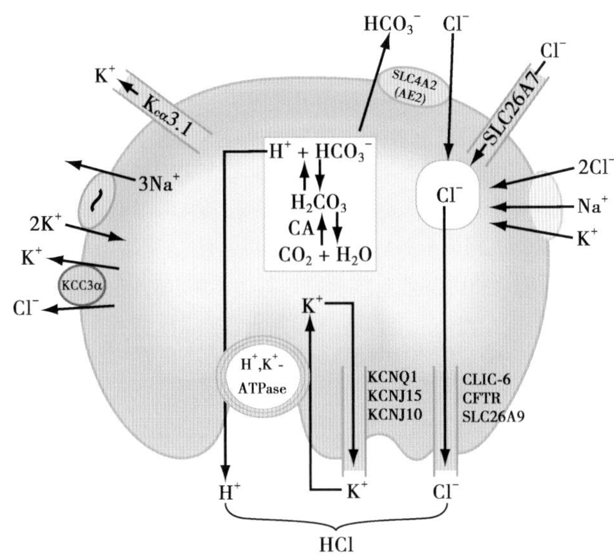

图 51.13　壁细胞中离子转运和盐酸（HCl）生成的示意图。胃酸的分泌需要一种功能性的 H^+、K^+-ATP 酶以及顶端和基底外侧的 K^+ 和 Cl^- 通道、转运蛋白和交换器。CO_2 水合形成 H^+ 和 HCO_3^- 产生酸，该反应由细胞质碳酸酐酶（CA）催化。在腔内 K^+ 存在的情况下，H^+、K^+、-ATP 酶将 H^+ 泵入胃腔内以交换 K^+。顶端 K^+ 通道（KCNQ1、KCNJ15 和/或 KCNJ10）提供 H^+、K^+-ATP 酶功能所需的 K^+。细胞内 K^+ 的来源是基底外侧 Na^+、K^+-ATP 酶（显示为～）和 NKCC1。对于分泌的每种 H^+、HCO_3^- 通过阴离子交换器（SLC4A2，或 AE2）穿过基底外侧膜退出细胞。与 H^+ 同时，Cl^- 通过氯化物细胞内通道-6（CLIC-6）、囊性纤维化跨膜调节因子（CFTR）和/或 SLC26A9 穿过管腔膜，形成中性 HCl，完成盐酸分泌。细胞内 Cl^- 的来源是基底外侧协同转运蛋白 NKCCl、交换蛋白 SLC4A2（AE2）和氯离子通道 SLC26A7 转运而来。最近，在基底外侧膜上发现了 2 个对酸分泌有负调节作用的钾离子通道：电中性 K^+，Cl^- 协同蛋白 KCC3α 和中间 Ca^{2+} 激活的 K^+ 通道 Kcα3.1。（From Chu S，Schubert ML. Gastric secretion. Curr Opin Gastroenterol 2012；28：587-93.）

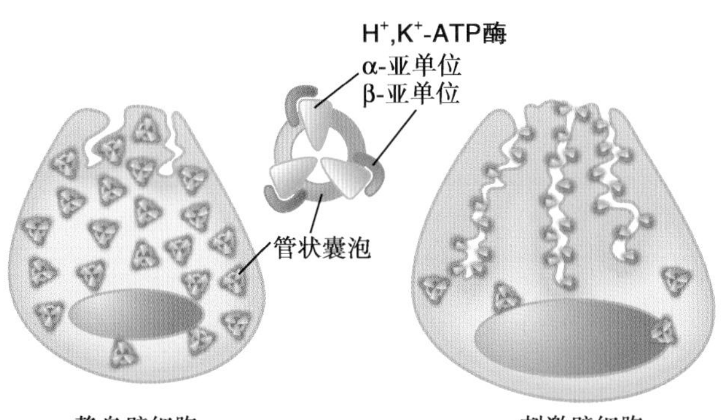

图 51.14　H^+，K^+-ATP 酶易位和活化的模式图。在静息状态下，H^+，K^+-ATP 酶被隔离在细胞质小管状囊泡内，无活性。当刺激时，小管状囊泡向顶端膜移动并与顶膜融合，形成广泛的微管状系统。H^+，K^+-ATP 酶易位到微管膜以及管腔 K^+ 的存在一起激活了该酶

子循环是由假定的腔内钾通道 KCNQ1/KCNE2、KCNJ10（Kir4.1）和 KCNJ15（Kir4.2）完成的[147,148]。KCNQ1 是一种电压激活的钾离子通道，当被小的调节亚单位 KCNE2 修饰时，导致它对电压不敏感，构成开放和酸激活的通道[149,150]。胃液（8～12mmol/L）中的钾离子浓度超过血浆钾离子浓度 2～4 倍。壁细胞的基底外侧膜可能含有对酸分泌有负调节作用的钾离子输出者（即电子中性钾离子共同转运体，KCC3a，以及中间 Ca^{2+} 激活的钾离子通道，Kca3.1）[151,152]。

对于每一个 H^+ 的分泌，都有一个 HCO_3^- 通过 SLC4A2，阴离子交换器 2（anion exchanger 2，AE2）穿过基底外侧膜（见图 51.13）[153]。由于这种 HCO_3^-/Cl^- 交换，壁细胞内的酸碱度在酸分泌过程中仅保持微碱性[154]。HCO_3^- 从壁细胞快速进入血液被称为碱性潮。其中一些 HCO_3^- 可能被胃表面上皮细胞吸收和分泌。

与 H^+ 同时，Cl^- 通过顶端氯离子通道（可能是氯离子胞内通道-6、囊性纤维化跨膜调节剂和/或 SLC26A9（见图 51.13））进入胃腔内[155]。氯离子通过基底外侧阴离子交换器（SLC4A2）、SLC26A7 通道和 Na^+-2KCl 共转运体-1（NKCC1）进入细胞（见图 51.13）[156-158]。

（七）质子泵抑制剂和阻断剂

1. 质子泵抑制剂

质子泵抑制剂（PPI）是胃酸激活的前体药物，共价结合于胃黏膜表面 ATP 酶的半胱氨酸上，从而达到抑制 H^+K^+-ATP 酶（也称为质子泵）的作用。目前的质子泵抑制剂（如奥美拉唑、兰索拉唑、雷贝拉唑、泮托拉唑和埃索美拉唑）由两个杂环部分组成，一个吡啶环和一个苯并咪唑环，由甲基磺酰基连接（图 51.15）。它们是弱碱（pKa 4 或 5），集中在体内 pH 小于 4 的酸性环境。分子的 pKa 指的是化合物接受或提供质子的意愿程度，基于对数标度，pKa 为 5 的化合物比 pKa 为 4 的化合物碱性强 10 倍。当一种化合物处于一个酸碱度等于其 pKa 的环境中时，一半的分子将被质子化，一半的分子将不被质子化。如果一种化合物，如 pKa 为 4 的质子泵抑制剂，放在一个酸碱度小于 1 的环境中，超过 99.9% 的分子将被质子化。质子泵抑制剂在非质子化形式下是膜渗透性的，在质子化形式下是相对不可渗透的。在血液（pH 7.4）中，质子泵抑制剂主要是非质子化的，因此容易进入细胞（达到血浆浓度峰值的时间，约 2 小时；消除半衰期≈1 小时），通过细胞质扩散，然后在分泌小管的酸性环境中质子化并被亚磺酰胺或亚磺酸捕获（图 51.16）[159]。由于 PPI 的基本 pKa 效应和"离子捕获"，使分泌小管中 PPI

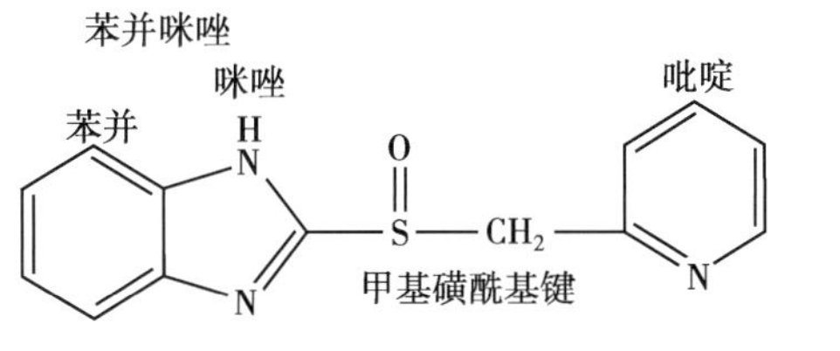

苯并咪唑
咪唑
苯并
吡啶
甲基磺酰基键

图 51.15　质子泵抑制剂的结构。质子泵抑制剂由两个杂环基团组成，一个苯并咪唑环和一个吡啶环，通过甲基磺酰基键连接。质子泵抑制剂是弱碱性（pKa 4～5），可在 pH<4 的体内酸性空间蓄积并活化。一旦在壁细胞小管内活化，质子泵抑制剂与插入的 H^+、K^+-ATP 酶 α 亚基内的某些半胱氨酸残基共价结合

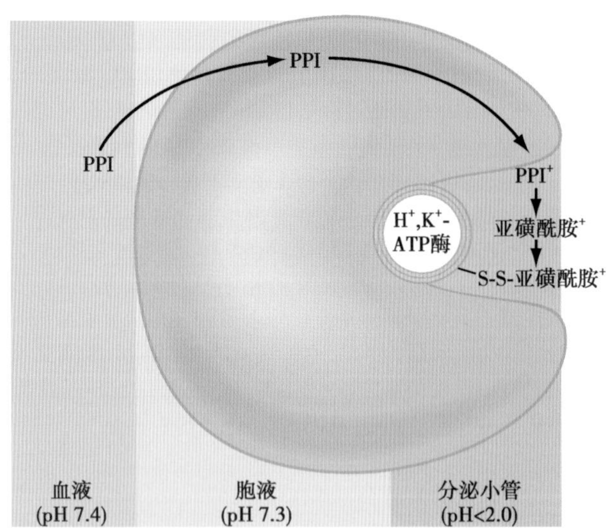

图 51.16 质子泵抑制剂(PPI)作用机制的模式图。质子泵抑制剂从血流到达壁细胞,通过细胞质扩散,并在分泌小管的酸性环境中蓄积。在小管内,质子泵抑制剂被质子化,并被捕获为亚磺酸,随后脱水为亚磺酰胺。亚磺酰胺通过二硫键与 H^+、K^+-ATP 酶的一个或多个半胱氨酸共价结合,抑制该酶活性。尽管所有 PPI 均与半胱氨酸 813 结合,但奥美拉唑也与半胱氨酸 892 结合,兰索拉唑与半胱氨酸 321 结合,泮托拉唑与半胱氨酸 822 结合

的浓度比血液中高 100 000~1 000 000 倍。亚磺酰胺迅速与 H^+,K^+-ATP 酶腔内暴露的 α 亚单位上的半胱氨酸反应,形成共价(电化学)二硫键(见图 51.15)[160]。所有质子泵抑制剂都与 α 亚单位的半胱氨酸 813 结合,奥美拉唑还与半胱氨酸 892 结合,兰索拉唑另与半胱氨酸 321 结合,泮托拉唑也与半胱氨酸 822 结合。因为只有顶端膜插入的 H^+,K^+-ATP 酶容易被质子泵抑制剂阻断,并且酸性环境(pH 4)是捕获质子泵抑制剂并将其转化为活性物质所必需的,所以当在基础(禁食)状态下给药或当酸分泌受到抑制时,质子泵抑制剂的效力会降低[161,162]。因为大多质子泵是在早餐时起作用的,所以建议在第一餐前 30 分钟至 1 小时服用质子泵抑制剂。如果需要更强的抑制作用,应在晚餐前服用额外剂量[163]。泵蛋白的重新合成使机体从抑制胃酸分泌中恢复(大鼠需 54 小时)。据推测,通过还原剂如谷胱甘肽还原半胱氨酸二硫键(大鼠 15 小时)也可能起到这种作用[164]。质子泵抑制剂抑制胃酸的生理后果是高胃泌素血症。胃泌素不仅是促胃分泌素,而且在正常组织和肿瘤组织中发挥促生长作用(见图 51.11)。高胃泌素血症可导致壁细胞和 ECL 细胞增生,在停止质子泵抑制剂后仍持续 2~3 个月[165]。临床结果是长期质子泵抑制剂停药后胃酸分泌反弹。这可能导致健康个体出现消化不良症状,加重 GERD 患者的反流症状,并引发十二指肠溃疡患者的症状[166]。在慢性严重高胃泌素血症患者中,少数 PPI 诱导的 ECL 增生可能会进展为异型增生和神经内分泌肿瘤(即 ECL 类癌;参见第 34 章)(参见图 51.11)[167-169]。在过去的 25 年中,胃神经内分泌肿瘤(NET)的发病率增加了 5 倍多,胃类癌来源于含组胺的 ECL 细胞,是胃中最常见的 NET(见第 34 章)。

尽管质子泵抑制剂已经彻底改变了胃酸相关性疾病的预后,并成为预防非甾体抗炎药和抗血小板药物引起的胃十二指肠溃疡和出血治疗的金标准,但最近有许多发表的文章提示 PPI 存在潜在的危害。潜在的严重副作用包括肠道微生物群的改变、细菌过度生长、细菌性腹膜炎、肠道感染、微量营养素缺乏、慢性肾病、认知功能障碍、心肌梗死、肺炎、骨折、药物相互作用和死亡[170]。相对有力的证据表明质子泵抑制剂与肠道微生物群的改变、微量营养素缺乏(如镁、维生素 B_{12}、铁和钙)和肠道感染有关。然而,支持其他有关的副作用证据不足,所有的资料都是回顾性观察性数据库研究,并不能确定其因果关系[171,172]。适当应用质子泵抑制剂时,益处远大于潜在的不利影响。GERD 患者,尤其是糜烂性食管炎和狭窄患者,以及非甾体抗炎药、阿司匹林和双重抗血小板治疗,所导致的溃疡相关出血风险增加的患者,应该选用质子泵抑制剂治疗。对于无适应证的患者,应停用 PPI。当开出长期处方时,应使用最低有效剂量的质子泵抑制剂,并定期重新评估其需求。

2. 钾离子竞争性酸阻断剂

钾离子竞争性酸阻断剂(如伏诺拉生和瑞伐拉赞)通过竞争性阻断钾结合位点来抑制壁细胞 H^+-K^+-ATP 酶的作用。与质子泵抑制剂相比,酸催化激活不是必需的,起效更快(第 1 天),生物利用度不受食物摄入的影响。伏诺拉生是一种吡咯衍生物,pKa 为 9,达到血浆浓度峰值的时间约为 2 小时,消除半衰期约为 7 小时[174]。虽然质子泵抑制剂和伏诺拉生在肝脏中都被细胞色素 P450(CYP450)酶代谢,但后者主要使用 CYP3A4,而质子泵抑制剂主要使用 CYP2C19。与 PPI 相比,伏诺拉生可在更大程度上抑制胃酸分泌,因此,血清胃泌素浓度高 1.5~2 倍。ECL 增生发生在人体内,胃泌素水平升高是否会导致人体内类癌肿瘤的增加仍有待确定。长期安全性尚不清楚,但肠道微生物群和细菌过度生长的变化已有报道,由于酸分泌受到明显抑制,肠道感染预计会增加。与 PPI 不同,伏诺拉生可抑制肾髓质集合管中的 H^+-K^+-ATP 酶,但其意义尚不清楚。在治疗消化性溃疡和预防非甾体抗炎药诱发的消化性溃疡(见第 53 章)、治疗 GERD 和根除幽门螺杆菌方面,其似乎与质子泵抑制剂一样有效。

(八) 对一次进食的综合反应

来自胃内外的刺激汇聚在胃肠神经元上,这些神经元是酸分泌的主要调节者。效应神经元包括胆碱能(ACh)和肽能(即 GRP 和 VIP)神经元。虽然胃黏膜内存在一氧化氮和过氧化氢酶神经元,但它们作为酸分泌调节剂的确切生理作用尚不清楚。效应神经元通过调节胃泌素、生长抑素和可能的组胺的分泌直接或间接地作用于靶细胞(见图 51.8 和图 51.10)。

在基础状态下,通过生长抑素对胃底/胃体(泌酸黏膜)中的 ECL(组胺)和壁(酸)细胞以及胃窦(幽门黏膜)中的 G(胃泌素)细胞的持续抑制作用,胃酸分泌被维持在较低的水平(见图 51.5、图 51.9 和图 51.10)。在进食期间,通过消除生长抑素的抑制作用,同时直接刺激酸和胃泌素的分泌,达到最大酸分泌,约为基础的 10 倍。这在很大程度上是通过胆碱能肠神经元的激活来实现的(见图 51.10)。对食物的关注、视觉、嗅觉和味觉占餐后总酸分泌的 50%[175]。对食物的

预期激活中枢神经元,其信息输入通过迷走神经传递到胃和幽门黏膜中的胃胆碱能肠神经元[176]。中枢神经系统的组成部分包括迷走神经的背侧运动核、孤束核和下丘脑。在胃底/体内,胆碱能肠神经元释放乙酰胆碱直接刺激壁细胞,也可通过消除生长抑素对壁细胞和 ECL 细胞的抑制性旁分泌影响而间接刺激壁细胞[56,102]。由此产生的组胺增加通过壁细胞上的 H_2 受体直接刺激酸分泌,并通过介导生长抑素分泌抑制的 H_3 受体间接刺激酸分泌(见图 51.10)[56,177]。因此,组胺通过 H_3 受体起作用,通过抑制生长抑素分泌来增强促胃分泌素刺激酸分泌的能力。胆碱能神经元的净效应是抑制所有旁分泌抑制作用(即生长抑素)和增强壁细胞上的旁分泌刺激作用(即组胺通过 H_2 受体起作用)。有一些证据表明,PACAP 肠神经元可能参与酸分泌的调节,可能是通过刺激 ECL 细胞分泌组胺,但其确切的生理作用尚不清楚[111-113,178-181]。

在胃窦中,胆碱能肠神经元通过预期进餐而被激活,直接刺激胃泌素分泌,也通过抑制生长抑素分泌而间接刺激胃泌素分泌(见图 51.10)[42,43,182-194]。在生理浓度下,胃泌素直接刺激壁细胞,更重要的是,通过增强组胺的分泌间接刺激壁细胞[195,196]。

当食物进入胃时,同样的胆碱能神经元被胃扩张进一步机械激活,并被食物的蛋白质成分化学激活[191,192,197,198]。最初,摄入的食物充当分泌酸的缓冲剂。由此导致的酸度降低(即 pH 增加)进一步抑制生长抑素的分泌,从而增加胃泌素的分泌[101,192]。蛋白激活直接刺激胃泌素分泌的 GRP 神经元(见图 51.10)。G 细胞上已发现有钙敏感受体和 L-氨基酸受体(GPRC6A),提示 G 细胞可直接感知胃腔蛋白及其分解产物(见图 51.10)[199-201]。应该注意的是,抑制生长抑素的分泌可产生最佳的胃泌素反应。

当食物从胃中排空时,许多旁分泌和神经通路被激活,以恢复生长抑素在胃底/胃体和胃窦中的抑制作用,从而抑制胃酸的分泌(见图 51.10)。第一,连接胃泌素和胃窦生长抑素细胞的刺激旁分泌途径被激活,其作用是在释放胃泌素后恢复胃窦生长抑素的分泌[83]。第二,通过预期进餐以及蛋白质和胃扩张,胆碱能神经元的激活较少。第三,随着胃扩张减少,VIP 神经元优先被激活,刺激生长抑素分泌[191]。第四,随着食物的缓冲能力丧失,胃窦和胃底生长抑素细胞(通过感觉 CGRP 神经元)暴露于腔内酸的完全刺激作用。第五,小肠释放的胃肠激素如 CCK,刺激生长抑素分泌。胃底和胃窦生长抑素分泌的增加减弱了胃酸和胃泌素的分泌,恢复了消化间期的基础状态。这种状态的特征是连续的生长抑素细胞对 ECL 细胞(组胺)、壁细胞(酸)和 G 细胞(胃泌素)的持续抑制(见图 51.9 和图 51.10)。这种抑制的减少足以再次引发胃酸分泌。

(九) 幽门螺杆菌诱发的胃酸分泌紊乱

幽门螺杆菌急性感染导致胃酸过少[202-206],而慢性感染导致胃酸过少或过多(图 51.10 和图 51.17),这取决于感染的严重程度和感染部位。对理解幽门螺杆菌在胃中定植并可能导致溃疡的机制提供了一些见解。

急性幽门螺杆菌感染期间胃酸分泌的减少被认为有利于

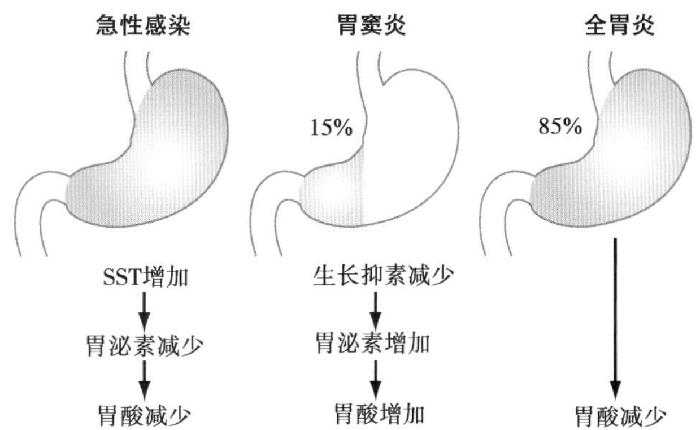

图 51.17 Hp 感染对胃酸分泌影响的模式图。急性 Hp 感染与生长抑素(SST)增加有关,从而使胃泌素和胃酸分泌减少。慢性感染可能与胃酸分泌减少或增加有关,这取决于胃炎的严重程度和分布。大多数慢性感染 Hp 的患者表现为全胃炎,并出现胃酸分泌减少。少数慢性感染患者表现为以胃窦为主的胃炎,这些患者易患十二指肠球溃疡,由于胃窦 SST 分泌减少和随后胃泌素分泌的相应增加,产生胃酸量增加。(From Schubert ML, Peura DA. Control of gastric acid secretion in health and disease Gastroenterology 2008;134:1842-60.)

细菌的存活及其在胃中的定植[207]。幽门螺杆菌抑制胃酸分泌的机制是多因素的,包括细菌成分(如空泡毒素、脂多糖或酸抑制因子)对壁细胞(可能还有 ECL 细胞)的直接抑制作用,以及细胞因子、激素、旁分泌变化对壁细胞功能的间接抑制和神经调节机制作用[208-211]。幽门螺杆菌本身可干扰质子泵转录和翻译,以及插入壁细胞顶端膜[212,213]。它还引起宿主分泌至少 2 种细胞因子(IL-1β 和肿瘤坏死因子-α),直接抑制壁细胞分泌。急性感染 Hp 的大鼠,其胃黏膜中幽门螺杆菌可激活 CGRP 感觉神经元,与已激活的生长抑素相结合,从而抑制胃泌素、组胺和胃酸的分泌(见图 51.10)[206,215]。神经通路的激活可解释,初次定植于胃黏膜表面的幽门螺杆菌可导致胃酸分泌下降。

另一方面,幽门螺杆菌的慢性感染可能与胃酸分泌减少或增加有关,这取决于胃炎的严重程度和分布(见图 51.17)[216]。大多数慢性感染幽门螺杆菌的患者表现为全胃炎(见第 52 章),并产生低于正常量的胃酸[217]。初期胃酸分泌减少是由于幽门螺杆菌本身的产物或更可能是炎症过程的产物对壁细胞功能的抑制,如前面讨论的急性感染[218,219]。这一过程通常随着 Hp 的根除而逆转[220-222]。在这类患者中,幽门螺杆菌可以预防 GERD、Barrett 食管和食管腺癌,并增强质子泵抑制剂的抗分泌作用[223,224]。在幽门螺杆菌阴性的患者中,停止长期(即>8 周)质子泵抑制剂治疗可能会导致反跳性胃酸分泌过多,这可能会出现 GERD 症状或加重 GERD 病情,特别是在巨大裂孔疝患者中更容易出现这些现象[225,226]。胃酸分泌过多持续至少 8 周,可能是因为高胃泌素血症而导致壁细胞和 ECL 细胞数量增加[227]。但幽门螺杆菌感染患者在停止质子泵抑制剂后无胃酸反跳现象,其原因可能是由于幽门螺杆菌以及炎症浸润产生的细胞因子抑制了酸的分泌,从而掩盖了反弹。随着时间的推移,慢性感染幽门螺杆菌的患者可能会出现胃底腺体萎缩和壁细胞丢失,导致不可逆的胃酸缺乏(见第 52 章)。

第 52 章中讨论的自身免疫性胃炎是一种泌酸黏膜的炎

症性疾病,其特征是针对壁细胞质子泵的自身抗体,随后壁细胞减少[228,229]。H^+,K^+-ATP 酶是部分幽门螺杆菌感染患者的主要自身抗原,针对这些抗原的抗体可能在萎缩性胃炎后期发展中起一定作用。推测这种抗体的产生是因为幽门螺杆菌脂多糖和质子泵之间有相似的抗原。这两种蛋白都含有 Lewis 表位[230]。在美国普通人群中,自身免疫性胃炎的患病率约为 2%,但在患有其他自身免疫性疾病(如 1 型糖尿病、甲状腺疾病和外周血单核细胞增多症)的患者中,其患病率增加了 3~5 倍[231]。

应该注意的是,只有 10%~15% 的慢性感染幽门螺杆菌的患者胃酸分泌增加。这些患者有以胃窦为主的炎症,并易患十二指肠溃疡(见第 52 和 53 章)。胃酸分泌增加被认为是由于胃窦生长抑素含量减少,基础和刺激胃泌素分泌增加(见图 51.16)[232-235]。生长抑素分泌减少的确切机制尚不清楚,但可能涉及炎症和/或幽门螺杆菌产生的 N-甲基组胺(一种选择性 H_3 受体激动剂)诱导的细胞因子[236,237]。人们可以推测 H_3 受体激动剂可以扩散穿过胃窦黏膜与胃窦生长抑素细胞上的 H_3 受体相互作用。导致生长抑素分泌抑制,从而刺激胃泌素分泌[57]。此外,白细胞介素-8 和血小板活化因子在幽门螺杆菌感染的黏膜中上调,能够刺激分离的 G 细胞释放胃泌素[238,239]。

三、胃酸分泌的测定

(一) 适应证

胃酸分泌检测可评估胃产生胃酸的基础和最大能力。大多数十二指肠溃疡患者和几乎所有胃泌素瘤(Zollinger-Ellison 综合征)患者的胃酸分泌增加,而慢性萎缩性胃炎、恶性贫血和胃腺癌的胃酸分泌非常低或缺乏。胃酸分泌试验在临床上越来越少被应用,但它可能有助于高胃泌素血症(如胃泌素瘤)患者的诊断和治疗,以及术后复发性消化性溃疡患者迷走神经切断术不完全的诊断。显示空腹胃酸分泌情况或空腹胃 pH 可排除胃酸缺乏是空腹血清胃泌素浓度升高的原因。胃泌素瘤患者表现为高胃泌素血症,基础酸分泌量增加(见第 34 章)。胃分泌试验也可能有助于评估新的抗酸分泌药物的抑酸作用,并可能为难治性 GERD 和消化不良患者的治疗方案调整提供依据。

(二) 方法

吸出胃液是测定人体胃酸分泌最常用的方法。传统方法是将一鼻胃管放入禁食者胃内合适的部位。可通过透视或注射 100mL 水后回收 90mL 以上来确定位置是否合适。通过负压吸引收集胃液。当胃管定位合适时,只有 5%~10% 的胃液不被收集,进入十二指肠。碳酸氢盐的中和作用,及微量酸扩散回黏膜,导致对真实分泌速率的小幅低估。最近,有一种内镜技术来测量胃泌素瘤患者的酸分泌。在这种技术中,所有的胃内容物被吸出并丢弃,然后在内镜直视下收集单个 15 分钟的胃液样本[240]。虽然用电极或无线胶囊测量胃 pH 的方法越来越多地被使用,但是应该注意的是,这种技术并不能定量评估胃酸的产生量,因此,其测定值不一定与传统的吸出技术的检测值一致。

胃液样品中的 H^+ 浓度可通过两种方法中的一种来测定。首先,样品可以在体外用碱(如氢氧化钠)滴定。将一定体积的胃液滴定至任意酸碱度终点(如 7)所需的碱毫摩尔(mmol)代表样品的"可滴定"酸度,单位为 mmol/L。另一种方法是用电极测量样品的酸碱度。因为酸碱度电极测量的是氢离子的活性而不是浓度,所以有必要将活性转化为使用胃液中 H^+ 活度系数表的浓度[241]。用这两种方法中任何一种测定出样本 H^+ 浓度(单位:mmol/L)后,再乘以样本体积(单位:L),即可测定采集期间的酸量(如 mmol/h 或 mmol/kg 体重/h)。

(三) 基础胃酸排出量

基础酸分泌量(basal acid output,BAO)是避免刺激的条件下评估静息状态下的胃酸分泌。收集连续 4 个 15 分钟的时间段所测酸量的总量,并用每小时的 H^+ mmol 数表示基础胃酸分泌。男性基础胃酸排出量的正常上限约 10mmol H^+/h,女性约 5mmol H^+/h(表 51.1)[242]。基础胃酸排出量的数值在同一个人身上也是每小时都在波动的。基础胃酸排出量的最低值出现在早上 6 点到 11 点之间,基础胃酸排出量的最大值出现在下午 2 点到 11 点之间。这种变化也与周期性胃运动活动有关,胃运动复合波期基础胃酸排出增加[243]。

(四) 最大胃酸排出量和胃酸峰值排出量

最大胃酸排出量(maximal acid output,MAO)和胃酸峰值排出量(peak acid output,PAO)是用来估计外源性促分泌剂如五肽胃泌素(皮下或肌内注射 6μg/kg 或持续静脉注射 6μg/kg/h)刺激下的胃酸排出量。五肽胃泌素是一种人工合成的类似于胃泌素的物质,含有生物活性的 C 端序列。可能的副作用有脸红、恶心、腹痛、头晕和心悸。然而许多国家不再生产五肽胃泌素。

MAO 是 4 个连续 15 分钟采集周期的酸输出之和。PAO 的计算方法是将 4 个测试周期中记录的 2 个最高排出量的总和乘以 2。MAO 的预期范围为每小时 5~50mmol H^+,PAO 为每小时 10~60mmol H^+。男性和吸烟者的 MAO、BAO 含量较高,这与壁细胞数量(即壁细胞总数)相关。健康受试者和疾病患者 MAO 的典型结果见表 51.1。

表 51.1　健康和疾病中胃分泌试验的典型结果

	基础胃酸分泌量 (BAO)/(mmol H^+/h)		最大胃酸分泌量 (MAO)/(mmol H^+/h)	
	平均	范围	平均	范围
健康受试者				
男性	2.5	0~10	25	7~50
女性	1.5	0~5	15	5~30
十二指肠溃疡				
男性	5.0	0~15	40	15~60
女性	3.0	0~15	30	10~45
胃溃疡				
男性	1.5	0~8	20	5~40
女性	1.0	0~5	12	3~25
胃泌素瘤				
男女合计	0.5	10~90	65	30~120

（五）假喂食刺激酸排出

可通过假喂食来研究胃酸分泌的头相，对美食的想法、视觉、嗅觉和味觉通过迷走神经传递到胃肠神经元，刺激胃酸排出[175,244]。假性喂养，咀嚼食物，然后吐出，约 50% 会出现 PAO。思维和味觉似乎比视觉和嗅觉起着更重要的作用。胆碱能和 GRP 神经元也参与其中，因为阿托品或选择 GRP 拮抗剂可以消除这种反应[245]。假喂养刺激酸排出可用于诊断术后复发性消化性溃疡患者的迷走神经是否完全切断[246]。

（六）膳食刺激胃酸排出

体内连续胃内滴定法是一种用于测量膳食刺激胃酸排出的研究工具[247,248]。它测量胃酸排出的胃期和小肠期。在胃内最合适的部位放置双腔管，并将缓冲到 pH 5.5 或 5 的均质膳食注入胃中。从一个胃腔中取少量胃内容物，测量 pH，然后将内容物返回胃。第二个腔用于在进食时注入碳酸氢钠以维持胃 pH。维持胃内容物 pH 恒定所需的碳酸氢钠量是衡量餐后酸分泌反应的指标。进食后胃酸分泌迅速增加，接近 PAO。

四、胃酸分泌增加的相关疾病

十二指肠溃疡患者表现为基础和刺激的胃泌素和胃酸的产生增加（见表 51.1）[249]。众所周知，大多数十二指肠溃疡是由胃窦感染 Hp 引起的（见第 52 章），这种感染是导致这些患者体内胃酸分泌紊乱的原因。在 Hp 感染的十二指肠溃疡患者中，用壁细胞泌酸功能指标的五肽类胃泌素可刺激 PAO 增高，就如同内源性胃泌素功能性反应指标的 GRP 刺激可引起 PAO 增加一样[234,250,251]。Hp 感染对生长抑素分泌抑制可能是这些变化的根本原因（见图 51.10 和图 51.17）。根除 Hp 既能恢复生长抑素的分泌，又能随着时间的推移使基础的和受刺激的胃泌素和酸的分泌降低到正常水平，从而为十二指肠溃疡提供永久性治愈[233,234,250,252-254]。

与十二指肠溃疡相比，胃溃疡患者即使感染 Hp，其基础和刺激性酸的产生却正常或减少（见表 51.1）。这表明胃黏膜防御的改变可能具有重要的病理生理学意义（见第 53 章）。根据其胃溃疡部位及是否并发有十二指肠溃疡将胃溃疡进行分类[255]。Ⅰ型溃疡发生在胃体内，一般以低酸分泌为特征。这些结果可能反映了更严重和更广泛的泌酸黏膜炎症和功能性壁细胞团减少。Ⅱ型溃疡发生在胃窦，以低、正常或高酸分泌为特征。Ⅲ型溃疡发生在幽门 3cm 内，常伴十二指肠溃疡，以高酸输出为特征。Ⅳ型溃疡发生在胃贲门，以低酸分泌为特征[256]。因此，胃溃疡离幽门越远，胃酸分泌就越少。

有以胃酸分泌过多和随后的消化性溃疡为特征的其他少见疾病（见第 53 章）。如全身性肥大细胞增多症，由于肥大细胞数量增加而产生高组胺水平，持续刺激壁细胞分泌酸[257]。部分毕Ⅱ术后的患者保留的部分胃窦组织可被碱性分泌物刺激，导致生长抑素分泌减少，胃泌素增多，胃酸分泌增加，吻合口溃疡形成[80,110,258]，任何原因导致的慢性高钙也可导致酸分泌过多，因为钙直接刺激 G 细胞分泌胃泌素及壁细胞分泌酸[259,260]。

如第 34 章所讨论的，最典型的以胃酸分泌过多为特征的疾病是胃泌素瘤[261-263]。BAO 几乎总是高于 15mmol/h，并且 BAO/PAO 比值通常为 0.6 或更高（见表 51.1）。由胃泌素瘤合成的胃泌素分泌入血液中，随着血液循环到达胃黏膜，与泌酸的壁细胞及产生组胺的 ECL 细胞上的 CCK-2 受体结合，诱导胃酸分泌和黏膜的增生。黏膜增生的临床表现为壁细胞和 ECL 细胞增生和皱襞肥大。虽然正常人体主要分泌 G17，其次是 G34，但胃泌素瘤患者主要分泌 G34，其次是 G17，并且胃泌素浓度明显增高。

胃泌素瘤的诊断和治疗在第 34 章已详细讨论。促胰液素试验诊断胃泌素瘤的基本原理是在正常情况下，胃窦生长抑素细胞能抑制 G 细胞分泌胃泌素。促胰液素直接刺激 G 细胞，同时通过刺激生长抑素的分泌间接抑制 G 细胞；后者的作用通常占主导地位，促胰液素对胃泌素的刺激程度不显著（图 51.18）。由于胃泌素瘤不存在有功能耦合的生长抑素细胞，促胰液素的作用仅仅是刺激胃泌素瘤细胞分泌胃泌素[264-266]。几乎所有的胃泌素瘤也含有生长抑素受体，选用^{111}In-DTPA 苯丙氨酸奥曲肽扫描，使生长抑素受体显像，这个方法是胃泌素瘤定位的首选方法，其对原发性肿瘤的敏感性为 71%，特异性为 86%，对转移性疾病的检测灵敏度为 92%[267,268]。PPI 是首选的抗酸分泌疗法，在大多数胃泌素瘤患者中能控制其胃酸分泌及预防并发症[269]；PCAB 可能是另一种替代方案。

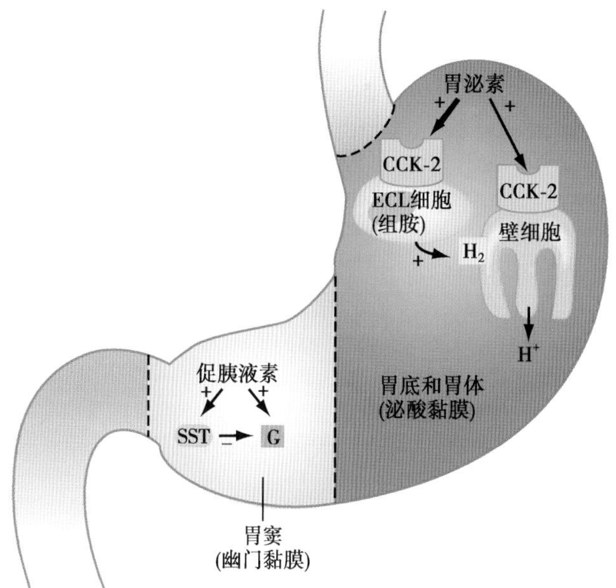

图 51.18　Zollinger-Ellison 综合征（ZES）患者胃泌酸黏膜中胃泌素和幽门黏膜中促胰液素作用的示意图。胃泌素由胃泌素瘤合成并分泌到血液中，通过分泌胃酸的壁细胞和分泌组胺的肠嗜铬样（ECL）细胞上的胆囊收缩素 2 型（CCK-2）受体发挥作用，增加胃酸分泌并诱导细胞增殖。在胃窦中，外源性胰泌素［即胰泌素刺激试验（见正文和第 34 章）］通常直接刺激胃泌素分泌，同时刺激生长抑素（SST）的分泌而抑制胃泌素分泌，导致很少或无胃泌素释放。然而，在 ZES 患者中，由于胃泌素瘤不含功能偶联的 SST 细胞，胰泌素的作用仅是刺激肿瘤分泌胃泌素。（From Hung PD，Schubert ML，Mihas AA. Zollinger-Ellison syndrome. Curr Treat Options Gastroenterol 2003；6：163-70.）

大约25%的胃泌素瘤患者有MAN-I,这是一种常染色体显性遗传病,以胰腺内分泌肿瘤、甲状旁腺功能亢进和垂体腺瘤为特征(见第33章)。它是由编码核蛋白Menin的*MEN-I*基因突变引起的临床综合征。Menin存在于G细胞中,具有抑制胃泌素基因表达的作用[270]。

五、胃蛋白酶原分泌

胃蛋白酶原属于胃天冬氨酸蛋白酶家族,是一种不活跃的多肽原酶,称为酶原。它们主要在主细胞中合成,但也在颈部黏液细胞中合成。胃蛋白酶原在胃腔内被胃酸转化为胃蛋白酶,其中含有2个活性位点的天冬氨酸残基。一旦这个反应开始,胃蛋白酶可以自催化胃蛋白酶原转化为胃蛋白酶[271]。胃蛋白酶在pH为1.8至3.5时具有最佳活性,在pH为5时出现可逆失活,在pH为7时出现不可逆性失活。胃酸不仅为消化活性提供了一个最佳pH,而且它本身也可使食物蛋白变性,使其更容易被消化水解。因此,胃酸和胃蛋白酶协同工作,促进消化食物蛋白。如前所述,部分消化的蛋白质刺激胃泌素,从而分泌胃酸[272]。最近的数据表明,胃蛋白酶可能对杀灭摄入细菌也有重要作用[17,273]。

胃蛋白酶原被分离成7个同工酶。在pH为5时电泳向阳极迁移最快的5个组分(胃蛋白酶原1到胃蛋白酶原5)在免疫学上类似,称为Ⅰ组胃蛋白酶原(PG Ⅰ;旧称"胃蛋白酶原A")[274]。PG Ⅰ在泌酸黏膜的主细胞和黏液细胞中表达。位于PG Ⅰ之后的是2种免疫学上类似的同工酶原,胃蛋白酶原6和胃蛋白酶原7,称为Ⅱ类胃蛋白酶原(PG Ⅱ;旧称"胃蛋白酶原C")。PG Ⅱ约占胃蛋白酶总含量的20%,在泌酸黏膜和幽门黏膜以及十二指肠Brunner腺中表达。

胆碱能肠神经元释放的乙酰胆碱是胃蛋白酶原分泌最重要的生理刺激物。ACh通过主细胞上的M_1和M_3毒蕈碱受体作用,增加胞质钙浓度[275]。钙反过来激活细胞质激酶、磷酸酶和一氧化氮合酶,诱导胃蛋白酶原的分泌[276]。其他能够通过钙信号通路刺激主细胞分泌胃蛋白酶原的因子包括缩胆囊素、胃泌素和GRP[277-280]。增加主细胞内cAMP的因子,如异丙肾上腺素、促胰液素、血管活性肠肽和组胺,也会增加胃蛋白酶原的分泌。就像激活酪氨酸激酶的因子,如表皮生长因子、转化生长因子-α促进胃蛋白酶分泌一样[279]。此外,胃扩张通过结合一氧化氮(NO)胆碱能途径增加胃蛋白酶原分泌入胃腔内[281]。胃蛋白酶原的分泌抑制剂包括生长抑素、神经肽Y、PYY和IL-1β。因此,根除Hp这种通过产生IL-1β促进宿主炎症反应的细菌,可以恢复胃蛋白酶原的分泌[282]。最佳的胃蛋白酶原分泌也需要一个功能性的钠-2氯化钾协同转运体(NKCCl)[157]。

血清PG Ⅰ浓度与MAO相关;血清胃蛋白酶原越来越多地被用于无创诊断胃萎缩(见第52章)[283,284]。因此,血清PG Ⅰ小于30μg/L或血清PG Ⅰ/PG Ⅱ比值≤3.0被用作无创检测胃黏膜萎缩[287,288]。因为高胃泌素血症是胃酸缺乏的生理反应,空腹血清胃泌素浓度超过400pg/mL也可能提示胃萎缩的存在。利用界值曲线分析大规模日本人群的血清PG Ⅰ、PG Ⅱ、PG Ⅰ/PG Ⅱ和胃泌素测量值结果,这些数据显示,如果区分了Hp阳性和阴性状态,萎缩性胃炎的诊断准确性可进一步提高[289]。因此,PG Ⅰ、PG Ⅱ、其比值和空腹胃泌素已被用作评估萎缩程度的血清学标记[285,286-288]。

应该注意的是,PPI治疗后人血清PG Ⅰ可升高,Hp感染后其血清PG Ⅱ也会升高[290-292]。PG Ⅰ和PG Ⅱ均经肾脏过滤代谢,但肾功能不全患者血清PG Ⅰ浓度升高高于PG Ⅱ浓度[293,294]。此外,亚洲和西方人群在PG Ⅰ和PG Ⅱ浓度与酸分泌相关性方面可能存在差异。

因为PG是由胃分泌的,它们在非胃组织中存在可提示为病理状况。例如,食管中胃蛋白酶的存在可以表明胃食管反流的存在;它存在于气道中可能表示咽喉反流。一些数据支持呼吸消化道的上皮细胞摄取胃蛋白酶,这可能参与致癌作用[295]。

六、胃脂肪酶分泌

胃脂肪酶由胃泌酸黏膜的主细胞分泌,通过水解生成游离脂肪酸、甘油二酯和2-单甘油酯来促进食物中甘油三酯的消化。胃脂肪酶的性质与胰脂肪酶有很大的不同。胃脂肪酶的最适pH为4.5~5.5(胰脂肪酶为6.5~7.4),且不需要辅酶。此外,308残基的N-糖基天门冬酰胺对消化性蛋白水解的保护作用,使胃脂肪酶在酸性胃液(pH=2)中保持其活性,尽管胃液有很高的消化性[296,297]。

胃脂肪酶的激活剂和抑制剂类似于胃蛋白酶原的分泌。据报道,衰老会减少胃脂肪酶的分泌,尽管相关数据还存在争议[298]。在人类中,饮食中脂肪含量的增加会导致胃脂肪酶分泌的相应增加[299]。餐后胃脂肪酶分泌量比胰脂肪酶少。但是,胃脂肪酶的活性等于或大于胰脂肪酶。因此,胃脂肪酶能够消化食物中10%~25%的甘油三酯[300]。外分泌性胰腺功能不全的患者胃脂肪酶的分泌量会增加3~4倍,可部分但不完全弥补胰脂肪酶的缺失(图51.19)[301]。有一种反馈机

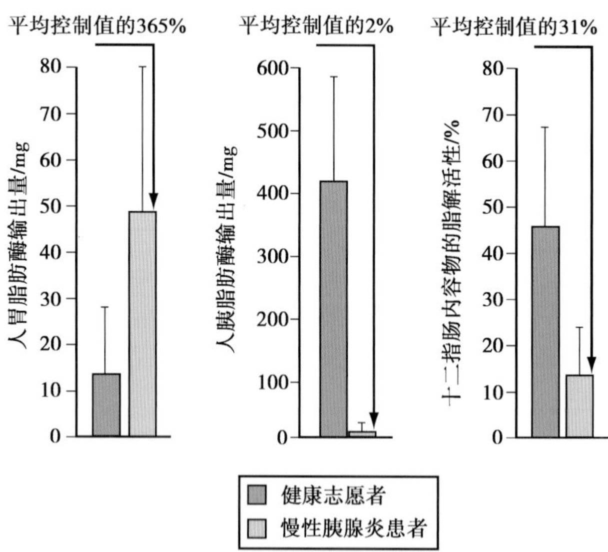

图51.19　健康志愿者和慢性胰腺炎伴外分泌功能不全(慢性胰腺炎)患者中人胃脂肪酶(左图)、人胰脂肪酶(中图)和十二指肠内容物中脂解活性(右图)的相对输出量。注意,尽管慢性胰腺炎患者的人胃脂肪酶输出量增加,但总体升高幅度不足以完全纠正十二指肠脂解活性的降低。(From Carrière F, Grandval P, Renou C, et al. Quantitative study of digestive enzyme secretion and gastrointestinal lipolysis inchronic pancreatitis. Clin Gastroenterol Hepatol 2005;3:28-38.)

制是小肠中的脂肪通过激素途径抑制胃脂肪酶的分泌，GLP-1 是主要的参与介质[302]。

七、内因子分泌

内因子（intrinsic factor，IF）是一种 50kD 糖蛋白，由人体壁细胞分泌，部分由主细胞分泌，是吸收钴胺素（维生素 B_{12}）所必需的因子[303]。

虽然前面讨论的胃酸分泌的所有刺激物（如胃泌素、组胺和乙酰胆碱）和抑制剂（如生长抑素）对 IF 分泌有类似的影响，但 IF 的分泌并不是与酸分泌特异性耦合的。例如，PPI 抑制酸的分泌，对基础 IF 分泌或刺激后的 IF 分泌没有显著的影响[304]。然而一些报告指出长期使用 PPI 可能会降低血清钴胺素浓度，这可能是由于胃酸促进食物蛋白质消化释放钴胺素的功能受到抑制[305,306]。钴胺素的推荐每日摄入量仅为 2μg/天；人体总贮存量约为 2 500μg。因此，由抗酸分泌疗法导致的钴胺素缺乏症是罕见的，这是由于 PPI 对酸的抑制不完全，同时机体钴胺素的总储存量很高[12,307,308]。

钴胺素从食物到组织的输送，始于通过胃蛋白酶的 pH 依赖活性，从食物蛋白质中释放钴胺素，然后钴胺素与分泌到胃液中的 2 种结合蛋白结合：IF 和转钴胺素蛋白（haptocorrin，R 结合蛋白）[309,310]。转钴胺素蛋白也存在于唾液和胆汁中，与 IF 相比，在酸性胃腔中钴胺素与之结合更强烈，因此，大多数钴胺素最初与转钴胺素蛋白结合。在十二指肠，钴胺素通过胰蛋白酶从转钴胺素蛋白中释放出来，然后游离钴胺素与 IF 结合。IF-钴胺素复合物对胰腺蛋白水解具有抵抗性，并最终与远端回肠黏膜上的特定受体结合。这种受体（cubilin）在微绒毛间隙中表达，介导 IF-钴胺素复合物的内吞作用[311]。一旦进入回肠细胞，IF 被溶酶体酶降解，钴胺素与转钴胺素（transcobalamin）结合。钴胺素-运钴胺素复合物释放到循环中，通过受体介导的内吞作用进入细胞。进入细胞后，钴胺素与转运蛋白分离并转化为其活性形式甲基钴胺素和 5-脱氧腺苷钴胺素。这些活性形式是蛋氨酸合成酶和甲基丙二酰辅酶 A 变异酶的辅酶，它们分别参与同型半胱氨酸甲基化为蛋氨酸和线粒体中支链氨基酸和奇链脂肪酸的分解代谢[312]。

经肠外给予大剂量非放射性钴胺素后，再口服放射性钴胺素，IF 缺乏症患者在 24 小时尿液收集中排泄出的放射性钴胺素比正常对照组少得多（Schilling 试验，第一部分）。如果 IF 与放射性钴胺素一起口服给药，则尿放射性钴胺素排泄正常（Schilling 试验，第二部分）。钴胺素缺乏除了 IF 缺乏有关外，可能还与下面这些原因有关：胃酸缺乏症或胃酸减少（食物蛋白中钴胺素的消化性水解减少）、细菌过度生长（细菌竞争钴胺素）、胰腺功能不全（转钴胺素蛋白-钴胺素复合物的胰蛋白酶裂解受损）、回肠受体缺陷（cubilin 突变）、回肠炎或回肠切除（IF-钴胺素吸收位点缺失）[313-315]。

IF 的分泌远远超过钴胺素吸收所需的量。因此，在大多数胃酸少的患者中，持续低量 IF 分泌足以防止钴胺素缺乏。恶性贫血（PA）患者确实会出现钴胺素缺乏。2% PA 患者年龄超过 60 岁[316]。病理［自身免疫性化生性萎缩性胃炎（见第 52 章）］表现为慢性炎症，主要是淋巴细胞浸润泌酸黏膜，并伴有壁细胞和主细胞的丢失。发病机制包括促炎 Th1 $CD4^+$ T 淋巴细胞直接攻击壁细胞 H^+，K^+-ATP 酶的 α-和 β-亚基，并出现针对 H^+，K^+-ATP 酶或 IF 的循环自身抗体[317-321]。Hp 慢性感染可能在某些患者的免疫应答中起主要作用。有人提出，Hp 诱导的炎症导致遗传易感个体对自身抗原（如 H^+，K^+-ATP 酶）的耐受性下降，或者由于 Hp 脂多糖和 H^+，K^+-ATP 酶之间存在有交叉抗原而获得抗体，这两者都含有 Lewis 表位[228,230,322]。90% 的 PA 患者存在针对 H^+，K^+-ATP 酶的抗体，但随着自身免疫性胃炎的发展，该比例可下降至 55%～80%，这可能是因为 Hp 的清除和抗原驱动的丧失[317-322]。遗传因素，如 IF 基因中的 Glu→Arg（Q5R）突变，也可能使个体易患 PA[323]。

慢性萎缩性胃炎所致钴胺素缺乏症的治疗方法是补充维生素 B_{12}，可以每月注射 1 毫克，也可以每日高剂量口服 1～2mg。高剂量的口服是有效的，因为少量的钴胺素可以被动吸收而不需要 IF[1,324]。

八、碳酸氢盐分泌

与十二指肠 HCO_3^- 分泌相比，对胃中 HCO_3^- 分泌调控的研究较少。由于同时大量分泌 H^+，胃 HCO_3^- 分泌的确切功能尚不确定。然而，HCO_3^- 的分泌与保护性上皮前碱性层的形成有关（见图 51.2）。

由于大量 H^+ 的存在，胃 HCO_3^- 分泌量的测量受到了阻碍，因此需要使用有效的抗分泌化合物来消除尽可能多的胃酸[325]，或使用不受酸存在影响的测量方法。测量 HCO_3^- 分泌量的一种方法是使用内置 pH 和 CO_2 电极，其中 HCO_3^- 浓度使用 Henderson-Hasselbalch 方程计算[326,327]。

胃的 HCO_3^- 分泌是一个能量依赖的过程。这一发现表明，在 HCO_3^- 分泌过程中，胃电位差几乎没有变化，这表明 HCO_3^- 转运是通过电中性离子交换机制进行的，可能是 HCO_3^- 交换 Cl^-[328]。尽管一些阴离子交换体、溶质载体和阴离子转运体已经定位于胃细胞，包括 AE2、AE4、SLC4A2、SLC4A4、SLC26A6、SLC26A9 和 PAT1，但几乎没有证据表明胃表面细胞确实分泌 HCO_3^-[329-355]。HCO_3^- 分泌的确切细胞尚不清楚，但 H^+ 分泌过程中部分 HCO_3^- 分泌的来源实际上可能是壁细胞。如前所述，对于每个 H^+ 的分泌，HCO_3^- 离子通过负离子交换体 SLC4A2 穿过基底外侧膜离开壁细胞[153]（见图 51.13）。这种 HCO_3^- 可能碱化灌注表面上皮细胞的血液，被碳酸氢钠共转运体所吸收（NBC1 和 NBC2）。然后由上皮细胞分泌，以保护上皮细胞免受腔内酸的侵害[333]。然而，对于表面细胞来说，壁细胞可能不是 HCO_3^- 的唯一来源，因为 PPI 对胃 H^+ 分泌的明显抑制并不能显著减少十二指肠溃疡患者胃 HCO_3^- 的分泌[334]。

前列腺素 E_2 类似物刺激胃 HCO_3^- 分泌[335,336]，阻断内源性前列腺素（PG）合成可减少胃的 HCO_3^- 分泌[337]。在小鼠和大鼠中，参与刺激胃 HCO_3^- 分泌的前列腺素 E 受体亚型为 EP1[338-340]。PG 刺激的 HCO_3^- 分泌对局灶性上皮损伤的反应显然依赖于阴离子转运体 SLC26A9，因为在 SLC26A9 敲除小鼠中这一反应过程消失了[341]。老年人胃黏膜 PG 合成和 HCO_3^- 分泌均下降。最近研究提示，气态介质 NO、前列腺素的硫化氢和辣椒素敏感的传入神经一起参与了胃 HCO_3^- 分泌的调节[345,346]。

九、黏液分泌

胃表面有一种牢固的黏性黏液凝胶。它由 95% 的水和

5%的广泛交联黏蛋白组成，黏蛋白是 MUC 基因的产物[347,348]。超微结构研究显示了 2 种不同的黏蛋白类的交替层，即 MUC5AC（由表面和胃小凹上皮细胞分泌）和 MUC6（由颈部和腺体细胞分泌）。胃保护化合物香叶基香叶基丙酮(geranylgeranylacetone)增加大鼠胃黏膜 MUC6 表达[349]，胃保护化合物拉夫替丁(lafutidine)和瑞巴派特(rebamipide)增加人体黏液厚度和黏蛋白含量[350,351]提示黏液凝胶可能参与了黏膜防御。此外，Hp 感染抑制 MUC1 的分泌，并在富含 MUC5AC 的凝胶层内积累和破坏[352,353]。MUC5AC 分泌在感染 Hp 的胃癌患者的一级亲属中增加，表明黏液分泌可能是对生物体更严重炎症反应的标志[354]。

黏液凝胶厚度具有动态变化性（图 51.20）。在活啮齿动物中可连续、非侵入性地测量黏液凝胶厚度，其方法是通过交替测量聚焦在表面上皮细胞和黏液凝胶表面的荧光标志物（如用碳颗粒或荧光微球描绘），或测量黏液在胃腔表面和上皮细胞表面微吸管之间的垂直移动[355-358]。

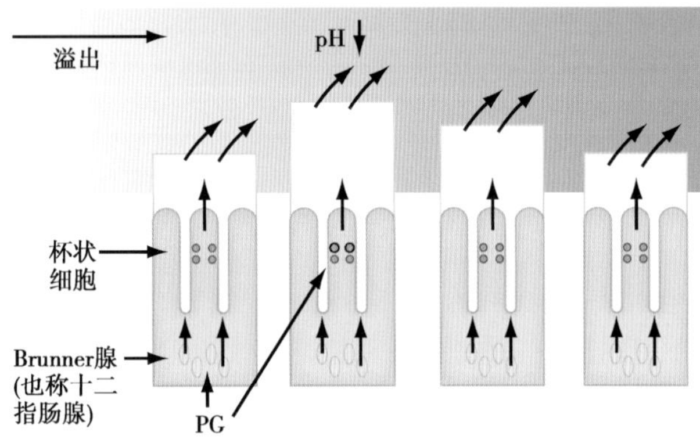

图 51.20　十二指肠黏液凝胶厚度对腔内酸反应的动态调节。在左起第 1 图中，碱性黏液分泌和脱落进入管腔的速率是平衡的。管腔内酸导致杯状细胞和 Brunner 腺体的黏液分泌突然胞外暴发，使凝胶增厚（第 2 图）。新分泌的黏液以更高的速率进入管腔中，形成新的稳定状态凝胶厚度（第 3 图和第 4 图）。(Adapted from Kaunitzand and Akiba, Keio J Med 2002;51:29-35.[397])

胃黏膜表面的 pH 梯度已经在包括人类在内的多物种中被观察到[356]。在大多数情况下，组织表面是相对碱性的，在离组织表面较远的地方逐渐变酸性。这种梯度靠活跃的上皮碳酸氢盐分泌维持[359]。尽管大多数使用微电极测量胃黏膜表面的 pH 接近中性，但最近使用对 pH 敏感荧光染料结合体外共聚焦显微镜测量了豚鼠和青蛙的表面 pH 接近 4[360,361]。表面 pH 梯度的稳态超出黏液凝胶层的厚度，这一现象提示，在黏液与水腔界面，或上皮表面与腔内内容物界面上形成的未搅拌层，也可以通过限制未搅拌层内的对流混合来增强黏膜防御[356]。几乎没有数据支持上层黏液是质子的重要扩散屏障的假说[362-365]。荧光珠对胃黏液层的物理研究发现与肠道黏液相比，胃黏液具有更牢固的黏附内层。对黏蛋白核心蛋白的蛋白质组学分析证实，胃黏液主要由 *MUC5AC* 基因产物组成，胃黏膜黏蛋白与胃肠道其他部分分泌的黏蛋白 O-聚糖模式存在显著差异[367,368]。

三叶因子(trefoil factor, TFF)肽是与黏蛋白共同分泌的[369]。TFF 是 7~12kD 的多肽，具有 3 个内部二硫键的共同结构，产生 3 个内部环的标志性“三叶草”结构，被命名为 TFF1、TFF2 和 TFF3。TFF 具有对胃蛋白酶的抵抗性，能够在胃腔内完整存活[370]。TFF1 储存在胃小凹及表面黏液细胞中，TFF2 储存在胃腺黏液细胞中，TFF3 储存在肠杯状细胞中[371-375]。大鼠胃液中 TFF2 的浓度约为 10μm[371,376]。

三叶肽的定位和与黏蛋白的协调分泌表明它们也可能参与黏膜防御[373,377,378]。支持这一观点的证据包括：①给予胃保护剂后，TFF1 表达增加[379]；②在黏蛋白溶液中加入 TFF2 显著提高了黏蛋白溶液的黏度和弹性[380,381]；③长期使用 PPI 治疗的大鼠可增加胃分泌物中 TFF2 的浓度，同时促进修复以及预防腔内有害物质引起的损伤[382]；④*TFF2-/-*基因敲除小鼠胃腺细胞缩短，上皮迁移减少，净酸分泌增加，使用非选择性 COX 抑制剂吲哚美辛 12 小时后，病变数量增加了 4 倍[383]，而且黏膜损伤后表面碱化减弱[384]。

TFF 蛋白也与胃癌的发病机制有关（见第 1 和 54 章）。在人类中，TFF1 表达降低与加速胃癌进展和生存期差有关[385]。在小鼠中，敲除 *TFF1* 基因后，可增加对胃癌前病变和恶性病变的易感性[386]。Hp 感染对 TFF2 表达的影响尚不确定，有 1 篇报道显示 TFF2 表达增加，另 1 篇报道显示 TFF2 表达降低[387,388]。

不同黏液蛋白类型对便秘患者的临床意义也在研究中，便秘患者胃黏液分泌率和黏度均有所下降[389]。

十、胃液中的胃癌生物标志物

随着新技术的出现，如逆转录聚合酶链反应测定非编码小分子核糖核酸 RNA 如微小 RNA(miR)和长链非编码 RNA(lncRNA)，与质谱、红外光谱、气相色谱法等其他分析方法的结合，开辟了胃分析的新领域。微量物质可以量化，也可以用于诊断或作为生物标志物。

已经有研究报道 lncRNA、miR 和色氨酸代谢产物在胃癌诊断中的检测特征[390-394]。这些研究是利用在诊断性内镜检查中收集的少量胃液样本进行的。lncRNA 在血浆、肿瘤组织和胃液中的表达水平与肿瘤分期相关，胃液中 lncRNA 的表达水平也随肿瘤分期的变化而变化。在一项体外研究验证了 lncRNA 与胃癌有关这一假设，发现 lncRNA-RMRP（线粒体 RNA 加工内切酶的 RNA 成分）对 miR-206（参与细胞周期素介导的细胞增殖）有“海绵”样吸附抑制作用[393]。在胃癌和胃炎患者胃镜下获得的胃液中，报道了色氨酸代谢产物的改变。作者将观察到的变化归因于犬尿氨酸途径的上调，推测这种物质的代谢变化可能是生物标志物鉴定的基础[391]。由于 PG 的表达与胃癌相关，所以胃液中 PG Ⅰ/Ⅱ结合胃液中黑色素瘤相关基因(MAGE)的浓度[395]对胃癌检测具有较高的特异性和敏感性[396]。

（王俊雄 译　王立　袁农 校）

参考文献

第 52 章　胃炎和胃部疾病

Mark Feldman, Pamela J. Jensen, Colin W. Howden 著

章节目录

一、定义 …… 739
二、急性胃炎 …… 739
三、慢性胃炎 …… 740
（一）幽门螺杆菌胃炎 …… 740
（二）慢性萎缩性胃炎（胃萎缩） …… 746
（三）贲门炎 …… 749
四、其他感染性胃炎 …… 749
（一）病毒性胃炎 …… 749
（二）细菌性胃炎 …… 750
（三）真菌性胃炎 …… 751
（四）寄生虫性胃炎 …… 751
五、肉芽肿性胃炎 …… 752
（一）结节病（肉样瘤病） …… 752
（二）黄色肉芽肿性胃炎 …… 752
六、独特的胃病变 …… 752
（一）胶原性胃炎 …… 752
（二）淋巴细胞性胃炎 …… 753
（三）嗜酸性粒细胞性胃炎 …… 753
七、炎性肠病性胃炎 …… 753
（一）克罗恩病 …… 754
（二）溃疡性结肠炎 …… 754
八、深在性囊性胃炎 …… 754
九、过敏性胃炎 …… 755
十、反应性胃病 …… 755
（一）药物、毒素和违禁药物 …… 755
（二）胆汁反流 …… 756
（三）应激 …… 756
（四）辐射 …… 756
（五）移植物抗宿主病 …… 756
（六）缺血 …… 757
（七）脱垂 …… 757
十一、增生性胃病（包括 Ménétrier 病） …… 757
十二、门静脉高压性胃病 …… 758
十三、鉴别诊断 …… 758
十四、治疗 …… 758
（一）幽门螺杆菌感染 …… 758
（二）其他类型的胃炎和胃病 …… 761

一、定义

患者、临床医生、内镜医师和病理学家对胃炎的定义往往不同。一些人将其定义为一种综合征，另一些人将其定义为胃的异常内镜外观，还有一些人将其定义为胃的显微镜下黏膜的炎症。首选胃炎的最后一种定义，并在本章中使用，胃的其他非炎症性疾病被称为胃病。

组织学胃炎与症状之间的关系不大。事实上，许多胃炎患者是无症状的。显微镜下的异常和胃镜下异常之间的关系也是不精确的。在一项对 400 例患者的研究中，尽管 14% 的患者胃镜检查正常，但仍存在组织学胃炎；另有 20% 的患者胃镜检查异常，而无组织学上的胃炎改变[1]。后一种患者（胃镜检查异常而无胃炎）常有反应性胃病（后文讨论）。

必须进行胃活检才能诊断胃炎。胃镜活检的潜在适应证可能包括因消化不良接受 EGD 检查的患者[2]，胃镜下有胃黏膜的糜烂、溃疡、胃皱襞厚、胃息肉或肿块以及诊断幽门螺杆菌（Hp）感染的患者（稍后讨论）。应在胃窦进行两次活检（小弯和大弯）；一次从角切缘进行；另外两次从胃体进行（小弯和大弯）。应将来自不同区域的活检样本置于单独的容器中，并应在编录表格中为病理学家注明活检部位的位置。每次活检都是临床医师和病理学家进行交流临床数据、内镜检查结果和组织病理学的极好机会。病理学家在没有了解临床背景的情况下解释活检时，可能会发生错误。

悉尼分类系统试图统一内镜和组织学胃炎和胃病的术语[3]。然而，悉尼系统的复杂性和经常不能获得足够数量的活检标本，使其难以广泛应用于临床，但可以用于临床研究。本章提供了胃炎和胃病的病因学分类。

二、急性胃炎

以胃内中性白细胞致密浸润为特征的急性胃炎罕见。这种罕见性与更常见的“活动性”胃炎不同，在这种胃炎中，中性粒细胞可与慢性炎性细胞（淋巴细胞、浆细胞）一起存在，如 Hp 胃炎（见后文）。大多数形式的急性中性粒细胞性胃炎是由于侵入性微生物感染所致。

蜂窝织炎（化脓性）胃炎是一种胃黏膜下层和固有肌层的感染，通常不感染黏膜层[4-19]。已鉴定出多种类型的侵袭性微生物，包括革兰氏阴性杆菌、厌氧菌、革兰氏阳性球菌（包括 A 组链球菌）和真菌（如毛霉菌病，见后文）。胃蜂窝织炎可酷似肿块。食管也可能受累，甚至是感染的明显来源。感染可扩散到邻近的肝脏和脾脏并形成脓肿。急性蜂窝织炎/坏死性胃炎与多种疾病相关，包括最近大量饮酒、呼吸道感染、艾滋病和其他免疫功能低下状态，包括肝移植。

蜂窝织炎性胃炎的一种特别严重的类型是气肿性胃炎，是由于胃受到产气微生物的感染（如产气荚膜梭菌、大肠埃希菌和金黄色葡萄球菌）所致。这种胃炎在胃壁和门静脉系统常有气体存在（图 52.1）。影像学检查（平片，CT）显示气泡与胃的外形一致，常表现为囊状气泡。尽管可从蜂窝织

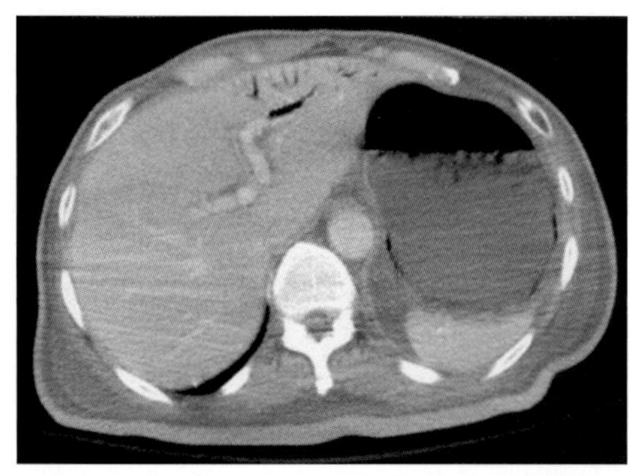

图 52.1 气肿性胃炎 CT。一例 67 岁男性糖尿病伴冠状动脉疾病和既往卒中患者的腹部 CT 影像，其因突发恶心、呕吐和腹痛从养老院入院。查体：全腹弥漫性压痛。CT 显示充满液体的胃后壁有曲线样气体，以及门静脉气体。使用广谱抗生素成功治疗，2 周后重复扫描发现气肿消退。(Courtesy T. Ynosencio, MD. Baylor Universlty Medical Center, Dallas, TX.)

炎或气肿性胃炎中完全恢复，但有时候可发展为胃（和食管）气性坏疽并具有致死性。气肿性胃炎的危险因素包括近期胃十二指肠手术、摄入腐蚀性物质、胃肠炎、或胃肠道梗死。

蜂窝织炎性或气肿性胃炎患者通常表现为脓毒血症，表现为急性上腹痛、腹膜炎、化脓性腹水、发热和低血压。

术前可通过腹部平片、超声或 CT 诊断。胃镜检查时伴或不伴活检和胃内容物培养可确定诊断。大体上，可见胃壁厚而水肿，有多处穿孔，黏膜可显示颗粒状、绿黑色渗出物。显微镜下，水肿的黏膜下层显示大量的多形核细胞浸润和大量革兰氏阳性和/或革兰氏阴性细菌，以及血管内血栓形成，黏膜可显示大面积坏死。蜂窝织炎性胃炎的死亡率接近 70%，可能是因为它罕见和难以诊断，也可能是因为治疗启动太晚。早期联合针对最常见微生物的全身性广谱抗生素（大肠埃希菌和其他革兰氏阴性杆菌、厌氧菌和 A 组链球菌以及金黄色葡萄球菌），万古霉素和哌拉西林/他唑巴坦是一种经验性治疗方案，可以使用。

急性蜂窝织炎性胃炎可与粒细胞白血病和中性粒细胞减少症所致胃炎的临床表现不同。尽管不像中性粒细胞减少性盲肠炎或小肠结肠炎那样常见，但中性粒细胞减少性胃炎可能是一个孤立疾病。其他形式的急性胃炎在后面讨论（见感染性胃炎）。

三、慢性胃炎

慢性胃炎可能在临床上无症状，但比急性胃炎更常见。其患病率在发达国家呈下降趋势[20]。这些慢性胃炎（包括 Hp 胃炎）的主要重要性与它们是其他疾病的风险因素有关，如消化性溃疡病（PUD）和胃肿瘤，包括腺癌和淋巴瘤（MALToma），在其他章节中将详细讨论。非幽门螺杆菌慢性胃炎也不少见，大多数病例尚不清楚其病因。非 Hp 胃炎在非裔美国人中的发生率低于其他人种，并且与美国退伍军人人群中的质子泵抑制剂（PPI）使用相关[21]。慢性胃炎可分为 3 种类型：通常是由于幽门螺杆菌感染引起的弥漫性胃窦炎、周围肠化生性萎缩性胃炎（environmental metaplastic atrophic gastritis, EMAG）和自身免疫性肠化生性萎缩性胃炎（autoimmune metaplastic atrophic gastritis, AMAG）（图 52.2 和图 52.3）。

（一）幽门螺杆菌胃炎

幽门螺杆菌（Hp）是一种革兰氏阴性螺旋状或螺旋状有鞭毛的杆菌。感染 Hp 通常会引起弥漫性胃窦炎（见图 52.3A）。Hp 胃炎最初累及黏膜浅层。在某些情况下，尤其是在儿童期，感染是短暂的，但感染通常会导致慢性活动性胃炎，这基本上是一种未经治疗的终身疾病。Hp 感染诱导的趋化因子导致中性粒细胞和其他细胞（活动性炎症），与慢性炎症特征的细胞（淋巴细胞、浆细胞和巨噬细胞）共存的持续性急性炎性浸润。尽管有这种强大的宿主免疫反应，但这种细菌在于大多数感染者中持续存在[22]。在一些急性感染病例中导致 Hp 清除的宿主因素在很大程度上仍不清楚[23,24]。

一种以含有 Russell 小体的浆细胞黏膜浸润为特征的 Hp 胃炎（鲁塞尔小体胃炎）已有描述[25,26]。内镜下可识别的一种 Hp 胃炎是结节性胃炎，从胃中根除该微生物后可消退[27-29]。结节性胃炎/胃病可通过其鸡皮样外观识别，这些内镜表现也可见于其他疾病，包括克罗恩病、梅毒性胃炎、淋巴细胞性（静脉曲张样）胃炎、胶原性胃炎（均在后面讨论）和 AA-淀粉样变性[30]。

1. 流行病学、危险因素和传播

Hp 感染是人类最常见的慢性细菌感染。据估计，世界上超过 50% 的人口感染了这种细菌，包括发展中国家 70% ~ 80% 的人口。基因序列分析表明，人类感染的时间已经超过 6 万年，与他们第一次从非洲移民的时间相对应[31]。

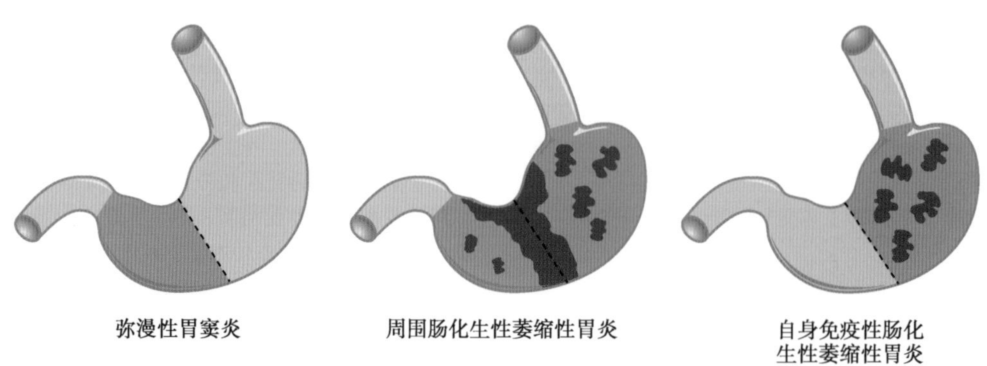

图 52.2 慢性胃炎的局部分布图。在周围肠化生性萎缩性胃炎和自身免疫性肠化生性萎缩性胃炎的示意图中，较暗的区域代表局灶性萎缩和肠上皮化生区域

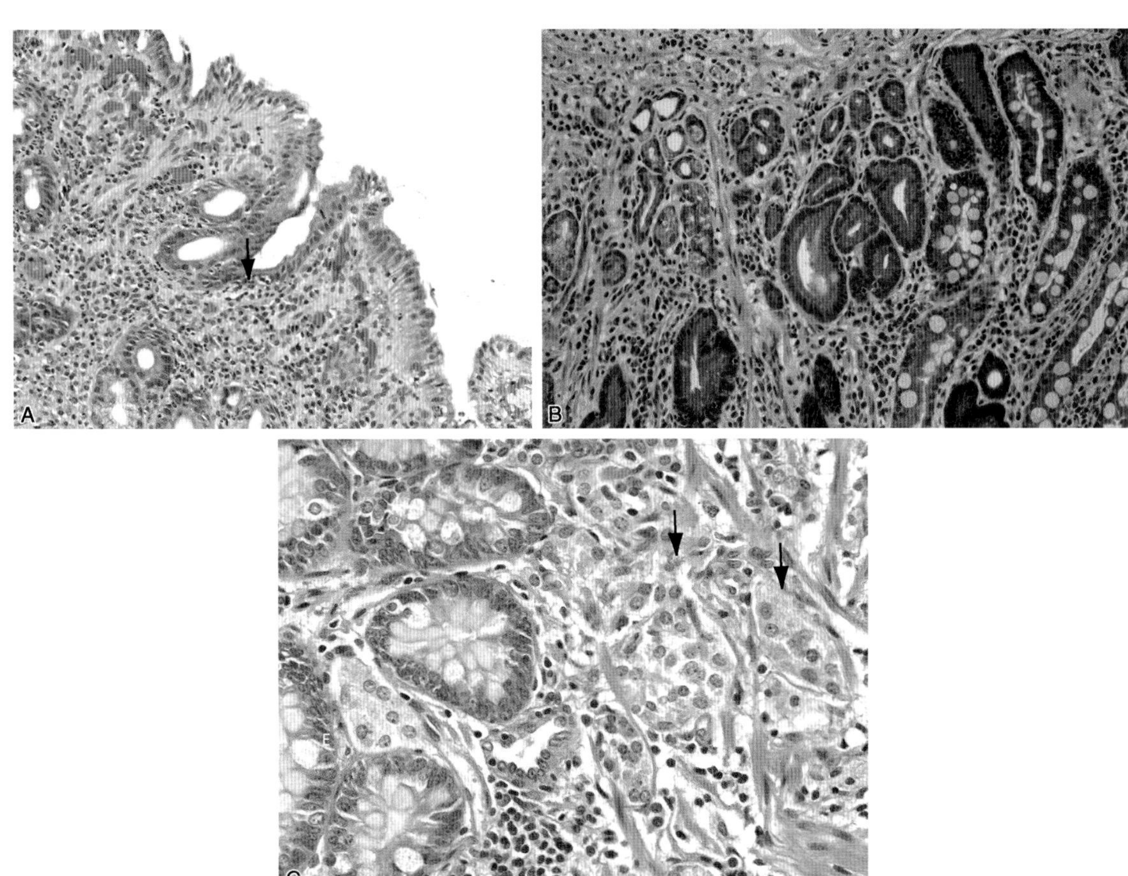

图 52.3　慢性胃炎的组织病理学(正常组织学见第 49 章)。A,弥漫性胃窦胃炎。固有层内的慢性炎症和浸润胃小凹上皮的中性粒细胞。该病变是 Hp 感染的特征(箭)(HE 染色,×400)。B,周围肠化生性萎缩性胃炎。注意几个腺体内衬杯状细胞(HE 染色,×200)。C,自身免疫性肠化生性萎缩性胃炎,伴杯状细胞化生和肠嗜铬样细胞巢(箭)(HE 染色,×400)

感染的一个关键危险因素是儿童期所处的社会经济地位。感染通常在幼年时获得,特别是在发展中国家,大多数儿童在 10 岁前受到感染[32,33]。在儿童早期,细菌自发清除很常见,但往往伴随后再感染。在大龄儿童和成人中,感染通常持续存在。因此,在世界发展中地区到 20~30 岁时 Hp 感染率可超过 80%。在发达国家,如美国,幼儿也可能获得 Hp,随着自发清除,再感染的机会较低,因此,持续性感染较少[33,34]。事实上,Hp 感染的血清学证据在 10 岁以前的儿童中并不常见,但在 18~30 岁的成人中上升至 10%,在 60 岁或以上的成人中进一步增加至 50%[33]。这种感染率随年龄增长而增加,最初被认为是在整个成人生活中持续获得。然而,新发成人感染和再感染相当罕见,特别是在发达国家,估计每年不到 0.5%的病例发生再感染。即使在发达国家,流行病学证据也支持儿童期获得性感染。因此,当地任何年龄组 Hp 感染的频率反映了特定出生队列在生命早期获得细菌的比率。在美国,白人中任何年龄组内的感染均低于非裔美国人和西班牙裔美国人[35]。西班牙裔移民及其第一代子女比其第二代后代更有可能携带 Hp[36]。这些差异可能与生命早期与获得性感染有关的因素有关。

住房密度、家庭拥挤的条件、兄弟姐妹的数量、共用一张床、缺乏热水或自来水与较高的感染率有关[33,37]。在日本,Hp 感染率的下降似乎与战后国家经济进展及卫生条件和卫生设施的改善相平行。在 1950 年以前出生的日本人中,70%以上的人被感染,而 1950 年至 1960 年出生的人占 45%,1960 年至 1970 年出生的人占 25%[38]。目前日本儿童感染并不常见。在美国也观察到类似的患病率下降,这表明随着发达国家当前出生队列到达老年,与 Hp 感染相关性疾病如 PUD 将会减少[39]。

对双胞胎的研究支持 Hp 感染的遗传易感性。因为在不同家庭喂养的同卵双胞胎比单独喂养的异卵双胞胎具有更大的感染一致性[40]。然而,共同成长的双胞胎比单独成长的双胞胎具有更高的 Hp 感染一致性,这表明环境因素对于儿童期的获得也很重要。

人类似乎是 Hp 的主要宿主。Hp 在人与人之间传播的精确方式仍不清楚,可能有多种机制起作用。细菌从胃-口、粪-口、或可能的口-口暴露传播,似乎是人与人之间传播的最可能解释[32,41]。感染的家族内聚集性(通常具有基因相同的 Hp 菌株)也支持人与人之间的传播[33]。与未感染个体相比,感染个体更有可能感染配偶或子女。对同胞间传播的支持来自报告感染可能性与家庭中儿童数量相关的研究,如果年长的兄弟姐妹也被感染,年幼的儿童则更容易被感染[33]。在 6 个拉丁美洲国家进行的一项研究表明,家庭拥挤、与 4 名或 4 名以上的儿童一起生活是感染的危险因素[17]。母婴传播的可能性也很大[34,42]。

细菌经胃-口和粪-口传播似乎是 Hp 获得进入人类宿主的主要机制。该细菌可从呕吐物、雾化呕吐物和腹泻粪便中培养出来，提示传播的可能性[43]。与粪便和唾液相比，呕吐物中的微生物负荷高 100 倍；在呕吐过程中，雾化呕吐物中的微生物也存在至 1.2m 处。在急性胃肠道疾病期间暴露于感染的家庭成员，尤其是呕吐，似乎是感染的风险因素[44]。在急性病期间，通过接触感染的呕吐物或感染儿童的反流物质，可能发生自然传播[44]。这种接触可以解释在婴儿日托环境中发生的母亲/儿童 Hp 感染和假定的儿童间传播的高度一致性[45]。

特别是在发展中国家，受 Hp 污染的水可能作为 Hp 的环境来源，因为微生物可以在水中存活数天。在感染流行地区的市政水样中可发现 46 个 Hp DNA，但 PCR 检测到的 Hp 是否是有活力的生物体还有待证实[31]。在 Hp 感染率较高的国家，在河流和溪流中游泳、饮用未经处理的溪水或食用未煮熟蔬菜的儿童更有可能携带 Hp，为生物体的环境（水源性）来源提供了进一步的间接证据。

细菌通过口-口接触传播的频率尚不清楚。尽管在牙菌斑、牙周袋和唾液中可以鉴定出微生物，但患病率较低，微生物计数也是如此[47,48]。因此，口腔是否可以作为 Hp 的来源或储存库是值得怀疑的。此外，职业暴露于牙菌斑、牙周袋和口腔分泌物的牙医和口腔卫生学家，Hp 感染的感染率没有增加[27]。在发达国家，感染经口-口传播给配偶似乎也不常见。

感染的胃液可作为细菌传播的来源[49,50]。在使用各种消毒不充分的胃器械、内镜及内镜附件的过程中，也发生了医源性感染[32]。胃肠病医生和护士获得 Hp 的风险似乎增加[51]。强制性的普遍预防措施、洗手、标准化设备消毒，以及使用视频内镜将仪器通道重新定位远离口腔，可减少这种职业性和医源性传播。

虽然人类是 Hp 的主要宿主，但家猫、圈养灵长类动物和绵羊也可以隐藏这些微生物。有可能这些动物实际上是从人类来源获得了它们的 Hp。从猫唾液和胃液中分离出活菌，提示有传播给人类的可能[32]。Hp 单倍型在非洲的猫种中持续存在，这表明感染可能在遥远的过去的某个时间点已过渡到人类[51]。

2. 发病机制

Hp 的一个独特之处是，尽管这种病原体存在于胃里，但它还是会引发疾病。然而，胃 Hp 感染本身不足以完全解释广泛的相关胃十二指肠疾病。致病性和临床结果取决于细菌和宿主因素。因此，Hp 的毒力既与允许定植和适应胃环境的细菌特性有关，也与宿主的病理生理学改变有关。描述不同 Hp 菌株基因组的研究，促进了我们对该生物体以及可能影响疾病发病机制的潜在细菌基因表达模式的理解[52-54]。

Hp 胃炎的发病机制复杂，尚不完全清楚，详细描述超出本章的范围。只讨论关键的致病因素，感兴趣的读者可以参考其他来源[55-77]。

Hp 在其身体的一端含有 6~8 根鞭毛，鞭毛介导的运动是 Hp 成功定殖宿主所需的少数特征之一[55]。该生物体的鞭毛可使 Hp 快速迁移到胃黏液层下方更有利的胃位置。

Hp 暴露于低胃 pH 水平可增加编码尿素酶的细菌基因的表达[55]。尿素酶有助于 Hp 适应酸性胃环境，当其尿素酶将尿素分解成 CO_2 和氨（NH_3）时，使细菌附近发生更中性的 pH，NH_3 与 H^+ 反应产生铵离子（NH_4^+）[56]。

Hp 对胃型黏膜表现出严格的趋向性，包括存在胃上皮化生的胃肠道非胃区。相反，Hp 不定植于发生肠化生性改变的胃上皮（见后文），可能是因为宿主肠化生性上皮产生的抗菌因子选择对抗定植。这种可能性得到了以下发现的支持：Hp 很少定植于胃腺黏膜的较深部分，在那里发现了抗菌 O-聚糖[57]。肠化生也可能与胃酸降低/胃酸缺乏有关，可促使胃与其他（非 Hp）种类的细菌过度生长。

Toll 样受体（toll-like receptor，TLR）是一个模式识别受体家族，对各种细菌分子具有特异性[63,43]。TLR 是宿主先天免疫系统的组成部分[44]。来自 Hp 的脂多糖 PS 通过 TLR4 和 TLR2.2[64-66,244]，刺激胃上皮细胞和单核细胞反应。

Hp 和胃上皮细胞之间的关键相互作用是由一段被称为 cag 致病基因岛（cag pathogenicity island，cag PAI）的细菌 DNA 介导的。cag PAI 内的基因编码Ⅳ型分泌装置 cagE，该装置允许该细菌其他大分子物质，如 cag A 直接递送到宿主细胞中[53,57]。cag PAI 在人类慢性 Hp 胃炎的发病机制中起重要作用[53,68]。与 cag PAI 阴性菌株相比，携带 cag PAI 的 Hp 与白细胞介素（IL）-8 表达增加、黏膜炎症、消化性溃疡和细胞凋亡相关[69,70]。与感染野生型菌株的沙鼠相比，只感染缺乏 cagE 的突变 Hp 菌株的蒙古沙鼠表现出更轻的胃炎、更少的消化性溃疡、更少的肠上皮化生（less intestinal metaplasia，IM）和更少的胃癌[71]。来自不同地理位置 Hp 群体的不同 cagA 蛋白，似乎在不同的人体内被宿主细胞酪氨酸磷酸化，导致对细胞内信号产生不同的影响[78-85]。cagA 的这种异质性可能导致不同的宿主反应，这可以解释在 Hp 相关疾病中观察到的一些地理差异。尽管 cagA 蛋白的酪氨酸磷酸化可能很重要，但它不是该分子调节宿主反应的唯一机制[86,87]。

所有 Hp 菌株都具有 vacA 基因，超过一半的菌株产生空泡化细胞毒素 VacA[53,73]。VacA 通过与细胞蛋白酪氨酸磷酸酶的相互作用附着在宿主上皮细胞上[72]。因此，当暴露于分泌 VacA 的 Hp 时，前蛋白酪氨酸磷酸酶缺陷的小鼠不会发生胃溃疡[74]。在 Hp 的 vacA 基因的 5' 信号区（s 区）和中间区（m 区）已检测到不同的 vacA 等位基因[75]。s 区以等位基因 s1（可进一步区分为 s1a、s1b、s1c）或等位基因 s2 存在，而 m 区以等位基因 m1 或 m2 存在。通过等位基因组合指定 VacA 的产生（如 s1/m1、s1/m2、s2/m1 和 s2/m2）。特殊的 vacA 等位基因（s1 和 m1）与消化性溃疡[75]和诱导宿主上皮细胞凋亡有关[76]。

其他细菌毒力因子也与胃腺癌的风险增加有关。然而研究表明，这些细菌因素中的任何一种都会直接导致癌症，但事实证明这些研究是徒劳的。这些发现支持了这样一种观点：即任何增加宿主对感染的炎症反应的细菌或宿主因素，都可能增加胃癌的风险，并且黏膜炎症、细胞损伤和胃萎缩的程度是个体患者癌症风险的最佳决定因素[77]。

胃上皮细胞除了是 Hp 感染的靶标外，还在宿主对 Hp 感染的反应中起着不可或缺的作用。上皮细胞对 Hp 的反应包括形态改变[88]、紧密连接复合体的破坏[89]、产生细胞因子[67]、增殖增加、通过凋亡增强细胞死亡，以及诱导与感染伴随的细胞应激相关的许多宿主基因[23]。

感染 Hp 的上皮细胞的基因表达受转录因子调节，特别是核因子-κB(NF-κB)。如第 2 章所述，NF-κB 调节多种促炎性细胞因子和细胞黏附分子的表达，以应对感染或局部细胞因子环境。胃上皮细胞 NF-κB 活性增强与中性粒细胞浸润强度和黏膜 IL-8 水平相关[48,67]。鉴于 IL-8 基因[90]某些多态性与黏膜 IL-8 表达增加、炎症和与胃癌相关的其他癌前变化相关，该通路特别令人感兴趣。Hp 感染似乎通过各种信号机制激活胃上皮细胞系中的 NF-κB，其中包括有丝分裂原活化蛋白激酶[49,66,68,91]。有丝分裂原活化蛋白激酶级联调节广泛的细胞功能，包括增殖、炎症反应和细胞存活[69,92-94]。

氧化应激在 Hp 感染过程中也调节宿主基因表达[95,96]。活性氧如羟基自由基(—OH)对宿主 DNA 的氧化被认为通过诱导 DNA 损伤在恶性变中起因果作用。出于这个原因，人们越来越关注抗氧化剂在癌症预防或治疗中的作用，因为 Hp 感染与组织抗氧化剂清除剂抗坏血酸水平降低有关。此外，有证据表明，富含抗氧化剂[97]或异硫氰酸酯类的“营养保健品”，如萝卜硫素[98]，可能通过减少炎症和减轻细菌负荷，来拮抗氧化应激和保护宿主免受胃癌的侵袭。对蒙古沙鼠进行的体外和体内研究表明，抗氧化剂化合物谷胱甘肽的前体 N-乙酰半胱氨酸，如果在 Hp 感染后早期给药，可以减少 Hp 胃炎[99]，但该化合物是否会减少癌变尚不确定。

表达外炎性蛋白 A(outer inflammatory protein A，OipA)的 Hp 菌株与细菌密度增加、黏膜 IL-8 水平升高[100]和中性粒细胞浸润以及更严重的临床后果相关[101]。

来自 Hp 细胞壁的肽聚糖(胞壁质)可通过 cag PAI 编码的 cagE 转位到胃上皮细胞。一旦进入宿主细胞，核苷酸结合寡聚化结构域-1 就会识别这种胞壁质，提供了细菌感知的新机制[102]。如前所述，胞壁质与核苷酸结合寡聚化结构域-1 的结合，可导致 NF-κB 的激活和随后编码促炎分子的各种宿主基因的表达。

Hp 中性粒细胞激活蛋白促进中性粒细胞与内皮细胞黏附，刺激中性粒细胞和单核细胞趋化，在质膜上形成烟酰胺腺嘌呤二核苷酸磷酸氢氧化酶复合物，随后产生活性氧中间物[86,103]。在 Hp 胃炎存在的炎症环境中，肿瘤坏死因子-α(TNF-α)和干扰素-γ(IFN-γ)可增强 Hp 中性粒细胞激活蛋白对神经营养细胞的作用。上皮细胞发生凋亡后，吞噬细胞清除死亡细胞。吞噬细胞吞噬坏死的上皮细胞可能是 Hp 能激活宿主反应的另一个重要机制[23,2]。

中性粒细胞和巨噬细胞的募集和激活引起其他炎症介质的释放。Hp 感染时胃黏膜发生诱生型一氧化氮合酶(iNOS)表达增加[23]。产生的一氧化氮(NO)与渗入中性粒细胞产生的超氧阴离子(O_2^-)反应，形成过氧亚硝基阴离子($ONOO^-$)，一种强效的氧化剂和硝化剂。NO 和 $ONOO^-$ 具有抗菌作用，但不受控制或不适当的产生，也可能在 Hp 感染期间观察到的胃黏膜细胞损伤中发挥作用。此外，Hp 尿素酶对尿素的分解代谢产生 NH_3 和 CO_2，后者可通过与过氧亚硝基阴离子反应形成中间产物 $ONOOCO_2^-$，然后形成硝酸盐，迅速中和过氧亚硝基阴离子的杀菌活性。因此，尿素酶可能通过中和一些宿主细胞反应有利于 Hp 的定植，但这一机制也增强了 $ONOO^-$ 的硝化潜力，可能有利于宿主细胞 DNA 的突变。

细菌尿素酶在巨噬细胞中诱导的细胞因子包括 TNF-α 和 IL-6，89[104]，IL-6 也由热休克蛋白 60.9[105]诱导上皮细胞分泌的细胞因子与固有层中炎症细胞释放的细胞因子互补。完整细菌可以诱导产生趋化因子，募集 T 细胞产[106,91]以及 IL-12[92,93,107,108]和 IL-18[94,109]细胞因子，有利于选择 Th1 细胞，具有细胞因子分泌的特征模式。Th1 细胞通过产生 IFN-γ 和 TNF-α 促进细胞介导的免疫反应，而 Th2 细胞产生 IL-4、IL-5、IL-10 和转化生长因子(TGF-β)。Th2 细胞可促进黏膜对蠕虫和其他寄生虫的 IgA 或 IgE 反应，以及减轻 Th1 细胞因子引起的炎症反应。先前的研究表明，Hp 感染的胃黏膜是先决条件，有利于 Th1 的发育而不是 Th2 细胞的发育[92,107]。

Hp 感染引起的 T 细胞(如 Th1 细胞)激活可能与更严重的炎症和胃十二指肠疾病有关。在 Hp 感染患者的黏膜中发现活化的 $CD4^+$ T 淋巴细胞产生的细胞因子 IL-17 水平升高[110,111]。IL-17 又诱导胃上皮细胞表达 IL-8，从而增强中性粒细胞的募集。IL-17 激活转录因子也可能导致 Hp 感染过程中观察到的众多其他促炎细胞因子和酶，如 IL-1β、TNF-α 和 COX-2 水平升高。Th1 细胞产生的 IFN-γ 和 TNF-α 可增加上皮中许多基因的表达，包括 IL-8。这些细胞因子也能增强细菌结合[66]，它们也可能增加细菌负荷[112]。在动物模型中，Th1 细胞增加上皮细胞凋亡[38]以及炎症、腺体萎缩和异型增生倾向[113]。TNF-α、IFN-γ 和 IL-1β 也上调胃上皮细胞 Fas 抗原表达[114]。由于 Th1 细胞比 Th2 细胞表达更高水平的 Fas 配体(FasL)，Hp 感染过程中 Th1 细胞的相对增加，可能通过 Fas-Fas 配体(FasL)相互作用诱导上皮细胞死亡[114,115]。观察到胃黏膜中质子泵(H^+，K^+-ATP 酶)特异性 Th1 细胞通过 Fas-FasL 相互作用杀死靶上皮细胞，并可能在自身免疫性胃炎中作为效应细胞，这一观察结果支持了这一观点(稍后讨论)[116]。

IgA 抗体通常在胃肠道中产生(见第 2 章)，高度适应黏膜保护，在不激活补体级联反应和引起有害量的细胞损伤和炎症的情况下产生保护性免疫。Hp 感染时产生 IgA 的浆细胞数量增加。然而，还检测到产生 IgG 和 IgM 的浆细胞数量也增加，以及活化的补体。识别 Hp 的单克隆抗体可与人和鼠胃上皮细胞发生交叉反应[117,118]。将这些抗体转移到受体小鼠可诱导胃炎发生[117]。识别黏膜相关淋巴组织淋巴瘤(MALToma)个体热休克蛋白的 B 细胞转移也可诱导胃炎[119]。

除少数例外，除非用抗生素进行一些干预，否则 Hp 的感染在宿主的一生中会持续存在。这一观察结果导致了免疫耐受是否损害免疫的研究。一些细菌因素，包括尿素酶和过氧化氢酶，阻碍了宿主对感染的固有反应[22]。此外，Hp 产生的精氨酸酶可抑制 NO 的产生，这可能有利于细菌的存活[120]，而 Hp 的强毒株损害细胞的吞噬功能[121]和黏液的生成[122]。VacA 毒素可通过抑制抗原呈递途径损害巨噬细胞的细菌抗原呈递[123]。此外，Hp 可产生模拟宿主分子的分子，如 Lewis 抗原，理论上这些分子可以刺激 T 细胞释放细胞因子，有助于避免自身免疫反应。然而，如前所述，与 Hp 感染相关的细胞因子谱并不是在耐受环境中预期会发生的。例如，IL-4、IL-10 和 TGF-β(可介导抗炎作用)的表达水平与促炎性 Th1 细胞因子如 IFN-γ 和 TNF-α 不同[23]。由于感染的胃黏膜以慢性活动性炎症为特征，即使不能预防慢性炎症反应，如果已经发生耐受,也可能有利于持续性感染。

控制炎症程度的宿主基因组区域的遗传异质性与胃癌的发生相关(见第 54 章)[124]。控制 IL-1[125] 区域的多态性与 Hp 感染者胃酸减少和胃癌的发生率增加有关,并降低十二指肠溃疡复发的发生率[126]。IL-1 表达的增加可能不仅驱动炎症,还会导致先于胃癌发生的已知生理变化,因为 IL-1 可强效抑制胃酸的分泌(见第 51 章)。其他调节 Hp 炎症反应的基因,包括 IL-10、TNF-α 和 IL-8,也与导致癌症的一系列事件有关[127,128]。

在 Hp 感染的个体中,空腹和膳食刺激的血清胃泌素水平升高是有据可查的[3]。Hp 感染对受感染个体胃酸分泌的净效应是可变的,然而,这取决于 Hp 感染的持续时间和分布以及胃底腺黏膜有无萎缩(见第 51 和 53 章)。Hp 感染还可减少胃黏蛋白分泌和黏膜疏水性,这种异常在根除感染后可以逆转。在 Hp 感染过程中,由于 Hp 感染的直接作用和伴随的炎症反应,共同增加了上皮细胞增殖和程序性细胞死亡,上皮屏障功能发生改变[23]。

前面讨论的 Hp 胃炎宿主发病机制中的细菌(Hp)相关因素总结在框 52.1 中。环境因素在 Hp 宿主相互作用中具有调节作用。如吸烟、高盐饮食和各种环境诱变剂等因素可严重影响黏膜损伤的程度和进展速度。例如,在日本,1965 年至 1995 年间胃癌的发病率下降了 60%。尽管最常见的 Hp 菌株的毒力没有变化。这种急剧下降归因于社会变化,如冷藏(与盐保存相比)、饮食西方化和吸烟减少[77]。

框 52.1 与胃炎发病机制有关的 Hp 的某些组分
Cag 致病岛(PAI),包括 CagA 和 CagE
鞭毛
Hp-中性粒细胞激活蛋白(HP-NAP)
脂多糖
外部炎性蛋白 A(Oip A)
肽聚糖(胞壁质)
脲酶
空泡毒素 A(VacA)

3. 诊断

有内镜检查和非内镜检查都可用于诊断 Hp 感染。这类技术可直接(胃组织学检查、粪便细菌抗原测定和细菌培养)或间接(尿素酶检测或抗体反应)检测 Hp[129,130]。选择合适的方法取决于临床情况、人群感染率、检测前感染概率、检测的可用性和成本。近期使用抗生素或 PPI 可能会影响某些检测的结果[131]。常用的诊断试验及其优缺点总结见表 52.1。

表 52.1 Hp 感染的检测方法

内镜检查	优点	缺点
活检尿素酶	快速出结果	需要内镜检查
	在未使用 PPI 或抗生素的患者中,准确性高	治疗后或使用 PPI 的患者内镜检查不太准确
	无额外的病理学成本	
组织学检查	优异的灵敏度和特异性,特别是通过特殊的免疫染色,提供了关于胃黏膜的额外信息	昂贵的(内镜和病理学成本) 观察者之间存在一些差异 准确度受 PPI 和抗生素使用的影响
细菌培养	特异度≈100% 可进行抗生素敏感性试验	难以培养 方案无法广泛使用
		昂贵
非内镜检查		
血清学检测(定性或定量 IgG)	广泛可用的 廉价	如果 Hp 流行率较低 阳性预测值(PPV)较差
	阴性预测值(NPV)高	治疗后无效
尿素呼气试验(^{13}C 或^{14}C)	识别活动性感染	可用性和报销不一致
	准确性(PPV,NPV)不受 Hp 流行率影响	准确度受 PPI 和抗生素使用的影响
	在治疗前和治疗后均有用	^{14}C 检测有小辐射剂量
粪便抗原检测	识别活动性感染	可用数据较少
	准确度(PPV,NPV)不受 Hp 流行率的影响	准确性受 PPI 和抗生素使用影响
	治疗前和治疗后均有用	

PPI,质子泵抑制剂。

(1) 内镜检查

没有必要仅为诊断 Hp 感染而进行胃镜活检。当胃镜检查有临床指征时,有 3 种方法可识别胃活检标本中的 Hp:活检尿素酶检测、组织学检查和培养。方法的选择取决于临床实际情况、成本、可用性和检测准确性[125]。对于每种方法,都要从胃窦和胃体部获取 1~2 次活检。

最初建议进行活检尿素酶检测,因为该方法效率高、成本相对较低且通常准确[131,132]。通过将胃活检组织置于含有尿素和 pH 试剂(如酚酞)的培养基中,检测胃活检材料的脲酶活性。Hp 尿素酶水解尿素,释放氨,产生碱性 pH,导致酚酞试验培养基颜色变化[129]。检测结果可在几分钟至几小时内呈阳性。市售的几种尿素酶检测试剂盒,仅在培养基(琼脂凝胶或膜垫)和检测试剂方面存在差异[129]。这些试剂盒通常是廉价的,但在西方中心,可能会增加与获得胃组织样本相关的成本费用(例如,编码诊断性内镜检查)。然而,活检尿素酶检测的成本低于组织学检查。活检尿素酶试验的敏感性和特异性分别为 90%~95% 和 95%~100%[129,133]。胃部的血液[134]或使用抗生素、含铋化合物或抗酸分泌药物(尤其是 PPI)可能对准确度产生负面影响[135]。因此,在服用抗分泌药物的个体中,尿素酶试验阴性不能排除 Hp 感染,这是转诊接受内镜检查的常见情况。为了提高此类患者的敏感性,可以考虑停用可能存在问题的药物,并推迟内镜检查至停药后 2 周(如果可能),并可尝试检测胃窦和胃体的多个(>2)活检样本。

胃黏膜组织学评估一般不是诊断 Hp 所必需的,但它可以提供关于黏膜炎症严重程度的信息(见图 52.3A),以及用于检测 Hp 相关的癌前病变如化生、(慢性)萎缩性胃炎(后文讨论)和异型增生[129]。组织学检查一直被认为是鉴定 Hp 感染的金标准,报道的敏感性和特异性分别高达 95% 和 98%[136]。然而,胃内微生物的分布和密度可能不同,存在取样误差的可能性,尤其是在服用抗分泌药物的患者中。生物体的检测常见于标准的 HE 染色,但可用 Giemsa 染色、银染色、Genta 等特殊染色或特异性免疫组化染色进行改进(图 52.4)[130,136,137]。

黏膜活检的培养是困难的,因为 Hp 的生长苛求复杂的营养物质且生长缓慢,需要专门的培养基和生长环境[129,130]。培养 Hp 在美国当代实践中并不常规可用。在培养胃黏膜活检组织进行 Hp 检测时,应在活检钳暴露于福尔马林前获得组织。然后将组织置于仅含几滴生理盐水或适当培养基的容器中,以在转运至当地或异地微生物学检测机构期间保存好标本[130]。虽然一般不推荐进行黏膜培养,但培养联合抗生素敏感试验可指导难治性感染患者的后续治疗,认识到体外敏感性试验并不总能预测临床治疗结果[130,138]。

(2) 非内镜检查

血清学检测是临床上最流行的非侵入性检测方法,以其方便、费用相对较低而被使用。如前所述,感染会激发全身免疫反应,酶联免疫吸附试验技术可以检测多种细菌抗原的 IgG 血清抗体[129,130]。IgA 和 IgM 抗体检测的可靠性较低,不推荐使用[129]。基于实验室的全血检测试剂盒可在 30 分钟内提供结果,并允许进行"服务点"检测。虽然血清学检测相对便宜、无创,并且非常适合初级保健机构,但 Hp 在检测人群中的流行率影响其准确性[131]。血清学检测的敏感性一般相当高(90%~100%),但其特异性各不相同(76%~96%)。因此,在感染不太常见的人群中(包括美国),血清学检查的阴性预测值较高,但阳性预测值不高,假阳性结果较多。在开始 Hp 根除治疗前,建议在低患病率人群中使用另一种检测,如尿素呼气试验或粪便抗原检测(稍后讨论)。即使在成功治疗 Hp 感染后,血清学仍可保持阳性数月或更长时间,因此,血清转化(即从阳性结果至阴性结果)虽然是治疗成功的特异性结果,但不是检测根除的实用方法[139]。

尿素呼气试验(urea breath testing, UBT)可检测活动性 Hp 感染,有助于作出诊断和记录成功的治疗[131]。UBT 依赖于用碳同位素标记的口服给药尿素的细菌水解,无论是非放射性^{13}C 还是放射性^{14}C(图 52.5)。尿素水解生成氨和标记 CO_2($^{13}CO_2$ 或$^{14}CO_2$),可在呼气样本中检测到[140]。非放射性^{13}C 检测被推定用于儿童,同时也适用于孕妇需要检测的罕见病例,但一般不建议在妊娠期进行 UBT,因为妊娠期间 Hp 的治疗很少适用。^{14}C 检测的辐射剂量较低(1μC),相当于 1 天的背景辐射暴露。UBT 的特异性超过 95%,使得假阳性结果不常见。该检测的敏感性为 88%~95%,在接受 PPI、铋剂或抗生素等抗分泌治疗的患者中有假阴性结果。为了提高诊断准确性,最好在 UBT 前 1~2 周停用 PPI、铋剂和抗生素。UBT 在胃切除患者中不准确。

粪便抗原检测是一种检测 Hp 抗原的免疫测定方法,是诊断活动性 Hp 感染和确认治疗后根除效果的另一种非侵入性方法。粪便抗原检测的总体敏感性和特异性与 UBT 相当(分别为 94% 和 97%)。快速 Hp 粪便抗原检测可用于门诊访视期间的检测。但其准确性略低于传统的实验室的粪便检

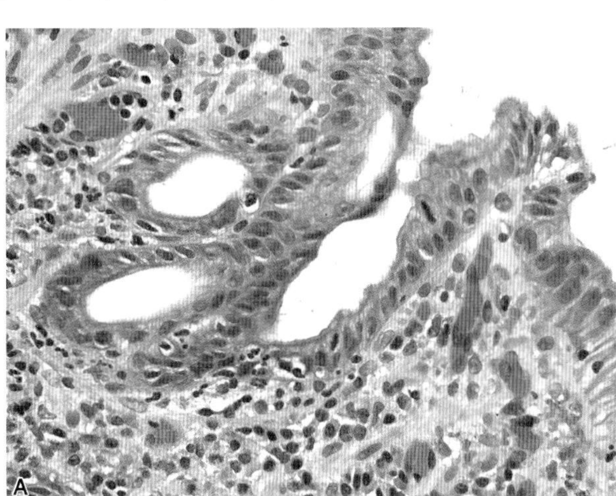

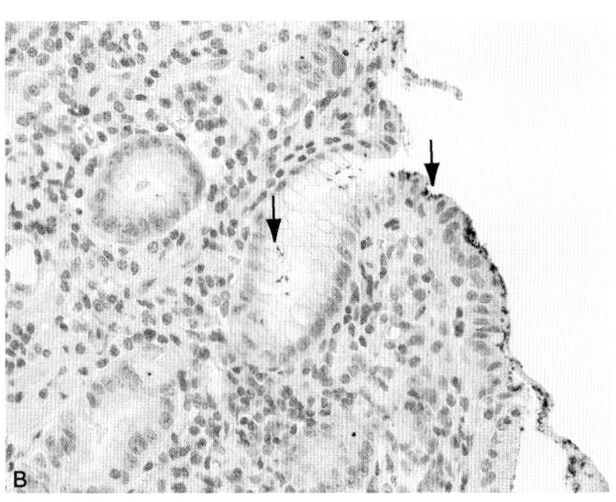

图 52.4　Hp 胃炎的组织病理学。A,活动性慢性胃炎伴弥漫性淋巴浆细胞炎症和中性粒细胞浸润胃小凹上皮(HE 染色,×400)。B,Hp 的免疫组化显示沿胃上皮表面的微生物(箭)(免疫组织化学染色,×400)

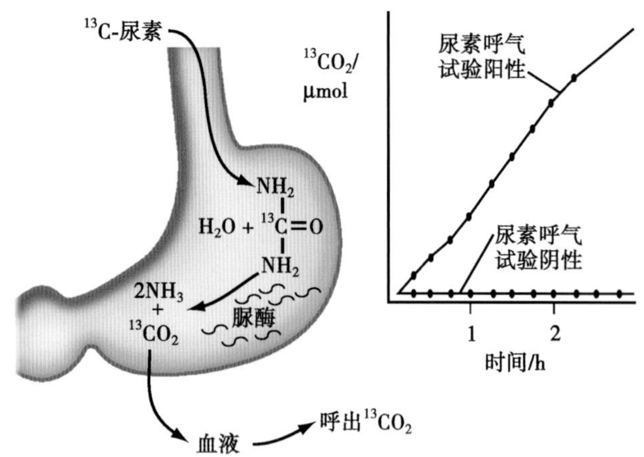

图 52.5 尿素呼气试验(更完整的描述见正文)。(From Walsh JH, Peterson WL. Drug therapy: the treatment of Hp infection in the management of peptic ulcer disease. N Engl J Med 1995;333:984-91.)

测[141]。PPI、铋剂和抗生素的使用也可降低粪便检测的敏感性,可降低细菌负荷,因此,在使用粪便抗原检测时,建议采用与 UBT 早期相似的预防措施。

PCR 是检测 Hp 和检测抗生素耐药基因的敏感方法,但在临床常规诊断中尚不适用[142]。在社区环境中鉴定胃活检、粪便或饮用水中的细菌,在流行病学或传播研究中对微生物进行分型,以及检测抗生素耐药基因,这对于研究目的是有用的。

当有临床指征时,适合通过 UBT 或粪便抗原检测确认感染已成功根除。现行的美国治疗指南(稍后讨论)建议,所有感染者都应接受检测,以确认成功根除感染[143,144]。欧洲指南支持对所有接受 Hp 根除治疗的个体进行非侵入性检测,以确认根除情况。只有在临床需要重复操作的情况下,才需要进行治疗后内镜检查和活检。在此类患者中,采集胃的多个区域样本进行活检,对于避免遗漏由于先前抗生素和抗分泌药物改变细菌密度和分布而导致的持续性感染非常重要。这些检测不应在治疗结束后 6 至 8 周内进行,因为早期检测可能产生假阴性结果。此外,可能影响检测结果的药物,如 PPI,应在检测前停用至少 1~2 周,以提高检测的准确性。与 Hp 感染相关的慢性炎症可能需要数月,有时在根除微生物后需要一年以上的时间才能消退,因此不应将其在活检材料中的存在解释为持续性感染。

(二) 慢性萎缩性胃炎(胃萎缩)

正如第 49 章所讨论的,胃黏膜具有快速的更新率,由祖细胞(干细胞)衍生的新细胞取代脱落到管腔或被破坏的细胞。这一过程保持了泌酸的和胃窦黏膜腺体的厚度和不同的细胞群。在慢性胃炎过程中,细胞丢失的速度可能超过干细胞替代丢失细胞的能力,导致黏膜变薄。这通常伴有来源于峡部干细胞的上皮化生[145]。这种黏膜变薄和伴随的化生(最常见的是肠化生,但有时是假性幽门、胰腺、鳞状上皮或纤毛化生),如果伴有慢性炎症,则称为慢性萎缩性胃炎或胃萎缩。慢性萎缩性胃炎可为局部性或弥漫性,常呈斑片状(见图 52.2)。它是异型增生和胃癌的重要风险因素(见第 54 章)[146,147]。

在慢性萎缩性胃炎(胃萎缩)中[148-168],胃腺体内的特殊细胞(如壁细胞和主细胞)丢失,导致其分泌产物减少或缺失,如内因子(IF)、盐酸(胃酸过多或胃酸缺乏)以及胃蛋白酶原,从而增加不良后果的风险,如维生素 B_{12} 吸收不良、产气细菌过度生长和肠道感染等。

一个国际胃肠病学家和病理学家小组[可操作的与胃癌风险联系的胃炎评估(OLGA)]试图对慢性萎缩性胃炎进展为胃癌的风险进行分期[169]。识别出 OLGA 阶段 0~Ⅳ(表 52.2)。OLGA 系统是基于胃癌风险与胃腺萎缩程度有关的假设[170-173]。也有人提出 IM,IM 比胃萎缩更容易被病理学家识别,可以用来代替胃萎缩(OLGIM)[174,175]。然而,在识别胃癌高风险患者时,关注 IM 而不是胃萎缩的程度可能不太敏感[176]。京都分类系统也用于评估癌症风险,尤其是在日本[177]。IM 亚型分为完全型(小肠型)或不完全型(结肠型)的预后价值尚不确定,尽管文献综述表明不完全型(结肠型)的癌症风险更高,特别是如果肠杯状细胞主要含有磺黏蛋白而不是唾液酸黏蛋白时[178]。

表 52.2 慢性胃炎癌症风险的 OLGA 和 OLGIM 分类

OLGA 分期					
萎缩		体部(胃体及胃底黏膜)			
		无	轻度	中度	重度
胃窦*	无(0)	0	Ⅰ	Ⅱ	Ⅱ
	轻度(1)	Ⅰ	Ⅰ	Ⅱ	Ⅲ
	中度(2)	Ⅱ	Ⅱ	Ⅲ	Ⅳ
	重度(3)	Ⅲ	Ⅲ	Ⅳ	Ⅳ
OLGIM 分期					
肠上皮化生		体部(胃体及胃底黏膜)			
		无	轻度	中度	重度
胃窦	无(0)	0	Ⅰ	Ⅱ	Ⅱ
	轻度(1)	Ⅰ	Ⅰ	Ⅱ	Ⅲ
	中度(2)	Ⅱ	Ⅱ	Ⅲ	Ⅳ
	重度(3)	Ⅲ	Ⅲ	Ⅳ	Ⅳ

*胃窦包括来自胃角的活检结果。

Modified from Rugge M, Correa P, Di Mario F, et al. OLGA staging for gastritis: a tutorial. Dig Liver Dis 2008;40:650-8; and Capelle LG, de Vries C, Haringsma J, et al. The staging of gastritis with the OLGA system by using intestinal metaplasia as an accurate alternative for atrophic gastritis. Gastrointestinal Endoscopy 2010;71:1150-8.

公认的两种类型的慢性萎缩性胃炎(图 52.2,图 52.3B 和 C):EMAG,也称为多灶性萎缩性胃炎和 AMAG,也称为弥漫性胃体萎缩性胃炎。在疾病谱的两端,可以通过临床、实验室、内镜和组织学特征来区分这些类型(表 52.3)。然而,在许多情况下,由于重叠特征,EMAG(通常是由于慢性 Hp 感染引起)和 AMAG(通常是由于针对壁细胞各种抗原的自身反应性 T 细胞和 B 细胞/浆细胞引起)之间的区别模糊不清。例如,在 EMAG 中,随着时间的推移,Hp 可能会从胃中消失,因为胃上皮细胞被化生肠上皮所取代,尽管血清 IgG 抗体作为 Hp 既往感染的标志物可能会持续存在。同样,有人提出,

表 52.3　AMAG 和 EMAG 的特征

AMAG↔AMAG/EMAG	Overlap↔EMAG
内因子抗体，壁细胞	Hp 胃炎（当前，既往）
其他自身免疫性疾病	可能可逆（Hp Rx）
胃窦不受累	胃窦受累
血清 PG Ⅰ↓及 PG Ⅰ/PG Ⅱ比值↓	血清 PG 水平变化更大
高胃泌素血症（可标记）	血清胃泌素正常或轻度升高
胃类癌	

AMAG，自身免疫性肠化生性萎缩性胃炎；EMAG，多灶性萎缩性胃炎；Overlap，重叠；PG，胃蛋白酶原。

通过分子模拟，Hp 抗体可与壁细胞抗原如 H^+，K^+-ATP 酶（质子泵）的 α 和 β 链发生交叉反应，从而形成 AMAG[179,180]。首先由 Correa 推广的肠上皮化生、异型增生和胃癌的这一演变顺序，现已被广泛接受，并在第 54 章中讨论。虽然对胃 IM 患者进行内镜监测的作用仍存在争议，但有些人提倡[147,181]。胃镜检查时可显示胃上皮化生和异型增生，特别是采用窄带成像技术和色素内镜等增强成像方法时（图 52.6）[147]。

1. 多灶性萎缩性胃炎

多灶性萎缩性胃炎（EMAG）是以胃窦和胃体均受累伴腺体萎缩和 IM 为特征（图 52.3B）。为了使病理学家能够诊断 EMAG，内镜医师从胃窦、角切迹和胃体获得至少 2 份活检标本非常重要。[本章译者注解：病理取材方面建议 5 块活检：距幽门 2~3cm 的胃窦处取 2 块（1 块取胃小弯远端，另 1 块取胃大弯远端），距贲门 8cm 处的胃体取 2 块（1 块取胃小弯，另 1 块取胃大弯），1 块取胃角]累及胃体的萎缩性胃炎可能伴有假性幽门上皮化生，其中黏膜类似胃窦黏膜，但胃蛋白酶原Ⅰ（PG Ⅰ）仍可被染色，PG Ⅰ是一种通常在胃体黏膜中表达的酶原。也可能发生其他类型的化生（胰腺、鳞状和纤毛型）。

胃镜检查可因黏膜变薄而见黏膜苍白，表面光亮，黏膜下血管明显（图 52.6）。然而，内镜在诊断慢性萎缩性胃炎方面既不敏感也无特异性，尤其是在 50 岁以下的患者中[148]，放大内镜和自动荧光成像视频内镜在检测萎缩方面可能更敏感[146,147]。

EMAG 的发病机制是多因素的，但 Hp 感染起着最重要的作用，约 85% 的患者被牵连。EMAG 可发生于 Hp 感染者的生命早期。遗传和环境因素，尤其是饮食也很重要。某些人群易患 EMAG，包括非裔美国人、斯堪的纳维亚人、亚洲人、西班牙裔、中南美洲人、日本人和中国人。在中国已经开展了基于性别、一般健康状况、癌症家族史和饮食/饮酒的模型，对 EMAG 患者的胃癌风险进行分层，并确定是否需要筛查胃镜检查[149]。IM 是异型增生和胃癌（通常为肠型）的风险因素（见第 54 章）。据估计，胃肠化生病变中胃肿瘤（异型增生、癌症）的发生率为每年 1%，尽管这些新发肿瘤病变大多为异型增生病变而非浸润性癌[151]。根据上皮的形态和产生的黏蛋白类型，胃黏膜的 IM 可分为 3 种亚型[178]。

2. 自身免疫性肠化生性萎缩性胃炎

自身免疫性肠化生性萎缩性胃炎（AMAG），也称为弥漫性胃体萎缩性胃炎，是胃体腺体的自身免疫性破坏。AMAG 是恶性贫血的病理过程，恶性贫血是一种自身免疫性疾病，通常发生在北欧或斯堪的纳维亚背景患者和非裔美国人中。可能与其他自身免疫性疾病有关，尤其是自身免疫性甲状腺炎。尽管一些 AMAG 患者是无症状的，但许多患者主诉消化不良伴餐后不适[182]。

AMAG 患者表现出胃酸缺乏或胃酸过少、高胃泌素血症伴胃窦 G 细胞增生，继发于胃酸减少或缺乏，以及血清 PGI 浓度低伴血清 PGI/PGII 比值低[183,184]。受累患者通常具有抗壁细胞抗原和 IF 的循环抗体；IF 抗体对 AMAG 的敏感性较低，但特异性较高，而抗壁细胞抗原抗体的敏感性较高，但特异性较低。一般认为自身反应性 T 细胞和随后 B 细胞/浆细胞产生的针对 H^+，K^+-ATP 酶（ATP4A 和 ATP4B）的 α 和/或 β 链的自身抗体被认为在 AMAG 的发病机制中起作用[185]。假性幽门化生（有时称为解痉多肽表达化生）和胰腺腺泡样化生也是 AMAG 的特征[186]。

组织学上，广泛 IM 的萎缩腺体局限于胃体黏膜（图 52.3C）[187]。萎缩通常是局灶性的，保留的相对正常的泌酸黏膜岛可在内镜或影像学上出现息肉样（假息肉）。罕见情况下，AMAG 进展为弥漫性（完全性）胃萎缩。高胃泌素血症是胃酸缺乏的结果，与肠嗜铬样细胞增生和胃类癌有关[152]（在第 34 章中更详细地讨论）。

AMAG 患者中经常存在壁细胞抗原抗体，最显著的抗体是 H^+，K^+-ATP 酶。这些抗体也可以在各种其他自身免疫性疾病患者中检测到，包括 1 型糖尿病[154-156]和自身免疫性甲状腺疾病（Graves 病和桥本甲状腺炎）[157,158]，解释了这些疾病与恶性贫血的相关性。在 1 型糖尿病患者中，发生 AMAG 的风险增加了 3~5 倍，一些学者通过胃镜和黏膜活检对 1 型糖尿病患者进行了筛查。AMAG 还与自身免疫性胰腺炎以及乳糜泻/疱疹样皮炎相关[162,188]。

在 AMAG 患者中，胃黏膜内慢性炎性浸润中存在的一部分 $CD4^+$ 淋巴细胞在 H^+，K^+-ATP 酶的作用下增殖。大多数 $CD4^+$ 细胞分泌 Th1 细胞因子，如 IFN-γ 和 TNF-α，为 B 细胞免疫球蛋白的产生提供帮助，并增强穿孔素介导的细胞毒性，以及 Fas-Fas 配体介导的细胞凋亡。这些因素共同作用可能导致 AMAG 的腺体破坏。

许多 AMAG 患者存在 Hp 的循环抗体和/或在其胃泌酸黏膜中可检测到 Hp。由此可见，Hp 可能在 AMAG 的发病机制中起一定作用[189]。似乎产生 cagA 和 VacA 的 Hp 菌株最有可能引起 AMAG。这些特殊的 Hp 菌株通常是 s1m1 VacA 亚型，也表达 Lewis 血型抗原 X 和 Y[190]。Hp 上的 Lewis 抗原可能有助于伪装生物体，因为这些抗原也存在于人胃上皮细胞上。有人提出，当 Hp 产生 Lewis 抗原 X 和 Y 的抗体时，它们与上皮细胞上的相似抗原发生交叉反应，导致 AMAG（分子模拟）。如果随着时间的推移，这类患者发展为慢性萎缩性胃炎伴 IM，则活动性 Hp 感染率将会下降。

阻断程序性死亡受体（如 PD-1）的免疫检查点抑制剂更常用于癌症患者，据报道，其中一种药物尼鲁单抗（nivolumab）可引起自身免疫性出血性胃炎[191]。

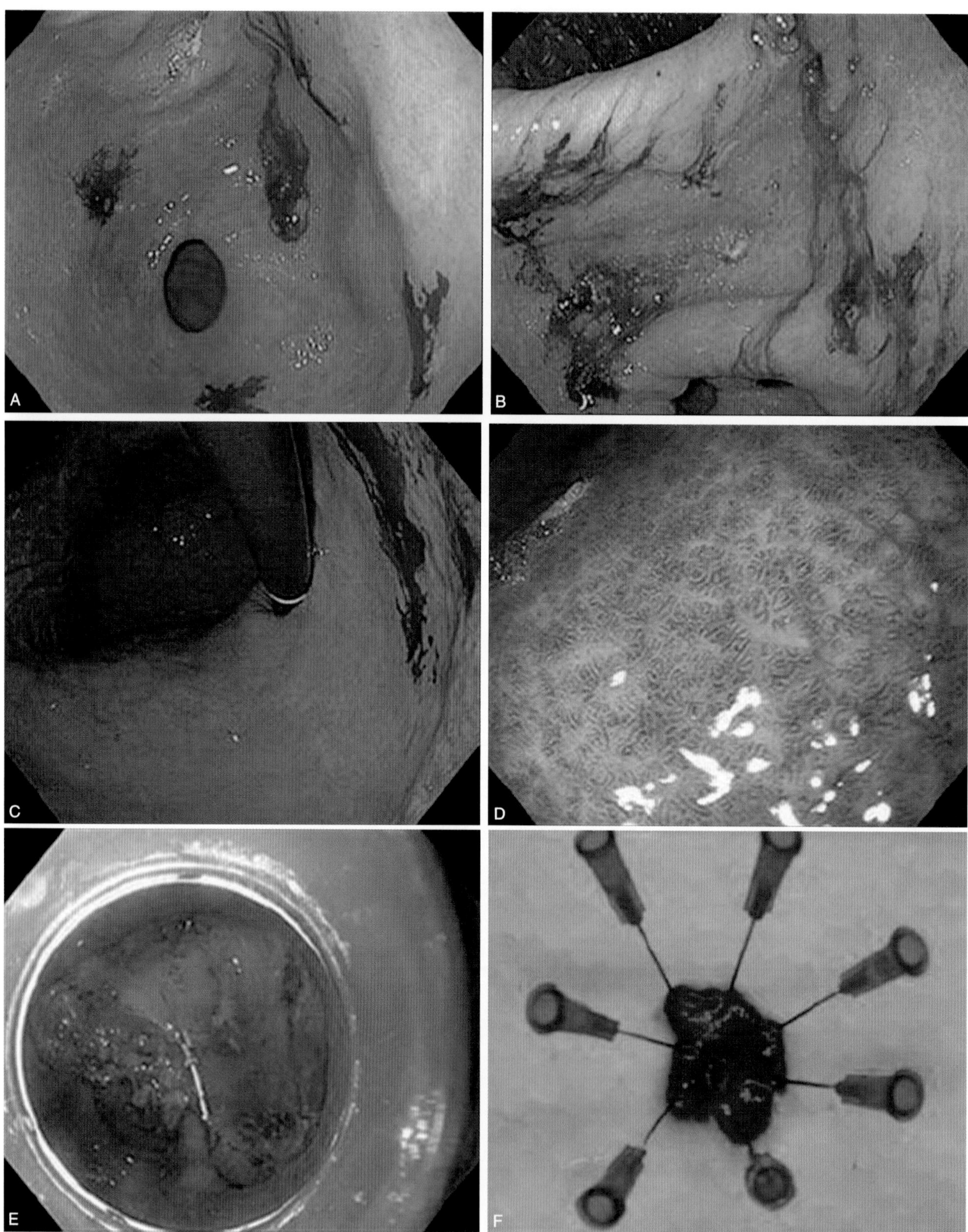

图 52.6　化生性萎缩性胃炎患者的内镜图。注意胃窦(A)、切缘(B)和胃体部小弯侧(C)缺乏皱襞。活检部位显示局部出血。突出黏膜血管模式的窄带成像(D)未提示异型增生,0.8%靛胭脂染色也未提示异型增生(未显示)。注意胃窦部 2.5cm 的异型增生上皮区域(E);异型增生区域已被标记(F),预期进行内镜黏膜下切除术。(From Gomez JM, Wang AY. Gastric intestinal metaplasia and early gastric cancer in the west;a changing paradigm. Gastroenterol Hepatol 2014;10:369-78, with permission.)

(三) 贲门炎

在贲门部,食管和胃黏膜的鳞柱状交界处下方通常有一小圈胃腺体(见 49 章)。在正常志愿者的内镜研究中,大多数人在该区域有贲门型黏膜;其余有泌酸黏膜及其特殊的壁细胞和主细胞[192]。贲门型黏膜炎症(贲门炎)被归因于 Hp 和胃食管反流病(GERD)。健康志愿者发生的贲门炎主要是由于感染 Hp 所致。然而,在诊断性内镜检查期间发现贲门炎的患者中,仅 11% 存在 Hp。诊断性内镜检查人群中,贲门炎的严重程度与食管下段 24 小时酸暴露相关[193]。慢性萎缩性贲门炎伴 IM 被认为是胃食管交界处腺癌的前兆(见第 46~48 和 54 章)。

四、其他感染性胃炎

除了 Hp 感染性胃炎(最常见和最重要的胃部感染)和急性蜂窝织炎性胃炎(尽管罕见但危及生命)之外,还有许多其他可导致发病的感染性胃炎。

(一) 病毒性胃炎

1. 巨细胞病毒

巨细胞病毒(CMV)是一种可以感染胃的人类疱疹病毒(HHV5)。尽管胃 CMV 感染可能发生在免疫功能正常的宿主,但感染通常发生在免疫功能低下的宿主[194]。实体器官或造血细胞移植(见第 36 章)、艾滋病(见第 35 章)、癌症或服用免疫抑制药物(尤其是糖皮质激素)的患者感染风险增加。

胃 CMV 感染的患者可出现上腹痛伴发热和非典型淋巴细胞增多[195]。气相色谱成像可显示胃皱襞明显增厚,胃窦僵硬变窄,提示浸润的胃窦肿瘤。胃镜检查可发现增厚的出血皱襞,胃窦黏膜充血水肿,覆有多发性溃疡,提示胃恶性肿瘤、黏膜下胃窦肿物或消化性溃疡。也可能发生类似于 Ménétrier 病(后文讨论)伴蛋白丢失性胃病的肥厚型和/或息肉样胃炎,尤其是儿童,包括一例 CMV/Hp 合并感染[196]。

黏膜活检标本检查显示炎性碎片、慢性活动性胃炎和含有 CMV 包涵体的增大细胞,提示存在活动性感染(图 52.7A)。"猫头鹰眼"核内包涵体是常规 HE 组织学标本中 CMV 感染的标志,可见于血管内皮细胞、黏膜上皮细胞和结缔组织基质细胞。也可出现多个颗粒状、嗜碱性胞浆包涵体(见图 52.7B)。当 HE 染色切片中难以发现典型包涵体时,CMV 的免疫组化染色可能有所帮助。通常采用静脉注射更昔洛韦或膦甲酸钠治疗,如可行,同时减少免疫抑制剂的使用。在艾滋病患者中,需要行抗逆转录病毒治疗,以预防 CMV 感染复发。

2. 其他疱疹病毒

由单纯性疱疹病毒-1(HHV-1)或水痘-带状疱疹病毒(HHV-3)引起的胃炎罕见[197,198]。感染者通常在幼年时出现初始感染,之后病毒保持较低水平直至再激活。再激活与癌症(包括淋巴瘤)、放疗和/或化疗药物的使用有关。这些疱疹病毒性胃炎的典型免疫功能低下患者可能出现恶心、呕吐、腹痛、发热、寒战、疲乏和体重减轻。气钡双重对比 X 线片显示鹅卵石样、轮廓参差不齐的浅溃疡和充满钡的交错缝隙网络,与溃疡区域相对应。胃镜检查发现多发的、小的、隆起的溃疡斑块或线状、浅表溃疡,呈纵横交错状,使胃呈鹅卵石样外观。应在内镜检查时进行刷检细胞学和活检。刷检细胞学的优点是可对更大面积的黏膜进行取样。大体上,溃疡呈多发性小溃疡,大小均匀。显微镜下,细胞学涂片和活检标本显示非特异性活动性炎症,含有散在的多核细胞,含有模糊(毛玻璃样)核内包涵体。HHV-1 和 HHV-3 在组织中显示相同的组织学特点,故需要对适当的拭子或组织标本进行免疫组化、病毒培养或 PCR,以鉴别这两种病毒感染[198]。用阿昔洛韦治疗是合理的,但价值尚未得到证实。

EB 病毒(EBV)(HHV-4)不存在于正常胃黏膜中,但几乎一半胃炎患者胃中可以出现 EBV[199]。EBV 是否是这些病例中胃炎的原因尚不确定。EBV 感染与深囊性胃炎(稍后讨论)和胃癌有关[200]。急性 EBV 感染引起的传染性单核细胞增多症可导致胃淋巴样增生伴异型淋巴细胞[201]。

3. 麻疹

由麻疹病毒引起的麻疹有许多胃肠道症状,包括罕见的胃炎。特征性组织学类型是胃上皮细胞和基质细胞内存在大量多核巨细胞,伴背景轻度慢性炎症[202]。

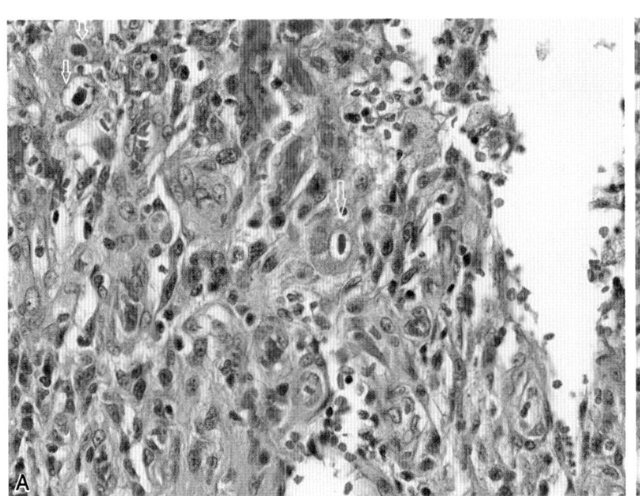

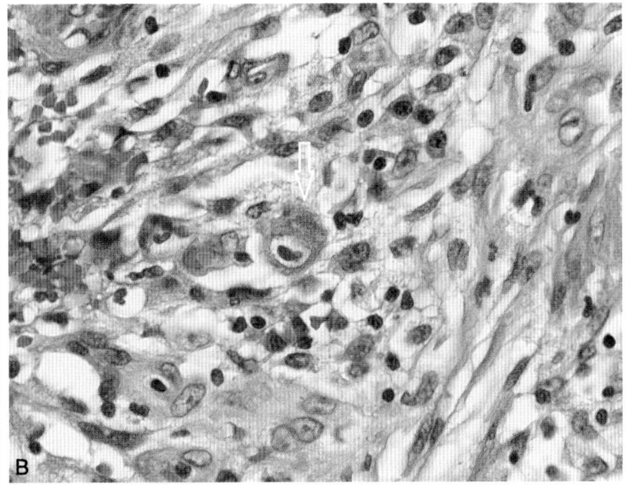

图 52.7 巨细胞病毒性胃炎的组织病理学。A,胃溃疡伴肉芽组织,含有几种 CMV 包涵体(箭)(HE 染色,×600)。B,典型 CMV 感染细胞伴巨细胞,形成典型的 Cowdry A 型核包涵体和颗粒状胞浆包涵体(HE 染色,×600)

(二) 细菌性胃炎

1. 分枝杆菌感染

胃感染结核分枝杆菌罕见[203]。患者通常表现为腹痛、恶心和呕吐、结核性胃溃疡引起的胃肠道出血、贫血、发热和体重减轻。胃结核可能与胃出口梗阻有关。影像学检查可见胃增大、胃窦狭窄、变形及幽门前溃疡。上消化道胃镜检查显示溃疡、肿块或胃出口梗阻。十二指肠结核也可引起胃出口梗阻[204]。大体检查时,胃部表现为多个小的黏膜糜烂、溃疡、浸润肿块(肥大型)、硬化性炎性病变、或从幽门周围淋巴结扩展或从其他邻近器官侵犯造成的幽门梗阻。活检显示干酪样肉芽肿,含有朗汉斯巨细胞和罕见的仅用抗酸染色可见的微小杆菌。第84章讨论了治疗。

虽然鸟分枝杆菌复合群(鸟分枝杆菌、胞内分枝杆菌、嵌合体分枝杆菌)感染是艾滋病患者中常见的机会性感染(见第35章),但很少涉及胃。显微镜下,胃黏膜显示大量含有许多抗酸杆菌的泡沫状组织细胞。治疗采用大环内酯类抗生素(克拉霉素或阿奇霉素)加利福平和乙胺丁醇。

2. 放线菌病

原发性胃放线菌病是一种少见的、慢性、进行性、化脓性疾病,以形成多个脓肿、引流瘘管以及丰富的肉芽组织和致密纤维组织为特征[205]。胃放线菌病的症状包括发热、上腹痛、上腹部肿胀、腹壁脓肿伴瘘管和上消化道出血。放射学研究经常提示恶性肿瘤或消化性(胃)溃疡。内镜检查提示为局限性、溃疡性胃癌,可通过内镜活检作出诊断。

大体上,切除的胃显示胃壁有一个大的、界限不清的溃疡性肿块。显微镜下,多发性脓肿显示感染因子以色列放线菌,这是一种通常存在于口腔内的革兰氏阳性丝状厌氧菌。在含有脓液的肿块活检或引流窦活检可发现该菌提示放线菌病。如果仅通过组织学检查识别疾病,则预后良好。建议使用青霉素或阿莫西林/克拉维酸进行长期(6~12个月)大剂量抗生素治疗。

3. 梅毒

美国一期和二期梅毒的发病率不断上升,2016年报告的病例超过27 000例,与2015年的病例报告和小病例相比增加了17.6%[206]。系列强调了胃肠病学家和病理学家对梅毒的千变万化表现保持警惕并熟悉疾病组织病理学模式的重要性[207,208]。二期或三期梅毒的胃受累在临床上很少被认识,其通过内镜活检标本检查的诊断鲜有报道。应该认识到胃内梅毒的特征,从而可以在疾病进展和造成永久性残疾之前,为有效的抗生素治疗提供机会。梅毒性胃炎可与肝炎和直肠炎同时发生[207]。胃梅毒可发生在HIV感染的情况下。

患者通常表现为消化性溃疡的症状,常伴有上消化道出血。与胃梅毒酷似的疾病包括消化性溃疡、胃腺癌、淋巴瘤、结核和克罗恩病。早期二期梅毒的急性胃炎可产生放射学最早可检测到的体征,表现为皱襞不同程度增厚,可变为结节状,伴或不伴溃疡。可出现胃中部狭窄("沙漏"胃)(图52.8A)。内镜下可见大量浅表、不规则溃疡,上覆盖白色渗出物,周围有红斑(见图52.8B),周围黏膜也可呈结节状。内镜检查也可显示明显水肿的胃皱襞。

大体上,胃可增厚收缩,可呈多发性匐行性溃疡。胃部分切除标本可显示致密、粗大的黏膜皱襞及数目较多的小黏膜溃疡。显微镜下,活检显示重度胃炎伴固有层致密浆细胞浸

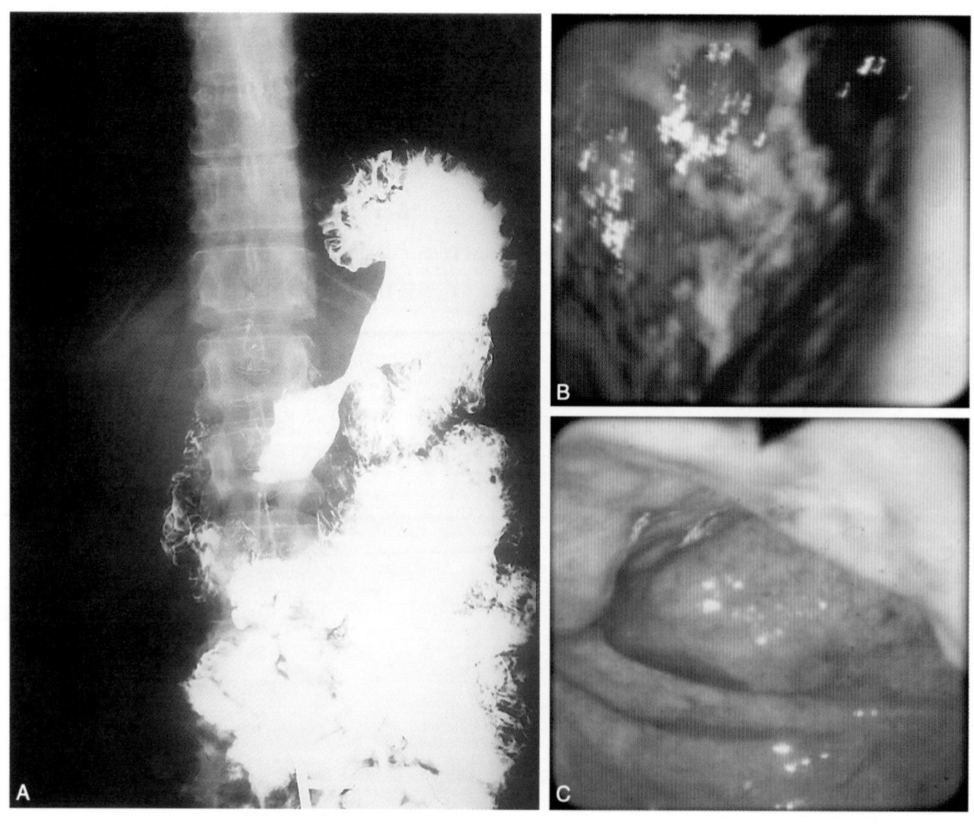

图52.8 胃梅毒(梅毒性胃炎)。上消化道系列胶片(A)显示胃中部狭窄("沙漏"胃)伴胃窦部畸形。另一例胃梅毒患者青霉素治疗前(B)和治疗后4周(C)的内镜表现。(Courtesy Mark Feldman,MD,Dallas,TX.)

润、不同数量的中性粒细胞和淋巴细胞浸润、腺体破坏、血管炎和肉芽肿。Warthin-Starry 银染色或改良 Steiner 银浸渍染色可显示大量螺旋体。血清性病研究实验室和梅毒螺旋体免疫荧光检查可呈阳性，PCR 可检测梅毒螺旋体基因。青霉素治疗效果非常好（见图 52.8C）。

4. 其他细菌

海尔曼尼螺杆菌是螺旋状的细菌，也是慢性活动性胃炎的罕见原因。这种感染可能是胃黏膜相关淋巴组织淋巴瘤（MALT 瘤）的风险因素[209]。这些生物最初被称为人类胃螺旋菌，比 Hp 长，且有多个螺旋。其中一种海尔曼尼菌种，即毕氏螺杆菌，已从人胃黏膜中分离得到[210]。与 Hp 一样，用 Giemsa 试剂可以染色的另一种微生物是猪肠弯曲杆菌[211]。这些非 Hp 弯曲杆菌的临床意义仍有待确定。

（三）真菌性胃炎

1. 念珠菌病

胃溃疡的真菌定植念珠菌属并不少见[212]。对于这种定植是否具有任何临床意义，或者微生物实际上是否加重并使胃溃疡持续存在，目前仍存在争议。内镜下，与典型的胃溃疡相比，与白色念珠菌定植相关的胃溃疡直径往往更大，更常被怀疑为恶性。还可观察到弥漫性浅表糜烂。放射学研究显示微小的阿弗他样糜烂，这是胃念珠菌病中最早可检测到的 X 线改变。阿弗他溃疡可进展为深线性溃疡。

胃肠道真菌定植常见于基础恶性肿瘤患者和接受抗生素或糖皮质激素治疗的免疫功能低下患者，也可能发生于免疫功能正常的患者。胃腔内酵母微生物的大量生长（酵母牛黄）是胃外科手术的潜在并发症，通常是消化性溃疡手术的并发症。胃部念珠菌感染也可发生于酒精中毒患者。

肉眼可见，胃黏膜有微小糜烂、广泛点状、线状溃疡或胃溃疡。显微镜下，坏死的纤维素样碎片层显示酵母菌或假菌丝。在 HE 染色中可以看到微生物；然而，可能需要特殊染色，如过碘酸希夫（PAS）染色或乌洛托品银染色。通常是不需要治疗卡氏念珠菌属本身，但如果怀疑有症状的念珠菌病，可以用氟康唑治疗，但其疗效未得到证实。

2. 组织胞浆菌病

进展性播散性组织胞浆菌病罕见，最常发生在非常年轻的人、老年人或免疫缺陷者。播散性组织胞浆菌病可累及胃肠道的任何部位，但胃部受累并不常见[213]。肥厚的胃褶皱、酷似胃腺癌的肿块、或胃溃疡可能与胃组织胞浆菌病有关。X 线检查可显示胃环状浸润病变。内窥镜检查可显示胃皱襞扩大和发红。活检标本显示混合性慢性炎性浸润内有非干酪样肉芽肿。乌洛托品银染色将突出显示许多小的（2~5μm）圆形至椭圆形酵母形式，偶有出芽，与荚膜组织胞浆菌相容。静脉注射两性霉素 B 脂质体治疗，然后给予伊曲康唑治疗≥12 个月是适当的[214]。

3. 毛霉菌病

胃毛霉菌病（也称合子菌病或藻菌病）是一种罕见的、高致死性真菌感染[215]。风险因素包括营养不良、免疫抑制、抗生素治疗和严重的代谢性酸中毒，通常是糖尿病酮症酸中毒。大多数患者表现为上消化道出血或胃溃疡[216]。胃毛霉菌病可以分为侵袭性和非侵袭性（定植）。蕈状真菌对胃和血管壁的深层侵犯是前者的特征（见前面的急性胃炎部分）。腹痛是最常见的主诉。在非侵袭型中，真菌定植于浅表黏膜，而不引起炎症反应。

大体上，受累患者的手术标本显示累及黏膜和胃壁的出血性坏死。显微镜下，组织中存在直角分枝的无分隔 10~20μm 的菌丝，并浸润到血管壁。治疗方法是切除受累胃的坏死部分。侵袭性胃毛霉菌病几乎总是致命的。

4. 曲霉菌病

急性曲霉菌性胃炎罕见，可具有高度侵袭性[217]。

5. 隐球菌病

隐球菌累及胃和十二指肠可能与免疫受损的宿主有关，包括艾滋病合并隐球菌性脑膜炎的患者[218]。

6. 红曲霉病

这种形式的真菌性胃炎是通过食用干燥咸鱼获得的，并可导致侵袭性真菌感染[219]。

（四）寄生虫性胃炎（另见第 113 和 114 章）

1. 隐孢子虫病

隐孢子虫病可能很少累及胃部[220]。

2. 贾第鞭毛虫病

蓝氏贾第鞭毛虫很少能感染胃[221]。有人认为滋养体感染与慢性萎缩性胃炎以及其相关的胃酸过低有关。

3. 类圆线虫病

胃很少受类圆线虫的影响[222]。该微生物可能定植在完整的胃黏膜上，也可能与出血性消化性溃疡有关。大多数患者免疫功能低下。可出现外周血嗜酸性粒细胞增多。可通过内镜活检、粪便检查或十二指肠抽吸物检查来确诊。播散性类圆线虫病（过度感染）可迅速致死。如果可行，治疗包括伊维菌素和减少免疫抑制的应用（见第 114 章）。

4. 异尖线虫病

摄入含有异尖线虫属线虫幼虫的生海鱼后，可发生侵袭性异尖线虫病（以前称为异尖线虫病）。大多数病例是在日本确诊的。虫体可移行到胃、小肠或结肠[223]。通常，患者表现为上腹疼痛或完全无症状。慢性胃异尖线虫病可导致胃穿孔。一些患者表现为轻度的外周血嗜酸性粒细胞增多。内镜检查可显示坚硬、淡黄色黏膜下肿块伴糜烂。影像学检查可发现充盈缺损，提示胃肿瘤。

大体上，胃显示多发性糜烂灶伴出血和胃壁小的 5~10mm 的胃病变。显微镜下，胃切片显示出明显的嗜酸性肉芽肿性炎症伴胃内形成脓肿和肉芽组织。嗜酸性脓肿内可含有直径 0.3mm 的小蠕虫，即为幼虫型。如果内镜检查不能检测到幼虫，可通过血清学检查确诊。治疗方法是内镜下清除线虫，然后给予阿苯达唑。据报道，含有甲酚木酯的非处方药可成功地缓解相当严重的急性消化不良症状[224]。

5. 蛔虫病

虽然胃蛔虫病很少见，但可发生由蛔虫病引起的慢性、间歇性胃出口梗阻[225]，胃蛔虫病也与上消化道出血有关，内镜检查显示胃和十二指肠内有数条蛔虫[225]。治疗方法是内镜下摘除，然后给予甲苯达唑或阿苯达唑（见第 114 章）。

6. 钩虫病

有据报道内窥镜发现、捕获和从胃内取出钩虫美洲钩虫[226]。

7. 毛细线虫病

据报道毛细线虫病引起的嗜酸性胃炎，可能与摄入生鱼有关[227]。

五、肉芽肿性胃炎

多种肉芽肿性疾病可影响胃[228,229]。在儿童中，最常见的是克罗恩病（图 52.9），稍后在第 115 和 116 章中讨论。在成人中，结节病（见第 37 章）和克罗恩病是最常见的疾病。螺旋体（如梅毒螺旋体）、分枝杆菌（如结核分枝杆菌）、真菌、寄生虫和细菌 *T. whipplei* 杆菌（见第 109 章）感染也可引起肉芽肿性胃炎、黄色肉芽肿性胃炎（见后文）、异物、淋巴瘤、朗格汉斯细胞组织细胞增多症（胃嗜酸性肉芽肿）、嗜酸性肉芽肿伴多血管炎（以前称为 Churg-Strauss 综合征）、儿童慢性肉芽肿病及罕见肉芽肿伴多血管炎（见第 37 章）。

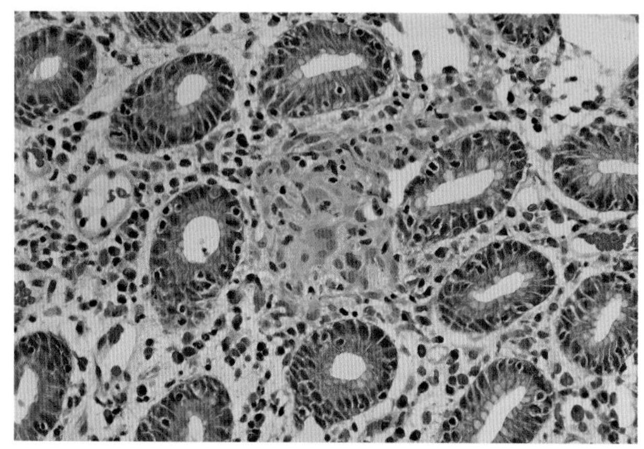

图 52.9　一例克罗恩病患者肉芽肿性胃炎的组织病理学。固有层内存在非干酪样肉芽肿（HE 染色，×200）

也会发生孤立的特发性肉芽肿性胃炎。其中一些“特发性”病例最终可能演变为克罗恩病或结节病。其他“特发性”肉芽肿性胃炎的病例似乎是由于 Hp 感染引起的，在适当的抗生素治疗后可能会缓慢消退，有时会留下黏膜变色[230]。

（一）结节病（肉样瘤病）

结节病是一种全身性肉芽肿疾病，有时累及胃肠道、肝脏和脾脏（见第 37 章）。胃窦是结节病最常见的胃肠道受累部位，约有 10% 的病例受累[231]。在其他器官无肉芽肿性疾病的情况下，不能诊断为肉芽肿性胃炎。受累患者通常在 30~50 岁，典型表现为上腹痛、恶心、呕吐和体重减轻。偶尔出现大量胃肠道出血。胃结节病可导致幽门出口梗阻、胃酸缺乏和恶性贫血。在 X 线上，胃结节病可酷似弥漫性胃腺癌（“皮革状胃”）或 Ménétrier 病。

内镜检查可发现胃远端狭窄，有多处幽门前溃疡或糜烂、萎缩，胃皱襞粗大呈弥漫性鹅卵石样外观，或黏膜正常伴有镜下肉芽肿。胃结节病患者手术标本显示胃壁增厚，有糜烂和溃疡灶。显微镜下，尽管肉芽肿可能是坏死性的，但黏膜检查通常显示多发性非干酪样肉芽肿[232]。由于胃肠道组织中存在的肉芽肿是一种非特异性的结果，因此应进行特殊的染色以排除肉芽肿性感染，特别是 TB。在某些情况下，可能难以鉴别胃结节病与胃克罗恩病或孤立的特发性肉芽肿性胃炎。

糖皮质激素治疗是治疗胃结节病的基础（见第 37 章）。胃大部切除术适用于阻塞和严重出血的患者。

（二）黄色肉芽肿性胃炎

黄色肉芽肿性胃炎（xanthogranulomatous gastritis，XGG）是一种罕见的胃炎，全球报道的病例不足 15 例。XGG 的特征是泡沫状组织细胞明显增生，并混有急慢性炎性细胞、多核巨细胞和纤维化。破坏性炎症和纤维化过程可扩展至邻近器官，类似胃肿瘤，或与胃肿瘤共存[233-235]。已报道 XGG 与胃放线菌病相关[236]。

六、独特的胃病变

（一）胶原性胃炎

胶原性胃炎罕见，可与胶原性十二指肠炎、胶原性结肠炎、淋巴细胞性结肠炎、乳糜泻和/或自身免疫性疾病有关[237-243]。在儿童和青少年中也有报道，通常是一种孤立现象。在一个系列中，确定了 2 种临床模式。在儿童和年轻成人中，表现贫血和上腹痛症状本身归因于胃炎。在老年人中（年龄 35~77 岁）表现的症状通常是由于共存乳糜泻或胶原性结肠炎引起的腹泻[242]。

上胃肠道（UGI）钡剂造影可显示胃体部黏膜表面异常，呈马赛克样，与黏膜结节相对应。内镜检查可发现多处不同程度的离散性黏膜下出血、胃糜烂和沿胃体胃大弯的粗糙皱襞。胃体和胃窦活检标本发现常含有夹带毛细血管的固有层上皮下区域有斑片状、慢性、浅表性胃炎、局灶性萎缩和 20~75μm 厚的不规则胶原沉积（图 52.10）。通常存在表面上皮的微小糜烂，炎性浸润主要由浆细胞、上皮内淋巴细胞和嗜酸

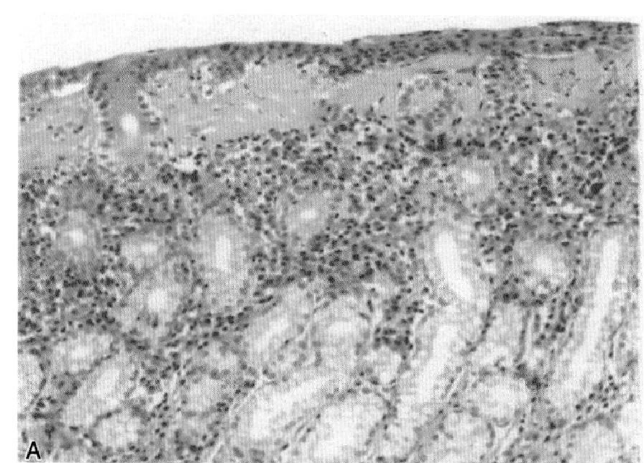

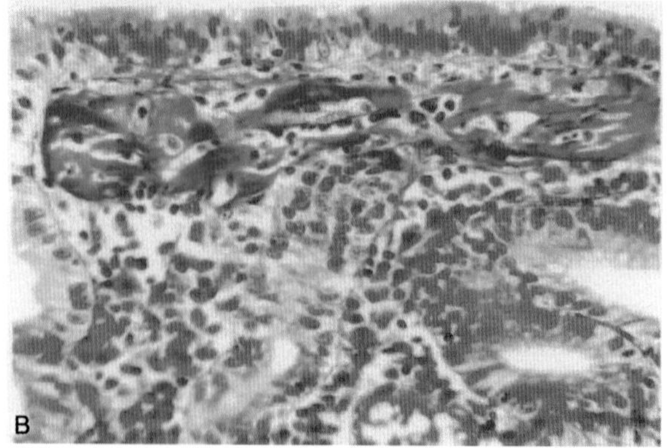

图 52.10　胶原性胃炎的组织病理学（A，HE 染色，×200；B，Masson 三色，×400）。胶原带上皮下增厚明显。（From Wang HL, Shah AG, Yerian LM, et al. Collagenous gastritis: an unusual association with profound weight loss. Arch Pathol Lab Med 2004;128:229-32）。

性细胞组成，以及黏膜肌层的显著肥大。对这种情况的病因、自然史和适当治疗知之甚少。

（二）淋巴细胞性胃炎

淋巴细胞性胃炎[244]以表面和胃小凹上皮致密的淋巴细胞浸润为特征（图 52.11A）。淋巴细胞性胃炎与一种被称为内镜下形式的痘疹样胃炎有关，以结节、皱襞增厚和糜烂为特征[245]。成人淋巴细胞性胃炎通常见于 Hp 感染患者。此类患者的 Hp 根除治疗可显著改善胃上皮内淋巴细胞浸润、胃体炎症和消化不良症状。淋巴细胞性胃炎与胃淋巴样增生的关系尚不明确，后者也与 Hp 感染有关。胃黏膜相关淋巴样组织淋巴瘤（MALToma）患者由于 Hp 感染，淋巴细胞性胃炎的患病率明显增加。因此，淋巴细胞性胃炎可能是 Hp 感染患者胃 MALToma 的先驱病变（见第 32 章和第 54 章）。

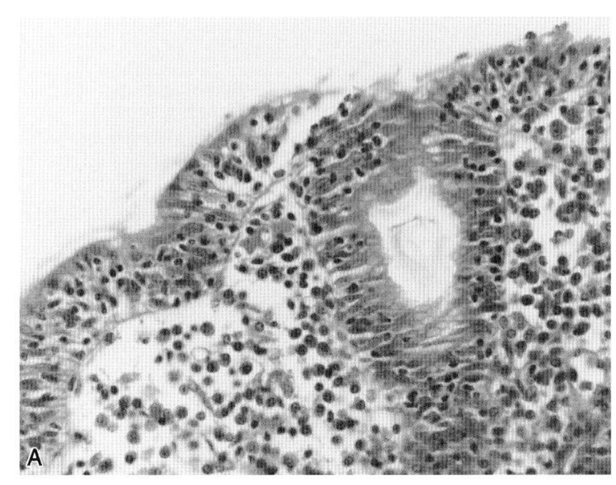

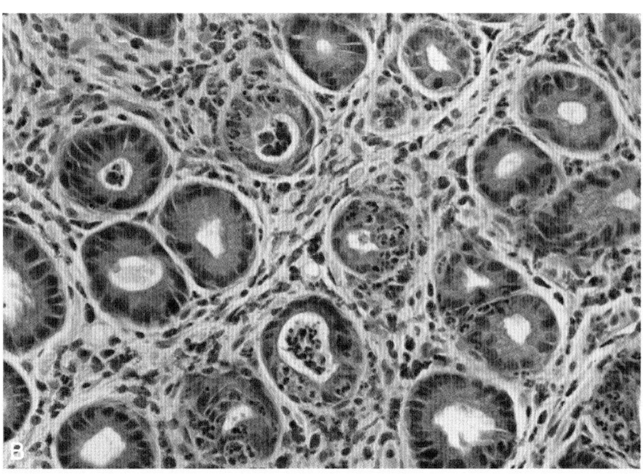

图 52.11　淋巴细胞性胃炎（A）和嗜酸性胃炎（B）的组织病理学。A，胃窦黏膜的高倍视图显示大量深染的单核细胞，伴上皮内淋巴细胞明显增多（HE 染色，×400）。B，在固有层内和胃腺壁及管腔内观察到大量嗜酸性粒细胞。患者还出现外周血嗜酸性粒细胞增多（HE 染色，×400）。（Courtesy Pamela Jensen，MD，Dallas，TX.）

令人信服的证据表明，淋巴细胞性胃炎可能是乳糜泻的表现，也是乳糜泻更严重和更早发病形式的标志（见第 107 章）[245,246]。在开始无麸质饮食后，这些患者的淋巴细胞性胃炎缓慢消退。其他淋巴细胞性胃炎的相关病因包括：乳糜泻、HIV 感染、克罗恩病、常见的多种免疫缺陷和药物治疗[247]。

淋巴细胞性胃炎的内镜检查显示黏膜皱襞较厚、结节状和阿弗他糜烂（疣状胃炎）[245,248]。胃活检显示浆细胞和淋巴细胞浸润导致固有层扩大，伴有罕见的中性粒细胞。这些表现可仅见于胃窦黏膜，或仅见于胃体黏膜，或两者兼有。黏膜表面和浅层小凹上皮显示有明显的 CD3+T 淋巴细胞上皮内浸润，上皮变平，顶端黏蛋白分泌丧失。

淋巴瘤样胃病[249,250]是由于 $CD56^+$ 自然杀伤淋巴细胞浸润胃，类似胃淋巴瘤。大多数病例是在日本报告的，在日本，对健康个体的癌症内镜筛查很常见。在 10 例成人（年龄 46~75 岁）系列中，病变表现为约 1cm 隆起结节。往往无胃部症状。大多数淋巴瘤样病变无需治疗即可消退，但病变有时会复发。尚未有死亡报告。

X 连锁淋巴增生性疾病也可发生慢性活动性胃炎[251]。

（三）嗜酸性粒细胞性胃炎

嗜酸性粒细胞性胃炎是嗜酸性粒细胞性胃肠炎的常见组成部分[252-254]，这是一种病因不明的罕见疾病，是以胃肠道嗜酸性粒细胞浸润、外周血嗜酸性粒细胞增多和胃肠道症状为特征，没有已知的嗜酸性粒细胞增多的原因（例如寄生虫感染、牛奶蛋白过敏）或其他炎症性胃肠道疾病（如炎症性肠病）。嗜酸性粒细胞性胃肠炎在第 30 章中有更详细的讨论。

嗜酸细胞性胃炎和嗜酸细胞性胃肠炎一样，根据受累胃壁的层次（即黏膜病、肌层病和浆膜下病）进行分类。胃肠道黏膜受累可导致腹痛、恶心、呕吐、体重减轻、贫血和蛋白丢失性胃病。肌层受累一般会产生胃出口梗阻症状[253]。罕见的浆膜下嗜酸性粒细胞疾病患者可发生嗜酸性腹水。

胃的影像学检查可显示黏膜皱襞增厚、结节或溃疡。胃镜检查可发现外观正常的黏膜或充血、水肿的黏膜，表面糜烂或胃皱壁肿胀的。嗜酸性粒细胞性胃炎可能模似胃癌。胃黏膜活检对诊断至关重要，表现为明显的嗜酸性粒细胞浸润、嗜酸性小凹脓肿、坏死伴大量中性粒细胞和上皮再生（见图 52.11B）。异常嗜酸性粒细胞浸润定义为：每高倍视野至少有 20 个嗜酸性粒细胞，可以是弥漫性的，也可以是多灶性的。有人提出对下列病例诊断为嗜酸性粒细胞性胃炎，嗜酸性粒细胞浸润黏膜表面、小凹上皮、较深的黏膜或黏膜下层，或与黏膜损伤的其他特征相关（例如小凹增生或结构紊乱伴显著慢性或活动性炎症）[252]。有必要对胃进行全层活检，以诊断肌肉疾病。可以进行穿刺术来诊断浆膜疾病。

如第 30 章中所讨论的，在排除了其他与外周嗜酸性粒细胞增多相关的全身性疾病（如嗜酸性粒细胞增多性肉芽肿伴多囊性-嗜酸性粒细胞增多症综合征、寄生虫感染）后，伴有致残性胃肠道症状的患者，可使用糖皮质激素进行有效治疗。胃出口梗阻患者可能需要内镜治疗（如球囊扩张）或手术干预。

七、炎性肠病性胃炎

胃炎在成人，尤其是克罗恩病和 UC 儿童患者中被越来越认识到[255-257]。炎症性肠病相关胃炎中最常见的 2 种组织学异常是慢性非活动性和慢性活动性胃炎。胃黏膜局灶性增厚的胃炎和 Hp 胃炎在这些患者中较少见。局灶性增厚的胃炎特征是胃小凹和腺体周围有微小的淋巴细胞和巨噬细胞(组织细胞)的聚集,通常也有中性粒细胞浸润(图 52.12)。局灶性增厚胃炎有时可见于克罗恩病,但在 UC 中不常见。

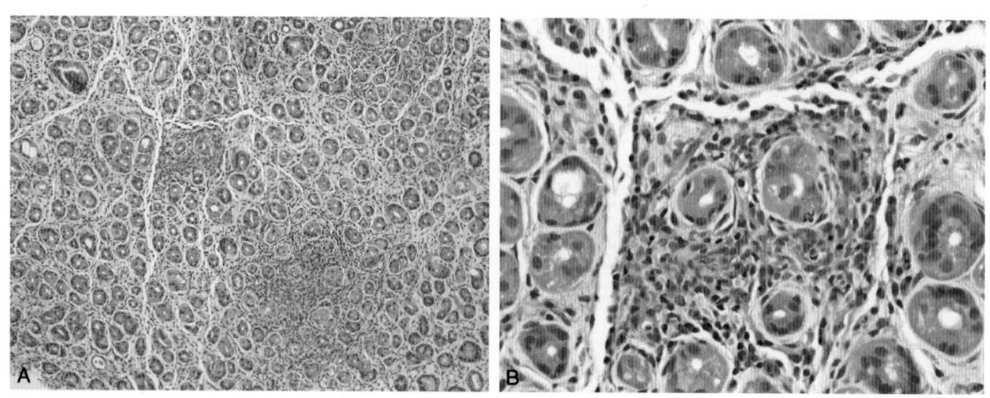

图 52.12　局灶性增强胃炎的组织病理学。A,胃黏膜低倍视图,显示边界不清的炎性细胞结节(HE 染色,×100)。B,高倍视图显示淋巴细胞、嗜酸性粒细胞和中性粒细胞的混合浸润,局灶性浸润腺体上皮(HE 染色,×400)

(一) 克罗恩病

累及胃的克罗恩病(Crohn disease)并不常见[258],通常与肠道疾病一起发生(见第 115 和 116 章)。虽然罕见病例可能孤立于胃或胃和十二指肠,但对孤立性胃克罗恩病的诊断应谨慎[259]。对此类患者进行密切随访,适用于随后发生下消化道克罗恩病或其他肉芽肿性疾病,如结节病。

胃克罗恩病的症状是非特异性的,包括恶心和呕吐、上腹痛、厌食和体重减轻。胃的放射学对比研究显示胃窦皱襞增厚、胃窦狭窄、浅溃疡(口疮)或较深的溃疡。邻近小肠或结肠病变节段的胃部受累最好通过影像学检查来显示。内镜检查可更好地观察黏膜缺损,其特征为黏膜发红、形状不规则的溃疡和黏膜破坏模式的糜烂。结节性病变经常发生,并且在结节顶部常有糜烂。非典型性鹅卵石样表现可能与裂隙样溃疡包围的结节有关。肿胀的皱襞,被线状沟纹或糜烂性裂隙穿过,被称为"竹节样"征[260]。与克罗恩病相关的胃溃疡或糜烂最常见于胃窦和幽门前区,与溃疡倾向于圆形或椭圆形的消化性溃疡不同,克罗恩病的溃疡和糜烂通常为匐行性或纵向的。

胃克罗恩病的黏膜活检或手术标本的显微镜下特征可以是,但并不总是,像回肠或结肠的显微镜特征(见第 115 和 116 章)。它们包括肉芽肿性炎症(见上文关于肉芽肿性胃炎的章节)、透壁性慢性炎症、匐行性或纵向溃疡和明显的黏膜下纤维化(见图 52.9)。内镜下正常的胃窦黏膜中可出现肉芽肿。如前所述,局灶性增厚胃炎也很常见(见图 52.12)。

克罗恩病胃炎的治疗应以临床症状为依据,而不仅仅是通过黏膜活检证实胃炎来治疗的。目前尚缺乏药物治疗胃和十二指肠克罗恩病的双盲随机对照临床试验。PPI 治疗应作为有症状患者的首选方法。尚未在对照临床试验中证明糖皮质激素、氨基水杨酸盐、免疫抑制剂(如硫唑嘌呤)和生物制剂(如抗 TNF-α 药物)的有效性,但有英夫利西单抗治疗成功报告[259]。对药物和内镜治疗无效的胃出口梗阻,可以通过胃肠吻合术进行治疗,理想情况下最好是在腹腔镜下进行。克罗恩病的治疗将在第 115 章和 116 章中详细讨论。

(二) 溃疡性结肠炎

溃疡性结肠炎(UC)中胃炎的患病率低于克罗恩病,尤其是局灶性增厚胃炎的患病率,但高于无炎症性肠病的对照组[255,256]。 在大约 5% 的 UC 病例中,胃的内镜下表现异常,与直肠和结肠的内镜下表现相似(见第 115 章和第 116 章)。此类伴有"溃疡性胃炎"的 UC 患者的特征为:①胃组织病理学与结肠组织病理学相似;②对抑酸药物(H2RAs 或 PPI)几乎无反应;③溃疡性胃炎对 UC 标准治疗的反应。所有溃疡性胃炎 UC 患者不是患有全结肠炎,就是进行了直肠结肠切除术,后者中的许多人还患有结肠袋炎[261,262,276]。据推测,UC 治疗常用的抗炎药物如糖皮质激素,可能掩盖了一些患者的溃疡性胃炎。

八、深在性囊性胃炎

深在性囊性胃炎(gastritis cystica profunda,GCP)是一种罕见的胃假性肿瘤,表现为胃腺体囊肿样扩张,穿过黏膜肌层,进入黏膜下层[263-270]。这种病变可能是部分胃切除术与 PUD 胃空肠吻合术的并发症,通常发生在胃肠吻合术部位。GCP 也可能发生在未手术的胃部,与 Ménétrier 病[263]和胃癌有关[264-267]。内翻增生样胃息肉可能是 GCP 的一种变体。胃息肉切除术后 GCP 也可能是医源性的[268]。

壁细胞顶端 K^+ 流出通道的 β 亚基的靶向缺失,导致侵袭性胃癌小鼠出现 GCP 样病变[269]。

一般认为,黏膜内的损伤和炎症会导致黏膜肌层断裂和上皮迁移至黏膜下层[270]。如果存在,GCP 中的胃部症状是非特异性的。胃成像和内镜检查通常显示模拟恶性肿瘤的多发性外生胃肿块。EUS 可通过显示病变的囊性性质来协助诊断。GCP 的诊断应导致对胃癌的全面彻底检查。无胃癌的 GCP 患者是否需要内镜监测后续癌症发展尚不明确。

GCP 可在黏膜下注射后以抬高病变，通过圈套息肉切除术取出。还报告了 GCP 的内镜黏膜下剥离术，切除了共存的早期胃癌[264]。在某些情况下，需要手术切除。

大体上，胃黏膜表面显示多个结节和外生性肿块。切面胃壁较厚，存在多个囊肿。显微镜下黏膜呈小凹状增生，囊性腺体经破坏的黏膜肌层伸入至黏膜下层，很少伸入固有肌层（图 52.13）。与慢性炎症有关，扩张的腺体之间有展开的肌束。

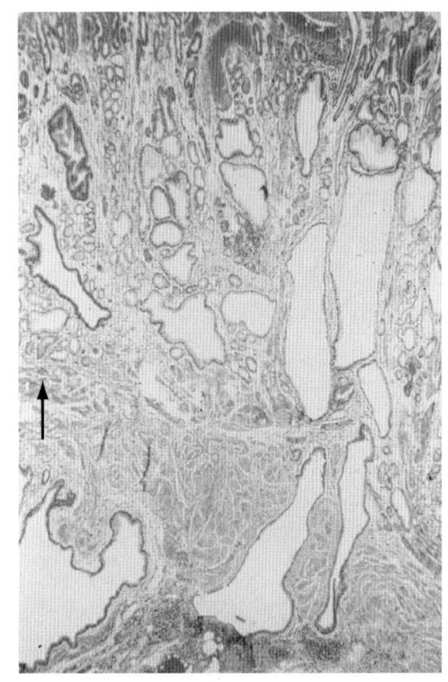

图 52.13　深在性囊性胃炎的组织病理学。可见许多胃腺的囊性扩张，延伸穿过黏膜肌层（箭），类似胃癌（HE 染色）

九、过敏性胃炎（另见第 10 章）

对牛奶蛋白过敏的婴儿，临床表现为呕血和黑便，在胃镜检查时可见广泛的胃炎和胃病[271]。这些婴儿的胃黏膜活检可显示中性粒细胞和嗜酸性粒细胞性胃炎伴黏膜出血。相反，通过以下方法诊断为食物过敏的儿童，开放消除激发试验的胃炎发病率不高于无食物过敏的儿童[272]。

十、反应性胃病

胃黏膜上皮细胞可能受到多种机制的损伤，这些机制不会产生显著的炎症浸润。这种损伤导致上皮快速恢复（表面重修）和小凹增生的细胞再生。由于缺乏炎性细胞，上述病变最好称为反应性胃病。尽管有时仍使用较旧的术语"急性糜烂性胃炎"。约 15% 的胃黏膜内镜活检发生反应性胃病。其发生率随年龄的增长而增加，意想不到的是，其发生率随着胃肠道其他部位的炎症而增加[273]。

内镜下表现为反应性胃病的患者胃黏膜表现为一系列红色条纹[274]、上皮下出血、黏膜糜烂，甚至急性溃疡。急性糜烂和溃疡常为多发性，由于血红蛋白暴露于胃酸中，这些病变的基底常染成深褐色。

大体上，大多数胃糜烂和急性胃溃疡表现为直径 1～2mm 的界限清楚的出血性病变。如果损伤严重，病变之间的黏膜可出现严重出血。显微镜下，糜烂显示浅层固有层坏死。急性溃疡是延伸至黏膜肌层的坏死区域。小凹增生是上皮再生的标志（图 52.14）。常合并细胞核不典型的腺体可误诊为异型增生，甚至癌。在黏膜坏死、细胞碎片和肉芽组织背景下诊断肿瘤应极其谨慎。由于活检程序本身可能引起组织出血，因此，上皮下出血应占活检标本的四分之一以上，被视为有显著出血。在一些反应性胃病患者中，正电子发射断层摄影扫描期间胃可能会"发光"[275]。

反应性胃病（急性糜烂性胃炎）的最常见原因将在后面讨论。

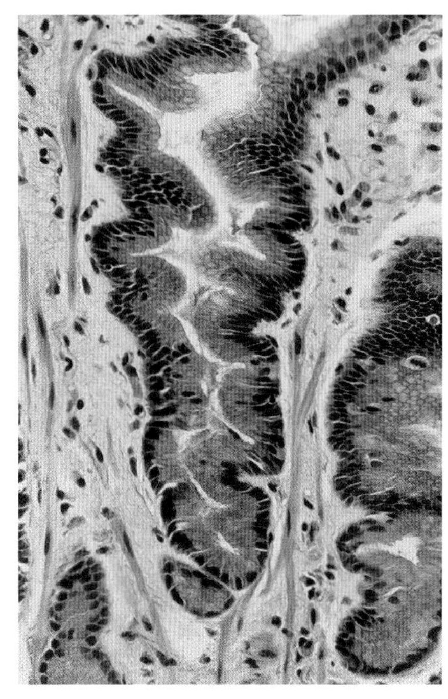

图 52.14　小凹增生的组织病理学，通常见于反应性胃病。胃小凹陷呈细长的螺旋状外观（HE 染色）

（一）药物、毒素和违禁药物

摄入阿司匹林和/或非阿司匹林非甾体抗炎药（NSAIDs），包括 COX-2-选择性抑制剂，是反应性胃病非常常见的原因[276]。NSAIDs 胃病与 PUD 之间的关系在第 53 章中讨论。表 52.4[277-284] 中列出了其他可能损伤胃的药物。碳酸镧（Fosrenal）是一种用于终末期肾病患者的磷酸盐结合剂，产生的磷酸镧可沉积在胃黏膜中，引起白斑和组织细胞增多症[284]。多种毒素和违禁药物可损伤胃，其中乙醇是最常见的毒素。急性摄入乙醇后，内镜检查经常观察到上皮下出血，活检标本上一般无明显的黏膜炎症（图 52.15）。酒精和阿司匹林（或 NSAIDs）的联合作用比单独使用任何一种药物引起的胃黏膜损伤更大。由于使用高纯度可卡因引起的出血、胃溃疡和幽门或幽门前穿孔已被充分描述[285]。表 52.4 列出了毒素诱导的反应性胃病的其他一些原因。

表 52.4　可能引起反应性胃病的一些药物、毒素和违禁药物

药品	毒素和违禁药物
阿司匹林、其他 NSAIDs 和 COX-2 抑制剂	腐蚀性的/腐蚀性物品(见第 28 章)
双膦酸盐类(如阿仑膦酸钠)	可卡因
溴西泮(静脉注射苯二氮䓬类药物)	乙醇
肿瘤化疗药物	重金属(如硫酸汞)
氟化物	氯胺酮(吸入用于娱乐用途)
铁补充剂	硒
磷酸钠(肠道准备剂)	

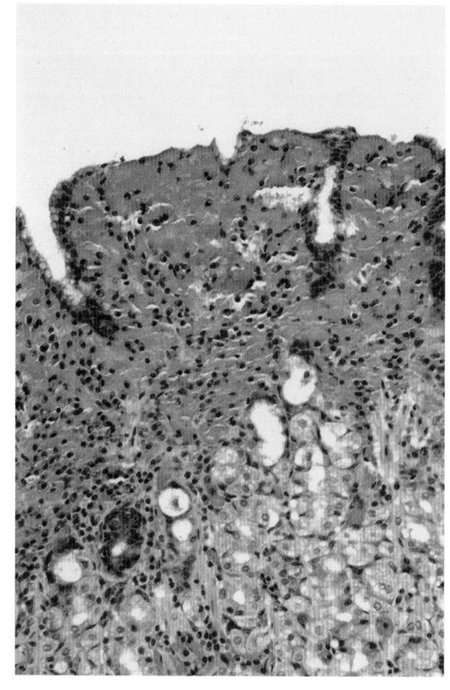

图 52.15　酒精性胃病的组织病理学。出血局限于黏膜的浅表部分,缺乏炎性细胞(HE 染色)

(二) 胆汁反流

胆汁反流到胃在 PUD(见第 53 章)、胃癌和肥胖症手术后很常见[286-288]。胆汁反流性胃病也可能发生在胆囊切除术或胆道括约肌切开术后,该手术允许十二指肠持续暴露于胆汁中,有可能发生十二指肠胃胆汁反流[289]。

在未接受手术的成人或儿童患者中也可观察到胆汁反流性胃病[275,290]。例如,有消化不良症状、胃镜检查可见红色条纹和组织学上有反应性胃病的成人患者胃内常有胆汁[275]。经证实的胆汁反流患儿主要表现为小凹增生[290]。胆汁反流性胃病最终可能导致 IM[289]。

胆汁反流性胃病的诊断可能具有挑战性,因为许多胃内有胆汁的患者没有症状。因此,需要结合临床、内镜和组织学检查结果。诊断标准尚未得到普遍认可。根据组织学(存在 IM 和组织水肿以及不存在 Hp 和慢性炎症)提出了胆汁反流的指标。使用该指标,发现胃食管反流病(GERD)患者的胆汁反流性胃病的患病率高于对照组[291]。一种更直接的方法是使用胃探针来评估胃中的胆红素浓度(Bilitec 2000)[292],但这是对十二指肠胃反流而不是胃病的检测。

胆汁反流性胃病患者的内镜检查可见胃黏膜肿胀、发红、糜烂和胆汁染色。在既往接受过胃切除术的患者中,共存的 Hp 胃炎是否恶化或减轻内镜检查异常尚不确定[293,294]。活检标本显示小凹增生、囊腺扩张、可能被误诊为异型增生或癌的非典型腺体,以及缺乏急性和慢性炎性细胞。IM[289]甚至胃萎缩也可导致并可能增加胃残留胃癌的风险(见第 54 章)。不幸的是,由于严重的胆汁性胃病而进行的胆汁分流手术不能逆转 IM 或胃萎缩。因此,在因胃癌或消化性溃疡进行初始胃手术时,应构建 30cm Roux-en-Y 支或进行约 10~12cm 等(同向)蠕动空肠间置(插入)术是值得的,以试图预防胆汁反流性胃病和随后的肠化生和萎缩性改变。

完整胃或手术胃的胆汁性反流性胃病的治疗也具有挑战性,并非基于大量对照临床试验[295-299]。在一项胆囊切除术后胆汁反流性胃病的随机试验中,PPI 雷贝拉唑(每日 20mg)、抗酸剂铝碳酸镁(每次 1g,每日 3 次),尤其是其组合改善了症状和胃组织病理学异常,以及通过胆汁监测仪监测评估的胆汁反流减少[299]。硫糖铝也已在一些研究中成功使用,但在其他研究中未能成功使用[296,298]。在大多数临床试验中,未给予安慰剂,而是将药物治疗与单独观察进行比较。胆汁反流性胃病的其他药物治疗还包括熊去氧胆酸和考来烯胺[295,297]。最近的一项非随机研究发现,熊去氧胆酸似乎优于 PPI[288]。

在药物治疗失败的患者中,如果症状严重,建议手术治疗。对于迷走神经干切断术和胃空肠吻合术后出现胆汁反流性胃病或食管炎的患者,建议拆除胃空肠吻合术。对于既往接受过 Billroth Ⅱ 胃切除术和胃空肠吻合术的患者,可以进行 Roux-en-Y 分流术。在先前未手术的 Roux-en-Y 胆道分流术和未手术患者中的长期结果良好[300,301]。

(三) 应激

严重的物理或热创伤、休克、败血症或头部损伤后,胃黏膜的糜烂和急性溃疡可能迅速发生。这些通常被称为应激性溃疡,将在第 53 章中进行讨论。

(四) 辐射

外部电离辐射对胃造成的损伤可分为急性(<6 个月)或慢性(>1 年)(见第 41 章)[302,303]。人们认为辐射诱发胃病的耐受水平约为 4 500cGy。当胃剂量≥5 500cGy 时,大多数患者将出现胃病和/或胃溃疡形成的临床证据。肝动脉灌注钇-90 微球选择性内放射治疗肝细胞癌(见第 96 章)也可导致反应性胃病。放射性胃溃疡通常为单发性,直径 0.5~2cm,位于胃窦部。报告了需要内镜治疗以控制出血的大量出血性胃病。

(五) 移植物抗宿主病

移植物抗宿主病(graft-versus-host disease,GVHD)最常发生在同种异体骨髓移植后,实体器官移植后较少见(见第 36 章)。急性 GVHD 发生在移植后第 21~100 天之间,而慢性

GVHD 发生在第 100 天之后。急性 GVHD 通常累及胃肠道（尤其是肠道）。

胃 GVHD 表现为恶心、呕吐、上腹痛，无腹泻。GVHD 中的 EGD 可显示黏膜缺失、糜烂或水肿。在无腹泻患者以及有或无腹泻但直肠乙状结肠活检标本正常的患者中，可能需要胃黏膜活检来诊断 GVHD，尤其是当这些患者有 UGI 症状时。然而，一般而言，在诊断急性 GVHD 方面，直肠乙状结肠活检比胃（或十二指肠）活检更敏感[304]。胃 GVHD 的基本病理损害包括胃黏膜颈部区域的单细胞（凋亡小体）坏死。坏死包括充满核破裂碎片和细胞质碎片的上皮内空泡。2014 年美国国家卫生研究院（NIH）会议最近更新了受急性和慢性 GVHD 影响的主要器官系统的组织病理学诊断标准。在胃内，通过每个活检切片的细胞凋亡病灶大于或等于一个来确认诊断。长期 GVHD 的特征为腺体破坏、溃疡和/或黏膜下纤维化。炎症通常是极轻微的[305]。

（六）缺血

在慢性肠系膜缺血患者中可观察到与反应性胃病一致的组织学改变（见第 38 章）[306]。慢性缺血性反应性胃病以及慢性缺血性胃溃疡可能继发于慢性肠系膜功能不全或与动脉粥样硬化栓塞相关[307,308]。从事剧烈体力活动的运动员，特别是长跑运动员，可能会出现反复发作的缺血性反应性胃病和慢性胃肠道出血伴贫血[309]。

（七）脱垂

胃贲门黏膜在干呕和呕吐时可脱出进入食管腔内而受伤[310]。钡剂检查和食管镜检查可显示脱垂的胃黏膜。脱垂、充血的黏膜可显示糜烂和浅表溃疡。一项研究显示，在脱垂性胃病患者中，病理性胃食管酸反流的发生率较高[311]。

十一、增生性胃病（包括 Ménétrier 病）

增生性胃病是一种罕见的疾病，其特征为与上皮增生相关的巨大胃皱襞[312]。已经确定了两种临床综合征：即 Zollinger-Ellison 综合征（在第 34 章中讨论）和 Ménétrier 病及其更罕见的变体，称为增生性、高分泌性胃病。图 52.16A 和 B

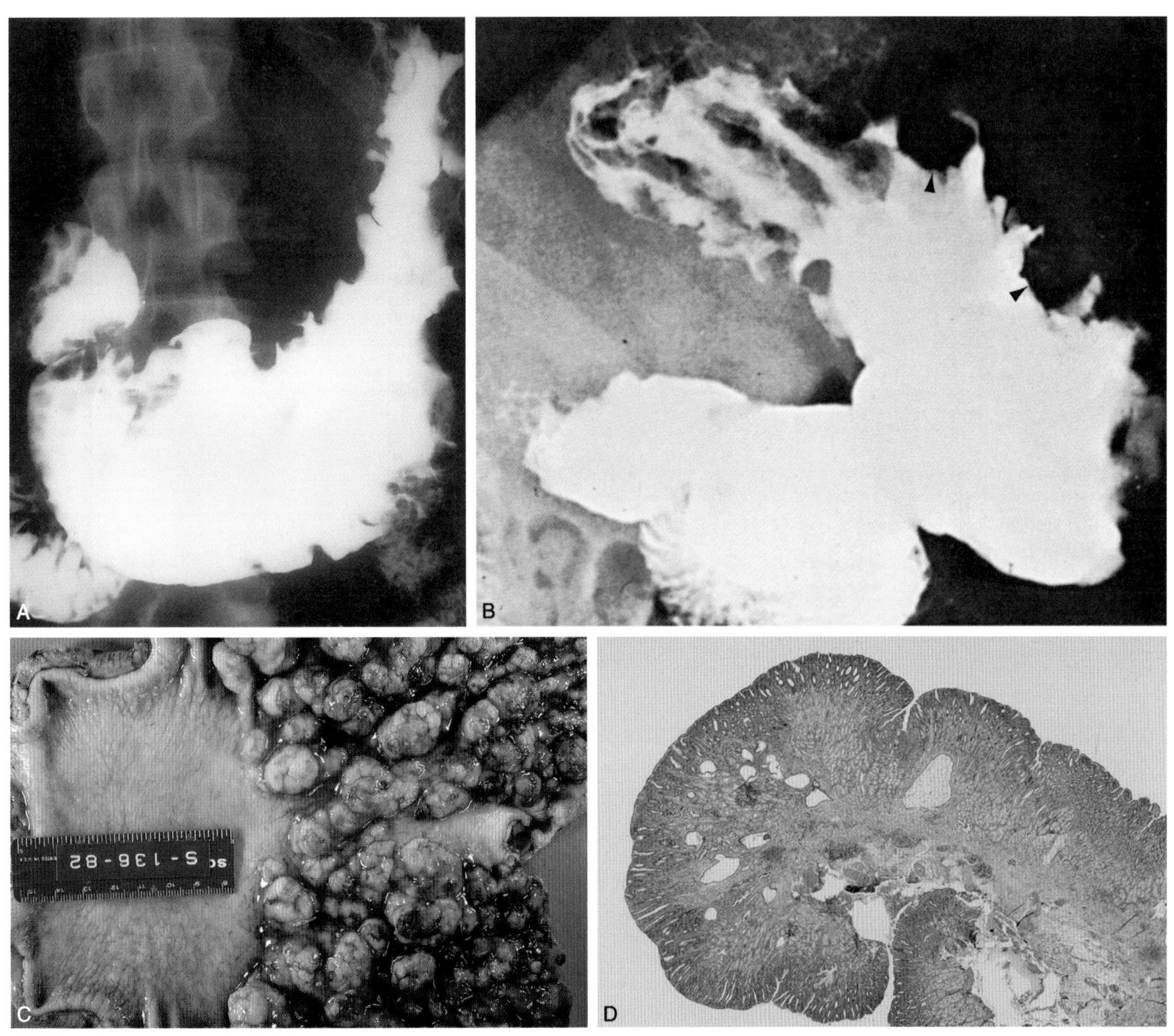

图 52.16　伴有巨大胃皱襞的增生性胃病的放射学和组织病理学示例。A，Zollinger-Ellison 综合征患者上消化道系列的胶片。B，Ménétrier 病患者上消化道系列的胶片。C，一例 Ménétrier 病患者全胃切除术标本（右：胃体，显示增生黏膜和脑回状皱襞；左：胃窦，相对正常）。D，Ménétrier 病组织病理显示皱襞增大伴胃小凹增生，腺体囊状扩张，轻微胃炎

显示了这两种情况下胃皱襞肥大。Ménétrier 病的胃皱襞增大是由于小凹细胞增生、水肿和不同程度的炎症所致。

Ménétrie 病通常但不总是与蛋白丢失性胃病（见第 31 章）和胃酸过少有关，而其罕见的增生性、高分泌的变异型与胃酸分泌增加或正常以及壁细胞和主细胞增生有关，伴有或不伴有过多的胃蛋白丢失。Ménétrier 病与 Hp、CMV 和 HIV 的感染有关[313-315]。

比 Ménétrier 病和 Zollinger-Ellison 综合征更常见的其他疾病也可引起胃皱襞肥大[312]，包括胃恶性肿瘤（腺癌、淋巴瘤）、肉芽肿性胃炎、胃底静脉曲张和嗜酸性胃炎。此外，据报告厚皮性骨膜病（原发性肥大性骨关节病）可引起类似于 Ménétrier 病的肥大性胃病[316,317]，与原发性干燥综合征（SjÖgren 综合征）相同[318]。

Ménétrier 病患者可出现体重减轻、上腹痛、呕吐、厌食、消化不良、呕血和大便隐血试验阳性等。Ménétrier 病可能是自限性的，10 岁以下或发生在产后的患者可完全消退。CMV 感染可引起儿童期的 Ménétrier 病[196]。

Ménétrier 病的胃癌的风险似乎增加（见第 54 章）[319]。该病的一种纤维化变体可酷似皮革状胃癌[320]。

Ménétrier 病患者的黏膜显示为不规则的肥大皱襞，累及整个胃体。黏膜还显示肿胀、海绵状外观，被折痕细分为类似脑沟回样的图像。当 EUS 显示胃壁第二层增厚时（深层黏膜，正常为低回声），可怀疑 Ménétrier 病，并可通过内镜黏膜剥离术进行组织学确认[321,322]。已描述了类似于多发性增生性胃息肉的 Ménétrier 病息肉样变体。

Ménétrier 病患者的胃切除标本通常显示为大的息肉样胃皱襞或大的脑沟回样胃皱襞，胃窦保留（见图 52.16C）。在没有胃切除术的情况下，需要进行全层胃黏膜活检，以充分评估增生性胃病患者的胃组织学。Ménétrier 病和增生性高分泌性胃病的主要镜下特征是小凹增生伴囊性扩张（见图 52.16D）。在典型的 Ménétrier 病中，壁细胞和主细胞可能减少，并被黏液腺取代。

Ménétrier 病的病因尚不清楚，尽管一些病例无疑是由 CMV 或 Hp 的胃部感染引起的。在 29 岁和 35 岁的同卵双胞胎男性中，同时患有这种疾病表明了有遗传成分[323]。与幼年息肉病相关的 SMAD4 种系突变可导致混合性肥大/息肉样胃病[324]。表面黏液细胞增生可能是由于局部过度产生 TGF-α 使胃黏膜 EGF 信号增强所致[325]。有人提出了幼年息肉病综合征和 Ménétrier 病的一元化假说[324]。作者假设一种机制 Hp 感染与 TGF-β-SMAD4 通路失活和 TGF-α 过度表达有关[325]。有人认为 UC 与 Ménétrier 病之间是有关联的[326]。

增生性胃病的理想治疗方法尚不清楚，因为该病如此罕见，缺乏对照试验。可能会自发消退，尤其是儿童。更昔洛韦可用于伴有 CMV 胃炎的 Ménétrier 病患儿。应寻找并治疗 Hp 感染。

如果存在，使用抗分泌药物（H2RAs 或 PPI）可以改善症状[327]，尤其是如果患者患有 Zollinger-Ellison 综合征或正常胃泌素血症的增生性、高分泌的 Ménétrier 病变异型。胃分泌抑制药物可能通过加强细胞间紧密连接来减少胃蛋白流失。一些 Ménétrier 病患者对西妥昔单抗（爱必妥）[326]，一种抗 EGF 受体的单克隆抗体输注有反应（表 52.5）。还有一些患者对生长抑素类似物奥曲肽有反应[328,329]。部分或全胃切除适用于严重并发症，包括难治性或复发性出血、梗阻、严重低蛋白血症、异性增生或癌症进展。

表 52.5　在一家研究机构接受治疗的 7 例患者中静脉输注西妥昔单抗对 Ménétrier 病病程的影响[326,341]

患者	西妥昔单抗治疗持续时间（月或周期）	最近的组织学	治疗后状态
1	18	最低 FH	停止治疗
2	15	最低 FH	停止治疗
3	40	最低 FH	仍在接受治疗
4	9	正常	胃切除术
5	24	发育不良 治疗后 12 个月病变停止	胃切除术
6	9	FH	胃切除术
7	8	FH	胃切除术

FH，胃小凹增生。

十二、门静脉高压性胃病

这种情况代表了肝硬化患者胃肠道失血的一个重要原因。胃黏膜活检显示血管扩张和充血，但无明显程度的炎性浸润或反应性胃病（见第 20 和 92 章）。

十三、鉴别诊断

能模拟胃炎和胃病的最重要的疾病是胃息肉（肿瘤性和非肿瘤性）和胃恶性肿瘤（见第 32 和 54 章）。尽管 CT 标准在区分胃炎/胃病和胃恶性肿瘤方面很有用[330]，但内镜检查和由病理学专家审查的胃活检是最有用的诊断程序。反应性胃病（急性糜烂性胃炎）患者在正电子发射断层摄影扫描期间，偶尔可见胃摄取氟脱氧葡萄糖增加，尤其是胃的近半部分，不应与肿瘤混淆[275]。证明 B 细胞克隆性（如通过免疫染色）也有助于区分胃边缘区淋巴瘤与慢性淋巴细胞性胃炎或淋巴瘤样胃病。

十四、治疗

（一）幽门螺杆菌感染

最近关于幽门螺杆菌感染治疗的建议来自多伦多共识会议和美国胃肠病学会（ACG）的更新指南[143,144]。尽管某些治疗原则已得到普遍认可，但世界各地对幽门螺杆菌感染的治疗各不相同。世界不同地区的具体建议通常反映了抗菌药物的可用性和耐药模式以及当地对某些幽门螺杆菌相关结局（如胃癌）的担忧。幽门螺杆菌感染管理的主要指南反映了总体管理的一致性，但存在地区差异[331-361]。历史上，推荐的幽门螺杆菌治疗方案通常包括 PPI 加 2 种抗生素治疗 10~14

天。但是，最近的建议已经转向标准的 14 天治疗持续时间，因为较短的治疗持续时间与有效性降低相关。然而，鉴于随机对照试验没有足够的证据支持对特定治疗持续时间的强烈建议，治疗持续时间具有了一定的灵活性。此外，目前通常推荐 PPI 和 3 种抗生素或抗菌药物的四联组合[144]。

治疗依从性可能是一个问题，因为需要使用多种药物，并且经常发生与药物相关的轻微副作用。应告知患者可能发生的轻微不良反应（如腹泻、味觉障碍、痉挛），以及在整个疗程中同时服用所有处方药的重要性。与抗生素的耐药性和当地生态相关，治疗成功率因国家和国家内地区的不同而异[334,335]。来自休斯敦的一项研究，对 5 种抗生素的耐药率如表 52.6 所示。不到 50% 的病例幽门螺杆菌菌株对所有 5 种抗生素均敏感[351]。

表 52.6　休斯敦 135 株幽门螺杆菌耐药性分析

抗菌药物	耐药菌株%（95% CI）
阿莫西林	0
克拉霉素	16%（10%～23%）
左氧氟沙星	31%（23%～39%）
甲硝唑	20%（13%～27%）
四环素	1%（0～2%）

From Shiota S, Reddy R, Alsarra A, et al. Antibiotic resistance of Helicobacter pylori among male United States veterans. Clin Gastro Hepatol 2015; 13: 1616-24.

理想情况下，个性化治疗方案应以了解感染个体患者的微生物的特定 Hp 抗生素耐药模式为指导。然而，这些信息在当代美国实践中通常不可用，因为很少有实验室提供微生物培养和抗生素敏感性评估。因此，了解患者个体的个人抗生素应用史并对当地抗生素耐药性模式有一些了解是非常重要的[336]。一些地区日益严重的抗生素耐药问题正在推动未来新型方案的开发。

1. 初始治疗

2017 年更新的 ACG 实践指南中纳入了多种方案作为幽门螺杆菌感染的初始治疗[143]。表 52.7 总结了每种方案的推荐强度和证据质量。建议采用各种“初始”治疗，以便临床医生在为个体患者选择最佳方案时具有一定的灵活性，如对患者的既往抗生素应用史有一些了解。仅对少数主要治疗方案提出了强烈建议。尽管并非所有目前可用的 PPI 都获得美国 FDA 批准作为幽门螺杆菌感染治疗方案的一部分，但没有证据表明这类药物在疗效方面存在任何差异。

克拉霉素三联疗法包括克拉霉素 500mg、阿莫西林 1 000mg 和 PPI 标准剂量每日 2 次，联合给药 14 天。真正对青霉素过敏的患者应接受甲硝唑 500mg，每日 3 次，代替阿莫西林（有关青霉素过敏试验详见后文）。尽管克拉霉素三联疗法曾是幽门螺杆菌感染最常见和最推荐的治疗方案，但由于克拉霉素耐药率升高，该治疗方案已成为不利方案。然而，回顾性收集的单个美国中心的数据发现，15 年期间的根除率约为 79.5%，未观察到疗效随时间推移明显降低[143]。尽管 ACG 仍认为它是“主要”治疗方案之一，但不应提供给既往接受过克拉霉素（或另一种大环内酯类药物，如阿奇霉素）治疗幽门螺杆菌感染或其他适应证的患者。此外，不建议在 Hp 对克拉霉素的局部耐药率估计为 15% 或更高的地区使用（例如，见休斯敦的表 52.8）。克拉霉素耐药性最好被认为是一种绝对现象，不能通过增加剂量来克服。

表 52.7　2017 年 ACG 关于幽门螺杆菌感染治疗的临床指南中推荐的一线治疗方案总结

一线方案	组成部分	持续时间/d	推荐程度	证据等级	备注
克拉霉素三联疗法	PPI，克拉霉素 500mg 和阿莫西林 1 000mg，每日 2 次（或者，如果对青霉素过敏，则使用甲硝唑 500mg 每日 3 次代替阿莫西林）	14	条件性	低（持续时间，中度）	避免既往接触过大环内酯类药物的患者使用。避免在局部克拉霉素耐药率≥15% 的地区使用
含铋剂的四联疗法	PPI 每日 2 次，次枸橼酸铋或次水杨酸盐每日 4 次，四环素 500mg 每日 4 次和甲硝唑 250 至 500mg 每日 3 或 4 次	10～14	强烈	低	特别推荐用于既往接触过大环内酯类药物或对青霉素过敏的患者
伴随治疗	PPI，克拉霉素 500mg，阿莫西林 1 000mg 和硝基咪唑类药物 500mg，每日 2 次	10～14	强烈	非常低	硝基咪唑类药物可以是甲硝唑或替硝唑
序贯疗法	PPI 和阿莫西林 1 000mg，均为每日 2 次 PPI，克拉霉素 500mg 和硝基咪唑类 500mg，均为每日 2 次	5～7 5～7	条件性	低（持续时间，非常低）	硝基咪唑类药物可以是甲硝唑或替硝唑
混合疗法	PPI 和阿莫西林 1 000mg，均为每日 2 次 PPI，克拉霉素 500mg、阿莫西林 1 000mg 和硝基咪唑类 500mg，均为每天 2 次	7 7	条件性	低（持续时间，非常低）	硝基咪唑类药物可以是甲硝唑或替硝唑
左氧氟沙星三联疗法	PPI 每日 2 次，左氧氟沙星 500mg 每日 1 次，和阿莫西林 1 000mg 每日 2 次	10～14	条件性	低（持续时间非常低）	—
左氧氟沙星序贯疗法	PPI 和阿莫西林 1 000mg，各每日 2 次 PPI 和阿莫西林 1 000mg，每日 2 次，左氧氟沙星 500mg，每日 1 次，硝基咪唑类 500mg，每日 2 次	5～7 5～7	条件性	低（持续时间，非常低）	硝基咪唑类药物可以是甲硝唑或替硝唑

PPI，质子泵抑制剂。

Adapted from Checchi S, Montanaro A, Pasqui L, et al. L-thyroxine requirement in patients with autoimmune hypothyroidism and parietal cell antibodies. J Clin Endocrinol Metab 2008; 93: 465-9.

表 52.8 2017 年 ACG 幽门螺杆菌感染治疗临床证据等级指南推荐的抢救治疗方案总结

补救治疗方案	持续时间/d	建议	证据等级	备注
含铋剂的四联疗法（见表 52.7）	14	强烈	低	适用于含克拉霉素方案初始治者疗失败的患者
左氧氟沙星三联疗法（见表 52.7）	14	强烈	中度（持续时间，低）	适用于含克拉霉素方案初始治疗失败的患者
伴随治疗（见表 52.7）	10~14	条件	极低	
利福布汀三联疗法	10	条件	中度（持续时间，极低）	PPI 每日 2 次、利福布汀 300mg 每日 1 次和阿莫西林 1 000mg 每日 2 次
高剂量双联治疗	14	条件	低（持续时间，极低）	PPI 和阿莫西林 750mg，每日 4 次

ACG，美国胃肠病学会。

Adapted from Checchi S，Montanaro A，Pasqui L，et al. L-thyroxine requirement in patients with autoimmune hypothyroidism and parietal cell antibodies. J Clin Endocrinol Metab 2008；93：465-9.

以铋剂为基础的四联疗法是另一种推荐的主要治疗选择。包括铋盐（如次水杨酸铋或次枸橼酸铋）、四环素、甲硝唑和 PPI 联合治疗 10~14 天。由于该方案既不含克拉霉素，也不含阿莫西林，因此适用于既往使用过大环内酯类、居住在大环内酯类高耐药地区（≥15%）的患者以及真正对青霉素过敏的患者。最近缺乏四环素仿制药的可用性限制了该方案的应用。然而，这个问题现在应该已经得到解决。克拉霉素耐药的存在并不影响以铋剂为基础的四联疗法的有效性。含有次枸橼酸铋 140mg、甲硝唑 125mg 和四环素 125mg 的复方胶囊，可能有助于简化患者以铋剂为基础四联疗法。在两项独立研究中，接受其中 3 种联合胶囊每日 4 次和 PPI 每日 2 次治疗 10 天的患者的根除率与标准 10 天克拉霉素三联疗法相当（88% vs 83%）[345]，并且与 7 天克拉霉素三联疗法相比疗效显著更高[346,347]。

伴随治疗（也称为非基于铋的准药物治疗）是克拉霉素，阿莫西林、甲硝唑（或替硝唑）和 PPI 构成的四联组合。尽管它是 2017 ACG 指南中推荐的主要治疗之一，但最近没有基于美国的临床试验评估其有效性。最佳治疗持续时间尚不确定，各项研究使用 3~14 天。目前的建议是，应在 10~14 天内给药。

序贯治疗包括两步方案，每次持续 5~7 天。第一步，PPI 与阿莫西林单独给药。第二步中，PPI 与克拉霉素和硝基咪唑类药物（通常是替硝唑，也可是甲硝唑）合用。这种方法是在欧洲发展起来的，在那里得到了广泛的采用。尚未在北美进行的试验中对其进行广泛评价，但未发现其优于其他方案。尽管使用了克拉霉素，但最初认为其治疗克拉霉素耐药的幽门螺杆菌菌株的有效性有限，在一项早期荟萃分析中[362]，序贯疗法根除了 76.9% 的克拉霉素耐药菌株，而克拉霉素三联疗法为 40.6%。然而，最近一项更新的荟萃分析发现，与 14 天标准三联疗法或 10~14 天含铋剂的四联疗法相比，序贯疗法无显著优势[363]。与其他治疗相比，其相对复杂性，以及来自北美试验的关于其与其他治疗相比缺乏优效性的有限证据，限制了其作为一线治疗选择的实用性和吸引力。

还开发了各种"混合"方案，基本上包括序贯和伴随治疗的一些要素的组合，复杂性相应增加。例如，一种方法包括给予 PPI 和阿莫西林治疗 7 天，然后在接下来的 7 天给予 PPI、阿莫西林、硝基咪唑类和克拉霉素。尽管在亚洲的研究表明其有效且与高水平的治疗依从性相关。但在北美尚未进行将该方法与其他方案进行比较的试验研究。

除以铋剂为基础的四联疗法外，前面列出的所有方案均包括克拉霉素。鉴于克拉霉素的耐药性问题，已经开发出用替代抗生素替代克拉霉素的方案用于一线治疗。最常评价的克拉霉素替代药物是左氧氟沙星。包括这种氟喹诺酮类抗生素的治疗方案通常与 PPI 和阿莫西林联合使用。在北美，左氧氟沙星三联疗法尚未被正式评价为一线治疗。然而，来自世界各地的研究表明，其疗效与克拉霉素三联疗法相似，但局部抗生素耐药率限制了其有效性。左氧氟沙星也在各种序贯方案中进行了研究，在这些方案中，左氧氟沙星基本上取代了克拉霉素。然而，在北美进行的试验中并未对其进行评估。在一项美国随机对照试验中，发现左氧氟沙星、奥美拉唑、硝唑尼特和多西环素的联合治疗优于克拉霉素为基础的三联疗法[364]。目前还没有关于该方案的进一步试验报告。

在采用表 52.7 中描述的治疗方案的患者中，50% 的患者可能会发生与治疗相关的不良反应，但通常是轻微的，不需要中止治疗。一些常见的不良反应包括使用甲硝唑和克拉霉素引起的味觉改变和胃肠道不适，以及使用阿莫西林引起的过敏反应和腹泻。此外，不应给儿童或有生育能力的女性开四环素。幽门螺杆菌治疗的不良反应已被广泛报道[337,338]。咨询患者预期轻微不良反应可能会改善患者的依从性[340]。

2. 补救治疗

初始治疗高达 25% 的患者幽门螺杆菌感染治疗失败。治疗失败的最重要预测因素是抗生素耐药性和治疗依从性差。由于治疗后患者的上消化道症状是根治成败的不可靠指标，所以建议所有患者在治疗后重新检测[143]。治疗后检测应采用活动性感染检测，如尿素呼气试验或粪便抗原检测，感染治疗后应始终避免血清学检测。只有实施常规治疗后测试程序，临床医生才能在实践中对根除治疗的成功率有一些了解。一线方案治疗失败的患者应使用补救方案重新治疗。一般而言，患者不应接受既往使用过的联合治疗，尤其是含克拉霉素或左氧氟沙星的联合治疗。

对于在以克拉霉素为基础的主要方案治疗后发生持续性感染的患者，建议以铋剂为基础的四联疗法或以左氧氟沙星为基础的三联疗法重新治疗。表 52.8 总结了关于补救治疗方案的建议。

全世界对用于治疗幽门螺杆菌的抗生素的原发性耐药性差异很大。在美国，甲硝唑和克拉霉素的耐药率分别高达到

40%和11%。然而,最近关于美国境内幽门螺杆菌抗菌药物耐药性的可靠数据仍然很少。甲硝唑和克拉霉素的耐药性随着患者年龄的增长而增加,女性比男性更常见,耐药率也存在地区和种族差异。幽门螺杆菌对四环素和阿莫西林的耐药性仍然极为罕见(<1%)[336,356,357]。从美国男性退伍军人样本中分离出的幽门螺杆菌菌株的耐药率报告见表 52.6。阿莫西林耐药频率较低,强调了该抗生素在治疗幽门螺杆菌感染中的重要性。与克拉霉素和左氧氟沙星不同,允许将阿莫西林纳入补救治疗,即便其是初始失败方案的一部分。然而,这也突出了当代美国临床实践中阿莫西林"过敏"的问题。高达 10%的美国成年人群可能声称对青霉素过敏,这通常妨碍阿莫西林作为幽门螺杆菌感染治疗方案的一部分。然而高达90%的人青霉素过敏皮试阴性[365],表明并非真正的过敏。因此,理想情况下,Hp 感染一线治疗失败且有青霉素"过敏史"的患者应转诊至过敏专科医生进行正式的过敏试验。如果发现为非过敏性,可以安全地选择基于阿莫西林的补救治疗(见表 52.8)。

抗生素耐药性显著影响以克拉霉素为基础的三联疗法的成功,但在铋剂为基础的治疗方案中不太重要。克拉霉素耐药始终影响治疗结果,而当在适当方案中使用甲硝唑时,甲硝唑耐药似乎更多的是体外现象而不是体内现象。尽管最近的证据表明,甲硝唑耐药可能影响序贯治疗的疗效[343]。克拉霉素的耐药性似乎是绝对的,通过增加剂量不容易克服。核糖体 RNA 23S 链保守环(*A2143G*、*A2142G* 和 *A2142C*)内的 3 种细菌点突变之一,可干扰核糖体大环内酯类结合并导致克拉霉素耐药性[131]。其中 *A2143G* 突变似乎对治疗的不良反应影响最大,可能是三联疗法失败的主要原因。由于特定突变的检测在临床上不可用,因此如果克拉霉素通过培养和敏感性试验怀疑或证实耐药,则建议使用不含大环内酯类的治疗方案。相反,对甲硝唑的耐药性似乎是一种相对现象,在大多数情况下可以通过使用较高的剂量(500mg)或将药物与铋剂联合来克服。阻止甲硝唑还原为其活性代谢物的细菌点突变是导致耐药性的原因[131,334]。

幽门螺杆菌感染复发包括再感染(新菌株)和复发(原始菌株)。复发倾向于在治疗后第一年占主导地位,此后真正的再感染。复发可能与 6~8 周根除后的诊断试验结果为假阴性有关。在对全球文献的批判性综述中,总体年幽门螺杆菌复发风险范围从发达国家的 3.4%(95%可信区间,3.1~3.7)到发展中国家的 8.7%(95%可信区间,8.8~9.6)[358]。在美国和西欧,成人再感染并不常见,每年可能低于 1%。正如本章前面提到的,再感染倾向于、更常见于儿童,特别是在原发感染自发清除后,据报道,生活在世界 Hp 高流行地区的成人再感染更高[359]。迄今为止,在 7 个拉丁美洲社区进行的最大的比较 Hp 根除试验中,总体一年复发率为 11.5%,各研究中心的复发范围从 6.8%到 18.1%[360,361]。

在过去的几十年里,已经报道了 Hp 感染与几种非胃十二指肠疾病的相关性[366],包括免疫性血小板减少性紫癜[367,368]和缺铁性贫血[369]。在这种情况下可考虑对此类患者进行治疗。

3. 预防 HP 感染

在 4 000 名初治未感染的 6~15 岁中国儿童中,接种 3 剂口服疫苗,使用 Hp 尿素酶的 B 亚单位(与大肠埃希菌不耐热肠毒素的 B 亚单位融合作为辅剂),在疫苗接种后第 1 年自然获得的 Hp 感染减少了 72%。在疫苗接种后的第 2 和 3 年,该 Hp 疫苗的有效性降至约 55%[370]。该口服疫苗与安慰剂疫苗具有相似的不良反应特征。预计在 Hp 感染高流行的地理区域进行其他疫苗试验。

同时在中国一个慢性胃炎和胃癌患病率极高的地区进行的病例对照研究发现,摄入绿茶可使胃炎和胃癌的发病风险降低近 50%[371]。

(二)其他类型的胃炎和胃病

如果可以确定的话,非 Hp 胃炎和胃病的治疗取决于基础病因。对有症状的特发性非 Hp 胃炎患者的拟定治疗包括"胃保护"药物[372,373],但在美国尚无此类药物获批用于治疗非 Hp 胃炎或胃病。

(王俊雄 译,王立 刘军 校)

参考文献

第 53 章　消化性溃疡疾病

Francis K. L. Chan, James Y. W. Lau 著

章节目录

一、流行病学 …… 762
二、病因和发病机制 …… 762
（一）幽门螺杆菌感染 …… 763
（二）阿司匹林和其他非甾体抗炎药的应用 …… 763
（三）其他导致溃疡和特发性溃疡的原因 …… 764
三、临床特征和诊断 …… 764
四、活动性消化性溃疡的药物治疗 …… 766
（一）治疗药物 …… 766
（二）幽门螺杆菌（Hp）相关溃疡 …… 767
（三）非甾体抗炎药引起的溃疡 …… 767
（四）其他原因的溃疡和特发性溃疡 …… 768
五、难治性消化性溃疡 …… 768
六、溃疡的预防 …… 768
（一）抗酸药 …… 768
（二）H_2 受体拮抗剂（H_2RA） …… 768
（三）米索前列醇 …… 769
（四）质子泵抑制剂（PPI） …… 769
（五）环氧化酶-2 抑制剂（COX-2 抑制剂）（替代非甾体抗炎药） …… 769
（六）风险评估与药物选择 …… 770
七、并发症及其治疗 …… 770
（一）出血 …… 770
（二）穿孔 …… 773
（三）梗阻 …… 774
八、应激性溃疡 …… 775

胃肠道溃疡可定义为黏膜内层有≥5mm 的破损，内镜检查时有明显的深度或组织学检查证实病变达到黏膜下层。糜烂是指小于 5mm 的黏膜损伤。溃疡和糜烂之间的区别是比较主观的。消化性溃疡（PUD）是指由多种原因引起胃十二指肠的溃疡。这些病变之所以被称为"消化性"，是因为胃蛋白酶在酸性 pH 环境下水解（见第 51 章），在黏膜损伤中起主要作用，而与刺激物无关。

之前数十年的研究集中在胃酸分泌的作用以及压力、性格类型和遗传学在 PUD 发病机制中的影响。组胺-2（H_2）受体的发现和 H_2 受体拮抗剂（H_2RAs）[1]，以及随后的质子泵抑制剂（PPI）的开发，使 PUD 治疗发生了重大变化。幽门螺杆菌（Hp）的发现及其在 PUD 中的作用（见第 52 章）将 PUD 从一种慢性、复发性疾病转变为一种可治愈的疾病[2]。至今 Hp 感染仍然是世界上 PUD 发病的一个重要原因。在发达国家，尤其是在老龄人口中，频繁使用非甾体抗炎药（NSAIDs），包括用于治疗心血管疾病的小剂量阿司匹林已成为 PUD 的主要原因。

一、流行病学

在过去的两个世纪里，PUD 的流行病学发生了显著变化。在 1840 年至 1890 年之间出生的连续队列中，PUD 的患病和死亡风险增加，然后下降[3]。胃溃疡（GU）的发病高峰在 19 世纪上半叶，随后十二指肠溃疡（DU）的发病高峰在 19 世纪下半叶。Sonnenberg 提出了出生队列效应来解释消化性溃疡发病率和死亡率的峰值。在儿童或青少年时期感染 Hp，在晚年表现为消化性疾病。随着时间的推移，人群中的 Hp 感染率逐渐下降，感染人群也逐渐从年轻人转向老年人。DU 和 GU 的发病率随着 Hp 感染率的下降而下降，这可能是卫生条件改善，以及食品和水供应更加安全的结果。

在发达国家，根据医生诊断 PUD 的年发病率波动在 0.14% 到 0.19%；而医院诊断 PUD 的年发病率则较低，波动在 0.03% 至 0.17%。经医生诊断的 PUD 的患病率为 0.12%～4.7%，经医院诊断的患病率为 0.1%～2.6%[4]。PUD 的患病率有很大的地域差异。在一项纳入中国上海 1 022 名志愿者（平均年龄 48 岁）的内镜检查中，PUD 的患病率为 17.2%，其中 93% 感染了 Hp[5]。

PUD 最常见的并发症是出血。据报道，人群中 PUD 年出血率为（19～57）/10 万人（约 0.02%～0.06%）。消化性溃疡穿孔（PULP）的发生率低于出血，据报道每 10 万人中有 4～14 例（0.004%～0.014%）[6]。近年来，随着无并发症 PUD 病例数的下降，消化性溃疡并发症的发生率也在下降。Laine 及其同事[7]使用一个全国住院数据库来计算 2001 年至 2009 年期间胃肠道并发症的年发病率和死亡率。在此期间，消化性溃疡出血的发生率从 48.7/10 万降至 32.1/10 万。在同一时期，年龄和性别调整后的上消化道出血死亡率从 3.8% 降至 2.7%。2009 年，上消化道出血的死亡率（2.45%）明显低于上消化道穿孔的死亡率（10.7%）。在一项纳入了 403 567 名中国台湾患者的基于人群的队列研究中，有并发症的消化性溃疡的住院率在 10 年间显著下降[8]；因此，每年因 DU 出血而住院的比例从 108/10 万下降到 40/10 万，因 DU 穿孔而住院的比例从 9.8/10 万下降到 5.8/10 万。GU 出血和穿孔的年住院率也有类似的下降，分别从 117/10 万降至 61/10 万和 11/10 万降至 6/10 万。

二、病因和发病机制

PUD 的主要危险因素是 Hp 感染和 NSAIDs 的使用（图

53.1)，并且正如后文将讨论的，许多 PUD 患者同时具有这两种危险因素。但另一方面，PUD 患者也可能没有这两种危险因素（Hp 阴性、NSAIDs 阴性溃疡）；部分后一类患者有其他病因，如胃泌素瘤（ZES；见第 34 章），此外为特发性溃疡。

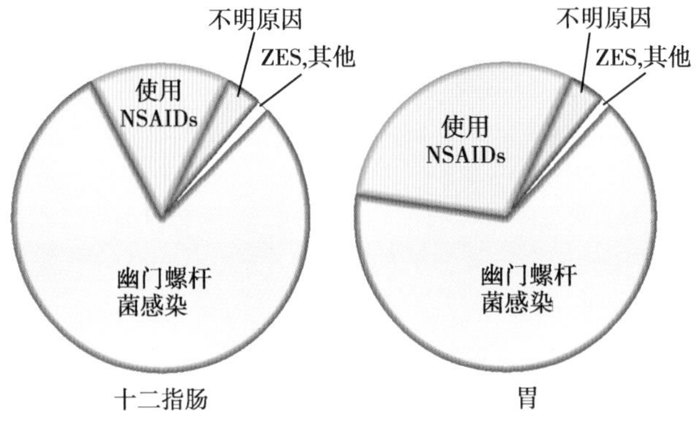

图 53.1　图示消化性溃疡（PUD）病征。所示比例为基于西方国家研究的粗略近似值。Hp 感染和 NSAIDs 使用对消化性溃疡的相对影响在不同人群中差异很大，在人群内，随着年龄和社会经济地位的不同而变化。此外，由于 NSAIDs 的使用和 Hp 感染往往同时存在，因此图中描绘的分离有些人为。NSAIDs，非甾体抗炎药；ZES，胃泌素瘤

（一）幽门螺杆菌感染

Hp 感染的患病率在世界各国之间差异很大（见第 52 章）。由于检验方法、抽样人群的不同，2009 年到 2011 年的一系列研究表明，Hp 的感染率波动在 7%～87%。美国以及欧洲的一些国家 Hp 感染的患病率最低（7%～33%）[9]。日本和中国的患病率为 56%～72%。总体来看，Hp 的感染率在下降。Feinstein 和他的同事研究了 1998 年到 2005 年美国医院消化性溃疡住院记录[10]，随着消化性溃疡年住院率下降（71.1/10 万人下降至 56.5/10 万人），Hp 感染相关性疾病的住院率也在下降（35.9/10 万人下降至 19.2/10 万人）。消化性溃疡出血患者 Hp 感染率仍然很高。Sanchez-Delgado 和他的同事总结了 71 项研究，其中包括 8 496 名消化性溃疡出血患者，其 Hp 感染率是 72%。出血后检测 Hp 的机会增多与 Hp 检出率升高有关[11]。

如第 51 和 52 章所示，10%～20% 感染 Hp 的患者出现以胃窦病变为主的胃炎，从而引起胃酸分泌增多，增加了患 DU 的风险。胃酸分泌过增多导致十二指肠胃酸负荷过高，引起十二指肠球部胃上皮化生[12]。部分专家认为，化生上皮被胃中的 Hp 感染，形成局灶性“十二指肠炎”（严格意义上来说是胃炎），有时伴黏膜糜烂与溃疡形成。

大部分 Hp 感染的患者都存在广泛的胃炎，累及胃窦和胃底黏膜，导致胃酸分泌减少[13]，易出现胃溃疡。在这些人中，黏膜防御机制减弱（如第 51 章所示），而非胃酸高分泌，导致胃溃疡形成。第 52 章讨论了 Hp 基因及其编码蛋白质在 PUD 发病机制中的作用。

（二）阿司匹林和其他非甾体抗炎药的应用

阿司匹林单用或者阿司匹林联合血小板腺苷二磷酸抑制剂，如氯吡格雷（双抗疗法）是预防心血管事件的基础用药。在美国，NSAIDs 的使用率达到总人口的 11%。NSAIDs 的常规应用增加了 5～6 倍消化道出血风险[14]。NSAIDs 的使用者中，1%～40% 因为溃疡相关的严重并发症住院[15]。同时服用阿司匹林和 NSAIDs 的患者，并发症发生率更高。丹麦一项基于人群的研究表明，单独应用低剂量阿司匹林的患者发生消化道出血的比值比 2.6%，同时服用 NSAIDs 的患者中，比值比增加至 5.6%[16]。西班牙一项关于因 NSAIDs 相关不良胃肠道事件住院的死亡率的全国研究中，归因于使用 NSAIDs/阿司匹林的死亡率为 15.3/10 万人，而普通人群的死亡率为 2.5/10 万人[17]。

胃和十二指肠黏膜有数个避免胃酸和胃蛋白酶损伤的保护机制（参见第 51 章）。NSAIDs 引起黏膜损伤的机制包括破坏黏液磷脂、细胞膜，以及解偶联线粒体氧化磷酸化，但大多数证据表明 NSAIDs 通过抑制前列腺素的合成损伤胃和十二指肠黏膜[18]。COX 异构体：COX-1 和 COX-2 负责前列腺素的合成。COX-1 在胃中表达，能够帮助维持胃上皮细胞以及黏膜屏障的完整性。COX-2 在正常的胃中不表达，但会受炎症过程产生的细胞因子的影响而迅速表达。传统的 NSAIDs 如布洛芬对 COX-1 和 COX-2 同工酶的抑制作用大致相同。COX-1 抑制剂减少了前列腺素的合成，削弱黏膜防御系统。动物实验发现中性粒细胞黏附于胃壁微血管，在 NSAIDs 引起的损伤中发挥着重要的作用。中性粒细胞黏附后释放无氧自由基、蛋白酶，阻塞毛细血管血流。抑制中性粒细胞黏附能减弱 NSAIDs 诱导的损伤。此外，2 种气体介质，一氧化氮（NO）以及硫化氢（H_2S）有助于维持胃黏膜屏障。NO 和 H_2S 增加黏膜的血供，刺激黏液分泌，抑制中性粒细胞黏附[19]。与母体药物相比，释放 NO 和 H_2S 的 NSAIDs 衍生物已被证明可以预防胃损伤。胃酸发挥着次要但也是非常重要的作用，能将浅表黏膜病变转化为更深的损伤，干扰血小板的聚集，延缓溃疡愈合[20]。

Hp 感染会影响接受 NSAIDs 治疗的患者发生 PUD 的风险。一项 meta 分析表明，在长期应用 NSAIDs 的患者中，合并 Hp 感染将 PUD 出血的风险增加了 6 倍，而在仅有 Hp 感染和单独使用 NSAIDs 使用的患者中，上述风险分别增加了 1.79 倍和 4.85 倍[21]。一项最新的 meta 分析支持上述观点[22]。对于即将开始应用 NSAIDs 治疗的患者，根治 Hp 能够降低溃疡发生率[23,24]。一项系统综述表明，检测或者根除 Hp 能够降低应用 NSAIDs 患者消化性溃疡发生的风险[25]；然而，仅仅根除 Hp 不足以预防溃疡风险高的 NSAIDs 使用者的消化性溃疡出血[26,27]。

有证据表明 Hp 感染可增加应用小剂量阿司匹林的患者发生 PUD 的风险。近期有消化性溃疡出血的 Hp 感染患者，继续应用小剂量阿司匹林治疗，如能成功根除 Hp，则能将溃疡再出血的风险降到很低，这与阿司匹林/奥美拉唑联合治疗的效果相似[26]。而在继续服用 NSAIDs 的溃疡出血患者中，根治 Hp 并不能达到很低的再出血风险。在一个长期的前瞻性队列研究中[28]，合并 Hp 感染且服用小剂量阿司匹林（≤160mg/d）的患者，在消化性溃疡出血后恢复服用阿司匹林，根除 Hp 之后的再出血风险低，该风险与近期开始服用阿司匹林的既往无消化性溃疡患者的风险相似（每 100 患者・年出血<1 次）。相反，没有 Hp 感染（既往或现症）的出血性溃

疡，同时接受阿司匹林治疗的患者，继续应用阿司匹林肠溶片治疗的再出血风险高（每 100 患者·年出血>5 次）。

（三）其他导致溃疡和特发性溃疡的原因

吸食可卡因和甲基苯丙胺者可出现胃和十二指肠的深溃疡，甚至穿孔，可能是由于这些物质导致黏膜缺血[29]。双膦酸盐疗法和胃十二指肠溃疡相关[30]，虽然临床上更关注双膦酸盐导致食管损伤。应用糖皮质激素发生 PUD 的风险较小[31]。但糖皮质激素合用 NSAIDs 比单独应用 NSAIDs 发生 PUD 的风险高[32]。选择性 5-羟色胺再摄取抑制剂抗抑郁药的使用与 PUD 之间存在微弱的关联，尤其在同时应用 NSAIDs 的患者中。

吸烟、精神压力、A 型性格、酗酒也是 PUD 的危险因素。虽然这些因素会导致消化性溃疡，但是不能单独致病。Hp 感染是混杂因素，而早期的研究并未提及。

PUD 的一个不常见的病因是胃泌素瘤（参见第 34 章）[33]。系统性肥大细胞增多症（参见第 37 章），是另一个不常见的原因。肥大细胞分泌组胺作用于组胺受体，导致胃酸分泌过多，从而引发胃十二指肠多发溃疡[34]。消化性溃疡还与 α_1 抗胰蛋白酶缺乏、慢性阻塞性肺部疾病、慢性肾脏病相关。其他疾病，如胃癌、胃淋巴瘤、克罗恩病，也会在消化道出现酷似消化性溃疡的溃疡。消化性溃疡的罕见原因，包括嗜酸粒细胞性胃肠炎、病毒（如巨细胞病毒）感染、免疫功能缺陷患者的白塞病、海尔曼幽门螺杆菌感染以及胃黏膜异位的 Meckel 憩室。

随着全球范围内 Hp 感染率下降，特发性溃疡占比上升。北美的一项研究表明，超过 10% 的消化性溃疡与 Hp 和 NSAIDs 应用无关。特发性溃疡的发病率是否上升仍然存在争议。有人认为，由于 Hp 感染率下降，特发性溃疡的比例相对升高，而不是特发性溃疡的真实发病率升高。然而，一些前瞻性数据表明，特发性溃疡出血的绝对发病率增加了 4 倍。重要的是，相比于有 Hp 溃疡病史的患者，特发性溃疡出血患者的再出血风险增加 4 倍，死亡率增加超过 2 倍[35]。

三、临床特征和诊断

无并发症的 PUD 患者的主要症状是上腹部疼痛。典型的疼痛和饥饿相关，发生在夜间，进食或者服用抑酸剂后常可缓解。患者经常诉消化不良，如腹胀和早饱。部分患者主诉胃灼热，可能伴或不伴糜烂性食管炎。长期 NSAID 使用者，多为老年人，可出现溃疡出血或穿孔，而无上述溃疡症状。

胃镜是诊断无并发症消化性溃疡的首选方法（图 53.2 A 和 B）。胃镜比影像学检查（如上消化道钡餐造影）具有更高的敏感性和特异性。然而，胃镜检查费用高，并且有并发症风险（参考第 42 章）。所以，可根据一些因素决定疑似 PUD 的患者是否需行胃镜检查。正如本章后面以及第 20 章所述，急性消化道出血的患者需行内镜检查以明确诊断，并实施内镜下治疗。此外，上腹痛考虑 PUD 的患者，一旦出现体重减轻、反复呕吐等报警症状时，需警惕胃部的恶性疾病，此时也需要行胃镜检查（框 53.1）。如果胃镜下发现胃溃疡或者十二指肠溃疡，应取胃黏膜活检做快速尿素酶试验来诊断 Hp 感染（参见第 52 章）。由于存在胃癌风险，应从胃溃疡的边缘取活检。如果胃溃疡活检显示良性，通常会在 8 周之后复查胃镜以确认胃溃疡是否愈合，因为有 4% 的首次胃镜显示良性溃疡的患者之后复查发现为恶性病变[36,37]。

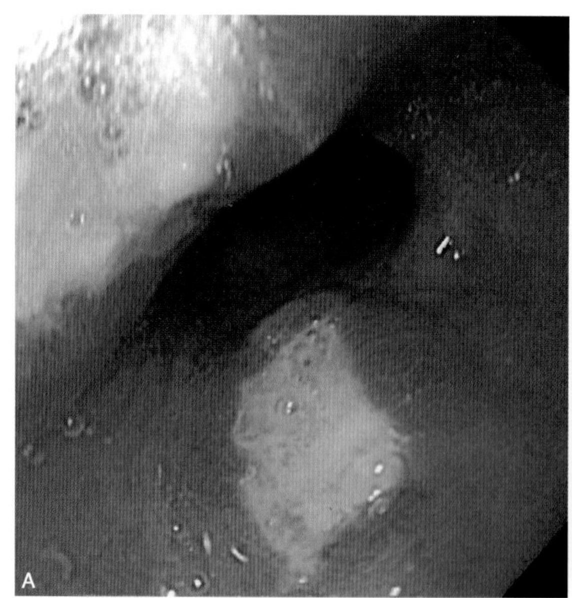

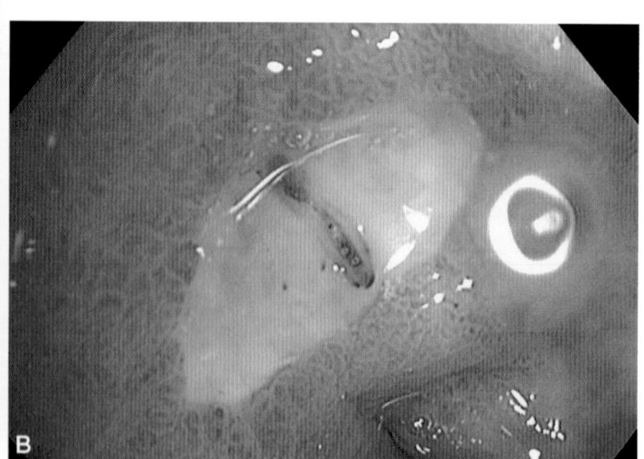

图 53.2　A，使用（非甾体抗炎药）NSAIDs 的患者基于较为清洁的胃窦胃溃疡的内镜视图。感染 Hp 检测均为阴性。B，Hp 快速尿素酶试验阳性患者十二指肠溃的内镜视图。无 NSAIDs 使用史

框 53.1 有上消化道症状的患者的警报特征*
年龄大于 55 岁的新发消化不良患者
有上消化道癌家族史
急性或慢性胃肠道出血,包括不明原因的缺铁
黄疸
左侧锁骨上淋巴结病(Virchow 淋巴结)
可触及腹部肿块
持续性呕吐
进行性吞咽困难
不明原因的体重减轻
*出现这些特征提示需尽快行胃镜和其他检查,以确定明确诊断(见第 14 章)。

消化不良性的上腹症状包括上腹痛或者上腹不适,在临床很常见,占家庭医生就诊的 2%~5%(参见第 14 章)[38]。由于对所有消化不良患者都进行快速胃镜检查的成本高昂,且不切实际,因此建议将其他两项非胃镜检查策略(除上消化道造影之外,该检查对 PUD 的敏感性和特异性较低)作为疑诊 PUD 患者的初始诊疗步骤(图 53.3),即:①"检测-治疗",基于无创 Hp 感染检测,一旦发现 Hp 感染,则进行根除治疗;②经验性抑酸治疗,通常使用 PPI。

Gisbert 和 Calvet[39] 回顾相关文献总结出 Hp"检测-治疗"策略可治愈大多数消化性溃疡、预防大多数胃肠道疾病。改善小部分 Hp 相关性功能性消化不良患者的症状。8 项随机对照试验(RCT)对比了"检测-治疗"策略与"内镜主导"策略。这些试验检测 Hp 的方法不同,年龄的上限从 45 岁到 55 岁不等。一些研究用血清学检测诊断 Hp 感染,其特异性低于^{13}C 呼气试验(参见第 52 章)。不同研究人群中的 Hp 检出率为 23%~53%。经过 12 个月的随访,两组人群消化不良症状的比例相似。8 项试验中有 7 项报道了费用数据,"检测-治疗"策略的费用较低,因避免了许多内镜操作。Ford 和同事对 5 项 RCT 共 1 924 名患者进行了 meta 分析,发现尽快行胃镜检查的患者在 12 个月,消化不良症状缓解效果略优于接受"检测-治疗"策略的患者[风险比,0.95;95% 可信区间(CI),0.92~0.99],可能归功于结果正常的胃镜对患者有一定的安慰效应[40]。

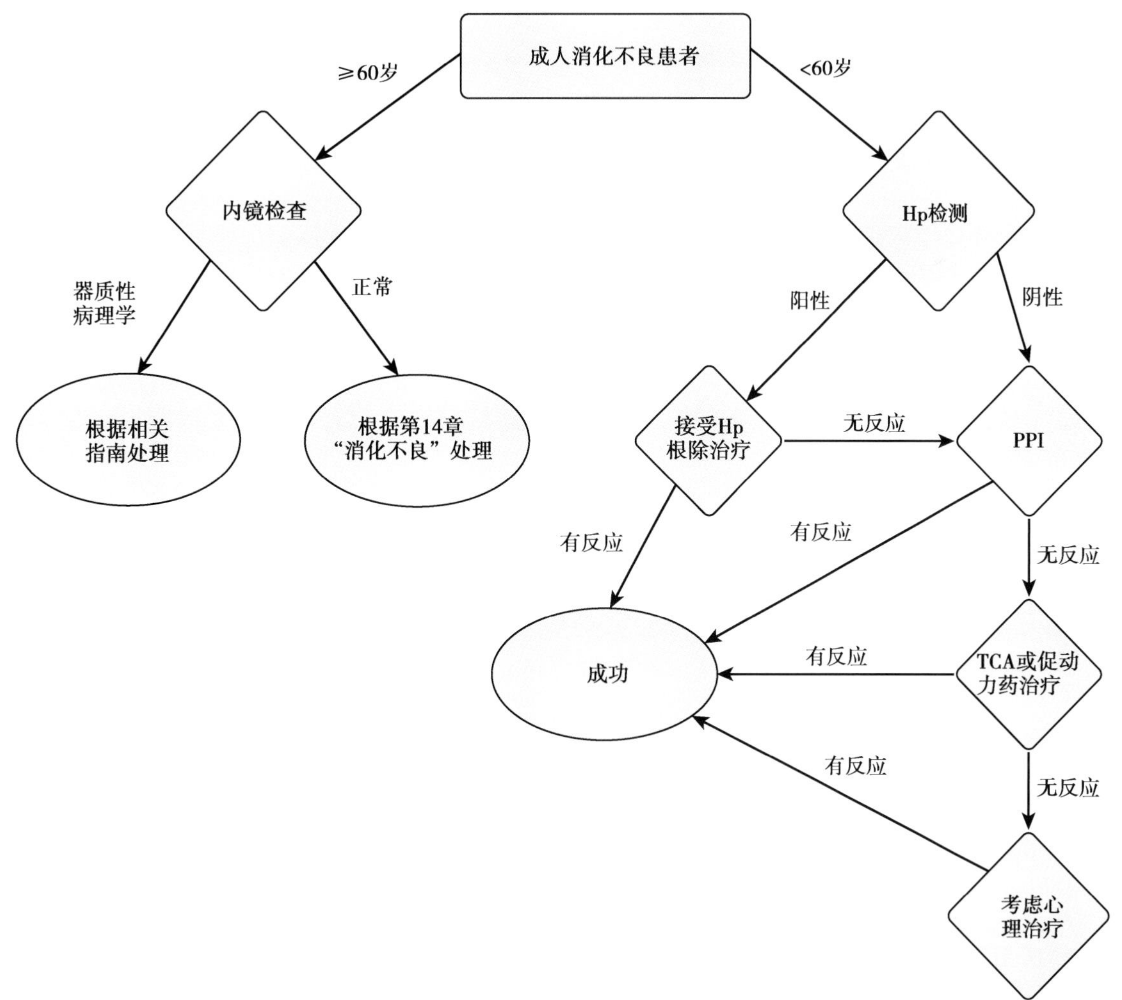

图 53.3 美国胃肠病学会(ACG)和加拿大胃肠病学会(CAG)对未确诊消化性溃疡诊治的指南流程图。这也是目前对疑似 PUD 患者的管理方法。TCA,三环类抗抑郁药物;PPI,质子泵抑制剂。(Adapted from Moayyedi P, Lacy BE, Andrews CN, et al. ACG and CAG clinical guideline: management of dyspepsia. Am J Gastroenterol 2017;112:988-1013)

根据美国胃肠病学会(ACG)/加拿大胃肠病协会(CAG)联合指南,推荐小于60岁不明原因的消化不良患者应当进行无创的Hp检测,阳性时根除Hp。Hp阴性或根除Hp后症状无缓解的患者应当进行PPI试验性治疗。如果PPI治疗无效,可以应用三环类抗抑郁药物或促胃肠动力治疗。上消化道恶性肿瘤如胃癌的发病率随着年龄的增长而升高,因此,非胃镜的管理策略目前主要应用于具有上腹部症状的年轻人。尽快行胃镜检查的年龄界限存在争议,很大程度上取决于该人群上消化道癌症的流行病学。在西方国家,上消化道癌症在年轻人群中不常见,因此常以50岁或55岁为界值。60岁以上,新出现提示消化性溃疡的上腹部症状的患者应当行胃镜检查。在亚洲和东欧,胃癌发病率远高于西方国家,胃镜检查年龄应更年轻。

2017年ACG/CAG有关消化不良的联合指南推荐小于60岁不明原因的消化不良患者,应当进行无创Hp检测,阳性时治疗[39,41]。Hp阴性或根除Hp治疗无效的患者应当进行PPI试验性治疗。如果PPI治疗无效,可以应用三环类抗抑郁药物或促胃肠动力治疗(参见第14章和图53.3)。在Hp中高流行地区,“检测-治疗”策略更优。2017年Maastricht会议共识推荐不明原因的消化不良患者行“检测-治疗”策略。这一决策基于地区Hp流行病学特性和成本效益考虑[40,42]。“检测-治疗”策略不适用于出现报警症状的人群或老年人群。然而,一篇纳入了15项研究的综述质疑了这些报警症状(参见表53.1)预测恶性肿瘤(与PUD或非溃疡性消化不良相反)的能力[43]。不同研究中报警症状诊断恶性肿瘤的敏感性波动在0%到83%。

四、活动性消化性溃疡的药物治疗

多种药物可用于治愈活动期DU和GU。

(一) 治疗药物

1. 抗酸药

抗酸药可以中和胃酸,但是其促进溃疡愈合的能力较弱。大多数内科医生不推荐抗酸药作为治愈溃疡的主要药物,但可以用来缓解消化不良的症状。含镁抗酸药的最常见不良反应为腹泻。相反,含铝及钙抗酸制剂会导致便秘。慢性肾脏病患者应谨慎应用所有抗酸药,因含镁抗酸药会导致高镁血症,含钙抗酸药可导致高钙血症,含铝抗酸药具有神经毒性[44]。

2. 抗分泌药物

无并发症的Hp溃疡不需要常规应用抑制胃酸分泌的药物,因为即使没有抑酸治疗,在成功根除Hp后其溃疡可以愈合;然而,抑制胃酸分泌药物在非Hp感染的消化性溃疡患者中发挥重要作用。第34章讨论了抑酸药在治疗胃泌素瘤方面发挥的作用。

(1) H_2 受体拮抗剂

H_2 受体拮抗剂(H_2RAs)竞争性抑制组胺刺激胃酸分泌(参见第51章),显著抑制基础及餐后胃酸分泌[45]。夜晚应用 H_2RAs 可有效抑制夜间胃酸分泌[46]。口服 H_2RAs 吸收良好,且吸收不受进餐影响。口服后1~3小时血药浓度达峰值。H_2RAs 能够通过血脑屏障、胎盘屏障[47,48]。口服之后,一些 H_2RAs(西咪替丁,雷尼替丁,法莫替丁)经肝脏首次代谢后生物利用度下降35%~60%。而尼扎替丁无肝脏首过效应,口服后其生物利用度将近100%。H_2RAs 在肝脏代谢,肾脏排泄。当肌酐清除率小于50mL/min时,建议减少 H_2RAs 用药剂量。透析不会去除血液中大量的 H_2RAs,因此,透析患者无须调整 H_2RAs 剂量。肝脏衰竭患者无需降低剂量,除非合并有慢性肾脏疾病。H_2RAs 耐药快且常见[49],耐药机制不清。

H_2RAs 安全,可耐受。一项对随机临床试验的meta数据分析表明:H_2RAs 和安慰剂的总体不良反应率没有显著性差异[50]。然而,在个案报道和非对照病例系列中描述了 H_2RAs 的一些不良反应。西咪替丁有微弱的抗雄激素作用,偶致男性乳房发育、阳痿[51]。

西咪替丁和雷尼替丁都与肝脏细胞色素P-450(CYP)混合功能氧化酶系统结合,能够抑制其他经此途径代谢的药物清除,如华法林,茶碱,苯妥英钠,碘卡因,奎尼丁[52]。相反,法莫替丁、尼扎替丁对CYP系统没有显著影响。

(2) 质子泵抑制剂

质子泵抑制剂(PPI)通过抑制胃壁细胞的 H^+-K^+-ATP酶来抑制胃酸分泌(参见第51章)。该药是前体药,必须由酸激活才能抑制 H^+-K^+-ATP酶。有趣的是,前体药PPI也是酸不稳定的化合物,口服给药必须有肠溶衣或抗酸药以避免被胃酸降解[53]。肠溶PPI的吸收可能不稳定,口服给药后2~5小时才能达到血药浓度峰值。虽然PPI血浆半衰期短(≈2小时),但是由于PPI前体药的活性代谢产物与 H^+,K^+-ATP酶共价结合,其抑酸作用持久。PPI主要由肝脏代谢,但有严重肾脏、肝脏损伤的患者也不需要调整剂量。CYP2C19具有基因多态性,PPI代谢涉及其中的一种同工酶。大约25%的亚洲人和3%的白人缺乏CYP2C19活性。这种基因多态性导致奥美拉唑、兰索拉唑和泮托拉唑的血药浓度明显升高,而雷贝拉唑不受影响[36,37,54]。

PPI在酸性环境下才能浓集激活,因此主要与活化的质子泵结合。食物刺激后,60%~70%的质子泵被激活泌酸;因此,饭前即刻服用PPI更有效。推荐在早餐前服用PPI[55]。和 H_2RAs 不同,尚未发现对PPI治疗的抑酸作用的耐药性。

质子泵抑制剂通过提高胃的pH,可以影响一些药物的吸收。然而,这种pH效应在临床上很少有重要的影响,除非PPI与酮康唑或地高辛一起给药[55-57]。酮康唑的吸收需要借助胃酸,如果同时应用了PPI,这种抗真菌药物可能不会被有效吸收。如果患者同时需要PPI和抗真菌治疗,建议选择酮康唑以外的药物。相反,胃pH升高有利于地高辛的吸收,使地高辛血药浓度升高。对于同时接受PPI和地高辛治疗的患者,临床医生应考虑监测地高辛血药浓度。

因为PPI是由CYP系统代谢的,所以它们有可能改变其他通过CYP酶清除的药物的代谢。PPI与氯吡格雷之间的潜在相互作用已引起广泛关注。氯吡格雷是一种非阿司匹林抗血小板前体药物,可被肝脏CYP2C19和其他CYP激活为其活性代谢产物。PPI通过竞争性抑制CYP2C19降低了氯吡格雷的抗血小板作用。对观察性研究进行的meta分析表明,在同时接受PPI和氯吡格雷治疗的患者中,包括心源性死亡在内的主要不良心血管事件显著增加[58,59]。然而，PPI 和氯吡格雷使用的相关性尚未得到前瞻性研究和大规模随机对照试验的证实[60,61]。尽管研究结果不一致，美国和欧洲的监管机构已经发出警告，反对在接受氯吡格雷治疗的患者中同时使用某些 PPI。

关于长期使用 PPI 的安全性，还有一些其他方面的担忧。到目前为止，PPI 的使用与许多疾病相关，包括骨质疏松、低镁血症、胃癌、肠道感染、间质性肾炎、肺炎、痴呆和 NSAID 相关肠病。目前，还没有确凿的证据表明这些疾病归因于 PPI 的使用[62]。但可能会出现新的证据，表明两者之间存在因果关系。与此同时，应该禁止在没有明确指征的情况下长期应用 PPI。

（3）钾竞争性酸阻滞剂

在酸分泌途径的最后阶段，钾离子竞争性酸阻滞剂（P-CAB）可与钾离子竞争抑制壁细胞中的 H^+，K^+-ATP 酶（见第 51 章）[63]。与 PPI 不同，P-CAB 是酸稳定的，不需要酸性环境来激活（即不需要前体药物）。到目前为止，沃诺拉赞（vonoprazan）是唯一在日本和其他一些国家上市的 P-CAB。其首剂就可发挥接近最大的抑制作用，并持续 24 小时[63]。在两个 3 期随机对照试验中，沃诺拉赞（每天 1 次，20mg）对胃溃疡和十二指肠溃疡愈合方面的治疗效果不逊于兰索拉唑（每天 1 次，30mg）[64,65]。另外两项随机试验显示，在预防长期使用 NSAIDs 和小剂量阿司匹林相关的溃疡复发方面，沃诺拉赞（10mg 和 20mg）与兰索拉唑（15mg）同样有效[66]。

3. 黏膜保护剂

硫糖铝是硫酸化蔗糖的复合铝盐。当暴露在胃酸中时，硫酸盐阴离子可以静电结合到受损组织中的带正电荷的蛋白质上[67,68]。硫糖铝（1g，每天 4 次）在十二指肠溃疡的愈合方面与 H_2RAs 一样有效，并被美国食品药品管理局（FDA）批准用于这一适应证。由于硫糖铝溶解性差，所以很少（<5%）被人体吸收，该药基本通过肠内途径排出。由于缺乏全身吸收，硫糖铝基本没有全身毒性。硫糖铝对慢性肾病患者体内铝蓄积的影响还没有得到充分的研究，在这一人群中最好避免使用硫糖铝。该药与其他药物之间重要的相互作用似乎很少见。如果将硫糖铝与其他药物分开给药，也可以规避其相互作用。

胶体铋制剂，如胶体次枸橼酸铋和次水杨酸铋（如 Pepto-Bismol），在治愈消化性溃疡方面具有中等疗效，但机制尚不清楚[69]。铋盐与黏液形成复合物，可覆盖于溃疡表面。另外认为铋剂可诱导黏膜前列腺素合成和碳酸氢盐分泌增加。铋剂对 Hp 具有抗菌活性，美国 FDA 已批准铋与其他药物联合用于治疗 Hp 感染（见第 52 章）。铋剂在很大程度上不能被吸收，并从粪便中排出。结肠细菌将铋盐转化为硫化铋，从而使粪便变黑。微量的铋被上消化道吸收，在随后 3 个月或更长时间随尿液缓慢排出。短期标准剂量使用铋剂，其毒性风险很小；然而，如果长期大剂量服用铋剂，特别是在慢性肾脏疾病患者中，则有可能出现铋剂相关脑病并出现神经精神症状。

米索前列醇是 FDA 批准的一种前列腺素 E_1 类似物，用于预防 NSAID 导致的消化性溃疡[70]。该药不仅增强黏膜防御机制，还通过抑制组胺刺激的环状 3'，5'-环磷酸腺苷（AMP）的产生来抑制胃酸分泌[71]。口服吸收良好，米索前列醇的血药浓度在大约 30 分钟后达到峰值，血清半衰期约为 1.5 小时。该药不影响肝脏 CYP450。米索前列醇的代谢物从尿液中排出，但慢性肾脏疾病患者没有必要减少应用剂量。剂量相关性腹泻是其最常见的不良反应，发生率高达 30%，限制了米索前列醇的应用。腹泻与前列腺素引起的肠道电解质和水分泌增加和/或肠道转运时间加快有关。与食物一起服用米索前列醇可能会减少腹泻。米索前列醇能刺激子宫平滑肌，因此禁用于可能妊娠的女性。

（二）幽门螺杆菌（Hp）相关溃疡

第 51 章详细讨论了 Hp 感染的治疗（表 51.2 和表 51.3）。众所周知，根除 Hp 感染不仅可以治愈消化性溃疡，还可以预防溃疡的复发和并发症[72-75]。由于 Hp 感染占十二指肠溃疡病例的 80%～90%，因此对十二指肠溃疡患者进行 Hp 检测是必要的。如果内镜诊断十二指肠溃疡，应该行胃黏膜活检检测 Hp 感染。有充分证据提示 10～14 天的 Hp 根除治疗足以治愈十二指肠溃疡，因此通常不需要额外的抗胃酸分泌治疗。对于无并发症的患者，不推荐在抗生素治疗后，常规进行随访内镜检查来记录愈合情况，并在胃镜时进行检测以证明 Hp 根除。然而，可用尿素呼气试验等无创检查方法来确认 Hp 根除。对胃溃疡患者行 Hp 根除治疗 7～14 天后是否需要抗胃酸分泌治疗存有一定争议。1 周无酸抑制的抗菌治疗可有效地治愈 Hp 相关性胃溃疡[72]。在对胃溃疡愈合试验的一项 meta 分析中，Hp 根除治疗和溃疡愈合药物的治疗效果相似[73]；然而，在有巨大溃疡或有并发症的胃溃疡患者中，额外的抑酸治疗可以促进溃疡的愈合。建议对这类患者进行内镜随访检查，以记录愈合情况，排除恶性肿瘤，并确认是否成功根除 Hp。

（三）非甾体抗炎药引起的溃疡

1. H_2 受体阻滞剂（H_2RA）

常规剂量的 H_2 受体阻滞剂在治疗 NSAID 相关性十二指肠溃疡方面比胃溃疡更有效。如果患者继续服用 NSAIDs，有关 H_2 受体阻滞剂治愈消化性溃疡的数据有限。因此，H_2 受体阻滞剂不是需要持续 NSAID 治疗的溃疡患者的首选药物。

2. 质子泵抑制剂（PPI）

目前的证据[76-78]显示质子泵抑制剂在治愈 NSAID 引起的消化性溃疡方面优于标准剂量的 H_2 受体阻滞剂。在一项对持续服用 NSAIDs 的消化性溃疡患者使用艾司奥美拉唑（20 或 40mg/d）或雷尼替丁（150mg，每天 2 次）的随机对照研究中，8 周时溃疡愈合率在艾司奥美拉唑组为 85% 和 86%，在雷尼替丁组为 76%[78]。在另一项对持续服用 NSAIDs 的 NSAID 相关性胃溃疡患者的研究中，8 周时溃疡愈合率在兰索拉唑 15mg/d 和 30mg/d 治疗的患者中，分别为 69% 和 73%，而在雷尼替丁（150mg，每日 2 次）治疗组的患者中只有 53%。

3. 米索前列醇

在持续服用 NSAID 的溃疡患者中，米索前列醇在 8 周的溃疡愈合率为 67%，而安慰剂组的溃疡愈合率只有 26%[79]。然而，米索前列醇在治愈 NSAID 相关溃疡方面的疗效不如

PPI。一项随机试验将足量米索前列醇(200μg,每天4次)与奥美拉唑(每天20或40mg)对比,用于持续接受NSAID治疗的十二指肠溃疡或胃溃疡患者[80]。8周后,DU愈合率在奥美拉唑治疗的两个剂量组都为89%,而在米索前列醇治疗组只有77%。与之类似的,GU愈合率在接受20mg奥美拉唑治疗组为87%;在接受40mg奥美拉唑治疗组为80%;在米索前列醇治疗组为73%。虽然目前米索前列醇很少用于治疗或预防消化性溃疡,但两项随机试验表明,米索前列醇对服用NSAIDs和小剂量阿司匹林时出现不明原因出血患者的小肠溃疡和糜烂的愈合是有效的[81,82]。

(四) 其他原因的溃疡和特发性溃疡

如果确定消化性溃疡的病因不是Hp感染或NSAID使用(如胃泌素瘤),则应治疗潜在的疾病(见第34章)。特发性、非Hp、非NSAID溃疡的治疗依赖于抗胃酸分泌疗法,通常是长期给予PPI(维持治疗),就像在中高危患者长期使用抑酸药预防NSAID引起的溃疡一样(见下文)。

五、难治性消化性溃疡

大多数消化性溃疡在抑酸治疗8周内痊愈。然而,在少数但相当轻微的患者中,尽管进行了常规治疗,溃疡仍然存在。这种溃疡即为难治性。难治性消化性溃疡没有标准化的定义,这使得研究之间的比较变得困难。在一些顽固性溃疡患者中,溃疡的症状持续存在,并可能很严重。在另一些患者,顽固性溃疡没有症状,只有在内镜检查时才能发现(例如,在8周的随访内镜检查中评估胃溃疡的愈合情况)。

对于经过常规治疗后而溃疡后而未愈合的患者,临床医生应考虑以下问题:

- 患者是否遵守了治疗计划?
- 溃疡是否穿透胰腺、肝脏或其他器官?
- 是否有Hp感染?如果已经应用了抗生素治疗,应该对患者进行检测,以明确Hp是否已经根除。如果还没有诊断和治疗过Hp,应进行检测诊断和治疗。同时应考虑到Hp检测可能有的假阴性结果(见第52章)。
- 患者是否还在服用NSAID?NSAID的使用可能会被隐瞒。应仔细询问关于非处方NSAIDs(包括小剂量阿司匹林)的使用情况,如有可能应停止使用NSAIDs。
- 患者是否抽烟?如果是,应强烈建议其戒烟。
- 溃疡治疗的时间是否足够?大的溃疡比小的溃疡需要更长治疗时间才能愈合。巨大溃疡(如>2cm)在抑酸治疗12周以上仍持续存在时,才被认定为是难治的。
- 有证据提示高胃酸分泌性疾病吗?有胃泌素瘤或Ⅰ型MEN家族史,或有慢性腹泻、甲状旁腺功能亢进症引起的高钙血症,或溃疡累及球后十二指肠或空肠近端,提示胃泌素瘤的诊断(见第34章)。
- 最后,病变真的是消化性溃疡吗?原发性或转移性肿瘤、感染(如巨细胞病毒)、可卡因使用、嗜酸性胃肠炎和克罗恩病均可导致与消化性溃疡相似的胃和十二指肠溃疡。应适当考虑和排除这些疾病。

真正难治性消化性溃疡的治疗选择包括更长的抗胃酸分泌治疗疗程,通常应用之前PPI剂量的两倍。尽管现在不常见,但对于有症状的难治性或穿透性溃疡,仍可能需要择期手术治疗。本章稍后将讨论手术方案。

六、溃疡的预防

大多数关于溃疡预防的研究都以内镜终点(而不是临床终点)来评估各种方案的有效性。内镜下溃疡被定义为直径为5mm或更大的,有一定深度的局限性黏膜缺损[83]。然而,许多研究将溃疡的标准放宽到直径为3mm的扁平黏膜破损。小溃疡和糜烂的区别有一定的主观性,易产生观察者间的偏倚。这些内镜下微小病变的临床相关性尚不确定。据推测内镜检查结果与溃疡并发症风险处于中低水平的患者的临床结局大致相关。目前还不清楚内镜检查的结果是否可以推广到高危患者。由于很少有前瞻性试验结果来评估溃疡预防用药的真正临床疗效,临床判断主要依赖于内镜观察的数据。

对于Hp相关溃疡,在根除了Hp之后无需溃疡预防(见前面和第52章)。因此,大多数溃疡预防方案的应用,都与预防中高度溃疡风险患者的NSAID相关性溃疡有关。表53.1列出了NSAID引起溃疡的危险因素。可减少NSAID所致溃疡进展的药物将在后面讨论。溃疡预防也经常应用于特发性溃疡患者。在列出的药物中,只有抗胃酸分泌剂是预防特发性溃疡的常用药物。

表53.1 非甾体抗炎药相关溃疡的风险因素*

风险因素	风险比
有复杂的溃疡病史	13.5
使用多种非甾体抗炎药(包括阿司匹林、COX-2抑制剂)	9
使用大剂量非甾体抗炎药	7
使用抗凝剂	6.4
无并发症的溃疡病史	6.1
年龄>70岁	5.6
幽门螺杆菌感染	3.5
使用糖皮质激素	2.2

*并非所有的非甾体抗炎药均具有相同的风险。

(一) 抗酸药

许多临床医生给服用NSAIDs的患者开抗酸剂作为辅助治疗,既是为了缓解消化不良症状,也是为了预防溃疡(希望如此);然而,抗酸剂在预防NSAID引起的溃疡方面并没有被证明有效。抗酸药可能会掩盖消化不良的症状,从而产生一种预防溃疡的错觉,并增加长期NSAID治疗导致无症状性溃疡并发症的风险。服用NSAIDs且有溃疡风险的患者应避免服用抗酸药。

(二) H_2受体拮抗剂(H_2RA)

如前所述,使用标准剂量的H_2RA不能有效预防NSAID引起的胃溃疡[84,85],还有可能是有害的。一项对服用NSAID

患者的随机试验的系统回顾研究[85]得出结论，每天使用两倍标准剂量的 H_2RA 可显著降低内镜下 NSAID 相关的十二指肠溃疡和胃溃疡的风险。然而，大剂量 H_2RA 是否能预防 NSAID 所致溃疡的并发症尚不清楚。相反，与对 NSAIDs 相关溃疡的预防相比，H_2RA 对小剂量阿司匹林相关溃疡的预防似乎更有效。在一项对应用小剂量阿司匹林有溃疡复发出血风险患者的 12 个月多中心随机试验中，应用 PPI 和应用 H_2RA 的再出血发生率没有显著差异[89]。

（三）米索前列醇

米索前列醇预防 NSAID 所致溃疡的疗效已经在随机对照试验中进行了评估[86,87]。对这些试验的系统回顾显示，各种剂量的米索前列醇（每天 400～800μg）都可以降低 NSAID 引起的内镜下溃疡的风险[85]。然而，只有足量的米索前列醇（每天 800μg）才能减少溃疡并发症的发生[86]。在一项对接受 NSAIDs 治疗的类风湿性关节炎患者进行的随机双盲试验中，米索前列醇（200μg，每天 4 次）将胃肠道并发症的发生率降低了 40%（安慰剂组为 0.95%，米索前列醇组为 0.57%）。然而，在这项试验中，接受米索前列醇治疗的患者中，多达 30% 的患者出现了胃肠道不适，这限制了米索前列醇的临床应用。尽管内镜研究表明，小剂量的米索前列醇，如每次 200μg，每天 2 或 3 次，可以预防 NSAID 引起的溃疡，其副作用比足量应用较小[86]，但如此低剂量的米索前列醇并不能预防溃疡并发症[88]。

（四）质子泵抑制剂（PPI）

PPI 显著降低内镜下十二指肠溃疡和胃溃疡风险[85]。有研究在接受 NSAIDs 治疗的患者中，将 PPI 的疗效与 H_2RAs 和米索前列醇进行了比较。两项为期 6 个月的研究将奥美拉唑每天一次 20mg 与标准剂量雷尼替丁（150mg，每天两次）和半量米索前列醇（200μg，每天两次）进行比较[76,80]。奥美拉唑在预防内镜下溃疡方面比标准剂量雷尼替丁更有效，与半量米索前列醇相当。在预防 NSAID 相关性溃疡方面，奥美拉唑相对于雷尼替丁的优势在于大幅减少了内镜下 DU。事后分析显示，奥美拉唑比雷尼替丁增加的保护作用大多发生在 Hp 感染者中。另一项内镜研究比较了大剂量米索前列醇（200μg，每天 4 次）和 2 个剂量的兰索拉唑（每天 15mg 和 30mg）在长期服用 NSAID，有 GU 病史，但没有 Hp 感染的患者中，对溃疡的预防作用[88]。米索前列醇在预防胃溃疡方面比任何一种剂量的兰索拉唑都有效，但由于米索前列醇组的撤药率较高，其与兰索拉唑相比没有实际优势。在一项预防内镜下溃疡的头对头研究中，比较了 2 个剂量泮托拉唑和 20mg/d 奥美拉唑在服用 NSAIDs 的类风湿性关节炎患者中的作用，结果显示服用泮托拉唑 20mg、泮托拉唑 40mg 和奥美拉唑 20mg 患者的 6 个月无溃疡概率分别为 91%、95% 和 93%[89]。

两项相同的多中心随机临床试验比较了 6 个月期间，艾司奥美拉唑（20mg 或 40mg）与安慰剂在使用 NSAIDs 或 COX-2 抑制剂的患者中预防溃疡的效果。两项研究中的患者均为 Hp 阴性，年龄超过 60 岁，有胃溃疡或十二指肠溃疡病史。总体而言，服用安慰剂、艾司奥美拉唑 20mg 和艾司奥美拉唑 40mg 的患者溃疡发生率分别为 17.0%、5.2% 和 4.6%[90]。

PPI 是否能降低 NSAID 相关性消化性溃疡出血的风险主要基于观察性研究和 1 项针对高危患者的随机试验。一项大规模的病例对照研究发现，在长期使用 NSAID 的患者中，PPI 治疗可以显著降低上消化道出血的风险（相对危险度，0.13；95% CI，0.09～0.19）[91]。这项随机试验比较了长期（6 个月）奥美拉唑疗法与 1 周根除 Hp 疗法，在预防 Hp 感染患者复发溃疡出血方面的效果，这些患者近期有 NSAID 相关性溃疡出血史并且持续使用萘普生[92]。在接受 Hp 根除治疗的患者中，18.8% 出现了复发性溃疡出血，而接受奥美拉唑治疗的患者中，这一比例仅为 4.4%。

（五）环氧化酶-2 抑制剂（COX-2 抑制剂）（替代非甾体抗炎药）

COX-2 抑制剂有望在保证 NSAIDs 疗效的同时将其胃肠道毒性降至最低[93-97]。一项对随机试验的系统综述结果显示，与非选择性 NSAIDs 相比，COX-2 抑制剂引起胃十二指肠溃疡（相对风险，0.26；95% CI，0.23～0.30）和溃疡并发症（相对风险，0.39；95% CI，0.31～0.5）的风险显著降低，因胃肠道症状停药的发生率也减少[94]；然而，COX-2 抑制剂减少溃疡发生的作用，可被小剂量阿司匹林的联合应用所抵消[59]。

目前的证据表明，在有溃疡风险的患者中，COX-2 抑制剂与联合使用非选择性 NSAIDs 和 PPI 一样有效。一项随机对照研究比较了联合应用 NSAID 双氯芬酸和奥美拉唑与塞来昔布在 Hp 阴性或既往行 Hp 根除的患者中，二级预防溃疡出血的效果[95]，两组患者在 6 个月内再次出血的比例相似（双氯芬酸/奥美拉唑组为 6.4%，塞来昔布组为 4.9%）。虽然这两种疗法的溃疡出血发生率差不多，但随后的随访内镜显示，每组患者中都有 20%～25% 在 6 个月内镜检查时发现了溃疡复发。这些研究结果表明任何一种治疗方法都不能消除极高危患者再次出血的风险。在一项为期 13 个月的随机双盲试验中，比较了单用塞来昔布和联用塞来昔布/艾司奥美拉唑在有 NSAID 相关性溃疡出血史的患者中预防溃疡复发出血的作用。或结果显示单用塞来昔布组有 8.9% 的患者出现溃疡复发出血，而联合治疗组没有溃疡复发出血（$P=0.0004$）[96]。

尽管 COX-2 抑制剂改善了胃的安全性，但与这类新的 NSAIDs 相关的心血管风险成为人们非常关注的问题。在 VIGOR 研究中[97]，接受罗非昔布治疗的患者急性心肌事件的发生率比接受萘普生治疗的患者高 4 倍，尽管绝对发生率较低。这种观察到的心肌梗死发生率的差异是否与萘普生的抗血小板特性及罗非昔布的促血栓作用有关，还存有争议。关于 COX-2 抑制剂心血管风险的进一步数据来自两项有关结肠息肉预防的长期研究，分别使用了罗非昔布［Vioxx 的预防腺瘤性息肉研究（APPROVE）］[98]和塞来昔布［塞来昔布预防腺瘤的研究（APC）］[99]。在 APPROVE 研究中，18 个月的中期数据表明，每天接受 25mg 罗非昔布治疗的患者发生严重心血管事件的风险是安慰剂组患者的两倍。2004 年，鉴于这一意外发现，罗非昔布自动退出了全球市场。在 APC 研究中，33 个月的中期数据显示，每天两次 400mg 大剂量应用塞来昔布显著增加了严重心血管事件的发生率（风险比为 1.9；

95% CI,1~3.3)。MEDAL 项目是对 3 项试验的心血管血栓事件的预先指定的汇总分析,在这些试验中,骨关节炎或类风湿性关节炎患者被随机分配应用依托考昔(每天 60mg 或 90mg)或双氯芬酸(每天 150mg)。在平均 18 个月治疗后,两组患者的心血管血栓事件发生率相似[100]。

目前的证据表明,除了足量萘普生(1 000mg/d)外,不仅 COX-2 抑制剂,非选择性 NSAIDs 也会增加心血管血栓的风险。COX-2 抑制剂随机试验的 meta 分析显示(数据主要来自罗非昔布和塞来昔布),与安慰剂相比,所有 COX-2 抑制剂都增加了心血管血栓形成的风险(风险比,1.42;95% CI,1.13~1.78)。这在很大程度上归因于心肌梗死风险的增加,而其他血管事件的差异很小。塞来昔布对心血管血栓事件的影响呈剂量依赖性增加。重要的是,COX-2 抑制剂和非选择性 NSAIDs 在心血管血栓风险方面没有显著差异,只有萘普生(500mg,每天 2 次)是唯一的例外。在一项观察性研究的 meta 分析中,大剂量罗非昔布(≥25mg,每天 1 次)、双氯芬酸和吲哚美辛与心血管血栓事件的增加有关,而塞来昔布并没有显著增加心血管血栓形成的风险,尽管不能排除当剂量超过 200mg/d 时风险增加的可能[101]。在一项大规模、随机、非劣效性的试验中,比较了塞来昔布和萘普生、布洛芬在心血管风险升高的关节炎(主要是骨关节炎)患者中的安全性[102],纳入了超过 2.4 万名患者,平均治疗时间为 20 个月,平均随访期为 34 个月。研究发现,塞来昔布(平均约 200mg/d)在心血管安全性方面不逊于布洛芬(约 2 000mg/d)或萘普生(约 850mg/d)。接受塞来昔布治疗的患者发生不良胃肠道事件的风险明显低于使用萘普生或布洛芬的患者。服用塞来昔布的患者发生不良肾脏事件的风险也明显低于服用布洛芬的患者;然而,在研究期间持续服用小剂量阿司匹林的患者比例尚不清楚,而且很少患者有消化道出血的病史。因此,尚不清楚塞来昔布相对于萘普生或布洛芬的优势是否可以外推到合并服用阿司匹林并有高消化道出血风险的患者。在另一项对心血管风险和胃肠道不良事件风险均高,需要合并使用低剂量阿司匹林和 NSAID 患者为期 18 个月的随机试验中,塞来昔布联合 PPI 在降低溃疡复发出血的风险方面优于萘普生联合 PPI[103,108]。

(六) 风险评估与药物选择

NSAIDs 的安全处方应该基于对每个患者胃肠道和心血管风险的评估。对于心血管风险较低的患者,治疗方法可以根据胃肠道风险水平进行分级,如下所示(表 53.2):

表 53.2 根据胃肠道和心血管风险,推荐降低 NSAIDs 相关溃疡风险的建议

	胃肠道风险*		
	低	中	高
低 CV 风险	最低有效剂量的 NSAID	NSAID+PPI 或塞来昔布单药	塞来昔布+PPI
高 CV 风险†	萘普生或塞来昔布,联合 PPI	萘普生或塞来昔布,联合 PPI	塞来昔布联合 PPI(如果单纯止痛药失败)

*低胃肠道风险表示无风险因素(见表 53.1);中度胃肠道风险表示有 1 或 2 个风险因素;高胃肠道风险表示有≥3 个风险因素、既往有并发症的溃疡或伴随使用低剂量阿司匹林或抗凝剂。所有需要 NSAIDs 治疗的有溃疡病史的患者均检测 Hp,如果存在感染,应给予根除治疗(见第 52 章)。

†高 CV 风险表示需要使用预防性低剂量阿司匹林进行严重 CV 事件的一级预防或二级预防。CV,心血管;NSAIDs,非甾体抗炎药;PPI,质子泵抑制剂。

- 溃疡风险低:无危险因素。没有危险因素的患者(见表 53.1)使用 NSAIDs 后出现溃疡并发症的风险非常低(≈1%/年)。合理使用 NSAIDs,包括避免大剂量应用 NSAIDs,以及在最低有效剂量下使用致溃疡性较低的 NSAIDs(如布洛芬、双氯芬酸)是一种经济有效的方法。
- 中度溃疡风险:1~2 个危险因素。这些患者应该在 NSAIDs 治疗的同时接受抗溃疡药物(PPI 或米索前列醇)的联合治疗。单独使用塞来昔布与上述联合治疗一样有效。

溃疡风险高:3 个或更多的危险因素,溃疡并发症史,或同时应用小剂量阿司匹林、糖皮质激素或抗凝治疗。一般来说,在这些患者中应该避免使用 NSAIDs,这不仅是因为溃疡并发症的高风险,还因为存在合并症时溃疡并发症的严重后果。如果急性自限性关节炎(如痛风)需要短期抗炎治疗,可以考虑使用糖皮质激素(不同时使用 NSAIDs),因为单用糖皮质激素不会增加溃疡的风险。如果慢性关节炎需要规律抗炎治疗,塞来昔布和 PPI 的联合应用可提供最好的胃肠道保护。

对心血管高危患者的定义仍然没有统一的界定。美国心脏协会建议,对于心血管事件的 10 年风险在 10% 或以上的所有看上去健康的男性和女性,都应该考虑服用阿司匹林[104]。如果关节炎患者已经在服用阿司匹林进行二级预防,或者根据美国心脏协会指南需要阿司匹林进行一级预防,我们则认为他们有显著的心血管风险。由于 COX-2 抑制剂和大多数非选择性 NSAIDs 具有潜在的心血管危害,如果可能,心血管风险较高的患者应该避免使用这些药物。布洛芬可能通过与血小板 COX-1 竞争性结合而减弱阿司匹林的心脏保护作用,因此应避免同时使用布洛芬和小剂量阿司匹林。如果 NSAIDs 对心血管高危患者是必要的,目前的证据表明,可以考虑使用中等剂量的塞来昔布(200mg/d)或萘普生。联合使用 NSAIDs(如萘普生)和小剂量阿司匹林的一个主要缺点是显著增加溃疡并发症的风险;因此,塞来昔布和小剂量阿司匹林联合使用,可能是长期需要 NSAIDs 治疗,而又有高胃肠道并发症和高心血管不良事件风险患者的最佳选择。

由于 Hp 感染增加了 NSAIDs 使用者溃疡并发症的风险,长期服用 NSAIDs 的有消化性溃疡病史的患者应该接受 Hp 检测,如果有 Hp 感染应根除 Hp。

七、并发症及其治疗

(一) 出血

急性上消化道出血是消化性溃疡最常见的并发症,已经

在第 20 章详细讨论。消化性溃疡仍然是急性上消化道出血的首要原因[105]。共识小组建议采用多学科的方法进行治疗出现上消化道出血的患者[106]。急性上消化道出血患者应在就诊时立即进行评估。容量复苏应优先于内镜检查。如果有肝病特征,应警惕食管胃底静脉曲张出血,而非溃疡出血的可能。这一区别既具有预测预后的意义,也具有管理意义。静脉曲张出血的死亡率高于溃疡出血。如果有静脉曲张出血的可能性,应在内镜检查前采取特殊措施,例如使用血管活性药物(如奥曲肽)和抗生素(如头孢噻肟)预防感染性并发症,如自发性细菌性腹膜炎(见第 92 和 93 章)。

1. 内镜治疗

早期内镜检查通常被定义为在患者入院后 24 小时内进行胃镜检查(EDG)。在有活动性上消化道出血迹象的患者中,紧急内镜检查可明确诊断并提供可能的干预措施。随机对照试验表明,对再出血风险低的患者行早期内镜检查可以缩短住院时间,减少资源消耗,并便于门诊患者的管理[107-109]。对 18 项比较了内镜治疗和单用药物治疗的临床试验进行 meta 分析后显示,在进一步出血的发生率[优势比(OR) 0.35; 95% CI 0.27~0.46],手术(OR 0.57; 95% CI 0.41~0.81),以及更重要的,死亡率(OR 0.57;95% CI 0.37~0.89)方面,内镜治疗具有优势[110]。

国际共识小组[104]建议使用预后评分来指导对患者的治疗。Rockall 评分系统是使用内镜检查前后的临床参数来预测死亡率的综合评分。该评分来自英国国家审计收集的数据[109]。另一方面,Glasgow Blatchford 评分(GBS)仅使用临床参数来预测是否需要干预,并根据患者的血红蛋白水平和血尿素氮浓度、入院时的脉搏和收缩压、是否存在黑便或晕厥,以及心脏或肝衰竭的证据来计算[110]。GBS 是最广泛验证的评分,与临床结局相关。

在一项 3 012 例患者的多中心前瞻性研究中[111],在预测是否需要干预或死亡方面,GBS 评分是 4 项中最好的评分。受试者操作曲线下面积(AUROC)为 0.86 的干预或死亡。GBS 评分为 1 似乎是门诊管理的阈值。但是,GBS 评分未定义临界值,高于该临界值,必须进行紧急内镜检查。相当大比例的低至中位评分患者需要内镜治疗。

在行 EGD 时,溃疡出血的内镜下征象不仅确定消化性溃疡为出血来源,而且本身也是患者结局的预后因素(见第 20 章)。常用的命名法是根据 Forrest 和 Finlayson 的原始描述[112]修改的版本。Laine 和 Jensen[113]总结了没有内镜治疗的前瞻性试验中与出血病灶相关的进一步出血、手术和死亡率。

- Ⅰ型:活动性出血:
  Ⅰa:喷射性出血(图 53.4)
  Ⅰb:渗出性出血(见图 53.4)
- Ⅱ型:近期出血的柱头:
  Ⅱa:无出血可见裸露血管(见图 53.4)
  Ⅱb:黏附性血凝块(见图 53.4)
  Ⅱc:扁平色素沉着(见图 53.4)
- Ⅲ型:清洁的基底溃疡

具有活动性出血和无出血的裸露血管的溃疡("突起的变色"或"哨兵血凝块")需要内镜治疗(见第 20 章)。

有"黏附性血凝块"溃疡的内镜治疗存在争议。黏附性

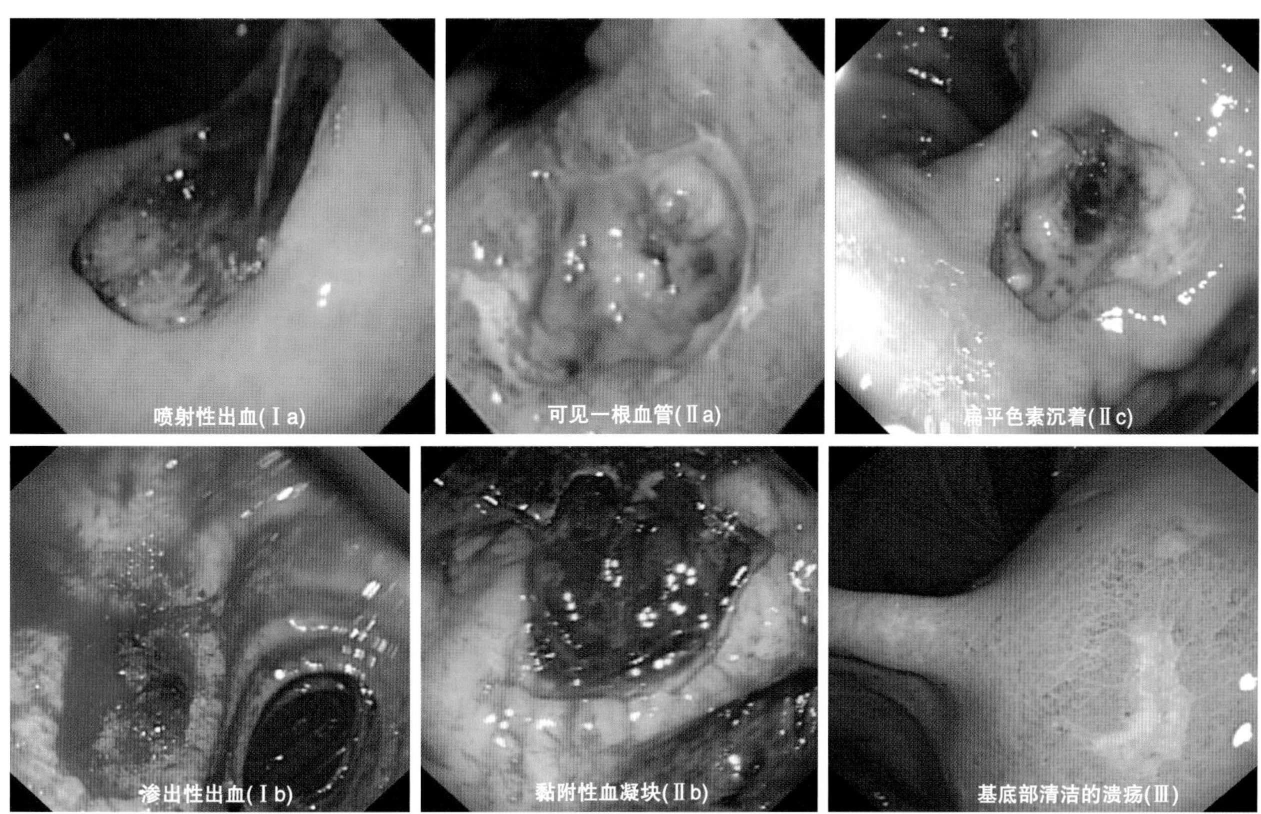

图 53.4　使用 Forrest 分类的出血性消化性溃疡的内镜表现

血凝块的定义随着内镜冲洗力度的不同而异。两项随机对照研究[114,115]和一项 meta 分析[116]比较了药物治疗和内镜治疗有"黏附性血凝块"的溃疡患者,得出结论,在清除血凝块后对其下方血管进行内镜治疗,可以将再出血的风险从 30%降低到 5%。

哨兵血凝块通常是裸露血管的同义词[117]。它代表纤维蛋白凝块,可以堵塞被侵蚀动脉的裂缝。当溃疡开始愈合时,血凝块溶解,在溃疡底部留下平坦的色素沉着,最终从溃疡底部消失。出血血管的这种演变通常不到 72 小时。具有扁平色素沉着或清洁基底部的溃疡通常不需要内镜治疗。

最近,加州大学洛杉矶分校的一个研究小组报告了他们使用内镜多普勒探头探查溃疡基底的经验。在 163 名具有不同内镜下出血征象的出血性溃疡或近期出血患者的前瞻性队列中,在具有轻微出血征象的溃疡中发现了多普勒信号(黏附性血凝块 68.4%,扁平色素沉着 40.5%)[118]。在随后纳入了 148 名消化性溃疡出血患者的随机对照试验中,Jensen 及其同事[119]将多普勒探头引导止血与标准内镜止血进行了比较。使用多普勒探头引导治疗的 30 天再出血率较低(11.1% vs 26.3%,$P=0.02$)。

内镜治疗方式在第 20 章中有更详细的讨论,而所使用的方法在这里进行简要的讨论。

(1) 注射方法

内镜下将稀释的肾上腺素注射到出血的消化性溃疡中,通过容积填塞和局部血管收缩起作用。这项技术很容易学习,而且不会对组织造成损害。另外,稀释的肾上腺素不会诱发血管血栓形成。单独注射稀释肾上腺素后再出血的患者比例为 20%~30%。注射稀释的肾上腺素可以清楚地看到出血的血管,然后应该联合热凝或夹子封闭该血管。在一项 meta 分析中[120],肾上腺素注射后加用第二种止血方法显著降低了再出血率[危险比(RR)0.57,0.43~0.76]、急诊手术率(RR 0.68,0.5~0.93)和死亡率(RR 0.64,0.39~1.06)。治疗结果的改善似乎在有活动性出血的溃疡(Forrest Ⅰ型溃疡)中更为明显。单纯注射稀释的肾上腺素不再被认为是充分的治疗方法。应该增加诱导动脉血栓形成的第二种治疗方法。

(2) 热凝方法

热凝方法包括接触和非接触方法。接触热凝方法更常用。常用的接触式热探头是有加热器探头和双极探头。术语热凝固一词强调了对血管进行牢固的机械压迫的必要性。当产生热能紧密黏接动脉管腔时,通过压迫阻断血流可降低"散热"效应。主要的非接触式方法是氩等离子体凝固(见第 20 章)。

(3) 机械方法

夹闭血管止血的机械方法应用广泛。在翻转内镜状态下切线应用夹子治疗十二指肠球后壁或胃小弯溃疡出血在技术上可能存在困难。在比较内镜治疗方式的 meta 分析中,止血夹的止血率优于单独注射,与热凝固相当[108,121]。

最近,一项多中心随机对照试验在 66 例难治性出血性溃疡患者中比较了内镜吻合夹系统(over-the scope-clips,OTSC)与标准内镜下止血夹和热凝方法的使用[122]。使用 OTSC 与进一步出血率降低相关(15.2% vs 57.6%)。OTSC 由形状记忆性镍钛合金制成,直径高达 13mm 的,能够在更广泛的区域内进行强大的组织压缩。现行标准是在预先注射或不注射肾上腺素的情况下,使用内镜止血夹或热凝固。当其他方式失败时,OTSC 似乎是一种有用的急救方法。

2. 抗分泌治疗

消化性溃疡出血的抗胃酸分泌治疗的原理是基于胃蛋白酶活性和血小板聚集均具有 pH 依赖性的事实。当纤维蛋白或血小板栓塞出血动脉的裂缝时,溃疡会停止出血。当胃 pH 超过 4 时,胃蛋白酶失活,阻止血凝块的酶消化。胃 pH 为 6 或更高对于凝块稳定和止血至关重要。Labenz 及其同事[123]研究了接受大剂量奥美拉唑(静脉推注 80mg,随后 8mg/h)或大剂量雷尼替丁(静脉推注 50mg,随后 0.25mg/kg/h)治疗的胃溃疡或十二指肠溃疡患者的胃 pH。奥美拉唑 99.9% 的时间里胃 pH 超过 6,而接受雷尼替丁的患者,只有不到 50% 的时间胃 pH 超过 6(GU 患者 46% 的时间和 DU 患者 20% 的时间)。PUB 研究是一项国际多中心研究,入组了 764 例溃疡出血患者。该研究评估了内镜止血后大剂量埃索美拉唑在出血性消化性溃疡中的应用。PPI 将 30 天内复发性出血的发生率由 11.6%降至 6.4%。此外,接受 PPI 治疗的患者需要进一步内镜治疗、输血和手术的人数较少[124]。

比较使用 PPI 与安慰剂或 H_2RA 的随机试验的 Cochrane 系统综述得出结论,使用 PPI 治疗可显著降低复发性出血和手术的发生率,但未降低总死亡率[125]。在活动性出血或无出血可见血管患者的亚组分析中,使用 PPI 治疗观察到死亡率显著降低(OR 0.53;95% CI,0.31~0.91)。

使用 PPI 的最佳剂量和 PPI 给药的常规仍存在争议。比较内镜下止血后使用小剂量至大剂量 PPI 的随机对照试验(RCT)的 meta 分析纳入了包括出血性溃疡伴轻微出血病灶和基底部清洁的溃疡[126]。大多数研究不足以证明小剂量和大剂量 PPI 之间的等效性。一个国际共识小组继续支持使用大剂量的 PPI,特别是在高风险患者中[104]。

在一项大规模随机研究中,对内镜检查前先期使用静脉输注 PPI 进行了研究[127]。对有明显上消化道出血征象的患者随机接受大剂量 PPI 输注和安慰剂。该队列中的大多数(60%)患者在 EGD 时发现消化性溃疡出血。该研究表明,早期 PPI 输注降低了消化性溃疡患者的内镜下出血病灶分期,从而减少了内镜治疗的需求;因此,PPI 组在次日早晨 EGD 期间观察到的活动性出血或近期出血的主要病灶溃疡较少。PPI 输注后溃疡开始愈合,第二天观察到基底部清洁溃疡显著增多。这项研究具有节约成本的意义,因为预先使用静脉 PPI 所需的内镜治疗较少。在等待内镜检查的患者中,开始 PPI 治疗是合理的。

3. 手术治疗

有效的内镜干预和改进的药物治疗大大减少了急诊溃疡手术的需求。在美国,控制溃疡出血的手术率持续下降(从 1993 年的 13.1%下降到 2006 年的 9.7%),而内镜治疗率上升(12.9%到 22.2%)[128]。在 2006 年的一项英国国家审计中,出现上消化道出血的 4 478 名患者中只有 2.3%需要手术。手术后死亡率为 29%[129]。内镜治疗无法控制或内镜治疗后再出血的难治性溃疡出血患者需要手术治疗。内镜止血治疗后再出血的独立预测因素,包括血流动力学不稳定、并发有其他疾病、内镜下有活动性出血、巨大溃疡、十二指肠球后壁溃疡或胃小弯溃疡[130]。通常情况下,可以尝试再次行内镜止血。一项将再次内镜治疗与手术治疗进行比较的随机对照试验表明,再次内镜止血的有效率为 75%,且与操作相关的并发症的发生率较低[131]。

溃疡出血的急诊手术方式是有争议的。一些外科医生认为,单独缝合溃疡并联合抑酸治疗,比行胃切除术或迷走神经切断术这类"标准"手术更安全。根除 Hp 和 PPI 为外科医生减少了手术量。

在内镜止血和 PPI 输注时代之前,发表了两项比较最小手术和标准性手术的随机对照试验[132,133]。一项英国多中心研究,在出血胃溃疡或十二指肠溃疡患者中比较了最小手术量(单独缝合血管或溃疡切除加静脉 H_2RA 治疗)与标准性溃疡手术(迷走神经切断术和幽门成形术或胃部分切除术)。该试验被中止,因为分配到最小手术组的患者中,致死性复发性出血的发生率较高(62 例患者中有 7 例,其中 6 例死亡)。在接受标准溃疡手术的 67 例患者中,4 例再次出血,无死亡[132]。在法国外科研究协会进行的一项试验中,十二指肠溃疡患者随机接受锁边缝合加迷走神经切断引流或部分胃切除术[133]。在缝合和迷走神经切断术组,60 名患者中有 10 名(17%)发生复发性出血;10 名复发性出血患者中有 6 名需要转为毕氏Ⅱ式(Billroth Ⅱ式)胃切除术。在分配接受部分胃切除术的 60 名患者组中,仅 2 名(3%)发生再出血,均在保守治疗后恢复。在一项意向治疗分析中,未观察到总死亡率和十二指肠瘘发生率的差异。这两项随机对照试验表明,单纯缝合加或不加迷走神经切断术与较高的复发性出血相关。排除溃疡或在胃溃疡的情况下,溃疡切除对于预防复发性出血很重要。在对来自美国高校外科医生国家手术质量改进计划的数据进行的一项综述中,与迷走神经切断术后切除或引流(39/283,13.8%)相比,接受简单缝合或溃疡切除(106/498,21.3%)的患者的 30 天死亡率更高。本回顾性分析存在明显的偏倚[134]。

4. 血管造影介入治疗

对于消化性溃疡出血的患者,血管造影栓塞出血动脉是一种替代手术的方法。对 6 项比较血管造影介入治疗和手术的回顾性研究进行汇总分析,发现介入治疗后再出血率较高(51/178, 29% vs 36/241, 15%; RR 1.82; 95% CI 1.20 ~ 2.67)[135]。死亡率无显著差异(17% vs 23%)。在具备放射技能的情况下,通常会在手术前尝试血管造影术介入治疗。最近的一项随机对照研究将内镜止血后增加血管造影栓塞与标准治疗进行了比较,结果并未证实预防性栓塞治疗在减少死亡率方面有优势[136]。在符合方案分析中,内镜加栓塞术的再出血率明显较低(6/96,6.2%,vs 14/123,11.4%)。在对大于或等于 15mm 溃疡的亚组分析中,栓塞将出血率从 23.1%减少到 4.5%。作者建议,对于有大量出血的大溃疡,应考虑在内镜止血后进行血管造影栓塞。

(二) 穿孔

胃溃疡或十二指肠溃疡穿孔(图 53.5)是一类外科急症,可能是消化性溃疡的最初表现,特别是在应用 NSAIDs 的患者中。溃疡穿孔有接近 30%的死亡率。患有严重合并症和未及时手术的老年人预后最差。临床表现是腹膜炎,但在年龄较大和免疫功能低下的患者中,临床体征可能会不典型(见第 39 章)。

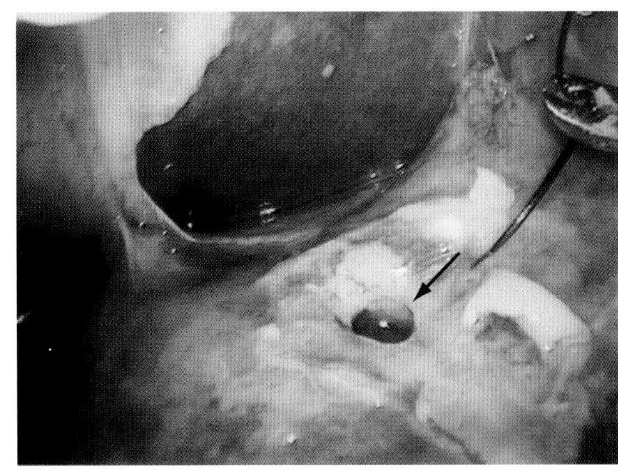

图 53.5　十二指肠穿孔的腹腔镜视图(箭)。邻近腹膜有纤维素性渗出

1. 药物治疗

标准化的围手术期处理方案可以改善预后。在丹麦的一项多中心研究中(n=2 619)[137],PULD 试验显示,对脓毒症进行积极而有针对性的治疗,更重要的是,在发病后 6 小时内进行手术,在有严格处理方案的 117 家医院中,死亡率为 17%,在 512 家未采用方案的医院中,死亡率为 27%。其他措施包括目标导向的补液治疗,一般呼吸和循环支持,静脉应用广谱抗生素,以及插入双通道鼻胃管(NG)和尿管。手术后常规静脉应用 PPI。

溃疡穿孔的非手术治疗应尽量少用。它包括 NG 吸引术、肠外应用抗生素和静脉补液。在一项随机对照试验中,Croft 和同事[138]对可疑消化性溃疡穿孔诊断的患者随机进行保守治疗或立即手术治疗。内科治疗组和外科治疗组的总体并发症发生率和死亡率(5%)较低,且相似。在 40 名接受保守治疗的患者中,11 名患者在 12 小时内没有好转,并接受了手术。11 例中有 3 例发现癌穿孔(2 例胃和 1 例乙状结肠)。该研究结果强调了对非手术治疗的普遍反对意见:穿孔部位的不确定性,胃肠道肿瘤穿孔的可能性,以及减弱的功能使自发性闭合不太可能。老年人对脓毒症的耐受性差。确定性治疗的任何延误都会导致不良的结果。

2. 手术治疗

胃十二指肠溃疡穿孔的死亡率很高。一项对 2011 年至 2013 年丹麦的溃疡穿孔手术的回顾性研究显示,在 726 名患者中,90 天的死亡率为 25.5%。124 名患者(17.1%)需要再次手术,其中约三分之一是因为持续性漏[139]。

Boey 和同事[140]发现术前休克、重大内科疾病和穿孔超过 12 小时是重要的不良预后因素。PULP 评分是最近从丹麦 11 家医院接受手术的 2 668 名患者队列中得出的。评价项目包括年龄大于 65 岁,活动性恶性肿瘤或获得性免疫缺陷,肝硬化,糖皮质激素使用,穿孔超过 24 小时,休克,血清肌酐水平升高,以及美国麻醉医师协会(ASA)评分大于 1。PULP 评分可准确预测溃疡穿孔患者的死亡(AUROC 为 0.83)[141]。然而,该评分尚未在丹麦以外的中心得到验证。

消化性溃疡穿孔手术治疗的争论集中在腹腔镜和开腹修补之间的选择，以及穿孔闭合后是否需要进行标准溃疡手术（以及选择哪种标准手术）。十二指肠穿孔和胃穿孔的治疗也不同。使用大网膜补片简单闭合十二指肠或幽门旁溃疡穿孔已被广泛应用。

对3项随机对照试验（2项来自香港和1项荷兰的LAMA研究）的meta分析表明，消化性溃疡穿孔的腹腔镜修补术与开腹手术治疗相比，在腹部脓毒症性并发症（OR 0.66；95% CI，0.3~1.47）和肺部并发症（OR 0.43；95% CI，0.17~1.12）方面更有优势[142]；因此，腹腔镜修补术至少应被认为不逊于开腹修补术。然而，在这些随机对照试验中可能存在选择偏倚。风险较高的患者（延迟就诊、休克和严重合并症的患者）可能更适合开腹手术。较大的穿孔（>10mm）提示有相当大的溃疡，也应该通过开腹手术进行处理；这类患者通常需要胃切除。

胃溃疡穿孔约占消化性溃疡穿孔的20%。流行病学数据显示，在穿孔性溃疡中胃溃疡的比例升高，特别是在使用NSAIDs的老年患者中。胃溃疡穿孔的患者更有可能年龄较大，并有严重的合并症，这使得他们的预后较差。像十二指肠溃疡穿孔一样，对于胃溃疡穿孔的手术选择也存在争议。幽门前区域的小穿孔应简单缝合。小弯胃角切迹处胃溃疡的最佳治疗方法应包括胃窦切除和小弯溃疡切除，然后进行毕Ⅰ式或Ⅱ式重建。迷走神经切断术的作用尚不清楚。胃溃疡穿孔一期切除的倡导者认为，胃切除术后的死亡率没有增加，术后溃疡相关并发症的发生率降低。支持一期切除的论据还包括恶性溃疡的可能性。约6%的穿孔性胃溃疡为恶性[143]。在纳入了287例胃溃疡穿孔的回顾性研究中，仅接受补片闭合的患者中有21.5%的患者死亡，而接受胃切除术的患者中有24.3%的患者死亡[144]。

在Hp相关性溃疡中，根除Hp可以减少修补术后溃疡的复发。在一项来自香港的随机对照试验中，99名溃疡穿孔修补术后的患者随机行根除Hp治疗或PPI治疗。1年后，接受Hp根治的患者复发率显著降低（4.8% vs 38.1%）[145]。对5项随机对照试验的meta分析显示，在十二指肠溃疡穿孔的患者中，简单封闭穿孔加上Hp根除与简单封闭穿孔相比，Hp根除后一年溃疡复发率为5.2%，而未根除Hp患者的溃疡复发率为35.2%。这些数据支持在大多数十二指肠溃疡穿孔中使用简单封闭[146]。

（三）梗阻

胃出口梗阻现在是消化性溃疡的少见并发症。其临床表现包括恶心、餐后呕吐、腹胀、疼痛、早饱，以及对可能存在的胃出口梗阻患者的诊断方法，已在第15和50章中讨论。胃出口梗阻应提示临床医生注意可能的恶性肿瘤（见第54章）。

1. 药物治疗

梗阻性消化性溃疡的患者通常有容量丢失。呕吐物中液体、氢离子和氯离子的丢失会导致低氯血症、低钾血症及代谢性碱中毒。应对患者使用生理盐水进行容量复苏，在尿量充足后补钾。对于严重营养不良患者，应考虑肠外营养。用大口径NG管对胃进行减压可以缓解呕吐，帮助监测液体流失，并使胃恢复张力。大量非胆汁染色的抽出液有助于区分胃出口梗阻和高位小肠梗阻。静脉PPI的使用减少了胃酸的排出量，使液体和电解质的管理变得更容易。PPI疗法还能促进溃疡愈合，减轻炎性水肿，并有助于治疗梗阻。这种治疗对大约一半的患者有效。在活动性溃疡和水肿的患者中改善尤其明显。因此，手术应被推迟到进行充分保守治疗之后。其他可能影响手术指征的因素包括慢性溃疡，既往溃疡并发症史，以及患者的年龄和医疗条件。此外，许多权威人士主张在手术前进行内镜扩张。

2. 内镜治疗

内镜球囊扩张术已成功地应用于消化性溃疡引起的胃出口梗阻患者（图53.6）[147-149]。在内镜检查中，通过一根带柔性尖端的胆道型导丝穿过狭窄。然后，将低顺应性的球囊通过导丝，在内镜可视下进行扩张。优先选择球囊扩张，因为充气后的球囊可产生均匀的径向力，这在理论上比使用传统扩张器所产生的纵向剪切力更有优势。该手术通常在X线引

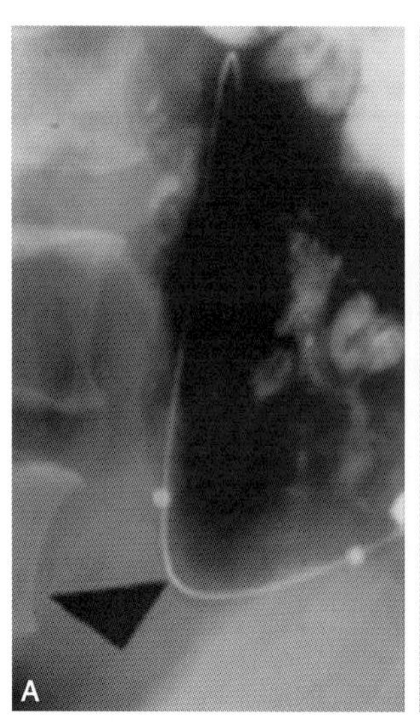

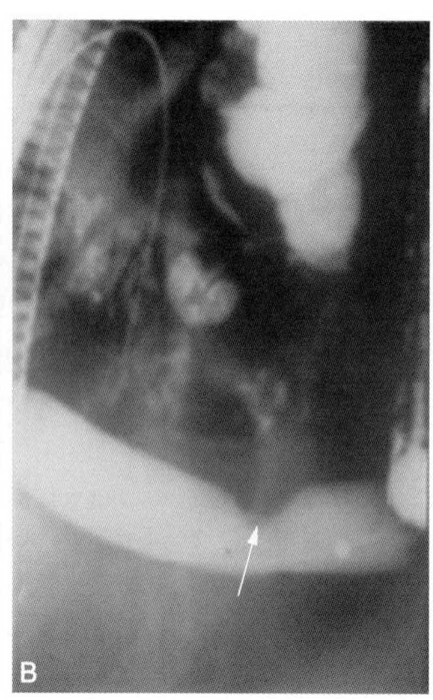

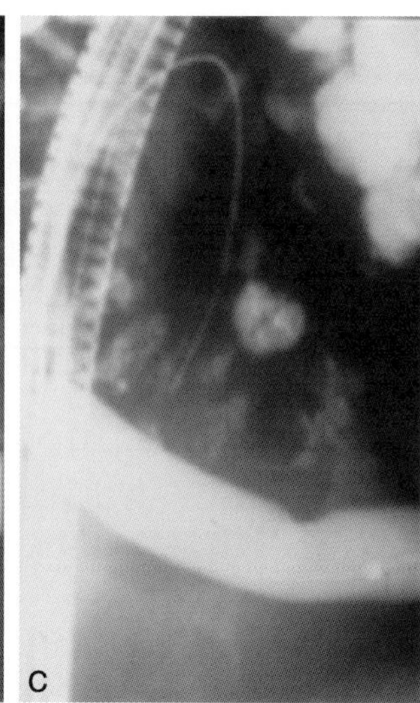

图53.6 由溃疡引起的幽门梗阻的内镜下扩张。该手术在X线透视引导下进行。采用3.7mm治疗通道的双通道内窥镜。A，首先用胆型导丝穿过狭窄。沿导丝将整个范围内的球囊穿过狭窄处。B，观察到代表狭窄（箭）的腰部，在球囊充盈时几乎消失（C）

导下进行。最好在两三个疗程内逐步扩张狭窄部位。球囊到底要扩张至多少直径大小比较合适尚不清楚，许多权威机构建议扩张至 15mm，通常可以缓解症状。然而胃动力减退也会引起类似于梗阻的相应症状。球囊越大，穿孔的风险越大。内镜系列报道 78% 至 100% 的患者梗阻症状在扩张后立即缓解。在一小部分 Hp 感染的患者中，球囊扩张后行 Hp 根除治疗可使症状持续缓解[150]。

3. 手术治疗

已有多种手术被应用于梗阻性十二指肠溃疡、幽门管溃疡和幽门前溃疡。包括迷走神经切断术和引流术（胃空肠吻合术或幽门成形术），或胃窦切除术。少见的幽门前胃溃疡梗阻的首选手术方式是先行胃窦切除，然后行毕氏 Ⅰ 型胃十二指肠吻合术。

八、应激性溃疡

应激相关胃和十二指肠黏膜损伤（应激性溃疡）是危重患者的一种并发症，通常在重症监护室（ICU）接受治疗。应激性溃疡的病因可能与黏膜缺血，以及休克或低心输出量引起的内脏灌注不足有关。幸运的是，只有一小部分应激相关黏膜病变的患者有临床上明显的消化道出血。在一项队列研究中[151]，2 252 名 ICU 患者，只有 1.5% 出现了临床上严重的出血。应激性溃疡出血的独立预测因素是呼吸衰竭（OR 15.6）和凝血功能障碍（OR 4.3）。2015 年，一项针对 1 034 名 ICU 患者的前瞻性研究[152]显示，2.6% 的患者发生了临床上严重的消化道出血。那些有 3 种或 3 种以上并发疾病、肝病、接受肾脏替代治疗以及器官衰竭评分较高的患者为应激性溃疡出血的高危患者。ICU 中的创伤性脑损伤和烧伤患者也属于发生消化道出血的高危人群。在不同的研究中，似乎有不同的出血预测因素。肠内营养的使用可以中和胃酸，防止消化道出血。

PPI、H_2RA 和硫糖铝是用于预防应激性溃疡的药物。在对 57 个随机对照试验（$n=7\ 293$）进行的 meta 分析中，Alhazzani 及其同事[153]发现，PPI 在预防临床严重消化道出血方面比 H_2RA（OR 0.38）、硫糖铝（OR 0.30）或安慰剂（OR 0.24）更有效。然而，与 H_2RA（OR 1.27）、硫糖铝（OR 1.65）和安慰剂（OR 1.52）相比，PPI 增加了院内获得性肺炎的风险。有人担心抑酸治疗使患者容易发生院内感染，可能与肠道菌群失调有关[154]。一项欧洲多中心随机研究纳入了 3 298 名 ICU 患者，给予 40mg 静脉 PPI 或安慰剂，发现 90 天死亡率在两组间相似（31.1% vs 30.4%）。不良事件（胃肠道出血、艰难梭菌感染、肺炎或心肌缺血）的发生率相似（21.9% vs 22.6%）。PPI 组临床严重消化道出血事件的发生率较低（2.5% vs 4.2%）[155]。

（王俊雄 译，　王立 校）

参考文献

第 54 章　胃腺癌和其他胃肿瘤

Michael Quante, Jan　Bornschein 著

章节目录

一、流行病学 …… 776
二、病因学和发病机制 …… 777
（一）幽门螺杆菌感染 …… 778
（二）饮食危险因素 …… 780
（三）吸烟 …… 780
（四）酒精 …… 780
（五）肥胖 …… 781
（六）遗传因素 …… 781
三、肿瘤遗传学 …… 782
四、癌前状态 …… 784
（一）慢性萎缩性胃炎 …… 784
（二）肠化生和异型增生 …… 784
（三）胃息肉 …… 786
（四）既往胃切除术史 …… 786
（五）消化性溃疡病 …… 786
（六）Ménétrier 病 …… 786
五、筛查与监测 …… 786
六、预防 …… 787
（一）根除 HP …… 787
（二）阿司匹林和其他非甾体抗炎药(NSAID)，包括(环氧化酶-2)抑制剂(COX-2) …… 787
（三）他汀类药物 …… 787
（四）抗氧化剂 …… 788
（五）其他饮食因素 …… 788
七、临床特征 …… 788
八、诊断 …… 788
（一）内镜 …… 788
（二）CT 胃造影 …… 789
（三）血清标志物 …… 789
九、分类与分期 …… 790
（一）超声内镜检查 …… 790
（二）CT 和 PET 成像 …… 791
（三）腹腔镜腹腔灌洗 …… 791
（四）其他成像方式 …… 791
（五）新辅助治疗后的再分期 …… 791
十、预后与治疗 …… 791
（一）外科手术 …… 792
（二）内镜黏膜切除术和内镜黏膜剥离术 …… 792
（三）化疗 …… 792
（四）放化疗 …… 793
（五）腹腔内化疗 …… 793
（六）不能切除的疾病 …… 793
十一、其他胃肿瘤疾病 …… 794

尽管胃癌在许多工业化国家的发病率在下降，但其仍然是世界上与癌症相关死亡的主要原因。在本章中，我们主要讨论胃腺癌，它占胃恶性肿瘤的大部分。

一、流行病学

胃癌是世界上癌症死亡的第三大原因[1]，尽管总发病率在下降[2]。在西方国家，胃癌的发病率在过去一个世纪里急剧下降。在美国胃癌的死亡率自 1950 年以来下降了 87%，在欧洲也有类似的趋势[3]。在美国胃癌的发病率已降至约 7.6 例/10 万人[4]，而早在 1945 年，胃癌仍是男性癌症死亡的主要原因[5]。

胃癌发病率有很大的地域差异，远东地区的发病率最高。东欧、中美洲和南美洲的发病率也很高，北美、北非、南亚和澳大利亚的发病率最低[6]。尽管过去在工业化国家中胃癌很常见，但最新的流行病学数据表明，超过 70% 的胃癌新发病例在发展中国家，这反映出发达国家的胃癌发病率下降速度更快[1]。

在美国中位诊断年龄为 70 岁[4]。在胃癌高发国家日本，平均确诊年龄大约提前了 10 年，这可能反映了由于广泛筛查而导致的时间前置的偏倚。男性胃癌的发病率大约为女性的两倍（表 54.1）[1]。美国黑人胃癌的发病率几乎是白人的两倍。美洲原住民和西班牙裔发生胃癌的风险也高于白种人。与非交界性胃癌相反，食管胃交界处腺癌（EGJ，以前称为“贲门癌”）的发病率正在上升[2]。根据美国监测、流行病学和最终结果（Surveillance, Epidemiology, and Ends Results, SEER）数据库，这些交界性癌现在占美国胃癌的 27%，而在 1975 年仅为 10%[4]。

胃癌有许多饮食、环境和遗传风险因素（框 54.1）。但主要的危险因素仍然是幽门螺杆菌（Hp）感染和相关的慢性活动性胃黏膜炎症（见第 52 章）。

表 54.1　2012 年每 10 万人口胃癌发病率和死亡率（经年龄调整）

	发病率		死亡率	
	男	女	男	女
发达国家	15.6	6.7	9.2	4.2
发展中国家	18.1	7.8	14.4	6.5

Data from Torre LA, Bray F, Siegel RL, et al. Global cancer statistics, 2012. CA Cancer J Clin[Internet]. 2015; 65: 87—108. Available from http://WWW.ncbi.nlm.nih.gov/pubmed/25651787

框 54.1 胃腺癌的危险因素

确定的：
腺瘤性胃息肉*
慢性萎缩性胃炎
吸烟史
异型增生*
EBV(EB 病毒)
胃手术史(尤其是 Billroth Ⅱ)
HP 感染
肠上皮化生
遗传因素：
胃癌家族史(一级亲属)*
家族性腺瘤性息肉病(伴胃底腺息肉)*
遗传性非息肉性结直肠癌
Juvenile 息肉病(幼年型息肉病)
Peutz-Jeghers 综合征*
很可能的：
高盐摄入
胃溃疡病史
肥胖(限于贲门腺瘤)
恶性贫血史*
经常使用阿司匹林和其他 NSAID(保护性)
使用鼻烟
可能的：
高硝酸盐饮食
大量饮酒
大量摄入抗坏血酸盐(维生素 C)(保护性)
大量摄入新鲜水果和蔬菜(保护性)
低社会经济地位
Ménétrier 病
他汀类药物使用(保护性)
可疑的：
绿茶消费量高(保护性)
增生和胃底腺息肉

*建议对具有该危险因素的患者进行癌症监测。

二、病因学和发病机制

胃癌可采用 Laurén 分类细分为两种不同的组织学亚型，具有不同的流行病学和预后特征(图 54.1)[7]。肠型胃癌的特征是形成类似腺体样管状结构，其特征与肠腺相似。这种类型的胃癌与环境和饮食风险因素的联系更为密切，往往是胃癌高发地区的主要形式，也是目前全球范围内正在下降的胃癌组织学形式。弥漫型胃癌缺乏腺体结构，由浸润胃壁的内聚性差的细胞组成。其在全世界范围内被发现的频率相同，发生在较年轻的人群中，其预后比肠型胃癌差。弥漫型胃癌广泛累及胃可导致胃壁僵硬和增厚，这种情况被称为皮革状胃(Zinitis plastic)。弥漫型胃癌的另一个关键特征是具有印戒细胞，即一种特殊的充满黏蛋白的细胞，在肠型腺癌中不存在。但也存在混合表型，包含主要以肠型或弥漫型为特征的异质区域。

胃腺癌也分为近端肿瘤(EGJ 和胃贲门区)和远端或非交界型肿瘤(胃底、胃体和胃窦)。根据 Siewert 分类法(依据肿瘤所在位置分类)，交界型癌可进一步分为Ⅰ型(EGJ 上方 1~5cm)、Ⅱ型(交界处上方 1cm~交界处下方 2cm)和Ⅲ型(交界处下方 2~5cm)肿瘤[8]。远端食管腺癌、EGJ 腺癌和非交界型远端胃癌亚组的遗传和细胞起源之间没有明确的区别[9]。有趣的是，随着 Hp 感染率的降低，非交界型肿瘤不断减少，而更多的近端肿瘤在不断增加。在小鼠模型中，甚至有人推测 Barrett 食管相关食管癌和 EGJ 癌起源于胃贲门[10]。来自基因表达谱的新数据表明，病理外观和临床行为的差异可能是由于存在独特的分子表型。胃癌基因组图谱的特征显示酪氨酸激酶受体表达中存在多种改变，酪氨酸激酶受体与其配体和下游效应分子结合代表了未来药物开发的潜在途径。

癌症基因组图谱(Cancer Genome Atlas，TCGA)联盟，根据大约 300 种胃癌的基因组图谱提出了 4 种胃癌亚型[11]。这种分类与包括表观基因组、转录组和蛋白质组分析在内的不同平台高通量数据的聚类有很好的相关性。到目前为止，支持该拟定分类的生物相关性的数据很少。而之前对胃癌的转录组分析证明了具有不同预后结果或对全身治疗反应不同的表型簇[12,13]。

一般认为，肠型胃癌是通过多步骤过程发生的，在这个过程中，正常黏膜依次转化为过度增生的上皮、随后是化生过程导致腺体萎缩、异型增生、进而发生癌。在结肠癌中，转变的每一步都与特定的基因突变相关的证据很强[14]，但胃癌遵循遗传事件的可比序列的证据一直缺乏。然而，在肠型胃癌和结直肠癌中，DNA 突变似乎是随着时间的推移在正常人胃的干细胞中建立的，并且在肠上皮化生中，这些突变通过涉及隐窝裂变和腺体单克隆转化的过程通过胃扩散[15]。肠型胃癌的发病机制是一个多步骤的过程，这一论点主要得到以下观察结果的支持：在肠型癌症患者和胃癌高发国家中，慢性萎缩性胃炎和肠上皮化生的发生率均较高(见第 52 章)[16,17]。这种由 Pelayo Correa 及其同事开发的肠型胃癌多步骤模型[18]，假定存在最终导致胃癌发生的癌前变化的时间顺序。肠型胃癌的发生和发展的一个共同特征是胃黏膜的慢性炎症。Hp 感染是胃部炎症的主要病因和胃癌的主要病原体(见第 52 章)。在一部分患者中，炎症过程导致萎缩性胃炎的发生(腺体组织缺失)，随后进展为肠上皮化生、异型增生、早期胃癌、最终进展为晚期胃癌(图 54.2)。尽管动物模型表明，在高度异型增生发生前的所有阶段均可能逆转，但对于无法再阻止肿瘤进一步进展的人类“不可返回点”的定义仍存在争议[19,20]。如最近的 meta 分析所示，根除 Hp 有可能预防胃癌[21,22]。如果干预时胃黏膜没有癌前状态(腺体萎缩、肠上皮化生)，根除 Hp 的预防作用更明显[23]。根除 Hp 可阻止癌前状态的进一步进展，甚至可有一定程度的消退[24]。尽管目前认为肠化生的存在最有可能标志着“不可返回点”，但如果存在晚期病变(例如早期胃癌内镜切除术后)甚至可影响 Hp 的根除[25]。与结肠癌观察到的情况不同，参与这一进展的每一步的确切基因仍未明确。尽管如此，新一代测序技术已表明，EGJ 的胃癌和癌的基因改变比结肠癌存在更多的异质性[26,27]。此外，胃癌的癌前阶段在内镜检查过程中不如结肠癌容易识别，许多胃癌具有非常异质性，含有大量的间质细胞。据报道，这些基质细胞，还包括已知促进肿瘤生长的与癌

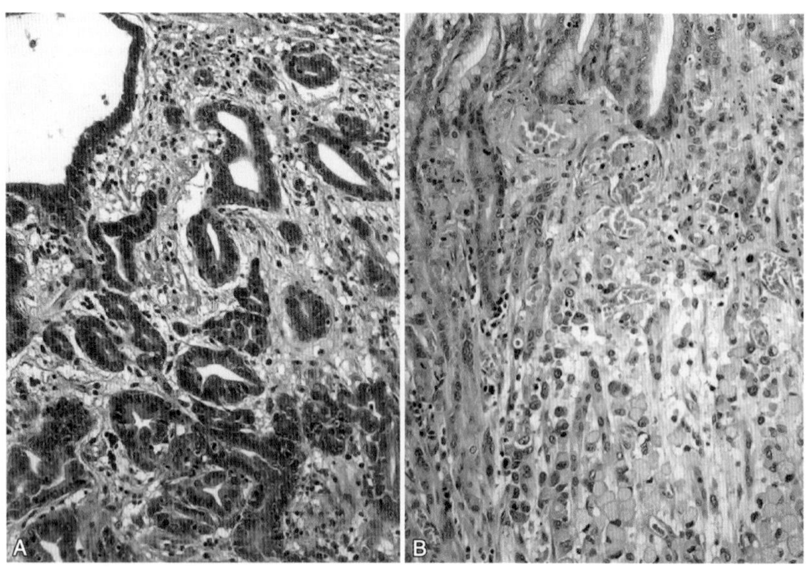

图 54.1　两种类型胃癌的组织病理学。A,肠型胃腺癌的特征为形成酷似肠腺的腺体样管状结构。B,弥漫型胃癌是含有单个侵袭性肿瘤细胞,通常含有丰富的黏蛋白,缺乏任何腺体样结构。HE 染色。(Courtesy Rhonda K. yantiss,MD,Boston,Mass.)

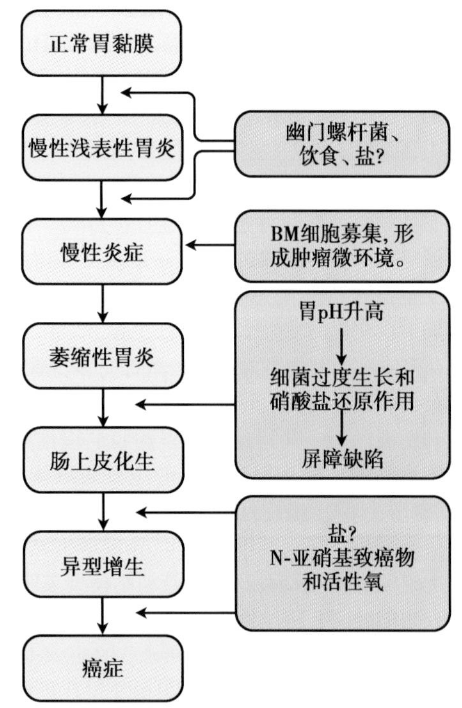

图 54.2　胃腺癌病理事件的 Correa 路径。在高分化的肠型胃癌中,组织病理学研究表明,慢性 Hp 感染在数十年内进展为慢性胃炎、萎缩性胃炎、肠上皮化生、异型增生和癌症。癌症的发展归因于慢性炎症引起的 DNA 改变。这与骨髓源性免疫细胞和间充质细胞(BM 细胞)的募集和形成有利于肿瘤发生的微环境有关。上皮细胞增生与凋亡之间的不平衡,以及在萎缩和胃酸缺乏的情况下,具有硝酸还原酶活性的肠道细菌在胃内定植,促进致癌性亚硝胺的形成,导致致癌基因变异的积累。以胃体为主的萎缩,或特殊胃腺细胞(如壁细胞和主细胞)的丢失,可能是进展为癌症的关键起始步骤。(From Fox JG, Wang TC. Lnflammation, atrophy, and gastric cancer. J Clin lnvest 2007;117:60-9.)

症相关的成纤维细胞,表现出明显的遗传和表观遗传变化,可能混淆对肿瘤的分析[28,29]。这一特征使得难以鉴定胃癌中特定基因突变的时间。目前,慢性炎症在弥漫型胃癌中的作用,以及如图 54.2 中所提出的肠型胃癌通路的相似性(如果有的话)仍有待明确。与两种组织学亚型相关的一个共同因素,是与 Hp 感染的强相关性,已证明 Hp 感染可直接修饰参与 DNA 损伤修复(DDR)通路的基因[30]。DDR 相关基因的修饰是胃癌发生的常见事件[31]。

(一) 幽门螺杆菌感染(另见第 52 章)

幽门螺杆菌(Hp)是一种革兰氏阴性微需氧细菌,感染全球近一半人口,被认为是胃癌的主要病原体。事实上,国际癌症研究机构(世界卫生组织的一个分支)已将幽门螺杆菌归类为 1 类(或确定)致癌物。在研究的每个人群中均发现了 Hp 感染,以发展中国家和东亚大部分地区的患病率较高[32,33]。

慢性 Hp 感染的自然史包括 3 种可能的结果[34]:①单纯性胃炎,患者通常无症状;②十二指肠溃疡表型,有 10%～15% 的受感染者发生;③胃溃疡/胃癌表型。胃癌发生的风险与背景胃炎的类型不同,但一般而言,导致低酸状态的胃体显性胃炎主要与风险增加相关。而 Hp 诱导的十二指肠溃疡病与高胃酸排出量以及发生胃癌的风险降低有关[35]。研究提示 Hp 感染者每年感染比率中有 1%～3% 发展为慢性萎缩性胃炎[18,36,37]。因此,那些在遗传上易患萎缩性胃炎的患者,Hp 感染也很可能易患胃癌。尽管 Hp 感染与弥漫型胃癌和肠型腺癌均相关,但我们在本章主要关注肠型腺癌形成的机制,因为对它们的研究更多。Hp 感染与黏膜相关淋巴组织淋巴瘤的相关性将在第 32 章中讨论。

Hp 感染引起的胃腺癌发生的风险增加取决于多种因素,包括宿主遗传因素、细菌菌株(包括细菌毒力因素)、感染持续时间以及是否存在其他环境危险因素(如不良饮食习惯、吸烟)。在日本队列研究中,仅感染 Hp 的患者在随访期间发生了胃腺癌(2.9 vs 0;$P<0.001$)[38]。来自中国的另外队列研究也报告了类似的结果[39,40]。在西方国家,Hp 感染与胃癌的相关性似乎仅局限于非交界性肿瘤[41]。然而有数据表明,Hp 也可能与 Siewert Ⅲ型交界性癌以及潜在的Ⅱ型肿瘤亚组有关[42,43]。

毒力强的细菌菌株、基因载体宿主和有利的胃环境的组合,可能是胃癌发生的必要条件。目前,对人类宿主的遗传易感因素的研究主要是基于单个基因,但新一代测序等新技术将会增强对宿主遗传因素的鉴定。然而,最重要的因素似乎是 Hp 感染引起的慢性炎症,从而导致胃黏膜上皮屏障功能受损,因而增加了其他致病因素(如不良饮食)的影响。炎症环境的几个方面被认为是致癌物,它们包括氧化应激增加和氧自由基形成,导致 DNA 损伤,CD_4^+T 细胞和骨髓细胞增加,促炎性细胞因子生成增加,这些均导致细胞更新加速,细胞凋亡减少,以及出现错误的或不完全 DNA 修复的可能性[44]。事实上,最近的研究表明,DNA 修复机制缺陷的动物,在慢性感染 Hp 后表现出更严重的胃黏膜异型增生[45]。如前所述,Hp 能够直接修饰 DDR 相关基因及其功能[30]。因此,迄今为止的证据清楚地表明,诱导螺杆菌相关疾病最重要的辅助因子是宿主免疫反应。事实上,慢性炎症与大量非胃癌有关。

胃黏膜的慢性炎症似乎是进展为胃癌的必要条件。在人类感染中很难研究其疾病机制,因此,我们对螺杆菌生物免疫应答的大部分理解,是来自在小鼠模型中进行的工作。不同近交系的小鼠对感染有不同程度的疾病易感性反应,几种基因敲除模型有助于阐明免疫应答的个体成分在疾病中的作用。

对 C57BL/6 易感小鼠品系的遗传操作促进了详细的研究,从而使人们更深入地了解促进小鼠胃癌的遗传因素,特别是适应性免疫应答的作用。例如淋巴细胞缺陷小鼠的胃螺杆菌感染不会导致组织损伤、细胞谱系改变或化生-异型增生-癌序列[46,47]。相反,B 细胞缺陷小鼠的感染(保留了正常的 T 细胞反应)会导致严重的萎缩和化生,与感染螺杆菌的野生型小鼠相同[47]。总之,这些研究强调了 $CD4^+$T 淋巴细胞在协调胃肿瘤中的关键作用。

易感小鼠品系,如 C57BL/6,能产生强烈的 Th1 型免疫反应(辅助性 T 细胞 1 型,表达 γ-干扰素和白细胞介素-12),而耐药菌株如 BALB/c,具有极化 Th2 应答(表达 IL-4 和 IL-5)[48,50]。Th2 应答与保护黏膜免疫受损伤相关,尽管无法消除细菌定植,事实上,通常与较高的细菌定植率有关。小鼠品系如 C3H 具有混合 Th1/Th2 细胞因子谱,表现出中间疾病,表明免疫应答内的细胞因子相互作用形成疾病的连续体,而不是离散的疾病状态。最近 Th17 细胞(表达 IL-17),已被证明是 Hp 诱导胃炎的重要组成部分[51]。尽管复合免疫环境最有可能决定疾病的表现,但单个细胞因子可能在疾病的易感性和预防中发挥作用。在幽门螺杆菌感染过程中,Th1 细胞因子 IFN-γ 可促进或抑制炎症驱动的胃癌,提示有一种更特异的免疫应答负责癌症促进或监测。尽管过去的研究表明 IFN-γ 可能促进胃肿瘤的发展,但最近发现在 IL-1β 和猫属螺杆菌依赖性致癌物模型中,胃中低水平的 IFN-γ 过度表达能够抑制胃癌[52,53]。此外,IFN-γ 被证明可以抵消 Th17 细胞的发育[53]。因此,肿瘤微环境中相同细胞和细胞因子的不同组成,可以形成一个有利于或抑制致癌物的星座。另一方面,缺乏 IL-10 细胞因子(一种抑制免疫反应的细胞因子)的小鼠对感染反应表现为严重的萎缩性胃炎[46-50]。最近遗传小鼠模型说明了 IL-6/IL-11 家族细胞因子在胃癌发生中的重要性[54]。

野生型菌株内免疫应答操作证实了 Th1/Th2 应答在致病中的核心作用。例如感染肠道蠕虫(多形螺旋线虫)会使免疫反应向 Th2 极化倾斜,并保护 C57BL/6 宿主免受螺杆菌诱导的萎缩和化生[55]。这种小鼠模型模拟了在非洲地区观察到的寄生虫感染状态和反常的低胃癌-高幽门螺杆菌感染率,可能解释了这种明显的不一致性。小鼠中的这些观察结果导致了非洲和拉丁美洲的人类研究,证实了胃癌发病率低的地域对 Hp 具有更高的 Th2/Th1 免疫应答[56,57]。一般而言,在血清 IgE 水平较高且蠕虫肠道寄生率在 50% 以上的地区,发现 Th2 型应答增加。这些发现进一步强调了宿主对感染反应的重要性,并表明操纵遗传预定的宿主细胞因子谱,以应对环境挑战可能会减少或加剧疾病过程的可能性。

对人体组织的研究也表明,Hp 的定植程度取决于多种因素,如调节性 T 细胞(Treg)的存在和活性或初始(幼稚)壁细胞数量(反映胃体的酸分泌能力)[58-60]。Tregs 与细菌定植增加[61]、慢性炎症改变[62]和免疫抑制细胞因子如 IL10、IL17、TGF-β 的表达有关[59,63]。在胃癌的情况下,Tregs 在胃黏膜和外周血中均增加[64-66]。Th1/Th2 衍生细胞因子的比值在无症状胃炎中最高,表现为胃萎缩、肠上皮化生和上皮内瘤样变向胃腺癌进展的稳定下降趋势。这与外周血中 Treg 细胞区室的同时增加,以及有利于 Treg 介导的慢性炎症的 CagA 阳性菌株的持续存在有关[67]。虽然 Hp 感染与胃癌的关系并不平行,但异型增生和浸润性癌的发生往往发生在 Hp 定植率显著下降或在某些情况下完全从胃中消失的时候。胃癌几乎总是发生在长期胃黏膜萎缩和低胃酸的情况下,这种情况容易导致肠道细菌过度生长。尽管针对 Hp 的抗生素根除治疗能延缓和抑制小鼠胃癌的发展[20,68],但抗生素不仅能根除 Hp,还可以根除定植于萎缩和低酸胃中的其他微生物。事实上,与定植常规菌群的 Hp 感染的 INS-GAS 小鼠相比,用 Hp 感染其他无菌 INS-GAS 小鼠导致进展为胃癌的时间延迟[69]。因此,Hp 可能只是导致胃癌进展的初始或最普遍的微生物因素。Ferreira 等最近报道,胃腺癌患者的胃微生物群与慢性胃炎患者有明显差异[70]。显性胃微生态失调的特征是,微生物多样性降低和 Hp 丰度降低以及包括肠道共生菌在内的细菌属的过度表达。关于这些发现,同样令人感兴趣的是,在癌症发生之前,Hp 在人类以及小鼠中主导了其他更为多样的胃微生物群系[71]。

由于 Hp 基因组内的点突变、插入、缺失和碱基对替换,Hp 菌株之间存在大量的遗传多样性。几种菌株可能感染单个个体,现有菌株可发生突变,并随时间而变化[72,73]。尽管存在这种遗传多样性,但一些基因被认为是胃癌的危险因素,包括 *cag* 致病岛、*vacA* 基因和 *babA2* 基因,是迄今为止其他因素中相关性最强和研究最广泛的。

Hp 基因组有 165 万个碱基对,编码约 1 500 个基因,其中三分之二已被赋予生物学作用[74]。剩余三分之一基因组的功能仍不清楚,但利用 DNA 微阵列或全基因组测序技术进行全基因组分析,将在不久的将来给出 Hp 基因组的广阔前景。导致癌变的因素包括:能够使细菌有效地定植于胃黏膜的因素、激发更具侵袭性的宿主免疫应答的因素,以及影响宿主细胞生长信号通路的因素。

向胃上皮细胞的运动是 Hp 生存策略的重要特征,这是由几个因素保证的。螺旋运动由 FlaA 和 FlaB 蛋白介导的,这两种蛋白旨在导航较厚的胃黏液。此外,Hp 产生 Hp1069 一种公认的胶原酶,可修饰细胞外基质和黏液层,从而降低黏稠度并允许细菌渗透[75,76]。此外,Hp 还表达多种基因,这些基因有助于缓冲胃酸,以维持相对中性的 pH。这包括由 7 个基因组成的尿素酶基因簇,其中 UreA/UreB 复合物(包括尿素酶)编码 10% 的 Hp 蛋白,对其生存至关重要。

Cag 致病岛约为 40kb,包含 31 个基因。该岛的末端基因 *cagA* 常被用作整个 cag 位点的标记。与 cagA 阴性(cagA-)株相比,cagA 阳性(cagA+)株炎症更严重,萎缩程度更高,进展为胃腺癌的概率更大[77-80]。估计其相对风险范围从 2 到高达 28.4[34]。许多邻近 cagA 的基因编码 4 型分泌系统(TFSS),通常被视为将细菌蛋白(如 cagA)注射到宿主细胞中的分子针。cagA 被注射到宿主细胞中,在那里它被 Src 和 c-Abl 激酶磷酸化,这一惊人的发现提出了 cagA 可以直接促进生长、迁移和转化的可能性。事实上,Hp cagA 转基因表达诱导小鼠胃肠和造血系统肿瘤[81]。在致病岛内的其他基因(*cagE* 或 *picB*、*cagG*、*cagH*、*cagI*、*cagL*、*cagM*)也被认为对疾病很重要,因为它们似乎是体外上皮细胞细胞因子释放所必需的,尽管它们似乎对免疫细胞细胞因子活化的影响不大[82-84]。这些发现可能解释了 cagA-菌株在体内减弱的炎症反应和较低的癌症风险[85-88]。

cagA 的细胞内磷酸化发生在某些谷氨酸-脯氨酸-异亮氨酸-酪氨酸-丙氨酸(glutamate-proline-isoleucine-tyrosine-alanine,EPIYA)基序上。描述了 4 个不同的 EPIYA 基序(EPIYA-A、-B、-C 和-D),其流行率因地理区域而异[89,90]。这些基序进一步影响 cagA 诱导的免疫应答以及相关的癌症风险。在一个 EPIYA-C 片段的情况下,胃癌的比值比接近 7.3,在 2 个或 2 个以上片段的情况下,胃癌的比值比可能高达 51[91,92]。同时,进一步的 cagPAI 相关基因的遗传变异已被证实与胃癌相关[93]。

所有 Hp 菌株均携带 *vacA* 基因,该基因编码造孔形成、空泡毒素,但表达因等位基因变异而不同。大约 50% 的 Hp 菌株表达 vacA 蛋白,vacA 蛋白已被证明在体外是一种非常强大的 T 细胞活化抑制剂[94]。尽管 vacA 和 cagA 映射到 Hp 基因组内的不同位点,但 vacA 蛋白通常在 cagA+菌株中表达。VacA 有多种形式,s1m1 菌株具有高度产毒素性。其他细菌毒力因子如 cagE,可能在细胞凋亡和宿主炎症反应的调节中发挥作用,从而促成疾病表现。事实上,"强毒株"(cagA+、cagE+和 vacA+、s1m1)比"非强毒株"(cagA-、cagE-和 vacA-)似乎是更有效的促炎介质诱导剂,这可能解释了 cagA+毒株与胃癌有更高的相关性[95]。

(二) 饮食危险因素

许多饮食因素被认为是胃癌的危险因素。胃癌发病率的下降与冷藏的广泛使用和伴随的新鲜水果和蔬菜摄入量的增加,以及腌制和咸味食品的摄入量的减少相吻合。冷藏时间超过 10~20 年与胃癌发生的风险降低相关[18]。较低的温度降低了新鲜食物中细菌、真菌和其他污染物的比率,以及细菌形成亚硝酸盐的速度。此外,大量摄入长期保存的食物可能与胃癌风险增加相关[96],可能是由于盐、硝酸盐和多环芳香胺的含量增高。

高硝酸盐摄入的影响受到了广泛的关注。当硝酸盐被细菌或噬菌体还原为亚硝酸盐时,它们可与其他含氮物质反应,形成 N-亚硝基化合物,是已知的有丝分裂原和致癌物。在大鼠中,已证明 N-亚硝基化合物可引起胃癌。然而,试图将 N-亚硝基暴露与胃癌风险联系起来的研究目前尚无定论,这也许反映了硝酸盐摄入量不一定与亚硝化水平相关的事实[97]。瑞典一项队列研究发现,与高硝酸盐饮食摄入相关的胃癌风险增加了近 2 倍[96]。然而,来自欧洲的单独大型队列研究并没有证明硝酸盐摄入量与胃癌风险之间的相关性[98,99]。

与胃癌发生有关的另一个因素是高盐饮食(腌制食品、酱油、干咸鱼和咸肉)。在螺杆菌感染的情况下,高盐摄入与人和动物中较高的萎缩性胃炎发生率相关,并增加了动物模型中亚硝化食物的致突变性[18,100]。高盐饮食与胃癌风险增加约 1.5~2 倍相关[101]。队列研究和病例对照研究也发现,与加工肉类摄入相关的胃癌风险增加[96,102]。可能的机制包括较高的细菌负荷、Hp-cagA 表达上调、细胞增殖和 p-21 表达增加[100,103,104]。Hp 感染与胃癌的饮食危险因素之间存在明显的交互作用,与仅存在其中一个危险因素的个体相比,大量摄入红肉或加工肉类的 Hp 阳性受试者的危险增加不成比例[105]。

流行病学研究在水果和蔬菜消费以及胃癌风险方面的结果不一致[106-109]。其他被认为是胃癌潜在危险因素的食物或饮食因素,是大量摄入油炸食物、高脂肪食物、大量摄入红肉和黄曲霉素[102,110-112]。大量摄入新鲜鱼类和抗氧化剂的饮食可能具有保护作用(另见后文)[111,113-115]。然而,尚无足够的数据对这些影响因素作出明确的结论。

(三) 吸烟

长期以来烟草一直被确定为致癌物,大量的流行病学研究表明,吸烟与胃癌之间存在关联[116]。来自欧洲和亚洲的几项大型队列研究报告,吸烟者患胃癌的风险显著增加[117-119]。最近一项 meta 分析发现,与从不吸烟者相比,当前吸烟者在贲门或非贲门区域发生胃癌的风险增加了 1.5~2 倍[120]。作者还报告了吸烟量越多,与胃癌风险的相关性越高。

鼻烟是一种无烟烟草制品,作为香烟的替代品推广,据报道可降低致癌亚硝胺的水平。然而,瑞典一项队列研究的结果表明,在常规鼻烟使用者中,非贲门区胃癌的风险增加了 1.4 倍[121]。同时实验研究证明,鼻烟暴露也会增加 Hp 感染小鼠的胃癌发生率[122]。

(四) 酒精

大多数流行病学研究未能证明饮酒与贲门或非贲门胃癌之间的相关性[119,123,124]。然而,几项 meta 分析显示,大量饮酒与胃癌风险之间存在较小却显著的相关性(选定亚组中 RR,1.16~1.87)[125-128]。尽管其中一些分析提示交界性癌的风险高于远端胃癌,但一些作者陈述了相反的效应。总体而言,风险增加似乎是中度的,并受多种因素(包括吸烟和体力活动)的影响。有趣的是,酒精摄入可能会增加某些乙醇脱氢酶基因多态性患者,发生胃癌的风险[129]。

(五) 肥胖

肥胖是许多胃肠道恶性肿瘤公认的风险因素[130]。BMI 增加与轻度至中度胃贲门癌风险增加相关,但与非贲门癌无关[131-134]。美国国立卫生研究院-美国退休人员协会(National Institutes of Health-American Association of Retired Persons, NIH-AARP)饮食和健康队列研究的结果表明,病态肥胖(定义为 BMI≥35)以及腰围过大与胃贲门癌风险增加 2~3 倍相关,但与非贲门癌无关[135]。来自荷兰的一项单独队列研究也发现,随着 BMI 的增加,患贲门癌的风险也增加[131]。最近对 391 456 例患者的 EPIC 队列数据进行的分析中,其中 124 例发生食管癌和胃腺癌,193 例贲门癌和 224 例非贲门胃癌均与 BMI 无关[136]。肥胖和贲门癌风险之间的可能关联,可能是由促炎性细胞因子和腹腔内内脏脂肪产生的脂肪因子介导的[137]。

(六) 遗传因素

与大多数恶性肿瘤一样,遗传和环境因素在胃癌的发病机制中起着重要作用。通常认为,肠型胃癌主要是由于环境因素(即 Hp 感染),而弥漫性胃癌被认为主要是遗传性恶性肿瘤。然而,在肠型胃癌的情况下,因为主要的环境因素、Hp 感染、也往往表现出家族聚集性,所以将相对值分配给环境和遗传因素是复杂的。尽管如此,在未来胃癌类型可能更倾向于根据基因改变进行分类,并分为具有不同致癌机制和临床行为的分子亚组,而不是组织学类型[138]。

总体而言,10%的胃癌病例似乎表现出家族聚集性[139],即使在控制了 Hp 感染状态后,家族史也可能是一个独立的风险因素[140,141]。在一项对胃癌患者亲属的队列研究中,经 Hp 感染校正后,兄弟姐妹患胃癌的风险增加了 2 倍[142]。在一项来自日本的病例对照研究中,阳性家族史与女性患胃癌的概率(odds)显著增加相关(OR,5.10),但与男性无关[143]。来自斯堪的纳维亚的一项研究表明,双胞胎患胃癌的相对风险显著增加(单卵双胞胎 RR 为 9.9%,双卵双胞胎 RR 为 6.6%),这导致研究人员推算出遗传因素占胃癌的 28%,而共享环境因素占 10%,非共享环境因素占 62%[144]。最近一项包含超过 8 万人的 32 项研究的 meta 分析报告,有阳性胃癌家族史的受试者的汇总相对危险度增加 2.35(95% CI 1.96~2.81);如果一级亲属有胃癌家族史,则被诊断为胃癌的风险甚至更高(RR 2.71,95% CI 2.08~3.53)[145]。

在肠型胃癌所见的家族聚集性中,可能与宿主对 Hp 感染的免疫反应中起作用的遗传因素有关。来自韩国的数据表明,有胃癌家族史的个体,常同时患有 Hp 感染和相关的萎缩性胃炎或肠上皮化生[146]。在一项来自苏格兰的病例对照研究中,与对照组相比,胃癌患者亲属的萎缩和胃酸过少的患病率更高,但 Hp 感染率相似[147]。更高的萎缩患病率仅限于 Hp 感染的患者,提示这些患者可能对 Hp 表现出更强烈的免疫反应。在许多模型系统中,胃萎缩的发生与强烈的 Th1 免疫应答有关[50,55,148]。因此,推测胃萎缩和胃癌的候选疾病易感基因,可能是参与 Hp 感染固有的和适应性免疫应答的基因。炎症由一系列促炎和抗炎细胞因子调节,一些基因多态性已被描述影响细胞因子应答。随着最近开始的新一代测序方法,我们也许能够确定胃癌发病率增加的家族,是否具有更致癌免疫应答的遗传倾向。

其中一个因子是 IL-1β,一种重要的促炎性因子和强效的酸分泌抑制剂。事实上,在 Hp 感染的情况下,促炎性 IL-1 基因簇多形态(编码 IL-1β 的 *IL-1B* 和编码其天然存在的受体拮抗剂 IL-1RA 的 *IL-1RN*)与肿瘤进展之间存在关联。研究显示,携带 *IL-1β-31* C* 或-*511* T* 和 *IL-RN* 2/** 2 基因型的个体发生 Hp 依赖性胃酸过低和胃癌的风险更高[149]。与非炎症基因型相比,这些基因型进展为癌症的风险增加在 2~3 倍范围内。初步报告,在其他研究中也得到证实[150-154]。随后 Hwang 及其同事[155]证明 *IL-1B-511T/T* 基因型或 *IL-1RN* 2* 等位基因携带者的黏膜 IL-1β 水平高于非携带者,并证实了-*511T/T* 基因型与严重胃部炎症和萎缩之间的关联。IL-1β 致癌作用的重要性现已在转基因研究中得到证实,在转基因小鼠中,人 IL-1β 的胃特异性表达导致自发性胃部炎症和癌症,这与骨髓源性抑制细胞早期募集到胃相关[156]。值得注意的是,在 Barrett 食管以及食管和 EGJ 肿瘤的小鼠模型中,IL-1β 在食管鳞状上皮中的表达,也导致食管炎和贲门干细胞扩增形成胃食管肿瘤,这支持 Barretts 相关腺癌起源于类似胃癌表型的胃癌假说[10]。

肿瘤坏死因子(TNF-α)和白细胞介素-10(IL-10)的基因多态性与胃癌风险的其他相关性已有报道。TNF-α 和 IL-10 的促炎基因型分别与非贲门胃癌的风险增高 2 倍相关。当 *IL-1B* 和 *IL-1RN* 的促炎基因型结合时,具有 3 种或 4 种高危基因型的患者发生胃癌的风险增加了 27 倍[157]。其他的研究表明,TOII 样受体-4(*TLR-4*)基因的多态性也会增加患胃癌的风险。*TLR-4*+896G 多态性携带者发生胃酸过低的比值比增加了 11 倍,胃萎缩和炎症明显更严重[158]。越来越多的证据表明,胃癌的遗传倾向可能在很大程度上取决于 TLR 和细胞因子对慢性幽门螺杆菌感染的反应。TLR1 的多态性似乎可预防胃癌的发生(OR 0.4;95% CI 0.22~0.72),并且与下游细胞因子信号转导的改变进一步相关[159,160]。

最常见的遗传性胃癌是弥漫型胃癌,这种胃癌见于编码细胞黏附分子 E-钙黏蛋白的基因 *CDH1* 存在种系突变的情况下。发现新西兰一个大的家系存在 E-钙黏蛋白基因的种系突变,另外几个家系中也有类似突变的报道,均为弥漫型胃癌[161-164]。*CDH1* 突变个体的胃癌发病年龄小于 40 岁,但可具有高度变异性,估计发生胃癌的终生风险接近 70%[165,166]。种系 *CDH1* 突变也与家族性小叶乳腺癌有关[167,168]。

胃癌家族聚集性的一小部分可归因于其他癌症综合征。家族性非典型性息肉病患者,胃腺瘤的患病率为 35%~100%,其患胃癌的风险比普通人群高近 10 倍[169]。在这一特定患者群中的异型增生病变经常来自胃底腺息肉,并在幼年时发生[170-171]。胃底腺息肉在其他方面不倾向于进展为异型增生。遗传性非息肉病性结直肠癌(hereditary nonpolyposis colorectal cancer,HNPCC)综合征患者,发生胃癌的风险约为11%,主要为肠型胃癌,诊断时平均年龄为56岁[172]。幼年型息肉病患者的胃癌发病率约为12%~20%[173,174]。除了前面描述的种系基因改变外,外显子测序等新一代测序技术导致了参与胃癌发生的新分子和机制的检测。在8%~10%的胃癌患者中,在*ARID1A*基因(也称为*BAF250a*、*SMARCF1*或*OSA1*)中发现了体细胞突变,*ARID1A*基因是SWI-SNF染色质重塑复合物的一个辅助亚基,参与DNA修复、分化和发育过程[175-178]。值得注意的是,EBV感染的癌症在73%的患者中显示*ARID1A*突变。此外,*ARID1A*突变与*TP53*突变呈负相关,并与*PIK3CA*突变同时发生。*ARID1A*改变的患者无复发生存期更长,表明这些癌症属于具有不同致癌机制以及临床行为的分子亚群[175-178]。对体细胞拷贝数畸变分析还显示了显著扩增的基因,包括在胃癌和胃食管癌中的治疗靶向激酶,如*ERBB2*、*FGFR2*、*EGFR*和*MET*。

三、肿瘤遗传学

虽然萎缩和肠上皮化生与胃癌风险相关,但通过这些阶段的直接细胞进展尚未得到最终证实。事实上,胃癌很可能起源于胃黏膜内的干细胞或祖细胞,而不是直接来自终末分化的化生性细胞。几十年来,研究者一直试图解开导致胃癌发生和进展的突变,以揭示类似于结直肠癌中所见的获得性突变的逻辑进展。然而,胃癌并不像结直肠癌进展那样遵循模式,胃癌中没有明确的突变线性序列,基因改变存在更大的异质性。

尽管对大型高通量数据的初步研究主要集中在转录组分析上[179-181],但更先进的基因组测序技术的出现,能够对胃癌的突变图谱进行全基因组分析[182-184]。国际联合体中多个研究小组的共同努力,使对大型队列的多级组数据进行更全面的综合分析成为可能[9,13,138]。TCGA联盟提供了大约300个胃癌的5个不同平台上的综合数据。他们证明了不同水平的基因组数据以及表观遗传变化和转录组甚至蛋白质组分析之间聚类的良好相关性[138]。基于他们的聚类分析,作者提出了胃癌的4组分类:第一组(EBV)与EBV感染有关,表现出显性表观遗传超甲基化谱(EBV)。第二组(MSI)微卫星不稳定性(MSI)呈阳性,与结直肠癌MSI亚组相似。其余肿瘤分为低突变率和低拷贝数畸变频率的一组(GS),称为“基因组稳定”亚型,高突变率和进一步相关基因组改变的一组(CIN),称为“染色体不稳定”型。值得注意的是,GS组主要包括弥漫型肿瘤,而CIN组则代表更多的肠型癌症。这些亚型在位置上的分布存在一些差异,CIN肿瘤在近端位置的比例更高,这一点后来也被证实适用于食管腺癌[9]。这种分类的临床相关性,是通过编码靶向治疗方法中使用的信号通路的基因的显性变化模式提出的。亚洲癌症研究组在他们的3 000例胃癌队列中遵循了类似的方法,尽管比TCGA更关注转录组数据[13]。因此,Cristescu等预先提出了相似的4组分类,也报告了作为该4组预后预测因素的特性。该分类在几个独立队列中得到验证,包括TCGA患者组。这些综合研究中描述的实际基因组变化与之前发表的结果一致。

非整倍体在胃癌中很常见(60%~75%),但细胞遗传学研究未能发现任何一致的染色体异常。比较基因组杂交研究表明,染色体臂4q、5q、9p、17p和18q表现出DNA拷贝数的频繁减少,而染色体臂8q、17q和20q通常表现出DNA拷贝数增加[185]。

人们普遍认为*TP53*是胃癌中最常见的突变基因(占胃癌的60%~70%),*Ras*、*APC*和*Myc*的突变罕见[186,187]。APC位点的杂合性缺失更为常见。另一个高频率(≈60%)发现的基因异常,是染色体3P上的抑癌基因脆性组氨酸三联体基因(*FHIT*)的缺失或抑制。抑制进入细胞周期的基因,如*p16*和*p27*,在近一半的胃癌中表现出表达减弱[188-193]。*p27*表达缺失与预后较差相关[188,190]。*p16*表达缺失最常见于分化较差的癌,但对预后没有可测量的影响[194]。*p16*和*p27*的表达减少发生在检测不到的突变的情况下,被认为继发于高甲基化[192]。其中许多种癌症表现出许多启动子区域的高甲基化,包括*MLH1*启动子区域,并表现出高水平的微卫星不稳定性(MSI-H)表型(见第1章)。多个抑癌基因已被证明在胃癌中发生甲基化。新出现的证据表明,这些表观遗传变化,包括整体低甲基化和启动子高甲基化,发生在胃癌的早期。此外,肿瘤相关基质成纤维细胞似乎也发生了DNA甲基化变化,提示肿瘤微环境的重要作用。

已经论述了许多生长因子通路的过度表达或扩增,包括*COX-2*(70%)、肝细胞生长因子/分散因子(*HGF/SF*)(60%)、血管内皮生长因子(*VEGF*)(50%)、*c-met*(50%)、乳腺癌-1(*AIB-1*)扩增(40%)和β-连环蛋白(25%)(表54.2)[195]。据

表54.2 胃腺癌的异常基因

异常	基因变化的频率/%
微卫星不稳定性	15~50
DNA非整倍体	60~75
缺失/抑制	
p53	60~70
FHIT(脆性组氨酸三联基因)	60
APC(结肠腺癌性息肉病基因)杂合性缺失	50
DCC(结直肠癌基因缺失)杂合性缺失	50
高甲基化导致表达减少	
p16	≈50
TFF1(人三叶因子1基因)	≈50
p27	<50
MLH1(人MUTL同源1基因)	15~20
E-cadherin(E-钙黏蛋白)	50
扩增/过度表达	
COX-2(环氧化酶-2)	70
HGF(肝细胞生长因子)	60
VEGF(血管内皮生长因子)	50
C-met	50
AIB-1(乳腺癌-1扩增)	40
Beta-catenin(β-连环蛋白)	25
EGFR(EGF受体基因)	15
突变	
P13K(磷脂酰肌醇3激酶基因)	25
PTPRT(蛋白-酪氨酸磷酸酶受体基因)	17

报道,约 15% 的胃癌同时过表达 EGF 和 EGF 受体(EGFR),这与自分泌机制一致。在所分析的胃癌中,高达 25% 发现了编码磷脂酰肌醇 3-激酶(PI3K)催化亚基的基因 *PIC3A* 突变[196]。此外,同一实验室在 17% 的胃癌中发现了编码人蛋白酪氨酸磷酸酶(PTP)的基因突变,其中蛋白酪氨酸酶磷酸酶受体类型(PTPRT)改变最频繁[197]。

胃特异性肿瘤抑制基因 *TFF1*(trefoil factor 1 三叶因子 1)和 RUNX3(Runt 相关转录因子 3)目前已被确定,可能代表胃癌通路的"守门人",是进一步研究的合乎逻辑的靶标[198,199]。在约 50% 的胃癌中描述了 *TFF1* 的缺失,*TFF1* 基因敲除小鼠发生自发性胃窦肿瘤。*TFF1* 的突变也有描述,这些通过包括 PI3-激酶和磷脂酶-C[200] 表达的信号通路增强胃癌细胞侵袭能力被 STAT-3 抑制,STAT-3 的激活也正在成为导致胃癌的关键通路[54]。RUNX3 很有可能通过诱导 P21 和 Bim 抑制胃上皮生长,减弱 Wnt 信号,并在 82% 的胃癌中发生改变[201]。研究这些基因及其对胃癌表型的贡献,将对我们理解疾病进展很有价值。

继发于 DNA 错配修复基因缺陷的二核苷酸重复序列中的 MSI(微卫星不稳定),如 *MLH1* 和 *MLH2*(mutL 同源基因 1 和 2),主要与结直肠癌的发生有关,尤其是 HNPCC 综合征(遗传性非息肉病性结直肠癌)。HNPCC 综合征患者的胃癌发病率为 11%,提示 MSI 也可能在胃癌的发生发展中起一定作用[172]。MSI 见于 15%~50% 的散发性胃癌中,其中肠型胃癌的患病率较高[202-207]。低水平微卫星活性(如 MSI-低)在胃癌患者中 40% 的肠上皮化生区域发现[207],在腺瘤性息肉中发现 14%~20%[205,207,208]。MSI-H 仅发生 10%~16% 的胃癌中。MSI 与 *TP53* 突变、高分化-中高分化组织学和在胃远端位置的发生频率较低相关。检查 MSI 对患者生存率影响的研究显示结果不一致[208,209]。当研究结果综合在一起时,似乎 MSI 确实在胃癌的发病机制中发挥作用,很可能在肠上皮化生发生之前(见图 54.2),最常见的原因是 *MLH1* 启动子的甲基化。

关于弥漫型胃癌的遗传学数据越来越多[138,184]。已发现一些遗传性弥漫型胃癌家系携带 E-cadherin 基因(*CDH1*)的种系突变[161-163,210,211]。然而,*CDH1* 突变也被描述为散发性弥漫型胃癌的主要特征。支持 E-钙黏蛋白(E-cadherin)在胃癌发病机制中作用的进一步证据表明,51% 的胃癌发生 E-钙黏蛋白表达的抑制,在弥漫型胃癌中发现的百分比更高[212]。此外,E-钙黏蛋白低表达与较高的淋巴结转移率和生存率降低相关[213,214]。胃癌中 *CDH1* 突变率总体较低。因此,在胃癌中观察到的 E-钙黏蛋白的表达下降很可能继发于 *CDH1* 启动子的高甲基化,这种高甲基化发生在 50% 的胃癌和 83% 的弥漫型胃癌中[215]。E-钙黏蛋白是一种跨膜蛋白,通过 α-和 β-连环蛋白与肌动蛋白细胞骨架连接,建立细胞极性并介导同嗜性细胞相互作用[216,217]。E-钙黏蛋白的表达下降被认为促进了癌细胞与其细胞基质的解离,增强了胃癌细胞的迁移和侵袭。在 68% 的胃癌中 α-连环蛋白的表达也降低或缺失[218]。因此,E-钙黏蛋白似乎是作为一种肿瘤抑制基因,可能在弥漫型胃癌的发病机制中起重要作用。在弥漫型胃癌中常见的其他改变是:Wnt 相关基因的改变以及 Ras 同源基因家族成员 A 基因(*RHOA*)的改变,这似乎是该组织学亚型所独有的[184]。

也许与胃腺癌进展过程中获得的基因改变同样重要的是问题,"这些变化发生在什么靶细胞中?"一个细胞要积累自主生长所必需的遗传变化的数量,它必须是长寿的。由于这些原因,目前的认识是:一个常驻的组织干细胞是基因突变的靶标,成为"癌干细胞"——能够自主生长并具有转移的潜能。最近,在小鼠中进行的几项简明的遗传谱系追踪研究,建立了能够区分两种不同类型的胃肠道干细胞的标记。隐窝基底柱状细胞(CBC)是表达 Lgr5 和 CD133(Prom-1)的快速循环干细胞[219,220]。绒毛蛋白转基因可鉴定位于胃窦腺体亚群下三分之一的多能祖细胞[221],而在胃窦部也可以鉴定出多个肠道干细胞标记。有趣的是,Lgr5 在一些胃窦腺体和贲门中显示出家系标记[220]。慢循环细胞,通常在胃窦隐窝的+4 位置发现(即从隐窝底部向上计数的第四上皮细胞),其特征是 Bmi1 和 Tert 的明显表达[222,223]。尽管这两种类型的细胞在功能上是相互联系的[224],但它们确切的层级关系仍有待确定。Sigal 及其同事证明了 Lgr5 阳性胃干细胞直接依赖 CagA 激活,从而报道了幽门螺杆菌感染诱导胃癌发生的进一步机制[225]。同一研究组还提出上皮细胞过度增殖和腺体增生的协调,作为对基质腔隙细胞(主要是涉及幽门螺杆菌诱导 Wnt 信号的肌成纤维细胞)感染的反应[226]。

在胃泌酸腺体中,胃干细胞的增殖区位于峡部、胃腺体的中部,细胞被认为是双向迁移以供应覆盖胃小凹的胃表面黏液细胞,以及构成腺体底部的胃壁细胞和酶原细胞[227]。胃体干细胞尚未确定,前面讨论的标志物均未标记胃腺体峡部内的任何特异性细胞。最近,通过谱系追踪研究显示祖细胞(如 Krt19+和 TFF2+细胞)可标记不同的胃祖细胞[228,229]。通常,柱状化生对 TFF2 和 Krt19 呈阳性。鉴于肠上皮化生发生在胃黏膜和食管,类似的干细胞产生这两者是合理的。无论其定位(CBC 或+4 位置)或功能如何,胃肠道干细胞均依赖于干细胞微环境的信号,如隐窝周围的肌成纤维细胞和邻近的分化上皮[230]。干细胞维持和增殖所需的重要信号通路包括 Wnt、Notch、骨形态发生蛋白(BMP)和刺猬通路(Hedgchog pathways)[231]。

关于局部基质微循环与上皮细胞相互作用的理论知识越来越多。胃癌细胞生物学行为的调节因子是癌症相关的成纤维细胞,其已被证明可改变转化生长因子 β(TGFβ)依赖性信号,增加细胞运动性,因此具有侵袭性[232,233]。肿瘤浸润淋巴细胞及其邻近区域的密度,也改变了肿瘤的侵袭性,因此对胃腺癌或 EGJ 腺癌患者的预后结果有影响[234,235]。该因素部分反映在全身炎症水平上[236]。全身性炎症可部分由内脏脂肪组织介导,已证实网膜脂肪细胞通过激活肿瘤细胞中的 P13K-Akt 信号转导增强胃癌的侵袭性[237]。

除了来自体外(vitro)和体内(vivo)模型的有价值的数据外,对下一代高通量和测序数据进行"虚拟显微切割"的方法,有希望增进我们对不同细胞组分网络及其对肿瘤起始、促进和进展(包括侵袭性和转移行为)影响的了理解(图 54.3)。

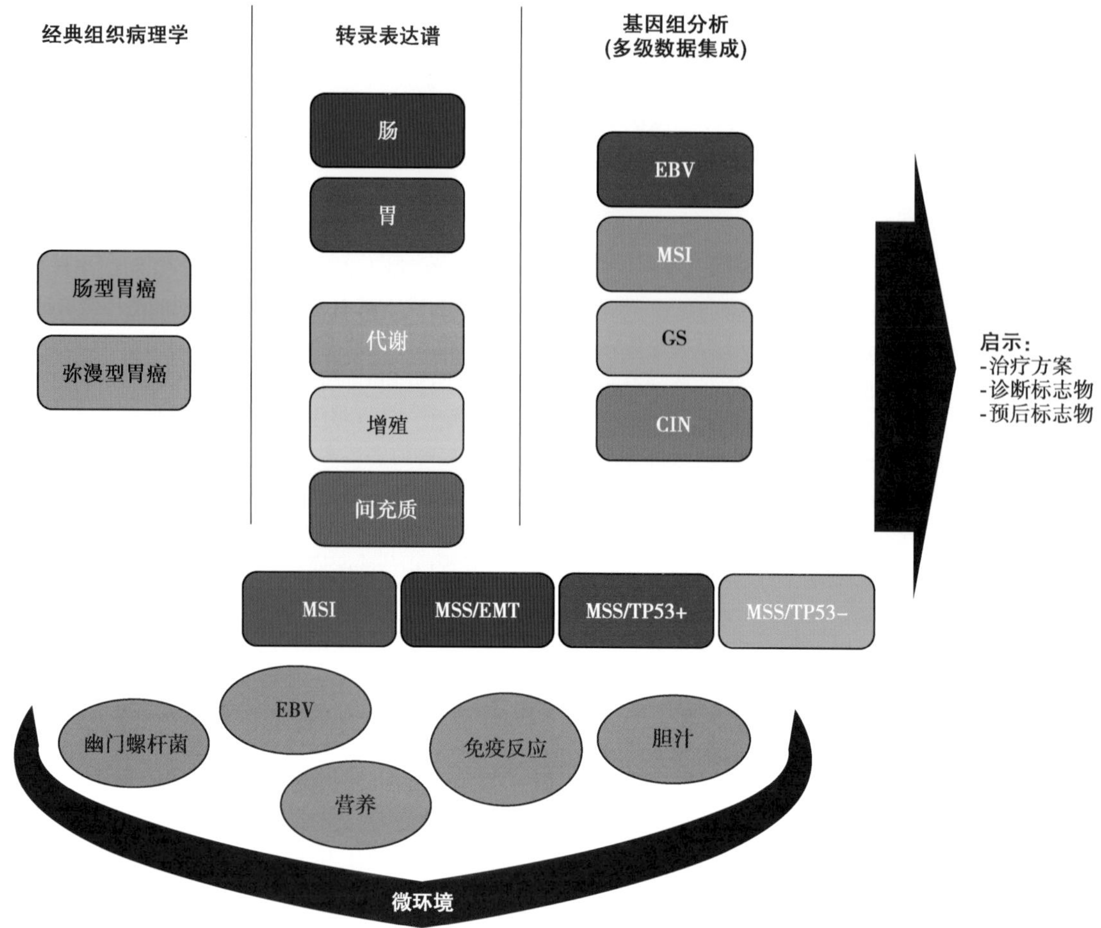

图 54.3 胃癌的分子分层。本图概述了胃癌亚型的最新概念。这些分类来源于转录本谱高通量研究以及下一代测序收集的数据,超越了经典的组织病理学分类(左)。早期的转录数据表明,在通路分析(中间、底部)启用更多的功能解释之前,二分法组表现出与经典 Lauren 类型(中间、顶部)相似的特征。最近的概念通常基于多层次的数据整合,但仍然主要来源于基因数据,如 TCGA 方法(EBV,EB 病毒;MSI,微卫星不稳定性阳性癌;GS,基因组稳定性癌;CIN,染色体不稳定性癌)或来自亚洲癌症研究组(ACRG)方法(MSI,微卫星不稳定性阳性癌;MSS/EMT,微卫星稳定伴上皮间质转化的转录标记;MSS/TP53+,微卫星稳定伴 *TP53* 突变;MSS/TP53-,微卫星稳定伴野生型 *TP53*)。一个特别的兴趣在于了解驱动每个表型的因素,主要是与肿瘤微环境的相互作用

四、癌前状态

(一) 慢性萎缩性胃炎

慢性萎缩性胃炎定义为:在胃的适当区域中特殊腺体组织的损失,是一种确定的形态学变化,沿着胃癌发展的顺序发生[238]。萎缩性胃炎每年进展为胃癌的发生率约为 0.1%~1.0%[239-243]。胃内萎缩性胃炎的程度与进展为癌症的风险相关[244-246]。大量研究已经证明,只有在基线时有广泛黏膜萎缩性变化的患者,在长期随访期间发展为胃腺癌[247]。

萎缩性胃炎有两种形式(见第 52 章)。最常见的是环境多灶性萎缩性胃炎(MAG),与 HP 感染有关,更可能与化生有关。HP 感染的存在可使萎缩性胃炎发生的风险约增加 10 倍[248]。萎缩性胃炎流行率存在相当大的地区差异。与西方国家相比,亚洲地区患病率约增加 3 倍[248,249]。萎缩性胃炎的第二种形式是自身免疫性化生性萎缩性胃炎(AMAG),与抗壁细胞和内在因子抗体有关。这种形式的萎缩局限于胃体和胃底。自身免疫性化生性萎缩性胃炎与恶性贫血和胃癌风险增加相关,尽管不如 HP 诱导的 MAG 多见,因炎症程度很可能较轻[240,250]。

在胃萎缩的情况下,胃癌风险增加的潜在机制可能与低酸输出(胃酸过少或胃酸缺乏)有关,低酸输出易导致非幽门螺杆菌细菌过度生长,更多地形成 N-亚硝基化合物,及胃腔内抗坏血酸分泌减少[251]。此外,循环胃泌素水平升高是对酸输出减少的反应。胃泌素是一种已知的胃黏膜细胞生长因子,胃泌素的持续升高可能导致细胞异常生长及增加肿瘤进展的风险[252,253]。

(二) 肠化生和异型增生

按 Filipe 组的分类[254],肠上皮化生(IM)可细分为 3 类。Ⅰ型(完全型)IM 含有分泌唾液酸黏蛋白的杯状细胞和成熟的非分泌性吸收细胞。Ⅰ型 IM 不是胃癌的风险因素。Ⅱ型(不完全型)IM 含有少量(如果有的话)吸收细胞、处于不同分化阶段的分泌中性或酸性唾液酸黏蛋白的柱状"中间"细胞,以及分泌唾液酸黏蛋白和/或偶尔分泌硫酸黏蛋白的杯状细胞。Ⅲ型(不完全型)的分化程度低于Ⅱ型,中间细胞主要分泌硫酸黏蛋白,杯状细胞分泌唾液酸和/或硫酸黏蛋白。Ⅱ型或Ⅲ型 IM 与胃癌发生风险增加约 20 倍相关[255,256]。在

随访 5 年内,有 42% 的Ⅲ型 IM 患者发生早期胃癌,提示 IM 是肠型胃癌的癌前病变[256]。荷兰对 92 250 例患者进行的一项大型全国队列研究发现,胃 IM 患者的癌症年进展率为 0.25%[243]。然而,癌症是起源于IM 区域还是 IM 是否仅仅代表了较高胃癌风险的一个标志物仍不清楚,主要是由于这种情况的局灶性和斑片状外观所致。与萎缩性胃炎的情况一样,HP 感染者 IM 的患病率亚洲(≈40%)比西方国家高[248,249]。尽管人们普遍认为 IM 与肠型胃癌的风险增加相关,但弥漫型胃癌患者的非肿瘤胃黏膜 IM 患病率也较高[257,258]。

如前所述,最近的多项研究提示,肠上皮化生不是胃癌唯一可能的前体病变。尽管关于与胃癌风险增加相关的黏膜谱系变化的顺序和联系方面存在争议,但人们普遍认为分泌酸的壁细胞的损失(也称泌酸萎缩)是诱导化生的先决条件。胃底的胃窦化或胃底存在化生性腺体,其一般表型与胃窦或幽门腺相似(也称为假性幽门化生),通常与肠型胃腺癌相关,这种表型也被称为表达解痉多肽的化生(SPEM)[259],其特征是胃底存在三叶因子 2(TFF2 或解痉多肽)免疫反应阳性细胞,其形态特征类似于胃窦深层腺细胞。在美国、日本和冰岛的 3 项研究中,观察到 SPEM 与 90% 以上的切除胃癌相关[259-261]。来自小鼠的数据表明,幽门螺杆菌诱导的 TFF2 表达与胃黏膜相同隔室中的 $CD44^+$ 肿瘤干细胞相关,因此可能促进进一步的恶性进展。SPEM 和肠上皮化生可能与假定的胃癌前病变具有同等的重要性。然而,这些化生是否能进展为异型增生或肿瘤仍有待确定。另外,肠上皮化生可能反映了黏膜在面对慢性感染和炎症时进一步良性尝试增加修复。

胃异型增生和腺癌的组织学评估,是基于 2000 年国际胃肠道病理学家会议共识的结果——维也纳分类(表 54.3)[262]。胃异型增生的患病率在低风险地区低至 0.5%[263],高风险地区为 20%[264]。前瞻性研究表明,低级别异型增生可能在高达 60% 的病例中消退,然而有 10%~20% 进展为高级别异型增生(图 54.4)[265-267]。高级别异型增生很少消退,并且与每年 2%~6% 进展为胃癌的年发生率相关[267,268]。在一项荷兰前瞻性队列研究中,高级别异型增生与进展为胃癌的风险增加 40 倍相关[211]。高级别异型增生通常与同时性癌相关,可以是单灶性或多灶性的病灶[269]。

表 54.3　胃异型增生 Padov 国际分类系统

类别	定义	组织学描述
Ⅰ	正常	正常胃结构,无或轻微炎性浸润
	反应性小凹增生	一般结构保存完好,但有上皮细胞增生、细胞核增大和有丝分裂象
	肠上皮化生	Ⅰ型:与小肠形态相似,有吸收性肠上皮细胞、刷状缘清晰和形态良好的杯状细胞 Ⅱ型:不完全肠化生伴不规则黏液空泡,无刷状缘,难以识别吸收性肠上皮细胞;细胞主要分泌唾液酸黏蛋白 Ⅲ型:细胞主要分泌硫酸黏蛋白,其他与Ⅱ型相同
Ⅱ	异型增生不确定	不能辨别细胞是肿瘤还是非肿瘤细胞,通常表现活检标本不足,存在结构扭曲和细胞核异型性
Ⅲ	非侵袭性肿瘤	表型肿瘤上皮,局限于基底膜内的腺体结构;包括腺瘤
Ⅳ	疑似侵袭性癌	可分为“低级别”和“高级别”肿瘤上皮,无法明确识别侵袭性癌
Ⅴ	侵袭性癌	浸入性癌

Adapted from Rugge M, Correa P, Dixon M, et al. Gastric dysplasia: the Padova International Classification. Am J Surg Pathol 2000; 24: 167-76.

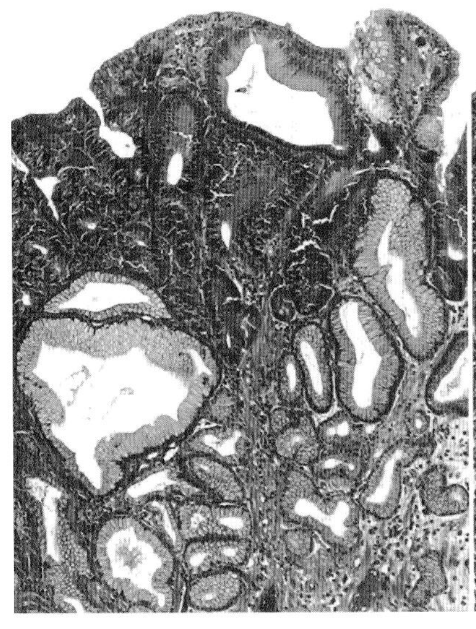
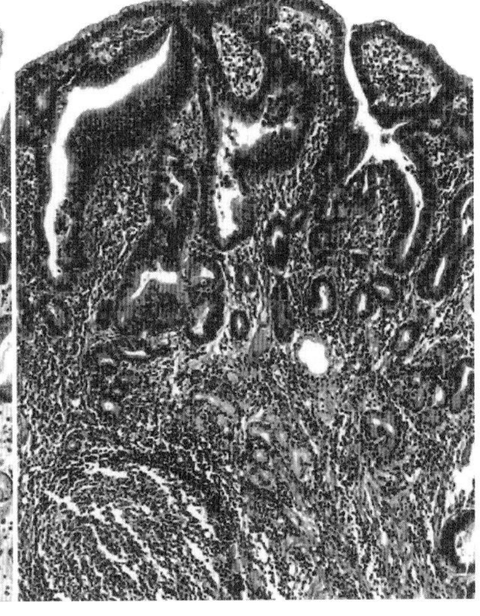

图 54.4　胃异型增生的组织病理学。左侧:低级别异型增生的特征是肿瘤性上皮细胞增生,伴细胞核假复层化和深染,无结构改变。右侧:高级别异型增生的特征是有更为严重的细胞学异常和结构异常,包括不规则融合或筛板状腺体和乳头状。(HE 染色)

(三) 胃息肉

一般人群中胃息肉的患病率约为 0.8% ~ 2.4%[270,271]。胃息肉主要包括胃底腺息肉(≈50%)、增生性息肉(≈40%)和腺瘤性息肉(≈10%)[271,272]。

胃底腺息肉的临床病程一般是良性的,在 PPI 使用的时代其检出率越来越高。在接受上消化道内镜检查的 599 例连续患者系列中,使用 PPI 超过 5 年与胃底腺息肉风险增加近 4 倍相关[273]。这些息肉的恶变率通常很低(≈1%),仅局限于大于 1cm 的息肉[274]。胃底腺息肉良性性质的一个显著例外是家族性腺瘤性息肉病。本组胃底腺息肉的患病率为 51% ~ 88%,其中超过 40% 的病例存在异型增生[170,171]。

增生性息肉通常是良性的、多发性的,常见于慢性炎症性疾病(例如慢性萎缩性胃炎)、恶性贫血、慢性胃窦炎、溃疡和糜烂附近观察到,尤其是在胃肠道造口术部位。随着时间的推移,息肉可能消退、保持稳定或体积增大,并且在根除 HP 后通常会消退。男性和女性受影响同样,息肉通常出现在成年的中期或后期[275]。发生恶变的罕见增生性息肉常有异型增生或肠上皮化生区域,典型者形成分化良好的肠型癌[274]。

与其他胃息肉相比,胃腺瘤发生恶变的比率较高。当胃腺瘤随后进行连续内镜检查和活检时,大约有 11% 的病例在 4 年内由异型增生进展为原位癌[276]。胃息肉内镜活检可伴有明显的取样误差[277]。英国胃肠病学会于 2010 年发表了关于胃息肉管理的指南[278],其中的建议是:①所有胃息肉至少应进行活检;②所有的胃腺瘤、有症状的息肉和伴有异型增生的息肉都应切除;③如存在 HP 感染,应在增生性或腺瘤样息肉患者中根除 HP。应根据个体情况决定监测间隔。

(四) 既往胃切除术史

据一些研究小组报告,针对良性疾病的胃部手术,可使患者从术后 20 年开始易患胃癌的风险更高[279-282]。对那些 50 岁之前接受手术者来说风险最大,也许反映了手术与癌症发展之间需要有一段长期缓慢发展的时期[281]。癌症倾向于发生在胃侧的手术吻合口或其附近;很少发生在吻合术的肠侧[283]

已经提出了许多理论,来解释在手术吻合部位形成癌症的倾向增加。它们包括胃酸过低导致细菌过度生长、亚硝酸盐生成增加、胆盐和胰酶(强效的胃刺激物)的慢性肠胃反流,以及由于胃窦激素水平低(包括胃泌素)引起的剩余胃黏膜萎缩[18,284,285]。采用胃空肠吻合术 Billroth Ⅱ型手术更易发生癌症,其发生率是采用胃十二指肠吻合术 Billroth Ⅰ型手术的 4 倍,表明胆汁反流可能是一个重要的易感因素[280]。HP 感染和相关的肠上皮化生在胃切除术后胃癌中的发现频率低于非手术胃的远端胃癌[286]。目前尚不清楚在癌症发病率较低的地区,对该患者人群进行胃癌筛查是否具有成本效益。随着 HP 根除治疗和 PPI 治疗的出现,消化性溃疡病的胃切除数量急剧下降,显著降低了作为胃癌风险因素的胃切除术后状态的影响。

(五) 消化性溃疡病(另见第 53 章)

大量流行病学研究表明,在有胃溃疡病史的患者中,患胃癌的风险持续增加。在一项队列研究中,瑞典成年人平均随访 9 年,有胃溃疡病史的与胃癌风险增加 1.8 倍相关[287]。有趣的是,十二指肠溃疡病史与胃癌发生风险降低相关。在美国退伍军人的病例对照研究中重复了这些发现[288]。这些相关性仅局限于非贲门胃癌;胃溃疡病史与贲门癌之间无相关性[288]。目前尚不清楚胃溃疡本身是否易患癌症。增加的风险可能是由感染 HP 介导的,Hp 可导致萎缩性胃炎、肠上皮化生和癌症。

(六) Ménétrier 病(另见第 52 章)

在病例报告的回顾中,15% 的 Ménétrier 病患者伴有胃癌[289],包括记录了从异型增生进展为癌症的数例病例[290,291]。由于 Ménétrier 病罕见,很难以任何可控的方式研究其与胃癌的关系,因此也无法提出关于内镜监测的建议。

五、筛查与监测

大多数关于胃癌筛查的文献来自东亚,那里的胃癌患病率是世界上最高的[292]。自 1960 年以来,日本一直在使用上消化道钡剂检查进行大规模筛查,如果发现任何可疑病变,则进行内镜检查,这仍然代表了基于当前日本癌症筛查指南的推荐方法[293]。日本研究人员报道,该筛查方法的敏感性为 66% ~ 90%,特异性为 77% ~ 90%[294]。然而,调查研究表明,在临床实践中,上消化道内镜检查是亚洲应用最广泛的胃癌筛查方法[259]。

不足为奇的是,来自日本的研究也表明,筛查可以在早期阶段诊断胃癌,一项研究报告了超过一半的筛查病例被诊断为Ⅰ期癌[296]。来自日本公共卫生中心队列的长期随访数据显示,接受筛查的受试者死于胃癌的风险降低了近 50%[297]。来自日本的另一项单独队列研究发现,在参与胃癌筛查的人群中,胃癌死亡风险降低了 25% ~ 35%[298]。然而,所有原因导致死亡的风险降低程度相似,在预防胃癌死亡方面,与筛查相关的真实获益程度存在一定程度的不确定性。

血清胃蛋白酶原(PG)的检测越来越多地用于筛查胃癌前病变风险最高的患者。胃产生两种胃蛋白酶原:PGⅠ和 PGⅡ。在慢性萎缩性胃炎中,由于胃主细胞数量减少,PGⅠ的产生减少,而 PGⅡ水平保持相对恒定,有时甚至可以在炎症反应中升高(见第 52 章)。因此,低血清 PGⅠ水平(<70mg/L)和低 PGⅠ/PGⅡ比值(<3.0)均可用于萎缩性胃炎患者的鉴别[292]。一项大型前瞻性队列研究表明,基线 PGⅠ、PGⅠ/PGⅡ和 HP 抗体水平的联合检测,可成功地识别进展性胃癌风险最高的患者,这些患者可能适合转诊内镜检查[299-302]。

在高危人群中(如亚洲老年男性),采用上消化道内镜进行筛查可能具有成本效益[303]。然而,在胃癌发病率较低的人群中,筛查产生相同程度的有益影响的可能性较小。欧洲共识指南建议对诊断为广泛胃黏膜萎缩的患者进行内镜监测[304]。建议这些患者每 3 年进行一次胃镜检查。尽管初步分析认为这种方法具有成本效益,但目前正在进行前瞻性随机试验以支持这一策略[305,306]。美国最近的 meta 分析表明,当应用于具有进一步危险因素的选定个体时,这种策略只能在低发病率的西方国家才具有成本效益[307]。

六、预防

鉴于胃癌的致命性及其与慢性感染和炎症的关系，人们广泛关注胃肿瘤性病变“化学预防”的可能性。研究最多的方法是根除 HP，但也考虑补充抗氧化剂和使用非甾体抗炎药（NSAID）和环氧化酶 2 抑制剂（COX-2 抑制剂）。

（一）根除 HP

根除 HP 可降低随后发生胃癌的风险。毫无疑问，多种器官系统的慢性炎症可导致恶性肿瘤，根除 HP 可以减轻或缓解胃部炎症，可导致氧化应激和细胞增殖下降[308]。此外，涉及根除长爪沙鼠胃螺杆菌生物的有限研究表明，根除感染可部分逆转萎缩和化生，抑制进展为胃癌[309]。一项对小鼠的研究证实了化生的可逆性和早期根除 HP 预防胃癌的作用。随着以后的再根除，癌症进展的速度减慢，死亡率显著下降[19]。

然而，目前尚缺乏通过人体前瞻性随机试验，明确证明 HP 根除的防癌作用。这在一定程度上是由于需要纳入大量的高危患者，以在胃癌事件的罕见终点方面达到足够的把握度，在一定程度上是由于伦理问题，将患者随机分配至研究组，使其不接受 1 类致癌物的治疗。解决第一个问题的一种方法是，检查根除 HP 对癌前状态的影响，如胃萎缩和肠上皮化生。因此，大多数研究显示了在预防胃病进展方面的有益作用[310-314]。在一项来自中国的 587 例 Hp 感染患者的随机、安慰剂对照试验中，接受 Hp 根除治疗与肠上皮化生进展风险显著降低相关（比值比，0.63）[314]。相反，在墨西哥成年人中进行的一项随机安慰剂对照试验，未显示根除 HP 对预防肠化生组织学进展的益处[313]。

在 1 630 例“健康”HP 阳性个体中进行的一项前瞻性、随机安慰剂对照试验，试图确定在中国高危人群中根除 HP 是否会降低胃癌的发病率。尽管在接受 HP 根除治疗的患者组中没有观察到总体组获益，但在研究开始时没有癌前病变（胃萎缩、肠化生或异型增生）的患者亚组中，胃癌发生率降低。根除组中的一些患者可能已经超过了前面提到的“无回报点”（point of no return），此时细胞改变已经充分积累以促进癌症的发生[315]。最近对随机试验的 meta 分析发现，根除 HP 与胃癌风险显著降低 35% 相关[22]。

鉴于相关多灶性异型增生的高发生率，在早期胃癌治疗后根除 HP 甚至可能是有益的。在 Fukase 等对切除的早期胃癌患者进行的一项开放性随机对照试验中，根除 HP 与发生异时性胃癌（即不同时发生的）的风险降低相关（比值比，3.35；95% CI，0.016 1～0.775）。尽管结果相互矛盾，但最近的 meta 分析支持 Fukase 和其同事的初步调查结果[316,317]。

在西方国家，由于 HP 感染率较低，胃癌发病率不断下降，因此胃癌预防工作尚未得到广泛开展。然而，Parsonnet 及其同事的成本效益模型表明[318]，如果假设治疗 HP 感染可以预防 30% 的可归因胃癌，那么筛查和治疗 HP 感染在预防胃癌方面具有潜在的成本效益，特别是在高危人群中。来自英国的一项分析也得出结论，根除 HP 是具有成本效益的[319]。

另一种选择是基于人群的 HP 感染的疫苗接种。但已证明开发出有效的疫苗，以及定义正确的疫苗接种时间点是很困难的。尽管最近的一项研究显示了令人鼓舞的结果，但目前尚不清楚临床适用的疫苗是否会在不久的将来获得[320]。

（二）阿司匹林和其他非甾体抗炎药（NSAID），包括（环氧化酶-2）抑制剂（COX-2）

在其他作用中，阿司匹林和其他 NSAID 抑制环氧化酶。COX-1 在胃肠道中呈组成性表达。在正常胃肠黏膜中通常未观察到 COX-2 表达，但在多种上皮恶性肿瘤（包括胃癌）中可诱导 COX-2 表达[321,322]。COX-2 的表达与人和小鼠癌症模型中的侵袭性细胞生长相关[323-326]，并发现在 70% 的胃癌中过表达[327]。在这种情况下，COX-2 可以潜在地促进肿瘤的生长、抑制细胞凋亡、增加血管生成。据报道，COX-2 在癌前病变中的表达升高，包括肠上皮化生和异型增生，根除 HP 后 COX-2 的表达似乎降低[328]。

多项流行病学研究表明，使用 NSAID 与胃癌风险降低之间存在一致相关性[329-332]。在一项来自洛杉矶县的病例对照研究中，使用 NSAID 超过 5 年与非贲门胃癌的风险降低相关（比值比，0.61），并且存在显著的 NSAID 剂量相关效应[330]。一项使用英国全科医生研究数据库的巢式病例对照研究发现，长期使用非阿司匹林类 NSAID 可降低胃癌风险（比值比为 0.65），但使用阿司匹林对胃癌风险没有影响[332]。这项研究与最近在英国进行的队列研究形成对比，该队列研究纳入了来自英格兰和苏格兰的 3 833 例胃癌患者和 4 654 例食管癌患者[333]。在这些队列中，长期使用阿司匹林与胃癌诊断后的癌症特异性死亡率无关（汇总校正 HR，1.06；95% CI，0.85～1.32）。另一方面，近期 meta 分析报告了任何 NSAID 的使用与胃癌风险降低之间存在显著的相关性（RR，0.78；95% CI，0.72～0.85），阿司匹林和非 ASANSAID 的结果大致相似，且对非贲门胃癌的影响略微明显[334]。

在一项 HP 阴性肠上皮化生患者的随机对照试验中，接受 COX-2 选择性抑制剂——罗非昔布和安慰剂治疗的患者，2 年后肠上皮化生的消退率没有差异[335]。这项试验受到随访期相对较短和使用癌前终点的限制。在 HP 感染和组织学显示为慢性萎缩性胃炎（或更严重）的患者中，进行的一项单独的随机对照试验中，HP 根除和使用 COX-2 选择性抑制剂塞来昔布 24 个月者，均导致组织学消退改变，但未观察到叠加效应[336]。在比较使用与不使用阿司匹林治疗的各种结局的随机试验进行的总结分析中，随访 10～20 年的研究报告显示，那些使用阿司匹林治疗的患者胃癌风险降低（比值比 0.42）[337]。有必要在高危患者中进行进一步的试验，以确定 NSAID 是否对胃癌的预防有效。

（三）他汀类药物

他汀类药物是一类广泛使用的羟甲基戊二酸单酰辅酶（AHMG-COA）抑制胆固醇的药物，在许多流行病学研究中发现，与各种恶性肿瘤风险降低相关。他汀类药物除了具有降低胆固醇的特性外，还具有抗增殖和促凋亡的作用[338]。来自中国台湾的一项基于人群的病例对照研究发现，服用处方他汀类药物的患者胃癌风险显著降低（比值比 0.68），在他汀类药物累计使用最高的患者中,观察到胃癌风险降低更大[339]。在一项对来自韩国的糖尿病患者进行的单独病例对照研究中,他汀类药物使用史与胃癌的发病率降低 80% 相关[340]。来自荷兰的一项药学数据库研究发现,使用他汀类药物与任何类型癌症的风险降低显著相关,然而,与胃癌无显著相关性,尽管病例数量相对较少[341]。meta 分析表明他汀类药物在胃癌风险方面的总体有利特征,显示风险降低范围在 32%~44%之间[342,343]。有趣的是,西方或亚洲队列之间在该效应方面无统计学显著差异。

未来在胃癌高危患者中对各种他汀类药物进行随机对照试验,将有助于确定这类药物作为化学预防剂的作用。

(四) 抗氧化剂

慢性炎症状态如 HP 胃炎可导致衍生于氧和氮的自由基生成[344]。这些自由基可通过许多不同的方式促进癌变,包括直接损伤 DNA 和抑制 DNA 修复机制、抑制细胞凋亡和激活细胞增殖途径。类胡萝卜素、维生素 C 和 E 等抗氧化剂与活性氧和氮结合,以中和其损伤作用。

流行病学数据支持抗氧化剂摄入量增加与胃癌风险降低之间的关系[345-349]。一项来自日本的巢式病例对照研究中,低血浆 β 胡萝卜素水平与胃癌风险增加相关[347]。来自韩国的一项病例对照研究发现,硝酸盐/抗氧化剂摄入比率升高与胃癌风险增加相关[348]。在瑞典的一项队列研究中,高水平的维生素 A 及 α 和 β 胡萝卜素的摄入与胃癌风险降低 50% 相关[349]。最近一项关于 α 和 β 胡萝卜素摄入影响的 meta 分析,分析了 13 项病例对照和 8 项队列研究的数据,并报告了病例对照和队列研究之间各自结果的不一致性[350]。

随机对照试验显示,补充抗氧化剂对胃癌发生风险的影响不一致。在胃癌前病变(非萎缩性或萎缩性胃炎、肠上皮化生或异型增生)患者中进行的抗氧化剂(维生素 A、C 和 E)的随机安慰剂对照试验中,补充抗氧化剂既未导致组织学进展减缓,也未增加组织学消退[351]。在中国进行的一项随机对照试验也发现,联合补充维生素 C、E 和硒对萎缩性胃炎、肠上皮化生、异型增生或癌症联合终点的患病率没有影响[352]。在中国一般人群营养干预试验的 10 年随访中,发现接受硒、维生素 E 和 β 胡萝卜素联合治疗的受试者胃癌死亡率降低[353]。有趣的是,Li 等对 2013 年的可用数据系统性分析中报告,尽管高膳食摄入维生素 C、维生素 E 以及 α 和 β 胡萝卜素导致胃癌风险降低,但这些因素的实际血液水平与胃癌风险无关[354]。鉴于缺乏令人信服的化学预防作用以及 β 胡萝卜素和维生素 A 疗效试验的结果,其中接受 β 胡萝卜素和维生素 A 的受试者患肺癌的风险增加[355],尚不推荐补充抗氧化剂预防胃癌。这与最近关于补充硒对癌症有预防作用的 Cochranemeta 分析一致[356]。尽管观察性研究的一些数据表明胃癌部位特异性风险小幅降低,但研究是具有异质性的,需要前瞻性随机对照试验来支持这一假设。

(五) 其他饮食因素

绿茶在亚洲国家被广泛饮用,被认为具有预防上消化道癌症的作用。绿茶中的多酚和其他代谢物质,如表没食子儿茶素、没食子酸酯(epigallocatechin-3-gallate,EGCG)和其他没食子儿茶素,具有多种抗肿瘤作用,包括诱导细胞凋亡、抑制肿瘤细胞生长和增殖以及降低 COX-2 的表达[357-359]。EGCG 还具有抗氧化特性,也可能具有抗炎特性[360,361]。尽管病例对照研究显示胃癌风险与绿茶消费量呈负相关,但队列研究基本上没有显示出两者之间的相关性[362,363]。一项来自日本的队列研究确实报告了,高绿茶摄入量的女性患胃癌的风险降低,但男性的风险没有变化[364]。最近一项观察者研究的 meta 分析表明,长期大剂量摄入绿茶可略微降低胃癌的风险[365],但在缺乏前瞻性对照试验的情况下,不推荐绿茶作为胃癌的化学预防。关于食用大蒜的影响,也有类似的结果[366]。

坚持地中海饮食有可能将胃癌风险和相关死亡率降低近 30%(RR 0.72;95% CI 0.60~0.86)[367]。最近的一项模型计算预测,到 2025 年,增加水果和蔬菜的摄入量将预防相对较高比例的胃癌病例,主要是在发展中国家[368]。

七、临床特征

早期胃癌在高达 80% 的病例中无症状。当症状确实出现时,它们往往酷似消化性溃疡疾病。进展期胃癌最常见的症状是体重减轻(≈60% 的患者)和腹痛(≈50% 的患者)[369]。其他症状表现包括恶心、呕吐、厌食、吞咽困难、黑便和早饱。胃窦和幽门部肿瘤可发生幽门出口梗阻,贲门部肿瘤可因食管下括约肌受累而引起吞咽困难,发生假性贲门失弛缓症(见第 44 章)[370]。罕见发生副肿瘤综合征。曾有血栓性静脉炎(Trousseau 征)、神经病变、肾病综合征和 DIC 的报道[371-373]。皮肤副肿瘤综合征也不常见,包括腋窝色素沉着斑(黑棘皮病;见第 25 章)以及突发的脂溢性皮肤病(老年疣)和瘙痒(Leser-Trélat 体征)[374]。

体格检查通常无明显异常。恶病质和肠梗阻体征是最常见的异常表现。偶尔可以发现上腹部肿块、肝大、腹水和下肢水肿[375]。在癌症进展到晚期之前,实验室检查一般很少有阳性发现。溃疡性肿块的慢性出血可引起粪便隐血试验阳性和贫血,可能发生低蛋白血症。转氨酶值,特别是血清碱性磷酸酶水平,可能继发于肝转移而升高。

33% 的病例在诊断胃癌时已发生转移[376]。最常见的转移部位是肝脏(40%)和腹膜[377]。其他扩散部位包括脐周淋巴结(Sister joseph 结节)、左锁骨上前哨淋巴结(Virchow 淋巴结)、道格拉斯囊(Blumer 直肠架)和卵巢(Krukenberg 瘤)。也有报道胃癌转移至肾、膀胱、脑、骨、心脏、甲状腺、肾上腺和皮肤[375]。有转移性疾病的不寻常表现的报道,如骨转移引起的肩手综合征、眼眶和视网膜转移引起的复视和失明,以及因 Krukenberg 瘤引起的女性男性化[378-381]。

八、诊断

(一) 内镜

内镜是目前诊断胃癌的首选方法(图 54.5A)。当发现不愈合的胃溃疡时,建议从溃疡边缘和基底部至少取 6~8 块活检标本[382]。美国胃肠病学会(AGA)建议对 55 岁以上新发消化不良症状的患者和 55 岁以下有“报警”症状(体重减轻、反复呕吐、吞咽困难、出血证据、贫血)的患者进行上消化道内镜检查[383]。PPI 经验性治疗和根除 HP 仍不能缓解症状的消化不良患者,也应及时接受内镜检查评估。这些建议的基础是 55 岁以下个体的胃癌发病率较低。基于患者的基线胃癌风险,在隐匿性出血和结肠镜检查正常的患者中,上消化道内镜检查检测胃癌的诊断率将有所不同。

在日本和其他胃癌高患病率地区,色素内镜、放大内镜和窄带成像被单独或联合用于辅助检测早期胃癌(见图 54.5B)。研究发现,明显的不规则黏膜表面和血管模式与异型增生和癌的存在相关[384]。对自发荧光和共聚焦显微内镜等新技术,在早期胃肿瘤诊断中的应用也正在进行研究[385,386]。据报道,钡剂研究对晚期胃癌的检出敏感性为 60%~70%,特异性为 90%[387]。然而,上消化道钡剂系列检查,在很大程度上已被上消化道内镜检查所取代,成为诊断胃癌的首选初始检查。

已经开发了一种基于内镜所见外观的早期胃癌分类系统[388]。其目的是评估早期病变黏膜下浸润的风险和淋巴结扩散的风险(图 54.6)。有 3 种类型:包括浅表息肉样病变(0~1 型)、浅表扁平/凹陷型病变(0~Ⅱa、b 和 c 型)以及浅表挖空(深凹陷)病变(0~Ⅲ型)。最常见的亚型是 0~Ⅱc 型,即非息肉样凹陷型病变[388]。该分类系统在日本最常使用。在日本内镜黏膜切除术和内镜黏膜剥离术经常用于治疗早期胃肿瘤。

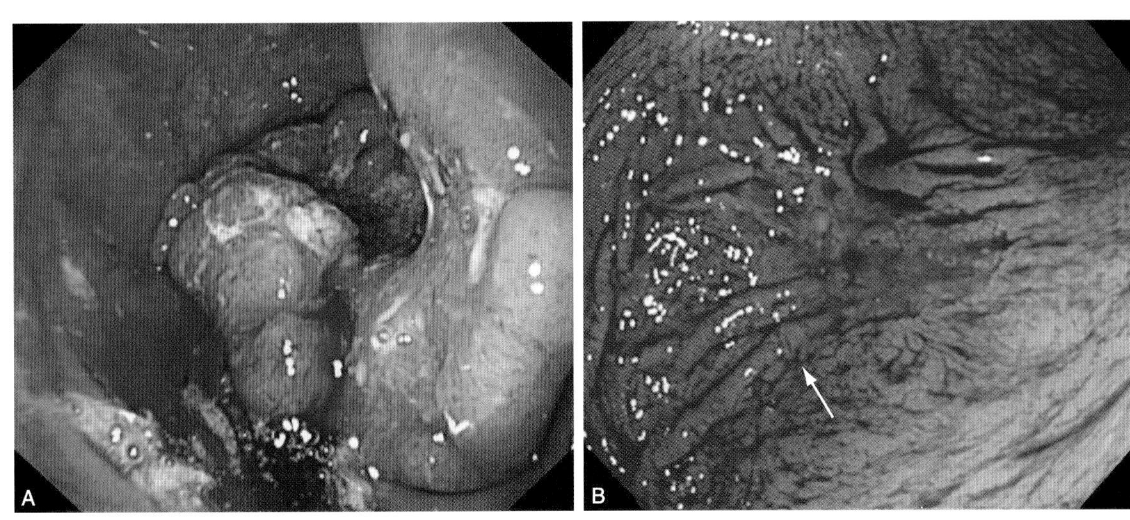

图 54.5 胃癌内镜检查示例。A,溃疡性胃腺癌肿块病变;B,彩色内镜观察的浅表凹陷型早期胃癌。用靛胭脂红染色突出显示(箭头)。(A,With permission from the Gastrolab Endoscopy Archives. The Wasa Workgroup on lntestinal Disorders,2008[Accessed 14 Oct 2008,at http://www. Gastrolab. net/pa-269. htm];B,from Toyoda H,Tanaka K,Hamada Y,et al. Endoscopic diagnosis of hypopharyngeal,esophageal and gastric neoplasm. Dig Endosc 2006;18:S41-3.)

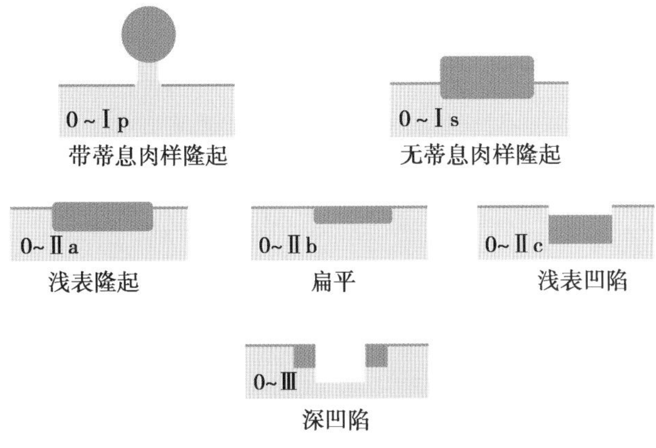

图 54.6 胃肿瘤病变主要分型示意图:息肉型(Ⅰp 和Ⅰs);非息肉样(Ⅱa、Ⅱb 和Ⅱc)和非息肉样挖空型(深凹陷型)(Ⅲ)。(From the Paris endoscopic classification of superficial neoplastic lesions:esophagus,stomach,and colon:November 30 to December 1,2002. Gastrointest Endosc 2003;58:S3-43.)

(二) CT 胃造影

虽然 CT 结肠成像作为结肠息肉和结肠癌的筛查方式的潜在作用获得了显著的关注,但 CT 胃造影也被研究用于早期胃癌的诊断。在一项来自韩国的 39 例早期胃癌患者的研究中,CT 胃造影成像检查的灵敏度为 73%~76%,观察者之间可靠性良好的($K=0.84$)[389]。迄今为止,仅使用这种成像模式进行了小规模的研究,CT 胃造影成像还不能推荐用于研究范围之外的筛查。

(三) 血清标志物

到目前为止,尚未发现对胃癌诊断具有较高敏感性和特异性的可靠血清标志物。在萎缩性胃炎和肠上皮化生患者中报告了低血清 PGⅠ水平、PGⅠ与 PGⅡ的低比值和高胃泌素血症,但对胃癌的检测结果好坏参半[390,391]。在一项对 17 000 例日本男性的研究中,PG 检测阳性(定义为 PGⅠ<50μg/L,PGⅠ/PGⅡ<3.0)结合上消化道系列检查,仅在 0.28% 的受试者中确定了胃癌,然而这些癌症中 88% 为早期癌症[392]。此外,仅通过 PG 检测确定的 89% 癌症为早期胃癌。该检测的局限性在于诊断胃癌的特异性较低[393]。因此,目前正在使用血清 PG 评估,来识别从进一步诊断检测(如通过内镜检查)中获益的癌前病变患者。

血清 CEA 和糖类抗原(CA)19-9 均已被广泛研究用于胃

癌的诊断。这些标志物对早期胃癌的敏感性尤其低[394]，其水平升高也见于其他上皮恶性肿瘤。这些肿瘤标志物在复发性胃癌中经常升高，尤其是在手术切除前水平升高的患者中[395]。然而，这些标志物的诊断质量仍然很低，它们可能作为预后指标发挥作用，因为 CEA 和 CA19-9 均与胃癌患者不利的临床病理学特征和不良结局相关[396,397]。其他研究已经确定，TGF-β1、CA 72-4、肿瘤 M2-丙酮酸激酶和肝细胞生长因子是胃癌的潜在标志物[398-401]，但对于 CEA 和 CA19-9，临床应用可作为预后指标，尤其是手术治疗后复发的预后指标[402]。

除了经典的血清标志物外，最近的重点是所谓的液体活检，主要是评估循环肿瘤细胞和循环肿瘤 DNA。富集和测序方法的最新进展使我们能够分析这些因素，即使不需要侵入性组织采样，也可以提供突变谱和肿瘤异质性的信息[403]。尽管关于诊断准确性和作为预后标志物的价值的数据仍然不一致，但指导靶向治疗的潜在用途变得更有意义。一个突出的例子是通过分析循环血浆 DNA 来评估 Her2 扩增[404,405]。这种方法有可能克服组织分析中的肿瘤异质性和抽样误差的问题[406]。

九、分类与分期

已有几种分类系统来进一步定义胃癌和预测预后。如前所述（见图 54.1）胃癌可分为肠型和弥漫型，胃癌也可分为早期和进展期病变。早期胃癌是指一种侵袭不超过黏膜下层，无论淋巴结是否受累。这种形式的癌症在远东地区，特别是日本的患病率更高，预后十分有利。亚洲报告的 5 年生存率大于 90%，比西方国家的 80% 要高[407-410]。

胃癌最常用的临床分期分类系统是 TNM 系统，由国际抗癌联合会（UICC）和美国癌症联合委员会（AJCC）制定使用[411,412]。在 TNM 分期系统中，T（tumor，肿瘤）表示肿瘤穿透深度（图 54.7）：T1a 表示肿瘤侵犯黏膜层或固有层；T1b 表示侵犯黏膜下层；T2 表示侵犯到固有肌层；T3 表示侵犯到浆膜下结缔组织；T4a 表示侵犯到浆膜（脏腹膜）；T4b 表示侵犯到邻近器官或结构。N（Nodes 淋巴结）表示淋巴结受累程度：N0 表示无淋巴结受累；N1 表示 1~2 个淋巴结受累；N2 表示 3~6 个淋巴结受累；N3 表示 7 或 7 个以上淋巴结受累。M（metascasis，转移）表示存在转移：M0 表示无转移；M1 表示远处转移，包括肿瘤周围细胞学检查阳性（表 54.4）。在最近的 AJCC（美国癌症联合委员会）分期手册中，贲门癌（距离 GE 交界处 5cm 以内，并越过 GE 交界处的肿瘤）现在与食管和 GE 交界处肿瘤一起归类[412]。最近的研究是根据胃癌生物学特征重新分类。将肿瘤生物学纳入分期分类系统的前景令人感兴趣，尽管这需要未来的验证研究。

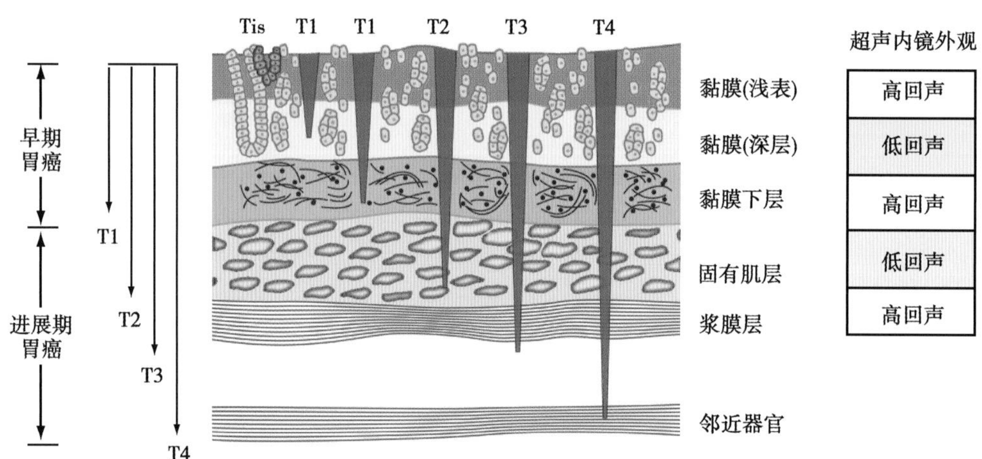

图 54.7　胃腺癌浸润深度分类（T 分类）。在 TNM 分类中，T 表示浸润深度：Tis 表示原位癌；T1 表示肿瘤局限于黏膜（T1a）和黏膜下层（T1b）；T2 表示肿瘤侵犯固有肌层而未侵犯浆膜层；T3 表示肿瘤穿透浆膜下结缔组织，而未累及脏腹膜或邻近组织结构；T4 表示肿瘤侵犯浆膜（脏腹膜），可能累及邻近器官和组织。在早期胃癌中，肿瘤仅局限于黏膜和黏膜下层（T1），无论淋巴结是否受累

表 54.4　根据胃癌 TNM 分类的临床分期

	N0	N1	N2	N3	M1（Any N）
Tis	0	—	—	—	—
T1	ⅠA	ⅠB	ⅡA	ⅡB	Ⅳ
T2	ⅠB	ⅡA	ⅡB	ⅢA	Ⅳ
T3	ⅡA	ⅡB	ⅢA	ⅢB	Ⅳ
T4a	ⅡB	ⅢA	ⅢB	ⅢC	Ⅳ
T4b	ⅢB	ⅢB	ⅢC	ⅢC	Ⅳ

is，原位；M，转移；N，淋巴结受累；T，肿瘤。

*From Brierley JD, Gospodarowicz MK, Wittekind C, editors. TNM Classification of Malignant Tumours. 8th ed. Hoboken, NJ: Wiley-Blackwell; 2017.

胃癌的准确分期对治疗决策具有重要意义。超声内镜（EUS）是胃癌分期研究最多的方法，仍然是评估肿瘤浸润深度和淋巴结受累的首选检测方法。然而，CT 和 MRI 检查图像质量的改善，使这些研究成为 EUS 检查的潜在替代和辅助手段。

（一）超声内镜检查

超声内镜（EUS）可显示胃壁的 5 层。浅表层胃黏膜表现为第一层回声（高回声），深层黏膜表现为第二层低回声；黏膜下层表现为第三层回声（高回声），固有肌层表现为第四层低回声；浆膜表现为第五层回声（高回声）。EUS 还可以识别和活检黏膜下病变，如胃淋巴瘤和间质瘤。这些病变通常涉及黏膜下层和固有肌层增厚，在钡剂检查或内镜检查中表现

为胃皱襞增厚。根据 EUS 对胃癌分期的 meta 分析结果，EUS 区分 T1 ~ 2 与 T3 ~ 4 肿瘤的灵敏度为 86%，特异性为 91%[413]。认别黏膜内病变(T1a)的灵敏度为 83%，特异性为 79%。EUS 可能对识别内镜黏膜切除术或内镜黏膜剥离术适合的早期胃癌病变特别有用[414](图 54.8)。在 N 分期方面，EUS 对胃周围淋巴结的检出率与 CT 分期相当[415,416]。与肿瘤浸润深度相比，EUS 在淋巴结状态评估中的准确性略低，区分阳性和阴性淋巴结状态的灵敏度为 69%，特异性为 84%[413]。N 分期的一个特别困难在于许多小淋巴结也可隐藏转移灶，因此可能发生低估。

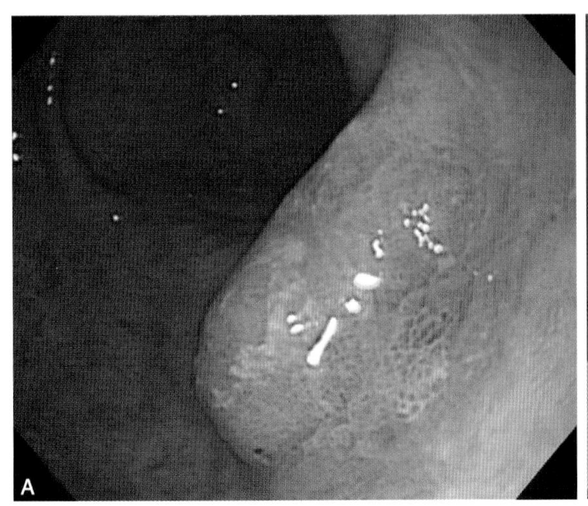

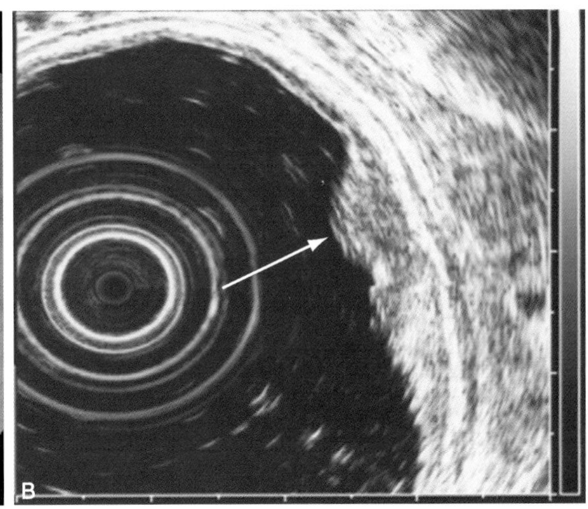

图 54.8　早期胃癌分期。A，早期胃癌的内镜图像显示胃窦后壁有一个 25mm 的突出肿块。B，病灶 EUS 图像，显示黏膜低回声团块(箭头)，黏膜下层完整。(From Kim JH, Song KS, Youn YH, et al. Clinicopathologic factors influence accurate endosonographic assessment for early gastric cancer. Gastrointest Endosc 2007;66:901-8.)

(二) CT 和 PET 成像

CT 和正电子发射断层显像(PET)成像技术的进步极大地提高了 CT 对胃肿瘤分期的诊断能力。虽然多排螺旋 CT(MDCT)的研究不如 EUS 广泛，但它可以将胃壁视为 3 层(内层对应黏膜、中间层对应黏膜下层、外层对应固有肌层和浆膜层)，但外层有稍高的衰减。在 T 和 N 两个分期方面似乎与 EUS 具有相当的准确性。胃肿块与邻近器官之间脂肪平面的缺失提示肿瘤侵袭。MDCT 对总体 T 分期的准确率为 77% ~ 91%，对判别浆膜受累的准确率为 83% ~ 100%[417,418]。使用 MDCT 对 N 分期的准确率可高达 89%[419,420]。与所有其他成像模式一样，CT 难以识别小于 5mm 的淋巴结转移。目前 CT 检查的作用主要是检测远处转移灶，并作为 EUS 评估局部淋巴结是否受累的补充。目前尚不清楚 EUS 或 MDCT(或两者联合)对胃癌 T 和 N 分期是否具有优越性，其基础技术仍在不断发展和完善。

不推荐单独使用 PET 扫描作为胃癌分期的唯一成像检查，主要是因为大多数胃腺癌的 FDG(F-18 氟脱氧葡萄糖)摄取量较低，并且也存在假阳性(见第 52 章)[421]。然而，在最初分期为局限性胃癌的患者中，PET/CT 联合应用可使转移性疾病的检出率增加了 10%，从而改变临床管理方法[422]。

(三) 腹腔镜腹腔灌洗

大约一半的胃癌转移患者的肿瘤累及腹膜[377]。目前的成像技术如 EUS 和 CT 对检测腹膜播散的能力有限。事实上，高达三分之一看似可切除的疾病患者，在腹腔镜检查分期时证实有腹膜扩散的迹象[423]。美国国家综合癌症网络指南建议，对考虑新辅助化疗的看似可切除的疾病患者进行腹腔镜检查和腹腔灌洗[424]，然而，美国采用这种做法的速度缓慢。一项使用 SEER 医疗保险数据的研究发现，只有 8% 接受过任何手术的胃癌患者接受了腹腔镜检查[425]。

(四) 其他成像方式

钆 MRI 成像模式也用于胃癌分期。它的优点与 CT 相似(能够发现远处转移)和缺点(需要充分的胃扩张)。MRI 对 T 分期的准确率为 90% ~ 93%，对 N 分期的准确率为 91% ~ 100%[417]。然而，鉴于研究数量较少，目前尚不提倡将 MRI 作为胃癌分期的首选检测方法。

(五) 新辅助治疗后的再分期

新辅助化疗后胃癌再分期的准确性显著降低。EUS 对 T 和 N 再分期的准确率均低于 50%，CT 治疗后分期也报告了同样令人失望的结果[426]。然而，使用术前临床分期评估新辅助放化疗的反应，可能与总生存期和无病生存期密切相关[427]。因此，再分期主要用于排除远处转移，作为手术可切除性评估的一部分。

十、预后与治疗

总体而言，美国胃癌的 5 年生存率为 27%(而结肠癌为 64%)[4]。TNM 分类用于将疾病分为 4 个临床阶段(Ⅰ ~ Ⅳ)，以预测接受胃切除术治疗患者的预后(见表 54.4)。日本研究的生存率数据通常优于西方国家，这可能是因为日本偏好扩大淋巴结切除术，或者是因为“低估”少于西方国家[428]。有数据表明，肿瘤体积较大(>5cm)可能与较差的生存率独立相关，与淋巴结状态或总体肿瘤分期无关[429]。

（一）外科手术

外科手术切除仍是胃癌主要的治疗方法。但单纯手术后的生存率较差（5 年时为 20%～50%），因此必须努力改善该组患者的疗效，采用围手术期化疗或术后（辅助）放化疗。此外，手术切除往往能最有效地缓解症状，尤其是梗阻症状。在某些情况下，诊断也需要手术，如活检结果阴性的难以愈合的胃溃疡，以及持续性幽门出口梗阻疑诊胃窦癌时。大多数胃癌患者应尝试外科手术治疗。然而，由于在广泛的弥漫型胃癌（皮革胃）、巨大转移性疾病、腹膜后浸润或腹膜转移癌的情况下，或者患者有严重的共病，预后可能非常差，因此使手术切除的价值受到质疑。手术和腹腔镜检查尤其有助于癌症的分期。腹腔镜检查可以帮助确定原发肿瘤的可切除性、腹腔沉积物和新辅助治疗的适宜候选人。腹腔镜腹腔灌洗已被用于检测腹腔内游离的癌细胞。腹腔镜灌洗阳性与最终发生明显腹膜转移显著相关[430]。

一般而言，全胃切除术适用于近端胃肿瘤和弥漫型胃癌，部分胃切除术适用于远端胃肿瘤。法国和意大利进行的大型、随机多中心试验比较了次全胃切除术与全胃切除术治疗胃窦腺癌，结果发现 5 年生存率或手术死亡率无差异[431,432]。一些中心认为进行完整的脾切除术和胃切除术。然而，几项回顾性和前瞻性研究发现，同时进行脾切除术会增加发病率，对生存率没有影响或更差[433,434]。

伴随胃切除术的淋巴结切除术范围，多年来一直是一个有争论的话题。日本提倡比西方同行（D1 切除）更广泛的淋巴结清扫（D2 切除），并认为具有更高的生存率。D2 切除需要切除腹腔干和肝十二指肠韧带的淋巴结，以及 D1 手术中采集的胃周淋巴结。报道的生存率的差异可能反映了日本早期胃癌的发病率要高得多。在日本进行的更广泛的淋巴结清扫可能会发现更多的阳性淋巴结，使 N0 分期的日本患者的生存率似乎高于其潜在"低估"的西方患者。来自荷兰的一项大型多中心随机试验报告，与更保守的 D1 淋巴结清扫术相比，D2 淋巴结清扫术的 5 年生存率没有显著改善，而且术后死亡和并发症更多[435]。在随后对这些患者进行的 15 年随访中，研究者报告总体生存期无显著差异，但 D2 切除组的胃癌相关死亡率显著降低（37% vs D1 组 48%）[436]。英国一项包含 400 例患者的随机试验同样显示，更广泛的手术无任何益处，D1 切除术的 5 年生存率为 35%，D2 切除术的 5 年生存率为 33%[433]。目前，数据不足以支持日本以外的医疗中心实行扩大淋巴结切除。为了防止"低估"，目前的建议是推荐至少切除 15 个淋巴结的 D1 淋巴结切除术[437]。

（二）内镜黏膜切除术和内镜黏膜剥离术

内镜技术的进步使得内镜黏膜切除术（EMR）和内镜黏膜剥离术（ESD）可以作为早期胃癌（EGC）选择的根治疗法。这项技术在日本和韩国已广泛用于治疗肠型早期胃癌。研究表明，只有 3.5% 的 EGC 小于 2～3cm 的患者有淋巴结受累，使得这些病变适合接受局部治疗。大于 4.5cm 的病灶扩散到黏膜下层的概率大于 50%，与"阳性"淋巴结有关，因此内镜下可切除的可能性较小[438]。

对胃癌行 EMR 治疗提出了以下标准：①经 EUS 检查癌位于黏膜，淋巴结未受累；②病灶轻度隆起（Ⅱa 型）时肿瘤最大小于 2cm，肿瘤平坦或轻度凹陷（Ⅱb 或Ⅱc 型），无溃疡瘢痕时肿瘤最大小于 1cm；③无多发性胃癌或同时发生的腹部癌的证据；④癌为肠型的[439]。尽管有这些指导原则，EMR 通常不可能整块切除大于 1.5～2.0cm 的病灶，而分块切除 EGC 与根治性切除率下降有关[440]。

ESD 是日本开发的一种技术，可以整块切除较大的 EGC，以及选定的黏膜下浸润性肿瘤。实行 ESD，先进行黏膜下注射，然后使用内镜下电刀切除整块肿瘤（图 54.9）[441]。内镜下预测 EGC 的 T 分期不如结肠病变准确，病变边缘不太明显。此外，与结肠病变不同，在胃黏膜内发现淋巴管，胃部病变不遵循腺瘤-癌转化序列。由于这些差异，ESD 整块切除提供了准确组织学分期和 EGC 潜在治愈的最佳机会。除 R0 切除外，ESD 对浸润深度和淋巴血管受累进行更精确的组织病理学评估，并对淋巴结转移的风险进行适当评估。如果术前评价未发现局部淋巴结受累，则可切除更大的浅表病变。日本已制定了早期胃癌 ESD 的扩展标准：①无溃疡的任何大小的黏膜肠型癌；②有溃疡的小于 3cm 的黏膜肠型癌；③小于 3cm 的黏膜下肠型癌和黏膜下浸润小于 500μm[442,443]。随着该 ESD 经验的增加，目前报告的整块切除率已超过 90%，局部复发率低于 3%[441]。由于部分病灶切除的体积较大，胃穿孔的风险相对较高（2%～6%）[444,445]。然而早期识别出的穿孔，通常可以使用内镜夹闭合进行保守治疗[441]。胃 ESD 的西方指南包括绝对标准和扩展标准，这取决于病变的大小和形态。最近来自西方中心的胃 ESD 研究显示了与东方中心相当的结局，尤其是在关键终点方面，例如 R0 切除和并发症。在一项由一家西方转诊中心的 191 例 ESD 切除的 EGC 的前瞻性观察性研究中，观察到整块和 R0 切除率分别为 98.4% 和 90.2%（对于符合指南标准的病变）以及 89.0% 和 73.6%（对于符合扩展标准的病变）。对于 EGC 但淋巴结受累风险较高且不适合外科胃切除术的患者，ESD 联合腹腔镜淋巴结清扫术可能是一种替代方法[446]。尚无比较手术与内镜切除术治疗早期胃癌的发表的随机临床试验。

（三）化疗

在西方国家，大约 75% 的胃癌患者在确诊时疾病已扩散到胃周围淋巴结或有远处转移[447]。早期阶段的患者，通常采用手术结合以治愈为目的的围手术期化疗进行治疗。已经进行了大量的临床试验，来评价胃癌根治性切除术后辅助化疗的作用[448]。大多数研究都尚无定论，但这些试验的一系列 meta 分析表明，接受辅助化疗的患者死亡风险降低了 15%～20%[449,450]。基于顺铂或表柔比星的辅助化疗的随机试验在很大程度上未显示出获益[451,452]。一线化疗的最佳方案尚待明确。三药联合方案是否比潜在毒性较低的二联方案更有效是一个争议点。历史上临床试验包括食管癌、EGJ 和胃腺癌。尽管 Chau 及其同事证实食管和 EGJ 腺癌的预后稍好，但 3 组患者的总生存率或缓解率无统计学差异，综合这些情况可能隐藏了密切相关的位置依赖性结局[453]。然而，TCGA 中食管癌和胃癌的新特征表明，这些肿瘤在分子水平上存在较大的差异，因此应该采取不同的治疗方法，至少在不同的治疗试验中进行探讨。欧洲癌症研究和治疗组织的专家小组对 GE 交界处附近肿瘤的差异化治疗和分期建议进行了区分。食管胃交界部腺癌（AEG）Ⅰ、Ⅱ型肿瘤建议术前放化疗。对于 AEG Ⅲ型（贲门）肿瘤，建议围手术期化疗为最佳选择。

新辅助化疗似乎对可切除疾病患者有益。在英国 MAGIC

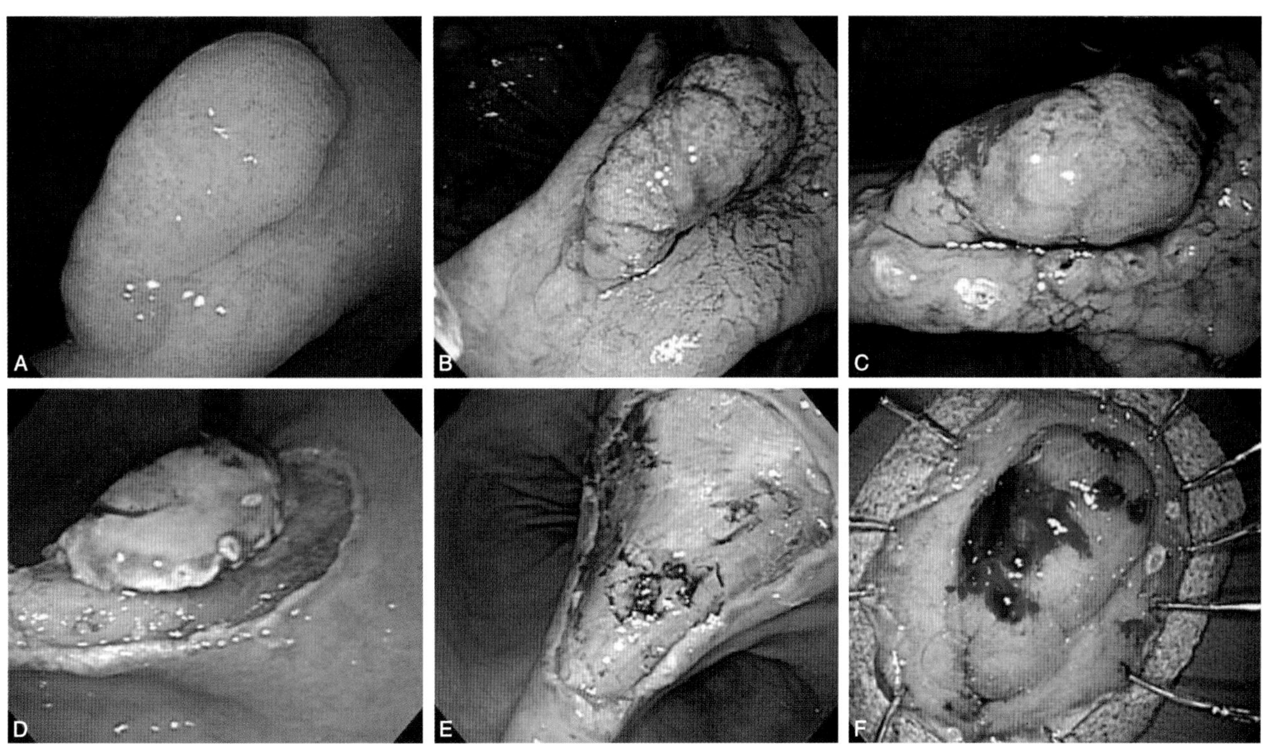

图 54.9 早期胃癌内镜黏膜下剥离术(ESD)。A,传统内镜检查,显示胃角部早期胃癌 0~Ⅰp 型(EGc,0~Ⅰp 型)。B,内镜下观察,喷洒靛蓝胭脂红以增强病灶边缘清晰度。C,病灶周边的正常组织用针刀做了标记。D,用绝缘尖头高频电刀在标记点周围做圆周切割。E,对病灶进行黏膜下整体剥离后显示出基底部。F,切除标本浸入福尔马林前,将标本拉伸固定在木板上。(From Lee IL,Wu cs,Tung SY,et al. Endoscopic submucosal dissection for early gastric cancers;experience from a new endoscopic center in Taiwan. J Clin Gastroenterol 2008;42;42-7)

试验中,503 例胃、胃食管或远端食管癌患者被随机分配接受单纯手术或新辅助化疗表柔比星、顺铂和 5-氟尿嘧啶(5-FU)后手术治疗。与单纯手术相比,新辅助化疗组 5 年无进展生存期(36% vs 23%)和总生存期显著改善[454]。因此,术前新辅助化疗被认为是胃癌手术前的标准治疗选择。在最近的 FLOT4-A10 试验中,与表柔比星、顺铂、氟尿嘧啶或卡培他滨(ECF/ECX)相比,多西他赛、奥沙利铂和氟尿嘧啶/亚叶酸钙(FLOT)围手术期化疗,显著改善了可切除胃癌患者的无进展生存期和总生存期(OS),提示 FLOT 是胃或胃食管交界部腺癌患者围手术期治疗的首选方案。

(四) 放化疗

手术切除后联合放化疗,看来能有效改善胃癌无进展生存期和总生存期。组间试验 0116(Intergroup Trial 0116)随机分配 603 例胃癌或胃食管癌患者,接受单纯手术或手术后 5-FU、甲酰四氢叶酸和放射治疗。单纯手术组受试者的中位生存期较短(27 个月 vs 36 个月),总生存期和无复发生存期更短[455]。本研究结果发表后,辅助放化疗成为美国的标准治疗,尽管最佳化疗方案尚不明确。新辅助放化疗应用的早期研究,以及最近尚未发表的试验也显示了可喜的结果[456]。

(五) 腹腔内化疗

由于全身化疗对胃癌腹膜转移的治疗在很大程度上是无效的,因此对于肿瘤切除后治愈但显微镜下证实残留病变可能性大的患者,可以考虑进行腹腔内(IP)化疗。在一项对 248 例胃癌患者的随机试验中,与单纯手术相比,术后高温腹腔内化疗与总体生存率的改善相关[457]。Ⅲ期和Ⅳ期疾病、浆膜浸润和淋巴结转移患者的治疗获益最明显。尽管第二项临床试验报告了相似的结果[458],但其他研究未能证明高温 IP 化疗的获益[459,460]。一项对可切除胃癌患者进行 IP 化疗研究的 meta 分析报告,接受高温 IP 化疗的患者死亡风险显著降低(比值比,0.60)[461]。目前高温 IP 化疗的使用应仅限于注册参加临床试验的患者。根据在旧金山举行的 2018 年胃肠道癌症研讨会上公布的数据,1989 年至 2014 年间,在法国 19 个中心接受治疗的 180 例患者,接受了肿瘤细胞减灭术联合腹腔热灌注化疗,与单纯手术切除相比,97 例胃癌伴腹膜癌患者的总生存期有所改善。

(六) 不能切除的疾病

遗憾的是,高达三分之一的胃癌患者在确诊时患有不可手术切除的疾病[376]。对无远处转移的局部晚期胃癌进行化疗,可导致肿瘤缩小至可成功根治性切除的程度[462,463]。即使无法进行根治性手术,与该组患者的最佳支持治疗相比,化疗也显示出可改善生存期和生活质量[464]。因此无法手术的局部晚期和/或转移性(Ⅳ期)疾病患者应考虑进行全身治疗(化疗),与单纯的最佳支持治疗相比,可改善生存期和生活质量。

Wagner 及其同事[465]的 meta 分析证明,联合化疗对患者的生存率获益较小但具有显著性,联合治疗方案的中位生存期为 8.3 个月,单药治疗的中位生存期为 6.7 个月。正如预期的那样,联合治疗方案的毒性增加,因此,联合化疗应只考虑体能状态良好的患者。一般采用铂类和氟尿嘧啶类的二联组合，关于三联方案的效用仍存在争议。虽然晚期胃癌没有单一的标准治疗，但有一些证据来自 meta 分析。在Ⅲ期试验中与生存期延长相关的药物有顺铂、多西他赛和曲妥珠单抗，曲妥珠单抗是一种干扰 HER2/neu 受体的单克隆抗体。HER2 被扩增，是 7%～34% 胃癌中肿瘤发生的关键驱动因素。在 ToGA Ⅲ期多中心随机研究中，HER2 过度表达的胃癌患者接受化疗和曲妥珠单抗治疗，中位总生存期为 13.8 个月，而单独接受化疗的患者为 11.1 个月[466]。除了拉帕替尼双重阻断剂 EGFR/HER2 之外，使用新型抗 HER2 靶向药物帕妥珠单抗和 T-DM1 进一步操纵该通路，可能会产生阳性结果。因此，应进行 HER2 过表达的肿瘤评估，对每例 HER2+胃腺癌患者，应考虑在姑息性化疗的基础上加用曲妥珠单抗（图 54.10）。相反，在未经选择的患者中，靶向表皮生长因子受体（EGFR）通路联合化疗迄今为止尚未取得成果。同样使用抗血管生成单克隆抗体贝伐珠单抗，在一项大规模的全球随机试验中也未成功[467-471]。仔细选择患者亚群将成为未来临床试验的关键因素。

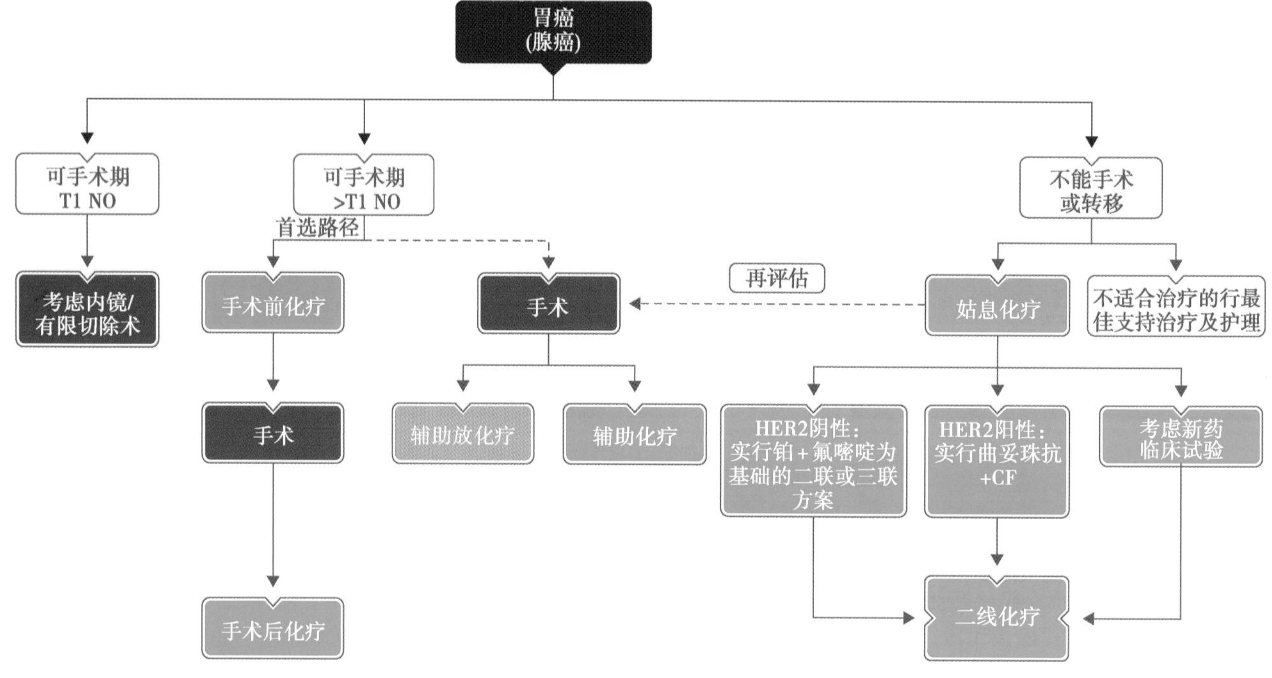

图 54.10　胃癌治疗流程。(Taken from Smyth EC, Verheij M, Allum w, et al. Gastric cancer: EMSO Clinical practice guidelines for diagnosis, treatment, and follow-up. Ann Oncol 2016;27(suppl 5):v38-v49.)

多项随机临床试验证明了，以多药顺铂为基础方案的疗效[472,473]。一项使用 EOX 方案（表柔比星、奥沙利铂和卡培他滨的较新临床试验发现其疗效不低于以顺铂为基础的方案，中位生存期为 11.2 个月[474]。EOX 方案的益处是奥沙利铂和卡培他滨分别替代顺铂和 5-Fu，使其更方便、易于给药、且副作用可能更少。二线化疗也可作为最佳支持治疗的辅助治疗，但同样未确定标准治疗方案。多烯紫杉醇或伊立替康单药治疗已被证明优于最佳支持治疗[475-477]，最近的一项研究显示伊立替康并不优于每周一次的紫杉醇。因此，可考虑将伊立替康或紫杉烷类的紫杉醇，单药治疗作为晚期胃癌患者的二线治疗选择[478]。抗 VEGFR-2 单克隆抗体雷莫昔单抗（ramucirumab）在 2 项随机Ⅲ期试验中显示出活性。作为一种单药，其在二线治疗中的生存获益与细胞毒性化疗相当，而雷莫昔单抗联合紫杉醇与紫杉醇单药相比也具有生存获益。

晚期胃窦远端或幽门胃癌患者有发生胃出口梗阻的风险。根据试验情况，进行胃空肠吻合术手术，以缓解症状并允许继续肠内营养。随着内镜支架的出现，跨越梗阻肿瘤的十二指肠支架置入术已成为缓解症状的一种非手术替代方法。评价胃空肠吻合术与支架置入术的研究的文献综述结果，发现技术成功率为 96%～100%，早期和晚期并发症以及持续症状无差异[479]。再发梗阻症状以支架置入更为多见。结论是胃空肠吻合术和内镜下支架置入术都是缓解恶性胃出口梗阻的可接受选择。如何决策，应根据个体的临床状况以及外科或内镜专业知识技能的可用性作出决定。

十一、其他胃肿瘤疾病

胃淋巴瘤、胃肠基质瘤和神经内分泌肿瘤（类癌）见第 32～34 章。乳腺癌、黑色素瘤、肺癌、卵巢癌、肝癌、结肠瘤和睾丸癌均可发生胃转移。其中以乳腺癌最为常见[480]。其他可累及胃的罕见恶性肿瘤包括卡波希肉瘤（见第 35 章）、肌间神经鞘瘤、血管球瘤、小细胞癌和壁细胞癌[481-484]。胃的其他良性肿瘤包括脂肪瘤、残留胰腺（异位胰腺）（见第 55 章）、黄色瘤和胃底腺囊肿。

（施海韵 译　袁农 校）

参考文献

第七部分　胰腺

第 55 章　胰腺解剖学、组织学、胚胎学和发育异常

Megha S. Mehta, Bradley A. Barth, Sohail Z. Husain 著

章节目录

一、胰腺的历史 …… 795
二、解剖学 …… 796
（一）胰管结构 …… 796
（二）血液循环 …… 797
（三）淋巴引流 …… 797
（四）神经支配 …… 797
三、组织学和超微结构 …… 797
四、胰腺的发育 …… 800
（一）胚胎和胎儿发育 …… 800
（二）转录因子和外源信号 …… 801
（三）胰腺损伤时胚胎因子的重现 …… 801
五、发育异常 …… 802
（一）环状胰腺 …… 802
（二）胰腺分裂 …… 802
（三）异位胰腺组织 …… 803
（四）胰腺发育不全 …… 803
（五）先天性囊肿 …… 804
（六）胰胆管畸形愈合 …… 804

一、胰腺的历史

尽管胰腺作为器官早已为人所知，但其关键的消化功能直到最近才被证实[1,2]。在公元前 300 年左右，希腊医生 Herophilos 首次描述了胰腺。在公元 1 世纪末，另一位希腊权威，以弗所（土耳其古城）的 Rufus 将这个器官命名为"胰腺"。这个词的字面意思是"所有的肉或肉"，将其与骨或软骨区分开来。不幸的是，由 Galen 在同一时间或 Rufus 之后不久给予器官"kalikreas"的名字，意思是"美丽的肉体"，但没有被采纳。尽管如此，Galen 认为胰腺起着支持和保护覆盖在上面的血管的作用。在犹太律法的中心文本《塔木德》（*Talmud*）中，胰腺被称为"肝脏的手指"。Vesalius 认为这个器官是胃的垫子。1642 年，Wirsung 描述了人类的胰管。1664 年，de Graaf 从狗的胰瘘中发现了胰腺分泌物。

近 200 年后才发现了胰腺分泌物的消化作用。1834 年的 Eberle、1836 年的 Purkinje 和 Pappenheim 及 1844 年的 Valentin 分别观察到胰液乳化脂肪、蛋白水解蛋白及消化淀粉的功能。伯纳德（Bernard）随后利用胰瘘制剂的分泌物证明了胰液的联合消化作用。1876 年，Kuhne 引入了"酶"一词，并首先分离出胰蛋白酶。酶的概念很快导致了胰淀粉酶和脂肪酶的鉴定。1889 年，Pavlov 的学生 Chepovalnikoff 在十二指肠黏膜中发现了肠激酶，一种对激活胰蛋白酶和随后的其他消化蛋白酶级联反应至关重要的酶。

1895 年，巴甫洛夫的另一名学生 Dolinsky 通过向十二指肠内注入酸来刺激胰腺分泌，这导致 1902 年 Bayliss 和 Starling 发现了分泌素，这是有史以来发现的第一种激素[3]。

在 1869 年，Langerhans 首次描述了胰腺的组织结构。此后不久，Heidenhain 发现，随着喂食后胰腺腺泡细胞的颗粒区域消失，胰液中的酶活性反向增加；他正确地得出结论，这些颗粒中含有消化酶前体或酶原。1875 年，Friedreich 首次对胰腺疾病进行了系统的描述，随后 Fitz 于 1889 年对急性胰腺炎进行了经典的叙述[4]。

在 1905 年，胰腺首次引起诺贝尔委员会的注意，当时 Ivan Pavlov 因其在消化生理学方面的工作而获奖，他特别强调胃和胰腺的神经调节。1923 年，加拿大人 Frederick Banting 和 John Macleod 因成功从狗的胰腺中纯化胰岛素而获奖。值得注意的是，医学生 Charles Best 是共同的发现者，并与 Macleod 分享了奖金。1946 年，John Northrop 因其纯化结晶形式酶的工作而共同分享诺贝尔奖。在胰酶中，他成功地使胰蛋白酶、糜蛋白酶和羧肽酶结晶。

1958 年，Frederick Sanger 因确定胰岛素的结构而获得了他的第一个诺贝尔奖。然而，Sanger 最著名的是他在 1980 年获得的第二个诺贝尔奖，因为他开发了一种 DNA 测序的签名方法。1974 年，George Palade、Albert Claude 和 Christian de Duve 一起因在细胞生物学方面的开创性发现而获得诺贝尔奖。Palade 使用胰腺腺泡细胞，结合新开发的差速离心、电子显微镜和脉冲追踪技术，描述了核糖体沿内质网（粗面内质网）在合成蛋白质和蛋白质通过高尔基体进入分泌途径中的作用[5]。1977 年，Rosalyn Yalow 因开发肽类激素的放射免疫测定法而获奖，其中原型为胰岛素。她和 Solomon Berson 共事，但在诺贝尔奖颁发前，她不幸去世。最近，Günter Blobel 因其利用胰腺腺泡细胞发现控制细胞内蛋白转运的内在信号机制而于 1999 年获得了诺贝尔奖。以上这些奖项展示了胰腺方面的研究是如何推进重大科学发展的。

二、解剖学

胰腺是一个柔软、长条形、扁平的腺体，长约 12～20cm[6]。成人的胰腺重约 70～110g。胰腺表面呈粗糙的分叶状，被细微的结缔组织覆盖，没有外包膜。胰腺位于腹膜后，大约位于 L1～L2 腰椎水平。胰头在右侧，位于十二指肠的弯曲处，胰腺其余部分结构斜置于后腹部，其尾部一直延伸到脾脏胃面(图 55.1)。

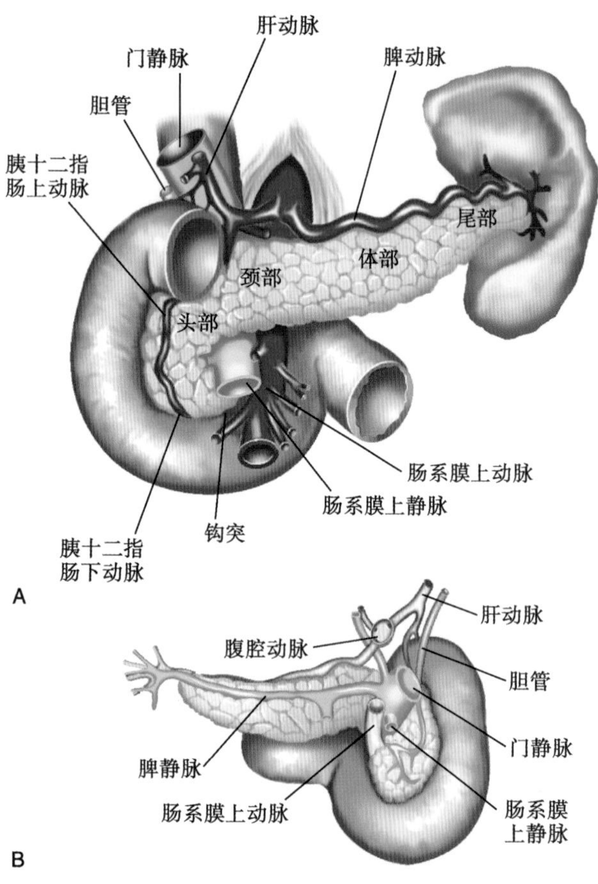

图 55.1 胰腺的解剖关系。A，正面图。B，背面图

胰头的前面紧邻幽门、十二指肠球部和横结肠。后面与右肾的肾门及内侧缘、下腔静脉和右肾血管、右性腺静脉、右膈脚毗邻。

钩突(舌状突起)是胰腺组织的延伸，从胰头下部伸出，向上并向左延伸。钩突位于主动脉和下腔静脉的前方，表面覆盖有胰颈下的肠系膜上血管。钩突的大小和形状变化很大，也可能出现无该结构的情况。

胰颈是腺体一处狭窄区域，从胰头向左侧延伸，连接胰头和胰体。该区域长约 1.5～2cm，宽约 3～4cm。胰颈的后方是门静脉与肠系膜上静脉和脾静脉的汇合处。前面部分被幽门和小网膜覆盖。胰颈向右延伸至从胃十二指肠动脉分出的胰十二指肠前上动脉水平。

胰体总体向左侧延伸，位于主动脉前方，腹膜后方，由小网膜与主动脉相连。胰体的前面被大网膜覆盖，分隔胃和胰腺。胃的胃窦和胃体以及横结肠系膜贴于胰体前面。胰体后方与主动脉、肠系膜上动脉起点、左膈脚、左肾、左肾上腺和脾静脉相邻。胰体的中线部分覆盖于腰椎前，使得胰腺此区域最易受到腹部创伤。胰体横向通过并与胰尾延伸，无明确边界。胰尾结构多样，其末端可至脾门。胰尾被大致定义为肠系膜血管左侧缘的中间部分延伸到胰腺末端的结构。胰尾尖端位于腹膜内，位于肾脾韧带间。胰腺与后腹部重要结构的关系见图 55.2。

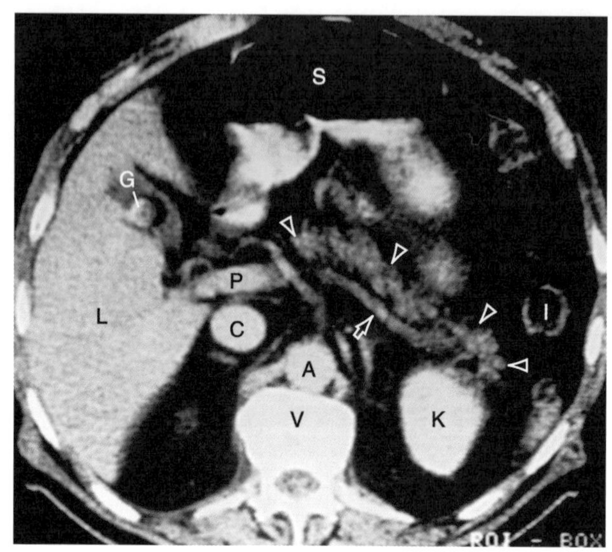

图 55.2 CT 显示胰腺与其他腹内结构的正常解剖关系。胰腺的边界用箭头表示。脾静脉用箭头表示。A，主动脉；C，腔静脉；G，偶发胆结石；I，小肠；K，左肾；L，肝脏；P，门静脉；S，胃；V，椎骨。(Courtesy M. P. Federle MD.)

(一) 胰管结构

主胰管(Wirsung 管)起始于胰尾部，由与腺体小叶相吻合的小管形成。它由左向右延伸，并随分支导管的汇入而扩大。导管位于胰尾、胰体的上下缘之间，稍靠后。主胰管在到达胰头前，朝向尾部和后方。胰管在十二指肠大乳头水平与胆管交汇(图 55.3A)。

Wirsung 管和胆总管经十二指肠大乳头开口于十二指肠。十二指肠壶腹是胰胆乳头内的共同通道，胰胆管在此处汇合，由包膜相分隔。十二指肠壶腹的长度平均为 4.5mm，直径约为 1～12mm[7,8]。由 3 个圆形肌束组成，统称为 Oddi 括约肌，包裹于胰胆管及肝胰壶腹之外。Wirsung 管与胆管之间的结构关系比较复杂[9-11]。大体解剖及 ERCP 研究发现，人群中约 2/3～3/4 的胆胰管有共同通道，而约 1/5 的胆胰管互相分离，不到 1/10 的胰胆管之间被网膜隔开。共同通道较长或胰胆畸形融合会增加胰腺炎或胆道癌的风险。

大约 70% 的人有单独的附属胰管(Santorini 管)，即副胰管结构(见图 55.3A)[12]。副胰管位于胆管的前方，开口于十二指肠小乳头，小乳头位于大乳头近端的十二指肠降部。高达 10% 的人主胰管与十二指肠大乳头之间出现中断，胰液只能引流经小乳头进入十二指肠，这种变异称为胰腺分裂(见图 55.3B)。胰管系统中可能存在着多种变异。

主胰管在胰头处最宽，随着向胰尾延伸逐渐变细[13]。目前普遍认为胰管宽度上限为胰管头部(5mm)、体部(4mm)和尾部(3mm)，不同年龄段儿童的胰管宽度有所不

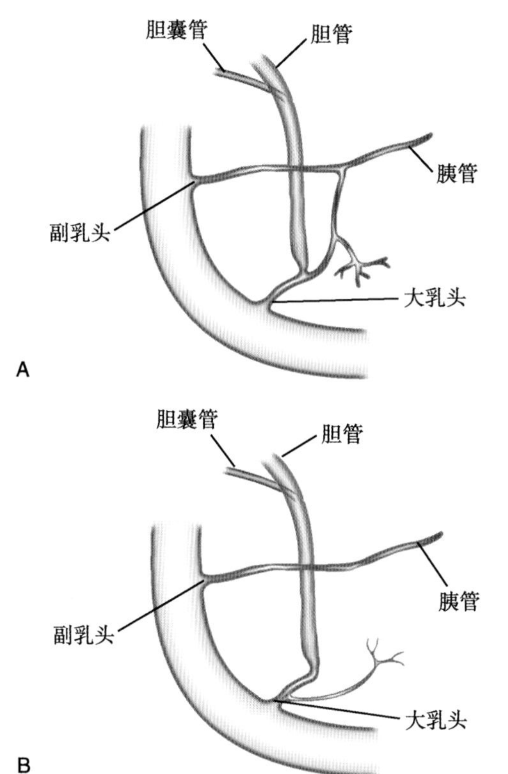

图 55.3　胰管系统的解剖结构。A，最常见的结构。大部分胰腺分泌物与胆汁一起通过主乳头排空到十二指肠。大约70%的成人胚胎背侧胰管的近端部分保持通畅，并通过副胰管进行排空。B，胰腺分裂。胚胎背侧和腹侧胰管未能融合。大部分胰腺分泌物通过副乳头排空。只有来自钩突和部分胰头（来源于胚胎腹侧胰腺）的胰腺分泌物通过主乳头引流

同（表 55.1）[14-17]。了解胰管的正常大小范围可为慢性胰腺炎等主因胰管扩张或狭窄引起的疾病提供依据。

表 55.1　美国不同年龄段儿童胰管平均大小

年龄/岁	胰管大小/mm（平均值±SD）
1~3	1.13±0.15
4~6	1.35±0.15
7~9	1.67±0.17
10~12	1.78±0.17
13~15	1.92±0.18
16~18	2.05±0.15

Data from Chao, H-C, Lin S-J, Kong M-S, et al. Sonographic evaluation of the pancreatic duct in normal children and children with pancreatitis. J Ultrasound Med 2000;19:757-63.

（二）血液循环

胰腺有丰富的血液供应，主要来自腹腔动脉和肠系膜上动脉的分支[6]。胰头及周围十二指肠由 2 条胰十二指肠动脉弓供应。由腹腔动脉分出的肝总动脉，进而分出前、后胰十二指肠上动脉，前、后胰十二指肠下动脉由肠系膜上动脉分支形成。胰腺所有的主要动脉全部走行于胰管后方。

脾动脉走行于胰体、胰尾的后方，及胰腺上缘的上方和下方。它发出背胰动脉，通常在发出胰下动脉后与后上弓相连。

胰尾动脉起源于胃网膜左动脉或脾动脉。它与脾动脉、胰大动脉和其他胰动脉分支相连。丰富的血液循环使胰腺能够通过感知血糖浓度和控制胰岛其他激素的释放，迅速发挥关键的内分泌功能，以维持血糖稳态。

一般情况下，胰腺的静脉血管分布与动脉相似。它汇入门静脉系统，门静脉系统是由肠系膜上静脉和脾静脉在胰腺颈部后方交汇处汇合形成的。门静脉位于胰腺的后方和下腔静脉的前方。胆总管位于门静脉前方，肝动脉位于胆总管左侧。脾静脉起源于脾门，在胰尾后方弯曲，位于脾动脉下方，沿胰腺后表面向右弯曲。胰静脉流经胰腺的颈部、体部和尾部并与脾静脉相连。胰十二指肠静脉与相应的动脉毗邻并汇入脾静脉或门静脉。由于脾静脉与胰腺的解剖关系密切，累及胰体和胰尾的炎症性疾病或肿瘤性疾病可进一步导致脾静脉阻塞。这会导致脾门处的静脉阻塞，进而使静脉血液回流不畅，通过胃短静脉和胃网膜左静脉，导致胃静脉曲张。

（三）淋巴引流

淋巴管将表面的淋巴网引流至局部淋巴结，一般与较大的血管相邻近[18]。它们由小的腺泡周围和小叶周围毛细血管网，汇入胰腺血管旁的大导管。上淋巴管沿胰腺上缘与脾血管紧密相连，而下淋巴管则与胰下动脉相连。上、下淋巴管收集胰尾和胰体的左半部分至脾门的淋巴结。上淋巴管收集胰颈和胰体右半部邻近胰头上缘的淋巴结。这些淋巴结也有来自前后胰腺表面的分支。胰颈和胰体的其余部分向右引流。总之，密集的血管和淋巴管网络，以及肿瘤诱导血管和淋巴管形成的能力，为胰腺癌的转移提供了充足的条件[19]。

（四）神经支配

胰腺的内脏传出神经经迷走神经和内脏神经受肝丛、腹腔神经丛支配。迷走神经的输出纤维通过这些神经丛而不产生突触，终止于位于大脑小叶间隔的副交感神经节，胰腺节后纤维支配腺泡、胰岛和导管。交感传出神经节前神经元的胞体起源于胸腰椎脊髓的外侧灰质。神经节后交感神经元的主体位于腹部的大神经丛中。节后纤维只支配血管。自主神经纤维，传出纤维和传入纤维，均位于胰腺血管附近。迷走神经还包含一些内脏传入纤维。

三、组织学和超微结构

胰腺是一种复合的小结节状腺体，其轮廓与唾液腺相类似。小叶在大体检查中可见，由包括导管、血管、淋巴管和神经在内的结缔组织隔膜连接。外分泌部分的基本亚单位是腺泡，基部是一球状暗染色分泌细胞团，称为腺泡细胞（图 55.4）。球形腺泡与杯状颈相连，杯状颈由称为导管细胞的小管上皮细胞组成。腺泡的内腔形成分泌管的末端。通过逆行注射乳胶制成的具有腐蚀性的导管系统模型显示，泡管腔内有一个不断增大的广泛的导管网络，引流胰腺分泌物，经小叶内、小叶间、叶间，最后进入主胰管（图 55.5）[20]。胰管系统无横纹，由柱状上皮排列。可偶见杯状细胞和嗜银细胞。较大的导管壁厚，由结缔组织和弹性纤维组成。内分泌部分由

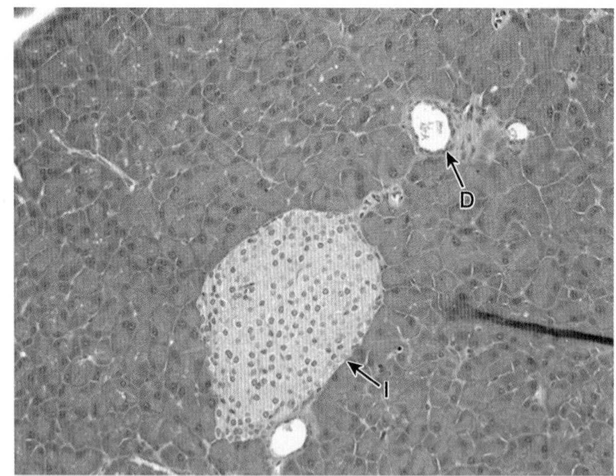

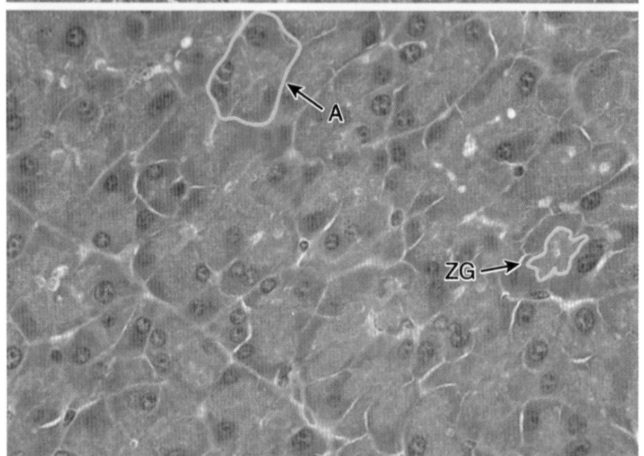

图 55.4　胰腺组织学。上图，胰腺低倍组织切片，显示导管(D)和胰岛(I)(HE 染色)。下图，高倍切片，显示许多腺泡(A)，其中含有嗜酸性酶原颗粒(ZG)。(Courtesy Abrahim l. Orabi.)

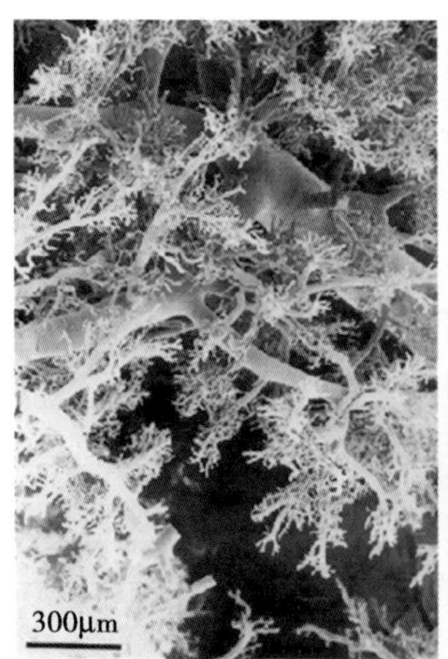

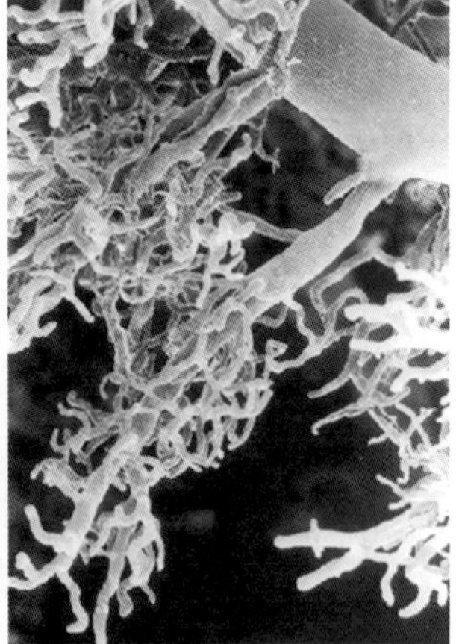

图 55.5　用乳胶填充胰管并消化胰腺组织后获得的胰腺外分泌导管系统的扫描电子显微图。导管系统的最小胚根与腺泡相连。右侧图为放大的图像。(From Ashizawa N, Watanabe M, Fukumoto S, et al. Scanning electron microscopic observations of 3-dimensional structure of the rat pancreatic duct. Pancreas 1991;6:542-50.)

朗格汉斯胰岛组成，在 H & E 染色上，胰岛是球状的淡染细胞簇。对胰腺各个主要的实质细胞的详细描述，揭示了胰腺显著的结构-功能关系。

光镜下，腺泡细胞为高大的锥体或柱状上皮细胞，它们基部宽阔，位于基底层，顶端集中于中央腔。在静息状态下，大量嗜酸性酶原颗粒充满细胞顶端。细胞的基部有 1 或 2 个位于中心的球形核和嗜碱性细胞质。高尔基复合体位于细胞核和酶原颗粒之间，镜下可为一个清晰的无染色区域。

电镜下可见腺泡细胞的亚细胞结构(图 55.6)。腺泡细胞最具有特征性的是集中在顶端的致密的酶原颗粒。紧密连接在细胞顶端形成一条带状带，由相邻细胞的外膜小叶相联系产生。这些连接防止分泌物从导管回流到细胞间隙[21]。间隙连接点允许小分子在细胞间流动，分布在细胞的外侧膜上，由较大的盘状膜斑相连接形成。

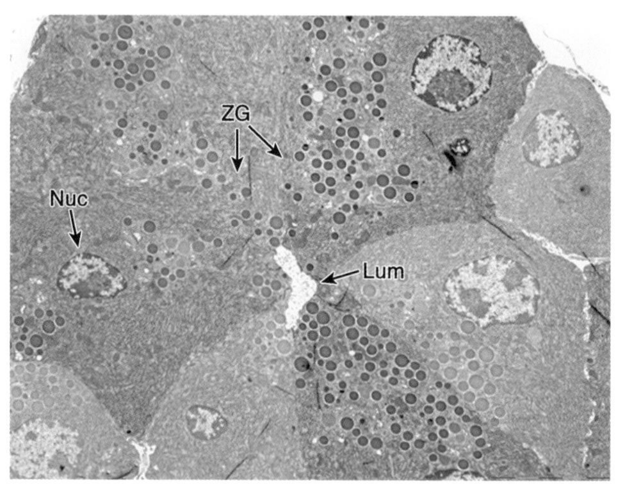

图 55.6　胰腺腺泡的电子显微照片，显示中央管腔(Lum)周围的腺泡细胞。腺泡细胞核(Nuc)和酶原颗粒(ZG)易于识别(×3 200)。(Courtesy Abrahim l. Orabi.)

线粒体是细长的圆柱形结构，横截面呈椭圆形，包含发育良好的嵴和基质颗粒(图 55.7)。它们集中在腺泡细胞的酶原颗粒周围、细胞核内和基底外侧膜[22]。粗面内质网约占细胞体积的 20%[23]。它占据腺泡细胞的大部分基部，在顶端与酶原颗粒交错。这种丰富的粗面内质网使腺泡细胞合成的蛋白质比体内任何其他实质细胞都多[24]。高尔基复合体由扁平的膜状小囊以及含有絮状电子致密物质的小囊泡组成。高尔基体在分泌蛋白的运输和成熟的凝缩液泡中形成酶原颗粒方面起着重要的作用。

研究表明，发酵原颗粒含有 12~15 种不同的消化酶，约占颗粒蛋白质的 90%[25]。腺泡细胞在进食后会发生周期性的形态变化[26]。进餐后，酶原颗粒通过一种特殊形式的调节分泌(称为序贯复合胞吐)迅速排空到腺泡管腔[27,28]。在这种情况下，酶原颗粒与顶端质膜发生初始融合，随后发生连续的颗粒-颗粒融合事件，将多个小泡以串珠形式连接到顶端管腔。这一过程解决了从细胞相对较小区域快速排空大量颗粒物的问题。

腺泡细胞的顶膜仅占总质膜的一小部分，但其表面的几个长度约为 0.2μm 并延伸到腺泡腔的短而细微绒毛(图 55.8)，使其表面积扩大。细丝形成微绒毛的轴以及顶端质膜下的网络。管腔通常含有电子密度高的絮状物质，即分泌的消化酶。形态不同的细胞，称为中心腺泡细胞，桥接腺泡细胞

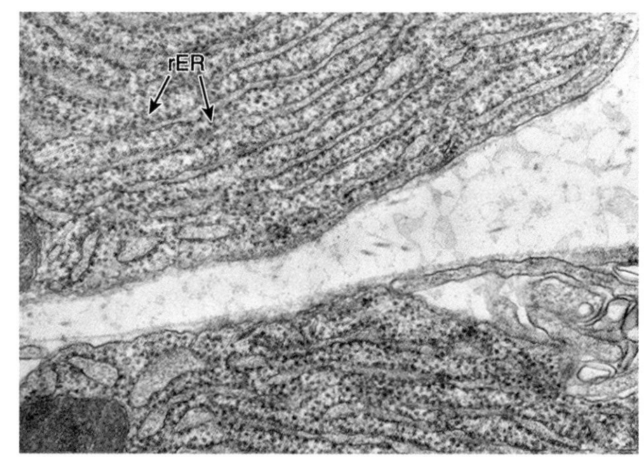

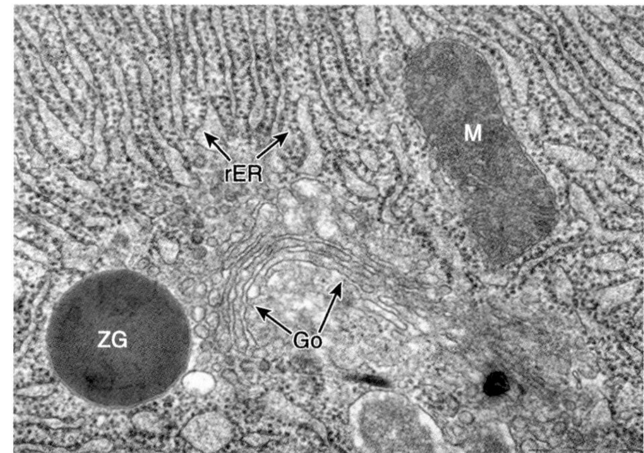

图 55.7　腺泡细胞部分的电子显微照片。上图代表基底外侧区域，显示粗面内质网（rER）片层。下图还显示了高尔基复合体（Go）、线粒体（M）和酶原颗粒（ZG）（×43 000）。（Courtesy Abrahim l. Orabi.）

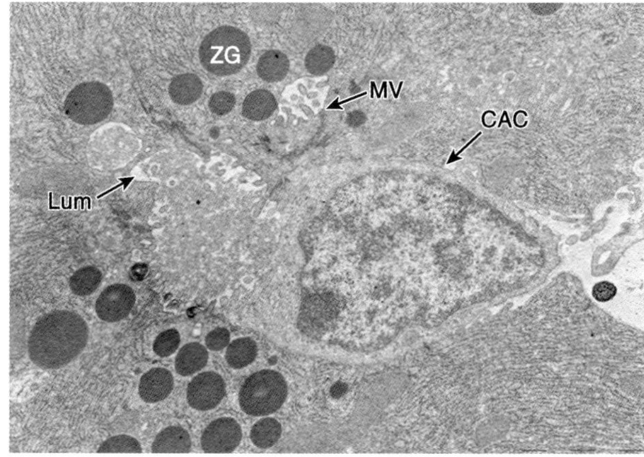

图 55.8　中心腺泡细胞（CAC）和中央管腔周围腺泡细胞（Lum）的电子显微照片（×9 000）。MV，微绒毛；ZG，酶原颗粒。（Courtesy Abrahim l. Orabi.）

和导管上皮。这些中心腺泡细胞在 H&E 染色上呈淡染，比腺泡细胞小。

沿着腺泡细胞的基底表面，但不在相邻细胞之间延伸的是薄基底层。下面是胶原纤维和丰富的毛细血管网。来自交感神经和副交感神经系统的传出神经纤维穿过基底膜，终止于腺泡细胞附近。胶原纤维和其他细胞外基质蛋白由一种不太常见的驻留细胞类型——胰腺星状细胞（pancreatic stellate cell，PSC）分泌[29]。在静止状态下，PSC 具有维持胰腺微结构以及促进腺泡细胞分泌的基本功能。然而，在胰腺损伤和炎症过程中，处于激活状态的 PSC，转化为肌成纤维细胞样细胞，帮助补充恢复所需的基质，甚至可以作为兼性祖细胞。对于持续性损伤，由于细胞外基质蛋白沉积增加，它也可以通过诱导纤维化而引起损害，从而导致慢性胰腺炎（见第 59 章）。PSC 还参与提供胰腺癌周围丰富的基质环境，从而限制肿瘤治疗的效果。最后，PSC 还可以伴随癌细胞到达转移部位，加速癌症的进展[30]。

对于持续性损伤，它还可能通过诱发纤维化而造成伤害。由于细胞外基质蛋白沉积增加，导致慢性胰腺炎（见第 59 章）。PSC 还参与在胰腺腺癌周围提供丰富的基质环境，这可以限制癌症治疗的效果。最后，PSC 还可以伴随癌细胞转移到其他部位以促进癌症进展。

导管细胞具有电子透明细胞质，其中细胞器较少[31]。细胞质通常含有大量游离核糖体，这些核糖体存在于小而圆的线粒体中。线粒体的普遍存在对于导管细胞执行其主动离子转运的主要功能是必要的[32]。腺泡细胞分泌少量富含氯化钠的液体，而导管细胞吸收氯化物，并主动分泌碳酸氢盐和水，以提供大部分胰液。分泌到肠道的碳酸氢盐中和胃酸，并为消化酶功能提供最佳缓冲 pH。导管细胞内的几种酶和多种离子通道协调着碳酸盐和水的净分泌。它们包括碳酸酐酶和 CFTR。前一种酶可以用来标记导管细胞。CFTR 的严重缺陷导致胰腺发育过程中的胰管阻塞和胰腺外分泌的宫内破坏，并形成囊肿和纤维化；因此该疾病的名称被称为“囊性纤维化”（见第 57 章）。

在人类胰腺中，朗格汉斯岛大约有 100 万个。胰岛由多边形内分泌细胞的吻合索组成（见图 55.4）。每个胰岛直径约 0.2mm，比腺泡大得多，由与外分泌腺相连的细结缔组织纤维与周围外分泌组织隔开。每一个胰岛都被一个由开孔内皮细胞排列的丰富毛细血管网所包围和穿透。毛细血管排列在门脉系统中，将血液从胰岛输送到腺泡细胞（图 55.9）。胰岛

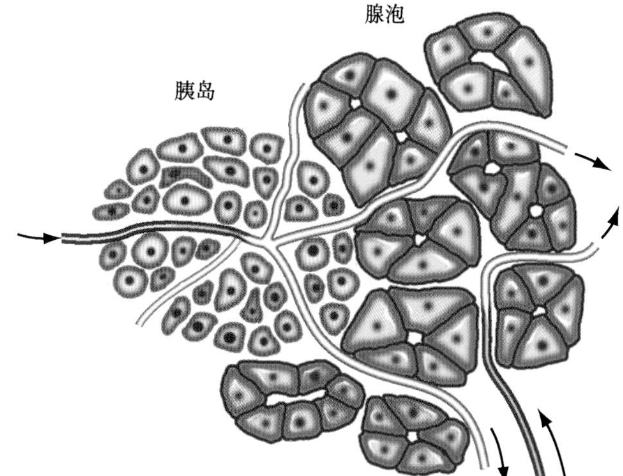

图 55.9　显示外分泌胰腺双重血供的胰岛腺泡门脉系统示意图。（From Goldfine ID，Williams JA. Receptors for insulin and CCK in the acinar pancreas：Relationship to hormone action. lnt Rev Cytol 1983；85：1.）

腺泡-门脉系统由进入胰岛的传入小动脉组成,形成毛细血管团,并作为传入外分泌组织的传出毛细血管离开胰岛[33-35]。与其相伴行的动脉系统直接向外分泌胰腺供血,通过门脉系统,胰岛素等胰腺激素在外分泌胰腺上发挥其局部作用。朗格汉斯岛周围的腺泡细胞(岛周腺泡)在形态和生化上与远处的腺泡(远岛腺泡)不同。岛周腺泡有较大的细胞、细胞核和酶原颗粒区,以及不同比例的一些消化酶。这些差异似乎与腺泡细胞表达胰岛素受体以及胰岛素影响腺泡生长和分泌的发现有关。

内分泌胰腺有 5 种主要的细胞类型。β 细胞最多,约占胰岛的 50%~80%,它们分泌胰岛素和胰淀素。PP 细胞,又称 F 细胞,占 10%~35%,分泌胰多肽和肾上腺髓质素。α 细胞占 5%~20%,分泌胰高血糖素。剩下的 5%由分泌生长抑素的 δ 细胞和分泌胃泌素的 ε 细胞组成。其他罕见的胰岛亚群产生其余激素,如甘丙肽。

四、胰腺的发育

(一) 胚胎和胎儿发育

胰腺起源于后肠内胚层[36]。两芽形成:1 个背芽和 1 个双裂腹芽。大约在妊娠 1 个月后,前肠外翻成一层覆盖的间充质,形成了背芽的第一个形态学证据。大约 1 周后,一个腹芽形成作为肝憩室的出口。腹芽双叶起源,左腹芽逐渐退化[37]。背芽和腹芽都经历了茎部的伸长和分枝的形态发生。妊娠 37~42 天,随着十二指肠的生长,腹侧胰腺围绕十二指肠旋转并与背侧胰腺融合(图 55.10)。

胰腺背侧形成胰尾、胰体和胰头的上部。还形成背侧胰管,包括主胰管(Wirsung 管)的远端和整个副胰管(Santorini 管)。腹侧胰腺形成钩突和胰头的下部。腹胰的腹管形成了主胰管的近端。如前所述,与腹芽和背芽相对应的两个导管系统有 10%的人无法融合。在这种情况下,副胰管作为胰液引流的主要管道发挥作用。胰腺分裂的临床意义将在后文讨论。若腹侧胰腺未能完全围绕十二指肠旋转,或左腹芽持续存在,可导致环状胰腺,也将在后文讨论。

胰腺背腹芽融合后,胰腺的细胞结构迅速繁殖。值得注意的是,3 种功能不同的实质细胞类型,即腺泡细胞、导管细胞和胰岛细胞都是从同一胰腺祖细胞谱系分化而来。Rutter 及其同事的经典研究将胰腺分化过程描述为两个不同的阶段[38]。第一个阶段,称为初级转变,是指预分化细胞向原分化状态的转化,其中存在低水平的胰腺特异性蛋白。第二阶段,即第二个过渡期,以胰腺细胞数量和胰腺特异性蛋白合成的急剧增加以及外分泌和内分泌分化的加速为标志。胰腺腺泡细胞在这个阶段合成其特有的丰富的内质网和密集的顶端定位酶原颗粒[39]。虽然背侧胰腺出现在腹侧之前,但根据这两个阶段的表现,两者的外分泌分化功能似乎为同时发育[40]。

在内分泌细胞的个体发育中,最初胰高血糖素阳性 α 细

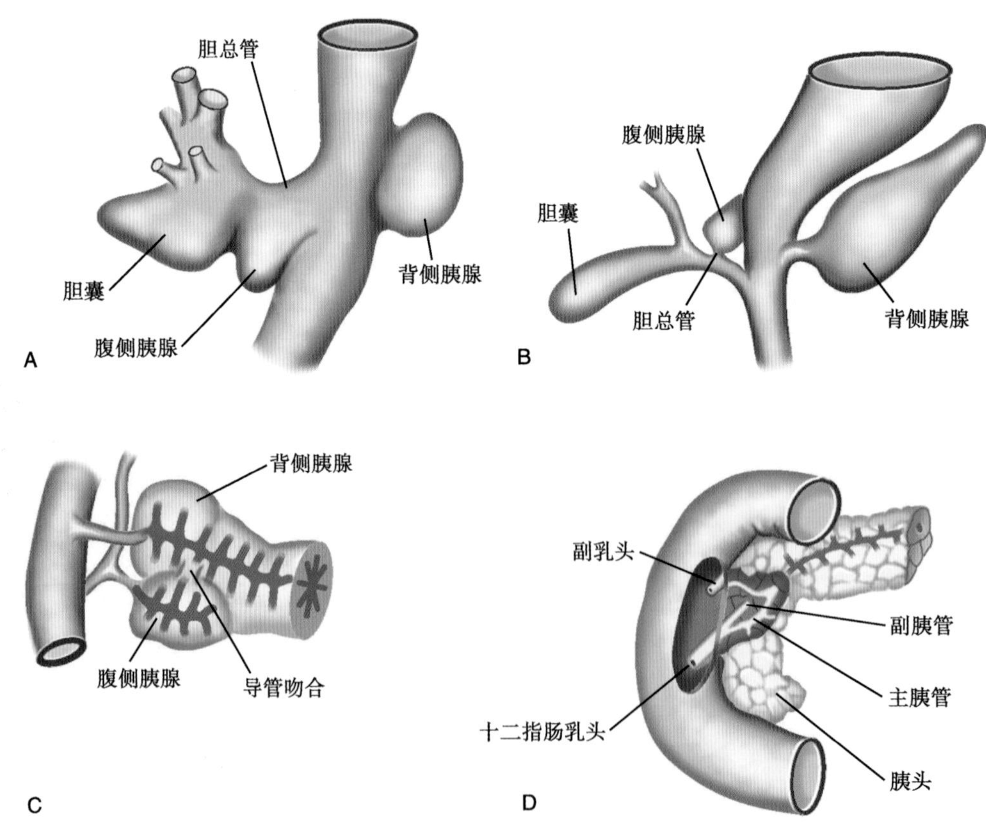

图 55.10 胰腺胚胎发育阶段。A,妊娠 4 周左右,前肠形成背芽和腹芽。B,约 6 周时,腹侧胰腺向较大的背侧胰腺延伸。C,到约 7 周时,背侧和腹侧胰腺发生融合,开始导管吻合。D,出生时胰腺为单一器官,导管吻合完整。(Modified from Arey LB. Developmental anatomy: a textbook and laboratory manual of embryology. 7th ed. Philadelphia: WB Saunders; 1974.)

胞占优势[41]。在第二次转变之后，胰岛素阳性β细胞的数量超过了所有其他内分泌细胞类型。此外，内分泌谱系发生了显著的转变。虽然它们最初是上皮细胞，但研究表明，在发育的这一点上，这些细胞并非平行于基底膜进行分裂，而是开始垂直于基底膜进行分裂，最终形成胰岛单位[39]。新定向的细胞后代失去了与管腔的紧密连接。内分泌谱系最终经历了一个完整的上皮细胞到间充质细胞的转化过程，这是一个至今在发育生物学中堪称奇迹的过程，同时也在癌症生物学中提出了转移这个主要问题[42]。

（二）转录因子和外源信号

引导胰腺发育的序列和信号因子在脊椎动物物种间似乎惊人的相似，主要区别在于器官形成的时间方面。事实上，我们大部分的认识来源于对小鼠发育过程的描述，以及利用转基因小鼠进行谱系追踪实验的能力。尽管如此，我们仍然需要通过对人类状况的观察来确认动物的发育模型[43]。这一领域的研究正在迅速发展；此文中，我们重点介绍一些值得注意的发展机制。

胰腺的形态变化以及胰腺祖细胞的生长、繁殖和分化是由来自两个不同来源的分级信号协调的：胰腺细胞的基因组内，特别是由一系列转录因子[44]，以及与成熟胰腺相邻的组织结构，都将被讨论。

转录因子是与特定 DNA 序列结合的蛋白质[45]。它们的作用是激活或抑制转录所必需的 RNA 聚合酶的募集。转录因子是根据其 DNA 结合域来分类的。本文对胰腺发育中的几个关键转录因子进行了综述。

胰-十二指肠同源异型盒基因抗原 1（Pdx1），也称为胰岛素启动因子 1（Ipf1）或胰岛/十二指肠同源盒-1（Idx1），是最早的胰腺特异性转录因子，可在胚胎发育第 5 周，即胚芽形成之前检测到。因此 Pdx1 可作为早期胰腺祖细胞标志物[46,47]。胰腺发育方面研究常以胰腺特异性表达的 Pdx1 基因启动子为靶点。例如，在腹侧前肠，Pdx1 的表达促进了腹侧胰腺的发育；相比之下，无 Pdx1 的 *Sox17* 基因表达促进了邻近肝外胆管的发育。小鼠[48]和人类[49]中的缺失 Pdx1 可导致胰腺发育不全（稍后讨论），这一结论突出了 Pdx1 在形态学发育中的重要性。Pdx1 缺乏使胰腺上皮无法对间充质促生长信号做出反应[50]。在成年后，Pdx1 主要在β细胞中表达，维持β细胞的特性，并结合与激活胰岛素启动子[46,51]。使成年小鼠β细胞中的 Pdx1 失活可导致糖尿病[52]。因此 Pdx1 是正常胰腺发育以及β细胞所必需的。

胰腺特异性转录因子 1（Ptf1）的α亚单位，也称为 p48，是一种基本的螺旋-环-螺旋型蛋白。它作为 Ptf1 这种三聚体蛋白复合物的一部分，发挥调节外分泌相关基因表达的作用[53]。这一亚单位最初与 Pdx1 共同表达于 3 种胰腺前体细胞中，后期仅于腺泡细胞中表达[54,55]。小鼠的 Ptf1α 缺陷可导致胰腺发育不全，外分泌系统完全不发育，但仍可产生异位内分泌细胞[56]。在人类谱系中，Ptf1α 的截断性单核苷酸碱突变可导致胰腺和小脑发育不全[57]。

人类同源异型盒基因 9（Hlxb9）也被称为运动神经元和胰腺同源异型盒 1（Mnx1），早在脊索和胰腺内胚层的第八体节阶段就表达了。Hlxb9 基因缺陷小鼠的背侧胰腺发育不全，腹侧胰腺仅有轻微缺陷[58,59]；然而，在抑制 Pdx1 表达的情况下，Hlxb9 的持续表达也会导致胰腺发育受损[60]。Hlxb9 的双向作用结果表明，在胰腺发育过程中，转录因子在时间及空间上精准且平衡的表达，对胰腺的正常发育至关重要。成熟胰腺中 Hlxb9 仅表达于β细胞中。[58,59]

神经生长素 3（Ngn3）是一种基本的螺旋-环-螺旋型转录因子，是表达 Pdx1 的祖细胞分化为内分泌谱系的标志[61]。值得关注的是，Ngn3 的表达在祖细胞开始分化为内分泌细胞后逐渐下调[62]。Ngn3 完全缺失的小鼠体内缺乏胰腺内分泌细胞。相比之下，Ngn3 畸形突变的患者由于 Ngn3 的肠道丢失导致肠内分泌细胞缺失而发生严重的先天性腹泻，但他们不会死于新生儿糖尿病[63]。综上所述，结果表明内分泌细胞的正常分化依赖于 Ngn3 的低水平表达[64]。

Gata4 和 Gata6 是锌指转录因子家族的一部分，调控多种内胚层器官的细胞增殖和分化[65]。*GATA4* 或 *GATA6* 的突变将导致人类胰腺发育不全。最近的研究发现 Gata6 表达于多能干细胞中。此外，Gata4/6 在维持胰腺特性中的作用已通过小鼠模型进行证实；由于失去了 Gata4/6 介导的对音猬因子（Shh）的抑制作用，腹侧和背侧胚芽仅发育成胃肠道[66]。诸多近期研究证实了 Gata6 在功能性β细胞分化中的作用[67]。

其他涉及外分泌范畴的转录因子包括腺泡细胞的 Mist1 和导管细胞的 Sox9。内分泌通路的转录因子有 MafA、isl1、Brn-4、NeuroD、Nkx6. 1、Nkx2. 2、Pax4、Pax6 和 Arx。

胰腺发育除受到转录因子的影响外，还受控于邻近组织结构中信号蛋白的表达水平。胚胎发育早期，中胚层的 Wnt 信号（见第 1 章）和成纤维细胞生长因子 4（FGF4）信号受到抑制，以维持内胚层胰腺的特异性[68,69]。此外，中胚层视黄酸信号可改善胰腺发育的前后位置[70-72]。

胰腺的背侧和腹侧与其各自结构的关系使得它们可以有不同的定义。在胚胎发育早期，脊索与胰腺背侧相接并控制其发育。去除脊索可阻断背芽中胰腺外分泌和内分泌标志物的表达，而脊索与内胚层的联合培养可启动并维持胰腺基因的表达[73]。来自脊索的信号通过抑制抗胰腺因子 Shh 的表达来实现胰腺背侧特异性，而 Shh 使 PDX1 的表达成为可能。[74-75]相反，胰腺腹侧的发育依赖于邻近心脏间质中提取的 FGF 信号。[76]与胰腺相邻的其他新生器官（如心脏）中信号因子的表达也对胰腺发育过程进行调节。胚胎发育后期，背主动脉和卵黄静脉等内皮组织会影响胰腺的发育[77,78]。除了内胚层与内皮细胞的接触可促进胰腺背侧出芽外，血管内皮细胞分泌 1-磷酸鞘氨醇也可促进这一过程[79]。

胰腺间充质细胞分泌的生长因子对内胚层器官原基的发育至关重要[80]。胰腺祖细胞的生长因 FGF-10 等间充质及间充质因子的存在，从分化状态转变为增殖状态。胰腺的最终大小取决于早期胚胎阶段的原始祖细胞数量，这一发现表明维持胰腺祖细胞增殖状态的重要性[81]。胰腺的发育同样受到基质成分的影响。例如，β细胞的数量会因神经嵴细胞迁移至胰腺而受到影响[82]。相反，胰腺细胞也可能向邻近组织细胞传递功能信号。

（三）胰腺损伤时胚胎因子的重现

胰腺发育的几个特点在两个临床条件下进行了总结。在第一种情况下,在胰腺损伤的恢复过程中(例如,急性胰腺炎发作后),一些胚胎转录因子从残留的腺泡细胞中重新出现,形成新的导管复合体,称为腺泡-导管化生。这一过程出现于胰腺组织恢复和再生之前[83]。在第二种情况下,胰腺导管腺癌及其癌前病变、胰腺上皮内瘤变,除 Notch(胰腺 *Kras* 基因增效突变的前提下)[84]等胚胎基因的被迫表达或通过抵消β-连环蛋白等信号通路外,是类似于从腺泡到导管的化生过程[85]。因此,了解胰腺的发育过程,对于帮助我们制定促进胰腺恢复的治疗计划、认识胰腺的异常现象甚至胰腺癌的发生过程是重要的。

另一个与胰腺发育相关的新兴研究领域是寻找有助于胰腺更新和再生的干细胞龛或胰腺祖细胞[86]。恢复和理解胰腺异常甚至某些形式的胰腺癌是如何发生的。已知腺泡细胞通常在适应性生长的过程中进行分裂[87],但一些研究表明,部分存活的腺泡细胞会发生腺泡-导管化生,而这种新的导管复合体是其他胰腺细胞类型新生的祖细胞。部分研究团队认为原代导管细胞是兼性祖细胞[88,89]。近期研究分离出可表达标志物 ALDH1(醛脱氢酶)的中心泡细胞,这些细胞可分化为外分泌细胞和内分泌细胞[90]。有人认为,在电子显微镜下可以看到一个全新的腺体,突出胰腺管腔,称为胰管腺,起着干细胞龛的作用[91]。如前所述,甚至有观点认为像 PSC 等间充质细胞也可成为祖细胞。这些新的观点揭示了胰腺内部的因素和细胞的复杂环境以维持胰腺完整性,及调节胰腺在胚胎早期发育之后的更新和再生。

五、发育异常

(一) 环状胰腺

环状胰腺是一种先天胰腺发育异常,指部分胰腺在十二指肠壶腹前部形成一条带状结构,导致完全或部分肠梗阻(图 55.11)。对患者进行腹部影像学检查或尸检的回顾性研究表明,环状胰腺的发生率估计分别在 1/1 000[92-94]和 3/20 000[95,96]。

充足证据表明环状胰腺的发病机制与遗传因素有关。病例报道环状胰腺可发生于兄弟姐妹[97]或同卵双胞胎[98]中,在都被诊断为环状胰腺的母亲及其孩子身上同时检测到表达 utrophin 基因(*UTRN*)的染色体 6q24.2 存在微重复[99]。

此外,环状胰腺更常见于其他先天异常,如 21-三体、心脏缺陷、器官旋转不良、十二指肠闭锁、泌尿生殖系统异常和气管食管瘘等患者中[100,101]。*Hh* 基因在胰腺器官发生中的作用已在本章前文中阐明。*Shh* 和 *Ihh* 基因缺陷的小鼠模型中环状胰腺发生率为 42% ~85%[102,103]。

尽管环状胰腺通常在产前或婴儿期被确诊,但仅仅认为它是婴儿期疾病是错误的。第二个确诊高峰为 40~70 岁的成年人[101],与儿童相比,成人的症状明显不同。未经产前超声进行鉴别的患儿往往表现为非胆汁性呕吐或喂养不耐受。不同的是,成人常表现为腹痛、胰腺炎、胆道梗阻,或伴有恶心、呕吐和腹胀[101]。儿童环状胰腺需经腹部 X 线片、超声或上消化道相关检查以提供诊断依据。而对于成年患者,CT 扫描、MRCP 或 ERCP 为更常用的检查手段。环状胰腺的诊断常常是在剖腹手术中做出的。

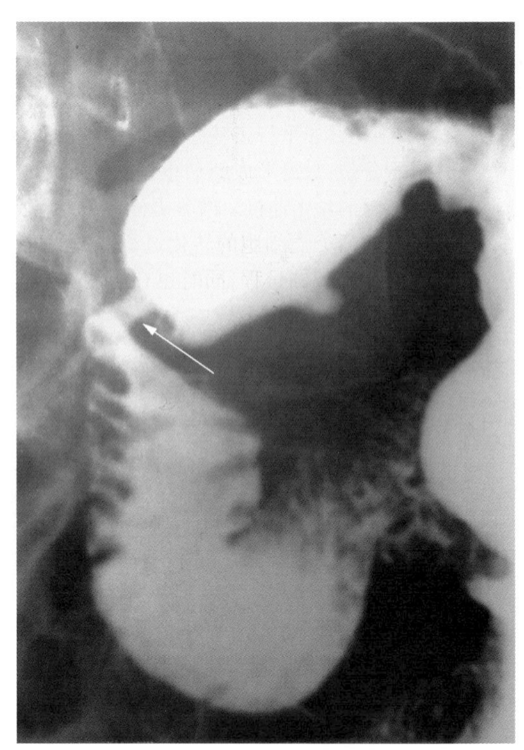

图 55.11　上消化道钡剂造影系列的胶片显示十二指肠中段狭窄(箭)伴有近端扩张,结果与环状胰腺相一致。CT 扫描发现环状胰腺,并在手术中证实。(Courtesy Michael Federle, MD.)

在这些病例中,十二指肠吻合术可作为肠梗阻的有效治疗方式,并被认为是患儿和部分成人患者的首选治疗方法。与儿童相比,成人需要进行复杂的胰腺手术的概率更高[100,101]。行手术修复的患儿,成年后出现急性或反复发作胰腺炎的风险增加[101,104]。在患有环状胰腺的成人中,胰胆肿瘤的风险显著增加[102,105],已有相关报道表明该病患者患十二指肠癌的风险增加[106]。因此,应加强对这一类人群的进行癌症早期筛查及监测。

(二) 胰腺分裂

胰腺分裂(pancreas divisum, PD)是由于在胚胎形成过程中,背侧和腹侧胰管未能融合所致(图 55.12),导致大多数外分泌分泌物从副胰管和小乳头相对较小的背侧导管引流。胰腺分裂有 3 种不同类型[107]。有 71% 的胰腺分裂患者发生典型或完全分裂,其中背侧导管和腹侧导管之间的融合完全失败。第二种类型的胰腺分裂称为显性型或背侧导管胰腺分裂,其中无腹侧导管,发生在 6% 的分裂患者中。最后一种类型为不完全胰腺分裂,其中腹侧胰管和背侧胰管之间仍然有一个小的交通,发生在 23% 的患者。

尸检研究中发现,有 5% ~10% 的人群患胰腺分裂,与通过 ERCP 这一手段进行检查的检出率相近[108-110]。几十年前,科顿研究表明 26% 的复发性胰腺炎患者,通过 ERCP 评估胰腺炎病情时被检出患胰腺分裂,这体现了胰腺分裂与胰腺炎的因果关系[111]。2011 年的一项基于 MRI 的横断面研究表明,PD 应是慢性和复发性胰腺炎的危险因素[112]。

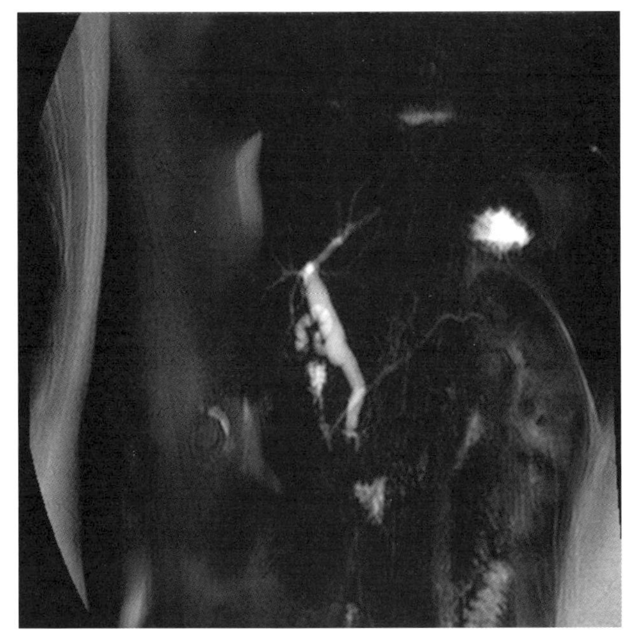

图 55.12　复发性胰腺炎、胰腺发裂和 1 型胆总管囊肿患儿的 MRCP 成像

然而，近期研究表明，*SPINK1* 和 *CFTR* 这两个基因的突变，与有症状的 PD 患者之间存在一定的联系，表明 PD 与其他胰腺疾病的危险因素相关，促使胰腺疾病进一步发展[113,114]。然而，最近的一项系统评价发现 PD 和胰腺疾病之间没有明确的相关性[115]。目前暂未明确 PD 是胰腺疾病的病因还是加重胰腺疾病的危险因素。在 2011 年的一篇与 PD 相关的壶腹癌病例报告中也对 PD 的致癌可能性进行了描述，随后的一篇回顾性综述表明，7.8% 的 PD 患者有胰胆肿瘤[116,117]。

胰腺分裂可通过逆行性胰胆管造影、EUS、腹部 CT 或 MRCP 等辅助检查进行诊断。虽然逆行性胰胆管造影被认为是诊断 PD 的金标准，但近期研究表明[118]，促胰液素增强 MRCP 可作为一种有潜力的辅助检查方式，其灵敏度为 73.3%，特异度为 96.8%；无促胰液素的 MRCP 不具诊断效能。仅有一少部分 PD 患者因解剖结构异常出现症状，但在一些复发性急性胰腺炎和慢性胰腺炎患者中，内镜或手术治疗似乎可以缓解症状（见 59 章）。

在 2008 年，对 57 例 PD 患者进行回顾性数据研究显示，在中位随访 20 个月后，76% 的复发性急性胰腺炎患者、42% 的慢性胰腺炎患者及 33% 的单纯疼痛患者的临床症状有所改善[119]。2009 年的一项数据研究再次评估了 145 名接受十二指肠小乳头内镜治疗的 PD 患者的长期预后。在中位随访 43 个月时 53% 的复发性急性胰腺炎患者、18% 的慢性胰腺炎患者和 41% 的伴有胰腺型疼痛的患者临床表现得到改善[120]。Kanth 等在对 528 例复发性急性胰腺炎患者的系统回顾中发现，内镜治疗是一种有效的手段。[121] 另一项最近的系统综述对比了内镜和手术治疗的作用，并得出结论：尽管两种方法都能改善症状，但手术治疗的效果更好，手术治疗及内镜治疗的症状改善率分别为 72% 和 62.3%[122]。

（三）异位胰腺组织

异位胰腺组织，通常称之为异位胰腺，根据尸检资料显示，该病发病率为 0.6%～13.7%。异位胰腺与正常胰腺之间无任何解剖或血管联系。异位胰腺最常出现于胃（图 55.13）、十二指肠、空肠近端和回肠。少数情况下，也可出现于 Meckel 憩室（6%），甚至出现于脐、胆管、胆囊、脾门、结肠或阑尾中。[123] 异位胰腺组织很少有临床意义，但已有导致胰腺炎[124]、溃疡伴出血[125]、肠套叠[126]和恶性肿瘤[127,128]的病例。在影像学上，异位胰腺表现为一个平滑、广基底的黏膜下肿物，约 45% 的患者有典型的中央凹陷。EUS 用于术前准确鉴别胃肠道间质瘤和异位胰腺[129]，EUS 的典型特征包括胃窦位置、黏膜凹陷、3～4 层组织、病变导管[130]。必要时，如果症状明显或需要病理证据，内镜下使用圈套器进行结扎及切除术可以安全地切除病变[131]。手术切除可作为另一种治疗选择，但在是否切除偶然发现的异位胰腺组织方面仍存在争议，有病例报告显示，异位胰腺有一定的恶变潜能[132]。

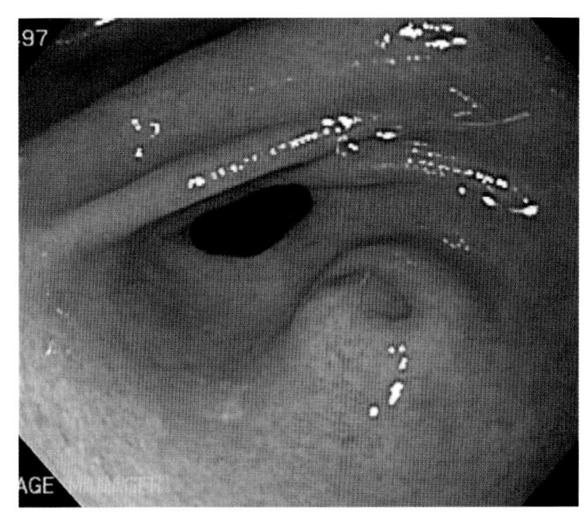

图 55.13　一名 8 岁男孩胃窦内异位胰腺的内镜视图。注意中央凹陷

（四）胰腺发育不全

胰腺发育不全是一种罕见的情况，既可以是完全的，也可以是部分的。具有靶向胰岛素启动因子 1（*IPF1*）基因突变的纯合子小鼠出生时没有胰腺，且研究表明，胰腺发育不全的患者可存在 *PDX1* 和 *PTF1A* 基因突变[49,57,133]。最近有重要研究表明，在 27 名胰腺发育不全患者的队列中有 15 名患者存在 *GATA6* 基因突变[134]。

完全胰腺发育不全大多可致命，由于患儿患有糖尿病和吸收不良，同时由于缺乏胰岛素，这种重要的宫内生长因子，该病患儿可出现宫内生长迟缓[135,136]。部分胰腺发育不全，或背侧胰腺发育不全，由于仍有功能性胰腺组织的存在，临床表现可能并不显著。背侧胰腺发育不全，也称先天性短胰腺，与多脾综合征和胃肠道旋转不良[137]、肾脏异常[138]和异位有关[139]。最近的一项研究对一种与青年成熟期发病的糖尿病相关的新表现型进行了报道，这种糖尿病是由 *PDX1* 的变异引起的[140]。胰腺发育不全应通过临床表现进行初步诊断，并通过 MRI 进行进一步证实。

(五) 先天性囊肿

先天性胰脏囊肿是罕见的,可出现于任何年龄段人群,甚至在产前超声波常规检查也可以确诊[141,142]。囊肿为单发或多发,与胰液聚集的区别在于上皮细胞的存在。囊肿被认为是由于胰腺导管系统发育异常而形成的。通常随着永久性导管的发育,胚胎导管会退化;然而,若胚胎导管持续存在时,它们会发生堵塞和积液,导致先天性囊肿[143]。

临床表现不定,从影像学检查偶然发现到触及腹部肿块,可表现为伴有或不伴有呕吐、胆道梗阻或急性胰腺炎。孤立性胰腺囊肿通常是肠内多发囊肿,可能完全位于胰腺实质内,并可与胰管相通[144]。多发胰腺囊肿多发生于有相关异常表现的患者中,可见于系统性疾病,如 von HippelLandau 综合征、Ivemark Ⅱ综合征或多囊肾[145,146]。对 15 例先天性胰腺囊肿患者回顾性研究中,大多数在 2 岁前出现,30% 的病例发现相关的异常表现[147]。先天性胰腺囊肿多位于胰体和胰尾(62%),胰头较少(32%)[148]。手术治疗可完全切除囊肿。胰头囊肿可以在必要时使用内镜或手术引流以解决。

(六) 胰胆管畸形愈合

胰胆管畸形汇合(pancreaticobiliary malunion,PBM)是一种先天畸形,由于胆汁和胰液的排泌管道之间没有间隔而形成共同通道所致(图 55.14)。PBM 可伴有胆管扩张。两根导管的异常汇合常发生在十二指肠壁以外;因此 Oddi 括约肌作用于胆胰管的舒缩作用消失,使胰腺外分泌物可进入胆道系统,胆汁也可进入胰管。最近的数据表明,在共同通道大于等于 5mm 的患者胆汁中可以检测出淀粉酶浓度明显升高[149]。若淤积的胆汁与反流的胰液混合,混合处胆管肿瘤发病风险将在患者成年期升高[150]。胆道肿瘤最常见于胆囊内;然而,若患者存在先天胆道扩张,则胆管肿瘤的发病风险也会增加至 32.1%,而没有胆道扩张的患者胆道肿瘤的发病率为 7.3%[151]。反之同理,胆汁反流到胰腺也会增加急性胰腺炎的发病风险。

PBM 分为 3 种类型:pb 型,指胰管汇入胆管;bp 型,指胆管汇入胰管;以及 Y 型,指胆管与胰管有长达 15mm 甚至更长的共同通道[152,153]。大量研究表明,bp 型和 pb 型为最常见的 PBM 类型[154,155]。大约 15% 的复发性胰腺炎患儿存在这种异常[155],且胆管囊肿通常也与 PBM 有关(两组实验结果分别为 94% 和 100%)[55,154]。胰胆管畸形愈合可以通过传统胆道造影(ERCP、术中胆管造影或经皮胆管造影)、MRCP 或螺旋 CT 扫描进行诊断。诊断金标准仍为传统胆道造影。

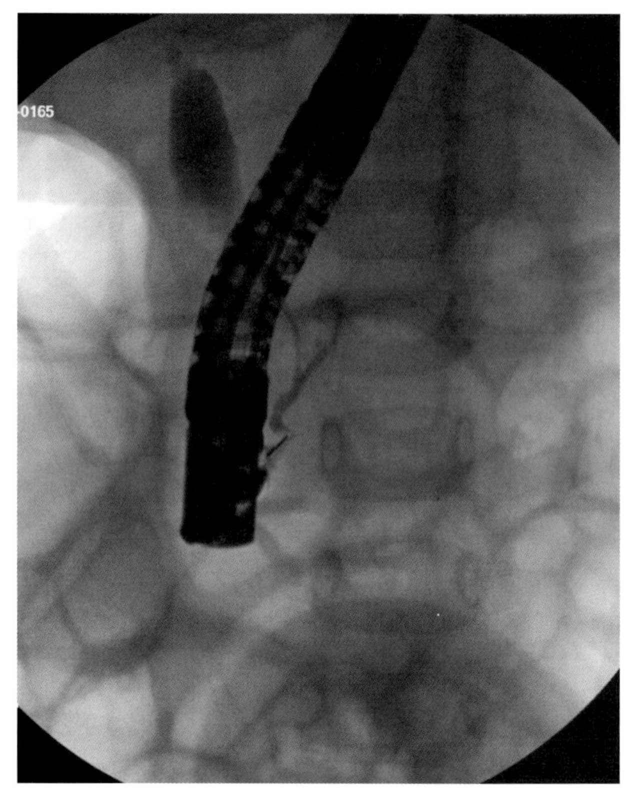

图 55.14　一例 4 岁女性的 ERCP 显示胆总管囊肿和长共同通道。继发于急性和慢性胰腺炎的胆总管狭窄穿过胰头

研究表明,胰胆汇合异常的患者发生胆道恶性肿瘤的风险有所增加。62.5% 的成人胆囊癌患者、50% 的胆囊腺肌瘤病患者和 33.3% 的胆管癌患者存在胰胆管汇合畸形[154]。此外,PBM 患者较非 PBM 患者,出现胆管癌的时间会早 15~20 年[150]。在日本,PBM 患者无论伴有或不伴有胆管囊性扩张,其胆囊癌发病率均较高[156]。PBM 患者胆囊黏膜的细胞增殖活性增加,儿童期早期亦是[157]。尽管对于 PBM 患者的管理方式随不同人种而发生变化[158-160],但由于存在这种异常表现的患者癌症风险均升高,推荐采用胆囊切除术、胆管切除术和肝空肠吻合术进行治疗[156,161]。

(施海韵 译,孙明瑜　李鹏 校)

参考文献

第 56 章 胰腺分泌

Stephen J. Pandol 著

章节目录

一、功能性解剖 …… 805
二、外分泌物的组成 …… 806
（一）无机成分 …… 806
（二）有机成分 …… 807
三、主要消化酶的功能 …… 807
（一）淀粉酶 …… 807
（二）脂肪酶 …… 807
（三）蛋白酶 …… 808
四、消化酶的合成与运输 …… 808
蛋白质合成的调控 …… 808
五、酶分泌的细胞调节 …… 808
六、器官生理学 …… 809
（一）消化间期的分泌 …… 809
（二）消化分泌 …… 809
（三）反馈调节 …… 810
七、胰腺分泌功能试验 …… 810
（一）直接试验 …… 811
（二）间接试验 …… 812

很长一段时间以来，胰腺外分泌引起了生理学家和其他科学家的极大兴趣；实际上，20 世纪之交在胰腺中首次证明了激素的作用[1]。胰腺是集蛋白的合成和运输[2]，离子和水的分泌[3,4]，以及这些过程中包含的信号转导[5]机制的主要器官。本章简要描述了当前对胰腺外分泌生理学的认识。

一、功能性解剖

胰腺外分泌的功能单元由腺泡及其引流小管组成（图 56.1）[6]。导管上皮细胞延伸至腺泡管腔，中心腺泡细胞位于导管上皮延伸至腺泡中（见第 55 章）。中心腺泡细胞在为胰腺细胞谱系提供祖细胞方面起着关键作用[7,8]。导管引流进小叶间导管，继而排入主胰管系统。

腺泡（acinus）可以是球形或管状，如图 56.1 所示，或者可以具有其他一些不规则形状[6]。腺泡细胞专门用于合成、储存和分泌消化酶。刺激酶分泌的激素和神经递质的受体位于其基底外侧膜上[5]。细胞的底部包含细胞核以及丰富的粗面内质网（rough endoplasmic reticulum，RER），用于蛋白质合成（图 56.2，左）。细胞的顶端区域含有储存消化酶的酶原颗粒。腺泡细胞的顶面还具有微绒毛。在微绒毛内和在顶质膜下面的细胞质中是丝状肌动蛋白网，参与酶原颗粒内容物的胞吐作用[9]。分泌物进入腺泡腔。腺泡细胞之间的紧密连接

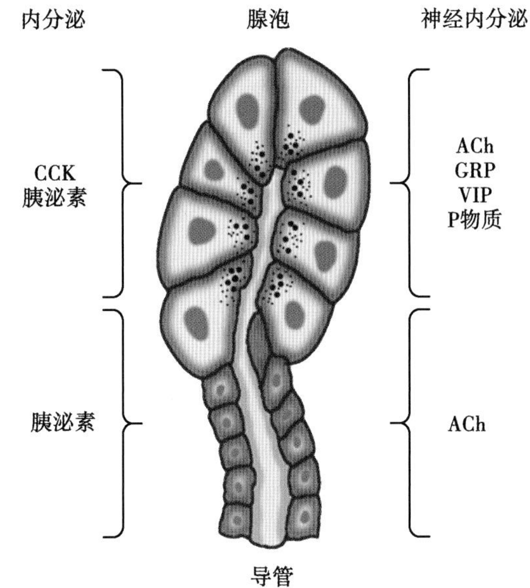

图 56.1 肠消化期间胰腺外分泌的调节。外分泌受内分泌和神经内分泌途径调节。此外，内分泌和神经内分泌介质对腺泡和导管的分泌调节不同。对于腺泡，胆囊收缩素（CCK）、胰泌素、乙酰胆碱（ACh）、胃泌素释放肽（GRP）、血管活性肠肽（VIP）和 P 物质调节分泌［信号机制（第二信使）如图 56.6 所示］。胰泌素和 ACh 是胰腺导管分泌碳酸氢盐的主要调节因子（参与导管分泌的转运蛋白如图 56.4 所示）。（Adapted from Gorelick F，Pandol SJ，Topazian M. Pancreatic physiology，pathophysiology，acute and chronic pancreatitis. Gastrointestinal Teaching Project，American Gastroenterological Association；2003.）

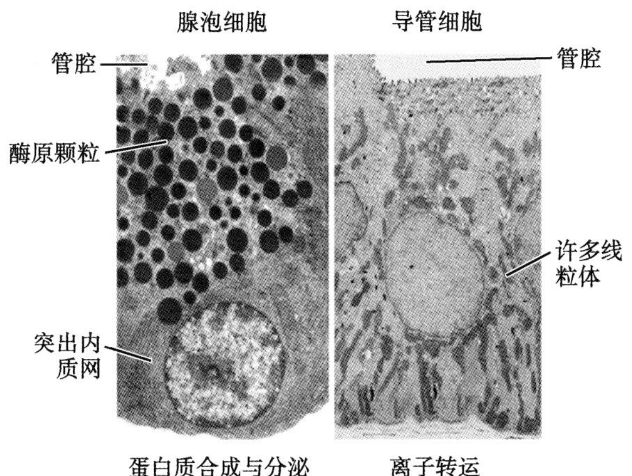

图 56.2 外分泌细胞的超微结构。外分泌细胞的超微结构反映了其特殊功能。胰腺腺泡细胞（左）和导管细胞（右）均被极化，具有明确的顶端（管腔）、外侧和基底区域。胰腺腺泡细胞有明显的基底粗面内质网，用于合成消化酶，顶端有酶原颗粒，用于存储和分泌消化酶。胰管细胞含有许多线粒体，用于产生其离子转运功能所需的能量。（Adapted from Gorelick F，Pandol SJ，Topazian M. Pancreatic physiology，pathophysiology，acute and chronic pancreatitis. Gastrointestinal Teaching Project，American Gastroenterological Association；2003.）

在细胞的顶端周围形成一条有屏障作用的带，阻止例如消化酶这样的大分子通过[10]。连接复合物也提供水和离子的细胞旁通道。

腺泡细胞之间的另一种细胞间连接是间隙连接。这些相邻细胞之间特有的质膜起着小孔的作用，允许小分子（分子量 500~1 000Da）通过。间隙连接允许细胞之间的化学物质和电子的交流。例如，钙信号在腺泡细胞之间协调影响着消化酶的分泌[11,12]。

导管上皮由柱状细胞和锥状细胞组成，并含有丰富的线粒体，这是离子运输所需能量产物所必需的（见图 56.2，右）。导管细胞和中心棘突细胞都含有碳酸酐酶，这对于它们分泌碳酸氢盐很重要[3]。

二、外分泌物的组成

（一）无机成分

胰腺外分泌液的主要无机成分是水、钠、钾、氯化物和碳酸氢盐（图 56.3）。水和离子分泌的目的是将消化酶输送到肠腔，并帮助中和排入十二指肠的胃酸。用促胰液素刺激过程中分泌的胰液澄清、无色、呈碱性且与血浆等渗。流速从静止（消化间）状态下的平均流速 0.2 或 0.3mL/min 增加到餐后刺激过程中的 4.0mL/min。每日总分泌量为 2.5L。胰液的渗透压与流速无关。然而，当胰腺受到促胰液素（更大体积输出的主要介质）的刺激时，碳酸氢盐和氯化物的浓度会相互改变（见图 56.3）。

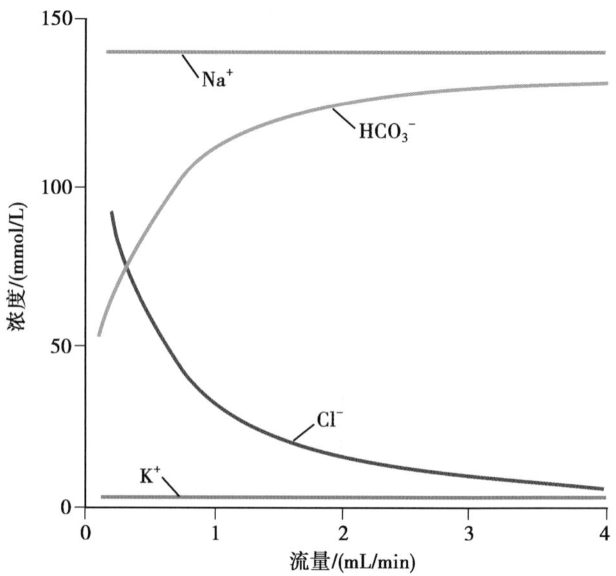

图 56.3 胰腺碳酸氢盐和其他电解质的分泌。随着刺激（即一餐），胰腺分泌物的流量增加。此外，随着流速的升高，胰液中氯化物和碳酸氢盐的浓度发生显著变化。碳酸氢盐浓度升高导致碱性分泌。碳酸氢盐来自胰腺导管上皮细胞。与腺泡细胞相反，导管分泌大量含有高浓度碳酸氢盐的液体。与导管分泌相比，腺泡细胞的分泌量被认为是较小的，随着胰腺刺激的增加，离子浓度接近导管分泌物的浓度。值得注意的是，来自胰腺、胆道系统和十二指肠黏膜的碱性分泌物可中和从胃输送到十二指肠的酸性分泌。这种 pH 中性环境对于最佳的消化酶和肠黏膜功能非常重要。（Adapted from Gorelick F，Pandol SJ，Topazian M. Pancreatic physiology，pathophysiology，acute and chronic pancreatitis. Gastrointestinal Teaching Project，American Gastroenterological Association；2003.）

促胰液素通过结合其在导管细胞基底外侧膜上的受体来刺激分泌，从而激活腺苷酸环化酶并增加环状单磷酸腺苷（cAMP）；而乙酰胆碱通过结合其受体并提高细胞内钙离子浓度来做到这一点[3]。促胰液素刺激的初始步骤涉及腔膜上依赖 cAMP 和依赖 Ca^{2+} 的氯离子（Cl^-）通道活化以及基底外侧膜的 K^+ 通道活化（图 56.4）[3,13]。依赖 cAMP 的 Cl^- 腔通

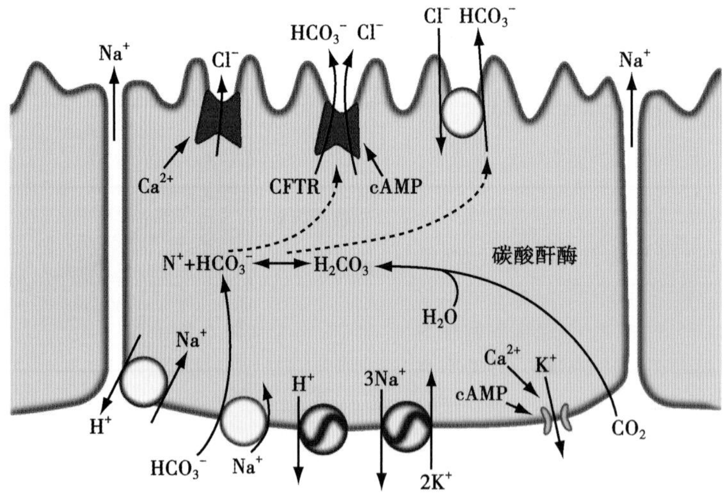

图 56.4 胰管细胞的离子转运。HCO_3^- 通过两种机制递送用于最终分泌。其一是膜可扩散的 CO_2 在碳酸酐酶的作用下，催化转化为 HCO_3^- 和 H^+，H_2CO3 脱水酶使 CO_2 水合，从而形成 H_2CO_3，然后解离为 HCO_3^- 和 H^+。胰管细胞富含碳酸酐酶。在另一种情况下，Na^+ 和 HCO_3^- 在基底外侧膜上共转运。然后，HCO_3^- 通过囊性纤维化跨膜转导调节因子（CFTR）和 Cl^--HCO_3^- 阴离子交换均可用于顶端分泌。Na^+ 和 H_2O 通过细胞间连接输送到管腔。H^+ 通过基底外侧 Na^+、H^+ 反向转运和 H^+-ATP 酶从细胞中清除，以维持细胞内 pH 恒定。通过增加细胞环磷酸腺苷（cAMP）水平（胰泌素）和钙水平（乙酰胆碱）的激动剂（即胰泌素和乙酰胆碱）增加顶端 Cl^- 和 HCO_3^- 通道以及基底外侧 K^+ 通道的通透性，来激活分泌。（Adapted from Gorelick F，Pandol SJ，Topazian M. Pancreatic physiology，pathophysiology，acute and chronic pancreatitis. Gastrointestinal Teaching Project，American Gastroenterological Association；2003.）

道是囊性纤维化跨膜转导调节因子(CFTR)[13,14]。cAMP 激活该通道导致 Cl^- 分泌到管腔中,并与 Cl^--HCO_3^- 的反向运输联动,导致腔内的 Cl^- 交换为 HCO_3^-。有证据表明 CFTR 也直接参与 HCO_3^- 的分泌[3,4,15,16]。在导管细胞的基底外侧表面上有 Na^+、H^+ 反向运输,Na^+、HCO_3^- 同向运输,2 个 ATP 酶(H^+-ATPase 和 Na^+,K^+-ATPase)和一个 K^+ 通道。总之,这些转运蛋白可促进 HCO_3^- 在根尖表面的分泌,并在导管细胞内维持中性 pH[17]。Na^+ 和水被分泌到导管系统中,以抵消 HCO_3^- 分泌所产生的电势和渗透压。CFTR 功能完全缺失的突变在儿童时期会导致外分泌胰腺的破坏,而部分功能的突变则会在以后的生活中导致胰腺炎[18]。此外,最近的研究表明,酗酒和吸烟会导致 CFTR 功能受到抑制从而引起胰腺炎[19,20]。

(二) 有机成分[21-24]

人的胰腺具有合成蛋白质(主要是消化酶)的能力。框 56.1 列出了主要的蛋白水解酶、淀粉分解酶、脂解酶和核酸酶等消化酶。某些酶以多种的形式存在(如阳离子胰蛋白酶原、阴离子胰蛋白酶原和中胰蛋白酶原)。能够消化胰腺的酶储存在胰腺中,并作为不活跃的前体形式分泌到胰管中。如图 56.5 所示,这些酶的激活发生在肠腔中,其中一种肠糖蛋白肽酶肠激酶通过去除(水解)分子的 N 端六肽片段(Val-Asp-Asp-Asp-Asp-Lys)来激活胰蛋白酶原[21]。然后,催化其他非活性前酶的活化。

除消化酶外,腺泡细胞还分泌胰蛋白酶抑制剂:胰分泌胰蛋白酶抑制剂。这种 56 个氨基酸组成的肽通过与酶在催化位点附近形成相对稳定的复合物,而使胰蛋白酶失活[25]。胰蛋白酶是在胰腺或胰液中自发形成的,抑制剂的作用是使胰蛋白酶失活并促进其降解,从而防止胰腺炎等疾病的发生[26]。

框 56.1　胰腺腺泡细胞分泌产物

酶原*
阴离子胰蛋白酶原
阳离子胰蛋白酶原
糜蛋白酶原(A 和 B)
激肽原
中胰蛋白酶原
前羧肽酶 A(1 和 2)
前羧肽酶 B(1 和 2)
弹性蛋白酶原
前磷脂酶 A_2

酶
淀粉酶
羧酸酯酶
脱氧核糖核酸酶
脂肪酶(甘油三酯脂肪酶)
核糖核酸酶
甾醇脂酶

*列出的酶原储存在胰腺中,并以无活性的酶原形式分泌到十二指肠腔中。如果这些酶在胰腺中具有活性,它们将会消化胰腺。其他酶,如淀粉酶和脂肪酶,以其活性形式存储和分泌。

Adapted from Gorelick F, Pandol SJ, Topazian M. Pancreatic physiology, pathophysiology, acute and chronic pancreatitis. Gastrointestinal Teaching Project, American Gastroenterological Association; 2003.

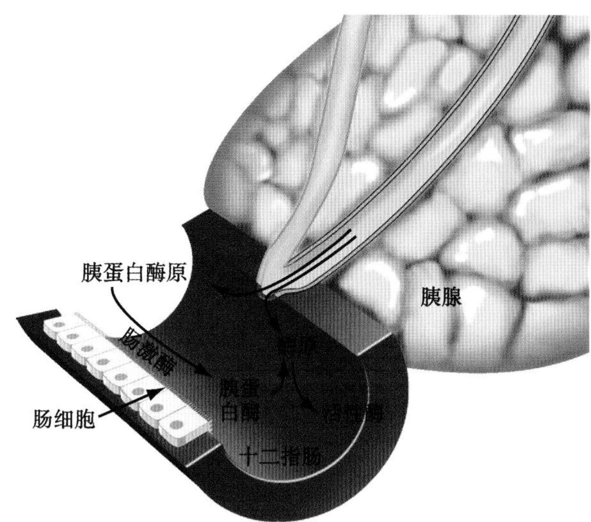

图 56.5　酶原活化位点。胰蛋白酶原、糜蛋白酶原、弹性蛋白酶原、羧肽原酶和磷脂酶原 A2 储存在胰腺中,并以无活性的酶原形式分泌到十二指肠腔中。其他酶,如淀粉酶和脂肪酶,以其活性形式存储和分泌。后一种酶的活性形式对胰腺没有影响,因为它不含淀粉或甘油三酯(TG)。无活性酶原的激活发生在十二指肠腔中。在那里,刷状缘酶肠激酶将分泌的胰蛋白酶原转化为胰蛋白酶。然后,胰蛋白酶原和其他酶原通过胰蛋白酶的蛋白水解裂解转化为活性形式。(Adapted from Gorelick F, Pandol SJ, Topazian M. Pancreatic physiology, pathophysiology, acute and chronic pancreatitis. Gastrointestinal Teaching Project, American Gastroenterological Association; 2003.)

三、主要消化酶的功能

(一) 淀粉酶

人淀粉酶由胰腺和唾液腺分泌。这些酶消化饮食中的淀粉和糖原。人唾液淀粉酶和胰淀粉酶具有相同的酶活性。但是,它们的分子量,碳水化合物含量和电泳迁移率有所不同[27]。唾液淀粉酶可在口腔中启动消化,并可能占淀粉和糖原消化的很大一部分,因为它在与食物一起被输送到胃和小肠时起着持续性的作用。在胃中,可以通过进餐,以及唾液和胃黏液的碱性环境来缓冲分泌的胃酸的影响,从而保护淀粉酶活性。唾液和胰淀粉酶的作用都是水解每一个碳 1 和氧之间连接处的 1,4-糖苷键。淀粉酶消化的产物是麦芽糖和麦芽三糖(分别为 2-和 3-α-1,4-连接分子)和含有 1,6-糖苷键的 α-糊精,因为淀粉中的 1,6-糖苷键不能被淀粉酶水解。肠细胞的刷状缘酶将淀粉酶消化产物完全水解为葡萄糖。最终产物葡萄糖通过 Na^+ 偶联转运,转运到整个肠吸收性上皮细胞(见第 102 章)[28]。

(二) 脂肪酶

胰腺分泌 3 种脂肪酶:脂肪酶(或 TG 脂肪酶)、原磷脂酶 A2 和羧酸酯酶(见框 56.1)。唾液(舌)和胃脂肪酶也有助于脂肪的消化,但幅度较小(参见第 50 章)。胰腺脂肪酶结合在 TG 油滴的油-水界面上,在那里它将 TG 分子水解成从碳 1 和 3 释放的 2 个脂肪酸分子,进而一个单甘酯和一个脂肪酸在碳 2 处酯化成甘油[21,29]。胆汁酸和脂肪酶对于脂肪酶的活性很重要。胆汁酸有助于 TG 的乳化,以扩大脂肪酶作用的表面积,它们与脂肪酸和甘油单酸酯形成胶束,进而从油水界面除去这些产物。辅脂肪酶被认为与脂酶和胆汁盐形成复合物。该三元复合物锚定脂肪酶,并使其在更亲水的环境中能够作用于油滴的疏水表面。磷脂酶 A_2 催化磷脂酰胆碱碳 2 处的脂肪酸酯键的水解[23]。这种裂解导致游离脂肪酸和溶血磷脂酰胆碱的形成。羧基酯酶具有广泛的特异性,可裂解胆固醇酯、脂溶性维生素酯、TG、甘油二酯和甘油单酯。胆盐对这种酶的充分活动也很重要[30]。

(三) 蛋白酶

胰腺分泌多种蛋白酶原,在十二指肠被胰蛋白酶激活(见框 56.1)。胰蛋白酶,糜蛋白酶和弹性蛋白酶是切割与特定氨基酸相邻的特定肽键的内肽酶[21]。胰液中还含有羧肽酶,羧肽酶是在蛋白质的羧基末端切割肽键的外肽酶。

胃蛋白酶和胰蛋白酶的联合作用导致寡肽和游离氨基酸的形成。这些寡肽可以被肠细胞刷状缘酶进一步消化(见第 102 章)。游离的氨基酸和寡肽通过一组与 Na^+ 和 H^+ 偶联转运蛋白跨肠黏膜转运[31]。有趣的是,在消化过程中只有某些氨基酸(主要是必需氨基酸)可以在管腔中测量,这表明蛋白酶的组合作用不是随机的,是由各个蛋白酶的特异性组合产生的。这些氨基酸在刺激胰腺分泌,抑制胃排空,调节小肠蠕动和引起饱腹感方面具有更大的作用。因此,蛋白酶作用的特定模式导致了胃肠道中几个器官的生理调节。

四、消化酶的合成与运输

消化酶的合成发生在 RER 的内部空间中(见图 56.2,左)[2,32]。信号假说解释了将细胞信使 RNA(mRNA)转化为可输出蛋白的机制。该假说的主要特征是核糖体亚基附着在 mRNA 上,并在新生蛋白质的 NH2 末端启动疏水性"信号"序列的合成。然后,该复合物附着在内质网的外表面,并且信号序列将被合成的蛋白质定向进入内质网的管腔。

新合成的蛋白质可在内质网中发生修饰,包括二硫键的形成,磷酸化,硫酸化和糖基化[33]。在内质网中也发生构象变化,影响蛋白质的三级和四级结构。RER 中加工过的蛋白质被转运到高尔基复合体,在那里发生进一步的转译后修饰和浓缩[34]。为了使蛋白质在各个区室之间发挥适当的功能和转运,需要重要的构象特异性。被叫作伴侣蛋白和折叠酶的蛋白促进了这些构象特异性。当 RER 对蛋白质合成的需求增加时或当细胞应激导致蛋白质解折叠时,RER 通过增加分子伴侣和折叠酶的合成来作出反应,停止蛋白质的合成,甚至使用未折叠蛋白反应(unfolded protein response,UPR)的机制来降解未折叠的蛋白质[33]。通过将蛋白质保持在适当的构象,UPR 可以维持蛋白质在细胞区室之间的正常运输。重要的是,最近的研究表明,过量饮酒和吸烟介导胰腺炎的机制之一是通过改变 RER 中的蛋白质折叠并抑制 UPR 来实现的[35-37]。

高尔基复合体还具有将新合成的蛋白质分类和靶向到各种细胞区室中的重要功能。消化酶被运输到酶原颗粒,而溶酶体水解酶被分类到溶酶体[32,38,39]。与酶原颗粒相比,对溶酶体的分类机制有了更好的理解。对于溶酶体途径,在蛋白质以顺式-高尔基体形式存在期间,将 6-磷酸甘露糖基团添加到蛋白质的寡糖链上。6-磷酸甘露糖基团充当特定受体的识别位点。溶酶体酶 6-磷酸甘露糖与其受体的相互作用导致形成囊泡,该囊泡将该复合物转运至溶酶体,从而递送酶。在溶酶体中,酶从受体解离,继而循环回到高尔基体。消化酶是通过胞吐作用分泌的[2]。胞吐作用包括分泌颗粒向顶端表面移动,识别质膜部位进行融合以及融合后颗粒膜-质膜-膜部位的裂变。研究已证明肌动蛋白-肌球蛋白[40-43]、可溶性 N-乙基马来酰亚胺敏感因子附着蛋白受体(SNARE)蛋白[44,45]和鸟肽三磷酸结合蛋白在这些过程中的作用[42,46,47]。激动剂受体产生的细胞内信号与这些实体相互作用,通过酶原颗粒的胞吐作用介导消化酶的分泌。

蛋白质合成的调控

之前已部分阐明了调节胰腺外分泌中消化酶表达的机制。研究解决了以下两个问题:第一,消化酶在胰腺中的特异性表达是什么原因? 第二,饮食营养素的变化如何改变特定消化酶的合成? 第一个问题的答案是,消化酶(如淀粉酶、糜蛋白酶和弹性蛋白酶)的基因在其 5' 侧翼核苷酸序列中含有增强子区域,该区域调节其 mRNA 的转录,称为胰腺共有元件[48-51]。胰腺转录因子-1 选择性存在于外分泌胰腺中,并与该区域结合,是这些消化酶的表达所必需的[52,53]。因此,胰腺转录因子-1 至少代表一种解释胰腺中消化酶表达的差异调节因子。关于第二个问题,大量研究表明,特定消化酶的相对合成速率随饮食摄入量而变化。例如,富含碳水化合物的饮食会导致淀粉酶的合成增加,而导致糜蛋白酶原的减少[54];富含脂质的饮食会增强脂肪酶的表达[55];富含酒精的饮食会降低淀粉酶的表达[56]。证明淀粉酶基因的表达受胰岛素和饮食的调节[56]。引起这种适应的机制仅被部分理解,包括转录和转录后调节[54]。

五、酶分泌的细胞调节

通过体外制备来自小动物的分散的腺泡细胞和腺泡,证实了神经体液刺激腺泡细胞的机制。涉及使用人体组织的研究是有限的,但在外分泌胰腺的生理和病理生理研究中非常重要[57-59]。

通过使用放射性标记的配体和特异性拮抗剂,已在几种物种的制剂中鉴定出胆囊收缩素(CCK)、乙酰胆碱、胃泌素释放肽(GRP)、P 物质、血管活性肠肽(VIP)和促胰液素的受体。此外,已经通过克隆和测序阐明了每种受体类型的分子结构[60,61]。每种都是 G 蛋白偶联受体,具有 7 个疏水域,被认为是跨膜区段(见第 4 章)。这些受体位于腺泡细胞的基底外侧质膜上。

腺泡细胞上的受体根据刺激-分泌耦联的方式分为两类(图 56.6)。第一类是 VIP 和胰泌素。这些药物与腺泡细胞的相互作用导致腺苷酸环化酶的激活和细胞 cAMP 的升高,进而通过 cAMP 依赖性蛋白激酶 A 激活胞吐作用和酶分泌[62]。第二类是乙酰胆碱、CCK、GRP 和 P 物质。这些激动剂的作用包括刺激膜磷酸肌醇的细胞代谢和通过动员细胞内

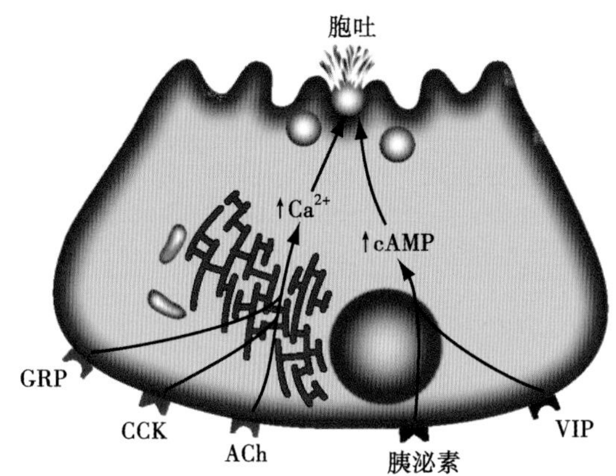

图 56.6 受体介导的分泌。刺激消化酶分泌的胰腺腺泡细胞激动剂通过 2 种不同的途径发挥作用。在一种途径中，激动剂如胃泌素释放肽（GRP）、胆囊收缩素（CCK）和乙酰胆碱（ACh）通过细胞钙（Ca^{+}）的增加介导分泌。在另一种途径中，激动剂如血管活性肠肽（VIP）和胰泌素通过增加细胞环磷酸腺苷（cAMP）介导分泌。联合激动剂刺激后，细胞钙和 cAMP 同时增加对分泌具有协同效应。也就是说，观察到的反应大于单独作用的单个激动剂的累加反应预期的反应。（Adapted from Gorelick F, Pandol SJ, Topazian M. Pancreatic physiology, pathophysiology, acute and chronic pancreatitis. Gastrointestinal Teaching Project, American Gastroenterological Association; 2003.）

储备提高细胞内游离钙浓度（$[Ca^{2+}]_i$）[63,64]。具体来说，激动剂--受体相互作用导致磷脂酶 C 介导的磷脂酰肌醇 4,5-二磷酸水解为 1,2-二酰基甘油和肌醇 1,4,5-三磷酸酯（IP_3）。IP_3 又从内质网存储中释放钙。钙释放到细胞质中导致介导分泌反应的游离钙浓度迅速升高[65]。钙释放到细胞质中也是由兰尼碱受体和与兰尼碱受体相互作用的信号介导的，如钙和脂肪酸辅酶 A（CoA）酯[66,67]。参与细胞内钙释放的其他分子为环二磷酸腺苷--核糖和烟酸腺嘌呤二核苷酸磷酸[68,69]。

细胞内增加$[Ca^{2+}]$介导分泌的机制尚未确定，但涉及钙调蛋白依赖性蛋白激酶和肌动蛋白-肌球蛋白相互作用，SNARE 蛋白和鸟苷三磷酸结合蛋白如前所述。这些试剂对酶分泌的持续刺激还取决于细胞外钙的内流[70]。内流机制涉及内部内质网及其钙存储以及与质膜通道相连的一组支架蛋白之间的复杂相互作用[71]。钙流入所必需的质膜通道由 Orai-1[72] 的亚基组成。Orai-1 通道在胰腺炎的治疗中的重要性正在显现，因为该通道在实验性胰腺炎中被高度激活，而对 Orai-1 的抑制降低了胰腺炎的严重程度[73]。

酶分泌的胞内机制还可以通过 1,2-二酰基甘油和蛋白激酶 C[74]，以及花生四烯酸来调节[75]。cAMP 激动剂和磷酸肌醇钙激动剂也会使细胞蛋白发生特定的磷酸化和去磷酸化[76]。这些机制在分泌中的确切作用尚未确定。

腺泡细胞对通过 cAMP 和钙变化起效的激动剂组合的最终酶分泌反应超过了这两种单独反应的总和。这种组合的一个例子是 VIP 或促胰液素与乙酰胆碱。这种增强反应的确切机制尚不清楚，但它可能在生理上发挥作用，从而产生大量的分泌。

六、器官生理学

人的胰腺外分泌发生在禁食（消化间期）状态和进食（消化）后。当消化道上部的食物被清除时，消化的分泌模式开始。对一个每天吃 3 顿饭的人来说，消化模式从早餐后开始，一直持续到一天的晚些时候，在消化道清除了晚餐后。

（一）消化间期的分泌

胰腺在消化间期的分泌模式是周期性的，并遵循迁移肌电复合体的规律（migrating myoelectric complex, MMC；参见第 99 章）[77,78]。这种规律每 60～120 分钟出现一次，酶分泌的激增与胃和十二指肠（即第二和第三阶段）蠕动增强的时间段有关。在 MMC 的Ⅱ期和Ⅲ期中，除了胰腺酶的分泌外，十二指肠中碳酸氢盐和胆汁的分泌（继发至部分胆囊收缩）也增加了（见第 64 章）。底层机制涉及胆碱能神经系统以及胃动素和胰多肽[78,79]。消化间期阶段的胰腺分泌是 MMC"管家"功能中的一部分（见第 99 章）。

（二）消化分泌

与胃分泌一样，胰腺外分泌随着进食分为 3 个阶段：头期、胃期和肠期。

迷走神经调节外分泌的头期。通过测量假喂食（咀嚼和吐出食物）刺激的外分泌，可以评估人类对胰腺外分泌的头期刺激程度。一项研究[80]表明，假性喂养刺激胰腺酶分泌，其分泌率高达最大分泌率的 50%，当酸性胃分泌物被阻止进入十二指肠时，碳酸氢盐分泌物却没有增加。当胃分泌物进入十二指肠时，胰酶的分泌率上升到最大值的约 90%，碳酸氢盐也被分泌出来。这些结果表明，头部刺激可特异性地增加胰腺中腺泡的分泌，而十二指肠中较低的 pH（来自胃酸）会增加腺泡的分泌，并引起导管中的碳酸氢盐分泌。

乙酰胆碱无疑是介导头期胰腺分泌的主要神经递质，因为胆碱能拮抗剂能极大地减少甚至在某些情况下消除假喂养刺激的胰腺分泌[81,82]。在胰腺中发现含有肽 VIP、GRP、CCK 和脑啡肽的神经末梢。对于 VIP 和 GRP，支持这些肽在分泌性头期中作用的数据最有力[83,84]。在动物的迷走神经刺激下，这两种肽均被释放到胰腺静脉流出物中。此外，如前所述，腺泡细胞具有介导酶分泌的 GRP 和 VIP 受体（见图 56.6）。导管上皮还通过分泌水和碳酸氢盐对 VIP 作出反应[84]。

胃期胰腺的分泌是由于食物刺激作用于胃。主要的刺激是胃胀，它主要引起酶的分泌，而很少分泌水和碳酸氢盐。胃底或胃窦的球囊扩张可通过胃胰迷走神经反射而导致少量，富含酶的分泌[85]。

当胃液和餐食进入十二指肠时，各种腔内刺激物通过神经和体液机制作用于肠道黏膜，刺激胰腺分泌。胃的 3 个过程——酸、胃蛋白酶和脂肪酶的分泌、消化和排空——与胰腺分泌的肠期机制紧密相关。当食糜开始从胃进入小肠时，肠期就开始了。它是由激素和肠胰迷走神经反射介导的。

与头和胃期相比，在肠期有显著的导管分泌。导管内分泌是由肠腔中的氢离子引发的。当管腔的 pH 小于 4.5[86,87]时，分泌素由十二指肠黏膜的肠内分泌 S 细胞释放。释放的促胰液素的量以及胰腺分泌的体积取决于输送到十二指肠的可滴定酸的负荷。用特异性抗分泌素抗体免疫中和胰液素可使膳食刺激的胰腺体积和碳酸氢盐分泌减少多达 80%[88]。

抗分泌素抗体也能抑制食物刺激酶分泌多达 50%,这表明促胰液素还具有以下作用:可能通过增强激动剂(如乙酰胆碱)的作用来分泌酶。因此,完全的膳食刺激反应是由多种介质的组合产生的。

在肠期,消化酶的胰腺分泌是由长度超过 8 个碳的管腔内脂肪酸,这些脂肪酸的单甘油酯,肽,氨基酸和少量葡萄糖介导的[89]。最有效的刺激人类胰腺分泌的氨基酸包括苯丙氨酸,缬氨酸,蛋氨酸和色氨酸[90]。胰腺对肽和氨基酸的反应与灌注到肠道的总负荷有关,而与浓度无关[91,92]。

肠道刺激引起的酶分泌反应的介质是神经和体液(图 56.7)。迷走神经干切断术和阿托品显著抑制酶(和碳酸氢盐)对肠道氨基酸和脂肪酸的低负荷以及生理浓度的 CCK 输注的反应[93,94]。这些结果表明,迷走神经反射可介导酶的分泌并增加碳酸氢根。分泌素刺激分泌。

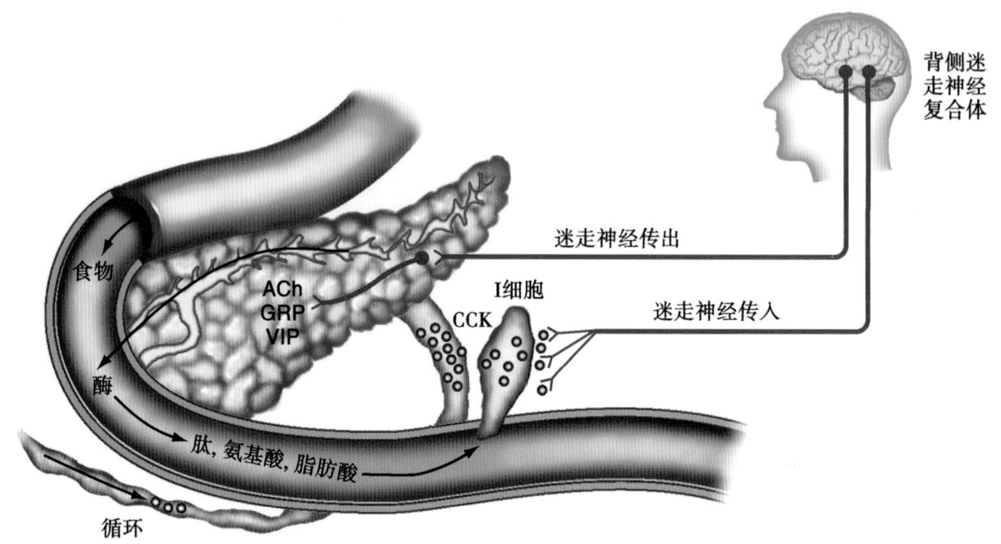

图 56.7 图示说明了介导涉及胆囊收缩素(CCK)的膳食刺激胰腺分泌的几种神经和激素途径。首先,输送到十二指肠中的肽、氨基酸和脂肪酸等膳食营养物质刺激 CCK 从含 CCK 的 I 细胞局部释放到 I 细胞基底外侧表面周围的区域。释放的 CCK 激活迷走神经传入神经元,将信号传递到背侧迷走神经复合体,在那里感觉信息被整合,迷走神经传出被激活。迷走神经传出与胰腺神经节神经元形成突触。反过来,通过神经递质乙酰胆碱(ACh)、胃泌素释放肽(GRP)和血管活性肠肽(VIP),产生于胰腺神经节的效应神经元激活胰腺实质细胞的分泌。除激活神经通路外,I 细胞释放的 CCK 进入全身循环,并可能作为胰腺腺泡细胞上的激素引起分泌。(Adapted from Gorelick F, Pandol SJ, Topazian M. Pancreatic physiology, pathophysiology, acute and chronic pancreatitis. Gastrointestinal Teaching Project, American Gastroenterological Association; 2003.)

CCK 是肠期膳食刺激酶分泌的主要体液介质。CCK 的循环浓度随进餐而增加[89],主要的循环形式为 58 个氨基酸大小(CCK-58)[95]。CCK 通过脂肪和蛋白质的消化产物从小肠上部黏膜释放,小部分由淀粉消化产物释放[89]。

为了解释胆碱能途径和 CCK 之间的相互作用,以解释胆碱能抑制作用对肠期胰腺分泌的显著影响,研究发现 CCK 激活了十二指肠黏膜中的传入神经元[96]。这些传入神经元激活了迷走神经反射,引起胰酶的分泌,如图 56.7 所示。

当标准营养物质进入十二指肠时,先前描述的膳食肠道阶段分泌机制的要素被激活。然而,刺激的幅度随营养物质的类型和输送部位的不同而变化[97-100]。例如,与标准膳食相比,要素膳食(蛋白质、氨基酸和低脂肪)的输送导致胰腺酶分泌减少,营养物质输送到空肠比输送到十二指肠引起胰腺分泌减少。此类信息对于为胰腺疾病(例如急性或慢性胰腺炎)患者提供营养的策略至关重要。对于急性胰腺炎,胰腺的刺激会加剧疾病的严重性。在慢性胰腺炎中,胰腺受到刺激会加剧疼痛(参见第 58 和 59 章)[101]。

(三) 反馈调节

在动物中,从肠中转移胰液会导致胰腺分泌增加[102]。另一方面,已发现腔内消化酶在动物和人类中均抑制胰腺消化酶的分泌[103,104];CCK 参与了这一调控[104],由此引出了管腔内调节酶分泌的因子包括消化酶的概念。假设在进餐期间,当胰蛋白酶被膳食蛋白质占据时,由于无法利用胰蛋白酶来引起反馈抑制,因此胰腺分泌得以增强。饭后,胰蛋白酶和其他消化酶在肠腔中游离,并抑制肠 CCK 释放和胰酶的分泌。

以上假设描述了 CCK 释放因子介导了胰蛋白酶的这种作用。一种是由胰腺分泌的称为监控肽的蛋白质[103]。另一种称为腔内 CCK 释放因子[105]。监控肽和腔内 CCK 释放因子均导致 CCK 从肠内分泌 CCK 细胞(I 细胞)释放到血液中。这些释放因子可能是酶分泌的生理反馈机制的介质。据信,当胰蛋白酶未与膳食蛋白结合时,上述胰蛋白酶的作用是由于胰蛋白酶使 CCK 释放因子降解所致(参见第 4 章图 4.5)。

七、胰腺分泌功能试验

为了诊断诸如慢性胰腺炎和胰腺癌等疾病,已设计了各种检测来测量胰腺的分泌功能(表 56.1)[106-108]。值得注意的是,可能存在的胰腺疾病(即慢性胰腺炎)对于此处描述的测试功能影响很小。

表 56.1 胰腺分泌功能试验

试验	描述	优点	缺点	临床适应证
直接分泌	测量静脉胰泌素给药后十二指肠内容量和 HCO_3^- 分泌量	提供最灵敏和最特异的胰腺外分泌功能测量	需要十二指肠插管和激素静脉给药；未广泛使用	检测到轻度、中度或重度胰腺外分泌功能障碍
CCK	测量静脉 CCK 给药后十二指肠输出的淀粉酶、胰蛋白酶、糜蛋白酶和/或脂肪酶			
胰泌素和 CCK	测量静脉胰泌素和 CCK 给药后的体积、HCO_3^- 和酶			
间接(需要十二指肠插管)				
Lundh 测试餐	口服试验餐后十二指肠胰蛋白酶浓度的测定	不需要激素静脉给药	需要十二指肠插管，测试餐和正常解剖结构，包括小肠黏膜；未广泛使用	当无法进行直接检查时(例如，由于可用性有限)，可检测中度或重度胰腺外分泌功能障碍
间接(无管)				
粪便脂肪测试	摄入已知脂肪量的食物后测量粪便中的脂肪	提供脂肪泻的定量测量	需要足够的膳食脂肪摄入和粪便采集；仅检测重度胰腺功能障碍	检测重度胰腺外分泌功能障碍和脂肪泻
粪便糜蛋白酶	测量粪便中的糜蛋白酶或弹性蛋白酶 1	不需要静脉注射，试管或口服底物给药	对检测轻度或中度功能障碍不敏感	检测重度胰腺外分泌功能障碍
粪便弹性蛋白酶 1				
NBT-PABA	随餐口服 NBT-PABA 或荧光素二月桂酸酯，然后测量血清或尿液中的 PABA 或荧光素	为重度胰腺功能障碍提供简单的测量	不得检测轻度或中度功能障碍；小肠黏膜疾病患者的结果可能异常	检测重度胰腺外分泌功能障碍

荧光素二月桂酯
CCK，胆囊收缩素；NT-PABA，N-苯甲酰基-L-酪氨酰-对氨基苯甲酸。

胰腺功能的检测已适应于内镜检查，可能包括胰液中蛋白质和蛋白质修饰的测量[109-111]。功能检测分为两大类：直接检测和间接检测。胰腺分泌功能的直接检测包括在静脉注射促分泌剂或联合促分泌剂后收集胰腺分泌液。胰腺分泌功能的间接检测包括：①摄入营养物质后测量十二指肠样品中的胰酶；②消化酶对被摄入底物的作用产物；③粪便中的胰酶。应使用哪种胰腺功能检查取决于临床问题以及检查的特征和可用性。胰腺外分泌具有非常大的功能储备。直到通过 CCK 刺激的消化酶分泌所测定的功能降低至正常水平的 5%～10%，才会发生消化和吸收不良[112]。因此，许多依赖于消化酶将摄入的底物转化为可测量产物的测试对胰腺疾病并不敏感，除非存在中度至重度胰腺功能不全。因此，静脉注释胰腺促分泌剂后测量十二指肠分泌产物具有最大的灵敏度和特异性。直接检测的主要缺点是需要十二指肠插管，并不是所有的中心都能熟练正确地进行这项研究。此外，成像技术的改进用于诊断胰腺疾病大大减少了这些检查的使用。然而，在某些情况下，直接进行胰腺功能检查可能有助于诊断胰腺疾病。重要的是，尽管影像学已取得进展，但慢性或复发性急性胰腺炎的诊断仍然存在困难，可能难以确诊(参见第 58 和 59 章)，仍然需要利用胰腺液相关的功能并开发新的测量方法(如炎性生物标志物)是一个重要进展[110,113,114]。

(一) 直接试验

直接试验为测量胰腺功能提供了黄金标准。分泌的刺激最常被描述为使用促胰液素、CCK 或两者的组合。该组合可提供有关腺泡和导管细胞分泌物的完整信息。在经典描述中，需要进行胃和十二指肠插管。胃插管需要清除胃分泌物，因为胃分泌物会干扰测量胰腺分泌的水和碳酸氢盐。低 pH 也可能改变胰腺酶的活性。十二指肠管用于输注不可吸收的标志物和收集胰腺分泌物。使用不可吸收的标志物(例如钴胺素或聚乙二醇)可以在不需要完全抽吸分泌物的情况下对分泌物进行定量。直接功能检测基于以下原理：水，碳酸氢盐和酶的分泌的最大值与胰腺的功能有关。从历史上看，促胰液素试验(静脉注射促胰液素，并测量体积和碳酸氢盐)可提供有关胰腺在各种临床环境中的功能信息[106-108]。给予 CCK 和消化酶分泌的测量也已成功地用于证实胰腺功能不全[115]首选的试验是基于胰泌素静脉注射给药和使用内镜抽吸胰腺分泌物，每隔 45～60 分钟测量胰液中碳酸氢盐的峰值浓度[111,116-118]。合成胰泌素(SecroFlo, ChiRhoClin, Inc.)的剂量为 0.2μg/kg，在 1 分钟内注射。在 15 分钟收集过程中测量碳酸氢盐浓度，持续 1 小时。还可测定淀粉酶、胰蛋白酶、糜蛋白酶和脂肪酶[115,119-121]。当功能正常时，开发炎症标志物的测量指标可能对确定胰腺中是否存在炎症很有价值。

（二）间接试验

1. Lundh 测试餐[122]

这项膳食测试主要具有历史意义，旨在确定膳食对胰腺分泌的影响。Lundh 测试餐现在很少在临床实践中使用，但可能用于研究环境受试者摄入 300mL 液体测试膳食，其中包括奶粉、植物油和葡萄糖（6% 脂肪、5% 蛋白质和 15% 碳水化合物）。进餐后，每隔一段时间从插管的十二指肠吸出样品，以测量消化酶浓度。通常只测量胰蛋白酶的活性，然而增加脂肪酶或淀粉酶测定可能会提高测试灵敏度。该测试不适用于患有黏膜疾病（如腹腔疾病）或胃十二指肠解剖结构发生变化（如在进行迷走神经切断和引流手术或 Billroth Ⅱ 胃切除术之后）的患者。Lundh 试验餐与分泌素 CCK 试验的比较表明，后者对检测轻度胰腺疾病更敏感，而这些试验在较晚期胰腺疾病中更适用[106]。

2. 粪便脂肪测量

当刺激的脂肪酶输出下降至正常值的 5%～10% 以下时，就会发生脂肪泻[112]。因此，在摄入脂肪量充足（70～100g/d）的受试者中，测量 72 小时粪便中的脂肪含量被认为是一种诊断脂肪泻的有效手段。正常情况下，摄入的脂肪有 7% 或更少出现在粪便中。对单个粪便中的油脂进行简单的定性显微镜检查几乎与定量测量脂肪一样敏感[106,123]。由于脂肪泻仅发生在晚期胰腺疾病中，因此粪便脂肪测量在轻中度疾病的诊断中没有用（见第 59 章）。

3. 粪便糜蛋白酶和弹性蛋白酶 1 测量

多年来，粪便糜蛋白酶测量已被用作胰腺功能的间接测试，尤其是用于确定囊性纤维化患者的胰腺功能不全[106,108]。这种测量对晚期胰腺功能不全患者的敏感度约为 85%，而对于轻度和中度胰腺功能不全患者则相对不敏感。

粪便胰腺弹性蛋白酶 1 测量广泛应用于临床实践，在胰腺功能不全的患者中出现异常，但在慢性胰腺炎引起的轻度或中度胰腺疾病的患者中可能是正常的[124-126]。

总而言之，本文所述的几种检查方法能够检测伴有胰腺外分泌不足和脂肪泻的严重胰腺疾病。然而，只有直接检测才能识别出轻度胰腺疾病患者。最近的内镜改进提升了直接功能检测。此外，在胰腺炎中发生的炎症蛋白和蛋白修饰的特定测量方面将取得进展。

（施海韵 译，孙明瑜　李鹏 校）

参考文献

第 57 章　胰腺遗传性疾病和小儿胰腺疾病

David C. Whitcomb，Mark E. Lowe 著

章节目录

一、背景 …… 813
二、定义和术语 …… 814
（一）胰腺生物学和疾病模型 …… 815
（二）非胰腺炎的腺泡细胞功能障碍/衰竭 …… 820
（三）导管细胞相关的胰腺炎发病机制 …… 821
（四）导管细胞生理学和导管相关性胰腺炎概述 …… 821
（五）CF 跨膜传导调节因子（*CFTR*）变体 …… 822
（六）钙敏感受体基因变体 …… 826
三、修饰炎症、进展为慢性胰腺炎和修饰表型的基因 …… 826
（一）*CLDN2-MORC4* …… 826
（二）SLC26A9：CF 疾病严重程度修饰基因 …… 827
（三）CF 相关的糖尿病风险 …… 828
四、遗传学与患者管理的整合 …… 828
五、小儿胰腺炎 …… 829
（一）急性胰腺炎 …… 829
（二）复发性急性胰腺炎和慢性胰腺炎 …… 830
六、胰腺孟德尔遗传疾病的临床管理 …… 830
（一）囊性纤维化 …… 830
（二）遗传性胰腺炎 …… 836
（三）家族性胰腺炎 …… 838
（四）Schwachman-Diamond 综合征 …… 838
七、罕见的遗传综合征与胰腺病理学 …… 839
（一）Johanson-Blizzard 综合征 …… 839
（二）Pearson 骨髓-胰腺综合征 …… 840
（三）胰腺发育不全 …… 840
（四）其他罕见综合征 …… 840
八、复发性急性和慢性胰腺炎相关的家族性代谢综合征 …… 841
（一）家族性甲状旁腺功能亢进伴高钙血症 …… 841
（二）乳糜微粒血症综合征 …… 841

一、背景

精准医学的新模式为理解胰腺疾病提供了一个强有力的框架，并导致对疾病机制的新见解。该框架在临床和转化科学方面取得了一系列突破。目前，国际社会已就促进精准医学的慢性胰腺炎（chronic pancreatitis，CP）新的机制定义达成了共识[1]，一个国际共识小组还得出结论，CP 传统的定义和诊断标准是基于识别胰腺不可逆的纤维化，排除了早期 CP 的诊断，对靶向治疗几乎没有指导意义[2]。因此，需要一种新的模式来改善胰腺疾病的管理。

本章重点介绍遗传学作为决策医学的一个关键组成部分，以 CP 的机制定义为基础，重点强调了孟德尔疾病和影响胰腺的复杂遗传条件。迅速扩展的遗传信息已组织成系统和模型，并在可能的情况下与临床管理考虑因素相联系。本章将概述目前已知影响人类健康的许多关键基因和遗传综合征的知识。在可能的情况下，讨论将超越遗传学，讨论胰腺疾病精准医学的原则，并指导临床医生对已确诊、疑似、早期或复杂胰腺疾病患者使用遗传学数据。

传统（20 世纪，西医）模式是基于疾病的细菌理论，其中只有一种因素引起特定疾病。在细菌理论模型中，使用临床病理学标准定义特定的疾病。一种疾病可进一步归类为一种综合征，由通常一起出现的一组症状和体征组成，用于描述和诊断疾病。将疾病定义为综合征并不需要了解或解决病因、机制、自然病程或干预措施的效果。

1963 年至 1989 年期间，在 3 次“Marseille 研讨会”中，国际上努力定义胰腺炎，尤其是 CP[3-5]。由于活体患者的胰腺组织获取具有挑战性，1984 年开发了一种更实用的临床方法，使用成像标准作为纤维化的替代指标，称为剑桥评分[6]。CP 被定义为“胰腺持续的炎症性疾病，以不可逆的形态学改变为特征，典型者引起疼痛和（或）永久性的功能丧失”[6]。随后的定义和诊断标准遵循了这种方法。然而，临床病理学方法对 CP 的潜在机制知之甚少。因此，在使用细菌理论范式（如 Koch 假设）中规定的“科学方法”进行了约 100 年的研究后[7]，1995 年承认 CP 仍然是一个发病机制不确定、临床过程不可预测和治疗不明确的神秘未知过程[8]。1996 年发现阳离子胰蛋白酶原基因（*PRSS1*）的突变引起遗传性胰腺炎（hereditary pancreatitis，HP），其表型为复发性急性胰腺炎（recurrent acute pancreatitis，RAP）和 CP，与常见的胰腺炎性疾病相似[9,10]，将遗传学的概念引入胰腺炎症性疾病。然而，这一概念并不符合 CP 的传统定义，也不符合证明不可逆纤维化的诊断标准。在其他疾病相关基因中额外遗传风险变异的发现，进一步挑战了胰腺疾病的临床病理学框架。这些事实，再加上后面描述的新的观察结果，表明对胰腺炎等复杂疾病的传统方法是不够的。

卫生保健专业人员和患者，根据内镜逆行胰胆管造影（ERCP）或 CT 等成像程序检测到的组织纤维化认识到胰腺炎传统方法的很多缺点。第一，从出现症状到疾病诊断的时间往往为 5~10 年或更长时间[11,12]。在这段时间内患者可能患有 RAP 和进行性疼痛，接受多次昂贵的侵入性诊断测试，并可能寻求可能不符合其长期利益的放射治疗[2]。第二，单独使用影像学诊断“早期”CP 是不可能的，因为早期纤维化

的敏感表现对 CP 没有特异性[2,13,14]。第三,使用临床病理评估的临床病程,包括疾病轨迹、并发症和结局是不可预测的[8,15]。第四,治疗往往是基于症状,而不是针对潜在的问题,因此即使在治疗期间,疾病通常仍会继续进展[2,7]。由于 CP 是一种影响多种途径的复杂疾病,选择“纤维化”作为定义疾病和衡量进展的主要生物标志物是有问题的。具体而言,纤维化的成像特征与疼痛[16]、胰腺外分泌功能[17-22]、糖尿病[13,23]或疾病进展[14,15]的相关性不佳,这些都是这些患者的主要临床问题。

对于复杂的胰腺炎等综合征的早期诊断和持续治疗需要一个新的模式[7]。复杂疾病需要 2 个或 2 个以上独立因素相互作用才能引起疾病,而单个因素既不是引起疾病的必要条件,也不足以单独引起疾病。对于胰腺炎等复杂疾病,需要精准的医学辅助诊断,因为多种病因可导致相同的病理学,相同的病理学可导致不同的结果,且治疗效果不可预测。胰腺疾病的精准医学关注的是潜在机制,而不是由临床病理学标准、建模和疾病模拟定义的人群中的病例对照相关性,而不是病理学特征分类,并为个体而不是人群提供指导。这种方法依赖于了解疾病的生物学基础,需要使用包含相关的生物学机制以及患者特异性变异的疾病模型,并寻求在多种条件下预测多个变量的影响,而不是识别单个致病因素。尽管将有用的模型整合到相关模型中,将精准医学应用于许多疾病仍然是一个未来的概念,但现在精准医学用于胰腺疾病是可能的。

胰腺是精准医疗的一个重要用例,因为胰腺是一个简单的腺体,只受少数环境和代谢因素的影响[7]。胰腺只有 3 种特化细胞:腺泡、导管和胰岛。每种细胞类型都有一个主要功能,其分子机制已得到很好的描述。此外,由于胰腺的腹膜后位置(在一定程度上免受创伤)、受括约肌保护的导管系统(防止与肠腔环境直接接触)和血液供应(防止来自肠道的门静脉血液),保护胰腺免受与大多数环境损害的直接接触。另外胰腺在外源性解毒或清除废物方面不起主要作用,因此它通常也能免受大多数有毒化合物的影响。由于缺乏强有力的、独立的环境因素或其他因素直接引起胰腺的复杂炎症性疾病,如 CP,突出了致病性遗传变异和疾病修饰因子等其他因素单独或联合的重要性。对分子机制的了解,包括蛋白质、编码蛋白质的基因以及患者现有条件和环境背景下的调节机制,为精准医疗提供了基础。对成人和儿童特发性 RAP 和 CP 中的多个基因进行基因检测,对临床诊断和治疗这些疾病具有重要的意义[24-27]。使用新的工具和方法,将简单和复杂的基因发现与临床症状、生物标志物和进展阶段整合到临床实践中,会带来额外的好处。精准医学还超越了遗传学的范畴,考虑到个体对环境(内部和外部)和生活方式的暴露[28,29]。它努力通过对潜在促成因素的更精确测量,重新定义我们对疾病的发生和进展、治疗反应和健康结局的理解[28,29]。尽管对于大多数疾病,精准医学的广泛采用和应用仍然存在许多障碍[30],但 CP 和相关模型的新机制定义,现在已使胰腺炎症性疾病的精准医疗成为可能。

剩下的一些挑战包括需要考虑的大量基因变异,包括疾病修饰因子,以及遗传实验室责任人的专业知识,他们为复杂的非孟德尔和非癌症条件生成临床报告,并需要接受解剖学或实验室病理学或孟德尔遗传学培训,而不是患者的护理培训。由于大多数 RAP 患者和(或)早期 CP 患者没有单一的病因,明显的家族史、区分家族特征或病理特征,因此缺乏定义和诊断疾病或提供临床管理指导的传统背景。需要新的整合方法和有用的工具来更充分地受益于精准医疗的新机遇。

二、定义和术语

精准医学:也称个性化或个体化医疗,在这里被定义为一门破译致病根源,以及使用靶向治疗以最小化功能障碍和最大化健康的学科。对于复杂疾病,将疾病定义为常规或正常功能的破坏,而疾病是一种损害器官或系统正常功能的病理状态,通常通过辨别症状和体征来表现。胰腺获得性疾病表明,尽管存在潜在的疾病,但器官或系统在未发生疾病的情况下仍能充分发挥功能。然而,在特定的易感基因或修饰基因或调控区域内存在致病性种系突变表明,自受孕以来,特定生物系统内存在潜在的功能性疾病,在特定条件下需要适当的反应。在某些情况下,如损伤或应激使系统超过耐受的阈值,细胞或腺体不能再代偿导致病理后果的疾病。致病基因变异、新陈代谢、环境应激或损伤组合的病理后果启动并驱动疾病的治疗过程。因此,在没有疾病的情况下,致病基因变异代表着风险,而在存在疾病的情况下,致病基因变异有助于确定疾病发病机制。

胰腺炎症性疾病:大多数具有临床意义的胰腺疾病都是复杂的炎症性疾病,分为急性胰腺炎(acute pancreatitis, AP)[31,32]、RAP[24,25]和 CP[1,24,33]。此外,还有一些罕见的孟德尔综合征以不同的方式影响胰腺(如胰腺外分泌功能不全),但这些遗传性疾病的分期和管理通常遵循更复杂的胰腺疾病的方法。

急性胰腺炎(AP):AP 是由突发性胰腺损伤触发的事件,随后是连续的炎症反应(见第 58 章)。RAP 定义为具有遗传、环境、创伤、形态学、代谢、生物和/或其他风险因素的个体,在经历了 2 次或 2 次以上有记录的 AP 发作(间隔至少 3 个月)后发生的起源于胰腺内的多种不同急性炎症反应的综合征[25]。

慢性胰腺炎(CP):CP 是一个具有持续性和进展性病理阶段的过程,通常开始为 AP 或 RAP,以免疫系统介导的胰腺破坏和广泛的腺体纤维化和萎缩结束(见第 59 章)[6,24,33-35]。CP 的新机制定义包括先前已确诊和晚期 CP 的充分描述特征,包括胰腺萎缩、纤维化、疼痛综合征、导管扭曲和狭窄、钙化、胰腺外分泌功能障碍、胰腺内分泌功能障碍和异型增生[1]。

此外,CP 的本质首次被定义为“具有遗传、环境和(或)其他风险因素的个体,对实质损伤或应激产生持续病理反应的胰腺病理纤维炎症综合征”[1]。该定义与涵盖患者一生的渐进模型(图 57.1)相关联[1]。该定义还特别将 CP 与腺泡或导管细胞的正常损伤→炎症→消退→再生序列的变异与损伤或应激源特异性联系起来,为 RAP 的紊乱和导致 CP 提供特

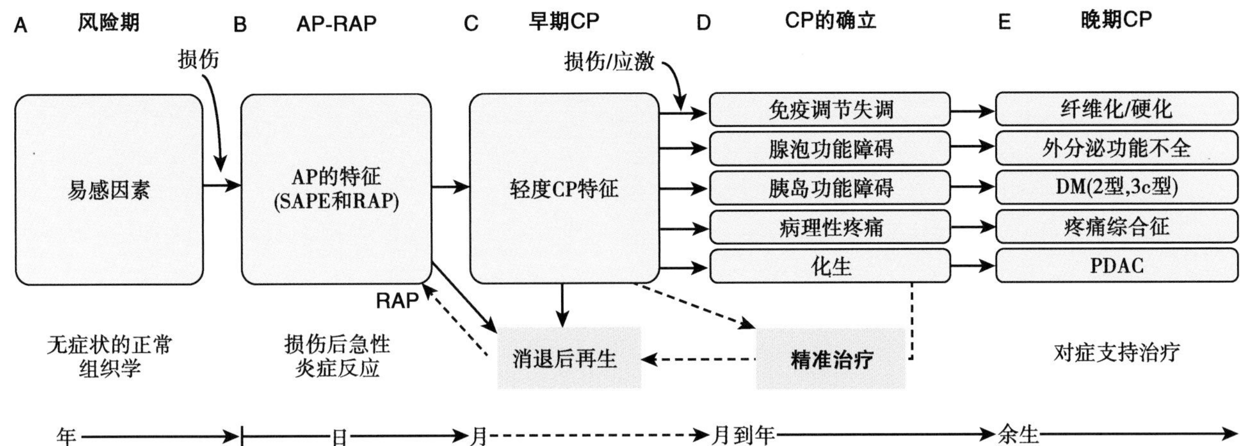

图 57.1　胰腺炎临床分期的进展模型。胰腺炎的 5 个临床阶段（A 到 E）由疾病的临床症状和生物标志物定义。该过程反映了对损伤→炎症→消退→再生序列的正常和异常反应。一个阶段内症状复发并进展至下一阶段的风险由与复发性损伤或应激相关的遗传和环境风险因素决定。C 期，即早期 CP，无法通过传统的影像学标准进行诊断，但可使用整合患者的临床状况、风险水平和相关生物标志物的精准医学方法来预估 CP 的可能性[2]。D 期和 E 期反映了对特定细胞类型的持续性（可能是永久性的）损伤和功能障碍，包括产生过度纤维化的星状细胞、腺泡细胞、导管细胞、胰岛细胞、神经细胞和再生细胞的化生等慢性炎症细胞。由于细胞类型具有不同的功能障碍风险水平，不同病例之间 CP 的特征不同。预防和治疗方法是针对 C 期和 D 期（虚线），可挽救正常的功能。E 期是指功能丧失，需要对症治疗（如疼痛管理）或替代治疗（如 PERT、胰岛素）。AP-RAP，急性胰腺炎-复发性急性胰腺炎；CP，慢性胰腺炎；DM，糖尿病；PDAC，胰腺导管腺癌；PERT，胰酶替代疗法；SAPE，前哨急性胰腺炎事件。（From Whitcomb DC, Frulloni L, Garg P, et al. Chronic pancreatitis: an international draft consensus proposal for a new mechanistic definition. Pancreatology 2016;16:218-224.）

异性。新的定义与一个渐进模型相关联，该模型将 AP 作为前哨急性胰腺炎事件（sentinel acute pancreatitis event, SAPE）[36,37]，将 RAP 作为进展为 CP 的重要近端风险因素。渐进模型也预期早期 CP，这不能通过 CP 的传统定义来诊断[2,38]。因此，在 RAP 和（或）早期 CP 患者出现成熟和晚期 CP 的共同特征之前，以及早期治疗最有可能有效时，导致 CP 的过程有可能在早期发现[2]。RAP25 和 CP 的新定义并不相互排斥，两种综合征可同时存在[39]。

遗传性胰腺炎（HP）：HP 是指一个家族中的 RAP 或 CP，其中胰腺炎表型似乎是通过常染色体显性模式表达的致病基因突变遗传的[40,41]。携带引起常染色体显性胰腺炎的基因突变（如 *PRSS1* p. N29I, p. R122H）但无明确家族史的胰腺炎个体也患有 HP。

家族性胰腺炎：该术语是指在一个家族中发生的任何原因导致的胰腺炎，考虑到家族的规模和定义人群中胰腺炎的发生率，其发生率高于仅偶然预期的发生率。家族性胰腺炎可能由或不由遗传缺陷引起。

热带性胰腺炎（TP）：TP 以前被定义为发生在热带地区的一种早期发病的非酒精性 CP[42]，通常聚集在家庭成员中，并且可能具有复杂的遗传基础[43,44]。随着对复杂遗传学知识的不断增长，术语“热带胰腺炎”一词可能会过时。

累及胰腺的孟德尔综合征：这些疾病是遵循经典孟德尔遗传模式的胰腺疾病，被认为是常染色体显性（如 HP；见前文）或常染色体隐性［如囊性纤维化（CF）］遗传病。如 CF、先天性胰腺脂肪瘤病［Shwachman-Diamond 综合征（SDS）］、Johanson-Blizzard 综合征（JBS）等，它们通常影响胰腺以外的多个器官。Pearson 综合征（骨髓-胰腺综合征）是一种罕见的线粒体 DNA（mtDNA）断裂综合征，伴有胰腺外分泌功能障碍和母系遗传。

复杂胰腺疾病：这些是不遵循孟德尔单基因遗传学模式的胰腺疾病。大多数 CP 病例都是复杂的遗传疾病。根据定义，当多种因素必须同时发生才能表达表型时，就会建立复杂的胰腺疾病，并且可能涉及 2 个或 2 个以上基因（多基因疾病）、基因-环境相互作用或多种因素的组合。复杂的遗传无序与加性遗传效应不同，在加性遗传效应中，其中 2 个单独基因位点的遗传效应等于其个体效应的总和。在多基因疾病中，来自 1 个以上基因的致病等位基因以共生方式引起疾病，而单独的突变基因均不致病。修饰基因不会引起疾病，相反，它们会改变疾病过程的特定方面或赋予遗传疾病独特的表型特征。

（一）胰腺生物学和疾病模型

图 57.1 显示了 CP 的进展模型，组织遗传和环境的风险以及修饰因素、临床特征、生物标志物和并发症，以应对损伤→炎症→消退→再生序列的功能障碍[1]。一些患者在未经历所有步骤的情况下出现了 CP 的证据，但该模型仍可以计算出大多数患者复杂的风险特征和进展概率。该模型对各阶段的损伤或进展机制是不可知的，只要它包括显著的损伤和（或）应激以及炎症。后期并发症纤维化、胰腺外分泌功能不全、糖尿病、各种慢性疼痛综合征和癌症风险并不能相互替代，而是代表与胰腺相关的不同细胞类型或系统的疾病特征。

CP 有许多独立和联合的危险因素，一旦炎症过程启动，这些因素就会成为致病因素（见图 57.1，阶段 A 期）。TIGAR-O 是一类发病因素的首字母缩略词，包括毒物-代谢、特发性、遗传性、自身免疫性、复发性急性或重症 AP 和梗阻性原因[33]。更新后的 TIGAR-O 列表（框 57.1）整理了个体中发现的主要发病因素，说明大多数患者都具有多种风险因素。TIGAR-O 方法还使用修改后的首字母缩略词，集成到 M-ANNHEIM 分类系统中[45]。

框 57.1 TIGAR-O 第 2 版胰腺炎病因分类

毒物-代谢

- 与酒精有关的
  - 1~2 杯/d(低风险)
  - 3~4 杯/d(中度风险)
  - 5 杯或以上/d(高风险)
  - >偶尔——进展风险高
- 吸烟
  - 既往吸烟者(中度风险)
  - 目前吸烟者(易感性和进展高风险)
- 高钙血症
  - 甲状旁腺功能亢进症
  - 其他 NOS
- 高甘油三酯血症
  - 临床诊断-散发性或遗传学未知(见下文)
- 慢性肾衰竭
- 药物(见框 57.2 及第 58 和 59 章)
- 毒素
  - 氧化应激产物
  - 有机化合物(如 DBTC)
  - 其他,NOS
- 其他
  - 辐照后
  - 其他,NOS

特发性

- 早期发性(<35 岁)
- 晚发性(≥35 岁)
- 热带(已过时)
  - 热带钙化性胰腺炎
  - 纤维钙化性胰腺糖尿病
- 其他,NOS

遗传性

- 疑似(无基因分型或基因分型有限)
- 常染色体显性遗传(孟德尔遗传)
  - *PRSS1* 突变(遗传性胰腺炎)
  - 羧酸酯脂肪酶(CEL)——MODY 8 表型
  - 其他,NOS
- 常染色体隐性遗传(孟德尔遗传)
  - *CFTR*,2 种重度反式变体(囊性纤维化)
  - *CFTR*,<2 种重度反式变体(CFTR-RD)CFTR
  - *SPINK1* 2 种致病性反式变体
  - 其他,NOS
- 复杂的遗传学——任何上述未包括的疾病机制:
  - 具有致病性钙敏感受体(*CASR*)变体
  - 具有致病性 *CEL* 变体(非 MODY 8)
  - 具有致病性 *CFTR* 变体
  - 具有致病性 *CTRC* 变体
  - 具有致病性 *SPNK1* 变体
  - 其他,NOS
- 修饰基因(病原体相关变异)
  - *CLDN2*
  - *SLC26A9*
  - *GGT1*
  - *ABO*——B 血型
  - 乳糜泻相关致病变异体
  - 其他,NOS
- 高甘油三酯血症综合征(病原体相关变异)
  - *LPL*——脂蛋白脂酶缺乏症
  - *APOC2*——载脂蛋白 C-Ⅱ缺乏症
  - 其他家族性乳糜微粒血症综合征(FCS)
  - 多因素乳糜微粒血症综合征(MCS)
  - 其他,NOS
- 罕见的非肿瘤性胰腺遗传变异相关综合征
  - Shwachman-Diamond 综合征
  - Johanson-Blizzard 综合征
  - 线粒体,包括 Pearson 骨髓-胰腺综合征。
  - 其他,NOS

自身免疫性胰腺炎与免疫相关疾病

- 孤立性自身免疫性慢性胰腺炎
  - AIP Ⅰ型(仅限于胰腺)
  - AIP Ⅱ型
- 与胰腺炎相关的免疫系统疾病
  - IgG4 相关疾病(包括Ⅰ型 AIP);
  - 克罗恩病相关的胰腺炎
  - 溃疡病相关的胰腺炎

复发性和重症急性胰腺炎

- 复发性急性胰腺炎
- 坏死后(重症急性胰腺炎)
- 损伤亚型
  - 胆源性胰腺炎
  - 创伤性-伴有胰腺坏死
  - 缺血性或围手术期
  - 血管疾病
  - 未确定,或 NOS

梗阻性

- 胰腺分裂
- Oddi 括约肌功能障碍或狭窄
- 主胰管结石
- 广泛的胰腺钙化
- 局部肿块(不包括促纤维增生反应)
- 导管狭窄——包括创伤性,无胰腺坏死
- 壶腹前十二指肠壁囊肿
- 其他,NOS

TIGAR-O 第 2 版风险分类。该列表更新了 Etemad 和 Whitcomb33 于 2001 年提出的第 1 版,以反映新的发现和对旧类别的澄清。患者通常具有列表中导致急性和慢性胰腺炎复发的多种风险因素。应记录每例患者的所有相关病因。2001 年版的主要变更包括:根据酒精和吸烟暴露进行的风险分层,高甘油三酯血症的进一步定义包括遗传风险,发病年龄限制为特发性(使热带胰腺炎成为历史类别),更新基因谱,重点关注孟德尔和复杂的炎症性疾病,并指定修饰基因、乳糜泻基因和高甘油三酯血症基因。更新了自身免疫性疾病分类。通过区分损伤亚型更新了 RAP 重度 AP 类别,特别包括胆源性胰腺炎和其他腺泡外细胞和导管外细胞病因。所用缩略语见正文。CFTR,CF 跨膜传导调节因子;NOS,未另行说明。(Modifications by Whitcomb,2018 年)

1. 饮酒和吸烟

饮酒和吸烟是成人 AP、RAP 和 CP 的重要定性和定量风险因素。单独饮酒和吸烟不足以引起 RAP 或 CP,但在胰腺炎背景下,无论是在症状发作或诊断时,还是从该时间点开始,均显著增加了疾病严重程度和进展的风险。酒精可以被建模为有或无酗酒的受试者,通过每天饮酒量/每周饮酒天数、按 3 分量表(<2 次/d、2~5 次/天或>5 次/d),或其他标准化量表建模来衡量是否酗酒,并在一生中建模[46,47]。吸烟可以分为从不吸烟(一生中吸烟<100 支)或曾经吸烟(吸烟>100 支)、既往或当前吸烟者,并通过每天吸烟的包数和吸烟的年包数进行量化[46,47]。在北美胰腺炎研究Ⅱ(North American Pancreatitis Study Ⅱ,NAPS2)[48-50]中使用这种方法证明,CP 的风险只发生在每天 5 杯酒精饮料的阈值或以上,吸烟与 CP 的风险呈剂量依赖性相关,与饮酒无关。因此,酒精和吸烟的影响是累加和(或)相乘的。酒精和吸烟的影响在男性和女性之间,以及在欧洲和非洲祖先之间存在差异[46,47]。此外,暴露的数量和时间可以计算修饰基因对饮酒者和吸烟者 CP 风险的影响[51,52]。

2. 前哨急性胰腺炎事件(SAPE)

CP 的 SAPE 模型旨在整合导致 CP 的致病因素,指出 CP 是一种获得性疾病,无症状受试者多年来存在各种 CP 的风险,需要"事件"来启动病理过程,临床上公认的 AP 通常是最明显的事件[36]。术语"哨兵"一词是指医生在预测未来可能需要立即采取行动以避免病理损伤方面的作用。该"事件"的后果是激活免疫系统,吸引单核细胞(成为固有巨噬细胞),激活星状细胞(负责纤维化),以及表观遗传或适应性变化,增加胰腺对 RAP 的敏感性,并驱动导致 CP 特征性表现的病理过程[53]。提出 SAPE 模型[48-50]作为 CP 的坏死-纤维化模型的替代方法[54],因为大多数 CP 患者从未患有 AP 伴明显胰腺坏死。此外,HP[9,10]的疾病机制与 CP 的蛋白栓/结石模型不相容[55]。因此,SAPE 模型作为一个框架,可以分析 RAP 和 CP 的多种病因和进展阶段的影响,以及研究有或无 AP 病史的 CP 患者之间在致病因素上的差异。

多队列研究表明,SAPE 模型适用于大多数 CP 患者[56]。从 AP 进展为 CP 的风险由环境和遗传因素进一步定义[51,57-60]。因此,SAPE 模型在进展模型中起着重要作用,即在患有胰腺疾病的背景下预测胰腺炎的时间和性质。

3. 腺泡:胰腺外分泌功能单位模型

虽然医生通常将胰腺外分泌部分视为一个单元,但胰腺炎的病因和机制通常始于腺泡细胞或导管内。这种区分对于针对性治疗和制定管理计划非常重要。

腺泡和导管细胞组成功能单位,称为腺泡(腺泡的复数)(见第 55 章)。腺泡和导管的简化模型如图 57.2 所示。腺泡(顶部)是腺泡细胞的局部组织,顶端膜朝向胰管最上游的管腔。导管(底部)是由导管细胞组成的组织,形成从每个腺泡中心延伸到十二指肠管腔的管道。这里没有显示对复杂胰腺疾病各方面的神经、血管、胰岛、免疫细胞和支持组织,的都非常重要,因为 AP 的启动起源于其中许多影响腺泡细胞或导管的因素相互影响,是一种复杂的疾病易感机制,在不同的受试者中具有不同的危险因素组合。

4. 腺泡细胞功能障碍和疾病

腺泡细胞构成了大部分胰腺实质肿块,直接或间接导致了大多数胰腺炎症性疾病,因为其产物是导管内容物的主要贡献者。胰腺腺泡细胞的主要功能是合成和分泌胰腺消化酶

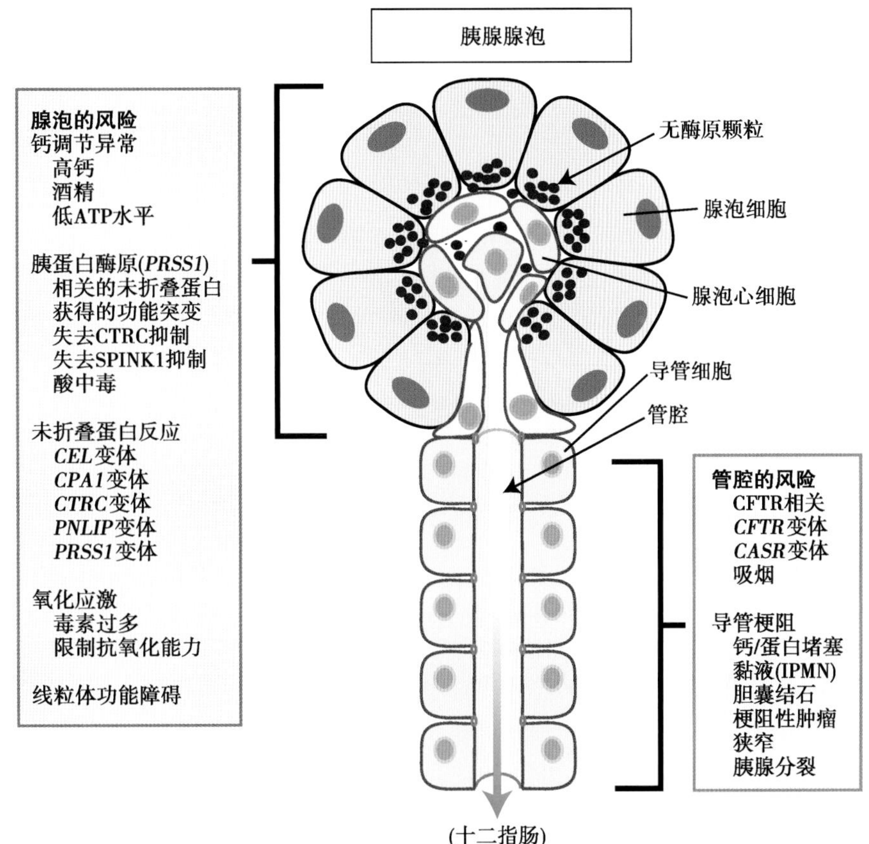

图 57.2　胰腺腺泡。概述了一个胰腺腺泡模型,展示了单个腺泡细胞与顶膜酶原颗粒和形成最终通向十二指肠导管的导管细胞之间的关系。中心腺泡细胞具有导管细胞生理学,但定位于腺泡内。胰腺炎风险通常可归因于腺泡(左侧列表)或导管(右侧列表)。(Illustration property of David C Whitcomb,used with permission)。IPMN,导管内乳头状黏液性肿瘤;CFTR,CF 跨膜传导调节因子。其他缩略语见正文

(见第 56 章)。该过程包括在粗面内质网(rough endoplasmic reticulum,RER)中合成一系列胰腺酶原蛋白(酶原),将正确折叠的蛋白运送到高尔基体进行分类并包装在酶原囊泡中,将酶原囊泡运送到顶端,和酶原顶端分泌到胰管中(图 57.3)。该过程需要大量的能量用于蛋白质合成和离子(如钙)在细胞间的转运。

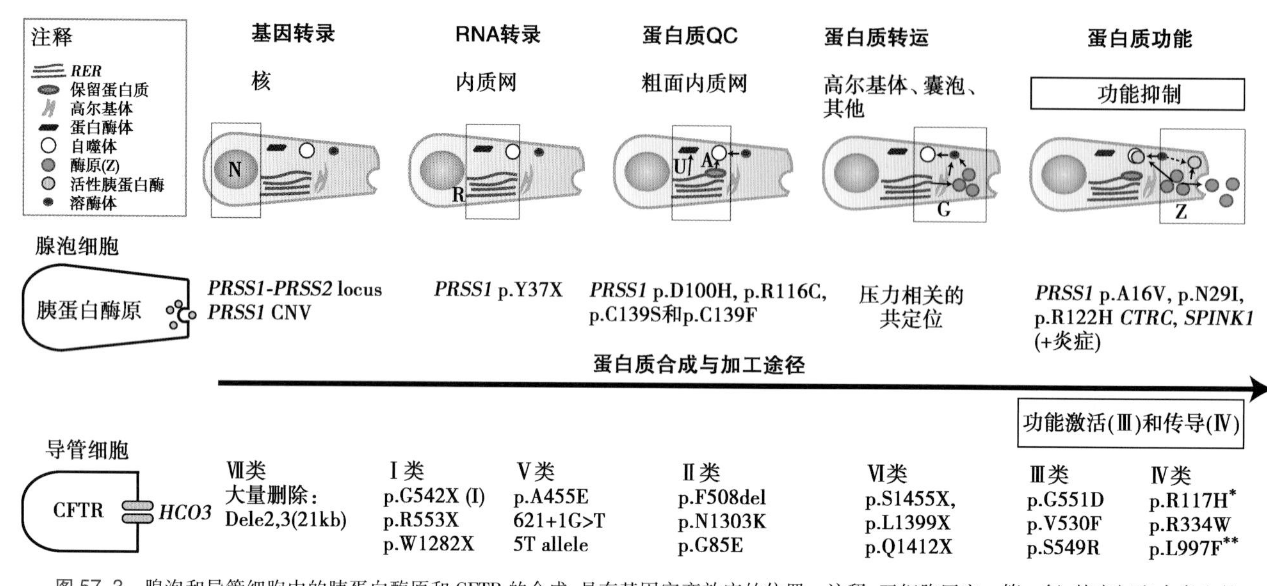

图 57.3 腺泡和导管细胞中的胰蛋白酶原和 CFTR 的合成,具有基因突变效应的位置。注释:亚细胞区室。第一行:特定间室内发生的一般细胞过程。第二行:腺泡细胞的描述,表明导管细胞中平行的各种区室和活性的亚细胞位置(未显示)。第三行:腺泡细胞生物学。基因转录产生 RNA。*PRSS1-PRSS2* 启动子变异会降低基因转录,而拷贝数变异(CNV)会增加转录本的数量。基因翻译发生在核糖体(R)和粗面内质网(RER)中。截断突变(X)导致 RER 中 RNA 向蛋白质的翻译失败。蛋白质质量控制(蛋白质 QC)检测泛素化(U)并转移到蛋白酶体再循环成氨基酸的有缺陷或未折叠的蛋白质。如果蛋白质形成复杂的聚集体阻塞了 RER,则 RER 的阻塞部分被切除并发生自噬(A)。蛋白质运输开始于高尔基体,并以酶原颗粒(Z)继续。胰蛋白酶原可被激活为胰蛋白酶,分子错误分类、酶原颗粒与溶酶体(L)融合或应激条件,尤其是功能获得性 *PRSS1* 突变[酶原颗粒或混合隔室中的活性胰蛋白酶(黄色液泡)]。CTRC 和 SPINK1 与胰蛋白酶原合成和分选,并提供对胰蛋白酶的保护。SPINK1 在应激时被上调,以提供额外保护。蛋白质功能通常延迟,直到酶原从腺泡细胞中释放出来并转运到十二指肠。第四行:导管细胞生物学。*CFTR* 变体由功能基因(Ⅰ类至Ⅶ类)组织,而不是改变加工的亚细胞位置。最近提出了一种新的Ⅶ类[145],用于导致无(或减少)RNA 转录的变体。无义和剪接位点变异体完全(Ⅰ类)或部分(Ⅴ类)破坏翻译成功能性蛋白。引起错误折叠和从 RER 中清除的非同义氨基酸替换通常为Ⅱ类。一些变体改变了顶膜上转运和保留的各个方面,作为Ⅵ类变体。一些变体导致顶端表面的 CFTR 分子无功能(Ⅲ类)或对一般阴离子电导、碳酸氢盐(**)或两者(*)的功能减弱。CFTR,CF 跨膜传导调节因子。(Illustration property of David C. Whitcomb, used with permission)

维持腺泡细胞内的低钙浓度对于保护它们免受过早的胰蛋白酶原活化至关重要。腺泡细胞钙可通过神经激素过度刺激而升高[61,62],高细胞外钙浓度[63]、打开顶膜钙通路的胆汁酸反流[64,65]、长期大量饮酒降低刺激诱导的 AP[66] 阈值、线粒体损伤[67],以及调节细胞内钙的其他因素[68]。任何增加腺泡细胞钙的过程都将通过钙依赖性胰蛋白酶原激活和稳定机制容易诱发 AP[68]。

5. 胰蛋白酶依赖性胰腺炎途径

AP 和 CP 可通过几种机制从腺泡细胞内触发和驱动。胰蛋白酶是触发 AP 的关键。胰蛋白酶是主要的消化酶,因为它能将自身和所有其他酶原激活为其活性形式(见第 56 章)胰腺内消化酶的激活导致自身消化、免疫激活分子的释放和免疫系统组分的直接交叉激活,进一步放大了对损伤的免疫反应[37,69]。

胰蛋白酶在 AP 中的重要性,通过对实验 AP 具有抗性的基因工程胰蛋白酶"敲除"小鼠来说明[70]。因此,尽可能地减少胰腺内不受控制的胰蛋白酶活性的产生对于保护患者免受 AP 的影响至关重要。

腺泡细胞合成胰蛋白酶作为前酶胰蛋白酶原,胰蛋白酶原是一种酶原,通常在到达十二指肠之前保持无活性,并被十二指肠酶肠激酶激活。阳离子胰蛋白酶原(PRSS1)是胰蛋白酶原的主要形式(≈65%),其次是阴离子胰蛋白酶原少(PRSS2,≈30%)和中糜蛋白酶(PRSS3,≈5%)。

胰蛋白酶原分子有 2 个球状结构域,通过单个连接链连接(图 57.4)。胰蛋白酶原的激活通常发生在肠激酶或胰蛋白酶将 8 个氨基酸的肽[胰蛋白酶原活化肽(未显示)]从胰蛋白酶原裂解形成胰蛋白酶时。

胰蛋白酶原也有 2 个位点,使其被蛋白分解酶消化。胰蛋白酶可通过另一种胰蛋白酶分子在 Arg122-Val123 肽键或另一种消化酶糜蛋白酶 C(CTRC)在 Leu81-Glu82 肽键裂解而被消化[71,72]。

胰蛋白酶原分子还具有 2 个钙结合袋,可确定胰蛋白酶原分子是否会被胰蛋白酶激活(在高钙浓度下)或被胰蛋白酶破坏(在低钙浓度下)。因此,局部钙浓度是胰蛋白酶激活和失活之间的关键开关[73]。

胰蛋白酶原可通过自动激活(通过钙升高和细胞 pH 降低促进)、通过另一种胰蛋白酶、通过其他细胞区室(如溶酶体)中的其他酶和/或其他机制过早激活为胰蛋白酶[74-76]。此外,根据对特发性 RAP 患者的研究、细胞生物学研究、动物模型和体外实验,推导出了在错误的时间控制错误地点胰蛋

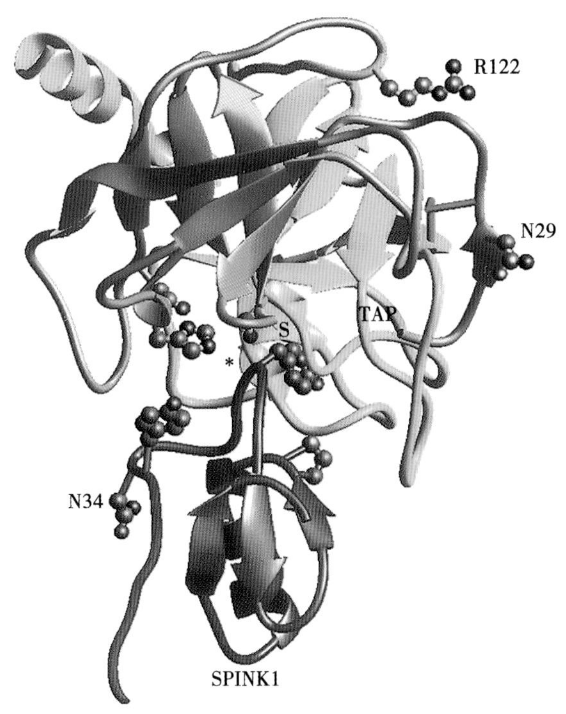

图 57.4　基于 X 射线晶体学的阳离子胰蛋白酶原(PRSS1)和胰腺分泌性胰蛋白酶抑制剂(SPINK1)模型。阳离子胰蛋白酶原分子包含 2 个球状结构域(蓝色和黄色),由连接侧链连接(图顶部)。胰蛋白酶原被激活为胰蛋白酶,通过胰蛋白酶原活化肽(TAP)裂解,允许三维构象变化,特异性口袋(S)开放和活性位点的高效酶活性(*)。说明了与遗传性胰腺炎相关的 2 个主要 *PRSS1* 突变(N29,R122)的位置。注意 R122 在连接胰蛋白酶原 2 个(蓝色和黄色)球状结构域的侧链中的位置。显示 SPINK1 分子(红色)与胰蛋白酶结合。说明了与特发性和家族性胰腺炎相关的主要 *SPINK1* 突变 N34 的位置。(Figure courtesy Drs. Andrew Brunskill and William Furey)

白酶活性的多种机制。

6. 胰蛋白酶依赖性胰腺炎途径

泛胰腺腺泡细胞表达的基因内的多种基因变异体通过对胰蛋白酶损伤的不等效保护增加了胰腺炎的风险[37,77-79]。AP 是渐进模型中 RAP(即 SAPE)的第一个警告信号。大部分与 AP 相关的遗传变异与胰蛋白酶依赖性途径有关(见图 57.3)。因此,易患 AP 的遗传因素也使受试者易患 RAP 和 CP。然而,来自腺泡细胞内的其他风险因素可通过通常独立于胰蛋白酶依赖性胰腺炎途径的途径引起 CP(稍后讨论)。

(1) PRSS1:阳离子胰蛋白酶原遗传变异体。研究现阳离子胰蛋白酶原基因的功能获得性突变可引起 HP[9]。两种已充分描述的 *PRSS1* 变体 p. N29I 和 p. R122H 可引起常染色体显性遗传性 HP(稍后讨论)。第三种变体 p. A16V 具有相似但较弱的胰腺炎易感风险[80,81]。图中 p. R122H 和 p. N29I 突变的位置显示与图 57.4 中的活性位点有关。在图 57.3 的胰蛋白酶致病模型中。功能获得性突变位于与钙依赖性胰蛋白酶调节相关的区域,可能促进胰蛋白酶原激活或延缓胰蛋白酶原失活,与钙浓度无关。功能获得性突变通常导致常染色体显性遗传模式;2 个胰蛋白酶原等位基因中只有 1 个必须编码超功能胰蛋白酶时才能引起胰腺炎,从而表现出表型。

另外两个遗传学证据说明了胰蛋白酶在 RAP 和 CP 发生中的重要性。首先,*PRSS1* 位点的二重化导致拷贝数变异,也通过剂量效应易患 HP[82,83]。其次,*PRSS1-PRSS2* 基因位点上的非编码启动子区变体减少了胰蛋白酶原的表达,并且对与胰蛋白酶相关的多种病因的 RAP 和 CP 具有保护作用,包括酒精性 RAP 和 CP[51,84-86]。

(2) PRSS2:阴离子胰蛋白酶原遗传变异体。阴离子胰蛋白酶原(PRSS2)是胰腺胰蛋白酶原的一种形式,通常以阳离子胰蛋白酶原的一半量表达,尽管在某些情况下该比例可能发生变化。迄今为止,尚未发现功能获得性突变。然而,功能缺失突变 *PRSS2* p. G191R 与胰腺炎的保护有关[87,88]。该突变将精氨酸(R)引入 *PRSS2* 的表面环,使其成为胰蛋白酶介导的立即降解的靶标。即使在高钙浓度下也易破坏 PRSS2,保护天然自溶位点,可能降低总胰蛋白酶水平,因此具保护作用。

(3) SPINK1:胰腺分泌性胰蛋白酶抑制剂基因突变。胰腺分泌性胰蛋白酶抑制剂[PSTI 或丝氨酸蛋白酶抑制剂,Kazal 型(SPINK1)]是一种由 56 个氨基酸组成的肽,是胰蛋白酶的自杀抑制剂,它不可逆地阻断胰蛋白酶的活性位点(见图 57.4)。SPINK1 由胰腺腺泡细胞与胰蛋白酶原一起合成,与胰蛋白酶原共定位在酶原颗粒中。在胰腺内,SPINK1 是抵抗过早激活的胰蛋白酶原最重要的防线之一[9,89]。

SPINK1 的表达与胰蛋白酶原的表达无关。SPINK1 是一种急性期反应物,血清浓度随全身炎症而显著升高[90,91]。在胰腺正常情况下,胰蛋白酶原表达水平是胰腺所有基因中最高的,而 SPINK1 水平非常低,导致其抑制效力非常有限[92]。伴随着胰腺炎症,SPINK1 的表达显著增加到胰蛋白酶原的数倍[92],可能导致游离胰蛋白酶活性显著降低。

SPINK1 p. N34S 变异体存在于全世界 1%~4% 的大多数人群中[89,93]。该变异体导致 SPINK1 功能丧失。p. N34S 氨基酸替换本身是良性的,但标志着干扰基因表达的复杂单倍型[94]。*SPINK1* 基因的其他几个变体也被描述过[95]。例如,大于 C 型致病变体的 *SPINK1* IVS3+2T 引起外显子跳跃[96],最常见于亚洲血统个体[97-99]。

SPINK1 变异在儿童早发性 RAP 和 CP 中很常见[89,100],在家族性胰腺炎[93]、TP[43,44] 和酒精性 CP[101,102] 中常见,通常是多基因胰腺炎相关基因型的一个特征[60,103-105]。因此,致病性 *SPINK1* 变异可能与通过胰蛋白酶依赖性胰腺炎途径的胰腺炎的任何病因有关。使用受试者 *SPINK1* 变异频率的多重荟萃分析检验该假设,按不同的近端病因学风险分类[106]。*SPINK1* p. N34S 在与胰蛋白酶依赖性途径[特发性 CP(OR 15)和热带 CP(OR 19)]相关的胰腺炎病因中(高比值比,或 OR)中作用最强。而在其他病因中作用较弱[如酒精相关性胰腺炎(OR 5)]。因此,突变型 *SPINK1* 不能预防胰蛋白酶相关的复发性胰腺损伤。因此,在未受影响的个体中,*SPINK1* 突变的重要性极小,而在 RAP 受试者中,特别是当与 *PRSS1* 或 *CFTR* 突变相关时,*SPINK1* 突变的影响是非常重要的。

SPINK1 究竟是 CP 的易感基因还是修饰基因目前存在争议,因为 *SPINK1* 变异相对常见,在其他胰蛋白酶激活遗传变异的背景下致病。但部分个体具有纯合子或复合杂合子致病 *SPINK1* 基因型,而无其他明显的致病因素。在这些情况下,

复合致病性 *SPINK1* 变体的影响似乎是致病原因（见隔离酶和其他消化酶相关缺陷）。

（4）CTRC：糜蛋白酶原 C 变体。CTRC 是一种钙依赖性丝氨酸蛋白酶，与其他酶原一起在胰腺腺泡细胞中合成。对 CTRC[71,72,107] 的功能研究表明，CTRC 在胰蛋白酶降解中起主要作用，CTRC 的功能缺失突变破坏了这一机制。Rosendahl 及其同事[71] 对 *CTRC* 基因进行了候选基因分析，确定了多个、罕见的功能缺失突变，CP 患者比对照组更常见。重要的是，他们证明了 CTRC 变体 p. R29Q、p. G214R 和 p. S239 C 损害功能[108]。这种变异是罕见的，很少在临床上见到[52]。

第一个关于胰腺炎的全基因组关联研究（GWAS）确定了 *CTRC* 基因位点与胰腺炎之间的强关联[51]。该效应不在 CTRC 蛋白本身内，尽管复杂的单倍型包括编码区的 p. G60G 同义变异[52]。尽管致病性 c. 180 C 大于 T（p. G60 G）等位基因在一般人群中很常见（约占等位基因的 11%），但它与并发致病性 *CFTR* 变异体或 *SPINK1* p. N34S 显著相关［总计 22. 9% vs 16. 1%（10. 2% 无酗酒），OR = 1. 92，95% CI = 1. 26～2. 94，P = 0. 002 3］，与酒精性和非酒精性 CP 病因显著相关（20. 8% vs 12. 4%，OR = 1. 9，95% CI = 1. 30～2. 79，P = 0. 000 9）[52]。在波兰[109]、法国[110] 和印度的 CP 患者中也观察到 CTRC p. G60G 变异的极高患病率[111]。这些发现表明，高危复杂单倍体型干扰了 CTRC 在降解胰腺内胰蛋白酶中的正常和重要作用，可能是通过改变基因表达[52]。

CTRC p. G60G 单倍型在酒精性泛胰腺炎中的作用尤为重要。酒精和吸烟一般同时发生，但 *CTRC* c. 180T（p. G60G）在 CP 中的频率，而不是 RAP，在从不饮酒者-曾经吸烟者（22. 2%）中比曾经饮酒者-从不吸烟者（10. 8%）中更高，这表明吸烟而不是酒精可能是这种相关性的驱动因素[52]。

胰蛋白酶依赖性胰腺炎途径也影响儿童。对波兰儿童人群中高危 CTRC p. G60G 单倍型的分析发现患病率和效应量非常高，次要等位基因频率（MAF）为 32%（而对照组为 10%），OR 为 23（P<0. 001）[109]。在其他人群中的作用需要进一步分析。

7. 蛋白质错误折叠依赖性胰腺炎途径

胰腺消化酶的 DNA 测序确定了许多引起蛋白质非同义突变的遗传变体。进一步研究它们在这种情况下的相对频率，和对照群体以及细胞系中的功能研究发现，当氨基酸替换导致蛋白质错误折叠并增加 RER 应激时，变异体具有致病性[112]。细胞激活状态、基因表达水平、错误折叠程度和在 RER 内聚集倾向均影响未折叠蛋白反应（unfolded protein response，UPR）的活化[113-116]。

蛋白质合成是资源利用最高的细胞过程之一，尤其是在蛋白质分泌细胞中。真核细胞需要一个巨大的、复杂的和高度调节的系统来监测蛋白质合成，根据所需营养物质的可用性和细胞应激来增加或减少整体蛋白质合成[117-119]。被称为分子伴侣的特殊蛋白确保新合成的蛋白正确折叠，不聚集，并进入正确的亚细胞区室。分子伴侣首先被鉴定为是“热休克蛋白”，因为它们在热应激后被显著上调，使蛋白质变性，触发合成更多的蛋白质折叠支持分子。还维持了复合蛋白降解系统，包括降解特定错误折叠蛋白的泛素-蛋白酶体系统，以及降解较大蛋白聚集体和细胞碎片的自噬系统。增加 RER 中未折叠蛋白量的条件触发了 UPR，UPR 由协调的翻译和转录程序组成，旨在降低蛋白质合成速率，增加热休克蛋白的合成，并启动细胞自噬和凋亡。线粒体中也存在类似的过程。最近对胰腺腺泡细胞的研究表明，不受调节的胰蛋白酶活性（来自 Spink3 基因敲除小鼠[120]）、强烈的 UPR 反应、自噬途径的功能障碍和（或）腺泡细胞线粒体功能障碍均导致自噬功能受损，并且是 AP 和 CP 多种近端病因发病机制中的主要促成因素[76,119-121]。然而，实验模型和人类疾病之间的转化需要更多的研究去验证。

（1）**错误折叠的消化酶**：PRSS1，羧肽酶 A1，CTRC，PNLIP。腺泡细胞主要是蛋白质合成细胞，其合成的主要蛋白质是酶原。越来越多的病例报告称，新蛋白质的错误折叠似乎是疾病的主要机制，这包括胰蛋白酶原（*PRSS1*）[115]、羧肽酶 A1[116,122]、*CTRC*[123]、胰腺甘油三酯脂肪酶（*PNLIP*）[124] 和其他罕见突变[112,114]。这些致病性变体需要 DNA 测序来检测和功能研究来表征，因为许多计算机模拟的硅严重分子对于检测这种特定类型的功能障碍是不准确的。也有可能在 CP 病程早期识别这些疾病，并重新利用针对未折叠蛋白引起的其他疾病开发药物，帮助管理这些疾病。

（2）CEL：羧酸酯脂肪酶变体和 EL-CELP 融合蛋白。CEL 是一种消化酶，通过与其独特结构和相邻假基因（*CELP*）有关的几个复杂过程引起胰腺病理改变。发现两个挪威糖尿病和胰腺外分泌功能障碍家系存在 *CEL* 基因外显子 11 的突变[125]。外显子 11 编码人 CEL 羧基端不同数量的串联重复序列。这两个家族均有常染色体显性遗传性糖尿病，通常在 40 岁以前被诊断。所有突变携带者粪便弹性蛋白酶水平均较低，检测的 10 例受试者脂肪吸收系数均较低，脂溶性维生素水平降低。所有家族成员均无 AP 病史。尸检时，发现一名家庭成员的胰腺萎缩和纤维化，组织学检查显示明显的纤维化和黏液化生。第二项使用 MRI 的研究显示，当糖尿病出现在亲属中时，受累儿童在通常年龄之前就表现出胰腺脂肪瘤病的证据[125]。因此，*CEL* 基因变异引起 CP。组织培养研究表明，*CEL* 变异体形成细胞内聚集体触发不适应性 UPR 导致凋亡细胞死亡，是 CP 发生的病理生理学基础[114,126]。

约 1% 的成人有 CEL 及其假基因 CELP 的重组等位基因。杂交基因编码 *CEL* 近端区域和 *CELP* 远端的预测嵌合蛋白，包括 *CELP* 串联重复区域的可变数量[127]。杂交等位基因在北欧特发性 CP 人群中富集 5 倍以上，表明它是 CP 的遗传风险变异体。3 个亚洲人群中均不存在重组等位基因[128]。

（二）非胰腺炎的腺泡细胞功能障碍/衰竭

Shwachman-Diamond 综合征（又称中性粒细胞减少伴胰腺功能不全）：SDS 是一种常染色体隐性遗传的多系统孟德尔疾病、是以胰腺外分泌功能不全（exocrine pancreatic insufficiency，EPI）为特征，而不是胰腺炎、周期性中性粒细胞减少症、骨畸形和其他特征[129,130]。发现一个以前未被表征的致病基因，并命名为 Shwachman-Bodian-Diamond 综合征基因（*SBDS*）[129]。基因产物参与核糖体成熟，这一过程是许多细胞类型的关键。此外，其他基因如 *DNAJC21*、*SRP54*、*EFL1* 和其他的突变似乎会引起类似的综合征[131-134]。疾病和临床综合征的分子机制将在后面讨论。

Johanson-Blizzard 综合征(UBR1)(又称鼻翼育不良、甲状腺功能减退、胰源性胃液缺乏和先天性耳聋综合征)：Johanson-Blizzard 综合征是一种常染色体隐性遗传的多系统孟德尔综合征，其特征是从子宫内便开始出现的胰腺外分泌功能破坏，尽管较轻的病例可能在以后的生命中出现[135,136]。Johanson-Blizzard 综合征是由编码 E3 泛素连接酶之一的 *UBR1*[137] 突变引起的，该酶通常通过蛋白酶体(对细胞内氨基酸的生成至关重要的系统)从细胞中去除和降解各种胞质消化酶[117]。Johanson-Blizzard 综合征的临床谱将在后面进一步描述。

(三) 导管细胞相关的胰腺炎发病机制

胰管系统具有 2 个重要功能。首先，它将每个腺泡连接到十二指肠以输送胰腺消化酶。其次，产生大量碳酸氢钠来中和胃盐酸。碱性胰液还可保护胰腺免受胰腺消化酶的预先激活，以及可能的其他保护功能。

有 2 种一般病理状态将导管与胰腺炎联系起来(见图 57.2)。第一种是导管细胞不能按需生成足够的富含碳酸氢盐的液体。第二种是导管阻塞(见图 57.2 和框 57.1)。因此，低头压、高远端阻力或两者联合可导致流量减少。

(四) 导管细胞生理学和导管相关性胰腺炎概述

近端(上游)导管细胞的主要功能是分泌富含碳酸氢盐的液体，将酶原冲出胰腺并进入十二指肠。富含碳酸氢盐的液体具有 2 个关键功能。首先，胰腺碳酸氢钠分泌在进入十二指肠时起到缓冲胃的酸分泌作用。涉及十二指肠激素分泌素释放的反馈机制与胃的盐酸分泌完美匹配碳酸氢盐分泌(见第 4 和 56 章)。其次，导管中的碳酸氢钠保持碱性 pH，有助于保持胰蛋白酶原处于非活性确认状态。导管细胞碳酸氢盐的分泌似乎进一步受到导管细胞上蛋白酶激活受体以及钙离子传感器和其他与损伤和炎症相关的受体的调节。

碳酸氢盐的分泌过程包括阴离子[氯化物和(或)碳酸氢盐]，穿过导管细胞基底侧膜向顶膜的能量依赖性转运，然后分泌到导管中(图 57.5)。由于导管腔内添加了阴离子增加了导管内的负电势，吸引带正电荷的钠离子进入导管细胞间的管腔内，从而发生分泌[138-140]。添加钠和氯化物/碳酸氢盐可增加溶质浓度和渗透压，并将水吸入导管。导管是一个“死胡同”，随着静水压的增加，溶液被挤出腺泡、导管和胰腺，进入十二指肠。

当导管冲洗机制失效，产生胰蛋白酶，激活其他酶原，随

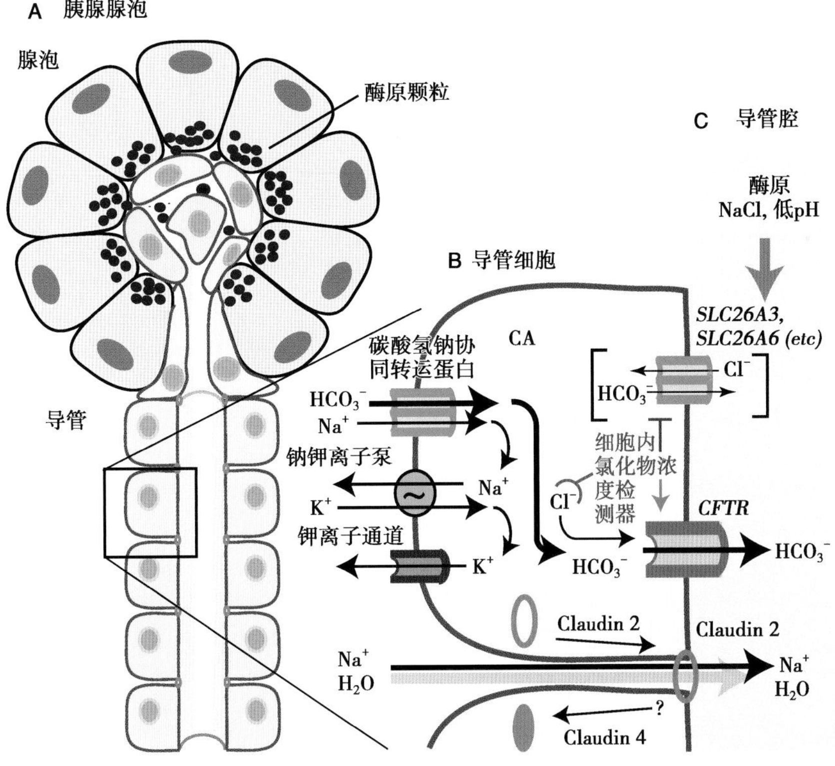

图 57.5　导管细胞和碳酸氢盐分泌。A，胰腺腺泡显示导管和导管细胞的解剖位置。B，具有胰腺碳酸氢钠分泌所需的关键转运蛋白和通道的单个导管细胞的放大视图。碳酸氢盐(HCO^-)主要使用碳酸氢钠协同转运蛋白(NBC)沿电离梯度被拉入导管细胞。钠离子(N^+)梯度由钠-钾泵(NK 泵)维持，而膜电位由钾离子(K^+)通道调节。随着导管细胞活化，CFTR 打开，基于电化学梯度，氯化物(Cl^-)和碳酸氢盐(HCO^-)开始穿过顶膜(B 组和 C 组的连接处)，达到稳态浓度。因为膜电位是负的(如−60mV)，Cl^- 和 HCO^- 都是阴离子(负电荷)，因此离子流的初始方向是细胞到管腔。同时，很可能在紧密连接处 Claudin 4 被 Claudin 2 取代，形成 Na^+ 和 H_2O 的细胞旁通道。在狭窄的管腔内加入阴离子可增加离子浓度和负电荷，将钠和水吸入管腔内，迫使液体流出导管进入十二指肠。由于上游液体被钠和碳酸氢盐取代，氯化物浓度下降。随着细胞内氯化物的损失，WNK1(细胞内氯化物浓度检测器)与 CFTR 相互作用，将其转化为碳酸氢盐传导通道，并抑制 SLC26A6 氯化物-碳酸氢盐交换器，以限制氯化物的进一步损失。当 CFTR 关闭时，系统恢复到静息状态。CFTR，CF 跨膜传导调节因子。(Illustration property of David C Whitcomb，used with permission)

后开始损伤时,就会触发 AP 和 CP。这种失败最著名的例子是胆结石阻塞胰管引起的胆汁性 AP。除梗阻外,胰腺对 AP 敏感,当 *CFTR* 突变时分泌减少,或当存在有利于胰蛋白酶激活的条件时,不能激活 CFTR 和冲洗导管。吸烟等环境因素也会降低导管细胞功能,减少液体分泌,部分是通过引起 CFTR 的内化[141,142]。吸烟和其他环境因素也可能引起黏蛋白积聚或蛋白质堵塞而发病[55,143]。综上所述,导管疾病产生了一个"管道"问题,需要与腺泡细胞相关机制不同的管理策略。

(五) CF 跨膜传导调节因子(*CFTR*)变体

CFTR 基因是调节胰管细胞功能的最重要的分子。双等位基因严重致病性基因突变导致的功能性 CFTR 分子丢失导致 CF,CF 是导管细胞唯一已知的主要、孟德尔(常染色体隐性遗传)遗传病。人近端(上游)胰管细胞利用 CFTR 分泌碳酸氢盐,且没有其他选择一因此 CFTR 的缺失导致胰腺的损伤,这与基因型直接相关。胰腺也是 CF 患者最先衰竭的器官,早期 CP 合并假性囊肿和纤维化导致名称为"胰腺囊性纤维化",现简称为 CF。较轻的突变和包括 CFTR 突变在内的复杂基因型,引起仅局限于一个或多个器官的 CF 样疾病,被称为 CFTR 相关疾病,即 CFTR-RD。

CFTR 分子形成在呼吸系统上皮细胞、汗腺、消化道黏膜、胆道上皮、胰管细胞和其他位置表达的调节离子通道。在生理条件下,通过 CFTR 传导的主要阴离子是氯化物,在某些条件下是碳酸氢盐。*CFTR* 基因包含 24 个外显子和 3 个剪接变体,编码 1 480 个氨基酸的单一蛋白。CFTR 分子有 12 个跨膜结构域、2 个核苷酸结合结构域(NBD1 和 NBD2),一个具有多个磷酸化位点的调节结构域(R 结构域)(图 57.6)。引起各结构域内氨基酸替换的遗传变异决定了不同类型的功能障碍,这些功能障碍进一步分为不同的类别(后文)。

当导管细胞被胰泌素或血管活性肠肽(作用于增加细胞内环磷酸腺苷的基底外侧受体)激活时,可刺激 CFTR 介导的胰液分泌(见第 56 章)。环磷酸腺苷激活蛋白激酶 A 介导的 R 结构域不同位点的磷酸化,随后通过 CFTR 通道增加阴离子传导(如氯化物、碳酸氢盐)。胆碱能药物或其他增加细胞内钙的激动剂对导管细胞的刺激也能增强阴离子分泌。

CFTR 遗传变异分类:CFTR 遗传学在 CFTR 功能紊乱中起主要作用,其临床疾病特征反映了性别、修饰基因、环境因素、代谢状态、生活方式和合并症等其他因素的影响。虽然已知约有 2 000 个 CFTR 变异体(www.cftr2.org),占 CF 或 CFTR-RD 临床病例的绝大多数,但不足 100 例。在具有北欧血统的人群中,仅约 20 种变体的 MAF 高于 0.1%,仅 p.F508del、p.G551D、p.W1282X 和 p.N1303K 的 MAF 大于 1%[144]。其他人群在 CF 患者中(包括美国)观察到的顶级变体的等位基因患病率低得多,其中 ExAC 和 TOPMED 数据库中的 MAF 变体,与 p.F508del(rs113993960)相关,为 0.004~0.007,而 pG542X(rs113993959)为 0.000 3 至 0.000 4,pG551D(rs75527207)为 0.000 1~0.000 3,p.W1282X(rs77010898)为 0.000 3 至 0.000 4,p.N1303K(rs80034486)为 0.001~0.002,p.R5553X(rs74597325)为 0.000 1,p.R117H(rs78655421)为 0.001 5~0.001 6(严重程度不同,取决于与 5T 等位基因的连锁)。根据对患者表型的影响,将 CFTR 变体分类为重度、轻度可变、临界的或良性。根据对蛋白生成、稳定性和通道功能的影响,还将 CFTR 变体分为 5 个机制类别(表 57.1)。Ⅰ类变体包括导致截断、无功能蛋白的提前终止密码子。由于蛋白质错误折叠或其他特征,Ⅱ类变体导致加工缺陷,包括 p.F508del。Ⅲ类变体改变 CFTR 通道调节,被认为是门控突变,因为通道不能开放或保持开放。Ⅳ类变体影响 CFTR 通道传导,使离子流通过通道发生,但水平显著降低。Ⅴ类变体由于外显子跳跃(如 IVS8-T5 等位基因引起外显子跳跃率高)或引起稳定性下降,改变了细胞表面功能性 CFTR 的量。Ⅰ~Ⅲ类功能为重度,没有或极少的功能 CFTR 蛋白到达细胞表面。Ⅳ级和Ⅴ级在功能上是轻度可变和临界的,因为 CFTR 蛋白到达质膜但不能充分发挥作用。现已经提出了Ⅵ类,代表细胞膜的快速分子更新,Ⅶ类代表影响 mRNA 生成的变体[145]。与蛋白质合成和加工途径相对应的功能类别如图 57.3(底行)所示。

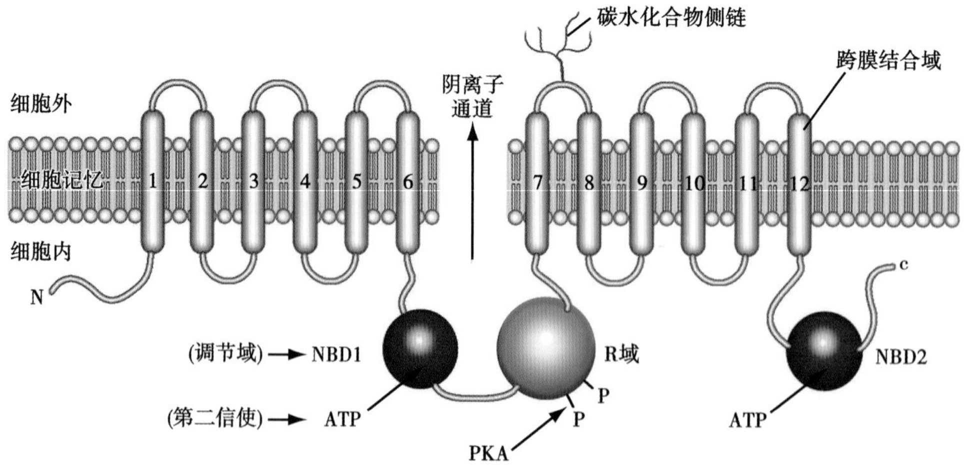

图 57.6 CFTR 结构域。CFTR 分子是一种通过胰管细胞顶端细胞膜形成调节阴离子通道的单一肽。CFTR 至少存在 2 种构象(单通道和双通道)。该分子通过 12 个跨膜结构域(编号 1~12)定位于细胞膜中。至少有 3 个主要调控结构域,包括核苷酸结合结构域 1 和 2(NBD1,NBD2)和一个调控结构域(R 结构域)。一些第二信使系统直接与这 3 个调节结构域相互作用,包括 ATP 和 PKA。钙、细胞内谷氨酸和其他第二信使系统或因子(图中未显示)也调节 CFTR 的各个方面。CFTR,CF 跨膜传导调节因子;PKA,蛋白激酶 A

表 57.1 *CFTR* 突变的分类、效应和潜在治疗

种类	突变(示例)	缺陷(占正常的百分比)	胰腺功能障碍	治疗/批准的
Ⅰ	W1282X G542X R553X R1162X	合成	严重	通读
Ⅱ	F508del A561E N1303K G85E	成熟 0.5% 0.0% 0.2% 0.5%	严重	校正(+) 是(使用增效剂)
Ⅲ	G551D S549R S549N G1244E G1349D	激活 3.2%	严重	增效剂 是 是 是 是
Ⅳ	R117H R334W R347H R347P A455E	传导 20.0% 3.9% 1.0% 5.6%	轻度	增效剂 是 是 是
Ⅴ	A455G 3 849+10kbC>T 2 789+5G>A 621+3A>G 711+3A>G	丰度	轻度	增效剂 是 是
Ⅵ	A455G 3 849+10kbC>T 2 789+5G>A 621+3A>G 711+3A>G	稳定	轻度	稳定剂
Ⅶ	Del2,3(21kb) 1 717-1G>A 1 898+1G>A	无蛋白	严重	无法挽救

用于说明每个 CFTR 功能类别中的变体和美国获批治疗的示例新疗法和扩展适应证正在持续开发和批准过程中,因此治疗决策应基于最新更新指南。

CFTR 基因型:基因型是 CFTR 位点 2 个等位基因的组合。定义了细胞中 CFTR 的整体功能,一个等位基因遗传自父亲,另一个遗传自母亲。CFTR 变异体可以在一个或两个等位基因上,功能严重的变异体必须在两个等位基因上引起 CF。如果一个严重的变异在一个等位基因上,那么这个人通常是无症状的,被认为是携带者——即使细胞 CFTR 功能降低了大约 50%。如果一个人具有 3 个或 3 个以上 CFTR 基因变异,那么其中至少有 2 个必须在同一等位基因上(称为复杂等位基因)。在同一等位基因上的变体被认为是顺式的,而在相反等位基因上的变体被认为是反式的。如果有多个致病性 CFTR 变体都是顺式的,那么该人是 CFTR 变体携带者,将无症状。除非在反式等位基因上有未鉴定的变体(如第Ⅶ类),或者他们有涉及其他基因和环境因素的复杂紊乱。

CFTR 功能表型:CF 患者受累的许多器官具有替代途径和保护机制,可最大限度地减少 CFTR 功能完全丧失的影响。胰腺和汗腺是两个例外,它们具有良好的基因型-表型相关性。由于一个 CFTR 拷贝的完全丢失没有表型,双等位基因致病性 CFTR 变体的相对严重程度由最不严重的变体定义。因此,具有两种严重 CFTR 基因型的个体可能具有典型的、伴胰腺功能不全(pancreatic insuffciency,PI)的早发性 CF,而具有一种严重和一种轻度可变 CFTR 基因型的个体可能具有较轻形式的 CF、发病年龄较晚、胰腺功能充足(pancreatic sufficiency,PS)[146]。然而,胰腺并不容易研究,因此在个体中检测 CFTR 功能通常是通过汗液氯化物检测来完成的。

CFTR 变体功能的测量:在大约 2 000 个 CFTR 变体中,根据患者表型,当未分类变体与已知的重度变体反式时,绝大多数暂时归类为重度、轻度可变、临界或良性。CFTR 蛋白功能最准确的测量指标是进行定点突变,在多种实验条件下,在优化的细胞系统中测试突变体 CFTR 的通透性和电导特性[147,148]。这些信息提供了对蛋白质序列改变变异体影响的直接功能洞察。每个等位基因(反式)上最具损伤性的变异体的总和应该可以假设地预测患者疾病的严重程度。虽然这种方法是一个有用的近似值,但许多其他因素有助于发挥功能包括复杂单倍型中的其他致病变异、CFTR 和各种器官内其他分子的机制作用、修饰因子、表观遗传学、环境因素等。因此,即使在基因型相似或相同的患者中,例如同卵双胞胎[149]也可能存在广泛的表型特征或严重程度。此外,由于 CF 患者的临床症状谱可以与其他非 CF 疾病重叠,CF 或 CFTR-RD 的诊断不仅需要临床环境、家族史和(或)CFTR 基因型,还需要检测患者的 CFTR 功能。

碳酸氢盐缺陷型 CFTR 变体(CFTR-BD):通过关注一个器官对疾病进行表型分析可能导致将变异归类为良性,而它们与其他器官的疾病密切相关。这是一类与胰腺炎相关的 CFTR 变异体的情况,但研究者在观察因肺部疾病转诊的患者时将其归类为良性。上皮细胞具有一种称为 WNK1 的内部氯化物浓度监测受体,可调节多个离子通道、转运蛋白和泵的活性[150]。WNK1 直接调节 CFTR,动态改变渗透性和电导特性,从氯化物型通道到碳酸氢盐型通道[151]。LaRusch 及其同事[148]基于这个范例和以前的数学模型,证明了 CFTR 依赖性碳酸氢盐分泌在人类胰腺中的关键作用[138]。他们从 NAPS2 研究中筛选了 984 例表型良好的胰腺炎病例,从 81 例先前描述的胰腺炎患者 CFTR 变异体中,筛选出具有碳酸氢盐缺陷电导(CFTR-BD)的 CFTR 的候选突变。与典型 CF 无关的 9 种变体(CFTR p. R74Q, p. R75Q, p. R117H, p. R170H, p. L967S, p. L997F, p. D1152H, p. S1235R 和 p. D1270N)与胰腺炎相关(OR 1.5, $P=0.002$)。克隆变体并在 EK 293T 细胞中检测氯化物和碳酸氢盐传导性,尽管氯化物正常,但在 WNK1 存在的情况下,碳酸氢盐渗透性和传导性显著降低。三维模型表明,碳酸氢盐传导缺陷可能是由至少 4 种机制引起的(图 57.7)。分子动力学模拟表明 CFTR 通道的物理限制和动态通道调节的改变。由于其他一些器官使用 CFTR 分泌碳酸氢盐,NAPS2 队列进一步评估了慢性鼻窦炎(因为黏液水合需要碳酸氢盐)以及男性不育,因为碳酸氢盐是输精管发育[避免先天性双侧输精管缺如(congenital bilateral absence of the

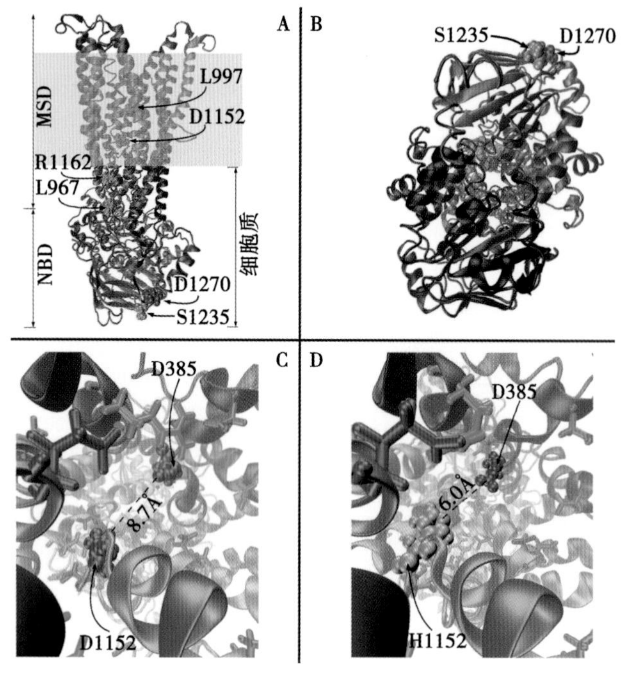

图 57.7 CFTR 结构——碳酸氢盐变体(CFTR-BD)。A 和 B,显示了来自侧面和底部的 CFTR 分子,残基 1-859 为黑色,残基 860-1480 为蓝色,CFTR-BD 变体为红色,阴影区域表示质膜的位置。CFTR-BD 变体的不同位置表明存在多种机制,包括通道阻塞、NBDs 相互作用改变、细胞内信号改变和(或)其他机制。C,是通过向下观察通道筒观察的野生型 p. D1152 的预测位置。D,是致病性变体 p. H1152 的预测位置。C 和 D,显示了 CFTR p. D1152H 通过物理阻塞较大碳酸氢根离子孔隙对碳酸氢盐电导的影响。p. D1152H 周围的电荷分布用红色带负电荷的残基和绿色带正电荷的残基突出显示。D 中的变体残基 H1152(青色)可向通道中心移动,从而导致通道直径收缩。Å,以 AngstrÖms 测量的野生型和变体残基位置的通道直径;MSD,跨膜结构域;NBD,核苷酸结合结构域。(From LaRusch J, Jung J, General IJ, et al. Mechanisms of CFTR functional variants that impair regulated bicarbonate permeation and increase risk for pancreatitis but not for cystic fibrosis. PLOS Genetics 2014;10[4]:e1004376.)

vas deferens, CBAVD)]和精子存活所必需的。研究发现 CFTR-BD 变异体显著增加鼻-鼻窦炎(OR 2.3, $P<0.005$)和男性不育症(OR 395, $P<0.0001$)的风险。此外,杂合子 CFTR-BD 变异体加 SPINK1 p. N34S 变异基因型与胰腺炎密切相关,无鼻窦炎和不孕效应[104,148]。

汗液氯化物检测:汗液氯化物检测仍然是 CFTR 功能的最可靠、标准化和广泛可用的功能检测,因为正常的汗腺功能直接依赖于 CFTR 功能,并且因为与 CF 疾病发病相关的大多数其他腺体和器官相对无法获得[152]。汗腺由产生等渗盐溶液的外分泌腺和连接汗腺至皮肤表面的汗腺导管组成。CFTR 和上皮钠通道(ENaC)在外分泌腺尤其是导管中表达,它们吸收氯化物和钠,产生低渗(低钠和氯化物浓度)溶液(汗液),在不损失电解质的情况下蒸发汗液使身体降温。正常情况下,汗液中氯化物的浓度低于 20mmol/L,但水平随着分泌速率的增加而增加,有一些人中浓度可达到近 60mmol/L[152]。

在囊性纤维化(CF)的患者中,氯化物的浓度比正常高 3~5 倍,静息浓度高于 60mmol/L,刺激氯化物水平接近 120mmol/L。重度、引起 CF 的突变杂合子受试者的汗液氯化物检测通常几乎正常[152]。值得注意的是,对一些临床囊性纤维化和汗液氯化物检测非常异常的患者进行广泛的基因检测,只有一种可识别的致病基因 CFTR 变体(它们似乎是杂合子),表明其他强烈影响 CFTR 功能的重要因素尚未确定。目前诊断囊性纤维化的临床指南包括汗液氯化物浓度≥60mmol/L,以及与囊性纤维化一致的临床特征(包括新生儿筛查阳性,NBS)和(或)阳性家族史[153]。具有囊性纤维化特征且中间汗液氯化物测试结果为 30~59mmol/L 的患者仍可能患有囊性纤维化[153]。仅影响碳酸氢盐传导性的 CFTR 变异体患者可能被汗液氯化物检测遗漏。

汗液氯化物检测在评估可能未确诊 CF 或 CFTR-RD 的有症状患者中也可能很重要。CFTR-RD 包括 RAP 和 CP、CBAVD、播散性支气管扩张和硬化性胆管炎,它有可单独出现或结合其他特征[154-156]。当发现不明原因的 RAP 和(或)早期 CP 患者可能具有致病源性 CFTR 变体时,确定其是否具有 CP 或 CFTR-RD 的临床验证的功能试验是汗液氯化物试验。特异性靶向 CFTR 功能的新疗法的可用性突出了诊断 CF 或 CFTR-RD 的重要性(后文)。虽然胰泌素刺激的胰腺功能检测也可测量 CFTR 功能,但结果的解释受到进展性胰腺疾病胰液中碳酸氢盐浓度降低和环境因素(如吸烟)的干扰[157-159]。

囊性纤维化基金会临床护理指南建议进一步评价中间汗液氯化物水平,如图 57.8 所示。该算法从"囊性纤维化的临床表现"开始,可能包括美国 NBS 期间免疫无反应性胰蛋白酶原水平升高,但汗液氯化物检测结果居中的患者[160]。这种方法也可能对仅影响胰腺的 CTRF-RD 有用,但这种方法在成人 RAP 或 CP 人群中的应用尚未见报道。

新生儿 CF 筛查——CRMS/CFSPID:绝大多数 NBS 和中间汗液氯化物检测结果的婴儿在不确定的时间内保持无疾病状态。因此,在美国,这些婴儿被归类为 CF 跨膜传导调节因子相关代谢综合征("代谢综合征"反映的是账单代码问题,而不是任何代谢特征),在其他国家被归类为 CF 筛查阳性、非确定性诊断(CF screen positive, inconclusive diagnosis, CFSPID)[160]。美国/欧洲共识小组统一的新定义将 CRMS/CFSPID 定义为一种婴儿的特征,该婴儿 CF 的 NBS 检测呈阳性,并且(a)汗液氯化物低于 30mmol/L,2 个 CFTR 突变,其中至少 1 个具有不明确的表型结果;或者(b)中间汗液氯化物值(30~59mmol/L)和 1 或 0 个引起 CF 的突变[160]。CF 的突变在 CFTR2 数据库中进行了一般性定义,其他变异被归类为具有不同临床后果的突变(MVCC,如Ⅳ类或Ⅴ类),非 CF 突变,当与另一个 CF 突变反式突变时,不会导致 CF(不排除突变可能导致类似轻度 CF 或 CFTR-RD 的 CF 样临床特征)、意义不明的变体或良性[156]。我们建议由有资质的医生进行遗传咨询和随访临床评估,并建议进一步检测[160]。

CFTR 疾病机制:CF 的医学方法稍后介绍,而 CFTR 在疾病中的机制在此讨论。两个 CFTR 等位基因的严重突变导致 CFTR 功能的完全或几乎完全丧失导致 CF。CF 的分子后果包括不能充分水合黏液和其他大分子,导致黏性物质和浓缩腺体蓄积。这种情况导致胰腺和呼吸系统的器官进行性破坏,以及肝脏、肠道、汗腺和上皮细胞分泌发挥重要生理

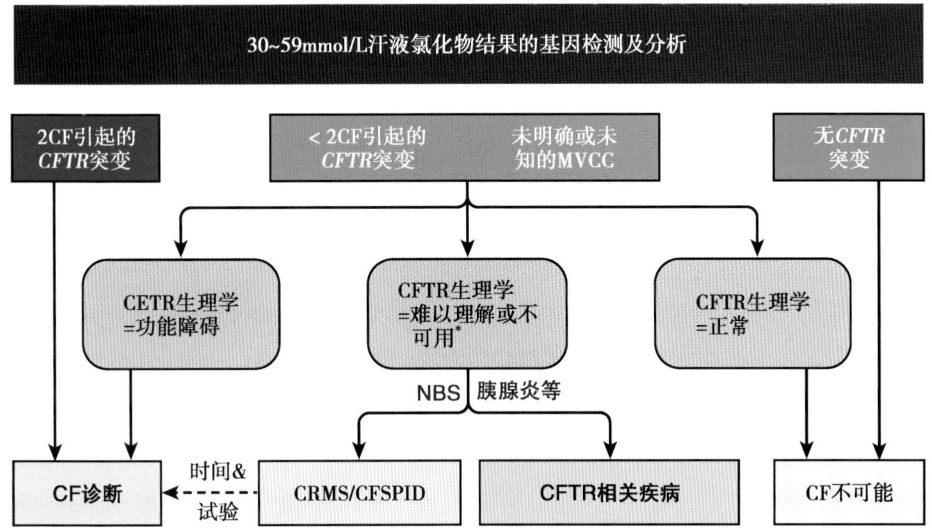

图 57.8　囊性纤维化(CF)和囊性纤维化跨膜传导调节因子(CFTR-RD)的诊断指南。诊断为囊性纤维化、CRMS/CFSPID 和 CFTR-RD。CP 的主要临床表现包括新生儿筛查(NBS)结果阳性、CF 的体征和症状和/或 CF 的家族史。评估从汗液氯化物检测开始。汗液氯化物大于 60mmol/L 的可诊断为 CF,低于 29mmol/L 则不太可能诊断 CF(未显示)。汗液氯化物 30~59mmol/L(蓝条)代表中间范围,应考虑扩展 *CFTR* 基因分析和/或功能分析。如果 *CFTR* 基因检测确定了一种致病性 *CFTR* 变异和/或 MVCCs 和/或未定义的变异,则需要 CFTR 生理学检测(NPD 或 ICM)来定义 CF、CRMS/CFSPID(婴儿)、CFTR 相关疾病(通常为大龄儿童或成人)或另一种非 CF 疾病的最终分类。请注意,CRMS/CFSPID 类别(浅黄色框)并不排除最终的 CF 诊断,因为临床特征可能随着时间的推移或进一步检测而发展(虚线箭示)。虚线箭是单向的,因为 CF 的诊断在患者及其家属的心目中几乎不可能消除。复杂基因型包括一种 *CFTR* 变异加另一种致病性变异(例如,在 SPINK 1、CTRC)的患者可能是胰腺炎的高危人群,但患 CF 的风险较低,通过 NPD 或 ICM 可能接近正常的 CFTR 生理学,因为这测量的是总体基因型,而不是每个等位基因产物的功能(归类为 CF 不太可能,浅蓝色方框)。CRMS/CFSPID,囊性纤维化相关代谢综合征/囊性纤维化筛查阳性(包括诊断);ICM,肠道电流测量;MVCC,不同临床结果的突变;NPD,鼻腔电位差。* CF 综合征的临床症状和体征见正文。(Modified form Farrell PM, White TB, Ren CL, et al. Diagnosis of cystic fibrosis: consensus guidelines from the Cystic Fibrosis Foundation. J Peds 2017; S4-S15e. 1. Illustration property of David C Whitcomb, used with permission.)

作用的其他部位的功能障碍。如前所述,胰腺具有双重风险,因其大多数蛋白质是酶原,胰蛋白酶激活将导致复发性损伤,并最终通过进行性纤维化破坏胰腺。在囊性纤维化患儿中,由胰蛋白酶介导的胰腺损伤和破坏与此模型一致,因为囊性纤维化的病理机制是假性囊肿形成和纤维化,而不是单独的萎缩(正如导管阻塞所预期的)[161]。囊性纤维化患儿的胰腺损伤似乎与发育中的腺泡细胞中胰蛋白酶原的表达大致平行,从妊娠 16 周开始,浓度逐渐增加,直至患儿出生,并在出生后 6 个月内水平显著升高[162,163]。由此产生的组织学结果具有儿童和成人发病的终末期 CP 的许多特征,但也有明显的扩张导管,表现为多个充满蛋白的囊肿(图 57.9)。

具有致病性 *CFTR* 变异个体的总体临床表现取决于 *CFTR* 组合突变的性质、缺陷基因操作的遗传背景(如修饰基因)和环境因素[156,161,164]。约 70%~90% 的非西班牙裔白人 CF 患者携带 p. F508del。不同的突变是其他种族和祖先群体共有的,包括 3120+1G 大于 A,这是非洲裔美国人第二常见的 CF 等位基因(9.5%~3%)[165],西班牙裔美国人常见的 p. R334W 突变,以及德系犹太人的 p. W1282X 突变(~45%)[156,166,167]。

携带 2 个 *CFTR* 重度反式突变的患者通常会出现 CF 的经典特征,汗腺中的氯化物水平升高、胰腺功能不全、复发性和慢性肺部感染以及男性 CBAVD。重度 CF 的复杂表现还包

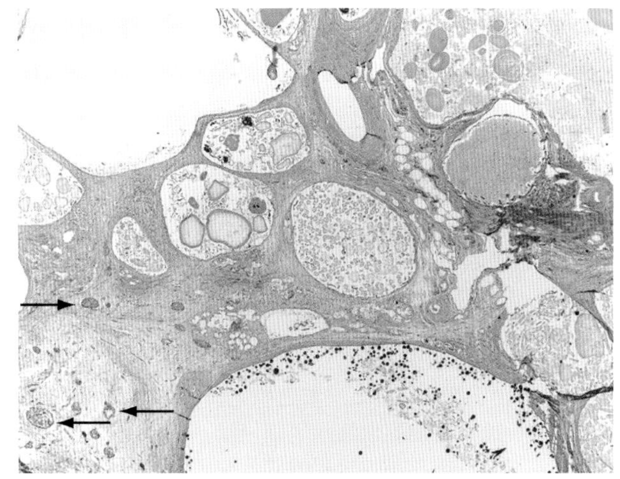

图 57.9　来自一例具有 CF 严重特征的儿童尸检的胰腺组织病理学。没有残留的正常导管或腺泡。相反,可见扩张的导管和有浓缩物质的"囊肿"。其他 CF 病例跨越了该图像与其他形式胰腺炎伴腺泡萎缩、纤维化和慢性炎症所见慢性胰腺炎之间的范围。箭头显示残留胰岛。(From Whitcomb DC, Cystic fibrosis-associated pancreatitis. In: Beger HG, Warshaw A, Buchler MW et al, editors. The pancreas: an integrated textbook of basic science, medicine and surgery. Oxford: Blackwell; 2008.)

括胎粪性肠梗阻、远端肠梗阻综合征(distal intestinal obstruction syndrome,DIOS)、胆囊功能障碍、肝硬化和其他胃肠道问题。

一例重度 *CFTR* 突变(Ⅰ~Ⅲ类,如 p. F508del)和一个轻度可变 *CFTR* 突变(Ⅳ类或Ⅴ类,如 p. R117H 或 p. R334W)患者通常因 CFTR 功能不完全丧失,氯化物和(或)碳酸氢盐电导部分降低,以及随后的残余导管细胞功能而伴有 PS-CF,导致腺泡细胞存活[138,146]。这种 CFTR 功能异常的残余胰腺实质使 PS-CF 患者成为 AP 和 RAP 的高危人群,发生率为 22%[146]。这些患者更有可能只有一部分表达 CFTR 的器官受到影响,表现出的症状可能发生在生命较晚的时候(青少年或 20 多岁)。

环境和修饰基因变异:CF 的许多特征不能用 *CFTR* 序列的变异来解释。相反,这些特征是由特定的环境因素或修饰基因引起的[156,161]。环境因素,如呼吸系统的细菌定植、烟草烟雾、营养不良[168]和环境过敏原[169]都会导致肺部疾病的严重程度。其他主要因素是修饰基因,这些修饰基因强有力地导致 *CFTR* 基因型明显相同的患者具有广泛的临床特征[156,167,170]。1998 年 2 组实验[171,172]证明致病性 *CFTR* 变异在特发性和酒精性 CP 中也非常常见,这表明 *CFTR* 突变可能是更复杂性状的一部分[104,173]。由于杂合子致病性 *CFTR* 变异体在欧洲血统人群中很常见,并且由于 CF 儿童(无 CF 的专性 *CFTR* 突变携带者)的父母与正常人群相比,似乎没有增加 AP 或 CP 的发病率[174],很可能需要一种特异性靶向胰腺的第二因子[37,173]。在早发性特发性胰腺炎中,第二个因素可能是 *SPINK1*、*CTRC* 或 *CASR* 的遗传变异、胰腺分裂等解剖因素、环境因素或其他机制[99,103-105,148,175]。尽管仍然需要对这些患者进行高质量的治疗试验,但问题是"管道"问题之一,应该考虑恢复丧失的 CFTR 功能和(或)降低胰液流动阻力的方法。

(六) 钙敏感受体基因变体

钙在胰腺生理和病理生理中起着多重作用。一方面,腺泡内细胞钙的调节对于预防胰腺损伤至关重要[176,177],而增加胰管中钙的浓度会增加持续胰蛋白酶激活和沉淀为含钙结石的风险。钙敏感受体基因(*CASR*)是 G 蛋白偶联受体超家族的膜结合成员。CaSR 在钙稳态中起重要作用,反映在其参与钙稳态的甲状旁腺和肾小管细胞表达中。CaSR 已在人胰腺腺泡和导管细胞以及各种非外分泌组织中被鉴定出[178],尽管其在胰腺中的功能意义尚未确定。通过扩展十二指肠生理学,CaSR 在胰管中的可能作用是合理的,注意到 CaSR 与 CFTR 在分泌碳酸氢盐的上皮细胞中共表达[179]。CaSR 激活剂量依赖性地升高细胞内钙水平,引起钙依赖性 CFTR 碳酸氢盐分泌以及调节参与该过程的其他分子[179]。在 *CASR* 中已描述了 170 多种与家族性低钙尿症高钙血症、新生儿重度原发性甲状旁腺功能亢进、常染色体显性低钙血症和相关高钙血症或低钙血症疾病相关的功能性突变(激活和失活)[180]。常见的 *CASR* 变异 p. R990G、p. A986S 和 p. Q1011E 与各种人群的尿石症和高钙尿症密切相关[181]。

2003 年,Felderbauer 等[182]调查了一个家族性胰腺炎和 *SPINK1* p. N34S 变异的家族。然而,这些家庭成员中只有 2 人患有 CP,并且都被发现有一个新的 *CASR* c. 518T>C 突变,与高钙血症有关。随后在印度 TP 患者[183]以及美国散发性和酒精性 CP 患者中发现了其他 CASR 变异体(伴或不伴 *SPINK1* 突变)之间的相关性,其中 *CASR* p. R990G(rs1042636)变异体使相对风险分别增加了 2 倍和 3 倍[184](给出 rs 编号,因为氨基酸编号可能会根据所使用的 *CASR* 转录本而发生变化)。在一个法国队列中[185]也发现了多个罕见的 *CASR* 变异,在多个中国胰腺炎患者中发现了 p. A986S 变异(rs1801725)[186]。*CASR* p. Q1011E(rs1801726)也被广泛研究,但在胰腺疾病中的明确作用尚未确定。在不同人群中发现不同的 CASR 多态性是耐人寻味的,但似乎推测的轻度高钙血症是胰腺炎的辅助因子,而不是一个独立的危险因素,如在高钙血症动物模型中所见[63,187],或作为具有 *SPINK1* 或 *CFTR* 或其他因素的复杂功能基因型的一部分。降低 CaSR 功能的 *CASR* 变体也可能导致胰腺疾病,因为 CaSR 也作为十二指肠的氨基酸受体,将肠腔营养物质与随后刺激胰酶分泌的胆囊收缩素释放联系起来[188]。

三、修饰炎症、进展为慢性胰腺炎和修饰表型的基因

在与损伤和炎症反应相关的基因中发现了许多致病性遗传变异。这些变体的致病作用似乎不是通过引起损伤,而是通过改变机体对其他病因引起的损伤或炎症的反应所致。

(一) *CLDN2-MORC4*

Claudin 2 是由 *CLDN2* 编码的紧密连接分子。Claudins 封闭上皮细胞之间的空间,标记顶侧和基底侧膜之间的转换,并控制水和电解质的细胞旁流量。人类基因组最多有 27 个 Claudin 蛋白家族,一般分为"紧密"封闭 Claudin(如 1、3、5、11、14、19)和"渗漏"孔形成 Claudin(如 2、10、15、17)[189]。Claudin 2 在主动分泌/吸收或炎症过程中插入紧密连接以交换"密封"Claudins,形成对钠和水具有渗透性的孔隙[189-191]。

第一个 GWAS 在 *CLDN2* 基因位点上发现了一个大的复杂单倍型之间的强相关性,该单倍型从跨膜 *CLDN2* 的 *TBC1D8B*——*RIPPLY* 基因延伸到 rs7057398 和 rs12688220[51] 定义的 *MORC4* 基因。风险等位基因在对照人群中普遍存在(欧洲约 26%,亚洲人约 36%,非洲祖先约 2%),提示它可能是一种疾病严重程度修饰因子。与该位点的相关性与胰腺炎风险已在多个非非洲祖先群体的多项研究中重复[84-86,192]。Claudin-2 在胰管和腺泡细胞中表达,在 AP 中表达上调[51,193]。*CLDN2* 编码区无突变与疾病风险相关[51,194]。MORC4 是一种 CW 型锌指蛋白,可能的转录因子在大多数细胞中低水平表达,但在睾丸和胎盘中高水平表达[195,196]。胰腺中 *MORC4* 的表达似乎并不能改变胰腺炎[51],需要进一步的研究来确定胰腺疾病中可能的致病性。尚不清楚 *RIPPLY1* 和 *TBC1D8B* 在胰腺中的表达[51]。

CLDN2 位点(也称为 *CLND2-MORC4* 位点)需要按性别对群体进行单独分析,因为它位于 X 染色体上。男性拥有一条染色体(半合子基因型),女性拥有 2 条染色体(纯合子或杂合子基因型)。使用 NAPS2 队列 Whitcomb 及其同事[51]将男性风险等位基因携带者建模为纯合子(男性半合子频率为 0.26),女性为风险等位基因的真正纯合子(女性纯合子频率

为 0.07)，表明这可能有助于解释男性 CP 风险高于女性的原因。Giri 等人计算了纯合子和杂合子 rs12688220 风险等位基因的 OR 值分别为 14.62 和 1.51[86]。按酒精和非酒精病因比较 CP 亚群，*CLDN2* 高危单倍型显示与酒精密切相关($P=4\times10^{-7}$)，高危等位基因单倍型见于 26% 的对照组、32% 的非酒精相关病因组和 43% 的酒精相关胰腺炎组[51]，且与女性(OR 1.71)[84]相比，在男性中的作用更强(OR 2.66)[84]。

CLDN2 在精准医疗中的重要性源于等位基因在大多数人群中的高频率，以及风险等位基因与酒精的强烈相互作用。尽管还需要进一步的工作来更好地理解其潜在的机制，这些数据对于胰腺炎和饮酒患者的风险分层和咨询是有用的。

高甘油三酯血症相关基因变异

高甘油三酯血症是 AP、AP 严重程度及 CP 的危险因素。脂蛋白脂肪酶基因(lipoprotein lipase gene，LPL)的致病变体作为与胰腺炎相关的高甘油三酯血症疾病的原型。甘油三酯(triglyceride，TG)本身不具有直接毒性，但其被脂肪酶(包括胰脂肪酶)水解后可产生饱和脂肪酸和不饱和脂肪酸，具有促炎性，对胰腺和其他器官具有高水平毒性[197,198]。

根据空腹血清甘油三酯水平对患者进行分类[199]。正常水平低于 150mg/dL(1mmol = 88.6mg/dL)，高甘油三酯血症分为轻度(150~199mg/dL)、中度(200~999mg/dL)、重度(1 000~1 999mg/dL)和极重度(≥2 000mg/dL)[199]。重度高甘油三酯血症患者罹患胰腺炎的终生风险约为 5%，极重度者约为 10%~20%，明显高于一般人群约 0.5%~1% 的终生风险[200]。虽然发生 AP 的风险主要见于重度或极重度高甘油三酯血症(见第 58 章)，但在实践中，血清 TG 的水平随饮食变化显著，故门诊患者的 TG 水平与 AP 早期观察到的 TG 水平之间并没有很好的相关性[201]。

TG 水平与 AP 的严重程度及并发症直接相关。

在来自美国宾夕法尼亚州匹兹堡市 400 例 AP 患者的单中心研究中，持续性器官衰竭的发生率与 TG 水平成比例增加，低于 150mg/dL 时约为 17%，150~199mg/dL 时约为 30%，200~999mg/dL 时约为 39%，高于 1 000mg/dL 时约为 48%[202]。在多变量分析中，TG 水平为 200~999mg/dL 和大于 1 000mg/dL 时，持续性器官衰竭的风险分别增加 OR2.6 和 4.9[202]。在中国的江西南昌 1 539 例 AP 患者中也观察到类似的趋势[203]。高甘油三酯血症 AP 的风险与未经治疗/控制不佳的糖尿病、酗酒、妊娠、用药和遗传因素相关[200]。因此，高甘油三酯血症 AP 代表了一种复杂的基因-环境和可变风险的复合物，有可能通过精准医学评估和靶向治疗进行管理。

高甘油三酯血症的遗传学涉及 TG 水平高达数千的一些家族性综合征，更复杂的情况需要遗传和环境条件的组合考量。家族性高脂血症，以前分为 Fredrickson Ⅰ型、Ⅴ型和Ⅳ型，常与 RAP 有关。Ⅰ型高脂血症现被称为家族性乳糜微粒血症综合征(familial chylomicronemia syndrome，FCS)，是一种常染色体隐性遗传病，与 *LPL* 或其他基因的致病变异有关。

LPL：*LPL*[207]突变导致的脂蛋白脂肪酶缺乏[204-206]引起约 80% 的 FCS 病例。血清 TG 浓度和乳糜微粒显著升高支持 LPL 缺乏症的诊断，当患者无 AP 发作时，可通过静脉注射肝素试验[206]证实此诊断。

其他血脂异常基因：FCS 还可见于载脂蛋白 C-Ⅱ(*APOC2*)[205]、*APOA5*、糖基磷脂酰肌醇锚定的高密度脂蛋白结合蛋白 1(*GPIHBP1*)、脂肪酶成熟因子 1(*LMF1*)等其他基因的功能缺失突变，以及存在 LPL 酶的循环抑制剂[208,209]。此外，Johansen 和他的同事[210]对血脂异常/高甘油三酯血症患者进行了 GWAS 研究，并在几个基因中确定了与疾病密切相关的常见变异，包括 *APOA5*、*GCKR*、*LPL* 和 *APOB*。

目前已知许多家族性或散发性高甘油三酯血症的患者都有一种复杂的综合征，称为多因子乳糜微粒血症综合征(MCS)。MCS 患者可能同时存在杂合子功能缺失突变和(或)TG 升高基因的可能致病的频繁变异，从而产生作为一种复杂遗传疾病的重度高甘油三酯血症[211]。最近一个专家小组建议定义 FCS 评分来区分 FCS 和 MCS，并推测这将有助于确定谁有 AP 的风险[211]。然而，这一推测尚未得到充分的检验。

家族性高脂血症和 CP 的关系复杂，代表了高甘油三酯血症性 AP 患者的一个子集。在 521 例表型良好的 CP 患者的 NAPS2-CV 队列中，医生确定 4% 的病例的主要病因是高甘油三酯血症，另外 13% 的病例是风险因素，表明 CP 伴高甘油三酯血症的风险增加约 2~6 倍[49]。在匹兹堡大学 121 例血清 TG 水平≥500mg/dL 的 AP 患者的另一项研究中，平均随访 64.7±42.8 个月后，16.5% 的患者确定为 CP[212]。综上所述，CP 似乎可在家族性高甘油三酯血症的最严重、长期和控制不佳的病例中发生，这些病例适合 AP 的反复发作(例如具有遗传性 LPL 缺陷的患者)以及复杂的高甘油三酯血症和 AP 患者。

(二) SLC26A9：CF 疾病严重程度修饰基因

遗传修饰基因在胰腺疾病中的作用在 CF 中有明确的定义。在 CF 患者中进行的遗传相关性研究已经确定了许多修饰基因，这些修饰基因在新生儿筛查 CF 和 CF 相关糖尿病(CF-related diabetes，CFDM)时与更严重的胰腺疾病相关，如下文所述[213,214]。CF 中最强的修饰基因之一是溶质载体家族 26 成员 9 基因(*SLC26A9*)，一种多功能离子转运蛋白，作为氯离子/碳酸根离子交换、氯离子通道和氯化钠协同转运[215]发挥作用，最初在 GWAS 研究中被确定为主要的 CFDM 修饰基因[213]。

SLC26A9 在唾液腺、胃和肺中高浓度表达，在肾脏、十二指肠、胰腺和其他器官中表达水平较低。SLC26A9 对胰腺功能并不关键；基因敲除小鼠的主要表型是胃酸分泌完全丧失，而不是胰腺功能障碍，这表明该通道/转运蛋白在胃酸分泌中起着至关重要的作用[215]。然而，SLC26A9 与 CFTR 在许多分泌液体的上皮细胞中合作，CFTR 功能的丧失和 SLC26A9 功能的降低都会导致更严重的 CF 表型[213,214,216,217]。CF 患者和携带高危 *SLC26A9* 基因变异患者的胰腺疾病更严重[214,216,218]以及，胎粪性肠梗阻[214]、肺功能障碍[217]和其他影响的风险更高[216,219]。此外，携带致病性 *SPC26A9* 变体的患者患糖尿病(DM)的风险很高，因为 GWAS 研究确定了人类基因组所有位点中 CF 和 DM 之间的相关性最高的 *SLC26A9* SNP[213]。虽然很明显，其他溶质载体家族基因和其他基因也会改变 CF、其他综合征和具有明确病理特征的疾病，但 *SLC26A9* 代表了一种与特异性人类疾病无关，但会使多种功能失调的细胞和器官系统恶化的遗传变异的原型。有机会靶向这些修饰基因来改善患者疾病的严重程度是未来研究的目标。

（三）CF 相关的糖尿病风险

在非 CF 的胰腺疾病中，DM 代表了一种常见的、可变的和潜在的严重并发症，可能具有多种遗传和环境风险，以及解剖学机制。由于 CP 胰腺严重、终末期破坏或手术切除部分或全部胰腺实质伴胰岛细胞量专性减少所致的非 1 型、非 2 型 DM 被称为 3cDM 型。然而，20%～30% 的 RAP 或早期 CP 患者也患有 DM，可能是由于修饰基因或其他因素，而不是整个胰岛的丢失。为了研究 DM 的非遗传风险因素，研究人员使用 NAPS2 队列比较了伴或不伴糖尿病的 CP 患者的人口统计学和疾病特征[23]。风险特征与 2 型 DM 人群对照相似，如果患者有 DM 家族史、具有非洲血统、且超重（OR 1.62）或肥胖（OR 2.8），则更有可能发生 DM。通过钙化、萎缩和既往胰腺手术测量的结果，CP 的严重程度也会影响风险，EPI 也是一个显著的风险（OR 1.9）[23]。血统和家族史显著影响风险的事实表明，遗传修饰基因有助于 CP 患者 DM 的发生。

四、遗传学与患者管理的整合

精准医学方法通过使用新技术增加了医疗保健行业的多学科培训和护理。第一个技术进步是对医疗保健信息的组织和标准化，用于详细跟踪患者疾病历程中的所有特征、检测和生物标志物，框架化并与其他重叠或不同疾病和结局的患者进行比较[220,221]。为了使这些信息充分有用，患者和各种医疗保健服务提供者必须随时提供这些信息[30]。第二是推进成像技术，提供疾病病理和疾病分期的结构和功能证据。第三是"组学"革命，在特定的临床背景下，可以在患者中测量数以百万计的分析物。这些"组学"中最重要的是破译患者的整个基因组，这在他们整个生命过程中不会改变，包含了对特定基因、蛋白质产物、细胞类型和生物系统如何可能在不同条件下工作的强大预测意义。第四，需要提供与新的计算和分析工具相关的研究和人口数据集的可用性，为丰富的数据集提供背景和比较，以推进生物医学发现[220-222]。第五，需要简单和复杂的疾病模型来组织单个患者内的变量，并确定疾病驱动因素、疾病分期、疾病活动度、并发症易感性和治疗目标[1,2,7]。幸运的是，通过基因检测可以很容易地检测到与 *CFTR* 突变相关的胰管分泌缺陷等简单模型，并且已经证明了有效的靶向治疗策略[223]。最后，"智能手机"和其他设备允许患者连续跟踪和记录他们的病情和对治疗的反应，并更充分地参与他们的医疗保健[30]。由于不常见疾病的风险和特征的独特组合很少，因此也需要新的方法来分析这些复杂疾病的特征，如 N-of-one 试验，以收集、组织和评估特定干预在规定条件下是否有效的证据[39,224]。

管理胰腺疾病的共识建议包括早期诊断和结构化纵向护理[2,225,226]。对于早期 CP 的诊断尚未达成共识，尽管一致认为它的存在很重要[2,38]。由于早期、轻度、非钙化或微小变化 CP 的诊断是复杂的，一些专家建议应使用"占位符"诊断可能的 CP 或"证据不足"对患者进行随访[227]。对疑似或证实 CP 患者的评估和随访期间，临床数据收集和记录应标准化[225]。追踪胰腺疾病各组分的功能很重要，因为影像学、外分泌腺功能、内分泌功能、疼痛和癌症风险之间没有很好的相关性。

对疑似或确诊的胰腺炎患者的初步评估应涉及风险因素（家族史和遗传、环境暴露和临床环境，如既往 AP 发作）、鉴别诊断、症状和体征以及营养和胰腺结构和功能的基线指标。家族史（最好使用标准化的家族树）应包括胰腺炎、胰腺癌（pancreatic cancer，PC）、糖尿病和高甘油三酯血症，并考虑以往的基因检测结果。如果未进行基因检测，或变体组检测不充分，则应在适当的遗传咨询后安排扩展的基因检测。应量化饮酒史和吸烟史。应记录拟人化指标，包括身高、体重、血压和心率。需要使用标准化技术和报告对胰腺进行高质量的成像[228]，并且正在出现更好的标准化和报告结构和物理特征的方法，例如使用弹性成像或使用胰泌素刺激的磁共振胰胆管造影（secretin-stimulated magnetic resonance cholangiopancreatography，sMRCP）诊断纤维化的功能[24,229-231]。实验室检查应包括血清脂溶性维生素（A、D、E、K）、维生素 B_{12}、矿物质和微量元素水平、基线骨密度和糖尿病筛查（如空腹血糖、血红蛋白 A1c，如果异常则转诊）[225,232]。营养和炎症的常用指标包括总蛋白、白蛋白、离子钙、前白蛋白、骨钙素、硒、C 反应蛋白和血脂全套检测[233]。还应包括胰腺外分泌功能检查。尽管对最佳方法尚未达成共识，但通常使用人粪便弹性蛋白酶-1 检测（成形粪便）、胰泌素刺激的胰腺功能检测（在无 *CFTR* 突变的情况下）或血清胰蛋白酶原水平（无疼痛发作的患者）。疼痛评估使用多维量表测量其强度、性质和位置、频率以及疼痛对情绪或活动水平的影响[226]。作为基线评估的一部分，如果之前未提供，患者应接受基因检测咨询。孟德尔疾病的基因检测对于识别受累家族成员的致病变异、明确病因和预后、以为高危家族成员和计划生育提供信息具有实用性。然而，复杂的遗传疾病需要额外的考虑，合格的遗传咨询师在评估过程中的作用与孟德尔疾病不同[234]。风险变异的基因检测也可能明确疾病的病因、结局和管理策略。这些对于在其他风险因素背景下进行解释尤为重要。应在检测前明确告知患者，使其了解获益、风险（如人寿保险）和限制，并提供知情同意书[234]。患者在检测后还应该接受咨询，使其了解识别的内容以及对其及其家人的意义（并提供其检测结果）。许多基因检测公司都提供这种服务。

应至少每年对患者进行一次评估，评估和记录与胰腺炎相关症状的变化或住院间隔、新出现的症状（尤其是可能提示癌症的症状）、功能异常[外分泌和（或）内分泌功能不全]、影像学形态学变化（如果进行过）和实验室检查[225,235]。应询问患者是否有提示 EPI 的症状，包括腹部胀气、腹胀、排便频繁（尤其是进食后）、体重减轻和存在脂肪泻[225]。CP 患者应至少每年筛查一次脂溶性维生素、矿物质和微量元素的营养缺乏，并监测骨密度，并根据骨折风险评估进行治疗[225]。尽管没有足够的数据推荐对 CP 患者进行常规 PC 筛查，但临床医生应追踪新发糖尿病、无痛性黄疸、体重减轻或新发的放射到背部的腹部疼痛等症状。

新的和已确立的药物和治疗方法的出现，可以被重新利用并用于胰腺疾病，需要继续检验并应用于特定的问题[39,223]。随着时间的推移，系统收集个体患者推荐的措施将有助于研究和优化这些治疗的使用。

五、小儿胰腺炎

一度被认为不常见的小儿胰腺疾病的发病率似乎正在增加。医生意识的增强似乎是小儿胰腺疾病增加的主要原因[236]。AP 发生于包括婴儿在内的所有儿科年龄段[237,238]。成人 AP 的常见原因是过量饮酒和胆结石,这些原因在儿童中较少见到。大多数儿童的 RAP 和 CP 病例具有结构或遗传基础(框 57.2)[60,100,239]。易患 AP 的遗传因素似乎与 CP 相关的遗传因素相似,将在以下章节中详细讨论。

框 57.2　儿童获得性胰腺炎的病因

创伤	柯萨奇病毒-B 病毒
内镜逆行胰胆管造影	埃可病毒
药物	肠道病毒
α-甲基多巴	EB 病毒
锑(五价的)	甲型肝炎病毒
硫唑嘌呤	疱疹病毒
偶氮水杨二钠	甲型流感
西咪替丁	钩端螺旋体病
阿糖胞苷	疟疾
地达诺斯	麻疹
红霉素	流行性腮腺炎
雌激素	支原体病
呋塞米	狂犬病
糖皮质激素	风疹
异烟肼	伤寒
静脉注射脂肪乳剂	**胆道疾病**
拉米夫定	**胰腺分裂**
左旋天冬氨酸酶	代谢疾病
6-巯基嘌呤	囊性纤维化
氨基水杨酸	高钙血症
甲硝唑	高甘油三酯血症
喷他脒	蛋白质-热量营养不良
普鲁卡因	瑞氏综合征
利福平	**家族性疾病**
柳氮磺胺吡啶	**混杂原因**
磺胺类药	先天性部分脂肪代谢障碍
舒林酸	糖尿病酮症酸中毒
四环素	过敏性紫癜
丙戊酸	热带胰腺炎
扎西他滨	川崎病
感染	十二指肠溃疡穿孔
艾滋病/艾滋病毒相关	系统性红斑狼疮
蛔虫病	

(一) 急性胰腺炎

病因:急性胰腺炎(AP)(定义见前文)是一种具有多种病因的突发性胰腺炎症性疾病(见框 57.2)。儿童中最常见的已知病因是胆道疾病(10%~30%)、药物(25%)、全身性疾病(33%)、创伤(10%~40%)、代谢性疾病(2%~7%)和 HP(5%~8%),13%~34%的病例为特发性[240]。发病率的很大差异是由于在儿童 AP 诊断不足时进行的研究造成的。其中一些病例发生在具有高危基因改变的儿童中,尤其是 *SPINK1* 和 *CFTR* 突变的胰腺特异性组合[241]。基因检测稍后讨论,通常在反复发作后和排除其他常见原因后进行。

创伤:创伤是 AP 的一个原因,即使胰腺被其腹膜后位置很好地保护免受轻微损伤。创伤通常是钝性的,与其他腹腔脏器的损伤有关,并在损伤后不久变得明显,尽管损伤显然可能先于胰腺炎的表现或再识别数周。在严重受伤或受虐待的儿童中,通常胰腺损伤容易被忽视。

结构异常:随着 MRI 和 MRCP 等成像技术的提高,结构异常被更早地识别出。胰腺分裂是最常见的解剖结构异常,但也观察到多种其他胆管和胰管的结构异常(见第 55 章)。

ERCP 术后胰腺炎是多个系列中发生胰腺炎的一个重要原因[242,243],并且在儿童进行 ERCP 的任何地方均可观察到该病因。MRCP 的广泛使用极大地减少了诊断性 ERCP 的使用,尽管 ERCP 在治疗干预中仍然是非常有价值的(见第 61 章)。

胆道疾病:胆石性胰腺炎在儿童中较成人少见,这可能反映了青春期前胆石症相对少见[60]。必须考虑到这一诊断,与年龄大小无关。

药物治疗:药物仍然是儿童 AP 的常见原因,尽管在鉴别诊断中也必须考虑处方用药的基础疾病[244,245]。最近的研究发现丙戊酸盐是与儿童胰腺炎最常见的相关药物,其次是门冬酰胺酶、泼尼松或 6-巯基嘌呤[242,243,246,247]。在接受任何药物治疗的儿童中发生持续性腹部疼痛应提示药物性胰腺炎的可能性。仅通过记录胰腺疾病、停药后改善和重新给药时疾病复发证实了这一点。

感染:感染,特别是病毒感染[248],经常与儿童胰腺炎有关。肠道病毒,尤其是柯萨奇病毒,与特发性 AP 有关[249]。在 EBV 感染的儿童中有胰腺炎的报道[250]。腮腺炎的儿童患有胰腺炎时常以腹痛和血清淀粉酶值升高为表现,归因于腮腺炎病毒感染[251]。已有多份病例报告中记录了肺炎支原体感染和 AP,有时在一周或两周后发生 AP[248]。虽然在美国不常见,但蛔虫病是南非和印度等地区儿童胰腺炎最常见的原因之一,在胰管内可发现蠕虫。胰腺炎在 HIV/AIDS 患者中很常见,可能是由于药物所致,并与高脂血症和(或)线粒体毒性有关(见框 57.1 和框 57.2,以及第 35 章)。

全身性疾病:在 2 项研究中,溶血性尿毒综合征是 AP 最常见的全身性原因[242,243]。尽管任何原因引起的尿毒症都是胰腺损伤的风险因素,但其机制尚不清楚,可能是多因素的。SLE[252] 和川崎病[253] 与胰腺炎相关。当患儿对其他治疗无反应或似乎有不明原因的急性炎症过程时,应在 ICU 考虑 AP。AP 也常见于器官移植后(见第 36 章)。在糖尿病酮症酸中毒[242,243,254] 和各种先天性代谢缺陷中偶尔观察到胰腺炎[255]

获得性代谢紊乱。与儿童胰腺疾病发生相关的最常见的代谢紊乱是蛋白质-卡路里营养不良。在严重营养不良的儿童中,胰酶分泌往往受损,而体积和碳酸氢盐分泌却得以保留。据说恶性营养不良后胰腺功能的恢复比消瘦后更快,但无论哪种情况,胰腺疾病都可能导致恢复期吸收不良。对营养不良儿童进行积极的早期再喂养与具有临床意义的胰腺炎的发生有关。营养不良曾被认为是导致 TP 的主要促成因素,但现在这一点受到质疑,因为 TP 主要是在营养良好的患者中观察到,通常存在基因突变[42,44,256]。

临床特征:AP 的诊断是基于突然发生的典型腹痛综合征,伴有血清淀粉酶或脂肪酶升高至正常水平上限的至少 3

倍(见第 58 章)[31,257,258]。疼痛通常在上腹部,进食时加重,可伴有恶心、呕吐,偶见黄疸。通常出现一过性发热。在婴儿和幼儿中,可能会出现呕吐、发热、易怒、腹胀等症状[237]。正常血清淀粉酶值随年龄增长而增加,这可能是由于胰腺异构淀粉酶延迟出现所致,胰腺异构淀粉酶通常在 3 个月前不存在,往往直到 11 个月时才被检出,即便如此,也要到 10 岁才能以成人水平存在。而唾液异构淀粉酶出现得更早,成熟得也更早。

AP 初次发作后,约 10% 的儿童可出现复发性 AP[243]。复发性 AP 患者最常见的诊断是结构异常,或家族性胰腺炎或复杂的遗传风险[60,100,243]。医师应该进行仔细的评估,以确定或排除可逆的原因,以防止进一步发作,并降低发生 CP 及其并发症的风险[235]。

(二) 复发性急性胰腺炎和慢性胰腺炎

复发性急性胰腺炎(RAP)和慢性胰腺炎(CP)曾经被认为是罕见的,许多 RAP 和 CP 患儿正在被报道。腹部成像水平的改善、医生的意识以及患病率的可能变化证明 CP 是儿童的一个主要医疗问题,而且成本非常高[259]。

最近一项关于儿童 RAP 和 CP 的多国横断面研究[国际儿科胰腺炎研究组:寻找一种治疗方法(International Study Group of Pediatric Pancreatitis: In Search for a CuRE, INSPPIRE)]为 CF 以外的儿科复杂的胰腺疾病提供了新的见解[100]。在初始队列的 301 例病例中,儿童的年龄平均值和标准差为 11.9±4.5 岁,57% 为女性。146 例患者记录了 CP,其中 84% 报告了既往复发的 AP 病史。西班牙裔儿童比 CP 更易患 RAP。大约 48% 的 RAP 患者与 73% 的 CP 患者发现至少 1 个胰腺炎相关基因突变($P<0.001$)。如果儿童在 *PRSS1*(OR 4.2)或 *SPINK1*(OR 2.30)中有致病性变异,则其更可能表现为 CP 而不是 RAP[100]。胰腺炎相关性腹痛是前一年内 81% 的 RAP 或 CP 患儿的主要症状,CP 组以急诊科就诊、住院以及内科、内镜和手术干预多见[100]。

儿童比成人更少暴露于 AP 和 CP 的环境风险因素中,尤其是长期饮酒和吸烟。根据年龄,评估 INSPPIRE 队列中 RAP 或 CP 儿童的人口统计学和临床信息的风险因素[60]。342 例中首诊年龄小于 6 岁患儿占 38%,6~11 岁占 32%,≥12 岁占 30%。早期发病与 *PRSS1* 和 *CTRC* 的致病性基因变异、AP 或 CP 家族史、胆管囊肿或慢性肾功能衰竭有关[60]。晚发性 RAP 和 CP 与高甘油三酯血症、溃疡性结肠炎、自身免疫性疾病或药物使用相关[60]。晚发型患儿也更易急诊就诊($P<0.05$)或合并糖尿病($P<0.01$)[60]。

对新发 AP、RAP 和 CP 患者的评价建议正在不断发展。INSPPIRE 联盟最近对 RAP 和 CP 的因果评价提出了一系列建议[235]。他们建议对解剖、代谢和遗传原因进行系统评价,包括汗液氯化物检测或 *CFTR* 基因检测(即使新生儿 CF 筛查结果为阴性)、*RSS1*、*CTRC* 和 *SPINK1* 基因检测以及乳糜泻筛查[235]。还应评价 EPI 及相关维生素和营养缺乏、糖尿病和并发症的检测[235]。

六、胰腺孟德尔遗传疾病的临床管理

对胰腺功能至关重要的几个基因表现出遗传变异和多态性,导致孟德尔胰腺疾病,通常有多系统受累(表 57.2)。

表 57.2 胰腺外分泌及相关基因的遗传性和先天性疾病

疾病	缺陷基因或蛋白质(遗传特征)
胰腺外分泌功能不全	
胰腺发育不全(见第 55 章)	*PDX1* 或 *PTF1A*(隐性)
囊性纤维化	$CFTR^{sev}/CFTR^{sev}$(隐性)
Shwachman-Diamond 综合征	*SBDS* 隐性
Johanson-Blizzard 综合征	*UBR1* 隐性
Pearson 骨髓-胰腺综合征	线粒体 DNA(线粒体)
孤立性酶缺乏症	见正文
胰腺炎	
遗传性	*PRSS1*(常染色体显性遗传) *CEL*
家族性	*SPINK1*/*SPINK1*(常染色体隐性) $CFTR^{sev}$ 或 $CFTR^{bl}$/SPINK1(复合)
CFTR-RD	$CFTR^{sev}/CFTR^{m-v}$(隐性)
散发的	*CTRC*(复合) *CASR*(复合)
修饰基因	*CLDN2* *SLC26A9*(CFTR 相关的)
高甘油三酯血症	脂蛋白脂肪酶(显性基因)
	载脂蛋白 C-Ⅱ

添加了之前表 57.2 中的脚注,并将 *CEL*、*PRSS1*、*CLDN2*、*SLC26A9* 添加到该脚注中,这些在章节中进行了定义。

(一) 囊性纤维化

囊性纤维化(CF)是白人人群中最常见的致死性遗传缺陷,见于 1/2 500~1/3 200 活产婴儿。与欧洲血统的儿童相比,非洲、美洲原住民、亚洲、东印度人或中东背景的儿童发病率低[260]。预后显著改善,CF 患者的预测中位生存期延长到 47 岁以上[261]。尽管如此,死亡时的中位年龄约为 30 岁。在这里,我们重点关注胰腺上囊性纤维化跨膜传导调控因子(*CFTR*)基因突变的表现,胃肠病学家也对肠道、肝胆和营养问题进行了较简短的讨论(表 57.3)。

表 57.3 CF 患者中选定胃肠道表现的频率*

器官	表现	所有患者中的发生频率/%	成年人中的发生频率/%
胰腺	总胃液缺乏	85~90	85~90*
	糖耐量异常	20~30	20~30
	部分或正常功能	10~15	10~15
	胰腺炎	1~2(所有 CF) 22%(PS-CF)	2~3
	糖尿病	4~7	4~7
肠道	胎粪性肠梗阻	10~25	
	直肠脱垂	1~2	
	远端肠梗阻综合征	3	18
	肠套叠	1	1~2

表 57.3　CF 患者中选定胃肠道表现的频率*（续）

器官	表现	所有患者中的发生频率/%	成年人中的发生频率/%
肝脏	脂肪肝	7	20~60
	局灶性胆汁性肝硬化	2~3	11~70
	门静脉高压症	2~3	28
胆道	胆囊异常、无功能或小胆囊	25	5~20
	胆结石	8	10~25
	胆管狭窄	1~20	1~20
食管	胃食管反流病	未知	80

*发生频率可能取决于基因型。
CF，囊性纤维化；PS-CF，CF 伴胰腺功能不全。

临床特征：在美国，超过 60% 的 CF 患者是通过新生儿筛查确诊的[261]。2016 年，所有患者诊断时的中位年龄为 4 个月，67% 在出生后第一年诊断。所有患者中约 10% 在 10 岁以后确诊，少数在 40 岁以后确诊。

通过新生儿筛查确定的大多数婴儿在筛查时症状轻微或无症状。在筛查出 CF 阳性的婴儿中，大多数在证明汗液氯化物浓度升高（表 57.4）或在特定检测方案中证明鼻生物电学反应异常后很容易得到证实。如果执行得当，这些检测是可靠的。但是，在新生儿、营养不良、使用某些药物或汗液不足的患者中，可能会观察到假阳性和假阴性结果（见表 57.4）。因此，大多数专家坚持使用在 CF 中心经常使用的标准化方法进行检测。

表 57.4　汗液试验（毛果芸香碱定量电泳）：高汗液电解质水平的适应证和条件

适应证	高汗液电解质水平疾病
患 CF 的兄弟姊妹	CF
慢性肺部症状	外胚层发育不良
持续性咳嗽	糖原贮积病，1 型
反复呼吸道感染	肾上腺功能不全
支气管炎	家族性甲状旁腺功能减退
支气管扩张	岩藻糖苷贮积症
肺叶肺不张	垂体后叶激素抵抗性尿崩症
发育停滞（生长发育不良）	黏多糖贮积症
直肠脱垂	家族性胆汁淤积综合征
鼻息肉病	环境剥夺综合征
新生儿肠梗阻	急性呼吸系统疾病（喉炎、会厌炎、病毒性肺炎）
胎粪性肠梗阻	
婴儿早期黄疸	慢性呼吸系统疾病（支气管肺发育不良）
儿童或青少年肝硬化	
门静脉高压症	α_1-抗胰蛋白酶缺乏症
患有无精症或无精症的成年男性	
中暑	
低蛋白血症	
低凝血酶原血症	

CF，囊性纤维化。

由于 CF 患者新的表型和基因型信息的激增，CF 基金会选择了一个国际共识委员会提供的 CF 诊断建议[153]，在很大程度上认识到许多患者有 *CFTR* 相关异常但没有 CF[262]。该小组得出结论，对于新生儿筛查阳性且 *CFTR2* 突变列表中有 2 个 CF 突变的患者、或 CF 或胎粪性肠梗阻的症状和体征，可作出 CF 的推定诊断，但必须通过汗液氯化物试验阳性（>60mmol/L）来确诊。指南将非 CF 患者分为 2 组：分别为 CFTR 相关代谢综合征（CRMS）和 CFTR 相关疾病（CFTR-RD），如前所述。

框 57.3 列出了 CF 的临床特征，表 57.3 列出了 CF 的各种胃肠道表现的发生频率。早期临床特征是消化不良或 CFTR 突变所致的其他胰腺和肠道表现（稍后讨论）。一些儿童疾病和 *CFTR* 突变之间的表型-基因型关系通常是惊人的，在超过 85% 表现为 PI 的儿童和大多数表现为胎粪性肠梗阻的婴儿中检测到严重的 *CFTR* 突变[164]。

框 57.3　CF 的临床表现

上呼吸道	糖尿病
鼻窦炎	钙化
黏膜肥大、鼻息肉	消化不良伴脂肪泄，粪溢
下呼吸道	维生素缺乏
肺不张	**肝、胆管**
肺气肿	黏液分泌过多
感染支气管炎、支气管肺炎、支气管扩张、肺脓肿。	胆结石、胆囊萎缩
	局灶性胆汁性肝硬化
呼吸衰竭，右心衰竭	门静脉高压±食管静脉曲张
胃肠	脾功能亢进
胆盐缺乏	**生殖**
胰腺功能不全	女性：阴道黏液黏度增加，受精减少
GERD	男性：不育；输精管、附睾和精囊缺失
PUD	**骨骼**
胎粪性肠梗阻	骨龄延缓
肠扭转	脱矿质
腹膜炎	肥大性肺骨关节病
回肠闭锁	**眼**
远端肠梗阻综合征	静脉怒张
便秘	视网膜出血
肠套叠	**其他**
直肠脱垂	通过皮肤过量损失盐，导致盐耗竭
胰腺	中暑
胰腺炎	顶泌汗腺肥大
营养衰竭	

CF，囊性纤维化。

CF 患者出生时肺功能正常，但在新生儿期后 CF 相关的发病率和死亡率中占很大一部分。肺部疾病的严重程度取决于已知和未知因素。遗传和环境因素与 CF 的肺功能变化成比例[263]，在具有相同 CFTR 基因型的患者中，肺部疾病的严重程度存在广泛差异。环境因素可能包括铜绿假单胞菌的慢性感染、营养状况、烟草烟雾和环境过敏原[169]，而遗传因素包括炎症反应基因[264,265]和修饰基因的变体[266-268]。

胰腺病理学：大多数（85%~90%）CF 患者表现为胰腺外分泌功能障碍的证据[146,269]。尽管 CF 婴儿的胰腺功能障碍最初可能表现得很轻微，但通常会进展为胰腺外分泌功能衰竭。当严重受累时，胰腺会出现萎缩、囊性纤维化和脂肪变性。组织学上，胰腺小导管和中心腺泡细胞的增生和最终坏死、连同浓缩的分泌物一起，导致胰腺小导管堵塞，随后侵蚀腺泡，引起上皮变平和萎缩（见图 57.9）。囊性间隙充满了富含钙的嗜酸性凝结块。阻塞的腺泡周围可能存在轻度炎症反应，进行性纤维化逐渐分离并取代胰腺小叶。朗格尔汉斯岛在大多数情况下是幸免的，直到过程的晚期并集中在萎缩的胰腺中。钙化虽然罕见，但在 X 线片上可能很明显。US、MRI 和 CT 可记录胰腺疾病的进展。胰腺可以表现为正常、不完全或完全的脂肪瘤病（最常见）、囊性或大囊性或表现为萎缩的胰腺[270]。胰腺异常与外分泌功能障碍程度的相关性较差[2]。

胰腺外分泌功能不全（EPI）和胰腺炎。囊性纤维化患者通常有胰腺功能不全（PI），这是一个由肠道病理、高热量需求和食欲不振混合的问题。脂肪和蛋白质消化障碍伴粪便丢失是 CF 的主要胰腺表现，尽管不同患者的严重程度可能存在相当大的差异。PI 组的脂肪泻和氮质泻通常大于黏膜吸收不良组。只有当脂肪酶和胰蛋白酶的分泌降至正常值的 10% 以下时，才能识别胰腺外分泌功能不全[271]。大多数 CF 患者表现为这种模式的胰腺功能不全。在婴幼儿期未出现胰腺功能完全丧失的患者中，RAP 可能使 CF 的病程复杂化。胰腺炎在老年患者中往往更成问题[146]。

胰腺内分泌功能障碍和糖尿病。据报道，30%～75% 的囊性纤维化患者出现葡萄糖不耐受，高达 10% 的年轻患者出现具有临床意义的糖尿病。囊性纤维化相关糖尿病（CF-related diabetes mellitus，CFRD）随着年龄的增长而发展。在 20 岁时，30% 的囊性纤维化患者需要胰岛素，40% 的 CF 患者在 30 岁前需要胰岛素[272]。囊性纤维化相关的糖尿病的病因和表现与典型的 1 型或 2 型糖尿病不同，可能反映了朗格尔汉斯岛的破坏，与其他形式的 CP 相似。然而，内分泌缺陷的严重程度落后于外分泌缺陷，因为胰岛相对幸免，直到胰腺破坏的晚期（见图 57.9）。囊性纤维化相关的糖尿病与呼吸和营养状况的恶化、晚期微血管并发症的发展和死亡率增加相关[273]。专家强调需要多学科团队方法，以及使用高能量饮食（超过每日推荐摄入量的 100%），并适当调整胰岛素剂量[273]。为维持充足的营养，可能需要夜间肠内喂养。还应仔细考虑治疗选择，以最大化地增加内源性肠促胰岛素，优化代谢，保留 β 细胞功能，并降低 PC 风险[232]。

1. 胰腺功能障碍的治疗

（1）胰酶补充剂：营养是 CF 的主要挑战（见“营养管理”）。治疗 CF 胰腺外分泌功能衰竭引起的消化不良，需要将活性消化酶随餐一起递送至近端小肠（见第 59 章）。可以使用多种胰腺制剂，但不同的产品的酶活性差异很大，对于一些 CF 患者来说，脂肪酶活性降低仍然是一个问题。肠溶性微球是首选的替代形式，因为其可保护消化酶免受胃酸破坏（pH<4），并且是有效的。必须考虑微球的大小。如果大多数微球太大（>1mm），则微球/酶的排空可延迟到食物完全进入小肠之后。还应考虑 H_2 受体阻滞剂（H2RA）或质子泵抑制剂（PPI），以及未包被或肠溶胰酶补充剂，尤其是因为有助于中和胃酸的胰腺和十二指肠碳酸氢盐转运系统被破坏时。与其他形式的胰腺功能不全相反，CF 患者十二指肠和胆管树内的碳酸氢盐分泌也受损，导致十二指肠 pH 显著低于正常值[274,275]。因此，在没有抑酸作用的情况下，未包被的酶容易被胃酸灭活，肠溶产品可能不会释放其内容物[274]。应避免使用含有碳酸钙或氢氧化镁的抗酸剂，因为它们可能干扰胰酶补充。

CF 患者胰腺外分泌功能不全的初治疗包括胰酶替代治疗，剂量范围为每餐 500～2 000U 脂肪酶活性/kg 体重，餐前即刻给药，并与零食同服[276]。通常将剂量推进至 1 000～2 500U 脂肪酶活性/kg 体重，但最终剂量取决于年龄、胰腺功能不全的程度、脂肪摄入量和选择的市售制剂。治疗的充分性通常根据临床依据确定。频繁大量的脂肪泻、过度腹胀和排气、食欲亢进或生长速度不足是治疗不充分的体征。即使采用优化治疗，脂肪吸收也可能无法恢复正常。在很大程度上，脂肪吸收不能正常化可能反映了异常肠黏膜对脂肪酸的摄取减少[277]。

胰酶替代制剂通常会引起婴儿口周和肛周刺激。尽管微球制剂较少见。因为胰腺提取物的嘌呤含量较高，一些服用大量胰酶制剂的患者可能发生高尿酸尿。高剂量胰酶给药后报告了结肠狭窄和纤维化结肠病，导致停用所有高剂量的胰酶制剂。纤维化结肠病于 1994 年首次被认识[278]，到 1996 年几乎消失了[279]。

（2）维生素补充剂：脂肪消化障碍和吸收不良可导致 CF 患者脂溶性维生素的缺乏（维生素 A、D、E、K）[233,280]。在 CF 患者中，维生素 A 的缺乏很少引起临床异常或眼睛和皮肤的问题，但维生素 A 水平过高会损害儿童的呼吸和骨骼系统，并干扰其他脂溶性维生素的代谢[281]。然而，由于目前没有关于补充维生素 A 的随机对照研究，因此无法得出 CF 人群需补充维生素 A 的结论[281]。可能发生维生素 D 缺乏，影响钙稳态、骨矿化、炎症、情绪和其他骨骼外效应。维生素 D 水平受饮食摄入、日光照射和遗传的影响，缺乏维生素 D 比单纯摄入更为复杂[233,282,283]。补充剂可能有效，根据血清测量结果，建议对个体患者进行维生素 D 的替代治疗[284,285]。维生素 E 缺乏在 CF 儿童中很常见，可引起溶血性贫血、小脑性共济失调和认知困难等多种疾病[286]。与对照组相比，水溶性维生素 E 的治疗可以显著改善血清维生素 E 水平，但研究尚未证明其对治疗的临床获益[286]。维生素 K 缺乏伴凝血功能障碍可发生在任何年龄。其临床表现从轻度瘀斑或紫癜增加到灾难性出血不等，并影响骨形成。每天补充 1mg 维生素 K 似乎可以改善骨钙素水平，骨钙素是骨代谢的一个标志物，一项系统性综述中没有发现补充维生素 K 的危害[287]。所有 CF 患者应每日接受多种维生素制剂，许多患者需要补充维生素 A、D、E、K，并且对于 EPI 患者，应加用胰酶替代治疗（pancreatic enzyme replacement therapy，PERT）[233,239]。每年监测脂溶性维生素的血清浓度对 CF 儿童很重要，建议每年监测一次[239]。

2. 肠道表现

由于 CFTR（囊性纤维化跨膜传导调控因子）在肠细胞顶膜表达，因此囊性纤维化会显著影响胃肠道[288]。远端回肠阻塞综合征、肠套叠、阑尾炎、慢性便秘、结肠肠壁增厚、纤维化结肠病、肠积气、胃食管反流病和消化性溃疡病已有描述[270]。

(1) **病理学**:囊性纤维化患者的小肠黏膜腺体腔内可能含有不同数量的浓缩分泌物,但很少有杯状细胞数量增加。阑尾常受累,但很少引起阑尾炎或肠套叠[289]。十二指肠 Brunner 腺可表现为上皮衬里细胞扩张、变平,管腔内有串状分泌物。老年囊性纤维化患者的小肠黏膜常表现为广泛扩张的充满黏液的隐窝,黏液常呈层状或可从裂隙隐窝中挤出。隆起的杯状细胞似乎挤掉了中间的柱状上皮。固有层中可能存在不同的细胞浸润。囊性纤维化中的黏膜更丰富,着色更强烈,并含有更多的弱酸基团和蛋白质。

(2) **影像学特征**:囊性纤维化的胃肠道影像学特征差异很大[270]。影像学检查通常是针对特定症状进行的,可以检测到与囊性纤维化相关和不相关的病变。婴儿胎粪性肠梗阻和儿童和成人的囊性纤维化 DIOS(后文描述)是例外,它们具有清晰的影像学表现[270,290,291]。

(3) **肠道病理生理学**:小肠黏膜的改变引起肠道生理功能紊乱。各种研究已证明,胰腺外分泌功能不全没有明显的吸收缺陷,或者在充分的胰腺替代治疗后吸收缺陷仍然存在。

基础和刺激后的十二指肠碳酸氢盐分泌在很大程度上依赖于功能性囊性纤维化跨膜电导调控因子。囊性纤维化患者也存在同样的碳酸氢盐双重分泌异常,这在一定程度上解释了囊性纤维化患者十二指肠近端餐后 pH 的降低,即使是在胰腺刺激后[275]。与小肠和呼吸道不同,结肠的囊性纤维化跨膜电导调节因子缺陷不能被任何其他氯化物通道所代偿[292]。因此,结肠功能缺陷与囊性纤维化跨膜传导调节因子密切相关。

囊性纤维化患者的乳糖酶缺乏伴乳糖吸收不良仅反映了正常的种族和年龄相关表型。然而,成人型低乳糖酶血症和乳糖吸收不良患者的骨密度可能降低[293]。

(4) **胎粪性肠梗阻**:胎粪性肠梗阻可:以是无并发症的,也可以是复杂的。复杂性胎粪性肠梗阻包括肠阻塞伴节段性肠扭转、闭锁、坏死、穿孔、胎粪性腹膜炎(全身性)和巨大胎粪假性囊肿形成[294,295]。无并发症的胎粪性肠梗阻的特征性表现为远端回肠狭窄,呈串珠状,是由浓缩胎粪的蜡样、灰色颗粒引起,超过该颗粒远的结肠仍处于空虚状态。多达一半的胎粪性肠梗阻病例在肠穿孔后并发肠扭转、闭锁、或胎粪外渗至腹膜腔引起的胎粪性腹膜炎,这在临床上可能仅表现为腹腔内钙化、胎粪假性囊肿、广泛粘连性胎粪性腹膜炎或胎粪性腹水。胎儿肠扭转和血管受损可能引起闭锁。

特征性影像学表现为肠袢不均匀扩张,气液平面缺失或减少[270,290,291,296]。黏性胎粪中滞留的小气泡可能分散在整个远端小肠中[297]。钡灌肠显示小结肠,可勾勒出回肠远端阻塞的胎粪块轮廓(图 57.10)。腹腔钙化反映了胎粪性腹膜炎,胎粪性假性囊肿可取代正常肠袢。

胎粪性肠梗阻通常在出生后 48 小时内表现出典型的肠梗阻体征,而婴儿身体状况良好。复杂性胎粪性肠梗阻甚至更早出现,婴儿的病情更加严重。羊水过多是一种常见的产前表现。当开始喂养时,可出现伴或不伴腹胀的胆汁性呕吐。胎粪性腹膜炎的婴儿通常表现为腹部触痛、发热和休克的附加体征[297]。囊性纤维化的家族史有助于确立诊断。通过腹壁,尤其是右下腹,可以看到并可触及扩张的、坚硬的、橡皮状

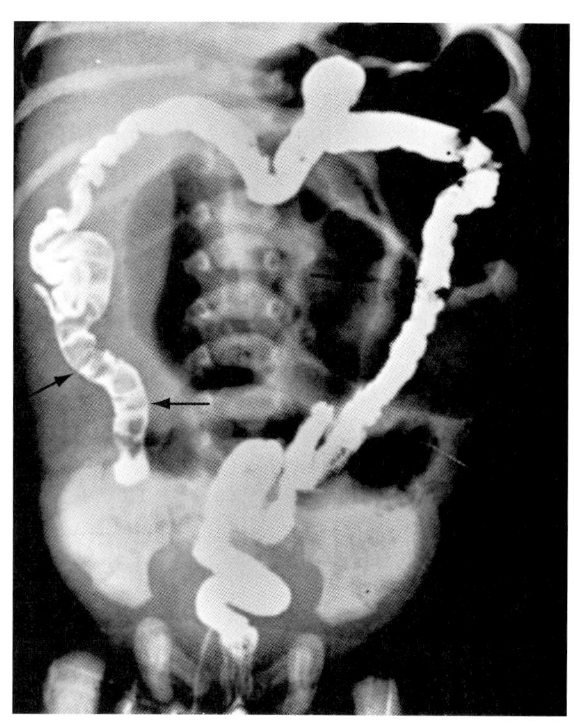

图 57.10　一例胎粪性肠梗阻婴儿的钡灌肠检查胶片,显示小结肠以及回肠远端胎粪(箭)。还观察到小肠袢扩张

肠袢。

CFTR 变异的基因筛查,应在产前超声检查有胎粪性肠梗阻,如肠强回声或腹膜钙化异常证据的患者中进行[297]。如果结果表明 CFTR 基因型正常,遗传咨询应关注测试限度和扩大鉴别诊断,而在一个或多个父母或孩子中检测致病性 CFTR 等位基因,应导致更专注于对囊性纤维化的咨询[297]。

胎粪性肠梗阻一直被认为是致命的,直至 1948 年,第一批患者通过手术成功治疗。最近的报道表明,手术死亡率非常低,无并发症的胎粪性肠梗阻的长期生存率接近 90%[297]。复杂性胎粪性肠梗阻需要手术治疗[298]。

术中和术后使用了各种冲洗液溶解和排出异常胎粪。N-乙酰半胱氨酸(Mucomyst)通过裂解黏蛋白分子中的二硫键来降低黏蛋白溶液的黏稠度,聚山梨醇酯 80(Tween 80)是一种温和的工业洗涤剂和防腐剂,现在普遍认为是安全有效的。对于大多数无并发症的胎粪性肠梗阻的婴儿,通过使用稀释的泛影葡胺(泛影葡胺,泛影酸钠)或全浓度碘海醇或碘他拉葡胺Ⅱ进灌肠给药,以非手术方式缓解肠梗阻,可缩短住院时间并减少早期呼吸道并发症[294,297]。这些灌肠剂均为高渗性(1 900mOsm/L),通过将水从婴儿体内吸引出来使结肠内容物水合而发挥作用[294]。灌肠剂回流到回肠末端对于缓解肠梗阻至关重要[294]。然而,水溶性高渗性灌肠剂可能引起危险的液体和电解质变化,尤其是在小的患病婴儿中,它们可引起结肠穿孔。此外,最近使用泛影葡胺灌肠剂的病例系列的成功率仅为 36%~39%[294]。诊断性钡灌肠应先于治疗性泛影葡胺灌肠。存活超过 6 个月的 CF 和胎粪性肠梗阻婴儿与任何 CF 患者的预后相同,且不倾向于有更严重的疾病。

(5) **远端肠梗阻综合征(DIOS)**:DIOS 是 CF 患者的回肠末

端和近端结肠内黏性粪便引起的完全性或不完全性肠梗阻[299,300]。囊性纤维化患者中DIOS的发病率和患病率低于3%。欧洲最近的发病率为5~12次发作/(1 000患者·年)[300,301]。欧洲儿科胃肠病学和营养学会囊性纤维化工作组将DIOS定义为"腹痛和(或)腹胀的短期病史(数天)和回盲肠内的粪便肿块,但无完全性梗阻体征"[301]。与DIOS相比,囊性纤维化中的便秘被定义为"腹痛和(或)腹胀,或在最近几周至几个月内排便频率下降和(或)在最近几周或几个月内粪便硬度增加,而使用通便剂后症状缓解"[301]。

液体分泌的减少和肠内容物水合的减少以及脂肪和营养物质消化延迟或不足是DIOS的原因,可能是由于营养物质介导的回肠破裂激素(如肽YY)释放诱导的肠道转运缓慢所致[302]。DIOS的其他风险因素包括重度基因型、脱水、胎粪性肠梗阻或DIOS病史、器官移植和囊性纤维化相关糖尿病[299,300]。引起胎粪性肠梗阻的修饰基因的可能作用尚未在DIOS中得到充分阐述。肠套叠和较少见的肠扭转可能使DIOS复杂化。

DIOS可能是囊性纤维化的表现症状。在DIOS中出现由异常肠内容物引起的部分或完全性肠梗阻的临床谱:①便秘或粪便嵌塞引起的复发性和痉挛性腹痛;②软的、可触及的盲肠部肿块,最终可能自行排出;③回肠末端、右半结肠或两者中均有坚硬的、油灰状粪便物质引起的完全性梗阻。急性发作的胆汁性物质呕吐伴进行性绞痛性腹痛和(或)腹部X线检查显示小肠内液平面是DIOS伴完全性肠梗阻的体征[299]。粪便团块可在钡灌肠中识别,但可能必须与盲肠肿瘤和阑尾脓肿相鉴别。腹部-盆腔CT通常显示近端小肠显著扩张,远端回肠中有浓缩的粪便物质[299]。DIOS的鉴别诊断包括便秘、阑尾炎、阑尾脓肿或黏液囊肿、肠套叠、克罗恩病、肠粘连、肠扭转、纤维化结肠病和恶性肿瘤[299]。

DIOS的治疗在很大程度上是经验性的[299,301,303]。曾经是一个外科问题,现在简单的DIOS通常对医疗管理有反应,现在需要手术的患者不到5%[300,304]。在考虑手术之前,应尝试对每例患者进行一种以上治疗方式的逐步治疗试验[303]。积极的药物治疗包括常规口服剂量的胰酶和大便软化剂,包括:聚乙二醇[304],口服或直肠给予10% N-乙酰半胱氨酸,必要时加用泛影葡胺灌肠,尽管缺乏来自预防或治疗的随机试验的高质量证据[305]。口服N-乙酰半胱氨酸、增加胰酶剂量和乳果糖维持治疗已成功用于预防该综合征的复发。使用平衡肠道灌洗液治疗这种疾病也可能是有益的。聚乙二醇维持治疗因其疗效好、副作用少而得到不断普及。

3. 肝脏和胆系的表现

囊性纤维化肝病(CF liver disease,CFLD)涵盖了在囊性纤维化患者中观察到的许多肝异常,包括肝脂肪变性、血清转氨酶水平升高、胆管疾病、新生儿胆汁淤积、多小叶肝硬化和局灶性胆汁性肝硬化[306,307]。2016年,肝脏疾病占囊性纤维化死亡的2.7%[261]。在一项大型法国队列中,囊性纤维化肝病的发生率每年增加约1%,至25岁时达到32.2%[308]。此外,重度囊性纤维化肝病的发生率仅在5岁后增加,30岁时增加至10%[308]。囊性纤维化肝病和严重囊性纤维化肝病的危险因素是:男性、新生儿肝病、严重CFTR基因型,胰腺外分泌功能不全,胎粪性肠梗阻病史和修饰基因[216,308-310]。其他风险因素可能使囊性纤维化患者易患肝胆疾病,一些特征与非酒精性脂肪变性的非囊性纤维化患者重叠[310]。

一项关于囊性纤维化肝病儿童的研究表明,这些患者比无肝病的年龄和性别匹配的对照组具有更严重的囊性纤维化表型[311]。2016年,报告了胆结石(0.6%)、肝硬化(2.8%)、非肝硬化性肝病(3.9%)、急性肝炎(0.1%)、肝脂肪变性(0.4%)和其他肝病(2.0%)[261]。另一项研究发现28%的囊性纤维化成年患者有肝硬化,其中三分之二伴有门静脉高压[312]。伴有PS的CF患者肝脏异常的患病率明显较低。

肝损伤试验可中度升高,并随病程波动。高达20%的囊性纤维化合并胰腺功能不全的患者血清ALT质升高,40%~50%的患者血清转氨酶水平间歇性升高。许多囊性纤维化患者的空腹胆汁酸水平升高,这可能是本病肝功能较敏感的指标之一。

CF和EPI患者胆汁酸代谢紊乱。粪便胆盐丢失率高,通常接近回肠切除患者的水平(见第64章)。胰酶替代治疗可改善脂肪吸收,从而减少粪便胆汁酸排泄和脂肪泻。在不存在胰酶的情况下,胆汁酸池的周转率分数增加,总胆汁酸池的大小减小[313],然而,胆汁脂质组成和饱和指数接近胆石症患者的水平[314]胰酶补充剂治疗可使异常的胆汁脂质水平恢复正常。

胆囊和胆道:约25%的CF患者胆囊和胆道异常,与年龄、临床病程或肝脏病理无关。在23%的患者中发现了微小胆囊,在8%患者中发现了结石或胆泥。来自囊性纤维化登记研究的数据表明,只有约0.3%的囊性纤维化患者最终需要胆囊手术[261]。

小胆囊是常见的,特征是含有厚的无色"白色胆汁"。上皮衬里细胞内存在黏液,黏膜下立即可见存在大量充满黏液的囊肿。胆囊管可萎缩或被黏液堵塞。黏液栓不会造成肝管或胆管阻塞,但导管内结石有时会引起梗阻症状,并易引发胆管炎。

4. 其他临床表现

男性生殖器异常:尽管男性生殖不是消化系统并发症,但不育是与重度或轻度CFTR变异相关的最敏感表型之一,并与CFTR相关胰腺炎重叠,包括碳酸氢盐电导缺陷变异(如前所述)。

男性生殖道最明显的变化发生在附睾、输精管和精囊。睾丸网完整。精索的多个组织切片很少在一个以上水平显示通畅。除这些缺陷外,与睾丸下降相关的异常也显著增加,如腹股沟疝、睾丸鞘膜积液和隐睾。由于这些变化,大约97%患有CF的男性不育。这些缺陷可见于出生后不久的男婴,可能有助于支持不典型病例CF的诊断。

对临床上不怀疑患有CF的先天性输精管缺如患者进行评估,发现CFTR突变频率较高[315]。在仅发现先天性输精管缺如的男性中,高达70%在CFTR的至少1个等位基因中存在可检测的突变。RNA转录的改变也可能与这种缺陷有关,因为在先天性输精管缺如的男性中,突变体5T可减少野生型CFTR的功能性信使RNA转录,频率较高[315]。通过CFTR分泌碳酸氢盐对精子至关重要,CFTR-BD变体男性可能发生不育[148]。本组男性无CF的其他表现,归类为CFTR-RD[154]。

癌症风险：随着囊性纤维化患者年龄的增长，癌症风险增加。癌症往往发生在 30 岁，累及食管、小肠和大肠、胃、肝、胆道、胰腺或直肠[316,317]。最近在美国进行的一项为期 20 年的研究中，近 420 00 例患者证明消化道癌症的风险增加，尤其是在移植后[318]。这项相同的研究也发现淋巴细胞性白血病和睾丸癌的风险增加，但黑色素瘤的风险降低。发病机制尚不确定，但在囊性纤维化患者以及其他原因导致的 CP 患者中也观察到 PC 风险增加[317,319]。随着囊性纤维化患者的生存率不断增加，应牢记这种癌症风险的增加[320,321]。对于有不明原因主诉的青少年和成年人，尤其是与腹部器官相关的主诉时，应评价其是否患有隐匿性恶性肿瘤。最近一个关于囊性纤维化患者结直肠癌筛查的共识小组建议在 40 岁时进行结肠镜检查，并根据个体结果进行随访筛查[322]。器官移植受者应接受应从 30 岁开始筛查结直肠癌。

5. 营养管理

营养目标：在常规临床环境中，囊性纤维化患者的营养管理是基于营养需求评估的（见第 5 章），考虑儿童年龄和成人 BMI 的年龄、身高、体重和人体测量学、肺病的严重程度以及厌食、PI 和黏膜功能障碍[239,323]。理想情况下，应鼓励适合年龄的饮食（为健康人群参考卡路里摄入量的 1.1~2 倍），提供充分的 PERT（如有指征，可进行胃酸抑制），以尽可能实现正常的脂肪平衡[239]。许多囊性纤维化中心也鼓励高热量、高脂肪和不限盐的饮食。营养在肺功能中的作用很重要，因为 BMI≥第 50 百分位数的患者往往肺功能（FEV_1）在正常的 80% 以内[239,323]。

2005 年，囊性纤维化基金会修订了营养分类指南，删除使用理想体重百分比来定义营养衰竭。在 2008 年对该指南进行了审查和更新[323]。对于 2 岁以下的儿童，身高体重百分位数应维持在第 50 百分位数或以上。直到 20 岁，建议 BMI ≥第 50 百分位数。还建议女性的 BMI 应≥22kg/m^2，男性的 BMI 应≥23kg/m^2。2016 年 ESPEN-ESPGHAN-ECFS 关于囊性纤维化婴儿、儿童和成人营养管理的指南中也给出了类似的建议[239]。

囊性纤维化患者中的营养不良可由多种因素导致，这些因素可增加营养损失、减少能量摄入和增加能量消耗。营养损失增加主要与基础胰腺功能不全相关，但也受到糖尿病控制不佳、呕吐和（或）反流、肠内黏液过多和胆盐分泌不足等状况的影响。能量摄入既可受到疾病并发症的影响，也可受到心身问题、心理社会问题、压力和治疗不依从的影响，尤其是儿童和青少年[239]。严重的呼吸道症状可伴有厌食、恶心和呕吐。胃肠道症状或并发症，如腹痛、胃食管反流伴胸痛、厌食和呕吐可导致热量摄入减少。在一些患者中，临床抑郁、身体疲劳、嗅觉障碍（食物不开胃）和身体形象改变可导致摄食量减少。能量消耗增加也经常伴随囊性纤维化患者的严重呼吸系统疾病，可能与以下变量相关：包括慢性感染、发热、呼吸功增加和支气管扩张药物的使用[239]。囊性纤维化患者的最佳饮食摄入量大于健康儿童和成人的推荐膳食营养素供给量（RDA）。为了预防或延缓营养缺乏的发生，ESPEN-ESPGHAN-ECFS 营养指南建议患者在饮食中注意大量营养素的平衡，并注意足以预防或延缓肌肉质量和功能损失的蛋白质和脂肪的摄入。一般而言，能量摄入量应适合年龄，并支持正常体重，注意个体间的范围较宽，约为健康人群参考摄入量的 1.1~2 倍。还建议在饮食中摄入电解质，根据需要进行补充；补充脂溶性维生素；并为胰腺功能不全患者开具 PERT 处方[239]。在囊性纤维化患者中使用 PERT 可挽救生命，但给药更具经验性，可能无法很好地转化为 CP 和胰腺外分泌功能不全成人患者的剂量。最近对婴儿囊性纤维化患者（长达 12 个月）的共识建议是：摄入 2 000~4 000U 脂肪酶/120mL 配方奶粉或估计的母乳摄入量，以及食物中约 2 000U 脂肪酶/g 膳食脂肪[239]。对于 1~4 岁的儿童，使用 2 000~4 000U 脂肪酶/g 膳食脂肪，根据需要增加剂量（最大剂量为 10 000U 脂肪酶/kg/d）[239]。对于 4 岁以上儿童和成人，从 500U 脂肪酶/kg/餐开始，向上滴定至最大剂量 1 000~2 500U 脂肪酶/kg/餐，或 10 000U 脂肪酶/kg/d，或 2 000~4 000U 脂肪酶/g 膳食脂肪，与所有含脂肪的膳食、零食和饮料同服[239]。对于 70kg 的囊性纤维化患者，这相当于 70 000~175 000U 脂肪酶/餐，这与一项双盲、随机、安慰剂对照的胰酶胶囊平行组试验中 72 000U 脂肪酶单位/餐有效改善脂肪吸收系数的剂量相似（3 Creon 24 000）[324]。

肠内管饲：即使没有随机试验的支持证据，肠内管饲仍然是囊性纤维化患者营养不良的常见治疗方法。约 10% 的囊性纤维化患者需要补充管饲[261]。比利时最近一项关于肠内管饲的回顾性 CF 登记研究表明，肠内管饲改善了 BMI z 评分并稳定了 FEV_1[325]。该结果与既往研究一致，显示营养状况和肺功能之间存在相关性[323]。重要的是，登记研究发现，直到患者的营养和肺部状态显著低于整体 CF 队列时，才开始管饲。该观结果表明，需要更好的预测性计划和等待营养失败的早期标志物。

胃食管反流病症状的存在和严重程度可能影响对管饲首选途径的选择。一些青少年学习每晚通过软硅橡胶喂养管，以便给予鼻饲。一些家庭和患者可能首选胃造瘘口喂养，尤其是年幼儿童。在首次出现营养失败体征时，即应进行胃造口术或空肠造口术喂养。标准配方通常耐受性良好。鼓励夜间输注以促进白天的正常饮食模式。最初，30%~50% 的估计热量需求应在夜间提供。对有肠内营养管的患者，可使用不含酶补充剂的极低脂肪、元素配方，并应通过连续输注的方式给予[326]。对于标准配方，在补料期间提供胰酶替代治疗的方法是可变的。一种含有固定化脂肪酶的新型在线检测药盒提供了另一种有吸引力的选择[327,328]。接受肠内喂养的患者应在至少 2 个不同的夜晚，通过测量喂养后 2~3 小时和喂养结束时的血糖水平来监测碳水化合物不耐受。可能需要胰岛素来预防高血糖症，在急性疾病、糖皮质激素治疗和其他健康状态变化期间应调整胰岛素剂量。在某些情况下，可能需要肠外营养，但应保留用于急性支持，并尽快恢复某种形式的肠内营养。

用靶向药物治疗 CFTR 功能性变体：在通过递送 DNA 或蛋白质增加肺中功能性 CFTR 来治疗囊性纤维化的大量努力未能为人类提供持久的改善后，努力转向恢复内源性 CFTR 的功能[329]。研究人员使用具有数千个小分子的高通量筛选，确定了改善内源性、突变型 CFTR 功能的化合物[330]。其中一种化合物 VX-770 或依伐卡托（ivacaftor）（Kalydeco）的首个靶向治疗针对第三种最常见的囊性纤维化引起突变

p. G551D。VX-770 通过改变突变型 CFTR 的门控功能来增加通道开放的概率，从而增加 Cl^- 的分泌，改善 p. G551D CFTR 的功能[331]。在Ⅱ期和Ⅲ期临床试验中，VX-770 改善了第 1 秒呼气容积(FEV_1)的预测值，降低了汗液氯化物浓度，并降低了肺急性加重的频率[332,333]。对治疗后未出现早期应答的受试者子集进行随访，结果显示其具有长期临床获益[334]。VX-770 被 FDA 批准用于具有导致 CFTR 门控功能障碍的多种突变患者[335-337]。该人群不包括携带最常见致病变体 CFTR p. F508del 的患者。该变体导致 CFTR 折叠、转运、膜稳定性和氯离子通道活性的多种缺陷。通过将 VX-770 与 VX-809(lumacaftor)(一种促进 CFTR 折叠的小分子)结合来解决该问题。该联合用药可部分挽救 p. F508del CFTR 功能[338]。联合治疗的临床试验显示 p. F508del CFTR 纯合子患者的临床结局有所改善，该治疗已获得 FDA 批准[339]。然而，一般而言，CFTR 增强子和校正子的作用似乎不是突变特异性的。相反，药物反应的强度与增强药物 ivacaftor、校正药物 lumacaftor 和 ivacaftor-lumacaftor 联合治疗的残留 CFTR 的功能高度相关，并且这些效应是累加的[340]。大约有一半符合条件的囊性纤维化患者联合使用 ivacaftor 和 luma-caftor 治疗[261]。其他小分子复方制剂正在开发或试验中，可能会导致疗效改善[341]。

预后：根据国家囊性纤维化登记研究数据估计的生存统计量通常令人困惑，因为不同的组在报告生存数据时使用不同的方法和术语[342]。2012 年至 2016 年期间在美国出生的患者的中位预测生存期的最新估计值为 42.7 岁[261]。对于达到 40 岁的患者，预测的中位生存期几乎为 60 岁。尽管如此，在 2016 年死于囊性纤维化的 373 人中，他们的中位年龄仅为 29.6 岁。大多数发病和死亡与慢性肺部疾病有关，67% 的死亡是由于呼吸系统或心肺疾病引起的[261]。营养支持、胰酶替代和积极治疗肺部疾病在改善生活质量和持续时间方面的相对作用仍在研究中。伴有 PS 的 CF 患者的肺部状态优于伴有 PI 的 CF 患者，提示该疾病具有异质性，并且通过更好的营养和治疗可以提高生存率。

随着生存率的提高，囊性纤维化患者面临的问题可能会改变，并开始蔓延到护理人员的领域，主要关注囊性纤维化成年人的问题。这些医学问题包括胰腺炎、营养不良、肝硬化伴门静脉高压、糖尿病及其长期并发症、骨量减少和生殖问题，以及所有在儿童期常见的问题。在囊性纤维化登记研究的 2016 年报告中，老年患者的骨病、胃食管反流病、鼻窦疾病、哮喘、焦虑和抑郁的患病率较高。囊性纤维化相关糖尿病在成人中比在儿童中更常见(35.1% vs 6.4%)。成人肺部疾病比儿童更严重，营养不良仍然是囊性纤维化成人患者的一个问题，尽管营养状况总体上有所改善[261]。越来越多的患者需要评估消化道的潜在恶性肿瘤，并评估肝病或其他并发症，这将需要胃肠病专家的特别关注。

(二) 遗传性胰腺炎

遗传性胰腺炎(HP)是一种 RAP 综合征，常导致 CP，在胰腺炎表型似乎通过常染色体显性模式表达的致病基因突变遗传的家族个体中发生[9,343]。最常见的原因是阳离子胰蛋白酶原基因(*PRSS1*)的功能获得性突变，其改变了通常由钙控制的调节结构域(见图 57.4)。大多数 *PRSS1* 突变的家族来自美国和欧洲，少数来自日本和南美洲，但没有来自南亚的。大多数(65%~81%)但并非所有具有常染色体显性遗传模式的胰腺炎家族均具有 *PRSS1* 突变[344,345]。

临床特征：*PRSS1* 突变引起的 HP 表型特征局限于胰腺，因为胰腺是胰蛋白酶原表达的主要位点。主要表型是 RAP，一部分患者进展为 CP，所有并发症与其他形式的 CP 相同。

急性胰腺炎：急性胰腺炎(AP)的发作通常是 HP 患者发病的信号。在美国 181 例症状的 *PRSS1* 突变携带者的家族/队列中，首次诊断为胰腺炎的中位年龄为 7 岁(四分位距，3~16；范围 < 1~73)[12]。在法国，EUROPAC 研究中，PRSS1 p. R122H 和 PRSS1 p. N29I 的中位症状发作时间分别为 10 年(范围 1~73)[346]、10 年及 14 年[344]。AP 和 RAP 的诊断和治疗与其他类型胰腺炎相同(见第 58 章)。发作的严重程度各不相同。一些家庭似乎比其他家庭有更严重的发作和并发症[10,347]。绝大多数发作持续不到 7 天，受累患者平均年发作 2 次(p. R122H)或 1.4 次(p. N29I)。p. R122H 的住院率(每年 0.33)显著高于 p. N29I 突变的住院率(每年 0.19)[344]。不常见的、长期、持续性或冒烟型 AP(病情进展缓慢而无临床症状的 AP)患者可能住院数周或数月。

基因突变携带者胰腺炎表型的外显率不完全(≈80%)[12,344,346,348]。表观不完全外显率和可变表达似乎是由遗传和环境因素共同决定的[349]。例如，在携带其他突变(如 *PRSS1* 加 *SPINK1*)的患者中观察到发病年龄更早和临床病程更严重[350]。

AP 的第一次发作是 RAP 循环开始的信号。HP 患者尚无特定的预防性治疗来阻止其进展或将发作的严重程度降至最低。通常推荐少食多餐，避免高脂肪饮食，并使用抗氧化剂和维生素。必须避免饮酒和吸烟。在一项对 14 例 HP 合并 CP 患者的研究中，血清超氧化物歧化酶水平显著高于其他家庭成员、人群对照或 7 名非 HP 患儿，血清维生素 E 和硒水平显著低于其他家庭成员、人群对照或 7 例非 HP 患儿[351]。一项使用抗氧化剂和维生素的小型开放标签试验似乎减少了 HP 家族中疼痛发作的天数[352]。在另一项钙离子通道阻滞剂氨氯地平的初步研究中，4 例接受治疗的患者的镇痛药使用和症状评分降低[353]。

慢性胰腺炎：慢性胰腺炎(CP)的发病目前难以确定，但在 HP 中估计了症状发作(通常是 AP 的症状)和外分泌/内分泌功能衰竭之间的时间(图 57.11)。在 EUROPAC 研究中，10 岁时胰腺外分泌衰竭的累积风险为 2.0%，20 岁时为 8.4%、40 岁时为 33.6% 和 70 岁时为 60.2%[344]。在法国和美国也观察到相似的结果[12,346]。

疼痛：疼痛是 HP 最令人痛苦和最使人衰弱的特征之一。疼痛体验具有高度变异性，表明存在多种修饰因素[226,354]。一般而言，在 RAP 或 CP 背景下，持续疼痛的患者通常具有更多的疼痛相关残疾/失业和显著较低的生活质量评分[355,356]。持续性胰腺疼痛信号可导致疼痛集中和慢性疼痛综合征，使患者虚弱，并与高卫生资源使用相关[354,355,357,358]。重度神经性疼痛患者也可能有神经肥大和神经密度增加的手术结果[359,360]。在药物、内镜或既往手术治疗失败的 CP 或 RAP

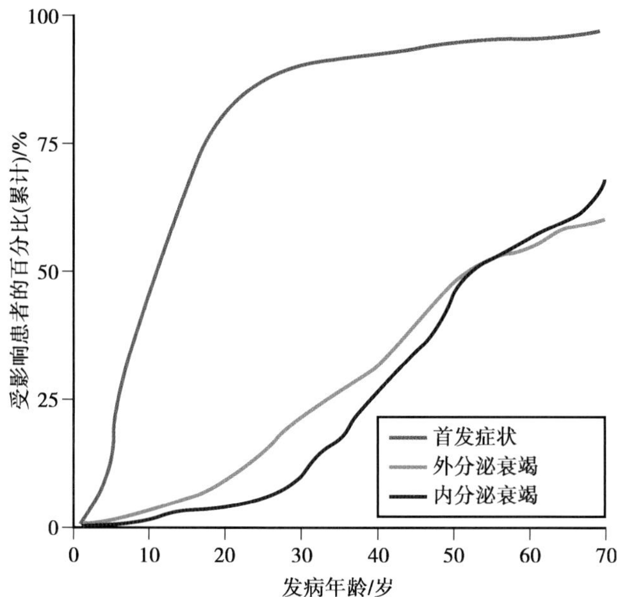

图 57.11　遗传性胰腺炎(HP)患者症状发作的年龄。由于 *PRSS1* R122H 突变导致遗传性胰腺炎的受试者通常发病年龄较早(20 岁之前),尽管首发症状可能发生在老年患者中。一部分受试者出现外分泌和(或)内分泌功能衰竭,通常发生在首次出现症状后 20～30 年。(From Howes N, Lerch MM, Greenhelf W, et al. Clinical and genetic characteristics of hereditary pancreatitis in Europe. Clin Gastroenterol Hepatol 2004;2:252-61.)

导致生活质量受损的患者出现难治性疼痛的情况下,应将全胰腺切除联合胰岛自体移植(total pancreatectomy with islet autotransplantation, TPIAT)视为一种潜在有效的治疗方法[361]。值得注意的是,如果 *PRSS1* 变异患者年龄较小且病程较短,则接受胰岛自体移植的预后较好,这可能是因为纤维化较少、胰岛产量较好[362]。在专家中心,根据医学结果研究健康调查简表(SF-36)的平均身体健康总评和心理健康总评数据,胰岛自体移植患者的平均健康相关生活质量有非常显著的改善[363]。尽管正在做进一步的工作来确定与疼痛和靶向治疗相关的环境和遗传因素,但目前的证据表明,早期手术有助于降低中枢性疼痛的可能性[354]。

糖尿病:在 EUROPAC 研究中,10 岁时内分泌衰竭的累积风险为 1.3%,20 岁时为 4.4%,30 岁时为 8.5%,到 50 岁时为 47.6%(见图 57.11)[344]。同样,26% 的法国 HP 患者患有糖尿病,中位发病年龄为 38 岁[346]。内分泌衰竭(糖尿病)的累积发病率在 50 岁以后继续增加,尤其是在至少一项研究中 p. N29I 变异者[344]。

胰腺癌:HP 患者中胰腺癌(PC)的发生率显著增加[12,344,364,365]。胰腺癌似乎在胰腺炎发作后约 30～40 年发生[364,366,367]。70 岁时胰腺癌的初始估计累积风险为 40%(95% CI:9%～71%)[364,368]。在法国,50 岁和 75 岁时男性胰腺癌的累积风险分别为 11% 和 49%,女性为 8% 和 55%[365]。然而,另外两项年龄较大、队列较大的研究发现 70 岁时的累积风险较低——EUROPAC 研究为 18.8%[344],美国为 7.2%[12]。

PC 发病率高的原因尚不清楚。*PRSS1* 基因似乎在散发性胰腺癌中不起作用[369],和我们目前对胰蛋白酶生物学的认识,没有为胰蛋白酶如何作为癌基因或其他癌症相关因子提供理论基础。相反,由不受调控的胰蛋白酶原活化引起的复发性胰腺损伤和随后的炎症反应似乎提供了具有致癌性的环境[367,370]。然而,尽管在 HP 患者中胰腺上皮内瘤变(pancreatic intraepithelial neoplasia, PanIN)病变经常发生且发生在早期,但它们似乎与钙化、纤维化或炎症的程度无关[371]些进展,胰腺癌的治疗选择有限,尽管最近取得了一些进展,但预后仍然较差。最有效的方法是预防,认识到早发性胰腺炎是胰腺癌最强的已知风险因素之一。导致胰腺癌的高危生活方式是吸烟,吸烟会使胰腺癌的风险增加一倍[321]。这种风险加倍在 HP 患者中变得至关重要,HP 患者的胰腺癌潜在风险已经是一般人群风险的 50 倍。事实上,吸烟使 HP 患者经年龄和性别校正的 OR 增加了 1 倍,吸烟者诊断胰腺癌的中位年龄早 20 岁[364]。除吸烟外,糖尿病似乎是 HP 患者发生胰腺癌的危险因素[365]。

虽然 HP 家系有较高的癌症风险,但尚未建立有效的筛查方法。在胰腺炎患者解剖结构扭曲的腺体中早期发现胰腺癌是困难的。因此,专家小组的共识指南建议,如果处于胰腺癌风险年龄范围内的个体正在考虑胰腺手术,则应考虑全胰腺切除术[372]。年轻患者可接受胰岛自体移植,但由于存在移植恶性肿瘤细胞的风险,胰岛自体移植在长期 CP 老年患者中的作用尚不确定[361,373]。

诊断:在 1996 年以前,HP 的诊断纯粹基于临床标准,包括家族谱系的检查。阳离子胰蛋白酶原基因突变 *PRSS1* p. R122H 和 p. N29I 的发现为分子诊断打开了大门[9,173]。尽管大多数具有 RAP 和 CP[和(或)糖尿病或胰腺癌]常染色体显性模式的家族将具有功能获得性 *PRSS1* 突变,但高达 20% 的 HP 家系将不具有可识别的 *PRSS1* 突变[12,344,346]。*PRSS1* 重复变异也与 HP 相关[82,83,374]。诊断需要其他特发性 AP 或 RAP 的临床体征,以及与 HP 相关的强家族史或与 *PRSS1* 变异[41]。

基因检测:基因检测结果在患者的一生中保持不变,对未来的后代和其他家庭成员有影响,并可能影响社会和生殖选择、就业和保险[41,375]。因此,临床医生必须充分理解检测的意义,准备好为患者提供检测前和检测后的遗传咨询(或将患者转诊至遗传咨询师),并确保在检测前获得知情同意[41,375]。*PRSS1* 突变检测的原因包括验证临床怀疑、帮助患者了解或验证其病情,并帮助个体评估其患胰腺炎和最终患胰腺癌的风险。遗传信息也可能有助于作出人生决策,以尽量减少疾病风险(如生殖、饮食、酒精、吸烟)。鉴定已确定的胰腺炎相关基因突变对加快昂贵和长期的儿童 RAP 的评估是有价值的,并且可能排除进一步评估成人胰腺炎的不明原因。

在正确应用现代技术的情况下,基因检测在识别特定突变方面的阳性和阴性预测值几乎是完美的[234,376]。对检测结果的判读及其对患者意义的解释仍然是关键问题。预后可以从前面的临床讨论中用一般术语来概述,注意到存在显著的变异性,并且未来治疗在预防不良结局方面的有效性尚不清楚。最后,突变阳性个体有 50% 的概率将突变传递给每个孩子。

临床上未受影响的人的阳性检测结果被认为是胰腺炎风险增加的原因,该风险可能随着年龄的增长而降低。在一个已知*PRSS1*基因突变家系的阴性检测结果基本上消除了这种遗传形式胰腺炎的风险。如果之前未在家族中发现突变，则认为未受影响个体的阴性检测结果无信息，因为无法区分受试个体是否无遗传风险或是否遗传了不同的胰腺炎易感基因突变。应始终通过商业基因检测实验室获得最新信息。遗传咨询信息可通过国家遗传咨询师协会或美国遗传咨询委员会获得[376]。

儿童基因检测提出了独特的问题[376]。与成人患者不同，儿童在法律上不能提供知情同意。因此，对儿童的决定基本上留给了父母或法定监护人。对于7岁及以上的儿童，父母或法定监护人可以提供基因检测的知情同意书，但这些年龄较大的儿童也应同意进行检测。检测儿童*PRSS1*基因突变的主要原因是帮助确定不明原因胰腺炎的原因，或确认有HP高危儿童的疑似胰腺炎，从而限制进一步的调查。不鼓励对无症状儿童进行检测，因为目前在识别年轻携带者方面没有明确的医学益处。据报道，饮酒、高脂肪食物和情绪压力会促发胰腺炎发作，而且吸烟会增加患胰腺炎和胰腺癌的风险，因此一些看护人员提倡进行基因检测以鼓励突变阳性的年长儿童避免这些过度的行为。然而，避免食用高脂肪食物、酒精和烟草对所有儿童来说都是的极好一般健康建议，因此，没有强制进行检测的理由。在任何一种情况下，都必须仔细考虑年龄较大儿童推迟测试或继续测试以缓解他们自身焦虑和更多地了解他们自身健康的个人意愿。

（三）家族性胰腺炎

家族性胰腺炎的初始症状发生在年轻时（如<20岁），更可能与强烈的遗传风险相关。常染色体显性遗传模式通常是由于功能获得性*PRSS1*突变引起（见上文）。常染色体隐性遗传疾病的最常见原因与纯合子或复合杂合子*CFTR*突变（通常包括一个或多个Ⅳ类或Ⅴ类突变）和（或）*SPINK1*突变或更复杂的基因型相关。

（四）Schwachman-Diamond 综合征

Schwachman-Diamond综合征（SDS）是一种罕见的常染色体隐性遗传疾病，与*SBDS*基因[129]和可能的其他基因（如*DNAJC21*、*ELF1*和*SRP54*）的突变有关的[130]。SDS的特征是EPI出现血液学异常（如周期性中性粒细胞减少）、骨骼缺陷和身材矮小（见表57.4）[130,377-379]。胰腺外分泌功能障碍和周期性中性粒细胞减少症见于大多数患者[130,377,379]。中性粒细胞减少症定义为中性粒细胞绝对计数低于1 500/mL[130]。报告了许多其他特征（框57.4）。然而，对北美SDS登记研究中37例患者的回顾表明，中性粒细胞减少是就诊时最常见的血液学异常（81%），而仅有一半（51%）的患者表现为中性粒细胞减少和脂肪泻[380]。该登记研究由血液科医生领导，因此这些数据可能反映了一些选择、检测或转诊偏倚。高达三分之一的患者发生骨髓增生异常综合征和急性白血病。

重度SDS病例出现在婴儿期，伴有吸收不良，发育停滞或复发性感染。由于胰腺、血液和其他特征的表达多变，轻度病例的诊断可能会延迟[377,380,381]。已经确认了数百个家庭，其中大多数只有一个受影响的成员[378]。

框57.4　Shwachman-Diamond 综合征的临床特征（发生率）

胰腺
外分泌胰腺发育不全（91%～100%）
脂肪泻（55%～88%）
血液学
中性粒细胞减少（88%～100%）
胎儿血红蛋白水平升高（80%）
白细胞减少症（52%）
贫血（42%～66%）
全血细胞减少（44%）
血小板减少（24%～34%）
骨髓增生异常综合征（8%～33%）
白血病（12%）
骨骼
干骺端软骨发育不全（44%）
胸廓发育不良（32%）
长骨管缺陷（?）
短肋或肋骨外翻（?）
其他（<5%）
生长
正常生长速度的身材矮小（常见）
其他
精神运动发育迟滞（常见）
肝脏生化检测水平异常（常见）
心肌异常（尸检时为50%）
智力低下（33%）
糖尿病（<5%）
肝大（<5%）
肾小管功能障碍（?）
牙齿异常（?）
鱼鳞病（?）

SDS遗传缺陷：与SDS连接的主要基因是*SBDS*基因。该基因有5个外显子，编码250个氨基酸的预测蛋白，参与核糖体成熟和相关系统[382]。大多数SDS病例的遗传缺陷是由正常*SBDS*基因与无功能假基因（命名为*SBDSP*）之间的基因转换导致蛋白产物功能障碍所致[129,382]。*SBDSP*假基因DNA编码与*SBDS*基因编码的同源性为97%。最初在原始家族中发现了14种截然不同的突变，最常见的是转换突变183-184TA→CT和258+2T→C；183-184TA→CT引入了一个过早的终止密码子，p. K62X，而258+2T→C破坏供体剪接位点。目前已发现*SBDS*中40多种新的遗传变异为复合杂合基因型，具有常见的基因转换等位基因之一[382]。未描述p. K62X变体的纯合子，表明存活需要功能性SBDS蛋白。不到10%具有SDS临床特征的患者没有*SBDS*突变。其中一些个体在*DNAC21*中具有双等位基因遗传变异体，其蛋白产物有助于60S核糖体亚基的成熟[131]。

*SBDS*编码一个高度保守且广泛表达的29kD蛋白。与来自60S核糖体亚基的鸟苷三磷酸酶延伸因子6一起，SBDS的功能是启动翻译[383-385]。此外，SBDS可能参与调节端粒酶对端粒的募集，从而有助于维持端粒长度[386]。遗传缺陷导致胰腺腺泡细胞缺陷，伴有酶基因合成和PI显著减少，而不是对胰腺炎的易感性。缺乏SBDS表达也会影响髓系分化，增加骨髓衰竭和急性髓系白血病的风险[380]。SBDS缺乏小鼠

模型显示,该蛋白是胰腺发育和功能所必需的[387]。SBDS 缺陷的人胚胎干细胞和诱导多能干细胞在体外表现出胰腺外分泌和造血分化缺陷,细胞凋亡增强,培养上清液中蛋白酶水平升高,可以通过转基因拯救恢复 SBDS 蛋白表达或通过向培养基中补充蛋白酶抑制剂逆转缺陷,表明蛋白酶介导的自身消化有助于 SDS 的发病机制[388]。阿塔鲁伦(ataluren)是一种抑制无义突变的药物,最初开发用于治疗囊性纤维化、在从 SDS 患者获得的造血细胞中恢复 SBDS 表达并刺激髓系分化[389]。

临床特征:SDS 的临床特征为胰腺和血液系统。现在可以通过整合高危家族的基因型和表型类型,来证实广泛的特征和严重程度。

胰腺功能不全:SDS 的临床特征通常在出生后第一年变得明显[163,377,381,390]。重度胰腺功能不全(PI)、脂肪泻和发育停滞是常见的症状,但并非总是存在或诊断所必需[377,380,381,391]。如果基因检测不能诊断[392],正常的汗液氯化物浓度(或 CFTR 功能的其他正常测量值)可以帮助区分 SDS 和 CF[163]。胰腺病变似乎开始于子宫内泛胰腺腺泡的发育障碍[163]。肉眼观察,胰腺呈脂肪状,可能较小或正常大小。广泛的脂肪瘤样改变导致 CT、MRI 或 US[393,394] 腹部成像时的特征性改变(图 57.12),但这些成像结果并不总是存在[380]。主胰管和胰岛正常,胰腺腺泡组织有广泛的脂肪替代[163]。胰腺外分泌功能的一系列评估显示酶分泌的持续缺陷,但近半数患者在 4 岁后显示出与年龄相关的中度改善,导致 PS[377,381],一些胰酶(如胰蛋白酶)比其他酶(如淀粉酶)恢复更多。

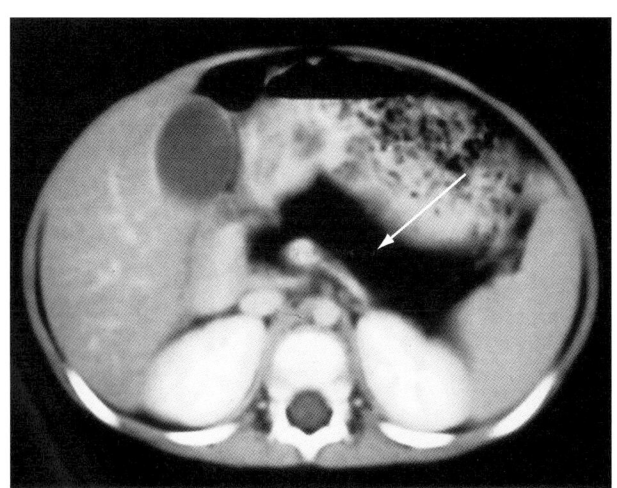

图 57.12　Shwachman-Diamond 综合征患者胰腺 CT 表现。请注意,胰腺(箭)保留了典型的大小和形状,但它富含脂肪,因此表现为极低密度结构。(Image courtesy professor Peter Durie)

血液学表现:中性粒细胞减少相关感染也是 SDS 早期和潜在的严重问题。中性粒细胞减少在三分之二的患者中以周期性方式发生,经检测,中性粒细胞似乎有迁移和趋化受损[395]尽管它们仍然可以形成脓肿[130]。SDS 患者易受各种细菌、病毒和真菌感染,而中性粒细胞减少症患者的感染率高于预期[130,379]。常见的感染包括中耳炎、鼻窦炎、肺炎、骨髓炎、尿路感染、皮肤和软组织感染以及淋巴结炎[130,396]。高达 80% 的患者发生正色素性、正红细胞性贫血[130]。有时会出现血小板减少。全血细胞减少患者的预后最差[377]。而所有 SDS 患者的中位生存年龄为 35 岁,全血细胞减少患者的中位预期寿命仅为 24 岁。全血细胞减少症在平均年龄 6 岁时出现,有 10%~25% 的患者发生[396]。高达三分之一的 SDS 患者发生骨髓增生异常综合征,约 10%~25% 的患者发生白血病,通常为急性髓系白血病[377,379,381,395]。

生长和发育:SDS 儿童的出生体重通常较低(2.9±0.5kg,第 25 百分位数)[377],到 6 月龄时,平均身高和体重通常低于第 5 百分位数。此后,生长速度表现正常[377]。身材矮小与营养无关[163,379]。可能存在一些临床上明显的骨骼异常。例如,44% 的患者干骺端软骨发育不良和骨发育不全明显,尤其是股骨头和胫骨近端[130,163]。胸廓发育不良,如漏斗胸、窒息性胸廓发育不良、肋骨外翻和其他骨骼畸形也有报道[130,163,377,397]。大多数患者的身高和体重保持在第 3 百分位数以下,尽管一些成人达到身高的第 25 百分位数[163]。男性和女性可能受到相同的影响,但男性比女性更有可能接受彻底的调查,导致轻度的确定偏倚[378,381]。

治疗:SDS 患者治疗胰腺外分泌缺陷比囊性纤维化更为直接,因为胰腺和十二指肠中的碳酸氢盐分泌不受到影响。胰酶替代治疗应以减少脂肪泻和改善体重增加为目标。如囊性纤维化中所述,可能还需要脂溶性维生素、中链硫酸三甘氨酸(中链 TG)和其他高热量补充剂。

SDS 患者通常由血液科医生领导的多学科团队进行随访。在粒细胞减少症期间,应评估是否发热,并使用适当的抗菌药物治疗。重度中性粒细胞减少症或疑似有重度感染的患者应住院并接受静脉注射抗生素治疗,直至病情好转[379]。对于出现重度中性粒细胞减少症的复发性侵袭性细菌和(或)真菌感染,应考虑长期使用 G-CSF[379]。患者可能对低剂量 G-CSF 的间歇性给药方案有反应(例如,2~3μG/kg,每 3 天一次),或可能需要连续给予更高剂量[379]。造血干细胞移植仍然是严重再生障碍性贫血或恶变的 SDS 个体的唯一治愈性疗法[130]。出血或重度贫血发作可能需要输血或输注血小板[379]。应监测髋关节疾病,如发生进展应进行手术干预。在这种情况下使用重组人生长激素还没有进行系统的研究,但有轶事报道显示出加速生长的疗效。

七、罕见的遗传综合征与胰腺病理学

(一) Johanson-Blizzard 综合征

Johanson-Blizzard 综合征是一种罕见的常染色体隐性遗传综合征,与泛素-连接酶 E3(*UBR1*)基因突变有关[137,398,399]。该综合征的胰腺成分以胰腺功能不全和生长受限为特征,伴胰腺脂肪瘤样转化而非 AP。*UBR1* 中的大多数突变是无义突变、移码突变、剪接位点突变或导致无活性蛋白的小框内缺失[399]。一些患者存在错义突变或小的框内缺失,导致较轻的表型[135,399,400]。最近的一项研究在 Johanson-Blizzard 综合征患者中发现了 *UBR1* 的外显子缺失或重复,从而扩展了这种疾病的基因型[401]。泛素-连接酶 E3

属于细胞内蛋白质降解系统的 N 端规则途径。已知在胰腺炎期间可触发自身消化的消化丝氨酸蛋白酶是 *UBR1* 的特异性底物，当 *UBR1* 因功能缺失突变而存在缺陷时，消化丝氨酸蛋白酶在胰腺中表达上调[137,399]。作为主要和最一致的人类表型，胰腺外分泌功能不全是子宫内胰腺炎的结果，导致腺体完全破坏，尽管情况并不总是如此。Johanson-Blizzard 综合征的胰腺受累可能是轻度的，直到生命后期才明显[136]。*UBR1* 的小鼠基因敲除表现出与人类表型非常相似的特征，包括生长受限、颅面异常和胰腺外分泌功能不全。与野生型动物相比，小鼠腺泡细胞损害了胆囊收缩素受体刺激的兴奋-分泌偶联，对实验性胰腺炎更敏感，在病程中对更严重的全身炎症反应更敏感。这些发现与细胞内不能降解各种细胞溶质消化酶相一致。

与 SDS 患者和囊性纤维化患者不同，Johanson-Blizzard 综合征患者保留了导管输出液体和电解质[402]。它们还具有胰蛋白酶、辅脂酶和总脂肪酶的腺泡分泌减少，血清免疫反应性胰蛋白酶原水平较低，与原发性腺泡细胞缺陷一致[402]。组织学上，胰管和胰岛被保留，但被结缔组织包围，腺泡完全缺失。除胰腺腺泡细胞缺损伴吸收不良外，该综合征还表现为鼻翼成形不全、耳聋、甲状腺功能减退、侏儒症、恒牙缺失、心脏异常、泌尿生殖系统畸形、中线外胚层头皮缺陷和肛门闭锁或前肛门[136,399,401]。SDS 中没有血液学异常[402]。到目前为止，*UBR1* 变异与 CP 的相关性仍在研究中[399,403]。

（二）Pearson 骨髓-胰腺综合征

Pearson 骨髓-胰腺综合征是一种罕见的常染色体显性线粒体 DNA（mtDNA）断裂综合征，以难治性铁粒幼细胞性贫血伴骨髓前体空泡化为特征，常伴胰腺外分泌功能障碍[404,405]。其他受影响器官系统包括肾脏（肾小管病变、氨基酸尿、范可尼综合征）、肝脏（肝大，细胞溶解和胆汁淤积）、内分泌腺（糖尿病、肾上腺功能不全）、神经肌肉系统和心脏[405-407]。生化特征包括乳酸酸中毒、血浆瓜氨酸和精氨酸水平低以及尿液中瓜氨酸升高、乳酸/丙酮酸尿症、柠檬酸循环中间产物增多，偶尔还会出现与柠檬酸循环中关键酶和其他线粒体功能丧失相一致的酮尿症[405]。

该综合征患者在婴儿期可有输血依赖性大细胞性贫血，但所有其他骨髓细胞系似乎均正常。胰腺功能不全是由泛纤维化而非腺泡细胞的脂肪替代所致，如 SDS，更可能与糖尿病相关。该综合征在儿童早期死亡率较高，存活的患者发生多系统进行性受累，包括肝脏、肾脏、肠道和皮肤，均有线粒体异常。

Pearson 骨髓-胰腺综合征的分子缺陷最初被确定为线粒体 DNA 的 4 977 个碱基对缺失，包括编码 NADH 脱氢酶、细胞色素氧化酶和 ATP 酶的基因部分[408]。目前已经发现了多种其他线粒体缺陷[406,409]，这些缺失似乎两侧有核苷酸重复序列[409]。Cherry 及同事[410]证实，与对照多能干细胞相比，具有缺失线粒体 DNA 高负荷的多能干细胞在体外培养时，在生长、线粒体功能和造血表型方面存在差异。疾病的临床特征和严重程度似乎与器官分布和异常线粒体 DNA 的比例相关[406,411]。存活患者可能出现其他线粒体 DNA 缺失综合征的特征。没有特殊治疗来纠正这些异常。

（三）胰腺发育不全

胰腺发育不全极为罕见，详细讨论见第 55 章[412,413]。心脏畸形、胆囊发育不全和肠道畸形也常见于这些患者。肠旋转不良通常导致胰腺钩突发育不全，很可能是与十二指肠旋转相关的发育问题[414]。

胰腺发育不全的鉴别诊断包括新生儿一过性糖尿病、胰腺发育不良、囊性纤维化、SDS、Johanson-Blizzard 综合征和其他罕见疾病。然而，在胰腺发育不全中，严重的内分泌和外分泌缺陷持续存在，血清 C 肽和胰高血糖素水平检测不到，影像学检查（如 MRI）胰腺缺失。这些儿童被视为患有 1 型糖尿病（接受胰岛素治疗）和重度胰腺外分泌功能不全（接受胰酶补充治疗）。通过正确的诊断和治疗患者有可能生存。

背侧胰腺的部分胰腺发育不全也极为罕见（见第 55 章）。与胰腺完全发育不全不同，患者可无症状，或也可表现为胆管梗阻、胰腺炎或糖尿病[415]。腹侧胰腺缺失和发育不全也极为罕见。在携带编码肝细胞核因子 1 同源盒 B（HNF-1B）基因突变的患者中，已经描述了胰腺腹侧和背侧的缺失[416]。

（四）其他罕见综合征

已确定影响胰腺的其他罕见综合征。例如无脾伴囊性肝、肾和胰腺（Iverson 综合征），发生肾、肝和胰腺的“发育不良”（在发育紊乱的意义上）无其他异常[417]。组织学上，胰腺有扩张的、大的、形状不规则的导管，周围有同心松散的间充质及其明显的实质纤维化和萎缩区[417]。

分离酶和其他消化酶相关缺陷

脂肪酶：先天性胰脂肪酶缺乏是一种罕见的疾病，伴随着其他酶的不同保存[418-420]。在脂肪酶缺乏症患者中，一直未发现该基因突变，直到最近报告了 2 例患有 *PNLIP* 新突变的兄弟[421,422]。男性和女性均会受累。这种疾病的最早和最具特征性的表现似乎是粪便排出异常量的且容易分离的油，这通常是造成脏污的原因。仅偶尔观察到发育停滞，无全身表现。2 例已知 *PNLIP* 突变即 p. Thr221Met 的兄弟有 CP 的临床证据[422]。疾病的机制似乎是蛋白质错误折叠和 RER 应激[124]。

这些患者十二指肠内容物内胰脂肪酶活性低或无。胰蛋白酶和淀粉酶活性在某些患者有所降低，但其他外分泌汗腺功能参数（包括辅酯酶和磷脂酶 A 活性、碳酸氢盐和容量分泌）通常是正常的。任何残留的脂肪酶活性均被认为是由舌或胃脂肪酶活性引起的结果。

除其功能缺失外，未检测到免疫反应性脂肪酶[418]，表明完全不存胰脂肪酶或发生影响免疫原性和功能的主要结构变化。对外源性胰酶治疗的反应欠佳，常需限制膳食脂肪，以避免油性便和大小便失禁。

辅脂酶：在近亲结婚和非近亲结婚的男性后代中描述了辅脂酶缺乏症[423,424]。这些患者表现为稀便和脂肪泻，但生长和发育正常。辅脂酶活性显著降低，其他胰酶分泌正常。十二指肠内滴注纯化的辅脂酶可显著改善脂肪吸收。在与

CF 和 SDS 相关的 PI 患者的研究中，脂肪泻仅发生在脂肪酶和辅脂酶分泌分别减少至平均正常值的 2% 以下和 1% 以下时[425]。迄今为止，CLPS 中没有与辅脂酶缺陷相关的遗传变异。

L-丝氨酸蛋白酶抑制剂 Kazal 1 型(SPINK1)缺乏症：2 例 *SPINK1* 纯合子变体患者表现为婴儿型胰腺外分泌功能不全[426]。两名患者均有 *SPINK1* 的功能缺失遗传变异。1 例患者 SPINK1 完全缺失，另 1 例患者的 Alu 元件倒置插入到 *SPINK1* 的 3'-未反式区域，导致编码 SPINK1 的 mRNA 水平检测不到。每例患者的胰腺均显示弥漫性脂肪变性。显然，糖尿病不是该综合征的特征，因为这两名患者仅接受胰酶替代治疗效果良好。Spink3（*SPINK1* 的小鼠同源物）缺陷小鼠的胰腺发育正常，直至交配后 15.5 天[120]。然后，它们的胰腺腺泡细胞进行性丢失，直到 14.5 日龄死亡，推测是由于营养不良所致。总之，这些发现表明，SPINK1 和 Spink3 在胰腺腺泡细胞的存活或再生中具有关键功能，与它们更广为人知的抑制胰蛋白酶的功能不同。

肠激酶缺乏：尽管自 1969 年首次发现肠激酶以来，很少出现先天性肠激酶（肠肽酶）缺乏的报告[427]，但根据其在兄弟姐妹中的记录表明其具有家族性[428]。2 个家系的 DNA 测序显示 2 个受累兄弟姐妹无义突变的复合杂合性以及第二个家系患者无义突变和移码突变的复合杂合性[429]。这些患者表现为吸收不良、低蛋白血症和严重的生长受限。评价包括正常淀粉酶和脂肪酶活性，但十二指肠中胰蛋白酶活性极低，汗液电解质浓度正常。加入外源性肠激酶可激活肠腔胰蛋白酶原。小肠形态及双糖酶水平正常。在接受疑似 PI 评价的婴儿中有 1%~2% 的先天性肠激酶缺乏症被辨别出，尽管最近没有新患者的报告[428]。成人期随访显示，婴儿期出现的体重增加不良消退，即使未进行胰酶替代治疗，患者也无胃肠道症状[429]。

与肠激酶缺乏相关的脂肪泻可能与磷脂酶的继发性缺乏有关，磷脂酶的激活需要胰蛋白酶，而胰蛋白酶又被肠激酶激活。囊性纤维化和 SDS 患者的终末内肠激酶活性增加，但黏膜肠激酶活性正常[428]。肠激酶水平和活性理论上也可能随着显著的小肠黏膜损伤而下降。然而，即使在未经治疗的乳糜泻中，也有黏膜正常和肠腔内肠激酶活性正常的报道[430]。

八、复发性急性和慢性胰腺炎相关的家族性代谢综合征

（一）家族性甲状旁腺功能亢进伴高钙血症

高钙血症可能通过胰蛋白酶原激活和胰蛋白酶稳定与 AP、RAP 和 CP 有关[185,431]。大多数原因是主要代谢紊乱，如原发性甲状旁腺功能亢进、恶性肿瘤如多发性骨髓瘤、维生素 D 毒副作用、结节病、全胃肠外营养和围手术期体外循环中大剂量钙的输注所致[431-435]。

已对高钙血症性 AP 的遗传风险进行了研究。对 CASR 基因的研究表明，需要 CASR、SPINK1 和（或）CFTR 变异体以及酒精或其他因素的组合来靶向胰腺，作为 RAP 和 CP 的复杂疾病结果，因为单独的 CASR 突变并不充分[182-184,436]。但一名 CYP24A［一种编码线粒体 24-羟化酶的基因，可使 1,25(OH)2D 失活］功能缺失突变的女性在妊娠期间发生高钙血症、肾结石、肾钙质沉着症和 AP[437]，尽管 AP 发作在该综合征患者中似乎并不常见[438]。

（二）乳糜微粒血症综合征

家族性乳糜微粒血症综合征和多因素乳糜微粒血症综合征已在前面讨论了。

致谢

作者感谢 Celeste Shelton CGC 博士、Mark Haupt 医学博士和 Brandon Blobner 博士对本章的批判性评论所作的贡献。

（施海韵　译，闫秀娥　刘军　校）

参考文献

第 58 章　急性胰腺炎

Santhi Swaroop Vege 著

章节目录

一、疾病的发病率及负担 …… 842
二、定义 …… 843
三、病程 …… 844
四、发病机制和病理生理学 …… 844
五、诱发因素 …… 846
（一）梗阻 …… 847
（二）乙醇和其他毒物 …… 847
（三）药物 …… 848
（四）代谢障碍 …… 849
（五）感染 …… 850
（六）血管疾病 …… 850
（七）创伤 …… 850
（八）ERCP 术后 …… 850
（九）术后状态 …… 851
（十）遗传和基因疾病 …… 851
（十一）混杂病因 …… 851
（十二）有争议的病因 …… 852
六、临床特征 …… 852
（一）病史 …… 852
（二）体格检查 …… 853
七、鉴别诊断 …… 853
八、实验室诊断 …… 853
（一）胰酶 …… 853
（二）普通血液学检查 …… 855
九、影像学诊断 …… 855
（一）腹部平片 …… 855
（二）胸部影像 …… 855
（三）腹部超声 …… 855
（四）EUS 和 ERCP …… 855
（五）CT …… 855
（六）MRI …… 856
十、鉴别酒精性和胆石性胰腺炎 …… 856
十一、疾病严重程度的预测方法 …… 856
（一）评分系统 …… 857
（二）CT …… 857
（三）胸部影像 …… 858
十二、治疗 …… 858
（一）第一周初始治疗 …… 858
（二）静脉补液和电解质复苏 …… 858
（三）呼吸监护 …… 859
（四）心血管监护 …… 860
（五）代谢并发症 …… 860
（六）抗生素 …… 860
（七）急诊 ERCP …… 860
（八）营养 …… 860
（九）其他非介入治疗 …… 861
（十）介入治疗 …… 861
（十一）其他并发症 …… 862
（十二）急性胰腺炎的长期后遗症 …… 863
（十三）腹腔间隔室综合征 …… 863
（十四）混杂并发症 …… 863

一、疾病的发病率及负担

急性胰腺炎(acute pancreatitis,AP)的患者数量及经济负担日益增加,目前已成为胃肠道疾病住院最主要的原因之一[1]。诸多研究表明世界范围内其发病率不断上升[2],通常在每 10 万人中有 20 到 40 人发病。来自欧洲的研究表明尽管各地区的潜在病因不同,但总体呈上升趋势。例如,胆石和酒精分别是欧洲南部及东部的主要病因,而欧洲北部和西部的胆石-酒精比例则基本相同[2]。同样一项来自急诊的研究也表明在 6 年时间里因 AP 就诊的人数上升 12%,住院人数上升 15%,并且 AP 成为 2012 年第 12 位急诊最常见的消化道疾病[3]。急诊的就诊次数及其带来的花费增加可能是由饮酒相关的年轻患者增加以及慢性胰腺炎急性加重所引起的。基于世界范围内的人群队列研究表明,AP 和胰腺癌分别是最常见和最致命的胰腺疾病[4]。儿童病例数的大幅上升也与 AP 发病率的增长有关[5],推测这种增长可能和成人一样,也是由于超重相关的胆结石所致。然而,由于轻症患者可能被遗漏以及 10%重症患者在诊断前可能已死亡,预测的发病率并不准确[6]。相反,许多因其他原因而出现血清淀粉酶和(或)脂肪酶轻度升高的腹痛患者则被错误地诊断为 AP。

AP 发病率的上升似乎也伴随着花费的增加[7]。2014 年在美国,除了消化道出血和胆石症,AP 占据出院诊断的前三位。当年 279 145 例的入院病例中,30 日再入院率和死亡率分别为 14.3% 和 0.7%。医疗花费为 26 亿美元。同年,在美国有 2 834 例 AP 直接相关致死和 5 392 例间接由于 AP 死亡的病例,令 AP 成为第 14 位致死的消化道疾病。虽然从 1997 年至 2012 年住院时长和死亡率已经下降,但是平均住院费用增长了 120%,达到近 34 000 美元[8]。AP 的总死亡率从数年前的>10% 大幅下降至近几年<2%[1,7,9]。余下部分将主要阐述基于最近循证文献的临床管理，而不是对于该话题的百科全书式的描述。

二、定义

20 年来，参与治疗 AP 患者的医生们一直以 1992 年亚特兰大共识作为主要参考[10]，但由于随后对该疾病各个方面的进展，最近有必要对共识进行修订[11]。虽然生理学上 AP 定义为一种可累及其他邻近组织或远处器官系统的胰腺急性炎症过程。但目前将 AP 定义为患者需满足以下 3 条标准中的 2 条[11]：①症状（例如急性发作的上腹和（或）左上腹疼痛，常放射至背部）与胰腺炎相符；②血清淀粉酶或脂肪酶水平高于三倍实验室参考值上限；③影像学检查与胰腺炎相符，通常使用 CT 或 MRI。

若无 CT、MRI、EUS 或 ERCP 提示慢性胰腺炎，胰腺炎通常被归类为急性。如果发现存在上述影像描述，胰腺炎被归类为慢性，任何急性胰腺炎的进一步发作均视为是慢性胰腺炎的加重（见第 59 章）。然而表现为慢性胰腺炎急性发作的患者同样适用全部 3 条标准。

一旦 AP 的诊断成立，则将患者进行疾病严重程度分类。2012 年亚特兰大标准修订版[11]（框 58.1）将严重程度分为轻度、中重度和重度。轻度急性胰腺炎为最常见的类型，没有相关器官衰竭及局部或全身并发症，通常在第一周内缓解。中重度急性胰腺炎[12]被定义为存在一过性器官衰竭（持续时间<48 小时）和（或）局部并发症。重度急性胰腺炎被定义为存在持续性器官衰竭（持续时间>48 小时）。局部并发症包括急性胰周液体积聚、急性坏死物积聚（胰腺坏死和胰周坏死，无菌性或感染性）、假性囊肿和包裹性坏死（walled-off necrosis，WON；无菌性或感染性；图 58.1 和图 58.2）。其他被认可的重度胰腺炎的标志包括纳入 Ranson 的 11 个非胆石性胰腺炎标准中的 3 个或更多[13]和急性生理学和慢性健康状况评价Ⅱ（acute physiology and chronic health evaluation Ⅱ，APACHE-Ⅱ）评分大于 8 分[14]。

尽管在最初的亚特兰大分类中[10]，略去了一些令人困惑的词语，如蜂窝织炎（对于不同的专科医生意义不同）和出血性胰腺炎。术语出血性胰腺炎（hemorrhagic pancreatitis）并不是坏死性胰腺炎的一个同义语。若在病程的早期出血，可能是由于严重的炎症过程导致的静脉出血。迟发或严重的出血

框 58.1　2012 年急性胰腺炎亚特兰大分类修订
轻度急性胰腺炎
无器官衰竭
无局部或全身并发症
中重度急性胰腺炎
一过性器官衰竭（<48 小时）和（或）
局部或全身并发症*不伴持续性器官衰竭
重度急性胰腺炎
持续性器官衰竭（>48 小时）——单器官或多器官
*局部并发症为胰周液体积聚、胰腺坏死和胰周坏死（无菌性或感染性）、假性囊肿和坏死性包裹（无菌性或感染性）。

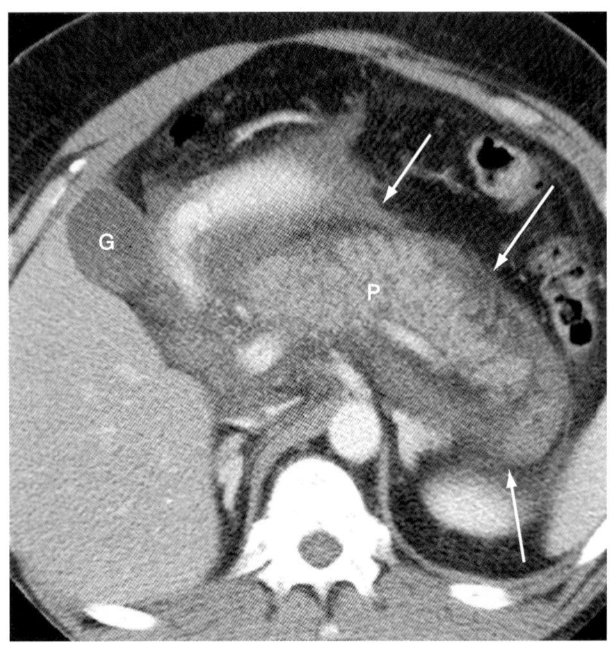

图 58.1　CT 提示急性间质性胰腺炎伴胰腺弥漫水肿（P）和胰腺周围炎症改变（箭）。胰腺灌注良好，无坏死表现。G，胆囊

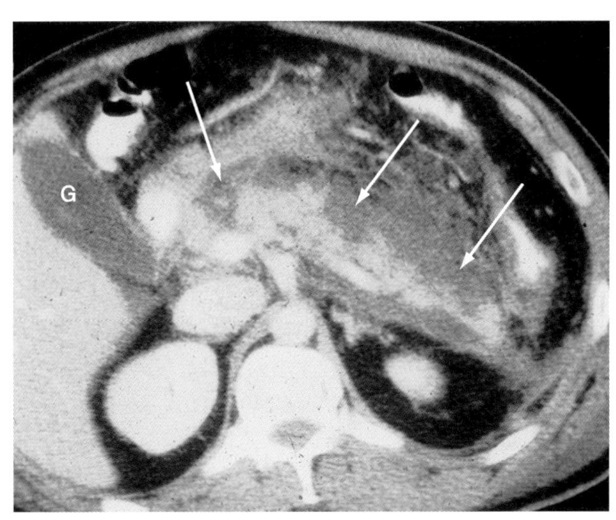

图 58.2　CT 提示急性胰腺坏死伴局部胰腺实质区域（箭）灌注减低及胰周炎症。估计胰腺坏死区域小于 30%。G，胆囊

更多地与假性动脉瘤形成相关，导致出血性积聚和腹腔积血。间质性胰腺炎占到了 75%～80% 病例，增强 CT 扫描显示胰腺灌注良好且不伴低密度区或非灌注区。术语轻度（mild）和间质性（interstitial）胰腺炎通常可以互换，两者都与轻度病程有关。根据修订的亚特兰大分类，坏死性胰腺炎包括胰腺和（或）胰周坏死。大约 45% 的坏死性胰腺炎同时累及胰腺和胰腺周围组织，另外 45% 病例是孤立性胰腺周围坏死，单纯胰腺坏死仅占 5%[15]。当 CT 扫描≥30% 胰腺实质低密度或无增强时可诊断胰腺坏死。胰腺周围的低密度区可认为是急性胰周液体积聚，若积聚越过如 Gerota 筋膜等筋膜平面时，则应当考虑为急性胰周坏死物积聚而不是单纯的液体积聚。大约 30%～50% 的 AP（主要是间质性胰腺炎）存在可吸收的胰周液体积聚。在大约 4 周后，如果急性胰周液体积聚仍存在

且形成囊壁,则被称为"假性囊肿"。因为大多数液体积聚可以吸收,故真正的假性囊肿并不常见,尽管大多数持续存在的液体积聚常被宽松地描述为"假性囊肿"。假性囊肿可邻近或远离胰体部,有时可在盆腔或胸腔等处看到这些富含酶的充满液体的囊。即使在 CT 上假性囊肿表现为液体伴低回声,当假性囊肿存在于胰体部时,通过 MRI 或 EUS 可发现囊内的胰腺坏死碎片。这种"假性囊肿"更准确的名称应为坏死物积聚。坏死物积聚也可能在胰周,若在 4 周后形成囊壁则被称为包裹性坏死。在最初的亚特兰大分类中定义的术语胰腺脓肿(pancreatic abscess)已被删去,因为它通常是感染性坏死的最终结果,也很罕见。同样地,由于没有干预的自发感染罕见,也不推荐使用感染性假性囊肿一词。

所有这些术语中,最重要的是区别胰腺坏死和假性囊肿。包裹性坏死是在 5~6 周后胰腺坏死物液化[16],与假性囊肿类似,形成囊壁。虽然假性囊肿中常含有液体,但胰腺坏死尽管早期形成包裹,其中含有的大量坏死碎片只有到 5~6 周后才液化。因碎片通常较厚且似橡胶般黏稠,不建议过早抽吸包裹性坏死(早于 4 周)。4 周后可采用类似于假性囊肿的治疗方法,如手术、内镜或经皮引流(见第 61 章)。

框 58.2 与重度急性胰腺炎相关的因素

患者特征

年龄>55 岁[11,13,210,327]

肥胖(BMI>30kg/m^2)[313]

意识状态改变[223,224]

共患病[11]

全身炎症反应综合征(SIRS)[11,20,217,223,224]

- 下列满足 2 条或更多(SIRS 标准)
- 脉搏>90 次/min
- 呼吸频率>20 次/min 或 $PaCO_2$<32mmHg
- 体温>38℃或<36℃
- 白细胞数>12 000/mm^3 或 4 000/mm^3 或>10% 杆状核

实验室发现

BUN>20mg/dL 或 BUN 水平进行性升高[225]

血清肌酐水平上升[314]

血细胞比容>44% 或进行性上升[231]

影像学发现

胸腔积液[195]

肺部浸润[11]

多部位或广泛胰外液体积聚[203]

BMI,体重指数;BUN,血尿素氮水平。

三、病程

AP 有两个显著的阶段。第一阶段通常持续 1 周,以可引起器官衰竭的全身性症状为特征。胰腺炎症可能会导致全身炎症反应综合征(systemic inflammatory response syndrome, SIRS)。在这个阶段感染性并发症并不常见[17]。发热、心动过速、高血压、呼吸窘迫和白细胞增多常与 SIRS 有关(框 58.2);呼吸、循环和肾功能衰竭通常与持续性 SIRS 有关。在一些早期研究中,并发症也包括了消化道出血、肝衰竭和凝血功能障碍,但由于较罕见且相关数据较少,修订后的亚特兰大分类中已删除。在第一天或者 1 周内可以观察到大多数的器官衰竭,此时应作为重度胰腺炎考虑(和治疗)该患者。如果器官衰竭超过 48 小时,则应确诊为重度胰腺炎。如果在 48 小时内器官衰竭缓解且有局部并发症,该病例可归为中重度急性胰腺炎。如果没有发现局部并发症,修订后的亚特兰大分类仍然将该患者归为中重度急性胰腺炎;然而其最初表述是患者伴有局部并发症但没有器官衰竭[12]。未来分类可能分别针对仅有单纯液体积聚、短暂器官衰竭和既往共病加重的患者进行分型,而非均归为中重度急性胰腺炎。

第二阶段通常在 7 天后开始,以局部并发症及相应的继发感染为特征。第一阶段出现的器官衰竭可能持续且常伴有感染性坏死,从而影响后期发病率和病死率。根据定义,除了少数患者有不伴器官衰竭或局部并发症的持续腹痛,轻度 AP 与第二阶段无关。通常在约 5% 的间质性胰腺炎(通常与轻度胰腺炎同义)患者中由于细胞因子介导的 SIRS 而出现器官衰竭;如果器官衰竭持续存在,则考虑 AP 为重度。

AP 的第一阶段通常持续一周。在该阶段,疾病的严重程度与因腺泡细胞损伤引起 SIRS 而导致的胰腺外器官衰竭直接相关。包括血小板活化因子(platelet activating factor, PAF)、TNF-α、核因子 κB(nuclear factor κB, NF-κB)和大量的白细胞介素(interleukin, IL)(见第 2 章)在内的多种细胞因子参与该过程。第一周内,炎症早期阶段动态演变,胰腺和胰腺周围出现不同程度的缺血或水肿,表现为不可逆的坏死和液化,或出现胰腺内和胰腺周围液体的积聚。胰外器官衰竭的严重程度常与胰腺和胰周变化的程度成比例。然而,器官衰竭可能独立于胰腺坏死而发展[16],相反胰腺坏死的患者可能也并没有器官衰竭的证据。器官衰竭的发展似乎与全身炎症反应级联反应持续存在有关(稍后讨论)。

大约 75%~80% 的 AP 患者有(间质性胰腺炎)并且没有进入第二阶段。然而约 20% 的患者中,由于与坏死过程相关(坏死性胰腺炎),病程可延长至数周至数月。第二阶段的死亡率与多种因素的共同作用有关,包括器官衰竭继发的无菌性坏死、感染性坏死、重度坏死过程引起局部并发症或手术/微创干预引起的并发症[18-20]。

AP 的死亡率有两个高峰。美国和欧洲的大多数研究表明约半数的死亡出现在第一二周,常因多器官衰竭[18-20]。死亡可非常迅速,例如在苏格兰大约四分之一的死亡出现在入院后 24 小时,三分之一在 48 小时内[20]。疾病的第二周后,患者死于多器官衰竭相关的胰腺感染。一些欧洲的研究报道,感染有非常高的晚期死亡率[21]。尚不清楚这是与胰腺坏死相关的内源性感染,还是与因感染并发症所行的手术干预有关。较之于年轻健康的患者,高龄多基础病的患者有更高的死亡率。那些患病后存活的患者,严重的胰腺坏死可能会导致慢性胰腺炎及其所有并发症(见第 59 章)[21]。

四、发病机制和病理生理学

针对 AP 发病机制发表的大多数数据来自于动物模型。虽然胆石和酒精在人类中可能造成了 60% 或更多的 AP,但并没有针对这 2 种诱发因素的动物模型。用来诱发动物模型中胰腺炎的雨蛙肽和牛磺胆酸盐并不能造成人类的胰腺炎。尽管有这些局限性，动物模型中 AP 的解剖和生化异常与人类相似。无论病因，一旦 AP 过程启动，造成局部和全身并发症的继发过程均类似。这很重要，因为意味着如果有药物可以治疗该急性病，它应在极早期起效并且在早期阻止该过程。

AP 发病机制的始动步骤是在腺泡细胞内足量的胰蛋白酶原转化为胰蛋白酶，清除活化胰蛋白酶的正常机制受到破坏（见图 57.3）。胰蛋白酶反之促进酶原的转化，包括胰蛋白酶原和弹性蛋白酶的惰性前体，磷脂酶 A_2（phospholipase A_2，PLA_2）和羧肽酶，进而激活酶类（见第 56 章）。胰蛋白酶同样可以激活补体和激肽系统。可以在自消化胰腺的同时，释放更多酶类而形成恶性循环。通常而言，少量的胰蛋白酶原可以在胰腺内自发活化，但胰内保护性机制可以迅速清除胰蛋白酶。胰分泌性胰蛋白酶抑制剂（现称 SPINK1）结合并灭活大约 20% 胰蛋白酶活性。其他清除胰蛋白酶的机制包括中胰蛋白酶，Y 酶以及可以分解和灭活其他胰蛋白酶分子的胰蛋白酶自身。胰腺同样含有非特异性抗蛋白酶如 α_1-抗胰蛋白酶和 α_2-巨球蛋白。另外的保护机制是：腺泡细胞通过合成时的胞内间隔、转运、来自溶酶体的消化酶之间经过高尔基体时的分离等方法分隔胰酶，这十分重要，因为组织蛋白酶 B 可以将胰蛋白酶原激活为胰蛋白酶。低浓度的腺泡细胞内钙聚集同样进一步阻止了胰蛋白酶的自身激活。

在实验性胰腺炎中，10 分钟内出现了胰蛋白酶的激活，并且大量胰蛋白酶[22]和不断聚集的胰蛋白酶原激活肽（trypsinogen activation peptide，TAP）在胰腺内蓄积[23,24]。当胰蛋白酶原被激活成胰蛋白酶时会生成 TAP，并且在血浆、尿液和腹水中聚集的 TAP 与胰腺炎症反应严重程度相关，并与腺泡细胞的坏死和胰腺内出血关系最为密切[25,26]。

腺泡细胞损伤后胰酶在溶酶体内的共定位是关于 AP 发病机制的一个亮点假说，但是两者的相关性并不明确。胰蛋白酶原的激活发生在腺泡细胞受到生化和形态学损伤之前，这与溶酶体酶（如组织蛋白酶 B）和消化酶（包括不稳定液泡中的胰蛋白酶原）的共定位有关[26,27]。完全抑制组织蛋白酶 B 可以在体外阻止缩胆囊素类似物雨蛙肽所诱导的胰蛋白酶原激活[28]，从而支持了共定位假说。因此完全抑制组织蛋白酶 B 可以预防或治疗 AP。然而酶的共定位也可能出现而不造成明显腺泡细胞损伤[29]。

其他两种实验性 AP 的特点是：①当酶持续合成时，早期阻断胰酶分泌；②破坏腺泡细胞和小叶内胰管（pancreatic duct，PD）细胞的胞间屏障。这种屏障的破坏促进了胰酶从腺泡细胞和管腔向间质的外渗。这种现象可能可以解释间质水肿的快速发展和胰酶在血清内的进行性聚集[30]。

正如在第 57 章中讨论的，与遗传性胰腺炎相关的基因突变同样支持了胰酶原在胰内激活是 AP 发病机制的中心这个假说[30-32]。在遗传性胰腺炎的患者中，突变的胰蛋白酶（通常是 R122H 或 N29I 突变）造成胰蛋白酶耐降解或胰蛋白酶原过早激活（功能获得突变），导致了胰腺的自消化及 AP 发作。*CFTR* 基因的突变同样与胰腺炎有关（见第 57 章）。*CFTR* 阴离子通道允许氯和碳酸氢盐分泌入胰管，从而允许大量释放的酶和酶原“井喷式”进入十二指肠（见第 56 章）。已经描述了超过 1 200 种 *CFTR* 突变，其中一些较为严重而一些较轻微。纯合子严重突变可能会产生黏稠浓缩的酸性胰液，进而导致儿童时期的导管梗阻和胰腺功能不全。带有一个主要或次要突变的杂合子可能由于腺泡或导管细胞功能的变化（如碳酸氢盐电导率变化），而发生急性复发性或慢性胰腺炎。最近，与胰腺分裂有关的 CFTR 突变被认为在 AP 的发病机制中有协同效应。虽然大多数有胰腺分裂的患者（总人群的 7% 到 10%；见第 55 章）从不发展为胰腺疾病，但那些同样有 *CFTR* 转运体功能障碍的人可能有发展为胰腺炎的风险[33]。第三个与胰腺炎相关的基因异常是 *SPINK1* 基因的突变[34]。如前所述，*SPINK1* 通过抑制过早活化的胰蛋白酶来保护腺泡细胞。该基因的突变可能限制了该蛋白的活性，但确切机制仍不明确。

胆石相关性胰腺炎的发病机制仍不明确（见第 65 章）。可能诱发胆石性胰腺炎的因素包括胆汁反流入胰管[35,36]、壶腹部结石阻塞胰管或一过性结石造成的水肿[37]。当远端胆管和胰管形成共同通道，胆石嵌顿于十二指肠乳头时，可能发生胆汁逆流入胰管。另一种可能是，近期胆石通过的损伤致 Oddi 括约肌功能不全，胆汁可能自十二指肠逆流入胰管。

就实验而言，胆汁逆流入胰管会造成胰腺的损伤，尤其是当胆汁被感染或与胰酶混合时。胆汁和胰酶的混合增加了主胰管的渗透性，而这与胰腺实质炎症有关[38]。不过共同通道理论也稍有问题，因为胰管压力总是高于胆管压力，从而使得胆汁不太可能逆流入胰管。胆汁自十二指肠反流也不太可能，因为在明显容易反流的情况下，并不会发生胰腺炎，如内镜下括约肌切开术后或外科括约肌成形术后。

对于胆石性胰腺炎机制的一个热门理论是在远端胆管嵌顿的结石阻塞胰管而增加了胰内压力，因此损伤了导管和腺泡细胞。一项在负鼠身上进行的实验支持了该理论[36]，其观察到结扎胰管造成了严重的坏死性胰腺炎，并且在 3 天内对导管系统的降压可防止发展为腺泡细胞坏死和严重炎症[37]。

AP 的病理生理起始于腺泡损伤，如果不加以控制，会导致局部炎症并发症、全身炎症反应甚至脓毒症。病理生理机制包括微循环损伤、白细胞趋化、促炎和抗炎细胞因子释放、氧化应激、胰液渗漏至胰腺区域和细菌易位至胰腺和全身循环。

胰酶的释放可损伤血管内皮、间质和腺泡细胞[39-41]。腺泡损伤导致了内皮黏附分子的表达（如 VCAM-1），进一步促进了炎症反应[42]。在实验性 AP 的早期出现了包括血管收缩、毛细血管淤滞、局部氧饱和度下降和进行性缺血等微循环改变。这些异常情况增加了血管通透性且导致腺体的水肿（水肿性胰腺炎或间质性胰腺炎）。血管损伤可以导致局部微循环衰竭并增加对胰腺的损伤。尚不确定缺血再灌注损伤是否在胰腺出现[41]。受损胰腺组织的再灌注可能会导致自由基和炎症细胞因子的释放和入血，从而造成进一步损伤。在动物和人类胰腺炎的早期阶段，补体激活和后续 C5a 的释放在巨噬细胞和多形核白细胞的归巢中起着重要作用[43,44]。活化的粒细胞和巨噬细胞在 NF-κB 等转录因子的作用下释放促炎细胞因子，包括 TNF、IL-1、IL-6、IL-8 和 PAF。促炎细胞因子经常伴随着抗炎细胞因子（IL-2、IL-10、IL-11）的产生[45]，这些细胞因子发挥下调炎症的作用。其他的炎症介质还包括花生四烯酸代谢物（前列腺素、PAF 和白三烯）、一氧化氮、蛋白水解酶和脂肪分解酶，以及超过内源性抗氧化系统清除能力的过量活性氧。这些物质同样与胰腺微循环相作用,从而增加血管通透性,进一步诱发血栓形成和出血以及后续的胰腺坏死。最近的一项研究表明减少腺泡细胞的谷胱甘肽聚集可能会导致氧化应激的增加和更严重的胰腺炎[42]。同时,腺体的缺血和严重炎症可以造成主级和次级胰管的破坏,导致胰腺内部和周围的局部液体积聚,最终形成假性囊肿[46,47]。

一些有严重胰腺损伤的患者可发展为全身并发症,如发热、急性呼吸窘迫综合征(acute respiratory distress syndrome,ARDS)、胸腔积液、肾功能衰竭、休克、心肌抑制和代谢并发症。SIRS在AP的患者中常见,可能是由发炎胰腺中活化的胰酶(磷脂酶、弹性蛋白酶、胰蛋白酶)和细胞因子(TNF、PAF)释放入门脉循环所介导的[48]。细胞因子到达肝脏后激活肝库普弗细胞,而其又反之诱导肝脏表达和分泌细胞因子进入全身循环。这会造成急性期蛋白合成(如C反应蛋白[C-reactive protein,CRP]、IL-6)并且可能导致SIRS以及对肾、肺和其他器官的损伤,导致多器官功能障碍和衰竭[49]。

活化磷脂酶A(卵磷脂酶)可以消化肺表面活性物质主要成分卵磷脂,并可能会诱发ARDS。急性肾衰竭可以用血容量不足和低血压来解释。心肌抑制和休克可能继发于血管活性肽和心肌抑制因子的释放。代谢并发症包括低钙血症、高脂血症、伴或不伴酮症酸中毒的高血糖、低血糖。低钙血症的发病机制是多因素的,包括低白蛋白血症(最重要的原因)、低镁血症、钙皂形成、激素失衡(如包含甲状旁腺激素、降钙素和胰高血糖素)、游离脂肪酸-白蛋白复合物结合钙离子、细胞内钙离子转运和全身对内毒素的全身暴露[50]。

血行播散或肠道细菌易位进入淋巴均能出现胰腺感染(感染性坏死和感染性假性囊肿)。因为存在复杂的免疫学和形态学屏障,一般情况下不会出现细菌易位。然而在AP中,这些屏障遭到破坏,造成局部和全身感染[51]。肠道缺血继发于血容量不足和胰腺炎诱发的肠内动静脉短路,可能是肠道细菌穿透肠道屏障的原因[52]。在犬的实验性胰腺炎中,肠腔内大肠埃希菌易位到肠系膜淋巴结和远端位置[53]。在猫实验性胰腺炎中,将结肠包裹在防水袋中可以防止结肠细菌易位入胰腺[54]。

最近更多的研究给出了有力的证据:虽然胰蛋白酶原活化为胰蛋白酶似乎是胰腺炎中炎症级联反应中不可或缺的第一步,但是维持胰腺炎症依赖于损伤相关分子和模式介导的细胞因子激活,从而导致共栖(肠道)生物易位入循环,以及其诱导的腺泡细胞内固有免疫应答。相当意外的是,这些研究揭示的固有反应包括了核苷酸结合寡聚结构域1(nucleotide-binding oligomerization domain 1,NOD1)的激活反应,这种NOD1的反应在NF-κB和Ⅰ型干扰素的激活和产生中起到至关重要的作用。因此最近的进展挑战了长期以来以胰蛋白酶为中心的对胰腺炎的认识。现在越来越清楚地知道在腺泡细胞内,强烈的炎症信号机制对于胰腺炎的发病至关重要,这可能解释了胰腺炎中强烈的全身炎症反应[58]。

有证据逐渐表明吸烟是AP的一个独立危险因素。Barreto使用逐步分析方法,回顾了香烟烟雾中各种代谢物对胰腺成分(外分泌、内分泌、神经激素、星形细胞、导管系统)的影响,并且强调了它们引起AP的已知和潜在机制[55]。

在不同的AP动物模型中,线粒体功能障碍以及作为其下游主要效应因子的自噬受损在AP的发展中起着重要作用。特别是该通路增强亲环蛋白D和ATP合酶的相互作用,介导了L-精氨酸诱导的胰腺炎——一种机制未知的重度AP模型。恢复线粒体和(或)自噬功能的策略可能被开发用于治疗AP[56]。

五、诱发因素

AP有很多不同的病因,然而要确定每一特定患者的病因往往很困难。例如,一名有饮酒史和胆石的患者,两个因素中之一甚至两者均可能是AP的病因。如果在这个患者中血清ALT水平升高,则可能更多地考虑是由胆石引起。然而每个患者都必须通过彻底的病史询问和体格检查、实验室和影像学检查来确定病因。在被称为"特发性AP"之前,需要完善如促胰液素刺激MRCP、EUS和基因检测等更特异的检查和规程。虽然目标是逐渐减少被归为特发性胰腺炎的病例比例,但并不适合将某些无明确证据引起AP的情况列为急性胰腺炎的原因(例如Oddi括约肌功能障碍,胰腺分裂等)。

虽然胆石和酒精可能是绝大多数AP的原因,许多其他因素也在不同程度上诱发AP(框58.3)。虽然以下部分描述了AP的少数病因,但是一些不常见病因可能与多个因素共同作用。例如关于胰腺分裂是否是AP的病因一直有相互矛盾的研究,然而有研究表明在胰腺分裂的患者中胰腺CFTR基因突变可能会诱导胰腺分裂的患者容易发展为AP[33,58]。随着我们对该病认识的深入,明确的病因无疑会增加,被诊断为"特发性"的病例有望不断减少。

框58.3 可能诱发急性胰腺炎的因素

梗阻
- 胆石
- 肿瘤
- 寄生虫
- 十二指肠憩室
- 环状胰腺
- 胆总管囊肿

酒精/其他毒物/药物
- 乙醇
- 甲醇
- 蝎毒
- 有机磷类杀虫剂
- 药物(见框58.4)

代谢异常
- 高甘油三酯血症
- 糖尿病
- 高钙血症

感染

血管疾病
- 血管炎
- 胰腺血管栓塞
- 低血压/缺血

创伤

术后状态

ERCP术后(见框58.5)

遗传/家族/基因

争议性

胰腺分裂

Oddi括约肌功能障碍

混杂因素

自发性

(一) 梗阻

1. 胆结石

胆石是导致胰腺炎的最常见的梗阻性因素(见第 65 章),并引起约 40% 到 60% 的胰腺炎病例[57,59],然而只有 3% 到 7% 的胆石患者出现胰腺炎。胆石好发于女性,因此胆石性胰腺炎在女性中更常出现。因为小结石比大结石更容易通过胆囊管引起壶腹梗阻,所以当结石直径小于 5mm 时(比值比 4:5)[60],AP 更常出现。胆囊切除术和胆道结石清除可以预防复发证实了该因果关系[61]。48 小时内出现血清 GGT≥40U/L、ALT≥150U/L 和脂肪酶≥15 倍正常上限的三联征已被用来作为儿童急性胆源性胰腺炎的一个简单临床预测指标。当患儿以上指标数值低于 2 或 3 个阈值时不太可能出现胆道因素所致的 AP[62]。AP 在孕妇中罕见,多数见于妊娠晚期,胆石为最常见病因[63]。胆石和酒精分别是南欧和东欧的主要病因,而北欧和西欧胆石-酒精作为病因的比例相当[2,64]。

2. 胆泥和微结石症

胆泥(biliary sludge)是胆囊胆汁中的黏性悬浮液,可能含有小(<3mm)结石(如微结石)[65]。因为小结石可以隐藏在胆泥中,两者常一起被描述为胆泥和微结石。在大多数患者中胆泥无症状。其通常是由胆固醇一水化物结晶或胆红素钙颗粒组成[65]。超声下胆泥产生不伴声影的可移动低回声,并且位于最靠近胆囊的层面。与延长禁食或全肠外营养(total parenteral nutrition,TPN)有关的功能性胆汁淤积,或远端胆管梗阻中出现的机械性淤积都可能形成胆泥。此外,头孢菌素类抗生素头孢曲松钠在胆汁内的浓度过高时,也可以形成胆泥,但该过程很少造成结石[66]且停药后胆泥可溶解。胆泥和结石可以解释 22% 的肝移植后迟发性 AP[67]。关于 EUS 在特发性胰腺炎中作用的一项系统评价发现,大约 40% 经腹超声、CT 甚至 ERCP 归为"特发性"的病例 EUS 诊断具有胆石症、胆泥或微结石[70]。虽然在特发性 AP 的患者中常常发现胆泥,两个非对照性研究的结果证明了两者之间的致病关系,阐明了胆泥可以导致胰腺炎,并且胆囊切除术、乳头括约肌切开术或熊去氧胆酸(熊二醇)疗法减少了 AP 的反复发作[69,70]。在这两个研究中,推测为特发性胰腺炎的病例里,胆泥发生率为 67% 和 74%。然而其他的研究者只在不到 10% 的复发性 AP 患者中发现微结石或胆泥[71,72]。治疗选择包括胆囊切除术、熊去氧胆酸疗法、内镜下乳头括约肌切开术或密切观察。

3. 肿瘤

据推测,胰腺癌通过阻塞胰管而常造成急性和复发性 AP,且在 40 岁以上的人群中多见(见第 60 章)。AP 也同样增加了继发胰腺癌的风险。在最近一个 1 609 名 AP 患者的队列研究中,由胰腺癌引起 AP 的比例为 1.4%。在该队列中,如果 CA19-9 超过 200U/L 时,15.8% 的 AP 患者存在胰腺癌[73]。虽然从 AP 发展为慢性胰腺炎可能会增加后续胰腺癌的风险,但丹麦的一项基于人群的研究表明 AP 患者 2 年和 5 年绝对危险度分别为 0.68%(95% 置信区间:0.61%~0.77%)和 0.85%(95% 置信区间:0.76%~0.94%)[74]。中国的一项研究中,47 名出现 AP 的胰腺癌患者中大多数为轻度 AP,胰腺癌作为病因诊断的中位时间为 101 天[75]。在 1 年内诊断为胰腺炎的病例中胰腺癌的合并比值比(pooled OR)最高(合并比值比=23.3;95% 置信区间:14.0~38.9),并且少于 2/5/10 年的风险分别为 3.03(95% 置信区间:2.41~3.81)、2.82(95% 置信区间:2.12~3.76)和 2.25(95% 置信区间:1.59~3.19)。胰腺炎,尤其是慢性胰腺炎,与胰腺癌风险显著升高有关,并且该风险随着胰腺炎诊断年限增长而下降[76]。以该方式出现的最常见的肿瘤是导管内乳头状黏液瘤[77],一项综述发现导管内乳头状黏液瘤(包括分支胰管型和主胰管型)占 AP 病因的 12%~67%。其他部位来源的胰腺转移癌(肺、乳腺)也可造成胰腺炎[78]。主乳头的大腺瘤偶尔也是梗阻性胰腺炎的病因(见第 69 章)。

4. 其他病因

其他罕见的与 AP 相关的梗阻性情况将在其他章节讨论,包括胆总管囊肿[79]、十二指肠憩室[80]、环状胰腺[81]和阻塞胆胰管的寄生虫病,如蛔虫病[82]和华支睾吸虫病[83]。蛔虫病梗阻胰管是儿童 AP 的主要病因(60%)[84],并且在印控克什米尔地区引起了 23% 的 AP 病例[85],为克什米尔第二大常见 AP 病因[83]。

(二) 乙醇和其他毒物

1. 乙醇

乙醇是胆石之外第二常见的 AP 病因,至少 30% 的 AP 病例由其引起[76]。发达国家中乙醇是慢性胰腺炎的第一大病因,但需要长期的乙醇摄入(每日超过 4 到 5 标准杯并持续至少 5 年),而这类人群患有 AP 的终生风险仅为 2%~5%[1]。急性和慢性胰腺炎之间的关系非常复杂,尤其是酒精性慢性胰腺炎。经典的观点是,酒精可导致慢性胰腺炎,而且临床上出现 AP 表现的饮酒患者已有潜在的慢性胰腺炎[86]。但在 20 世纪 90 年代,Ammann 等质疑了该假说,他们对一组急性胰腺炎患者进行了一段时间的随访,并且通过手术病理表明了急性期到慢性期的过程[87]。这一系列证据提示酒精并不是通过潜在的慢性胰腺炎而在早期引起 AP,而是通过"坏死-纤维化假说"导致慢性胰腺炎。一些尸检研究同样证明在很大一部分患者中,酒精性 AP 的发生并不伴有潜在的慢性胰腺炎。然而,一项包含 21 名酒精性 AP 行手术治疗的病例系列研究表明,6 例首次发作的患者中在第一次发病时都已患有慢性胰腺炎[88]。因此,对于酒精性 AP 是否仅见于已有慢性胰腺炎改变的腺体中的争论持续不休。一些近期研究(包括基于人群的研究和在儿科患者中的研究)和 meta 分析明确地阐述了在某些患者中 AP 到复发性 AP 再到慢性胰腺炎的过程[89-91]。一篇 meta 分析报道了 10% 首次发作 AP(所有病因)的患者和 36% 复发性 AP 的患者进展为慢性胰腺炎,并且酒精、吸烟和男性是这种进展的危险因素[92]。然而这种现象并没有解决关于 AP 首次发作是否已存在慢性胰腺炎的争论,而仅限于随后慢性胰腺炎的临床检测。

慢性胰腺炎的不同机制包括:

(1) 坏死-纤维化序列,由 Comfort 等提出[93.94],设想纤维化由 AP 反复发作导致,也可能是亚临床反复发作。AP 初期的炎症和坏死造成了导管周围区域的瘢痕,瘢痕形成导致导管阻塞,使得导管内淤积和继发结石形成。支持这一理论的组织病理学研究显示,在 AP 缓解期中小叶周围轻度的纤维化,随后出现了明显的纤维化伴导管变形。这被认为是一个在反复发作的 AP 中出现的阶梯式进展。Amman 及其同事的临床研究中也支持了该理论[87]。在他们的研究中,对 254 名第一次酒精性胰腺炎发作后的患者进行前瞻性随访,发现慢性胰腺炎的发作频率和严重程度与慢性胰腺炎的进展速度有直接关联。

(2) 酒精对腺泡细胞的直接代谢毒性效应。

(3) 由于自由基的氧化应激。

(4) 前哨急性胰腺炎事件(Sentinel Acute Pancreatitis Event,SAPE)假说认为慢性胰腺炎最多见的原因是二重打击模型。该模型认为 AP 单次发作造成炎症细胞的浸润和胰腺星状细胞的激活,并在具有高危因素的易感人群中进一步导致纤维化[95]。如果刺激因素被消除(如某种药物),那么胰腺会回归正常。如果没有去除(如酒精),腺泡细胞则继续分泌细胞因子以响应氧化应激,并且星状细胞继续被激活以构建基质和胶原。该模型使用前哨事件,代表了疾病修饰疗法(disease modifying therapy)时代的到来。

上述的理论和动物模型不能完全解释人类酒精性胰腺炎的发展。很可能一部分患者会通过如前哨急性胰腺炎事件等机制从急性酒精性胰腺炎发展为慢性胰腺炎,但剩下患者可能会发展为一种未知的惰性纤维炎症反应,并最终在临床上表现为 AP。更重要的是,无明显结构性损伤的酗酒人群发生 AP 这一现象提示,对于那些有饮酒史的特发性胰腺炎患者可能被不恰当地归为酒精性 AP。对临床医生来说,要认识到较之于 AP,酒精更容易引起慢性胰腺炎。持有怀疑态度可能对评估那些初始考虑为酒精性急性胰腺炎但胰腺无明显结构性损伤患者有所帮助。

2. 其他毒物

甲醇[96],有机磷类杀虫剂[97]和特立尼达蝎(Trinidad scorpion)[98]的毒液已经被报道可诱发 AP,后两种毒物的机制被认为是对胰腺的过度刺激。吸烟被证明是 AP 的一个独立危险因素[99-101]。尽管美国的一项人群研究表明吸烟为非胆石性 AP 的危险因素[102],但令人惊讶的是,中国台湾的研究报告了吸烟与风险增加并不相关[102]。另一研究发现吸烟与较低的 AP 诊断年龄和较高的复发率有关[103]。

(三) 药物

药物是 AP 一个不常见但重要的病因。尽管报道认为药物引起的 AP 占全部病例的 1%~4%,但大多缺乏说服力。药物引起的 AP 可能仅占小于 1%的病例[104]。虽然超过 120 种药物可能与 AP 有关,但大多来自零星的病例报告,对于没有明显病因的 AP 患者,临床医生务必小心,不应轻易认定为某种药物导致。许多已发表的病例报告都有不合适的 AP 诊断标准、无法排除更多常见病因或缺乏对药物的再试验等综合问题。此外,许多病例报告还包含了那些在 AP 发生前使用了很长时间(>6 个月)的药物,但这并不合适。药物诱发的胰腺炎往往发生在开始使用药物后的 4 到 8 周内。由于缺乏精心设计的临床试验,临床医生很大程度上依赖于已发表的病例判断可能引发 AP 的药物。

药物诱发的胰腺炎很少伴有药物反应的临床或实验室证据,如皮疹、淋巴结病和嗜酸性粒细胞增多症。虽然药物再试验阳性是对因果关系的最好证据,但是由于许多有特发性胰腺炎或胆道微结石的患者常有 AP 的反复发作,所以并不足以论证其因果。因此,在胰腺炎的复发中停用和重新使用药物诱发可能只是一种巧合而不是因果关系。虽然缺乏药物再试验,但是如果在众多病例报告中开始使用一种药物和 AP 发作之间有一致的潜伏期则应当高度怀疑。框 58.4 展示了已发表的具有有力证据的导致 AP 的药物,那些是具有再试

框 58.4　与急性胰腺炎有关的药物 *

对乙酰氨基酚
5-氨基水杨酸复合物(柳氮磺吡啶、奥沙拉嗪、美沙拉秦)
L-天冬酰胺酶
硫唑嘌呤
贝那普利
苯扎贝特
大麻素
卡托普利
卡比马唑
西咪替丁
氯氮平
可待因
阿糖胞苷
氨苯砜
去羟肌苷
地塞米松
依那普利
红霉素
雌激素
氟伐他汀
呋塞米
氢氯噻嗪
氢化可的松
异环磷酰胺
干扰素-α
异烟肼
拉米夫定
赖诺普利
氯沙坦
葡甲胺
甲巯咪唑
甲基多巴
甲硝唑
6-巯基嘌呤
奈非那韦
炔诺酮/雌醇
喷他脒
普伐他汀
普鲁卡因胺
吡硫醇
辛伐他汀
磺胺甲嘧啶
磺胺甲噁唑
葡萄糖酸锑
舒林酸
四环素
磺胺甲噁唑/甲氧苄啶
丙戊酸

*仅列出 1 类和 2 类药物。1 类药物:2 篇或更多病例报告发表,缺少其他急性胰腺炎病因,至少 1 篇报告有激发试验。2 类药物:4 篇或更多病例报告发表,缺少其他急性胰腺炎病因,至少 75%发表病例有一致的潜伏期。

From Badalov N, Baradarian R, Iswara K, et al. Drug induced acute pancreatitis: an evidence based approach. Clin Gastroenterol Hepatol 2007;101;454-76.

验证据或可预测潜伏期的药物[104]。通过上报 FDA 不良事件报告系统，一些药物可能造成 AP。然而不良事件报告系统高度依赖临床医生提交药物监测报告(Medwatch reports)，而该系统又具有报告偏倚。来自瑞典的一项基于人群的研究发现增加 AP 相关药物的使用，对 AP 的发作、严重程度或复发的流行病学变化，没有重大影响[105]。

药物诱发的胰腺炎有很多的潜在致病机制。最常见的是超敏反应，它常常在开始用药的 4 到 8 周后出现且与剂量不相关。药物再使用时，AP 可在数小时至数天内复发。药物可能通过该机制作用的例子有 5-氨基水杨酸、甲硝唑和四环素。第二种机制推测可能是毒性代谢物堆积造成胰腺炎，多数在使用后数月发生。该分类的例子有丙戊酸和去羟肌苷。可能引起高甘油三酯血症的药物(如噻嗪类、异维甲酸、他莫昔芬)同样在该分类中。最后，一小部分药物可能有内在毒性，过量服用可能会导致胰腺炎(红霉素、对乙酰氨基酚)。近年来有大量文献提到了越来越多用于治疗 2 型糖尿病的二肽基肽酶-4 抑制剂(DPP-4 抑制剂)导致 AP 的风险。但已发表的报道在风险问题上相互矛盾。最近的一篇对 13 项研究的 meta 分析表明使用 DPP-4 抑制剂患 AP 风险稍高。然而，在队列研究中并未观察到这种风险[106]。因此需要进一步的临床试验来证实该发现。在有高心血管风险的 2 型糖尿病患者人群中，无论有无胰腺炎既往史，相比安慰组，使用利拉鲁肽(一种 GLP-1 受体拮抗剂)治疗的患者 AP 发生较少，然而利拉鲁肽与血清淀粉酶脂肪酶升高有关，但并不能预测后续 AP 事件的发生[107]。一项对 2 型糖尿病患者的大样本 meta 分析表明 AP 风险增加了 2 倍[108]。

一般来说，药物诱发的胰腺炎通常较轻且为自限性。诊断只有在除外酒精、胆石、高甘油三酯血症、高钙血症和肿瘤(合适年龄人群中)才能成立。一些药物在随机临床试验中表现出较高的致 AP 频率(如 6-巯基嘌呤有 3%～5% 和去羟肌苷有 5%～10%)[111]，但是一些药物被错误地归为病因且不再使用，仅仅是因为挫败的临床医生没有发现其他病因。对于一些药物(如他汀类)，这种停用可能是有害的。主要基于没有明确的病因学证据和基于仅有 1 篇或更少的先前发表的病例报告，临床医生应该审慎地诊断药物诱导的 AP。最后，没有证据证明任何药物能造成慢性胰腺炎。

(四) 代谢障碍

1. 高甘油三酯血症

高甘油三酯血症可能是在继胆石和酗酒后第三大常见病因，无论任何地区，基本占 2%～5%[1] 至 20% 病例。一项包含 1 340 名患者的对 31 项研究的 meta 分析表明高甘油三酯血症能占到 AP 全部病例的 9%，并且显著高甘油三酯血症的患者 14% 将发展为 AP。高甘油三酯血症同样与超过一半的妊娠期胰腺炎有关。血清 TG 浓度超过 1 000mg/dL(11mmol/L)可能促发 AP。然而更多近期研究提示可能需要更高血清 TG 才能促发 AP，也许需超过 2 000mg/dL 且伴有由于乳糜微粒浓度升高而致的明显乳糜(乳白色)血[110]。

高甘油三酯血症的致病机制尚不明确，但是胰脂肪酶原位释放游离脂肪酸可能会损伤胰腺腺泡细胞或内皮细胞[91]。游离脂肪酸的释放引起游离自由基损伤，并且直接损伤细胞膜[92]。

大多数有高乳糜微粒血症的成年人有轻型基因遗传性Ⅰ型或Ⅴ型高脂蛋白血症和一种其他已知能升高血脂的情况[如酒精滥用、超重、糖尿病、甲状腺功能减退、库欣病、妊娠、肾病综合征和药物治疗(雌激素[111] 或他莫昔芬、糖皮质激素、噻嗪类或 β 肾上腺素能阻滞剂)]。有 3 种典型类型的患者发展为高甘油三酯血症性胰腺炎。第一种是有高甘油三酯血症病史的控制不佳的糖尿病患者。第二种是入院时发现高甘油三酯血症的饮酒患者。第三种(15% 到 20%)是由药物和饮食引起的高甘油三酯血症，无糖尿病、无饮酒、无肥胖的人群。如果在药物暴露之前有高甘油三酯血症背景，药物诱发 AP 更有可能出现。

大多数酒精滥用的人会出现一定程度但短暂的血清 TG 水平升高。这种情况像是一种并发现象，并非他们胰腺炎的原因[112]，因为酒精本身不仅损伤胰腺(见前文)还以剂量依赖的方式升高血清 TG 浓度。有严重高甘油三酯血症的酗酒患者常伴有原发性脂蛋白代谢遗传障碍。

与其他病因相比，高脂血症是否会导致更严重疾病尚不清楚[113]。另一方面，对 15 项研究(1 564 名患者)的一项 meta 分析发现，较之于非高甘油三酯血症病因，高甘油三酯血症的患者预后更差[114]。在高甘油三酯血症患者中，血清淀粉酶和(或)脂肪酶水平可能在起病时并不会大幅升高(见后文)。

2. 糖尿病

糖尿病增加了发展为 AP 的风险[108]。这种风险可能是由于糖尿病人群中胆石和高甘油三酯血症的患病率增加。在一项对 2 型糖尿病患者的大型研究中(LEADER，Liraglutide Effect and Action in Diabetes：Evaluation of Cardiovascular Outcome Results)，有接近 25% 的患者血清脂肪酶和淀粉酶升高，但不伴有 AP 症状。临床医生在评估 2 型糖尿病患者的腹部症状时必须注意该数据[115]。糖尿病患者由于并发血脂障碍导致胆汁胆固醇过饱和，生成胆固醇过饱和结晶，从而易造成胆石(见第 65 章)。同样地，有长期糖尿病的患者通常发展为胆囊胆汁淤积，从而导致胆固醇结晶沉淀和胆石。流行病学研究已经证明了在糖尿病人群中 AP 的风险增加[116-118]。因为常有如肥胖和潜在共病等多种已知的发展为重症的危险因素，糖尿病人发展为重度胰腺炎的风险更高[12]。

3. 高钙血症

任何原因导致的高钙血症很少与 AP 相关。提出的机制包括在胰管腔内的钙盐沉积和胰腺实质内胰蛋白酶原向胰蛋白酶的钙激活[119]。在慢性高钙血症中 AP 的低发病率表明其机制可能不是血清钙水平导致胰腺炎(如血清钙的急性升高)。对大鼠的急性钙灌注导致了胰蛋白酶原向胰蛋白酶的转换、高淀粉酶血症和剂量依赖的 AP 形态学改变。

不到 0.5% 的原发甲状旁腺功能亢进引起 AP，并且在甲状旁腺功能亢进的患者中 AP 发病率在 0.4% 到 1.5%(第 37 章)[120]。有趣的是在一项基于社区的研究中，甲状旁腺功能亢进患者中，AP 发生的风险并没有增加，同样也没有因果关系[121]。胰腺炎也极少与其他导致高钙血症的原因一起发生，包括有代谢性骨病、全肠外营养、结节病、维生素 D 毒性和体外循环期间高剂量灌注钙等。

（五）感染

虽然许多感染原被认为是 AP 的病因[83]，但从发表的报道通常不能建立一个明确的因果关系。感染原引起 AP 的诊断需要 AP 的证据、活动性感染的证据和缺少其他更可能造成 AP 的病因。目前已知 AP 与病毒（流行性腮腺炎病毒、柯萨奇病毒、甲乙丙肝病毒和如巨细胞病毒、水痘带状疱疹病毒、单纯疱疹病毒和 EBV 等许多疱疹病毒）、减毒麻疹，腮腺炎，风疹病毒的疫苗、细菌（支原体、军团菌、钩端螺旋体、沙门菌、结核分枝杆菌和布氏杆菌）、真菌（曲霉菌、念珠菌）、寄生虫（弓形虫、隐孢子虫、蛔虫、华支睾吸虫）有关。华支睾吸虫和蛔虫通过阻塞主胰管而造成 AP。在有 AIDS 的患者中（见第 35 章），包括巨细胞病毒、念珠菌属、新型隐球菌、刚地弓形虫和可能的鸟分枝杆菌复合群等感染原可能造成 AP[83]。

（六）血管疾病

胰腺缺血很少造成 AP。在大多数病例中较轻，但是也能出现致死性坏死性胰腺炎。血管炎（如 SLE[122]、结节性多动脉炎）[123]、经腹主动脉造影术后胆固醇斑块的动脉粥样硬化栓塞[124]、术中低血压[125]、失血性休克[127]、麦角胺过量和肝细胞癌经导管动脉栓塞术等都可能造成缺血。同样缺血也是一种体外循环后胰腺炎的解释。在猪中，心包填塞引起的心源性休克由于激活肾素-血管紧张素系统，造成了血管痉挛和选择性胰腺缺血[127]。在长跑运动员中出现的 AP 也可能有缺血的基础[128]。

（七）创伤

穿透伤（枪伤或针刺伤）或钝器伤都能损伤胰腺[129]。钝器伤是脊椎对胰腺挤压的结果，如在汽车事故中方向盘造成的挤压。在钝器伤中，因为需要基于胰腺损伤的程度制定手术计划，所以术前确定有无胰腺损伤很重要。第二，即使没有邻近器官的严重创伤，也可能需要手术或内镜治疗胰腺导管的损伤。

创伤性胰腺炎的诊断很困难，并且需要高度怀疑。创伤可以是轻度挫伤，也可以是很重的挤压伤或腺体的横断，后者常出现在腺体跨越脊椎的部位。横断伤能造成急性胆管破裂和胰性腹水。与其他邻近的腹腔内结构不同，基于腹痛和腹部压痛的特征决定有无胰腺损伤是不可能的。无论有无胰腺损伤，腹部创伤患者中血清淀粉酶或脂肪酶活性都可能会增加。

诊断胰腺创伤高度依靠 CT、MRI 或 MRCP，可能显示挫伤或被膜下血肿所致的部分腺体肿大，胰腺炎症性改变，以及如果有导管破裂等形成的肾周间隙前部的积液。即使是明显的胰腺创伤，前 2 天内 CT 也可能正常。如果临床高度怀疑胰腺损伤或者 CT、MRI 扫描显示异常，需行 ERCP 决定有无胰管的损伤。如果胰管无明显损伤且无较大的腹腔内损伤，则不建议手术。然而如果 ERCP 发现胰管横断伴胰性液体外渗且无其他腹腔内损伤，跨越损伤部位的胰管支架可能有效[130]。通过合适的清创术能够处理胰腺的严重损伤。十二指肠或胆管的合并伤可以通过胆道分流、胃空肠吻合术和用于营养的空肠造口术治疗。胰腺创伤术后患者中大约三分之一会出现胰外瘘。奥曲肽减少胰腺分泌，可能对胰腺损伤后有益[131]。

如果没有其他结构（局部血管、肝、脾、肾、十二指肠和结肠）的严重损伤，胰腺创伤的预后良好。然而导管损伤可能会瘢痕化并且造成主胰管狭窄，导致阻塞性慢性胰腺炎。

（八）ERCP 术后

AP 是 ERCP 最常见也是最让人担心的并发症，具有一定的发病率和偶然死亡率（见第 42 章）。无症状的高淀粉酶血症出现在 35%～70% ERCP 术后[133]。临床胰腺炎可发生在 5% 的诊断性 ERCP 和 7% 的治疗性 CP 患者中；在怀疑 Oddi 括约肌功能障碍（sphincter of Oddi dysfunction，SOD）和既往有 ERCP 术后胰腺炎（post-ERCP pancreatitis，PEP）的患者中可高达 25%[133]。

最近一项对含 108 项随机对照试验（randomized controlled trial，RCT），含有对照组或单臂研究，涵盖 13 296 名患者的系统评价报告了 PEP 总发病率为 9.7%，死亡率为 0.7%。8 857 名患者描述了 PEP 的严重程度：5.7%、2.6% 和 0.5% 患者分别有轻度、中度和重度胰腺炎。在 2 345 名高风险患者中，PEP 的发病率为 14.7%（轻、中、重度分别为 8.6%、3.9% 和 0.8%，死亡率为 0.2%）。北美、欧洲和亚洲 RCT 研究中 PEP 发病率分别为 13%、8.4% 和 9.9%。2000 年之前和之后的 ERCP 术后胰腺炎的发病率分别为 7.7% 和 10%[134]。

导致 PEP 的机制复杂且尚未完全明了。PEP 被认为是多因素的，包括化学、流体力学、酶、机械和热力等因素，而不是某种单一发病机制。虽然预测哪些患者会出现 PEP 存在不确定性，但是一些独立或共同作用的危险因素被认为是 PEP 的预测因子（框 58.5）[135,136]。识别这些 PEP 的危险因素对认识到哪些病例中应当尽可能避免 ERCP，或者考虑保护性内镜措施或药物干预是至关重要的。

框 58.5 增加 ERCP 术后胰腺炎风险的因素
患者相关
年轻，女性，怀疑 Oddi 括约肌功能障碍，复发性胰腺炎史，ERCP 术后胰腺炎史，血清胆红素水平正常
过程相关
胰腺导管内注射，困难插管、胰腺括约肌切开、预切开、球囊扩张
术者或技术相关
实习生参与、不使用导丝的导管、高风险步骤中使用胰管支架失败

通常来说，患者胆管或胰管异常的可能性越大，发生 PEP 的可能性就越小[138]。Cheng 构建了一个含 160 个变量的数据库，在美国中西部前瞻性的评价来自 15 个中心的超过 1 000 名患者[134]。他们的研究强调了包括年龄、SOD、既往 PEP 史等患者因素，以及胰管内注射、副乳头括约肌切开术和术者经验等技术因素的作用。最有可能发展为 PEP 的是怀疑有胆总管结石且血清胆红素正常，但进行了括约肌切开却没有找到结石的女性患者。在此部分人群中，27% 发展为 PEP。MRCP 和 EUS 不会造成胰腺炎，能够为这些病例提供有用的信息（可能如 ERCP 一样准确），建议作为这些患者首选的初始评估方法。在一项对 2 715 例治疗性 ERCP 的研究中，发现内镜医生的经验减少了患者和操作相关的 ERCP 术

后并发症相关风险因素[138]。

通过在术后评估血清淀粉酶或脂肪酶可以早期识别 PEP[139,140]。在一项包含 231 名患者的研究中，2 小时血清淀粉酶和脂肪酶在区分非胰腺炎性腹痛和 PEP 方面，比临床评估更准确。术后 2 小时血清淀粉酶值超过 276IU/L（参考范围，30～70IU/L）和脂肪酶超过 1 000IU/L（参考范围，45～100IU/L）几乎对 PEP 有 100% 阳性预测值[141]。最近，Ito 及其同事发现如果血清淀粉酶在 3 小时后正常，只有 1% 患者发展为 PEP，而如果淀粉酶超过 5 倍正常值上限则有 39% 发展为 PEP[142]。因为 PEP 可能会在操作后 24 小时出现，因此单独一项血清淀粉酶或脂肪酶并不能指导患者是否患有 PEP。然而，存在腹痛而血清淀粉酶和（或）脂肪酶正常时可以除外 AP。

虽然人们对开发一些预防 PEP 的药物很感兴趣，很少有研究能证明某种药物值得广泛使用。很多药物如硝酸甘油、硝苯地平、喷洒型利多卡因和注射用肉毒杆菌等没有显示任何优势。蛋白酶抑制剂加贝酯在一些小规模试验中表现出一些益处但是非常昂贵[144]。在许多研究中通过生长抑素抑制胰酶外分泌并无优势，其类似物奥曲肽仅减少了高淀粉酶血症。

明确能减少术后胰腺炎风险的 3 种主要方式包括预防性胰腺支架、术前静脉输液和非甾体抗炎药（NSAIDs）直肠给药。放置胰腺支架可以明确减少高风险患者 PEP 的风险[144]。放置胰管支架已经成为预防术后胰腺炎高危患者的标准方法。胰管支架有效可能是因为预防了插管诱发的水肿，后者可引起胰管阻塞；其原理在于 ERCP 插管和烧灼可导致术后壶腹水肿和痉挛，而后者造成梗阻及 AP。一些研究和 meta 分析确证了高风险 PEP 患者中预防性放置胰管支架可以获益。预防性胰管支架为 3Fr 或 5Fr，长度可短于 5cm 或长于 5cm，用于临时放置以度过 2～3 天的壶腹水肿期。超过 70% 的支架在壶腹水肿的 3～4 天内提供胆汁和胰液流出的通路，之后会自行脱落。如果一周后 X 线片提示支架无移位，则通常需要在 14 天内应用内镜取出。因为留置超过 14 天能造成慢性导管损伤，所以需要取出支架。一项有 43 595 次 ERCP 操作的瑞典国家注册数据表明较之于短和细的支架，直径>5Fr 和长度>5cm 的胰管支架可能有更好的保护效果[145]。但并不能确定置入的胰管支架确切型号（除了材料、长度和直径），所以需审慎对待他们的结论。如果没有行预防性胰管支架的患者出现 PEP，或者如果支架移位而患者出现严重症状，急诊补救性 ERCP 重新放置或更换胰管支架可能是治疗早期 PEP 的一种新方法，并且和临床胰腺炎快速缓解和血清淀粉酶脂肪酶水平降低有关[146]。已经证明通过导丝先行引导造影导管或乳头切开胆胰管插管能够减少胰腺炎的风险，并且有相对高的（约 98%）插管成功率（见框 58.5）[147]。一项对困难插管患者的 meta 分析提示单独使用双导丝技术（double guidewire technique，DGT）似乎会增加 PEP 的风险，而且与其他技术相比在实现胆道插管方面没有任何优势。胰管支架可能减少使用 DGT 时 PEP 的风险[55]。与 NSAID 直肠给药共同作为围手术期干预，其影响尚不明确。

减轻局部炎症反应方面，NSAID 的效果最确切。一项对 602 名行高风险 ERCP 患者的多中心、双盲、安慰剂对照 RCT 研究证实，术后吲哚美辛直肠给药显著减少了 PEP 的发生[148]。已经有许多关于给予高风险患者和所有行 ERCP 患者的 NSAIDs 类型（如双氯芬酸或吲哚美辛），以及直肠给药的时机（如术前或术后，如果内镜医生感觉因为操作会有 PEP 高风险）的研究发表。两项 meta 分析总结出吲哚美辛直肠给药只对高风险患者有用，术前应用也同样有效[148,149]。另一项 meta 分析显示对所有患者 ERCP 术前吲哚美辛直肠给药并不增加术中出血[150]，研究也表明了直肠应用吲哚美辛对 ERCP 操作时间不定的患者有益[151]。最近的 meta 分析表明了术前或术后 NSAIDs 直肠给药对所有接受 ERCP 治疗的患者有效[152]。因此，吲哚美辛为主的 NSAIDs 直肠给药明确有效，除非有特殊禁忌证，建议在所有 ERCP 患者术前均给药。

应用生理盐水或乳酸林格液静脉扩容在 AP 的早期治疗中非常重要（稍后讨论），一些研究报道了两种液体在预防 PEP 中的优势。给药时机在不同研究中不尽相同：基于患者和操作本身的 PEP 风险因素，在术前或术中开始并且持续到术后的不同时期。一项对围手术期静脉容量管理的系统评价显示有证据证明静脉容量管理对 PEP 有预防作用，但研究的异质性妨碍了肯定结论的得出[153]。需要足够有力的随机试验来评估围手术期容量管理的预防效果。另一项系统评价报道了在围手术期积极使用乳酸林格液能减少 PEP 的总发病率、中到重度胰腺炎和高淀粉酶血症的发生，减少住院时间以及减轻疼痛[154]。这项 meta 分析也指出了一些关于围手术期使用静脉容量管理的缺陷，尤其是在接受直肠 NSAIDs 的患者中有无额外效果。此外也并未调查两者联合的成本效益。为了解决这些缺陷，正在筹备一项足够有效的随机对照试验来评价液体管理计划和液体类型能否在接受预防性直肠 NSAIDs 的患者中进一步减少 PEP[155]。通过这项正在进行的试验，希望能更好地明确预防性胰管支架、NSAIDs 直肠给药、围手术期液体治疗以及 3 种方式联合在 PEP 预防中的作用。

（九）术后状态

术后胰腺炎也见于胸腔或腹腔手术后[156]。0.4%～7.6% 体外循环手术后出现胰腺炎[125,157]。27% 行心脏手术患者出现高淀粉酶血症并且 1% 发展为坏死性胰腺炎[115]。体外循环术后胰腺炎的特殊风险包括术前肾功能不全、术后低血压和术中氯化钙的使用等。6% 的肝移植后出现胰腺炎[158]。术后胰腺炎的死亡率据称比其他形式的胰腺炎更高（高达 35%）。增加术后胰腺炎死亡率和发病率的因素有诊断延迟、低血压、药物（如硫唑嘌呤/围手术期氯化钙使用）、感染和共患病。术后胰腺炎同样应该被视为胰腺手术后的特殊并发症。

（十）遗传和基因疾病

遗传性胰腺炎是一种有可变外显率的常染色体显性疾病，已在第 57 章中讨论。

（十一）混杂病因

AP 很少伴有克罗恩病[160]。近期一项来自丹麦的病例对照研究发现在克罗恩病和溃疡性结肠炎患者中 AP 分别有

4倍和1.5倍增加。一些专家将这种增加归于如5-氨基水杨酸/柳氮磺吡啶以及唑嘌呤类(硫唑嘌呤/6-巯基嘌呤,见框58.4)等药物的使用。支持特发性IBD和胰腺炎的假设包括:胰腺炎是IBD的一种肠外表现,十二指肠克罗恩病能引起胰液梗阻,克罗恩病中的肉芽肿性炎症能累及胰腺,或者与自身免疫性胰腺炎相关。阿尔伯塔省的克罗恩病患者数据库报道了有6.2%服用唑嘌呤类的患者出现AP[161]。乳糜泻(celiac disease)[162]同样被认为与胰腺炎有关,但这种关系仍不明确。乳糜泻患者由于小肠屏障异常,使得肠腔的淀粉酶被过量吸收,导致高淀粉酶血症。在伴有腹痛的乳糜泻患者中,血清淀粉酶的升高多见于AP时[163]。重度烧伤后的患者中也能出现胰腺炎[164]。

自身免疫性胰腺炎(详见下一章)少见并发AP或复发AP,如2型,与粒细胞上皮病变有关[165]。研究者揭示有复发性自身免疫性胰腺炎的患者通常无典型的血清IgG4升高,常见于年轻女性患者[166]。

如在第53章中讨论的,消化性溃疡(peptic ulcer disease,PUD)(穿透性十二指肠或胃溃疡)能累及胰腺,造成可能致命的胰腺炎。尽管已并不常见,也应在适当情况下将穿透性溃疡作为胰腺炎的病因考虑[167]。

(十二) 有争议的病因

1. 胰腺分裂

胰腺分裂作为最常见的胰腺先天畸形,见于5%~10%的普通健康人群中,绝大部分从不出现胰腺炎(见第55章)。关于其他正常导管解剖的胰腺分裂是否是急性复发性胰腺炎病因的争论仍在持续[168]。胰腺分裂人群患胰腺炎的机制可能是胰液流经副乳头时的相对性狭窄。支持胰腺分裂是胰腺炎病因的论点包括:①来自ERCP转诊中心的各种数据表明,与正常人相比,因复发性胰腺炎转诊的患者有更高的胰腺分裂发生率;②多个观察系列报道了内镜下括约肌切开术或放置越过副乳头的支架,减少了复发性胰腺炎的发生率[169];③有小型随机对照研究提示,胰腺分裂并接受导管支架1年的患者比未接受的患者发生胰腺炎的频率更低[170]。不支持这种关联的论点包括:①有研究表明胰腺分裂的患者中胰腺炎发病率与普通人群相当[171];②观察性报道有一些缺陷,如随访时间不够长(通常仅1~2年)以及复发性AP是变异性很大的疾病[151];暗该单一对照研究[170]有缺陷,它是仅包含19名患者的非盲法试验。并且由于他们AP发作间期存在多次腹痛发作,所以可能为慢性胰腺炎。此外,考虑到证据不足,对胰腺分裂患者进行内镜治疗造成PEP风险较高,因此内镜下治疗胰腺分裂的风险获益比是存疑的。

与普通人群或由其他病因导致的AP患者相比,胰腺分裂和急性复发性胰腺炎的患者中基因异常的发生率相同[171]或更高[172]。例如,发展为AP的胰腺分裂患者似乎有更高的CTFR突变的发生率[173]。鉴于有研究报道了AP和胰腺分裂的患者中SPINK-1和CFTR突变的关联,有专家提出,胰腺分裂人群患有特发性胰腺炎(急性或急性复发性)不仅与胰腺分裂相关,而且也与基因异常相关。这一观察结果以及经副乳头内镜治疗与大量并发症(如狭窄)相关的发现,提示对胰腺分裂和AP患者进行侵入性治疗应慎重。也应积极探寻AP发作的其他病因。因此,仅存在胰腺分裂可能并不足以诱发AP,其他因素也可能是促使AP发病的必要因素(见该节对基因因素的讨论)[174]。

2. Oddi括约肌功能障碍(见第63章)

Oddi括约肌功能障碍(SOD)同样是AP的一个可疑病因。研究发现复发性AP患者中最常见的异常为SOD(通常定义为基础胰腺括约肌压力>40mmHg),大约在35%~40%的患者中出现。支持SOD为AP病因的主要论点为,许多观察研究报道了内镜下胰腺括约肌切开术或外科括约肌成形术减少了胰腺炎的反复发作[174]。反对SOD为AP病因的论点包括:①缺乏治疗这种疾病的前瞻性盲法对照试验;②观察性报道随访时间短;③ERCP、Oddi括约肌测压和疑似SOD患者的胰腺括约肌切开与胰腺炎高风险(25%~35%)有关;④特发性复发性胰腺炎的自然病史极其多变,可能会掩盖治疗的细微效果[175];⑤缺乏确定胰管括约肌压力正常范围的相关数据[175]。虽然可以考虑特发性复发性AP能否归为2型SOD,大量患者胆囊切除术后腹痛,但是没有客观证据表明3型SOD诊断后行ERCP、Oddi括约肌测压和胆管和(或)胰管括约肌切开会更容易出现胆胰疾病。对于3型SOD患者,已经发表了一项大型严格的多中心RCT(EPISOD试验)[176]。该试验总结出,胆囊切除术后腹痛患者,接受ERCP及测压、括约肌切开,与假括约肌切开术相比较,并没有减少因疼痛造成的失能。这些发现并不支持在这种患者中行ERCP和括约肌切开术。

六、临床特征

AP临床表现与其他急腹症相似,故而难以通过病史和体格检查诊断(框58.6)。

框58.6 急性胰腺炎的鉴别诊断
胆源性疼痛
急性胆囊炎
空腔脏器穿孔(如消化性溃疡穿孔)
肠系膜缺血或梗死
肠梗阻
心肌梗死
主动脉夹层
异位妊娠

(一) 病史

大多数AP发作时开始出现腹痛。胆源性疼痛可能预示进展为AP。胰腺炎的疼痛通常累及整个上腹部,也可能在中上腹右上腹,而局限于左侧较为罕见。下腹疼痛可能是由胰腺渗出快速扩散至左半结肠所致。

疼痛发作迅速,但是并不像内脏穿孔那么突然,通常在10~20分钟内达到最大强度。偶尔疼痛会逐渐加重并且在几小时后达到高峰。疼痛持续,并且可达到中等至非常严重的程度。改变体位几乎不能减轻疼痛,通常呈难以耐受、持续的钻痛。一半患者疼痛呈束带样放射至背部。若疼痛持续仅数小时后即消失,提示非胰腺炎性疾病,如胆源性疼痛或消化性溃疡等。5%~10%的患者发作时无疼痛感,该症状可能是严重致死的特征[6]。

90%的患者伴恶心和呕吐。呕吐可能很严重并持续数小时,可能伴有干呕且疼痛不缓解。呕吐可能与剧烈疼痛或炎症累及胃后壁有关。

(二) 体格检查

阳性体征因严重程度而异。轻度胰腺炎患者可能不会有急性病的体征。腹部压痛可能较轻且无腹肌紧张。在重症胰腺炎中,患者为重症病容并且由于胃、小肠或结肠梗阻,常有以上腹为著的腹膨隆。几乎所有患者上腹部有压痛,可以通过轻触或轻叩腹部引出。腹肌紧张以上腹部为著。与不适的程度相比,压痛和肌紧张可能比预计的要轻。弥漫性腹膜炎的板状腹少见,但可以出现板状腹,这种情况难以与内脏穿孔相鉴别。肠鸣音可能减弱或者消失。

其他腹部体征可能包括出血性渗出物至相应部位所致的一侧或双侧胁腹部的瘀斑[Gray Turner 征(图 58.3A)]或围绕脐周的瘀斑[Cullen 征(图 58.3B)],发生率低于 1%,且预后较差。胰性渗出物至腹壁可造成罕见的硬质红斑(brawny erythema)。病程中可触及的上腹部肿块可能为假性囊肿或较大的炎性团块。

一般体格检查,尤其在重症胰腺炎中,如果有第三间隙液体丢失和全身毒性,可能会发现明显异常的生命体征。通常脉搏在 100~150 次/min(窦性心动过速),血压在开始时高于正常(可能因为疼痛),当第三间隙液体丢失和血容量不足时下降。体温开始时可能正常,但是在 1~3 天内由于严重的腹膜后炎症和胰腺炎症介质的释放,体温可能会升高至 38.3~39.4℃[177]。

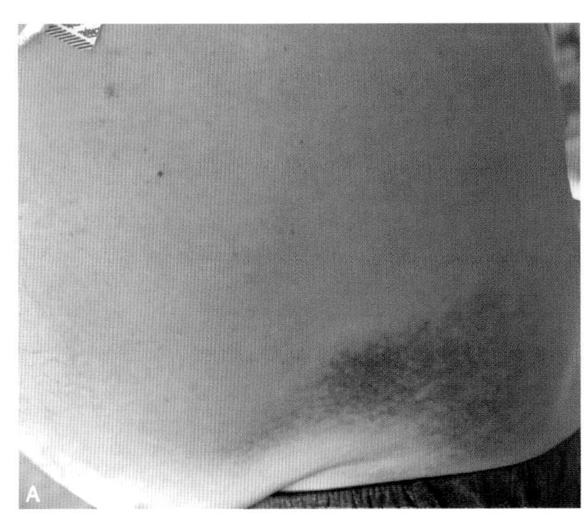

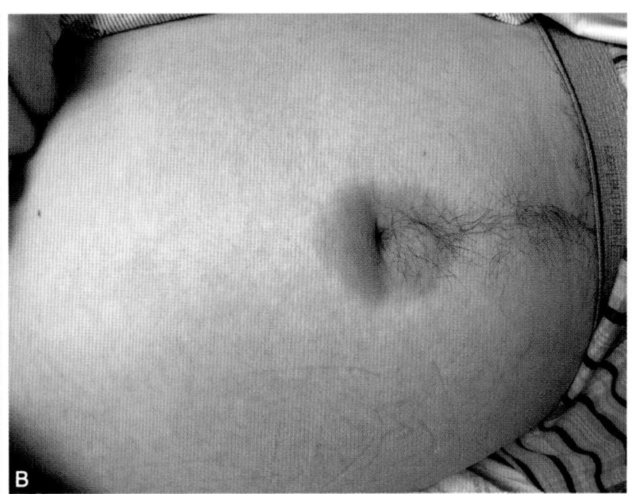

图 58.3 A,Grey Turner 征:腹痛 1 周继而出现急性胆源性坏死性胰腺炎的一名 57 岁男性左侧腹部瘀斑。B,Cullen 征:患酒精性胰腺炎的一名 40 岁男性脐周区域的瘀斑和皮下水肿。(Courtesy of Dr. Shilpa Sannapaneni, Dallas, TX)

如果膈下炎性渗出引起呼吸时疼痛,可能会出现呼吸浅促。呼吸困难可能伴有胸腔积液、肺不张、ARDS 或者心力衰竭。胸部检查可能发现由于腹痛导致膈肌不敢活动而导致的膈肌运动受限,叩诊呈浊音,胸腔积液时肺底呼吸音减弱。同样由于酒精戒断、低血压、电解质失衡(如低钠血症、低氧血症)、发热或胰酶对中枢神经的毒性效应,可能出现定向障碍、幻觉、激惹和昏迷[178]。如果出现结膜黄染,可能是胆总管结石(胆石性胰腺炎)、胰头部水肿或共患肝病造成的胆管梗阻所导致。

AP 患者中可出现少见的可伴多关节炎的皮下结节性脂肪坏死性脂膜炎(PPP 综合征,见第 25 章)[179]。皮下脂肪坏死为 0.5cm~2cm 的红色触痛结节,常出现在四肢远端,但也可出现在头皮、躯干或臀部。有时先于腹痛或不伴腹痛,但通常在发作时出现,随临床改善而消失。

一些体格检查指出了 AP 特殊的病因。肝大、蜘蛛痣和掌鞘增厚提示酒精性胰腺炎。发疹性黄色瘤和视网膜脂血症提示高甘油三酯血症性胰腺炎。腮腺疼痛和肿胀提示流行性腮腺炎。高钙血症时可出现带状角膜病变(一种角膜外侧缘的浸润)。视网膜微栓塞可能导致典型的眼底疾病,包括失明在内的视觉障碍,即 Purtscher 视网膜病变,该病变见于除 AP 外的许多疾病中[180]。

七、鉴别诊断

胆源性腹痛与 AP 相似,常位于上腹且较严重,但通常只持续数小时而不是数日(见第 65 章);消化性溃疡穿孔为突发、逐渐弥漫的疼痛伴板状腹,活动时疼痛加重。可出现恶心和呕吐,但在疼痛发作后不久消失(见第 53 章);肠系膜缺血或梗死在临床多见于患有房颤或粥样硬化性疾病的老年人,突发与体格检查不符的疼痛、便血及恶心呕吐。可存在轻度到中度的腹部压痛,并且尽管疼痛剧烈,但板状腹可能并不明显(见第 118 章);肠梗阻为周期性疼痛,腹部膨隆显著,持续呕吐且可能含有粪便,多可闻及肠鸣音亢进(见第 123 章)。其他情况详见在框 58.6 列出的 AP 的鉴别诊断。

八、实验室诊断

(一) 胰酶

通常来说,AP 的诊断依据为血液中血清淀粉酶或脂肪酶至少3倍升高[181]。

1. 血清淀粉酶水平

健康人约40%~45%的有活性的血清淀粉酶来源于胰腺,其他来源包括唾液腺等。可以利用简单的分析技术分离来自胰腺和唾液腺的淀粉酶。胰腺疾病胰腺(P)-同工酶增加,测定P-同工酶能够提高诊断准确性。然而这种检测手段并不常用。

由于血清总淀粉酶检测迅速并且廉价,故而成为诊断AP的常用方法。发病后6~12小时内升高并快速地从血液中清除(半衰期10小时)。由肾脏清除的血清淀粉酶可能不足25%,其他清除途径尚不清楚。通常发病第一天就出现血清淀粉酶升高,并且在无并发症的情况下可持续3~5天,检测灵敏度至少可达85%。致死性胰腺炎患者中[6],在轻症或在慢性胰腺炎基础上发作时(由于胰腺残留很少的腺泡细胞),或者在AP恢复期间淀粉酶在循环中被清除时,血清淀粉酶水平可能正常或少许上升,该水平可能在几天内快速回归正常。在高甘油三酯血症相关的胰腺炎中,血清淀粉酶也可能假性正常[182],因为淀粉酶抑制剂可能与TG升高有关。在这种病例中,对血清进行连续稀释通常能发现淀粉酶升高。高淀粉酶血症也见于许多情况,并不是特异地出现于胰腺炎。事实上,在血清淀粉酶升高的患者中,一半可能并没有胰腺疾病[181]。血清淀粉酶浓度在AP中通常超过正常值上限的2~3倍,而其他原因所致的高淀粉酶血症常低于该水平[183]。然而血清淀粉酶水平并不能百分百鉴别疾病,血清淀粉酶水平升高是胰腺炎的支持性指标,而不是决定性指标。此外还存在一些持续性高淀粉酶血症的人群不伴有任何临床症状,可能是巨淀粉酶血症(稍后讨论)或家族性胰源性高淀粉酶血症所致[184]。导致高淀粉酶血症的非胰腺疾病包括正常产生淀粉酶的其他器官的病理过程(如唾液腺、输卵管)。而且如卵巢乳头状囊腺瘤、良性卵巢囊肿和肺癌等肿瘤,产生和分泌唾液腺(S型)同工酶,也能够造成高淀粉酶血症。肠内P型同工酶漏出并被腹膜吸收,可能可以解释在肠梗死或消化道穿孔患者中的高淀粉酶血症。肾功能衰竭减少了对酶的清除,能够使血清淀粉酶增加至4~5倍正常值上限[185]。较之于腹膜透析,血液透析的患者往往血清淀粉酶水平更高。在有慢性肾脏病的患者中,肌酐清除率和血清淀粉酶水平并没有明显的负相关,并且约三分之一有明显肾功能不全(低肌酐清除率)的患者胰酶水平正常。

血清淀粉酶水平慢性升高(不伴尿淀粉酶)可见于巨淀粉酶血症。在这种情况下,正常的血清淀粉酶与一种免疫球蛋白或异常血清蛋白结合,形成过大且难以被肾小球滤过的复合物,因而有更长的血清半衰期[185]。巨淀粉酶血症可能被错误地诊断为胰腺疾病,但无其他临床后果。在AP中,尿淀粉酶清除率肌酐清除率比值(amylase-to-creatinine clearance ratio,ACCR)可能从大约3%增加至大约10%[186],但是即使较轻的肾功能不全也会干扰ACCR的准确性和特异性。除了诊断低ACCR的巨淀粉酶血症,尿淀粉酶测定和ACCR在临床上并不使用。巨淀粉酶血症同样也能够在血液样本中被直接测定。孟乔森综合征(Munchausen syndrome)中,用唾液故意污染尿液,能够增加尿淀粉酶,但血淀粉酶却正常。这种情况能够通过测定尿中S型淀粉酶而排除。

急诊室使用脂肪酶替代检测套餐医嘱中的淀粉酶,在维持患者服务质量和针对腹痛患者的医生选择方面,是一种减少额外检测和花费的有效工具[187]。淀粉酶检测快速而易于操作,可能在床旁临床诊断方面有潜在的应用,尤其是在乡村和偏远地区等实验室设备受限的地方[188]。

2. 血清脂肪酶水平

在AP诊断的灵敏度方面,血清脂肪酶与血清淀粉酶相似,至少有85%[181]。然而较之于淀粉酶,脂肪酶对胰腺炎可能有更好的特异性。例如唾液腺疾病、产淀粉酶肿瘤、输卵管炎等的妇科疾病和巨淀粉酶血症等非胰源性疾病中,血清淀粉酶升高而血清脂肪酶正常。血清脂肪酶总是在疾病的第一天上升并且持续时间比血清淀粉酶更长,这令其有稍高的敏感度[189]。结合淀粉酶和脂肪酶结果并不能增加诊断准确性,并且会增加花费。

在检测特异性方面,脂肪酶面临与淀粉酶一样的问题。无胰腺炎时,血清脂肪酶可能在肾功能不全时有小于2倍正常值的上升[190]。在类似AP的急性消化道疾病中[191],可能通过缺血、发炎或穿孔的肠道吸收,血清脂肪酶有小于3倍正常水平的上升。很少有胰源性腹部疾病,如小肠梗阻等,能够使脂肪酶(和淀粉酶)高于3倍正常值。一些人认为检测血清脂肪酶比血清淀粉酶更好,因为其敏感性与淀粉酶相似,且特异性更佳,然而也有人认为没有明确的优势[9]。

许多正常人群可能存在几乎无临床意义的血清淀粉酶和(或)脂肪酶的升高[192]。与无糖尿病患者相比,糖尿病患者似乎存在不明原因导致的脂肪酶中位数升高[193]。在该前瞻性研究中揭示了有20%的2型糖尿病患者有血清脂肪酶升高,并且有2%的患者在无症状的情况下血清脂肪酶也有超过3倍的升高。然而,当评估血清淀粉酶时,仅发现5%的2型糖尿病患者水平升高,但没有患者的水平升高达到3倍以上。尽管这些发现的意义尚不明确,但是近来的一项研究认为胰酶的低水平上升可能与慢性胰腺炎中胰腺导管的持续改变有关[194]。虽然需要进一步的研究,但是在没有其他AP的临床表现的情况下,不应该对淀粉酶和脂肪酶水平上升的无症状患者进行广泛的评估。

临床还可以检测血清脂肪酶亚型,例如胰腺来源的脂肪酶。然而,在小型研究中发现该亚型的检测并不优于常规脂肪酶,但临床需要时可作为补充检测项目[195]。一项来自澳大利亚和新西兰的研究发现用AP患儿第一天的脂肪酶升高预测危重症,敏感度可达82%,但特异度仅有53%[196]。另外一项研究同样报道了脂肪酶早期7倍升高对于预测小儿AP危重症的敏感度、特异度、阳性和阴性预测值及阳性和阴性似然比分别为85%、56%、46%、89%、1.939和0.27[197]。高脂肪酶血症的总阳性预测值为38%。因为相对低的阳性预测值,在危重患者中,内科医生应当谨慎解读其脂肪酶3倍升高的高脂肪酶血症。更高的脂肪酶临界值可提高其在AP中的诊断价值,并且减少了不必要的影像学检查。伴脂肪酶升高的非AP患者最常见的第一诊断包括休克、心搏骤停和恶性肿瘤[198]。非胰腺来源的血清脂肪酶水平升高最常见于肝功能衰竭和肾功能衰竭[199]。最近一项研究指出脂肪酶(91%)相较于淀粉酶(61%)敏感度更高,且其特异度>91%。对于疑似AP的患者,脂肪酶应当取代淀粉酶作为一线实验室检查指标[200]。一项 Cochrane 系统评价关注了持续严重上腹痛或弥漫性腹痛的急性发作患者,评估其血清淀粉酶、血清脂肪酶、尿胰蛋白酶原-2 和尿淀粉酶单独或联合诊断 AP 的诊断准确度,发现有 25% 的假阴性率和 10% 假阳性率[201]。对于预测有不耐受经口进食高风险的患者,重新进食前血清脂肪酶水平超过 2.5 倍的正常值上限可能是一个潜在有用的阈值[202]。

3. 其他胰酶水平

在急性胰腺炎症中,淀粉酶和脂肪酶以外的其他胰腺消化酶也可释放入全身循环并且已被用于诊断 AP。它们包括 PLA_2、胰蛋白酶/胰蛋白酶原、羧酸酯酶、羧肽酶 A、辅脂肪酶、弹性蛋白酶、TAP、尿和血清胰蛋白酶原-2 和核糖核酸酶。但其中没有任何一种单独或联合检测在诊断上优于血清淀粉酶或脂肪酶,且大多数不能进行检测。

(二) 普通血液学检查

在重症胰腺炎中,白细胞数常显著升高,但一般不意味着感染。血糖可能升高并伴有血清胰高血糖素升高。血清 AST、ALT、碱性磷酸酶和胆红素同样可能升高,尤其是在胆石性胰腺炎中,胆管结石或许能够解释这种异常。然而在 AP 中胰腺炎症本身也可能部分阻塞远端胆管。血清转氨酶可帮助鉴别胆源性和酒精性胰腺炎(见后文)[203]。

AP 患者中常见血钙下降,主要与血清白蛋白下降有关。正如之后会讨论的一样,因为钙与富含白蛋白的血管内液结合运输并渗透至腹膜,所以钙减少可以提示疾病严重程度。血钙减少并不是由于皂化。平均红细胞体积能辅助鉴别非酒精性和酒精性 AP[204]。由于酒精对骨髓中红细胞形成有毒性效应,酗酒患者可能有更高的平均红细胞体积。AP 患者血清 TG 水平升高,但在饮酒、未控制的糖尿病或 TG 代谢障碍时也会出现 TG 升高。

九、影像学诊断

(一) 腹部平片

腹部 X 线片所见范围可能从轻症中的无异常到小肠节段的局限性肠梗阻[“哨兵袢(sentinel loop)”]或者更严重疾病中的结肠切割征(colon cutoff sign)。此外,腹部平片有助于排除其他引起腹痛的原因,例如肠梗阻和穿孔。空腔消化道在腹部平片上的影像取决于胰腺渗出的范围和位置。胃的异常是由于网膜囊中的渗出造成了胃向前移位,并伴有胃的轮廓与横结肠分离。小肠异常是由于小肠系膜附近的炎症引起,包括一个或多个空肠袢(哨兵袢)、回肠末端或盲肠或者十二指肠的梗阻。广泛性肠梗阻可在严重疾病中发生,可能存在空腔胃肠道的其他异常。十二指肠降部可能被增大的胰头部所拉长或占据。此外,渗出扩散至结肠的特定部位可能造成该部分结肠痉挛,以及痉挛远端无充气(结肠切割征)或痉挛近端结肠扩张。以胰头为主的胰腺炎倾向于渗出扩散至近端横结肠,造成结肠痉挛以及升结肠扩张。弥漫性胰腺炎症倾向于渗出扩散至结肠下缘以及出现不规则结肠袋形。从胰尾部到毗邻降结肠的膈结肠韧带的渗出可能造成降结肠的痉挛和横结肠的扩张。其他腹部平片所见可能提供病因或严重程度的线索,包括钙化胆石(胆石性胰腺炎)、胰腺结石或钙化(慢性胰腺炎急性加重)和腹水(重症胰腺炎)。腹膜后气体提示胰腺脓肿可能。

(二) 胸部影像

30% AP 患者出现胸部影像的异常征象,包括单侧膈抬高、单/双侧胸腔积液、继发于限制性呼吸运动的基底或盘状肺不张、肺部浸润。胸腔积液可能出现在双侧或局限于左侧,只出现在右侧者罕见[205]。入院时发现有胸腔积液和(或)肺部浸润的 AP 患者提示可能有严重疾病[206]。在最早的 7~10 天内,同样可能出现 ARDS 或心力衰竭的征象。心包积液罕见。

(三) 腹部超声

在住院的前 24 小时一般用腹部超声来寻找胆石、胆总管结石所致的胆管扩张及腹水。由于富含蛋白的液体从血管内渗出至腹腔,中至重度的 AP 患者中腹水常见。超声可见胰腺弥漫性增大和低回声(存在 25%~35% 可能性:肠内气体掩盖了胰腺)。少见的情况下有灶性低回声区域。慢性胰腺炎可能也有如导管内或实质的钙化以及胰管的扩张等超声表现。超声并不是评估胰腺炎症胰外扩散程度或者胰腺坏死的良好影像学手段,因此不用于确定胰腺炎的严重程度。AP 患者可以凭借超声来评估假性囊肿的发展(稍后讨论)。胆总管结石由于气体干扰,可能在急性发作时无法诊断,肠道气体减少后或许能够被发现。未来或许能够应用胰腺的超声造影评估 AP 严重程度[207]。

(四) EUS 和 ERCP

在 AP 发作时及发作后数周,EUS 对胰腺成像可显示典型的低回声异常信号,与慢性胰腺炎和恶性肿瘤难以区分。在 AP 早期阶段,EUS 能有效地用来探查胆总管结石,以避免胆管无结石时的 ERCP。EUS 同样能够通过胰腺回声质地的改变,预测 AP 的严重程度[79]。一项针对中度或不确定的胆总管结石风险的患者的 RCT 发现,为确诊胆总管结石而行的 EUS,可以使几乎一半病例避免进行不必要的 ERCP[208]。在入院时完成的 EUS 能够可靠地探测到胰腺坏死,如胆总管结石等共存的疾病[209]以及预测死亡率[210]。在特发性 AP 中,近年来的指南和综述建议在 8~12 周后行 EUS 以寻找病因,如胆总管微结石、造成梗阻的近胰管小肿瘤、以 AP 发作为表现的慢性胰腺炎,以及一些 CT 扫描遗漏的解剖学异常等[211]。一项研究提示在评估特发性 AP 时,确定胰腺炎病因方面 EUS 比 MRCP 有更高的诊断准确性(64% vs 34%)[212]。

(五) CT

CT 是诊断 AP 及其腹腔内并发症的最重要影像学检查[213]。CT 的主要适应证为:①排除其他严重腹腔内疾病(如肠系膜梗死或消化性溃疡穿孔);②AP 严重程度分级;③明确有无胰腺炎并发症出现(如消化道或肝、脾、肾等邻近脏器及血管受累)[214]。螺旋 CT 是最常用的技术。条件允许的情况下,应在给予患者口服造影剂,然后静脉注射造影剂后进行扫描,以识别胰腺坏死的区域。如果胰腺灌注正常,则认为是间质性胰腺炎(见图 58.1)。AP 发生后 48~72 小时后,可能出现静脉造影后充盈缺损的胰腺坏死(见图 58.2)。

在大鼠 AP 模型胰腺炎发作时给予碘造影剂导致坏死增加[215],提示在 AP 病程早期使用静脉造影剂可能增加胰腺坏死,然而并没有其他动物模型支持该理论。以人为研究主体的数据结果是相互矛盾的。目前两项回顾性研究表明早期的对比增强 CT 使胰腺炎恶化[215],但并没有被第三项回顾性研究印证[216]。

非增强 CT 可将 AP 的严重程度分为 5 个等级(A~E)(稍后讨论)[203]。虽然胰腺中存在气体提示胰腺产气微生物感染,但也能与无菌性坏死(图 58.4)伴肠道微穿孔或邻近假性囊肿进入胰腺同时发生[217]。而且绝大多数胰腺感染经 CT 扫描时并未发现气体。

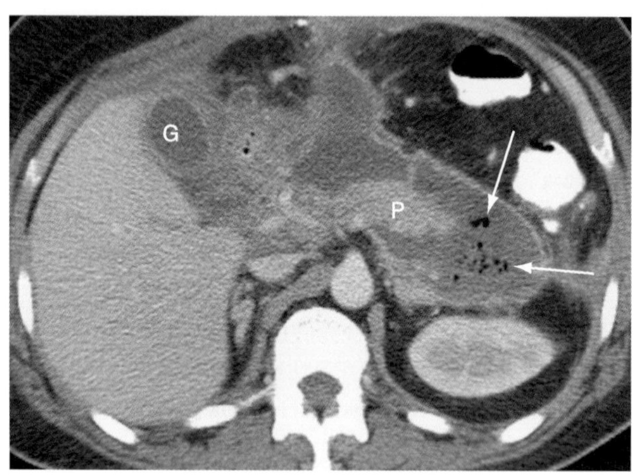

图 58.4 CT 提示急性坏死性胰腺炎。含有无菌性坏死所致气泡(箭头)的胰周炎症环绕胰腺。患者没有相应临床表现故较不考虑脓肿。G,胆囊;P,胰腺

灌注 CT 扫描是近期发展起来的,较之于传统 CT 扫描,其通过静脉内放射性造影剂的灌注更早地发现坏死[86]。一项来自日本的多中心研究提示灌注 CT 除了能早期发现胰腺坏死,也能预测持续性器官衰竭[218]。另一项发展起来的技术为减影 CT,其中减色图(subtraction color map)是从非对比和对比 CT 中生成的。这项技术较之于传统 CT 扫描,同样能够早期发现坏死[219]。

(六) MRI

MRI 如 CT 一样提供了关于胰腺炎严重程度的信息。然而 MRI 能更好地对坏死残余进行显影,在评价液体积聚方面比 CT 更有优势[220]。在发现胆总管结石方面,MRI 比 CT 更好,效果与 EUS、ERCP 相同[221]。MRI 同样在勾勒胰管、展示胰管破坏及不连续等损伤、提示胰管结石等方面比 CT 有优势。MRCP 对比剂钆[222]能够造成肾源性系统性纤维化[223]。然而在有肾功能损害的患者中出现肾源性系统性纤维化的风险非常低,并且新的药剂并不与该疾病相关联。MRI 比 CT 更难进行且更昂贵。MRI 也要求患者在图像采集过程中保持静止,往往也需要比螺旋 CT 需要更长的时间。在高风险胆总管结石的患者中,MRCP 常常在 ERCP 前进行,并且需要更长的住院时间、更高的影像学费用以及倾向于更高的住院花费[224]。MRCP 前使用静脉促胰液素能让胰管有更好的显影[225],已证明在对特发性胰腺炎和复发性胰腺炎患者的评估中十分有用[225,226]。因此,尽管 MRI 和 MRCP 在 AP 的管理中有确切的作用,但也需要意识到其局限性。

十、鉴别酒精性和胆石性胰腺炎

酒精性和胆石性胰腺炎的鉴别诊断十分重要,因为去除这些病因可以预防后续胰腺炎发作。酒精性胰腺炎在 40 岁左右的男性中发生频率更高,通常在大量饮酒 5 到 10 年后出现首次临床发作。与之相比,胆源性胰腺炎在女性中更常见,首次临床发作常在 40 岁之后。AP 反复发作提示酒精性 AP,但未被发现的结石也能引起复发性胰腺炎。在没有行胆囊切除术的急性胆源性胰腺炎出院患者中,30% 到 50% 在出院不久后出现复发性胰腺炎(平均出现复发胰腺炎时间 108 天)[227]。因此胆源性胰腺炎中切除胆囊十分重要。

实验室检查有助于鉴别两者。血清 ALT 浓度超过 150IU/L(≈3 倍升高)对胆石性胰腺炎的特异度为 96%,阳性预测值为 95%,但敏感度仅有 48%[205]。也可以检测血清 AST 浓度,但是总胆红素和碱性磷酸酶浓度在鉴别胆石性胰腺炎和酒精性胰腺炎或者其他病因方面,帮助不大。关于高血清脂肪酶与淀粉酶比值能否区分酒精和其他病因的报道不一[228,229]。

应该对每名首次 AP 发作的患者行常规腹部 B 超,以寻找胆囊、胆总管中的结石和肝外胆管梗阻的证据。然而,腹部超声常遗漏胆管结石,且大多数结石在急性发作时排出。ERCP 仅适用于那些结石伴持续性胆管梗阻所致的重度 AP 患者,以及术中无法清除胆石的患者。在大多数有胆源性胰腺炎的患者中,胆总管结石可排出且不需要进一步评估。虽然在同次住院行腹腔镜胆囊切除时,胆管可以通过手术胆管造影成像,但大多数患者并不需要。

许多临床医生喜欢在术前对胆管进行评估,但造成胆源性胰腺炎的大多数结石已经排出,并不清楚哪些人需要进行评估。对于轻中度风险胆总管结石的患者,当 PEP 的风险超过 ERCP 的受益时(正常宽度胆管和肝功能化验正常)ERCP 并不合适。然而,如果胆管已经扩张和(或)肝功能检测指标升高,则有理由在术前进一步评估。虽然 EUS 是探测胆管结石的一种准确方法并且被推荐在胆囊切除术前评估胆管,但是这种情况下很少需要使用它[230]。它应该作为一种针对那些怀疑有结石残留但不能进行 MRCP 的患者的保留手段。MRCP 具有很好的诊断准确性,但作为一种非侵入式检测,如果临床医生考虑胆总管结石存在的可能性较低时,常作为首选。如果在术中发现胆总管结石,可以在术中取出或术后内镜下清除结石[231]。在清除胆总管结石方面,腹腔镜探查胆管与术后 ERCP 同样安全有效[232]。

十一、疾病严重程度的预测方法

根据修订后的亚特兰大分类,AP 按严重程度可分为 3 级:轻度、中重度和重度,轻度 AP 约占 80%。在病程早期

24~72 小时内预测严重程度非常重要，尤其在入院和最初 24 小时内。如果预测提示疾病为中度或重度，有利于与患者沟通疾病的病程；将他们分诊至重症监护病房（ICU）或普通监护病房（step-up unit）；当有具体的干预措施可实施时，尽早干预。过去数年里提出了多种临床表现、实验室检查特征和评分系统用来预测重度 AP。预测中重度 AP 的研究相当有限，其中包括修订后的亚特兰大标准[233]。然而尽管有大量的文献，但是目前仍没有完善的预测方法。由于很大一部分 AP 患者并不发展为中重度或重度疾病，因此大多数预测方法阴性预测值非常高但无良好的阳性预测值。两个前瞻性队列研究报道了现有的评分系统已经达到了它们在预测 AP 中持续性器官衰竭的最高效能。将多种预测原则组合能够提高准确性，但会更加繁杂，因而限制了临床使用。除非有新的方法学进展，否则我们对 AP 严重程度的预测已经无法再有所进步[234]。一篇最近的系统评价关注了持续性器官衰竭（重度 AP）和感染性胰腺坏死的预测方法，发现可以使用血尿素氮水平来预测入院 48 小时后的持续性器官衰竭，使用降钙素原预测确诊为胰腺坏死患者中的感染性胰腺坏死[234]。并未发现有合适的方法来预测入院 48 小时内持续性器官衰竭[235]。我们迫切需要的，是一个对于中重度或重度 AP 有着高阳性预测值的系统或参考标准。同时，最近关于 AP 早期管理的 AGA 技术评审指出，未发现使用可改善临床结果的预测工具进行的研究[236]。因此，建议在临床实践中采用临床判断和多种预测工具。同理，在同一技术评审的 meta 分析中没有包含预测严重程度的特殊方法。因此以下将简要列出许多预测方法，并补充一些被广泛研究方法的额外信息。目前大多数系统多在研究目的和比较不同队列方面显示出更大的作用，而不是在指导临床诊疗中。

近来的指南和综述建议，入院时应结合以下预测因素进行临床判断：高龄（>60 周岁）、BMI、Charlson 合并症指数、腹腔积液或入院胸片中的浸润、血细胞比容升高、尿素氮水平升高、血清肌酐升高、48 小时 CRP>15mg/dL[1,211,237]。

血清淀粉酶和脂肪酶的升高程度与严重程度无关。然而，据报道，在儿科 AP 中，脂肪酶升高 7 倍可预测严重疾病，其敏感性、特异性、阳性和阴性预测值分别为 85%、56%、46% 和 89%，阳性和阴性似然比分别为 1.939 和 0.27[197]。在慢性胰腺炎基础上叠加的 AP，其严重程度通常轻于没有慢性胰腺炎的 AP。当 AP 与慢性胰腺炎叠加时，体重减轻，高龄和合并症可预测基于人群研究的严重性[237]。急性胆源性胰腺炎中的线阵超声内镜表明了 AP 严重程度与弥漫性实质水肿、紧贴实质周围和（或）腹膜后游离的液体积聚，以及胰腺周围水肿之间的显著关系，也同样预测了死亡率[238]。一个大型的官方数据库显示，转运的 AP 患者有更严重的疾病和更高的总死亡率，而在校正疾病严重程度后死亡率相似。疾病严重程度、保险状态、种族和年龄都会影响转运 AP 患者的决定[239]。

近几年报道了大量预测 AP 严重程度的临床和实验室方法。它们包括降钙素原[240]、TNF-α[241]、血小板生成素[242]、羧肽酶-B 激动肽[243]、多形核弹力蛋白酶、PLA_2、儿童 AP 中的 D-二聚体[244,245]、更高的尿 β2 微球蛋白比 saposin B 比率[246]、铁调素[247]、可溶性 B7-H2（sB7-H2）[248]、肽素（copeptin）[249]、IL-6[250]、IL-17、IL-23[251]、褪黑素[252]、抗胰岛素蛋白（resistin）[253]、低血清脂质浓度[254]、平均血小板体积[255]、前蛋白酶（presepsin）[256]、可溶性尿激酶型纤溶酶原激活物受体（soluble urokinase-type plasminogen activator receptor）[257]、尿中性粒细胞明胶酶相关脂质运载蛋白（urinary neutrophil gelatinase-associated lipocalin）[258]、LP-PLA2 基因多态性 V279F 和 R92H[259]、TLR3 和 TLR6 中的基因多态性[260]、内脏脂肪组织增加[261]、基质金属蛋白酶-8[262]、IL13/IFN-γ 比[263]、抗凝血酶Ⅲ[264]、高内脏脂肪伴低骨骼肌体积[265]、住院心率变异性[266]及其他。

入院时存在 SIRS 及在 48 小时内 SIRS 的持续存在增加了发病率和死亡率。在一项研究中，25% 持续性 SIRS、8% 一过性 SIRS 和 1% 无 SIRS 的患者最终死亡[267]。

尽管现在严重程度是根据 AP 的器官衰竭或解剖并发症（例如胰腺坏死）的存在来定义的，但已经开发出使用临床标准的前瞻性系统来确定疾病的严重程度。这些系统包括 Ranson 和 APACHE 评分[13,14]。不幸的是这些评分系统（下文讨论）十分复杂并需要多个参数。此外这些系统在发病后的 48 小时内并不准确。

（一）评分系统

APACHEⅡ已经是多年来最有效的系统，并且后续没有评分系统能比其更优。但是 APACHE Ⅱ很复杂，所以很少应用于临床实践中。大多数研究使用 8 分或更高作为 AP 的标准。Ranson 及同伴总结了最初 48 小时内 11 个有预后意义的表现。最初列表[13]主要是在酒精性胰腺炎患者中分析的，并且在 8 年后为胆石性胰腺炎进行了调整[268]。通常认为 3 分或更高意味着重度 AP。Imrie 或 Glasgow 评分[269]是一个英国常用的相对简化版列表（8 条标准）。在布列根和妇女医院胰腺中心进行了一系列前瞻性和回顾性研究[270-272]。该研究在一个囊括了超过 200 家医院约 3 700 名患者的大型数据库的基础上进行。在包括确证研究在内的仔细分析后，他们明确了一个仅包括 5 个变量的简化系统，能够准确地在疾病病程的早期预测严重程度。这个评分系统被称为 BISAP（AP 严重程度床旁指数，Bedside Index for Severity in AP），每个参数为 1 分——尿素氮（BUN）超过 25mg/dL、精神状态受损（Impaired mental status）、SIRS、年龄（Age）大于 60 周岁以及胸腔积液（Pleural effusion），总分为 5 分。4 或 5 分的 BISAP 评分提示发展为器官衰竭的风险增加 7 倍到 12 倍。BISAP 并不优于 APACHEII。其他评分系统包括无害 AP 评分（harmless AP score）[273]、日本 AP 严重程度评分[274]和 PANC 3 评分[275]。

目前没有任何的评分系统优于 APACHE Ⅱ，但是它的不足在于过于复杂。简单的 SIRS 评分和其他复合评分系统同样有效，并且简单、廉价、入院即行[125]。SIRS 被定义为有下列 4 条标准中的两条或更多：心率>90 次/min、直肠温度<36℃或>38℃、白细胞数<4 000/mm^3 或>12 000/mm^3、呼吸频率超过 20 次/min 或动脉 PCO_2<32mmHg（见框 58.2）。

（二）CT

CT 发现的大量液体积聚和（或）广泛胰腺坏死与危重症相关。Balthazar 报道了 37 名 CT 评级 D 级或 E 级的患者中有

5 名死亡(13.5%)，而 51 名 B 级或 C 级患者中无一死亡(表 58.1)[213]。使用 CT 严重程度指数(CT severity index，CTSI 评分；见表 58.1)，评分为 0～6 分的 77 名患者中 3 名死亡(3.8%)，11 名评分为 7～10 分的患者中有 2 名死亡(18%)。较之于死亡率，CT 分级评分与局部并发症(假性囊肿和脓肿)相关性更好。37 名 D 级或 E 级评分的患者中 54% 出现局部并发症，然而 51 名评分为 A 级到 C 级的患者中仅有 2 名(5.9%)有这种问题[213]。因此，数据并不能证实 CTSI 比 A 级到 E 级评分更具预测性。文献中对于 CT 显示的坏死程度能否预测器官衰竭尚存争议[11,12,16,245-247]。改良 CTSI 有助于对炎症和坏死的简易评估，其中同样包括对胰外并发症的评估[276]。

表 58.1　Balthazar CT 分级系统和 CT 严重程度指数(CTSI)

Balthazar 等级	定义	分值
A	符合轻度胰腺炎的正常胰腺	0
B	腺体局部或弥漫增大，包括轮廓不规则和密度不均但不伴胰腺周围炎症	1
C	B 级加上胰腺周围炎症	2
D	C 级加上相关单个液体积聚	3
E	C 级加上 2 个或多个胰腺周围液体积聚或者胰内或腹膜后气体	4
CTSI = Balthazar CT 分级系统加上坏死评分*		
	坏死评分	分值
	不存在坏死	0
	至多 33% 胰腺坏死	2
	33%～50% 坏死	4
	>50% 坏死	6

*CTSI 最高可达到的分值：4(Balthazar E 级)+6(>50% 坏死)= 10 分。

(三) 胸部影像

在入院 72 小时内胸部影像(或 CT)记录到的胸腔积液与危重症相关[205,206]。

十二、治疗(见图 58.5)

(一) 第一周初始治疗

目前尚无治疗 AP 的特效药，治疗指南主要针对支持治疗和并发症的治疗。因为有很好的支持治疗，包括 ICU 护理和更多对后续并发症的有效疗法，在世界不同区域内 AP 死亡率已经从大约 10% 降至 5% 或更低。患者通常持续禁食直到恶心、呕吐消失。然而这种概念已经有很大变化，目前治疗的关键在于肠道唤醒而不是肠道休息[277]。通过给予早期经口进食，肠道黏膜屏障得以保留，并防止细菌从肠腔转移到循环中。缓解疼痛也是早期管理的一个重点。常使用患者控制型麻醉泵给药的阿片类镇痛药，是最广泛使用的药物[278]，如芬太尼和氢吗啡酮等。阿片类的剂量需仔细管控并且根据现行需要调整日常基础量。虽然已经报道吗啡会增加 Oddi 括约肌张力并且使血清淀粉酶升高[279]，但是尚未显示将其用于缓解胰腺炎的疼痛会对临床结局不利。鼻胃管并不常规使用，因为其在轻度胰腺炎中无益。它仅在治疗胃或十二指肠梗阻或难治性恶心呕吐时使用。同样的，常规使用质子泵抑制剂或 H2RA 并没有显示益处。

有早期器官衰竭征兆的如低血压(静脉容量管理后收缩压仍小于 110mmHg)、呼吸衰竭(使用鼻导管或面罩最大限度氧气补充治疗后氧饱和度小于 90%)或肾功能不全[最大容量管理后血清肌酐仍超过 2mg/dL(176.8μmol/L)]的患者应该通过密切关注生命体征和尿量来仔细看护。呼吸急促不应该认为是由于腹痛所致。建议监测血氧饱和度以及必要时检测动脉血气，而低氧血症时必需予氧气支持。任何出现早期器官功能不全表现的患者应当考虑转入 ICU，但在不同的中心进入 ICU 的指征并不相同。虽然在美国许多患者是基础性管理(除非需要呼吸或血压支持)，但在美国以外早期器官衰竭征兆(如氧气需求逐渐增加、静脉输液以维持血压或肾脏替代治疗等)是进入重症或普通监护病房的指征。

(二) 静脉补液和电解质复苏

随着疾病早期炎症的进展，富含蛋白质的血管内液体大量渗入腹膜腔和腹膜后腔，导致血液浓缩和肾脏灌注减少，BUN 水平随之升高，随后血清肌酐水平升高。而后对胰腺的灌注压力降低导致微循环改变，从而导致胰腺坏死。因此，入院时血细胞比容超过 44% 或未能在 24 小时内降低是坏死性胰腺炎的预测指标[280]，且 BUN 的升高或持续上升与死亡率增加有关[272]。血细胞比容和 BUN 这些血管内容量的标志物与 AP 严重程度的关系意味着对其进行拮抗也是正确的。因此早期大量静脉补液对于血管内复苏而言最重要，目标是提供足够的血管内容量以减少血细胞比容和 BUN，从而增加胰腺灌注。这是多年来 AP 中广泛研究的管理策略之一。虽然在这些指南和综述中对这种静脉容量管理方面存在显著差异，但是血管容积管理已经被专家和许多指南广泛推荐[9,211,280-282]。Haydock 等在一项系统评价中发现这种管理的重要部分中，最高等级证据非常少[283]。这种容量管理包括多个方面：液体类型、给予的总量、频率、时机、持续时间和对治疗的监测力度。新西兰的一项国家调查发现在 AP 中静脉内容量管理有很大不同，这并不奇怪，积极的容量管理多在器官衰竭时进行并且没有遵循已发表的指南[284]。乳酸林格液被推测可以减少胰腺中细胞内酸中毒，从而降低胰蛋白酶活性。一项小型的 RCT 研究展示了乳酸林格液对减少 SIRS 评分和 CRP 水平方面比生理盐水更优，但是在重要的临床结果中未显示出区别[285]。

一项 AGA 技术评审[237]报道了对许多关于 AP 早期静脉内容量管理合格研究的 meta 分析："总之，没有足够的证据表明使用各种参数来指导输液的目标导向治疗，可降低持续的单个或多个器官系统衰竭、感染性胰腺(周围)坏死或 AP 致死的风险。同样没有 RCT 证据证明存在某种特殊类型的液体疗法(如乳酸林格液)能够减少死亡风险或者持续性单个或多个器官衰竭。在常规静脉液体中添加羟乙基淀粉并不能

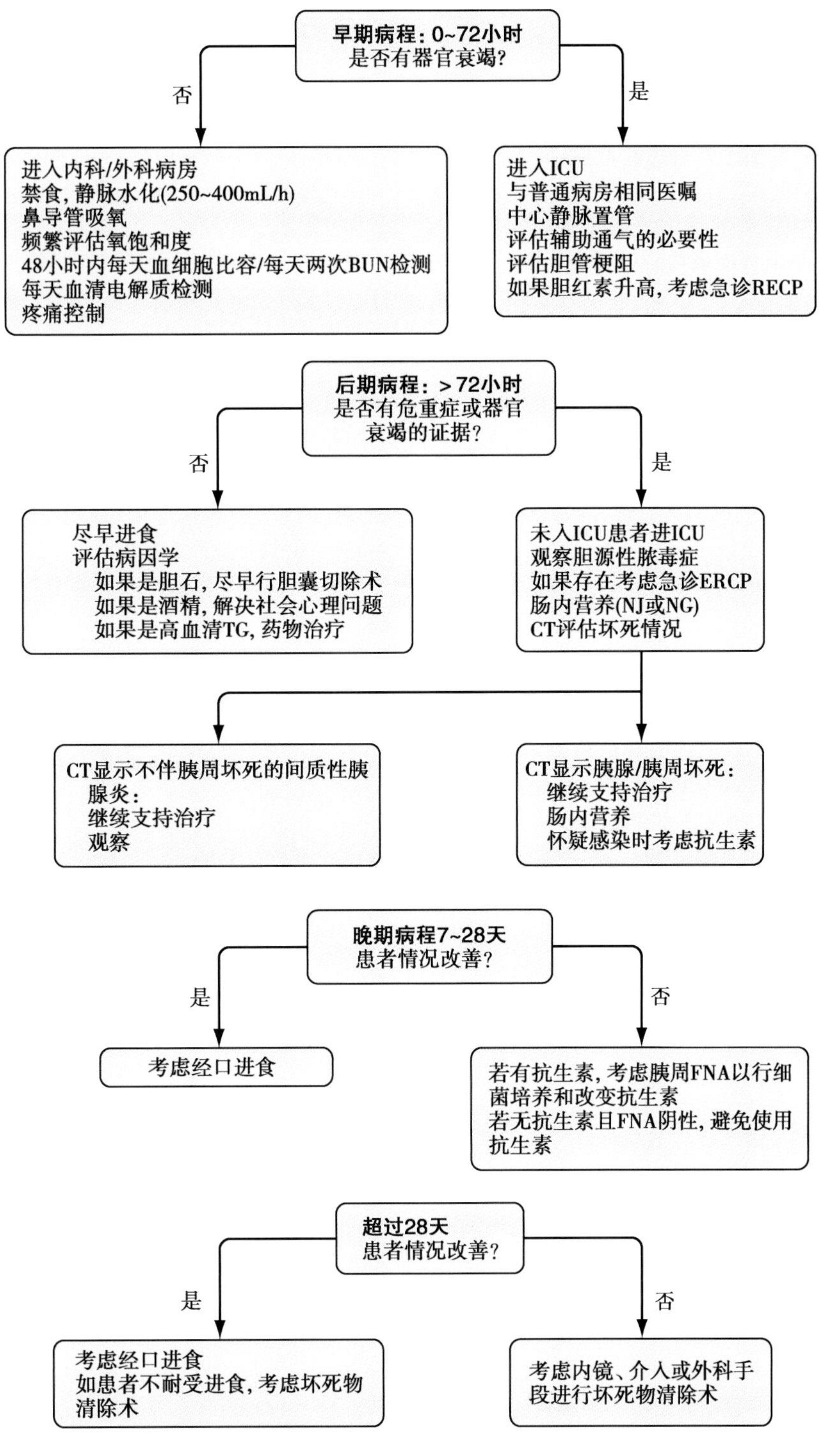

图 58.5　对于急性胰腺炎病程中不同阶段的管理原则。BUN，血尿素氮；NJ，鼻空肠

减少死亡风险并且可能增加 AP 中持续性器官系统衰竭的风险。”基于这项 meta 分析，随附的 AGA 指南推荐了以液体管理为目标导向的治疗，但是也警告其证据质量很低，未来的试验必须解决此类疗法在 AP 早期管理中很多方面的问题[286]。尽管存在这些实际性的限制，但建议最好在入院最初 24 小时内，以每小时 5~10mL/kg 体重或每小时 250~500mL 的乳酸林格液进行补充。除了对容量负荷过重的临床监测，每小时尿量、血细胞比容下降和 BUN/血清肌酐水平也能用来指导这种治疗，而且不需要进行侵入性监测。不应该使用如羟乙基淀粉等药物。

（三）呼吸监护

由于影响 AP 患者的低氧血症常见且顽固，目前的指南建议在所有 AP 患者中初始常规使用鼻导管吸氧[287]。

最好通过鼻导管或储氧面罩补充氧气，以使氧饱和度保持在 90% 以上。如果鼻导管或面罩给氧无法纠正低氧血症或有乏力及临界呼吸储备不足，需要尽早进行无创正压通气或气管内插管及辅助机械通气。

非重力依赖区的肺超声能可靠地探测 AP 中呼吸功能障碍的演变。这种简单的床旁技术有望成为严重程度分层的手段[288]。ARDS 与严重呼吸困难、进行性低氧血症和死亡率增加有关，通常出现在疾病的第 2～7 天（但同样可在入院时出现），并有持续性的肺泡毛细血管通透性增加，引起间质水肿。胸部 X 线片可能显示多肺叶的肺泡浸润。治疗方法是通过气管插管进行呼气末正压通气，通常采用低潮气量以防止肺容积伤。没有特殊的治疗能够预防或减轻 ARDS。据报道，ARDS 早期的无创正压通气[288]和连续性肾脏替代治疗对 AP 中的 ARDS 治疗同样有效[289]。康复后肺的结构和功能通常恢复正常。

（四）心血管监护

严重 AP 的心脏并发症包括心力衰竭、心肌梗死、心律失常和心源性休克。可能会出现心脏指数的增加和总外周阻力的降低，并且对晶体液输注有反应。如果适当的液体复苏后低血压持续存在，可能需要静脉给予升压药。

（五）代谢并发症

可能在严重胰腺炎的前几天出现高血糖症，但通常会在炎症消退后消失。血糖产生波动，此时应谨慎给予胰岛素。新西兰的一项研究中指出，在 AP 病程早期瘦素水平与持续高血糖相关[290]。低钙血症主要是由于血清白蛋白降低。富含白蛋白的血管内液渗出至腹膜和腹膜后，以及在急性期减少白蛋白合成的负相反应物效应（negative phase reactant effect）都会导致白蛋白丢失，白蛋白丢失造成通常与白蛋白结合的钙减少。因这种丢失是非电离的，所以低钙血症大都无症状且不需要特殊治疗。但是可能出现血清离子钙的减少并且造成神经肌肉应激性升高。如果共存低镁血症，会抑制甲状旁腺素的释放，这种情况下补充镁可使血钙恢复正常。镁耗尽的病因包括尿、便或呕吐物中镁的丢失或脂肪坏死区域镁的沉积。一旦血清镁正常，并且血钾正常且未给予洋地黄，神经肌肉应激性的症状和征象就可能需要静脉注射葡萄糖酸钙。静脉输注钙会增加钙与心肌受体的结合，置换钾离子并且可能造成严重的心律失常。

（六）抗生素

抗生素有时会在 AP 中作为预防性治疗手段（在有明确证据的感染前）或作为已确诊感染的治疗。胰腺和胰周组织的坏死（坏死性胰腺炎）能够出现感染（感染性胰腺坏死）并增加死亡率[291,292]。抗生素在已确诊的胰腺或胰外部位感染中的作用毋庸置疑。亚胺培南、氟喹诺酮类（环丙沙星、氧氟沙星、培氟沙星）和甲硝唑是可以在胰腺组织中达到最高抑菌浓度的药物，然而它们在预测为中重度或重度的 AP 中或在已确诊的坏死性胰腺炎中的预防性作用还有很大争议。大多数指南并不推荐预防性抗生素[237]。

将来需要有足够大样本量的研究来评估预防性抗生素治疗在预测为中重度或重度的 AP 中或在已确诊的坏死性胰腺炎中的益处。需要评估在特殊亚型中，使用抗生素可能的益处，如伴或不伴器官衰竭的广泛坏死等。

（七）急诊 ERCP

关于早期清除可能嵌顿的胆石能否改善胆源性胰腺炎预后的问题一直留有争议。由于结石引起的壶腹水平阻塞是急性胆源性胰腺炎的主要机制，因此适合通过 ERCP 清除结石以帮助患者康复。胆源性胰腺炎患者在胆囊切除术之前可以急诊或限期进行 ERCP。急诊 ERCP 有多种定义：24 小时、48 小时或 72 小时以内。对于轻度胆源性急性胰腺炎，标准的治疗方案是同期腹腔镜胆囊切除术，治疗前可选用 ERCP 或术中胆道造影。最近的指南建议对胆管炎患者，或由肝功能指标升高和（或）影像上提示存在胆总管结石而导致持续性胆道梗阻的患者，应在 72 小时内行急诊 ERCP[9,211]。一篇报告表明在急性胆源性胰腺炎中，如果患者有胆管炎、总血清胆红素>85. 5mmol/L（5mg/dL）、临床情况恶化（疼痛加重和白细胞数升高和生命体征恶化）或影像上明确胆总管结石，应在 24h 或 48h 内行急诊 ERCP[293]。

最近的 AGA 技术评审报道了一篇在 935 例急性胆源性胰腺炎患者中行急诊 ERCP 的 8 个 RCT 的 meta 分析[237]。这篇报道发现急性胆源性胰腺炎中行急诊 ERCP 对单器官或多器官衰竭、感染性胰周坏死、坏死性胰腺炎的出现率或死亡率并没有改善。在仅有的一项针对少量胆管炎患者的研究中指出，是否进行急诊 ERCP 并没有区别。对于胆管炎患者而言，ERCP 是标准治疗方案，最近的研究试图将这些患者排除在外。然而由于不同的研究中对胆管炎的定义多种多样，从而使阐述变得十分困难。急诊 ERCP 可以稍减少住院时间。因此可以谨慎地得出结论，在胆源性胰腺炎中急诊 ERCP 的作用可能主要是针对有胆管炎的患者。为了获取好的证据，该报告建议将来的试验应该着力于确定急诊 ERCP 在胆管炎、明确的胆源性梗阻、定义明确的推测为重度 AP 等 3 个亚组中是否有作用。

（八）营养

多年来保持患者禁食是治疗 AP 患者的原则。然而禁食会对肠道黏膜屏障产生不利影响，并促进了肠腔内细菌易位至胰腺等腔外组织，从而导致发病率和死亡率增加。因此某些中心践行了通过营养引起肠蠕动而不是通过禁食使肠静止的概念[277]。普遍观察到，大多数轻度（或间质性）胰腺炎患者在 5 天内出院。两项关于轻症患者的报道表明早期再进食能改善预后并能更早出院[294,295]。但另一方面，对 3 项研究的 meta 分析表明早期再进食延长了住院时间[296]。

一项研究解决了有关血清淀粉酶或脂肪酶水平升高是否会影响临床医生延长再进食时间的问题：116 名有 AP 的患者在临床医师决策下进食，有 21% 在再进食 250kcal/d 时出现疼痛[297]。如果血清脂肪酶水平有 3 倍以上的升高，再进食时临床复发率为 39%，而淀粉酶小于 3 倍升高的患者复发率为 16%。此外，大多数 3 倍血清脂肪酶水平升高的患者再进食时疼痛没有复发。另外一项 meta 分析报道了 2. 5 倍或更高的血清脂肪酶与经口进食不耐受有关[202]。为了明确早期进食的作用，有试验比较了不同进食方案的区别，其中包括禁食、流食、软质饮食、低脂固体饮食和完全固体饮食。研究者同样关注了胰酶正常后进食和立即开始进食的差异。

RCT 报道称轻度 AP 不用遵循标准禁食原则，可以立即开始进食[294]，即使最初就进行完全固体饮食[295]。并且其他人报道称可以进行低脂固体饮食和流食[296]，或者软质饮食和低渣流食[297]，而无须等待疼痛减轻或胰酶正常。甚至在重度 AP 中，早期少量经口进食的患者也可以显著地减少感染、干预需求、ICU 和住院时间[298]。基于 11 项 RCT，一篇 AGA 技术评审和 AGA 指南建议所有 AP 患者（轻度、中重度和重度）在可耐受时早期进食（通常在 24 小时内）[94,135]。然而若有明显的恶心呕吐或肠梗阻则需要等其减轻。

在推测为重度、确证为中重度、重度和坏死性胰腺炎、部分轻度 AP 中，TPN 的目的是让肠道休息。对 11 项 RCT 的 meta 分析表明较之于肠内或经口进食，TPN 增加了单器官或多器官衰竭和感染性坏死的风险[237]，并且 AGA 指南基于中等质量的证据给出了强推荐，如果 AP 患者不能耐受长期经口进食，肠内营养较 TPN 更优[286]。因此目前 TPN 在 AP 中的指征是针对长期不能经口进食且不能肠内营养或不耐受的患者。甚至在明确的坏死性胰腺炎或推测为重度 AP 中，已经表明可以尽快地进口进食且不需要人工营养（即肠外或肠内营养）。一些报道表明在推测为重度或明确坏死性胰腺炎中，在首个 24 小时中早期开始肠内营养可能会有益处。然而一项 RCT 认为与 3 天后按需肠内营养相比，并不支持在推测为重度 AP 的患者中尽早进食，3 天后对这类患者进行按需肠内营养更佳。通常需要 3 到 5 天来确立中重度或重度 AP 的诊断，因此在这段时间内，如果不能经口进食则可以考虑鼻胃管或鼻腔肠管喂养[299]。已经很明确鼻胃管和鼻腔肠管喂养的效果相等：对 3 项 RCT 的 meta 分析并没有显示 2 种肠内营养的形式有任何区别[237]。然而这些试验中存在许多方法学问题，并且在一项试验中所用的鼻空肠途径实际是幽门后喂养。鼻空肠喂养有许多理论优势，尤其是通过回肠制动机制（ileal brake mechanism）而给胰腺提供更多休息。因此目前指南推荐对长期不能经口进食的 AP 患者使用鼻胃管或鼻腔肠管喂养。

总而言之，无须考虑 AP 患者严重程度，只要无明显呕吐就能立即开始轻质流食。如果进食不会加重疼痛或造成呕吐，可以快速过渡到低脂饮食。对于那些 3~5 天后由于呕吐或疼痛加重而不能够耐受任何形式经口进食的患者，可通过鼻胃管给予低脂饮食；如果仍不能耐受可以给予幽门后喂养。应当避免使用 TPN。

（九）其他非介入治疗

在一项试验中提示[300]，住院期间进行单次简短的戒酒辅导比后续门诊咨询辅导更能减少总住院次数。这一方法也得到了其他研究的支持，研究表明这种咨询辅导对某些慢性酒精相关性疾病有益。另一项近期研究表明在住院期间的简短干预是不够的，尤其是在酒精使用障碍筛查量表（Alcohol Use Disorders Identification Test，AUDIT）评分显示重度酗酒和高复发率的年轻人群中[301]。一项 4 年的随访研究观察到，在住院期间进行简短戒酒辅导后急性酒精性胰腺炎的高复发率。同样，戒烟辅导也很重要。

（十）介入治疗

1. 胆囊切除术

包括急诊 ERCP（24~72 小时），胆囊切除术前胆石选择性 ERCP 以及作为最终治疗的胆囊切除术。第 61 章已经讨论了急诊 ERCP 的作用。

如果在胆源性胰腺炎发作时未行胆囊切除术，6 周内 AP 的复发率为 18%[302]。过去手术医师担心手术时的腹部炎症而不在 AP 发作时处理胆囊。然而在轻度、间质性胰腺炎患者中，胆囊切除术的经验不断积累，在最近指南中推荐对轻度和间质性胰腺炎的病例同次住院时行胆囊切除术[9,211]。这些指南同样推荐了在中重度到重度（坏死性）胰腺炎中等待和进行后续的胆囊切除术的间隔时间。这些推荐各有不同，包括从炎症减退到发作 6 周后所有的液体积聚稳定。一项最近的 RCT 将急性胆源性胰腺炎患者随机分组，并比较了 72 小时内行胆囊切除术和 25~30 天后行胆囊切除术之间的区别，发现早期手术明显减少了胰胆管的并发症和再入院，而死亡率没有区别（见之前的讨论），转为开腹胆囊切除术的概率也没有区别。对不能耐受胆囊切除术的高风险患者以及等待胆囊切除术间期的坏死性胰腺炎患者中，胆道括约肌切开术能预防 AP 进一步发作，但不能预防如胆源性疼痛和急性胆囊炎等胆源性事件。一项最近的报告观察到，被错误诊断为轻度、间质性胰腺炎而行同次住院胆囊切除术的患者，较之于年龄和性别匹配但未行同次住院胆囊切除术的坏死性胰腺炎患者而言，他们坏死性胰腺炎的后续演化有更差的结局（如感染性胰腺坏死）[303]。如果患者被诊断为急性间质性胆源性胰腺炎，并且正在评估是否进行同样的入院胆囊切除术，若是在胆囊切除术前白细胞计数升高，则应重复进行 CT 扫描以发现首次 CT 扫描未显示的坏死性胰腺炎。

2. 胰液积聚的干预治疗

通常在 2~4 周之间，胰腺液体积聚界限逐渐清晰并形成囊壁。由于此时急性胰腺（胰周）液体积聚通常已经吸收，因而持续存在且形成囊壁的通常为 WON 而非假性囊肿（图 58.6）。仅仅存在这些局部并发症并不是干预的指征。大约有三分之二的坏死性胰腺炎患者不进行任何干预也能缓解。微创引流或清创的指征已经被进一步明确，包括感染性胰腺

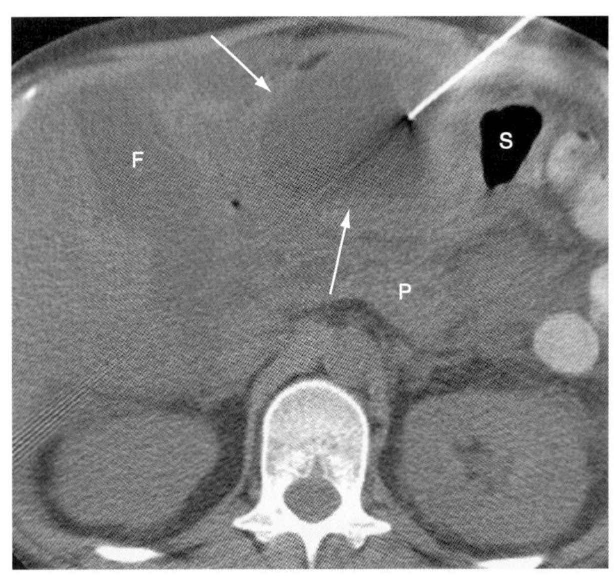

图 58.6 CT 显示包裹性胰腺坏死。可见 5.4cm 充满脓液的积液（箭），管腔内可见抽吸针尖。脓肿位于胰腺前方（P）和胃内侧（S）。存在右肝下积液（F）

(胰周)坏死、消化道或胆管梗阻、持续的不适主诉伴体重减轻和衰弱、胰管离断综合征(disconnected PD syndrome)以及如空腔脏器穿孔或瘘管等并发症。一项关于 AP 有症状假性囊肿,采取内镜引流与外科囊肿胃造口术对比的 RCT 发现,外科手术并不比内镜治疗更优。然而,内镜治疗可能使住院时间缩短、患者身心更健康和花费减少[304]。长期以来,对于有液体积聚感染迹象或临床状况恶化的患者,采用开腹坏死物清除术治疗胰腺液体积聚。随后一项 RCT 提示早期手术(2 周内)会增加死亡率和发病率[305],并且随后的建议中强调了在液体集聚形成囊壁后手术,而这通常需要约 4 周。

推荐坏死物清除术类型包括留置导管闭式持续冲洗、坏死物清除术及不冲洗闭式引流、坏死物清除术及被膜切开。较之于开放式手术坏死物清除术,大量报道更支持如经皮、腹膜后电视辅助、腹腔镜、内镜或联合方法等微创治疗,因为其产生更低的死亡率和发病率[306]。一项 RCT 展示了从经皮引流开始,随后电视辅助腹膜后引流的微创阶梯方式较之于手术坏死物清除术的优势[307]。一项 meta 分析发现虽然微创途径确实比开放式坏死物清除术有特定的优势,但一项 RCT 和 3 篇其他报告结果的异质性,提示需要更高质量的试验[308]。随后同组的另一 RCT 阐明了内镜干预比外科坏死物清除术更有优势。同一研究组最近的 RCT 比较了内镜干预和内窥镜腹膜后干预,内镜干预减少了住院时间以及如瘘管等并发症的发生,但有相似的死亡率和其他主要并发症发生率[310]。

胰管离断综合征是大量胰体坏死在近端和远端节段中断胰管的一种情况。常通过初始时胰腺中部坏死、坏死区域持续性液体积聚、同一区域 ERCP 见完全截断以及胰腺远端节段可及增强而确立该诊断。根据最初的报道,该并发症需要在液体积聚内长期猪尾导管引流(经腹或经十二指肠),最近的报道证实了这一建议[311]。最近一项包含 167 名患者的大型系列报告,较之于无离断胰管的患者,这些患者通常需要混合干预(hybrid intervention)(内镜下超声引导的多通道/双模态技术,内镜下/经皮窦道坏死物清除术)[312]。虽然自膨式金属支架能在短期内使用 3 周,但是后续的治疗应该是从胃至液体积聚的单入口或使胰性分泌物更好排出的多通道猪尾管。

在世界范围内,抽吸或清创胰腺液体积聚最常使用的微创技术是经皮引流。然而近几年内镜治疗变得非常流行。虽然腹腔镜治疗在完成操作上有优势,通常 1 次完成并且同时解决了如胆囊切除术等其他问题。但是这种方法并不被许多腹腔镜外科医师接受且关于这种方法的文献相当有限。同样还不清楚应该首选早期引流和后续清创及坏死物清除术[313-315],还是前期清创及坏死物清除以缩减治疗环节。

(十一) 其他并发症

1. 胃肠道出血

胃肠道出血可能是胰腺炎的炎症导致的(框 58.7),或者是与胰腺炎局部炎症不直接相关的损伤引起的,如消化性溃疡或食管贲门黏膜撕裂(Mallory-Weiss tear)。前者被认为是由于释放的活化酶对血管结构的刺激作用,或炎性残余或液体积聚使周围结构压迫性坏死所致。据报道,脾动脉,脾静脉或门静脉破裂,死亡率很高。[317]。使用放射性介入技术进行暂时性治疗,并随后进行更确切的外科结扎术或切除术。胰腺急性和慢性的炎症过程能够导致邻近的脾静脉形成血栓,从而导致伴或不伴食管静脉曲张的胃底静脉曲张。这些静脉曲张破裂而导致大量出血(见第 20 和 92 章)。静脉曲张破裂的治疗可以通过内镜下静脉曲张套扎或脾切除术而治愈。假性囊肿可合并假性动脉瘤形成,这通常可以在动态对比增强 CT 上(图 58.7)见到。如果出血可选择动脉造影及栓塞来治疗。假性动脉瘤在坏死性胰腺炎中出现的频率越来越高,且在消化道出血前。当发现假性动脉瘤时,在出血前对其进行治疗很重要,因为它并不具备像常规动脉一样的三层结构,所以很容易破裂。据报道,介入放射学和栓塞术取得了高度成功[318]。如果没有成功,那在进行开放性手术之前可以进行经皮凝血酶注射,尽管目前该方法很少在临床上应用。胰管出血少见,在慢性胰腺炎中更常见(见第 59 章)。坏死物清除术后出血常见,可能是因过度的清创,或血管结构旁放置或使用不顺畅的引流管,或长期使用金属支架而引起。

框 58.7　急性胰腺炎的并发症

局部性
- 假性囊肿
- 无菌性坏死(胰周,胰腺,或两者都有)
- 感染性坏死(胰周,胰腺,或两者都有)
- 脓肿
- 消化道出血
  - 胰腺炎相关
    - 脾动脉破裂或脾动脉假动脉瘤破裂
    - 脾静脉破裂
    - 门静脉破裂
    - 脾静脉血栓形成导致胃食管静脉曲张出血
    - 假性囊肿或脓肿出血
    - 坏死物清除术后出血
  - 非胰腺炎相关
    - 食管贲门黏膜撕裂
    - 酒精性胃病
    - 应激性胃黏膜病变
- 脾脏并发症
  - 梗死
  - 破裂
  - 血肿
  - 脾静脉血栓形成
- 小肠或结肠瘘管形成或梗阻
- 肾积水

系统性
- 呼吸衰竭
- 肾功能衰竭
- 休克
- 高血糖
- 高钙血症
- 弥散性血管内凝血
- 脂肪坏死(皮下结节)
- 视网膜病变
- 精神病

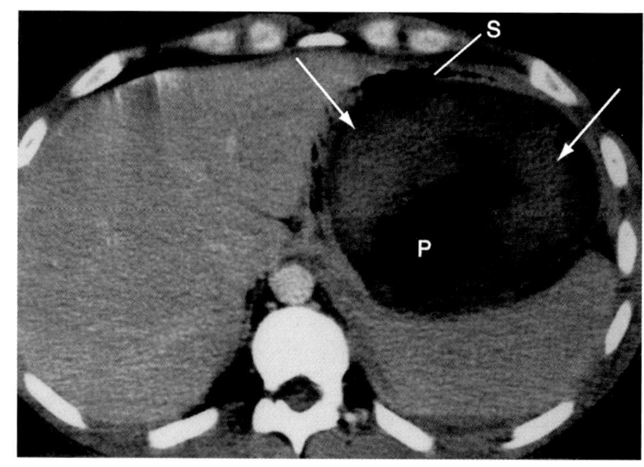

图 58.7　CT 显示胰腺假性囊肿伴急性出血。可见 10cm 胰腺假性囊肿(P),内含有高密度(CT 值 45HU)物质(箭),表示急性出血。假性囊肿压迫胃(S)。这些发现在手术时得到证实

2. 脾脏并发症

胰腺炎的脾脏并发症包括脾假性囊肿、脾静脉血栓形成、脾梗死和脾坏死、脾破裂、血肿[319]。部分并发症可能会危及生命并且需要紧急脾切除术(见框 58.7)。内脏静脉血栓形成在 AP 患者中的发生率为 1.8%[320]。如果没有出血并发症,抗凝对患者来说是安全的;如果没有潜在的高凝状态,推荐使用 3~6 个月的抗凝药[321]。

3. 肠压迫或瘘管形成

自胰尾部炎性残余的压迫性坏死能够阻塞或与小肠或大肠形成瘘管,最常见的部位是左半结肠。常为手术治疗。

(十二) 急性胰腺炎的长期后遗症

AP 发作后常见外分泌和内分泌功能不全。一项系统评价发现,在急性事件后的 12 个月内,有 15% 的 AP 患者出现了新的糖尿病发作,并且 5 年内风险达到 2 倍以上[322]。40% 新诊断的糖尿病前期或糖尿病患者在 AP 发生后出现了胰腺外分泌功能不全[323]。一项最近的 meta 分析显示 10% 的 AP 患者和 36% 的复发性 AP 患者之后会发展为慢性胰腺炎[92]。

(十三) 腹腔间隔室综合征(见第 11 章)

腹腔间隔室综合征(abdominal compartment syndrome,ACS)被定义为与器官功能不全或衰竭相关的持续腹腔内压超过 20mmHg(通过膀胱内压力记录导管证实)[324]。因为 AP 中广泛地使用大量静脉容量补充而使更多的液体渗入腹膜后,所以 ACS 的发病率可能会增加[249]。一项系统评价发现 38% 的 AP 患者出现 ACS[325],其中 11% 接受了经皮引流作为初始治疗,74% 接受了开腹减压。ACS 与 AP 的死亡率和发病率增加有关。另一篇综述认为在重度 AP 伴器官衰竭的患者中,ACS 是一种伴发现象(epiphenomenon)而不是器官衰竭的原因[326]。

(十四) 混杂并发症

胰性脑病包含 AP 患者出现的多种中枢神经系统症状,包括激惹、幻觉、意识错乱、定向障碍和昏迷。类似的综合征可能出现在酒精戒断和其他可能的病因中,如电解质紊乱(如低钠血症)或低氧血症。Purtscher 视网膜病变(散在火焰状出血伴棉绒斑)能造成暴盲[181],其被认为是由于脉络膜和视网膜动脉的微栓塞所致。

(程卓　闫秀娥 译,鲁晓岚 校)

参考文献

第 59 章　慢性胰腺炎

Chris E. Forsmark 著

章节目录

一、流行病学 …… 865
二、病理学 …… 865
三、病理生理学 …… 865
四、病因学 …… 867
（一）酒精 …… 867
（二）吸烟 …… 867
（三）热带性胰腺炎 …… 867
（四）遗传学 …… 868
（五）自身免疫性胰腺炎 …… 868
（六）梗阻 …… 872
（七）其他因素 …… 872
（八）特发性 …… 872
五、临床特征 …… 873
（一）腹痛 …… 873
（二）脂肪泻（胰腺外分泌功能不全）…… 874
（三）糖尿病（胰腺内分泌功能不全）…… 875
六、体格检查 …… 875
七、诊断 …… 875
（一）胰腺功能检测 …… 876
（二）胰腺结构检测（影像学）…… 877
八、诊断策略 …… 881
九、治疗 …… 881
（一）腹痛 …… 881
（二）消化不良和脂肪泻 …… 885
（三）糖尿病 …… 886
十、并发症 …… 886
（一）假性囊肿 …… 886
（二）消化道出血 …… 887
（三）假性动脉瘤 …… 887
（四）脾静脉血栓形成所致静脉曲张出血 …… 888
（五）胆管梗阻 …… 888
（六）十二指肠梗阻 …… 888
（七）胰瘘 …… 888
（八）恶性肿瘤 …… 889
（九）动力障碍 …… 889

慢性胰腺炎是包含了多种病因而最终出现相同表现的一种综合征。传统慢性胰腺炎的定义是基于胰腺组织学上慢性和不可逆的损伤。慢性胰腺炎的组织学特征表现为慢性炎症、纤维化以及最终导管、外分泌（腺泡细胞）及内分泌（朗格汉斯岛）的破坏（图 59.1），并产生不同程度的症状以及腺体结构和功能上的紊乱。组织学标准在临床上使用价值有限。胰腺组织对临床医师来说很难获取。一些患者可能有慢性胰腺炎的组织学证据，但是并没有这种疾病造成的症状或并发症。此外慢性胰腺炎的组织学特征通常较局限，即使可以获取小的活检也可能遗漏该疾病。最后，这种组织学特征并非独有，在其他情况下（如正常衰老、社交性饮酒、吸烟、长期存在的糖尿病等）也可见到。慢性胰腺炎同样能基于临床特征［腹痛、外分泌功能不全（脂肪泻）或内分泌功能不全（糖尿病）］或者包括超声（US）、计算机断层扫描（CT）、超声内镜（EUS）、磁共振成像（MRI）、磁共振胰胆管造影（MRCP）、内镜逆行胰胆管造影（ERCP）在内的影像学来定义。基于影像学方法来定义慢性胰腺炎也不完美，因为可能需要疾病发展多年才会出现能够通过这些方法探测到的形态学改变。在临床过程的早期，许多影像学所见可能确实是正常或接近正常的。早期诊断慢性胰腺炎，可以有一些有效疗法，但通常十分困难甚至几乎不可能[1]。依赖影像学表现的诊断标准明确了疾病存在及严重程度，综合了诊断和分级标准。这种分级系统同样会混杂所有病因，因此会掩盖影响临床医师判断的重要不同。

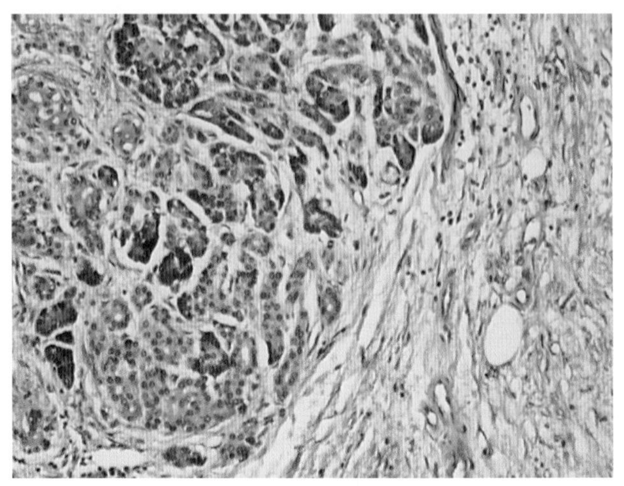

图 59.1　慢性胰腺炎的组织学表现。可见腺泡组织被破坏，代之以广泛的纤维化和相对保留的胰岛。（HE 染色）

尽管事实上许多证据表明许多患者有从急性胰腺炎到慢性胰腺炎的演化（见第 58 章），这些定义仍是进行了一种潜在的假设：急性胰腺炎和慢性胰腺炎是完全不同的两种疾病。在现代发病机制模式中，急性胰腺炎是发展为慢性胰腺炎必要的第一步。认为这 2 种情况是一类因素的不同终点可能更为准确：急性胰腺炎是一种事件，而慢性胰腺炎是不同发展速度和结局的持续过程。

考虑到病因的重要性，获取胰腺组织困难以及现有可用的诊断工具缺乏敏感性，最好将慢性胰腺炎定义为一种综合征[1,2]。这种综合征具有包括危险因素、基因背景、症状、胰腺内分泌及外分泌紊乱、影像学上的结构改变以及可能获取的组织学在内的一系列特征。不同患者中这些特征可能变化很大，且像所有综合征一样，单纯某一种特征的存在不足以进行诊断。

一、流行病学

慢性胰腺炎可以在多至 5% 的尸检中被证实[3,4]。相似但不太明显的组织学特征更为常见[5,6]。因为这些个体可能在存活时并没有慢性胰腺炎的临床症状，通过这种类型的尸检数据来确定慢性胰腺炎的患病率可能具有误导性。即使长期适量饮酒也可在没有症状及临床特征时出现慢性胰腺炎的组织学改变[7-9]。同样地，衰老、吸烟、慢性肾脏病和长期糖尿病能够造成难以与慢性胰腺炎区分的胰腺组织学改变[5,6,10]。因此单独通过组织学或尸检数据进行诊断会高估有临床意义的慢性胰腺炎发病率。

在一些回顾性研究中估计慢性胰腺炎年发病率为 5/100 000～12/100 000[11-16]。在美国，发病率大约 5/100 000～8/100 000[14,17,18]，并且似乎随时间推移在逐渐增加。慢性胰腺炎的患病率大约 50/100 000[14-20]。在大多数研究中，酒精滥用占到全部慢性胰腺炎病例的半数及以上[14]。这些流行病学数据说明地区之间存在大量差异[14,18,20]。这种发病率的差异部分是由于不同人群中饮酒量的差异，但是另一方面可能仅反映了采用不同诊断手段和标准。

慢性胰腺炎在男性中多见，且多数在中年出现，大多数患者被诊断时年龄超过 40 岁[14-17]。慢性胰腺炎耗损大量医疗支出及住院率。大约非公立医院每年有 26 000 次住院将慢性胰腺炎列为第一诊断；每年超过 80 000 次住院中将慢性胰腺炎作为出院诊断之一[14,19,21-24]。慢性胰腺炎的预后不尽相同，且常基于慢性酒精性胰腺炎患者持续酗酒或伴随吸烟史[14,17,19]。可以通过是否需要就医、住院或通过并发症发展、生存质量下降或死亡来估计其预后。

关于慢性胰腺炎患者生存质量的数据[25-30]表明存在腹痛和持续酗酒（在慢性酒精性胰腺炎患者中）的结果对生存质量产生主要的负面影响，较之于普通人群这些患者生存质量进行性下降也并不意外[30]。疼痛是生存质量下降的主要原因，并且持续的疼痛，即使比间断疼痛程度更轻，也有很大负面影响[29,30]。慢性胰腺炎患者死亡率受持续的吸烟及酗酒影响[14,17]。在一项较大的多中心研究中，标化死亡率比值为 3.6∶1（即诊断慢性胰腺炎的患者死亡的比例是年龄匹配对照的 3.6 倍），生存率在吸烟或患慢性酒精性胰腺炎的老人中有最显著的下降[31]。持续饮酒增加了额外 60% 的死亡风险。在其他研究中也观察到了死亡风险有类似比率增加[17,32]。总的来说，慢性胰腺炎患者 10 年生存率约 70%，20 年生存率约 45%。造成慢性胰腺炎患者死亡的原因通常并不是胰腺炎本身，而是伴随的其他临床情况，如吸烟、持续饮酒、胰腺癌和术后并发症[14,32]。

二、病理学

不同病因的慢性胰腺炎随着疾病的进展常有类似病理发现（见图 59.1）。这种损伤在早期慢性胰腺炎中常多变且不均匀。可以见到小叶间纤维化区域，且纤维化通常延伸至导管结构。纤维化区域可见淋巴细胞、浆细胞、巨噬细胞和肥大细胞浸润[33,34]。导管可能存在嗜酸性蛋白栓。在受影响的小叶中，纤维化包裹并替代了腺泡细胞。除非在疾病的极晚期，否则胰岛受损通常不严重。也可能见到如水肿、急性炎症和腺泡细胞或脂质坏死等急性胰腺炎表现。随着疾病进展，小叶内和小叶间的纤维化逐渐扩大。胰腺导管出现纤维化进展、狭窄形成和扩张等异常表现。导管蛋白栓可能会钙化并且阻塞主胰管。导管上皮可能变为立方形并出现萎缩或鳞状上皮化生，或者完全被纤维所取代。激活的胰腺星状细胞被认为可能和纤维化有密切关系。

大多数长期慢性胰腺炎患者中都可以发现这些组织学特征。尤其是包括小叶周围纤维化和导管化生在内的许多变化在没有慢性胰腺炎的高龄患者和长期糖尿病患者中也很常见。慢性梗阻性胰腺炎（与肿瘤或狭窄引起的主胰管梗阻有关）组织学改变略有不同，局限于梗阻上游的腺体，且蛋白质沉淀和导管内结石并不常见[34]。

自身免疫性慢性胰腺炎可表现出 2 种独特的组织学模式[35-38]。第一种模式（1 型）中可见包括浆细胞在内的大量淋巴浆细胞浸润，且免疫球蛋白 G 亚型 4（IgG4）染色通常呈阳性。影响大、小静脉的梗阻性静脉炎和旋涡（席纹状）纤维化模式也是其特征。这种特征称为淋巴浆细胞硬化性胰腺炎。1 型自身免疫性胰腺炎被认为是 IgG4 相关性疾病的一种表现[39]。第二种模式（2 型）的特征是中性粒细胞浸润，且缺少 IgG4 阳性的浆细胞，其被称作特发性导管中心性慢性胰腺炎。随着时间的推移，这种形式可能表现出更多终末期慢性胰腺炎的表现，并与其他形式的慢性胰腺炎难以区分。

三、病理生理学

慢性胰腺炎的病理生理过程尚未完全阐明。病理生理过程必须最终解释慢性胰腺炎的特征，包括实质细胞丧失，慢性炎症和纤维化的持续存在等。因此提出的任一机制必须包含对细胞坏死或凋亡、炎症细胞活化的启动和维持以及胰腺星状细胞纤维增生的解释[2]。像所有其他器官一样，胰腺对损伤的反应是有限的。并且虽然各种病因不可能都有相似的病理生理学，但最终组织学结果是相似的。关于疾病的机制研究由于人体组织难以获得以及动物模型相对缺乏而受到影响[40]。

关于酒精性慢性胰腺炎的研究最为广泛[41-44]。没有一种理论能充分解释为什么重度酗酒者中只有不到 5% 的人患慢性胰腺炎。基因差异可能确实起到重要作用（第 57 章）。酒精经肝脏和胰腺代谢。在肝脏中酒精氧化代谢的主要最终产物是乙醛。胰腺中通过另一种途径产生脂肪酸乙醇酯（fatty acid ethanol ester,FAEE)。酒精及 FAEE 之类的代谢物对胰腺腺泡细胞有直接的损伤作用。在动物模型和人类慢性酒精性胰腺炎中,可以见到氧化应激和标志自由基产生的膜脂质过氧化增加。此外,FAEE 能够诱导腺泡细胞中胞质内钙持续升高,而该机制在胰腺炎的其他实验性病因中也存在[40]。酒精也可能导致腺泡细胞对胆囊收缩素(cholecystokinin,CCK)等生理刺激[40]或吸烟等病理暴露[45,46]的敏感性增加。吸烟和饮酒的相互作用是日益认识到的慢性胰腺炎危险因素[14,45]。动物模型中慢性酒精摄入也会让腺泡细胞对生理应激敏感性增加,或上调参与细胞死亡的酶的表达和多种活性基因的表达。酒精能促进胰腺炎引起的炎症反应[41,42]。除酒精对腺泡细胞的这些多重影响外,还有酒精对导管细胞的损伤。最后,酒精及其代谢产物似乎能刺激胰腺星状细胞[41,45,47-49]。这些细胞如在肝脏中一样,似乎是纤维化的最终共同途径[48,49]。

胰腺星状细胞被发现与腺泡相关。通常可在腺泡周围发现,并有较长的细胞质突起并延伸到腺泡细胞,但也有少量存在于血管和导管中。可通过细胞质中存在维生素 A 脂滴来识别静止的胰腺星状细胞。它们在活化时呈星状或肌纤维母细胞外观,并表达平滑肌肌动蛋白及丢失脂滴。这种活化对于细胞开始分泌细胞外基质并在腺体内产生纤维化是必要的。胰腺星状细胞的活化可由酒精或其代谢产物之一引起,但也可由胰腺腺泡细胞坏死后释放的炎性细胞因子和活性氧引起[47-49]。此外,生长因子(血小板源性生长因子、转化生长因子-β1)、激素、细胞内信号分子、转录因子、血管紧张素Ⅱ等均可激活胰腺星状细胞。在人类和动物组织中都在急性胰腺炎的广泛坏死和炎症区域中发现活化的胰腺星状细胞。这些活化的胰腺星状细胞产生维持活化的自分泌因子。除了在细胞外基质的分泌和调节中发挥作用外,胰脏星状细胞还可以对刺激产生反应而增殖,迁移到炎症区域,并参与吞噬作用。在酒精性(和其他形式)慢性胰腺炎中,可能通过多种机制产生胰腺星状细胞的活化。

慢性饮酒还可能通过其他机制造成慢性胰腺炎。长期饮酒导致胰液富含蛋白质而体积小、碳酸氢盐量少。这些特征有利于在慢性酒精性胰腺炎演变早期就存在蛋白质沉淀的形成。这些沉淀可能会钙化,进而导致胰管结石的形成,进一步对结石上游的导管和实质造成损伤。然而在大多数患者中,这些蛋白质沉淀和导管结石似乎不会引起最初的胰腺损伤,但可能会促进疾病进展。

有几种关于慢性胰腺炎的病理生理学假设试图将这些观察结果组合成连贯的模型。一种假说认为导管阻塞(狭窄或结石引起)是慢性胰腺炎的病因而不是结果。这种导管梗阻假设与大多数临床和实验证据不一致,且人类的慢性胰腺炎也有一些例外(如慢性阻塞性胰腺炎等罕见情况)。第二种模型,毒性代谢假说主要关注酒精及其代谢物(吸烟或其他毒素)的作用以及它们破坏胰腺和活化胰腺星状细胞的能力。第三种提出的模型是坏死-纤维化假说,该假说认为伴有细胞坏死或凋亡的反复或严重的急性胰腺炎发生后,以纤维化取代坏死组织的愈合过程最终导致了慢性胰腺炎的发展。最后一个假设的重要支持证据来自一些自然病程的研究,这些研究表明酒精性胰腺炎急性发作更严重和更频繁的患者更常发展为慢性胰腺炎[50-53]。通过对人类和动物模型的观察进一步夯实了急性胰腺炎的多次临床或亚临床发作可导致慢性胰腺炎的这一概念[1,2]。

尚不清楚为何只有小部分(<5%)的长期酗酒者会发展为慢性胰腺炎。许多可能的解释包括存在重要的共毒素,遗传或表观遗传背景差异,或胰腺微环境差异。吸烟是慢性酒精性胰腺炎发生的一个非常重要的辅助因子[1,2,14,54-60]。慢性酒精性胰腺炎发病率也存在难以解释的种族差异[13,61,62]。几种形式的慢性胰腺炎中发现了多种突变,提示复杂的遗传背景造成了对慢性胰腺炎的相对易感性(见第 57 章)。已经识别出囊性纤维化跨膜传导调节因子(*CFTR*)、阳离子胰蛋白酶原基因(*PRSS1* 基因)、丝氨酸蛋白酶抑制剂 Kazal 1 型(*SPINK1*,一种胰蛋白酶抑制剂)、糜蛋白酶 C、钙敏感受体基因、羧肽酶 A-1(*CPA1*)、羧基酯脂肪酶、claudin-2(*CLDN2/MORC*)和其他多种基因的突变[63]。这些突变和更多有待鉴定的突变本身可能足以产生胰腺炎(目前只有 *PRSS1* 满足这一要求)或者可能只会诱发疾病。在第 57 章详细讨论了这些突变,在这里将其作为目前发病机制模型的基础可能有所帮助。这一方式的概念为复杂的遗传背景提供了对疾病的易感性[1,2,64,65]。这种遗传背景可能包括编码消化酶、蛋白酶-酶抑制剂、离子通道、紧密连接蛋白的基因突变,其他各种影响环境毒素的代谢(如烟草、酒精)基因突变,在炎症或纤维化作用的基因,以及其他未发现的基因。只有一种突变(在遗传性胰腺炎家系中的 *PRSS1* 功能获得突变)足以在大多数或所有携带它的人群中引起胰腺损伤,但即使这样也会导致疾病严重程度不同。发现的大多数突变主要是造成了疾病的易感性[63]。在这种复杂的多基因背景下覆盖了一些环境因素,如长期饮酒、吸烟,或一些导致胰腺炎初发的因素(如胆结石、高甘油三酯血症)。它们增加了腺泡、导管和星状细胞的生理应激。这种压力可能不足以造成损伤,但也可能造成细胞损伤、坏死或凋亡。坏死的初发事件可能是腺泡细胞内消化酶的过早激活,或环境因素的毒性作用,也可能是其他潜在病因。坏死之后出现炎症,这种坏死-炎症过程可能会继续进展或消退。这一事件本质上是急性胰腺炎的发作,但它可能有或没有症状。对部分人而言进展可能永远不会超过这个阶段且逐渐缓解。在另一部分人群中,持续的细胞代谢和氧化应激(二次打击)或其他一些触发因素可导致腺泡和导管细胞持续或反复地损伤并伴有坏死。而这解释了反复发作急性胰腺炎人群患慢性胰腺炎的风险较高[66]。与肝脏相同,这一过程与星状细胞的活化和细胞外基质的产生有关,最终形成纤维化。纤维化可能通过引起额外的腺泡细胞缺血并继续推动这一过程而开始恶性循环。这种假设在理论上可以解释多种形式的慢性胰腺炎。这种构架似乎符合不断发表的实验和临床数据。并且是一种有用的慢性胰腺炎的病理生理学思路:一种与不同基因易感性、多种疾病诱因、多种中间修饰因子相关的疾病,以及造成胰腺损伤和纤维化的相似的最后共同通路,而最终伴器官衰竭。这些基因易感性、环境因子和修饰因子对疾病的发展既不是必要的也不是必需的,但是在患者个体中促进了疾病发展[67]。

四、病因学(框 59.1)

(一) 酒精

框 59.1　慢性胰腺炎的病因分类

毒物代谢性	IgG4 相关性系统疾病,2 型
酒精	**复发性和急性重症胰腺炎**
烟草	坏死后(重症坏死性胰腺炎后)
高钙血症	血管性疾病/缺血
高甘油三酯血症	**梗阻**
慢性肾衰	良性胰管梗阻
特发性	创伤性狭窄
热带性钙化性胰腺炎	急性重症胰腺炎后狭窄
胰腺纤维钙化性糖尿病	壶腹部梗阻
早发特发性	Oddi 括约肌狭窄
迟发特发性	乳糜泻
基因性	克罗恩病
常染色体显性	恶性胰管梗阻
遗传性胰腺炎(*PRSS1* 突变)	壶腹部癌
常染色体隐性或修饰基因	十二指肠癌
CFTR 突变	胰腺导管腺癌
SPINK1 突变	导管内乳头状黏液瘤
糜蛋白酶 C 突变	**无症状胰腺纤维化**
Claudin 突变	长期饮酒
钙敏感受体基因	衰老
羧基酯脂肪酶	慢性肾脏病
其他	糖尿病
自身免疫性胰腺炎	放疗病史
IgG4 相关性系统疾病,1 型	

Ig,免疫球蛋白 G;PRSS1,阳离子胰蛋白酶原基因;SPINK,丝氨酸蛋白酶抑制剂 Kazal 1 型基因。

在西方国家,酒精至少是 50% 慢性胰腺炎的病因[14,16,45,59,60,68-71]。慢性酒精性胰腺炎的风险随着饮酒量增加呈对数增长,并且没有不发生疾病的最低阈值[14,45]。酒精约占慢性胰腺炎归因风险的 40%,并且酒精似乎增加了其他慢性胰腺炎病因造成胰腺损伤的风险[14,66,71]。在普遍饮酒的国家可能很难确定是否酒精确实导致了疾病。在几乎所有慢性酒精性胰腺炎患者中,在发展为慢性胰腺炎之前至少需要 5 年(大多数患者超过 10 年)每天摄入超过 4~5 杯酒[14,59,60]。一些研究表明,适量饮酒实际上可能有保护作用[60]。男性比女性更容易患慢性酒精性胰腺炎,可能是由于饮酒更多或其他基因因素[63]。只有 2% 到 5% 的酗酒者最终发展为慢性胰腺炎,这表明有其他重要的辅助因素[14,45]。潜在的辅助因素包括基因多态性和突变[63,72],高脂和高蛋白质饮食[73,74],饮酒类型或摄入方式[14,74-76],相关抗氧化剂或微量元素的相对缺乏[77,78]和吸烟[14,55-60,79,80]。其中吸烟可能有最强关联。在一些研究中,90% 的慢性酒精性胰腺炎患者同时也是长期吸烟者[14,57-60,79,80]。吸烟似乎也容易使胰腺钙化快速进展[81,82]。发生酒精性胰腺炎的风险也存在种族差异,这表明可能在环境毒素或酒精的解毒能力或其他遗传或表观遗传因素的上存在一定差异。虽然慢性酒精性胰腺炎风险在黑人中较高,但自述式调查的数据表明饮酒或吸烟的黑人的比例与白种人相似[14,61,62]。

许多酒精引起的慢性胰腺炎患者早期可能有持续 5~6 年的急性胰腺炎反复发作,随后发展为慢性疼痛或外分泌或内分泌功能不全[66]。基于几项关于自然病程的大型研究,认为大多数首次发作急性酒精性胰腺炎的患者已有组织学上的慢性胰腺炎。然而即使随访时间很长,高达 40% 的急性酒精性胰腺炎患者不会发展为临床上可识别的慢性胰腺炎(钙化和外分泌或内分泌功能不全),且可能不会复发[14,73,75,83-86]。虽然他们可能没有发展成可识别的慢性临床疾病,但基于尸检研究和功能研究[87]而言,这些患者很可能有慢性胰腺炎的组织学证据。尽管一些研究表明,疾病可能会在停止饮酒后不久发作[60,76,89],但大量饮酒似乎与急性发作没有关联[88]。

并非所有慢性酒精性胰腺炎患者都有胰腺炎急性发作。少于 10% 的患者在没有腹痛的情况下出现外分泌或内分泌功能不全[14,68-70]。一些表现为慢性疼痛的患者并无前驱急性疼痛发作。酒精性胰腺炎发作后戒酒虽然不能阻止外分泌不全和内分泌不全的进展,但可以减缓其速度[14]。未发展为明显慢性胰腺炎的患者停止饮酒似乎确实能减少其急性酒精性胰腺炎复发的可能[85]。

慢性酒精性胰腺炎的预后相对较差,且死亡率通常高于其他病因的慢性胰腺炎[14,17,31,32]。生活质量也大幅下降。虽然疼痛通常会持续数年之后自动缓解。许多患者可能在数年后出现外分泌和/或内分泌功能不全。在一项大型自然病程研究中,48% 的患者发病后出现外分泌功能不全,中位数为 13.1 年,而 38% 的患者在发病后出现内分泌功能不全,中位数为 19.8 年[69]。59% 的患者在诊断后发生弥漫性胰腺钙化,中位数 8.7 年。其他研究发现钙化、外分泌和内分泌功能不全的发展更为迅速和频繁[68]。

(二) 吸烟

暴露在烟草烟雾中会引起动物胰腺的损伤[40,46]。每天一包以上的吸烟者有 3 倍以上的患病风险[14,54-60]。吸烟可能占到慢性胰腺炎归因风险的 25%,并且对同时饮酒的人尤其有害[14,58,60,79,80]。吸烟在慢性酒精性胰腺炎患者中很常见,且与胰腺钙化风险增加有关,慢性胰腺炎临床发作后戒烟可降低后续钙化的风险[14,54,59,60,81,82,90]。强有力的证据已经表明吸烟是慢性胰腺炎的一个独立危险因素[14-18,57-60]。吸烟也与慢性胰腺炎患者更容易继发胰腺癌以及总死亡率升高有关[14-18,31,32]。

(三) 热带性胰腺炎

尽管其发病率正在下降,热带性胰腺炎仍是印度西南部某些地区较常见的慢性胰腺炎形式之一。在非洲、东南亚和巴西等其他地区也有少量报道。热带性胰腺炎通常是一种少年和青年疾病,平均发病年龄为 24 岁[91-96]。超过 90% 的患者在 40 岁前发病。在流行地区(印度南部)调查的总体流行率为 1/500~1/800[93]。在印度南部,过去热带性胰腺炎约占慢性胰腺炎的 70%,而酒精则是北部更主要的原因。最近有报道指出热带胰腺炎有向发病年龄增大、营养不良较轻,和糖尿病不太严重等转变的趋势[94-96]。最近的综述也指出酒精和吸烟正在逐渐成为印度慢性胰腺炎的最常见原因[94-96]。

热带性胰腺炎的典型表现为腹痛、严重营养不良和外分泌或内分泌功能不全。一个显著的特征是糖尿病倾向,并且内分泌功能不足似乎是慢性热带性胰腺炎(通常被归类为糖尿病特殊病因,称作胰腺纤维钙化性糖尿病)不可避免的后果。外分泌功能不全也很常见。90% 以上的患者会出现巨大胰腺结石,其病理特征是巨大的导管内结石伴明显的主胰扩张及腺体萎缩。

热带性胰腺炎的病理生理学机制尚不清楚,但最近的分析指出其有很强的基因成分,*SPINK1*、*CFTR*、*CTRC* 和 *CLDN2/MORC* 突变最常见[97-99]。已提出的疾病环境诱因包括蛋白质-热能营养不良、微量元素和微量营养素缺乏伴有氧化应激(通过外源性生物制剂、工业污染物、饮食或营养缺乏)、存在于木薯(树薯——一种主要的饮食组成)中的氰苷、病毒和寄生虫感染以及其他因素。

(四) 遗传学

只有一种突变确定引起慢性胰腺炎:遗传性胰腺炎家系中的 *PRSS1* 突变[63,64,67,98]。所有其他已识别的突变(第 57 章讨论)和基因多态性应被认为是辅助因素,如增加对环境毒素的易感性的突变或者增加疾病进展速度或严重程度的修饰基因。多态性和突变共同作用决定了对疾病的易感性。已明确的最常见的突变包括 *PRSS1*(阳离子胰蛋白酶原)、*SPINK1*(胰蛋白酶抑制剂)和 *CFTR* 基因,不太常见的突变包括糜蛋白酶 C、*CPA1*、羧基酯脂肪酶和 claudin-2(*CLDN2/MORC*)。一些研究表明,某些不太严重的 *CFTR* 基因突变和 *SPINK1* 突变可能与“特发性”慢性胰腺炎有关。在多达一半的特发性慢性胰腺炎患者中发现了 *CFTR* 基因突变[63,100],这远高于该人群中的预期比例。对这些数据的分析表明,一条染色体上较严重的 CFTR 突变与另一条染色体上较轻微的 *CFTR* 突变的组合与慢性胰腺炎尤其相关(见第 57 章)。这些突变引起或促进慢性胰腺炎的机制有几种潜在途径[101,102],包括导致腺泡细胞内消化酶(如 PRSS1,SPINK1)活化的胰蛋白酶依赖途径;由于液体和碳酸氢盐流动性不足造成导管梗阻(如 CFTR);蛋白质错误折叠导致内质网应激(如 CPA1)。对这些突变和其他突变基因已有商业化基因检测。

(五) 自身免疫性胰腺炎

自身免疫性胰腺炎(autoimmune pancreatitis,AIP)是指对类固醇治疗有反应的两种不同的(框 59.2)胰腺慢性炎症和纤维化疾病[35-39,103,104]。1 型 AIP 患者的胰腺有包括浆细胞和 CD4 阳性 T 细胞等免疫细胞密集浸润。在 1 型 AIP 中,有许多浆细胞(图 59.2A)表面表达 IgG4。许多 1 型 AIP 患者中也能看到血清 IgG4 水平升高。IgG4 不能交联抗原且不能激活经典补体级联反应,也一直没有明确 IgG4 的特异性靶点。尚不明确 IgG4 是否参与了疾病的发病机制,并且有资料提示它可能在 AIP 及相类似情况的 IgG4 相关性疾病的患者中具有抗炎作用[105]。实验证据表明存在含有体液免疫和细胞免疫的复杂机制[35,39,103]。在胰腺中可见到纤维化、硬化和闭塞性静脉炎等特征,并且和 1 型 AIP 的致密慢性炎症浸润有关[35-38]。虽然这种炎性浸润见于胰腺,但类似的浸润也见于胆管、唾液腺、腹膜后、淋巴结、肾、前列腺、壶腹和一些偶发器官[39,103,106-108]。活检标本中每高倍视野见到超过 10 个 IgG4 阳性浆细胞则支持 1 型 AIP 诊断[36-38,103,108],但该数量基于活检组织会有所变化。纤维化通常呈席纹状,或类似车轮辐条的回旋状,致密炎细胞浸润闭塞静脉通路。这种模式被称作淋巴浆细胞坏死性胰腺炎。

框 59.2 1 型和 2 型自身免疫性胰腺炎的特征

特征	1 型 AIP	2 型 AIP
组织学	淋巴浆细胞浸润	导管周围淋巴浆细胞及中性粒细胞浸润
	导管周围致密浸润且导管上皮无损伤	中性粒细胞破坏导管上皮(粒细胞性上皮损伤)
	席纹状纤维化	少见闭塞性静脉炎
	闭塞性静脉炎	无 IgG4 阳性细胞
	大量(>10 个/HPF)IgG4 阳性细胞	
	纤维炎性过程可能延展至胰周区域	
平均发病年龄	60~70 岁	40~50 岁,但年轻人和儿童也可发病
性别优势	男性	相等
常见临床表现	梗阻性黄疸(75%)	梗阻性黄疸(50%)
	急性胰腺炎(15%)	急性胰腺炎(33%)
胰腺影像学	胰腺弥漫性肿大(40%)	胰腺弥漫性肿大(15%)
	胰腺局灶性肿大(60%)	胰腺局灶性肿大(85%)
IgG4	血清中升高(约 2/3 患者)	不相关
	受累组织中染色阳性	
其他器官受累	胆道狭窄	不相关
	涎腺炎	
	腹膜后纤维化	
	假瘤	
	肾	
	肺	
	其他	
伴随疾病		炎症性肠病
长期预后	常复发	少见或不复发

AIP,自身免疫性胰腺炎;HPF,高倍视野;Ig,免疫球蛋白 G。

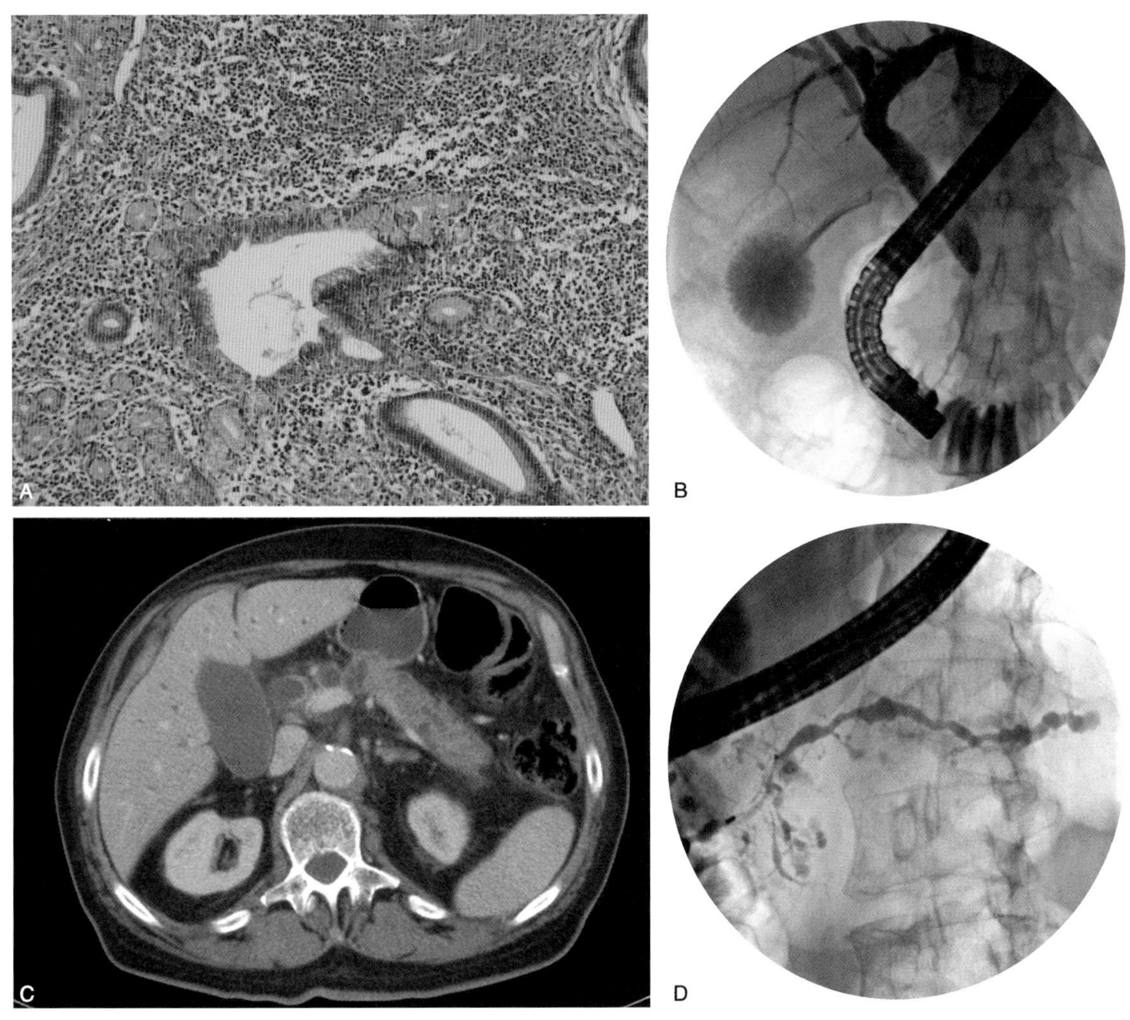

图 59.2　自身免疫性胰腺炎。A，胰腺切除标本的组织病理学显示累及较大胰管的淋巴浆细胞浸润（苏木精伊红染色）。B，胆管造影显示累及胆管胰腺内部分的光滑性狭窄。C，CT 显示胰管扩张，无胰腺实质萎缩。D，胰腺造影：显示胰管中度扩张，呈弥漫性不规则区，狭窄、扩张交替区。胰头有一个更明显的狭窄区域。（C. Mel Wilcox，MD，Birmingham，AL.）

虽然 1 型 AIP 可能表现为胰腺单独受累，但更常伴随胰腺外表现，出现这种情况被称作 IgG4 相关性疾病（图 59.2 和图 59.3）[39,103,106-108]。已明确的最常见胰腺外表现包括胆管狭窄、肺门淋巴结病、硬化性涎腺炎、腹膜后纤维化和肾小管间质性肾炎[107,108]。这些器官的组织活检会表现出类似的富含 IgG4 阳性浆细胞的炎性浸润。至少 60% 的 1 型 AIP 患者可能在胰腺病变之前、之后或同时出现其他器官受累[103,107,108]。Mikulicz 综合征（涎腺和泪腺中可见大量 IgG4 阳性单核细胞浸润），Küttner 瘤（颌下腺）、Riedel 甲状腺炎、嗜酸性血管中心纤维化（眼眶和上呼吸道）、多灶性纤维硬化病、炎性假瘤及纵隔和腹膜后纤维化，以及主动脉周围炎、炎性主动脉瘤、特发性小管间质性肾炎等大量疾病，已经被归为 IgG4 相关性疾病的临床表现[39,106-108]。

第二种类型以一种名为特发性导管中心性胰腺炎的不同组织学模式为特征，称为 2 型 AIP。尽管 2 型 AIP 在西方国家更为常见，但也不如 1 型常见，占所有 AIP 病例的不到 20%[103]。2 型 AIP 表现为胰腺伴微脓肿的中性粒细胞浸润（粒细胞-上皮性病变），闭塞性静脉炎罕见（表 59.1）[36,37]。2 型 AIP 局限于胰腺，与胰腺中 IgG4 阳性浆细胞浸润无关，也与血清中 IgG4 水平升高无关。然而，2 型 AIP 可能与潜在的炎症性肠病相关（15%～30% 的 2 型 AIP 患者）。

1 型 AIP 多见于男性（2∶1），且通常中年或更大年龄起病[39,103]。超过 85% 的患者在 50 岁以后起病，平均发病年龄为 70 岁。2 型 AIP 在更年轻的时候起病，甚至可能在青年和儿童中发病。这两种类型的 AIP 最常见的初始表现是由于胰内胆管梗阻造成的无痛性梗阻性黄疸（见图 59.2B）。胰腺增大压迫胆管或胆道浸润（IgG4 胆管炎）均可造成黄疸。一种较不常见的初始表现是急性胰腺炎，但这是 2 型 AIP 中最常见的类型。其他症状可能包括体重减轻、呕吐和葡萄糖不耐受。虽然疼痛少见，但可能出现腹痛和背部放射痛。这些临床特征加上影像学检查显示弥漫性或局灶性胰腺肿大（见图 59.2C），常常被怀疑为胰腺癌。在对怀疑胰腺癌而接受胰腺切除术，但切除标本中未发现恶性肿瘤患者的研究中，有多达 10% 显示有 AIP 的证据[109,110]。在 1 型 AIP 中，也可能由于胆道近端狭窄发生黄疸或胆汁淤积：易累及肝门区的类型则类似原发性硬化性胆管炎（PSC）的表现。这种模式不仅与 PSC 相似，也与胆管癌相似。与典型 PSC 不同，这种疾病通常与炎症性肠病无关且对激素敏感。1 型 AIP 常见的其他临床

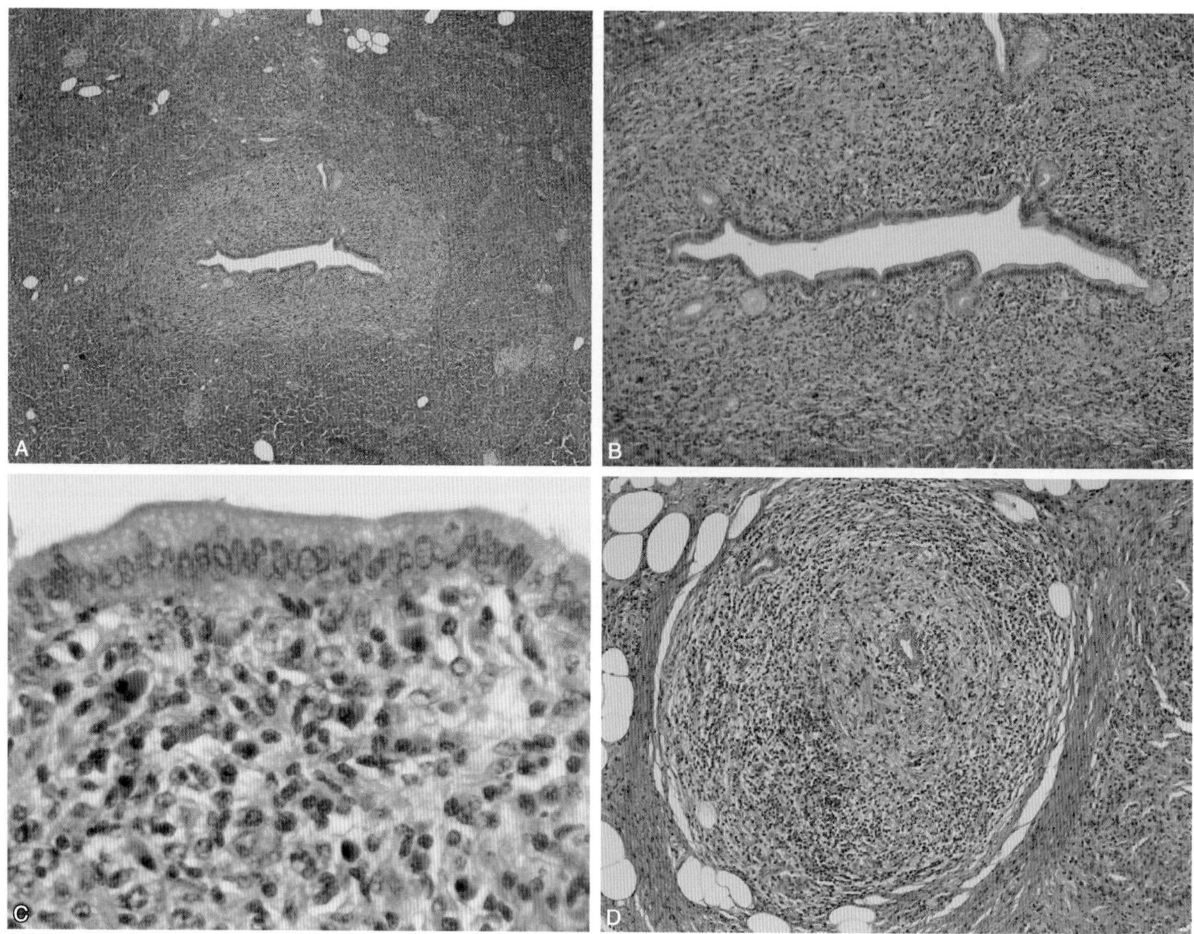

图 59.3 淋巴浆细胞硬化性胰腺炎，是自身免疫性胰腺炎中最常见的一种。A，袖套样导管周围淋巴浆细胞浸润，周围胰腺实质正常(HE 染色，×20)。B，导管周围浸润明显(HE 染色，×200)。C，胆管周围富含浆细胞的混合浸润(HE 染色，×200)。D，另一例袖套样浸润伴导管周围纤维化(HE 染色，×20)。(Courtesy Dr. Pamela Jensen, Dallas, TX.)

表 59.1 1 型自身免疫性胰腺炎的国际共识诊断标准

标准	1 级证据	2 级证据
P：胰腺实质影像(parenchymal imaging)	典型影像：胰腺弥漫肿大伴延迟强化 伴或不伴胰腺环状强化	不确定影像：节段或局灶增强伴延迟强化
D：导管影像(ductal imaging)(ERCP 或 MRCP)	长狭窄(大于胰管长度的 1/2)，或不伴上游胰管扩张的多个狭窄	节段或局灶胰管狭窄，不伴显著的(>5mm)上游胰管扩张
S：血清学(serology)	IgG4>2 倍正常值上限	IgG4 1~2 倍正常值上限
OOI：其他器官受累(other organ involvement)	胰腺外器官受累的组织学证据(至少下列 4 条中的 3 条) 显著的淋巴浆细胞浸润伴纤维化 席纹状纤维化 闭塞性静脉炎 大量 IgG4 阳性细胞 或 胰腺外器官受累的影像学证据(任一) 节段或多个近端或近端及远端胆管狭窄 腹膜后纤维化	胰腺外器官受累的组织学证据，包括胆管或壶腹部活检 显著的淋巴浆细胞浸润和大量 IgG4 阳性细胞 或 体检或影像学证据 涎腺或泪腺对称性增大 与 AIP 一致的肾脏受累
H：胰腺组织学(histology of pancreas)	组织活检或切除标本中的淋巴浆细胞性硬化性胰腺炎(至少 3 条) 不伴粒细胞的导管旁淋巴浆细胞浸润 闭塞性静脉炎 席纹状纤维化 大量(>10 个/HPF)IgG4 阳性细胞	组织活检中的淋巴浆细胞性硬化性胰腺炎(至少 2 条) 不伴粒细胞的导管旁淋巴浆细胞浸润 闭塞性静脉炎 席纹状纤维化 大量(>10 个/HPF)IgG4 阳性细胞
Rt：激素反应(response to steroids)	快速(2 周)影像学可见的缓解或胰腺/胰外表现显著改善	

表 59.1　1 型自身免疫性胰腺炎的国际共识诊断标准(续)

诊断	诊断主要基础	影像学证据	间接证据
确诊 1 型 AIP	组织学	典型/不确定	
	影像学	典型	除 D 以外任一 1 级/2 级证据
		不确定	2 个及以上 1 级证据
	激素反应	不确定	1 级 S/OOI 或 1 级 D+2 级 S/OOI/H
可能 1 型 AIP		不确定	2 级 S/OOI/H+Rt

2 型 AIP 诊断需要典型影像学表现及组织学证实或共存炎症性肠病,并且激素治疗有效。

AIP,自身免疫性胰腺炎;HPF,高倍视野;IgG4,免疫球蛋白 G 亚型 4。

From Chari ST, Kloeppel G, Zhang L, et al. Histopathologic and clinical subtypes of autoimmune pancreatitis: the Honolulu consensus document. Pancreatology 2010;10:664-72; Shimosegawa T, Chari ST, Frulloni L, et al. International consensus diagnostic criteria for autoimmune pancreatitis: Guidelines of the International Association of Pancreatology. Pancreatology 2011;40:352-8.

表现包括硬化性涎腺炎(通常表现为双边对称的唾液腺肿胀),腹膜后纤维化(最常表现为输尿管被压迫所致的肾盂积水),肾脏占位,小管间质性肾炎,淋巴结病(尤其是纵隔、颈部和腹部),前列腺炎、硬化性胆囊炎,间质性肺炎和肝、肺、前列腺和垂体的假瘤[103,108]。

1 型和 2 型 AIP 胰腺的影像学特征相似。腹部 US 通常显示胰腺弥漫性增大、低回声。EUS 上表现类似。CT 最常见的表现为弥漫增大的腊肠样胰腺(见图 59.2C),造影剂延迟和时间延长[35,38,103,109,111]。一些患者在延迟相中胰腺周围可能出现囊样低密度边缘,也可能有类似于胰腺肿块的局灶性肿大。如连续延伸至腹膜后或腹膜后血管周围的纤维化和炎症等其他 CT 表现也可能被怀疑是癌症。胰腺 MRI 也可能表现为弥漫性胰腺肿大,典型的表现是 T1 加权信号减弱而 T2 加权信号增强[103,111]。MRCP 对识别胆道梗阻和可视化 AIP 中可能的异常胰管很有帮助[38,108,111,112]。EUS 可表现为弥漫性增大的低回声腺体[113]。对腺体使用 EUS 引导的细针穿刺通常没有诊断价值[114],尽管有通过 EUS 引导的组织活检进行诊断的病例报道[115]。

两种类型 AIP 的特征之一是弥漫性或节段性胰管不规则和狭窄(见图 59.2D)。导管可能呈弥漫性狭窄和线状,也可为导管的狭窄部分和正常或扩张部分交替出现[38,103,111,116]。MRCP 通常能够识别胰管异常,但如果胰管呈线状并弥漫受累的话可能无法显示胰管。ERCP 能更好地显示胰管[116],但与 MRCP 相比 ERCP 的风险和成本更高。一些患者可能有更局限的节段性或孤立性胰管狭窄,这种模式更倾向于恶性。关于行二次 ERCP 的一些研究表明,在没有糖皮质激素治疗时存在从节段性进展为弥漫性病变。随着时间的推移,尤其是对于未经治疗或复发的患者,疾病可能会最终停止并导致胰腺萎缩和钙化。此时与其他形式的慢性胰腺炎无法区分。日本的研究指出,在所有评估为慢性胰腺炎的患者中高达 6%患有 AIP,总体患病率估计为 4.6/100 000[39,117],几乎没有其他的流行病学估计。

通常根据临床和影像学特征考虑该病。在一半到三分之二 1 型 AIP 病例中,实验室评估可有以 IgG4 为主的血清免疫球蛋白升高。虽然有各种使用的临界值,目前的共识和诊断指南以 IgG4 水平超过正常上限的 2 倍为参考[38,103]。血清 IgG4 升高并非 AIP 特异性的,也偶在胰腺癌患者中见到。也已报道了包括抗核抗体、抗乳铁蛋白抗体、抗碳酸酐酶Ⅱ抗体、抗平滑肌抗体、类风湿因子和抗线粒体抗体在内的其他多种自身抗体。这些自身抗体不如 IgG4 敏感,因此在诊断方面效果较差。在 2 型 AIP 患者中缺少这些血清学标志物。

存在几种 1 型 AIP 的诊断系统。一次国际共识会议制定了目前在全世界广泛使用的标准[38]。提出的国际共识标准见表 59.1。其使用包括胰腺和胰管影像,血清学,其他器官受累,组织学(如果可行),和激素试验反应在内的 5 个标准。该系统可根据现有标准的组合,将患者分为确诊或可能的 1 型 AIP。值得注意的是,1 型 AIP 可以在不需要胰腺活检的情况下得到相对准确的诊断,而 2 型 AIP 的诊断几乎总是需要的胰腺活检或切除。因为胰腺癌远比 AIP 常见,AIP 的准确诊断与胰腺癌相鉴别特别重要[109,110,118-120]。恶性肿瘤的特征性表现包括胰管扩张,单部位胰管高度狭窄伴腺体上游萎缩,或 CT 影像上低密度局灶性肿块。不幸的是,这些影像学特征并不是高度敏感和特异的,要区分 AIP 和胰腺癌可能需要胰腺组织活检、激素试验或胰腺切除术。在开始糖皮质激素治疗试验之前,应努力除外恶性肿瘤。但在某些情况下并不可能,潜在恶性肿瘤的可能性仍然存在。典型情况可能是中年男性存在梗阻性黄疸伴胰头肿大,ERCP 和 EUS 的组织取样尚不能确定。这种情况下,糖皮质激素治疗试验可能和延误恶性肿瘤的最终诊断有关。然而,糖皮质激素治疗作用通常在 2~4 周内明显,并且如果随访密切,这样的试验也是合理的。

慢性自身免疫性胰腺炎可在几个月内迅速进展,从最初症状发展到终末期慢性胰腺炎。有证据表明早期糖皮质激素治疗可以预防后续的并发症[103,121]。糖皮质激素治疗通常会有相当显著的改善,症状和影像学异常都能迅速缓解。尽管推荐 0.6~1mg/kg,糖皮质激素的剂量并没有明确建议[103,108,121]。最常见的起始剂量是每天 40mg 泼尼松。应审慎地在 2~4 周时重复胰腺成像,以评估临床和影像学反应。一旦疗效明确(通常在 4 周后),通常以每周 5~10mg 的速度逐渐减少泼尼松的剂量,并且总治疗时间为 10~12 周。尽管在 4 周内可以见到下降,但在数月内可能不会出现完全的血清学反应(血清 IgG4 正常)。30%~50%的 1 型 AIP 患者在糖皮质激素治疗后复发[103,121]。复发通常包括复发性胆道梗阻伴胆汁淤积性肝酶指标升高或明显黄疸。如果有的话,2 型 AIP 患者很少复发。1 型 AIP 的复发可以通过重复糖皮质激素治疗,然后通过低剂量(例如,5~10mg/d)维持泼尼松来控制。

硫唑嘌呤等免疫调节剂已被用于激素依赖患者以减少和

停止激素的使用，并取得了不同程度的成功[121]。对于使用硫唑嘌呤复发或不能耐受的患者继续使用激素是有效的，利妥昔单抗可用于难治性病例[103,108,121]，糖皮质激素治疗不仅可以改善胰腺结构异常，而且可以改善胰腺外分泌和内分泌功能（以及如果受累涎腺功能）。基于治疗开始时已纤维化和萎缩的程度不同，功能的改善程度不同。很少见到切除术（如胰十二指肠切除术）后的临床复发。

（六）梗阻

由肿瘤、瘢痕、胰管结石、十二指肠壁囊肿或Vater乳头或副乳头狭窄引起的主胰管慢性梗阻可在梗阻上游实质内引起慢性胰腺炎。胰管梗阻也可能是其他类型的慢性胰腺炎的重要原因（例如酒精引起的慢性胰腺炎中蛋白质沉淀阻塞小或大胰管分支）。然而慢性阻塞性胰腺炎是指由主胰管单独（通常）的显著缩窄或狭窄引起的独有情况。许多情况可造成慢性阻塞性胰腺炎。腺癌、胰岛细胞瘤、导管内乳头状黏液瘤或壶腹肿瘤引起的肿瘤阻塞可导致主胰管获得性狭窄（见第60章）。在急性胰腺炎严重发作后，特别是与胰腺坏死相关的发作后，可能出现良性狭窄（见第58章）。胰腺的钝性和穿透性创伤可导致胰管狭窄，最常见于胰管与脊柱相交之处的腺体中部。其中每个过程都与阻塞部位上游腺体的慢性胰腺炎有关。慢性阻塞性胰腺炎的病理表现为弥漫性小叶间和小叶内纤维化，通常在受累区域均匀对称分布。

胰腺分裂是一种常见的正常变异，大约见于4%～11%的人群（见第55章）。在胰腺分裂患者中，副乳头可能不足以使胰液自由地流入十二指肠，从而可能导致胰腺炎急性发作。目前不认为胰腺分裂是慢性胰腺炎的主要原因。大量的自然病程研究未能明确胰腺分裂与急性或慢性胰腺炎之间的关系。发展为胰腺疾病的胰腺分裂患者，往往不是受胰腺分裂影响，而是同时存在可能是胰腺炎原因的潜在基因突变[122,123]。和胰腺分裂相同，Oddi括约肌功能障碍常不被认为是慢性胰腺炎的原因，而是急性或复发性急性胰腺炎的原因。对于慢性胰腺炎和Oddi括约肌功能障碍或胰腺分裂患者，难以预测其括约肌消融的反应，但通常效果较差。由于认识到这种情况下括约肌消融通常缺乏效果，外科教科书早已警告不要单独将括约肌成形术作为慢性胰腺炎的治疗方法。

（七）其他因素

1. 复发或急性重症胰腺炎

慢性胰腺炎可在通常伴有胰腺坏死或需要清创的急性胰腺炎严重发作后出现。任何病因的轻型急性胰腺炎反复发作都可能最终导致胰腺内慢性炎症发展，胰腺星状细胞的活化和慢性胰腺炎。高甘油三酯血症即其中一个例子。血清甘油三酯数值高于10g/L往往导致重度急性胰腺炎。许多患者会反复出现急性炎症的临床和亚临床发作，并且一些患者最终发展为慢性胰腺炎[124,125]。

在急性胰腺炎首次发作之后，大约10%的患者会被诊断为慢性胰腺炎[14,52]。慢性胰腺炎的预测因子包括多次复发、吸烟和饮酒[14,50-53]。在任何病因导致的重度急性胰腺炎合并胰腺实质坏死的患者中，也可能出现慢性胰腺炎的特征（见第58章）[14,126-129]。值得注意的是胰腺外分泌和内分泌功能不全可能更常见。大约25%的患者在急性胰腺炎发作后会发展为胰腺外分泌功能不全，饮酒常为病因，重症坏死性胰腺炎是主要的预测因子[129]。大约三分之一的患者在急性胰腺炎发作后出现糖尿病或糖尿病前期，但其危险因素不像胰腺外分泌功能不全那样确定[130]。综合这些数据表明，急性胰腺炎后继发慢性胰腺炎的发生率比通常认为的更高。

在严重胰腺坏死后，特别是在那些接受坏死组织清除术的患者中可出现包括外分泌和内分泌功能不全的慢性胰腺炎。在一项研究中，未行坏死组织清除术的胆源性坏死性胰腺炎患者其外分泌功能不全和内分泌功能不全的发生率低于做过该手术的患者（外分泌和内分泌功能不全分别为13% vs 58%和26% vs 75%）[126]。因此，即使没有行坏死组织清除术，重症坏死性胰腺炎也可能导致慢性胰腺炎并导致外分泌和内分泌功能不全。在坏死性胰腺炎康复后，可观察到高达80%的患者的胰腺功能检测持续下降[126]。残留胰管狭窄在重度急性胰腺炎后也很常见，它们也可能促进狭窄上游腺体中慢性胰腺炎的发展。在另一些病例中，长期迁延不愈的临床过程最终可导致慢性胰腺炎。

2. 无症状胰腺纤维化

在一些情况下，在没有慢性胰腺炎临床表现时就可见到尤其是包括纤维化在内的慢性胰腺炎组织学证据。老年人的胰腺内可能发生类似慢性胰腺炎的组织学改变[3-6]。在这些患者中ERCP也可显示与慢性胰腺炎一致的胰管改变[131,132]。这些结构变化通常与胰腺功能紊乱或慢性胰腺炎的临床特征不相符[132]。没有慢性胰腺炎临床症状的长期饮酒者通常有慢性胰腺炎的组织学证据[7,8]。

血液透析患者中急性胰腺炎发病率更高，一些证据表明慢性胰腺炎在这一人群中也可能也有更高的发病率。影像学和尸检数据显示，高达五分之一的患者在没有临床症状时表现出与慢性胰腺炎一致的变化[133,134]。慢性肾功能衰竭似乎经常产生无症状的胰腺纤维化。胰腺形态和功能改变在长期糖尿病患者中也很常见[10]。尤其是1型糖尿病患者中胰腺比正常情况下要小[10,135]。在通过ERCP进行的研究中，40%～50%的糖尿病患者胰管异常，伴有提示慢性胰腺炎的异常情况[136,137]。在由粪便弹性蛋白酶测定所确定的胰腺功能[10,138]，或更正式的直接胰腺功能测定中[139]，有40%～50%的患者存在异常。尚不清楚是糖尿病导致了胰腺的变化，还是相反情况，这种关联的原因不明。由于胰岛素是外分泌胰腺的营养因子，以及糖尿病可产生微血管病变，胰岛素缺乏和长期糖尿病可以共同解释胰腺损伤。虽然对胰腺结构和功能的这些测量结果可能存在，但它们通常并不能解释症状，因而对这些患者不应常规使用胰酶治疗[10]。吸烟是慢性胰腺炎的一个重要危险因素，尸检研究显示，吸烟会导致特别是小叶内纤维化的胰腺纤维化[140]。

结合这些观察表明，各种疾病和正常损耗（如正常老化，长期酒精摄入，吸烟）对胰腺可能产生类似于组织学标准下慢性胰腺炎一样的损伤，但不足以引起症状，也没有严重到需要将这些患者贴上疾病的标签。这个概念将在“诊断”部分进一步讨论。

（八）特发性

特发性胰腺炎占所有慢性胰腺炎病例的10%到

30%[14,59,62,141,142]，但取决于人群和地域。特发性疾病在女性中尤为常见；在一些研究中，它是女性最常见的病因[141]。然而，许多患者可能被误诊为特发性疾病。考虑到没有可靠方法来确定酒精摄入量，也没有对胰腺炎而言的最低绝对摄入阈值。其中部分患者肯定多少会受到酒精毒性的影响。类似地，一些已知或未知基因异常的患者中可有特发性的病例[98,100-102,143,144]，特别是在青年时期发病的患者[144]。一些我们以前认为是特发性的疾病反而是自身免疫性疾病。在以往的许多研究中，吸烟并没有被纳入潜在病因，因此吸烟也可能占这些患者中相当大比例的病因。因此大多数关于这一情况的研究可能涉及几种不同病因的病例，导致解释关于特发性慢性胰腺炎的文献比较困难。

慢性特发性胰腺炎有两种形式，一种发病早，主要出现在二三十岁，另一种发病晚，出现在六七十岁[69,142]。早发慢性特发性胰腺炎的平均发病年龄在 20 岁左右，性别比例似乎相等。疼痛作为其主要表现，在高达 96% 的患者中出现，高于酒精中毒或迟发性慢性胰腺炎的发病率。胰腺钙化、外分泌功能不全和内分泌功能不全（如糖尿病）在发病时极为罕见（<10%），并且其后发展非常缓慢。该病中平均 25 年出现胰腺钙化，26 年出现外分泌不全，27.5 年出现内分泌不全[69]。慢性胰腺炎的并发症（假性囊肿、脓肿、胆道梗阻和十二指肠梗阻）约在 20% 的患者中发生，而 60% 的患者最终需要手术治疗（主要因腹痛）。因此，早发慢性特发性胰腺炎是一种以剧烈疼痛为特征，但在结构（钙化）或功能（外分泌或内分泌功能不足）方面的发展非常缓慢的疾病。因为大多数可用的诊断工具依赖于这些结构或功能异常，所以这种结构或功能异常的延迟可能使诊断相当困难。

迟发性慢性特发性胰腺炎较少表现为疼痛。在记录最好的病例系列中[69]，尽管 75% 的患者最终出现疼痛，只有 54% 的患者以疼痛起病。中位发病年龄为 56 岁，同样地，发病率在男性和女性中相同。外分泌不全（22%）和内分泌不全（22%）在诊断时并不少见，并最终分别出现在 46% 和 41% 的病例中。外分泌不全和内分泌不全发生的中位时间分别为 16.9 年和 11.9 年。生命表分析提示，经过很长时间随访（>30 年），最终 75% 将发展为外分泌功能不全，50%～60% 将发展为内分泌功能不全，90% 将发展为弥漫性胰腺钙化[69,145]。因此，该疾病往往有一个相对无痛并伴有通常发展为胰腺钙化，外分泌功能不全，内分泌功能不全的过程。衰老本身可与胰腺实质和导管内结构变化发展相关，这些变化与慢性迟发性胰腺炎难以区分[132]，因此并非总能清楚地鉴别正常衰老和迟发性慢性特发性胰腺炎。

五、临床特征

（一）腹痛

腹痛是慢性胰腺炎患者最常见的临床问题，也是最影响患者生活质量的症状[30,146]。严重的疼痛会降低食欲，限制食物的摄入，导致体重减轻和营养不良。慢性严重疼痛导致生活质量急剧下降[25-30,146]，社会功能丧失，可能麻醉镇痛药成瘾[147,148]，自杀率增加[149]。在美国，大约一半的慢性胰腺炎患者接受了阿片类药物治疗。顽固性疼痛是慢性胰腺炎患者住院、内镜干预和手术的最常见原因。疼痛没有特征性的单一模式，通常被描述为上腹部的疼痛，并伴有背部的放射。疼痛常被描述为深部、穿透样、钻痛，常伴有恶心和呕吐。可以通过前坐或前倾、卧于一侧的膝胸位，或下蹲并将膝盖紧贴胸部来缓解。疼痛餐后加重且常在夜间发生。

腹痛的自然病程各不相同且难以预测。例如，许多慢性胰腺炎患者最初表现为疼痛发作，中间穿插着相对缓解的时期。在急性疼痛发作的间期，这样的患者可能被认为是复发性急性胰腺炎。随着时间的推移，疼痛可能变得更持续，导致慢性胰腺炎的诊断更加明确。值得注意的是，特别是在长期的慢性胰腺炎中，疼痛发作时淀粉酶或脂肪酶水平可能不会升高。有些患者可出现逐渐加重的持续性腹痛，有些患者则无腹痛。疼痛一旦出现，通常会随时间在性质、严重程度和时机上发生变化。根据慢性胰腺炎的病因不同，50%～90% 的患者在疾病过程中会感到疼痛[14,25-30,150-154]。一些观察性研究记录了一些患者随着时间推移会疼痛减轻，尽管疼痛减轻的时机和程度在不同的研究中有所不同。在一项研究中，疼痛缓解似乎最常发生在发展为弥漫性胰腺钙化、外分泌功能不全和内分泌功能不全的时期[68]。其他研究没有发现同样的相关性，但许多研究已经注意到疼痛随着时间有不太明显的逐渐消退的趋势[69,70,150-154]。大约一半患者的疼痛可能最终会减轻。因疼痛或并发症而进行的手术缓解了一部分患者的疼痛，但在很长时间的随访中，也可以在接受药物治疗的患者中看到类似比例的疼痛缓解[68,155]。然而，并不能准确预测某一患者的疼痛模式，是随着时间推移疼痛可能加重、还是稳定或好转。对任何慢性胰腺炎治疗效果的判断必须考虑到这种极其不同的疼痛自然病史[156-159]。

有多种慢性胰腺炎疼痛的可能原因，但可以归结为以下两个主要机制：①胰腺内压力升高、缺血和炎症；②周围和中枢感受性神经的损伤和功能改变。在许多包括慢性胰腺炎在内的慢性疼痛中，也可以将疼痛分为伤害感受性疼痛（由于对非神经组织的实际或接近损伤，造成伤害感受器的激活）和神经性疼痛（由躯体感觉神经系统的损伤或疾病引起的疼痛）[156,157,160]。

1. 缺血和炎症所致压力增加

胰腺导管或实质内压力增加导致组织缺血是一种被提出的疼痛机制。多项临床和实验证据表明，胰管或胰腺实质内压力升高是胰源性疼痛发生的重要原因。慢性胰腺炎患者因慢性疼痛而进行手术时，胰腺导管和组织压力通常会升高[161-163]。在一些慢性胰腺炎疼痛患者中，也有报道通过 ERCP 测量的胰管压力升高[164,165]。胰管引流术可使胰管压力降至正常水平，并可减轻疼痛[161-163]。然而，有腹痛和无腹痛的患者胰管压力可能相同[165]，并且内镜支架置入后压力的降低与疼痛缓解无关[166]。

胰管内压力升高可能与主胰管或侧支的胰管梗阻有关。存在胰管狭窄和上游胰管扩张可能是对于压力增加及其导致的疼痛的一组患者的准确预测指标。然而，胰管狭窄或胰管扩张与疼痛之间没有关系[156,157,167,168]。尽管如此，胰管扩张或胰管狭窄的患者最有可能通过内镜或手术治疗缓解疼痛。

压力升高引起疼痛的机制尚不明确，但可能与胰腺组织缺血有关。在慢性胰腺炎动物模型中,胰腺压力升高与胰腺血流减少、组织氧供和间质 pH 相关。在这些模型中,胰腺促分泌剂导致胰腺血流进一步减少(而不是正常预期的增加),毛细血管充盈减少,并加剧组织缺血。这些观察结果与间隔室综合征的观察结果一致[162]。对接受手术的慢性胰腺炎患者的小型研究也表明,胰腺组织的 pH 低于非慢性胰腺炎患者[169]。ERCP 时使用铂电极进行测量,慢性胰腺炎患者的胰腺血流量也低于对照组[170]。因此由于刺激胰腺分泌而加重的组织缺血可能是组织压力升高引起疼痛的机制。

胰腺炎症随着炎症介质的释放也可能导致疼痛。特别是受损腺泡细胞释放的胰蛋白酶和固有肥大细胞释放的类胰蛋白酶可激活蛋白酶激活受体 2(PAR-2),使瞬时受体电位香草醛活性纤维的反应变得敏感,释放 P 物质作为疼痛信号转导的关键分子[156,160]。值得注意的是,在疼痛发作时,可能不会出现血清脂肪酶或淀粉酶水平升高或急性胰腺炎症的影像学证据。

2. 周围神经和中枢神经的改变

需要通过痛觉神经元发出的信号来感知疼痛。慢性胰腺炎患者的形态学研究显示胰腺内神经的直径和数量,与神经和神经节相关的炎症细胞灶,神经鞘损伤均有增加[156,160,171,172]。破坏神经鞘可能令炎症介质进入神经元中。不管是胰腺内部还是周围的局部问题引起疼痛,感知疼痛信息都需要与中枢神经系统进行交流。胰腺的神经支配是复杂的,有内脏、躯体和自主神经。胰腺的伤害感受性感觉传入神经的树突与交感神经一起从胰腺到达腹腔神经节,尽管此时没有突触。这些树突状纤维继续和左、右内脏大神经汇合在一起,到达交感干神经节,然后到达位于脊髓 T_5 至 $T_9 \sim T_{10}$ 节的背根神经节的第一个细胞体。这些背根神经元的突起通常在进入脊髓背角之前下行和上行几个脊髓节段。传入的疼痛纤维可能在这些连接中穿过中线,从而解释了胰腺疼痛多位于中线。来自第一级背根神经节细胞体的轴突有两条不同的通路。一些投射到脊髓背角,并可能释放多种介质,包括 P 物质、降钙素基因相关肽和谷氨酸等到达二级神经元,这些二级神经元通过脊髓丘脑白质束投射到丘脑。这些神经元可能与投射到躯体感觉皮层(用于疼痛的认知整合)以及边缘系统和下丘脑(用于疼痛的情感和自主整合)的三级神经元建立突触。投射的第二种途径包括与脊髓同一水平的突触,其交感传出细胞体向下投射内脏神经到腹腔神经丛,第二级交感神经元投射回胰腺。迷走传入神经也可能携带来自胰腺的有害刺激(尤其是牵张)。

这些通路的有害刺激可以有多种机制。压力、缺血、炎症、热和其他经典刺激都能激活这些通路。炎症介质的积累和神经损伤会使神经敏感,出现高反应[156,160,173]。慢性胰腺炎患者的小叶间和小叶内神经束中伤害感受性神经递质(如 P 物质、降钙素基因相关肽)增加[160,173]。胰腺内神经和炎症细胞之间空间上的密切关系支持了神经免疫相互作用的补充机制。在慢性胰腺炎疼痛的患者和慢性胰腺炎动物模型中可见神经生长因子和一种受体(TrkA)的表达[173,174]。神经生长因子是参与致敏作用的关键分子之一[173,174]。如胰蛋白酶等内源性蛋白酶,也可以激活胰腺感觉神经元并使其敏感,这一过程通过蛋白酶激活受体-2(PAR-2)介导。PAR-2 的另一种激活物是肥大细胞产物类胰蛋白酶[160,173]。有趣的是,肥大细胞常见于慢性胰腺炎患者的胰腺组织标本。尽管数据表明,胰腺神经附近产生致敏因子,改变了感觉神经元的形式和功能,慢性胰腺炎中炎症细胞及其产物和胰腺内神经元相互作用的确切机制尚不完全清楚。

此外,来自其他类型慢性疼痛研究的大量证据表明,慢性外周神经损伤或炎症导致脊髓和中枢神经系统的伤害感受处理过程改变。慢性疼痛可产生一种中枢敏感性的疼痛状态,在这种状态下,消除疼痛的最初来源可能不能缓解疼痛[156,160,175,176]。这种情况下,疼痛可能是对非伤害性或生理刺激(痛觉异常)的反应,也可能是对疼痛刺激的过度反应(痛觉过敏)。这些现象取决于脊髓水平和大脑的变化。大量研究证实慢性胰腺炎患者中枢神经系统结构和功能改变[156,160,177,178]。这些变化包括痛觉输入的中央处理改变,痛觉阈值改变,以及大脑微观及宏观结构改变。相比于正常健康对照,慢性胰腺炎患者中的变化包括岛叶、继发性躯体感觉皮层和扣带皮层的重组、并伴有这些神经网络的神经元异常兴奋[160]。也有包括内脏疼痛处理区域的皮质体积厚度减少,脑电图异常,以及大脑功能 MRI 异常在内的许多结构变化被记录[156,160]。痛觉过敏和痛觉异常背后的中枢神经系统重组和可塑性可能是限制疼痛治疗效果的主要因素。这一事实在全胰腺切除术后仍有胰腺疼痛的患者身上表现得更为明显。疼痛是复杂的,所有患者并不只有一种单一机制,这意味着没有一种单一治疗是有效的。

3. 疼痛的其他原因

除了这两种主要机制外,还应考虑其他各种导致疼痛的因素。慢性胰腺炎的并发症本身也可能引起疼痛。这些并发症包括十二指肠梗阻、胆管梗阻、假性囊肿和继发胰腺癌。这些通常有特定的治疗方法。通过 CCK 产生的胰腺过度刺激也被推测为疼痛的一个潜在原因,因为在慢性胰腺炎中血清 CCK 水平可能升高,并且 CCK 对胰腺的刺激可能增加腺体内的压力或者促进非顶部的基底外侧分泌酶。降低血清 CCK 水平是一种使用非肠溶胰酶来减轻疼痛的潜在机制。

(二) 脂肪泻(胰腺外分泌功能不全)

人的胰腺有大量的外分泌储备。脂肪泻通常在胰腺脂肪酶分泌减少到最大输出量 10% 以下时才会发生[179]。因此,脂肪泻是慢性胰腺炎极晚期的一个特征,这时大部分腺泡细胞受损或破坏,但也可能见于胰管堵塞、胰腺手术后、急性坏死性胰腺炎发作后。晚期慢性胰腺炎会出现脂肪、蛋白质和碳水化合物消化不良。当蛋白酶分泌少于正常的 10% 时,也会发生蛋白泻(蛋白质消化不良)。受累患者可能出现腹泻和体重减轻。有些患者可能会观察到大量恶臭粪便,甚至可能注意到明显的油滴排出。与小肠疾病相关的吸收不良不同,水样腹泻、过量气体和腹部绞痛在慢性胰腺炎患者中并不常见。这种差异可能是由于慢性胰腺炎和外分泌不足患者比乳糜泻等小肠疾病患者能更好地保留碳水化合物吸收以及小肠和结肠功能。即使粪便中有明显脂肪丢失,大多数患者每天也只排出 3 或 4 次粪便,有些患者可能只排出 1 次。

一般来说,脂肪消化不良比蛋白质或碳水化合物消化不良更早,更严重。有几种对这一现象的解释。第一,尽管胃脂肪酶能够水解高达 20%的膳食脂肪，脂肪消化主要依靠胰脂肪酶和共脂肪酶。第二，与胰蛋白酶或淀粉酶等其他胰酶的分泌相比，脂肪酶分泌随着慢性胰腺炎的进展更早、更大幅度地减少。第三，脂肪酶比其他胰酶对酸性破坏更敏感。在慢性胰腺炎中，碳酸氢盐分泌减少，十二指肠 pH 下降，脂肪酶更容易失活。第四，除了脂肪酶失活外，十二指肠低 pH 还容易导致胆盐的沉淀，从而阻止混合微粒的形成，进一步干扰脂类的消化吸收。第五，脂肪酶比其他消化酶对胰蛋白酶的消化和降解更敏感。

据报道，慢性胰腺炎发生外分泌不足的中位时间低至 5 年[68]，但大多数研究报告了在发生脂肪泻前更长的患病时间。在一项大型自然病程研究中，慢性酒精性胰腺炎患者发生外分泌不足的中位时间为 13.1 年，迟发性慢性特发性胰腺炎患者为 16.9 年，早发性慢性特发性胰腺炎患者为 26.3 年[69]。在很长时间的随访中，大约 50% 至 80% 的慢性胰腺炎患者最终会出现外分泌不足[68-70,145]。

尽管存在消化不良，但体重显著下降的情况并不常见。患者通常会增加热量摄入以弥补粪便丢失。此外，胃脂肪酶（酸稳定）可部分弥补胰脂肪酶的缺失[180]。尽管慢性胰腺炎患者的静息能量消耗普遍增加，但体重通常保持不变。体重减轻最常见于由于疼痛、恶心或呕吐导致的无法充分经口进食的疼痛发作时。伴随疾病如小肠细菌过度生长（SIBO，见第 105 章）或胰腺或胰外恶性肿瘤也可能导致体重减轻。最后，体重减轻可能发生在经济困难、存在慢性严重酒精中毒或失去社会支持的患者中，因为这些可能导致热量和蛋白质摄入不足。显著的体重减轻应该引起对这些潜在原因的调查。更轻微的体重减轻和其他消化不良并发症更常见[181-186]。

在慢性胰腺炎和脂肪泻患者中可出现脂溶性维生素缺乏[182-187]。慢性胰腺炎患者存在明显的维生素 D 缺乏、骨质减少和骨质疏松[185-189]。研究表明，40%的患者骨质减少，25%的慢性胰腺炎和脂肪泻患者骨质疏松[188]。水溶性维生素和微量营养素缺乏较不常见，通常只认为是摄入不足的结果。尽管维生素 B_{12} 的吸收需要未受损的胰腺功能来降解膳食钴胺素中的 R 因子，但维生素 B_{12} 缺乏在慢性胰腺炎患者中相当罕见。

除了上述代谢影响外，存在外分泌不足也与慢性胰腺炎患者总体死亡率增加有关[190,191]。

（三）糖尿病（胰腺内分泌功能不全）

与外分泌功能不全一样，内分泌功能不全是长期慢性胰腺炎的后果，尤其在胰腺切除术后和热带性（纤维钙化性）胰腺炎中常见。胰岛细胞在慢性胰腺炎中似乎对破坏相对耐受（见图 59.1）[192]。发生糖尿病不仅仅是由于胰岛的进行性破坏导致 β 细胞的丢失，其机制要复杂得多[193-197]。

多种因素使慢性胰腺炎（和胰腺癌）糖尿病不同于经典的 1 型或 2 型糖尿病，胰源性糖尿病被定义为 3c 型糖尿病[197]。3c 型糖尿病的特点是低水平的胰岛素和负向调节激素（特别是胰高血糖素和胰多肽），酮症罕见，以及频繁治疗引起的低血糖[193-197]。大约一半发展为糖尿病的慢性胰腺炎患者最终需要胰岛素[195]。与 1 型糖尿病不同的是，产生胰岛素的 β 细胞和产生胰高血糖素的 α 细胞都受到了损伤。这种组合由于缺少胰高血糖素的代偿性释放，增加了过度强化胰岛素治疗导致长期严重低血糖的风险[194,198]。

在慢性胰腺炎晚期患者中，糖尿病几乎与脂肪泻一样常见。在一项研究中，酒精性、迟发特发性、早发特发性慢性胰腺炎患者发生糖尿病的中位时间分别为 19.8 年、11.9 年和 26.3 年[69]。其他研究指出有 6～10 年的更短的中位时间[68,70,199,200]。最终在长期随访中，不同 CP 病因有 40%～80% 的慢性胰腺炎患者有糖尿病[68,69]。接受胰腺手术的慢性胰腺炎患者有较高的外分泌和内分泌功能不全的发生率[201-203]。与慢性胰腺炎相关的糖尿病患者中，微血管病并发症和病程相似的 1 型糖尿病患者同样常见[194,204]。

六、体格检查

很少有慢性胰腺炎的诊断性或特异性体格检查。患者可能出现营养不良伴肌肉减少症，并可能表现为轻度至中度腹部压痛。在病情较严重的患者中，体重减轻和营养不良的情况可能更为明显。可触及的肿块提示为假性囊肿，但少见。同时存在酒精性肝病或胰头胆管受压时可表现为黄疸。在慢性胰腺炎或并存慢性肝病所致门静脉高压的患者中，可发现由于脾静脉血栓形成而可触及脾。在一些 AIP 患者中，可能发现共存的自身免疫性特征，如涎腺肿大或淋巴结病。

七、诊断

有多种可用于慢性胰腺炎的诊断试验。这些诊断性检查通常分为检测胰腺功能异常的检查和检测胰腺结构异常的检查（表 59.2）。在更详细地考虑这些检查之前，最好记住在几乎所有患者中，慢性胰腺炎是一种缓慢进展的疾病。在早期胰腺中，慢性炎症、细胞坏死和凋亡、胰腺星状细胞活化等都有进展，但这些慢性胰腺炎的特征仅在组织学上可见。随着纤维化的进展和组织的丧失和破坏，疾病变得更加明显。可能需要几年甚至几十年的时间才出现胰腺结构或功能的异常，甚至根本不出现[1,2,67-70,104,205]。在已经出现明显功能或结构异常的晚期疾病中，所有现有的诊断试验都是最准确的。相反，在早期或进展较少的慢性胰腺炎中，所有诊断试验多少都不准确。

表 59.2 对慢性胰腺炎可行的诊断试验*

胰腺结构检测	胰腺功能检测
EUS	直接激素检测（使用促胰液素和/或胆囊收缩素刺激）： 采用经口十二指肠管 采用内镜
MRI 及 MRCP，使用或不使用促胰液素刺激	粪便弹性蛋白酶
CT	血清胰蛋白酶原（胰蛋白酶）
ERCP	粪便糜蛋白酶
经腹 US	粪便脂质
腹部 X 线平片	血糖水平

*每列中排序以估算的敏感性降序排列。

CT，计算机断层扫描；ERCP，内镜逆行胰胆管造影；EUS，超声内镜；MRCP，磁共振胰胆管造影；MRI，磁共振成像；US，超声。

慢性胰腺炎的功能异常包括外分泌功能不全(消化不良和脂肪泻)和内分泌功能不全(3c 型糖尿病)。此外,一些诊断性测试检测胰腺的最大刺激分泌能力,而其在外分泌或内分泌功能衰竭之前就会出现异常[205,206]。用于诊断的结构异常包括主胰管内的改变(扩张、狭窄、不规则、胰管结石)、胰管分支(扩张、不规则)或胰腺实质(腺体分叶、回声改变、囊肿、结石、萎缩等)。慢性酒精性胰腺炎、慢性遗传性胰腺炎、热带性胰腺炎和迟发性慢性特发性胰腺炎的患者最容易出现这些功能或结构的异常,虽然这一过程可能需要数年时间。这些变化在早发性慢性特发性胰腺炎患者中发展特别缓慢甚至有时根本没有[1,67,69,205]。

要确定这些诊断试验的敏感性、特异性和准确性,就需要将试验结果金标准进行比较,这种金标准需要是某种可以提供可靠、确定的证据以证明疾病存在与否。在慢性胰腺炎的情况中,该金标准是胰腺组织学检查(见图 59.1)。不幸的是,整个腺体的组织学变化并不一致[33],因此活检标本的结果可能具有误导性。更重要的是,获得胰腺组织是有风险的,而且很少,仅仅为了诊断而进行。此外,在有衰老、社交性饮酒、吸烟和糖尿病因素而无慢性胰腺炎临床特征的患者中,也可能有类似的组织学发现[4-10,132]。鉴于缺乏功能性的金标准,金标准的替代包括其他诊断测试或长期随访。大多数研究没有对诊断为早期慢性胰腺炎或可能为早期慢性胰腺炎(诊断试验不是明确阳性患者)的患者进行足够长的监测,以确定是否存在慢性胰腺炎。金标准的另一种潜在替代是一些其他诊断试验,事实上,新的诊断试验常与 ERCP、EUS、CT、MRI 和胰腺功能试验或这些试验的组合相比较。

在慢性胰腺炎和存在极晚期结构或功能异常的患者中,几乎没有其他疾病能模仿这些异常,基本上所有诊断试验都是准确的。早期、晚期或轻微变化的慢性胰腺炎患者中情况截然不同,因为缺乏容易识别的结构或功能异常,在疑似慢性胰腺炎患者中情况更是如此[1,205,207]。在这种情况下,只有灵敏度最高的试验才有可能建立诊断,而缺乏金标准可能导致诊断混乱和难以做出结论。除了在敏感性和特异性的基础上选择诊断试验,临床医生必须考虑检测的可行性、花费和风险以达到诊断信息最大及伤害最小。在此将对每个可用的诊断工具进行讨论。

(一) 胰腺功能检测

胰腺功能测试可分为两种,一种是通过测量胰酶或碳酸氢盐的输出量来直接测量胰腺功能,另一种是间接测量释放的酶(通过其对底物的作用或其在血液或粪便中的水平)。

1. 直接检测

直接激素刺激试验被认为是对慢性胰腺炎最敏感的功能试验[1,205-208]。这些检查需要在十二指肠放置导管或内窥镜,刺激胰腺分泌物(通常用促胰液素,但有时用 CCK),收集胰腺分泌物进行分析(输注促胰液素时为碳酸氢盐浓度,输注 CCK 时用酶的分泌)。一些研究将这些激素刺激试验的结果与胰腺组织学进行了比较,总的敏感性在 67% 到 88% 之间[209-211]。一项最大的研究比较了 108 名患者中组织学和促胰液素-CCK 联合检测[209]。刺激后碳酸氢盐输出量与慢性胰腺炎的组织学严重程度呈线性相关。虽然在 69 例组织学正常或不确定的患者中,碳酸氢盐平均峰值浓度在正常范围(>80mmol/L),但在轻度、中度和重度组织学慢性胰腺炎患者中,碳酸氢盐平均峰值浓度分别为 70、63 和 50mmol//L。本研究中激素刺激试验的总灵敏度为 67%,特异度为 90%,总准确度为 81%。当仅局限于 29 例有中度或重度慢性胰腺炎组织学改变的患者进行分析时,激素刺激试验的灵敏度上升到 79%。在同一组 29 例患者中,ERCP 的敏感性为 66%。

与 ERCP 相比,直接激素刺激试验似乎对诊断慢性胰腺炎更敏感。胰腺功能检测的灵敏度为 74%~97%,特异度为 80%~90%[208-217]。在这些研究中,这两种测试在大约四分之三的患者中具有一致性,而一些研究表明一致性更高。大多数研究也注意到结构异常逐渐增多和激素刺激试验结果的进行性异常之间的普遍的相关性,尽管关系并不确切。这些研究多数也能鉴别出结果不一致的患者,即 ERCP 时异常和激素刺激试验结果正常的患者,以及 ERCP 时正常和激素刺激试验结果异常的患者。在 4 项研究中,激素刺激试验结果异常而 ERCP 正常的患者比例为 3%~20%[210-215]。3 项小型研究对这些仅根据激素刺激试验结果异常进行诊断的患者进行了随访,并在随访中发现 90% 的患者出现了慢性胰腺炎的进展[217-219]。这些数据指出,直接的胰腺功能测试似乎能够鉴别出一组慢性胰腺炎患者,他们有受刺激时分泌功能的异常,但(当时)还没有 ERCP 可识别的结构异常。相反,大多数这些研究也报道了激素刺激试验结果正常和 ERCP 异常的患者。这类患者通常不太常见,在一些研究中平均不到 10%。在一小群这样的患者的长期随访中发现 0~26% 发展为慢性胰腺炎[217-219]。这些研究指出在两项试验结果不一致的情况下,激素刺激试验似乎比 ERCP 更敏感和更特异[220,221]。

一些专家认为,在直接的胰腺功能测试产生可靠的阳性结果之前,胰腺需要有 30% 到 50% 的损伤。尽管直接胰腺功能试验在理论上有优势,但仍有一些局限性。第一,在提供检测的机构之间没有很好地标准化。第二,因只有极少数转诊中心可以使用这些试验,所以大多数临床医生在诊治慢性胰腺炎患者时无法使用它们。第三,患者很难在没有注射镇静剂的情况下忍耐放置口十二指肠管长达一个小时或更长时间。第四,精确测量碳酸氢盐浓度或酶输出量可能具有挑战性。曾在接受毕Ⅱ式胃切除术的患者,糖尿病、腹腔疾病和肝硬化患者,以及近期急性胰腺炎发作后恢复的患者中报告了假阳性结果。直接胰腺功能检查对常用的诊断方法(如 CT 或 MRI)未证实的结构和功能异常,或当这些影像学结果不明确并推测慢性胰腺炎患者最有用。这种类型的试验在排除怀疑有慢性胰腺炎的慢性腹痛患者中最有用,并可以让这些患者免受贴上慢性胰腺炎的标签及其负面影响,避免了 ERCP 等诊断性检查的风险[1,205,207,220]。

有多种让患者更容易耐受(通过镇静)以及使用更广泛的改良的直接胰腺功能测试。一种改良是在 ERCP 时直接在胰管中放置导管(即所谓的导管内促胰液素试验)来收集胰腺分泌物。该检测通常只采集 15 分钟的胰腺输出量,以尽量减少 ERCP 导致胰腺炎的可能性。它不是标准化的并且可能是因为收集时间太短,似乎不像标准直接胰腺功能测试那样准确[222]。一种常见的胰腺功能检测方法是使用镇静和标准上消化道内窥镜代替常规的口十二指肠管,并使用常规医院实验室来分析碳酸氢盐输出量。避免了例如在非麻醉患者中放置收集管,以及需要专用实验室通过反滴定法来测量碳酸氢盐浓度等限制了标准直接胰腺功能测试的广泛应用。与导管内促胰液素检查不同,这种内镜下改良检查虽然不完全准确,但几乎与标准的直接胰腺功能检查一样准确[206,220,223-225]。这项试验最初的描述是每 15 分钟定时抽吸十二指肠液,共收集 60 分钟。对保持患者镇静和占用内镜室来说这是一段很长的时间,尽管可能可以缩短试验和只收集在促胰液素注射后 30 分钟和 45 分钟的样品[206,226,227]以使灵敏度减少最小。该测试的另一种改变是以 CCK 作为促分泌剂,测量脂肪酶的输出量,而不是碳酸氢盐的输出量[228]。这种改变似乎比基于促胰液素的胰腺功能检测更不准确。与传统的胰腺功能检测一样,内镜下的胰腺功能检测与 ERCP 等替代诊断检测相比较[229],总体一致率为 86%,并且内镜下胰腺功能检测具有很高的阴性预测价值。无论是传统的还是内镜下的胰腺功能检查,其价值在于高灵敏度和由此产生的除外慢性胰腺炎的能力[205,220,225,230]。目前的做法是给予 0.2μg/kg 的重组促胰液素,通过 Dreiling 管或内镜收集样品超过 45~60 分钟,每 15 分钟等分或取样。对液体样品进行碳酸氢盐浓度分析;将所有样品碳酸氢盐浓度小于 80mmol/L 定义为异常结果。

2. 间接检测

由于直接胰腺功能检测的复杂性、不适性和有限的可行性而产生了开发间接胰腺功能检测的想法。间接试验通常测量血液或粪便中的胰酶。口服底物后收集血液、呼吸或尿液中的代谢物以测量对胰酶的影响,这种方法曾经被考虑或仅用于研究。

(1) 血清胰蛋白酶原

可以在血液中测量血清胰蛋白酶原(通常称为血清胰蛋白酶)并粗略估计胰腺功能。晚期慢性胰腺炎伴脂肪泻患者可发现血清胰蛋白酶原水平异常降低[231]。血清胰蛋白酶在其他形式的脂肪泻患者中不会降低,但可在胰管梗阻(包括恶性梗阻)患者中见到低水平的血清胰蛋白酶原。该测试可通过商业实验室进行,但都有不同的正常范围。

(2) 粪便胰酶

粪便中糜蛋白酶或弹性蛋白酶的低浓度可反映这些胰酶不能被充分输送到十二指肠。两者都可以在随机的粪便样本中检出。粪胰糜蛋白酶在大多数慢性胰腺炎和脂肪泻患者中含量较低。粪糜蛋白酶可通过商业实验室检测。有报道在其他吸收不良情况(乳糜泻、克罗恩病)、大便被稀释的腹泻疾病和严重营养不良中也有假阳性结果。因为该检查在无脂肪泻的患者中通常是正常的,它只有在晚期慢性胰腺炎中呈阳性才可靠。粪弹性蛋白酶-1 与粪糜蛋白酶相比具有明显的优势,它在通过粪便时更稳定,更容易测定。粪便中浓度低于 200μg/g 则认为异常,提示胰腺外分泌功能不全。低于 100μg/g 粪便被认为是胰腺外分泌功能不全的证据。该检测在较晚期的慢性胰腺炎中相当准确[191,207,232,233]。粪弹性蛋白酶-1 在其他如短肠综合征和小肠细菌过度生长等引起腹泻的疾病中会被稀释,从而导致其假性降低。该测试应在固体或半固体粪便标本上进行。在美国,参考实验室可进行粪便弹性蛋白酶测定。

(3) 粪便脂肪排泄

丧失 90% 胰脂肪酶的分泌能力后就会发生脂肪消化不良。胰脂肪酶的功能评估是测定收集 72 小时的粪便中粪便脂肪的排泄量。虽然理论上很简单,但在实践中很难进行。患者必须至少在试验前 3 天和试验后 3 天遵循含有 100g/d 脂肪的饮食,并且很难完全收集样本。健康情况下,粪便中的脂肪应少于 7g(摄入量的 7%)。测定粪便脂肪需要准确知道饮食中脂肪的含量,而这很难被确定。粪便脂肪的定性分析也可以用随机粪便标本苏丹Ⅲ染色法进行。每高倍视野中发现超过 6 个脂滴被认为是阳性结果,但与粪便脂肪排泄一样,患者必须摄入足够的脂肪以产生可被测量的脂肪泻。粪便苏丹Ⅲ染色仅在有大量脂肪泻的患者中才呈阳性[207,208]。

(二) 胰腺结构检测(影像学)

1. 腹部平片

对慢性胰腺炎而言,腹部平片上发现弥漫的(并非局灶)胰腺钙化较为特异。胰腺的囊性肿瘤和胰岛细胞肿瘤以及胰周血管可见到局灶钙化。钙化发生在慢性胰腺炎自然病程的晚期,发展可能需要 5~25 年的时间[69,70,145]。钙化在酒精性、迟发性特发性、遗传性和热带性胰腺炎中最常见,在早发性特发性胰腺炎中较少见。在吸烟的患者中更常见到慢性胰腺炎临床病程以及随后的钙化进展增快[53-58,84,85,234]。钙化形成后并非一成不变,事实上随着时间的推移,钙化可能会增加或减少[234,235]。

2. 腹部 US

US 已作为诊断慢性胰腺炎的工具被广泛研究。因为许多患者的胰腺(特别是胰头)由于被覆肠道气体或因体型而不能充分显示,所以这种方法受到一定限制。慢性胰腺炎的 US 表现为胰管扩张、胰管结石声影、腺体萎缩、腺体边缘不规则、假性囊肿、实质回声改变(见表 59.2)。大多数研究表明,其敏感度为 50%~80%,特异度为 80%~90%[236]。在一项比较经腹 US 与 CT、ERCP 和 EUS 的研究中,US 的准确性为 56%[237]。在该研究中,其他诊断检查显示胰腺正常的患者中,有 40% 的患者胰腺出现了一些异常(如胰腺实质回声改变)。日本一项包含 130 000 次腹部 US 检查的大型筛查性研究发现,在缺乏慢性胰腺炎临床特征的情况下,存在回声增强,胰管轻度扩张,小囊腔,甚至导管钙化[238]。这些异常大部分不能归因于慢性胰腺炎,而应是衰老。这些研究表明,正常人的 US 表现有很大的波动,并且如果可见的变化较轻,正常(或与年龄相关)的变异与慢性胰腺炎二者很难区分。尽管相对便宜和安全,腹部 US 检查在评估疑似慢性胰腺炎的患者中并不普遍有用。正常胰腺或中等或明确的晚期慢性胰腺炎变化有诊断价值,但轻度慢性胰腺炎的改变就不那么特异,必须根据临床病史和患者的年龄来解读。US 在筛查慢性胰腺炎并发症(如假性囊肿或胆管梗阻)和评估其他可能类似慢性胰腺炎症状的情况(如胆道疾病)中是有用的。

3. CT

CT 对慢性胰腺炎的总敏感度在 75%~90% 之间,特异度在 85% 或以上[236,237,239]。CT 基本上可以对所有患者的胰腺进行成像,因此较之于 US 有很大的优势。表 59.3 概括了慢性胰腺炎的 CT 诊断异常。大多数关于慢性胰腺炎的诊断性 CT 的研究并没有使用最先进的 CT 技术。与所有诊断检查一样,CT 在实质性结构改变后的晚期慢性胰腺炎中最准确(图 59.4)。虽然 CT 比 US 昂贵且会使患者暴露于电离辐射,但

表 59.3　US 或 CT 的慢性胰腺炎分级

等级	US 或 CT 发现
正常	在可见到完整腺体的高质量成像上无异常发现
可疑	下列中的 1 种： 体部胰管轻度扩张(2~4mm) 胰腺增大≤2 倍正常
轻中度	前述发现中的 1 种加上下列至少 1 种： 胰管扩张(>4mm) 胰管不规则 囊腔(单个或多个)<10mm 实质回声/密度不均 导管壁回声增强 胰头或胰体轮廓不规则 实质局灶坏死或缺失
重度	轻度/中度特征加上下列中 1 种或多种： 囊腔(单个或多个)>10mm 导管内充盈缺损 结石/胰腺钙化 导管梗阻(狭窄) 重度导管扩张或不规则 邻近器官侵犯

Adapted from Sarner M, Cotton PB. Classification of pancreatitis. Gut 1984; 25:756.

CT,计算机断层扫描;US,超声。

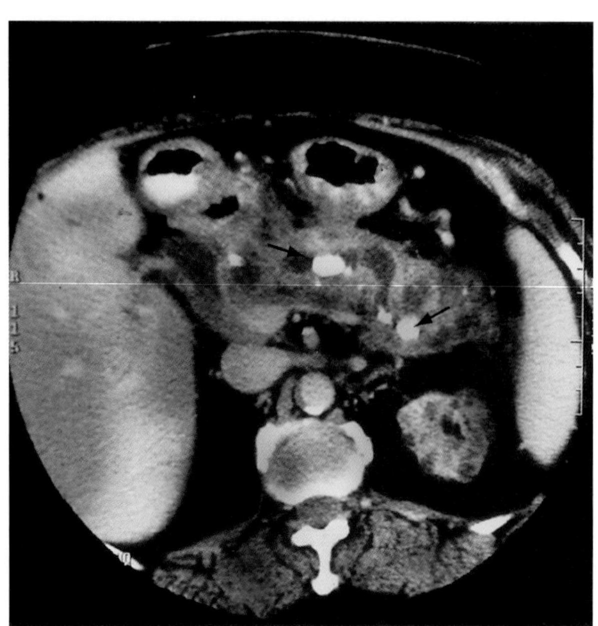

图 59.4　CT 显示在长期慢性胰腺炎中明显扩张的胰管内有数个大的、致密钙化的结石(箭)

其更敏感与特异。胰腺脂肪化的意义尚不明确[240,241]。这种情况被称为脂肪性胰腺、胰腺脂肪代谢障碍、非酒精性脂肪性胰腺病等,可能与代谢综合征、肥胖、衰老或其他未知因素有关,其本身并不是慢性胰腺炎的特异性发现。

4. MRI

在慢性胰腺炎患者中,MRI 联合 MRCP 与 CT 一样准确,甚至可能更准确[236,239,242]。约 90% 的病例 MRCP 结果与 ERCP 结果一致[220,225]。MRCP 与 ERCP 在胰管较小的区域(胰尾和侧支)或胰管改变较细微时不那么一致。促胰液素可以改善对胰管的显像[236,242-245]。此外,使用钆作为造影剂可以增加信号强度(通常在 T1 成像上)和动脉增强率,可能会提高对腺体的成像能力[242,246]。最后,在注射促胰液素(secretin injection,S-MRCP)MRCP 过程中,可以定性或半定量地评估胰腺到十二指肠的液体输出量,从而估计胰腺的分泌功能[242,247,248]。促胰液素 MRCP 已经与内镜下的胰腺功能检测进行了比较[248]。在胰腺功能检查正常的 23 例患者中,MRCP 显示异常的有 8 例,提示促胰液素 MRCP 可能有显著的假阳性率。一些分析表明,不测量碳酸氢盐浓度而仅测量促胰液素刺激后的液体体积的话很不准确因而不能用于临床[249]。一项研究还比较了一组因非钙化性慢性胰腺炎而接受全胰腺切除术的患者的 MRI 所见和组织学结果[250]。使用 2 个 MRI 特征作为临界仅达到 65% 的敏感度和 89% 的特异度。对慢性胰腺炎的最强预测因素是胰管不规则、T1 加权信号增强和促胰液素刺激后十二指肠充盈。磁共振图像分析的进展将继续改善 MRCP 的图像质量,以期在未来精确度与 ERCP 相当。然而像 ERCP 一样,MRCP 对于没有明显导管异常的患者也不准确。尽管 MRI 已经广泛应用,但并不是所有的中心都有能力进行高质量的 MRCP 或 S-MRCP。

5. ERCP

胰管造影被认为是对胰腺结构最特异和敏感的检查。在给予治疗方面(如胰管支架植入术、结石取出术)它也比之前讨论的所有诊断试验都有优势。然而,其缺点是 ERCP 是最危险的诊断试验,至少有 5% 的患者出现并发症(某些亚组高达 20%),死亡率为 0.1% 至 0.5%。在大多数关于慢性胰腺炎患者的研究中,ERCP 的敏感度在 70%~90% 之间,特异度在 80%~100% 之间[231,236,237]。因此,慢性胰腺炎可以存在没有任何可见的胰管内改变[1,209,219,221,229,236,251,252]。

表 59.4 列出了 ERCP 中慢性胰腺炎的诊断性特征。这是 30 多年前举行的国际共识会议上制定的[253,254]。诊断基于主胰管和侧支的异常。ERCP 对疾病晚期患者具有高度的敏感性和特异性。大量胰管扩张伴有交替狭窄(串珠样表现)是极晚期慢性胰腺炎的特征(图 59.5)。较不明显的胰脏造影变化则不太明确和特异(图 59.6)。ERCP 的准确解读需要有高质量的研究(充盈到第二级分支,没有明显的运动伪影)和获取高分辨率 X 线图像的能力。许多胰腺造影不满足这些适于研究的标准。胰腺导管充盈不足可能会表现为导管边缘不规则(导致慢性胰腺炎的过度诊断),或者无法描绘侧支充盈不足的改变(导致慢性胰腺炎的诊断不足)。

表 59.4　慢性胰腺炎的经内镜逆行胰管造影的剑桥分级

等级	主胰管	侧支
正常	正常且胰管充盈至侧支	正常
可疑	正常	<3 个异常
轻度	正常	≥3 个异常
中度	异常	≥3 个异常
重度	异常并有下列中的 1 种： 大囊腔(>10mm) 梗阻或狭窄 充盈缺损 重度扩张或不规则	≥3 个异常

Adapted from Axon ATR, Classen M, Cotton PB, et al. Pancreatography in chronic pancreatitis; international definitions. Gut 1984;25:1107-12.

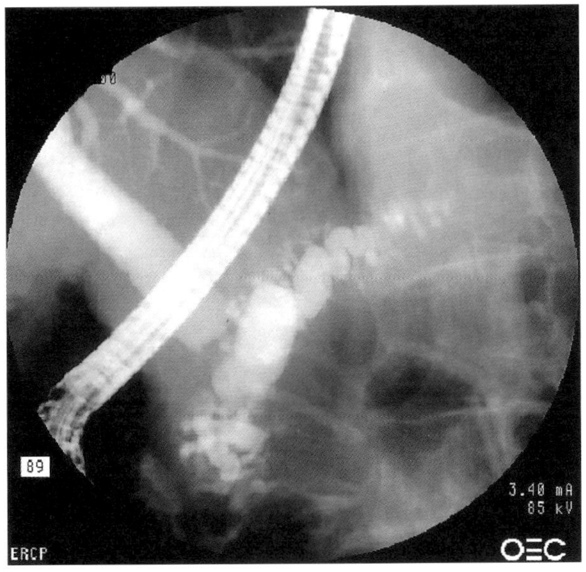

图 59.5　内镜逆行胰管造影显示胰管明显扩张，并且狭窄和扩张交替出现。这种"湖链"样外观是慢性胰腺炎的诊断

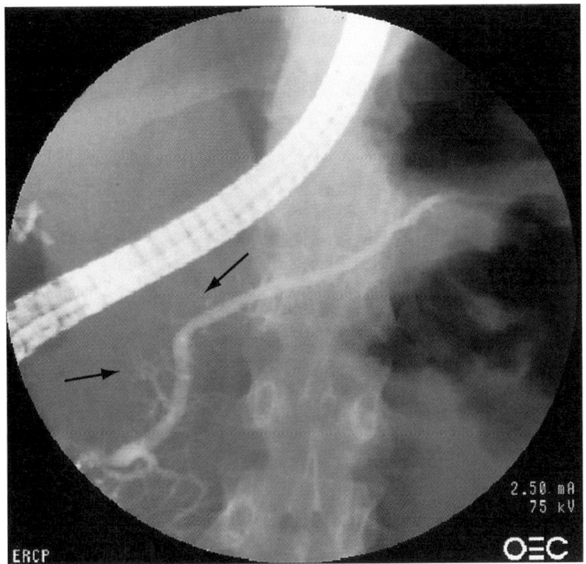

图 59.6　内镜逆行胰管造影显示，直接胰腺功能(胰泌素)检测提示慢性胰腺炎的患者，仅在侧支(箭)有细微改变。这些细微的发现通常不足以明确诊断慢性胰腺炎

在其他情况下也可见到慢性胰腺炎特有的胰管异常。最常见的是衰老对胰管的影响。虽然在正常的衰老过程中很好地保留了胰腺功能，但胰管可能会出现明显的异常。它们包括主胰管及其侧支的局灶性或弥漫性扩张，出现囊腔，甚至导管结石[131,132,221,255,256]。在之前提到的大型 US 筛查研究中，认为 50% 的钙化和 80% 以上的导管扩张和囊性病变不是因为慢性胰腺炎，而是由衰老引起的。这些变化是否是生命正常损耗的后果尚不明确。急性胰腺炎发作后也可能出现暂时的胰管改变，可能需要数月时间才能恢复[221]。胰腺癌胰管内可出现类似慢性胰腺炎的病变。最后，放置胰管支架可在胰管内产生类似慢性胰腺炎的新发异常，而这种异常在支架移除后可能不会完全消失[221,257,258]。用于预防 ERCP 术后胰腺炎等目的，放置临时的、极小口径的胰腺支架似乎很少产生这些导管改变[259]。

在观察者间和观察者内都有很大可能对 ERCP 的解读存在明显差异[221]。最初的共识会议确定了胰管扩张、异常胰管轮廓和异常侧支等异常，但没有定义绝对标准来区分正常和异常或正常变异[254]。在一项研究中，74 份尸体胰腺造影报告被提交给 6 名有经验的内镜医师[131]，要求他们判断这些胰腺造影图片是否证实了慢性胰腺炎以及异常的严重程度。之后判断与胰腺组织学的相关性。所有 6 名内镜医师都正确地识别出 5 名慢性胰腺炎患者。在剩下的 69 名受试者中，并无慢性胰腺炎的组织学证据。根据观察者的不同，主要基于主导管和侧支的轻度异常，42% 到 98% 的胰腺造影被认为有慢性胰腺炎。由于胰腺与年龄相关的变化导致了错误的解读。另一项研究试图通过在 3 个不同的场合向 4 名内镜专家提供 51 张胰腺造影图片来评估观察者内部的变化[260]。在 47% 到 95% 的病例中，每个内镜医师的 3 份报告结果都是一致的(观察者内部变异率高达 53%)。在 ERCP 评估中，观察者内和观察者间的变化大多不是因为明显的异常，而与对轻度或细微的胰腺造影变化的解读有关。这是与 ERCP 作为诊断工具相关的最本质性的临床问题；微小或较轻的胰管异常非特异，并不是慢性胰腺炎的可靠标志。考虑到 ERCP 的风险和有可用的胰管成像替代方法(MRCP 或 EUS)，ERCP 不应该被用作慢性胰腺炎患者的诊断工具。只有在计划治疗时才应使用 ERCP。

6. EUS

EUS 可以通过克服腹部 US 成像的问题(如肠腔内的干扰气体)，对胰腺实质和胰管进行非常详细的检查。传统诊断系统[最低标准术语(minimal standard terminology, MST)]是基于胰腺导管和实质的异常(表 59.5)。这些特征可以单独分类为无、最小、中等或广泛，但通常在实践中只按是否存在进行评分，并使用存在特征的总数作为分数。该试验的敏感性和特异性由定义慢性胰腺炎的阈值总评分决定。使用的阈值分数范围很大，从 1 到 6 不等。大多数研究使用 3 个或 3 个以上的特征来定义阳性结果[236,251,261-263]。第二个诊断系统称为 Rosemont 标准也用于慢性胰腺炎的 EUS 诊断(见表 59.5)。其通过专家共识所制定，并且包括主要和次要标准，以尝试对严重程度进行半定量。对这些新标准的初步研究没有记载观察者间一致性或测试准确性方面的改进[239,261-264]。

表 59.5　EUS 诊断慢性胰腺炎

标准 MST EUS 分级系统		EUS 诊断 Rosemont 标准	
实质异常	点状高回声	主要特征	点状高回声伴声影(主要 A)
	高回声条索		主胰管结石(主要 A)
	分叶状轮廓		蜂窝状小叶(主要 B)
	囊肿		
导管异常	主胰管扩张	次要特征	非蜂窝状小叶
	主胰管不规则		点状高回声不伴声影
	管壁高回声		条索影
	可见侧支		囊肿
	钙化		主胰管轮廓不规则
			主胰管扩张
			管壁高回声
			侧支扩张
在标准 EUS 系统中,每项发现计相同分,总分为发现的总数量。在 Rosemont 系统中,诊断分层如下:			
与慢性胰腺炎一致		1 个主要 A 特征和≥3 个次要特征或 1 个主要 A 特征和 1 个主要 B 特征或 2 个主要 A 特征	
推测为慢性胰腺炎		1 个主要 A 特征和<3 个次要特征或 主要 B 特征和≥3 个次要特征或 >5 个次要特征	
不确定是慢性胰腺炎		3~4 个次要特征或 主要 B 特征和<3 个次要特征	
正常		≤2 个次要特征	

EUS,超声内镜;MST,最低标准术语。

在少数患者中已将 EUS 与胰腺组织学进行了比较。一项研究在 71 例怀疑慢性胰腺炎而接受手术治疗的患者中比较了 EUS 特征和组织学[265]。使用超过 3 个 EUS 标准的临界值,EUS 的敏感度为 83%,特异度为 57%。在一个有更多进展期慢性胰腺炎组织学证据的亚组中,其敏感度为 83%,特异度为 80%。没有某一 EUS 标准比其他任何标准能更好地预测纤维化,但 EUS 标准的数量与疾病的组织学严重程度之间存在普遍的相关性。另一项对 42 例胰腺手术前接受 EUS 检查的患者(主要是癌症患者)的研究发现,临界值超过 4 个 EUS 标准,敏感度为 90%,特异度为 86%[266]。一项针对 25 名患者的研究指出,胰腺纤维化与 EUS 评分相关,EUS 异常(≥4 项标准)有 84% 敏感度[267]。一项研究比较了 50 例进行全胰腺切除术治疗非钙化慢性胰腺炎的慢性腹痛患者中的 Rosemont 标准和组织学[268]。MST 系统与 Rosemont 系统相关性较好,但两者与组织学相关性较差。在该分析中,超过半数的 Rosemont 评分正常的患者有慢性胰腺炎的组织学证据,而有"不确定"特征的患者中有 80% 是慢性胰腺炎,几乎所有具有"提示"特征的患者都是慢性胰腺炎。一项使用 EUS 引导的胰腺穿刺活检的研究发现 EUS 与组织学一致性较差,但获得的组织学标本很小而并不能代表整个腺体[269]。

约有 80% 患者中 EUS 和 ERCP 一致[221,236,251,270-274]。EUS 也与标准/导管内直接胰腺功能检测进行了比较。在这些研究中,这些检测的一致性差别很大,从 10% 到 90% 不等[221,225,251,273-275]。这种变化一部分与疾病的严重程度和疾病谱偏倚有关。在疾病进展期的患者中一致性最好。在一项研究中,EUS 对晚期慢性胰腺炎(ERCP 的典型表现和胰腺功能异常检查)的敏感性良好(超过 3 项标准的敏感度为 73%,特异度为 81%),但对进展较少的慢性胰腺炎敏感度仅为 10%[275]。

EUS 检查结果与其他诊断检查结果不一致的大多数例子中,通常是 EUS 检查结果异常而其他检查正常[276]。说明了 EUS 的特异性问题。特异性是由选择的临界值决定的,而会被其他类似于慢性胰腺炎 EUS 表现的临床情况所降低。这可能是一个实质性难题,因为常可遇见慢性胰腺炎的 EUS 改变。近期急性胰腺炎发作引起的水肿可使导管边缘和小叶内间隔更加明显,从而降低特异性[251]。通过 EUS 可观察到胰腺中类似于慢性胰腺炎变化的与年龄相关的改变[277]。在没有慢性胰腺炎临床表现的情况下,长期饮酒和吸烟也可产生类似的变化[251,278-280]。在一项研究中,39% 的不明原因消化不良患者具有 5 个或 5 个以上的慢性胰腺炎 EUS 特征,对照组中 34% 具有 3 个或 3 个以上的特征[281]。这些患者中的全部或大多数存在或将发展为慢性胰腺炎似乎不太可能。

慢性胰腺炎的 EUS 诊断是基于 US 图像的解读。在这种解读中,观察者间只有中度的差异[251,282]。与 ERCP 不同的是,观察者内的一致性似乎很高[283]。在缺乏其他诊断试验提供确凿信息的情况下,存在 3 个或 4 个(或更少)EUS 特征是否足以作出慢性胰腺炎的最终诊断还有待确定[221,225,276,284,285]。由于缺乏有用的金标准,解决该问题需要对患者进行长时间的随访,并且一些研究显示 EUS 对于最终发展为明确的慢性胰腺炎的预测能力有限[276]。包括造影剂的使用、数字图像分析和 EUS 弹性成像等。EUS 成像进展正在研究中,但尚未显示其能提高诊断准确性[285],而且这些技术可能在评估胰腺肿块病变方面最适用[110]。

EUS 对晚期慢性胰腺炎患者具有较高的准确性(图 59.7)。对慢性胰腺炎而言,EUS 评分大于 5(按照 MST 标

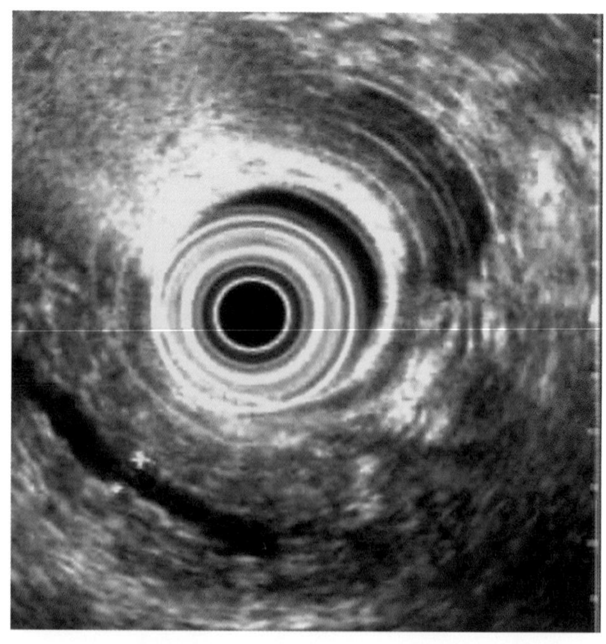

图 59.7　慢性胰腺炎患者胰体部的 EUS 影像。在扩张胰管上的标志物显示高回声边缘,这是慢性胰腺炎的诊断特征之一。这些标志物周围的实质显示高回声链和病灶,这是慢性胰腺炎的其他特征。EUS,超声内镜

准)具有相对特异性。完全正常或接近正常的 EUS(0-2 条标准)不像慢性胰腺炎[284,285]。EUS 评分为 3 或 4 应被认为不确定,需要根据患者的临床表现进行解读,并考虑到酒精、烟草、年龄和其他可出现类似慢性胰腺炎变化的相关情况(糖尿病、慢性肾病)的影响。

八、诊断策略

常由于腹痛综合征而怀疑为慢性胰腺炎的诊断,较少的原因是考虑有外分泌(腹泻、脂肪泻、体重减轻)或内分泌功能不全(糖尿病)。在怀疑有外分泌或内分泌功能不全的亚组中,疾病很可能存在很长时间,大多数可用的诊断试验能够发现这种相对较晚期的疾病。因为其他情况可能与慢性胰腺炎相似(胰腺恶性肿瘤、导管内乳头状黏液瘤、囊性肿瘤),有必要行高质量的断层成像检查以除外这些可能疾病。使用多排探测器技术或胰腺特异的高质量 CT 扫描或有 MRCP 的 MRI 是最好的初始诊断检查[221,225,284,285]。这些患者可能已经做了常规的腹部 CT(通常是通过急诊),但没有高质量的 CT(或 MRI+MRCP),所以如果以前的报告质量较低,值得重新进行。如果 CT 或 MRI 不能证明慢性胰腺炎,则接下来应该使用灵敏度最高的检查。由于直接胰腺功能检查还没有被广泛应用,下一步行 EUS 是最合理的。如果 EUS 检查结果不明确,可行的话进行激素刺激胰腺功能检测[1,221,284]。这可能需要将患者转诊到进行功能测试的中心。ERCP 不应用作诊断目的。如果对诊断仍有疑问,定期随访并重新评估可能是唯一的诊断方法。需要新的诊断学生物标志物,并且大量关于鉴别慢性胰腺炎及其并发症发展的预测因素的研究正在进行[286]。

九、治疗

(一) 腹痛

腹痛是慢性胰腺炎最常见、最使人筋疲力尽也是最需要治疗的症状。对疼痛的初步评估应集中于能够识别出有特定治疗方法的相关情况。这些情况包括胰腺假性囊肿、十二指肠(可能还有胆管)受压、合并胰腺癌和胃轻瘫。断层成像除了识别类似慢性胰腺炎的其他诊断外,还有助于识别其中一些并发症。CT 或 MRI 可鉴别(或提示)是否存在特定可治疗的并发症外,对于鉴别胰腺结构异常(特别是胰管扩张)的患者非常有用。鉴别胰管扩张对于确定哪些患者最有可能受益于内镜或手术治疗很有用。关于疼痛治疗的随机试验很少,安慰剂对照试验更少,因此大多数干预措施的支持证据基础相当薄弱[158,159]。在已知的慢性胰腺炎疼痛试验中,这些患者的安慰剂效应至少是 20%[287]。

1. 药物治疗

(1) 镇痛药

大多数慢性胰腺炎患者需要某种形式的镇痛[147]。一些患者的疼痛可使用对乙酰氨基酚或阿司匹林来缓解,但是大多数患者需要更强效的麻醉药。使用这些药物有麻醉药上瘾的风险。成瘾的风险尚未确定,估计为 10%～30%[147],但可能更高。应当努力减少使用麻醉药品,但是对于有剧烈疼痛的患者不应停用麻醉药品。尽量减少麻醉药滥用和成瘾风险的策略包括让同一医生负责开处方、持续咨询、监测处方和定期随诊。疼痛门诊可能有帮助,也可能没有帮助。以非麻醉方式为主的疼痛治疗门诊对慢性胰腺炎患者最有用。如果非麻醉性药物无效,可以开始使用如曲马朵等效价较低的阿片类药物。曲马朵是一种具有 mu 型阿片激动剂和单胺能性质的双效镇痛药。治疗慢性胰腺炎时高剂量曲马朵与口服吗啡相当,但对肠道运动的影响较小[156,207,288]。一些患者需要使用更强效的麻醉药,但应遵循世卫组织疼痛缓解阶梯的标准指南[156,207]。在这种情况下,集中精力将患者疼痛控制到可接受的水平而非完全缓解,并逐渐增加剂量或药效是有益的。对于需要更强效麻醉药的患者,也可以考虑使用辅助药物。许多患者存在抑郁,同时存在的抑郁症降低了疼痛阈值。慢性胰源性疼痛可导致伤害感受性神经元中异常的脊髓门控,这是一种中枢敏感的疼痛状态,伴有痛觉过敏和痛觉异常[156,173-176]。三环类抗抑郁药可以是有用的辅助药物,不仅因为它们可以治疗抑郁症和潜在地调节中枢疼痛,而且它们对疼痛有直接影响并增强麻醉药的效果。5-羟色胺再摄取抑制剂(SSRI)和 5-羟色胺和去甲肾上腺素再摄取抑制剂(如度洛西汀)等其他抗抑郁药也可能有这种效果[156,157]。最后,加巴喷丁类(电压门控 N 型钙通道 a_2d 亚基抑制剂)中的加巴喷丁和普瑞巴林作为麻醉药的辅助药物用于各种慢性疼痛状态。在一项对需麻醉药控制疼痛的慢性胰腺炎患者的随机试验中,多至每天两次 300mg 剂量的普瑞巴林减少了患者的疼痛[156,157,289]。可能有通过感觉测试来判定患者有痛觉过敏或痛觉异常的,以预测对加巴喷丁的反应[290]。加巴喷丁的副作用很常见,包括头晕和醉酒感。其他辅助药物尚未经过严格研究,但它们经常用于慢性胰腺炎持续剧烈疼痛的患者以改善疼痛治疗并将麻醉药的剂量和效力降至最低。鉴于对慢性胰腺炎疼痛的神经病理机制的认识逐渐深入,使用这些类型的药物似乎是合理的。没有关于这些患者使用医用大麻的数据。

(2) 戒烟和戒酒

长期酗酒会加速慢性胰腺炎患者胰腺功能障碍的进展,即使完全戒酒也不能阻止这个进程[89]。此外,持续的酗酒和吸烟也增加了死亡率[14,17,31]。因此,除了对腹痛的影响外,也有充分的理由鼓励患者停止饮酒和吸烟。大多数研究(但不是全部)已经证明,停止饮酒的患者疼痛或疼痛复发明显减少。在一篇对这些研究的总结中,疼痛在 26% 的戒酒患者中持续存在,而在那些继续饮酒的患者中这一比例为 53%[291]。在一项关于慢性胰腺炎自然病程的研究中,持续的酒精滥用与更高的疼痛复发风险相关[292]。这些数据支持戒酒对疼痛有一些有益的影响,但这种影响程度不是很高。戒烟似乎在预防烟草导致的疾病和减少继发性胰腺癌风险方面有更多的好处[14,17,52-55,293]。特别是在急性复发性胰腺炎的一个阶段停止吸烟可以降低随后发展为慢性胰腺炎的风险。

(3) 抗氧化剂

自由基损伤是酒精性和其他形式慢性胰腺炎所致胰腺损伤的机制之一。慢性胰腺炎(特别是酒精性胰腺炎)患者被证明有氧化应激和抗氧化能力降低[67,100,156,294]。氧化应激也是胰腺星状细胞的一种强激活因子[47-49]。有两项关于抗氧化剂的相对较大的安慰剂对照试验[295,296]。在印度的一项大型研究中,发现抗氧化剂组每月疼痛天数显著减少(每月少7.3天,而安慰剂组少3.2天)。该试验招募了相对年轻、体重过轻、主要患有特发性或热带性胰腺炎的受试者。试验中使用了硒、β-胡萝卜素、维生素C、维生素E和蛋氨酸的组合。来自英国的第二项试验[296]使用了更高剂量的相同抗氧化剂,但招募的人群年龄较大,没有营养不良,并且主要是由于酒精和吸烟所致的慢性胰腺炎。尽管血清抗氧化剂水平有所改善,但该试验证明抗氧化剂治疗没有任何益处。所有可获取证据的综述表明,总体疼痛评分略有降低[297]。因此,抗氧化剂的整体作用是有限的,并且在美国没有广泛使用[298]。

(4) 胰酶疗法

胰腺分泌受十二指肠内胰蛋白酶和营养物质的反馈控制。使用胰酶来减轻疼痛是基于这些药物激活该反馈控制系统以减少胰腺分泌。将蛋白酶输送到十二指肠或空肠近端可抑制胰腺分泌。这种作用是由于在该段小肠的蛋白酶能够破坏肠道CCK释放因子来减少CCK的释放,而肠道CCK释放因子是存在营养物质时CCK释放的主要刺激物之一。在慢性胰腺炎患者中,缺乏运输到十二指肠的蛋白酶可以使更多的CCK释放因子逃脱变性。因此可以预期十二指肠内的CCK释放因子水平和血清CCK水平升高。较高水平的循环CCK可以刺激胰腺的分泌,这种刺激可能通过提高胰腺导管或组织压力或者胰管阻塞时迫使消化酶进入间质而导致胰腺疼痛。口服胰酶可通过在十二指肠提供可以使CCK释放因子变性的活化丝氨酸蛋白酶,恢复胰腺分泌的正常反馈抑制,从而减少过度刺激及减轻疼痛。

如第56章所述,胰腺分泌的体积和碳酸氢盐不受十二指肠内存在的蛋白酶的控制。此外,胰腺的分泌受体液和神经的控制。因此通过口服酶补充剂以抑制胰酶释放不太可能产生完全抑制分泌的效果,而且对分泌的影响程度因人而异。这种可以控制胰酶分泌的反馈控制系统的存在,在非慢性胰腺炎的人群和一些慢性胰腺炎患者中都有所记录[299]。这种反馈系统失调的一个标志可能是慢性胰腺炎患者,尤其是伴有疼痛的患者血清中CCK的升高。血清CCK升高仅见于一些慢性胰腺炎患者。很可能就像所有推测的疼痛原因一样,这种反馈失调可能只对一部分患者重要。

几个小型随机、前瞻性、双盲试验试图描述口服胰酶减少慢性胰腺炎患者疼痛的有效性。两项使用非肠溶(片剂)形式酶的研究表明有好处[300,301]。另外四项使用肠溶微球制剂的研究没有显示出任何益处[302-305]。这些研究之间的差异可能反映了患者的选择,也可能反映了酶制备的不同选择(表59.6)。小肠的反馈敏感部分似乎位于最近端,肠溶制剂在到达更远端小肠之前可能不会释放大部分蛋白酶。因此非肠溶的酶比较适用于将丝氨酸蛋白酶充分运输到十二指肠。结合了两种酶研究的分析得出了酶并不能减轻疼痛的结论[306,307],但是考虑到上述讨论的机制,这种结合分析方法在这种情况下可能并不合适。尽管如此,酶被广泛用于治疗这些患者的疼痛[298]。由于非肠溶酶可被胃酸失活,因此需要同时使用抑制胃酸或中和胃酸的药物。在2个证实有效的研究中,病情较轻的患者(无胰管扩张、钙化、脂肪泻)、女性、慢

表59.6　治疗慢性胰腺炎的酶制剂

产品	剂型	脂肪酶含量/每片或每粒(USP单位)
Creon	猪肠溶胶囊	3 000,6 000,12 000,24 000,36 000
Zenpep	猪肠溶胶囊	3 000,5 000,10 000,15 000,20 000,25 000,40 000
Pancreaze	猪肠溶胶囊	4 200,10 500,16 800,21 000
Pertzye	猪肠溶及碳酸氢盐	4 000,8 000,16 000
Viokace	猪非肠溶药片*	10 440,20 880

*非肠溶制剂需要与组胺-2受体拮抗剂或质子泵抑制剂共用以避免胃酸使胰酶变性

每餐胰酶总剂量需要依据反应进行滴定,但通常每餐需要40 000~90 000单位脂肪酶,零食时为其半量。该剂量应该在进餐时平均分散。

性特发性胰腺炎患者的反应最好。在美国只有一种非肠溶包被制剂。每日4次约150 000单位剂量的蛋白酶(2片Viokace 20 800,每日4次,随餐和夜间服用)。在弥漫性钙化或胰管扩张的晚期慢性胰腺炎患者中,尽管这些患者常由于胰腺外分泌功能不全而需要酶替代,但是治疗疼痛的试验很少成功。

2. 内镜治疗(见第61章)

内镜治疗的主要目的是通过解除胰管梗阻来改善胰管引流。内镜治疗仅限于胰管解剖结构可治疗的一组患者。这些患者通常是胰管扩张(>5mm)伴有单一或显性狭窄,或者胰头部梗阻性结石及上游胰管扩张。然而,重要的是,需要记住一些胰管扩张的患者很少或没有临床症状[168],并且胰管扩张并不一定与胰管压力升高相关。腺体上游或尾部的狭窄和结石由于离内镜头端太远,通常不适合内镜治疗。具体的内镜治疗方法有胰括约肌切开术、支架置入和取石术(有时伴有碎石术)。因为它们通常一起进行,每种治疗方法的单独作用难以量化。

(1) 胰管括约肌切开术

需要放置更大口径的胰管支架和胰管结石取出时需要进行胰管括约肌切开术。可以使用拉弓式括约肌切开术,也可以在小口径胰管支架上使用针刀括约肌切开术[308]。这两种技术的使用取决于当地的偏好。主乳头胰腺括约肌切开术仅适用于因长期瘢痕性括约肌狭窄而导致慢性阻塞性胰腺炎(一种罕见的慢性胰腺炎)的患者。没有证据支持Oddi括约肌功能障碍是慢性胰腺炎的病因或诱发原因[309],并且其对急性复发性胰腺炎的作用仍有争议[310,311]。没有数据支持Oddi测压法和测压指导疗法在慢性胰腺炎患者中的作用。在极少数情况下,胰腺分裂患者会出现明显的背侧胰管上游扩张和慢性胰腺炎。在这种情况下,支架联合乳头括约肌小切开是有用的,但是没有背侧胰管扩张的慢性疼痛时乳头括约肌小切开治疗是无效的。此外,症状性胰腺炎和胰腺分裂患者通常有潜在的可以解释胰腺炎的基因突变[122,123],从而使得内镜治疗的作用和效果更加难以定义。

(2) 支架置入

在第61章中详细讨论了胰管支架置入,它最常用来扩张或越过梗阻性狭窄(图59.8)。专科中心的一些关于支架治

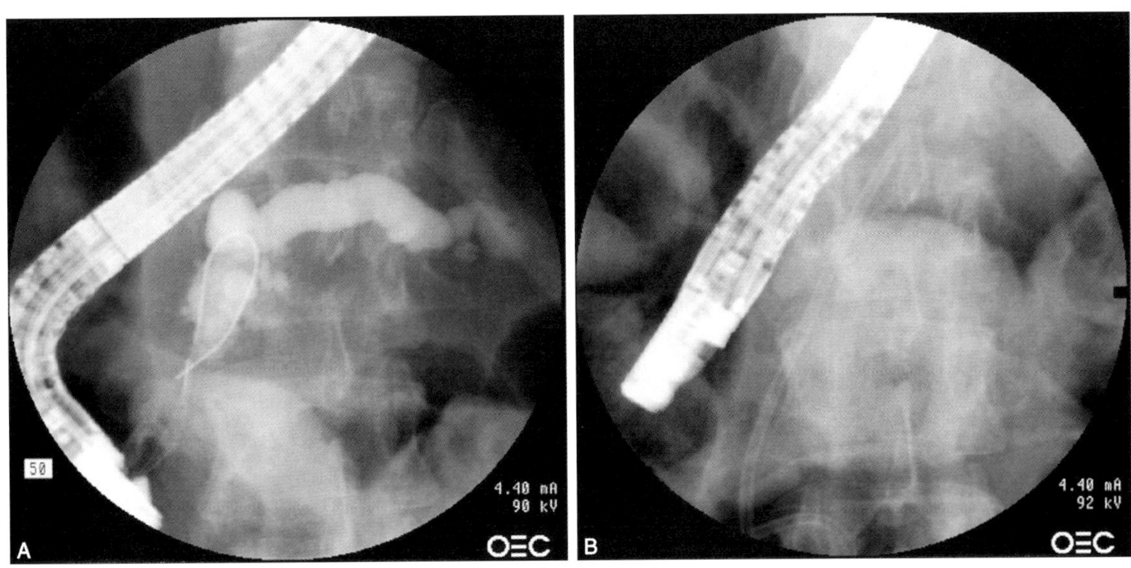

图 59.8　慢性胰腺炎患者的内镜逆行胰胆管造影(ERCP)。A,可见扩张的胰管,胰头有单一明显狭窄及上游扩张。B,已在狭窄处置入支架

疗的回顾性病例系列报告了近 90% 的内镜治疗成功率(成功放置支架)和大约一半到三分之二的患者疼痛改善[312-314]。内镜治疗的高成功率反映了这些中心高度的专业性和严格的患者选择,但成功的内镜治疗不一定能减轻疼痛。最大的多中心报告涉及 1 000 多名患者,因胰头部单一明显狭窄而行支架置入的患者在平均随访时间 4.9 年时,57% 的患者疼痛明显改善,其他 19% 患者有疼痛显著改善但仍需要继续内镜治疗[313]。约 20% 的患者出现支架治疗的并发症,死亡率为 0.6%[312-314]。最常报道的并发症是支架堵塞(疼痛反复发作、急性胰腺炎发作或其他并发症)、支架内移位(可能需要手术取出)和胰管穿孔。在这些患者中会出现支架引起的新的胰管狭窄,但通常没有临床意义(与先前正常的胰管中出现狭窄的患者不同)。

有人可能会认为,放置支架后疼痛缓解的患者可能是胰管压力高的患者,而支架治疗降低了压力。在一项测定支架置入术后疼痛缓解和胰管压力的研究中,9 名压力正常的患者中有 3 名在支架置入结束时仍有疼痛,而 4 名胰管持续高压的患者术后没有疼痛[165]。支架置入后无论胰管直径(胰管压力降低的替代标志)是否降低,疼痛改善都是相似的,而且疼痛缓解可能不受支架阻塞的影响[166]。对于支架治疗的反应似乎不能从测量胰管内压力或初始胰管直径来预测。因此通常是基于症状而不是引流的管腔直径来决定是否移除支架。即使在专业中心,大约有 1/4 的患者因内镜治疗失败而需要手术[166,312-314]。有 1/3 至 1/2 的患者在有最初的临床疗效后症状再发。

(3) 清除胰管结石

内镜下清除胰管结石比较困难,并且只有在小部分患者中能够做到。多发性结石、大结石、胰体和尾部结石、侧支结石、嵌顿结石或狭窄胰管后结石通常不能进行内镜技术治疗。切除大或嵌顿的结石需要使用以体外冲击波碎石(ESWL)或胰管内碎石装置为主的碎石术。胰管结石的存在与疼痛没有密切的关系,许多胰管结石患者没有疼痛。大多数回顾性病例报告的成功率都是可行内镜下取石的已筛选患者。在一项包含 3 189 名患者的 27 项关于 EWSL 的已发表研究的分析中,完全胰管清除的概率为 16%～88%[315],平均约为 71%。在其余 22% 的患者出现了部分胰管清除,并且在随访时约 20% 的患者出现结石复发[315]。在这项研究分析中通过多项指标测量疼痛缓解,随访时 53% 没有疼痛,33% 有改善但仍轻度疼痛,10% 有持续的严重疼痛。因此,症状改善的速度大于完全结石清除的比率。在一项比较了单独 ESWL 与 ESWL 后内镜取石的随机试验中,两组患者的疼痛缓解效果相似[316]。在本试验中,随访 2 年 ESWL 组疼痛复发率为 38%,ESWL 加内镜组为 45%。ESWL 加内镜组的治疗费用是 3 倍。这些数据表明,体外冲击波碎石可能能够减小结石的大小使其不再产生梗阻,或者除了破碎胰腺结石外,还对胰腺的疼痛有其他方面影响。一些指南推荐 ESWL 可以单独作为治疗大于 5mm 的胰管结石的慢性胰腺炎患者疼痛的适宜方法。碎石术并发症[156,285]少见,发生率低于 10%[315]。现在也有一些设备可以在小型镜下进行胰管镜检查,也可以直观地进行碎石术。关于这种方法有效性的数据有限[317]。

(4) 联合内镜治疗

虽然刚才通过单独的内镜技术讨论了内镜治疗,但经常需要联合这些治疗方法来治疗慢性胰腺炎患者。而这部分患者是那些胰管解剖正常的患者,因此仅代表慢性胰腺炎患者的一部分。在大型的病例系列中使用了各种评价疼痛缓解的方法,约三分之二的患者成功地通过内镜进行了治疗[156,285,313,314,318]。有一些小的随机试验比较了内镜和外科治疗对胰管解剖正常的慢性胰腺炎的疗效。一项试验将 72 例患者随机分为内镜治疗(胰腺括约肌切开术、支架治疗或结石取出)和外科治疗(胰管引流或胰腺切除术)两组[319]。在 1 年的随访中,疼痛缓解率相似。然而在 5 年的随访中,86% 的手术组和 61% 的内镜组疼痛部分缓解或没有疼痛。此外手术组体重增加更多,糖尿病发病率也有类似结果。该实验的不足之处在于没有积极地行最佳的内镜治疗(有些患者只接受了胰管括约肌切开术),并且手术疗法可能比经典疗法更积极(80% 接受了胰腺切除术),以及方法学略欠缺。

该试验采用伪随机化，且没有进行意向性分析。第二项随机试验比较了更积极的内镜手术（包括ESWL）和更常规的外科手术（胰空肠吻合术或改良Puestow手术）[320,321]。由于手术组有更好的结果，该试验在只有39名患者入组时提前停止。在中位随访2年后，随机接受手术的患者在生活质量评定方面有更低的疼痛评分和较好的身体健康状况。在32%的内镜组和75%的外科组中，疼痛完全或部分缓解。在5年的随访中，相比5%的手术组患者，68%的内镜组患者需要额外的内镜或手术治疗来缓解疼痛，手术组在疼痛缓解方面有持续的优势[321]。两组患者的生活质量和残余胰腺功能相近。尽管数量较少，但这些数据表明手术治疗比内镜治疗更有效且更持久[322]。应该与正在考虑治疗方法的患者讨论该结论。许多患者仍然会选择内镜治疗以避免手术。只有一小部分慢性胰腺炎和特殊胰管解剖患者可以接受内镜治疗，包括胰管扩张（通常为5mm）以及胰头梗阻性狭窄或结石。如胆管狭窄和假性囊肿等内镜下治疗并发症将在后面及第61章讨论。

3. 手术治疗

最常因药物治疗失败的顽固性腹痛而考虑进行慢性胰腺炎的手术治疗。这些患者的其他手术指征包括累及邻近器官或结构的并发症（十二指肠、脾静脉或胆道并发症），内镜或影像学介入失败的假性囊肿，胰内瘘，以及已广泛评估但仍要除外的恶性肿瘤。治疗疼痛的手术选择有胰管引流、全部或部分胰腺切除术，以及两者兼用。手术方式的选择在很大程度上取决于胰管的解剖结构、疼痛可能的发病机制、相关并发症以及当地的手术偏好和熟练度[285,323-325]。

导管引流术技术要求最低，并且保留的胰腺实质最多。该手术的基本原理是缓解胰管梗阻和降低胰管内压，从而减轻疼痛。胰管引流手术通常需要胰管扩张到5mm以上，这一直径相对容易识别和吻合[323]。在胰管扩张且胰头无炎性肿块的患者中可以考虑该操作。最常见的手术是胰管空肠端侧吻合术或Partington-Rochelle改良Puestow术。该术式纵向切开胰管，再用Roux-en-Y吻合术将其与小肠的旷置端吻合。该端侧也可用于减压任意共存的假性囊肿。若手术需要，可以切开导管狭窄以及轻松地取出结石。在没有胰管扩张的情况下也可以进行该手术（正常导管的Puestow术或V型成形术），但认为其缓解疼痛的效果较差[324]。这项手术可以在腹腔镜下进行。改良Puestow手术死亡率极低[323]。

没有比较改良Puestow术与其他手术治疗的随机试验。在经过筛选的患者中，约有四分之三患者的疼痛可以立即缓解[232-325]。在长期随访中，约有一半的患者持续感到疼痛缓解。这种有效性下降的原因尚不清楚，但可能是吻合口闭合、起源于胰头其他未引流节段的疼痛或其他疼痛原因的进展（神经炎症、中枢神经系统敏感、十二指肠或胆管阻塞等）。因此需要权衡简单低风险的手术和随时间逐渐严重的疼痛。外分泌和内分泌功能通常不受手术本身的影响，但似乎和未手术患者一样持续下降。

为了克服简单引流术早期较低和晚期较高的失败率，发展出了胰管引流术与胰腺切除术相结合的方法。由于许多外科医生认为胰头是疾病的先导部位，所以研究主要集中在头部。常规的纵向胰空肠吻合术不能完全减压腺体头部胰管，Santorini导管，以及引流钩突支。一些患者可能伴有胰腺头部的炎性肿块，使得胰头部的胰管引流更加困难。此外对于有胰头较大的炎性肿块压迫和梗阻十二指肠或胆管的患者而言，可能需要切除胰头。处理这些问题的方法包括胰头切除术（胰十二指肠切除术[Whipple手术]，保留十二指肠的Whipple手术，或保留十二指肠的胰头切除术[DPPHR]）以及胰管引流联合局部切除全部胰头或部分胰头[325]。值得注意的是，胰腺切除术等外科手术术后疼痛的改善并不是因为更好地引流了胰头部的胰管，而部分原因可能是在扩大切除的过程中去除了胰腺的内脏传入神经。

Whipple切除术或保留十二指肠的Whipple切除术可使65%~95%的患者减轻疼痛[285,323]。Whipple术通常用于仅局限于胰腺头部的患者，特别是胰腺有大量炎性肿块并考虑为恶性的患者。相关的胆道或十二指肠梗阻，在这些伴有胰头炎性肿块的患者中更常见，并且也可以在切除时治疗。这些手术的发病率和死亡率高于单纯的胰管引流术。尽管大中心的死亡率低于3%，但在多达一半的病例中出现术后早期并发症（主要是正常胃动力破坏和胰漏）。如果炎症肿块阻塞或压迫大动脉或静脉，手术死亡率较高。

已经发展出一些术式可以不像传统Whipple术一样破坏胃肠道生理来切除全部或部分胰腺头部，并限制被切除胰腺组织的数量。DPPHR是Beger术的变体，手术方法是切除胰头但保留十二指肠，并用旷置的Roux-en-Y空肠端覆盖该部位以引流胰、胆道分泌物[326]。随后对该手术进行了改进，以避免对门静脉和肠系膜上静脉周围剥离（以及相关的出血风险），并限制了胰腺组织（特别是胰岛细胞）被切除的数量。在Frey进行的一种改良中，只取出少量的胰头且不破坏胆管和胰周血管[327]。这种方法中增加了胰体部和尾部胰管的纵向切口，并在空肠的长吻合口上覆盖开放的胰管和取出的胰头部。第三种手术称为Berne术，采用无纵向胰管切开的胰头切除术，但在十二指肠和胰后血管旁留下一狭长的胰腺组织[328]。

有几项随机试验和荟萃分析比较了Whipple术和DPPHR（Frey或Beger术）[323,329,330]。在短期随访中，这些手术在缓解疼痛方面有相同的效果，在接受Whipple术的患者中有更多的糖尿病。在长期随访中，DPPHR的这一优势可能会丧失。然而比较Beger术和Frey术的随机试验显示了相似的术后并发症、疗效和长期生活质量。术后并发症比简单改良的Puestow手术更常见，但短期和长期疼痛缓解效果都更好。在美国，少数外科医生接受过此类DPPHR的培训。对于良性和恶性胰腺疾病，腹腔镜和机器人辅助的手术方法都是可行的[331,332]。慢性胰腺炎术后发生的并发症因手术方式的不同而各异。它们包括胰瘘、伤口感染、胃排空延迟、腹腔内脓肿、胰腺炎、胆管炎和胆漏。

尚不明确手术的最佳时机。过去认为手术是当其他疗法（药物和内镜）不足以缓解疼痛时考虑的和最后的选择。一些分析建议在患者出现痛觉过敏和/或阿片类药物依赖之前尽早手术更好[333,334]。正在进行一项随机试验来评估这一观点[335]。

慢性胰腺炎的外科治疗也可能涉及一些不常用的手术。以胰腺体部胰管损伤后合并上游阻塞性慢性胰腺炎为代表，在一些疾病局限于胰体尾的患者中可以考虑切除胰体尾。全或近全胰切除术同时自体胰岛细胞移植的应用越来越频繁。常在顽固性疼痛且胰管未扩张的患者中考虑该治疗。因为术前通常没有明确的慢性胰腺炎影像学证据，这些患者必须被准确诊断为慢性胰腺炎[220,230,250,268]。自体胰岛细胞移植如果成功，可以保留足够的胰岛以避免糖尿病。实践中大约 40% 的患者达到了不依赖胰岛素，80% 患者疼痛缓解[336,337]。术后糖尿病的风险取决于胰腺切除术时的胰岛细胞分泌量。有过胰腺手术史的患者胰岛分泌量降低[336-338]。全胰腺切除术和胰岛细胞自体移植也用于儿童胰腺炎（特别是遗传型）。目前，它仍然主要是一种对于其他方式失败并有剧烈疼痛的患者的补救手术。

在护理慢性胰腺炎而接受手术的患者时，谨记外分泌和内分泌功能不全可能是手术和疾病进展的结果很重要。尤其是外分泌功能不全因为可能症状很轻微，所以无法被发现。在 30%～40% 进行简单的引流术的患者和三分之二进行胰腺切除术的患者中可能发生脂肪泻[191-339]。胰腺术后使用胰酶补充剂可以更好地吸收营养，大多数（或全部）慢性胰腺炎患者术后应考虑使用胰酶补充剂。慢性胰腺炎手术后发生内分泌功能不全（糖尿病）也很常见，但并非常态，主要是胰腺切除和疾病进展的结果。

4. 神经阻滞和神经松解术

腹腔丛传递包括胰腺在内的上腹部器官的内脏传入冲动。发自腹腔丛的内脏大神经，内脏小神经和内脏最小神经穿过横膈膜到达脊髓。阻止伤害感受性刺激传递的尝试收效甚微。可以通过 CT 或 EUS 引导技术进行腹腔神经丛阻滞（通常联合使用糖皮质激素和长效局部麻醉剂如布比卡因等）和腹腔神经丛神经松解术（使用无水乙醇注射），但较之于 CT 引导下进行，EUS 引导更安全、有效、持久[340-342]。尽管有这些优势，EUS 引导下腹腔神经丛阻滞由于其反应不可预测以及作用短暂而很少被使用[343]。腹腔神经丛松解术已用于胰腺癌，但不推荐用于慢性胰腺炎患者。目前的指南不推荐腹腔神经丛阻滞或神经松解术治疗慢性胰腺炎疼痛[156,207,285]。

干扰内脏神经的传导也可能阻断中枢对痛觉输入的感知。这种方法通常包括切除一侧或两侧的内脏大神经，并可以通过胸腔镜手术进行。胸腔镜内脏神经切除术后 1 年的疼痛缓解率平均约为 50%，随着随访时间延长下降至 25%[344,345]。反应缺乏可能是由于有多个脊髓水平接受内脏神经传入，以及内脏神经根数量有巨大差异，从而使得完全切断神经很困难。很少进行这种治疗。

另一种减少痛觉的方法关注于中枢神经系统和疼痛感知上。这包括如上所述的中枢作用药物如 SSRI 和加巴喷丁类的治疗，也包括脊髓刺激和经颅磁刺激大脑疼痛中心[156,346,347]。这些都是新方法，但是其整体效果仍有待确定。

5. 疼痛的治疗

有很多方法可以治疗疼痛。第一步是确立正确的诊断，这对进展较慢的慢性胰腺炎可能具有挑战性。应谨慎评估可能引起疼痛的且有特殊治疗手段的并发症，如胃、十二指肠或胆道梗阻、假性囊肿或继发癌症[207,348]。在开始治疗之前，量化疼痛的严重程度、特征和时间性质，以及对生活质量的影响是有帮助的。对于大多数患者来说，首先应该尝试进行正规的逐步戒酒和戒烟计划以及使用低效镇痛药进行药物治疗。尽管在减轻疼痛方面支持胰酶和抗氧化剂有效的数据有限，但是可能会尝试添加其作为药物治疗的一部分。对于反应不充分的患者，应考虑使用更强效的麻醉性镇痛药和辅助药物（SSRI 或加巴喷丁）。如果无效，决定下一步治疗取决于是否有大于 5mm 的胰管扩张。对于胰管扩张的患者，应考虑内镜或手术治疗。选择内镜或手术治疗以及手术治疗的类型，取决于患者选择，可行的治疗手段和胰腺解剖。考虑到全胰切除术和胰岛细胞自体移植仅适用于特定患者，对于无扩张胰管的患者适合持续药物治疗。

（二）消化不良和脂肪泻

虽然慢性胰腺炎患者可能会出现脂肪、蛋白质和碳水化合物消化不良，但脂肪消化不良是其主要临床问题。据估计，每餐中 90 000USP 单位的脂肪酶应该足以消除脂肪泻[171,191,207]。这相当于大约 10% 的胰腺脂肪酶输出的正常下限。许多因素限制了市售酶补充剂的有效性。胰酶补充剂的酶含量各不相同。市售制剂的脂肪酶含量为每片 3 000～40 000USP 单位。目前有 5 种品牌产品可购买（见表 59.6），且没有通用形式的胰酶。

大部分脂肪酶由于被胃酸变性或被蛋白酶破坏而不能以活性形式到达小肠。大多数市售的肠溶酶制剂使用的微球太大而无法与食物同步地从胃中排出。这些肠溶微球也可能在到达远端空肠或回肠之前不会释放其酶内容物，并且远端不利于脂肪有效的消化和吸收。最后，酶制剂的效价相对较低，所以每餐和零食时都必须服用许多药片或药丸。这一要求会对依从性产生很大的负面影响。并且这些药物都比较昂贵，患者每个月花费高达 2 000 美元。这些因素都影响了对脂肪泻的有效治疗。即使在临床研究中，也不常见到将脂肪消化功能纠正到正常水平[349]。

管理脂肪泻的目标是确保在每餐饭的餐前和餐后时期至少有 90 000USP 单位的脂肪酶。由于许多患者仍有残存的胰腺分泌，且胃脂肪酶可部分弥补胰脂肪酶的缺失，因此不必每个患者都给予该量。通常 40 000～50 000USP 单位作为起始剂量，根据效果向上加量。包括在胰腺手术或因慢性胰腺炎行切除术的风险最高的患者在内[329]，对许多患者的治疗不足[191,350-352]。如果选择非肠溶制剂，则必须同时使用 H2 受体拮抗剂或质子泵抑制剂抑制胃酸。通常通过临床参数来衡量酶补充的有效性，包括粪便性状改善，便中可见脂肪减少，体重增加。通常不需要在治疗开始前和治疗期间进行 72 小时粪便脂肪分析以证明其有效性，但对于那些没有出现预期反应的患者可以考虑该手段。定期评估脂溶性维生素（特别是维生素 D）的缺乏情况，并通过骨密度测试评估是否存在骨质减少或骨质疏松很重要[182-191,207,352]。适宜的酶治疗可改善营养状况、体重、生活质量，并且可能改善死亡率[190]。对慢性胰腺炎的饮食建议通常是极低脂饮食，也有许多其他饮食。没有证据表明哪种饮食方式更不容易引起疼痛，并且极低脂饮食可能会导致脂溶性维生素缺乏加重。应当采用有益于心脏健康的或地中海式饮食，并避免食用会引起症状的食物。

对酶疗法治疗脂肪泻失败有几种可能的解释。最常见的是剂量不足，通常是由于患者不依从必要的药物效价和药量。换一种效价更高的制剂以减少服用药物数量可能会有帮助。

如前所述,采用非肠溶制剂的患者应给予抑酸剂并且确保服用。肠溶制剂通常不与减少胃酸的药物共用。一些患者使用的肠溶制剂可能会在小肠中段或远端释放酶,这种延迟释放可能不足以有效地治疗脂肪泻。部分患者加用抑制胃酸的药物可以促进这些肠溶制剂在小肠近端开放,改善脂肪消化,对于治疗无效的患者也可以考虑使用。酶应该在进食过程中分散摄入[191,352]。如果反应仍不满意,从一种方案改为另一种(例如从肠溶制剂改为非肠溶制剂+抑酸药)或将脂肪酶剂量提高到每餐 90 000USP 单位以上可能有用。如果所有这些措施都没有达到预期的效果,那么应当寻找其他可能会产生吸收不良的病因,比如乳糜泻或 SIBO 可能是某些患者的特殊问题[353,354]。这些患者的 SIBO 机制尚不清楚,但可能与小肠运动异常(由疾病或麻醉性镇痛剂引起)、广泛使用质子泵抑制剂治疗促进胃内细菌过度生长、既往胰腺和肠道手术以及胰液杀菌能力降低等有关。最后,如果所有这些措施都失败了,可以使用吸收不需要脂解(因此也不需要脂肪酶)的中链甘油三酯代替膳食脂肪。

(三) 糖尿病

应当对慢性胰腺炎患者定期监测糖尿病发展,应每年测定空腹血糖水平和糖化血红蛋白[194,207]。可以通过测定 C 肽水平估计残余功能性 β-细胞数量。尽管许多患者可能由于胰岛破坏而患有糖尿病,但这些患者中大约一半的糖尿病患病风险来自 2 型糖尿病的经典危险因素[355]。糖尿病是慢性胰腺炎患者死亡的独立预测因素。微血管进行性病变或更严重的并发症,如治疗引起的低血糖(特别是营养不良等胰高血糖素储备不足的患者),可导致患者死亡或患病。酮症酸中毒少见。一些患者对口服降糖药如磺酰脲类、噻唑烷二酮类、二甲双胍或其他药物有反应。首选二甲双胍,因为有间接证据表明它可以降低继发性胰腺癌的风险[195]。然而通常需要胰岛素,慢性胰腺炎患者对胰岛素的需求往往低于 1 型糖尿病患者。过分尝试严格控制血糖可能会导致治疗性低血糖的严重并发症[198]。只有在高甘油三酯血症性胰腺炎的患者中应尝试严格控制血糖,因为其糖尿病通常是原发疾病,而严格控制血糖后才可能控制血脂。对于长期糖尿病患者,需要适当监测肾病、视网膜病变和神经病变。

十、并发症

(一) 假性囊肿

假性囊肿是一种含有胰液的充满液体的有壁囊腔。发生在 25% 的慢性胰腺炎患者中且最常见于慢性酒精性胰腺炎[356-359]。假性囊肿最常见的症状是腹痛,大多数有症状的患者都会出现腹痛。少见的可表现为可触及的肿块、恶心和呕吐(由于压迫胃或十二指肠)、黄疸(由于压迫胆管)和出血,有患者可无症状。至少一半患者中可见血清脂肪酶和淀粉酶的升高,并且血脂肪酶或淀粉酶的持续升高可提示存在假性囊肿。假性囊肿通常通过影像学检查,包括 US、CT、MRI 和 EUS 来诊断。CT 和 MRI 的优势是可以显示假性囊肿的包膜,以判断包膜的成熟程度,并确定假性囊肿与胃和十二指肠的关系,这对选择治疗方式很有帮助。MRI 还可以提供一些额外的关于积聚内容物特征的信息,特别是主要是液体还是液体固体混合物。出现在胰腺外的假性囊肿很少含固体物质[360]。从而可以与取代正常胰腺并含有液体和固体物质的包裹性坏死进行鉴别。尽管约 70% 的假性囊肿与胰管相连,并不需要为了诊断而行 ERCP[357,358]。ERCP 与大约 15% 无感染的假性囊肿发生机会感染相关,所以只有紧急治疗并且给予了抗生素后才应该进行该操作。

假性囊肿在慢性胰腺炎中的自然病程尚未完全明确。总的来说,20% 到 40% 病例中出现了假性囊肿的并发症。并发症包括压迫胰周大血管、胃或十二指肠,感染,出血以及瘘管形成。许多假性囊肿无症状或并发症。与急性胰腺炎相关的液体积聚和假性囊肿不同,慢性胰腺炎背景下发生的囊肿自行减小要少见得多。尽管如此,也并非所有患者都需要治疗。对于症状轻微或无症状且无并发症的患者应采取保守治疗[357,358,361]。有症状或复杂的假性囊肿需要治疗。慢性胰腺炎的假性囊肿在诊断时通常已经成熟(CT 或 MRI 上可见肉芽组织包膜),不需要为了使囊肿包膜成熟而推迟治疗。

对有症状的,复杂的,或迅速增大的假性囊肿而言,可以通过外科,经皮或内镜治疗。如果能找到安全入路,可以经皮导管引流假性囊肿。不推荐对慢性胰腺炎合并胰腺假性囊肿进行经皮引流,通常认为由于这种囊肿和液体积聚的下游胰管梗阻有关,导致沿管路的瘘管形成、假性囊肿复发以及拔管后慢性瘘管的风险都高得难以接受。尽管经皮引流术的长期成功率不明,但肯定相对较低。几乎都会出现拔管后液体再次积聚。并发症出现概率通常小于 10%～15%,包括出血、腔内感染及沿管路的引流瘘管形成。

如果可以通过乳头或胃或十二指肠壁到达液体积聚,可以通过内镜治疗假性囊肿。选择的路径取决于假性囊肿的位置。对于位于胰头部与胰管相连的小假性囊肿,可采用经乳头引流术。所有其他可以行内镜治疗的患者,根据部位的不同,可采用内镜下囊胃造瘘术或囊空肠造瘘术,通常报道的成功率为 80%～90%[361-364]。许多中心将内窥镜治疗作为一线治疗,并发症的发生率约为 10%[361-364]。大多数并发症与透壁支架放置有关,包括出血(可能大量)、穿孔和未曾感染的液体积聚出现感染。使用 EUS 评估肠腔和假性囊肿之间的大血管,并直接引导穿刺以避开邻近血管、减少并发症。如果进行内镜治疗,抗生素预防和手术前备术是必不可少的。支架通常情况下放置数周或更长时间,以对假性囊肿进行减压。尽管大多数可行,但并非所有假性囊肿都可以接受内镜治疗。内镜治疗的长期成功率尚不明确,但似乎与手术一样良好。

外科治疗通常包括囊肿减压至小肠袢或胃中,通常一起进行胰管引流手术(如改良的 Puestow 手术)。手术治疗的长期成功率约为 90%,手术死亡率低于 3%。尽管假性囊肿术后复发率只有 10%,但在长期随访中,一半患者可能会再次出现疼痛。所有假性囊肿的治疗方法都是如此,因为慢性胰腺炎所致的疼痛在没有假性囊肿的情况下也可能发生。对于那些存在微创内镜或经皮治疗严重并发症的患者也有必要进行手术治疗。囊胃造瘘术和囊空肠造瘘术可以在腹腔镜下进行[365]。一项小型前瞻性随机试验比较了 EUS 引导的假性囊肿引流术和开腹囊胃造瘘术,发现假性囊肿复发率无差异,且内镜治疗与更短的住院时间、更好的生活质量和更低的费用相关[366]。没有研究直接比较腹腔镜和内镜技术[367,368]。

已经注意到假性囊肿下游胰管狭窄(朝向十二指肠)或胰管严重破坏通常与经皮引流失败有关。这些特征预示拔管后会立即复发。除非这些解剖问题得到解决,否则内镜治疗也容易出现类似的问题。MRCP 可用于识别有胰管狭窄或严重破坏且复发风险增加的患者。虽然不是所有中心的常规方法,但可以考虑进行 EUS 引导的假性囊肿引流联合 ERCP(之前或之后即刻)。ERCP 的目的是识别胰管狭窄或大的胰管破坏,并进行支架桥接治疗。这可能会减少拔除经肠假性囊肿支架后假性囊肿的复发风险。在一些不能进行该操作的患者中,将永久留置经肠支架[362-364],但这种方法的长期安全性尚不清楚。

假性囊肿占所有胰腺相关囊性积聚的 90%。包裹性胰腺坏死(在一部分急性胰腺炎中)在 CT 上表现为囊性,但治疗方法与假性囊肿不同[360]。还有许多囊性肿瘤可以类似假性囊肿的表现,尤其是囊性肿瘤(见框 59.3 和第 60 章)。

框 59.3 胰内囊性积聚	
假性囊肿(70%~90%)	
囊性肿瘤(10%~15%)	黏液性囊腺瘤和囊腺癌
	导管内乳头状黏液瘤
	浆液性囊腺瘤
	浆液性囊腺癌
	实性假乳头状瘤
	腺泡细胞囊腺癌
	绒毛膜癌
	畸胎瘤
	胰岛细胞瘤囊性变
	胰腺导管腺癌
真性囊肿(少见)	胰腺多囊病(孤立或与多囊肾病有关)
	von Hippel-Lindau 病
	单纯囊肿
	皮样囊肿
多囊性损伤(非常少见)	淋巴上皮样囊肿
	子宫内膜囊肿
	与囊性纤维化有关的巨囊
	潴留囊肿
	寄生囊肿(细粒棘球绦虫或猪带绦虫)

(二) 消化道出血

慢性胰腺炎背景下可有多种因素导致消化道出血。有些与慢性胰腺炎无关,如贲门黏膜撕裂出血、食管炎、消化性溃疡和并发酒精性肝硬化引起的静脉曲张。另一些则是胰腺炎的直接结果,最显而易见的是胰腺假性囊肿、假性动脉瘤出血,以及门静脉或脾静脉血栓形成。

假性囊肿壁可出血。囊壁的小血管(静脉、毛细血管或小动脉)出血,可导致假性囊肿增大并进一步使这些小血管破裂[369]。血液可能残留在假性囊肿内,也可能通过自发性假性囊肿减压而进入胃肠道或进入胰管(胰性血液),最终进入肠腔[370]。假性囊肿壁的小血管出血通常量小,但常因假性囊肿增大而引起腹痛加重。

(三) 假性动脉瘤

假性动脉瘤是假性囊肿对动脉肌性血管壁的酶促及压力消化的结果。假性动脉瘤可以破裂至假性囊肿中(使假性囊肿转变为较大的假性动脉瘤),也可以直接破裂到相邻脏器、腹腔或胰管。5%~10% 伴假性囊肿的慢性胰腺炎病例可能并发假性动脉瘤出血,尽管在接受血管造影的慢性胰腺炎患者中,可能在高达 21% 的患者中发现假性动脉瘤[369,371,372]。胰腺手术后也可见到假性动脉瘤。许多内脏动脉可能受累,以脾动脉最常见,其次是胃十二指肠动脉或胰十二指肠动脉。一旦发生出血,死亡率至少为 40%,并且和失血严重程度及其他同时存在的情况都相关。虽然假性囊肿死亡罕见,但超过一半的假性囊肿死亡是出血所致。

假性动脉瘤出血可能是间歇、缓慢的,也可能是急性、大量的。常见表现是腹痛(由于假性囊肿增大),不明原因贫血以及明显的消化道出血(如果血液可以通过假性囊肿或胰管到达肠腔)。在许多病例中,最初会发生自限性出血(所谓的前哨出血),数小时或数天之后会出现大量活动性出血。最初的自限性出血可能是由于出血瞬间填塞了假性囊肿。在胰腺炎或已知假性囊肿的患者中,存在不明原因失血或任何量的消化道出血应立即提高对假性动脉瘤警惕。如果在上消化道出血的情况下怀疑有假性动脉瘤,应立即进行上消化道内镜检查。如无明显出血部位,应考虑假性动脉瘤的形成。很少有从壶腹部渗出的血液(胰性血液),但没有该发现并不除外假性动脉瘤。

下一步评估应是紧急 CT 扫描并静脉注射造影剂。初始非增强图像上假性囊肿内的高密度物质高度提示假性动脉瘤,静脉注射造影剂后,低密度假性囊肿内可见圆形乳浊状结构(图 59.9)。最好避免口服造影剂以避免干扰必要时的血

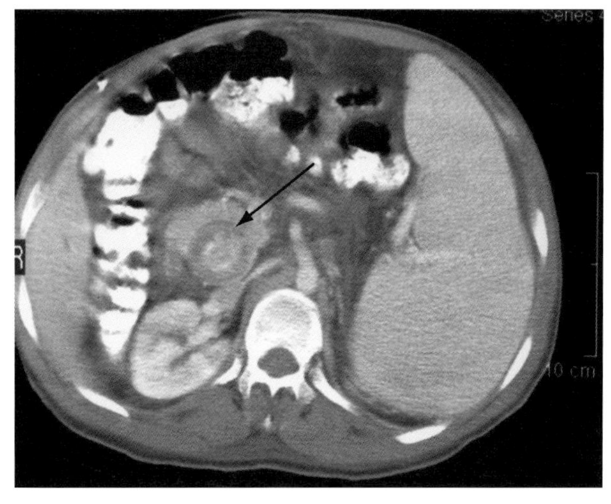

图 59.9 CT 扫描显示静脉内注射造影剂后不透明的假性囊肿,包括假性动脉瘤(箭)

管造影。在大多数中心,CT 发现假性动脉瘤后立即进行血管造影以确定并栓塞假性动脉瘤。一旦识别假性动脉瘤,无论是否引起出血都应该进行治疗。血管造影栓塞或支架植入术已经在很大程度上取代了一次性手术[371,372],后者仅适用于上述治疗失败的病例。

(四)脾静脉血栓形成所致静脉曲张出血

静脉曲张出血可使慢性胰腺炎复杂化,因为两者都与酒精性肝硬化或脾静脉(以及较少发生的门静脉)血栓形成有关。脾静脉血栓形成是最常见的,可产生区域性或左侧门静脉高压症[373]。脾静脉可通过胃短静脉到胃左静脉进行减压,在贲门和胃底产生明显的静脉曲张。根据静脉解剖,也可能出现食管静脉曲张,但食管静脉曲张一般比胃静脉曲张小。这种情况下胃静脉曲张的自然病程尚不清楚,但出血的总体风险低于肝硬化食管静脉曲张[369]。胃静脉曲张出血的概率约为 10%或更低[373]。因此在无出血的情况下不需要治疗。如发生出血,可通过脾切除术治愈。利用氰基丙烯酸盐注射或其他技术,可内镜下控制胃静脉曲张出血。

(五)胆管梗阻

远端胆管被胰头后部包绕。胰头的炎症和纤维化,以及此处的肿瘤或假性囊肿,会压迫胰腺内胆管,导致肝脏化验异常、黄疸、胆源性疼痛或胆管炎。约 10%的患者会出现有症状的胆管梗阻。肝脏化验结果显示胆汁淤积,CT 或 US 检查显示胆管扩张,或两者均存在都可考虑存在胆管狭窄。ERCP 特征性表现为远端胆管长锥形狭窄(图 59.10)。

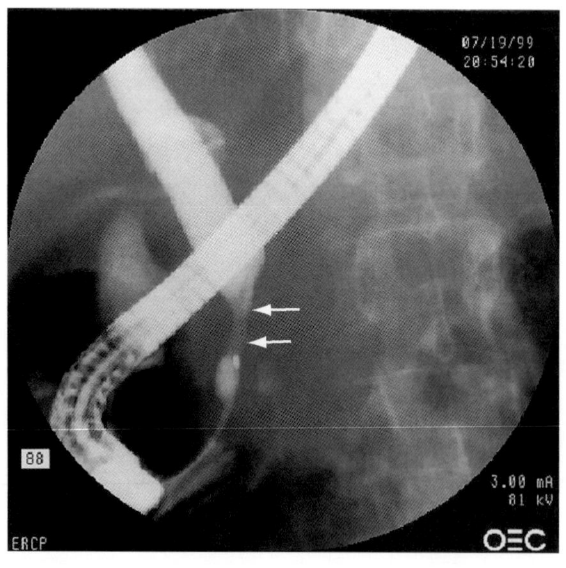

图 59.10　逆行胆管造影显示一例慢性胰腺炎患者胆管通过胰头时光滑狭窄(箭)

发生胆管炎是治疗的绝对指征。存在肝脏化验异常或黄疸并非单一因素所致,因为受影响最多的是酗酒患者,而酒精性(或本身存在的)肝病也会导致肝脏化验显著异常。临床、生化甚至放射学表现并不总能区分胆道狭窄和原有肝脏疾病[374]。必要时可行肝脏活检以确定治疗方案。无症状的胰内胆管狭窄,在没有症状、黄疸或进行性肝脏化验异常的情况下,通常可以密切随访。如果担心出现继发性胆汁性肝硬化,应进行肝活检。对于黄疸或胆源性疼痛的患者,在没有其他解释(即原有肝脏疾病)的情况下,应进行治疗。胆管梗阻的最终治疗通常包括胆总管空肠吻合术或胆总管十二指肠吻合术等胆道旁路手术。这些患者许多可能有胰头部的炎性肿块并进行随后的切除(Whipple 术或保留十二指肠的胰头切除术)。一项研究表明,手术减压成功后,由慢性胆道梗阻引起的肝纤维化可能会减少[375]。虽然内镜下塑料支架治疗慢性胰腺炎所致的胆道梗阻通常暂时有效(见第 61 章),但长期的成功率相对较低[376]。放置一个或多个塑料支架治疗胆道梗阻相对简单,但长期管理复杂,需要数月至数年更换多个支架,并且支架移位和梗阻较为常见。长期内镜下支架治疗通常需要使用多个塑料支架或全覆膜金属支架,治疗时间为 6~12 个月[377,378]。患者的长期反应远低于胆道旁路手术。慢性胰腺炎患者出现胆管狭窄也可能是胰腺恶性肿瘤发展的信号[110]。在这种情况下 EUS 可用于鉴别良恶性狭窄。

(六)十二指肠梗阻

大约 5%慢性胰腺炎患者存在有症状的十二指肠狭窄。最常见的原因是胰头部常伴有炎性肿块的纤维化。慢性胰腺炎中存在胰腺恶性肿瘤也可有同样表现[110]。十二指肠梗阻的症状包括恶心、呕吐、体重减轻和腹痛,可并发胆管梗阻。因为十二指肠狭窄的范围在内镜检查时常常被低估,最好是用口服造影剂的 CT 或上消化道钡餐检查进行检查。由于狭窄程度可能随着炎症部分缓解而改善,可以尝试试验性保守治疗。保守治疗失败的患者需要手术治疗。最简单的方法是通过腹腔镜行胃空肠吻合术,并可以与胆管和/或胰管引流术(胰管空肠侧吻合术)相结合。对于有较大的胰头炎性肿块[323-325]或怀疑恶性肿瘤的患者,也可考虑行保留十二指肠的胰头切除术或 Whipple 术。

(七)胰瘘

1. 外瘘

胰外瘘常是手术或经皮治疗慢性胰腺炎或假性囊肿的后果[379,380]。据估计,通过完全肠道休息和肠外高营养,可治疗约一半的该类型瘘管。最常见的并发症是脓肿和出血。有证据表明,每 8 小时皮下注射 100μg 奥曲肽,可加速此类瘘的闭合。即使使用奥曲肽,成功的药物治疗也需要数周时间。在胰管破裂处内镜放置支架可以有效地迅速关闭瘘管。尽管可能同时需要对腹腔内液体积聚经皮引流,高达 75%的胰内瘘可通过内镜技术有效治疗[379,380]。对于内镜治疗失败或不能进行的患者,手术治疗包括胰腺切除术(如果瘘管在尾部)或瘘管空肠吻合术,即将瘘管覆于空肠旷置端[379]。

2. 内瘘

胰内瘘主要发生在假性囊肿破裂后或胰腺外伤后的慢性胰腺炎中。液体可流向腹腔(胰性腹水)或胸膜腔(胰性胸腔积液),或者少见地流向相邻的空腔脏器(胃、十二指肠或结肠)。在 MRCP 上通常可以发现瘘管的位置和走行。根据液体积聚的部位,患者可能并无慢性胰腺炎症状的相关主诉,但可能会出现腹胀或气短。虽然这种瘘发生于晚期慢性胰腺炎,但可能没有近期明确有症状的胰腺炎病史。诊断可以通过测定相关积液中升高的淀粉酶来建立，通常超过 4 000U/L。

全肠道休息、肠外高营养、腹穿或胸穿、奥曲肽等保守治疗对部分胰内瘘有效[379]。如果漏出是在胰体或胰头，覆盖瘘管部位的胰管支架非常有效。在某些情况下，仅用一个短的胰管支架连接壶腹就足以治愈瘘管。如果漏出是在胰尾仍应行内镜治疗，但效果较差。如果瘘来自完全阻塞的胰管上游（不包括胰尾综合征）则无效。在这种情况下，需要切除或外科引流远端胰腺，并在术前使用 MRCP 明确导管解剖以制定手术计划。

（八）恶性肿瘤

所有类型的慢性胰腺炎中胰腺癌风险都很高（见第 60 章）。慢性胰腺炎患者一生中罹患胰腺癌的概率约为 4%，估计相对危险度为 13[14,31,32,381]，其中遗传性胰腺炎患者、吸烟者和同时患有糖尿病的患者罹患胰腺癌的风险最高[14,197,381-384]。

目前尚无鉴别单纯慢性胰腺炎与慢性胰腺炎合并腺癌的完全可靠的方法。症状和体征可能相似（腹痛、体重减轻、黄疸）。在没有广泛转移的情况下，如 CT、US 甚至 ERCP 等影像学检查可能无法确立诊断。EUS 最为准确，但在已经存在回声质地改变的病变胰腺内发现一个小的低回声肿瘤很困难。然而当病变很小时，EUS 在检测共存的恶性肿瘤方面优于 CT。EUS 还具有可以对任何可疑病变进行直接组织活检的明显优势。

肿瘤标志物可能有助于区分慢性胰腺炎和癌症。CA19-9 是胰腺腺癌最常用的肿瘤标志物，在 70%～80% 的胰腺腺癌患者中升高[385]。胆道梗阻和胆管炎也可使 CA19-9 升高。尽管这些技术在遗传性胰腺癌和遗传性胰腺炎的家系中可能有用，但并不值得在一般的慢性胰腺炎患者中使用。一些患者可能需要腹腔镜或剖腹探查来确定是否存在共存的胰腺癌。在通过手术切除除外恶性肿瘤的良性假瘤患者中，常能发现慢性自身免疫性胰腺炎的变化[38,110]。

在慢性胰腺炎患者中胰腺外的癌症也有增加。这些癌症，特别是上消化道和肺部的癌症，可能与同时吸烟的影响有关[14,17,31,32]。

（九）动力障碍

慢性胰腺炎患者中可见胃轻瘫和十二指肠动力障碍[386,387]，其可能是由于胃周炎症、慢性胰腺炎相关的激素变化（如血浆 CCK 升高）、胰腺重建手术，或麻醉性镇痛药副作用。因为胃轻瘫可能产生与慢性胰腺炎难以区分的症状，并可能干扰胰酶的有效排泌，所以在临床上很重要[387]。早饱、恶心、呕吐、体重减轻者应考虑胃轻瘫。

（程卓　译，闫秀娥　李鹏　校）

参考文献

第 60 章　胰腺癌、囊性胰腺肿瘤和其他非内分泌胰腺肿瘤

Bijal Modi, G. Thomas Shires 著

章节目录

一、胰腺癌 ······ 890
(一) 流行病学 ······ 890
(二) 病理学 ······ 891
(三) 临床特征 ······ 893
(四) 诊断 ······ 893
(五) 分期 ······ 896
(六) 治疗 ······ 896
二、胰腺囊性肿瘤 ······ 900
(一) 黏液性囊性肿瘤 ······ 901
(二) 浆液性囊腺瘤 ······ 902
(三) 导管内乳头状黏液性肿瘤 ······ 903
(四) 实性假乳头状瘤 ······ 904
三、其他胰腺肿瘤 ······ 905

一、胰腺癌

最常见的起源于胰腺的恶性肿瘤是导管腺癌[1]。胰腺癌是一种高度致死性恶性肿瘤，占美国所有癌症病例的3%，但占所有癌症死亡病例的7%。预计2017年大约有53 760例新发病例和43 090例死亡病例[2]。尽管与其他恶性肿瘤相比，其发生率相对较低，它是男性和女性癌症死亡的第四大原因。预计到2030年将成为癌症死亡的第二大原因[1]。新诊断的胰腺癌的5年生存率仍为8%[3]。许多因素使早期发现和早期检测和更好的治疗选择方案成为一个持续的挑战。

(一) 流行病学

1. 发病率

在2003—2014年期间，美国胰腺癌(pancreatic cancer, PC)的发病率保持稳定，白种人群中略微升高[4]。胰腺癌是一种衰老性疾病，诊断时的中位年龄为71岁，许多病例在65岁之前确诊。45岁以前很少见。50岁以后其发病率急剧上升。与白人相比，黑人中的发生率较高，男性略占优势[4]。

2. 高危人群

存在许多与胰腺癌发生相关的风险因素。某些风险因素是不变的：高龄、男性、种族和家族史。其他风险因素是随着时间积累或为环境因素(肥胖、吸烟、酗酒、慢性胰腺炎)。绝大多数胰腺癌为散发性。大约5%~10%的病例与家族性胰腺癌综合征相关，定义为有2个或者2个以上一级家庭成员患有胰腺癌的病例。家族性胰腺癌综合征患者往往在诊断时更年轻(中位年龄64~65岁)[5]。表60.1总结了与胰腺癌风险增加相关的一些遗传综合征。胰腺癌风险增加与许多遗传基因突变相关：*BRCA2*、*CDKN2A*、*ATM*、错配修复酶不稳定(如Lynch综合征、*PALB2*、*STK11*、*PRSS1*和*SPINK2*中存在)。*CDKN2A*和*BRCA2*是与遗传性胰腺癌相关的最突出的遗传性基因突变，其中*BRCA2*突变代表是最常见的基因突变[5,6]。

表 60.1　与胰腺癌风险增加相关的病史特征和遗传综合征

病史	基因突变	相对风险	70 岁时的个体风险
没有	无	1	0.5%
乳腺癌	*BRCA2*	3.5~10	5%
	BRCA1	2	1%
FAMMM 综合征	*TP16*(*CDNK2A*)	20~34	10%~17%
≥3 个患有胰腺癌的 FDR	未知	32	16%
遗传性胰腺炎	*PRSS1*	50~80	25%~40%
Peutz-Jeghers 综合征	*STK11/LKB1*	132	30%~60%
HNPCC 综合征	*MLH1*, *MSH2*, 其他	未知	<5%
年轻患胰腺癌	*FANC-C*, *FANC-G*, 其他	未知	未知
X 家族	Palladin	未知	未知

FAMMM，家族性非典型多发性痣黑色素瘤；FDR，一级亲属；HNPCC：遗传性非息肉病性结直肠癌；X，研究家族性胰腺癌的单亲家庭。

Modified from Hruban R, Pitman M, Klimstra D. Ductal adenocarcinoma. AFIP atlas of tumor pathology. Tumors of the pancreas. Washington, D. C.: American Registry of Pathology; 2007. pp 111-64.

家族性非典型多发性痣黑色素瘤(familial atypical multiple mole melanoma, FAMMM)是一种由肿瘤抑制基因*CDKN2A*突变定义的常染色体显性疾病。正常情况下，*CDKN2A*编码p16蛋白，阻止视网膜母细胞瘤基因的磷酸化和活化。FAMMM患者存在患黑色素瘤和胰腺癌的风险[7]。

遗传性胰腺炎(见第57章)，通常由PRSS的常染色体显性突变引起，与74岁时接近50%的胰腺癌发病率相关[8]。其他非遗传性形式的慢性胰腺炎患者发生胰腺癌的可能性也更高。吸烟和饮酒是可能协同慢性胰腺炎影响肿瘤发展的危险因素[9]。携带*STK11*基因突变的Peutz-Jeghers综合征个体，在第126章讨论，到65~70岁患胰腺癌的累积风险为11%~36%[10]。

由于疾病发生率低、成像所需的成本和专业知识以及成像模式的灵敏度相对较低，对胰腺癌进行筛查是一项困难的任务。提高筛查阳性预测值的最有效机制是识别高危人群。目前，家族史和确定的基因突变的存在是识别高危人群的最有效机制[11]。患有胰腺癌的一级亲属（first-degree relative，FDR）的数量严重影响个体的癌症风险。有 2 个受影响一级亲属的患胰腺癌的风险增加了 6.4 倍，有 3 个受影响一级亲属的，患胰腺癌的风险增加了 32 倍[12]。

2013 年国际胰腺癌筛查癌症联盟（International Cancer of the Pancreas Screening，CAPS）已经同意，有 3 个或者 3 个以上血缘亲属患有胰腺癌，至少有 1 个一级亲属受累的个体，应考虑进行筛查。至少有 2 个受影响的一级亲属的患者也应考虑进行筛查。有 2 个受累血缘亲属的胰腺癌个体，至少有 1 个一级亲属，可考虑进行筛查。应考虑对特定突变患者进行筛查，应考虑对 Peutz-Jeghers 综合征（不考虑家族史）和 BRCA2/PALB2/p16/Lynch 综合征患者（FDR 伴 PC）进行筛查。公认确定的筛查方式包括磁共振成像（MRI）/磁共振胰胆管造影（MRCP）和超声内镜（EUS）[13]。启动筛查的年龄尚无共识，尽管 AGA 建议遗传性胰腺炎患者在 35 岁开始筛查，或家族性胰腺癌患者在指示病例年龄前 10 年开始筛查[14]。

一项包括 309 名 35 岁以上的无症状高危亲属的筛查注册研究，首先行 MRCP 检查，如果发现了病变，再进行 EUS 检查。在完成了至少一项初步筛查的 109 名亲属中，有 9 人经 EUS 确认发现明显异常。对高危亲属的总体诊断率为 8.3%（图 60.1）[15]。另一种策略是使用唾液中的 mRNA 生物标志物来识别分子变化的特定图谱。使用 4 个 mRNA 生物标志物的逻辑回归模型可以从非肿瘤中区分出来可切除的胰腺癌，敏感性为 90%，特异性为 95%[16]。

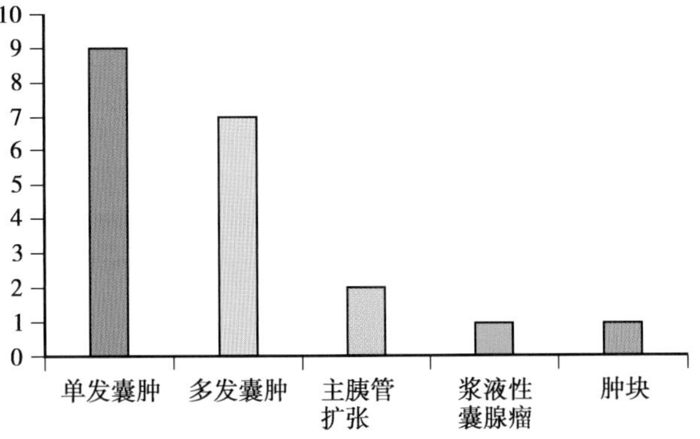

图 60.1　35 岁以上胰腺癌患者无症状、高危亲属中初始胰腺横断面成像阳性结果的分布。6 名亲属接受了手术切除，2 名患有 IPMN，2 名患有原位癌（1 名患有 PanIN 2，另 1 名患有 PanIN 3），1 名患有 T3N0 PC，1 名患有浆液性囊性肿瘤。IPMN，导管内乳头状黏液性肿瘤；PaNin，胰腺上皮内瘤变。（Modified from Ludwig E，Olson SH，Bayuga S，et al. Feasibility and yield of screening in relatives from familial PC families. Am J Gastroenterol 2011；106：946-54）。

3. 环境因素

胰腺癌最重要的环境因素，也可能是唯一确定的环境因素就是吸烟。Meta 分析显示吸烟者胰腺癌的相对危险度（relative risk，RR）为 1.7。戒烟后 10 年胰腺癌的风险仍有增加。危险度呈剂量依赖性，每天每增加 5 支烟则危险度增加[17]。所有胰腺癌患者中吸烟占到了病因的 20%～25%[18]。

肥胖与胰腺癌发病率的增加有关。2012 年世界癌症研究基金小组将体重、腰围和腹部体重的增加与胰腺癌直接联系了起来[19]。随着体重指数的增加，胰腺癌的风险持续增加[20]。

膳食成分作为环境危险因素对胰腺癌的影响似乎比最初在人口研究中发现的要小。有一些证据表明，大量摄入红肉或者加工肉类可能会轻微增加胰腺癌发病的风险[21]，而最近的研究并不支持叶酸的保护作用[22]。支持食用水果和蔬菜对预防胰腺癌有保护作用的病例对照研究证据有限[23,24]。

糖尿病与患胰腺癌风险增加相关[25]。超过 10 年的长期糖尿病，与胰腺癌风险增加有关。队列分析表明，与年龄匹配的无糖尿病患者相比，糖尿病患胰腺癌的风险增加 8 倍[26]。四分之一的患者在诊断时是糖尿病患者。另外 40% 有糖尿病前期血糖升高[27]。糖尿病与肿瘤诱发之间的因果关系尚不清楚。胰岛细胞减少和小肿瘤负荷并不足以引起大多数胰腺癌患者的内分泌功能不全，而在接受肿瘤切除术的患者中，糖耐量有时也会改善[28]。与其他口服降糖药不同，用于 2 型糖尿病的 GLP-1 模拟药物（如依赛纳替德）和 GLP-1 代谢抑制剂（例如 DPP4 抑制剂，如西格列汀）与胰腺癌风险增加近 3 倍有关[29]。

（二）病理学

正如第 55 章所述，在正常胰腺中发现了不同类型的上皮细胞：①腺泡细胞，约占腺体体积的 80%；②导管细胞，占 10%～15%；③内分泌胰岛细胞，约占 1%～2%。超过 95% 的胰腺恶性肿瘤来自于腺体的外分泌成分（导管和腺体细胞），其特征与腺癌一致。内分泌肿瘤仅占胰腺肿瘤的 1%～2%，将在 34 章讨论。非上皮性胰腺恶性肿瘤极为罕见[30]。最近的胰腺癌基因组测序最终生成一个完整的组织-分子分类系统。世界卫生组织胰腺外分泌瘤的分类仍然广泛使用（框 60.1）[31]。

框 60.1　WHO 对原发性胰腺外分泌肿瘤的分类

Ⅰ. 良性
- ⅰ. 浆液性囊腺瘤
- ⅱ. 黏液性囊腺瘤
- ⅲ. 导管内乳头状黏液腺瘤
- ⅳ. 成熟囊性畸胎瘤

Ⅱ. 临界（恶性潜能不确定）
- ⅰ. 黏液性囊性肿瘤伴中度异型增生
- ⅱ. 导管内乳头状黏液性肿瘤伴中度异型增生
- ⅲ. 实性假乳头状瘤

Ⅲ. 恶性
- ⅰ. 导管腺癌
- ⅱ. 破骨细胞样巨细胞瘤
- ⅲ. 浆液性囊腺癌
- ⅳ. 黏液性囊腺癌（非侵袭性或侵袭性）
- ⅴ. 导管内乳头状黏液性癌（非侵袭性或侵袭性）
- ⅵ. 腺泡细胞癌
- ⅶ. 胰母细胞瘤
- ⅷ. 实性假乳头状癌
- ⅸ. 各种其他癌症

Data from Hruban R，Pitman M，Klimstra D. Ductal adenocarcinoma. AFIP atlas of tumor pathology. Tumors of the pancreas. Washington，D. C.：American Registry of Pathology；2007. pp 111-64.

胰腺导管腺癌占胰腺肿瘤的85%~90%[30,31]。尸检显示60%~70%的肿瘤位于胰腺头部,5%~10%在体部,10%~15%在尾部。肉眼所见这些肿瘤表现为质硬肿块,边界模糊,与周围胰腺及胰腺周围组织混杂在一起。胰头癌的平均大小为2.5~3.5cm,而胰体癌和胰尾癌的平均大小为5~7cm。肿瘤大小的差异与近端肿瘤比远端肿瘤的症状和体征出现更早有关。

位于胰头部的肿瘤常阻塞远端的胆管和胰管,这些梗阻常分别导致黄疸和慢性胰腺炎的症状。胰腺的病理改变包括导管扩张和胰腺实质的纤维化萎缩。有些肿瘤可累及壶腹部及十二指肠。在诊断时几乎均会发现向胰腺外和后腹膜组织浸润,并可导致门静脉或肠系膜上血管和神经的侵犯。胰腺尾部的肿瘤与胆道和胰管梗阻无关。远端肿瘤的胰腺外浸润可侵犯脾脏、胃、结肠的脾曲或左侧肾上腺。在晚期患者中,转移到淋巴结、肝脏和腹膜非常常见。肺、胸膜和骨则较少受累[32]。

显微镜下,导管腺癌分为分化良好,中度分化或低分化[30]。高分化肿瘤表现为不规则的管状肿瘤腺体,轻度细胞异型性,有丝分裂活性低和显著的黏蛋白生成。分化的丧失是由于细胞没有排列成腺体结构,细胞异型性和有丝分裂活性增加,黏蛋白的产生停止。一些使用多变量分析的研究表明,组织学分级与切除后的生存率相关[33]。

导管腺癌会引起强烈的纤维增生反应,这是它们在大体检查中为什么很硬的原因。与慢性胰腺炎相比,导管内钙化是唯一很少被发现的。肿瘤以外的胰管可表现为乳头状增生或黏液细胞肥大。这些发现的意义尚不清楚。肿瘤在显微镜下淋巴管和神经周围间隙侵袭非常明显。胰头肿瘤转移到胰十二指肠的淋巴结非常常见。局部晚期进展可看到腹腔干和腹主动脉旁淋巴结受累。

几种免疫组化化学标记对产生黏液的肿瘤有诊断价值。包括胰腺腺癌。其中比较著名的标志物是MUC1、MUC3、MUC4、CEA、CA199、DuPan2和CA125[30]。这些标志物不能区分胰腺和胰腺外来源的肿瘤,限制了他们评估未知原发灶的肝转移肿瘤的有效性。然而,它们在区分肿瘤学和非肿瘤性导管改变,以及区分导管、腺体跑或神经内分泌肿瘤方面特别有用。细胞角蛋白是鉴别腺泡、导管和胰岛细胞肿瘤的其他有用的标志物。尽管所有导管腺癌染色可见细胞角蛋白7、8、18和19,但大多数腺泡和神经内分泌肿瘤细胞角蛋白7不染色[30]。

分子病理学和遗传学改变

胰腺肿瘤的发生是一系列复杂事件的结果。很可能是细胞内多次基因突变与细胞外微环境改变的共同作用。胰腺癌被认为从一种非恶性前体病变,即胰腺上皮内瘤变(PanIN),经过进行性细胞和细胞核非典型增生逐步发展为侵袭性胰腺癌。随着时间的推移,这种组织病理学进展是通过一系列潜在的遗传性和获得性基因改变介导的(表60.2)[34]。最近,胰腺腺癌的基因测序也涉及其中SWI/SNF的染色质混合重组改变,特别是染色质*BRG1*。当合并*KRAS*时,*BRG1*可导致导管内乳头状黏液瘤和侵袭性腺癌[35]。

*KRAS*基因是一种致癌基因,其激活突变是胰腺腺癌中最常见的基因突变。在30%的早期肿瘤和95%的晚期肿瘤中检测到*KRAS*的激活突变[34]。

表60.2 胰腺癌中常见受影响的信号通路和这些通路中最常见的受影响基因

信号通路	受影响基因(染色体区域)
细胞凋亡	*TP53*(17p)
DNA损伤修复	*TP53*(17p)
G_1/S期转变	*CDKN2A*/p16(9p) *CCND1*(11q13)
细胞-细胞黏附	
侵袭调节 整合素信号通路 嗜同性细胞 黏附力	*CDH1*(16q22)
胚胎信号通路 Notch通路 Hedgehog通路 Wnt通路	-
MAPK信号传导 c-Jun氨基末端激酶 ERK TGF-β信号传导	*K-ras2*(12p) *SMAD4/DPC4*(18q)

Adapted from Ottenhof N, de Wilde R, Maitra A, et al. Molecular characteristics of pancreatic ductal adenocarcinoma. Pathol Res Int 2011;2011:620601.

*KRAS*的突变导致了丝裂原活化蛋白激酶和AKT通路的结构性激活和失调,导致细胞增殖和存活失控[36]。

*KRAS*密码子12突变已被证实是正常组织从非恶性肿瘤病变,Pan-IN,并过渡到侵袭性腺癌的早期获得性突变[37]。由于*KRAS*在胰腺瘤变中较为常见,其靶点是潜在的检测手段,也有可能是治疗靶点。

*CDKN2A*是一种肿瘤抑制基因,是一种获得性突变。通常发现在晚期而不是早期的Pan-IN突变。*CDKN2A*基因产物p16的丢失与不受控制的细胞周期蛋白D1激活有关。*P16*基因产物的丢失与进行性组织异型增生有关[38]。肿瘤抑制基因*SMAD4*和*TP53*的突变几乎均在高级别胰腺上皮内瘤变中发现。*TP53*蛋白产物p53在DNA修复和凋亡中是不可或缺的。*TP53*的缺失导致可能受损的细胞无法控制生长[39]。

肿瘤细胞向侵袭性恶性肿瘤的进展通常是通过获得突变后克隆进化发生的。如前所述,有许多突变与*KRAS*突变同时发生:*CDKN2A/p16*、*TP53*和*SMAD4*。基因工程小鼠模型已经在实验中总结了这种病变谱。例如,胰腺上皮内瘤变从1级到3级发展为浸润性癌与不断增加的基因突变有关(图60.2)[40]。要更好地理解一系列事件,不仅需要分析单个细胞的改变,还需要分析细胞间的相互作用和微环境的作用。人类胰腺腺癌的全球基因组测序揭示了肿瘤遗传学的极端复杂性,但确实确定了12个核心细胞通路和过程,每个通路和过程在多达100%的肿瘤中都发生了改变[41]。

许多疾病患者的基因组测序显示,转移性人群有别于原发癌的遗传异质性。对这些突变时间的定量分析显示,从突变开始到原发癌细胞的诞生,有10年的时间间隔。另外病变

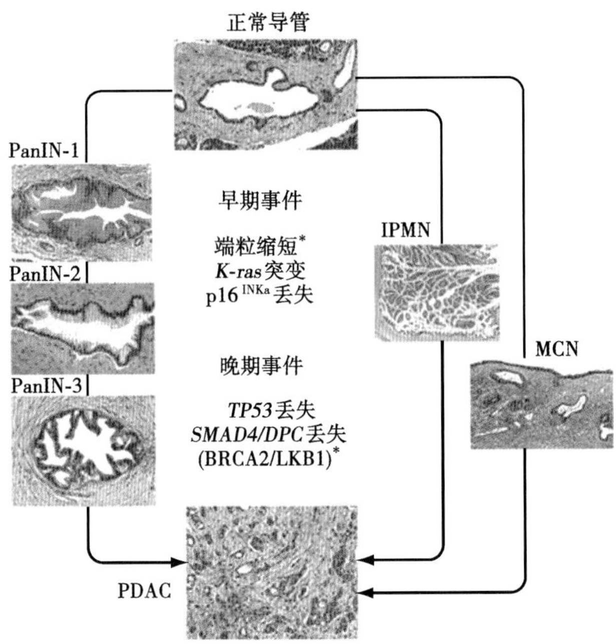

图 60.2 参与胰腺进展为腺癌的胰腺前体病变和遗传事件。图中为 3 种已知的人胰腺导管腺癌（PDAC）前体病变：PanIN、MCN 和 IPMN。左侧为 PanIN 分级方案；分级增加（1～3）反映异型性增加，最终导致明显的 PDAC。右侧显示了 MCN 和 IPMN 向 PDAC 的潜在进展。胰腺癌中记录的基因改变也发生在 PanIN 中，在 MCN 和 IPMN 中的程度较轻，具有明显的时间顺序，尽管这些改变与特异性组织病理学特征的获得无关。列出了各种遗传事件，并分为主要发生在 PDAC 进展早期或晚期的事件。星号表示并非所有前体病变共有的事件（例如，在 PanIN 中记录端粒缩短和 *BRCA2* 丢失，在 PDAC 和 IPMN 子集中记录 LKB1 丢失）。IPMN，导管内乳头状黏液性肿瘤；MCN，黏液性囊性肿瘤；PanIN，胰腺上皮内瘤。（From Hezel AF, Kimmelman AC, Stanger BZ et al. Genetics and biology of pancreatic ductal adenocarcinoma. Genes Dev 2006;20:1218-49.）

转移需要大约 5 年的时间，随后直至患者死亡又约 2 年时间[42]。4 个主要驱动基因的数量与无病生存期和总生存期显著相关，这是独立于传统临床分期的重要信息。这些数据表明，使用现有的诊断和治疗方案，对于这种预后不佳的疾病，诊断和最终干预的时间窗还要长很多[43]。

组织学上一直以来描述的胰腺癌的间质纤维化可能允许肿瘤生长并阻碍治疗药物的输送。基质的乏血供，各种细胞因子和其他免疫调节剂为未来的治疗指明了方向，而局部炎症是一个比较关键的因素[44]。已经发现炎症相关基因的遗传多态性与临床有关。炎症通路基因 *MAPK8IP1* 和 *SOCS3* 中的单核酸多态性与 10 个月或者 6 个月的生存优势有关。相对来说，这类患者一般携带 1 个次等位基因。而携带 2 个次等位基因者，一般生存优势有 2 年[45]。

（三）临床特征

大多数胰腺癌患者在病程后期出现症状。缺乏早期症状导致诊断延迟，大多数患者诊断时已为无法切除的肿块或已经有转移。胰头肿瘤会在疾病早期出现症状。相比之下，胰腺体尾部的肿瘤的特征则是“沉默”。只有在广泛的局部生长或者广泛的转移发生后才会有身体上的表现。临床症状和体征可以为胰腺肿瘤的可切除性提供线索（表 60.3）[46]。

表 60.3 不可切除（姑息性）和可切除（切除）胰腺癌患者的人口统计学特征及表现的症状和体征

	姑息组（N=256）	切除组（N=512）
人口统计学特征		
年龄，平均/岁	64.0	65.8
男性/女性	57%/43%	55%/45%
种族	91%白种人	91%白种人
症状和体征/%		
腹痛	64	36*
黄疸	57	72*
体重减轻	48	43
恶心/呕吐	30	18*
背痛	26	2*

*P=0.001，与姑息组相比。

Modified from Sohn T, Lillemoe K, Cameron J, et al. Surgical palliation of unresectable periampullary adenocarcinoma in the 1990s. J Am Coll Surg 1999;188:658-66.

胰腺肿瘤常表现为胆道梗阻，如黄疸、尿色加深、大便颜色变浅或白陶土样大便、皮肤瘙痒、巩膜黄染、胰腺炎和胆管炎。由于胰头肿瘤靠近胰管，梗阻症状较早出现。体/尾部肿瘤的患者当发现时一般处于疾病的进展期。伴有胰管梗阻的患者也可以出现胰腺外分泌不足，表现为脂肪泻和营养吸收不良。

疼痛是许多胰腺癌患者的主要症状。疼痛主要是因为腹腔或肠系膜上动脉丛的神经被侵犯所引起的[47]。疼痛程度低，常呈钝痛，位于上腹部的隐痛。疾病进展期，疼痛可局限于背部中间或者偏上的位置。这种疼痛也可能发生在餐后，导致患者减少能量的摄入，最终导致体重减轻和恶病质。

其他非特异性症状包括恶心、疲劳、厌食和体重减轻。这些症状可能是由于肿瘤累及十二指肠，引起局部梗阻所致，但也可能不是。胰腺癌可以引起不同程度的胰腺炎和糖尿病。约 85% 的胰腺癌患者在确诊时患有糖尿病和糖耐量异常，其中 55%～85% 是在肿瘤确诊 2 年前确诊的[48]。急性胰腺炎则不太常见。肿瘤导致的胰管阻塞可引起高脂血症，临床上常见轻度急性胰腺炎，对于没有其他病因的老年患者，应引起临床的注意。

（四）诊断

1. 超声（US）和计算机断层扫描（CT）

经腹 US 通常是许多有黄疸的胰腺癌患者首选的检查方法。US 有助于评估胆结石的存在和确定胆道扩张。CT 是疾病诊断和分期的首选方法。这项技术的最近的改进，通过更快更薄的断层扫描成像大大提高了分辨率。多期成像技术可获得造影前、胰腺实质峰期和肝门脉峰期的图像。早期显示肿瘤，延迟可更好地观察血管关系和肝转移情况[49]。CT 对胰腺癌的总体敏感性为 86%～97%，但对小于 2cm 的病变的敏感性接近 77%[48]。

胰腺的 CT 检查方法包括使用静脉和口服造影剂的双相

扫描。第一阶段，动脉早期阶段，在静脉造影剂注射25秒获得扫描，并为手术提供可视化的动脉解剖[50]。第二次动脉（胰腺）期扫描是在静脉造影剂使用40秒后进行的。此时正常胰腺得到最大程度的强化，可以识别非强化肿瘤病变（图60.3A）。第三步，在注射静脉造影剂70秒后进行门静脉期扫描，可以准确检测肝转移，并评估肿瘤累及门静脉和肠系膜静脉（图60.3B）。

长期以来胰腺肿瘤不可切除的CT标准如下：①远处转移（如肝、腹膜或者其他位置）；②包绕了腹腔干或肠系膜上动脉；和/或③门静脉或肠系膜上静脉闭塞。尽管静脉重建可以挑战这个标准。CT检查肿瘤侵犯血管的灵敏度为55%～97%。特异性为91%～100%。关于可切除性，CT的敏感性为76%～92%，特异性为82%～100%[48]。

根据这些CT标准，一些预计有可能切除的患者（5%～15%）在腹腔镜检查中发现有不可切除的病变[51]。另一组按照CT标准可切除的患者在探查手术中发现不可切除，通常是由于T4病变。这类患者显然不能从手术探查中获益，而且通过术前影像学来识别仍然是一个挑战。

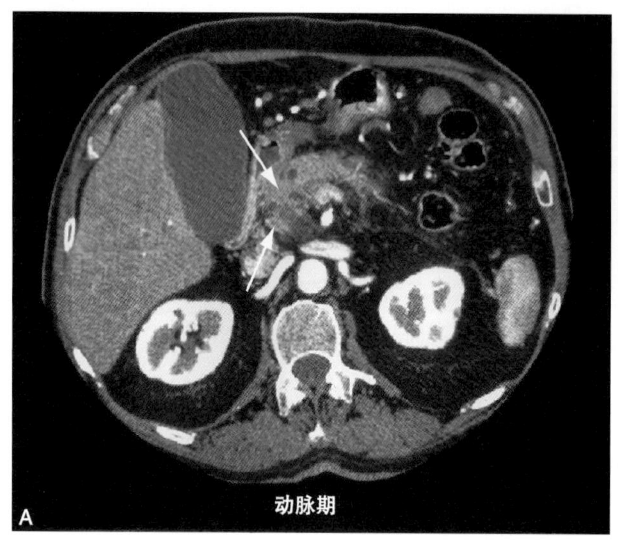

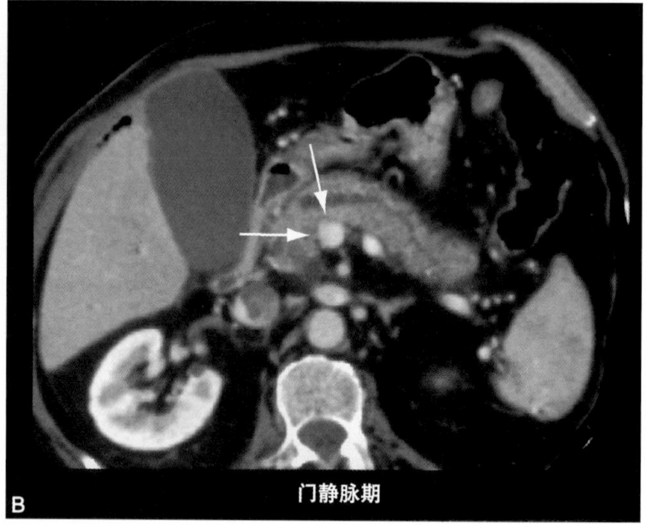

图60.3　胰腺癌患者的胰腺CT扫描。A，动脉期显示胰头部无强化病变（箭）。B，静脉期显示门静脉周围未受累的脂肪平面（箭）

2. 内镜逆行胰胆管造影（ERCP）

ERCP是诊断壶腹周围各种肿瘤的重要工具[52]。大多数肿瘤来自胰腺（85%），很少来自远端胆管（6%）、壶腹（4%）或者十二指肠（4%）。内镜逆行性胰胆管造影可以看到胰胆树，以区分良性（如结石）和恶性梗阻原因。ERCP上的双管征，表现为胆道和胰管狭窄，在许多胰腺癌患者中常见（图60.4）。

在ERCP的时候可以通过活检和刷检来获取组织样本。在病源量大的中心可以使用专门的导管镜检查胆道病变。胆管远端肿瘤也可以通过刷检进行常规细胞学或者遗传学分析[53]。大多数专家推荐一种联合方法，包括刷检和活检，以提高ERCP诊断的敏感性[50]。比较EUS引导下细针穿刺活检（EUS-FNA）和ERCP的细胞学数据有限。回顾性数据显示，与单纯ERCP相比，EUS-FNA具有更高的敏感性、特异性和准确性，且危险性更小[54]。在具备EUS的中心，ERCP更多地用于置入支架来缓解胆管梗阻和进行姑息治疗。

3. 超声内镜（EUS）

自20世纪90年代早期以来，EUS一直是诊断胰腺癌最准确的单一检测方法[55]。EUS可通过胃和十二指肠检查胰腺，许多研究显示，在检测胰腺肿物方面，比CT具有更高的特异性和敏感性（图60.5）。在过去10年里，CT扫描技术的进步，增加了空间分辨率和多平面重建和薄层选择，提高了评估血管侵犯和预测肿瘤可切除性的敏感性和准确性。回顾性和前瞻性观察数据表明，EUS在诊断胰腺癌和MDCT相比具有更高的准确性[56,57]，直到采用最先进的成像技术进行前瞻性、头对头的比较研究，EUS仍然是检测小肿瘤最敏感的方法。行EUS-FNA细胞学检查，通过提高对最敏感的成像方式的特异性，提高了总体的准确性[58]。

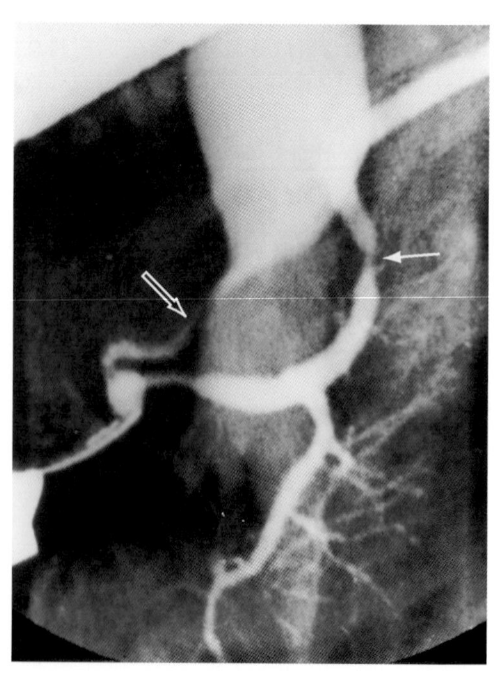

图60.4　ERCP显示胰腺癌患者的胆管狭窄（空心箭）和胰管狭窄（实心箭）。胆管狭窄近端胆管明显扩张

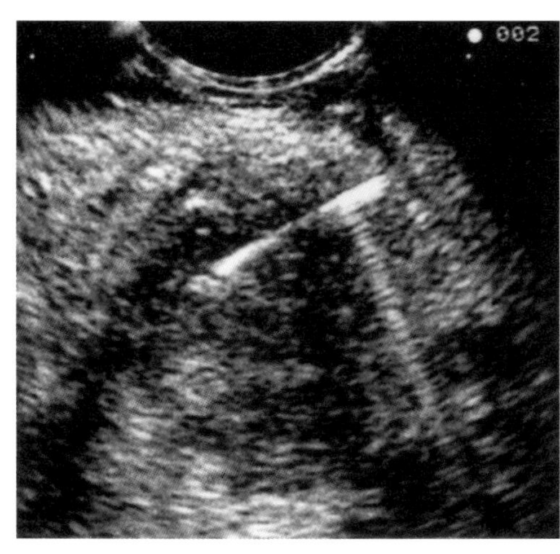

图 60.5 胰腺癌超声内镜(EUS)图像,显示肿瘤活检时的穿刺针

EUS 在小的,可能可切除的病变上,显示出了显著的优势。EUS 在检测小于 3cm 的肿瘤方面比 CT 或 MRI 具有更高的敏感性[59]。EUS 可以非常有利于评估临床怀疑胰腺癌但多层螺旋 CT 未能发现的病变。回顾性数据显示,对于临床怀疑为胰腺癌但 CT 图像上未显示肿块的胰腺癌患者,其诊断具有较高的敏感性和准确性[60]。

EUS 高度依赖操作者,在达到熟练使用前需要积累丰富的经验[61]。EUS-FNA 假阳性率极低,然而,在手术最关注的病灶中,相对较高的假阴性率仍会使得患者考虑是否决定手术[62]。在适当的临床环境中,细胞学检查阴性不妨碍探查。最后,EUS 不能提供关于转移性疾病的信息,需要补充 CT 或 MRI 来完成疾病的治疗前分期。

目前 EUS 在一些疑似胰腺癌患者的评估中仍占有重要的地位,但并非所有患者都需要 EUS。除非怀疑是不同类型的肿瘤,否则对于 CT 标准可切除的具有典型表现的患者,不太可能改变其手术决定。在可切除的交界性病变中,EUS 还可以对手术切除和新辅助治疗的患者进行分层,或将患者纳入新辅助治疗的扩大研究中。

4. 磁共振成像(MRI)

最近 MRI 的多项发展使得其在胰腺肿瘤评估中的应用越来越多,最近的几项研究显示其结果可与 CT 相媲美[63]。大于 1.5T 的高场强、肝脏特异性造影剂和弥散加权成像,这些都有助于改善成像。与 CT 相比,MRI 提供了更强的软组织对比,从而在检测非轮廓改变损伤方面具有更高的灵敏度[64]。

典型胰腺癌的表现是一个有不同密度的、边缘不清晰的肿块。在脂肪抑制 T1 信号时,肿瘤通常呈现低密度,而在 T2 加权像上,肿瘤的强度是可变的。多序列采集对于原发肿瘤和任何远处疾病的全面评估都是必需的[65]。MRI 能够较好地评估 CT 等衰减病灶、小肿瘤,胰头肿大和实质的局灶性浸润[64]。Java 语言描述:CT 上等衰减的病灶可能只是如胰腺萎缩或者胰管扩张的次要征象。但在 MRI 上可以看到 79.2% 的敏感性[66]。使用钆对比增强 MRI 和 MRA 技术可以证明肿瘤侵犯血管,评估病变可切除性的敏感性和 CT 相当[63]。但与 CT 不同,MRI 不涉及辐射,使用无碘造影剂,可用于肾功能不全者,罕见肾毒性。

MRCP 也可以在做 MRI 时获得。MRCP 使用重 T2 加权像,强调含液体的结构,如胰管、囊肿和胰周积液。所获得的图像与 ERCP 所获得的图像高度相似,并且很容易显示胰管梗阻、扩张和结石。与 ERCP 相比,MRCP 是无创的,不需要在胰胆管中注射造影剂,避免了可能出现的过敏反应、胰腺炎、感染等并发症。MRCP 不能进行治疗或诊断干预,需要内镜治疗或活检的患者不能从 MRCP 中获益。

5. 正电子发射断层摄影/计算机断层扫描(PET/CT)

PET 是一种无创成像工具,它可提供肿瘤的代谢和半定量数据,而不是单纯的形态学信息。这种诊断方法是基于与正常胰腺实质相比,肿瘤细胞对放射性标记葡萄糖的更多摄取。静脉给予放射性葡萄糖类似物^{18}F-FDG,然后通过 PET 扫描仪检测 FDG 的摄取情况。联合 PET/CT 与同步非造影 CT 一起进行,以增强空间解释。PET 扫描通常不能显示正常的胰腺。相反,胰腺癌则表现为胰腺床有摄取增加的局灶区域。肝转移也可能表现为肝脏内的"热点"。由于缺乏解剖细节,PET 扫描作为一种胰腺癌的诊断方式没有明确的作用。最近的一项研究显示,与对比度增强的多探头 CT 相比,PET/CT 对 PC 的检出率无明显优势[67]。当瘢痕组织或术后变化可能难以与复发性癌性瘤区分时,PET/CT 也可用于评估胰腺切除术后的肿瘤复发[68]。最后,PET/CT 可有益于评估肿瘤对初次或新辅助化疗的反应,这可能导致改变临床治疗决策[69]。

6. US 和 EUS 引导下细胞学检查

胰腺的 FNA 细胞学检查一直是胰腺肿瘤患者治疗的重大进展之一。CT 引导下活检已经使用了 30 多年,被认为是一种安全、可靠的技术,具有合理的灵敏度和几乎没有假阳性的结果。EUS 引导下 FNA 的经验显示了相似的结果。即使在无梗阻性黄疸的胰腺肿块患者中,诊断准确率也可高达 97.6%[70]。当患者被认为患有不可切除或转移性胰腺癌时,CT 或 EUS 引导下的 FNA 活检适用于疾病的组织学确认,除非需要进行姑息性手术。即使慢性胰腺炎的诊断被合理的排除,恶性肿瘤的证据也可能排除胰腺的其他罕见良性疾病,如结核和结节病。FNA 细胞学检查和免疫组化检查通常可以区分腺癌和其他胰腺肿瘤如神经内分泌瘤和淋巴瘤,可能导致采用不同的治疗方案。

在有经验的外科医生手中,除非患者正在进行新辅助研究,否则组织学诊断不是大多数具有适当临床和 CT 结果和潜在可切除肿瘤的患者,进行手术的先决条件。假阴性率足够高,导致 FNA 阴性结果不能明确地排除恶性肿瘤。CT 引导下的细针穿刺活检或 EUS-FNA 最有可能遗漏更小的、有效可治愈的肿瘤。不改变治疗方案的诊断测试会显著增加治疗成本和延迟外科手术干预的时间[71]。

7. 血清肿瘤标志物

多种多样的肿瘤标志物已经被提出用于胰腺癌,但目前唯一具有使用价值的是血清 CA199。虽然不适合筛查,但它是胰腺癌诊断、预后和治疗检测的一个有价值的辅助手段。

对于胰腺癌的诊断,CA199 的敏感性和特异性随着阈值的不同而不同。该肿瘤标志物的主要警惕的是阳性预测值低,特别是在无症状个体中。一项研究表明,37U/ml 水平是鉴别良恶性胰腺疾病最准确的临界点。在这个水平上，报道的敏感性和特异性仅为 77% 和 87%[72]。黄疸的存在，特别是胆管炎，在没有恶性肿瘤（假阳性结果）的情况下可以发现非常高的 CA199 值。另外，少量 Lewis 血型阴性（Le[a-]，Le[b-]）的患者不表达 CA199 抗原（5%～10%人群），可能导致假阴性结果[73]。

CA199 水平确实对可切除疾病有预后价值。术前高水平的 CA199 已经被证明在分期腹腔镜检查时具有更高的隐匿性转移的可能[74]。当前美国临床肿瘤学会（ASCO）指南不使用 CA199 水平作为可切除性的标志。最近一项对 260 例接受手术切除的胰腺癌患者的研究发现，6 个月内 CA199 正常化的患者的平均生存期是那些持续升高患者的两倍（29.9 个月 vs 14.8 个月，$P=0.0004$）。术后水平高于 90U/mL 的患者不能从新辅助化疗中获益[75]。一项对转移性疾病患者的化疗试验发现，CA199 的降低与有效率、无进展生存期和总生存期的增加相关[69]。未来的实验应包括 CA199 测量，以进一步验证其在预测结果中的作用。

（五）分期

美国癌症联合委员会（American Joint Committee on Cancer，AJCC）的胰腺癌分期系统见表 60.4[76]，该系统于 2010 年最后一次修订，未进行进一步修改以区分不可切除（T4、Ⅲ期和Ⅳ期）和可切除疾病（T1～3、Ⅰ期和Ⅱ期）。分级系统仍存在一些不足。首先，如果不进行手术干预，就无法对淋巴结状态进行准确评估，这一缺陷可能导致对不适合剖腹手术患者的局部晚期疾病的低估。其次，在确定临床分期时，并未考虑具有重要预后意义的切除边缘。由于这些和其他缺点，AJCC 分期系统的临床适用性有限[77]。

胰腺癌的分期基于 4 个不同患者组的识别。第一组涉及表现为转移性疾病的患者。手术对这些患者没有益处，其生存期短，化疗是其姑息治疗措施以外的主要治疗方式。第二组包括局部晚期不可切除疾病但无转移的患者。这些患者可能从新辅助放化疗中受益，根据其治疗反应，可能是后续手术探查的候选者[78]。第三组被定义为临界可切除组，更有可能从新辅助治疗中获益[79]。第四组由明确可切除疾病的患者组成。除非入组一项实验性新辅助治疗方案，否则应提倡立即手术治疗。

胰腺癌患者的最低分期检查应该包括体格检查以及腹部和骨盆的 CT 或 MRI。如前所述，多期对比 CT 或 MRI/MRA 在识别不可切除疾病方面相当且极其准确[63,66]。在临界病例和术前治疗计划中，EUS 可通过进一步评估血管浸润和组织采样来补充 CT，然而，CT 成像不能正确预测 25%～30%患者的可切除性[80]。在大多数情况下，遗漏的病灶超出了目前放射学成像的分辨率，包括肝、腹壁、胃、肠或网膜的腹膜表面。这种肿瘤播散的成功检测取决于腹腔探查和直视检查，目前只能通过腹腔镜或剖腹手术实现。

已发表的数据表明，约 25%经 CT 证实为局部疾病的患者，也有疑似转移的植入物[79]。对于其中许多这类患者，腹腔镜检查可以避免不必要的手术探查来评估肿瘤的可切除性。分期程序仅增加了几分钟计划的治疗手术时间，并与简单的诊断性腹腔镜检查联合活检可疑结节。收集腹腔冲洗液

表 60.4　TNM 系统和美国癌症联合委员会（AJCC）胰腺癌分期

肿瘤（T）			
TX	无法评估原发肿瘤		
T0	无原发性肿瘤证据		
Tis	原位癌[包括Ⅲ级胰腺上皮内瘤变（PanIN）]		
T1	肿瘤局限于胰腺，最大范围≤2cm		
T2	肿瘤局限于胰腺，最大范围>2cm		
T3	肿瘤超出胰腺，但未累及腹腔干或肠系膜上动脉		
T4	肿瘤累及腹腔干或肠系膜上动脉（不可切除的原发肿瘤）		
淋巴结转移（N）			
Nx	无法评估局部淋巴结		
N0	无局部淋巴结转移		
N1	局部淋巴结转移		
远处转移（M）			
MX	无法评估远处转移		
M0	无远处转移		
M1	远处转移		
AJCC 分期			
0 期	Tis	N0	M0
ⅠA 期	T1	N0	M0
ⅠB 期	T2	N0	M0
ⅡA 期	T3	N0	M0
ⅡB 期	T1	N1	M0
	T2	N1	M0
	T3	N1	M0
Ⅲ期	T4	N1	M0
Ⅳ期	任何 T	任何 N	M1

From Greene FL，Compton C，Fritz A，et al. Exocrine pancreas. AJCC cancer staging manual. 7th ed. New York：Springer-Verlag；2010. pp 241-47.

用于第二次麻醉暴露的细胞学分析的热情减弱，因为阳性灌洗似乎不能预测生存率，尽管这可能随着新辅助化疗方法的探索而改变。CT 扫描和选择性分期腹腔镜检查的结合增强了对转移性、局部不可切除和可切除胰腺癌患者的识别，并有助于根据不同的治疗方案对患者进行分层。目前胰腺癌的诊断和分期的流程应包括对所有胰腺体部和尾部肿瘤患者（其中非疑似转移的频率接近 50%）和胰头部肿瘤大于 2cm 的患者进行腹腔镜检查，因为腹腔镜检查的成功率与原发肿瘤的大小成正比[81]。

（六）治疗

1. 手术治疗

手术切除是胰腺癌最有效的治疗方法[82]，绝大多数患者为晚期，只有大约 15%～20% 的患者可以接受胰腺癌切除[79,80,83]。不幸的是，即使在最理想的情况下，接受辅助化疗的胰腺癌切除患者的中位生存率也只有 20～23 个月[84]。R0

切除，无受累淋巴结和肿瘤大小是最有力的预后指标[85,86]。

局部晚期的疾病的手术适应证目前处于不断变化的状态，尽管任何手术干预的目标应该是 R0 切除。目前美国国家综合癌症网络(NCCN)指南对可切除的定义是：无动脉(肝总、肠系膜上、腹腔干)受累者，且无 SMV-PV 受累，或小于等于 180°包绕且无静脉不规则改变[86]。远处受累，通常表现为恶性腹水或肝脏转移、腹膜或腹主动脉周围淋巴结转移，是切除的绝对禁忌证。

相对的手术禁忌证包括肠系膜上静脉或门静脉的包绕或闭塞，或疾病直接浸润至腹腔干、肠系膜上动脉、腔静脉或主动脉。近年来，血管切除和重建的应用越来越广泛，因为对于局部晚期病变，如果直接向静脉浸润是唯一的限制，就可以通过选择适宜患者行手术切除达到 R0 的切除目标[87]。

术前常规 ERCP 和胆道支架置入以减轻黄疸，并没有显示可以降低术后的病发率和死亡率。而且该行为可能增加手术感染并发症的可能[88]。多项研究表明，胰十二指肠切除术死亡率的增加与高胆红素血症有关。然而，胆道系统支架置入术和随后肝功能检查的改善并没有被证明可以降低死亡率[89]。因此，对于可切除肿瘤(经 CT 评估)的患者，并不推荐常规的术前胆道支架植入术。严重黄疸和预期延迟手术，以及进入术前(新辅助)治疗的黄疸患者可以进行暂时性胆道引流。对于体弱多病无法承受手术或疾病无法被切除的患者，内镜胆道支架，最好是可膨胀的金属支架，可以提供很好的姑息治疗[90,91]。

胰腺癌最常见的手术是保留幽门胰十二指肠切除术(图 60.6)，主要切胰头、十二指肠、远端胆管和近端空肠，并进行胰空肠吻合[92]。提倡行全胰腺切除术治疗导管腺癌以避免胰瘘的出现。然而，全胰切除术的概念在很大程度上已被放弃，因为曾具有相当高的发病率的胰空肠吻合术并发症治疗，已得到改善。对于其他侵袭性较弱的原发性胰腺肿瘤，如胰腺内乳头黏液性肿瘤和胰腺内分泌肿瘤，全胰切除术可能对体积较大的局部病变有益。外分泌不足很容易治疗，糖尿病治疗的持续改进使得脆性糖尿病的挑战在无胰腺状态不那么困难。标准 Whipple 手术的其他扩展，如扩大腹膜后淋巴结切除术，并没有显示出明显的生存获益。基于术中冰冻切缘的观察，将胰腺切除范围扩大到传统的胰颈解剖已进行全面评估。初始是 R1 边缘，但后续附加切除达到了 R0 永久切除，与 R1 切除的患者相比，生存率无变化[93]。多项随机临床试验表明，手术时间延长，出血增加，术后死亡率增加，但生存期没有提高[94-99]。

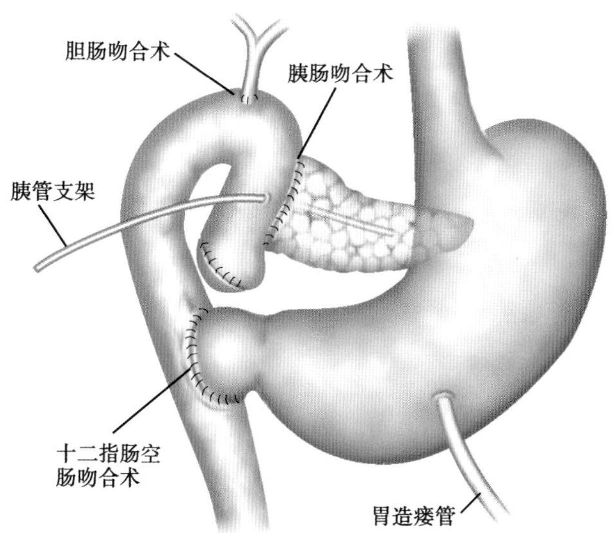

图 60.6　保留幽门的胰十二指肠切除术示意图。胰腺支架显示在胰管中。(From Jimenez RE, Fernandez-del Castillo C, Rattner DW, et al. Outcome of the pancreaticoduodenectomy with pylorus preservation or with antrectomy in the treatment of chronic pancreatitis. Ann Surg 2000;231:293-300.)

以前，胰十二指肠切除术(Whipple 手术)与高发病率和死亡率相关。当今许多大数据显示死亡率低于 3%，在过去的 50 年里，并发症也随之减少[100]。尽管在手术切除方面有了显著的改进，但术后并发症的发生率仍然高达 30% ~ 60%[101]。胰瘘在历史上是 Whipple 手术最常见的并发症，见于大约 22% ~26% 的患者中[102]。许多潜在的内源性和外科危险因素已被评估为胰瘘的危险因素：年龄、性别、体重指数、糖尿病、心血管因素、疾病部位、残余胰腺结构、胰管大小、吻合方法和术中出血量。瘘管的诊断可以通过 CT 或 US 显像[103]。治疗包括持续积极的营养支持，采用肠内营养而不是肠外营养。与肠外营养相比，肠内营养治疗效果更好，瘘口关闭更快，瘘口关闭率更高，康复更快[104]。结果的改善也与胰腺外科中心的发展有关。在那里，胰腺外科医生可以发展更专业的技术。一项使用 20 世纪 90 年代医疗保险数据库的研究表明，比较小病人量(每年<1 例)医院与大病人量(每年>5 例)医院行胰十二指肠切除术的死亡率，死亡率增加了 4 倍[105]。关于医疗机构病人量作为胰十二指肠切除术死亡率的独立预测因子的争议仍在继续。来自行政数据来源的各种研究没有达成明确的共识。总体而言，自 20 世纪 90 年代以来，美国高风险手术的死亡率有所下降，原因有几个。外科医生的个人经验，而不是每年的外科机构或外科医生的病人量，可以决定手术结果[106]。在最近的一项研究中，重要的死亡率预测因子是年龄、身体状态和营养不良，而不是住院患者人数[107]。微创和机器人技术已经被用于试图降低胰十二指肠切除术的发病率。到目前为止，这些手术在特定的患者中，在主要发病率和死亡率方面有相同的结果，住院时间稍短，被较高的再住院率抵消。手术时间延长(427 分钟 vs 360 分钟)和费用并没有被瘘形成率的降低或胃排空延迟所抵消[108]。

新技术的实行增加了手术时间。美国外科医师协会国家手术质量改善项目发现，较长的手术时间与较差的围手术期结果独立相关。所有的疾病随着手术时间的增加而逐步增加。与已知的术前危险因素无关[109]。这些发现表明手术时间是质量改善的相关风险参数。

尽管预后有所改善，但胰腺切除术在美国仍未被充分应用于胰腺癌的治疗。Bilimoria 和他的同事利用 1995 年至 2004 年的国家癌症数据库对早期胰腺癌患者进行了队列研究，发现有 38.2% 的潜在可切除疾病的患者没有进行手术[110]。年龄超过 65 岁、黑人、社会经济地位低、受教育程度低、肿瘤位于胰头的胰腺癌患者是不太能接受手术治疗的。研究还报道了Ⅰ期疾病患者胰腺切除术与那些不行手术者相比,平均生存期为19.3个月和8.4个月(图60.7)。一项研究强调了手术的可获得性是生存的一个预测因素。该研究发现了29%的黑人患者从未接受过手术评估。而那些接受过手术评估的人,仍然不太可能接受手术治疗。尽管在未经调整的模型中,黑人患者的生存率太低了,但在校正之后,种族对生存率没有显著影响[111]。这些数据可能反应了对胰腺手术有效性的一种虚无主义态度和医疗保健选择的可获得性差异。

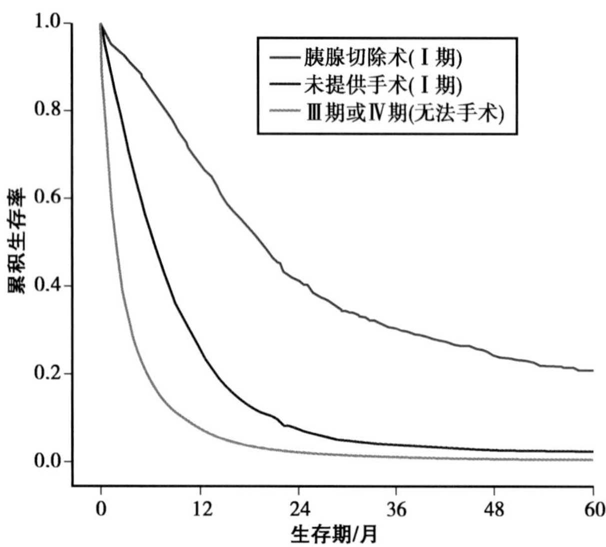

图60.7 胰腺癌5年生存率比较(比较3组患者):因临床Ⅰ期疾病行胰腺切除的患者(n=2 746);虽是临床Ⅰ期疾病但未行胰腺切除的患者(n=3 644);以及未接受手术的Ⅲ或Ⅳ期疾病患者(n=68 521)。(Modified from Bilimoria K, Bentrem DJ, Ko CY, et al. National failure to operate on early stage pancreatic cancer. Ann Surg 2007;246:173-80.)

最后,胰腺癌的预后仍然很差,即使在适当选择的患者进行潜在的治疗性手术后也是如此。手术后5年生存率约为25%[112],患者根据临床分期,中位生存期在12.7~24.1个月[113]。尽管手术相关的早期死亡率降低,1年生存率提高,但长期生存率在30年里是相似的[114]。最近在外科技术和围手术期护理方面的进展可能已经达到了让生存获益的极限。单纯的外科手术受到了肿瘤生物学行为和完整切除的解剖边界的限制。显微边缘可能是肿瘤生物学的一个标志,而不仅仅是手术不充分的一个反应[115,116]。长期疗效的改善有待于多模式治疗的共同努力,可能是由免疫治疗和快速发展的分子靶向治疗来推动[44,45]。

2. 辅助和新辅助治疗

对于15%~20%可切除肿瘤的患者,生存期仍然较短,5年生存率为10%~30%,随着时间的推移,采用更好的手术技术、改善术后护理和辅助治疗可能会提高生存率。疾病复发的风险因素包括边缘阳性、淋巴结受累、高度恶性的肿瘤和原发性肿瘤大小大于2.5cm[117,118]。辅助治疗是指术后预防癌症复发的治疗。胰腺癌最常见的复发是远处转移性疾病,仅15%的复发发生在局部肿瘤床上[119]。这导致了关于除化疗外辅助放射治疗作用的持续争论。

从1980年至2000年,辅助放化疗(即化疗与放疗同时进行)是潜在根治性胰腺癌切除术后的标准治疗。这些建议是基于1974年至1982年间胃肠道肿瘤研究组(Gastrointestinal Tumor Study Group, GITSG)进行的一项小型研究的结果[120]。该研究将43例术后患者随机分为2个组,一组为单独观察组,另一组为放化疗组(用4 000Gy外照射)。同时推注5-氟尿嘧啶(5-FU)作为放射增敏剂。治疗组的中位生存期为21个月,显著长于未治疗组的11个月中位生存期。GITSG研究因其样本量小且缺乏统计学把握度而受到批评,然而,挪威胰腺癌实验组的另一项单独研究显示了相似的结果,并支持辅助治疗的生存获益[121]。

1999年欧洲癌症研究和治疗组织(European Organization for Research and Treatment of Cancer, EORTC)的一项研究结果对这一结论提出了质疑[122]。与GITSG的研究设计相似,EORTC将114例术后患者随机分为观察组或放化疗组(4 000cGy外照射和同步连续输注5-FU)。治疗组的中位生存期仅比观察组长4.5个月(分别为17.1个月和12.6个月),该差异无统计学意义。同样,两组预计的2年生存率也无显著差异(分别为37个月和23个月)。

2001年欧洲胰腺癌研究组(ESPAC-1试验)公布了一项更大的289例患者的研究结果后,引发了进一步的争议[123]。ESPAC-1研究设计复杂,将术后患者随机分为4组:观察组、化疗组、放化疗组或放化疗加化疗组。结果显示,接受放化疗和未接受放化疗患者的中位生存期无差异(分别为15.5个月和16.1个月)。即使对于切除边缘阳性的患者,被认为是最适合辅助放化疗的候选者,这种治疗也没有对生存率产生影响。在对仅接受化疗的患者亚组分析中,2年生存率为30%,这表明单独化疗有益。ESPAC-1试验的结果通过其大样本量得到了验证,但引起了很大的争议,批评主要指向该研究的错综复杂的随机化方案、中断的放疗过程和用于统计分析的数据汇集。

早期的研究显示,吉西他滨治疗胰腺癌比5-FU更有效。RTOG 9704评价了在以5-FU为基础的放化疗之前给予吉西他滨,随后再次给予吉西他滨。该试验显示加用吉西他滨后,可改善5年生存率(22% vs 18%),但该差异不具有统计学意义[124]。

许多人质疑辅助放射治疗本身的作用,因为这种方式主要用于降低局部复发的风险。虽然现代放疗技术提高了放疗质量,限制了毒副反应,但大多数患者仍死于转移性疾病。因此,仅使用化疗进行研究(表60.5)。其中规模最大的是CONKO研究,该研究将368例术后患者随机分配至吉西他滨单药组或无治疗组。该试验显示中位生存期从20.2个月提高到22.8个月,5年生存率从9%提高到21%[125]。2017年,ESPAC-4试验发布,在730例患者中比较了辅助吉西他滨/卡培他滨联合方案与吉西他滨单药方案。结果显示联合治疗组的中位总生存期为28.0个月,而单药组为25.5个月[126]。

不幸的是,没有试验明确地比较单独辅助化疗与化疗加放疗。RTOG 0848目前正在招募接受吉西他滨/厄洛替尼辅助治疗的切除胰腺癌患者,随后通过观察或5-FU/放射治疗或卡培他滨/放射治疗进行随访。国家癌症中心网络的现行指南建议,辅助治疗可以是单独的化疗或化疗加放化疗[127]。一些中心目前正在使用新辅助治疗,定义为手术前给予的治

表 60.5　术后辅助治疗试验中胰腺癌切除患者的中位生存时间、2 年生存率和 5 年生存率

治疗	中位时间/月	2 年生存率/%	5 年生存率/%
GITSG	21	24	19
EORTC	17.1	30	20
ESPAC-1	20.1	30	21
CONKO-001	22.1	34	22.5
RTOG(5-FU 组)	16.9	22	18
RTOG(吉西他滨组)	20.6	31	22

5-FU,5-氟尿嘧啶。

Adapted from Regine WF, Winter KA, Abrams RA, et al. Fluorouracil vs gemcitabine chemotherapy before and after fluorouracil-based chemoradiation following resection of pancreatic adenocarcinoma: a randomized controlled trial. JAMA 2008;299:1019.

疗。这种方式在临界可切除患者中获得了更大的认可,否则这些患者存在切缘阳性切除的风险。临界可切除患者的定义各不相同,但通常包括无远处转移证据的肠系膜血管受累患者组。公认的,新辅助治疗的潜在获益是增加可切除疾病患者接受化疗的可能性,降低临界可切除疾病的分期,增加切缘阴性切除的可能性,并潜在地避免了对表现为亚临床转移性疾病患者的手术,并治疗微转移性疾病。新辅助治疗的选择包括放疗、化疗、序贯治疗、同步治疗或混合方案。已经报告或目前正在招募许多研究(表 60.6)。由于缺乏随机数据,新辅助治疗仍被认为是研究性的。NCCN 和 ASCO 指南均认为临界状态疾病的新辅助治疗方案是合理的治疗选择。

3. 姑息性手术

世界卫生组织定义的姑息治疗目标是"实现患者及其家属的最佳生活质量"。恶性肿瘤的早期干预与生活质量和寿命的改善有关[128]。

表 60.6　胰腺囊性肿瘤的流行病学和生物学特征

肿瘤	性别	生命的高峰 10 年	囊性肿瘤/%	恶性潜能和自然史
浆液性囊腺瘤	女性	第 7 年	32~39	切除是治愈性的;浆液性囊腺癌极为罕见
黏液性囊性肿瘤	女性	第 5 年	10~45	无论上皮异型增生的程度如何,切除均可治愈;存在浸润性腺癌时预后不良
导管内乳头状黏液性肿瘤	男女相等	第 6~7 年	21~33	仅显示腺瘤性和临界细胞异型性的病变预后良好;存在浸润性腺癌时预后不良
实性假乳头状瘤	女性	第 4 年	<10	伴罕见淋巴结和淋巴结外转移的惰性肿瘤;完全切除时预后极佳
囊性内分泌肿瘤	男女相等	第 5~6 年	<10	与实体神经内分泌肿瘤相似(见第 33 章)
导管腺癌伴囊性变	男性略多	第 6~7 年	<1	预后不佳,与实体腺癌相似
腺泡细胞囊腺癌	男性	第 6~7 年	<1	与实体型相似;侵袭性肿瘤的预后略好于导管腺癌

Modified from Brugge W, Lauwers G, Sahani D, et al. Cystic neoplasms of the pancreas. N Engl J Med 2004;351:1218-26.

80% 的患者在病程中出现梗阻性黄疸。历史上,胆肠旁路手术是标准实践。然而,由于胃/十二指肠梗阻的风险较高,这种治疗模式不再受欢迎[129]。在过去 10 年中,内镜和经皮入路已变得司空见惯(见第 61 和 70 章)。姑息性外科旁路术的使用显著下降,因为术前成像检查对不可切除或隐匿性转移性疾病患者的探索较少。在内镜姑息治疗的同时,使用薄层横截面成像的计算机断层扫描技术的改进,减少了亚临床不可切除疾病患者接受手术[130]。姑息性内镜手术的耐受性良好,可在门诊进行。在经验丰富的医生手中,内镜下胆道和十二指肠支架置入的成功率高于 90%,与手术相关的死亡率较低[131]。内镜与手术缓解梗阻性黄疸患者的生存率差异,可能反映了内镜治疗患者的合并症更多和功能状态更差[132]。

有两种类型的胆道支架可供使用:塑料支架和自膨式金属支架。塑料支架是短期使用的首选,需要每 3 个月更换一次,以预防支架闭塞或胆管炎的并发症。与塑料支架相比,自膨式金属支架和硅胶覆膜支架改善了长期通畅率,并且在长期应用中更耐用,例如在接受新辅助放化疗的患者中[133,134]。由于覆膜金属支架在手术时易于取出,对于可能成为手术候选者的患者来说,不再需要塑料支架[135]。

传统上,十二指肠梗阻是通过胃空肠吻合术进行手术治疗的。在接受手术证实的、不可切除的壶腹周围肿块切除术的无症状患者中,进行预防性外科旁路手术与不进行旁路手术的结局比较证实,预防性胃空肠吻合术可降低晚期胃出口梗阻的风险,术后并发症或住院时间无差异[136]。当然,在这种情况下的任何研究都有其固有的偏见,因为合并症较少和功能状况较好的患者很可能会接受外科手术干预。使用自膨式金属支架缓解恶性十二指肠梗阻已显示成功,这种方式在未来可能会越来越多地使用[131,137]。在胆道或十二指肠应用中,因支架功能障碍的再入院比手术旁路术失败更常见,但手术旁路术患者的住院总天数并未减少[138]。

无法手术的胰腺癌疼痛是一个常见的问题,80% 的受累患者出现重度疼痛[139]。阿片类药物给药难以控制不能手术的胰腺癌患者的疼痛,并与许多毒性相关。腹腔神经丛阻滞或腹腔神经丛松解术可通过手术、经皮或 EUS 引导进行。通过 EUS 进行的化学神经松解术在改善疼痛方面的有效率为 73%[140]。发现单次注射是足够的,具有相似的应答率[141]。一项前瞻性腹腔镜研究显示疼痛评分降低,但功能等级无改善[142]。胸部内脏神经切除术是阻断这种疼痛途径的替代方法[143]。这些手术的有效性是中等的,最大的随机试验是在

接受 EUS 进行癌症诊断和分期的患者中进行的。这项研究显示了显著的疼痛缓解,但吗啡消耗量、生活质量改善或生存率未显著降低(见第 61 章)[144]。

4. 晚期疾病的治疗

(1) 远处转移性疾病

单药化疗已成为转移性胰腺癌的主要治疗方法。吉西他滨一直是转移性 PC 的标准治疗;然而,有效率很低,只有 6%~10%[145,146]。吉西他滨获得批准是基于一项具有里程碑意义的试验,该试验表明,吉西他滨能够减轻疾病相关症状,包括疼痛和体重减轻[147]。在这项试验后的数年里,其他联合化疗、靶向治疗或免疫治疗的研究没有显示统计上显著的生存改善。2007 年,一项针对吉西他滨(单独使用或联合使用埃罗替尼)的随机 3 期临床研究首次显示,联合治疗比单独使用吉西他滨具有统计上显著的生存优势[148]。联合埃罗替尼后,中位生存期从 5.91 个月提高到 6.24 个月。许多人质疑 10 天中位生存期的增加是否具有临床意义。治疗的进一步进展随着一项研究的发表而到来,该研究将病人随机接受 FOLFIRINOX(叶酸、氟尿嘧啶、伊立替康、奥沙利铂)与吉西他滨的治疗[149]。该试验显示,联合治疗的生存率有显著提高,从 6.8 个月提高到 11.1 个月(图 60.8)。可以推测,该方案的毒性明显高于单独使用吉西他滨。2013 年的一项研究表明,吉西他滨联合白蛋白结合型紫杉醇(nabpaclitaxel)可将吉西他单用 6.8 个月的生存率提高到联合使用 8.5 个月[150]。目前对转移性疾病患者的治疗建议包括:对于一般状况良好、耐受联合治疗的患者,可采用 FOLFIRINOX 或联合使用吉西他滨+白蛋白-紫杉醇;对于耐受联合治疗的患者,不能耐受联合治疗的患者,则单独使用吉西他滨。

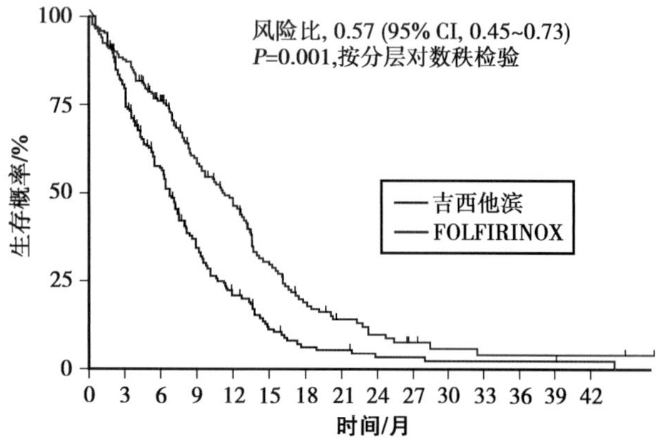

图 60.8　根据吉西他滨或 FOLFIRINOX 治疗,转移性胰腺癌患者总生存率的 Kaplan-Meier 估计值。(Modified from Bilimoria K, Bentrem DJ, Ko CY, et al. National failure to operate on early stage pancreatic cancer. Ann Surg 2007;246:173-80.)

(2) 不可切除/临界可切除非转移性疾病

临界可切除病变是由于邻近或直接累及静脉和/或动脉血管系统,而不可能通过 R0 切除的局部疾病。尚未明确定义该患者人群的治疗。对于定义为临界可切除的癌症,NCCN 建议避免直接手术和新辅助化疗和/或放化疗的多模式治疗。关于临界可切除疾病新辅助治疗的意见主要基于回顾性数据。数据显示缓解率、可切除性和 R0 切除均有所增加[151,152]。使用新辅助 FOLFIRINOX 或吉西他滨/白蛋白结合型紫杉醇联合或不联合序贯放化疗治疗临界或局部晚期疾病的近期研究获得了令人印象深刻的结果,切除患者的可切除率为 60.80%,R0 切除率为 80%~90%[153-163]。接受手术切除的患者与接受初次手术切除的患者的历史比较相比,无进展生存率和总生存率相似[164]。需要更多的前瞻性数据来阐述新辅助治疗的真实风险和获益。

对就诊时明显无法切除的疾病,传统治疗方法被定义为化疗和放化疗。尸检系列表明,30% 的 OT 患者死于局部进展的并发症,而不是转移性疾病[165]。许多研究使用化疗、放化疗或序贯治疗作为控制疾病或潜在降低疾病分期的方式。这些研究由异种性研究人群和年龄较大、疗效较差的化疗方案定义[166]。目前正在研究使用与较高缓解率相关的吉西他滨/白蛋白结合型紫杉醇或 FOLFIRINOX 方案。

放射治疗的真正益处尚不明确。一项由 43 例接受化疗或放化疗的局部晚期胰腺癌患者的 GITSG 试验证明了联合治疗方案的 10 周生存获益,代价是严重毒性[167]。最近两项使用同步放化疗试验均显示了严重的毒性,然而,FFCD 试验显示中位生存期缩短,而 ECOG 试验则显示相应同步放化疗组的生存期获益[168,169]。最后,LAP 07 试验将患者随机分配至诱导吉西他滨组和吉西他滨/厄洛替尼组。在最初入组的 442 例患者中,269 例在诱导化疗后表现稳定,并被随机分配到相同剂量化疗继续组或卡培他滨/放疗组。最终数据表明,总生存期无差异,以增加毒性为代价改善了放疗组的局部控制[170]。基于上述研究和其他研究,美国肿瘤学会建议对局部晚期疾病进行诱导化疗,并考虑对诱导治疗后无进展的患者同步进行放化疗[171]。

较新的治疗方式,包括更好地定义治疗领域和剂量探索,允许在维持剂量强度的同时改善毒性。由于淋巴结扩散的风险约为 30%,因此通常在放疗野中包括淋巴结引流池[172]。为了尽量减少毒性,目前的研究是将放疗定位在原发肿瘤,避免选择性淋巴结照射[173]。调节强度的放射治疗允许在肿瘤区域周围进行放射治疗雕刻[174]。最近,立体定向放射治疗(stereotactic body radiation therapy, SBRT)已显示出前景,并可设定新标准。SBRT 以适当的方式在有限剂量下使用每个治疗分次的高剂量,Ⅱ期数据显示局部控制率高,毒性控制良好。目前尚无比较 IMRT 与 SBRT 的研究[175]。

二、胰腺囊性肿瘤

胰腺囊性肿瘤相对少见,占胰腺肿瘤的 10% 以下[176]。由于横断面成像的广泛可用性和分辨率的提高,胰腺囊性病变的诊断急剧增加[177]。MRI 系列发现患病率高达 20%[178],70 岁以上患者的累计患病率为 40%。最近对一家机构 8 年期间进行的 24 000 例腹部 CT 和 MRI 研究进行了回顾,发现 1.2% 的患者存在胰腺囊肿,其中 60% 可能为囊性肿瘤[179]。黏液性囊性肿瘤(mucinous cystic neoplasm, MCN)、浆液性囊腺瘤[浆液性囊性肿瘤(serous cystic neoplasm, SCN)]和胰腺导管内乳头状黏液瘤(IPMN)占胰腺原发性囊性肿瘤的 80% 以上。准确地识别这些病变很重要,因为它们与胰腺假性囊肿相似,并且在手术治疗后具有较高的治愈率(见第 59 章)。

发现胰腺囊性病变后的患者评估,应首先排除胰腺假性囊肿。临床结果往往指导进一步的研究。与囊性肿瘤相反，假性囊肿缺乏上皮内衬，代表由炎症或阻塞破坏的导管外渗的胰腺分泌物的聚集（参见第 58 和 59 章）。假性囊肿患者常有急性或慢性胰腺炎或腹部外伤史，而大多数囊性肿瘤患者缺乏此类前期因素。与囊肿性肿瘤相比，支持诊断为假性囊肿的特征包括 CT 或 MRI 上缺乏中隔、形成小腔、固体成分或囊壁钙化。对于假性囊肿，ERCP 或 MRCP 传统上显示囊肿与主胰管相通。对假性囊肿液的评估显示高水平的淀粉酶，这对于囊性肿瘤是不典型的，除非它们与胰管有交通。

如果可以被排除胰腺假性囊肿的诊断，随后的评估应侧重于识别那些由于实际或潜在的恶性肿瘤而需要手术切除的肿瘤。与导管腺癌相反，具有恶性潜能的囊性肿瘤生长缓慢，即使在恶性变性的情况下也有良好的预后报告。具有恶变潜能的肿瘤包括 MCN、IPMN、实性假乳头状瘤（solid pseudopapillary tumor，SPT）和囊性胰岛细胞瘤。相反，浆液性囊腺瘤几乎普遍为良性，它们约占所有胰腺囊性肿瘤的三分之一。最初的挑战是将良性和潜在恶性囊性肿瘤区分开（见后文）。更困难的任务是将癌前病变和侵袭性肿瘤区分开，以避免老年人、高危患者的过度治疗，并以成本-有效的方式集中监测成像，以促进安全的手术策略。

首选的诊断检查是腹部 MRI 和 MRCP。如果无法完成 MRI，则使用 CT 胰腺成像是一种很好的替代方法。这些成像技术能够进行肿瘤定位，有时还能够区分假性囊肿和囊性肿瘤。ERCP 可用于诊断 IPMN，并允许通过刷检获取活检样本。EUS 可对囊壁进行详细定性，识别分隔、乳头或壁结节等精细结构（图 60.9）。此外，使用 EUS 还可以对囊肿内容物进行 FNA。囊液分析有助于评价囊性肿瘤（表 60.7）[176]。

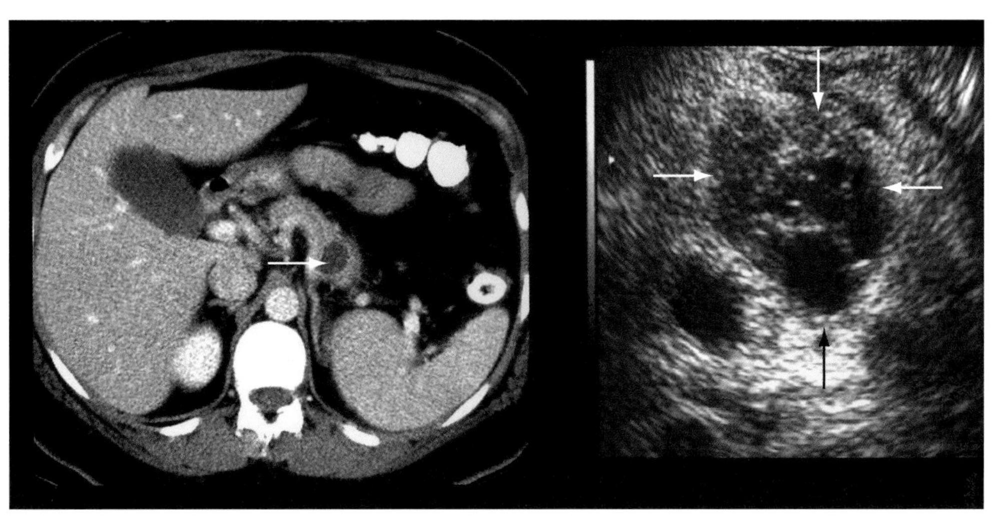

图 60.9　影像学检查显示胰腺尾部黏液性囊性肿瘤。左侧，CT 上囊肿清晰可见（箭）。右侧，超声内镜（EUS）图像显示 CT 上不清楚的中隔和囊肿内分房。箭表示 EUS 所描述的肿瘤。EUS 允许对囊液体进行采样

表 60.7　胰腺各种囊性病变囊液分析

参数	假性囊肿	浆液性囊腺瘤	黏液性囊腺瘤（良性）	黏液性囊腺瘤（恶性）	导管内乳头状黏液瘤
黏度	低	低	高	高	高
淀粉酶水平	高	低	低	低	高
CEA 水平	低	低	高	高	高
CA724	低	低	中等	高	中等到高
细胞学结果	组织细胞	具有富含糖原细胞质的立方体细胞	柱状黏液上皮细胞，异型性不同	腺癌细胞	柱状黏液上皮细胞，异型性不同

CEA，癌胚抗原。

（一）黏液性囊性肿瘤

黏液性囊性肿瘤（MCN）是一种罕见的胰腺囊性肿瘤，在大多数系列中比 IPMN 和 SCNs 少见[180]。一些研究表明，MCN 的患病率约为 IPMN 的一半[181,182]。MCN 以女性为主，女性与男性的比例为 20∶1，95% 以上的病例局限于腺体的体部和尾部。它们是单发的、含有黏蛋白的、多房或单房病变，纤维化壁较厚（图 60.10）[183]。

当中年女性腹部 CT 或 MRI 显示胰腺体部或尾部囊肿时，应怀疑 MCN。MCN 是一种边界清楚、薄壁的单发性囊肿，可为单房或多房。它们缺乏与主胰管的交通，与 IPMN 不同[184]。EUS 适用于临床和成像时特征偏离这种经典模式。EUS 比 MRI 或 CT 能更详细地识别分隔和囊壁结节，并可进行囊壁活检和囊液抽吸分析。囊肿液分析通常显示黏稠的黏液样物质，黏液淀粉酶水平低，肿瘤标志物（CEA）升高，细胞学检查可见黏液上皮细胞。这些发现有助于区分 MCN 与浆液性

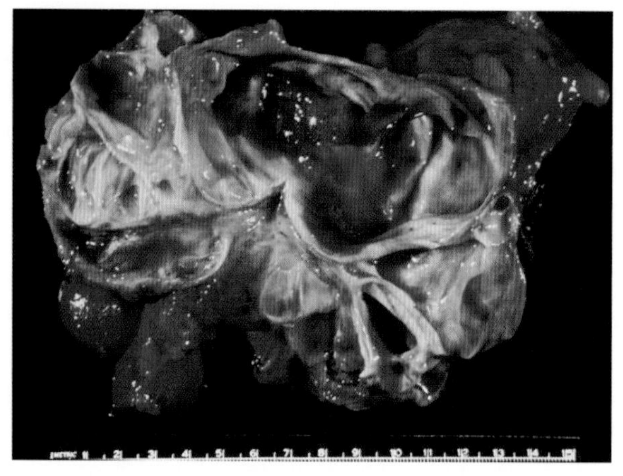

图 60.10 胰腺尾部多房黏液性囊性肿瘤

囊腺瘤(低液体 CEA)和 IPMN(高液体淀粉酶)(见表 60.7)。

多年来,黏液性囊性肿瘤被误认为是 IPMN,反之亦然。这导致了对黏液性囊性肿瘤真实的临床和病理特征的混淆。国际胰腺协会提出了将黏液性囊性肿瘤和 IPMN 准确区分的指南[185]。这一指南要求肿瘤内组织学上存在卵巢型基质,以确诊 MCN。根据这一标准,MCN 和 IPMN 现在被认为是两种不同的肿瘤,具有不同的遗传学、生物学行为和预后[183]。

黏液性囊性肿瘤以女性为主,男女比例为 20∶1,95% 以上的病例局限于腺体的体部和尾部。它们是单发的、含黏蛋白的、多房性或单房性病变,纤维化壁较厚。就诊时的平均年龄为 50 岁。在老年患者中,大多数患者主诉主要为腹痛或可触及的肿块。由于 CT 和 MRI 的广泛应用,越来越多的肿瘤被偶然发现。

由于 MCN 固有的恶性潜能,建议对所有 MCN 进行手术切除。考虑到大多数肿瘤位于腺体的体部或尾部,胰体尾切除加或不加脾切除是首选术式。腹腔镜手术是可接受的,失血量更少,住院时间更短,手术时间、发病率和死亡率没有差别[186,187]。考虑到淋巴结转移很少,因此没有必要切除紧邻胰腺淋巴结以外的淋巴结。在小病变或良性病变的情况下,可进行剜除术,无局部复发风险,无死亡率。在低风险肿瘤中,为了保留实质并避免胰腺功能不全,暂时性瘘管的显著风险是可以接受的[188]。中央胰腺切除术还可以保留胰腺功能,允许完全切除侵犯主胰管的病变,防止安全剜除[189]。

良性或临界黏液性囊性肿瘤的 5 年生存率非常高,据报道治愈率为 100%[185,188]。鉴于黏液性囊性肿瘤从未是多灶性的,切除的非侵袭性肿瘤患者不需要长期监测。对于侵袭性黏液性囊性肿瘤,切除肿瘤的 5 年生存率范围为 30%~63%[183,188]。

(二) 浆液性囊腺瘤

浆液性囊腺瘤主要是良性肿瘤,几乎没有恶性行为的风险。浆液性囊腺瘤的临床表现与黏液性囊性肿瘤相似,多发生于女性(75%)胰腺体部或尾部,平均年龄 62 岁[190]。还注意到与希佩尔-林道综合征(von Hippel-Lindau 病)的相关性。历史上,大多数患者表现为模糊的腹痛或不适,但当肿瘤增大达到较大尺寸时(10~25cm),有相当数量的患者出现可触及的肿块。目前,大多数是在评估其他未相关疾病期间检查到的偶然发现的无症状肿瘤[191]。

肉眼观察,浆液性囊腺瘤由边界清楚的胰腺肿瘤组成,在横断面上表现为由纤细的纤维间隔分隔的数目较多的微小囊肿,呈蜂窝状(图 60.11)[192]。囊肿内充满透明的水样液体,

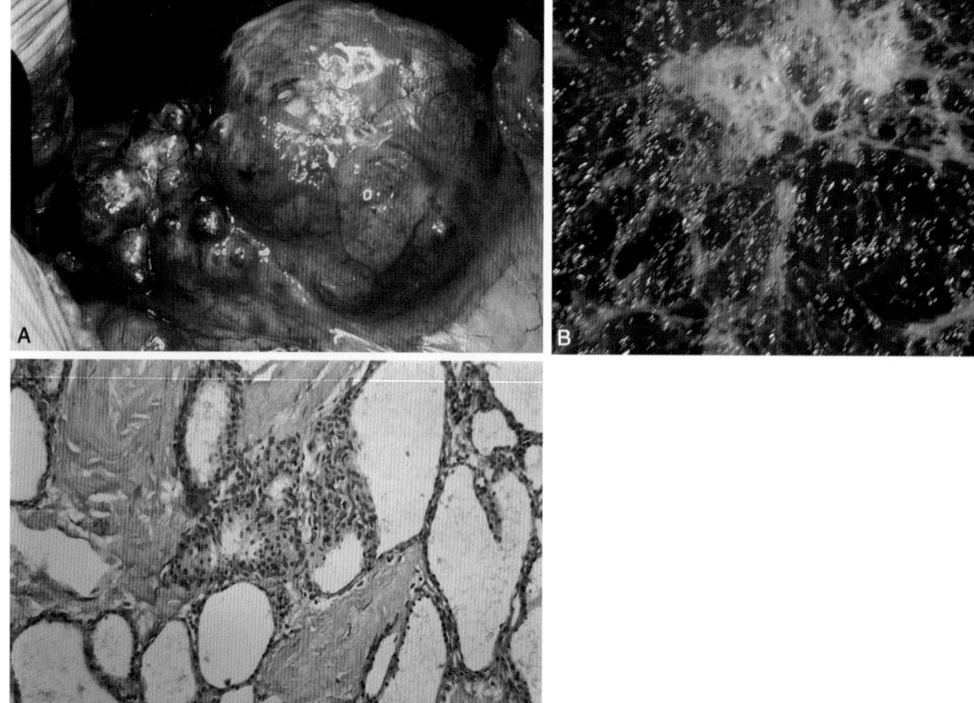

图 60.11 胰尾部浆液性囊腺瘤。A,手术时,大部分胰腺实质已被囊性肿瘤所取代。B,切面可见多个囊肿,中央有纤维化瘢痕。C,组织病理显示含浆液的囊肿,内衬富含糖原的单一立方细胞(HE 染色)

通常排列在可能钙化的中央星状瘢痕周围。CT 特征性图像是中央呈“阳光照射样”钙化的海绵状肿块，但这一情况仅发生在 10% 的患者中（图 60.12A）[176]。EUS 可能比 CT 能更好地分辨蜂窝结构（见图 60.12B）。发生大囊性变异，提示肿瘤可发生囊性变，导致与假性囊肿或 MCN 混淆[193]。囊液分析特征性地显示低黏度，低水平的 CEA，细胞学检查呈阴性（见表 60.7）。

与黏液性囊性肿瘤不同，浆液性囊腺瘤被认为是良性肿瘤。也有浆液性囊腺癌的罕见病例报告，但占已知病例的 3% 以下[194]。手术切除是症状性病变的首选治疗方法。切除的方法取决于肿瘤的位置，包括带或不带脾切除术的远端全胰切除术、Whipple 手术、中胰切除术、或剜除术。

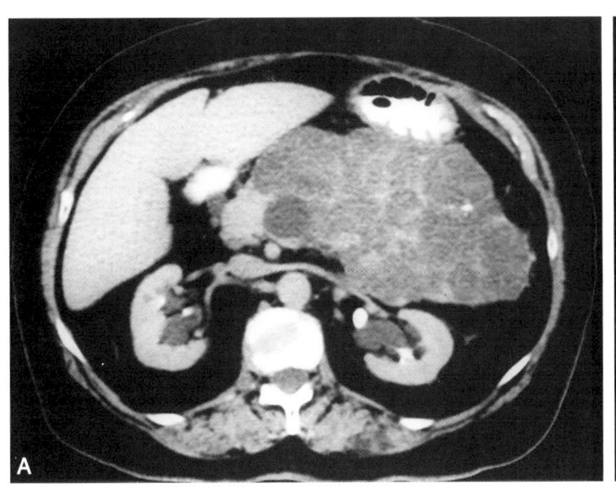

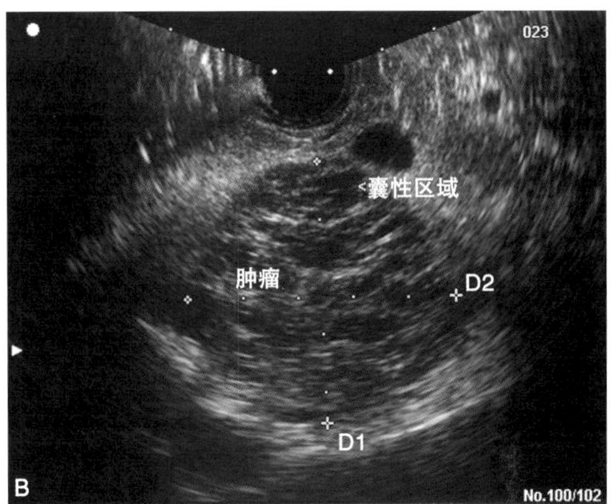

图 60.12　影像学检查显示胰腺体尾部浆液性囊腺瘤。A，CT 显示其海绵状外观和钙化。B，超声内镜（EUS）显示 4.5cm×4.8cm 浆液性囊腺瘤呈蜂窝状外观。（Courtesy Michael Nunez，MD，Dallas TX.）

如果无症状，浆液性囊腺瘤可以安全地观察。但观察有肿瘤持续生长的风险，可能导致出血、占位效应引起梗阻性黄疸、胰腺管梗阻伴外分泌不足或胃出口梗阻等并发症[195]。记录了两种不同的增长模式，分为缓慢（每年 1mm）和较快速（每年 5mm）[196]。就诊时肿瘤的大小并不是快速生长的有用决定因素。另一组患者平均随访 42 个月，发现肿瘤大小与随后的生长速率相关[197]。尽管几乎所有无症状患者都可以安全地进行监测成像，但新出现的症状、症状恶化或肿块迅速增大时，应提高对浆液性囊腺癌的怀疑指数并考虑手术治疗[198]。位于胰腺头的大直径肿瘤更易表现出侵袭性行为，需要切除[199]。

（三）导管内乳头状黏液性肿瘤

自 1982 年对其进行首次报道以来，由于横断面成像的使用增加，IPMN 的发病率迅速上升[200]。大多数 IPMN 是偶然诊断的，真实患病率未知，在 70 岁以上患者中的患病率范围为 0.000 8%～10%[201,202]。人们对该病及其与慢性胰腺炎鉴别的认识提高，加上诊断成像技术的改进，导致识别和报告的“新”病例激增。关于这些肿瘤已应用了多种术语，包括黏液性导管扩张症、导管内产黏蛋白肿瘤、导管内囊腺瘤、胰管绒毛状腺瘤和导管内乳头状肿瘤。然而，自 1996 年以来，世卫组织和武装部队病理研究所都统一将该实体称为 IPMN[203]。

主胰管的 IPMN 代表主胰管内乳头状肿瘤，表现为黏蛋白高分泌，常导致胰管扩张和慢性阻塞性胰腺炎（图 60.13）。IPMN 被认为是癌前胰腺病变，组织学上其上皮可显示单个肿瘤内从增生到癌的区域。根据其组织学特征，IPMN 通常分为以下几组：良性（腺瘤）、交界性和恶性[203]。恶性组根据延伸是否超过基底膜，进一步细分为非浸润性（原位癌）和浸润性癌。恶性肿瘤在主胰管 IPMN 中占 64%，在分支胰管 IPMN 患者中占 18%[204]。

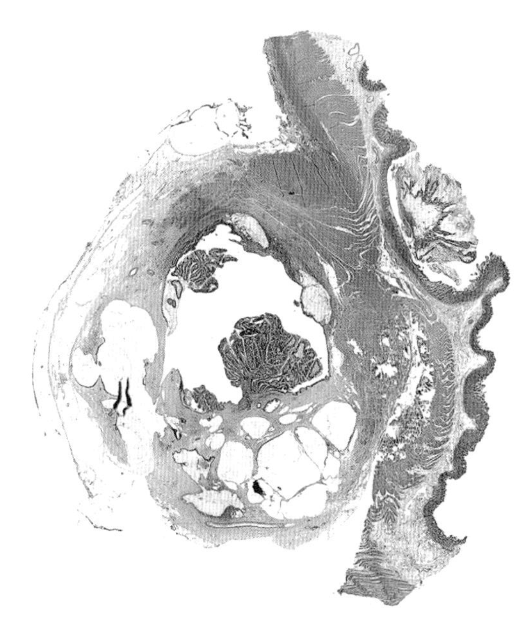

图 60.13　恶性导管内乳头状黏液性肿瘤的组织病理学视图。胰管内有乳头状肿瘤生长。注意胰腺周围的黏蛋白湖。图片右侧为十二指肠，其右上方为黏液性肿瘤局灶性侵犯十二指肠（HE 染色，低倍）

临床上，IPMN 在男性和女性中的发生频率相等，诊断时的中位年龄约为 65 岁。大约 75% 的患者有症状，腹痛和体重减轻是最常见的主诉。20% 的患者有复发性胰腺炎病史，约 25% 的患者有急性胰腺炎。没有一组症状允许术前识别

IPMN 的恶性变体，然而，恶性肿瘤患者年龄更大，更有可能出现黄疸或新发糖尿病[205]。

对 IPMN 患者的评估包括腹部 CT 或 MRI、MRCP，以及目前较少见的 ERCP。CT 常显示胰管扩张，伴或不伴相关囊性肿块。胰管扩张常令人印象深刻，在 CT 上可酷似 MCN（图 60.14）。MRI 发现恶性与良性或交界性 IPMN 相比，壁结节（60% vs 4%）和壁增强（74% vs 21%）更常见[206]。通过 ERCP 进行的评估通常显示 Vater 壶腹扩张伴黏液挤出，这一发现对主胰管 IPMN 具有特异性。胰管造影时的其他表现包括主胰管扩张、黏稠黏液或肿瘤结节引起的充盈缺损（图 60.15）和囊性区域与主胰管之间相通。

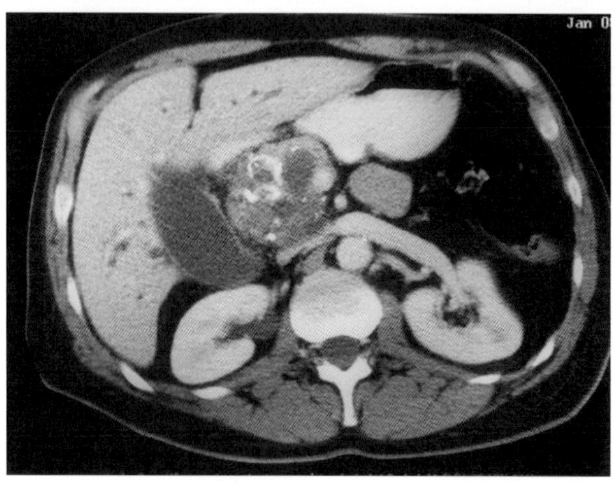

图 60.14　CT 显示累及胰头的导管内乳头状黏液性肿瘤（IPMN）

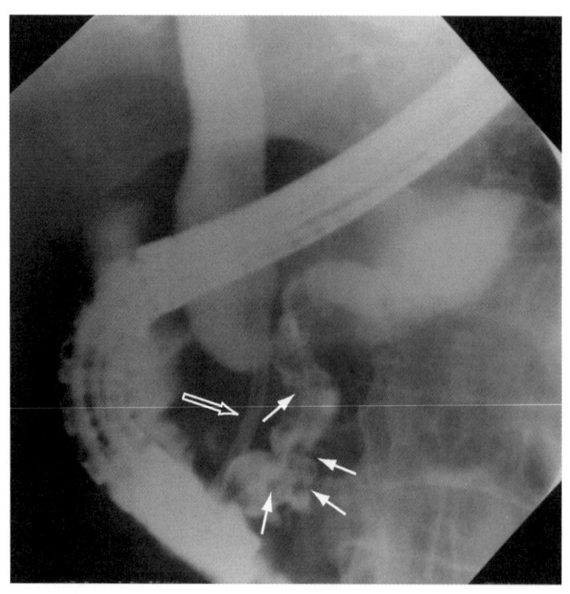

图 60.15　内镜逆行胰胆管造影（ERCP）显示导管内乳头状黏液性肿瘤。近端胰管可见多个充盈缺损（实线箭）。还可见使用支架治疗的胆道梗阻（空心箭）

IPMN 的充分治疗需要胰腺切除，可成功缓解症状并防止肿瘤进展为浸润性癌。胰十二指肠切除术是大多数患者的首选治疗方法，因为胰头的 IPMN 占优势，但胰体尾切除术适用于胰体或尾部的病变。术中冰冻切片是排除切缘恶性肿瘤的必要手段，但切缘低度异型增生不应导致全胰切除术。

残余胰管异型增生不能预测浸润性疾病的发生或生存率的降低[207]。证实了 IPMN 作为遗传缺陷的概念，边缘的不典型增生与残余腺体的复发有关，但这不是在切除边缘[208]。当 IPMN 累及整个胰管系统时，全胰腺切除术是唯一的治愈性手术选择。

IPMN 切除后的预后很好，根据初次切除时是否存在浸润进行预测，5 年疾病特异性生存率至少为 75%。与浸润性组织学患者预后较差相关的因素包括：淋巴结转移、淋巴血管浸润、神经周围浸润和切缘阳性[209]。胰腺残端的疾病复发常见于切除无浸润性 IPMN 后。一项研究发现 21% 的患者在中位随访 46 个月时复发[208]。良性 IPMN 切除后，新发 IPMN 和浸润性癌的患病率均随时间增加。在平均随访 73 个月期间，153 例边缘阴性患者中有 20% 复发，31 例中有 3 例患有浸润性癌症[207]。另一个机构发现浸润性肿瘤在 1 年、5 年和 10 年时的估计复发机会分别为 0%、7% 和 38%[210]。这些数据强调了无限期密切监测和术后成像，对即使没有侵袭性肿瘤的患者的重要性。胰腺局部疾病复发的患者可从完成胰腺切除术中获益[205,210]。

（四）实性假乳头状瘤

胰腺的实性假乳头状瘤（SPT）是 1934 年首次报道的一种罕见肿瘤，占胰腺囊性肿瘤的 10% 以下[176]。女性比男性更易受累（比例为 10∶1）。一般来说，这是一种 30 多岁年轻女性的疾病，50 岁以上的成人报告的病例非常少（5%）[211]。在文献中可以找到几个儿科系列，这些患者（年龄范围 1～18 岁）至少占所有已知病例的 20%[212]。

最常见的临床表现是腹痛，见于 67%～81% 的患者[213,214]。第二常见的是腹部巨大肿块，这是 35% 患者的主诉。至少 15% 的肿瘤是偶然发现的，通常在常规体检或创伤后评估期间发现的[211]。至于胰腺其他囊性病变，用 CT 或 MRI 评估（图 60.16）和对 EUS-FNA 的考虑为指导临床治疗提供了足够的信息[215,216]。

大多数（60%）假乳头状肿瘤见于胰腺体部和尾部。肿瘤在发病前可能相当大，34% 的患者肿块直径大于 10cm。大体上，小的肿瘤相对实性，而较大的变体表现为明显的囊性变。显微镜下观察到实性、假乳头状和出血性假囊性区域的混合物。可见均匀的肿瘤细胞被血管玻璃样的基质分隔[217]。

尽管大多数实性假乳头状瘤表现为良性行为，但这些肿瘤被认为是恶性潜能不确定的病变。对已发表系列的大型荟萃分析发现实性假乳头状癌的发生率为 20%[211]。目前诊断恶性肿瘤的标准包括：神经周围浸润、血管浸润、邻近组织浸润或转移[211]。最常见的转移部位是肝脏，就诊时 5%～10% 的患者可见转移性疾病。

尽管以女性为主，但在 SPT 中未发现与雌激素受体的相关性。胰腺癌发生中的其他常见突变基因，如 *K-ras* 和 *TP53*，在这些肿瘤中也不存在。相反，实性假乳头状瘤表现出 E-钙黏蛋白（E-cadherin）的异常表达（见第 1 章）。虽然正常细胞表现为细胞膜内 E-钙黏蛋白表达，但 100% 的 SPT 表现为细

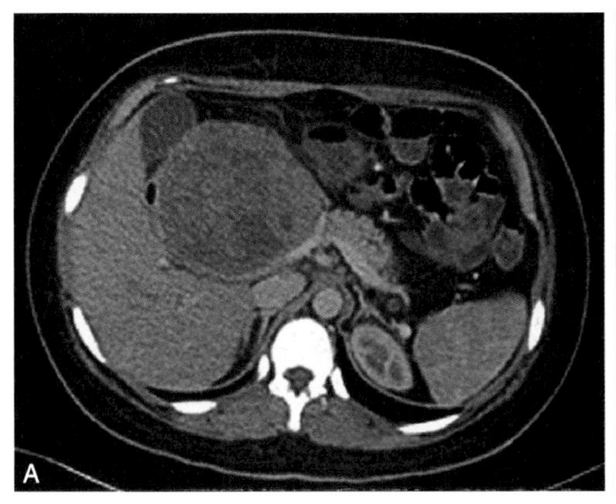

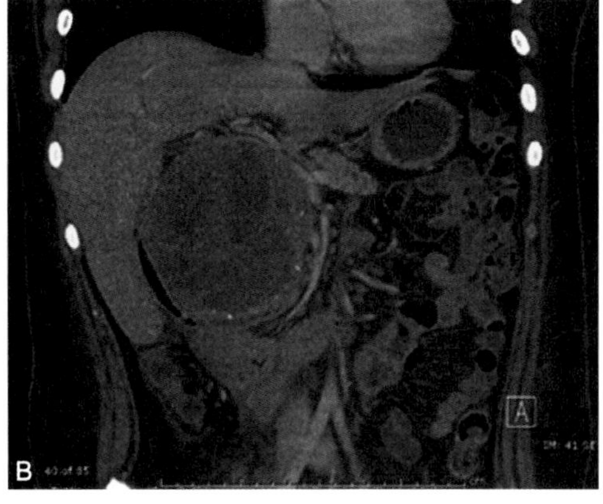

图 60.16　横断面图像(A)和冠状 CT 图像(B)显示一名 16 岁女性胰腺广泛实性假乳头状瘤。在使用股总静脉移植物替代门静脉长段和受累肠系膜上静脉后,进行 R0 切除

胞内 E-cadherin 表达完全缺失或 E-cadherin 异常定位于细胞核[218]。这些发现与 E-cadherin 基因的突变无关,而是与 β-连环蛋白(β-catenin)、p120 等伴侣分子的异常表达有关[219]。分子研究发现 90% 的病例 β-catenin 基因外显子 3 发生点突变[220]。这一发现具有诊断价值,细胞间黏附的丧失可能有助于解释在这种肿瘤中观察到的囊性变。

总体而言,SPT 是一种生长非常缓慢的肿瘤,总体生存率高于 90%。完全切除是首选的治疗方法,在可能的情况下也建议切除同时性或间期转移灶[214,221]。在一项多机构回顾性研究中,所有患者在 R0 切除后的 5 年生存率均为 100% 的[213]。也有延长生存期的报道,即使存在转移性疾病[211,221]。关于实性假乳头状瘤的辅助治疗没有重要的数据可用。

2018 年,美国胃肠病学会(ACG)发布了关于本节讨论的各种胰腺囊性病变诊断和治疗的最新指南[222]。

三、其他胰腺肿瘤

胰腺的其他非内分泌肿瘤包括腺泡细胞癌、淋巴瘤和肉瘤。腺泡细胞癌极为罕见,约占胰腺肿瘤的 1%~2%。临床表现可能与胰腺导管腺癌难以区分。腺泡细胞癌的 CT 表现与导管腺癌有一定的区别,包括无胆道或胰管扩张的大肿瘤,外生形态和增强的包膜[223]。少数患者(10%~15%)可表现为脂肪酶高分泌综合征,临床观察到高血清脂肪酶水平和周围脂肪坏死[224]。脂肪酶高分泌综合征常出现在肝转移中,被认为是一个不利的预后因素。

总的来说,腺泡细胞癌被认为是侵袭性恶性肿瘤,50% 的病例有肝转移;然而,预后似乎比导管腺癌好。在最近的一项基于监测、流行病学和最终结局(Surveillance, Epidemiology, and End Results, SEER)数据库的腺泡细胞癌研究中,不可切除疾病患者的 5 年生存率为 22%,可切除疾病患者的 5 年生存率为 72%[225]。在有限转移的患者中,包括同步和异时肝切除术在内的积极治疗方法与局限性切除患者的生存率相同[226]。

原发性胰腺淋巴瘤占胰腺恶性肿瘤不足 0.7%,占所有结外非霍奇金淋巴瘤的不足 1%(见第 32 章)[227]。非霍奇金淋巴瘤继发累及胰腺更为常见。原发性胰腺淋巴瘤患者无周围或纵隔淋巴结病变,无肝或脾受累,白细胞计数正常[228]。流式细胞术的 FNA 活检在诊断中具有较高的准确性[229]。诊断原发性胰腺淋巴瘤是很重要的,因为治疗主要是非手术的(见第 31 章)。治疗通常包括化疗和放疗的结合,文献报道治愈率接近 30%[230]。少数小肿瘤(被认为是癌)患者仅接受手术治疗,生存率很好。肿瘤极少转移到胰腺,最常见的是肾癌。

胰腺内分泌肿瘤的讨论见第 34 章。

(郑炜　译,闫秀娥　李鹏　校)

参考文献

第 61 章　胰腺疾病的内镜治疗

Ryan Law，Todd H. Baron 著

章节目录

一、急性胰腺炎 …… 906
二、急性胰腺炎的局部并发症 …… 906
（一）假性囊肿 …… 907
（二）包裹性坏死 …… 907
（三）复发性急性胰腺炎 …… 909
三、慢性胰腺炎 …… 910
（一）胰管内镜治疗 …… 910
（二）假性囊肿 …… 911
（三）胆道狭窄 …… 911
（四）顽固性疼痛 …… 911
四、胰管漏 …… 911
五、胰腺癌 …… 912
六、胰腺囊肿 …… 912

自 1974 年首次报道内镜逆行胰胆管造影（ERCP）和经内镜胆管括约肌切开术以来，ERCP 技术取得了许多进展。包括超声内镜检查（EUS）、计算机断层扫描（CT）和 MRCP 在内的微创诊断方式已取代了诊断性 ERCP。然而，治疗性 ERCP 仍可用于胰腺疾病的治疗，并不断发展。本章综述了急性胰腺炎及其并发症的内镜治疗，以及复发性急性胰腺炎、慢性胰腺炎、胰腺癌、胰腺囊肿的内镜治疗。

一、急性胰腺炎

当患者出现急性胰腺炎时，内镜检查的作用仅限于 2 种情况：第一，胆石性胰腺炎患者（见第 58 和 66 章）；第二，通过肠内喂养提供营养支持（见第 6 章）。胆石性胰腺炎是一过性或持续的胆泥嵌塞或壶腹部共同通道内的结石引起。ERCP 和胆管括约肌切开术通过移除嵌顿结石和随后缓解胰腺导管梗阻来改善胆石性胰腺炎的预后。对急性胆石性胰腺炎患者的早期研究表明，在入院 72 小时内进行 ERCP 和括约肌切开术可改善临床重度急性胰腺炎患者的预后[1]。但是，meta 分析并没有证明早期常规 ERCP 可显著影响死亡率和胰腺炎的局部或全身并发症，且与预测的严重程度无关。然而，目前的建议支持在同时患有胆管炎或胆道梗阻的患者中应考虑早期 ERCP[2]。因此，ERCP 最好用于根据高胆红素血症和临床胆管炎证据怀疑有胆道梗阻的患者，因为在血清胆红素正常的情况下，壶腹部不太可能被梗阻[3-6]。可以评估重度胆源性胰腺炎患者胆管结石的微创成像模式包括 CT、MRCP[7] 和 EUS[8]。这些检查有助于在发现胆管结石时选择 ERCP 患者，并防止不必要的 ERCP 和潜在不良事件的风险[9,10]。如果在 ERCP 治疗急性胆石性胰腺炎期间未发现胆管结石，则尚无数据指导是否应进行经验性胆管括约肌切开术。括约肌切开术可降低胆囊切除术前急性胰腺炎和胆管炎复发的风险[11]。然而，轻度胆源性胰腺炎的早期腹腔镜胆囊切除术（3 天内），无须等待转氨酶恢复正常，可以改善预后，减少后续 ERCP 的需求[12]。事实上，早期胆囊切除术被认为是标准治疗[13]。在未接受胆囊切除术的患者中，ERCP 联合胆道括约肌切开术降低了胆石性胰腺炎复发的风险[14]。

基于随机前瞻性研究，证据支持对重度急性胰腺炎患者进行早期肠内营养。与肠外营养相比，肠内营养的成本更低，感染并发症更少（见第 6 章）。鼻胃管喂养似乎与放置在 Treitz 韧带外的管一样有效[15]，尽管后者更适用于因严重十二指肠水肿导致胃潴留而无法耐受鼻胃管喂养的患者。在急性胰腺炎的情况下，有多种内镜技术可用于放置鼻空肠营养管，包括经鼻内镜的方式[16-21]。

二、急性胰腺炎的局部并发症（也见第 58 章）

有多种局部并发症可以作为急性胰腺炎的并发症出现，并有明确的命名[22]，包括胰周积液、胰腺和胰周坏死（无菌或感染），以及假性囊肿和包裹性坏死（walled-off necrosis，WON；无菌或感染）。分界清楚的症状性和/或感染性积液靠近（对向）胃或十二指肠壁的患者，可接受内镜引流治疗[23]。急性胰周积液在急性胰腺炎病程的早期形成，通常无需治疗即可自行吸收。急性假性囊肿是急性胰腺炎的后遗症，至少需要 4 周才能包裹，且无明显的固体碎屑。急性胰腺假性囊肿通常是胰腺导管漏的结果（图 61.1）。另外，随着时间的推移，胰腺和胰周脂肪坏死区域可能液化而成为假性囊肿[24]。尽

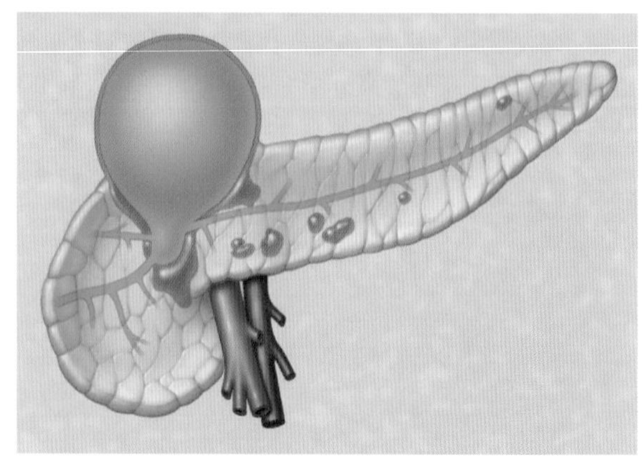

图 61.1　急性胰腺假性囊肿形成机制的示意图。主胰管的局限坏死导致富含酶液体蓄积的渗漏

管假性囊肿包裹至少需要 4 周的时间,但必须认识到,在一些有明显早期急性胰腺坏死(>30% 坏死)的患者中,胰腺和胰周坏死可能演变为影像学上类似假性囊肿的集合[25]。这些采集物中含有大量的固体碎屑,使用典型的假性囊肿引流方法对其进行内镜治疗通常会导致感染性并发症,因为污染和固体碎屑的清除不充分[26-28]。

(一) 假性囊肿

急性假性囊肿引流适用于治疗可能感染或可能无感染的症状性假性囊肿[29]以及影像学检查显示的进行性增大。急性假性囊肿的症状和体征包括腹痛(通常因进食而加重)、体重减轻、胃出口梗阻、梗阻性黄疸和胰漏,这些可能导致胰源性腹水或胰瘘[30]。假性囊肿可通过十二指肠乳头(经乳头)、胃或十二指肠壁(经壁)或通过这些方式的组合引流[31,32]。

1. 经十二指肠乳头引流

如果假性囊肿与主胰管相连,无论是否行胰括约肌切开术,放置胰管支架都是有效的,特别是对于较小的假性囊肿(<5~6cm),因为这些假性囊肿无法通过其他腔道排出[33,34]。支架的近端(指向胰腺尾部)可以直接进入假性囊肿,将漏出区域从漏出处上游连接到胰管,或者完全位于漏出处的下游。跨越胰漏架桥是首选的方法,因为它可以恢复胰管的连续性,而且看起来更有效(图 61.2)[35,36]。经乳头引流避免了经腔道引流可能发生的出血或穿孔。然而,在胰管正常的患者中,胰管支架可能会导致主胰管形成瘢痕[37]。

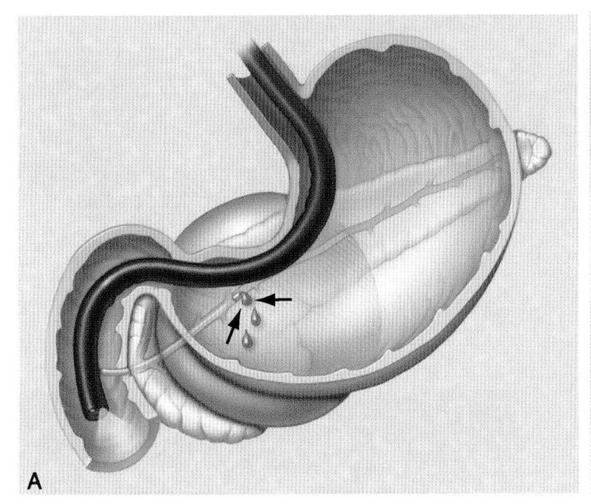

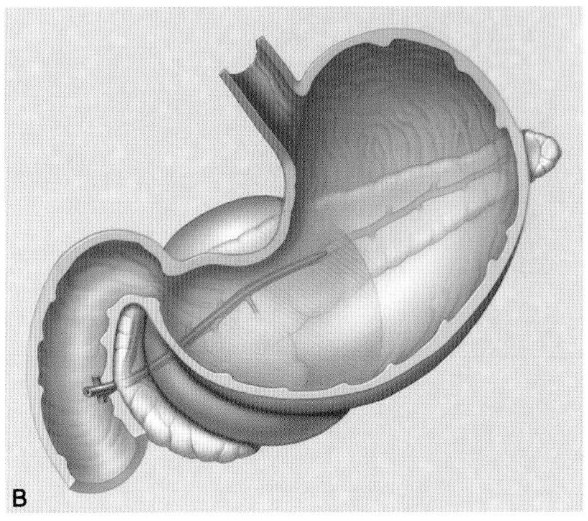

图 61.2 胰腺假性囊肿经乳头引流示意图。A,显示主胰管侧支渗漏的胰腺图片(箭头)。B,在渗漏处放置胰管支架

2. 经腔道引流

假性囊肿经腔道引流目前尚无固定的方法。经腔道引流是通过不使用电灼针或使用电灼装置[如针刀、囊肿切开刀、电烧强化腔道贴壁型金属支架(lumenapposing metal stent, LAMS)]进入积聚处进行[38]。在预防出血和穿孔等不良事件方面,EUS 引导的引流优于非 EUS 引导的引流[39]。虽然 EUS 引导引流相对于非 EUS 引流的优势尚未得到明确证明[40],但有数据支持常规应用 EUS 引导下跨壁引流[40-43],特别是在非 EUS 引导下引流失败的情况下[44]。EUS 引导下的穿刺成功率超过 95%,且不良事件发生率低[45-48]。传统上,一旦成功进入假性囊肿腔,需要应用扩张球囊将穿刺路径扩张至直径 8~10mm,以便放置 1 或 2 个 10Fr 的双猪尾支架(图 61.3)[49]。自膨胀覆膜金属支架已经被用来代替塑料支架,或者作为塑料支架的补充[50-52]。一种新型的 LAMS 最近被开发出来,以减轻传统引流技术的局限性[53]。两个美国食品药物管理局(FDA)获批的 LAMS 支架推送系统可用于胰腺液体积聚的治疗,一方面需要通过传统的引流技术置入支架(步骤 1,穿刺;步骤 2,留置导丝;步骤 3,穿刺路径扩张;步骤 4,支架释放),另一方面是尖端装有电灼刀,允许同时穿刺和扩张,随后放置支架,在某些情况下不需要留置导丝。

经过简单的内镜下引流后,在手术后 4~6 周后行 CT 随访。当影像学证实假性囊肿消失后,内镜移除所有的内支架经。内镜下胰腺假性囊肿引流术的成功率、复发率和不良事件发生率差异较大,这可能是因为许多已发表的报告异质性较大,包括急性和慢性假性囊肿以及“胰腺脓肿”的患者。此外,一些患者接受了经乳头引流术,另一些接受了经腔道引流术,还有一些同时接受了两种干预。尽管如此,累计引流成功率约为 75%~90%,不良事件发生率约为 5%~10%,假性囊肿复发率为 5%~20%[54,55]。

(二) 包裹性坏死

胰腺坏死是失活的胰腺实质,通常伴有胰周脂肪坏死。早期可通过 CT 增强扫描发现无强化的胰腺实质区域。胰腺坏死常伴有主胰管的严重破坏。几周后,坏死区域继续进展和扩大,包含了液体和固体碎片(图 61.4)。这种晚期胰腺坏死最初称为系统性胰腺坏死[30],但现在通常称为包裹性坏死。这些术语用来区分晚期坏死和早期(急性)期胰腺坏死。WON 的 CT 表现可能被误诊为急性假性囊肿[25,28,56,57]。

无菌性 WON 引流的指征和时机是有争议的。在包裹完全形成之后,才能进行内镜下引流。无菌 WON 引流的适应证为急性胰腺炎发作后 4 周或 4 周以上出现顽固性腹痛、胃出口梗阻或营养不良(如持续全身疾病、厌食和体重下

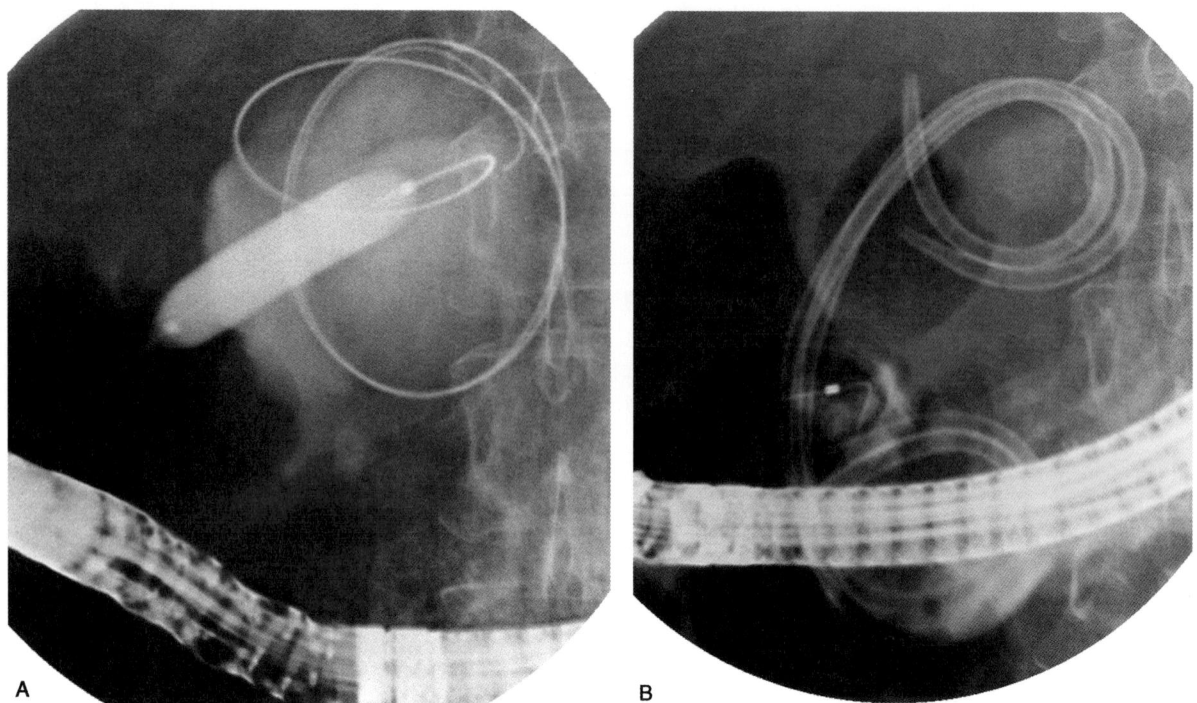

图 61.3　胰腺假性囊肿的内镜下经十二指肠引流。A，进入假性囊肿，导丝盘绕于囊肿内。扩张球囊已经通过十二指肠壁充盈。B，囊肿内已置入两枚双猪尾支架

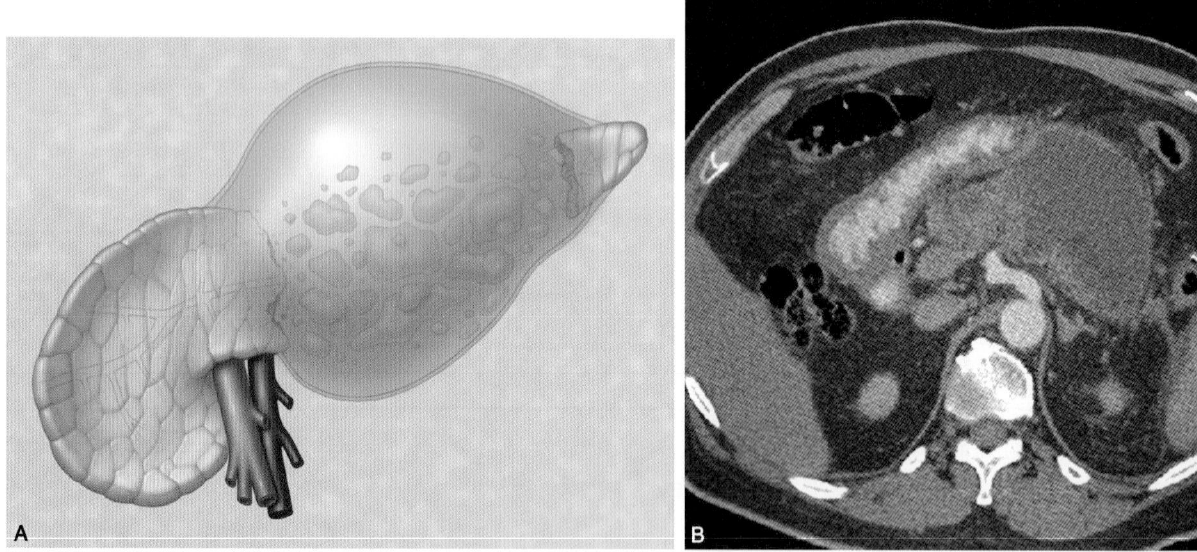

图 61.4　A，包裹性（机化的）胰腺坏死（WON）示意图。B，WON 患者的 CT。采用直接坏死组织切除术成功进行了内镜治疗（见图 61.5）

降）[58]。由于内镜下引流 WON 技术难度较大，不良事件发生率较高，且往往涉及病情较重的患者。因此应当慎重考虑无菌情况下内镜干预 WON[28,59]。内镜下引流的替代治疗方案包括肠外或肠内空肠营养和非内镜下引流方法，如经皮引流和外科引流，包括微创手术[58]。所选择的治疗方案通常基于当地的技术水平和共患疾病的严重程度。理想情况下，这些患者最好采用多学科治疗方法。

由于需要排出固体物质，腔镜下引流 WON 的方法不同于假性囊肿的引流。内镜的方法已经有了显著提高。一般来说，因为不能清除固体碎片，单纯经乳头入路是不够的。最常用的是经腔道引流的方法，因为它可以清除液化物质和固体碎片。早期的经腔道引流技术包括使用经鼻灌洗管和跨壁支架一起放置，以冲洗固体碎片[28,60]。另一种方法是使用经皮内镜胃造瘘管，以提供一种将冲洗管置入坏死腔内的方法，并避免经鼻胆管引流引起的不适[28,61,62]。一般来说，已不再常规使用经鼻囊肿引流管冲洗。

一种清除坏死碎片的方法是直接进行内镜下坏死清创术。通过使用大直径气囊（最高可达 20mm）扩张穿刺通道，或通过预先放置的 LAMS，然后通过前视内镜直接进入坏死腔（图 61.5）[28,63,64]。然后使用圈套、抓取钳和其他配件来清

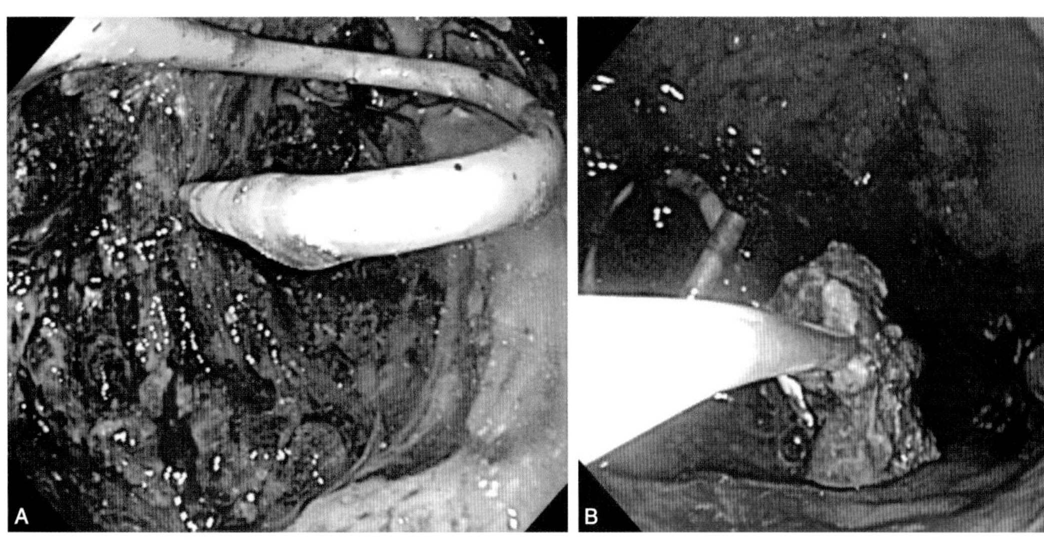

图 61.5 在图 61.4.A 中描述的患者中进行的直接内镜下坏死切除术。A,从坏死腔内部的内镜视图;观察到留置的猪尾支架和周围坏死碎片。B,用圈套器经胃后壁将坏死的实质性物质从腔内抽出

除固体碎片[65]。一项回顾性研究表明,这种方法优于冲洗方法[66]。然而,经常需要重复手术来清除残留的坏死物质,并尝试治疗可能的胰管破坏,以防止胰管断裂。目前治疗 WON 的策略包括放置大直径的 LAMS(以便液体流出,并在必要时方便直接内镜下进行坏死清除)(图 61.6 和 61.7)[67]。直接内镜下坏死清创术并不是常规手术,而用于那些不能改善病情或表现出临床恶化的患者。

胰腺坏死的引流与较高的不良事件发生率和较长的住院时间有关[41],而急性胰腺炎的假性囊肿患者往往严重胰管异常相对较轻,较少复发。

感染性胰腺坏死是引流的指征。在内镜干预前,可能需要经皮细针穿刺(FNA)来确定细菌状况[68]。

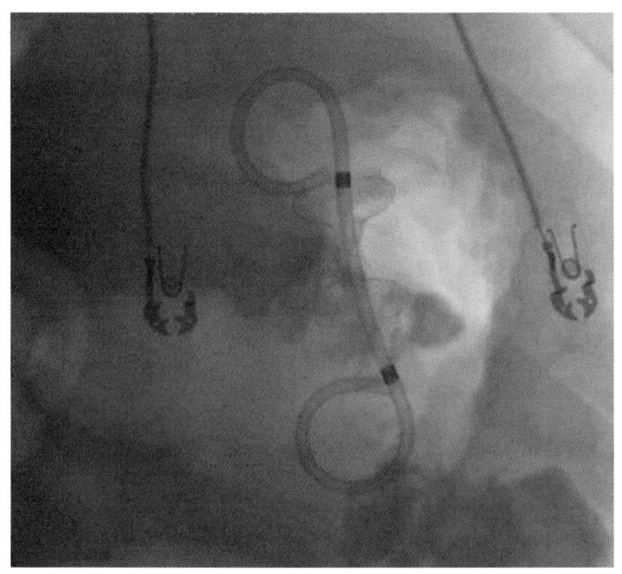

图 61.6 将管腔贴壁金属支架(LAMS)置入胰腺积液处,以促进引流后的 X 线透视图像。在 LAMS 内还可以看到双猪尾塑料支架,以防止支架移位或出血等不良事件

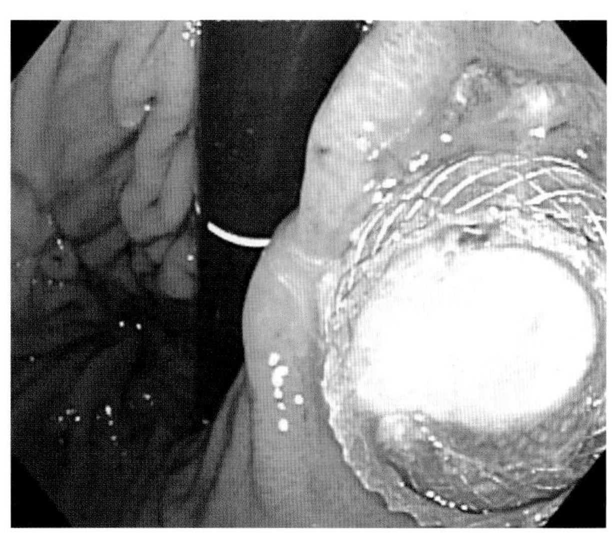

图 61.7 EUS 引导下将与管腔匹配的金属支架置入胰液积聚处,并随后引流脓性物质的内镜图像

(三) 复发性急性胰腺炎

复发性急性胰腺炎的诊断和治疗均具有挑战性。大约 10% 的病例无法确定疾病的病因[69,70]。其他章节讨论的多种因素可能与急性胰腺炎的反复发作有关,包括酒精、微结石、Oddi 括约肌功能障碍(SOD)、胰腺分裂、遗传性胰腺炎、囊性纤维化和其他基因突变、胆总管囊肿、环状胰腺、胆胰管汇流异常、壶腹病变、胰腺肿瘤和自身免疫性胰腺炎。

EUS 被认为是评估急性胰腺炎复发可能原因的重要工具[71]。EUS 可检测到胆胰管系统胆结石、胆泥和微结石[72],从而指导胆囊切除术或治疗性 ERCP 的实施。此外,自身免疫性胰腺炎的诊断可基于影像学表现并经 EUS-FNA 或活检证实[73,74]。在经过彻底的临床、实验室评估和 EUS 检查后排除其他不明原因的急性复发性胰腺炎的患者中,ERCP 结合胰管压力测定测量胰腺括约肌压力,从而诊断胰腺 SOD[75,76]。随后的胆管和胰腺括约肌切开术(当发现括约肌

压力升高时)可防止胰腺炎的复发。值得注意的是,胰腺 SOD 在复发性胰腺炎中的作用是有很大争议的。

胰腺分裂见于高达 10% 的人群中(见第 55 章),它是由背侧胰管和腹侧胰管融合失败造成的[77]。胰腺分裂是胰腺炎的原因之一,这一说法尚存争议[78],但在一部分患者中可能是由于小乳头对胰液的引流不畅造成功能性梗阻。胰腺分裂可以通过 CT、MRI 或 EUS 诊断[79]。促胰液素 MRCP 可预测小乳头功能性梗阻患者[80]。可通过小乳头插管证实胰腺分裂,也可以通过静脉注射促胰液素来完成。内镜下小乳头括约肌切开术对无慢性胰腺炎广泛改变的患者可减少或防止急性胰腺炎的进一步发作[81-83]。

三、慢性胰腺炎(见第 59 章)

对有症状的慢性胰腺炎患者可进行多种内镜干预(框 61.1)[84]。

框 61.1 慢性胰腺炎的内镜治疗
胰腺括约肌切开术
胰管结石取出术
胰管狭窄扩张术
胆管狭窄扩张
胰管漏导致腹水或胸腔积液的治疗
胰腺假性囊肿引流术
放置胆道和胰腺支架

(一) 胰管内镜治疗

胰管狭窄和胰管结石常同时存在,造成主胰管梗阻,并可导致腹痛、慢性胰腺炎基础上合并急性胰腺炎。胰管狭窄的内镜治疗是通过球囊或导管扩张,然后放置 1 个或更多的胰管塑料支架(图 61.8)[64,84,85]。可以更换支架并保持固定一段时间。

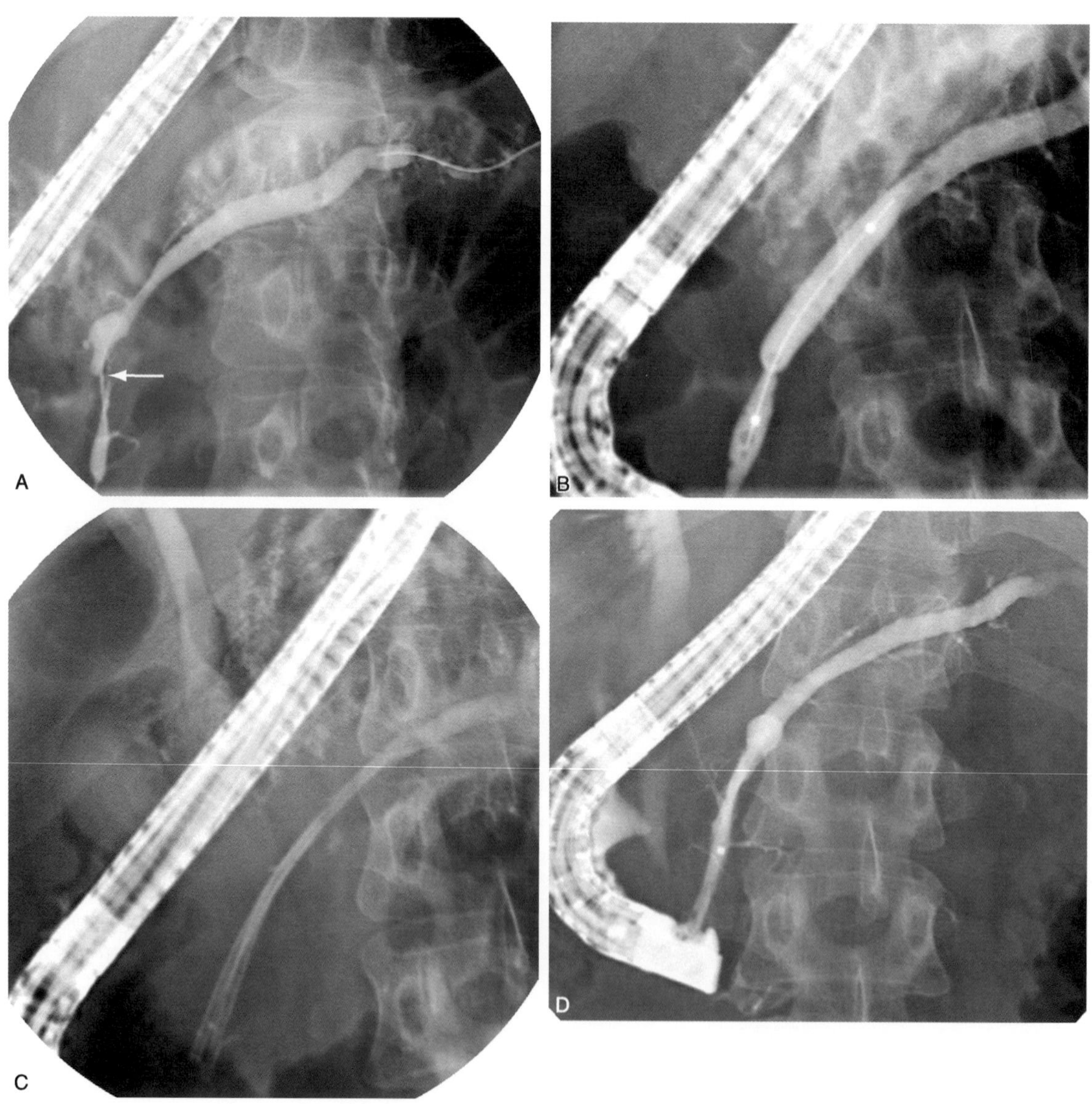

图 61.8 胰管狭窄的内镜治疗。A,初始胰腺造影片显示胰头狭窄(箭头)伴上游胰管扩张。B、狭窄的球囊扩张(注意腰部)。C,置入 2 个并排塑料支架。D,随访胰腺造影显示狭窄改善

在成人中，由于结石已钙化且经常嵌顿于侧支及狭窄的胰管内，因此采用标准的胆道结石取出技术进行胰管括约肌切开术及胰管结石取出很少能成功。如果可行的话，可以在内镜下取出或不取出结石之前行体外冲击波碎石术来粉碎结石[84,86-88]，如果需要取出大的、梗阻性结石，体外振波碎石必不可少。胰管镜引导下的胰管内碎石术（激光或液电碎石）也被用于碎石和取出阻塞的结石[89]。胰腺内镜治疗初次技术成功率很高[90]。在一些病例报道中，三分之二的患者在不需要手术的情况下取得了长期的临床成功，并且每年因疼痛住院率显著降低[86,91]。

对疼痛性梗阻性慢性胰腺炎患者进行了两项前瞻性随机研究，比较内镜治疗和手术治疗[92,93]。内镜治疗需要更多的操作次数，疼痛改善在手术组中更常见。然而，这两项研究都存在局限性，即在一项研究中缺乏体外冲击波碎石，而在另一项研究中缺乏创伤性较小的内镜狭窄治疗[94]。

如果由于胰头内无法通过的结石或狭窄而无法经乳头入路治疗胰管阻塞时，可以在 EUS 引导下行经胃胰管穿刺术[95]。可行会师技术或经胃或经十二指肠胰管支架置入[96,97]。

（二）假性囊肿

慢性胰腺炎假性囊肿的形成机制与急性胰腺炎假性囊肿不同。正如第 59 章所讨论的，慢性胰腺炎假性囊肿是慢性胰腺炎和由纤维性狭窄或结石引起的下游胰管梗阻的后遗症（图 61.9）[98]。这导致胰管爆裂（胰漏）和胰液积聚。这些积聚不含固体碎片，通常也不是急性炎症过程的结果。内镜下治疗慢性胰腺假性囊肿的方法与早期治疗急性假性囊肿的方法相似。主要的区别是如果不治疗潜在的胰管异常则可能导致复发[99,100]。

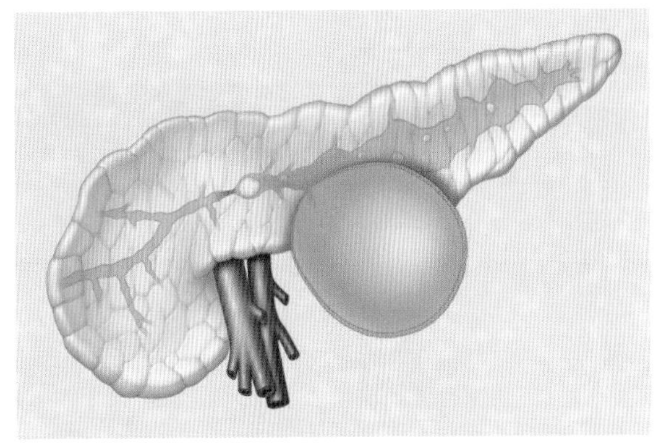

图 61.9　慢性胰腺假性囊肿形成机制示意图。主胰管梗阻导致上游渗漏和假性囊肿形成

（三）胆道狭窄

胰头内的纤维化可以包绕远端胆管，导致胆道狭窄的形成。可能的后遗症包括肝纤维化（继发性胆汁性肝硬化）和胆管炎。通过球囊扩张和内镜下置入多个平行的塑料支架或一个全覆膜自膨胀金属支架（self-expandable metal stent，SEMS）可以消除胆道狭窄[85,101-103]。非钙化性慢性胰腺炎患者对胆道狭窄扩张的反应优于钙化性胰腺炎患者。内镜下置入胆道支架可用于治疗慢性胰腺炎所致的良性胆道狭窄，有以下几种情况：①术前放置以缓解黄疸和胆管炎；②慢性胰腺炎基础上并发急性胰腺炎，之后发生胆道梗阻时的支架临时置入；③难治性狭窄的长期治疗[104]。放置全覆膜 SEMS 并在 3~6 个月移除后，可以解决高达 80% 的由慢性胰腺炎引起的胆道狭窄。必须强调的是，SEMS 未经 FDA 批准治疗良性胆道疾病，而且有可能很难或不能移除。未覆膜的 SEMS 不应用于慢性胰腺炎继发的良性胆道狭窄。

（四）顽固性疼痛

慢性胰腺炎顽固性疼痛的患者可以从 EUS 引导下的腹腔神经丛阻滞中获益。不幸的是，这种效果是短暂的，需要辅助其他治疗；因为治疗效果有限，这种由疼痛专家或 EUS 提供的治疗并没有被广泛使用[105,106]。

四、胰管漏

胰漏和胰管中断可作为急性或慢性胰腺炎的后遗症（见第 58 和 59 章），以及胰腺手术（图 61.10）和创伤后的后遗

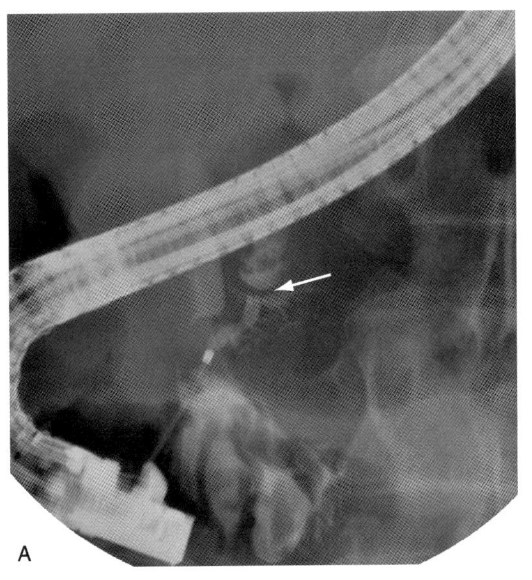

图 61.10　慢性胰腺炎所致胰管漏的内镜治疗。A，胰头狭窄（箭）

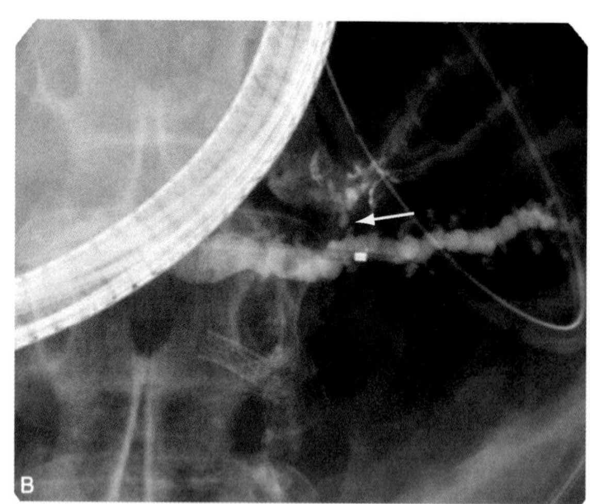
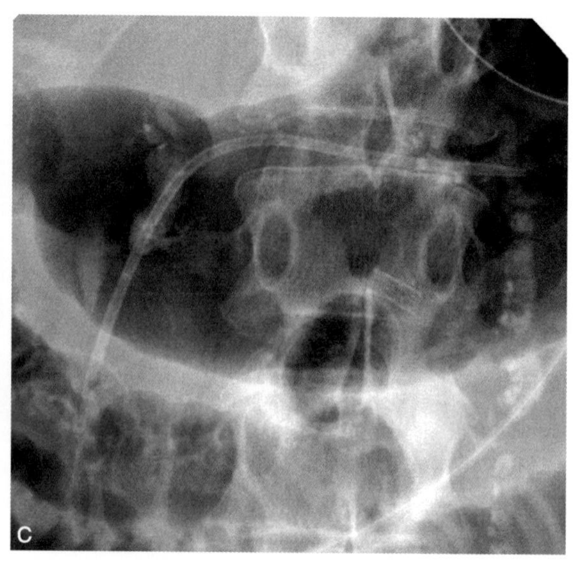

图 61.10(续)　B,狭窄上游侧支泄漏(箭)。C,在泄漏部位放置胰腺支架

症。胰腺的尾部、体部或头部都有可能出现渗漏。液体可向外侧(脾脏方向),向内侧十二指肠或胆管,进入小网膜囊,或进入纵隔或腹部,分别形成胸腔积液和腹水。

外瘘(胰腺皮肤瘘)通常发生在胰腺手术或经皮胰液积聚引流后。通过是否流出高淀粉酶胰液来鉴别外瘘。

大多数胰腺手术后发生的胰漏通过外科留置引流管来控制。随着时间的推移,这些渗漏会逐渐闭合,内镜治疗一般只针对持续性或难治性渗漏[107,108]。在没有手术引流的情况下,可以进行内镜治疗有症状的渗漏。与临床症状加重或症状相关的内漏需要干预[109]。

胰漏的内镜干预与胰腺假性囊肿和坏死相似。在大量胰液积聚的情况下,可进行跨壁引流,伴或不伴经乳头治疗。这将在内部控制胰漏。在没有胰液积聚的情况下,治疗方法是经胰管置入支架以促进胰管内引流[30,110,111]。

经乳头治疗的目的是跨越胰漏部位进行支架桥接[35],但当胰漏发生于胰尾切除术后或漏出的部位位于胰尾时,经乳头治疗不可行。在这种情况下,支架的前端位于胰漏位置的下游。

在有外引流的患者中,改行内镜治疗以去除引流管,其成功与否取决于与内引流支架的大小相比,外引流管的大小。内镜成功置入支架后,缩小、夹紧或移除外部引流管可促进内引流和瘘管闭合。各种各样的胶合剂已经被用于封闭胰瘘和胰漏[112],尽管这些药物没有得到 FDA 的批准,且有可能阻塞主胰管。

五、胰腺癌(参见第 60 章)

胰腺癌的内镜下治疗主要包括通过 ERCP 经乳头置入胆道支架来减轻恶性胆道梗阻(见第 60、69 和 70 章)。对某些患者,在胰管内放置支架可以减轻胰管阻塞引起的腹痛[113]。此外,部分胰腺癌患者合并胰管梗阻可发展为假性囊肿或胰漏;跨越胰管狭窄置入胰管支架是有用的。15% ~ 20% 的胰腺癌患者因十二指肠肿瘤侵袭而导致胃出口梗阻[114,115]。内镜下放置非覆膜的 SEMS 是一种有效的姑息治疗方法,与旁路手术相比,它能更快地恢复经口肠内营养,但增加了再堵塞的风险,需要再次介入治疗[116,117]。EUS 引导的胃肠吻合术是一种新的非手术治疗胃出口梗阻的方法,它应用 LAMS 将胃与十二指肠或空肠吻合[118]。恶性胆道和十二指肠梗阻的联合姑息治疗也是可行的[97,119,120,121]。可以通过使用无水乙醇在 EUS 引导下阻断腹腔神经丛,使神经节永久消融来治疗胰腺癌腹痛。这种治疗看起来是有效和可持续的[104,105]。EUS 引导下置入放疗标记物可用于胰腺癌放射治疗。金标记被放置在肿瘤边缘的几个位置,以帮助在图像引导的放射治疗中定位[122]。

六、胰腺囊肿

如第 60 章所述,胰腺囊肿和囊性肿瘤种类繁多。CT、MRI 和 EUS 可以区分和指导观察或手术治疗[123,124]。越来越多的数据表明,EUS 对特定类型的囊肿注射治疗在未来可能是一种有用的非手术方法[125]。

(郑炜 译,闫秀娥　李鹂 校)

参考文献

第八部分 胆道

第 62 章 胆道解剖学、组织学、胚胎学、发育异常和小儿疾病

Jonathan R. Strosberg, Taymeyah Al-Toubah 著

章节目录

一、肝脏和胆道的胚胎学 …… 913
二、解剖和组织学 …… 915
（一）胆管 …… 915
（二）胆囊 …… 916
三、发育异常 …… 917
（一）肝外胆管 …… 917
（二）胆囊 …… 917
四、婴幼儿胆道疾病的处理方法 …… 917
（一）一般特征 …… 917
（二）诊断 …… 918
五、小儿胆管疾病 …… 919
（一）胆道闭锁 …… 919
（二）自发性胆管穿孔 …… 922
（三）胆汁栓塞综合征 …… 923
（四）先天性胆总管畸形 …… 923
（五）肝纤维囊性疾病 …… 924
（六）非综合征性小叶间胆管缺乏 …… 925
（七）综合征性小叶间胆管缺乏 …… 925
（八）原发性硬化性胆管炎 …… 927
（九）慢性胆汁淤积 …… 928
六、小儿胆囊疾病 …… 928
（一）胆石症 …… 928
（二）结石性胆囊炎 …… 930
（三）非结石性胆囊炎 …… 930
（四）急性胆囊积液 …… 931
（五）胆囊运动障碍 …… 931

本章回顾了胆管及胆囊的胚胎学和解剖学特征，重点是有助于诊断和治疗胆道疾病以及了解这些结构的异常和先天畸形的信息。婴幼儿和儿童的胆道疾病被认为是因为许多在生命早期发生的疾病是由于形态发生异常或对发育过程产生不利影响所致。

一、肝脏和胆道的胚胎学

肝脏由 2 个原基发育而来（图 62.1）：肝憩室和原始横隔（参见第 71 章）[1,2]。心脏中胚层的近端表达成纤维生长因子（fibroblast growth factor，FGF）1、2 和 8 及骨形成蛋白，诱导前肠内胚层发育为肝。前肠卵黄囊颅腹交界的内胚层细胞增殖形成肝憩室，并沿着腹侧生长入原始横隔。周围的中胚层和外胚层通过来自中胚层组织的信号，如骨形成蛋白、Wnt 和 FGF 蛋白家族的配体，参与了内胚层向肝母细胞的特异性分化。当完成细胞分化并迁移至原始横隔后，肝母细胞在妊娠第 26~32 天完成增殖并形成肝芽[1,3]。前内胚层和肝憩室生成同源结构域转录因子——造血干细胞表达同源盒（Hhex）、Prospero 同源盒蛋白 1（Prox1），后两者是肝母细胞迁移至原始横隔，为肝脏生长和形态发生的关键因子[4,5]。另外一个同源结构域蛋白，Hlx 是肝母细胞增殖的关键因子。当胚胎发育至 5mm 时，可以清楚地分辨出憩室的实心头端（肝）和空心尾端两部分。大部分肝分化为肝细胞索和肝内胆管。肝细胞核因子（HNF）4 驱动肝细胞进一步分化和上皮细胞向典型肝窦结构转化[6]。

双分化潜能的肝母细胞表达甲胎蛋白和肝细胞的各种标志物，如白蛋白、角蛋白以及胆管细胞的标志物（细胞角蛋白 19，CK19）。转录因子性别决定区 Y 框蛋白 9（SOX19），是肝憩室表面上皮细胞中最早表达的胆管特异性标志物。肝母细胞进入原始横隔后其表达立即消失，但是整个胆系发育过程中，SOX19 表达会再次出现[1]。这些早期分子改变一般出现在妊娠第 18 天，相当于胚胎 2.5mm 时。同源异型盒基因 *Hbex* 在肝母细胞分化和胆管形态发生中起着决定性的作用[5]。转化生长因子（TGF）-β、Wnt、FGF、Hippo、GATA、FOXA、ONECUT2 和 HNF3/叉头转录因子家族和 HNF6 等也是消化道内胚层形成和分化中所必需的[3,4]。原始横隔由间充质细胞和来源于卵黄静脉的毛细血管丛组成。妊娠第 3~4 周即胚胎 3~4mm 时，逐渐增长的肝憩室以上皮形式插入原始横隔。

肝内胆管由门脉分支附近的原始肝细胞发育而来[2,4]。肝门部首先发育，之后通过一系列不对称性的重塑过程向外

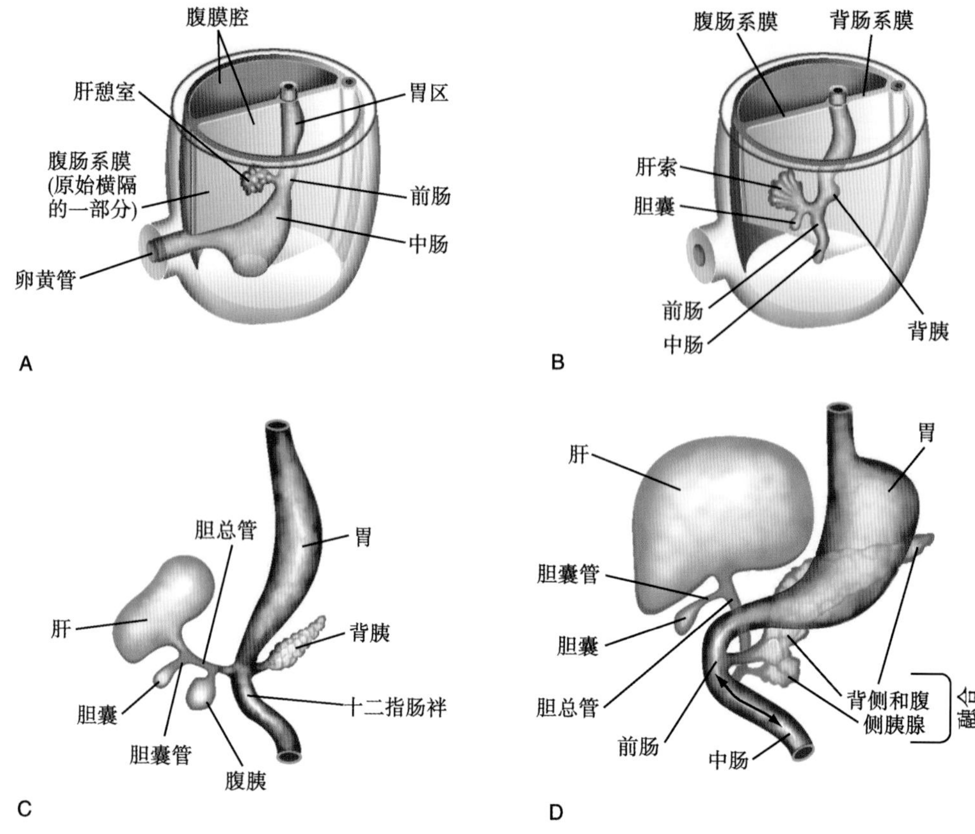

图 62.1　肝脏、胆囊、肝外导管、胰腺和十二指肠的胚胎发育阶段。A,4 周。B 和 C,5 周。D,6 周。(From Moore KL. The developing human. Philadelphia:WB Saunders;1973.)

周延展[5,6]。胆管细胞与基底膜关系密切,提示胆管细胞形态发生信号主要来源于细胞外基质,包括层粘连蛋白和Ⅳ型胶原[7,8]。门脉分支远端的肝细胞最早呈环状向胆管细胞转化。第二层原始肝细胞通过类似的转化在门脉周围形成环形裂缝,两侧覆以胆管上皮细胞[9]。上述转化形成双层外壁圆柱形结构,具有狭缝状的管腔和胆管腔,在妊娠第 9 周时可被检测到。因此小叶间和小叶内胆管网状结构发育自有限的板状空间。门脉周围间充质分泌 TGF-β,并形成 TGF-β 活性从门脉至实质由高到低的梯度差异[10]。间充质同时产生 Jagged1,通过细胞连接激活 Notch2 信号通路参与胆管细胞分化。TGF-β 和 Notch 联合其他信号分子,共同刺激胆管板的双层胆管细胞序贯性不对称分化[10]。Wnt 家族的分泌因子也参与肝母细胞向胆管细胞的分化调节。胆管发育循双轴进行:沿径向轴形成胆管,并沿肝门向肝小叶外周呈轴向延伸长度。

在胚胎 10mm 阶段,这些与成人毛细胆管形态相似的双壁分支管状结构穿过肝索。这些结构不同于成人,因为它们由 6 个或更多肝细胞而不是 2 个肝细胞所包围。抗角蛋白抗体免疫组化检测证实,胆管上皮细胞(胆管细胞)是由原始肝细胞分化而来。妊娠第 20~25 周,肝细胞 CK8 和 CK18 活性增加并表达 CK19,启动向胆管细胞表型的转化[10]。胆管细胞-间充质细胞连接在胆管形成中具有重要作用。在胆管板向胆管转变的过程中,门脉肌成纤维细胞显著延展并包绕新生成的胆管。门脉周围结缔组织、类固醇激素和基底层在胆管分化中也可能具有重要作用。胆管板结构需要通过一个重吸收过程(可能是通过凋亡)进行广泛的重塑,以形成胆管围绕门静脉的特征性吻合体系。原始肝内胆管细胞中持续表达启动凋亡的蛋白,特别是 Fas 反基因和 c-Myc[11],同时表达受损和凋亡细胞的标志物 Lewis 抗原。抑制凋亡的 Bcl-2 蛋白在早期肝内胆管细胞中未见表达,但是后期可检测到。发育期胆管板 3D 结构重建显示,胆管板重构大约发生在妊娠第 11 周,由肝门启动,并向肝周延展[10]。大部分重构在短期内完成,但是到妊娠 40 周仍有一些小的门静脉分支周围没有独立胆管伴行,而是被(不连续的)胆管板包绕。胆管板畸形是儿童胆管疾病的共同特征,可发生于胆管形态发生的各个阶段,包括胆管板重构缺陷,肝母细胞向胆管板细胞分化异常,和原始胆管结构成熟异常[10,12]。

肝总管、胆总管、胆囊管和胆囊发育自邻近肝和腹侧胰腺的腹侧前肠,与腹侧胰腺源自同一区域,但是与肝并不相同。肝外胆管系统发育早于肝内胆管,起源于表达转录因子胰腺-十二指肠同源异型盒 1(Pdx1)的祖细胞[13]。转录因子 Sox17 决定了 Pdx1 向胰腺还是肝外胆管系统转录。Notch 家族的转录因子发状分裂相关增强子 1(Hes1),也参与了肝外胆管系统和腹侧胰腺的适当转录调节[1]。

原始肝外胆管维持了与胆管板(肝内胆管起源)的延续性[7]。与传统的胆管发育概念不同,妊娠过程中并没有胆管腔内胚层闭塞这一"固化期"。胚胎发育至 16mm 时,胆囊管和胆囊近端为空心结构,但是胆囊底仍被残留的上皮栓部分堵塞,直至妊娠 3 个月时胆囊才通畅。后续直至出生的发育主要是持续性的生长。胆囊的特征性折叠发生于妊娠快结束时，并在新生儿期继续适度发育。胆汁分泌始于妊娠第 4 个月，之后胆管系统持续储存胆汁，并分泌至肠腔，使肠内容物(胎粪)变为墨绿色。

二、解剖和组织学

(一) 胆管

成人肝脏小胆管和大胆管总长度在 2 千米以上。定量计算机辅助三维成像测算显示，人体肝脏肉眼可见的胆管系统平均容积为 20.4cm^3[14,15]。研究显示，胆管细胞顶端表面微绒毛和纤毛的存在，可将平均内表面积($398cm^2$)放大约 5.5 倍，并在胆管细胞功能调节中起重要作用。微绒毛和纤毛运动活跃，可在促胰液素等激素的刺激下，显著改变胆汁流动和其成分[16,17]。肝内小胆管的一个普遍特征是其与门脉血管和淋巴管结构关系紧密，使不同腔隙间的选择性物质交换成为可能。小胆管和大胆管细胞超微结构相似，但是功能存在明显差异[17]。例如，肝内大胆管参与促胰液素调节的胆汁分泌，小胆管并不参与[18]。此外，促胰液素受体和 CO_2 交换 mRNA 仅在肝内大胆管表达[17]。

胆汁分泌始于胆管树最小分支的微胆管[19]，相邻肝细胞顶端表面形成微胆管的特殊的基底膜，微胆管、肝细胞之间利用相互连接形成一个多边形通道网络[19]。胆汁流入由基底膜、肝细胞和胆管细胞共同排列组成的终末小胆管(Hering 管)[15]，并沿 Hering 管流入小叶周围和小叶间胆管[20,21]。这些终末小胆管的内径在 15~20μm 以下，管腔内覆以立方上皮细胞。终末端的一个或多个梭形胆管细胞可与肝细胞共用一个管腔，当逐渐靠近门脉时，转变为 2~4 个立方上皮细胞排列成行[19]。胆汁由小叶中央细胞沿肝门三管系统(从肝腺泡的 3 区至 1 区)流动(见第 71 章)。当发生慢性肝外胆管梗阻时，终末胆管细胞增殖[21]。

小叶间胆管紧密包绕在门脉分支周围形成丰富的吻合网络结构[22-24]，其直径在 30~40μm，由腔内侧富含微绒毛的单层立方或柱状上皮构成(图 62.2)[19]。这些细胞高尔基体突出并富含小泡，这些小泡可能通过胞吐和内吞参与细胞质、胆汁和血浆之间的物质交换[19]。当靠近肝门时，小叶间胆管直径变大，并在壁内出现平滑肌纤维。平滑肌纤维的存在，为胆管造影中显示的该水平胆管狭窄提供了形态学基础[24]。随着管腔逐渐增宽，上皮逐渐增厚，周围结缔组织层逐渐增厚并富含弹性纤维。这些胆管进一步汇合形成肝门部肝内大胆管，直径达到 1~1.5mm，并进一步汇合形成主肝管。

0.5~2.5cm 长的左肝管和右肝管在肝门部汇合形成肝总管(图 62.3)[25,26]。95% 以上左肝管和右肝管在肝外汇合，肝内汇合或者胆囊管汇入右肝管前均未汇合者少见[26]。主肝管离开肝门后走行于肝十二指肠韧带的 2 层浆膜内，并通过这种纤维组织鞘与邻近血管相连。成人肝总管长约 3cm，通常在右侧与胆囊管汇合，形成胆总管(或简称胆管)[26]。胆囊管与肝总管汇合处的长度和角度变化较大。70% 的患者胆囊管直接汇入胆总管，也有胆囊管走行于胆管的前面或后面，并在其内侧与胆管汇合之前绕其旋转[25]。胆囊管也可平行于肝总管走行 5~6cm，并在十二指肠第一部分自后方汇入。

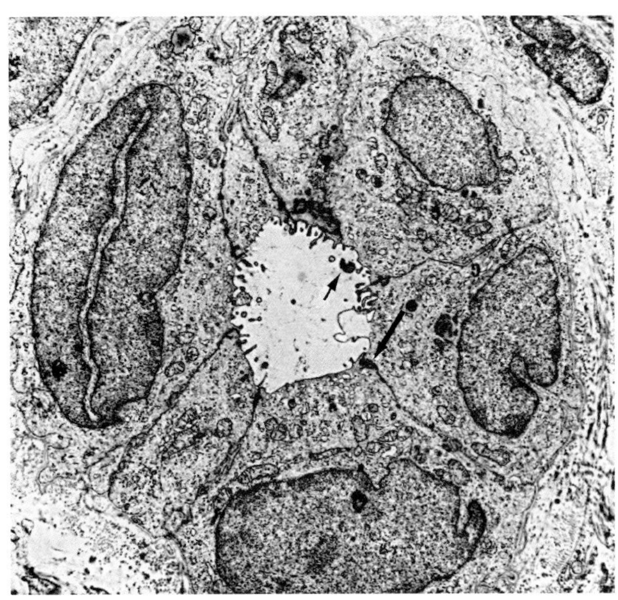

图 62.2　小叶间胆管的超微结构。导管内衬一层立方上皮细胞，通过紧密连接(长箭头)连接，并在其管腔表面显示微绒毛结构(短箭头)。(From Jones AL, Springer-Mills E. The liver and gallbladder. In: Weiss L, editor. Modern concepts of gastrointestinal histology. New York: Elsevier; 1984. p 740.)

在人体中，肝门处的肝内大胆管(直径 1~1.5mm)具有许多不规则的侧支和囊袋(直径 150~270μm)，定向在一个平面上，在解剖学上与横裂相对应[19]，还发现侧枝胆管上较小的囊袋。许多侧枝胆管的末端以盲囊结束，但其他侧枝胆管特别是肝门部胆管之间存在相互交通。在胆管分叉处，几个主要胆管的侧枝相连形成胆管丛。这些结构的功能意义尚不清楚。盲袋可能具有储存或调节胆汁成分的功能，而胆管丛为大胆管之间物质交换提供了解剖基础。

肝门的解剖结构对外科医生尤其重要(另见第 71 章)。肝门的纤维结缔组织板包括包绕门静脉脐部的脐板、胆囊床的囊板和覆盖静脉韧带的 Arantian 板[26]。肝门板矢状切面的组织学检查显示丰富的结缔组织，包括神经纤维、淋巴管、小毛细血管和小胆管。界板系统中的胆管与肝外胆管相对应，其长度在每个节段中各不相同[26]。

与结肠类似，胆囊、胆总管壁也由黏膜层、黏膜下层和肌层构成[24]。胆管壁黏膜层由单层柱状上皮构成，黏膜下层规律分布可分泌黏液的管状腺，开口于黏膜表面。胆总管长 6.0~8.0cm，走行于小网膜中，位于门静脉前方和肝固有动脉右侧[26]。胆管直径平均在 0.5~1.5cm[21]，肝外胆管壁由单层结缔组织和少量平滑肌纤维混合而成。仅胆囊颈、胆管末段具有明显的平滑肌结构。胆总管在后腹膜内经十二指肠上部后方，走行于十二指肠沟和胰头后方，并斜行进入十二指肠降部后内侧肠壁，与主胰管汇合形成 Vater 壶腹(见图 62.3)[25]。壶腹部黏膜明显隆起形成十二指肠乳头。10%~15% 患者胆管和胰管分别开口于十二指肠。胆管在与胰管结合前逐渐变细至 0.6cm 或更细[26]。

当胆管和胰管穿入十二指肠壁时，环形和纵行肌均增厚构成 Oddi 括约肌(见图 62.3 和第 63 章)[27]。其结构变异很大，但通常由以下几个部分组成：①胆管括约肌，环绕于胆总

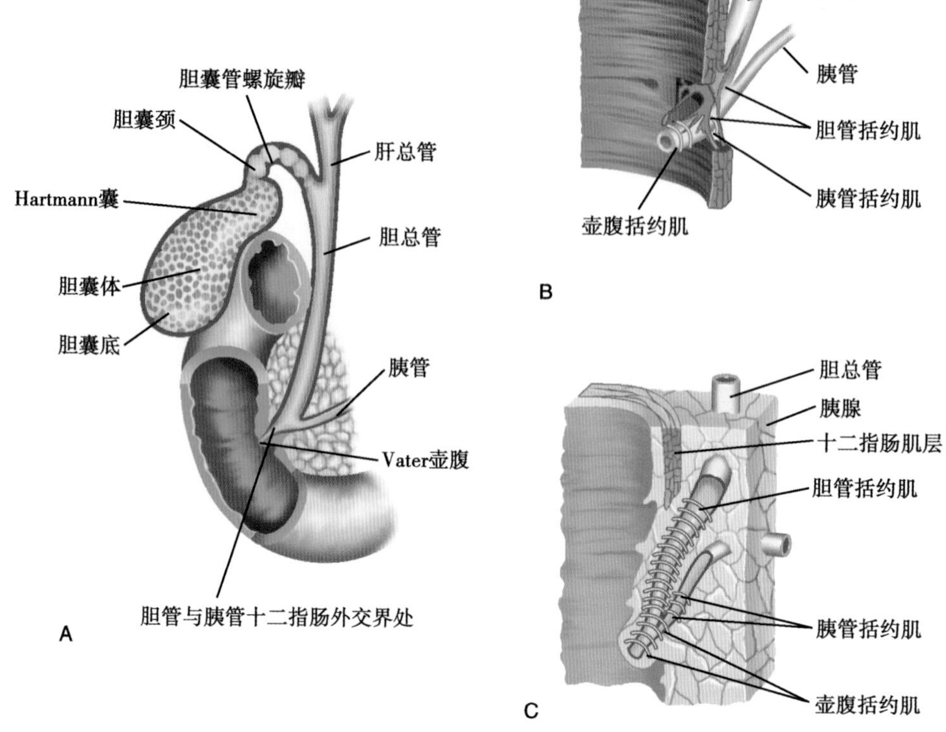

图 62.3　胆囊、肝外胆道和胆总管十二指肠交界处(A)的示意图,以及胆管和胰管交界处(B)和 Oddi 括约肌(C)的放大视图。(From Lindner HH. Clinical anatomy. East Norwalk, CT: Appleton & Lange; 1989, copyright McGraw-Hill.)

管与胰管汇合部上方胆总管的肌纤维;②胰管括约肌,约 1/3 人群存在胰管括约肌,包绕于十二指肠段内汇入壶腹之前的胰管周围;③纵束,跨越胆管和胰管间隙的纵行肌束;④壶腹括约肌,围绕在 Vater 壶腹周边疏松环形纤维外的纵行肌纤维[24]。胆总管括约肌收缩使胆管腔变小,阻止胆汁流出。纵束收缩使胆管变短,促进胆汁流入十二指肠。壶腹括约肌收缩使壶腹缩窄,可防止肠内容物反流至胆管和胰管。然而,由于胆管和胰管共同开口于壶腹部,括约肌收缩可能导致胆汁反流入胰管[27]。

肝内和肝外胆管高度依赖动脉供氧,大量肝固有动脉和胃十二指肠动脉的分支血管网供应胆管[22,24,28]。胆管十二指肠上段由其下方的十二指肠后动脉和上方的肝右动脉供应。这些血管的损伤可造成胆管缺血和狭窄[25]。

肝内和肝外胆管由相互交通的静脉丛引流[21,22],胆管内网状静脉丛位于胆管内壁,胆管旁静脉丛位于胆管外并与其平行。

大量毛细血管丛穿越门脉分支并包绕在胆管周边[22,28]。血液流经胆管周围血管丛,通过门静脉的小叶间分支流入肝窦。通过血液和胆汁之间蛋白质、无机离子和胆汁酸的双向交换,胆管周围血管丛可调节胆汁分泌。由于血液流动的方向(从大血管流向小血管)与胆汁流动的方向相反,因此,胆管周围血管丛可使胆汁中重吸收成分逆流至肝细胞内。

肝内动脉、静脉、胆管和肝细胞受肾上腺能和胆碱能神经支配。在自主神经系统中存在多种调控肽,如酪氨酸神经肽、降钙素基因相关肽、生长抑素、血管活性肠多肽、脑啡肽、铃蟾肽等。受酪氨酸神经肽调控的肝外胆管,可通过自分泌或旁分泌机制调控胆汁流动。

肝、胆囊和胆总管近端的淋巴管流入肝门淋巴结[24]。胆管下端引流的淋巴管流入胰头周围淋巴结。

(二) 胆囊

胆囊(见图 62.3)位于肝右叶下缘的胆囊窝内[29],主要功能是浓缩和储存胆汁,并控制胆汁流入十二指肠以协助脂肪消化(参见第 64 章)[24,29]。成人胆囊为 3cm 宽,7cm 长的梨形可扩张结构,可储存 30ml~50ml 胆汁[29]。胆囊周围包裹着一层薄薄的由平滑肌细胞组成的肌层,内表面大量褶皱结构增加了其吸收面积。胆囊前面覆盖着一层与肝包膜融合的外膜,后部和顶端覆盖着脏腹膜。胆囊由底部、体部、漏斗部和颈部四部分组成[24],胆囊底前壁位于右腹直肌外侧缘和第九肋软骨交点,胆囊底体后壁分别与横结肠、十二指肠紧邻,因此当胆囊穿孔时结石可轻易穿透上述脏器[29,30]。胆囊体向颈部移行过程中逐渐变细构成胆囊漏斗部,其底面接近颈部的突起称为 Hartmann 囊。胆结石嵌顿于 Hartmann 囊时,阻塞胆囊管而引起胆囊炎[29],当炎症严重时可阻塞邻近的胆总管(Mirizzi 综合征)(参见第 65 章)。

胆囊颈部与胆囊管相连并汇入胆管(见图 62.3)[29]。胆囊管长约 4cm,与胆囊表面柱状上皮、黏膜固有层、肌层和浆膜相连续。胆囊颈部黏膜形成海斯特氏螺旋瓣,调节胆汁流入及流出胆囊。

胆囊由肝右动脉的分支胆囊动脉供血[29,31]。胆囊动脉在胆囊颈部附近分为两个分支:一个是供给浆膜面的浅分支,另一个是供给胆囊内壁的深分支,但是其起源和走行变异较多[29]。由于胆囊动脉是终末动脉,胆囊特别容易因炎症或肝动脉血流减少而引起缺血性损伤和坏死。

胆囊静脉回流胆囊和胆囊管的血流并汇入门静脉,偶有直接进入肝血窦[24,29]。胆囊的淋巴管与格利森氏囊的淋巴管相连,其浆膜下和黏膜下淋巴流入胆囊颈部附近的淋巴结[24]。胆囊的交感神经来源于腹腔神经丛,与肝动脉和门静脉的分支一起伴行。胆囊引起的内脏性疼痛经由交感神经纤维传导,主要投射到右季肋部、上腹部和右肩胛部。胆囊运动由两条迷走神经分支支配[24]。

胆囊黏膜由大量折叠成嵴和皱褶的单层柱状上皮构成。胆囊壁由黏膜层、固有层、肌层和浆膜层组成[32],其中肌层较厚,由纵横交错的纵向和螺旋平滑肌纤维组成。小管泡状腺体见于胆囊颈部区域,参与黏液的分泌[29,32]。Rokitansky-Aschoff 窦是胆囊表面上皮的内陷,可通过肌层延伸[24]。这些结构可能是炎症的来源,最有可能是由于细菌在内陷的停滞和增殖。Luschka 管可沿胆囊的肝表面观察到,并直接开口于肝内胆管而不是胆囊腔内。这些结构被认为代表了一种发育异常,当它们存在于胆囊中时,可能是导致胆囊切除术后胆漏的来源[29]。

三、发育异常

(一) 肝外胆管

副胆管是只引流特定肝叶或肝段的畸形胆管,可以直接连接胆囊、胆囊管、左、右肝管或胆总管[25,33]。在罕见情况下,右肝管直接与胆囊或胆囊管相连,术前胆管造影需警惕这种变异的可能性,以防术中横断或结扎胆管。

胆管重复畸形罕见,多数为相互独立的胆管分别引流左右肝叶,并开口于十二指肠[25]。

胆囊引流和走行变异较常见[25],胆囊管重复畸形亦有发生。多数胆囊管缺失见于胆囊发育不全的患者(见后),极少数单纯胆囊管缺失,胆囊与胆总管直接相连。

(二) 胆囊

多数胆囊结构异常不引起临床症状,但偶尔可诱发胆汁淤积、胆囊炎和胆囊结石[25,33]。胆囊结构或位置异常所引发的疾病,鉴别诊断较困难。

胆囊发育不全可独立存在或与其他先天畸形同时发生[33],尸检阳性率在 0.04% ~ 0.13%,多由于胆囊芽发育不全或空泡化异常。发育过程中实体内胚层索的不完全空泡化可导致胆囊或胆囊管的先天性狭窄,胆囊壁内可出现前肠内胚层来源的多种异位组织,如胃、肝、肾上腺、胰腺和甲状腺。

双胆囊是一种罕见的畸形,发病率为 1/10 000 ~ 5/10 000[33,34]。两个胆囊共用同一个胆囊管,形成一个 Y 形管道,或者每个胆囊都有一个单独的胆囊管,并分别汇入胆总管[25]。胆囊三体也是一种罕见的先天性异常[35]。多发胆囊通常是由于胆结石、胆泥淤积、胆囊炎或肿瘤性病变才被发现。双叶胆囊、胆囊憩室均是罕见的发育异常。胆囊形态发生过程中,胆囊芽空泡化不完全时,单个胆囊可被分隔为多个腔室[34]。胆囊憩室和分隔导致胆汁淤积,并可促进胆结石的形成。

胆囊位置畸形报道较多[34],如左侧胆囊,位于镰状韧带左侧,肝左叶下方,可能是由于胚芽从肝憩室向左侧而不是向右侧迁移所致[25]。也有学者提出左侧胆囊是由左肝管独立发育而来,而右侧正常胆囊退化。另一种位置异常为肝内胆囊,可能是由于尾芽向前推进比颅芽更远并被颅侧结构包裹。当尾芽运动落后于颅芽时,就会产生游离胆囊。在这种情况下,胆囊被腹膜完全覆盖,并通过肠系膜将胆囊或胆囊管悬吊于肝脏下表面,引起胆囊活动异常并易于发生扭转。虽然发生率很低,胆囊亦可位于腹壁、镰状韧带或腹膜后[34]。

折叠胆囊有多种形式,如底部弯曲形成"倒圆锥形帽"样外观[34],通常位于浆膜后位置。这种异常通常认为是由于胚胎窝内胆囊异常折叠造成的。发育早期窝内胆囊异常折叠可导致胆囊体部与漏斗部的扭结,虽然不会导致临床症状,但会干扰影像学判断。

四、婴幼儿胆道疾病的处理方法

(一) 一般特征

胆汁淤积性肝病是由于肝细胞胆汁形成异常或肝内和肝外胆道胆汁引流不畅所致。其中许多疾病是由于个体发育缺陷或出生后不能适应宫外环境所致。框 62.1 提供了影响胆道的疾病列表,这些疾病同时发生于婴幼儿和年长儿童,本章后面将讨论这些疾病。重点是新生儿胆管疾病和年长儿童胆道疾病的独特方面。许多新生儿胆汁淤积性肝病的一般特征是相似的,小儿肝病的核心问题是鉴别肝内胆汁淤积和肝外胆汁淤积(表 62.1)[36]。代谢性或感染性肝病的治疗和胆道异常的手术治疗都需要早期诊断。即使无法进行有效的治疗,患有进行性肝病的婴儿和儿童在转诊接受肝移植治疗之前,也可从慢性肝病的最佳营养支持和管理中获益。

框 62.1 婴幼儿和儿童胆道疾病

胆管疾病
同种异体移植物排斥
胰腺疾病(炎症或肿瘤)引起的胆管梗阻
胆栓综合征
胆道蛔虫病
Caroli 病
胆总管囊肿
囊性纤维化(CF)
肝外胆道闭锁
移植物抗宿主病
特发性胆管狭窄(可能是先天性的)
肝内胆管缺如(综合征性或非综合征性)
创伤后胆管狭窄
硬化性胆管炎(炎症性肠病相关,免疫缺陷相关,新生儿)
自发性胆管穿孔
胆管内外肿瘤
胆囊疾病
无结石性胆囊炎
急性胆囊炎
急性胆囊积液
异常
胆石症
慢性胆囊炎
肿瘤

表 62.1　各种新生儿胆汁淤积疾病的相对频率

疾病	发生率/%
新生儿特发性肝炎	30~35
肝外胆道闭锁	30
α_1-抗胰蛋白酶缺乏症	7~10
肝内胆汁淤积综合征(Alagille 综合征、进行性家族性肝内胆汁淤积症、其他)	5~6
肝炎(CMV,风疹,HSV,其他)	3~5
胆总管囊肿	2~4
细菌性脓毒症	2
内分泌疾病(甲状腺功能减退症,全垂体功能减退症)	≈1
半乳糖血症	≈1
先天性胆汁酸代谢缺陷	≈1
其他代谢紊乱	≈1

CMV,巨细胞病毒;HSV,单纯疱疹病毒。

由于肝胆系统功能不成熟的原因,在新生儿期出现胆汁淤积性黄疸的不同疾病的数量可能多于其他任何生命时期(见框 62.1)[37,38]。基因组测序发现了以前被标记为特发性新生儿肝炎的新缺陷。婴儿肝功能不全,无论何种原因,通常与胆汁分泌功能衰竭和胆汁淤积性黄疸有关。尽管胆汁淤积可以追溯到肝细胞或胆道系统水平,但在实践中,在损伤的初始和后续部位方面,疾病之间可能存在相当大的重叠。例如,胆管上皮损伤通常是巨细胞病毒感染引起的新生儿肝炎的显著特征。胆道机械性梗阻总是产生肝功能不全,在新生儿中可能与肝实质异常有关,如肝细胞巨细胞转化。巨细胞——新生儿肝脏损伤的常见非特异性表现——是否反映了胆道梗阻的有害作用,或者是肝细胞和胆管上皮是否在个体发育过程中被一种常见的因子损伤,如对两种细胞均具有趋向性的病毒,目前尚不清楚。新生儿胆汁淤积症通常伴随的另一个常见组织学变量是胆管缺如或小叶间胆管数量减少[39]。这一发现在 Alagille 综合征患者中可能是最重要的,也可能是许多其他疾病的偶发特征,包括特发性新生儿肝炎、先天性巨细胞病毒感染和 α1-抗胰蛋白酶缺乏症。连续肝活检通常显示每个门管区胆小管数量进行性减少,并伴有不同程度的相关炎症和纤维化。

(二) 诊断

在大多数患有胆汁淤积性肝病的婴儿中,这种情况出现在出生后的前几周。鉴别结合高胆红素血症与新生儿常见的非结合生理性高胆红素血症或偶尔与母乳喂养引起的长期黄疸的鉴别非常重要[40]。对于 14 天以上有黄疸的新生儿,必须考虑肝脏或胆道疾病的可能性(另见第 77 章)。完全性胆道闭锁患儿的粪便无胆色(呈白陶土色),但在不完全性或进展性胆道梗阻早期,粪便颜色可表现为正常或仅有间歇性色素沉着。必须排除危及生命但可治疗的疾病,如细菌感染和许多先天性代谢缺陷。外科手术在解除胆道闭锁或胆总管囊肿的胆道梗阻方面能否成功,取决于早期诊断和手术。

评价胆汁淤积性肝病婴儿的方法见框 62.2。初步评估应及时确定是否存在胆汁淤积性黄疸,并评估肝功能不全的严重程度。可能需要更详细的研究,并应以病例的临床特征为指导。无须对每例患者进行所有相关的诊断试验。超声检查可及时确诊黄疸新生儿的胆总管囊肿,因此,无须排除肝脏疾病的感染和代谢原因。已经提出了许多常规和专门的生化测试和成像程序来区分婴儿肝内和肝外胆汁淤积,从而避免了不必要的手术探查[40,41]。标准肝脏生化测试通常显示血清直接胆红素、转氨酶、碱性磷酸酶和脂质水平的不同程度升高。不幸的是,由于至少 10% 的肝内胆汁淤积症婴儿的胆汁分泌功能衰竭,这足以导致诊断试验结果与提示胆道闭锁的结果重叠,因此没有一项试验证明是具有令人满意的鉴别价值[42]。粪便中胆色素的存在一般可除外胆道闭锁,但胆汁淤积患者排出的分泌物或脱落的上皮细胞所致的粪便着色,可能会产生误导。

框 62.2　婴儿胆汁淤积症的评估

病史和体检

家族史、妊娠、是否存在肝外异常和大便颜色的详细信息

确定肝脏疾病是否存在和严重程度的试验

分级血清胆红素分析

肝脏生化检查(AST、ALT、碱性磷酸酶、5′-核苷酸酶、GGTP)

肝功能检查(凝血酶原时间、部分凝血活酶时间、凝血因子、血清白蛋白水平、血清氨水平、血胆固醇水平、血糖)

感染测试

血常规

血液、尿液和其他可疑部位的细菌培养

病毒培养

血清学检测(HBsAg,TORCH,EBV,细小病毒 B19,HIV,其他)

腹水穿刺术

代谢和遗传研究

α_1-抗胰蛋白酶水平和表型(如果水平降低)

代谢筛查(尿液和血清氨基酸、尿液有机酸)

尿液还原性物质

红细胞半乳糖-1-磷酸尿苷酰转移酶活性(Gal-1-PUT)

血清铁和铁蛋白水平

汗液氯化物分析

甲状腺激素,促甲状腺激素(根据指征评价垂体功能减退)

尿液和血清中胆汁酸和胆汁酸前体的分析

Alagille 综合征和进行性家族性肝内胆汁淤积的遗传学研究

影像学检查

肝脏和胆道超声(首先)

肝胆闪烁显像

磁共振胰胆管造影

先天性感染的长骨和颅骨以及肺和心脏疾病的胸部 X 线摄影

经皮或内镜下胆管造影术(罕见指征)

侵入性检查

疑似贮积病的骨髓检查和皮肤成纤维细胞培养

十二指肠插管以评估液体中的胆色素

经皮肝活检(用于光学和电子显微镜检查、酶学评价)

剖腹探查术和术中胆管造影

HBsAg,乙型肝炎表面抗原;STS,梅毒血清学检查;TORCH,弓形虫病,其他,风疹,巨细胞病毒,疱疹。

超声检查可用于评估肝脏的大小和回声。即使在新生儿中，高频实时超声通常也可以确定胆囊的存在和大小，检测胆管和胆囊中的结石和淤泥，并显示胆道系统的囊性或阻塞性扩张。也可识别肝外异常。

门静脉周围的三角形索状物或带状回声（厚度≥3mm），代表门静脉头侧的锥形纤维化团块，似乎是胆道闭锁早期诊断的特异性超声表现[43,44]。胆囊“鬼影”三联征定义为：胆囊长度小于 1.9cm；缺乏光滑或完整的回声黏膜衬里，壁不清晰；轮廓不规则或呈小叶状，已被提出作为胆道闭锁的附加标准。

CT 提供的信息与超声相似，但由于暴露于辐射、缺乏用于对比的腹内脂肪以及需要大剂量镇静或全身麻醉，不适用于 2 岁以下的患者。

磁共振胰胆管造影（MRCP）用 T2 加权涡轮自旋回波序列进行成像，广泛用于评估所有年龄组的胆道。在 1999 年的一项研究中，MRCP 可靠地显示了正常新生儿的胆管和胆囊。在一些胆道闭锁患者中，胆管不显影和小胆囊的显示是特征性的 MRCP 表现。另一项研究发现，MRCP 描绘肝外胆道闭锁的准确率为 82%，敏感性为 90%，特异性为 77%。与以前的报道相反，MRCP 也出现假阳性和假阴性结果。严重肝内胆汁淤积症与胆道闭锁的鉴别可能很困难[46]，因为 MRCP 勾画肝外胆道的能力取决于胆汁流量。MRCP 可以准确地确定胆总管囊肿，并已成为原发性硬化性胆管炎诊断的首选术式。

使用肝胆闪烁显影剂如 ^{99}mTc 亚氨基二乙酸衍生物可能有助于区分肝外胆道闭锁和其他原因引起的新生儿黄疸[45]。不幸的是，1997 年的一项研究表明，50% 小叶间胆管缺乏但无肝外梗阻的患者中，放射性核素的胆汁排泄缺失[47]。在特发性新生儿肝炎的患者中，25% 也证实无胆汁排泄。然而，该方法仍可用于评估胆囊积水或胆石症患者的胆囊管的通畅性。

内镜逆行性胰胆管造影（ERCP）可用于评估肝外胆道梗阻患儿，并已在患有胆汁淤积的新生儿中成功实施[41]。操作者在婴儿中完成该手术需要相当多的技术专业知识。大多数新生儿需要全身麻醉才能获得满意的检查。经皮经肝胰胆管造影术可能对选定患者的胆道可视化有价值[48]，但该技术在婴儿中比在成人中更难进行，因为肝内胆管更细，并且大多数发生在婴儿中的疾病不会导致胆道扩张。介入性 ERCP 常用于扩张胆管狭窄和取出儿童胆总管结石。

经皮肝活检在评估胆汁淤积患者中特别有价值，即使是最小的婴儿，也能在镇静和局部麻醉下进行[49]。例如，90%～95% 的患者可根据临床和组织学标准诊断为肝外胆道闭锁。当对诊断的怀疑持续存在时，可以通过小切口开腹术和手术胆管造影术直接检查胆道的通畅性。在包含 646 例患者的 11 项研究中使用的各种诊断方法的 meta 分析中，经皮肝活检的准确率优于所有非侵入性方法，汇总的敏感性为 98%（95% CI，96%～99%），特异性为 93%（95% CI，89%～95%），阳性预测值为 93.0%，阴性预测值为 97.7%[50]。肝活检在显示药物或病毒引起的胆管缺乏或胆道损伤方面也很有价值。

五、小儿胆管疾病

（一）胆道闭锁

胆道闭锁的特点是由于全部或部分肝外胆管破坏而导致胆汁流完全阻塞[51]。作为基础疾病过程的一部分或由于胆道梗阻，伴随的肝内胆管损伤和纤维化也有不同程度的发生[52]。

1. 流行病学

在美国该病的发生率为 1/10 000～1/15 000 例活产婴儿，约占新生儿胆汁淤积性黄疸的 1/3（见表 62.1）。它是肝脏疾病死亡的最常见原因和儿童转诊肝移植的原因（约占所有病例的 50%）[53]。胆道闭锁的病因尚不清楚，这种疾病不是遗传性的，有几次报道称双卵和同卵双胞胎不一致的胆道闭锁。在一项 461 例法国患者的研究中，无法证实季节性、时间聚类或时间空间聚类[54]。家族性病例报告罕见，在大多数情况下，均没有提供肝外胆道的详细组织学描述，以排除与重度肝内胆汁淤积相关的胆管狭窄或发育不全。在 1997 年至 2002 年进行的美国多州病例对照国家出生缺陷预防研究中，非西班牙裔黑人母亲所生的婴儿比非西班牙裔母亲所生的婴儿风险更大[55]。

2. 病因和发病机制

已经提出了几种机制来解释肝外胆道的进行性闭塞，目前有如下几种假说[56]。没有证据表明胆道闭锁是由于胚胎发育过程中胆管形态发生或再通失败的结果。临床特征支持这一概念，即在大多数情况下，胆道损伤发生在胆道形态发生后，通常发生在出生后。缺血造成肝外胆管损伤的假说，几乎没有证据支持。支持潜在的毒素诱导损伤是基于以下发现：在家畜和斑马鱼模型中，摄入植物异黄酮与胆道闭锁的发生相关[57]。巨细胞病毒（CMV）、C 组轮状病毒、EB 病毒（EBV）、呼肠弧病毒 3 的先天性感染偶尔被涉及其中[56]。在一项研究中，56% 的胆道闭锁患者对 CMV 的反应中产生干扰素（IFN）-γ 的肝 T 细胞显著增加，而对其他病毒和对照组的反应极小，因此提示在一些患者中，围生期 CMV 感染是胆管损伤的一个合理的启动因子[58]。

全基因组关联和其他基因组研究已确定 GPC1 为胆道闭锁的易感基因[59]。该基因编码 glypican 1-a 硫酸乙酰肝素蛋白多糖，调节 Hedgehog 信号和炎症。与对照组相比，胆道闭锁患者的肝脏样本胆管细胞顶端 GPC1 水平降低。另一项全基因组关联研究确定了位点 10q24.2 上胆道闭锁的易感位点，该位点与 X-脯氨酰氨肽酶 P1（*XPNPEP1*）和 *ADD3* 具有强关联性[59]。*XPNPEP1* 在胆管上皮细胞中表达，并参与炎症介质的代谢。*ADD3* 编码内收蛋白，一种膜骨架蛋白，在调节上皮细胞-细胞黏附中起作用，并在胎儿肝脏中高表达。

对胆道闭锁患儿肝脏的互补 RNA 进行基于寡核苷酸基因芯片分析，已证实参与淋巴细胞分化和炎症的基因的协调激活[60]。在小鼠模型和胆道闭锁患者中，越来越多的证据表明，自身免疫、细胞、体液、先天免疫失调以及 T 调节细胞功能的作用（见第 2 章）[61]。在遗传易感宿主中，产前或围生期病毒感染可能引起胆管细胞凋亡、抗原释放和肝内和肝外胆管 MHC-Ⅱ类分子异常表达[56]。病毒、天然或改变的胆管抗原被巨噬细胞或树突细胞吞噬和处理，递给幼稚 T 细胞，使其活化。活化的 CD4⁺T 细胞引起 IFN-γ 诱导的巨噬细胞反应和细胞毒性 CD8⁺T 细胞和 B 细胞的活化。活化的巨噬细胞释放炎症介质（包括肿瘤坏死因子（TNF）-α、一氧化氮和活性氧），浆细胞释放自身抗体，CD8⁺ T 细胞释放颗粒酶、穿孔素和 IFN-γ，通过凋亡或坏死途径导致胆管细胞损伤（见第 1 章和第 72 章）。胆道闭锁婴儿中负责控制 T 细胞介导的病原体免疫应答的 CD4⁺T 细胞调节性 T 细胞（Treg）亚群缺乏，这种缺乏可能加重胆管损伤[56]。肝星状细胞（肌成纤维细胞）和成纤维细胞被激活，从而引起肝内和肝外胆管纤维化。由此引起的胆管细胞损伤、炎症和纤维化导致胆管完全梗阻。上述机制是如何相互协调的，为什么疾病只发生在出生后的最初几个月，为什么少数围生期病毒感染的婴儿会发生胆道闭锁，以及为什么在移植的肝中疾病不会复发，这些都是尚未回答的问题。

胆道闭锁的循环炎症标志物持续存在，大部分不受门肠吻合术的影响（见后文），1 型辅助性 T 细胞（Th1）效应因子白介素-2（IL-2）和 IFN-γ，一些 2 型辅助性 T 细胞（Th2）效应因子（白细胞介素-4）以及巨噬细胞标志物（TNF-α）明显进行性升高。还发现可溶性细胞黏附分子 sICAM-1 和 sVCAM-1 的表达增加，可能反映了循环炎症和免疫活性细胞持续募集到肝脏和胆道系统中[62]。这种免疫反应是由病毒感染诱导的，还是反映了对感染或环境暴露的遗传程序化反应，目前仍不清楚。

10%～25%的患者发生肝外异常，包括心血管缺陷、多脾、旋转不良、内脏转位和肠道闭锁[63,64]。一些有内脏异位的患者，包括胆道闭锁和多脾的婴儿，发现存在 *CFC1* 基因的功能缺失突变[65,66]。该基因编码一种 CYPTIC 的蛋白，在形态发生过程中参与建立左右轴。相反，对胆管闭锁和内脏异位婴儿的有限研究中没有发现 *INV* 基因的突变，*INV* 基因也参与决定偏侧性[67]。在对患有所谓“胚胎型”胆道闭锁的婴儿肝组织进行的微阵列分析中，发生肝外畸形和早发发生胆汁淤积性黄疸，染色质完整性和功能相关基因的独特表达模式（Smarca-1，Rybp 和 Hdac3）和 5 个印记基因（*Igf2*、*Peg3*、*Peg10*、*Meg3* 和 IPW）的过表达被发现，意味着未能下调影响肝脏和其他器官发育的胚胎基因程序[68]。*Jagged1*［Alagille 综合征的基因缺陷（见后文）］）错义突变已在 102 例胆道闭锁患者的 9 例中得到确认，胆道闭锁患者预后不良[69]。

3. 病理学

肝脏活检标本的组织病理学发现对胆道闭锁患者的治疗非常重要[51,53]。在病程早期，肝脏结构一般仍存在，表现为不同程度的胆管增生、胆管及细胞内胆汁淤积、汇管区水肿和纤维化（图 62.4）[53]。汇管区胆栓高度提示大胆管梗阻。此

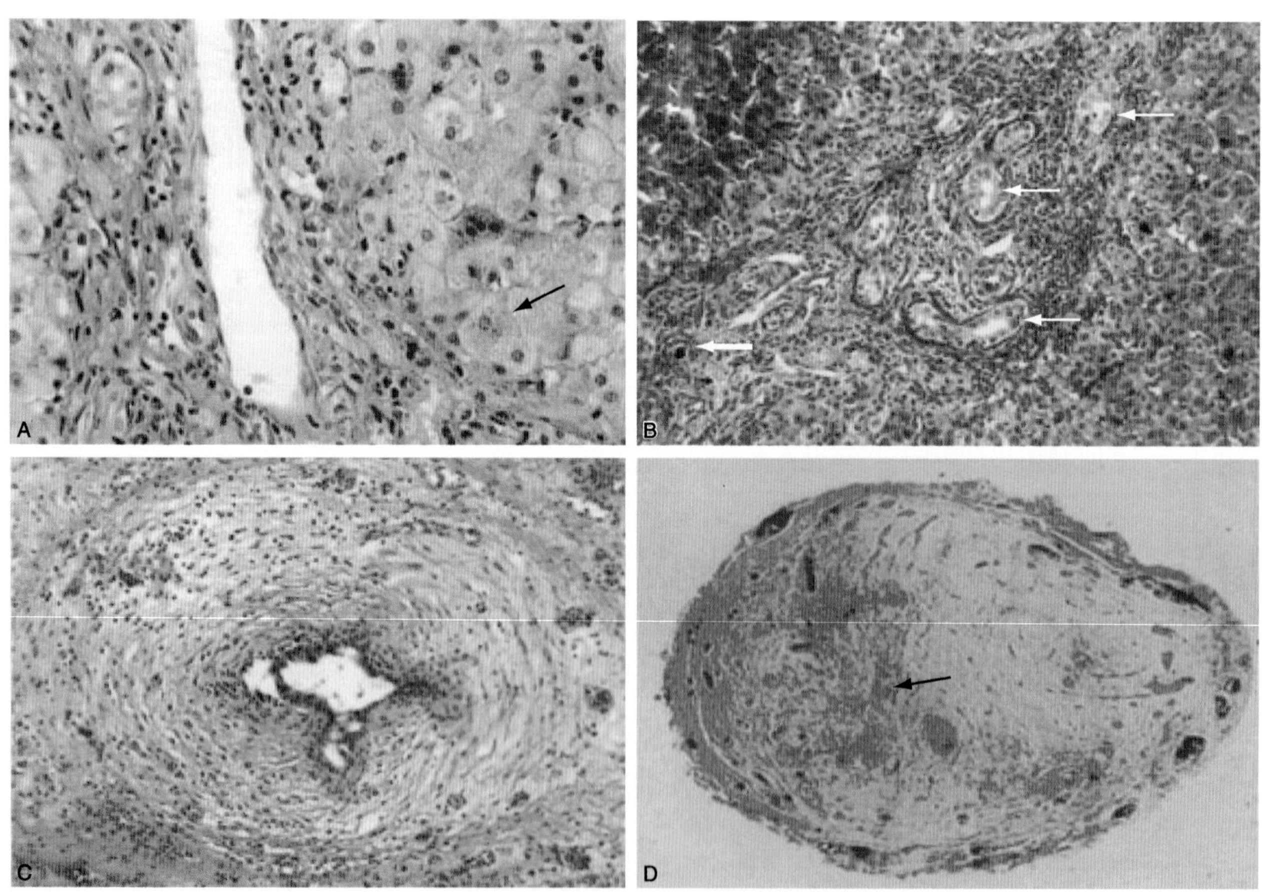

图 62.4　胆道闭锁时肝脏和肝外胆管的组织学表现。A，肝细胞和小管内胆汁淤积，多核巨细胞（箭头）和门管区炎症（HE 染色，×400）。B，门脉道扩张伴门脉纤维化，胆管增生（细箭头），胆管内有胆栓（粗箭头）（Masson 三色，×250）。C，肝门部近端肝总管，胆管上皮脱落，胆管壁向心性纤维化，导管周围淋巴细胞浸润，管腔狭窄但通畅（HE 染色，×150）。D，残余胆管，管腔完全闭塞（箭头），管壁向心性纤维化（HE 染色，×40）。（From Sokol RJ，Mack C，Narkewicz MR，Karrer FM. Pathogenesis and outcome of biliary atresia：current concepts. J Pediatr Gastroenterol Nutr 2003；37：4-21. Used with permission.）

外，小叶内胆管上皮细胞出现不同程度损害，包括水肿、空泡化，甚至脱落进入管腔。汇管区有不同程度的炎症细胞浸润，25%患者可出现与新生儿肝炎程度相似的肝细胞巨细胞化。小叶内胆管偶尔呈胆管板样，提示胆道闭锁患者存在产前发育阶段的胆管重构异常[70]。无论是否恢复胆汁流通，发病初期或出生后几个月内即出现胆汁性肝硬化。

胆道闭锁肝外胆管的解剖变异多样，Kasai 提出了一个实用的描述分类[72]。根据闭锁的部位，分为 3 个主要类型。Ⅰ型为胆总管闭锁，近端胆管通畅。Ⅱ型累及肝管，肝门部胆管囊性扩张。在Ⅱa 型闭锁中，胆囊管和肝管通畅，而在Ⅱb 型闭锁中，胆囊管和肝管也发生闭塞。这些类型的胆道闭锁可经手术治愈，但遗憾的是仅占所有病例的 10%。90%或以上的患者为Ⅲ型闭锁，肝总管、左肝管、右肝管、胆囊管均闭锁，同时肝门部胆管无囊性扩张，整个肝门部均为锥形的致密纤维组织，大约 80%的患者胆囊也在一定程度上受累。Ⅲ型闭锁则没有未闭的肝内胆管或扩张的肝门部胆管以供胆肠吻合，因此也被称为“不可纠正的”闭锁。

至少一部分肝外胆管的完全纤维闭塞是纤维残留物显微镜检查中发现的一致特征[72]。胆道的其他节段可显示管腔伴胆管上皮细胞不同程度的变性、炎症和导管周围组织纤维化（见图 62.4）。在大多数患者中，肝内延伸至肝门的胆管在出生后的第 1 周内是畅通的，但逐渐被破坏，推测是由损伤肝外胆管的相同过程和胆道梗阻的影响所致。在超过 20%的患者中，发现了与导管板畸形中观察到的相似的同心管状导管结构，表明疾病过程干扰了胆道的正常重塑。

4. 临床特征

大多数胆道闭锁婴儿是在正常妊娠后足月出生的，出生体重正常[73]。女婴比男婴更常受累。围生期病程通常不显著，出生后体重增长和发育正常。在生理性高胆红素血症期后，父母或医生观察到黄疸。长期黄疸时可能被错误地归因于母乳喂养[74]。任何 14 天以上有黄疸的新生儿，必须考虑肝脏或胆道疾病的可能性。已确诊的胆道闭锁患儿的粪便是无胆色的（白陶土色），但在病程早期，粪便可能表现为正常颜色或间歇性的着色。在中国台湾，通过使用给予父母的粪便颜色卡来筛查胆道闭锁，减少了用于评价胆汁淤积的晚期转诊的数量[75]。

肝脏典型肿大，右肋缘下 2~6cm 可触及质韧边缘[53]。脾脏通常在病程早期不肿大，但随着门静脉脉高压的发展而增大。最初不存在腹水和水肿，但维生素 K 缺乏可导致凝血功能障碍。

实验室检查最初发现胆汁淤积的证据，血清总胆红素水平为 6~12mg/dL，其中至少 50%为结合胆红素[53]。2011 年的一项研究显示，超过一半的胆道闭锁患儿在出生后不久直接胆红素水平升高，提示围生期发病[76]。血清转氨酶、GGTP 和碱性磷酸酶水平中度升高。

5. 治疗

胆道闭锁诊断初步检查通常包括经皮肝活检，以获得胆道梗阻的组织学证据（胆管增生、胆管阻塞、门脉纤维化）。当临床、病理及影像学结果提示胆道闭锁的可能性时，有必要进行剖腹探查和手术胆管造影术以记录梗阻部位，并直接尝试手术治疗[52,77]。肝门胆管近端部分或囊性结构通畅，允许在约 10%的患者中与肠段进行传统吻合。在大多数近端肝外胆管闭塞的患者中，首选的手术方法是 Kasai 开发的肝门肠吻合术（图 62.5）[78,79]。横断远端胆管，将纤维胆管残端剥离至门静脉分叉上方区域[80]。然后在该水平向后和向外侧进行剥离，横断组织的纤维锥与肝脏表面齐平，从而暴露可能含有残留显微镜下胆管的区域。该手术通过在横断组织的裸露边缘周围吻合空肠 Roux-en-Y 袢完成，为胆道引流提供通道。应避免多次尝试重新探查和翻修无功能的胆管[81]。糖皮质激素和 UDCA 作为利胆剂的辅助治疗在术后被广泛应用[82,83]，但在一项前瞻性双盲随机对照研究中，糖皮质激素并没有降低 Kasai 门肠吻合术后肝移植的需求[48]。

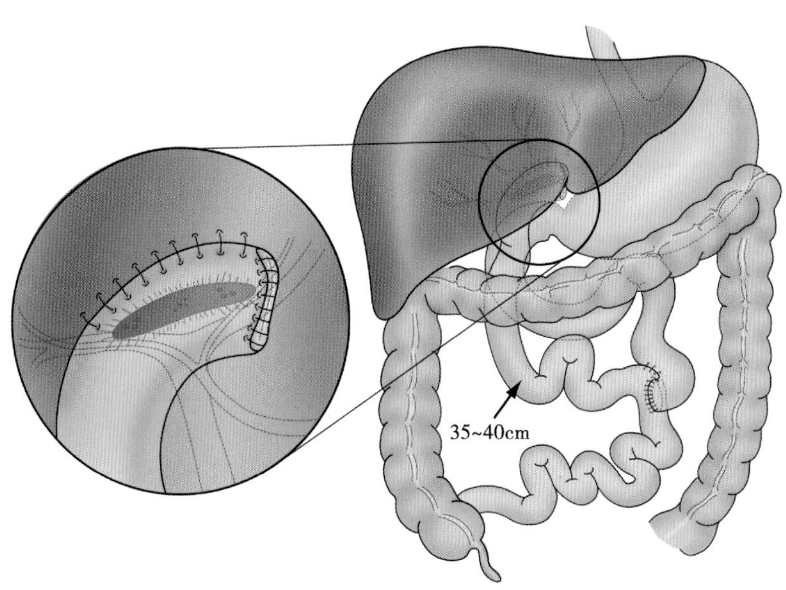

图 62.5　胆道闭锁的 Kasai 手术。手术切除闭锁的肝外胆管和来自肝门的纤维组织锥后，对肝门进行 35~40cm 的 Roux-en-Y 吻合。该夹层可发现多个小但通畅的胆管，并引流至，Roux 肠袢。左侧显示了空肠袢与肝门吻合的放大图。（Figure drawn and kindly provided by Dr. Frederick Ryckman，Cincinnati，OH.）

6. 预后

未经治疗的胆道闭锁预后极差，通常在两年内死于肝衰竭[85]。来自美国众多小儿外科医生和医疗实践机构的数据显示，在接受 Kasai 手术的 670 名患者中，实际 5 年存活率为 48%（图 62.6）[86]。来自欧洲、日本和美国的几个大型系列显示了相似或略好的结果[87-90]。2003 年来自日本胆道闭锁注册研究的一份报告中，Kasai 手术后 57% 的患者黄疸消退，总体 5 年和 10 年生存率分别为 75.3% 和 66.7%[87]。截至报告发表时，108 例患者中的 57 例在没有接受肝移植的情况下已存活 10 年。在法国确定的 10 年期间（1986—1996 年）所有胆道闭锁患者系列中，采用 Kasai 手术和必要时肝移植治疗的患者的总体生存率为 68%[88]。未接受肝移植患者 10 年生存率为 29%，这一数字与作者从 750 例已发表病例中汇编的 31% 相似。儿童肝病研究网络（Childhood Liver Disease Research Network，ChiLDReN）是在美国和加拿大研究胆道闭锁的多中心联盟，报道了 219 例胆道闭锁的儿童，这些儿童在 Kasai 门肠吻合术后约 10 年仍存活，其肝脏为自体肝脏。这些患者中 98% 以上有慢性肝病的临床或生化证据[89]。因此，胆管闭锁儿童从 Kasai 门肠吻合术中获得长期益处，尽管大多数儿童存在持续性肝功能不全。进行性胆汁性肝硬化可能导致肝衰竭死亡或需要肝移植，尽管明显成功地恢复了胆汁引流。

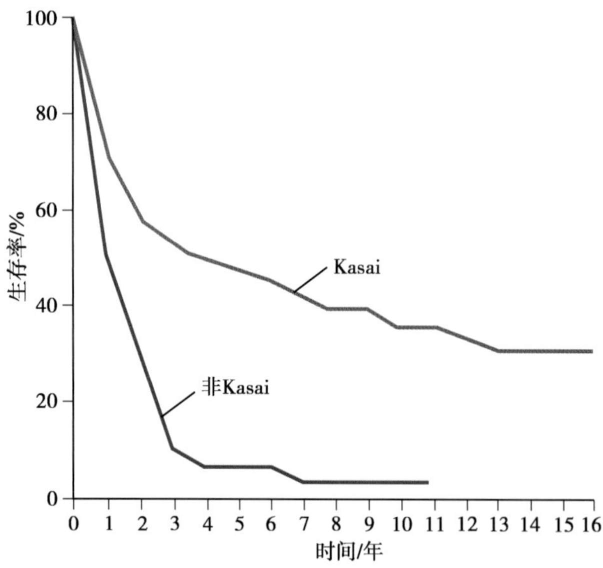

图 62.6　670 例接受 Kasai 门肠吻合术（蓝线）的肝外胆道闭锁婴儿和 88 例未接受手术或仅接受胆道闭锁剖腹探查术（红线）的肝外胆道闭锁婴儿的存活率。平均随访时间为 5 年。两组间生存率差异具有统计学显著性（$P=0.001$）。（From Karrer FM，Lilly JR，Stewart BA，et al. Biliary atresia registry：1976 to 1989. J Pediatr Surg 1990；25：1076-80.）

已发现几个因素导致了门肠吻合术后的不同结局。手术时患者的年龄是最关键的[87,88,91]。在几个系列中，80%～90% 的婴儿在出生后 60 天内转诊接受手术，胆汁流量得以重建[87,92]。在 90 天后的诊断中，黄疸仍然有可能消退，但即使是在肝移植时代，长期存活率也会受到影响[91]。在美国对 244 名婴儿进行的一项前瞻性研究中，肝门闭锁、胆总管完全闭锁、胆道闭锁脾畸形综合征、腹水和结节性肝病患者的移植或死亡风险增加[93]。在法国的一项大型研究中，影响总生存期的独立预后因素为进行 Kasai 手术和手术时年龄小于 45 天[88]；肝外胆管完全闭锁和多脾综合征的结局不太有利。手术中心的经验也很重要[88]。

影响预后的因素包括 Kasai 门肠吻合术后 3 个月时的血清总胆红素水平。如果 kasai 术后 3 个月时总胆红素≤2mg/dL，则可以预测患者在出生后 2 年内不需要肝移植。如果该时间点的总胆红素≥6mg/dL，则 2 年内需要肝移植的可能性很高[94-96]。至少为 150～400μm 的肝门前胆管结构，特别是内衬有柱状上皮的胆管结构，并不始终与良好的预后相关[94,97]。实质性肝细胞损伤，表现为肝活检标本上小叶排列紊乱和巨细胞转化，与不良预后相关。肝活检标本中存在导管板畸形也预示着 Kasai 门肠吻合术后胆汁流动不畅。胆汁分泌量与在切除的肝门标本中确定的胆管总面积相关[98,99]。潜在胆管和肝脏疾病的进展速度也限制了生存率[51,100]。这种疾病并不局限于肝外胆道，可能与肝内胆管的进行性炎症和破坏以及最终肝硬化有关[51]。上行性细菌性胆管炎复发，最常见于术后前 2 年内，可导致持续的胆管损伤，甚至导致再次梗阻[101]。胆管炎主要发生于有一定程度胆汁引流的婴儿，可能是由于肝门部通畅的胆管提供了上行感染的途径。预防性口服抗生素通常用于预防 Kasai 门肠吻合术后复发性胆管炎，但这种方法的对照试验尚未进行[102]。生长障碍与 2 岁时需要肝移植或死亡相关。对于胆汁引流良好和肝脏合成功能保留的患者，单纯食管静脉曲张破裂出血并不是紧急肝移植的绝对指征[103,104]。

在 Kasai 门肠口吻合术后不能成功恢复胆汁流动、转诊过晚（可能在 120 日龄或以后），以及尽管进行了胆汁引流但最终仍发生终末期肝病的儿童中，肝移植至关重要[88,105,106]。在美国，大约 80% 的胆道闭锁患者在 18 岁时需要肝移植，胆道闭锁占儿童所有肝移植的 40%～50%。由于腹腔内粘连和遇到的各种肠道重建，Kasai 门肠吻合术在技术上使肝移植更加困难[107]。然而，使用减小尺寸的同种异体肝移植和活体相关供体，预期一年生存率可超过 90%（见第 97 章）[105,108,109]。

（二）自发性胆管穿孔

自发性胆管穿孔是一种罕见但伴有明显胆汁淤积的婴幼儿疾病[110]。穿孔通常发生在胆囊管和胆管的交界处。原因尚不清楚，目前有证据表明可能与胆汁浓缩或狭窄造成的胆管远端梗阻有关[111]。穿孔部位的先天薄弱和感染引起胆管壁损伤也是可能的原因之一。自发性胆管穿孔可合并Ⅰ型、Ⅵ型先天性胆总管囊肿和急性胰腺炎。

大多数婴儿在穿孔前看起来是健康的。临床症状（黄疸、白陶土大便、尿色加深和腹水）通常发生在出生后的最初几个月内[111]，也可表现为呕吐和体重增长停滞。进行性腹胀是常见的特征，脐疝或腹股沟疝时可能呈现胆汁样颜色的腹水。

典型的生化改变为血中结合胆红素轻至中度增高伴转氨酶轻度升高。腹腔穿刺可见清亮、胆汁颜色的无菌腹水。超声检查提示腹水或右上腹局限性的液体积聚，胆管无扩张。肝胆闪烁扫描显示同位素在腹腔内部位不固定的积聚[111]。

穿孔的位置依赖术中胆管造影来确定[112]。手术方式包括简单的胆汁性腹水引流，和穿孔部位的修复[112]。如果穿孔与胆管梗阻有关，则可能需要通过胆囊空肠吻合术进行引流。门静脉血栓形成已被报告为一种并发症，可能与胆汁的刺激作用或压迫门静脉的胆汁瘤有关。

（三）胆汁栓塞综合征

浓稠浓缩的胆汁和黏液的栓子也可引起胆管梗阻[113,114]。健康的婴儿也会受到影响，但这种情况更常见于不能进食和需要长期胃肠外营养的患病早产儿。发病机制可能涉及胆汁淤积、禁食、感染和胆红素负荷增加。与严重溶血相关的胆汁淤积或胆汁浓缩综合征可能是胆栓综合征的变体，但随着预防和治疗 Rh 和 ABO 血型不合的方法的出现，目前并不常见。临床表现可能类似于胆道闭锁。超声可显示肝内胆管扩张。诊断通常需要剖腹探查和手术胆管造影。只需单纯的冲洗胆管即可治愈[115]。

（四）先天性胆总管畸形

1. 流行病学和分类

胆总管畸形并不是真正的囊肿，因为它们不是包裹的上皮化结构。由于历史原因，这些先天性异常将继续被称为胆总管囊肿，但病因可能具有异质性，并且具有共同的局灶性或弥漫性肝外胆管扩张伴不同程度的肝内胆管受累[116,117]。胆总管囊肿不是家族性的，女性儿童比男性儿童更常见。妊娠期和老年患者均有报道，但约三分之二的患者在 10 岁之前就医。

Todani 及其同事们提出的分类方法被频繁引用（图 62.7）[118,119]。Ⅰ型囊肿：有几种Ⅰ型囊肿，占病例的 80%～90%，表现为胆管节段性或弥漫性梭形扩张。Ⅱ型囊肿：由真正的胆总管憩室组成。Ⅲ型囊肿：包括胆管十二指肠内部分扩张，或胆总管囊肿。Ⅳ型囊肿：可分为Ⅳa 型（肝内、肝外胆管多发性囊肿）和Ⅳb 型（肝外胆管多发性囊肿），Ⅳb 型变异不常见，或可能与Ⅰ型重叠。Ⅴ型囊肿：又称 Caroli 病，包括肝内胆管系统的单个或多个扩张，其是否应被视为胆总管囊肿的一种形式尚不确定[119,120]。

西方人群中Ⅰ型和Ⅳ型胆总管囊肿的发病率估计为 1/100 000～1/150 000。在一些亚洲国家，发病率可能高达 1∶10 000。胆总管憩室（Ⅱ型囊肿）和胆总管囊肿（Ⅲ型囊肿）发病率明显低，约 1/10 000 000[116,117]。

2. 病因学

胆总管畸形的原因尚不明确[117]，可能的机制包括先天性胆管壁较薄，胆管胚胎发育期间上皮细胞增殖异常，以及先天性胆管梗阻[116,121]。有学者已经提出了与其他梗阻性胆管疾病（如胆道闭锁）的关系，但尚未得到证实。在 33 例胆总管畸形患者的基因测序研究中，未检测到单基因缺陷，但发现 21 种潜在损伤性新生致病变异，即使在复合杂合子状态下也可能影响肝胆道的发育过程[122]。已有报道称，胰胆管畸形愈合（胰管和胆管异常愈合）的发生率较高（40%），这可能导致胰腺分泌物回流至胆道（见第 55 章）[123]。这一过程可能导致发育中的胆管进行性损伤，随后出现无力和扩张。胆总管囊肿可能与其他发育异常有关，包括结肠闭锁、十二指肠闭锁，肛门闭锁，胰腺动静脉畸形，多隔膜胆囊，室间隔缺损、主

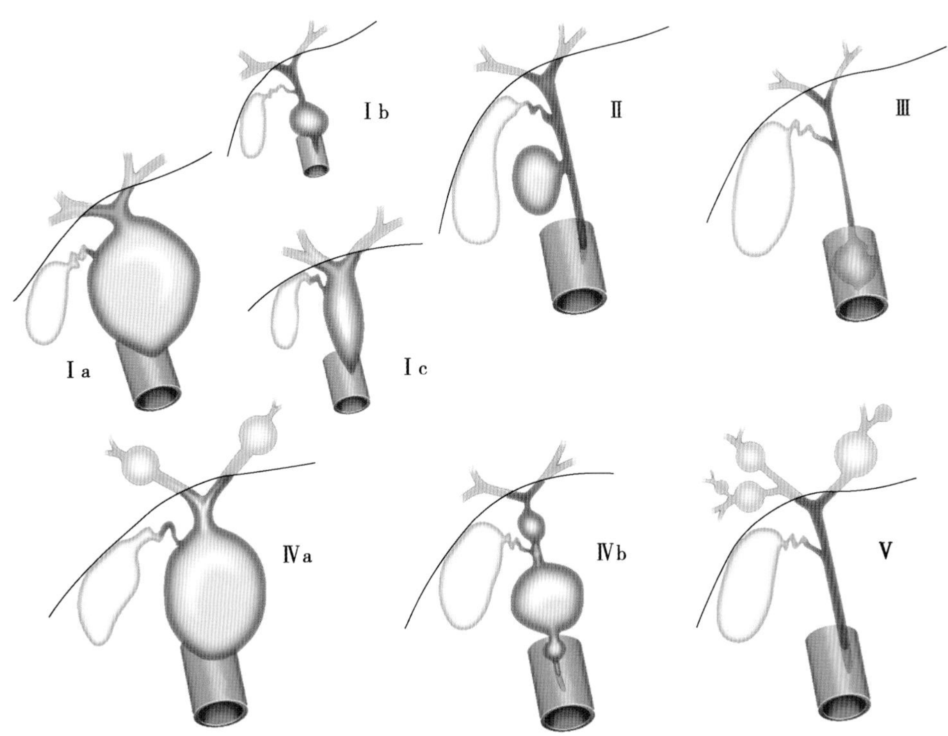

图 62.7　根据 Todani[119] 及其同事的胆总管畸形分类。Ⅰa，胆总管扩张；Ⅰb，节段性扩张；Ⅰc，弥漫性扩张；Ⅱ，胆总管憩室；Ⅲ，胆总管囊肿；Ⅳa，多发性囊肿（肝内和肝外胆管）；Ⅳb，多发性囊肿（肝外胆管）；Ⅴ，肝内胆管单个或多个扩张（Caroli 病）。（From Savader SJ，Benenati JF，Venbrux AC，et al. Choledochal cysts：classification and cholangiographic appearance. AJR 1991；156：327-31.）

动脉发育不全、胰腺分裂、胰腺发育不全、肝脏局灶性结节性增生和先天性门静脉缺如。在一些常染色体隐性遗传性多囊患者中也发现胆总管囊肿(见第 96 章)[124]。

3. 病理学

扩张的胆管段由纤维壁组成,可无上皮衬里或低柱状上皮[117]。可出现轻度慢性炎症。多伴有胆管末端的完全炎性梗阻常见于胆总管囊肿的婴儿。

受累新生儿肝脏活检标本显示大导管梗阻的典型特征[117],结果可能与肝外胆道闭锁中观察到的结果相似。门脉区水肿、胆管增生和纤维化突出。在长期胆管梗阻的老年患者中可观察到胆汁性肝硬化的模式。囊壁癌可能在青春期发生(见第 69 章)[125,126]。

4. 临床特征

婴儿型胆总管囊肿病必须与新生儿其他形式的肝胆疾病相鉴别,特别是胆道闭锁[116]。该病常出现在出生后的最初几个月内,多达 80% 的患者有胆汁淤积性黄疸和无胆色便[117]。可能发生呕吐、易激惹和发育停滞。体格检查发现肝脏肿大,约半数患者可扪及腹部包块。在出生后诊断的 72 例患者中,50 例(69%)表现出黄疸,25 例与腹痛相关,3 例可触及腹部肿块;13 例(18%)仅表现为腹痛,2 例(3%)仅有可触及腹部肿块。在 2008 年的系列研究中,成年人以腹痛为主(97% vs 63%;$P<0.001$),儿童则以黄疸为主(71% vs 25%,$P=0.001$)[126]。在老年患者中,上腹痛可能是由于胰腺炎所致。反复发作的胆管炎可引起间歇性黄疸和发热。在不到 20% 的患者中观察到"腹痛、黄疸、可触及腹肿块"的典型三联征。

胆总管囊肿可发生自发性穿孔,特别是当胆汁流受阻时。由于胆汁引流不畅、胆泥、蛋白质栓、脂肪酸和钙组成的结石造成的胆道梗阻,由于胆道梗阻,在出生后的几个月内可发生进行性的肝脏损伤[127]。

5. 诊断

超声检查是胆总管畸形最佳的诊断手段(图 62.8)[45,128]。研究表明,产前超声可用于胎儿胆总管囊肿检测。妊娠期间连续超声检查可监测胆总管囊肿的演变。对于年龄较大的儿童,经皮肝穿胆管造影(PTC)或 ERCP 有助于确定胆总管囊肿的解剖特征,胆管病变起始部位(胆胰管汇流异常),肝内和肝外受累程度(胆管狭窄和结石)[128]。MRCP 检查用于评估胆管囊肿和畸形的程度,以及胆胰管汇流异常[129]。与 ERCP 相比,MRCP 对成人轻度胆管畸形、小的胆总管囊肿诊断效果较差[130]。在临床实践中,大多数小儿外科医生依赖术中胆管造影判断肝内和肝外受累的程度[117]。

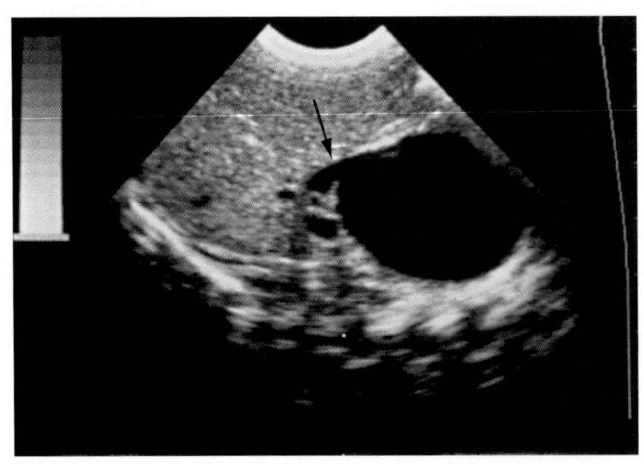

图 62.8　超声显示胆汁淤积婴儿的Ⅰ型胆总管囊肿。该横断扫描显示右上限可见一巨大囊性肿块。箭头所示为囊肿与胆管的连接点

6. 治疗

首选的治疗方法是手术切除囊肿并重建肝外胆道[117,119],腹腔镜手术在多数情况下是可行的。胆道引流通常采用胆管空肠 Roux-en-Y 吻合术完成。切除囊肿可减少胆汁淤积并降低胆管炎和胆管癌的风险。据报道,癌症的总体风险为 10%~15%,Ⅰ型和Ⅳ型风险最高,且随着年龄的增长而增加。只有在复杂的解剖结构不允许完全切除时,才应做单纯的减压内引流。长期随访至关重要,因为初次手术后数年可能发生复发性胆管炎、结石、吻合口狭窄和胰腺炎等。

(五) 肝纤维囊性疾病

肝纤维囊性疾病是一种罕见的先天性疾病,表现为肝内非阻塞性囊性或梭形胆管扩张[131,132]。在单纯形式中,称为 Caroli 病,扩张通常是节段性和囊状的,与结石形成和复发性细菌性胆管炎相关。最常见的一种类型为 Caroli 综合征,与先天性肝纤维化(CHF)典型的门管区病变有关[132-134]。也可能存在肝外胆管扩张(胆总管囊肿)。肾脏受累以两种形式发生,肾小管扩张伴 Caroli 病发生,这两种疾病均可与常染色体隐性遗传性多囊肾病(*ARPKD*)或罕见的常染色体显性遗传性多囊肾病相关。在 ARPKD 患者中发现了多囊肾和肝病 1 基因(*PKHD1*)的突变(见第 96 章)[136]。该基因编码一种被称为纤维蛋的大分子蛋白(4 074 个氨基酸),导致肝脏和肾脏中的主要结构异常。该蛋白与肝细胞生长因子受体具有相同的结构特征,似乎属于一个蛋白超家族,参与调节细胞增殖、黏附和排斥。纤维囊蛋白定位于肾上皮细胞和胆管细胞的初级纤毛上,提示纤毛功能障碍与囊肿发生有关。Joubert 综合征、Meckel-Gruber 综合征、Bardet-Biedel 综合征、Jeune 综合征和磷酸甘露糖苷酶缺乏症(一种先天性糖基化病)是影响初级纤毛结构或功能成分的其他罕见遗传疾病。可能与 CHF 相关。

1. 病理学

肝内囊肿与胆道相连,内衬可溃疡或过度增生的上皮[131]。囊肿内可含有浓缩的胆汁、结石和脓性物质。

肝活检标本可发现正常组织或急性或慢性胆管炎的特征。可能存在汇管区水肿和纤维化。在与 CHF 相关的病例中,可以预期与导管板畸形相关的结果,汇管区胆管管腔在中心血管化结缔组织核心周围形成一个上皮内衬的圆形裂隙,或一系列胆管管腔在中心周围呈圆形排列。

2. 临床特征

患者通常在儿童期和青春期因肝脏肿大和腹痛而就医[135,136]。这种疾病在新生儿中表现为肾脏疾病或胆汁淤积[136]。胆管的囊状或梭形扩张易导致胆汁淤积,从而形成胆泥和胆结石。细菌性胆管炎发作时可出现发热和间歇性黄疸。在与 CHF 相关的病例发现肝脾大,受累患者可因食管静脉曲张出血[131]。有时可触及多囊肾。

CHF 可能有几种形式。门静脉高压表现最常见于儿童时期的食管静脉曲张出血。胆管炎型表现为胆汁淤积和复发性胆管炎。混合型则同时具有门静脉高压和胆管炎的特征。胆道疾病可以非常隐匿,甚至是潜伏的,很难通过肝脏生化检测或影像学检查确定。

在一项 73 例 CHF 和 ARPKD 患者(年龄 1~56 岁,平均 12.7 岁)的前瞻性研究中,26 例患者在生命早期出现与肝脏相关的初始症状[133],60%的 5 岁以下儿童出现脾大。血小板计数是门静脉高压严重程度的最佳预测指标。70%的患者存在胆道异常(40%为 Caroli 综合征,30%为单纯性胆总管扩张)。肝脏和肾脏严重程度的变异性不能用特异性 PKHD1 突变来解释。在一篇对 ARPKD 肝脏并发症的综述中,根据文献汇编,788 例患者中 45%记录有门静脉高压,54%[1]记录有复发性胆管炎[34]。由于 CHF 中的胆道异常,即使在无 Caroli 综合征的情况下也可发生胆管炎。

肝生化检查结果可能正常,或血清胆红素、碱性磷酸酶和转氨酶水平轻度到中度升高[132-134]。肝脏合成功能良好不受影响,但囊性胆管内反复感染和胆道梗阻最终可导致肝衰竭。最大浓缩能力降低是最常见的肾功能异常检测结果,血尿素氮和血清肌酐水平的不同升高,反映了潜在肾脏疾病的严重程度[136]。

3. 诊断

超声、MRCP、CT 在显示肝内胆管囊性扩张有重要价值[133,137,138]。肝脏回声增强反映了该疾病的基础纤维化。可探及肾囊肿或肾乳头强回声。经皮或内镜下胆管造影(图 62.9)通常显示正常胆管伴节段性囊性肝内胆管扩张[139]。在罕见情况下,该过程可能仅限于肝脏的一个叶。诊断 CHF 很少需要肝活检。

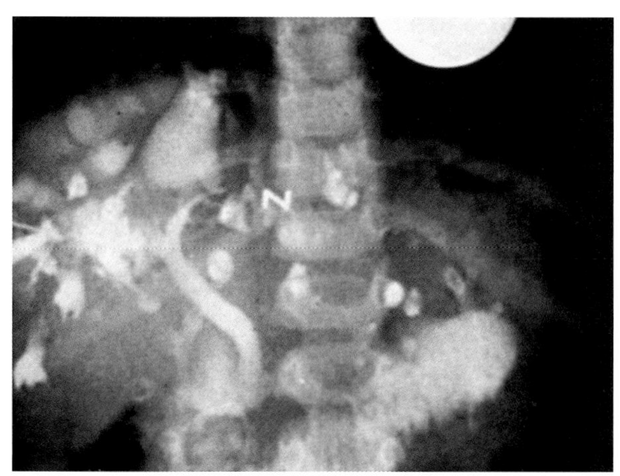

图 62.9 Caroli 病的胆管造影表现。经皮胆管造影术显示整个明显增大的肝脏有多个囊性病变。囊性病变与胆管连接。肝外胆管正常。(From Kocoshis SA, Riely CA, Burrell M, Gryboski JD. Cholangitis in a child due to biliary tract anomalies. Dig Dis Sci 1980;25:59-65.)

4. 预后和治疗

临床病程常并发胆管炎反复发作[136,139],可发生败血症和肝脓肿。在持续性或反复性感染的情况下,预后较差。结石常发生在囊性扩张的胆管内,可使胆管炎的治疗复杂化。广泛肝内胆管结石患者可出现顽固性腹痛。通过手术、内镜或碎石术取石结石通常是不可行的。肝部分切除术适用于局限于单叶的疾病[140]。单纯手术引流通常无效,可能使后期肝移植复杂化。UDCA 治疗已成功用于溶解肝内胆管结石。在异常胆管内可发生胆管癌[141]。在 CHF 和 Caroli 病患者中,门静脉高压和静脉曲张出血可能占主导地位[136]。在一些伴有多囊肾的患者中,会发生终末期肾病。对于有广泛疾病和常见并发症(如难治性胆管炎)的患者,肝移植是一种选择[142]。

(六) 非综合征性小叶间胆管缺乏

小叶间胆管的缺乏可能是特发性胆汁淤积婴儿和儿童中的孤立和无法解释的结果,也可能是一组异质性疾病的特征,包括风疹和巨细胞病毒的先天性感染以及遗传疾病,如 α_1-抗胰蛋白酶缺乏和先天性胆汁酸代谢异常[143,144]。在 Williams 综合征和 Noonan 综合征的一些病例中也存在胆管缺乏[145,146]。小叶间胆管缺乏的定义为小叶间胆管数量与汇管区数量的比值小于 0.4[10,147]。应在肝活检标本上检查至少 10 个汇管区,以确保存在小叶间胆管缺乏。这种结构异常也被称为“肝内胆管闭锁”或“肝内胆管发育不全”,然而,这些术语意味着比目前更深入地了解胆管缺乏的发病机制。病例可能来自真正的胆管发育不全,但更多的是由于活动性损伤和胆管丧失所致[10,147]。胆管缺乏的发生可能没有相关的其他发育异常,也没有记录的宫内感染或遗传疾病,但这种特发性的非综合征性小叶间胆管缺乏的病因可能是异质性的,具有极其多变的临床特征和预后[144]。胆汁淤积通常在婴儿早期发生,可能与进行性肝病有关。

新生儿期以后发生的胆管缺乏常被称为胆管消失综合征。肝脏损伤可能是进行性的,导致死亡或肝移植。这种疾病的病因具有异质性,包括感染、缺血、药物不良反应、自身免疫性疾病、同种异体排斥和恶性肿瘤。阿莫西林-克拉维酸和甲氧苄啶/磺胺甲噁唑是与胆管消失综合征相关的药物(见第 88 章)[148]。

(七) 综合征性小叶间胆管缺乏

综合征性小叶间胆管缺乏(Alagille 综合征或肝动脉发育不良)是家族性肝内胆汁淤积症中最常见的一种,这种疾病的特征是以慢性胆汁淤积、小叶间胆管数量减少和各种其他先天性畸形为特征[149,150]。

1. 病因学

家系研究已经建立了具有不完全外显率和可变表达率的常染色体显性传播方式[151]。在一些患者中检测到 20 号染色体短臂的部分缺失,并导致 Alagille 综合征基因的鉴定。在大约 94%的受累者中发现了 *jagged1*(*JAG1*)基因突变,包括总基因缺失以及蛋白截断、剪接和错义突变[152]。*JAG1* 编码 Notch 信号通路中的配体,参与发育过程中细胞命运的决定[153]。在 *JAG1* 突变阴性的 Alagille 综合征患者中,发现了编码 Notch2 受体基因的突变[154]。与 *JAG1* 突变患者相似,Notch2 受体基因突变患者表现出受累系统高度可变的表达性,但通常患有肝脏疾病。编码血小板反应蛋白 2 的 *THBS2* 已在全基因组关联研究中被确定为严重肝脏疾病的候选遗传修饰因子。血小板反应蛋白 2 在小鼠肝脏的胆管和汇管区表达,并影响 Jag-Notch 信号通路[155]。

JAG1 全基因缺失的患者和基因内突变的患者之间似乎没有表型差异。该疾病可能仅影响一个家族成员,此类疾病可能代表 JAG1 基因的自发突变。另外,基因表达的变异性可能很大,以至于受影响最小的家庭成员没有被诊断出来。1994 年对 43 位先证者收集的 33 个家系进行分析,证实了 Alagille 综合征为常染色体显性遗传,认为外显率为 94%,15% 的病例为散发的,但表达性各不相同,26 人(包括 11 个同胞兄弟姐妹)病情较轻[156]。

2. 病理学

小叶间胆管缺乏是本病的特征性改变,即小叶间胆管数量与汇管区数之比显著降低(<0.4)[148]。出生后前几个月的组织学特征可能与新生儿肝炎的组织学特征重叠,均表现为肝细胞气球样变、可变的胆汁淤积、门脉区炎症和巨细胞转化。通常,在初始肝活检标本中,小叶间胆管的数量不会减少,但胆管损伤可能明显,包括与小叶间胆管相连的汇管区细胞浸润、胆管上皮淋巴细胞浸润和核固缩以及胆管周围纤维化表现。个体患者的连续活检标本最初可显示胆管增生,随后在生命后期出现胆管缺乏(图 62.10)[157]。小叶间胆管缺乏通常在 3 个月后明显,也可能存在轻度门静脉周围纤维化,但进展为肝硬化并不常见。肝外胆管通畅,但通常伴狭窄或发育不良。超微结构研究证明,胆色素在高尔基体外凸间隙溶酶体和囊泡附近的细胞质中积聚。胆小管的结构通常正常,但在某些情况下,也可能表现为扩张,微绒毛变钝和缩短。

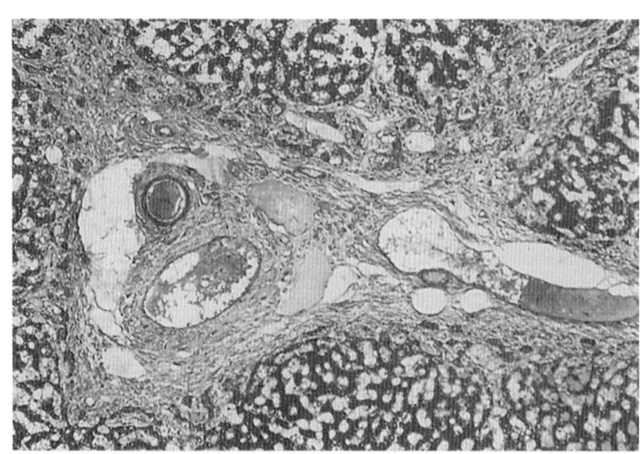

图 62.10 综合征性小叶间胆管缺乏(Alagille)的组织学特征。在低倍显微镜照片中显示肝脏的门脉三联征,有明显的肝动脉和静脉,但没有胆管(Masson 三色染色)。(From Portmann BC, Roberts EA. Developmental abnormalities and liver disease in childhood. In: Burt AD, Portmann BC, Ferrell LD, editors. MacSween's pathology of the liver. 6th ed. London: Churchill Livingstone Elsevier; 2012. p 121.)

3. 发病机制

有关胆管缺乏和胆汁淤积的发病机制尚不清楚,肝胆疾病如何与在其他器官系统中发现的多种先天性异常相关也是未知的。Jag1 突变纯合子小鼠在胚胎形成早期死于出血,并表现出胚胎和卵黄血管重塑缺陷[158]。人胚胎发育期间 JAG1 在血管系统和其他间充质和上皮组织中的强表达,提示异常血管生成与 Alagille 综合征的发病机制有关,特别是小叶间胆管缺乏。在人类胚胎中,JAG1 在远端心脏流出道和肺动脉、大动脉、门静脉、视泡、耳囊泡、鳃弓、后肾、胰腺和心系膜;主要支气管分支周围;以及神经管中表达[159]。所有这些结构在 Alagille 综合征中均受累。许多 JAG1 突变产生提前终止密码子,其中许多突变产生截短的蛋白,对 Notch 信号发挥结构域负面影响[160]。尽管 Alagille 综合征异常的血管基础似乎是可能的,但导致胆管缺乏的确切机制仍不清楚。Notch 信号在胆管上皮细胞的分化中具有重要作用,并在肝内胆管发育过程中对其小管的形成至关重要[161]。有证据表明,出生后肝脏生长过程中胆管缺乏分支和延长,导致外周胆管缺乏和胆汁淤积[162]。

值得注意的是,这种疾病在新生儿期可发生严重的胆汁淤积,即使小叶间胆管的数量不减少。相反,在生命后期,当根据临床和生化标准判断胆汁淤积可能不太严重时,肝活检标本上可能无法检测到小叶间胆管。

4. 临床特征

95% 的患者存在不同程度的慢性胆汁淤积[151,163]。在新生儿期可观察到黄疸和白陶土样大便,多数在 2 岁内即变得很显著,强烈瘙痒一般在 6 个月大时出现[149]。肝和脾常肿大。出生后几年内可在手指伸肌表面、掌纹和腘窝处发现黄色瘤。婴幼儿期即可发现畸形面容(图 62.11),并随着年龄的增长而变得更加典型[150]。前额宽大,眼窝深陷且间距很大,下颌骨小而尖,使脸部呈现三角形样外观,同时颧骨低平,耳朵突出。Alagille 综合征伴有多种表型的肝外异常。1999 年汇总的 92 例病例分析显示,胆汁淤积发生率为 96%,心脏杂音发生率为 97%,蝶形椎发生率为 51%,后胚胎环(虹膜和角膜中胚层发育不全)发生率为 78%,特征性面容发生率为 96%[163]。身材矮小是一个常见的特征,但慢性胆汁淤积的严重程度只是一部分原因。血中生长激素结合蛋白水平升高,使这些患者对生长激素不敏感[164]。15%~20% 患者存在轻至中度智力障碍。大多数患者有先天性心脏病,外周肺动脉狭窄发生率约 90%[163,165]。全身血管多发畸形,且血管畸形与颅内出血风险相关。骨异常包括骨龄减小、远节指(趾)骨变短和椎弓缺陷(如蝶状椎体、半椎体、椎根间距变小)。眼科检查可发现眼部异常,包括后胚胎环、视网膜色素沉着和

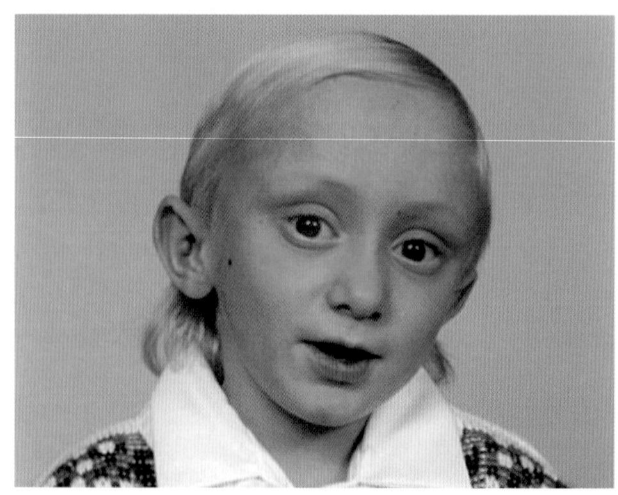

图 62.11 综合征性小叶间胆管缺乏的面部外观。(Photograph courtesy Dr. Binita Kamath, Philadelphia, PA.)

虹膜束。肾异常和性腺功能减退也有报道[151,164]。

血总胆红素水平(通常为 2~8mg/dL)在婴儿期升高,其后呈间歇性升高[163,166],结合胆红素约占 50%。血清碱性磷酸酶、GGTP 和 5'-核苷酸酶水平可显著升高,一定程度上与胆汁淤积程度相对应。血清转氨酶水平轻度至中度升高。血清胆固醇水平在 200mg/dL 或更高,甘油三酯在 500~1 000mg/dL 之间。血清总胆汁酸浓度显著升高,但血清、尿液和胆汁中的胆汁酸谱与其他胆汁淤积性疾病没有本质区别。

5. 预后和治疗

临床病程以不同程度的胆汁淤积为特征,有时因并发病毒感染使病情恶化。瘙痒、皮肤黄色瘤和与维生素 E 缺乏有关的神经肌肉症状可导致发病。治疗包括提供足够的热量摄入,预防或纠正脂溶性维生素缺乏,以及缓解瘙痒的对症措施(见第 21 和 91 章)。长期预后取决于肝脏疾病和相关畸形的严重程度[165]。Alagille 课题组长期随访结果显示,80 例该病患者中有 21 例死亡,但仅 4 例死于肝病[149]。部分胆道外分流术可有效治疗药物治疗无效的无肝硬化患者的严重瘙痒和高胆固醇血症[167,168]。在另一项 92 例患者系列中,死亡率为 17%[163]。显著增加死亡率的因素包括肝脏疾病或肝移植(25%)、复杂的先天性心脏病(15%)和颅内出血(25%)。本病可发展至肝癌[169]。5 岁以下儿童血清总胆红素水平高于 6.5mg/dL、结合胆红素高于 4.5mg/dL、胆固醇高于 520mg/dL,提示很可能与远期严重肝病有关[170]。在一项对 268 例患者的回顾性综述中,血管异常(如颅内动脉瘤)占死亡率的 34%[171]。基于这些研究,所有患者的 20 年预期寿命为 75%,不需要肝移植的患者约为 80%,需要肝移植的患者约为 60%。在一项 168 例肝病患者的研究中,10 年和 20 年时,自体而非移植肝患者的精算生存率分别为 51% 和 38%,总生存率分别为 68% 和 62%[172]。新生儿胆汁淤积性黄疸与自体肝脏的存活率较相关。肝移植的生存率和候选者可能受到相关心血管异常严重程度的限制。在 UNOS 数据库中因 Alagille 综合征移植的 467 例儿童中,Alagille 综合征患者的 1 年和 5 年生存率显著低于胆道闭锁患者(分别为 82.9% 和 78.4% vs 89.9% 和 84%)。Alagille 综合征患者死于移植物衰竭、神经系统疾病和心脏并发症的发生率显著高于胆道闭锁患者[173,174]。

(八) 原发性硬化性胆管炎

原发性硬化性胆管炎(PSC)是一种罕见的进行性胆道疾病,以肝内和肝外胆管系统炎症和纤维化为特征,最终导致胆汁性肝硬化[175,176]。流行病学研究报告北美儿童的 PSC 患病率为 15 例/100 万儿童[177]。这里仅讨论对婴幼儿和儿童特别重要的 PSC 方面(PSC 的详细讨论见第 68 章)。

PSC 是一种病理过程,发生在无胆总管结石或胆管手术史的情况下。硬化性胆管炎在新生儿期可能不常见,随后可能出现在自身免疫(PSC)特征,通常与炎症性肠病(IBD)有关,也可能与其他疾病有关,包括朗格汉斯细胞组织细胞增多症、免疫缺陷、银屑病和 CF(称为继发性硬化性胆管炎的病因)。在成人中,还必须排除胆管癌,然而在儿童中很少报告该并发症。一项对 781 名 PSC 患儿的多中心分析显示,61% 为男性,76% 患有 IBD,33% 与自身免疫性肝炎重叠,13% 患有小胆管 PSC。发病 10 年后发生门静脉高压和胆道并发症者分别占 38% 和 25%[178]。

在新生儿期有 PSC 发病的报道[179],在这种情况下,在出生后 2 周内可观察到胆汁淤积性黄疸和无胆色便。其表现特征与肝外胆道闭锁几乎相同,但经皮胆道造影显示胆道系统通畅,肝段分支稀疏、狭窄和肝内胆管局灶性扩张。可能累及肝外胆管。黄疸在 6 个月内自行消退,但在儿童期以后,所有患者均具有胆汁性肝硬化和门静脉高压症一致的临床和生化特征[179]。与成人和年长儿的 PSC 不同,新生儿的 PSC 与肠道疾病无关。

新生儿鱼鳞病和硬化性胆管炎是一种独特的综合征,由编码紧密连接蛋白 claudin-1 的 CLDN1 基因突变引起。在这种疾病中,胆汁淤积被认为是由于 claudin-1 的缺失,导致细胞旁通透性增加和继发于细胞旁胆汁反流引起的胆管损伤[180]。肝脏疾病的严重程度差异很大[181]。UDCA 治疗可能有益,并可能延缓疾病的进展。肝移植不影响疾病的皮肤病表现,但可作为进展期肝病的备用治疗措施。

IBD 相关 PSC 通常发生在 UC 患者中[178,]但在克罗恩病患者中已有病例报道。肠道症状可在 PSC 诊断前出现,与 PSC 同时出现,或在 PSC 诊断后数年出现。与成人相同,肠道疾病的治疗(包括结肠切除术),并不影响 PSC 的进展。乳糜泻也与 PSC 相关[182]。

经胆管造影证实,朗格汉斯细胞组织细胞增生症中可出现与 PSC 相似的病变,这一过程是由于组织细胞浸润和汇管区进行性瘢痕形成引起的,导致肝内胆管扭曲变形。胆汁淤积可发生在朗格汉斯细胞组织细胞增多症的诊断之前,但多数是在诊断之后才被发现[183]。儿童朗格汉斯细胞组织细胞增多症可累及多个器官,包括尿崩症、骨病变、皮肤病变、淋巴结病和突眼。化疗不影响胆道疾病的进程。在一些进展为终末期肝病的儿童中,肝移植已获得成功[184]。

硬化性胆管炎似乎发生在一些具有各种细胞和体液免疫缺陷的儿童中。隐孢子虫和巨细胞病毒同时存在于其中一些患者的胆道中,以及 AIDS 成人中(见第 35 章)[185]。相关感染的治疗尚未证实对胆道疾病的影响。

免疫球蛋白 IgG4 相关硬化性胆管炎伴有血清 IgG4 水平升高,是一种多系统纤维炎性疾病的胆道表现,其中受累器官具有 IgG4 阳性细胞的特征性淋巴浆细胞浸润(见第 68 章)。在儿童中罕有报道,通常与自身免疫性胰腺炎有关(见第 59 章)。与 PSC 相反,该病与 IBD 无关,通常表现为梗阻性黄疸,对糖皮质激素治疗有反应[186]。

通常,成人 PSC 患者表现出乏力、体重减轻、瘙痒、右上腹疼痛和间歇性黄疸。在儿童中,临床表现变化较大,最常见的症状是腹痛、黄疸和嗜睡[176,177]。体格检查有时发现肝肿大,可伴有脾大、结膜黄疸,罕见腹水。

PSC 没有明确的诊断试验,诊断是基于生化、组织学和影像学数据的综合[182]。PSC 患儿血清碱性磷酸酶和 GGTP 水平常升高,血清转氨酶水平仅轻度升高[187,178]。不到一半的儿童患者出现高胆红素血症。一些患者中可能发现血清自身抗体,包括抗核抗体和平滑肌抗体[187]。三分之二患儿可检出具有核周荧光的非典型 ANCA。由于 CF 的胆道表现与 PSC 相似,因此应考虑 CFTR 基因突变的基因检测(见第 57 章)。

在肝活检标本中，组织学结果可能提示 PSC，但通常不具有诊断价值。在疾病后期可能出现特征性的同心圆导管周围（"洋葱皮"）纤维化，但通常仅发现新生导管增殖和纤维化[188]。

鉴别 PSC 与自身免疫性肝炎可能有困难，特别是肝活检标本中存在循环非器官特异性自身抗体和存在肝脏疾病特征的情况下。在 25%～30% 的病例中儿童可发生重叠综合征，同时伴有肝和胆汁淤积的血清肝脏生化检查结果，以及自身免疫性肝炎和 PSC 的组织学特征（见第 90 章）[175]。血清学表现包括 ANA、平滑肌抗体、抗肝肾微粒体 1 型抗体和核周 ANCA 的存在[189]。

PSC 的诊断是通过胆管造影确定的[190]。MRCP 是肝内和肝外胆管可视化的首选检查方法，与 ERCP 检查结果相当，且侵入性显著低于 ERCP[190]。可发现肝内和肝外胆管形态的不规则，包括交替狭窄和产生串珠状外观的扩张区域。在新生儿期后出现症状的患者中，肝内胆管受累占主导地位。偶尔可见导管外显性狭窄或乳头狭窄。胆管造影正常的小管 PSC，有 10%～15% 的儿童出现 PSC 的组织学特征[178,191]。

儿童 PSC 的预后有待观察。疾病的临床过程多变，但通常是进行性的[176,178]。在 1994 年对 56 名患儿系列的研究中，从出现症状开始的中位生存期大约为 10 年，与成人报告的结果相似[192]。在另一项 52 名儿童的研究中，无肝移植者的中位生存期为 12.7 年[176]。对发病前生存因素的分析表明，年龄较大、脾大和凝血酶原时间延长提示预后不良[193]。也可发生肝细胞癌，但成人 PSC 的重要并发症胆管癌在儿童中很少有报道[178]。

儿童 PSC 的治疗效果不理想[194]。没有对照试验令人信服地表明任何药物治疗可改善 PSC 组织学特征并延长其生存期。在成人和儿童中，应用 UDCA 治疗可改善临床症状和肝脏生化检查异常，但尚未证实治疗对生存期的长期获益，且高剂量对成年 PSC 患者有害[177,194]。在有限的研究中，口服万古霉素对儿童伴发的 PSC 和 IBD 是一种有效的治疗方法，可能与其作为抗生素的作用及其免疫调节特性有关[195]。可能需要对胆管显性狭窄进行内镜扩张治疗。

对于进展为终末期肝病、复发性细菌性胆管炎或难治性瘙痒的患者，肝移植是一种重要的选择。儿童的长期结果似乎与因其他适应证接受移植的年龄匹配的儿童相当，移植后远期效果无明显差别[196]。10%～27% 的 PSC 患者移植后复发[176,196]。

（九）慢性胆汁淤积

胆汁淤积性肝病对儿童的营养状况、生长和发育产生不利影响，最终影响发病率和死亡率。对于患有慢性（有时是进行性）胆汁淤积性肝病的儿童，治疗重点是促进生长发育，尽量减少不适[197]。

60% 慢性肝病的儿童无法避免出现蛋白质-能量营养不良导致的生长障碍[197-199]。胆汁淤积儿童常出现脂肪泻，是由于长链甘油三酯的脂肪降解、溶解和肠道吸收受损所致。中链甘油三酯在肠道吸收前不需要胆汁酸盐的溶解，因此，商业配方以口服形式提供能量或补充油脂。

胆汁淤积患儿脂溶性维生素缺乏引起的疾病多数可以预防[200]。因为易于给药和预期有效，在胆道闭锁婴儿中进行了聚乙二醇 1000-多种脂溶性维生素混合液性制剂能否促进吸收的前瞻性研究。然而，尽管口服该制剂，胆道闭锁和持续性胆汁淤积的婴儿化验仍提示脂溶性维生素不足。对于胆道闭锁特别是血清总胆红素水平大于 2.0mg/dL 的婴儿，需要单独补充相应维生素并严密监测[201]。

由于维生素 D 缺乏可引起代谢性骨病（佝偻病和病理性骨折），每天必须供给充足的维生素 D_2（5 000IU/d）或 25-羟维生素 D_3［3～5μg/(kg·d)］。还可能需要补充元素钙［50～100mg/(kg·d)］和磷［25～50mg/(kg·d)］。即使血 25-羟维生素 D 水平正常，胆汁淤积患儿仍存在骨矿质量减少，可能与肝脏胰岛素样生长因子-1 生成不足有关[202]。

缺乏维生素 A 的患者可出现干眼症、夜盲症和皮肤增厚。需要口服维生素 A 补充剂，每天 5 000～25 000 国际单位[200]。

维生素 K 缺乏和相关的凝血异常可以通过口服水溶性维生素 K 治疗，剂量为每次 2.5～5mg，每周两次，最多每天 5mg。口服无反应或出血严重的患儿需要肌注维生素 K（参见第 94 章）[203]。

慢性维生素 E 缺乏可能产生一种致残性退行性神经肌肉综合征，其特征为反射消失、眼肌麻痹、小脑共济失调、周围神经病变和脊髓后角功能异常[200]。2 岁内即可发病。由于高脂血症患者的血清维生素 E 水平可能会假性升高，因此血维生素 E 与血脂的比值对于患者维生素 E 含量的评估更为准确。例如小于 12 岁以下儿童维生素 E 缺乏的标准是比值小于 0.6。儿童可能对大剂量的标准维生素 E 制剂［150～200IU/(kg·d)］无反应。肌内注射 *dl*-α-维生素 E（50mg/d）或水溶性维生素 E 制剂，聚乙二醇 1000 维生素 E 琥珀酸酯［15～25IU/(kg·d)］是有效的[200]。

黄色瘤和瘙痒也可引起很明显的不适。3 月龄时可出现瘙痒[204]。大多数瘙痒症治疗的成功取决于胆管是否通畅，使胆汁酸和其他胆汁成分能够进入肠腔。胆道转流手术已被成功地用于减轻肝内胆汁淤积患者的顽固性瘙痒[204,205]。抗生素利福平通过上调生物转化和胆汁排泄途径，以及利胆剂 UDCA 已被用于治疗瘙痒，并取得了不同程度的成功[206-208]。有证据表明阿片受体介导的中枢源性起源参与瘙痒的发生，阿片受体拮抗剂如纳曲酮对一些其他药物治疗无效的严重瘙痒患者有效。但是药物副作用、戒断症状和缺乏儿童用药经验限制了这些药物的普遍应用。不可吸收的阴离子交换树脂考来烯胺可结合肠腔中的胆汁酸、胆固醇和其他潜在的毒性物质[206-208]。考来烯胺可降低血脂水平，并结合与瘙痒发病机制有关的物质，早餐前或餐前分次给药 0.25～0.5g/(kg·d)，可以缓解严重瘙痒和黄色瘤[204]。但是考来烯胺口感很差，药物浓缩后可能引起肠梗阻，还可导致高氯血症酸中毒。一种新型的胆汁酸螯合剂考来维伦[209]，其胆汁酸结合效果优于考来烯胺，且口感更好，但它在胆汁淤积性肝病中的应用受到限制（见第 64 和 91 章）。皮肤瘙痒也可采用紫外线 B 光治疗。

六、小儿胆囊疾病

（一）胆石症

1. 流行病学

胆石症在健康儿童中并不常见，通常发生在有诱发条件的患者中[210-213]。对 1 570 人(年龄 6~19 岁)的超声检查调查中,仅在 2 例女性受检者中检查出胆囊结石,年龄为 13 岁和 18 岁[214,215]。研究人群中无人接受过胆囊切除术。胆石症的总患病率为 0.13%(女性为 0.27%)。多数病例是在接近青春期时发病,但胆结石在任何年龄都有报道,包括胎儿期。婴幼儿和儿童以色素性胆结石为主。与胆石症风险增加的病症见表 62.2。对 2 项包含 605 例儿童患者的大系列数据的综合分析提供了信息[216,217],53%的患者报告了症状,18%的患者出现了并发症(如胰腺炎、胆总管结石、急性结石性胆囊炎)作为胆石症的首发指征。在 60%患者中可确定基础疾病和风险因素[216,217]。肥胖作为儿童胆石症的风险因素发挥着越来越重要的作用[218]。

表 62.2 儿童胆石症发生的危险因素

危险因素	举例
溶血性疾病	遗传性球形红细胞增多症
	镰状细胞病
	地中海贫血
新生儿或先天性疾病	胆总管囊肿
	坏死性小肠结肠炎
	肠外营养
	早产儿
遗传性疾病	*ABCB4* 突变(MDR3 缺陷)
	ABCB11 突变
	ABCG5/G8 突变
	囊性纤维化(CF)
	Gilbert 综合征
	21 三体
营养状况	胰岛素抵抗
	肥胖
系统性疾病	克罗恩病
	肝病和肝硬化
	脓毒症
药物	头孢菌素
	利尿剂
外科手术	心脏手术(体外循环溶血)
	回肠切除术
	新生儿肠切除术
其他	胆管运动障碍
	癌或白血病治疗

ABC,ATP 结合盒;MDR,多重耐药。

Modified from Svensson J, Makin E. Gallstone disease in children. Semin Pediatr Surg 2012;21:255-65.

2. 发病机制

对胆结石发病机制的深入讨论见第 65 章,在婴儿和儿童期某些因素可能具有更大的重要性[213,219]。据报道,患有结石性胆囊炎的早产儿发病率增加,这些早产儿通常经历一段长时间的禁食,而不能频繁刺激胆囊收缩,并且需要长时间的胃肠外营养。其中许多患者的医疗过程复杂,包括频繁输血、败血症发生、腹部手术、利尿剂和麻醉性镇痛药的使用。在这种情况下,对胆结石的有限分析通常显示,存在混合性胆固醇-胆红素钙结石。在危重婴儿中,从常见的胆囊增大、膨胀、充满胆泥到最终发生胆石症,可能存在一个连续统一体。与成人一样,患有疾病或既往切除回肠末端的儿童胆结石的发病率增加。在 2007 年的一个系列研究中,30 例患有胆结石的儿童中有 24%有碳酸钙结石,而碳酸钙结石以前被认为是罕见的[220]。

黑色素胆结石通常见于慢性溶血性疾病患者[221]。这些结石主要由胆红素钙组成,含有大量结晶性碳酸钙和磷酸盐。在镰状细胞病中,胆结石的风险随着年龄的增长而增加,至少 14%的 10 岁以下儿童和 36%的 10~20 岁儿童会发生胆结石(见第 37 章)[222]。作为 Gilbert 综合征(一种慢性非结合型高胆红素血症)基础的尿苷二磷酸葡萄糖醛酸转移酶 1A1(*UGT1A1*)基因启动子的多态性(见第 21 章)似乎是一个主要的遗传风险因素,其增加了镰状细胞病患者胆结石的发生频率,并导致其胆结石发病年龄提前[223]。

导致儿童胆石症的遗传因素目前尚未明确。编码胆汁胆固醇转运蛋白 ATP 结合盒(ABC)G5/G8 和磷脂转运蛋白(*ABCB4*)的基因多态性仅限于成人胆石症(见第 65 章)。核受体亚家族 1,H 组,成员 4(*NR1H4*)基因,编码核胆盐受体法尼醇(farnesoid)X 受体,是胆固醇胆石易感性的另一个候选基因。低磷脂相关胆石症的发生与 *ABCB4* 突变(多重耐药 3 缺陷)和导致症状性和复发性胆石症的低胆汁磷脂浓度相关。患者可表现为肝内胆管结石、胆泥或沿胆道的微结石[224]。

婴儿梗阻性黄疸也可由褐色色素胆石症引起[225,226]。褐色色素结石由不同比例的胆红素钙、磷酸钙、棕榈酸钙、胆固醇和有机物质组成。非结合胆红素在总胆色素中占很大比例。在一些情况下,胆汁具有较高的 β-葡萄糖醛酸酶活性,并且在培养物中生长了大量的多种细菌。据推测,色素性胆结石是在这些胆道细菌感染的婴儿中自发形成的。

没有明确胆石症病因的患者更可能是女性、老年人和肥胖者,有胆囊疾病家族史,出现成人样症状的可能性更大。493 例肥胖儿童中有 10 例检出胆囊结石(2%;女孩 8 例,男孩 2 例)[227]。这些患者以胆固醇性胆结石为主。通过对皮马印第安人的仔细研究,人们对胆结石的发病机制有了深入的了解。皮马印第安人胆固醇性胆结石的发病率极高。在 13 岁以下的皮马印第安人中尚未检测到高度饱和的胆汁,但在青春期生长发育过程中,两种性别的胆汁饱和度均显著增加[228]。在该人群中,胆汁酸池大小的性别相关差异开始于青春期,随着年龄的增长,年轻男性表现出胆汁酸池的大小显著增加,而年轻女性仅表现出轻微增加。由于胆固醇性胆结石与较小的胆汁酸池相关,因此,胆汁酸池大小在两性之间的差异也可能是胆固醇性胆结石发病率在青春期开始出现性别相关差异的原因。

长期使用大剂量头孢曲松(第三代头孢菌素),与胆囊内钙-头孢曲松盐沉淀物的形成有关,这一过程也称为胆道假性结石，在接受该药物治疗严重感染的患儿中，有 30%～40% 可出现这种情况[229]。患者可主诉腹痛，并表现出肝内胆汁淤积的体征。超声检查可见胆汁污泥和胆囊沉淀物。该问题通常在停药后自行消退。

3. 临床特征

胆结石以发生在胆囊中为主，儿童胆管结石的发病率低于成人，且多数患者无明显症状。一般是在检查其他问题或具有胆石症高风相关因素进行筛查时发现的[213]。患者可主诉不同严重程度的间歇性腹痛，在年长儿中疼痛可能局限于右上腹，而婴儿定位不明确。体格检查一般无明显异常。右上腹压痛提示胆囊炎，如结石移位至胆囊颈部并阻塞胆囊管时发生胆囊炎。婴儿可能表现出烦躁不安易怒、胆汁淤积性黄疸和无胆色粪便[213]。

肝脏生化检查一般正常[213]。腹部平片可显示结石，取决于结石的钙含量。超声检查被认为是胆结石最敏感和最特异的影像学诊断方法。肝胆闪烁显像是一种有价值的辅助手段，胆囊不显影提示了急性胆囊炎的证据（见后文）。

4. 治疗

有症状或胆囊无功能的患者，胆囊切除术仍是首选的治疗方案[213]。儿童和 10 个月以上婴儿可采用腹腔镜胆囊切除术[230]。基于临床表现和术中情况，必要时可行术中胆管造影和胆管探查。在年龄较大的儿童和青少年，如果腹腔镜胆囊切除术前明确诊断胆总管结石，则应在术前先完善内镜下括约肌切开术和取石。

无症状且没有生化异常（“隐性结石”）的结石，治疗更为困难。流行病学调查和成人胆结石放射性碳年代测定显示，胆结石形成至出现症状之间有超过十年的时间[231]。对于有溶血或回肠疾病等合并疾病的患者，胆囊切除术可与其他外科手术同时进行。为了预防胆囊炎和胆总管结石等并发症的发生，慢性溶血性贫血和无症状胆石症患儿常规接受腹腔镜胆囊切除术[232]。合并肝病、严重肥胖、囊性纤维化患儿胆囊切除术手术风险大，是否手术需依据临床情况决定。在这种情况下，患者应该被告知疾病的性质和可能发生的症状。在婴儿中有胆石症甚至胆总管结石自发性消退的报道。在一项超声随访研究中，有症状的儿童中有 16.5% 的胆结石消失，婴儿中有 34.1% 的胆结石消失[216]。此外，婴儿结石很少复发，因此胆囊切除术不是必需的。但是，梗阻性胆汁淤积患儿有出现脓毒症和胆管炎的风险，必须行胆囊切除术[213]。

儿童可能出现胆道微结石及相关的临床症状，其胆道影像学检查通常正常。超声内镜检查可发现胆囊微结石。腹腔镜胆囊切除术基本可治愈[233]。

儿童胆结石替代治疗（例如，口服胆汁酸制剂溶石治疗，冲击波碎石术）的经验有限。UDCA 对胆色素结石为主的效果有限，但对多重耐药 3 基因缺陷的患者有意义[224]。UDCA 对 10 例囊性纤维化患儿的 X 线阳性结石治疗无效[234]。

（二）结石性胆囊炎

胆石症可能与急性或慢性胆囊炎有关（见第 65 章）[210,211,213]。急性胆囊炎常因结石嵌顿在胆囊管内而引起。继发于胆汁引流不畅，液体积聚的胆囊内压力进行性升高、结石的存在和胆汁酸的化学刺激作用可导致进行性炎症、充血和血管损伤，甚至可发生胆囊梗死、坏疽和穿孔。梗阻的胆囊腔内细菌增殖可促成该这过程，导致胆源性败血症。

慢性结石性胆囊炎比急性胆囊炎多见，可以隐匿发生，也可在急性胆囊炎数次发作后发生。胆囊上皮通常会出现溃疡和瘢痕。

1. 临床特征

急性发作的右上腹痛是急性胆囊炎的主要症状[235]，婴儿疼痛定位不明显，可伴有恶心和呕吐。儿童黄疸发生率高于成人（50%）。起病急骤，可出现呼吸变浅和发热，特别是合并细菌感染时。右上腹压痛、反跳痛多阳性，Murphy 氏征可阳性。

慢性胆囊炎起病时腹痛多不明显，主要表现为反复发作的上腹部不适。年龄较大的患儿可表现出不能耐受高脂肪食物。64% 不伴有胆囊或胆管梗阻的胆石症儿童可出现右上腹痛，可能主要是慢性胆囊炎引起。体格检查可正常或呈胆囊区压痛，Murphy 征阳性。

急性胆囊炎时白细胞计数多升高，以中性粒细胞升高为主[213]。血清胆红素和碱性磷酸酶水平可能升高。血清转氨酶水平可正常，升高时提示肝细胞损伤，可发生在急性胆总管梗阻早期。

在慢性胆囊炎患者中，全血细胞计数和肝脏生化检查一般均正常。当出现急性或慢性的临床症状时，腹部平片可发现右上腹的钙化灶[213]。腹部超声检查对诊断胆囊结石非常有价值，可显示胆囊壁增厚，还可能显示继发于胆囊结石移位引起的胆管阻塞导致的胆道扩张。MRCP 可显示相似的结果，但通常婴儿和幼儿需要在全身麻醉下进行[236]。在急性病患者中很少需要肝胆闪烁显像，但在评估慢性胆囊炎患者的胆囊功能障碍方面可能有价值。

2. 治疗

急性炎症期患者需应用静脉补液、镇痛药和广谱抗生素。一旦容量不足得到纠正，感染控制后应尽早行胆囊切除术[237]。高风险患者急性炎症期可尝试经皮经肝胆囊穿刺引流，外科手术结果好（参见第 66 章）。术中需行胆管造影以除外胆总管结石，必要时可行胆总管探查。儿童胆囊切除术时行腹腔镜胆管探查术治疗胆总管结石非常安全，多数患者胆管结石均可清除[238]。

胆囊切除术也是治疗慢性结石性胆囊炎的首选方法，腹腔镜下胆囊切除术适用于多数患者[239,240]。

（三）非结石性胆囊炎

非结石性胆囊炎是一种无胆结石的急性胆囊炎症（见第 67 章）[241]。儿童中并不常见，与感染或严重的全身疾病有关。病原体包括链球菌（A 组和 B 组）、问号钩端螺旋体、革兰氏阴性菌（如沙门菌、志贺菌和大肠埃希菌）及寄生虫感染（如蛔虫、蓝氏贾第鞭毛虫）。该病在甲型肝炎或戊型肝炎感染中很少发生。免疫功能低下的患者，应考虑贝氏等孢球虫、巨细胞病毒、隐孢子虫、曲霉菌、念珠菌属等病原体感染[242]。无结石性胆囊炎可发生于腹部创伤之后，在系统性血管炎患者中也可观察到，包括结节性多动脉炎、系统性红斑狼疮、过敏性紫癜、变应性肉芽肿性血管炎和川崎病。然而在这些情况下，也可能仅为无炎症的胆囊扩张。胆囊管先天性狭窄或炎症或肿大的淋巴结外部压迫与儿童疾病有关。

非结石性胆囊炎的发病机制是多因素的，胆汁淤积和局部缺血引起胆囊黏膜损伤，最终导致胆囊坏疽、积脓和穿孔。

急性非结石性胆囊炎的临床表现包括右上腹或上腹痛、恶心、呕吐、发热和偶发的黄疸[243]。右上腹压痛、反跳痛阳性，有时可触及肿大的胆囊。因为潜在的合并症可能掩盖病情，婴儿、危重患者查体阳性可能不明显。

肝脏生化检查可能出现碱性磷酸酶和结合胆红素水平升高。白细胞数量增多。超声检查发现增大、壁厚、膨胀的胆囊，其内可见胆泥但不含结石[243]。亦可见到胆囊周围积液或壁内积气。

一些儿童可能出现慢性右上腹痛、恶心或呕吐的症状[241]。白细胞计数及肝脏生化检查结果一般正常。大多数患者通过放射性核素肝胆扫描证实胆囊功能异常。这些患者一般存在慢性胆囊炎症，需要行胆囊切除术。

许多非结石性胆囊炎患者对胃肠减压、静脉输液和抗生素等非手术治疗有反应，临床症状和影像学结果消退。胆囊壁厚度和张力进行性增加、胆囊内持续无声影物质或胆泥淤积和胆囊旁积液的患者，需行胆囊切除术[241,243]。在剖腹手术可确诊。胆囊通常是发炎的，胆汁可培养出致病细菌或含有寄生虫。胆囊可发生坏疽。病情危重但没有发生穿孔或坏疽时，经皮胆囊穿刺引流术可作为替代治疗方法。

（四）急性胆囊积液

婴幼儿和儿童可发生非结石性、非炎性胆囊膨胀[244,245]，胆囊没有炎症，胆汁培养通常是无菌的。与急性非结石性胆囊炎不同，急性胆囊积液预后良好。在没有机械压迫的情况下，胆囊管周围淋巴结可发生弥漫性肠系膜淋巴结炎。在某些病例中可观察到与其他感染（如猩红热和钩端螺旋体病）的暂时性关系[246]。急性胆囊积液与川崎病和过敏性紫癜有关[247]。与非结石性胆囊炎类似，该疾病可发生在长期接受胃肠外营养的儿童中，在某些情况下，无法确定病因。

急性胆囊积液与急性发作的痉挛性腹痛有关，通常伴有恶心和呕吐[247]。可能出现发热和黄疸。右上腹通常有压痛，可触及膨胀的胆囊。

肝脏生化检查水平可能轻度升高。白细胞计数可能升高。其中一些变化可能是由于相关疾病所致，如猩红热或川崎病。超声检查显示胆囊肿大、膨胀，但无结石。

许多患者在剖腹手术时确诊为急性胆囊积液[247]。如果胆囊出现坏疽，则必须行胆囊切除术。胆囊壁病理检查通常显示水肿和轻度炎症。胆汁培养物通常是无菌的。基于这些特点，部分术者选择简单的胆囊造瘘术而不是胆囊切除术来治疗急性胆囊积液[247]。但急性胆囊积液一般采取非手术治疗，重点是支持治疗和并发疾病的处理。在大多数患者中，特别是完全胃肠外营养但之前已开始肠道喂养的儿童，胆囊积液可自行消退。超声检查在确定诊断和跟踪胆囊膨胀的自发消退方面是很有用的。本病预后良好。胆囊功能在大多数情况下有望恢复正常[247]。

（五）胆囊运动障碍

胆囊或胆道运动障碍是儿童慢性腹痛的原因之一。根据餐后腹痛、无胆石症和胆囊收缩素刺激的肝胆闪烁成像显示胆囊射血分数异常，可作出诊断。在一些报告中，胆囊切除术后的疼痛缓解程度存在差异[248]。胆囊射血分数低于 35% ~ 50% 即为异常，是手术治疗的指征（见第 63 和 67 章）。然而，关于儿童胆道运动障碍的诊断标准尚未达成共识，症状通常与功能性消化不良重叠[249]。

在 107 名进行胆囊切除术的儿童中，62 名（58%）儿童的胆囊运动障碍是最常见的手术指征[250]。在另一项已发表的报告中，排除了其他常见的胃肠道疾病后，51 名因胆囊运动障碍接受腹腔镜胆囊切除术的儿童，38 名可进行随访的患者中，有 27 名（71%）的症状完全缓解[251]。恶心、上腹痛和胆囊射血分数低于 15% 的存在是可靠地预测胆囊切除术获益的因素（阳性预测值为 93%）。27 例症状完全缓解的患儿中，仅 10 例（41%）发现慢性胆囊炎的组织学证据，提示其并不是成功结局的独立预测因素。这些患者存在慢性炎症表明他们可能患有慢性非结石性胆囊炎，而不是胆囊动力障碍。

（王迎春　译，闫秀娥　刘军　校）

参考文献

第 63 章 胆道运动功能和功能障碍

B. Joseph Elmunzer, Grace H. Elta 著

章节目录

一、解剖和生理学 …… 932
二、胆囊功能性疾病 …… 932
三、Oddi 括约肌功能障碍 …… 933
（一）定义 …… 933
（二）流行病学 …… 933
（三）临床特点 …… 933
（四）分类 …… 933
（五）诊断 …… 934
（六）治疗 …… 935
四、胰腺炎中的 Oddi 括约肌功能障碍 …… 936
（一）特发性复发性急性胰腺炎 …… 936
（二）慢性胰腺炎 …… 936

一、解剖和生理学

胆囊呈梨形，存储胆汁并具有可扩张性，可排放胆汁至十二指肠消化食物（参见 62 章）。它位于肝下表面，由底部、体部和颈部 3 个部分组成，在消化间期和餐后规律充盈、排空。上消化道内食物的存在刺激胆囊收缩素（cholecystokinin，CCK）分泌，调控胆汁排入十二指肠肠腔。

Oddi 括约肌（sphincter of Oddi，SO）由多层平滑肌纤维组成，嵌入十二指肠壁内肌层但功能与之不同，并形成长约 4～10mm 的高压带（参见第 62 章）。Oddi 括约肌由 3 部分组成：①壶腹括约肌，很短，包绕于胆胰管汇合后的共同通道之外；②胰管括约肌，较短，包绕主胰管起始部；③胆管括约肌，最长，包绕胆总管远端（图 63.1）。纵肌束是跨越胆管和胰管间隔的肌束。Oddi 括约肌首先为屏障功能主要起阻断作用，在消化间期通过紧张性收缩，限制胆汁流动。其次为泵功能，通过节律性收缩控制胆汁流入十二指肠腔，可能起到远端胆管的管家功能。Oddi 括约肌参与移行性复合运动，在强烈的十二指肠收缩前期和收缩过程中，胃动素诱发括约肌收缩的频率和幅度增加。

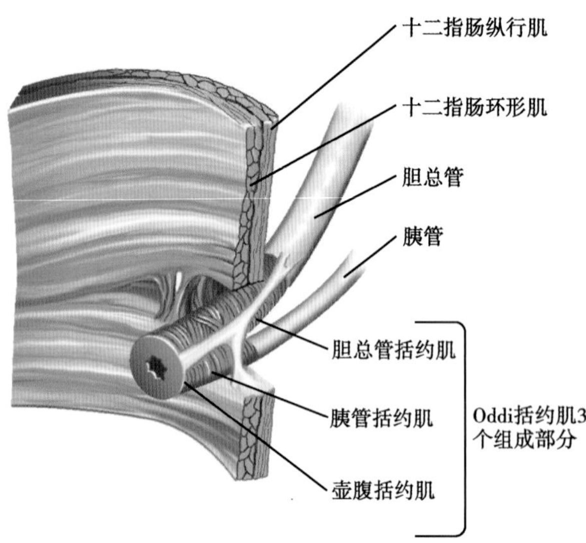

图 63.1 Oddi 括约肌解剖图谱。Oddi 括约肌由 3 个部分组成：壶腹括约肌（包绕短的胆胰共同通道），胰管括约肌和胆管括约肌（最大部分）

胆道运动受复杂的神经激素调节，包括交感神经、副交感神经、脊神经和肠神经[1]。几乎所有的肠神经系统中的神经递质均在胆道中发现。胆囊和 Oddi 括约肌之间的反射通路，调控胆汁的流动[2]。

二、胆囊功能性疾病

尽管非结石性胆囊疼痛归因于运动紊乱，但并无确切依据。胆囊胆汁淤积易导致胆泥和结石的形成，但胆囊功能障碍（或运动障碍）即在无结石或胆泥的情况下出现胆囊排空延迟，这是否可导致胆道症状尚不清楚。根据一项小样本随机对照试验（RCT）和部分观察性研究的结果，胆囊排空延迟预示胆囊切除术后疼痛可缓解[3-6]，但是这一结论仍存在争议[7-8]。胆囊排空延迟可见于正常无症状人群，功能性胃肠病患者中更常见[9-10]。它似乎也与许多不相关的疾病有关，如肥胖和糖尿病。运动障碍可能是胆囊炎症的重要原因，许多非结石性胆囊切除标本中均存在炎症，但是根据慢性胆囊炎[4]的组织学诊断来确定症状来源于胆囊一直存在争议[11]。

9 项 meta 分析[7]和 23 项研究的系统回顾[8]得出结论，现有的证据均不支持将胆囊造影作为胆囊切除术后症状缓解的预测因素（参见第 67 章）。然而，其他较小的 meta 分析表明，胆囊切除术对有症状的胆囊功能障碍患者有效，具有统计学意义[12,13]。尽管这种诊断存在争议，但在美国，胆囊功能障碍是胆囊切除术的主要原因，占成人患者的 20%，儿童则为 50%[14,15]。事实上，美国胆囊切除术治疗非结石性胆道疼痛的频率是其他发达国家的 3.5 倍，这表明胆囊切除术被过度应用[16]。

具有典型胆源性疼痛但是经皮腹部超声检查未见胆结石征象的患者，应接受超声内镜检查评估有无胆泥或微结石的存在。如果超声内镜检查未见异常，患者具有典型的胆源性疼痛症状，不需要进一步的检查，因为许多胆源性疼痛、超声检查没有结石且胆囊运动正常的患者在胆囊切除术后症状缓解[17]。如果疼痛不典型，患者可能存在功能性腹痛综合征，不应进行手术。如果临床症状既不典型，也不是典型的非胆源性疼痛，患者需在静脉应用 CCK 下行胆囊闪烁扫描，评估

胆囊排空情况,尽管正如前面提到的,这个测试来预测胆囊切除术后症状缓解情况仍备受争议。

一个多学科共识专家小组全体一致同意,需要一个大型、多中心 RCT 来比较手术和保守治疗对典型胆源性腹痛、胆囊超声检查正常、CCK 胆囊闪烁显像异常患者的疗效[18]。虽然正如前面所提到的,CCK 胆囊闪烁显像主要用于评估非典型症状,专家建议将其用于无症状发作或正在住院时具有典型胆源性腹痛(罗马Ⅳ共识意见,参见第 12、14、22 和 67 章)的患者。一项包含 93 名胆囊排空差的患者的前瞻性研究表明,具有典型胆源性腹痛患者胆囊切除术的效果显著优于那些非典型症状患者(优势比为 22.3,$P<0.001$)[19]。与之相反,一些研究表明,非典型症状患者在不进行胆囊切除术的情况下,症状可自发性改善[20]。专家小组也不建议单纯基于输注 CCK 诱发疼痛而作出临床决策[18]。

三、Oddi 括约肌功能障碍

(一) 定义

Oddi 括约肌功能障碍(SOD)是一种发生在 Oddi 括约肌水平的良性非结石性梗阻性疾病。SOD 依据发病机制可分为 2 个亚型:①SO 狭窄(或壶腹狭窄),为纤维化、炎症或两者同时引起的继发性梗阻;②SO 运动障碍,为括约肌痉挛引起的间歇性梗阻。这两种机制在 SO 的功能障碍并不是相互排斥的。壶腹狭窄一词通常与 SO 狭窄亚型互换使用。

(二) 流行病学

未切除胆囊患者中,经测压证实的 SO 高压发生概率尚不明确。无论是否存在腹痛或血清转氨酶水平升高,40% 的胆囊结石患者可见 SO 基础压升高[21]。81 名胆源性疼痛且胆囊完整但无结石的患者中,有 70% 存在胆囊排空延迟、SOD,或两者兼有[22]。相比之下,无症状且无胆囊结石的 50 名志愿者中,SO 基础压均低于 30mmHg[23]。

胆囊切除术后持续或复发性胆源性疼痛患者中,SO 高压的研究较多,但结果受纳入标准的影响。10% ~ 20% 的胆囊切除术后患者,仍然存在与术前相似的胆源性疼痛[24],最常见的解释是术前症状并不是由胆囊疾病引起。这类患者最有可能的原因是功能性胃肠病,如肠易激综合征或功能性消化不良,9% ~ 14% 的胆囊切除术后疼痛患者中存在 SOD[25]。当排除了胆囊切除术后其他原因引起的疼痛,并在更仔细的筛选组中经 Oddi 括约肌压力测定(SO manometry,SOM)证实,SOD 发病率为 30% ~60%[26]。

(三) 临床特点

SOD 表现为以下 3 种情况:①胆囊切除术后持续或复发性的胆源性疼痛;②复发性特发性(原因不明)的胰腺炎;③具有胆源性腹痛但胆囊完好且没有胆石症。SOD 通常呈自发性,但肝移植术后[27]、艾滋病[28]、长期应用阿片[29]、或高脂血症患者发病率增高(表 63.1)[30]。

表 63.1 SOD 相关临床情况

可能性	胆囊切除术后胆源性疼痛
很可能	胆囊完好的胆源性疼痛
可能	肝移植后
	AIDS 合并病毒和原虫感染
	慢性胰腺炎
	高脂血症
	特发性复发性急性胰腺炎
	应用阿片类制剂

AIDS,获得性免疫缺陷综合征;SOD,Oddi 括约肌功能障碍。

虽然胆道型 SOD 可见于所有年龄,但中年女性最常见,占患者总数的 75% ~ 90%。临床表现为典型的胆源性腹痛,位于上腹或右上腹,程度重,可向背部或右肩胛区放射。腹痛呈阵发性,每次持续 30 分钟以上,每年至少发作一次[31]。罗马Ⅳ会议共识基于专家经验和意见,提出了 SOD 的诊断标准[32]。尽管这些标准可能有助于筛选出能从治疗干预中获益的患者,但仍需要进一步的前瞻性研究证实。

因为 ERCP 是唯一可靠的诊断和治疗 SOD 的方法,且有很大的操作风险,寻找能够准确预示 SOD 和括约肌切开效果的临床特点至关重要。有限的研究显示,间歇性腹痛伴有恶心和呕吐,并且在胆囊切除术后至少 1 年没有疼痛的患者 ERCP 治疗可能有效[33]。疼痛发作时血清转氨酶水平的一过性升高支持 SOD 的诊断[34]。胃排空延迟、每日应用阿片类药物和年龄小于 40 岁与括约肌切开术(见后)效果差有关[35]。但是这些预判因素并没有经过严格验证,除了肝功升高,均无法在临床实践中发挥明显作用。一项正在进行的多中心前瞻性队列研究(the RESPOnD Study)旨在严格确定接受 ERCP 的疑诊 SOD 患者的特征,最终目的是严格寻找与治疗反应相关的临床和操作特点。

(四) 分类

Milwaukee 分类系统是在依据诊断标准将疑诊胆道型 SOD 患者分为 3 类的基础上进行了修正。该系统被应用于临床实践,因为它可以预测胆道括约肌切开的结果(表 63.2)。

表 63.2 胆道型 SOD 改良 Milwaukee 和罗马Ⅳ诊断系统

改良 Milwaukee	罗马Ⅳ	特征
胆道Ⅰ型	SO 狭窄	胆源性腹痛
		胆管直径>9mm
		血清谷丙转氨酶或谷草转氨酶升高
胆道Ⅱ型	胆道括约肌功能障碍	胆源性腹痛 上述客观标准中的一项
胆道Ⅲ型	功能性疼痛	仅有胆源性腹痛

SO,Oddi 括约肌;SOD,Oddi 括约肌功能障碍。

根据改良后的 Milwaukee 分类系统，Ⅰ型 SOD 为胆源性疼痛，血清转氨酶（转氨酶或碱性磷酸酶）升高［超过正常上限（upper limit of normal，ULN）的 1.1 倍］，胆管扩张直径大于 9mm。Ⅱ型 SOD 为胆源性疼痛、转氨酶升高或胆管扩张。Ⅲ型 SOD 为胆源性疼痛，但没有任何其他客观检查异常。这种分类系统不要求转氨酶升高与疼痛发作相关，尽管这种相关性可能是治疗有效的一个预测因素[34]。

类似的胰腺型 SOD 分类系统将在后文阐述[36]。Ⅰ型胰腺型 SOD 具有胰源性腹痛、至少一次血淀粉酶或脂肪酶升高至 1.1 倍 ULN 和胰管扩张（胰头部>6mm，体部>5mm）；Ⅱ型胰腺型 SOD 具有胰源性腹痛和其他两项异常之一；Ⅲ型胰腺型 SOD 仅有胰源性腹痛。然而，目前这种分类系统并没有证据支持，目前只在不明原因的复发性胰腺炎患者中考虑胰腺型 SOD 的诊断。

2014 年发表的一项具有里程碑意义的多中心 RCT（EPISOD 研究）显示，疑诊Ⅲ型 SOD 患者不能从 ERCP 和括约肌切开术中获得中期或长期益处[37]。在该研究的基础上，结合现有的全部研究数据，罗马共识委员会和其他学者均提出需要对 SOD 亚型进行重新分类[38]。在新分类系统下，Ⅲ型 SOD 被取缔，因为它并不来源于括约肌功能障碍。这些患者具有小肠消化间期运动活性异常[39]，和十二指肠（而非直肠）扩张引起的十二指肠内脏痛觉过敏[40]，提示存在功能性腹痛综合征。

传统Ⅰ型 SOD，同时具有转氨酶升高和胆管扩张的患者，存在 SO 水平的机械性胆道梗阻，现归类于 SO 狭窄。传统Ⅱ型 SOD，患者存在至少一过性的胆道梗阻，有 SO 痉挛因素参与，现归类于胆管括约肌功能障碍（functional biliary sphincter disorder，FBSD）。这种新的分类系统更好地体现了我们目前的认知程度，但需要明确 SO 狭窄和 FBSD 之间重叠的部分。为了更好地定义这种新的分类系统，需要收集更严格的临床数据进行前瞻性验证。

（五）诊断

1. 无创性检查

疑诊 SOD 的患者首先需完善肝功、血淀粉酶、脂肪酶和腹部影像学评估，如腹部超声、CT 或 MRCP。体格检查多正常，但可能存在轻微右上腹或上腹压痛。常常同时进行标准检查（常规内镜和影像学检查）和其他腹痛常见原因（如 GERD、NAFLD 和 IBS）的实验性治疗。

SOD 的无创性诊断检查包括胆道闪烁显像、脂肪餐/CCK/促胰液素刺激的超声检查、促胰液素刺激的 MRI 和 EUS。这些检查的诊断性能在很大程度上得到了 SOM 的验证，后者曾作为 SOD 诊断的金标准，现在被发现存在诸多不足（见下文）[37,41]，限制了其在临床实践中的应用。

胆道闪烁显像可用于评估胆汁排入十二指肠的流量，可用于 SOM 检查前的筛查[42]。虽然胆管扩张和重度胆道梗阻的患者闪烁显像通常阳性，但对于 SO 造成的低度或间歇性胆道梗阻，闪烁显像敏感性较差[43]。在富含脂质的饮食或静脉注射 CCK 后，如果 SO 功能障碍，胆管可能在压力刺激下扩张，腹部超声可以检测到这种变化。胆囊切除术后患者中，与 SOM 相比，脂肪餐刺激的超声检查对 SOD 诊断的敏感性为 21%，特异性为 97%[44]。与之相似，在静脉注射促胰液素后胰管扩张，可用来诊断胰管括约肌功能障碍（见后）。在复发性胰腺炎患者中，与 SOM 相比，促胰液素刺激的超声检查对 SOD 诊断敏感性为 88%，特异性为 82%[45]。

促胰液素刺激的磁共振胰管造影也被用于评估特发性复发性急性胰腺炎患者有无胰管阻塞。初步研究显示，与 SOM 相比，其特异性高，但敏感性低[46,47]。同样，复发性胰腺炎且经 SOM 证实存在 SOD 的患者中，促胰液素刺激的 EUS 诊断敏感性有限[48]。

因此，无创性检查对 SOD 诊断准确性有限，不足以依赖其作出临床决策，目前还不能作为诊断依据。

2. 有创性检查

ERCP 仍然是 SOD 诊断和治疗的金标准，尽管术后并发症以疑诊 SOD 者发生率最高。如果没有实施预防性干预，其 ERCP 术后胰腺炎发生率超过 25%，风险增加了 3 倍以上[49]。虽然短时间预防性留置胰管支架和术前肛塞 NSAIDs 可降低 ERCP 术后胰腺炎的风险[50-52]，SOD 患者 ERCP 术后仍有明显的并发症发生率和偶发死亡事件。因此，ERCP 应仅用于症状严重、风险效益比获益明显的人群。虽然 EUS 和 MRCP 可作为安全的 ERCP 替代影像学检查方法，以除外结石、肿瘤和胰腺分裂，但他们不能用于 SOD 的诊断（和治疗）。偶尔，壶腹内肿瘤可呈与 SOD 类似的表现。如果在内镜下括约肌切开术后壶腹部出现多余的组织，需取活检[53]。

3. SOM

尽管手术中或经皮途径亦可实施 SOM，但一般在 ERCP 过程中进行。Geenen 等对疑诊Ⅱ型胆道 SOD 的患者进行了一项具有里程碑意义的随机对照试验[54]，证明 SOM 可预测内镜下括约肌切开术后疼痛是否改善。SO 基础压>40mmHg 的患者，其术后症状改善率为 91%，而基础压升高括约肌切开假手术组症状改善率仅 25%。而 SO 压力正常的患者，括约肌切开术后症状改善率仅 42%，与假手术组效果类似（33%）。另一项针对 SO 压力升高Ⅱ型胆道 SOD 患者的对照研究，也得出了类似的结论[55]。该研究中，括约肌切开组 11/13 例患者得到了临床改善，而假手术组为 5/13。除 SO 基础压增高之外，其他 SOM 结果异常的患者，包括 Oddi 括约肌收缩过速（相位波频率增加）、逆行收缩增加和 CCK 矛盾运动反应，括约肌切开手术或假手术疼痛改善无差异。

虽然这些早期的研究对临床实践产生了重大影响，但将 SOM 作为诊断工具越来越受到质疑。一些非对照研究提出更容易测定的指标，如转氨酶升高和胆道扩张能够更好地预测括约肌切开的疗效[56]。另外一些研究显示 SOM 对 SOD 诊断有很高的特异性，但敏感性差；敏感性差可能是 42% 的 SOM 正常的Ⅱ型胆道 SOD 患者在括约肌切开术后症状亦缓解的原因。此外，Ⅰ型胆道 SOD 患者 SOM 异常率仅 65%～85%，但括约肌切开术后症状缓解率在 90% 以上，可能也是 SOM 敏感性较低引起的[57]。SOM 敏感性低的另一种可能原因是，压力测定只能测定一个时间点，而 Oddi 括约肌痉挛是间歇性发作的，测压时可能并没有发生痉挛。两项研究表明，症状持续但首次 SOM 正常的患者中，40%～60% 第二次 SOM 异常[58,59]。前文提到的 EPISOD 研究中，SOM 对结果不具备预测性和可重复性[37,41]。

因此,SOM 在临床实践中逐渐被舍弃[60]。一般用于诊断传统的Ⅱ型胆道 SOD 或胰腺 SOD(见后),或用于评估既往括约肌切开术后症状复发患者残留括约肌的存在。SO 基础压异常在胆胰管通常均有,但也可仅有胆管括约肌或胰管括约肌[61]。在血清转氨酶水平升高的患者 SO 基础压升高多局限于胆管括约肌,而胰腺炎患者多局限于胰管括约肌[62]。对于临床指征为胆源性疼痛而非特发性胰腺炎,且 SOM 正常的患者,一些专家建议完全避免胰管干预,以减少术后胰腺炎的概率。以往其他专家曾建议对所有患者均同时进行胆管、胰管括约肌切开术,以解除胆胰管的高压,不考虑临床指征是胆源性疼痛还是特发性胰腺炎。然而,临床试验的结果并不支持"双括约肌切开术"治疗 SOD[37,63]。当因特发性复发性胰腺炎行 SOM 并准备实施胰管括约肌切开术时,需要明确是否存在胰管括约肌压力测定异常,以评估胰管括约肌切开术的急性(ERCP 术后胰腺炎)和远期(胰管括约肌再狭窄引起的胰腺炎或腹痛)风险,但这一做法也正在发生变化。综上,需要进一步的研究来明确 SOM 的适应证和作用。

4. 其他基于 ERCP 的诊断干预措施

试验性放置胰管或胆管支架以预测括约肌切开术的效果,SO 肉毒杆菌毒素注射均曾被尝试作为 SOD 的替代性诊断方法[64,65]。虽然初步结果显示这些方法有一定的实用性,但是操作步骤复杂、伴随风险多和支架导致的胰管损伤限制了其在临床的广泛开展。后续仍需要进一步研究这些方法在 SOD 诊断中的价值。

(六) 治疗

1. 药物治疗

拟诊或确诊 SOD 患者饮食和药物治疗的研究很少。有学者建议低脂饮食以减少胰胆刺激,目前没有数据证实这一说法。硝苯地平、硝酸盐、奥曲肽、解痉药、5 型磷酸二酯酶抑制剂、经皮神经刺激和电刺激均被证实可降低 SO 基础压,但缺乏充分的临床数据。两项短期、安慰剂交叉对照研究表明,75% 拟诊或确诊 SOD 的患者口服硝苯地平后,疼痛显著降低[66,67]。然而,随后的一项研究表明,与安慰剂相比,缓释硝苯地平没有改善临床症状,但增加了心血管副作用[68]。一项应用硝酸盐治疗 SOD 的前瞻性研究以摘要形式发表,显示其可以减轻疼痛,但应用也受到副作用的限制[69]。另一个前瞻性研究显示,曲美布汀(一种解痉药)联合硝酸盐(舌下或经皮肤)改善 SOD 相关疼痛的速度与括约肌切开类似[70]。显然,还需要更多的研究来确定药物治疗对 SOD 的作用,鉴于 SOD 为良性病,在进行括约肌切开治疗前,所有症状较轻的 SOD 患者都应首先尝试药物治疗。试验性解痉药或低剂量三环类抗抑郁药(降低内脏高敏感)应用较多。有 FBSD 和严重腹痛的患者药物治疗有效可能性较小,可首先考虑内镜治疗。

2. 括约肌切开术

可以考虑诊断为 SOD 的最常见原因是胆囊切除术后患者仍存在胆源性腹痛。SOM 异常的上述患者,90%~95% 传统Ⅰ型胆道 SOD(括约肌狭窄)和 85% 传统Ⅱ型 SOD(FBSD)患者在括约肌切开术后得以缓解腹痛。SOM 正常时,90%~95% Ⅰ型胆道 SOD 患者仍可在括约肌切开术后得以缓解疼痛。因为 SOM 结果可能误导判断(14%~35% SOM 正常),SOM 不是判断Ⅰ型胆道 SOD 患者是否进行括约肌切开术的指征,而应行经验性内镜下括约肌切开治疗。

Ⅱ型胆道 SOD 且 SOM 正常的患者中,35%~42% 括约肌切开术后疼痛缓解。虽然症状改善率与假治疗对照组相似,但真正的临床疗效可能仅见于少数患者。因此,尽管Ⅱ型 SOD 且 SOM 异常是括约肌切开术的指征之一,Ⅱ型 SOD 患者依据 SOM 结果、作出是否行括约肌切开的决策越来越受到质疑。基于上述实验结果及 SOM 的局限性,多数专家主张传统Ⅱ型 SOD(FBSD)患者直接行经验性胆道括约肌切开术,而不参考 SOM 的结果。这种策略的优点是那些 SOM 正常但括约肌切开术后症状可改善的患者得到了治疗机会,但是同时伴随着操作相关并发症风险的增加,如出血和穿孔。决策分析模型证实,Ⅱ型 SOD 患者由经验丰富的 ERCP 术者直接行括约肌切开术的获益高于基于 SOM 的治疗策略[71]。经验性括约肌切开术在 FBSD 患者中的风险能否被临床和经济获益所抵消,需要进一步前瞻性研究来明确。

传统Ⅲ型 SOD 患者的治疗一直存在争议。基于明显不利的风险-效益比,许多治疗性内镜医师均避免在这些患者行 ERCP 下压力测定。与预期结果一致,EPISOD 研究的结果证实了 ERCP 在胆囊切除术后疼痛患者的治疗中没有作用,也没有客观的发现。

很少有研究关注具有胆源性疼痛、胆囊完好且无胆结石的 SOD 患者。究竟胆囊切除术后的病理生理改变导致 SOD,还是 SOD 患者更可能因为其临床症状而接受胆囊切除术,目前尚不清楚。胆囊切除术后可暴露潜在的亚临床 SOD 患者,因为其去除了 SO 痉挛时可用以蓄积肝外胆管系统内容物的储存池[72]。此外,在胆囊切除术中,从胆囊经由胆囊管到 SO 的神经被切断,可能导致 SO 运动改变[73]。然而,也有少数研究显示 SOD 可见于胆囊完整的患者。一项小的病例研究显示,胆囊完整但 SO 高压的患者,括约肌切开术后疼痛长期缓解率可达到 43%;另外一些患者在胆囊切除术后症状最终得到改善[74]。显然,如何评估和治疗这一具有挑战性的患者群体,仍有待进一步研究。

3. 胆道括约肌切开术失败

框 63.1 列出了 SOD 患者胆道括约肌切开术效果不佳的可能原因。最可能的原因疼痛不是胰胆源性的,而是由肠道运动异常或内脏高敏感引起[40]。或者是胆道括约肌切开程度不足,或发生再狭窄[75]。进一步内镜下胆道治疗,或外科括约肌成形术的临床效果不详。

框 63.1　推测 SOD 患者胆道括约肌切开术后疼痛缓解失败的可能原因

初次括约肌切开不充分
非胆胰源性疼痛,特别是功能性胃肠道疾病
再狭窄的发生
胰腺造影正常的隐性慢性胰腺炎

SOD,Oddi 括约肌功能障碍。

括约肌切开术后症状缓解的患者,再次出现术前类似的症状时,可接受二次 ERCP 明确切开是否充分,以及是否发生再狭窄,尽管这些患者的最初反应也可能是因为安慰剂效应。

在没有胰腺异常的情况下,残余胰管括约肌高压引起持续疼痛尚存在争议。一些专家提倡初次 ERCP 即行"双括约肌切开术"来预防这一问题,尽管其再干预率(因持续性或复发性疼痛)与以往单个括约肌切开术的对照组并无差异[76]。

最后,一些拟诊 SOD,胆道括约肌切开术治疗无效的患者,可能是由于"微小改变"的慢性胰腺炎。EUS 可见慢性胰腺炎相关的实质和导管改变(参见第 59 章)[77]。

四、胰腺炎中的 Oddi 括约肌功能障碍

(一) 特发性复发性急性胰腺炎

SO 引流不畅可导致胰管压力短暂或持续性升高,导致胰腺实质损伤和继发炎症。虽然因结石或肿瘤引起的胰管梗阻可引起急性胰腺炎,但在首次发作的特发性胰腺炎中,是否为 SO 狭窄或痉挛引起胰管梗阻所致尚不明确。对于胰腺炎反复发作,特发性胰腺炎的反复发作可能导致胰管括约肌纤维化和/或炎症,进一步诱导或促进之后的反复发作。不管是否是真正的诱发原因,31%~78%特发性复发性急性胰腺炎(idiopathic recurrent acute pancreatitis,IRAP)患者存在 Oddi 括约肌压力升高[36,63,78]。

ERCP 通常在转诊中心应用于经标准评估、超声内镜和/或 MRCP 检查无法解释的 IRAP 患者的诊断和治疗。现有数据表明,以 ERCP 为基础的干预措施可消除或减少 50%~60%患者的胰腺炎复发[63,79,80]。然而,这一结论尚需严格的验证,且需权衡 ERCP 相关的高操作风险。一次不明原因的胰腺炎发作,甚至隔几年的两次发作,都不足以作为施行 ERCP 操作的理由,因为许多患者不会再次发作[78]。

拟行内镜治疗的患者,其症状多较重,极度渴求接受 ERCP。由于这类患者更易发生并发症,ERCP 成本和风险高,需要设立严格的 ERCP 和 EUS 假干预组 RCT 研究从方法学上为 IRAP 治疗决策制定提供依据。

IRAP 患者进行 ERCP 时,不同专家间存在操作差异,但证据较薄弱。常用的策略包括胆管和胰管双测压(随后进行选择性括约肌切开),经验性胆道括约肌切开和胰管测压,或经验性双括约肌切开(基于测压结果的不准确性)。一项随机试验表明,胰管压力异常的患者,单纯胆管括约肌切开(由于切开共同通道括约肌,也可以减少胰管内压力)与双括约肌切开效果相同[63]。尽管该研究存在不足,但其结果很有意义,因为胰管括约肌切开短期及远期并发症发生率极高,包括乳头再狭窄(偶可导致比原来的问题更严重的过程)。因此一些内镜医师在 ERCP 操作时调整了他们对经验性胆道括约肌切开术的做法仅行胆管括约肌切开,保留了胰腺测压和内镜治疗以应对胆道治疗反应不足、术后效果不佳时才考虑胰管压力测定和内镜下胰管括约肌切开。显然,IRAP 的 ERCP 诊断和治疗尚需要更多的研究,任何 ERCP 治疗 IRAP 的随机试验都应该比较胆道和双括约肌切开术,并将测压结果与括约肌消融反应相关联。

10%~30%常规筛查除外胆胰管系统解剖异常等病因(胆囊或胆管结石、胆泥;未发现的胰腺或壶腹肿瘤;胰管异常如胰腺分裂、胆胰管汇合异常;慢性胰腺炎)的急性胰腺炎患者,在考虑诊断胰腺型 SOD 之前,须先行 EUS 检查。总的来说,现有的研究显示,EUS 可能会揭示 30%~80%其他检查无阳性发现急性胰腺炎患者的病因,且受到患者胰腺炎发作次数和胆囊是否完好的影响[81,82]。

胆囊完整且反复不明原因胰腺炎发作的患者,胆道微结石是最有可能的原因,可行胆道括约肌切开或胆囊切除术(见第 58 和 65 章)[83]。尽管 EUS 对胆道微结石诊断准确性更高,但由于胆管括约肌切开可同时处理 EUS 无法诊断的 SOD 和胆道结晶,因此多选择胆管括约肌切开。

(二) 慢性胰腺炎

40%~87%慢性胰腺炎患者存在 SOD[84]。SOD 是慢性炎症的结果,还是其在慢性胰腺炎的发病机制中单独发挥作用,目前尚不明确。非对照研究显示,内镜下胰管括约肌切开术可以改善约 50%慢性胰腺炎伴胰管内高压患者的疼痛[85,86]。然而,由于缺乏充分的证据,是否向慢性胰腺炎和反复发作的急性炎症或仅伴有慢性疼痛或不伴有慢性疼痛的患者提供 ERCP 和 SOM,仍有待确定。在某些情况下,其他治疗如胰管结石取出和狭窄扩张,需要先行胰管括约肌切开术。总的来说,SOD 在慢性胰腺炎中的作用有限。

(王迎春　闫秀娥 译,鲁晓岚 校)

参考文献

第 64 章　胆汁分泌和肠肝循环

Peter Fickert, Paul A. Dawson 著

章节目录

一、胆汁酸合成和代谢 …… 938
二、肠肝循环 …… 941
三、肝内胆汁酸转运和胆汁分泌 …… 942
（一）非胆汁酸依赖性胆汁 …… 942
（二）胆肝分流通路 …… 943
（三）肝内胆汁酸转运 …… 943
（四）肝窦 Na⁺依赖性胆汁酸摄取 …… 945
（五）肝窦非 Na⁺依赖性胆汁酸摄取 …… 945
（六）肝窦胆汁酸流出 …… 945
（七）毛细胆管胆汁酸转运 …… 945
四、肠道和肾胆汁酸转运 …… 945
（一）肠道胆汁酸转运 …… 945
（二）肾胆汁酸转运 …… 945
（三）分子机制 …… 946
五、肠肝循环障碍 …… 946
（一）胆汁酸合成 …… 946
（二）胆汁酸和胆脂跨膜转运 …… 946
（三）胆汁酸生物转化（早期解离和脱羟基作用） …… 948
（四）胆汁酸循环 …… 948
六、针对胆汁酸的治疗 …… 949
（一）胆汁酸替代治疗 …… 949
（二）熊去氧胆酸 …… 949
（三）胆汁酸受体激动剂和拮抗剂 …… 949
七、胆汁酸螯合剂和转运抑制剂 …… 949

胆汁的形成对于肠道脂质消化吸收、胆固醇稳态和脂溶性外源物、药物代谢及重金属在肝脏的排泄是必不可少的[1]。胆汁的形成过程依赖于胆汁酸的肝脏合成和毛细胆管分泌。胆汁酸是胆汁中主要的有机阴离子，维持肝脏胆汁形成对正常肝功能至关重要。胆汁酸也经历了有效的肠肝循环，小肠重吸收胆汁中的大部分胆汁酸，回到肝脏并被肝细胞分泌。因此，胆汁酸合成、胆道分泌或肠道重吸收的紊乱对胆汁形成和肝脏及胃肠道生理功能有着深远的影响。胆汁酸合成和肠肝循环中的关键酶、转运子和调节因子的确认，提高了我们对胆汁形成或分泌异常所致的遗传性和获得性疾病的认识[2]。此外，近期发现胆汁酸可作为配体，通过细胞核和 G 蛋白偶联受体信号通路发挥作用，有助于对胆汁酸相关肝胆和肠道疾病的发病机制和治疗方案提供新的见解。本章主要论述胆汁酸及其功能、合成、分泌和肠肝循环。现有的针对胆汁酸的治疗方法也有一定涉及。

胆汁成分复杂，为富含脂质的胶束溶液，与血浆渗透压相同，主要由水、无机电解质和有机溶质如胆汁酸、磷脂[主要是磷脂酰胆碱（phosphatidylcholine，PC）]、胆固醇和胆色素等组成（表 64.1）。胆汁中亦含有细胞外囊泡，携带肝细胞或胆管细胞衍生蛋白、脂质和 RNA 分子[3]。图 64.1 显示了胆汁中主要有机溶质的相对含量。肝脏每天分泌胆汁约 500～600mL，其中含量最高的有机成分是胆汁酸。肝毛细胆管细胞膜分泌胆汁酸和其他溶质形成渗透压梯度，使水和其他小分子溶质渗透入胆道间隙。在健康人体内，毛细胆管分泌足量并浓缩的胆汁酸，肝细胞内胆汁酸浓度在较低的微摩尔水平，而毛细胆管内浓度在 1 000μmol/L 以上。胆汁酸经毛细胆管分泌后沿胆道下行，储存并集中于胆囊。进食后，胆囊收

表 64.1　肝胆汁成分

组分	浓度
电解质和矿物质/（mmol/L）	
钠	140～160
钾	3～8
氯	70～120
碳酸氢盐	20～50
钙	1～5
磷酸盐	1～2
金属/（μmol/L）	
镁	1～3
铁	18～52
铜	12～21
有机成分/（mmol/L）	
胆汁酸	5～50
胆红素（总）	1～2
磷脂（卵磷脂）	0.5～20.0
胆固醇	0.5～1.0
谷胱甘肽	3～5
葡萄糖	0.2～1.0
尿素氮	2.2～6.5
蛋白质/（g/dL）	0.2～3.0

人胆汁测量值引自 Albers CJ, Huizenga JR, Krom RA, et al. Composition of human hepatic bile. Ann Clin Biochem 1985;22:129-32; Keulemans YC, Mok KS, de Wit LT, et al. Hepatic bile versus gallbladder bile: a comparison of protein and lipid concentration and composition in cholesterol gallstone patients. Hepatology 1998;28:11-6; and Ho KJ. Biliary electrolytes and enzymes in patients with and without gallstones. Dig Dis Sci 1996;41:2409-16.

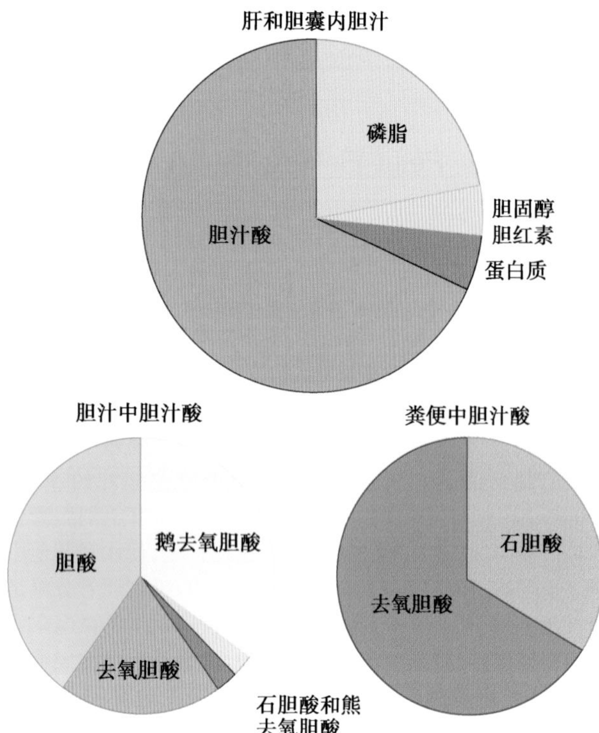

图 64.1　上图，健康人体肝胆胆汁的典型溶质组成。胆汁酸是胆汁中的主要溶质，约占 67%。磷脂约占胆汁的 22%，胆固醇 4%，胆红素 0.3%，蛋白质 4.5%。胆汁中胆汁酸组成见左下角图。胆汁酸、鹅去氧胆酸和去氧胆酸占胆汁中胆汁酸含量的 95% 以上，几乎所有胆汁中胆汁酸均为结合胆汁酸。胆汁石胆酸和熊去氧胆酸的比例不同，但很少超过 5%。胆汁中的大多数石胆酸以硫酸化形式存在。当以治疗剂量给药时，熊去氧胆酸在胆汁中的比例可升高到 40%。粪便中胆汁酸组成见右下图。粪便中胆汁酸几乎均为非结合胆汁酸。因为结肠中存在细菌水解酶，主要由脱羟基胆汁酸、去氧胆酸和石胆酸组成（见图 64.2）

缩并将胆汁排入十二指肠。然后胆汁酸沿着小肠流动，在小肠中促进脂肪的消化和吸收，激活肠道受体，并刺激肠道激素的产生。近端小肠重吸收较少，末端回肠为主要的重吸收部位。重吸收的胆汁酸通过门静脉血运返回肝脏，再经肝血窦膜转运作用重新分泌进入胆汁[4]。

胆汁酸在肝脏和胃肠道中具有多种生理功能。首先，胆汁酸诱导肝脏分泌胆汁和脂质（磷脂和胆固醇）。胆汁酸从血液向毛细胆管的矢量运动产生渗透性水流，这是胆汁形成的主要决定因素。第二，胆汁酸有助于膳食中脂肪的消化，是肠道吸收胆固醇和脂溶性维生素所必需的。它们还通过溶解膳食中的脂质和脂类消化产物，形成混合胶束来促进膜孔扩散并运输到肠黏膜，从而协助肠道吸收。脂溶性维生素（A、D、E 和 K）的吸收依赖于胆汁酸胶束的存在，胆汁酸合成、肝脏分泌或肠肝循环的紊乱均可导致脂溶性维生素缺乏。胆汁酸除了在膳食脂肪吸收中发挥重要作用外，还可能通过加速蛋白质变性和随后的胰蛋白酶消化来促进蛋白质的肠道消化。第三，胆汁酸通过整合作用维持体内胆固醇平衡。胆汁酸是小肠吸收胆汁和膳食中胆固醇所必需的。与之相反，胆汁酸同时通过多种途径促进体内胆固醇的清除。例如，胆固醇分解代谢为胆汁酸的量与粪便中排泄的胆汁酸量基本平衡，这一途径占每天胆固醇清除量的一半。胆汁酸还可促进胆道胆固醇分泌，从而促进其经肠道排泄。最后，肠腔内胆汁酸可作为胆固醇受体，结合肠道内胆固醇并直接排泄[4,5]。胆汁酸通过直接抑菌作用或胆汁酸-脂肪酸混合胶束参与肠道抗菌防御系统。胆汁酸还通过结合肠道内的受体诱导抗菌因子的产生，增强黏膜屏障的完整性，从而减少小肠细菌的易位和炎症反应[5,6]。除了抗菌作用外，胆汁酸亦参与肠道微生态的构成[7]。反之，肠道微生态也参与胆汁酸的代谢和生物转化，从而显著改变胆汁酸库的物理化学和信号特性[8,9]。肠道内胆汁酸-微生态相互作用调节个体代谢，参与代谢综合征、非酒精性脂肪肝和肝硬化等疾病的并发症或病情进展。结合胆汁酸以钙盐形式完全可溶，从而可减少不溶性钙沉淀的产生，阻止胆管和胆囊结石形成。胆汁酸还通过防止肠源性高草酸尿来抑制肾结石的产生[7,10]。胆汁酸同时具有激素样作用，通过细胞核和 G 蛋白偶联受体来调节其肠肝循环和代谢。此外，胆汁酸信号通路也有助于肝脏代谢、肠道运动和脂肪、葡萄糖、蛋白质及能量稳态的调节[11-14]。

一、胆汁酸合成和代谢

胆汁酸在肝腺泡中央周围肝细胞中由胆固醇合成。在这个过程中，亲脂化合物胆固醇被转化为水溶性产物。人类新合成的胆汁酸为胆酸（cholic acid，CA；3，7，12-三羟基胆汁酸）和鹅去氧胆酸（chenodeoxycholic acid，CDCA；3，7-二羟基胆汁酸）（图 64.2）。新合成的胆汁酸被称为初级胆汁酸，以区别于细菌代谢产生的次级胆汁酸。表 64.2 阐述了胆汁酸在人体内的合成和更新动力学。在正常生理条件下，肝脏合成的胆汁酸量为 0.2～0.6g/d，但小肠切除后最高可达 4～6g/d。肝脏胆汁酸合成涉及到两个主要途径，“经典”中性途径（胆固醇 7α 羟化酶通路）主要合成 CA 和“替代”酸性途径（氧甾酮 7α 羟化酶通路）主要合成 CDCA[2]。在经典途径中，胆固醇 7α 羟化酶［细胞色素 P450 7A1（CYP7A1）］直接将胆固醇转化为 7α-羟基胆固醇。在替代途径中，胆固醇首先在侧链上被 C-24、C-25 或 C-27 固醇羟化酶羟基化，生成 24，25 或 27-羟基胆固醇，以 27-羟基胆固醇为主，然后由氧甾醇 7α 羟化酶（CYP7B1）作用。

胆汁酸生物合成是一个涉及 17 种不同酶的复杂过程，可分为 2 组[2]。第一组修饰甾醇环，第二组修饰甾醇侧链。经典途径中，首先对甾醇环进行修饰，之后才是侧链；而替代途径中先进行侧链修饰，或与甾醇环修饰同时进行。在两种主要的生物合成途径中，在数量上成人以经典（CYP7A1）途径为主。遗传性 *CYP7A1* 基因突变的成年患者，胆汁酸合成量下降了 90%，为这一结论提供了依据。新生儿可能以替代途径为主，因为新生儿 CYP7A1 表达水平低，且遗传性 *CYP7B1* 突变的儿童存在严重胆汁淤积性肝病。

经典途径的限速步骤是 CYP7A1 酶。多项实验均证实胆汁酸可反馈抑制 CYP7A1，在给予疏水胆汁酸后胆汁酸的合成降低，而在回肠切除或给予胆汁酸螯合剂后，胆汁酸肠肝循环受损其合成增加[15]。CYP7A1 通路的负反馈调控分子机制涉及肝脏和小肠，并已被阐明。在主要途径中，胆汁酸作为回肠上皮细胞法尼酯 X 受体（farnesoid X receptor，FXR）的配体，

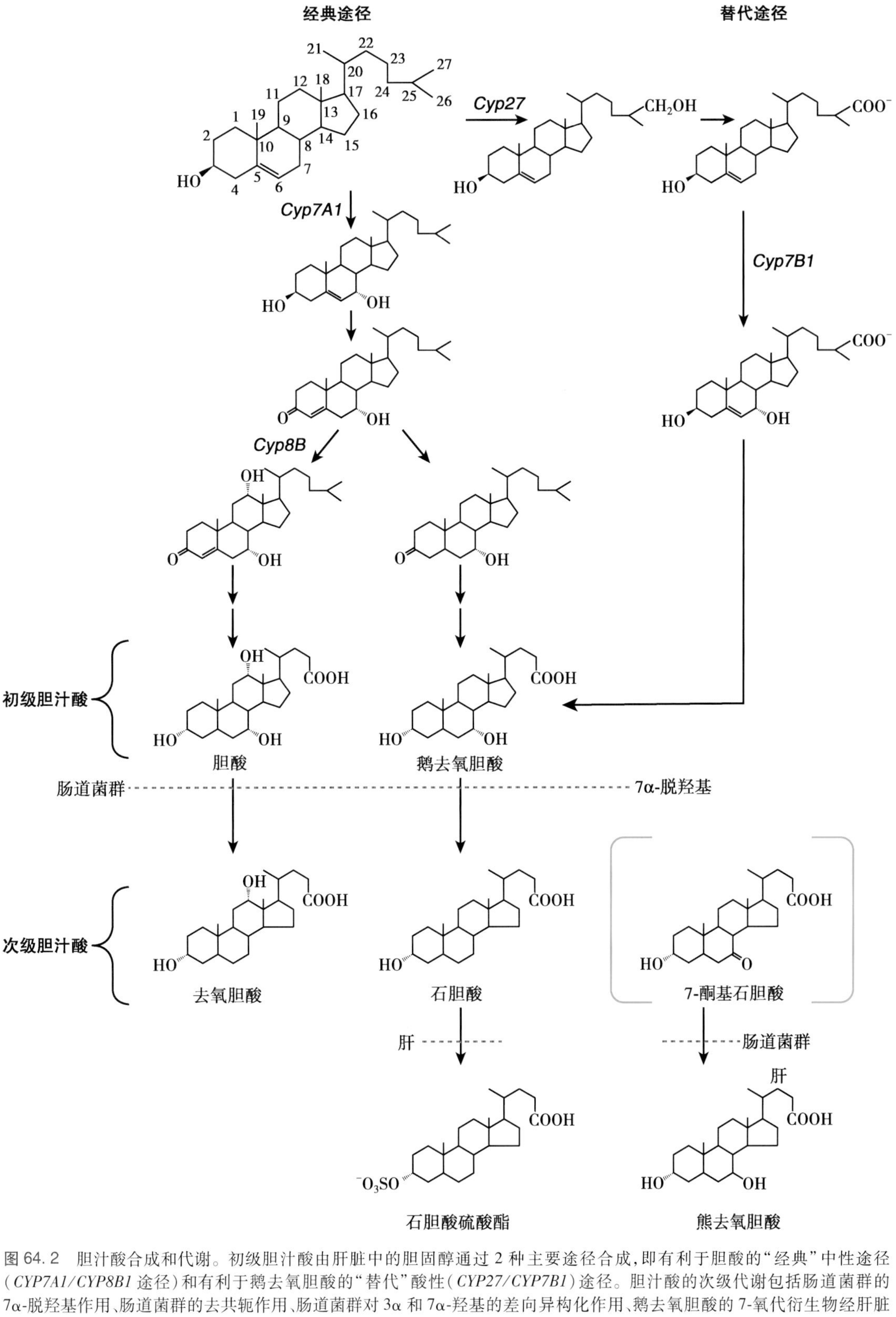

64

经典途径

替代途径

Cyp27

Cyp7A1

Cyp7B1

Cyp8B

初级胆汁酸

胆酸

鹅去氧胆酸

肠道菌群 7α-脱羟基

次级胆汁酸

去氧胆酸

石胆酸

7-酮基石胆酸

肝

肠道菌群

肝

石胆酸硫酸酯

熊去氧胆酸

图 64.2　胆汁酸合成和代谢。初级胆汁酸由肝脏中的胆固醇通过 2 种主要途径合成，即有利于胆酸的“经典”中性途径（*CYP7A1/CYP8B1* 途径）和有利于鹅去氧胆酸的“替代”酸性（*CYP27/CYP7B1*）途径。胆汁酸的次级代谢包括肠道菌群的 7α-脱羟基作用、肠道菌群的去共轭作用、肠道菌群对 3α 和 7α-羟基的差向异构化作用、鹅去氧胆酸的 7-氧代衍生物经肝脏还原成 7-氧代石胆酸以及 3β-羟基胆汁酸的肝脏再差向异构化作用。胆汁酸也主要在 C-3 位被肝脏和肾脏硫酸化。CYP，细胞色素 P450；CYP7A1，胆固醇 7α-羟化酶；CYP7B1，羟甾醇 7α-羟化酶；CYP8B1，甾醇 12α-羟化酶；CYP27，甾醇 27-羟化酶。（Adapted with permission from Dawson PA. Bile formation and the enterohepatic circulation. In: Johnson LR, Ghishan FK, Kaunitz JD, et al, editors. Physiology of the gastrointestinal tract. 5th ed. London: Academic Press; 2012. p 1466.）

表 64.2 健康受试者中个体胆汁酸池大小和动力学

胆汁酸	含量/mg	分次更新率/(/d)	肝脏合成/(mg/d)	每日初级胆汁酸流入量/(mg/d)
胆酸	500~1 500	0.2~0.5	120~400	—
去氧胆酸	250~800	0.1~0.4	0	40~200
鹅去氧胆酸	500~1 200	0.2~0.4	100~250	—
石胆酸	50~150	0.8~1.0	0	50~100
总量	1 300~3 650	—	220~650	90~300

胆汁酸池大小、更新、合成和每日输入的测量值引自 Vlahcevic ZR, Miller JR, Farrar JT, et al. Kinetic and pool size of primary bile acids in man. Gastroenterology 1971;61:85-90;Cowen AE, Korman MG, Hofmann AF, et al. Metabolism of lithocholate in healthy man. Ⅱ. Enterohepatic circulation. Gastroenterology 1975;69:67-76;Everson GT. Steady-state kinetics of serum bile acids in healthy human subjects:single and dual isotope techniques using stable isotopes and mass spectrometry. J Lipid Res 1987;28:238-52;Berr F, Pratschke E, Fischer S, et al. Disorders of bile acid metabolism in cholesterol gallstone disease. J Clin Invest 1992;90:859-68;Hulzebos CV, Renfurm L, Bandsma RH, et al. Measurement of parameters of cholic acid kinetics in plasma using a microscale stable isotope dilution technique:application to rodents and humans. J Lipid Res 2001;42:1923-9.

诱导合成内分泌多肽激素——成纤维细胞生长因子-19(fibroblast growth factor-19, FGF19;啮齿类动物的同源基因是FGF15)。FGF19 分泌进入门静脉血流,并作用于肝细胞表面受体[β-klotho 蛋白和 FGF4 受体(FGFR4)的复合物],抑制CYP7A1 表达和胆汁酸合成。FGF19 调控途径之外,肝细胞内胆汁酸还通过 FXR 信号通路,间接在转录和转录后机制抑制 CYP7A1 mRNA 的表达[16,17]。在转录水平上,FXR 上调孤儿核受体微小异源二聚体伙伴基因(small heterodimer partner, SHP)的表达,从而干扰了 CYP7A1 表达所需的肝细胞核因子 4α(hepatocyte nuclear factor 4α, HNF4α)和肝受体同源物 1(liver receptor homolog 1, LRH-1)的活性。在转录后水平,FXR 上调 RNA 结合蛋白 ZFP36L1 的表达,从而促进 CYP7A1 mRNA 的更新。这些复杂的分子调控机制将胆汁酸合成与肠道和肝脏胆汁酸水平的变化联系起来。

替代途径的主要调控机制为转录后水平。这涉及到类固醇合成快速调节蛋白(StAR)家族成员将胆固醇输送到线粒体内膜(甾醇 27-羟基化位置)。然而,胆汁酸亦可在转录水平调控替代途径。胆汁酸通过 FXR 诱导 MAP bZIP 转录因子 G[之前称为 v-maf 肌腱膜纤维肉瘤癌基因同源物 G(musculoaponeurotic fibrosarcoma oncogene homolog G, MafG)],抑制胆汁酸合成替代途径中重要基因的转录,如 *CYP27A1* 和 *CYP7B1*,但不影响 *CYP7A1* 的表达[18]。表 64.3 总结了调节胆汁酸生物合成和肠肝循环的受体和蛋白因子。

在分泌到毛细胆管之前,CA 和 CDCA 都通过在其侧链上添加甘氨酸或牛磺酸而 N-酰基化,这个过程通常称为结合。结合胆汁酸亲水性更强,侧链酸性强度增加,本质上是将弱酸(非结合胆汁酸 pKa≈5.0)转化为强酸(甘氨酸结合物 pKa≈3.9;牛磺酸结合物 pKa≈2.0)。与甘氨酸或牛磺酸结合的主要功能,是减少胆汁酸在肠肝循环中通过细胞膜的被动扩散。因此,有效地摄取和输出结合胆汁酸需要特定的细胞膜载体。与非结合胆汁酸相比,结合胆汁酸在酸性 pH 下溶解性更高,在高浓度钙存在时更不易发生沉淀。结合的最终结果是维持胆道、胆囊和小肠腔内胆汁酸的高浓度,以促进脂质的溶解、消化和吸收。遗传性胆汁酸结合障碍的患者存在脂溶性维生素吸收不良和脂肪泻,对补充结合胆汁酸如甘胆酸治疗反应良好,揭示了胆汁酸结合修饰的生理意义[19,20]。

表 64.3 参与胆汁酸合成和肠肝循环调节的蛋白质和基因

蛋白(基因)	蛋白在胆汁酸代谢中的作用
FXR(*NR1H4*)	胆汁酸活化的核受体;调控胆汁酸合成、转运和代谢
HNF4α(*NR2A1*)	核受体;正向调节 CYP7a1 表达和胆汁酸合成
LRH-1(*NR5A2*)	核受体;正向调节 CYP7a1 表达和胆汁酸合成
SHP(*NR0B2*)	核受体;拮抗 HNF4α 和 LRH-1,从而负反馈抑制肝胆汁酸合成;调控胆汁酸转运和代谢
PXR(*NR1I2*)	胆汁酸和外源物激活的核受体;参与次级胆汁酸解毒作用
VDR(*NR1I1*)	维生素 D 和胆汁酸激活的核受体;参与 LCA 解毒作用
CAR(*NR1I3*)	外源物激活的核受体;参与次级胆汁酸解毒作用
MafG(*MAFG*)	转录因子;负向调节胆汁酸合成和转运
FGFR4(*FGFR4*)	膜受体;负反馈调节 CYP7A1 和胆汁酸合成
ZFP36L1(*ZFP36L1*)	RNA 结合蛋白;负向调节 CYP7a1 表达和肝胆汁酸合成
β-klotho(*KLB*)	与 FGFR4 组成膜共同受体;使肝脏对 FGFR4-FGF19 通路具有特异性;负反馈调节 CYP7A1 和胆汁酸合成
FGF19(*FGF19*)	蛋白生长因子;胆汁酸刺激后由回肠、肝、胆囊分泌;通过 FGFR4:β-klotho 复合物调节肝胆汁酸合成
TGR5(*GPBAR1*)	胆汁酸活化的 G 蛋白耦联受体;介导胆汁酸的全身作用;调节肠道动力、代谢

CAR,组成型雄甾烷受体;FGF19,成纤维细胞生长因子 19;FGFR4,成纤维细胞生长因子受体 4;FXR,法尼酯 X 受体;HNF4α,肝细胞核因子 4;LCA,石胆酸;LRH-1,肝受体同源物 1;MafG,MAF bZIP 转录因子 G(以前称为 v-MAF 禽肌腱膜纤维肉瘤癌基因同源物 G);PXR,孕烷 X 受体;SHP,小异源二聚体伴侣;TGR5,Takeda G 蛋白耦联受体;VDR,维生素 D 受体;ZFP36L1,锌指蛋白 36 样 1。

肠道微生物的胆汁酸代谢始于小肠。虽然大多数分泌到小肠的结合胆汁酸被完整有效地重吸收,但肠道细菌来源的胆汁酸水解酶会将小肠内约 15% 胆汁酸上的甘氨酸或牛磺酸去除。这些非结合胆汁酸可以进入结肠,或在小肠经被动或主动吸收后返回肝脏，并重新与甘氨酸或牛磺酸结合，并与新合成的胆汁酸一起重新分泌到胆汁中。这一肠道解离和肝脏再结合的过程是胆汁酸代谢的常规途径。肠道菌群对胆汁酸的另一种修饰是对 α-羟基进行异构化，生成相应的 β-羟基衍生物（“异”胆汁酸），如异石胆酸和异去氧胆酸[21]。虽然在某些个体的盲肠或结肠内容物中可能存在大量异胆汁酸，但这些源自肠道的异胆汁酸尚未得到广泛的研究，其生理或临床意义仍不清楚。7α 羟基 CDCA 可在肠道菌群作用下异构为 3α，7β-二羟胆酸——熊去氧胆酸（UDCA）[22]。UDCA 从肠道被吸收后，与肝脏中的甘氨酸或牛磺酸结合，作为胆汁酸池的次要成分循环，通常少于 5%。需要注意的是，UDCA 除了作为一种次要的次级胆汁酸由肠道微生物产生外，还可用于治疗各种类型的胆汁淤积性肝病（参见第 91 章）[23]。

一部分循环中的胆汁酸在小肠未被重吸收并进入结肠，在结肠中基本完全解离。结肠内一小部分细菌能够有效地去除 C-7 位羟基（7α 脱羟基），从而将 CA 转换为脱氧胆酸（deoxycholic acid，DCA，C3 和 C12-二羟基胆酸），将 CDCA 转换为石胆（lithocholic acid，LCA，C3-单羟基胆酸），如图 64.2 所示[22]。尽管肠道微生物催化的其他胆汁酸修饰，如解离、异构和氧化作用可以被肝脏中的酶逆转，但是胆汁酸的 C7 位点不会出现再羟基化[24]。因此，细菌对胆汁酸的 C7 位脱羟基作用对胆汁酸池组成和特性的形成特别重要。结肠可重吸收大约 50% 转换出的 DCA 以及一部分 LCA。返回肝脏后，DCA 与甘氨酸或牛磺酸重新结合，并与初级胆汁酸一起循环，而 LCA 则重新结合并硫酸化[25]。肠肝循环中的胆汁酸在肝内重新结合非常迅速，因此几乎所有内源性胆汁酸（主要是 CA、CDCA、DCA 和 UDCA）都以结合形式存在。结肠中细菌对胆汁酸的解离和脱羟基作用也非常迅速，因此粪便中主要含有非结合次级胆汁酸，和少量（<15%）其他类型胆汁酸（参见图 64.1）[26]。

人体内次级胆汁酸代谢有几条途径，包括 β-羟基异构胆汁酸在肝脏的反向异构，7-氧石胆盐在肝脏还原成 CDCA 或 UDCA，以及胆汁酸的羟基化、葡萄糖醛酸化或硫酸化（参见图 64.2）[25]。胆汁酸硫酸化或葡萄糖醛酸化后肠道和肾脏重吸收减少，在循环胆汁酸池中迅速消失。硫酸化对 LCA 的代谢尤为重要。未修饰的 LCA 具有内在的肝毒性，硫酸化 LCA 的 3-羟基位可使其外排增加，从而起到重要的保肝作用[27]。除了硫酸化或葡萄糖醛酸化作用外，胆汁酸甾环的其他位置也可发生羟基化，包括 C-1、C-2、C-4 或 C-6。成人正常生理条件下，这些多羟基胆汁酸通常处于非常低的水平。但是这些不寻常的胆汁酸种类在新生儿、减重手术后和胆汁淤积性肝病患者中水平较高。肝脏第 1 期、第 2 期负责羟基化和硫酸化胆汁酸的酶，其表达由 LCA 或利福平等药物在转录水平调控，机制包括外源性激活核受体-孕烷 X 受体（pregnane X receptor，PXR）和组成性雄激素受体（constitutive androsterone receptor，CAR）（参见第 88 章）。

二、肠肝循环

肠肝循环由肝脏、胆道、胆囊、小肠、门静脉循环及结肠和体循环（较小程度上）组成（图 64.3）。机制上看，胆汁酸的肠肝循环由储存室（胆囊和小肠）、瓣膜（Oddi 括约肌和回盲瓣）、机械泵（小肠）和化学泵（肝细胞、胆管细胞和回肠上皮细胞）组成。

胆汁酸高效的肠道重吸收和肝脏摄取使其能够有效地循环和保存，在很大程度上限制了胆汁酸进入肠道和肝胆系统。空腹时，胆汁酸沿着胆道向下移动，并在胆囊中浓缩 10 倍左右，导致小肠、门静脉、体循环和肝脏中胆汁酸水平较低。然而，肝胆汁酸分泌量保持恒定，未进入胆囊的那部分胆汁酸的肠肝循环仍在继续。进食后，结肠黏膜释放胆囊收缩素，作用于胆道并松弛 Oddi 括约肌，刺激胆囊收缩。胆囊内浓缩的混合胶束（胆汁酸、磷脂和胆固醇）经胆道进入小肠。在肠腔内，这些胶束通过刺激胰脂肪酶对甘油三酯的作用促进脂肪的消化和吸收，溶解长链饱和脂肪酸等水解产物，并将这些疏水性脂质穿过静止的水层运送到黏膜表面。在消化较多食物时，胆囊仍然收缩，肝脏分泌的胆汁酸可绕过胆囊直接进入十二指肠。在此期间，小肠腔内胆汁酸浓度可达 5~10mmol/L，远高于形成胶束所需的约 1.5mmol/L 的阈值。在消化间期，Oddi 括约肌收缩，胆囊松弛，使分泌入胆汁的胆汁酸多数进入胆囊并存储。胆汁酸可通过激活 G 蛋白偶联受体 TGR5 直接调控，或刺激回肠合成和释放 FGF19（松弛胆囊的多肽激素）来间接调控这一过程[28]。总的来说，胆汁酸的肠肝循环在消化过程中加速，而在两餐之间和夜间禁食期间会减慢。胆囊切除术后，这种节律性胆汁酸分泌仍然存在。当胆囊缺失时，禁食期间胆汁酸储存于近端小肠，通过肠移行性复合运动驱动远端肠腔内胆汁酸池（参见第 99 章）。进食后，小肠收缩加速并推动储存的胆汁酸到远端回肠，原地重吸收并返回肝脏以供再次分泌入胆汁。

胆汁酸的肠肝循环非常高效，仅不到 10% 的肠道胆汁酸不能被重吸收，经粪便排出。胆汁酸在小肠内被动重吸收并主动转运至回肠末端[29]。成人肠肝循环中胆汁酸池大小约为 2~4g。每餐胆汁酸池循环 2~3 次，肠道每天可重吸收 10~30g 胆汁酸。每天不能重吸收的量约 0.2~0.6g，并经粪便排出。肝脏内胆固醇转化为胆汁酸可平衡粪便排泄丢失的量，以维持胆汁酸池的大小。表 64.2 总结了人体内胆汁酸转化的动力学。

胆汁酸的肠肝循环是有利的，因为它可以蓄积大量具有清洁作用的分子，并可在一天中消化一餐或多餐时反复使用。回肠主动转运系统和肠肝循环的存在，使肝脏胆汁酸分泌与合成相互独立，从而提高了肠道营养物质消化吸收的效率。由于胆汁酸分泌刺激肝内胆汁分泌，维持肠肝循环也可促进胆汁的持续分泌。胆囊的存在保证了胆汁酸生物合成与肠内运输的相互独立，其浓缩并储存胆汁酸后，以可控的方式将高浓度胆汁酸释放到十二指肠。回肠胆汁酸转运系统和胆囊是互补的，两者并不重叠，它们协同作用来储存胆汁酸。当回肠胆汁酸转运系统缺失而仅有胆囊时，分泌至肠道的胆汁酸不能被充分重吸收。胆囊排空之后必然会有一段不应期，在这段时间内胆汁酸供应不足，无法促进脂质的有效消化和吸收。不应期一直持续到肝合成新的胆汁酸并恢复胆汁酸池。

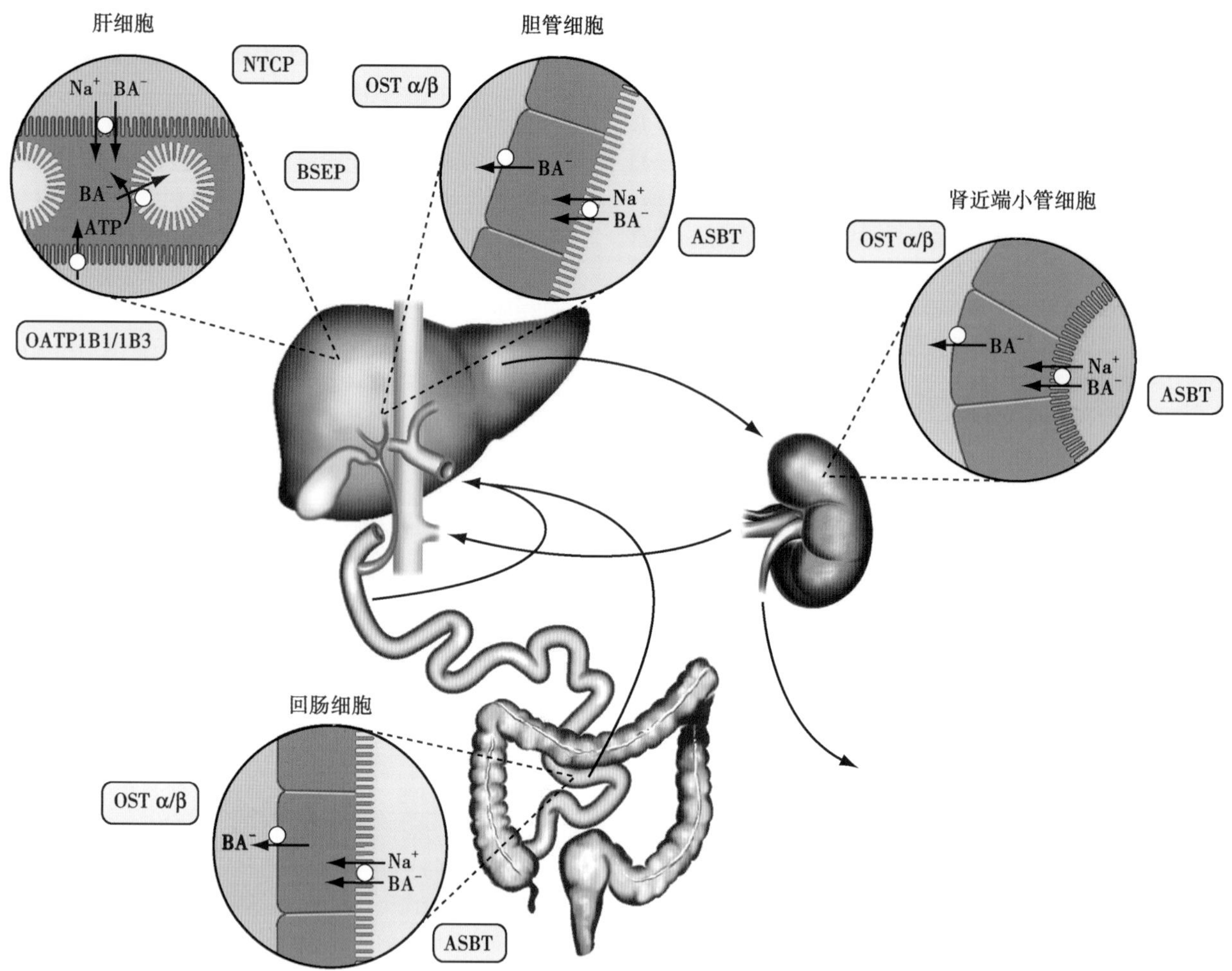

图 64.3　胆汁酸的肝肠循环。显示负责胆汁酸(BA)跨各种上皮细胞转运的单个转运蛋白,包括肝细胞、胆管细胞、回肠细胞(回肠上皮细胞)和肾近曲小管细胞。A^-,阴离子;ASBT(基因符号 *SLC10A2*),顶端胆汁酸转运蛋白;BSEP(*ABCB11*),胆盐输出泵;NTCP(*SLC10A1*),Na^+-牛磺胆酸共转运多肽;OATP,有机阴离子转运多肽;OST,有机溶质转运蛋白。(Adapted with permission Shneider BL. Intestinal bile acid transport:biology,physiology,and pathophysiology. J Pediatr Gastroenterol Nutr. 2001;32:407-17.)

三、肝内胆汁酸转运和胆汁分泌

肝细胞和胆管上皮细胞(胆管细胞)分泌具有渗透活性的无机和有机溶质,进入毛细胆管间隙和胆道腔内形成胆汁,应用甘露醇或赤藓醇作为惰性标志物进行了相关研究。肝毛细胆管胆汁形成可分为两部分:胆汁酸依赖的胆汁(胆汁与胆汁酸分泌相关)和非胆汁酸依赖的胆汁(胆汁归因于活性无机电解质和其他溶质的分泌),分别约占基础自发性胆汁的 60% 和 40%[1]。肝内依赖 ATP 的载体将胆汁主动分泌至毛细胆管腔内,形成较大的聚合物和混合胶束,无法沿毛细胆管壁周围的细胞旁连接弥散回肝内。化合物如结合胆汁酸通过泵作用跨越毛细胆管细胞膜产生胆汁,被称为初级溶质。除胆汁酸外,初级溶质还包括谷胱甘肽、结合胆红素、重金属以及各种代谢物和外源物的结合物。水、血电解质、钙、葡萄糖、氨基酸、碳酸氢盐和其他小分子溶质随渗透梯度流入毛细胆管称为二级溶质。初级溶质的促胆汁分泌活性,定义为每分泌一定量的溶质所引起的胆汁量。每分泌 1μmol 天然胆汁酸,其促胆汁分泌活性为 8~40μL。肝细胞和胆管上皮分泌的胆汁酸以外的其他初级溶质,如谷胱甘肽和碳酸氢盐也有参与胆汁的形成。毛细胆管内新分泌胆汁在胆管内运输过程中,被胆管细胞修饰,包括:①对葡萄糖、氨基酸和胆汁酸等溶质的吸收;②水通过特定通道(水通道蛋白)和细胞旁流动;③分泌溶质,如碳酸氢盐和氯化物。不同物种间胆管分泌所占比重存在差异,人类约为胆汁流量的 30%,而在动物(如大鼠)中不到 10%[1]。

(一) 非胆汁酸依赖性胆汁

胆汁酸外其他初级溶质的分泌也参与肝毛细胆管内胆汁分泌,主要是还原性谷胱甘肽(glutathione,GSH)和碳酸氢盐(HCO_3^-)。毛细胆管通过多重耐药相关蛋白 2(MRP2)通路,依赖 ATP 分泌 GSH 和 GSH 结合物。GSH 以高浓度分泌入胆汁,GGTP 和二肽酶在腔内分解代谢 GSH 进一步提高了溶质浓度,增加毛细胆管内胆汁形成的渗透驱动力。除了依赖 ATP 的有机阴离子分泌至胆汁外,肝细胞和胆管细胞可通过 HCO_3^-/Cl^- 阴离子交换剂 AE2 不依赖 ATP 分泌 HCO_3^-,对于不依赖于胆汁酸的胆汁也很重要。这种 HCO_3^- 分泌发生在胆管上皮细胞受到各种激素和神经肽刺激之后,如促胰液素、血管活性肠肽和胆汁酸[30]。

（二）胆肝分流通路

“胆肝分流”这一理论由 Alan Hofmann 首先提出，是指胆汁中非结合二羟基胆汁酸被胆管细胞被动吸收，然后通过静脉回流至肝脏，并被肝细胞吸收后再次分泌至胆汁的循环。吸收质子化的非结合胆汁酸分子可产生 HCO_3^-，它与肝内再分泌的胆汁酸一起生成富含碳酸氢盐的胆汁。这个理论可以很好地解释：在给予治疗剂量的非结合 C-24 二羟基胆汁酸（如 UDCA）或非结合短侧链的 C-23 胆汁酸类似物（如 norUDCA）后，可观察到胆汁流量增加[31]。尽管这一理论在概念上是合理的，并且与现有的数据基本一致，但胆肝循环的肝内定位和其被动属性，使其难以被进一步研究或证实。此外，由于在正常生理条件下，胆管内胆汁基本均为结合胆汁酸，最初认为非结合胆汁酸胆肝分流所引起的胆汁流量变化是微不足道的。随后发现胆道上皮细胞表达顶端钠依赖性胆汁酸转运蛋白（ASBT；基因符号 *SLC10A2*）和有机溶质转运蛋白 OSTα-OSTβ（基因符号 *SLC51A* 和 *SLC51B*），使结合胆汁酸的胆肝分流成为可能。然而，该通路在人类中的意义仍有待确定。事实上，ASBT 在胆道上皮的作用可能是协助胆管细胞测定胆汁中胆汁酸的浓度，以激活细胞信号通路，而不是转运大量胆汁酸[32]。

（三）肝内胆汁酸转运

90% 以上分泌到胆汁中的胆汁酸来源于循环池。肝细胞必须有效地将胆汁酸从门静脉血液中转运至胆汁，才能保障这一进程的顺利进行。胆汁酸经过这一跨肝细胞转运后被浓缩，是由肝窦和毛细胆管质膜上一系列特定的转运系统实施的，包括初级（atp 依赖）、二级（Na^+梯度依赖）和三级（OH^-或 HCO_3^-依赖的阴离子交换）转运。不同情况下，胆汁酸通过肝脏的流量和参与的肝细胞数量不同。空腹时门静脉周围肝细

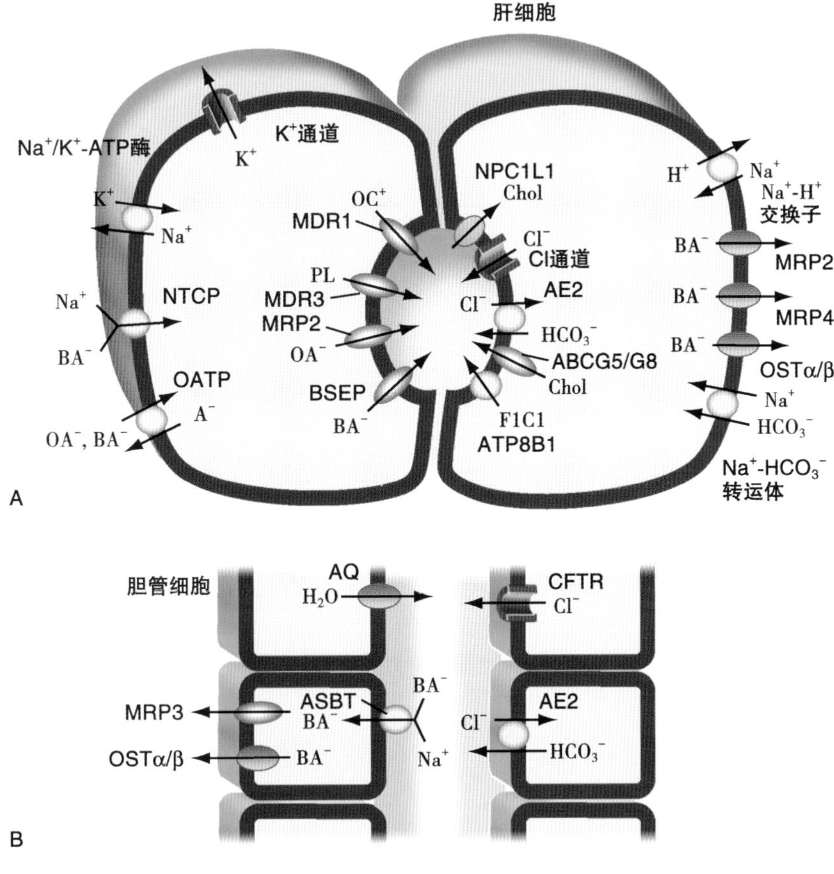

图 64.4 肝细胞和胆管细胞与胆汁酸分泌相关的重要转运蛋白。在肝细胞的窦状隙膜上，Na^+-牛磺胆酸共转运多肽（NTCP；基因符号 *SLC10A1*）介导结合胆汁酸的摄取。通过 NTCP 的胆汁酸钠依赖性摄取是由 Na^+/K^+-ATP 酶产生的内向钠梯度差驱动的，而膜电位部分由 K^+ 通道产生。非 Na^+ 依赖性胆汁酸摄取由有机阴离子转运多肽 OATP1B1（*SLCO1B1*）和 OATP1B3（*SLCO1B3*）介导。肝窦状膜还包含 Na^+-H^+ 交换器和 Na^+-HCO_3^- 协同转运蛋白（同向转运蛋白）。在毛细胆管膜上，胆汁酸通过胆盐输出泵（BSEP；*ABCB11*）分泌，而硫酸化或葡萄糖醛酸化的胆汁酸则通过多重耐药相关蛋白 2（MRP2；*ABCC2*）分泌。毛细胆管膜还表达 ATP 依赖性输出泵，将磷脂（多重耐药蛋白 3、*MDR3*、*ABCC3*）、胆固醇和植物甾醇（*ABCG5/ABCG8*）以及药物代谢产物（MDR1；*ABCB1*）转运至胆汁。毛细胆管膜也表达 ATP 非依赖性转运蛋白，包括输入甾醇、氯离子通道的 Niemann-Pick C1 样 1（NPC1L1）蛋白和分泌碳酸氢盐的氯化物-碳酸氢盐阴离子交换异构体 2（AE2）。FIC1（*ATP8B1*）是进行性家族性肝内胆汁淤积 1 型中突变的 P 型 ATP 酶。在大胆管的胆管细胞内，结合胆汁酸被顶端 Na^+ 依赖性胆汁酸转运蛋白（ASBT；*SLC10A2*）吸收。然后胆汁酸可能通过异聚转运蛋白 OSTα-OSTβ 或 ATP 依赖性载体 MRP3（*ABCC3*）从基底外侧表面进入肝动脉循环。胆管细胞还表达其他多种对修饰胆汁很重要的载体，包括 CFTR，分泌碳酸盐的 AE2⁻和促进水运动的多种水通道蛋白亚型。A^-，阴离子；BA^-，胆汁酸阴离子；Chol，胆固醇；OA^-，有机阴离子；OC^+，有机阳离子；PL，磷脂。（Adapted with permission from Wagner M, Zollner G, Trauner M. New molecular insights into the mechanism of cholestasis. J Hepatol 2009;51:565-80.）

胞(最靠近门静脉)对胆汁酸的摄取最高,进食后则以肝腺泡的远端肝细胞为主。相反,新合成胆汁酸的产生和分泌主要在中央静脉周围肝细胞(最靠近中央静脉)。因此,门静脉周围肝细胞运输的胆汁酸比例最高,是胆汁酸依赖胆汁的主要驱动因素。

健康人门静脉血液中胆汁酸的浓度为20~50μmol/L。肝脏对胆汁酸的吸收通常表现为分段摄取或首过摄取,与通过肝血窦后一次可排出的胆汁酸比例相一致。肝血窦分段摄取胆汁酸的比例为50%~90%,且保持恒定,不受体循环中胆汁酸浓度的影响。肝分段摄取比例与胆汁酸结构和白蛋白结合相关,亲水性结合胆汁酸如结合 CA 的摄取量最高(80%~90%),非结合疏水性蛋白结合胆汁酸如 CDCA 的摄取量最低(50%~60%)。由于肝脏的快速鉴别清除作用,体循环中总胆汁酸的浓度很低,空腹和餐后分别为 2~5μmol/L 和 5~15μmol/L,且体循环中胆汁构成与全身其他部位并不一致[33]。

维持胆汁酸肠肝循环的主要转运蛋白如图 64.3 和图 64.4 所示,其特性见表 64.4。由于其对胆汁分泌的重要性,胆汁酸转运蛋白研究较多,然而肝窦状隙和毛细胆管膜还表达可转运其他内源性和外源性化合物的转运蛋白[34]。

表 64.4　参与胆汁形成和胆汁酸肠肝循环的转运蛋白的位置和功能

转运蛋白(基因)	位置	功能
肝细胞	**胆汁酸依赖的胆汁**	
NTCP(*SLC10A1*)	基底外侧膜	Na^+依赖的胆汁酸和外源物摄取
OATP1B1(*SLCO1B1*)	基底外侧膜	非 Na^+依赖的胆汁酸和外源物摄取
OATP1B3(*SLCO1B3*)	基底外侧膜	非 Na^+依赖的胆汁酸和外源物摄取
Na^+,K^+-ATP 酶	基底外侧膜	分泌 2 Na^+并与 3 K^+交换
BSEP(*ABCB11*)	毛细胆管膜	ATP 依赖的胆汁酸外排
MDR3(*ABCB4*)	毛细胆管膜	ATP 依赖的磷脂酰胆碱外排
ABCG5/ABCG8	毛细胆管膜	ATP 依赖的甾醇外排
NPC1L1	毛细胆管膜	甾醇向内转运
FIC1(*ATP8B1*)	毛细胆管膜	ATP 依赖的氨磷脂翻转
	非胆汁酸依赖胆汁	
OATP1B1,1B3,2B1	基底外侧膜	非 Na^+依赖的有机阴离子、阳离子和中性类固醇转运
MRP2(*ABCC2*)	毛细胆管膜	ATP 依赖的葡萄糖醛酸、谷胱甘肽和硫酸结合物
	窦状隙胆汁酸外排	
MRP3(*ABCC3*)	基底外侧膜	ATP 依赖的胆汁酸、葡萄糖醛酸结合物外排
MRP4(*ABCC4*)	基底外侧膜	ATP 依赖的谷胱甘肽和胆汁酸外排
OSTα-OSTβ(*SLC51A*,*SLC51B*)	基底外侧膜	胆汁酸外排
胆管细胞	**胆管分泌**	
Aquaporin 1(*AQP1*)	顶端膜	水转运
Aquaporin 4(*AQP4*)	基底外侧膜	水转运
AE2(*SLC4A2*)	顶端膜	Cl^-交换以分泌 HCO_3^-
CFTR(*ABCC7*)	顶端膜	Cl^-分泌
ASBT(*SLC10A2*)	顶端膜	胆汁酸摄取(胆肝分流)
回肠上皮细胞		
ASBT(*SLC10A2*)	顶端膜	Na^+依赖的胆汁酸摄取
NPC1L1	顶端膜	类固醇向内转运
OSTα-OSTβ(*SLC51A*,*SLC51B*)	基底外侧膜	胆汁酸外排
MRP3(*ABCC3*)	基底外侧膜	胆汁酸外排

ABC,ATP 结合盒;AE2,氯化物-碳酸氢盐阴离子交换异构体 2;ASBT,顶端 Na^+胆汁酸转运蛋白;BSEP,胆盐输出泵;FIC1,进行性家族性肝内胆汁淤积 1 型中突变的 P 型 ATP 酶;MDR,多重耐药蛋白;MRP,多重耐药相关蛋白;NPC1L1,尼曼匹克 C1 样 1;NTCP,Na^+-牛磺胆酸共转运蛋白;OATP,有机阴离子转运多肽;OST,有机溶质转运蛋白;SLC,溶质载体。

（四）肝窦 Na^+ 依赖性胆汁酸摄取

肝窦（基底外侧）膜结合胆汁酸的摄取主要（>80%）由二级（Na^+ 依赖）转运系统介导，依赖于基底外侧膜维持 Na^+ 外高内低梯度的 Na^+/K^+-ATP 酶驱动。虽然对结合胆汁酸非常重要，但 Na^+ 依赖转运只占非结合胆汁酸（如 CA 和 UDCA）摄取的一半以下。肝细胞钠耦合胆汁酸摄取的主要转运蛋白是 Na^+-牛磺胆酸联合转运多肽（NTCP；基因符号 *SLC10A1*）。遗传性 NTCP 基因缺陷患者血浆中结合胆汁酸水平显著升高（25~100 倍），但没有黄疸、瘙痒或其他肝病表现[35,36]。除了作为肝内胆汁酸重吸收的主要转运体之外，NTCP 可作为肝细胞表面受体与 HBV 和 HDV 结合，并协助病毒进入细胞内（参见第 79 和 81 章）[37]。NTCP 的 267 位丝氨酸突变为苯丙氨酸（c. 800C>T；rs2296651；p. Ser267Phe）为自然突变之一，可导致胆汁酸转运活性基本丧失。这种变异在亚洲人群中最多见（次等位基因频率 3.1%~9.2%），其辅助病毒进入细胞的能力亦减弱，从而降低 HBV 易感性。基于这些发现，目前已有靶向 NTCP 的病毒进入抑制剂的研究，来阻断新生 HBV 感染或降低慢性 HBV 感染患者的病毒载量。

（五）肝窦非 Na^+ 依赖性胆汁酸摄取

非结合胆汁酸如 CA 主要由有机阴离子转运多肽（organic aniontransporting polypeptide，OATP；基因符号 *SLCO*，其中"SLC"和"O"分别表示溶质载体和 OATP）基因家族成员以不依赖 Na^+ 的方式摄取。与 NTCP 和 ASBT 等 Na^+ 联合转运体不同，OATP 介导的溶质摄取驱动来源尚不清楚，且其转运可能是双向的。可能的转运机制包括协助扩散和电中性交换，将溶质摄取与 HCO_3^- 或谷胱甘肽流出相耦合[38]。人 OATP1B1（基因符号 *SLCO1B1*；旧称 OATP-C）和 OATP1B3（基因符号 *SLCO1B3*；旧称 OATP8）主要在肝脏表达，负责大部分非 Na^+ 依赖性胆汁酸清除。然而，除了胆汁酸之外，OATP1B1 和 OATP1B3 也运输其他各种有机阴离子和溶质，包括葡萄糖醛酸胆红素（参见第 21 章），类固醇代谢产物（雌二醇-17β-葡萄糖醛酸盐，脱氢表雄酮硫酸盐，和硫酸雌酮），花生四烯酸类（前列腺素 E_2、血栓素 B_2 和白三烯 C_4），诊断性染料[如溴磺酚酞和吲哚菁绿（indocyanine green，ICG）]和药物（如利福平、他汀、地高辛和非索非那定）。值得注意的是，人类 12 号染色体上相邻基因 *SLCO1B1* 和 *SLCO1B3* 的联合缺失会导致 Rotor 综合征，这是一种 Dubin-Johnson 综合征之外的，罕见的良性遗传性高结合胆红素血症[39]。尽管并未测定 OATP1B1/OATP1B3 缺陷患者的血浆非结合胆汁酸清除率，但在同源 Oatp1a/1b 基因缺陷的小鼠中，肝脏对非结合胆汁酸清除率受损，但是结合胆汁酸清除不受影响[39]。此外，单纯 OATP1B3 缺陷即可引起 ICG 清除延迟，导致血中 ICG 潴留（浓度升高），而肝功化验和肝穿刺病理正常[40]。由于胆汁酸池以结合胆汁酸为主，而肝细胞对结合胆汁酸摄取以 Na^+ 依赖性方式为主，这些宽谱特异性 OATPs 可能对非胆汁酸代谢产物和外源物质的肝脏清除更为重要。事实上，OATP 基因的遗传多态性影响药物代谢，并与部分药物毒性有关[41]。

（六）肝窦胆汁酸流出

肝细胞基底外侧膜（肝窦）转运非结合、结合或修饰后（硫酸化、葡萄糖醛酸化、多羟基化）胆汁酸进入迪塞氏间隙，由异聚有机溶质转运蛋白 OSTα-OSTβ，MRP 家族成员包括 MRP3（基因符号 *ABCC3*）、MRP4（基因符号 *ABCC4*）和其他载体介导。结合和非结合胆汁酸外排至肝血窦后，被运送到更多的中心周围肝细胞，进行再摄取并分泌入胆汁[42]。这一过程动态地从肝小叶 2 区和 3 区募集更多的肝细胞，以维持胆汁酸清除和分泌进入胆汁，从而保护门静脉周围脆弱的 1 区肝细胞。此外，肝细胞第 1 期或第 2 期代谢产生的修饰后胆汁酸也通过基底外侧膜排出进入体循环，被肾脏过滤并随尿液排出。这些肝保护机制，包括下调肝胆汁酸摄取的主要转运蛋白，是对胆汁酸超载继发反应的重要组成部分[43]。

（七）毛细胆管胆汁酸转运

由于胆汁酸具有潜在的去清洁还原作用，其肝细胞摄取和外排必须严格平衡，否则细胞内蓄积可导致细胞毒性。不管其摄取机制如何，重吸收和新合成的胆汁酸都被 ATP 依赖的胆汁酸盐外排泵（bile salt export pump，BSEP；基因符号 *ABCB11*）运送至毛细胆管细胞膜，并分泌至胆汁。2 型进行性家族性肝内胆汁淤积症（progressive familial intrahepatic cholestasis type 2，PFIC2；一种以胆汁酸分泌受损为特征的肝脏疾病）患者存在 *ABCB11* 突变，证实了 BSEP 是毛细胆管细胞膜主要的胆汁酸转运蛋白（参见第 77 章）[44]。尽管胆汁酸是 BESP 的主要底物，但许多其他化合物如环孢素、利福平、曲格列酮、波生坦和格列本脲等药物，亦可与 BSEP 结合，直接竞争性拮抗 BESP 与胆汁酸的结合，减少胆汁酸输出，这可能是某些药物导致肝损伤的重要机制（参见第 88 章）[45]。

四、肠道和肾胆汁酸转运

（一）肠道胆汁酸转运

多个研究均显示，回肠末端是胆汁酸重吸收的主要部位。在回肠之前肠腔内胆汁酸浓度几乎没有下降，而回肠切除术后患者存在胆汁酸吸收不良。原位灌注肠段胆汁酸吸收测定显示，回肠胆汁酸转运系统效率很高，足以重吸收全部胆道外排的胆汁酸。回肠主动转运是结合胆汁酸重吸收的主要途径，特别是亲水性强和牛磺酸结合的胆汁酸。在近端小肠，部分甘氨酸结合胆汁酸被质子化，当消化过程中腔内 pH 短暂变为酸性环境时，可通过非离子被动扩散吸收。此外，小肠和结肠的肠道菌群作用下代谢产物可生成疏水性非结合胆汁酸，具有弱酸性，作为溶质可经被动扩散吸收。

（二）肾胆汁酸转运

部分（10%~50%，取决于胆汁酸种类）门静脉循环中的胆汁酸，未经过肝脏首过式重吸收，直接流入体循环。胆汁酸与血浆蛋白的结合降低了肾小球滤过，并最大限度地减少胆汁酸经尿排出。健康肾脏每天大约滤过 100μmol 的胆汁酸。值得注意的是，由于高效的肾小管重吸收能力，只有 1~2μmol 胆汁酸从尿中排出。即使在血浆胆汁酸浓度显著升高的胆汁淤积性肝病患者中，24 小时尿非硫酸化胆汁酸排泄量也远低于肾小球滤过量。随后的研究证实，肾小球滤过的胆汁酸被肾小管主动重吸收，导致胆汁淤积性肝病患者血清胆汁酸浓度升高。与回肠一样，肾近端小管上皮表达 Na^+ 浓度梯度驱动的转运蛋白，作为保存胆汁酸的挽救机制。

（三）分子机制

胆汁酸在回肠刷状缘膜囊泡被 Na^+ 胆汁酸转运蛋白（apical sodium-dependent bile acid transporter，ASBT；基因符号 *SLC10A2*）主动转运至细胞内。通过克隆肝脏、胆道、回肠和肾脏组织中 Na^+-胆汁酸联合载体，阐明了这些组织间胆汁酸转运系统的关系。肝脏和回肠分别表达不同但相关的 Na^+-胆汁酸联合转运蛋白 NTCP 和 ASBT，而回肠上皮细胞、肾近端小管细胞和胆管细胞表达 ASBT。ASBT 介导的顶端刷状缘膜囊泡胆汁酸重吸收的驱动力包括细胞内负电位、外高内低的 Na^+ 浓度梯度和细胞周围 Na^+ 从肠道黏膜下层回流到管腔[46]。ASBT 可以运输所有主要种类的胆汁酸，但不能运输修饰过的胆汁酸或不相关的溶质。ASBT 基因突变可导致原发性胆汁酸吸收不良（一种与肠道胆汁酸吸收不良和脂肪泻相关的疾病），提示大多数人体肠道胆汁酸重吸收是由 ASBT 介导的[47]。

回肠胆汁酸结合蛋白（ileal bile acid binding protein，IBABP；基因符号 *FABP6*）是脂肪酸结合蛋白家族成员之一，在回肠上皮细胞胞质中含量丰富。尽管不是必需的，IBABP 缺陷小鼠的回肠胆汁酸重吸收存在部分缺陷，提示 IBABP 参与了胆汁酸的跨细胞转运[48]。回肠上皮细胞、胆管细胞和肾近端小管细胞基底外侧膜上负责胆汁酸输出的转运蛋白已经被确定。异聚有机溶质转运蛋白 OSTα-OSTβ 表达于回肠上皮细胞、肝细胞、胆管细胞和肾近端小管细胞的基底外侧膜上，负责转运胆汁酸以及多种有机阴离子和药物。遗传性人 OSTβ 基因（*SLC51B*）突变已被确定为先天性慢性腹泻的原因之一，与 ASBT 突变患者观察到的表型相似[49]。

五、肠肝循环障碍

胆汁淤积被定义为胆汁形成异常，通常分为肝内胆汁淤积（肝细胞水平上胆汁形成的功能缺陷）和肝外胆汁淤积（胆道内胆汁流动受阻）。胆汁酸和其他有机溶质的肝脏转运受损是遗传性和获得性胆汁淤积性肝病的一个显著特征。肠肝循环障碍一般分为以下 4 类：①胆汁酸形成障碍（合成和接合）；②胆汁酸跨膜转运障碍（重吸收和分泌）；③涉及细菌转化的异常（去结合和去羟基化）；④器官或器官间的运动障碍（胆汁酸循环）[50]。

罕见的遗传性胆汁酸合成障碍的特异性诊断，依赖于通过快原子轰击质谱和电喷雾多级串联质谱等方法进行体液（尿、血液、胆汁）分析[2]。表现为 CA 和 CDCA 显著减少或完全缺失，胆汁、血清和尿液中的非典型胆汁酸浓度显著升高。空腹血清胆汁酸升高也被认为是妊娠期肝内胆汁淤积（intrahepatic cholestasis of pregnancy，ICP）的早期特征。然而，仅测量血清总胆汁酸浓度而不分析单个胆汁酸和胆汁酸中间体，在诊断或治疗大多数肝病和胆汁酸吸收不良方面，与常规肝功化验相比，似乎没有什么优势。靶向或全外显子测序已被用于诊断与胃肠道或肝脏疾病相关的遗传性胆汁酸合成和转运异常[49,51]。

（一）胆汁酸合成

由胆固醇合成胆汁酸是维持肠肝循环中胆汁酸池所必需。尽管遗传性合成缺陷很罕见，但这些疾病说明了胆汁酸合成对正常肝脏和肠道功能的重要性。胆汁酸合成异常包括经粪便排泄耗尽胆汁酸池，丧失胆汁酸依赖的胆汁，胆道排出胆固醇和外源物减少，脂肪和脂溶性维生素吸收不良，细胞毒性胆汁酸合成中间体蓄积。据报道，参与胆汁酸生物合成的 11 种酶和 1 种转运蛋白存在遗传缺陷，包括胆固醇 7α 羟化酶（*CYP7A1*）、甾醇 27 羟化酶（*CYP27A1*）、氧甾醇-7α 羟化酶（*CYP7B1*）、3β 羟基-Δ5-C27-类固醇氧化还原酶（*HSD3B7*）、Δ4-3-氧甾醇 5β-还原酶（*AKR1D1*）、2-甲基酰基复合酶-A-消旋酶（*AMACR*）、酰基辅酶 A 氧化酶 2（*ACOX2*）、D-双功能蛋白（*HSD17B4*）、类固醇载体蛋白 X（*SCP2*）、胆汁酸辅酶 A 连接酶（*SLC27A5*）、胆汁酸复合酶 A：氨基酸-N-酰基转移酶（*BAAT*）、过氧化物酶体 ATP 结合盒（ABC）转运体 2（*ABCD3*）。除了这些特定的缺陷，过氧化物酶体生物发生异常的疾病如 Zellweger 综合征，也会影响胆汁酸的合成，因为胆汁酸侧链修饰发生在过氧化物酶体中（参见第 77 章）。

单个酶的缺陷通常不足以阻止所有胆汁酸的产生，因为存在多种合成途径。临床上，胆汁酸合成缺陷的患者通常表现为脂肪泻、生长迟缓、脂溶性维生素吸收不良相关的后遗症以及轻至重度肝病。尽管在一些其他类型的胆汁淤积中，血清 GGTP 水平升高，但胆汁酸合成障碍所致的胆汁淤积患者中，GGTP 水平通常是正常的，这与酶缺陷发生在毛细胆管分泌之前有关。根据突变性质和受影响的合成通路步骤不同，胆汁酸合成障碍临床严重程度不同，最严重的为新生儿胆汁淤积性肝病或后期的神经系统疾病。例如，脑腱黄瘤病（CTX）是一种罕见的遗传性疾病，是由线粒体酶类固醇 27-羟化酶（*CYP27A1*）突变引起的。在 CTX 中，胆汁酸合成的替代途径被阻断，胆汁酸的产生减少但没有完全消除。CTX 可在婴儿早期即出现胆汁淤积性肝病，但一般表现为后期进行性神经紊乱、过早动脉粥样硬化、白内障和腱黄瘤。报道最多的胆汁酸合成障碍是 3β 羟基-Δ5-C27-类固醇氧化还原酶（*HSD3B7*）缺陷，同时影响胆汁酸合成的经典途径和替代途径。本病的特点是进行性肝内胆汁淤积和异常胆汁酸的蓄积。临床表现包括高非结合胆红素血症、黄疸、血清转氨酶升高、脂肪泻、脂溶性维生素缺乏、瘙痒和生长不良。疾病的进展不同，但最终多数患者进展至肝硬化和肝衰竭。胆汁酸替代疗法（早期口服胆汁酸如 CA），已被证实对胆汁酸合成障碍有效，但对 Zellweger 综合征作用有限（参见第 77 章）[52,53]。

（二）胆汁酸和胆脂跨膜转运

越来越多的疾病被发现与胆汁酸和有机溶质转运的重要基因突变有关[54]。表 64.5 汇总了这些疾病，包括 PFIC、良性复发性肝内胆汁淤积（benign recurrent intrahepatic cholestasis，BRIC）、ICP、低磷脂相关胆石症（low phospholipid-associated cholelithiasis，LPAC）、Dubin-Johnson 综合征、Rotor 综合征、谷固醇血症、原发性胆汁酸吸收不良和各种形式的先天性腹泻。

表 64.5 遗传性转运蛋白缺陷相关的肠肝循环疾病

疾病	转运蛋白缺陷	缺陷蛋白(基因)	临床特征
进行性家族性肝内胆汁淤积			
1 型	氨磷脂	FIC1(*ATP8B1*)	进行性胆汁淤积,血清胆汁酸水平升高,瘙痒,低或正常的血 GGTP 水平,胰腺炎,肠吸收不良,听力受损
2 型	胆汁酸	BSEP(*ABCB11*)	进行性胆汁淤积,黄疸,巨细胞形成,小叶或门脉纤维化,肝胆恶性病变,低或正常的血 GGTP 水平
3 型	磷脂酰胆碱	MDR3(*ABCB4*)	胆汁淤积,胆管明显增殖和门脉周围纤维化,血 GGTP 水平升高
良性复发性肝内胆汁淤积			
1 型	氨磷脂	FIC1(*ATP8B1*)	周期性胆汁淤积,血胆汁酸水平升高,瘙痒,低或正常的血 GGTP 水平,吸收不良,听力受损
2 型	胆汁酸	BSEP(*ABCB11*)	周期性胆汁淤积,胆石症,低或正常的血 GGTP 水平,肝脾大
LPAC	磷脂酰胆碱	MDR3(*ABCB4*)	胆石症,肝内高回声灶,胆管纤维化,血 GGTP 水平升高
妊娠期肝内胆汁淤积			
	磷脂酰胆碱	MDR3(*ABCB4*)	妊娠 3 个月出现的胆汁淤积,流产和早产,血 GGTP 水平升高
	胆汁酸	BSEP(*ABCB11*)	妊娠 3 个月出现的胆汁淤积,流产和早产,血 GGTP 水平正常
Dubin-Johnson 综合征			
	有机阴离子结合物	MRP2(*ABCC2*)	黄疸,良性高结合胆红素血症
Rotor 综合征			
	有机阴离子结合物	OATP1B1(*SLCO1B1*) OATP1B3(*SLCO1B3*)	黄疸,良性高结合胆红素血症,嗜胆阴离子如 BSP 和 ICG 清除延迟
谷固醇血症			
	胆固醇,植物甾醇	*ABCG5*,*ABCG8*	黄色瘤,高胆固醇血症,冠状动脉性心脏病
原发性胆汁吸收不良			
	胆汁酸	ASBT(*SLC10A2*) OSTβ(*SLC51B*)	慢性腹泻,脂肪泻,脂溶性维生素吸收不良

ABC,ATP 结合盒;ASBT,顶端 Na^+胆汁酸转运蛋白;BSEP,胆盐输出泵;BSP,溴磺酚酞;FIC1,进行性家族性肝内胆汁淤积 1 型中突变的 P 型 ATP 酶;ICG,吲哚菁绿;LPAC,低磷脂相关胆石症;MDR,多重耐药蛋白;MRP,多重耐药相关蛋白;OST,有机溶质转运蛋白。

PFIC 1 型(PFIC1,既往称为 Byler 病)主要表现为血清 GGTP 水平低或正常的患者中,出现慢性肝内胆汁淤积和粗颗粒状胆汁。PFIC1 患者的基因缺陷被定位到 18 号染色体上,与类似但疾病表型较轻的 BRIC 定位在同一区域。联合检索发现一种 P 型 ATP 酶,命名为 FIC1(基因符号 *ATP8B1*),是导致 PFIC1、某些形式的 BRIC 和 Greenland 家族性胆汁淤积症的致病基因。P 型 ATP 酶不同于 ABC 转运蛋白,为一个大的家族,包括离子泵如 Na^+/K^+-ATP 酶、Ca^{2+}-ATP 酶和铜转运 Wilson 病基因产物。对 PFIC1 和 BRIC 患者 *ATP8B1* 突变谱的分析显示,该基因的突变类型和位点与临床严重程度相关。BRIC(1 型 BRIC)以更无害的 *ATP8B1* 错义突变为主,而 PFIC1 以无意义、框架移位和大的缺失突变为主[44]。FIC1 为氨磷脂(磷脂酰丝氨酸)翻转酶,可维持细胞质膜内部和外部之间磷脂的不对称分布,其活性依赖于辅助蛋白 CDC50A(促进了 FIC1 向细胞质膜运动)的共同表达[55]。在人类中,FIC1 蛋白在许多组织中表达,包括胰腺、小肠、膀胱、肾上腺、胃、前列腺和内耳。FIC1 在肝外组织的表达和活性可能导致 PFIC1 患者出现高频腹泻,胰腺炎,细菌性肺炎、汗液电解质异常,和听力受损,且这些症状即使肝移植后仍不能改善[56,57]。尽管 FIC1 缺乏导致胆汁淤积的作用机制仍有待阐明,*ATP8B1* 突变小鼠的实验结果显示,氨磷脂翻转酶活性的丧失使毛细胆管膜更容易受到疏水胆汁酸的损害。PFIC1 和 BRIC 1 型的治疗药物包括 UDCA、利福平和补充脂溶性维生素。对于药物治疗无效的患者应行手术治疗,建议采用部分胆汁外分流术(partial external biliary diversion,PEBD)[58]。对于没有进展至肝硬化的患者,PEBD 可以改善生长和肝功能,同时减少瘙痒和减缓肝纤维化的进展。肝移植可缓解 PFIC1 患者的胆汁淤积,但不能改善,甚至可能加重肝脏脂肪变性[58]。

PFIC 2 型(PFIC2,也称为 BSEP 缺乏症)与胆汁酸分泌减少、进行性胆汁淤积、低或正常血清 GGTP 水平、小叶和门脉纤维化、肝巨细胞转化、肝组织学检查胆管增生缺乏相关。该疾病已被定位到染色体 2q24，缺陷基因（*ABCB11*）编码毛细胆管 BSEP 蛋白。*ABCB11* 突变影响 BSEP 蛋白的合成、细胞内转运或稳定性，BSEP 蛋白缺失或其在毛细胆管细胞膜表达的缺失者，病情更重，治疗效果差[59]。

PFIC2 患者表现为婴儿高血清胆汁酸水平、难治性瘙痒、肠道吸收不良、发育不良和胆汁淤积，最终在成年前即出现肝硬化和终末期肝病。胆汁淤积之外，严重的 BSEP 缺乏会显著增加肝胆系统恶性肿瘤的风险，包括肝癌和胆管癌[56,57]。PFIC2 的治疗与 PFIC1 类似，包括营养支持、补充脂溶性维生素、UDCA、利福平和 PEBD，可缓解轻型患者的症状。作为分子伴侣辅助特定错义突变 BSEP 折叠或具有靶向性的药物，可能有一定的治疗作用[60]。最终，大多数重型患者都需要接受肝移植。但是，由于 BSEP 抑制性抗体的产生，PFIC2 患者在肝移植后仍存在复发性低 GGTP 型胆汁淤积[61]。

PFIC 3 型（PFIC3，也称为 MDR3 缺陷）与其他 PFIC 亚型截然不同。这些患者的血清 GGTP 水平明显升高，肝脏组织学检查显示广泛的胆管增生和门静脉及门静脉周围纤维化[62]。最常见的临床表现包括胆汁淤积、瘙痒、黄疸、肝大、脾大和门静脉高压，且胆管癌风险高。PFIC3 源于 MDR3（基因符号 *ABCB4*）缺陷，编码毛细胆管细胞膜 ABC 转运蛋白，主要功能为将 PC 分泌到胆汁[63]。在 PFIC3 中，肝胆汁酸分泌没有直接受影响，但 PC 转运显著减少，造成胆汁中 PC 含量大大减少。在胆汁中，PC 通常与胆汁酸形成混合胶束，并起到缓冲其具有细胞毒性的清洁属性。在没有胆磷脂的情况下，疏水胆汁酸的毒性会引起胆汁淤积性肝损伤[64]。除了儿童 PFIC3 发病早，临床表现重之外，*ABCB4* 纯合子或杂合子变异临床表现较轻，可能直到成年才有症状。例如，*ABCB4* 杂合子或较轻的突变型与 LPAC 和 ICP 相关（参见表 64.5 和第 40 章）。PFIC3 的药物治疗包括 UDCA 和利福平，但对于大多数 PFIC3 患者来说，远期效果不佳，需肝移植方可治愈。

除了进行性肝内胆汁淤积之外，*ABCB11* 错义突变可见于较轻型类似 BRIC 的患者（见前文和表 64.5）。与 *ATP8B1* 突变相关的 BRIC 不同，由 *ABCB11* 突变引起的 BRIC 患者不会出现胰腺炎等肝外症状，更容易形成胆结石。基于这些发现和参考 PFIC 的遗传分型原则，BRIC 可分为 1 型和 2 型，分别对应 *ATP8B1* 和 *ABCB11* 突变。与 ABCB11 突变症状较轻，更易发展至 ICP[65]。

大多数 PFIC 涉及的干细胞毛细胆管细胞膜转运体和临床特征均已在前文进行描述。其他可表现为 PFIC 相似症状的基因突变和相应临床表现包括：①紧密连接蛋白 TJ2，表现为低水平或正常 GGTP 型胆汁淤积；②胆汁酸活化的核受体 FXR，表现为新生儿胆汁淤积和终末期肝病；③肌球蛋白 5B（*MYO5B*），可引起微绒毛包涵体病，表现为低水平或正常 GGTP 型胆汁淤积但没有复发性腹泻；④UNC-45 肌球蛋白伴侣 A（*UNC45A*）。

（三）胆汁酸生物转化（早期解离和脱羟基作用）

肠道菌群介导的胆汁酸降解始于小肠，在小肠淤滞和小肠细菌过度生长的患者中，胆汁酸降解增加。由于非结合胆汁酸溶解性低于甘氨酸或牛磺酸结合胆汁酸，其在肠腔内沉淀或滞留在溶液中被被动吸收。因此细菌过度降解降低了小肠腔内胆汁酸浓度，使可与小肠内脂质膳食形成混合胶束的胆汁酸减少。在健康人体内，结肠内也存在胆汁酸降解，非结合胆汁酸通过 7α-脱羟基作用生成 DCA 和 LCA，这些次级胆汁酸与胃肠道和肝脏疾病相关。不同个体胆汁中 DCA 的水平差异很大，从几乎检测不出到超过胆汁酸含量的一半。DCA 的产生受结肠胆汁酸 7α-脱羟基细菌含量和结肠通过时间的调控，因此饮食和影响肠道运动的因素均有作用[22]。

（四）胆汁酸循环

1. 胆道梗阻和胆瘘

胆结石或胆管癌等原因引起的胆道梗阻导致肝内胆汁酸潴留，可能引起肝细胞坏死或凋亡。部分潴留的胆汁酸被硫酸化修饰，硫酸化和未硫酸化的胆汁酸最终都从肝细胞返回进入体循环。尽管尿中胆汁酸的排泄增加，血浆中胆汁酸的浓度仍上升 20 倍以上。当胆道完全梗阻时，胆汁酸不能分泌至小肠，导致小肠对脂溶性维生素吸收不良和脂肪泻，同时无法形成次级胆汁酸，基本无粪便胆汁酸排泄。

胆瘘患者胆汁酸进入小肠后即发生分流。由于胆汁酸合成受负反馈的控制，分流后负反馈减少，胆汁酸的合成显著上升，最高可达 20 倍。肝脏功能不受影响，但由于最大胆汁酸合成量（4~6g/d）低于正常肠肝循环情况下的胆汁酸合成量（12~18g/d），通过肝脏的胆汁酸流量显著减少。与胆道梗阻一样，小肠内胆汁酸浓度降低，导致脂溶性维生素吸收不良。膳食脂肪的吸收，特别是含有长链饱和脂肪酸的膳食甘油三酯的吸收也减少。

2. 胆囊切除术

尽管移除了储存和浓缩胆汁酸的重要部位，但胆囊切除术对胆汁酸分泌的总体影响很小，胆汁酸稳态也没有实质性改变[66]。在没有胆囊的情况下，空腹时胆汁酸储存在小肠中。进食后胆汁酸池移至回肠末端，在那里被主动重吸收，并通过门静脉循环返回肝脏。有报道显示 CA 脱羟基化为 DCA 增多，这可能是由于空腹状态下胆汁酸的肠肝循环增加所致。腹泻是胆囊切除术后最常见的症状之一[67]。在这些患者中，胆汁酸池移至小肠的量超过回肠转运能力或控制肝脏胆汁酸合成的肠-肝信号通路，从而导致胆汁酸腹泻[68]，胆汁酸螯合剂治疗有效（见下文）。

3. 回肠切除术

回肠末端切除可引起肠道胆汁酸吸收不良。如果切除范围较短（<100cm），对胆汁酸代谢的影响很小，因为增加的肝胆汁酸合成平衡了粪便中的丢失量。大量未吸收的胆汁酸进入结肠，抑制肠液中水分吸收或诱导肠细胞分泌，从而导致轻度水样腹泻[68]。口服胆汁酸螯合剂可以缓解症状。切除 100cm 以上的回肠（包括回盲瓣）时，肝胆汁酸分泌减少，因为最大合成量明显低于正常的肝分泌速率。胆汁酸池量随着时间流逝逐渐缩小，胶束减少和小肠黏膜表面积的缩小，导致肠道脂肪吸收不良。结肠脂肪酸流量增加，抑制水分吸收，导致严重腹泻，且对胆汁酸螯合剂反应较差。如果腹泻量极大并伴有其他营养物质吸收不良，则可诊断为短肠综合征，治疗极其复杂且效果差。在一些病人，脱脂饮食后粪便重量和频率

减少。其他治疗还包括给予结合胆汁酸、谷氨酰胺和生长因子如胰高血糖素样肽-2 的类似物[69]。

4. 胆汁酸引起的腹泻

肠肝循环有效地保存胆汁酸，从而维持胆汁酸的流动和足够的腔内胆汁酸浓度，使胶束溶解和脂质吸收。胆汁酸引起的症状性腹泻（bile acid-induced diarrhea，BAD；分 4 类；参见第 16 章）是由于肠道主动转运障碍，最常见的原因是回肠切除或涉及回肠的疾病如克罗恩病（1 型）。以下疾病也与胆汁酸引起的腹泻相关，如慢性胰腺炎、乳糜泻、糖尿病、CF 和非甾体抗炎药（NSAIDs）的使用（可引起远端肠道溃疡和狭窄）。常见且诊断不足的胆汁酸相关腹泻见于腹泻型 IBS 和功能性腹泻（类型 2）[68]。在这些患者中，有证据表明胆汁酸腹泻主要是由于肝脏胆汁酸合成过多，而不是回肠吸收缺陷。从机制上讲，这可能与调节肝胆汁酸合成的肠-肝信号通路和 FXR-FGF19 通路的改变有关（参见第 16 章）。胆囊切除术后腹泻也是胆汁酸腹泻的一种（3 型）。最后，ASBT 基因突变也可引起罕见的先天性或初级胆汁酸吸收不良（4 型），这些患者早在婴儿期即出现慢性腹泻、脂肪泻，脂溶性维生素吸收不良，和生长不良。然而，ASBT 突变并不是造成绝大多数胆汁酸腹泻的原因[70]。

过量的胆汁酸进入结肠增加了局部二羟基胆汁酸的浓度，后者改变电解质平衡和加速肠道运输，从而引起腹泻。结肠中的水分输送对肠道液体和电解质平衡的调节至关重要，是腹泻的最终决定因素。胆汁酸通过肌醇 1，4，5-三磷酸和钙依赖机制，明显增加了灌注结肠中氯的分泌，从而在结肠水运输中发挥作用。三羟基胆汁酸对其没有影响，而二羟基胆汁酸在高浓度时诱导净分泌，在低浓度时阻碍液体和水的吸收。要诱导净分泌，胆汁酸必须：①具有适当的结构（疏水二羟基胆汁酸，DCA 或 CDCA）；②水相中高浓度（>1.5mm）；③存在于 pH 适宜的碱性环境中（粪便 pH>6.8）。

六、针对胆汁酸的治疗

（一）胆汁酸替代治疗

胆汁酸替代疗法是用来纠正胆汁酸缺乏（罕见的先天性胆汁酸合成障碍或胆汁酸池耗竭）。在胆汁酸合成受损而接合功能（酰胺化）正常的患者中，补充非接合 CA 可以抑制细胞毒性胆汁酸前体的合成，恢复肠肝循环中的初级胆汁酸输入，可以达到远期获益[52]。然而，在那些罕见的胆汁酸结合缺陷的患者中，需要使用结合胆汁酸（如甘胆酸）进行治疗[20]。虽然 UDCA 可用于多种其他适应证，但在此情况下不推荐单独使用 UDCA，因为它不能抑制内源性细胞毒性胆汁酸前体的合成。对于严重胆汁酸吸收不良或短肠综合征的患者，胆汁酸替代疗法可部分纠正近端小肠的胶束溶解和脂肪吸收障碍。

（二）熊去氧胆酸

由于其安全性和无肝细胞毒性，熊去氧胆酸（UDCA）仍然是最常用的胆汁酸治疗方案[71]。口服后 UDCA 蓄积并最终可达循环胆汁酸池的 40%，取代更疏水的内源性胆汁酸。UDCA 最早是被美国食品药品管理局（FDA）批准用于胆结石溶石治疗，但由于腹腔镜胆囊切除术的良好效果，应用并不广泛。然而，由于减肥手术后症状性胆石症发病率逐渐增加，UDCA 被用于预防术后胆石症的发生，不过有轻度的复发率[72]。FDA 批准胆汁酸替代疗法用于 PBC 治疗（参见第 91 章）。对于 PBC 患者，UDCA 刺激胆道 HCO_3^- 分泌，从而减轻胆汁酸所致的胆管损伤，延缓胆管纤维化进展，降低肝移植率并提高生存率[73]。UDCA 治疗对 ICP 有一定疗效，对低磷脂相关胆石症等其他疾病也有良好的效果[74,75]。此外，对于 UDCA 单药治疗效果不佳的 PBC 患者，联用贝特类降脂药或 FXR 激动剂奥贝胆酸（见后文）可有效地改善胆汁淤积[76,77]。

norUDCA 是 UDCA 侧链上少了一个碳原子的化学类似物。经过这种修饰后，norUDCA 不能与牛磺酸或甘氨酸结合，显现出显著的胆肝分流。norUDCA 可改善 MDR2/Abcb4 敲除小鼠（PSC 动物模型）的胆管周围纤维化，并在 PSC 患者的 2 期临床试验中取得成功[78]。

（三）胆汁酸受体激动剂和拮抗剂

胆汁酸合成和运输调节因子的确定，以及设计出胆汁酸受体的配体，不仅有利于研发新的药物（如奥贝胆酸、FGF19 类似物）来治疗胆汁淤积性肝病，也使胆汁酸和其衍生物，在代谢综合征及并发症的脂肪、葡萄糖、蛋白质和能量稳态调节中的治疗作用再次得到重视（参见第 87 章）[31]。FXR 激动剂奥贝胆酸可以改善从未治疗过或 UDCA 治疗反应不佳 PBC 患者的胆汁淤积（参见第 91 章）[79]。不良反应包括瘙痒和血浆高密度脂蛋白水平降低[80]。

七、胆汁酸螯合剂和转运抑制剂

胆汁酸螯合剂是一种带正电的聚合树脂，它在肠道内与胆汁酸相结合，以降低水相胆汁酸浓度和肠道保存胆汁酸的效率。对于轻度胆汁酸腹泻患者，胆汁酸螯合剂通过降低结肠中游离胆汁酸的浓度来缓解症状。胆汁酸螯合剂还可减轻胆汁淤积患者的瘙痒，可能是通过降低体循环中胆汁酸或其他胆道阴离子成分的浓度，不过临床证据较薄弱，而且疗效很有限[81]。除了考来烯胺和考来替泊等较老的制剂，已研发出胆汁酸结合能力更强的新型胆汁酸螯合剂。考来维仑是 FDA 批准的一种新型胆汁酸螯合剂，用于治疗高胆固醇血症和改善成人 2 型糖尿病的血糖控制。

除了结合树脂在腔内与胆汁酸直接结合之外，还可直接抑制回肠 ASBT 来降低胆汁酸。在日本，一种 ASBT 抑制剂已被批准用于治疗慢性便秘，而其他几种有效的 ASBT 抑制剂正在试验或临床开发阶段，将用于治疗胆汁淤积性肝病[82,83]。

（王迎春 闫秀娥 译，鲁晓岚 校）

参考文献

第 65 章　胆囊结石疾病

David Q. -H. Wang, Nezam H. Afdhal 著

章节目录

一、胆结石类型 …… 950
二、流行病学 …… 950
（一）风险因素 …… 951
（二）防护性因素 …… 953
三、胆汁的成分和异常 …… 954
（一）胆汁的物理化学特性 …… 954
（二）胆汁脂类的肝脏分泌 …… 956
四、病理生理学 …… 957
（一）肝脏胆汁胆固醇分泌过多 …… 957
（二）胆固醇快速成核和结晶 …… 958
（三）原核与抗核因子失衡 …… 958
（四）胆囊功能失调 …… 959
（五）肠道因素 …… 960
（六）胆结石的生长 …… 960
五、遗传学 …… 960
六、色素结石 …… 964
（一）黑色素结石 …… 964
（二）褐色素结石 …… 964
七、自然史 …… 965
（一）无症状结石 …… 965
（二）糖尿病患者的结石 …… 966
（三）症状性结石 …… 966
（四）特殊患者群体 …… 966
八、诊断 …… 968
（一）超声 …… 969
（二）超声内镜 …… 969
（三）口服胆囊造影术 …… 970
（四）胆道闪烁显像术 …… 970
（五）逆行胰胆管造影 …… 971
（六）CT 与 MRI …… 971
九、临床疾病 …… 972
（一）胆源性疼痛与慢性胆囊炎 …… 972
（二）急性胆囊炎 …… 972
（三）胆总管结石 …… 974
（四）胆管炎 …… 975
十、罕见并发症 …… 976
（一）气肿性胆囊炎 …… 976
（二）胆囊肠瘘 …… 977
（三）Mirizzi 综合征 …… 977
（四）瓷化胆囊 …… 977

胆固醇性胆结石是西方国家发病率最高、且医疗费用花费最高的消化系统疾病之一。至少有 2 000 万美国人（约占成年人的 12%）患有胆结石[1-11]。由于肥胖症高发，与胰岛素抵抗和代谢综合征相关的胆石症发病率逐步上升，每年约有 100 万的新发病例出现[12-14]。虽然许多胆结石“无症状”，但其中约有三分之一最终会出现症状和并发症[15]。估计每年有 70 万例胆囊切除术用于治疗胆石症，其医疗费用每年超过 60 亿美元[2]。此外，由于难以避免的胆石症相关并发症每年有 3 000 人死亡（占总死亡人数的 0.12%）[1]。在美国，胆石症患者的心血管疾病发病率、癌症发病率和总死亡率均有所增加[16]。

一、胆结石类型

根据化学成分和外观，胆结石可分为 3 种类型：胆固醇结石、胆色素结石和罕见类型结石[3,4,17]。在美国和欧洲国家，大部分胆结石（约占 75%）为胆固醇结石[15]，其主要是由胆固醇单水合物结晶和不规则胆红素钙沉淀组成，通常还包括碳酸钙或磷酸盐。这些结石常被分为纯胆固醇结石或含有 50% 以上胆固醇（按重量计）的混合型结石。剩下的胆结石是主要含有胆红素钙的色素结石，分为两类：黑色结石（约 20%）和棕色结石（约 4.5%）。罕见类型的胆结石（约 0.5%）包括碳酸钙结石和脂肪酸钙结石。胆结石也按其位置分为肝内结石、胆囊结石和胆管结石（胆总管结石），其中，肝内结石主要是棕色结石，胆囊结石主要是胆固醇结石，也有小部分黑色结石，胆管结石多由混合型的胆固醇结石组成。

二、流行病学

鉴于统计学分析的特点，对胆结石患病率的调研比胆结石发病率更普遍。患病率通常定义为在任一时间点或时间段内胆结石病例数除以有结石风险的人群。发病率通常定义为一段时间内新发的胆结石病例数除以有结石风险的人群。因此，至少在 2 个不同的时间（即在时间间隔的开始和结束时）进行胆结石的检查才能确定发病率。相比之下，患病率可以通过仅在一个时间点进行采样（例如通过超声筛查或尸检中）来确定。

虽然对特定人群中胆结石的真实发病率的统计并非易事，已经有一项大规模调研对丹麦人群中的胆结石发病率进行了统计[18]。30、40、50 和 60 岁的丹麦男性胆结石的 5 年发病率分别为 0.3%、2.9%、2.5% 和 3.3%，而丹麦女性分别为 1.4%、3.6%、3.1% 和 3.7%。可以发现女性在 30 岁和 40 岁时，其发病率高于男性，但随着年龄的增长，这种差异会逐渐

缩小。由于其与丹麦人群及其他群体预计的发病率一致，在某种程度上可以反映遗传因素和环境因素对特定人群胆结石形成有相互作用[19]。意大利的一项研究是通过对 Sirmione 镇原本无胆结石的患者进行 10 年的随访得到的胆结石发病率[20]。该研究表明，每年的新发病例占 0.5%。尽管在 Sirmione 镇的横断面研究显示，患者年龄，女性患者，分娩次数，肥胖和高甘油三酯血症与胆结石有关，但在纵向研究中对胆结石形成的危险因素进行多因素分析后仅提示年龄和肥胖为危险因素。

不同人群中胆结石的发生率存在显著差异，这表明遗传因素在胆固醇结石的发病机制中起着至关重要的作用。致病因素可能是多种多样的，并因人群而异。大量相关研究发现，在 20~55 岁女性中胆结石的患病率为 5%~20%，在 50 岁之后为 25%~30%。男性的患病率大约是同龄女性的一半。

超声筛查或尸检数据通常用于估计不同人群中胆结石疾病的患病率，如图 65.1 所示。虽然超声筛查不能区分胆固醇与胆色素结石，但 70%~80% 的胆囊结石都被认为是胆固醇结石。

有研究通过口服胆囊造影(oral cholecystography，OCG)对美洲印第安人的胆结石患病率进行统计[21]。经过充分研究发现南亚利桑那州的印第安人胆结石患病率很高，在 25 岁以上的女性为 70%。而后，采用超声对全国 20~74 岁具有代表性的人群进行筛查，其中包括墨西哥平民、西班牙裔美国白人、非西班牙裔美国白人和非西班牙裔美国黑人。横断面研究显示其患病率在某些美洲原住民部落(如印第安人)中最高，西班牙裔美国人高于白人，在美国黑人中最低[14]。

美洲印第安人是胆固醇性胆结石发病风险极高的人群，其他高危人群包括北美和南美的美洲原住民及斯堪的纳维亚人，他们中有 50% 的人于 50 岁时出现胆结石。相比之下，非洲人群体中胆结石的风险最低。在亚洲人群体中，胆结石的患病率处于中等水平。在某些特定群体中，胆结石患者的一级直系亲属其胆结石的可能性是对照组的 4.5 倍，这也证明了遗传易感性。

(一) 风险因素

1. 年龄和性别

流行病学和临床研究发现，胆固醇性胆结石在儿童和青少年中很少发生，且其患病率在男女群体中均随年龄呈线性增长，在 70 岁的女性群体中其患病率接近 50%[22,23]。此外，老年人发生胆囊结石并发症的风险更高，而 65 岁以上患者手术死亡率则往往高得令人难以接受。瑞典和智利的老年女性其胆汁胆固醇饱和度较年轻对照组明显升高，并且年龄与肝胆汁胆固醇的分泌水平呈正相关[24,25]。在动物中，已证明衰老会使胆汁分泌和胆固醇的肠道吸收增加，肝脏合成分泌胆盐减少，胆囊收缩力降低，从而导致胆固醇胆结石形成增加[26]。

流行病学调查与临床研究表明，在所有年龄段的患者中，女性形成胆固醇胆结石的可能性是男性的两倍。这种差异始于青春期，并一直持续到生育年龄，这是由于女性性激素的作用所致[15]，性别差异使肝脏对雌激素的反应不同，影响胆固醇的代谢。人类和动物研究表明，雌激素会增加肝脏胆汁胆固醇的分泌，增加胆固醇结石的发生风险，从而导致胆汁中胆固醇饱和度增加[27-30]。

2. 饮食

流行病学调查发现，胆固醇结石普遍存在于西方饮食的人群中，这些饮食中含有大量的热量、胆固醇、饱和脂肪酸、精制碳水化合物、蛋白质、盐及少量纤维。在北美、南美以及欧洲人群中，胆固醇结石疾病的患病率明显高于亚洲和非洲人群[3,31]。多项临床研究发现，中国胆固醇结石发病率增加与中国传统饮食西化有关[32]。在日本，胆固醇结石曾经很罕见，但是自 20 世纪 70 年代以来，西式饮食习惯的引入导致其发病率明显增加[33]。

3. 妊娠和分娩次数

妊娠是发生胆汁淤积和胆结石的危险因素[34]。在妊娠

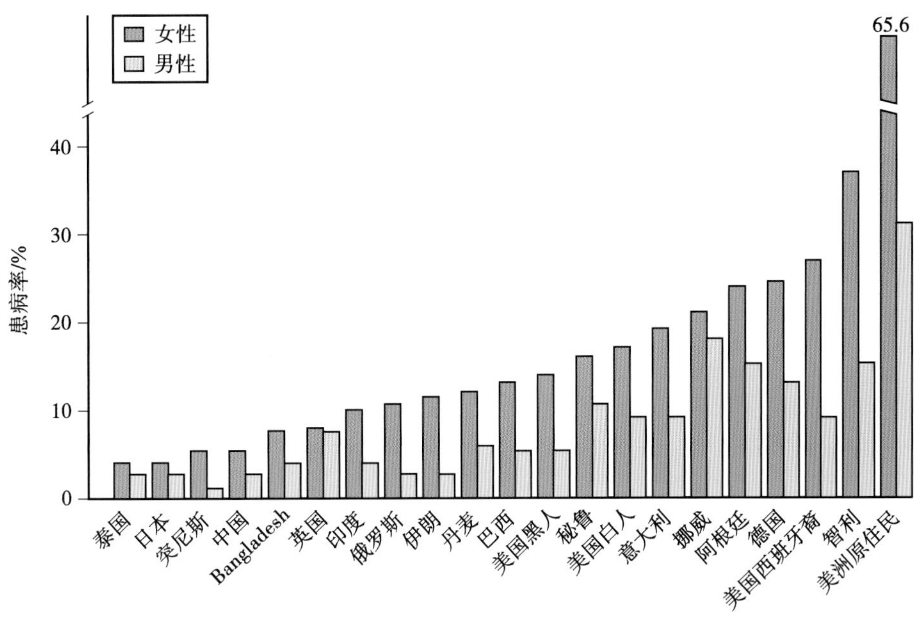

图 65.1　基于美国的调查，18 个国家中按性别列出的胆固醇性结石的患病率

期间，由于雌激素水平的显著增加使肝脏胆固醇分泌增加和胆汁过饱和，导致胆汁更易形成结石。此外，胆囊运动功能受损，胆囊体积增大，胆汁淤积增加，这更促进了胆囊中胆汁淤积及结石的形成[35]。孕激素浓度升高也会使胆囊运动性降低。由于性激素，尤其是雌激素的血浆浓度随妊娠时长呈线性增长，因此在妊娠晚期，胆结石形成的风险极高。分娩次数增多，尤其对年轻女性群体而言，可能是胆结石形成的一个危险因素。

4. 快速减肥

众所周知，快速体重减轻是胆固醇结石形成的危险因素[36]。约50%接受胃旁路手术的肥胖患者于手术后6个月内形成胆泥，最终形成胆结石。对严格控制饮食的患者，其胆结石发生率也可达25%。此外，这些患者中约40%会在6个月内出现与胆结石有关的症状。快速减肥导致胆结石形成的机制是在限制热量时肝脏胆汁胆固醇分泌增加，胆囊产生黏蛋白增多及胆囊运动功能受损。在该高危群体中，可以通过预防性使用UDCA来预防胆结石。据报道，每天服用600毫克UDCA，可以将超低能量饮食的肥胖患者的胆结石患病率从28%降至3%（见下文）[37]。

5. 全胃肠外营养

全胃肠外营养（TPN）与胆石症和非结石性胆囊炎的发展有关。在行TPN后的3周之内，由于禁食时间长，胆囊内形成胆汁淤积。此外，由于Oddi括约肌不能松弛使胆汁优先流入胆囊。大约45%的成人和43%的儿童在接受全胃肠外营养3~4个月后形成胆结石[38,39]。由于接受TPN的患者经常会存在严重的健康问题，不适合行腹部手术，因此，如果没有禁忌证，对结石的预防应采取预防性治疗。对长期静脉TPN治疗的患者每天静脉输注八肽胆囊收缩素（CCK）是安全且有效的预防结石的方法[40]，对接受TPN治疗的患者应常规使用。

6. 胆汁淤积

胆汁淤积是胆固醇和胆色素结石发病的关键中间阶段，因为其可促进板状胆固醇单水合物晶体的结晶和聚集，以及胆红素钙的沉淀，最终形成肉眼可见的结石[41,42]。另外，胆汁淤积可诱发急性胆囊炎、胆管炎和急性胰腺炎，也与许多诱发胆结石形成的情况有关，包括妊娠、体重快速下降、脊髓损伤、长期全胃肠外营养和奥曲肽治疗[3]。虽然胆汁淤积在大多数情况下可逆，但在12%~20%的个体中此种情况会持续存在或消失后重新出现，最终导致胆结石[43]。持续胆汁淤积患者使用UDCA治疗可降低胆汁淤积临床并发症的发生率（见下文）。

7. 药物

（1）雌激素

大多数（但并非全部）的临床研究表明，绝经前妇女使用口服避孕药类固醇和结合雌激素会使胆固醇胆结石的患病率增加1倍[15,44]。此外，法国一项针对45 984名绝经后妇女的大型研究发现，使用激素替代疗法会增加胆囊切除术的风险［危险比（HR），1.10］，但仅限于接受雌激素抵抗治疗的女性（HR，1.38）[45]。对绝经后妇女应用雌激素治疗以及对男性前列腺癌患者采用雌激素治疗也有类似的增加结石风险的效果[44,46]。因此，目前已提出雌激素是胆固醇结石形成的重要危险因素。在小鼠模型中，肝雌激素α受体（而非β）在雌激素的胆固醇胆结石形成中起关键作用[29]。被雌激素激活的肝雌激素α受体通过刺激胆固醇调节元件结合蛋白2（sterol-regulatory element binding protein-2，SREBP-2）途径对胆固醇生物合成产生负反馈调节，进而在胆固醇生物合成途径中激活SREBP-2反应基因[30]。这一改变导致肝脏分泌新合成的胆固醇增加，胆汁过饱和，使固体胆固醇单水晶体更易析出形成胆结石。此外，对小鼠的遗传分析表明，G蛋白偶联受体30（G protein-coupled receptor 30，GPR30）作为一种新的雌激素受体，也是一种被称为*Lith18*的胆结石基因。GPR30与雌激素α受体在结石形成上有协同作用，能促进雌激素诱导的胆结石形成[47]。此外，雌激素还能降低血浆低密度脂蛋白（LDL）水平，增加血浆高密度脂蛋白（HDL）浓度。血浆低密度脂蛋白水平的降低是肝脏低密度脂蛋白受体表达增加的结果，会提高血浆低密度脂蛋白的清除率。肝脏对低密度脂蛋白摄取的增加也可能导致胆汁中胆固醇的分泌增加，高水平的雌激素会导致胆囊动力减退，从而导致胆汁淤滞。

（2）降脂药物

降脂药物能调节胆固醇和胆盐代谢的关键途径，因此可能会影响胆结石的形成。氯贝丁酯是与胆结石形成有关的降脂药，能通过降低胆固醇7α-羟化酶（经典途径胆盐合成的限速酶）的活性，诱导胆汁中胆固醇过饱和并降低胆盐浓度（参阅第64章）[48]。3-羟基-3-甲基戊二酰辅酶A（3-hydroxy-3-methylglutaryl coenzyme A，HMG-CoA）还原酶抑制剂（他汀类药物）能降低胆汁胆固醇的饱和指数（cholesterol saturation index，CSI），但其在预防或治疗胆结石疾病中的作用仍需进一步研究[49]。有效的胆固醇吸收抑制剂依泽替米贝可预防胆固醇胆结石的形成，促进胆结石易感C57L小鼠的胆结石的溶解，其也可作为胆结石患者有效的胆甾醇去饱和剂[50,51]。考来烯胺和烟酸则与胆结石的形成没有关系。

（3）奥曲肽

当使用生长抑素类似物奥曲肽治疗肢端肥大症时，会增加胆结石的患病率，大约28%的肢端肥大症患者会形成胆结石。接受奥曲肽治疗的肢端肥大症患者会导致胆囊运动功能障碍，肠蠕动缓慢，结肠脱氧胆酸的形成和吸收增加[52]，这些均会促进胆固醇结石的形成。

（4）头孢曲松

第三代头孢菌素头孢曲松的作用时间长，其大部分能从尿液中排出。但是，约有40%的药物以未代谢的形式分泌到胆汁中，其浓度达到血浆中浓度的100~200倍并超过其在胆汁中的饱和溶解水平。一旦超过其饱和水平，头孢曲松将与钙络合形成不溶性盐，进而导致胆泥淤积的形成。据报道，在接受大剂量头孢曲松（60~100mg/kg/d）的儿童中，有43%会形成胆泥淤积，其中约19%的患者会出现胆道症状[53]。停用头孢曲松后，胆泥通常会消失。

8. 脂肪代谢异常

流行病学调查显示，血浆高密度脂蛋白水平与胆固醇结石的发病率呈负相关[54]。相比之下，高甘油三酯血症与胆结石患病率的增加呈正相关[55]。这些看似独立的变量实际上是相互关联的，因为高甘油三酯水平往往随着体重的增加而增加，而与血浆高密度脂蛋白水平呈负相关。有趣的是，血浆中高总胆固醇和低密度脂蛋白胆固醇水平不是胆结石形成的危险因素。

9. 系统性疾病

(1) 肥胖与胰岛素抵抗

肥胖是众所周知的胆石症危险因素，随着世界范围内肥胖症的流行和胰岛素抵抗发生率的增加，胆结石的患病率也在上升[56,57]。一项针对肥胖女性的大型前瞻性研究显示，BMI 与胆石症患病率之间存在很强的线性关系[58]。在这项研究中，BMI 最高(>45kg/m^2)的女性患者其胆结石风险比非肥胖女性高 7 倍。肥胖会使肝脏向胆汁中分泌的胆固醇增加，这可能是与肝脏中 HMG-CoA 还原酶的酶活性升高以及胆固醇合成增加有关。因此，与非肥胖者相比，肥胖者胆囊中的胆汁更易形成结石。在肥胖患者组中观察到其胆汁中胆固醇与可溶性脂质(胆汁酸和磷脂)的比例更高，这容易导致胆固醇结晶和胆结石形成。肥胖患者的胆囊运动能力受损，促进了黏蛋白的分泌和积累以及胆固醇结晶的形成。对肥胖与非肥胖者，其促成核和抗成核因素对胆囊胆汁中胆固醇结晶和胆结石形成的影响仍值得进一步研究。

(2) 糖尿病

由于高甘油三酯血症和肥胖症均与糖尿病有关，并且由于糖尿病患者胆囊的运动能力常受到损害[59]，因此长期以来，人们一直认为糖尿病患者发生胆结石的风险增高，然而，尚不能证明糖尿病是胆结石的独立危险因素。由肝脏特异性胰岛素受体破坏导致的肝胰岛素抵抗小鼠更容易患胆固醇结石[60]。肝脏胰岛素抵抗可经叉头转录因子 FoxO1 途径增加肝脏胆固醇转运蛋白 Abcg5 和 Abcg8 的表达继而促进肝脏胆汁胆固醇的分泌。它还能减少胆盐合成酶的表达，特别是氧甾醇 7α-羟基化酶，进而对胆盐结石的形成造成影响。

(3) 回肠疾病

回肠末端疾病或切除已被作为胆结石形成的危险因素。例如，克罗恩病患者的肠道胆盐吸收常受到损害，使其胆结石风险增加[61]。回肠末端特殊胆盐转运蛋白(例如回肠顶端钠依赖性胆汁酸转运蛋白)的丢失可能导致粪便中胆盐排泄过多，胆盐储存变小，从而增加胆固醇结石的风险。这些变化也可能导致胆色素结石的形成，因为胆盐向结肠的递送增加会使未结合胆红素产生溶解增加，从而增加胆汁中胆红素的浓度[62]。

(4) 脊髓损伤

脊髓损伤与胆结石的高患病率有关，据报道，此类患者中约 31% 患有胆结石，其胆道并发症的年发生率为 2.2%。尽管脊髓损伤患者胆结石并发症发生率比普通人群的胆结石发生率高至少 2 倍，但相对危险度仍较低，因此不建议行预防性胆囊切除。目前对于脊髓损伤与胆结石形成之间关系的机制尚不清楚。虽然这些患者胆囊松弛功能受到损害，但进餐引起的胆囊收缩是正常的。因此，仅仅是由于胆汁淤积引起的胆结石风险增加可能性不大。

(5) 非酒精性脂肪性肝病

胆石症和非酒精性脂肪肝病(NAFLD)在正常人群中均非常普遍，并且经常在同一类人群中共存(见第 87 章)。流行病学和临床研究指出，这两种疾病之间存在一定的相关性，两者间相似的危险因素会对非酒精性脂肪肝和胆石症的自然病史产生影响，另外非酒精性脂肪肝的确是胆固醇胆石症的独立危险因素。虽然许多临床研究已经证明非酒精性脂肪肝和胆结石疾病之间的关系，但其结果多样[63-68]。有研究者对肥胖手术前患有 NAFLD 的肥胖症患者其胰岛素抵抗(用稳态模型评估)、肝纤维化、非酒精性脂肪性肝炎(NASH)和胆结石疾病之间的关系展开研究[67]。发现在患有胆囊疾病的病态肥胖患者中 NASH 的患病率为 18%。1988 年至 1994 年，美国进行了第三次大型的国家健康与营养调查(National Health and Nutrition Examination Survey, NHANES)，共调查 12 232 名受试者，并指出胆石症(胆结石的患病率为 7.4%，胆囊切除术的施行率为 5.6%)与 NAFLD 之间的相关性为 20.0%[63]。胆囊切除组(48.4%)和胆结石组(34.4%)的 NAFLD 患病率明显高于无胆结石组(17.9%)。这些发现表明，两种情况都与代谢紊乱相关，例如肥胖，胰岛素抵抗，血脂异常和代谢综合征。

(6) 乳糜泻

乳糜泻是一种慢性小肠自身免疫性肠病，是由遗传易感个体对膳食中麸质不耐受引起的(见第 107 章)。临床研究发现，在乳糜泻患者开始无麸质饮食之前，由于肠道疾病引起的近端小肠 CCK 释放缺陷，导致脂肪饮食后胆囊的排空功能受损[67-72]。CCK 的缺乏会显著增加胆固醇结石的发生，这与胆囊和小肠的运动障碍有关[73]。由于无麸质饮食可以有效改善乳糜泻，因此乳糜泻患者的早期诊断和治疗对于预防 CCK 缺乏对胆道和肠道功能的长期影响至关重要。当在饮食中重新添加麸质时，乳糜泻患者会有临床症状及组织病变的复发。此外，一些患者对无麸质饮食的反应不佳。乳糜泻患者应常规接受超声检查，以确定是否保留有胆囊的运动功能以及是否有胆泥(胆结石的前兆)。肠道 CCK 分泌受损是乳糜泻和胆固醇结石之间的关键点[74]。由于对乳糜泻患者胆结石患病率的流行病学调查，以及乳糜泻对胆结石发病机制影响的临床研究的缺乏，对乳糜泻是否是胆石症的独立危险因素目前仍未知。

(二) 防护性因素

1. 他汀类药物

两项大型病例对照研究发现他汀类药物的使用与降低胆结石疾病的风险有关。第一项研究比较了 27 035 例需要进行胆囊切除术的胆结石患者和 106 531 例对照组，结果显示长期使用他汀类药物(>20 张处方和使用他汀类药物>1.5 年)是可以降低胆结石疾病的风险的[75]。他汀类药物的使用能降低因胆石症行胆囊切除术发生率[调整后的优势比(OR)，0.64]。在丹麦进行的一项针对 32 494 例胆石症患者和 324 925 名对照的人群研究中也得出了类似的结果[76]。与对照组相比，当前以及既往服用他汀类药物(>20 张处方)的患者胆石症风险的优势比分别为 0.76 和 0.79。

2. 抗坏血酸

豚鼠胆结石的发展与抗坏血酸(维生素 C)的缺乏有关，这一发现使人们开始对抗坏血酸与人胆结石之间的关系进行研究。在第三次 NHANES 中的 7 042 名女性和 6 088 名男性中，血清抗坏血酸水平与有或无临床症状的胆结石有相关性[77]。在女性人而非男性群体中发现，血清抗坏血酸水平每升高一个标准偏差，临床上胆囊疾病的患病率就会降低13%。

3. 咖啡

在对46 000名健康专业男性人员进行的为期10年的跟踪调查中发现，每天坚持喝2到3杯普通咖啡的受试者其有症状胆结石的可能性降低约40%[78]。每天喝4杯或更多咖啡会更有益（相对风险0.55），但无咖啡因的咖啡并没有益处。一项有81 000名女性的队列研究也对普通咖啡的类似益处进行了报道[79]。

三、胆汁的成分和异常

（一）胆汁的物理化学特性

1. 胆汁的化学成分

胆汁中的3种主要成分包括胆固醇、磷脂和胆盐，胆色素含量较少。胆固醇占胆汁和胆结石中固醇的95%，其余的5%是胆固醇前体和来自植物和贝类的膳食固醇。胆汁中胆固醇酯的浓度可忽略不计，其少于胆结石中总固醇的0.02%。最主要的磷脂是卵磷脂（磷脂酰胆碱），占总磷脂的95%以上。其余由脑啡肽（磷脂酰乙醇胺）和微量的鞘磷脂组成。磷酸胆碱头基和疏水尾含有2个长脂肪酰基链。胆汁卵磷脂在*sn*-1位置存在饱和的C-16酰基链，在*sn*-2位置存在不饱和的C-18或C-20酰基链。胆汁中卵磷脂的主要分子类型（及相应的频率）的含量分别为16∶0~18∶2（40%~60%）、16∶0~18∶1（5%~25%）、18∶0~18∶2（1%~16%）和16∶0~20∶4（1%~10%）。卵磷脂主要在肝细胞的内质网中由二酰甘油通过胞苷二磷酸胆碱途径合成。常见的胆盐通常包含4个具有极性羟基官能团的稠合烃环甾体核，以及与甘氨酸或牛磺酸酰胺键连接的脂族侧链。在胆汁中，超过95%的胆酸盐是5β，C-24羟化的酸性类固醇，它们以约3∶1的比例通过酰胺键连接至甘氨酸或牛磺酸，占正常人胆汁重量的三分之二，其亲水（极性）区域是甘氨酸或牛磺酸的羟基和共轭侧链，疏水（非极性）区域是环状甾体核。由于它们既具有亲水性表面又具有疏水性表面，因此是高度可溶的，类似洗涤剂的两亲分子。由于当其超过临界胶束浓度时具有自组装成胶束的能力，其具备高水溶性。

初级胆酸盐是胆固醇经肝分解代谢产物，由胆酸盐（三羟基胆盐）和鹅去氧胆酸盐（二羟基胆盐）组成（参见第64章）。次级胆酸盐是通过回肠和结肠中的肠道细菌的作用从初级胆汁盐类衍生而来的，包括脱氧胆酸盐、熊去氧胆酸盐和石胆酸盐。最重要的转化反应是初级胆盐的7α-脱羟基化反应，由胆酸盐生成脱氧胆酸盐，再由鹅去氧胆酸盐生成胆酸石酸盐。另一个重要的转化反应是鹅去氧胆酸盐的7α-脱氢反应，生成7α-氧代石胆酸盐。这种胆盐不会积聚在胆汁中，而是通过肝脏或细菌还原代谢，形成鹅去氧胆酸盐（主要在肝脏）或其7β-同分异构体熊去氧胆酸盐（主要由结肠中的细菌）。

胆色素是微量溶质，是某些卟啉的代谢产物。其重量约占胆汁的0.5%。它们主要是含有微量卟啉和未结合胆红素的胆红素结合物。胆红素可以与葡萄糖醛酸分子结合，使其溶于水。在人体胆汁中，胆红素单葡萄糖醛酸苷和二葡萄糖醛酸苷是主要的胆色素。其他胆色素包括木糖、葡萄糖和葡萄糖醛酸的单缀合物和双缀合物以及它们的各种同缀合物和异缀合物。

胆汁中也存在蛋白质和无机盐。白蛋白是胆汁中含量最丰富的蛋白质，其次是免疫球蛋白G和M，载脂蛋白AⅠ、AⅡ、B、CⅠ和CⅡ，转铁蛋白和α2-巨球蛋白。其他已被发现但在胆汁中未定量检测的蛋白质包括表皮生长因子、胰岛素、结合珠蛋白、CCK、溶酶体水解酶和淀粉酶，无机盐包括钠、磷、钾、钙、铜、锌、铁、锰、钼、镁和锶。

2. 胆汁脂质的物理状态

胆固醇几乎不溶于水，胆固醇溶于胆汁的机制很复杂，因为胆汁是一种水溶液。胆汁中2种主要类型的大分子聚集体是胶束和囊泡，可极大地增强胆固醇在胆汁中的增溶作用。

胆盐可溶于水溶液，因为它们是两亲性的，即同时具有亲水和疏水区域。胆盐的这种独特性质是取决于其羟基和侧链的数量和特征，以及特定水溶液的组成。当胆汁盐浓度超过临界胶束浓度时，胆盐单体可自发聚集形成简单的胶束，简单胶束（直径≈3nm）是小的、圆盘状和热力学稳定的聚集体，可溶解胆固醇。

它们还可以溶解并结合磷脂形成混合胶束，与简单胶束溶解相比，能溶解至少二倍量的胆固醇。混合胶束（直径4~8nm）是由胆盐、磷脂和胆固醇组成的大的、热力学稳定的聚集体，其大小取决于胆盐和磷脂的相对比例。混合胶束是脂质双层结构，其胆盐和磷脂的亲水基团排列在双层的“外部”，与水性胆汁相接触，而疏水基团排列在“内部”。因此，胆固醇分子可以溶解在双层的内部，远离外部的水区。可溶解的胆固醇量取决于胆盐的相对比例，当磷脂与胆盐的摩尔比在0.2~0.3之间时，胆固醇的最大溶解度出现。此外，当胆汁中总脂质浓度增加时，胆固醇在混合胶束中的溶解度增强。

当用准弹性光散射光谱和电子显微镜检查胆汁模型和天然胆汁时，发现除了胶束，囊泡还溶解胆汁中的胆固醇。胆汁囊泡是单层球形结构，含有磷脂、胆固醇和少量胆盐。囊泡明显大于简单或混合胶束（直径40~100nm），但远小于由多层球形结构组成的液晶（直径约500nm）。由于囊泡大量存在于肝胆汁中。因此可由肝细胞分泌。在新鲜采集的不饱和胆汁样本中经常检测到单层囊泡，并且与过饱和胆汁中发现的单层囊泡在外形上难以区分。稀释的肝胆汁（其中从未形成固态胆固醇晶体和胆结石）始终与胆固醇过饱和，这是因为囊泡溶解的胆汁胆固醇的量超过了混合胶束中的溶解量。富含胆固醇的囊泡在稀释胆汁中非常稳定，这与肝胆汁中没有胆固醇结晶一致。单层囊泡可以融合并形成大的多层囊泡（也称为脂质体或液晶）。在浓缩的胆囊胆汁中固态胆固醇一水合物晶体可能从多层囊泡中集结成核。

囊泡是相对静态的结构，受多种因素影响，包括胆汁脂质浓度以及胆固醇、磷脂和胆盐的相对比值，而胆汁中这三种重要脂质的相对浓度受其肝脏分泌率的影响，会随禁食和进食而变化。例如，在禁食期间，胆汁胆盐的肝输出量相对较低，因此，胆固醇与胆盐的比例增加，导致囊泡中携带的胆固醇多于胶束中携带的胆固醇。相比之下，进食后肝脏分泌胆汁的胆盐增加，使更多的胆固醇溶解在胶束中而不是囊泡中。另外，当胆汁酸盐的浓度较低时，尤其是在稀胆汁中，囊泡相对稳定，仅部分囊泡被转化为胶束。相反，随着胆囊胆汁浓缩，其胆汁盐浓度增加，囊泡可能会完全转化为混合胶束。因为可以从囊泡转移到混合的胶束中的磷脂比胆固醇多，所以残留的囊泡会被重塑，并且相对于磷脂，可能会含有更多的胆固醇。如果剩余的囊泡中胆固醇与磷脂的比例相对较低(<1)，则囊泡稳定，但是若其比例大于 1，囊泡会变得越来越不稳定。这些富含胆固醇的囊泡可能会将一些胆固醇转移到胆固醇含量较低的囊泡或胶束中，或者可能融合或聚集形成更大(直径约 500nm)的多层囊泡(即脂质体或液晶)。在偏振光显微镜下，液晶通常以具有马耳他十字形状的特征性双折射的圆形脂滴的形式出现。其本质上是不稳定的，可能会形成固态的板状胆固醇水合物晶体，该过程称为胆固醇成核。因此，胆固醇晶体成核会使囊泡中所含胆固醇量减少，但胶束中并没有减少，而囊泡是成核所需胆固醇的主要来源。

在正常生理条件下，胆汁在胆道内逐渐浓缩，使胆盐浓度逐渐接近其临界胶束浓度。当这种情况发生时，胆汁开始改变由肝细胞分泌到胆汁中的富含磷脂的囊泡的结构。这些相互作用是一系列复杂分子重排的开始，最终导致单一和混合胶束的形成。在过饱和胆汁中，肝细胞小管膜上的富含磷脂的囊泡会通过两种途径形成富含胆固醇的囊泡。因为胆汁酸盐比胆固醇溶解磷脂能力更强，所以当胆汁酸盐先从富含磷脂的囊泡中直接提取磷脂分子时，会形成富含胆固醇的囊泡。另一种途径是通过胆汁酸盐快速将富含磷脂的囊泡溶解，并产生含有过量胆固醇的不稳定混合胶束，这些胶束结构重排并最终形成富含胆固醇的囊泡。

3. 胆汁的相图和胆固醇在胆汁中的溶解度

在 20 世纪 60 年代，Small 及其同事对四元胆汁系统模型中胆固醇的最大溶解度(饱和度)极限进行确定，该系统由不同比例的胆固醇，磷脂，胆汁盐和水组成[80-82]。胆汁中 3 种脂质的相对比例(以摩尔百分比计)对确定胆固醇的最大溶解度起关键作用。当在固定的总脂质浓度下将这 3 种脂质的相对比例绘制在三角坐标上时，可以确定胆固醇在任何特定溶质浓度下的溶解度[77]。三角坐标图还说明了胆汁中胆固醇的物理相。例如，图 65.2 所示的相图其总脂质的特异浓度为 7.5g/dL，即人胆囊胆汁的典型特征[83,84]。肝内胆汁的典型总脂浓度为 3g/dL，其相界会存在不同，其胶束区更小，所有相界都向左移动，而其右侧扩大为两相区(即图 65.2 中的 E 区)。总脂浓度对胶束区胆固醇溶解的影响解释了为什么在同一受试者中，肝内胆汁比胆囊胆汁更容易出现胆固醇饱和。这是因为肝内胆汁中含有大量相对稳定的胆固醇-磷脂囊泡，所以在肝内胆汁中不会出现固态的板状胆固醇晶体。

也可用平衡相图预测在平衡相中出现固态胆固醇晶体[85]。虽然平衡过程是在肝细胞分泌胆汁并流入胆道后开始的，但向胆固醇晶体的转变只发生于胆囊胆汁中。例如，在不饱和胆汁中，所有胆固醇都可以溶解在单一和混合胶束中，并且相对胆汁脂质成分位于相图的胶束区域。相反，在过饱和胆汁中胆固醇不能被单一和混合胶束完全溶解，其胆汁中脂质成分位于相图胶束区域之外。在这种情况下，胆汁中高囊泡胆固醇浓度和高总脂质浓度可以共同产生固相。因此，

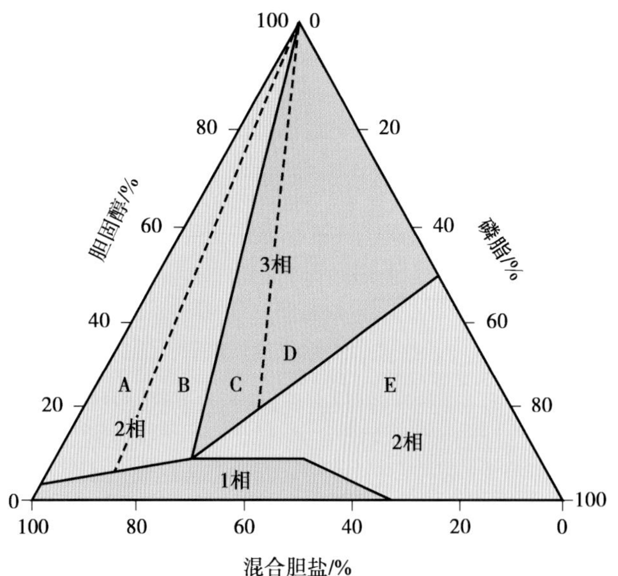

图 65.2 胆固醇-磷脂(卵磷脂)-混合胆盐系统(37℃，0.15mol/L NaCl，pH 7.0，总脂质浓度 7.5g/dL)的平衡相图，显示了结晶区域的位置和构型。组分以摩尔百分比表示。底部的单相胶束区由实线包围，在其上方，两条实线将两相区与中心三相区分开。根据胆汁中存在的固体和液体结晶序列，通过虚线将左侧 2 相和中心 3 相区域划分为区域 A 至 D。相数量代表示平衡状态。结晶区域 A 和 B 的相为胆固醇一水化物结晶和饱和胶束区；区域 C 和 D 的相为胆固醇一水化物晶体、饱和胶束和液晶；区域 E 的相为可变成分的液晶和饱和胶束。值得注意的是温度降低(37℃→4℃)，总脂质浓度(7.5g/dL→2.5g/dL)和胆盐疏水性(3α，12α→3α，7α→3α，7α，12α→3α、7β-羟基化牛磺酸结合物)逐渐改变所有结晶途径以降低磷脂含量，延缓结晶和降低胶束胆固醇的溶解度。这些变化产生了一系列新的具有扩大区域 E 的凝聚相图。(Reproduced with permission from Wang DQ, Carey MC. Complete mapping of crystallization pathways during cholesterol precipitation from model bile: influence of physical-chemical variables of pathophysiologic relevance and identification of a stable liquid crystalline state in cold, dilute, and hydrophilic bile salt-containing systems. J Lipid Res 1996;37:606-30.)

在典型的生理脂质比例即在平衡状态下，胆固醇晶体以饱和的单一胶束和混合胶束存在，或者以饱和胶束和囊泡的形式存在，这些胶束和囊泡可以形成多层透明液态晶体。胆盐和磷脂的浓度比以及胆盐和磷脂的总体亲水-疏水平衡也会影响胆汁的最终物理状态。

在胶束区内(见图 65.2)，胆汁是一种清澈、稳定的不饱和溶液，这是因为所有胆固醇都可以在热力学稳定的单一胶束和混合胶束中溶解。在胶束区的边界线上，胆汁因用尽了所有对胆固醇的增溶能力且胶束中无法再继续容纳其他胆固醇而达到饱和。在胶束区之外，过量的胆固醇不能被胶束溶解使胆汁过饱和[82,86]，并以一种以上的相(胶束，液晶和固体晶体)存在，因此其溶液看起来是浑浊的。显然，在胶束区之外时，相对稳定的单层胆固醇-磷脂囊泡可溶解大量胆固醇。术语“亚稳定区”是指相图中胆汁中的胆固醇在过饱和下的情况下即使经过很多天也可能不会形成固态胆固醇晶体的区域(胶束区上方附近)。该相图还表明，当胆汁中胆固醇的量超过胆汁酸盐与磷脂溶解的量时，固态板状胆固醇晶体就会在胆汁中沉淀。此外，胶束区外沿与胆固醇顶点相连的轴线

的距离比例常被用于计算 CSI(结石指数)[86]。因此,可以定量检查胆汁中胆固醇的饱和度。胆汁样本的 CSI 可以直接从相图中估算,也可以使用公式进行计算。CSI 是胆汁样品中胆固醇的实际含量与可以溶解在其中的胆固醇的最大含量之比。CSI 为 1 的胆汁已饱和;饱和指数小于 1 的胆汁是不饱和的;饱和指数大于 1 的胆汁是过饱和的。饱和度也可以通过将饱和指数乘以 100 来表示,称为饱和百分比。例如,在胶束区的边界处,胆汁饱和,而 CSI 为 100%。过饱和胆汁的 CSI 高于 100%,不饱和胆汁的 CSI 低于 100%。CSI 值还可用于预测胆汁中脂质颗粒的比例以及亚稳态和平衡的物理状态。

(二) 胆汁脂类的肝脏分泌

1. 胆汁中分泌的脂质来源

用于胆汁分泌的肝脏胆固醇水平的供应取决于胆固醇输入和输出的平衡及其在肝脏的代谢(图 65.3)(另见第 64 和 72 章)。输入量与肝脏从血浆脂蛋白(LDL>HDL>乳糜微粒残留物)中吸收的胆固醇(未脂化及脂化的)量和从头合成的肝脏胆固醇量有关。输出量与胆固醇在肝脏中转化为胆固醇酯(形成新的 VLDL 和储存)的量和转化为初级胆汁酸盐的胆固醇量有关。胆汁中相当一部分胆固醇也可自饮食中获得后通过载脂蛋白 e 将乳糜微粒残留物传递到肝脏。在低胆固醇或无胆固醇的情况下,胆汁中含有来自肝脏的新合成胆固醇和以几种不同方式入肝的预合成胆固醇。胆汁中大约 20% 的胆固醇来自肝脏的生物合成,80% 来自肝脏内的预合成胆固醇池。肝脏胆固醇的从头合成以醋酸为底物,受限速酶 HMG-CoA 还原酶的调节,这种酶可以根据肝脏的整体胆固醇平衡进行上调或下调,而其活性的增加会导致胆汁中胆固醇的过度分泌。预合成胆固醇的主要来源是肝脏摄取的血浆脂蛋白(主要是通过肝细胞基底膜上的高密度脂蛋白(HDL)和低密度脂蛋白(LDL)受体。与它们在胆固醇逆向转运中的主要作用相一致,HDL 颗粒是胆固醇的主要脂蛋白来源,是胆汁分泌的靶目标。在高胆固醇饮食条件下,膳食胆固醇通过肠道淋巴循环途径以乳糜微粒和乳糜微粒残留物的形式进入肝脏,乳糜微粒被血浆脂蛋白脂肪酶和转氨酶水解后进入肝脏。同时肝脏中新胆固醇的合成降低,仅占胆汁胆固醇的 5%。总体而言,肝脏可以系统地调节体内胆固醇的总量,任何过量的胆固醇都能得到有效的处理。

尽管胆汁中磷脂来源于肝细胞的细胞膜,但其组成与肝细胞膜的组成明显不同。肝细胞膜含有磷脂酰胆碱(卵磷脂)、磷脂酰乙醇胺、磷脂酰肌醇、磷脂酰丝氨酸和鞘磷脂。分泌到胆汁中的磷脂酰胆碱分子的主要由肝脏合成,一部分胆汁中的磷脂酰胆碱也可以来源于 HDL 颗粒的磷脂层。人体每天约有 10~15g 磷脂被分泌到胆汁中。

超过 95% 的胆盐在分泌到胆汁后,会通过肠肝循环返回肝脏,其主要通过主动转运从回肠末端吸收,如通过顶端钠依赖性胆汁酸转运蛋白和有机物转运蛋白 α 和 β(见第 64 章)。因此,肝脏中新合成的胆盐仅参与一小部分胆汁分泌(<5%),并补偿因未被肠道吸收而在粪便中丢失的胆盐量。当胆盐的肠肝循环被手术、疾病或药物(例如胆盐结合树脂如胆甾胺)部分或完全中断时,胆盐经粪便排泄会增加。肠肝循环的完全中断导致肝脏中胆盐合成的增多,同时使胆盐分泌速率调至正常值的 25%。在滑面内质网内和外两种途径中

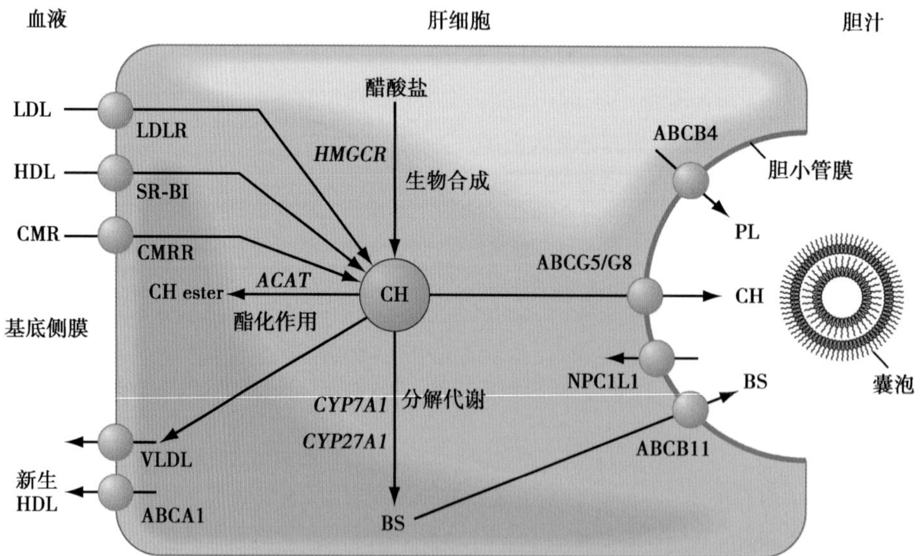

图 65.3　肝细胞水平胆固醇的摄取、生物合成、分解代谢和胆汁分泌。肝脏对胆固醇的摄取是由低密度脂蛋白(LDL)受体、高密度脂蛋白(HDL)的 B 类Ⅰ型清道夫受体(SR-BI)和乳糜微粒残粒(CMR)的乳糜微粒残粒受体(CMRR)介导。乙酸盐生物合成肝胆固醇(CH)受限速酶 3-羟基-3-甲基戊二酰辅酶 A 还原酶(HMGCR)的调节。部分胆固醇被酰基辅酶 A-胆固醇酰基转移酶(ACAT)酯化,储存在肝脏中。一些胆固醇用于形成分泌到血液中的极低密度脂蛋白(VLDL)。ABC 转运蛋白 ABCA1 可能直接或间接地将胆固醇和磷脂转运至细胞表面,在那里它们似乎形成与载脂蛋白中的两亲性 α-螺旋相互作用的脂质结构域。这种相互作用溶解了这些脂质,并产生了从细胞中解离的新生 HDL 颗粒。一部分胆固醇通过经典和替代途径合成胆盐(BS),分别由两种限速酶胆固醇 7α-羟化酶(CYP7A1)和甾醇 27-羟化酶(CYP27A1)调节。通过 3 种脂质转运蛋白(ABC)(分别为 ABCG5/G8、ABCB11 和 ABCB4),测定通过小管膜的胆汁胆固醇、胆盐和磷脂(PL)的肝脏分泌。Niemann-Pick C1 型类似蛋白 1(NPC1L1)可能在将胆固醇从肝胆汁带回肝细胞中的作用较弱。小管内显示一个囊泡

新合成的胆固醇均作为胆盐合成的底物，通过胆固醇 7α-羟化酶催化该过程的第一步。在一般情况下，胆盐合成主要以新合成的胆固醇作为底物。当长期应用 HMG-CoA 还原酶抑制剂（如他汀类药物）抑制胆固醇的从头合成时，源自血浆脂蛋白的预合成的胆固醇将会替代新合成的胆固醇。

2. 胆汁脂质分泌

有研究在新鲜的肝脏胆汁中检测到胆盐能刺激肝脏分泌囊泡[87,88]。在特定条件下培养时，大鼠肝细胞在相邻细胞之间的交界处与独立的"胆小管"形成连接。通过使用激光散射技术发现暴露在胆盐环境下的胆小管内有囊泡形成。此外，标本快速固定技术和电子显微镜为肝内小管外膜表面囊泡的形成和分泌提供了直接形态学证据[89,90]。大多数胆盐是以单体形式进入小管内，而胆汁磷脂和胆固醇以单层囊泡形式进入（见图 65.3）。一项对谷甾醇血症的分子遗传学研究（见第 64 章）表明，胆汁内胆固醇从肝细胞小管膜流出是一种蛋白质介导的过程。两种质膜蛋白-ATP 结合盒（ATP-binding cassette，ABC）甾醇转运蛋白 ABCG5 与 ABCG8 能促进胆固醇排除。这一过程对胆汁形成的意义已经在转基因小鼠中得到证实，在肝脏中人 *ABCG5* 和 *ABCG8* 基因的过表达会增加胆囊胆汁中胆固醇的含量[91-95]。尽管胆结石的患病率降低，但在 *Abcg5/g8* 双敲除小鼠以及致石性饮食的 *Abcg5* 或 *Abcg8* 单敲除小鼠中仍能观察到胆结石的形成[91-95]。这些结果证明存在不依赖 ABCG5/G8 胆汁分泌途径且在胆固醇结石中形成的作用。NPC1L1 蛋白在肝细胞的小管膜以及肠上皮细胞的顶膜中表达，而其在肝脏的表达水平低于小肠。这些结果表明，肝脏 NPC1L1 在调节胆汁内胆固醇的分泌方面作用较弱[96]。此外，B 类Ⅰ型清道夫受体（SR-BⅠ）定位于肝细胞的窦状间隙和小管膜。而在转基因和基因敲除后的小鼠喂食杂粮食物时，胆汁分泌胆固醇量与肝脏表达 SR-BⅠ的水平和其对肝血窦中将分泌到胆道中的 HDL 胆固醇的摄取成比例[97-98]。然而，SR-BⅠ的减少不影响小鼠胆结石的形成。这些结果表明，尽管 HDL 胆固醇是基础状态下胆汁胆固醇的主要来源，但乳糜微粒残留物中胆固醇的摄取似乎是小鼠饮食刺激下胆固醇生成过程中胆汁胆固醇分泌过多的主要原因[97]。

Abcb4 基因的缺失能完全抑制小鼠胆汁中磷脂的分泌[99]，这表明 ABCB4 可能负责磷脂酰胆碱从肝细胞小管的内质（内）到外质（外）的转运或"流动"，同时 ABCB4 也可能在外膜小叶内形成富含磷脂酰胆碱的区域。尽管小管膜的胞质内小叶富含胆固醇和鞘磷脂，并且可拮抗胆盐的渗透，但胆盐可促进胆汁胆固醇和磷脂酰胆碱的囊泡分泌。由于小管空间内的洗涤剂样胆盐分子可与小管膜相互作用，胆盐可优先分配到这些区域中以使膜不稳定并释放富含磷脂酰胆碱的囊泡。人类 *ABCB4* 基因突变会导致进行性家族性肝内胆汁淤积症 3 型以及低磷脂相关性胆石症的分子缺陷发生（见第 77 章）[100,101]。

胆盐包括在肝脏中新合成的胆盐和经历肠肝循环的胆盐。虽然其分泌与胆盐输出泵 ABCB11 有关，但胆盐分泌的确切分子机制尚不清楚（见第 64 章）[102,104]。虽然肝脏可直接分泌胆盐并影响胆固醇磷脂囊泡的分泌，但胆盐分泌是否在分子水平上与胆固醇和磷脂分泌相关目前尚不清楚。胆盐分泌和胆固醇分泌之间的关系呈曲线变化：在低胆盐分泌速率（通常<10μmol/h/kg）下，每个胆盐分子以更高的速率分泌胆固醇。尽管正常受试者的胆汁盐分泌率并不低，但长期禁食期间，夜间由于肝脏无法通过增加胆汁盐合成来充分补偿合成，患者胆盐分泌率可能会降低，并且胆盐损失很大，如胆瘘或回肠切除时发生的那样。在胆盐分泌率升高时，例如在进食期间和之后，胆汁胆固醇饱和度会低于用餐间期。在实验动物中发现胆汁分泌的有机阴离子不影响胆盐分泌，但能抑制肝脏将磷脂和胆固醇分泌到胆汁中，因为有机阴离子能与胆盐结合并阻止胆小管膜间相互作用。

四、病理生理学

图 65.4 展示了导致胆固醇胆结石形成的 5 个主要因素之间的相互作用：①某些遗传因素，包括 *LITH* 基因；②肝脏胆汁胆固醇分泌过多；③胆囊运动减弱；④胆固醇的快速相变；以及⑤某些肠道因素。这些缺陷共同作用促成胆固醇晶体成核与结晶，并最终导致胆固醇结石的形成。

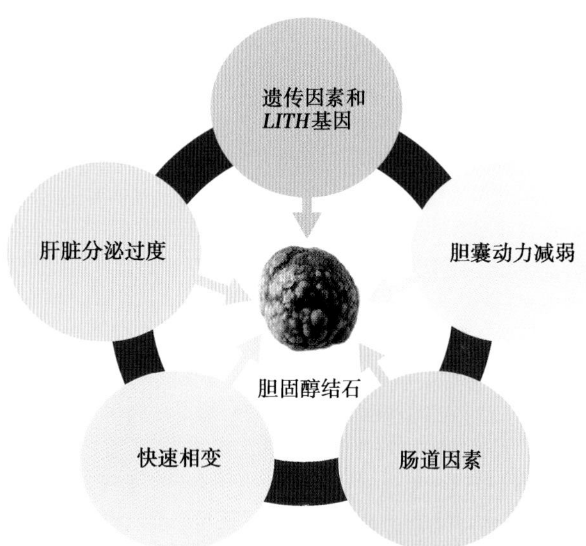

图 65.4　5 个主要因素共同促进胆固醇性胆结石的形成。这 5 个因素是：遗传因素和 *LITH*（胆结石）基因、肝脏胆固醇分泌过多、胆囊动力减弱、快速相变以及肠道因素。目前提出的假设是：肝脏胆汁胆固醇分泌过多是胆固醇结石的主要因素，部分是复杂的遗传倾向性的结果。下游效应包括胆囊动力不足与快速相变（见图 65.2）。胆囊动力不足的一个主要结果是胆盐（肠道因素）肝肠循环动力学的改变。肠道因素的改变导致胆固醇吸收增加以及胆盐吸收减少，从而导致胆盐的肝肠循环异常和胆汁胆盐池的缩小。胆囊运动功能减弱不仅促进了胆固醇的成核和结晶，而且还使胆囊保留固体板状胆固醇一水合物晶体。尽管在小鼠模型中发现了大量候选 *LITH* 基因，并发现了许多人类 *LITH* 基因，但其对胆结石发病机制的贡献还需要一步的研究（见表 65.1）

（一）肝脏胆汁胆固醇分泌过多

肝脏胆汁胆固醇分泌过多是胆固醇结石发病机制的主要成因。根据定义，过饱和的胆汁中具有无法在平衡状态时被胆盐和磷脂溶解的胆固醇。胆固醇过饱和的原因有以下：

①肝脏胆汁胆固醇分泌过多;②胆汁胆盐或磷脂相对正常的胆固醇分泌量减少;或③胆固醇分泌过多,加上溶解性脂类分泌不足。随着时间的推移,假设存在异质促成核因子(通常是黏蛋白凝胶),胆固醇过饱和则将诱导胆汁中生成固体的板状胆固醇单水结晶沉淀,随后结晶体凝结发展成为成熟的肉眼可见的结石。

(二)胆固醇快速成核和结晶

胆固醇成核和结晶是一个渐进的过程,其中过饱和的胆汁中不断出现固体的板状胆固醇单水结晶沉淀。可通过偏振光学显微镜在先前已表现为无晶体("各向同性的")的胆汁样本中观察到这种结晶体[105]。胆固醇结石患者与某些普通对照组患者的胆汁都有胆固醇过饱和的表现,因此胆固醇的过饱和程度并非判断胆结石的可靠指标。另一方面,胆囊胆汁的各向同性相的快速体外胆固醇成核与结晶也可将胆固醇结石患者的致石性胆汁与非胆结石对照患者的过饱和胆固醇胆汁区分开来[105]。前文所讨论的胆固醇、磷脂与胆盐的相图(见图65.2)往往用于研究亚稳态中间产物形成时的相变。另外,基于磷脂相对胆盐的比率、总脂质浓度、胆盐种类(亲水性与疏水性)、温度和CSI,可识别出5种结晶途径[83,106]。并且这些结晶途径已经在新鲜的人类与小鼠胆囊胆汁中得到了证实[83,106,107]。图65.2展示了磷脂与胆固醇相混合的胆盐模拟胆汁体系,用A~E分别指示5种不同的结晶途径,每种均代表了不同的相变序列,包括无水胆固醇途径和诱导固态板状胆固醇单水结晶的液晶途径[83,106]。某些途径中也会出现瞬态弧状晶体,与无水胆固醇晶体相一致[108,109]。无水胆固醇在水相环境中发生沉淀的缘由尚不明确,但它们的途径特殊,似乎来源于单层,而非多层脂质体。

在这些途径中,关键点是单层脂质体,其核心包含了液态的无水胆固醇分子,恰好反映了内部成核。事实上,当胆汁进入胆囊时,这些早期的泡状"核"已经开始了一连串的成核反应。基于视频增强的偏振光显微镜观察结果,目前的胆固醇成核与结晶模式表明胆囊泡一定是融合或至少是聚集在一起形成胆固醇单水结晶。由于胆固醇成核与结晶显然是在囊泡中开始的,因此囊泡的稳定性便决定了胆汁的稳定性。不稳定的囊泡可融化、聚集并生长成为多层液晶结构(脂质体),此时则能从溶液中析出胆固醇结晶。此外,准弹性光散射光谱的证明表明,固体的胆固醇晶体成核是由体外富含共轭脱氧胆酸盐的胆汁中的过饱和胶束直接发生,而没有任何的中间囊泡或液晶相。

在磷脂含量最低的胆汁中(见图65.2,区域A),首先出现了与无水胆固醇密度相一致的弧状结晶(d=1.030g/mL),而后经由螺旋形与管状结晶形成板状胆固醇单水结晶(d=1.045g/mL)[83,108,109]。磷脂含量较高时(区域B),胆固醇单水结晶出现相对弧状结晶与其他中间结晶更早。若磷脂含量达到正常生理水平(区域C),在早期的液晶(d=1.020g/m)出现后,便形成胆固醇单水结晶,再出现弧状与其他中间结晶。磷脂含量继续升高(区域D),液晶之后便仅出现胆固醇亿水结晶。达到最高磷脂摩尔分数时(区域E),液晶非常稳定,不形成固体结晶。降低温度(37℃→4℃),降低脂质浓度(5g/dL→2.5g/dL),降低胆盐疏水性(3α,12α→3α,7α→3α,7α,12α→3α,7β-羟基化牛磺酸轭合物),会逐渐使所有结晶途径向低磷脂含量转变,并减少胶束胆固醇溶解及延缓结晶化[83,106]。

人体胆囊胆汁中的胆固醇结晶途径和顺序与合适的物理化学条件下的匹配模型胆汁样本中完全一致,并且在模型胆汁样本中观察到的5个序列中有3个在人体和小鼠胆囊胆汁中也有发现[106]。值得注意的是,在人类成石性胆汁中的变相动力快于完全相同的模型胆汁样本,部分原因极大可能是胆固醇、次级胆盐和黏液糖蛋白水平升高的综合性影响的结果[84]。此外,胆脂、无机盐和蛋白因子对于稳定过饱和的胆汁也有着重要影响。阻碍胆固醇成核与结晶的非蛋白因素包括:①总脂质浓度低于3g/dL;②胆盐池疏水性降低;③胆盐相对磷脂比率降低;④囊泡中胆固醇对磷脂的比率降低;以及⑤总钙离子浓度降低。同理,相反的因素则促进胆固醇成核与结晶[110]。

(三)原核与抗核因子失衡

即使CSI值相似,胆结石患者的胆囊胆汁中的胆固醇结晶也显著快于对照组。这些发现表明,成石性胆汁中可能含有促成核介质,加速了结晶化;抑或是正常胆汁中含有抗成核介质,阻碍了结晶化。此外,胆汁中也可能同时包含促结晶物质与抑制物质,两者间的失衡导致了胆固醇结石患者的胆囊胆汁的快速胆固醇结晶[111,112]。

研究表明黏蛋白是促使胆固醇结晶的首要胆汁蛋白[113]。胆囊中产生黏蛋白的细胞分泌黏蛋白,作为正常生理状态下的黏液膜上的保护层。黏蛋白或黏液糖蛋白是由蛋白核心与许多碳水化合物侧链构成的大分子[114]。黏蛋白的一个重要特性在于其能够生成高浓度的凝胶相,该凝胶相与溶性相相比明显具有更强的黏度。

胆囊黏蛋白是0-连接糖蛋白中的一个异构家族,可分为两类:上皮黏蛋白与凝胶形成黏蛋白[115]。由黏蛋白基因1(*MUC1*)、*MUC3*与*MUC4*生成的上皮黏蛋白无法聚积,仅仅是位于上皮细胞顶面上的完整膜糖蛋白[116-119]。形成凝胶的黏蛋白MUC2、MUC5AC和MUC5B则由专门的胆囊黏蛋白生成细胞所分泌,为下层黏膜提供保护性涂层[116-119]。其可产生二硫键稳定性齐聚物或聚合体,这一现象反映了其黏弹特性。不同器官上的黏蛋白在碳水化合物侧链、蛋白质组成和电荷方面都有着区别,但特性却大体相同。黏蛋白具有与大量水分子相结合的亲水域。整个黏蛋白是带电荷的,同时也能够吸引其他带电物质,如钙离子。另外,黏蛋白分子上的疏水域(位于糖蛋白核心上的非糖基化区域)则允许脂质(如胆固醇、磷脂和胆红素)相结合。

胆囊黏蛋白在胆结石形成的初期有着重要的作用,是促进天然胆汁和模型胆汁胆固醇结晶的促成核剂。胆囊黏蛋白的分泌过盛是形成胆结石的先决条件,并且在多种胆结石动物模型的胆囊胆汁中也均可观察到胆囊黏蛋白含量上升[107,113,120]。此外,研究人员在胆结石上也发现到了黏蛋白,其作为结石生长的基质[121]。研究发现,胆结石中的黏蛋白以呈放射状或叠层式从无定形的中心向外围延伸。此外,黏蛋白也是胆囊中胆泥的主要成分,且有研究表明胆泥是胆结石的前兆。因此,可提出黏蛋白在胆结石形成上的2个作用:

①作为加速饱和胆汁中胆固醇成核与结晶的促成核剂；以及②作为结石生长期间固体胆固醇单水结晶沉淀的支架。

胆囊与胆管中的黏蛋白形成细胞所分泌出的黏液糖蛋白合成可能会受到来自含花生四稀酸的胆汁磷脂的黏膜前列腺素的调节[114]。在胆结石形成期间，胆囊过度分泌黏蛋白，这主要是饱和胆汁中某些成分刺激的结果。随后，黏蛋白聚合物的碳水化合物组主动与水结合形成凝胶。黏液糖蛋白核心中的疏水性多肽也可与胆汁中的胆红素和钙相结合。最终生成的不溶于水的凝胶糖蛋白和胆红素钙的混合物，其为胆固醇单水结晶成核提供了表面，并为结石的生长提供了支架。

胆囊中黏蛋白的分泌和积累由多个黏蛋白基因所决定。对 *Muc1* 基因进行靶向断裂可降低小鼠胆囊内的 MUC1 黏蛋白水平，从而降低胆固醇结石风险[122]。此外，*Muc1* 基因敲除小鼠在摄入致石性饮食后，胆囊 Muc5ac 凝胶形成黏蛋白基因的表达水平显著下降。因此，胆固醇结晶和胆结石形成也会有所减缓。以上研究结果表明，*Muc1* 与 *Muc5ac* 基因间相互作用可能会影响胆囊内黏蛋白的分泌与聚积。再者，在人类 *MUC1* 转基因的小鼠上观察到，胆囊上皮 MUC1 黏蛋白的增加可促进胆固醇胆结石形成，主要原因是其促进了小鼠胆囊胆固醇吸收与削弱了胆囊动力。这种促成石机制与凝胶分泌黏蛋白的机制完全不同[123]。综上，研究结果支持了这样一个理论，即对胆囊中凝胶分泌黏蛋白和上皮糖蛋白的分泌与聚积进行抑制可完全预防胆固醇结石的形成。

许多与刀豆球蛋白 A 琼脂糖可逆结合的糖蛋白也可以加速胆固醇结晶[124]，包括氨肽酶 N、免疫球蛋白、α_1 酸性糖蛋白、磷脂酶 C、纤维粘连蛋白和结合珠蛋白。其他促成核剂包括两亲的阴离子型多肽（APF）/钙结合蛋白、白蛋白-脂质复合物和Ⅱ型磷脂酶 A_2。此外胆汁中的非蛋白成分也可促成胆固醇结晶。胆汁中的钙与胶束和囊泡相结合，通过加速富含胆固醇的囊泡融合，实现对胆固醇结晶的促成反应。胆汁中的钙盐经过钙盐和胆固醇的过饱和作用，也可能促成胆固醇结晶，而黏蛋白的存在则更能加速这种作用。胆固醇结晶的形成速度随胆汁中脱氧胆酸盐的含量而变化，并与脱氧胆酸盐对胆脂质的相平衡关系的影响有关。胆汁中胆固醇的过饱和程度也决定了胆固醇结晶化的速度。

研究已确定了几种胆固醇结石抑制剂，包括载脂蛋白 AⅠ与Ⅱ、120-kd 糖蛋白、15-kd 蛋白，以及分泌性免疫球蛋白 A 及其重轻链[125-127]。载脂蛋白 AⅠ与 AⅡ可延长在过饱和模型胆汁中检测到晶体的时间。两者存在于一部分人类胆汁中，可抑制胆固醇成核与结晶。使用亲水性胆汁酸 UDCA 在胆囊切除术前进行 3 个月的治疗可延长在胆固醇结石患者的胆汁中检测到结晶体的时间，从而说明 UDCA 可作为抗成核因子[83,128-130]。UDCA 通过稳定囊泡，亦有可能是通过增强囊泡对载脂蛋白 AⅠ的吸收结合，以发挥其效用。

此外，通过凝集素亲和层析检测到健康人类胆囊胆汁中具有潜在的抗成核因子，其属于一种微酸性糖蛋白，分子大小为 120kD。该蛋白通过附着在结晶面上的最快速生长的微域和干扰溶质的进一步附着，从而实现对固体胆固醇结石生长的抑制效果。目前，尚不明确的抗成核因子仅存在 1 种或多种，以及它们如何抑制胆固醇结晶的形成，但已有研究提出单层囊泡是抗成核因子的关键作用点。

综上，虽然研究认为许多除黏蛋白凝胶外的胆囊蛋白是影响胆汁胆固醇成核与结晶的促成核或抗成核因子，但它们对于体内（如体内存在）胆固醇结石的发病机制仍不明确。再者，无论是在正常或异常的胆囊和肝脏胆汁中，可溶性胆汁糖蛋白的分解不会影响到检测到胆固醇单水结晶的时间，并且可溶性的胆囊蛋白在胆固醇结晶方面可能也并不具备病理生理作用。

（四）胆囊功能失调

正常生理条件下的胆囊全天会频繁地进行收缩，在进食间期，胆囊储存肝胆汁（健康个体的平均空腹量为 25～30mL）。进餐后，胆囊释放不定量的胆汁，这取决于神经激素的反应程度[131]。许多研究使用肝胆道闪烁摄影与超声（US）发现胆囊在进餐后会立即排空并再次补充[131]。相比之下，在胆固醇结石患者体内常观察到空腹胆囊体积较大、排空不完全和残余胆囊体积较大；无论其体内的结石大小，还是仅有单纯的成石性胆汁。在同时患有胆固醇结石和胆囊动力异常的患者中，其胆囊壁上的炎症通常较轻，并不足以引起胆囊动力受损。此外，消化期间的胆囊充盈不良直接导致从肝部输送更大比例的成石性胆汁至小肠，导致肝肠循环与胆盐疏水性提升。这些观察结果表明，胆囊动力不足的患者其胆囊的充盈与排空也会受到影响[131,132]。临床研究证明了胆囊动力不足与胆固醇结石有着紧密联系，在胆色素结石患者（空腹状态下没有胆囊体积较大和胆囊炎症）中也有发现轻度的胆囊动力不足[133]。胆固醇结石患者在接受成功的体外冲击波碎石术和口服胆汁酸溶解疗法（见下文）后，不存在结石的胆囊仍存在胆囊动力不足的现象[134,135]。研究发现，即便在未患有胆结石的健康个体中，胆囊排空的缺陷程度也与胆囊胆汁中的胆固醇含量比例成正比。这些研究结果表明，胆囊壁上过量的胆固醇分子可能具有损伤肌肉功能的效果。

体外研究发现，与对照组相比，胆固醇结石患者的胆囊功能异常，其无法与激动剂相结合[如 CCK 与质膜 CCK-1 受体（CCK-1R）的相结合]，分离出的平滑肌细胞收缩出现变化，分离出的平滑肌条和整个胆囊的收缩能力下降。其中响应激动剂结合的信号转导出现障碍。与胆固醇相关的收缩功能障碍在早期是可逆的，其出现的主要原因是胆囊平滑肌细胞膜上积累了过多的胆汁胆固醇。这种机制似乎解释了动物模型的胆汁中出现胆固醇过饱和时，为什么胆囊排空障碍会早于胆结石形成之前。此外，胆固醇结石患者的胆囊肌细胞上的平滑肌收缩能力似乎并未受到损伤。这些研究结果支持了胆囊内腔的胆固醇吸收上升与胆囊平滑肌功能障碍有关的假设。这种变化可引起肌质膜胆固醇含量增加，进而使肌质膜硬化。因此，当 CCK 与其在成石性胆囊中的平滑肌细胞上的受体相结合时，无法激活 G 蛋白，胆囊动力受损[136,137]。

胆囊动力减弱可先于胆结石形成。胆囊功能障碍所引起的胆囊淤积提供了胆囊糖蛋白凝胶中胆固醇晶体成核与胆结石生长的必要时间[138,139]。此外，胆囊内腔中形成的黏稠的黏蛋白凝胶可在物理上影响胆囊排空，从而促成胆囊动力减弱；亦可能发生于胆囊管。尤其是当胆泥中含有钙、色素、胆盐和糖蛋白时，其可以作为促进胆固醇成核与结晶或胆红素钙沉淀的滋生地。长期接受 TPN（见前文）的患者患胆结石风险较高,也反映了胆泥淤积对于胆结石形成的重要性[140]。譬如,40%接受 TPN 的克罗恩病患者都患有胆结石,但仅患有克罗恩病而未接受 TPN 的患者中仅有 27%患有胆结石。在 TPN 期间,由于不存在 CCK 释放的刺激因素(食物摄入),胆囊不会完全排空。结果导致胆囊中的胆汁便形成淤塞与胆泥,从而促成胆结石的形成。每日静脉注射 CCK 可避免胆囊动力不足,并降低形成胆泥与结石的风险。此外,利用 US 检测到的胆囊排空放缓与胆囊体积增大往往发生于妊娠和口服避孕药期间,这也是胆结石形成的 2 个危险因素(见前文)[28,29]。

胆囊胆汁浓度升高虽可提升胆固醇的可溶性,但也促进了胆汁中胆固醇成核与结晶,从而加速胆结石的形成[141,142]。除胆汁浓缩外,正常胆囊也可使胆汁酸化。酸化将提升钙盐(如胆红素盐和碳酸盐)的可溶性,而钙盐则是胆固醇成核与结晶的促成剂。因此,胆汁酸化不良促进胆结石的形成。

健康个体中,胆囊上皮细胞对胆固醇、磷脂和胆盐的不同吸收比率可降低胆汁中胆固醇的饱和度。然而,胆固醇患者的胆囊上皮已经失去了对胆汁胆固醇和磷脂的选择性吸收能力[143,144]。胆囊对脂质的吸收障碍使胆汁在储存过程中持续保持胆固醇过饱和的状态,从而促成了胆结石的形成[145]。胆囊吸收胆固醇的物理化学结果与动脉粥样硬化斑块的情况相似。情况可能如下,胆囊黏膜从过饱和的胆汁中不断吸收胆固醇分子[146],因为胆囊缺乏中间黏膜肌层和黏膜下层,未酯化的胆固醇分子迅速扩散到固有肌层。基于胆囊显然无法自主合成将胆固醇传输至血浆的脂蛋白,过量的未酯化的胆固醇分子只能通过酯化和储存作用,或是反扩散回到胆汁中来脱离胆囊黏膜和平滑肌[147]。在成石性条件下,胆固醇分子反扩散到胆汁中是无法实现的,因为胆囊胆汁持续处于饱和状态。因此,胆囊黏膜酰基辅酶 A-胆固醇酰基转移酶(ACAT)会酯化大多数胆固醇分子但并不能酯化全部的胆固醇分子。与动脉粥样硬化斑块相似,黏膜和肌膜显然已经出现胆固醇饱和,且与胆固醇酯微滴共存。另外,未酯化的胆固醇分子将插入肌细胞膜脂双层之间,这一过程将改变磷脂分子的物理状态(可由其刚性提升反映出来)。因此,胆囊动力功能受损时响应 CCK 的信号转导显著下滑。同时,从致石性胆汁中吸收过量的胆固醇分子直接刺激了胆囊黏膜与固有膜的增殖和炎症[131]。

(五)肠道因素

肠道胆固醇吸收效率高与近交系小鼠的胆固醇结石高患病率有着密切联系,易患胆结石的 C57L 小鼠的肠道胆固醇吸收也明显比具有胆结石抗性的 AKR 小鼠更高[148]。这些观察结果表明,饮食中胆固醇摄入量高和肠道胆固醇吸收率高是形成胆固醇结石的 2 个独立的危险因素。C57L 与 AKR 小鼠乳糜微粒残体胆固醇之间的新陈代谢差异可能是 C57L 产生成石性胆汁的成因,且从小肠吸收到的胆固醇为(以成石性饮食喂养的)小鼠的胆汁胆固醇分泌过多提供了重要来源[149]。肠动力变化也是胆结石形成的重要因素。小肠转运延迟或障碍与 CCK-1 受体敲除小鼠的肠道胆固醇吸收增强、胆汁胆固醇分泌增加和胆结石形成有关[149]。在部分胆固醇结石患者中,研究发现肠动力障碍与胆汁胆固醇升高有着联系。人体与小鼠研究发现了肠动力受损、脱氧胆酸盐与胆汁成石性之间的因果关系的证据。临床研究表明,以奥曲肽(一种已知的促成胆固醇结石疾病的危险因素)治疗肢端肥大症患者会导致结肠传输时间延长、胆汁脱氧胆酸盐浓度提升和胆固醇结晶快速沉淀[150-153]。此外,与未患有结石的个体对照相比,胆固醇结石患者的盲肠中的 7α-脱羟基酶活性提高与革兰氏阳性厌氧细菌数量的上升与胆汁脱氧胆酸盐水平上升有关[154]。胆汁脱氧胆酸盐和胆固醇浓度可通过抗生素治疗降低,其可降低残余 7α-脱羟基酶的活性。与具有抗性的 AKR 小鼠对比,易患胆结石的 C57L 小鼠的胆汁脱氧胆酸盐水平较高,这与胆固醇过饱和与胆结石形成有关[107,155]。已有研究提出,慢性肠道感染是胆固醇结石发病机制的潜在危险因素。一项小鼠研究表明,基于肠肝内螺杆菌(非 Hp)的远端肠道感染是过饱和胆汁中出现胆固醇成核与结晶的重要诱因[156,157]。此类螺杆菌也在患有慢性胆囊炎的智利患者中有所发现[158]。不过,慢性肠道感染是否对胆固醇结石的形成具有直接的致病作用还有待进一步研究。在克罗恩病患者和接受过肠切除或全结肠切除的患者中,其胆囊胆汁中均含有过饱和的胆固醇,而胆固醇结晶易于沉淀与形成结石[159]。在这些患者中,其胆盐的肝肠循环出现障碍,从而极大地降低了肝脏胆汁胆盐分泌,胆汁中的胆固醇可溶性也下降。再者,克罗恩病可导致肝肠胆红素循环障碍;胆汁中胆红素水平升高,胆红素钙沉淀,从而为胆固醇成核与结晶提供了病灶[62,160]。

(六)胆结石的生长

基于胆囊内存在胆固醇结晶而不存在胆结石的患者的研究发现,由胆固醇结晶发展至结石并不全是结晶化的过程。结石生长应是胆结石形成的第 2 个关键阶段,起因是胆囊排空延迟。在胆囊内同时发现多个结石的情况下,这些结石通常大小相等,证明该结石是与胆固醇结晶同时发生的,且结石的生长速度相同。相反,若结石的大小不一,则表明结石产生于不同时期。结石中心处的无定形物质包含胆红素、胆盐、黏液糖蛋白、碳酸钙、磷酸盐、铜和硫,它们为胆固醇成核与结晶提供了所需的病灶。固体板状胆固醇单水结晶往往聚集在该病灶周围。病灶的形成和随后的结石生长则可以通过黏蛋白、其他胆囊蛋白以及胆固醇过饱和来确定。结石的生长是一个不连续的过程,时常被胆红素钙和碳酸钙环的沉淀打断。由于胆固醇单水结晶通常以不定形组群随机聚积,呈放射状或同心状成层,因此胆固醇结石通常是由嵌入有机基质内的朝放射或水平方向的胆固醇晶体组成。而在结石外部,胆固醇单水结晶往往与表面垂直[161]。整个胆结石的形成过程中,黏蛋白提供了胆结石生长的基础。此外,同心的色素环将具有不同轴向方位的胆固醇单水结晶进行分层。这些环的化学成分与胆结石中心部分相似,可能反映了胆红素钙、其他钙盐与黏液糖蛋白的环状沉淀。

五、遗传学

关于人体胆固醇结石疾病的遗传组分的证据大多是间接性的,并且是基于地理和种族差异,或是家族与孪生子的研究[21,162-169]。皮马人和其他某些美洲北部和南部的印第安人显然具有遗传易感性,这类人罹患胆结石的风险最高(≈48%)[21,162-169]。相比之下,美国与欧洲白种人群的大体患病率约为 20%,非洲人群患病率最低(<5%),亚洲人的患病率居中,为 5%~20%(见图 65.1)。虽然已确定了许多有关胆结石形成的独立危险因素(如年龄、性别、分娩、肥胖、胰岛素抵抗、某些药物与快速减重)[26,30,60,170-172],但其中没有任何一个因素能够解释不同人群对胆结石患病率的显著差异,因此侧面说明了该疾病病因学具有遗传因素[5,6]。

患病个体的兄弟姐妹和其他家庭成员的胆结石患病率比其配偶或不相关对照组个体的患病率高得多,为 3∶1[164]。Gilat 等[166]使用 US 筛查患者的一级亲属,发现一级亲属的患病率是 21%,匹配的对照组的患病率为 9%。Sarin 等[167]同样观察到病患亲属的患病率比对照组高五倍。此外,胆固醇结石患者的姐姐的空腹十二指肠胆汁中的胆固醇过饱和程度高于对照组[168]。同卵成对双胞胎的胆固醇合成速率、胆汁饱和水平和胆结石发病率也远高于双卵男性双胞胎[169]。然而,即便是观察到以上种种结果,大多数案例中都未发现符合孟德尔定律的遗传模式。

实际上,针对具有不同患病率但生活在同一环境中的种群进行研究理论上能够捕捉到该疾病的遗传机制。但不幸的是,两个种群之间的联姻使得原始遗传背景在数代之内迅速流失,因此也给此类研究带来了困难。基于系谱数据,有研究调查了 32 组墨西哥裔美国家庭对症状性胆囊疾病的遗传易感性,估算得到的遗传可能性(即,由于基因影响的该特征的表型方差比例)为 44%[173]。在对美国 358 个家庭,1 038 个个体进行方差成分分析后,确定了症状性胆囊疾病的遗传可能性为 29%[174]。另外,瑞典一项针对 43 131 对双胞胎所进行的一项大型研究为遗传因素在胆固醇结石发病机制方面的作用提供了确凿证据[175]。在该研究中,单卵双胞胎的同病率显著高于双卵双胞胎,其中遗传因素占双胞胎之间表型变异的 25%。

Lin 等[176]的一项研究首次证明了人类胆结石可能是由于单基因缺损。根据其报告,在 232 名墨西哥裔美国人中,一种胆固醇 7-α-羟化酶(*CYP7A1*)基因的变异只在男性中出现,而未在女性个体上发现。CYP7A1 是一个非常有趣的候选基因,因为它能够对肝胆盐合成的经典途径上的限速酶进行编码,而胆盐是形成胆汁和保证胆固醇分子可溶于胆汁中的简单与混合胶束的必要物质。Pullinger 等在 2 名男性同型结合子中发现了 *CYP7A1* 另一个单基因缺陷与对 HMG-COA 还原酶抑制剂有抗性的血胆脂醇过多有关的胆固醇结石存在联系[178]。

ABCB4 基因能够对肝细胞小管膜上的磷脂酰胆碱转运蛋白进行编码,该基因的错义突变是某种胆石症的基础[99,178]。该疾病的主要特征是肝泥、胆囊胆固醇结石、轻度慢性胆汁淤积、胆汁内高胆固醇/磷脂比,以及胆囊切除术后症状复发[179-181]。肝脏由于 Abcb4 基因缺失所引起的胆汁磷脂质不足是小鼠患胆固醇结石疾病的关键危险因素。它通过扰乱液晶途径,从而极大地降低胆汁中的胆固醇可溶性,同时经由无水结晶途径加速胆固醇结晶[182]。这些发现为具有 ABCB4 变异的患者体内快速形成胆固醇结石的病理生理机制提供了新的观点,正是 *ABCB4* 的变异导致了这种与磷脂有关的胆石症,这是一种罕见的由单基因变异所诱发的胆系疾病。此外,在肝内胆管结石病(亚洲常见病例)的患者中,*ABCB4* 表达减低与磷脂酰胆碱转运蛋白水平减低同时出现,且胆汁中的磷脂浓度也出现显著下降(见第 68 章)[163]。此外,与对照组相比,胆结石患者中的 HMG-CoA 还原酶活性提升,CYP7A1 活性下降。针对该疾病,高胆固醇肝内胆管结石的形成可能是由于在胆固醇合成增多而胆盐合成减少的情况下,肝脏胆汁磷脂分泌下降所导致。

由于胆囊动力减弱会促进胆结石形成,因此调节胆囊动力的 CCK 与 *CCK-1R* 基因也是可能的胆石症相关基因[137,171]。*CCK-1R* 的遗传变异与胆结石风险有关,且在极少数肥胖胆结石患者中发现了 *CCK-1R* 异常剪接(预计可导致受体功能异常)[184,185]。然而,在胆结石患者中寻找 *CCK-1R* 基因变异和多态性的尝试始终未取得成功[186]。

一些研究报告称,载脂蛋白(*APO*)*E* 与 *APOB* 基因和胆固醇酯转运蛋白(三者均参与血浆中的胆固醇载运)的某些多态性与胆结石形成有关。*APOE* 基因的多态性的研究是胆结石患者基因多态性研究中最为普遍的,但关于 ε4 等位基因对胆结石的预防作用却一直没有定论[187-191]。ε2 等位基因似乎可以预防胆结石,并且肠道对膳食胆固醇的吸收程度也随着 APOE 异构体(ε4>ε3>ε2)而变化。同时,携带 *APOE2* 表型的个体的胆固醇的粪便排泄往往比携带 APOE 或 APOE4 的个体要高[192]。在一项关于胆囊疾病患者体内 *APOB*、*APOA Ⅰ* 和胆固醇酯转运蛋白基因位点的多态性的研究中,发现与另一组 HDL 降低因子有关的胆固醇酯转运蛋白基因的多态性与胆固醇结石有关[193]。此外,研究还指出 *APOB* 基因的 *X*+等位基因与胆固醇结石风险上升有着联系[194]。一项将大样本的德国胆结石患者队列作为对象的全基因组关联研究[195]与一项针对患病同胞对的连锁分析[196]确定了干细胞小管膜上的固醇载体 ABCG5 和 ABCG8 是胆结石的危险因素。随后,许多研究均表明,ABCG8 变异(T400K、D19H、A632V、M429V 和 C54Y)和 ABCG5 变异(Q604E)是欧洲、亚洲、智利和西班牙人群患胆结石的重要风险因子[197-203]。

表 65.1 是目前确定的 *LITH* 基因和人类胆固醇和胆色素结石主要候选基因类别的总结概要[31]。虽然已在人体内观察到某些候选基因,但它们在胆固醇胆结石形成方面作用仍有待进一步的研究。大体上,促成胆固醇结石形成的基因包括:①肝,肠黏膜脂质转运蛋白;②肝,肠黏膜脂质调节酶;③肝,肠黏膜胞内脂质转运蛋白;④肝,肠黏膜脂质转录因子;⑤肝脂蛋白受体及相关蛋白;⑥胆囊激素受体;以及⑦胆汁黏蛋白,进行编码的基因。

基于小鼠与人体研究,关于肝脏胆汁胆固醇分泌过多是由多个 *LITH* 基因诱导的理论早已提出;其中,胰岛素抵抗作为代谢综合征的一部分与促胆结石形成的环境因子相互作用,从而导致该表型的出现[204-206]。这些研究充分表明,胆固醇结石疾病是由多个 *LITH* 基因所导致,且胆结石疾病在小鼠与人类上均具有明显的遗传易感性特征。

表 65.1　截至 2019 年已鉴定的人类胆石结石基因（*LITH*）和基因产物

基因符号	基因名称	染色体定位	基因变异	遗传模式			潜在机制
				罕见的单基因	家族性寡基因	常见的多基因	
胆固醇结石							
脂质膜转运蛋白							
ABCG5/G8	ATP 结合盒式转运蛋白 G5/G8	2p21	ABCG8 p. D19H（rs1188753）	–	–	+	↑胆汁胆固醇分泌
ABCB4	ATP 结合盒式转运蛋白 B4	7q21. 1	多个	–	+	–	↓胆汁磷脂分泌
ABCB11	ATP 结合盒式转运蛋白 B11	2q24	多个	+	–	–	↓胆汁胆盐分泌
SLC10A2（*IBAT*）	溶质载体家族 10-2 成员 2（回肠钠依赖性胆汁酸盐转运体）	13q33	c. 378-105A>G（rs9514089）	–	+	+	↓肠道胆盐吸收
SLCO1B1（*OATP1B1*）	溶质载体有机阴离子转运蛋白家族成员 1B1	12p12	p. P155Thr（rs11045819）	–	–	+	↓肠道胆盐吸收
TM4SF4	跨膜蛋白 4	3q25. 1		–	TBD	TBD	超家族成员 4
脂质调节酶							
CYP7A1	胆固醇 7α-羟化酶（胆固醇 P450 7A1）	8q11-q12	启动子 SNP-204A>C	+	–	+	↓经典途径中胆盐生物合成的限速酶
UGT1A1	胆红素 UDP-葡糖醛酸基转移酶	2q37	启动子 A（TA）7TAA	–	–	+	↑肝部胆红素结合
SULT2A1	磺基转移酶	19q13. 33	rs2547231	–	–	+	？胆盐家族 2A-成员 1 与硫酸盐结合与解毒
GCKR	葡糖激酶	2p23. 3	rs1260326	–	–	+	↑糖代谢变化 ↑胆固醇合成调节蛋白
细胞内脂质调节转运蛋白							
CETP	胆固醇酯转运蛋白	16q12-q21	RFLP	–	–	+	↑HDL 分解代谢提升引起的肝胆固醇摄入
脂质调节转录因子							
NR1H4（*FXR*）	核受体 1H4（法尼醇 X 受体）	12q23. 1	启动子 SNPs-1G>T and -20647T>G，IVS7-31A>T	–	–	+	↓胆固醇向胆盐转换 ↑胆汁胆固醇分泌
脂蛋白受体及相关基因							
APOA1	载脂蛋白 A1	11q23-q24	−75G>A，RFLP	–	–	+	↑胆固醇逆转运提升后的胆汁胆固醇分泌
APOB	载脂蛋白 B	2p24-p23	c. 2488C>T，c. 4154G>A	+	–	+	↑肝 VLDL 合成降低后的胆汁胆固醇分泌
							↑肠道胆固醇吸收
APOC1	载脂蛋白 C1	19q13. 2	RFLP	–	–	+	↑APOC1 残粒样微粒胆固醇
LRPAP1	LDL 受体相关蛋白关联蛋白质 1	4p16. 3	内含子 5 嵌入/删除（rs11267919）	–	–	+	↑通过 LRP 从乳糜微粒残体中的肝胆固醇摄入
激素受体							
CCK1R（*CCKAR*）	缩胆囊素 1 受体（CCKA 受体）	4p15. 1-p15. 2	RFLP	+	–	+	↓胆囊和小肠动力
ESR2（*ERβ*）	雌激素受体 2	14q23. 2	c. 1092+3607（CA）$_n$	–	–	+	↑肝胆固醇的生物合成
AR	雄激素受体	Xq12	c. 172（CAG）$_n$	–	–	+	↓胆囊动力
ADRB3	β_3-肾上腺素受体	8p12	p. R64W（rs4944）	–	–	+	↓胆囊动力

表 65.1 截至 2019 年已鉴定的人类胆石结石基因(*LITH*)和基因产物(续)

基因符号	基因名称	染色体定位	基因变异	遗传模式			潜在机制
				罕见的单基因	家族性寡基因	常见的多基因	
黑色素结石							
ANK1	锚蛋白 1	8p11.1	多种	−	+	−	球形红细胞症→溶血
CFTR (*ABCC7*)	CF 跨膜调节蛋白	7q31.2	Δq31	+	−	−	↑胆红素肝肠循环 ↓胆汁 pH ↑胆盐粪便排泄
G6PD	葡糖-6-磷酸脱氢酶	Xq28	多种	+	+	+	↑溶血
GPI	葡糖-6-磷酸异构酶	19q13.1	p.Leu339Pro		TBD		TBD
PKLR	丙酮酸激酶	1q21	p.R510Q		TBD		TBD
HBA1/2	血红蛋白 α 链混合物	16p13.3	HbH	−	+	+	α-地中海贫血/β-地中海贫血中度/轻度镰状细胞疾病→溶血
HBB	血红蛋白 β 链混合物	11p15.5	p.E26K(HbE) p.E6V(HbS)			TBD	TBD
UGT1A1	胆红素 UDP-葡糖醛酸基转移酶	2q37	启动子 A(TA)7TAA	−	−	+	↑肝胆红素结合
胆管结石							
COMT	邻苯二酚-O-甲基转移酶	22q11.21	外显子 4-76C>G(rs4818)	−	−	+	↑雌激素水平
CXCR2	趋化因子(C-X-Cmotif)受体 2	2q35	c.811C>T(rs2230054) c.1235T>C(rs1126579)	−	−	+	TBD
IL8	白介素-8	4q13-q21	-351A>T(rs4073)	−	−	+	↑IL8 表达→炎症
NOS2	一氧化氮合成酶 2	17q11.2-q12	外显子 16+14C>T (rs2297518)	−	−	+	TBD
RNASEL	核糖核酸酶 L	1q25	外显子 1-96A>G (rs486907)	−	−	+	TBD

LRP,低密度脂蛋白受体相关蛋白;RFLP,限制性片段长度多态性;SNP,单核苷酸多态性;TBD,待定;UDP,二磷酸尿苷。
Adapted with permission from Krawczyk M, Wang DQ, Portincasa P, et al. Dissecting the genetic heterogeneity of gallbladder stone formation. Semin Liver Dis 2011;31:157-72.

肝细胞小管膜上的多个 ABC 转运蛋白中的 1 型转运蛋白的表达和功能的变化可影响胆结石形成,其途径是通过诱导胆脂分泌和胆汁成分发生改变。此外,可对多个脂蛋白受体进行解码的基因的变异、决定 HDL 和 LDL 摄入的相关蛋白的基因变异、几个通过肝细胞胞液转运胆脂的胞内蛋白的基因变异,以及调节肝胆固醇与胆盐代谢和胆脂分泌的转运因子的基因变异均可以诱导胆固醇结石的形成。可影响 CCK 与 CCK-1R(见前文)与黏蛋白的分泌和特性的基因突变也在胆结石的发病机制中扮演着重要的角色。一项大规模的病例对照研究[207]发现,肝胆固醇的生物合成增多和胆固醇的粪便排泄增加可发生于胆固醇结石之前,并是某些胆结石高危种族人群的关键代谢特征。该研究有力证明,通过抑制肝合成与肠道胆固醇吸收使胆汁胆固醇排出量降低可作为胆结石高危人群中的遗传缺陷亚群的治疗策略[208]。

肠黏膜脂质转运蛋白、脂质调节酶、胞内脂质转运蛋白和脂质调节转运因子的调节因素可影响肠道原本的胆固醇含量,而肠道内的胆固醇对肝脏胆汁分泌存在影响。肠道因素对于小鼠结石的作用的直接证据来源于一项针对 ACAT2-敲除小鼠的研究[209]。由于 *Acat2* 基因的缺失,小肠内的胆固醇酯合成出现不足,从而极大地影响了肠道胆固醇吸收,并形成对饮食性胆固醇结石的抗性。此外,有效的胆固醇吸收抑制剂依折麦布可通过有效降低肠道的胆固醇吸收和肝汁胆固醇分泌来实现对胆结石的抵御力,并通过减少小鼠的胆汁过饱和度来保护胆囊动力[50,210]。同时,依折麦布也能够极大地降低胆汁胆固醇饱和度并减缓胆结石患者胆汁中的胆固醇结晶化[50]。因此,肠道胆固醇吸收或乳糜微粒残体的肝摄取降低可降低胆汁胆固醇分泌和饱和程度。此外,可对回肠的顶端钠依赖性胆汁酸盐转运蛋白(ASBT)、胞质型回肠脂质结合蛋白(ILBP)与有机溶质转运蛋白 α 和 β(α 和 β,OSTα 和 β)进行编码的基因可促进胆结石形成,原理是通过降低回肠胆汁酸转运和改变胆汁酸池及其成分;这一结论基于对非肥胖女性胆结石患者与对照组之间的比较得出(见第 64 章)[211,212]。ASBT 基因(基因符号:*SLC10A2*)中的单核苷酸多态性 rs9514089 已证明是人类胆石症的易感性影响因素[213],不过 *rs9514089* 基因型在致胆结石风险上的效果并未在索布人身上出现[214]。因此有待进一步地研究针对更大规模的队列评估 *SLC10A2* 遗传变异对于胆结石形成的危险因素。

六、色素结石

尽管目前对黑色素与棕色素胆结石的发病机制的了解并不如胆固醇结石,并且两种类型的色素结石都有着自己独特的发病机制,不过两者的形成都是由于胆红素代谢异常,且其着色也均是胆红素沉淀的结果[215-217]。大体而言,无论是哪种色素结石的患者,其胆汁中都存在过量的未结合的胆红素,类似于胆固醇结石患者胆汁中胆固醇过饱和[218]。此外,两种类型的色素结石主要由胆色素构成,并具有供黏蛋白糖蛋白形成的基质。不同的是,在黑色结石中,色素主要是具有高度不可溶性的胆红素钙的交联聚合物,而棕色素结石的主要色素是单体胆红素钙。另外,两种色素结石的放射密度、在胆道所在位置,以及地理分布也均有所不同。

表 65.1 对关于色素结石的易感基因的研究结果进行了总结。多个候选基因均通过提高胆红素的肠肝循环促成色素结石的形成。吉尔伯特(Gilbert)综合征患者具有慢性轻度升高的未结合胆红素血症,但不存在肝疾病或明显的溶血,这是由于胆红素尿苷二磷酸葡糖醛酸基转移酶 1(基因符号:*UGT1A1*)表达降低所致,原因是该酶的基因启动子区域异常(见第 21 章)[219]。一项全基因组关联研究确定了 *UGT1A1* 基因变异是人类胆结石疾病的主要危险因素[220]。*UGT1A1* 启动子变异可提高镰状细胞疾病或囊性纤维化患者对色素结石的易感性[221-224]。一项回归分析表明,血清胆红素水平和胆结石的患病率与镰状细胞疾病患者中的 *UGT1A1* 启动子中[TA]的重复次数有着强烈联系;每重复一次,血清胆红素的水平就提升 21%,胆石症的风险就上升 87%[222]。再者,连锁不平衡变异情况下的 *UGT1A1* 基因变异与形成胆固醇结石的风险有关。这些研究结果表明,胆汁中含有过饱和的胆红素是形成色素和胆固醇结石的危险因素。如上文所述,提高的胆汁胆红素水平与增多的胆汁中胆红素钙沉淀为胆固醇成核与结晶提供了关键性的病灶。

CF 患者感染胆结石的概率为 10%~30%,比之年龄匹配对照组的患病率高了 5%,但胆囊胆固醇的饱和程度在患有或不患有胆结石的个体中并无差异。实际上,CF 患者的胆结石大体属于黑色素结石(即由胆红素钙组成,加上适量的胆固醇混合物),但很少会出现症状。在患 CF 的小鼠(ΔF508 突变)模型中,粪胆盐流失增加引起肝胆汁中疏水性胆盐含量增加并促进胆红素的肠肝循环[225]。这些变化则诱使血胆红素过多,同时使所有胆红素轭合物和非结合胆红素的水平明显升高,从而导致胆汁中的非结合胆红素中的二价金属盐发生水解与沉淀。此外,胆囊胆汁 pH 降低与胆汁中胆红素钙离子产物水平的增加则提高了胆汁中胆红素过饱和的可能性,从而形成黑色素胆结石。胰十二指肠同源盒基因-1(*Pdx1*)是形成适当的十二指肠主乳头、胆系周围的腺体与胆管产黏蛋白细胞,以及维护围生期间壶腹周围的十二指肠上皮细胞的必要因素(见第 62 章)。在 *Pdx1* 敲除小鼠中,十二指肠主乳头缺失导致肠胆反流与胆汁感染,从而形成棕色素结石,且采用抗生素治疗可极大地降低棕色素胆结石的出现概率[226]。

(一)黑色素结石

黑色素结石形成于无感染的胆囊中,尤其是慢性溶血性贫血患者(如 β-地中海贫血、遗传性球形红细胞症和镰状细胞疾病)、无效性红细胞生成(如恶性贫血)患者、伴随过量胆盐溢出至大肠的回肠疾病(如克罗恩病)患者、扩大回肠切除术患者,以及肝硬化患者中。这些变化往往伴随着回肠胆盐浓度升高,引起非结合胆红素可溶性增加,从而提升胆汁中的胆红素浓度,最终导致黑色素结石的形成[227]。所生成的非结合胆红素形成胆红素钙沉淀,从而形成结石[228]。这种结石的成分要么是纯粹的胆红素钙,要么是由非结合胆红素、胆红素钙、钙和铜组成的类似聚合物的混合物。黏蛋白糖蛋白在黑色素结石中的质量可占 20%,且在黑色素结石中未发现常规的结晶体结构。

在肝脏分泌方面,胆红素首先经 UGT1A1 单葡糖或双葡糖醛酸化,随后由 ABC 转运蛋白 C2(ABCC2);也叫作多药耐药相关蛋白(MRP2)分泌(见第 64 和 77 章)。在正常生理条件下,非结合胆红素无法分泌至胆汁中。虽然胆红素糖蛋白葡糖苷酸会经内源性 β-葡萄糖醛酸酶水解,但非结合胆红素也仅能形成不足 1% 的总胆色素,这主要是由于内源性 β-葡萄糖醛酸酶的活性受到胆道中 β-葡萄糖二酸 1,4-内酯的抑制[229,230]。因此,黑色素胆结石的统一的致病因素是肝分泌过量的胆红素轭合物(尤其是单葡糖醛酸苷)进入胆汁中。在存在溶血的情况下,肝分泌的胆红素轭合物会提升 10 倍。非结合单氢化胆红素是通过内源性 β-葡萄糖醛酸酶形成的,在过饱和的条件下会与钙同时发生沉淀。在水解速率为 1% 的条件下,非结合胆红素浓度大幅度提高,往往会大大超过胆汁中的胆红素可溶解度。胆汁酸化缺陷可由胆囊炎症或黏蛋白凝胶中的唾液酸和硫酸盐缓冲能力下降所致。缓冲能力的下降会加速碳酸钙和磷酸钙的过饱和,不过这种情况不会发生于低 pH 的情况下。此外,目前未能在黑色素结石患者中观察到胆囊动力缺陷。

(二)褐色素结石

褐色素结石的主要成分是非结合胆红素的钙盐,以及不等量的胆固醇、脂肪酸、色素与黏蛋白糖蛋白,以及少量的胆盐、磷脂质和细菌残留。褐色素结石介于红棕色与深棕色之间,亮度低,可轻易与黑色素结石区分开来。它们的形状往往是不规则的,偶尔可以形成球形。它们中多数呈现为黏稠淤泥状,部分有端面形成。与其他胆结石相比,褐色素结石要么光滑,要么粗糙,表面不具光泽,质地柔软易碎,质量较轻。其切面大多是层状构造(薄层状)或无定形状,不具备胆固醇结石的辐射状晶体结构。褐色素结石似乎始终呈现出薄层状的横截面,富含胆红素钙与富含棕榈酸钙的薄层相交替。

褐色素胆结石不仅会形成于胆囊中,更普遍存在于胆道的其他部分,尤其在肝内胆道。褐色素结石的形成需要有与胆道感染(尤其是大肠杆菌感染)相关的结构性或功能性胆汁淤积作为先决条件[231]。此类结石病在亚洲人群中的患病率非常高，而亚洲也是华支睾吸虫和蛔虫感染的常发地区，因此寄生虫因素被认为是褐色素结石形成的核心（见第 84 章）[232]。胆汁淤积使细菌感染以及胆管中的黏蛋白聚积和细胞骨架聚积更易发生。胆汁淤积的诱因可能是由于寄生虫及其卵细胞所导致的胆管狭窄和细菌感染[233]。随着褐色素结石易发的亚洲人群的胆道感染发生率下降，其患胆固醇胆结石与色素结石的比率也有所变化。在日本，褐色素结石的发病率自 20 世纪 50 年代后由 60% 降至 24%，其他亚洲国家也均有类似的报道[234-236]。

肠道细菌可产生 β-葡萄糖醛酸酶、磷脂酶 A1 与共轭胆酸水解酶。β-葡萄糖醛酸酶的会导致从葡糖醛酸胆红素中产生非结合胆红素；磷脂酶 A1 从磷脂质中释放棕榈酸与硬脂酸；儿胆酸水解酶从甘氨酸或牛磺酸结合胆盐中生成非结合胆盐。在一定程度上，电离的饱和脂肪酸、非结合胆红素与非结合胆盐可以钙盐的形式发生沉淀。黏蛋白凝胶则会聚集这些复合物沉淀，并促进其生长成为肉眼可见的褐色素结石。图 65.5 中呈现了可能的褐色素结石的形成机制。在正常生理条件下，胆汁中的胆红素基本以胆红素葡糖苷酸的形式存在，其在水介质中具有可溶性。胆汁中同样也含有来源于组织中的 β-葡萄糖醛酸酶，其产生于肝脏中，活性也会受到 β-葡萄糖二酸 1,4-内酯的抑制。当出现大肠杆菌感染时，细菌 β-葡萄糖醛酸酶的浓度会大幅度提升，并超过 β-葡萄糖二酸 1,4-内酯的抑制阈值。因此会导致胆红素葡糖苷酸经过水解产生非结合胆红素与葡糖醛酸；前者具有水溶性，并在其羧基自由基中与钙结合形成胆红素钙，从而导致褐色素结石的形成。

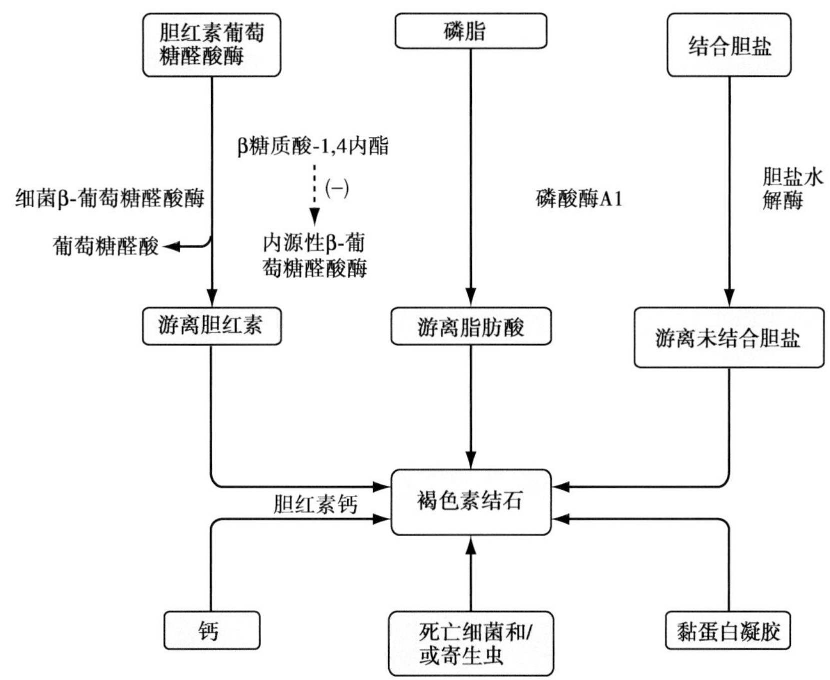

图 65.5　褐色素结石发病机制的建议。在正常生理条件下，非结合胆红素不分泌到胆汁中。即便内源性 β-葡萄糖醛酸酶可适度水解胆红素葡糖醛酸苷，但非结合胆红素占总胆色素的 1% 以下。主要是因为 β-葡萄糖醛酸酶的活性受到胆道系统中 β-葡萄糖醛酸-1,4-内酯的抑制。然而，过量细菌 β-葡萄糖醛酸酶的存在克服了 β-葡萄糖醛酸-1,4-内酯的抑制(−)作用，导致胆红素葡萄糖醛酸水解为游离胆红素和葡萄糖醛酸。游离胆红素与钙结合生成水不溶性胆红素钙。此外，磷脂酶 A1 从磷脂中释放游离脂肪酸，如棕榈酸与硬脂酸，而胆盐水解酶可从甘氨酸或牛磺酸结合胆盐中产生非结合胆盐。死亡细菌和/或寄生虫可作为加速胆红素钙沉淀的核。胆囊中的黏蛋白凝胶可以捕获这些复杂的沉淀物，并促进其生长为肉眼可见的结石

七、自然史

胆结石的自然史通常在 2 组不同的患者中进行描述，即有症状和无症状的患者。尸检研究清楚地表明，绝大多数胆结石患者是无症状的，并且仍然如此。确定无症状结石患者（以及有症状结石患者）并发症的真实发生频率，对于提供合理的、具有成本效益的治疗建议至关重要（见后文）。不幸的是，关于胆结石自然史的信息很少，并且存在一些差异[237-239]。

（一）无症状结石

Gracie 和 Ransohoff[237] 的研究改变了我们对胆石症病程和适当治疗的理解[237]。他们监测了 123 名密歇根大学教学教员 15 年，在常规筛查中发现他们患有胆结石后，在随访 5 年、10 年和 15 年时，分别有 10%、15% 和 18% 的患者出现症状，但没有患者出现严重并发症。研究人员认为，无症状胆结石患者在 5 年内每年发生胆源性疼痛的发生率约为 2%，然后随时间逐年降低。本研究中仅 3 例患者出现胆道并发症，所有并发症之前均有胆源性疼痛发作。事实上，胆源性疼痛不是胆道并发症，而是 90% 既往无症状胆结石患者的初始表现症状[237]。因此，在无症状结石患者中，并发症的发生频率较低，不必进行预防性的胆囊切除。

随后的研究报告称，最初无症状性胆结石患者出现胆源性疼痛和并发症的发生率略高[238]，但只有一项是长期前瞻性研究[239]。罗马胆石症流行病学和预防小组（Group for Epidemiology and Prevention of Cholelithiasis，GREPCO）报告了 151 例胆结石受试者的病程，其中 118 例在进入研究时无症状。在最初始无症状者中，2 年时胆源性疼痛的发生频率为 12%，4 年时为 17%，10 年时为 26%，10 年时胆道并发症的累计率为 3%[239]。

在 1987 年的一项研究中，1 371 例挪威未行胆囊切除术的患者中有 285 例（21%）意外发现了胆囊结石[240]。24 年后，一项随访研究纳入了 134 例胆结石患者[241]。89 例患者中有 25 例在超声上存在胆结石（总体 28%；女性 31%，男性 25%），随访时发现胆结石的初始大小和数量与结石持续性之间无相关性。134 例患者中的 9 例（7%）接受了胆囊切除术，91 例患者中的 5 例在随访前已死亡（6%）。随访期间，有 44% 的患者出现腹痛，29% 出现功能性腹痛。这项研究再次说明了无症状胆结石疾病的频繁消退与相对良性的性质。

（二）糖尿病患者的结石

糖尿病患者向来被认为是胆结石并发症的高风险人群。然而，糖尿病患者胆结石的自然史与非糖尿病患者中观察到的模式相同。对胰岛素抵抗糖尿病患者的前瞻性研究显示，随访 5 年后，15% 的无症状患者出现了症状[242]。此外，其并发症和死亡率与非糖尿病胆结石患者研究中的结果相当。因此，不建议对胰岛素抵抗的糖尿病患者和无症状胆结石患者行预防性胆囊切除术。

（三）症状性结石

胆结石的主要症状是胆源性疼痛（绞痛），描述为右上腹疼痛，通常放射至背部，伴或不伴恶心与呕吐。疼痛通常不是真正的绞痛（见第 11 章），几乎从不伴有发热。有症状胆结石的自然病程比无症状胆结石更具侵袭性。美国国家胆结石合作研究表明，在进入研究前一年的无并发症的胆源性疼痛的患者中，复发性胆源性疼痛的发生率为每年 38%[243]。其他研究人员报告症状性胆结石患者每年的复发性胆源性疼痛发生率高达 50%[244]。如前所述，有症状的胆结石患者也更容易发生胆道并发症。胆道并发症的风险估计为每年 1%～2%，并认为随时间的推移保持相对恒定[245]。因此，在出现胆道症状后，应向患者提供胆囊切除术。在手术风险较高的患者中，替代方法是密切观察，因为 30% 的患者不会再发生胆源性疼痛。

（四）特殊患者群体

胆结石的临床表现示意图见图 65.6，更详细的总结见表 65.2[246-250]。在第 58 章中讨论了胆源性胰腺炎。尽管对无症状胆结石的标准方案是观察，但一些无症状胆结石患者发生并发症的风险可能增加，可能需考虑预防性的胆囊切除术。

胆管癌和胆囊癌的风险增加与某些胆道疾病和某些种族（如：美洲原住民）相关（见第 69 章）。风险因素包括胆总管囊肿、肝内胆管囊性扩张症（Caroli 病）、胰胆管畸形愈合（也称为胰管和胆管的异常愈合，其中胰管引流到胆管中）、大型胆囊腺瘤与瓷化胆囊（见第 55、62 和 67 章）。胆管癌风险增加的患者更适合接受预防性胆囊切除术。如果计划实施腹部手术治疗其他适应证，则应进行附带性的胆囊切除术。

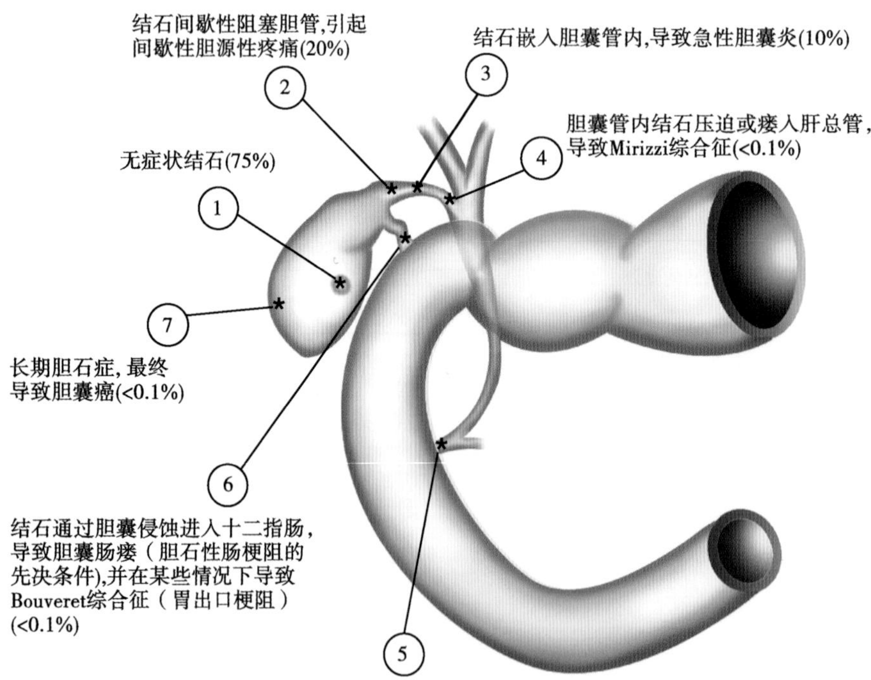

图 65.6　胆结石自然史和并发症的示意图。百分比表示基于自然史数据，胆结石患者发生并发症的近似频率。最常见的结局是结石患者终生无症状（1）、胆源性疼痛（2）、急性胆囊炎（3）、胆管炎（5）、胰腺炎（5）是最常见的并发症。Mirizzi 综合征（4）、胆囊肠瘘（6）、Bouveret 综合征（6）和胆囊癌（7）并不常见。（百分比之和>100%，因为急性胆囊炎患者通常有既往胆源性疼痛发作）

表 65.2 胆结石疾病的病理生理学、临床表现、诊断和治疗[a]

	胆源性疼痛	急性胆囊炎	胆总管结石	胆管炎
病理生理学	间歇性胆囊管阻塞 胆囊无急性炎症	胆管嵌顿结石 胆囊急性炎症 继发细菌性感染≈50%	结石从胆囊经胆囊管通过或形成于 BD 中 BD 间歇性阻塞	BD 中存在结石导致胆汁淤积 停滞的胆汁中细菌重复感染 早期出现菌血症
症状	上腹或右上腹内脏痛，疼痛位置不易确定，在 15 分钟内痛感逐渐提升，持续 1~6 小时，常伴有恶心 发作频率数日至数月不等 结石与排气、腹胀、胃肠胀气和消化不良无关	75% 的病例出现胆源性疼痛发作 上腹内脏痛变为右上腹、背部、右肩，以及胸腔（较为罕见）疼痛 常伴随恶心呕吐 疼痛持续时间超过 6 小时，长于普通胆源性疼痛	无症状 症状（若存在）常无法与胆囊性疼痛相区分 易导致胆管炎和急性胰腺炎	70% 的患者具有 Charcot 三联征（疼痛、黄疸与发热） 疼痛可能较轻且短暂，常伴随寒战 精神错乱、嗜睡与谵妄表明有脓毒症
体征	发作期间，轻度至中度上腹/右上腹压痛，残余的轻度压痛感可持续数日 通常查体正常	发热，通常低于 38.9℃，除非并发坏疽或穿孔 右肋下压痛，伴吸气停滞（墨菲征） 33% 的患者的胆囊可触及，尤其是首次发作的患者 20% 患者出现轻度黄疸；老年人发生率更高	若为间歇性堵塞，体征通常完全正常 黄疸伴随疼痛表示存在结石；无痛性黄疸与可触的胆囊及表示具有恶性肿瘤	95% 的患者有发热 90% 有右上腹压痛 80% 有黄疸 15% 有腹膜刺激征 低血压与精神错乱（与 Charcot 三联征共同形成 Reynolds 五联征）同时存在，且提示存在革兰氏阴性脓毒症
实验室检查结果	通常正常 血清胆红、碱性磷酸酶或淀粉酶水平升高表示同时存在胆管（BD）结石	常见杆状核白细胞增多 血清胆红素水平可为 2~4mg/dL，此外，即便不存在胆管结石或肝内感染，氨基转移酶和碱性磷酸酶水平也会升高 即使不存在胰腺炎，血清淀粉酶和脂肪酶也会轻度升高 若血清胆红素>4mg/dL 或淀粉酶或脂肪酶显著升高，应怀疑存在胆管结石	BD 梗阻患者中可见血清胆红素和碱性磷酸酶水平升高 血清胆红素水平>10mg/dL 提示存在恶性梗阻或溶血 血清氨基转移酶或淀粉酶（或脂肪酶）水平的短暂快速升高提示有结石通过	80% 的患者有白细胞增多，但其余可能白细胞数正常，伴有或不伴有杆状核白细胞 80% 的患者血清胆红素水平>2mg/dL 血清碱性磷酸酶水平通常出现升高 血培养通常呈阳性，尤其是在寒战或发热高峰期间抽取的；半数患者的血培养中生长出 2 种细菌
诊断性研究（关于成像检查的详情见表 65.3）	US 口服胆囊造影 Meltzer-Lyon 试验（见第 67 章）	US 肝胆显像 腹部 CT	ERCP EUS MRC 经皮 THC	ERCP 经皮 THC
自然史	初次发作后，30% 的患者没有更多的症状 其余症状的发生率以每年 6% 的速度上升，严重并发症的发生率以每年 1%~2% 的速度上升	50% 的病例无需手术即可在 10 天内自然缓解。 未经治疗，有 10% 的病例因局部穿孔而复杂化，1% 的病例因游离穿孔和腹膜炎复杂化	自然病程尚不明确，但其并发症比无症状胆囊结石更常见与更严重	如未及时明确诊断，死亡率非常高，死亡由败血症导致 BD 紧急减压（一般通过 ERCP 进行）可大大提高生存率
治疗（见第 66 和 70 章）	可选择性采用腹腔镜胆囊切除术，可进行术中胆道造影（IOC） 如 IOC 显示存在结石，可采用 ERCP 或胆总管切开探查术移除结石	腹腔镜胆囊切除术，可进行 IOC（如可能）；或采用开腹胆囊切除术 如 IOC 显示存在结石，可采用 ERCP 或 BD 切开探查术移除结石	采用 ERCP 移除结石，多数病例采用传统腹腔镜胆囊切除术	采用紧急 ERCP 移除结石，或至少进行 BD 紧急减压 使用覆盖革兰氏阴性菌、厌氧菌与肠球菌的抗生素 后续行胆囊切除术

[a] 有关胆源性胰腺炎的讨论，见第 58 章。

BD，胆管；IOC，术中胆道造影术；MRC，磁共振胰胆管造影；THC，经肝胆管造影；US，超声。

镰状细胞病患者更常见色素胆结石，且往往无症状。在此情况下，不建议实施预防性胆囊切除术，但如果因其他原因行腹部手术，应考虑附带性胆囊切除术。一些权威机构建议，如果存在胆结石，对患有遗传性球形红细胞增多症的无症状年轻患者联合进行预防性脾切除术和胆囊切除术。

接受减重手术的病态肥胖人群发生胆结石并发症的风险较高（见第 7 和 8 章）。这些患者患胆结石的频率大于30%。建议在减重手术的同时，进行附带性的预防性胆囊切除术。

一些研究人员提出，等待心脏移植的同时期胆石症患者，应接受预防性胆囊切除术，无论是否存在胆道症状，因为他们移植后出现胆结石并发症的风险增加[251]。然而，一项在肾移植受者中解决该问题的回顾性研究得出的结论是，在出现症状后，胆结石的并发症可以安全地进入老年期[252]。

八、诊断

影像学检查在诊断胆结石及相关疾病方面扮演着举足轻重的角色。表 65.3 展示了可用于胆道评估的众多成像技术[253-256]。每种影像都有着自己的优势与局限性，且不同方法的相对成本和对于患者的相对风险有着极大差异。除超声外，在评估可疑胆结石疾病患者时不应采用其他任何常规的方法。相反，诊断评价应基于个体的症状、体征和实验室研究结果理性地逐步进行（见下文）。

表 65.3　胆道的影像学检查

技术	检查结果/评价	
US（超声）	胆石症	结石表现为胆囊内腔可活动的独立的强回声灶，伴随声影。胆泥表现为层叠回声，不伴声影 结石>2mm 时，敏感度>95% 结石呈现声影时，特异性>95% 极少情况下，充满结石的胆囊可能是收缩的且不易被观察到，呈现出 WES 征（wall-echo shadow） 胆囊结石的最佳单项检查
	胆总管结石	≈50%的病例中可在 BD 中观察到结石，另外≈25%的病例可根据 BD 扩张推断是否存在胆结石，从而进一步确定 可确定 BD 结石存在，但无法排除结石
	急性胆囊炎	检测到结石时，超声莫菲氏征（使用超声探头引起胆囊局部压痛）在检测急性胆囊炎的阳性预测值>90% 胆囊周围积液（不存在腹水）和胆囊壁厚度>4mm（不存在低白蛋白血症）属于非特异性发现，但提示了急性胆囊炎的存在
EUS（超声内镜）	胆总管结石	高精度地确定与排除 BD 结石 EUS 与 ERCP 诊断的一致性≈95%；许多研究表明 EUS 的敏感性高于 ERCP 特异性≈97% 阳性预测值≈99%；阴性预测值≈98%；精确度≈97% 当经验丰富的操作员操作时，EUS 可替代 ERCP 排除 BD 结石，尤其是轻度或中度临床怀疑的条件下 胆总管结石轻度或中度临床可能性的患者可考虑
口服胆囊造影术*	胆石症	结石表现为可移动的充盈缺损 胆囊显影时，敏感性和特异性超过 90%，但有 25%的检查无显影，可能是结石以外的多种原因所致 胆囊浑浊显影提示胆囊管通畅 可用于评估非结石性胆囊疾病（如胆固醇贮积病和腺肌病；见第 67 章）
胆道闪烁显像（肝胆闪烁显像；羟基亚氨基二乙酸或二异丙基亚氨基二乙酸扫描）	急性胆囊炎	评估胆囊管的通畅度 可在 3~60 分钟内显示胆囊、BD 和小肠放射性的普通扫描 阳性结果定义为胆囊未显像，肝的放射性核素残留进入 BD 或小肠 敏感性≈95%，特异性≈90%；危重症禁食患者可能呈现假阳性结果 利用胆囊收缩素刺激，可确定胆囊的“排出分数”，并帮助评估非结石性胆源性疼痛患者（见第 67 章） 可大体排除急性胆囊炎的普通扫描
ERCP（内镜逆行胰胆管造影）	胆总管结石	BD 结石的标准诊断方法，其敏感性与特异性≈95% 在重症胆管炎时，使用 ERCP 取出结石（或至少排出感染的胆汁）可挽救生命，同时也降低了在胆囊切除术中使用胆总管切开探查术的必要 建议高度胆总管结石临床可能性患者采用
	胆石症	在造影剂逆流入胆囊中后，结石表现为充盈缺损，敏感性≈80%，但 US 仍是确定结石症的主要手段
MRC（磁共振胰胆管造影）	胆总管结石	快速无创的检查手段，可提供与 ERCP 相当的详细的胆管和胰管影像 敏感性≈93%，特异性≈94%，与 ERCP 持平 可有效用于检测非扩张胆管，尤其是胆总管下段，使用 US 无法对其进行良好的显影 可同时检测邻近结构，如肝与胰 建议轻度或中度胆总管结石临床可能性的患者采用
CT	胆结石并发症	不太适用于检测单纯的结石，但非常适合检测并发症，如脓肿、胆囊或 BD 穿孔，以及胰腺炎 螺旋 CT 被证明是排除 BD 结石的一种非侵入性手段；一些研究表明，CT 与口服胆囊造影剂联用可提高诊断准确性

*不经常采用；BD，胆管。

针对胆道的影像检查中显然不涉及腹部平片。虽然腹部平片是评估腹痛患者的一种有效手段，但其缺乏敏感性和特异性。仅 50% 的色素结石和 20% 的胆固醇结石含有足够的钙，从而使其可见于腹部平片中。由于西方国家中 80% 的胆结石都是胆固醇结石，因此使用 X 线检查就仅能检测到 25% 的结石了。在评价是否患有某些不常见的胆结石并发症（如气肿性胆囊炎、胆囊肠瘘与胆石性肠梗阻）或检测瓷化胆囊方面，腹部平片就更无用武之地了（见前文）。

（一）超声

自 20 世纪 70 年代引入超声（US）以来，它就一直是诊断胆石症的主要影像学手段。US 所需时间短，仅需禁食一夜或 8 小时，不涉及电离辐射，操作简单，可提供精确的解剖信息。且具有便携性，可置于危重患者床旁[238]。

胆结石的诊断依赖于对胆囊腔中的物体反射声波从而产生的声影的检测（图 65.7A）。结石具有可移动性，通常聚积于胆囊中一个独立的区域。现代 US 可探测到直径小至 2mm 的结石。但体积更小的结石无法检测到，或可能与胆泥（不产生声影的分层式的回声影像）相混淆[257]。

US 在探测胆囊中大于 2mm 的结石时的敏感性高于

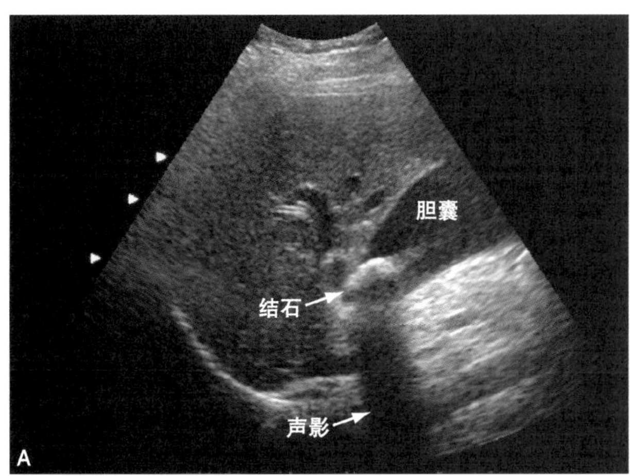

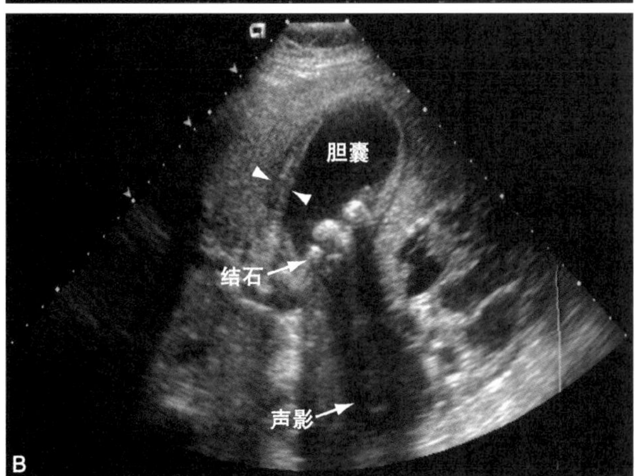

图 65.7　（A）胆石症的典型超声表现。胆囊（GB）腔内存在胆结石，其后方有声影。随着患者的重新定位，结石将移动，从而排除胆囊息肉的可能性。（B）急性胆囊炎背景下的胆石症。胆囊腔内可见多发胆囊结石，伴有相关的声影。此外，胆囊壁增厚（箭头）。（Courtesy Julie Champine，MD，Dallas，TX.）

95%[258]。若结石产生声影，其特异性则高于 95%。极少情况下，结石周围的胆囊成熟瘢痕和胆囊收缩会妨碍对胆囊或结石的定位，这也提示胆囊癌的可能性。充满结石的胆囊收缩时会呈现出“双边影”或“WES 征”的信号，探查时立即可见到胆囊壁、结石与声影。若无法使用超声诊断识别到胆囊，可采用额外的影像学检查，如口服胆囊造影术和腹部 CT。

US 是诊断胆囊胆结石的标准方法，但在检测胆管（胆总管）结石方面，其特异性明显降低[259]。由于胆总管下段贴近于十二指肠，肠腔内的气体常常会干扰 US 影像，因此无法探查胆管全长[260]。因此，仅 50% 的胆管结石可借助 US 精确探测到[254]。然而，在未进行胆囊切除术的情况下，若发现胆管扩张，也可以推断有结石堵塞胆管。由于内镜逆行胰胆管造影（ERCP）发现 US 结果假阴性出现的频率较高，所以将胆管直径的正常值上限从 10mm 降至 6mm。即便如此，通过 US 表现出的胆管扩张推断胆总管结石的敏感性也仅为 75%。

US 在诊断急性胆囊炎的方面极为有效[261]。胆囊周围出现积液（不存在腹水时）和胆囊壁厚超过于 4mm（不存在低白蛋白血症）即表明患有急性胆囊炎（见图 65.7B）。不幸的是，在重症监护的患者中，常在不具有其他胆囊疾病证据的患者身上频繁观察到此类非特异性发现[261]。更具特异性的发现应是超声莫菲氏征，超声医师可在超声探头下引起胆囊局部压痛。

引出超声莫菲氏征的程度取决于操作医师，且需要患者敏感性较高。在存在胆结石的条件下，超声莫菲氏征出现即表明急性胆囊炎的阳性预测值高于 90%[262]。另外，US 也可在鉴别诊断中帮助定位其他腹部疾病，如脓肿和假性囊肿。

（二）超声内镜

超声内镜（EUS）可高精度地检查胆总管结石。与 US 相比，EUS 更具侵入性，价格更高，但优势在于能够从胃肠内腔中对胆管进行显影，在这方面的能力可与 ERCP 相持平。胃肠道内超声显像比经腹的 US 具有几个优势，包括与胆管距离更近、分辨力更高，以及不受肠道气体或腹壁层的干扰（图 65.8）。在几组研究中，EUS 在诊断胆道结石方面的阳性预测值为 99%，阴性预测值为 98%，精确率为 97%；这与 ERCP 相当[263,264]。若使用 EUS 发现胆道结石，则有必要采取内镜治疗；若高度怀疑胆总管结石，可将 ERCP 作为初步检查。然而，几项比较 EUS 与 ERCP 的研究发现，两种技术均可准确确认和排除胆总管结石，EUS 在安全性和成本方面均具有优势[265-267]。

研究还发现，EUS 在检测是否存在胆管结石方面优于 MRC（见后文）。在临床怀疑胆总管结石的患者中，采用 EUS 的主要优势在于能够避免不必要的 ERCP 和括约肌切开术，后两者并非没有风险。采用 EUS 确定是否有 ERCP 指征可避免大量的 ERCP，并减少并发症。一项基于随机对照试验的回顾性研究对 EUS 引导下的 ERCP 和单纯的 ERCP 在检测胆管结石方面进行了比较[268]。与随机接受单纯 ERCP 的对照组相比，随机接受了 EUS 的患者中有 67% 不必采用 ERCP，且出现并发症和胰腺炎的比率更低（分别为 0.35 和 0.21）。在 213 例患者中，仅 2 例使用 EUS 未能检测到胆管结石（0.9%）。因此，EUS 在在排除胆管结石方面被认为是一项

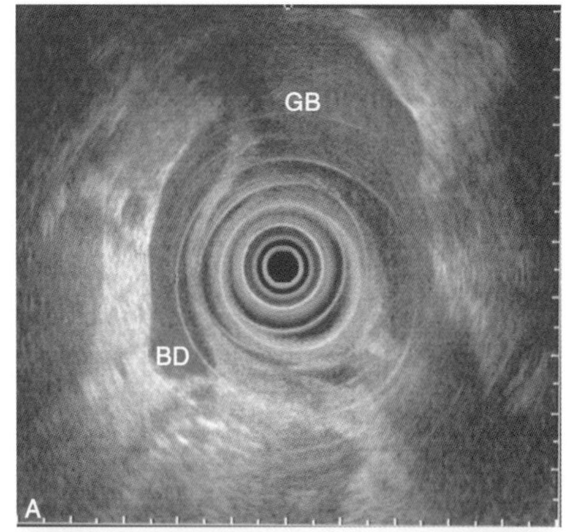

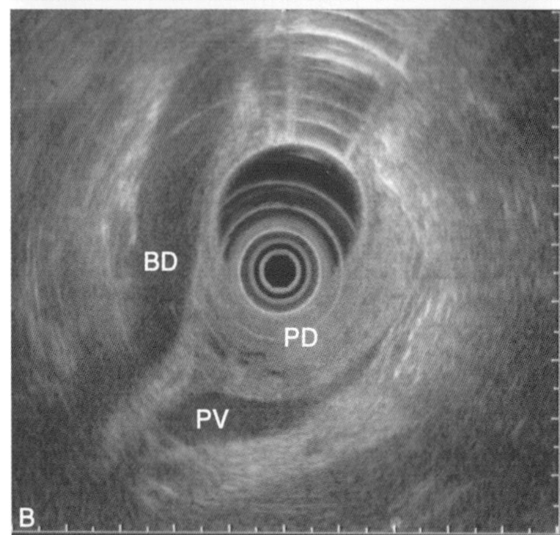

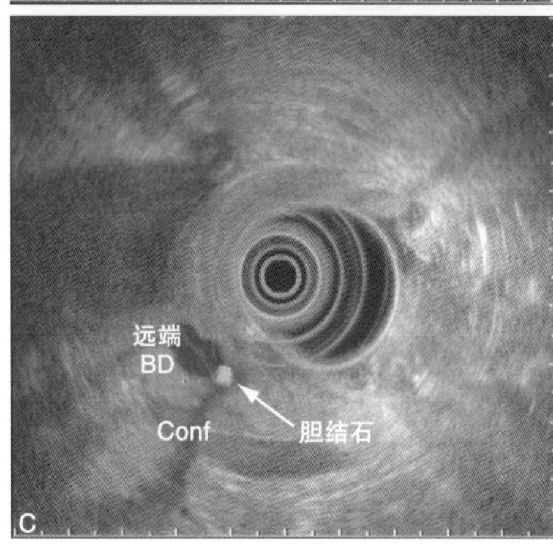

图 65.8　放射状扇形扫描内镜的 EUS，显示胆总管结石。显示胆管（BD）延伸至胆囊（GB）水平（顶部）和远端（A 和 B）。BD 的最大直径为 12mm（B），胆管远端变细至直径 7mm（C）。在远端 BD 内，胆结石清晰可见（C）。注意：相邻结构与 BD 的接近度以及 EUS 解析这些结构的难易程度。Conf，门静脉和脾静脉汇合处；PD，胰管；PV，门静脉

合适的检查手段，尤其是针对轻度或中度结石验前概率的患者。

（三）口服胆囊造影术

作为曾经胆囊影像学检查的主流医学手段，由于存在多种应用局限性，如今已作为检测胆囊结石的辅助性手段[254]。其唯一有用的临床适应证是在 US 无法明确诊断的情况下，用于评估考虑进行医疗溶石或碎石的患者（见第 66 章）[269]，以及评估有未知胆囊疾病（如腺肌病和胆固醇贮积病）的患者。

（四）胆道闪烁显像术

胆道闪烁显像术（核素肝胆动态显像）是针对胆囊和胆道的一种放射性核素显像，能够有效地评估疑似急性胆囊炎的患者[270]。通过确定胆囊管的通畅率，胆道闪烁显像可快速（90 分钟内）排除腹痛患者患急性胆囊炎的可能性[271,272]。该方法可在急诊情况下针对非空腹患者使用，检查前需进行发射 γ 射线的^{99m}Tc 标记羟基亚氨基二乙酸（HIDA）或二异丙基亚氨基二乙酸（DISIDA）的静脉注射，注射后药物会快速的经肝脏吸收并分泌到胆汁中[254]。如图 65.9 所示，注射后的连续扫描通常应在 30~60 分钟内显示出胆囊、胆管和小肠的放射显像[216]。以往，使用此技术对黄疸患者进行显像具有限制性，但使用 DISIDA 可允许针对血清胆红素达 20mg/dL 的患者进行胆道显影。

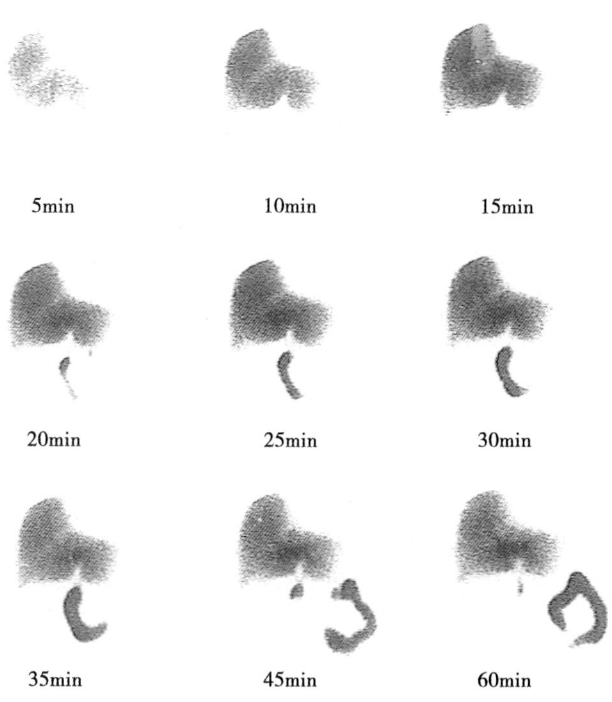

图 65.9　胆道闪烁显像显示急性胆囊炎特征性的胆囊管梗阻。γ-发射放射性同位素标记的二异丙基亚氨基二乙酸经静脉注射后迅速被肝脏摄取（5 分钟时），并排泄到胆汁中（20 分钟时）。连续图像显示同位素迅速进入十二指肠（45 分钟时）并在小肠远端通过，但从未集中在胆囊中。若胆囊未能在 30~60 分钟内显示为热点构成阳性结果，意味着胆囊管梗阻

异常或“阳性”扫描结果定义为胆囊无显影，放射性分泌物进入胆管或小肠。此检查方法在检测急性胆囊炎方面的精确度为 92%，高于 US。在禁食或危重患者中常出现假阳性结果，此类患者的胆囊动力低于正常水平。胆囊动力的下降导致更多的水分被吸收，从而使胆汁凝胶化。在危重患者中，胆汁淤积和肝细胞功能异常使放射性核素显像剂清除率下降。虽然因胆管梗阻所引起的胆囊不显影是急性胆囊炎的特征，但胆囊周围肝脏的放射性核素摄取也是有用的第二特征[273]。

在部分患者中(如:慢性胆囊炎、肝疾病或胆总管结石的患者),采用放射性核素扫描进行胆囊显影需要延迟数个小时,且应在 4 小时(或更久)后再次进行扫描,以确定未患有急性胆囊炎。针对危重患者,这种需延迟等待胆囊显影是有问题的,但针对 60 分钟内胆囊未显影的患者可通过静脉注射Ⅳ型硫酸吗啡解决延迟等待的问题。吗啡可增加 Oddi 括约肌内的压力,从而促进胆汁流入胆囊(若不存在胆管梗阻)。

注射吗啡 30 分钟后,进行第二次扫描,如胆囊显影,则可排除胆管梗阻,进而排除急性胆囊炎。但在约半数的危重患者中可能出现胆囊不显影,即使是注射吗啡后,这会导致胆道闪烁显像结果假阳性。

胆道闪烁显像目前仍作为评估疑似急性胆囊炎危重患者的主要方法,但额外使用 CCK 注射可有效辨别非结石性慢性胆源性疼痛的患者,从而避免采用诊断性的胆囊切除术(见第 67 章)。胆道闪烁显像的另一重要作用是无创检测是否有胆汁从胆管中溢出,这是胆囊切除术的并发症之一(见第 66 章)[274]。

(五) 逆行胰胆管造影

逆行胰胆管造影(ERCP)是检测胆总管结石最有效的疗法[275];此技术将在第 70 章中更详细地论述。存在结石的胆管表现为充盈缺损,检测敏感度为 95%(图 65.10)[276]。注意,应谨慎避免将气体意外注入到胆道中[277],因为气泡可在 ERCP 中出现胆结石样表现。ERCP 检测胆管结石的特异性约为 95%。

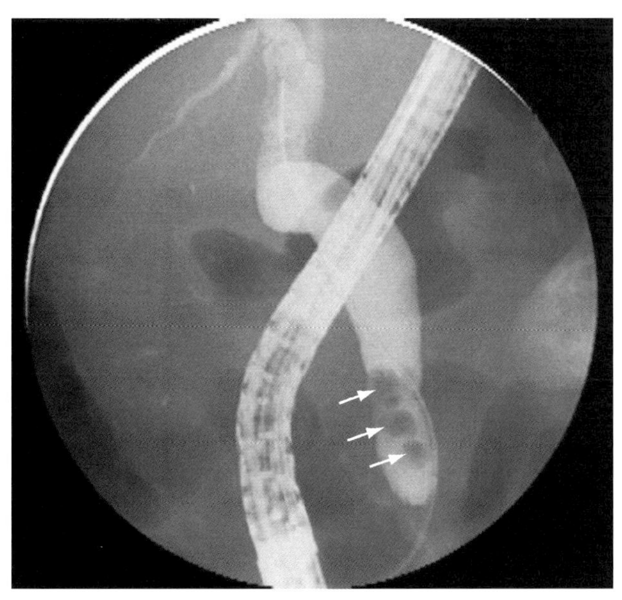

图 65.10　ERCP 显示胆总管结石伴胆管扩张至 15mm 和 3 个代表结石的充盈缺损(箭)

ERCP 改变了胆总管结石的治疗方法[278]与其他胆管疾病患者的治疗带来的革命性的变化(见第 70 章)。随着 EUS 和 MRC 被越来越多地应用,ERCP 在诊断胆总管结石方面的作用也出现了极大的改变。国立卫生研究院的一项会议共识建议,仅在高度怀疑胆总管结石的患者中(即,有必要采用治疗性干预时)使用 ERCP。若仅单独诊断胆总管结石,EUS 和 MRC 的精度与 ERCP 不相上下[279]。

(六) CT 与 MRI

CT 主要用于检测胆石症和胆总管结石患者的并发症,如急性胆囊炎的胆囊周围液体积聚、胆囊壁气体(表明患气肿性胆囊炎)、胆囊穿孔和脓肿(图 65.11)。也有研究通过口服胆囊造影剂利用螺旋 CT 胆管造影术(CT cholangiography,CTC)检测胆总管结石[280,281]。虽然 CTC 在检测胆管结石的方面仍弱于 ERCP,但却能够反映出周围其他部分的病理异常[282]。MRC 在胆道显影和胆结石的检测中极为有效。该方法尤其适用于检测胆管未扩张情况下的肝外胆管远端部分的异常;该部分通常无法通过经腹 US 良好地显像[239]。随着腹腔镜胆囊切除术的问世,急需一项简单快速,且易于使用的除外胆管结石的无创检测手段。MRC 可以高敏感的检测胆管结石,并形成胆管三维影像(图 65.12)[266,267]。一篇系统性综述将 MRC 与诊断性 ERCP 在检测胆总管结石的方面进行了比对,结果显示 MRC 的敏感性为 93%,特异性 94%[268]。

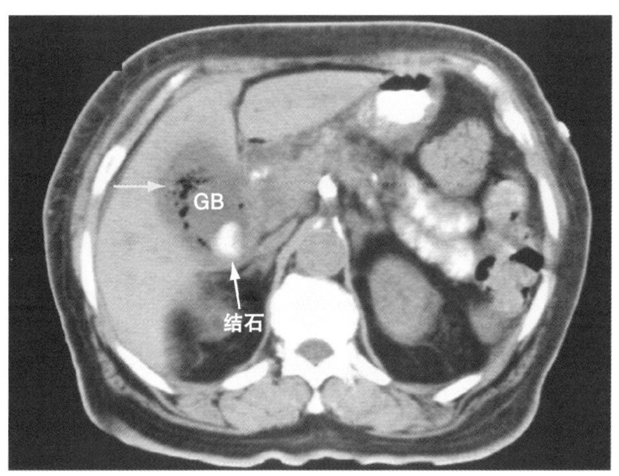

图 65.11　腹部 CT 显示气肿性胆囊炎伴相关胆石症。胆囊(GB)内存在由产气微生物继发感染引起的气泡(黄色箭)。(Courtesy Julie Champine, MD, Dallas, TX.)

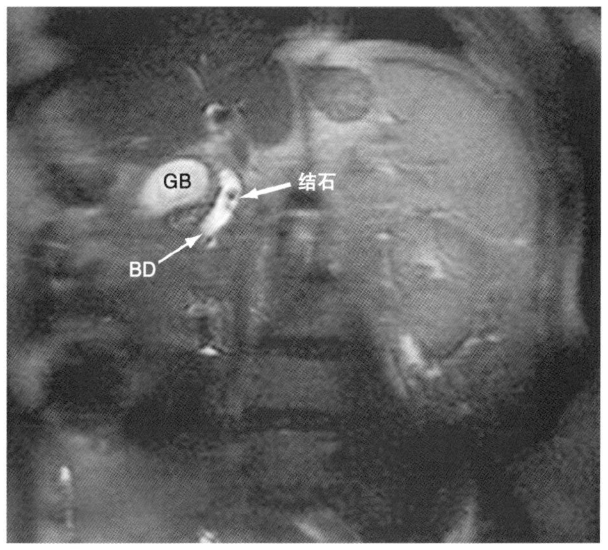

图 65.12　MRC 显示胆总管结石。胆囊(BD)内有 2 个充盈缺损,即为胆结石。(Courtesy Julie Champine, MD, Dallas, TX)

九、临床疾病

（一）胆源性疼痛与慢性胆囊炎

胆源性疼痛是胆石症最常见的症状，约75%的胆结石疾病患者因为偶发性腹痛而就医。在胆结石并发症（如急性胆囊炎）患者中，通常会在并发症发作前的几个月内反复出现腹部疼痛。

1. 发病机制

胆源性疼痛是由于一个或多个结石间歇性地阻塞胆囊管所致。胆源性疼痛并不一定伴随胆囊管梗阻所致的胆囊发炎。另外，应避免使用“慢性胆囊炎”来描述胆源性疼痛，因为“慢性胆囊炎”就表示存在慢性炎症，这在某些患者中并不存在。实际上，胆源性疼痛的剧烈程度和频率与胆囊病理变化并无关联[285]。在胆源性疼痛患者中，所观察到的最常见的组织学改变是胆囊壁轻度纤维化，伴慢性炎性细胞浸润，但黏膜完整。胆源性疼痛的反复发作也与胆囊瘢痕、萎缩和胆囊 Rokitansky-Aschoff 窦（壁内憩室）有关。在约10%的胆源性疼痛患者中，可从胆囊胆汁或胆结石本身培养出细菌，但认为细菌感染不会引起这些症状（见第67章）。

2. 临床特征

本质上，胆源性疼痛来自内脏，因此难以明确具体疼痛点[286]。在典型病例中，患者出现发作性上腹痛，多数位于上腹部或右上腹，但有时也发生于腹部其他位置。进食可刺激疼痛发作，但多数病例中并无该现象。在发作时间方面，在减肥和明显缺乏体力活动（如：长时间卧床）的情况下更容易引发胆源性疼痛。

过去常用的“胆绞痛”应属于用词不当，因为胆源性疼痛是持续性的，而非断断续续的，应当明确“绞痛”的定义。胆源性疼痛的痛感会在15分钟到1小时内逐渐达到顶峰，并持续1或数小时，随后逐渐缓解。在三分之一的病患中，疼痛会突然停止。若疼痛持续超过6小时，则提示急性胆囊炎可能，而非单纯的胆源性疼痛（见第11章）。

以发作频率从高至低排序，患者分别会在上腹部、右上腹、左上腹和腹部其他部位或下腹部感觉到剧痛。因此，非右上腹的疼痛可排除胆石疾病这种概念是错误的。在半数的患者中，疼痛会蔓延至肩胛骨、右肩或下腹部。胆源性疼痛常伴随出汗，恶心，也可出现呕吐；但胆源性疼痛引发的呕吐不如肠梗阻和急性胰腺炎那样持久。与其他类型腹痛患者一样，胆源性疼痛患者常常表现为不安和亢奋。

胆结石患者常见的嗳气、腹胀、胃肠胀气和消化不良很大可能与结石无关。这些非特异性症状出现频率与非胆结石人群相似。因此，症状仅为消化不良和其他非特异性上消化道症状的胆结石患者不建议实施胆囊切除术。胆源性疼痛患者的体格检查通常正常，在发作时可存在轻度或中度的胆囊压痛，且在发作后的几天内可能持续存在轻度压痛。

3. 诊断

在单纯胆源性疼痛患者中，实验室检查通常正常。若血清胆红素、碱性磷酸酶和淀粉酶水平升高，则表明胆总管结石并存。

大体上，只建议胆源性疼痛患者应首选且只应选择 US 对右上腹进行影像学检查。虽然 US 的诊断精确度极高，但由于大量患者都会因为多种原因行 US 检查，所以偶尔也会遗漏掉具有临床重要性结石，并导致正确诊断的延迟[255]。鉴于胆源性疼痛具有相对良性的自然病程，对 US 结果阴性的患者进行随访观察是安全的，可对再次出现症状的患者进行进一步的检查[287]。

4. 鉴别诊断

反复发作的上腹症状需鉴别的疾病包括反流性食管炎、消化性溃疡、胰腺炎、肾绞痛、憩室炎、结肠癌、IBS、神经根病和心绞痛（见第11章）。通常情况下，仔细询问病史可有助于缩小鉴别诊断范围。在一项针对1 008例因为胆结石而接受胆囊切除术患者的研究中，与胆源性疼痛（偶发性胆囊疼痛）相关的临床表现是偶发性疼痛（通常每月1次或更低频率），疼痛可持续30分钟至23小时，发生于傍晚或夜间，症状开始于手术1年前或更近的时间[288]。黄色肉芽肿性胆囊炎是一种罕见的慢性胆囊炎的侵袭性变异，其特征是胆囊壁上出现灰黄色的结节或条痕，这是富含脂质的巨噬细胞的表现；同时也可能表现为急性黄疸。

5. 治疗

复发性单纯胆源性疼痛且已证明有胆结石的患者通常行选择性腹腔镜胆囊切除术（见第66章）进行治疗。急性胆源性疼痛也可通过注射哌替啶进行缓解，同时可服用酮咯酸或双氯芬酸。有研究称，预防性地服用阿司匹林可预防胆结石的形成和胆结石患者急性发作，但长期服用其他非甾体抗炎药对预防胆结石形成无效[280,281]。

（二）急性胆囊炎

急性胆囊炎是结石疾病最常见的并发症。急性胆囊炎的主要标志是与胆囊壁炎症相关的腹痛、右上腹压痛、发热和白细胞增多。在约90%的病例中，其根本原因是胆囊出口被胆囊管、胆囊颈或 Hartmann 袋中的结石梗阻所致[291]。对于其余10%的病例，胆囊炎的发生并不伴有结石（无结石胆囊炎；见第67章）。由结石引起的急性胆囊炎通常发生在年轻健康女性，且预后良好。但急性无结石胆囊炎常出现于危重患者，伴随高发病率与死亡率。

1. 发病机制

急性胆囊炎发病通常是由于结石嵌入胆囊管并引起慢性梗阻，并不是单纯胆源性疼痛的暂时性梗阻[291]。胆囊腔中的胆汁淤积导致胆囊黏膜受损，随后释放胞内酶并激活一系列的炎症介质。

在动物研究中，胆囊管结扎后，结果往往是胆囊内容物被逐渐吸收，而不引发炎症[292]；此时，需要在梗阻的胆囊中留置导管注射刺激物（如：浓缩胆汁或溶血卵磷脂）或导管引起损伤，才会出现急性胆囊炎。研究认为，磷脂酶 A 由胆结石导致损伤的黏膜所释放，其将卵磷脂转换为溶血卵磷脂。正常胆囊的胆汁中不存在溶血卵磷脂，但见于急性胆囊炎患者的胆囊内容物中[293]。在动物模型中，向胆囊中注射溶血卵磷脂可诱发急性胆囊炎，伴随蛋白质分泌升高与水分吸收下降，以及和前列腺素 E 和 $F_1\alpha$ 合成增加相关的白细胞浸润。研究发现，注射吲哚美辛（一种 cox 抑制剂）可阻断该炎症反应。针对从胆囊切除术中获取到的人体组织的研究证明，存在炎症的胆囊中产生的前列腺素有所提高。此外,已证明向急性胆囊炎患者静脉注射吲哚美辛或口服布洛芬可降低胆囊内压力和缓解疼痛[293]。

关于前列腺素在急性胆囊炎发展中的作用的支持性证据来自一项前瞻性研究,研究中出现胆源性疼痛的患者被随机分配于接受双氯芬酸(一种前列腺素合成酶抑制剂)治疗或(无药用效果的)安慰剂治疗[294]。最终,接受安慰剂治疗的40 例患者中有 9 例发生急性胆囊炎,而 20 例接受双氯芬酸治疗的患者的胆源性疼痛均得到缓解。这些数据表明,与胆囊管梗阻相关的 1 个或多个腔内因素会损伤胆囊黏膜,并刺激前列腺素合成。因此导致的液体分泌和炎性改变则诱发新一轮的黏膜损伤和炎症[294]。

约半数急性胆囊炎患者的胆囊胆汁中可培养出肠杆菌[295]。但目前并不认为细菌是急性胆囊炎的诱发因素。

2. 病理学

若于急性胆囊炎发作前数日进行检查,常可发现胆囊肿胀,并有结石嵌入胆囊管中[296]。打开胆囊后,可观察到炎症渗出物,偶尔可见脓液。疾病发作后,常见的胆汁色素会被吸收,并被稀薄的黏液状液体、脓液或血液所取代。急性胆囊炎发作后若长期不进行治疗,且胆囊管持续梗阻,胆囊腔中则将充满清澈的黏液状液体,这种现象称为胆囊积水。

急性胆囊炎的组织学改变范围包括从伴随水肿的急性炎症至胆囊壁坏死或穿孔。令人意外的是,组织学改变与患者症状的严重程度几乎没有联系[296]。若针对急性胆囊炎患者行胆囊切除术后未发现结石,则应仔细从组织结构上检查样本,寻找脉管炎或胆固醇栓塞的证据,因为这些系统性疾病可表现为无结石性胆囊炎(见第 37 章)。

3. 临床特征

约 75% 的急性胆囊炎患者曾有胆源性疼痛发作(见表 65. 2)[297]。通常情况下,此类患者若出现长时间疼痛症状,则应警惕非单纯胆源性疼痛的可能性。当胆源性疼痛超过 6 小时,应考虑急性胆囊炎。

与单纯胆源性疼痛相反,多数患者的体征可提示急性胆囊炎的诊断。急性胆囊炎患者常出现发热,但体温一般不超过 38. 9℃,除非胆囊出现坏疽或穿孔(图 65. 13)。20% 的急性胆囊炎患者会出现轻度黄疸,而老年患者则为 40%。患者的血清胆红素水平一般低于 4mg/dL[298]。胆红素高于该值则表示有胆总管结石的可能性,在 50% 的急性胆囊炎和黄疸患者中可出现这种情况。急性胆囊炎患者出现黄疸的另一个病因则是 Mirizzi 综合征,这与肝总管的炎性梗阻有关(见下文)。

三分之一患者腹部查体可表现出右肋下压痛并可触及胆囊;在初次发作急性胆囊炎的患者中更容易触及胆囊。胆囊炎反复发作通常会导致胆囊瘢痕与纤维化,从而使胆囊无法扩张。虽然原因不明,但患者的胆囊通常可在正常解剖位置的外侧触及。

急性胆囊炎一个相对具特异性的体征是墨菲征(Murphy sign)[297]。在右肋下触诊期间,患者深吸气可使检查者的手触及发炎的胆囊,并导致疼痛或吸气停止。在适当的临床背景下,墨菲征的存在可以作为急性胆囊炎的可靠指标,虽然胆结石仍应通过 US 进行检查。

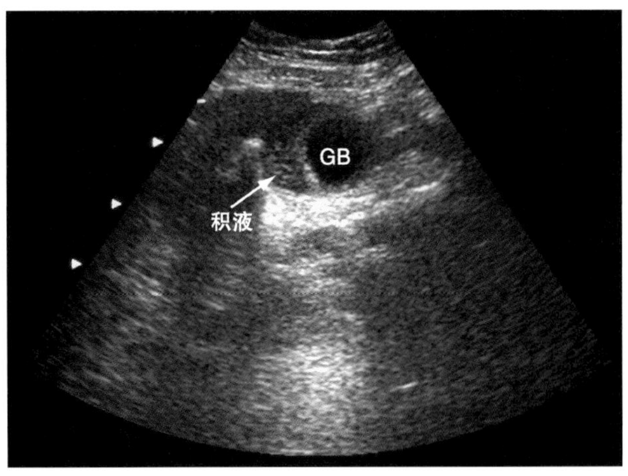

图 65. 13　US 显示胆囊(GB)附近有复杂的液体聚积,并伴随胆囊穿孔。(Courtesy Julie Champine, MD, Dallas, TX)

4. 自然史

在不加以治疗的情况下,急性胆囊炎引发的疼痛感会在 7~10 天内逐渐缓解[299]。而在住院治疗时,患者的症状常在 48 小时内缓解。一项研究表明,未出现并发症的急性胆囊炎的患者约 87% 可自行缓解,但 7% 的患者可能出现坏疽性胆囊炎,6% 出现胆囊积脓,3% 出现胆囊穿孔,以及少于 1% 的患者出现气肿性胆囊炎[300]。

5. 诊断

也许是因为过于常见,急性胆囊炎往往是有腹部症状患者首先鉴别诊断的疾病;若仅考虑临床标准,其实有些诊断过度。一项前瞻性研究针对 100 名右上腹疼痛和压痛的疑似急性胆囊炎的患者进行了研究,发现仅三分之二的病例诊断正确。因此,临床医生必须使用实验室和影像学检查来确定存在急性胆囊炎,同时除外并发症(如坏疽和穿孔),并寻找其他有类似临床表现的可能病因。

表 65. 2 呈现了急性胆囊炎最常见的实验室检查结果[299]。急性胆囊炎患者中,常见以未成熟中性粒细胞为主的白细胞升高。因为在鉴别诊断中经常将急性胆囊炎诊断为胆管结石伴胆管炎,因此应格外注意肝脏生化检查结果[298]。即便没有胆管梗阻,急性胆囊炎也往往会引起血清转氨酶和碱性磷酸酶水平轻微升高。如前文所述,血清胆红素的水平也会因为急性胆囊炎而轻微提升(2~4mg/dL),甚至血清淀粉酶和脂肪酶也会出现非特异性的升高。血清胆红素值高于 4mg/dL 或淀粉酶值高于 1 000U/L 往往提示急性胆囊炎与胆管结石或急性胰腺炎共存,且应进行进一步的检查。

当血白细胞升高超过 15 000/mm^3 时,尤其在伴有严重疼痛、高热(体温>38. 9℃)和寒战的情况下,应考虑化脓性胆囊炎(积脓症)或胆囊穿孔,这种情况需进行紧急外科手术。这类进展性的胆囊疾病也可能出现在局部和全身临床表现不明显的情况下。

在有右上腹疼痛和压痛的危重患者中,US 是最有效的影像学检查,它能够精确地确定是否存在胆结石,且可作为体格检查的补充。超声莫菲氏征(定义为探头下胆囊局部压痛)在检查急性胆囊炎时的阳性预测值大于 90%;其诱发条件是存在胆结石、操作员技巧熟练,以及患者本身较为敏感[301]。

此外,US 能够发现提示急性胆囊炎存在的非特异性表现,如胆囊周围出现积液和胆囊壁增厚(大于 4mm)。若患者患有腹水或低白蛋白血症,上述两个表现在检查急性胆囊炎时便缺乏特异性[255,302]。

由于胆结石的患病率较高,许多表现为急性腹痛(如急性胰腺炎和消化性溃疡并发症)的非胆道疾病的患者都会有偶然发现的或与临床无关的胆结石。而采用胆道闪烁显像可极为有效地排除急性胆囊炎,这可以帮助临床医师专注于急性腹痛患者的非胆源性病因[248]。正常的胆道闪烁显像在注射同位素后的 30~60 分钟内呈现出胆囊、胆管和小肠的显影。除非特殊情况,正常的胆道闪烁显像结果可除外由胆结石所致的急性胆囊炎。许多研究表明,闪烁扫描显像在检测急性胆囊炎方面的敏感性与特异性约为 94%。然而,其敏感性与特异性在肝疾病患者或接受肠外营养或禁食的患者中会显著下降。这些情况往往会导致假阳性,表现为不患有急性胆囊炎患者的胆囊中不出现同位素。若阳性结果定义为胆囊中不出现同位素,则假阴性结果定义为在患有急性胆囊炎的情况下,胆囊内充满同位素(这种情况实际上是不可能发生的)。因此,闪烁显像检查不应作为对胆囊炎疑似患者的首次影像学检查手段,而应作为针对已确定存在胆结石,且可能存在其他导致急性腹部疼痛的非胆系因素的患者的后续影像学检查[303]。

对急性胆囊炎患者行腹部 CT 的最大收获在于能够检查其是否存在并发症,如气肿性胆囊炎和胆囊穿孔。同时,CT 可排除其他可产生类似临床表现的腹内因素。譬如,腹部 CT 在检查气腹、急性胰腺炎、胰腺假性囊肿、肝或腹腔内脓肿、阑尾炎和空腔内脏梗阻或穿孔的方面具有高度敏感性。腹部 CT 不建议用于明显患有急性胆囊炎的患者,但如果诊断不确定或手术最佳时间不能确定,CT 检查则非常关键。

6. 鉴别诊断

在急性胆囊炎的鉴别诊断中应主要考虑的疾病包括阑尾炎、急性胰腺炎、肾盂肾炎或肾结石、消化性溃疡、急性肝炎、肺炎、肝脓肿或肝癌,以及淋球菌性肝周炎或衣原体肝周炎。在建议患者进行胆囊切除术之前应考虑以上可能性。

7. 治疗

疑似急性胆囊炎的患者应住院治疗。患者常因呕吐或食欲不佳而导致血容量减少,此时应静脉输注液体或电解质。若患者腹部膨隆或持续呕吐,应禁食,并留置鼻胃管。

在无并发症急性胆囊炎患者中,无需常规给予抗生素。抗生素仅建议在患者出现感染中毒表现或怀疑出现并发症(如胆囊穿孔或气肿性胆囊炎)的时候使用。研究指出,广谱抗生素的作用范围通常可覆盖革兰阴性菌和厌氧菌,有多种可行的治疗方案。最常用的方案包括哌拉西林-他唑巴坦,头孢曲松钠+甲硝唑或左氧氟沙星+甲硝唑。

急性胆囊炎的确定疗法是胆囊切除术。已证明在腹腔镜下行胆囊切除术在治疗急性胆囊炎时是安全且有效的(见第 66 章)[304]。

(三) 胆总管结石

胆总管结石是指胆管内发生结石。与胆囊中的结石一样,胆管内的结石可多年无症状,已知胆管内的结石可安静地进入十二指肠,也许是经常发生的。与胆囊结石不同的是,胆囊结石在临床上通常表现为相对良性的反复发作的胆源性疼痛,当胆管结石引起症状时,往往表现为危及生命的并发症,如胆管炎和急性胰腺炎(见第 58 章)。因此,在发现胆总管结石后,通常应进行干预取出结石(见第 70 章)。

1. 病因学

结石可能是从胆囊进入胆管或在胆管中重新形成。大体上,来自同一例患者的所有结石,无论来自胆囊或胆管,都属于同一类型,要么为胆固醇结石,要么为胆色素结石。胆固醇结石只会来自胆囊,任何在胆管中发现的胆固醇结石一定是在胆囊中形成然后移动到胆管的。黑色素结石(与衰老、溶血、酗酒和肝硬化有关)也形成于胆囊,但极少会移动到胆管。胆管中的大部分色素结石均为柔软的褐色素结石。胆汁中磷脂和胆红素在细菌的作用下,重新在胆管中形成褐色素结石(见前文)[305]。褐色素结石常导致胆管狭窄,且往往伴随胆管炎。褐色素结石也见于肝内胆管结石和复发性化脓性胆管炎患者(见第 68 章)[306]。

15% 的胆囊结石患者存在胆管结石。与之相对,有胆管结石的患者中 95% 存在胆囊结石[307]。对于接受胆囊切除手术后几个月或几年内出现胆总管结石的患者,难以再确定结石是在先前的治疗中被忽略了,还是后续形成的。实际上,胆管中胆色素结石的形成也是内窥镜下括约肌切开术的一个晚期并发症[308]。在一项针对超过 400 名行内窥镜下括约肌切开术患者的长期预后的研究中,发现胆管结石的累积复发率为 12%;所有的复发的结石均为棕色素结石。这一研究结果表明,括约肌切开术将导致慢性细菌定植,从而促进胆红素的游离和色素结石沉淀。

胆管中的结石通常停留在 Vater 壶腹的下端。胆管梗阻使近端胆管压力上升,导致胆管扩张。正常的胆管压力为 10~15cmH_2O,在完全梗阻后上升至 25~40cmH_2O。当压力超过 15cmH_2O,胆汁流速会降低,并在达到 30cmH_2O 时停止流动。

在约 75% 的病例中,胆管可扩张到能通过 US 或腹部 CT 检测到。但在曾患复发性胆管炎的患者中,因胆管出现纤维化,无法扩张。此外,部分胆总管结石患者的胆管因为梗阻程度较轻(为轻度或中度)而无法检查到。

2. 临床特征

胆总管结石的发病主要是源于胆道梗阻,胆道梗阻使胆道压力升高,胆汁流量减少。梗阻的发生速度、范围和胆汁的细菌污染量是决定产生症状的主要因素。急性梗阻通常引起胆源性疼痛和黄疸,而梗阻在数月内逐渐发展,最初可表现为瘙痒或单纯黄疸[309]。如果细菌增殖,可能导致危及生命的胆管炎(见后文)。

如果胆管梗阻是间歇性的,则患者体格检查结果通常是正常的。当梗阻持续数日至数周时,可观察到轻度至中度黄疸。无疼痛的深度黄疸,特别是可触及胆囊(Courvoisier 征),提示胆管肿瘤性梗阻,即使患者胆囊内有结石。对于长期胆管梗阻,可能导致继发性胆汁性肝硬化,导致出现慢性肝病的体格检查结果。

如表 65.2 所示,实验室检查结果可能是确定胆总管结石存在的唯一线索[310]。随着胆管梗阻,血清胆红素和碱性磷酸酶水平均出现升高。由于排泄受阻,胆红素在血清中蓄积,而由于小管上皮合成酶增加，碱性磷酸酶水平升高。碱性磷酸酶水平的升高比胆红素水平的升高更快，且先于胆红素水平的升高[311]。血清胆红素水平的绝对高度与梗阻程度成正比，但碱性磷酸酶水平的高度与梗阻程度或梗阻原因无关。在胆总管结石病例中，血清胆红素水平通常在 2~5mg/dL 范围内[242]，很少超过 12mg/dL。血清转氨酶或淀粉酶水平短暂出现"峰值"提示胆管结石进入十二指肠。据报道，肝脏相关生化检查在检测胆总管结石方面的总体敏感性为 94%；血清 γ-谷氨酰转肽酶水平升高最常见，但在临床实践中可能无法评估[311]。

3. 自然史

关于无症状胆管结石自然史的信息很少。在许多患者中，这些结石持续数月或数年无症状，但现有证据表明，无症状胆管结石自然史的良性程度低于无症状胆囊结石[309,312]。

4. 诊断

实际上，仅 50% 的病例可应用 US 对胆管结石进行显像[259]，而胆管扩张大于 6mm 的病例中 76% 可有效显像。US 可确定，或至少表明，胆管结石的存在，但不能绝对排除胆总管结石。在这种情况下，EUS 的优势就在于能够更精确地对胆管进行显像，但比常规 US 更具有侵入性。EUS 排除或明确胆总管结石的敏感性和特异性约为 98%，可与 ERCP 相持平[263]。

ERCP 是诊断和治疗胆管结石的标准方法[313]，其敏感性和特异性约为 95%。但在临床考虑胆总管结石可能性较低时，应首先采用侵入性较低的 EUS 和 MRC 检查（见前文）[279]。

经皮经肝胆管造影（transhepatic cholangiography，THC）也是可以用于明确胆总管结石的精确检查方法。THC 技术最适用于有肝内胆管扩张的情况，且主要在 ERCP 无法进行或操作失败的情况下采用。

腹腔镜 US 可在胆囊切除术期间胆囊移除之前进行。腹腔镜 US 检测胆总管结石的精确度与外科胆管造影术相当，因此便不需要再使用后者进行评估[314]。

5. 鉴别诊断

由于胆总管梗阻所导致的症状难以与胆囊管梗阻所导致的症状相区分。因此，胆源性疼痛永远是具有完整胆囊的患者的鉴别诊断的关键点。黄疸或肝脏生化测试结果异常往往高度提示疼痛源于胆总管而非胆囊。

在黄疸患者中，胆总管恶性梗阻或胆总管囊肿所致的梗阻在临床上可能与胆总管结石无法区分（见第 62 和 69 章）。对于伴随右上腹疼痛和肝脏生化检查结果异常的 HIV 阳性患者[315]，应考虑与 AIDS 相关的胆管疾病和乳头狭窄（见第 35 章）。

6. 治疗

由于胆总管结石经常引发严重并发症，如胆管炎和急性胰腺炎，因此建议几乎所有的胆总管结石患者都接受治疗[316]。对此，最优的治疗方案应根据患者症状的严重程度、是否存在合并的医学问题、当地专家的水平和胆囊是否已切除来决定。

在行腹腔镜胆囊切除术期间意外发现胆总管存在结石是外科医生面临的一大难题。部分外科医生可能会尝试对胆管进行腹腔镜下探查。在一些情况下，手术将改为开腹胆囊切除术同时行胆总管探查术，但这种方式不仅会带来更高的并发症发病率，也延长患者的住院时间。或者腹腔镜胆囊切除术可按原计划进行，之后患者接受 ERCP 治疗移除胆道结石。若是成功行 ERCP，可治愈疾病，但若未能通过 ERCP 移除结石，就面临就是必须接受第三次手术，即胆总管探查术的风险。总之，内镜医师水平越高，外科手术医师就越倾向于行腹腔镜胆囊切除术后通过内镜治疗移除胆管结石[316]。

在手术风险极高的患者中，可通过内窥镜移除胆管结石而不行胆囊切除术。这种方案尤为适合老年患者或同时患有其他严重疾病的患者[317]。仅 10% 的患者会因症状复发需要进行胆囊切除术。关于胆结石的外科治疗和内窥镜治疗分别在第 66 章和 70 章中进行更详细的论述。

（四）胆管炎

在所有常见的胆结石并发症中，最严重与最致命的是急性细菌性胆管炎。由于胆管压力上升会导致细菌快速经肝脏进入血液，最终形成败血症。此外，胆管炎的诊断往往有困难（尤其是在关键的疾病早期），这是因为缺乏提示胆管是败血症源头的临床表现[34]。表 65.2 中罗列了可帮助诊断早期胆管炎的症状、体征和实验室检查数据。

1. 病因学和病理生理学

在约 85% 的病例中，胆管炎是由嵌顿在胆管中的结石导致胆汁淤积所致[318]。其他可导致胆管炎的胆管梗阻疾病包括肿瘤（见第 60 和 69 章）、胆管狭窄（见第 68 和 70 章）、寄生虫感染（见第 68 和 84 章），以及胆胰管汇流异常（见第 62 章）。此次讨论仅针对由胆管中胆结石所引起的胆管炎。

胆管梗阻是导致胆管炎的必要因素，但它不足以直接引起胆管炎。胆管炎发生于大多数胆总管结石患者和几乎所有胆管创伤后狭窄患者中，但仅在 15% 的肿瘤性胆管梗阻患者中出现。其最可能的原因是，在胆总管结石和胆管狭窄的大多数患者中，已含有细菌的胆管会被阻塞，但这一情况极少出现在肿瘤性梗阻患者中。恶性梗阻往往比胆管狭窄或胆管结石导致的梗阻更彻底，但很少会导致十二指肠内容物中的细菌逆行到胆管中[319]。

最常见的从胆汁中培养出的细菌种群包括大肠杆菌、克雷白氏杆菌、假单胞菌、变形杆菌和肠球菌。另外，在约 15% 的胆汁样本中发现厌氧菌种群，如脆弱拟杆菌和产气荚膜梭菌。厌氧菌的出现往往伴随着需氧菌，尤其是大肠埃希菌。胆管炎所导致的发热和寒战就是由胆管内细菌引发的菌血症所致。细菌从胆汁中回流到肝静脉血的程度直接与胆道压力成正比，因而也与梗阻程度成正比[303]。因此，通常可通过胆管减压来有效治疗该疾病。

2. 临床特征

Charcot 三联征是胆管炎的标志，包括右上腹疼痛、黄疸与发热（见表 65.2）。仅 70% 的患者会表现出所有的 3 个症状[319]。胆管炎所导致的疼痛可能出乎意料的轻微与短暂，但通常会伴随发冷与寒战。精神错乱、嗜睡和谵妄主要出现在老年患者中。在重症化脓性胆管炎中，可出现与 Charcot 三联征共存的精神状态变化与低血压，常称为 Reynolds pentad 五联征。

体格检查方面，发热较为常见，在 95% 的患者出现，且往往超过 38.9℃。90% 的患者出现右上腹压痛，但仅 80% 的患者可通过临床体征发现黄疸。值得注意的是，仅在15%的患者中出现腹膜刺激征。同时出现低血压与精神异常提示革兰氏阴性菌感染。在被忽略的重症胆管炎病例中，肝内脓肿可作为晚期并发症出现（见第84章）。

实验室检查结果通常能够帮助明确菌血症起源于胆道系统。尤其应注意，80%患者的血清胆红素水平超过2mg/dL。若胆红素水平起初为正常，则不应考虑胆管炎的诊断[314]。另外，在80%的患者中，白细胞总数升高。而在许多白细胞总数正常的患者中，外周血涂片检查发现未成熟中性粒细胞明显增多。血清碱性磷酸酶水平也通常会出现升高。另外，在患者同时患有胰腺炎的情况下，血清淀粉酶水平也出现升高。

在大多数病例中，血培养可培养出肠道微生物，尤其是在患者寒战发热高峰期间取得的培养样本。血液中发现的微生物与胆汁中的始终相同。

3. 诊断

针对胆管炎的主要影像学诊断方法与胆总管结石一致。50%的病例通过US可观察到结石[191]，但约75%的病例可通过胆管扩张推测存在胆结石（见表65.3）。US结果正常无法排除临床表现提示为胆管炎的患者存在胆总管结石的可能性[303]。

腹部CT在排除胆结石并发症方面具有较好的表现，如急性胰腺炎和脓肿，但常规腹部CT无法除外胆管结石。如前文所述，EUS和MRC在检查和除外胆总管结石方面的准确度要远高于CT。

ERCP是诊断胆总管结石和胆管炎的决定性检查手段。此外，ERCP可引流压力升高的感染性胆汁，从而挽救生命。若无法行ERCP，可进行经皮THC（见第70章）。

4. 治疗

在疑似细菌性胆管炎的情况下，应立即取得血培养样本，并针对可能存在的致病微生物进行有效的抗生素治疗[320]。在轻症病例中，使用单一的药物（如每6~8小时静脉输注2.0g的头孢西丁）便足够。重症病例则应采取更强的抗感染方案［如庆大霉素、氨苄西林、甲硝唑或广谱药物（如每6小时静脉注射3.375g的哌拉西林）；如怀疑存在耐药菌，则每8小时静脉输注1g的美罗培南］。

患者的状况在治疗后6~12小时内出现改善。在多数案例中，感染会在2~3天内得到控制，伴随体温下降、不适感缓解和血白细胞水平降低。在此类病例中，可依照具体需求决定最终的治疗方案。然而，若在6~12小时的严格观察后发现患者一般情况恶化，伴随体温升高、疼痛加重、精神错乱或低血压，则应立即进行胆管减压治疗[320]。如果可行，可选择ERCP下取石作为治疗方案，或至少通过胆道支架行胆管减压。大量对照研究将ERCP下胆道减压与急诊手术和胆总管探查术进行比对，发现通过内窥镜治疗的患者的并发症发生率和死亡率明显较低[316]。关于胆管炎的外科治疗和内镜治疗将分别在第66和77章中详细论述。

十、罕见并发症

表65.4列举了胆结石疾病几种罕见并发症的临床表现、诊断和治疗。

表65.4　胆结石疾病的罕见并发症

并发症	发病机制	临床特征	诊断/治疗
气肿性胆囊炎	产气微生物（魏氏梭菌、大肠杆菌和厌氧性链球菌）导致的胆囊壁继发性感染 常发于老年糖尿病患者；可不伴结石（见第67章）	症状和体征与重症急性胆囊炎相似	腹部平片可显示胆囊窝处有气体 US和CT在确定气体方面敏感性更高 可通过静脉输注抗生素（针对厌氧菌）治疗，同时早期行胆囊切除术 发病率与死亡率高
胆囊肠瘘	结石（通常是大型结石）侵蚀胆囊壁进入邻近肠道；常见于十二指肠，其次是结肠结肠肝曲、胃和空肠	症状和体征与急性胆囊炎相似，但有时瘘无临床症状 当结石>25mm，尤其在老年女性患者中，可导致肠梗阻或"胆石性肠梗阻"；梗阻最常发生的部位为回肠末端 较少出现胃出口梗阻（Bouveret综合征）	腹部平片显示胆道内存在气体和/或胆石性肠梗阻，以及右下腹钙化结石 上消化道造影可能显示存在瘘管 有单个结石通过形成的瘘可能自然闭合 可采用胆囊切除术和瘘管闭合手术治疗 胆石性肠梗阻需急诊剖腹手术；诊断常常延误，导致死亡率≈20%
Mirizzi综合征	结石嵌顿在胆囊颈或胆囊管，对肝总管形成外源性压迫，伴随炎症或瘘管	黄疸与右上腹疼痛	ERCP显示肝内胆管扩张，以及肝总管外源性压迫，可能伴随瘘管 外科手术前的诊断十分重要，可以指导手术，并最小化胆管损伤风险
瓷化胆囊	胆囊壁内钙化，通常伴随结石	胆囊壁钙化本身无症状，但胆囊钙化属于晚期并发症（≈20%；见第69章）	腹部平片或CT显示胆囊壁内钙化 采用预防性胆囊切除术预防癌变

（一）气肿性胆囊炎

气肿性胆囊炎患者的临床表现与无并发症的急性胆囊炎患者相同；但气肿性胆囊炎的胆囊壁会出现由产气微生物继发感染引起的气泡。在腹部平片、US和腹部CT上，胆囊窝区可见明显的气囊（见图65.12）[321]。气肿性胆囊炎常发于无胆结石的糖尿病患者或老年男性，其起始原因可能是胆囊动脉粥样硬化伴缺血（见第67章）。由于该病胆囊穿孔的风险较高，因此有必要进行厌氧菌覆盖的紧急抗生素治疗和早期胆囊切除术。

（二）胆囊肠瘘

当结石通过胆囊壁（通常是胆囊颈部）侵蚀并进入中空内脏时，就会发生胆囊肠瘘。进入肠管的最常见入口点是十二指肠，其次是结肠肝曲、胃和空肠。症状最初与急性胆囊相似，尽管有时结石可能进入肠道直接排出体外，而不引起任何症状[322]。由于胆道无压力过高的表现，因此胆管炎并不常见，尽管胆囊和胆管有细菌种植。根据胆道积气的影像学证据怀疑胆囊肠瘘的诊断，并可通过上消化道或下消化道的钡剂造影检查证实。通常直到手术时才能确定瘘的精确解剖位置。

若胆石直径超过 25mm，则可能表现为小肠梗阻（胆石性肠梗阻）（尤其是老年女性），回盲部是最常见的梗阻部位[323]。在这种情况下，腹部平片可显示胆道积气、小肠扩张和右下腹巨大胆石的病理特征。然而不幸的是，胆石性肠梗阻的诊断通常被延误，导致的死亡率约为 20%。Bouveret 综合征（又称胆石性肠梗阻）的特征是，通过胆囊十二指肠瘘迁移的大型胆石嵌塞于十二指肠导致的胃出口梗阻[324]。

（三）Mirizzi 综合征

Mirizzi 综合征是一种罕见的并发症，嵌入胆囊颈部或胆囊管的结石外压迫肝总管，导致黄疸、胆管梗阻，在某些情况下还会出现瘘管[325,326]。通常胆囊收缩并含有结石。ERCP 通常显示肝总管的特征性外源性压迫。传统上通过开放性胆囊切除术进行治疗，尽管已经成功地进行了内镜下支架植术和腹腔镜胆囊切除术。术前对 Mirizzi 综合征的诊断很重要，可以避免胆管损伤（见第 66 章）[327]。

（四）瓷化胆囊

严格地说，瓷化胆囊（定义为胆囊壁的壁内钙化）不是胆结石的并发症，但在这里提及，是因为癌有发展为胆囊钙化晚期并发症的显著趋势（特别是胆囊壁局灶性而非弥漫性钙化）[328]。通过腹部平片或腹部 CT 可诊断瓷化胆囊，可见胆囊壁壁内钙化。在偶尔的人中，钙过度分泌到胆汁中导致“钙乳”胆汁或“石灰”胆汁，可以模拟瓷化胆囊的成像特征。预防性胆囊切除术，最好是通过腹腔镜方法，适用于预防癌症的潜在发展，否则可能发生在高达 20% 的病例中（见第 69 章）[329]。

（王迎春　周明新 译，鲁晓岚　闫秀娥 校）

参考文献

第 66 章　胆结石疾病的治疗

Robert E. Glasgow 著

章节目录

一、内科治疗 …… 978
（一）溶石治疗 …… 978
（二）体外冲击波碎石术 …… 980
二、手术治疗 …… 981
（一）开腹胆囊切除术 …… 981
（二）腹腔镜胆囊切除术 …… 982
三、治疗方式的选择 …… 985
四、治疗适应证 …… 985
（一）无症状胆结石 …… 985
（二）胆源性疼痛与慢性胆囊炎 …… 985
（三）急性胆囊炎 …… 985
（四）胆源性胰腺炎 …… 987
（五）特殊问题 …… 987
五、胆总管结石 …… 989
（一）术前存在的胆总管结石 …… 989
（二）胆囊切除术中发现的胆总管结石 …… 989
（三）胆囊切除术后发现的胆总管结石 …… 990
六、胆管损伤和狭窄 …… 990
七、胆囊切除术后综合征 …… 991
（一）胆总管结石 …… 992
（二）胆囊管残留 …… 992
（三）Oddi 括约肌功能紊乱 …… 992
八、胆结石、胆囊切除术与癌症 …… 992
（一）胆道癌 …… 992
（二）结直肠癌 …… 992

目前有多种方法用于治疗有症状的胆结石患者，随着内镜、放射及化学性疗法的技术的提升，胆石症患者的整体诊疗有了不少进步，但手术治疗仍是其最重要的治疗方式。腹腔镜胆囊切除术仍是治疗胆源性疼痛及胆石症相关并发症如急性胆囊炎、胆源性胰腺炎和胆总管结石等的标准治疗方案（亦见第 65 章）

一、内科治疗

1873 年由意大利学者 Schiff 首次提出采用药物治疗的方式治疗胆石症[1]。1876 年，弗吉尼亚州的学者 Dabney 首次报道采用胆汁酸能有效治疗胆结石，这一结果在 1937 年被明尼苏达州的 Rewbridge 进一步证实[2,3]。尽管前期有类似报道，但药物溶石的治疗方法一直到 20 世纪 70 年代大宗临床系列研究被报道后才开始被接受。同样也有采用溶剂接触反应溶解胆结石及经皮胆囊切开取石技术的报道，但这些措施的治疗效果尚未证实优于口服药物溶石、冲击波碎石及腹腔镜胆囊切除术的效果，目前已不被采用。目前，常见的非手术方式治疗胆结石的主要方案为口服熊去氧胆酸（ursodiol，UDCA），单独用药或辅以体外冲击波碎石。

虽然非手术治疗在经筛选的受试者群体中被证明有效，但只适用于少数受试者，其治疗效果只有对结石较小且在透 X 线的胆固醇结石有效。大量混有胆色素及胆盐的混合性结石可溶性较低。另外，长期药物治疗结石只有对易形成结石疾病导致的暂时性结石有效。对于大多数患者来说，胆结石形成意味着胆汁脂质排泄失衡，胆囊胆汁淤积或胆系感染（见第 65 章）。在这些患者中，有 30%～50% 的患者在溶石后的 5 年内复发[4-6]。因此，选择合适的治疗方案必须综合考虑结石的种类、症状的严重程度、结石相关的体征、胆囊的功能以及患者自身一般情况等。

（一）溶石治疗

口服药物溶石的原理是逆转导致胆固醇结石形成的条件，即胆汁与胆固醇的过饱和状态（见第 65 章）。当结石中的胆固醇能被周围介质溶解时，胆固醇结石便会溶解。鹅去氧胆酸和 UDCA 都是通过减少胆汁内胆固醇分泌使胆汁去饱和来溶解胆结石。其通过胶束增溶，形成液晶相或两种机制同时进行以促进胆固醇从结石中溶解。鹅去氧胆酸作为第一种被用于溶石的胆汁酸，由于其存在腹泻、升高血清转氨酶和胆固醇水平等副作用而被弃用。UDCA 有很好的耐受性且目前已应用于口服溶石的治疗中。通过随机对照后发现，单独应用 UDCA 或联合应用 UDCA 及鹅去氧胆酸均有效[6-8]。

结石的溶解速度是一种动态过程，包括：①热力动力学，包括胆汁的去饱和程度和胆汁中 UDCA 的浓度；②动能，包括胆汁的涡流；③结石的面积体积比值。口服药物溶石以热力动力学为作用目标[9]。由于小结石的面积体积比较小，因此口服药物溶解的反应速度更快，更有效。但口服药物溶石并不能解决胆囊内胆汁淤积的问题[10]。虽然一些促胃肠动力药物如 α-肾上腺素拮抗剂、克拉霉素和多潘立酮等已被证明能增强胆囊的运动，但已有研究证明它们对预防和治疗胆结石是无效的[11-13]。

1. 患者选择

选择患者进行口服药物溶石需要考虑胆结石的阶段、胆囊功能以及结石的特点，具体选择标准见框 66.1。对无并发症的胆结石患者可考虑口服药物溶石，包括胆源性疼痛程度轻或偶发的患者。对无症状患者，由于其绝大多数病史中无临床症状，因此不建议进行溶石治疗或手术治疗。对存在重度或频繁发作的胆源性疼痛患者以及存在胆结石并发症（包

框 66.1　口服胆汁酸溶解疗法的选择标准
胆石症分期
有症状(胆源性疼痛)但无并发症
胆囊功能
口服胆囊造影显示胆囊混浊(胆囊管未闭)
刺激胆囊闪烁显像结果正常(胆囊排空正常)
胆囊功能超声检查结果正常(餐后胆囊排空正常)
结石特点
射线可透的
CT 上与胆汁呈等密度或低密度、无钙化的结石
直径≤10mm(最佳<6mm)

括胆囊炎、胰腺炎及胆管炎)的患者,不建议口服溶石治疗,而应尽早手术治疗(见下文)。

另外,胆囊必须有功能且胆囊管必须通畅才能使不饱和的胆汁及结石自胆囊排出。通常采用口服胆道造影剂来评估胆囊管的通畅程度。也已开始应用胆囊刺激闪烁显像及超声检查来评估胆囊管通畅程度及胆囊功能。

结石的性质对溶石治疗的效果起重要作用。口服药物溶石仅对胆固醇结石有效果。虽然对结石成分的评估有一定的困难,但普通 X 线片或 CT 影像上结石的显像表现可作为一定的参考。胆固醇结石在平片上是不显影的,在 CT 上表现为低密度或等密度影,缺乏结石钙化表现[14]。在口服胆囊造影剂过程中,由于胆固醇结石的比重小于或等于含有造影剂的胆汁的比重,会使结石漂浮。虽然结石数量并不会对口服药物溶石的成功率产生影响,但只有当患者结石占据胆囊一半以上的体积时才考虑进行治疗。而且虽然口服药物溶石对直径≤10 毫米的结石均有效果,但其对直径小于 5 毫米的结石治疗效果最佳[15,16]。最佳的口服药物溶石的结石类型如图 66.1 所示。

2. 治疗方法

熊去氧胆酸(UDCA)是口服药物溶石的首选药物,每天按 10~15mg/kg 体重的剂量进行服用。考虑到患者的依从性问题,晚间给药的效果比餐前给药更好[17]。与鹅去氧胆酸不同,UDCA 具有良好的耐受性且无明显的副作用。治疗应持续到至少间隔 1 月进行 2 次超声检查,结果证实结石溶解。如果患者不能耐受药物或在治疗过程中出现胆结石并发症,抑或是 6 个月后结石未能溶解或 6 个月后仅部分溶解,2 年内

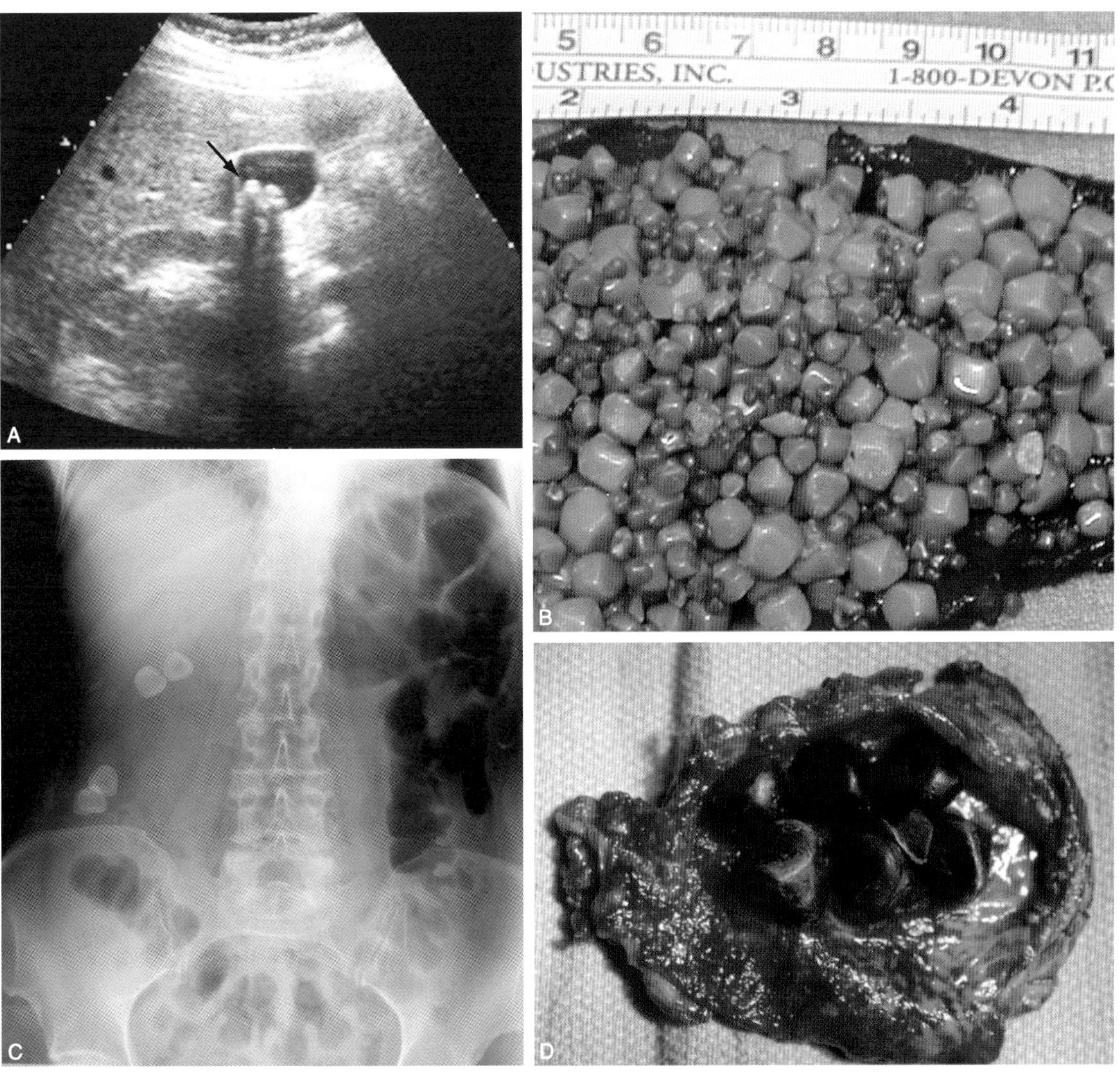

图 66.1　A 和 B,适合口服溶石治疗的胆结石;A,超声显示小胆结石(箭);B,多发性小胆固醇结石。C 和 D,口服溶解治疗不适宜的胆结石;C,平片上不透放射的胆结石;D,大的色素性胆结石

没有完全溶解者，应停止治疗。

3. 疗效

20%～70%使用UDCA的患者结石能完全溶解。有报告提示疗效的差异受不同患者、胆汁酸剂量、治疗时间和用于诊断结石是否溶解的技术的影响。一项关于药物溶石随机试验的meta分析显示约有37%的患者结石溶解[8]。结石的溶解率上：大于10mm的结石为29%，小于10mm的结石为49%，小于5mm的结石为70%。溶解速度因患者而异，平均每月0.7mm[9]。在结石完全溶解之前，患者的症状便会得到改善。另外，有报道称长期的治疗可以降低胆源性疼痛和急性胆囊炎的风险，而不仅仅是由于结石溶解[16]。虽然是对合适的患者进行药物溶石，但口服药物溶石后5年内结石复发率率为50%，大多数于最初的2年内复发[5,18]。这一结果也指出与胆结石形成相关的其余因素如胆汁淤积及反复感染等并不是通过药物溶石治疗可以解决的。单发结石患者复发的风险比多发性结石患者低。

（二）体外冲击波碎石术

体外冲击波碎石术的基本原理是通过减小结石的面积体积比进而提高口服药物溶石的疗效，减小结石大小，使小结石及碎屑直接自胆囊排入肠道而不引起相关症状。该技术是将聚焦的高压声波传入胆结石进行碎石。目前已开发出四种类型的碎石机：液电式、压电式、电磁式及最近的激光式碎石机。不管能量源如何，碎石机所发出的冲击波都是通过体液介质最终传递至软组织，在通过软组织的过程中，能量并没有显著降低，最终会通过结石并对其前后壁产生压力和张力，使结石表面形成气穴，最终导致结石碎裂。影响碎石效果的因素包括结石的大小、结石的微晶结构及结石自身结构。虽然结石的成分不会影响碎石的成功率，但考虑到只有胆汁酸疗法能有效溶解胆固醇结石，因此二者可联合使用。

1. 患者选择

由于冲击波碎石术通常与口服药物溶石相结合，因此冲击波碎石术的患者选择标准与口服药物溶石治疗相似，见框66.2。需要结合胆囊造影、胆囊功能超声及胆囊刺激显像对胆囊功能及胆囊管的通畅性检查的结果。冲击波碎石仅适用于轻度且无并发症的胆源性疼痛患者，对妊娠及抗凝治疗患者，不能行冲击波碎石治疗。冲击波碎石也可治疗孤立且尺寸小于2cm的结石[19,20]。由于只有胆固醇结石能通过口服药物溶石进行有效清除，因此结石需具备如X线可透过等影像学特点以证实为胆固醇结石。

框66.2 体外冲击波碎石术的选择标准

胆石症分期

有症状（胆源性疼痛）但无并发症者

胆囊功能

口服胆囊造影显示胆囊混浊（胆囊管未闭）

刺激胆囊闪烁显像结果正常（胆囊排空正常）

胆囊功能超声检查结果正常（餐后胆囊排空正常）

结石特点

射线可透的

CT上与胆汁呈等密度或低密度、无钙化的结石

直径<20mm

2. 治疗方法

患者通常给予药物镇静、镇痛或麻醉处理，取俯卧位以尽可能缩小冲击波源与结石间的距离，消除肠内气体及肋缘的干扰。通过超声对碎石区进行定位和监测[21]。通常需要多次碎石以实现碎石效果最大化，影响碎石成功率的因素包括结石的破碎程度及胆囊的排空情况[22-24]。碎石结果取决于结石自身特点及冲击波的能量大小。与结石相关的几个重要特点包括结石的大小和数量，以及它们的构成和钙含量[25]。冲击波的能量，单次冲击波所含的脉冲数量和脉冲频率等也会影响成功率[26,27]。每日应按体重口服UDCA 10～15mg/kg进行溶石，尤其是当存在残留结石大于2mm，胆囊功能差或碎石术后的3～6个月内胆囊内有未能清除的小碎片时。图66.2是一个联合治疗成功的案例。

3. 疗效

患者在第6和12个月后不再发生结石的概率分别为47%～77%及68%～84%[20,22,28-32]。随访资料显示，3年、5年和10年结石复发率分别为27%、41%和54%[33]。结石的复发通常与易成石胆汁以及胆囊运动功能障碍有关，而与患者自身差异如性别，年龄和体重等无关。提示碎石治疗可能失败的因素包括大于16mm的结石，多发结石以及CT提示结石密度大于84Hu者[34]。复发性结石通常较小且多发，常会引起胆源性疼痛。碎石术后联合应用UDCA效果并不理想[35]。

冲击波碎石的副作用包括冲击波接触部位的皮下瘀斑（8%）、血尿（4%）和肝血肿（<1%）。未发现有长期肝生化功能异常者。大约三分之一的患者出现胆源性疼痛，5%的患者出现胆囊管堵塞，结石排出相关并发症如胆源性胰腺炎等的发生率不到2%[22]。

冲击波碎石在老年人中比年轻人有更高的应用价值，多发结石患者的应用价值低于单发结石患者。与UDCA联合应用时，冲击波碎石与小结石患者的开腹胆囊切除术具有一样的应用价值，而对于有较大结石患者，其应用价值较低[36,37]。冲击波碎石与腹腔镜胆囊切除术相比，接受腹腔镜胆囊切除术的患者术后6个月在生活质量上得到了更大的提升，而那些接受冲击波碎石的患者则存在更高的复发率和伴发胆道相关症状发生率[38]。

4. 胆管结石

体外冲击波碎石也可应用于治疗胆总管结石，已有文献证明体内液电碎石有效。这些治疗方案仅适用于常规内镜取石失败（见第70章），机械碎石术或胆管结石手术治疗（见下文）失败的患者。冲击波碎石术的适应证包括：胆管内嵌顿的大结石，不适于内镜下取石患者，肝内结石，胆管狭窄上游的结石，胆囊管内残余结石，以及与Mirizzi综合征（肝总管受压）相关的胆管结石（见第65章）。冲击波治疗胆管结石的患者与单纯胆囊结石患者的筛选标准相似。

胆管结石的取石成功率达70%～90%[39-44]。大部分患者在治疗结束后须于内镜下取出较大的结石碎块。10%的患者出现轻度一过性胆道出血，4%的患者术后出现胆源性脓毒症。其他并发症与胆囊结石碎石术后的并发症相似。由于可能存在并发脓毒症的可能，需行术前内镜检查，使用鼻胆管或

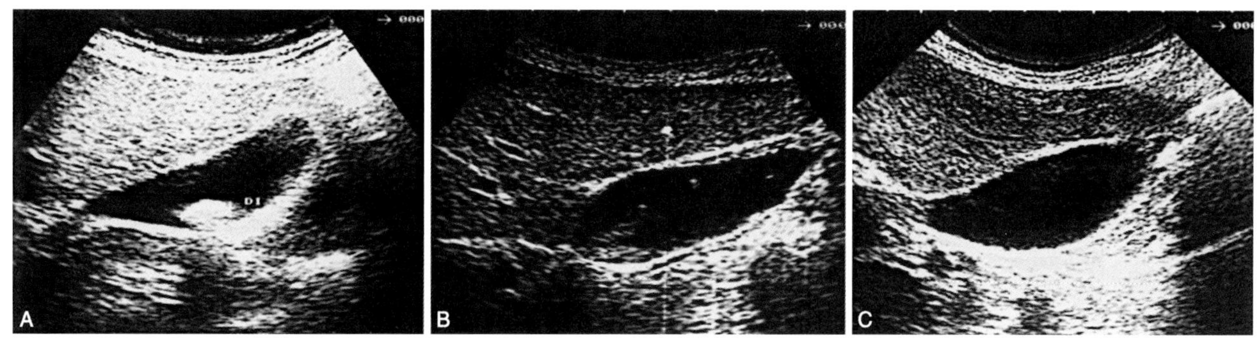

图 66.2　体外冲击波碎石术前(A)、术后 1 天(B)和术后 6 周(C)单发结石胆囊的超声。碎石后 1 天可见多个小结石碎块(B),碎石后 6 周消失(C)

经皮胆道引流。使用抗生素能有效减小胆源性脓毒症的发生风险。

二、手术治疗

在美国每年有约 700 000 例胆囊结石患者接受胆囊切除手术,绝大多数手术在腹腔镜下进行。例如,2005 年在犹他州进行的 7 888 例胆囊切除术中有 96% 是腹腔镜下胆囊切除术,4% 是开腹手术。通过对全国医院出院患者数据库 1997—2006 年的病例回顾后发现,仅有 12% 的胆囊切除术是开腹进行的[45]。在所有腹腔镜手术中,中转开腹的手术率为 5%～10%[46,47]。对复杂胆结石症患者,如急性胆囊炎、胆源性胰腺炎及胆总管结石患者,相较于单纯结石的患者,更适合进行开腹胆囊切除手术或腹腔镜中转开腹[46]。尽管目前患者治疗越来越主张微创化,但对存在胆结石相关并发症的患者,开腹行胆囊切除术仍非常重要。

(一) 开腹胆囊切除术

KarlLangenbuch 是柏林的一名外科医生,于 1882 年第一次开展胆囊切除术。自此,胆囊切除术由于能有效缓解临床症状及术后病发率低而成为治疗胆结石的主要方法。在前瞻性研究中发现,90%～95% 的胆囊切除术患者的术后症状得到了明显且完全的缓解[48,49]。胆囊切除术在缓解胆源性疼痛方面的效果比非特异性胃肠道症状(如消化不良和胃肠胀气等)的缓解效果更好。

1. 技术操作

开腹胆囊切除术自首次报道以来其手术方法无明显更改,医生需站在患者的右侧,自右肋缘下方 2 横指处做(Kocher)切口。又或者可采用腹正中切口,在进行腹腔探查并剥离胆囊粘连组织后以逆行的方式自胆囊基底部至胆囊颈部哈氏囊处分离,将胆囊从胆囊窝中解剖出来。在游离胆囊时,需仔细注意胆囊动脉及胆管的辨别。胆道造影能用于寻找胆道结石并确定其解剖结构。将胆囊管和胆囊动脉结扎后分离。另一种方法是自 Calot 三角处进行分离,步骤同腹腔镜下胆囊切除术相似(见下文),先将胆囊自肝脏游离后进行切除。Calot 三角是胆囊管、肝总管及肝脏下缘构成的区域,在该区域下进行相关结构的解剖和辨别,损伤胆管的风险较小。步骤完成后,进行关腹。胆囊切除术后的患者很少进行腹腔闭式引流。

2. 效果

多年来,开腹胆囊切除术的风险有所降低。在 1932 年之前,35 373 例行胆囊切除术的患者其总死亡率只有 6.6%[50],到 1952 年,这一比率下降至 1.8%[51]。胆囊切除术的总死亡率平均约为 1.5%。因胆源性疼痛而选择手术治疗的患者死亡率较低,平均不足 0.5%(表 66.1)[52-54]。急性胆囊炎患者行急诊胆囊切除术且需要行胆管探查时,死亡率高出数倍(见表 66.1)。此外,死亡率与患者年龄成正比(图 66.3)。根据丹麦 1977 年至 1981 年全部胆囊切除术患者进行分析,50 岁以下患者选择胆囊切除术死亡的风险为 0.028%[53];80 岁以上患者的死亡率上升到 5.56%。美国的情况同样类似,自 1932 年至 1978 年间,在纽约医院康奈尔医学中心接受胆囊切除术的 11,808 名患者中,50 岁以下的患者因慢性胆囊炎行择期胆囊切除术的死亡风险为 0.1%,50 岁或以上的患者死于择期胆囊切除术的风险为 0.8%[54],1989 年加州和马里兰州 42 474 例胆囊切除术患者的死亡率为 0.17%[55]。在该研究中,65 岁以下患者的死亡率为 0.03%,而 65 岁及以上患者的死亡率高于 0.5%。同样,老年患者的发病率、平均住院时间和平均住院费用明显高于年轻患者。胆囊切除术后的患者的死亡常与心血管疾病,尤其是急性心肌梗死相关。

表 66.1　开腹胆囊切除术的死亡率与临床表现的关系

参考病例	年份	患者数量	胆囊切除术患者的临床表现(死亡率)		
			胆源性疼痛	急性胆囊炎	胆管探查术
52	1962—1966	28 621	1.5%	3.5%	N/A
53	1977—1981	13 854	0.4%	1.6%	2.3%
54	1932—1978	11 808	0.5%	2.9%	3.5%
55	1989	42 474	0.02%	0.26%	N/A

N/A,不能提供。

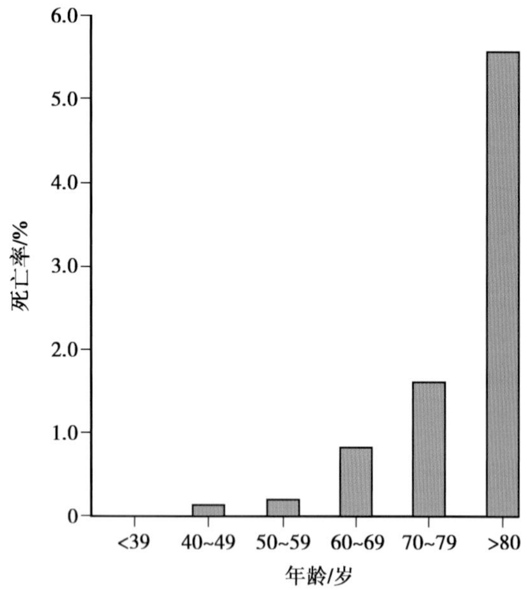

图 66.3　年龄与开腹胆囊切除术死亡率的关系。数据包括 1977 年至 1981 年间在丹麦接受手术的所有患者。(Data from Bredesen J, Jorgensen T, Andersen TF, et al. Early postoperative mortality following cholecystectomy in the entire female population of Denmark, 1977-1981. World J Surg 1992;16:530-5).

开腹胆囊切除术的术后并发症并不常见。在一项针对 20 世纪 60 年代接受胆囊切除术的 28 621 名患者进行的大型研究中，其并发症发生率为 4.0%[52]。后续研究证实围手术期发病率为 4.0%～5.0%[56-58]。大多数并发症相对较轻，如伤口感染或血肿、尿潴留或尿路感染以及肺不张等。与胆囊切除术密切相关的并发症包括胆漏、胆道损伤和急性胰腺炎。在这些并发症中，胆道损伤是最严重的并发症，常需要内镜治疗，在某些情况下，还需要进行复杂的外科手术进行修复。另外，胆道损伤可导致良性胆管狭窄和胆道梗阻，可能会继发胆汁性肝硬化和肝功能衰竭。开放性胆囊切除术中胆道损伤的发生率尚不确切，大约每 200～600 例中有 1 例[59,60]。一般来说，胆道损伤是可预防的，其通常是由于手术经验不足、对胆道解剖结构的变化认识不足或对正常解剖结构认知错误等造成的。异常大量出血、严重炎症和急诊手术对这些并发症的影响并不如想象中那么大。

(二) 腹腔镜胆囊切除术

在 20 世纪 80 年代后期首次被报道后，腹腔镜胆囊切除术被迅速应用于治疗胆结石并发症。与开腹胆囊切除术相比，该微创手术的优点包括较低的并发症发生率和死亡率，以及患者可以较早恢复正常活动。从历史角度看，腹腔镜胆囊切除术是腹腔镜诊断过程中的产物，也是妇科医生在早期腹腔镜手术中努力的成果。腹腔镜胆囊切除术的发展基于小型摄像机和其他特殊医疗设备的发展。仪器和设备的进步大大增加了在大多数胃肠疾病尤其是胆石症的治疗中应用微创手术的安全性和实用性。

1. 技术操作

腹腔镜胆囊切除术在全身麻醉下进行。对于单纯胆石症患者，包括有胆源性疼痛的患者不建议常规使用预防性抗生素[61]。对急性胆囊炎和胆管炎等有胆结石潜在感染并发症风险的患者，以及有慢性症状或高龄患者，须于术前应用抗生素。弹力袜可用于降低下肢血栓栓塞的风险。通过采用二氧化碳诱导气腹来为观察腹腔脏器及为器械操作提供空间，该气体不可燃且生理无害。气腹可以通过封闭技术实现，其先通过小切口将 Veress 针插入腹膜，然后放置手术套管针，或者通过开放性方法小切开后在直视下放入手术套管针。气腹建立后，自脐部放入套管针，并放置腹腔镜。其余 3 个套管分别放在上腹部，以便放置手术装置和牵拉器械。

目前对腹腔镜胆囊切除术最确切的描述是其作为一种“相对安全的手术”方法[62]，如图 66.4 所示。在此入路中，在进行胆道造影或分离胆囊管和动脉之前，先解剖整个胆囊三角，显露胆囊管和动脉、胆囊漏斗部以及胆囊和胆囊管的交界处。助手通过将胆囊底向头侧牵拉，置于肝脏前方并将漏斗部向外侧牵拉。主刀医生自上腹部切口进行操作，解剖游离胆囊管和胆囊动脉。对胆囊管与胆囊的连接处应特别注意，以确保胆管的游离没有被遗忘。通过向胆囊管插入导管进行胆道造影，如果胆道造影显示解剖结构正常且没有胆总管结石征象，则可将导管移除，并用金属夹夹闭分离胆囊管和胆囊动脉。而后将胆囊从胆囊床中解剖游离出来，通常在游离后放入标本回收袋内经脐部切口取出。胆囊从肝脏剥离的过程中要尽量小心避免胆囊穿孔，因为胆囊结石和胆汁的外漏会增加术后发热和腹腔内脓肿形成的风险[63]。手术结束时抽空气腹并缝合关闭手术切口。

在 20 世纪 10 年代，一些外科医生使用单切口进行腹腔镜胆囊切除术，手术医生仅通过脐部的手术切口放置腹腔镜和手术器械。与传统的四孔腹腔镜手术相比，该方式更加美观，但单切口手术时间较长，费用较高，伤口并发症和疝的发生率较高，胆道损伤的发生率较高，尚未被广泛接受[64-66]。

2. 胆道造影的基本原理

腹腔镜胆囊切除术中行胆道造影有两个目的。其一，胆道造影能检测到未发现的胆道结石。其二，胆道造影能证实胆道解剖结构。在腹腔镜胆囊切除术出现之前，在胆囊切除术中常规行胆道造影的价值一直存在争议，一些外科医生对何时选择应用该技术存在争议[67]。该争议在腹腔镜时代仍然存在。常规使用胆道造影因其获益相对较小、不能识别所有残留结石、偶尔出现假阳性结果、增加成本和风险等因素而受到指责。尽管如此，在所有胆石症患者中发生胆管结石者占 8%～16%。在胆囊切除术患者中使用胆道造影检测出之前未发现的胆管结石的概率约为 5%，而胆管解剖异常的检出率为 12%[68]。在腹腔镜胆囊切除术中，二维成像和无法触及肝门部结构这两个问题使胆囊管-胆总管连接处的分辨成为难题。在对任何重要结构进行分离之前，胆道造影在胆管解剖结构显影方面都起着特别重要的作用。来自澳大利亚和瑞典的大规模人群调查研究表明，常规术中胆道造影能有效地减少发生严重胆道损伤的风险[69,70]。常规进行胆道造影时，腹腔镜胆囊切除术中胆道损伤的发生率为 0.2%～0.4%，而不进行造影时为 0.4%～0.6%[71]。当该费用与胆管损伤后所需的相关费用联系起来时，常规行胆道造影具有较高的性价比[72]。此外，常规行胆道造影能及早地确定术中可能发生胆管损伤的风险[73]，从而在发生胆道损伤时提高修复率。

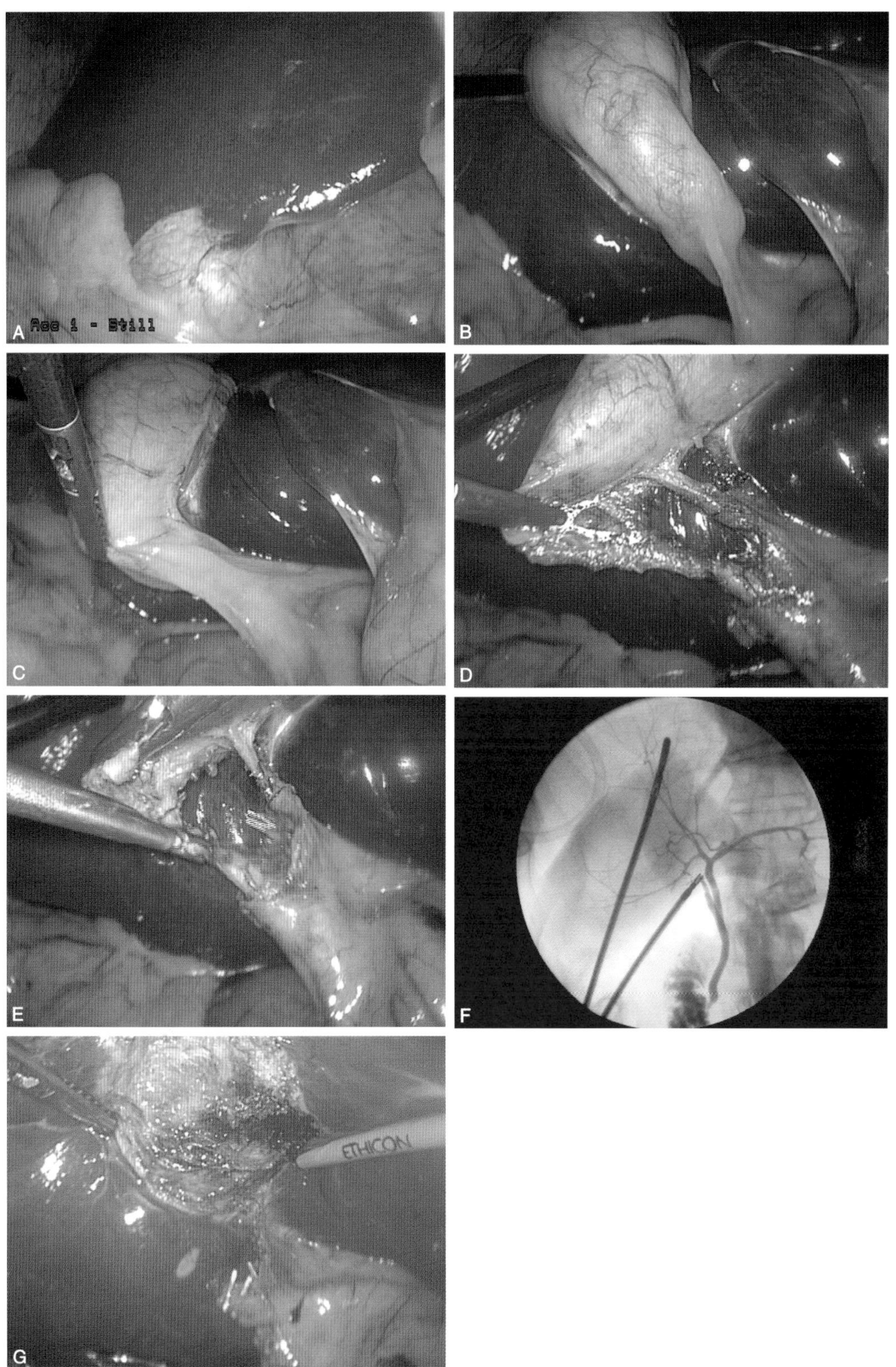

图 66.4　腹腔镜胆囊切除术。A,原位胆囊。B,向右肩及头侧方向牵拉胆囊底,显露胆囊漏斗部。C,将漏斗部向右下腹侧牵拉,游离胆囊三角,胆囊三角即胆囊管、胆囊边缘和肝边缘交界的区域。D,将覆盖在胆囊三角前部和后部的腹膜分离,暴露出“关键的安全视野”。E,胆囊管中的胆道造影导管。F,胆管造影正常。G,通过电灼法用电钩将胆囊自胆囊窝中取出

尽管这些结果都支持常规行胆道造影，但大多数外科医生考虑到存在未发现胆道结石的概率较低且胆管损伤较少，选择性地采用胆道造影。当病史提示有胆道结石可能时（例如胰腺炎，胆管炎，肝生化检查异常，术前影像学检查检出胆管结石）或术中须确认胆道解剖结构时，应行胆道造影检查。

3. 效果

几项大型研究介绍了腹腔镜胆囊切除术的经验（表66.2）[74-83]。一项对美国腹腔镜胆囊切除术经验的回顾性研究发现胆囊切除术后死亡率为0.06%。在国际上，其手术相关死亡率为0%～0.15%。在美国，有2.2%的患者需要中转开腹，而在国际上该比率为3.6%～8.2%，通常是由于炎性反应使肝门部结构解剖困难。主要术后并发症发生率约5%，胆道损伤的发生率为0.14%～0.5%。手术时间为1～2个小时不等，其中大多数患者选择行日间手术或门诊手术，绝大多数患者于术后一周内恢复包括工作在内的所有日常活动。

表66.2 腹腔镜胆囊切除术的疗效观察

编号	病例数	发病率/%	死亡率/%	胆管损伤/%	转换率*/%
74	3 319	6.7	0.15	0.33	5.2
75	6 076	4.3	0.12	0.86	6.8
76	13 833	4.3	0.14	0.59	5.3
78	2 201	4.3	0	0.14	4.3
79	114 005	5.4	0.06	0.5	2.2
80	33 563	8.5	0.09	0.2	3.5
81	56 591	N/A	N/A	0.42	N/A
82	3 285	10.1	0.2	0.25	3.6
83	22 953	14.6	0.3	0.3	5.3

*开腹胆囊切除术。

在美国，尚不存在也不可能存在将腹腔镜胆囊切除术与开腹胆囊切除术的结果进行比较的随机的前瞻性研究。患者对腹腔镜手术方法的追捧以及手术医生对该手术方式的迅速掌握使得对这两种手术进行直接对照比较变得困难。来自美国的非随机数据和其他国家的小样本随机试验均支持腹腔镜手术优于开放手术的观点[52,84-88]。在这些研究中，腹腔镜优点主要包括缩短住院时间，减轻疼痛，术后并发症少，术后康复时间短以及成本低廉等。人群调查研究结果提示腹腔镜技术引入后，胆囊切除术相关的死亡率大幅下降（表66.3）[89]。

表66.3 引入腹腔镜胆囊切除术之前（1989年）和之后（1992年）马里兰州的胆囊切除术相关死亡率

变量	1989	1992	%变化
胆囊切除术数量	7 416	9 993	+35
每千人胆囊切除术的粗略比率	1.57	2.04	+30
手术死亡率/%	0.84	0.56	-33
死亡数量	62	56	-10

Data from Steiner CA, Bass EB, Talamini MA, et al. Surgical rates and operative mortality for open and laparoscopic cholecystectomy in Maryland. N Engl J Med 1994;330:403-8.

与开腹手术相比，腹腔镜胆囊切除术优点明显，但并发症发生率高，尤其是胆道损伤。尽管目前尚不清楚世界范围内胆道损伤的准确发生率，但有2条证据表明其发生率较过去有所下降。首先，地区性研究表明，随着腹腔镜胆囊切除术整体手术经验的提升，胆道损伤率降低（图66.5）[90,91]。然而奇怪的是，随着外科医生个人手术经验的提升，胆道损伤的发生并没有继续下降，而是趋于稳定[91-93]。虽然胆道损伤更常见于外科医生初期实行腹腔镜手术时，但经验丰富的外科医生仍会发生胆道损伤，尽管其发生率较低。随着整体手术经验的增加，腹腔镜胆囊切除术的胆道损伤的发生率已接近开腹胆囊切除术。此外，自腹腔镜胆囊切除术应用伊始，前往转诊三级医疗中心接受治疗的胆道损伤患者的数量有所下降[94]。在美国，腹腔镜胆囊切除术的应用增长非常迅速，且可能已经超出医学教育系统对所有从业者进行充分培训的能力要求。可用“学习曲线”解释最初相对较高的胆管损伤率，这也可作为引入医疗实践的其他新技术的警醒示例。

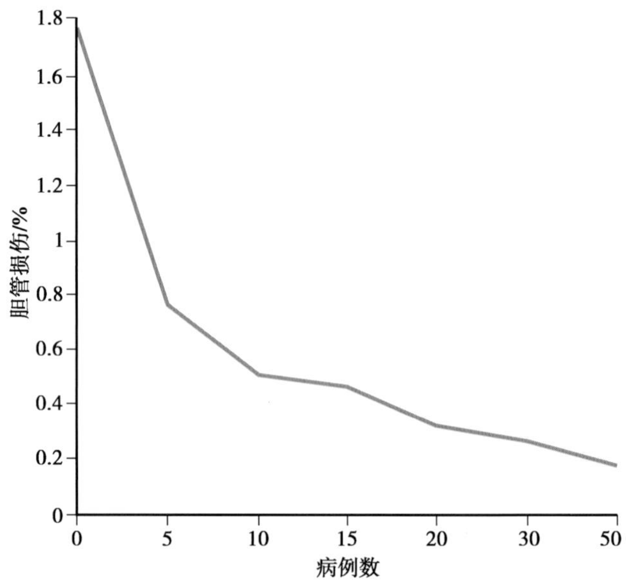

图66.5 腹腔镜胆囊切除术中外科医生的经验对胆管损伤风险的影响。随着经验的积累，胆管损伤风险明显下降，归因于“学习曲线”。（Data adapted from Moore MJ, Bennett CL. The learning curve for laparoscopic cholecystectomy. The Southern Surgeons Club. Am J Surg 1995;170:55-9.）

与历史上开腹胆囊切除术的使用率相比，腹腔镜胆囊切除术治疗胆石症的应用频率增加引起了人们的关注。在宾夕法尼亚州的一个特定的保健维护组织人群中，胆囊切除术的比率从1988年每千名参与者中1.35例（采用腹腔镜手术之前）增加到1992年的每千人2.15例（采用腹腔镜手术后）[95]。未发现同期疝修补术或阑尾切除术的有类似的比例变化。同样，来自马里兰州的数据显示，当地居民施行胆囊切除术的比率从1987年的1.69/1 000下降到1989年的2.17/1 000[89]，苏格兰地区的数据显示，实行胆囊切除术的年龄标化率增加了20%[96]。目前对手术应用量增加的原因尚不清楚，很可能与胆囊切除术的适应证的扩大有关，例如将非结石性胆囊疾病纳入胆囊切除术的适应证（参见第67章）。该领域的专家共识认为,患者在选择胆囊切除手术方案时不应因腹腔镜手术的实用性进行改变。

三、治疗方式的选择

有临床症状的胆石症患者治疗方法选择时的影响因素包括胆石症的分期、结石的特点、胆囊功能和患者的偏好。对于单纯性胆源性疼痛的患者,治疗方法包括手术和口服药物溶石并/或不并碎石术。无论结石的数量、大小和种类如何,外科手术在处理胆泥淤滞和成石胆汁的根本原因方面都具有一定的优势。虽然口服药物溶石对部分患者有效,但腹腔镜胆囊切除术的低并发症发生率抵消了非手术治疗的所有潜在优势。此外,非手术治疗由于治疗的持续时间长,且结石复发的可能性高,因此对部分患者不适用。患者的选择对治疗方案的选择也有重要影响。有些患者不能耐受行胆囊切除术或全身麻醉,抑或选择不做手术,仅对这些患者选择行药物治疗。其他有胆结石并发症的患者,应进行腹腔镜胆囊切除术。对于有胆结石并发症的患者,无论是否行胆道造影,腹腔镜胆囊切除术是首选治疗方法;对于行腹腔镜胆囊切除术风险大的患者,可考虑行开腹下胆囊切除术。

四、治疗适应证

(一) 无症状胆结石

对无症状胆石症患者的治疗需考虑疾病的既往病史,参见第 65 章。一般来说,无症状胆囊结石患者较少发生危及生命的并发症,而与结石有关的症状仅在少部分患者中出现[97-101]。当无症状患者出现临床症状时,其最初常表现为单纯的胆源性疼痛。事实上,大多数发生胆结石并发症的患者都有胆源性疼痛的先兆[102]。决策分析法计算结果表明,对无症状患者行胆囊切除术的风险与预防未来发生严重胆结石后遗症的受益率相近[103]。这些计算是基于开腹胆囊切除术的结果得出的;胆囊结石严重后遗症的发生率是基于对中西部一所重点大学的一组男性教师的长期随访结果得出的。目前尚不清楚这些数据是否适用于当前更倾向选择行腹腔镜胆囊切除术的女性患者群体。而对于所有无症状患者来说,选择预防性胆囊切除与仅对有症状患者行胆囊切除术相比没有明显获益[104,105]。此外,研究对健康相关生活质量的分析也不支持对无症状患者行胆囊切除术[106]。

在某些亚组中,使用预防性胆囊切除治疗无症状胆囊结石的可能利大于弊。例如,美洲本土居民中胆石症与胆囊癌发病率的高相关性足以证明预防性胆囊切除是合理的[106]。在接受心脏和肺移植的患者中,胆石症并发症的发病率很高而且可能需要预防性胆囊切除[107,108]。奇怪的是,存在无症状胆囊结石的肾移植患者其胆石症相关并发症的发生风险较低,因此,可不考虑行预防性胆囊切除术(见下文)[109,110]。儿童胆石症并发症的风险可能超过胆囊切除术的风险(见下文)。对进行减重手术或其他类型腹部手术的无症状患者,不需要行胆囊切除术[111]。

有观点认为糖尿病患者极易形成胆结石并合并其他结石并发症。因胆石症相关并发症行急症手术的糖尿病患者其术后并发症发病率和死亡率也极高。不过这一假说目前尚未被证实,因为如高脂血症、肥胖、心血管疾病和慢性肾脏疾病等其他变量也混杂其中[112]。因此,对存在无症状胆石症的糖尿病患者没必要行预防性胆囊切除术[113]。相关数据证明,对出现症状的糖尿病患者,由于其发展为坏疽性胆囊炎的风险增高,需进行早期干预[114]。因此,糖尿病患者相较于非糖尿病患者而言,其胆结石相关并发症的严重程度更严重。

(二) 胆源性疼痛与慢性胆囊炎

1. 患者选择

多数胆道疾病的手术是为了缓解因胆囊管一过性梗阻引起的症状诸如间歇性上腹部疼痛、恶心和呕吐,又被称为胆源性疼痛(旧称"胆绞痛")(见第 11 和 65 章)。组织学上,慢性胆囊炎患者的胆囊通常(但不总是)表现出慢性胆囊炎的特有征象如纤维化和单核细胞浸润。此外,胆源性疼痛患者比结石无症状患者更容易发生胆结石并发症,对这类有症状患者可行胆囊切除术。与其他任何手术一样,必须对症状缓解和未来预防并发症方面的潜在获益与手术风险进行权衡。幸运的是,胆囊切除术的生理影响较小,即使是老年人和消瘦的患者也可以安全地进行手术。在肝硬化失代偿的患者中,胆囊切除术的风险明显升高[115]。只有在症状严重、出现并发症或肝硬化得到很好代偿的情况下,才可进行该手术[116,117](见第 73 和 74 章)。对单纯胆源性疼痛患者行胆囊切除术治疗时,围手术期常规应用抗生素较少[118]。

2. 评价

胆源性疼痛的诊断通常是根据临床病史得出(见第 11 和 65 章)。但体格检查较少能发现胆石症的重要体征;大多数单纯的胆源性疼痛患者在疼痛发作期间无压痛。少数几种术前常规实验室检查是必要的,但是如果手术医生需要选择性而不是对每一个患者进行常规胆管造影,则应进行肝脏生化检查,以筛选出漏诊的胆总管结石。大多数胆源性疼痛患者的影像学评估方法仅限于超声检查,其诊断胆囊炎的敏感性(95%)和特异性(98%)均较高,对胆囊炎症表现如胆囊壁增厚、胆囊周围积液增多以及胆管扩张等也有一定的诊断价值。其他辅助检查,包括口服造影剂胆囊造影、MRCP、ERCP 或 CCK 闪烁显像等对证实怀疑有胆结石但彩超检查阴性的特殊患者的诊断,以及对怀疑有复杂胆石症的患者评估是较为有效的。对存在非典型的消化道症状的患者可采用 EGD、CT 或联合应用对其他消化道疾病进行鉴别排除,如食管炎,消化道溃疡或隐匿性肿瘤等。

(三) 急性胆囊炎

急性胆囊炎患者的治疗应先行静脉补液,恢复组织灌注和电解质平衡。由于有 40% 以上的患者胆汁及胆囊壁细菌培养呈阳性,因此需静脉抗生素治疗[119]。头孢菌素如头孢西丁对轻中度患者可获得较为满意的疗效,但对更严重患者,应使用广谱抗生素,如哌拉西林他唑巴坦或第三代头孢菌素联合甲硝唑。若怀疑为坏疽性或气肿性胆囊炎,应联合应用一种有效的抗厌氧菌药物。如果通过手术解决了发病诱因,对轻中度胆囊炎患者术后不需要抗生素治疗[119]。对于感染严重、术中发生化脓性胆囊穿孔或坏疽性胆囊炎的患者，术后应继续使用抗生素。

后续处理取决于诊断的明确程度、疾病的严重程度以及患者的整体状况。如果胆囊炎症状严重且出现胆囊穿孔等并发症，应急诊行胆囊切除术。如果症状性质未明，需行手术明确诊断。相反的，对患有心力衰竭等合并症的老年患者，其治疗多选择非手术治疗。

曾经对典型的急性胆囊炎患者行胆囊切除术的时机选择一直存在争议，多项前瞻性随机对照临床试验对急性胆囊炎早期（发病 3 天以内）和延迟（6~8 周后）手术的策略进行对比（表 66.4）[85,120-126]。其数据分析表明，对于一般患者而言，优先选择早期手术治疗可以减少住院总时间和费用，减少术后并发症发生率，同时也能预防急性胆囊炎加重导致死亡[127]。早期手术似乎并未显著增加胆囊切除术的主要并发症如胆管损伤的发生风险。

表 66.4 急性胆囊炎早期与延迟开腹或腹腔镜胆囊切除术：7 项随机试验的综合结果

胆囊切除术的时机	患者人数	死亡率/%	胆管损伤	平均住院总时间/d	治疗失败*
早期†	378	0	0	9.6	N/A
延迟‡	364	2.0	0	17.8	26%

*失败定义为急性症状恶化，需要早期手术者。

†就诊当天内。

‡6~8 周后。

N/A，无数据。

Data from Johansson M，Thune A，Nelvin L，et al. Randomized clinical trial of open versus laparoscopic cholecystectomy in the treatment of acute cholecystitis.

Br J Surg 2004；92：44-9. Jarvinen HJ，Hastbacka J. Early cholecystectomy for acute cholecystitis：a prospective randomized study. Ann Surg 1980；191：501-5. Lahtinen J，Alhava EM，Aukee S. Acute cholecystitis treated by early and delayed surgery. A controlled clinical trial. Scand J stroenterol 1978；13：673-8. Linden WVD，Sunzel H. Early versus delayed operation for acute cholecystitis. A controlled clinical trial. Am J Surg 1970；120：7-13. Lo CM，Liu CL，Fan ST，et al. Prospective randomized study of early versus delayed laparoscopic cholecystectomy for acute cholecystitis. Ann Surg 1998；227：461-7. McArthur P，Cuschieri A，Sells RA，Shields R. Controlled clinical trial comparing early with interval cholecystectomy for acute cholecystitis. Br J Surg 1975；62：850-2. Lai PB，Kwong KH，Leung KL，et al. Randomized trial of early versus delayed laparoscopic cholecystectomy for acute cholecystitis. Br J Surg 1998；85：764-7.

尽管最初对将腹腔镜胆囊切除术治疗急性胆囊炎的安全性存在担忧，但其在大多数情况下是可行的。在处理腹腔炎症较重的患者时会存在对胆囊三角形的分辨与解剖受限或凝血障碍等情况。在这些情况下，可能需要另一种替代全胆囊切除术的方法，如腹腔镜下次壶腹旷置术，壶腹缝合术或使用开放式手术[128]。胆道造影在急性胆囊炎患者中尤为重要，其可确定导管的解剖结构。腹腔镜胆囊切除术在处理胆源性疼痛患者时有着切口疼痛轻，住院时间缩短和更快地恢复工作等优点，也可用于急性胆囊炎患者。

对于有严重合并症（如肝衰竭、呼吸衰竭或心力衰竭）的高危患者，胆囊造口（胆囊引流术）应优于胆囊切除术。对大多数患者而言，经皮穿刺技术已取代了胆囊造口手术。对急性胆囊炎发作后好转的患者，若其整体情况允许，可进行腹腔镜胆囊切除术。也可以通过胆囊造瘘管去除残留的结石，患者同样可以获得预期的治疗效果。在行胆囊造瘘治疗的所有患者中约有一半患者出现复发性胆道症状[129]。图 66.6 展示了一例患者通过经皮胆囊造瘘术获得最佳治疗的例子。经皮胆囊造瘘术适用于高手术风险患者，并不受急性胆囊炎的严重程度或胆囊的影像学表现的影响。最近，内镜下胆囊跨壁引流术已被证明与经皮引流同样有效，其可以对不适合手术治疗的患者的胆囊进行减压[130]。在此操作中，通过放置连接胆囊及内脏（通常是十二指肠）的腔内支架将胆汁引流。

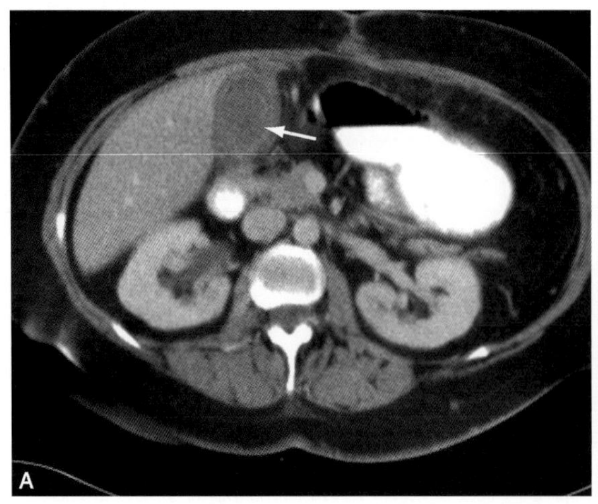

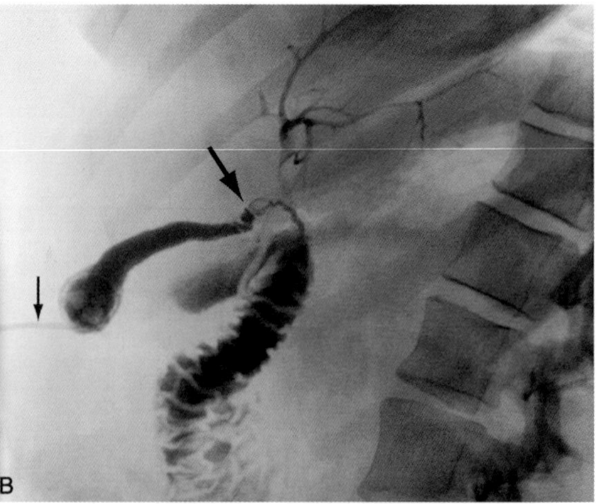

图 66.6 一例 47 岁女性严重急性胆囊炎患者的影像学检查，并发内脏穿孔术后多系统器官衰竭导致 ICU 住院时间延长。A，CT 显示急性胆囊炎伴胆囊壁增厚和胆囊周围积液（箭）。B，通过经皮胆囊造口术后（小箭）进行的胆管造影显示胆囊结石嵌顿在胆囊颈部（大箭）。胆囊造瘘管留在原位，患者临床得到改善

如果患者将来有可能行手术治疗，则不应行内镜下透壁引流术，因为除切除胆囊外，手术还需要修复十二指肠孔。

急性胆囊炎患者与是否患有糖尿病与感染并发症如败血症的发生频率显著相关[131]。对糖尿病患者应尽快行胆囊切除术治疗。同样，老年人发生急性胆囊炎的临床常常表现看似较轻，但隐匿性重度急性胆囊炎例如坏疽性或气肿性胆囊炎的发生率则较高。发生坏疽性或气肿性胆囊炎相关的影响因素包括男性、糖尿病、心血管疾病和初始 WBC 计数超过 15 000/mm^3。与糖尿病患者一样，老年患者应于疾病早期行胆囊切除术以确保及时控制感染。不建议在腹腔镜胆囊切除术后常规使用外科引流导管治疗急性胆囊炎，这可能是无益甚至有害的[131]。

1. 非结石性胆囊炎

在没有胆结石的情况下发生的急性胆囊炎被称为非结石性胆囊炎（见第 67 章）。其最常发生于因其他严重疾病（如创伤、烧伤或重大手术）的住院患者身上。在门诊患者中，以外周血管疾病成年男性患者发病风险最高[132]。另外非结石性胆囊炎也可能会使艾滋病患者的治疗复杂化（请参阅第 35 章）[133]。

目前对非结石性胆囊炎的病理生理机制尚不清楚，禁食、胆囊血供改变、因子Ⅻ的活化、前列腺素和内毒素引起的胆汁淤滞等均可能产生影响（见第 67 章）。胆囊中的泥沙常会阻塞胆囊管。坏疽，积脓和胆囊穿孔等使非结石性胆囊炎的病程更加复杂化，而并不能使结石性急性胆囊炎的病程复杂化。在一些文献中，这些并发症的发生率可达到 75%[134]。胆囊切除术一直是非结石性胆囊炎治疗的主要治疗方法。当怀疑存在坏疽、积脓或胆囊穿孔时，将胆囊及时切除至关重要。然而对一些患者而言，由于其存在有其他潜在疾病，手术风险高，因此可在初期采用超声引导下经皮胆囊造瘘术，多数患者能通过该方式获得痊愈。在胆道造影提示存在腹腔内败血症或持续性胆囊管阻塞时，需要行胆囊切除手术治疗。

2. 气肿性胆囊炎

气肿性胆囊炎是一种罕见的疾病，其特征性是由于胆囊壁受到产气细菌尤其是厌氧菌的感染（见第 65 章）。糖尿病被认为是引起该疾病的危险因素，而坏疽和穿孔通常也使该病的病程复杂化。气肿性胆囊炎的患者应在体液及电解质水平稳定后立即行腹腔镜胆囊切除术。应使用针对革兰氏阴性杆菌和厌氧细菌的抗生素。

（四）胆源性胰腺炎

对胆源性胰腺炎患者的病理生理及临床表现的讨论见第 58 和 65 章。胆源性胰腺炎患者的最初治疗包括液体复苏、肠道休息并监测并发症。大多数患者病情相对较轻，行保守治疗后可在 1 周内得到临床愈合。

对急性胰腺炎的患者早期应通过超声检查确定是否合并胆石症。如确诊，一般在患者出院前行腹腔镜胆囊切除术。在过去，胆源性胰腺炎发病早期行胆囊切除术有很大的风险。因此常将手术时间推迟 1 到 2 个月，以便炎症消退。其主要缺点是有高达一半患者在观察期有继发胰腺炎的可能。现在人们逐渐意识到，可于胰腺炎临床症状消失同期进行胆囊切除术[135,136]。该方法缩短了总的病程和住院时间[136]。此外，还能防止胰腺炎复发。根据国际胰腺病学会的建议，应于胆囊切除术中行胆道造影术以排除胆管残留结石风险[137]。

对严重或坏死性胰腺炎患者，应将胆囊切除术推迟数周，以便：①患者从胰腺炎的后遗症中恢复；②肝十二指肠韧带的炎性反应减轻，以便术中能安全进行解剖；③对确诊胰腺假性囊肿的小部分患者，可能需要其他外科治疗。对于合并胆管炎或持续胆汁淤积致重症胰腺炎的患者，可经内镜切开括约肌行胆管清除术[138]。这种方法比早期胆管探查手术的并发症发生率低（见第 70 章）。

（五）特殊问题

1. 妊娠期胆石症

有时胆囊疾病会于妊娠期首发或加重。在这种情况下，最常见的临床表现是胆道疼痛加重和急性胆囊炎。由胆总管结石引起的黄疸和急性胰腺炎很少见。对有症状的患者只能选用超声检查评估有无胆道疾病。考虑到传统放射成像和放射性核素扫描的潜在致畸作用，在孕期无法应用。

过去，由于担心妊娠前 3 个月和妊娠晚期行手术治疗会发生流产和早产等并发症，因此不建议在妊娠期间行胆囊切除手术。另外，由于以往担心套管针对子宫的潜在损伤，以及气腹对胎儿循环功能的影响不明，认为妊娠是腹腔镜手术的绝对禁忌证。现在麻醉和抑制宫缩等药物的改进使妊娠期间的腹部手术变得更安全。几项大型病例研究表明，在妊娠期进行胆囊切除术对胎儿和产妇的发病率影响较小[139,140]。尽管如此，仅在必要时才会于孕期行腹腔镜胆囊切除术。其手术适应证包括复杂的胆结石疾病如急性胆囊炎和胆源性胰腺炎、潜在疾病对孕妇构成威胁时或者当母亲无法提供足够的营养时，在这些情况下，潜在疾病对妊娠产生的风险超过了手术对妊娠的风险。由于妊娠早期流产及致畸的风险较高以及妊娠晚期可能发生早产，因此妊娠中期行手术治疗最为安全。

2. 儿童期胆结石病

胆石症在儿童的发病率似乎有所升高。约 20% 的患者是因慢性溶血导致胆色素结石形成[141]。长期禁食和全肠外营养作为重要的危险因素被逐渐重视。而回肠疾病或肠切除病史也会增加胆结石发生风险。儿童胆石症的治疗必须考虑结石的类型（胆色素结石或胆固醇结石），是否有症状以及其他潜在风险如全胃肠外营养（TPN）的影响。所有有症状的胆结石患者都需要行胆囊切除术，目前对无症状胆结石的治疗尚不明确。部分接受全肠外营养婴儿的胆结石会在重新进行经口喂养后消失。因此，对该情况下的无症状婴儿进行 12 个月的观察是合理的。对胆结石持续存在和无症状胆色素结石（不能自发溶解）的患者最好采用腹腔镜胆囊切除术治疗。

3. Mirizzi 综合征

Mirizzi 综合征是指胆囊管内结石持续压迫造成的肝总管梗阻。最初 Mirizzi 综合征包括两种类型[142]。在Ⅰ型中，肝总管被一个存在于胆囊颈部或胆囊管内的巨大的结石压迫，其继发的相关炎症可能会导致肝外胆管中段的阻塞和狭窄。Ⅱ型是指结石侵犯肝总管形成胆囊胆管瘘。Mirizzi 综合征很少见，在所有接受胆囊切除术的患者中发生率仅有 1%，多数患者出现反复发作的疼痛、发热和黄疸。超声检查通常提示胆囊结石合并胆囊缩小、肝外胆管解剖正常以及肝内胆管中度扩张，应用 MRCP 和 ERCP 有助于显示肝管解剖结构。典型的表现是肝内胆管扩张，胆管大小正常，常与胆囊管汇入肝总管水平发生梗阻。其梗阻症状及周围的炎性表现可能与肝门部胆管癌（Klatskin 瘤）相混淆（见第 69 章）。

对胆囊切除困难的患者应考虑 Mirizzi 综合征的可能。对Ⅰ型 Mirizzi 综合征的治疗可采取胆囊切除术并或不并胆管探查。对存在严重炎症反应的患者，由于很难辨认其解剖结构，最好选择行胆囊部分切除术联合术后内镜下乳头括约肌切开探查以确保胆管结石的清除。对Ⅱ型 Mirizzi 综合征的治疗应考虑肝总管和胆管损伤的程度。为指导手术治疗，Ⅱ型 Mirizzi 综合征已被重新分类为Ⅱ、Ⅲ和Ⅳ型。当瘘管累及范围不足胆管的三分之一时，为Ⅱ型；累及三分之一至三分之二时，为Ⅲ型（图 66.7）；累及范围超过三分之二时，为Ⅳ型。Ⅱ型和Ⅲ型 Mirizzi 综合征可以根据需要选择行部分胆囊切除术、结石清除及胆总管成形术。对Ⅳ型 Mirizzi 综合征存在的巨大缺损需要行肝总管空肠 Roux-en-Y 吻合术进行修复[142]。

4. 胆石性肠梗阻

胆石性肠梗阻是一种罕见的肠梗阻，是由巨大的胆结石嵌顿在肠腔内引起的。Bouveret 综合征是指胆结石嵌顿在十二指肠远端或幽门部导致的胃出口梗阻的症状。胆结石性肠梗阻为机械性梗阻而非动力性肠梗阻，正如“肠梗阻”的字面含义一样。患者平均年龄一般超过 70 岁，女性多见。在 70 岁以下的患者中，胆石性肠梗阻的发生率不到 1%，而在 70 岁或以上的患者中，胆石性肠梗阻的比例接近 5%[143]。其症状为典型的机械性肠梗阻表现，包括腹痛、呕吐和腹胀，仅小部分患者有急性胆囊炎的症状，但有半数患者自述有胆结石病史[144]。

40% 的患者肝脏生化检测异常，转氨酶升高，但黄疸较少见。大多数患者的腹部平片显示肠道积气影，符合肠梗阻一般特点。大约一半的患者存在胆道积气，少数患者可见异位的胆结石。有时采用上或下消化道钡餐造影检查能确定梗阻或瘘管的位置，但多数情况下该检查不需要进行。采用超声检查可帮助胆石症的诊断，并可对瘘管进行观察。

胆石性肠梗阻的病理生理学定义是指通直径超过 2.5cm 的胆结石通过胆囊肠瘘进入并阻塞肠腔。瘘管最常见于开口于十二指肠，结肠少见。当胆结石沿肠管顺行向下通过时，会间歇性地阻塞管腔。完全性肠梗阻最常于回肠发生，可能是因为其管腔最窄。由于结石在通过肠管的过程中症状会不断反复，因此其阻塞具有“滚动”的特点。

治疗应首先进行补液和恢复电解质平衡，然后行开腹探查术。腹腔镜探查也是可行且有效的。当通过小肠切开术取

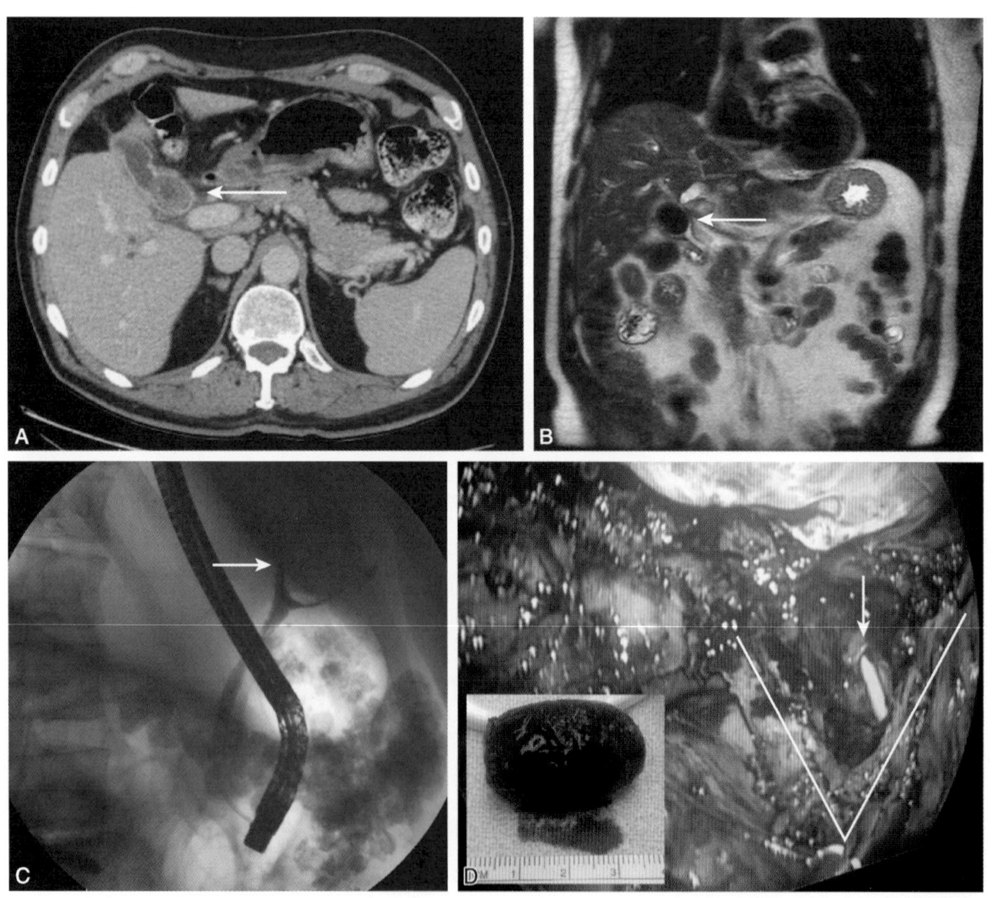

图 66.7　Ⅲ型 Mirizzi 综合征。A，CT 显示胆囊漏斗部嵌顿巨大胆囊结石（箭）。B，MRCP 显示胆囊漏斗部嵌顿巨大胆囊结石（箭）。C，ERCP 显示肝总管被腔内巨大胆囊结石阻塞，与胆囊胆总管瘘相符（箭）。D，手术中取下的胆囊前壁照片，其余胆囊内侧壁边缘以白线突出显示。可见肝总管和胆囊漏斗部内侧壁之间有一个瘘口（含 ERCP 术中放置的蓝色胆道支架）（箭），肝总管完整性破坏近 50%，符合Ⅲ型 Mirizzi 综合征。插图显示了致病的 3cm 胆结石

出结石后肠梗阻症状可得到缓解，此时应注意探查是否存在其他结石可能。只有在发生肠穿孔或肠缺血时才需行肠切除术。并不需要行胆囊切除术同时闭合胆囊肠管瘘来阻断胆囊与邻近十二指肠之间的连接，因为胆囊可通过瘘管减轻结石所致的压力升高。更重要的是，该手术操作复杂而且合并症多，许多瘘管会随着时间自行关闭[144]。这种高风险人群的死亡率很高，平均 15%～18%，5%的患者结石性肠梗阻可能复发。

5. 偶然的胆囊切除术

一些情况下会在进行另一种手术前或术中发现胆结石的情况，针对该情况，需要在术前规划时考虑到存在附带胆囊切除的可能并在手术知情同意书中进行描述。附带胆囊切除术的目的是预防部分有症状的胆石症继续发展而出现临床症状如术后早期的急性胆囊炎。另有文章指出部分手术如行胃切除术或胃旁路手术的肥胖患者会存在后续内镜或外科手术治疗胆结石并发症困难的情况（见第 8 和 53 章）。不过正如预期一样，胆囊切除术会增加术后并发症的风险。是否选择附带胆囊切除术是基于获益及风险进行评估的。

如前所述，典型的胆结石患者往往无症状。在长期随访中发现这些人中有 18%～35%后续出现症状[97,103,104]。对部分群体，其风险更高。结石较大（>2.5cm）和胆囊壁钙化（瓷化胆囊）的患者发生急性胆囊炎、胆石性肠梗阻和胆囊癌的风险较高，这类患者具有行附带胆囊切除术的指征[145-147]。对于因慢性溶血继发色素性胆结石的镰状红细胞病患者，由于区分镰状细胞危象与急性胆囊炎的临床表现较困难，因此也有行胆囊切除术的指征[148]。同样，其他溶血性贫血患者，如 β 地中海贫血患者等发生胆结石的风险很高，而且其中很大一部分会出现症状[149]。如果对溶血性贫血患者行脾切除术，那么对其中的无症状结石患者行胆囊切除术是有指征的。最后，在行胆囊切除术外的腹腔镜手术时，如果含有结石的胆囊被留在原位，术后胆道症状发生率高。某项研究发现在 68 例行腹腔镜手术的有无症状胆结石患者中，54%术后出现症状，22%在术后 30 天内需行胆囊切除术治疗[150,151]。

在行腹部手术后另行附带胆囊切除术的发生率较低[152]。如果患者身体健康，所行手术顺利，且术中暴露充分，可于下一次手术时行附带胆囊切除术，包括结肠切除术。老年患者的风险并没有增加。而附带胆囊切除术可能会在某些情况下增加术后伤口感染的风险[153]。

五、胆总管结石

在对有胆道症状患者进行检查时，胆囊切除术期间或胆囊切除后探查胆囊结石时，都可能发现胆总管结石。其治疗方案有几种，包括口服药物溶石、介入放射技术联合内镜技术以及手术等（见第 70 章）。根据结石的临床特点（黄疸、胆管炎、胰腺炎或无症状）、胆囊状况、患者的年龄和一般情况选择合适的治疗策略。其他需考虑的因素包括外科手术、内镜和放射科专家的专业水平。

（一）术前存在的胆总管结石

当患者术前已发现胆总管结石时，可通过内镜下括约肌切开术清除胆管内结石，然后进行腹腔镜胆囊切除术。另一种方法是开腹或腹腔镜下胆囊切除术联合胆管探查术。行腹腔镜胆囊切除术和内镜下取石术时行腹腔镜下胆管探查术的频率低于行开腹胆囊切除手术时行开腹下胆管探查术的频率[154]。通过经胆囊管进入或直接切开胆管进行腹腔镜下胆管探查是一项对技术要求较高的手术，即使是由经验丰富的外科医生进行操作，其胆管结石清除的成功率也仅为 83%～97%[155-157]。决策分析及随机对照研究的结果发现，行腹腔镜下胆囊切除术联合经胆囊或经胆管胆道探查的患者与术前行内镜下取石后再行腹腔镜下胆囊切除术患者相比，其并发症发病率和死亡率更低，住院时间更短，康复更快，手术次数更少[154-156]。对于是否仅采用手术治疗很大程度上取决于外科医生及其团队的经验和技术。如果外科医生缺乏足够的培训经验及接受过培训的团队和设备，则应首选两阶段（手术联合内镜）的治疗方法。

（二）胆囊切除术中发现的胆总管结石

如果在腹腔镜胆囊切除术中通过胆管造影发现之前未探查到的胆总管结石，可选择以下 3 种方式处理：①中转为开腹胆管探查；②腹腔镜下胆管探查；③腹腔镜胆囊切除术后进行内镜下括约肌切开并清除结石。这些选项的选择流程如图 66.8 所示。其影响因素包括：胆道结石的数量和位置，受累胆管的病理学表现，以及外科及内镜医师的操作经验。腹腔镜胆囊切除术联合术后内镜下括约肌切开取石的效果对大多数患者来说都是令人满意的，同时还具备微创手术的优点。从技术方面讲，内镜下括约肌切开成功率较低，对于 5%～10%的患者，即使是熟练的内镜医师将胆管结石完全清除的概率也只有 84%～89%[158]。对这类患者常需要行二次手术。越来越多的经验表明，腹腔镜胆管探查是安全有效的，其结石清除率平均为 95%，手术死亡率为 0.5%[155,158-160]。与内镜

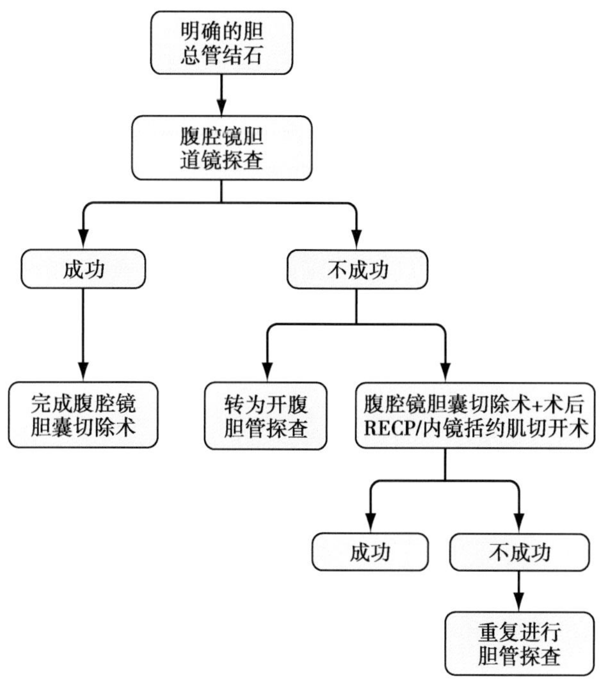

图 66.8 腹腔镜胆囊切除术中意外发现的胆管结石处理的流程。ERCP/ES，内镜逆行胰胆管造影/内镜下括约肌切开术

下括约肌切开术相比，腹腔镜胆管探查术在疗效，成本和安全性方面更有优势[161]。

与开腹下胆管探查一样，腹腔镜胆管探查首选经胆囊途径进行胆管探查，并通过胆囊管切口取出结石。在极少数情况下，如结石太大或位于胆囊管与胆总管交接处的上方时，则需要切开胆总管探查，该方式包括对胆管的探查和直接胆管切开取出结石，对胆管切口必须用缝合线封闭，通常放置T管以防止胆管狭窄，特别是当胆管很细时，在没有T管的情况下在缝合后很可能产生难以扩张的狭窄。因此，胆管细小是直接切开探查的禁忌证。对结石清除不完全患者也可放置T管，以允许介入科医师进行胆道减压和经皮取石。

（三）胆囊切除术后发现的胆总管结石

对既往接受胆囊切除术的患者若发现胆总管结石后最好通过内镜下括约肌切开并结石取出术进行治疗。如果近期行胆管探查后留有T管，通常可以通过T管对结石进行影像学检查协助取出。在这种情况下很少需要手术，但如果需要，通常会进行开腹胆管探查，因为胆囊切除术后已不存在经胆囊管进入胆管的通路。

六、胆管损伤和狭窄

良性胆管狭窄通常是由胆囊切除术中的医源性损伤所导致的。少数狭窄是慢性胰腺炎，PSC，既往胆管手术史（包括切除和移植）和胆总管结石导致的。胆囊切除术中胆管的损伤可能是由于对胆管解剖结构的了解不充分；夹子、缝线或电凝的位置不准确；在调整胆囊管位置时使胆管过度牵拉；以及牵拉和暴露得不充分等。这些损伤通常发生在一些顺利进行的胆囊切除术中，并且外科医生可能不会注意到其发生。

胆管损伤有3种类型。第一种类型是胆囊切除术后胆管完全闭塞，黄疸在术后早期迅速出现。第二种类型是由于肝外胆管的横断，胆囊管结扎放置无效或移位导致的胆汁性腹水，或胆囊窝因胆囊-肝管分裂或Luschka胆管离断导致的胆漏。胆漏通常与肝下间隙的感染性胆汁积相关。第三种类型是由于部分胆管梗阻导致疼痛，黄疸或胆管炎间歇性发作，通常在胆囊切除术后2年内发生。3种损伤模式如图66.9所示。

在腹腔镜胆囊切除术后早期，临床医生应警惕任何出现持续性腹痛、恶心和发热的患者发生胆道损伤的可能。对胆囊切除术后患者早期或晚期出现胆道梗阻症状进行鉴别诊

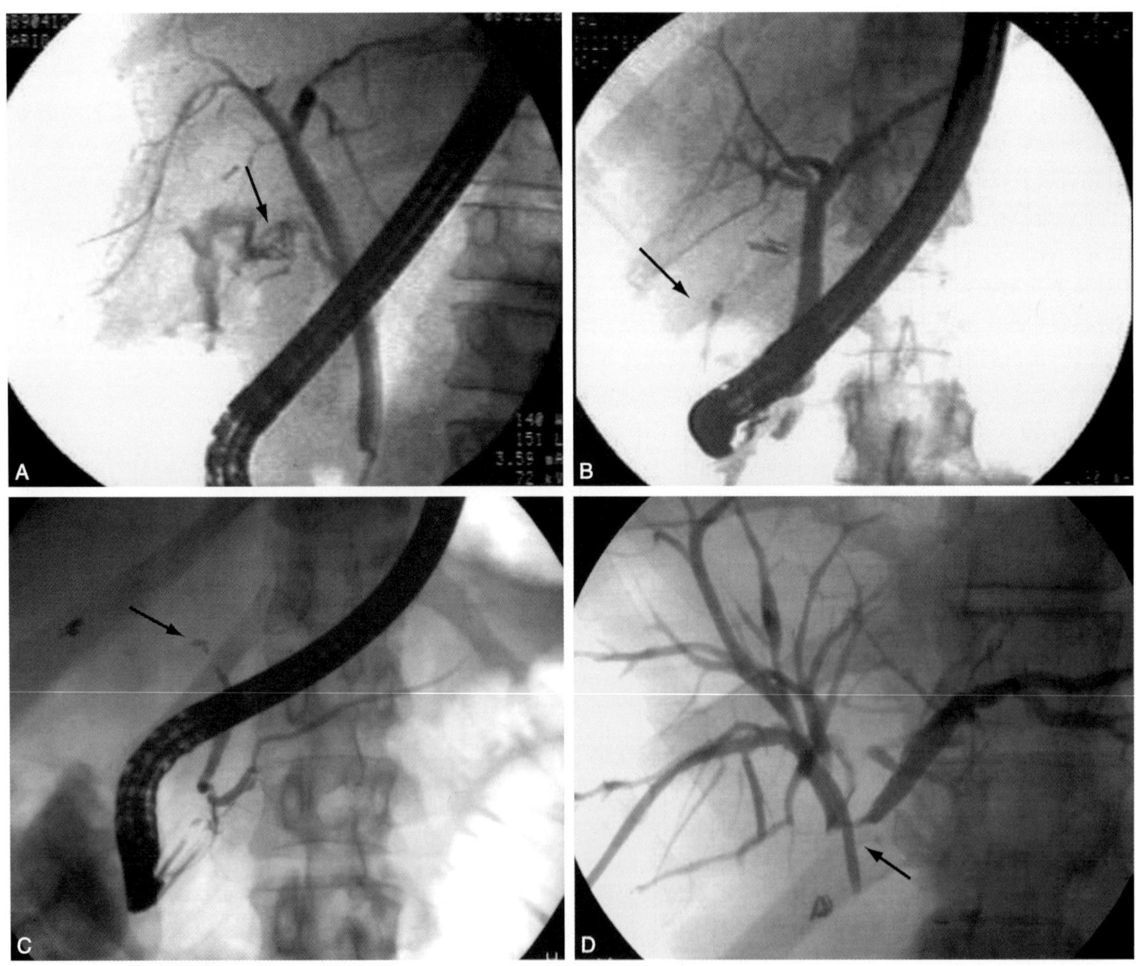

图66.9　腹腔镜胆囊切除术中胆管损伤的3种常见类型。对于第一种类型（A和B），患者可能表现为胆囊管残端漏导致的胆汁瘤或胆汁性腹水（A中的箭）或Luschka管导致的胆漏（B中的箭）。对于第二种类型（C和D），患者表现为黄疸，伴或不伴有胆漏，这是继发于因胆管被误认为是胆囊管而切除的结果。这些问题通常涉及肝管汇合部损伤和肝右动脉损伤。C，ERCP显示手术夹堵塞胆管（箭）；D，经肝胆管造影图显示肝管汇合部被切除（箭）

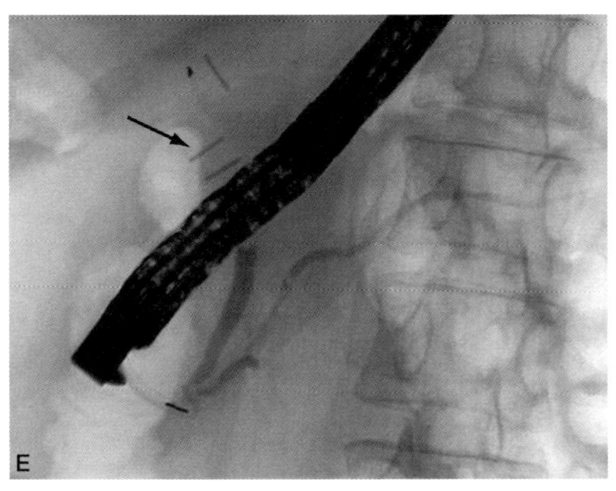

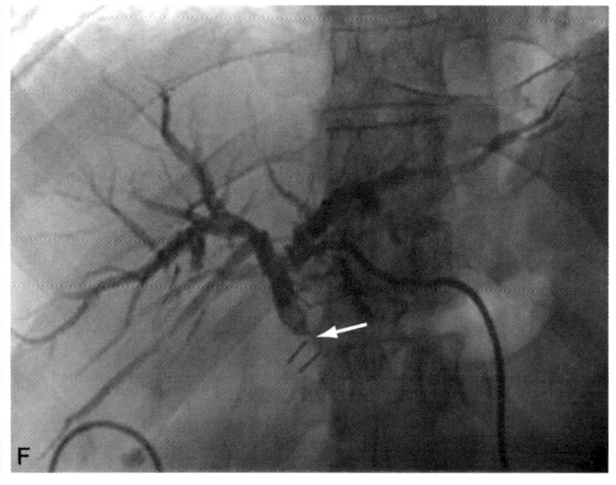

图 66.9(续) 第三种类型(E 和 F),患者表现为由放置在胆管而不是胆囊管上的手术夹或热损伤导致的狭窄引起的黄疸。E,ERCP 显示手术夹导致的狭窄(箭);F,经肝胆管造影显示对应的胆管狭窄(箭)

断,主要为胆道狭窄和胆总管结石。由于症状,体征和肝脏生化检查水平可能相同,因此这两者在临床上可能难以区分。

对疑似胆道损伤和/或狭窄患者的评估通常首选彩超对扩张的胆管、肝下积液或胆管瘤进行观察。在术后早期,采用锝标记的放射性核素扫描可以迅速且无创地显示胆道通畅程度并排除胆漏。若上述检查提示存在胆道损伤,应采用 ERCP 对病变进行鉴别。治疗的首要目的是通过经皮穿刺对胆汁积聚进行引流以控制肝下间隙感染,同时通过内镜下或经肝途径进行胆管引流(见第 70 章)。当感染控制且胆道引流后,需要通过 ERCP 经肝胆管造影以确定解剖结构和制定修复计划。

大多数胆管损伤或术后良性狭窄的患者最好行手术治疗。虽然有许多手术进行了报道,但切除受损胆管联合行端侧 Roux-en-Y 胆总管空肠吻合术或肝肠吻合术的效果最佳。修复成功的标准为:完全切除损伤或狭窄段、吻合口无张力、采用可吸收的精细缝线在吻合口完成黏膜之间完全吻合并保证近端胆管无瘢痕形成以及保持胆管血供。手术治疗良性胆道狭窄的死亡率平均为 0%~2%,其死亡风险与肝硬化、肾功能衰竭、难治性胆管炎、年龄和营养不良等危险因素直接相关。胆道修复术对治疗良性胆管狭窄效果良好,治愈率约 85%~98%[162-165]。而在高位狭窄或肝硬化患者中其疗效较差。对于高位狭窄患者,可能需要特殊的技术来对炎症过程中未受影响的健康胆管组织进行吻合,也有可能需要切除肝脏。复发性狭窄的治疗是一个技术性难题,但仍有 75% 的患者获得了满意的结果[166]。对术后胆道狭窄可采用内镜或经皮球囊扩张伴或不伴支架植入术治疗,前提需考虑残余胆管是否被破坏。良性术后狭窄通常可以通过放置可取出的塑料支架进行内镜下治疗。虽然内镜治疗常需分成多个阶段进行,但在合适的患者身上可以获得良好的结果(见第 70 章)。目前尚没有前瞻性的随机对照研究对手术、内镜和放射介入学方法进行对比。在一项非随机试验中,88% 的肝空肠吻合术患者实现了术后胆管长期通畅,相比之下,接受球囊扩张但未使用支架的患者有 55% 获得了术后胆道长期通畅[167]。该研究对术后死亡率未进行报道。鉴于由经验丰富的外科医生行肝空肠吻合术可以获得良好的长期效果和低死亡率,所有适合的胆道狭窄患者都应首选手术治疗。对存在胆汁性肝硬化、严重的合并症以及狭窄复发率高的患者最好行非手术治疗。

七、胆囊切除术后综合征

胆囊切除术后综合征是指在胆囊切除术后出现的类似于胆道疼痛的腹部症状(另见第 63 和 65 章)。该术语具有一定误导性,因为它包括了广泛的胆道和非胆道疾病,很少与手术本身相关。胆囊切除术后此类症状的发生率为 5%~40%[49,168-171]。最常见的术后症状是消化不良、胃肠胀气和腹胀,以胆囊切除术后早期多见。其他症状有持续性的右上腹痛或上腹痛。也有一小部分患者表现为严重腹痛、黄疸或呕吐;与轻度或非特异性症状的患者相比,这类患者更有可能发现不同的可治疗的病因。如果症状出现在术后早期,必须怀疑继发于医源性胆道损伤的胆汁性腹膜炎。

胆囊切除术后症状的鉴别诊断包括肠外疾病如心肌缺血、非胆汁性胃肠道疾病如消化性溃疡、胆道疾病如胆总管结石、功能性疾病如肠易激综合征和精神疾病等(框 66.3)。临床医生必须仔细考虑疼痛的非胆道原因的可能性,并适当地指导评估。

框 66.3 胆囊切除术后腹痛的原因分析

胆道疾病	胃食管反流病
胆管狭窄	肠易激综合征
胆道恶性肿瘤	肠道恶性肿瘤
胆总管结石	腹腔内粘连
胆总管囊肿	肠系膜缺血
胆囊管残余	消化性溃疡
Oddi 括约肌功能紊乱	**肠外疾病**
胰腺病因	冠状动脉疾病
胰腺炎	肋间神经炎
假性囊肿	神经系统疾病
恶性肿瘤	精神疾病
其他胃肠道疾病	外伤性神经瘤
食管运动障碍	

（一）胆总管结石

胆管结石是胆囊切除术后症状的最常见原因。它们可能是胆囊切除术时被忽视的残留结石，也可能是较少见的主要在胆管形成的结石。胆总管结石的自然病史尚不清楚，但在一些患者中，这些结石显然可引起胆源性疼痛、黄疸、胰腺炎或胆管炎。临床表现提示胆总管结石的诊断。肝脏生化检查值，尤其是碱性磷酸酶水平可能升高。超声可显示胆管扩张，而结石显影并不常见。MRCP 和 ERCP 可以证实胆管结石的存在，并排除其他可能性，如胆管狭窄或肿瘤。采用内镜下括约肌切开取石术可治愈大多数患者[172]。

（二）胆囊管残留

在一些患者中，胆囊切除术后症状的原因可能是由于胆囊管残留（或残端）或一小部分胆囊残留的病理学改变导致的[173,174]。已知的一些异常包括胆囊管结石、瘘管、肉芽肿和神经瘤，合并胆管结石常见。尽管这种综合征的存在一直存在争议，但在一项随机试验中，胆囊切除术中完全切除胆囊管的术后后遗症少于部分胆囊管留在原位的标准手术技术[175]。在腹腔镜胆囊切除术的时代，胆囊管离胆囊起始部更近，以最大限度地降低因胆囊管插入肝总管时的剥离而导致胆管和右肝动脉损伤的风险；因此，胆囊管残端综合征的发生率可能更高[176]。MRCP 和 ERCP 可用于描述疑似胆囊管残余病变患者的胆道解剖结构。其治疗方法是手术切除胆囊管残端。

（三）Oddi 括约肌功能紊乱

对胆囊切除术后疼痛患者出现 Oddi 括约肌结构或功能异常的发生率高达 10%（见第 63 章）[177,178]。其结构异常为括约肌狭窄，其特点是导致基础括约肌压力升高的某固定部位的括约肌狭窄，该狭窄可能是由外伤引起的，如胆结石、器械刺激、胰腺炎或感染等。而功能性或运动性障碍则包括胆道或 Oddi 括约肌运动障碍、壶腹部痉挛或新近的括约肌功能紊乱。由于平滑肌强制性或周期性收缩，胆道测压时可发现括约肌压力升高。目前对该紊乱的病因尚不清楚，而且在许多情况下对其结构或功能性异常不能区分，所以更倾向于使用 Oddi 括约肌功能紊乱这一通用名称。

Oddi 括约肌功能紊乱的临床表现包括胆源性疼痛、黄疸和胰腺炎。其典型表现为 ERCP 下显示胆管扩张和造影剂排空延迟（>45 分钟）。通过其胆源性疼痛症状、肝脏生化检测指标异常程度和胆管扩张程度可有效预测内镜下括约肌切开手术的效果[179]。对于未明确诊断的患者，应进行胆道测压。其治疗方法为内镜下括约肌切开术，部分特定的患者可能需行括约肌成形术和分隔成形术（见第 63 章）[180]。

八、胆结石、胆囊切除术与癌症

许多研究表明，胆囊结石及胆囊切除术与胆囊、胆管、胃、结肠、乳腺和子宫等不同器官的癌症的发生有关。目前尚不清楚胆囊疾病及其治疗与这些恶性肿瘤之间是否存在因果关系。常见的环境因素，也许是饮食因素，都可能会对这些疾病的发病产生影响。另一方面，胆结石患者胆汁成分的改变会对癌症的发展产生影响。另外，胆囊切除术增加了胆汁酸的肝肠循环，增加了黏膜在具有潜在致癌作用的次级胆汁酸如脱氧胆酸中的暴露水平（见第 64 章）。

（一）胆道癌

与胆结石关系最密切的癌症是胆道自身的癌症，尤其是胆囊癌（见第 69 章）。大多数胆囊癌患者都有胆结石病史，流行病学资料显示这两种疾病之间有很强的相关性。胆结石较大者相比结石较小者、多发性胆结石患者相比单一胆结石患者，以及在美国原住民中，其胆囊癌的发生风险更高[181-183]。胆囊壁钙化或瓷化胆囊也与胆囊癌相关[184]。胆结石和胆管癌之间统计学相关性较小，同时研究发现行胆囊切除术的患者的发生癌症的风险低于未经治疗的患者[185,186]。

（二）结直肠癌

20 世纪 80 年代早期的研究发现胆囊切除术与后续出现的结直肠癌（尤其是右半结肠癌）之间存在统计学关系[187-189]。发生结直肠癌的风险虽然在统计学上具有显著性，但仍然很低（相对风险为 1.5～2.0）。后续研究对这种联系提出了质疑，并将其归因于胆结石而非胆囊切除术，同时也发现在胆囊切除术后很快便出现结直肠癌的发病率升高，提示它们之间不具有因果关系（见第 127 章）[190,191]。对于有明确手术指征的患者，上述因素不应成为阻碍胆囊切除术的参考因素。

（周明新　闫秀娥 译，黄永辉 校）

参考文献

第 67 章　非结石性胆源性疼痛、急性非结石性胆囊炎、胆固醇贮积病、腺肌瘤病和胆囊息肉

Karin L. Andersson, Lawrence S. Friedman 著

章节目录

一、非结石性胆源性疼痛 …… 994
（一）定义和临床特征 …… 994
（二）流行病学和病理生理学 …… 994
（三）诊断和治疗 …… 994
二、急性非结石性胆囊炎 …… 995
（一）定义 …… 995
（二）流行病学 …… 995
（三）发病机制 …… 995
（四）临床特征 …… 995
（五）诊断 …… 995
（六）治疗 …… 996
三、胆固醇贮积病 …… 997
（一）定义 …… 997
（二）流行病学 …… 997
（三）病理学 …… 998
（四）发病机制 …… 998
（五）临床特征 …… 998
（六）诊断 …… 998
（七）治疗 …… 998
四、腺肌瘤病 …… 998
（一）定义 …… 998
（二）流行病学 …… 999
（三）病理学 …… 999
（四）发病机制 …… 1000
（五）临床特征 …… 1000
（六）诊断 …… 1000
（七）治疗 …… 1001
五、胆囊息肉 …… 1001
（一）定义 …… 1001
（二）流行病学 …… 1001
（三）病理学 …… 1001
（四）临床特征和诊断 …… 1002
（五）自然史 …… 1002
（六）治疗 …… 1003

虽然胆结石及其并发症是导致胆囊切除的主要原因[1]，但也有 15% 的胆囊切除术无胆结石[2]。在这些患者中，多数胆囊切除术是为了治疗两种不同临床综合征的其中一种：非结石性胆源性疼痛或非结石性胆囊炎。如表 67.1 所示，非结石性胆源性疼痛多见于年轻女性，多为门诊患者，可类似于结石性胆源性疼痛。急性非结石性胆囊炎常见于卧床或病情危重的老年男性，多合并血管疾病。由于这两种疾病的临床表现和预后有很大的不同，所以本章节将它们分开讨论。另外，阐述 3 种无症状胆囊疾病——胆固醇贮积病、腺肌瘤病和胆囊息肉。

表 67.1　非结石性胆源性疼痛和急性非结石性胆囊炎的比较

	非结石性胆源性疼痛	急性非结石性胆囊炎
流行病学	女性多见(80%)	男性多见(80%)
	青年或中年门诊患者	病情危重的老年 ICU 患者
	危险因素与胆石症类似(例如肥胖和多胎妊娠)	危险因素包括存在动脉粥样硬化、近期手术史和血流动力学不稳定
临床表现	与结石性胆源性疼痛同样的阵发性右上腹或上腹痛	原因不明无法定位病灶的败血症，迅速进展为坏疽和穿孔
	体格检查多为正常	查体或许能发现体温升高；仅有 25% 的患者存在右上腹压痛
	实验室检查多为正常	可能有白细胞增多和高淀粉酶血症
诊断标准	超声显示胆囊多为正常，无结石表现	见表 67.2
	用 CCK 刺激后胆道闪烁显像测量 GBEF 或许可以明确能在胆囊切除术后获益的患者	
治疗方案	对于典型的胆源性疼痛或 GBEF<35% 且存在持续症状提示没有潜在功能性胃肠病的患者，可考虑择期胆囊切除术	对于坏疽或穿孔，应施行急诊胆囊造瘘术或急诊胆囊切除术
疾病预后	好，发作能自发缓解或在胆囊切除术后改善	差，与潜在的并发疾病有关，死亡率在 10%~50%

GBEF，胆囊喷射分数。

一、非结石性胆源性疼痛

(一) 定义和临床特征

胆源性疼痛(或胆绞痛)的典型表现是剧烈的、突发的上腹或右上腹痛,在15分钟内疼痛程度逐渐加重,持续发作30分钟或更长时间,之后慢慢缓解。对于“胆源性”最典型的表现是右侧季肋部疼痛,可放射至右肩[3]。疼痛的发作多由进食引起,可能伴有坐立不安、恶心或呕吐。在发作间期,除可能会残留上腹部压痛之外,体格检查多为正常。

当患者有相关病史并且超声确认胆结石时,处理方法直截了当——选择胆囊切除或较少尝试的药物溶石(见第65和66章)。相比之下,非结石性胆源性疼痛的治疗很困难。这些患者的临床表现和胆源性疼痛的表现与胆石症患者相似,但是超声检查中胆囊正常,血清肝脏酶学和胰腺酶学水平正常[4,5]。非结石性胆源性疼痛可能源于一系列重叠的疾病,包括慢性非结石性胆囊炎和胆囊运动障碍(胆道运动障碍),它们具有相同的临床症状,但切除后的胆囊病理表现却有所不同。对于非结石性胆源性疼痛的患者,胆囊切除术后临床症状的改善尚不确定。

(二) 流行病学和病理生理学

超声阴性的胆源性疼痛在人群中很常见,男性约7%,女性约20%[6]。非结石性胆源性疼痛多见于年轻女性。在一项100多名患者的研究中,83%为女性,平均年龄约为30岁[5]。

非结石性胆源性疼痛的病因尚不清楚,但是间接证据表明几种不同的病因可能导致相同的临床表现。与胆结石患者或无胆道症状的对照组相比,非结石性胆源性疼痛患者受刺激后十二指肠中的胆汁在胆汁酸和磷脂方面浓度更低[7]。低胆汁酸浓度可能与此类患者中胆囊的延迟或不完全收缩有关。磷脂含量的降低支持胆磷脂水解为游离脂肪酸进而诱发炎症的假说。

在非结石性胆源性疼痛的患者中,年轻的育龄期女性占绝大多数。这种与胆石症的流行病学特点近乎相同的情况提示这两种疾病具有相似的危险因素。一些研究显示近一半的非结石性胆源性疼痛患者在切除的胆囊标本中能发现微小结石[8],这表明起初的超声是假阴性。一些研究显示部分非结石性胆源性疼痛患者在切除的胆囊中有胆固醇贮积病的组织学证据(见后文)[9]。虽然是偶然发现的病理学表现,但是在一些患者中胆固醇贮积可能会破坏正常的胆囊收缩功能并导致胆源性疼痛。在其他患者,切除的胆囊有明显的炎症,为慢性非结石性胆囊炎的表现[10]。

非结石性胆源性疼痛被胃肠病学国际工作委员会列为功能性胃肠疾病[罗马Ⅳ分类(见第122章)],这意味着诊断不需要病理学改变[4]。在胆囊组织学正常的患者中,胆囊收缩和Oddi括约肌松弛之间不协调或胆囊运动障碍(也称为功能性胆囊疾病)可引起胆源性疼痛(见第63章)。对于胆囊正常的患者,非结石性胆源性疼痛和其他功能性肠病之间的紧密联系提示内脏高敏感可能是引起胆源性疼痛的常见原因[6]。

(三) 诊断和治疗

如前所述,非结石性胆源性疼痛的症状可能与胆石症难以区分。细致回顾患者的主诉,明确这些症状是胆源性疼痛,而不是消化不良、烧心、腹部绞痛或腹胀[3]。如果这些症状符合胆源性疼痛,应与影像科医生共同详细回顾超声检查的结果。超声不太可能遗漏大于2mm的胆结石(超声发现结石的敏感性超过95%),但是只关注排除结石,则可能会忽略胆囊疾病的其他超声证据。对于有典型胆道症状而超声检查阴性的患者,用EUS、MRCP或促胰液素增强MRCP进一步评估胆道可能会获益[11]。胆囊腺肌增生症或胆固醇小息肉的患者可能也会有胆源性疼痛,而胆囊切除术能缓解疼痛(见下文)。对于胆源性疼痛而超声检查结果正常的患者,决定胆囊切除术的时机和适应人群是一种挑战(见第63章)。

刺激胆道闪烁显像

虽然仍有争议,但是通过胆道闪烁显像计算胆囊喷射分数(gallbladder ejection fraction,GBEF)是一种确定哪些非结石性胆源性疼痛的患者会从胆囊切除术获益的方法(另见第63章)。静脉注射放射性标记的亲肝胆系统制剂(如^{99m}Tc-二异丙基亚氨基二乙酸),使其在胆囊内浓缩,之后缓慢注射CCK刺激胆囊收缩(超过30分钟),计算机辅助伽马摄像机测量胆囊收缩前后的活动。GBEF定义为活动变化值除以活动基线值。对健康志愿者的研究显示正常GBEF的均值为75%且几乎都超过35%[5]。脂肪餐是相比于CCK更省钱的替代方法,它利用经口摄入脂肪(通常是对半混合的牛奶)来刺激胆囊的生理收缩,GBEF的正常值往往低于CCK刺激后的正常值[12,13]。

只有不到一半的非结石性胆源性疼痛的患者GBEF降低,大多数GBEF降低的患者在随访3年后仍有症状。如果对这些患者进行胆囊切除术,组织学证据显示慢性胆囊炎约占90%,胆囊管狭窄占80%,胆固醇贮积病占30%[12]。胆囊切除术后长期症状缓解率在GBEF异常的患者中超过50%[5,14,15],但是也有50%的患者没有接受手术同样有临床症状缓解[16]。在一项对GBEF低于35%且症状不典型的患者进行的研究中,30%的患者临床症状自行消失,持续发作的患者中57%在胆囊切除术后症状消失[17,18]。一项随机对照试验评估了胆囊切除术治疗GBEF降低的胆源性疼痛的效果,所有11名接受胆囊切除术的患者在平均54个月的随访期内均有症状消失,不手术组的10名患者仍有症状[5]。

尽管是良性的,但是GBEF正常的非结石性胆源性疼痛患者有一个可变的病程。有些患者发现非胆源性因素,另一些患者的症状会随着时间而消退。虽然术后症状缓解率与GBEF降低的患者胆囊切除术后相当,但是胆囊切除术一般不推荐用于GBEF正常的非结石性胆源性疼痛患者[19]。GBEF多用于评估非结石性胆源性疼痛,但是它并不是预测胆囊切除术疗效的可靠因素。一般来说,在胆囊切除之后,典型的胆源性疼痛比不典型的症状(如腹胀或消化不良)更容易缓解。这个观察结果提出了一个问题,即是否应根据症状而决定是否手术,而不是闪烁造影检查。建议在决定手术前进行一段时间的观察或药物治疗,以使症状有可能得到缓解。

刺激胆道闪烁显像在早期用于评估胆源性疼痛患者(有时在超声无法证实胆结石后立即进行),非胆源性或自限性疾病没有被排除,导致该检查的阳性预测值下降[20]。GBEF降低对于功能性胆囊疾病并无特异性,也可见于无症状的健康人、IBS 和服用影响胃肠动力的药物(包括钙通道阻滞剂,口服避孕药和 H2 受体拮抗剂)。相关症状高度提示非结石性胆源性疼痛且排除其他诊断之后,应该进行该项检查。胆源性疼痛的患者在超声检查正常时应进行血清肝脏生化、胰腺酶学和上消化道内镜检查,以排除导致临床症状的其他原因[21]。如果这些检查不能提供另一种解释,患者应再观察几个月以使症状有自发缓解的可能,之后再进行胆道闪烁显像。对于有不典型症状或其他功能性胃肠病症状的患者,应考虑对内脏高敏感的治疗(见第 12、14、22 和 122 章)。

非结石性胆源性疼痛的诊断具有不确定性,随之而来的是此类患者胆囊切除术的比例急剧增加,尤其是在年轻人群、有保险的人群以及应用腹腔镜手术之后。在同一人群中,因胆石症而行胆囊切除术的比例已经有所下降[22]。

二、急性非结石性胆囊炎

(一) 定义

急性非结石性胆囊炎是胆囊在无结石的情况下发生的急性炎症。由结石引起的急性胆囊炎在第 65 章讨论。“非结石性胆囊炎”曾受到质疑,因其错误地提示该病只是单纯的无结石性胆囊炎。相反,“坏死性胆囊炎”则能反映出该疾病特有的病因、病理和预后[23]。

(二) 流行病学

在美国,5% ~ 10% 的胆囊切除术和急性非结石性胆囊炎有关。对外伤或烧伤术后以及住院患者施行的胆囊切除术,超过一半是因为非结石性胆囊炎[24]。在一个病例系列研究中,0. 19% 的外科 ICU 患者出现了非结石性胆囊炎,占所有急性胆囊炎的 14%[25]。

急性非结石性胆囊炎很少在没有外伤或应激的情况下出现,尤其是儿童[26]、合并血管病变的老年患者[27]、骨髓移植受者、化疗患者[28]和艾滋病患者[29]。在某些情况下能找到特殊的感染因素,如免疫功能低下患者中的沙门菌[30]、金黄色葡萄球菌[31]、免疫缺陷患者中[25]的巨细胞病毒、寨卡病毒[32]和儿童中的 EB 病毒[26]。系统性血管炎如结节性多动脉炎、系统性红斑狼疮、过敏性紫癜和嗜酸性肉芽肿性多脉管炎(Churg-Strauss 综合征)可出现急性非结石性胆囊炎,多由胆囊缺血损伤所致[33]。在阿仑单抗治疗多发性硬化的过程中也观察到几例急性非结石性胆囊炎病例[34]。急性非结石性胆囊炎也越来越多地见于没有任何危险因素的健康人[35,36]。急性非结石性胆囊炎患者多为老年人,而结石引起的胆囊炎患者则多为年轻女性[25]。

(三) 发病机制

大多数急性非结石性胆囊炎见于长时间禁食、卧床和血流动力学不稳定的情况。虽然正常情况下胆囊上皮是一种坚固的组织,但是会持续暴露于体内最有害的物质之一:浓缩的胆汁酸液。在正常的一天中,胆囊会多次排空浓缩的胆汁,然后重新充满稀释的肝脏胆汁(毒性可能较小)。随着禁食时间的延长,胆囊不能接受 CCK 刺激而排空,浓缩的胆汁会淤积在胆囊腔内[37]。另外胆囊上皮有较高的能量代谢需求,以吸收胆汁中的电解质和水分。卧床、禁食和内脏血管收缩(常因 ICU 中的感染性休克所致)的患者可能会发生胆囊上皮的缺血性和化学性损伤[38]。一项研究比较了因胆结石切除的胆囊与因急性非结石性胆囊炎切除的胆囊的微循环情况,结果显示非结石性胆囊炎的胆囊内毛细血管几乎没有充盈,这表明微循环紊乱和缺血可能在其发病机制中起重要作用[39]。

因子Ⅻ的不适当激活(在动物中证实能诱发胆囊炎症[40])和胆囊壁中前列腺素的局部释放[41,42]也与非结石性胆囊炎的相关组织损伤有关。在动物模型中,吲哚美辛能通过抑制前列腺素的合成来减轻组织的破坏。急性非结石性胆囊炎中胆囊上皮紧密连接蛋白的表达不同于结石性胆囊炎,这可能反映了胆囊壁通透性增加在全身炎症反应中的作用[43]。胆囊黏膜感染的细菌,一般是革兰氏阴性肠道细菌和厌氧菌[44],是急性非结石性胆囊炎的继发事件,而不是引起最初损伤的原因。

在年轻患者中,关于急性非结石性胆囊炎发病率上升的一个假说是肥胖以及随之而来的胆囊壁脂肪的增加,在动物模型中证实这会干扰胆囊的排空。在一项研究中,16 位急性非结石性胆囊炎患者的胆囊壁脂肪明显多于无胆囊炎的正常人[45]。

(四) 临床特征

急性非结石性胆囊炎的临床表现与急性结石性胆囊炎不同。虽然右上腹痛、发热、胆囊局限压痛和白细胞增多可能在典型病例中很明显(例如年轻的门诊患者),但是老年术后患者常缺乏部分或全部这些特征[46]。75% 的病例中起初没有与右上腹痛相关的症状或体征。不明原因的发热、低血压、白细胞增多或高淀粉酶血症可能是唯一线索。

与典型的结石性胆囊炎相比,急性非结石性胆囊炎的病程更呈现为暴发性。在确诊时,至少一半的患者有胆囊炎的并发症,如坏疽或胆囊局限性穿孔[47,48]。胆囊积脓和胆管炎可能会使胆囊细菌性重复感染的病例更加复杂。该病常见于体弱患者同时并发症进展迅速,死亡率很高,从 10% 到 50% 不等,而结石性胆囊炎的死亡率只有 1%。如此高的死亡率使得一些研究者建议,对于在 ICU 中那些无法找到脓毒症原因的危重患者,应考虑经验性胆囊造瘘术[49]。

(五) 诊断

急性非结石性胆囊炎并发症发展迅速,早期诊断对于降低死亡率至关重要。不幸的是,由于缺乏和胆囊相关的特异性临床表现,加上混杂有前期手术或外伤相关的临床表现,早期诊断非常困难。对于老年高危患者,高度警惕胆源性脓毒症才有希望实现早期诊断和治疗。表 67. 2 描述了急性非结石性胆囊炎的几种诊断标准。

表 67.2　急性非结石性胆囊炎的诊断标准

方法	表现
临床评估	如果存在右上腹压痛则支持诊断,但75%的病例没有 不明原因发热、低血压、白细胞增多或高淀粉酶血症经常是唯一的发现
超声	无腹水和低白蛋白血症(血清白蛋白<3.2g/dL)时胆囊壁增厚(>4mm) 超声检查时 Murphy 征阳性(超声定位胆囊时压痛最明显) 胆囊周围积液 能床边检查是一个主要优势
CT	无腹水和低白蛋白血症时胆囊壁增厚(>4mm) 胆囊周围积液,浆膜下水肿(无腹水时),胆囊壁内气体或黏膜坏死 排除其他腹腔内疾病的最佳检查手段,但需要将患者搬运至扫描机器处
肝胆闪烁显像	放射性核素正常排入胆管和十二指肠但胆囊未显影提示急性胆囊炎 危重症卧床患者因为胆汁黏稠可能假阳性 急性胆囊炎的排除诊断优于确诊

1. 超声

超声应用广泛并且易于床旁进行,在疑似急性非结石性胆囊炎的评估中具有优势[50]。3 种提示胆囊疾病的超声表现为:①无腹水或低白蛋白血症时胆囊壁增厚(>4mm);②超声 Murphy 征阳性(超声定位胆囊时压痛最明显);③胆囊周围积液。胆囊壁增厚(图 67.1)对胆囊炎并无特异性,但在适当的临床情况下提示胆囊受累,需进一步评估。超声 Murphy 征依赖于检查者,也需要患者配合,阳性是胆囊炎症的可靠标志[51]。胆囊周围积液提示疾病进展。超声诊断急性非结石性胆囊炎的敏感性为 67%~92%,特异性在 90% 以上[50]。

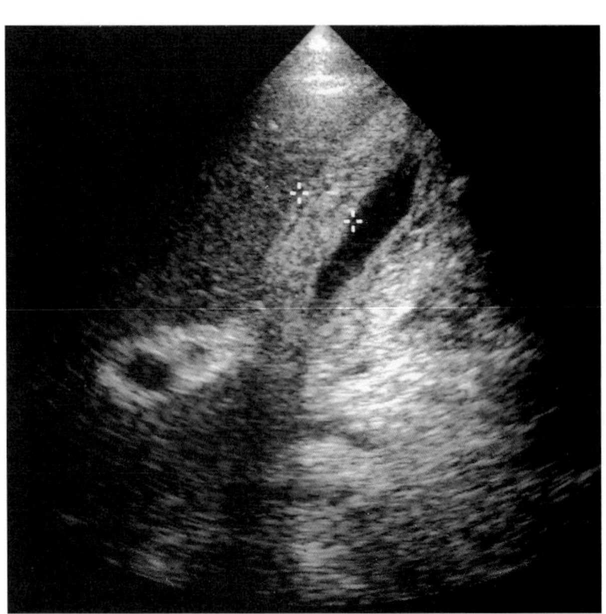

图 67.1　超声显示胆囊壁增厚至 17mm(星号所示),这是急性非结石性胆囊炎的特征。当超声探头压在腹部胆囊上方时,出现压痛点(超声 Murphy 征)。诊断经手术得到证实。(Courtesy David Hurst,MD,Dallas,TX.)

研究人员提出了一种超声评分系统用以提高危重患者超声诊断的准确性[52]。胆囊扩张或胆囊壁增厚各加 2 分,胆囊壁"条纹状"增厚(低回声层和高回声层交替出现)、胆汁淤积和胆囊周围积液各加 1 分。6 分或更高的分数能准确预测出现非结石性胆囊炎。

一个研究小组评估了在 ICU 中常规应用超声早期发现非结石性胆囊炎的效果。在一组 53 例机械通气患者中,3 例男性通过超声检查和临床表现诊断为急性非结石性胆囊炎,然而 30% 的非结石性胆囊炎患者也探查到胆囊的异常表现。应当在急性非结石性胆囊炎高风险的患者中进行超声检查[53]。

2. CT

胆囊炎的 CT 表现与超声相似,包括胆囊壁增厚(>4mm)、胆囊周围积液、浆膜下水肿(无腹水)、胆囊壁内气体和黏膜坏死脱落。经手术证实这些征象预测急性非结石性胆囊炎的敏感性和特异性超过 95%。在发现腹腔其他可能引起发热或腹痛的疾病方面,CT 优于超声[54]。不过 CT 的一个明显缺点是不能在床边进行检查,而这对于许多危重患者来说是必需的。一些研究者强调 CT 是对超声的补充,可以在超声正常的高危患者中发现胆囊疾病。

3. 肝胆闪烁扫描显像

对临床表现提示急性胆囊炎的患者,肝胆闪烁扫描显像有助于排除胆囊管梗阻。在正常情况下,静脉注射的放射性核素吸收到肝脏、分泌入胆汁、浓缩至胆囊(在扫描仪器上呈现为"热点"),最后排泄进入十二指肠。胆囊管阻塞的阳性结果为放射性核素正常进入十二指肠,但是胆囊未充盈。在结石性胆囊炎的发病机制为结石阻塞胆囊管,闪烁扫描显像提示胆囊充盈排除了胆囊炎[55]。

肝胆闪烁扫描显像诊断急性非结石性胆囊炎的准确性较差。胆囊水肿在闪烁显像时会出现类似于结石性胆囊炎的梗阻表现。急性非结石性胆囊炎患者经常会长时间禁食,会导致胆汁浓缩、黏稠,在胆囊管中流动性变差,在肝胆闪烁扫描显像中出现假阳性。大多数急性非结石性胆囊炎(与结石性胆囊炎相比)没有胆囊管阻塞,肝胆闪烁扫描显像也可能出现假阴性[56]。该检查的敏感性超过 90%,但是对于禁食,危重患者缺乏特异性,主要用于排除而不是确诊急性非结石性胆囊炎。一项对危重患者进行超声和胆道闪烁扫描显像的研究发现胆道闪烁扫描显像对急性非结石性胆囊炎的早期诊断有帮助,单独的超声不能及早决定是否需要手术[57]。

为了提高准确性,研究人员建议使用吗啡增强胆道闪烁扫描显像,静脉注射吗啡(0.05~0.1mg/kg),增加胆汁通过 Oddi 括约肌的阻力。如果胆囊管通畅,就会"强制充满"胆囊,减少检查结果的假阳性[58]。虽然这项检查可以排除胆囊炎,但是不适用于危重患者。

(六)治疗

急性非结石性胆囊炎会迅速发展为坏疽和穿孔,需要尽早识别和干预。支持治疗包括恢复血流动力学稳定,合并胆道感染时应用抗生素覆盖革兰氏阴性肠道菌和厌氧菌。

1. 外科胆囊切除术和胆囊造瘘术

急诊开腹和胆囊切除术曾是急性非结石性胆囊炎的治疗方法(见第 66 章)。之后腹腔镜胆囊切除术成为标准的手术方式。由于患者病情不稳定无法耐受麻醉和手术，近年来逐渐应用影像引导下的经皮胆囊造瘘术[59,60]。如有必要，在病情稳定后行胆囊切除术。

2. 经皮胆囊造瘘术

对外科手术风险高危的患者进行超声引导下经皮经肝穿刺置入胆囊造瘘引流管联合静脉抗生素，在一些研究中取得良好结果[49,61,62]。85%～90% 的患者治疗有效，10% 的患者出现并发症。胆囊造瘘术的短期死亡率较高，反映的是基础疾病的高死亡率，不是手术的高死亡率。多数急性非结石性胆囊炎患者能耐受经皮穿刺引流，如果引流后胆管造影正常就拔除引流管，之后不需要胆囊切除术[61,62]。

3. 经乳头或经壁内镜下胆囊造瘘术

部分怀疑为急性非结石性胆囊炎的危重患者有大量腹水或不可纠正的凝血障碍，不适合超声引导下经皮胆囊造瘘术。这些患者可能会受益于内镜治疗，在 ERCP 时通过不透 X 线的弯头导丝沿着胆管壁选择性进插入胆囊管。如果导丝成功穿过胆囊管的螺旋瓣，在胆囊内放置猪尾支架，另一端通过鼻胆管引出或留在十二指肠内引流（“双猪尾”支架）[63]。如果不进行括约肌切开术，出血的风险很低。由于胆囊靠近胃肠道，EUS 引导下经管壁置入自膨胀覆膜金属支架也是治疗非结石性胆囊炎的方法，成功率为 97%[64]，常用于晚期肝病和腹水患者，比经皮手术疼痛少。

经 ERCP 胆囊插管的成功率为 90%，对胆囊内黏稠的黑色胆汁和胆泥进行引流和灌洗，大多数危重患者的临床情况会有好转。内镜技术比超声引导下置入胆囊造瘘管更繁琐和昂贵，适用于不能耐受经皮手术或合并凝血障碍的患者[65]。

三、胆固醇贮积病

（一）定义

胆固醇贮积病是一种胆囊上皮的获得性组织学异常，特征是上皮巨噬细胞内胆固醇酯和甘油三酯的过度积聚（图 67.2）[66]。虽然在术前可能怀疑此诊断，但是临床医生多在胆囊手术切除后发现这种病变。

胆固醇贮积病和胆囊腺肌症（见后文）归类于“胆囊增生性疾病”，这个术语在 1960 年提出，用来描述具有共同特征的胆囊疾病。此类疾病没有炎症表现，却存在黏膜异常增生、胆囊造影时造影剂过度积聚和排泄[67]。这一概念的支持者认为在没有胆结石的情况下，胆源性疼痛可以用某种“胆囊增生性疾病”解释。由于缺乏共同的病因和特异性临床表现，建议放弃这一术语。

（二）流行病学

根据大体观察诊断标准或显微镜下诊断标准，5%～40% 的尸检标本有胆固醇贮积病。在一项纳入 1 300 例尸检的大规模研究中，用显微镜检查每个胆囊后发现 12% 有胆固醇贮积病[68]。在外科手术切除的胆囊中，18% 有胆固醇贮积病，比尸检标本高 50%[69]。因为没有临床症状，胆固醇贮积病的发病率尚不清楚。

胆固醇贮积病与胆固醇结石有相似的易感人群和流行病学特征[70]，不过这两种疾病独立发生，不一定同时存在。与胆结石一样，胆固醇贮积病少见于儿童，多见于 60 岁以下女

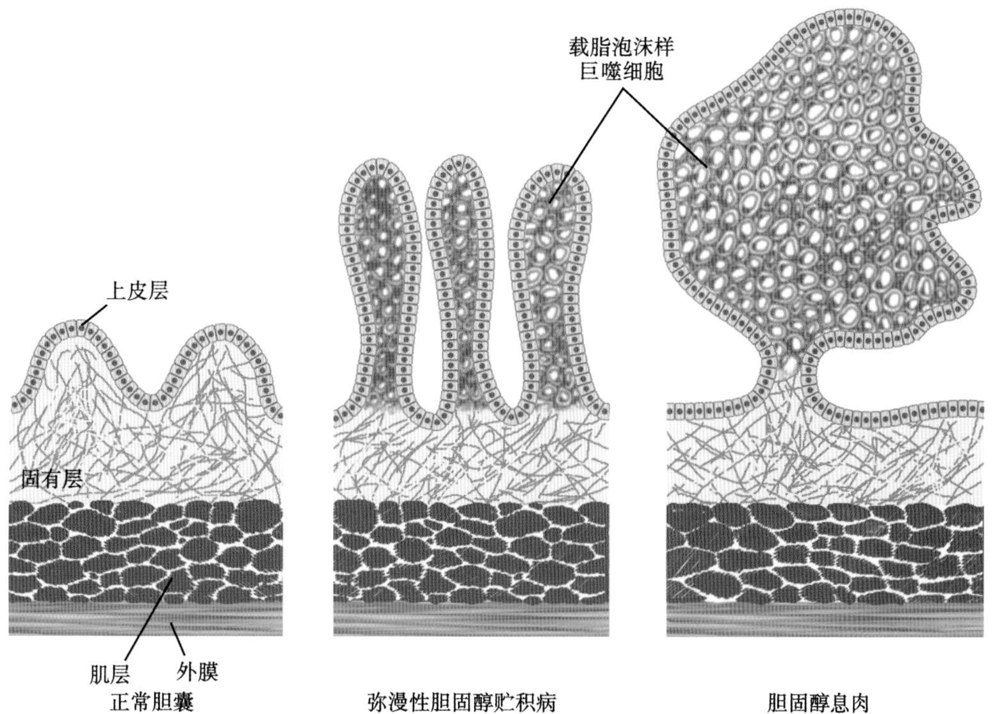

图 67.2　正常胆囊、弥漫性胆固醇贮积病和胆固醇息肉的示意图。注意富含脂质的泡沫样巨噬细胞在弥漫性胆固醇贮积病和胆固醇息肉中的分布。弥漫性胆固醇贮积病（中间图；另见图 67.3）占病例的 80%，一般无症状。胆固醇息肉（右图）见于 10% 的胆固醇贮积病病例，是典型的小而易碎的赘生物，有溃疡或自发从黏膜上脱落的倾向。弥漫性胆固醇贮积病合并胆固醇息肉占病例的 10%。尽管通常无症状，但这些息肉与胆源性疼痛甚至急性胰腺炎相关

性。性别差异在60岁以后不明显。如果类比于胆固醇结石，西方国家的患病率更高，但是目前尚无种族、民族或地理上的差异。肥胖可能是危险因素，减肥手术切除的胆囊中有38%存在胆固醇贮积病[71]。

（三）病理学

胆固醇贮积病的病理学定义是胆囊黏膜内脂质（胆固醇酯和甘油三酯）的沉积。脂质沉积的4种类型如下[66]：

弥漫性：脂质分布于除胆囊管之外的整个胆囊上皮。这种类型占80%。

胆固醇息肉：多余的脂质局限于上皮的一个或多个区域，最终形成突入胆囊腔内的赘生物。孤立性胆固醇息肉占10%。

弥漫性胆固醇沉积合并胆固醇息肉：弥漫性胆固醇沉积的背景下出现胆固醇息肉。这种类型占10%。

局灶性胆固醇沉积：过多的脂质沉积局限于黏膜的一小片区域。

1. 大体标本观察

当开腹或腹腔镜检查胆囊时，20%的病例可依据半透明的胆囊浆膜诊断胆固醇贮积病。切开胆囊后观察黏膜有淡黄色线状纵向条纹，呈现为“草莓样胆囊”（黏膜是胆汁样颜色而不是红色）。在手术切除胆囊诊断胆固醇贮积病时，50%的病例中也发现胆结石。如果在尸检时诊断胆固醇贮积病，只有10%发现结石[68]，表明这是相互独立的两种疾病。

2. 显微镜下观察

无一例外均有黏膜增生，50%的病例中有明显的增生表现。增生为绒毛状，显著特征是细长的绒毛内有大量巨噬细胞，每个巨噬细胞都充满脂滴，具有泡沫细胞的特征性外观（图67.3）。在轻症中泡沫细胞限于绒毛的尖端（肉眼观察时所见的线状条纹），严重时泡沫细胞充满整个绒毛并溢出到黏膜下层。细胞外脂质沉积很少见，胆汁中偶见黄色的细小颗粒（脂质小体）是游离的泡沫细胞团。

（四）发病机制

胆固醇酯和甘油三酯沉积的原因尚不清楚[72]。一个假说是胆固醇来源于血液[73]或机械因素阻碍胆囊排空导致的脂质局部沉积[74]。胆囊上皮在组织胚胎学上类似于肠道吸收细胞，能从胆汁中吸收胆固醇[75,76]。胆囊胆汁中的胆固醇处于吸收的理想物理状态（混合胶束）。但问题在于为什么再吸收的胆汁胆固醇被酯化，然后以胆固醇沉积的形式储存在泡沫巨噬细胞中[77]。同胆固醇结石一样，胆固醇贮积病多见于胆汁中胆固醇过饱和的胆囊[78]。胆固醇异常沉积的两种疾病（胆固醇贮积病和结石）可能有共同的致病机制（如异常胆汁的分泌），但是在患者中常各自独立进展，这取决于其他因素，如胆汁中成核蛋白的存在和胆固醇的黏膜酯化率[79]。胆固醇贮积病与血清胆固醇水平升高无关[70]。

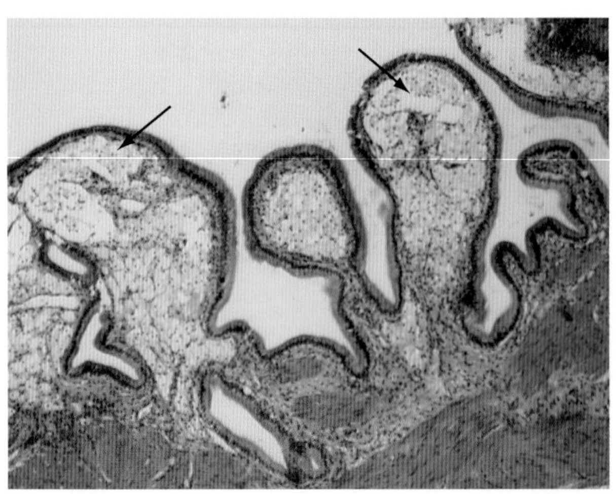

图67.3　弥漫性胆固醇贮积病的组织病理学。注意增生、细长的绒毛和泡沫状巨噬细胞（箭）（HE染色）。（Courtesy Pamela Jensen，MD，Dallas，TX.）

（五）临床特征

从未有胆道症状的患者在尸检时却容易发现胆固醇贮积病，这表明此类疾病一般没有临床表现。个别患者有类似于胆源性疼痛的右上腹或上腹钝痛或隐痛，在胆囊切除术后诊断为胆固醇贮积病，而不是结石或胆囊炎。在接受胆囊切除术的非结石性胆源性疼痛患者中，病理发现胆固醇贮积病的患者疼痛缓解的可能性高于非胆固醇贮积病患者[9]。

一项回顾性研究分析了近4 000例手术切除的胆囊标本，55例为非结石性胆固醇贮积病[80]。研究发现近一半的胆固醇贮积病出现原因不明的复发性胰腺炎，推测微小的胆固醇息肉脱离胆囊壁，短暂阻塞Oddi括约肌，从而引发急性胰腺炎。在术后随访5年，胰腺炎未复发。相关研究人员[81,82]建议在特发性胰腺炎的鉴别诊断中应考虑胆固醇贮积病（具体地说是胆固醇息肉）。一项纳入6 868例胆囊切除术的回顾性研究对此提出了质疑，18%（1 053例）有胆固醇贮积病，在排除胆结石后没有患者出现胰腺炎[83]。

（六）诊断

超声或胆囊造影很难发现弥漫性胆固醇沉积（如前述，占80%）。较大息肉的超声表现是胆囊腔内单一或多个固定的无阴影的回声[84]。多数息肉很小（2～10mm）。EUS能准确识别胆固醇息肉，表现为特征性高回声点状聚集[85]。在胆囊造影中，息肉表现为在不透明的胆囊腔内那些小而圆的透明，在胆囊部分排空和压迫腹部后最明显。

（七）治疗

胆囊切除术前难以诊断胆固醇贮积病，一般无需治疗。少数由超声或胆囊造影诊断的息肉样胆固醇贮积病，没有胆道症状的话也不需要干预。如果患者出现胆源性疼痛或胰腺炎，需要胆囊切除术[80]。目前没有治疗胆固醇贮积病的药物。

四、腺肌瘤病

（一）定义

胆囊腺肌瘤病（一个含义模糊的术语）是一种获得性的增生性病变，特征是表面上皮过度生长凹入增厚的肌层，甚至更深[86]。文献有许多不同的术语，最常见的是腺肌瘤（病变局限于胆囊底部）、Rokitansky-Aschoff窦（多见，但在解剖学上不准确）和腺肌症[87]。该病变是良性的，与胃肠道其他部位的腺瘤上皮无关。单纯的腺肌瘤病没有恶变倾向。

（二）流行病学

因诊断标准的不同和是否检查切除的或尸检的胆囊标本，胆囊腺肌瘤病的患病率有很大差异。一项大规模研究纳入了超过 10 000 例的胆囊切除术后标本，Shepard 和同事[88] 仅发现 103 例腺肌瘤病，发病率约为 1%。女性多于男性，比例为 3∶1，发病率随年龄增加而上升。没有种族和地理的流行病学差异。

（三）病理学

回顾胆囊和 Rokitansky-Aschoff 窦的正常组织学结构有助于理解腺肌瘤病的病理（图 67.4）。与小肠不同，胆囊没有黏膜肌层，固有层直接毗邻肌层。在儿童时期，上皮层形成皱褶，由固有层支撑。随着年龄的增长，上皮层的凹陷可能会深入到肌层，形成 Rokitansky-Aschoff 窦。切除的胆囊中约 90% 有这种获得性病变[86]。若 Rokitansky-Aschoff 窦深入呈分支状并伴有肌层增厚（肥大），则诊断为腺肌瘤病。Rokitansky-Aschoff 窦破裂是罕见的黄色肉芽肿性胆囊炎的病理学基础，胆囊参与了含脂巨噬细胞的炎症过程（见第 65 章）。

1. 大体标本观察

胆囊腺肌瘤病可累及整个胆囊（弥漫型或广泛型腺肌瘤病），更常见的是局限于胆囊底部（多称为腺肌瘤）。罕见的情况是局限于胆囊壁的一个环形节段（节段型腺肌瘤病），引起管腔狭窄和哑铃状胆囊（图 67.5）。胆囊壁受累部分会增厚至

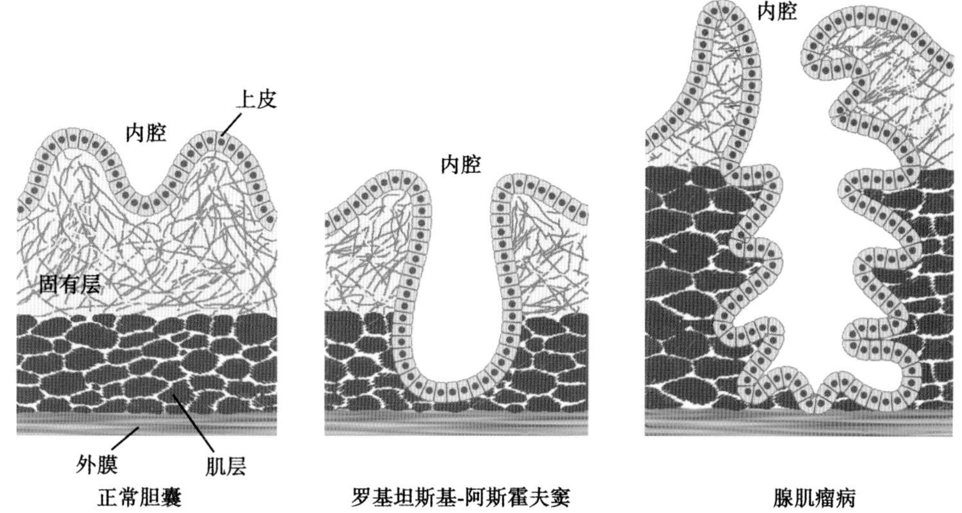

图 67.4　正常胆囊、Rokitansky-Aschoff 窦和腺肌瘤病。约 90% 的切除胆囊中存在 Rokitansky-Aschoff 窦，由上皮内陷到肌肉层形成微小的壁内憩室组成。它们本身没有临床意义。腺肌瘤病的组织学诊断要求 Rokitansky-Aschoff 窦较深，呈分支状，伴有肌肉层肥大

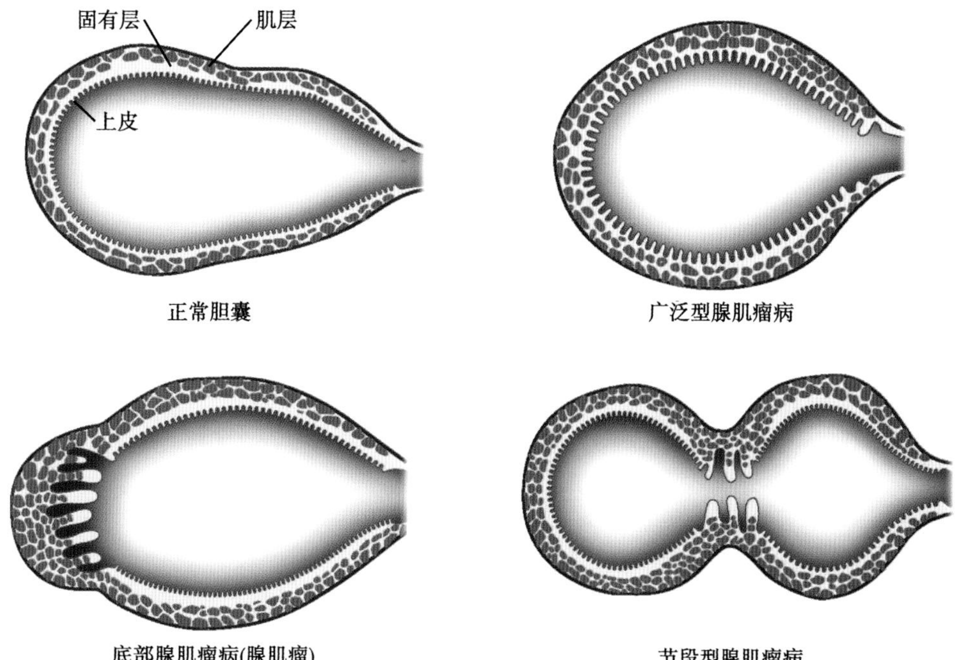

图 67.5　腺肌瘤病不同类型的示意图。大多数病例局限于胆囊底部（在这种情况下，病变被称为腺肌瘤），广泛型和节段型少见，腺肌瘤直径通常为 10～20mm，主要局限于壁内或也可突入腔内形成息肉状病变

10mm 以上，肌层是正常厚度的 3～5 倍。切面观察 Rokitansky-Aschoff 窦有明显的囊性扩张，可能充满色素碎片或结石。

2. 显微镜下观察

肌层增生，上皮内偶有肠化生，多伴有轻度慢性炎症。

（四）发病机制

腺肌瘤病的发病机制尚不清楚。机械性梗阻（如结石、胆囊管扭结、先天性隔膜）引起胆囊腔内压力增加，导致 Rokitansky-Aschoff 窦囊性扩张，之后出现肌层增生和腺肌瘤病[86]。与结肠憩室一样，Rokitansky-Aschoff 窦好发于肌层最薄弱的地方（穿支血管的部位）。然而并不都能有胆囊流出道梗阻的证据，只有 60% 的腺肌瘤病有结石[88]。一些研究者认为腺肌瘤病是慢性炎症的结果，同样炎症也并不一直存在，尤其是病变局限于底部时[89]。另一些研究者观察到腺肌瘤病与胰胆管汇流异常有关（见第 55 章和第 62 章）。在一项研究中，一半的腺肌瘤病合并胰胆管异常汇合[90]，在另一项研究中，三分之一的胰胆管汇流异常合并腺肌瘤病[91]。这两种特殊疾病在发病机制上的联系尚不明确。

（五）临床特征

同胆固醇贮积病一样，腺肌瘤病多没有症状，通常在尸检或手术切除时偶然发现。如前所述，在胆囊切除后发现腺肌瘤病的病例中，一半以上存在胆结石，这部分病例的症状可以归因于结石。非结石性腺肌瘤病引起的症状与胆石症相关的胆源性疼痛较易区分。

在极少数情况下，胆囊腺癌与腺肌瘤病相关（图 67.6）[92]，但是恶性肿瘤往往远离腺肌瘤病的区域，因此可能是巧合而不是因果。然而，一些腺肌瘤病所在的胆囊部位出现胆囊腺癌的病例报道造成了超声或胆囊造影的诊断不确定性[93]。一项回顾性研究分析了 3 000 多个切除的胆囊标本，结果显示伴节段型腺肌瘤病的胆囊发生胆囊癌的频率（6.4%）明显高于偶发。研究者建议应将节段型腺肌瘤病考虑为潜在的癌前病变[94]。对节段型腺肌瘤病伴胆囊癌的二次回顾研究显示从增生到恶变的标本在细胞学上有一系列的异型性，这提示存在肿瘤进展的过程[95]。

偶然发现的单纯的胆囊腺肌瘤多为良性。如果怀疑伴有肿块性病变（特别是>10mm 或节段型腺肌瘤），必须对胆囊进行充分的影像学检查，同时考虑胆囊切除术。

（六）诊断

如前所述，多在胆囊切除和胆囊的直接检查之后才能诊断腺肌瘤病。如果存在一些特定的放射学和超声的表现，也能作出术前诊断。

在胆囊造影中（见第 65 章），构成 Rokitansky-Aschoff 窦的壁内憩室可能充满造影剂，并产生特征性的不透光点，平行于胆囊腔的边缘[96]。局限性的底部腺肌瘤病（腺肌瘤）表现为底部的充盈缺损，节段型腺肌瘤病表现为胆囊腔环周性狭窄（图 67.7）。与胆固醇贮积病一样，检查时胆囊排空部分造影剂同时适当按压利于腺肌瘤病的放射学成像[96]。

超声在评估胆囊方面基本取代胆囊造影，但是对于腺肌瘤病的诊断缺乏特异性。胆囊壁增厚（>4mm）不是腺肌瘤病的特异性表现，也见于许多其他疾病（如肝病伴腹水）[97]。对腺肌瘤病的放射学、超声以及病理学的研究发现胆囊壁的弥漫性或节段性增厚伴壁内憩室（圆形无回声灶）能准确预测腺肌瘤病[98]。如果壁内憩室（扩张的 Rokitansky-Aschoff 窦）充满胆泥或微小结石，病变可能出现回声伴声影或混合伪影[99]。超声造影对腺肌瘤病有较好的敏感性[100]。EUS 表现为多发微囊肿，是 Rokitansky-Aschoff 窦扩大之后的特征性表现[85]。腺肌瘤病在 CT 和 MRI 上的表现包括胆囊壁层不同程度地增强[101]、在增厚的胆囊壁内发现 Rokitansky-Aschoff 窦[102]以及浆膜下脂肪增生[103]。一项研究纳入了 20 例手术证实为腺肌瘤病的患者，在术前接受了超声、螺旋 CT 和 MRI 检查，这 3 种诊断方法的准确率分别为 66%、75% 和 93%[104]。对于诊断不确定的患者，MRI 是鉴别腺肌瘤病与胆囊恶性病变的最准确手段[105]。在一个病例报告中，无癌症组织学证据的腺肌瘤病造成了 18-氟脱氧葡萄糖 PET 假阳性，原因可能和相关的炎症活动有关[106]。

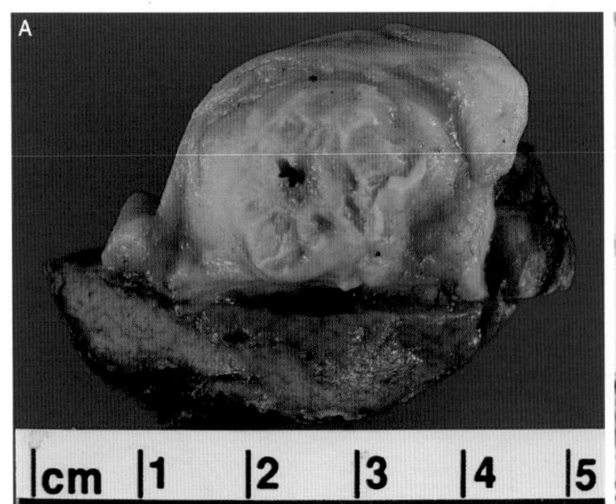

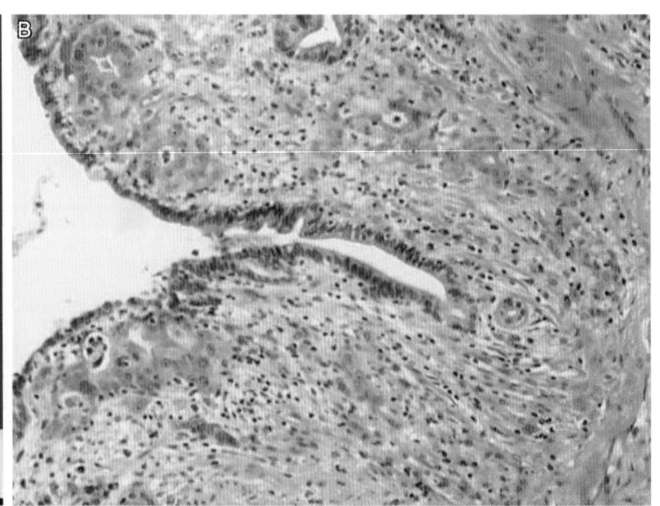

图 67.6　A，胆囊腺肌瘤病合并腺癌的大体病理学表现；B，组织病理显示胆囊中分化腺癌破坏腺肌瘤病的黏膜（HE 染色）。（Courtesy Aviva Hopkowitz，MD，Dallas，TX.）

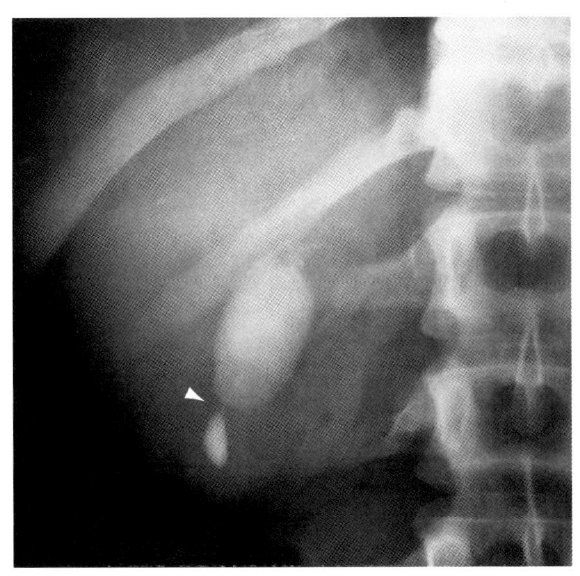

图 67.7　口服胆囊造影显示 28 岁男性餐后上腹痛放射至背部的节段性腺肌瘤病。该胶片显示了与腺肌瘤病相关的胆囊壁环形节段(箭头),其导致管腔收缩。尽管不存在胆结石,但进行了胆囊切除术,患者的症状得到缓解。(Courtesy W. J. Kilman, MD, Dallas, TX.)

(七) 治疗

腺肌瘤病在没有胆道症状时不需要治疗。如果患者出现胆源性疼痛,放射或超声检查提示腺肌瘤病合并结石,需要行胆囊切除术。棘手的临床情况是患者有临床症状,怀疑是腺肌瘤病却没有结石[93]。此时,腺肌瘤病范围越广泛或表现越严重,症状越可能与胆囊病变有关,患者将受益于胆囊切除术。除非影像学显示可能有肿块或节段型腺肌瘤病,否则担心恶变不是手术的理由。

五、胆囊息肉

(一) 定义

"胆囊息肉"用于描述胆囊腔内的黏膜突起[107]。大部分胆囊息肉由脂质沉积或炎症所致,而不是肿瘤。虽然缺少能明确息肉性质的组织学证据,但是临床医生需要根据息肉的影像学表现、患者的特点和症状等间接信息来判断息肉是否为恶性以及是否需要切除胆囊。

(二) 流行病学

胆囊息肉的发生率(基于病理学或影像学的定义)为1%~4%[108],在某些人群中可能高达 5%~10%。胆囊息肉通常在胆囊切除术时偶然发现,随着影像学检查的广泛应用,胆囊息肉的诊断也日益增多。

(三) 病理学

如表 67.3 所示,胆囊息肉分为非肿瘤性息肉(占所有胆囊息肉的 95%)或肿瘤性息肉[109]。

表 67.3　胆囊息肉的类型

组织学类型	相对发生率/%	肿瘤性	大小/mm	息肉数目	注解
胆固醇息肉(胆固醇贮积病的息肉样形式)	60	否	2~10	多发(均数为 8)	可能相互分离,临床表现同胆结石一样,可能引起胆源性疼痛、胆管梗阻或胰腺炎 若患者无临床表现,不需要手术
腺肌瘤(腺肌瘤病的局限形式)	25	否	10~20	1	常局限于胆囊底部,呈半球形突入腔内,大部分局限于肌壁 若患者有临床症状或不能排除肿瘤,需要手术
炎性息肉	10	否	5~10	50%病例为 1;50%病例为 2~5	由肉芽组织和纤维组织组成,伴随淋巴细胞和浆细胞浸润固有层 不需要手术
腺瘤	4	是	5~20	三分之二病例为 1,三分之一病例为 2~5	罕见,仅见于 0.15%切除的胆囊 通常有蒂,一半的病例伴有结石 胆囊内唯一具有癌前病变可能性的息肉;从腺瘤发展为癌的概率比结肠息肉要低得多 癌变的腺瘤直径都大于 12mm,小于 10mm 的可以超声随访 大小为 10~18mm 的息肉,腹腔镜胆囊切除术是最好的手术选择 大于 18mm 的息肉,应开腹而不做腹腔镜胆囊切除术,浸润性癌可能性大,可能需要扩大切除
混杂肿瘤	<1	是	5~20	1	罕见(见正文),息肉的发生率<0.10%

1. 胆固醇息肉

胆固醇息肉是胆囊息肉最常见的类型，也是含脂泡沫状巨噬细胞浸润固有层引起的胆固醇贮积病的一个亚型。胆固醇息肉的发病机制见胆固醇贮积病的章节（见前文）。胆固醇息肉通常很小（直径<10mm），是通过一根薄而质脆的柄附于黏膜的带蒂息肉[109]。在手术切开胆囊时，经常会发现游离的微小胆固醇息肉漂浮在胆汁中[110]。虽然在 20% 的病例中可能是单发的，但在一个病例系列研究中胆固醇息肉的平均数目是 8[111]。多发息肉一般是胆固醇息肉，预示为良性。

2. 腺肌瘤

位于胆囊底部的胆囊腺肌瘤病可表现为突入腔内的半球形隆起，类似息肉。这种病变称为腺肌瘤，但不是肿瘤性病变。腺肌瘤的发病机制见"腺肌瘤病"一节（见前文）。病变的大小通常约为 15mm，局限于胆囊的肌层[109]。

3. 炎性息肉

炎性息肉是由淋巴细胞和浆细胞浸润形成肉芽组织或纤维组织组成的微小固定病变。平均 5～10mm。50% 为单发息肉，其余为 2～5 个[109]。几乎都是在胆囊切除时偶然发现炎性息肉。

4. 腺瘤

胃肠道的腺瘤性息肉非常多见，但是胆囊腺瘤很少见，在切除的胆囊标本中仅有 0.15% 左右的发生率[112]。

腺瘤的典型表现是单发、带蒂的息肉，直径在 5～20mm，可出现在胆囊的任何部位。当为多发息肉，约三分之一的病例有 2～5 个息肉。在组织学上分为乳头状和非乳头状。前者由高柱状上皮细胞覆盖的分枝状的结缔组织组成，后者由纤维间质包裹的腺体增生组成。在极少数情况下，整个胆囊黏膜会发生腺瘤化改变，出现无数微小的黏膜息肉，称为多中心乳头状瘤病。值得注意的是，一半的腺瘤性息肉病例会出现胆结石[109]。

不同于在结肠中腺瘤多于腺癌，在胆囊中腺瘤比癌更少见（比例为 1∶4）。从腺瘤发展为腺癌的概率尚不明确。在日本 1 600 多例的胆囊切除术中，18 例发现胆囊腺瘤[113]，其中 7 个腺瘤含有癌性病灶。79 例发现浸润性癌，15（19%）例在癌组织内发现残留的腺瘤组织，这提示最初的病变可能是腺瘤。值得注意的是，所有包含癌性病灶的腺瘤都大于 12mm，提示大的腺瘤可能是癌前病变。

5. 混杂息肉

虽然各种各样的良性病变都可能表现为胆囊息肉，但是这些病变比较少见。纤维瘤、平滑肌瘤和脂肪瘤在胃肠道其他部位很常见，然而在胆囊中罕见。神经纤维瘤、类癌[114]和胃腺体异位更少见[115]。总的来说，胆囊非腺瘤性肿瘤性息肉的发生率低于 1/1 000[109]。

（四）临床特征和诊断

胆囊息肉一般不会引起症状，通常在因结石行胆囊切除术或因其他适应证行影像学检查偶然发现。在特殊情况下，息肉（没有胆结石）会由于症状而经超声或放射学检查诊断。这些临床症状类似于胆源性疼痛，但是可能缺乏典型的表现（例如剧烈的、突发的上腹或右上腹痛，在 15 分钟内逐渐加重，持续数小时后慢慢缓解）。良性胆囊息肉会造成急性非结石性胆囊炎或胆道出血，但相对罕见[116]。

超声诊断胆囊息肉的准确率一般为 80%，没有胆结石时准确率更高。然而，在经超声诊断为胆囊息肉的患者中，三分之一在胆囊切除术时没有发现息肉。一项研究纳入了 213 例超声检查怀疑胆囊肿瘤而行胆囊切除术的患者，83% 的影像学上≤5mm 的病变在病理检查中并不存在[117]。

胆囊息肉的组织学类型不能仅依据临床加以区分。超声和胆囊造影也不能准确预测组织学类型（图 67.8）[97]。虽然经腹超声对息肉的敏感性高达 80%，但对息肉类型的准确性低至 20%[118,119]。EUS 是诊断胆囊息肉更为敏感和特异的方法。一项比较经腹超声与 EUS 的研究发现 EUS 鉴别息肉类型的准确率超过 90%[120]。多项研究表明一种包含息肉的大小、数目、形状、回声和息肉边界的 EUS 评分系统能预测胆囊息肉的肿瘤风险，EUS 的彩色多普勒血流也可预测恶性肿瘤[120-123]。术前用 18 氟脱氧葡萄糖 PET 准确预测胆囊息肉患者存在胆囊恶性肿瘤的情况也有病例报告[124]。

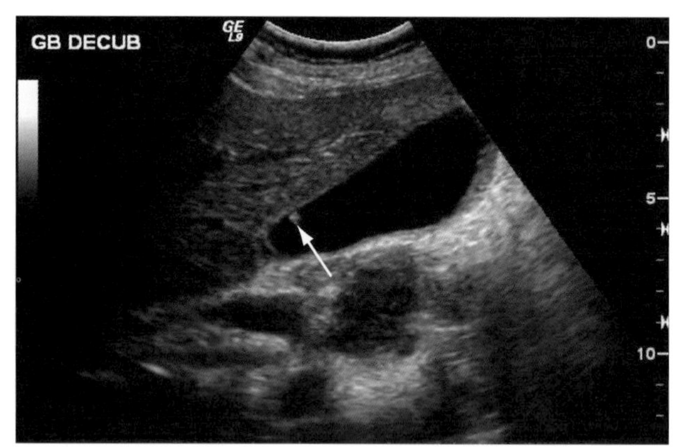

图 67.8　超声检查（右纵向视图）显示胆囊息肉。1 例 55 岁女性患轻度胆源性疼痛。超声显示 4mm 管腔的充盈缺损（如箭所示），其后无声影，固定于胆囊壁上。这些发现与胆囊息肉一致，尽管组织学不能从超声图预测。胆囊切除术后发现有多发性胆固醇息肉，其中一个异常大。（Courtesy R. S. Harrell, MD, Dallas, TX.）

其他研究评估了恶性肿瘤的临床和影像学预测因素。除息肉大小（>10mm）以外，年龄超过 60 岁是肿瘤的最强预测因素。并发胆结石也有较高的恶性肿瘤风险[125]。单发息肉和有症状的息肉比多发息肉和无症状息肉更有可能是恶性。

（五）自然史

一些探讨未经治疗的胆囊息肉的自然史的研究表明大多数息肉属于良性，可以采用"观察和等待"的方法[126]。一项来自 Mayo Cinic 的研究，纳入了约 200 名胆囊造影显示为胆囊息肉但是没有随即行胆囊切除术的患者[127]。经过 15 年的随访，只有不到 10% 的患者出现需要手术治疗的症状，均没有胆囊癌。

一项研究在 5 年内对 109 例息肉小于 10mm 的患者进行每年或半年一次的超声检查。在此期间，没有患者发生胆囊癌，超过 88% 的患者没有出现息肉的增长[128]。

另一项研究纳入 224 例胆囊息肉患者，其中 95% 在超声检查中预测是胆固醇息肉,其余的是"不确定的良性息肉样病变"[129]。经过平均 9 个月的随访,所有最初是良性的息肉没有变化或者在胆囊切除术后证实为良性。三分之二的不确定的良性息肉样病变在胆囊切除后证实是腺瘤或癌。这些结果表明大多数胆囊息肉是良性的,高风险息肉通常有一个可识别的特征,如较大的体积。

其他研究表明以直径 10mm 作为胆囊切除术临界值可能过高,起初大小为 6~9mm 的息肉很少出现胆囊癌前病变或恶性病变[130,131]。一项来自中国的研究纳入了 1 446 名经超声检查发现息肉并随后行胆囊切除术的患者,然后分析了恶性肿瘤的预测因素[132]。该研究中息肉类型的发生率为:胆固醇息肉占 87.1%,良性非胆固醇息肉 11.2%,恶性息肉 1.7%。大多数良性非胆固醇息肉为腺瘤,超过一半的息肉小于 10mm。研究发现年龄超过 50 岁、存在临床症状、大于 10mm 和胆结石是恶性息肉的独立预测因素。虽然有 8mm 的单发息肉为恶性息肉,但是大多数恶性息肉(83%)大于 15mm。这些数据表明有症状的大息肉,尤其在合并胆结石时,应行胆囊切除术。然而,应用这些数据在低风险人群中治疗小的、无症状的息肉比较困难。研究建议对于无高危特征的息肉定期进行 5 年的影像学随访,根据息肉大小确定检查的频率。

另一项大规模研究纳入 1 204 例经影像学检查诊断为胆囊息肉的患者,在诊断之后接受胆囊切除术($n=194$)或随访($n=1\,010$)[133]。息肉平均大小为 6.9mm。在 2 年的随访中,28% 的患者出现息肉增长。恶性息肉明显大于良性病变,平均大小分别为 27.5mm 和 12.3mm。值得注意的是,恶性息肉中有 5% 只有 3~5mm,8% 为 5~10mm。研究的结论是手术是 3~10mm 息肉的最终治疗方法。但是在本研究中患者是根据风险选择手术的,如息肉增长或怀疑恶性。因此预计到相对较高的恶性风险,在该研究中 20% 为恶性。这项研究也包括有症状的患者和胆结石患者,所以可能存在其他已知的恶性肿瘤风险预测因素和胆囊切除术的指征。

(六) 治疗

有胆源性疼痛以及胆囊息肉和结石的患者应行择期胆囊切除术。对于没有并发胆结石的胆囊息肉,如何决定更为复杂。对于这些患者来说,手术取决于症状的严重程度、症状是否源于胆道以及息肉的超声表现(特别是大小)。

由于 10mm 或更大的息肉发生癌变的可能性更大,对于这种大小的无症状息肉,拟行手术的患者可考虑择期腹腔镜胆囊切除术[134-136],低风险的患者可以定期超声检查监测息肉大小(每 6 个月一次)或者 EUS 进一步检查[134,136]。大于 18mm 的息肉有很高的恶性风险,如有可能应及时行胆囊切除术。一项研究发现这种大小的病变可能为累及胆囊浆膜的晚期浸润性癌,需要比腹腔镜更广泛的手术范围[137]。因此,研究者建议对于这些胆囊大息肉样病变采用开腹胆囊切除术。

如何处理 6~9mm 的息肉存在争议。在这些低风险人群中,定期监测息肉的生长或变化是明智的。有研究建议在首次发现这种息肉之后 3~6 个月行腹部超声检查,排除快速增长的肿瘤,然后每隔 6~12 个月检查。监测的最佳持续时间尚不明确。鉴于体积小却有肿瘤的风险,其他研究建议对这种大小的息肉行胆囊切除术,但这种方法比较激进[138,139]。

现在许多专家建议对于小于 6mm 的无症状息肉无需常规监测,因为这种大小的息肉在大规模研究中证实是良性[139]。过去专家曾建议所有<10mm 的息肉在诊断之后 6~12 个月复查,然后每隔 6~12 个月复查 1~2 年,以确认息肉大小是否变化[140]。更保守的放射学指南建议监测 5 年,6~9mm 的息肉每年复查,小于 6mm 的息肉在 1 年、3 年和 5 年复查[141]。

胆囊息肉监测的最佳方式需要明确。英国的一项成本效益分析报告称每 6 个月对所有胆囊息肉进行一次超声检查,20 年的费用估计为 970 万美元。假设所有的肿瘤性息肉都变成恶性(这一过程尚未得到充分证明),超声检查每年可能会挽救约 5.4 个生命。鉴于胆囊癌的罕见性,对全部胆囊息肉进行监测的费用可能不合理。将范围限制在 5~10mm 的息肉可能会提高成本效益[142]。

对于胆囊小息肉的随访不适用于 PSC,在 PSC 中胆囊息肉样病变的恶性风险高达 60%(见第 68 章)。在这一高危人群中,小于 10mm 的息肉建议胆囊切除术。

(刘文正　闫秀娥 译,黄永辉 校)

参考文献

第 68 章　原发性和继发性硬化性胆管炎

Cynthia Levy, Christopher L. Bowlus 著

章节目录

一、原发性硬化性胆管炎 ………………………………… 1005

（一）流行病学 ………………………………………… 1005

（二）病因和发病机制 ………………………………… 1005

（三）临床、实验室和影像学特征 …………………… 1008

（四）诊断 ……………………………………………… 1011

（五）鉴别诊断 ………………………………………… 1012

（六）自然史和预后模型 ……………………………… 1012

（七）并发症 …………………………………………… 1014

（八）治疗 ……………………………………………… 1016

二、继发性硬化性胆管炎 ………………………………… 1019

（一）IgG4 相关性硬化性胆管炎 …………………… 1019

（二）复发性化脓性胆管炎 …………………………… 1019

硬化性胆管炎是一种胆汁淤积性疾病，特征为慢性的肝内外胆管的局部炎症、纤维化和破坏。呈现慢性、进行性进展的过程，而持续性胆管损伤可导致胆管梗阻、胆汁性肝硬化和肝功能衰竭以及相关的并发症。Delbet 于 1924 年首次报道了硬化性胆管炎[1]，多年来都被视为一种罕见疾病，但是在 20 世纪 70 年代内镜逆行胰胆管造影（ERCP）以及磁共振胆管成像（MRC）技术的出现提高对硬化性胆管炎真实发病率的认识，也促进了对自然病程的研究。但是，硬化性胆管炎的很多方面仍是未知的，最为明显的是缺乏对病因的详细认识和明确有效的药物治疗方案。

许多不同的疾病在胆管造影时有“硬化性胆管炎”的表现，即胆管系统弥漫性狭窄和节段性扩张。这种征象在原发性硬化性胆管炎（primary Sclerosing Cholangitis，PSC）中最为典型，这是一种经常与炎症性肠病（IBD，包括溃疡性结肠炎或克罗恩病）相关的疾病。PSC 也可能与各种纤维化、自身免疫性和浸润性疾病有关，不过这些关联是否意味着共同的发病机制或者表象尚不清楚。继发性硬化性胆管炎（secondary sclerosing cholangitis，SSC）指的是一种因已知疾病或损伤引起的类似于 PSC 的综合征（表 68.1）。

表 68.1　继发性硬化性胆管炎的原因

儿科	良性	恶性
胆道闭锁	自身炎症性疾病	壶腹癌
囊性纤维变性（CF）	嗜酸性胆管炎	胆管癌
先天性胆管异常	肥大细胞胆管炎	胆囊癌
组织细胞增生症 X	结节病	肝细胞癌
鱼鳞病合并硬化性胆管炎	医源性胆管损伤	淋巴瘤
新生儿硬化性胆管炎	胆囊切除术	转移癌
原发性和继发性免疫缺陷	肝移植（吻合口和非吻合口狭窄）	胰腺癌
家族性进行性肝内胆汁淤积 3 型	感染性	
镰状细胞病	AIDS 胆管病	
	复发性化脓性胆管炎	
	血管性	
	动脉内化疗	
	缺血性胆管病	
	门脉高压性胆道病	
	血管炎	
	其他	
	胆管炎性假瘤	
	胆石症（Mirizzi 综合征）	
	慢性胰腺炎	

一、原发性硬化性胆管炎

PSC 起初认为是肝外胆管的“闭塞性胆管炎”，伴有胆管壁的弥漫增厚和管腔狭窄[2]，好发于 30~40 岁之间的男性，并且与溃疡性结肠炎密切相关。但是随着不同临床情况下不同亚型的出现，PSC 表现出越来越多的特征。经典的 PSC，如今多称为“大胆管型 PSC”，多见于男性（男女比例为 3∶2），60%~80% 的病例与 IBD 并存，典型的表现为胆汁淤积。典型的 IBD 是一种轻度的无症状且伴有回肠炎的全结肠炎，但直肠不受累。尽管在北半球 PSC 与 IBD 之间的相关性似乎更大，但是无 IBD 的 PSC 也在增加。大胆管型 PSC 的自然史从快。速恶化到缓慢发展均有。据报道，该类患者在无肝移植的情况下的平均生存期为 12 年（早期报道）至 20 多年[3-5]。大胆管型 PSC 最为常见，也是研究最为深入的一个类型，与 HLAA*01、B*08、DRB1*03 单倍型之间存在密切相关性。

“小胆管型 PSC”的患者较少，他们的临床表现、生化和组织学特征与 PSC 相符，但缺乏 PSC 典型的胆管造影表现。小胆管型 PSC 在所有 PSC 中的比例在 5%~20%[6-9]。在一些情况下，诊断需要同时合并有 IBD。在 HLA 单倍型方面，不伴 IBD 的小胆管型 PSC 与大胆管型 PSC 相比存在差异，这说明两者本质不同[10]。在过去，这部分的患者归类为 AMA 阴性的原发性胆汁性肝硬化（PBC）或者自身免疫性胆管病。在 3 项对小胆管型 PSC 的长期随访研究中，12% 至 17% 的患者进展为经典的大胆管型 PSC[6-8]。在 63~126 个月的中位随访期内，患者均未出现胆管癌，并且小胆管型 PSC 组的生存期也优于经典 PSC 对照组[6-8]。

根据诊断标准的不同，1%~53.8% 的 PSC 可能会与自身免疫性肝炎（Autoimmune hepatitis，AIH）相重叠。使用 AIH 诊断的标准化评分系统（见第 90 章），7.5% 的 PSC 是“确诊”或“疑似”AIH，但是 PSC-AIH 重叠综合征的诊断标准未能达成共识[11,12]。这些患者可能表现为血清转氨酶水平显著升高，组织学也与 AIH 一致，或者表现为典型的 AIH，之后随着硬化性胆管炎的发展而出现胆汁淤积。在某些病例中，免疫抑制剂治疗可能对 PSC-AIH 重叠综合征有效。重要的是，包括抗核抗体（ANA）和平滑肌抗体（Smooth muscle antibodies，SMA）在内的自身抗体多见于不合并 AIH 的 PSC。此外，在 MRC 检查中 10% 或以上的 AIH 可能具有与 PSC 相一致的胆管成像特征[13,14]。

需要重点关注的群体为儿童和非高加索人种的 PSC 患者。儿童 PSC 与成人 PSC 有许多相同的特征，即男性占优势和与 IBD 密切相关[10]。然而，儿童 PSC 似乎对药物治疗更敏感（见下文），与 AIH 的重叠率更高，有时称为“自身免疫性硬化性胆管炎”[15]。大多数 PSC 的研究在北欧人群或北欧后裔人群中进行，导致 PSC 被认定是一种高加索人的疾病。然而，非裔美国人 PSC 的发病率和患病率至少与高加索人一样高[16-18]。在非裔美国人中，男性的优势不那么明显而且 IBD 的发病率较低。尽管 HLA-B8 与 PSC 的相关性均见于高加索人和非裔美国人，HLA-DR3 与 PSC 的相关性却只见于欧洲人，少见于非裔美国人[17]。

（一）流行病学

PSC 的临床表现复杂而且诊断标准各异，许多发表的研究本身存在转诊偏倚，因此 PSC 的真实的发病率和患病率很难确定。大型队列研究的数据显示在北美和北欧地区，PSC 的年发病率约为 1/100 000~1.5/100 000，年患病率约为 6/100 000~16/100 000[19-21]。在世界其他地区 PSC 患病率的评估数据有限，但一般认为会较低[22]。相关研究可能低估了真实世界中 PSC 的患病率，因为早期数据是在磁共振成像（MRI）和磁共振胰胆管造影（MRCP）广泛应用之前收集的，研究基于特定人群，而且缺乏 PSC 特定的国际疾病分类代码。

尽管 PSC 可以发生在任何年龄段，但多见于 25~45 岁之间，确诊时的中位数年龄在 36~39 岁[4,5,20,23]。虽然三分之二为男性，但是性别差异在不合并 IBD 的亚组中并不明显[23]。女性在确诊 PSC 时的年龄通常大于男性。PSC 也与不吸烟有关，但是这种作用是否独立于 IBD 仍然有争议[24-26]。在女性中，咖啡和激素治疗能降低发生 PSC 的风险[27,28]。

（二）病因和发病机制

PSC 的病因和发病机制尚不清楚。遗传、环境和免疫因素可能在疾病易感性中起关键作用，疾病的进展可能取决于胆汁淤积。目前最引人注意的发病机制模型是将 PSC 视为一种在遗传易感人群中由于暴露于环境或有毒触发因素（如细菌的细胞壁产物）而诱发的免疫反应。任何关于 PSC 发病机制的理论都必须能够解释与 IBD 的密切联系、阐述肠道和肝脏之间的独特关系以及营养物质、胆汁酸和免疫细胞的作用。

1. 遗传因素

相关研究已经证实遗传因素在 PSC 发病机制中的重要性，PSC 患者兄弟姐妹的患病风险会增加 9~39 倍，并且与特定的 HLA 单倍型有关[29]。早期的研究确认了 PSC 与 HLA B8 和 DR3 之间的密切相关性，随后的研究在数千名患者全基因组相关研究的基础上发现了更多的疾病基因[30-38]。经过充分验证，已经确认了 20 多个风险基因（表 68.2），但这也仅占衡量 PSC 易感性的小部分。多数确认的位点与其他免疫介导的疾病有关，包括 UC 和 CD[35]。此外，基于 PSC 和其他免疫介导疾病之间存在重叠的遗传关联（即所谓的多效性）的假设，初步确认了 33 个基因。

虽然取得了上述进展，但是与 HLA 单倍型的关联性仍是最重要的问题。由于 HLA B8 和 DR3 在不合并 PSC 的 IBD 患者中并没有过度表达，上述的发现并不能简单地用 PSC 和 IBD 之间的相关性进行解释。随后的分子基因分型研究表明，与 PSC 关联度最强的扩展 HLA 单倍型如下[17,39-41]：

B*08:01；

DRB1*03:01-DQA1*05:01-DQB1*02:01；

DRB1*13:01-DQA1*01:03-DQB1*06:03；

DRB1*15:01-DQA1*01:02-DQB1*06:02；

DRB1*01:01-DQA1*01:01。

与预防 PSC 发生相关的单倍型包括：

DRB4*01:03-DRB1*04:01-DQA1*03-DQB1*03:02；

DRB4*01:03-DRB1*07:01-DQA1*02:01-DQB1*03:03；

DRB4*02:02-DRB1*11:01-DQA1*05:01-DQB1*03:01。

表 68.2　PSC 的风险等位基因

染色体	多态性	比值比	候选基因	参考
确认				
1	rs3748816	1.21	*TNFRSF14*,*MMEL1*	34
2	rs6720394	1.6	*BCL2L11*	31
2	rs7426056	1.3	*CD28*,*CTLA4*	35
2	rs7556897	0.85	*CCL20*	347
2	rs4676410	1.38	*GPR35*	36
3	rs3197999	1.33	*USP4*,*MST1*	35
3	rs80060485	1.44	*FOXP1*	38
4	rs17032705	1.18	*NFKB1*	347
4	rs13140464	1.3	*IL2*,*IL21*	35
6	**rs3099844** **rs2844559**	**4.8** **4.7**	***HLA-B***	30
6	rs56258221	1.23	*BACH2*	35
10	rs4147359	1.24	*IL2RA*	35
11	rs7937682	1.17	*SIK2*	35
11	rs663743	1.20	*CCDC88B*	38
12	rs11168249	1.15	*HDAC7*	35
12	rs12369214	0.85	*RFX4*,*RIC8B*	347
12	rs3184504	1.18	*SH2B3*,*ATXN2*	35
16	rs725613	1.20	*CLEC16A*	38
16	rs11649613	1.19	*CLEC16A*	357
18	rs1452787	0.75	*TCF4*	36
18	rs1788097	1.15	*CD226*	35
19	rs60652743	1.25	*PRKD2*,*STRN4*	35
21	rs1893592	1.22	*UBASH3A*	38
21	rs2836883	1.28	*PSMG1*	35
可能				
2	rs7608910	1.12	*PUS10*	38
2	rs11676348	1.14	*TGR5*,*CXCR2*	38
8	rs2042011	0.92	*RN7SKP226*	38
10	rs2497318	0.01	*EIF2S2P3*	38
10	rs10748781	1.13	*NKX2-3*	38
11	rs559928	0.88	–	38
16	rs7404095	0.91	*PRKCB*	38
18	rs12968719	1.12	*PTPN2*	38
19	rs679574	1.10	*FUT2*	38

*最重要的多态性用粗体显示。
PSC,原发性硬化性胆管炎。

仅在合并 IBD 的患者中,HLA-B*08 和 DRB1*13:01 与小胆管型 PSC 相关,这提示小胆管型 PSC 和大胆管型 PSC 之间存在遗传相关性[10]。然而,包括 HLA-B*07 和 HLA-DRB1*15 在内的 HLA 却仅仅只和与免疫球蛋白(Ig)G4 升高的 PSC 患者之间存在密切相关性[42]。

在 PSC 中识别致病基因或与 HLA 相关的致病基因仍是很大的挑战。该区域的精细定位和变异对 HLA-DR 多肽结合槽的影响的模型表明,HLA-DR β 链上 37 和 86 位残基的变化会影响Ⅱ类呈递分子多肽抗原的结合[40]。其他研究表明 HLA-C 和 HLA-B 突变与 PSC 亦相关,可作为自然杀伤(NK)细胞上的杀伤免疫球蛋白受体(killer immunoglobulin receptor,KIR)的抑制性配体[43,44]。此外在Ⅲ类区域发现了独立于

HLA 的 *NOTCH4* 基因[39]。值得注意的是,迄今为止的基因研究仅限于北欧人群。在非裔美国人(HLA-DR3 少见)中,PSC 与 HLA-B8 密切相关,与 HLA-DR3 无关[17]。

除 HLA 之外,全基因组研究发现至少还有 22 个其他基因与 PSC 相关,其中的多数基因参与先天和获得性免疫反应(特别是 T 细胞应答)[35,37]。仅有一半左右的 PSC 相关基因同样与 UC、CD 或两者有关联。虽然 PSC 与 IBD 的遗传相关性很强($r=0.56$),但与 UC 的相关性要弱得多($r=0.29$),与 CD 的相关性没有统计学意义($r=0.04$)[38]。网络分析还没有识别出任何共同的功能通路,能提示一种同时适用于 IBD 和 PSC 的特殊机制。许多 PSC 相关的基因也与经典的自身免疫性疾病有关(多效性),如类风湿性关节炎和 1 型糖尿病。尽管取得了这些进展,但是只有不到 10% 的 PSC 遗传特性能用已确认的基因解释。

涉及 PSC 疾病进展的遗传修饰因子的研究更少。几项研究探讨了 HLA 单倍型和临床结局的关系,不过由于研究队列规模较小,结果并不一致。一项对 3 402 例 PSC 患者的全基因组关联研究的数据分析没有发现临床事件发生时间与 HLA 单倍型之间的关联。不过 PSC 与 6 号染色体上的 rs853974 之间存在显著相关性,与 GG 和 AG 基因型相比,AA 基因型具有保护作用(风险比分别为 0.46 和 0.55)[45]。Rs853974 多态性位于 R-Respondin 3(*RSPO3*)基因附近,而 *RSPO3* 基因在胆管细胞中呈高水平表达,这提示该基因在 PSC 疾病进展中可能有潜在作用。

2. 免疫因素

尽管 PSC 的免疫学基础有很充分的临床和遗传学证据,但导致 PSC 的确切靶点和免疫应答仍不明确。目前尚不清楚 PSC 是类似于经典自身免疫性疾病,即特定自身抗原所致的靶向组织破坏,还是类似于自身炎症性疾病(如 IBD),即存在对肠道菌群抗原的先天异常免疫应答,该机制能激活获得性免疫反应。一种将 IBD 和 PSC 关联的假说是,PSC 由细菌或类似于病原体的分子模型(如脂多糖)触发,这些物质通过存在炎症反应和渗透性增加的肠道进入门脉循环("肠瘘症")(见第 2 章)。类似于病原体的分子模型通过模式识别受体(包括 Toll 样受体和 CD14)激活巨噬细胞、树突状细胞和 NK 细胞,导致细胞因子的分泌。IL-12 反过来激活 NK 细胞,并通过 TNF-α、IL-1β 和 CXCL8 促进淋巴细胞的聚集和激活。NK 细胞可能被 MHC Ⅰ类基因链相关产物 MICA 和 MICB 激活,MICA 和 MICB 是应激诱导蛋白,可通过 NKG2D 受体促进 NK、NKT 和 γδT 细胞的细胞毒作用。

巨噬细胞在 PBC 中会特异性聚集在窦状隙和窦周隙。作为先天免疫反应向获得性免疫反应转变的关键细胞,巨噬细胞可能在 PSC 中发挥重要作用。与正常人相比,PSC 患者肝脏汇管区 CD68 和(或)髓过氧化物酶阳性细胞的数量明显增多[46]。此外,遗传学研究证实,巨噬细胞刺激蛋白 1 作为一种巨噬细胞的循环前蛋白和抑制因子,与 PSC 的易感性相关。GPBAR1 是巨噬细胞、胆管上皮细胞(和肠上皮细胞中胆汁酸的细胞表面受体,能有效抑制巨噬细胞的功能[47-49]。值得注意的是,*GPBAR1* 基因变异降低或取消了编码蛋白功能,这与 PSC 之间存在相关性[50]。

尽管遗传学研究证实 PSC 涉及获得性免疫反应,但是获得性免疫反应异常在 PSC 中所起的作用所知甚少。在 PSC 患者中,免疫组化显示浸润肝脏的细胞主要由未激活的记忆性 $CD8^+$T 细胞组成,这些 T 细胞会在汇管区周围表达肠道整合素 α4β7。T 细胞还与黏膜相关 T 细胞一起定位于纤维化区域,这些 T 细胞大量存在于肝脏之中,不仅具有识别细菌抗原的能力,还能够产生 IL-1 和 IL-17 等细胞因子[51]。值得注意的是,PSC 外周血单核细胞在粪肠球菌或白色念珠菌刺激后能够发生更为显著的 IL-17 反应,PSC 肝脏中有大量产生 IL-17A 的细胞[52]。

与健康人群和 PBC 或 UC 相比,PSC 的外周调节性 T 细胞(regulatory T cells,Tregs,用于免疫激活的重要介体)数量明显减少,其中 PSC 风险等位基因 *IL2RA* 基因纯合子减少的幅度最大[53]。PSC 外周 Tregs 的功能同样受损。PSC 患者肝脏中的 Tregs 的数量相比于 PBC 患者也出现明显减少,不过 PSC 和 UC 重叠时,外周血 $CD4^+$ $CD25^+$ T 细胞的比例高于单纯 UC[54,55]。应该注意的是,先前的研究已经证实 PBC 和 UC 患者的外周和组织中 Tregs 的比例低于对照组,这表明 Tregs 的变化可能是炎症性疾病的一个普遍特征[56,57]。

CD28 是诱导 T 细胞活化、存活和增殖的协同刺激分子,而编码 CD28 的基因与 PSC 之间存在相关性。PSC 患者肝脏中 $CD4^+CD28^-$ T 细胞多于外周。此外与 PBC、NASH 和健康人相比,PSC 患者肝脏中 $CD4^+CD28^-$ T 细胞也更多见[55]。这些 $CD28^-$ T 细胞是一类处于激活状态的记忆细胞,细胞内储存细胞毒分子,并能通过表达黏附分子和趋化因子受体以促进组织浸润和胆管定位,在体外也能激活胆管上皮细胞。

3. 淋巴细胞转运

随着对肝脏和肠道淋巴细胞转运共同机制认识的不断深入,IBD 和 PSC 之间的联系得到了更好的阐述。PSC 可能在全结肠切除术后数年发生。有证据表明,PSC 肝脏中会表达通常局限于肠道的黏附分子和趋化因子受体,导致肠道来源的淋巴细胞重新聚集[58-61]。在肠道系统中,淋巴细胞的重新聚集需要肠道相关淋巴组织中树突状细胞的激活,导致淋巴细胞表达整合素 α4β7 和趋化因子受体 CCR9,它们分别依赖于细胞黏附分子-1(MAdCAM-1)和趋化因子配体 25(CCL25)[62]。在 PSC 中不仅门静脉和肝窦内皮细胞表达 MAdCAM-1 和 CCL25,肝脏组织中 $CCR9^+$淋巴细胞比 PBC 也会发生特异性增加。此外,PSC 肝脏中接近 20% 的淋巴细胞表达 CCR9,而在正常或 PBC 患者肝脏中表达 CCR9 的淋巴细胞不到 2%[60]。MAdCAM-1 在肝脏的表达可能需要血管黏附蛋白 1(一种在人体肝脏表达的对氨基脲敏感的胺氧化酶)对甲胺的脱氨作用进行介导[63]。在 TNF-α 存在的情况下,甲胺能够诱导肝内皮细胞表达功能性 MAdCAM-1,这与 PSC 淋巴细胞与肝血管的黏附性增加有关。

4. 生态失调

对 PSC 肠道和胆道微生物群的研究可能有助于解释 PSC 肠道和肝脏之间的重要联系。一些研究记录了 UC 和 CD 中肠道细菌、噬菌体和真菌的组成改变,最常见的是种群多样性的减少以及种群构成的某些特定改变(这些发现会联想到自身免疫的"卫生假说")。慢性肝病患者,尤其是晚期肝硬化患者,也经常出现生态失调。此外,胆汁酸对 PSC 和 IBD 的肠道微生物群有显著影响[64]。不过迄今的研究表明,PSC 的肠道菌群与IBD不同[64-72]。事实上，与单纯IBD相比，PSC合并IBD的微生物群和单纯PSC的关系更密切。除肠道菌群外，PSC的胆道菌群也可能发生改变。岩藻糖基转移酶2基因(*FUT2*)参与蛋白糖基化，基因变异会导致FUT2蛋白缩短，即所谓的非分泌因子，与PSC和CD有关。有趣的是，PSC胆汁中的微生物因*FUT2*基因型不同而异，其中厚壁菌显著增加，而变形菌明显下降。实验证据表明生态失调是PSC的原因而不是结果，在Mdr2缺失的硬化性胆管炎小鼠模型中，无菌小鼠的血清碱性磷酸酶、谷草转氨酶和胆红素水平高于常规饲养小鼠[73]。此外，肝纤维化、胆管炎症和胆管减少在无菌环境中更为严重。在无菌环境中，初级胆汁酸无差异，次级胆汁酸也无差异。尽管研究没有确定微生物群的具体变化，但是提示胆汁酸和肠道细菌之间可能存在相互作用，使PSC的病情恶化。

5. 毒性胆汁理论

虽然遗传学证据不支持胆汁作为PSC的起始因素，但是一些证据表明胆汁在PSC的进展中发挥重要作用。胆汁由胆汁酸、胆红素、胆固醇、磷脂和蛋白质组成的混合物，有多种保护这些物质的机制(见第64章)。PSC时胆汁成分改变、胆汁流量减少和胆管压力升高都可能破坏正常的稳态，形成毒性胆汁。稀释和碱化(即所谓的"碳酸氢盐伞")能保护胆管上皮细胞不受胆汁的影响。磷脂酰胆碱和胆固醇混合形成的胶团也能阻止胆汁酸的毒性作用。这些机制会因为维持胆汁酸/磷脂比率[MDR3(多药耐药蛋白3)或BSEP(胆盐输出泵)]或者碳酸氢盐排泄和胆汁水合作用[CFTR或AE2(阴离子交换蛋白2)]的转运蛋白受损而遭到破坏。此外，PSC中常见的胆汁淤积现象可能导致中毒性胆汁的形成和胆管损伤的加重。

支持毒性胆汁酸理论的证据主要来自Mdr2缺失的小鼠[74-76]。靶向阻断Mdr2会导致胆管硬化、肝内外胆管狭窄和扩张、洋葱皮样胆管周围纤维化以及胆管局灶性闭塞，这些变化类似于人类的原发性或继发性硬化性胆管炎[74]。在人类中，Mdr2(MDR3或ABCB4[ATP结合亚家族B，成员4])的变异与常染色体显性遗传的妊娠肝内胆汁淤积症和胆囊疾病相关，也和罕见的常染色体显性遗传的进展性家族性肝内胆汁淤积症3型相关(见第64章)。此外一些罕见的基因突变也与硬化性胆管炎有关[77,78]，但是遗传学研究尚未发现*ABCB4*基因突变与PSC易感性之间存在任何联系[79]。血清胆红素水平正常的PSC患者胆汁中胆汁酸和脂类排泄正常，提示毒性胆汁理论可能只在PSC的晚期发挥作用[79,80]。

6. 胆管上皮细胞

胆管上皮细胞(biliary epithelial cell，BEC)在PSC发病机制中的作用尚不清楚，但通过了解BEC在免疫细胞募集和激活中的作用，发现BEC是积极的参与者，并不是无辜的旁观者。当被激活时，BEC表达大量受体、细胞因子和趋化因子，这些可以协调许多免疫过程。除表达MHC Ⅱ类抗原外，BEC还表达CD1d，并能向NK T细胞递呈脂类抗原[81]。CD1d在PSC中表达下调。Toll样受体在BEC上也有表达，部分PSC血清中发现的针对BEC的IgG可诱导培养BEC上TLR4和TLR9的表达[82]。事实上，用含有抗BEC抗体的PSC血清处理BEC时能诱导粒细胞-巨噬细胞集落刺激因子、IL-1β和IL-8的分泌。然而，这些抗BEC抗体的靶点仍不清楚。BEC表达的黏附分子如细胞内黏附分子-1也可能在T淋巴细胞的募集中发挥作用[83]。

7. 感染和抗原因素

一些研究试图识别肠道中的感染性或其他抗原性因素，这些因素可能通过门静脉系统和"肠瘘"进入肝脏并引发PSC，但迄今仍未取得成果。大多数PSC患者胆汁培养呈阳性，但似乎主要与内镜操作有关[84]。此外有研究显示PSC和PBC的BEC中有细菌内毒素的积聚[85]。

(三) 临床、实验室和影像学特征

1. PSC和IBD

PSC和IBD之间关系密切，但仍有未知。虽然早期研究表明80%的PSC患者合并IBD，但是后续数据显示这一比例在65%~70%[4,19-21]。PSC合并IBD时，约80%为UC，不到20%为CD[4,19-21]。相反，在所有UC中，合并PSC的比例为2.4%~4.0%，而在CD中为1.4%~3.4%[25,86]。IBD合并PSC时结肠受累更广泛，全结肠炎中PSC的发生率约为5.5%，而远端结肠炎中仅为0.5%[86]。PSC与局限于小肠的CD没有相关性。可能存在种族差异性，非裔美国人中PSC合并IBD的比例为58.8%~60.5%，日本人中为21.1%[17,18,87]。

与IBD的其他肠外表现(如葡萄膜炎和结节性红斑)不同，PSC的进展通常独立于IBD[88]，UC在行全结肠切除术后数年还可能被确诊为PSC[89,90]。PSC多具有广泛性结肠炎，无论归类为UC还是CD，临床上一般都处于静止期[91-93]。右半结肠的炎症要比左半结肠更明显。此外，接受过直肠结肠切除术和回肠袋-肛门吻合术的PSC发生贮袋炎的频率更高[94-96]。与PSC相关的CD通常局限于结肠，多无狭窄或瘘管形成。与UC相比，CD出现全结肠炎的概率较低，这可以解释为什么CD合并PSC明显低于UC。

虽然早期研究显示，IBD和非IBD的患者之间在组织学[97]或胆管造影[98]上没有差异，但后续研究表明IBD的存在和类型会影响PSC的预后。合并UC的PSC发病年龄更早，肝胆管癌、肝移植和死亡的发生率更高[23,99]。

一些没有明显IBD症状的患者可能会在结肠中发现亚临床组织学改变，或者可能在以后发展为临床上的结肠炎[88]。因此需要高度警惕IBD的出现，建议对所有新确诊为PSC的患者行结肠镜检查同时随机进行结肠黏膜活检。

2. 症状

PSC初始的临床表现多种多样，从无症状的血清碱性磷酸酶水平升高到失代偿性肝硬化伴黄疸、腹水、肝性脑病或静脉曲张出血。最常见的症状包括黄疸、乏力、瘙痒和腹痛[100-104]。其他相关症状包括发热、寒战、盗汗、睡眠障碍和体重减轻(表68.3)。越来越多的PSC能在无症状或早期阶段得到诊断。大量研究表明，15%~44%的PSC在诊断时是无症状的[6,100,102-105]。这可能是因为IBD患者常规进行肝脏生化检查以及广泛应用MRCP和ERCP评估血清碱性磷酸酶水平升高。

PSC的症状通常表现为间歇性发作，瘙痒、黄疸、腹痛和发热通常伴随不同时间的无症状期[106]。原因可能为微结石和胆泥引起的暂时性胆管梗阻，导致胆汁淤积从而诱发急性炎症反应。

表 68.3　PSC 确诊时最常见的症状和体征

症状	比例/%
乏力	65~75
腹痛	24~72
瘙痒	15~69
发热/盗汗	13~45
无症状	15~44
体重下降	10~34
体征	
黄疸	30~73
肝大	34~62
脾大	32~34
色素沉着	14~25
腹水	4~7

PSC,原发性硬化性胆管炎。

Data from Wiesner R, Grambsch P, Dickson E, et al. Primary sclerosing cholangitis: Natural natural history, prognostic factors and survival analysis. Hepatology 1989;10:430-6; Farrant J, Hayllar K, Wilkinson M, et al. Natural history and prognostic variables in primary sclerosing cholangitis. Gastroenterology 1991;100:1710-17; Broome U, Olsson R, Loof L, et al. Natural history and prognostic factors in 305 Swedish patients with primary sclerosing cholangitis. Gut 1996;38:610-15; Okolicsanyi L, Fabris L, Viaggi S, et al. Primary sclerosing cholangitis: Clinical presentation, natural history and prognostic variables: An Italian multicentre study. Eur J Gastroenterol Hepatol 1996;8:685-91; Feldstein A, Perrault J, El-Youssif M, et al. Primary sclerosing cholangitis in children: A long-term follow-up study. Hepatology 2003;38:210-17; Porayko M, Wiesner R, LaRusso N, et al. Patients with asymptomatic primary sclerosing cholangitis frequently have progressive disease. Gastroenterology 1990;98:1594-602.

3. 体格检查

PSC 患者的体格检查可能正常,尤其是无症状的患者。如有异常,最常见的是肝大、黄疸和脾大(见表 68.3)。皮肤的异常也较为多见,包括色素沉着、瘙痒引起的抓痕和黄色瘤。随着肝病的进展,还可能出现蜘蛛痣、肌肉萎缩、外周水肿、腹水和其他晚期肝病的体征(见第 74 章)[100,101]。

4. 实验室检查

PSC 的生化标志是血清碱性磷酸酶水平的慢性升高,多为正常上限的 3~5 倍。然而在经胆管造影证实为 PSC 的患者中,高达 6% 的碱性磷酸酶水平正常[107,108]。在某些病例中,尽管血清碱性磷酸酶水平正常,但是肝脏活检显示组织学分期已经为晚期阶段[108]。除了儿童、急性胆管炎或重叠 AIH[11,109,110],血清转氨酶水平升高的幅度很少超过正常上限的 4~5 倍。血清胆红素水平经常波动,可能正常也可能升高,主要为结合胆红素的升高。血清白蛋白水平降低和凝血酶原时间延长反映了晚期肝病患者的肝脏合成功能障碍。此外,营养不良和潜在的 IBD 可能会降低血清白蛋白水平。与胆汁淤积相关的维生素 K 吸收不良可能是凝血酶原时间延长的原因之一。胆汁淤积的其他非特异性后果包括血清铜、血清铜蓝蛋白升高、肝脏铜沉积、尿铜排泄增加和血清胆固醇水平的升高。

多数 PSC 会有一些免疫标志物和血清自身抗体,但并不具有特异性。高球蛋白血症常见,50% 的患者血清 IgM 水平升高,IgG 和 IgA 水平也可能升高[100]。PSC 患者体内能检测到自身抗体[111]。低滴度的 ANA 阳性率为 24%~53%,SMA 阳性率为 13%~20%,但是 AMA 阳性率不到 10%[112]。最常见的是 ANCA(c-ANCA 或 p-ANCA)[113],阳性率为 65%~88%,可能会对异种抗原产生反应[114,115]。这些抗原主要为中性粒细胞核膜蛋白,相应的抗体被称为抗中性粒细胞核抗体[116]。ANCA 不是 PSC 的特异性抗体,也常见于 IBD 和 AIH[116]。在挪威人群中,ANCA 阳性与低患病年龄、低胆管癌发生率和高 HLA-B*08 和 DDRB1*03 阳性率有关[117]。不同于肉芽肿性多发性血管炎,p-ANCA 的滴度与 PSC 的疾病活动性或严重程度无关[113]。此外,自身抗体也不能提示是否合并 IBD。66% 的 PSC 有抗心磷脂抗体阳性,有研究认为该抗体的滴度与疾病严重程度相关[117,112]。ANA、p-ANCA 和 SMA 在儿童中的阳性率分别为 50%、66% 和 45%[109]。总而言之,虽然 PSC 中自身抗体的阳性率很高,但是这些抗体和疾病的发病机制、预后或疗效之间的联系尚未证实(见下文)。因此,检测自身抗体对于 PSC 而言临床价值有限。

5. 影像学

ERCP、MRCP 或经皮经肝穿刺胆管造影(transhepatic cholangiography,THC)能确定 PSC 的诊断,同时提供病变分布和病变程度的信息。特征性的胆管造影表现为胆管的多发性狭窄和扩张。狭窄的区域、正常或接近正常内径的区域以及狭窄后扩张的区域相互穿插,于是胆管呈现为典型的"串珠状"征象。狭窄的节段多表现为短的、环状或带状(图 68.1),晚期可看到较长的融合性狭窄。局部扩张的胆管可呈囊状或憩室状。主要的局灶性狭窄区域称为显性狭窄,常发生在肝管分叉处[118]。有时肝内胆管的弥漫性受累可能会有一种类似于"修剪后的树枝样"外观,与各种原因所致肝硬化时见到的弥漫性肝内胆管萎缩难以区分,不规则的胆管壁结构或合并肝外胆管受累会支持 PSC 的诊断。

约 75% 的病例均有肝内外胆管的异常,15%~20% 表现为孤立性肝内胆管受累[86,102,119],孤立性肝外胆管异常较为罕见,约为 6%,甚至更少[105,107,119]。15% 可能累及胆囊管和胆囊,但在常规胆管造影中并不明显[120],41% 存在非特异性胆囊异常,包括胆囊壁增厚、胆囊增大、胆石症、胆囊炎和胆囊肿块性病变[121],很少出现与慢性胰腺炎相似的胰管异常[122]。77% 合并有非特异性门脉周围的淋巴结病变,但并不提示有恶性可能[123,124]。

MRI 和 MRCP 是诊断 PSC 的首选[118,125,126],并且已经发表了指南指导如何规范化应用的[127]。除了鉴别诊断,MRI 还可以根据肝脏异常形态、脾脏大小、门静脉高压特点、肝脏实质和胆管强化模式提供预后信息[119]。MR 弹性成像可与 MRCP 和 MRI 相结合,对肝纤维化进行分期(见第 74 章)[128]。有研究将振动控制瞬时弹性成像应用于 PSC,结果显示肝脏硬度测量与纤维化的阶段相关,对晚期纤维化和肝硬化的诊断准确性优于 AST/血小板比率、FIB-4 评分和 Mayo 风险评分(见第 74 章和第 80 章)[129]。PSC 中纤维化分期的最佳肝脏硬度临界值分别为≥7.4kPa(F1)、≥8.6kPa(F2)、≥9.6kPa(F3)和≥14.4kPa(F4)。

6. 组织学

肝外胆管的大体和组织学标本均显示胆管壁弥漫性增厚

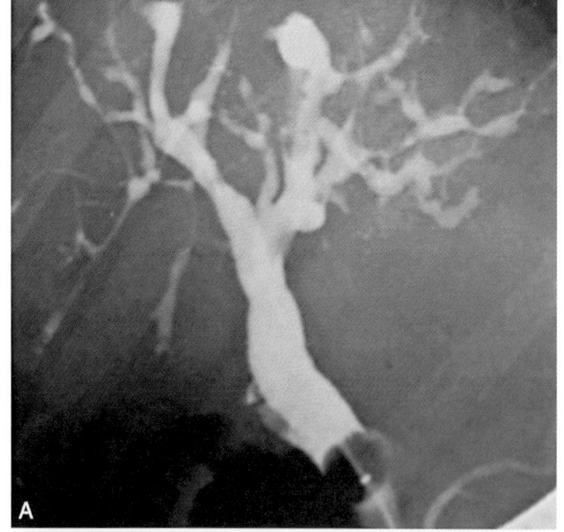

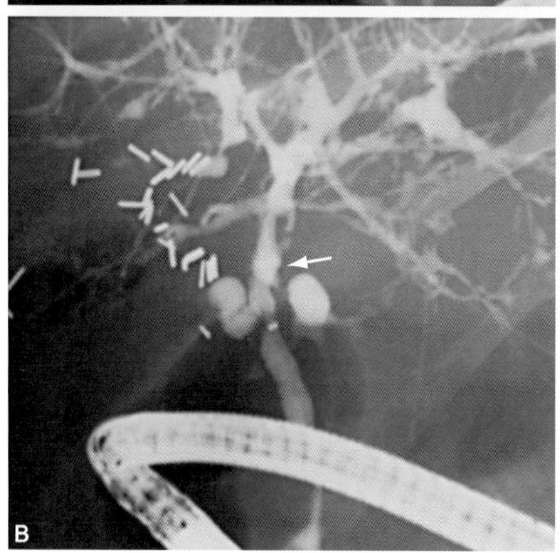

图 68.1 2 例原发性硬化性胆管炎(PSC)患者内镜逆行胰胆管造影(ERCP)的胶片。A,通过球囊导管注入造影剂的 ERCP(见于胆管远端)。肝内胆管主要受累,表现为分枝减少,呈“修剪样”,弥漫性节段性狭窄的胆管与正常或轻度扩张的胆管交替出现(胆管扩张),导致“串珠样”外观。B,影像学特征包括肝内胆管弥漫性不规则、多发性短狭窄和胆管扩张、胆总管壁小憩室(箭头)和既往胆囊切除术的组织夹

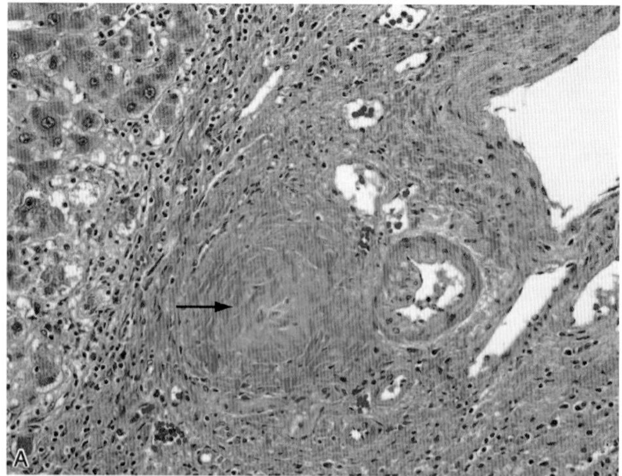

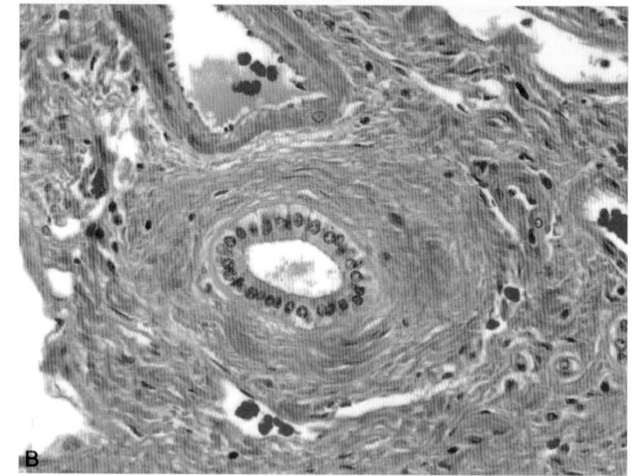

图 68.2 原发性硬化性胆管炎(PSC)的肝脏组织病理学。A,肝段胆管因纤维化而闭塞(箭头),显示“纤维闭塞性胆管炎”(HE 染色,×200)。B,中等大小的胆管周围有同心性纤维化,呈洋葱皮样外观(HE 染色,×400)。(Courtesy Matthew Yeh, MD, PhD, Seattle, Wash.)

和纤维化。纤维化伴有混合性炎症浸润,可累及胆管上皮组织和腺体[130,131]。有研究描述了胆管腺体的大量增生并伴有神经细胞增殖[132]。肝移植时切除的 PSC 肝脏标本显示胆管存在薄壁囊状扩张(胆管扩张),与胆管造影时出现的“串珠状”表现相一致[133]。

PSC 的肝脏活检结果多种多样,但没有特异性的诊断标准。PSC 典型的胆管病变是一种纤维闭塞性的过程,可能导致中等大小的胆管周围出现同心性纤维化,类似于“洋葱皮”(图 68.2)。然而,不到一半的活检标本会有这种现象[130,131]。小叶间的胆管分支可能会出现完全阻塞,导致纤维闭塞性胆管炎。只有 5%~10% 的活检标本中存在这种现象,但这是确诊 PSC 的重要依据[133]。在这个过程中,胆管上皮可能退化和萎缩,完全被纤维索取代。其他特征性的组织病理学表现包括胆管增生、胆管周围炎和胆管减少。炎症程度可能不同,但通常是基于门脉区域在胆管周围的淋巴细胞、浆细胞和中性粒细胞的混合,也可见淋巴滤泡和淋巴细胞聚集[132,133]。

PSC 的许多组织学表现无特异性,在其他疾病中也会存在,有时候会难以区分 PSC 和 PBC。在一项研究中,只有 28% 的患者能通过组织学检查鉴别是 PSC 还是 PBC[134]。当存在淋巴细胞界面性肝炎时,与 AIH 的鉴别可能很困难,主要因为这两种疾病都有高丙种球蛋白血症和自身抗体[11,135]。当出现严重的胆汁淤积时,肝脏中铜积聚可能很严重,类似于肝豆状核变性(见第 76 章)[136]。

如 METAVIR 和 Ishak 评分这些常用于慢性病毒性肝炎的组织学分期系统(见第 74 章和 80 章),在 PSC 中尚未得到充分研究。目前在 PSC 中应用最广泛的是由 Ludwig 和同事在 1981 年提出的分期系统[137],与 PBC 大致相同(见第 91 章)。1 期(门脉期):病变局限于门静脉,包括门脉炎、结缔组织扩张和胆管炎。2 期(门脉周围期):特点是炎症和纤维化范围扩大,出现界面性肝炎(“块状坏死”)和门脉周围纤维化。不同程度的胆管梗阻会导致不同程度的胆管增生和胆管炎。3 期(间隔期):特点是纤维间隔不同的门脉汇管区相互连接,偶见桥接性坏死。4 期(肝硬化期):进展为胆汁性肝硬化。随着病情进展,炎症可能消退,但是会有明显的局部胆管增生。

用于慢性病毒性肝炎组织学分期的 Ishak 系统评分在 0~6 分之间,但是在 PSC 中的研究比较有限[138-141],而 METAVIR 纤维化分期在 PSC 中的研究则更少[129]。Nakanuma 和同事

提出的 PBC 分期系统[142]，包括纤维化、胆管减少和胆汁淤积（以地衣红阳性颗粒测量）。Nakanuma 分期实际是上述 3 个特征的得分总和：1 期为 0 分，2 期为 1~3 分，3 期为 4~6 分，4 期为 7~9 分。虽然 Nakanuma、Ishak 和 Ludwig 组织学分期均与 PSC 的无移植生存率和肝移植时间有关，但是 Nakanuma 分期的相关性最强，纤维化程度和地衣红阳性颗粒沉积是最具鉴别性的特征[140,141]。

只有一项研究分析了 PSC 的组织学分期在观察者之间的一致性[140]。6 位病理学家对 119 例活检标本使用 Ludwig、Ishak 和 Nakanuma 系统进行评分，结果表明有很好的一致性。Ludwig、Ishak 和 Nakanuma 纤维化评分系统的 kappa 指数（κ）分别为 0.62、0.64 和 0.67。值得注意的是，Nakanuma 综合评分系统的一致性只有中等（$\kappa=0.56$）。此外，Ishak 分期和 Ludwig 分期高度相关（$r=0.93$，$P<0.001$）。

以肝脏活检作为终点，一项观察性研究和几项临床试验分析了组织学分期随时间的变化。在唯一的关于组织学进展的纵向观察性研究中，Angulo 和同事们对 107 例 PSC 患者的 307 份肝脏活检标本进行分析，活检间隔时间中位数为 11 个月。使用 Markov 模型，他们估计 2 期患者在 1 年、2 年和 5 年的进展率分别为 42%、66% 和 93%[143]。在 1 年、2 年和 5 年后，从 2 期进展到 4 期（胆汁性肝硬化）的概率分别为 14%、25% 和 52%。不过 15% 的患者观察到分期的回落。

与观察性研究不同，临床试验以固定的时间间隔进行前瞻性活检，减少了治疗偏倚。总体而言，这些研究没有发现组织学分期在 1~5 年内有显著变化[144-146]。无论临床认为是进展、好转或无变化，多数患者的组织学分期没有相应改变，进展或好转的比例接近[138,147-152]。关于 simtuzumab 的随机对照试验对 PSC 组织学纤维化的发展进行了最为详细的评估，simtuzumab 是一种抗赖氨酸氧化酶类 2 的单克隆抗体（见下文）。225 名 PSC 患者参加了一项为期两年的随机试验，使用 simtuzumab 或安慰剂，在起始和之后每年进行肝脏活检[139]。无论分组如何，平均的肝脏胶原含量都在 4.5%~6.3%，在 2 年的疗程中没有发生明显变化。活检标本也通过 Ishak 系统进行了纤维化分期，在 216 例肝活检标本中，74 例（34%）无变化，80 例（37%）至少进展了一期，62 例（29%）至少回退了一期。在 191 例无肝硬化的患者中，30 例（16%）在 2 年内进展为肝硬化。

（四）诊断

PSC 的诊断尚无统一标准。PSC 的诊断需要基于临床、生化、血清学、组织学和典型的胆管造影，同时排除硬化性胆管炎的继发性因素。典型的胆管造影表现为多灶性狭窄和胆管扩张。狭窄的区域中穿插着正常或接近正常胆管直径的区域以及狭窄后扩张的区域。孤立性肝外胆管受累罕见，仅有肝内胆管改变为 20%~28%。显性狭窄是指胆总管直径小于 1.5mm 或左右肝管分叉后 2cm 以内胆管直径小于 1.0mm，累积发生率为 36%~57%。接近 90% 的 PSC 有胆囊异常，其中 8%~26% 能发现胆管结石[153]。

以前 ERCP 是诊断 PSC 的标准检查，可能也是最敏感的检查，但是有高达 10% 的出血、穿孔、感染和胰腺炎的风险[118,154]。得益于图像质量的改进和无创的优势（图 68.3），MRCP（或 MRC）在诊断上已经基本取代了 ERCP。一项包括

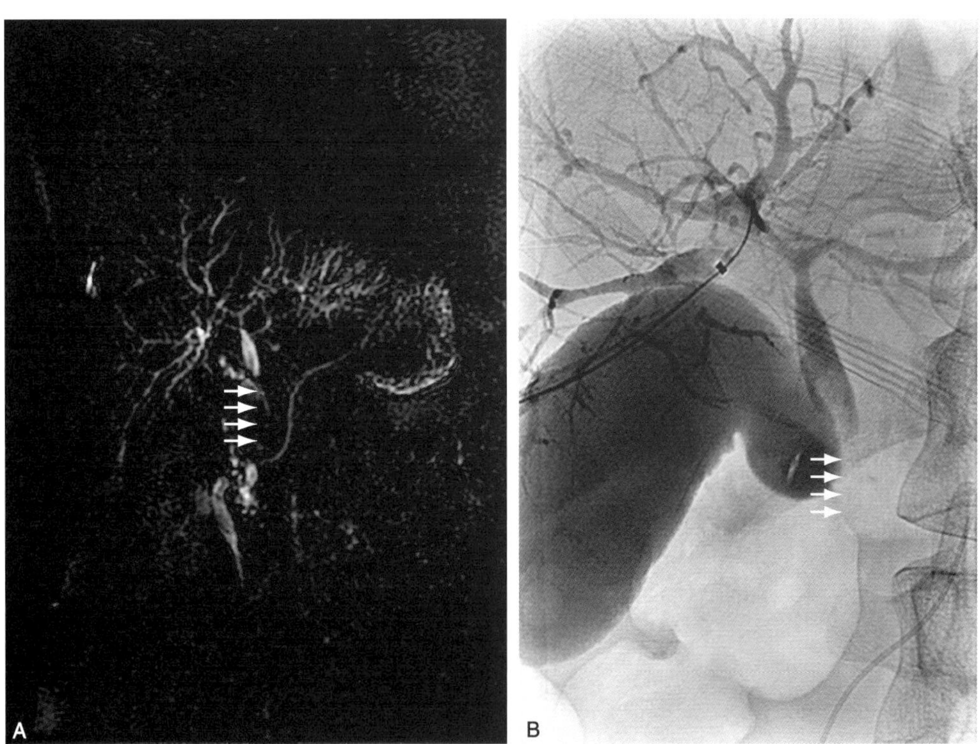

图 68.3　A，原发性硬化性胆管炎（PSC）患者的重建磁共振胰胆管造影（MRCP）图像。肝内胆管基底部弥漫性异常，表现为“枯树枝样和串珠状”外观。在远端胆管水平（箭）存在明显狭窄，表现为 MRI 上信号缺失。B，同一位患者的经皮胆管造影。远端胆管狭窄（箭）伴胆囊明显增大，提示狭窄累及胆囊管。在远端胆管癌患者中也观察到类似的结果

6 项大型研究的荟萃分析发现，MRC 在大多数 PSC 具有足够的敏感性和特异性，因此是更合适的一线诊断方法[155]。不过如果高度怀疑 PSC，而 MRC 是阴性或不明确，则应该进行 ERCP[118]。此外，ERCP 可用于进一步诊断和治疗，包括细胞刷检、胆管内活检和超声、胆道镜和共聚焦内镜诊断胆管癌以及球囊或导管扩张治疗狭窄、胆管支架、括约肌切开和取石。经皮 THC 也可用于诊断和治疗，但是需要经皮肤穿刺。如果肝内胆管扩张不明显，技术上可能比较困难（见第 70 章）。

MRC 对 PSC 的诊断预测值相对较高，建议 IBD 和肝脏生化提示为胆汁淤积的患者行 MRC 评估肝胆系统（见第 21 和 73 章）。超声或 CT 可能有助于规划进一步的诊断和治疗策略，但是不足以诊断 PSC。如果 MRC 成像良好却仍不能诊断 PSC，则应考虑肝活检明确有无小胆管型 PSC 或者其他肝脏疾病。ERCP 用于诊断不明、怀疑恶性肿瘤或者计划对狭窄进行扩张治疗的患者（图 68.4）。

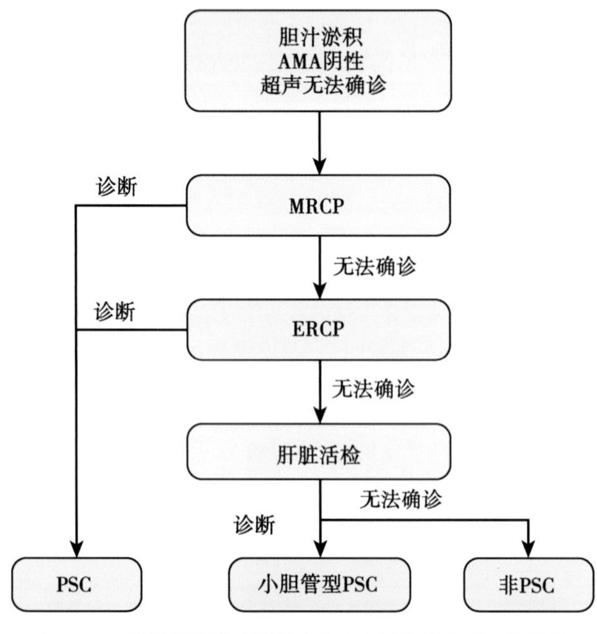

图 68.4 原发性硬化性胆管炎（PSC）的诊断流程。患者典型表现为胆汁淤积，超声可排除胆汁淤积的常见原因，抗线粒体抗体（AMA）阴性一般可以排除原发性胆汁性肝硬化（PBC）。在排除继发性硬化性胆管炎的前提下，磁共振胰胆管造影（MRCP）可诊断 PSC。如果 MRCP 不能诊断，则应进行内镜逆行胰胆管造影（ERCP）和/或肝活检以确诊 PSC 并排除胆汁淤积的其他原因，如 AMA 阴性的 PBC

（五）鉴别诊断

如果患者合并 IBD 同时胆管造影有硬化性胆管炎的特点，那么 PSC 的诊断可以成立。但是必须排除硬化性胆管炎的继发因素，尤其是在没有合并 IBD 的情况下（表 68.4）。虽然 PSC 和 SSC 有不同的特征，但是尚不能通过这种差异作出准确的诊断（见表 68.1）[118]。

胆总管结石和胆管癌可能与 PSC 同时发生，或者独立于 PSC 出现。在存在多发胆总管结石或弥漫性胆管癌的情况下，很难诊断潜在的 PSC。非 PSC 相关的肝硬化的胆管造影有时可能与 PSC 混淆，然而非 PSC 的肝硬化的胆管造影多表现为肝内胆管广泛逐渐变细，而没有胆管不规则或狭窄。

表 68.4 PSC 和 SSC 的胆道造影特征

疾病	特征
急性细菌性胆管炎	肝内外胆管多发灶性狭窄，胆管轻度扩张、憩室样突起，像"修剪过的树木"
AIDS 相关的胆管病	多处的肝内胆管狭窄、结石和胆源性脓肿
腐蚀性胆管炎（如氟尿苷）	近端肝内胆管狭窄、胆管坏死、胆管瘤、脓肿、胆管铸型综合征
IgG4 相关性硬化性胆管炎	局限性肝内胆管狭窄，胆管壁不规则
缺血性胆管病	远端胆管狭窄，乳头炎，非结石性胆囊炎
门静脉高压性胆道病	多发灶中央型胆管狭窄，胆管壁增厚、管腔可见，胰腺异常类似于自身免疫性胰腺炎
PSC	中央型胆管和肝外胆管异常

IgG4，免疫球蛋白 G4。
PSC，原发性硬化性胆管炎。

作为一种慢性胆汁淤积性疾病，PBC 与 PSC 有一些共同的临床特征（见第 91 章）。然而，PBC 多见于中年女性，与 IBD 无关，与高滴度的 AMA 有关。虽然这两种疾病的肝脏组织学可能有重叠（见上文）[134]，但是应用胆管造影很容易鉴别这两种疾病。尽管晚期 PBC 患者也可表现为肝内胆管平滑变细，但没有胆管不规则狭窄，也没有肝外胆管狭窄。AMA 阴性的 PBC 可能很难与小胆管型 PSC 区分，因为两者的血清学和胆管造影可能重叠，但人口统计学和组织学特征不同。此外，PBC 特异性抗核抗体（如抗 gp210 和抗 sp100）有助于诊断 AMA 阴性 PBC（见第 91 章）[156]。IgG4 硬化性胆管炎，也称为 IgG4 相关性胆管炎，有时见于自身免疫性胰腺炎，也需排除（见下文）[157]。

（六）自然史和预后模型

PSC 是一种有多种临床表型的异质性疾病，不同的进展速度可导致一种或多种可能的结局。尽管在个别患者中可能不进展或不明显，但是 PSC 一般分为以下 4 个临床阶段：

- 亚临床期：患者可能有 PSC 的胆管造影证据，但是血清肝脏生化指标正常，也没有临床症状。这些患者多是通过影像学偶然发现或长期 IBD 进行筛查而确诊[107,158]。MRI 随访发现亚临床期的 PSC 进展缓慢。
- 无症状期：患者无症状，但生化指标异常，典型表现为血清碱性磷酸酶水平升高，伴有不同程度的胆红素和转氨酶水平升高。
- 症状期：出现胆汁淤积或肝脏损伤症状，或两者兼有。多出现瘙痒、乏力、胆管炎和黄疸。
- 失代偿期肝硬化：终末期肝病不断恶化的症状和并发症，如腹水、脑病和静脉曲张出血。

这种疾病进展模型为了解 PSC 不同的自然史提供了一个有用的框架。

1. 无症状 PSC

在已发表的队列研究中，15% ~ 44% 是无症状 PSC[102,103]。一些研究指出无症状 PSC 通常有一个良性病程。

由 305 位瑞典 PSC 患者组成的队列中，44% 没有症状，在 69 个月的中位随访期内，只有 22% 出现了症状[102]。整个队列的中位生存期为 12 年，无症状患者明显优于有症状患者。相比之下，Porayko 和同事[105]对 45 名无症状的 PSC 进行了中位数 6.25 年的随访，13 位患者(31%)出现了肝功能衰竭，导致肝移植或死亡。总体而言，24 位患者(53%)出现症状，34 位患者(76%)出现进展性肝病，有新的症状或体征、胆管造影结果恶化或进展性肝脏组织学异常。在这项研究中，无症状患者 7 年无肝衰竭的中位生存率估计为 71%，显著低于基于年龄、性别和种族匹配的美国对照人群。这些研究之间疾病进展的差异可能是由于患者群体的不同、转诊偏倚、"无症状"的定义和临床随访时间的不同。

2. 有症状 PSC

确诊时有症状的患者预后一般比无症状的差[106]。有症状的患者在确诊时临床分期可能更提前，生化检查和胆管造影的异常更多，肝脏活检标本的组织学分期更高。Farrant 和同事记录了 126 位 PSC 患者的自然史，84% 有症状，中位随访 5.8 年，估计中位生存期为 12 年。瑞典的一项大型研究也有类似的发现，研究开始时即有症状的患者，其生存期(9.3 年)明显低于无症状的患者[102]。

3. 总体预后

PSC 的总体预后随着时间的推移发生了变化。目前尚不清楚这是因为疾病行为的改变、轻症病例的及时诊断还是抽样更具代表性。例如，荷兰一项对 174 位 PSC 患者的研究表明[159]，PSC 的总体预后好于之前的研究，中位预期生存期为 18 年。本研究中生存期提高的原因尚不清楚，但数据主要来自 20 世纪 90 年代，而此前其他研究的数据来自 20 世纪 70 年代和 80 年代。虽然在此期间治疗的进步并不显著，但 20 世纪 90 年代的早期诊断可能导致了选择上的差异，这似乎影响了结果。与这项研究一致的是，一项来自荷兰的包括 590 位患者的大型人群研究，预估非移植中心的中位无移植生存期为 21.2 年，而移植中心随访的患者中位无移植生存期为 13.2 年，这表明存在明显的转诊偏倚[4]。与这些发现一致的是，在国际 PSC 研究小组注册的 7 000 多位患者的中位无移植生存期为 14.5 年，其中包括几十年前确诊的患者和所有来自专科中心的患者[23]。相比之下，一份 800 多位患者的登记报告估计无移植的中位生存期为 21 年[5]。

一般来说，确诊时高龄、男性、大胆管型 PSC(而不是小胆管型 PSC)、合并 UC(而不是 CD 或无 IBD)会增加肝移植或死亡的可能[23]。越来越多的证据表明血清碱性磷酸酶水平是 PSC 的预后标志物。多项研究表明血清碱性磷酸酶水平持续保持正常或至少低于正常上限的 1.5 倍一般不会有肝脏失代偿、肝移植、肝脏相关死亡和胆管癌等临床结局[160-164]。

4. 小胆管型 PSC

3 项研究对小胆管型 PSC 的临床随访情况进行了初步调查。83 位联合队列中的患者与 157 位年龄和性别匹配的大胆管型 PSC 进行了比较[9]。22% 的小胆管型 PSC 在中位时间 7.4 年内进展为大胆管型 PSC。20 位大胆管型 PSC 出现胆管癌，仅有 1 例小胆管型 PSC 进展为大胆管型 PSC 后又出现胆管癌。此外，小胆管型 PSC 平均无移植生存期更长(13 年 vs 10 年)。因此，在某些病例中小胆管型 PSC 可能代表了早期 PSC，并进展为大胆管型 PSC，但小胆管型 PSC 似乎与胆管癌无关，小胆管型 PSC 的长期生存率更高。

5. 小儿 PSC

PSC 在儿童中也呈一个渐进的过程。在一项纳入 36 个机构的 781 名 PSC 患儿的大型国际研究中，确诊时的中位年龄为 12 岁，39% 为女性，76% 合并 IBD[109]。87% 为大胆管型 PSC，1/3 合并 AIH。确诊 PSC 时，5% 出现门静脉高压并发症，10 年后增加至 38%。5 年和 10 年的无移植生存率分别为 88% 和 70%。8 位患儿在确诊后平均 6 年出现胆管癌。

6. 预后模型

对自然史的研究能够了解可能影响 PSC 预后的特定的临床、生化和组织学表现。虽然早期的研究分析了导致 PSC 生存率较低的单个因素，但随后的研究使用了多因素回归分析，如 Cox 分析，开发出更复杂的数学模型来预测生存。1989 年，Wiesner 和同事提出了第一个模型[100]，该模型基于年龄、血清胆红素、血红蛋白、是否合并 IBD 以及组织学分期。该模型确定了 3 个危险组(低、中、高)，预测的生存曲线类似于观察的生存曲线。此后，其他模型相继出现，并对原有的 Mayo Clinic 模型进行了修订(表 68.5)。最新的 Amsterdam-Oxford 模型是基于 692 名 PSC 的数据建立的[165]。该模型使用 7 个变量，包括 PSC 亚型、诊断时年龄、白蛋白、血小板、AST、碱性磷酸酶和胆红素，用于在诊断后的最初几年内预测长期无移植生存情况。

表 68.5 PSC 自然史模型中使用的生存独立预测因子和预后指数公式

Mayo Clinic 模型[100]	King's College 模型[101]	Multicenter 模型[349]	Revised Mayo 模型[349]	Amsterdam-Oxfor 模型[165]
生存预测				
年龄	年龄	年龄	年龄	年龄
胆红素	肝大	胆红素	胆红素	胆红素
组织学分级	组织学分级	组织学分级	白蛋白	白蛋白
血红蛋白(Hgb)	脾大	脾大	谷草转氨酶(AST)	谷草转氨酶
炎症性肠病(IBD)	碱性磷酸酶		静脉曲张出血	碱性磷酸酶
				血小板
				原发性硬化性胆管炎亚型(PSC)

表 68.5 PSC 自然史模型中使用的生存独立预测因子和预后指数公式(续)

Mayo Clinic 模型[100]	King's College 模型[101]	Multicenter 模型[349]	Revised Mayo 模型[349]	Amsterdam-Oxfor 模型[165]
预后指数公式*				
R=0.06×年龄+0.85×$\log_e$[min(胆红素或10)]+4.39×$\log_e$[min(Hgb 或 12)]+0.51×组织学分级+1.59×IBD	R=1.81×肝大+0.88×脾大+2.66×log(碱性磷酸酶)+0.58×组织学分级+0.04×年龄	R=0.535×loge(胆红素)+0.486×组织学分级+0.041×年龄+0.705×脾大	R=0.03×年龄+0.54×$\log_e$(胆红素)+0.54×$\log_e$(AST)+1.24×静脉曲张出血−0.84×白蛋白	PI=0.323×PSC 亚型+0.018×确诊时年龄−2.485×白蛋白+2.451×血小板+0.347×AST+0.337×总胆红素
注解:				
3 个确定的风险级别:低、中、高	-	基于 426 名患者的数据	基于 5 个中心 529 名患者的数据;不需要肝活检	基于 692 名患者

*年龄的单位是年;白蛋白的单位是 g/dL;碱性磷酸酶的单位是 U/L;谷草转氨酶的单位是 U/L;胆红素的单位是 mg/dL;血红蛋白的单位是 g/dL。如果存在炎症性肠病、肝大、脾大或静脉曲张出血,则数值为 1;如果不存在,则数值为 0。如果是大胆管的原发性硬化性胆管炎亚型为 1,如果是小胆管的原发性硬化性胆管炎亚型为 0。min,最小值;PI,预后指数;PSC,原发性硬化性胆管炎;R,风险评分。

Child-Pugh 分级也可用于预测 PSC 患者的生存期(见第 92 章)。Shetty 和同事发现在 PSC 相关的肝硬化中 Child-Pugh 分级为 A 级、B 级和 C 级的 7 年生存率分别为 89.8%、68% 和 24.9%(Kaplan-Meier 分析)[166]。然而,随后的评估表明 Child-Pugh 分级的准确性低于修订的 Mayo 风险模型,特别是对于早期 PSC[167]。

目前还缺乏一种纳入胆管造影的有效的 PSC 预后模型。2002 年,Ponsioen 和同事将基于 ERCP 肝内和肝外胆管病变类型和严重程度的 Amsterdam 胆管造影分期系统纳入一个模型计算预后指数[168]。胆管造影分期与生存率负相关,证实了胆管造影对于预后的价值。最近,一个法国团队通过三维 MRI 和 MRCP 记录了 PSC 在影像学上的病程,同时创建了一个预测病程的评分[119]。与疾病进展相关的变量包括肝内胆管扩张、肝脏形态异常和门静脉高压(如果 MRI 没有使用钆),以及肝脏形态异常和实质强化不均(如果 MRI 使用钆)。但是观察者之间的差异使 ERCP 和 MRCP 的解读变得复杂,使每个变量的实际评分变得困难。

尽管在各种自然史模型中使用的数学公式繁琐,但这些模型在 PSC 的临床管理中很有用。通过比较预测生存率和现有的肝移植后生存率,可以决定肝移植时机。然而,具有不同预后变量的多种模型在临床实践中的应用可能是混乱的。这些模型也可能没有考虑到可能影响 PSC 预后的其他临床事件,如胆管癌或静脉曲张出血。进一步完善这些预后模型,包括对特定的预后变量的使用达成共识,可能终会阐明它们在临床实践中的作用。

(七) 并发症

1. 胆汁淤积

PSC 可能会出现与慢性胆汁淤积相关的并发症(见第 21 和 91 章)。瘙痒是最常见的症状之一,会对患者的生活质量产生不利影响[5,169-172],可能会出现严重的抓伤和疲劳。慢性胆汁淤积性瘙痒的发病机制尚不清楚,治疗反应也不一致(见第 91 章)。胆汁淤积时血浆和组织中胆汁酸的积聚可能是引起瘙痒的潜在原因,经典的治疗方法是口服胆汁酸结合树脂(如消胆胺)。然而,并非所有血清胆汁酸水平升高的患者都会瘙痒,而且胆汁酸升高的程度和瘙痒的强度之间并不存在相关性。尽管胆汁酸水平相对稳定,但是瘙痒却多为间歇性发作。一些证据表明胆汁淤积与内源性阿片类药物水平的增加有关。在动物模型中,胆汁淤积与血浆内源性阿片类药物水平升高之间存在相关性[173]。在人类中,胆汁淤积患者在使用阿片类拮抗剂后可能会出现阿片类药物戒断症状。此外,小型临床试验表明具有阿片类拮抗剂特性的纳洛酮和纳曲酮可以缓解胆汁淤积性瘙痒[174,175]。

尽管证据水平很低,但是 5-羟色胺、组胺和孕酮代谢物浓度的升高也与瘙痒的发病机制有关,最近,溶血磷脂酸成为一种重要的神经递质,参与胆汁淤积性瘙痒的调节。自体趋化因子是一种溶血磷脂酰胆碱合成溶血磷脂酸的酶,与胆汁淤积性瘙痒的存在、程度以及对治疗的有效性相关[176]。

营养缺乏可能使晚期 PSC 的慢性胆汁淤积复杂化。脂溶性维生素 A、D、E 和 K 的肠道吸收特别受影响,可能与肠道结合胆汁酸浓度降低有关,在一项临床试验研究中,维生素 A、维生素 D 和维生素 E 缺乏的比例分别为 40%、14% 和 2%,准备接受肝移植的患者里维生素 A、维生素 D 和维生素 E 缺乏的比例分别为 82%、57% 和 43%[177]。伴随疾病如 IBD、慢性胰腺炎和乳糜泻也可能导致肠道吸收不良,临床表现有夜盲(维生素 A 缺乏症)和凝血障碍(维生素 K 缺乏)。

代谢性骨病(也称肝性骨营养不良)在 PSC 中常被低估。代谢性骨病有两种类型:骨软化症和骨质疏松症。随着营养管理的改善,骨软化症(骨矿化减少)相对罕见,而胆汁淤积患者的大多数骨病是骨质疏松。PSC 患者的骨密度明显低于年龄和性别匹配的对照组[178],有三分之一的髋关节或脊柱骨密度低于 1.0 标准差,非椎体脆性骨折的发生率相对较高(18%)[179]。PSC 和其他慢性胆汁淤积性肝病骨密度损失的发病机制尚不清楚。肠道维生素 D 的吸收不良可能不是主要的异常,因为血清维生素 D 水平正常,补充维生素 D 通常不会对骨质疏松的严重程度产生显著影响。长期伴随 IBD 是该人群骨质疏松的独立危险因素,糖皮质激素的使用加剧骨质疏松。

2. 胆结石

与正常人群相比，胆石症在 PSC 中更为常见。胆结石，通常是色素性胆红素钙结石，在 PSC 中的发病率约为 25%（见第 65 章）[121]。胆道狭窄易导致胆汁淤积、胆泥和结石形成。超声对胆管内结石的灵敏度仅为中等。因此，PSC 合并胆汁淤积或黄疸恶化的患者应接受诊断性 ERCP（预期有治疗干预），以鉴别是胆结石还是狭窄或胆管癌。

3. 胆管癌

胆管癌是起源于胆管上皮的恶性肿瘤，是 PSC 的一种严重并发症（见第 69 章）。PSC 是胆管癌的癌前状态，类似于 UC 与结肠癌的关系。PSC 患者一生中发生胆管癌的风险在 5%~20%，在诊断为 PSC 后的第一年风险最大，之后是每年 0.5%~1.5% 的风险[4,23,180,181]。肿瘤最常见于肝总管和肝门周围，但可能仅累及胆管、肝内胆管和胆囊管。从肝移植出现之后，胆管癌成为 PSC 死亡的主要原因。PSC 发生胆管癌的危险因素包括年龄、男性、大胆管型 PSC 和 UC，而小胆管型 PSC、CD 或不合并 IBD 似乎是保护因素[23,180-183]，血清碱性磷酸酶水平正常或接近正常可能也是保护因素[184,185]。

PSC 中胆管癌的发病机制尚不清楚。虽然胆管癌可能出现在 PSC 的任一阶段，但是慢性炎症容易导致上皮异型增生，增加恶变的风险。促炎症细胞因子可能在刺激 DNA 氧化损伤和 DNA 修复过程失活中有一定作用。

当 PSC 患者有黄疸加重、体重减轻或腹痛等临床情况恶化的表现时，应怀疑胆道恶性肿瘤，不过良性显性狭窄也可能会有相同的表现。在 PSC 中诊断胆管癌是一个特殊的挑战。胆管造影中恶性胆管狭窄可能与 PSC 难以区分（图 68.5）。胆管癌呈匍行性生长而不是孤立的肿块，因此 CT 或 MRI 横断面成像对胆管癌的敏感性较低。

糖链抗原 19-9（CA19-9）是普遍用于检测胆管癌的血清标志物。CA19-9 是一种糖脂，在许多不同的癌症中都有表达，在胆汁淤积时可能也会升高。一项研究以 129U/mL 为最佳临界值的敏感性为 78%、特异性为 98%，另一项研究以 20U/mL 为临界值的敏感性为 78%、特异性为 67%。此外，CA19-9 需要表达 Lewis 血型抗原，而 5%~10% 的人群缺乏这种抗原。岩藻糖基转移酶基因 *FUT2* 和 *FUT3* 的变异会影响血清 CA19-9 水平。根据这些基因型调整不同的临界值会提高 CA19-9 的敏感性[186]。

在胆管癌的诊断中难以获取足够的组织样本。ERCP 细胞刷检对胆管癌的诊断有很高的特异性，但灵敏度不到 60%[187,188]。胆管内活检有望提高胆管恶性肿瘤的检出率，但尚未得到证实。早期研究表明，细胞刷检联合活检能将恶性肿瘤的诊断灵敏度提高到 70%[189]。特殊的技术（如荧光原位杂交）能提高细胞学检查的灵敏度，以更好地识别异倍体[190,191]。3、7 或 17 号染色体拷贝数的增加和（或）9p21 的缺失将细胞学的灵敏度提高到 89%[192,193]。一种包括细胞学、活检和 FISH 的诊断方法的总体灵敏度为 82%，特异度为 100%，阳性预测值为 100%，阴性预测值为 87%[194]。EUS、胆管内超声和胆道镜检查等其他检查可以提高组织取样的诊断准确性（见第 69 章）。

合并胆管癌预后不佳，确诊后中位生存期为 5 个月[195,196]。

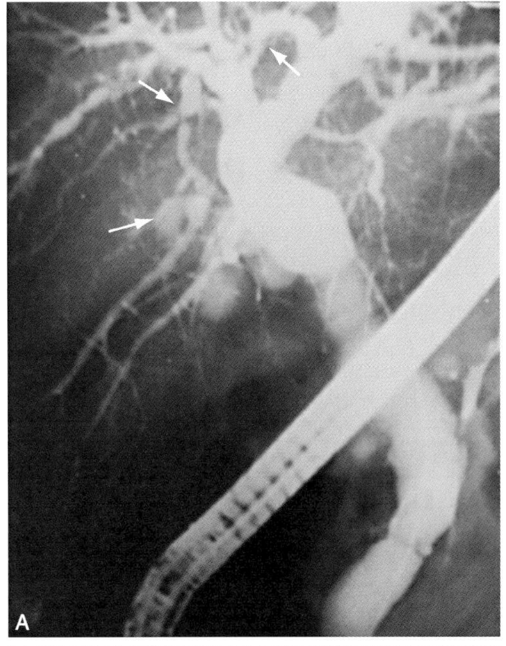

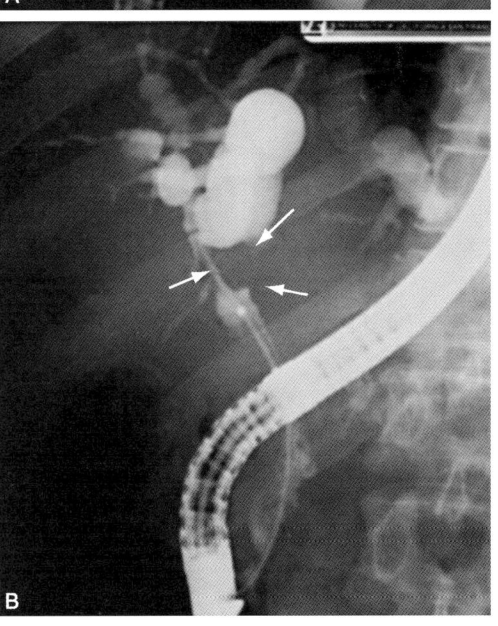

图 68.5　原发性硬化性胆管炎（PSC）合并胆管癌的胆管造影进展。该例 43 岁男性，有 3 年轻度溃疡性结肠炎病史，表现为皮肤瘙痒和血清碱性磷酸酶升高。A，最初内镜逆行胰胆管造影（ERCP）检查显示轻度弥漫性 PSC 改变，无并发症。肝内胆管存在多处短的环形狭窄和胆管扩张（箭示），胆管有单个短的环形狭窄。胆囊管未充盈。B，出现进展性黄疸和体重快速下降 7 个月后，行第 2 次 ERCP。发现有一个 2cm 的肿块阻塞肝总管（箭示）。一根造影导管穿过肿块，梗阻近端左主干肝内胆管明显扩张，右主干肝内胆管完全闭塞

由于肝移植术后胆管癌的复发率高，胆管癌患者很少会成为肝移植的候选（见第 69 章）。此外，在接受肝移植的 PSC 中，高达 10% 可能会发现隐匿性胆管癌。

在 PSC 中筛查胆管癌仍有争议，没有强有力的证据表明会改善生存期。然后在 PSC 中胆管癌的发生率很高而且后果严重，一些指南因此建议每年行 CA19-9 联合超声检查或 MRCP[126]。

PSC 也有患胆囊癌的高风险，出现肝硬化时 HCC 风险

同样增加。虽然之前在 PSC 中胆囊癌发病率为 3%~14%[197]，但一项对 7 000 多名 PSC 的分析显示 PSC 胆囊癌和 HCC 的发病率均只有 0.8%[23]。尽管如此，北美和欧洲的专业协会仍建议每年行腹部超声筛查胆囊癌（见第 69 和 96 章）[198,126]。

4. 结肠肿瘤

越来越多的证据表明，UC 合并 PSC 发生结肠肿瘤（异型增生或癌）的风险明显高于单独的 UC[4,199,200]。UC 增加了结肠异型增生和结肠癌的风险（见第 116 章），病程和严重程度是最强的相关危险因素。在荷兰一项对 590 例 PSC 的研究发现在确诊 PSC 之后的 10 年、20 年和 30 年，重度异型增生或结直肠癌的累积风险分别为 3%、7% 和 13%，与年龄和性别匹配的人群相比，PSC 合并 UC 发生结直肠癌的风险增加 9 倍，与 UC 对照组相比增加 10 倍[4]。与 UC 相比，PSC 合并 IBD 发生结直肠癌的年龄更小，结肠镜检查能有效降低结直肠癌相关死亡率。美国和荷兰的一项大型纵向协作研究对 1 911 例结肠 IBD 施行了进展期结肠肿瘤的评估。虽然各组炎症程度和轻度异型增生的发生率没有差异，PSC 合并 IBD 发生进展期结直肠癌的风险比无 PSC 的 IBD 增加 2 倍[200]。年龄增加以及结肠炎症活动同样是结直肠癌的独立危险因素。此外，诊断为轻度异型增生的 PSC 合并 IBD 发生进展期肿瘤的风险也高了 2.5 倍。PSC 合并 UC 更有可能在结肠中同时存在异型增生。一项系统回顾纳入了 14 项监测 UC 和轻度异型增生的研究，结果表明 PSC、隐性异型增生、远端和多部位轻度异型增生与进展为结直肠癌有关[201]。无 IBD 的 PSC 发生结直肠癌的风险似乎没有增加[4]。

PSC 为何会增加结肠肿瘤的风险尚不清楚。UC 发生异型增生和肿瘤的患者的粪便胆汁酸浓度更高[202]，所以结肠内高浓度的次级胆汁酸对于肿瘤的发生可能起一定的作用。PSC 合并 UC 患者右半结肠癌的发生率高于单独 UC 患者，进一步支持了上述理论。PSC 合并 IBD 的肠道菌群组成与不合并 PSC 的 IBD 相比有显著差异，胃球菌属和梭杆菌属的微生物多样性和丰富度降低[66,67,71]。PSC 合并 IBD 的肠道菌群与粪便胆汁酸之间可能有独特的联系[64]。

结肠次级胆汁酸浓度升高可能解释了熊去氧胆酸（UDCA）预防结肠肿瘤的机制。有两项研究显示在 PSC 合并 UC 的患者中 UDCA 的使用降低了结肠异型增生或结肠癌的风险[203,204]。UDCA 可能会降低结肠中次级胆汁酸的浓度，影响蛋白激酶 C 亚型的表达、花生四烯酸代谢和 COX-2 的表达，从而起到预防结肠肿瘤的作用[205-208]。一项巢式队列研究纳入了关于 UDCA 的大剂量、双盲、安慰剂对照试验，结果却发现 UDCA 增加了结直肠肿瘤的风险[209]。鉴于这些相互矛盾的数据，目前不推荐 UDCA 用于 PSC 合并 IBD 患者结直肠肿瘤的化学预防[126]。

合并 UC 的 PSC 应从确诊 PSC 开始每隔 1~2 年进行结肠异型增生或结肠癌的监测[126]。与 UC 一样，在多部位行黏膜活检（见第 116 章）。虽然使用染色内镜的靶向活检有效提高了肿瘤检出率，但是随机活检发现肿瘤的概率增加 20%，随机活检与染色内镜应该联合进行[210]。因为仍有结肠肿瘤的风险，在肝移植后也要继续监测[211-213]。未发现 IBD 的患者在确诊 PSC 时应当行结肠镜检查，需多点活检排除结肠炎。如果活检结果阴性，每隔 5 年复查结肠镜[214]。

5. 造瘘口静脉曲张

在因 IBD 行直肠结肠切除和回肠造瘘术的 PSC 患者中，四分之一可能会出现造瘘口静脉曲张[215]。这些静脉曲张可能会自发出血和剧烈出血。注射硬化、弹簧圈栓塞、造瘘口翻修和经颈静脉肝内门腔内支架分流等止血治疗（见第 92 章）起初有效[216-218]，然后出血普遍会反复发生，肝移植是缓解门静脉高压和治疗肝脏疾病的有效方法。

（八）治疗

除肝移植外，尚无 PSC 的特效治疗，肝脏失代偿前的治疗目标是治疗并发症，如细菌性胆管炎和瘙痒、预防骨质疏松和营养不良以及早期诊断恶性肿瘤，包括胆管癌、胆囊癌和结肠癌。一旦肝病进展，就应开始进行肝移植的评估。

1. 基础疾病的药物治疗

关于 PSC 虽然进行了多种药物的研究，但只有少数有意义的随机、安慰剂对照试验（表 68.6）。无论在临床、生化、组织学还是在数学风险评分中，不同研究里定义的终点均有很大差异。临床试验应该有关于替代终点的共识，这样能提高药物研发的可能[219,220]。然而，目前还没有药物可以改变 PSC 的自然病程。

UDCA 是 PSC 中研究最广泛的药物[221-228]。在胆汁淤积的情况下 UDCA 发挥有益作用的机制包括保护胆管细胞免受疏水性胆汁酸的细胞毒性、刺激肝脏胆汁分泌、保护肝细胞免受胆汁酸诱导的细胞凋亡以及诱导抗氧化（见第 91 章）[229,230]。大多数临床试验显示血清肝脏生化指标有所改善，但是没有一项试验证明 UDCA 能有生存获益或者延迟肝移植的时间。此外，UDCA 并不能延缓乏力、瘙痒或胆管癌的发展。

标准剂量的 UDCA 并没有表现出令人满意的效果，因此多项研究所采用的 UDCA 剂量为 30mg/(kg·d)，为 PBC 推荐剂量的两倍[225-228]。一项研究纳入了 219 名来自斯堪的纳维亚半岛的患者，随机接受 17mg/(kg·d) 的 UDCA、23mg/(kg·d) 的 UDCA 或安慰剂，为期 5 年，结果显示各组的无肝移植生存期之间并没有差异。该研究未能招募到足够的试验人数，仅有 18 位患者达到研究终点，这反映出了 PSC 临床试验的困难。然而，在一项前瞻性、安慰剂对照的随机试验中，UDCA 剂量为 25~30mg/(kg·d)，为期 6 年，结果显示大剂量 UDCA 导致死亡、肝移植和静脉曲张的风险更高[231]。研究的额外分析表明肝脏生化指标得到改善的患者可能会获得一些临床益处[163,164]，停用 UDCA 会导致瘙痒、肝脏生化指标和 Mayo 风险评分（见上文）均发生恶化[232]。

一些调节胆汁酸的新药在改善肝脏生化指标方面有良好的初步结果，包括 nor-UDCA，UDCA 的 C_{23} 同系物[233]，在前期研究中表现出较好的抗胆汁淤积、抗炎和抗增殖特性[234]，毒性低于 UDCA。在欧洲的一项多中心二期临床试验中，无论之前是否使用过 UDCA，nor-UDCA 均能改善血清碱性磷酸酶水平[235]。正在研究中的药物还包括能调节胆汁酸稳态和其他代谢过程的受体激动剂。

表 68.6　PSC 药物治疗的随机对照试验*

药物	年份	N	治疗	试验周期	结果	参考文献
秋水仙碱	1995	84	秋水仙碱(1mg) 安慰剂作对照	36 个月	组织学、肝脏生化或临床结果均无改善	350
UDCA	1997	105	UDCA(13~15mg/kg/d) 安慰剂作对照	24 个月	对治疗失败的(包括死亡、肝移植、肝硬化、组织学进展超过 2 期、失代偿期肝硬化、肝脏生化或有症状的进展)无改善 改善肝脏生化指标	148
UDCA	2001	26	UDCA(20mg/kg/d) 安慰剂作对照	24 个月	改善肝脏生化指标,减少组织学进展和胆管造影进展	138
UDCA 和甲硝唑	2004	80	UDCA/甲硝唑(600~800mg/d) UDCA/安慰剂作对照	36 个月	改善肝脏生化指标、Mayo 评分(表 68.5)和组织学进展,未见胆管造影改善	150
UDCA	2005	219	UDCA(17~23mg/kg/d) 安慰剂作对照	60 个月	非移植生存率、肝脏生化指标和生存质量均无改善	351
UDCA	2008	31	UDCA(10、20、30mg/kg/d)	24 个月	改善肝脏生化指标和风险评分(仅高剂量)	151
UDCA	2009	150	UDCA(28~30mg/kg/d) 安慰剂作对照	60 个月	无收益,反而增加了不良事件的发生	146
万古霉素或甲硝唑	2013	35	万古霉素(125 或 250mg/d),甲硝唑(250 或 500mg, tid)作对照	3 个月	万古霉素或低剂量的甲硝唑改善肝脏生化指标和 Mayo 风险评分	243
nor-UDCA	2017	161	nor-UDCA(500、1 000 或 1 500mg/d) 安慰剂作对照	12 周	降低碱性磷酸酶水平(降低 12.3%~26.0%,而安慰剂则增加 1.2%)	235

*超过 20 例受试者的试验。
PSC,原发性硬化性胆管炎;UDCA,熊去氧胆酸。

PSC 的免疫学机制使得免疫抑制治疗成为一种似乎合理的选择。然而无论口服或鼻胆管灌注,糖皮质激素没有明确的益处[236,237]。一项纳入 21 例 PSC 的非对照初步研究显示口服布地奈德没有疗效却导致明显的骨量丢失[237]。在一项小规模前瞻性对照研究中,为期两年的甲氨蝶呤和安慰剂相比没有生化、组织学或胆道造影的差异[238]。一项关于他克莫司的研究表明在一年之后 PSC 的生化指标有明显改善,但是胆管造影或组织学没有改变[239]。英夫利昔单抗和依那西普都是 TNF-α 抑制剂,对 PSC 均无疗效[152,240]。

抗生素的疗效尚不明确,仍在不断研究中。在一项纳入 14 例儿童 PSC 的研究中口服万古霉素能改善肝脏生化指标,在无肝硬化的患儿中尤为显著[241]。该研究发现口服万古霉素能改善肝脏组织学和影像学表现,同时增加转化生长因子-β(TGF-β)和调节 T 细胞的水平,这提示可能涉及一种免疫调节机制[242]。口服万古霉素 12 周后,成人 PSC 的血清碱性磷酸酶水平也有一定程度的下降[243]。虽然有这些阳性结果,但是肠道菌群改变带来的潜在危害可能会限制抗生素的广泛应用。

其他处于研究阶段的方法还有抗纤维化治疗,但迄今没有研发出让患者获益的药物。针对多种通路的联合治疗可能有效。关于各种药物(如硫唑嘌呤、糖皮质激素、UDCA 和抗生素)的联合治疗的研究数据有限、结果混杂[244,245,150],一些研究认为无效,另一些显示在少数患者中有组织学的改善。此外,联合治疗会增加药物不良反应的风险。

2. 并发症的药物治疗

PSC 治疗的重要组成部分之一是对相关并发症的管理,包括瘙痒、营养不良和细菌性胆管炎。瘙痒的处理同其他胆汁淤积性疾病一样(见第 91 章),包括避免热和其他刺激加重瘙痒。阴离子交换树脂(消胆胺、盐酸考来替泊或考来维仑)是一线治疗,不过患者的依从性可能会有问题,因为药物的口感差、容易导致便秘和影响其他药物的吸收。利福平对于保守治疗和树脂治疗无效的患者来说是一种有效和安全的选择[246]。阿片类拮抗剂(纳洛酮和纳曲酮)对胆汁淤积性瘙痒有效,但是可能会出现自限性阿片类戒断症状[174,175,247,248]。选择性 5-羟色胺再摄取抑制剂的疗效有限[249]。对这些治疗无反应、经内镜或经皮引流无效(见后文)的患者需要血浆置换或鼻胆管引流。肝移植可以治疗顽固性瘙痒,不过除非有合适的活体供者,否则不太可行。

脂溶性维生素水平和 INR 可用于筛查 PSC 相关的营养不良。大多数患者可以口服维生素,而严重的肠道脂肪吸收不良的患者需要胃肠外途径补充维生素。维生素 D 缺乏导致骨量减少,严重程度与肝病的程度无关[250]。PSC 应该在确诊时就进行筛查,之后每隔 2 到 3 年进行一次。如果骨量减少，及时补充维生素 D(1 000IU/d) 和钙(1~1.5g/d)，双膦酸盐则用于骨质疏松的治疗[125]。INR 延长的原因可能是晚期肝病而不是维生素 K 缺乏，不过对于凝血障碍的患者，需进行口服维生素 K 试验(见第 94 章)。

每年约有 10% 的 PSC 出现细菌性胆管炎，这是常见的并发症之一。除自发性细菌性胆管炎之外，PSC 在接受各种胆管相关器械操作之后发生胆管炎的风险同样很高，应使用抗生素预防感染，常用药物包括氟喹诺酮、头孢菌素或 β-内酰胺酶抑制剂，疗程为 5~7 天。PSC 中细菌性胆管炎的诊断标准尚不明确。在东京指南(见第 65 章)中急性胆管炎的诊断依赖于异常的肝脏生化指标，不适用于 PSC。PSC 相关的细菌性胆管炎症状不明显，若患者有发热、白细胞增多、右上腹疼痛或肝脏生化指标恶化时需警惕。虽然反复发作会导致患者体质虚弱，但是细菌性胆管炎并没有增加 PSC 患者等待肝移植时死亡的风险[251]。每 3-4 周交替使用阿莫西林-克拉维酸、环丙沙星和(或)甲氧苄啶/磺胺甲噁唑可使复发性胆管炎患者获益。

3. 内镜治疗

对于有明确适应证的患者，内镜治疗能减轻黄疸、瘙痒和腹痛，缓解胆汁淤积，减少细菌性胆管炎的发作，促进胆汁流动。理论上胆管的长期通畅可以延缓疾病的进展，预防胆汁性肝硬化。涉及 PSC 内镜的多是一些小规模、回顾性和非对照研究，因此不推荐常规使用内镜治疗。

已经或怀疑有显性狭窄的患者最有可能从内镜治疗中获益。显性狭窄的定义是肝外胆管直径≤1.5mm 或者左右肝管分叉 2cm 以内肝内胆管直径≤1mm[252]，合并出现黄疸、瘙痒、胆管炎或腹痛等情况。显性狭窄降低非移植生存率[253]，多项研究表明显性狭窄行内镜治疗(球囊扩张联合或不联合支架临时置入)之后临床表现、生化指标和胆管造影均有明显改善[254-258]。括约肌切开术存在争议，可能导致远端胆管进一步硬化、增加细菌性胆管炎的风险和围手术期出血的风险(尤其是肝硬化)，但是对于需要多次 ERCP 和困难插管的患者，括约肌切开术能预防 ERCP 术后胰腺炎。

胆汁淤积进展时应考虑合并胆总管结石可能。30% 的病例 ERCP 可能会漏诊微小结石，会将其视为符合 PSC 的胆管壁不规则[259]。直视胆道镜可以发现微小结石，必要时可进行碎石治疗。直视胆道镜有助于评估显性狭窄并进行靶向活检，提高了诊断的准确性[260]。

球囊扩张联合胆管支架可能增加并发症的风险[261,154]。指南建议避免常规置入胆管支架，如果有严重狭窄，推荐短期置入(<2 周)[118,126]。重要的是，PSC 在 ERCP 之前需要使用抗生素预防感染，在 ERCP 之后继续治疗 3~5 天。

3 项研究表明对显性狭窄的内镜治疗可延缓疾病的进展。Baluyut 及其同事[262]对 63 例 PSC 进行了病情分级和球囊扩张治疗(置入或不置入支架)，中位随访时间为 34 个月，5 年的生存率优于修订 Mayo 风险评分预测值(见表 68.5)。Stiehl 和同事[263]对 52 例接受 UDCA 治疗时出现显性狭窄的 PSC 进行内镜下球囊扩张和临时的支架置入，无肝移植的生存率在 3 年、5 年和 7 年均优于多中心模型评分的预测值(见表 68.5)。这项研究的后续数据表明球囊扩张能改善 PSC 的无肝移植生存率[264]。Gluck 及其同事[265]的一项回顾性研究也证实接受内镜治疗的患者在 3 年和 4 年的生存率优于修订的 Mayo 模型评分预测值。

PSC 的内镜治疗有局限性，ERCP 术后发生并发症的风险增加，如胰腺炎、胆管炎、穿孔或胆汁淤积加重，总体发生率在 7.3%~10%[265]。弥漫性肝内胆管狭窄无法从内镜治疗中获益，并且 ERCP 术后胆管炎的风险高[263]。专家操作并且把握好 ERCP 的适应证(如黄疸、瘙痒或胆管炎，也就是那些最有可能受益的人群)会降低患者的风险(见第 70 章)[266]。鉴于相关研究的局限性，常规内镜治疗狭窄仍然存在争议。

4. 经皮治疗

经皮 THC 联合球囊扩张或(和)支架置入，也可用于治疗 PSC 的胆管狭窄。这种方法有出血和胆汁性腹膜炎的风险，也会增加患者的不适感。当内镜治疗存在禁忌证或失败之后才推荐经皮 THC(见第 70 章)。

5. 外科手术治疗

(1) 胆道手术

随着内镜治疗的进步和肝移植的出现，胆道手术已经很少用于 PSC。常用的术式是切除狭窄段之后行肝肠吻合术或胆肠吻合术[267-269]。PSC 和肝硬化患者的术后死亡率很高。此外，胆道手术会使以后的肝移植手术复杂化。目前，对 PSC 进行胆道手术的适应证很少，只适用于早期 PSC 和胆管狭窄却不接受内镜或经皮介入治疗的少数患者。

(2) 肝移植

肝移植是唯一能够明确改变 PSC 自然病程的治疗，肝移植后患者的生活质量改善[270,271]。和其他肝病一样，失代偿期肝硬化和门静脉高压并发症是适应证(见第 97 章)。复发性胆管炎、顽固性瘙痒和早期肝门部胆管癌是少见的适应证。自 2005 年以来在美国 PSC 接受肝移植的比例一直稳定在 4.0%~4.8%[272]。早期研究认为 PSC 肝移植时应进行 Roux-en-Y 胆管吻合术，这一说法近来受到质疑。相关研究发现，胆管间吻合术后胆管炎和迟发性非吻合口狭窄的发生率更低，患者生存率和移植肝脏存活率类似(见第 97 章)[273-275]。

PSC 肝移植术后患者的生存率和移植肝脏的存活率都很好[276-278]。1 年、5 年和 10 年的生存率分别为 93.7%、86.4% 和 69.8%，相应的移植肝脏存活率分别为 83.4%、79.0% 和 60.5%[276]。PSC 在肝移植后的总体生存率优于其他肝脏疾病[279,280]。接受肝移植的 PSC 预后不良的相关因素包括高龄、血清白蛋白水平降低、肾功能衰竭、肝硬化 Child-Pugh C 级和器官共享联合网络(UNOS)状态[279,281,282]。

胆管癌会影响 PSC 肝移植的效果。早期研究表明在供体偶然发现胆管癌时，受体的生存率很低，1 年生存率为 30%[283]。基于这些研究基础，胆管癌是肝移植的禁忌。另一项研究证实胆管癌患者肝移植的预后不佳，但是在移植时偶然发现的小胆管癌患者有较好的生存率[278]。随后的研究表明胆管癌患者肝移植之后 1 年和 5 年生存率分别为 65%~82% 和 35%~42%[284,285]。一项纳入美国 12 个中心的合作研究显示，肝移植前接受外照射、近距离放疗、放射增敏治疗和(或)化疗的 5 年无复发存活率为 65%(见第 69 章)[286]。

肝移植后胆管狭窄复发较为常见，可能是 PSC 复发的表现。除此之外，胆管狭窄的潜在原因还包括 ABO 血型不相容、肝动脉闭塞、慢性胆管缺失性排斥反应、Roux-en-Y 相关性胆管炎和缺血。复发性 PSC 的诊断标准为符合典型胆管造影改变,肝脏组织学为纤维性胆管炎、纤维闭塞性病变、胆管纤维化或胆汁性肝硬化,同时排除其他胆管狭窄的危险因素(如肝动脉闭塞、ABO 血型不相容、移植后排斥反应)或在移植后 90 天内发生非吻合口狭窄[287]。依据这些严格的标准,肝移植后 PSC 的复发率在 2.6~9.1 年间为 5.7%~59.1%[277,278,288-291]。虽然有多种危险因素(如移植前的活动性 IBD 和他克莫司),但是均未证实。一些研究表明肝移植前切除结肠降低 PSC 复发[289,292,293],但是尚无有效治疗或预防肝移植后 PSC 复发的方法。一项英国的研究显示 PSC 复发后移植肝脏衰竭或死亡的风险增加[292]。三分之一的复发性 PSC 病情会持续进展,导致死亡或再次移植。

肝移植对 IBD 的病程和结肠癌变的影响是一个有待深入研究的领域。在不同的研究中肝移植后 IBD 的病程各异[90,277,294-297]。一项来自 Mayo Clinic 的研究纳入了 151 例 PSC 合并 IBD,在肝移植时均有完整的结肠,虽然存在移植相关的免疫抑制,在中位数为 10 年的随访期间 37.1%的患者需要升级 IBD 的治疗,57.6%的患者病情稳定,5.3%的患者病情好转[298]。该研究发现他克莫司导致 IBD 恶化,硫唑嘌呤则具有保护作用。在 84 例移植时不合并 IBD 的 PSC 中,26.2%后续出现 IBD,霉酚酸酯可能增加了 IBD 的风险。一项大规模单中心研究显示肝移植增加结肠切除的风险[299],但是其他研究结果却与之相反。UC 在肝移植后结直肠肿瘤的风险增加[213,214,277],虽然尚未在所有研究中得到证实,但是建议 PSC 合并 UC 在肝移植之后每年进行结肠镜检查。

二、继发性硬化性胆管炎

其他疾病可能导致胆管出现与 PSC 相似的特征,统称为继发性硬化性胆管炎(SSC)(见表 68.1)。SSC 常见于胆囊切除术或肝移植后的胆管缺血或损伤。在腹腔镜胆囊切除术的应用早期,医源性胆管损伤率从 0.1%~0.2%(开腹胆囊切除术)上升至 0.8%~1.4%[300]。不过随着腹腔镜的广泛应用,两种术式的胆管损伤率已经相似[301]。既往 26%的 AIDS 合并有胆管病,多见于 CD4 计数低于 100/mm^3 的患者,但是随着 AIDS 治疗的进步,AIDS 相关胆管病变得罕见。隐孢子虫、微孢子虫、巨细胞病毒和其他微生物从感染者的胆汁中分离出来(见第 35 章)[302-305]。相比之下,肝移植后胆管狭窄的发生率在增加,这与边缘供者、心源性原因死亡后供者以及部分肝移植(如活体肝移植)有关,吻合口狭窄的发生率为 5%~25%,非吻合口狭窄的发生率为 10%~15%[306]。

SSC 的其他原因包括结节病、嗜酸性胆管炎和 IgG4 相关性硬化性胆管炎[189]。当包虫囊肿与胆管相通时[308],胆管暴露在治疗药物之中(如氟尿嘧啶和甲醛)[307],可产生 SSC 的胆道造影表现(见表 68.4 及第 84 和 88 章)。

结节病经常累及肝脏,在一些罕见病例中会导致胆汁淤积,表现出类似于 PSC 的特征[309]。嗜酸性胆管炎是一种罕见的疾病,其特征是大量嗜酸性粒细胞的透壁性浸润[310]。肥大细胞对胆管的浸润在引起 SSC 的各种疾病中很常见,例如在一个病例中 SSC 是由系统性肥大细胞增多症引起[311]。

毒素和血管损伤也可能导致 SSC。肝移植术后肝动脉血栓形成[312]和危重(烧伤和脓毒症)患者也可能发生 SSC[313]。罕见的结节性多动脉炎影响肝动脉血流从而引起 SSC 也有报道[314]。尽管外源性胆管压迫、门静脉胆管病变和门静脉海绵样胆管病合并肝外门静脉阻塞并不属于 SSC,但在影像上可能具有相似的表现[315]。

(一) IgG4 相关性硬化性胆管炎

IgG4 相关性硬化性胆管炎,又称 IgG4 相关性胆管炎或 IgG4 硬化性胆管炎,是 IgG4 相关性疾病在胆道系统的表现,特征是 IgG4 阳性的淋巴细胞和嗜酸性粒细胞浸润,并伴有闭塞性静脉炎和绒毛膜样纤维化[316]。IgG4 硬化性胆管炎的发病机制是抗原诱发的免疫反应,促使 B 细胞产生 IgG4,同时激活 T 细胞分泌促纤维化细胞因子[317]。长期暴露在溶剂和工业气体与 IgG4 硬化性胆管炎有关,表明环境因素可能导致一种诱发免疫反应的新抗原[318]。包括 IL-4 和 IL-13 在内的 2 型 T 辅助细胞(Th2)细胞因子以及转化生长因子-β 和 IL-10 的产生,由浆细胞来源的 RANKL(核因子 kappa-B 配体的受体激活物)介导,进而抑制 T 细胞的增殖并诱导 Th2 的分化[319,320]。

IgG4 相关性硬化性胆管炎多发于年龄大于 60 岁的群体,以男性为主。常见胰腺或其他器官(涎腺炎)的受累,但与 IBD 无关。由于罕见,IgG4-SC 的患病率和发病率尚不清楚。

IgG4 相关性硬化性胆管炎的表现可能与 PSC 或胆管癌类似,容易漏诊(见表 68.4)[118,321-323]。因此所有疑似 PSC 或胆管癌的病例都应和 IgG4 相关性硬化性胆管炎鉴别,尤其是不合并 IBD 的老年男性。诊断应基于组织学、影像学、血清学、其他器官受累以及对糖皮质激素治疗的反应,符合 HISORt 标准[324]。虽然大约 10%的 PSC 血清 IgG4 水平升高,但往往低于 IgG4 相关性硬化性胆管炎。高于正常上限的 4 倍以上是 IgG4 相关性硬化性胆管炎的特异性表现[325]。30%的 IgG4 相关性硬化性胆管炎的血清 IgG4 水平没有升高。如果在主乳头或胆管活检中发现大量 IgG4 阳性淋巴细胞(>20 个/HPF),支持 IgG4 相关性硬化性胆管炎的诊断[157,326,327]。

治疗类似于自身免疫性胰腺炎,包括糖皮质激素,超过 95%的患者对糖皮质激素有反应[321]。然而会经常复发,可以使用硫唑嘌呤或其他免疫抑制剂进行长期维持治疗。肝硬化或胆管癌少见,远期预后良好。

(二) 复发性化脓性胆管炎

复发性化脓性胆管炎(Recurrent pyogenic cholangitis,RPC)是 1930 年由 Digby 首次报道的一种 SSC,Cook 和同事将其定义为以反复出现细菌性胆管炎、肝内色素结石和胆管狭窄为特征的综合征,可能导致慢性肝病和胆管癌[328,329]。RPC 又被称为肝内胆管结石病。虽然 RPC 的患病率一直在下降,但在东南亚仍然常见,也同样发生于西方国家的移民之中。男女比例相同,农村和较低的社会经济地位似乎是危险因素[330,331],这表明流行病学的变化可能与蛋白质含量更高的西式饮食有关;改善卫生条件,减轻与华支睾吸虫和蛔虫相关的疾病负担,认为这些感染是 RPC 的诱因(见第 84 章)。

华支睾吸虫、后睾吸虫和蛔虫的感染与 RPC 流行之间存在密切相关性。然而,与普通人群相比,RPC 发生寄生虫感染的频率没有增加,约一半的 RPC 没有感染的证据[332-334],亚洲一些 RPC 流行区华支睾吸虫的感染率很低[335]。细菌感染也是 RPC 的原因之一,门脉菌血症可能与胃肠道感染和细菌移位、社会经济地位低下和营养不良有关[331]。低饱和脂肪饮食可能会降低胆囊收缩能力,促进结石形成。

1. 临床特征和诊断

RPC 经常出现急性细菌性胆管炎的症状,包括发热、右上腹痛和黄疸,也称为 Charcot 三联征(见第 65 章)。患者也可能出现腹痛或胰腺炎。RPC 的影像表现具有特征性,大多数患者(75% ~ 80%)有肝内结石,主要累及左肝管(图 68.6)[336]。胆管扩张很常见。肝内中央胆管不成比例地扩张,周围胆管突然变细和衰减。胆管结石导致肝内胆管扩张和下游胆管狭窄[337]。胆管造影术(经皮穿刺或内镜)可以定位肝内结石和狭窄,放置引流管或取出结石。MRCP 能发现全部扩张的胆管和 98% 的局灶性胆管狭窄和胆管内结石,胆管造影只能发现 44% ~47% 的节段性胆管异常。MRCP 是首选的诊断方法[338]。研究显示在 82 例胆管癌合并 RPC 中,胆管癌多位于胆管结石的萎缩段伴有门静脉闭塞或狭窄[339]。

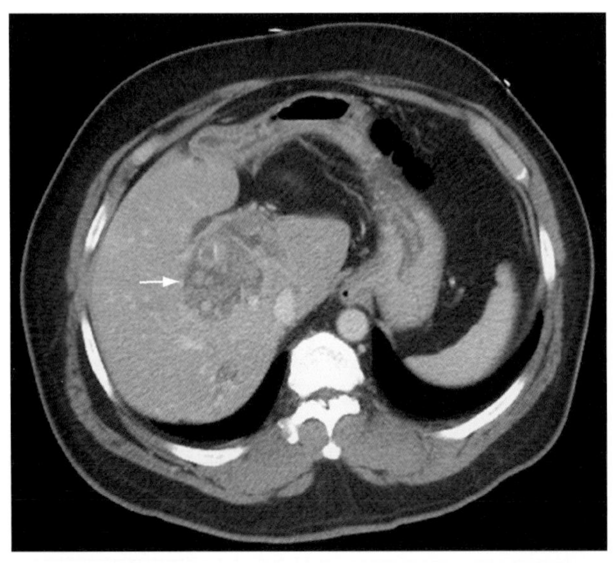

图 68.6 有复发性化脓性胆管炎病史患者的 CT。注意右侧肝内胆管重度扩张伴明显的胆管内结石(箭示)

首次发作胆管炎合并肝内结石和狭窄的患者应该检查华支睾吸虫和后睾吸虫,尤其是来自或去过流行地区的患者。感染 4 周后粪便中出现虫卵[337],收集粪便后鉴定粪便样本中的虫卵可以诊断寄生虫感染,十二指肠液或胆汁也能检测虫卵或完整的虫体。外周嗜酸性粒细胞增多可能与血清 IgE 水平升高有关[340]。

2. 治疗

一旦获得血液或胆汁培养的阳性结果,立即开始抗生素治疗。有活动性寄生虫感染证据的患者需要抗寄生虫药治疗(见第 84 章)。

在胆管炎和肝内外胆管扩张的患者中,ERCP 是首选的治疗方法。无论是否鼻胆管引流或经皮胆管引流,ERCP 联合括约肌切开用以清理胆管结石(见第 70 章)。一些研究回顾分析了各种非手术方式在 RPC 急性期的数据。Sperling 和同事比较了 41 例 RPC 的治疗效果[336],62% 只接受诊断性 ERCP 的 6 患者出现复发,接受治疗性 ERCP 或手术治疗的患者中复发率只有一半。治疗性 ERCP 对肝外胆管受累的患者特别有效,与手术相当。左右肝管同时受累的患者往往需要更多的影像学检查、经皮胆管造影以及内镜或外科手术[341]。

肝空肠吻合术是治疗 RPC 患者肝内结石的常用术式[342]。腹腔镜胆道旁路手术证实是一种可行且有效的治疗方法[343,344]。

3. 预后和并发症

RPC 的自然病程尚不明确。复发性胆管炎患者在 3 年复发率为 25%,5 年复发率为 37%[345]。继发性胆汁性肝硬化可能持续进展,需要肝移植。胆管癌与 RPC 相关,累计发生率为 3% ~9%(见第 69 章)[346]。

(刘文正 闫秀娥 译,鲁晓岚 校)

参考文献

第 69 章　胆管、胆囊和壶腹部肿瘤

Sumera H. Rizvi, Gregory J. Gore 著

章节目录

一、胆管癌 …… 1021
（一）流行病学 …… 1021
（二）病因学 …… 1022
（三）病理学 …… 1022
（四）发病机制 …… 1023
（五）临床特征和诊断 …… 1023
（六）分期 …… 1026
（七）治疗 …… 1027
二、胆囊癌 …… 1028
（一）流行病学 …… 1029
（二）病因学 …… 1029
（三）病理学 …… 1029
（四）发病机制 …… 1030
（五）临床特征和诊断 …… 1030
（六）分期 …… 1031
（七）治疗 …… 1031
三、壶腹癌 …… 1032
（一）流行病学 …… 1032
（二）病因 …… 1032
（三）病理学 …… 1032
（四）发病机制 …… 1032
（五）临床特征和诊断 …… 1033
（六）分期 …… 1033
（七）治疗 …… 1034
四、胆道的其他肿瘤 …… 1034

胆道恶性肿瘤占胆道肿瘤的绝大部分，其分为 3 类：①肝内和肝外胆管癌；②胆囊癌；③Vater 壶腹癌[1]。在美国和其他西方国家，胆道恶性肿瘤很少见。根据在胆管内的解剖位置，胆管癌可进一步分为肝内、肝门部和远端胆管癌。但是，在世界上某些地区，它们的患病率很高，使其成为这些地区癌症死亡的主要原因。胆管癌具有高度侵袭性，且远期预后不良。

一、胆管癌

胆管癌是一种上皮性癌，具有由肝内和肝外胆管来源的胆管上皮的分化特征[2]。这是最常见的胆道肿瘤和第二常见的原发于肝脏的恶性肿瘤[仅次于肝细胞癌（HCC）（参见第 96 章）]。自 20 世纪 70 年代以来，胆管癌在全世界范围内的发病率一直在上升[3-6]。

根据在胆管内的位置，胆管癌分为肝内、肝门和远端胆管癌三种亚型，每种解剖亚型都有其独特的流行病学、发病机制、危险因素、治疗和预后[2]。肝内胆管癌发生在肝实质内和二级胆管的上方（参见第 62 章），肝门周围或肝门部胆管癌发生在二级胆管和胆囊管的汇入部位之间，远端胆管癌发生在胆囊管的汇入部位的下方（图 69.1A）[2]。肝门部胆管癌也称为 Klatskin 肿瘤（见图 69.1B），在临床上根据 Bismuth-Corlette 分型被分为Ⅰ～Ⅳ型。Ⅰ型累及肝总管远端至左右肝管汇合处；Ⅱ型累及左右肝管汇合处；Ⅲa 型累及左右肝管汇合处，并向上延伸至右肝管。Ⅲb 型累及左右肝管汇合处并向上延伸至左肝管；Ⅳ型呈多灶性或累及左右肝管汇合处，并沿左右肝管向上延伸。胆管癌的自然病程呈侵袭性，诊断后中位生存期不到 24 个月[7]。

（一）流行病学

胆管癌是最常见的胆道癌症和第二大最常见的原发性肝脏恶性肿瘤[8]。虽仅占所有恶性肿瘤的 2%，但它在常见的 GI 恶性肿瘤中排第九位。肝胆恶性肿瘤分别占世界和美国总癌症相关死亡率的 13% 和 3%，这些死亡中有 10%～20% 是由胆管癌引起的[9]。

胆管癌全球各地发病率不同。在东南亚的发病率最高，按年龄校正后的发病率高达每 10 万人口 113 例，而澳大利亚的发病率最低，低至每 10 万人口 0.1 例[10,11]。在美国，研究发现按年龄校正后的胆管癌发生率存在种族差异，其中亚裔和西班牙裔患者的发生率最高（分别为 3.3/100 000 和 2.8/100 000），而非洲裔美国人的发生率最低（2.1/100 000）[8]。男性的胆管癌的发病率和年龄校正后的死亡率高于女性[8]。在世界范围内，诊断的平均年龄约为 50 岁[8,10]。在西方工业化国家中，大多数病例是在 65 岁以上的患者中诊断出来的，而胆管癌在 40 岁之前罕见，但原发性硬化性胆管炎（PSC）患者除外（参见第 68 章）[8,10]。

大多数胆管癌位于肝门部（50%～60%）或远端（20%～30%），而肝内胆管癌仅占所有胆管癌的大约 20%[12]。自 20 世纪 80 年代以来，已有多项研究表明肝内胆管癌的发生率增加，而肝门部和远端胆管癌的发生率则随之下降[13]。这个趋势在一定程度上可能是由于将肝门部肿瘤误分类为肝内肿瘤所导致的。根据美国的“监测、流行病学和最终结果”数据库，在 1990 年至 2001 年之间，按年龄校正后的肝内胆管癌的发病率增加，而肝门部和远端胆管癌的发病率在此期间有所下降。《国际疾病分类-肿瘤学》（*International Classification of Disease for Oncology*）第 2 版将 Klatskin 肿瘤归类为肝内肿瘤。而在 2001 年出版的第 3 版中，将 Klatskin 被重新分类为肝外肿瘤[3,13]。

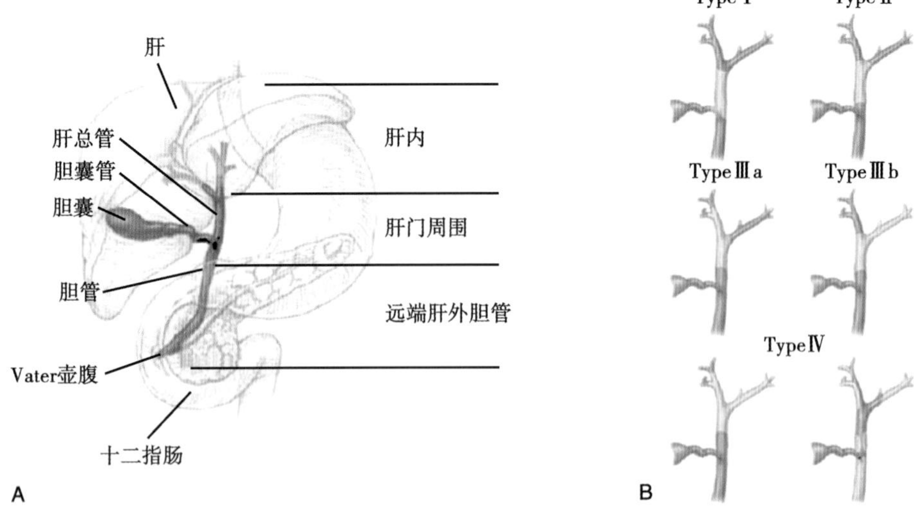

图 69.1　胆管癌的分类。A,肝内,肝门周围和远端胆管癌的解剖学分类。B,肝门周围胆管癌的 Bismuth-Corlette 分类为Ⅰ~Ⅳ型。肿瘤用黄色表示,正常胆管用绿色表示。(Modified from Blechacz BR, Komuta M, Roskams T, Gores GJ. Clinical diagnosis and staging of cholangiocarcinoma. Nat Rev Gastroenterol Hepatol 2011;8:512-22.)

(二) 病因学

在大多数病例中,胆管癌的病因尚不清楚。目前已经确定了几个风险因素(框 69.1)。这些危险因素的特点是与炎症和胆汁淤积有关。然而,探索危险因素与胆管癌相关性的研究通常受到洲际和洲内异质性以及癌症登记不准确的限制,例如胆管癌与其他胆道恶性肿瘤和 HCC 的分类。

框 69.1　胆管癌的危险因素
确定的危险因素
Caroli 病
胆总管囊肿
胆石症
泰国肝吸虫感染
原发性硬化性胆管炎
钍造影剂
可能的危险因素
胆肠引流操作
肝硬化
华支睾吸虫感染
大量饮酒
丙型肝炎
毒素(二噁英,聚氯乙烯)

1. 已确定的危险因素

尽管存在几种已知的胆管癌危险因素,但大多数病例为散发,并且没有已知危险因素。PSC 是胆管癌的最常见危险因素之一(参见第 68 章)。但是,只有 10% 的胆管癌归因于 PSC。在 PSC 患者中,胆管癌的年发病率为 0.6%~1.5%,30 年累积发病率为 20%[5]。对新诊断的 PSC 应重视对胆管癌的怀疑,27%~37% 的胆管癌是在诊断 PSC 后的第一年内发现的[5]。还发现了其他胆管疾病是导致胆管癌的危险因素。患有 Caroli 病和胆总管囊肿(尤其是Ⅰ型和Ⅳ型)的患者胆管癌的风险增加了多达 50 倍,终生发病率为 6%~30%(参见第 62 章)。切除囊肿可减少但不能消除胆管癌发展的风险[9]。肝脏结石合并反复发作化脓性胆管炎的患者发生胆管癌的风险为 10%(参见第 68 章)[14]。在胆肠引流过程中反复发作细菌性胆管炎也与胆管癌的发展有关[14]。胆管癌的其他危险因素包括在东亚地区流行的胆道感染泰国肝吸虫和华支睾吸虫(参见第 84 章)[15]。诸如钍造影剂(过去曾用作放射造影剂)和二噁英等致癌物也与胆管癌风险增加有关(参见第 89 章)[16]。

2. 可能的风险因素

胆管癌与炎症性肠病(溃疡性结肠炎或克罗恩病)之间的关联存在争议,并且可能受 PSC 是否存在和持续时间的影响。因此,尚不清楚炎症性肠病是否会给 PSC 患者带来胆管癌的额外风险[8]。胆管癌和病毒性肝炎之间的关联研究显示出洲际差异性。肝内胆管癌与丙型肝炎病毒和乙型肝炎病毒感染及肝硬化有关,而肝门部胆管癌仅与肝硬化有关(参见第 96 章)[6,8,17]。肥胖,糖尿病和非酒精性脂肪性肝病与胆管癌风险增加有关,但数据不一致[8,18]。在西方工业化国家中,这些疾病的发生率一直在上升,这一趋势可能解释了这些国家正在上升的肝内胆管癌的发病率。大量饮酒与肝内、肝门部和远端胆管癌有关,被认为是可能的危险因素[8,17,18]。

(三) 病理学

胆管癌是一种寡细胞的、高度促结缔组织增生的肿瘤。肉眼上,肝内胆管癌可分为 3 种亚型:肿块型、导管周围浸润型和导管内生长型。肿块型是肝内胆管癌最常见的类型,占 85% 以上病例[20,21]。

肿块型倾向于侵入肝实质,在晚期阶段侵入淋巴管,而导管周围浸润型则通过淋巴管沿 Glisson 鞘扩散[21]。肉眼上,肝门部胆管癌具有导管周围浸润型,结节型或导管内生长型三种模式,最常见的是导管周围浸润型。因为肝门部胆管癌对胆汁有趋向性,所以最初的生长模式通常是导管周围型,并且随着肿瘤的进展,形成了肿块,导致肿块形成和导管周围浸润[22,23]。导管内乳头状腺癌沿胆道黏膜浅表扩散,而无纤维肌壁层深层浸润，预后较非乳头状癌好[19]。经常观察到这种类型转移到区域和胰腺周围淋巴结。从组织学上讲，90%的胆管癌是腺癌。其他组织学类型包括肠型腺癌、透明细胞腺癌、印戒细胞癌、腺鳞癌、鳞状细胞癌和小细胞癌[24]。

（四）发病机制

胆管癌的发病机制很复杂，可能与微环境中的炎症、环境因素以及肿瘤细胞的遗传畸变（获得性和种系）有关。大多数现有资料都与遗传畸变有关，包括转录组分析、拷贝数变异、DNA 甲基化、microRNA 分析和体细胞突变[25-28]。关于遗传畸变的最详细的资料是《癌症基因组图谱》(*The Cancer Genome Atlas*)对胆管癌的集成基因组分析，其中的胆管癌主要是肝内胆管癌，并且肝吸虫和肝炎病毒均阴性[28]。在这些肿瘤中发现了抑癌基因的失活突变，包括 *ARID1A*、*ARID1B*、*BAP1*、肿瘤蛋白 p53(tumor protein p53, *TP53*)、磷酸酶和肌腱蛋白同源物(phosphatase and tensin homolog, *PTEN*)，以及癌基因异柠檬酸脱氢酶(isocitrate dehydrogenase, *IDH*) 1 和 2、*BRAF* 和 *KRAS*[28]。各不相关的致癌危险因素可能会影响胆管癌的体细胞畸变模式。例如，肝吸虫相关的胆管癌具有较高的 *TP53* 突变频率，而 *IDH1*、*IDH2* 和 *BAP1* 突变在非肝吸虫相关的胆管癌中更常见[28]。

胆管癌的所有的基因组改变因解剖亚型而异。肝内胆管癌中成纤维细胞生长因子受体(fibroblast growth factor receptor, *FGFR*) 1～3、*IDH1*、*IDH2* 和 *BAP1* 的分子畸变频率较高，而 *ARID1B*、*PBRM1* 及蛋白激酶环状 AMP 激活的催化亚基 α(*PRKACA*)和 β(*PRKACB*)在远端和肝门部胆管癌中突变频率更高[26]。类 E74 的 ETS 转录因子 3(*ELF3*)的失活突变优先发生在远端胆管癌中(表 69.1)[29]。

表 69.1　胆管癌的分子畸变

胆管癌亚型	分子畸变
肝内	*FGFR2* 基因融合
	异柠檬酸脱氢酶(*IDH*) 1/2 突变
	Mcl-1 扩增
	MET-肝细胞生长因子(HGF)过表达
	BAP1 失活突变
	ARID1A 失活突变
	PTPN3 激活突变
	KRAS 激活突变
	PIK3CA 激活突变
肝门部	*HER2* 扩增
	ERBB2 遗传畸变
	蛋白激酶环状 AMP 激活的催化亚基 α(*PRKACA*)和 β(*PRKACB*)基因融合体
	KRAS 激活突变
	PIK3CA 激活突变
远端	类 E74 的 ETS 转录因子 3(*ELF3*)失活突变
	ERBB3 突变
	KRAS 激活突变
	PIK3CA 激活突变

FGF 信号转导异常导致癌症发生，见于包括胆管癌在内的一系列恶性肿瘤中。受体酪氨酸激酶 *FGFR2* 的基因融合导致其不依赖配体的激活。在 11%～14%的肝内胆管癌中存在 *FGFR2* 基因融合[30-32]。这些基因融合的发现值得注意，因为它们通常是驱动突变的目标。*IDH* 突变是胆管癌中相对普遍的遗传畸变，在 23%～28%的肝内胆管癌中可观察到[33,34]。IDH1 和 IDH2 是催化反应的酶，导致生成 α-酮戊二酸。*IDH* 和 *IDH2* 的点突变导致 2-羟基戊二酸增加，这是一种合成代谢物，可促进恶性肿瘤的广泛表观遗传畸变[34,35]。目前正在进行 FGFR、IDH1 和 IDH2 的小分子抑制剂治疗胆管癌的临床试验。

（五）临床特征和诊断

胆管癌的诊断具有挑战性，因为其通常表现隐匿，并且诊断研究的结果通常是非特异性的。目前需要采用多学科方法，包括临床评估以及实验室、内镜和影像学研究(图 69.2 和图 69.3)[36]。

肝内胆管癌主要表现为腹痛和全身症状，例如恶病质、不适和疲劳。在大多数情况下，肝门部和远端胆管癌表现为继发于恶性胆道梗阻的无痛性黄疸。在 10%的患者中，细菌性胆管炎是最初出现的症状。体格检查可发现萎缩-肥大同时存在，表现为对侧可触及未受累的肝叶肥大，并伴有受累的肝

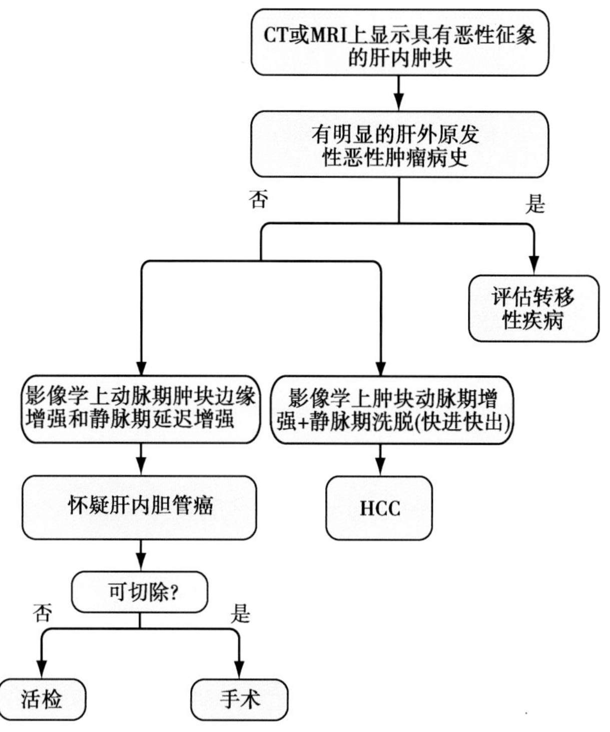

图 69.2　肝内胆管癌的诊断流程。在肝内肿块病变和无已知肝外原发性恶性肿瘤的情况下，应进行肝脏 CT 或 MRI 的动态成像。动脉期肿块整个增强和门静脉期的“洗脱”提示肝细胞癌(HCC)。在整个动脉期肿块的对比边缘增强和延迟的门静脉增强应引起对肝内胆管癌的怀疑；在这种情况下，应确定肿瘤的可切除性。如果认为病变是可完全切除的，无须进行活检，将患者转诊进行手术切除。如果认为肝内胆管癌无法切除，应进行活检以确诊并指导适当的治疗

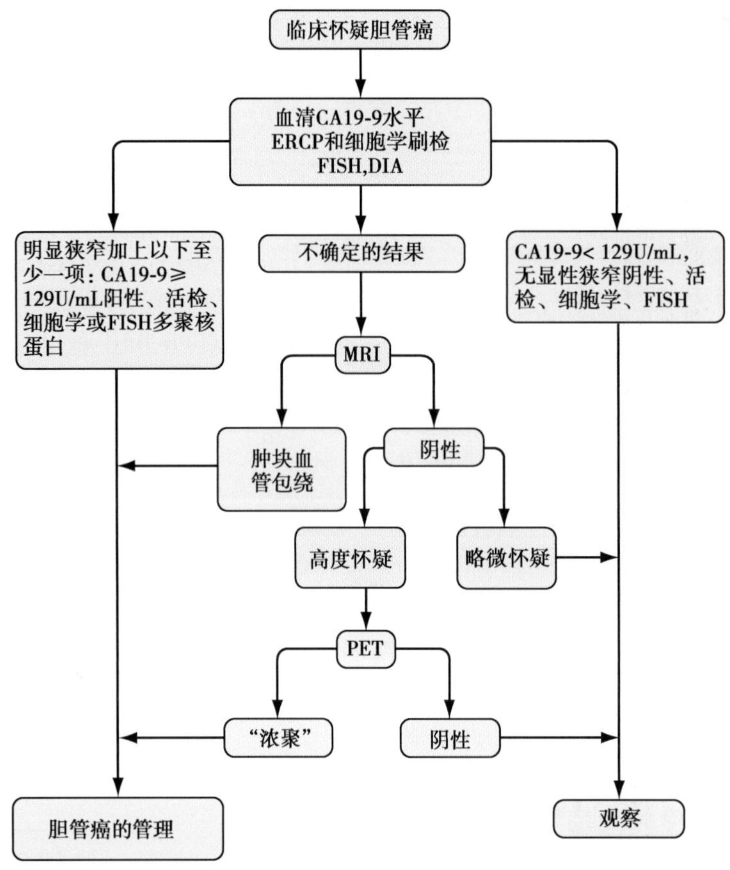

图 69.3　肝门周围胆管癌的诊断流程。对临床上疑似肝门周围胆管癌的病例,应检查血清 CA19-9 水平、ERCP 和对内镜下获得的恶性外观区域的胆管刷检进行常规以及分子细胞学分析。如果这些检测结果是正常或为阴性,建议对患者进行密切随访。胆管癌的治疗应通过识别显性狭窄、血清 CA19-9 水平高于 129U/mL、活检或细胞学检查结果为癌或多聚核蛋白阳性。在不确定的病例中,建议进行肝脏钆增强磁共振(MRI)检查。如果发现肿块或血管包绕,应开始胆管癌的治疗。如果 MRI 检查为阴性,但临床仍怀疑胆管癌,则可进行正电子发射型计算机断层显影(PET)检查。如果在 PET 上发现"浓聚"(阳性结果),应开始胆管癌的治疗。如果 PET 结果为阴性,建议对患者密切随访。如果 MRI 结果为阴性,并且认为不太可能发生胆管癌,则应对患者进行定期随访。DIA,数字图像分析;FISH,荧光原位杂交

叶萎缩,其原因是血管被包绕和胆管梗阻。

实验室检查可能表现为梗阻性胆汁淤积。对不明原因狭窄的病例,需应用血清学和胆管样本排除免疫球蛋白 G4(IgG4)相关性胆病(参见第 59 和 68 章)。胆管癌中最常用的血清肿瘤标志物是 CA19-9。在 PSC 患者中,当临界值为 129U/mL 时,CA19-9 诊断胆管癌的敏感性和特异性分别为 79% 和 98%。在没有 PSC 的患者中,灵敏度为 53%,临界值为 100U/mL[37]。高水平的 CA19-9 水平(>1 000U/mL)与转移性胆管癌有关[37]。需要注意的是,在红细胞或体液中不表达 Lewis 抗原的患者(约占一般人群的 5%~10%)血清 CA19-9 水平检测不到[39]。在细菌性胆管炎和胆总管结石的患者中偶尔会观察到 CA19-9 明显升高(参见第 65 章)。同样需要注意的是,多达三分之一的血清 CA19-9 水平升高的患者没有胆管癌。

1. 肝内胆管癌

肝内胆管癌通常表现为肝脏的肿块。在存在肝硬化的情况下,很难区分肝内胆管癌和 HCC。在评估直径大于 2cm 的肝内病变时,动态 CT 和 MRI(图 69.4)有助于区分胆管癌和 HCC,相比 HCC,前者表现为静脉、动脉和延迟静脉期的进行性增强,而后者表现为静脉期洗脱[40a]。肝内胆管癌的特征是在动态 CT 或钆增强 MRI 早期出现初始边缘或外周动脉强化,并在延迟期出现进行性向心性强化[41,42]。

CT 主要用于术前判断;它提供血管和其他解剖结构的信息,在评估可切除性的准确性是 60%~88%[43]。CT 对检测淋巴结 N2 转移的敏感性(见下文)仅为 54%[43]。在肝内胆管癌评估中,PET/CT 的敏感性和特异性分别为 95% 和 83%[44]。对于肝内胆管癌,组织学诊断应局限于不能切除的病例,因为与 HCC 的区分会影响治疗的选择。

2. 肝门周围和远端胆管癌

胆管造影是肝门周围和远端胆管癌的基本诊断工具,它同时可提供解剖学信息和组织学诊断。可以采用多种方法,包括 ERCP、经皮经肝穿刺胆道造影(transhepatic cholangiography,THC)和磁共振胰胆管造影(MRCP)(图 69.5)。选择 ERCP 还是经皮 THC 取决于可疑胆道狭窄的位置、当地医生是否具备专业知识,和该技术是否可到达狭窄部位。无论是 ERCP 还是经皮 THC 都提供了关于胆道内肿瘤扩散的信息,并对恶性胆道梗阻进行细胞学取样和治疗干预。MRCP 不能进行此类干预,但是这项技术无创,并且提供了关于肿瘤范

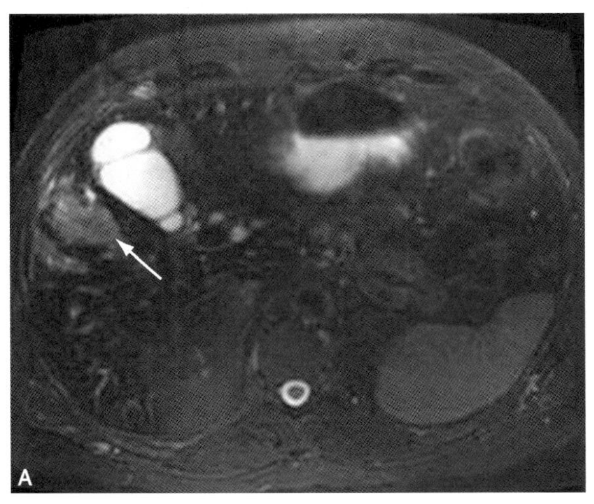

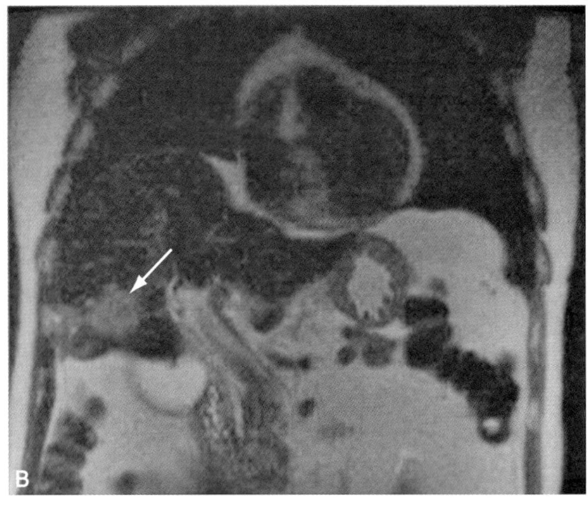

图 69.4　肝内胆管癌的成像。此为一例肝内胆管癌患者使用氧化铁进行的钆增强磁共振成像。箭指向 T2 加权图像中的肿瘤。A，轴向视图。B，冠状位视图

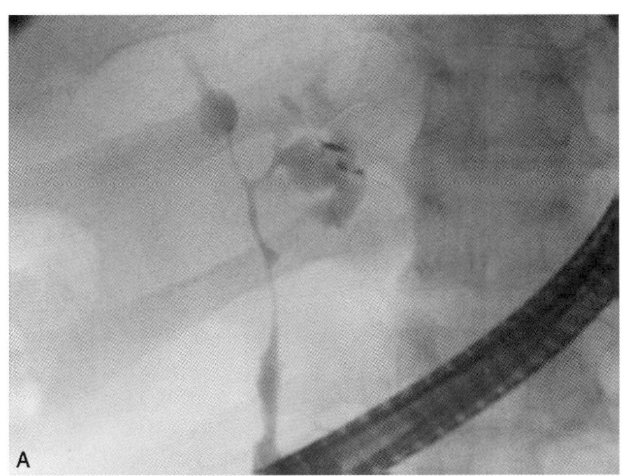

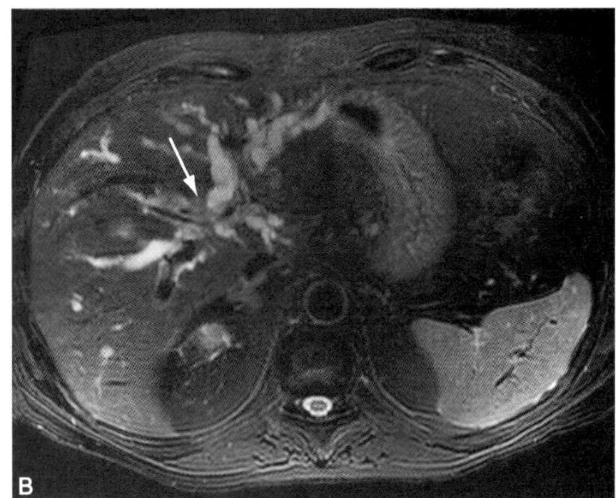

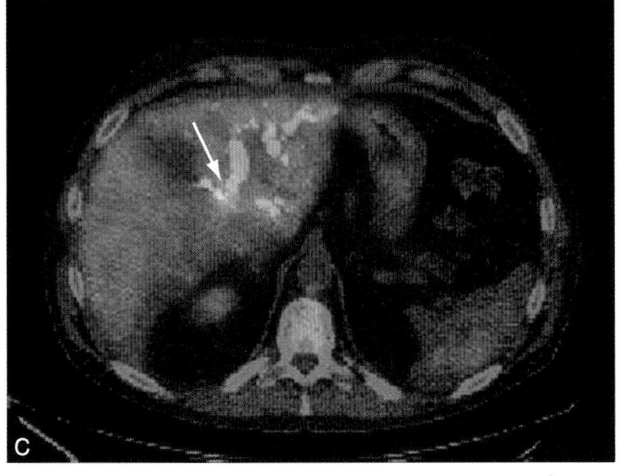

图 69.5　肝门周围胆管癌的影像学。A，肝门周围胆管癌患者 ERCP 的胶片显示出与 Bismuth-Corlette Ⅳ型一致的显性胆道狭窄。B，同一患者氧化铁钆增强 MRI。箭指向 T2 加权图像上观察到的胆道肿瘤。C，同一患者 PET/CT 扫描。增强区域（箭）为胆道肿瘤

围、血管包绕、原发肿瘤与周围结构的关系，以及肝内和肝外转移等额外信息[45]。在胆道造影之前应进行断层成像，以帮助指导有关胆道引流的决策。MRI 和 MRCP 是目前评估肝门周围胆管癌胆管肿瘤侵犯程度的最佳影像学技术，而 CT 在检测血管强化和评估可切除性方面具有优势[46]。对于肝门周围胆管癌，PET 的敏感性和特异性分别仅为 69% 和 67%，检测局部淋巴结转移的敏感性仅为 13% ~ 38%[47,48]。在炎症环境中可以观察到 PET 结果假阳性[44]。因此，它在肝门周围病变的应用应限于在其他检查完成后，其范围和其他特征（包括恶性肿瘤）尚不确定的情况下。远端胆管癌肿块型并不常见，在临床研究中常与肝门周围胆管癌合并。因此，应采用与肝门周围胆管癌相同的实验室和影像学标准。

超声内镜检查(EUS)可以提供更多关于肿瘤大小和与周围结构相关的解剖位置的信息。与CT或MRI相比,EUS的肿瘤检出率更高,尤其是远端胆管癌[50]。此外,EUS还提供了关于局部淋巴结的信息,并允许通过FNA对淋巴结进行取样。但是,非常不鼓励通过EUS对原发病灶进行活检,因为这可能会导致肿瘤细胞扩散,尤其是在准备进行肝移植的情况下[51]。对于大多数恶性肿瘤而言,值得进行胆管癌的组织诊断;然而,由于肿瘤的寡细胞特性,病理诊断具有挑战性。组织很难获得,炎症引起的细胞反应性改变常常使诊断复杂化。最常见的收集肝门周围和远端胆管癌肿瘤组织的技术是ERCP过程中行细胞学刷检[51a]。虽然常规细胞学检查有很高的特异性(100%),但它受到低敏感性(43%)的限制[52]。荧光原位杂交(fluorescence in situ hybridization,FISH)已被证明可以提高细胞学诊断胆管癌的敏感性和特异性,无论患者是否患有PSC[49]。因为染色体不稳定是癌症的一个标志,FISH检测被用于通过使用荧光标记的DNA探针来评估染色体畸形(染色体的增加或损失)。优化后的FISH探针(针对1q21、7p12、8q24、9p21位点)增加了胰胆恶性肿瘤检测的敏感性和特异性(分别为93%和100%)[54]。

诊断胆管癌的新技术包括胆管镜、导管内超声和共聚焦激光显微内镜[55]。在少数患者中进行的有限的前瞻性研究表明,与不明原因狭窄的胆道刷检相比,胆管镜检查活检的诊断准确性有所提高[55]。因此,因这些技术还没有在临床实践中常规开展,应在上述方法仍未确诊的高度怀疑胆管癌病例中进行。

(六) 分期

恶性肿瘤的分期系统旨在为预后和治疗提供指导。肝内、肝门部和远端胆管癌有几种分期系统;不幸的是,这些方法都不是最优的。2009年,美国癌症联合委员会(American Joint Committee on Cancer,AJCC)/国际癌症控制联盟(Union for International Cancer Control,UICC)对TNM系统进行了修改,为每种胆管癌类型指定了一个单独的分期系统[47,57]。已有新的和有前景的分期系统开发出来,但是仍需要验证[19,57a]。

肝内胆管癌的独立预后因素包括肿瘤数量、血管侵犯和淋巴结转移[58]。肝内胆管癌有3种分期系统,其主要区别在T分期,3种分期系统分别为:①AJCC/UICC TNM分期系统;②肝癌研究组的日本分期系统;③国家癌症中心的日本分期系统[19]。在这3种分期系统中,只有AJCC/UICC TNM分期系统(表69.2)显示了分期与生存期的相关性,但该系统受限于需要对Tis(原位癌)和T4分期进行组织诊断[57,59]。

肝门部胆管癌的独立预后因素包括肿瘤分型、淋巴结转移和手术切除边缘阴性(R0)。肝门部胆管癌的4个主要分期系统是Bismuth-Corlette分型[60,60a]、纪念斯隆-凯特琳癌症中心(Memorial Sloan-Kettering Cancer Center,MSKCC)分期系统[61]、AJCC/UICC TNM分期系统[57]和梅奥诊所分期系统[63]。Bismuth-Corlette分型是为指导外科治疗而制定的,并不是一个分期系统,它不能提供预后,也不与手术结果相关。虽然MSKCC分期系统(表69.3)显示T分期与R0、N2和M1状态相关,但不能可靠地区分可切除和不可切除的疾病。与其他3个使用手术信息的系统不同,梅奥临床分期系统(表69.4)基于诊断时的非手术信息,因此梅奥临床分期系统可用于预测不可切除患者的生存期。此外,与AJCC/UICC系统相比,该系统能更好地预测预后,这由更大的一致性统计数据来佐证(表69.5)[63]。远端胆管癌的独立预后因素包括肿瘤浸润的深度、淋巴结转移、周围神经、微血管和胰腺的侵犯以及R0切除。与其他类型的胆管癌相比,这种类型的胆管癌更容易观察到淋巴结转移。AJCC/UICC TNM分期系统是远端胆

表69.2　肝内胆管癌的TNM和AJCC/UICC分期系统TNM发期标准

TNM分期	标准		
Tx	原发肿瘤无法评估		
T0	无原发肿瘤的证据		
Tis	原位癌(导管内肿瘤)		
T1a	孤立性肿瘤≤5cm,未侵犯血管		
T1b	孤立性肿瘤>5cm,无血管侵犯		
T2	伴血管侵犯的单发肿瘤或多发肿瘤,无论有无血管侵犯		
T3	肿瘤穿透脏腹膜		
T4	肿瘤直接侵犯肝外的局部结构		
Nx	局部淋巴结无法评估		
N0	无局部淋巴结转移		
N1	有局部淋巴结转移		
M0	无远处转移		
M1	有远处转移		
AJCC/UICC分期	**肿瘤**	**淋巴结**	**远处转移**
0	Tis	N0	M0
ⅠA	T1a	N0	M0
ⅠB	T1b	N0	M0
Ⅱ	T2	N0	M0
ⅢA	T3	N0	M0
ⅢB	T4 任何T	N0 N1	M0 M0
Ⅳ	任何T	任何N	M1

AJCC,美国癌症联合委员会;UICC,国际癌症控制联盟。

表69.3　肝门区胆管癌的MSKCC分期系统

分期	标准
T1	肿瘤累及左右肝管汇合处±单侧向二级胆管延伸
T2	肿瘤累及左右肝管汇合处±单侧向二级胆管延伸并且同侧门静脉受累±同侧肝叶萎缩
T3	肿瘤累及左右肝管汇合处+双侧延伸至二级胆管或单侧延伸至二级胆管+对侧门静脉受累或门静脉主干或双侧门静脉受累

MSKCC,纪念斯隆-凯特琳癌症中心。

表 69.4　梅奥诊所的肝门区胆管癌分期系统

分期	标准
Ⅰ	单个肿块且≤3cm ECOG 体力状态评分 0 血清 CA 19-9 水平(U/mL)<1 000 无血管包绕 无转移
Ⅱ	单个肿块且≤3cm ECOG 体力状态评分 1~2 血清 CA 19-9 水平(U/mL)<1 000 存在血管包绕 无转移
Ⅲ	单个肿块且>3cm 或有多个肿块 ECOG 体力状态评分 0~2 血清 CA 19-9 水平(U/mL)≥1 000 存在淋巴结转移
Ⅳ	ECOG 体力状态评分 3~4 腹膜(或其他器官)转移

ECOG,美国东部肿瘤协作组。

表 69.5　肝门区胆管癌的 TNM 和 AJCC/UICC 分期系统 TNM 分期标准

TNM 分期	标准		
Tx	原发肿瘤无法评估		
T0	无原发肿瘤的证据		
Tis	原位癌		
T1	肿瘤局限于胆管内,并延伸至纤维组织的肌层		
T2a	肿瘤侵入胆管壁外的脂肪组织		
T2b	肿瘤侵犯邻近的肝实质		
T3	肿瘤侵袭门静脉或肝动脉的单侧支		
T4	肿瘤直接侵犯肝外的局部结构		
Nx	局部淋巴结无法评估		
N0	无局部淋巴结转移		
N1	区域淋巴结转移(≤3 个淋巴结)(包括肝门、胆囊管、胆总管、肝动脉、胰十二指肠后、门静脉淋巴结)		
N2	区域淋巴结转移(≥4 个淋巴结)		
M0	无远处转移		
M1	有远处转移		
AJCC/UICC 分期	**肿瘤**	**淋巴结**	**远处转移**
0	Tis	N0	M0
Ⅰ	T1	N0	M0
Ⅱ	T2a-b	N0	M0
ⅢA	T3	N0	M0
ⅢB	T4	N0	M0
ⅢC	任何 T	N1	M0
ⅣA	任何 T	N2	M0
ⅣB	任何 T	任何 N	M1

AJCC,美国癌症联合委员会。UICC,国际癌症控制联盟。

管癌唯一的分期系统(表 69.6)。如前所述,与以前的版本相比,将肝门部与远端胆管癌分开是一个进步,对 T 分期的重新定义也是如此。这种分期系统提供了需要验证的预后信息,但不能指导治疗。

表 69.6　远端胆管癌的 TNM 和 AJCC/UICC 分期系统 TNM 分期标准

TNM 分期	标准		
Tx	原发肿瘤无法评估		
Tis	原位癌		
T1	肿瘤局限于胆管内,并延伸至纤维组织的肌层		
T2	肿瘤侵入胆管壁外的脂肪组织		
T3	肿瘤侵犯邻近的肝实质		
T4	肿瘤侵袭门静脉或肝动脉的单侧支		
Nx	局部淋巴结无法评估		
N0	无局部淋巴结转移		
N1	区域淋巴结转移(≤3 个淋巴结)(包括肝门、胆囊管、胆总管、肝动脉、胰十二指肠后、门静脉淋巴结)		
N2	区域淋巴结转移(≥4 个淋巴结)		
M0	无远处转移		
M1	有远处转移		
AJCC/UICC 分期	**肿瘤**	**淋巴结**	**远处转移**
0	Tis	N0	M0
Ⅰ	T1	N0	M0
ⅡA	T1	N1	M0
ⅡA	T2	N0	M0
ⅡB	T2	N1	M0
ⅡB	T3	N0-1	M0
ⅢA	T1	N2	M0
ⅢA	T2-3	N2	M0
ⅢB	T4	N0-2	M0
Ⅳ	任何 T	任何 T	M1

AJCC,美国癌症联合委员会;UICC,国际癌症控制联盟。

(七) 治疗

1. 肝内胆管癌

(1) 手术切除和肝移植

胆管癌唯一治愈的治疗方法是手术切除。21 世纪以来,由于对患者的精心选择,手术结果有了显著改善,手术死亡率较低,R0 切除术率较高[60a]。单发肝内胆管癌可通过肝段或肝叶切除术来治疗。高达 54% 的患者在就诊时已不能切除,大约 30% 的患者术前评估可以切除但在手术时发现不能切除。术后复发率高达 62%[64]。肝内胆管癌切除术后的 5 年生存率在 22% 到 42% 之间,63% 的患者可做到 R0 切除[65]。

据报道 R0 切除后 5 年生存率为 40%～63%。手术相关的发病率和死亡率分别为 35% 和 5%[12,66]。生存率与 R0 切除、阴性淋巴结转移状态(N0)、单发肿瘤、年龄更小、体力状态更好呈正相关[12,64,65,67]。新辅助治疗和辅助治疗均未获得统计学上显著的生存获益[65,67]。因为预后不佳,传统上肝内胆管癌被认为是肝移植的禁忌证。然而,在合并非常早期肝内胆管癌(单发肿瘤直径≤2cm)的肝硬化患者中,肝移植可能是一种选择[68]。在一项研究中,极早期的肝内胆管癌患者的 5 年生存率为 65%,而晚期患者(单个肿瘤>2cm 或多灶性病变)的患者则为 45%[69]。

(2) 局部治疗

对于不能切除的晚期肝内胆管癌患者,局部治疗是一种替代治疗方案。晚期肝内胆管癌患者经动脉化疗栓塞术(transarterial chemoembolization, TACE)的平均总生存率为 12～15 个月[70]。使用钇-90 微球经动脉放射栓塞的安全性和有效性与 TACE 相当[71]。

2. 肝门周围和远端胆管癌

在无 PSC 的情况下,手术切除也是肝门周围和远端胆管癌的首选治疗方法(框 69.2)。肝门周围胆管癌的切除可采用肝叶或扩大的肝叶和胆管切除术,并进行局部淋巴结清扫术和 Roux-en-Y 型肝空肠吻合术。有时可以通过术前门静脉栓塞实现切除,这会导致对侧肝叶代偿性增生。由于残余肝的体积增加,这项技术使扩大肝部分切除术具有可行性[62]。远端胆管癌的外科手术治疗通过 Whipple 切除术进行。N0 患者在 R0 切除后的五年生存率是:肝门周围胆管癌为 20%～67%,远端胆管癌为 27%～37%。结果在 20 世纪初有所改善[62,73]。不幸的是,R0 可切除率通常小于 50%[62,67]。肝门周围胆管癌的手术死亡率约为 10%,远端胆管癌的手术死亡率为 3.0%[12,67,72,73]。无论是辅助化疗还是新辅助化疗或放疗都没有被证明是有效的,因此,不推荐在切除肝门周围或远端胆管癌患者中使用[74]。

框 69.2 肝门区胆管癌不可切除的标准
一侧肝叶萎缩伴对侧门静脉分支被包绕
单叶萎缩伴对侧二级胆管根部受累
双侧门静脉支包绕
双侧肝动脉包绕
远处淋巴结转移
肝门部胆管癌,Bismuth-Corlette Ⅳ型
肝内或远处转移
原发性硬化性胆管炎
严重的合并症

在 PSC 患者中,胆管癌的手术切除可能会伴有肝功能衰竭或二次胆管癌,且有在胆肠吻合区发展的趋势[75,76]。因此,认为 PSC 和肝门周围胆管癌是不可切除的,应考虑行肝移植而不是切除术。在过去,肝移植并不是肝门周围胆管癌患者的选择,因为移植后的 5 年生存率只有 23%～26%[75]。随后,开发了新的肝移植方案,包括新辅助外照射放射治疗和同时全身 5-氟尿嘧啶化疗,随后是近距离放射治疗和口服卡培他滨维持化疗,直到移植。成功完成该治疗方案的患者的 5 年和 10 年无复发生存率分别为 65% 和 59%,移植后的复发率和全因死亡率分别为 20% 和 22%[77]。对于无 PSC 的患者,选择标准包括肝门周围肿瘤直径小于 3cm,无肝内或肝外转移以及不可切除性。

3. 化疗、放射治疗和靶向治疗

目前还没有治疗胆管癌的根治性药物。各种化疗药物,如吉西他滨、其他抗代谢药物、紫杉烷、铂类似物、蒽环类药物和丝裂霉素已被评估为单一或联合治疗方法。FDA 批准的唯一治疗胆管癌的化疗药物是吉西他滨。2010 年,Advanced Biliary Cancer-02(ABC-02)试验显示,与单用吉西他滨相比,吉西他滨-顺铂联合治疗 3 个月的总体生存率和无进展生存率有统计学意义。在联合治疗组中,唯一更严重的副作用是血液毒性。然而,肝硬化患者不包括在试验中[78]。因此,吉西他滨联合顺铂已成为非肝硬化患者不可切除胆管癌的治疗标准[79]。

目前没有大型随机对照试验评估不可切除胆管癌的放射治疗的益处。因此,放射疗法的使用仍存在争议[2]。

靶向药物用于治疗其他癌症,如肝细胞癌和肾细胞癌,显著延长了患者的生存期。针对胆管癌的靶向药物(即 FGFR 和 IDH 抑制剂)正在进行临床试验评估。需要对以生存为主要终点的胆管癌患者进行大型随机对照试验,而不仅仅是肿瘤反应。

4. 姑息治疗

胆管癌患者常伴有胆汁淤积、腹痛和恶病质,这些都限制了患者的生活质量。因此,姑息治疗在胆管癌患者治疗中非常重要。恢复胆道引流的方法包括内镜、经皮和外科技术。内镜和经皮方法是基于胆道支架的放置(参见第 70 章),而外科方法通过胆总管或肝空肠吻合术建立一个旁路。类似的内镜和手术方法的效果相近,但是手术的死亡率、手术相关并发症的发生率和住院时间要高一些[79]。是否采用内镜或经皮胆道支架取决于恶性狭窄的解剖位置(参见第 70 章)。虽然单侧胆汁引流通常已经足够,但双侧胆汁引流与生存率的增加有关[80,81]。在放置支架之前,横断面成像至关重要,它可以避免试图对萎缩的肝叶或无法进行充分引流的肝叶进行内镜下引流。不经引流而逆行注射造影剂,有很高的医源性细菌性胆管炎风险,并可能非常严重。建议恶性胆道梗阻患者早期进行干预,因为当血清总胆红素水平大于 10mg/dL 时,血清胆红素水平正常化的时间将从 3 周增加到 6 周,时间增加了一倍[82]。

建议采用外照射放射和术中或导管内近距离放射治疗作为姑息治疗[83]。然而,目前还没有大型的前瞻性随机对照试验为这些技术在胆管癌中的应用提供足够的证据。虽然有一些回顾性研究表明 TACE 可以提高生存率,但目前还没有大型的前瞻性随机对照试验证明 TACE 或其他局部胆管癌治疗的有效性[84]。

二、胆囊癌

胆囊癌是第二大最常见的原发性胆道恶性肿瘤和第五大最常见的消化道恶性肿瘤。与其他胆道恶性肿瘤一样,在大多数情况下,胆囊癌在晚期才被诊断出来,只有三分之一的病例在手术探查前被诊断为胆囊癌[85]。胆囊癌的生长速度要快于胆管癌,一般而言,胆囊癌的诊断要晚于壶腹癌(见后文)。胆囊癌不适合药物或放射疗法,而手术切除是唯一可能治愈的疗法。不幸的是，在诊断时只有少数患者适合外科手术。胆囊癌的预后很差，5 年生存率为 0～10%，中位生存期不到 6 个月。目前已有人提倡更积极的手术方法。

（一）流行病学

胆囊癌的分布具有地域异质性，女性的发病率是男性的 2～3 倍[86,87]。诊断时的平均年龄为 65 岁，发病高峰出现在 70 和 80 岁。全球胆囊癌发病率最高的地区是印度北部和智利中南部，按年龄标准化的发病率，女性为 27/100 000，男性为 12/100 000[86]。亚洲和某些东欧国家（如波兰）的发病率也很高[88]。胆囊癌在西欧国家和美国很少见，1973 年至 2009 年，按年龄校正的发病率为每 10 万人中 1.4 人[89]。在美国，女性胆囊癌的发病率明显高于男性（1.7/100 000 vs 1/100 000）[87]。与白种人相比，美洲原住民和阿拉斯加原住民胆囊癌的发病率明显更高（种族发病率比率，男性为 4.5，女性为 5.4）[90]。全球胆囊癌的发病率与胆石症的发病率相当（参见第 65 章）。总体而言，自 1990 年以来，美国大多数种族的胆囊癌发病率都有所下降（非裔美国人的发病率一直保持稳定）[87,91]。在欧洲、加拿大和日本也观察到了类似的趋势[92]。虽然有人猜测发病率的下降可能与同期胆囊切除术的数量增加有关，但尚未发现胆囊切除率与胆囊癌发病率之间的联系[93,94]。2000 年至 2005 年，美国胆囊癌的年龄校正死亡率为每 10 万人中 0.7 人，自 1990 年以来总体下降[7]。据报告，智利南部的死亡率最高（每 100 000 人中有 35 人死亡）[95]。

（二）病因学

胆囊癌的病因尚不清楚，但目前认为是多因素的。胆囊癌的几种危险因素见框 69.3。胆囊癌的主要危险因素是胆石症（参见第 65 章）。在 65%～90% 的胆囊癌患者中发现了胆结石。胆石症高发人群也是胆囊癌高发人群。智利的尸检研究表明，胆石症患者患胆囊癌的风险增加 7 倍，而美国的流行病学研究仅观察到胆石症患者患胆囊癌的风险轻微增加 3 倍[94,95]。实际上，仅有 1%～3% 的胆石症患者会发展成胆囊癌，而 20% 的胆囊癌患者没有胆石症的证据。因此，不建议在无症状的胆结石患者中进行预防性胆囊切除术来预防胆囊癌。据报道胆囊癌的风险与胆结石的大小和数量之间呈正相关，但也可能反映了胆石症的持续时间[96]。没有观察到不同类型的胆结石发生胆囊癌风险的差异。瓷化胆囊（胆囊壁广泛钙化）是胆囊癌的经典但有争议的危险因素[97]。尽管有报道称瓷化胆囊患者的胆囊癌风险增加，但其风险可能仅限于选择性黏膜钙化（Ⅱ型和Ⅲ型瓷化胆囊）的患者，而不限于弥漫性黏膜钙化（Ⅰ型）的患者[98]。

胆囊腺瘤性息肉是胆囊癌的另一个危险因素（参见第 67 章）。患病风险与息肉的大小、类型和生长速度呈正相关。腺瘤性息肉大于 1cm，无蒂并伴有胆结石，体积迅速增大，多普勒超声显示动脉血流或有症状的患者发生恶性转化的风险增加，应进行预防性胆囊切除术[97,99]。胰胆管汇流异常或胰胆管系统异常汇合（anomalous union of the pancreaticobiliary ductal system，AUPBD）与胆囊癌的发生有关（参见第 55 章）[100]。在这种先天性缺陷中，胰管和胆管在十二指肠壁外形成一条长长的共同通道。这种异常在亚洲，特别是日本最为普遍，它会导致胆汁淤积和胰腺分泌物反流进入胆囊，并导致黏膜的慢性炎症。在 AUPBD 患者中，胆道癌症，尤其是胆囊癌的发生频率很高，某些系列报道其发生频率约为 50%[100]。然而，根据是否存在相应的胆管扩张，该频率可在 10% 到 38% 之间变化[101]。伴有胆总管囊肿的患者胆囊癌的发生率低于无胆总管囊肿的患者[101]。诊断为胆囊癌时，AUPBD 患者通常比非 AUPBD 患者年轻 10 岁，并且胆石症的发生率较低[101]。由于胆囊癌的风险显著增加，数个日本肝胆肿瘤协会建议对 AUPBD 患者进行预防性胆囊切除术[97,101]。

PSC 与胆囊癌相关，有研究报道，高达 20% 的 PSC 患者会发生胆囊腺癌，40%～60% 的 PSC 患者的胆囊肿块为恶性肿瘤[102]。因此，PSC 和任何大小的胆囊肿块患者都应进行胆囊切除术或密切监测胆囊癌（参见第 67 章和第 68 章）。

胆囊腺肌症的特征是在固有肌层形成囊肿的基础上合并黏膜显微内陷（Rokitansky-Aschoff 窦）（参见第 67 章）。日本一项大型研究显示，60 岁及以上的胆囊局部腺肌症患者发生胆囊癌的频率较高[103]。一般而言，胆囊腺肌症被认为是一种良性疾病。

与胆囊癌相关的其他疾病包括炎症性肠病、肝内胆管异型增生和胆管癌[102]。已证明伤寒沙门氏菌或副伤寒的慢性携带者罹患胆囊癌的风险增加[104]。其他细菌，如大肠杆菌和 Hp，也与胆囊癌有关，但数据尚无定论。胆囊癌患者的一级亲属发生这种恶性肿瘤的相对风险为 13.9[105]。暴露于黄曲霉毒素（一种已知的肝致癌物）与胆囊癌有关[106,108]。血浆中黄曲霉毒素加合物含量较高的患者与血浆中黄曲霉毒素加合物含量较低的患者相比，其发生胆囊癌的比值比为 7.61[107,108]。在胆囊癌的动物模型中还发现了其他致癌物，包括 3-甲基胆蒽、邻氨基偶氮甲苯和亚硝胺。其他潜在的致癌物质包括芥子油、自由基氧化产物和次级胆汁酸。肥胖被认为是胆囊癌的一个危险因素，尤其是女性[109]，但还没有证据证明肥胖症是独立于胆石症的危险因素。

框 69.3　胆囊癌的危险因素

黄曲霉毒素
致癌物质*
胆管癌
胆石症（结石大小>1cm）
慢性伤寒沙门氏菌或副伤寒带菌者
有患胆囊癌的一级亲属
炎症性肠病
肝内胆管发育不良
Lynch 综合征
胰胆管汇流异常
瓷化胆囊
PSC
年龄≥60 岁的患者合并胆囊腺肌症

*甲基胆蒽，邻氨基偶氮甲苯，亚硝胺，可能还有其他物质。
PSC，原发性硬化性胆管炎。

（三）病理学

80% 到 95% 的胆囊癌是腺癌；大多数为中度至高分化[110]。腺癌进一步分为乳头状、管状和结节状，其中乳头状腺癌是侵袭性最低的类型[111]。按频率排列，较不常见的类型包括未分化癌或未分化癌、鳞状细胞癌和腺鳞癌。罕见类型包括类癌、小细胞癌、恶性黑素瘤、淋巴瘤和肉瘤[111]。60%的胆囊癌位于胆囊底部,30%在体部,10%在胆囊颈部[110]。与胆管癌相似,乳头状胆囊癌的浸润和转移扩散到淋巴结的可能性较低[111]。胆囊癌通过直接浸润、淋巴或血行转移、神经周围浸润、腹腔内或导管内浸润等途径传播。肿瘤细胞的扩散取决于胆囊生理淋巴丛,包括沿胆道的一级淋巴结(胆囊管、胆管、肝管),其次是胰十二指肠淋巴结,以及沿肝总动脉和腹腔干的淋巴结。54%~64%的患者有淋巴结转移,且与浸润的深度相关。由于静脉引流,胆囊癌易累及肝床,主要进入肝段Ⅳb和Ⅴ(参见第71章),并且解剖上的相近,可直接侵犯肝脏。在24%的病例中观察到神经周围扩散,19%的病例中观察到导管内扩散。

(四) 发病机制

胆囊癌可由黏膜异型增生或原位癌发展为腺癌,或由与结肠癌相似的腺瘤-癌序列发展而来(参见第127章)[112-114]。在手术切除的胆囊标本中,异型增生灶和原位癌常在胆囊癌旁发现,被认为是侵袭性腺癌的癌前病变[88]。异型增生发展为癌的时间估计为10~15年[113]。主要致病因素是炎症。全外显子组和靶向基因测序研究已经协助确定了胆囊癌的突变情况。这些分析表明,胆囊癌与胆管癌在遗传学上不同[115,116]。在一个队列中,全外显子组和超深层测序在35.8%的病例中鉴定出ErbB蛋白家族的突变[115]。此外,ErbB途径突变的病例的预后更差。同样,包括胆囊癌在内的胆管癌症的分子特征表明,在胆囊癌中表皮生长因子受体(epidermal growth factor receptor,*EGFR*)家族基因(*EGFR1*、*ERBB2*、*ERBB3*)频繁激活,以及体细胞端粒酶逆转录酶(telomerase reverse transcriptase,TERT)启动子突变[26]。在不同系列的胆囊癌中,有47.1%~59%的患者报道了抑癌基因*TP53*的突变[115,116]。*PIK3CA*的激活突变在5.95%~12.5%的胆囊癌中被报道[116,117]。*PIK3CA*突变导致PI3K通路-AKT通路的激活,该通路介导了一系列恶性肿瘤的发生。胆囊癌中遇到的其他遗传异常包括*CDKN2A/B*丢失(5.9%~19%)和*KRAS*突变(4%~13%),以及*ARID1A*(13%)和*NRAS*(6.3%)的突变[116]。

(五) 临床特征和诊断

47%~78%的患者在先前认为是良性疾病的胆囊切除术中偶然发现胆囊癌,反映了这种恶性肿瘤最初的临床隐匿性[118]。偶然诊断的胆囊癌在诊断时通常比症状性癌分期更早,并且有更好的中位生存率[118]。常见的临床表现包括胆道或腹部疼痛,以及继发于胆管直接侵犯或有肝十二指肠韧带转移的黄疸。体重减轻、腹胀或其他因压迫或者侵袭邻近器官而引起的症状表明疾病更加严重。

CEA和CA 19-9是胆囊癌最常用的肿瘤标志物[119]。在4.0ng/mL时,血清CEA水平升高的敏感性和特异性分别为50%和93%。截至20U/mL时,血清CA 19-9水平升高的敏感性和特异性分别为79%和79%[119,120]。这些测试有助于诊断,但不应依赖于此,因为在炎症、其他胃肠道肿瘤和妇科恶性肿瘤中,这些标志物的水平可以升高。此外,还有一部分人不产生CEA。腹部超声通常是出现上述症状的患者首先进行的影像学检查之一。超声诊断胆囊癌的灵敏度和准确性分别为85%和80%,早期癌症,特别是无蒂息肉,可能会漏诊。典型的胆囊癌影像学表现包括胆囊壁的局灶性或弥漫性增厚,起源于胆囊壁的大于2cm的腔内肿块,以及取代或掩盖胆囊并经常侵犯邻近器官的肝下肿块(图69.6)。提示胆囊恶性病变的表现包括不规则的、不对称的壁厚大于1cm,管腔内大于1cm的结节状或光滑肿块,固定在胆囊壁上,不会因患者的活动而移位,也没有声影。在不确定的情况下,多普勒超声

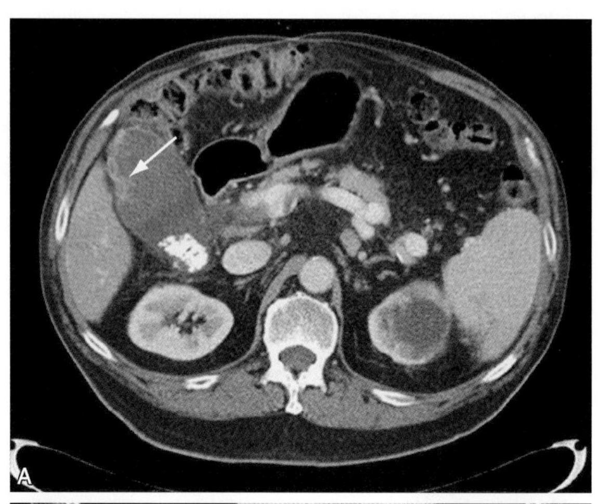

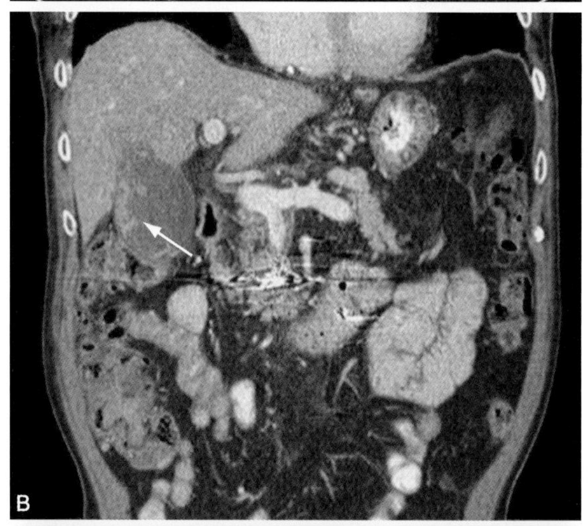

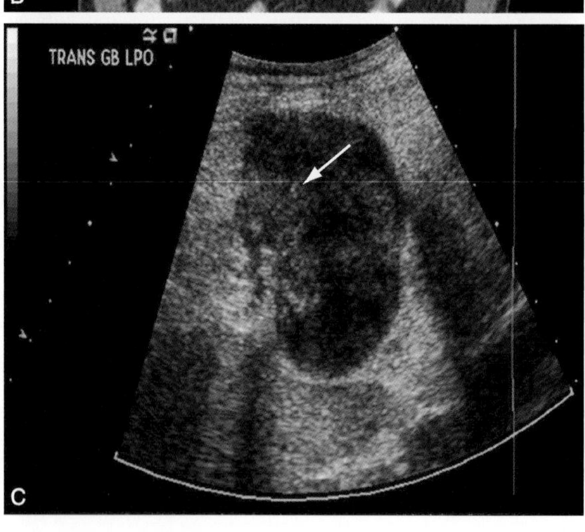

图69.6 胆囊癌成像。A,腹部的轴向CT视像。胆石位于胆囊肿块下方(箭)。B,同一患者冠状位。C,同一患者超声显示起源于胆囊壁并突入管腔的巨大肿块(箭)

可以尝试根据彩色信号、血流速度和阻力指数(动脉血流阻力的测量)的模式来鉴别胆囊病变的良恶性[121]。

如果超声检查结果不确定,则 MRI 和 CT 有助于诊断。螺旋 CT 在评估局部范围方面具有 83%~86%的准确性,在 T2 和更高分期准确性更好(见后文),因此有助于术前规划[122,123]。PET 在胆囊癌中的作用正在发展中,并不是常规检查[124]。PET 检测胆囊癌的敏感性仅为 75%~78%[125,126]。它的主要作用是发现远处转移,从而导致疾病治疗的改变[44]。

(六) 分期

胆囊癌分期系统包括 Nevin-Moran 分期系统和日本胆道外科学会分期系统。最常用的分期系统是 AJCC 和 UICC 描述的 TNM 系统(表 69.7)。基于 TNM 的分期系统与生存率相关。已报告的 0、Ⅰ、Ⅱ、ⅢA、ⅢB、ⅣA 和ⅣB 期胆囊癌患者的 5 年生存率分别为 80%、50%、28%、8%、7%、4% 和 2%。在 2018 版 AJCC/UICC 分期系统中,T2 期分为 T2a(肿瘤位于胆囊腹膜侧)和 T2b(肿瘤位于胆囊肝侧)[57]。在比较不同的预后和治疗研究时,重要的是要考虑到应用的分期系统版本的差异。

表 69.7　胆囊癌的 TNM 和 AJCC/UICC 分期系统

TNM 分期	标准		
Tx	原发肿瘤无法评估		
T0	无原发肿瘤的证据		
Tis	原位癌(导管内肿瘤)		
T1a	肿瘤侵袭固有层		
T1b	肿瘤侵犯固有肌层		
T2a	肿瘤侵犯腹膜侧的肌肉周围结缔组织,未累及浆膜		
T2b	肿瘤侵犯肝侧的肌肉周围结缔组织,但不直接向肝内扩散		
T3	肿瘤穿透浆膜 和/或 肿瘤直接侵入肝脏 和/或 肿瘤侵袭其他邻近器官(如胃、十二指肠、结肠、胰腺、网膜、肝外胆管)		
T4	肿瘤侵入门静脉或肝动脉 或 肿瘤侵入≥2 个肝外器官或结构		
Nx	局部淋巴结无法评估		
N0	无局部淋巴结转移		
N1	局部淋巴结转移(≤3 个淋巴结)		
N2	局部淋巴结转移(≥4 个淋巴结)		
M0	无远处转移		
M1	有远处转移		
AJCC/UICC 分期	**肿瘤**	**淋巴结**	**远处转移**
0	Tis	N0	M0
Ⅰ	T1	N0	M0
ⅡA	T2a	N0	M0
ⅡB	T2b	N0	M0
ⅢA	T3	N0	M0
ⅢB	T1-3	N1	M0
ⅣA	T4	N0-1	M0
ⅣB	任何 T	N2	M0
	任何 T	任何 N	M1

AJCC,美国癌症联合委员会;UICC,国际癌症控制联盟。

(七) 治疗

手术是胆囊癌唯一有可能治愈的治疗方法[127]。只有 15%~47%的患者在诊断时可以进行手术切除,因为大多数病例的病情已经进展到晚期。手术禁忌证包括多发性肝转移或远处转移、大血管侵犯或大血管包绕、恶性腹水和身体状态差[110]。直接侵犯结肠、十二指肠或肝脏并不被认为是手术切除的绝对禁忌证。手术治疗的目标是 R0 切除,外科治疗的目标是 R0 切除,定义为切缘阴性和淋巴结清扫后显微镜下仅累及一个水平的淋巴结。胆囊癌的 R0 切除术已被证明与生存率相关,并显著提高 5 年生存率[118,128]。然而,在接受手术探查或再探查的患者中,只有 36%~49%的患者实现了 R0 切除术[118,128]。

有治疗目的的外科手术包括:①单纯胆囊切除术;②扩大或根治性胆囊切除术,附加切除大于 2cm 的胆囊床,并在十二指肠第二部分、胰头、腹腔轴后方行肝十二指肠韧带淋巴结清扫术;③扩大的胆囊切除术,肝段或肝叶切除;④扩大的胆囊切除术,广泛切除主动脉旁淋巴结;⑤扩大的胆囊切除术,包括胆管切除术或胰十二指肠切除术。手术方法取决于肿瘤的范围。只有不到 10%的胆囊癌患者被诊断为 Tis 和 T1a 期肿瘤。在这个阶段,可以通过单纯胆囊切除术治疗胆囊癌,其 5 年生存率达到 85%~100%。一些报道也赞成对 1b 期胆囊癌行单纯胆囊切除术,并报告了单纯或根治性胆囊切除术后的生存率相近[129,130]。然而,高达 15%的 1b 期胆囊癌患者的淋巴结转移呈阳性,而 1a 期胆囊癌患者的这一比例为 2.5%[131]。同时,单纯胆囊切除术(与根治性切除相比)的术后复发率更高;因此,建议 1b 期胆囊癌行根治性胆囊切除术[131-134]。

T2 期肿瘤侵犯固有肌层需要根治性胆囊切除术,5 年生存率为 59%~90%,而单纯胆囊切除术的 5 年生存率为 17%~40%[135-137]。值得注意的是,T2 胆囊癌的肿瘤浸润风险和癌症扩散方式与肿瘤是位于胆囊的肝侧还是腹膜侧有关。合并肝侧肿瘤的 T2 胆囊癌患者比合并腹膜侧肿瘤的患者有更高的血管侵犯、神经侵犯和淋巴结转移率(分别为 51% 和 19%、33% 和 8%、40% 和 17%)[138]。因此,根据肿瘤在胆囊腹膜侧或肝侧的位置,更新的 AJCC/UICC 分期系统已将 T2 期胆囊癌分为 T2a 和 T2b[57]。

T3 和 T4 期肿瘤(侵犯浆膜的肿瘤)的手术方法存在争议。一些研究显示,对于 T3 和 T4 期肿瘤,根治性胆囊切除术后 5 年生存率没有益处,但其他研究则报告 5 年生存率分别为 15%~63% 和 7%~25%[139]。由于胆囊癌的预后较差,并且有可能生存获益,并且延长了直至复发的生存期,因此许多中心建议对这些晚期胆囊癌采取根治性手术方法。

当在腹腔镜过程中诊断出胆囊癌时,应将手术改为开腹手术,并应切除腹腔镜打孔部位,因为在医源性播散后,肿瘤可能在这些部位复发[140]。进一步的手术治疗取决于肿瘤的分期,如图 69.7 所示。当胆囊癌是在手术后确诊时,进一步的治疗取决于肿瘤的分期和手术标本边缘肿瘤的存在与否。对于 T1 期、T2 期、T3 期和 T4 期肿瘤,在初始标本中再次探查发现残余肿瘤的可能性分别为 50%、61%、85% 和 100%[118]。新辅助或辅助治疗不能提供生存获益,不推荐使用[65,118]。

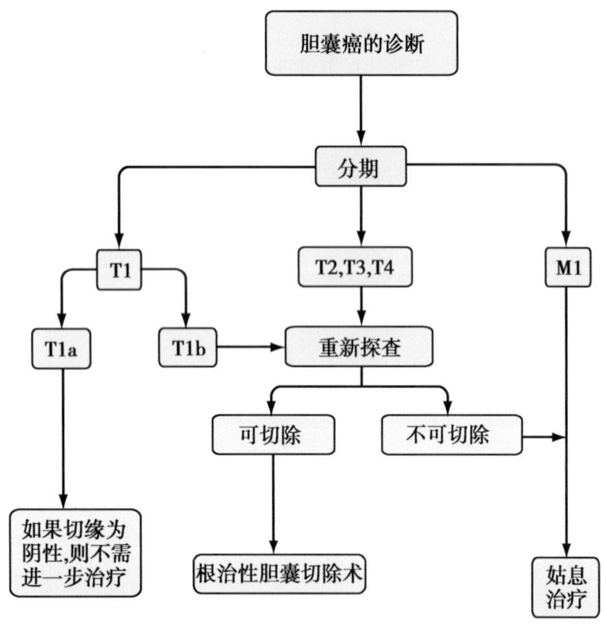

图 69.7 腹腔镜胆囊切除术术中或术后发现胆囊癌的处理流程。如果病理检查发现胆囊切除术标本为 T1a 期肿瘤,手术切缘阴性,则不需要进一步治疗。若发现肿瘤为 T1b 期或切缘恶性组织阳性,则需重新探查进一步切除。同样发现胆囊癌为 T2 期、T3 期、T4 期的患者应行手术再探查。如果再次探查发现胆囊癌可切除,应行根治性胆囊切除术。如果无法切除,则需姑息治疗。当术后分期显示转移扩散时,姑息治疗是必需的。M,转移分期;T,肿瘤分期。(Modified from Misra S, Chaturvedi A, Misra NC, Sharma ID. Carcinoma of the gallbladder. Lancet Oncol 2003;4:167-76.)

不能切除的胆囊癌患者的标准治疗是吉西他滨联合顺铂化疗。该建议主要基于 ABC-02 试验(见前文),该试验包括 149 例胆囊癌患者,显示总生存期改善了 3.6 个月,与胆管癌相似[78]。在较小的研究中评估了其他化疗药物和吉西他滨为基础的联合疗法[与奥沙利铂、5-氟尿嘧啶(5-FU)或卡培他滨]和靶向药物(西妥昔单抗、厄洛替尼或贝伐单抗),但未能显示出优于吉西他滨和顺铂联合用药,因此仍然是不可切除胆囊癌的一线治疗。通常认为胆囊癌对放疗不敏感[79]。

三、壶腹癌

Vater 壶腹癌属于壶腹周围癌家族。该家族包括十二指肠癌、Vater 壶腹癌、远端胆管癌和胰腺癌(参见第 60 章)。壶腹癌是壶腹周围癌的第二大常见类型(仅次于胰头癌)。区别不同类型的壶腹癌很重要,因为壶腹癌通常比其他类型的癌症诊断得更早,因此处于可切除的阶段,从而有更好的预后[141]。

(一) 流行病学

壶腹癌较少见,在所有胃肠道癌症中占不到 1%,在壶腹周围癌中占 4%~8%。据估计,每年的发病率为每 10 万人中有 0.6 人[141,142]。发病高峰在 70 岁以上。男性略占多数,男女比例为 1.48∶1[143]。已经观察到种族差异性,绝大多数患者是白种人,其次是西班牙裔和亚洲裔患者。非裔美国人在美国的发生率是最低的[141]。自 1970 年以来,壶腹癌的发病率每年在美国增加 0.9%[143]。

(二) 病因

虽然在大多数病例中,壶腹癌的病因尚不清楚,但有几种情况与这种恶性肿瘤有关,大多数是病例报告或小宗病例系列报告。家族性腺瘤性息肉病(familial adenomatous polyposis, FAP)是壶腹癌发生的重要危险因素(参见第 126 章)[144]。壶腹周围癌是 FAP 患者第二大致死原因(仅次于结肠癌)。通常,壶腹周围癌比结直肠癌发生得晚,但与散发性壶腹癌相比,发生得早[144]。因此,建议 FAP 患者根据十二指肠息肉病的程度,每隔 6 个月~4 年定期筛查上消化道肿瘤(息肉或癌)[144]。同样,在患有 Gardner 综合征(FAP 的一种变异)患者中,壶腹癌的发生率也有所增加(参见第 126 章)[145]。Lynch 综合征(遗传性非息肉性结直肠癌)似乎不易患壶腹癌(参见第 127 章)[146]。据报道,其他易患壶腹癌的遗传疾病包括 1 型神经纤维瘤病和 Muir-Torre 综合征[147,148]。如在胆管癌中一样,慢性肝吸虫感染是壶腹癌的危险因素(参见第 84 章)[142]。

(三) 病理学

Vater 壶腹是一个解剖复杂的区域,包括乳头、胆胰共同通道、远端胆管和远端主胰管。从肉眼上看,壶腹癌可分为以下 3 类:①壁内突出(壶腹内);②壁外突出(壶腹周围);③溃疡性壶腹[142]。溃疡型通常在晚期得到诊断,并且有最高的淋巴结转移率。与解剖学多样性一致,壶腹具有不同的组织学细胞类型,如胰胆管共同通道上皮、胆管上皮、胰管上皮或十二指肠黏膜、Brunner 腺和胆道壁上异常的胰腺腺泡。细胞异型性最常见的部位是胆胰共同通道,其次是胰管、十二指肠上皮和 Brunner 腺[149]。壶腹肿瘤中 75% 为腺癌,20% 为良性腺瘤,5% 为神经内分泌肿瘤[150]。腺癌占壶腹恶性肿瘤的 90%,其余包括不常见的类型,如黏液、印戒细胞和未分化癌[150]。组织病理学上,90% 的壶腹腺癌可分为胰胆型和肠型[151,152]。根据组织学亚型、尾侧同源结构域转录因子 2(caudal-type homeodomain transcription factor 2, CDX2)和黏蛋白 1(Mucin 1, MUC1)免疫组织化学染色对壶腹癌的组织分子表型可能有一定的预测价值。在两个不同的系列中,胰胆管组织分子表型(CDX2 阴性,MUC1 阳性)患者的预后比肠道表型(CDX2 阳性,MUC1 阴性)患者更差[153-155]。然而,随后的一项研究并没有明确这两种亚型之间的预后差异[156]。

(四) 发病机制

大多数壶腹癌遵循腺瘤-癌序列,30%~91% 的壶腹癌中可见残存的腺瘤组织[142]。尽管癌前病变可从肠以及胰胆管的组织发展而来,但是肠型癌通常从腺瘤发展,而胰胆管和溃疡性癌通常缺乏癌前病变[142]。肠型和胆胰型有明显的分子改变。*KRAS* 改变在胰胆管型中更常见,而腺瘤性息肉病结肠基因改变在肠型中更常见[157]。其他的基因畸变包括 *TP53* 突变、*ERBB2* 扩增和 *CDKN2A* 缺失[157]。根据对壶腹癌的深入基因组分析,驱动基因突变的频率在肠型和胆胰型之间不同,尽管常见的突变有显著的重叠,包括 *KRAS*、*TP53*、*Smad4* 和 *CTNNB1*[158]。值得注意的是,*ELF3* 已被鉴定为壶腹癌中一种新的突变驱动肿瘤抑制基因。*ELF3* 是 ETS 转录因子家族的成员,编码 E26 转化特异性转录因子,它的失活突变存在于 10%~12% 的壶腹癌中[29,158]。*ELF3* 失活促进上皮细胞的运动和侵袭[158]。

(五) 临床特征和诊断

与其他壶腹周围和胆道恶性肿瘤一样,壶腹癌在 70%~82% 的病例中最初表现为梗阻性黄疸。尤其是胆胰壶腹部癌,起病就表现为梗阻性黄疸[151]。由于其解剖位置,胆汁淤积症比其他壶腹周围及胆道恶性肿瘤发展得更早,因此在诊断时的可切除率更高。无黄疸患者可表现为细菌性胆管炎。很少有患者因胆管梗阻及肿瘤出血导致无胆色素粪便,而出现"银色粪便"。当怀疑梗阻性胆管炎时,进一步的诊断评估与其他胆道恶性肿瘤相似。免疫组织化学分析表明 CEA 和 CA 19-9 在肿瘤中高表达[159]。血清 CEA 和 CA19-9 浓度升高分别见于 11%~29% 和 41%~63% 的壶腹癌患者。在单变量但非多变量分析中,这些血清肿瘤标志物的升高与肿瘤复发和无病生存率降低相关[159,160]。

通常,壶腹癌是通过内镜检查来诊断的,依据肉眼和活检标本的结果(图 69.8)。随后的诊断性检查主要针对可切除性的评估和转移的检测。对于其他胆道癌和壶腹周围癌,通常使用 CT 和 MRI 等成像技术[161]。在 MRI 结合 MRCP 影像上,壶腹癌通常在 T2 加权像上表现为一个离散的低密度肿块。有时,肿瘤可表现为胆管周围不规则增厚或隆起至十二指肠。常可见胆管和胰管同时扩张("双管征")或仅见胆管扩张,仅见胰管扩张的情况很少见[161]。在常规磁共振成像基础上增加弥散加权成像可以提高壶腹癌的检出率[162]。通常,EUS 被用于术前评估。其检测邻近器官侵犯的准确率为 80%~90%,检测血管侵犯的敏感性和特异性分别为 73% 和 90%[163,164]。PET 在壶腹部肿瘤中的作用尚未得到很好的研究。

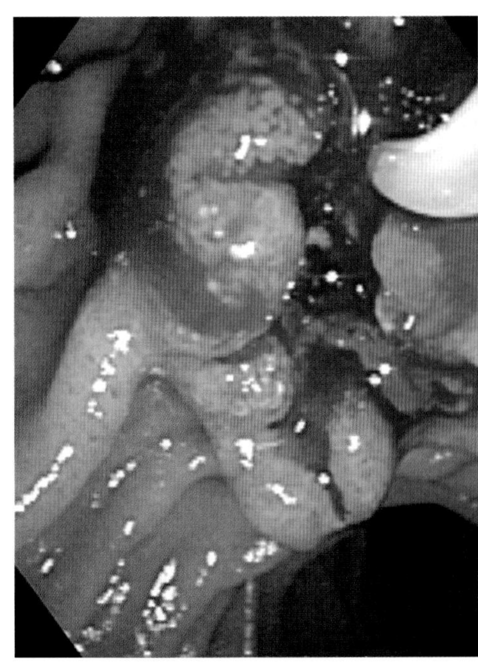

图 69.8　壶腹癌的内镜表现。在进行括约肌切开术后,在 Vater 壶腹部置入导管进行胆道引流

(六) 分期

根据 AJCC/UICC TNM 分类对壶腹癌进行分类(表 69.8)[57]。据报道,0、ⅠA、ⅠB、ⅡA、ⅡB、Ⅲ和Ⅳ期的 5 年存

表 69.8　壶腹癌的 TNM 和 AJCC/UICC 分期系统

TNM 分期	标准
Tx	原发肿瘤无法评估
T0	无原发肿瘤的证据
Tis	原位癌
T1a	肿瘤局限于壶腹或 Oddi 括约肌
T1b	肿瘤侵袭 Oddi 括约肌以外和/或十二指肠黏膜下层
T2	肿瘤侵袭十二指肠固有肌层
T3a	肿瘤侵袭胰腺(≤0.5cm)
T3b	肿瘤向胰腺内延伸>5cm 或 肿瘤浸润胰腺周围软组织,不累及腹腔干或肠系膜上动脉 或 肿瘤侵犯十二指肠浆膜,不累及腹腔干或肠系膜上动脉
T4	肿瘤累及腹腔干、肠系膜上动脉和/或肝总动脉
Nx	局部淋巴结无法评估
N0	无局部淋巴结转移
N1	局部淋巴结转移(≤3 个淋巴结)
N2	局部淋巴结转移(≥4 个淋巴结)
M0	无远处转移
M1	有远处转移

AJCC/UICC 分期	肿瘤	淋巴结	远处转移
0	Tis	N0	M0
ⅠA	T1a	N0	M0
ⅠB	T1b-2	N0	M0
ⅡA	T3a	N0	M0
ⅡB	T3b	N0	M0
ⅢA	T1-3	N1	M0
ⅢB	T4	任何 N	M0
	任何 T	N2	M0
Ⅳ	任何 T	任何 N	M1

AJCC,美国癌症联合委员会;UICC,国际癌症控制联盟。

活率分别为 49%、40%、44%、33%、26%、16% 和 4%。在单变量分析中，T 分期可以预测生存率，但在多变量分析中，T 分期不能预测生存率[151,165]。然而，据报道，淋巴结转移的风险随着 T 分期的增加而增加。总体而言，42% 到 60% 的患者在手术时被发现有淋巴结转移[166,167]。淋巴结受累率是总体生存率的一个负预测因子，淋巴结阳性患者的 5 年生存率为 9%~47%，而淋巴结阴性患者的 5 年生存率达到 59%~63%[159,168]。多因素分析显示，其他独立的生存预测因素包括淋巴管侵犯、神经侵犯、晚期和胆胰管类型的肿瘤[151,159,169]。

（七）治疗

手术切除是治疗壶腹癌的唯一方法。然而，与其他胆道恶性肿瘤不同的是，77%~93% 的壶腹癌在确诊时是可切除的[166,170]。标准的手术方式是胰十二指肠切除术。在没有淋巴结转移的情况下预后良好，5 年存活率为 59%~78%[171-173]。淋巴结转移的情况下，预后明显变差，5 年生存率为 16%~25%[171-173]。淋巴结包膜外侵犯可导致预后进一步恶化，5 年生存率仅为 9%。据报道，淋巴结微转移是一个不利的预后因素，建议对切除的淋巴结进行免疫组化分析[174]。局部手术或内镜下乳头切除术已有报道，但不推荐，因为复发率高于胰十二指肠切除术[1]。无论是否接受放疗，对术前化疗的患者进行的回顾性分析未显示出死亡率改善或 5 年总生存率的改善[175]。因此，新辅助治疗在壶腹癌中的作用有待进一步研究。

两个大型随机对照试验评估了辅助化疗和放化疗的优势。Johns Hopkins-Mayo 诊所的合作研究显示，淋巴结阳性患者接受以 5-FU 为基础的辅助性放化疗的结果有显著改善，5 年存活率从 6% 提高到 28%[173]。同样，欧洲胰腺癌研究小组-3 壶腹周围癌试验报告提出，接受 5-FU 加亚叶酸辅助治疗的患者的中位生存期为 58 个月，接受吉西他滨治疗的患者的中位生存期为 71 个月，而未接受辅助化疗的患者的中位生存期为 41 个月；在对独立的预后因素进行校正后，辅助化疗的益处达到了统计学意义[176]。随后的 meta 分析报告了相互矛盾的结果，其中一项显示接受辅助放化疗的患者的死亡风险（风险比为 0.75）显著降低[177]。另一组显示辅助治疗没有生存获益[178]。然而，辅助化疗或放化疗可能对部分壶腹癌患者有作用，尤其是那些淋巴结阳性的患者。

尚未在大型随机对照试验中对化疗或放疗对不能切除的壶腹癌患者的益处进行评估。治疗试验包括了各种类型的壶腹周围癌患者，包括前面描述的 ABC-02 试验中的 20 名壶腹癌患者[78]。在缺乏足够数量的不能切除的壶腹癌患者的随机对照试验的情况下，化疗和放疗的作用没有明确的定义。

姑息治疗应致力于减轻肿瘤相关并发症，以提高患者的生活质量为目标。梗阻性胆汁淤积症是发病的主要原因，通常可以通过内镜或经皮胆道支架置入，或通过类似于其他胆道或壶腹周围恶性肿瘤的外科旁路手术来进行姑息性治疗。

四、胆道的其他肿瘤

其他肿瘤疾病可累及胆道（框 69.4）。有必要将其纳入胆道肿瘤的鉴别诊断，因为对不同肿瘤类型的处理不同。神经外胚层起源的肿瘤，如类癌（参见第 34 章）和副神经节瘤，是罕见而且典型的无功能肿瘤[179]。它们通常位于 Vater 壶腹中。有时，类癌在肝外胆道中发展，主要在胆管中。患者通常是女性和年轻人。胆道原发性类癌占所有胃肠道类癌的不到 1%，通常与类癌综合征无关[180,181]。大约三分之一的患者在诊断时有转移。治疗选择手术切除，预后一般较好[182-184]。副神经节瘤患者经常出现消化道出血，只有 25% 出现黄疸。据估计，它们的恶性潜能为 33%，一些研究人员建议将胰十二指肠切除术作为首选治疗方法[185]。颗粒细胞瘤是神经源性的，罕见，只有少数病例被报道过。通常，它们位于肝外胆管，特别是在胆囊管和胆管的交界处[186]。当它们位于肝门时，有时可引起胆道梗阻[186]。由于它们是良性的，切除通常

框 69.4　腺癌以外的胆道肿瘤
胆囊
良性
腺瘤
颗粒细胞瘤
间充质瘤（脂肪瘤、平滑肌瘤、血管瘤、淋巴管瘤）
副神经节瘤
恶性
腺鳞癌
神经内分泌肿瘤（类癌）
小细胞癌
梭形细胞肉瘤样癌
其他（血管肉瘤，癌肉瘤，Kaposi 肉瘤，平滑肌肉瘤，恶性纤维组织细胞瘤，黑色素瘤，转移性肿瘤，非霍奇金淋巴瘤，横纹肌肉瘤）
腺瘤样变
腺肌瘤/腺肌瘤病
胆固醇息肉
异位（胃、胰腺、肝脏、肾上腺、甲状腺）
炎性息肉
胆管
良性
腺纤维瘤
腺瘤
腺肌瘤
肝前肠纤毛囊肿
囊腺瘤和囊腺癌
颗粒细胞瘤
错构瘤
神经瘤
浆液性囊腺瘤
单发或多发囊肿
恶性
胚胎性（葡萄状）横纹肉瘤
白血病
淋巴瘤
黑色素瘤
转移性肿瘤
神经内分泌肿瘤（良性肿瘤）
副神经节瘤
癌前病变
异型增生（上皮内瘤变/不典型增生）
胆管导管内乳头状黏液瘤（胆道乳头状瘤病）

可以治愈[187]。少数情况下，肝外胆管神经瘤在胆囊切除术后发生[188]。胆囊中已发现间质肿瘤，如脂肪瘤，平滑肌瘤，血管瘤和淋巴管瘤。一般来说，间质肿瘤极少见，仅限于病例报告。淋巴管瘤通常是无症状和偶然发现的。但是，它们可以增大并导致腹痛或黄疸。超声、CT 和 MRI 结合 MRCP 有助于术前诊断。通常，淋巴管瘤表现为多房、充满液体和具有薄壁和间隔的囊性肿块，注射造影剂后信号密度增强[189]。大多数报道的病例都成功地通过手术切除治疗，如果肿瘤位于胆囊内，则行胆囊切除；如果肿瘤位于 Vater 壶腹区域，则通过内镜切除[190-193]。Vater 壶腹区也有错构瘤的报道，并通过内镜成功切除[194]。

胆囊异位可由胃、胰腺、肝脏、肾上腺或甲状腺组织引起。出血等临床并发症极为罕见[195,196]。良性胆道病变包括腺瘤、囊腺瘤、腺纤维瘤、囊肿和颗粒细胞瘤。子宫腺肌瘤多见于 Vater 壶腹。囊腺瘤多见于女性，主要表现为腹痛。主要见于肝内胆管，超声表现为囊壁和间隔的乳头状突起。它们被认为是癌前病变，因为它们有可能转化为囊腺癌。因此，首选的治疗方法是完全切除[197-199]。

胆管癌以外的胆道恶性肿瘤包括囊腺癌、淋巴瘤和恶性黑色素瘤。这些恶性肿瘤主要发生在肝外胆管。囊腺癌在形态上可与胆管细胞癌相区别[200]。它们很少位于胆囊内[201]，症状无特异性，CT 和 MRI 有助于诊断。首选的治疗方法是手术切除[201]。胆道恶性黑色素瘤并不常见，应该立即进行皮肤黑色素瘤的检查，因为已经报道了转移到胆管的病例[202,203]。淋巴瘤有时会累及肝外胆道，常被误诊为胆管癌[204,205]。一般来说，胆道淋巴瘤罕见，仅占淋巴瘤的不到 1%[205,206]。滤泡性淋巴瘤起源于肝外胆管和胆囊的报道很少。通常，这些肿瘤是在切除后诊断出来的。胚胎性胆道横纹肌肉瘤在成人中极为罕见，但在儿童中是该解剖部位最常见的恶性肿瘤[207]。在手术前常被误诊为胆总管囊肿[208]。完全手术切除的可能性极小，建议采用多学科方法进行治疗。胆道横纹肉瘤的预后良好，报道的 5 年存活率高达 78%[209]。

胆管癌的癌前病变包括高级别不典型增生和胆管内乳头状黏液性肿瘤（intraductal papillary mucinous tumor of the bile duct，IPNB）。高级别胆管不典型增生可能是胆管癌的先兆，特别是在 PSC 患者中[210-213]。高级别异型增生的患者比低级别异型增生或无异型增生的患者更容易发生多体性荧光原位杂交[211]。在 PSC 相关的胆管细胞癌中描述了一种化生-异型增生-癌序列[212]。然而，高级别异型增生的 PSC 患者的治疗仍然是一个挑战。在美国，通常使用保守的方法，包括使用连续 MRCP 和/或 ERCP 进行观察和密集监视。在有良好器官分配的国家，肝移植已被认为是治疗 PSC 中出现的高级别异型增生的首选方法[210]。

IPNB 包括胆管内乳头状胆管癌和胆管乳头状瘤、胆管内乳头状黏液性肿瘤等前驱病变[214]。胆管乳头状瘤是一种具有高度恶性潜能的罕见疾病，其特征是胆道内大量的乳头状腺瘤[215]。临床表现包括反复腹痛、黄疸和急性胆管炎。由于 IPNB 是一种弥漫性/多灶性实体，MRCP 或 ERCP 可用来描述其在胆道内的范围[216]。IPNB 患者应该考虑手术切除，因为这些病变具有很高的恶性潜能[217]。

（周宇航　闫秀娥 译，黄永辉 校）

参考文献

69

第 70 章 胆道疾病的内镜和放射治疗

Theodore W. James, Todd H. Baron 著

章节目录

一、胆道影像学 …… 1036
（一）经腹超声检查 …… 1036
（二）磁共振胰胆管造影与多排螺旋 CT 胆道成像 …… 1036
（三）超声内镜诊断 …… 1037
（四）内镜逆行胰胆管造影 …… 1038
（五）超声内镜引导下胆管引流 …… 1038
二、内镜治疗 …… 1039
（一）胆管结石 …… 1039
（二）胆漏 …… 1040
（三）原发性硬化性胆管炎 …… 1040
（四）良性胆管狭窄 …… 1041
（五）不明原因的胆管狭窄 …… 1042
（六）恶性胆道狭窄 …… 1043
（七）Oddi 括约肌功能障碍 …… 1044
（八）外科手术所致的解剖改变 …… 1044
（九）不良事件 …… 1044
三、经皮经肝穿刺胆管造影术 …… 1045
（一）技术 …… 1045
（二）术后胆道狭窄 …… 1046
（三）原发性硬化性胆管炎 …… 1046
（四）胆管漏 …… 1046
（五）胆管损伤 …… 1046
（六）胆管结石 …… 1046
（七）恶性胆道梗阻 …… 1047
四、经皮胆囊造瘘管置入术 …… 1048
五、经皮和内镜联合的治疗方法 …… 1049

胆道疾病的内镜治疗和放射治疗齐头并进。内镜治疗是应用内镜逆行胰胆管造影（ERCP）和超声内镜（EUS）引导的技术。ERCP 主要由接受过胃肠病规范培训的内镜医师执行，但在一些中心也由外科医生操作。ERCP 是技术要求最高的内镜手术之一，对于复杂病例的成功处理，其学习曲线很陡峭。EUS 引导下治疗几乎完全由受过胃肠病培训的内镜医生完成，随着新的适应证的出现，其应用范围也在不断扩大。胆道的放射治疗是由介入放射科医师通过经皮途径进行的。这 3 种方法应该被视为互补而不是竞争。决定采用内镜或放射学方法往往是基于当地的专业水平；其他考虑因素包括医生的转诊模式、胆道内病变的位置、一种方法的失败以及由于手术而改变的解剖结构。

一、胆道影像学

胆道影像对于制定胆道疾病患者的治疗方法至关重要，无论采取内镜还是经皮的方法，都是如此，本文将对此进行简要讨论。

（一）经腹超声检查

胆道的非侵入性影像通常先用经腹超声，它可以提供肝脏的整体图像，几乎随处可用。没有辐射，也不需要造影剂。可以很容易显示肝内胆管扩张，也可记录胆管的大小。超声还提供胆囊成像和胆结石检测（参见第 65 章）。其对胆总管结石的诊断具有较高的特异性，但敏感性不超过 68%，往往低于 50%[1-3]。如果结石较小且胆管不扩张，则敏感性会降低。超声检测肝外胆管梗阻的准确率很高（78%～98%）；然而，胆总管结石的验前概率极大地影响了其应用[4]。当结合临床和实验室评估使用时，超声可以区分肝实质疾病和肝外胆管阻塞，具有合理的敏感性和高特异性（参见第 21 章）。但超声在确定梗阻程度和原因方面的准确度较低，分别为 27%～95% 和 23%～88%[2]。此外，超声在区分梗阻的良恶性病因方面能力有限。在肥胖患者中，这些局限性可能会很明显，因为超声波需要穿透的距离增加，从而降低了图像的分辨率和深度。超声的进展包括三维和四维成像[5]、造影剂的使用[6]和弹性成像（参见第 74 章）。

（二）磁共振胰胆管造影与多排螺旋 CT 胆道成像

磁共振胰胆管造影（MRCP）是一种 MRI 方法（因此是非侵入性的），它依赖于胆汁的高 T2 信号，在图像上产生高强度的明亮信号。固体物质，如胆总管结石，会在胆管内出现界限清楚的暗色充盈缺损。MRI 不需要口服或静脉注射造影剂。对于胆总管结石的检测，MRCP 的灵敏度为 81%～100%，特异性为 96%～100%，总体诊断准确率高（图 70.1）[7-9]。假阳性结果可能来源于胆道积气。此外，MRCP 在显示良性和恶性狭窄方面有很高的准确性[10,11]，并可对肝内胆管进行全面评估。对于怀疑肝移植（LT）后有胆道并发症的患者（参见第 97 章），可采用静脉注射锰福地吡三钠（Teslascan, Amersham Health, Princeton, NJ）。该药主要在胆汁中排泄，可提高肝移植后胆漏和狭窄的影像敏感性[12]。此外，MRI 可以使用静脉造影剂，如钆酰胺（Omniscan, GE Healthcare, UK）或钆喷酸二葡胺（Magnevist, Bayer Healthcare, Leverkusen, Germany 或 MultiHance, Bracco, Princeton, NJ），用于检测肝脏、肝门周围或胰腺的肿块病变的特点。MRI 的禁忌证包括心脏起搏器、自动植入式心律转复除颤器和某些类型的脑动脉瘤夹。需要引起

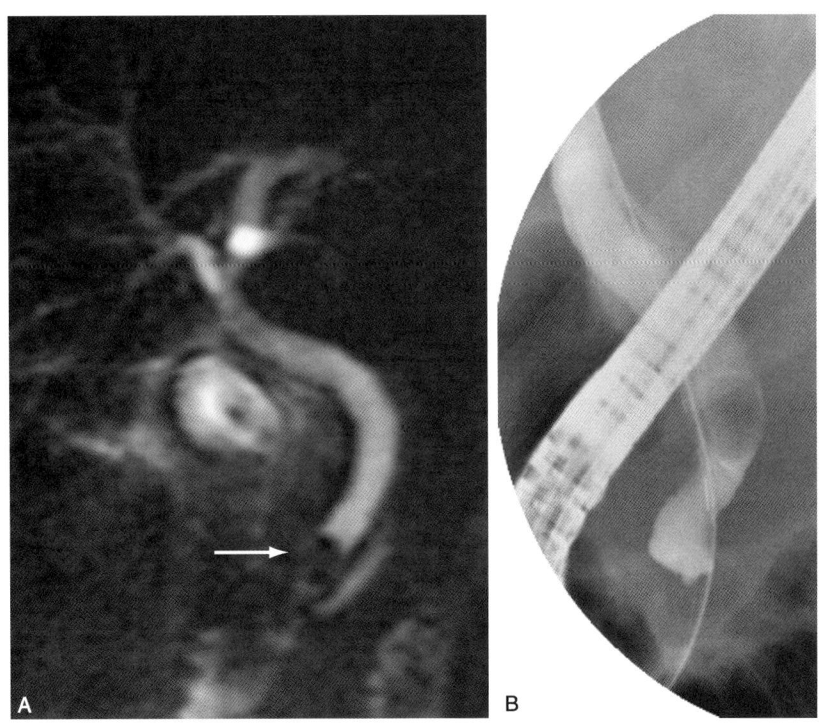

图 70.1　磁共振胰胆管造影（MRCP）和内镜逆行胰胆管造影（ERCP）上的胆总管结石。A，MRCP 显示远端胆管充盈缺损（箭示）。B，具有相同充盈缺陷的相应 ERCP 图像

注意的是钆静脉造影剂可能会诱发肾性系统性纤维化，这是一种罕见的硬皮病样疾病，表现为皮肤硬化和影响多个器官的纤维化改变。病因尚不清楚，但报告显示，既往患有肾脏疾病（肾功能衰竭）的患者风险最大[13,14]。在肾功能不全的患者中避免使用钆和使用更低的剂量可以降低风险[15]。

多排螺旋 CT 胆道成像（multidetector CT cholangiography，MDCT）是一种以 CT 为基础的成像方法。MDCT 结合了快速容积采集和薄层成像。水被用作胆道的口服造影剂，也可使用静脉碘化造影剂。在横断面上获得的图像可以在矢状面或冠状面重建，并进行三维重建。静脉造影剂不会在胆汁中排泄，而是增强邻近的内脏结构，如肝脏、胰腺和其他软组织。因此，胆管表现为低密度的结构，如果扩张的话，则更容易显示。在涉及肝脏和胆管的恶性肿瘤手术切除后，由于 MDCT 具有较高的空间分辨率和显示吻合口小肿瘤复发的能力，因此 MDCT 优于 MRCP[16]。MDCT 对胆管狭窄诊断的敏感性和特异性分别为 85.7% 和 100%[17]。MDCT 对胆管结石的诊断也有很高的敏感性和特异性，但当结石较小或与胆汁密度相似时，诊断准确率会大大降低[18]。MDCT 的缺点是患者暴露于电离辐射和注射造影剂的潜在有害影响。

（三）超声内镜诊断

诊断性超声内镜检查（EUS）使用的是超声内镜，它的尖端有一个超声换能器，向周围组织发射高频声波。根据成像需求以及是否可能需要针吸活检，选择环扫 EUS 或线阵 EUS。胆道的 EUS 检查可以通过经胃或经十二指肠的途径进行。除了胰胆管外的结构，经胃扫查可提供胰颈、胰体、胰尾以及胆囊和左肝内胆管的图像，而经十二指肠扫查可提供胰头、胆囊、壶腹和胆管的图像。在 EUS 上，胆总管结石表现为高回声灶并伴有声影（图 70.2）。EUS 检测胆总管结石的灵敏度和特异度分别为 95% 和 97%[19,20]，且对判断肝外胆道梗阻的原因有很高的准确性，灵敏度为 97%，特异度为 88%。EUS 可区分恶性梗阻的不同原因。特别是对于胰腺肿瘤的诊断，EUS 比 CT（5%～77%）、经腹 US（50%～67%）、MRI（50%～67%）和 ERCP（90%）更敏感（93% 到 100%）（参见第 60 章和第 61 章）。EUS 比 ERCP 的创伤性小，没有相关的辐射或造影剂暴露。EUS 与 FNA 结合，可以对肿块和淋巴结进行组织诊断。在某些患者中，尤其是有 MRI 禁忌证和病态肥胖的患者，EUS 可能优于 MRCP。对于外科术后解剖结构改变的患者，尤其是具有 Roux-en-Y 和 Billroth Ⅱ 解剖结构，内镜无法推进到感兴趣的区域以提供图像，MRCP 可能优于 EUS。对于有症状的胆石症和不确定的胆管结石患者，EUS 和 MRCP

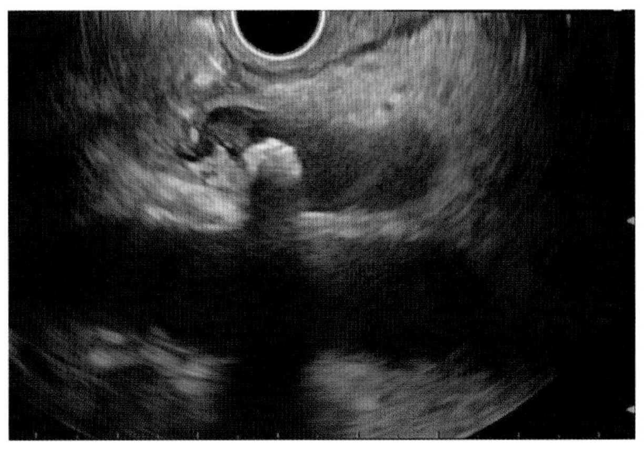

图 70.2　EUS 图像显示胆总管结石。注意胆管中三分之一处的单个结石。结石与 EUS 探头之间具有强回声界面，声后有声影

都是可接受的术前影像检查方式[21]。

(四) 内镜逆行胰胆管造影

内镜逆行胰胆管造影(ERCP)已经从单纯的诊断发展到几乎完全为治疗性操作。ERCP 通常使用中度镇静剂[22],尽管在美国的大多数中心,ERCP 是在麻醉下进行的,特别是在病情较重的患者和预计复杂的病例中。在 ERCP 中接受丙泊酚麻醉的患者可能比接受其他形式的全身麻醉的患者恢复时间更快[23]。ERCP 采用侧视十二指肠镜,可以识别大乳头。胆管插管是在内镜和透视引导下进行的。各种导管、导丝和支架可以用来进行治疗干预。目前认为诊断性 ERCP 已过时,但对疑似 SOD 患者行测压(参见第 63 章)以及在其他影像学检查无法诊断的情况下可能诊断为 PSC 有所保留(参见第 68 章)[24-26]。

(五) 超声内镜引导下胆管引流

在三级中心,超声内镜引导下胆管引流(EUS-guided biliary drainage,EUS-BD)已逐渐成为标准 ERCP 失败或无法进行 ERCP 的患者胆道减压的替代方法[27-30],可能会在由于手术改变解剖结构、胃出口梗阻、壶腹周围憩室或无法将导丝通过胆道梗阻等情况下应用[31,32]。虽然传统上在 ERCP 失败的情况下进行经皮经肝穿刺胆管引流,但它与高发病率和生活质量降低有关(见后文)[33]。EUS-BD 最常见的方法是经胃至肝内胆道系统和经十二指肠至肝外胆道系统。治疗方法包括 EUS 引导下胆总管十二指肠造瘘术(EUS-guided choledochoduodenostomy,EUS-CD)、EUS 引导下胆囊十二指肠造瘘术、EUS 引导下肝肠造瘘术(EUS-guided hepaticoenterostomy,EUS-HE)和 EUS 引导下对接引流术(EUS-guided rendezvous,EUS-RV),这些需要熟练掌握 EUS 和 ERCP 的技术。

EUS-CD 包括在 EUS 引导下用 FNA 针经十二指肠穿刺肝外胆管,然后将导丝送入胆道,扩张胆道,在十二指肠第一部分的近端放置支架[34,35]。已经介绍了各种进入胆道和瘘管扩张方法,每种方法的选择取决于机构和内镜医生的偏好。一项关于 EUS-CD 的 meta 分析发现,EUS-CD 的技术成功率为 94%,早期不良事件(adverse event,AE)(即并发症)的发生率为 19%[36]。自膨胀金属支架通常比塑料支架更受欢迎,因为它可以防止胆汁外漏,提高耐久性和通畅性。

EUS 引导下的胆囊十二指肠造瘘术既可用于不适合接受胆囊切除术的患者初次胆囊引流,也可用于二次胆囊引流,以便拔除先前放置的临时经皮胆囊造瘘管。该手术包括通过十二指肠壁对胆囊颈部进行 FNA 穿刺,然后将导丝置入胆囊内。通常情况下,用双蘑菇头金属支架在器官之间建立吻合,降低支架移位风险(图 70.3)。通常在金属支架内放置塑料猪尾支架,以防止支架堵塞[37]。

EUS-HE 包括经胃或经空肠(在手术改变解剖结构的情况下)FNA 穿刺左肝内胆管的一个分支,然后将导丝推进胆道系统并放置支架(图 70.4)[38]。彩色多普勒可用于探测穿刺路径血管,从而避开这些血管,并通过抽吸胆汁和/或注射造影剂进行胆道造影来确认进入胆道。EUS-HE 可作为明确的治疗方法,如用于恶性胆道梗阻的姑息治疗,用于术前减压,或作为下游治疗的入口,包括顺行支架置入术[39,40]。

EUS-RV 用于 ERCP 失败的病例,作为辅助插管和/或在再次尝试 ERCP 时放置导丝的手段。步骤包括在 EUS 引导下从胃或十二指肠穿刺胆道系统,然后进行胆道造影和向胆道系统放置导丝[41]。导丝穿过壶腹部进入十二指肠。经透视确认导丝到位后,撤出超声内镜和穿刺针,同时保持导丝位置不变。接下来可以执行以下两种方法中的一种。在第一种方法中,在导丝旁插入十二指肠镜,并向壶腹部推进,在那里找到导丝并用于辅助插管。或者,可以用钳子或圈套抓住导丝的远端,通过治疗钳道或与内镜一起通过口腔取出;然后将带有导丝的十二指肠镜推进到壶腹。无论采用哪种方法,最终目的都是通过内镜解除梗阻[42-44]。对于存在壶腹周围大憩室的患者,该技术对于胆管插管和结石清除是最有用的。

EUS-BD 模式的选择取决于患者和提供者的特征,并往往

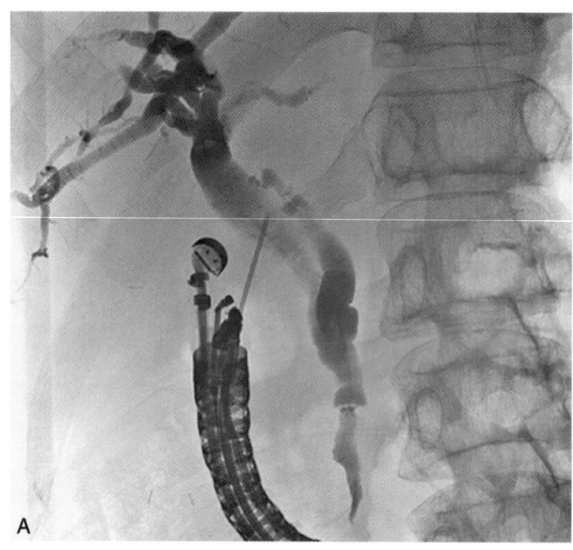

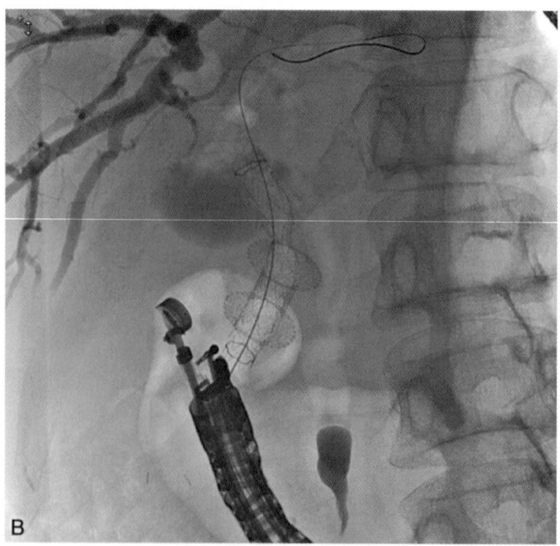

图 70.3 一例转移性黑色素瘤所致恶性胆道梗阻患者,EUS 引导下胆总管十二指肠吻合术(CD)的 X 线透视图像。A,X 线图像显示通过 19 号针头将造影剂注入胆道中。在胆管远端可见狭窄。B,显示管腔对合的金属 CD 支架在适当位置的 X 线片。通过 CD 支架将一个 10mm×6cm 全覆膜金属支架置入胆管,在全覆膜金属支架内置入一个 7Fr 塑料支架

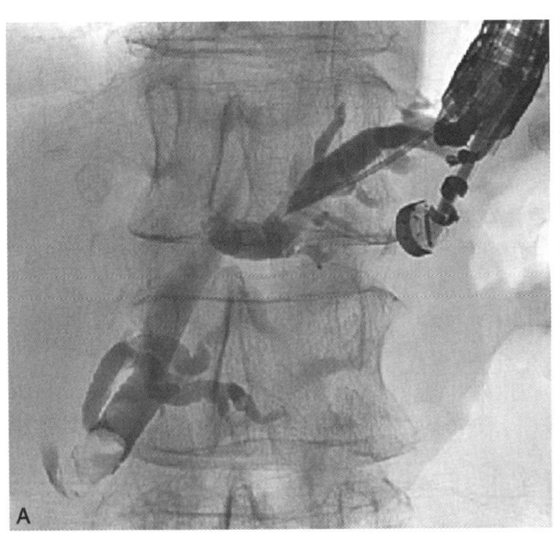

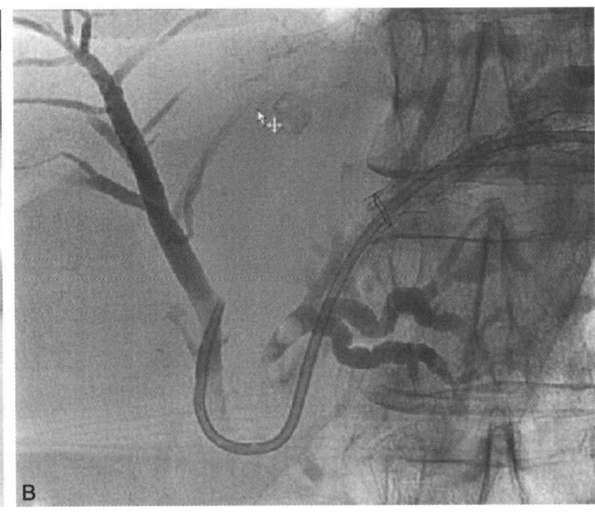

图 70.4　一例在腹腔镜胆囊切除术中胆管损伤后接受肝管空肠吻合术的患者，在 EUS 引导下肝胃吻合术（HG）的 X 线透视图像。A，X 线片图像显示通过 19 号针头将造影剂注入胆道。在肝管空肠吻合口近端可见梗阻性结石。B，显示 HG 支架就位的 X 线片。通过 HG 支架，在球囊扩张后穿过左右肝管分叉将 7-Fr 塑料支架置入右侧胆管系统

由内镜医生的偏好决定。有人建议，如果可以到达壶腹，应首先尝试 EUS-RV，如果导丝不能推进到所需位置，则应将 EUS-CD 或 EUS-HE 作为挽救方法[45]。如果无法接近壶腹，最初可以尝试 EUS-CD 或 EUS-HE。在 ERCP 失败的患者中，这两种方法似乎同样有效和安全[46]。越来越多的证据表明，当内镜医生对 EUS 和 ERCP 具有同样的丰富经验时，EUS-BD 可能等同于 ERCP，作为恶性胆道梗阻的主要治疗方法[47,48]。

二、内镜治疗

（一）胆管结石

ERCP 通常在已知有胆总管结石或至少中度可疑胆总管结石的患者中施行（参见第 65 章）[49]。对于胆囊结石且几乎不怀疑胆总管结石的患者，首选无创影像检查（MRCP、MDCT）或 EUS，以最大限度地降低 ERCP 并发症的可能性[7]。对于临床怀疑胆总管结石程度较低且计划行胆囊切除术的患者，可以行术中胆道造影术，如果发现结石，则可以进行腹腔镜探查和取石。然后，ERCP 可以用于没有取出结石的患者[8]。

标准的取石方法是内镜下胆管括约肌切开术，以便扩大乳头，随后用球囊或取石网篮取出结石（图 70.5）。采用这种方法，80% 以上的结石可以成功取出[50]。较大的结石可能需要其他的取出技术（稍后讨论）。括约肌预切开术，即在插管和/或导丝引导前在乳头上做一个切口，可用于传统方法插管失败的病例，由熟练的内镜医生操作时，不会增加 AE 的

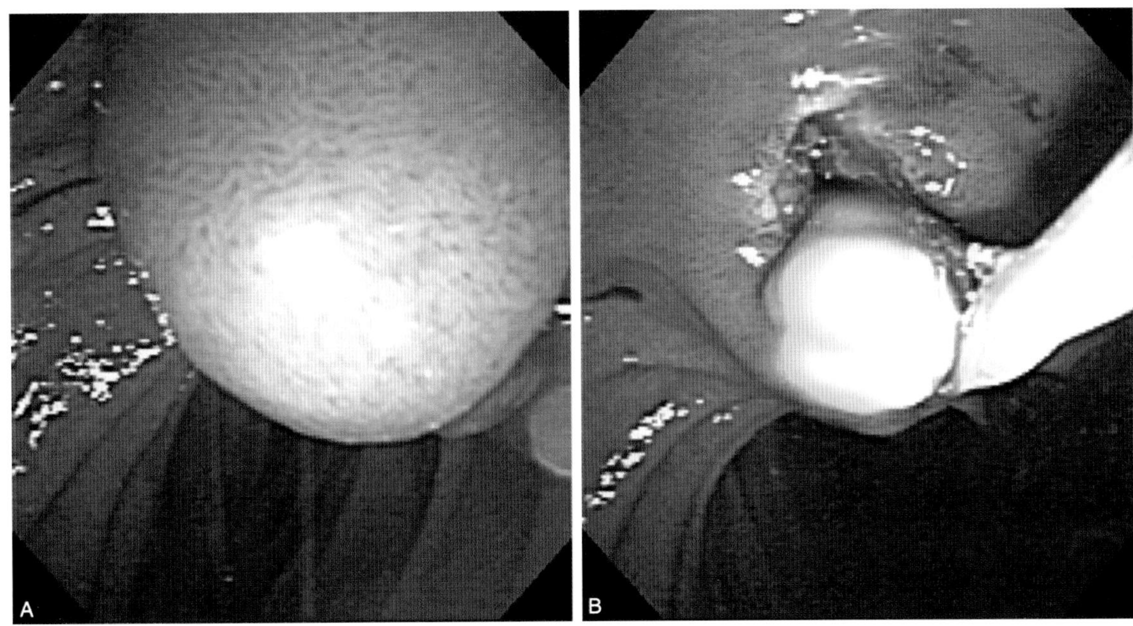

图 70.5　取出胆管结石期间的内镜图像。A，可见与嵌顿结石一致的乳头隆起。B，内镜下括约肌切开术后，取出结石

风险[51]。

胆道括约肌切开术的替代方法是球囊乳头扩张术（球囊括约肌成形术），可使用小直径球囊（4～8mm）[52]。该技术作为一种保留 Oddi 括约肌功能的方法，尤其是年轻患者。采用球囊或网篮技术取出结石。大多数关于球囊括约肌成形术的文献来自美国以外的国家。两项关于球囊括约肌成形术与括约肌切开术的随机试验的 meta 分析显示，球囊括约肌成形术的胰腺炎发生率和机械碎石的需要量明显较高，但出血的风险明显低于括约肌切开术[53,54]。在美国，唯一一项比较球囊括约肌成形术和括约肌切开术的随机试验提前结束，因为有 2 名年轻患者死于 ERCP 术后的胰腺炎[55]。然而，括约肌成形术仍然是凝血障碍患者[53]、合并肝硬化的患者（特别是 Child-Pugh C 级患者）[53]（参见第 74 和 92 章）和解剖结构改变的患者[如 Billroth Ⅱ 胃空肠造口术（参见第 53 章）]的一种替代方法，在这些患者中，括约肌切开术在技术上存在困难[53]。在这种情况下，应采用预防性放置胰腺支架和给予直肠吲哚美辛等措施，以降低胰腺炎的风险[56,57]。

清除大的胆管结石（定义为任意直径≥1.5cm），除了前面介绍的技术外，可能还需要其他技术才能成功清除。其中一种技术是碎石术。碎石术的一种形式是机械碎石术，将结石装在专门的大网篮里捕获并粉碎（图 70.6）[58]。结石碎片使用标准的取石技术取出。另一种形式的碎石术是胆管内碎石术，它是通过使用激光或液电导管在胆道镜直视下进行碎石[59]。有必要进行直接观察，以确保碎石装置是针对结石而不是胆管壁。胆道括约肌切开术和大直径（12～20mm）球囊扩张术相结合已被用于清除大结石并减少机械性碎石的使用。这种大直径扩张方法似乎是安全的，并且不增加 ERCP 后胰腺炎的风险[60]。如果大的结石无法取出，则放置胆道支架以缓解梗阻[61]。然后可以选择性地进行其他手术，以清除残留结石。

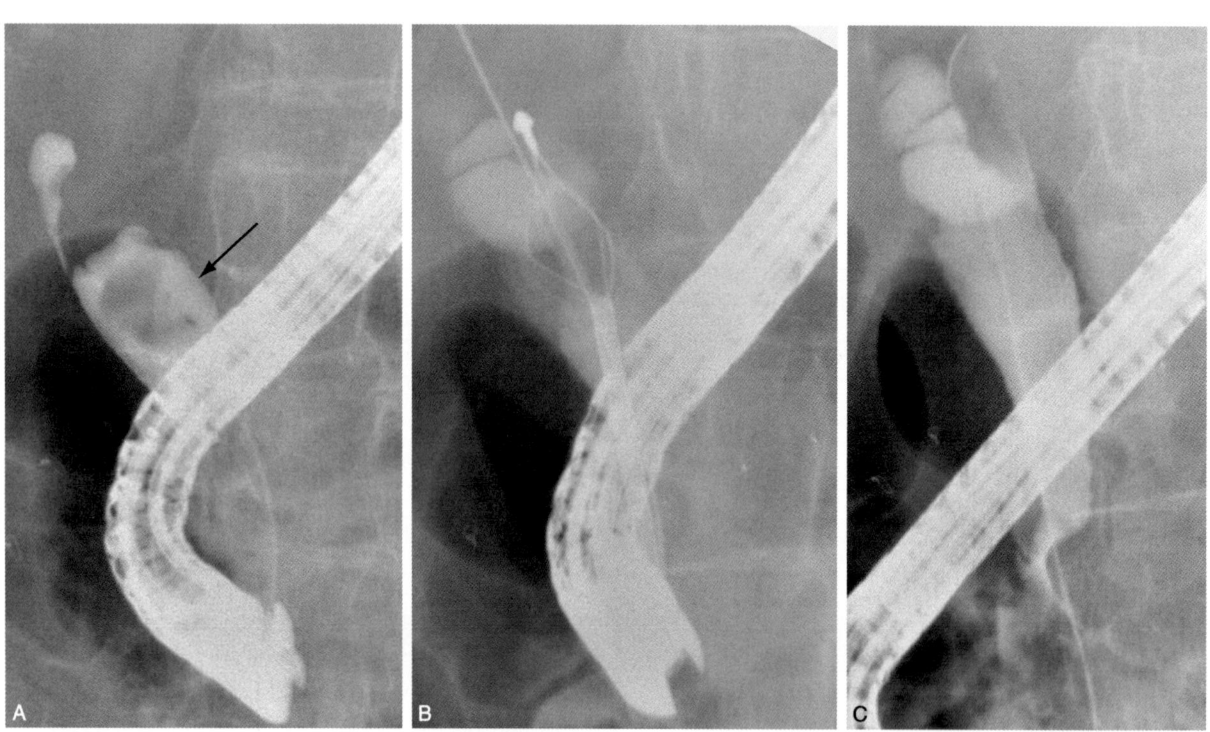

图 70.6　胆管结石的机械碎石术。A，内镜逆行胆管造影显示大结石（箭示）。B，碎石网篮粉碎结石。C，随访胆管造影显示结石从胆管中清除

（二）胆漏

如前所述，胆漏是由术后并发症和创伤引起。腹腔镜胆囊切除术的胆管损伤发生率为 0.06%～0.3%[62]。最常见的情况是，胆囊切除术后胆漏来自胆囊管或 Luschka 管（参见第 62 章）。这些较小的渗漏通常可以通过仅仅进行胆管括约肌切开术或放置塑料胆道支架（7～10Fr）或两者兼备来处理[63]。这种方法将胆汁从渗漏处转移到十二指肠，并抵消了胆道括约肌的高压作用。更复杂的渗漏通常需要放置一个或多个大直径塑料胆道支架，并结合胆管括约肌切开术（图 70.7）[64]。使用可拆卸的、覆膜的自膨胀金属支架（self-expanding metal stent，SEMS）治疗难治性渗漏临床也有效[65,66]。

（三）原发性硬化性胆管炎

原发性硬化性胆管炎（PSC）患者可以从内镜治疗显性狭窄或胆管结石中获益（参见第 68 章）[67]。显著胆管狭窄患者通常表现为进行性胆道梗阻；但胆管癌的症状与良性显性狭窄的症状之间存在相当大的重叠[68]。因此，PSC 患者必须始终考虑到胆管癌的可能。常规的刷检细胞学检查在这些患者中的敏感性较低，但荧光原位杂交已被证明对检测胆管癌有较高的敏感性（参见第 69 章）[69]。然而，在没有显著狭窄的情况下，特异性很低[70]。胆道镜（胆管镜）可以提高这些患者恶性肿瘤的检出率[71]。基于探针的共聚焦激光内镜已用于诊断不明原因的胆管狭窄[72]。这项技术需要注射荧光素造

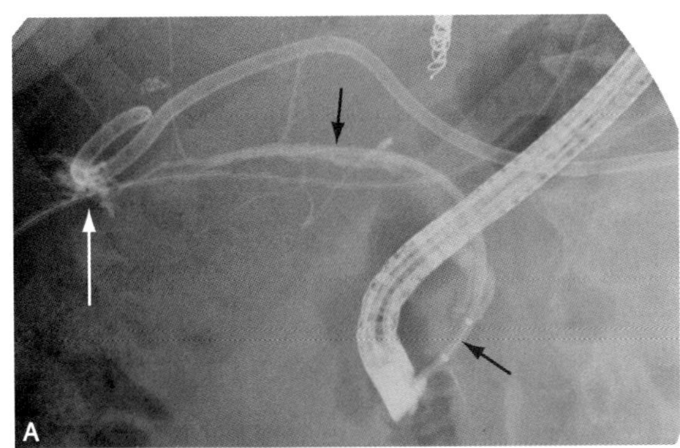

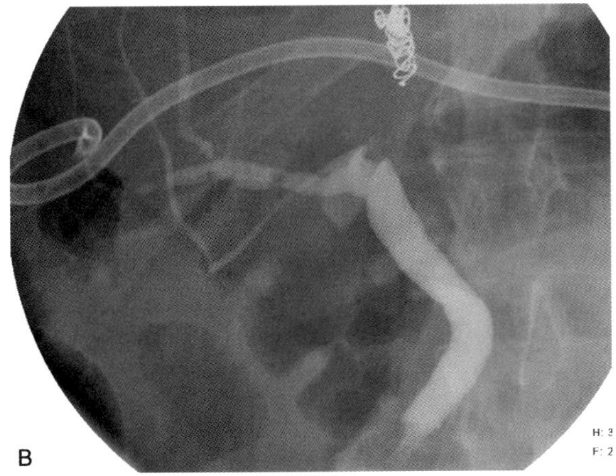

图 70.7　经内镜治疗的肝切除术后肝内胆漏。A,在经皮引流管附近观察到造影剂外渗(长箭示);放置内部胆道支架(短箭示)。B,随访胆管造影显示胆漏消失

影剂,并使用专门的探针,可以实现细胞层面的实时可视化。目前已经提出了使用基于探针的激光内镜检查的说明标准;然而,在常规推荐这种技术之前,还需要更多的数据[73]。

内镜下治疗显著狭窄包括球囊扩张,通常结合短期(<8周)放置大口径(10Fr)支架(图 70.8)。内镜治疗后的终点包括临床、生化和放射学的改善,成功率从 65% 到 100% 不等[74]。

(四) 良性胆管狭窄

良性胆管狭窄由多种疾病引起(框 70.1),对治疗的反应因病因而异。内镜治疗包括 X 线引导下进行球囊扩张,然后放置胆道支架。内镜治疗的目标是长期胆道减压;然而,如果微创方法无效,内镜治疗也可作为外科手术的桥梁[75]。内镜支架可以是塑料的,也可以是全覆膜的 SEMS。未覆膜 SEMS 会造成不可逆的组织增生和支架嵌入,妨碍取出,因此不用于良性胆管狭窄的治疗。相反,全覆膜 SEMS 可以临时放置,可用于良性胆管狭窄的治疗[76]。置入单个塑料支架相对容易,且成本效益比较高;然而,这一优势因通畅时间短和长期成功率低而被抵消。另一种方法是使用多个大口径塑料支架(10~11.5Fr),定期置入胆道,最长可达 1 年(图 70.9)[77-79]。与塑料支架相比,SEMS 具有更大的直径和更高的通畅率,并且解决狭窄所需的内镜治疗次数更少。使用大直径(10mm)的覆膜 SEMS 可能是多个塑料支架的替代方案;随着时间的推移 SEMS 使得狭窄扩张,通常在 3~6 个月后移除,尽管一些数据表明,它们可能会保持原位长达一年[80]。使用这种方法的结果令人鼓舞,但在良性疾病中使用 SEMS 仅限于慢性胰腺炎引起的良性胆管狭窄,而且仅限于有限的停留时间[81]。慢性胰腺炎会导致远端胆管狭窄,这种狭窄通常难以通过单一塑料支架进行内镜治疗,尤其是钙化性慢性胰腺炎患者(参见第 59 章)[82]。如前所述,可以放置多个塑料支架。覆膜 SEMS 已被批准用于治疗慢性胰腺炎引起的胆管狭窄[83]。

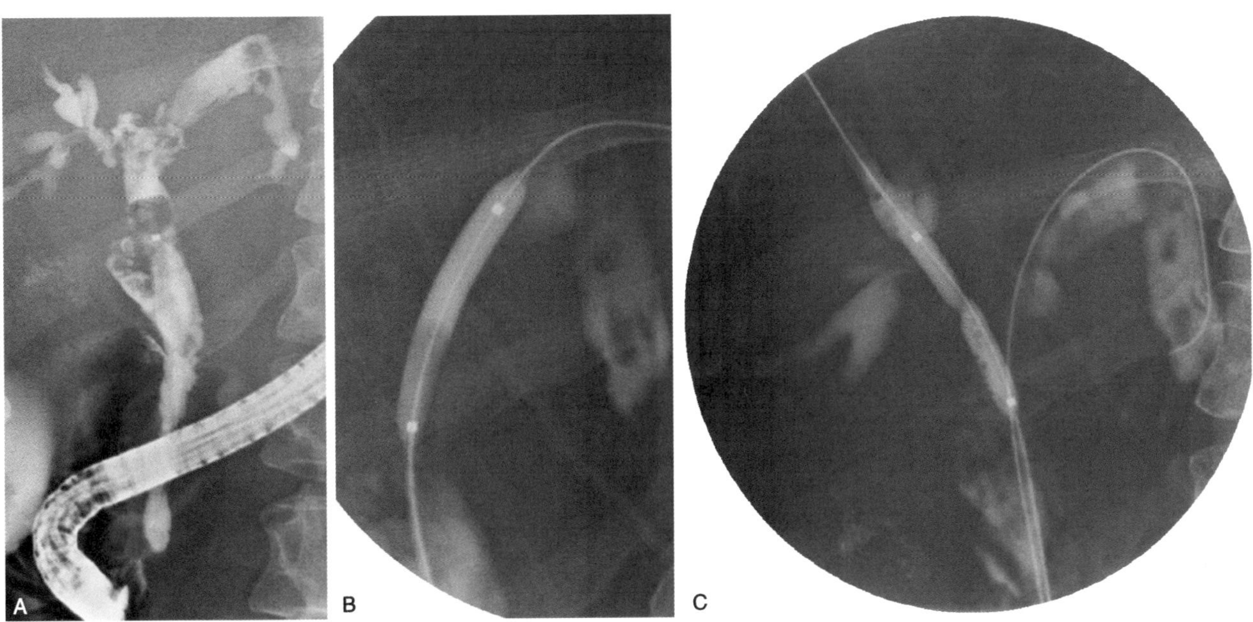

图 70.8　原发性硬化性胆管炎(PSC)的内镜治疗。A,胆管造影显示左右肝管不规则狭窄伴肝内胆管结石。B,左肝管球囊扩张。C,右肝管球囊扩张

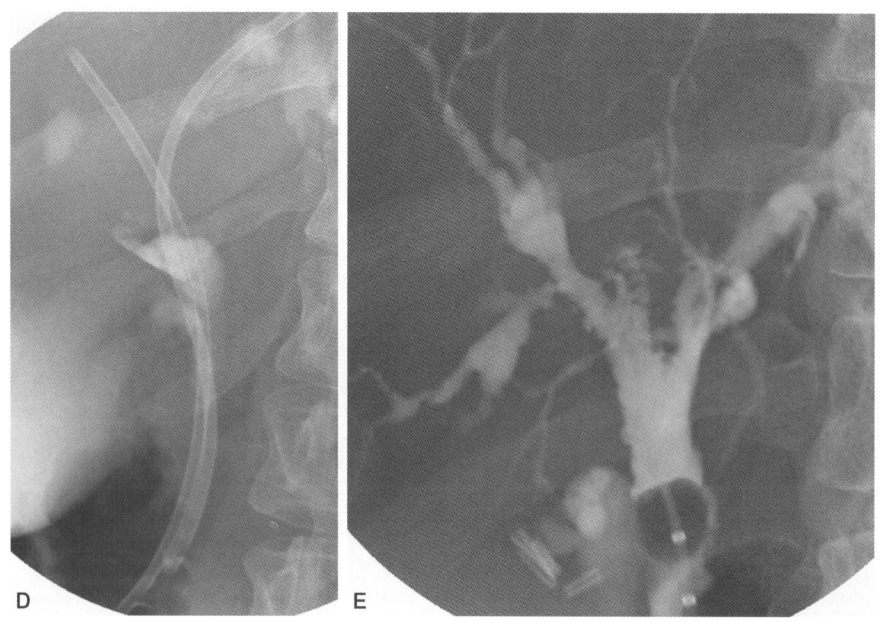

图 70.8(续)　D,置入双侧塑料胆管支架。E,采用球囊阻塞技术的随访胆管造影显示明显改善

框 70.1　良性胆道狭窄的主要原因	
慢性胰腺炎	腹腔镜胆囊切除术
手术后	肝移植
胆管切除与胆总管吻合术	原发性硬化性胆管炎

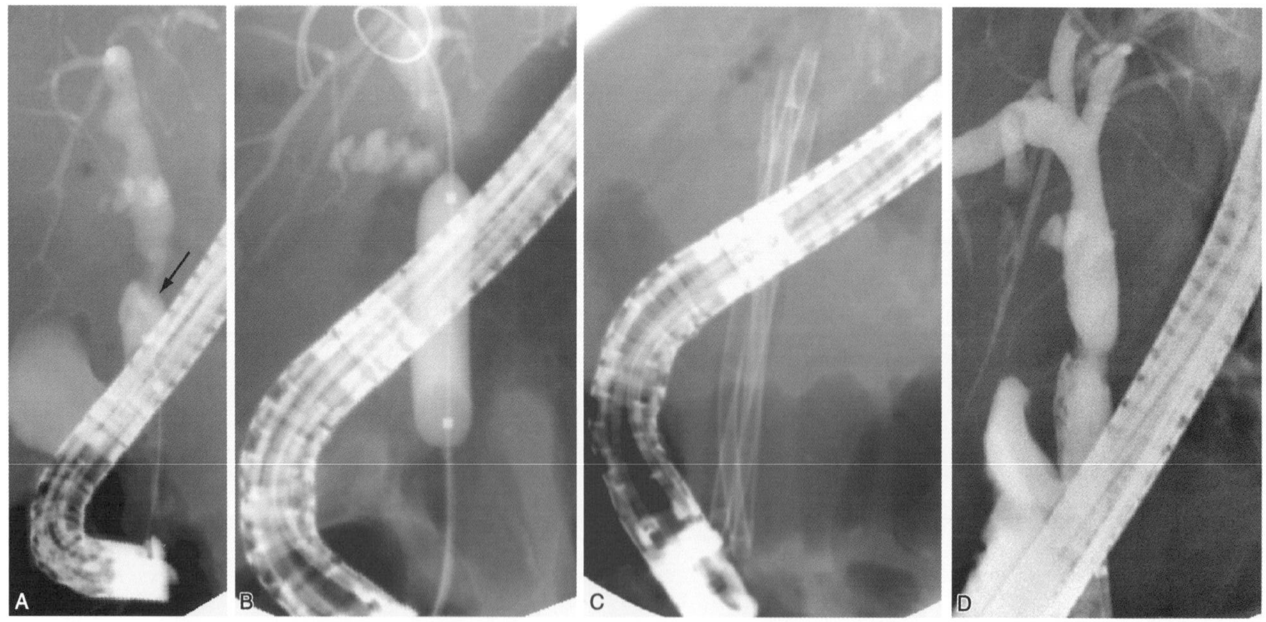

图 70.9　使用多个支架进行胆总管吻合口狭窄的内镜治疗。A,胆管造影显示吻合口狭窄(箭示)。B,狭窄处球囊扩张。C,放置多枚塑料支架。D,随访胆管造影显示改善

(五) 不明原因的胆管狭窄

基于影像结果和组织取样,一些胆道狭窄不容易区分良性或恶性。ERCP 的组织取样技术包括导丝引导的胆管刷检细胞学和胆管内活检[43,84]。其他可用于评估不明原因狭窄的技术包括 EUS、胆管内超声[84]、胆道镜检查(有或没有定向活检)[85]和基于探针的共聚焦激光内镜检查[84]。有一小部分患者,诊断仍不明确,有些患者只有在长期随访或手术探查、切除时才能确定最终诊断,或在 PSC、LT 的情况下才能确定。

（六）恶性胆道狭窄

内镜下解除恶性胆道梗阻可以通过经乳头途径，放置大口径塑料支架（10-Fr）或 SEMS 穿过恶性狭窄，也可以通过 EUS，结合 EUS-BD，如 CD 或 HE 来实现。采用的方法取决于狭窄的位置（肝总管远端分叉处、肝周或肝门）和解剖学限制，如胃出口梗阻或外科手术后改变的胆道或消化道解剖（参见第 69 章）。

1. 远端胆管狭窄

胰头癌是引起远端胆管梗阻的最常见原因（参见第 60 第 61 章）。对于计划进行手术切除（胰十二指肠切除术）的已知胰腺癌患者，不鼓励术前常规 ERCP 进行胆道减压。一些研究表明，这种方法并不能改善手术效果，而且增加了 ERCP 的总发病率和 AE（并发症），可能会延迟或影响手术切除[86]。术前 ERCP 的适应证包括急性胆管炎和严重瘙痒[87]。此外，在进行新辅助化疗时，由于手术切除的时间通常会延长，并且需要降低血清胆红素水平以允许化疗，因此适用于支架放置。在这种情况下，使用短长度的 SEMS（覆膜或无覆膜）似乎是最好的选择；数据显示，与 SEMS 相比，放置塑料支架时，接受术前化学放射治疗的胰腺癌患者的支架闭塞率较高[88]。在手术切除时，未覆膜 SEMS 与肿瘤一起被切除。与放置塑料支架相比，无论可切除性如何，在胰腺癌患者中放置 SEMS 都可能具有成本效益[89-91]。

ERCP 联合胆道支架置入是一种成熟的姑息性手术过渡的替代方法，可以作为门诊手术安全进行[92]。在 SEMS 出现之前，对远端胆道梗阻进行了使用塑料支架内镜治疗和手术的对比研究。塑料支架的主要局限性是由于细菌生物膜或植物物质的反流而导致支架闭塞[93]。因此，在手术和内镜的对比研究中，内镜组的初始住院时间较短，但被后续需要住院和重复 ERCP 以处理支架堵塞所抵消。标准大口径塑料支架的闭塞中位时间约为 3 个月。支架闭塞会导致黄疸复发，通常伴有胆管炎。使用 SEMS 克服了细菌生物膜的问题，随机对照试验显示 SEMS 的通畅率优于塑料支架（图 70.10）[94]。尽管 SEMS 的成本明显提高，但无论预期存活率如何，使用 SEMS 都是划算的[95]。未覆膜的 SEMS 闭塞一般很容易通过放置塑料支架或在现有支架内放置新的 SEMS 来处理。覆膜金属支架的开发是为了防止肿瘤过度生长和组织增生引起的闭塞；一项 meta 分析表明，覆膜支架的通畅率为 304 天，而无覆膜支架为 141 天[96]。覆膜 SEMS 与较高的支架移位率和可能增加的急性胆囊炎风险相关[97,98]。

2. 肝门周围胆管梗阻

肝门周围胆管狭窄可能是由胆管癌或转移性疾病引起的。肝门周围肿瘤获得充分姑息治疗的临床成功率低于远端胆管肿瘤[99]。缓解肝门狭窄的主要考虑因素之一是，只在一侧放置支架（单侧）还是在左右肝内胆管放置支架（双侧）。双侧内镜下支架置入术的技术成功率较低。大多数肝门周围梗阻的患者在只引流一侧肝脏（单侧引流）时将得到充分的缓解；因为没有进入对侧，降低了污染对侧的风险[100]。左、右胆管系统均注入造影剂的患者需要双侧支架置入，以防止不可控制的胆管炎[101]。在 ERCP 前，腹部 CT 可能会发现肝脏一叶萎缩，ERCP 时应特别避开此叶，因为造影剂污染后需要引流以防止胆管炎，但太不可能帮助缓解。另外，MRCP 可以在 ERCP 前明确胆道解剖结构。

与塑料支架相比，金属支架是否能延长肝门周围肿瘤的姑息治疗时间，这一点并不确定，就像远端胆管狭窄的情况一样（见前文）。在 17 例 Bimuth Ⅱ 型和Ⅲ型肝门周围胆管癌行

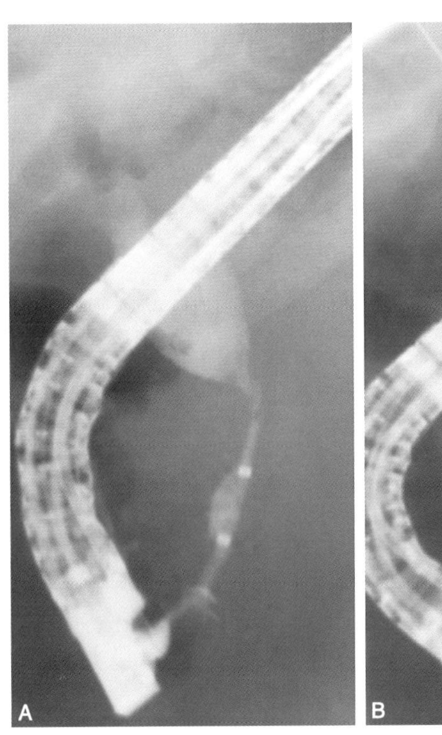

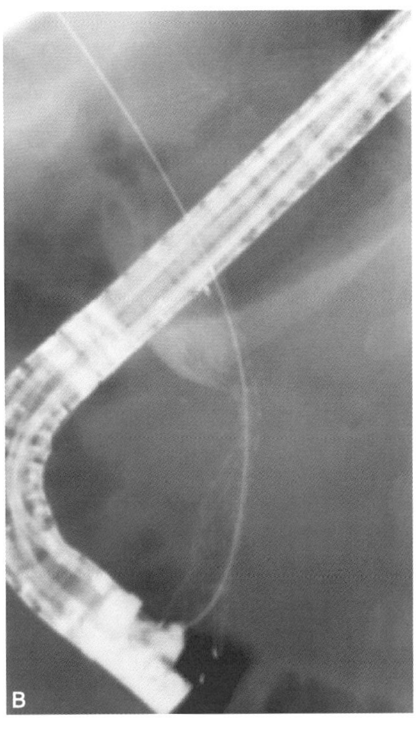

70.10　内镜下缓解不可切除胰腺癌引起的梗阻性黄疸。A，胆管造影显示远端胆管梗阻性狭窄。B，自膨式金属支架展开后即刻的薄膜影像

金属支架置入术的前瞻性单臂试验研究中（参见第 69 章），支架中位通畅率为 12 个月[102]。一项非比较性的单臂研究显示，在大多数（69%）不可切除的肝门部周围胆管癌患者中，插入 Wall stent（一种金属支架）是安全可行的，并能成功实现缓解，而不需要进一步的胆道再介入[103]。在一项对使用塑料支架或金属支架治疗肝门周围肿瘤患者的前瞻性观察队列研究中，放置金属支架的患者术后并发症发生率和需要经皮引流的比例明显降低[104]。这一发现表明，金属支架对肝门周围胆管梗阻的疗效与对远端胆管梗阻的疗效相同[105]。

很少有关于内镜和经皮途径治疗肝门周围肿瘤的比较研究（见后文）。一项关于仅使用 SEMS 治疗肝门周围胆管癌的内镜和经皮治疗结果的研究发现，经皮放置 SEMS 组的胆道减压成功率显著高于经内镜放置 SEMS 组[106]。无论采用哪种手术，最初胆道引流成功的患者，其中位生存期都比胆道引流失败的患者长得多。此外，在胆道减压成功后，两组患者的中位生存期和支架通畅时间相似。

综上所述，对于无法切除的肝门周围胆管癌患者行 ERCP 姑息治疗，合理的做法是在引流侧局限性注射造影剂，进行单侧支架置入。一个支架，无论是塑料的还是金属的，通常足以达到缓解的目的[107]。然而，SEMS 似乎比塑料支架具有更好的缓解作用[108,109]。最后，从内镜的角度来看，肝门周围肿瘤在技术上比非肝门肿瘤更难成功引流。

光动力疗法（photodynamic therapy，PDT）已被用于不能切除的肝门周围胆管癌患者的姑息治疗，这些患者在内镜下放置塑料支架后，黄疸仍不能缓解[110]。与历史对照组相比，使用 PDT 可显著改善胆汁淤积、生活质量和存活率[111,112]，并且可长期维持[113]。相关研究是在美国以外的国家进行的，这些国家容易获得更小、更灵活的激光纤维。尽管如此，光动力疗法在美国的试验已经显示出令人振奋的结果[114-116]。胆管癌的光动力疗法一般局限于精通这一治疗的某些中心。不幸的是，PDT 的成本已经急剧上升，以至于往往无法实施。

胆管内射频消融术也被用于治疗胆管癌[117]。直径为 10-Fr 的柔性探针可以通向狭窄处，并与标准的外科电发生器一起使用。初步数据很有希望，该技术有可能取代 PDT[118,119]。

（七）Oddi 括约肌功能障碍

根据不同程度的影像和实验室异常，Oddi 括约肌功能障碍（SOD）在历史上被分为Ⅰ型、Ⅱ型和Ⅲ型（参见第 63 章）[120,121]。所有类型都以间歇性胆源型腹痛为特征。Oddi 括约肌测压可以在 ERCP 期间进行，方法是向胆管或胰管内灌注水或插入固态测压导管，分别测量胆管或胰管的括约肌压力。SOD Ⅰ型（括约肌狭窄）与实验室检查结果的客观异常（通常在发作时）以及影像学检查中肝外胆管的异常扩张有关。SOD Ⅱ型（括约肌功能障碍）与实验室检查结果异常或胆管扩张有关。SOD Ⅲ型仅以疼痛为特征，然而，由于缺乏客观结果支持其存在，这一诊断在临床实践中已基本不用[122]。

随着人们对 SOD 认识的改变，对这种疾病的治疗也发生了实质性的变化。Cotton 及其同事的 EPISOD 研究是一项大型随机临床试验，研究对象是胆囊切除术后疼痛且胆道梗阻的客观证据很少或没有客观证据的患者，患者随机接受括约肌切开术或假干预治疗[26]。在这项研究中，内镜下括约肌切开术在预防腹痛复发方面的效果实际上比假干预更差。因此，不建议 SOD 患者进行常规 ERCP，当然也不建议仅有疼痛的患者在没有客观异常结果的情况下进行 ERCP。胆囊切除术后疼痛的患者应评估疼痛的其他病因或先前手术的潜在并发症。

（八）外科手术所致的解剖改变

在过去，手术改变上消化道解剖结构的患者曾接受过经皮途径来研究胆道。遇到的最困难的解剖结构是 Roux-en-Y 胃旁路术后（参见第 8 章）。在这类患者中，替代的方法包括独特的内镜技术[123]、EUS 引导下方法[124]或者联合内镜和腹腔镜辅助方法[125]。在手术改变解剖结构的患者中，到达胆道的内镜方法通常涉及使用较长的内镜，包括球囊辅助和螺旋肠镜。这种方法的缺点包括手术时间长、技术成功率低、前视镜和用于治疗干预的附件少[126]。随着治疗性 EUS 的兴起，扩大了内镜在外科解剖结构改变的患者中治疗胆道梗阻的选择范围，并可能优于小肠镜辅助治疗。在一项对存在外科解剖改变和胆道梗阻患者的研究中，小肠镜辅助 ERCP 的技术成功率为 65.3%，EUS-BD 的技术成功率为 98%[127]。由于单纯的内镜手术技术要求高，劳动强度大，因此通常只在三级中心进行。

另一种方法是腹腔镜手术，在外科医生的协助下，将十二指肠镜通过套管针经腹腔插入到被排空的胃中，其技术成功率高达 98%[128]。这种方法需要多个专科的协调，并需要对设备进行消毒，而且由于手术室内的透视质量通常较低，因此这种方法具有挑战性。由于进入腹腔部位的脓肿形成率相对较高，使这种方法更加复杂[129]。尽管存在这些限制，腹腔镜辅助 ERCP 仍是经皮经肝穿刺胆管造影术（transhepatic cholangiography，THC）的常用替代方法（见后文），并可能是没有新型 EUS 疗法中心的首选方法。

（九）不良事件

ERCP 可能发生五种主要不良事件[130]：镇静剂相关、胰腺炎、出血、穿孔和感染。由于患者选择和操作者技术和经验的差异，ERCP 术后胰腺炎的发生率有所不同。高危患者是年轻、健康女性，尤其是那些已知或怀疑患有 SOD 的患者[131]。老年人和患有慢性胰腺炎或胰腺癌者术后胰腺炎的概率较低。在主胰管内预防性放置支架降低了高危患者发生胰腺炎风险，几乎消除了重症胰腺炎的风险[132]。胰管支架置入术一般在胆管插管困难或不慎插入胰管时推荐使用[133]。已证明经直肠给予预防性非甾体抗炎药（NSAIDs）可以降低 ERCP 后胰腺炎的风险[134]，可能优于预防性支架或支架与直肠 NSAIDs 联合使用[135,136]。胆管括约肌切开后可能发生出血。括约肌切开术后出血的危险因素包括凝血障碍和在括约肌切开 72 小时内进行抗凝治疗[137]。不到 1% 的患者发生十二指肠穿孔，可能需要手术治疗，特别是在十二指肠一侧壁受损的情况下[138,139]。感染主要发生在 ERCP 术后胆道引流不充分的患者。这些患者包括广泛肝内 PSC 或晚期肝门周围肿瘤，以及因胆道梗阻而接受支架置入失败的患者。内镜医师 ERCP 操作量少似乎也与成功率较低和 AE 发生率较高有关(另见第 42 章)[140]。因此,目前正在努力建立 EUS 和 ERCP 的标准化培训,以及评估操作熟练程度的方法[141]。

三、经皮经肝穿刺胆管造影术

经皮 THC 是一种有创性的诊断检查,必要时可用于治疗。鉴于有一系列无创的影像学检查,经皮 THC 很少用于诊断。可以用于胆道梗阻减压、取石、狭窄球囊扩张以及经肝引流管或支架置入。该手术一般用于因胆肠 Roux-en-Y 吻合术、胃旁路手术或肝外胆管狭窄不能通过内镜行 ERCP 的患者(见前文)。在一些机构,复杂的肝门周围肿瘤患者优先行经皮胆道引流以解除胆道梗阻。2% ~4% 的病例会发生与手术相关的严重 AE,如出血、脓毒症或胆漏[142]。手术一般可以在中度镇静的情况下进行[143]。通常预防性使用静脉广谱抗生素[144]。

(一) 技术

经皮 THC 前回顾 CT 和 MRI 结果有助于确定最佳路径(即从右侧或左侧)和主要扩张胆管的位置,并有助于避免无意中穿越邻近结构,如结肠。使用经腹超声引导,从剑突下入路的方法,只需极少的穿刺次数,即可轻松进入左侧扩张的胆管[145]。然而,最常用的是标准的右侧入路,从肋间入路进行,通常是通过第十肋间隙以下的腋中区。多次穿刺会增加气胸或胆源性胸腔积液的风险。

无论从哪一侧开始,在透视引导下将 22 号针向肝门中央推进,并在缓慢抽出穿刺针时轻轻注入造影剂。最初使用这种小的穿刺针可减少肝脏创伤以及出血的可能性,尽管可能需要多次进针才能插入胆管,特别是在胆管没有扩张的情况下。超声引导或 CT 引导可辅助进入未扩张的胆管[146,147]。

胆管插管成功后,可以进行诊断性胆管造影。由于狭窄或结石与胆道其他部位不相通,孤立的胆管可能需要通过额外穿刺进行疏通。如果该手术只是诊断性的,胆道梗阻不明显,则只需将针拔出。但如果胆道系统存在梗阻,则应郑重考虑穿过梗阻,并留置减压“外-内”引流管,对梗阻的胆道系统置之不顾,可能导致穿刺部位的胆汁渗漏。使用肝门部肝内胆管作为最终通路可以降低肝动脉损伤的风险。如果最初插管的导管位置过于靠近中心(肝动脉较大的分支倾向于更中心),则应该选择更靠外的通路进入胆管。通常,需要使用第二根穿刺针刺穿更外周的管道,而第一根穿刺针则用于使这种新的、更安全的通路管道变得不透明和可视化。然后将一根 0.018 英寸的“微型”导丝通过针头进入胆道,并沿导丝用扩张导管来逐级“扩大”通路。一旦通路建立,则可穿过梗阻并放置外-内引流管(图 70.11)。这些引流管的引流孔位于梗阻水平之上;远端猪尾留置在小肠内。导管的大小通常在 8~12Fr 范围内。较大的导管可能会产生更好的减压效果,但必须注意不要放置特别大的导管,以免阻塞较小胆道的引流,尤其是在 PSC 的情况下,许多阻塞的胆道没有扩张。如果在初次尝试时无法穿过梗阻,可在胆道梗阻近端留置引流管(外引流),在经过几天的引流后,可以通过这个通道后续尝试穿过梗阻。这种延迟往往可以使炎症减轻,增加导管随后内置的可能性。一般情况下,外-内引流管进行外置引流,直到发热或胆道淤血消失。将引流管外端关闭,以进行内引流,可减少每天 1L 以上的胆汁流失,并防止相关的脱水或电解质异常。初次手术中获得的胆汁样本可以送去做培养或细胞学检查。

经皮 THC 的禁忌证是凝血障碍。一般来说,INR 小于 1.8,血小板计数大于 50 000/mm^3 时,认为该手术是安全的(参见第 94 章)。通常在手术前需要即刻纠正任何异常情况。肝脏和穿刺点之间有明显的腹水会增加胆汁渗漏的风险,而曲折的胆道置管过程可能会导致导管的错位或未来操作的困

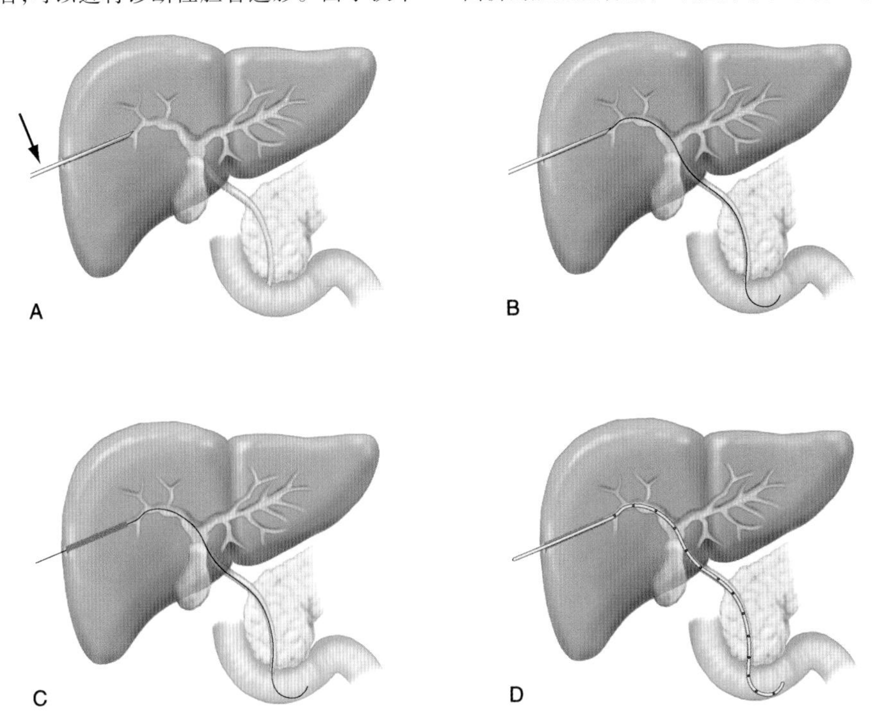

图 70.11　经皮经肝穿刺胆管造影术示意图。A,识别外周胆管,并用穿刺针进入外周胆管(箭示)。B,将导丝通过穿刺针穿过阻塞病变进入十二指肠。C,退出穿刺针。D,沿导丝插入内-外引流导管

难。在有大量肝周腹水的情况下,可以进行术前穿刺抽水或在手术过程中使用超声引导在肝脏旁放置一个小型临时腹腔引流管。胆道脓毒症避免胆管过度扩张以及手术过程中限制操作次数可以使胆道脓毒症降到最低。一旦放置了导管,就可以用于进一步操作或干预的通道。

在初次胆道减压后,应避免进一步干预,直到发热和脓毒症消退。手术后的初始 24~48 小时内,需要密切监测患者。导管周围、导管内或消化道大量出血提示可能损伤肝动脉[148]。肝动脉假性动脉瘤可能会延迟发生,有时会在最初手术后 1 周或 2 周后出现。如果持续出血导致血红蛋白水平大幅下降或血流动力学不稳定,应在发现受损血管后进行肝血管造影和栓塞术。在初次手术后,或在随后的操作过程中,导管或胆管中的少量血液通常是自限性的,并在 1 到 2 天内消失。

(二) 术后胆道狭窄

术后狭窄可能发生于腹腔镜胆囊切除术、肝大部切除术和 LT 后的胆管吻合处,或因缺血或复发性 PSC 在肝内胆管发生狭窄(参见框 70.1 及第 66、68 和 97 章)。应用胆道损伤的 Strasberg 分类(涵盖所有术后胆道损伤)或 Bismuth 分类(专门针对肝门部狭窄)来描述术后胆道狭窄(参见第 69 章)[149,150]。可以通过内镜或经皮穿刺来扩张术后或其他良性胆道狭窄,或通过外科放置 T 管的成熟技术(参见第 66 章)来实施。T 管的成熟通常需要 6 周,因此,在此之前不能移除外引流管。

在没有胆管炎或脓毒症临床症状的情况下,经皮 THC 和胆道球囊扩张术可以同时进行。留一个 8 或 10Fr 的经肝导管,患者在 6 周后再次进行胆道造影术,此时如果胆管狭窄 30%或更多,则进行进一步的狭窄扩张。然后将导管逐级增大到 12Fr,以促进直径较大的狭窄的愈合。如果狭窄在随访中消失,可以拔除导管;否则,在 6~8 周后应进行类似的手术。

在已发表的一项最大的长期随访研究中,对 85 例良性胆管狭窄患者进行了经皮胆管球囊扩张术[151]。随访的 75 例患者中,84 个胆道狭窄进行了 112 次治疗和 205 次经皮手术。狭窄球囊扩张 8~12mm。每隔 2 到 14 天重复一次,直到胆道造影显示造影剂自由引流至小肠,且无残留狭窄。外-内引流管引流平均保留 14~22 天,如果在夹闭引流管时感觉良好且胆道造影正常,则将其取出。从技术上讲,所有的手术都是成功的。共有 52 名、11 名、10 名和 2 名患者分别接受了 1 次、2 次、3 次和 4 次扩张。主要并发症发生在 2%的手术中:2 例膈下脓肿,1 例肝动脉假性动脉瘤和 1 例胆道出血。第一次治疗后 5 年、10 年、15 年、20 年和 25 年未发生临床显著再狭窄的概率分别为 0.52、0.49、0.49、0.41 和 0.41,第二次治疗后分别为 0.43、0.30、0.20、0.20 和 0.20。吻合口和非吻合口狭窄的再狭窄率差异无统计学意义。总体而言,75 例患者中有 56 例(75%)成功地接受了经皮治疗。

LT 后,经皮 THC 用于治疗胆管与胆管吻合术的并发症,尤其是在实施了肝管空肠吻合术的患者;后者通常不能通过内镜途径到达吻合口(参见第 97 章)。肝空肠吻合术适用于儿童、PSC 患者和因胆管间(胆总管间)的胆道吻合术及活体肝移植并发症而再次手术的患者[152]。对于胆管间吻合口和肝管空肠吻合口狭窄的治疗,经皮治疗具有较高的非手术成功率[153-155]。此外,对于那些通过 ERCP 可以接近胆管但内镜方法失败的患者中,经皮途径通常是成功的[156]。

(三) 原发性硬化性胆管炎

现在大多数原发性硬化性胆管炎(PSC)的非手术治疗都是通过 ERCP 进行(参见前文和第 68 章)。过去,经皮治疗显著狭窄采用球囊扩张,然后放置胆道引流管 2~3 个月,对治疗 PSC 患者的胆道梗阻症状非常有效[157],但对于黄疸超过 6 个月的患者,由于肝实质功能障碍,效果较差。之后,文献中仅有经皮治疗 PSC 的病例报告[158]。根据我们的经验,经皮治疗对内镜无法解决的显著狭窄患者有效(图 70.12)。在这种情况下,经皮穿入的导丝或导管可以留在十二指肠内,以便于以后的内镜检查(见后文)。

(四) 胆管漏

在病因上胆管漏几乎总是发生在手术后,并且发生于吻合口(例如,在肝移植后)和非吻合口部位。后者包括肝切除和腹腔镜损伤后肝和胆管的切缘表面。经皮治疗可能包括引流腹腔内的游离胆汁和局部聚积的胆汁(胆汁贮留囊型包块),以及在渗漏部位上方或横跨渗漏部位放置胆道引流管,以使大多数病例能成功闭合[159-161]。

无论是与经皮穿刺治疗相结合,还是作为经皮治疗的替代方法,ERCP 在胆管漏的治疗中都是有效的,其解决率可达 90%或更高[162-163]。手术可采用单纯括约肌切开[164,165]、并或不并括约肌切开术的塑料胆道支架置入[166-168],以及放置全覆膜 SEMS[169,170]。无论采用哪种方法,ERCP 的治疗机制都与胆管和十二指肠的压力平衡有关,从而使胆汁可以顺利流入十二指肠[170]。

(五) 胆管损伤

腹腔镜胆囊切除术的广泛开展导致胆总管损伤发生率增加(参见第 66 章)。胆管损伤的其他原因包括胆管探查、腹部手术或创伤引起的胆管损伤。经皮经肝穿刺胆管放置胆道引流管可作为损伤的主要治疗方法,也可作为手术修复的辅助手段[172]。Misra 及其同事对 51 名腹腔镜胆囊切除术胆管损伤后接受经皮胆道治疗的患者进行了 10 年的回顾性评估;45 名患者在转诊前接受了手术修复。总体而言,51 例患者中,46 例最初经皮治疗,5 例在肝管空肠吻合术失败后经皮治疗。平均随访 76 个月,非手术经皮球囊扩张治疗的总成功率为 58.8%。

(六) 胆管结石

胆管结石可以通过 ERCP(见前文)内镜下处理,也可以通过胆囊造瘘管、经皮放置引流管或外科 T 管(见后文)经皮处理。胆囊引流管或 T 管的管道在使用前大约需要 6 周时间才能成熟。在许多情况下,胆管结石可以通过顺行路径扩张乳头的方法清除[174,175]。可能需要机械碎石的结石被冲入十二指肠。经皮导管更换数天后取出。采用这种方法,所述结石清除率达到 94%或更高[174,176]。在某些情况下,特别是在复杂的肝内结石的情况下,小口径胆道镜可以通过成熟的经皮通道。然后使用各种技术将结石击碎,成功率很高(参见第

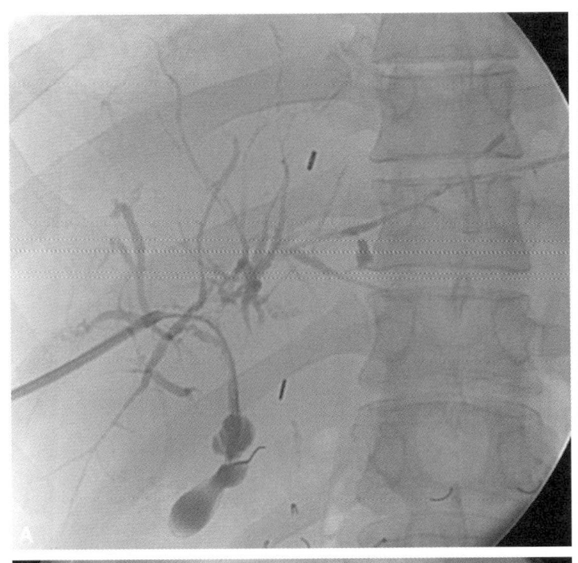

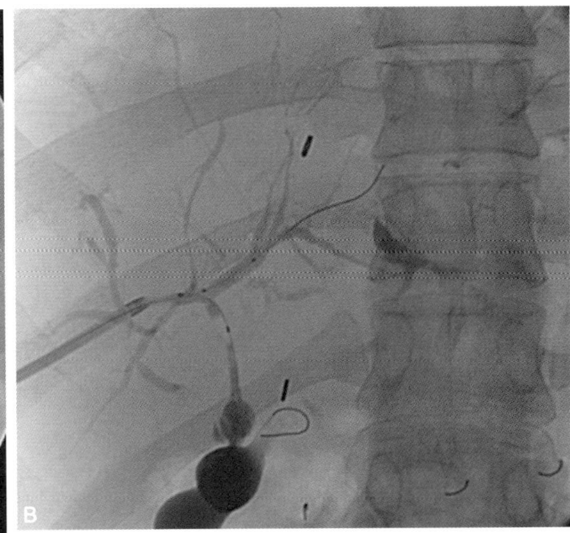

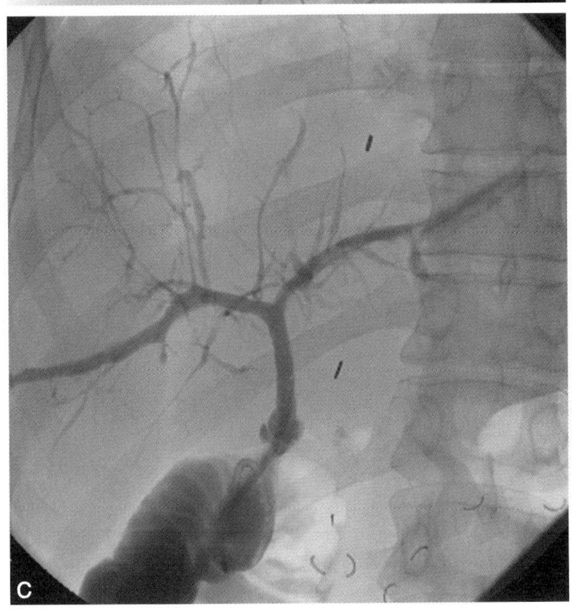

图 70.12　肝管空肠吻合术患者肝移植后复发性原发性硬化性胆管炎的经皮治疗。A，首先穿刺针穿刺将导丝引入空肠。B，左、右肝管球囊扩张。C，留置内-外胆道导管进行后续的胆道造影

66 章）[177,178]。

（七）恶性胆道梗阻

无论是手术前还是姑息治疗，均可经皮放置支架来缓解恶性胆道梗阻。支架由硬质塑料或自膨胀的金属组成。SEMS 的设计是为了避免细菌生物膜造成的闭塞，而细菌生物膜常见于塑料支架，导致需要重新干预（见前文）。

远端胆管狭窄（如胰头癌导致）最好通过 ERCP 进行治疗（见前文），因为根据一项较早的随机试验，内镜下支架置入比经皮支架置入痛苦更少，并发症也更少[179]。然而，在这些患者中，经皮支架置入很容易实现，在内镜治疗失败或不充分的情况下，可能需要进行经皮支架置入术[180]。由于大口径（≥10Fr）支架需要扩张一条穿过肝脏的通道，而这通常无法一次完成，因此在支架最终内置之前，往往需要多次介入放置塑料支架。在如此积极的扩张过程中发生的出血，往往需要维持外置管以排出胆道内的血液。与塑料支架相比，经皮放置 SEMS 可显著延长支架通畅率，减少再次介入的必要，并缩短住院时间[181]。此外，经皮放置 SEMS 的优势在于可以使用小直径的预置推送系统，因此经皮通道不需要扩张，并且可以一步到位地插入支架[181,182]。在一项内镜与经皮姑息治疗恶性胆道梗阻的随机试验中，金属胆道支架一次性经皮放置，塑料支架经内镜放置，经皮放置 SEMS 与胆道再发梗阻的发生率降低 34%[183]，尽管这些差异可能与支架的类型有关，而不是与入路有关。

内镜下解除肝门周围胆管梗阻（如由肝门周围胆管癌或 Klatkin 肿瘤引起的）比解除远端胆管梗阻更困难（见上文）。一些研究表明，经皮途径治疗这些肿瘤优于内镜方法，术后胆管炎的发生率更低[106,183]。

覆膜 SEMS 旨在通过减少肿瘤生长和组织增生导致的闭塞来提高支架的通畅性。研究已经取得了可喜的结果[184,185]，尽管还没有关于通过经皮途径放置覆膜支架和无覆膜支架的随机试验发表。

四、经皮胆囊造瘘管置入术

急性结石性胆囊炎的标准治疗方法是胆囊切除术(参见第65章和第66章)。即使腹腔镜胆囊切除术问世,仍有一些患者不适合做手术。经皮胆囊造瘘管置入术是治疗这些患者的一种微创方法,可以在局部麻醉剂或适度镇静的情况下进行。置入后可使胆囊立即减压。放置期间获得的胆汁样本可用于指导抗菌治疗,该管还可用于胆道造影,以确认胆囊管是否梗阻,如果胆囊管通畅,则为胆管梗阻。经皮胆囊治疗作为老年人或不适合手术者的非手术方法,可用于治疗严重的急性结石性胆囊炎,并可避免急诊手术,允许随后进行腹腔镜胆囊切除术[185-188]。

经皮胆囊造瘘管置入术的使用受到几个因素的影响,包括患者的不适、外置管的管理以及相关的并发症,包括脱出、蜂窝织炎、瘘管形成和感染。因此,最好将其作为临时的解决方案[189]。虽然经皮胆囊造瘘管放置的目的通常是为胆囊切除术提供一个桥梁,或在临床改善后可能移除,但当手术风险过高时,如潜在的医疗合并症和/或存在移除引流管后胆囊炎复发的风险增加等情况下,该管可能成为永久性的。在这些情况下,长期经皮引流管置入可能会导致严重的疼痛、不便和外观受损,并降低患者的生活质量[190]。

对于因上述原因造成胆囊造瘘管拔除困难的病例,可以采用EUS引导下的胆囊内引流的治疗方法[191]。这种方法是在EUS引导下从胃或十二指肠穿刺胆囊,然后放置双蘑菇头金属支架,在器官之间建立吻合[192,193]。在此操作后,可拔除经皮引流管,而不会有胆囊炎复发的风险。

另外,可以通过经皮处理胆囊、胆囊管或胆管中的结石。可以扩张成熟的经皮穿刺通道,然后将结石取出(图70.13)。肝内胆囊和小且萎缩的厚壁胆囊不适合这种方法。尽管经皮

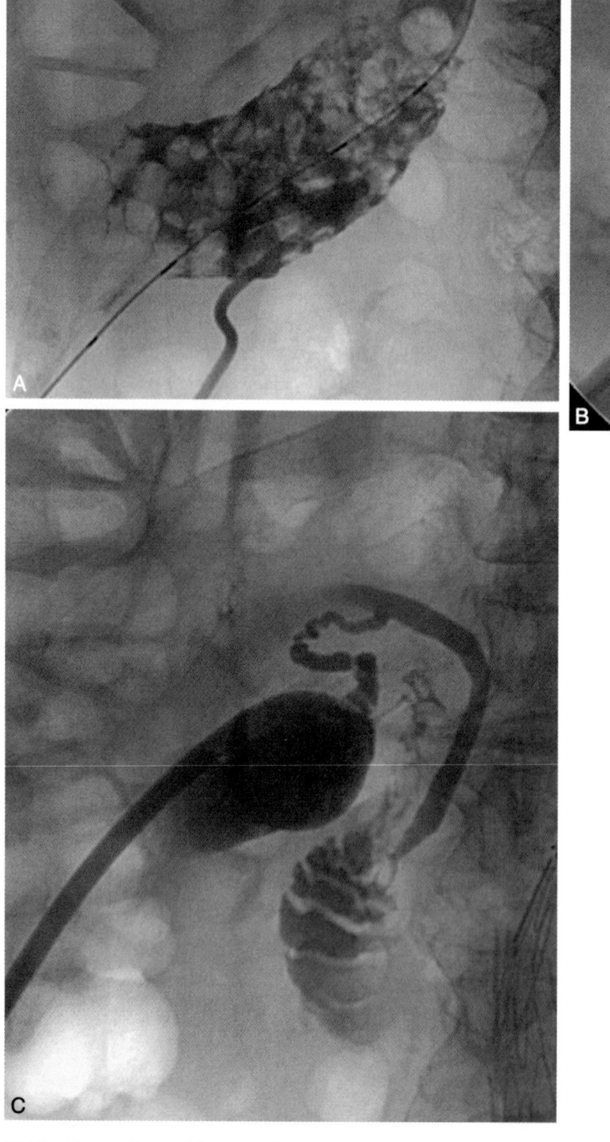

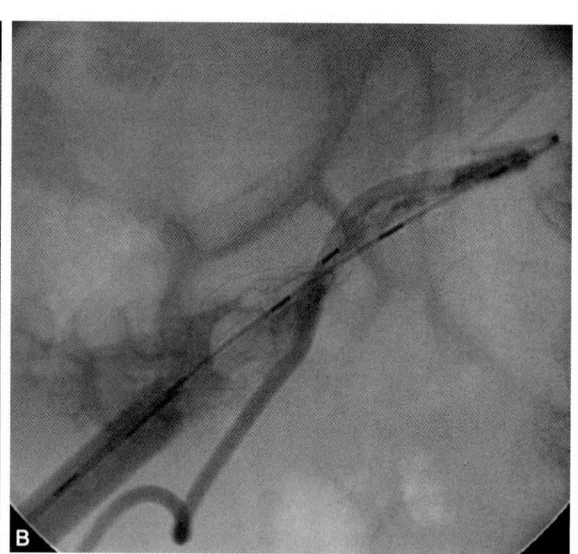

图70.13 经皮治疗结石性胆囊炎。A,将经皮导管置入胆囊。显示存在多发性胆结石。B,大口径导管可取出结石。C,证实胆结石完全清除

取石的成功率很高，但结石仍可能复发[194]。

重症监护室的患者面临的另一个挑战是疑似急性非结石性胆囊炎的处理(参见第 67 章)。引出 Murphy 征非常困难，几乎不太可能，尤其是对插管或反应迟钝的患者。延迟诊断和治疗可能导致胆囊坏疽和穿孔，并导致死亡。对于临床高度怀疑急性非结石性胆囊炎的患者，应经皮放置胆囊引流管。如果胆囊是患者临床问题的根源，胆囊造瘘管保留 6 周后，成熟窦道形成，造瘘管方可安全取出。在一项研究中，55 名疑似急性非结石性胆囊炎的危重患者接受了经皮胆囊引流管置入术，24 小时内临床改善率为 58.7%，72 小时内临床改善率为 95.7%[195]。胆囊造瘘管拔除后的急性非结石性胆囊炎 8 年间的复发率低于 3%[196]。

五、经皮和内镜联合的治疗方法

在某些情况下，虽然 ERCP 不成功，但仍需在内镜下进入胆管，可采取经皮-内镜联合的方法，即所谓的会师技术(图 70.14)[197]。一个例子是同时存在十二指肠大憩室和胆管结石的患者。如果憩室阻碍了通过内镜进入胆道，可经皮将一根导丝穿入十二指肠；然后将患者带到 ERCP 室，并重复 ERCP。用钳子抓取导丝，并将附件穿过导丝，从而实现括约肌切开和取石。类似的方法可以在 EUS 引导下进行导丝放置(见前文)[198]。大多数恶性狭窄不需要这种技术，如果内镜方法失败，完全可以通过经皮的方法进行治疗。

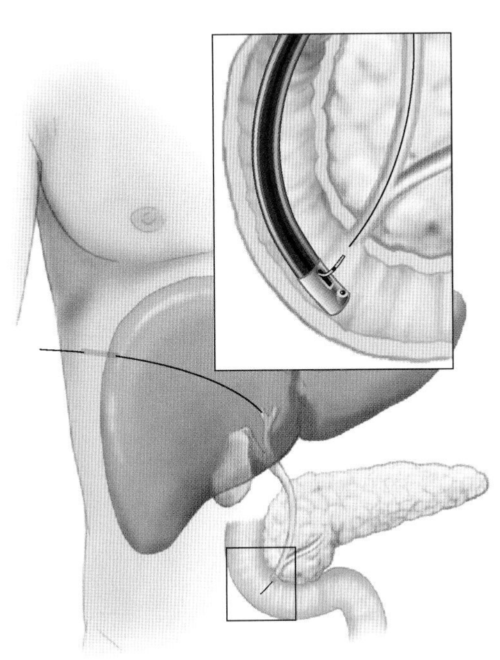

图 70.14　经皮和内镜联合入路进入胆道的示意图。经皮将导丝穿入十二指肠并通过内镜进行识别(插图)，然后用圈套器抓住导丝，将其穿过内镜并从口中拉出，从而提供进入胆道的通道

(周宇航　闫秀娥 译，黄永辉 校)

参考文献

索引

^{18}F-FDG-PET 扫描 671
2 型糖尿病 30
5-羟色胺 44,113
5-羟色胺$_4$受体激动剂 192
5-羟色胺拮抗剂 192
5-羟色胺能通便剂 258
Addison 病 520
AIMS65 评分 269
ALPINES 失调 198
Barrett 食管 655
Bazex 综合征 347
Blatchford 评分 269
Boerhaave 综合征 189,631
Bouveret 综合征 988
Budd-Chiari 综合征 572
Burkitt 淋巴瘤 427
B 型 Niemann-Pick 病 521
Cajal 间质细胞 241,691,696,698
Cameron 病变 280,362
Carney-Stratakis 综合征 445
Carney 三联征 444
Castleman 病 558
Celiac 病 30
CFTR 基因型 823
Chagas 病 247,617,634
Child-Pugh 分级 1014
Churg-Strauss 综合征 510
Cori 循环 62
Crohn disease 754
CT 877
CT 结肠成像术 285
CT 严重程度指数 858
Cullen 征 348
Dieulafoy 病变 280,538
Dieulafoy 样病变 358
DNA 修复基因 9
EBV 感染 485
EoE 403
ERCP 878
ERCP 术后胰腺炎 829
EUS 879
Fabry 病 521
Fitz-Hugh-Curtis 综合征 549,554
Forrest 分类 271
Gaucher 病 521
G 蛋白偶联受体 37
H_2 受体拮抗剂 766
Heller 肌切开术 624
HELLP 综合征 567
Hp 感染 174,279
Hp 感染检测 277
Huntington 病 523
IgE 15
IgG4 相关性疾病 511
IgG4 相关性硬化性胆管炎 1019
IgM 14
Ishak 评分 1010
Ivor-Lewis 食管胃切除术 674
Jackhammer 食管 616,625
Johanson-Blizzard 综合征 839
Klippel-Trenaunay 综合征 544
Laurén 分类 777
Lebrikuzumab 单抗 407
Lenta 胆管炎 494
Lundh 测试餐 812
L-丝氨酸蛋白酶抑制剂 Kazal 1 型（SPINK1）缺乏症 841
Mallory-Weiss 综合征 189,280,631
MALT 淋巴瘤 420
MALT 型边缘区 B 细胞淋巴瘤 425
McKeown 食管胃切除术 674
Meckel 憩室 292
Mirizzi 综合征 977,987
MRI 145,878
Murphy 征 147
Ménétrier 病 414,757
M 细胞 15
NAFLD 92
NK-1 受体拮抗剂 192
NUTRIC 评分 76
Obalon 球囊系统 105
Oddi 括约肌 932
Oddi 括约肌功能紊乱 992
Oddi 括约肌功能障碍 852,933,1044
Orbera 胃球囊 105
Osler-Weber-Rendu 病 343,543
OTSC 血管夹 277
OTSC 止血夹 277
Parkes Weber 综合征 545
Pearson 骨髓-胰腺综合征 840
PFIC 2 型 947
PFIC 3 型 948
PPP 综合征 347
PYTHON 73
P 物质 42
ReShape 胃球囊 105
RFA 660
Rosemont 标准 879
Schwachman-Diamond 综合征 838
SMAD4 8
Southern 印迹试验 421
Stevens-Johnson 综合征 341
Swansea 标准 569
Tangier 病 521
tLESR 抑制剂 649
TNM 系统 790
TP53 8
T 细胞分化 19
Von Hippel-Lindau 病 451
Waldenström 巨球蛋白血症 515
Waldeyer 环淋巴瘤 430
Wilkie 综合征 522
Wilson 病 572
Zenker 憩室 352
α-地中海贫血/X 连锁精神发育迟缓综合征蛋白 450
α 重链疾病或地中海淋巴瘤 427

A

阿片类肠道疾病 159
阿片类药物解毒 160
阿司匹林 655,659
阿特金斯饮食 93
癌干细胞 6
癌基因 6
癌前状态 776,784
癌症 75,79
癌症与肿瘤基因组学 11
艾洛比昔巴特 259

艾滋病相关腹膜炎 549,554
安非他酮 94
安非他酮/纳曲酮 94
氨基酸 38,54
奥利司他 95
奥曲肽 278

B

靶向治疗 678
白斑 334
白塞病 338,510
白色念珠菌 632
败血症 63
半月线疝 371
包裹性坏死 843,907
饱腹感 113,708
饱腹感测试 710
暴发性肝衰竭 495
暴食症 115
杯状细胞 17
钡剂灌肠 285
被动型大便失禁 225
贲门失弛缓症 615,616,623
贲门炎 749
苯并咪唑衍生物 191
鼻肠管通路 77
鼻胃管 630
必需氨基酸 54
必需脂肪酸 55
必需脂肪酸缺乏症 55
闭眼征 157
蓖麻油 256
壁腹膜 549
壁细胞胞内途径 730
扁平苔藓 341
便秘 121,238,488,716
辩证行为疗法 123
标记红细胞扫描 268
标准药物治疗 159
表皮生长因子 47
病毒性肝炎 570
病毒性胃炎 749
哺乳动物西罗莫司靶蛋白(mTOR) 450
不明原因腹泻 211
不明原因胃肠道出血 289
不透射线标志物 249

C

草莓舌 333
长物体 383
肠壁囊样积气 505
肠壁囊样积气症 219
肠病相关性T细胞淋巴瘤 429
肠道导向催眠治疗 159
肠道定向催眠疗法 319
肠道菌群 215
肠道溃疡 489
肠道气体 213
肠道微生物群 24,89
肠肝循环 941
肠激酶缺乏 841
肠内管饲 835
肠内喂养 84
肠内营养 72,77
肠内营养制剂 84
肠腔内容物 241
肠切除术后腹泻 209
肠上皮化生 784
肠上皮细胞 16
肠神经肽 40
肠神经元发育不良 246
肠衰竭 72
肠外营养 72,85
肠系膜囊肿 558
肠系膜上动脉动脉瘤 542
肠系膜上动脉压迫综合征 522
肠系膜上动脉综合征 121,188,547
肠型胃癌 781
肠移植 487
肠易激综合征 208,308,716
超敏反应 174
超声 969
超声内镜 592,671,790,894,969
超声内镜引导下胆管引流 1038
超重 96
成人肥厚性幽门狭窄 693
成人型Still病 505
成纤维细胞生长因子 47
痴呆 80
迟发型皮肤超敏试验 68
迟发性皮肤卟啉症 349
迟发性倾倒综合征 75
耻骨直肠肌 224
充气扩张术 624
重复嗳气 217
抽吸治疗 105
出血 591,648,762,770
出血性胰腺炎 843
处方药 649
穿孔 590,591,648,762,773
传递介质 39
传统染色内镜 667
创伤后膈疝 365
创伤性膈疝 365
唇部肿瘤 331
唇炎 331
瓷化胆囊 977
磁共振成像 228,895
次要亚型 408
刺激胆道闪烁显像 994
刺激性栓剂 257
刺激性泻药 256
卒中 79
促动力药 649
促胃动力剂 177
促分泌泻药 257
簇状细胞 18
催眠疗法 159
错构瘤 681

D

大便失禁 221
大胆管型PSC 1013
大麻素 46,192
大麻素剧吐综合征 188
大疱性表皮松解症 340
大容量腹泻 198
代谢性骨病 1014
单纯疱疹病毒 485,633
单纯疱疹病毒性肝炎 570
单纯性胃炎 778
单核细胞增多症样综合征 489
单基因自身免疫综合征 490
单气囊内镜 294
胆道癌 992
胆道闭锁 919
胆道出血 281
胆道恶性肿瘤 1021
胆道梗阻 893
胆道闪烁显像 934
胆道闪烁显像术 970
胆道狭窄 911
胆肝分流 943
胆固醇快速成核和结晶 958
胆固醇息肉 1002
胆固醇贮积病 997
胆管 915
胆管癌 1012,1015,1021
胆管梗阻 301,888
胆管结石 1039,1046
胆管漏 1046
胆管上皮细胞 1008
胆管损伤 990,1046

胆管炎 592,975
胆红素 296
胆碱能药物 258
胆结石 147,847,950
胆结石病 565
胆漏 1040
胆绿素还原酶 296
胆囊 916,917
胆囊癌 1028
胆囊肠瘘 977
胆囊功能失调 959
胆囊管残端综合征 992
胆囊切除术 996
胆囊切除术后综合征 991
胆囊收缩素 40,866
胆囊息肉 1001
胆囊腺肌瘤病 998
胆囊炎 592
胆囊运动障碍 931
胆囊造瘘术 996
胆泥 847
胆石性肠梗阻 988
胆石性胰腺炎 856
胆石症 928,1015
胆盐输出泵 300
胆胰分流术 98
胆源性疼痛 972,985,994
胆源性胰腺炎 987
胆汁反流 756
胆汁栓塞综合征 923
胆汁酸 938
胆汁酸螯合剂 949
胆汁酸替代疗法 949
胆汁酸性腹泻 209
胆汁酸循环 948
胆汁淤积 946,952,1014
胆汁脂质分泌 957
胆总管结石 301,974,989,992,1012
弹性假黄瘤 344
蛋白酶 808
蛋白异常血症 515
蛋白质 38
蛋白质-能量营养不良 63,64
蛋白质丢失性胃肠病 411
蛋白质能量营养不良 52,63
氮排泄量 55
氮平衡 54,55
氮质血症 55
导管内乳头状黏液性肿瘤 903
导管阻塞 866
低 FODMAP 食谱 252
低β脂蛋白血症 521
低蛋白血症 413
低度十二指肠黏膜炎症 174
低灌注症状 142
低碳水化合物饮食 93
低限制性饮食 406
低脂饮食 93
骶神经刺激 235,260
地图舌 333
地中海饮食 93
递质释放模式 34
癫痫 61
电刺激 234
电外科学 588
淀粉酶 807
淀粉性腹膜炎 555
淀粉样变 344,525
淀粉样变性 338
凋亡 3
丁酰苯类 191
动静脉畸形 540
动力障碍 889
动脉瘤 540
动作电位 698
毒性代谢假说 866
毒性胆汁酸理论 1008
独特的胃病变 752
杜氏肌营养不良症 523
短肠综合征 55,72,359
对比成像 618
钝挫性损伤 631
钝性物体 383
多巴胺 44
多巴胺 D2 受体拮抗剂 191
多步骤形成 5
多发性内分泌肿瘤综合征 1 型 450
多发性硬化 522
多发性硬化症 245
多骨硬化性组织细胞增生症 515
多库酯钠 257
多排螺旋 CT 671
多配体蛋白聚糖 412
多普勒内镜探头 272
多器官功能障碍综合征 553
多器官衰竭 73
多形性红斑 341
多灶性平滑肌瘤 558
多灶性萎缩性胃炎 747

E

鹅去氧胆酸 259
呃逆 165,559
恶心 182
恶性胆道梗阻 1043,1047
恶性非上皮肿瘤 679
恶性黑色素瘤 679
恶性萎缩性丘疹病 343
恶性营养不良症 64
恶性肿瘤 889
蒽醌类 256
儿茶酚胺 44
耳鼻咽喉疾病 643
二苯基甲烷衍生物 256
二次内镜检查 278
二代测序 11

F

发育 308
发育异常 802,917
反刍 642
反刍疾病 116
反刍综合征 188
反复嗳气 217
反馈调节 810
反流 167,352
反流机制 637
反应性胃病 739,755
防护性因素 953
放化疗 793
放射性肝病 584
放射性核素成像 268,285
放射性核素扫描 145
放射性直肠炎 288
放线菌病 750
非编码 RNA 9
非出血性裸露血管 275
非胆汁酸依赖性胆汁 942
非梗阻性黄疸 305
非霍奇金淋巴瘤 432,513
非结石性胆囊炎 930,987
非酒精性脂肪性肝病 30,953
非糜烂性疾病 647
非特殊性喂养或进食障碍 115
非特异症状 893
非甾体抗炎药 629
非综合征性小叶间胆管缺乏 925
肥大舌 334
肥大细胞增多症 345
肥胖 29,75,88,781
肥胖与胰岛素抵抗 953
分泌性腹泻 196,198
分枝杆菌 750

分子诊断 11
芬特明/托吡酯 93
吩噻嗪类 191
粪便白细胞检查 204
粪便抗原检测 745
粪便糜蛋白酶测量 812
粪便潜血试验 294
粪便嵌塞 247
粪便软化剂 257
粪便渗漏 236
粪便渗漏型 225
粪便特征 201
粪便胰酶 877
粪便胰腺弹性蛋白酶 1 测量 812
粪便隐血试验 204
粪便脂肪测量 812
粪便脂肪排泄 877
粪便脂肪排泄量 204
蜂窝织炎(化脓性)胃炎 739
否认排便 247
匐行性皮疹 350
辐射 739,756
辐射损伤 545
辅酶 60
辅脂酶缺乏症 840
辅助放射治疗 440
辅助性放化疗 678
腐蚀物摄入 385
负氮平衡 55
复发或急性重症胰腺炎 872
复发性阿弗他口腔溃疡 337
复发性腹痛 152
复发性化脓性胆管炎 1019
复发性急性胰腺炎 813,830,909
复发性呕吐 186
复合性腹泻 196
复苏 265
复杂性消化不良 171
复杂胰腺疾病 815
副交感神经 596
副肿瘤性天疱疮 340
副肿瘤性肢端角化病 347
副肿瘤综合征 512
腹部 US 877
腹部创伤超声重点评估 145
腹部平片 877
腹部脏器膨出 559
腹侧壁疝 371
腹股沟疝 367,369
腹膜 549
腹膜分散平滑肌瘤病 558
腹膜假黏液瘤 557
腹膜囊肿 557
腹膜肿瘤 555
腹腔动脉瘤 542
腹腔干压迫综合征 547
腹腔灌洗 791
腹腔间隔室综合征 149,863
腹腔镜 560
腹腔镜胆囊切除术 982
腹腔镜腹腔灌洗 791
腹腔镜检查 791
腹腔镜手术 355
腹腔内化疗 793
腹腔内脓肿 389
腹腔内粘连 555
腹腔细菌清除率 551
腹水 501
腹水及腹膜炎 508
腹痛 478,488,499,881
腹泻 194,474,488,490
腹型癫痫 522
腹型偏头痛 522
腹胀 218
腹主动脉瘤 149,540

G

钆 MRI 成像模式 791
改变生活方式 649
钙敏感受体基因 826
干呕 182
干燥综合征 332,508
甘露醇 255
肝病 74
肝胆闪烁扫描显像 996
肝淀粉样变性 526
肝动脉栓塞 467
肝动脉血流阻力指数 494
肝豆状核变性 299,572
肝窦阻塞综合征 492
肝放射性栓塞 468
肝静脉血栓形成 572
肝静脉压力测定 494
肝门静脉高压症 571
肝门区胆管癌 1027
肝门周围胆管癌 1024,1025
肝门周围胆管梗阻 1043
肝内胆管癌 1023,1024,1027
肝内胆汁酸转运 943
肝糖原 62
肝外胆管 917
肝细胞性肝癌 584
肝纤维囊性疾病 924
肝移植 468,486,1018
肝硬化 501
肝脏胆汁胆固醇分泌过多 957
肝脏浸润性疾病 300
肝脏受累 508
肝脏移植后妊娠 572
肝脏真菌感染 490
感觉测试 622
感染后功能性消化不良 174
感染性胆管炎 489
感染性结肠炎 287
感染性休克 143
肛管超声内镜检查 228
肛管成像检查 228
肛管塞 234
肛管直肠疾病 478
肛裂 289
肛门镜检查 284
肛门括约肌 223
肛门受累 507
肛门直肠测压 226,251
肛门直肠感觉受损 224
肛门直肠生物反馈 259
肛周疼痛 490,500
高氨血症 74
高胆红素脓毒症综合征 489
高锝酸盐闪烁显像 268
高分辨率测压 619
高钙血症 245,849
高甘油三酯血症 827,849
高尿酸血症 91
高收缩性食管 616,617,625
高温腹腔内化疗 793
高硝酸盐 780
膈肌裂孔 354
膈疝 360
膈上憩室 354
膈下脓肿 395
各种假定机制 160
根除 Hp 感染 177
梗阻 246,774,872
梗阻性黄疸 305
公共卫生观点 239
功能性腹痛 308
功能性腹痛综合征 154
功能性腹泻 208
功能性脑成像 159
功能性呕吐 187
功能性胃肠病 306,308
功能性胃肠道疾病 121,152,158

功能性消化不良 171,716
功能性消化不良的治疗 177
功能性幽门梗阻 715
功能性肿瘤 451
共病的心理障碍 154
钩虫病 751
姑息性内镜治疗 677
孤立的幽门压力波 704
孤立性非结合高胆红素血症 298
孤立性直肠溃疡综合征 244
股疝 367
骨关节炎 92
骨盆疝和会阴疝 372
骨髓外造血 514
骨髓纤维化 514
固定性幽门梗阻 715
固有层淋巴细胞 19
固有淋巴样细胞 20
瓜尔胶 253
灌肠剂 257
光学染色内镜 667
光学相干断层扫描术 668
过度活动综合征 403
过敏性结肠炎 403
过敏性嗜酸粒细胞性直肠结肠炎 132
过敏性胃肠病 414
过敏性胃炎 755
过敏性紫癜 509

H

海绵状血管瘤 540
含铁血黄素沉着症 517
汗液氯化物检测 824
核细胞 19
核医学检查 391
核原癌基因 7
褐色素结石 964
黑便 262
黑棘皮病 92,347
黑毛舌 333
黑色素结石 964
恒径小动脉畸形 280
横膈膜疾病 549,559
横纹肌活动肌电图 251
红霉素 720
红曲霉病 751
红细胞异常 515
呼气试验 709
壶腹癌 1032
花粉-食物过敏综合征 131
滑动性食管裂孔疝 360
滑脱肋骨综合征 154
化疗 776,792
化疗栓塞 468
化疗诱导的食管炎 629
化学性结肠炎 591
化学致癌 10
坏疽性胆囊炎 147
坏疽性脓皮病 342
坏死-纤维化假说 866
坏死松解性游走性红斑 518
环境多灶性萎缩性胃炎 784
环磷酸腺苷 37
环型胰腺 694
环咽嵴 614,623
环氧化酶-2 抑制剂 769
环状胰腺 802
黄疸 296
黄色肉芽肿性胃炎 752
回避性/限制性摄食障碍 116
回肠造口术后腹泻 209
蛔虫病 751
会阴下降综合征 224,244
昏迷 495
混合性结缔组织病 509
活动性出血 265,273
活动性动脉出血 273
活检尿素酶检测 744
获得性代谢紊乱 829
获得性神经病变 247
霍奇金淋巴瘤 513

J

饥饿 62,708
机会性感染 472
机械方法 772
机械辅助通气 69
肌酐-身高指数 68
肌筋膜疼痛综合征 153
肌萎缩侧索硬化 614
肌营养不良 246,523
基础胃酸排出量 734
基底洁净溃疡 277
基因组不稳定性 657
激素 33
极端年龄 151
急迫型大便失禁 225
急性肠梗阻 185
急性肠系膜缺血 149
急性出血性直肠溃疡综合征 289
急性胆囊积液 931
急性胆囊炎 147,972,985
急性胆源性疾病 147
急性放射性肠炎 575
急性非结石性胆囊炎 995
急性腹痛 139,145,153
急性腹痛的类型 144
急性腹泻 198,201,207
急性坏死物积聚 843
急性坏死性溃疡性牙龈炎 335
急性或亚急性肝细胞损伤 299
急性假性囊肿 907
急性阑尾炎 146
急性镰状细胞性肝内胆汁淤积症 516
急性呕吐 183,188
急性排斥反应 487
急性脾隔离症 515
急性脾梗死 515
急性憩室炎 148
急性生理学和慢性健康状况评价 843
急性食管坏死 634
急性胃肠道出血 263
急性胃炎 739
急性细菌性胆管炎 1020
急性胰腺炎 73,148,565,814,829,842,906
急性胰周液体积聚 843
急性移植物抗宿主病 495
急性中性粒细胞性胃炎 739
脊髓病变 246
脊髓损伤 236,522,953
脊柱关节病 511
计算机断层扫描 145
继发性(外科)腹膜炎 551
继发性硬化性胆管炎 1019
家庭功能障碍 158
家族性地中海热 511
家族性非典型多发性痣黑色素瘤 890
家族性肝内胆汁淤积1蛋白 300
家族性甲状旁腺功能亢进伴高钙血症 841
家族性乳糜微粒血症综合征 827
家族性胃肠道间质瘤 445
家族性腺瘤性息肉病 786
家族性胰腺炎 815,838
甲磺酸伊马替尼 441
甲基纤维素 253
甲状旁腺功能减退 520
甲状旁腺功能亢进 520
甲状腺功能减退 245,519
甲状腺功能亢进 519
甲状腺髓样癌 95,520
贾第鞭毛虫病 751

钾竞争性酸阻滞剂 767
钾离子竞争性酸阻断剂 732
假体旁肠瘘 542
假喂食刺激酸排出 735
假性贲门失弛缓症 618
假性肠梗阻 186,716
假性动脉瘤 887
假性囊肿 843,886,907,911
尖锐物体 381
间接测热法 52
间皮瘤 557
间歇性禁食 93
间歇性能量限制 93
剪切波超声弹性成像 494
减肥手术 76
减肥术后营养缺乏 76
减瘤手术 441,468
碱性磷酸酶 61
建立成功的医患关系 157
建立治疗关系 317
浆膜炎综合征 501
浆母细胞性淋巴瘤 432
浆液性囊腺瘤 900,902
交感神经 596
胶囊技术 709
胶囊内镜 589
胶囊式内镜检查 293
胶原性胃炎 752
焦点心理动力学治疗 123
接受性松弛 702
结肠传输闪烁扫描显像 249
结肠传输时间 249
结肠镜 590
结肠镜检查 267,284,285
结肠镜息肉切除术 288
结肠憩室 286
结肠切除术 260
结肠神经内分泌肿瘤 464
结肠受累 507
结肠息肉 288
结肠腺瘤性息肉病基因 8
结肠血管扩张 289
结肠炎 287
结肠造口术 235,260
结肠肿瘤 288,1016
结缔组织疾病 511
结构性疾病试验 249
结核分枝杆菌 634
结核性腹膜炎 151,554
结节病 527,752
结节病胃肠道受累 528
结节性多动脉炎(PAN) 507
结节性多动脉炎 343,349,509
结节性红斑 342
结节性硬化症 451
结节性再生性肝增生 501
结石性胆囊炎 930
结直肠癌 31,369,992
结直肠异物 384
紧急内镜检查 265
进食障碍 112,247
进行性系统性硬化症 343,544
近贲门憩室 356
近端肿瘤 777
经腹超声 1036
经颈静脉肝内门体分流术 283
经口出口缩窄术 104
经口内镜下肌肉切开术 624
经口内镜下食管括约肌切开术 593
经皮穿刺脓肿引流术 393
经皮穿刺造口 79
经皮胆囊造瘘管置入术 1048
经皮胆囊造瘘术 997
经皮经肝穿刺胆管造影术 1045
经皮胫神经刺激 236
经皮内镜下胃空肠造口术 81
经皮内镜下胃造口术 80
经腔道引流 907
经十二指肠乳头引流 907
经食管超声心动图 630
精神疾病 310
精神心理障碍 247
精神药理学治疗 318
精准医学 814
颈部黏液细胞 686
净吸水率 194
静脉曲张出血 282,888
静脉曲张硬化治疗导致的食管损伤 629
静息电位 698
静息能量消耗 52
酒精 780,867
局灶性住院溃疡 279
巨大肥厚性胃病 414
巨舌 334,525
巨噬细胞 20
巨细胞病毒 633
巨细胞病毒感染 487
聚碳酸钙 253
聚乙二醇 255

K

卡波西肉瘤 336
开腹胆囊切除术 981
抗T细胞抗体 488
抗毒蕈碱药 192
抗恶心、呕吐疗法 721
抗反流屏障 635,636
抗反流手术 653
抗分泌药物 766
抗分泌治疗 772
抗生素类 628
抗生素治疗 392
抗酸药 766
抗胸腺细胞球蛋白 488
抗氧化剂 788,881
抗组胺药 192
科萨科夫(Korsakoff)痴呆 74
颗粒细胞瘤 680
可耐受上限 56
可屈式乙状结肠镜检查 284
可溶性和不溶性混合纤维 253
克隆扩增 6
克鲁兹锥虫 634
克罗恩病 73,342,754
空肠憩室 359
口服补液 73,206
口服胆囊造影术 970
口服冷冻治疗 491
口服耐受性 21
口干症 332
口腔白斑 334
口腔感觉障碍 332
口咽吞咽困难 162,613,622
夸希奥科病 64
矿物油 257
奎尼丁 629
溃疡 648
溃疡病 101
溃疡近期出血 265
溃疡性Zenker憩室 353
溃疡性结肠炎 342,754
括约肌切开术后出血 282
括约肌填充剂 234

L

阑尾神经内分泌肿瘤 463
阑尾炎 565
阑尾周围脓肿 395
蓝色橡皮泡痣综合征 344
蓝色橡皮疱痣综合征 292,544
狼疮蛋白丢失性肠病 414
朗格汉斯细胞组织细胞增生症 514
酪酪肽 113

雷拉莫林 259
类癌综合征 465
类风湿性关节炎 503
类天疱疮 340
类圆线虫病 751
累及胰腺的孟德尔综合征 815
冷球蛋白血症 510
离子通道偶联受体 37
离子吸收不良 253
立体定向放射治疗 900
立体定向体放疗 582
利拉鲁肽 94
利那洛肽 257
联合内镜治疗 883
镰状红细胞性胆管病 516
镰状细胞性贫血 515
良性胆管狭窄 1041
良性非上皮性肿瘤 680
良性前列腺增生 369
良性上皮性肿瘤 679
裂纹舌 333
临床 Rockall 评分 269
淋巴结清扫术 674
淋巴瘤 418,679,905
淋巴瘤样胃病 753
淋巴细胞性胃炎 753
淋巴细胞转运 1007
淋巴引流 797
淋巴组织增生性疾病 487
磷酸盐灌肠剂 257
鳞状细胞癌 336,625
鳞状细胞癌变异体 678
鳞状细胞乳头状瘤 679
流行病学 154
硫酸乙酰肝素蛋白 412
瘘管 103
滤泡性淋巴瘤 426
氯化钾 629
氯卡色林 94
氯离子通道激活剂 257
卵叶车前子 253
裸露血管 273

M

麻疹 749
麻醉包 383
麻醉性肠综合征 159
马方综合征 511
埋藏缓冲器综合征 83
埋藏综合征 589
慢波 696
慢传输型便秘 243
慢性嗳气 217
慢性病毒性肝炎 501
慢性肠系膜缺血 153
慢性胆囊炎 972
慢性胆汁淤积 928
慢性胆汁淤积性疾病 1012
慢性放射性肠炎 575
慢性分泌性腹泻 204
慢性腹壁疼痛 153
慢性腹痛 152
慢性腹泻 198,202,207
慢性肝病 571
慢性肝细胞疾病 300
慢性功能性疼痛 154
慢性假性肠梗阻 359
慢性呕吐 186,189
慢性渗透性腹泻 205
慢性水样腹泻 200
慢性特发性腹痛 154
慢性疼痛行为 154
慢性疼痛综合征 156,159
慢性胃肠道失血 264
慢性胃炎 740
慢性萎缩性胃炎 746,784
慢性炎性腹泻 205
慢性炎症性腹泻 200
慢性炎症性疾病 315
慢性胰腺炎 73,813,814,830,864,910,936
慢性胰腺炎假性囊肿 911
慢性脂肪性腹泻 200,206
慢性阻塞性肺疾病 524
毛霉菌病 751
毛细线虫病 751
毛细血管瘤 539
毛状白斑 334
梅毒 750
梅毒螺旋体 634
梅克尔憩室 292
酶偶联受体 37
美泊珠单抗 401
门静脉高压性胃病 281,546,758
门静脉血栓 486
门控理论 155
门脉高压性脑病 74
门体分流手术 283
弥漫型胃癌 781
弥漫性大 B 细胞淋巴瘤 425
弥漫性食管痉挛 625
弥漫性胃窦炎 740
弥漫性胃体萎缩性胃炎 747
迷走神经病变 614
糜蛋白酶原 C 变体 820
糜烂性食管炎 647
秘密服用泻药 326
免疫功能低下 151
免疫球蛋白 A 14
免疫缺陷性相关淋巴瘤 431
免疫增殖性小肠疾病 427
免疫治疗 678
膜电位 698
膜型节段性缺损 688
墨菲征 147,973

N

纳曲酮 94
难治性低血压 267
囊性纤维化 824,830
囊性纤维化肝病 834
囊性胰岛细胞瘤 901
脑-肠神经轴 156
脑-肠轴 310
脑-肠轴功能失调 155
脑-肠轴功能障碍 154
脑血管意外 522
内分泌 34
内分泌疾病 517
内镜检查 618,635,644
内镜减重手术 593
内镜减重治疗 104
内镜逆行胰胆管造影 894,1038
内镜黏膜剥离术 792
内镜黏膜切除术 661,792
内镜黏膜下剥离术 593
内镜切除术 675
内镜下出血病灶 278
内镜下黏膜活检 671
内镜下袖状胃成形术 105,109,110
内镜下支架置入术 794
内镜下止血 268,273,287,588
内镜消融 660
内镜消融治疗 675
内镜止血夹 268
内镜治疗 721,1018
内疝 373
内因子 100
内因子分泌 737
内源性初级传入神经元 707
内脏超敏反应 155
内脏传入信号 156
内脏动脉瘤 541

内脏敏感 155
内脏疼痛 312
内脏信号放大 312
内脏性疼痛 139
能量储存 113
能量存储 51
逆行胰胆管造影 971
黏附血凝块 273,276
黏膜 597
黏膜保护剂 767
黏膜活检的培养 745
黏膜免疫 13
黏膜免疫系统 15
黏膜撕裂 189
黏膜下层 598
黏膜相关淋巴组织 420
黏液分泌 737
黏液性囊性肿瘤 900,901
念珠菌病 335,751
鸟苷酸环化酶 C 激动剂 257
尿素呼气试验 745
凝血功能障碍 517
脓毒症 524
虐待史 156,157

O

呕吐 182
呕吐反射回路 183
呕血 262

P

帕金森病 245,523,614
帕内特细胞 17
排便功能 242
排便协同失调 224
排便训练 259
排便障碍 243
排便障碍手术 261
排粪造影 228,250
排空不全 224
排气障碍 218
派尔斑 15
派尔集合淋巴结 15
膀胱压力 149
旁分泌 34
疱疹病毒感染 335,487
疱疹性几何学舌炎 334
疱疹样皮炎 134,350
盆腔脓肿 395
盆腔脂肪增多症 549,557
皮肤和胃肠道的寄生虫病 350
皮肤胃电图 189
皮肤转移瘤 348
皮肌炎 343,346
脾动脉瘤 541
脾破裂 591
平滑肌疾病 246
平滑肌瘤 680
平台电位 698
平坦黑色出血斑 276
苹果酸舒尼替尼 442
葡萄糖耐量 54
葡萄糖依赖性促胰岛素多肽 42
普卡那肽 258
普鲁卡必利 258

Q

其他特殊性喂养或进食障碍 115
“脐结肠炎”腹泻综合征 498
脐疝 371
气管食管瘘 598
气囊辅助肠镜 589
气体爆炸 591
气肿性胆囊炎 976,987
气肿性胃炎 739
起搏电位 696
起搏频率 699
起搏区域 700
起源和组织化学特征 448
憩室病 75,286
憩室固定术 353
憩室周围脓肿 395
牵涉性疼痛 142
铅中毒 335
前列腺素 D2 受体 407
前皮神经卡压综合征 153
前哨急性胰腺炎事件 817
前神经切除术 154
腔内憩室 358
腔内阻抗测量 622
腔外憩室 357
强碱 386
切开 689
切口疝 369
倾倒综合征 75,717
清除紊乱 115
清除胰管结石 883
清髓性预处理 491
球囊扩张 1018
球囊排出实验 228,251
球囊压塞 282
球形气压调节器(恒压器)试验 710
曲霉菌病 751
躯体-腔壁性疼痛 142
躯体症状障碍 310,324
趋化因子 22
全基因组测序 657
全身炎症反应综合征 844
全外显子测序 657
全胃肠外营养 54,952
缺铁性贫血 295
缺血 757
缺血性结肠炎 287
缺血性胃轻瘫 714

R

热带性胰腺炎 815,867
热接触探头 268
热量补充与避免高血糖症 54
热凝方法 772
热探头疗法 273
热效应 52
人格特征 310
人工神经网络评分 269
人际关系治疗 123
人乳头瘤病毒 633
人乳头瘤病毒感染 336
人体测量学 67
人为癌症 327
人为腹泻 326
人为疾病 321
人为贫血 327
人为胃肠道出血 327
人为性腹泻 211
认知分析治疗 123
认知行为疗法 319
认知行为治疗 123,159
妊娠 151
妊娠剧吐 187,563
妊娠期胆石症 987
妊娠期胆汁淤积症 565
妊娠期恶心呕吐 186
妊娠期黄疸 301
妊娠期急性脂肪肝 569
容积激光显微内镜 668
容量清除 639
溶石治疗 978
溶血性尿毒综合征 517
肉毒毒素 259
肉毒毒素注射 623
肉瘤 679,905
肉芽肿性肝病 527
肉芽肿性胃炎 752

肉芽肿性血管炎 510
蠕动缺失 616,617,625
乳果糖 255
乳糜泻 30,133,953
乳头旁憩室 357
入口斑 604
瑞戈非尼 443
瑞利珠单抗 401
润滑剂 257

S

三羧酸循环 55
三叶因子 47
瘙痒 349
色素结石 964
山梨醇 255
闪烁扫描法 709
闪烁显像 710
疝 559
膳食刺激胃酸排出 735
膳食替代饮食 93
上腹壁疝 371
上皮-间充质转化 6
上皮内淋巴细胞 19
上胃肠道 262
上胃肠道出血 269
上胃肠道恶性肿瘤 281
上消化道穿孔 588
上行性胆管炎 147
上行性内脏疼痛传递 155
舌痛 332
舌下免疫治疗 136
舌炎 332
社会心理环境 309
社会支持 310
射频消融 468
深部肠镜检查 294
深在性囊性胃炎 754
神经传递 34
神经递质 33,43,311
神经激肽-1受体拮抗剂 192
神经节细胞减少症 246
神经内分泌肿瘤 446
神经生理学检测 229
神经系统 224
神经系统疾病 186
神经系统支配 700
神经纤维瘤病1型 344,451
神经性贪食症 115
神经性厌食症 114
神经支配 797
神经阻滞和神经松解术 885
肾/胰腺移植 485
肾上腺功能不全 520
肾移植 485
渗漏 102,103
渗透性腹泻 195,198
渗透性泻药 253
生长激素释放肽 43
生长抑素 42,278,728
生长抑素类似物 399,458,466,469
生长抑素受体成像 467
生长抑素受体显像 438
生长因子受体 6,46
生理调节 308
生理学测量 249
生态失调 1007
生物-心理-社会模式 155
生物电阻抗分析法 68
生物反馈疗法 232
生物利用度 56
生物心理社会模式 307
生物医学模式 306
声门痉挛 189
十二指肠闭锁和狭窄 693
十二指肠梗阻 888
十二指肠及壶腹神经内分泌肿瘤 464
十二指肠溃疡 762
十二指肠溃疡表型 778
十二指肠憩室 357
十二指肠腔内憩室 358
十二指肠胃反流 641
十二指肠重复囊肿 695
十二指肠转位 98
实际体重 53
实体瘤 558
实体器官移植 483
实性假乳头状瘤 901,904
食管 608
食管癌 663
食管钡剂造影 647
食管闭锁 598
食管壁内假性憩室 355
食管测压 189,647
食管超敏反应 625
食管穿透性损伤 631
食管动力障碍 613
食管反流试验 645
食管感觉 611
食管和胃肠道受累 507
食管环 603
食管裂孔疝 280,360,639
食管鳞状细胞癌 663
食管黏膜活检 644
食管黏膜撕裂症 280,631
食管旁疝 360
食管蹼 604
食管蠕动 608
食管酸清除 639
食管体部憩室 354
食管吞咽困难 162
食管胃交界处 610
食管下括约肌松弛 611
食管腺癌 664
食管血管瘤 681
食管炎 279
食管源性胸痛 165
食管远端痉挛 616
食管重复畸形 602
食糜 696
食物蛋白诱导的肠病 133
食物蛋白诱导的小肠结肠炎综合征 132
食物过敏 127,403
食物或药物不耐受 170
食物嵌塞 381
食物热效应 52
食物性腹泻 208
食欲 113
嗜酸性粒细胞生长因子 407
嗜酸性粒细胞相关胃肠道疾病 403
嗜酸性粒细胞性结肠炎 401,409,488
嗜酸性粒细胞性食管炎 131,401,404
嗜酸性粒细胞性胃肠炎 132,403
嗜酸性粒细胞性胃炎 753
嗜酸性粒细胞增多性胃肠疾病 401
嗜酸性肉芽肿伴多发性血管炎 409
嗜酸性肉芽肿性多血管炎 510
嗜酸性胃肠炎 693
噬血细胞性淋巴组织细胞增多症 515
手术后腹泻 209
手术后胃轻瘫 714
瘦素 43,113
舒尼替尼 469
术后恶心呕吐 186
术后吞咽困难 618
述情障碍 157
树突状细胞 20
衰老 3
双膦酸盐类 629
双气囊内镜 294
双气囊小肠镜 294
水电解质代谢紊乱 190
水痘-带状疱疹病毒 485

水合状态 66
水疱样大疱性皮肤病 340
水溶性维生素 60
水样泻 198
水肿 413
睡眠障碍 643
顺序神经电刺激 721
死亡结构域相关蛋白 449
速激肽 42
酸袋 639
酸性制剂 386
酸抑制试验 644
隧道式留置 CVC 86

T

他汀类药物 787
胎儿性多毛症 347
胎粪性肠梗阻 833
肽受体放射性核素放射治疗 469
贪食症 325
碳水化合物 55
碳酸氢盐缺陷型 CFTR 变体 823
糖酵解 55
糖链抗原 19-9 1015
糖尿病 54,91,245,517,849,875,953
糖尿病性胃轻瘫 713
糖皮质激素 192
糖异生 62
套细胞淋巴瘤 425
套扎治疗 268
特发性分泌性腹泻 211
特发性复发性急性胰腺炎 936
特发性高氨血症 495
特发性胃轻瘫 715
特殊患者群体 966
特殊类型脓肿的引流 395
特殊药物 628
特殊饮食 87
疼痛 893
疼痛的下行调节 155
疼痛敏感性 158
疼痛信号的去抑制 154
疼痛阈值 158
体格检查 157
体内细胞量 68
体外冲击波碎石术 980
体重减轻 66
体重指数 67
替加色罗 258
天疱疮 340
条件必需氨基酸 54
调强放疗 579
铁过载 491,502
通畅性胶囊系统 590
头颈部癌症 79
透壁撕裂 189
突变型甲状腺素转运蛋白 525
推进式肠镜检查 293
推进式小肠镜 294
吞气症 217
吞咽困难 161,352,473
吞咽疼痛 473
吞咽痛 164
吞咽诱导的食管下括约肌松弛 637
托吡酯 93
脱垂 757
唾液腺疾病 332

W

外分泌物 806
外科手术切除 792
外科胃底折叠术 652
外瘘(胰腺皮肤瘘) 912
外源信号 801
外周静脉穿刺的中心静脉导管 86
外周作用促动力药 190
完全的节段性缺损 688
顽固性疼痛 911
网膜梗死 559
网膜阑尾炎 559
危重症 76
微创食管切除术 674
微量营养素 56
微量元素 60
微生物-微生物信号 28
微生物群 10
微生物群-肠-脑轴 29
微型营养评定 70
韦卢斯特拉格 259
韦尼克(Wernicke)脑病 74
韦尼克脑病 100
维持疗法 651
味觉 38
味觉减退 333
味觉障碍 333
胃 683
胃癌 776
胃嗳气 217
胃闭锁 688
胃部术后腹泻 209
胃残余容积 77,84
胃肠道饱腹多肽 113
胃肠道出血 101,489,496
胃肠道过敏 131
胃肠道间质瘤 433,436
胃肠道内镜检查 265
胃肠道异物 377
胃肠道转移瘤 511
胃肠动力障碍 186
胃肠间质瘤 680
胃肠瘘 396
胃肠外营养制剂 85
胃肠胀气 217
胃出口梗阻 183,794
胃促动力药 192
胃促生长素 708
胃蛋白酶原 736
胃底和幽门松弛剂 721
胃底腺息肉 786
胃底折叠术 355
胃电刺激 193
胃电刺激器 721
胃电疗法 721
胃动力 121
胃动素 43
胃动素受体激动剂 192
胃窦十二指肠测压 709,711
胃窦血管扩张症 281,545
胃感觉活动 706
胃和食管癌 170
胃饥饿素 113,193
胃肌电活动 696,710
胃畸胎瘤 691
胃空肠吻合术 786,794
胃快速排空 717
胃溃疡/胃癌表型 778
胃溃疡 762
胃淋巴瘤 420
胃弥漫性大 B 细胞淋巴瘤 423
胃泌素 40,727
胃泌素瘤 453
胃内球囊 105
胃扭转 365
胃排空测量 189
胃排空率 709
胃排空延迟 173,641
胃旁路术 97
胃平滑肌细胞内电记录 696
胃起搏 721
胃憩室 356,690
胃轻瘫 186,713
胃蠕动 709
胃神经肌肉功能 696

胃神经肌肉疾病 711
胃神经内分泌肿瘤(胃 NET) 460
胃神经支配 685
胃十二指肠测压 189
胃十二指肠吻合术 786
胃石 384
胃食管反流 167,635
胃食管反流病 92,170,337,403,563,716
胃受累 507
胃束带术 98
胃酸分泌 640
胃酸峰值排出量 734
胃体和胃窦促动力剂 720
胃萎缩 746
胃息肉 786
胃脂肪酶 736
胃重复畸形 690
胃灼热 166,642
胃灼热与肠易激综合征重叠 172
萎缩性舌 334
文化信仰 158
吻合口溃疡 101
握拳测力法 68
无功能性胰腺神经内分泌肿瘤 459
无线动力胶囊 249
无线视频胶囊式内镜 267
无症状胆石症 985
无症状结石 965
无症状胰腺纤维化 872
戊型病毒性肝炎 570

X

吸入性肺炎 189
吸烟 89,780,816,867
息肉病综合征 345
息肉切除术 288
息肉切除术后电凝综合征 591
硒 788
系统性肥大细胞增多症 513
系统性红斑狼疮 343,414,507
系统性疾病 953
系统性淋巴瘤所致的肝脏受累 512
系统性硬化病 506
系统性硬化症 246
细胞毒性化疗 470
细胞因子 46,315
细胞增殖 1
细菌性胃炎 750
细菌学 390
狭窄 102
下丘脑-垂体-肾上腺轴 312
下胃肠道 262
下胃肠道出血 283
下行抑制系统 155
下行抑制性疼痛通路 156
下咽憩室 614,623
先天性胆总管畸形 923
先天性高神经节细胞增多症 246
先天性膈疝 363
先天性和牵引性食管憩室 354
先天性静脉畸形肢体肥大综合征 544
先天性囊肿 804
先天性食管狭窄 601
先天性胃畸形 688
先天性无神经节细胞症 246
先天性胰脂肪酶缺乏 840
先天性幽门缺失 693
先兆子痫 566
纤维血管息肉 680
显微镜下结肠炎 208
线粒体 55
腺苷 46
腺瘤 679
腺泡 805
腺泡细胞癌 905
腺泡细胞功能障碍和疾病 817
消化不良 61,169,885
消化道出血 479,887
消化分泌 809
消化性溃疡 170,270,762
消化性溃疡病 564,786
消化性溃疡穿孔 148,762
消化性食管狭窄 648
消融术 677
小肠 Dieulafoy 病变 292
小肠梗阻 147,578
小肠镜 589
小肠淋巴瘤 425
小肠憩室 292
小肠神经内分泌肿瘤 462
小肠受累 507
小肠细菌过度生长 503
小胆管型 PSC 1013
小儿胰腺炎 829
小容量腹泻 198
小胃 690
小细胞癌 678
哮喘 642
心理健康转诊 159
心理困扰 310
心理社会因素 175
心理社会资源 158
心理因素 310
心理治疗 122,159
心血管疾病 525
心脏射频消融术 630
新辅助放化疗 678
新辅助放疗 678
新辅助化疗 677,792
新辅助治疗 440
信号转导相关癌基因 7
行为特征 157
胸神经根病 154
胸痛 642
熊去氧胆酸 949,979
休克 142
袖状胃切除术 97
序贯治疗 760
选择性腹泻综合征 208
血隔离症 516
血管发育不良 290,537
血管和淋巴管新生 10
血管活性肠肽 41
血管活性肠肽瘤 458
血管扩张 290,531
血管瘤 539
血管神经性水肿 151
血管通路装置 86
血管性血友病 290
血管炎 507
血管异常 602
血管造影 268,287
血管造影介入治疗 773
血管造影术 285
血管造影栓塞 278
血红素加氧酶 296
血流动力学 142
血清蛋白 68
血清淀粉酶 854
血清素 44
血清胃蛋白酶原 786
血清胰蛋白酶原 877
血清脂肪酶 854
血清肿瘤标志物 895
血栓性血小板减少性紫癜 517
血小板衍生生长因子 47
血液喷雾剂 277
血液系统恶性肿瘤 512
血液循环 797
血友病 517
血脂紊乱 91
寻常型天疱疮 340

Y

牙龈口炎 335
牙龈肿大 335
亚急性腹痛 153
亚麻籽 253
严重胃肠道出血 262
炎性肠病性胃炎 753
炎性腹泻 198
炎性肌病 508
炎性纤维性息肉 679
炎症性肠病 30,336,403,564
盐水、自来水和肥皂水灌肠 257
眼咽型肌营养不良 614
阳离子胰蛋白酶原基因 819
腰疝 372
药物性肝损伤 495
药物引起的肝毒性 505
药物治疗 158
要素饮食 406
夜间进食综合征 115
一过性食管下括约肌松弛 611,637
一氧化氮 45
伊马替尼 440
衣原体腹膜炎 554
医学治疗 93
医源性淋巴增殖性疾病 431
依维莫司 469
胰胆管畸形愈合 804
胰岛素瘤 451
胰岛素样生长因子 47,517
胰多肽 113
胰多肽家族 42
胰高血糖素 41
胰高血糖素瘤 457
胰高血糖素样肽 1 113
胰高血糖素样肽 72
胰管结构 796
胰管结石 910
胰管括约肌切开术 882
胰管离断综合征 862
胰管漏 911
胰管狭窄 910
胰瘘 888
胰酶疗法 882
胰泌素 40
胰内瘘 888
胰外瘘 888
胰腺 795
胰腺癌 890,912
胰腺导管内乳头状黏液瘤 900
胰腺发育不全 803,840
胰腺分裂 802,852
胰腺分泌功能试验 810
胰腺功能检测 876
胰腺功能障碍 832
胰腺和胆囊受累 508
胰腺假性囊肿 900
胰腺淋巴瘤 430
胰腺孟德尔遗传疾病 830
胰腺囊性肿瘤 900
胰腺囊肿 912
胰腺内分泌功能不全 875
胰腺外分泌功能不全 874
胰腺星状细胞 866
胰腺炎 95,592
胰腺炎症性疾病 814
胰性脑病 863
胰源性出血 281
移行性复合肌电活动 700
移植后淋巴增殖性疾病 431
移植物抗宿主病 487,497,756
遗传 90
遗传性出血性毛细血管扩张症 291,343,543
遗传性肛门内括约肌肌病 246
遗传性胃癌 781
遗传性胰腺炎 813,815,836,851,890
遗传易感性 174
乙酰胆碱 43,723,728
乙酰辅酶 A 55
异尖线虫病 751
异食癖 116
异位胃黏膜 604
异位胰腺组织 803
异型增生 658
抑酸药物 177,277
抑郁症 247
意识控制丧失 245
癔球症 164
阴离子转运蛋白 297
饮酒 816
饮食疗法 406
饮食因素 11
饮食治疗 721
饮食咨询 721
隐孢子虫病 751
隐匿性呕吐 327
隐匿性胃肠道出血 262
隐球菌病 751
应对 310
应激 311,756
应激性溃疡 279,775
婴儿肠绞痛 132
婴儿肥厚性幽门狭窄 691
婴儿期过敏性结肠炎 409
营养不良 63
营养风险评分 76
营养风险筛查 76
营养化学感应 38
营养康复 124
营养品 722
营养评估 117
营养评估技术 66
营养缺乏 100,190,338
营养性消瘦症 64,65
营养性侏儒症 64,65
硬化性胆管炎 1004
硬化治疗 268
硬皮病 544
幽门括约肌测试 710
幽门螺杆菌感染 420,763,778
幽门螺杆菌胃炎 740
幽门螺杆菌相关性胃炎 414
幽门张力增加 704
疣状癌 678
有丝分裂灾难 574
与多排螺旋 CT 胆道成像 1036
原发性胆汁性肝硬化 300
原发性腹膜炎 549,554
原发性肝淋巴瘤 430
原发性结直肠淋巴瘤 430
原发性渗出性淋巴瘤 432
原发性硬化性胆管炎 927,1005
原核与抗核因子失衡 958
原位肝移植 486
远端肠梗阻综合征 833
远端胆管癌 1024
远端胆管狭窄 1043
远端或非交界型肿瘤 777
远端食管痉挛 617,618

Z

再喂养低磷血症 124
再喂养综合征 86
早期倾倒综合征 75
造口狭窄 102
造瘘口静脉曲张 1016
增强胃调节作用的药物 180
增生性胃病 757
增殖性脓性口炎 342
增殖性疣状白斑 334
诈病 325

张力蛋白同源物 450
掌跖角化病 346
胀气综合征 217
针刺疗法 721
真菌感染 485
真菌性动脉瘤 542
真菌性腹膜炎 555
真菌性胃炎 751
镇静 587
正常传输型便秘 243
正氮平衡 55
症状性结石 966
支架置入 882
支气管炎闭塞综合征 487
脂肪代谢异常 952
脂肪瘤 681
脂肪酶 807
脂肪酸乙醇酯 865
脂肪吸收不良 61
脂肪泻 198,874,885
脂类 55
脂联素 113
脂溶性维生素 60
脂质 38
脂质代谢紊乱 520
直肠 224
直肠超敏反应 156
直肠刺激 159
直肠感觉测试 228
直肠感觉减弱 244
直肠静脉曲张 289
直肠溃疡 289
直肠敏感性和感觉测试 251
直肠膨出 243
直肠前突 243
直肠神经内分泌肿瘤 463
直肠脱垂 244
直接激素刺激试验 876
直接经皮空肠造口术 83
直接抗病毒药 490,495
植入式血管通路装置或“端口” 86
止血喷雾剂 268
酯质肉芽肿瘤样增生病 515
质子泵抑制剂 650,731,766
治疗计划 158
致癌生长因子 6
致癌信号通路 9
致幻毒品 157
痔疮 289
中臂肌围 67
中链甘油三酯 73
中枢介导的腹痛综合征 154
中枢敏化 154
中枢情绪区域 159
中枢去抑制 156
中枢神经系统的作用 156
中枢神经系统疾病 522
中枢疼痛调节失调 156
中枢性放大 313
中枢作用止吐药 190
中心静脉导管 86
中心静脉导管并发症 86
肿瘤代谢 10
肿瘤浸润深度 671
肿瘤微环境 9
肿瘤抑制基因 6,7
肿瘤转移的生物学特征 10
中毒性表皮坏死松解症谱 341
中毒性巨结肠 488
重度肥胖 96
重症肌无力 523,614
周期性呕吐综合征 187
周围肠化生性萎缩性胃炎 740
主动脉瓣狭窄 290
主动脉肠瘘 282,542
主观总体评估 70
主细胞 686
主要矿物质 56
住院患者腹泻 210
住院患者溃疡出血 279
转化生长因子-α 47
转化生长因子-β 47
转录因子 801
转移瘤 680
锥体外系(运动)障碍 523
锥体外系反应 61
自发性胆管穿孔 922
自发性食管破裂综合征 631
自发性食管血肿 632
自发荧光成像 668
自分泌 34
自然杀伤T细胞肠道淋巴瘤 430
自身免疫性肠化生性萎缩性胃炎 740,747
自身免疫性肝病 572
自身免疫性肝炎 505
自身免疫性化生性萎缩性胃炎 784
自身免疫性慢性胰腺炎 865
自身免疫性胰腺炎 868
自由基 788
自主神经功能测试 189
自主神经系统功能障碍 523
纵行肌 609
总能量消耗 52
综合征性小叶间胆管缺乏 925
阻塞性睡眠呼吸暂停 92
组胺 45
组胺2受体拮抗剂 650
组织胞浆菌病 751
组织抵抗力 640
最大胃酸排出量 734

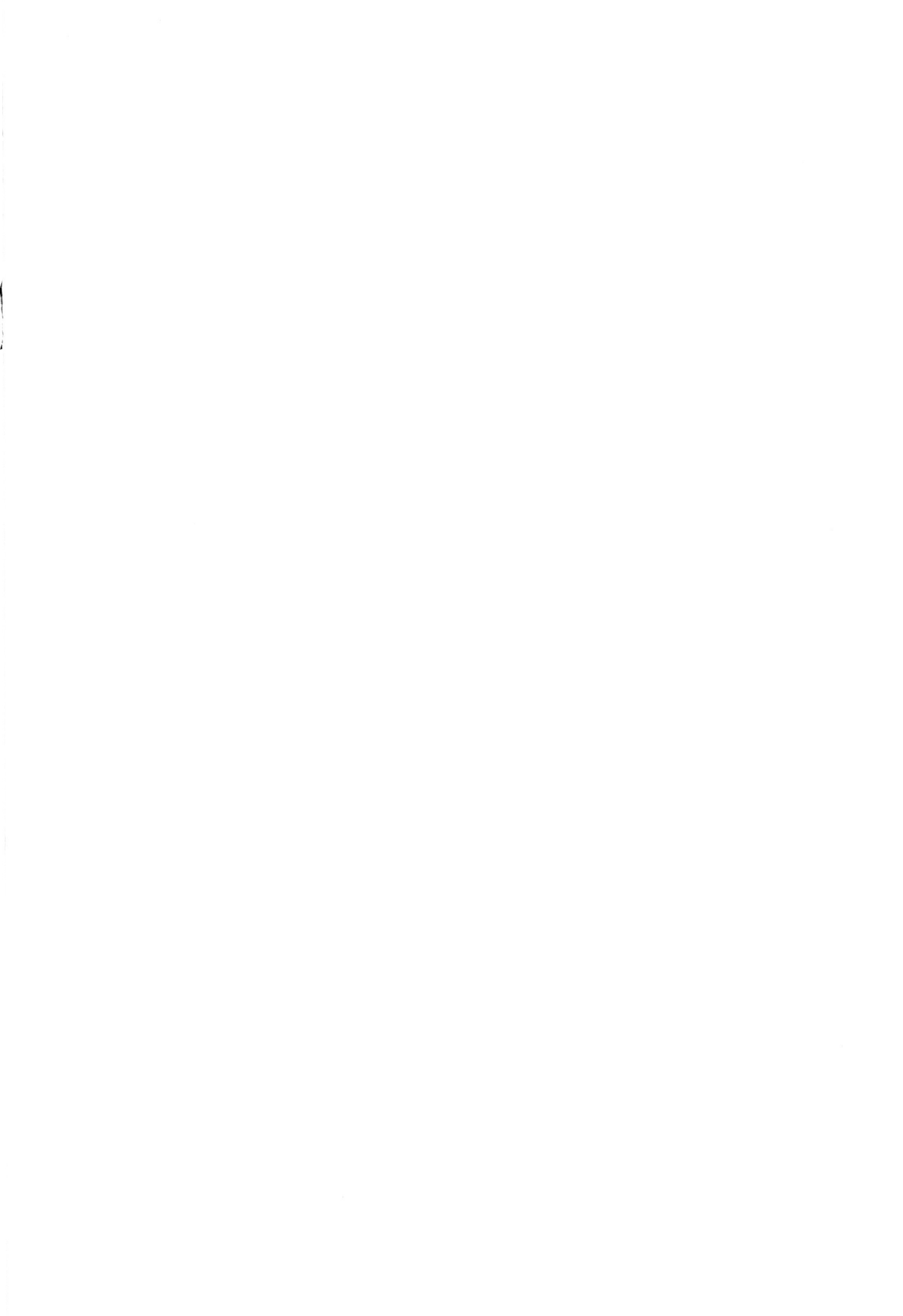